COMPREHENSIVE TEXTBOOK OF PSYCHIATRY/VI

VOLUME 1
SIXTH EDITION

SENIOR CONTRIBUTING EDITOR

Robert Cancro, M.D., Med.D.Sc.
Professor and Chairman, Department of Psychiatry, New York University School of Medicine; Director, Department of Psychiatry, Tisch Hospital, the University Hospital of New York University Medical Center, New York, New York; Director, Nathan S. Kline Institute for Psychiatric Research, Orangeburg, New York.

CONTRIBUTING EDITORS

Dennis P. Cantwell, M.D.
Joseph Campbell Professor of Child Psychiatry, University of California at Los Angeles School of Medicine; Director of Residency Training, Division of Mental Retardation and Child Psychiatry, Neuropsychiatric Institute and Hospital, Los Angeles, California.

Allen Frances, M.D.
Professor and Chairman, Department of Psychiatry, Duke University Medical Center, Durham, North Carolina.

Jack A. Grebb, M.D.
Clinical Associate Professor of Psychiatry, The University of Illinois at Chicago College of Medicine, Chicago, Illinois.

Lissy F. Jarvik, M.D., Ph.D.
Professor of Psychiatry and Biobehavioral Sciences, University of California at Los Angeles School of Medicine; Distinguished Physician (Emeritus), West Los Angeles Veterans Affairs Medical Center, Los Angeles, California.

Joel Yager, M.D.
Professor and Associate Chair for Education, Department of Psychiatry and Biobehavioral Sciences, University of California Los Angeles School of Medicine; Associate Chief of Psychiatry for Residency Education, West Los Angeles Veterans Medical Center, Los Angeles, California.

FRONT COVER: *The illustration is a computer-generated transaxial SPECT superimposed on an MR scan from a human subject demonstrating the precise anatomical distribution and concentration of benzodiazepine receptors in the cortical—particularly occipital—regions of the brain. (Figure courtesy of Robert T. Malison, M.D., and Erik G. Miller, CORITech Inc., New Haven, Connecticut.) For a discussion of neuroimaging see Section 1.10 on Principles of Neuroimaging by Robert T. Innis, M.D., Ph.D., and Robert T. Malison, M.D.*

COMPREHENSIVE TEXTBOOK OF PSYCHIATRY/VI

VOLUME 1
SIXTH EDITION

EDITORS

HAROLD I. KAPLAN, M.D.

Professor of Psychiatry, New York University School of Medicine
Attending Psychiatrist, Tisch Hospital, the University Hospital of the New York University Medical Center
Attending Psychiatrist, Bellevue Hospital Center
Consultant Psychiatrist, Lenox Hill Hospital
New York, New York

BENJAMIN J. SADOCK, M.D.

Professor and Vice Chairman, Department of Psychiatry, New York University School of Medicine
Attending Psychiatrist, Tisch Hospital, the University Hospital of the New York University Medical Center
Attending Psychiatrist, Bellevue Hospital Center
Consultant Psychiatrist, Lenox Hill Hospital
New York, New York

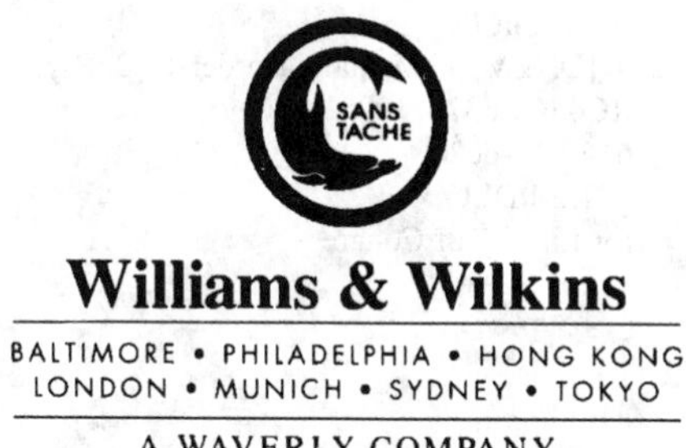

Williams & Wilkins

BALTIMORE • PHILADELPHIA • HONG KONG
LONDON • MUNICH • SYDNEY • TOKYO

A WAVERLY COMPANY

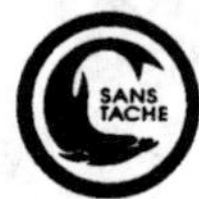

Editor: David C. Retford
Managing Editor: Kathleen Courtney Millet
Production Coordinator: Barbara J. Felton
Copy Editor: Hockett Editorial Service
Designer: JoAnne Janowiak
Illustration Planner: Lorraine Wrzosek
Project Editor: Lynda Abrams Zittell, M.A.

Williams & Wilkins
351 West Camden Street
Baltimore, Maryland 21201-2436, USA
800-638-0672

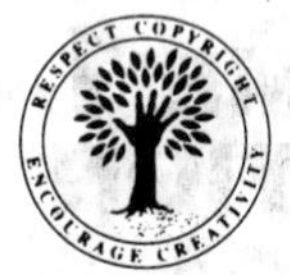

Notice. The indications and dosages of all drugs in this book have been recommended in the medical literature and conform to the practices of the general medical community. The medications described do not necessarily have specific approval by the Food and Drug Administration for use in the diseases and dosages for which they are recommended. The package insert for each drug should be consulted for use and dosage as approved by the FDA. Because standards for usage change, it is advisable to keep abreast of revised recommendations, particularly those concerning new drugs.

Printed in the United States of America

First Edition 1967
Second Edition 1975
Third Edition 1980
Fourth Edition 1985
Fifth Edition 1989

Library of Congress Cataloging-in-Publication Data

Comprehensive textbook of psychiatry/VI / editors, Harold I. Kaplan, Benjamin J. Sadock.—6th ed.
p. cm
Includes bibliographical references and index.
ISBN 0-683-04532-6 (hard cover)
1. Psychiatry. I. Kaplan, Harold I. II. Sadock, Benjamin J.
[DNLM: 1. Mental Disorders. 2. Psychiatry. WM 100 C737 1995]
RC454.C637 1995
616.89—dc20
DNLM/DLC
for Library of Congress 95-10275
CIP

95 96 97 98 99
1 2 3 4 5 6 7 8 9 10

Dedicated to our wives,
Nancy Barrett Kaplan
and Virginia Alcott Sadock,
without whose help and sacrifice
this textbook would not have been possible

PREFACE

This is the sixth edition of the *Comprehensive Textbook of Psychiatry* to be published. Work began on the first edition in 1965, so this edition represents the 30th anniversary of the founding of this textbook. The editors wish to acknowledge the more than 1500 psychiatrists and behavioral scientists who have contributed to the text over that time, whose efforts made this and previous editions possible.

A major change in psychiatry occurred since the last edition of the *Comprehensive Textbook* was published in 1989—a new classification of mental disorders appeared. In 1994 the fourth edition of *Diagnostic and Statistical Manual of Mental Disorders* (DSM-IV) was published by the American Psychiatric Association. DSM-IV is the official nomenclature used by psychiatrists and other mental health professionals and was prepared during the same time this textbook was written. Including the new nosology in this book required a prodigious effort that resulted in this being the first major textbook to discuss and critique the new terminology completely and to describe all mental disorders according to the current DSM-IV diagnostic criteria.

TEACHING SYSTEM

This textbook forms one part of a comprehensive system we have developed to facilitate the teaching of psychiatry and the behavioral sciences. At the head of the system is *Comprehensive Textbook of Psychiatry,* which is global in depth and scope; it is designed for and used by psychiatrists, behavioral scientists, and all workers in the mental health field. *Kaplan and Sadock's Synopsis of Psychiatry* is a relatively brief, highly modified, original, and current version useful for medical students, psychiatric residents, practicing psychiatrists, and mental health professionals. Another part of the system is *Study Guide and Self-Examination Review for Kaplan and Sadock's Synopsis of Psychiatry,* which consists of multiple-choice questions and answers; it is designed for students of psychiatry and for clinical psychiatrists who require a review of the behavioral sciences and general psychiatry in preparation for a variety of examinations. Other parts of the system are the pocket handbooks: *Pocket Handbook of Clinical Psychiatry, Pocket Handbook of Psychiatric Drug Treatment,* and *Pocket Handbook of Emergency Psychiatric Medicine.* Those books cover the diagnosis and the treatment of psychiatric disorders, psychopharmacology, and psychiatric emergencies, respectively, and are compactly designed and concisely written to be carried in the pocket by clinical clerks and practicing physicians, whatever their specialty, to provide a quick reference. Finally, *Comprehensive Glossary of Psychiatry and Psychology* provides simply written definitions for psychiatrists and other physicians, psychologists, students, other mental health professionals, and the general public. Taken together, those books create a multipronged approach to the teaching, study, and learning of psychiatry.

CHANGES IN THIS EDITION

FORMAT This edition has 650 more pages than the previous edition because of the inclusion of more written material, illustrations, and tables, including all the tables from DSM-IV. Color illustrations of all the major drugs currently used in psychiatry in their various dosage forms have been added and include all the latest drugs available in the United States.

Following the style of other major medical textbooks, internal citations of the literature have been eliminated. Contributors were asked to cite 30 to 40 major books, monographs, or articles in their fields and to include very current and up-to-date references where possible. Contributors were also asked to note the five most important references with an asterisk.

CASE EXAMPLES Nearly every diagnostic category and condition covered in DSM-IV is illustrated with a case example. Most come from the contributor's clinical experience, and some come directly from the American Psychiatric Association's new *DSM-IV Casebook.* When case studies from *DSM-IV Casebook* are used, the discussion section has been retained to provide useful information on differential diagnosis and treatment.

SECTIONS REWRITTEN BY NEW CONTRIBUTORS Most sections were completely rewritten for this edition. They include: Perception and Cognition; Aggression; Psychoanalysis; Erik H. Erikson; Theories of Personality and Psychopathology: Approaches Derived from Philosophy and Psychology; The Psychiatric Interview, History, and Mental Status Examination; Medical Assessment and Laboratory Testing in Psychiatry; Psychiatric Rating Scales; Classification of Mental Disorders; Schizophrenia: Genetics, Somatic Treatment, Psychosocial Treatment, Individual Psychotherapy; Schizoaffective Disorder, Schizophreniform Disorder, and Brief Psychotic Disorder; Mood Disorders: Epidemiology, Genetic Aspects, Psychodynamic Etiology, Clinical Features; Specific Phobia and Social Phobia; Obsessive-Compulsive Disorder; Posttraumatic Stress Disorder and Acute Stress Disorder; Somatoform Disorders; Factitious Disorders; Paraphilias; Gender Identity Disorders; Eating Disorders; Impulse-Control Disorders Not Elsewhere Classified; Adjustment Disorders; History, Classification, and Current Trends in Psychosomatic Medicine; Gastrointestinal Disorders; Obesity; Cardiovascular Disorders; Endocrine and Metabolic Disorders; Skin Disorders; Stress and Psychiatry; Behavior and Immunity; Consultation-Liaison Psychiatry; Malingering; Adult Antisocial Behavior and Criminality; Academic Problem and Borderline Intellectual Functioning; Psychiatry and Medicine; Psychiatric Aspects of Acquired Immune Deficiency Syndrome; Psychiatry and Reproductive Medicine; Death, Dying, and Bereavement; Other Psychiatric Emergencies; Behavior Therapy; Group Psychotherapy, Combined Individual and Group Psychotherapy, and Psychodrama; Family Therapy; Couples Therapy; Other Methods of Psychotherapy; Brief Psychotherapy; Electroconvulsive Therapy; Psychosurgery; Adulthood; Community Psychiatry;

Economics of Psychiatry; and Role of the Psychiatric Hospital in the Treatment of Mental Illness.

CHILDHOOD DISORDERS AND CHILD PSYCHIATRY

The chapters on child and adolescent psychiatry have been heavily rewritten. As in the adult areas the new organization is based on DSM-IV. The new sections include: Communication Disorder NOS; Feeding and Eating Disorders of Infancy and Early Childhood; Separation Anxiety Disorder and Anxiety in Children; Childhood or Adolescent Antisocial Behavior; and Identity Problem and Borderline Personality Disorders.

Sections completely rewritten include: Introduction and Overview; Normal Child Development; Normal Adolescent Development; Psychiatric Examination of the Infant, Child, and Adolescent; Mental Retardation; Learning Disorders, Motor Skills Disorder, and Communication Disorders, including Introduction and Overview, Reading Disorder, Mathematics Disorder, Disorder of Written Expression, Expressive Language Disorder, Mixed Receptive-Expressive Language Disorder, Phonological Disorder, and Stuttering; Pervasive Developmental Disorders; Attention-Deficit Disorders; Disruptive Behavior Disorders; Tic Disorders; Elimination Disorders; Selective Mutism; Reactive Attachment Disorder of Infancy or Early Childhood; Stereotypic Movement Disorder and Disorder of Infancy, Childhood, or Adolescence NOS; Mood Disorders and Suicide; Schizophrenia with Childhood Onset; Individual Psychotherapy; Group Psychotherapy; Pharmacotherapy; Partial Hospitalization; Residential and Inpatient Treatment; Psychiatric Treatment of Adolescents; Psychiatric Aspects of Day Care; Adoption; Physical Abuse, Sexual Abuse, and Child Neglect; Children's Reaction to Illness, Hospitalization, and Surgery; and Foster Care.

NEW SECTIONS

Neural sciences This chapter has been reorganized and updated to reflect the growing knowledge in the field. New sections in this edition include: Monoamine Neurotransmitters; Amino Acid Neurotransmitters; Basic Molecular Neurobiology; Population Genetics in Psychiatry; and Future Directions for Neuroscience and Psychiatry.

Sections that have been rewritten by new contributors include: Functional Neuroanatomy; Neuropeptides: Biology and Regulation; Intraneuronal Signaling Pathways; Applied Electrophysiology; Basic Science of Sleep; Principles of Neuroimaging; Psychoneuroendocrinology; Immune System and Central Nervous System Interactions; Chronobiology; and Genetic Linkage Analysis of the Psychiatric Disorders. Other rewritten and updated sections include: Neural Sciences: Introduction and Overview; and Basic Electrophysiology.

Neuropsychiatry and behavioral neurology A major expansion of the section on behavioral neurology and neuropsychiatry has been added to this book. Sections included for the first time include: Neuropsychiatry: Clinical Assessment and Approach to Diagnosis; Neuropsychiatric Aspects of Cerebrovascular Disorders and Tumors; Neuropsychiatric Aspects of Epilepsy; Neuropsychiatric Aspects of Head Trauma; Neuropsychiatric Aspects of Movement Disorders; Neuropsychiatric Aspects of Multiple Sclerosis and Other Demyelinating Disorders; Neuropsychiatric Aspects of Infectious Disorders; Neuropsychiatric Aspects of Endocrine Disorders; Neuropsychiatric Aspects of Headache; and Neuroimaging in Clinical Practice.

Biological therapies A major change first introduced in the sixth edition of *Kaplan and Sadock's Synopsis of Psychiatry* is incorporated into this textbook. Drugs used in the treatment of mental disorders are classified and discussed pharmacologically, rather than as antidepressants, antipsychotics, and the like. The editors use that unique format to provide the reader with an understanding not only of the general principles of psychopharmacology but also of the use of each psychotherapeutic drug according to its pharmacological activity as a discrete drug, rather than as one of a family of drugs. This edition adds information about the uses, precautions, interactions, and dosages of drugs and includes information on every drug recently introduced in the United States.

Geriatric psychiatry The chapters on geriatric psychiatry have been largely expanded to reflect the increasing importance of the subject to clinical psychiatry. Nearly every section is new to this edition or has been rewritten by a leading geropsychiatric expert.

DSM-IV The mental disorders discussed in this textbook are consistent with the nosology of DSM-IV. The inclusion of the DSM-IV nosology and diagnostic criteria means that almost every chapter dealing with clinical disorders has undergone a thorough and extensive revision. For example, DSM-IV no longer uses the term "organic mental disorders." An entirely new chapter in this textbook—Delirium, Dementia, and Amnestic and Other Cognitive Disorders and Mental Disorders Due to a General Medical Condition—has been written to reflect that change.

Other new sections include: Relational Problems; Noncompliance with Treatment; and Premenstrual Dysphoric Disorder. Previously included in one section are two new sections—Panic Disorders and Agoraphobia, and Generalized Anxiety Disorder.

SUBSTANCE-RELATED DISORDERS The topic of psychoactive substance-induced disorders—the term used in the revised third edition of DSM (DSM-III-R)—is now covered in an entirely new and expanded chapter of this textbook—Substance-Related Disorders—to reflect the DSM-IV organization. New sections include: Introduction and Overview; Amphetamine- (or Amphetaminelike)-Related Disorders; Caffeine-Related Disorders and Nicotine-Related Disorders; Cannabis-Related Disorders; Cocaine-Related Disorders; Hallucinogen-Related Disorders; Inhalant-Related Disorders; Opioid-Related Disorders; Phencyclidine- (or Phencyclidine-like)-Related Disorders; and Sedative-, Hypnotic-, or Anxiolytic-Related Disorders. In addition, Alcohol-Related Disorders has been rewritten by a new contributor and is updated to include all the changes and criteria in DSM-IV.

Other new sections New sections have been added to chapters, such as Contributions of the Psychosocial Sciences, Classification of Mental Disorders, and Other Psychotic Disorders. New sections include: Memory; Brain Models of Mind; Sociobiology and Its Application to Psychiatry; International Perspectives on Psychiatric Diagnosis; Schizophrenia: Epidemiology; Acute and Transient Psychotic Disorders and Culture-Bound Syndromes; Mood Disorders: Introduction and Overview; Neuropsychological and Neuropsychiatric Aspects of HIV Infection in Adults; Genetic Counseling; Psychiatric Rehabilitation; and Role of Examinations in Psychiatry.

UPDATED SECTIONS Every sixth edition contribution that was written by a previous contributor has been thoroughly updated. Each section represents the most current exposition of the subject. Those sections include such topics as: Piaget's Approach to Intellectual Functioning; Learning Theory; Sociology and Psychiatry; Epidemiology; Animal Research and Its Relevance to Psychiatry; Statistics and Experimental Design; Normal Human Sexuality and Sexual Dysfunctions; Homosexuality and Homosexual Behavior; Sleep Disorders; Personality Disorders; Respiratory Disorders; Musculoskeletal Disorders and Rheumatoid Arthritis; Psycho-oncology; Other Additional Conditions That May Be a Focus of Clinical Attention; Psychiatry and Surgery; Physical and Sexual Abuse of Adult; Suicide; Psychoanalysis and Psychoanalytic Psychotherapy; Hypnosis; Cognitive Therapy; Evaluation of Psychotherapy; Graduate Psychiatric Education; Legal Issues in Psychiatry; Ethics in Psychiatry; History of Psychiatry; and Future of Psychiatry.

THE CRISIS IN THE FUTURE OF PSYCHIATRY

The introduction of the American Health Security Bill (the Clinton plan) in 1993 served as a catalyst for dramatic change in the delivery of health care in the United States even though the bill was not enacted into law. In the vanguard of change were the insurance companies and the health maintenance organizations (HMOs), which are, in the main, managed care programs run by large profit-seeking corporations. Managed care has had serious and adverse effects on the practice of psychiatry. For example, most managed mental health care (MMHC) plans restrict the number of outpatient visits for psychotherapy to a small and unpredictable number of sessions, usually 5 to 20 a year. Although some types of psychotherapy can be conducted within that framework, other types (insight oriented) require frequent visits over an extended period. Before a patient can be referred to a psychiatrist, many HMOs require that the patient see a primary care physician (the so-called gatekeeper), sometimes for several weeks; during that time, the doctor may prescribe pharmacotherapy about which he or she may have limited knowledge. Drugs, rather than psychotherapy, become the treatment of choice even though many studies have found the superior efficacy of psychotherapy used in conjunction with drugs in the treatment of most mental disorders, particularly depressive disorders and schizophrenia. Persons who are emotionally well make fewer general medical visits than do persons with emotional disorders. Providing timely psychotherapy results in savings in the overall cost of general medical care.

Many HMOs require preauthorization by a panel of so-called behavioral health experts. This panel requires information about the intimate and private details of a person's life to authorize therapy. If the patient or doctor refuses to comply, permission for psychiatric treatment is usually denied. And even if the patient is permitted to enter therapy, the psychiatrist must send frequent written reports to the HMO about the treatment, which breaches the confidentiality and trust of the doctor-patient relationship. Patients usually must be treated by psychiatrists who are enrolled in their particular HMO. They forfeit the right to see a doctor of their own choosing. In the traditional fee-for-service system patients can seek treatment from any psychiatrist they choose and can seek a second or even a third opinion if they so desire. In an HMO the patient does not have these options. Capitation, another method of payment used by HMOs, is untested in psychiatry and may mean "de-capitation" of the field.

HMOs use from 15 to 30 percent of their revenues to pay for marketing, administration, and the distribution of profits to owners and investors—money that would otherwise be available for clinical care, research, and medical education. Health care in America is being "corporatized," and HMOs reap profits by often eliminating laboratory tests, referrals to specialists, and reducing length of hospital stay to questionable and dangerous proportions. For example, patients with major psychiatric disorders are being forced out of the hospital, often against their will and against the recommendation of their psychiatrists. HMOs also increase their profit margin by paying lower fees to doctors, and since the HMOs control the supply of patients, price control rules the system.

The issue of financial liability is another area of danger to doctors who work for HMOs. Psychiatrists (and other physicians) who sign contracts with HMOs must agree to accept complete liability if any adverse effects to the patient occur during the course of treatment. Consider this example: A psychiatrist wants to hospitalize a potentially suicidal patient, but the HMO refuses to pay for hospitalization or limits the number of days allowed in the hospital to fewer than the psychiatrist deems necessary. The psychiatrist can be sued for malpractice if the patient ultimately commits suicide because of premature hospital discharge mandated by the HMO. The HMO accepts no liability for any adverse outcome based on their decisions. The only alternative is for the psychiatrist to treat the patient for no fee or for the patient to pay for treatment out-of-pocket. Neither option is satisfactory.

Currently, the future of psychiatric treatment is of concern. Unfortunately, prejudice toward mental illness still exists in many quarters—political policy makers, insurance companies, the general public, and, sadly, the medical profession itself. Psychiatry and medicine are at a crossroad. It would be tragic to take the path that discards and negates the humanism that psychiatry has brought to medicine and the great advances that have been made over the past hundred years by Sigmund Freud and other great psychiatric clinicians and researchers.

ACKNOWLEDGMENTS

The production of this book was a major undertaking that involved the efforts of many coworkers. Lynda Zittell, M.A., Education Coordinator of the Department of Psychiatry at New York University School of Medicine, was key to the successful preparation and completion of this book. We thank her for her help. In addition, we wish to extend our thanks to Justin Hollingsworth, who worked with alacrity and was involved in every aspect of this textbook. Laura Marino, Justin Hartung, and Yolanda Howard assisted the editors and were helpful throughout. We also want to thank Rachel Youngman of Hockett Editorial Service for her extraordinary effort in the production of this book.

In the preparation of this textbook the editors have enlisted the help of five outstanding Contributing Editors, Jack Grebb, M.D., Clinical Associative Professor of Psychiatry at University of Illinois at Chicago, College of Medicine; Joel Yager, M.D., Professor of Psychiatry at the University of California School of Medicine at Los Angeles; Alan Frances, M.D., Professor of Psychiatry at Duke University Medical Center; Dennis Cantwell, M.D., Professor of Child Psychiatry at the University of California School of Medicine at Los Angeles; and Lissy Jarvik, M.D., Ph.D., Professor of Psychiatry at the University of California School of Medicine at Los Angeles. Dr. Grebb helped in the conceptualization and organization of the Neural Sciences chapter and consulted in all areas of biological and somatic psychiatry. He is also co-author of *Kaplan and Sadock's Synopsis of Psychiatry*, seventh edition. Dr. Yager helped in consulting on various areas of clinical psychiatry. Dr. Frances was helpful in advising the editors about DSM-IV, and Dr. Cantwell was instrumental in organizing and obtaining contributors for the section on child psychiatry. Lissy Jarvik, M.D., Ph.D., Professor of Psychiatry and Biobehavioral Sciences at the University of California School of Medicine at Los Angeles, assisted by Gary Small, M.D., Associate Professor of Psychiatry and Biobehavioral Sciences at that institution, deserve special mention and acknowledgment for their efforts in organizing the chapter on Geriatric Psychiatry. We thank our contributing editors for their help in coordinating and integrating the areas for which they were responsible. Both the editors and the field of psychiatry owe them a debt of gratitude for their outstanding help.

We especially want to thank Virginia Alcott Sadock, M.D., Clinical Professor of Psychiatry and Director of Graduate Education in Human Sexuality at New York University School of Medicine. As in all our previous books, she has served as an assistant to the editors and actively participated in every editorial decision. Her enthusiasm, sensitivity, comprehension, and depth of psychiatric knowledge were of immeasurable importance to the editors. She has ably represented not only the viewpoint of women in medicine and psychiatry but has also made many contributions to the content of this textbook. We are deeply appreciative of her outstanding help and assistance.

Others who helped in the production of this book and who deserve mention are Joan Welsh; Caroly Pataki, M.D.; Richard Perry, M.D.; Norman Sussman, M.D.; Phillip Kaplan, M.D.; Peter Kaplan, M.D.; Victoria Sadock; James Sadock; and Nancy B. Kaplan. We also thank Dorice Vieira, Head of Educational Services of the Frederick L. Ehrman Medical Library of the New York University School of Medicine, for her valuable assistance in this project.

We also take this opportunity to acknowledge those who have translated this and other works by the editors into foreign languages. Current translations include Italian, French, Portuguese, Spanish, Indonesian, Russian, Japanese, Polish, Greek, Turkish, and German, in addition to a special Asian and international student edition of *Synopsis*.

Robert Cancro, M.D., Professor and Chairman of the Department of Psychiatry at New York University School of Medicine, participated as Senior Contributing Editor of this edition. Dr. Cancro's commitment to psychiatric education and psychiatric research is recognized throughout the world. He has been a source of great inspiration to the editors and has contributed immeasurably to this and previous editions. Dr. Cancro is renowned as a researcher, clinician, and educator and is a much valued and highly esteemed friend and colleague.

Finally, we wish to express our deep appreciation to our 361 contributors, who worked with enthusiasm and who were cooperative in every aspect of this textbook.

Harold I. Kaplan, M.D.
Benjamin J. Sadock, M.D.

New York University Medical Center
New York City, 1995

CONTRIBUTORS

Susan F. Abbott, M.D. Clinical Assistant Professor of Psychiatry, State University of New York at Stony Brook School of Medicine, Stony Brook, New York; Research Fellow, American Suicide Foundation, New York, New York; Director, Adolescent Psychiatry, John T. Mather Memorial Hospital, Port Jefferson, New York.

Robert C. Abrams, M.D. Associate Professor of Clinical Psychiatry, Cornell University Medical College, New York, New York; Associate Attending Psychiatrist, New York Hospital-Cornell Medical Center, Westchester Division, White Plains, New York.

George K. Aghajanian, M.D. Professor of Psychiatry and Pharmacology, Yale University School of Medicine, New Haven, Connecticut.

W. Stewart Agras, M.D., F.R.C.P.(C) Professor of Psychiatry, Stanford University School of Medicine; Director, Stanford University Psychiatric Clinics, Stanford, California.

Hagop S. Akiskal, M.D. Professor of Psychiatry, University of California at San Diego School of Medicine; Director, International Mood Center, La Jolla, California; Director, Outpatient Psychiatric Services, San Diego Veterans Affairs Medical Center, San Diego, California.

George S. Alexopoulos, M.D. Professor of Psychiatry, Cornell University Medical College, New York, New York; Director, Cornell Institute of Geriatric Psychiatry, New York Hospital-Cornell Medical Center, Westchester Division, White Plains, New York.

Meenakshi Alreja, Ph.D. Assistant Professor of Psychiatry, Yale University School of Medicine, New Haven, Connecticut.

Kenneth Z. Altshuler, M.D. Stanton Sharp Professor and Chairman, Department of Psychiatry, University of Texas Southwestern Medical Center, Dallas, Texas.

Jambur Ananth, M.D., D.P.M., F.R.C.P.(C) Adjunct Professor of Psychiatry, University of California at Los Angeles School of Medicine, Los Angeles, California; Clinical Director, Department of Psychiatry, Harbor-UCLA Medical Center, Torrance, California.

George W. Arana, M.D. Professor of Psychiatry and Associate Dean of Clinical Affairs, Medical University of South Carolina; Executive Medical Director, Medical University of South Carolina Medical Center, Charleston, South Carolina.

L. Eugene Arnold, M.D. Professor Emeritus of Psychiatry, Ohio State University, Columbus, Ohio; Special Expert, Child and Adolescent Disorders Research Branch, Division of Clinical and Treatment Research, National Institute of Mental Health, Rockville, Maryland.

J. Hampton Atkinson, Jr., M.D. Adjunct Professor of Psychiatry, University of California at San Diego School of Medicine, La Jolla, California; Psychiatry Service, San Diego Veterans Affairs Medical Center, San Diego, California.

Lorian Baker, Ph.D. Research Professor of Child Psychiatry, University of California at Los Angeles School of Medicine, Los Angeles, California.

F.M. Baker, M.D., M.P.H. Associate Professor of Psychiatry, University of Maryland School of Medicine; Attending Psychiatrist, University of Maryland Hospital, Baltimore, Maryland; Consulting Research Scientist, Mental Disorders of the Aging Research Branch, National Institute of Mental Health, Bethesda, Maryland.

Jay M. Baraban, M.D., Ph.D. Associate Professor of Neuroscience, Psychiatry, and Behavioral Sciences, Johns Hopkins University School of Medicine, Baltimore, Maryland.

David H. Barlow, Ph.D. Distinguished Professor of Psychology, State University of New York at Albany; Director, Center for Stress and Anxiety Disorders, Albany, New York.

John J. Barry, M.D. Acting Assistant Professor of Psychiatry and Behavioral Sciences, Stanford University School of Medicine; Director, Evaluation and Consultation Clinic, Department of Psychiatry and Behavioral Sciences, Stanford University Medical Center, Stanford, California.

Aaron T. Beck, M.D. Professor Emeritus of Psychiatry and Director, Psychopathology Research Center, University of Pennsylvania School of Medicine, Philadelphia, Pennsylvania; President, The Beck Institute for Cognitive Therapy and Research, Bala Cynwyd, Pennsylvania.

Arthur L. Benton, Ph.D. Professor Emeritus of Neurology and Psychology, University of Iowa College of Medicine, Iowa City, Iowa.

Kate Berg, Ph.D. Deputy Scientific Director, National Center for Human Genome Research, National Institutes of Health, Bethesda, Maryland.

Sarah L. Berga, M.D. Associate Professor of Obstetrics, Gynecology, Reproductive Sciences and Psychiatry, University of Pittsburgh School of Medicine; Attending Physician, Magee-Women's Hospital, Pittsburgh, Pennsylvania.

Karen Faith Berman, M.D. Chief, Unit on Positron Emission Tomography, Clinical Brain Disorders Branch, Intramural Research Program, National Institute of Mental Health Neuroscience Center at St. Elizabeth's, Washington, DC.

William Bernet, M.D. Associate Clinical Professor of Psychiatry, Vanderbilt University School of Medicine; Medical Director, The Psychiatric Hospital at Vanderbilt, Nashville, Tennessee.

Hector R. Bird, M.D. Professor of Clinical Psychiatry, Columbia University College of Physicians and Surgeons; Deputy Director, Department of Child and Adolescent Psychiatry, New York State Psychiatric Institute; Attending Psychiatrist, Columbia-Presbyterian Medical Center, New York, New York.

Garth Bissette, Ph.D. Associate Professor of Psychiatry, Duke University Medical Center, Durham, North Carolina.

Barry Blackwell, M.D., F.R.C.Psych. Professor of Psychiatry, University of Wisconsin Medical School, Milwaukee Clinical Campus; Director, Behavioral Medicine, Sinai Samaritan Medical Center, Milwaukee, Wisconsin.

Ray Blanchard, Ph.D. Associate Professor of Psychiatry, University of Toronto Faculty of Medicine; Senior Psychologist, Gender Identity Clinic, Clarke Institute of Psychiatry, Toronto, Ontario, Canada.

Dan G. Blazer II, M.D., Ph.D. J.P. Gibbons Professor of Psychiatry and Dean of Medical Education, Duke University Medical Center, Durham, North Carolina.

Efrain Bleiberg, M.D. Seeley Professor of Psychiatry, Karl Menninger School of Psychiatry and Mental Health Sciences; Executive Vice President and Chief of Staff, The Menninger Clinic;

Training and Supervising Analyst, Topeka Institute for Psychoanalysis, Topeka, Kansas.

Peter B. Bloom, M.D. Clinical Professor of Psychiatry, University of Pennsylvania School of Medicine; Senior Attending Psychiatrist, Institute of Pennsylvania Hospital, Philadelphia, Pennsylvania.

Soo Borson, M.D. Associate Professor of Psychiatry and Behavioral Sciences, University of Washington School of Medicine; Attending Geropsychiatrist, University Hospital, Seattle, Washington.

James Robert Brasic, M.D., M.P.H. Research Assistant Professor of Psychiatry and Coordinator, Developmental Neurobiology Unit, Division of Child and Adolescent Psychiatry, Department of Psychiatry, New York University School of Medicine; Clinical Assistant, Department of Psychiatry, Bellevue Hospital Center, New York, New York.

Joel D. Bregman, M.D. Associate Professor of Psychiatry and Behavioral Sciences, Assistant Professor of Pediatrics, and Medical Director of Emory Autism Resource Center, Emory University School of Medicine, Atlanta, Georgia.

Robert W. Buchanan, M.D. Research Associate Professor of Psychiatry, University of Maryland School of Medicine; Chief, Outpatient Program, Maryland Psychiatric Research Center, Baltimore, Maryland.

Jack D. Burke, Jr., M.D., M.P.H. Professor and Head, Department of Psychiatry and Behavioral Science, Texas A&M University Health Science Center; Chairman, Department of Psychiatry, Scott and White Clinic and Hospital, Temple, Texas.

Vivien K. Burt, M.D., Ph.D. Assistant Professor of Psychiatry, University of California at Los Angeles School of Medicine; Associate Director of Residency Education and Director of Women's Life Center, Neuropsychiatric Institute and Hospital, Los Angeles, California.

Robert W. Butler, Ph.D. Assistant Professor of Neuropsychology, Cornell University Medical College; Assistant Attending Psychologist, Memorial Hospital; Assistant Member, Memorial Sloan-Kettering Cancer Center, New York, New York.

Eric D. Caine, M.D. Professor of Psychiatry and Neurology, University of Rochester Medical Center; Attending Psychiatrist, Strong Memorial Hospital, Rochester, New York.

Magda Campbell, M.D. Professor of Psychiatry, New York University School of Medicine; Attending Psychiatrist, Tisch Hospital, the University Hospital of the New York University Medical Center; Attending Psychiatrist, Bellevue Hospital Center, New York, New York.

Robert Cancro, M.D., Med.D.Sc. Professor and Chairman, Department of Psychiatry, New York University School of Medicine; Director, Department of Psychiatry, Tisch Hospital, the University Hospital of New York University Medical Center, New York, New York; Director, Nathan S. Kline Institute for Psychiatric Research, Orangeburg, New York.

Dennis P. Cantwell, M.D. Joseph Campbell Professor of Child Psychiatry, University of California at Los Angeles School of Medicine; Director of Residency Training, Division of Mental Retardation and Child Psychiatry, Neuropsychiatric Institute and Hospital, Los Angeles, California.

Daniel X. Capruso, Ph.D. Clinical Assistant Professor of Neurology, State University of New York at Buffalo School of Medicine and Biomedical Sciences; Clinical Neuropsychologist, Buffalo General Hospital, Buffalo, New York.

Gabrielle A. Carlson, M.D. Professor of Psychiatry and Pediatrics and Director, Child and Adolescent Psychiatry, State University of New York at Stony Brook School of Medicine, Stony Brook, New York.

William T. Carpenter, Jr., M.D. Professor of Psychiatry and Pharmacology, University of Maryland School of Medicine; Director, Maryland Psychiatric Research Center, Baltimore, Maryland.

Janice H. Carter-Lourensz, M.D., M.P.H., F.A.A.P. Assistant Professor of Child Psychiatry and Pediatrics, University of California at Los Angeles School of Medicine, Los Angeles, California.

Domenic A. Ciraulo, M.D. Professor of Psychiatry and Lecturer of Pharmacology and Experimental Therapeutics, Tufts University School of Medicine; Chief, Psychiatry Service, Department of Veterans Affairs Outpatient Clinic, Boston, Massachusetts.

Michael R. Clark, M.D. Assistant Professor of Psychiatry and Behavioral Sciences, Johns Hopkins University School of Medicine; Director, Consultation/Liaison Psychiatry, Johns Hopkins Hospital, Baltimore, Maryland.

Calvin A. Colarusso, M.D. Clinical Professor of Psychiatry, University of California at San Diego School of Medicine; Director, Child Psychiatry Residency Training Program, University of California at San Diego, La Jolla, California; Training and Supervising Analyst, San Diego Psychoanalytic Institute, San Diego, California.

Ralph Colp, Jr., M.D. Assistant Professor of Clinical Psychiatry, Columbia University College of Physicians and Surgeons; Senior Attending Psychiatrist, St. Luke's-Roosevelt Hospital Center, New York, New York.

Ian A. Cook, M.D. National Institute of Mental Health Research Fellow in Psychiatry, University of California at Los Angeles School of Medicine, Los Angeles, California.

Jeremy D. Coplan, M.D. Assistant Professor of Clinical Psychiatry, Columbia University College of Physicians and Surgeons, New York, New York.

Richard Coppola, D.Sc. Chief, Neuroimaging Unit, Clinical Brain Disorders Branch, National Institute of Mental Health Neuroscience Center at St. Elizabeth's, Washington, DC.

Patrick W. Corrigan, Psy.D. Assistant Professor of Clinical Psychiatry, University of Chicago Pritzer School of Medicine, Chicago, Illinois.

Paul T. Costa, Jr., Ph.D. Clinical Professor of Psychiatry, Georgetown University School of Medicine and Health Sciences, Washington, DC; Associate Professor of Medical Psychology, Johns Hopkins University School of Medicine; Chief, Laboratory of Personality and Cognition, Gerontology Research Center, National Institute on Aging, Baltimore, Maryland.

Joseph T. Coyle, M.D. Eben S. Draper Professor of Psychiatry and Neuroscience and Chairman, Department of Psychiatry, Harvard Medical School, Boston, Massachusetts.

Thomas J. Crowley, M.D. Professor of Psychiatry, University of Colorado School of Medicine; Attending Psychiatrist, University Hospital and Colorado Psychiatric Hospital, Denver, Colorado.

Jeffrey L. Cummings, M.D. Professor of Psychiatry, Biobehavioral Science, and Neurology and Director, Alzheimer's Disease Center, University of California at Los Angeles School of Medicine, Los Angeles, California; Chief, Behavioral Neuroscience Section, Psychiatry Service, West Los Angeles Veterans Affairs Medical Center, Los Angeles, California.

John F. Curry, Ph.D. Associate Professor of Psychiatry and Behavioral Sciences, Duke University Medical Center; Associate Professor of Psychology, Duke University, Durham, North Carolina.

David G. Daniel, M.D. Associate Clinical Professor of Psychiatry, George Washington University School of Medicine and Health Sciences; Director, Washington Clinic Research Center, Falls Church, Virginia; Guest Researcher, Clinical Brain Disorders

Branch, Intramural Research Program, National Institute of Mental Health Neuroscience Center at St. Elizabeth's, Washington, DC.

Jacques Darcourt, M.D. Professor of Biophysics Image Processing, Nice Medical School, Université de Nice Sophia Antipolis; Associate Director, Nuclear Medicine Department, Centre Antione Lacassagne, Nice, France.

Jonathan R.T. Davidson, M.D. Professor of Psychiatry and Director of Anxiety and Traumatic Stress Program, Duke University Medical Center, Durham, North Carolina.

Charles DeBattista, D.M.H., M.D. Clinical Fellow in Affective Disorders, Department of Psychiatry and Behavioral Sciences, Stanford University School of Medicine, Stanford, California.

Lynn H. Deutsch, D.O. Clinical Assistant Professor of Psychiatry, Georgetown University School of Medicine; Medical Officer, Commission on Mental Health Services, St. Elizabeth's Campus, Acute Psychiatric Hospital, Washington, DC.

Stephen I. Deutsch, M.D., Ph.D. Professor and Associate Chairman, Clinical Neurosciences, Department of Psychiatry, Georgetown University School of Medicine; Chief, Psychiatry Service, Department of Veterans Affairs Medical Center, Washington, DC.

Scott R. Diehl, Ph.D. Chief, Molecular Epidemiology and Disease Indicators Branch, Division of Epidemiology and Oral Disease Prevention, National Institute of Dental Research, Bethesda, Maryland.

David F. Dinges, Ph.D. Associate Professor of Psychology in Psychiatry, University of Pennsylvania School of Medicine; Co-Director, Unit for Experimental Psychiatry, Institute of Pennsylvania Hospital, Philadelphia, Pennsylvania.

Steven L. Dubovsky, M.D. Professor of Psychiatry and Medicine, Vice-Chairman for Clinical Affairs, Department of Psychiatry, University of Colorado School of Medicine, Denver, Colorado.

Michael F. Egan, M.D. Medical Director, National Institute of Mental Health Neuroscience Research Center at St. Elizabeth's; Senior Staff Fellow, Neuropsychiatry Branch, National Institute of Mental Health Neuroscience Center at St. Elizabeth's, Washington, DC.

John Richard Elpers, M.D. Professor of Clinical Psychiatry, University of California at Los Angeles School of Medicine, Los Angeles, California; Vice Chairman, Department of Psychiatry for Planning and Development; Director of Ambulatory Care Services, Harbor-UCLA Medical Center, Torrance, California.

Spencer Eth, M.D. Associate Professor of Clinical Psychiatry and Biobehavioral Sciences, University of California at Los Angeles School of Medicine; Clinical Professor of Psychiatry and the Behavioral Sciences, University of Southern California School of Medicine; Associate Chief of Psychiatry, West Los Angeles Veterans Affairs Medical Center, Los Angeles, California.

David Fassler, M.D. Clinical Associate Professor of Psychiatry, University of Vermont College of Medicine, Burlington, Vermont; Director, Child and Adolescent Psychiatry, Choate Health Systems, Woburn, Massachusetts.

Beverly J. Fauman, M.D. Associate Professor of Psychiatry, University of Maryland School of Medicine; Senior Psychiatrist, Walter P. Carter Center, University of Maryland Medical Systems, Baltimore, Maryland.

Fawzy I. Fawzy, M.D. Professor and Deputy Chair, Department of Psychiatry and Biobehavioral Sciences, University of California at Los Angeles School of Medicine; Deputy Director, Neuropsychiatric Institute and Hospital, Los Angeles, California.

Wayne S. Fenton, M.D. Associate Clinical Professor of Psychiatry and Behavioral Sciences, George Washington University School of Medicine and Health Sciences, Washington, DC; Medical Director, Chestnut Lodge Hospital; Director of Research, Chestnut Lodge Research Institute, Rockville, Maryland.

Jack M. Fletcher, Ph.D. Professor of Pediatrics and Neurosurgery, University of Texas Medical School at Houston; Professor, Department of Psychology, University of Houston, Houston, Texas.

Abby J. Fyer, M.D. Professor of Clinical Psychiatry, Columbia University College of Physicians and Surgeons; Co-Director, Anxiety Disorders Clinic, New York State Psychiatric Institute, New York, New York.

Glen O. Gabbard, M.D. Bessie Walker Callaway Distinguished Professor of Psychoanalysis and Education, Karl Menninger School of Psychiatry and Mental Health Sciences, The Menninger Clinic; Training and Supervision Analyst, Topeka Institute for Psychoanalysis, Topeka, Kansas; Clinical Professor of Psychiatry, University of Kansas School of Medicine, Wichita, Kansas.

Warren J. Gadpaille, M.D. Clinical Professor of Child Psychiatry and Medical Student Education, University of Colorado Health Sciences Center, Denver, Colorado.

Russell Gardner, Jr., M.D. Harry K. Davis Professor of Psychiatry and Behavioral Sciences, University of Texas Medical Branch, Galveston, Texas.

Paul E. Garfinkel, M.D., F.R.C.P.(C) Professor and Chairman, Department of Psychiatry, University of Toronto; President and Psychiatrist-in-Chief, Clarke Institute of Psychiatry, Toronto, Ontario, Canada.

Thomas R. Garrick, M.D. Professor of Psychiatry, University of California at Los Angeles School of Medicine; Chief, General Hospital Psychiatry, West Los Angeles Veterans Affairs Medical Center, Los Angeles, California.

T. Conrad Gilliam, Ph.D. Professor of Genetics and Development, Columbia University College of Physicians and Surgeons; Head, Molecular Genetics Unit, New York State Psychiatric Institute, New York, New York.

J. Christian Gillin, M.D. Professor of Psychiatry, University of California at San Diego, San Diego, California.

Michael J. Gitlin, M.D. Clinical Professor of Psychiatry, University of California Los Angeles School of Medicine; Director, Affective Disorders Program, Neuropsychiatric Institute and Hospital, Los Angeles, California.

Marion Z. Goldstein, M.D. Clinical Associate Professor of Psychiatry and Director, Division of Geriatric Psychiatry, State University of New York at Buffalo School of Medicine and Biomedical Sciences, Buffalo, New York.

Jack M. Gorman, M.D. Professor of Clinical Psychiatry, Columbia University College of Physicians and Surgeons; Chief, Department of Clinical Psychobiology, New York State Psychiatric Institute; Attending Psychiatrist, Presbyterian Hospital, New York, New York.

Irving I. Gottesman, Ph.D., F.R.C.Psych.(Hon.) Sherrell J. Aston Professor of Psychology and Professor of Pediatrics (Genetics), University of Virginia, Charlottesville, Virginia.

Gary L. Gottlieb, M.D. Clinical Professor of Psychiatry, University of Pennsylvania School of Medicine; Director and Chief Executive Officer, Friends Hospital, Philadelphia, Pennsylvania.

Igor Grant, M.D., F.R.C.P.(C) Professor and Vice Chairman, Department of Psychiatry, University of California at San Diego School of Medicine; Chief for Ambulatory Care, Psychiatry Service, San Diego Veterans Affairs Medical Center, San Diego, California.

Jack A. Grebb, M.D. Clinical Associate Professor of Psychiatry, The University of Illinois at Chicago College of Medicine, Chicago, Illinois.

John F. Greden, M.D. Professor and Chair, Department of Psychiatry and Research Scientist, Mental Health Research Institute, University of Michigan Medical Center, Ann Arbor, Michigan.

Alan I. Green, M.D. Associate Professor of Psychiatry, Harvard Medical School; Administrative Director, Commonwealth Research Center, Massachusetts Mental Health Center, Boston, Massachusetts.

Richard Green, M.D., J.D. Professor of Psychiatry Emeritus, University of California at Los Angeles School of Medicine, Los Angeles, California; Consultant Psychiatrist and Research Director, Gender Identity Clinic, Charing Cross Hospital, London, England.

David J. Greenblatt, M.D. Professor and Chairman, Department of Pharmacology and Experimental Therapeutics and Professor of Psychiatry, Medicine, and Anesthesia, Tufts University School of Medicine, Boston, Massachusetts.

Stanley I. Greenspan, M.D. Clinical Professor of Psychiatry, Behavioral Sciences, and Pediatrics, George Washington University School of Medicine and Health Sciences; Supervising Child Psychoanalyst, Washington Psychoanalytic Institute, Washington, DC.

John H. Greist, M.D. Clinical Professor of Psychiatry, University of Wisconsin Medical School; Distinguisted Senior Scientist and Co-Director, Lithium Information Center, Dean Foundation for Health, Research and Education, Madison, Wisconsin.

Richard L. Gross, M.D. Clinical Professor of Psychiatry and Behavioral Sciences, George Washington University School of Medicine and Health Sciences; Clinical Professor of Psychiatry, Georgetown University Medical Center; Attending Psychiatrist, Children's National Medical Center, Washington, DC.

Hillel Grossman, M.D. Assistant Professor of Psychiatry, Tufts University School of Medicine; Attending Psychiatrist, New England Medical Center, Boston, Massachusetts.

Frederick G. Guggenheim, M.D. Marie Wilson Howells Professor and Chairman, Department of Psychiatry and Behavioral Sciences, University of Arkansas for Medical Sciences, Little Rock, Arkansas.

John G. Gunderson, M.D. Associate Professor of Psychiatry, Harvard Medical School, Boston, Massachusetts; Director, Psychosocial Research, Training, and Consultations, McLean Hospital, Belmont, Massachusetts.

Thomas G. Gutheil, M.D. Professor of Psychiatry, Harvard Medical School; Co-Director, Program in Psychiatry and the Law, Massachusetts Mental Health Center, Boston, Massachusetts; Special Consultant, Risk Management Foundation of the Harvard Medical Institutions, Cambridge, Massachusetts.

Jodi Halpern, M.D., Ph.D. Robert Wood Johnson Clinical Scholar, Neuropsychiatric Institute and Hospital, Los Angeles, California.

Gregory L. Hanna, M.D. Assistant Professor of Psychiatry, University of Michigan Medical Center; Attending Psychiatrist, Child and Adolescent Psychiatric Hospital, Ann Arbor, Michigan.

M. Jackuelyn Harris, M.D. Associate Professor of Psychiatry, University of California at San Diego School of Medicine; Co-Director, Geriatric Psychiatry Program, San Diego Veterans Affairs Medical Center, San Diego, California.

James C. Harris, M.D. Associate Professor of Psychiatry and Behavioral Sciences, Pediatrics, and Mental Hygiene and Director of Developmental Neuropsychiatry, Johns Hopkins University School of Medicine, Baltimore, Maryland.

Donald P. Hay, M.D. Associate Professor of Psychiatry and Director of Geriatric Psychiatry Inpatient Program, Late Life Mood Disorders Program, and Geriatric Psychiatry Residency Program, St. Louis University School of Medicine, St. Louis, Missouri.

A. Scott Henderson, M.D., D.Sc., F.R.A.C.P., F.R.A.N.Z.C.P., F.R.C.P., F.R.C. Psych., F.A.S.S.A. Professor, The Australian National University; Director, National Health and Medical Research Council, Social Psychiatry Research Unit, Canberra, Australia.

Lionel Hersov, M.D., F.R.C.P., F.R.C.Psych., D.P.M. Royal Free Hospital and Tavistock Centre; Emeritus Consultant Psychiatrist, Bethlem Royal Hospital and Maudsley Hospital, London, England.

Jerry D. Heston, M.D. Associate Professor of Psychiatry and Medical Director, Child and Adolescent Day Treatment Program, University of Tennessee College of Medicine, Memphis, Tennessee.

Jonathan M. Himmelhoch, M.D. Professor of Psychiatry, University of Pittsburgh School of Medicine; Director, Research Affective Disorders Clinic, Western Psychiatric Institute and Clinic, Pittsburgh, Pennsylvania.

Charles H. Hinkin, Ph.D. Assistant Professor in Residence Department of Psychiatry and Biobehavioral Sciences, University of California at Los Angeles School of Medicine; Assistant Chief, Neuropsychology Assessment Laboratory, West Los Angeles Veterans Affairs Medical Center, Los Angeles, California.

Robert M.A. Hirschfeld, M.D. Titus H. Harris Distinguished Professor and Chair, Department of Psychiatry and Behavioral Sciences, University of Texas Medical Branch, Galveston, Texas.

Max Hirshkowitz, Ph.D. Associate Professor of Psychiatry, Baylor College of Medicine; Director, Veterans Affairs Medical Center Sleep Research Center, Houston, Texas.

Ralph E. Hoffman, M.D. Associate Professor of Psychiatry, Yale University School of Medicine; Director, Center for Biocognitive Studies, Yale Psychiatric Institute, New Haven, Connecticut.

Jimmie C. Holland, M.D. Professor of Psychiatry, Cornell University Medical College; Chief, Psychiatry Service and Wayne E. Chapman Chair in Psychiatric Oncology, Memorial Sloan-Kettering Cancer Center, New York, New York.

Syed Arshad Husain, M.D., F.R.C.Psych. Professor of Psychiatry and Child Health, University of Missouri-Columbia School of Medicine; Chief, Division of Child and Adolescent Psychiatry, University of Missouri School of Medicine, Columbia, Missouri.

Thomas Hyde, M.D., Ph.D. Director, Neurology Consultation Services, Clinical Brain Disorders Branch, National Institute of Mental Health Neuroscience Center at St. Elizabeth's, Washington, DC.

Steven E. Hyman, M.D. Associate Professor of Psychiatry and Neuroscience, Harvard Medical School; Director of Research, Department of Psychiatry, Massachusetts General Hospital, Boston, Massachusetts.

Robert B. Innis, M.D., Ph.D. Associate Professor of Psychiatry and Director, Neurochemical Brain Imaging Program, Yale University School of Medicine, New Haven, Connecticut.

Jerome H. Jaffe, M.D. Adjunct Clinical Professor of Psychiatry, University of Maryland School of Medicine, Baltimore, Maryland; Director, Office of Scientific Analysis and Evaluation and Associate Director, Center for Substance Abuse Treatment, Substance Abuse and Mental Health Services Administration, Rockville, Maryland.

Lissy F. Jarvik, M.D., Ph.D. Professor of Psychiatry and Biobehavioral Sciences, University of California at Los Angeles School of Medicine; Distinguished Physician (Emeritus), West Los Angeles Veterans Affairs Medical Center, Los Angeles, California.

Daniel C. Javitt, M.D., Ph.D. Assistant Professor of Psychiatry and Neuroscience and Director, Laboratory of Clinical and Experimental Electrophysiology, Department of Psychiatry, Albert Einstein College of Medicine of Yeshiva University; Director of

Schizophrenia Research Unit, Bronx Psychiatric Center, Bronx, New York.

James W. Jefferson, M.D. Clinical Professor of Psychiatry, University of Wisconsin Medical School; Distinguished Senior Scientist and Co-Director, Lithium Information Center, Dean Foundation for Health, Research and Education, Madison, Wisconsin.

Michael A. Jenike, M.D. Associate Professor of Psychiatry, Harvard Medical School; Associate Chief of Psychiatry for Research, Department of Psychiatry, Massachusetts General Hospital, Boston, Massachusetts.

Peter S. Jensen, M.D. Chief, Child and Adolescent Disorders Research Branch, Division of Clinical and Treatment Research, National Institute of Mental Health, Rockville, Maryland.

Dilip V. Jeste, M.D. Professor of Psychiatry and Neurosciences, University of California at San Diego; Director, Geriatric Psychiatry Clinical Research Center, San Diego Veterans Affairs Medical Center, San Diego, California.

Gloria Johnson-Powell, M.D. Professor of Child Psychiatry, Harvard Medical School; Director, Partnerships in Prevention, Judge Baker Children's Center, Boston, Massachusetts.

Rebecca M. Jones, M.D. Acting Assistant Professor of Psychiatry and Behavioral Sciences, University of Washington School of Medicine; Attending Psychiatrist, Harborview Medical Center, Seattle, Washington.

Leslie B. Kadis, M.D. Assistant Clinical Professor of Psychiatry, Langley Porter Neuropsychiatric Institute, University of California at San Francisco School of Medicine, San Francisco, California.

Balu Kalayam, M.D. Associate Professor of Clinical Psychiatry, Cornell University Medical College, New York, New York; Associate Attending Psychiatrist, New York Hospital-Cornell Medical Center, Westchester Division, White Plains, New York.

Harold I. Kaplan, M.D. Professor of Psychiatry, New York University School of Medicine; Attending Psychiatrist, Tisch Hospital, the University Hospital of the New York University Medical Center; Attending Psychiatrist, Bellevue Hospital Center; Consultant Psychiatrist, Lenox Hill Hospital, New York, New York.

Robert M. Kaplan, Ph.D. Professor of Family and Preventive Medicine and Chief, Division of Health Care Sciences, University of California at San Diego School of Medicine, La Jolla, California.

Diana Kaplan, Ph.D. Clinical Instructor of Child and Adolescent Psychiatry, New York University School of Medicine, New York, New York.

Ismet Karacan, M.D., Med.D.Sc. Professor of Psychiatry and Director, Sleep Disorders and Research Center, Baylor College of Medicine; Senior Attending, Psychiatry Service, Methodist Hospital; Active Staff, Texas Children's Hospital, Houston, Texas.

T. Byram Karasu, M.D. Silverman Professor and Chairman, Department of Psychiatry, Albert Einstein College of Medicine of Yeshiva University; Psychiatrist-in-Chief, Montefiore Medical Center, Bronx, New York.

Marvin Karno, M.D. Professor of Psychiatry, University of California at Los Angeles School of Medicine; Director, Division of Social and Community Psychiatry, Neuropsychiatric Institute and Hospital, Los Angeles, California.

Wayne Katon, M.D. Professor and Chief, Division of Consultation-Liaison, Department of Psychiatry and Behavioral Sciences, University of Washington School of Medicine, Seattle, Washington.

Ira R. Katz, M.D., Ph.D. Professor of Psychiatry and Director, Division of Geriatric Psychiatry, Medical College of Pennsylvania, Philadelphia, Pennsylvania.

Kenneth S. Kendler, M.D. Professor of Psychiatry and Human Genetics and Director, Psychiatric Genetics Research Program, Medical College of Virginia, Virginia Commonwealth University, Richmond, Virginia.

John S. Kennedy, M.D., F.R.C.P.(C) Assistant Professor of Geriatric Psychiatry, Vanderbilt University School of Medicine; Director, Inpatient Older Adult Psychiatry Service, Vanderbilt University Medical Center, Nashville, Tennessee.

Paulina F. Kernberg, M.D. Associate Professor of Psychiatry, Cornell University Medical College, New York, New York; Associate Attending Psychiatrist and Director, Child and Adolescent Psychiatry, The New York Hospital-Cornell Medical Center, Westchester Division, White Plains, New York.

Julie B. Kessel, M.D. Medical College of Pennsylvania, Philadelphia, Pennsylvania.; Forensic Research Unit, Norristown State Hospital, Norristown, Pennsylvania.

Ronald C. Kessler, Ph.D. Professor of Sociology and Program Director, Institute for Social Research, University of Michigan, Ann Arbor, Michigan.

Bryan H. King, M.D. Assistant Professor of Child and Adolescent Psychiatry, University of California at Los Angeles School of Medicine, Los Angeles, California.

Darrell G. Kirch, M.D. Professor of Psychiatry, Health Behavior, Pharmacology, and Toxicology and Dean, School of Medicine, Medical College of Georgia, Augusta, Georgia.

Laurel J. Kiser, Ph.D. Associate Professor of Psychiatry and Executive Director, Child and Adolescent Day Treatment Services, University of Tennessee College of Medicine, Memphis, Tennessee.

Herbert D. Kleber, M.D. Professor of Psychiatry, Columbia University College of Physicians and Surgeons; Director, Division on Substance Abuse, Columbia University College of Physicians and Surgeons and the New York State Psychiatric Institute; Attending Psychiatrist, Columbia-Presbyterian Hospital, New York, New York.

James A. Knowles, M.D., Ph.D. Assistant Professor of Psychiatry, Columbia University College of Physicians and Surgeons, New York, New York.

Melvin Konner, M.D., Ph.D. Samuel Candler Dobbs Professor of Anthropology, Emory University; Associate Professor of Psychiatry and Neurology, Emory University School of Medicine, Atlanta, Georgia.

John Y.M. Koo, M.D. Associate Professor of Dermatology, University of California at San Francisco School of Medicine; Director, University of California at San Francisco Psoriasis Treatment Center, Phototherapy Unit, and Dermatology Drug Research Unit, University of California at San Francisco Medical Center, San Francisco, California.

David J. Kupfer, M.D. Professor and Chairman, Department of Psychiatry, University of Pittsburgh School of Medicine; Director of Research, Western Psychiatric Institute and Clinic, Pittsburgh, Pennsylvania.

Asenath La Rue, Ph.D. Associate Professor of Psychiatry, University of New Mexico School of Medicine, Albuquerque, New Mexico; Associate Research Psychologist, Department of Psychiatry and Biobehavioral Sciences, University of California at Los Angeles School of Medicine, Los Angeles, California.

Melvin R. Lansky, M.D. Adjunct Professor of Psychiatry, University of California at Los Angeles School of Medicine; Training and Supervising Analyst, Los Angeles Psychoanalytic Institute, Los Angeles, California.

Michael R. Lavin, M.D. Instructor of Psychiatry, The New York Hospital-Cornell Medical Center, Westchester Division, New York, New York.

Eleanor P. Lavretsky, M.D., Ph.D. Research Psychopharmacologist, Neuropsychiatric Institute and Hospital, Los Angeles, California.

Lawrence W. Lazarus, M.D. Assistant Professor of Psychiatry and Director, Geropsychiatry Fellowship Program, Rush Medical College, Chicago, Illinois.

Barry D. Lebowitz, Ph.D. Chief, Mental Disorders of the Aging Research Branch, National Institute of Mental Health, Rockville, Maryland; Adjunct Faculty, Department of Psychiatry, Georgetown University Medical Center, Washington, DC.

Marguerite S. Lederberg, M.D. Clinical Professor of Psychiatry, Cornell University Medical College; Attending Psychiatrist, Memorial Sloan-Kettering Cancer Center, New York, New York.

Anthony F. Lehman, M.D. Professor of Psychiatry and Director, Center for Mental Health Services Research, University of Maryland School of Medicine, Baltimore, Maryland.

Gregory B. Leong, M.D. Associate Clinical Professor of Psychiatry, University of California at Los Angeles School of Medicine; Staff Psychiatrist, West Los Angeles Veterans Affairs Medical Center, Los Angeles, California.

Ira M. Lesser, M.D. Professor of Psychiatry, University of California at Los Angeles School of Medicine, Los Angeles, California; Director of Residency Training and Vice Chair for Academic Affairs, Department of Psychiatry, Harbor-UCLA Medical Center, Torrance, California.

Molyn Leszcz, M.D., F.R.C.P.(C) Assistant Professor of Psychiatry, University of Toronto Faculty of Medicine; Coordinator of Group Therapy, Baycrest Center for Geriatric Care; Coordinator of Group Therapy, Mount Sinai Hospital, Toronto, Ontario, Canada.

Andrew F. Leuchter, M.D. Associate Professor of Psychiatry, University of California at Los Angeles School of Medicine; Director, Quantitative Electroencephalography Laboratory, Neuropsychiatric Institute and Hospital, Los Angeles, California.

Harvey S. Levin, Ph.D. Professor of Neurological Surgery, University of Maryland School of Medicine, Baltimore, Maryland.

David A. Lewis, M.D. Professor of Psychiatry and Neuroscience, University of Pittsburgh School of Medicine; Attending Psychiatrist, Western Psychiatric Institute and Clinic, Pittsburgh, Pennsylvania.

Robert P. Liberman, M.D. Professor of Psychiatry, University of California at Los Angeles School of Medicine; Director, Clinical Research Center for Schizophrenic and Psychiatric Rehabilitation, Neuropsychiatric Institute and Hospital; Attending Psychiatrist, West Los Angeles Veterans Affairs Medical Center, Los Angeles, California; Attending Psychiatrist, UCLA-Camarillo State Hospital, Camarillo, California.

William L. Licamele, M.D. Clinical Professor in Psychiatry and Pediatrics, Georgetown University School of Medicine and Health Sciences; Director, Child and Adolescent Psychiatry, Georgetown University Hospital, Washington, DC.

Michael R. Liebowitz, M.D. Professor of Clinical Psychiatry, Columbia University College of Physicians and Surgeons; Director, Anxiety Disorders Clinic, New York State Psychiatric Institute, New York, New York.

Keh-Ming Lin, M.D., M.P.H. Professor of Psychiatry, University of California at Los Angeles School of Medicine, Los Angeles, California; Director, National Institute of Mental Health Research Center on the Psychobiology of Ethnicity, Harbor-UCLA Medical Center, Torrance, California.

John R. Lion, M.D. Clinical Professor of Psychiatry, University of Maryland School of Medicine, Baltimore, Maryland.

Mark S. Lipian, M.D., Ph.D. Assistant Clinical Professor of Psychiatry and Biobehavioral Sciences, University of California at Los Angeles School of Medicine, Los Angeles, California; Assistant Clinical Professor of Psychiatry and Human Behavior, University of California at Irvine College of Medicine, Irvine, California.

Alan A. Lipton, M.D., M.P.H. Clinical Professor of Psychiatry, University of Miami School of Medicine, Miami, Florida; Chief of Psychiatric Services, State of Florida Alcohol, Drug Abuse, and Mental Health, Tallahassee, Florida.

James E. Lubben, D.S.W., M.P.H. Associate Professor of Social Welfare, University of California at Los Angeles School of Public Policy and Social Research; Co-Director, Public Health and Social Work Faculty Development Program, California Geriatric Education Center, Los Angeles, California.

Jeffrey M. Lyness, M.D. Assistant Professor of Psychiatry, University of Rochester Medical Center; Clinical Director, Geriatrics and Neuropsychiatry Unit, Strong Memorial Hospital, Rochester, New York.

Wayne Macfadden, M.D. Clinical Assistant Professor of Psychiatry, University of Pennsylvania School of Medicine; Chief, Inpatient Detoxification Unit, Philadelphia Veterans Affairs Medical Center, Philadelphia, Pennsylvania.

Robert T. Malison, M.D. Assistant Professor of Psychiatry, Yale University School of Medicine; Chief of Neuroimaging, Clinical Neuroscience Research Unit, Abraham Ribicoff Research Facilities, Connecticut Mental Health Center, New Haven, Connecticut.

Alfred E. Mamelok, M.D., F.A.C.S. Clinical Associate Professor of Ophthalmology, Cornell Medical College; Attending Ophthalmologist, New York Hospital; Attending Surgeon and Chief of Uveitis Clinic, Manhattan Eye, Ear and Throat Hospital; Section Chief, Ophthalmology, Beth Israel Hospital, New York, New York.

Salvatore Mannuzza, Ph.D. Associate Professor of Clinical Psychology, Columbia University College of Physicians and Surgeons; Research Scientist, Anxiety Disorders Clinic and the Department of Psychology, New York State Psychiatric Institute, New York, New York; Senior Psychologist, Long Island Jewish Medical Center, New Hyde Park, New York.

Theo C. Manschreck, M.D., M.P.H. Professor of Psychiatry and Human Behavior, Brown University School of Medicine; Director of Laboratory for Clinical and Experimental Psychopathology, Director of Division of Public Psychiatry, and Director of Schizophrenia and Related Psychosis Research, Brown University, Providence, Rhode Island; Lecturer in Psychiatry, Harvard Medical School; Senior Psychiatrist, Massachusetts General Hospital, Boston, Massachusetts.

Stephen R. Marder, M.D. Professor of Psychiatry, University of California at Los Angeles School of Medicine; Chief, Psychiatry Service, West Los Angeles Veterans Affairs Medical Center, Los Angeles, California.

Maurice J. Martin, M.D. Professor of Psychiatry, Mayo Medical School; Senior Consultant in Adult Psychiatry, Mayo Clinic, Rochester, Minnesota.

Steven S. Matsuyama, Ph.D. Associate Director, UCLA Alzheimer Disease Center; Associate Research Geneticist, Department of Psychiatry and Biobehavioral Sciences, University of California, Los Angeles; Chief, Psychogeriatric Laboratory, and Research Geneticist, West Los Angeles Veterans Affairs Medical Center, Los Angeles, California.

Richard E. Mattison, M.D. Blanche F. Ittleson Associate Professor of Child Psychiatry and Director, Division of Child Psychiatry, Washington University School of Medicine, St. Louis, Missouri.

Ruth McClendon, M.S.W. Assistant Clinical Professor, Langley Porter Neuropsychiatric Institute, University of California at San Francisco, San Francisco, California.

Robert R. McCrae, Ph.D. Research Psychologist, Personality, Stress, and Coping Section, Gerontology Research Center, National Institute on Aging, Baltimore, Maryland.

J. Stephen McDaniel, M.D. Assistant Professor of Psychiatry and Behavioral Sciences and Instructor of Family and Preventive Medicine, Emory University School of Medicine; Medical Director, Psychiatric Services, Grady Health System Infectious Disease Program, Atlanta, Georgia.

Susan L. McElroy, M.D. Associate Professor of Psychiatry, University of Cincinnati College of Medicine; Co-Director, Biological Psychiatry Program, Department of Psychiatry, University of Cincinnati Medical Center, Cincinnati, Ohio.

Thomas H. McGlashan, M.D. Professor of Psychiatry, Yale University School of Medicine; Executive Director, Yale Psychiatric Institute, New Haven, Connecticut.

Richard D. McKee, Ph.D. Research Assistant, University of California at San Diego, La Jolla, California.

William T. McKinney, Jr., M.D. Asher Professor of Psychiatry and Behavioral Sciences, Northwestern University Medical School; Director, The Asher Center for the Study and Treatment of Depressive Disorders, Chicago, Illinois.

Francis J. McMahon, M.D. Postdoctoral Fellow, Department of Psychiatry, Johns Hopkins University School of Medicine, Baltimore, Maryland.

Susan E. McPherson, Ph.D. Assistant Clinical Professor of Psychiatry, University of California at Los Angeles School of Medicine; Director, Los Angeles Area Alzheimer's Outreach Program, Alzheimer's Disease Core Center, University of California at Los Angeles, Los Angeles, California.

Ismael Mena, M.D. Professor of Radiological Sciences, University of California at Los Angeles School of Medicine, Los Angeles, California; Director, Division of Nuclear Medicine, Harbor-UCLA Medical Center, Torrance, California.

Joseph Mendels, M.D. Honorary Professor of Human Behavior and Psychiatry and Professor of Pharmacology, Jefferson Medical College of Thomas Jefferson University; Medical Director, Philadelphia Medical Institute, Philadelphia, Pennsylvania.

Mario F. Mendez, M.D., Ph.D. Associate Professor of Neurology, University of California at Los Angeles Medical School; Director, Neurobehavior Unit, West Los Angeles Veterans Affairs Medical Center, Los Angeles, California.

W. Walter Menninger, M.D. Clinical Professor of Psychiatry, University of Kansas School of Medicine, Kansas City, Kansas; President and Chief Executive Officer, Menninger Foundation and Clinic; Instructor, Topeka Institute for Psychoanalysis, Topeka, Kansas.

Delinda E. Mercer, M.S. Counseling Psychologist, University of Pennsylvania, Philadelphia, Pennsylvania.

Kathleen Ries Merikangas, Ph.D. Associate Professor of Psychiatry and Epidemiology and Director, Genetic Epidemiology Research Unit, Yale University School of Medicine, New Haven, Connecticut.

Jon K. Meyer, M.D. Professor of Psychiatry, Psychoanalysis, and Family Medicine, Medical College of Wisconsin; Director, Psychotherapy Center, Columbia Hospital; Chief of Psychiatry, Froedtert Memorial Lutheran Hospital, Milwaukee, Wisconsin; Training and Supervising Analyst, Chicago Institute for Psychoanalysis, Chicago, Illinois.

Juan E. Mezzich, M.D., Ph.D. Professor of Psychiatry and Epidemiology, University of Pittsburgh School of Medicine, Pittsburgh, Pennsylvania; Honorary Professor, Cayetano Heredia Peruvian University, Lima, Peru.

Edwin J. Mikkelsen, M.D. Associate Professor of Psychiatry, Harvard Medical School; Medical Director, Mentor Clinical Care, Boston, Massachusetts; Consulting Child Psychiatrist, The Eunice Kennedy Shriver Center, Waltham, Massachusetts.

Andrew H. Miller, M.D. Associate Professor of Psychiatry and Behavioral Sciences, Emory University School of Medicine, Atlanta, Georgia.

Bruce L. Miller, M.D. Associate Professor of Neurology, University of California at Los Angeles School of Medicine; The French Foundation for Alzheimer Research, Los Angeles, California; Director, Medical Affairs, Attending Neurologist, Harbor-UCLA Medical Center, Torrance, California.

Mark J. Mills, J.D., M.D. Clinical Professor of Psychiatry and Biobehavioral Sciences, University of California at Los Angeles School of Medicine, Los Angeles, California; Principal, Forensic Sciences Medical Group, Rancho Santa Fe, California.

Paul C. Mohl, M.D. Professor of Psychiatry and Director of Psychiatric Residency Training, University of Texas Southwestern Medical Center, Dallas, Texas.

Steven O. Moldin, Ph.D. Assistant Professor of Psychiatry, Washington University School of Medicine; Assistant Professor of Psychology, Washington University; Director, Center for Psychiatric Genetic Counseling, Washington University Medical Center; Attending Staff Psychologist, Jewish, Barnes, and Renard Hospitals at the Washington University Medical Center, St. Louis, Missouri.

John J. Mooney, M.D. Assistant Professor of Psychiatry, Harvard Medical School; Senior Investigator, Neuropsychopharmacology/Psychiatric Chemistry Laboratory, Massachusetts Mental Health Center; Staff Psychiatrist, New England Deaconess Hospital, Boston, Massachusetts.

Constance A. Moore, M.D. Medical Director, Sleep Disorders and Research Center, Baylor College of Medicine; Director, Veterans Affairs Medical Center Sleep Diagnostic Clinic, Houston, Texas.

John E. Morley, M.B., B.Ch. Dammert Professor of Gerontology and Director, Division of Geriatric Medicine, St. Louis University Health Science Center; Director, Geriatric Research Education and Clinical Center, Veterans Affairs Medical Center, St. Louis, Missouri.

J. Craig Nelson, M.D. Professor of Psychiatry, Yale University School of Medicine; Director, Inpatient Psychiatry Services; Director, Geriatric Psychiatry Program, Yale-New Haven Hospital, New Haven, Connecticut.

Charles B. Nemeroff, M.D., Ph.D. Reunette W. Harris Professor and Chairman, Department of Psychiatry and Behavioral Sciences, Emory University School of Medicine, Atlanta, Georgia.

John C. Nemiah, M.D. Professor of Psychiatry, Dartmouth Medical School, Hanover, New Hampshire; Clinical Staff, Mary Hitchcock Memorial Hospital, Lebanon, New Hampshire; Professor of Psychiatry Emeritus, Harvard Medical School, Boston, Massachusetts.

Eric J. Nestler, M.D., Ph.D. Elizabeth Mears and House Jameson Professor of Psychiatry and Pharmacology and Director, Division of Molecular Psychiatry, Yale University School of Medicine, New Haven, Connecticut.

Jeffrey H. Newcorn, M.D. Associate Professor of Psychiatry and Pediatrics, Mount Sinai School of Medicine; Director, Division of Child and Adolescent Psychiatry, Mount Sinai Hospital, New York, New York.

Dorian S. Newton, Ph.D. Director, Mills College Counseling and Psychological Services, Oakland, California.

Peter M. Newton, Ph.D. Professor of Psychology, Wright Institute, Berkeley, California.

Grayson S. Norquist, M.D. Deputy Director of the Division of Epidemiology and Services Research and Associate Director for Services Research, National Institute of Mental Health, Rockville, Maryland.

Charles P. O'Brien, M.D., Ph.D. Professor and Vice Chairman of Psychiatry, University of Pennsylvania/Veterans Affairs Medical Center, Philadelphia, Pennsylvania.

Kristen M. Oeth, M.S. Lecturer, Department of Behavioral Neuroscience, University of Pittsburgh, Pittsburgh, Pennsylvania.

Martin T. Orne, M.D., Ph.D. Professor of Psychiatry, University of Pennsylvania School of Medicine; Director, Unit for Experimental Psychiatry and Senior Attending Psychiatrist, The Institute of Pennsylvania Hospital, Philadelphia, Pennsylvania.

Laszlo A. Papp, M.D. Associate Professor of Clinical Psychiatry, Columbia University College of Physicians and Surgeons; Director, Biological Studies Unit, New York State Psychiatric Institute; Director, Anxiety Disorders Program, Hillside Hospital, New York, New York.

Herbert Pardes, M.D. Lawrence C. Kolb Professor and Chairman, Department of Psychiatry, Columbia University; Director of Psychiatry, Columbia-Presbyterian Medical Center; Vice President for Health Sciences and Dean, Faculty of Medicine, Columbia University College of Physicians and Surgeons, New York, New York.

Barbara L. Parry, M.D. Associate Professor of Psychiatry, University of California at San Diego School of Medicine, La Jolla, California; Director, Psychiatric Emergency Room, Associate Director of Program in Consultation-Liaison Psychiatry and Behavioral Medicine, and Psychiatric Consultant of Medical Intensive Care Unit, University of California at San Diego Medical Center, San Diego, California.

Daisy M. Pascualvaca, Ph.D. Senior Staff Fellow, Laboratory of Psychology and Psychopathology, National Institute of Mental Health, Bethesda, Maryland.

Caroly S. Pataki, M.D. Clinical Assistant Professor of Psychiatry, New York University School of Medicine; Assistant Director of Training and Education of Child Psychiatry Fellowship Program, New York University Medical Center; Chief of Child and Adolescent Psychiatry, Lenox Hill Hospital, New York, New York.

Katharine A. Phillips, M.D. Instructor in Psychiatry, Harvard Medical School, Boston, Massachusetts; Assistant Psychiatrist, McLean Hospital, Belmont, Massachusetts.

Daniel A. Plotkin, M.D., M.P.H. Associate Clinical Professor of Psychiatry, University of California at Los Angeles School of Medicine; Medical Director, Gateways Hospital and Mental Health Centers, Los Angeles, California.

Ovide F. Pomerleau, Ph.D. Professor of Psychology in Psychiatry and Director, Behavioral Medicine Program, University of Michigan Medical Center, Ann Arbor, Michigan.

Harrison G. Pope, Jr., M.D. Associate Professor of Psychiatry, Harvard Medical School, Boston, Massachusetts; Chief, Biological Psychiatry Laboratory, Laboratories for Psychiatric Research; Psychiatrist, McLean Hospital, Belmont, Massachusetts.

Michael K. Popkin, M.D. Professor of Psychiatry and Medicine, University of Minnesota Medical School; Chief of Psychiatry, Hennepin County Medical Center, Minneapolis, Minnesota.

Charles W. Popper, M.D. Clinical Instructor in Psychiatry, Harvard Medical School; Consultant in Psychiatry, Children's Hospital Medical Center, Boston, Massachusetts; Attending Child and Adolescent Psychiatrist, McLean Hospital, Belmont, Massachusetts.

Joel A. Posener, M.D. Instructor in Psychiatry, Harvard Medical School, Boston, Massachusetts; Staff Psychiatrist, McLean Hospital, Belmont, Massachusetts; Staff Psychiatrist, Brigham and Women's Hospital and Massachusetts Mental Health Center, Boston, Massachusetts.

Robert M. Post, M.D. Chief, Biological Psychiatry Branch, National Institute of Mental Health, Bethesda, Maryland.

Arthur J. Prange, Jr., M.D. Boshamer Professor of Psychiatry, Research Scientist for the Brain and Development Research Center, and Director of the Mental Health Clinic Research Center, University of North Carolina School of Medicine; Attending Psychiatrist, University of North Carolina Hospitals, Chapel Hill, North Carolina.

Karl H. Pribram, M.D. Professor Emeritus, Stanford University, Stanford, California; James P. and Anna King University Professor and Eminent Scholar, Commonwealth of Virginia, Radford University, Radford, Virginia.

Patricia N. Prinz, Ph.D. Professor of Psychiatry and Behavioral Sciences, University of Washington School of Medicine, Seattle, Washington.

David B. Pruitt, M.D. Professor and Vice Chairman, Department of Psychiatry and Director, Division of Child and Adolescent Psychiatry, University of Tennessee Memphis College of Medicine, Memphis, Tennessee.

Peter V. Rabins, M.D., M.P.H. Professor of Psychiatry, Johns Hopkins University School of Medicine, Baltimore, Maryland.

Richard H. Rahe, M.D. Professor of Psychiatry and Biobehavioral Sciences, University of Nevada School of Medicine; Director, Veterans Affairs Medical Center Nevada Stress Center; Medical Director, Nevada Mental Health Institute, Reno, Nevada; Visiting Professor of Psychiatry and Military Psychology, Uniformed Services University of the Health Sciences, Bethesda, Maryland.

Jeffrey L. Rausch, M.D. Professor and Vice Chairman, Department of Psychiatry and Health Behavior, Medical College of Georgia; Attending Psychiatrist, Veterans Affairs Medical Center, Augusta, Georgia.

Darrel A. Regier, M.D., M.P.H. Director, Division of Epidemiology and Services Research, National Institute of Mental Health, Rockville, Maryland; Clinical Professor of Psychiatry, Georgetown University School of Medicine, Washington, DC.

William E. Reichman, M.D. Associate Professor of Clinical Psychiatry and Director, Division of Geriatric Psychiatry, Department of Psychiatry, Robert Wood Johnson Medical School, University of Medicine and Dentistry of New Jersey; Medical Director, Comprehensive Services on Aging (COPSA), Institute for Alzheimer's Disease and Related Disorders, University of Medicine and Dentistry of New Jersey Community Mental Health Center at Piscataway, Piscataway, New Jersey.

James E. Rosenberg, M.D. Chief Resident in Forensic Psychiatry, Neuropsychiatric Institute and Hospital, Los Angeles, California.

Judith Wilson Ross, M.A. Professor of Medicine, University of California at Irvine College of Medicine, Irvine, California; Associate, Center for Healthcare Ethics, St. Joseph Health System, Orange, California.

Richard B. Rosse, M.D. Associate Professor of Psychiatry, Georgetown University School of Medicine; Psychiatry Service, Department of Veterans Affairs Medical Center, Washington, DC.

Alec Roy, M.B. Assistant Chief of Psychiatry for Substance Abuse, East Orange Veterans Affairs Medical Center, East Orange, New Jersey; Professor of Psychiatry, New Jersey Medical School, University of Medicine and Dentistry of New Jersey; Newark, New Jersey.

Robert T. Rubin, M.D., Ph.D. Blue Cross of Western Pennsylvania Professor of Neurosciences and Professor of Psychiatry, Medical College of Pennsylvania and Hahnemann University; Director, Neurosciences Research Center, Allegheny-Singer Research Institute, Allegheny General Hospital, Pittsburgh, Pennsylvania.

David R. Rubinow, M.D. Clinical Director, National Institute of Mental Health; Chief, Section on Behavioral Endocrinology, Biological Psychiatry Branch, National Institute of Mental Health, Bethesda, Maryland.

A. John Rush, M.D. Betty Jo Hay Distinguished Chair in Mental Health and Professor of Psychiatry, University of Texas Southwestern Medical Center, Dallas, Texas.

Joel Sadavoy, M.D., F.R.C.P.(C) Associate Professor of Psychiatry, University of Toronto Faculty of Medicine; Psychiatrist-in-Chief, Joint Department of Psychiatry, Mount Sinai Hospital-Ontario Cancer Institute-Princess Margaret Hospital, Toronto, Ontario, Canada.

Benjamin J. Sadock, M.D. Professor and Vice Chairman, Department of Psychiatry, New York University School of Medicine; Attending Psychiatrist, Tisch Hospital, the University Hospital of the New York University Medical Center; Attending Psychiatrist, Bellevue Hospital Center; Consultant Psychiatrist, Lenox Hill Hospital, New York, New York.

Virginia A. Sadock, M.D. Clinical Professor of Psychiatry and Director of Graduate Education in Human Sexuality, New York University School of Medicine; Attending Psychiatrist, Tisch Hospital, the University Hospital of the New York University Medical Center; Attending Psychiatrist, Bellevue Hospital Center, New York, New York.

Rafael J. Salin-Pascual, M.D., Ph.D. Professor of Physiology, Departamento de Fisiologia, Faculatad de Medicina, Universidad Nacional Autonomona de Mexico, Mexico City, Mexico.

Alberto B. Santos, M.D. Professor of Psychiatry and Director of Residency Training, Department of Psychiatry and Behavioral Sciences, Medical University of South Carolina, Charleston, South Carolina.

Paul Satz, Ph.D. Professor of Medical Psychology, University of California at Los Angeles School of Medicine; Chief of Neuropsychology, Neuropsychiatric Institute and Hospital, Los Angeles, California; Director of Research, UCLA-Camarillo State Hospital, Camarillo, California.

Alan F. Schatzberg, M.D. Kenneth T. Norris, Jr., Professor and Chairman, Department of Psychiatry and Behavioral Sciences, Stanford University School of Medicine; Chief of Service, Stanford University Hospital, Stanford, California.

Stephen C. Scheiber, M.D. Adjunct Professor of Psychiatry, Northwestern University Medical School, Chicago, Illinois; Adjunct Professor of Psychiatry, Medical College of Wisconsin, Milwaukee, Wisconsin; Senior Attending Physician, Evanston Hospital, Evanston, Illinois; Executive Vice President, American Board of Psychiatry and Neurology, Deerfield, Illinois.

Joseph J. Schildkraut, M.D. Professor of Psychiatry, Harvard Medical School; Director, Neuropsychopharmacology/Psychiatric Chemistry Laboratory, Massachusetts Mental Health Center, Boston, Massachusetts.

Peter J. Schmidt, M.D. Chief, Unit on Reproductive Endocrine Studies, Section on Behavioral Endocrinology, Biological Psychiatry Branch, National Institute of Mental Health, Bethesda, Maryland.

Richard S. Schottenfeld, M.D. Associate Professor of Psychiatry, Yale University School of Medicine; Director, Substance Abuse Treatment Unit, Connecticut Mental Health Center; Chief Executive Officer, The APT Foundation, New Haven, Connecticut.

John E. Schowalter, M.D. Albert J. Solnit Professor of Child Psychiatry and Pediatrics and Professor of Psychiatry, Yale University School of Medicine; Attending Psychiatrist and Assistant Chief of Child Psychiatry, Yale-New Haven Hospital, New Haven, Connecticut.

Marc A. Schuckit, M.D. Professor of Psychiatry, University of California at San Diego School of Medicine; Director, Alcohol Research Center, San Diego Veterans Affairs Medical Center, San Diego, California.

S. Charles Schulz, M.D. Professor and Chair, Department of Psychiatry, Case Western Reserve University; Director, Department of Psychiatry, University Hospitals of Cleveland, Cleveland, Ohio.

Richard I. Shader, M.D. Professor of Pharmacology and Experimental Therapeutics, Tufts University School of Medicine, Boston, Massachusetts.

Steven S. Sharfstein, M.D. Clinical Professor of Psychiatry, University of Maryland School of Medicine; President, Medical Director and Chief Executive Officer, Sheppard and Enoch Pratt Hospital, Baltimore, Maryland.

Judith Shay, M.D. Assistant Professor of Psychiatry, Mount Sinai School of Medicine; Assistant Attending Psychiatrist, Mount Sinai Hospital; Director, Child Psychiatry Outpatient Clinic, Mount Sinai Medical Center, New York, New York.

M. Tracie Shea, Ph.D. Associate Professor of Psychiatry and Human Behavior and Director of Clinical Assessment and Training Unit, Brown University; Psychologist, Post Traumatic Stress Disorders Clinic, Veterans Affairs Medical Center, Providence, Rhode Island.

Daniel J. Siegel, M.D. Assistant Professor of Psychiatry, Department of Psychiatry and Biobehavioral Sciences, University of California at Los Angeles School of Medicine; Acting Director, Residency Training in Child and Adolescent Psychiatry, Neuropsychiatric Institute and Hospital, Los Angeles, California.

George M. Simpson, M.D. Professor of Research Psychiatry, Director of Clinical Research, University of Southern California School of Medicine, Los Angeles, California.

Elyse J. Singer, M.D. Associate Professor, University of California at Los Angeles School of Medicine; Staff Neurologist and Research Physician, West Los Angeles Veterans Affairs Medical Center; Attending Neurologist, University of California at Los Angeles Medical Center, Los Angeles, California.

Samuel G. Siris, M.D. Professor of Psychiatry, Albert Einstein College of Medicine of Yeshiva University, Bronx, New York; Director, Adult Psychiatric Day Programs, Hillside Hospital Division of the Long Island Jewish Medical Center, Glen Oaks, New York.

Gary W. Small, M.D. Associate Professor of Psychiatry and Biobehavioral Sciences, University of California at Los Angeles School of Medicine; Director, Geriatric Psychiatry Fellowship Program, Neuropsychiatric Institute and Hospital; Chief, Geriatric Psychiatry Program, West Los Angeles Veterans Affairs Medical Center, Los Angeles, California.

S. Mouchly Small, M.D. Professor and Chairman Emeritus, Department of Psychiatry, State University of New York at Buffalo School of Medicine and Biomedical Sciences; Director Emeritus, American Board of Psychiatry and Neurology; Attending Psychiatrist, Erie County Medical Center; Consultant, Buffalo Veterans Affairs Medical Center; Honorary Staff Psychiatrist, Buffalo General Hospital; Honorary Staff Psychiatrist, Children's Hospital, Buffalo, New York.

Buster Deangelo Smith, M.D. Instructor of Psychiatry, Medical College of Pennsylvania, Philadelphia, Pennsylvania.

G. Richard Smith, M.D. Professor, Vice Chairman, and Director of Centers for Mental Healthcare Research, Department of Psychiatry and Behavioral Sciences, University of Arkansas for Medical Sciences, Little Rock, Arkansas; Director, Health Services

Research and Development, John L. McCellan Memorial Veterans Hospital (North Little Rock), North Little Rock, Arkansas.

Solomon H. Snyder, M.D. Distinguished Service Professor of Neuroscience, Pharmacology, Molecular Sciences, and Psychiatry, Johns Hopkins University School of Medicine, Baltimore, Maryland.

Vicki M. Soukup, Ph.D. Assistant Professor of Neurology and Director, Neuropsychology Services, Department of Neurology, University of Texas Medical Branch, Galveston, Texas.

Robert L. Spencer, Ph.D. Assistant Professor of Psychology, University of Colorado, Boulder, Colorado.

Larry R. Squire, Ph.D. Professor of Psychiatry and Neurosciences, University of California at San Diego School of Medicine; Research Career Scientist, San Diego Veterans Affairs Medical Center, San Diego, California.

Peter Steinglass, M.D. Clinical Professor of Psychiatry, Cornell University Medical College; Executive Director, Ackerman Institute for Family Therapy, New York, New York.

Robert A. Stern, Ph.D. Assistant Professor of Psychiatry and Human Behavior, and Clinical Neurosciences, Brown University School of Medicine; Director, Neurobehavioral Research, Department of Psychiatry, Rhode Island Hospital, Providence, Rhode Island.

Anne Marie Stoline, M.D. Staff Psychiatrist, Sheppard and Enoch Pratt Hospital, Baltimore, Maryland.

Alan Stoudemire, M.D. Professor of Psychiatry and Behavioral Sciences, Emory University School of Medicine, Atlanta, Georgia.

James J. Strain, M.D. Professor and Director, Division of Behavioral Medicine and Consultation Psychiatry, Mount Sinai Medical Center, New York, New York.

Gordon D. Strauss, M.D. Professor of Psychiatry and Director, Graduate Medical Education, Department of Psychiatry and Behavioral Sciences, University of Louisville School of Medicine; Staff Psychiatrist, Louisville Veterans Affairs Medical Center, Louisville, Kentucky.

Margaret L. Stuber, M.D. Assistant Professor of Psychiatry and Director of Education for Child Psychiatry, University of California at Los Angeles School of Medicine; Director of Pediatric Consultation-Liaison, Center for the Health Sciences, University of California at Los Angeles, Los Angeles, California.

Mark D. Sullivan, M.D., Ph.D. Assistant Professor, Division of Consultation-Liaison, Department of Psychiatry and Behavioral Sciences and Attending Physician, Multidisciplinary Pain Center, University of Washington School of Medicine, Seattle, Washington.

Norman Sussman, M.D. Clinical Associate Professor of Psychiatry, New York University School of Medicine; Director, Psychopharmacology Research and Consultation Service, Bellevue Hospital Center, New York, New York.

Peter Szatmari, M.D. Associate Professor of Psychiatry, Faculty of Health Sciences, McMaster University; Consultant Psychiatrist, Chedoke Child and Family Centre, Chedoke-McMaster Hospital, Hamilton, Ontario, Canada.

Manuel E. Tancer, M.D. Associate Professor of Psychiatry and Behavioral Neurosciences and Director of Social Phobia Program, Mood and Anxiety Disorders Clinical Research Division, Wayne State University School of Medicine, Detroit, Michigan; Director of Research, Department of Psychiatry, Veterans Affairs Hospital, Allen Park, Michigan.

Kenneth Tardiff, M.D., M.P.H. Professor of Psychiatry and Public Health, Cornell University Medical College; Medical Director and Attending Psychiatrist, Payne Whitney Clinic-New York Hospital, New York, New York.

H. Gerry Taylor, Ph.D. Associate Professor of Pediatrics, Case Western University School of Medicine; Associate Professor of Pediatrics, Rainbow Babies and Children's Hospital, Cleveland, Ohio.

Thomas W. Uhde, M.D. Professor and Chairperson, Department of Psychiatry and Behavioral Neurosciences, Wayne State University School of Medicine; Chairman, Department of Psychiatry, Detroit Receiving Hospital; Psychiatrist-in-Chief, Detroit Medical Center, Detroit, Michigan.

Jerome V. Vaccaro, M.D. Associate Professor of Clinical Psychiatry and Director of Community Psychiatry, University of California at Los Angeles School of Medicine, Los Angeles, California.

Louis Vachon, M.D. Professor and Chairman, Division of Psychiatry, Boston University School of Medicine; Psychiatrist-in-Chief, Boston University Medical Center Hospital, Boston, Massachusetts.

Wilfred G. van Gorp, Ph.D. Associate Professor in Residence of Psychiatry and Biobehavioral Sciences, and Co-Director of Neuropsychology Post-doctoral Training, University of California at Los Angeles School of Medicine; Chief, Neuropsychology Assessment Laboratory, West Los Angeles Veterans Affairs Medical Center, Los Angeles, California.

Daniel P. van Kammen, M.D., Ph.D. Professor of Psychiatry, University of Pittsburgh Medical School; Chief of Staff, Highland Drive Veterans Affairs Medical Center, Pittsburgh, Pennsylvania.

William W. Van Stone, M.D. Emeritus Clinical Associate Professor of Psychiatry and Behavioral Sciences, Stanford University School of Medicine, Stanford, California; Chief of Treatment Services, Mental Health and Behavioral Sciences Services, Department of Veterans Affairs Medical Center, Washington, DC.

Jeff Victoroff, M.D. Assistant Professor of Neurology, University of Southern California School of Medicine, Los Angeles, California; Director of Neurobehavior and Director of Neuromedicine Clinic, Rancho Los Amigos Medical Center, Downey, California.

Michael V. Vitiello, Ph.D. Professor of Psychiatry, Behavioral Sciences, and Psychology and Associate Director, Sleep and Aging Research Program, University of Washington, Seattle, Washington.

Benedetto Vitiello, M.D. Head, Pediatric Psychopharmacology Program, Child and Adolescent Disorders Research Branch, National Institute of Mental Health, Rockville, Maryland.

Fred R. Volkmar, M.D. Harris Associate Professor of Child Psychiatry, Pediatrics, and Psychology, Child Study Center, Yale University School of Medicine; Attending Psychiatrist, Yale-New Haven Hospital, New Haven, Connecticut.

Thomas A. Wadden, Ph.D. Professor of Psychology in Psychiatry, University of Pennsylvania School of Medicine, Philadelphia, Pennsylvania.

William L. Webb, Jr., M.D. Professor of Psychiatry, University of Connecticut School of Medicine; Psychiatrist-in-Chief Emeritus, Institute of Living, Hartford, Connecticut (*deceased*).

Thomas A. Wehr, M.D. Chief, Clinical Psychobiology Branch, Intramural Research Program, National Institute of Mental Health, Bethesda, Maryland.

Daniel R. Weinberger, M.D. Chief, Clinical Brain Disorders Branch, Intramural Research Program, National Institute of Mental Health Neuroscience Center at St. Elizabeth's, Washington, DC.

Myron F. Weiner, M.D. Aradine S. Ard Chair in Brain Sciences, Vice Chairman for Clinical Services, and Chief of Geropsychiatry, Department of Psychiatry, University of Texas Southwestern Medical Center; Attending Physician, Zale-Lipshy University Hospital, Dallas, Texas.

Robert L. Williams, M.D. Professor Emeritus of Psychiatry and Neurology and Former Co-Director of Sleep Disorders and Research Center, Baylor College of Medicine; Former Chief of Psychiatry Service, The Methodist Hospital and St. Luke's Episcopal Hospital; Former Senior Attending, Texas Children's Hospital, Houston, Texas.

G. Terence Wilson, Ph.D. Professor of Psychology, Rutgers University, Piscataway, New Jersey.

William C. Wirshing, M.D. Associate Professor of Clinical Psychiatry and Biobehavioral Sciences, University of California at Los Angeles School of Medicine; Chief, Schizophrenia Treatment Unit and Director, Brentwood Movement Disorders Laboratory, West Los Angeles Veterans Affairs Medical Center, Los Angeles, California.

Eve J. Wiseman, M.D. Assistant Professor of Psychiatry, University of Arkansas for Medical Sciences; Chief, Special Treatment Section, John L. McClellan Memorial Veterans Hospital, Little Rock, Arkansas.

Normund Wong, M.D. Professor and Chairman, Department of Psychiatry, Walter Reed Army Medical Center; Psychiatry Consultant to the Office of the Surgeon General, Washington, DC; Professor and Vice Chairman, Department of Psychiatry, Uniformed Services University of the Health Sciences, Bethesda, Maryland.

George E. Woody, M.D. Clinical Professor of Psychiatry, University of Pennsylvania School of Medicine; Chief, Substance Abuse Treatment Unit, Philadelphia Veterans Affairs Medical Center, Philadelphia, Pennsylvania.

Richard Jed Wyatt, M.D. Chief, Neuropsychiatry Branch, National Institute of Mental Health Neuroscience Center at St. Elizabeth's, Washington, DC.

Joel Yager, M.D. Professor and Associate Chair for Education, Department of Psychiatry and Biobehavioral Sciences, University of California Los Angeles School of Medicine; Associate Chief of Psychiatry for Residency Education, West Los Angeles Veterans Medical Center, Los Angeles, California.

J. Gerald Young, M.D. Professor of Psychiatry, Director, Developmental Neurobiology Unit, Division of Child and Adolescent Psychiatry, New York University School of Medicine; Attending Psychiatrist, Tisch Hospital, the University Hospital of the New York University Medical Center; Attending Psychiatrist, Bellevue Hospital Center, New York, New York.

Sidney Zisook, M.D. Professor of Psychiatry and Associate Residency Training Director, University of California at San Diego School of Medicine, La Jolla, California; Director of Research and Education, University of California at San Diego Outpatient Psychiatric Services, San Diego, California.

Rebecca K. Zoltoski, Ph.D. Research Associate, Department of Psychology, Brock University, St. Catharines, Ontario, Canada.

Stephen R. Zukin, M.D. Professor of Psychiatry and Neuroscience and Director, Biomedical Psychopharmacology Laboratory, Albert Einstein College of Medicine of Yeshiva University; Director of Research, Bronx Psychiatric Center; Attending Psychiatrist, Montefiore Medical Center, Bronx, New York.

CONTENTS

VOLUME ONE

VOLUME TWO

Drugs Used In Psychiatry

This guide contains color reproductions of some commonly prescribed major psychotherapeutic drugs. This guide mainly illustrates tablets and capsules. A † symbol preceding the name of the drug indicates that other doses are available. Check directly with the manufacturer. *(Although the photos are intended as accurate reproductions of the drug, this guide should be used only as a quick identification aid.)*

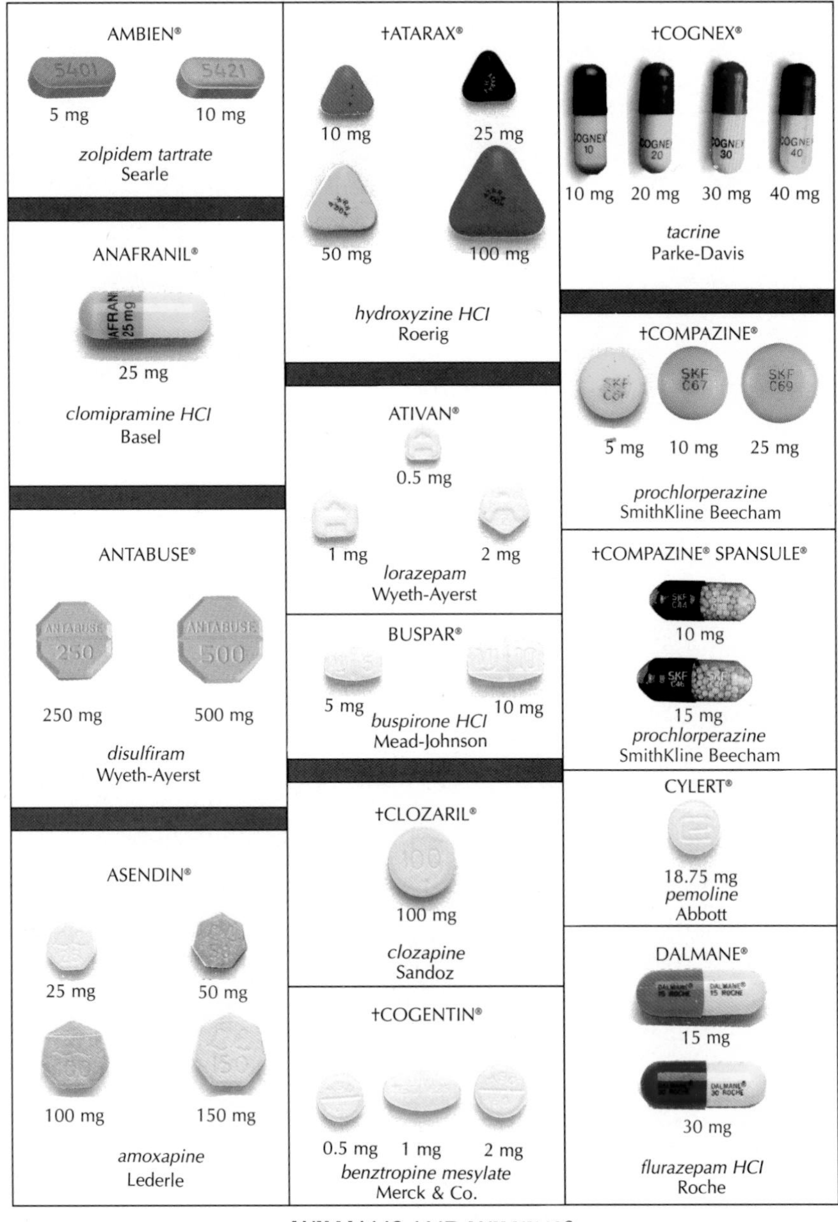

WILLIAMS AND WILKINS©

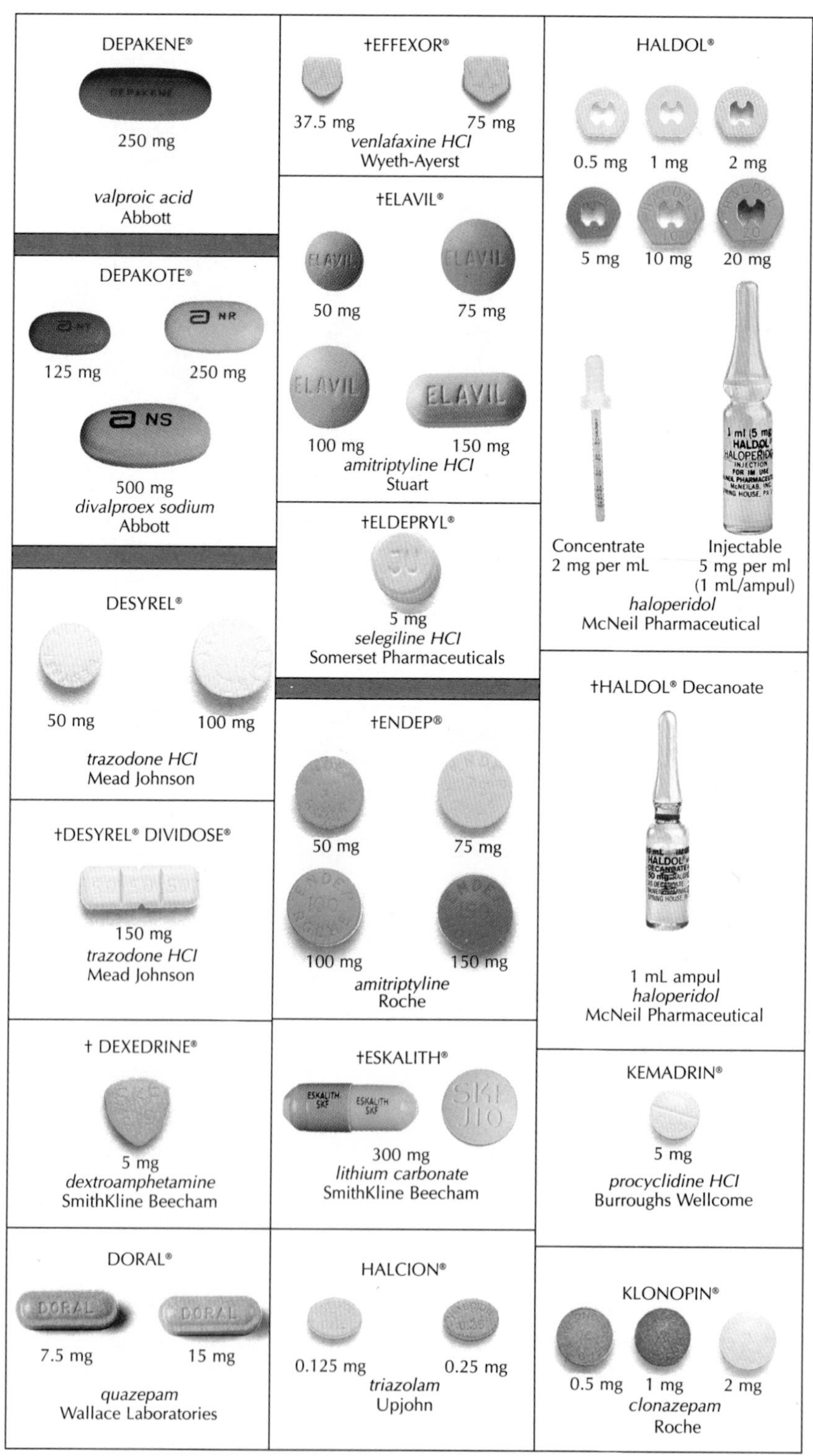
DEPAKENE®
250 mg
valproic acid
Abbott
DEPAKOTE®
125 mg
250 mg
500 mg
divalproex sodium
Abbott
DESYREL®
50 mg
100 mg
trazodone HCl
Mead Johnson
†DESYREL® DIVIDOSE®
150 mg
trazodone HCl
Mead Johnson
† DEXEDRINE®
5 mg
dextroamphetamine
SmithKline Beecham
DORAL®
7.5 mg
15 mg
quazepam
Wallace Laboratories
†EFFEXOR®
37.5 mg
75 mg
venlafaxine HCl
Wyeth-Ayerst
†ELAVIL®
50 mg
75 mg
100 mg
150 mg
amitriptyline HCl
Stuart
†ELDEPRYL®
5 mg
selegiline HCl
Somerset Pharmaceuticals
†ENDEP®
50 mg
75 mg
100 mg
150 mg
amitriptyline
Roche
†ESKALITH®
300 mg
lithium carbonate
SmithKline Beecham
HALCION®
0.125 mg
0.25 mg
triazolam
Upjohn
HALDOL®
0.5 mg
1 mg
2 mg
5 mg
10 mg
20 mg
Concentrate
2 mg per mL
Injectable
5 mg per ml
(1 mL/ampul)
haloperidol
McNeil Pharmaceutical
†HALDOL® Decanoate
1 mL ampul
haloperidol
McNeil Pharmaceutical
KEMADRIN®
5 mg
procyclidine HCl
Burroughs Wellcome
KLONOPIN®
0.5 mg
1 mg
2 mg
clonazepam
Roche

WILLIAMS AND WILKINS©

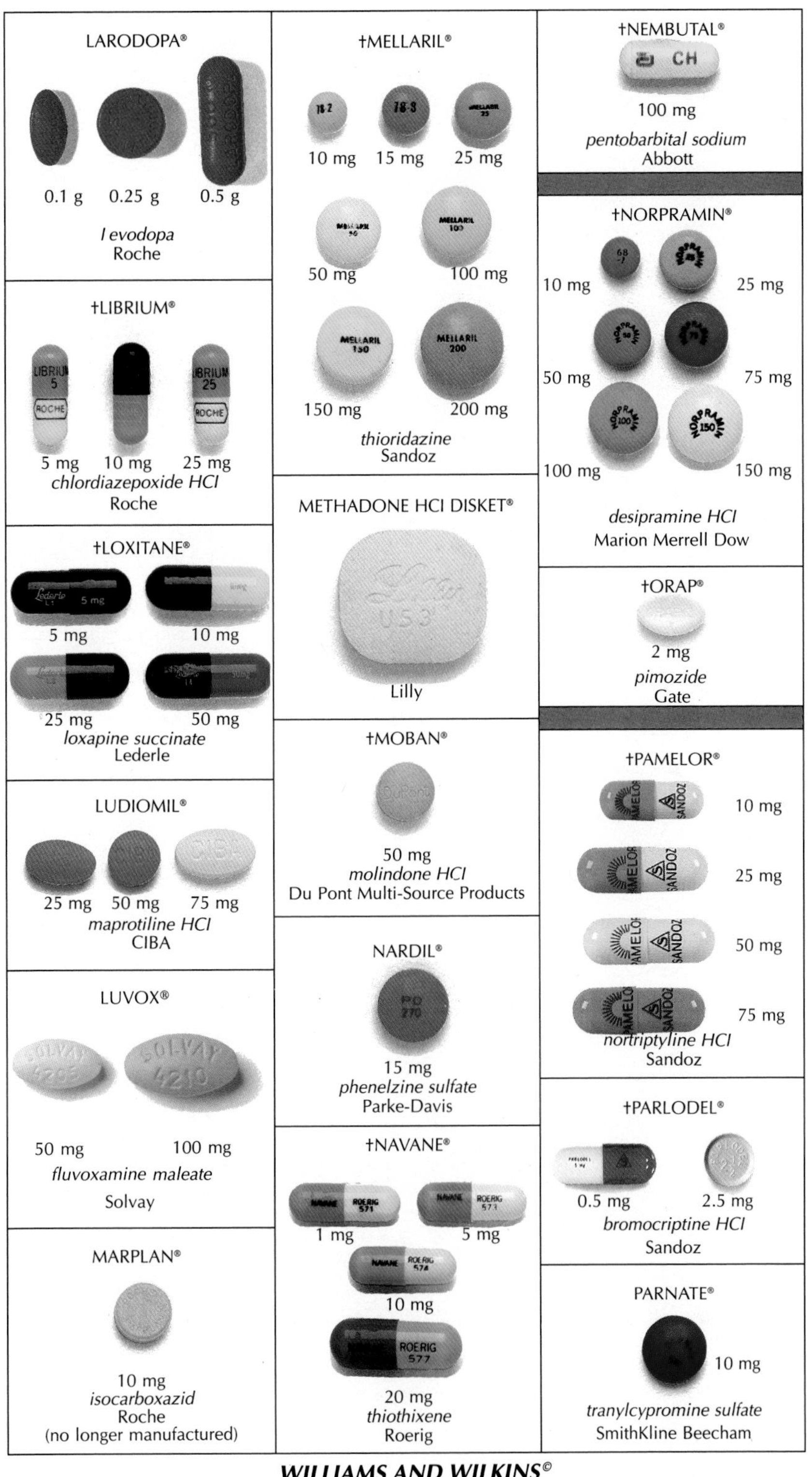
LARODOPA®
0.1 g 0.25 g 0.5 g
levodopa
Roche
†LIBRIUM®
5 mg 10 mg 25 mg
chlordiazepoxide HCl
Roche
†LOXITANE®
5 mg 10 mg
25 mg 50 mg
loxapine succinate
Lederle
LUDIOMIL®
25 mg 50 mg 75 mg
maprotiline HCl
CIBA
LUVOX®
50 mg 100 mg
fluvoxamine maleate
Solvay
MARPLAN®
10 mg
isocarboxazid
Roche
(no longer manufactured)
†MELLARIL®
10 mg 15 mg 25 mg
50 mg 100 mg
150 mg 200 mg
thioridazine
Sandoz
METHADONE HCl DISKET®
Lilly
†MOBAN®
50 mg
molindone HCl
Du Pont Multi-Source Products
NARDIL®
15 mg
phenelzine sulfate
Parke-Davis
†NAVANE®
1 mg 5 mg
10 mg
20 mg
thiothixene
Roerig
†NEMBUTAL®
100 mg
pentobarbital sodium
Abbott
†NORPRAMIN®
10 mg 25 mg
50 mg 75 mg
100 mg 150 mg
desipramine HCl
Marion Merrell Dow
†ORAP®
2 mg
pimozide
Gate
†PAMELOR®
10 mg
25 mg
50 mg
75 mg
nortriptyline HCl
Sandoz
†PARLODEL®
0.5 mg 2.5 mg
bromocriptine HCl
Sandoz
PARNATE®
10 mg
tranylcypromine sulfate
SmithKline Beecham

WILLIAMS AND WILKINS©

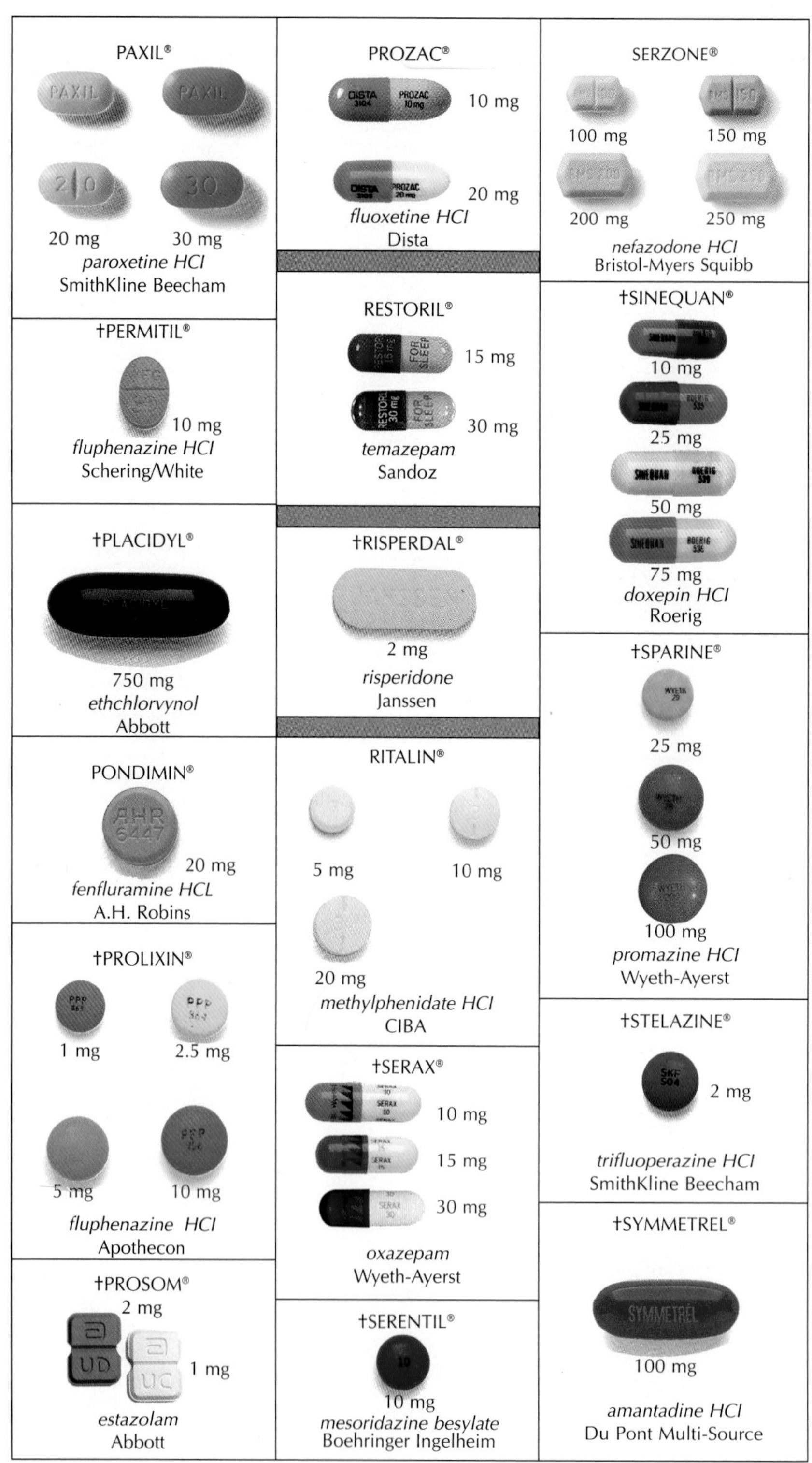
PAXIL®
PAXIL
PAXIL
20
30
20 mg
30 mg
paroxetine HCl
SmithKline Beecham
†PERMITIL®
10 mg
fluphenazine HCl
Schering/White
†PLACIDYL®
750 mg
ethchlorvynol
Abbott
PONDIMIN®
AHR 6447
20 mg
fenfluramine HCL
A.H. Robins
†PROLIXIN®
1 mg
2.5 mg
5 mg
10 mg
fluphenazine HCl
Apothecon
†PROSOM®
2 mg
UD
UC
1 mg
estazolam
Abbott
PROZAC®
DISTA 3104
PROZAC 10 mg
10 mg
20 mg
fluoxetine HCl
Dista
RESTORIL®
15 mg
RESTORIL 30 mg
FOR SLEEP
30 mg
temazepam
Sandoz
†RISPERDAL®
2 mg
risperidone
Janssen
RITALIN®
5 mg
10 mg
20 mg
methylphenidate HCl
CIBA
†SERAX®
10 mg
15 mg
30 mg
oxazepam
Wyeth-Ayerst
†SERENTIL®
10 mg
mesoridazine besylate
Boehringer Ingelheim
SERZONE®
BMS 150
100 mg
150 mg
200 mg
250 mg
nefazodone HCl
Bristol-Myers Squibb
†SINEQUAN®
10 mg
25 mg
SINEQUAN
50 mg
75 mg
doxepin HCl
Roerig
†SPARINE®
25 mg
50 mg
100 mg
promazine HCl
Wyeth-Ayerst
†STELAZINE®
SKF 504
2 mg
trifluoperazine HCl
SmithKline Beecham
†SYMMETREL®
SYMMETREL
100 mg
amantadine HCl
Du Pont Multi-Source
WILLIAMS AND WILKINS©

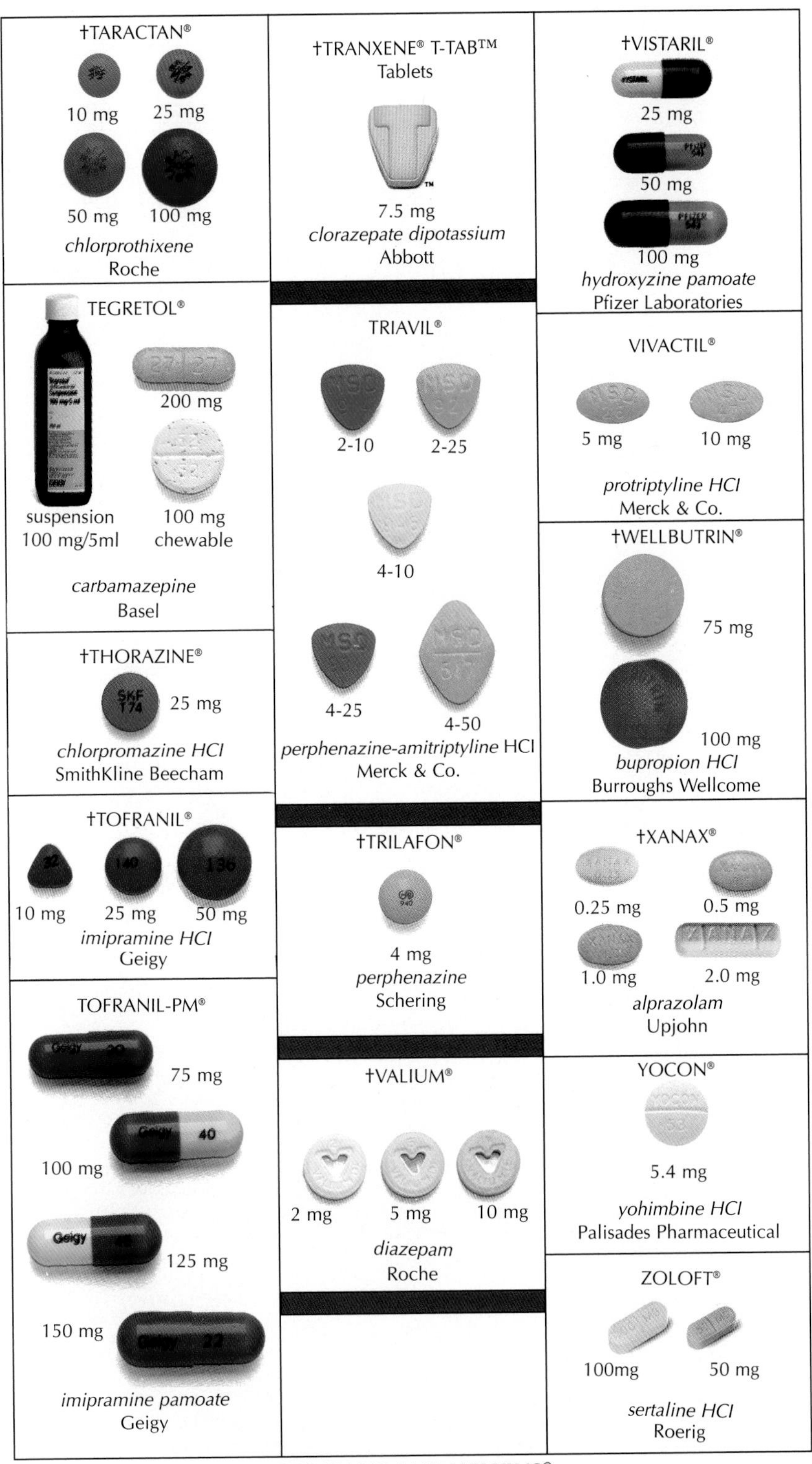
†TARACTAN®
10 mg
25 mg
50 mg
100 mg
chlorprothixene
Roche
†TRANXENE® T-TAB™
Tablets
7.5 mg
clorazepate dipotassium
Abbott
†VISTARIL®
25 mg
50 mg
100 mg
hydroxyzine pamoate
Pfizer Laboratories
TEGRETOL®
200 mg
suspension
100 mg/5ml
100 mg
chewable
carbamazepine
Basel
TRIAVIL®
2-10
2-25
4-10
4-25
4-50
perphenazine-amitriptyline HCl
Merck & Co.
VIVACTIL®
5 mg
10 mg
protriptyline HCl
Merck & Co.
†WELLBUTRIN®
75 mg
100 mg
bupropion HCl
Burroughs Wellcome
†THORAZINE®
25 mg
chlorpromazine HCl
SmithKline Beecham
†TOFRANIL®
10 mg
25 mg
50 mg
imipramine HCl
Geigy
†TRILAFON®
4 mg
perphenazine
Schering
†XANAX®
0.25 mg
0.5 mg
1.0 mg
2.0 mg
alprazolam
Upjohn
TOFRANIL-PM®
75 mg
100 mg
125 mg
150 mg
imipramine pamoate
Geigy
†VALIUM®
2 mg
5 mg
10 mg
diazepam
Roche
YOCON®
5.4 mg
yohimbine HCl
Palisades Pharmaceutical
ZOLOFT®
100mg
50 mg
sertaline HCl
Roerig

WILLIAMS AND WILKINS©

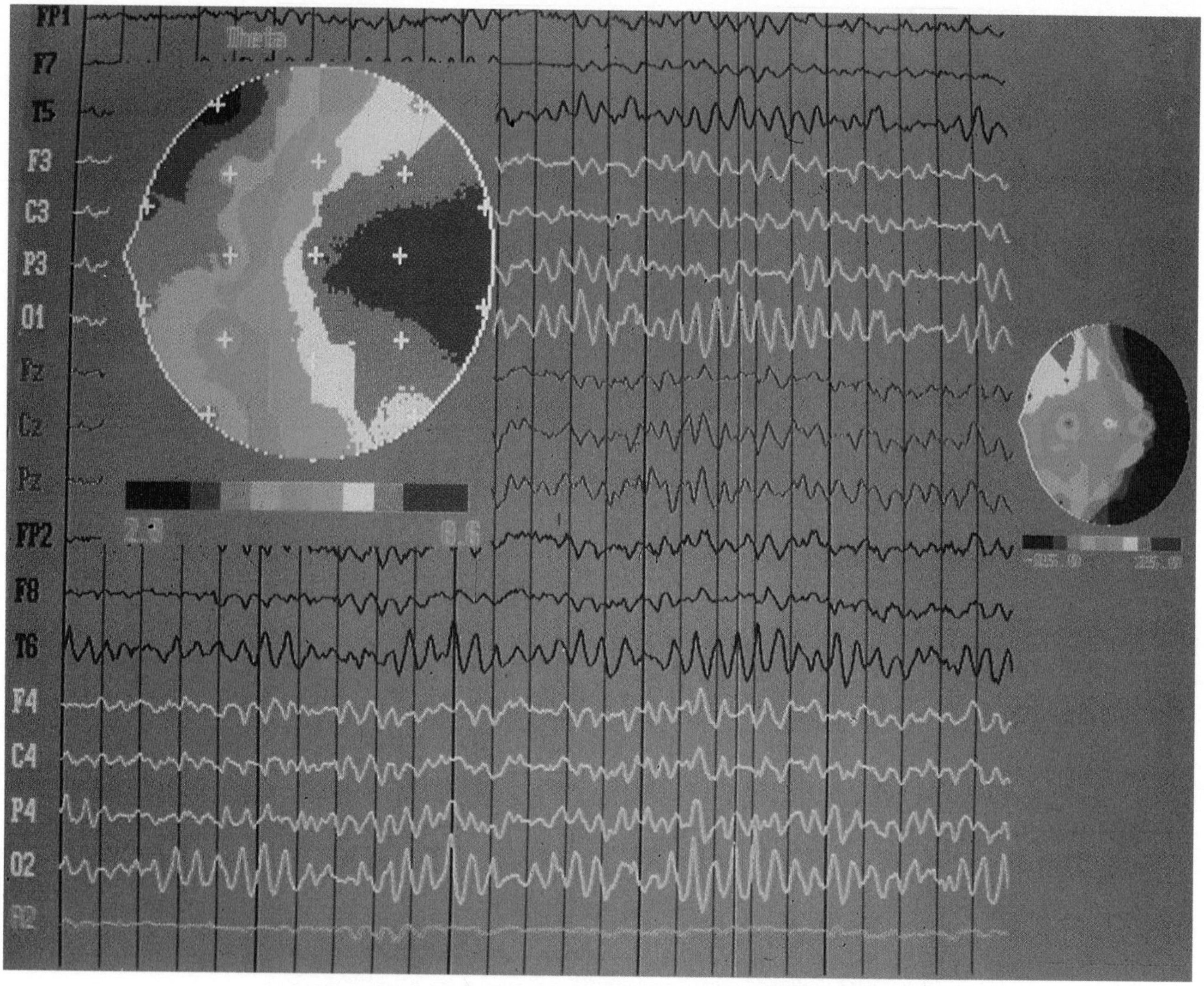

FIGURE 1.8-5 *Digital EEG recording and topographic map representation.*

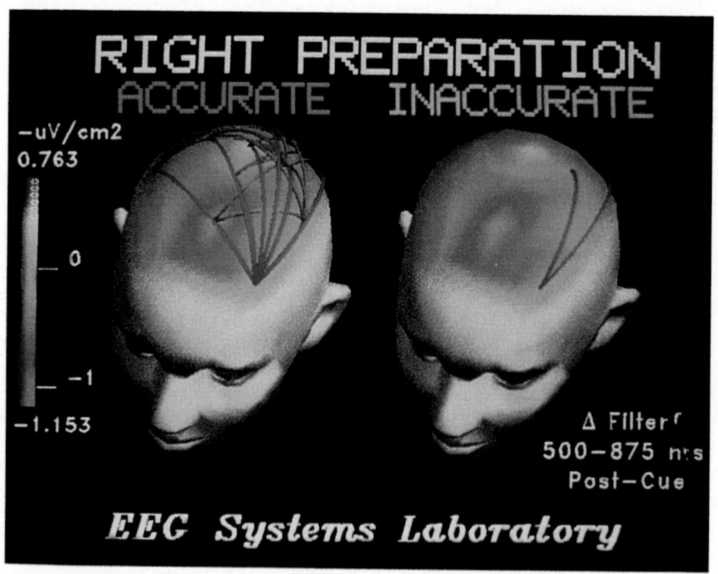

FIGURE 1.8-6 *Example of network from 124 lead recording.*

PLATE 1

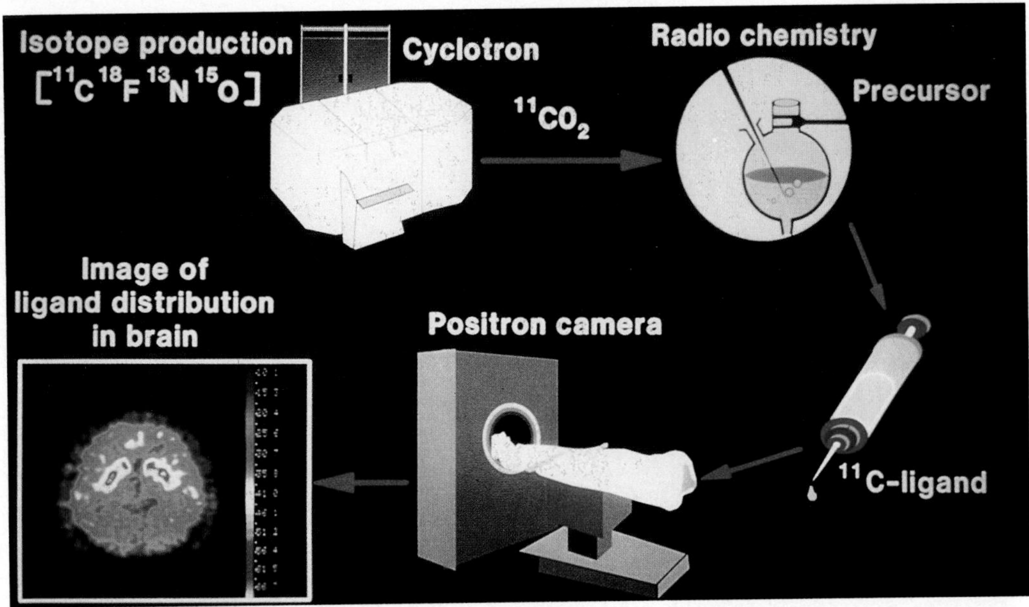

FIGURE 1.10-11 *Imaging of neuroreceptors by PET. The method involves the production of a positron-emitting nuclide, its incorporation into a radiopharmaceutical, injection of the radiopharmaceutical into a subject, and subsequent image reconstruction with the PET camera. The displayed PET image depicts the distribution of striatal dopamine D_2 receptors. SPECT imaging follows a similar procedure, except that the isotopes are longer-lived and can be produced by a distant central cyclotron facility (figure courtesy of G Sedvall). From G Sedvall, L Farde, F A Wiesel: Imaging of neurotransmitter receptors in the living human brain. Arch Gen Psychiatry* 43: 999. *Used with permission.*

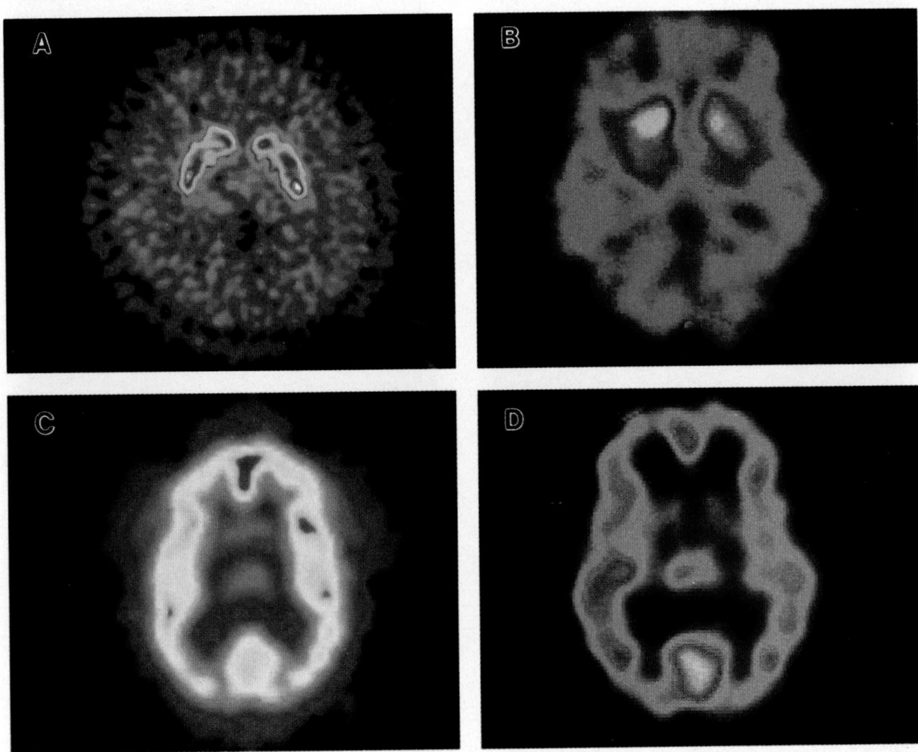

FIGURE 1.10-15 *Transaxial images showing the distribution of D_2 receptors in a human brain imaged with PET* (A) *using [C^{11}] raclopride (figure courtesy of Lars Farde) and with SPECT* (B) *using [I^{123}] iodobenzamide (figure courtesy of Robert Innis). Benzodiazepine receptors have been imaged with PET* (C) *using [C^{11}] flumazenil (figure courtesy of James Frost) and with SPECT* (D) *using [I^{123}] iomazenil (figure courtesy of the first author). For all images the frontal lobe is located at the top, and the occipital lobe is at the bottom of each photograph. D_2 receptors are highly concentrated in subcortical regions—the caudate and the putamen. Benzodiazepine receptors are present in several cortical regions, with the highest densities in the occipital cortex.*

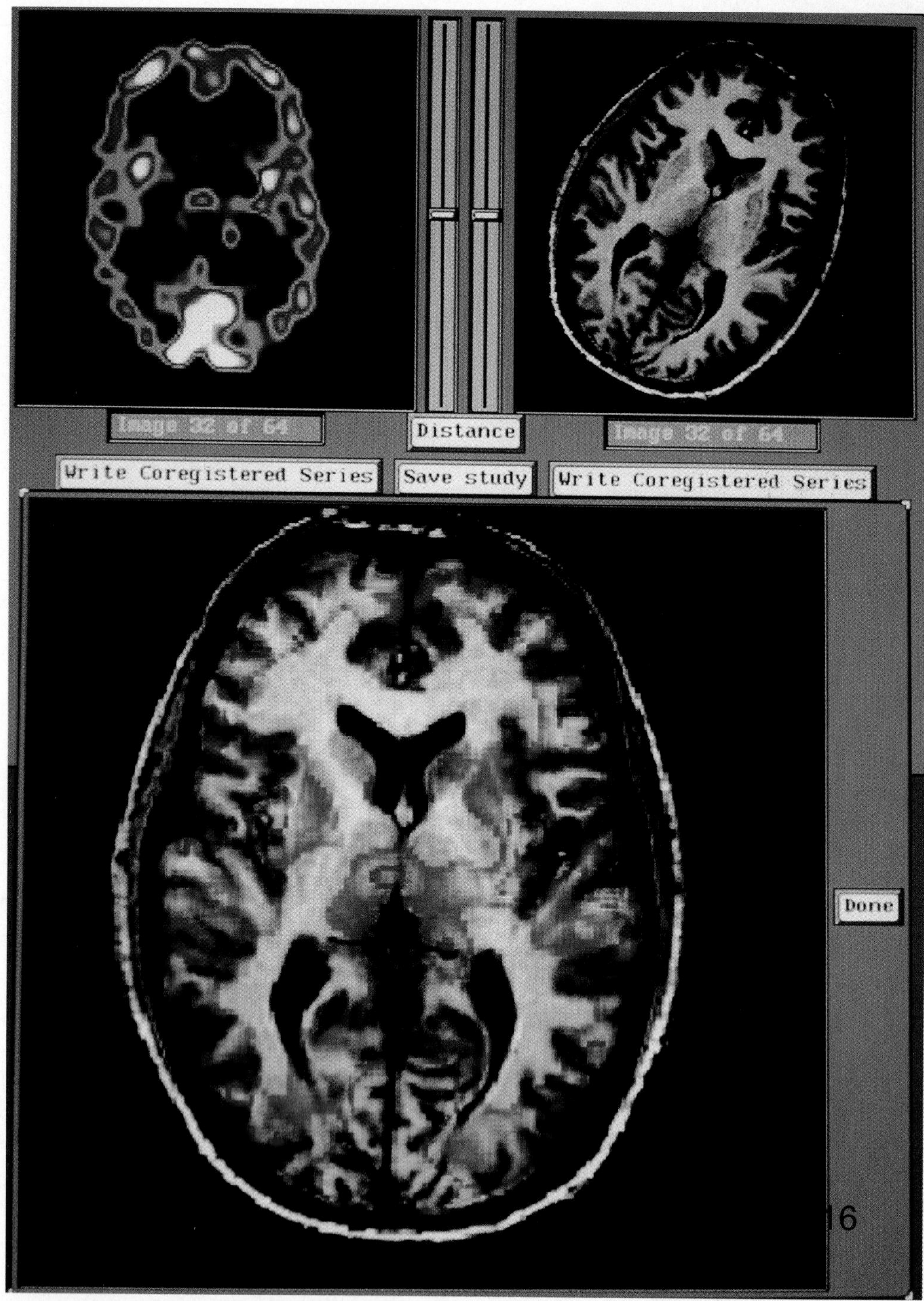

FIGURE 1.10-16 *Transaxial SPECT and MR images from a human subject studied with the benzodiazepine receptor radioligand, [I^{123}] iomazenil (figure courtesy of the second author and Erik G. Miller, CORITech Inc., New Haven, CT). Through a computer-assisted technique, the original three-dimensional MR image set (upper right) is mathematically transformed, interpolated, and resliced to match the SPECT series (upper left). The superimposed images (below) depict the precise anatomical distribution of [I^{123}] iomazenil, revealing highest concentrations of benzodiazepine receptors in cortical (particularly occipital) regions.*

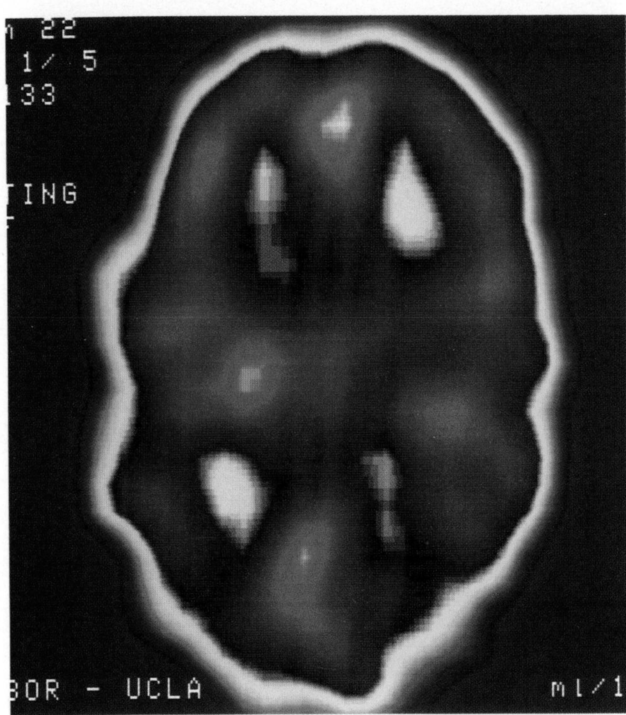

FIGURE 2.10-2 *Xenon 133 image of cerebral blood flow in a healthy elderly man. Blood flow ranges from 57 ml/100 g tissue a minute in the periventrical regions to 82 ml/100 g tissue a minute in the frontal and occipital regions.*

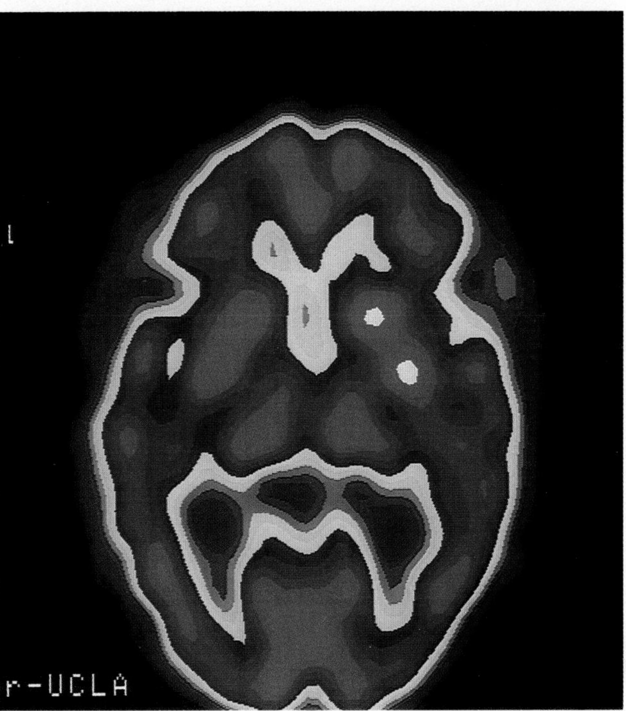

FIGURE 2.10-3 *SPECT of a normal subject using ^{99m}Tc-d,l, hexamethyl-propyleneamine-oxime (HMPAO). The color scale is set to maximum uptake with a shift to yellow at 66 percent maximum uptake and shift to green at 50 percent maximum uptake.*

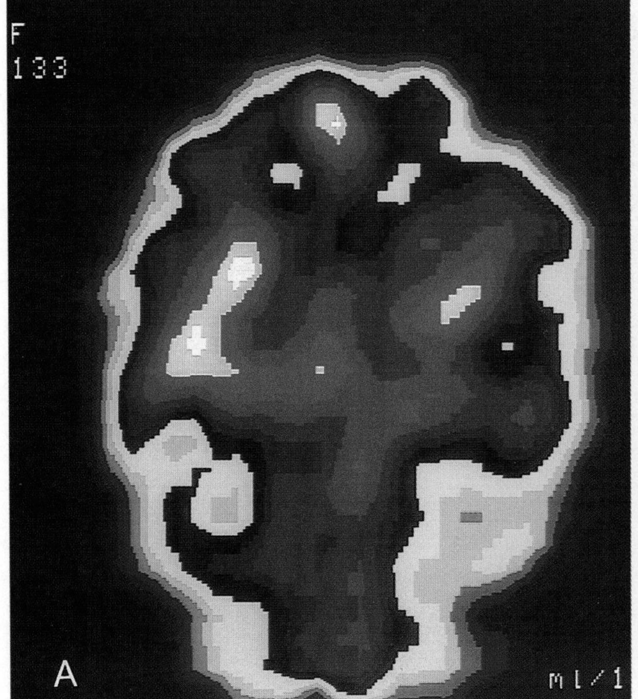

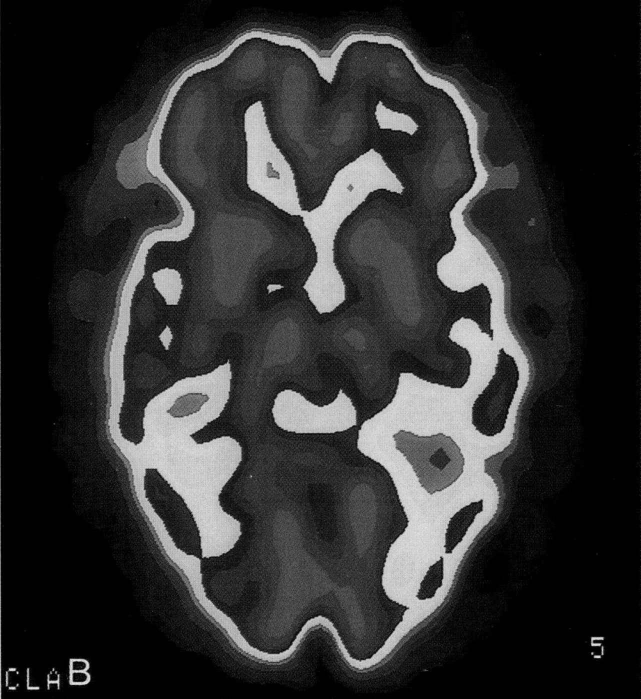

FIGURE 2.10-6A *Xenon 133 image of cerebral blood flow in a 69-year-old man with Alzheimer's disease. In the posterior temporal-parietal cortex blood flow is 18 to 25 ml/100 g tissue a minute whereas maximum flow occurs in the motor cortex at 46 ml/100 g tissue a minute.* B, *HMAPO SPECT from the patient in Figure 2.10-6A demonstrating a 50 percent reduction in blood flow in the posterior temporal-parietal cortex.*

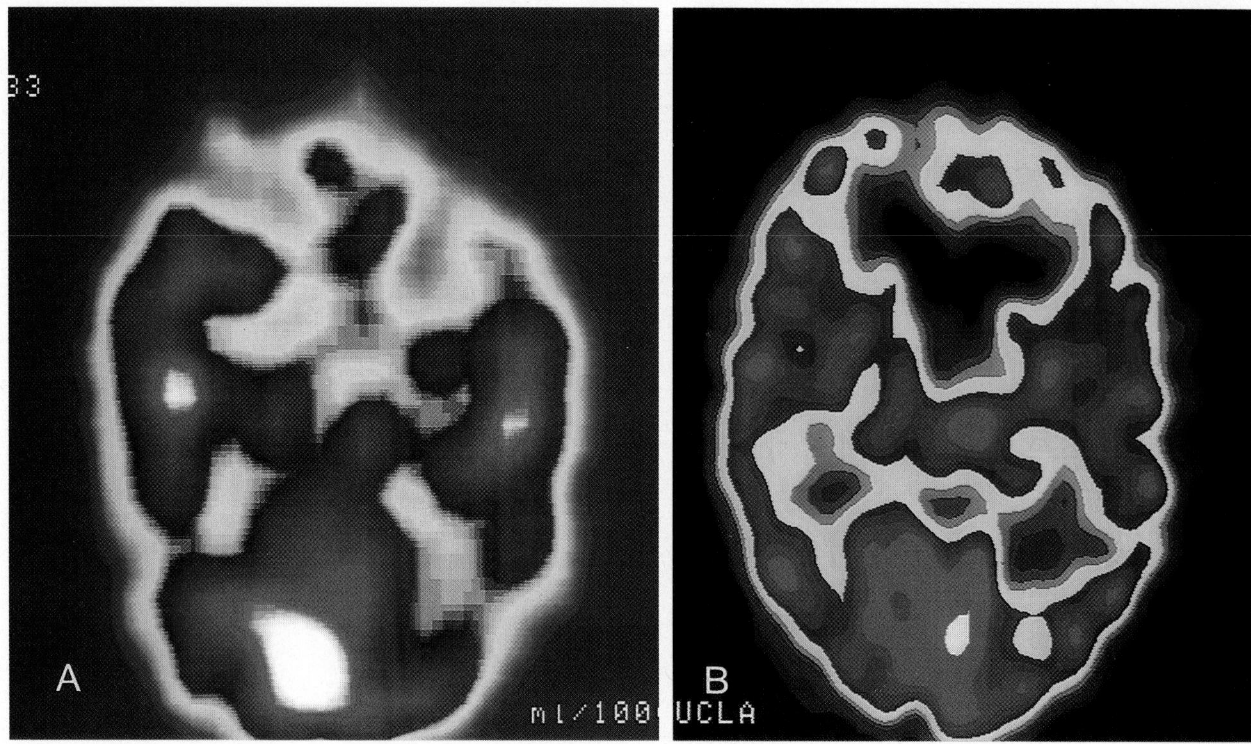

FIGURE 2.10-7A *Xenon 133 image of cerebral blood flow in a 52-year-old woman with a progressive frontal lobe degeneration. Blood flow ranges from 18 ml/100 g tissue a minute in the anterior frontal lobes to 74 ml/100 g tissue a minute in the occipital regions.* B, *HMAPO SPECT from the patient in Figure 2.10-6B demonstrating a 50 percent reduction in blood flow in the frontal regions.*

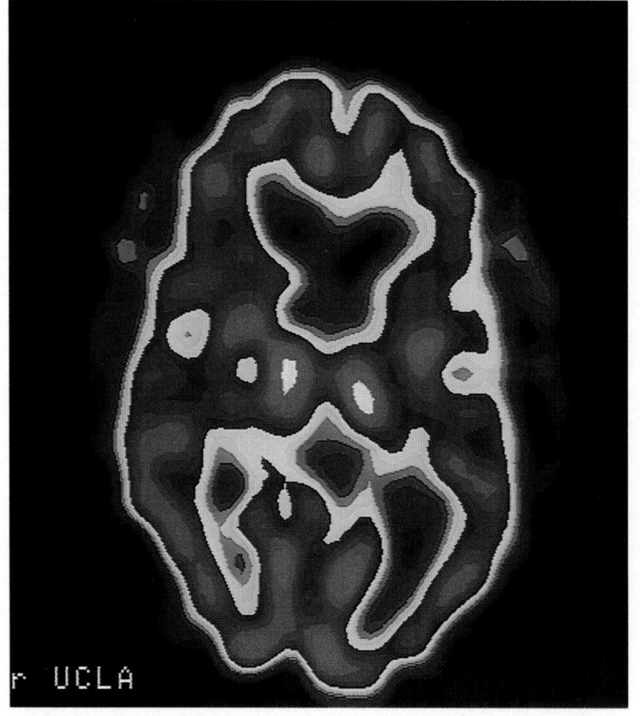

FIGURE 2.10-11 *HMPAO SPECT of a 46-year-old woman with dementia and chorea secondary to Huntington's disease. It shows marked hypoperfusion of both caudate regions.*

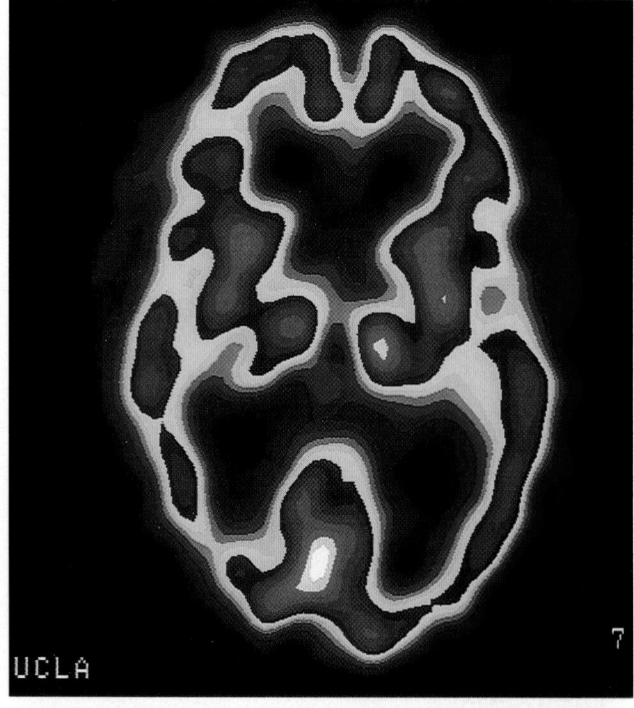

FIGURE 2.10-13 *SPECT of a patient with normal-pressure hydrocephalus that shows mild diffuse cortical and subcortical hypoperfusion.*

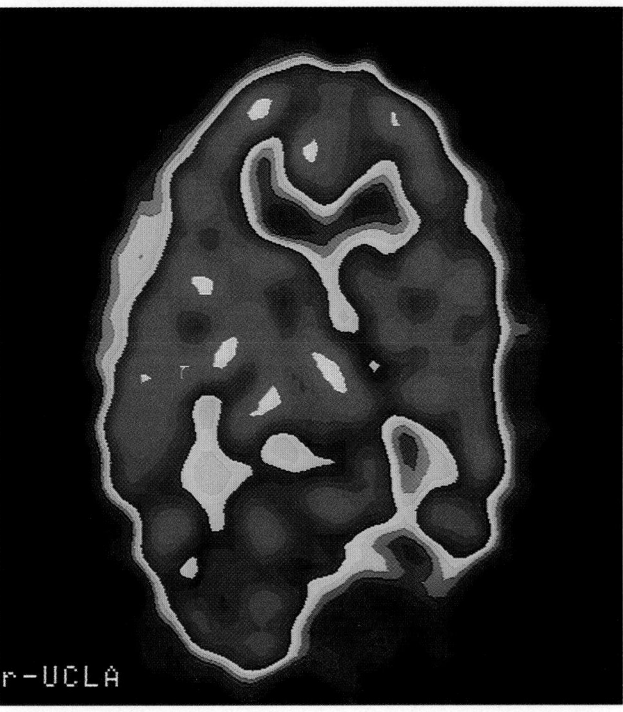

FIGURE 2.10-16 *HMPAO SPECT showing a 50 to 70 percent reduction in cerebral perfusion in the left occipital lobe in a patient with alexia without agraphia.*

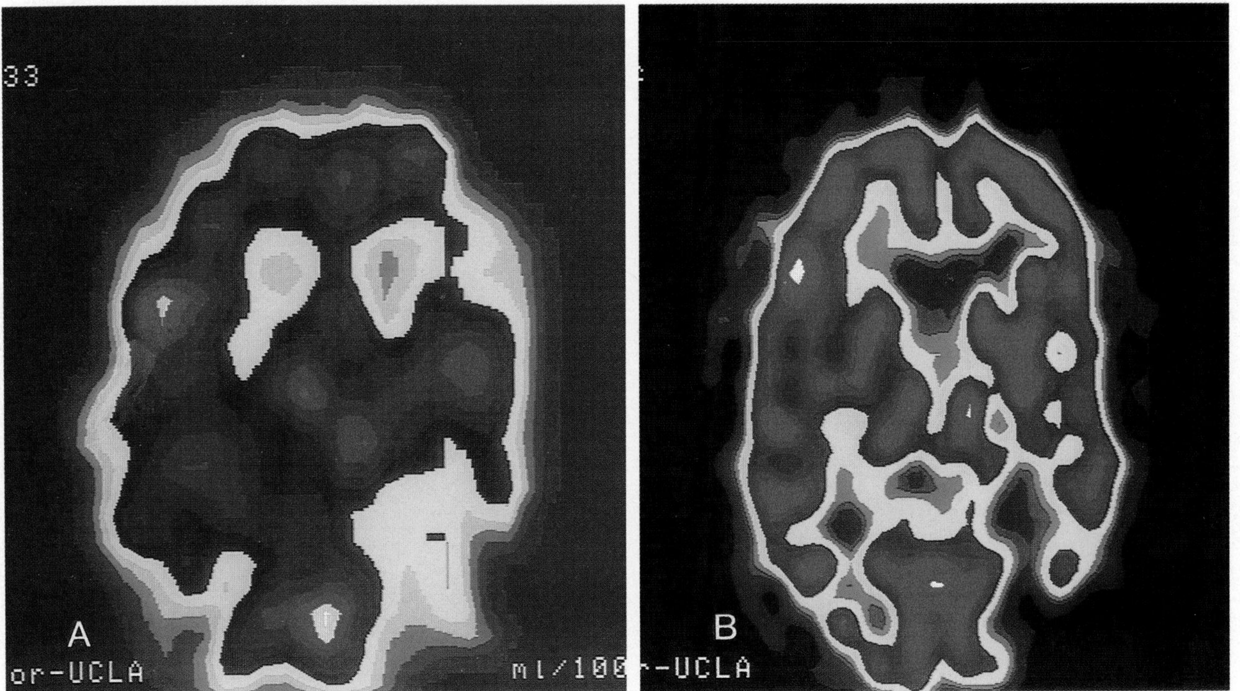

FIGURE 2.10-17A,B *Xenon 133 and HMPAO scans in a patient with vascular dementia show wedge-shaped areas of hypoperfusion in the left frontal and posterior parietal and right frontal areas.*

PLATE 6

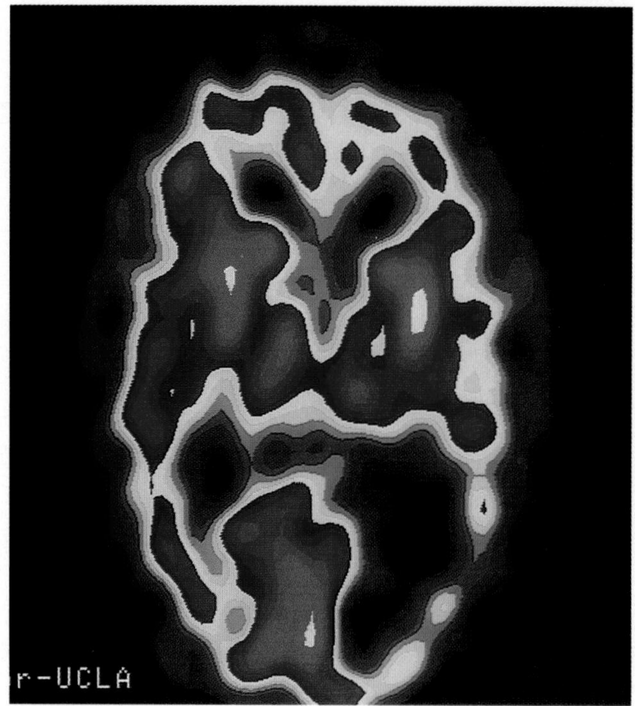

FIGURE 2.10-19 *HMPAO SPECT showing multifocal areas of hypoperfusion in a patient with chronic cocaine abuse.*

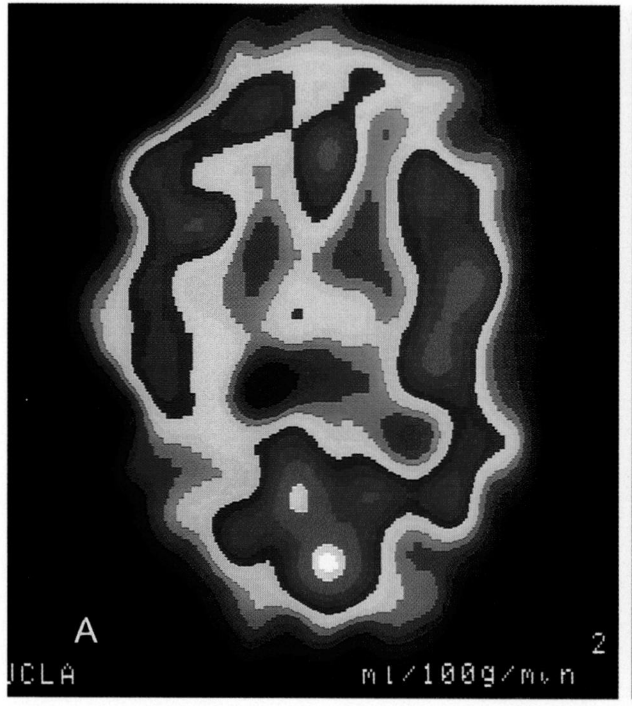

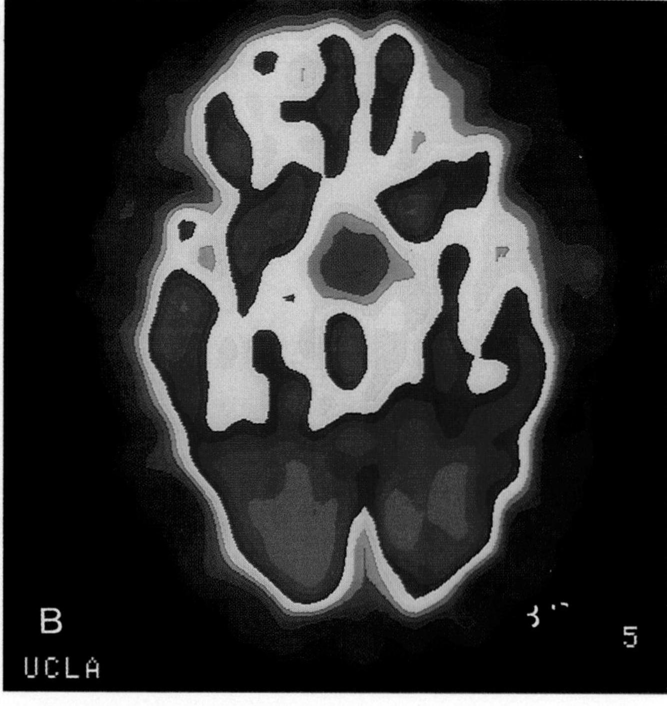

FIGURE 2.10-21A,B *Xenon 133 and HMPAO SPECT scans demonstrate bifrontal and bitemporal areas of hypoperfusion and a right posterior parietal contrecoup area of hypoperfusion.*

PLATE 7

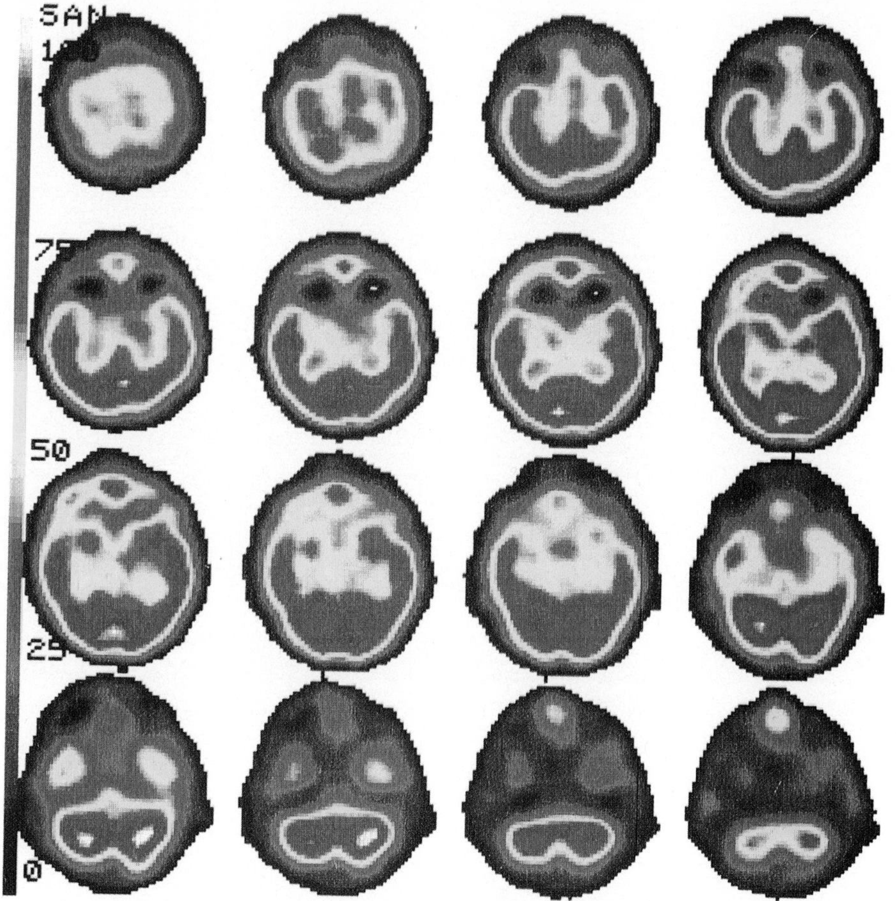

FIGURE 2.10-22 *HMPAO SPECT shows bifrontal hypoperfusion in a patient with a previous frontal leukotomy. Although only white matter fibers were cut the overlying cortex exhibits extensive hypoperfusion.*

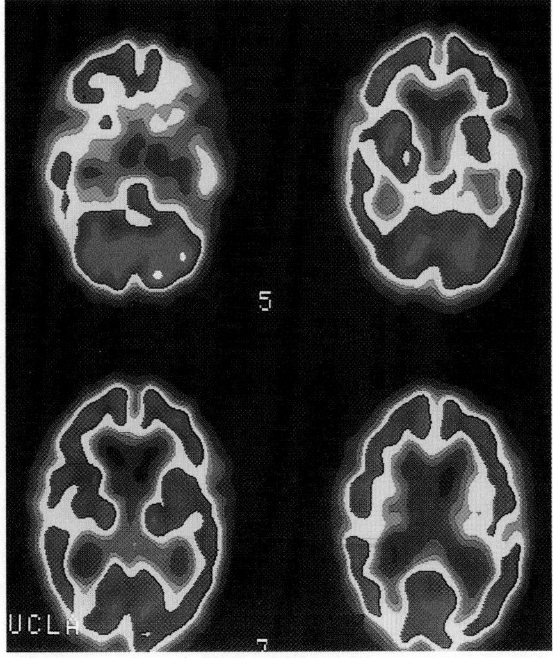

FIGURE 2.10-24 *HMPAO SPECT demonstrates severe left temporal and posterior left frontal hypoperfusion in a postictal woman with partial complex seizures.*

PLATE 8

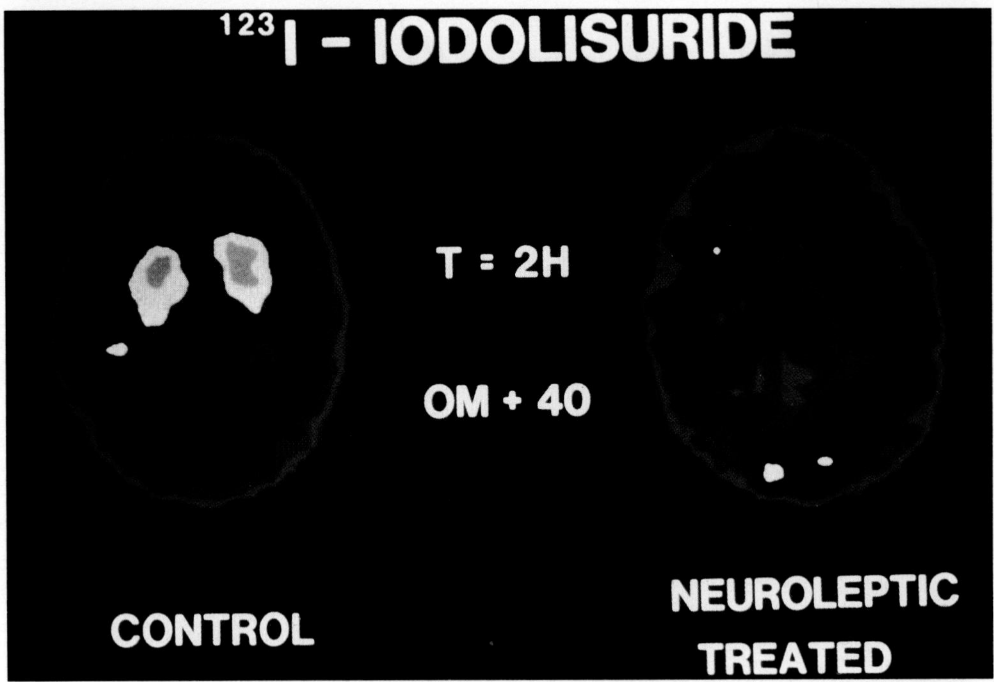

FIGURE 2.10-25 *Iodine 123-labeled lisuride SPECT. The D_2 agent shows extensive uptake in the basal ganglia, which is eliminated by preloading with the dopamine antagonist haloperidol (Haldol).*

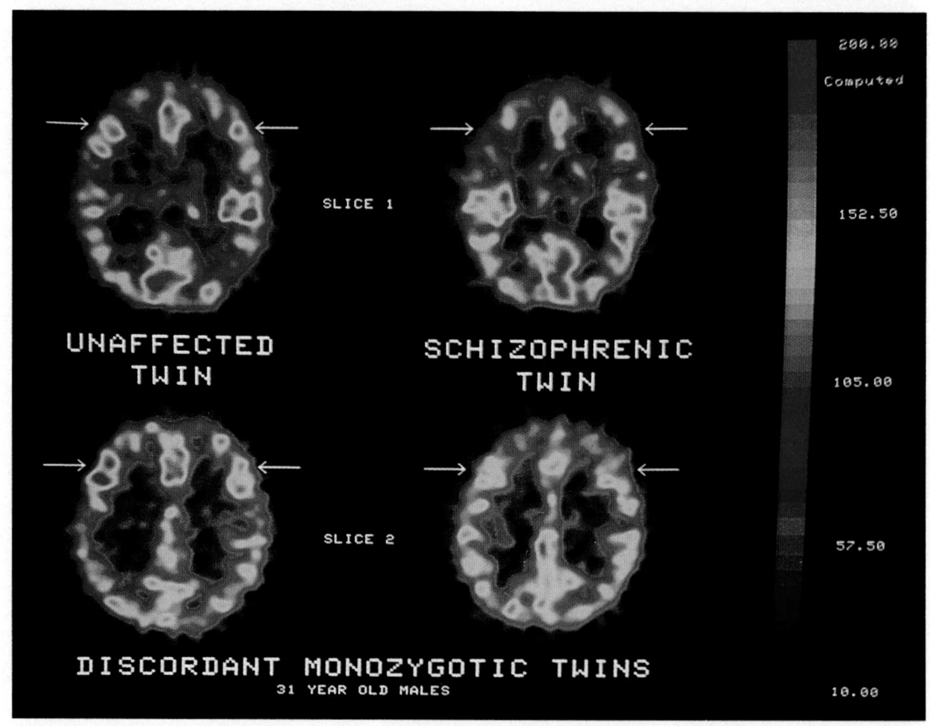

FIGURE 14.3-5 *Oxygen 15 water PET scans of a pair of monozygotic twins discordant for schizophrenia during performance of a prefrontal task. Two slices through the dorsolateral prefrontal cortex are shown for each twin; the more inferior slice is shown at the top. The affected twin is hypofrontal (that is, has less activity in dorsolateral prefrontal cortex [arrows]) compared with his well cotwin.*
* = P ≤ *.05 for between-group comparison of laterality index, a,b,c,d* = P ≤ *.05, .01, .005, .001, respectively, for within-group comparison of left versus right hemisphere relative CBF.*

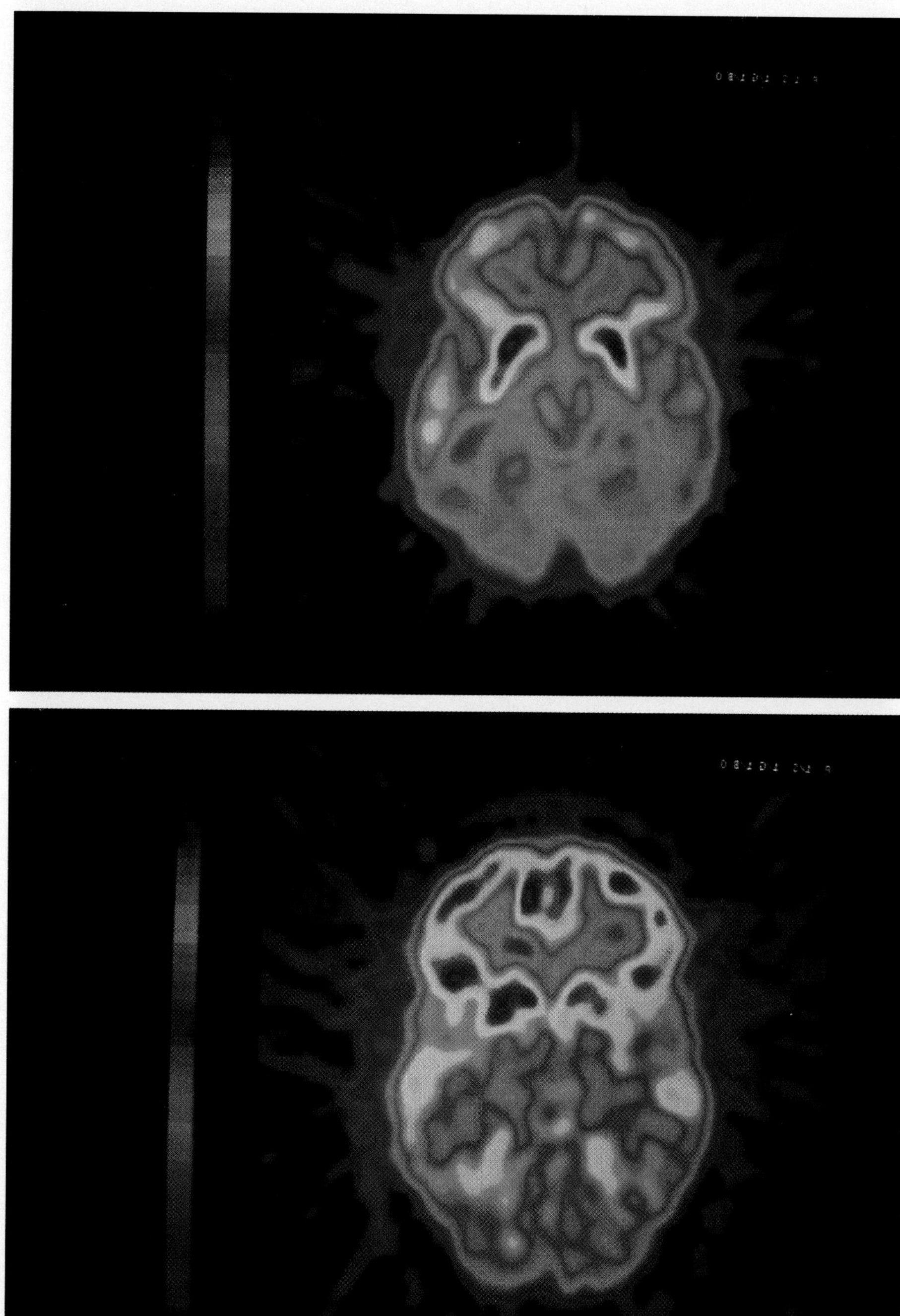

FIGURE 29.2a-2 *Positron emission tomographic scan using fluorodeoxyglucose of a patient with dementia due to HIV disease (above) and seronegative control subject (below). The scan of the seropositive patient is remarkable for hypermetabolism of the basal ganglia, particularly of the caudate, and cortical hypometabolism.*

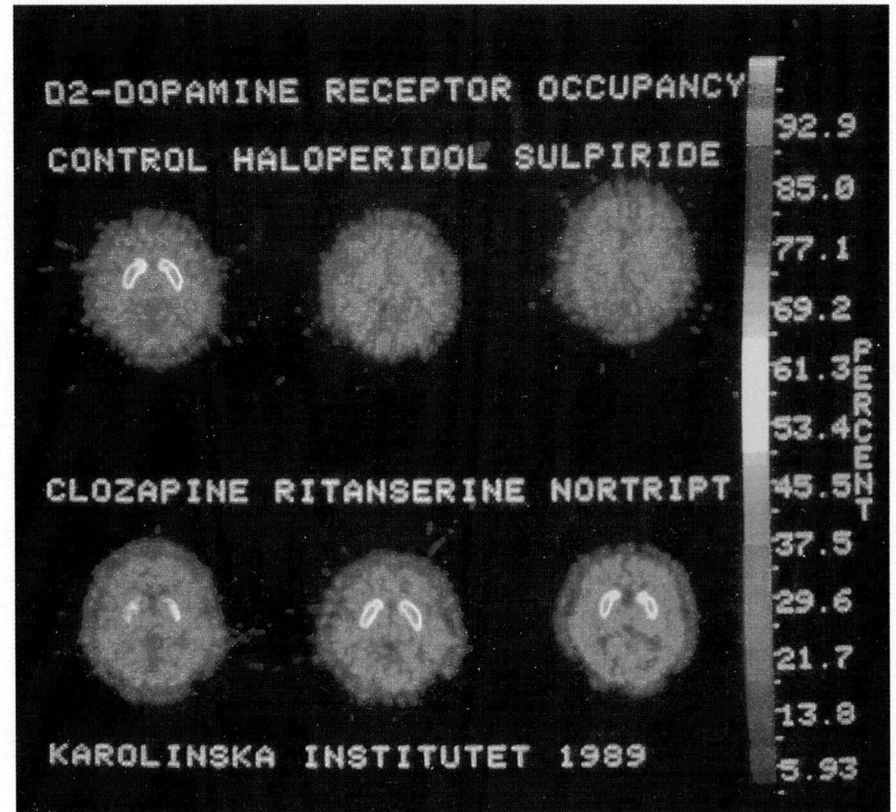

FIGURE 32.15-3 *PET-scan images of the brains of human subjects after administration of a tracer dose of [C^{11}] raclopride. The left upper panel shows an image from a healthy volunteer. Schizophrenic subjects treated with the antipsychotic drugs haloperidol, sulpiride, and clozapine show a marked reduction in the accumulation of radioactivity in the basal ganglia. Subjects treated with the 5-HT_2 antagonist ritanserine and the noradrenaline-uptake inhibitor nortriptyline do not show any reduction in the accumulation of radioactivity in the basal ganglia. From G Sedvall: PET imaging of dopamine receptors in human basal ganglia: Relevance to mental illness. Trends Neurosci* 13: *303, 1990. Used with permission.*

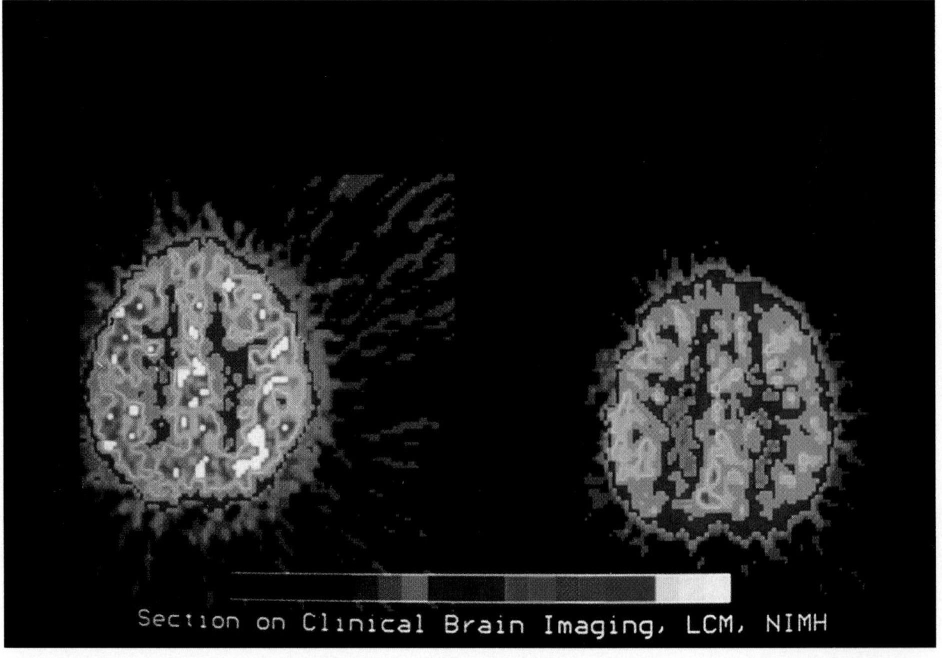

FIGURE 38-1 *Homologous slices from PET scans of an adult normal control (left) and an adult with ADHD (right) who is the parent of a child with ADHD. Red and orange areas represent high glucose metabolism; blue, violet, and lavender areas represent lower glucose metabolism (relation shown on bar). The adult with ADHD has a significant reduction in glucose metabolism in frontal and some other areas.*

CHAPTER 1 NEURAL SCIENCES

1.1 INTRODUCTION AND OVERVIEW

JACK A. GREBB, M.D.

INTRODUCTION

The advances in neural science research are, at an ever-increasing rate, expanding the knowledge base for psychiatry and affecting the clinical practice of the discipline. The next 16 sections of this chapter review both the old and the new in each of their fields. What most unifies the sections is the remarkable amount of information about newly discovered molecules, recently understood molecular pathways, and completely novel physiological mechanisms within the central nervous system (CNS). Those advances have three general effects. First, the new knowledge and ideas are challenging many aspects of existing knowledge and ideas. Second, the new knowledge is propelling the development of innovative and seemingly unconventional hypotheses. Third, the new knowledge is causing the previous or existing divisions and the distinctions among many basic science fields to weaken and fall, thus allowing for exciting interactional collaborations among the disciplines.

CHALLENGING THE OLD

Ideally, the process of scientific advancement should be seen not as challenging the old knowledge base but, rather, as editing and amending that base. In reality, however, scientific theories and philosophical positions can be held with a conviction equal to religious beliefs. Each of the next 16 sections presents new information that challenges currently held scientific dogma. Section 1.2, Functional Neuroanatomy, describes how recent studies of the motor system have challenged the classic division of the pyramidal (that is, the corticospinal) system from the extrapyramidal (that is, the basal ganglia) system. The authors conclude that the systems are not solitary and independent but, rather, related and dependent. Section 1.3, Monoamine Neurotransmitters, and Section 1.4, Amino Acid Neurotransmitters, introduce myriad neurotransmitter receptors. In the fifth edition of this textbook, the authors could write that there are two types of dopamine receptors, but in this sixth edition an author would have to write that there are five or six types of dopamine receptors, and many researchers believe other types are yet to be described. Moreover, in addition to the classic neurotransmitter categories—monoamine neurotransmitters (Section 1.3), amino acid neurotransmitters (Section 1.4), and neuropeptide neurotransmitters (Section 1.5)—novel neurotransmitters are also described in those sections. They include adenosine (Section 1.17), adenosine triphosphate (Section 1.17), nitric oxide (Sections 1.4 and 1.17), and the eicosanoids (Section 1.6). One novel putative neurotransmitter receptor that is not described in the following sections, but that represents an informative story, is the sigma receptor.

SIGMA RECEPTOR Only in the past few years has the sigma receptor been clearly distinguished from the phencyclidine (PCP) receptor. For many years, the literature showed an incomprehensible confusion because the benzomorphan opioids, such as pentazocine (Talwin), and PCP seemed to share the same receptor site. It is now clear that the principal site of action for PCP is the *N*-methyl-D-aspartate (NMDA) glutamate receptor, at which the binding of PCP results in an inhibition of calcium ion influx (Section 1.4). It is also now clear that there is a distinct set of sigma receptors.

Interest in the sigma receptors is keen because of the realization that several antipsychotic agents bind with high affinities to the sigma receptors. Those antipsychotic agents include haloperidol (Haldol) and remoxipride (Roxiam), an antipsychotic drug, until recently, under development that was reported to be associated with fewer extrapyramidal motor symptoms than the typical antipsychotics. Recently, it has been suggested that there are at least two types of sigma receptors. Basic researchers and pharmaceutical companies are actively synthesizing and testing novel sigma antagonists as potential antipsychotic agents.

BRINGING IN THE NEW

The identification of new receptors and the appreciation of new anatomical and intraneuronal pathways led naturally to the development of novel theories regarding physiological mechanisms. For example, in contrast to a model of mental illness based on too much dopamine or too little serotonin, the second and third messenger systems, including protein phosphorylation (Section 1.6), and the evolving understanding of molecular genetics (for example, immediate early genes) (Section 1.14), provide a much richer soil from which to sprout hypotheses.

Perhaps the key conceptual challenge of many of the discoveries is that the analysis of brain function needs to emphasize the regulation of neuronal processes. The implications of that approach are at least twofold. First, as researchers seek sites of pathology in the brains of mentally ill patients, they should try to design strategies that are capable of assessing abnormal regulation, not merely the presence or the absence of a particular function or molecule. Second, as researchers design novel treatments, they should consider how to modify the regulation of functions and not focus on turning neurons on and off. As a direct result of that approach, a significant research effort is now underway to design drugs that will affect regulatory processes within neurons (for example, protein kinases, gene expression), rather than to restrict the approach to affecting receptors located on the outside of neurons.

BRIDGING THE CONTEMPORARY

Not only is there a tendency to build walls between the new and the old, but there is also a tendency for walls to exist between distinct contemporary research efforts. Such walls are crumbling since it has proved to be advantageous for different disciplines to collaborate in their research efforts. For example, modern molecular techniques (Section 1.14) have resulted in the identification of many types of receptors, much to the glee of receptor-type biochemists. The identification of those types of receptors has allowed the biochemists to produce receptor type-specific antibodies, which can then be used by neuroanatomists to expose new neuronal pathways. Those discoveries, in turn, help guide the research of brain imagers. Eventually, the combined efforts of all those disciplines may lead to the identification of specific pathological processes in disease states and to the design of more precise treatment modalities for those illnesses.

OVERVIEW

NEUROANATOMY The organ of interest in psychiatry is the brain, and both the historical view and the contemporary view of the brain must start with its gross examination (Section 1.2, "Functional Neuroanatomy"). That gross examination is then followed by the labor-intensive task of trying to understand where every collection of cell bodies is, to which regions of the brain every neuron projects, and what the neurochemical constituents of every neuron are. Modern neuroanatomy has a goal every bit as grand as that for the human genome project (Section 1.17). The discoveries of modern neuroanatomy are challenging many of the previously believed tenets. In contrast to the descriptive approach of classic neuroanatomy, the emphasis of the new neuroanatomy is on functional systems in the brain. If a newly understood functional system breaks through the barriers described by classic neuroanatomy, so be it.

NEUROTRANSMITTERS The three principal neurotransmitter types in the brain are the monoamine neurotransmitters (Section 1.3), the amino acid neurotransmitters (Section 1.4), and the neuropeptide neurotransmitters (Section 1.5). However, other neurotransmitters (for example, nitric oxide, adenosine) do not fit neatly into that classification. Historically and certainly pharmacologically, the most important neurotransmitters have been the monoamine neurotransmitters—the catecholamines (dopamine, norepinephrine, and epinephrine), serotonin, acetylcholine, and histamine. Those neurotransmitters are the ones most commonly affected by the many drugs in the psychopharmacological armamentarium. The most exciting advances in the field of monoamine neurotransmitters are the identification of additional subtypes of receptors and the identification of subtypes of neurotransmitter reuptake pumps, since they, too, are the targets of psychopharmacological drugs (for example, tricyclic antidepressants). The identification of receptor and reuptake pump subtypes introduces the possibility of designing specific drugs that may have the desired therapeutic effects without the undesired adverse effects of currently available drugs.

By comparison with the amino acid neurotransmitters, the monoamine neurotransmitters account for only a small percentage of the neurons in the human brain. The regulation of the human brain is sometimes reduced to a balance between the inhibitory actions of γ-aminobutyric acid (GABA) and the excitatory actions of glutamate. That balance may be regulated by the effects of the monoamine and neuropeptide neurotransmitters. As with the monoamine neurotransmitters, researchers have identified subtypes of receptors and reuptake pumps for the amino acid neurotransmitters, thus allowing for the possible development of receptor-specific or reuptake pump-specific drugs. Two other areas in amino acid neurotransmitter research are the further research into the role of glycine as an excitatory amino acid neurotransmitter and research into a general role for amino acid neurotransmitters in pathological processes such as neurotoxicity and normal functions such as memory and learning.

The most striking aspect of the neuropeptide neurotransmitters is their sheer multitude. Furthermore, neuropeptides almost always coexist with other neurotransmitters (other neuropeptides, monoamine neurotransmitters, or amino acid neurotransmitters), thus adding to their complex role as potential modulators of neuronal activity. Out of the large number of peptides, however, the most exciting leads in research involve a role for corticotropin-releasing factor (CRF) in mood disorders and anxiety disorders, a role for somatostatin release-inhibiting factor (SRIF) in dementia of the Alzheimer's type and mood disorders, and a role for neurotensin (NT) and cholecystokinin (CCK) in schizophrenia.

SIGNAL TRANSDUCTION The process of *chemical neurotransmission* strictly refers to the release of a neurotransmitter by a presynaptic neuron, the travel of that neurotransmitter across some space (for example, the synaptic cleft), and the binding of that neurotransmitter to its specific receptor on a postsynaptic neuron (or an autoreceptor on a presynaptic neuron). The process of *signal transduction,* however, refers to the process by which an electrical signal (for example, the action potential) in the presynaptic neuron is translated into a chemical signal (for example, the release of a neurotransmitter) and how the chemical signal (for example, the interaction of a neurotransmitter and its receptor) is translated back into an electrical signal in the postsynaptic neuron. The two basic fields of study for the phenomenon are intraneuronal biochemistry (Section 1.6) and basic neuronal electrophysiology (Section 1.7).

Understanding of intraneuronal signaling pathways now includes the generation of second-messenger molecules, such as cyclic adenosine monophosphate (cAMP), which then activate a cascade of intraneuronal third, fourth, . . . nth messenger molecules. The mechanism for the cascade that is best elaborated is protein phosphorylation (Section 1.6), which is a reversible, posttranslational modification of a protein. The deletion or the addition of one or more phosphate groups to a protein changes the charge and the configuration of the protein and may result in a change in the function of that protein. Thus, protein phosphorylation can serve as a type of molecular on-off switch for protein function. In fact, protein phosphorylation more often modulates the function of a protein than it turns a specific function completely on or off. The identification of those multiple biochemical steps in signal transduction has presented research scientists with novel areas in which to seek pathophysiological processes and novel sites for therapeutic drug action.

The balance between external and internal concentrations of ions is the final summary of neuronal activity. That balance is achieved by a wide array of types of ion channels; some are regulated by neurotransmitters, and others are regulated by the voltage gradients directly. Many of the drugs of interest in psychiatry have their effects by acting directly on ion channels. The benzodiazepines act on $GABA_A$ receptors that are chloride ion channels. Phencyclidine acts on NMDA-type glutamate receptors that are calcium ion channels. Nicotine, the active ingredient in tobacco, acts on nicotinic acetylcholine receptors that are sodium and potassium ion channels. As with neurotransmitter receptors, the delineation of ion channel subtypes and the modulation of ion channel function by processes such as protein phosphorylation are among the most active areas of psychiatric research.

MEASURES OF TOTAL BRAIN FUNCTION Three of the sections in this chapter concern the function of the total brain. Applied electrophysiology (Section 1.8) describes techniques of clinical electrophysiology based, for the most part, on recording electrical activity through electrodes placed on the scalp. A subset of that discipline is the study of the basic science of sleep (Section 1.9), although the discipline of sleep research also reaches into many other fields, such as biochemistry and genetics. The section on neuroimaging (Section 1.10) describes several methods currently used in research settings to measure brain function, such as positron emission tomography (PET).

The most exciting new areas of research within the field of applied electrophysiology are quantitative electroencephalography (EEG), pharmacoelectroencephalography, and magnetoelectroencephalography (MEG). The techniques of quantitative EEG and MEG are noninvasive methods to measure aspects of brain function and may prove useful in psychiatric research when repeated measures of a single patient over time are indicated. In addition, especially with quantitative EEG, some researchers are developing the use of those techniques to aid in the classification and the diagnosis of psychiatric patients. Pharmacoelectroencephalography is the use of EEG-related technology to assess the response of patients to drug treatments; thus, clinicians may potentially be able to ascertain to which drugs a patient will respond and to ascertain early in a course of treatment to which drugs a patient will not respond. Sleep research has progressed from a time when sleep architecture was considered merely a marker for normal and abnormal brain function to the current time, when many researchers conceptualize the process of sleep as central to the maintenance of diverse normal brain functions, such as memory, learning, and mood regulation.

Brain imaging techniques can assess both structural and functional aspects of the brain. The principal structural techniques are computed tomography (CT) and magnetic resonance imaging (MRI). The principal functional techniques are positron emission tomography (PET) and single photon emission computed tomography (SPECT). The most novel area of research in brain imaging is magnetic resonance spectroscopy. For the moment, most techniques are limited to research applications, but certainly before the next century it is reasonable to predict that some of the techniques will find applications in the diagnosis and the treatment of psychiatric patients.

INTEGRATION AND MODULATION OF THE CNS The human body has three great communicative systems—the neural system, the immune system, and the endocrine system. All three systems communicate with each other, and a disease in one can cause dysfunctions in the others. The interactions between the endocrine system and the neural system (Section 1.11) and the interactions between the immune system and the neural system (Section 1.12) have been subjects of increasing interest in psychiatry, especially as the specific molecules that mediate those interactions have been discovered. Another common feature of the three systems is their regular change with time; neuronal function, immune responses, and the release of hormones all vary in a regular fashion with the day, the month, and the year. Chronobiology (Section 1.13) is the field of research that studies those temporal fluctuations.

Chronobiology is the study of the interaction of internal rhythms (for example, sleep and wakefulness) with external rhythms (for example, the seasons) and how that interaction of rhythms affects other bodily functions (for example, the CNS and the immune function). The sleep disorders, mood disorders, and eating disorders may all be taken to reflect abnormalities in the normal chronological rhythms. The appreciation of time in the assessment of those disorders has already led to novel, nonpharmacological treatment approaches for some of those conditions. The treatments include light therapy and manipulations of the sleep cycle.

One concept regarding hormones is that they provide behavioral programs for the rest of the body to follow. A slightly less powerful role for hormones is as a diffuse regulator of function. The power of hormones to affect behavior is shown by the psychiatric symptoms that can accompany hormonal dysfunctions (for example, adrenal and thyroid disorders). Endocrine abnormalities have also been studied as potential markers of both state and trait variables in psychiatric conditions.

In the 1980s and the 1990s the most striking demonstration of the interplay between the immune system and the CNS has been acquired immune deficiency syndrome (AIDS). In AIDS a virus that infects glial cells can result in many different behavioral disturbances (for example, dementia, depression, psychosis), in addition to its profound effects on immune function. Less obvious interactions between immunological insults and the CNS have now been hypothesized to be involved in schizophrenia, Alzheimer's disease, and Parkinson's disease.

GENETICS The techniques of molecular genetics and its discoveries and revelations have had profound effects on every discipline of psychiatric research. The concepts of basic molecular neurobiology are outlined in Section 1.14, and the concepts of population genetics in psychiatry are outlined in Section 1.15. The most direct interaction between those two areas of knowledge is the application of genetic linkage analyses to the study of psychiatric disorders (Section 1.16).

The basic process of genetics involves the *transcription* of deoxyribonucleic acid (DNA) into ribonucleic acid (RNA) and the *translation* of RNA into a protein. That is only the simplest statement of those processes; basic research has now revealed a complex system of regulation (for example, regulatory elements, transcription factors) for the steps of transcription and translation. The newly discovered molecules and pathways are further examples of new sites to study for pathology in disease states and plausible sites for treatment approaches. The field of basic molecular neuroscience has further enhanced the concept of signal transduction (Sections 1.6 and 1.7) inasmuch as both short-term and long-term neuronal regulation involves changes in gene expression. The alterations in gene expression occur both during development and in adulthood and may be the bases for abnormal and normal development and for abnormal and normal adaptation to stress. The molecular basis for the regulation of genetic expression includes such molecules as immediate early genes (for example, c-fos) and late response genes. Although such terms are still foreign in the psychiatric journals, it is safe to predict that they will predominate in the journals of the 21st century.

SUGGESTED CROSS-REFERENCES

Neuropsychiatry and behavioral neurology are discussed in Chapter 2; the neuropsychological aspects and the psychiatric aspects of AIDS are discussed in Sections 29.2a and 29.2, respectively; the neurochemical, viral, and immunological studies of schizophrenia are discussed in Section 14.4; the biochemical aspects of mood disorders are discussed in Section 16.3; biological therapies are discussed in Chapter 32; and Alzheimer's disease is discussed in Section 49.6a. The future of psychiatry is discussed in Section 53.2.

REFERENCES

Alper J S, Natowicz M R: On establishing the genetic basis of mental disease. Trends Neurosci *16:* 387, 1993.
Cotten M, Wagner E: Non-viral approaches to gene therapy. Curr Opinion Biotechnol *4:* 705, 1993.
Gur R E, Jaggi J L, Shtasel D L, Ragland J D, Gur R C: Cerebral blood flow in schizophrenia: Effects of memory processing on regional activation. Biol Psychiatry *35:* 3, 1994.
*Hobson J A: Sleep and dreaming. J Neurosci *10:* 371, 1990.
Javitt D C, Zukin S R: Recent advances in the phencyclidine model of schizophrenia. Am J Psychiatry *148:* 1301, 1991.
Jessell T M, Kandel E R: Synaptic transmission: A bidirectional and self-modifiable form of cell–cell communication. Neuron *10*(Suppl): 1, 1993.
Korsching S: The neurotrophic factor concept: A reexamination. J Neurosci *13:* 2739, 1993.
*Largent B L: Receptor mechanisms in schizophrenia: Possible role for the sigma receptor. In *Biological Basis of Schizophrenic Disorders,* T Nakazowa, editor, p 133. Japan Scientific Societies Press, Tokyo, 1991.
*Llinas R R, Pare D: Of dreaming and wakefulness. Neuroscience *44:* 521, 1991.
*Quirion R, Bowen W D, Itzhak Y, Junien J L, Musacchio J M, Rothman R B, Su T-P, Tam S W, Taylor D P: A proposal for the classification of sigma binding sites. Trends Pharmacol Sci *13:* 85, 1992.
*Winson J: The meaning of dreams. Sci Am *262*: 86, 1990.

1.2
FUNCTIONAL NEUROANATOMY

DAVID A. LEWIS, M.D.
KRISTEN M. OETH, M.S.

INTRODUCTION

This section reviews some of the major principles governing the anatomical organization of the human brain and illustrates those principles in the functional circuitry of several neural systems. The neural systems—the thalamocortical, basal ganglia, and limbic systems—were selected because of their particular relevance for neuropsychiatric disorders.

PRINCIPLES OF BRAIN ORGANIZATION

CELLS The human brain contains approximately 10^{11} nerve cells or *neurons.* In general, neurons are composed of four morphologically identified regions (Figure 1.2-1): (1) the cell body or *soma,* which contains the nucleus and can be considered the metabolic center of the neuron; (2) the *dendrites,* processes that arise from the cell body, branch extensively, and serve as the major recipient zones of input from other neurons; (3) the *axon,* a single process that arises from a specialized portion of the cell body (the *axon hillock*) and conveys information to other neurons; and (4) the *axon terminals,* fine branches near the end of the axon that form contacts *(synapses)* generally with the dendrites or the cell bodies of other neurons, release neurotransmitters, and thereby provide a mechanism for interneuronal communication.

The majority of the neurons in the human brain are considered to be multipolar in that they give rise to a single axon and several dendritic processes. Although there are a number of classification schemes for neurons in different brain regions, almost all neurons can be considered to be either projection or local-circuit neurons. *Projection neurons* have long axons and

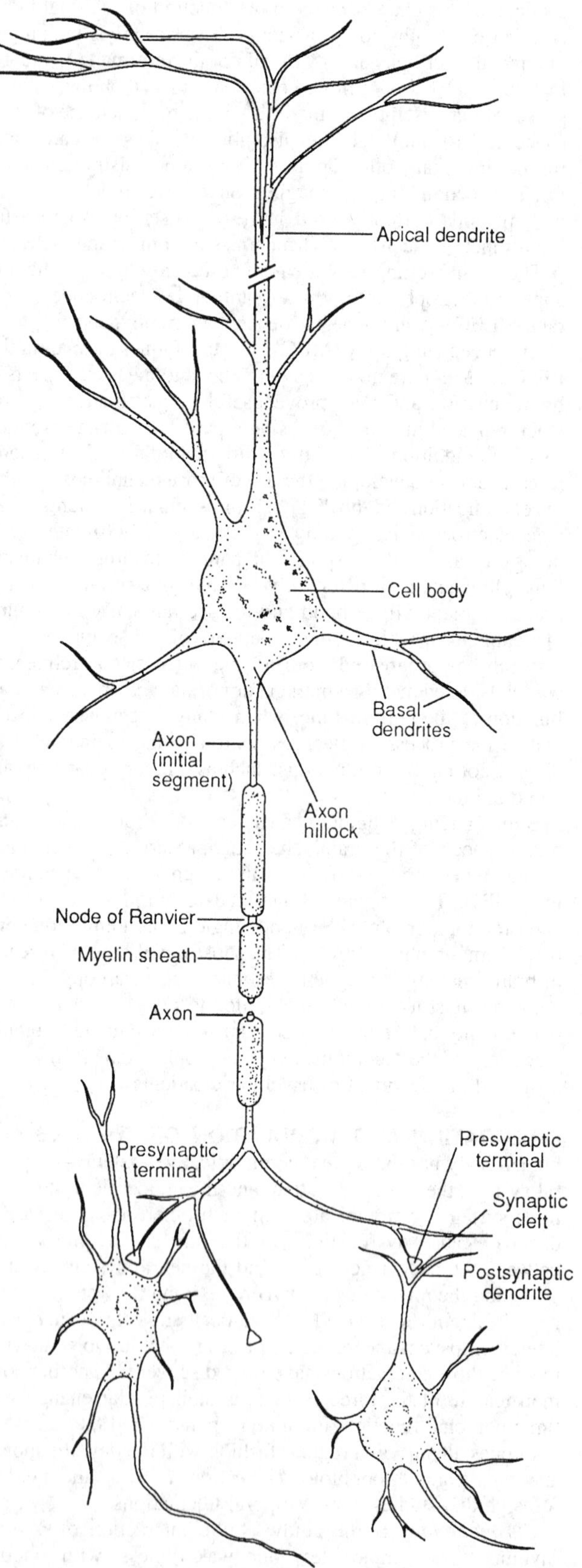

FIGURE 1.2-1 *Drawing of the major features of a typical neuron. (Adapted from E R Kandel: Nerve cells and behavior. In* Principles of Neural Science, *ed 3, E Kandel, J Schwartz, T Jessel, editors, p 19. Elsevier, New York, 1991.)*

convey information from the periphery to the brain (sensory neurons), from one brain region to another, or from the brain to effector organs (motor neurons). In contrast, *local-circuit* or *interneurons* have short axons and process information within distinct regions of the brain.

Neurons can also be classified according to the neurotransmitters they contain (for example, the dopaminergic neurons of the substantia nigra). Identification of neurons by their neurotransmitter content in anatomical studies provides a means for correlating the structure of a neuron with certain aspects of its function. However, neurotransmitters have defined effects on the activity of neurons, whereas complex brain functions, such as those disturbed in psychiatric disorders, are mediated by the coordinated activity of ensembles of neurons. Thus, the effects of neurotransmitters (or of pharmacological agents that mimic or antagonize the actions of neurotransmitters) on behavioral, emotional, or cognitive states must be viewed within the context of the neural circuits that they influence.

In addition to neurons, the brain also contains several types of *glial* cells, which are at least 10 times more numerous than the neurons. Although glial cells are not directly involved in information processing, they play several important roles in the nervous system. *Oligodendrocytes* and *Schwann cells,* found in the central and peripheral nervous systems, respectively, are relatively small cells that wrap their membranous processes around axons in a tight spiral. The resulting *myelin sheath* facilitates the conduction of action potentials along the axon. *Astrocytes,* the most numerous class of glial cells, appear to serve a number of functions, including participation in the formation of the blood-brain barrier, removal of certain neurotransmitters from the synaptic cleft, buffering of the extracellular potassium (K^+) concentration, and, given their close contact with both neurons and blood vessels, possibly a nutritive function. The third class of glial cells, the *microglia,* are actually derived from macrophages and function as scavengers, eliminating the debris resulting from neuronal death and injury.

ARCHITECTURE Neurons and their processes form groupings in a number of different ways, and those patterns of organization or architectures can be evaluated by several approaches. The pattern of distribution of the neurons, called *cytoarchitecture,* is revealed by aniline dyes that stain ribonucleotides, Nissl substance, in the nucleus and the cytoplasm of neuronal cell bodies. The Nissl stains demonstrate the relative size and packing density of the neurons and consequently reveal, for example, the organization of the neurons into the different layers of the cerebral cortex. In certain pathological states, such as Alzheimer's disease (called dementia of the Alzheimer's type in the fourth edition of *Diagnostic and Statistical Manual of Mental Disorders* [DSM-IV]), neuronal degeneration and loss results in striking changes in the cytoarchitecture of some brain regions (Figure 1.2-2).

The cytoarchitecture of the adult human brain is the product of a series of developmental processes that include neuronal genesis, migration, and differentiation. A disturbance in any of those processes may lead to distinctive changes in the cytoarchitecture. For example, in the brains of some schizophrenic patients, the layer II neurons of the entorhinal cortex, which normally gather into distinct clusters or islands (Figure 1.2-2A), have been reported to be located in deeper cortical layers. Although the validity of the reports awaits further confirmation, the observation may reflect an abnormality in the migration of the neurons during the second trimester of development.

Other types of histological techniques, such as silver stains, selectively label the myelin coating of axons and, consequently, reveal the *myeloarchitecture* of the brain. For example, certain regions of the cerebral cortex—such as area MT, a portion of the temporal cortex involved in processing visual information—can be identified by a characteristic pattern of heavy myelination in the deep cortical layers. The progression of myelination is highly region-specific, may not be complete for years after birth, and may be a useful anatomical indicator of the functional maturation of brain regions.

Immunohistochemical and other related techniques—which identify the location of neurotransmitters, their synthetic enzymes, or other molecules within neurons—can be used to determine the *chemoarchitecture* of the brain (Figure 1.2-3B). In some cases the techniques reveal striking regional differences in the chemoarchitecture of the brain that are difficult to detect in cytoarchitecture.

CONNECTIONS Every function of the human brain is a consequence of the activity of specific neural circuits. The circuits form as a result of several developmental processes. First, each neuron, either after it has migrated to its final location or in some cases before, extends an axon. The growth of an axon along distinct pathways is guided by molecular cues from its environment and eventually leads to the formation of synapses with specific target neurons. Although the projection of axons is quite precise, some axons initially produce an excessive number of axon branches or *collaterals* and thus contact a broader set of targets than are present in the adult brain. During later development the connections of particular neurons are focused by the pruning or elimination of axonal projections to inappropriate targets.

Within the adult brain the connections among neurons or neural circuits follow several important principles of organization. First, many but not all connections between brain regions are *reciprocal;* that is, each region tends to receive input from those regions to which it sends axonal projections. In some cases the axons arising from one region may directly innervate the reciprocating projection neurons in another region; in other cases local-circuit interneurons are interposed between the incoming axons and the projection neurons that furnish the reciprocal connections. For some projections the reciprocating connection is indirect, passing through one or more additional brain regions and synapses before innervating the initial brain region.

Second, many neuronal connections are either divergent or convergent in nature. A *divergent* system involves the conduction of information from one neuron or a discrete group of neurons to a much larger number of neurons that may be located in diverse portions of the brain. The locus ceruleus, a small group of norepinephrine-containing neurons in the brainstem that sends axonal projections to the entire cerebral cortex and other brain regions, is an example of a divergent system. In contrast, the output of multiple brain regions may be directed toward a single area, forming a *convergent* system.

Third, the connections among regions may be organized in a hierarchical or parallel fashion or both. For example, visual input is conveyed in a *serial* or *hierarchical* fashion through several populations of neurons in the retina to the lateral geniculate nucleus, to the primary visual cortex, and then progressively to the multiple visual association areas of the cerebral cortex. Within the hierarchical scheme, different types of visual information (for example, motion, form) may be processed in a *parallel* fashion through different portions of the visual system.

Finally, regions of the brain are specialized for different functions. For example, lesions of the left inferior frontal gyrus (Broca's area) produce a characteristic impairment in speech

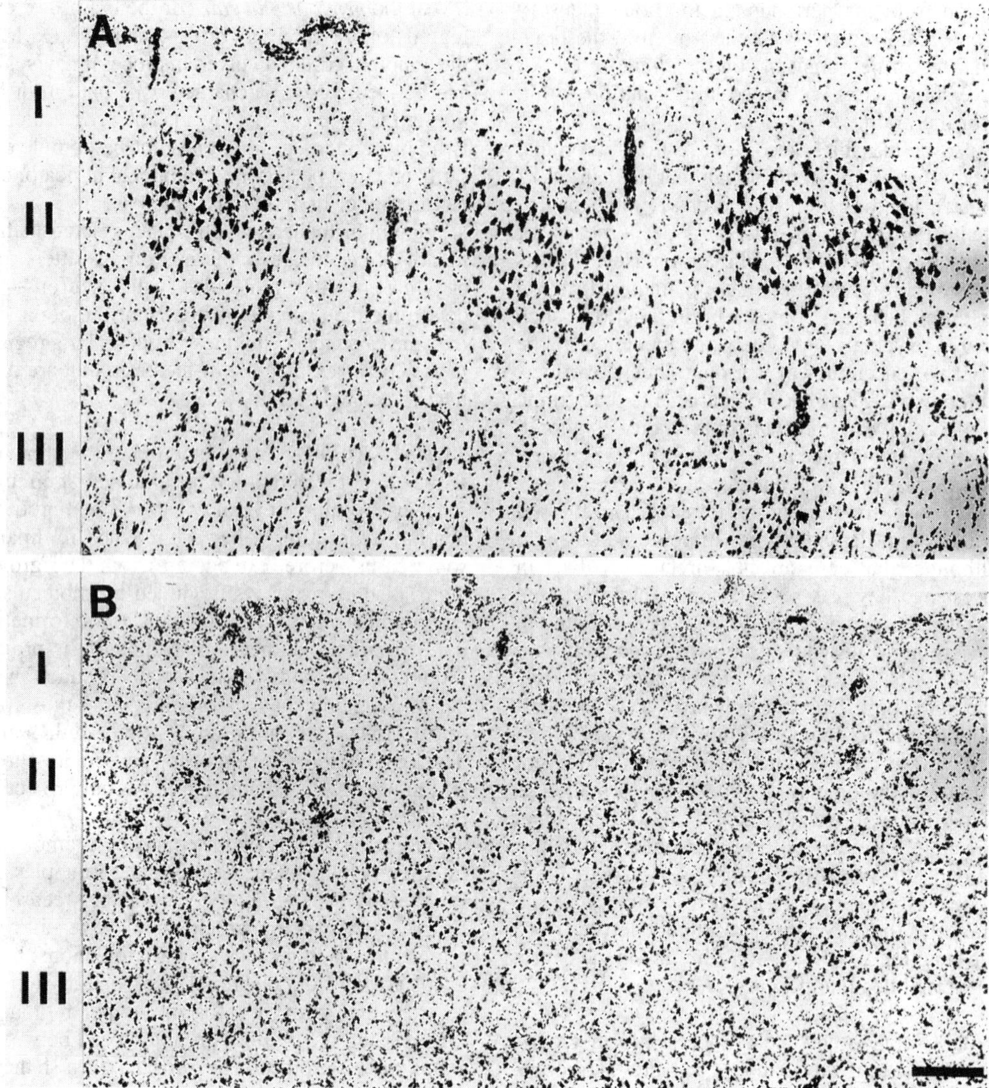

FIGURE 1.2-2 *Nissl-stained sections of the superficial layers of the intermediate region of human entorhinal cortex. In the control brain (A), layer II contains clusters or islands of large, intensely stained neurons. In Alzheimer's disease (B), the neurons are particularly vulnerable to degeneration, and their loss produces a marked change in the cytoarchitecture of the region. Roman numerals indicate the location of the cortical layers. Calibration bar (200 μm) applied to A and B. (Courtesy of M J Beall and M Brady, University of Pittsburgh.)*

production. However, speech is a complex faculty that depends not only on the integrity of Broca's area but also on the distributed processing of information across a number of brain regions through divergent and convergent, serial and parallel interconnections. Thus, the role of any particular brain region or group of neurons in the production of specific behaviors or in the pathophysiology of a given neuropsychiatric disorder cannot be viewed in isolation but must be considered within the context of the neural circuits connecting those neurons with other brain regions.

DISTINCTIVENESS OF THE HUMAN BRAIN Compared with the brains of other primate species, the human brain is substantially greater in size. In addition, not only has brain size increased overall, but certain areas of the human brain have expanded disproportionately. For example, the prefrontal cortex has been estimated to occupy only 3.5 percent of the total cortical volume in cats and 11.5 percent in monkeys but close to 30 percent of the much larger cortical volume of the human brain. Conversely, the relative representation of other regions is decreased in the human brain; for example, the primary visual cortex accounts for only 1.5 percent of the total area of the cerebral cortex in humans, but in monkeys a much greater proportion (17 percent) of the cerebral cortex is devoted to that region. Thus, the distinctiveness of the human brain is attributable both to its size and to the differential expansion of certain regions, particularly those areas of the cerebral cortex devoted to higher cognitive functions.

In addition, the expansion and the differentiation of the human brain is associated with substantial differences in the organization of at least certain elements of neural circuitry. For example, when compared with what is seen in rodents, the dopaminergic innervation of the human cerebral cortex is much more widespread and regionally specific. The primary motor cortex reçeives a dense dopaminergic innervation in both monkeys and humans, but that zone receives little dopaminergic input in rats. Those types of species differences indicate that there are limits to the accuracy of the generalizations made con-

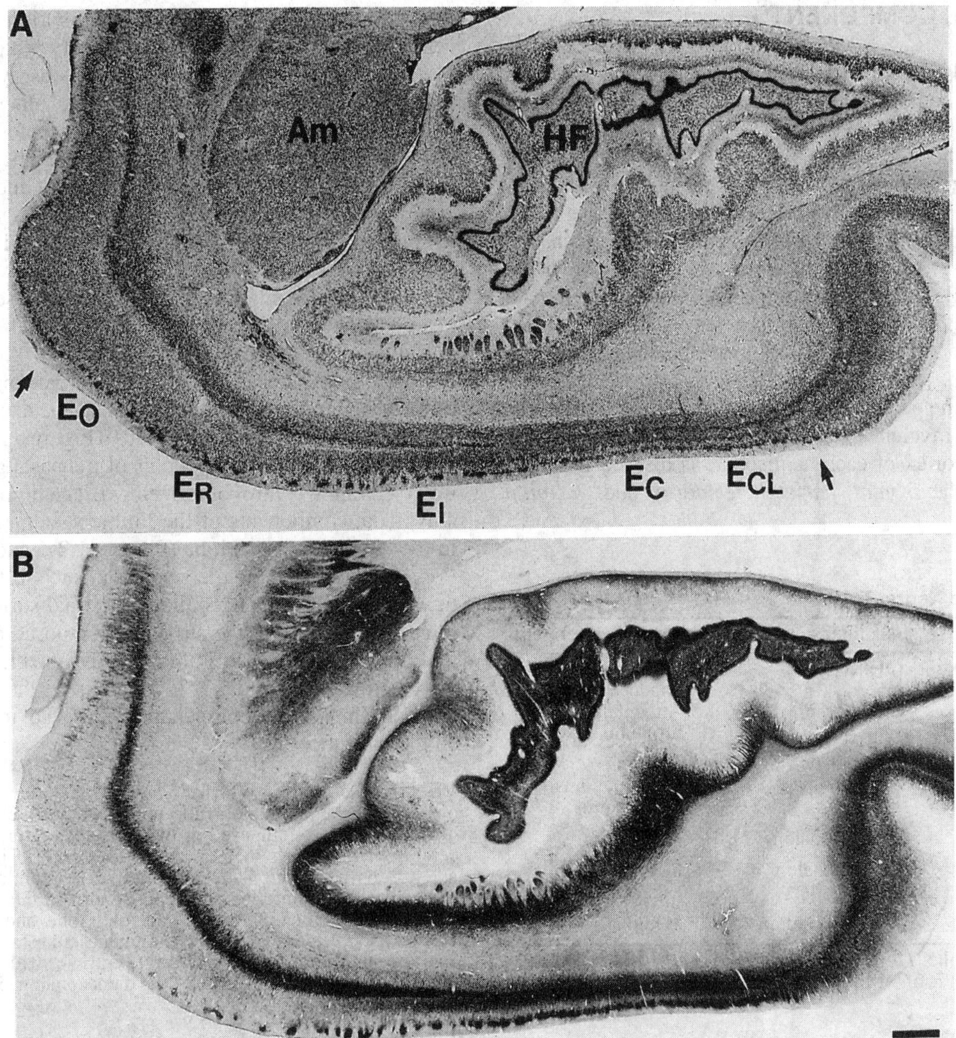

FIGURE 1.2-3 *Adjacent sagittal sections through the medial temporal lobe of the human brain labeled to reveal the cytoarchitecture (A-Nissl stain) and chemoarchitecture (B-nonphosphorylated neurofilament protein immunoreactivity) of the entorhinal cortex. Arrows indicate the rostral (left) and caudal (right) borders of the entorhinal cortex, and letters indicate some of its subdivisions. Substantial differences are evident in the cytoarchitecture and the chemoarchitecture of the subdivisions. Am indicates amygdala, HF indicates hippocampal formation. Calibration bar (2 mm) applies to both panels. (In M J Beall, D A Lewis: Heterogeneity of layer II neurons in human neocortex. J Comp Neurol* 321: *241, 1992. Used with permission.)*

cerning human brain function when using studies in rodents or even nonhuman primates as the basis for the inference. However, direct investigation of the organization of the human brain is obviously restricted and complicated by a number of factors. As indicated above, the expansion of the human brain is associated with the appearance of additional regions of the cerebral cortex. For example, the entorhinal cortex of the medial temporal lobe is sometimes considered to be a single cortical region, yet in the human brain the cytoarchitecture and the chemoarchitecture of that cortex differs substantially along its rostral-caudal extent (Figure 1.2-3). It is tempting to identify those regions by their location relative to other structures, but sufficient interindividual variability exists in the human brain to make such a topological definition unreliable. In the case of the entorhinal cortex, the location of its different subdivisions relative to adjacent structures, such as the amygdala and the hippocampus, varies somewhat across human brains. Therefore, in all studies, particularly those using the human brain, areas of interest must be defined in a manner that allows investigators to accurately identify the same region in all cases.

An additional limitation to the study of the human brain concerns the changes in morphology and biochemistry that can occur during the interval between the time of death and the freezing or fixation of brain specimens. In addition to the influence of the known postmortem interval, such changes may begin to occur during the agonal state preceding death. When comparing aspects of the organization of the human brain with that of other species, the researcher must try to account for changes that may have occurred in the human brain as a result of postmortem delay or agonal state. Furthermore, in the study of disease states, appropriate controls must be used, since differences in neurotransmitter content or other characteristics among cases could be a result of factors other than the disease state. Studies of the human brain in vivo —using such imaging techniques as positron emission tomography, magnetic resonance imaging, and magnetic resonance spectroscopy—circumvent many of those problems but are limited by a level of resolution that is insufficient for the study of many aspects of human brain organization.

STRUCTURAL COMPONENTS

MAJOR BRAIN STRUCTURES In the early stages of the development of the human brain, three primary vesicles can be identified in the neural tube: the *prosencephalon,* the *mesencephalon,* and the *rhombencephalon* (Table 1.2-1). Subsequently, the prosencephalon divides to become the *telencephalon* and the *diencephalon.* The telencephalon gives rise to the cerebral cortex, the hippocampal formation, the amygdala, and some components of the basal ganglia. The diencephalon becomes the thalamus, the hypothalamus, and several other related structures. The mesencephalon gives rise to the midbrain structures of the adult brain. The rhombencephalon divides into the *metencephalon* and the *myelencephalon.* The metencephalon gives rise to the pons and the cerebellum; the medulla is the derivative of the myelencephalon.

The cerebral cortex of each hemisphere is divided into four major regions; the *frontal, parietal, temporal,* and *occipital* lobes (Figure 1.2-4). The frontal lobe is located anterior to the central sulcus and consists of the primary motor, premotor, and prefrontal regions. The primary somatosensory cortex is located in the anterior parietal lobe; in addition, other cortical regions that are related to complex visual and somatosensory functions are located in the posterior parietal lobe. The superior portion of the temporal lobe contains the primary auditory cortex and other auditory regions; the inferior portion contains regions devoted to complex visual functions. In addition, some regions of the superior temporal sulcus receive a convergence of input from the visual, somatosensory, and auditory sensory areas. The occipital lobe consists of the primary visual cortex and other visual association areas.

TABLE 1.2-1
Derivatives of the Neural Tube

Primary Vesicles	Secondary Vesicles	Brain Components
Prosencephalon	Telencephalon	Cerebral cortex Hippocampus Amygdala Striatum
	Diencephalon	Thalamus Hypothalamus Epithalamus
Mesencephalon	Mesencephalon	Midbrain
Rhombencephalon	Metencephalon	Pons Cerebellum
	Myelencephalon	Medulla

Modified from J Nolte: *The Human Brain: An Introduction to Its Functional Anatomy,* ed 2, p 7. Mosby, St. Louis, 1988.

Beneath the outer mantle of the cerebral cortex are a number of other major brain structures, such as the caudate nucleus, the putamen, and the globus pallidus (Figures 1.2-5 and 1.2-6). Those structures are components of the basal ganglia, a system involved in the control of movement. The hippocampus and the amygdala, components of the limbic system, are located deep in the medial temporal lobe (Figures 1.2-6 and 1.2-7). In addition, derivatives of the diencephalon, such as the thalamus and the hypothalamus, are prominent internal structures; the thalamus is a relatively large structure composed of several nuclei that have distinct patterns of connectivity with the cerebral cortex (Figures 1.2-6 and 1.2-7). In contrast, the hypothalamus is a much smaller structure that is involved in autonomic and endocrine functions.

VENTRICULAR SYSTEM As the neural tube fuses during development, the cavity of the neural tube becomes the ventricular system of the brain. It is composed of two C-shaped *lateral ventricles* in the cerebral hemispheres that can be further divided into five parts: the anterior horn (which is located in the frontal lobe), the body of the ventricle, the inferior or temporal horn in the temporal lobe, the posterior or occipital horn in the occipital lobe, and the atrium (Figure 1.2-8). The *foramina of Monro* (interventricular foramina) are the two apertures that connect the two lateral ventricles with the *third ventricle,* which is found on the midline of the diencephalon. The *cerebral aque-*

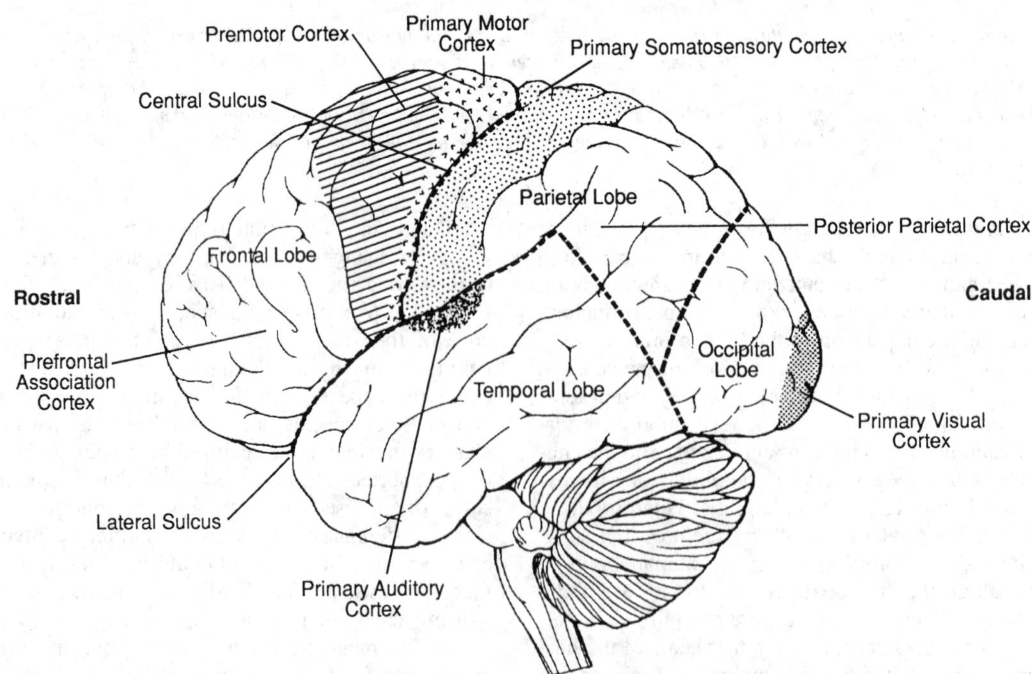

FIGURE 1.2-4 *Drawing of the lateral view of the human brain to show the location of the cortical lobes and select subregions. (Adapted from J P Kelly, J Dodd: Anatomical organization of the nervous system. In* Principles of Neural Science, *ed 3, E R Kandel, J H Schwartz, T M Jessel, editors, p 278. Elsevier, New York, 1991.)*

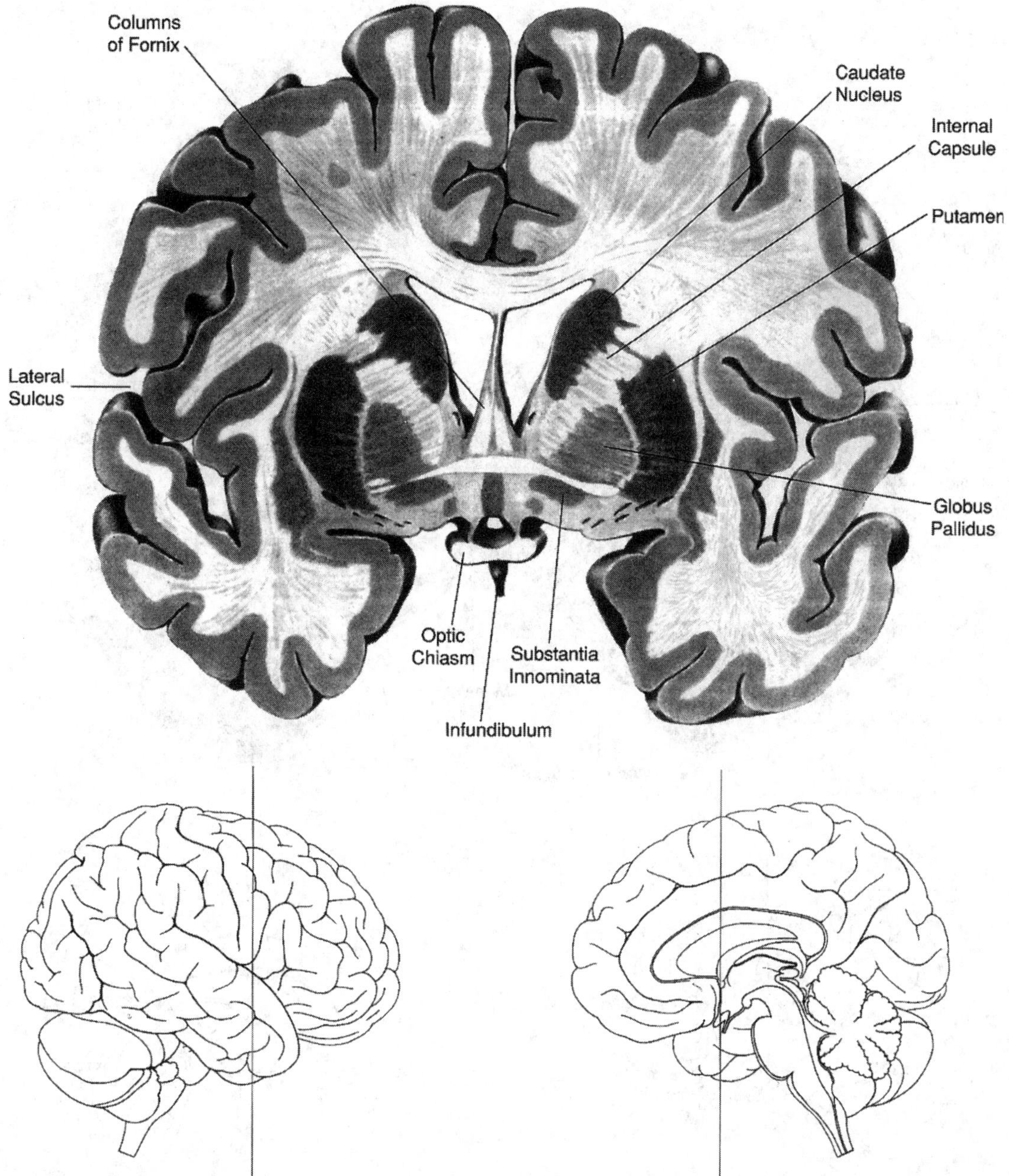

FIGURE 1.2-5 *Drawing of a coronal section through the optic chiasm of a human brain (6/5 x). The inset below indicates the level of the section. (Adapted from R Nieuwenhuys, J Voogd, C van Huijzen:* The Human Central Nervous System: A Synopsis and Atlas, *ed 3, p 70. Springer, New York, 1988.)*

duct connects the third ventricle with the *fourth ventricle* in the pons and the medulla.

The ventricular system is filled with cerebrospinal fluid (CSF), a colorless liquid containing low concentrations of protein, glucose, and potassium and relatively high concentrations of sodium and chloride. The majority (70 percent) of the CSF is produced at the choroid plexus located in the walls of the lateral ventricles and in the roof of both the third and fourth ventricles. The *choroid plexus* is a complex of ependyma, pia, and capillaries that invaginate the ventricle. In contrast to other parts of the brain, the capillaries in the choroid plexus are fenestrated, which allows substances to pass out of the capillaries and through the pia mater. The ependymal or choroid epithelial cells, however, have tight junctions between cells to prevent the leakage of substances into the CSF; that provides what is sometimes referred to as the *blood-CSF barrier*. In other parts of the brain, the endothelial cells of the capillaries exhibit tight junctions that prevent the movement of substances from the blood to the brain; that is referred to as the *blood-brain barrier*.

The CSF is constantly produced and circulates through the lateral ventricles to the third ventricle and then to the fourth ventricle. The CSF then flows through the medial and lateral apertures to the cisterna magna and pontine cistern and finally travels over the cerebral hemispheres to be absorbed by the arachnoid villi and released into the superior sagittal sinus. Disruptions in the flow of the CSF usually cause some form of hydrocephalus; for example, if an intraventricular foramen is occluded, the associated lateral ventricle becomes enlarged, but the remaining components of the ventricular system remain normal.

Several functions are attributed to the CSF: it serves to cushion the brain against trauma, to maintain and control the extracellular environment, and to spread endocrine hormones. Since the CSF bathes the brain and is in direct communication with extracellular fluid, it is pos-

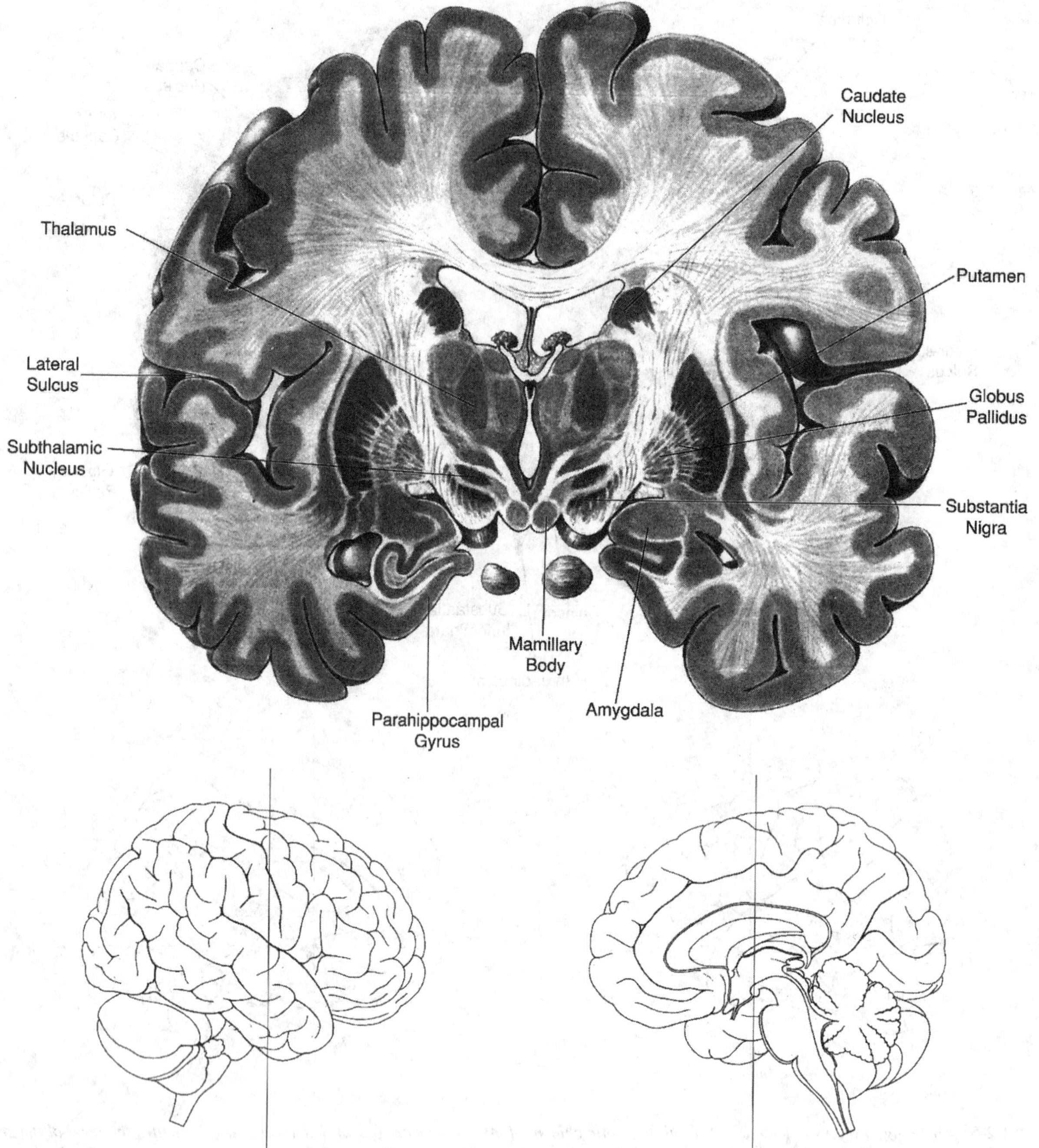

FIGURE 1.2-6 *Drawing of a coronal section at the level of the mamillary bodies (6/5 x). The inset below indicates the level of the section. (Adapted from R Nieuwenhuys, J Voogd, C van Huijzen:* The Human Central Nervous System: A Synopsis and Atlas, *ed 3, p 72. Springer, New York, 1988.)*

sible to measure the amount of certain compounds in the CSF as a correlate of the amount of that substance in the brain. For example, levels of homovanillic acid (HVA), a metabolite of the neurotransmitter dopamine, are thought to reflect the functional activity of that neurotransmitter. Thus, the concentration of HVA in samples of the CSF taken in a lumbar puncture may provide a picture of brain dopaminergic function. However, since the CSF bathes the entire brain, the CSF levels of HVA may not be a valid indicator of the activity of dopaminergic neurons in any particular brain area. Several studies have attempted to correlate CSF levels of HVA or other metabolites with levels of those metabolites in specific regions of human brains obtained at autopsy and in brain samples from nonhuman primates; the results of those studies are mixed and demonstrate that caution must be exercised in interpreting the findings of investigations that rely on CSF measurements as indicators of neurotransmitter activity.

FUNCTIONAL BRAIN SYSTEMS

The relation between the organizational principles and the structural components of the human brain are illustrated in three functional systems—the thalamocortical, basal ganglia, and limbic systems.

THALAMOCORTICAL SYSTEMS

Thalamus The largest portion of the diencephalon consists of the *thalamus,* a group of nuclei that serve as the major synaptic relay station for the information reaching the cerebral cortex. On an anatomical

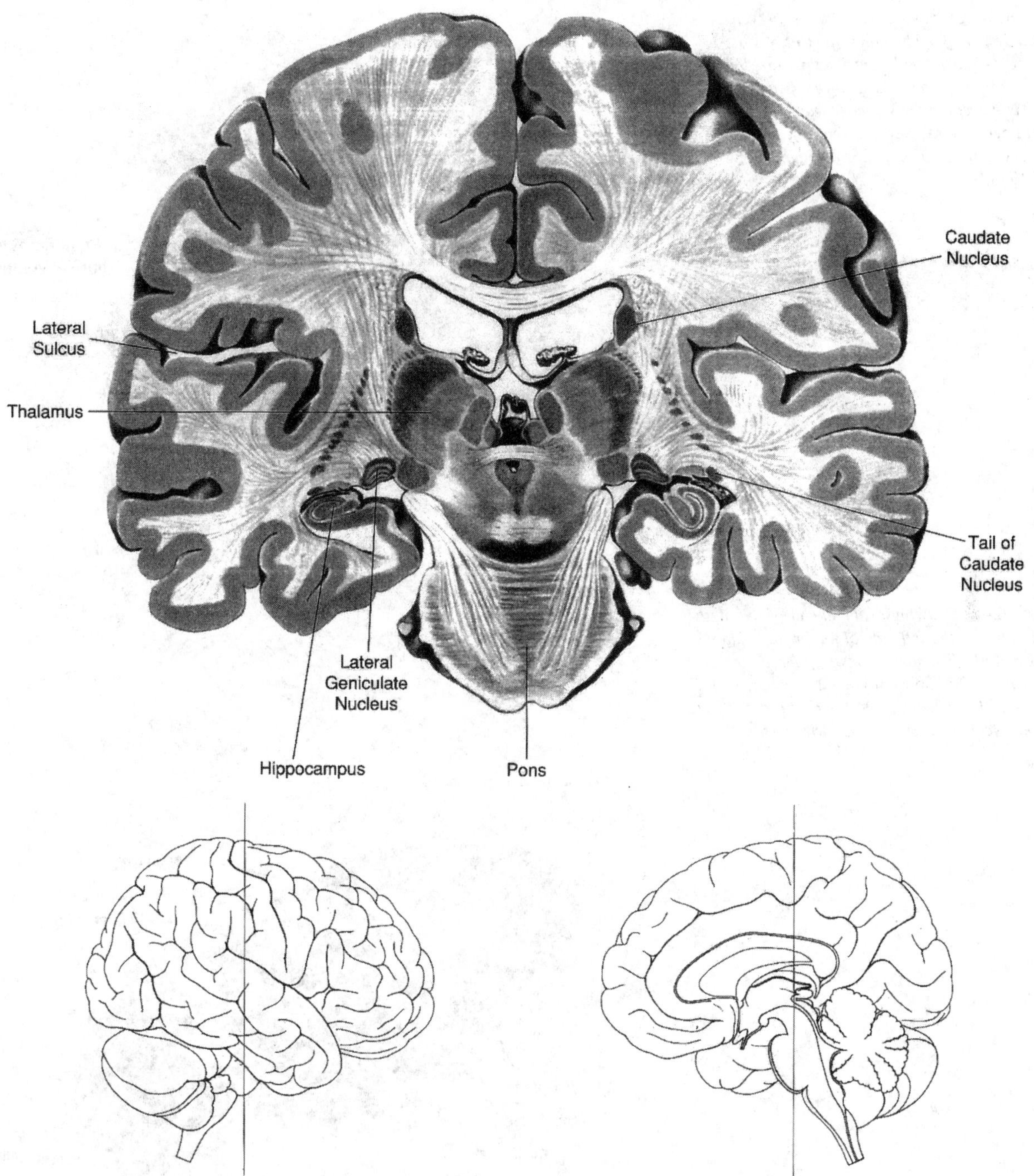

FIGURE 1.2-7 *Drawing of a coronal section through the posterior thalamus (6/5 x). The inset below indicates the level of the section. (Adapted from R Nieuwenhuys, J Voogd, C van Huijzen:* The Human Central Nervous System: A Synopsis and Atlas, *ed 3, p 74. Springer, New York, 1988.)*

basis the thalamic nuclei can be divided into six groups: anterior, medial, lateral, reticular, intralaminar, and midline nuclei. A thin Y-shaped sheet of myelinated fibers, the *internal medullary lamina,* delimits the anterior, medial, and lateral groups of nuclei (Figure 1.2-9). In the human thalamus the anterior and medial groups each contain a single large nucleus, the *anterior* and *medial dorsal nuclei.* The lateral group of nuclei can be further subdivided into dorsal and ventral tiers. The dorsal tier is composed of the *lateral dorsal,* the *lateral posterior,* and the *pulvinar nuclei;* the ventral tier consists of the *ventral anterior,* the *ventral lateral,* the *ventral posterior lateral,* and the *ventral posterior medial nuclei.* The lateral group of nuclei are covered by the *external medullary lamina,* another sheet of myelinated fibers. Interposed between those fibers and the internal capsule is a thin group of neurons forming the *reticular nucleus* of the thalamus. The *intralaminar nuclei,* the largest of which is the *central median nucleus,* are located within the internal medullary lamina. The final group of thalamic nuclei, the *midline nuclei,* cover portions of the medial surface of the thalamus. The midline nuclei of each hemisphere may fuse to form the interthalamic adhesion, which is variably present.

Thalamic nuclei can also be classified into several groups based on the pattern and the information content of their connections (Table 1.2-2). For example, *relay nuclei* project to and receive input from specific regions of the cerebral cortex. Those reciprocal connections apparently allow the cerebral cortex to modulate the thalamic input it receives. *Specific relay nuclei* process input either from a single sensory modality or from a distinct part of the motor system. For example, the lateral geniculate nucleus receives visual input from the optic tract and projects to the primary visual area of the occipital cortex. In contrast, *asso-*

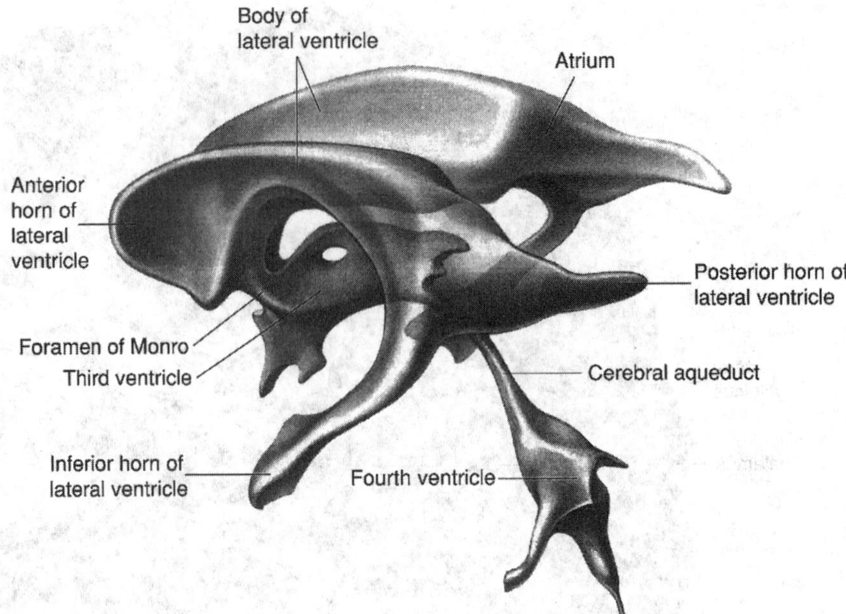

FIGURE 1.2-8 *Drawing of a cast of the ventricular system of the human brain (6/5 x). The C shape of the lateral ventricles within the cerebral hemispheres is shown. (Adapted from R Nieuwenhuys, J Voogd, C van Huijzen:* The Human Central Nervous System: A Synopsis and Atlas, *ed 3, p 26. Springer, New York, 1988.)*

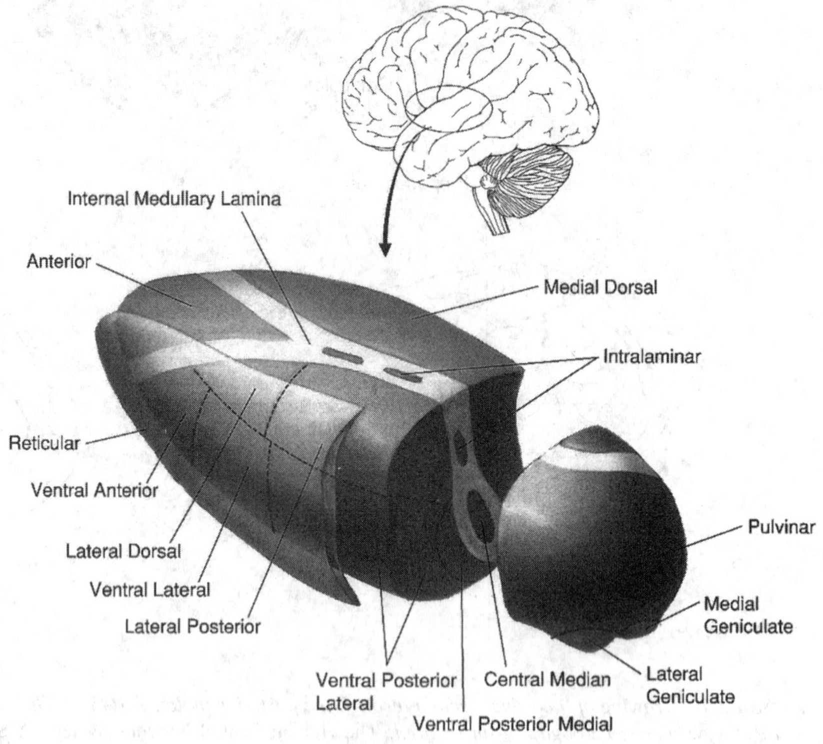

FIGURE 1.2-9 *Drawing of the nuclei of the thalamus as seen on the left side of the brain. (Adapted from J P Kelly: The neural basis of perception and movement. In* Principles of Neural Science, *ed 3, E R Kandel, J H Schwartz, T M Jessel, editors, p 291. Elsevier, New York, 1991. Used with permission.)*

ciation relay nuclei receive highly processed input from more than one source and project to larger areas of the association cortex. For example, the medial dorsal thalamic nucleus receives input from the hypothalamus and the amygdala and is reciprocally interconnected with the prefrontal cortex and certain premotor and temporal cortical regions. In contrast to relay nuclei, *diffuse-projection nuclei* receive input from diverse sources and project to widespread areas of the cerebral cortex and to the thalamus. The divergent nature of the cortical connections of those nuclei indicates that they may be involved in regulating the level of cortical excitability and arousal. Finally, the reticular nucleus is somewhat unique in that it receives input from collaterals of the axons that reciprocally connect other thalamic nuclei and the cerebral cortex. Each portion of the reticular nucleus then projects to that thalamic nucleus from which it receives input. That pattern of connectivity may indicate that the reticular nucleus samples both cortical afferent and efferent activity and then uses that information to regulate thalamic function.

Cerebral cortex The *cerebral cortex* is a laminated sheet of neurons, several millimeters thick, that covers the cerebral hemispheres. More than 90 percent of the total cortical area consists of the *neocortex,* which has a six-layered structure (at least at some point during development). The remainder of the cerebral cortex is referred to as the *allocortex* and consists of the *paleocortex* and the *archicortex,* regions that are restricted to the base of the telencephalon and the hippocampal formation, respectively.

TABLE 1.2-2
Connections of Thalamic Nuclei

Type	Nuclei	Principal Afferent Inputs	Major Projection Sites
Specific relay	Anterior	Mamillary body of hypothalamus	Cingulate cortex
	Ventral anterior	Globus pallidus	Premotor cortex
	Ventral lateral	Dentate nucleus of cerebellum	Motor, premotor cortices
	Ventral posterior lateral	Medial lemniscal and spinothalamic pathways	Somatosensory cortex
	Ventral posterior medial	Sensory nuclei of trigeminal nerve	Somatosensory cortex
	Medial geniculate	Inferior colliculus	Auditory cortex
	Lateral geniculate	Optic tract	Visual cortex
Association relay	Lateral dorsal	Unknown	Cingulate cortex
	Lateral posterior	Superior colliculus	Parietal cortex
	Pulvinar	Superior colliculus	Temporal, parietal, occipital cortices
	Medial dorsal	Amygdala and hypothalamus	Prefrontal cortex
Diffuse-projection	Midline	Reticular formation, hypothalamus	Basal forebrain, cortex
	Intralaminar	Reticular formation, spinothalamic tract, globus pallidus	Basal ganglia, cortex
	Reticular	Cerebral cortex, thalamus	Thalamus

This table does not include the cortical inputs to each thalamic nucleus. (Modified from J P Kelly: The neural basis of perception and movement. In Principles of Neural Science, *ed 3, E R Kandel, J H Schwartz, T M Jessell, editors, p 291. Elsevier, New York, 1991.)*

Within the neocortex, the two major neuronal cell types are the pyramidal and stellate or nonpyramidal neurons. *Pyramidal neurons,* which account for approximately 60 percent of all neocortical neurons, usually have a characteristically shaped cell body that gives rise to a single apical dendrite that ascends vertically toward the cortical surface. In addition, the neurons have an array of short dendrites that spread laterally from the base of the cell. Most pyramidal cells are projection neurons that are thought to use excitatory amino acids as neurotransmitters. In contrast, *nonpyramidal cells* are generally small, local-circuit neurons, many of which use the inhibitory neurotransmitter γ-aminobutyric acid (GABA).

Neocortical neurons are distributed across six layers of the neocortex; those layers are distinguished by the relative size and packing density of their neurons (Figure 1.2-10). Each cortical layer tends to receive particular types of inputs and to furnish characteristic projections. For example, afferents from thalamic relay nuclei terminate primarily in layer IV, whereas corticothalamic projections originate mainly from layer VI pyramidal neurons.

In addition to the horizontal laminar structure, many aspects of cortical organization have a vertical or columnar characteristic. For example, the apical dendrites of pyramidal neurons and the axons of some local-circuit neurons have a prominent vertical orientation, indicating that those neural elements may sample the input to or regulate the function of neurons in multiple layers, respectively. Afferent inputs to the neocortex from some brain regions also tend to be distributed across cortical layers in a columnar fashion. Finally, physiological studies in the somatosensory and visual cortices have shown that neurons in a given column respond to stimuli with particular characteristics, whereas those in adjacent columns respond to stimuli with different features.

The neocortex can be divided into two general types of regions. Regions with a readily identifiable six-layered appearance are known as the *homotypical cortex* and are found in association regions of the frontal, temporal, and parietal lobes. In contrast, some regions of the neocortex do not retain a six-layered appearance. Those regions, referred to as the *heterotypical cortex,* include the primary motor cortex, which lacks a defined layer IV, and primary sensory regions, which exhibit an expanded layer IV. The neocortex can be further divided into discrete areas, each area having a distinctive architecture, a certain set of connections, and a role in particular brain functions. Most subdivisions of the human neocortex have been based on cytoarchitectural features. The most widely used system is that of Korbinian Brodmann (Figure 1.2-11), who divided the cortex of each hemisphere into 44 areas. Although Brodmann's brain map has been extensively used in postmortem studies, many of the distinctions among regions are quite subtle, and the locations of the boundaries between regions may vary among persons.

Although a given cortical area may receive other inputs, it is heavily innervated by projections from particular thalamic nuclei and from certain other cortical regions either in the same hemisphere *(association fibers)* or the opposite hemisphere *(commissural fibers).* The patterns of connectivity make it possible to classify cortical regions into different types. *Primary sensory areas* are dominated by inputs from specific thalamic relay nuclei and are characterized by a topographic representation of visual space, the body surface, or the range of audible frequencies on the cortical surface of the primary visual, primary somatosensory, and primary auditory cortices, respectively. Those regions project in turn to nearby *unimodal association regions,* which are also devoted to processing information from a particular sensory modality. Output from those regions converges in *multimodal association areas,* such as the prefrontal cortex or the temporoparietal cortical regions. Neurons in those regions respond to complex stimuli and are thought to be mediators of higher cognitive functions. Finally, those regions influence the activity of the premotor and motor areas of the cerebral cortex that control behavioral responses.

Although that classification of cortical regions is accurate in many respects, it fails to account for some of the known complexities of cortical information processing. For example, somatosensory input from the thalamus projects to several distinct, topographically organized maps in the cerebral cortex. In addition, information flow within the cortex is not confined to the serial processing route implied in the classification scheme but also involves parallel processing streams, such as sensory input from the thalamus to both the primary and association areas.

Although this discussion has not distinguished between the cerebral hemispheres, certain brain functions, such as language, are localized to one hemisphere. The structural bases for the lateralization of function have not been determined, but some anatomical differences between the cerebral hemispheres have been observed. For example, a portion of the superior temporal cortex, called the planum temporale, is generally larger in the left hemisphere than in the right hemisphere. That cortical area, located close to the primary auditory cortex, appears to be involved in receptive language functions that are localized to the left hemisphere.

Functional circuitry The connections between the thalamus, the cortex, and certain related brain structures comprise three thalamocortical systems, each with different patterns of functional circuitry. Those three systems—sensory, motor, and association systems—are described separately here, but the three systems are heavily interconnected.

THALAMOCORTICAL SENSORY SYSTEMS Several general principles govern the organization of the thalamocortical sensory systems. First, sensory receptors transduce certain stimuli in the external environment to a neural impulse. The impulses ascend, often through intermediate nuclei in the spinal cord and the medulla, and ultimately synapse in specific relay nuclei of the thalamus.

Second, projections from peripheral sensory receptors to the thalamus and the cortex exhibit topography; that is, a particular portion of the external world is mapped onto a particular region of the brain. For example, in the somatosensory system, axons carrying information regarding a distinct part of the body synapse in a discrete part of the ventral posterior nucleus of the

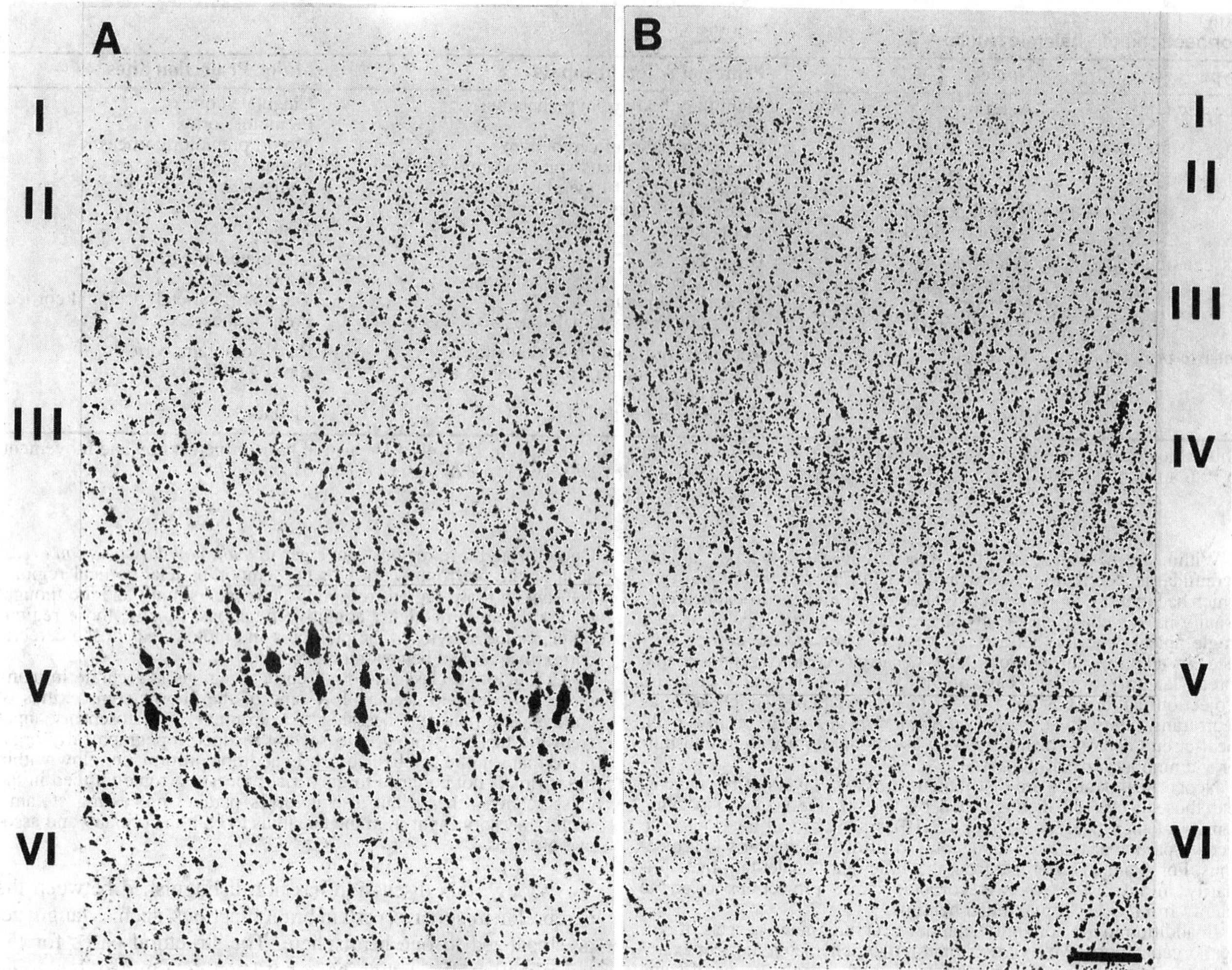

FIGURE 1.2-10 *Nissl-stained sections of (A) Brodmann's area 4 (primary motor cortex) and (B) area 41 (primary auditory cortex) from a control human brain. Roman numerals indicate the cortical layers. Marked differences in neuronal size and packing density between the layers of the two regions are evident. Calibration bar (200 μm) applies to A and B. (Courtesy of T Hayes and M Brady, University of Pittsburgh.)*

thalamus. Specifically, the ventral posterior medial nucleus receives inputs regarding the head, and the ventral posterior lateral nucleus receives inputs regarding the remainder of the body. The nuclei then project topographically to the primary somatosensory cortex, where several representations of the contralateral half of the body can be found. Those representations are distorted; regions heavily innervated by sensory receptors, such as the fingers, are disproportionately represented in the primary somatosensory cortex.

Third, in some cases, sensory inputs travel to the thalamus in a segregated manner according to the submodality of the information conveyed. The inputs are then processed in a parallel fashion; particular pathways may be exclusively devoted to processing a submodality. An example of such segregation is evident in the somatosensory system, where most fibers carrying tactile and proprioceptive information travel in the medial lemniscus, but pain and temperature information is conveyed to the ventral posterior thalamic nuclei through the spinothalamic tract. Although some tactile information is carried in the spinothalamic tract, the submodalities of pain and temperature are largely segregated from tactile and proprioceptive inputs as they ascend to the thalamus.

Finally, sensory pathways exhibit convergence; that is, primary sensory areas process sensory information and then project to unimodal association areas. Subsequently, the unimodal areas project to and converge in multimodal association areas. An illustration of convergence in sensory pathways is found in the somatosensory system. The primary somatosensory cortex, located in the anterior parietal lobe (Figure 1.2-12), has been divided into four regions on the basis of cytoarchitecture. Each of the cytoarchitectonic regions—numbered 1, 2, 3a, and 3b by Brodmann—contains a topographical representation of the body. The regions are heavily interconnected, and all project to the next level of somatosensory processing in area S-II. That type of projection, from one level of processing to a more advanced level, is termed a *feedforward* projection. The reciprocal connection, from the more advanced processing level back to the simpler level, is called a *feedback* projection. Both projections have distinct patterns of laminar termination: feedforward projections originate in the superficial layers of cortex (layer III) and terminate in layer IV; feedback projections originate in layers III, V, and VI and terminate outside layer IV. Further processing of somatosensory information occurs in higher-order somatosensory areas, such as area 7b of the posterior parietal cortex, which receive feedforward projections from S-II. Lesions of the posterior parietal cortex reflect the complexity of the information processed there; after a person has sustained a posterior parietal lesion, the ability to under-

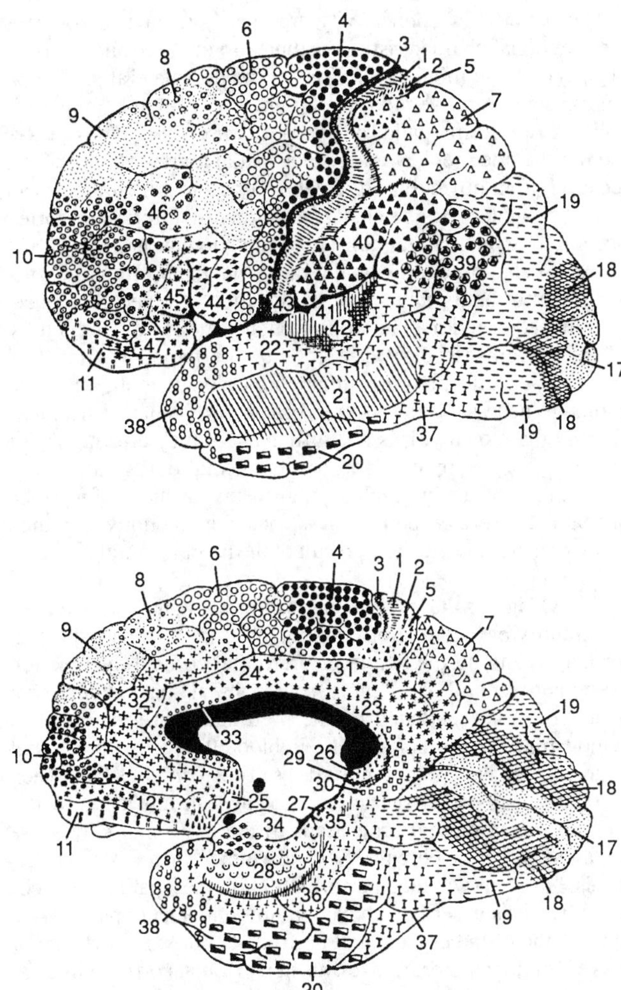

FIGURE 1.2-11 *Drawing of the cytoarchitectonic subdivisions of the human brain as determined by Brodmann. Top, lateral view; bottom, medial view.*

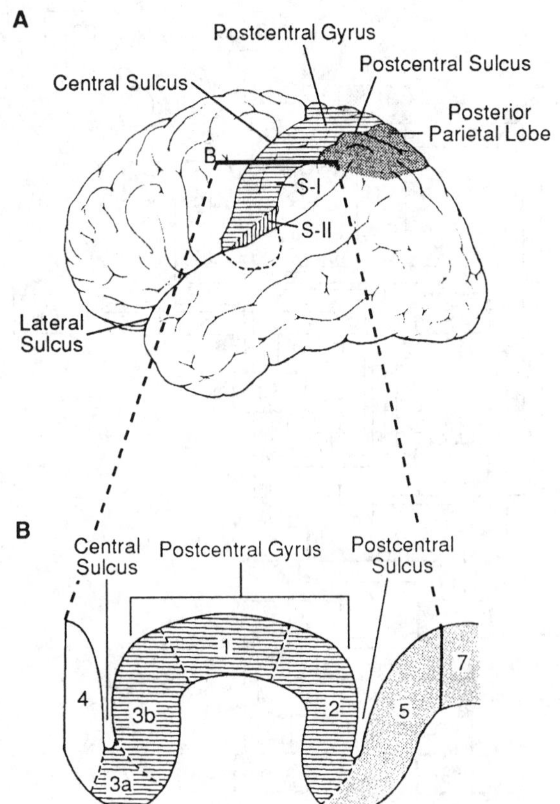

FIGURE 1.2-12 *Drawing of the location of the somatosensory cortices in the human brain. A: Somatosensory cortices are located in the anterior and posterior parietal cortex. B: Primary somatosensory cortex (S-I) is divided into four cytoarchitectonic regions, as shown on the drawing of the section taken at the level depicted in (A). (From J H Martin, T M Jessel: Anatomy of the somatic sensory system. In* Principles of Neural Science, *ed 3, E R Kandel, J H Schwartz, T M Jessel, editors, p 364. Elsevier, New York, 1991. Used with permission.)*

stand the significance of sensory stimuli is impaired, and extreme cases result in contralateral sensory neglect and inattention. However, the processing of somatosensory information within the cortex is clearly much more complex than what has been described here (Figure 1.2-13).

THALAMOCORTICAL MOTOR SYSTEMS The thalamocortical motor systems exhibit some unique organizational principles but also share many of the principles present in the sensory systems. First, in contrast to sensory systems, which primarily ascend from sensory receptor to cortical association areas, motor systems descend from association and motor regions of the cortex to the brainstem and the spinal cord. For example, the corticospinal tract originates in the layer V neurons of the premotor and primary motor cortices of the frontal lobe and terminates in the spinal cord to influence motor behavior.

Second, motor systems exhibit strong topography at both the thalamic and the cortical levels. For example, the corticospinal tract is organized so that a topographical respresentation of the contralateral half of the body is evident in the primary motor and premotor cortices. The representation of the body is disproportionate, with large regions of the motor cortex devoted to areas of the body involved in fine movement, such as the face and the hands.

Finally, there is a convergence of projections from several sensory association regions to the motor regions of the frontal cortex. For example, the premotor cortex receives a convergence of afferents from higher-order somatosensory and visual areas of the posterior parietal cortex, whereas afferents from the primary somatosensory cortex converge on the primary motor cortex. In addition to cortical input, the primary motor cortex receives afferents from the ventral lateral nucleus of the thalamus; that nucleus receives afferents predominantly from the cerebellum. The premotor cortex receives input from the ventral anterior thalamic nucleus, which receives much of its input from the globus pallidus.

The role of the primary motor cortex and the corticospinal tract in controlling movement in certain clinical disorders is often overshadowed by the known involvement of the basal ganglia in those movement disorders. For example, Parkinson's disease is characterized by a marked loss of the dopaminergic neurons in the mesencephalon. The neurons project to the striatum and to cortical regions, such as the primary motor cortex. Thus, in Parkinson's disease, a loss of dopaminergic innervation in the primary motor cortex may also play a role in the pathophysiology of the disease. In fact, studies of the motor cortex of parkinsonian patients have shown that the dopaminergic innervation of the motor cortex is depleted. Thus, the clinical features of Parkinson's disease may be the result of pathology in both the basal ganglia system and the primary motor cortex.

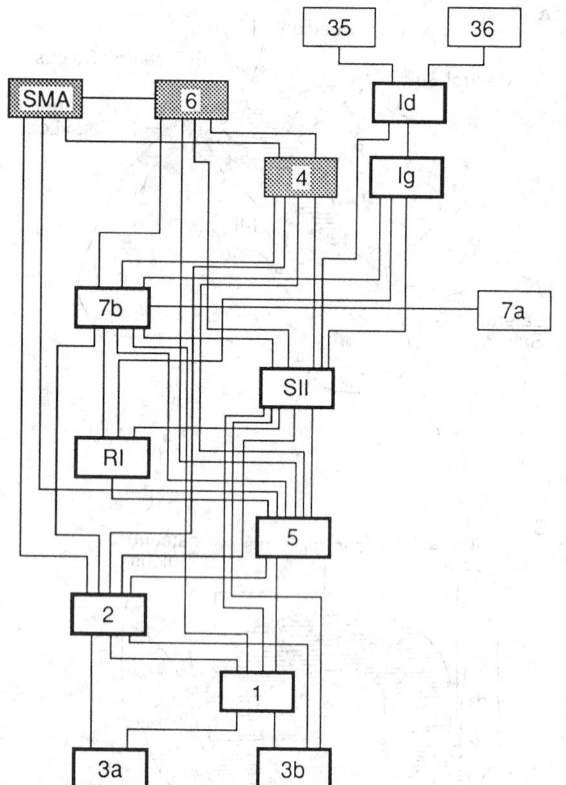

FIGURE 1.2-13 *A proposed organizational scheme of the connectivity among cortical areas involved in somatosensory information processing. Hierarchical assignments were made on the basis of feedforward and feedback patterns of connections, as described in the text. (For descriptions of those regions and additional details, D J Felleman, D C Van Essen: Distributed hierarchical processing in the primate cerebral cortex. Cereb Cortex* 1: *36, 1991. Used with permission.)*

THALAMOCORTICAL ASSOCIATION SYSTEMS The multimodal association areas of the cortex are organized according to several general principles. First, association regions receive a convergence of input from a variety of sources, including unimodal and multimodal association regions of the cortex, the association nuclei of the thalamus, and other structures. For example, the prefrontal cortex receives afferents from higher-order sensory cortices of the parietal and temporal lobes, the contralateral prefrontal cortex, the cingulate cortex of the limbic system, the medial dorsal nucleus of the thalamus, an association relay nucleus, and portions of the amygdala. The medial dorsal nucleus receives highly processed inputs from many sources, including some regions, such as the amygdala, that project directly to the prefrontal cortex. The redundant (direct and indirect) projections may serve to attach additional significance to certain inputs received by the prefrontal cortex.

Second, the projections that terminate in multimodal association regions exhibit a topographical organization. Since the information conveyed in those projections is highly processed, it does not appear that the topographical organization of the afferents is a representation of the external world. Nonetheless, a distinct pattern is present in the afferents received by association areas. For example, different cytoarchitectonic regions of the medial dorsal nucleus project to discrete regions of the prefrontal cortex. In addition, some of the cortical afferents received by the prefrontal cortex are topographically organized; certain regions of the prefrontal cortex predominantly receive highly processed information from one modality.

The patterns of connectivity are clearly related to some of the functional characteristics attributed to the prefrontal cortex. For example, in monkeys, lesions of the dorsolateral prefrontal cortex consistently produce an impairment in the monkey's ability to perform spatial delayed-response tasks. Those tasks require that the monkey maintain a spatial representation of the location of an object during a delay period in which the object is out of sight; it has been suggested that the prefrontal cortex plays a role in maintaining the spatial representation of the object. Such a function would require that the prefrontal cortex receive information regarding the location of objects in space, and, indeed, the dorsolateral prefrontal cortex is innervated by afferents from association regions of the parietal cortex that convey such information. Although the dorsolateral prefrontal cortex is necessary for the performance of delayed-response tasks in the monkey, it is not sufficient for the performance of the task. For example, lesions of the medial dorsal nucleus in the monkey result in similar impairments on the performance of spatial delayed-response tasks. Thus, the functions attributed to the prefrontal cortex are a result of the neural circuitry involving the region.

Knowledge of the integration of afferent inputs into the neural circuitry of certain prefrontal regions may also be important for understanding the nature of prefrontal cortical dysfunction in schizophrenia. For example, schizophrenic patients perform poorly on tasks mediated by the prefrontal cortex and fail to demonstrate the normal increase in blood flow to the prefrontal regions when engaged in those tasks. Those findings have been correlated with other measures that suggest, albeit indirectly, that the dopaminergic projections to the prefrontal cortex are impaired in schizophrenia. Several studies in nonhuman primates have shown that performance of the spatial delayed-response tasks described above requires an intact dopaminergic innervation of the dorsolateral prefrontal cortex. Knowledge of the role of dopaminergic afferents in prefrontal cortical circuitry may provide insight into at least certain aspects of the clinical features of schizophrenia.

BASAL GANGLIA SYSTEM The basal ganglia are a collection of nuclei that have been grouped together on the basis of their interconnections. The nuclei play an important role in movement and disorders of movement, such as dyskinesias.

Major structures The basal ganglia are generally considered to include the *caudate nucleus,* the *putamen,* the *globus pallidus* (referred to as the paleostriatum or pallidum), the *subthalamic nucleus,* and the *substantia nigra.* The term "striatum" refers to the caudate nucleus and the putamen together; the term "corpus striatum" refers to the caudate nucleus, the putamen, and the globus pallidus; and the term "lentiform nucleus" refers to the putamen and the globus pallidus together.

Although the above nuclei are generally agreed to belong to the basal ganglia, some controversy exists concerning whether other nuclei should be included in the definition of the basal ganglia. Some investigators believe that additional regions of the brain have anatomical connections that are similar to other components of the basal ganglia and should, therefore, be included in the term. Those additional regions are usually termed the ventral striatum and the ventral pallidum. The ventral striatum includes the nucleus accumbens, which is the region where the putamen and the head of the caudate nucleus fuse, and the olfactory tubercle. The ventral pallidum is a region that receives afferents from the ventral striatum and includes but is not limited to a group of neurons termed the substantia innominata. This section focuses on the structures generally accepted as belonging to the basal ganglia but also discusses additional structures when relevant to the functional anatomy of the system.

CAUDATE NUCLEUS The caudate nucleus is a C-shaped structure that is divided into three general regions. The anterior portion of the structure is referred to as the head, the posterior region is the tail, and the intervening region is the body (Figure 1.2-14). The caudate nucleus is associated with the contour of the lateral ventricles: the head lies against the frontal horn of the lateral ventricle, and the tail lies against the temporal horn. The head of the caudate nucleus is continuous with the putamen; the tail terminates in the amygdala of the temporal lobe.

PUTAMEN The putamen lies in the brain medial to the insula and is bounded laterally by the fibers of the external capsule and medially by the globus pallidus (Figures 1.2-5 and 1.2-6). As noted above, the putamen is continuous with the head of the caudate nucleus (Figure 1.2-14). Although bridges of neurons between the caudate nucleus and the putamen show the continuity of the nuclei, the two structures are separated by the fibers of the anterior limb of the internal capsule.

GLOBUS PALLIDUS In contrast to the caudate nucleus and the putamen, which are telencephalic in origin, the globus pallidus is derived from the diencephalon. The globus pallidus constitutes the inner component of the lentiform nucleus; with the putamen it forms a conelike structure, with its tip directed medially (Figures 1.2-5 and 1.2-6). The posterior limb of the internal capsule bounds the globus pallidus medially and separates it from the thalamus; the putamen borders the globus pallidus laterally. In the human the medial medullary lamina divides the globus pallidus into medial and lateral segments. (Figures 1.2-5 and 1.2-6).

SUBTHALAMIC NUCLEUS The subthalamic nucleus (of Luys) is also derived from the diencephalon. The large-celled nucleus lies dorsomedial to the posterior limb of the internal capsule and dorsal to the substantia nigra (Figure 1.2-6). Discrete lesions of the nucleus in humans lead to hemiballism, a syndrome characterized by violent, forceful choreiform movements that occur on the side contralateral to the lesion.

SUBSTANTIA NIGRA The substantia nigra is present in the midbrain between the tegmentum and the basis pedunculi and is mesencephalic in origin (Figure 1.2-6). The substantia nigra consists of two components: a dorsal cell-rich portion referred to as the pars compacta and a ventral cell-sparse portion denoted the pars reticulata. Most of the neurons in the pars compacta of the substantia nigra in humans are pigmented because of the presence of neuromelanin; those cells contain the neurotransmitter dopamine. The dendrites of the pars compacta neurons frequently extend into the pars reticulata, where they receive synapses from the neurons of the pars reticulata that use the inhibitory neurotransmitter GABA.

Internal organization

The caudate nucleus and the putamen are frequently referred to together because of their common characteristics. For example, both nuclei are telencephalic in origin and, in the rodent, are a continuous structure. In addition, they are composed of histologically identical cells. The majority (at least 70 percent) of the neurons in the striatum are medium-sized cells (10 to 20μm in diameter) that possess spines on their dendrites; those so-called medium spiny neurons are known to send their axons out of the striatum. In addition to medium spiny neurons, medium-sized cells without spines (medium aspiny neurons) are present, as are large cells with and without spines (large spiny neurons and large aspiny neurons). With the exception of the medium and large spiny cells, most other neurons are local-circuit neurons. That classification scheme is a simplified system that highlights the most salient features that distinguish the cells of the striatum; however, many authors further subdivide each category.

Although the neurons of the caudate nucleus and the putamen lack the notable cytoarchitectonic lamination of the cerebral cortex, an organization of the striatum has been elucidated. Immunohistochemical and receptor-binding studies have shown a discontinuity in the distribution of particular neurotransmitter-related substances that may have implications for the funtional circuitry of the basal ganglia. For example, in the striatum, zones that contain a low density of acetylcholinesterase (AChE) enzymatic activity are surrounded by regions rich in AChE activity. The AChE-rich regions are referred to as the *matrix,* and the AChE zones are termed either *striosomes* in the primate or patches in the rodent. The organization of several neuropeptide systems follows that organization. For example, the distributions of enkephalin, substance P, and somatostatin immunoreactivity show the compartmentalization of the striatum. In addition, in the rodent certain subtypes of dopamine receptors are present predominantly in one compartment as compared with the other. The discontinuous distribution of dopamine receptors may be clinically relevant to the use of antipsychotics, since many antipsychotic agents are dopamine-receptor antagonists that have differing affinities for dopamine-receptor subtypes. In addition, the distribution of some afferent systems terminating in the striatum follows the striosome-matrix organization. For example, afferents from the thalamus terminate preferentially in the matrix, rather than in the striosome.

Functional circuitry

Projections into, within, and out of the basal ganglia are topographically organized and maintain that topography throughout the processing circuits of the basal ganglia. The existence of such patterns of connectivity has resulted in the hypothesis that parallel, independent circuits exist in the basal ganglia that process information from functionally different regions of the brain and that subserve the many complex functions of the neural system.

INPUTS TO THE BASAL GANGLIA The striatum is the major recipient of the inputs to the basal ganglia. Three major afferent systems are known to terminate in the striatum: the corticostriatal, the nigrostriatal, and the thalamostriatal afferents (Figure 1.2-15). The corticostriatal projection originates from all regions of the neocortex, arising primarily from the pyramidal cells of layers V and VI. In many regions of the neocortex, the neurotransmitter involved is thought to be the excitatory amino acid glutamate. A topography governing corticostriatal projections has been found in the monkey. Afferents from the sen-

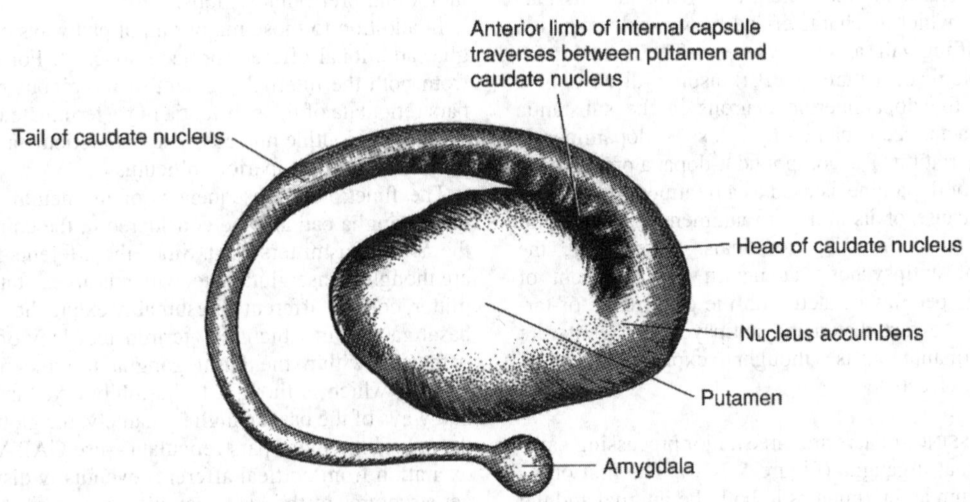

FIGURE 1.2-14 *Drawing of the right corpus striatum from the lateral view. The putamen obscures the more medial globus pallidus. (Adapted from M L Barr, J A Kiernan:* The Human Nervous System, *ed 5, p 208. Lippincott, New York, 1988.)*

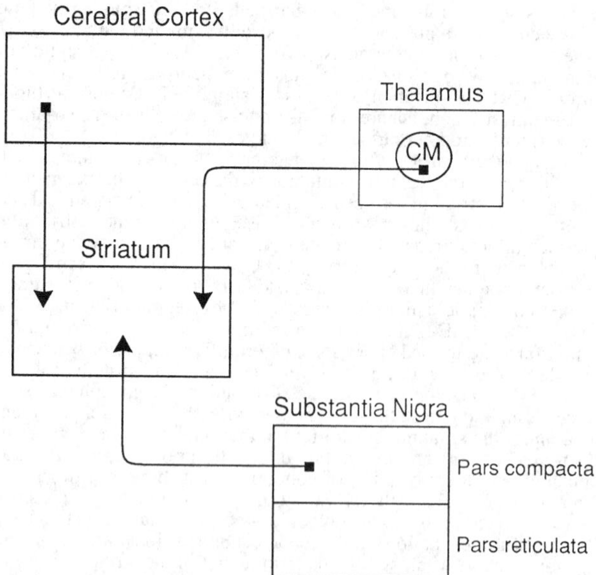

FIGURE 1.2-15 *Schematic drawing of the inputs into the basal ganglia system. Three major afferent systems have been identified: the corticostriatal, thalamostriatal, and nigrostriatal pathways.*

sorimotor cortex terminate predominantly in the putamen; association regions of the cortex terminate preferentially in the caudate nucleus. The prefrontal regions, in particular, provide a heavy input to the head of the caudate nucleus. In addition, afferents from the limbic cortical areas and from the hippocampus and the amygdala terminate in the ventral striatum. The second major class of afferents arises from the substantia nigra. Those fibers originate in the dopaminergic neurons of the pars compacta. The third afferent system originates in the thalamus. The thalamic nuclei providing the projection are the intralaminar nuclei, particularly the central median nucleus. The neurotransmitter of the pathway is not known at this time.

Other less substantial inputs also terminate in the striatum. Those inputs originate in the locus ceruleus and the raphe nuclei. The afferents from the locus ceruleus use the neurotransmitter norepinephrine, and the projections from the raphe nuclei contain serotonin.

Disruption of the input pathways of the basal ganglia has been associated with some movement disorders, such as Parkinson's disease, which is characterized by muscular rigidity, fine tremor, shuffling gait, and bradykinesia. The most consistent neuropathological feature of Parkinson's disease is a degeneration of the dopaminergic neurons in the substantia nigra pars compacta, accompanied by a loss of dopaminergic terminals in the striatum. The compound L-dopa, a precursor in the biosynthesis of dopamine, is used as a treatment for Parkinson's disease because of its ability to augment the release of dopamine from the remaining terminals. Conversely, the administration of antipsychotic agents in the treatment of schizophrenia has been associated with the occurrence of tardive dyskinesia; the fact that many antipsychotic agents are dopamine-receptor antagonists is thought to explain their movement-related side effects.

INTERNAL PROCESSING There are three major processing pathways within the basal ganglia (Figure 1.2-16). The first originates in the striatum and terminates in both the internal and the external segments of the globus pallidus and in the pars reticulata of the substantia nigra. The topography found in the afferent projection to the striatum appears to be maintained in that processing pathway. For example, the sensorimotor territories of the striatum project most heavily to the ventral portion of the globus pallidus, whereas association territories project to the dorsal regions of the globus pallidus. The second pathway is a projection from the external segment of the globus pallidus that terminates in the subthalamic nucleus. The third projection arises from the subthalamic nucleus and terminates in both segments of the globus pallidus and in the pars reticulata. Although most connections within the basal ganglia are unidirectional, a reciprocal projection is found between the external segment of the globus pallidus and the subthalamic nucleus.

The intrinsic circuitry of the basal ganglia is disrupted by a severe loss of neurons in the striatum in Huntington's disease. That autosomal-dominant disorder is characterized by progressive chorea and dementia. Although the location of the Huntington's disease gene has been identified as the short arm of chromosome 4, the cause of the selective degeneration of the striatal cells is not known. GABA and either enkephalin or substance P have been identified in neurons that are the earliest affected cells of the striatum. The termination of excitatory cortical afferents on those vulnerable cell populations has led to the hypothesis that the neurons may degenerate because of excitotoxic levels of glutamate transmission. Recent studies also indicate that cortical neurons are lost in Huntington's disease.

OUTPUT OF THE BASAL GANGLIA The internal segment of the globus pallidus is the source of much of the output of the basal ganglia (Figure 1.2-17). That segment of the globus pallidus provides a projection to the ventral lateral and ventral anterior nuclei of the thalamus and to the intralaminar thalamic nuclei—in particular, the central median nucleus. The pars reticulata of the substantia nigra also provides a projection to the ventral anterior and ventral lateral thalamic nuclei. Those portions of the ventral lateral and ventral anterior thalamic nuclei then project to the premotor and prefrontal cortices. As a result of the projections of the premotor and prefrontal cortices to the primary motor cortex, the basal ganglia are able to influence indirectly the output of the primary motor cortex. In addition, the cortical output of the basal ganglia exhibits marked convergence; that is, although the striatum receives afferents from all regions of the neocortex, the eventual output of the globus pallidus and the pars reticulata is largely conveyed, through the thalamus, to a much smaller portion of the neocortex, the premotor and prefrontal regions.

In addition to those major output pathways of the basal ganglia, additional efferent projections exist. For example, fibers from both the internal segment of the globus pallidus and the pars reticulata of the substantia nigra terminate in the tegmental pedunculo-pontine nucleus. The pars reticulata also furnishes a projection to the superior colliculus.

The functional consequences of the neural circuitry of the basal ganglia can also be considered in the context of some of the neurotransmitters used. Since the afferents from the cortex are thought to use glutamate, which is an excitatory neurotransmitter, cortical afferents presumably excite the structures of the basal ganglia in which they terminate. Many of the processing pathways within the basal ganglia use the neurotransmitter GABA, which is thought to be inhibitory. Finally, the output pathways of the basal ganglia—namely, the globus pallidus and the substantia nigra pars reticulata—use GABA as well. Thus, excitation from cortical afferents eventually disinhibits the target structures of the basal ganglia because of the back-to-back inhibitory pathways of the basal ganglia.

Historically, motor systems have been divided into pyramidal

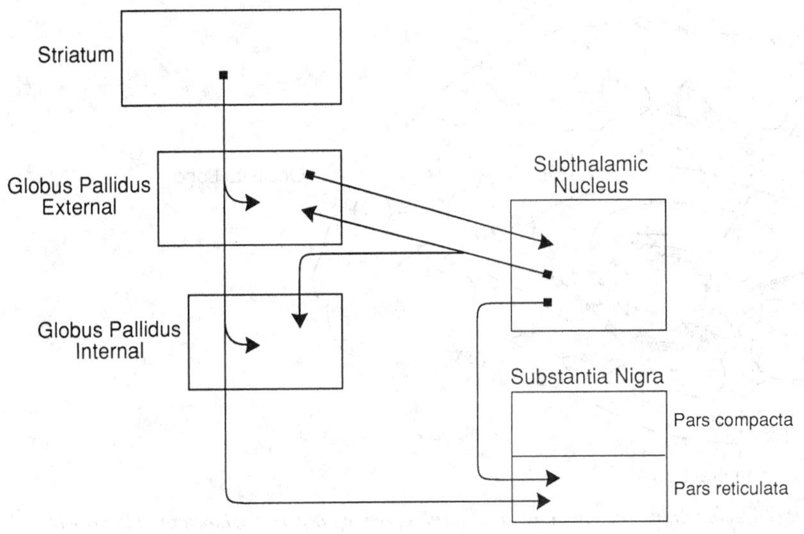

FIGURE 1.2-16 *Schematic drawing of the intrinsic circuitry of the basal ganglia. Afferents from the striatum terminate in both segments of the globus pallidus and in the pars reticulata of the substantia nigra. The subthalamic nucleus receives a projection from the external segment of the globus pallidus and projects back to both segments. Finally, the subthalamic nucleus projects to the substantia nigra pars reticulata.*

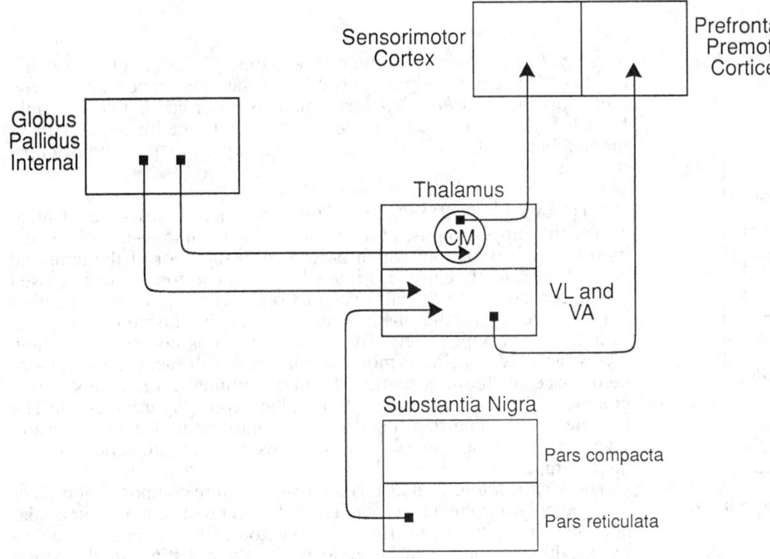

FIGURE 1.2-17 *Schematic drawing of the output of the basal ganglia system. The internal segment of the globus pallidus projects to the central median (CM), ventral lateral (VL), and ventral anterior (VA) nuclei of the thalamus. Those nuclei then project to sensorimotor, prefrontal, and premotor cortices. The substantia nigra pars reticulata also projects to the VL and VA nuclei.*

(corticospinal) and extrapyramidal (basal ganglia) components; that division is based on clinical findings suggesting that lesions of each system result in distinct motor syndromes. For example, lesions of the extrapyramidal system result in involuntary movements, changes in muscle tone, and slowness of movement; lesions of the pyramidal system lead to spasticity and paralysis. Because of those findings, the pyramidal and extrapyramidal systems were thought to independently control voluntary and involuntary movement, respectively. However, that division is no longer accurate for several reasons. First, other structures of the brain outside the traditional pyramidal and extrapyramidal systems, such as the cerebellum, are involved in the control of movement. Second, the pyramidal and extrapyramidal systems are not independent, but the neural circuits of those systems are interconnected. Finally, although the basal ganglia are important in the control of movement, the system also appears to be involved in other functions of the brain. For example, the cognitive dysfunction of Huntington's disease may be related to the striatal degeneration in that disorder. In addition, the basal ganglia may be involved in the pathophysiology of schizophrenia, since particular nuclei of the basal ganglia (for example, nucleus accumbens) may be a site of antipsychotic drug action. Further research will probably find conclusively that the basal ganglia subserve other functions in addition to the control of movement.

LIMBIC SYSTEM The concept of the limbic system as a neural substrate for emotional experience and expression has a rich but controversial history. More than 100 years ago Pierre Broca applied the term ''limbic'' (from the Latin *limbus* for border) to the curved rim of the cortex, including the cingulate and the parahippocampal gyri, located at the junction of the diencephalon and the cerebral hemispheres (Figure 1.2-18). In 1937 James Papez postulated, primarily on the basis of anatomical data, that the cortical regions are linked to the hippocampus, the mamillary body, and the anterior thalamus in a circuit that mediates emotional behavior (Figure 1.2-19). That concept was supported by the work of Heinrich Klüver and Paul Bucy, who demonstrated that temporal lobe lesions, which disrupt components of the circuit, alter affective responses in nonhuman primates. In 1952 Paul MacLean coined the term ''limbic system'' to describe Broca's limbic lobe and related subcortical nuclei as the neural substrate of emotion.

However, over the last 40 years it has become clear that some

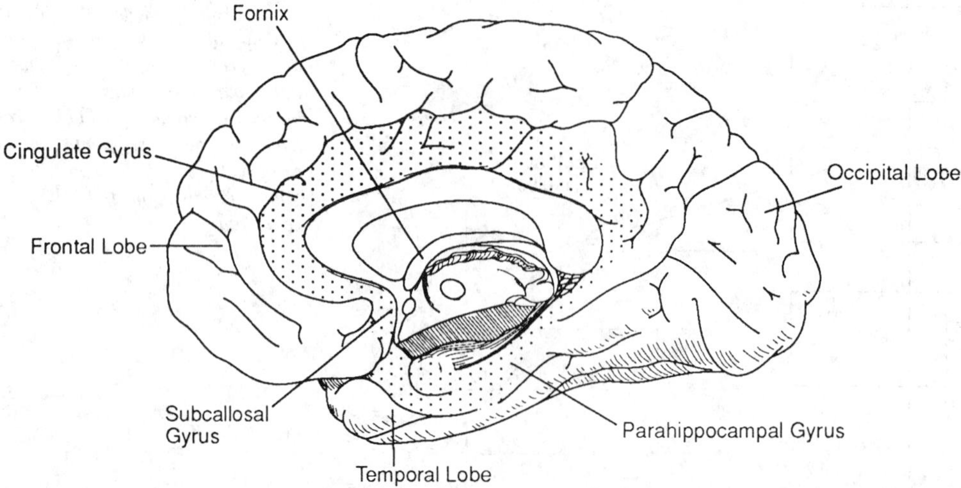

FIGURE 1.2-18 *The location of the limbic lobe (shaded area), containing the cingulate and parahippocampal gyri, is shown on this drawing of the medial surface of the human brain. (Adapted from I Kupfermann: Hypothalamus and limbic system: Peptidergic neurons, homeostasis, and emotional behavior. In* Principles of Neural Science, *ed 3, p 736, E R Kandel, J H Schwartz, T M Jessel, editors. Elsevier, New York, 1991.)*

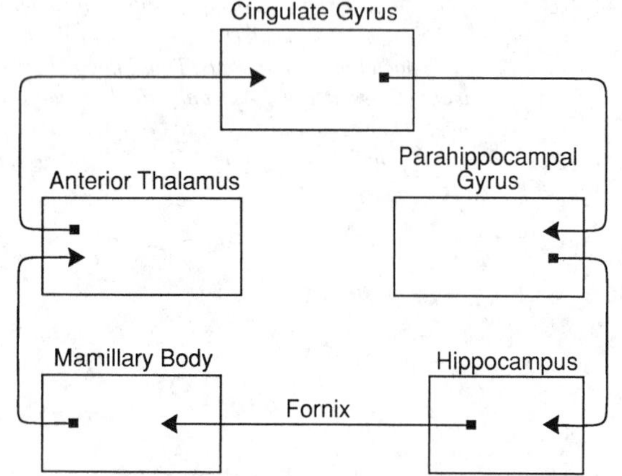

FIGURE 1.2-19 *A schematic drawing of the neural circuit for emotion as originally proposed by James Papez.*

limbic structures (for example, the hippocampus) are also involved in other complex brain processes, such as memory. In addition, expanding knowledge of the connectivity of traditional limbic structures has made it increasingly difficult to define the boundaries of the limbic system. Despite those limitations, the concept of a limbic system may still be a useful way to describe the circuitry that relates certain telencephalic structures and their cognitive processes with the hypothalamus and its output pathways that control autonomic, somatic, and endocrine functions.

Major structures As suggested above, there is no unanimity on the brain structures that constitute the limbic system. This section includes the brain regions that are most commonly listed as components of the limbic system: the cingulate and parahippocampal gyri (limbic cortex), the hippocampal formation, the amygdala, the septal area, the hypothalamus, and related thalamic and cortical areas.

LIMBIC CORTEX The limbic cortex is composed of two general regions, the cingulate gyrus and the parahippocampal gyrus. The *cingulate gyrus* includes several cortical regions that are heavily interconnected with the association areas of the cerebral cortex. The *parahippocampal gyrus,* located in the medial temporal lobe, contains several distinct cytoarchitectonic regions. One of the most important of those regions is the *entorhinal cortex,* which, as described below, not only funnels highly processed cortical information to the hippocampal formation but is also a major output pathway from the hippocampal formation.

HIPPOCAMPAL FORMATION Three distinct zones—the dentate gyrus, the hippocampus, and the subicular complex—constitute the hippocampal formation, which is located in the floor of the temporal horn of the lateral ventricle (Figure 1.2-7). Those zones are composed of adjacent strips of cortical tissue that run in a rostral-caudal direction but fold over each other mediolaterally in a spiral fashion, giving rise to a C-shaped appearance. The *dentate gyrus* is composed of three layers: an outer, acellular molecular layer, which faces the subarachnoid space of the hippocampal fissure; a middle layer composed of granule cells; and an inner polymorphic layer (Figure 1.2-20). The granule cells extend their dendritic trees into the molecular layer and give rise to axons that form the mossy fiber projection to the hippocampus.

The *hippocampus* is also a trilaminate structure composed of molecular and polymorphic layers and a middle layer that contains pyramidal neurons. On the basis of differences in cytoarchitecture and connectivity, the hippocampus can be divided into three distinct fields, which have been labeled CA3, CA2, and CA1. ("CA" is derived from the term "cornu ammonis," after the Egyptian deity Ammon, who was depicted with a ram's horns, which some early investigators thought described the shape of the hippocampus.) The white matter adjacent to the polymorphic layer of the hippocampus is known as the alveus. The axons in that structure contribute to the fimbria, which at the caudal end of the hippocampus becomes the crus of the *fornix.* Those bilateral structures converge to form the body of the fornix, which travels anteriorly and then turns inferiorly to form the columns of the fornix, which pass through the hypothalamus into the mamillary bodies (Figure 1.2-21). The *subicular complex* is generally considered to have three components—the presubiculum, the parasubiculum, and the subiculum—which together serve as transition regions between the hippocampus and the parahippocampal gyrus.

The components of the hippocampal formation have a distinct pattern of intrinsic connectivity that is largely unidirectional and provides for a specific flow of information (Figure 1.2-22). The major input to the hippocampal formation arises from neurons in layers II and III of the entorhinal cortex that project through the *perforant path* (that is, through the subiculum and the hippocampus) to the outer two thirds of the molecular layer of the dentate gyrus, where they synapse on the dendrites of granule cells. The mossy fiber axons of the granule cells then provide a projection to the pyramidal neurons of the CA3 field of the hippocampus. Axon collaterals from CA3 pyramidal neurons project within CA3 and, through the so-called Schäffer collaterals, to the CA1 field of the hippocampus. That region in turn projects to the subicular complex, which provides output to the entorhinal cortex, completing the circuit.

AMYGDALA Located in the medial temporal lobe just anterior to the hippocampal formation are a group of nuclei referred to as the amyg-

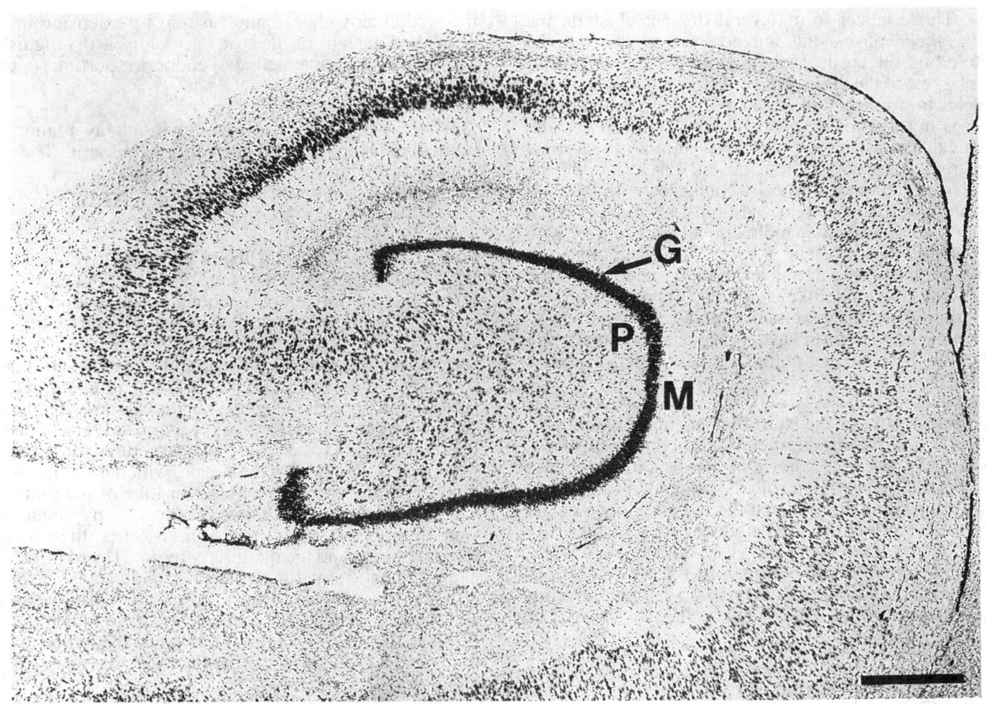

FIGURE 1.2-20 *Nissl-stained coronal section through the dentate gyrus of the human hippocampal formation. Medial is to the left. M, molecular layer; G, granular layer; P, polymorphic layer. Calibration bar equals 1.0 mm. (Courtesy of M Akil and M Brady, University of Pittsburgh.)*

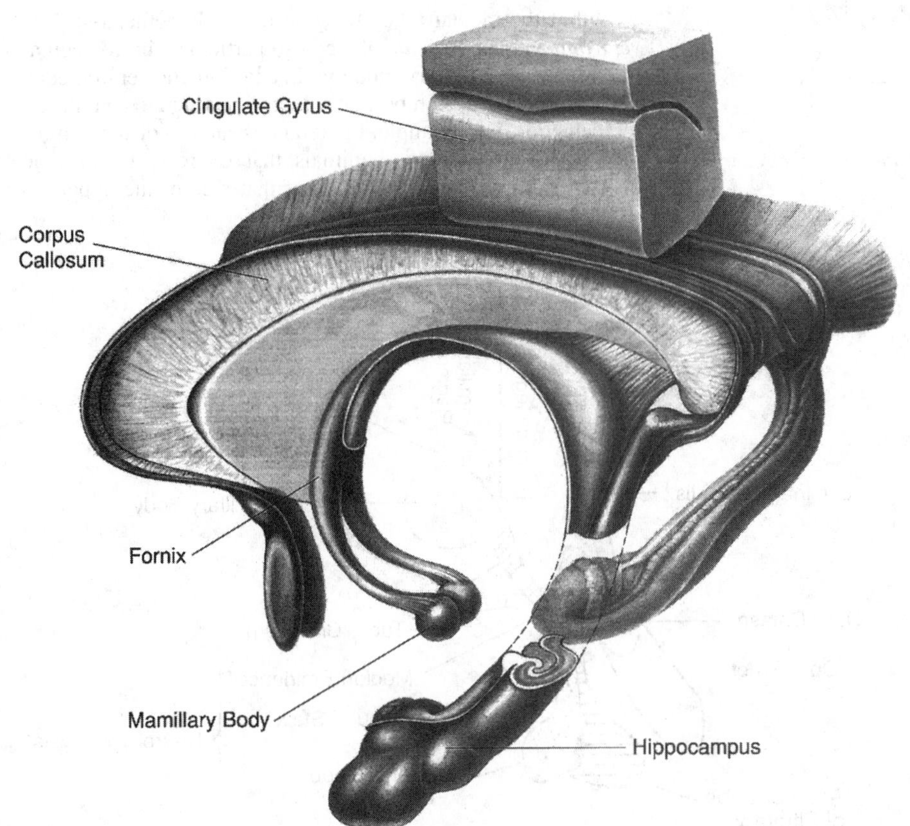

FIGURE 1.2-21 *Drawing of the fornix running between the hippocampal formation and the mamillary bodies. (Adapted from R Nieuwenhuys, J Voogd, C van Huijzen:* The Human Central Nervous System: A Synopsis and Atlas, *ed 3, p 28, Springer, New York, 1988.)*

dala (Figure 1.2-6). Those nuclei form several distinct clusters: the basolateral complex, the centromedial amygdaloid group, and the olfactory group, including the cortical amygdaloid nuclei. The *basolateral complex*, the largest of the three groups, differs from the remaining amygdaloid nuclei in a number of respects. Indeed, although the basolateral complex is not a laminated structure, its connectivity and some other anatomical characteristics are more similar to cortical regions than to the remaining amygdaloid nuclei. For example, the basolateral nuclei are directly and reciprocally connected with the temporal, insular, and prefrontal cortices. In addition, like some cortical regions, the basolateral complex shares bidirectional connections with the medial dorsal thalamic nucleus, and it receives projections from the midline and intralaminar thalamic nuclei. Finally, neurons of the basolateral complex with a pyramidallike morphology appear to furnish projections to the striatum that use excitatory amino acids as neurotransmitters. Thus, on the basis of those anatomical characteristics, one may hypothesize that the basolateral complex actually functions like a multimodal cortical region.

In contrast, the *centromedial amygdala* appears to be part of a larger structure that is continuous through the sublenticular substantia innominata with the bed nucleus of the stria terminalis. That larger structure, which has been termed the *extended amygdala,* consists of two major subdivisions. The central subdivision of the extended amygdala includes the central amygdaloid nucleus and the lateral portion of the bed nucleus of the stria terminalis. That subdivision is reciprocally connected with brainstem viscerosensory and visceromotor regions and with the lateral hypothalamus. In addition, it receives afferents from cortical limbic regions and the basolateral amygdaloid complex. In contrast, the medial subdivision of the extended amygdala, composed of the medial amygdaloid nucleus and its extension into the medial part of the bed nucleus of the stria terminalis, is distinguished by reciprocal connections with the medial or endocrine portions of the hypothalamus.

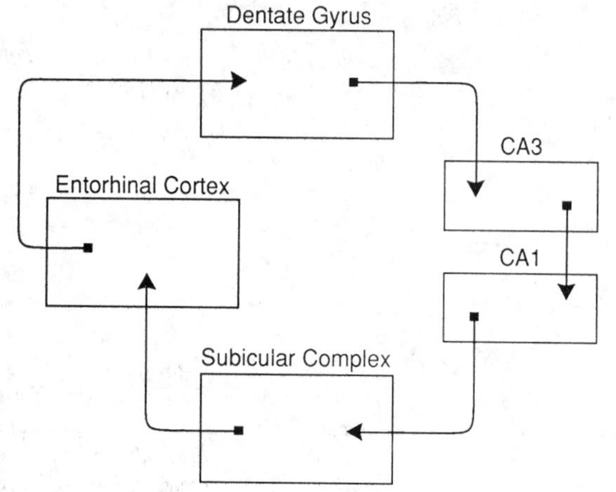

FIGURE 1.2-22 *Schematic drawing of the intrinsic neural circuitry of the hippocampal formation.*

SEPTAL AREA The septal area is a gray matter structure located immediately above the anterior commissure. The septal nuclei are reciprocally connected with the hippocampus, the amygdala, and the hypothalamus and project to a number of structures in the brainstem.

HYPOTHALAMUS The hypothalamus, a relatively small structure within the diencephalon, is a critical component of the neural circuitry regulating not only emotions but also autonomic, endocrine, and some somatic functions. In addition to its relations with other components of the limbic system, it is interconnected with various visceral and somatic nuclei of the brainstem and the spinal cord, and it provides an output that regulates the function of the pituitary gland. On its inferior surface, the hypothalamus is bounded rostrally by the optic chiasm and caudally by the posterior edge of the mamillary bodies. The area of the hypothalamus between those two structures, called the tuber cinereum, gives rise to the median eminence, which is continuous with the infundibular stalk and then the posterior lobe of the pituitary gland (Figure 1.2-23). On the basis of those features, the hypothalamus is subdivided from anterior to posterior into three zones: the supraoptic region, the tuberal region, and the mamillary region. (In addition, the preoptic area, a telencephalic structure located immediately anterior to the supraoptic region, is usually considered part of the hypothalamus.) Those three zones are also divided on each side into medial and lateral areas by the fornix as it travels through the body of the hypothalamus to the mamillary bodies. As shown in Table 1.2-3, the six parts of the hypothalamus contain different nuclei.

Those different nuclei subserve the diverse functions of the hypothalamus. For example, the *suprachiasmatic nucleus* receives both direct and indirect projections from the retina and appears to be important in the regulation of diurnal rhythms. The *supraoptic* and *paraventricular nuclei* contain large cells (magnocellular neurons) that send oxytocin-containing and vasopressin-containing fibers to the posterior neural lobe of the pituitary. In addition, some neurons of the paraventricular nucleus project to the median eminence, where they release neuropeptides, such as corticotropin-releasing factor, into the portal blood system. The neuropeptides then control the synthesis and the release of anterior pituitary hormones. The paraventricular nucleus also gives rise to descending projections that regulate sympathetic and parasympathetic autonomic areas of the medulla and the spinal cord.

Within the medial tuberal region of the hypothalamus, the *ventromedial* and *arcuate nuclei* also participate in the regulation of anterior pituitary function. In addition, the ventromedial nucleus may play an important role in reproductive and ingestive behavior. For example, bilateral destruction of the ventromedial nucleus produces animals that overeat and become obese, leading to the designation of that area of the hypothal-

FIGURE 1.2-23 *Drawing of the divisions of the hypothalamus. (Adapted from J Nolte:* The Human Brain: An Introduction to Its Functional Anatomy, *ed 2, p 250, Mosby, St. Louis, 1988.)*

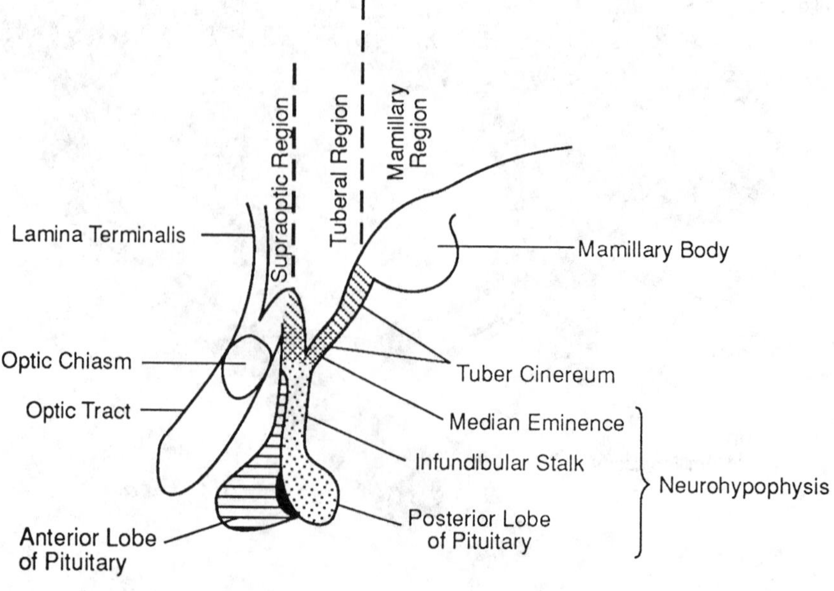

TABLE 1.2-3
Hypothalamic Nuclei

Region	Medial Area	Lateral Area
Supraoptic	Supraoptic nucleus Paraventricular nucleus Anterior nucleus Suprachiasmatic nucleus	Lateral nucleus Part of supraoptic nucleus
Tuberal	Dorsomedial nucleus Ventromedial nucleus Arcuate nucleus	Lateral nucleus Lateral tuberal nuclei
Mamillary	Mamillary body Posterior nucleus	Lateral nucleus

Modified from J Nolte: *The Human Brain: An Introduction to Its Functional Anatomy,* ed 2, p 251. Mosby, St. Louis, 1988.

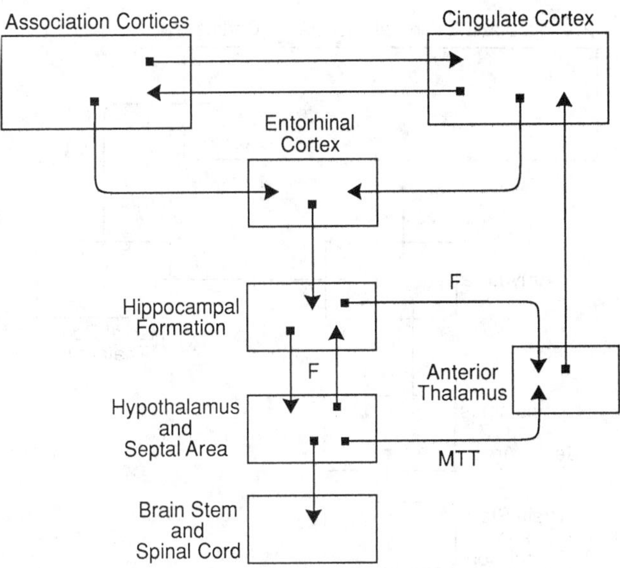

FIGURE 1.2-24 *Functional neural circuitry of the limbic system. This schematic diagram illustrates the manner in which the hippocampal formation and the anterior thalamus provide a mechanism for the integration of information between the cerebral cortex and the hypothalamus. F, fornix; MTT, mamillothalamic tract. (Adapted from J Nolte:* The Human Brain: An Introduction to Its Functional Anatomy, *ed 2, p 374, Mosby, St. Louis, 1988.)*

amus as the "satiety center." In contrast, lesions of the tuberal portion of the lateral hypothalamus result in a marked decrease in eating behavior, hence the designation of that region of the hypothalamus as the "feeding center." Although it is tempting to interpret those observations as meaning that those regions are the principal regulators of the indicated behavior, several caveats must be kept in mind. First, the observed behavioral change after a lesion or a stimulation of a brain region is likely to be the consequence of several different mechanisms. For example, the overeating after a ventromedial lesion may be due to disturbed autonomic regulation of gastric motility, and the observed obesity may be a consequence of metabolic alterations. Second, at least some components of the behavioral pattern resulting from hypothalamic stimulation can also be evoked by stimulating appropriate regions of the brainstem or other parts of the nervous system. Those types of findings reinforce the concept that hypothalamic nuclei are components of a complex neural circuit that, as a whole, is responsible for the observed behavior. As a corollary guideline, stimulation and lesion studies are rarely restricted to a single neuroanatomical structure. For example, manipulations of the lateral hypothalamus are likely to affect not only the lateral hypothalamic nucleus but also the medial forebrain bundle, which traverses that area. Finally, even restricted lesions frequently produce more than one behavioral change. For example, bilateral lesions of the ventromedial nucleus lead not only to overeating and obesity but also to the appearance of a rage response to what would normally be an innocuous stimulus.

The medial posterior section of the hypothalamus contains the *posterior nucleus* and the *mamillary bodies.* Within the mamillary bodies, the lateral and medial mamillary nuclei receive hippocampal input through the fornix and project to the anterior nuclei of the thalamus. The posterior nucleus shares reciprocal connections with the extended amygdala. That nucleus appears to be relatively more developed in primates than in rodents, suggesting that it plays an important but still to be clarified role in the human brain.

The lateral portions of the hypothalamus contain a relatively low density of neurons scattered among longitudinally running fibers of the medial forebrain bundle. That region is interconnected with multiple regions of the forebrain, the brainstem, and the spinal cord.

Functional circuitry The major structures of the limbic system are interconnected with each other and with other components of the nervous system in a variety of ways. However, several major output pathways of the limbic system are clearly defined. In one pathway (Figure 1.2-24) highly processed sensory information from the cingulate, the orbital and temporal cortices, and the amygdala is transmitted to the entorhinal cortex of the parahippocampal gyrus and from there to the hippocampal formation. After traversing the intrinsic circuitry of the hippocampal formation (described above), information is projected through the fornix either to the anterior thalamus, which in turn projects to the limbic cortex, or to the septal area and the hypothalamus. Those latter two regions provide feedback to the hippocampal formation through the fornix. In addition, the mamillary bodies of the hypothalamus project to the anterior thalamus. Finally, the hypothalamus and the septal area project to the brainstem and the spinal cord.

Another major pathway within the limbic system centers on output from the amygdala (Figure 1.2-25). In that pathway highly processed sensory information, primarily from the association regions of the prefrontal and temporal cortices, projects to the amygdala. Output from the amygdala is conducted through two main pathways. The *stria terminalis* accompanies the caudate nucleus in an arch around the temporal lobe and contains axons that project primarily to the septal area and the hypothalamus. The second major output route, the *ventral amygdalofugal pathway,* passes below the lenticular nucleus and contains fibers that terminate in a number of regions, including the septal area, the hypothalamus, and the medial dorsal thalamic nucleus. The medial dorsal nucleus in turn projects heavily to prefrontal and some temporal cortical regions.

Both of those pathways reveal how the limbic system is able to integrate the highly processed sensory and cognitive information content of cerebral cortical circuitry with the hypothalamic pathways that control autonomic and endocrine systems. In addition, the limbic system interacts with components of the basal ganglia system. For example, the ventral amygdalofugal pathway also projects to the nucleus accumbens (ventral striatum), the area where the head of the caudate nucleus fuses with the putamen (Figure 1.2-26). That region sends efferents to the ventral pallidum, an extension of the globus pallidus. That area in turn projects to the medial dorsal thalamic nucleus. The pathway indicates that the functions of the basal ganglia extend beyond the regulation of motor activities and shows the necessity of considering the function or dysfunction of particular brain regions in the context of all aspects of their circuitry.

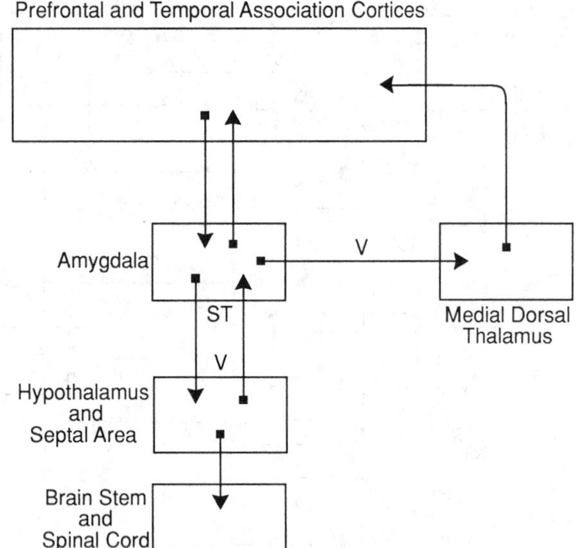

FIGURE 1.2-25 *Functional neural circuitry of the limbic system. This schematic diagram illustrates how the amygdala and the medial dorsal thalamus serve to integrate information processing between prefrontal and temporal association cortices and the hypothalamus. V, ventral amygdalofugal pathway; ST, stria terminalis. (Adapted from J Nolte:* The Human Brain: An Introduction to Its Functional Anatomy, *ed 2, p 375. Mosby, St. Louis, 1988.)*

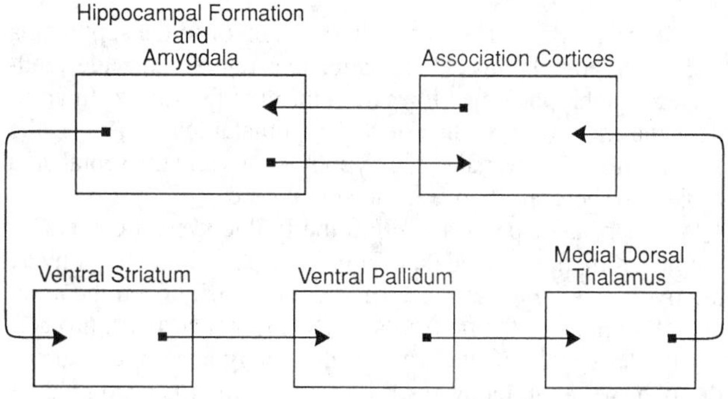

FIGURE 1.2-26 *Functional neural circuitry of the limbic system. This schematic drawing illustrates the interaction between the limbic system and certain components of the basal ganglia. (Adapted from J Nolte:* The Human Brain: An Introduction to Its Functional Anatomy, *ed 2, p 387. Mosby, St. Louis, 1988.)*

IMPLICATIONS

This section illustrates some of the major principles governing the organization of components of the human brain into functional neural systems. Those systems are formed by extensive and highly specific connections among certain anatomical structures, and the activation of those multiple connections gives rise to distinct behaviors, cognitions, and emotional states. Thus, knowledge of the anatomical organization of the functional systems is crucial for the development and testing of hypotheses regarding the biological bases of the signs and the symptoms of neuropsychiatric disorders.

SUGGESTED CROSS-REFERENCES

Section 1.6 discusses intraneural signaling pathways, Section 14.3 discusses brain structure and function in schizophrenia, Section 49.4d discusses central nervous system changes in normal aging, Section 49.5c discusses neuroimaging, and Section 49.6a discusses Alzheimer's disease and other dementing disorders.

REFERENCES

Akil M, Lewis D A: The dopaminergic innervation of monkey entorhinal cortex. Cereb Cortex *3:* 533, 1993.

Alheid G F, Heimer L: New perspectives in basal forebrain organization of special relevance for neuropsychiatric disorders: The striatopallidal, amygdaloid and corticopetal components of substantia innominata. Neuroscience *27:* 1, 1988.

*Alheid G F, Heimer L, Switzer R C: Basal ganglia. In *The Human Nervous System,* G Paxinos, editor, p 483. Academic Press, San Diego, 1990.

*Amaral D G, Insausti R: Hippocampal formation. In *The Human Nervous System,* G Paxinos, editor, p 711. Academic Press, San Diego, 1990.

Barbas H: Organization of cortical afferent input to orbitofrontal areas in the rhesus monkey. Neuroscience *56:* 841, 1993.

Barr M L, Kiernan J A: *The Human Nervous System: An Anatomical Viewpoint,* ed 5. Lippincott, Philadelphia, 1988.

Beall M J, Lewis D A: Heterogeneity of layer II neurons in human neocortex. J Comp Neurol *321:* 241, 1992.

Berman K F, Weinberger D R: The prefrontal cortex in schizophrenia and other neuropsychiatric diseases: In vivo physiological correlates of cognitive deficits. In *Progress in Brain Research,* vol 85, H B M Uylings, C G Van Eden, J P C De Bruin, M A Corner, M G P Feenstra, editors, p 521. Elsevier, Amsterdam, 1990.

Carpenter M B, Sutin, J: *Human Neuroanatomy,* ed 8. Williams & Wilkins, Baltimore, 1983.

Colonnier M: The electron-microscopic analysis of the neuronal organization of the cerebral cortex. In *The Organization of the Cerebral Cortex,* F O Schmitt, F G Worder, G Adelman, S G Dennis, editors, p 125. MIT Press, Cambridge, 1981.

Condé F, Lund J S, Jacobowitz D M, Baimbridge K G, Lewis D A: Local circuit neurons immunoreactive for calretinin, calbindin D-28k or parvalbumin in monkey prefrontal cortex: Distribution and morphology. J Comp Neurol *341:* 95, 1994.

DeFelipe J: Neocortical neuronal diversity: Chemical heterogeneity revealed by colocalization studies of classic neutrotransmitters, neuropeptides, calcium-binding proteins, and cell surface molecules. Cereb Cortex *3:* 273, 1993.

De Olmos J S: Amygdala. In *The Human Nervous System,* G Paxinos, editor, p 583. Academic Press, San Diego, 1990.

*Fellman D J, Van Essen D C: Distributed hierarchical processing in the primate cerebral cortex. Cereb Cortex *1:* 1, 1991.

Fuster J M: *The Prefrontal Cortex: Anatomy, Physiology and Neuropsychology of the Frontal Lobe,* ed 2. Raven Press, New York, 1989.

Gaspar P, Duyckaerts C, Alvarez C, Javoy-Agid F, Berger B: Alterations of dopaminergic and noradrenergic innervations in motor cortex in Parkinson's disease. Ann Neurol *30:* 365, 1991.

Goldman-Rakic P S: Cellular and circuit basis of working memory in prefrontal cortex of nonhuman primates. In *Progress in Brain Research,* vol 85, H B M Uylings, C G Van Eden, J P C De Bruin, M A Corner, M G P Feenstra, editors, p 325. Elsevier, Amsterdam, 1990.

*Goldman-Rakic P S: Circuitry of primate prefrontal cortex and regulation of behavior by representational memory. In *Handbook of Physiology: The Nervous System,* vol 5, J M Brookhart, V M Mountcastle, editors, p 373. American Physiological Society, Baltimore, 1987.

Graybiel A M: Neurotransmitters and neuromodulators in the basal ganglia. Trends Neurosci *13:* 244, 1990.

Groenewegen H J, Berendse H W: The specificity of the ''nonspecific'' midline and intralaminar thalamic nuclei. Trends Neurosci *17:* 52, 1994.

Hayes T L, Lewis D A: Hemispheric differences in layer III pyramidal neurons of the anterior language areas. Arch Neurol *50:* 501, 1993.

Jones E G: *The Thalamus.* Plenum, New York, 1985.

Jones E G, Powell T P S: An anatomical study of converging sensory pathways within the cerebral cortex of the monkey. Brain *93:* 39, 1970.

Kaas J H: Somatosensory system. In *The Human Nervous System,* G Paxinos, editor, p 813. Academic Press, San Diego, 1990.

Kandel E R, Schwartz J H, Jessell T M, editors: *Principles of Neural Science,* ed 3. Elsevier, New York, 1991.

Lopes da Silva F H, Witter M P, Boeijinga P H, Lohman A H M: Anatomic organization and physiology of the limbic cortex. Physiol Rev *70:* 2, 1990.

Nieuwenhuys R, Voogd J, van Huijzen C: *The Human Central Nervous System: A Synopsis and Atlas,* ed 3. Springer, New York, 1988.
Nolte J: *The Human Brain: An Introduction to Its Functional Anatomy,* ed 2. Mosby, St. Louis, 1988.
Pandya D N, Yeterian E H: Architecture and connections of cortical association areas. In *Cerebral Cortex,* vol 4, A Peters, E G Jones, editors, p 3. Plenum, London, 1985.
Papez J W: A proposed mechanism of emotion. Arch Neurol Psychiatry *38:* 725, 1937.
Rakic P: Specification of cerebral cortical areas. Science *241:* 170, 1988.
Russchen F T, Amaral D G, Proce J L: The afferent input to the magnocellular division of the mediodorsal thalamic nucleus in the monkey, *Macaca fascicularis.* J Comp Neurol *256:* 175, 1987.
*Saper C B: Hypothalamus. In *The Human Nervous System,* G Paxinos, editor, p 389. Academic Press, San Diego, 1990.
Webster K W: The functional anatomy of the basal ganglia. In *Parkinson's Disease,* G M Stern, editor, p 3. Johns Hopkins University Press, Baltimore, 1990.
Witter M P, Organization of the entorhinal-hippocampal system: A review of current anatomical data. Hippocampus *3:* 33, 1993.
Zeki S: *A Vision of the Brain.* Blackwell Scientific, Oxford, 1993.

1.3 MONOAMINE NEUROTRANSMITTERS

JAY M. BARABAN, M.D., Ph.D.
JOSEPH T. COYLE, M.D.

INTRODUCTION

Classic studies of the monoamine neurotransmitters identified those systems as the primary sites of action of antidepressant and antipsychotic agents. Accordingly, the systems have, for decades, dominated the biological theories of several major psychiatric disorders. In recent years, rapid progress has been made in defining at a molecular level the key components of the systems. For example, several monoamine uptake transporters thought to be the sites of action of antidepressants and psychostimulants have been cloned. Furthermore, the application of molecular biological approaches to monoamine receptors has unearthed an unexpected diversity of receptor subtypes. The likelihood that the new insights will stimulate the development of improved drug treatments and will facilitate investigations into the genetic basis of psychiatric disorders has injected renewed excitement into this field of research.

NEUROTRANSMITTER LIFE CYCLE

For monoamine neurotransmitters, synthesis proceeds by sequential enzymatic modification of simple, abundant precursor molecules, such as choline, tyrosine, and tryptophan. The completed neurotransmitters are stored within vesicles in the nerve terminal, are released into the synaptic cleft, and act on receptors located postsynaptically to transfer information across the synapse. In many cases they also interact with receptors located presynaptically on the nerve terminal to regulate the release process. Inactivation of monoamine neurotransmitters primarily involves a reuptake process that recycles the neurotransmitter or, in the case of acetylcholine, its immediate precursor.

CATECHOLAMINES The synthetic and degradative pathways for catecholamines are among the best understood of all neurotransmitters. The catecholamines include dopamine, norepinephrine, and epinephrine; dopamine and norepinephrine serve as precursors or as neurotransmitters in their own right, depending on the neuronal system. The catecholamine biosynthetic pathway is a tightly regulated sequence of enzymatic steps that ensures that a stable amount of neurotransmitter is available at the nerve terminal for release, regardless of varying activity levels of the neurons. Catecholamine synthesis is controlled within the nerve terminal, where the requisite enzymes are concentrated.

The initial and rate-limiting step in the synthesis pathway is tyrosine hydroxylase (Figure 1.3-1). Compared with the subsequent steps, the enzyme exhibits a relatively low velocity and is virtually saturated by its precursor, the nonessential amino acid L-tyrosine. Tyrosine hydroxylase converts tyrosine to the catechol dihydroxy-L-phenylalanine, L-dopa (levodopa [Larodopa]). That product is rapidly converted to dopamine by aromatic amino acid decarboxylase in the cytoplasm of catecholaminergic nerve terminals. The velocity of catecholamine synthesis is rigidly regulated at the tyrosine hydroxylase step. That enzyme is subject to end product inhibition; therefore, when catecholamines exceed the storage capacity of the vesicles within the nerve terminal, the excess free catecholamines inhibit the activity of tyrosine hydroxylase and thus prevent further synthesis. When catecholamine release is triggered by neuronal firing, that inhibition is removed. However, other factors come into play with increased demands for catecholamine release. Increases in the intracellular concentration of calcium, resulting from repeated nerve terminal depolarization, elicit the phosphorylation of tyrosine hydroxylase and increase the velocity of the enzyme. During periods of sustained increases in catecholaminergic neuronal activity, additional enzymes in the synthetic pathway are synthesized in the neuronal cell body and transported down to the terminal.

In the dopaminergic neurons, the final step in the synthesis pathway is the decarboxylation of L-dopa to dopamine. Noradrenergic neurons contain an additional enzyme located in the storage vesicle, dopamine-β-hydroxylase, which converts dopamine to norepinephrine. In the adrenal medulla and certain neuronal groups in the brain, an additional enzyme, phenylethanolamine-N-methyltransferase, catalyzes the conversion of norepinephrine to epinephrine. The amount of the enzyme in adrenal medullary cells is regulated by corticosteroids.

The primary mechanism for inactivation of synaptically released norepinephrine and dopamine is through the reuptake by a transport process concentrated on the nerve terminals. The transport is driven by the gradient of sodium ions across the neuronal membrane (high outside, low inside). The uptake systems for dopamine and norepinephrine have different pharmacological characteristics, with selective inhibitors available for each system, such as desipramine for norepinephrine uptake. In recent studies, distinct norepinephrine and dopamine uptake transporters have been cloned. Those transmembrane proteins share considerable homology with each other and with transporters for noncatecholamine transmitters, such as γ-aminobutyric acid (GABA) and serotonin. Anatomical localization of those transporter complementary deoxyrubonucleic acids (cDNAs) by in situ hybridization has provided graphic demonstration of the restricted expression of those genes to specific monoamine neurons. For example, norepinephrine neurons in the locus ceruleus only express the norepinephrine transporter. As those transporters are the primary sites of action of antidepressants and many stimulant drugs, such as cocaine, detailed knowledge of their molecular structure will probably facilitate studies of the regulation of those critical components of monoamine synaptic transmission. Furthermore, the possibility that genetic components of mood disorders or drug abuse are related to alterations in the coding or regulatory regions of transporter genes can now be investigated.

The catecholamines can also be enzymatically inactivated (Figure 1.3-2). Monoamine oxidase—an enzyme localized to the external membrane of the mitochondria, the power packs of the cells—plays a major role in catabolizing catecholamines that are free in the nerve terminal cytosol and unprotected by the storage vesicles. Catecholamines synthesized within the nerve terminal are sequestered in vesicles by an energy-dependent pump, thereby protecting them from catabolism by monoamine oxidase (MAO). Reserpine (Serpasil), an antihypertensive, inhibits the vesicular amine pump, causing the released catecholamines to be deaminated by MAO. Situated on the outer membranes of many different cell types is catechol-*O*-methyltransferase, which inactivates catecholamines that have diffused beyond the synaptic cleft by *O*-methylating one of the hydroxyl moieties. Unlike the catecholamine-synthesizing enzymes, which are restricted to catecholaminergic neurons, the catabolizing enzymes have a broad distribution in cells throughout the body. In fact, they serve a protective function because of their high activity in the gut and the liver by inactivating catecholamines and indirectly acting on sympathomimetics, such as tyramine and phenethylamine, that are contained within the diet. For patients treated with MAO inhibitors, that enzymatic barrier is inactivated. As a consequence, when those patients ingest food containing large amounts of tyramine, such as aged cheeses and meats, the tyramine has direct access to the general circulation, which releases norepinephrine from the sympathetic terminals, causing acute hypertension.

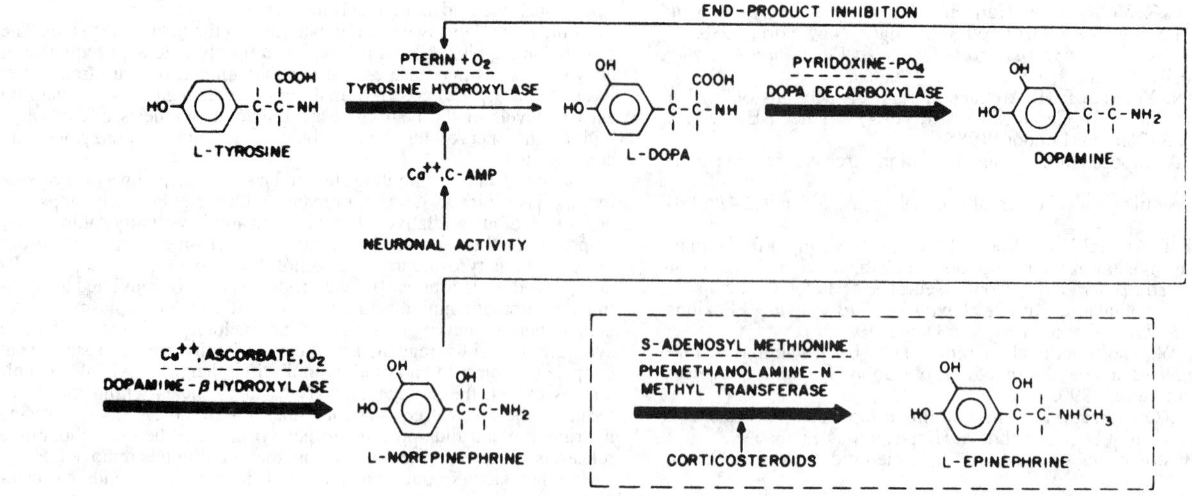

FIGURE 1.3-1 *Biosynthetic pathway for catecholamines.*

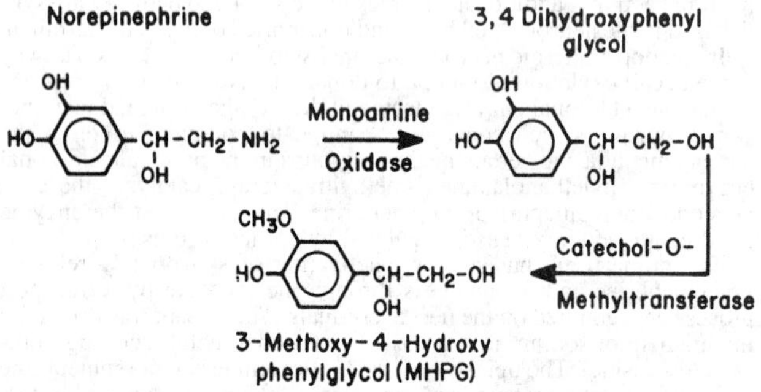

FIGURE 1.3-2 *Catabolism of norepinephrine.*

The ability of several psychostimulant drugs, such as amphetamine, to produce the release of vesicular catecholamines is thought to play a major role in their actions. Unlike tyramine, amphetamine, which is methylated on the carbon side chain, is resistant to degradation by MAO. Recent studies suggest that the releasing agents do not act through specific receptors. Instead, their ability to act as weak bases underlies their releasing properties. Intravesicular pH is typically acidic, a feature that is important for maintaining the catecholamine in a protonated form that cannot diffuse out of the vesicles. The accumulation of those weak base compounds in vesicles reduces the pH gradient and increases the efflux of those transmitters out of the vesicle into the cytoplasm of the nerve terminal. The weak base property of psychostimulants, which has been exploited clinically to hasten their excretion by urine acidification, appears to underlie their psychotropic effects.

SEROTONIN Serotonin (also called 5-hydroxytryptamine [5-HT]) is synthesized from the essential amino acid tryptophan, with tryptophan hydroxylase serving as the initial and rate-limiting step in the synthesis pathway (Figure 1.3-3). In contrast to L-tyrosine, the ambient levels of tryptophan are not saturating with regard to tryptophan hydroxylase. Thus, fluctuations in tryptophan levels in the blood and, therefore, in the brain can affect the amount of serotonin synthesized by serotonergic neurons. The ingestion of foods rich in tryptophan rapidly increases brain serotonin synthesis, which accounts for their mild sedating effects. After the hydroxylation of tryptophan, it is rapidly converted to serotonin by decarboxylation through aromatic amino acid decarboxylase. As with catecholaminergic neurons, the primary means to inactivate serotonin released into the synaptic cleft is through a high-affinity uptake process on serotonergic nerve terminals. That transport process is potently inhibited by tertiary tricyclic antidepressants, such as imipramine (Tofranil), and certain atypical antidepresdsants, such as fluoxetine (Prozac). As mentioned above, the cloning of the serotonin transporter has established that it is homologous to the catecholamine transporters. Those advances at the molecular level have also confirmed the selective expression of the transporter in 5-HT neurons and the marked selectivity of fluoxetine and its homologues, such as paroxetine, for the blockade of uptake at that site. Intracellular serotonin not protected by vesicular storage is catabolized by monoamine oxidase. Subtypes of MAO have been identified, with MAO_A acting primarily on serotonin and norepinephrine and MAO_B catabolizing primarily phenethylamines, including dopamine.

HISTAMINE The immunohistochemical visualization of histamine neurons in the brain has provided long-awaited confirmation of histamine's role as a neurotransmitter. The synthesis of histamine parallels that of other monoamines, inasmuch as it is produced from an amino acid precursor, histidine, by the enzyme histidine decarboxylase. As that enzyme is not saturated by circulating levels of histidine, the administration of histidine increases brain histamine levels. In neurons, histamine metabolism proceeds by methylation to form methylhistamine, which is further degraded by MAO.

ACETYLCHOLINE The life cycle of acetylcholine varies somewhat from the above-described scheme. The synthesis of acetylcholine is catalyzed by the enzyme choline acetyltransferase, which transfers an acetyl group from acetyl coenzyme A (CoA) to choline. Acetylcholine released into the synaptic cleft is rapidly catabolized by acetylcholinesterase, which is found in high concentrations on the external surfaces of cholinergic neurons, particularly in their synaptic cleft, and on the surfaces of many other cell types. That broad distribution of acetylcholinesterase keeps acetylcholine from diffusing from the synaptic cleft and activating, in an inappropriate fashion, distant cholinergic receptors. Cholinergic neurons possess a sodium-dependent high-affinity uptake process for choline, so the choline liberated by the breakdown of acetylcholine in the synaptic cleft is efficiently reused for acetylcholine synthesis. In fact, the high-affinity transport process for choline appears to be the rate-limiting step controlling acetylcholine synthesis. The velocity of the transport process is dynamically regulated on the basis of the antecedent activity of the cholinergic neurons. Thus, when cholinergic neurons are active in releasing acetylcholine, the velocity of the transport process increases to enhance the intracellular availability of choline.

MONOAMINE PATHWAYS

Anatomical studies of the monoamine pathways have identified several common features of their organization. Each of the systems originates in compact nuclei in the brainstem or the basal forebrain and send extensive projections throughout the brain. Those features have fostered the analogy to peripheral autonomic systems, suggesting that the monoamine systems act in a pervasive manner to set the tone of signal processing in target areas. However, the innervation pattern, although extensive, is not organized in a nonspecific manner. Each of the systems projects in a precise way to specific nuclei and to specific layers of the cerebral cortex. In addition, the distribution of specific receptor subtypes is also markedly heterogeneous, allowing the systems to elicit distinct effects in different regions or even on different cell types within the same area.

NOREPINEPHRINE The locus ceruleus is a tightly packed cluster of noradrenergic neurons located in the dorsal pons, which is the origin of the major norepinephrine innervation to the forebrain (Figure 1.3-4). Other norepinephrine neurons are distributed in the ventral brainstem and contribute a prominent innervation to the hypothalamus. The compact clustering of locus ceruleus neurons has facilitated the electrophysiological analysis of their activity, which has shown that the neurons are remarkably sensitive to a wide range of sensory stimuli. Those findings suggest that norepinephrine fibers that originate from the compact cluster to innervate essentially the entire central nervous system can broadcast information regarding a broad spectrum of incoming sensory stimulation.

SEROTONIN Serotonergic neurons are principally located in several clusters along the midline or the raphe of the brainstem (Figure 1.3-5). The dorsal raphe is located in the midbrain central gray matter on the midline just below the sylvian aqueduct; the nearby median raphe is situated more ventrally on the midline. Although those nuclei are adjacent, their projection patterns are clearly distinct, providing an illustration of the specifc

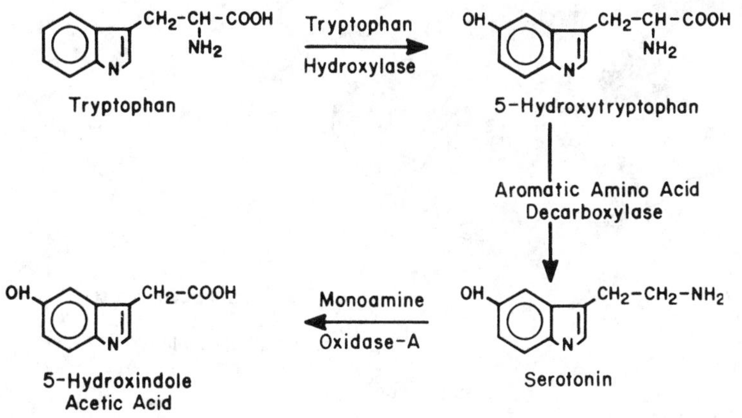

Tryptophan (CH_2-CH(NH_2)-COOH) —Tryptophan Hydroxylase→ 5-Hydroxytryptophan (OH; CH_2-CH(NH_2)-COOH)

5-Hydroxytryptophan —Aromatic Amino Acid Decarboxylase→ Serotonin (OH; CH_2-CH_2-NH_2)

Serotonin —Monoamine Oxidase-A→ 5-Hydroxindole Acetic Acid (OH; CH_2-COOH)

FIGURE 1.3-3 *Biosynthetic and catabolic pathway for serotonin.*

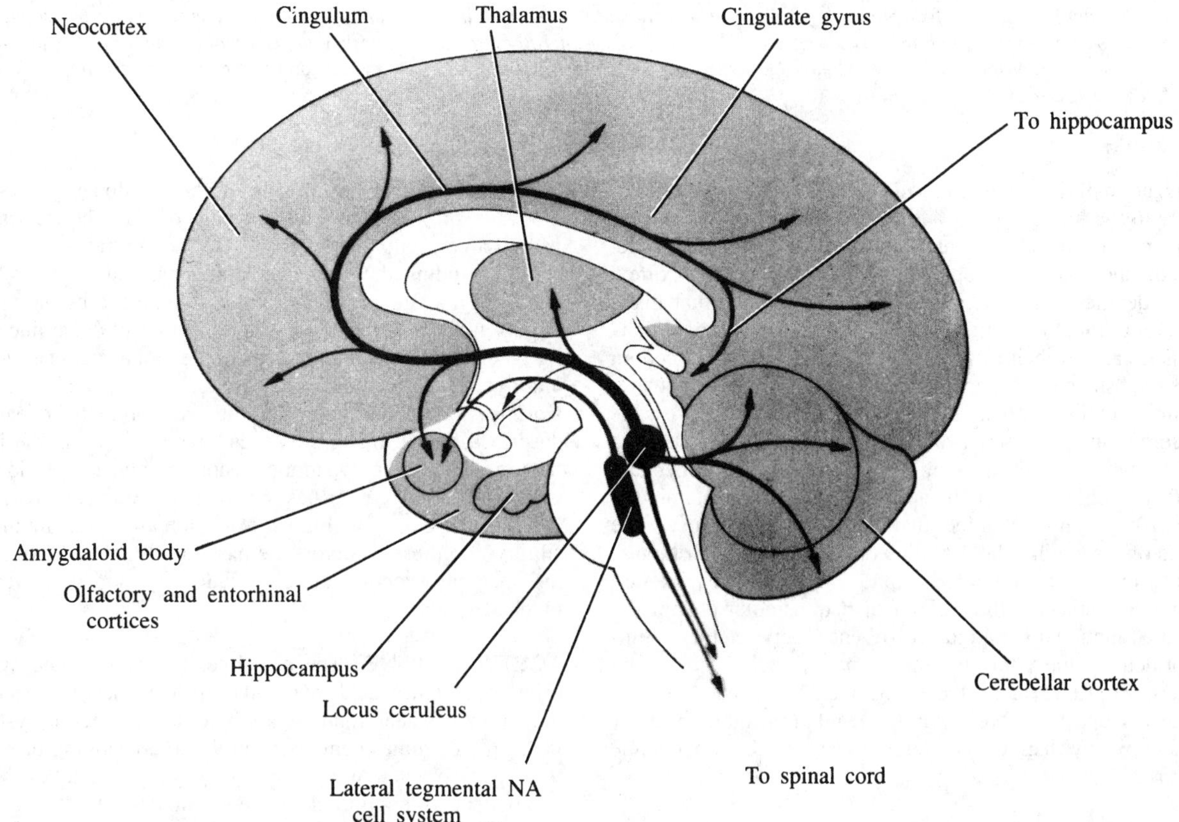

FIGURE 1.3-4 *Noradrenergic pathways. Locus ceruleus, which is located immediately underneath the floor of the fourth ventricle in the rostrolateral part of the pons, is the most important noradrenergic nucleus in the brain. Its projections reach many areas in the forebrain, the cerebellum, and the spinal cord. Noradrenergic neurons in the lateral brainstem tegmentum innervate several structures in the basal forebrain, including the hypothalamus and the amygdaloid body. (From L Heimer:* The Human Brain and Spinal Cord. *Springer, New York, 1983. Used with permission.)*

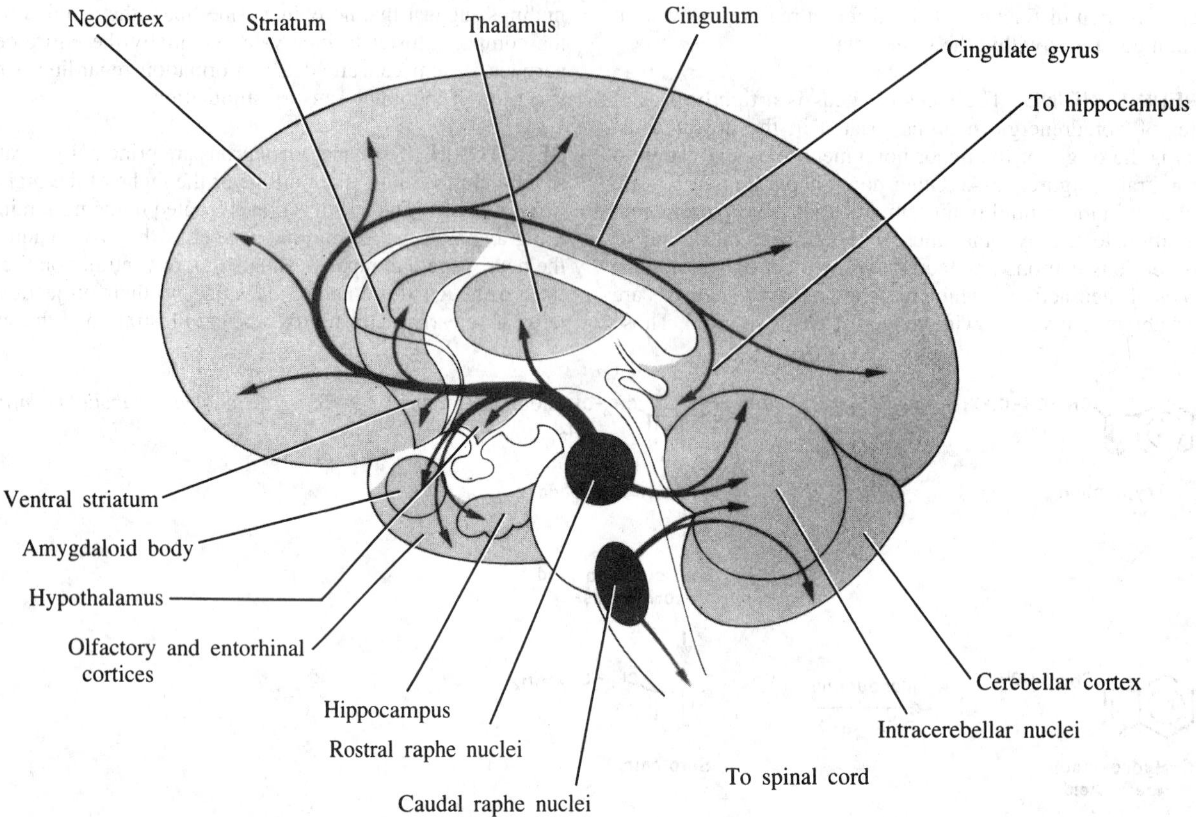

FIGURE 1.3-5 *Serotonergic pathways. The raphe nuclei form a more or less continuous collection of cell groups close to the midline throughout the brainstem, but for the sake of simplicity they have been subdivided into a rostral and a caudal group in the drawing. The rostral raphe nuclei project to a large number of forebrain structures. The fibers that project laterally through the internal and external capsules to widespread areas of the neocortex are not indicated in this highly schematic drawing. (From L Heimer:* The Human Brain and Spinal Cord. *Springer, New York, 1983. Used with permission.)*

organization of the system. The median raphe projects predominantly to the hippocampus, and the dorsal raphe projects predominantly to the striatum and the hypothalamus; both nuclei have distinct but overlapping projections to the neocortex. Recent detailed anatomical studies have suggested that fibers originating from those nuclei differ in their morphological characteristics and in their sensitivity to the toxic effects of certain abused substances. In particular, 3,4-methylenedioxymethamphetamine (MDMA) (ecstasy) appears to selectively affect the fine serotonin fibers emanating largely from the dorsal raphe neurons, whereas the thicker median raphe serotonin fibers are resistant. Similar distinctions apply to *p*-chloramphetamine, a derivative of amphetamine that preferentially induces the release of serotonin. Those findings indicate that, even though neurons located in the median raphe and the dorsal raphe are classified together on the basis of their transmitter phenotype, there are functionally important differences between them. Similar principles apply to other monoamine systems, as they do not appear to function in a monolithic fashion. Instead, growing evidence supports differences in the regulation and the activity of anatomically distinct subgroups in each of the monoamine systems.

DOPAMINE Dopamine projections stem largely from two clusters of dopamine neurons located in portions of the ventral midbrain referred to as the substantia nigra and the ventral tegmental area (Figure 1.3-6). The nigral dopamine neurons project mainly to the striatum and have, therefore, been implicated in the well-known motor side effects of dopamine receptor blockade produced by antipsychotic drugs. The ventral tegmental area group project largely to the ventral or limbic striatum, including the nucleus accumbens, and to other limbic areas, such as the prefrontal cortex, thought to be the primary targets underlying the antipsychotic actions of dopamine receptor blockade. Dopamine neurons in the arcuate and periventricular hypothalamic nuclei project to the pituitary and are responsible for the dopaminergic inhibition of prolactin release. As described below, major advances have occurred in the identification of multiple dopamine receptor subtypes. The localization of those receptors has shown preferential expression of certain subtypes in the limbic projection areas, raising the possibility that those receptors are particularly relevant to mediating the antipsychotic effects elicited by dopamine receptor blockade.

ACETYLCHOLINE The principle that monoamine systems originate in subcortical areas and project extensively throughout the cortex has been found to apply to the cholinergic system as well. Initial studies demonstrated that the lesioning of subcortical areas or their projection pathways depleted several key components of cholinergic nerve terminals—that is, acetylcholine, its synthetic enzyme choline acetyltransferase, and high-affinity choline uptake. The development of immunohistochemical techniques to visualize cholinergic neurons led to the identification of the source of the cholinergic innervations to the cortex as a cluster of neurons in the ventral forebrain, referred

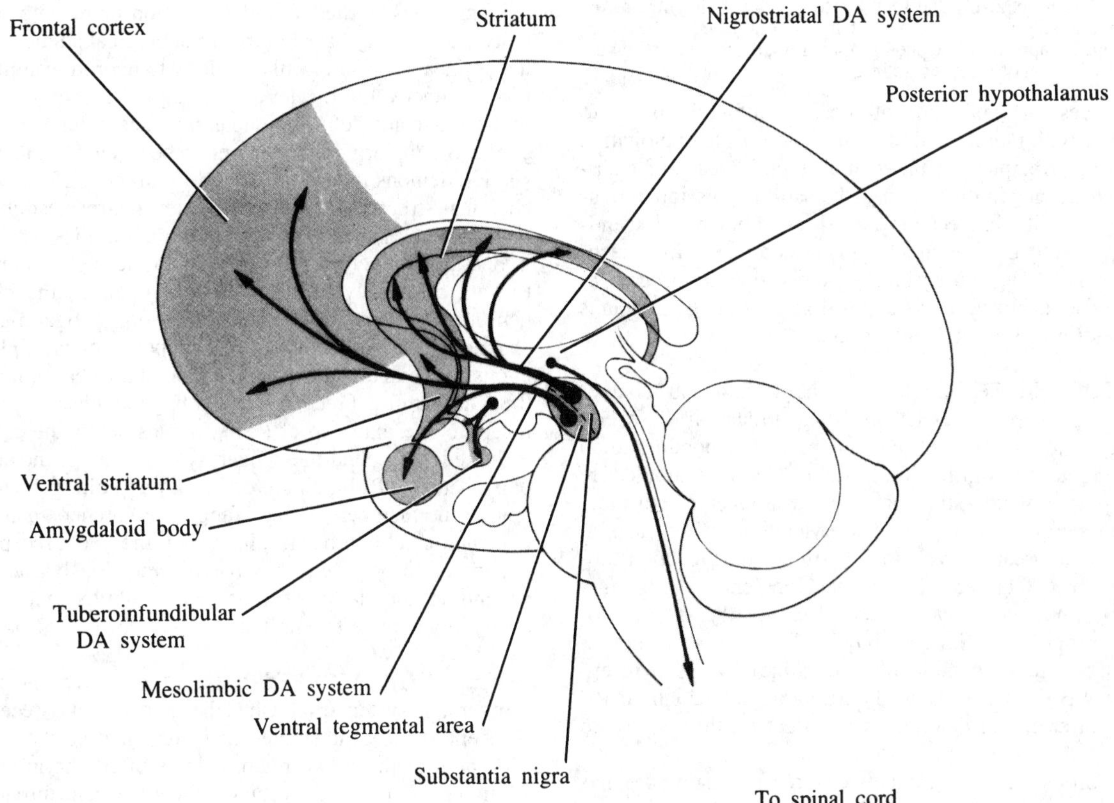

FIGURE 1.3-6 *Dopaminergic pathways. The nigrostriatal dopamine system originates in the substantia nigra and terminates in the main dorsal part of the striatum. The ventral tegmental areas gives rise to the mesolimbic dopamine system, which terminates in the ventral striatum, the amygdaloid body, the frontal lobe, and some other basal forebrain areas. The tuberoinfundibular system innervates the median eminence and the posterior and intermediate lobes of the pituitary; dopamine neurons in the posterior hypothalamus project to the spinal cord. (From L Heimer:* The Human Brain and Spinal Cord. *Springer, New York, 1983. Used with permission.)*

to as the nucleus basalis of Meynert. Additional clusters of cholinergic cells are present in the brainstem and account for thalamic cholinergic innervation. In contrast to the monoamine systems described above, which are composed primarily of neurons that send out long projections, the cholinergic system also contains a major group of interneurons found in the striatum, an area that is highly enriched in muscarinic cholinergic receptors. Those local interneurons play a major role in modulating striatal function and are presumably the site of action of anticholinergic agents used widely to treat the parkinsonianlike side effects of antipsychotics.

RECEPTORS

Neurotransmitter receptors are proteins located on the external surface of the neuronal membrane that detect neurotransmitters in the vicinity of the neuron and initiate a response to it. Binding of the neurotransmitter to the receptor triggers a cascade of events affecting neuronal activity. Inasmuch as the recognition site of the receptor is the focal point of neurotransmitter action, that aspect of receptor function has received a great deal of attention. The classic pharmacological approach to characterizing those sites entails evaluating the ability of compounds structurally related to the endogenous neurotransmitter to elicit or block a response. In that manner, receptor agonists and antagonists can be identified and their potencies evaluated.

The development of radioligand-binding techniques for neurotransmitter receptors has greatly facilitated the pharmacological characterization of receptor recognition sites. With that approach, the binding of drugs and neurotransmitter analogs to the recognition site is monitored directly by measuring their ability to compete with a radioactive compound or ligand for the receptor-binding site and thereby reduce the amount of the radioligand bound. The higher the affinity that a compound possesses for the recognition site, the lower the concentration required to inhibit receptor binding of the radioactive ligand. Two parameters widely used to characterize drug interaction with receptors are the K_d and B_{max}. K_d is defined as the concentration of drug needed to occupy half of the receptors. For example, haloperidol (Haldol), a high-potency antipsychotic, has a lower K_d and, therefore, a higher affinity for the D_2 dopamine receptor than does chlorpromazine (Thorazine), a low-potency antipsychotic. Estimates of receptor density in a tissue sample, often abbreviated as B_{max}, can also be obtained with radioligand-binding techniques by extrapolating the maximal number of sites available with increasing concentrations of radioligand.

The basic concepts of receptor-ligand interactions have been developed by studying brain homogenates incubated in physiological buffers in the presence of the radioactive ligand. However, the binding of radioactive ligands to receptors can also be studied in tissue slices or brain sections. A thin brain section affixed to a microscopic slide can be incubated in a physiological buffer containing the radioactive ligand, which binds to the appropriate receptors. The excess radioligand is then washed away by incubation in fresh buffer, leaving the specifically bound ligand attached to the receptors. In that way the distribution of radiolabeled receptors can be visualized at a microscopic level in the brain sections by exposing the sections to photographic film; at the precise cellular sites where a radioactive ligand is attached to the receptor, silver grains appear on the photographic film, thereby revealing the cellular distribution of receptors in brain tissue sections (Figure 1.3-7).

The successful application of receptor autoradiography to brain tissue with radioligands set the stage for the exploitation of the same principles for the visualization of receptor distribution in the living human brain with positron emission tomography (PET). With that technique, positron radiolabeled ligands are injected into the patient. By using computer-based techniques for resolving the radioactive emissions in space, relatively precise localization of the positron-emitting radioligands can be determined in the human brain.

RECEPTOR HETEROGENEITY Pharmacological characterization of receptors has led to the identification of several distinct receptors capable of recognizing and responding to an individual neurotransmitter (Table 1.3-1). Classic examples are norepinephrine, which stimulates both α-adrenergic receptors and β-adrenergic receptors, and acetylcholine, which acts at nicotinic and muscarinic receptors. Distinguishing receptor subtypes has been facilitated by the development of drugs that selectively antagonize one subtype and not the others. For example, propranolol (Inderal) blocks β-receptors but not α-receptors, whereas phentolamine (Regitine) blocks α-receptors but not β-receptors. Thus, the receptor subtype stimulated by a neurotransmitter determines its effect on the innervated neuron.

The ability to distinguish between receptor subtypes has refined the understanding of drug actions. For example, although it is well-known that antipsychotic drugs block the actions of dopamine, it has become clear that, of the two pharmacologically identified dopamine receptor subtypes, D_1 and D_2, the affinities of the antipsychotic drugs for the D_2 and not the D_1 subtype correlate closely with their clinical antipsychotic potency. Recent research on hallucinogens suggests that agonist activity at one of the receptors for serotonin, the 5-HT_2 receptor, accounts for the hallucinogenic activity of lysergic acid diethylamide (LSD) and mescalinelike drugs. Thus, with better definition of receptor subtypes, major advances are being made in the identification of the sites of psychotropic drug action. The availability of selective drugs also makes it possible to assess the involvement of particular receptor subtypes in the pathophysiology of psychiatric disorders.

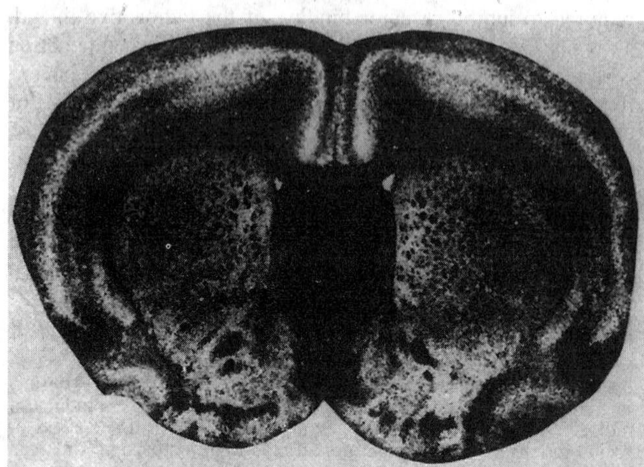

FIGURE 1.3-7 *Autoradiogram of 5-HT_2 receptor subtype, demonstrating heterogeneous distribution of the receptors thought to be the site of action of hallucinogens. (Photograph courtesy of M Blue.)*

In previous studies, the identification of receptor heterogeneity was entirely based on pharmacological studies; however, the application of molecular biology to neurotransmitter receptors has uncovered further complexity. In recent years, several of the classically defined monoamine transmitter receptors, such as the β-adrenergic receptor, have been cloned. Those initial studies demonstrated that, despite marked differences in the chemical structure of the transmittter, neurotransmitter receptors can be classified into two large superfamilies. The receptors in one group, exemplified by the nicotinic acetylcholine receptor, are essentially ion channels that open on the binding of neurotransmitters—thus, the designation "ligand-gated ion channels." Those receptors are composed of multiple homologous subunits that are arranged around the central ion pore. In the other family of receptors, including the muscarinic receptor, receptors are made up of a single transmembrane protein that is linked to second-messenger systems by guanosine 5′-triphosphate (GTP)-binding proteins. By exploiting the homology among the members of each family, researchers, using molecular biological approaches, have identified new receptors. The pursuit of that strategy has been tremendously successful in expanding knowledge of the receptor subtypes used by many of the monoamine transmitters.

ADRENERGIC RECEPTORS Early studies of the peripheral sympathetic system established the existence of α-receptors and β-receptors. Recent studies have revealed further important subtyping of those two major classes of adrenergic receptors. With regard to the β_1-receptor, the type concentrated in the heart, norepinephrine and epinephrine serve as agonists. The β_2-receptor exhibits greater sensitivity to epinephrine than to norepinephrine and to *N*-alkyl-substituted catecholamines, such as isoproterenol. In the brain, β_1-receptors appear to have a high degree of localization to neurons, whereas β_2-receptors are more concentrated on glia and blood vessels. Specific agonists and antagonists for the β-receptor subtypes are presently available. As mentioned above, the β-adrenergic receptors are linked to the GTP-binding protein, G_s, which stimulates adenylate cyclase, producing a cascade of cell-specific responses caused by the elevation of intracellular cyclic adenosine monophosphate (AMP).

The α-receptors have also been classified into two pharmacologically and physiologically distinct subtypes. The α_1-receptor, the receptor traditionally linked to smooth-muscle contraction and glandular secretion in the periphery, exerts its intracellular effects through a second-messenger system, the phosphoinositide system. The antihypertensive prazosin (Minipres) is a potent and specific inhibitor of the α_1-receptor. When activated, α_2-receptors are associated with a decrease in peripheral and central noradrenergic activity. In part, that decrease reflects the fact that α_2-receptors are coupled to a GTP-binding protein, G_i, that inhibits adenylate cyclase. In addition, presynaptic α_2-receptors on noradrenergic terminals inhibit the release of norepinephrine. The α_2-receptors have attracted considerable interest because clonidine (Catapres), a potent antihypertensive, has also been found to reduce the physiological symptoms of the withdrawal syndrome in persons addicted to opiates and nicotine.

DOPAMINERGIC RECEPTORS Classic pharmacological studies of dopamine receptors identified two distinct subtypes. The D_1 receptor exerts its physiological effects through the activation of adenylate cyclase by G_s. Although the transduction process mediating the effects of the dopamine D_2 receptor remains unclear, that receptor appears to be negatively coupled

TABLE 1.3-1
Classification of Monoamine Receptor Subtypes

Transmitters	Subtypes	Effectors	Comments
Dopamine	D_1	↑ cAMP	Stimulates transcription factor expression
	D_2	↓ cAMP	Site of action of typical antipsychotics
		↑ K^+ channels	
	D_3	? ↓ cAMP	Expressed in limbic system
	D_4	? ↓ cAMP	High affinity for clozapine
	D_5	↑ cAMP	Closely related to D_1
Norepinephrine	$\alpha_{1a,b,c}$	↑ PI	Antagonists lower blood pressure
	$\alpha_{2a,b,c}$	↓ cAMP	Decreases noradrenaline release
		↑ K^+ channels	
	$\beta_{1,2,3}$	↑ cAMP	
Histamine	H_1	↑ PI	Antagonists are classic antihistamines with sedative properties
	H_2	↑ cAMP	Antagonists are used in treating gastric ulcers
	H_3	?	Inhibits histamine release
Serotonin	5-HT_{1a}	↓ cAMP	Site of action of buspirone and related antianxiety drugs
		↑ K^+ channels	
	5-HT_{1b}	↓ cAMP	
	5-HT_{1c}	↑ PI	Similar to 5-HT_2
	5-HT_{1d}	↓ cAMP	
	5-HT_2	↑ PI	Site of action of hallucinogens
	5-HT_3	Directly linked to ion channel	Antagonists are potent antiemetic agents
	5-HT_4	↑ cAMP	
Acetylcholine	M_1	↑ PI	
		↑ cyclic GMP	
	M_2	↓ cAMP	Mediates vagal bradycardia
		↑ K^+ channels	
	M_3	↑ PI	
		↑ cyclic GMP	
	M_4	↓ cAMP	
	Nicotinic	Directly linked to ion channel	Distinct subtypes are found in brain

↑ cAMP—increases levels of cyclic AMP
↓ cAMP—decreases levels of cyclic AMP
↑ K^+ channels—opens potassium channels
↑ PI—stimulates phosphoinositide turnover
↑ cyclic GMP—increases levels of cyclic GMP
?—effector has not been clearly identified but may include the one listed

to adenylate cyclase through G_i. Although many antipsychotics have significant affinity for both dopamine receptor subtypes, several active drugs, such as haloperidol and molindone (Moban), are disproportionately weak antagonists of the D_1 receptor, suggesting that the D_2 subtype is the pertinent site for the therapeutic action of antipsychotics. Furthermore, the clinical potencies of many antipsychotic drugs of diverse chemical structures parallel their affinities for the D_2 receptors, as measured in vitro by radioligand-binding techniques. That correlation has prompted the widely accepted hypothesis that the D_2 receptor is the site of action of antipsychotics. The concomitant appearance of extrapyramidal neurological symptoms with antipsychotic treatment is also attributed to D_2 receptor blockade in the striatum.

The cloning in recent years of both the D_1 and D_2 receptor subtypes set the stage for searching for other homologous subtypes. The search has been fruitful, as several other dopamine receptor subtypes have been identified with distinctive pharmacological properties. Essentially, three D_2-like receptors have been cloned and are referred to either as D_2, D_3, and D_4 or as D_{2A}, D_{2B}, and D_{2C}. D_{2A} receptors appear to correspond to the classic D_2 receptors, expressed at high levels in the striatum, and display the expected pharmacological profile. The D_{2B} or D_3 receptor is more narrowly distributed than are D_{2A} receptors, with its expression found predominantly in limbic areas, such as the hypothalamus, and in the nucleus accumbens, suggesting that the D_{2B} or D_3 receptor may be particularly relevant to the antipsychotic actions of dopamine blockade. In addition to differences in anatomical distribution, pharmacological differences between the D_2 receptor subtypes have appeared as well, raising the possibility that selective antagonists can be developed. The D_4 or D_{2C} receptor has attracted considerable attention because it displays a high affinity for the atypical antipsychotic clozapine (Clozaril). In addition, like the D_3 receptor, the D_4 receptor appears to be preferentially expressed in limbic areas, rather than in the striatum. That distribution may account for the relatively low incidence of motor side effects associated with clozapine treatment.

The D_1 receptor subfamily, although not linked to antipsychotic agents, appears to play a key role in dopaminergic neurotransmission. To date, two D_1-like receptor subtypes have been cloned. One of them, the D_5 receptor, appears to be expressed outside the striatum, whereas the classic D_1 receptor is more uniformly distributed among the dopamine target areas. Clearly, the identification of numerous dopamine receptor subtypes provides fertile ground for developing and testing new hypotheses about the action of antipsychotic drugs and the pathophysiology of psychotic disorders.

SEROTONERGIC RECEPTORS At present, serotonin receptors have been divided into four classes. The hallucinogenic actions of lysergic acid diethylamide (LSD) have long been thought to involve interactions with brain serotonin systems, since both compounds share an indoleamine structure. Recent studies point to the 5-HT_2 receptor as the site of action of LSD, mescaline, and related hallucinogens. In animal model systems, selective 5-HT_2 receptor antagonists block behavioral responses to those compounds, and the affinities of a large series of hallucinogens for that receptor correlate closely with their human hallucinogenic potencies. The dense localization of 5-HT_2 receptors in cortical regions (Figure 1.3-7) suggests that the activation of that branch of the serotonergic system contributes to the hallucinogenic response, which has served as an intriguing model of clinical psychotic states.

Research on 5-HT_1 receptors has led to the further subdivision of that class into as least three receptor subtypes. Of particular interest to psychopharmacology have been studies relating the antianxiety action of buspirone (BuSpar), a nonbenzodiazepine anxiolytic, to its ability to stimulate 5-HT_{1a} receptors, Thus, more than one of the 5-HT receptors may be important sites of psychotropic drug action. In addition to the 5-HT_1 and 5-HT_2 groups, two other distinct subtypes have been identified, 5-HT_3 and 5-HT_4. The 5-HT_3 class is better understood, since highly potent and selective ligands are available for that subtype. In contrast to all the other monamine receptors, that receptor stands out as the only one identified to date that shares homology with the nicotinic receptor family. In other words, all the other monoamine receptors act through G-proteins. Only the nicotinic and 5-HT_3 receptors belong to the family of transmitter-operated ion channels. That receptors subtype has also attracted attention, since 5-HT_3 receptor antagonists appear to possess potential as therapeutic psychotropic agents in animal model studies. Members of that class are already used clinically as effective and potent antiemetic agents, since 5-HT_3 receptors are expressed at high levels in the area postrema of the brainstem. In forebrain regions, 5-HT_3 receptors are expressed at low levels, but behavioral studies in animals suggest activity in antianxiety and antipsychotic paradigms. The 5-HT_4 receptor has recently been identified as a pharmacologically distinct receptor mediating the stimulation of adenylate cyclase by serotonin.

HISTAMINERGIC RECEPTORS Both histamine H_1 and H_2 receptor subtypes are present in the brain. Classic antihistamines used for allergic symptoms are potent antagonists of H_1 receptors and exert marked sedative effects, presumably by blocking central H_1 receptors. Many phenothiazine antipsychotics are potent H_1 receptor blockers, and that property may underlie their prominent sedative effects. Cimetidine (Tagamet) and other H_2 receptor blockers are widely prescribed for their ability to suppress stomach acid secretion. Although cimetidine can produce an organic mental syndrome, especially in elderly patients, it remains to be determined whether that side effect stems from central H_2 receptor blockade. The H_1 and H_2 receptors provide an example of how different receptor subtypes allow an individual transmitter to affect distinct intracellular second-messenger systems; H_1 receptors stimulate the phosphoinositide system, whereas H_2 receptors activate adenylate cyclase. A third histamine receptor, referred to as H_3, has been identified by its distinct pharmacological profile. Stimulation of that receptor, thought to be expressed on histamine nerve terminals, suppresses histamine release.

CHOLINERGIC RECEPTORS Abundant pharmacological evidence points to the existence of multiple muscarinic receptor subtypes. For example, pirenzepine, a muscarinic acetylcholine receptor antagonist, is effective in inhibiting gastric acid secretion without causing tachycardia, suggesting that the classic anticholinergic responses are mediated by distinct muscarinic receptors. Furthermore, the stimulation of muscarinic acetylcholine receptors results in the regulation of multiple distinct intracellular signaling systems, including the activation of cyclic guanosine monophosphate (GMP) and phosphoinositide systems, and in the inhibition of adenylate cyclase. To date, multiple muscarinic receptor subtypes have been identified by using molecular biological techniques. They can be roughly subdivided into the pharmacologically defined M_1 and M_2 subtypes. The M_1 type, which is sensitive to pirenzepine, appears to be linked to the phosphoinositide intracellular system, whereas the M_2 receptor type appears to be negatively coupled to adenylate cyclase through a G_i protein. The development of specific agonists and antagonists for the brain muscarinic receptors has been prompted by the evidence that cortical and hippocampal cholinergic systems play an important role in cognitive functions, especially short-term memory. Consistent with the role of forebrain cholinergic neurons in cognitive functions, postmortem studies have revealed marked reductions in the presynaptic markers for cholinergic terminals in the hippocampus and the cortex and the loss of nucleus basalis cholinergic cell bodies in Alzheimer's disease.

SUGGESTED CROSS-REFERENCES

The electrophysiological actions of monoamines are discussed in Section 1.7. General concepts of neuronal signaling that apply to monoamines are presented in Section 1.6. Many of the molecular biology principles used in recent studies of monoamine systems are outlined in Section 1.14. The mechanism of action of antidepressants and antipsychotic agents are discussed in Sections 32.24 and 32.15, respectively.

REFERENCES

*Amara S G, Kuhar M J: Neurotransmitter transporters: Recent progress. Annu Rev Neurosci *16:* 73, 1993.

Bjorklund A, Lindvall O: Dopamine-containing systems in the CNS. In *Handbook of Chemical Neuroanatomy,* vol 2: *Classical Transmitters in the CNS,* A Bjorklund, T Hokfelt, editors, p 55. Elsevier, Amsterdam, 1984.

Burns R S, LeWit P A, Ebert M H, Pakenberg H, Kopin I J: The clinical syndrome of striatal dopamine deficiency: Parkinsonism induced by MPTP. New Engl J Med *312:* 1418, 1985.

*Cooper J R, Bloom F E, Roth R H: *The Biochemical Basis of Neuropharmacology,* ed 6. Oxford University Press, New York, 1991.

Fibiger H C, Vincent S R: Anatomy of central cholinergic neurons. In *Psychopharmacology: The Third Generation of Progress,* H Y Meltzer, editor, p 211. Raven, New York, 1987.

Frazer A, Hensler J G: Serotonin. In *Basic Neurochemistry,* ed 5, G J Siegel, B W Agranoff, R W Albers, P B Molinoff, editors, p 283. Raven, New York, 1994.

Green J P: Histamine. In *Basic Neurochemistry,* ed 5, G. J Siegel, B W Agranoff, R W Albers, P B Molinoff, editors, Raven, New York, 1994.

Maricq A W, Peterson A S, Brake A J, Myers R M, Julius D: Primary structure and functional expression of the $5HT_3$ receptor, a serotonin-gated ion channel. Science *254:* 432, 1991.

Nicoll R A: The septo-hippocampal projection: A model cholinergic pathway. Trends Neurosci *8:* 533, 1985.

Pacholczyk T, Blakely R D, Amara S G: Expression cloning of a cocaine and antidepressant-sensitive human noradrenaline transporter. Nature *350:* 350, 1991.

*Sibley D R, Monsma F J Jr: The molecular biology of dopamine receptors. Trends Pharmacol Sci *13:* 61, 1992.

*Sokoloff P, Giros B, Martes M P, Bouthenet M W, Schwartz J C: Molecular cloning and characterization of a novel dopamine D_3 receptor as a target for neuroleptics. Nature *347:* 146, 1990.

Sulzer D, Rayport S: Amphetamine and other psychostimulants reduce pH gradients in midbrain dopaminergic neurons and chromaffin granules: A mechanism of action. Neuron *5:* 797, 1990.

Taylor P, Brown J H: Acetylocholine. In *Basic Neurochemistry,* ed 5, G H Siegel, B W Agranoff, R W Albers, P B Molinoff, editors, p 231. Raven, New York, 1994.

*VanTol H H M, Bunzow J R, Guan H-C, Sunahara R K, Seeman P, Niznnik H B, Civelli O: Cloning of the gene for a human D_4 receptor with high affinity for the antipsychotic clozapine. Nature *350:* 610, 1991.

Weiner N, Molinoff P B: Catecholamines. In *Basic Neurochemistry,* ed 5, G J Siegel, B W Agranoff, R W Albers, P B Molinoff, editors, p 261. Raven, New York, 1994.

1.4
AMINO ACID NEUROTRANSMITTERS

DANIEL C. JAVITT, M.D., Ph.D.
STEPHEN R. ZUKIN, M.D.

INTRODUCTION

Amino acids are the most prevalent neurotransmitters in the mammalian central nervous system (CNS). Virtually all neurons in the CNS are activated by excitatory amino acid neurotransmitters and are inhibited by inhibitory amino acids. The amino acids that serve as neurotransmitters are all small, abundant, unbranched hydrophilic molecules. Although the amino acid neurotransmitters are present in high concentrations outside the brain, they are not actively transported into the CNS. The neurotransmitter pool, which is synthesized in situ, is, therefore, well insulated from fluctuations in serum amino acid levels. Whereas peptide neurotransmitters are present in concentrations on the order of picomoles per gram tissue and monoamine neurotransmitters are present in concentrations on the order of nanomoles, amino acid neurotransmitters are present on the order of micromoles.

Excitatory amino acids, of which glutamate is the most prevalent, are dicarboxylic in nature in that they possess two carboxylic acid groups. The inhibitory amino acids, γ-aminobutyric acid (GABA) and glycine, are monocarboxylic in that they possess only a single carboxylic acid group. The differential structure contributes to their functional specificity. Amino acid neurotransmitters mediate their actions predominantly at ligand-gated channel type receptors. Like the nicotinic receptors of a motor endplate, such receptors contain an integral ion channel and induce rapid, short-lasting alterations in membrane potential. Receptors linked to guanosine 5′-triphosphate (GTP)-binding proteins (G-proteins) have been described for excitatory amino acids and GABA and may play a modulatory role in CNS functioning.

EXCITATORY AMINO ACIDS

The ability of certain amino acids, such as glutamate and aspartate, to exert potent excitatory effects on cortical neurons was first observed in the late 1950s. Because of the high concentrations of glutamate in the CNS and the prominent role played by glutamate in intermediate metabolism, a specific neurotransmitter role for glutamate was not established until the early 1980s. The criteria for neurotransmitter status have now been fulfilled for glutamate. Other excitatory amino acids, including aspartate and homocysteate, may also act as neurotransmitters. Their roles relative to glutamate have not been established.

PRESYNAPTIC MECHANISMS

Synthesis Glutamate does not cross the blood-brain barrier. The pool of glutamate that participates in neurotransmission is synthesized in presynaptic nerve terminals and is separate from the metabolic pool. Whereas metabolic glutamate participates in the Krebs cycle and may be synthesized directly from glucose, neurotransmitter glutamate derives primarily from deamination of glutamine, which is inactive as a neurotransmitter. Glutamine is actively transported into the CNS and is plentiful extracellularly. Glutamine is taken up by presynaptic glutamatergic terminals by a specific, low-affinity, high-capacity uptake system. Glia serve as an intracellular reservoir system for glutamine and may contain concentrations that are 10-fold larger than the extracellular concentration.

Within the presynaptic terminal, glutamine is converted into glutamate by the action of a phosphate-activated glutaminase located within the mitochondria. Glutaminase activity serves as the rate-limiting step for glutamate synthesis. Glutaminase activity is inhibited by glutamate and ammonia, the products of the enzyme, and is stimulated by millimolar concentrations of calcium. As a result, the accumulation of ammonia in the brain during hepatic insufficiency or other metabolic disorders may lead to a clinically significant decrease in glutamate synthesis and release. GABA synthesis is less affected by alterations in glutaminase activity, so the accumulation of ammonia may lead to a net excess of inhibitory neurotransmission. The degree to which glutamate depletion accounts for the encephalopathic changes associated with liver failure remains to be determined.

After presynaptic release, glutamate is removed from the cleft by the actions of sodium-dependent transport pumps located on the nerve terminals and glia. Within glial cells, glutamate is reaminated to glutamine by adenosine 5′-triphosphate (ATP)-dependent glutamine synthetase. Glial glutamine diffuses into the extracellular space, where it is reabsorbed by glutamatergic terminals and reconverted to glutamate.

Anatomical Pathways Glutamatergic fibers give rise to the major afferent, intrinsic, and efferent pathways through the cortex (Figure 1.4-1). Many sensory organs—including the cochlea, the olfactory bulb, and the retina—use glutamate as their principal neurotransmitter. Large, myelinated, nonnociceptive primary somatosensory fibers may also use glutamate. Within the brain, thalamocortical fibers, which represent the main input to the cortex, are predominantly glutamatergic in nature. Virtually all pyramidal neurons in the cortex are glutamatergic. Pyramidal neurons constitute 60 to 80 percent of all the neurons in the cerebral cortex, and they mediate virtually all the cortical outflow. The dense, mutually facilitatory glutamate-mediated connections between pyramidal cells is a basic requirement for the extensive parallel information-processing operations of the cerebral cortex. Pyramidal neurons in the cortex project to both cortical and subcortical structures. The long corticospinal and corticobulbar tracts are glutamatergic in nature, as are many afferents to the cerebellum. The glutamatergic system is responsible for the bulk of the highly organized information flow through the brain. The role of other neurotransmitter pathways is primarily to regulate and modulate glutamate-mediated excitatory neuronal connections.

The corticostriatal pathway—which originates from the entire neocortex and projects to the ipsilateral caudate, the putamen, and, to a smaller extent, the nucleus accumbens—may be specifically implicated in the pathophysiology of schizophrenia.

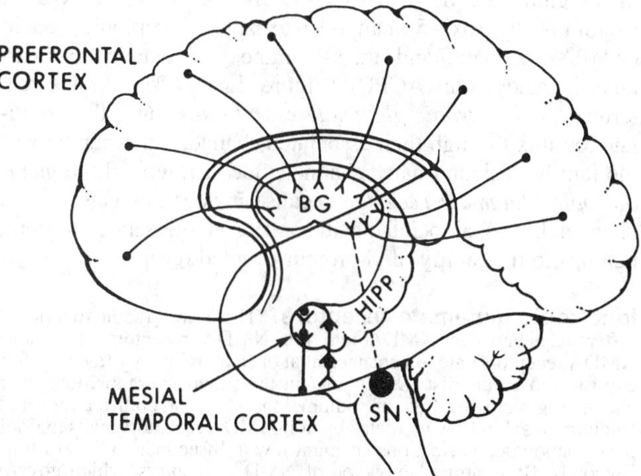

FIGURE 1.4-1 *Schematic diagram of cortical and hippocampal (HIPP) excitatory amino acid pathways (solid lines). Excitatory amino acid-containing neurons in the cortex exert descending control over the subcortical structures, including the basal ganglia (BG), that is behaviorally antagonistic to the control mediated by the ascending dopaminergic system (dashed line). In the mesial temporal cortex, excitatory amino acid-containing neurons give rise to the primary afferent, the intrinsic, and the efferent pathways of the hippocampal formation. (From D C Javitt, S R Zukin: The role of excitatory amino acids in neuropsychiatric illness. J Neuropsychiatry Clin Neurosci 2: 44, 1990. Used with permission.)*

Corticostriatal fibers impinge on the same intrinsic striatal neurons as the dopaminergic fibers of the nigrostriatal tract. Corticostriatal and nigrostriatal fibers exert behavioral effects that are essentially antagonistic. In experimental animals, corticostriatal ablation produces transient stereotypes similar to those induced by amphetamine, facilitates amphetamine-induced stereotypies and circling, and markedly inhibits haloperidol (Haldol)-induced catalepsy. The effects of corticostriatal ablation are not accompanied by increases in dopamine metabolite levels or by alterations in dopamine-receptor density. The functional dysregulation of dopaminergic neurotransmission induced by corticostriatal ablation may serve as a model for behavioral disorganization in schizophrenia. A similar system, the corticothalamic system, regulates information flow into the cortex. Abnormalities of corticothalamic neurotransmission may contribute to the sensory-gating abnormalities associated with schizophrenia.

Glutamatergic pathways in the hippocampus may be specifically relevant to the pathophysiology of dementing illness. Glutamatergic fibers give rise to the major afferent, intrinsic, and efferent pathways of the hippocampal formation. In Alzheimer's disease (called dementia of the Alzheimer's type in the fourth edition of *Diagnostic and Statistical Manual of Mental Disorders* [DSM-IV]) pyramidal neurons in the mesial temporal cortex and the subiculum are extensively damaged, leading to a virtual isolation of the hippocampus from the cerebral cortex. That disruption of hippocampal innervation may contribute to the memory deficits associated with Alzheimer's disease. In hypoxic and ischemic insults to the brain, the CA_3 region of the hippocampus may be selectively damaged. Disruption of the glutamatergic pathways within the hippocampus leads to severe disturbances in memory formation similar to those observed after a complete bilateral hippocampal ablation.

RECEPTORS Excitatory amino acids produce their CNS effects at distinct classes of receptors. Their nomenclature is based on their preferential activation by the prototypic synthetic glutamate derivatives *N*-methyl-D-aspartate (NMDA), α-amino-3-hydroxy-5-methyl-4-isoxazole propionic acid (AMPA), kainate, and trans-1-aminocyclopentane-1,3-dicarboxylic acid (trans-ACPD) (Figure 1.4-2). The first three, termed the *ionotropic glutamate receptors* because they regulate ion flux through their associated channels, are members of the family of ligand-gated channels; the last, termed the *metabotropic glutamate receptor* because it does not gate an ion channel but is associated with a second messenger system, belongs to the family of G-protein-coupled receptors.

Selective agonists

Quisqualate — Kainate — *N*-methyl-D-aspartate (NMDA)

Endogenous agonists

L-glutamate — L-aspartate

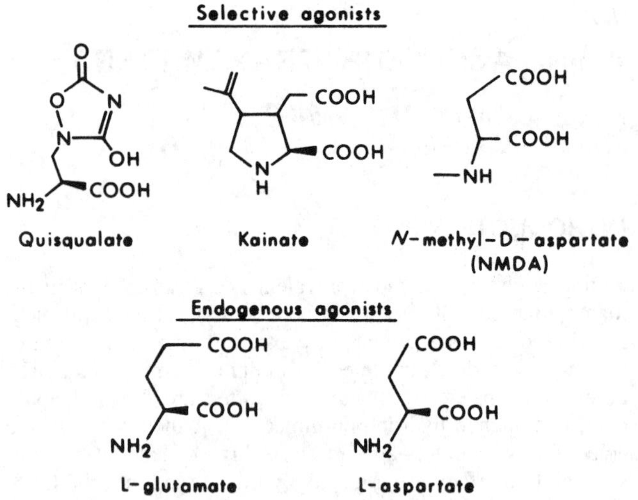

FIGURE 1.4-2 *Structures of the prototypical agonists for the non-NMDA (quisqualate, kainate) and NMDA ionotropic glutamate receptors and the endogenous excitatory amino acid neurotransmitters glutamate and aspartate. (From D C Javitt, S R Zukin: The role of excitatory amino acids in neuropsychiatric illness. J Neuropsychiatry Clin Neurosci* 2: *44, 1990. Used with permission.)*

Ionotropic glutamate receptors There are crucial functional differences between NMDA and non-NMDA receptors. The non-NMDA receptors gate ion channels that open in obligatory fashion after exposure to an agonist. Depending on the subunit composition, their channels govern the flux of sodium ions alone or both sodium and calcium ions. Ion flow mediated by non-NMDA receptors leads to brief postsynaptic depolarizations lasting a few milliseconds to tens of milliseconds. By contrast, activation of NMDA receptors, which govern calcium and sodium fluxes, gives rise to prolonged depolarizations lasting as long as 500 milliseconds. Another distinguishing characteristic of NMDA receptors is that, when neurons bearing them are at resting potential (inwardly negative), their channels are blocked by physiological concentrations of magnesium ion, and no ion fluxes can occur in response to an agonist. That magnesium block is voltage-dependent and can be relieved by neuronal depolarization caused by synaptic activity. Thus, ion flow through NMDA channels requires both presynaptic release of glutamate and postsynaptic neuronal depolarization through non-NMDA receptors. That unique property of NMDA-receptor channels allows them to selectively amplify non-NMDA-receptor-mediated synaptic responses that exceed a critical voltage or frequency. As the only receptors known to sense both presynaptic and postsynaptic activity, NMDA receptors satisfy the requirement of Hebbian associative learning a behavioral plasticity process whereby synaptic connections between concurrently activated presynaptic and postsynaptic neurons are strengthened. The high densities of NMDA receptors in the cortex and the hippocampus support that concept; their colocalization with AMPA receptors suggests that the two types of excitatory amino acid receptors act in concert. Activation of NMDA receptors triggers the process of long-term potentiation, which is postulated to underlie learning, memory formation, and developmental neuronal plasticity. Long-term potentiation is initiated by the entry of calcium ions through NMDA-receptor-gated channels. Calcium then triggers a cascade of biochemical events, including the production of nitric oxide (NO) by the activation of the enzyme NO synthase, which ultimately result in the long-term (weeks to months) strengthening of the involved synapse so that subsequent activation induces greater depolarization than that seen before long-term potentiation. NO is thought to be the retrograde messenger carrying the long-term potentiation signal from the postsynaptic aspect to the presynaptic aspect of the involved synapse.

Non-NMDA receptors The classification of the non-NMDA receptors has been a matter of considerable controversy over the years. In general, the results of electrophysiological experiments have supported the concept of a single type of non-NMDA ionotropic glutamate receptor, but radioligand-binding studies have suggested multiple types. The results of recent molecular cloning experiments have led to the identification of at least six distinct receptor proteins of about 100 kilodaltons (kd). Each of the proteins possesses four transmembrane domains. The regions forming the channel mouth in each case have a preponderance of negatively charged amino acids, in keeping with the cationic conductances gated by glutamate receptors. The intracellular domains contain mechanisms for the activation of protein kinases. The glutamate receptors $GluR_1$ to $GluR_4$ are thought to represent AMPA-receptor proteins and, when expressed, display a low affinity for kainate. By contrast, $GluR_5$ and $GluR_6$ are thought to represent kainate-receptor proteins and, when expressed, display a high affinity for kainate. Members of each of the groups have relatively low sequence identity with members of the other groups. The AMPA-selective subtypes can exist in alternate flip and flop forms on the basis of alternative splicing. The flop forms are expressed at low levels early in development and increase during maturation; the flip forms do not change during development. The presence of a flip module in a glutamate receptor causes dramatically enhanced sensitivity to activation by glutamate. Heterogeneity of native receptors presumably results from the assembly of multiple units of distinct subtypes in distinct brain regions and circuits. AMPA receptors consisting of $GluR_1$ or $GluR_3$ subunits form channels permeable to both sodium and calcium ions; if receptors also include $GluR_2$ subunits, they are permeable only to sodium ions and are blocked by calcium ions. Until now, pharmacological strategies for the study of non-NMDA glutamate receptors have been limited by a paucity of type-selective antagonists. The ability to express receptors assembled from specific subunits will now promote progress in that area.

NMDA receptors The NMDA type of glutamate receptor is the best characterized from a pharmacological standpoint. It possesses multiple regulatory sites (Figure 1.4-3). The binding of two molecules of glutamate is required to permit channel activation; the binding of glycine or similar amino acids (for example, D-serine) to a glycine-recognition site (distinct from the strychnine-sensitive inhibitory glycine receptor described below) is also required for activation to occur. An additional site has been identified at which polyamines, such as spermine and spermidine, enhance agonist-induced NMDA-receptor activation. Negative modulation of NMDA-receptor function can be induced by zinc ions, which are coreleased with glutamate from mossy fibers in the hippocampus, or by tricyclic antidepressants at concentrations above those achieved in clinical pharmacotherapy for depression. Ethanol, at doses relevant to its intoxicating effects, inhibits NMDA-receptor-gated ion flux significantly but has much less potent effects on non-NMDA glutamate receptors.

Two additional sites of particular importance are located within the NMDA-receptor-gated ion channel itself and, therefore, display both voltage-dependency and use-dependency. One site mediates the channel-blocking properties of the magnesium ion; the other, the phencyclidine (PCP) receptor, mediates the channel-blocking properties of PCP-like psychotomimetic drugs (Figure 1.4-4). Because their binding characteristics are sensitive to the functional state of the NMDA channel, PCP-receptor ligands have been used in radioreceptor assays as biochemical probes of NMDA-receptor function.

Results of recent molecular cloning experiments suggest that NMDA receptors are composed of multiple subunits and may be structurally similar to the non-NMDA and $GABA_A$ receptors. Koki Moriyoshi and colleagues reported cloning of a cDNA encoding a single protein, of relative molecular mass 105.5 kd, displaying electrophysiological and pharmacological properties of the NMDA receptor, including selective sensitivity to agonists, competitive antagonists, glycine-site agonists and antagonists, and zinc ions when expressed in *Xenopus* oocytes. Messenger ribonucleic acid (mRNA) for NMDAR1 or ζ1 was widely distributed throughout brain neuronal cells, and was found in virtually all neurons. That marked difference from the anatomical distribution of native NMDA receptors, and the fact that depolarizations induced by agonists in expressed NMDAR1 were much weaker than those induced following expression of presumed native receptors, were taken as evidence for the existence of additional subtypes of the NMDA receptor. Such additional subtypes have now been reported by two groups.

Hiroyuki Meguro and colleagues reported cloning of a novel mouse NMDA receptor subunit, termed ε1, with relative molecular mass of 163.267 kd. Although that subunit failed to cause expression of active NMDA receptors when expressed in *Xenopus* oocytes, coexpression with NMDAR1 resulted in active receptors with properties distinct from those expressed after injection of NMDAR1 alone. Anatomical distribution of the expression pattern of the ε1 subunit was distinct from that of the ζ1 subunit.

Most recently, Hannah Monyer and colleagues demonstrated three distinct cDNAs of rat brain encoding NMDA receptor subunits 2A, 2B, and 2C, with a high degree of homology among themselves but much lower homology with NMDAR1. A fourth subunit, 2D, was demonstrated by Kazutaka Ikeda and colleagues. On expression, each of those subunits formed a functional receptor channel only when coexpressed with NMDAR1. Anatomical localization of corresponding mRNAs indicated marked differences from NMDAR1 and among the distinct NMDAR2s. On expression by transfection in cultured cells, each of the distinct NMDAR2-NMDAR1 heteromers revealed distinct functional properties in terms of voltage sensitivity, kinetics, and affinities for agonists and antagonists.

At present the structures of the native NMDA receptor remain unknown. A number of additional subtypes of NMDA receptor subunits are expected to be cloned in the future, and there are likely to be a large number of distinct subunits with overlapping regional distributions. Only a combination of cloning techniques with detailed biochemical knowledge of mechanisms governing NMDA receptor activation and regulation and the regional variations in such mechanisms can successfully address the question of the nature of the native receptor.

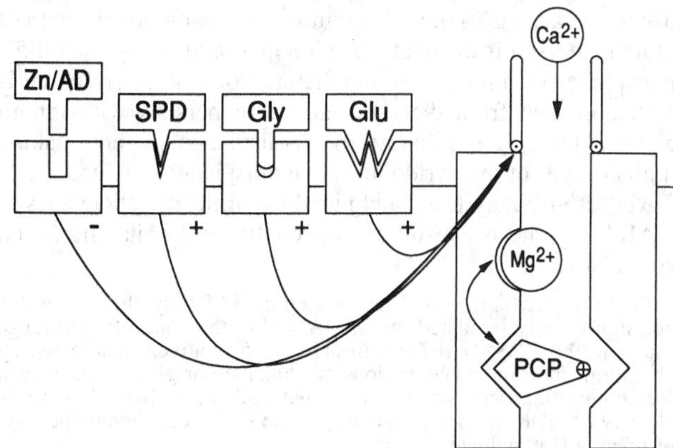

FIGURE 1.4-3 *Schematic structure of the NMDA receptor complex, showing the binding sites for glutamate (Glu), glycine (Gly), zinc (Zn), selected antidepressants (AD), phencyclidine (PCP), and the polyamines spermidine (SPD) and magnesium (Mg^{2+}). The opening of the channel allows calcium (Ca^{2+}) influx into the cell. (From D C Javitt, S R Zukin: Recent advances in the phencyclidine model of schizophrenia. Am J Psychiatry 148: 1310, 1991. Used with permission.)*

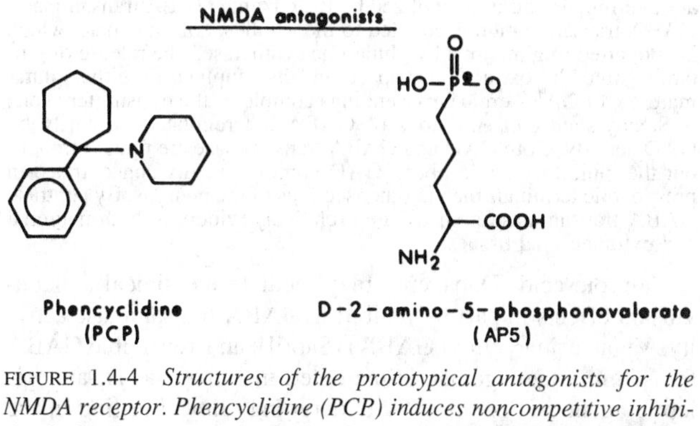

NMDA antagonists

Phencyclidine (PCP)

D-2-amino-5-phosphonovalerate (AP5)

FIGURE 1.4-4 *Structures of the prototypical antagonists for the NMDA receptor. Phencyclidine (PCP) induces noncompetitive inhibition by binding to a site located within the NMDA channel. D-2-Amino-5-phosphonovalerate (AP5) induces competitive inhibition by displacing glutamate from the NMDA recognition site. (From D C Javitt, S R Zukin: The role of excitatory amino acids in neuropsychiatric illness. J Neuropsychiatry Clin Neurosci 2: 44, 1990. Used with permission.)*

Metabotropic glutamate receptors The metabotropic glutamate receptor is distinct from the AMPA-kainate and NMDA receptors in belonging to the superfamily of G-protein-linked receptors, rather than to the superfamily of ligand-gated channels. The consequences of activating that class of glutamate receptor include the activation of phospholipase C and the production of inositol 1,4,5-triphosphate. The metabotropic glutamate receptor is found in glia as well as in neurons. Physiologically, the application of agonists or the synaptic release of glutamate onto metabotropic receptors produces a characteristic slow excitatory postsynaptic current. A role for the metabotropic glutamate receptor in long-term potentiation has been proposed.

CLINICAL APPLICATIONS

Excitotoxicity Glutamate and a number of its analogs have been shown to destroy CNS neurons by local or systemic application. Those toxic actions are mediated by excessive activation of postsynaptic NMDA or non-NMDA glutamate receptors, ultimately leading to the uncontrolled influx of calcium ions through open NMDA-receptor channels. Accordingly, such excitotoxicity can be blocked by glutamate-receptor antagonists. Calcium entry into neurons triggered by NMDA-receptor activation has as one of its consequences the activation of the enzyme nitric oxide synthase; the recent finding that inhibitors of that enzyme can prevent excitatory amino acid-induced neurotoxicity implicates nitric oxide as an important mediator of excitotoxicity.

Excitatory amino acids (such as monosodium glutamate) are present in the diet. Although the compounds do not readily penetrate the blood-brain barrier in healthy adults, the oral administration of monosodium glutamate destroys CNS neurons in immature animals, with particular damage to neurons in the brain regions lacking blood-brain barriers. Therefore, the question has been raised whether monosodium glutamate consumption by children may lead to neuroendocrinopathies by virtue of the excitotoxic damage to the arcuate nucleus of the hypothalamus.

Other dietary excitotoxins have been reported, including β-N-oxalylamino-L-alanine, which is associated with neurolathyrism, and β-N-methylamino-L-alanine, which is implicated in amyotrophic lateral sclerosis (ALS), parkinsonism, and dementia complex of Guam. Those correlations have raised the intriguing possibility that related excitotoxic mechanisms triggered by endogenous glutamate-receptor agonists in susceptible persons underlie such degenerative neuropsychiatric disorders as Alzheimer's disease, Huntington's disease, and ALS, in which excitatory amino acid concentrations in the CSF correlate with symptom severity. In experimental animals NMDA-receptor antagonists can prevent or limit neuronal damage induced by experimental seizures, hypoglycemia, hypoxia, ischemia, and CNS trauma.

Neurodevelopment NMDA receptors play a crucial role in several areas of neurodevelopment, including growth cone guidance during neuronal migration, dendritic spine formation and synapse elimination (synaptic pruning) during embryonic synaptogenesis, and cortical self-organization during early postnatal development. Several critical developmental processes, such as the development of ocular dominance columns in the visual system or spatial representation in the somatosensory system, depend on NMDA receptor-induced long-term potentiation and can be blocked by NMDA antagonists. NMDA receptor density is transiently enhanced during brain development and early in life. While that transient enhancement may play a critical role in brain development, it may also render the immature brain more sensitive than the adult brain to the excitotoxic effects of hypoxia, hypoglycemia, or environmental neurotoxins.

Schizophrenia Agents that block NMDA receptor, such as PCP, ketamine, or dizocylpine (MK-801) are collectively referred to as *dissociative anesthetics* because, at high doses, they induce a state in which subjects are awake but apparently dissociated from the environment. At subanesthetic doses those drugs induce a psychotic state that closely resembles schizophrenia and incorporates not only positive symptoms, but also negative symptoms and cognitive dysfunction. Recently, for example, it was demonstrated that infusion of subanesthetic doses of ketamine in normal volunteers induces perceptual alterations, impaired performance of frontal lobe tasks, such as the Wisconsin Card Sorting Test, and memory-encoding deficits similar to those observed in schizophrenia. Equivalent effects were noted in studies performed with PCP in the late 1950s and early 1960s. In controls the psychotomimetic effects of NMDA blockers are usually transient. Schizophrenic subjects and subjects with a constitutional predisposition to schizophrenia appear to be susceptible to the disorganizing effects of NMDA blockers and may show decompensations that persist for several weeks following a single, low dose. The ability of NMDA blockers to induce a psychotomimetic state that closely resembles schizophrenia has led to the development of the PCP-NMDA theory of schizophrenia, which suggests that endogenous dysfunction or dysregulation of NMDA receptor-mediated neurotransmission may play a crucial role in the pathogenesis of schizophrenia. Glycine, an allosteric potentiator of NMDA receptor-mediated neurotransmission, may significantly ameliorate negative symptoms and cognitive dysfunction in antipsychotic-resistant subjects, although NMDA receptor-based treatments of schizophrenia are limited by the lack of specific NMDA augmenting agents that reliably cross the blood-brain barrier. Mechanisms by which NMDA receptor dysfunction or dysregulation might occur in schizophrenia have not been determined. However, schizophrenia has been associated with a proliferation of glutamate immunoreactive fibers and alterations in NMDA and non-NMDA receptor density within specific brain regions, which suggests that there might be intrinsic abnormalities of the glutamate system. Abnormalities in the number and distribution of GABAergic neurons and receptors have also been reported, which suggests that glutamate dysfunction might also be secondary to disturbances in inhibitory feedback regulation.

INHIBITORY AMINO ACIDS: γ-AMINOBUTYRIC ACID

PRESYNAPTIC MECHANISMS

Synthesis The major excitatory and inhibitory transmitters in the brain differ by a single carboxyl group. GABA is synthesized in the brain primarily by the action of glutamic acid decarboxylase (GAD), which removes the α-carboxyl group of glutamate in an irreversible reaction that requires pyridoxal-5′-phosphate (vitamin B_6) as a cofactor. Normally, pyridoxine is well absorbed from dietary sources. In persons with inborn abnormalities of pyridoxine metabolism and in those taking high dosages of the pyridoxine antagonist isoniazid, inadequate GAD activity may lead to clinically significant deficiencies in GABA synthesis, resulting in confusion, irritability, and convulsions.

GAD activity is the rate-limiting step in GABA synthesis. GAD is not significantly regulated by GABA within the concentration range found in the CNS. GABA synthesis is also relatively unaffected by alterations in brain concentrations of glutamate or glutamine. In such metabolic conditions as hepatic encephalopathy, therefore, GABA levels may be relatively preserved, despite the sharp reduction in the level of releasable glutamate.

GABA is removed from the synaptic cleft by high-affinity transport proteins located on the presynaptic nerve terminals and glial cells. One member of a presumed family of GABA-reuptake proteins has recently been cloned from rat brain. Structurally, the GABA transporter appears to consist of a single protein with approximately 12 membrane-spanning regions. A highly homologous protein appears to be ubiquitously distributed in the human brain. The characterization of the GABA transporter may permit the development of clinically useful reuptake inhibitors.

Once GABA is taken up, reuse or metabolic conversion follows. GABA is absorbed into the mitochondria located in the glia or presynaptic terminals and is catabolized by the enzyme GABA transaminase. GABA transamination is coupled to the synthesis of glutamate, which is converted to glutamine by glutamine synthetase. The release of glutamine into the extracellular space and its reuptake by either glutamatergic or GABAergic nerve endings completes the transmitter cycle.

Steady-state concentrations of GABA are regulated primarily by GAD activity. Both GAD and GABA transaminase are found throughout the inhibitory nerve fibers. GAD is more heavily concentrated in presynaptic terminals than in other sections of the neurons. By contrast, GABA transaminase is distributed relatively widely in both neuronal and extraneuronal tissues.

Valproic acid (Depakene) may mediate its clinical anticonvulsant effects in part by inhibiting GABA transaminase activity. Vigabatrin (γ-vinyl GABA) (Sabril), an irreversible GABA transaminase antagonist, is marketed in Europe as an antiepileptic agent and is currently undergoing clinical testing in the United States. Vigabatrin has also been used experimentally for the treatment of tardive dyskinesia.

Anatomical pathways In the cortex GABA is localized primarily to intrinsic neurons that participate in local feedback loops. Those intrinsic inhibitory neurons constitute 20 to 25 percent of the total and exert a tonic inhibition on cortical pyramidal neurons to prevent uncontrolled excitatory activity. Destruction or degeneration of intrinsic cortical GABAergic neurons may play a fundamental role in the focal epilepsies. Several experimental brain lesions—including those produced by alumina gel, cobalt treatment, and hypoxia—lead to a selective loss of GABAergic neurons that may underlie the development of local seizure foci. However, in other models of epilepsy, GABAergic mechanisms appear to be normal, so GABAergic dysfunction may be sufficient but not necessary for epileptogenesis to occur.

About 20 percent of all cortical GABAergic neurons also show immunoreactivity for neuropeptide. The identified neuropeptides include somatostatin, neuropeptide Y, vasoactive intestinal peptide, cholecystokinin, substance P, and dynorphin. GABAergic neurons constitute the large majority of peptide immunoreactive neurons in the cortex.

In subcortical structures and the cerebellum, GABA is found in both intrinsic and projection neurons. GABAergic projection neurons are especially prevalent in the extrapyramidal motor system, where the majority of the efferent projections is inhibitory, rather than excitatory. GABAergic neurons from the dorsal striatum project to the pars reticulata of the substantia nigra as part of the striatonigral feedback pathway that regulates ascending dopaminergic neurotransmission. Striatal neurons also project to the internal segment of the globus pallidus, where they synapse on GABAergic efferent neurons that provide tonic inhibition to the subthalamic nuclei.

In Huntington's disease, there is selective degeneration of striatal GABAergic neurons projecting to the globus pallidus, leading to the overinhibition of the subthalamic nuclei and the expression of choreiform movements. Degeneration of the striatal GABAergic neurons also occurs after long-term antipsychotic treatment in a monkey model of tardive dyskinesia, suggesting that the same neuronal pathway may be implicated.

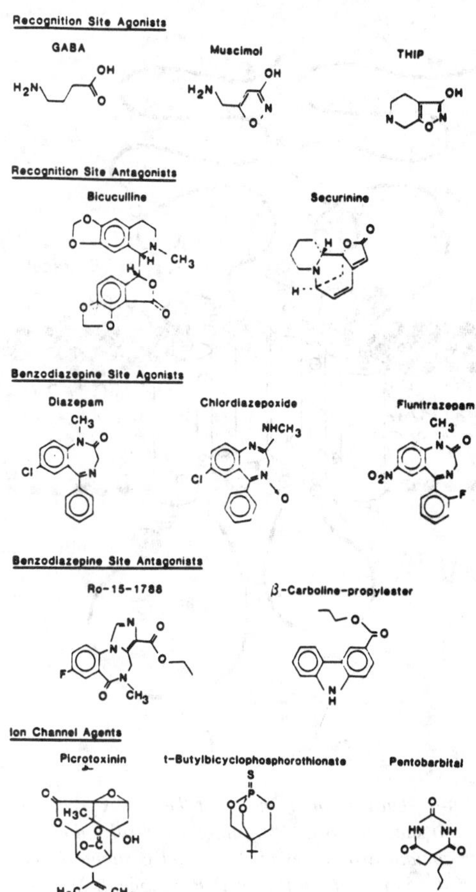

FIGURE 1.4-5 *Structure of the prototypical $GABA_A$ and benzodiazepine receptor agonists and antagonists.*

RECEPTOR MECHANISMS

$GABA_A$ receptors Two major types of GABA receptors have been identified by electrophysiological and neuropharmacological investigations. The first type, termed $GABA_A$, is a member of the ligand-gated channel family of synaptic receptors and is coupled to a chloride channel. Binding of GABA leads to a rapid opening of the $GABA_A$ channel and a brief current flow lasting milliseconds to tens of milliseconds.

At least three functional domains of the $GABA_A$ receptor complex have been identified: a GABA-recognition site, a channel site, and a benzodiazepine-receptor site. The $GABA_A$ receptor-associated benzodiazepine receptor, which exists only in the CNS, has been termed the central receptor to distinguish it from the peripheral receptor, which is present at highest concentration outside the CNS. The GABA-recognition site, the channel site, and the central benzodiazepine receptor are allosterically linked: binding to one site induces a complementary alteration in binding to the others. The structures of the prototypical ligands for each of the binding domains are shown in Figure 1.4-5.

GABA-RECOGNITION SITE The $GABA_A$ receptor consists of a number of subunits that surround a central channel (Figure 1.4-6). Binding of GABA to its recognition site induces a conformational shift of the receptor subunits such that anions may flow through the channel. The dose-response curve for stimulation chloride conductance by GABA is relatively steep, with a Hill coefficient close to two, suggesting that, on average, native $GABA_A$ receptors possess two independent GABA-binding sites. Occupation of both sites must occur before channel opening takes place.

$GABA_A$ agonists—including muscimol, progabide, and 4,5,6,7-tetrahydroisoxazolo [5,4c] pyridine-3-ol (THIP)—have been used experimentally for the treatment of epilepsy, Huntington's disease, and tardive dyskinesia with varying success. Unfortunately, the use of all available $GABA_A$ agonists is limited by peripheral toxicity. Bicuculline, a convulsant alkaloid, mediates its effects by displacing GABA from its binding site on the $GABA_A$ receptor complex in a competitive fashion.

CHANNEL SITE Agents that bind within the ion channel associated with the $GABA_A$ receptor complex may affect $GABA_A$-mediated neurotransmission independently of the GABA-recognition sites. Picrotoxin, a convulsant agent derived from the dried berries of the climbing shrub *Anamirta cocculus*, antagonizes $GABA_A$-receptor-mediated neurotransmission in a noncompetitive fashion by binding within the ion channel and preventing chloride flow. Cage convulsants, such as t-butylbicyclophosphorothionate, also induce potent convulsive effects by blocking $GABA_A$ channels, underscoring the critical role played by $GABA_A$ receptors in the maintenance of tonic inhibition of cortical pyramidal neurons.

Barbiturates compete for binding with picrotoxin. In the presence of anticonvulsant barbiturates, the duration of unitary ion channel openings is prolonged. At low dosages, barbiturates act primarily by potentiating the effects of administered GABA. At higher dosages, however, barbiturates may induce channel opening, even in the absence of GABA. Their ability to influence channel activity directly may be responsible for their greater propensity, relative to benzodiazepines, to induce severe CNS depression.

BENZODIAZEPINE RECEPTOR Benzodiazepine receptors are closely related to the GABA-recognition site of the $GABA_A$ receptor complex. Benzodiazepine-receptor agonists, such as diazepam (Valium) and clonazepam (Klonopin), increase the affinity of GABA for its binding site and make the complex more responsive to basal concentrations of GABA. Benzodiazepines induce a characteristic spectrum of neurobehavioral

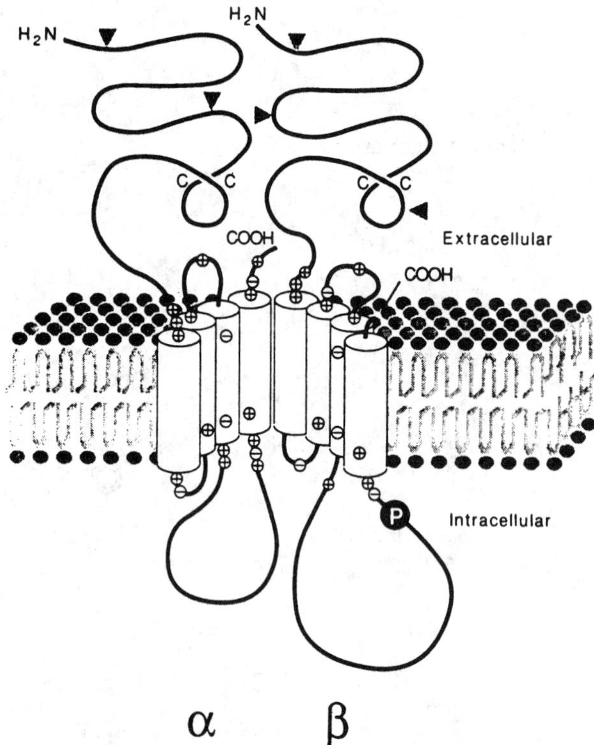

FIGURE 1.4-6 *Diagrammatic model of the $GABA_A$-receptor complex, showing two subunits (α and β) lining a central ion channel. Native receptors contain two copies of the α and β subunits and may also contain a third subunit, γ. (From P R Schofield, M G Darlison, N Fujita, D R Burt, F A Stephenson, H Rodriguez, L M Rhee, J Ramachandran, V Reale, T A Glencorse, P H Seeburg, E A Barnard: Sequence and functional expression of the $GABA_A$ receptor shows a ligand-gated receptor super-family. Nature* 328: *221, 1987. Used with permission.)*

effects, including anticonvulsant, muscle-relaxant, hypnotic-amnestic, and anxiolytic effects. Benzodiazepines induce their characteristic behavioral effects in the same rank order with which they bind to benzodiazepine receptors and stimulate $GABA_A$-receptor-mediated current flow, suggesting that their behavioral effects are attributable to their actions at the GABA-benzodiazepine receptor. A paradigm that has proved to be particularly sensitive for identifying active benzodiazepine derivatives is the conflict test, in which animals are punished for simultaneously rewarded behavior. Active benzodiazepines decrease the animals' sensitivity to the punishment. The potency with which benzodiazepine derivatives induce anticonflict effects in animals correlates well with their antianxiety and sedative-hypnotic potency in humans.

Benzodiazepine receptors associated with the $GABA_A$-receptor complex have been subtyped on the basis of their affinity for the triazolopyridazine CL218,872 relative to benzodiazepines, such as diazepam. Receptors showing high affinity for CL218,872 relative to diazepam were termed type 1 or ω_1 receptors while those showing equal affinity were termed type 2 or ω_2 receptors. Type 1 receptors are enriched relative to type 2 receptors in cerebellum. It was therefore hoped that selective benzodiazepine derivatives could be developed that retained their anxiolytic potency while having less propensity for inducing ataxia. Recently, additional benzodiazepine receptor subtypes have been identified on the basis of pharmacological and cloning studies. Regional differences in the ability of GABA to potentiate benzodiazepine binding have also been reported, which suggests that not all $GABA_A$ receptors possess a functional benzodiazepine binding site.

Inverse agonists and antagonists An unusual property of benzodiazepine receptors is their ability to mediate both the inhibition and the potentiation of $GABA_A$-receptor activation. Inhibitory agents, such as the β-carbolines, are classified as inverse agonists of the benzodiazepine receptor. Such agents induce anxiogenic, proconvulsant, and antiamnestic (nootropic) effects. Benzodiazepine-receptor antagonists inhibit the effects of both agonists and inverse agonists, restoring $GABA_A$ activity to the unmodified state. The first such compound to be described, flumazenil (Ro 15-1788) (Mazicon), is currently available for the treatment of benzodiazepine overdose.

Peripheral benzodiazepine receptors The complexity of characterizing the molecular targets of drugs is illustrated by the case of the peripheral benzodiazepine (also called ω_3) receptor. Early receptor-binding studies revealed a benzodiazepine-binding site unrelated to the $GABA_A$ receptor complex. The researchers hoped that agents that target the benzodiazepine-binding site would exert clinically useful and antianxiety effects without inducing CNS depression. However, they subsequently found that the non-$GABA_A$-receptor-associated site is widely distributed outside the brain, as well as within it. Outside the CNS, the site was designated the peripheral site to distinguish it from the $GABA_A$-receptor-associated site, which was termed the central site. Within the brain, peripheral receptors are concentrated in glial cells, rather than neurons. Furthermore, peripheral benzodiazepine-binding sites interact with compounds from a wide variety of chemical classes, and the rank order of potency with which ligands bind to the peripheral receptor does not correlate with their clinical potency as antianxiety agents. Thus, the interaction of benzodiazepines with the peripheral binding site does not appear to be relevant to their clinical effects.

The peripheral site should not be confused with either the benzodiazepine type 1 or the benzodiazepine type 2 subtypes of the central ($GABA_A$-receptor-associated) benzodiazepine receptor. The possibility that side effects of some benzodiazepines, especially endocrine effects, reflect interactions with the peripheral binding site is currently being explored. Recent studies suggest that the peripheral site is selectively associated with mitochondria. Whether the peripheral binding site represents a true receptor in the sense that its occupation is associated with a specific physiological response remains to be determined.

$GABA_A$-RECEPTOR STRUCTURE Initial insights into $GABA_A$-receptor structure were derived from the purification of native rat brain receptors. Those studies showed that $GABA_A$ receptors contain distinct α, β, and γ subunits. Receptors containing two copies of each of the α and β subunits possess all the properties of the native receptor except that they do not allow functional gating by benzodiazepines. The addition of a γ subunit confers the additional benzodiazepine sensitivity.

Partial sequencing of purified subunits has permitted the use of molecular cloning techniques to identify the genetic structure of $GABA_A$ receptors. $GABA_A$-receptor subunits show a high degree of homology with each other and with subunits from glycine and nicotinic acetylcholine receptors, suggesting that they all derive from a common ancestor. All have a typical structure consisting of four membrane-spanning regions that form the walls of the central channel.

An unexpected finding of the cloning studies has been the multiplicity of isoforms for each of the subunits. To date, at least six distinct isoforms of the α subunit, four isoforms of the β subunit, and three isoforms of the γ subunit have been identified. The α subunits appear to be the most critical in determining the affinity of the complex for GABA and benzodiazepine; the γ subunits appear to be necessary for conferring functional benzodiazepine sensitivity.

Thus, only receptor complexes incorporating a γ_2 subunit show sensitivity to benzodiazepines. Among such complexes, those incorporating α_2, $_3$, or $_5$ isoforms of the α subunit express benzodiazepine receptors that correspond to the pharmacologically defined type 1 (or ω_1) subtype. Those incorporating the α_1 isoform express type 2 (or ω_2) benzodiazepine receptors. Those incorporating α_4 or α_6 isoforms express benzodiazepine receptors that differ pharmacologically from both type 1 and type 2 benzodiazepine receptors.

The different subunit isoforms are differentially expressed in the brain. For example, in rat brain the α_1 isoform is ubiquitously distributed, but the α_2, α_3, α_5, and α_6 isoforms are concentrated in the pyramidal and granule cells of the hippocampal formation. The γ subunits appear to have a more restricted distribution than the α and β subunits, confirming the physiological demonstration that $GABA_A$ receptors in some brain regions may not be regulated by benzodiazepine. On the basis of the number of subunit isoforms isolated to date, there are more than 5,000 possible structures for a $GABA_A$ receptor containing two α, two β, and one γ subunit. Moreover, other combinations of subunits may be possible. Which structures dominate in vivo remains to be determined. The heterogeneity of $GABA_A$-receptor structure between and within brain regions may permit the development of novel drugs that are selective for specific subclasses.

$GABA_B$ Receptors The second type of central nervous system GABA receptor, the $GABA_B$ receptor, differs from the $GABA_A$ receptor in both structure and function. $GABA_B$ receptors are part of the family of *metabotropic receptors*. Those receptors consist of a single subunit possessing seven transmembrane domains. Most monoaminergic receptors are also included in the metabotropic family. Rather than being intrinsically linked to an ionophore, the receptors are coupled to G-proteins, through which they regulate several ion channels and effector mechanisms. $GABA_B$ receptors are insensitive to muscimol and bicuculline but display a high affinity for the β-*p*-chlorophenyl derivative of GABA, baclofen.

$GABA_B$ receptors were first demonstrated presynaptically on sympathetic and parasympathetic nerve terminals, where they act to inhibit neurotransmitter release. Subsequently, they have been demonstrated presynaptically on glutamate and GABA terminals in the CNS and postsynaptically on hippocampal cell dendrites. The $GABA_B$ receptors that regulate presynaptic glutamate release appear to be pharmacologically distinct from those that act as autoreceptors at GABA terminals. Most CNS regions contain both $GABA_A$ and $GABA_B$ receptors. $GABA_B$ receptors are heavily concentrated relative to $GABA_A$ receptors in the dorsal horn of the spinal cord, accounting for the clinical effectiveness of baclofen in the treatment of spasticity. $GABA_A$ and $GABA_B$ receptors are also differentially localized in the cerebellum.

$GABA_B$ receptors interact with several types of G-proteins and may be coupled to several different effector mechanisms, possibly even within the same neuron. In the hippocampus, postsynaptic $GABA_B$ receptors activate a potassium channel, leading to a late, slow hyperpolarization that inhibits neuronal activity. $GABA_B$-receptor activation may also inhibit voltage-dependent calcium channels, leading to a shortening of the action potential and to decreased presynaptic neurotransmitter release. Finally, $GABA_B$ receptors may regulate cyclic nucleotide turnover, leading to the modulation of intracellular second-messenger cascades.

CLINICAL APPLICATIONS

Anxiolytics and sedative-hypnotics The majority of currently available anxiolytic and sedative-hypnotic agents induce their effects by augmenting $GABA_A$ receptor-mediated neurotransmission. Barbiturates act primarily at the GABA channel site, whereas benzodiazepines act at the $GABA_A$-receptor-associated benzodiazepine receptor. Zolipidem (Ambien), a recently developed sedative-hypnotic, is an imidazopyridine and not a member of the benzodiazepine class. However, like benzodiazepines, it mediates its effect at the GABA-benzodiazepine receptor. The difference in the mechanism by which barbiturates and benzodiazepines interact with the GABA-receptor complex may account for the difference in the side-effect profile and, in particular, the much higher lethality of barbiturate overdose. Other atypical antianxiety agents, such as buspirone (BuSpar), may alter $GABA_A$ receptor-mediated neurotransmission indirectly by acting at non-GABAergic receptors on GABAergic neurons.

Movement disorders The injection of excitotoxins into the striatum, which leads to the degeneration of GABAergic striatonigral feedback neurons, induces choreiform movements similar to those seen in Huntington's disease or tardive dyskinesia. A similar loss of GABAergic striatonigral neurons has been observed in monkeys following prolonged exposure to antipsychotics. It has therefore been proposed that the loss of inhibitory feedback regulation to the substantia nigra may be responsible for the development of tardive dyskinesia in antipsychotic-treated subjects. Attempts to reverse symptoms of tardive dyskinesia with GABAergic agents, however, have been inconclusive.

Schizophrenia Schizophrenia has been associated with a decreased number and abnormal distribution of GABA neurons in cortex, particularly in supragranular cortical laminae. GABAergic neurons that show immunoreactivity for NADPH diaphorase (NO synthase) may be particularly affected. Increased GABA-receptor density has also been demonstrated, which may represent receptor upregulation secondary to decreased presynaptic GABAergic availability. Barbiturates and benzodiazepines are commonly used adjunctive agents to antipsychotics in the treatment of schizophrenia. It is unclear, however, whether such agents have specific antischizophrenic actions or whether their beneficial effects are solely related to their anxiolytic and sedative-hypnotic actions.

INHIBITORY AMINO ACIDS: GLYCINE

Glycine is the simplest amino acid in structure. Nutritionally classified as a nonessential amino acid, it comprises up to 5 percent of dietary protein. Glycine is a necessary intermediate in several metabolic pathways throughout the body. The vast metabolic pool of glycine contrasts with its sharply circumscribed role as a neurotransmitter. Glycine interacts with two distinct CNS systems: the inhibitory glycine receptor (termed the strychnine-sensitive glycine receptor because strychnine is its prototypical antagonist) is discussed here; the nonstrychnine-sensitive glycine-recognition site of the *N*-methyl-D-aspartate receptor is covered in the discussion of glutamate.

EVIDENCE FOR NEUROTRANSMITTER ROLE Glycine was first proposed to be a spinal inhibitory neurotransmitter on the basis of its enrichment in spinal gray matter relative to spinal roots or the brain as a whole. In spinal gray matter glycine is also present at higher concentration than are most other amino acids. Furthermore, the content of glycine in spinal gray matter but not that of other amino acids correlates with the number of interneurons remaining after ischemic damage to the cord. Although glycine is not specifically localized to synaptosomes (pinched-off nerve endings derived from fractionated neuronal tissue by differential centrifugation) or synaptic vesicles, it is found in high concentrations relative to other amino acids in a specific population of synaptosomes derived from the medulla and the spinal cord. Iontophoretically administered glycine decreases the excitability of spinal motor neurons and interneurons but not of cortical neurons. Furthermore, the application of glycine to the spinal cord mimics the effect of stimulation of the inhibitory interneurons.

PRESYNAPTIC MECHANISMS

Synthesis and metabolism Serine, which itself can be formed from glucose, is the chief precursor of glycine in nervous tissue through the enzyme serine transhydroxymethylase, which, together with D-glycerate dehydrogenase, is the best candidate for the rate-limiting enzyme governing CNS glycine synthesis. Glycine can also be formed from glyoxylate by a transaminase reaction with glutamate.

Transport into CNS Like other small amino acids—such as alanine, proline, and GABA—glycine does not readily penetrate into the CNS through the blood-brain barrier. By contrast, transport of glycine from the cerebrospinal fluid (CSF) to the blood is rapid and efficient. Thus, entry of glycine into the CNS depends on passive diffusion, and elevation of CNS levels can occur only when concentrations outside the CNS are significantly increased over their baseline physiological levels.

High-affinity synaptosomal uptake Sodium-dependent high-affinity uptake of glycine into synaptosomes has been demonstrated in both the neurons and the glia of central nervous tissue. High-affinity glycine uptake has been shown in the cortex, the cerebellum, the hypothalamus, the retina, the spinal cord, and the brainstem. Labeled glycine taken up through that system can be subsequently released by electrical or potassium stimulation.

POSTSYNAPTIC MECHANISMS

Strychnine-sensitive glycine receptor The glycine receptor gates a chloride channel. It is a ligand-gated channel that shares significant sequence homology and predicted transmembrane topology with subunits of the nicotinic acetylcholine receptor and with subunits of the $GABA_A$ receptor.

The glycine receptor consists of two homologous integral membrane-spanning polypeptide subunits termed α (48 kd_a) and β (58 kd_a). The ligand-binding site is on the α subunit. The glycine receptor is associated with a distinct 93 kd_a protein localized to the cytoplasmic face of glycinergic postsynaptic membranes, whose function is thought to involve synaptic topography or anchoring of the glycine receptor to cytoskeletal components.

The native glycine receptor has been deduced to be an $\alpha_3\beta_2$ oligopentamer surrounding the central pore defining the ion channel (Figure 1.4-7), consistent with the requirement of multiple molecules of glycine to activate the associated channel. A pentameric complex of transmembrane polypeptides around a central pore has been proposed as the fundamental quarternary structure defining the superfamily of ligand-gated channels.

Within the past several years considerable evidence for the heterogeneity of the glycine receptor has emerged. In rodent development, a neonatal spinal-cord isoform is present for two to three weeks after birth; the isoform displays reduced affinity for strychnine and a structurally distinct α subunit compared with the adult isoform. Recently, molecular cloning techniques have revealed the existence of multiple distinct glycine receptor α subunit genes. In addition to the originally described α subunit (now termed α_1), four variants have been described. The α_2 and α_{2*} variants are ligand-binding subunits of neonatal glycine receptors; α_3 and α_4 are expressed postnatally, the latter at very low levels. Functional expression in *Xenopus* oocytes has shown that rat or human α_1, α_2, or α_3 transcripts all result in the expression of glycine receptors that are blocked by strychnine at nanomolar concentrations; a rat α_{2*} variant sequence results in the expression of channels with a 500-fold weaker affinity for strychnine. That dramatic difference in strychnine sensitivity was shown on the basis of a single glycine-to-glutamate exchange within the α_2 polypeptide. Post-transcriptional processing as a mechanism governing glycine receptor heterogeneity has been shown in the form of alternative splicing of α subunits.

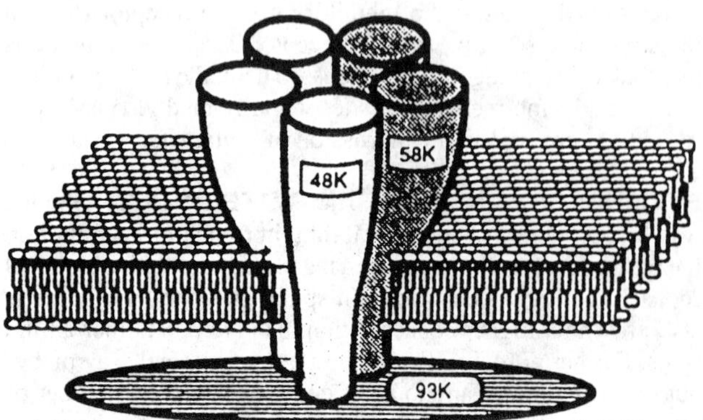

FIGURE 1.4-7 *Structure of the strychnine-sensitive glycine receptor complex, showing the subunit arrangement. (From D Langosch, C-M Becker, H Betz: The inhibitory glycine receptor: A ligand-gated chloride channel of the central nervous system. Eur J Biochem* 194: *1, 1990. Used with permission.)*

Pharmacology Agonists of the glycine receptor include both α-amino acids and β-amino acids. Among those, glycine itself is the most potent agonist, followed by β-alanine, taurine, L-alanine, L-serine, and proline. The known potent glycine receptor antagonists, displaying nanomolar affinities for the receptor, are strychnine, a plant alkaloid; RU5135, a steroid; and 1,5-diphenyl-3,7-diazaadamantan-9-ol. Behaviorally, blockade of the glycine receptor by antagonists produces hyperexcitation and convulsions. Biochemical characterization of the glycine receptor was initially achieved by means of a radioreceptor assay using [^{3}H]strychnine. The sodium-independent binding of that antagonist was displaced, apparently competitively, by agonist amino acids in rank order of their physiological potencies. Biochemical differences indicate that, although the binding domains of strychnine and glycine share considerable overlap, they are not identical.

Anatomical Distribution Quantitative autoradiographic studies of glycine receptors labeled with [^{3}H]strychnine autoradiography in mammalian CNS sections have uniformly shown a sharply limited regional distribution of the glycine receptor, with high levels found in the spinal cord and the brainstem. As increasingly sensitive and specific molecular probes have become available, that classical distribution has been called into question. For example, immunocytochemistry using monoclonal antibodies against the α-subunit antigen and the glycine-receptor-associated protein demonstrated low but significant immunoreactivity to be present in the olfactory bulb, the midbrain, the cerebellum, the spinal cord, and the brainstem. Recently, the use of a new monoclonal antibody directed against an epitope common to α subunit variants has revealed immunoreactivity in a number of high brain regions, including the cortex. The application of sequence-specific oligonucleotides for in situ hybridization in rat brain has shown that—although α_1 transcripts are found in the spinal cord, the brainstem and the colliculi—α_2 messenger ribonucleic acid (mRNA) is also detected in the hippocampus, the cortex, and the thalamus, and α_3 mRNA is detected in the olfactory bulb, the hippocampus, and the cerebellum. By contrast, β-subunit transcripts are expressed throughout the brain and the spinal cord. The basis of the marked discrepancy among anatomical distributions of β subunits, α subunits, and [^{3}H]strychnine binding is unknown. In principle, there could exist as yet unidentified α-subunit variants, or the β subunit may also be a component of ligand-gated channels other than the glycine receptor.

SUGGESTED CROSS-REFERENCES

Further information about the neuroanatomy of specific excitatory and inhibitory projections can be found in Section 1.2 on neuroanatomy. Further information on the receptor transduction mechanisms can be found in Section 1.7 on electrophysiology. Information regarding the contributions of specific cortical regions and pathways in schizophrenia can be found in Section 14.3 on brain structure and function and Section 14.4 on neurochemical, vital, and immunological studies in schizophrenia. The role of GABA benzodiazepine receptors in mood disorders is discussed in Chapter 16, and their role in anxiety disorders is discussed in Chapter 17. The clinical use of benzodiazepines is discussed in Section 32.7. The clinical use of

GABAergic agents in the treatment of epilepsy is discussed in Section 2.3 on neuropsychiatric aspects of epilepsy. For other drugs used to treat epilepsy see Section 32.11 on carbamazepine and Section 32.35 on valproate.

REFERENCES

*Akbarian S, Vinuela A, Kim J J, Potkin S G, Bunney W E Jr, Jones E G: Distorted distribution of nicotinamide-adenine dinucleotide phosphate-diaphorase neurons in temporal lobe of schizophrenics implies anomalous cortical development. Arch Gen Psychiatry *50:* 178, 1993.

Benes F M, Sorensen I, Vincent S L, Bird E D, Sathi M. Increased density of glutamate-immunoreactive processes in superficial laminae in cingulate cortex of schizophrenic brain. Cereb Cortex *2:* 503, 1992.

Benes F M, McSparren J, Bird E D, SanGiovanni J P, Vincent S L: Deficit in small interneurons in prefrontal and cingulate cortices of schizophrenic and schizoaffective patients. Arch Gen Psychiatry *48:* 996, 1991.

Benes F M, Vincent S L, Alsterberg G, Bird E D, SanGiovanni J P: Increased $GABA_A$ receptor binding in superficial layers of cingulate cortex in schizophrenics. J Neurosci *12:* 924, 1992.

Betz H: Glycine receptors: Heterogeneous and widespread in the mammalian brain. Trends Neurosci *14:* 458, 1991.

Betz H: Ligand-gated ion channels in the brain: The amino acid receptor superfamily. Neuron *5:* 383, 1990.

Biggio G, Costa E, editors: GABA and benzodiazepine receptor subtypes. Adv Biochem Psychopharmacol *46:* 1990.

Biggio G, Concas A, Costa E, editors: GABAergic synaptic transmission. Adv Biochem Psychopharmacol *47:* 22, 1992.

Bittiger H, Froestl W, Mickel S J, Olpe H-R. $GABA_B$ receptor antagonists: from synthesis to therapeutic applications. Trends Pharmacol Sci *14:* 391, 1993.

Burt D B, Kamatchi G L: $GABA_A$ receptor subtypes: From pharmacology to molecular biology. FASEB J *5:* 2916, 1991.

Carlsson M, Carlsson A: Interactions between glutamatergic and monoaminergic systems within the basal ganglia—implications for schizophrenia and Parkinson's disease. Trends Neurosci *13:* 272, 1990.

Cooper J R, Bloom F E, Roth R H: *The Biochemical Basis of Neuropharmacology.* Oxford University Press, New York, 1991.

Daly E C, Aprison M H: Glycine. In *Handbook of Neurochemistry,* A Lajtha, editor, vol 3, p 467. Plenum Press, New York, 1982.

Dawson V L, Dawson T M, London E D, Bredt D S, Snyder S H: Nitric oxide mediates glutamate neurotoxicity in primary cortical cultures. Proc Natl Acad Sci U S A *88:* 6368, 1991.

Dingledine R: New wave of non-NMDA excitatory amino acid receptors. Trends Pharmacol Sci *12:* 360, 1991.

Guastella J, Nelson N, Nelson H, Czyzyk L, Keynan S, Miedal M C, Davidson N, Lester H A, Kanner B I: Cloning and expression of a rat brain GABA transporter. Science *249:* 1303, 1990.

Hattori H, Wasterlain C G: Excitatory amino acids in the developing brain: ontogeny, plasticity and excitotoxicity. Ped Neurol *6:* 219, 1990.

Ikeda K, Nagasawa M, Mori H, Araki K, Sakimura K, Watanabe M, Inoue Y, Mishina M: Cloning and expression of the ε4 subunit of the NMDA receptor channel. FEBS Letters *313:* 34, 1992.

Ishii T, Moriyoshi K, Sugihara H, Sakurada K, Kadotani H, Yokoi M, Akazawa C, Shigemoto R, Mizuno N, Masu M, Nakanishi S: Molecular characterization of the family of the *N*-methyl-D-aspartate receptor subunits. J Biol Chem *268:* 2836, 1993.

*Javitt D C, Zukin S R: Recent advances in the phencyclidine model of schizophrenia. Am J Psychiatry *148:* 1301, 1991.

Javitt D C, Zukin S R: The role of excitatory amino acids in neuropsychiatric illness. J Neuropsychiatr Clin Neurosci *2:* 44, 1990.

*Javitt D C, Zylberman I, Zukin S R, Heresco-Levy U, Lindenmayer J P: Amelioration of negative symptoms in schizophrenia by glycine. Am J Psychiatry *151:* 1234, 1994.

*Kandel E R, Schwartz J H: Directly gated transmission at central synapses. In *Principles of Neural Science,* ed 3, E R Kandel, J H Schwartz, T M Jessel, editors, p 153. Elsevier, New York, 1991.

*Krystal J H, Karper L P, Seibyl J P, Freeman G K, Delaney R, Bremner J D, Heninger G R, Bowers M B Jr, Charney D S: Subanesthetic effects of the noncompetitive NMDA antagonist, ketamine, in humans. Psychotomimetic, perceptual, cognitive and neuroendocrine responses. Arch Gen Psychiatry *51:* 199, 1994.

Kuhse J, Becker C-M, Schmieden V, Hoch W, Pribilla I, Langosch D, Malosio M-L, Muntz M, Betz H: Heterogeneity of the inhibitory glycine receptor. Ann N Y Acad Sci *625:* 129, 1991.

Kvamme E, editor: *Glutamine and Glutamate in Mammals.* CRC Press, Boca Raton, Fla, 1988.

Langosch D, Becker C-M, Betz H: The inhibitory glycine receptor: A ligand-gated chloride channel of the central nervous system. Eur J Biochem *194:* 1, 1990.

McGeer P L, McGeer E G: Amino acid neurotransmitters. In *Basic Neurochemistry: Molecular, Cellular, and Medical Aspects,* G J Siegel, B W Agranoff, R W Albers, P B Molinoff, editors, p 311. Raven Press, New York, 1989.

Meguro H, Mori H, Araki K, Kushiya E, Kutsuwada T, Yamazaki M, Kumanishi T, Arakawa M, Sakimura K, Mishina M: Functional characterization of a heteromeric NMDA receptor channel expressed from cloned cDNAs. Nature *357:* 70, 1992.

Miller R J: Metabotropic excitatory amino acid receptors reveal their true colors. Trends Pharmacol Sci *12:* 365, 1991.

Monyer H, Sprengle R, Shoepfer R, Herb A, Higuchi M, Lomeli H, Burnashev N, Sakmann B and Seeburg P H: Heteromeric NMDA receptors: Molecular and functional distinction of subtypes. Science *256:* 1217, 1992.

Moriyoshi K, Masayuki M, Ishii T, Shigemoto R, Mizuno N, Nakanishi S: Molecular cloning and characterization of the rat NMDA receptor. Nature *354:* 31, 1991.

Olney J W: Excitotoxic amino acids and neuropsychiatric disorders. Annu Rev Pharmacol Toxicol *30:* 47, 1991.

Schofield P R, Darlison M G, Fujita N, Burt D R, Stephenson F A, Rodriguez H, Rhee L M, Ramachandran J, Reale V, Glencorse T A, Seeburg P H, Barnard E A: Sequence and functional expression of the $GABA_A$ receptor shows a ligand-gated receptor super-family. Nature *328:* 221, 1987.

Schwartz J H, Kandel E R: Synaptic transmission mediated by second messengers. In *Principles of Neural Science,* ed 3, E R Kandel, J H Schwartz, T M Jessel, editors, p 173. Elsevier, New York, 1991.

Seeburg P H: The TINS/TIPS Lecture: The molecular biology of mammalian glutamate receptor channels. Trends Neurosci *16:* 359, 1993.

Squires R F, editor: *GABA and Benzodiazepine Receptors.* CRC Press, Boca Raton, Fla, 1988.

Squires R F, Saedrup E: A review of evidence for GABAergic predominance/glutamatergic deficit as a common etiological factor in both schizophrenia and affective psychoses: more support for a continuum hypothesis of "functional" psychosis. Neurochem Res *16:* 1099, 1991.

Westbrook G L: Glutamate receptors and excitotoxicity. Res Publ Assoc Res Nerv Ment Dis *71:* 35, 1993.

Yamakura, T, Mori H, Masaki H, Shinoji K, Mishina M: Different sensitivities of NMDA receptor channel subtypes to noncompetitive antagonists. NeuroReport *4:* 689, 1993.

1.5
NEUROPEPTIDES: BIOLOGY AND REGULATION

GARTH BISSETTE, Ph.D.
CHARLES B. NEMEROFF, M.D., Ph.D.

INTRODUCTION

A neuropeptide, by definition, is a chain of two or more amino acids linked by peptide bonds and differs from other proteins only in the length of the amino acid chain. Over 100 unique biologically active peptide sequences have been purified from biological sources; their sizes range from two (carnosine and anserine) to over 40 amino acids (corticotropin-releasing factor [CRF] and growth hormone-releasing factor [GRF]). Most of the other known active peptides fall within these size limits. By convention peptides greater than 90 amino acids in length (about 10,000 daltons) are considered proteins. The principal examples discussed here are drawn from five different peptides. Their structures are shown in Table 1.5-1, and are written by convention from the amino terminus beginning on the left to the carboxyl terminus on the right. Those peptides are somatostatin (somatotropin release-inhibiting factor [SRIF]), thyrotropin releasing hormone (TRH), neurotensin, neuromedin N, and

TABLE 1.5-1
Selected Neuropeptide Structures

Name	Amino Acid Sequence
Thyrotropin-releasing hormone (TRH)	pGlu-His-Pro-NH_2 1 2
Somatostatin (SRIF-28)	NH_2-Ser-Ala-Asn-Ser-Asn-Pro-Ala-Met-Ala-Pro-Arg-Glu Arg Lys 1 SRIF-14 HO-Cys-Ser-Thr-Phe-Thr-Lys-Trp-Phe-Phe-Asn-Lys-Cys-Gly-Ala 4 5 4 5
Neurotensin	pGlu-Leu-Tyr-Glu-Asn-Lys-Pro-Arg-Arg-Pro-Tyr-Ile-Leu-OH 2 5 6 7
Neuromedin N	NH_2-Lys-Ile-Pro-Tyr-Ile-Leu-OH 4 4 6 7
Corticotropin-releasing factor (CRF) Rat/Human	Ser-Glu-Glu-Pro-Pro-Ile-Ser-Leu-Asp-Leu-Thr-Phe-His- Leu-Leu-Arg-Glu-Val-Leu-Glu-Met-Ala-Arg-Ala-Glu-Gln-Leu- Ala-Gln-Gln-Ala-His-Ser-Asn-Arg-Lys-Leu-Met-Glu-Ile-Ile-NH_2

Subscript numbers refer to points of known peptidase cleavage
1. Pyroglutamate aminopeptidase (E.C.-3.4.19.3)
2. Post Proline endopeptidase (E.C. 3.4.21.26)
3. Carboxypeptidase E (E.C. 3.4.17.10)
4. Metalloendopeptidase (E.C. 3.4.24.15)
5. Neutral endopeptidase (E.C. 3.4.24.11)
6. Metalloendopeptidase (E.C. 3.4.24.16)

CRF. Somatostatin, CRF, and TRH are hypothalamic-hypophysiotropic substances and, like neurotensin and neuromedin N, function in the central nervous system (CNS) as neurotransmitters or neuromodulators in ways that are often quite distinct from their effects on the endocrine axes. Neuropeptides have been implicated as chemical mediators in pathways subserving a variety of behavioral and physiological effects, including such diverse behaviors as thermoregulation, food and water consumption, sex, sleep, locomotion, memory, learning, and responses to stress and pain. Those actions have stimulated interest in the contribution of the peptidergic neuronal systems to the production of the symptoms and behaviors exhibited in such major psychiatric illnesses as psychoses, mood disorders, and dementias. In addition to their endocrine and neurotransmitter roles, many peptides and their receptors play active roles in development and often appear transiently in various anatomical regions or in such abundance that a trophic effect is postulated, an effect that does not necessarily remain once early development has been achieved. An example of this ontogenetic shift in concentrations is found in the distribution of messenger ribonucleic acid (mRNA) for somatostatin in developing rats. The mRNA exhibits more regional heterogeneity in developing rats than it does in adult animals, with the hypothalamic mRNA concentrations being much higher than the cerebrocortical expression.

Many of the known behavioral effects of neuropeptides are observed only after their direct injection into the CNS because most peptides apparently do not cross the blood-brain barrier in amounts sufficient to produce effects before being inactivated by serum and tissue enzymes that degrade them. The degradation is usually the result of the cleavage of specific amino acid sequences targeted by a specific peptidase designed for that purpose. Peptide fragments often possess full or partial biological activity at receptors and the relatively lengthy period of peptide-induced effects may be attributable to this delayed cessation of activity. The amount of neuropeptide that must be injected to elicit a physiological or behavioral effect is often criticized because endogenous neuropeptides exist in picomolar to femtomolar concentrations whereas nanomolar concentrations are often required to produce such effects. Such differences should be expected, however, when it is realized that the anatomical substrate mediating the behavior or effect may be quite far from the site of injection, that the preexisting endogenous peptide signal and its regulatory and feedback systems must be overwhelmed, and that a gauntlet of peptidases must be negotiated. Another disconcerting fact about neuropeptides is the propensity for a property or effect to be elicited by one or more apparently unrelated peptides. Although often frustrating and potentially confounding to researchers, that property can be explained by the ability of more than one sequence of amino acids to assume similar three-dimensional shapes and charge distributions, all of which may be recognized by the receptor, by the presence of multiple receptor types contained on neurons initiating the behavior and by possible similarities between second messenger transduction mechanisms activated by discrete and distinct peptide receptor types. This reliance on the tertiary structure for recognition is also used by the immune system, as well as by biological receptors. Because both descriptive (immunohistochemical) and quantitative (radioimmunoassay) methods for detecting the small concentrations of endogenous peptides rely on the immune system, it is always possible that a similarly shaped structure could confound the interpretation of immunoassay results. Thus descriptions of antisera specificity and amount of cross-reactivity with other potential ligands are critical to the proper evaluation of results. The dichotomy in methodology for detecting neuronal localization of peptide versus regional peptide concentration is also seen in the tools for peptide receptor identification by autoradiography (localization) and regional membrane preparations for receptor quantification (''grind and bind''). The analogous procedures for detecting peptide mRNA are *in situ* hybridization (localization) and Northern blot analysis or the polymerase chain reaction for regional mRNA quantification. All of the regional quantification techniques depend on dissection for ultimate detection resolution. Measurements of neuropeptide concentration changes do not indicate which of several mechanisms may be mediating the observed changes. Increases in concentration may represent increased synthesis and release, decreased release with continued synthesis, or decreased degradation. Attempts to verify peptide turnover may be made if the mRNA concentration, peptide concentration, receptor up-down-regulation, and degradative activity are known. Although methods to achieve each of these goals are now available, they have not yet been applied in combination to the same tissue sample.

Whereas the differences between neuropeptides and the classic chemical and amino acid neurotransmitters are often striking, their CNS effects are similar in that they primarily excite or inhibit discrete neurons upon direct application. As both of these effects may be observed among neurons from the same region, effects observed in one location cannot be generalized to either immediate or distal neurons. However, the onset of activity is often delayed for neuropeptides (seconds) as compared with the classic transmitters (milliseconds), whereas the duration of activity is relatively delayed for neuropeptides (minutes) as compared with most of the chemical and amino acid transmitters (seconds).

DISTRIBUTION

Neuropeptides are found throughout the CNS, as well as in various peripheral organs, such as the digestive tract, pancreas, and adrenal glands. Many CNS peptides, such as neurotensin and somatostatin, play dual roles in the brain and gut. The full extent of any communication between the CNS and gut systems employing the same peptide is not known with certainty, but may be considerable. Most of the CNS neuropeptides have been found predominately in neurons, but peptide receptors have been reported in glia.

Neuropeptides were originally purified from hypothalamic extracts and thus it is not surprising that some of the highest concentrations of certain neuropeptides are found in the hypothalamus. This is true for all four of the example peptides: TRH, CRF, somatostatin, and neurotensin. Those and many other neuropeptides also are widely distributed beyond the hypothalamus and may occur in either intrinsic interneurons or in longer projection neurons.

Immunohistochemical and retrograde tracing studies have focused on the locations and morphological types of the various neurons containing somatostatin. In the hypothalamus most of the somatostatin neurons terminating in the median eminence have been shown to have cell bodies mainly in the rostral periventricular nucleus, with some in the paraventricular nucleus and none in the arcuate nucleus. Thus the other hypothalamic regions (arcuate, suprachiasmatic, ventromedial) containing somatostatin neurons probably do not project to the median eminence and may be performing a regulatory or feedback function on neurons containing other hypothalamic releasing factors, such as GRF, CRF, TRH, or their afferents. In the cortex of rats somatostatin is found in some of the large stellate-shaped neurons and in abundance among the fusiform-shaped, nonpyramidal neurons of layers II to V, and particularly in layer V of the sensory cortex. In monkeys, however, layer III is where somatostatin is predominately located in visual, auditory, or association cortex, and cortical neurons containing somatostatin are usually oriented vertically in layers II to V and horizontally in layer VI. In human entorhinal cortex somatostatin neurons are abundant in the white matter underlying the cortex and are relatively uniformly distributed throughout the cortical layers, being absent only in the outer molecular layer. A recent comparison of human and monkey distribution of the prosomatostatin-derived peptides SRIF-28, SRIF-14, and SRIF-$28^{1\text{-}12}$ in the precortex found reduced staining of SRIF-28 in unperfused monkeys and human brain obtained five hours after death, indicating that the processing of peptides may continue after death unless halted biochemically. In the rat striatum somatostatin is extensively colocalized in neuropeptide Y-containing neurons, and although not influenced by lesions of the dopamine neurons innervating the striatum, somatostatin concentrations are increased by the destruction of cortical inputs. In the human hippocampus somatostatin neurons are arranged in a manner similar to that in rats and nonhuman primates, with cell bodies in the deep layers of the dentate gyrus producing fibers that terminate in the outer two thirds of the molecular layer. In the basal forebrain region of nonhuman primates, somatostatin is contained within small neurons of the nucleus basalis, which apparently communicate with the cholinergic neurons there. Those data indicate that the neuronal cell types and afferent and efferent connections of somatostatin-containing neurons vary widely among the different regions of the brain and that species differences occur with enough frequency to make direct extrapolations between species difficult.

Many neuropeptides have now been shown to be colocalized in neurons that also contain classic transmitters, other neuropeptides, or both. Neurotensin is found in neurons containing the dopamine synthetic enzyme tyrosine hydroxylase in the ventral tegmental area (VTA) and arcuate nucleus of the hypothalamus of rats. Recently this colocalization was shown to contain neurotensin in dense-core vesicles only in tyrosine hydroxylase staining cell bodies in the VTA whereas other nerve terminals that were stained for neurotensin did not contain tyrosine hydroxylase. That evidence is in disagreement with other evidence showing decreases in both dopamine and neurotensin after reserpine and the dual release of frontal cortex dopamine and neurotensin after electrical stimulation of the median forebrain bundle. Another subset of VTA neurons projecting to the frontal cortex has been shown to contain neurotensin, cholecystokinin (CCK), and tyrosine hydroxylase. Many other examples of colocalization have been cited, including reports of three to six peptides in a single neuron. TRH colocalization with another peptide, substance P, and a classic transmitter, serotonin, has been described for a population of neurons on the medial raphe nucleus and spinal cord. Corticotropin-releasing factor has been reported to be colocalized with three other neuropeptides (vasopressin, oxytocin, and neurotensin) in some neurons of the paraventricular nucleus of the hypothalamus in both rats and humans. Somatostatin has been found in γ-aminobutyric acid (GABA) neurons of the thalamus of cats and the cortex of rats and with neuropeptide Y in the striatum, hippocampus, and cortex. Colocalization reports may be more species specific than is generally realized, as the neurotensin-dopamine colocalization in the frontal cortex recently was noted to be absent in humans.

The two main methods for mapping peptides, immunohistochemistry and radioimmunoassay, are complementary in their determination of neuropeptide locations and concentrations, respectively, but they do not indicate which immunoreactive neuronal cell bodies are connected to the various immunoreactive terminal regions. Through the use of retrograde tracing methods and dual staining techniques, several pathways for certain peptides have now been delineated. They include projections of amygdala neurons containing neurotensin, somatostatin, or CRF to the parabrachial nucleus of the mesencephalon, and a neurotensin-containing projection from the lateral parabrachial nucleus back to the central amygdala has also been described. Two other neurotensin projections that have been observed in rats are those from the VTA to the nucleus accumbens and from the endopiriform nucleus and prepiriform cortex to the diagonal band area. This methodology has also led to the identification of TRH neurons in the paraventricular nucleus and bed nucleus of the stria terminalis as the origin of projections to the median eminence and septum, respectively. Lesion studies with excitotoxic amino acids or electrocoagulation have also demonstrated putative connections between discrete anatomical loci, such as the increased TRH immunoreactive concentrations in the nucleus of the solitary tract after bilateral electrolytic lesions of the TRH-containing paraventricular nucleus in rats. Although such work is beginning to elucidate the neuropeptide wiring diagram in mammalian brain, the association between discrete anatomical pathways containing a neuropeptide and the behaviors or effects observed after neuropeptide administration remains nascent. One of the best examples of this kind of association is seen in the response of CRF neuronal systems to stressful stimuli. The distribution of CRF neurons in the rat CNS is illustrated in Figure 1.5-1. In that paradigm radioimmunoassay studies have documented increased CRF content in the locus ceruleus and decreased CRF concentrations in the median eminence after a regimen of acute or chronic stress in rats. Other studies have shown that CRF-containing nerve terminals impinge upon noradrenergic neurons of the locus ceruleus and that exogenous CRF applied to those neurons increases their firing rate. Some of the noradrenergic locus ceruleus neurons, in turn, project to the hypothalamic paraventricular nucleus where their input increases CRF synthesis and release. Because CRF injection into the locus ceruleus elicits fearful or anxious behavior, one could postulate that the stress paradigm activates the CRF neurons terminating in the locus ceruleus noradrenergic neurons and that the increased CRF content in the locus represents an increased release of the CRF in this region onto the noradrenergic cell bodies. One can further postulate that the resulting increased noradrenergic signal, and perhaps other inputs to the paraventricular nucleus of the hypothalamus, mediates the stress-induced increased release of CRF from the median eminence, which is detected as decreased CRF concentrations. Thus, both an observed increase and decrease in regional CRF content can be hypothesized as resulting from an increased release of CRF with or without concomitant new synthesis of CRF to replace the released peptide. An alternative explanation for the apparent decrease in median eminence amounts of CRF after stress versus increased amounts in the locus ceruleus is that they are both released, but the CRF released from the median eminence is removed by the pituitary portal system whereas that in the locus ceruleus remains in the tissue that is dissected.

BIOSYNTHESIS

The biosynthesis of neuropeptides involves the transcription of mRNA sequences from DNA templates contained on the appropriate genes. In the past 10 years the application of molecular biological techniques has allowed the genes of many of the various peptides to be cloned and the complementary DNA probes constructed that allow mapping of the regions where the mRNA's coding for the peptide prohormone is located. A good example of the exploitation of such techniques is provided by TRH. Although TRH was the first of the hypothalamic releasing factors to be chemically identified, the TRH precursor was the last of the releasing-factor prohormones to be described. The gene for TRH in humans resides on chromosome 3; in the rat it consists of three exons (coding regions) separated by two introns (noncoded sequences). The first exon contains the 5′ untranslated end of the mRNA encoding the TRH preprohormone, the second exon contains the signal sequence and much

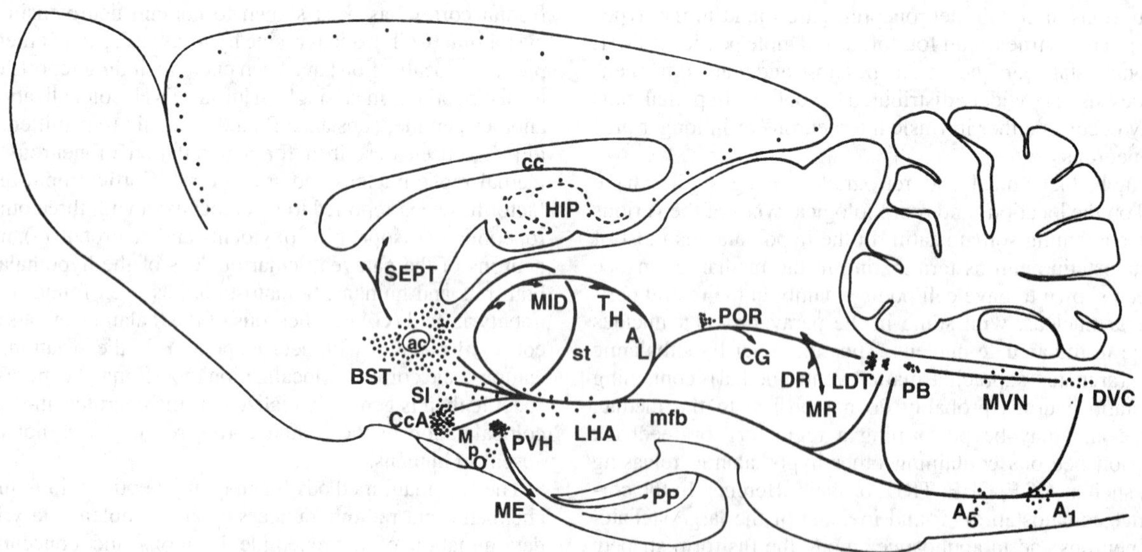

FIGURE 1.5-1 *Major CRF-stained cell groups (dots) and fiber systems in the rat brain. CC = corpus callosum; HIP = hippocampus; SEPT = septal region; AC = anterior commissure; BST = bed nucleus of the stria terminalis; SI = substantia innominata; CcA = central nucleus of the amygdala; MPO = medial preoptic area; PVH = PVN of hypothalamus; ME = median eminence; PP = posterior pituitary; LHA = lateral hypothalamic area; mfb = median forebrain bundle; MID THAL = midline thalamic nuclei; ST = stria terminalis; POR = perioculomotor nucleus; CG = central gray; DR = dorsal raphe; MR = median raphe; LDT = laterodorsal tegmental nucleus; LC = locus ceruleus; PB = parabrachial nucleus; MVN = medial vestibular nucleus; DVC = dorsal vagal complex; A_5, A_1 = noradrenergic cell groups. (Figure from L W Swanson, P E Sawchenko, J River, W W Vale: Organization of ovine corticotropin-releasing factor immunoreactive cells and fibers in the rat brain: An immunohistochemical study. Neuroendocrinology* 36: *165, 1983. Used with permission.)*

of the remaining amino terminal end of the precursor peptide, and the third contains the remainder of the sequence, including five copies of the TRH precursor sequence, the carboxy terminal region, and the 3′ untranslated region. Regions in the 5′ flanking sequence correspond to promoter regions and have sequence homologies with a glucocorticoid receptor binding site and the thyrotropin β subunit gene that may regulate the expression of the TRH gene. Although some disagreement about the sizes of the TRH precursors currently exists, the TRH prohormone has been mapped immunohistochemically to regions previously shown to exhibit TRH-containing cell bodies, including the paraventricular nucleus of the hypothalamus and the raphe nuclei, whereas the axons and terminals that have been identified as containing TRH do not stain as intensely for the precursor.

The neurotensin-neuromedin N gene was originally cloned from canine ileal mucosa, and complementary deoxyribonucleic acid (DNA) probes constructed against this form were used to clone the rat gene. The rat gene contains four exon sequences separated by three introns and spans approximately 10.2 kilobases. The neurotensin-neuromedin N sequence is contained in the fourth exon and the single copies of each peptide sequence are separated by a pair of dibasic residues. In pheochromocytoma (PC-12) neurons in culture, the neurotensin-neuromedin N gene is regulated by lithium, nerve growth factor, cyclic adenosine monophosphate (AMP) activators, and dexamethasone through their effects on a 5′ cis-regulating region. The distribution of the neurotensin-neuromedin N mRNA is generally the same as described for neurotensin-containing neuronal cell bodies, except in the hippocampus and subiculum, where few neurons stain immunohistochemically for neurotensin and yet an abundant amount of the neurotensin-neuromedin N mRNA is found.

The role of 5′ regulatory sequences on peptide genes has been well described for the somatostatin gene. The regulatory region in the somatostatin gene is upstream from the sequence coding the somatostatin mRNA and contains the palindrome sequence of eight base pairs that is found in other genes regulated by cyclic AMP. The promoter region acts on the downstream sequence as an enhancer for transcription and exhibits both distance and orientation sensitivity for the sequence being enhanced. This cyclic AMP response element demonstrates recognition sites for protein kinases A and C and casein kinase II, which may, in turn, regulate that activity.

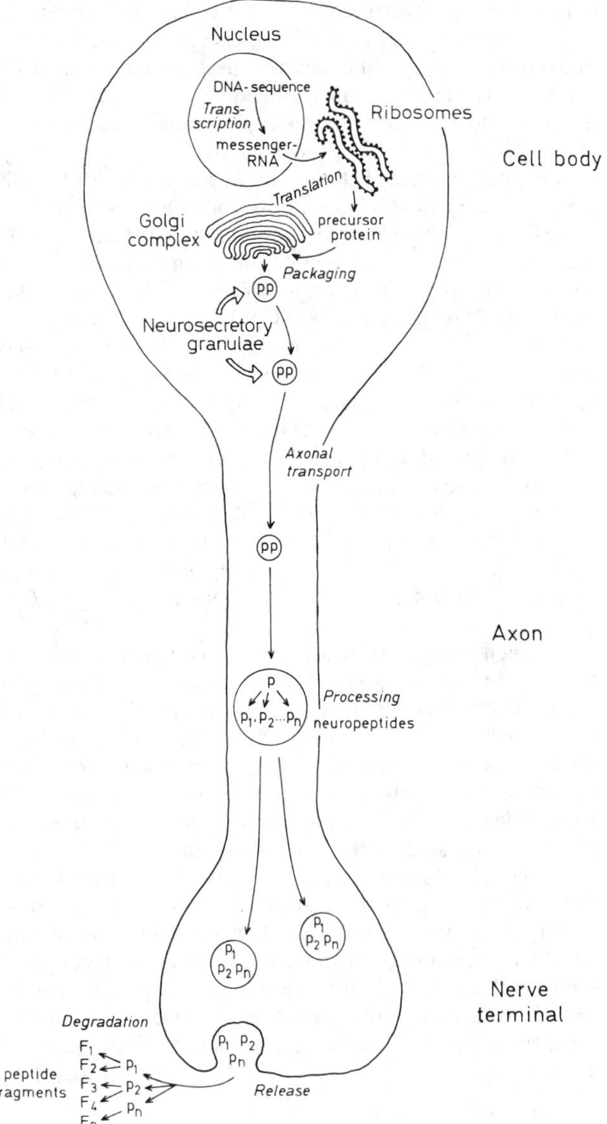

FIGURE 1.5-2 *The peptide neuron. The figure shows the main steps in the chain of events from the information stored in the DNA molecule to the peripherally detected peptide fragments. The DNA sequence in the nucleus is transcribed to the mRNA molecule for further transport to the endoplasmic reticulum, where a translation takes place to form a large precursor protein (preproprotein). That protein is prepared for the axonal transport by packaging into neurosecretory granulae within the Golgi complex. During the transport, the precursor protein is processed by specific cleavage enzymes into active and inactive peptide fragments. After release, the peptides are further degraded into smaller peptide fragments or constituent amino acids. (Figure from E Widerlov: The future of neuropeptides in psychiatry and neurology. In* Neuropeptides in Psychiatric and Neurological Disorders, *C B Nemeroff, editor. Johns Hopkins University Press, Baltimore, 1988. Used with permission.)*

PEPTIDE PROCESSING

As neuropeptides are first synthesized as larger precursor molecules, a wide variety of processes can come into play in the cleavage of the active peptide forms from the precursor (Figure 1.5-2). For example, somatostatin is first produced as a 116 amino acid prohormone called preprosomatostatin, and it contains a 24 amino acid signal sequence that is removed in the formation of the 92 amino acid prosomatostatin. It is further processed to either somatostatin-28 or somatostatin-14, and a major site of the processing step has been identified as the Golgi apparatus. The last processing step shows significant species differences, which should be considered when extrapolating between human and animal studies. For example, the 12 amino acid sequence of somatostatin-28 that is cleaved in the formation of somatostatin-14 is much more abundant in rodent brain than it is in humans. The joint actions of a basophilic aminoprotease and an endoprotease contained in secretory granules cleaves somatostatin-14 from somatostatin-28. Most active peptide sequences are flanked by dibasic amino acids (Arg and Lys), which act as cleavage sites for the carboxypeptidase-B types of enzymes. However, somatostatin-28 is cleaved at a single arginine from its prosomatostatin precursor. Related peptides are often contained in the same prohormone sequence, as is the case for neurotensin and neuromedin N. Those peptides are separated by a single pair of dibasic residues on their common mRNA and yet have distinctly different distribution patterns in the brain. Other tissues may also exhibit processing that is different from that of the brain, as is seen for neuromedin N in the mouse ileum. Multiple active peptide copies can also be contained in the prohormone structure as is noted with TRH, which has five complete copies in the mammalian 285 amino acid prohormone. Studies using antisera that recognize the intervening sequences between the five copies of TRH within the prohormone indicate that all five copies are liberated during processing. Prohormone processing can show regional differences within the brain, as is clearly seen for TRH. In the hypothalamus the main storage forms of TRH are TRH, pre-pro TRH (160-169), and pre-pro TRH (178-199), and two additional forms are found in the olfactory bulb region. The differences in the ratio of TRH to its prohormone precursor in various extraneuronal tissues also indicates widely varying regional differences in processing of the TRH precursors. Processing also can differ across the developmental spectrum, as has been reported for TRH. Hypothalamic TRH prohormone processing in mice was observed to accelerate during development based on the ratio of TRH to its precursors, and immunohistochemical staining or *in situ* hybridization autoradiography indicated that a significant amount of processing occurred during post-Golgi transport and storage.

Although many known peptides are complete and biologically active when cleaved from the prohormone, many others are subjected to posttranslational processing. Certain peptides have a metabolically blocked carboxy terminus that is often amidated. A glycine residue in the prohormone sequence often acts as the amide donor, and in the case of TRH is attached by a monoxygenase that is contained in secretory granules. TRH is further processed on the N-terminus where glutamine is cyclized by a glutamylcyclase. These alterations are usually effective in slowing degradation and are often required for biological activity, as is the case for TRH, which is usually inactive when the C-terminal amide is removed by proline endopeptidase to generate the free-acid structure. Other posttranslational processing events for active peptides include glycosylation and cyclization, which are often required for either biological activity or transport.

RECEPTORS

Neuropeptide receptors have undergone the same process of discovery and characterization that receptors for other neurotransmitters have enjoyed. The process begins with the pharmacological characterization of the receptor's physicochemical binding properties by assessing the affinity of various metabolically derived peptide fragments and the native molecule for the receptor binding site found in membrane preparations. Peptide receptor locations are mapped with radioactive or fluorescent tags that are inserted into peptide molecules, which often contain substituted amino acids at the most vulnerable peptidase cleavage sites. Once the peptide receptor is characterized pharmacologically, it is usually purified from some relatively enriched biological source tissue or brain region by affinity column chromatography. After it has been purified, binding parameters and activity are recharacterized for the reconstituted purified receptor protein and structural information can be obtained through X-ray crystallography. Now that it has become possible to purify mRNAs for peptide receptors, the induction of mutations should allow identification of the regions controlling ligand binding. The distribution of receptors mapped with autoradiographic techniques has been largely verified by in situ hybridization using receptor mRNA probes. That information will make it possible to design drugs specifically to fit those binding sites on the receptor, leading to the ability to manipulate peptide systems in ways that are currently enjoyed by the more classic neurotransmitters.

The process described has been closely followed in the purification of the neurotensin-neuromedin N receptor. Because neurotensin and neuromedin N share significant sequence homology, the latter is active in displacing ligands from the neurotensin receptor, but with approximately 20 times less potency. The neurotensin receptor was first characterized by photoaffinity labeling and cross-linking of radioiodinated ligands, which resulted in two labeled subunits of about 49 kd and 51 kd each from rat brain synaptosomes. The receptor was next solubilized and characterized for ligand affinity and binding capacity in mouse brain, which was followed by affinity column chromat graphic purification and confirmation of an aggregate molecular weight of approximately 100 kd. However, similar work with bovine cerebral cortex yielded a purified neurotensin receptor of approximately 72 kd, indicating that significant species differences may exist. The neurotensin receptor mRNA has been cloned, and regional in situ hybridization mapping studies indicate that its distribution is generally the same as was shown for the receptor using radioactive ligands and autoradiography. The location is particularly rich in dopamine cell body regions and some dopamine terminal regions, and thus it is not surprising that dopamine activity seems to regulate neurotensin receptor expression. Neurotensin receptors have been shown to be colocalized with enzymes that degrade both neurotensin and neuromedin N in primary cultures of neurons from the forebrains of 14-day-old mouse embryos.

Receptor populations for peptides exhibit changes in the numbers of binding sites on the basis of the amount of transmitter signal received and the input from second messenger feedback regulation. The up-regulation and down-regulation of peptide receptors has been most often demonstrated in the anterior pituitary, but has also been described for the cortex and other regions. Peptide receptor affinity for ligands usually remains stable in the face of this regulation of receptor number. Receptor expression fluctuates in various brain regions during development as well. Autoradiography has demonstrated high concentrations of somatostatin receptors in rat somatosensory cortex at day 16 of the embryo in the intermediate zone and a transient decrease in cortical plate somatostatin receptors at birth. Decreases to adult levels of somatostatin receptors in somatosensory cortex are achieved by 21 days after birth. Somatostatin receptors in the cerebellum of 13-day-old rats have been shown to be pharmacologically similar to those of adults in binding parameters. Several research groups have described different classes of somatostatin receptors on the basis of selective binding by various pharmacological ligands. Regional differences in the binding of somatostatin-28 and somatostatin-14 and their inability to desensitize each other's binding has indicated that separate receptor populations may exist for these two forms. Further evidence for distinct populations of SRIF-28 and SRIF-14 receptors is provided by their production of different second messenger effects and their opposite effects on potassium conductance in rat cortex. At the last count five different somatostatin receptor subtypes had been identified with molecular techniques.

Neuropeptide receptors have been associated with just about every type of second messenger signal transduction system that is currently known. Mechanisms using cyclic AMP; cyclic guanosine monophosphate; protein kinases A and C; sodium, potassium, and calcium channels; and inositol phosphate and diacylglycerol have all been identified as neuropeptide receptor signal transduction mechanisms. Such mechanisms offer a myriad of possible modulatory effects, from the amplification to the attenuation of postsynaptic signals, and contribute greatly to the integrative power of neural networks. Both the neurotensin receptor and the TRH receptor are internalized within the postsynaptic cell upon binding their endogenous ligand or the appropriate agonist, where portions of the complex may eventually be transported to the receptive cell's nucleus with regulatory effects. Specific receptor antagonists have been slow to develop, with opiate antagonists being the first example to be described. Altered molecular forms of native peptides, such as α-helical CRF, have been used with but limited success owing to size constraints on diffusion and their lack of ability to penetrate the blood-brain barrier.

The inability to block specific neuropeptide signals pharmacologically has severely hindered research into the roles of the endogenous peptides in various behaviors and physiological effects. The disadvantages of trying to decipher a substance's role in neurotransmission by examining only the effects of excess concentrations should be obvious to even casual observers.

PEPTIDASES

Peptides are degraded to smaller fragments, and eventually to single amino acids, by specific enzymes termed peptidases. As yet, peptides or their fragments have not been shown to be actively taken up by presynaptic elements as is the case for the monoamines. The enzymes may be found bound to post- or presynaptic neural membranes or in solution in the cytoplasm and extracellular fluid, and they are distributed widely in peripheral organs, serum, and cerebrospinal fluid (CSF), as well as in the CNS. They often have a metal ion among their subunit components; those components form the active site for cleavage of the target peptide sequence, and that active site often forms a three-dimensional cleft where the specific peptide bond cleavage occurs. There are several general classes of peptidases, with several distinct enzymes in each class. Those classes include the serine endopeptidases containing such enzymes as trypsin and chymotrypsin; the thiol peptidases, such as pyroglutamate amino peptidase and cathepepsin B and C; the acid proteases, such as pepsin and renin; the metalloendopeptidases, such as neural endopeptidase and angiotensin-converting enzymes; and the metalloexopeptidases, such as the aminopeptidases and the carboxypeptidases like enkephalin-convertase and carboxypeptidase A and B. These degradative enzymes are often the same as those used in processing but have different subcellular locations. An example is carboxypeptidase B, which cleaves the dibasic amino acid residues flanking the active peptide sequence in the prohormone during processing, or it can end activity at the receptor if the peptide contains dibasic amino acids in the active sequence, such as is seen for neurotensin. Peptidases have pH and temperature optimums for activity and can be inhibited by various chemicals or chelators or by amino acid substitution at vulnerable points in the peptide chain. Alterations in peptidase activity or concentration can contribute to alterations in the synaptic availability of a peptide, and the regulation of peptidase levels may be as exquisitely controlled as receptor number and peptide synthesis and release. Table 1.5-1 shows the potential cleavage points for neuromedin N, neurotensin, somatostatin, and TRH. Cleavage of the actively released form of the peptide usually ends biological activity, but examples abound of partial or complete receptor activation by partially metabolized peptides or their fragments.

The metabolism of TRH has been investigated fairly completely, principally because of the limited number of fragments that can be generated by a tripeptide. The principal cleavage enzymes are pyroglutamyl amino peptidase, which cleaves the cyclized glutamyl residue from the C-terminus and generates a histidine-proline (His-Pro) fragment. That factor spontaneously cyclizes into a diketopiperazine, the so-called cyclo His-Pro, after the N-terminal amide has been removed by the action of the proline endopeptidase. The active site of the pyroglutamyl amino peptidase enzyme has been shown to contain tyrosine, histidine, arginine, and possibly lysine residues, but does not contain serine, cysteine, aspartate, or glutamate. Regional differences in TRH degradation have been described, with spinal cord metabolism of TRH generating more deamidated TRH than cerebral cortex degradation. The half-life of TRH in serum is estimated at only two to three minutes and CSF is now known to contain pyroglutamyl amino peptidase activity. Neonatal CSF has less of such activity than does that of adults, and differences in subcellular localization of the enzyme in the adult hypothalamus (soluble fraction) and cerebral cortex (membrane bound) has been reported as well, with the brain activity of both forms decreasing during development. Both of those TRH peptidases have been detected in the cytosol of brain homogenates, but are found only in trace amounts in the soluble fraction of synaptosomes as most of their activity is associated with synaptosomal membranes. Thyroid hormones have been shown to regulate pyroglutamyl amino peptidase in the membrane-bound fraction but not in the soluble form, although in serum the peptidase does not appear to be influenced by thyroid hormones. Thus peptidases offer yet another opportunity for the integration and regulation of neuropeptide transmitter actions and synaptic availability. Because the present peptidase inhibitors are relatively nonspecific in their ability to block the various peptidases, there have been few attempts to influence peptide concentrations by pharmacological blockage of their associated peptidases. Captopril's (Capoten, Caposide) blockade of angiotensin-converting enzyme is one possible exception to that generality. It is expected that second and third generation peptidase inhibitors, with discrete peptidase and possibly regional specificity, will be developed that eventually may allow the truly elegant manipulation of endogenous neuropeptide concentrations.

NEUROENDOCRINE SECRETION

With the exception of neuromedin N, the example peptides are known to play major roles in pituitary endocrine regulation, including CRF-induced release of proopiomelanocortin products, such as adrenocorticotropic hormone (ACTH) and β-endorphin; TRH release of thyrotropin (thyroid-stimulating hormone, TSH) and prolactin; and somatostatin's (SRIF) inhibition of the release of growth hormone, thyrotropin, gonadotropins, and ACTH. Neurotensin, which is abundant in the hypothalamus and median eminence, may mediate the preovulatory release of luteinizing hormone and receive feedback for the induction of mRNA synthesis by estrogen. A sexually dimorphic distribution of the neurotensin-neuromedin N mRNA in the preoptic hypothalamus also supports such a role for neurotensin in rodents.

The peptides involved in neuroendocrine regulation have cell bodies residing in the hypothalamus that receive feedback from all levels of the endocrine axes. The complexity of those interactions has been well demonstrated for the hypothalamic-pituitary-thyroid axis (HPT) and the hypothalamic-pituitary-adrenal

(HPA) axis and have now been extended to the molecular level. The regulatory feedback of thyroid hormones onto the TRH synthesizing neurons of the paraventricular nucleus was first demonstrated with evidence of TRH concentration changes, reported to be reduced in the median eminence after thyroidectomy, but not in the rest of the hypothalamus, and which could be prevented by thyroid hormone replacement. The treatment of normal rats with exogenous thyroid hormone decreases TRH concentration in the paraventricular nucleus and the posterior nucleus of the hypothalamus. That effect was corroborated for the TRH prohormone as well, with median eminence levels of TRH prohormone being reduced by thyroidectomy and the precursor levels increasing toward normal amounts after thyroxine treatment. The TRH mRNA also exhibits such regulation by thyroid hormone as expected, with increased mRNA concentration in the paraventricular nucleus 14 days after thyroidectomy. Unilateral tri-iodothyronine implants prevent the increase in TRH mRNA that is seen on the contralateral untreated side in propylthiouracil-treated hypothyroid rats. The effects of thyroid hormones on TRH expression in the paraventricular nucleus of developing rats are not seen until between embryo day 20 and seven days after birth, although TRH mRNA is evident as early as embryo day 16. The ability of thyroid hormones to regulate TRH mRNA can be superseded by other stimuli that activate the HPT axis. In that regard repeated exposure to cold (which releases TRH from the median eminence) induces increases in the levels of TRH mRNA in the paraventricular nucleus despite concomitantly elevated concentrations of thyroid hormones. Further evidence of the different levels of communication of the HPT axis are seen in the ability of TRH to regulate the production of mRNA for the pituitary TRH receptor and for TRH concentrations to regulate the mRNA coding for both the α and β subunits of the thyrotropin (thyroid-stimulating hormone) molecule. The latter effect has been shown to be dependent on intracellular calcium and protein kinase C. The regulatory interplay also extends to the accessible pools of second messenger phosphoinositides, whose pool size is regulated by TRH receptor numbers. TRH-containing synaptic boutons have been observed in contact with TRH-containing cell bodies in the medial and periventricular subdivisions of the paraventricular nucleus, thus providing anatomical evidence for ultrashort feedback regulation of TRH concentrations there. Regional differences in CRF receptor regulation by corticosterone have also been reported, which have been shown to be partly due to differential glycosylation of the CRF receptor. The regulation of neuropeptide mRNA concentrations may be influenced by other neuropeptides, as well as by components of the particular endocrine axis normally associated with the particular peptide, as demonstrated by the ability of neuropeptide Y to increase hypothalamic CRF mRNA.

Because many endocrine systems are cyclic in their regulatory functions, it is not surprising that neuropeptides often exhibit rhythms in concentrations that are based on diurnal, lunar, and circumannual periodicities. Hypothalamic and extrahypothalamic regional concentrations of CRF exhibit increased concentrations in the afternoon relative to morning concentrations, and this increase can be attenuated by corticosterone only in the hypothalamus. Somatostatin, CRF, and TRH concentrations in the CSF of nonhuman primates exhibit daily fluctuations, and the monthly cycles in gonadotropins of mammals exhibiting estrus are well recognized. Circannual rhythms of neurotensin and somatostatin concentrations that are 180 degrees out of phase in rodent hypothalamus have been noted. Phases of mRNA concentration changes during development have been seen in CRF mRNA, which is present at gestational day 17, but decreases from day 19 to day 21, when concentrations again rise to attain adult levels by four days after birth. Other peptide mRNAs, such as somatostatin, do not exhibit such fluctuations during development, but do show differential distribution during ontogeny. Daily fluctuations in rat paraventricular nucleus CRF mRNA that were lowest during the period of highest plasma corticosterone levels during the 24-hour cycle have been reported.

NEUROPEPTIDES IN PSYCHIATRY

Human beings are less than ideal subjects for neuropeptide research for several reasons. The peripheral sources of many peptides, the relatively high concentration of serum peptidases, and the blood-brain barrier make serum concentrations of CNS neuropeptides difficult to interpret. The use of biopsy to assess tissue concentrations directly is not routinely repeatable, is limited to superficial structures, suffers from high morbidity, and would provide only a limited amount of information. Cerebrospinal fluid is thought to reflect extracellular fluid concentrations of transmitter substances, is in direct contact with the CNS and is screened from peripheral serum sources by the blood-brain barrier, and may be sampled across time. The limitations of CSF studies include a lack of information about the regional source of any concentration changes detected; the use of lumbar CSF, which is somewhat removed from higher CNS sources of peptides and subject to spinal cord peptide contributions to absolute concentrations; and the effects of previous drug treatments. Postmortem tissue studies of neuropeptide concentration changes in psychiatric disease are affected by agonal state, postmortem delay, previous drug treatment, and coexisting illnesses. Most of the data on CSF concentration changes or tissue concentration changes have been derived from comparisons between diagnostically defined psychiatric groups and control groups. However, the controls are often neurologically or psychiatrically impaired as well, and the accuracy and consistency of the diagnoses may be quite unreliable. In addition, the etiology of a diagnostic class of disease may differ among subjects in the same group. Even after matching for age, sex, or other demographic variables, genetic heterogeneity among human research populations results in individual variations of absolute peptide values that are often quite wide. Such variances severely reduce the power of group comparisons to detect alterations in peptide concentrations. The use of pretreatment and posttreatment CSF samples, or of samples taken during the active disease state versus when the patient is in remission, has begun to address the serious limitations in study design. For such progressive diseases as schizophrenia or Alzheimer's disease (called dementia of the Alzheimer's type in the fourth edition of *Diagnostic and Statistical Manual of Mental Disorders* [DSM-IV]), serial CSF samples may be a valuable indicator of disease progression or response to treatment. Even with these constraints, significant progress has been made in describing the effects of various psychiatric disease states on neuropeptide systems in the CNS.

Alzheimer's disease represents up to two thirds of the demented population encountered in clinical practice, and over half of the nursing home beds in the United States are currently occupied by such patients. The disease is characterized by a progressive, gradually worsening dementia that cannot be ascribed to metabolic disorders, pharmacological treatment, or infectious agents and is neuropathologically associated with above-normal numbers of senile plaques and neurofibrillary tangles as a result of the degenerative process. The first neurochemical deficit to be associated with Alzheimer's disease was reduced amounts of choline acetyltransferase containing nerve terminals in cortical regions as a result of degeneration of cholinergic neuronal perikarya in the nucleus basalis of Meynert in the substantia innominata of the basal forebrain. Within a few years of that finding somatostatin was found to be reduced in concentration in interneurons of the cortex of those patients. Subcortical regions containing somatostatin, such as the substantia innominata, hypothalamus, and bed nucleus of the stria terminalis, were usually spared, whereas somatostatin receptors in the cortex were decreased in number. In such regions as the hippocampus findings of somatostatin depletions were less consistent than in the cortex, but when depleted in the hippocampus, the somatostatin neurons colocalized with neuropeptide Y were spared. Somatostatin concentration in the CSF of patients with Alzheimer's disease has also been consistently found to be decreased, and this decrease has been correlated with the degree of cognitive impairment. Therapies that slow or partially reverse the dementia associated with Alzheimer's disease have been reported also to partially reverse the decrease in CSF somatostatin. However, somatostatin in CSF is also decreased in delirium, major depressive disorder, schizophrenia, multiple sclerosis, and dementia due to Parkinson's disease. Increased concentrations of a somatostatin cleaving peptidase have been described in certain cortical regions of the brain tissue of persons with Alzheimer's disease, raising the possibility that increased degradation of somatostatin may contribute to the decreases in somatostatin concentration observed in that disease. Treatment with somatostatin infusion, however, has not been successful in reversing the dementia. In experimental animals cysteamine depletion of hippocampus somatostatin leads to deficits in performance on tasks requiring retention of information, whereas chemical lesions of the substantia innominata lead to increased cortical concentrations of somatostatin and CRF. Those data have raised questions about whether the neuropeptide deficits precede, succeed, or occur in tandem with the cholinergic deficits seen in Alzheimer's disease, and whether the neurochemical systems and regions first exhibiting deficits are the site of the onset of pathology.

The CRF-containing interneurons of the cortex are also consistently depleted in Alzheimer's disease (Figure 1.5-3). As with somatostatin, subcortical areas containing CRF neurons may be spared, but, unlike somatostatin, CRF receptors are increased in number (up-regulated) with no change in affinity. Various research groups have reported the CRF concentrations in the CSF of such patients to be increased, decreased, or unchanged. Other peptides have been shown to be altered less consistently in Alzheimer's disease, such as substance P or neurotensin, whereas most peptides are reported to be unchanged, including TRH, vasoactive intestinal peptide, CCK, and the enkephalins. Many of those other relatively uninvolved peptides have been found in the neuritic plaques of patients' brain tissue, as well as neurites containing CRF and somatostatin. Only one peptide, galanin, is reported to be reliably increased in concentration in Alzheimer's disease. It is hoped that pharmacological compounds designed to activate the appropriate peptide receptors will allow new rational treatments to be assessed for that disease.

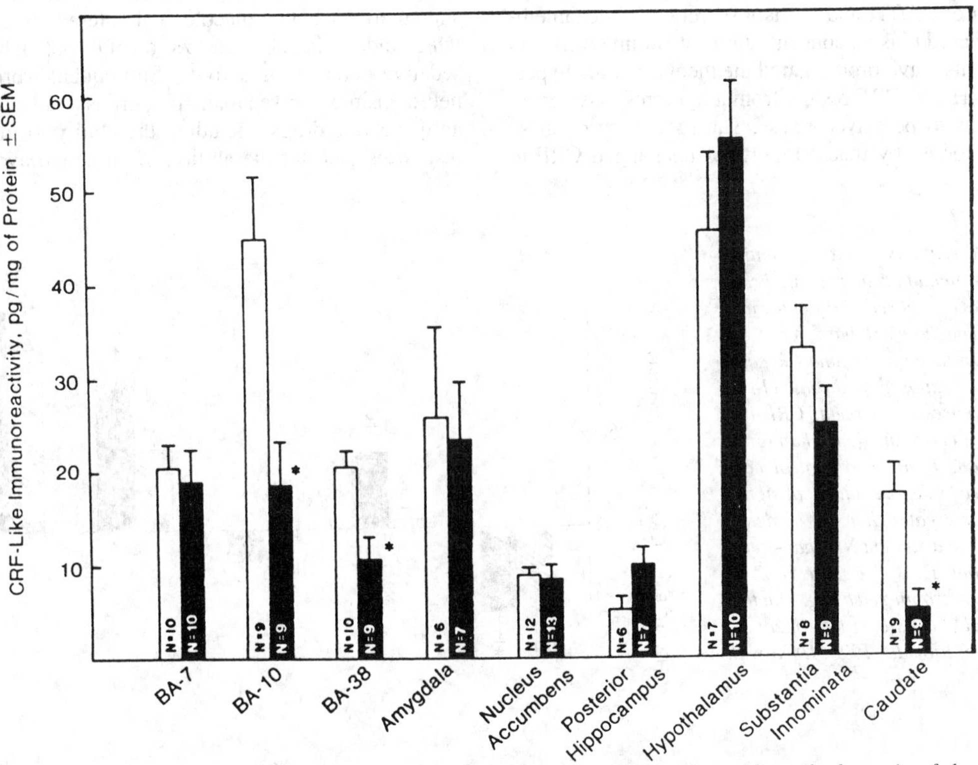

FIGURE 1.5-3 *Regional brain concentration of CRF-like immunoreactivity (CRF-LI) in patients with senile dementia of the Alzheimer's type (solid bars) and in control subjects (open bars). Number of samples from each brain region is shown inside respective bars. Concentration of CRF-LI is shown as mean ± SEM and is reported as picograms per milligram of protein. Statistical significance was sought by student's T-test and is represented by an asterisk, which indicates* P < *.01. (Figure from G Bissette, G P Reynolds, C D Kilts, E Widerlov, C B Nemeroff: Corticotropin-releasing factor-like immunoreactivity in senile dementia of the Alzheimer's type: Reduced cortical and striatal concentrations. JAMA 254: 3067, 1985. Used with permission.)*

MOOD DISORDERS As many aspects of mood disorders, particularly major depressive disorder, are similar to the behavioral and physiological effects of stressful stimuli on laboratory animals, it is not surprising that peptides that mediate responses to stress are altered in mood disorders. The HPA and HPT axes are both recruited by physiological and psychological stressors, such as hemorrhage stress, restraint stress, exposure to cold, and inescapable foot shock. Release of CRF and TRH from the median eminence and increases in messenger RNA for those peptides in the paraventricular nucleus have been demonstrated in laboratory animals after exposure to stressful stimuli, along with reciprocal desensitization of the receptors mediating release of the analogous pituitary hormones.

Regional alterations in CRF concentrations have been reported in animals exposed to acute and chronic stress (Figure 1.5-4), and CRF infusion directly into the CNS of animals results in behavioral alterations that resemble fear and anxiety and induces alteration in feeding, sleeping, sexual, and exploratory behaviors in ways that are similar to those reported by depressed patients. In human patients diagnosed with the most severe form of depressive disorder, melancholia, and with depression ratings that fall into the severe range, both CRF and TRH are increased in CSF, which may reflect increased hypothalamic or extrahypothalamic release of those peptides. The numbers of frontal cortex receptors for CRF have been reported to be decreased in suicides but unchanged, as was CRF concentration, in postmortem brain tissue of depressed patients. Additionally, the responses of the pituitary to exogenous challenges with TRH or CRF stimulation tests are blunted in the release of TSH or ACTH, presumably as the result of pituitary receptor down-regulation in a high proportion of severely depressed patients. Those data, together with the early escape from inhibition of ACTH and cortisol secretion by dexamethasone and increased plasma concentrations of serum cortisol in depressed patients, have promulgated the theory that the hypersecretion of TRH and CRF results from a hyperresponsiveness of those systems to perceived stress. The specificity of these findings is reinforced by recent reports of unchanged CRF in the CSF of patients with panic disorder and of decreased TRH in the CSF of underweight and recovering anorexic patients relative to controls. The reversal of most of these alterations with the successful treatment of depressive symptoms reinforces the concept that these alterations are state markers of depression rather than trait markers, and makes them potentially useful in assessing treatment response.

SCHIZOPHRENIA Both clinical and postmortem investigations of schizophrenic patients, as well as animal studies, have sought to elucidate the role of neuropeptides in the pathological manifestations of schizophrenia. Although severely constrained by diagnostic uncertainties and drug treatment effects, the research to date on the postmortem brain tissue of schizophrenic patients has not revealed major alterations of neuropeptide systems. A number of peptides (endogenous opioids, substance P, CCK, somatostatin) have been reported to be altered in the CSF of schizophrenic patients, but many of these findings either have not been independently reproduced or describe a marginally statistically significant difference in CSF peptide concentrations among groups of patients and controls with variance of over 100 percent around the mean. Further confounds are the effects of semichronic (weeks) treatment with antipsychotic drugs on peptide systems, which have been described for regional neurotensin, CCK, substance P, and somatostatin concentrations in laboratory animals. How much time is necessary to abolish those drug-induced alterations of neuropeptide system concentration changes is not known for humans, but may significantly exceed the two to three weeks of drug holiday used in most clinical studies.

The most likely candidate neuropeptide with evidence of selective alteration in schizophrenia is neurotensin. It was first shown to have pharmacological interactions with dopamine while undergoing characterization of its potent hypothermic and sedative potentiating activity. Subsequent work indicated that neurotensin possessed many properties that were also shared by antipsychotic drugs, including the ability to inhibit avoidance responses, but not the ability, in an active avoidance task, to

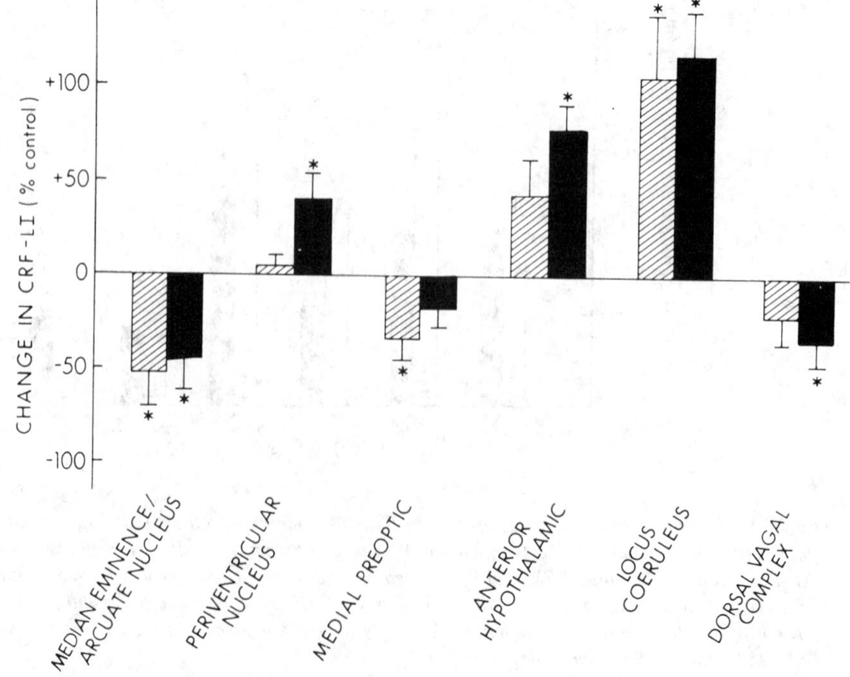

FIGURE 1.5-4 *Alterations in the concentration of CRF-like immunoreactivity in brain regions from rats exposed to acute and chronic stress. The hatched bars represent rats exposed to an acute stress and the solid bars represent rats exposed to chronic (14 d) stress. Values represent percent CRF-like immunoreactivity concentration change in these brain regions relative to control concentrations. Asterisks denote statistical significance equal to or greater than .05 as determined by ANOVA and student Newman-Keuls test. (Figure from E B De Souza, C B Nemeroff: Corticotropin-releasing factor: Basic and clinical studies of a neuropeptide. CRC, Boca Raton, Florida, 1990. Used with permission.)*

block the effects of indirect dopamine agonists or endogenous dopamine in the production of locomotor behavior and the ability to elicit increases in dopamine release and turnover after direct neurotensin injection. Unlike antipsychotics, neurotensin is not able to displace dopamine from its receptor. Neurotensin was shown to be colocalized in certain subsets of dopamine neurons and to be coreleased with dopamine in the mesolimbic and medial prefrontal cortex dopamine terminal regions that are implicated as the site of dopamine hyperactivity in schizophrenia. Antipsychotic drugs that act at dopamine and σ receptors increase the concentration of neurotensin in those dopamine terminal regions but not in other neurotensin-containing regions. That effect of antipsychotic drugs in increasing neurotensin concentrations persists after months of treatment and is accompanied by the expected increase in neurotensin mRNA concentrations, as well as by c-fos mRNA expression within hours of initial drug treatment. The altered regulation of neurotensin expression by antipsychotic drugs apparently extends to the peptidases that degrade the peptide, as recent reports have indicated decreased neurotensin metabolism in rat brain slices 24 hours after the acute administration of haloperidol.

With regard to schizophrenia, decreased neurotensin concentrations in their CSF have been reported for several populations of patients with that disorder as compared with controls or other psychiatric disorders. Although treatment with antipsychotic drugs has been observed to increase neurotensin concentrations in the CSF, it is not known whether this increase is causal or merely accompanies the decrease in psychotic symptoms seen with successful treatment. Postmortem studies have shown an increase in neurotensin concentrations in the dopamine-rich Brodmann's area 32 of the frontal cortex, but that may have been the result of premortem antipsychotic treatment. Other researchers have found no postmortem alterations in neurotensin concentrations of a wide sampling of subcortical regions. A recent comparison of the genomic sequence of the neurotensin-neuromedin N gene in schizophrenic patients compared with age- and sex-matched controls found no differences in the gene sequence. A critical test of the hypothesis that neurotensin may act as an endogenous antipsychotic-like substance awaits the development of a neurotensin receptor agonist that can be delivered from the periphery.

It is evident that the understanding of the neurobiology of neuropeptides has increased remarkably over the past several years. There is already considerable evidence that these neuroregulators are involved in both the pathophysiology of certain major neuropsychiatric disorders and the mechanism of action of some of the drugs used to treat those disabling illnesses. And, as further knowledge accrues, it is increasingly likely that neuropeptides will play a greater role in the development of diagnostic tests and novel treatments for the major psychiatric disorders.

SUGGESTED CROSS-REFERENCES

Psychoneuroendocrinology is discussed in Section 1.11, basic molecular neurobiology is discussed in Section 1.14, and neuropsychiatric aspects of endocrine disorders are discussed in Section 2.8.

REFERENCES

Banki C M, Arato M, Bissette G, Nemeroff C B: Elevation of immunoreactive CSF TRH in depressed patients. Am J Psychiatry *145:* 1526, 1988.

Banks W A, Kastin A J, Akerstrom V, Jaspan J B: Radioactively iodinated cyclo (His-Pro) crosses the blood-brain barrier and reverses ethanol-induced narcosis. Am J Physiol *264:* E723, 1993.

Bayer V E, Towle A C, Pickel V M: Ultrastructural localization of neurotensin-like immunoreactivity within dense core vesicles in perikarya, but not terminals, colocalizing tyrosine hydroxylase in rat ventral tegmental area. J Comp Neurol *311:* 179, 1991.

Bean A J, Adrian T E, Modlin I M, Roth R H: Dopamine and neurotensin storage in co-localized and non-colocalized neuronal populations. J Pharmacol Exp Ther *249:* 681, 1989.

Bean A J, Dagerlind A, Hokfelt T, Dobner P R: Cloning of human neurotensin/neuromedin N genomic sequences and expression in the ventral mesencephalon of schizophrenics and age/sex matched controls. Neuroscience *50:* 259, 1992.

*Benoit R, Esch F, Bennette H P J, Ling N, Ravazolla M, Orci L, Mufson E J: Processing of somatostatin. Metabolism *39* (2, Suppl): 22, 1990.

*Bissette G, Levant B, Nemeroff CB: Neurotensin and its possible significance in the pathophysiology of schizophrenia. In *Volume Transmission in the Brain: New Aspects in Electrical and Chemical Communication,* K Fuxe, L Agnati, editors. Raven, New York, 1990.

Bodenant C, Leroux P, Gonzalez B J, Vaudry H: Transient expression of somatostatin receptors in the rat visual system during development. Neuroscience *41:* 595, 1991.

Bruhn T O, Taplin J H, Jackson I M D: Hypothyroidism reduces content and increases in vitro release of pro-thyrotropin-releasing hormone peptides from the median eminence. Neuroendocrinology *53:* 511, 1991.

Bulant M, Beauvillain J C, Delfour A, Vaudry H, Nicolas P: Processing of thyrotropin-releasing hormone (TRH) prohormone in the rat olfactory bulb generates novel TRH-related peptides. Endocrinology *127:* 1978, 1990.

Bulant M, Delfour A, Vaudry H, Nicolas P: Processing of thyrotropin-releasing hormone prohormone (Pro-TRH) generates pro-TRH-connecting peptides. J Biol Chem *263:* 17189, 1988.

Burgunder J-M: Ontogeny of somatostatin gene expression in rat forebrain. Dev Brain Res *78:* 109, 1994.

Butler P D, Nemeroff C B: Corticotropin-releasing factor as a possible cause of comorbidity and depressive disorders. In *Comorbidity in Anxiety and Mood Disorders,* J D Maser, C R Clonibger, editors, p 413. American Psychiatric Press, Washington, 1988.

Campbell M J, Lewis D A, Benoit R, Morrison J H: Regional heterogeneity in the distribution of somatostatin-28 and somatostatin-28_{1-12}-immunoreactive profiles in monkey neocortex. J Neurosci *7:* 1133, 1987.

Chabry J, Gaudriault G, Vincent J, Mazella J: Implication of various forms of neurotensin receptors in the mechanism of internalization of neurotensin in cerebral neurons. J Biol Chem *268:* 17138, 1993.

Childs G V, Unabia G: Rapid corticosterone inhibition of corticotropin-releasing hormone binding and adrenocorticotropin release by enriched populations of corticotropes: Counteractions by arginine vasopressin and its second messengers. Endocrinology *126:* 1967, 1990.

Elde R, Schalling M, Ceccatelli S, Nakanishi S, Hokfelt T: Localization of neuropeptide receptor mRNA in rat brain: Initial observations using probes for neurotensin and substance P receptors. Neurosci Lett *120:* 134, 1990.

Fischer W H, Spiess J: Identification of a mammalian glutaminyl cyclase converting glutaminyl into pyroglutamyl peptides. Proc Natl Acad Sci USA *84:* 3628, 1987.

Funckes C L, Minth C D, Deschenes R: Cloning and characterization of mRNA encoding rat pre-pro-somatostatin. J Biol Chem *258:* 8781, 1983.

Gaspar P, Berger B, Febvret A: Neurotensin innervation of the human cerebral cortex: Lack of colocalization with catecholamines. Brain Res *530:* 181, 1990.

*Gershengorn M, Heinflink M, Nussenzveig D R, Hinkle P M, Pederson E F: Thyrotropin releasing hormone (TRH) receptor number determines the size of the TRH-responsive phosphoinositide pool. J Biol Chem *269:* 6779, 1994.

Gonzalez B J, Leroux P, Bodenant C, Vaudry H: Ontogeny of somatostatin receptors in the rat somatosensory cortex. J Comp Neurol *305:* 177, 1991.

Grigoriadis D E, De Souza E B: Heterogeneity between brain and pituitary corticotropin-releasing factor receptors is due to differential glycosylation. Endocrinology *125:* 1877, 1989.

Halbreich U: *Hormones and Depression.* Raven, New York, 1987.

Hauger R L, Millan M A, Catt K J, Aguilera G: Differential regulation of brain and pituitary corticotropin-releasing factor receptors by corticosterone. Endocrinology *120:* 1527, 1987.

Hayes T L, Cameron J L, Fernstrom J D, Lewis D A: A comparative analysis of the distribution of prosomatostatin-derived peptides in human and monkey neocortex. J Comp Neurol *303:* 584, 1991.

Hokfelt T, Everitt B J, Theodorsson-Norheim E, Goldstein M: Occurrence of neurotensin-like immunoreactivity in subpopulations of

hypothalamic, mesencephalic, and medullary catecholamine neurons. J Comp Neurol *222:* 543, 1984.
Hokfelt T, Fuxe K, Pernow B: *Progress in Brain Research, Vol 68. Coexistence of Neuronal Messengers: A New Principle in Chemical Transmission.* Elsevier, New York, 1986.
Hokfelt T, Tsuruo Y, Ulfhake B, Cullheim S, Arvidsson U, Foster G A, Shultzberg M, Schalling M, Arborelius L, Freedman J, Post C, Visser T: Distribution of TRH-like immunoreactivity with special reference to co-existence with other neuroreactive compounds. Ann NY Acad Sci *553:* 76, 1989.
Jolkkonen J, Lepola U, Bissette G, Nemeroff C B, Riekkinen P: CSF corticotropin-releasing factor is not affected in panic disorder. Biol Psychiatry *33:* 136, 1993.
Kasckow J, Nemeroff C B: The neurobiology of neurotensin: Focus on neurotensin-dopamine interactions. Regulatory Peptides *36:* 153, 1991.
Kislauskis E, Bullock B, McNeil S, Dobner P R: The rat gene encoding neurotensin and neuromedin N. J Biol Chem *263:* 4963, 1988.
Kitabgi P, Masuo Y, Nicot A, Berod A, Cuber J-C, Rostene W: Marked variations of the relative distributions of neurotensin and neuromedin N in micropunched rat brain areas suggest differential processing of their common precursor. Neurosci Lett *124:* 9, 1991.
Konkoy C S, Waters S M, Davis T P: Acute administration of neuroleptics decreases neurotensin metabolism on intact regional brain slices. J Pharmacol Exp Ther *269:* 555, 1994.
Krantic S, Martel J-C, Weissmann D, Pujol J-F, Quirion R: Quantitative radioautographic study of somatostatin receptors heterogeneity in the rat extrahypothalamic brain. Neuroscience *39:* 127, 1990.
Lee S L, Stewart K, Goodman R H: Structure of the gene encoding rat thyrotropin releasing hormone. J Biol Chem *263:* 5604, 1988.
Lesem M D, Kaye W H, Bissette G, Jimerson D C, Nemeroff C B: Cerebrospinal fluid TRH immunoreactivity in anorexia nervosa. Biol Psychiatry *35:* 48, 1994.
Martin J-L, Raynor C K, Gonzales C, Reisine T: Differential distribution of somatostatin receptor subtypes in rat brain revealed by newly developed somatostatin analogs. Neuroscience *41:* 581, 1991.
Mendez M, Cruz P, Joseph-Bravo P, Wilk S, Charli J L: Evaluation of the role of prolyl endopeptidase and pyroglutamyl peptidase I in the metabolism of LHRH and TRH in brain. Neuropeptides *17:* 55, 1990.
*Merchant K, Miller M A: Coexpression of neurotensin and c-fos mRNAs in rat neostriatal neurons following acute haloperidol. Mol Brain Res *23:* 271, 1994.
Moga M M, Gray T S: Evidence for corticotropin-releasing factor, neurotensin and somatostatin in the neural pathway from the central nucleus of the amygdala to the parabrachial nucleus. J Comp Neurol *241:* 275, 1985.
Mouri T, Itoi K, Takahashi K, Suda T, Murakami O, Yoshinaga K, Andoh N, Ohtani H, Masuda T, Sasano N: Colocalization of corticotropin-releasing factor and vasopressin in the paraventricular nucleus of the human hypothalamus. Neuroendocrinology *57:* 34, 1993.
Nemeroff C B, editor: *Neuropeptides in Psychiatric Disorders.* American Psychiatric Press, Washington, 1991.
Nussenzveig D R, Heinflink M, Gershengorn M C: Agonist-stimulated internalization of the thyrotropin-releasing hormone receptor is dependent on two domains in the receptor carboxyl terminus. J Biol Chem *268:* 2389, 1993.
Owens M J, Nemeroff C B: The physiology and pharmacology of corticotropin-releasing factor. Pharmacol Rev *43:* 425, 1992.
Panetta R, Greenwood M T, Warszynska A, Demchyshyn L L, Day R, Niznik H B, Srikant C B, Patel Y C: Molecular cloning, functional characterization and chromosomal localization of a human somatostatin receptor (somatostatin receptor type 5) with preferential affinity for somatostatin-28. Mol Pharmacol *45:* 417, 1994.
Rondeel J M M, Jackson I M D: Molecular biology of the regulation of hypothalamic hormones. J Endocrinol Invest *16:* 219, 1993.
*Sellar R E, Taylor P L, Lamb R F, Zabavnik J, Anderson L, Eidne K A: Functional expression and molecular characterization of the thyrotropin-releasing hormone receptor from the rat anterior pituitary gland. J Mol Endocrinol *10:* 199, 1993.
Sherman T G, Akil H, Watson S J: *The Molecular Biology of Neuropeptides: Discussions in Neuroscience,* vol 6. Elsevier Science, The Netherlands, 1989.
Suda T, Tozawa F, Iwai I, Sato Y, Sumitomo T, Nakano Y, Yamada M, Demura H: Neuropeptide Y increases the corticotropin-releasing factor messenger ribonucleic acid level in the rat hypothalamus. Mol Brain Res *18:* 311, 1993.
Tanaka K, Masu M, Nakanishi S: Structure and functional expression of the cloned rat neurotensin receptor. Neuron *4:* 847, 1990.
Torres H, Charli J-L, Gonzalez-Noriega A, Vargas M A, Joseph-Bravo P: Subcellular distribution of the enzymes degrading thyrotropin-releasing hormone and metabolites in rat brain. Neurochem Int *9:* 103, 1986.
Wang H L, Dichter M, Reisine T: Lack of cross-desensitization of somatostatin-14 and somatostatin-28 receptors coupled to potassium channels in rat neocortical neurons. Mol Pharmacol *38:* 357, 1990.
Whitnall M: Regulation of the hypothalamic corticotropin-releasing hormone neurosecretory system. Prog Neurobiol *40:* 573, 1993.
Wu P, Jackson I M D: Post-translational processing of thyrotropin-releasing hormone precursor in rat brain: Identification of 3 novel peptides derived from proTRH. Brain Res *456:* 22, 1988.
Zabavnik J, Arbuthnott G, Eidne K A: Distribution of thyrotropin-releasing hormone receptor messenger RNA in rat pituitary and brain. Neuroscience *53:* 877, 1993.
Zoeller R T, Kabeer N, Albers H E: Cold exposure elevates cellular levels of messenger ribonucleic acid encoding thyrotropin-releasing hormone in paraventricular nucleus despite elevated levels of thyroid hormones. Endocrinology *127:* 2955, 1990.

1.6 INTRANEURONAL SIGNALING PATHWAYS

ERIC J. NESTLER, M.D., Ph.D.
STEVEN E. HYMAN, M.D.

INTRODUCTION

Until relatively recently, synaptic transmission was conceptualized narrowly as a set of processes by which neurotransmitters, acting through their receptors, caused changes in the conductances of specific ion channels to produce excitatory or inhibitory postsynaptic potentials. According to that view, the human brain is a complex digital computer with its complexity derived largely from its wiring diagram. Over the past 20 years, however, it has become evident that neurotransmitters elicit diverse and complicated effects in target neurons, and that understanding has led to a more complete view of synaptic transmission. In most cases neurotransmitter-receptor interactions produce diverse effects on target neurons through a complex network of intracellular messenger systems involving G-proteins, second messengers, and protein phosphorylation. Those pathways are summarized in Figure 1.6-1.

Intracellular messenger pathways can be viewed as subserving three major functions in the nervous system. First, they mediate certain short-term aspects of synaptic transmission; those rapid actions of neurotransmitters on ion channels that do not involve ligand-gated channels are achieved through intracellular messengers. Second, they play the central role in mediating other actions of synaptic transmission; virtually all other effects of neurotransmitters on target neuron functioning, both short-term and long-term, are achieved through intracellular messengers (Figure 1.6-1). That role includes those long-term actions of neurotransmitters that are mediated through alterations in neuronal gene expression. Such a role for intracellular messengers is not limited to actions of neurotransmitters mediated by G-protein-linked receptors. Thus, although activation of ligand-gated ion channels leads to initial changes in membrane potential independent of intracellular messengers, activation of ligand-gated ion channels also leads to numerous additional (albeit slower) effects that are mediated by intracellular messengers. Third, by virtue of numerous interactions among the various intracellular messenger pathways, those pathways play the central role in coordinating a myriad of neuronal processes and adjusting neuronal function to environmental cues.

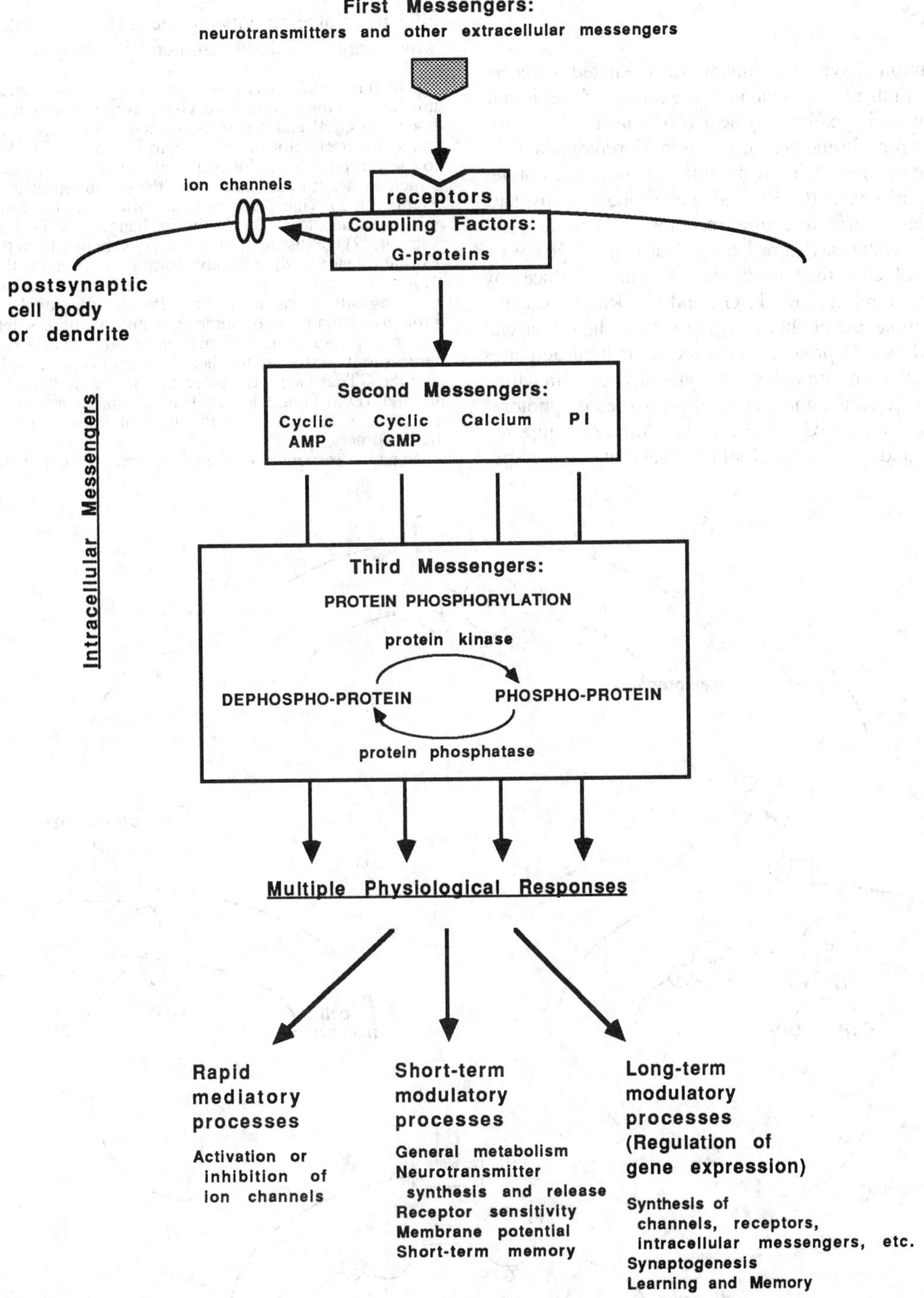

FIGURE 1.6-1 *The role played by intracellular messenger systems in synaptic transmission in the brain. Recent studies have focused on the involvement of intracellular messenger systems—involving coupling factors (termed G-proteins), second messengers (such as cyclic adenosine monophosphate [AMP], cyclic guanosine monophosphate [GMP], calcium, and the metabolites of phosphatidylinositol [PI]), and protein phosphorylation (involving the phosphorylation of phosphoproteins by protein kinases and their dephosphorylation by protein phosphatases)—in mediating multiple actions of neurotransmitters on their target neurons. The figure illustrates three major roles subserved by the intracellular messengers. In some cases, intracellular messenger pathways mediate the actions of some neurotransmitters in opening or inhibiting particular ion channels. However, intracellular messengers mediate most of the many other actions of neurotransmitters on their target neurons. Some actions are relatively short-lived and involve modulation of the general metabolic state of the neurons, their ability to synthesize or release neurotransmitter, and the functional sensitivity of their various receptors and ion channels to various synaptic inputs. Other actions are relatively long-lived and are achieved through the regulation of gene expression in the target neurons. Thus, neurotransmitters, through the regulation of intracellular messenger pathways and alterations in gene transcription and protein synthesis, alter the number and the types of receptors and ion channels in target neurons, the functional activity of the intracellular messenger systems in those neurons, and even the shape and the number of synapses that the neurons form. The figure is drawn to illustrate the amplification that intracellular messenger systems can give to neurotransmitter action. Thus, a single event of a neurotransmitter binding to its receptor (the first messenger level) can act through the other messenger levels to produce an increasingly wider array of physiological effects. (From S E Hyman, E J Nestler:* Molecular Foundations of Psychiatry, *p 45. American Psychiatric Press, Washington, 1993. Used with permission.)*

G-PROTEINS

With the exception of synaptic transmission mediated by receptors that contain intrinsic ion channels, the family of membrane proteins known as G-proteins may be involved in all other transmembrane signaling in the nervous system. G-proteins are so-named because of their ability to bind the guanine nucleotides guanosine triphosphate (GTP) and guanosine diphosphate (GDP). G-proteins serve to couple receptors to specific intracellular effector systems (Figure 1.6-2). Four major types of G-proteins are involved in the transduction of signals produced by neurotransmitter binding: G_s, G_i, G_q, and G_o. Rhodopsin, the light-sensitive molecule of photoreceptor cells in the retina, can also be viewed as a G-protein-linked receptor; light activates rhodopsin, which then, through a fifth type of G-protein called transducin (G_t), regulates the electrical properties of photoreceptor cells. Each type of G-protein is a heterotrimer composed of single α, β, and γ subunits. Distinct α subunits confer specific functional activity on the different types of G-proteins, which appear to share common βγ subunits.

The functional activity of G-proteins is shown schematically in Figure 1.6-2. In the resting state, G-proteins exist as heterotrimers that are bound to GDP and are unassociated with extracellular receptors or intracellular effector proteins (A in Figure 1.6-2). When ligand binds to the receptor, it produces a conformational change in the receptor, which causes it to associate with the α subunit of the G-protein (B in Figure 1.6-2). That association, in turn, alters the conformation of the α subunit and leads to (1) the exchange of GTP for GDP on the α subunit, (2) the dissociation of the βγ subunits from the α subunit, and (3) the release of the receptor from the G-protein (B and C in Figure 1.6-2). That process generates a free α subunit bound to GTP, which is biologically active and can regulate the functional activity of effector proteins within the cell. Some evidence, albeit less definitive, suggests that free βγ subunits may also have biological activity. The system returns to its resting state when the ligand is released from the receptor and the GTPase activity that resides in the α subunit hydrolyzes GTP to GDP (D in Figure 1.6-2). That action leads to the reassociation of the free α subunit with the βγ subunits to restore the original heterotrimers.

Synaptic responses mediated by ligand-gated channels and G-pro-

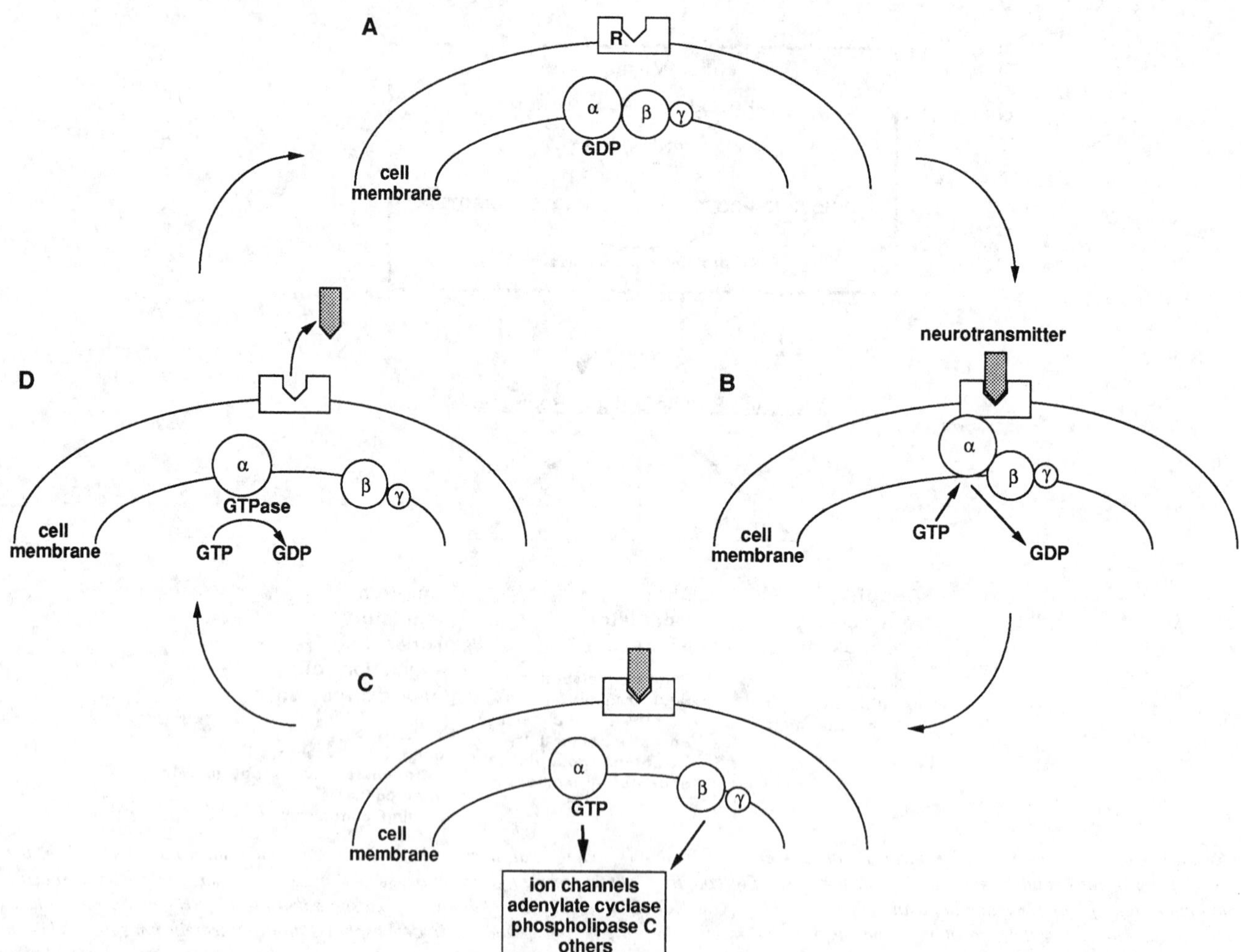

FIGURE 1.6-2 *G-protein function in the brain. (A) Under basal conditions, G-proteins exist in cell membranes as heterotrimers composed of single α, β, and γ subunits and are not associated physically with neurotransmitter receptors (R). In that situation the α subunits are bound to guanosine 5′-diphosphate (GDP). (B) On activation of the receptor by its ligand (such as a neurotransmitter), the receptor physically associates with the α subunit, which leads to the binding of guanosine 5′-triphosphate (GTP) to the α subunit and the displacement of GDP from the subunit. (C) GTP binding induces the generation of free α subunits by causing the dissociation of the α subunits from their βγ subunits and the receptor. Free α subunits, bound to GTP, are functionally active and directly regulate a number of effector proteins, which, depending on the type of α subunit and cell involved, can include ion channels, adenylate cyclase, and phospholipase C. Free βγ subunits may directly regulate some effector proteins. (D) GTPase activity intrinsic to the α subunit degrades GTP to form GDP. That action leads to the reassociation of the α and βγ subunits, which, along with the dissociation of the ligand from the receptor, leads to the restoration of the basal state. (From S E Hyman, E J Nestler:* Molecular Foundations of Psychiatry, *p 46. American Psychiatric Press, Washington, 1993. Used with permission.)*

tein-linked receptors have markedly different time courses. The direct effects of ligand-gated channels are usually extremely rapid and short-lived, typically being completed in less than one millisecond, whereas those mediated by G-protein-linked receptors are slower in onset (generally requiring at least 100 milliseconds to develop) and can be very long in duration (up to many minutes).

REGULATION OF ION CHANNELS G-proteins have been shown to couple neurotransmitter receptors to multiple types of intracellular effector proteins. In some cases G-proteins couple neurotransmitter receptors directly to ion channels (B in Figure 1.6-3). In that case it appears that the α subunit released from the G-protein-receptor interaction directly gates—that is, opens or closes—a specific ion channel. One of the best-established examples of that type of mechanism in the brain is the coupling of opiate, α_2-adrenergic, D_2-dopaminergic, muscarinic cholinergic, $5\text{-}HT_{1a}$-serotonergic, and γ-aminobutyric acid ($GABA_B$) receptors to the activation of an inward-rectifying potassium (K^+) channel through subtypes of G_o and G_i in many types of neurons. Some of those same neurotransmitter receptors have been shown to be similarly coupled to voltage-dependent calcium (Ca^{2+}) channels by the same types of G-proteins, although the channels are inhibited by the interaction. Other types of ion channels may also be coupled to neurotransmitter receptors by G-proteins.

REGULATION OF INTRACELLULAR SECOND MESSENGERS In many other cases G-proteins transduce the activation of neurotransmitter receptors into alterations in intracellular levels of second messengers in target neurons (Figure 1.6-1). Prominent second messengers in the brain include cyclic adenosine monophosphate (AMP), cyclic guanosine monophosphate (GMP), calcium, and the major metabolites of phosphatidylinositol (inositol triphosphate [IP_3] and diacylglycerol) and of arachidonic acid. As discussed above, altered levels of second messengers mediate the actions of neurotransmitter-receptor activation on some types of ion channels (C in Figure 1.6-3) and on numerous other physiological responses.

SECOND MESSENGERS

CYCLIC NUCLEOTIDES The first molecule shown to play a second-messenger role in cell function was cyclic AMP. Since its initial discovery more than 30 years ago, cyclic AMP has been implicated in mediating many actions of neurotransmitters and hormones on virtually every cell type, including neurons.

The molecular mechanism by which neurotransmitters regulate cyclic AMP levels is well established (Figure 1.6-4). G_s couples receptors (for example, β-adrenergic, D_1-dopamine, and vasoactive intestinal polypeptide [VIP] receptors) to adenylate cyclase, the enzyme responsible for the synthesis of cyclic AMP, such that the enzyme is stimulated by receptor activation. In contrast, G_i couples receptors (for example, opiate, α_2-adrenergic, and D_2-dopamine receptors) to adenylate cyclase, such that the enzyme is inhibited by receptor activation. Several forms of adenylate cyclase have been cloned. Those enzymes show different regional distributions in the brain and distinct regulatory properties. The enzymes differ in their ability to be regulated on binding free βγ complexes, and only certain forms are activated on binding calcium-calmodulin complexes.

Another cyclic nucleotide, cyclic GMP, has also been implicated as an intracellular second messenger in the brain and elsewhere, although its specific functions are less well established than cyclic AMP. Neurotransmitters appear to regulate cellular cyclic GMP levels by several mechanisms. In some cases, as with the atrial natriuretic peptide receptor, the enzyme guanylate cyclase (which catalyzes the synthesis of cyclic GMP) resides within the receptor protein. In other cases, nitric oxide appears to act as an intracellular second messenger in mediating the ability of certain neurotransmitters to activate guanylate cyclase (Figure 1.6-4). Those neurotransmitters are thought to elicit an increase in intracellular calcium levels (as described below), which activates nitric oxide synthetase, the enzyme responsible for the synthesis of nitric oxide. Nitric oxide then directly activates guanylate cyclase. In still other cases, it is conceivable, though not proved, that some neurotransmitter receptors are coupled by specific G-proteins to guanylate cyclase.

CALCIUM AND THE PHOSPHATIDYLINOSITOL SYSTEM On the basis of early studies showing that calcium mediates stimulus-secretion coupling in peripheral tissues, calcium has been shown to serve numerous second-messenger functions in virtually all cell types. The ways in which neurotransmitters alter intracellular calcium levels are more complex than those in which cyclic nucleotides act and involve two types of mechanisms that operate to different extents in different cell types (Figure 1.6-5). Neurotransmitter-receptor activation can alter the flux of extracellular calcium into neurons in a number of ways: (1) calcium can pass through ligand-gated channels, such as the nicotinic cholinergic and *N*-methyl-D-aspartate (NMDA)-glutamate receptors; (2) the conductance of specific voltage-gated calcium channels can be altered by direct coupling of receptors to the channels by G-proteins, such as with opiate receptors in certain cell types, as described above; (3) depolarization of a neuron by any means can activate voltage-

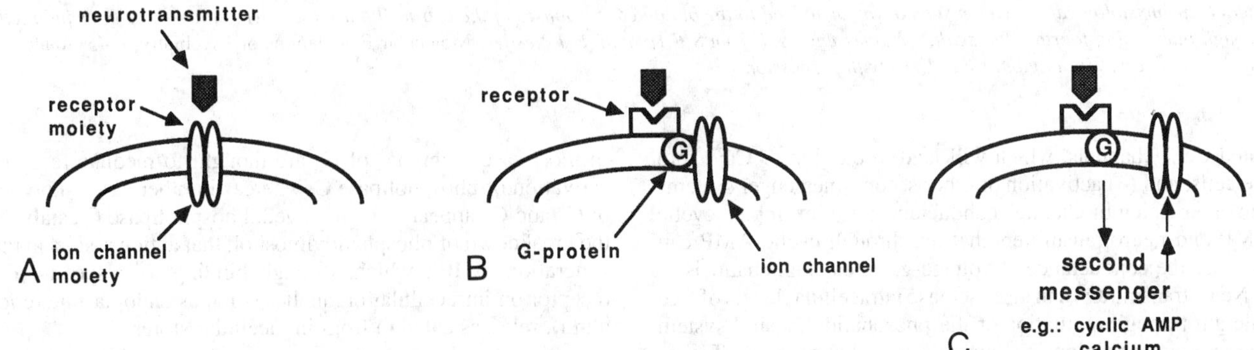

FIGURE 1.6-3 *Types of coupling of neurotransmitter receptors to ion channels. (From S E Hyman, E J Nestler:* Molecular Foundations of Psychiatry, *p 41. American Psychiatric Press, Washington, 1993. Used with permission.)*

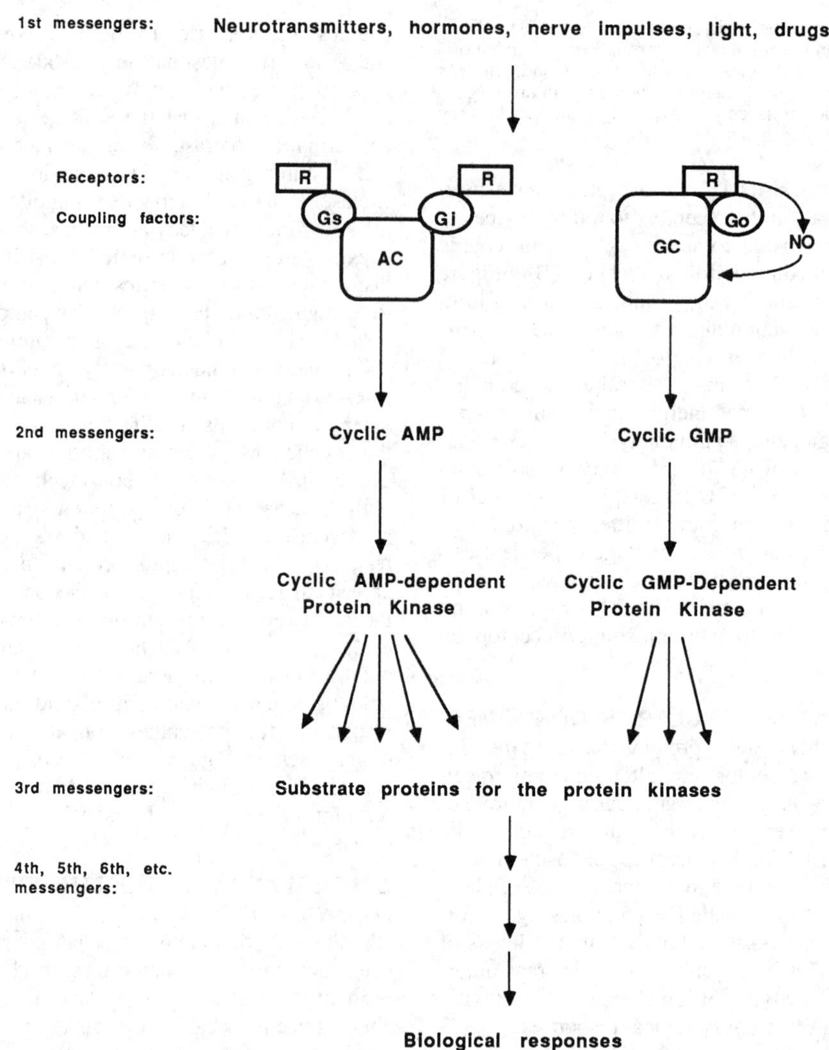

FIGURE 1.6-4 *Cyclic adenosine monophosphate (AMP) and cyclic guanosine monophosphate (GMP) second-messenger systems in the brain. Many of the effects of extracellular messengers, termed first messengers, on brain function are achieved through the cyclic AMP or cyclic GMP second-messenger systems. Most extracellular messengers influence the second-messenger systems through interactions with neurotransmitter receptors (R). However, some extracellular messengers, particularly drugs (for example, phosphodiesterase inhibitors, which inhibit the breakdown of cyclic AMP and cyclic GMP), can influence the second-messenger systems directly. G-proteins (G_s, G_i, and G_o) serve as coupling factors in that they mediate the ability of neurotransmitter receptors to activate or inhibit adenylate cyclase or possibly guanylate cyclase, the enzymes that catalyze the synthesis of cyclic AMP and cyclic GMP, respectively. The second messengers, in turn, activate specific types of protein kinases. The brain contains one major type of cyclic AMP-dependent protein kinase and one major type of cyclic GMP-dependent protein kinase, although subtypes of those enzymes are differentially expressed throughout the brain. The enzymes phosphorylate a specific array of substrate proteins, termed third messengers. Cyclic AMP-dependent protein kinase has a broad substrate specificity—that is, it phosphorylates many substrate proteins and mediates most of the numerous second-messenger actions of cyclic AMP in the nervous system. The substrate specificity of cyclic GMP-dependent protein kinase appears to be less broad than the substrate specificity of cyclic AMP-dependent protein kinase, although, by analogy with the cyclic AMP system, it probably mediates many of the second-messenger functions of cyclic GMP. Phosphorylation of the substrate proteins alters their physiological activity in such a way as to lead to the biological responses of the extracellular messengers either directly or indirectly through intervening fourth, fifth, sixth, etc., messengers. (From S E Hyman, E J Nestler:* Molecular Foundations of Psychiatry, *p 45. American Psychiatric Press, Washington, 1993. Used with permission.)*

gated Ca^{2+} channels, which will lead to the flux of Ca^{2+} into the cells; and (4) activation of other second-messenger systems can alter calcium-channel conductance; for example, cyclic AMP and neurotransmitters that act through cyclic AMP can increase the conductance of voltage-gated calcium channels.

Neurotransmitters can also increase intracellular levels of free calcium through regulation of the phosphatidylinositol system and subsequent actions on intracellular calcium stores (Figure 1.6-5). Thus, many types of neurotransmitter receptors are coupled through G-proteins to an enzyme termed phospholipase C. In most cases subtypes of G_q are thought to mediate receptor activation of phospholipase C, whereas in other cases subtypes of G_i and G_o appear to be involved. Phospholipase C catalyzes the breakdown of phosphatidylinositol; that action results in the generation of IP_3, which, through binding to a specific IP_3 receptor on intracellular organelles (such as endoplasmic reticulum), releases calcium from intracellular stores.

ARACHIDONIC ACID METABOLITES The prostaglandin and leukotriene system represents an additional family of intra-

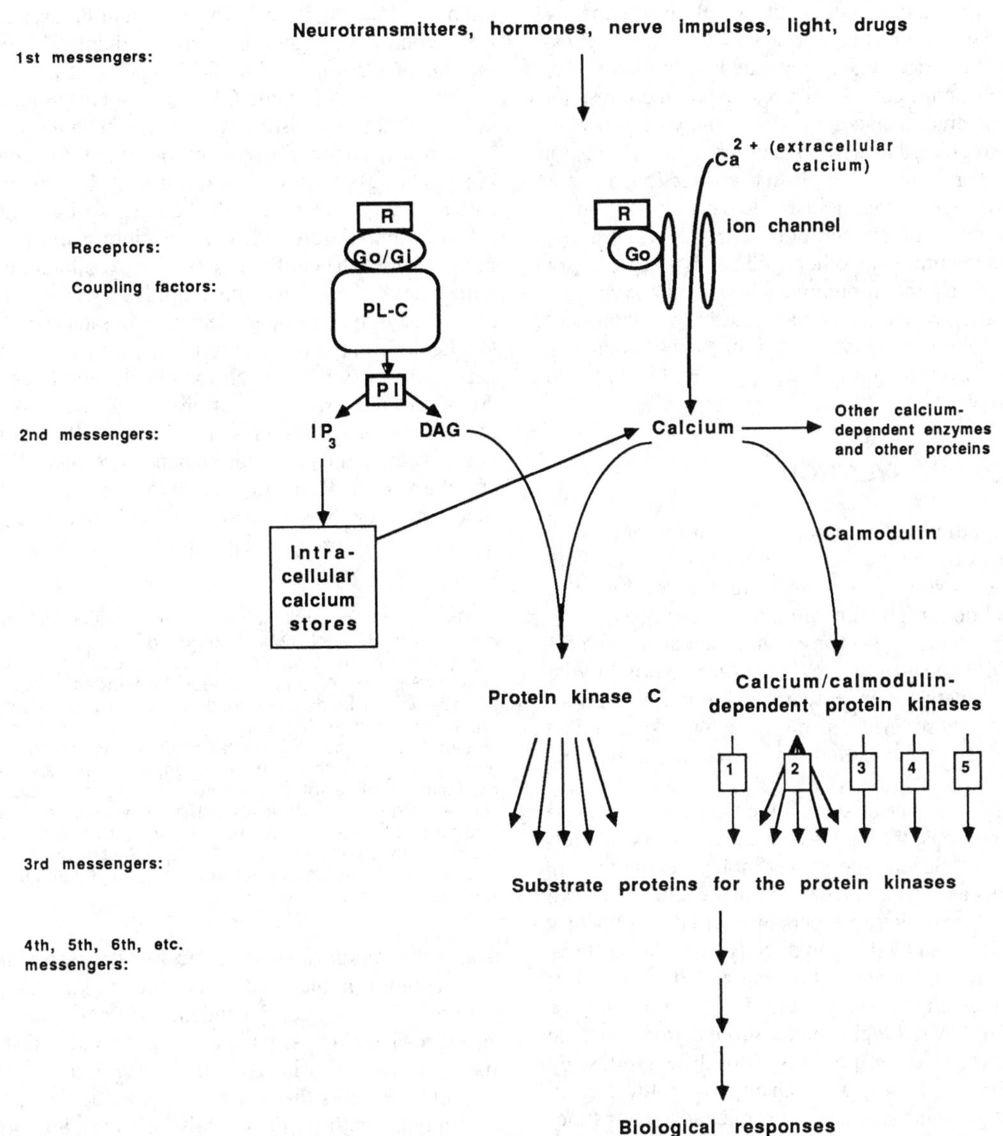

FIGURE 1.6-5 *Calcium and phosphatidylinositol second-messenger systems in the brain. Many of the effects of first messengers on brain function are achieved through the calcium and phosphatidylinositol second-messenger systems. As stated for the cyclic AMP and cyclic GMP systems in the legend for Figure 1.6-4, most actions of extracellular messengers on the second-messenger systems are achieved through interactions with neurotransmitter receptors (R). However, some drugs (such as calcium channel blockers and lithium [Eskalith]), can influence the second-messenger systems directly. G-proteins (G_i, G_o, and G_q) serve as coupling factors in that they mediate the ability of neurotransmitter receptors to regulate phospholipase C, which metabolizes phosphatidylinositol (PI) into the second messengers inositol triphosphate (IP_3) and diacylglycerol (DAG). IP_3 then acts to increase intracellular levels of free calcium (also a second messenger in the brain) by releasing calcium from internal stores. Increased levels of intracellular calcium also result from the flux of calcium across the plasma membrane through calcium and other ion channels, a flux stimulated by nerve impulses and certain neurotransmitters. G-proteins mediate many of the actions of neurotransmitters on such channels. The second messengers, in turn, activate specific types of calcium-dependent protein kinases, of which the brain contains two major classes. One class is activated by calcium in conjunction with the calcium-binding protein calmodulin and is referred to as calcium-calmodulin-dependent protein kinase. The brain contains at least five distinct types of that enzyme: (1–3) calcium-calmodulin-dependent protein kinases 1, 2, and 3; (4) phosphorylase kinase; and (5) myosin light chain kinase. The other major class of calcium-dependent protein kinases in the brain is activated by calcium in conjunction with diacylglycerol and various phospholipids and is referred to as calcium-diacylglycerol-dependent protein kinase or protein kinase C; at least seven closely related variants of the enzyme are present in the brain. Protein kinase C and calcium-calmodulin-dependent protein kinase 2 have broad substrate specificities (as indicated by the multiple arrows in the figure), and each probably mediates many of the numerous second-messenger actions of calcium in the nervous system. (The figure also illustrates that some of the second-messenger actions of calcium in the brain are mediated through proteins other than protein kinases.) Phosphorylation of substrate proteins or third messengers by those various calcium-dependent protein kinases alters their physiological activity in such a way as to lead to the biological responses of the extracellular messengers either directly or indirectly through intervening fourth, fifth, sixth, etc., messengers. (From S E Hyman, E J Nestler:* Molecular Foundations of Psychiatry, *p 51. American Psychiatric Press, Washington, 1993. Used with permission.)*

cellular messengers that appear to play a major role in the regulation of signal transduction in the brain and elsewhere mainly by modulating the generation of other second messengers. Prostaglandins and leukotrienes are generated as follows: An enzyme termed phospholipase A_2 cleaves membrane phospholipids to yield free arachidonic acid. The activity of phospholipase A_2 may be regulated by certain neurotransmitter-receptor interactions by G-proteins, although that connection remains speculative. Next, arachidonic acid is cleaved by cyclo-oxygenase to yield, after numerous additional enzymatic steps, several types of prostaglandins and other cyclic endoperoxides (for example, prostacyclins and thromboxanes) or by lipoxygenase to yield the leukotrienes. Those endoperoxides and leukotrienes exhibit varied biological activity in influencing adenylate cyclase, guanylate cyclase, ion channels, protein kinases, and other cellular proteins.

PROTEIN PHOSPHORYLATION

Protein phosphorylation is the major molecular currency with which protein function is regulated in response to extracellular stimuli. That view is supported by more than a generation of research. Thus, although proteins are known to be covalently modified in many other ways—for example, by adenosine 5′-diphosphate (ADP)-ribosylation, acylation (acetylation, myristoylation), carboxymethylation, tyrosine sulfation, and glycosylation—none of those mechanisms is as widespread and as readily subject to regulation by synaptic stimuli as phosphorylation.

Despite the large number of second messengers that can be activated within neurons, the signaling pathways work in a relatively uniform way. Second-messenger molecules may rarely have direct actions as effectors (for example, cyclic AMP can bind to and directly gate ion channels in neurons in olfactory epithelium, and Ca^{2+} can bind to and directly regulate the activity of several enzymes), but most of the known effects of intracellular second messengers are produced by stimulating the addition or the removal of phosphate groups from specific amino acid residues in target proteins. Phosphate groups, by virtue of their size and their charge, change the conformation of those substrate proteins and, in doing so, change their function. For example, a phosphorylated ion channel may open more or less readily, a phosphorylated neurotransmitter receptor may be inactivated, and a phosphorylated neurotransmitter synthesizing enzyme may act far more rapidly than before phosphorylation.

The regulation of protein function by phosphorylation plays a paramount role in signal transduction within the brain. In most cases neurotransmitters regulate protein phosphorylation through second-messenger-mediated activation of enzymes called protein kinases. Protein kinases transfer phosphate groups from adenosine triphosphate (ATP) to serine, threonine, or tyrosine residues in specific substrate proteins (Figures 1.6-4 and 1.6-5). In a smaller number of cases, neurotransmitters regulate protein phosphorylation through second-messenger-mediated regulation of protein phosphatases, enzymes that remove phosphate groups from proteins through hydrolysis. Each protein kinase and protein phosphatase acts on a specific array of substrate proteins.

PROTEIN KINASES

Second-messenger-dependent protein kinases Among the most prominent protein kinases in the brain are those activated by the second messengers cyclic AMP, cyclic GMP, calcium, and diacylglycerol. Those protein kinases are named for the second messengers that activate them. The brain contains one major class of cyclic AMP-dependent protein kinase and one major class of cyclic GMP-dependent protein kinase (Figure 1.6-4), although isoforms of those enzymes are now known. In contrast, two major classes of calcium-dependent protein kinases have been described (Figure 1.6-5). One is activated by calcium in conjunction with the calcium-binding protein calmodulin and is referred to as calcium-calmodulin-dependent protein kinase. The other is activated by calcium in conjunction with diacylglycerol and other lipids and is referred to as calcium-diacylglycerol-dependent protein kinase or protein kinase C. The brain contains several subtypes of each of those calcium-dependent enzymes, which exhibit different regulatory properties and are expressed differentially in neuronal cell types throughout the nervous system. Cyclic AMP-dependent protein kinase, calcium-calmodulin-dependent protein kinase type II, and the various forms of protein kinase C appear to be multifunctional enzymes in that they each phosphorylate a large number of substrate proteins and thereby influence a diversity of neuronal processes.

The mechanisms by which second messengers activate those protein kinases is well established. Each type of enzyme possesses a catalytic domain (the region that contains the active site that transfers a phosphate group from ATP to a substrate protein) and a regulatory domain (the region that binds the second messenger and confers second-messenger sensitivity to the enzyme). In the resting state the regulatory domain binds to and inhibits the catalytic domain. Binding of the second messenger to the regulatory domain alters its conformation and results in the release of the regulatory domain from the catalytic domain and, therefore, in catalytically active enzyme. For most enzymes the catalytic and regulatory domains reside within the same polypeptide chain, although for cyclic AMP-dependent protein kinase the two domains reside within distinct subunits termed regulatory and catalytic subunits.

Second-messenger-independent protein kinases The brain contains numerous types of protein kinases in addition to the second-messenger-dependent enzymes. They include protein tyrosine kinases, which phosphorylate substrate proteins specifically on tyrosine residues; casein kinases; and a number of protein kinases that appear to be associated physically and functionally with particular substrate proteins. Some of those protein kinases probably also play critically important roles in signal transduction in the brain, although the mechanisms involved are not as clearly established as for the second-messenger-dependent enzymes.

The best studied protein tyrosine kinases are those that are associated with plasma membrane receptors for many types of growth factors. Thus, receptors for insulin, epidermal growth factor, nerve growth factor, and many related growth factors possess protein tyrosine kinase enzyme activity within the receptor complex. Binding of the growth factors to the receptors leads to activation of the receptor-associated protein tyrosine kinase, which appears to mediate the physiological actions of those factors. The other major class of protein tyrosine kinases lacks that receptor domain. The mechanism underlying their regulation has remained elusive, although early evidence indicates that some of the enzymes may transiently become associated with specific receptors and thereby transduce extracellular signals into changes in intraneuronal function. Several lines of evidence suggest an important role for protein tyrosine kinases in brain-signal transduction. The enzymes are present in the adult brain at higher levels than in most other tissues, show striking regional differences throughout the brain, are enriched in synaptic fractions of brain along with a number of prominent substrate proteins, and can be regulated by depolarizing stimuli and glucocorticoid hormones in discrete regions of the central nervous system.

Another example of second-messenger-independent protein kinases are the MAP-kinases, first identified on the basis of their association with and phosphorylation of microtubule-associated proteins (MAPs). MAP-kinases have since been shown to phosphorylate a number of other proteins in the brain and elsewhere, including tyrosine hydroxylase. The mechanism by which the activity of MAP-kinases are regulated by extracellular signals has been established recently. The enzymes are activated by their phosphorylation by another protein kinase, called MAP-kinase kinase, which is, in turn, also activated on phosphorylation by MAP-kinase kinase kinases. The latter enzymes are subject to regulation by second messenger-dependent protein kinases and protein tyrosine kinases. Thus, the MAP-kinase pathway appears to be an important site on convergence of multiple signaling pathways.

PROTEIN PHOSPHATASES Less is known about protein phosphatases than about protein kinases, but the brain clearly contains several types of protein phosphatases that differ in their regional distribution in the brain and in their regulatory properties. Protein phosphatases can be divided into two major classes on the basis of the types of amino acids they dephosphorylate: serine-threonine phosphatases and tyrosine phosphatases.

By two known mechanisms neurotransmitters can influence protein phosphorylation through the regulation of protein serine-threonine phosphatases. In one mechanism a phosphatase referred to as calcineurin or phosphatase type 2B can be activated directly by binding calcium and calmodulin. Presumably, neurotransmitters that alter cellular calcium levels influence the phosphorylation of cellular proteins through alterations in calcineurin activity. The other mechanism is indirect and involves a class of proteins referred to as protein phosphatase inhibitors. The best known protein phosphatase inhibitors are phosphatase inhibitors 1 and 2 and dopamine and cyclic AMP-regulated phosphoprotein of 32 KD (DARPP-32), an inhibitor protein expressed in specific neuronal cell types in the brain. Those proteins are potent inhibitors of protein phosphatase type 1, and their phosphorylation by cyclic AMP-dependent protein kinase alters their inhibitory activity. Presumably, in neurons that contain those phosphatase inhibitors, neurotransmitters that alter cellular cyclic AMP levels influence the phosphorylation of cellular proteins through alterations in type 1 protein phosphatase activity.

PHOSPHOPROTEINS After the activation of protein kinases or alterations in protein phosphatase activity, the next step in intracellular signal transduction pathways involves regulation of the phosphorylation state of specific neuronal phosphoproteins. The phosphoproteins are referred to as third messengers. A large and increasing number of neuronal proteins have been shown to be regulated by phosphorylation. As shown in Table 1.6-1, brain phosphoproteins belong to every conceivable class of protein, indicating the widespread role of protein phosphorylation in the regulation of diverse aspects of neuronal function. That role includes the regulation of ion channel conductance, neurotransmitter receptor sensitivity, neurotransmitter synthesis and release, axoplasmic transport, elaboration of dendritic and axonal processes, and the development and maintenance of differentiated characteristics of neurons. As discussed below, phosphorylation of neuronal proteins plays a paramount role in the regulation of neural plasticity, including learning and memory. Moreover, protein phosphorylation mechanisms have been implicated in the pathophysiology of a growing number of neuropsychiatric disorders, particularly Alzheimer's disease and drug addiction.

TABLE 1.6-1
Classes of Neuronal Proteins Regulated by Phosphorylation

Enzymes involved in neurotransmitter biosynthesis and degradation
e.g., tyrosine hydroxylase
tryptophan hydroxylase

Neurotransmitter receptors
e.g., nicotinic acetylcholine receptor
β-adrenergic receptor
α_2-adrenergic receptor
$GABA_A$ receptor
muscarinic cholinergic receptor
glutamate receptor

Ion channels
e.g., voltage-dependent sodium, potassium, and calcium channels
ligand-gated channels
calcium-dependent potassium channels
nonspecific cation channel

Enzymes and other proteins involved in the regulation of second-messenger levels
e.g., G-proteins
phospholipases
adenylate cyclase
guanylate cyclase
phosphodiesterase
IP_3 receptor

Protein kinases
e.g., autophosphorylated protein kinases
(whereby most protein kinases phosphorylate themselves)
protein kinases phosphorylated by other protein kinases
(many examples)

Protein phosphatase inhibitors
e.g., Dopamine and cyclic-AMP Regulated Phosphoprotein of 32 KD
inhibitors 1 and 2

Cytoskeletal proteins involved in neuronal growth, shape, and motility
e.g., actin
tubulin
neurofilaments (and other intermediate filament proteins)
myosin
microtubule-associated proteins

Synaptic vesicle proteins involved in neurotransmitter release
e.g., synapsins I and II
clathrin
synaptophysin

Transcription factors
e.g., cyclic AMP-response element binding proteins (CREB)
immediate–early gene products (such as Fos, Jun, and Zif)
steroid and thyroid hormone receptors

Other proteins involved in DNA transcription or mRNA translation
e.g., RNA polymerase
topoisomerase
histones and nonhistone nuclear proteins
ribosomal protein S6
eIF (eukaryotic initiation factor)
eEF (eukaryotic elongation factor)
other ribosomal proteins

Miscellaneous
e.g., myelin basic protein
rhodopsin
neural cell adhesion molecules
myristoylated alanine-rich C kinase substrate (MARCKS)
growth-associated protein of 43 KD (GAP-43)

This list is not intended to be comprehensive but, instead, indicates the types of neuronal proteins regulated by phosphorylation. Some of the proteins are specific to neurons. The others are present in many cell types, in addition to neurons, and are included because among their multiple functions in the nervous system is the regulation of neuron-specific phenomena. Not included are the many phosphoproteins present in diverse tissues (including the brain) that play roles in generalized cellular processes, such as intermediary metabolism, and that do not appear to play roles in neuron-specific phenomena. (Modified from S E Hyman, E J Nestler: *Molecular Foundations of Psychiatry*. American Psychiatric Press, Washington, 1993. Used with permission.)

HETEROGENEITY IN BRAIN SIGNAL TRANSDUCTION PATHWAYS

Molecular biological studies have demonstrated extraordinary heterogeneity in intracellular messenger pathways, a degree of heterogeneity not suspected by classical biochemical, pharmacological, and physiological studies. For example, whereas biochemical and pharmacological studies indicated the existence of five types of G-proteins—G_s, G_i, G_o, G_q, and G_t—two types of cyclic AMP-dependent protein kinase, and just one type of protein kinase C, molecular cloning studies now indicate the existence of at least 15 distinct G-protein subunits, six distinct subunits of cyclic AMP-dependent protein kinase, and seven subtypes of protein kinase C. Such heterogeneity has been shown in each case to be due to a combination of the existence of numerous distinct genes for each of the proteins and alternative splicing of some common genes. In general, comparison of the individual subtypes of those proteins has indicated that they possess different regulatory properties and exhibit varying levels of expression in different neuronal cell types. That high degree of heterogeneity indicates still greater potential for functional specificity within and between neuronal cell types in the brain. In addition, such heterogeneity raises the possibility of developing drugs that interfere with specific subtypes of intracellular messengers; the drugs would represent novel approaches in the treatment of neuropsychiatric disorders.

NEURAL PLASTICITY

The human brain is remarkably plastic. It adapts to a wide variety of circumstances, forms memories of experiences, and learns procedures; it can become dependent on drugs or produce disabling psychopathology; and it can recover. The plasticity of the brain and, therefore, the ability to learn and adapt is at the heart of human evolutionary success in nature and of cultural evolution as well. What are the processes underlying the plasticity?

As discussed above, neurotransmitters elicit diverse types of physiological responses, in addition to simply producing rapid electrical changes, in target neurons. Those physiological responses include prolonged changes in the way in which the target neurons process subsequent synaptic information. The effects may be undetectable until the neuron is stimulated again by the same or other neurotransmitters.

Such modulatory actions of neurotransmitters form the biochemical and molecular basis of neural plasticity. Studies over the past 10 years have indicated that two general types of mechanisms are involved. One mechanism is protein phosphorylation, whereby modulation of neuronal function is achieved through phosphorylation-induced alterations in the functional state of a wide variety of neuronal proteins. Some examples include phosphorylation of ion channels (which alters the electrical excitability of target neurons), phosphorylation of neurotransmitter receptors (which alters the responsiveness of target neurons to synaptic inputs), and phosphorylation of neurotransmitter synthetic enzymes and of proteins that control neurotransmitter storage and release (which alters the ability of the neurons to influence their own target neurons).

The other general mechanism underlying neural plasticity is the regulation of neuronal gene expression. Changes in gene expression may produce quantitative and even qualitative changes in many of the protein components of neurons. Some examples include alterations in the number and the types of ion channels and receptors present on the cell membrane, levels of postreceptor signal transduction proteins expressed in neurons, and even the morphology and the number of synaptic connections they form. Regulation of neuronal gene expression by neurotransmitters is pervasive and occurs on a continual basis to fine-tune the functional state of neurons in response to complex synaptic inputs. Ultimately, the long-term effects of environmental factors on the brain, including long-term behavioral effects and long-term memory, are mediated through those complex processes involving regulation of protein phosphorylation and neuronal gene expression. Those biochemical and molecular changes lead successively to changes in the function or the efficacy of synapses, changes in the way individual neurons process information, and, ultimately, changes in communication among multicellular neural networks. Evidence accumulated over the past 20 years indicates ways in which phosphorylation alters the functional activity of specific proteins and establishes the precise mechanisms by which their phosphorylation, in response to neurotransmitters and other extracellular stimuli, mediates short-term and long-term effects of those extracellular stimuli on neuronal function (Figure 1.6-6). The mechanisms by which protein phosphorylation underlies the extraordinary plasticity evident in both the developing brain and the adult brain is considered in this section. The role of neuronal gene expression and of protein phosphorylation in the regulation of neuronal gene expression in mediating neural plasticity is covered in Section 1.14.

NEURONAL PROTEIN PHOSPHORYLATION To understand the exact mechanisms by which protein phosphorylation mediates neural phenomena, one must understand how it is that the addition of a phosphate group to a protein alters that protein's functional activity. Phosphorylation of a protein alters that protein's charge (phosphate groups are highly negatively charged), which can then also alter the protein's shape or conformation. When a protein's charge or conformation is altered, its intrinsic functional activity is likely to be changed (for example, the ability of an ion channel to open), or its ability to interact with other molecules is likely to be changed. Phosphorylation alters the affinity of certain proteins for other proteins, cofactors (in the case of enzymes), and other small molecules. For example, phosphorylation of tyrosine hydroxylase increases its affinity for its protein cofactor and thereby increases the rate at which it converts tyrosine to dopa; phosphorylation of the β-adrenergic receptor decreases its affinity for norepinephrine; phosphorylation of certain nuclear proteins alters their ability to initiate transcription of deoxyribonucleic acid (DNA).

The complexity of intracellular regulation is underscored by the now well-established observation that many, perhaps even most, proteins are phosphorylated on more than one amino acid residue by more than one type of protein kinase. That is referred to as multisite phosphorylation. Depending on the protein, phosphorylation of different residues can lead to similar or opposite changes in that protein's function. In some cases the phosphorylation of one residue can even influence the ability of the other residues to undergo phosphorylation.

The phosphorylation of neuronal proteins by more than one protein kinase probably integrates the activities of multiple intracellular pathways to achieve coordinated regulation of cell function. For example, the phosphorylation of tyrosine hydroxylase by cyclic AMP-dependent and calcium-dependent protein kinases enables neurotransmitters that act through the cyclic AMP and calcium systems to produce an integrated increase in catecholamine biosynthesis. That information further supports the view that protein phosphorylation is a final common molecular pathway through which multiple extracellular and intracellular signals converge to regulate neuronal function.

Regulation of receptors For all cases that have been investigated to date, neurotransmitter receptors, both presynaptic and postsynaptic, are regulated by phosphorylation (Table 1.6-1). Increasing evidence suggests that phosphorylation alters the functional activity of

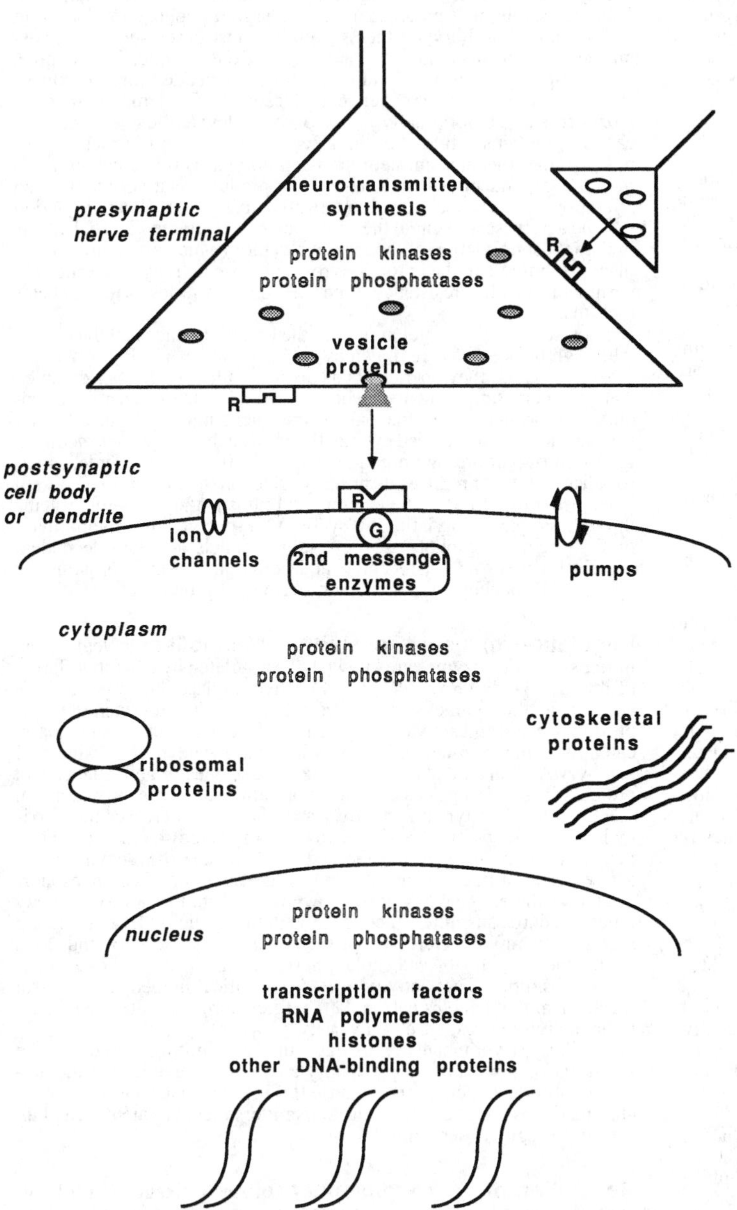

FIGURE 1.6-6 *Types of neuronal proteins regulated by phosphorylation. Virtually every class of protein and, therefore, every type of neural process are influenced through protein phosphorylation mechanisms. (From S E Hyman, E J Nestler:* Molecular Foundations of Psychiatry, *p 104. American Psychiatric Press, Washington, 1993. Used with permission.)*

receptors—for example, their ability to be activated by their endogenous ligand.

In many cases stimulation of a receptor by its own ligand leads to decreased (or increased) sensitivity of the receptor to subsequent stimulation, processes called homologous desensitization (or sensitization) of receptor function. In most cases studied to date, that action appears to be due to receptor-mediated activation of protein kinases leading to phosphorylation of the receptor. In other cases a receptor can be phosphorylated by a protein kinase activated by stimulation of another receptor type on the same cell. That action could lead to heterologous regulation of receptor function, in which receptor phosphorylation induced by one neurotransmitter/second-messenger system can influence the responsiveness of a neuron to other neurotransmitter/second-messenger systems. Most receptors probably exhibit both types of regulation and are phosphorylated by more than one protein kinase.

The best-studied example of receptor phosphorylation involves the β-adrenergic receptor. Activation of the β-adrenergic receptor leads, by coupling with G_s, to activation of adenylate cyclase and increased levels of cyclic AMP and of activated cyclic AMP-dependent protein kinase, which then phosphorylates the receptor on two serine residues in the region that interacts with G_s. In addition, the receptor is phosphorylated on several additional serine residues by another protein kinase physically associated with the receptor, termed β-adrenergic receptor kinase (or βark). That kinase can phosphorylate the receptor only when it is bound to the ligand—that is, the binding of the ligand to the receptor alters the receptor's conformation, and it is rendered a good substrate for the receptor kinase. Phosphorylation of the receptor by either protein kinase appears to desensitize the receptor to further activation by an adrenergic ligand in vitro and appears to play an important role in producing homologous desensitization of the receptor in vivo.

Phosphorylation of the β-adrenergic receptor can also be stimulated in response to activation of other receptors. For example, any neurotransmitter-receptor system that works through cyclic AMP can be expected to stimulate β-adrenergic receptor phosphorylation by cyclic AMP-dependent protein kinase and lead to receptor desensitization. Such phosphorylation mediates heterologous desensitization of the receptor.

Similar phosphorylation mechanisms have been reported to underlie homologous and heterologous desensitization of other G-protein-linked receptors. Notable examples include α-adrenergic and muscarinic cholinergic receptors.

Phosphorylation has also been shown to modulate the functioning of numerous ligand-gated ion channels, including the nicotinic acetylcholine, $GABA_A$, and glutamate receptors. The role of phosphorylation in regulating ligand-gated ion channels is best established for the nicotinic acetylcholine receptor, which is phosphorylated by cyclic AMP-dependent protein kinase, protein kinase C, and a protein tyrosine kinase. In each case phosphorylation of the receptor seems to increase the rate at which the receptor becomes desensitized to further stimulation by acetylcholine. Calcitonin gene-related peptide (CGRP) may be the neurotransmitter responsible for initiating cyclic AMP-dependent phosphorylation of the receptor at the neuromuscular junction. CGRP is colocalized with acetylcholine in motor neurons; release of

CGRP leads to the stimulation of adenylate cyclase, activation of cyclic AMP-dependent protein kinase, and phosphorylation and desensitization of the receptor. Since greater frequency of stimulation is required to release CGRP (compared with acetylcholine) from motor nerve endings, CGRP-mediated desensitization of the receptor may serve a negative feedback role on the function of the synapse during periods of intense stimulation.

Regulation of ion channels and pumps As with receptors, most ion channels can be phosphorylated by one or more protein kinases (Table 1.6-1). In most cases phosphorylation of the channels modifies their ability to open or close in response to their primary gating mechanism. One example is the L-type voltage-dependent Ca^{2+} channel, the type of channel inhibited by the dihydropyridine calcium channel blocker drugs, such as verapamil (Calan), used in cardiovascular medicine and occasionally in neuropsychopharmacology. When the L-type channel is phosphorylated by cyclic AMP-dependent protein kinase, it is rendered more likely to open in response to membrane depolarization. That mechanism plays an important role in the regulation of cardiac function: stimulation of β-adrenergic receptors by norepinephrine and epinephrine causes phosphorylation of the channel by increasing the levels of cyclic AMP and of activated cyclic AMP-dependent protein kinase. Because the phosphorylated L-type channel opens more, a greater amount of calcium enters the cell. In the heart that mechanism is responsible for catecholamine-induced increases in cardiac rate and contractility.

In some cases phosphorylation of ion channels may represent the primary gating mechanism that determines their opening or closing. One example of such a channel is a slowly depolarizing nonspecific cation channel identified in the rat locus ceruleus. That channel (or a closely associated protein) is phosphorylated by cyclic AMP-dependent protein kinase, which appears to initiate opening of the channel. The activity of the channel plays a central role in regulating the spontaneous—that is, pacemaker—activity of the neurons. The ability of various neurotransmitters—for example, vasoactive intestinal polypeptide and opioid peptides—to regulate the excitability of locus ceruleus neurons is mediated in part through alterations in the activity of that cation channel by cyclic AMP-dependent phosphorylation. Increasing evidence implicates such regulation of locus ceruleus excitability in setting levels of a person's attention span and vigilance and in mediating behavioral adaptations to stress and opiate addiction.

Most types of electrogenic pumps, which maintain stable levels of ions inside and outside the neuronal membrane, also undergo phosphorylation by second-messenger-dependent protein kinases. Those pumps include the Na^+/K^+-ATPase and the Ca^{2+}/Mg^{2+}-ATPase pumps. Phosphorylation and regulation of the activity of the Na^+/K^+-ATPase pump alter the rate at which the normal distribution of ions can be restored after a train of action potentials. That would be expected to alter the excitability of the neurons. Such a mechanism has recently been shown to operate in the brain, where dopamine and other neurotransmitters, through regulation of cyclic AMP-dependent protein phosphorylation, regulates activity of the Na^+/K^+-ATPase pump in target cells. One possibility is that neurotransmitter regulation of the Na^+/K^+-ATPase occurs indirectly through DARPP-32 (a phosphatase inhibitor); neurotransmitter activation of the cyclic AMP pathway leads to the phosphorylation and activation of DARPP-32, which then inhibits protein phosphatase I, leading to increased phosphorylation of the pump. Through that mechanism, the neurotransmitters can produce relatively long-lasting changes in the distribution of ions across the membrane, including changes in neuronal excitability. Phosphorylation and regulation of the activity of the Ca^{2+}/Mg^{2+}-ATPase pump, in a similar way, alter the excitability of neurons by influencing the ability of neurons to maintain the normal (low) levels of intracellular free calcium and to maintain healthy stores of calcium in intracellular organelles.

Regulation of intracellular messenger pathways Most of the protein components of intracellular messenger systems are themselves phosphoproteins—that is, substrates for protein kinases (Table 1.6-1). Extraordinarily complex cross talk between signaling pathways permits cells to coordinate their responses to environmental stimuli. Virtually every type of G-protein has been reported to undergo phosphorylation by a variety of protein kinases. Proteins that control the synthesis of the cyclic nucleotide second messengers (adenylate cyclase and guanylate cyclase) and the degradation of cyclic nucleotides (phosphodiesterases) are regulated by phosphorylation. Similarly, proteins that lead to increases in intracellular Ca^{2+} or phosphatidylinositol turnover (for example, phospholipase C, calcium channels, the IP_3 receptor) and proteins that decrease Ca^{2+} levels (for example, the Ca^{2+}/Mg^{2+}-ATPase pump) are regulated by phosphorylation. Moreover, phospholipase A_2, which generates arachidonic acid metabolites (such as prostaglandins) that modulate cyclic nucleotide and calcium levels, is also subject to phosphorylation. Many protein kinases are themselves phosphorylated and regulated by other protein kinases, and protein phosphatase type 1 is regulated by protein phosphatase inhibitor proteins, which themselves are regulated by phosphorylation. In addition, most—possibly all—protein kinases undergo autophosphorylation, in which they phosphorylate themselves. In most cases such autophosphorylation appears to facilitate activation of the enzyme. For example, autophosphorylation of calcium-calmodulin-dependent protein kinase II renders the protein independent of calcium. That means that the enzyme, activated originally in response to elevated levels of cellular calcium, remains active after the calcium levels have returned to normal. By that mechanism, neurotransmitters that activate calcium-calmodulin-dependent protein kinase II can produce relatively long-lived alterations in neuronal function. In other cases autophosphorylation may be a necessary event in the activation of the protein kinase. Defects in autophosphorylation of the insulin receptor (which, in addition to its insulin-binding site, has protein tyrosine kinase activity) underlies the peripheral insulin resistance seen in some famliies with diabetes mellitus.

Each second-messenger system in the brain influences all the others. Although the systems are drawn as distinct pathways in Figures 1.6-1, 1.6-4, and 1.6-5, they operate not as distinct pathways but as a complex web of interacting pathways. Thus, any time a neurotransmitter produces its primary effect on one second-messenger system, all other systems are also influenced eventually, with such interactions mediated for the most part through protein phosphorylation. For example, a neurotransmitter that produces its primary effect on the cyclic AMP system is expected to influence the calcium and phosphatidylinositol systems through the phosphorylation by cyclic AMP-dependent protein kinase of G-proteins, phospholipases, calcium channels, calcium-dependent protein kinases, the IP_3 receptor, and common substrate proteins for cyclic AMP-dependent and calcium-dependent protein kinases.

Regulation of neurotransmitter metabolism Neurotransmitter synthetic enzymes are known to be regulated by phosphorylation (Table 1.6-1). For example, tyrosine hydroxylase, the rate-limiting enzyme in the synthesis of the catecholamine neurotransmitters, is phosphorylated and activated by cyclic AMP-dependent protein kinase, calcium-calmodulin-dependent protein kinase, and protein kinase C and by MAP-kinase and probably other second-messenger-independent protein kinases. In most cases, phosphorylation increases the maximum velocity (V_{max}) of tyrosine hydroxylase (that is, it increases the maximal catalytic activity of a single enzyme molecule) or the affinity of the enzyme for its pterin cofactor (which makes the enzyme more active at subsaturating concentrations of the cofactor). Such phosphorylation of the enzyme has been shown to mediate the ability of many types of neurotransmitters (acting through the cyclic AMP and calcium systems) to rapidly increase tyrosine hydroxylase activity and, as a result, the capacity of catecholaminergic neurons to synthesize their neurotransmitter. That activity provides a critical homeostatic control mechanism that enables catecholaminergic neurons to alter their functional activity in response to a variety of synaptic inputs.

Similarly, tryptophan hydroxylase, the rate-limiting enzyme in the synthesis of serotonin, is phosphorylated and regulated by calcium-calmodulin-dependent protein kinase II. Such phosphorylation presumably mediates the ability of neurotransmitters that activate the calcium system to regulate serotonin biosynthesis in vivo.

Regulation of neurotransmitter release Regulation of calcium channel phosphorylation, described in the discussion of ion channels above, can alter the entry of calcium into nerve terminals and thereby the release of neurotransmitters from those terminals. Regulation of other types of channels can similarly alter neurotransmitter release by indirectly influencing the amount of calcium that enters the terminals during an action potential. However, additional important mechanisms regulate neurotransmitter release in the brain independent of ion channel phosphorylation. Those mechanisms appear to involve the phosphorylation of a family of synaptic vesicle-associated proteins (Table 1.6-1). Such regulation of neurotransmitter release is an important mechanism by which behavioral stimuli and psychotropic drugs modulate the strength of specific synaptic connections in the brain.

The best-studied synaptic vesicle-associated phosphoproteins are the synapsins. The synapsins comprise a family of phosphoproteins present in most synaptic terminals in the brain that are phosphorylated by cyclic AMP-dependent protein kinase and by calcium-calmodulin-dependent protein kinases I and II. Synapsin phosphorylation increases the amount of neurotransmitter released from nerve terminals in response to physiological stimuli. Phosphorylation of synapsins appears to augment neurotransmitter release by altering their binding affinity for synaptic vesicles and other cytoskeletal proteins. Such changes in synapsin-binding affinities are thought to regulate synaptic vesicle traffic within nerve terminals and, possibly, the process of exocytosis. Phosphorylation of the synapsins is regulated by a number of neurotransmitters, which influence cyclic AMP or calcium levels in nerve terminals, and appears to mediate the ability of those neurotransmitters to produce relatively long-lasting changes in the functional activity of those terminals. Phosphorylation of the synapsins also occurs in response to action potentials and probably represents one mechanism underlying posttetanic potentiation (PTP). PTP, a phenomenon described originally decades ago, occurs in most types of nerve terminals; a brief series of nerve impulses (referred to as a tetanus) increases the amount of neurotransmitter released by the terminals in response to a subsequent nerve impulse.

Regulation of neuronal growth and differentiation Protein phosphorylation also plays a critical role in cell growth, differentiation, and movement, although the details of the mechanisms remain obscure. Virtually all known cytoskeletal and contractile proteins are heavily phosphorylated by a number of protein kinases, and, in many cases, their functional activity is known to be altered by phosphorylation (Table 1.6-1). Specific types of protein kinases are induced in cells, including neurons, at precise points during the cell cycle. Similarly, specific types of protein kinases and substrate proteins are expressed in the brain at particular stages during development and differentiation. As mentioned above, virtually all growth factors that influence neural and nonneural cell types activate a class of receptors that possess protein tyrosine kinase activity within the receptor complex. Activation of that receptor-associated protein tyrosine kinase activity apparently leads to most and possibly all of the growth-promoting and differentiating effects of the factors. Neural cell adhesion molecules and proteins expressed specifically in axonal growth cones (the leading tips of growing axons), both of which are important for cell-cell interactions in the brain and the formation of synaptic connections, are also regulated by phosphorylation.

Regulation of gene expression Protein phosphorylation also plays a fundamental role in the regulation of neuronal gene expression, in a sense the ultimate end point of signal transduction in the brain. Such regulation appears to be achieved through the phosphorylation of a subset of the proteins that regulate transcription (Table 1.6-1).

MOLECULAR BASIS OF LEARNING AND MEMORY

Understanding how the brain learns and stores memories is a central goal of neurobiology. Each of the neurotransmitter and drug-induced changes in protein phosphorylation discussed above represents a form of molecular memory within individual neurons. In all likelihood, learning and memory at the level of the whole brain are mediated by complex accumulations of those basic types of changes to produce alterations in the function or the efficacy of synapses within particular neural systems. Changes in synaptic efficacy may be due to altered patterns of neurotransmitter release by the presynaptic neuron or to changes in the effect of the neurotransmitter on the postsynaptic cell. Since alterations in protein phosphorylation tend to be more readily reversible than are alterations in gene expression, regulation of the phosphorylation state of particular proteins may underlie short-term memory, whereas changes in gene expression leading to new protein synthesis may be required for longer-term memory. A goal of current research is to relate specific alterations in the phosphorylation or the expression of proteins to specific behavioral phenomena.

Long-term potentiation One candidate mechanism of memory that has received particular attention is long-term potentiation (LTP). Indeed, LTP occurring at synapses within area CA1 of the hippocampus represents the most widely studied form of activity-dependent synaptic plasticity in the mammalian nervous system. Hippocampal neurons have been intensively studied for several reasons. First, the hippocampus has a relatively simple and orderly architecture that permits physiological experimentation. Second, clinical-pathological correlations in humans after cerebrovascular disease, anoxic injury, and viral infections have demonstrated that the hippocampus is required for the formation of new memories. Bilateral hippocampal lesions, especially if they affect area CA1, are associated with an inability to learn new information.

LTP can be induced experimentally in vivo in area CA1 of the hippocampus by stimulating presynaptic fibers (the Schaffer collateral pathway) with a brief period of high-frequency electrical impulses that resemble impulse trains that can occur physiologically. The result of the tetanus is a marked and long-lasting enhancement in the functional responsiveness of postsynaptic cells to subsequent low-frequency stimulation; that is, depolarizing stimuli produce a much larger synaptic current after the induction of LTP than before. LTP induced in vivo in the CA1 region of hippocampus can last for weeks.

Hippocampal synapses that can express LTP use glutamate as their neurotransmitter. Glutamate receptor types (named for their selective agonists) include NMDA receptors and two types of non-NMDA receptors (kainate and quisqualate/α-amino-3-hydroxy-5-methyl-4-phosphonobutyrate [AMPA]). Activation of kainate and quisqualate-AMPA receptors causes increased permeability to sodium (Na^+) and, hence, depolarization of the postsynaptic neuron. NMDA receptors can permit entry of both Na^+ and Ca^{2+} but can be activated only by glutamate if the postsynaptic cell has been recently depolarized. Depolarization is required to relieve a block of the NMDA receptor channel by magnesium (Mg^{2+}). Thus, the NMDA receptor channel is both ligand-gated and voltage-gated.

In hippocampal CA1 neurons, LTP can only be activated if Ca^{2+} enters the postsynaptic neuron through NMDA channels. Compounds that selectively block the glutamate-binding site on NMDA receptors (such as D-2-amino-5-phosphonovalerate [APV]) or that block the NMDA receptor channel (such as menaquinone-801 [MK-801], recently renamed dizocilpine), block the initiation of LTP. Since Ca^{2+} entry into the postsynaptic cell depends on a close association between two events—prior depolarization of the postsynaptic cell and binding of glutamate to the NMDA receptor—NMDA receptors detect coincidences. A neural mechanism that detects coincident events (associations) is an attractive model of memory because association is the essence of classical conditioning in animals and of the inference of causal relations in humans.

Experimentally, the initiation of LTP can be separated from its long-term maintenance. For example, compounds that inhibit protein synthesis have no effect on the initiation of LTP in CA1 neurons but appear to block its maintenance. Some evidence indicates that entry of Ca^{2+} through NMDA receptor channels initiates LTP in CA1 neurons by activating protein kinases. Candidates include calcium-calmodulin-dependent protein kinase II and protein kinase C. Pharmacological inhibitors of those protein kinases inhibit the initiation of LTP.

Distinct processes underlie the maintenance of LTP. Once LTP is initiated, persistent activation of NMDA receptors or of postsynaptic calcium-dependent protein kinases is not required for its continued expression. Recent analyses have produced conflicting results as to whether the long-term increase in synaptic efficacy that characterizes LTP is due to a persistant alteration in presynaptic function—that is, a persistent increase in the amount of glutamate released on stimulation of presynaptic nerve terminals—or in postsynaptic function—that is, the magnitude of the response to glutamate binding. Presynaptic changes may reflect alterations in presynaptic protein kinases, voltage-gated channels, or proteins associated with synaptic vesicle function. Postsynaptic changes may reflect alterations in dendritic protein kinases, glutamate receptors, or even changes in gene expression within the postsynaptic neuron. Maintenance of LTP may require the generation of a signal in the postsynaptic neuron (such as nitric oxide) that is released from the neuron, crosses the synapse, and influences glutamate release presynaptically.

LTP has also been described at many other synapses in the brain. Different mechanisms may be involved in mediating the initiation and the expression of LTP compared with those established for the CA1 neuron of the hippocampus. For example, activation of NMDA receptors is not required for the production of LTP in CA3 hippocampal neurons.

SUGGESTED CROSS-REFERENCES

Genetics is discussed in Sections 1.15 and 1.16 and neurotransmitters in Sections 1.3 and 1.4. Neuroanatomy is discussed in Section 1.2.

REFERENCES

Alreja M, Aghajanian G K: Opiates suppress a resting sodium-dependent inward current in addition to activating an outward potassium current in locus coeruleus neurons. J Neurosci *13:* 3525, 1993.

Bekkers J M, Stevens C F: Presynaptic mechanism for long-term potentiation in the hippocampus. Nature *346:* 724, 1990.
*Berridge M J: Inositol triphosphate and calcium signaling. Nature *361:* 315, 1993.
Bertorello A M, Aperia A, Walaas S I, Nairn A C, Greengard P: Phosphorylation of the catlytic subunit of Na^+, K^+-ATPase inhibits the activity of the enzyme. Proc Natl Acad Sci USA *88:* 11359, 1991.
Blenis J: Signal transduction via the MAP kinases: Proceed at your own RSK. Proc Natl Acad Sci USA *90:* 5889, 1993.
Bliss T V P, Collingridge G L: A synaptic model of memory: Long-term potentiation in the hippocampus. Nature *361:* 31, 1993.
Bredt D S, Snyder S H: Nitric oxide, a novel neuronal messenger. Neuron *8:* 3, 1992.
Davis R J: The mitogen-activated protein kinase signal transduction pathway. J Biol Chem *268:* 14553, 1993.
*De Camilli P, Benfenati F, Valtorta F, Greengard P: The synapsins. Annu Rev Cell Biol *6:* 433, 1990.
Freissmuth M, Casey P J, Gilman A G: G-proteins control diverse pathways of transmembrane signaling. FASEB J *3:* 2125, 1989.
Gasic G P, Hollmann M: Molecular neurobiology of glutamate receptors. Annu Rev Physiol *54:* 507, 1992.
Greengard P, Valtorta F, Czernik A J, Benfenati F: Synaptic vesicle phosphoproteins and regulation of synaptic function. Science *259:* 780, 1993.
Hershey J W B: Protein phosphorylation controls translation rates. J Biol Chem *264:* 20823, 1989.
Huganir R L, Greengard P: Regulation of neurotransmitter receptor desensitization by protein phosphorylation. Neuron *5:* 555, 1990.
Hunter T, Cooper J A: Protein tyrosine kinases. Annu Rev Biochem *54:* 897, 1985.
Hunter T, Sefton B M, editors: *Protein phosphorylation. Parts A and B. Methods in Enzymology,* vols 200 and 201. Academic Press, New York, 1991.
*Hyman S E, Nestler E J: *Molecular Foundations of Psychiatry.* American Psychiatric Press, Washington, 1993.
Kacmarek L K, Levitan I B: *Neuromodulation: The Biochemical Control of Neuronal Excitability.* Oxford University Press, New York, 1986.
Kandel E R, Schwartz J H: Molecular biology of learning: Modulation of transmitter release. Science *218:* 433, 1982.
Korsching, S. The neurotropic factor concept: A reexamination. J Neurosci *13:* 2739, 1993.
Lefkowitz R J: G protein coupled receptor kinases. Cell *74:* 409, 1993.
Lefkowitz R J, Hausdorff W P, Caron M G: Role of phosphorylation in desensitization of the β-adrenoceptor. Trends Pharmacol Sci *11:* 190, 1990.
Madison D V, Malenka R C, Nicoll R A: Mechanisms underlying long-term potentiation of synaptic transmission. Annu Rev Neurosci *14:* 379, 1991.
Malinow R, Tsien R W: Presynaptic enhancement shown by whole-cell recordings of long-term potentiation in hippocampal slices. Nature *346:* 177, 1990.
Nestler E J: Molecular mechanisms of drug addiction. J Neurosci *12:* 2439, 1992.
Nestler E J, Duman R S: G-proteins and cyclic nucleotides in the nervous system. In *Basic Neurochemistry,* ed 5, G Siegel, B Agranoff, R W Albers, P Molinoff, editors, p 429. Raven, New York, 1994.
*Nestler E J, Greengard P: *Protein Phosphorylation in the Nervous System.* Wiley, New York, 1984.
Nestler E J, Greengard P: Protein phosphorylation and the regulation of neuronal function. In *Basic Neurochemistry,* ed 5, G Siegel, B Agranoff, R W Albers, P Molinoff, editors, p 449. Raven, New York, 1994.
Nicoll R A: The coupling of neurotransmitter receptors to ion channels in the brain. Science *241:* 545, 1988.
Nishizuka Y: Intracellular signaling by hydrolysis of phospholipids and activation of protein kinase C. Science *258:* 607, 1992.
Piomelli D, Greengard P: Lipoxygenase metabolites of arachidonic acid in neuronal transmembrane signalling. Trends Pharmacol Sci *11:* 367, 1990.
*Simon M I, Strathman M P, Gautam N: Diversity of G proteins in signal transduction. Science *252:* 802, 1991.
Zigmond R E, Schwarzschild M A, Rittenhouse A R: Acute regulation of tyrosine hydroxylase by nerve activity and by neurotransmitters via phosphorylation. Annu Rev Neurosci *12:* 415, 1989.

1.7 BASIC ELECTROPHYSIOLOGY

GEORGE K. AGHAJANIAN, M.D.
MEENAKSHI ALREJA, Ph.D.

INTRODUCTION

The emphasis of this section is on electrophysiology from the standpoint of the single neuron. The single neuron represents a fundamental nodal point for the integrative action of the nervous system as a whole. Reflected in the activity of single neurons are elementary processes occurring at the membrane level. The algebraic summation of elementary ionic membrane events underlies and explains the firing patterns of single neurons. Of relevance to psychiatry is the fact that many neurotransmitters and related psychotropic drugs are known to alter firing patterns by opening or closing specific types of ion channels. On a more global level, the activity of individual neurons can be viewed within the framework of neuronal networks and the behavioral, autonomic, and neuroendocrine processes served by those systems. This section presents an overview of cellular electrophysiology as a means of establishing links between basic biochemical and biophysical processes and clinically relevant issues, such as the action of psychotropic drugs on behavior.

ELEMENTS OF ELECTROPHYSIOLOGY

This section establishes a common language as a basis for communication between the expert and the nonexpert in electrophysiology. It also presents the basic principles and methods commonly used by electrophysiologists.

ION CHANNELS Ions, both negatively and positively charged, play a central role in the excitability of tissues. The lipoidal cell membrane serves as an electrical capacitor by separating the internal and the external ionic environments. The selective passage of one or another type of ion either into or out of the cell is made possible by specialized transmembrane proteins that form macromolecular pores, termed *ion channels.* The selective movement of ions through those channels causes excitation or inhibition, resulting in electrical signaling. The neuronal membrane in its resting state offers considerable resistance to the passage of ions, allowing for the establishment of a transmembrane potential; that potential difference or polarization is maintained by energy-dependent ion pumps, such as the sodium pump, which establish a negativity of the inside of the cell with respect to the extracellular space. The polarized neuronal membrane is, therefore, poised to respond electrically to changes in ionic permeability. The opening or the closing of ion channels produces a net flow of charge, resulting in a current that shifts transmembrane potential (E) in accordance with Ohm's law (E = IR) by altering the product of current (I), which in this case is carried by ions, and membrane resistance (R). In direct conformity with Ohm's law, an increased inward flow of positive ions (or an outward flow of negative ions) results in a decreased negativity of the transmembrane potential, an event termed *depolarization;* the reverse—that is, the increased negativity of the membrane potential—is termed *hyperpolarization.*

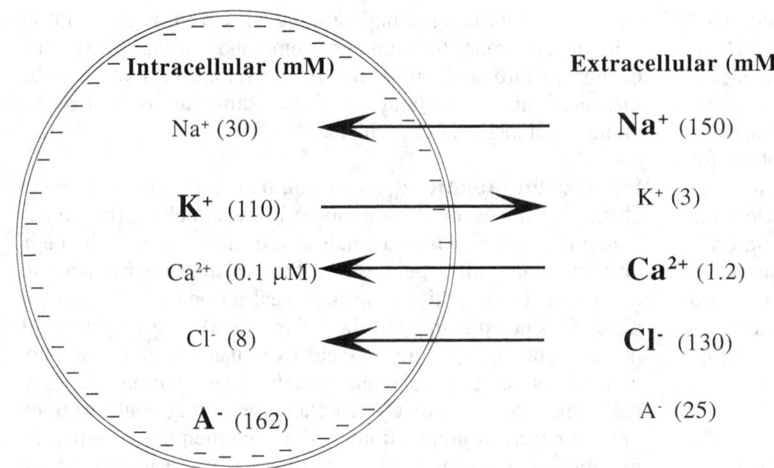

FIGURE 1.7-1 *The unequal distribution of ions in the intracellular and the extracellular compartments. The intracellular compartment has higher concentrations of potassium (K^+) and of the nondiffusible anions (A^-), whereas the extracellular compartment has higher concentrations of sodium (Na^+), calcium (Ca^{2+}), and chloride (Cl^-) ions. Arrows indicate the net direction of flow for each ion. Minus signs indicate the negativity of the intracellular compartment.*

Gating of ion channels Neuronal membranes are well endowed with ion channels that can be controlled by either electrical or chemical means. Although no channel is perfectly selective, channels tend to be identified by the predominant type of ions for which they have some degree of selective permeability. In that regard only four major ions need to be considered: sodium (Na^+), potassium (K^+), chloride (Cl^-), and calcium (Ca^{2+}). Ion channels are grouped into two broad categories, *electrically activated* (voltage-sensitive) and *ligand-gated,* depending on the manner in which they are gated—that is, opened or closed. Electrically activated channels are gated by changes in the transmembrane potential of the cell. The channels responsible for the action potential are of that kind, and they open when the membrane depolarizes to a critical level termed *spike threshold.* The channels involved in generating the action potential are primarily those selective for Na^+. In addition, voltage-sensitive Ca^{2+} channels become activated during the action potential. A second major type of ion channel is *chemically gated;* those channels are activated by neurotransmitter substances. However, the distinction between electrically activated and chemically activated channels is not absolute, and the function of many voltage-dependent channels can be modulated directly or indirectly by neurotransmitters.

Ion flow What are the electrophysiological consequences of the opening or the closing of ion channels? The answer to that question follows directly from the fact that energy-dependent pumping mechanisms establish an unequal distribution, inside to outside, of the four major ions that carry current in neurons (Figure 1.7-1). As a result, ions are in a position to flow down their concentration gradient; that situation creates a *diffusional potential* across a semipermeable membrane. The cell's transmembrane potential can either enhance or oppose the diffusional forces that drive the movement of ions. For a given ion, when the opposing membrane potential is equal to the diffusional potential, there can be no net flow of current; that is referred to as the *reversal* or *equilibrium potential* for that ion (in quantitative terms, that relationship is described by Nernst's equation). Na^+ and Ca^{2+} ions have a high outside-to-inside concentration ratio. Thus, at the *resting potential* of a typical neuron, which is normally negative inside with respect to outside by approximately −55 to −70 millivolts, the opening of Na^+ or Ca^{2+} channels results in an inward flow of those positive ions. At spike threshold (typically −55 millivolts), multiple voltage-sensitive Na^+ channels open in a kind of chain reaction to generate a massive but brief (0.1 to 2 millisecond) depolarization termed the *action potential* or *spike* (Figure 1.7-2); Ca^{2+} ions also enter the cell through their own voltage-sensitive channels during the action potential, particularly in the latter phase of depolarization. The entry of Ca^{2+} and Na^+ ions during the spike has several important implications: (1) Ca^{2+} functions as a major second messenger in the cell; (2) at the nerve terminal Ca^{2+} entry triggers the release of neurotransmitters; (3) Ca^{2+} activates a special kind of hyperpolarizing outward K^+ current (see below), which produces a potential called an *afterhyperpolarization,* so named because it comes after the spike (Figure 1.7-2). The afterhyperpolarization transiently diminishes cell excitability and thus serves an intrinsic negative feedback function.

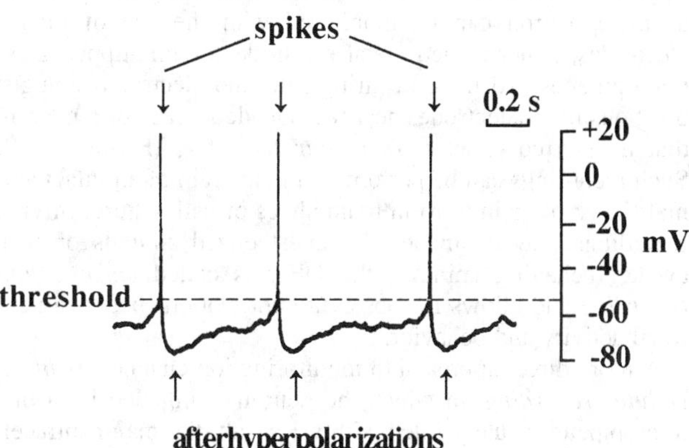

FIGURE 1.7-2 *An oscilloscope trace showing a repetitively firing neuron recorded intracellularly in vivo. This example was taken from a serotonergic neuron in the dorsal raphe nucleus of the rat midbrain. When the membrane potential reaches threshold in millivolts (approximately −55 mV), an all-or-none spike occurs. After each spike an afterhyperpolarization shifts the cell away from threshold into a more negative zone (near −80 mV). As the afterhyperpolarization decays, the cell again approaches spike threshold. (Trace supplied by G K Aghajanian.)*

The opening of Cl^- channels results in a hyperpolarizing effect because of the inflow of negative ions. Cl^- ions flow inward at resting potential, despite the inside negativity of the cell, because the high outside-to-inside ratio of Cl^- establishes a diffusional potential that exceeds the resting membrane potential. The opening of K^+ channels has a hyperpolarizing effect because of the outward flow of positive ions; the flow is outward because the diffusional potential of the high inside-to-outside ratio of K^+ ions exceeds the negativity of the membrane potential at resting levels. Conversely, the closing of K^+ channels, some of which may be open at rest (leakage channels), results in depolarization.

Thus, as depicted schematically in Figure 1.7-1, the existence of an unequal distribution of cations and anions accounts for the net direction and the magnitude of the current flow through the various ion channels. In terms of overall cell function, the net inward current resulting from the opening of Na^+ and Ca^{2+} channels (or the closing of K^+ channels) causes a depolarization with an increase in cell excitability or spiking; the net outward current caused by the opening of Cl^- or K^+ channels leads to hyperpolarization and a decrease in cell excitability or spiking.

BASIC TOOLS

Extracellular and intracellular recording *Firing rate* represents an integration at a cellular level of the multiple ion channel events that occur at the membrane level. The firing rate of a single neuron can be monitored with the use of microelectrodes, either etched metal electrodes or fine-tipped glass micropipettes. To measure firing rate, the electrophysiologist positions microelectrodes near the outside surface of a neuron; that is referred to as *extracellular recording* (Figure 1.7-3). Such recordings can be performed in the brain of an intact animal (in vivo) or in vitro in brain slices or cell culture. In vivo recordings may be made with anesthetized animals or with awake, behaving animals; the latter is called *chronic unit recording* and allows for observing correlations between neuronal activity and behavior.

A more direct approach to monitoring ion channels is *intracellular recording,* in which the neuron is impaled by a fine micropipette (usually filled with a K^+ salt, the major intracellular cation). By that means, transmembrane potentials or currents can be measured. Customarily, when membrane potential is recorded, current pulses of constant magnitude are periodically injected through the recording electrode to assess membrane *input resistance* (by Ohm's law, input resistance is equal to the voltage deflection recorded divided by the value of the constant-current test pulse). That is the *current-clamp* mode, which permits a direct assessment of membrane potential and membrane permeability, as indicated by changes in input resistance. An increase in input resistance indicates closing of channels, and a decrease indicates opening of channels.

An even more direct method for monitoring permeability changes in ion channels is the *voltage-clamp* technique. When intracellular recordings are made in the voltage-clamp mode, membrane voltage can be set at a given constant value, which is termed the *command voltage* (feedback circuits inject sufficient hyperpolarizing or depolarizing current through the intracellular electrode to maintain command voltage). By that means, inward and outward transmembrane currents can be measured directly without the confounding variables of membrane resistance and capacitance.

Patch-clamp recording One can detect the opening or the closing of a few or even a single ion channel by the *patch-clamp* method, in which a small area of neuronal membrane is brought against the opening of a fire-polished micropipette to form an extremely high-resistance seal termed a tight seal (or gigaseal, since it is in the billion ohm range). The validation of the existence of specific ion-selective channels and how they work rests on evidence obtained by that method. At first, researchers believed that patch-clamp recording could be done only in neuronal preparations with naked membranes—that is, membranes free of any glial covering—as occur in cell culture or in invertebrate ganglia. However, researchers have recently performed patch-clamp recordings in brain slices, applying the technique to the study of neurons within the context of a relatively intact local circuitry.

The patch-clamp method has four basic configurations: (1) cell-attached mode, (2) whole-cell mode, (3) inside-out mode, and (4) outside-out mode (Figure 1.7-4). In the *cell-attached* mode single-channel activity can be recorded from a patch of membrane that is contiguous with the cell interior. In the *whole-cell* mode the membrane patch is ruptured (usually with brief suction); communication is thereby established between the cell and the pipette interior. When the membrane patch is pulled away from the cell, the *inside-out* configuration is formed; the *outside-out* configuration is obtained when the electrode is pulled away from the cell while in the whole-cell mode. Each configuration has its special uses. Single-channel activity can be recorded in both inside-out and outside-out configurations. The whole-cell mode provides low-resistance access to the intracellular space, allowing accurate measurement of whole-cell currents and the rapid exchange of contents between the patch electrode and the cytosol, a process termed *intracellular dialysis.*

NEUROTRANSMISSION

NEURONAL ACTIONS PRODUCED BY NEUROTRANSMITTERS The two general methods for assessing the type of action a putative neurotransmitter may have on a given neuron are (1) the application of the exogenous transmitter candidate into the vicinity of the neuron while monitoring electrophysiological responses and (2) the stimulation of specific brain

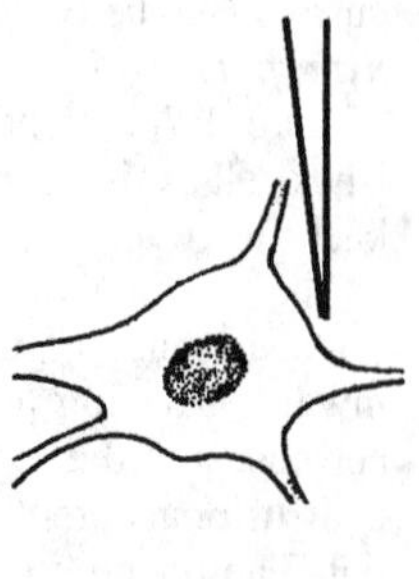

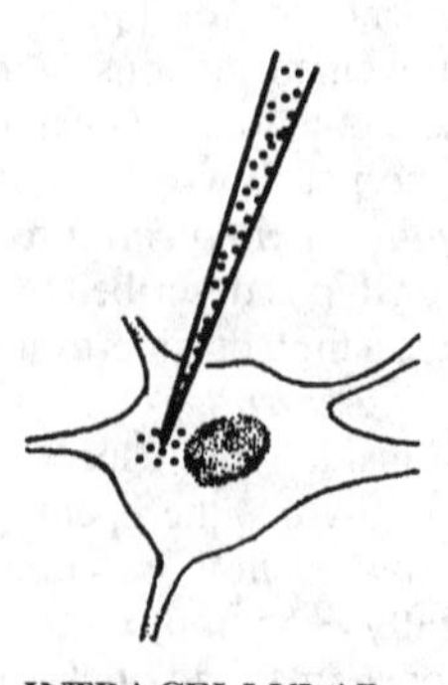

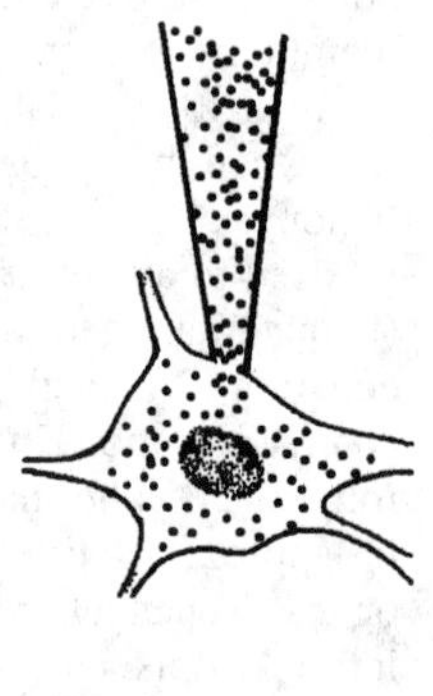

FIGURE 1.7-3 *The relation of the recording electrode to a neuron during extracellular, intracellular, and whole-cell recording. The sharp-tipped, high-resistance intracellular microelectrode impales the cell, but the pipette solution (represented by dots) mixes little with the intracellular contents. However, the low-resistance patch pipette used for whole-cell recording allows much mixing of the cell and the pipette contents (represented by a wide distribution of dots within the cell); therefore, whole-cell recording is a powerful tool for altering intracellular composition for the study of intracellular mechanisms.*

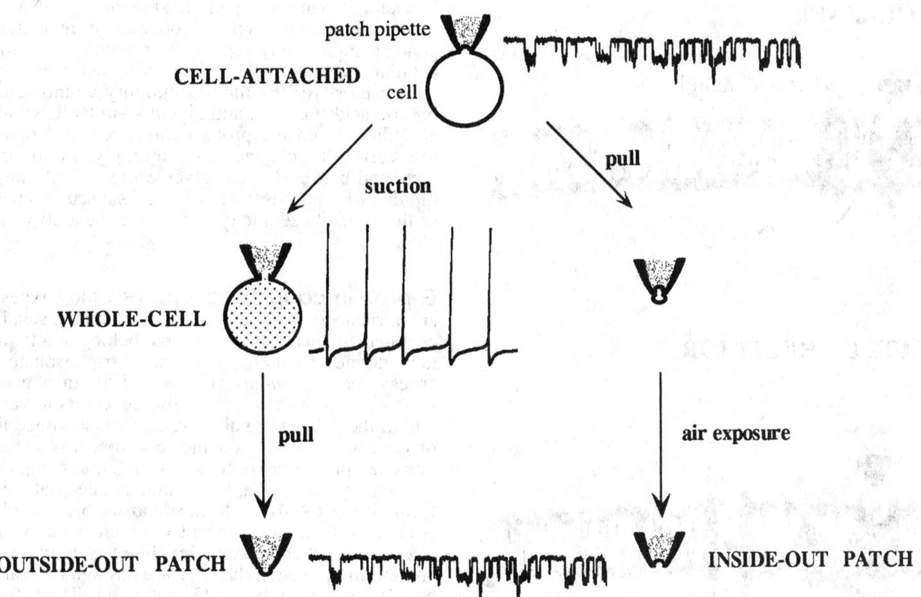

FIGURE 1.7-4 *The various configurations of patch-clamp recording. A patch pipette is brought close to the cell, and after a brief suction, a gigaseal is formed. Single-channel activity can be recorded from the patch of membrane enclosed within the pipette tip in the cell-attached mode (top panel). Alternatively, the patch of membrane can be ruptured by further suction to establish a whole-cell recording, in which spike activity can be recorded in a current-clamp mode; both voltage-gated and agonist-induced currents can be studied in the voltage-clamp mode (middle panel, left). The whole-cell configuration also allows the manipulation of the intracellular composition. The outside-out configuration can be obtained after establishing a whole-cell recording by simply pulling the pipette away from the cell (bottom panel, left). The inside-out mode is obtained by pulling the pipette away from the cell while it is still in the cell-attached mode; the vesicle so formed can be ruptured by exposing it to air (bottom panel, right); as a result, the inner side of the cell membrane faces the bath solution. Single-channel activity can be recorded in cell-attached, outside-out, and inside-out configurations.*

pathways that are thought to use the transmitter. Each of those approaches has its advantages and disadvantages in characterizing the effect of a presumed transmitter substance.

Actions elicited by microiontophoresis When a substance suspected of acting as a neurotransmitter is applied locally to neurons, excitatory or inhibitory effects on the firing rate may be observed. For several decades the most popular technique for applying neurotransmitters to central nervous system (CNS) neurons has been that of *microiontophoresis*. In essence, the technique involves the use of multibarreled micropipettes in which all the tips are in close approximation to one another; typically, one barrel is used to record neuronal spikes, and the other barrels are used to apply, by the passage of current, minute amounts of transmitter or drug ions in the direct vicinity of the recorded neuron. The procedure yields a useful characterization of the general type of response—that is, excitatory or inhibitory—produced by a substance when applied to a neuron.

Synaptic potentials The fact that a given neuron responds to an exogenous substance does not itself prove that it receives an endogenous input using that substance as a transmitter. Therefore, an essential part of the physiological characterization of a transmitter is to electrically stimulate and record within an anatomically and histochemically established pathway. Of greatest value is the monitoring of postsynaptic responses by intracellular recording. By that means, either depolarizing or hyperpolarizing potentials can be elicited in the postsynaptic cell; the depolarizing responses are termed *excitatory postsynaptic potentials* (EPSPs), and the hyperpolarizing responses are termed *inhibitory postsynaptic potentials* (IPSPs). EPSPs and IPSPs are characteristically small, graded potentials that can either elicit or abort the occurrence of an all-or-none spike; in any given instance the outcome depends on whether the integrated action of multiple EPSPs and IPSPs produces a net shift of the cell membrane potential toward or away from the spike threshold. The rates of rise and of decay are other important parameters of synaptic potentials. Some synaptic potentials are extremely rapid in onset and offset; others are slow in onset and of long duration. The physiological significance of a synaptic input can be viewed as a function of those rate characteristics: fast synaptic events transmit discrete messages; slow synaptic potentials alter cell excitability with respect to other inputs over relatively long periods of time and are in that sense modulatory.

COUPLING OF RECEPTORS TO ION CHANNELS Neurotransmitter receptors interact with ion channels either directly or indirectly through a sequence of intervening biochemical steps. In molecular terms those two modes of coupling are represented by the two major superfamilies of receptors: the *ligand-gated channels* and the *G-protein-coupled receptors*. Within each of those superfamilies are families of receptor subtypes for each transmitter substance. For example, the adrenoceptors constitute a family of receptor subtypes (for example, α_1, α_2, β_1, β_2), all of which belong to the G-protein-coupled receptor superfamily.

Ligand-gated channels The simplest and most direct form of coupling occurs when the transmitter recognition site (the receptor in the narrowest sense) is actually part of the protein complex that includes the ion channel itself (Figure 1.7-5). The classic example of that type of coupling is the nicotinic-cholinergic nonspecific cation channel of the skeletal neuromuscular junction. Acetylcholine-receptor sites are located on two of the five protein subunits that constitute that ion channel; when acetylcholine binds to those receptors, there is an immediate conformational change in the channel protein complex, resulting in a rapid and marked increase in permeability to Na^+ and to other cations. The great advantage of direct coupling is rapidity of response, which is of value in the transmission of excitatory impulses at the skeletal neuromuscular junction, where speed is of the essence.

In the CNS rapid, directly coupled excitatory neurotransmission is mainly served by a different class of substances, the excitatory amino acids, such as glutamate. The prominent action of the excitatory amino acids is to produce a rapid onset and a rapid offset of depolarization. Recently, with the cloning of a number of functionally expressed channel subunits, researchers have established that the amino-acid-receptor binding sites are situated on one or another subunit that forms the ion channel. In general, channels gated by excitatory amino acids are per-

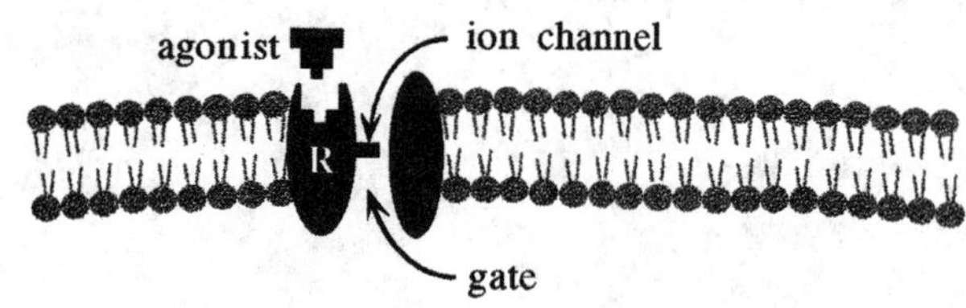

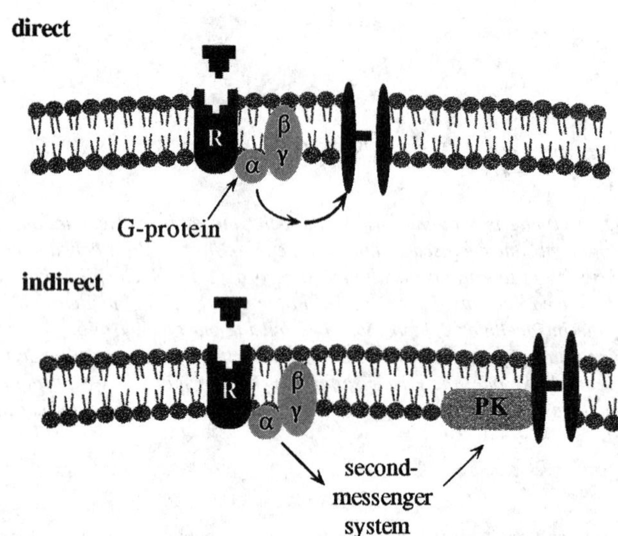

FIGURE 1.7-5 *Two major forms of coupling that can occur between receptors* (R) *and ion channels. The top panel shows a ligand-gated channel in which the receptor site is on the protein complex of the ion channel itself. The lower panels show G-protein coupling in which an intervening G-protein (the transducer) links the receptor to the ion channel. The linkage may be direct, in which the activated G-protein (α subunit) interacts with the ion channel (middle panel), or indirect, in which the G-protein couples through a second-messenger system (such as adenylate cyclase); the second messenger may then interact with the ion channel through a phosphorylation reaction catalyzed by a protein kinase* (PK). *Direct G-protein coupling and indirect G-protein coupling are not mutually exclusive mechanisms and may occur simultaneously to give rise to a dual form of coupling that can link a receptor to more than one type of channel.*

meable to Na^+, K^+, and—to a varying degree, depending on subunit composition—Ca^{2+}. The excitatory amino acids have been proposed as the principal transmitters for many primary sensory neurons and pyramidal tract neurons (upper motor neurons), where it is advantageous to have rapid transmission with minimum delay. In addition to those fast excitatory effects, the excitatory amino acids, acting through a different receptor, termed the *N*-methyl-D-aspartate (NMDA) receptor, produce a slow excitation by opening a special type of cation channel that has much greater permeability to Ca^{2+} than to Na^+ or K^+. In certain regions of the CNS, such as the hippocampus and the cerebral cortex, NMDA receptors play a critical role in the induction of long-term changes in synaptic efficacy—for example, long-term potentiation (LTP)—which may underlie certain forms of learning and memory. Two special characteristics of the NMDA channel are important for the induction of LTP: First, its permeability to Ca^{2+} plays an important role intracellularly in the induction of LTP. Second, at resting potential the NMDA channel is blocked by normal extracellular concentration of magnesium (Mg^{2+}); that blockade is voltage-dependent in that it is removed when the cell is concomitantly depolarized. Thus, when the cell is depolarized through one input, the resulting removal of Mg^{2+} blockade enhances ligand-gated opening of NMDA channels through another input. That type of cooperative interaction between two independent inputs may represent an analog of associative learning at a cellular level.

Receptors for the major inhibitory amino acids—that is, γ-aminobutyric acid (GABA) and glycine—in the CNS also appear to be situated directly on the protein complex that forms the ion channel—in this case, Cl^- channels. Accordingly, inhibitory responses (IPSPs) mediated by GABA and glycine in the CNS are characterized by the rapidity of their onset and offset. As discussed below, anxiolytic drugs of the benzodiazepine type enhance the ability of GABA to open Cl^- channels.

G-protein-coupled receptors Most types of receptors are not an intrinsic part of an ion channel but, instead, are coupled to ion channels by macromolecules that belong to a family of membrane proteins defined by their guanosine 5′-triphosphate (GTP)-binding properties—the *G-proteins* (Figure 1.7-5). In a general way G-proteins function as transducers, coupling receptors to various effector systems within the cell. Originally, researchers assumed that the only function of G-proteins was to couple receptors to second-messenger systems. For example, in heart cells β-adrenergic receptors acting through the stimulatory G-protein, G_S, stimulate adenylate cyclase to increase the formation of cAMP. In turn, adenosine 3′, 5′-cyclic phosphate (cAMP) is coupled to the opening of Ca^{2+} channels, which has an excitatory effect on heart cells. Acetylcholine has an opposing effect by causing an inhibition of adenylate cyclase through muscarinic receptors that are coupled to the inhibitory G-protein, G_i. Those two examples illustrate *indirect coupling* of receptors to ion channels through the stimulation or the inhibition of adenylate cyclase. However, new evidence, primarily of an electrophysiological nature, indicates that G-proteins can directly couple receptors to ion channels without involving any subsequent second messengers. The first evidence for *direct coupling* came from whole-cell and single-channel recordings in cultured heart cells. In heart cells, acetylcholine was known to have an inhibitory effect by activating an outward K^+ current. That does not involve any known diffusible second-messenger system but, rather, is mediated directly by G-proteins coupled to muscarinic cholinergic receptors.

Thus, acetylcholine acting through its G-protein-coupled muscarinic receptor has a dual action on heart cells: directly through an opening of K^+ channels and indirectly through a suppression of cAMP-mediated β-adrenergic excitation. Together, those effects explain the powerful suppressant effect of acetylcholine on cardiac activity.

As is often the case, peripheral systems such as the heart serve as a good model for neurotransmitter actions in the CNS. A large number of transmitter receptor systems point to evidence for G-protein coupling of signal transduction in the brain. The occurrence and the clinical implications of G-protein abnormalities are just beginning to be recognized in general medicine (for example, in pseudohypoparathyroidism). The possibility that such abnormalities may occur in psychiatric disorders remains to be explored.

CLASSIFICATION OF NEUROTRANSMITTERS

A single neurotransmitter not only may interact with more than one receptor subtype within the same superfamily but may also interact with receptor subtypes that belong to two different superfamilies. The first known example of that sort of crossing over was that of acetylcholine, which through its nicotinic receptor couples directly to a ligand-gated cationic channel and through its muscarinic receptor couples to a potassium channel or to adenylate cyclase through a G-protein. Now many more examples of such dual interactions are known. Within each receptor superfamily, a useful way of classifying neurotransmitters is according to the types of ion channels that they directly or indirectly regulate. That classification allows for a degree of simplification, since only four major types of ions—Na^+, K^+, Ca^{2+}, and Cl^-—are of concern. Much work in progress at this time is aimed at determining the types of channels that are affected by various transmitter substances in the CNS.

Table 1.7-1 summarizes data for the ligand-gated receptor superfamily. In addition to acetylcholine and the excitatory and inhibitory amino acids, one monoamine, serotonin (5-hydroxytryptamine[5-HT]), is included by virtue of the $5\text{-}HT_3$ receptor. As yet, no examples of neuropeptides have been discovered within the ligand-gated superfamily.

Table 1.7-2 summarizes data for the G-protein-coupled superfamily of neurotransmitter receptors. It includes at least one representative from each major class of transmitter substance, including acetylcholine, the monoamines, the excitatory and inhibitory amino acids, and the peptides. Across the various classes, inhibitory responses in most cases are mediated through an opening of K^+ (or closing of Ca^{2+}) channels, and excitatory responses are mediated through a closing of K^+ channels or the opening of nonspecific cation channels. Those differences are reflected in the types of G-proteins involved in the coupling. For example, the receptor subtypes known to couple through G_i and G_o are all linked to the opening of K^+ (or closing of Ca^{2+}) channels and are coupled negatively to adenylate cyclase. In contrast, the receptor subtypes linked to the closing of K^+ channels (muscarinic, α_1, 5-HT_2/5-HT_{1C}, substance P, and glutamate/metabotropic) activate the phosphoinositide second-messenger pathway through as yet unidentified, pertussis toxin-insensitive G-proteins.

PSYCHOTROPIC DRUG ACTION

The actions of most psychotropic drugs can be ascribed to interactions with one or another neurotransmitter system. That general finding is not surprising in view of the fact that chemical neurotransmission represents the predominant mode of interneuronal communication in the mammalian nervous system. Any aspect of the process of neurotransmission is a potential site for the interaction of a drug with a neurotransmitter: synthesis, storage, release, action on receptors, and inactivation (for example, uptake and catabolism). A drug effect may manifest itself rapidly (such as the immediate blockade of a transmitter at its receptor) or only after a delay of several weeks (such as a long-term up- or down-regulation of a receptor). In either case the ultimate effect of a drug is to promote or impede the ability of one or more given transmitters to gate ionic conductances.

TABLE 1.7-1
Ligand-Gated Channel Receptors

Neuro-transmitter	Receptor Subtype	Ion Channel	Physiological Response
Acetylcholine	Nicotinic	↑ Na^+/K^+	Fast excitation
Glutamate	AMPA	↑ Na^+/K^+	Fast excitation
	Kainate	↑ Na^+/K^+	Fast excitation
	NMDA	↑ $Ca^{2+}(Na^+/K^+)$	Slow excitation
Glycine	—	↑ Cl^-	Fast inhibition
GABA	$GABA_A$	↑ Cl^-	Fast inhibition
Serotonin	5-HT_3	↑ Na^+/K^+	Fast excitation

DRUGS AND LIGAND-GATED CHANNELS A diverse array of psychotropic drugs interact with receptor sites associated with ligand-gated channels. The drugs include (1) phencyclidine (PCP), which is a dissociative anesthetic with psychotomimetic properties that acts as a noncompetitive antagonist at NMDA receptors and (2) nicotine, which produces its reinforcing effects through its action on central nicotinic receptors. Therapeutically, the most commonly used drugs in the category are the benzodiazepine anxiolytics.

Anxiolytics The *benzodiazepines,* such as diazepam (Valium), constitute the major type of antianxiety (anxiolytic) drugs in clinical use today. The receptors that mediate the actions of benzodiazepines have a close association with $GABA_A$ receptors, a subtype of receptor for the inhibitory amino acid GABA. In turn, $GABA_A$ receptors are a constituent of a particular subset of Cl^- channels that they activate—that is, open. Together, the elements combine to form the benzodiazepine-receptor/GABA-receptor/Cl^--channel complex. Through that arrangement the benzodiazepines act indirectly (allosterically) to facilitate the ability of GABA to open Cl^- channels and, therefore, to produce inhibition at a cellular level. Thus, benzodiazepines, applied in small amounts by microiontophoresis to single neurons, have no effect by themselves but markedly enhance the inhibitory effects of GABA applied concurrently to the same neurons. As GABA represents the most prevalent inhibitory transmitter system in the brain, a facilitation of GABAs actions by benzodiazepines affects many kinds of inhibitory functions. Thus, the benzodiazapines have anticonvulsant and hypnotic properties, as well as antianxiety properties.

When benzodiazepines are used as anxiolytics, their hypnotic and anticonvulsant effects may be regarded as side effects. The abrupt cessation of long-term benzodiazapine treatment can result in withdrawal insomnia and convulsions, indicating the development of tolerance and dependence; that fact necessitates a tapering of drug dosage when patients are being withdrawn from benzodiazapines. On a single-cell level, tolerance to benzodiazepines is manifested by a reduced responsivity of neurons to GABA or in a reduction in the ability of benzodiazepines to facilitate inhibition mediated by $GABA_A$ receptors. Recently, a number of benzodiazapine-$GABA_A$ receptor subunits have been cloned. The marked differences in the regional expressions of

TABLE 1.7-2
G-Protein-Coupled Receptors

Neurotransmitter	Receptor Subtype	G-Protein	Ion Channel	Physiological Response
Acetylcholine	Muscarinic	?	↓ K^+[2]	Excitation
Serotonin	5-HT_{1A}	G_i/G_o	↑ K^+[1]	Inhibition
	5-HT_2/5-HT_{1C}	?	↓ K^+	Excitation
Norepinephrine	α_1	?	↓ K^+	Excitation
	α_2	G_i/G_o	↑ K^+[1]	Inhibition
	β	G_s	↓ K^+(AHP)	Excitation
Dopamine	D_1	G_s/G_{olf}	—	Variable
	D_2	G_i/G_o	↑ K^+	Inhibition
GABA	$GABA_B$	G_i/G_o	↑ K^+[1]	Inhibition
Somatostatin	—	G_i/G_o	↑ K^+	Inhibition
Substance P	—	?	↓ K^+	Excitation
Neuropeptide Y	—	G_i/G_o	↑ K^+[1]	Inhibition
VIP	—	G_s	↑ Cationic	Excitation
Opiate	μ, δ	G_i/G_o	↑ K^+[1]	Inhibition
Glutamate	Metabotropic	?	↓ K^+	Excitation

[1]Also a suppression of Ca^{2+} currents in dorsal root ganglion sensory neurons.
[2]Opens potassium channels and causes inhibition in a minority of neurons.

those subunits, as in the cerebellum versus the limbic cortex, raises the possibility that new classes of subtype-selective drugs can be developed that may, for example, avoid anticonvulsant and hypnotic side effects while retaining their anxiolytic activity.

DRUGS AND G-PROTEIN-COUPLED RECEPTORS A majority of drugs relevant to psychiatric practice are found within this category. Most known receptor subtypes are coupled through G-proteins, rather than ligand-gated channels (Tables 1.7-1 and 1.7-2). The greatest representation within the group is among the drugs that act, either directly or indirectly, on monoamine receptors; they include the antidepressants, the antipsychotics, and the hallucinogens. Only one category of drugs that act at peptide receptors, the opiates, is considered here. The underrepresentation of such drugs, despite the large number of neuropeptides, is explained in part by the facts that peptide analogs do not readily cross the blood-brain barrier and that few nonpeptide, systemically effective agents have been available until recently.

Antidepressants The three major classes of antidepressants are the tricyclics, such as imipramine (Tofranil); the monoamine oxidase inhibitors, such as phenelzine (Nardil); and the serotonin-specific reuptake inhibitors, such as fluoxetine (Prozac). Members of all three classes of drugs have immediate effects on the uptake or the accumulation of monoamines. Most tricyclic drugs and in some instances their metabolites rapidly block the reuptake of either serotonin or norepinephrine or both. The monoamine oxidase inhibitors induce an accumulation of monoamines by blocking a major enzyme responsible for the degradation of monoamines. The selective serotonin-uptake blockers are distinct from the tricyclic antidepressants in a number of respects, including a virtual absence of catecholamine-uptake-blocking activity, even of their metabolites. The monoamine-related actions of antidepressant drugs is an important underpinning of the monoamine hypothesis of depression. Stated in its most general form, the hypothesis proposes that depressive illnesses, particularly the major depressive disorders, arise from an impairment in either serotonergic function or noradrenergic function or both.

Any hypothesis of depression based on the mechanism of action of antidepressants must take into account the well-known delay (typically two to three weeks) from the onset of drug administration to therapeutic response. That protracted time is difficult to reconcile with the fact that the effects of drugs on amine uptake or metabolism are manifested within a matter of hours or days. Consequently, researchers have shifted away from the study of the short-term actions of the drugs to an examination of delayed effects that parallel the clinical course. Single-cell recordings in some postsynaptic regions of the rat brain have revealed that electrophysiological responses to serotonin, both inhibitory and excitatory, are progressively increased after one to two weeks of tricyclic drug administration. Usually, the inhibitory effects of serotonin are due to an opening of K^+ channels, and the excitatory effects are due to a closing of K^+ channels; evidence indicates that the receptors linked to the opening of K^+ channels belong to the serotonin$_{1A}$ (5-HT_{1A}) subtype. The enhancement of the electrophysiological actions cannot be explained by a blockade of serotonin uptake, since the enhancement is also produced by some atypical tricyclic drugs that do not block serotonin uptake. Studies suggest that serotonin-receptor sensitivity itself is somehow enhanced in a time-dependent fashion after long-term antidepressant administration.

The selective serotonin-uptake blockers, the newest class of antidepressant drugs introduced into clinical practice, do not operate through sensitizing postsynaptic response to serotonin. Instead, by maintaining high levels of serotonin extracellularly, they induce a delayed desensitization of inhibitory presynaptic serotonin receptors (serotonin autoreceptors); the monoamine oxidase inhibitors also appear to desensitize presynaptic serotonin receptors by that mechanism. As presynaptic receptors have a negative feedback influence on serotonin release, their desensitization results in an overall enhancement of serotonergic transmission. The possible relevance of serotonergic transmission to antidepressant drug action is underscored by recent clinical studies that show that a rapid depletion of the serotonin precursor tryptophan can induce a dramatic exacerbation of depression in drug-remitted patients.

Single-cell studies also reveal long-term changes in norepinephrine-receptor sensitivity: α_1-adrenoceptor responses are enhanced, and β-adrenoceptor responses are depressed. Those electrophysiological findings are in accord with biochemical studies that show a down-regulation of β-adrenoceptors after long-term antidepressant drug treatment. Whether those or other long-term alterations in receptor sensitivity contribute to the long-term therapeutic actions of the various classes of antidepressant drugs remains to be determined.

Antipsychotics Two major classes of antipsychotic drugs are the *phenothiazines,* such as chlorpromazine (Thorazine), and the *butyrophenones,* such as haloperidol (Haldol). Both types of antipsychotic drugs are potent dopamine-receptor antagonists, and the affinity of the drugs for dopamine receptors has a good correlation with clinical efficacy. On that basis, dopamine-receptor blockade may be responsible for antipsychotic activity. Parkinsonian side effects of the drugs are clearly attributable to a rapid blockade of dopamine receptors (D_2 and D_1 subtypes) in the extrapyramidal motor system. However, a true reduction in psychotic symptoms may be delayed for several weeks or more. Thus, as in the case of the antidepressant drugs, long-term adaptive changes may account for the delayed clinical response. One long-term change known to be induced by antipsychotic drugs is dopamine-receptor supersensitivity. That mechanism may be involved in the development of tardive dyskinesia, which is believed to be a manifestation of excessive dopaminergic transmission in the extrapyramidal motor system. However, as the emergence of tardive dyskinesia may be associated with an exacerbation of psychosis, dopamine-receptor supersensitivity per se cannot account for the antipsychotic activity.

An electrophysiological mechanism for delayed antipsychotic efficacy has been suggested on the basis of long-term studies in experimental animals. When antipsychotic drugs are administered for a short term, the rate of firing of single neurons in nigrostriatal and other dopaminergic pathways increases. However, when antipsychotic drugs are given over a period of weeks, the number of dopaminergic neurons whose firing can be detected becomes progressively reduced. Paradoxically, the quiescent cells are unable to fire not because they are hyperpolarized (that is, below spike threshold) but because they are in a state of *depolarization inactivation* (hyperdepolarization), which results from excessive depolarization. The precise mechanisms underlying the slow development of depolarization inactivation are not known. However, it is known that the induction of depolarization inactivation depends on the intactness of the neuronal feedback pathways that relay information from postsynaptic areas, such as the neostriatum, back to the dopaminergic cells of origin in the substantia nigra. The delayed reduction in the number of functional dopamine neurons correlates well with the delayed clinical response to antipsychotic drugs.

Possible actions of antipsychotic drugs at nondopamine receptors are also of interest. Virtually all the typical antipsychotic drugs have some degree of antagonist activity at a subset of serotonin receptors termed serotonin$_2$ (5-HT_2) receptors. Electrophysiological evidence shows that the effects of psychedelic hallucinogenic drugs are mediated through an agonist action at 5-HT_2 receptors (see below). The atypical antipsychotic drug clozapine (Clozaril), which does not induce extrapyramidal side effects or tardive dyskinesia, has a higher affinity for the 5-HT_2 and the closely related 5-HT_{1C} receptor than for the D_2 and D_1 dopamine receptor subtypes. On that basis the action of antipsychotic drugs at 5-HT_2 and 5-HT_{1C} receptors may be important in either promoting therapeutic effects or suppressing the development of side effects.

Clozapine has a relatively high affinity for a newly cloned dopamine receptor, the D_4 subtype. Of possible relevance to antipsychotic mechanisms is the fact that the D_4 receptor in limbic cortical regions has a relatively high expression, as compared with the extrapyramidal system, in which D_1 and D_2 receptors predominate. That differential distribution sets the stage for the development of a new generation of antipsychotic drugs selective for D_4 (and possibly also for 5-HT_2 and 5-HT_{1C}) receptors that avoid extrapyramidal side effects and other disabilities associated with D_2 and D_1 receptor blockade. Electrophysiological studies on D_4 receptors await the availability of such selective compounds.

Hallucinogens The *psychedelic* (mind-expanding) hallucinogens produce marked cognitive, affective, and perceptual disturbances while leaving orientation largely intact. The two major structural classes of hallucinogens are the *indolamines,* such as lysergic acid diethylamide (LSD), and the *phenethylamines,* such as mescaline. Because of the striking similarities of the clinical states produced by the two types of hallucinogens, a unitary mechanism has long been sought to account for the actions of the drugs on the nervous system. Apparently only one type of receptor has an affinity for both indolamine and phenethylamine hallucinogens, the 5-HT_2 receptor. For both classes of hallucinogens, radioligand-binding studies have shown a high correlation between hallucinogenic potency in humans and affinity for the 5-HT_2 receptor. That receptor is highly concentrated in or near layer 5 of the frontal and the occipital (visual) cortex in the human brain. Those regions of the brain are believed to serve cognitive and perceptual functions that are disordered by the hallucinogenic drugs. The 5-HT_2 receptors are located within a restricted subpopulation of interneurons in the cortex, presumably the critical site of action of the hallucinogenic drugs.

Electrophysiological studies in experimental rats have identified several neuronal systems that are affected in a like manner by the indolamine and the phenethylamine hallucinogens. The noradrenergic neurons of the locus ceruleus, which are diffusely activated by sensory stimuli applied anywhere on the body, are affected in a unique way by the drugs: the hallucinogens suppress their baseline firing while enhancing their responsivity to sensory stimuli. That pattern is specific to psychedelic hallucinogens; no other types of drugs are able to mimic the effect. In the cerebral cortex the hallucinogenic drugs produce a prolonged excitation of the subpopulation of interneurons that express 5-HT_2 receptors. All the shared physiological effects of the hallucinogens, including those in the locus ceruleus and the cerebral cortex, can be blocked by drugs that are highly selective antagonists of the 5-HT_2 receptor, such as ritanserin. As yet, the selective 5-HT_2 antagonists have not been tested for their ability to block the effects of hallucinogens in humans.

Anticholinergic deliriants Many chemical agents can induce a state of *delirium* characterized by confusion, disorientation, hallucinations, and short-term memory deficits. In some cases, deliriants act by causing a generalized metabolic dysfunction of the brain. However, the belladonna alkaloids, such as atropine and scopolamine, and their synthetic congeners can produce a delirium state by blocking one specific type of receptor in the brain, the muscarinic cholinergic receptor. In addition, other classes of psychotropic drugs, such as tricyclic antidepressants and low-potency antipsychotics, can produce clinically significant muscarinic receptor blockade to the extent that an overdose can present as a delirium.

Cholinergic neurons, arising from nuclei in the basal forebrain, have diffuse projections to regions of the brain that are believed to serve normal cognitive functions, such as the hippocampus and the neocortex. Electrophysiologically, the tonic release of acetylcholine onto postsynaptic neurons in those regions can be viewed as maintaining an optimal state of excitability. On a cellular level, acetylcholine, acting at muscarinic receptors, tonically enhances neuronal excitability by closing various types of K^+ channels. A blockade of muscarinic receptors leads to a reduction in the excitability of vast numbers of neurons in the hippocampus and the neocortex, resulting in a critical impairment in the ability of those neurons to process information arriving from other sources. If cholinergic transmission is restored by the administration of acetycholinesterase inhibitors, the delirium produced by antimuscarinic drugs can be reversed completely. A degeneration of cholinergic neurons has been implicated in the pathogenesis of Alzheimer's disease, which shares some of the characteristics of the antimuscarinic delirium. However, many other types of neuronal degeneration are present in Alzheimer's disease, and the relative importance of degeneration in the cholinergic system in the condition has not yet been determined.

Opiates Usually, opiates come within the purview of the psychiatrist within the context of drug dependence and drug withdrawal. Research on the cellular physiology of opiates has had practical clinical implications for the treatment of patients with opiate dependence. Opiate receptors are coupled through the pertussis-toxin-sensitive subset of G-proteins, such as G_i and G_o. Electrophysiological studies show that opiates generally have an inhibitory action on central nervous system neurons through the opening of K^+ channels or the closing of Ca^{2+} channels, both of which are G-protein-coupled. As discussed earlier, the opening of K^+ channels has a hyperpolarizing effect, thereby inducing the inhibitory effects mediated through opiate receptors. In addition, through G_i, which has an inhibitory coupling to adenylate cyclase, opiates can suppress the firing of noradrenergic neurons of the locus ceruleus that depend on endogenous cAMP for their repetitive activity. Opiate tolerance and opiate dependence in the locus ceruleus and several other regions of the brain and the spinal cord are associated with an up-regulation of the cAMP system at several points in the second-messenger pathway (for example, adenylate cyclase, cAMP-dependent protein kinase, and protein phosphorylation). The up-regulation, in part, accounts for the activation of firing that is induced in locus ceruleus neurons by the withdrawal of opiates. Behavioral studies in animals show that overactivity of the locus ceruleus plays a major role in mediating the aversive consequences of opiate withdrawal. Clonidine (Catapres), a drug that activates α_2 receptors, suppresses the overactivity of locus ceruleus neurons and ameliorates many of the symptoms of opiate withdrawal. The suppression of opiate withdrawal by clonidine can be explained by the fact that in locus ceruleus neurons α_2 receptors and opiate receptors are coupled to a common set of G-proteins and ion channels.

RELEVANCE TO PSYCHIATRY

The traditional inclination to regard electrophysiology as a discipline unto itself is rapidly changing, particularly in response to developments in molecular biology. Channels, receptors, and components of transducer systems are being cloned in large numbers and studied routinely by combined molecular, physiological, anatomical, and even behavioral approaches. Concepts and methods derived from electrophysiology, in conjunction with the other basic sciences, are being applied in an integrated way to clinical situations both diagnostically and therapeutically. For example, improved imaging techniques are being introduced in the diagnostic evaluation of psychiatric patients. Single photon emission computed tomography (SPECT) and positron emission tomography (PET) can reveal alterations in brain metabolism or receptor density in specific brain regions or systems. Such images reflect the state of activity or receptivity of clusters of individual neurons that operate within the labeled systems. Thus, a knowledge of electrophysiology at the single-neuron level is an essential component of the overall interpretation of information derived from brain imaging and other types of clinical assessment.

Similarly, knowledge derived from basic neurobiology is playing an increasingly important role in developing rational approaches to therapeutics. Most of the drugs currently in clinical use were arrived at by serendipity without a knowledge of mechanisms or pathophysiology. However, not all depressions, psychoses, and anxiety disorders are likely to be identical in cause or pathogenesis. Fine discriminations between pathophysiological subtypes will make it possible to select specific and efficacious treatments. For example, the drugs currently used in the treatment of schizophrenia have multiple neurochemical and physiological actions, no one of which may constitute the optimal therapy for a given type of patient. Moreover, extraneous actions of those drugs can induce serious and, occasionally, irreversible side effects, such as tardive dyskinesia. Even minor side effects can compromise the quality of life and have an adverse effect on patient compliance. In the future, drugs will have a greater selectivity for neurons that express receptor subtypes involved in the therapeutic actions, rather than side effects. Increasingly, the discriminating use of such drugs will require a familiarity with differential mechanisms of action at a basic biochemical and electrophysiological level.

SUGGESTED CROSS-REFERENCES

Applied electrophysiology is discussed in Section 1.8, neuroanatomy in Section 1.2, monoamine neurotransmitters in Section 1.3, amino acid neurotransmitters in Section 1.4, neuropeptides in Section 1.5, and intraneuronal biochemical signals in Section 1.6. Neuroimaging is discussed in Section 1.10 and molecular neurobiology in Section 1.14.

REFERENCES

Aghajanian G K: Central 5-HT receptor subtypes: Physiological responses and signal transduction mechanisms. In *Central Serotonin Receptors and Psychotropic Drugs*, C A Marsden, D J Heal, editors, pp 39–55. Blackwell Scientific, New York, 1992.

Aghajanian G K, Sprouse J S, Sheldon P, Rasmussen K: Electrophysiology of the central serotonin system: Receptor subtypes and transducer mechanisms. Ann NY Acad Sci *38:* 93, 1990.

Birnbaumer L, Abramowitz J, Brown A M: Receptor-effector coupling by G proteins. Biochim Biophys Acta *1031:* 163, 1990.

*Bloom F E, Kupfer D J, editors: *Psychopharmacology: The Fourth Generation of Progress.* Raven, New York, 1994.

*Cooper J R, Bloom F E, Roth R H: *The Biochemical Basis of Neuropharmacology*, ed 6. Oxford University Press, New York, 1991.

Dolphin A C: Nucleotide binding proteins in signal transduction and disease. Trends Neurosci *10:* 53, 1987.

*Hille B: *Excitable Membranes*, ed 2. Sinauer Associates, Sunderland, MA, 1992.

*Junge D: *Nerve and Muscle Excitation*, ed 3. Sinauer Associates, Sunderland, MA, 1992.

Kaczmarek L K, Levitan I B: *Neuromodulation*, Oxford University Press, New York, 1987.

*Kandel E R, Schwartz J H: *Principles of Neural Science*, ed 3. Elsevier, New York, 1991.

Meltzer H, editor: *Psychopharmacology: The Third Generation of Progress.* Raven, New York, 1987.

Nestler E J: Molecular mechanisms of drug addiction. J Neurosci: *12:* 2439, 1992.

Nicoll R: The coupling of neurotransmitter receptors to ion channels in the brain. Science *241:* 545, 1988.

Sakmann B, Neher E, editors: *Single Channel Recording*, Plenum, New York, 1983.

Shepherd G M: *Neurobiology*, ed 3. Oxford University Press, New York, 1994.

Snyder S H: *Drugs and the Brain.* Scientific American, New York, 1986.

Spiegel A M, Shenker A, Weinstein L S: Receptor-effector coupling by G proteins: Implications for normal and abnormal signal transduction. Endocr Rev *13:* 536, 1992.

1.8 APPLIED ELECTROPHYSIOLOGY

RICHARD COPPOLA, D.SC.
THOMAS HYDE, M.D., PH.D.

INTRODUCTION

Although it is clear that brain-behavior relations are mediated by neural activity, the essential associations between the central nervous system and the electroencephalogram (EEG) have only been established empirically. This empiricism has been vigorously pursued over several decades because the EEG remains the only entirely noninvasive functional "window on the brain." Psychiatry provided the initial interest in the electrical activity of the brain as reflected in the EEG. The main areas of focus in electroencephalography are in clinical applications and in basic brain research.

Changes in electrical activity reflect changes in the brain on at least two levels: (1) changes in the collective behavior of neurons, that is, the interaction among neurons; and (2) changes within the neuron, in cellular activity, metabolic or otherwise. Those changes may not only reflect pathological conditions in the brain but also represent important correlates of normal brain function. In addition, areas of brain activity remain inaccessible to the EEG, especially activity that is too localized or is spatially oriented in such a way that it cannot be measured at the scalp.

ORIGINS OF BRAIN ELECTRICAL ACTIVITY

CELLULAR BASIS OF ELECTRICAL ACTIVITY Action potentials of individual neurons are of very short duration, with small localized current flow. This localized flow is oriented such that activity over several cells is not summated. Synaptic events produce a greater current flow and are associated with a wider membrane area. Postsynaptic potentials (PSPs) result from depolarization or hyperpolarization of the postsynaptic membrane, depending on whether the synaptic activity was excitatory or inhibitory. Overall synaptic events depend on the collective behavior of a relatively large number of neurons. The PSPs thus reflect the number of interconnections among cells and the integration of activity over both time and space.

EEG It is generally accepted that the surface-recorded spontaneous electrical activity, the EEG, reflects voltages arising from extracellular current flow as a result of PSPs. In particular the large, vertically oriented pyramidal cells of the cortex probably contribute most from synchronous summated PSPs. The voltage distribution at the scalp results from the flow of current in a conductive medium, usually referred to as volume conduction. The signals are, however, modified by the intervening tissue layers and the complex geometry of the cortical folding.

EVOKED POTENTIALS Evoked potentials (EPs) reflect the specific activation of neurons, as opposed to the spontaneous activity recorded by the EEG at the scalp. This activation can be extrinsic as a result of sensory stimulation or intrinsic from cognitive factors. There are explicit fiber pathways and neural generators that can be associated with specific components, such as in brainstem evoked potentials (BSEPs).

EPILEPTIFORM ACTIVITY Epileptiform discharges are associated with paroxysmal depolarizing shifts synchronously occurring in collections of neurons. The extracellular current flow from these discharges is reflected in the characteristic sharp wave or spike at the scalp. Depolarization is followed by relatively long hyperpolarization, giving rise to the slow wave often recorded after the sharp wave discharge.

The underlying neuropathology of complex partial epilepsy appears to be disruptive of cellular processes leading to a postictal depression, whereas absence seizures (formerly known as petit mal) appear to be related to a more benign cellular process. Thus in absence seizures there is a relatively quick return to normal neuronal behavior after the seizure.

GENERATORS The electrical activity of the brain results from the flow of ions at the cellular level. This flow can be thought of as a current source, the simplest representation of which is a dipole. In this analogy the current sources can be thought of as the generators of the electrical and magnetic signals of the brain. Those sources can be biophysically described such that the voltage distribution at a distance from the dipole can be predicted; that is referred to as the forward problem. The location of a current source given the voltage pattern is the inverse problem. For any given voltage distribution an equivalent dipole can be computed. Whether this dipole has any physical reality or heuristic utility depends on the specific signals under investigation. There are situations in which dipole modeling leads to useful results concerning the underlying generators, but in general the complexities of the cortical convolutions, number of generators, synchronization, and location relative to the scalp overwhelm the problem.

RHYTHMIC ACTIVITY The EEG in many circumstances shows quasi-periodic wavelike potential fluctuations. Those signals may include normal spontaneous rhythms such as alpha and sleep spindles or pathological patterns seen during seizures or slow wave bursts.

Several examples of neuronal oscillatory behavior may relate to rhythms recorded at the scalp. There are populations of thalamic neurons with intrinsic rhythmic properties, and it has been theorized that through thalamocortical projections synchronous activity may be passed on to cortical areas. Evidence now exists that there are individual cells that can produce rhythmic activity even in the absence of synaptic input. Populations of such cells are able to sustain oscillatory behavior and in turn influence other populations of neurons.

Understanding the mechanisms of such oscillatory behavior involves models of the properties of the network as well as the dynamics of the individual elements. The strength and number of connections between cortical modules, their spatial arrangement, and many other parameters all determine the dynamic activity of the neocortex. The basic research interest in the EEG results from the general belief that the surface-recorded tracing is essentially reflective of these properties. Furthermore, emerging theories of neural organization suggest that that oscillatory activity forms the basis for processing and transmission of information in the brain.

STANDARD RECORDING METHODOLOGY

The electrical signal at the scalp is on the order of microvolts and requires considerable amplification to be recorded adequately. A differential amplifier with high input impedance is used to provide adequate signal-to-noise ratio. The gain is the number of times the voltage difference between the two input electrodes is amplified. Filter settings or time constants refer to the frequency response of the amplifier. The usual filter settings on amplifiers for clinical recording give a bandpass of 1 to 70 Hz.

Standard clinical recording relies on the placement of 19 electrodes over the scalp according to the International 10-20 System (Figure 1.8-1). That is a proportional measurement designed to normalize for head size with the intention that if electrodes are placed at proportionate distances from bony landmarks they will on average fall over intended cortical areas.

The exact number and placement of electrodes depends on the montages that are planned for actual recording (Table 1.8-1). There are two main forms of montage: bipolar and referential (sometimes mistakenly termed monopolar). The bipolar montage uses adjacent electrodes as the input pair for each differential amplifier. The referential montage uses the same electrode for one of the inputs on all channels. Montages are designed to aid in localization of various patterns of activity. The bipolar montage is useful for determining phase reversals of the EEG, whereas the referential montage aids specific localization.

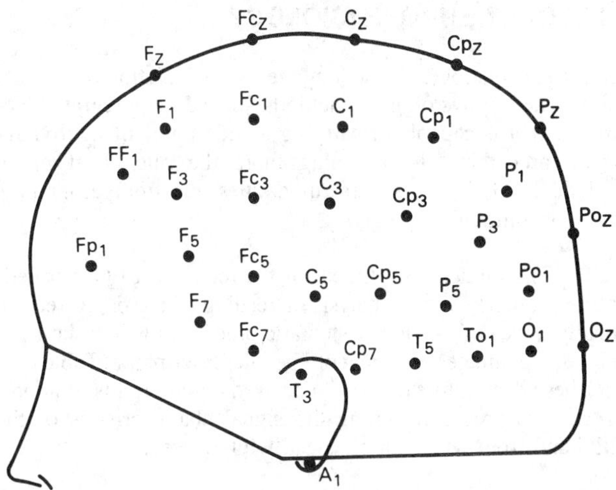

FIGURE 1.8-1 *Locations of electrodes on the scalp during standard clinical encephalography.*

TABLE 1.8-1
Recording Parameters and Terms

Gain	Degree of amplification
Filter	Frequency response
Bipolar	Recording between pairs of electrodes
Referential	All electrodes recorded to same reference
Montage	Actual set of electrodes used for recording

Recording is routinely made onto paper records by means of penwriters. Present computer systems allow direct recording onto digital media with or without concurrent paper record. Review may then be carried out on the computer display screen. The digital option is just now being accepted into clinical practice.

All recording methods are prone to a variety of artifacts that may stem either from the equipment or from the subject. Electrical noise, amplifier maladjustment, or pen maladjustment all lead to relatively obvious artifacts that affect the data throughout the record. The more troublesome artifacts are those generated by the subject and generally are due to head movements, muscle noise, or eye blinks that serve to obscure the actual data record.

The behavioral state of the subject should be either controlled or at least noted in order to allow for proper interpretation of the record. Increased slow activity is usual for a drowsy subject but would be abnormal in an otherwise supposedly alert subject. Alternately opening and closing the eyes allows for assessment of the reactivity of resting alpha rhythm and alpha blocking. Some forms of activation may be used during clinical recordings as an aid to unveiling underlying abnormalities. Those include hyperventilation and photic stimulation.

CLINICAL NEUROPHYSIOLOGY

Electroencephalography no longer exists in isolation from other clinical neurophysiological methods. Indeed the integrated laboratory that is capable of carrying a wide range of neurodiagnostic procedures is becoming more the rule. That might include EEG, EP in several modalities, electromyelography, and polysomnography.

EEG The clinical assessment of the recorded EEG proceeds from an orderly visual analysis or reading of the paper record. Ideally, this analysis is a systematic process in which the EEG record is evaluated in terms of specific descriptors (Table 1.8-2). These descriptors have been derived both in terms of appropriate measures considering the signal characteristics of the EEG and from what can be visually interpreted.

Amplitude The voltage of the EEG depends on the montage, frequency, and state of the subject among other variables. It is generally characterized along with the frequency (for example, low-voltage fast activity). The normal range for a scalp EEG is on the order of 10 to 100 microvolts (μV). Very low-voltage fast activity generally indicates a very disordered state, whereas high-voltage slow activity (other than sleep) can indicate encephalopathy.

Frequency The formal descriptive unit of frequency is the hertz (Hz), a measure of cycles per second. While the ongoing EEG may be rhythmic in nature it is generally of mixed frequency. In giving a description the frequency may be stated explicitly (for example, 2-Hz high-voltage waves). Generally, the frequencies are divided into bands referred to as delta (δ) (1 to 4 Hz), theta (θ) (4 to 8 Hz), alpha (α) (8 to 12 Hz), and beta (β) (13 to 20 Hz or higher). Quantitative analysis by computer signal processing requires very explicit definitions of the bands.

Waveform Wave morphology refers to the specific shape of the graphic elements as seen on the paper record. The α rhythm can appear almost sinusoidal, with well-formed waves. Spindles are generally formed of somewhat sharper waves. During sleep stages there is the development of large, slow waves that may or may not have symmetrical ascending and descending phases.

Topography Brainwave topography refers to the spatial distribution of specific activity over the scalp. The α rhythm, the predominant normal waking pattern, is usually maximal over the posterior regions. The salient features include the degree of synchrony (that is, how widespread the activity is and the symmetry or lack thereof). Most EEG patterns are fairly symmetric, marked asymmetry being suggestive of possible abnormality.

Reactivity It is important to note whether the EEG pattern is reactive to external stimuli, especially eye opening or closing by the subject.

TABLE 1.8-2
EEG Descriptors

Amplitude	Voltage of the EEG
Frequency	Cycles per second
Morphology	Wave shape
Topography	Spatial distribution
Reactivity	Eyes opened and closed
Symmetry	Homologous hemispheric locations

NORMAL BRAINWAVE DEVELOPMENT The development of the EEG follows a progression with age. Waking and sleeping patterns mature along a course that makes knowledge of the subject's age necessary for proper interpretation. That is especially true during infancy and childhood. The EEG attains an adult configuration when a person is 10 to 12 years of age.

NORMAL ADULT PATTERNS Recognizing the normal pattern of the EEG record in adults requires a knowledge of the usual rhythms in terms of the normative descriptors as well as the age and behavioral state of the subject.

A key feature of the normal pattern should be the occipital α rhythm. This rhythm is generally elicited with the patient in an eyes closed, relaxed, wakeful state, seen maximally over posterior regions with a moderate amplitude and frequency of 8 to 13 Hz. Any change from that relaxed state to either increased or decreased vigilance (arousal) will tend to attenuate the α rhythm. With levels of increased arousal, even that produced by eyes opening, the occipital α rhythm will often be replaced by more desynchronized, faster beta activity. A movement toward a more drowsy state will also produce a diminution of the α rhythm but now with an increase of slower, theta activity. Figure 1.8-2 illustrates that transition of states.

The regulation of the rhythmic pattern over time may in itself be a feature of a given person's EEG. Generally, in a healthy subject the EEG shows a stable pattern over time and may be used to assess changes in the state of the subject.

ABNORMAL PATTERNS Abnormalities of the EEG broadly fall into a few characteristic patterns. The main instances include slow waves, either focal or diffuse, and paroxysmal discharges including spikes and slow waves. In general, there is a rough correlation between the degree of EEG changes and the degree of behavioral impairment involved with dysfunction of the central nervous system. The initial EEG changes seen with very modest behavioral involvement, such as reduced attentional capacity, include slowing of the posterior α rhythm followed by a more widespread activity in the θ band and a decrease in reactivity. With continued behavioral impairment the EEG demonstrates loss of α and β activity with increased δ activity.

Any encephalopathy generally results in diffuse slowing of the EEG. Pathological processes that are more widespread contribute to a more diffuse pattern of EEG abnormality. Focal slowing (that is, δ or θ activity seen only in a relatively circumscribed region of the scalp recording) suggests the presence of a more focal structural abnormality. That abnormality might be the result of brain injury from trauma or a localized disease process, such as stroke or tumor.

Epileptiform activity consisting of sharp waves or spikes is the hallmark of underlying brain dysfunction (Figure 1.8-3). The process may be diffuse or may be the result of localized trauma. The behavioral manifestation depends on the brain region and the extent of the underlying abnormal process.

EVOKED POTENTIALS EPs represent neural activity in response to either internal or external events. They may be considered in two broad categories: sensory and cognitive. The sensory EPs relate to specifically physical sensory stimulation without behavioral involvement (Table 1.8-3). Cognitive EPs refer to recordings made where the subject has some type of processing task to perform in relation to the sensory input. Those are often referred to as event-related potentials (ERPs).

In clinical neurophysiology EPs are utilized mainly as a method to assess the functional integrity of well-defined sensory

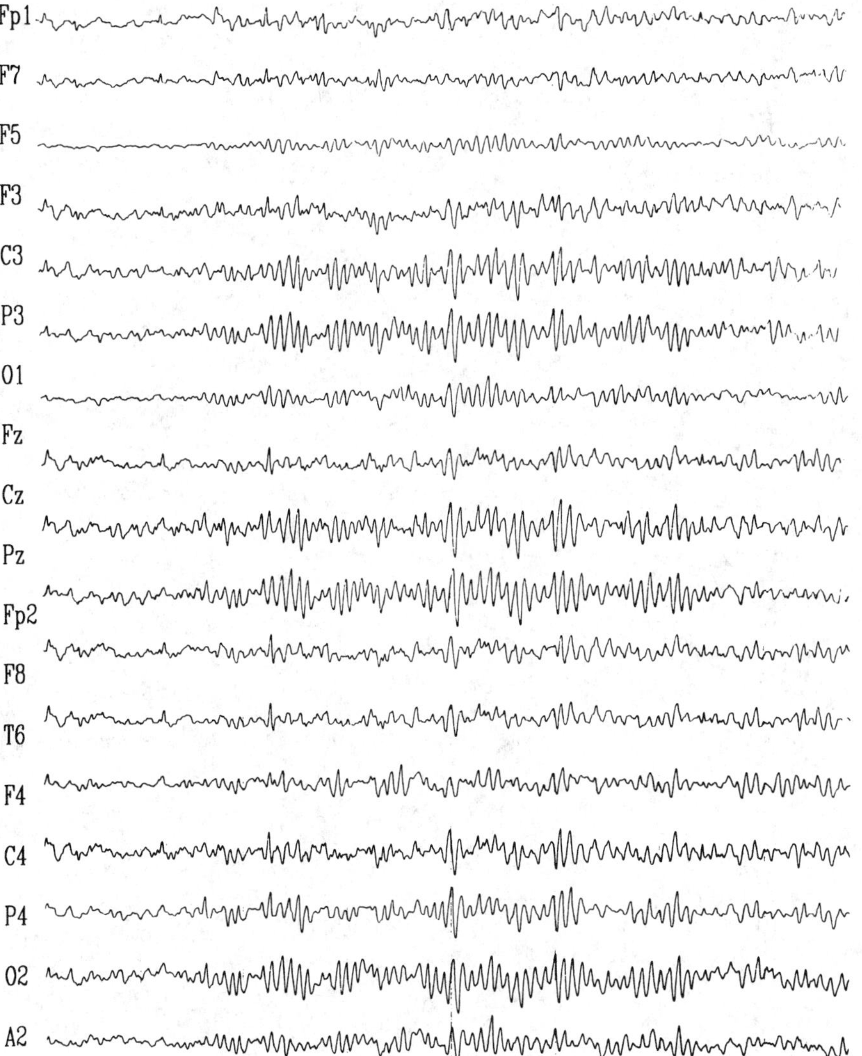

FIGURE 1.8-2 *Normal EEG, resting, eyes closed.*

pathways to the primary sensory projection areas of the cortex. There are four main types of EPs in this category: brainstem, auditory, somatosensory, and visual. Brainstem EPs are usually elicited by auditory stimuli presented at a fairly rapid rate and involve very short latency recording on the order of 10 milliseconds (ms). The main sensory modalities are tested with simple stimuli: usually click or tone pips for auditory, brief electric stimuli for somatosensory, and checkerboard or pattern reversal for visual stimuli (Figure 1.8-4).

EP Measures EPs are quantified in terms of measurements of specific peaks thought to represent the main components of the response. These peaks are labeled by their polarity and nominal latency. Thus, the visual EP P100 refers to a positive going peak at approximately 100 ms latency from the stimulus onset. In clinical neurophysiology a normal range has been established for the major responses. Abnormalities are noted by deviation from these norms and by deviations from the expected waveform pattern. EPs can be abnormal with respect to the time to evoke a particular peak or the amplitude of the peak. Conduction defects, as seen in demyelinating diseases such as multiple sclerosis, result in a delay in production of a peak. Amplitude asymmetries suggest focal abnormalities in the structures generating individual peaks.

APPLICATION TO NEUROPSYCHIATRY

Clinical neurophysiology that includes EEG and EP recording has as one of its key roles that of diagnostic exclusion (that is, to rule out specific organic disorders). The possible comorbidity of organic syndromes and idiopathic psychiatric conditions should also be considered.

A thorough electrophysiological evaluation should be strongly considered whenever any episodic event is noted in the presenting history. An EEG is clearly indicated as part of screening for a psychiatric patient whenever the history suggests any episodic behavior (including anxiety attacks and dissociative episodes) or a history of possible brain injury, loss of consciousness, or other neurological disturbance. In particular, the EEG is useful in assessment of the elderly patient, differentiating dementia from depression, and in assessment of the pediatric patient, differentiating attention-deficit disorders from absence seizures.

CLINICAL FINDINGS IN PSYCHIATRY In addition to the diagnosis of neurological comorbidity, the EEG results usually found in psychiatric patients include increased nonspecific EEG abnormalities, especially in patients with schizophrenia. However, there are no clinical findings that are of specific diagnostic

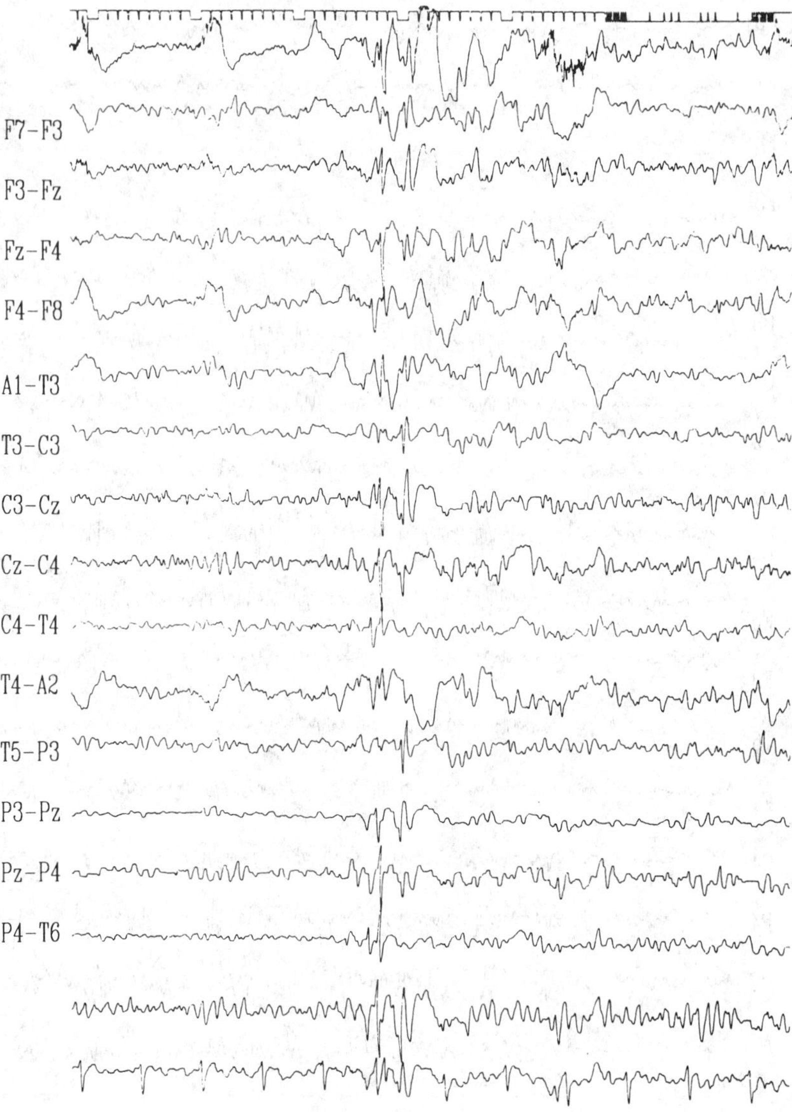

FIGURE 1.8-3 *Abnormal EEG study shows epileptiform activity.*

TABLE 1.8-3
Evoked Potentials

Brainstem—auditory
Visual—flash, checkerboard
Auditory—click
Somatosensory—electric

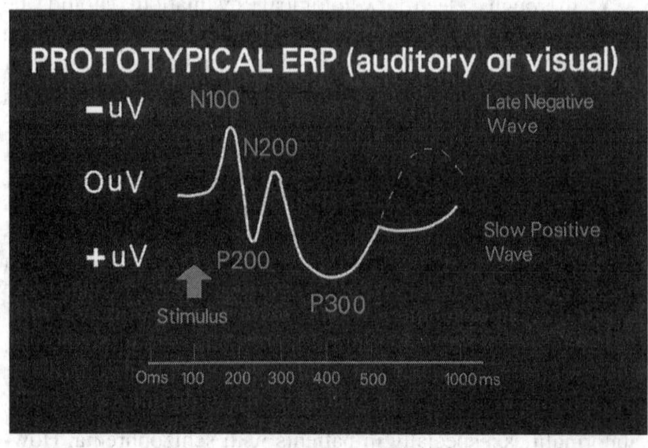

FIGURE 1.8-4 *Example of visual EP.*

utility in psychiatry. Electrophysiology does not provide any distinct pathognomonic signs in psychiatric applications. The main utility is one of exclusion of other underlying disorders.

The EEG may be useful in differentiating between depression and dementia in aged patients. Patients with dementing illnesses generally show a distinct deterioration of the EEG, usually with loss of the α rhythm and either increased δ or a pattern of low-voltage fast activity. Elderly patients with depression may show a maintenance of a posterior α rhythm, suggesting that a dementing process might not be part of the clinical picture.

ADVANCED METHODS A number of methodological advances beyond that used in standard clinical neurophysiology have widespread use in electrophysiological research. The development of cognitive psychophysiology has advanced research into the underlying neurophysiological mechanisms of cognition and behavior. Behavioral correlates that might follow from this research may be particularly useful to neuropsychiatry.

EVOKED POTENTIALS A number of EP paradigms are now almost routine in many laboratories that are not yet established as part of the clinical routine.

Sensory One of the early components of the response to auditory stimuli, such as clicks, is the P50. When presented in a conditioned paired click paradigm, the P50 to the second click of the pair is substantially reduced in healthy subjects. Several investigators have found that subjects with schizophrenia fail to show this reduction. That finding has been interpreted as a dysfunction of normal sensory gating (the modulation of incoming sensory signals). Similar recovery function paradigms, in which the response to the second of two paired stimuli is measured, have also been investigated with more equivocal results in other psychiatric diagnostic populations.

Cognitive Paradigms in cognitive psychophysiology have focused on two important responses: the N140 and the P300. The N140 is related to attentional processing and may be enhanced under conditions requiring selective attention for proper task performance. The P300 is related to information processing and is most noted in tasks requiring a behavioral response to target stimuli. Several patient populations show diminished P300 amplitude and increased latency. Those changes are generally interpreted as a disturbance in information processing because the latencies are well beyond the time frame of initial sensory pathways. The main limitation in the clinical application of cognitive EPs is the lack of specificity with regard to both the form of the cognitive disturbance and to the clinical population.

Readiness potentials Readiness potentials encompass several long latency components including the contingent negative variation (CNV), the motor readiness potential (MRP), or the *bereitschrafts* potential (BP). The typical CNV paradigm involves a warning stimulus followed at some time by an imperative stimulus usually requiring a response. The CNV is the slow negative shift that occurs during the one to two seconds between the stimuli.

QUANTITATIVE ELECTROPHYSIOLOGY

Both EEG and EP studies have been greatly extended with the recent advances in computer and graphic display technology. A number of different terms have been applied to the various newly evolved methods, including quantitative EEG (QEEG), computerized EEG mapping, and topographic brain mapping. Several directions are important. One of the driving forces behind the development of computerized transformations of EEG recordings was to provide quantitative analysis as an adjunct to the visual interpretation of EEG paper records. Most of the efforts in that direction have involved detailed frequency measurements, such as provided by spectrum analysis, which allows detailed quantification of both the frequency and the intensity of the electrical activity. A second direction has been the mapping of brain activity. The construction of color graphic displays of some measure recorded over the scalp surface has been popular (Figure 1.8-5). It is important to note, however, that just constructing a topographic map does not constitute an analysis of data. A third direction has been the increased density of recording electrodes with specific emphasis on localization.

DESCRIPTORS Quantitative methods for continuous EEG include various spectrum analysis measures. Those are primarily extensions of the visual methods that attempt to provide numerical measurements for the usual frequency domain parameters. Extensions to those descriptors include such terms as "coherence." That is a measure of the extent to which any two channels (electrodes) carry similar information and thus represent correlated activity. Research has focused on whether coherence is useful as a measure of the extent to which activity in different brain regions is related. Although many empirical studies have been carried out, underlying mechanisms contributing to coherence or useful behavioral correlates remain equivocal.

TOPOGRAPHIC MAPPING Methods of presenting EEG information in a graphical form having some resemblance to scalp or brain topography have garnered considerable attention. Most computerized EEG systems have a fixed schema or map on which the data for an individual subject are superimposed. In general such displays may be useful as schematic illustrations for ease in data presentation. There is, however, concern that such displays might be taken too literally in terms of localization of brain activity.

CLINICAL AND RESEARCH UTILITY Specific clinical advantage has yet to be unequivocally demonstrated for any of the quantitative or mapping techniques. Several scientific groups have organized to set guidelines for the development of those methods. Those groups have attempted to provide some standardization in order to further research in this field. The methods being employed are at present too diverse to lend themselves to rigorous organization. Therefore such guidelines are meant only to aid researchers in describing their work in a reliable fashion.

STATISTICAL CONSIDERATIONS One of the problems of QEEG has been the application of appropriate statistical methods to the complex multivariate designs that are usually employed. Often just the sheer number of statistical tests performed creates a difficulty. That is a problem of any large multivariable experiment but has been particularly of concern in this field because often the studies are completely empirical in nature. Some studies have demonstrated group differences between patients and controls or among different patient groups. The extension of these group findings to individual cases should not be the basis for individual diagnosis.

Several studies have utilized some form of discriminant analysis to classify individual subjects on the basis of multivariate measurements. However, the sensitivity and specificity of such methods are yet to be established.

PHARMACO-EEG

An application of quantitative electrophysiology that has seen considerable research application is the use of EEG to demonstrate and determine the effects of various pharmacological agents on the central nervous system. The main working hypothesis of this application is that if a drug has a behavioral effect then it will have a measurable effect on the EEG (Table 1.8-4). Measurable changes in the EEG owing to medication do not necessarily indicate a behavioral effect, but under that hypothesis an EEG effect is a necessary but not sufficient prerequisite.

Most pharmaco-EEG studies involve detailing changes in the EEG frequency spectrum with respect to drug administration. Work has shown that the major classes of psychoactive drugs have discriminable profiles of spectrum changes even for acute administration. A potential application is determining a patient's EEG response to a single test dose of a specific medication as a predictor of long-term efficacy for that patient.

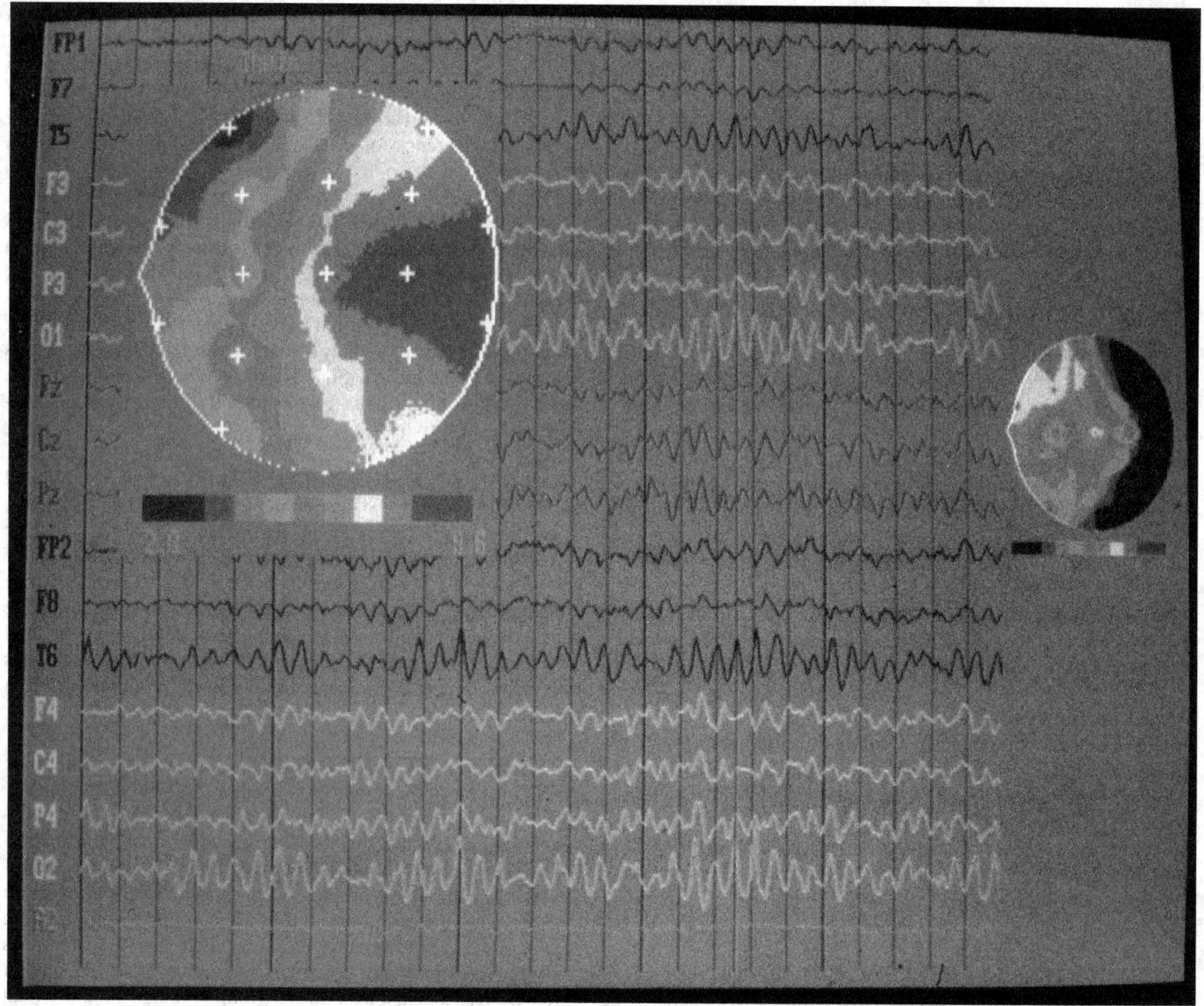

FIGURE 1.8-5 *Digital EEG recording and topographic map representation. (See Color Plate 1.)*

MAGNETOENCEPHALOGRAPHY

Magnetoencephalography (MEG) records the magnetic field resulting from the bioelectrical activity of the brain. Superconducting technology is necessary for the sensitivity required to detect the small magnetic field signal. The sophisticated instrumentation is at present at least an order of magnitude more expensive than EEG. Expansion to a larger number of channels with reduced cost can be expected; however, MEG will remain considerably more expensive than EEG.

Because the magnetic signal is not distorted by volume conduction in the same manner as the electrical signal recorded at the scalp it was hoped that MEG might provide better localization of the underlying sources of the neural activity. Studies have shown that the localization accuracy for MEG and EEG is comparable. However, MEG and EEG are sensitive to different aspects of brain structure and physiology. EEG dipole localization is much more dependent on detailed anatomy than MEG (that is, inaccuracies in head models will produce more significant errors in EEG localization). Another distinction is a differential sensitivity to the orientation of dipole current sources. The MEG can detect only the magnetic field from dipoles that are tangential to the skull; the EEG picks up signals from both tangential and radial sources. That difference can be especially useful in sorting out competing source configurations when MEG is utilized in conjunction with EEG.

TABLE 1.8-4
Characteristic Effects of Major Drug Classes on the EEG

Anxiolytics	Decrease of α and increase of β
Antidepressants	Increase of δ, decrease of α
Antipsychotics	Increase of θ

The main point in comparison is that the paradigmatic approach for both MEG and EEG is essentially the same because the same underlying neural activity gives rise to both the magnetic and the electric fields of the brain. Both technologies rely on an experimental model that hopes to relate brain function to neural activity. The usefulness of both modalities will depend on advances in localization methods. When combined with information from magnetic resonance imaging (MRI), considerable improvement in accuracy can be expected. In addition to cost there are practical differences between MEG and EEG relating to ease of application. With advanced mul-

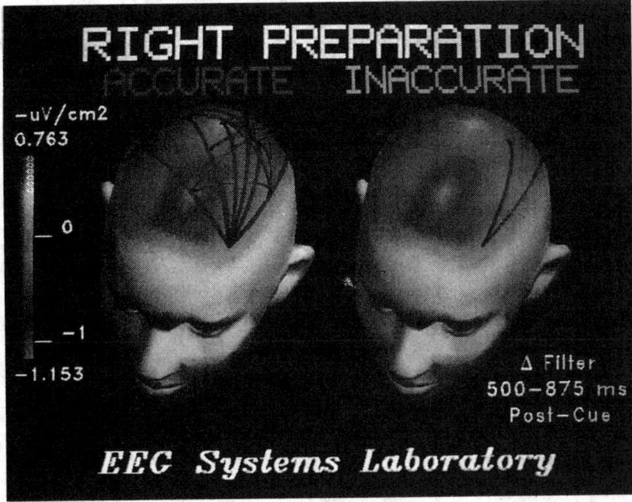

FIGURE 1.8-6 *Example of network from 124 lead recording. (See Color Plate 6.)*

tichannel whole-head systems MEG may have easier patient preparation. However, EEG will remain more portable and suitable for lengthy recordings.

NETWORK MODELS

Specific localization may be appropriate only in very special and limited circumstances. For example, in the case of brainstem evoked potentials, individual components of the waveform can be localized to the activity in specific brainstem nuclei. However, cognitive function, even of relatively simple form, probably requires a network of brain regions for its support. Several converging lines of research suggest a model of the brain as a parallel distributed processing mechanism. Implicit in such a model is the idea that the networks needed to sustain the functional behavior are necessarily dynamic.

The determination of such networks goes beyond the concept of localization manifested in most dipole modeling. Methods for elaborating such brain activity will require multielectrode recording, advanced data processing, and individualized structural brain models. Several research laboratories now have the capability for 64- and 128-channel recording (Figure 1.8-6). Specialized electrode nets and helmets have been designed to facilitate these studies. Combined with MRI structural information, the surface signals can be reconstructed as if they had been recorded on the cortex. It is then possible to study the interaction among the signals from different brain regions in relation to task demands in such a way as to determine whether those regions were functionally related. Because of the millisecond temporal resolution of electrophysiology the detailed dynamics of these regional interactions can be examined.

With those methods now under development improved resolution of the functional dynamics of brain activity can be expected. Application to cognitive function may reveal a better understanding of the neurophysiological substrate underlying the disturbances seen in neuropsychiatric disorders.

SUGGESTED CROSS-REFERENCES

Basic electrophysiology is introduced in Section 1.7 and sleep, including polysomnography, is discussed in Section 1.9.

REFERENCES

American Academy of Neurology: Assessment: EEG brain mapping. Neurology *39:* 1100, 1989.

American Academy of Neurology: Assessment: Magnetoencephalography (MEG). Neurology *42:* 1, 1992.

American Psychiatric Association Task Force: Quantitative electroencephalography: A report on the present state of computerized EEG techniques. Am J Psychiatry *148:* 961, 1991.

*Aminoff M J, editor: *Electrodiagnostics in Clinical Neurology,* 3rd ed., Churchill Livingstone, New York, 1992.

Blume W T, Kaibara M: *Atlas of Adult Electroencephalography.* Raven Press, New York, 1994.

Cohen D, Cuffin B N: EEG versus MEG localization accuracy: Theory and experiment. Brain Topography *4*: 95, 1991.

*Coppola R: Topographic mapping of multilead data. In *Event-Related Brain Potentials,* J W Rohrbaugh, R Parasuraman, R Johnson, editors, p 37. Oxford University Press, New York, 1990.

Daly D D, Pedley T A, editors: *Current Practice of Clinical Electroencephalography.* Raven Press, New York, 1990.

Fisch B J, Pedley T A: The role of quantitative EEG topographic mapping or 'neurometrics' in the diagnosis of psychiatric and neurological disorders: The cons. Electroencephalogr Clin Neurophysiol *73:* 5, 1989.

Gevins A S, Illes J: Neurocognitive networks of the human brain. Ann NY Acad Sci *620:* 22, 1991.

Gevins A S, Le J, Brickett P, Reutter B, Desmond J: Seeing through the skull: Advanced EEGs use MRIs to accurately measure cortical activity from the scalp. Brain Topography *4*: 125, 1991.

Gevins A S, Le J, Martin N K, Brickett P, Desmond J, Reutter B: High resolution EEG: 124 channel recording, spatial deblurring and MRI integration methods. Electroencephalogr Clin Neurophysiol *90:* 337, 1994.

Herrmann W M, Schaerer E: Pharmaco-EEG: Computer EEG analysis to describe the projection of drug effects on a functional cerebral level in humans. In *Clinical Applications of Computer Analysis of EEG and other Neurophysiological Signals,* F H Lopes da Silva, W S van Leeuwen, A Remond, editors, p 385, Elsevier, Amsterdam, 1986.

*International Pharmaco-EEG Group: Recommendations for EEG and evoked potential mapping. Neuropsychobiology *22:* 170, 1989.

John E R: The role of quantitative EEG topographic mapping or 'neurometrics' in the diagnosis of psychiatric and neurological disorders: The pros. Electroencephalogr Clin Neurophysiol *73:* 2, 1989.

John E R, Prichep L S, Easton P: Standardized varimax descriptors of event related potentials: Evaluation of psychiatric patients. Psychiatr Res Neuroimaging *55:* 13, 1994.

Lopes da Silva F H: Neural mechanisms underlying brain waves: From neural membranes to networks. Electroencephalogr Clin Neurophysiol *79:* 81, 1991.

*Neylan T C, Reynolds C F, Kupfer D J: Electrodiagnostic techniques in neuropsychiatry. In *Textbook of Neuropsychiatry,* S C Yudofsky, R E Hales, editors. American Psychiatric Press, Washington, DC, 1992.

Nuwer M R: Quantitative EEG: I. Techniques and problems of frequency analysis and topographic mapping. J Clin Neurophysiol *5:* 1, 1988.

*Nuwer, M R (chairman): IFCN guidelines for topographic and frequency analysis of EEGs and EPs. Report of an IFCN committee. Electroencephalogr Clin Neurophysiol *91:* 1, 1994.

Picton T W: The P300 wave of the human event-related potential, J Clin Neurophysiol 9: 456, 1992.

Pivik R T, Broughton R J, Coppola R, Davidson R J, Fox N, Nuwer M R: Guidelines for the recording and quantitative analysis of electroencephalographic activity in research contexts. Psychophysiology *30:* 547, 1993.

Rohrbaugh J W, Parasuraman R, Johnson R, editors: *Event-Related Brain Potentials: Basic Issues and Applications,* Oxford University Press, New York, 1990.

1.9 BASIC SCIENCE OF SLEEP

J. CHRISTIAN GILLIN, M.D.
REBECCA K. ZOLTOSKI, Ph.D.
RAFAEL SALIN-PASCUAL, M.D., Ph.D.

INTRODUCTION

Clinicians often evaluate patients who complain of sleeping too little, too much, or not well enough, or who have sleep-related behavioral disorders, such as sleepwalking, enuresis, or nightmares. The classification and treatment of those disorders have matured significantly in recent years. Furthermore, sleep disorders are particularly pertinent to psychiatrists and other mental health professionals because they are frequently associated with depression, anxiety, substance abuse, obsessive-compulsive disorder, psychosis, acute and chronic stress, and many other disorders.

PHENOMENOLOGY OF SLEEP AND WAKEFULNESS IN NORMAL HUMANS

SLEEP STAGES AND THEIR NORMAL ORGANIZATION

Most mammals have two major phases of sleep: rapid eye movement (REM) sleep and nonrapid eye movement (NREM) sleep. REM sleep is sometimes called dreaming or D sleep, since it is associated with dreaming, or paradoxical sleep, because the brain seems, paradoxically, to be activated during that state of sleep. NREM sleep conforms to traditional concepts of sleep as a time of decreased physiological and psychological activity. It is, therefore, sometimes called orthodox sleep or slow-wave, electroencephalogram (EEG) synchronized, or S sleep.

NREM sleep is further divided into four sleep stages on the basis of visually scored EEG patterns (Table 1.9-1 and Figure 1.9-1). Sleep normally begins with stage 1, a brief transitional phase, before progressing successively into stages 2 through 4. Stage 2 sleep is defined by the presence of sleep spindles and K complexes in the EEG. Stage 3 and stage 4 sleep, or delta sleep, are defined by the presence of delta waves in the EEG, a moderate (20 to 50 percent) and large (over 50 percent) proportion of an epoch of sleep, respectively.

REM sleep is characterized by an activated EEG, loss of tone in the major antigravity muscles, and periodic bursts of rapid eye movements. The REM latency is usually about 70 to 100 minutes in normal subjects, but may be significantly shorter in some patients with depression, eating disorders, borderline personality disorder, schizophrenia, alcohol-related disorders, or other psychiatric disorders. Thereafter, NREM and REM sleep oscillate with a cycle length of roughly 90 to 100 minutes. When it does occur, the percent of delta sleep is highest in the first NREM period of the night and declines with each successive NREM period. Most delta sleep occurs in the first half of the night, and most REM sleep in the second half.

REM sleep and NREM sleep differ in many psychological and physiological domains (Table 1.9-2). On a psychological level, REM sleep is associated with dreaming mentation, whereas NREM sleep is more likely to be associated with abstract thinking. Although autonomic functioning is often highly variable during REM sleep, it is usually slow and steady in NREM sleep. Studies in normal subjects suggest that the phase positions of the cortisol nadir and NREM sleep (stages 3 and 4) are influenced by genetic factors.

TERMS COMMONLY USED IN SLEEP LABORATORY STUDIES Many different measurements may be made of sleep, sleepiness, wakefulness, physiology, or performance in a sleep laboratory, depending on the purpose of the evaluation. In order to measure the stages of sleep, the subject is usually monitored by electrodes, which are attached to the scalp for recording an EEG, near the eyes for measuring eye movements, and on the chin (submental) muscles for recording muscle tone. In the clinical evaluation of a patient suspected of having a specific sleep disorder, various measurements may be made, including recordings of nasal and oral airflow by means of thermistors, electrocardiograms (ECGs), respiratory movements of the chest and abdomen, oxygen saturation, core body temperature (often rectal or tympanic membrane), muscle twitches of the legs (usually the anterior tibial muscles), penile erections, and esophageal pH (for gastroesophageal reflux) (Table 1.9-1).

Although most sleep laboratories use a common set of definitions for sleep stages, no commonly accepted definitions for some specific measures exist. For example, sleep onset is defined, depending on the laboratory, as the first epoch of stage 1, of stage 2, or of persistent sleep (that is, 9 minutes of sleep in a 10-minute period). Likewise, the first REM period may be defined as either the first epoch of REM sleep or the first period of persistent REM sleep (that is, three minutes). REM latency may either include or exclude wakefulness between sleep onset and the first REM period. Those variations in definitions do not usually make a great difference, but clinicians and researchers must be aware of them when comparing results and reports from different laboratories.

COMPUTER-ASSISTED ANALYSIS OF SLEEP RECORDS

Although visual scoring is still the standard method for identifying specific sleep stages, considerable progress has been made in using computers for this task. Some companies now market hardware and software designed to replace, or at least to assist, the sleep technician, and further advances can be expected in the coming years.

Two methods of EEG waveform analysis have received particular attention: spectral analysis and period-amplitude analysis. Spectral analysis uses fast Fourier algorithms to compute the cumulative or average power (μV^2) of specific frequency bands. That provides absolute measures of specific frequency components of the EEG in each epoch. Period-amplitude analysis computes the peak amplitude of each EEG wave and the time interval between zero crossings. It is particularly useful in estimating the amplitude and temporal distribution of transient phenomena in the EEG, such as delta waves, K complexes, and sleep spindles, but it may miss frequency components of the EEG that fail to produce zero crossings. Both methods measure slow-wave activity well.

MEASURES OF DAYTIME SLEEPINESS Excessive sleepiness is a common complaint in clinical practice and may be a sign of one of various treatable conditions, such as chronic partial sleep deprivation, certain sleep disorders (sleep apnea, narcolepsy, frequently interrupted sleep, sleep drunkenness), circadian rhythm disorders (phase-advance syndrome and phase-delay syndrome), certain medical conditions, and the effect of sedating medications. It should be distinguished from fatigue, which is often experienced as tiredness and a desire to sleep, but does not usually lead to sleep. The typical insomniac

TABLE 1.9-1
Technical Terms Commonly Used in Characterizing Sleep

Term	Definition
Alpha wave	EEG patterns (8–12 cps) typical of relaxed wakefulness, especially over the occipital cortex
Apnea index (AI)	Number of apneic events per hour of sleep; usually considered to be pathological if five or more
Cataplexy	Sudden, brief loss of muscle tone, in the waking state usually triggered by emotional arousal (laughing, anger, surprise), involving either a few muscle groups (e.g., facial) or most of the major antigravity muscles of the body. May be related to muscle atonia normally occurring during REM sleep. Associated with narcolepsy
Delayed sleep phase	A sleep disorder characterized by a persistently very late bedtime and onset of sleep (e.g., 4 AM) and a very late rising time (e.g., noon); extreme night owls
Delta wave	EEG pattern conventionally defined as ≥75 μV, ≥0.5 Hz; the amplitude tends to decrease with normal aging
Early morning awakening (EMA)	Time awake between the end of sleep and leaving one's bed
Electroencephalogram (EEG)	Electrical potential recordings taken from the scalp
Electro-oculogram (EOG)	Electrical recordings of eye movements
Electromyogram (EMG)	Electrical recording of somatic muscle tone
Hypopnea	A 50% or more reduction in respiratory depth for 10 seconds or more during sleep
K complex	An EEG wave characterized by an initial brief, low-amplitude component, followed by a high-amplitude, long-lasting component. Characteristic of stage 2 sleep
Maintenance of wakefulness test (MWT)	An objective method for determining daytime sleepiness; subject is instructed to remain awake while recumbent in the dark
Multiple sleep latency test (MSLT)	An objective method for determining daytime sleepiness; sleep latency and REM latency are determined for four or five naps (e.g., a 20-minute opportunity to sleep every two hours between 10 AM and 6 PM)
Nocturnal penile tumescence (NPT)	Quantitative measure of penile erections, which are normally present during REM sleep. May be used to evaluate complaint of impotence
NREM sleep	Stages 1, 2, 3, and 4 sleep
Periodic limb movements during sleep (PLMS)	Sleep-related periodic limb movements characterized by twitches of the big toe, ankle, or knee
PLMS index	Number of leg kicks per hour of sleep; usually considered pathological if five or more
Polysomnography	Detailed, sleep-laboratory-based, clinical evaluation of patient with sleep disorder; may include measures of EEG, eye movements, muscle tone at chin and limbs, respiratory movements of chest and abdomen, oxygen saturation, electrocardiogram (ECG), NPT, esophageal pH, as indicated
REM cycle length	Time from one REM period until the next
REM density	A measure of ocular activity during REM sleep
REM latency	Time from onset of sleep to onset of REM sleep. Declines with age from about 70–100 minutes in 20s to 55–70 minutes in elderly. Short REM latency has been associated with narcolepsy, depressive disorders, and a variety of clinical conditions
REM sleep	Rapid eye movement sleep. Characterized by low-voltage, relatively fast-frequency EEG, bursts of rapid eye movements, and loss of tone in the major antigravity muscles. Associated with dreaming
Respiratory disturbance index (RDI)	Number of apneas and hypopneas per hour of sleep
Sleep apnea	Sleep-related breathing disorder characterized by at least five episodes of apnea per hour of sleep, each more than 10 seconds in duration
Sleep efficiency	Percentage of time in bed spent in sleep. Usually above 90% in the young; declines somewhat with age
Sleep latency	Time from lights out to onset of sleep
Sleep spindle	An EEG wave characterized by 12–14-cps rhythm lasting about 0.5 second. Characteristic of stage 2 sleep
Stage 1 sleep	A brief transitional state of sleep between wakefulness and sleep, characterized by low-voltage, mixed-frequency EEG, slow eye movements. About 5% of normal sleep time
Stage 2 sleep	Usually about 45–75% of total sleep time. Characterized by K complexes and sleep spindles (12–14-cps rhythms) in the EEG
Stages 3 and 4 sleep	Sometimes referred to as delta sleep, based on amount of delta waves in EEG, 20–50% of an epoch (e.g., 30 or 60 seconds) for stage 3, more than 50% for stage 4. The amount per night declines from about 20–25% of total sleep time in teens to near zero in elderly
Total sleep time	Total time asleep (NREM + REM sleep)
WASO	Wake time after sleep onset

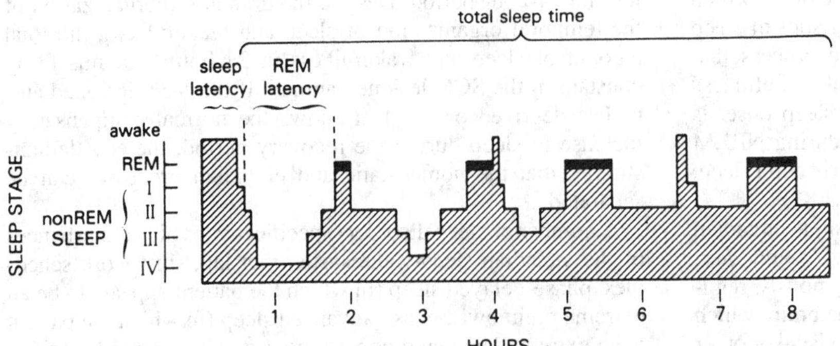

FIGURE 1.9-1 *Sleep pattern in a young adult during a normal night of sleep.*

TABLE 1.9-2
Comparison of NREM and REM Sleep

	NREM Sleep	REM Sleep
EEG	Spindles, K complexes, delta waves, synchronized	Low voltage, mixed frequency, sawtooth waves, activated
EOG	Quiescent or slow movements	Bursts of fast movements
EMG	Partial relaxation	Atonia of antigravity muscles
Intercostal muscles	Partial relaxation	Atonia
Genioglossus	Partial relaxation	Hypotonic
Blood pressure	Decreased, steady	Variable
Heart rate	Decreased, steady	Variable
Cardiac output	Decreased	Decreased
Cerebral glucose metabolism	Decreased	Unchanged or increased
Brain temperature	Decreased	Increased
Respiratory rate	Decreased	Variable
Ventilatory response to CO_2	Intact	Partially impaired
Genitalia	Infrequent tumescence	Tumescence
Mentation	Conceptual, abstract, infrequent dreaming	Perceptual, frequent dreaming
Pathology	Night terrors, somnambulism, panic attacks	Nightmares, REM sleep behavior disorder

patient, for example, complains about fatigue but has difficulty initiating and maintaining sleep. In contrast, the patient with true excessive daytime sleepiness readily and unwillingly falls asleep quickly at inopportune times and places, such as when driving, working, or meeting with friends. Persistent pathological sleepiness is clinically serious and may be associated with significant morbidity and mortality.

Daytime sleepiness can be assessed according to either subjective or objective criteria. During the routine review of symptoms, clinicians should ask about pathological daytime sleepiness, both of the patient and of others who have had an opportunity to observe the patient's levels of alertness and sleepiness. For a more detailed evaluation, clinicians can administer the Stanford Sleepiness Scale, a seven-point subjective scale ranging from one (maximum alertness) to seven (fighting to stay awake); it can be filled out by the patient, for example, every hour during the day to estimate subjective sleepiness and alertness.

Of the objective, laboratory-based methods for measuring daytime sleepiness, the Multiple Sleep Latency Test (MSLT) is the best known. Mean sleep latency is about 11 to 15 minutes for most healthy adults and about two to four minutes for patients with sleep apnea or narcolepsy. A second objective method for assessing alertness is the Maintenance of Wakefulness Test (MWT), in which the subject is asked to stay awake during four or five periods while lying in bed in the dark. Again, the latency to sleep is measured. Normal subjects can usually maintain wakefulness for about 18 minutes before falling asleep.

CIRCADIAN AND HOMEOSTATIC PROCESSES Sleep and wakefulness are strongly influenced by two separate processes: (1) one or more endogenous biological clocks, which change the propensity for sleep and the characteristics of sleep across the 24-hour day; and (2) a homeostatic process that increases the likelihood of sleep as the period of wakefulness lengthens. The duration of wakefulness before sleep onset is directly related to the amount of delta activity during NREM sleep. It is postulated that NREM sleep, particularly delta sleep, dissipates the effects of wakefulness.

The daily sleep-wake cycle is an example of a circadian rhythm (from the Latin *circa,* meaning "about," and *dies,* meaning "day"). Circadian rhythms are endogenously regulated by a biological clock or clocks located in the brain, which in turn are synchronized with the environment by visual or other clues (*Zeitgebers,* or time givers). For example, if humans (and members of some other species) live in an environment devoid of time cues, the length of the sleep-wake cycle and of other biological rhythms increases from about 24 hours to approximately 24.5 to 25 hours. That condition is called free-running. If, however, a 24-hour light-dark cycle of sufficient amplitude is imposed on this environment, subjects revert to a 24-hour sleep-wake cycle (that is, they are entrained to a 24-hour cycle).

Humans appear to have two peaks of daytime sleepiness, which are determined by the phase position of the circadian clock. The first, and obvious, one is at night in the normally entrained person; the second is in midafternoon (the siesta hour). Not surprisingly, automobile accidents caused by the driver's falling asleep at the wheel peak during the last half of the night and in the midafternoon. If the circadian temperature curve is used to index the phase position of the circadian oscillator, it is seen that the major period of sleepiness occurs near the nadir of temperature, that is, between 3 and 5 AM in normal circumstances. Both the duration of sleep and the type of sleep are strongly influenced by the phase position of sleep onset. People tend to awaken on the rising limb of the temperature curve; thus sleep tends to last longest when it starts near the peak of the curve. Furthermore, REM sleep is most likely to occur near the temperature nadir. Thus, REM latency is shorter and REM time is higher during morning naps as compared with afternoon or evening naps.

The suprachiasmatic nucleus (SCN) in the anterior hypothalamus maintains the 24-hour sleep-wake cycle and synchronizes it with environmental light-dark cycles. Lesions of the SCN in animals result in so-called arrhythmic rest-activity patterns, which no longer follow a circadian rhythm but are distributed as numerous short bouts of sleep and wakefulness during the 24-hour period. Despite the dramatic reorganization of the temporal organization of sleep and wakefulness, the total amount of sleep and wakefulness in 24 hours remains fairly constant in the SCN-lesioned animal. If the SCN-lesioned animal is deprived of sleep, it shows the normal compensatory increase in sleep during the recovery period, thereby demonstrating that the homeostatic and circadian processes can be separated.

A number of sleep disorders specifically involve disturbances of the circadian sleep-wake system: jet lag, shift-work schedules, phase-delayed sleep (in which the patient appears to be an extreme night owl), phase-advanced sleep (in which the patient is an extreme lark), and non–24-hour-day syndrome (in which the patient appears to free-run, with a period of about 25 hours between each sleep onset). A subjective scale for measuring morningness and eveningness, which is useful for clinical and research purposes, is available.

Because the length of the circadian sleep-wake cycle naturally tends to be greater than 24 hours, it is easier to shift sleep-wake rhythms when delaying or lengthening the cycle than when advancing or shortening it. For example, most persons cope with jet lag more easily when traveling west than when traveling east. It usually takes about one day to accommodate for each time zone traveled when moving in an easterly direction, and somewhat less when moving in a westerly direction. In addition, shift workers seem to feel better and perform better when going from a day to an evening to a night shift than from a day to a night to an evening shift. The appropriate administration of bright lights and darkness may ameliorate jet-lag and shift-work problems by hastening the resynchronization of the endogenous clock controlling sleep-wakefulness, temperature, and other psychobiological rhythms. For example, exposure to bright light in the evening and to darkness in the morning may help with jet lag when traveling west or with shift problems when changing from an evening to a night work schedule. In addition, the exogenous administration of melatonin may shift the phase position of the circadian oscillator and might eventually be useful for treating jet-lag, shift-work, and other circadian sleep-wake disorders in which rapid resynchronization of the biological clock is desirable.

Free-running in the natural environment has been implicated in two clinical sleep disorders. First, in certain blind persons the circadian oscillator is free-running even though the person tries to remain in a synchronized sleep-wake pattern. The drifting phase position of the circadian oscillator is shown by the free-running pattern of melatonin secretion (that is, the onset of melatonin appears approximately 45 minutes later each subjective day). As would be expected, those patients have a cyclic pattern of sleep disturbance with a period length of about three to four weeks as the circadian oscillator goes in and out of synchronization with the environment. Second, patients with the non–24-hour-day syndrome typically go to bed and arise about 30 to 45 minutes later each day (that is, they are free-running with a sleep-wake cycle of about 24.5 to 24.75 hours even though they live in the natural environment).

The flexibility of the circadian system appears to diminish with age in most persons. Thus the elderly usually suffer more from jet lag and shift-work schedules than do the young. In addition, the endogenous circadian oscillators tend to be phase advanced and to have less amplitude in the elderly as compared with the young. For example, the teenager typically likes to go to bed at around 2 AM and will sleep solidly until noon, whereas his or her grandparents retire by 9 PM, arise at around 6 AM after a night of shallow sleep, and nap in the midafternoon.

PHYLOGENY AND ONTOGENY OF SLEEP

PHYLOGENY Nearly all animals, even single-cell organisms, have a rest-activity cycle, but the circadian timing, amount, and type of sleep vary dramatically among species. A few species, such as the sloth, sleep as much as 20 hours a day, whereas others, such as the shrew, may not sleep at all. Some animals, including humans, are diurnal and sleep predominately at night. Other animals, such as the laboratory rat, are nocturnal and sleep predominately in the light. Still other species, such as the cat, are crepuscular and are active predominately at dawn and at dusk.

Among the higher animals, slow-wave sleep is present in birds, mammals, and some reptiles, suggesting an obligatory role for this sleep state. REM sleep is present in all marsupials and birds, as well as in some placental mammals and reptiles, but it is absent in the monotreme echidna, a primitive egg-laying mammal. Thus, it appears that NREM sleep evolved earlier than REM sleep, the former in association with homoiothermy and the latter with viviparity (live bearing).

Sleep patterns evolved as surviving species adapted to their environments. Predators that have secure environments, such as lions, generally sleep longer and more deeply than do prey that sleep in insecure environments, such as rabbits. Marine mammals, which must breathe while spending their lives in the water, have evolved interesting ways of sleeping. The blind Incus dolphin, which lives in turbid water, has to maintain almost continual activity; therefore, it apparently sleeps in numerous short periods, each averaging about 90 seconds. Some dolphin species exhibit unihemispheric sleep: while one hemisphere of the brain is in slow-wave sleep, the other is awake, with low-voltage, fast-frequency EEG waves. If one hemisphere is experimentally deprived of NREM sleep, it shows the expected increases in total sleep and delta sleep that accompany recovery from sleep deprivation of the whole brain. Likewise, some species of seals have also evolved hemispheric sleep, so that one side of the body maneuvers the head near the water surface in order to permit the animal to breathe occasionally as the other half of the brain sleeps. Further understanding of the anatomy and neurobiology of those and other species will provide insight into the mechanisms and functions of sleep.

ONTOGENY Sleep-wake states change dramatically across the life span, not only as to the amount of sleep, but also with regard to one's ultradian and circadian timing. The newborn human infant may average about 16 hours of sleep a day, of which about 50 percent is REM sleep. The duration of the REM sleep cycle is relatively short compared with that of the adult, and the sleep-wakefulness cycle is polyphasic, with numerous short bouts of sleep and wakefulness across the 24-hour period. During the first months of life, sleep-wake cycles gradually change as sleep at night and wakefulness by day become consolidated, although napping may continue into childhood. By the age of 3 or 4 years, a child's REM sleep will have fallen to the adult levels of about 20 to 25 percent and will remain in this range for the rest of life. Nevertheless, REM latency tends to decrease and the length of the first REM period to increase with age.

The amount of time spent in delta (stages 3 and 4) sleep each night peaks in early adolescence and gradually shortens with age until it nearly disappears in about the 60s. Young adults typically spend about 15 to 20 percent of total sleep time in delta sleep. By the age of 60 or 70, few persons have any delta-wave activity during sleep, with men tending to lose delta sleep at an earlier age than do women. The loss of delta sleep results more from a reduction in amplitude than from fewer slow (0.5 to 2 Hz) waves.

Sleep disturbances in the elderly After the age of 65, about one in three women and one in five men report that they take over 30 minutes to fall asleep. Wake time after sleep onset (WASO) tends to increase with age, perhaps because of the greater incidence of sleep-related breathing disorders (that is, mild apnea) and nocturnal myoclonus. Using the Apnea Index (AI) of five or more apneic episodes an hour as a cutoff criterion, prevalence rates are noted to range from 27 to 75 percent for older men and from 0 to 32 percent for older women. In general, the severity of apnea in older persons is mild compared with that seen in patients with clinical sleep apnea. Periodic limb movements during sleep (PLMS) are also common in the elderly, with prevalence rates ranging from 25 to 60 percent in various studies of the healthy elderly. Persons with PLMS are reported to sleep about an hour less per night than do controls without PLMS. Perhaps as a result, napping also increases with age, although it rarely accounts for a large proportion of total sleep time in healthy persons.

Average daily total sleep time actually increases slightly after the age of about 65, perhaps because time-in-bed increases with retirement. Greater numbers of elderly persons fall into either long-sleeping (nine hours or more) or short-sleeping (five hours or less) subgroups. It is noteworthy that death rates are higher in both long- and excessively short-sleeping persons. The reasons for that are still unknown, although there has been speculation that sleep apnea may contribute to increased mortality in the long-sleeping group.

Although the incidence of insomnia and certain other sleep-wake disorders tends to increase with age, clinicians should not assume that age explains those common complaints. Rather, the clinician must search for underlying conditions that can be treated, such as medical, neurological, psychiatric, situational, pharmacological, and circadian factors.

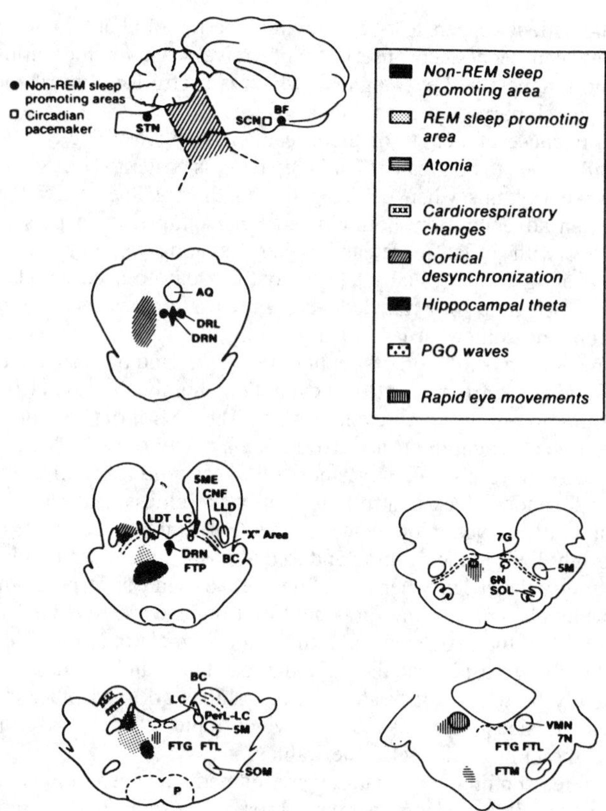

FIGURE 1.9-2 *Localization of NREM- and REM-sleep-promoting areas in the brain.*

NEUROBIOLOGICAL BASIS OF SLEEP

NEUROANATOMY OF SLEEP-WAKEFULNESS The neuroanatomy and neurophysiology of sleep and wakefulness are incompletely understood. Briefly, behavioral and cortical EEG activation depend on the reticular activating system, arising within the brainstem, and more rostral thalamic, hypothalamic, limbic, and cortical systems. The isolated brainstem can generate components of REM sleep, but NREM sleep is controlled by widespread anatomical areas. No specific neuroanatomical sleep center has yet been identified with certainty for the entire constellation of either REM or NREM sleep.

Reticular activating system The components of the ascending reticular activating system (ARAS) are critically important for the generation and maintenance of sleep-waking states (Figure 1.9-2). They reside in the oral pontine and mesencephalic tegmentum, including both noradrenergic cell bodies, such as the locus ceruleus (LC), and cholinergic cell bodies, such as the pedunculopontine tegmental (PPT) and lateral dorsal tegmental (LDT) nuclei. The LC neurons project rostrally through the mesencephalic tegmentum directly and diffusely to cortical areas and subcortical way stations; in addition, noradrenergic neurons project caudally into the brainstem and spinal cord. The PPT and LDT form the largest collection of cholinergic cells in the pontine tegmentum. They innervate the thalamus, hippocampus, hypothalamus, and cingulate cortex. In addition, histaminergic neurons in the posterior hypothalamus project to the cortex and maintain arousal. Glutaminergic neurons in subcortical and cortical structures may also play an important role in wakefulness and arousal.

Anatomical control of NREM sleep At least five anatomical sites have been implicated in the generation of NREM sleep: the basal forebrain area, the thalamus, the hypothalamus, the dorsal raphe nucleus, and the nucleus tractus solitarius (NTS) of the medulla. For example, lesions of the preoptic basal forebrain area produce hyposomnia lasting four to six weeks in rats and cats, whereas electrical stimulation and local warming of that region elicit both EEG and behavioral signs of sleep. In addition, some noncholinergic neurons in the basal forebrain discharge selectively during NREM sleep. The thalamus, in general, and the reticular neurons of the thalamus, in particular, appear to play an important role in the generation of cortical sleep spindles (12 to 14 cps) and delta waves (0.5 to 3 Hz, 75 μV or greater in humans) during NREM sleep. Researchers have suggested that thalamocortical cells are hyperpolarized by corticothalamic cells and are depolarized by cholinergic input from basal forebrain and the LDT-PPT and by possible noradrenergic, serotonergic, and excitatory amino acid input. The thalamocortical cells, which drive and synchronize the ensembles of cortical cells to produce the predominant EEG rhythms, change their rhythms from spindle frequencies to delta frequencies as they hyperpolarize. Although histaminergic cells in the posterior hypothalamus maintain arousal, the anterior hypothalamus may be involved in the induction of slow-wave sleep. The dorsal raphe nucleus, the origin of the serotonergic projections of the brain, also may be involved in the induction of sleep, at least inasmuch as either selective lesions or depletion of serotonin induces a dramatic insomnia lasting several days. Finally, the NTS was implicated by experiments in which medullary anesthesia or cooling of the fourth ventricular floor caused EEG activation. Low-frequency stimulation of that region produced EEG synchronization and behavioral sleep, whereas cells in the region increased their discharge rate during NREM sleep.

Neurological lesions associated with pathological somnolence, stupor, or coma have been noted in the midbrain and diencephalon, the oral pontine and midbrain tegmentum, and the posterior hypothalamus and subthalamus. A recently described syndrome of fatal insomnia was associated with degeneration of the thalamus, although it is doubtful that the insomnia resulted directly from such degeneration.

Anatomical control of REM sleep The major anatomical sites for control of REM sleep are in the brainstem. Transection and lesion studies suggest that the area of the midpons is necessary for REM sleep. Transection at the midpontine level produces a preparation with local signs of REM sleep (rapid eye movements, muscle atonia) caudal to the transection, whereas transections at the pontomedullary junction produce a preparation that does not show REM sleep signs in the medulla, but does show signs in the forebrain. Electrolytic and kainic acid lesions of the oral and caudal pontine tegmentum, including the LDT and PPT, eliminate or markedly reduce the amount of REM sleep.

A soldier ceased to have REM sleep after suffering a shrapnel wound, with a sliver lodging in the pontinemesencephalic region. Despite the documented loss of REM sleep over several years, the man apparently had no specific related problems.

As proposed in the reciprocal interaction model of REM sleep, cholinergic REM-on neurons in the LDT-PPT orchestrate the various events of REM sleep. They are inhibited by REM-off neurons in the LC and dorsal raphe. The REM-off cells decrease their discharge activity preceding a REM sleep episode and are at a very low level of activity, or silent, during REM sleep, thus disinhibiting the spontaneously active cholinergic neurons in the LDT-PPT. Serotonergic terminals, acting on 5-hydroxytryptamine type I (5-HT1_A) receptors on cholinergic cells, apparently hyperpolarize cholinergic burst cells, which may be responsible for pontine-geniculate-occipital (PGO) spikes, large monophasic electrical waves that appear just before and during REM sleep in cats and, presumably, in many species. Those data are consistent with the hypothesis that serotonergic neurons in the dorsal raphe inhibit PGO spikes; for example, they cease firing just before their appearance. Noradrenergic neurons in the LC may also inhibit REM sleep: not only are REM-off cells present, but the administration of α-methyl-para-tyrosine (AMPT), an inhibitor of tyrosine hydroxylase, the rate-limiting enzymatic step in the synthesis of catecholamines, shortens REM latency and increases REM sleep time in humans and animals.

Muscle atonia of REM sleep The muscle atonia of REM sleep is abolished by bilateral lesions of the pontine reticular region, just lateral to the LC (peri-LC α region) and its descending pathway to the bulbar reticular formation. Animals can ambulate during REM sleep and may show oneiric behavior, including locomotion and attack and fly-watching behavior, as if the animal were acting out a dream. Thus the muscle atonia of REM sleep is apparently mediated through nonmonoaminergic neurons of the peri-LC α, which project through tegmentoreticular tract projections to the bulbar magnocellular field and excite neurons in the reticular zone. That area, in turn, through projections in the ventrolateral reticulospinal tract, may induce muscle atonia by hyperpolarizing spinal motoneurons. Those mechanisms for atonia may be clinically relevant to two conditions characterized by abnormalities of muscle atonia: narcolepsy, in which patients experience sudden brief episodes of cataplexy, or loss of muscle tone, while awake; and REM sleep behavior disorder, in which patients maintain muscle tone during REM sleep and may act out their dreams.

BIOCHEMISTRY OF SLEEP-WAKEFULNESS The biochemistry of sleep also remains incompletely understood, although dramatic progress has been made in recent years (Table 1.9-3). Cortical and behavioral arousal mechanisms involve, at the very least, dopaminergic, noradrenergic, histaminergic, glutaminergic, and cholinergic neurons. Data implicating the latter systems have been briefly mentioned already. In addition, antihistamines, β-blockers, and, to some extent, anticholinergic agents are sedative. Neurotransmitter regulation of NREM sleep and REM sleep is complex. Although tryptophan has some value as a natural hypnotic, it should be emphasized that it or some contaminant has been connected with the eosinophilic myalgia syndrome, and it should not be recommended until its safety has been established.

Consistent with the concept that cholinergic neurons mediate cortical arousal and REM sleep, the administration of carbachol, neostigmine, and other cholinergic agonists in the medial pontine reticular formation induces REM sleep in cats. Researchers have discovered a hot spot in the peribrachial region of the cat, where a single injection of a cholinergic agonist will, after the delay of a day, significantly increase REM sleep for over 10 days.

REM sleep can be promoted and REM latency shortened in humans by cholinergic agonists, such as physostigmine (Antilirium, Eserine), arecoline, pilocarpine, and RS 86 (an experimental muscarinic agonist). Physostigmine-induced REM periods appear to be completely normal in their EEG, electro-oculogram (EOG), and electromyogram (EMG) patterns and, moreover, are associated with dreams that appear to be indistinguishable from those collected by arousing subjects from spontaneous REM periods.

Brain metabolism Consistent with the popular hypothesis that sleep is a time of rest and restoration, whole-body and brain metabolic rates decrease during NREM sleep as compared with both wakefulness and REM sleep. In contrast, and perhaps unexpectedly, the metabolic rate is about the same or is slightly increased during REM sleep as compared with wakefulness. Local cerebral metabolism has been studied in humans using the ^{18}F-fluoro-deoxyglucose (FDG) method with positron emission tomography (PET) or cerebral blood flow. No specific sleep center has yet been identified by those techniques. Perhaps in contradiction to the theory that dreaming is a right-hemisphere activity, the left hemisphere was metabolically more active than the right during REM sleep.

In recent years the relations between environmental and core body temperature, metabolism, and sleep have been investigated. Some investigators hypothesize that sleep and wakefulness have homeostatic effects on body and brain temperature. For example, it is known that the onset of NREM sleep tends to depress metabolic rate and to cool the brain and body. That may explain why delta sleep is increased after subjects are warmed in a hot tub or sleep in a moderately warm environment. Increased wakefulness in relatively cold environments may be explained by efforts to warm the body. Many patients with depressive disorders fail to show the drop in core body temperature during sleep and remain relatively hot.

Neuroendocrinology and neuroimmunology Some hormones and immune modulators are affected by the sleep-wake cycle. For example, plasma thyroid-stimulating hormone (TSH) rises during the evening hours and is inhibited by sleep onset. Growth hormone, however, is stimulated by sleep onset, particularly in association with delta sleep, and prolactin levels are increased throughout most of the sleep period. Luteinizing hormone is also increased during sleep, but only during adolescence. Although cortisol secretion increases during nocturnal

TABLE 1.9-3
Neurotransmitters and Neuromodulators That May Regulate Sleep-Wake States

Substance	Possible roles in regulation of sleep-wakefulness
Serotonin	L-tryptophan has hypnotic effects, increases delta sleep. Serotonergic neurons in DRN cease firing in REM sleep and may inhibit cholinergic neurons in LDT-PPT, PGO waves, and REM sleep
Norepinephrine	Noradrenergic neurons in LC cease firing in REM sleep and may inhibit REM sleep. Arousal
Acetylcholine	Cholinergic neurons in dorsal tegmentum orchestrate REM sleep, and together with basal forebrain inhibit cortical EEG synchronization through influence on thalamus
Dopamine	Mediates alerting effects of amphetamine and cocaine and sedating effects of antipsychotics. Sleepiness of narcolepsy may be related to decreased dopamine turnover
γ-aminobutyric acid (GABA)	Hypnotic and other effects of benzodiazepines may be mediated through enhancement of GABA
Adenosine	Appears to promote sleep. Alerting effects of caffeine may be mediated by blockade of adenosine receptors
Interleukins and other immune modulators	Interleukins promote slow-wave sleep in animals, and immune modulators may be increased in plasma at sleep onset in normal controls. NREM sleep measures may correlate with natural killer cell activity in humans
Prostaglandins	PDG_2 and PGE_2 increase sleep and wakefulness, respectively, in animals
Endogenous sleep factors	Putative hypnotoxins include delta-sleep-inducing substances—peptide (DSIP), uridine, argine vasotocin, muramyl peptides, and others

sleep, the increase is primarily driven by an endogenous circadian rhythm whether or not sleep occurs. Melatonin is released at night in the dark in entrained subjects, but its release also occurs independently of sleep and wakefulness. Some patients with depressive disorder have been reported to show blunted nocturnal TSH, melatonin, and growth hormone and elevated cortisol levels.

In keeping with traditional advice to get a lot of sleep when one is sick, sleep and the immune system apparently have mutually positive effects. Certain immune modulators, such as interleukins and tumor necrosis factor, may promote sleep. Sleep deprivation may depress immune measures in humans and animals. The interrelations between the brain and the immune system are an exciting area of research at this time.

DREAMING AND OTHER PSYCHOLOGICAL EXPERIENCES DURING SLEEP

Dreams are reported about 70 to 80 percent of the time when subjects are awakened from REM sleep. However, dreaming is not confined to REM sleep, but is reported after awakenings from NREM sleep about 10 to 20 percent of the time, especially after a few minutes of stage 1 sleep at sleep onset. Some kind of mental activity appears to occur throughout most sleep, and it may be the inability to turn off the mind during sleep that leaves many ruminative insomniac patients feeling as if they had never slept at all.

By most definitions, dreams involve a visual experience with a plot that evolves over time. They are experienced, if not always remembered, in full color and appear to take place in real time. Nevertheless, about one third of dreams often involve rapid shifts in time and place from one scene to the next; about 30 percent entail normally impossible acts, such as flying or talking with animals. Despite the often bizarre nature of dreams, most dreamers seem to accept the experiences uncritically as real at the time. Some persons, however, called lucid dreamers, are consciously aware that they are dreaming and can change the script of a dream as it takes place.

Although most persons spontaneously remember only one or two dreams during an average of about 10 hours of REM sleep a week, the variation in dream recall among them is impressive. Many say they rarely, if ever, dream; others say they dream nearly every night. Why such variation exists is not known. Dream recall does not appear to be related to the amount of REM sleep, but it may be correlated with the number or duration of waking episodes during the night. The memory for dreams is evidently increased if subjects are awakened directly from REM sleep and have an opportunity to think consciously about them. Even that explanation, however, is unsatisfying because the memory for dreams is strangely fleeting: nearly everyone has had the experience of awakening from a dream, thinking about it, and then later failing to recall the content even though remembering having had the dream. Although it is plausible to invoke psychological defenses—repression, suppression, and denial—for forgetting dreams, such explanations seem forced for dreams that are inherently interesting, bizarre, or exciting, or psychologically benign.

The classic nightmare occurs during REM sleep, but frightening experiences also may arise out of NREM sleep. The night terror, or incubus, for example, typically occurs during delta sleep in the first or second NREM period. Characterized by a sudden attack of fear, screaming, shortness of breath, and tachycardia, it may last for several minutes and be unresponsive to attempts to console the victim. In contrast to the nightmare, the patient rarely recalls specific content or visual images when awakened from a night terror and often has total amnesia for the entire episode the next day.

Many patients with panic disorder experience classic panic attacks during sleep, typically in NREM sleep during transitions between stages 2 and 3. Although patients with posttraumatic stress disorder often have terrifying nightmares and flashbacks, some of those events apparently occur during NREM sleep and are not typical REM sleep nightmares. That may explain why monoamine oxidase inhibitors, which can totally eliminate REM sleep, have had only modest success in treating such patients.

A more in-depth study of the phenomenology and neuroscience is now possible with the availability of interesting new approaches, based on functional brain imaging, the emerging neurophysiology of sleep, and cognitive neuroscience.

SLEEP DEPRIVATION

Historical evidence suggests that the general population in the United States sleeps less now than it did at the beginning of the century. With the invention of the electric light and central heating, the move from rural to suburban and urban life-styles, and the growth of international commerce and communication, periods of work and play have expanded to fill the last temporal frontier, nighttime. There is no doubt that many individuals are pathologically sleepy, either acutely or chronically, as a result of partial sleep deprivation or because of clinical disorders.

Excessive sleepiness is an important public health issue because it is responsible for many automobile and occupational accidents, and impaired performance, for example, by sleep-deprived physicians. Although the subjective report of insomnia should not be equated with objective sleep loss, prospective epidemiological studies have shown that persistent complaints of insomnia predict the later onset of depressive disorders.

Partial and selective deprivation of sleep and its different stages have been used to investigate the functions of sleep, but without completely satisfactory results. For example, volunteers have been kept awake for as long as 12 days. Total or partial sleep deprivation made them very sleepy, but it did not provoke either insanity or physical illnesses. The major effects were found to be psychobiological, primarily reductions in alertness, attention, information processing, motivation, and performance, especially for sustained, boring tasks or for highly complex tasks. In fact, many antidepressants and benzodiazepines selectively reduce REM sleep and delta sleep, respectively, but without harmful effects that are directly attributable to the REM or delta sleep deprivation.

Interruption of sleep continuity may be more disturbing for humans than loss of total sleep time. Frequent short breaks in sleep, even as brief as 15 seconds every 10 minutes, produce significant daytime sleepiness and dysphoria even when total sleep time is preserved. Such sleep interference is experienced by patients with bad coughs, painful arthritis, sleep apnea, or nocturnal myoclonus. As many patients do not remember those frequent, short interruptions, it is useful for the clinician to talk with a bed partner who can comment on sleep continuity.

In keeping with the homeostatic function of sleep, a rebound in total sleep time or in specific sleep stages usually follows deprivation of sleep or of a specific stage of sleep. After total and partial sleep deprivation, recovery sleep is characterized by short sleep latency and increases in sleep efficiency, delta sleep, and total sleep time.

After REM sleep deprivation, REM latency is shorter and REM sleep is increased for a few nights. Daytime sleepiness increases after sleep deprivation. In general, however, recovery from sleep deprivation does not require minute-by-minute compensation for lost sleep.

Overnight sleep deprivation depresses cerebral glucose metabolic rates within specific subcortical areas in the human brain, particularly the thalamus and midbrain white-matter areas, during wakefulness. That suggests that sleep deprivation depresses general arousal systems. However, selected areas of the brain may be spared when they are engaged in specific tasks at the time of the study, for example, visual areas when the subject has to perform a continuous visual performance task. In other words, during sleep deprivation the brain apparently reduces the number of parallel processing operations it can carry on simultaneously. That model is consistent with the general observation that sleep-deprived subjects can usually perform relatively well on focused tasks for short periods if they are sufficiently motivated. Less important activities or competing duties, however, may be neglected.

In contrast to the effects of relatively short-term sleep deprivation in humans, prolonged sleep deprivation in rats results in death. About three weeks of total sleep deprivation or about five weeks of selective REM deprivation is fatal. In those studies, experimental animals were awakened whenever they entered sleep or REM sleep, respectively, by turning a disk on which they lived. Control animals living on the other half of the same disk did not die. The cause of death was apparently related to a significant increase in overall metabolism in response to falling body temperature and increased food intake, but the exact mechanisms remain unknown.

Whether those results are applicable to humans is unknown. One researcher studied an extreme short sleeper, a 72-year-old woman who claimed to have slept only an hour a day since her late teens. Another investigator reported the case of a man who apparently stopped sleeping altogether for months, and who responded to treatment with serotonin precursors.

The question about the functions of sleep is still open. Various theories have stressed the themes of rest, recovery, or restoration; energy conservation and metabolic modulation; ecological and ethological processes that favor the survival of the species; instinctive behaviors; and enhancement of cognition and memory. However, there is little scientific support for those theories.

IMPLICATIONS FOR PSYCHIATRIC DISORDERS

Psychiatrists have long had a strong interest in sleep and dreaming. A constant question has been: Does sleep disturbance cause mental disorders or vice versa? In the last century, the English neurologist Hughlings Jackson said, "Find out about dreams and you will find out about psychosis." Somewhat later, Freud made dream interpretation one of the key elements of psychoanalytic theory and practice. Following the discovery of REM sleep in the early 1950s, psychiatrists and sleep researchers began to study the sleep patterns of schizophrenic and depressed patients, to test the hypothesis that hallucinations might represent waking dreams or some derangement of REM sleep, and to determine whether deprivation of REM sleep or sleep in general would be psychologically deleterious or beneficial.

The new neurobiology of sleep has important implications for our understanding of depressive disorders, some alcohol-related disorders, schizophrenia, eating disorders, borderline personality disorders, and other clinical conditions associated with short REM latency, increased REM sleep and increased REM density, and loss of stages 3 and 4 sleep.

The emerging concepts of sleep neurophysiology are consistent with the cholinergic-aminergic imbalance hypothesis of mood disorders, which proposes that depression is associated with an increased ratio of central cholinergic to aminergic neurotransmission. The characteristic sleep abnormalities of depressive disorders may reflect a relative predominance of cholinergic activity, originating within the LDT-PPT, in relation to noradrenergic and serotonergic activity, originating within the LC and DRN, respectively. Cholinergic projections from the dorsal tegmentum or basal forebrain to the thalamus may also suppress delta sleep. Consistent with the role of cholinergic mechanisms, depressed patients are significantly more sensitive, compared with normal controls, to the REM-sleep-inducing effects of muscarinic agonists, such as arecoline or RS 86. Antidepressant medications presumably reduce REM sleep either by their anticholinergic properties or by enhancing aminergic neurotransmission. Some drugs, such as the monoamine oxidase inhibitors, will entirely eliminate REM sleep when prescribed for two weeks or more at therapeutic doses. Intense and prolonged dreams often accompany abrupt withdrawal from antidepressant drugs, a reflection of a REM rebound following drug-induced REM deprivation.

Short REM latency has been found in some patients with schizophrenia, obsessive-compulsive disorder, eating disorders, narcolepsy, and borderline personality disorder. Both short REM latency and decreased delta sleep appear to be state and trait characteristics of depression. Short REM latency may also be a genetic marker for depressive disorders within families, and an indicator of a poor prognosis in recovered depressed and alcoholic patients.

Total sleep deprivation, partial sleep deprivation (especially in the last half of the night), and selective REM sleep deprivation have antidepressant effects on depressed patients. Unfortunately, the beneficial effects of sleep deprivation last only until the next sleep period, after which the patient typically awakens depressed again. Hence, sleep may be depressionogenic in some patients.

Many observations suggest that some depressed patients are overaroused, at least in some areas of the brain: the antidepressant effects of sleep deprivation, the loss of delta sleep and sleep continuity, elevated adrenocorticotropic hormone (ACTH) and cortisol, blunted nocturnal growth hormone, and increased core body temperature during sleep. Moreover, a preliminary PET study showed that cerebral glucose metabolism during the first NREM period was significantly elevated in depressed patients as compared with normal controls, and that depressed patients had some of the abnormalities during sleep that had previously been reported in other patients while awake, such as hypofrontality.

Consistent with the overarousal hypothesis, depressed patients who responded to sleep deprivation showed significantly elevated metabolic rates within the cingulate gyrus and amygdala before sleep deprivation as compared with both nonresponders and normal controls. After clinical improvement, metabolic activity normalized in responders and did not change in the two other groups.

If the clinical applications of sleep deprivation therapy in depressive disorders remain limited, the experimental and theoretical implications are intriguing. No other means is available to turn depression off and on so quickly and predictably as sleep deprivation and recovery sleep.

The clinical wisdom of the centuries, linking sleep to psychiatric disorders, has been reinforced by the revelations of modern neurobiology.

SUGGESTED CROSS-REFERENCES

Section 1.13 is devoted to the related issue of chronobiology. Chapter 23 discusses sleep disorders. Section 32.30 includes a discussion of sleep deprivation and sleep delay therapies. Section 49.6f focuses on sleep disorders in the elderly.

REFERENCES

*Benca R M, Obermeyer W H, Thisted R A, Gillin J C: Sleep and psychiatric disorders: A meta-analysis. Arch Gen Psychiatry *49:* 651, 1992.

Borbely A A, Tobler I: Endogenous sleep-promoting substances and sleep regulation. Physiol Rev *69:* 605, 1989.

Buchsbaum M S, Gillin J C, Wu J, Haslett E, Sicotte N, Dupont R, Bunney W E Jr: Regional cerebral glucose metabolic rate in human sleep assessed by positron emission tomography. Life Sci *45:* 1349, 1989.

Carskadon M A, Dement W C, Mitler M M: Guidelines for the multiple sleep latency test (MSLT): A standard measure of sleepiness. Sleep *9:* 519, 1986.

Daan S, Beersma D G M, Borbely A A: Timing of human sleep: Recovery process gated by a circadian pacemaker. Am J Physiol *246:* R161, 1984.

Datta S, Calvo J M, Quattrochi J J, Hobson J A: Long-term enhancement of REM sleep following cholinergic stimulation. NeuroReport *2:* 619, 1991.

Edgar D M, Dement W C, Fuller C A: Effect of SCN lesions on sleep in squirrel monkeys: Evidence for opponent processes in sleep-wake regulation. J Neurosci *13:* 1065, 1993.

Fischer-Perroudon C, Mouret J, Jouvet M: Sur un cas d'agrypnie (4 mois sans sommeil) au cours d'une maladie de Morvan. Effet favorable du 5-hydroxytryptophane. Electroencephalogr Clin Neurophysiol *36:* 1, 1974.

*Ford D E, Kamerow D B: Epidemiologic study of sleep disturbances and psychiatric disorders: An opportunity for prevention? JAMA *262:* 1479, 1989.

Franzini C: Brain metabolism and blood flow during sleep. J Sleep Res *1:* 3, 1992.

Gillin J C, Dow B M, Thompson P, Parry B, Tandon R, Benca R: Sleep in depression and other psychiatric disorders. Clin Neurosci *1*: 90, 1993.

*Gillin J C, Smith T L, Irwin M, Schuckit M: Increased pressure for REM sleep at admission to an alcohol treatment program predicts relapse at 3 months post-discharge in primary, nondepressed alcoholic patients. Arch Gen Psychiatry *51:* 189, 1994.

Gillin J C, Sutton L, Ruiz C, Kelsoe, J, Dupont R, Darko D, Risch S C: The cholinergic REM induction test with arecoline in depression. Arch Gen Psychiatry *48:* 264, 1991.

Gottschalk L A, Buchsbaum M S, Gillin J C, Wu J C, Reynolds C A, Herrera D B: Positron emission tomographic studies of the relationship of cerebral glucose metabolism and the magnitude of anxiety and hostility experienced during dreaming and waking. J Neuropsychiatry Clin Neurosci *3*: 131, 1991.

Hobson J A: Sleep and dreaming. J Neurosci *10:* 371, 1990.

Hoddes E, Zarcone V, Smyth H: Quantification of sleepiness: A new approach. Psychophysiology *10:* 431, 1973.

Holsboer F J, Spengler D, Heuser I: The role of corticotropin-releasing hormone in the pathogenesis of Cushing's disease, anorexia nervosa, alcoholism, affective disorders, and dementia. Prog Brain Res *93:* 385, 1992.

Horne J A, Ostberg O: Individual differences in human circadian rhythms. Biol Sand *71:* 506, 1985.

Irwin M, Smith T L, Gillin J C: Electroencephalographic sleep and natural killer activity in depressed patients and control subjects. Psychosom Med *54:* 10, 1992.

Janowsky D S, El-Yousef M K, Davis J M: A cholinergic-adrenergic hypothesis of mania and depression. Lancet *2*: 632, 1972.

Jones B E: Paradoxical sleep and its chemical/structural substrates in the brain. Neuroscience *40:* 637, 1991.

Kerkhofs M, Van Cauter E, Van Onderbergen A, Caufriez A, Thorner M O, Copinschi G: Sleep-promoting effects of growth-hormone-releasing hormone in normal men. Am J Physiol *264* (Endocrinol Metab *27:*) E594, 1993.

Keshavan M S, Tandon R: Sleep abnormalities in schizophrenia: Pathophysiological significance. Psychol Med *23:* 831, 1993.

Krueger J M, Obal F Jr: Growth-hormone-releasing hormone and interleukin-1 in sleep regulation. FASEB J *7*: 645, 1993.

Lavie P, Pratt H, Scharf B, Peled R, Brown J: Localized pontine lesion: Nearly total absence of REM sleep. Neurology *34:* 118, 1984.

Linkowski P, Van Onderbergen A, Kerhalofs M, Bosson D, Medlewicz J, Van Cauter E: Twin study of the 24-hour cortisol profile: Evidence for genetic control of the human circadian rhythm. Am J Physiol *264:* E173, 1993.

Livingston G, Blizard B, Mann A: Does sleep disturbance predict depression in elderly people? A study in inner London. Br J Gen Pract *43:* 445, 1993.

Luebke J I, Greene R W, Semba K, Kamondi A, McCarley R W, Reiner P B: Serotonin hyperpolarizes cholinergic low-threshold burst neurons in the rat laterodorsal tegmental nucleus *in vitro*. Proc Natl Acad Sci USA *89:* 743, 1992.

Meddis R, Pearson A J D, Lanford G: An extreme case of healthy insomnia. Electroencephalogr Clin Neurophysiol *35:* 213, 1973.

Mitler M M, Gujavarty K S, Browman C P: Maintenance of wakefulness test: A polysomnographic technique for evaluating treatment in patients with excessive somnolence. Electroencephalogr Clin Neurophysiol *53:* 658, 1982.

Nofzinger E A, Buysse D J, Reynolds C F III, Kupfer D J: Sleep disorders related to another mental disorder (nonsubstance/primary): A DSM-IV literature review. J Clin Psychiatry *54:* 244, 1993.

Oleksenko A I, Mukhametov L M, Polyakova I G, Supin A Y, Kovalzon V M: Unihemispheric sleep deprivation in bottlenose dolphins. J Sleep Res *1*: 40, 1992.

Shiromani P, Rapaport M H, Gillin J C: The neurobiology of sleep: Basic concepts and clinical implications. In *Psychiatry Update: The American Psychiatric Association Annual Review,* vol 6, R E Hales, A J Frances, editors, p 235. American Psychiatric Press, Washington, 1987.

Steriade M, McCarley R W: *Brainstem Control of Wakefulness and Sleep.* Plenum, New York, 1990.

Steriade M, McCormick D A, Sejnowski T J: Thalamocortical oscillations in the sleep and aroused brain. Science *262:* 679, 1993.

*Thorpy M J: *ICSD-International Classification of Sleep Disorders: Diagnostic and Coding Manual.* American Sleep Disorders Association, 1990.

Tobler I: Evolution and comparative physiology of sleep in animals. In *Clinical Physiology of Sleep,* R Lydic, J F Biebuyck, editors, p 21. American Physiological Society, Bethesda, 1988.

Wirz-Justice A: Biological rhythms in affective disorders. In *Fourth Generation of Progress,* F E Bloom, D J Kupfer, editors, p 22. Raven, New York, 1994.

Wu J C, Gillin J C, Buchsbaum M S, Hazlett E, Sicotte N, Bunney W E Jr: The effect of sleep deprivation on cerebral glucose metabolic rate in normal humans assessed with positron emission tomography. Sleep *14:* 155, 1991.

*Wu J C, Gillin J C, Buchsbaum M S, Hershey T, Johnson J C, Bunney W E Jr.: Effect of sleep deprivation on brain metabolism of depressed patients. Am J Psychiatry *149:* 538, 1992.

1.10 PRINCIPLES OF NEUROIMAGING

ROBERT B. INNIS, M.D., Ph.D.
ROBERT T. MALISON, M.D.

INTRODUCTION

Brain-imaging methods can, in general, be divided into those that provide information primarily on structure and those that provide information primarily on function. Thus, for psychiatric disorders that have a significant biological component, brain imaging may provide important clues to any associated structural or functional anomalies. Furthermore, by providing direct measurements of the brain, imaging offers advantages over indirect or peripheral measurements of central nervous system (CNS) function, such as plasma levels of neurohormones and neurotransmitter metabolites. Although no brain-imaging modality has a clearly defined clinical application in psychiatry at present, most are being actively studied as research procedures at many medical centers.

STRUCTURAL IMAGING

Although future advances may ultimately blur this distinction, computed tomography (CT) and magnetic resonance imaging (MRI) are fundamentally techniques of structural imaging that pictorially represent the spatial distribution of the intrinsic physical properties of brain tissue. In contrast to their now antiquated predecessors (conventional radiography, pneumoencephalography, and angiography), in which information about brain anatomy is largely inferred, CT and MRI probe the physical properties of neural tissues directly and noninvasively (Table 1.10-1).

COMPUTED TOMOGRAPHY In computed tomography (from the Greek *tomos* for cut) a highly focused source of external radiation is transmitted along multiple lines of trajectory through varying angles within a single plane of a subject's head. As X-rays pass through tissue they are attenuated as a result of interactions with tissue molecules and emerge with energy levels at a fraction of the original intensity. The nature of those tissue interactions involves both partial (Compton scattering) and complete (photoelectric) absorption of an X-ray's energy by electrons within individual atoms. As electrons absorb energy they are ejected from the atom; thus, X-rays are a form of ionizing radiation. The degree of energy absorbed by different tissues is proportional to their individual electron and physical densities. Attenuation values can be measured for various tissue types, including bone, brain tissue, and cerebrospinal fluid (CSF) (Table 1.10-2).

In contrast to conventional radiography, in which emerging X-rays are detected on film, CT scanners make use of highly sensitive scintillation crystal detectors. Detectors are positioned directly opposite the X-ray emitting source, and both rotate in synchrony through multiple views. That sensitivity allows the attenuation along many thousands of trajectories to be measured while maintaining safe levels of potentially harmful ionizing radiation. A series of images for a conventional head CT study requires roughly the same amount of radiation exposure to the patient as a routine chest radiograph. Because of the efficient design of modern CT scanners, a single-image slice (cross-sectional view) is acquired in a matter of seconds.

Once collected, attenuation information from individual trajectories is summed or back-projected for every imaging angle, thus creating a two-dimensional matrix of attenuation values (also referred to as CT numbers) for a given slice. The entire process is accomplished by use of an efficient computer algorithm (fast Fourier transformation), and is conceptually analogous to the simple childhood puzzle in which numbers in a square grid are inferred from their sums along each row. Individual matrix values are assigned corresponding shades of gray, white, and black, which are displayed as picture elements (pixels) on a video terminal; thus, an image of the brain's attenuation map is produced (Figure 1.10-1). That general method of image reconstruction is shared by many structural and functional imaging modalities. The final images produced are capable of an in-plane resolution of 0.8 mm, with slice thicknesses of approximately 5 mm.

As can be appreciated from the cross-sectional image depicted in Figure 1.10-1 CT scans enable one to distinguish among tissues when attenuation values differ. Therefore, bone is well delimited from fluid, which is well delimited from brain. That differentiation accounts for the widespread application of CT to measurements of ventricular and sulcal size in a host of neurological and psychiatric conditions. However, when CT values are similar, differences in contrast between different brain tissues (for example, gray and white matter) are difficult to discern (Table 1.10-1).

The current advantages of CT scanning are its widespread clinical availability and relative affordability compared with other imaging modalities, such as MRI. Its efficiency makes image acquisition fast, convenient, and relatively safe for patients. On the basis of its unparalleled capacity for imaging bony abnormalities and calcified tumors, CT remains the method of choice in many medical specialties today. For psychiatry, however, the intrinsic limitations imposed by relatively subtle differences in the attenuation values of different neural tissues are likely to restrict its future applications.

MAGNETIC RESONANCE IMAGING For imaging brain parenchyma, MRI has all but superseded CT as the modality of choice. The basis for the choice of MRI lies largely in its inherent versatility and the superior levels of contrast attained. In

TABLE 1.10-1
Comparison of Structural Imaging Modalities

Factor	Computed Tomography	Magnetic Resonance Imaging
Physical principle	X-ray attenuation	Hydrogen (proton) magnetic resonance
Tissue properties measured	Tissue (electron) density	T_1 and T_2 relaxation times; proton density
Imaging planes	Axial	Axial, coronal, and sagittal
Resolution (in plane)	< 1 mm	< 1 mm
Slice thickness	2–5 mm	1–3 mm
Tissue visualization		
Bone	Excellent	Invisible
Cerebrospinal fluid	Good	Excellent
Gray-white contrast	Poor	Outstanding
Cost	$400–$700	$800–$1,000

TABLE 1.10-2
Tissue Attenuation (CT) Values

Tissue	CT Value*
Air	−500
Water	0
Cerebrospinal fluid	+8
White matter	+15
Gray matter	+18
Bone	+200–500

*Relative attenuation values based on arbitrary units originally established by Godfrey Hounsfield.

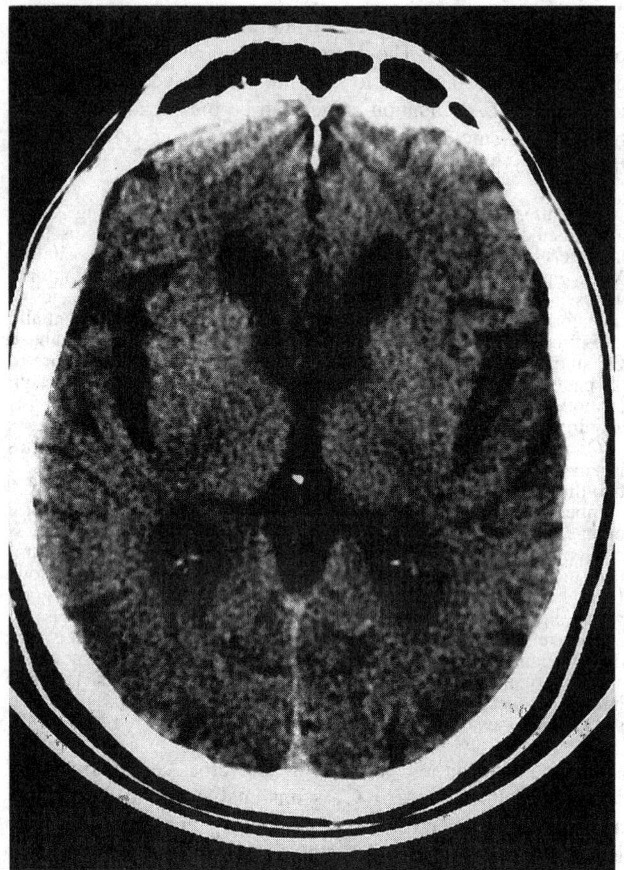

FIGURE 1.10-1 *Transaxial CT image of the brain at the level of the thalamus.*

fact, the level of image contrast and resolution is reminiscent of that seen in anatomical specimens (Figure 1.10-2).

Principles MRI relies on the basic observation that certain atomic nuclei behave like magnets. The simplest nucleus, that of hydrogen, contains a single proton. Because of the abundance of hydrogen nuclei in the body, their collective magnetic behavior provides the primary signal used in the production of MRI images. Much like a tiny bar magnet, a hydrogen nucleus possesses magnetic poles that derive from two intrinsic properties present in all such nuclei: (1) an unpaired proton or neutron and (2) nuclear spin. Just as a circular current of electricity produces a magnetic field perpendicular to its path, a spinning nuclear charge generates a magnetic field along its axis of spin.

The orientation of magnetic charges of individual hydrogen nuclei (hereafter also referred to as protons) is random in the body. If a strong external magnetic field is applied, however, nuclei align themselves parallel to the applied field, just as a compass needle aligns itself in the direction of the earth's magnetic field. By convention, that applied field is referred to as B_o. Once aligned, spinning nuclei take on a second motion, and they precess about B_o (Figure 1.10-3). The gyrating motion, like a wobbling top, enables the magnetic behavior to be probed. Nuclear precession has a measurable frequency, also known as the Larmor frequency (ω), which varies as a function of two factors: (1) atomic number and (2) the strength of B_o. Therefore, all hydrogen nuclei precess at the same ω when subjected to the same B_o. Similarly, magnetic species of differing atomic weights (for example, Li^7, C^{13}, F^{19}, P^{31}) present in the same B_o precess at characteristically different values of ω.

Even when protons are aligned with B_o and precess at the same rate no useful measurements are possible because the collective strength of the magnetic fields is immeasurably small relative to the large applied field, B_o, with which they are aligned. Moreover and equally important the precessing of nuclei is asynchronous (out of phase). If, however, nuclei are tipped away from the applied field momentarily, that collective behavior can be measured. Just as a compass needle is tipped away from magnetic north by the tap of a finger, protons can be tipped away from B_o by applying a pulse of energy of the same or resonant frequency as ω. On an atomic scale, such resonant frequencies lie in the radio-frequency spectrum. Because of the long wavelength, radio-frequency electromagnetism is nonionizing and poses no hazard to biological tissues.

After a radio-frequency pulse is applied, two important phenomena occur. First, as stated, protons are tipped away from the longitudinal axis of B_o. The amount of energy transmitted can be changed by varying the pulse duration, which determines the degree to which the protons are tipped. For example, a 90° pulse refers to the energy required to tip protons into the corresponding horizontal plane (Figure 1.10-4). Second, the radio-frequency pulse causes nuclei to precess in unison, and that synchronous behavior is known as phase coherence. At that point, with nuclei tipped out of the B_o axis and precessing in-phase, their collective magnetic behavior can be measured. The phenomena constitute the two most important tissue characteristics measured in MRI: T_1 and T_2 relaxation.

T_1 RELAXATION Measurement of magnetic resonance is possible because the altered situation of the tipped protons fails to prevail. Like the compass needle, which is deflected from north only transiently, individual nuclei flip back to their original state. In doing so, protons relinquish energy at the same radio-frequency used initially to tip them. Those radio-frequency waves are detectable by an external receiver. Thus, the gradual release of radio-frequency energy parallels the process by which protons reorient themselves with B_o. That process is referred to as longitudinal relaxation and is described by an exponential curve that increases with time as net magnetization in the longitudinal (B_o) axis returns to its original strength (Figure 1.10-4). The rate of longitudinal (also referred to as spin-lattice) relaxation is defined by the constant T_1, the time required for 63 percent of protons to return to the initial equilibrium state. T_1 is influenced by the chemical microenvironment of protons, the vast majority of which is in water. Therefore, insofar as the chemical environment of water varies in different brain tissues, T_1 varies with tissue type. The total amount of energy absorbed and subsequently emitted is a reflection of the total number of protons in the tissue. Hence, T_1 also contains information about a third measurable tissue parameter: proton density.

T_2 RELAXATION An understanding of transverse relaxation (T_2) relies on the concept of phase coherence. In the example of T_1, a 90° pulse was used to tip protons into the horizontal (transverse) plane. Immediately after excitation, nuclei precess in unison. Were conditions ideal and the magnetic field around all protons identical, precession would remain coherent indefinitely. In reality, nonuniformities exist in the magnetic field surrounding protons, and individual nuclei take on slightly faster or slower precessional frequencies. As each nucleus adopts a new rate, there is dephasing of the collective precessional frequency. That may be depicted graphically as the gradual dispersion of the transverse magnetization vector into multiple smaller vectors fanning out within the horizontal plane (Figure 1.10-5). The transverse component of magnetization is thereby weakened. In contrast to longitudinal relaxation, transverse (spin-spin) relaxation follows an exponential decay curve, and T_2 corresponds to the time required to lose 63 percent of initial signal strength. T_2 values are also specific to tissue type.

Pulse sequencing Because T_1 and T_2 relaxation times and proton densities are properties intrinsic to brain tissue, their measurement forms the basis of differentiating tissues in MRI studies. In contrast to CT, in which images reflect only a single parameter, X-ray attenuation, MRI is complex and versatile. Depending on how information is acquired, MR images give

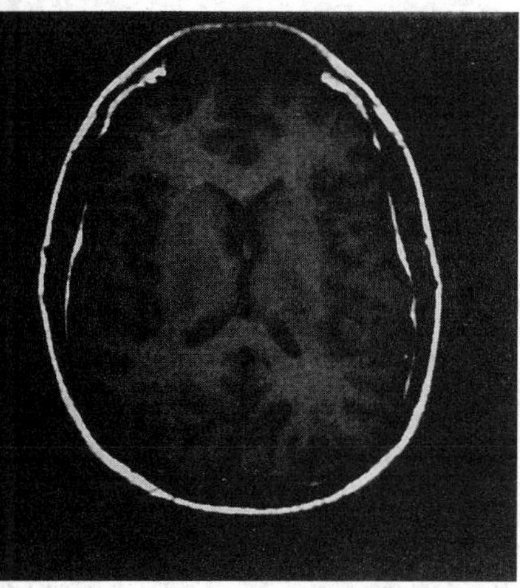
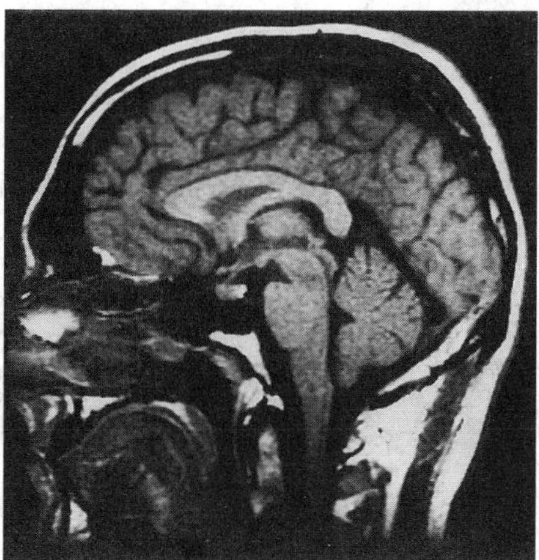
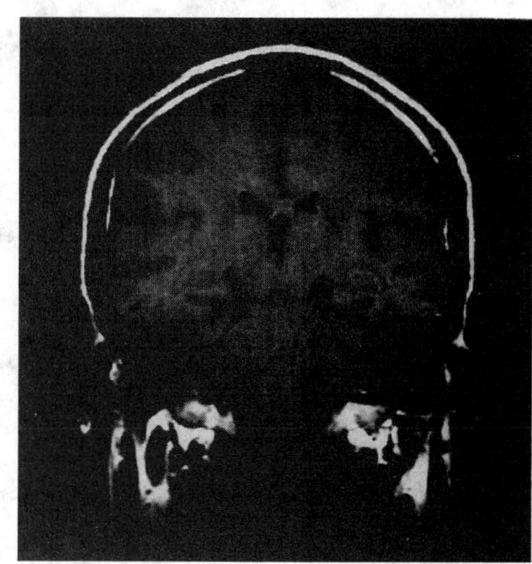

FIGURE 1.10-2 *Axial (left), sagittal (center), and coronal (right) MRI studies of the head acquired without repositioning the patient. In comparison to the CT scan in Figure 1.10-1, note the well-demarcated cortical gray matter on the axial MR image as well as the excellent visualization of brainstem and posterior fossa structures on the sagittal and coronal views. (Figure courtesy of R T Malison.)*

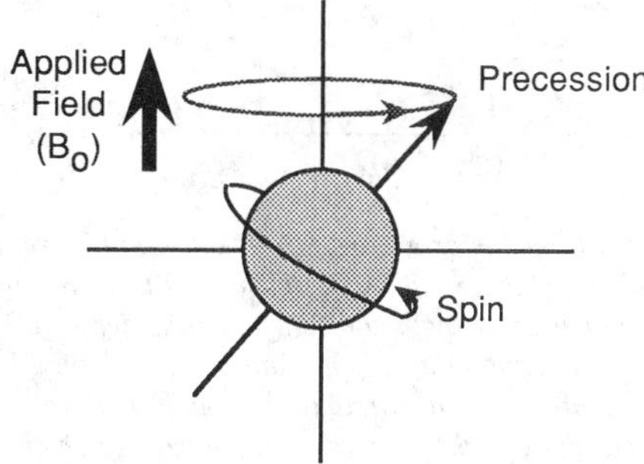

FIGURE 1.10-3 *The innate spin of the unpaired proton in the hydrogen nucleus produces a small magnetic field (depicted by an arrow along the axis pointed in the direction of its own magnetic north) perpendicular to the direction of spin. When placed in an external magnetic field (B_o), the proton field becomes aligned with the applied field and wobbles about B_o's axis in a motion known as precession. (Note that both motions describe a cone.) Precession occurs at a defined rate, known as the Larmor frequency, that varies with both the atomic weight of the nuclear species and the strength of the external field.*

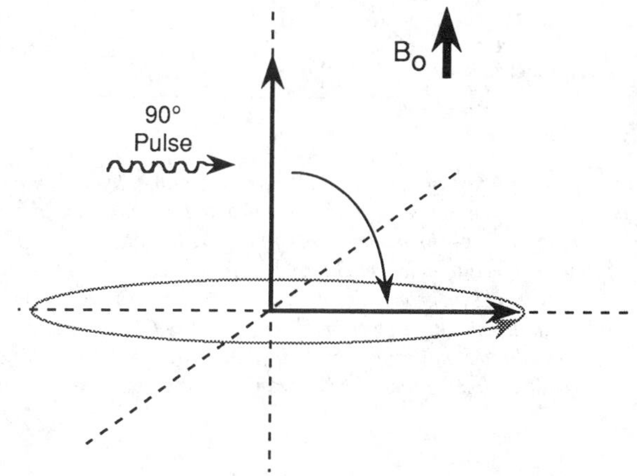

FIGURE 1.10-4 *In an applied magnetic field (B_o), hydrogen nuclei align in the same direction. Their collective strength may be depicted as a vector indicating the direction of net magnetic charge. When a resonant radio-frequency pulse of the same Larmor frequency as hydrogen is applied, that pulse tips the nuclei away from B_o. Here a 90° pulse displaces the net magnetization vector perpendicular to the axis of B_o. A circular path traced by the vector tip indicates the collective precession of hydrogen nuclei within the transverse plane.*

weight to one parameter over the others. Accordingly, MR images are referred to as T_1-, T_2-, or proton density-weighted, depending on which parameter most significantly contributes to image formation (Figure 1.10-6).

Information acquisition in MRI may be viewed as an interrogation of brain tissues. A question is asked in the form of a radio-frequency pulse, and the tissue replies in a similar radio-frequency language. How can the MRI device "hear" the specific language of an individual parameter when T_1 and T_2 relaxations are "speaking" simultaneously? As an analogy, imagine the following. Three children are bouncing on a trampoline. The judicious timing of the jump by the third child has the potential power of virtually doubling the height of one child's bounce while simultaneously nullifying the efforts of the other child. Similarly, image weighting in MRI is achieved by timing radio-frequency pulses in such a way as to enable one signal to stand out.

Pulse sequences are operator-controlled and fixed before image acquisition and depend on the desired weighting. The study of pulse sequencing is one of the most complex and rapidly progressing investigations in the field of MRI. For the interested reader, the following discussion of two basic imaging sequences (inversion recovery and spin-echo) provides an introductory explanation of how image weighting is possible.

INVERSION RECOVERY Inversion-recovery sequences elicit information primarily from the T_1 component of the magnetic resonance signal and are, therefore, said to be T_1-weighted. Such sequences consist of an initial 180° pulse followed by a 90° pulse. The initial excitation pulse inverts protons 180° in the applied field. Without a transverse component to their net magnetization, however, nuclei are immeasurable, and protons return silently to their original orientation. True to their characteristic relaxation times, different tissues recover from the initial inversion at different rates. Thus, by the time of the 90° measurement pulse, protons in different tissues are in relatively different states of recovery. Specifically, a tissue with short T_1 recovers rapidly and more fully than one with longer T_1. The time between excitation and measurement pulses is known as the inversion time (TI). That process is outlined in Figure 1.10-7. When nuclei recover completely, the sequence is repeated. The time between sequences is the repetition time (TR). TI and TR are operator-controlled, and each determines the final characteristics of image contrast. If TI is too short,

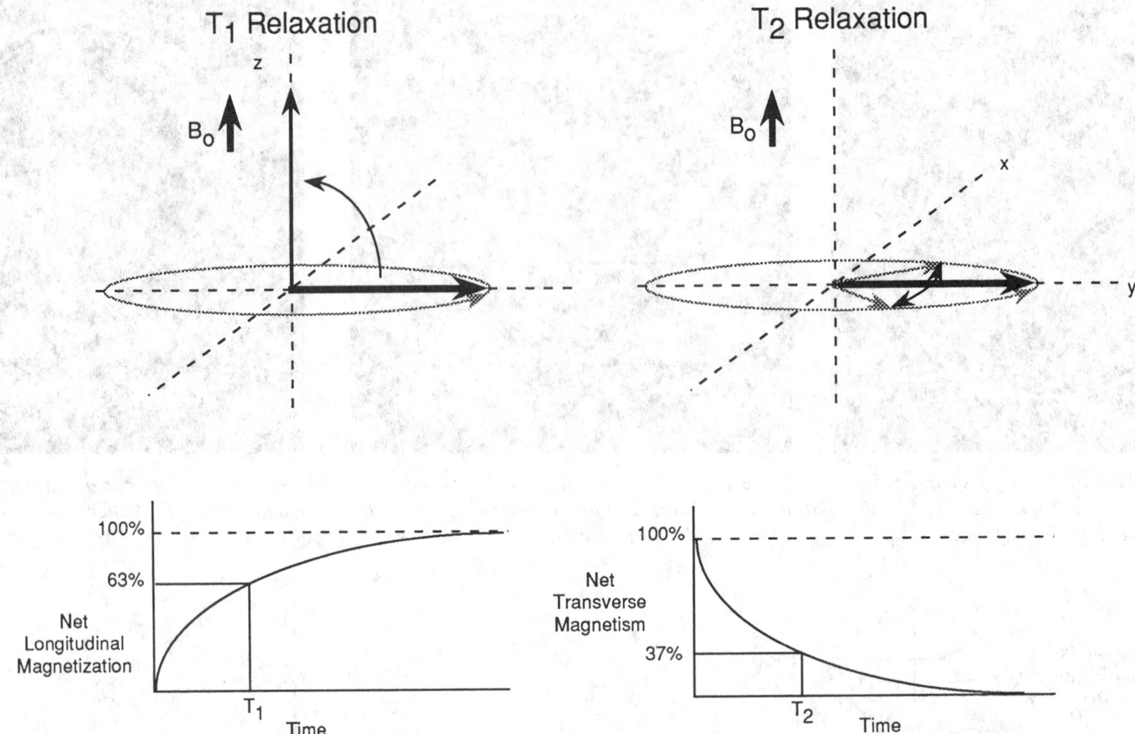

FIGURE 1.10-5 *Once tipped into the transverse plane, hydrogen nuclei undergo two simultaneous processes of relaxation. In T_1 relaxation the net magnetization in the transverse plane gradually diminishes as individual nuclei flip back to the vertical alignment with B_o. The rate of return of the longitudinal (z-axis) component of the magnetization vector is measured by the exponential growth constant T_1 and is depicted graphically as the time required to achieve 63 percent of the original equilibrium state. In T_2 relaxation, transverse magnetization is diminished by a second process, in which synchronously precessing nuclei lose coherence. Under the influence of local variations in magnetic field strength, nuclei gradually acquire slightly slower or faster precessional frequencies. That is shown schematically as the dispersion of the transverse magnetization vector into multiple smaller vectors that fan out within the x-y plane. In contrast to T_1, T_2 is an exponential decay constant and corresponds to the time required for the loss of 63 percent of transverse magnetization (to 37 percent of its original strength).*

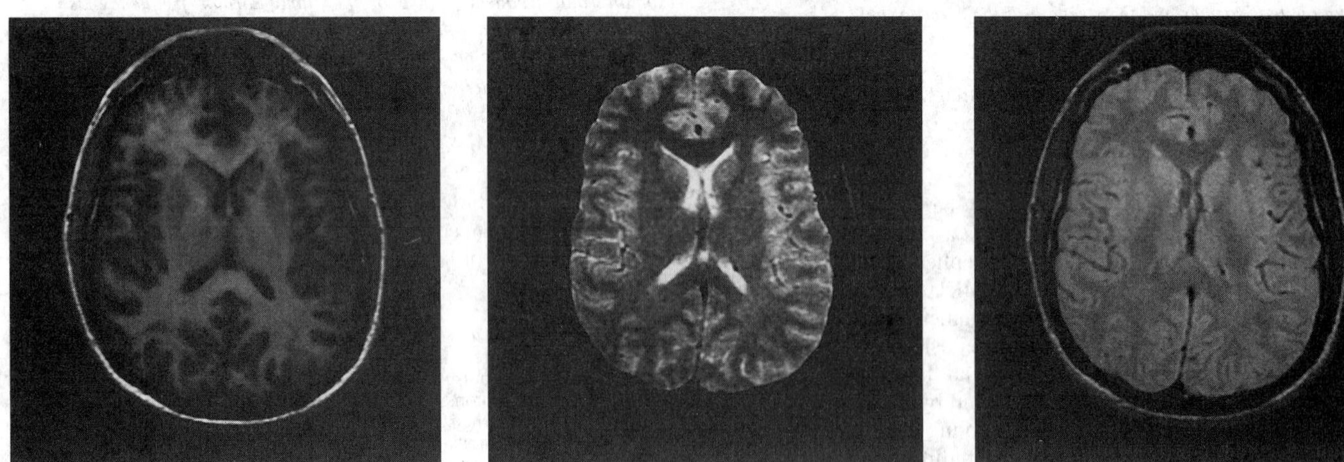

FIGURE 1.10-6 *T_1-weighted (left), T_2-weighted (center), and proton density-weighted (right) MRI studies obtained from the same axial plane. (Figure courtesy of R T Malison.) The T_1-weighted image was acquired using an inversion-recovery pulse sequence and demonstrates a characteristically high degree of contrast between gray and white matter. The increased signal intensity of cerebrospinal fluid produced by spin-echo pulse sequences is typical of T_2-weighted images. Thus, T_2-weighted images are often used clinically to detect subtle changes in brain fluid caused by many disease states. Proton density weighting produces lesser contrast between gray matter, white matter, and cerebrospinal fluid and is of limited utility. The images illustrate the absence of a universal color scale in MR imaging. (That is, the same brain structure can appear darker or lighter relative to other structures depending on the imaging sequence employed.)*

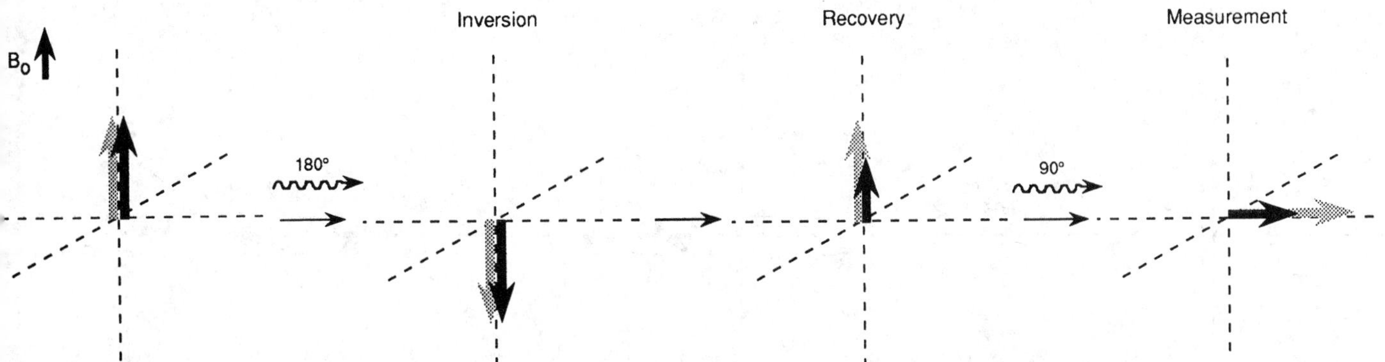

FIGURE 1.10-7 *Tissues with short T_1 relaxation times (light vector—white matter) may be distinguished from those with longer T_1 (dark vector—gray matter) by means of an inversion-recovery pulse sequence. An initial 180° radio-frequency pulse completely inverts nuclei in both tissues. Tissues with short relaxation times experience a quick return to their full longitudinal strength, whereas net magnetization in tissues with longer T_1 relaxation times lags behind. When a 90° pulse is applied before the second tissue recovers completely, a difference in transverse signal intensity is observed. Inversion-recovery sequences produce high levels of gray-white matter contrast, as illustrated in Figure 1.10-6.*

differences in recovery are slight, and image contrast is reduced. Conversely, if TI is too long, protons recover completely in all tissues, and contrast reflects only differences in proton density, which are relatively small compared with T_1. Therefore, one chooses TI and TR to maximize the differences in recovery between tissues of interest. Bright structures in T_1-weighted images correspond to areas of high signal intensities (short T_1—white matter), and dark structures possess weak signals (long T_1—CSF) (Figure 1.10-6). Inversion-recovery sequences excel in their ability to demarcate white and gray matter structures and are most widely use in anatomical studies of brain structure. Although their clinical indications are limited, T_1-weighted sequences are extensively used by researchers for morphological analyses of the brain in neuropsychiatric disorders.

SPIN-ECHO Spin-echo pulse sequences focus on the transverse component of proton relaxation and are referred to as T_2-weighted. T_2 relaxation refers to the gradual dephasing of the precessional frequencies of nuclei after an initial synchronizing radio-frequency pulse. That synchronous state is ultimately undermined by magnetic field inhomogeneities of two types: (1) those arising from molecules surrounding protons and (2) those arising from imperfections in the applied field. The former are innate properties of tissue type, and the latter are extrinsic and largely irrelevant. Nonetheless, both contribute to dephasing, and spin-echo sequences are made to try to eliminate the confounding influence of applied field inhomogeneities (denoted T_2*) on the measurement of actual or tissue-specific T_2.

Spin-echo pulse sequences rely on the same pulse identified earlier (180° and 90°) with one important difference: The order is reversed. Thus, protons are initially tipped into the transverse plane, where they precess in unison. Dephasing soon follows under the influence of T_2 and T_2*. What happens when the 180° pulse is administered? The analogy most commonly invoked is that of horses running on a racetrack. Initially aligned in the starting gate, horses gradually separate from the pack on the basis of their individual speeds. If midway during the race their direction were instantaneously reversed horses would race back toward the starting gate. If each horse maintained its original speed the horses would arrive at the gate together, as they had begun. In essence, the 180° pulse reverses the direction of dephasing nuclei so that they rephase. Because applied field inhomogeneities are fixed and T_2* is, therefore, constant, nuclei initially dispersing under those influences converge at the same rate. Their emergent signal is referred to as an echo because it returns in the absence of an applied pulse. That echo is weaker than the transverse component immediately after excitation because nuclei dephasing under local, inconstant inhomogeneities do not catch up and are not heard from. The signal loss between excitation and echo reflects true T_2 relaxation.

In addition to TR, the operator determines the time between excitation and echo (TE). The time interval between 90° and 180° pulses is designated *tau*. Because rephasing occurs at the same rate as dephasing, it follows that TE is twice *tau*. The principles of spin-echo are summarized in Figure 1.10-8. T_2-weighted images are commonly used because they often highlight subtle abnormalities within tissues. For example, spin-echo sequences provide dramatic pictures of multiple sclerosis plaques (Figure 1.10-9). Similar pathognomonic abnormalities in psychiatric illness have not been identified, and no comparable routine indication for MRI exists in psychiatric practice today.

Instrumentation and image production Most components of an MRI scanner follow logically from the physical principles just enumerated. The first prerequisite is the alignment of nuclei in an applied magnetic field; thus, all MRI scanners have a static magnet. To a large extent, the strength of the static magnet determines the quality of the images produced. Most scanners use superconducting magnets because of their strong fields, typically 0.5 to 1.5 tesla. Static magnets consist of circular coils surrounding the bed (gantry) of the machine. As electricity moves through the coils, a perpendicular magnetic field is produced that parallels the axis of the gantry. Unlike CT scanners, in which only the patient's head is inside the camera, the gantry of an MRI scanner is long, and the entire body of the patient lies within the bore of the magnet to ensure homogeneity of the applied field over the area of interest. Superconducting coils, because they lack resistance, perpetuate an electrical current indefinitely, and the fields produced are consistent. Because superconducting materials acquire that property only at very low temperatures, the coils are surrounded by liquid helium reservoirs at 4° Kelvin, which maintain the superconductivity.

MRI information is elicited in two stages. First, protons are perturbed by an applied radio-frequency pulse. Resonating protons then emit radio waves in a fashion characteristic of their tissue relaxation times. MRI scanners contain radio equipment in the form of both transmitting and receiving coils that interrogate and listen, respectively. Although sending and receiving information by radio waves are literally a household notion, the process by which MRI scanners spatially encode such complicated waveforms and thereby generate images is far less intuitive. Nonetheless, spatial information about protons relies on the same relation between precession and field strength. Specifically, it is possible to assign different resonant frequencies to protons by superimposing a magnetic gradient on the static field. Hydrogen nuclei thus precess at variable rates, depending on their positions in the gradient. Protons at the same point along the gradient (corresponding to a plane perpendicular to the direction of the gradient) share the same precessional frequency, whereas those in neighboring planes precess at correspondingly different rates. In that manner, a magnetic gradient permits a slice of tissue to be selectively excited. The coils used to produce the gradients are known as gradient magnets. The characteristic knocking heard during image acquisition emanates from those coils as they repetitively create and change gradient fields. By nature, gradients are easily produced in multiple directions. Thus, axial, coronal, and sagittal images are acquired without repositioning the patient. By changing gradients along different axes and exciting planes in a systematic fashion, one can gain a conceptual basis for understanding how images are produced. In actuality image production is more complex, and MRI scanners use techniques of frequency and phase encoding to gain two-dimensional information simultaneously.

The final stage of image production relies on computer processing and storage of data. Mathematical algorithms and Fourier transformations of a type similar to those used in CT scanning allow the efficient conversion of complicated waveforms obtained in multiple planes into a matrix of values corresponding to specific tissue properties. The smallest unit in such matrices corresponds to the smallest volume ele-

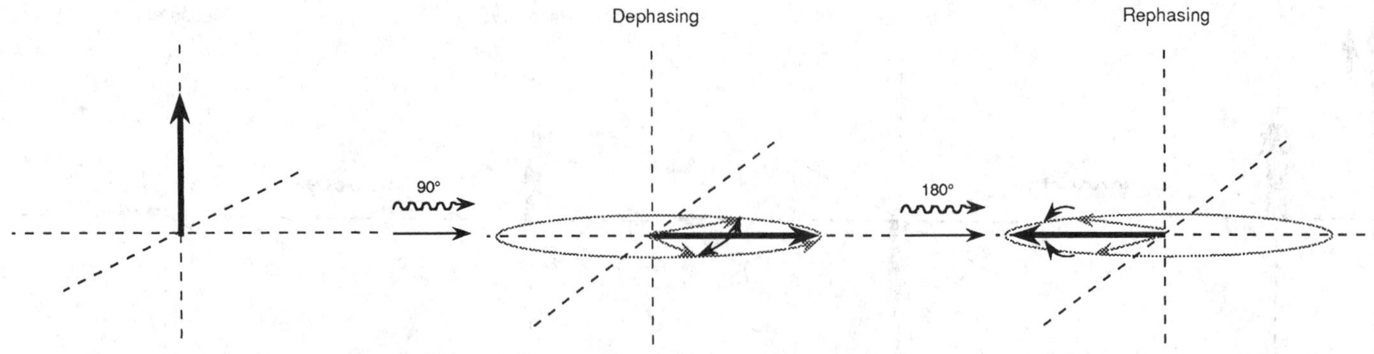

FIGURE 1.10-8 *In spin-echo pulse sequencing, net magnetization is tipped into the horizontal plane by an initial 90° pulse. Although nuclei initially precess in unison, dephasing occurs as a result of tissue-specific (T_2) and applied (T_2*) magnetic field inhomogeneities. A subsequent 180° pulse eliminates the degradation in transverse magnetization from T_2* by reversing the vectors so that they converge. With the rephasing of nuclei, an echo of the initial net transverse magnetization vector is heard, albeit somewhat more faintly because of the loss of signal by T_2 alone.*

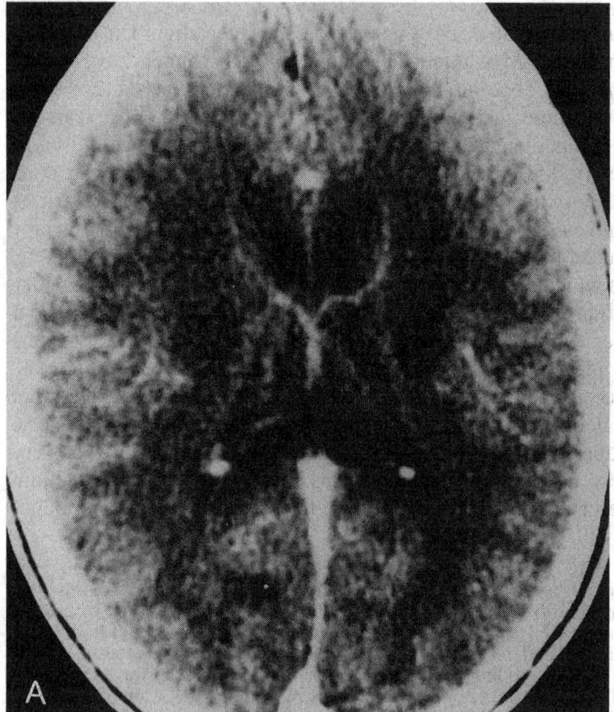

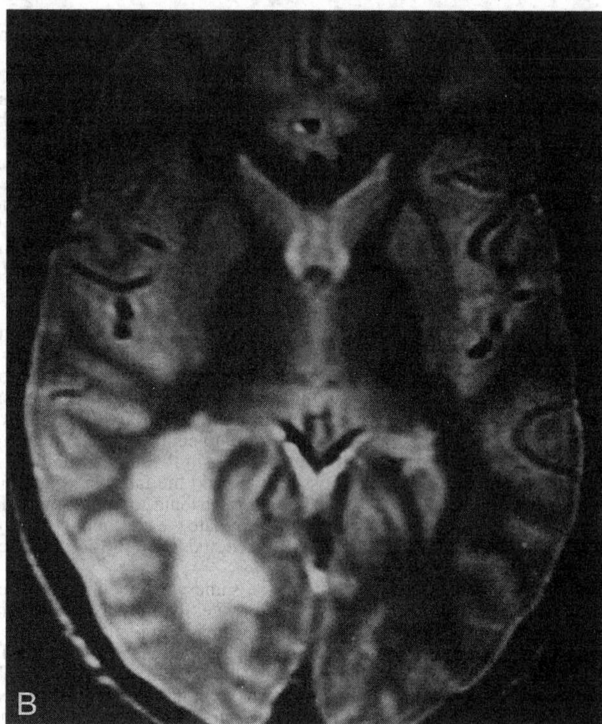

FIGURE 1.10-9 (A) *Transaxial CT image enhanced by intravenously administered contrast material in a patient with acute multiple sclerosis. The white matter regions throughout the slice are relatively uniform in appearance.* (B) *With a spin-echo pulse sequence, a T_2-weighted MR image at the same brain level in the patient reveals dramatic evidence of demyelination pathognomonic of multiple sclerosis. (Figure courtesy of S W Atlas. From* Magnetic Resonance Imaging of the Brain and Spine, *S W Atlas, editor, p 469. Raven, New York, 1991. Used with permission.)*

ment (voxel) of tissue resolved, which for modern scanners is on the order of a cubic millimeter.

FUNCTIONAL IMAGING

Although there is no universally accepted definition of functional imaging this section uses the term to refer to imaging modalities and methods that are used primarily to provide information on the neurochemistry, the metabolism, or the activity of the brain. Although the images may also provide information about brain anatomy they have lower resolution than CT and MRI and are not primarily used to provide structural information (Table 1.10-3).

MAGNETIC RESONANCE SPECTROSCOPY Magnetic resonance spectroscopy (MRS) provides a noninvasive means of assaying specific biologically relevant molecules in vivo. The chemical specificity of MRS is grounded in the same principles of magnetic resonance used by its structural imaging cousin, MRI. MRS does not expose the patient to radiation, and has a degree of safety similar to that of MRI. Especially for repeated studies, MRS may have significant advantages over other functional imaging modalities in the longitudinal study of neuropsychiatric disorders.

MRS differs considerably from MRI in ability to extract important information about the molecules in which nuclei reside. Because MRS measures a phenomenon known as chemical shift, it is sometimes referred to as chemical-shift spectroscopy. For example, MRS measures the inherent magnetic behavior of a variety of nuclear species contained naturally in biological compounds (for example, H^1, C^{13}, and P^{31}). Depending on atomic weight and magnetic field strength, each nuclear species precesses with a different Larmor frequency. For example, C^{13} precesses at a rate one quarter that of H^1 in an identical magnetic field. Differences in precession and excitatory radio-frequencies between nuclear species are relatively large, and easily separated, and are as distinctive as a signature. However, MRS depends on minor variations in precession manifested by individual nuclei of the same species. The differences derive from extremely small fluctuations in the magnetic field created by the chemical microenvironment of the nucleus. Depending on the organic molecule in which a nuclear species resides (or even depending on its relative position in the same molecule), the magnetic field it experiences is slightly modified, and so is its rate of precession. The physical basis of those variations lies in the movement of electrons in neighboring atoms. As electrons move, they create their own small regional magnetic fields that to a slight degree alter the magnetic field experienced by nuclei in their proximity. Because the spatial configuration of electrons is unique for a given molecule, precessing nuclei take on altered frequencies, which disclose their biochemical origins. Under the proper circumstances the various radio-frequency signals measured in MRS may be traced to specific chemical moieties.

An MRS spectrum is a graph of those signals as a function of their frequencies. An example of such a spectrum for P^{31} is given in Figure 1.10-10. Rather than a single radio-frequency peak for P^{31}, multiple peaks are shifted relative to one another. The differences in frequencies between individual peaks is extremely small and is expressed in parts per million (ppm) relative to a central radio frequency. As can be seen from the P^{31} spectrum, multiple phosphorus signals exist. Careful in vitro experiments have led to the identification of many of the corresponding in vivo peaks. Thus, the phosphorus contained in phosphocreatine has a different precessional frequency than that of inorganic phosphate. Similarly, the three P^{31} nuclei present in adenosine triphosphate each produce a distinct radio-frequency signal. Because the areas under individual phosphorus peaks relate to their relative tissue concentrations, functional information about intracellular metabolism, cell membrane recycling, and bioenergetic states may be inferred from such spectra.

For multiple reasons, MRS faces more stringent technical requirements than does MRI. Because the differences in resonant frequencies caused by chemical shifting are small, MRS requires a much greater uniformity in the applied magnetic field. That field uniformity is achieved by a process known as *shimming*. In addition, the applied magnetic fields used in MRS tend to be of greater strength—for example, 1.5 to 2.5 tesla. Those greater field strengths produce faster precessional frequencies, which result in proportionally larger and more discernible shifts between peaks. Although not universally true, MRS measurements are generally enhanced at high field strengths. In addition, the transmitting and receiving coils used in MRS must be capable of emitting and detecting a correspondingly broader range of radio-frequency waves. Despite those differences, many MRI scanners are currently capable of modifications that allow their use for MRS studies in conjunction with an MRS computer workstation.

One principal advantage of MRS is its chemical specificity. Furthermore, the simultaneous measurement of multiple chemical species is a unique advantage of MRS over other functional modalities. In addition, MRS is not limited to the study of molecules contained in organic compounds but is also capable of detecting certain endogenous ions (for example, Na^{23}) and exogenous nuclei of potential biological relevance (for exam-

TABLE 1.10-3
Comparison of Functional Imaging Modalities

Factor	Magnetic Resonance Spectroscopy	Positron Emission Tomography	Single Photon Emission Computed Tomography
Sensitivity	Poor (>10^{-6} M)	Extraordinarily high (<10^{-12} M)	Very high (<10^{-11} M)
Resolution of commercial devices	>10 mm	5–6 mm	7–8 mm
Isotopes	H^1, Li^7, C^{13}, F^{19}, Na^{23}, P^{31}	O^{15}, C^{11}, F^{18}	I^{123}, Tc^{99m}, Xe^{133}
$T_{1/2}$ of isotopes	Nondecaying	2, 20, 110 min	13, 6, 127 hour
Production of radionuclides	Naturally abundant (C^{13} and F^{19} supplied commercially)	On-site cyclotron	Commercial supplier or simple on-site generator
Cost of scan	\$600–\$1,000	ca. \$1,500–\$2,000	ca. \$400–\$1,000
Transmission scan for attenuation	N.A.	Typically performed	Not yet developed
Research uses			
Cerebral blood flow	No	Yes	Yes
Brain metabolism	Yes	Yes	Yes
Receptor imaging	No	>10-year track record	Active in past 3–5 years
Drug monitoring	Yes	Yes	Yes

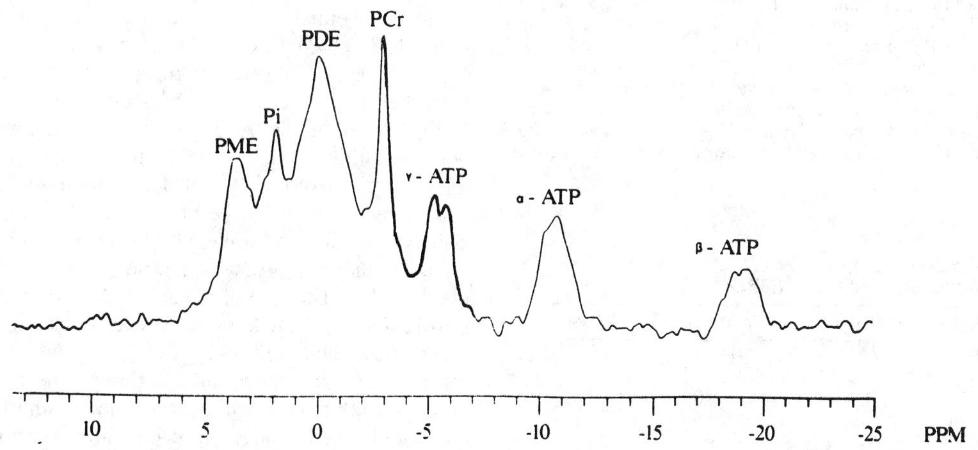

FIGURE 1.10-10 *P^{31} MRS spectrum obtained from the dorsolateral prefrontal cortex of a healthy human volunteer. Individual peaks correspond to the P^{31} signal of phosphomonoesters (PME), inorganic phosphate (Pi), phosphodiesters (PDE), phosphocreatine (PCr), and the three different phosphate moieties of adenosine triphosphate (ATP). The slight differences in resonant frequencies of the same nuclear species are known as chemical shifts and are measured in parts per million relative to a central radiofrequency. (Figure courtesy of M S Keshavan. From M S Keshavan, S Kapur, J W Pettegrew: Magnetic resonance spectroscopy in psychiatry: Potential, pitfalls, and promise. Am J Psychiatry* 148: *978, 1991. Used with permission.)*

ple, Li^7, F^{19}). In fact, the pharmacokinetic monitoring of tissue concentrations of both lithium and fluorinated pharmaceuticals (for example, trifluoperazine [Stelazine] and fluoxetine [Prozac]) with MRS represents a potentially promising technique in clinical psychopharmacology.

As with any imaging modality, MRS has intrinsic disadvantages. A central challenge in MRS remains the acquisition of a detectable signal from a defined volume of tissue in a reasonable period of time. Signals of the nuclei studied in MRS are fundamentally weak. A variety of factors are important in determining signal strength, including the intrinsic sensitivity of the nuclei, molecular mobility, isotopic abundance, and relative tissue concentrations.

Intrinsic sensitivity requires a clarification of an earlier principle. Magnetic nuclei actually acquire both parallel and antiparallel orientations in an applied field. The difference between the two populations, typically one nucleus in 10^7, accounts for the entire MRS signal. In practice, MRS is capable only of measuring substances present in biological tissues at concentrations greater than 0.5 mM. Because most neurotransmitters and many important brain metabolites are present physiologically only in nanomolar amounts, they are undetectable by MRS. One exception to that concentration barrier is the in vivo measurement of pH, in which nanomolar differences in hydrogen ion concentrations may be inferred from shifts in the chemical spectra of more concentrated metabolites. In addition, only molecules that are sufficiently mobile in solution generate signals strong enough to be measured. For both those reasons, in vivo measurements of receptor binding are areas where positron emission tomography (PET) and single photon emission computed tomography (SPECT) have clear superiority over MRS.

The natural abundance of magnetically active isotopes is also a determinant of signal strength. For example, virtually all the phosphorus contained in the human body is present in the form of P^{31}. For that reason, P^{31} is said to be 100 percent abundant. However, natural abundance varies among the elements (Table 1.10-4). For example, the majority of the body's carbon consists of the nonmagnetic isotope C^{12} (98.9 percent), and only the minority (1.1 percent) is magnetically resonant (C^{13}). Thus, the resonant signal of carbon-containing molecules is weak because of the relative scarcity of C^{13}. Necessity being the mother of invention, that difficulty in C^{13} MRS has been overcome by the development of enrichment techniques. Elegant studies using C^{13}-labeled glucose, for example, have allowed the direct measurement of glucose metabolism in vivo through observations of actual glycolytic intermediates (such as [C^{13}] lactate). In fact, the scarcity of C^{13} ultimately makes that powerful approach possible.

The net effect of poor signal strength has implications for two reciprocally related parameters of practical importance for MRS imaging: spatial and temporal resolution. Under ideal circumstances, useful MRS measurements may be acquired from a voxel (three-dimensional volume element of computer data) the size of a cubic centimeter in a matter of a few minutes for some species. For most nuclei, however, either longer times (10 to 30 minutes) or larger volumes (5 to 50 cc) are required to obtain a measurable signal above noise. PET and SPECT outperform MRS in regard to both temporal and spatial resolution. Nevertheless, spatial localization of MRS signals is one of the most active areas of current research. A variety of techniques now exist—including chemical shift imaging, depth-resolved surface coil spectroscopy, and image-selected in vivo spectroscopy—that allow the spatial encoding of MRS signals through the use of magnetic gradients.

TABLE 1.10-4
Sensitivity and Isotopic Abundance of Nuclei Detected by Magnetic Resonance Spectroscopy (MRS)

Isotope	Intrinsic Sensitivity[1]	Natural Abundance (%)[2]
H^1	100.00	99.98
Li^7	29.00	92.60
C^{13}	1.59	1.10
F^{19}	83.40	100.00
Na^{23}	9.24	100.00
P^{31}	6.64	100.00

[1]Relative sensitivity to detection by MRS.
[2]Extent to which an isotope constitutes the element under natural conditions.
Table courtesy of M S Keshavan, S Kapur, J W Pettegrew: Magnetic resonance spectroscopy in psychiatry: potential, pitfalls, and promise. From Am J Psychiatry *148:* 978, 1991. Used with permission.

Those methods represent an important integration of the biochemical information obtained by MRS with the anatomical information obtained from MRI. Although MRS "images" will never attain the level of resolution possible with MRI, their close relation may constitute an additional advantage for MRS in the realm of correlating brain function and brain structure.

PET AND SPECT Both PET and SPECT rely on the incorporation of a radioactive nuclide into a drug (called a radiopharmaceutical), which is typically injected intravenously into a patient. The subsequent uptake of the substance by the brain and the measurement of regional brain activities over time are analyzed to provide information about the neurochemistry, the metabolism, or the activity of the brain (Figure 1.10-11). As indicated in their names, both PET and SPECT represent emission methods, in which the source of activity is internal to the body, and should be distinguished from transmission methods, in which the source of activity is external to the body (for example, a chest X-ray is a typical transmission scan in which an external source of activity is directed at the body). Tissues and body cavities show differential absorption of the activity and cast graded shadows on a photographic film placed behind the subject. In contrast, the source of activity for PET and SPECT is internal to the body and derives from the physical decay of the radionuclide attached to the injected drug. The decay leads either directly or indirectly to the emission of high-energy photons that can penetrate the brain and the skull and can subsequently be measured in an external radiation-detection device, like a PET or SPECT camera. Those photons have high energies and are not part of the visible spectrum of electromagnetic energies. The cameras are equipped with computers that can reconstruct the original distribution of activities in a slice or a tomograph of the brain at multiple time points after the injection of the radiotracer substance. Thus, PET and SPECT are tomographic methods and should be distinguished from planar imaging (like a chest X-ray), which produces an image that is flat and in which all tissues through the thickness of the body are compressed.

How can knowledge of the time course and the distribution of radioactively labeled drugs in slices of the brain provide useful information about CNS function? The answer to that question relies heavily on the underlying physical principles.

PET The physical decay of PET radiopharmaceuticals involves the emission of a particle called a positron (designated as e^+ or β^+), which has the mass of an electron but a positive charge. The positron travels through the tissue a variable distance before colliding with an electron (e^-). That collision of matter and antimatter results in the annihilation of the two particles and the conversion of their combined masses into two high-energy photons of 511 KeV (thousand electron volts), which are simultaneously emitted at an 180° angle to each other. The average distance traveled by the positron is positively correlated with its energy, which varies for each radionuclide (Figure 1.10-12). The rate of decay of all radioisotopes, including positron-emitting nuclides, follows an exponential curve, which can be described with a half-life ($T_{½}$) value, the time required for half the radioactive atoms to decay. The $T_{½}$ values for typical positron-emitting nuclides is relatively short: from two minutes for O^{15} (an isotope of oxygen with an atomic weight of 15) to 110 minutes for F^{18}. The physical properties of positron emission determine the manner in which PET imaging can be used.

The emission of two photons at a 180° angle to each other provides the central basis for PET image reconstruction, the method of coincidence detection. The multiple crystals of the PET camera that detect the emitted photons use only those that are simultaneously acquired,

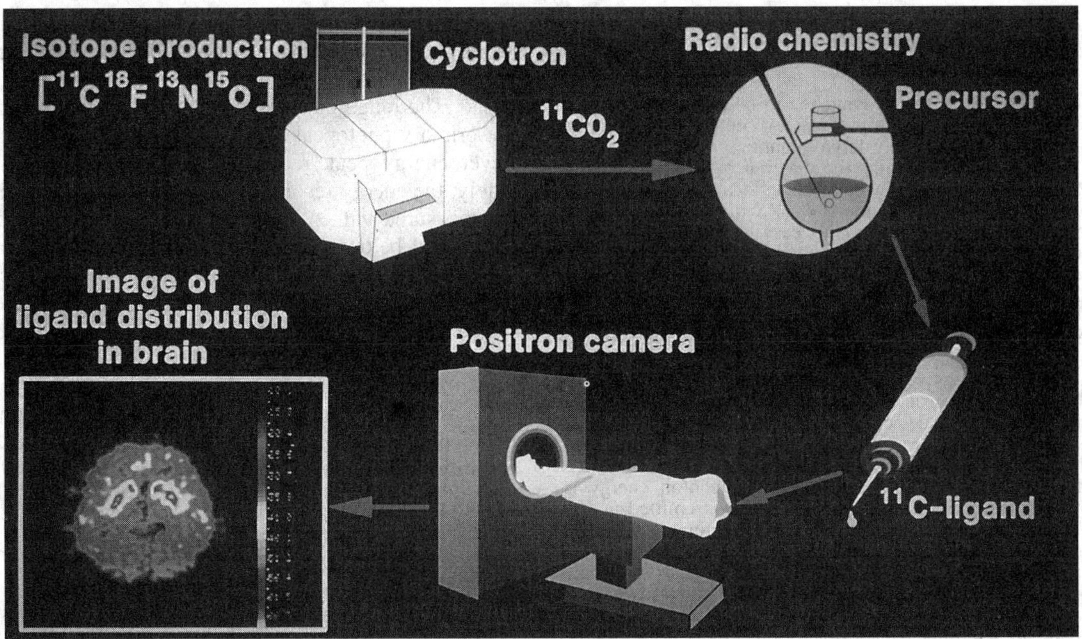

FIGURE 1.10-11 *Imaging of neuroreceptors by PET. The method involves the production of a positron-emitting nuclide, its incorporation into a radiopharmaceutical, injection of the radiopharmaceutical into a subject, and subsequent image reconstruction with the PET camera. The displayed PET image depicts the distribution of striatal dopamine D_2 receptors. SPECT imaging follows a similar procedure, except that the isotopes are longer-lived and can be produced by a distant central cyclotron facility. (Figure courtesy of G Sedvall. From G Sedvall, L Farde, F A Wiesel: Imaging of neurotransmitter receptors in the living human brain. Arch Gen Psychiatry 43: 999. Used with permission.) (See Color Plate 2.)*

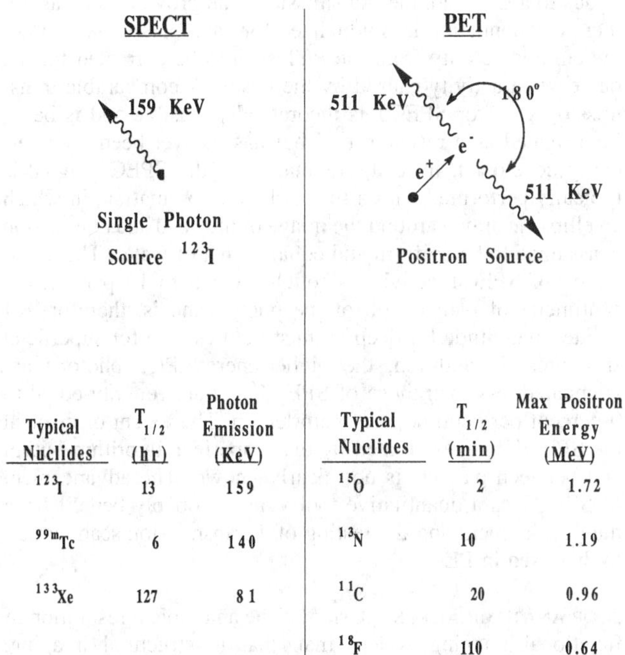

Typical Nuclides	$T_{1/2}$ (hr)	Photon Emission (KeV)
^{123}I	13	159
^{99m}Tc	6	140
^{133}Xe	127	81

Typical Nuclides	$T_{1/2}$ (min)	Max Positron Energy (MeV)
^{15}O	2	1.72
^{13}N	10	1.19
^{11}C	20	0.96
^{18}F	110	0.64

FIGURE 1.10-12 *Decay of a SPECT radiopharmaceutical results in the emission of a high-energy photon directly from the radionuclide. In contrast, decay of a PET radiopharmaceutical results in the emission of a positron (e^+), which travels a variable distance before encountering an electron (e^-), collision of which yields two 511 KeV photons at a 180° angle to each other. The distance traveled by the positron decreases the resolution of PET images when using the listed typical nuclides by 0.2 to 1.3 mm, with resolution measured as full width at half maximum. The long-lived SPECT radionuclides emit single photons of different energies, whereas the PET radionuclides consistently yield two photons of 511 KeV.*

which for present devices means within 3 to 10 nanoseconds of each other. Furthermore, the image reconstruction algorithm assumes that the emission occurred somewhere along the straight line connecting the two detectors. However, the physical principles of radioactive decay also lead to the method's limitations. Because the purpose of the imaging is to localize the radiopharmaceutical, rather than the site of annihilation of the positron, the anatomical resolution of PET is physically limited to a sphere with a radius approximately equal to the average distance traveled by the positron. For example, the decreased resolution for C^{11}-labeled compounds is because of the range of its positron is approximately 2 mm. In addition, the two emitted photons are not always exactly at a 180° angle to each other because the electron and the positron are not completely at rest when they annihilate. Thus, the accuracy of PET localization is physically limited by both the distance traveled by the positron and the deviations from the 180° angle.

The short $T_{1/2}$ values of the typically used positron-emitting nuclides generally require on-site production. As depicted in Figure 1.10-11, a PET center must usually have both a positron camera and a cyclotron for the production of radionuclides. For somewhat longer-lived isotopes (such as F^{18}, for which $T_{1/2}$ is equal to 110 minutes), a centrally located cyclotron could provide a radioisotope or a fully prepared radiopharmaceutical to several distant PET cameras. However, such central radiochemical facilities would likely remain unfeasible for short-lived isotopes such as O^{15}, for which $T_{1/2}$ is equal to two minutes. A cyclotron is expensive (approximate cost, $1 million to $2.5 million) and requires a highly skilled technical staff for operation and maintenance. In addition, the short $T_{1/2}$s of the positron emitters necessitate a rapid chemical synthesis of the injected radiopharmaceutical. Although a moderate number of radiopharmaceutical syntheses (for example, [F^{18}]fluorodeoxyglucose) have been automated and can be performed in robotically controlled hot cells, the majority of preparations is performed manually by radiochemists racing against the clock of nuclide decay.

SPECT The physical decay of a SPECT radiopharmaceutical involves the emission of a single photon directly from the radionuclide itself. The emissions are typically of lower energy than those for PET and include a primary emission of 159 KeV for I^{123} and 140 KeV for Tc^{99m} (a metastable isotope of technetium with an atomic weight of 99) (Figure 1.10-12). The half-lives of SPECT nuclides are typically longer than those used for PET and include a $T_{1/2}$ equal to 13 hours for I^{123} and six hours for

Tc^{99m}. As in PET, the physical properties of radionuclidic emission determine the manner in which SPECT can be applied.

Longer $T_{½}$ values allow the radionuclide to be manufactured at a central site and distributed to multiple imaging centers. For example, I^{123} can be produced in relatively large quantities by a commercial cyclotron facility, which then ships the material by express mail to multiple SPECT imaging centers, which can be located at distances of 3,000 miles or more away. Furthermore, Tc^{99m} can be produced from a molybdenum generator that is relatively easy to operate and that is located in the radiopharmacies of many nuclear medicine facilities. In addition, the longer $T_{½}$ values of SPECT radionuclides allow more time for the synthesis and the formulation of the radiopharmaceutical. Thus, the relatively long half-lives of SPECT radionuclides obviate the need for an expensive cyclotron and allow significantly more time for the preparation of the radiopharmaceutical.

The emission of a single photon implies that the image reconstruction algorithm must be intrinsically different from that of PET. SPECT cannot use the simultaneous detection of two gamma rays but, instead, uses collimation. A collimator is typically a block of lead with drilled holes that is placed between the source of activity and the camera's sodium iodide (NaI) crystal detectors. When the photon energy is absorbed by the crystal, light in the visible range is emitted and is detected by photomultiplier tubes. The holes in the collimator set limits on the possible locations of the source of the emission because the walls (septae) block those photons that enter at too sharp an angle (Figure 1.10-13). By viewing the source of activity from multiple angles, the reconstruction algorithm uses the same principles of back-projection as CT to determine the distribution of activity in the source (Figure 1.10-13).

The resolution of the camera is increased by use of longer and narrower holes in the collimator, but the total number of photons detected by the NaI crystal (that is, the overall sensitivity of the device) is correspondingly decreased. One of the implications of the emission of a single photon is an inherent trade-off between sensitivity and resolution in the design of the collimator. However, one of the advantages of single-photon emission is that the source of the activity comes directly from the nuclide itself rather than from an annihilation event at some distance from the radiopharmaceutical. In that regard, SPECT does not have a physical limit of anatomical resolution similar to that of PET; instead, its limits are determined by a complexity of factors, including scatter.

Physical constraints

SCATTER OF ACTIVITY The high-energy photons detected in both PET and SPECT imaging may deviate from a straight path by being scattered by the tissue. That so-called Compton scattering causes the photon not only to deviate from a straight path but also to decrease its energy by a transfer to electrons in the tissue. The range of energies detected by the camera includes the primary photopeak (for example, 159 KeV for I^{123}) and a lower energy peak representing scattered photons. Unfortunately, the energy resolution of present cameras is limited, and the measured values are distributed over a range of energies above and below the peak value. The photopeak and scatter windows overlap and are difficult to distinguish completely. Algorithms for subtracting the scatter component from the photopeak can partially correct the problem. However, the anatomical resolution of the final image is flawed to the extent that scattered photons are viewed by the image reconstruction program as coming from a source on a straight-line path. The scatter of photons is one of the factors that limit the anatomical resolution of both PET and SPECT images.

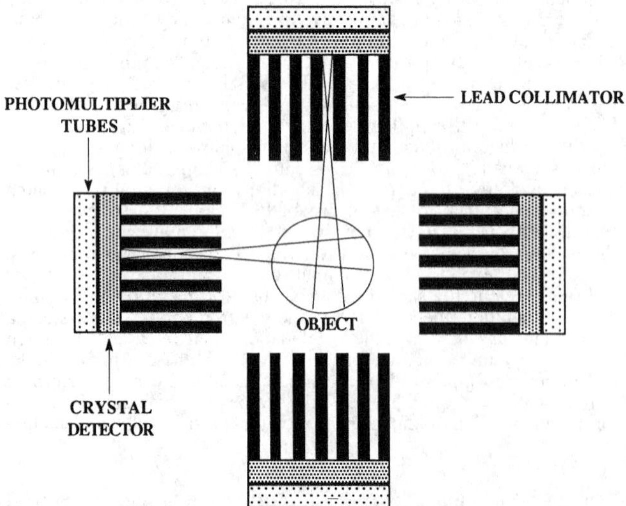

FIGURE 1.10-13 *The method of image reconstruction from back-projection in SPECT uses a collimator placed between the object and the crystal detector. The area of the object that is viewed by the underlying detector is decreased by having longer and narrower holes in the collimator. When the detector-collimator complex is moved around the object, multiple views are obtained, which provide the primary data for image reconstruction.*

ATTENUATION OF SIGNAL Only a portion of the activity emitted in the tissue actually escapes from the body, and some is completely absorbed or partially absorbed because of scatter. Thus, the emitted activity is attenuated by the tissue. Furthermore, attenuation is not uniform and is differentially affected by bone, air, fluid, and tissue. The problems caused by attenuation are evident in studies of individual patients when the operator attempts to measure absolute levels of tissue activity and are compounded when comparing studies of patients who have heads of different shapes and correspondingly variable attenuation maps. PET scans are fairly routinely corrected for attenuation by obtaining an initial transmission scan. Exactly analogous to a CT scan, the transmission scan provides a measurement of attenuation individualized for each person and allows the emitted activity from the PET scan to be corrected for the decrease in activity caused by the tissue. A comparable transmission scan for SPECT is theoretically feasible and is being investigated as a research tool but has not yet been commercially developed. Instead, attenuation of the SPECT signal is typically performed with a first-order approximation, in which an ellipse is drawn around the image of the head and attenuation is assumed to be uniform and equal to that of water. The attenuation of SPECT activity is roughly equal to 15 percent per centimeter of path length of the photon and is, therefore, of greater magnitude for deep brain structures than for superficial structures. In addition, the higher-energy PET photons are attenuated less than those of SPECT and are roughly equal to 9 percent per centimeter of path length. The extent of error in the SPECT images created by that imperfect algorithm within and between patients is not clearly known. The advancement of SPECT as a quantitative tool would probably benefit from the development and the testing of a transmission scan similar to that used in PET.

POOR ANATOMICAL RESOLUTION The anatomical resolution in functional imaging is less than that in structural imaging. Causes of the limited resolution include scatter of the photons and the engineering constraints on the number and the imperfections of the crystals and the associated electronic circuits. The definition of resolution derives from the ability to distinguish two separate points visually. The most commonly used numerical measure of resolution is the full width at half maximum (FWHM) of the line-spread function. Although the term sounds complex, it can be easily understood by considering the measured activities from two point sources with infinitely small dimensions (Figure 1.10-14). Viewed in only one axis, the measured activities should be two spikes with infinitely narrow

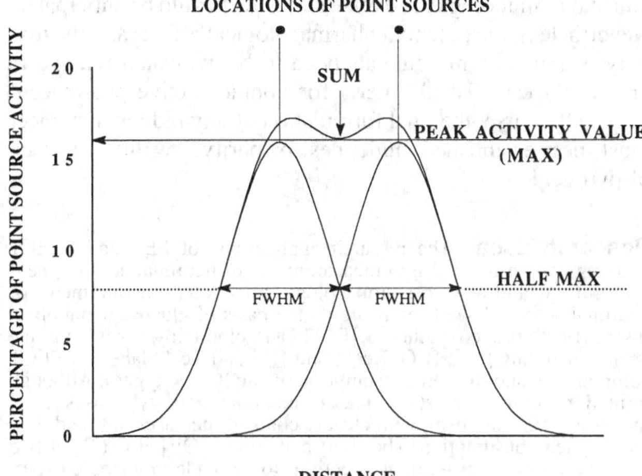

FIGURE 1.10-14 *The limited resolution of PET and SPECT cameras blurs the activity of single-point sources into adjacent regions with no activity. Viewed in just one dimension, a point source is visualized by the camera as a Gaussian curve. Resolution is defined as the width of the curve at half maximum measured peak levels (FWHM). For two point sources of equal intensity separated by a distance equal to the FWHM of the camera, the sum of the activities begins to show a modest decrease at the midpoint, which suggests that the original source had two points, rather than one.*

widths. Instead, the reconstructed image is blurred, and the curve of the activity typically follows a Gaussian function. The measured peak activity is much less than the actual activity in the point source, which has been blurred into adjacent regions with no activity. The resolution of the image is usually defined as the width of the curve at 50 percent of the maximum measured levels (FWHM) (Figure 1.10-14). The rationale for that definition can be appreciated by considering two point sources of equal activities and asking what distance is required to detect them as two separate points. The summed activities of the two point sources begin to show a modest decrease when the two points are separated by the distance equal to the FWHM (Figure 1.10-14).

The anatomical resolution of both PET and SPECT cameras has significantly improved over the past decade. The best commercially available PET devices have FWHM values of approximately 5 to 6 mm, and SPECT devices have FWHM values of 8 to 9 mm. A recently developed PET device at Lawrence Berkeley laboratories (University of California at Berkeley) is reported to have a resolution of approximately 3 mm.

PARTIAL VOLUME EFFECTS The limited anatomical resolution of PET and SPECT causes not only a blurred appearance in the images but also substantial errors in measurements. Regional activities are spread out or blurred over adjacent regions in all three dimensions. Using a pictorial analogy, tall, sharp peaks and deep, narrow valleys of activity are perceived by the camera as short, broad hills and shallow, wide troughs. That is, the measured activity from any individual volume element derives only in part from the actual activity in that volume but also from activity from surrounding areas. That so-called partial volume effect causes greater quantitative errors as the resolution decreases. The most important reason for improving the resolution of PET and SPECT cameras is not to acquire prettier pictures but to gain more accurate measurements of regional brain activities.

The errors created by partial volume effects may be simulated by scanning a phantom, which is typically a plastic cylinder with internal cavities of the same size and shape as the actual object to be studied. For example, blood flow in gray matter is approximately four times greater than that in white matter. Commercially available phantoms or models of the human brain have been carefully machined to re-create the geometry of gray matter so that when the phantom is filled with liquid containing a radioactive substance the gray matter has four times the amount of liquid as the white matter. For each particular camera, images of the phantom are used to estimate the appropriate recovery correction factor that should be applied to images of humans.

Partial volume effects may present a particular problem if the disorder being studied has both a structural abnormality and a functional abnormality. For example, PET and SPECT imaging of patients with Alzheimer's disease have shown decreased glucose metabolism and decreased blood flow in the temporoparietal regions. However, MRI studies have also shown a thinning of cortical gray matter in those same regions, with a resulting decrease in total gray matter volume. Because of partial-volume-effect errors, the functional images cannot be used to distinguish completely activity deriving from gray and white matter regions. Do Alzheimer's disease patients have decreased metabolism per gram of gray matter or decreased metabolism because the total mass of gray matter has decreased? That particular question is not completely answered, but it emphasizes the potential complications created by partial volume effects when the disorder being studied is associated with structural abnormalities that may by themselves modify the functional images.

PET versus SPECT Comparisons of the advantages and the disadvantages of PET and SPECT imaging methods seem inevitably to devolve into the single question of which is the better imaging modality. Unfortunately, the existing data do not justify a simple answer. PET and SPECT share many common advantages and disadvantages. Two major advantages of both methods are their high levels of sensitivity and chemical selectivity. For example, neurotransmitter receptors are present in relatively low concentrations of approximately 0.1 to 20×10^{-9} molar (M). MRI and MRS cannot study those targets because the limits of their sensitivities are in the range of 10^{-3} to 10^{-5} M. In contrast, PET, depending on the length of image acquisition, has sensitivity in the range of 10^{-12} to 10^{-13} M, and SPECT has roughly a 10-fold lower range. Thus, both PET and SPECT have adequate sensitivity for measurement of targets such as neuroreceptors, which are present in low concentrations. In addition, both use radiopharmaceuticals that may have high selectivity for targets in the brain—for example, a radioligand that binds exclusively to a particular receptor subtype.

Perhaps the two greatest disadvantages common to PET and SPECT are their limited anatomical resolution and the stringent requirements for a useful in vivo radiotracer. Limited resolution, leading to partial-volume-effect errors, has been discussed. In addition, many radioligands that are valuable tools in vitro may be useless as in vivo radiotracers. In general, a successful in vivo tracer must not be bound too tightly to plasma proteins, must be able to cross the blood-brain barrier, must not be metabolized too rapidly, and must not be too lipid-soluble. The design and the synthesis of useful radiopharmaceuticals can be difficult and has often been the rate-limiting step in both PET and SPECT imaging studies.

PET and SPECT share some of the greatest advantages and some of the greatest disadvantages of functional imaging modalities. But how do they compare with each other? Perhaps the major relative advantage of PET is its ability to provide quantitative information on brain function. The simultaneous emission of two photons provides intrinsic advantages for the accuracy of image reconstruction. The higher energy of its emission, compared with that of SPECT, leads to less scatter and less attenuation. Furthermore, the engineering of PET cameras is more advanced than that of SPECT cameras, and PET cameras can routinely use transmission scanning for attenuation correction. In contrast, the greatest relative advantages of SPECT are that it is easier to use and less expensive than PET. The longer-lived isotopes used do not require an on-site cyclotron and allow more time for radiosyntheses. In addition, the SPECT camera itself may cost only 20 to 25 percent of the cost of a PET device: $500,000 versus $2.5 million.

Both PET and SPECT technologies are in a period of rapid change, and the full capabilities of each have presumably not yet been achieved in engineering design, attenuation correction, image reconstruction, and synthesis of new tracers. In addition, the field of psychiatry has not yet clarified the specific questions to be answered by each. For those reasons the authors think that on the basis of existing data, there is inadequate evidence at present to include or exclude definitively either PET or SPECT as a clearly valuable tool for clinical care in the future. However, both methods are promising and justify research efforts for continued technical improvements, developments of applications, and comparisons of the two methods.

Safety Safety concerns regarding radiation exposure and pharmacological toxicity of the injected radiopharmaceutical are similar for PET and SPECT. Because functional imaging has no clearly established clinical usefulness in psychiatric disorders, it should be (but is, in fact, not always) limited to research studies. The U.S. Food and Drug Administration (FDA) has established limits of radiation exposure to various organs of the body and to the body as a whole that are applied to research studies and that are often lower than the exposures in routine clinical nuclear medicine procedures. Although FDA limits are thought to provide adequate safety, the long-term biological effects of ionizing radiation remain an area of active investigation and even controversy. A recent reanalysis of the radiation doses and the long-term effects of the atomic blasts in Hiroshima and Nagasaki suggests that the risks of low-dose radiation exposure (like that in PET and SPECT scans) may be greater than previously realized. For that reason, the FDA is likely to implement within the next one or two years a 2.5-fold lower radiation dose limit for research studies. Although many factors affect radiation dose estimates, including the amount of activity, type of emission, and residence time in the body, the shorter half-lives of PET radionuclides and the higher sensitivity of the PET method generally yield lower radiation burdens than a comparable SPECT study. The guideline is generally accepted to use doses of radiotracer that are as low as reasonably allowable to provide the desired results. Furthermore, the radiation exposures from typical PET and SPECT scans are thought to be reasonably safe within the context of the present knowledge of radiation biology.

Fortunately, the pharmacological toxicity of radiopharmaceuticals is often not even a significant issue. The sensitivity of functional imaging is so high that minuscule mass doses of a compound may be injected, although that small mass is associated with significant levels of radioactivity. For example, some radiopharmaceuticals are injected at doses (in milligrams per kilogram body weight) a million fold lower than the minimal dose needed to cause any pharmacological effect. In such situations, no pharmacological toxicity is expected, and only an unusual immunological adverse side effect could be anticipated. Nevertheless, the potential pharmacological effects and the toxicity of radiopharmaceuticals need to be evaluated relative to previously established criteria for nonradioactive pharmaceuticals. Of course, the final formulation of any radioactive tracer must meet established guidelines for purity, sterility, and lack of pyrogenicity.

Research uses The research applications of PET and SPECT imaging can be divided into measurements of neuronal activity, neurochemistry, and in vivo pharmacology. Functional measurements of neuronal activity have been made on the basis of glucose metabolism (using [F^{18}]fluorodeoxyglucose, [F^{18}] FDG), blood flow (using multiple agents including [O^{15}] H_2O, Xe^{133}, and I^{123}- and Tc^{99m}-labeled SPECT compounds), and oxygen consumption (using [O^{15}] oxygen). Although limited exceptions exist, increased neuronal activity causes local increases of metabolism, with closely coupled increases in blood flow and oxygen consumption. The short half-life of [O^{15}] H_2O ($T_{1/2}$ of two minutes) allows four to eight injections to be made in a single experimental setting to assess neuronal activity before and after a pharmacological or neuropsychological intervention. For example, studies localizing brain regions for cognitive functioning (such as word association) have been pioneered at the Washington University PET Center. Those studies may subsequently be applied to localize and measure the abnormal cognitive functioning found in psychiatric disorders. As another example, studies of brain glucose metabolism using [F^{18}]fluorodeoxyglucose have found decreased frontal lobe activity in patients with schizophrenia and the hypofrontality that is often associated with the disorder.

A large number of functional imaging studies of neuronal activity have used single photon-emitting isotopes of the noble gas xenon (Xe). Typically inhaled by passive rebreathing, the isotope Xe^{133} is a highly diffusable tracer; brain uptake and washout can be measured to provide estimates of cerebral perfusion. In contrast to other SPECT imaging agents, in which only relative estimates (that is, ratios of regional to whole brain blood flow) are possible, the Xe^{133} technique permits quantitative measurements (in milliliters per minute per brain volume) of regional cerebral blood flow. Although the application of that method to tomographic brain imaging was initially hampered by the intrinsically low photon energy of Xe^{133} (80 KeV), that relative disadvantage has been offset in recent years by the development of increasingly sensitive SPECT instrumentation. Researchers at the National Institute of Mental Health have used the Xe^{133} technique with great success in cognitive activation studies, including those involving functional activation of the dorsolateral prefrontal cortex by the Wisconsin Card Sorting Task.

A major advantage of the measures of neuronal activity is that they provide the final common result from multiple circuits and neurochemical systems on regional brain activities. However, a disadvantage of the measures is that they are relatively nonselective and do not distinguish terminal activity from cell body activity or increased activity of an excitatory versus an inhibitory neuronal system. For example, increased firing of inhibitory neurons is recorded in those images as increased neuronal activity, although the important functional implication may be postsynaptic inhibition in the target area.

Functional imaging of in vivo neurochemistry includes measurements of specific neurotransmitter circuits; the dopaminergic system is the most extensively studied system. That research was motivated in large part by the desire to apply the methods to the study of schizophrenia. The most widely publicized results are PET studies of the dopamine D_2 receptor. Using an almost irreversible radiotracer [C^{11}]N-methyl-spiperone, the Johns Hopkins PET Center has reported a 2.5-fold elevation of striatal D_2 receptors in drug-naive schizophrenic patients compared with healthy persons. In contrast and using the reversible tracer [C^{11}] raclopride, the Karolinska PET Center has reported that schizophrenic patients have normal densities of striatal D_2 receptors. The causes of those discrepant results are not known but may include the use of different radiotracers, methods of data analysis (kinetic versus equilibrium), and significantly different patient populations.

Neurochemical imaging can also provide information on aspects of neural transmission (Figure 1.10-15). In the dopaminergic system, imaging methods have been reported to measure the synthesis of the transmitter (with [F^{18}] fluoroDOPA), the synaptic release of the transmitter (by dopamine-induced displacement of D_2 radiotracers), the presynaptic dopamine transporter responsible for the reuptake of the transmitter, and probes for the enzyme monoamine oxidase involved in the metabolism of the neurotransmitter.

Pharmacologically oriented imaging studies either the radiolabeled drug itself or the actions of the drug with another radiolabeled probe that shares the same receptor. Examples of the first method include PET studies with [C^{11}] cocaine and [C^{11}] clozapine that have shown

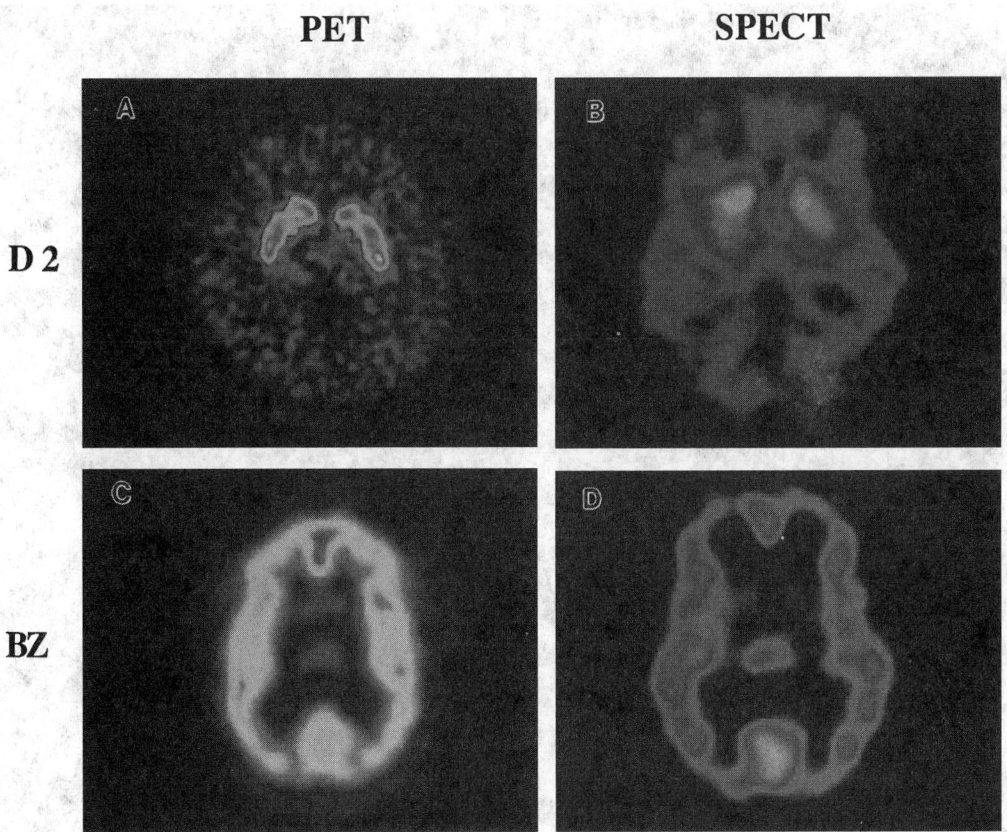

FIGURE 1.10-15 *Transaxial images showing the distribution of D_2 receptors in a human brain imaged with PET* (A) *using [C^{11}] raclopride (figure courtesy of Lars Farde) and with SPECT* (B) *using [I^{123}] iodobenzamide (Figure courtesy of Robert Innis). Benzodiazepine receptors have been imaged with PET* (C) *using [C^{11}] flumazenil (figure courtesy of James Frost), and SPECT* (D) *using [I^{123}] iomazenil (figure courtesy of the first author). For all images the frontal lobe is located at the top, and the occipital lobe is at the bottom of each photograph. D_2 receptors are highly concentrated in subcortical regions—the caudate and the putamen. Benzodiazepine receptors are present in several cortical regions, with the highest densities in the occipital cortex. (See Color Plate 3.)*

the kinetics of brain uptake and the regional distribution of those compounds. Examples of the second type are SPECT studies of the benzodiazepine receptor using [I^{123}] iomazenil in which displacement of the radiotracer by several benzodiazepine agents was analyzed to provide a measure of their in vivo potencies. Those studies were relatively long (up to seven hours) and took advantage of the relatively long $T_{1/2}$ of I^{123}.

Potential clinical uses PET and SPECT studies are generally thought to provide clinically useful information in selected neurological conditions, including localization of seizure focus in medication-refractory epilepsy, grading of brain tumors, localization and confirmation of cerebrovascular disorders, and diagnosis or confirmation of Alzheimer's disease. However, no comparable clinical usefulness has been demonstrated for any psychiatric disorder. The potential applications in psychiatry include the diagnosis and the monitoring of the course of illness (if reproducible biological markers are identified) and the monitoring of drug therapy (if such expensive methods are proved to be more valuable than plasma-drug levels). For the near future the major application of brain imaging in psychiatry will remain limited to research studies.

FUTURE DIRECTIONS

Brain imaging offers great potential to expand the knowledge of both the structural and the functional components of brain biology in psychiatric illnesses. The field has attracted significant attention because it is a direct and relatively noninvasive method by which to study the living human brain. At times, the potential applications often seem limited only by the ability to develop appropriate probes for specific neurochemical systems. However, the history of psychiatry, like that of other fields, is replete with methodological fads that are subsequently discredited and that disappear into obscurity. The presently fashionable interest in brain imaging requires significant effort in the development and the careful testing and validation of the methods so that they are not inappropriately applied.

Although the structural and the functional methods were considered separately here, significant progress is likely to be made in the integration of multimodality imaging. For example, coregistration of an MR image with a PET or SPECT scan of the same patient allows regions of interest to be clearly identified on the high-resolution MRI and allows data to be measured on the redirected region of interest applied to the high-sensitivity functional image. Significant progress in computer-directed coregistration methods has already been achieved (Figure 1.10-16), and future research may develop methods to use the anatomical information to correct the partial-volume-effect errors found in the functional images.

The radiation exposure associated with PET and SPECT imaging is presently considered reasonably safe. However, the development of MRI and MRS techniques that have no radiation risks would clearly be preferable. Dramatic progress in

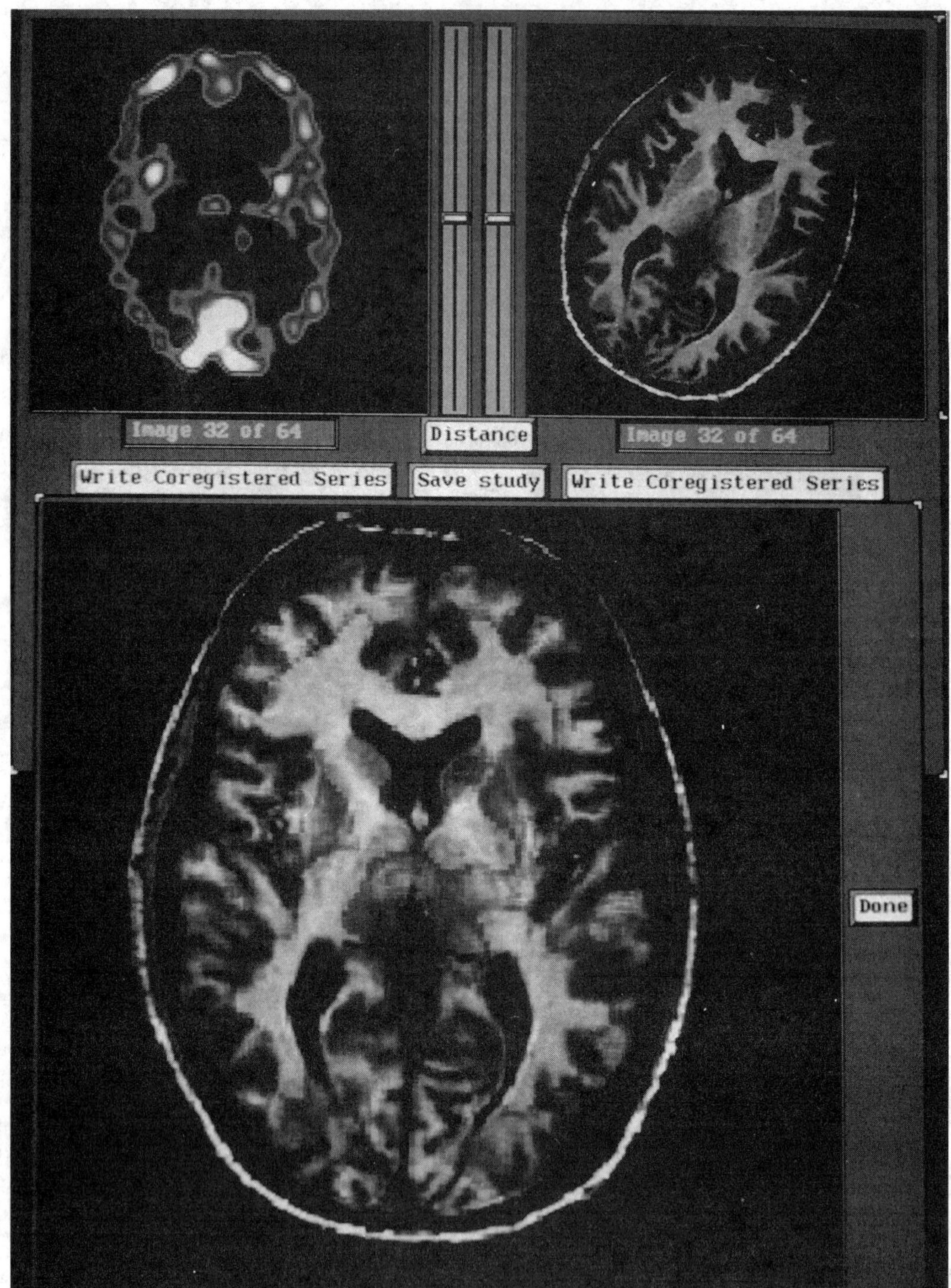

FIGURE 1.10-16 *Transaxial SPECT and MR images from a human subject studied with the benzodiazepine receptor radioligand, [I^{123}] iomazenil (Figure courtesy of the second author and Erik G Miller, CORITech Inc, New Haven, CT). Through a computer-assisted technique, the original three-dimensional MR image set (upper right) is mathematically transformed, interpolated, and resliced to match the SPECT series (upper left). The superimposed images (below) depict the precise anatomical distribution of [I^{123}] iomazenil, revealing highest concentrations of benzodiazepine receptors in cortical (particularly occipital) regions. (See Color Plate 3.)*

MRI instrumentation, computer software, and pulse-sequencing methods has brought image acquisition times of that structural modality into the dynamic range (hundreds of milliseconds). At the cutting edge of such developments, investigators at Massachusetts General Hospital have produced the first functional MR images of changes in cerebral blood volume after photic stimulation of the visual cortex. The trajectory of those advances suggests that future editions of this textbook will need to devote substantial attention to MRI as a functional imaging modality. In addition, MRS methods for the measurement of glucose metabolism may replace present functional methods. However, the higher sensitivity of functional imaging compared with MRI and MRS suggests that neurochemical targets present in low concentrations will continue to be measured by PET and SPECT.

SUGGESTED CROSS-REFERENCES

Brain-imaging techniques, including electroencephalography and magnetoencephalography, are discussed in Section 9.7. Neuroimaging in clinical practice is discussed in Section 2.10, and neuroimaging in geriatric assessment is discussed in Section 49.5c. The other sections in Chapter 1 discuss relevant neural sciences, particularly Section 1.2 on functional neuroanatomy and Sections 1.7 and 1.8 on applied electrophysiology.

REFERENCES

Abi-Dargham A, Laruelle M, Seibyl J, Rattner Z, Baldwin R M, Zoghbi S S, Zea-Ponce Y, Bremner J D, Hyde T M, Charney D S, Hoffer P B, Innis R B: SPECT measurement of benzodiazepine receptors in human brain with [^{123}I]iomazenil: Kinetic and equilibrium paradigms. J Nucl Med *35:* 228, 1994.

*Andreasen N C, editor: *Brain Imaging: Applications in Psychiatry.* American Psychiatric Press, Washington, DC, 1989.

Atlas S W, editor: *Magnetic Resonance Imaging of the Brain and Spine.* Raven, New York, 1991.

Belliveau J W, Kennedy D N, McKinstry R C, Buchbinder B R, Weisskoff R M, Cohen M S, Vevea J M, Brady T J, Rosen B R: Functional mapping of the human visual cortex by magnetic resonance imaging. Science *254:* 716, 1991.

Besson J A O: Magnetic resonance imaging and its applications in neuropsychiatry. Br J Psychiatry *157* (9, Suppl): 25, 1990.

David A, Blamire A, Breiter H: Functional magnetic resonance imaging: A new technique with implications for psychology and psychiatry [editorial]. Br J Psychiatry *164:* 2, 1994.

Farde L, Wiesel F A, Halldin C, Sedvall G: Central D_2-dopamine receptor occupancy in schizophrenic patients treated with antipsychotic drugs. Arch Gen Psychiatry *45:* 71, 1988.

Farde L, Wiesel F A, Nordstrom A L, Sedvall G: D_1 and D_2 dopamine receptor occupancy during treatment with conventional and atypical neuroleptics. Psychopharmacology *99:* 528, 1989.

Farde L, Wiesel F A, Stone-Elander S, Halldin C, Nordstrom A L, Hall H, Sedvall G: D_2 dopamine receptors in neuroleptic-naive schizophrenic patients. Arch Gen Psychiatry *47:* 213, 1990.

Fowler J S, Volkow N D, Wolf A P, Dewey S L, Schlyer D J, MacGregor R R, Hitzemann J L, Bendriem B, Gatley S J, Christman D: Mapping cocaine binding sites in human and baboon brain in vivo. Synapse *4*: 371, 1989.

*Hoffman E J, Phelps M E: *Positron Emission Tomography and Autoradiography: Principles and Applications for the Brain and Heart.* Raven, New York, 1986.

Innis R B, Al-Tikriti M S, Zoghbi S S, Baldwin R M, Sybirska E H, Laruelle M A, Malison R T, Seibyl J P, Zimmermann R C, Johnson E W, Smith E O, Charney D S, Heninger G R, Woods S W, Hoffer P B: SPECT imaging of the benzodiazepine receptor: Feasibility of in vivo potency measurements from stepwise displacement curves. J Nucl Med *32:* 1754, 1991.

Innis R B, Malison R T, Al-Tikriti M, Hoffer P B, Sybirska E H, Seibyl J P, Zoghbi S S, Baldwin R M, Laruelle M A, Smith E O, Charney D S, Heninger G, Elsworth J D, Roth R H: Amphetamine-stimulated dopamine release competes in vivo for [^{123}I] IBZM binding to the D_2 receptor in nonhuman primates. Synapse *10:* 177, 1992.

Innis R B, Seibyl J P, Scanley B E, Laruelle M, Abi-Dargham A, Wallace E, Baldwin R M, Zea-Ponce Y, Zoghbi S, Wang S, Gao Y, Neumeyer J L, Charney D S, Hoffer P B, Marek K L: Single photon emission computed tomographic imaging demonstrates loss of striatal dopamine transporters in Parkinson disease. Proc Natl Acad Sci USA *90:* 11965, 1993.

Jernigan T L: Techniques for imaging brain structure: neuropsychological applications. In *Neuromethods,* vol 17, *Neuropsychology,* A A Boulton, G B Baker, M Hiscock, editors, p 81. Humana, Clifton, NJ, 1990.

*Keshavan M S, Kapur S, Pettegrew J W: Magnetic resonance spectroscopy in psychiatry: Potential, pitfalls, and promise. Am J Psychiatry *148:* 976, 1991.

Lammertsma A A, Bench C J, Price G W, Cremer J E, Luthra S K, Turton D, Wood N D, Frackowiak R S J: Measurement of cerebral monoamine oxidase B activity using L-[^{11}C] Deprenyl and dynamic positron emission tomography. J Cereb Blood Flow Metab *11:* 545, 1991.

Laruelle M, Abi-Dargham A, Al-Tikriti M S, Baldwin R M, Zea-Ponce Y, Zoghbi S S, Charney D S, Hoffer P B, Innis R B: SPECT quantification of [^{123}I]iomazenil binding to benzodiazepine receptors in nonhuman primates. II. Equilibrium analysis of constant infusion experiments and correlation with in vitro parameters. J Cereb Blood Flow Metab *14:* 453, 1994.

Laruelle M, Baldwin R M, Malison R T, Zea-Ponce Y, Zoghbi S S, Al-Tikriti M S, Sybirska E H, Zimmermann R, Wisniewski G, Neumeyer J L, Milius R A, Wang S, Smith E O, Roth R H, Charney D S, Hoffer P B, Innis R B: SPECT imaging of dopamine and serotonin transporters with [^{123}I]β-CIT: Pharmacological characterization of brain uptake in nonhuman primates. Synapse *13:* 295, 1993.

Leenders K L, Salmon E P, Tyrrell P, Perani D, Brooks D J, Sager H, Jones T, Marsden C D, Frackowiak S J: The nigrostriatal dopaminergic system assessed in vivo by positron emission tomography in healthy volunteer subjects and patients with Parkinson's disease. Arch Neurol *47:* 1290, 1990.

Lock T, Abou-Saleh T, Edwards R H T: Psychiatry and the new magnetic resonance era. Br J Psychiatry *157* (9, Suppl): 38, 1990.

London E D: *Imaging Drug Action in the Brain.* CRC Press, Boca Raton, FL, 1993.

Lundberg T, Lindstrom L H, Hartvig P, Eckernas S A, Ekblom B, Lundqvist H, Fasth K J, Langstrom B: Striatal and frontal cortex binding of 11-C-labelled clozapine visualized by positron emission tomography (PET) in drug-free schizophrenics and healthy volunteers. Psychopharmacology *99:* 8, 1989.

Malison R T, Miller E G, Greene R, McCarthy G, Charney D S, Innis R B: Computer-assisted coregistration of multislice SPECT and MR images by fixed external fiducials. J Comput Assist Tomogr *17:* 952, 1993.

Mazziotta J C, Phelps M E: Positron emission tomography studies of the brain. In *Positron Emission Tomography and Autoradiography: Principles and Applications for the Brain and Heart,* M Phelps, J Mazziotta, H Schelbert, editors, p 493. Raven, New York, 1986.

Neumeyer J L, Wang S, Milius R A, Baldwin R M, Zea-Ponce Y, Hoffer E S, Al-Tikriti M, Charney D S, Malison R T, Laruelle M, Innis R B: [^{123}I]-2β-(4-iodophenyl)tropane: High-affinity SPECT radiotracer of monoamine reuptake sites in brain. J Med Chem *34:* 3144, 1991.

Oldendorf W H: *The Quest for an Image of Brain: Computerized Tomography in the Perspective of Past and Future Imaging Methods.* Raven, New York, 1980.

*Oldendorf W, Oldendorf W Jr: *MRI Primer.* Raven, New York, 1991.

Parker J A: *Image Reconstruction in Radiology.* CRC Press, Boca Raton, FL, 1990.

Petersen S E, Fox P T, Posner M I, Mintun M, Raichle M E: Positron emission tomographic studies of the cortical anatomy of single-word processing. Nature *351:* 585, 1988.

Pfefferbaum A, Zipursky R B: Neuroimaging studies of schizophrenia. Schizophr Res *4:* 193, 1991.

Prichard J W. Magnetic resonance spectroscopy of cerebral metabolism in vivo. In *Diseases of the Nervous System: Clinical Neurobiology,* ed 2, A K Asbury, G M McKhann, W I McDonald, editors, p 1589. Saunders, Philadelphia, 1991.

Rosen B R, Aronen H J, Kwong K K, Belliveau J W, Hamberg L M, Fordham J A: Advances in clinical neuroimaging: Functional MR imaging techniques. RadioGraphics *13:* 889, 1993.

Sedvall G, Farde L, Persson A, Wiesel F A: Imaging of neurotransmitter receptors in the living human brain. Arch Gen Psychiatry *43:* 995, 1986.

*Shulman R G, Blamire A M, Rothman D L, McCarthy G: Nuclear magnetic resonance imaging and spectroscopy of human brain function [review]. Proc Natl Acad Sci USA *90:* 3127, 1993.

Wong D F, Wagner H N, Tune L E, Dannals R F, Pearlson G D, Links J M, Tamminga C A, Broussolle E P, Ravert H T, Wilson A A, Toung J K T, Malat J, Williams J A, O'Tuama L A, Snyder S H, Kuhar M J, Gjedde A: Positron emission tomography reveals elevated D_2 dopamine receptors in drug-naive schizophrenics. Science *234:* 1558, 1986.

1.11 PSYCHONEUROENDOCRINOLOGY

DAVID R. RUBINOW, M.D.
PETER J. SCHMIDT, M.D.

INTRODUCTION

Psychoneuroendocrinology concerns itself with the relation between hormones and behavior. The relation is multifaceted. For example, hormones are capable of stimulating integrated behavioral responses, and hormone levels or dynamics may be altered by behavior or in a behavioral state-dependent fashion. In behavioral disorders, altered hormone levels or dynamics may serve as behavioral-state markers. Further, observed alterations in hormone activity may suggest central neuroregulatory systems that are pathophysiologically relevant and contribute to the phenomenology of the behavioral disorder. This section outlines the principles that underlie psychoneuroendocrinology and identifies the contribution of psychoneuroendocrinology to the understanding of behavior and of endocrine physiology.

BACKGROUND

HORMONES The mediators of interest in psychoneuroendocrinology are those cellular secretions that subserve intercellular communication. The secretions include a large array of substances with many functions, and the nature and the location of the function determine the class name applied to the substance. A *hormone* is a cellular substance that is secreted into the bloodstream and transported to a distant site, where it exerts its effects. A hormone that acts locally is called a *paracrine substance;* a hormone that regulates the function of the cell of origin has *autoregulatory* or *autocrine* effects. Neurons, like cells of the endocrine glands, are capable of secreting chemical substances involved in intercellular communication. Those substances that are released into the extracellular space by neurons and that cross a small gap (synapse) to act on other neurons are called *neurotransmitters.* Thus, the same substance (for example, norepinephrine or serotonin) may be called a neurotransmitter or a hormone, depending on whether it is released by a neuron or by an adrenal cell. In addition, many of the classic hormones have now been identified as coexisting in neurons with the classic neurotransmitters. Those hormones are often called *neuromodulators,* as they may modulate the effects of classic neurotransmitters; however, several of the neuromodulators appear to meet the criteria for a classic neurotransmitter, thus blurring the distinction between the terms. A *neurohormone* is a neuronal secretory product of specialized hypothalamic cells, neuroendocrine transducer cells, which convert an electrical signal *(neural impulse)* into a chemical signal *(hormone)* that is released from the median eminence into the portal hypophyseal bloodstream and carried to the pituitary to regulate the release of anterior pituitary hormones. Neurohormones, then, include the hypothalamic releasing (and release-inhibiting) factors—corticotropin-releasing hormone (CRH), growth hormone-releasing hormone (GHRH), somatostatin (somatotropin release-inhibiting factor [SRIF]), thyrotropin-releasing hormone (TRH), gonadotropin-releasing hormone (GnRH)—and oxytocin and vasopressin, hypothalamic hormones that are directly released from the posterior pituitary.

Several types of hormones exist: (1) *steroids,* which are derivatives of cholesterol that possess a four-ring structure and are synthesized primarily in the adrenals (glucocorticoids [cortisol] and mineralocorticoids [aldosterone]) and the gonads (estrogen, progesterone, testosterone), although steroids synthesized in the brain have recently been identified; (2) *peptides,* which are amino acid chains of about 40 or fewer amino acids, and proteins, which are long amino acid chains; (3) thyroid hormones; and (4) fatty acids.

CELLULAR MODES OF ACTION Steroids, in general, diffuse across the cell membrane and bind a receptor located in either the cytoplasm or the nucleus. The binding of the hormone to the receptor causes a change in the receptor (for example, phosphorylation) that enables the hormone-receptor complex to bind a part of the chromosomal deoxyribonucleic acid (DNA) that regulates gene expression or *DNA transcription* (formation of a ribonucleic acid [RNA] copy of a portion of the DNA). In addition to their effects on gene expression, steroid hormones may exert direct effects on the cell membrane (for example, alter ion flux or membrane potential) by several possible mechanisms. First, steroids or their metabolites can bind to and regulate the membrane receptors of other neuroregulators. Second, a membrane bound receptor for glucocorticoids has been identified, which is dissimilar to the classic intercellular glucocorticoid receptor. Third, steroids may modify the membrane lipid bilayer so as to increase or decrease the access of membrane receptors to their ligands. Those nongenomic mechanisms appear particularly important for the steroids that are synthesized in the brain (neurosteroids), such as the progesterone metabolites (and γ-aminobutyric acid [GABA]-A receptor modulators)—allopregnanolone and allotetrahydro deoxycorticosterone (DOC).

Peptides and proteins bind receptors that are located in the cell membrane. The ligand-bound receptor then activates or inhibits cellular second-messenger systems, such as cyclic adenosine monophosphate (cAMP) and phosphatidylinositol-diacylglycerol (PI-DAG), or regulates the opening and closing of membrane ion channels. A cascade of enzyme activations then occur, resulting in alterations in a number of cellular functions, including DNA transcription, cellular secretion, and response to other extracellular regulators.

Thyroid hormones are iodinated amino acids. Two tyrosines, each of which can bind two iodine atoms, join and form the two principal thyroid hormones, triiodothyronine (T_3 or liothyronine) and thyroxine T_4 or levothyroxine). T_3 is by far the more biologically potent hormone, both because it is less tightly bound to thyroid-binding protein (and hence more available to cells) and because it has a 10-fold greater affinity for the nuclear receptor for thyroid hormone. Despite the structural and biosynthetic dissimilarities between thyroid and steroid hormones, the thyroid hormone receptor is structurally similar to the steroid receptor and is part of the steroid-receptor superfamily, which includes the receptors for glucocorticoid, estrogen, testosterone, progesterone, and vitamin D, as well as thyroid hormone. Thyroid hormone, like the steroid hormones, appears to act by altering genomic transcription.

Eicosanoids are 20-carbon fatty acid derivatives of essential fatty acids (for example, arachidonic acid). Those substances—prostaglandins, thromboxanes, and leukotrienes—are powerful regulators of cellular activity that, because of their short half-lives, function primarily as autocrine or paracrine factors. The effects of the eicosanoids, which range from the regulation of hormonal and neural secretion to hormone-receptor modulation to chemotaxis, appear to be mediated, like the peptide hormones, by direct activation of membrane-bound second-messenger enzymes (for example, adenylate cyclase or phospholipase C).

HORMONE SECRETION AND REGULATION The brain endocrine system may exert its effects in several ways. First, brain hormones regulate peripheral hormone secretion through neuroendocrine axes (Figure 1.11-1). A typical neuroendocrine axis is shown in Figure 1.11-2. Under the control of neural inputs, a hypothalamic neuron secretes a neurohormone into the portal hypophyseal blood to regulate the release, by an anterior pituitary cell, of a second generation of hormones, which are released into the systemic circulation to act directly on cells (for example, growth hormone) or to stimulate the release of a third generation of hormones from peripheral endocrine organs. The secretion of the neurohormone or the releasing factor (or release-inhibiting factor in the case of SRIF) is in turn regulated by the second- or third-generation hormones. Second, neuromodulators that are either released locally in the extrahypothalamic brain or that are transported to the brain from peripheral sites are able to alter neuronal function in an integrated fashion, so as to produce changes in vegetative function and behavior. Thus, not only is the brain able, through the neuroendocrine axes, to regulate peripheral endocrine function, but the

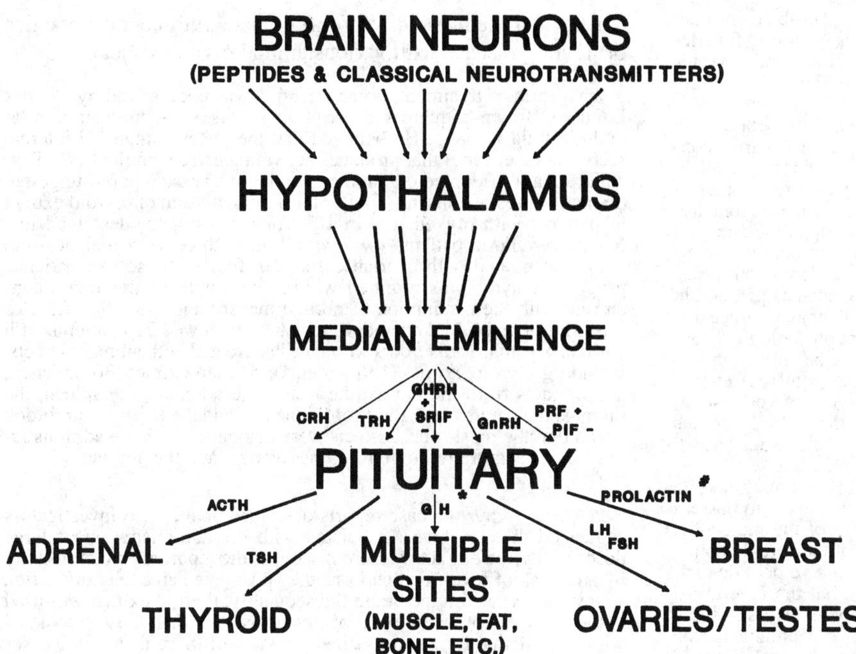

FIGURE 1.11-1 *Neuroendocrine axes. Neuroendocrine transducer cells in the hypothalamus secrete anterior pituitary regulatory factors into the portal hypophyseal blood system, which transports the factors from the median eminence to the anterior pituitary. The pituitary hormones that are released act at distant sites. (The feedback at the pituitary and the hypothalamus of the hormones secreted by the peripheral end organs is not shown.)*
#Unlike other anterior pituitary hormones, growth hormone has no specific end organ target.
**Unlike other anterior pituitary hormones, prolactin has no target gland negative feedback. Like growth hormone, prolactin release is regulated by both releasing factors (e.g., TRH) and release-inhibitory factors (e.g., dopamine).*

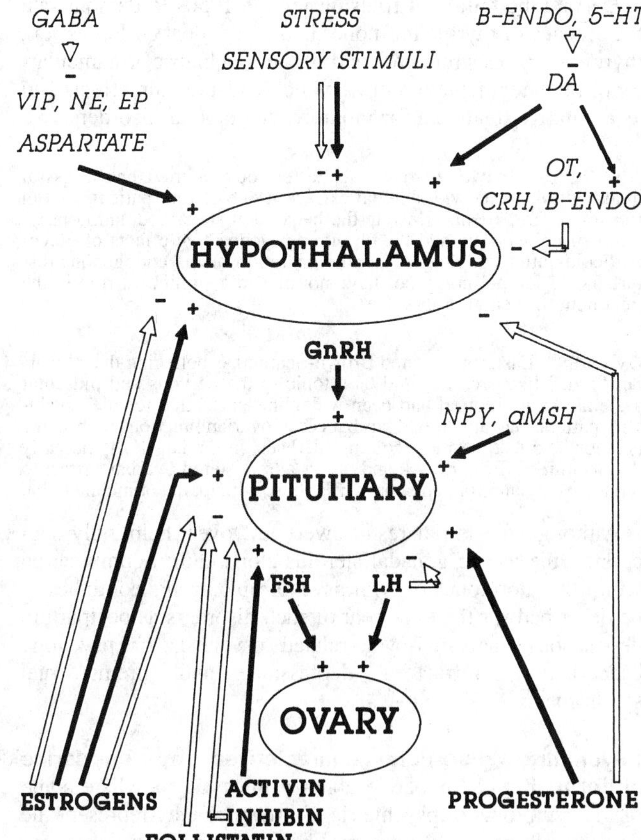

FIGURE 1.11-2 *The hypothalamic-pituitary-ovarian axis. Secretory products of the axis are in bold type, and modulators of the axis are in italics. Solid arrows indicate stimulation, and hollow arrows indicate inhibition. The ovarian products display feedback effects at both the pituitary level and the hypothalamic level.*

brain itself is the target for its own neuroregulatory secretions. Accordingly, some refer to the brain as the most prolific endocrine organ.

HORMONES AND BEHAVIOR

In addition to the widespread and selective distribution of hormones throughout the brain and their clear neuromodulatory function, the important role of hormones in behavioral regulation is suggested by three classes of observations: hormones as behavior regulators, structure-activity relations, and observed interrelations between endocrine and psychiatric disorders.

HORMONES AS BEHAVIOR REGULATORS Hormones are capable of activating neuronal aggregates in such a fashion as to orchestrate complex and coherent behaviors. The intracerebroventricular infusion of luteinizing hormone-releasing hormone (LH-RH) in rodents stimulates an integrated and complicated mating behavior; infusion of corticotropin-releasing hormone (CRH) activates and mediates the neuroendocrine, metabolic, circulatory, and behavioral components of the stress response. One investigator recently demonstrated that species-dependent pair bonding and affiliative behavior in small mammals called voles are mediated by oxytocin in the females and by vasopressin in the males.

STRUCTURE-ACTIVITY RELATIONS Elucidation of the process by which peptide hormones are synthesized and catabolized has revealed the regulatory potential of those chemical signals. In brief, intracellular chemical mediators stimulate or inhibit the reading of a segment of DNA by DNA polymerase and the generation (transcription) of a messenger RNA (mRNA) strand that is complimentary to the DNA segment. The mRNA is reassembled and modified in the nucleus and then transported to the cytoplasm, where it is read (translated) by the ribosome-protein complex and translated into a string of amino acids *(polypeptide)*. The polypeptide is then cut by enzymes to yield peptide hormones and subsequently may be further modified (posttranslational processing). In some cases the active hormone is a combination of two (dimer) or more peptide chains. Those chains may be identical (for example, activin) or different (for example, follicle-stimulating hormone [FSH], luteinizing hormone [LH], and thyroid-stimulating hormone [TSH], all of which share the same alpha chain but have different beta chains).

Four aspects of the process deserve amplification. First, peptides are cleavage products of larger prohormones. Those precursors may contain one copy or multiple copies of the peptide hormone or may contain multiple different peptide products. PreproTRH contains five copies of the TRH peptide; proopiomelanocortin contains the sequences for adrenocorticotropic hormone (ACTH), beta lipotropin, alpha melanocyte-stimulating hormone (MSH), and beta endorphin. The peptides liberated from the precursor reflect the activities of different enzymes, which in turn are regulated by intracellular factors, such as pH, and in a tissue-specific fashion. Thus, the same prohormone may produce different peptides in different tissues or under different physiological conditions. Similarly, the same genomic transcript may be spliced in different ways in a tissue-specific fashion so as to produce mRNA encoding different prohormones. The protachykinin gene gives rise to α-preprotachykinin, which yields substance P in the central nervous system (CNS), and to β-preprotachykinin, which yields substance P and substance K in the thyroid.

Second, metabolites of many peptides (ACTH, cholecystokinin [CCK], vasopressin, oxytocin, TRH, the endorphins) appear to possess striking biological activity. In addition, the activity of the metabolite may differ in potency, type, or direction from that of the parent peptide or sibling metabolites. For example, the nine-amino-acid peptide oxytocin interferes with learning and memory in rats, but the C-terminal tripeptide (three amino acids) fragment of oxytocin reverses some induced memory deficits. Moreover, although that tripeptide acts as a melanocyte-inhibiting factor, oxytocin has no effects on melanocytes, and the N-terminal pentapeptide (five amino acids) fragment of oxytocin is a melanocyte-stimulating factor. Similar metabolic modification of beta endorphin creates a hormone some believe to possess antipsychotic properties.

Third, minor differences in the formation or the structure of peptides can result in profound differences in activity. Vasopressin and oxytocin differ by two amino acids yet display opposite effects in a number of animal-learning paradigms; arginine vasotocin differs from oxytocin and vasopressin by only one amino acid but possesses its own unique set of activities.

Fourth, differences in the structure of peptide hormones determine the specificity of receptor-binding interactions and the susceptibility of the peptide to further metabolism. Subtle modification of a peptide (for example, acetylation) may protect the peptide from degradation, thus prolonging its duration of action and interfering with the formation of other potentially active metabolites. Alternatively, modification (for example, glycosylation) may eliminate the biological activity of the hormone, despite the fact that the measured level of the hormone is unchanged—that is, the assay recognizes the presence of the hormone, albeit biologically inactive. The role of peptide hormones in behavioral regulation is as complicated as the process of their biosynthesis and metabolism, for a disturbance of the process in any of a multitude of steps may result in an abnormal accumulation of biologically active peptides.

ENDOCRINE AND PSYCHIATRIC DISORDERS

Endocrine disturbances producing psychiatric disorders

A depression that in most respects is indistinguishable from major depressive disorder has been observed in association with both endogenous endocrine dysfunction (for example, Cushing's syndrome or hypothyroidism) and exogenous hormone administration (for example, glucocorticoids or thyroid hormones). Those behavioral disorders frequently (although not always) respond to the correction of the endocrine abnormality. Behavioral disorders have also been reported to be modulated by normal hormonal fluctuations across the menstrual cycle and precipitated by physiological, nontoxic levels of hormones (for example, progesterone). Since behavioral disorders are not uniform concomitants of endocrine disturbances, identification of those factors that predict or determine the behavioral response to normal or pathological hormone levels is critical to the understanding of the vulnerability to and pathogenesis of behavioral disturbances and psychiatric disorders.

Hormonal therapies for psychiatric disorders The therapeutic administration of hormonal preparations in both psychiatry and medicine dates from the late 19th-century practice of treating disease with various animal organ extracts.

That form of treatment, organotherapy, was popularized by Charles Edouard Brown-Séquard's description of his self-administration of orchitic fluid in 1889. He believed that the testes contain an internal secretion (spermine) that produces activating effects on the CNS. Psychiatry readily adopted organotherapeutics after case reports suggested dramatic cures of "insanity" after the administration of thyroid extract in patients with myxedema. In 1899 one investigator described five female psychotic patients (two with mania, three with melancholia) whom he treated with ovarian extract. In four of those five patients, psychiatric symptoms remitted within one month of treatment, concurrent with the resumption of normal menstruation. In 1900 Charles Easterbrook published a paper in which he reviewed 213 patients with various psychiatric disorders whom he had treated with animal extracts, including thyroid extract (130 patients), ovarian extract (36 patients), and extracts from the uterus, the testes, the adrenals, the spleen, the thymus, the parathyroid, the choroid plexus, and the brain. Easterbrook stated that the most robust effects were associated with the administration of extracts from the thyroid, the ovaries, and the adrenals.

THYROID After the case reports described above, two investigators suggested that the fever associated with the administration of large doses of thyroid extract was reminiscent of the reported cure of insanity by an attack of fever; on that basis they postulated an excitatory action of thyroid extract on the brain. Subsequently, thyroid extract was used in the treatment of many forms of psychosis other than those associated with myxedema. Easterbrook cited a review of more than 1,000 cases of treatment with thyroid extract for mental disorders, in which 17 percent recovered, 24 percent improved, and 59 percent showed no improvement. Easterbrook found only a 9 percent recovery rate in his series of 130 treatment-resistant patients. He stated that thyroid treatment was efficacious in female patients, however, particularly for insanities connected with childbearing. Easterbrook also described the efficacy of thyroid in the treatment of the manic state of *folie circulaire*.

Despite the failure of trials during the 1950s to demonstrate the efficacy of thyroid hormones in the treatment of depression, thyroid hormones remain a part of the psychiatric armamentarium in the augmentation of tricyclic antidepressant effects and as a putative treatment for rapid-cycling bipolar disorders.

ADRENALS In two separate trials Easterbrook reported the successful treatment of mania with adrenal extract in one of four patients and in four of seven patients. Despite the behavioral state-modulating properties of epinephrine and the observed psychoactive effects of glucocorticoids after the exogenous administration or the endogenous disturbances, adrenal hormones have not played a significant role in the treatment of mental illness.

OVARIES Easterbrook cited Brown-Séquard as believing that "ovarian fluid," like orchitic fluid, is a tonic to the nervous and muscular systems. In addition, it had been widely observed that female psychiatric patients had apparent disturbances of ovarian function and became amenorrheic just before becoming ill. Thus, in the late 19th and early 20th centuries, Easterbrook and others administered ovarian extract to female psychiatric patients, primarily those with mania or melancholia.

Although the initial results were not overwhelmingly successful, the use of gonadal steroids alone and in combination with other hormones or with psychotropic agents continues to be described for the treatment of such disorders as postpartum depression, menstrual-cycle-related psychosis or psychotic exacerbation, refractory depression, and premenstrual syndrome.

Psychiatric disorders characterized by endocrine abnormalities Endocrine abnormalities may mediate some of the symptoms of psychiatric disorders or may represent the downstream effects of a central chemical abnormality that produces both a psychiatric disorder and the endocrine abnormality. In the latter case the endocrine abnormality may provide a window into the brain, and knowledge of the physiological regulation of the hormone may suggest candidate systems for the pathological locus of the psychiatric disorder.

In general, three strategies have been used to study endocrine function in relation to psychiatric disorders. First, hormones are sampled cross-sectionally under basal conditions. Blood, cerebrospinal fluid (CSF), urine, saliva, and (in animal and postmortem studies) brain tissue have all been subjected to hormonal analyses with the hope that diagnostic group-related abnormalities (increases or decreases) in hormonal levels will be observed. One investigator observed increased plasma cortisol in depressed patients, a finding that initiated the ongoing search for the significance of hypothalamic-pituitary-adrenal (HPA) axis dysregulation in depression. In view of the dynamicity and the variability of endocrine secretion, single cross-sectional samples are of limited value.

A second strategy is that of sampling hormones (usually from blood or the CSF) over time to detect possible abnormalities of circadian secretion. Many hormones display characteristic patterns of secretion, peaks and valleys, over the course of the day. Those circadian patterns are centrally regulated, may be shifted or disturbed in the absence of a change in pulse secretion (for example, melatonin), and may evidence psychiatric disturbance-related neurodysregulation. The significance and the complexity of patterns of hormone secretion are discussed below.

A third strategy is that of provoking or challenging an endocrine system to determine if the response is normal. Several hypothalamic releasing factors (TRH, CRH, GHRH, GnRH) have been administered for that purpose, with the amount and the pattern of the stimulated pituitary hormone—TSH, ACTH, growth hormone (GH), FSH and LH—compared across diagnostic groups. Abnormal responses to those stimulation tests have been observed in several psychiatric disorders, particularly mood disorders. However, not all patients with a given psychiatric disorder display an abnormal response, nor is the abnormal response specific for any psychiatric disorder. The same is true for another dynamic test, the dexamethasone-suppression test, a challenge that measures the integrity of the CRH-ACTH-cortisol negative feedback system. Endocrine secretion is the product of multiple regulatory factors: physiological stimulators and inhibitors, circadian factors, stress, and peripheral feedback. Those multiple regulatory factors must be considered when one is attempting to infer what an abnormal hormone response reflects.

NEUROENDOCRINE MODULATION

A variety of factors may modulate the relation between hormones and behavior, illustrating the inadequacy of the conceptualization of the endocrine system as a system of chemical wires and circuits. Time, context, and control all appear to be capable of profoundly influencing the response to an endocrine signal.

TIME The timing of hormonal secretions is a critical component of the endocrine signal. For example, hormones such as GnRH and the gonadotropins (FSH and LH) are secreted in a pulsatile fashion, and much of their regulatory information and effect on their respective targets, the pituitary and the gonads, is conveyed by the pattern of pulsatility, its amplitude, and the interpulse interval. To attempt to infer the physiological significance of the hormone level independent of its pattern of secretion is tantamount to attempting to interpret a Morse code message that consists of only the total number of dots and dashes. If GnRH is administered in a pulsatile fashion to women with hypothalamic amenorrhea, normal ovulation and ovarian cyclicity will be restored. If it is administered continuously to normal women, anovulation and amenorrhea will result. Similarly, the rate of change of a hormone level may at times be more relevant than either the baseline or the poststimulation level. For example, ACTH secretion is inhibited by a glucocorticoid rate-dependent fast feedback system in which the rate of the rise of glucocorticoid, not the glucocorticoid level, is the factor that results in inhibition.

Several kinds of evidence suggest that prior exposure to a hormonal stimulus influences subsequent response to the same stimulus. In addition to the activating effects of hormones described earlier (that is, the direct and immediate cellular response to a hormone), organizational or long-term effects of hormone exposure have been observed. Neuropeptides affect many aspects of brain development (for example, neuronal proliferation, differentiation, organization of functional pathways), and alterations in hormone levels during development may alter brain structure and function and, consequently, behavior. For example, perinatal administration of opioids to rats produces an enduring increase in brain opiate receptors and long-term alterations in pain sensitivity in the adult animals. Similarly, perinatal administration of ACTH or an ACTH fragment (ACTH 4-10) enhances learning performance in adult animals and increases the spontaneous activity and aggression of adult animals when they are exposed to a novel environment. As many of the alterations observed in adult animals involve those behaviors that are ordinarily activated by the administered hormone, the developmental effects of perinatal hormones appear to be exerted on those neuronal systems that mediate the activational effects of the same hormone.

The significant effects of both the timing of a stimulus and the time elapsed after its application on subsequent response (to the same stimulus) are seen in studies of sensitization. Repeated administration of a stimulus may lead, over time, to profound long-term changes in behavioral or physiological response to the same stimulus; that is, the response to the stimulus grows and changes over time. It is not a cumulative response to repeated administration or stimulation, for without an obligatory passage of sufficient time between stimulations, sensitization does not occur. An example of hormonal sensitization in humans was provided recently by investigators who observed threefold increases in ACTH and beta endorphin after any of a series of infusions of the lymphocyte hormone interleukin-2 (IL-2) but who then observed almost 20-fold increases in IL-2-stimulated hormone levels when patients were reexposed to IL-2 after a treatment-free interval of as short as one week or as long as three months. Pharmacological sensitization and kindling (experimental epilepsy) studies ordinarily administer the stimulus repeatedly, but one investigator described a process of time-dependent sensitization in which the response to a stimulus changes simply with the passage of time after the initial administration of the stimulus. Thus, an exaggerated cortisol response to a stressor is seen if it was preceded by the administration of the stressor two weeks, but not two hours, earlier. Those studies suggest that responses to a stimulus change over time and provide a basis for understanding why differential responses to the same stimulus occur across individual persons.

CONTEXT The response to a hormonal stimulus depends on the context (both environmental and endocrine) in which it occurs. Vasopressin stimulates the absorption of water from the collecting duct in the kidney; however, that effect is inhibited by prostaglandin E_2, the level of which is directly related to the ambient glucocorticoid level. Estradiol may exert positive or negative feedback on its stimulatory hormone, FSH, in a menstrual cycle phase-dependent fashion. Gene expression can be stimulated or inhibited by glucocorticoids as a function of the ratio of two intracellular transcription regulators, c-fos and c-jun; that is, the intracellular context or state determines the response to a biological signal.

The environmental context may also determine the behavioral or physiological response to a biological stimulus. In a classic study, investigators observed that the behavioral response to an adrenaline infusion was entirely determined by the context (euphoria or anger) in which the person was placed. The adrenaline appeared to increase the intensity but not determine the quality of the experience. Other investigators observed context-dependent sensitization in which the repeated administration of high-dose cocaine sensitized both the behavioral and the biochemical (dopamine release in the nucleus accumbens) response to low-dose cocaine in rodents only if the low-dose cocaine was administered in the same cage as the high-dose cocaine; that is, if the animal received high-dose cocaine in a test cage and then received low-dose cocaine in the home cage, no sensitization was observed.

The endocrine environment may also provide a context that favors the facilitation or the extinction of certain behaviors. According to Donald Overton, in 1840 G. Combe anticipated the extensive literature on state-dependent learning when he wrote: ''Before memory can exist, the organs require to be affected in the same manner, or to be in a state analogous to that in which they were, when the impression was first received.'' Information learned in a particular context (for example, alcohol) is more efficiently retrieved if persons are in the same context at the time of retrial than if they are in a different state or context. Similarly, exogenous hormone administration (for example, progesterone) can create a context in which state-dependent learning can be demonstrated. The concept of state as a major determinant of the physiological or behavioral response to a stimulus (in which the output from a given input cannot be predicted without considering the context in which the events occur) has great explanatory potential for the variability of the behavioral and physiological responses to a given stimulus.

CONTROL The perception of control as a determinant of behavioral and physiological response is suggested by a variety of studies of the response to uncontrollable aversive stimuli. In those studies, animals developed a number of biological characteristics (depletion of forebrain norepinephrine, immune deficiencies—including decreased natural killer-cell activity and inability to reject implanted tumors—and opiate-mediated stress-induced analgesia) as a product of both repeated electrical shocks and the inability to terminate those aversive stimuli. Animals exposed to the same shocks at the same time but who were able to terminate the shocks by learning to press a lever did not experience the aforementioned biological changes.

The ability of perception of control to influence the response to a stimulus was demonstrated in a series of studies examining cerebral metabolic response (with a positron emission tomographic [PET] scan) to stimulation of reward centers in the brain, such as the medial forebrain bundle. The cerebral metabolic profile accompanying self-stimulation by the animal was different from that observed if the identical pattern of stimulation was exogenously administered.

The relation between biology and behavior (and perception) is clearly bidirectional. A series of studies demonstrated that both the endocrine response and the behavioral response to pharmacological and environmental challenges in primates are determined by the social status of the animal. In the squirrel monkey, for example, not only are plasma testosterone levels 2 to 50 times higher in the dominant male, compared with the subordinate male, but also the behavioral response to central oxytocin infusion is social status-dependent. The relation between hormones and behavior is far too complex to be adequately explained by simplistic unidirectional excess or deficiency models.

REPRODUCTIVE ENDOCRINOLOGY

The reproductive endocrine system offers a unique setting in which to investigate the relation between hormones and behavior for several reasons. First, the developmental neurobiological effects of the reproductive endocrine system have, in general, been studied more extensively than have those of other systems. Second, in addition to influencing neural organization, gonadal steroids modulate behavior, particularly (although not exclusively) a behavior—reproduction—that is critical for the survival of the species. Third, at least four relations between reproductive endocrine function and mood and behavioral disturbances have been observed and described (see below).

Although many of the neuroendocrine axes can adequately be described with cross-sectional stimulation and feedback loop diagrams, the female reproductive endocrine axis is a time-dependent endocrine cycle that requires, therefore, both cross-sectional and longitudinal schematization (Figures 1.11-2 and 1.11-3).

NORMAL CYCLING The first day of menstruation is, by convention, the first day of the menstrual cycle. Estrogen and progesterone levels are low then. GnRH is secreted in a pulsatile fashion from the hypothalamus and stimulates the secretion of FSH from the pituitary. FSH stimulates the secretion of estrogen from the ovarian follicles, resulting in the proliferation of the uterine lining. Estrogen and another ovarian hormone, inhibin, exert negative feedback on FSH release from the pituitary. At the end of the first menstrual cycle week, one follicle is selected and becomes the predominant follicle. That follicle undergoes maturation and secretes increasing amounts of estrogen.

The amplitude and particularly the frequency of GnRH pulses increase during the second menstrual cycle week, with the increasingly frequent GnRH pulses giving rise to a surge of LH secretion, the trigger for the expulsion of the egg from the follicle (ovulation) between 35 and 44 hours after the onset of the LH surge. Before the LH surge the rising estrogen levels through undetermined mechanisms suddenly exert a positive, rather than a negative, feedback on gonadotropin secretion and are responsible for triggering the LH surge. Ovulation marks the end of the follicular phase.

After ovulation and under the influence of LH stimulation, the remains of the ovarian follicle, the corpus luteum, secretes large amounts of progesterone and, to a smaller extent, estradiol. During that phase of the menstrual cycle, the luteal phase, the amplitude of the GnRH pulses increases, and the frequency greatly decreases under the influence of brain opiates. If fertilization and implantation of the egg do not take place, the corpus luteum atrophies. Progesterone levels precipitously decline, and that decline initiates the shedding of the uterine lining, menstruation, within approximately 14 days of ovulation. During the last few days of the luteal phase, declining estradiol levels remove the negative feedback on FSH secretion, thereby initiating the rise in FSH levels that will give rise to the next menstrual cycle.

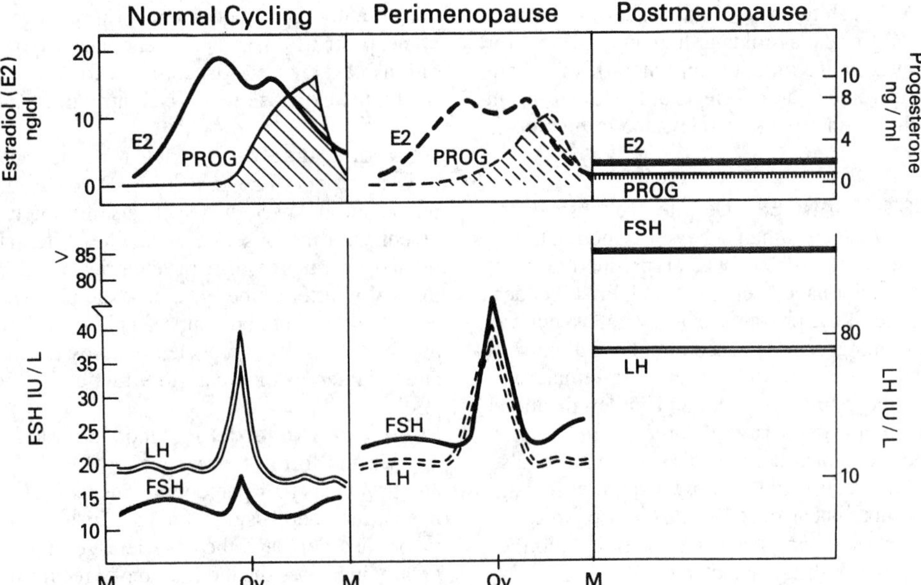

FIGURE 1.11-3 *Levels of the ovarian steroid estradiol (E2) and progesterone (PROG) (top) and the pituitary gonadotropic hormones follicle-stimulating hormone (FSH) and luteinizing hormone (LH) (bottom) at three phases of reproductive life. OV = ovulation; M = menses. The illustrated hormonal patterns for the perimenopause do not reflect intraindividual and interindividual variability in the frequency of ovulation and the length of the menstrual cycle during the phase.*

PERIMENOPAUSE AND MENOPAUSE As the number of viable ovarian follicles diminishes over the course of reproductive life, the ovary becomes progressively more insensitive to stimulation by FSH. As a consequence, FSH secretion is less restrained by estrogen negative feedback, and FSH levels begin to rise. That period of reproductive life is frequently, although not uniformly, characterized by increasing episodes of menstrual-cycle irregularity. When no remaining follicles can be recruited for oocyte development, estrogen levels remain low, no appreciable endometrial stimulation occurs, FSH and LH levels remain elevated, and menses ceases. That process, the *menopause,* is frequently defined retrospectively as the 12 months after the last menses.

The ratios of reproductive components and their levels change over the course of reproductive life. The perimenopause, for example, is characterized not only by increasing levels of FSH and decreasing levels of estrogen and progesterone but also by increased periods of estrogen exposure that is not opposed by progesterone, because of a decreased frequency of ovulation and subsequent luteal-phase development.

DEVELOPMENTAL NEUROBIOLOGY Gonadal steroids (estrogen, testosterone), like many steroids, have dramatic organizational effects; that is, exposure to gonadal steroids at a critical point in development produces long-term changes in brain morphology or function. Morphological changes consequent to perinatal exposure to gonadal steroids are seen at all levels of the CNS, including changes in the neuronal organelles; the size and the number of the neurons; the volume of the neuronal groups; the density of axonal arborization; the number, characteristics, and branching patterns of the dendrites; and the number and the patterns of synapses formed. Those effects of gonadal steroids on the central nervous system provide a basis for the *sexual dimorphisms*—that is, gender-related differences in brain structure or function. Sexual dimorphisms have been identified after comparing brain structure or function in females and males or the responses that occur after manipulating the gonadal steroid system. The organizational effects of exposure to gonadal steroids at critical developmental periods include the size (sexually dimorphic nucleus) or the existence (male nucleus of the ferret) of certain brain nuclei (both organized by androgens), cortical thickness and right-left cortical asymmetry (organized by androgens), the capacity to support cyclic gonadotropin secretion (eliminated by prenatal exposure to androgen), growth-hormone response to $alpha_2$ stimulation or autofeedback (androgen-dependent), reproductive or sexual behavior, and a variety of other nonreproductive behaviors (for example, play and aggression) that represent combinations of organizational and activational effects.

Three aspects of the organizational effects of gonadal steroids require emphasis. First, the reported sexual dimorphisms (morphological, physiological, behavioral) are species-dependent, with gender-related distinctions in humans far more subtle than those that appear in lower animals. Second, the effects are time-dependent and require exposure during specific windows of development. Prenatal androgen administration to a female ferret creates a male sexually dimorphic nucleus but does not alter mating behavior in the adult ferret, whereas postnatal administration does not influence the morphology of the sexually dimorphic nucleus but does result in male sexual behavior after reexposure to androgen during adulthood. Third, sexually dimorphic changes can include changes in both structure and function that no longer require the presence of the gonadal steroid beyond the critical period or changes in function that occur only on reexposure to the same steroid during adulthood.

In addition to the permanent, organizational effects, gonadal steroids have activational effects that are transient and do not require exposure during critical periods of development but that may display sexual dimorphism. Again, both structure and function are affected. Estrogen modulates (decreases) the protein constituents of cell membranes; those intramembranous particles and the patterns of brain synapses and dendritic spines vary in relation to estrogen levels in the estrus cycle of the rodent. In addition, estrogen increases the sensitivity to serotonin agonists and increases neuronal serotonin concentration and receptor density. Gonadal steroids bind neurons in a differential and regionally discrete fashion in the brain, where they act as major neuroregulators. To that extent, the behavioral effects of gonadal steroids display considerable redundancy and are not confined to single neuronal systems. For example, estrogen acts in the ventromedial nucleus to stimulate *lordosis behavior* (sexual receptivity) in the female rat by a variety of means: increasing receptor synthesis for progesterone, acetylcholine, oxytocin; increasing synthesis of enkephalin, LH-RH, and oxytocin; and increasing sensitivity to adrenergic stimuli.

Many of the above-described sexual dimorphisms occur in rodents, but some have been repeatedly identified in humans. For example, in some but not all studies, women have more cerebral blood flow and cerebral glucose metabolism than do men. Recent neuropsychological studies also suggest that men perform better than women in spatial tasks and worse than women in articulatory and fine-motor tasks, with those abilities varying over the menstrual cycle (and presumably with estrogen levels) in women. Although the role of the organizational and activational effects of gonadal steroids in human behavior (for example, cognition, vegetative function, and mood) is far from clear, the powerful neuromodulatory effects of those steroids in other species is such that their lack of relevance in humans is unimaginable.

BEHAVIORAL DISTURBANCES Despite the absence of specific mechanisms by which human behavior is modulated by gonadal steroids, at least four links between reproductive endocrine function and behavior have been identified. First, gender-related differences occur in the prevalence of several psychiatric disorders: males have a higher prevalence of antisocial personality disorder and alcohol-related disorders, and a female predominance exists in the eating disorders and in certain mood disorders, including major depressive disorder, rapid-cycling bipolar disorder, and mood disorder with seasonal pattern (also known as seasonal affective disorder). Those disparities in diagnostic prevalence do not appear to reflect differences in either health care-seeking behavior (and hence case identification) or in behavioral symptom-reporting characteristics.

Second, gender-related differences occur in response to psychopharmacological agents. Women are more susceptible than men to several psychotropic medication-induced side effects, such as tardive dyskinesia and tricyclic-induced mania, and the salutary therapeutic effects of the addition of T_3 to tricyclic antidepressants in partial responders or nonresponders are seen predominantly in women. In addition, both the endocrine response to pharmacological stimuli (for example, prolactin response to serotonin agonists) and the plasma levels of certain psychotropic agents, such as lithium carbonate, may vary as a function of the menstrual-cycle phase.

Third, gonadal steroids appear to exert psychotropic effects. In addition to the reports of the organotherapists mentioned above, recent studies have observed the successful treatment of psychiatric and behavioral disorders with gonadal steroids. Estrogen, for example, has been described as an efficacious adjunctive therapy in treatment-refractory depression in women, postpartum depression, and perimenopausal mood symptoms (even in the absence of estrogen-responsive hot flushes). Case reports suggest the efficacy of progesterone in patients with periodic psychosis. Gonadal steroid administration may also produce mood or behavioral symptoms. A premenstrual syndromelike symptom complex may appear in postmenopausal women when a synthetic progestogen is added to replacement estrogen, and many reports describe the appearance of marked depression, anxiety, irritability, or mood lability in association with oral contraceptives and postmenopausal hormonal replacement therapy. Anabolic androgenic steroid use is associated with cognitive, affective, and behavioral symptoms. To date, no clinical or biochemical factors enable one to predict reliably either the psychotoxic effects or the therapeutic effects of gonadal steroids in a given person.

Fourth, gonadal steroids may modulate the appearance or the severity of psychiatric disorders. For example, the menstrual cycle may interact with preexisting psychiatric disorders to influence their expression or timing. Case reports describe exacerbations during the luteal phase of the symptoms of several psychiatric disorders (major depressive disorder, schizophrenia, borderline personality disorder) and the menstrual-cycle entrainment of several psychiatric disorders, such as the periodic or atypical psychoses, which characteristically present with psychotic symptoms that are confined to the luteal phase. In addition to the modulatory effects of the menstrual cycle, periods of major reproductive endocrine change (for example, menarche, postpartum, and perimenopause) appear to represent conditions of increased susceptibility to the development or, more likely, the expression of psychiatric illness.

Menarchal disorders Menarche may interact with psychiatric disorders in several ways. Psychiatric disorders, such as mania and the periodic psychosis of puberty, may appear coincident with the onset of menarche. Alternatively, the gender-related prevalence of a psychiatric disorder may change dramatically after puberty. For example, eating disorders are equally prevalent in prepubertal boys and girls, but after puberty the female to male prevalence ratios for bulimia nervosa and anorexia nervosa increase to 9 to 1 and 19 to 1, respectively.

Postpartum disorders Mood disorders occur after childbirth in the form of depression (10 to 15 percent prevalence) and psychosis (0.1 percent prevalence). The best predictor of a postpartum depression is a past history or family history of mood disorders, and the experience of a postpartum depression greatly increases the likelihood of a recurrence (either puerperal or nonpuerperal). When psychosis, the severe form of puerperal mood disorder, occurs, the risk of a subsequent postpartum psychosis increases from 1 in 1,000 to between 1 in 4 and 1 in 7. Neither the phenomenology nor the prevalence of postpartum depression distinguishes it from the depression experienced by nonpregnant women in the same age group. However, the risk of psychiatric hospitalization in the month after pregnancy is sevenfold higher than the mean rate of hospitalization for the several years preceding pregnancy, and the risk of hospitalization for a psychotic disorder increases 25-fold. The puerperium, then, is a period of increased vulnerability to the expression of a mood disorder in those who may otherwise be predisposed to a mood disorder; the potential role of the dramatic hormonal changes during the puerperium is suggested by at least one report of the efficacy of estrogen in postpartum depression.

Menopausal disorders The relation between mood disorders and the menopause has been confounded by several methodological and conceptual problems. First, menopause in many studies is defined on the basis of age, rather than on the basis of a combination of clinical and hormonal measures, almost assuring the heterogeneity of women with respect to the critical variable, reproductive endocrine status. Second, the period of reproductive endocrine change that appears to be most relevant for mood change is the *perimenopause,* the time of decreasing ovarian sensitivity before the final menses (not the year after it, the definition of *menopause*). Third, many of the early descriptions of perimenopausal mood changes were similar to those of neurasthenia—increased worry, fatigue, decreased ability to cope—not depression, despite the relatively exclusive focus of psychiatry on involutional melancholia. Finally, controversy about the ability of the perimenopause to cause psychiatric syndromes obscures its possible role as a modulator of the expression of a psychiatric disorder. One investigator observed a bimodal peak for the onset of bipolar disorder in women (ages 20 to 30 and 40 to 50) but not in men; another investigator cited menopause as one of several factors that can induce the rapid cycling form of bipolar disorder.

Premenstrual syndrome Premenstrual syndrome (PMS) (called premenstrual dysphoric disorder in the fourth edition of *Diagnostic and Statistical Manual of Mental Disorders* [DSM-IV]) is a disorder that demonstrates the complexity of the relation between reproductive endocrine function and mood and behavior. Unlike other medical disorders, PMS is defined not so much by its symptoms as by the timing of the symptoms; that is, symptoms appear in the luteal phase of the menstrual cycle and then disappear soon after the onset of menstruation. The observed linkage of PMS to the menstrual cycle gave rise to causative hypotheses that posited an abnormality of gonadal steroids, of hormones or neurotransmitters that regulate or are regulated by gonadal steroids, or of neuroregulators that may mediate the effects of gonadal steroids on the CNS. The appearance in PMS of a variety of somatic symptoms (for example, bloating, abdominal swelling, and breast tenderness) that were believed to be normal concomitants of the luteal phase of the menstrual cycle (premenstrual molimina) further supported the belief that the symptoms of PMS (behavioral and somatic) must reflect abnormal reproductive endocrine function or differential sensitivity to and tolerance of gonadal steroid-induced physiological changes. To date, no disturbances of menstrual cycle hormonal function nor any luteal phase physiological abnormalities have been consistently identified to occur in PMS.

Even those differences in biological factors that have been identified in groups of patients with PMS compared with controls are not confined to the luteal phase but, rather, appear in both the follicular phase and the luteal phase. Those biological differences include the increased prevalence of abnormal TSH response to TRH, decreased slow-wave sleep, blunted growth hormone and cortisol response to L-tryptophan, phase-advanced temperature minima and offset of melatonin secretion, decreased red blood cell magnesium, and increased CRH-stimulated cortisol levels. If any of those biological findings are relevant to premenstrual syndrome, they must be related to the vulnerability to experience PMS symptoms but cannot by themselves explain the cyclic phenomena.

PMS, therefore, may reflect the occurrence of a trigger or cuing factor in the context of vulnerability to mood-state change. Without the special sensitivity or susceptibility, changes in gonadal steroids would not trigger entry into the PMS symptomatic state. That model is consistent with the best evidence to date for the relevance of gonadal steroids in premenstrual syndrome, the reported elimination of premenstrual syndrome by the suppression of ovarian cyclicity through medical or surgical means.

Evidence that PMS cannot be the product of reproductive endocrine events during the mid to late luteal phase has been provided by the authors, who observed the typical premenstrual syndrome symptom constellation in the context of an experimentally produced follicular phase. In the study the administration of a progesterone blocker with or without an ovarian-stimulating hormone (human chorionic gonadotropin) effectively blinded women with PMS to their menstrual cycle phase and showed that the elimination of the mid to late luteal phase had no effect on the subsequent characteristic appearance of PMS. Those findings suggest that PMS represents an autonomous mood state disorder that is linked to or entrained by but not caused by the menstrual cycle or, alternatively, represents a behavioral state that is triggered (but not caused) by hormonal events occurring earlier in the menstrual cycle than the mid luteal phase. The authors think that the relation between hormonal change and behavior and that the variability in the occurrence and the expression of behavioral disorders will be most fruitfully explored by attempting to define the interaction between mood state-triggering factors and the context that determines their effects.

SUGGESTED CROSS-REFERENCES

Section 1.5 discusses the processing of neuropeptides in detail, and Section 1.14 provides information on molecular biology techniques and transcriptional and translational processes involved in the synthesis of peptide and protein hormones. Section 9.7 describes the dexamethasone-suppression test and other tests. Chapters 16, 17, and 14 contain information on the hypothalamic-pituitary-adrenal axis, the hypothalamic-pituitary-thyroid axis, and the hypothalamic-pituitary-gonadal axis, respectively, and their relations to mood disorders, anxiety disorders, and schizophrenia. Sections 29.5 and 15.4 discuss in detail premenstrual dysphoric disorder and postpartum psychotic syndromes, respectively.

REFERENCES

Albert D J, Walsh M L, Jonik R H: Aggression in humans: What is its biological function? Neurosci Biobehav Rev *17:* 405, 1993.

Angst J: The course of affective disorders: II. Typology of bipolar manic-depressive illness. Arch Psychiatr Nervenkr *226:* 65, 1978.

*Antelman S M, Caggiula A R, Kocan D, Knopf S, Meyer D, Edwards D J, Barry H III: One experience with "lower" or "higher" intensity stressors, respectively, enhances or diminishes responsiveness to haloperidol weeks later: Implications for understanding drug variability. Brain Res *566:* 276, 1991.

Board F, Persky H, Hamburg D A: Psychological stress and endocrine functions: Blood levels of adrenocortical and thyroid hormones in acutely disturbed patients. Psychosom Med *18:* 324, 1956.

Denicoff K D, Durkin T M, Lotze M T, Quinlan P E, Davis C L, Listwak S J, Rosenberg S A, Rubinow D R: The neuroendocrine effects of interleukin-2 treatment. J Clin Endocrinol Metab *69:* 402, 1989.

*Dores R M, McDonald L K, Steveson T C, Sei C A: The molecular evolution of neuropeptides: Prospects for the '90s. Brain Behav Evol *36:* 80, 1990.

Easterbrook C C: Organo-therapeutics in mental diseases. Br Med J *2:* 813, 1900.

Insel T R: Oxytocin—a neuropeptide for affiliation: Evidence from behavioral, receptor autoadiographic, and comparative studies. Psychoneuroendocrinology *17:* 3, 1992.

Kendell R E, Chalmers J C, Platz C: Epidemiology of puerperal psychoses. Br J Psychiatry *150:* 662, 1987.

Kukopulos A, Reginaldi D, Laddomada P, Floris G, Serra G, Tondo L: Course of the manic depressive cycle and changes caused by treatments. Pharmacopsychiatry *13:* 156, 1980.

*Martin J B, Reichlin S: *Clinical Neuroendocrinology.* Davis, Philadelphia, 1987.

Mellon S H: Neurosteroids: Biochemistry, modes of action, and clinical relevance. J. Clin Endocrinol Metab *78:* 1003, 1994.

Overton D A: State dependent learning and drug discrimination. In *Handbook of Psychopharmacology,* L L Iversen, S D Iversen, S H Snyder, editors, p 59. Plenum, New York, 1984.

Pfaff D W: Patterns of steroid hormone effects on electrical and molecular events in hypothalamic neurons. Mol Neurobiol *3:* 135, 1989.

Pfaff D W, Schwanzel-Fukuda M, Parhar I S, Lauber A H, McCarthy M M, Kow L-M: GnRH neurons and other cellular and molecular mechanisms for a simple mammalian reproductive behaviors. Recent Prog Horm Res *49:* 1, 1994.

Plotsky P M, Meaney M J: Early, postnatal experience alters hypothalamic corticotropin-releasing factor (CRF) mRNA, median eminence CRF content and stress-induced release in adult rats. Mol Brain Res *18:* 195, 1993.

Porrino L J: Neurochemical studies of brain reward systems. Abstr 26th Annu Meeting, Am Coll Neuropsychopharmacol, 1987.

Post R M: Transduction of psychosocial stress into the neurobiology of recurrent affective disorder. Am J Psychiatry *149:* 999, 1992.

Rondeel J M M, Jackson I M D: Molecular biology of the regulation of hypothalamic hormones. J Endocrinol Invest *16:* 219, 1993.

Rubinow D R: The premenstrual syndrome: New views. JAMA *268:* 1908, 1992.

Schmidt P J, Nieman L K, Grover G N, Muller K L, Merriam G R, Rubinow D R: Lack of effect of induced menses on symptoms in women with premenstrual syndrome. N Engl J Med *324:* 1174, 1991.

*Tallal P, McEwen B S: Neuroendocrine effects on brain development and cognition. Psychoneuroendocrinology *16:* 1, 1991.

Truss M, Beato M: Steroid hormone receptors: Interaction with deoxyribonucleic acid y and transcription factors. Endocr Rev *14:* 459, 1993.

Weiss S R, Post R M, Pert A, Woodward R, Murman D: Context-dependent cocaine sensitization: Differential effect of haloperidol on development versus expression. Pharmacol Biochem Behav *34:* 655, 1989.

Winslow J T, Insel T R: Social status in pairs of male squirrel monkeys determines the behavioral response to central oxytocin administration. J Neurosci *11:* 2032, 1991.

*Yen S S C, Jaffe R B: *Reproductive Endocrinology: Physiology, Pathophysiology, and Clinical Management,* ed 3. Saunders, Philadelphia, 1991.

1.12
IMMUNE SYSTEM AND CENTRAL NERVOUS SYSTEM INTERACTIONS

ANDREW H. MILLER, M.D.
ROBERT L. SPENCER, Ph.D.

INTRODUCTION

Until recently, the immune system, through a complex interplay of cellular interactions and soluble mediators, was considered to be autoregulated. However, new data has provided evidence that the central nervous system (CNS) may play an important role in the modulation of the immune response under physiological conditions. Furthermore, immune cells have been found to produce soluble factors that may have significant effects on brain function. Those findings highlight the importance of interdisciplinary efforts that combine the knowledge and the techniques of the neurosciences and immunology and indicate that neural-immune interactions may contribute to the maintenance of bodily homeostasis and the development of disease.

OVERVIEW OF IMMUNE SYSTEM

The immune system has the capacity to protect the body from the invasion of foreign pathogens, such as viruses, bacteria, fungi, and parasites. Moreover, the immune system can detect and eliminate cells that have become neoplastically transformed. Those functions are accomplished through highly specific receptors on immune cells for molecules derived from invading organisms and a rich intercellular communication network that involves direct cell-to-cell interactions and signaling between cells of the immune system by hormones called *cytokines.* The body's absolute dependence on the efficient functioning of the immune system is illustrated by the less than one-year survival rate of untreated infants born with severe combined immunodeficiency disease and the devastating opportunistic infections and cancers that arise during acquired immune deficiency syndrome (AIDS).

CELLS AND TISSUES The immune system must be able to survey all tissues of the body for the presence of infectious agents or neoplastic cells and to mobilize its effector components to specific sites in the body where infectious agents may invade. Therefore, an important requirement of the immune system is that it be systemic and mobile. Cells of hematopoietic origin largely accomplish that function. Immune cells, like all other blood cells, are derived from hematopoietic precursor stem cells, which in the adult originate in the bone marrow. The stem cells are pluripotent and are capable of differentiating into any one of the various mature hematopoietic cells. There are two major paths of differentiation that appear to be regulated in part by cytokines and other hormones (Figure 1.12-1). The lymphoid path leads to the formation of the mature lymphocytes—B cells, T cells, and natural killer (NK) cells; the myeloid path of differentiation leads to the other cells of the blood (some of which participate in the immune response), including the monocytes and the granulocytes, which include neutrophils, eosinophils, and basophils. Monocytes and basophils may further differentiate into macrophages and mast cells, respectively, which take up residence in tissues throughout the body.

Lymphocyte maturation occurs in *primary immune tissues.* In humans the bone marrow serves as the primary site for B cell maturation, and the thymus is the primary site for T cell maturation. An important part of the maturation process is the screening out of cells that are reactive to the body's own constituents *(self-reactive).* On maturation, lymphocytes exit the primary immune tissues and circulate through the bloodstream and the lymphatic system into and out of the secondary immune tissues, including the spleen and widely distributed lymph nodes. *Secondary immune tissues* provide a structure for interactions between different immune cells and circulating pathogens.

NATURAL AND ACQUIRED IMMUNITY The immune system is often divided on a functional basis into two separate categories: natural or innate immunity and specific or acquired immunity (Table 1.12-1). The components of natural immunity act in a relativelynonspecific manner against pathogens or infected cells and may be evolutionarily more primitive than the specialized B and T lymphocytes that mediate specific immunity. Operationally, however, the two modes of immunity interact and cooperate.

Natural immunity The cells mediating natural immunity do not require prior activation to be functional and, therefore, provide an important first line of defense against infectious agents during the early stages of an immune response. Phagocytic cells and natural killer cells are examples of immune cells mediating nonspecific immunity. Phagocytic cells, such as macrophages, destroy extracellular pathogens (for example, bacteria and parasites) by engulfing and degrading them. Natural killer (NK) cells destroy virally infected cells by binding to them and releasing cytolytic factors, including perforin and the cytokine tumor necrosis factor (TNF). NK cells also have the ability to recognize and destroy some neoplastically transformed host cells, especially those of hematopoietic origin, thus providing some protection against cancer. Complement factor proteins, produced by the liver, provide an important humoral component in nonspecific immunity. Those functionally linked proteins interact with one another in a highly regulated manner and subserve many of the effector functions of the immune system, including cell lysis, opsonization, activation of inflammation by attracting inflammatory cells (chemotaxis) and stimulating those cells to release chemical mediators of inflammation, and neutralization of antigen-antibody complexes that could damage tissues.

Acquired immunity T and B lymphocytes are the crowning achievement of immune cell specialization and evolution. Those cells account for both the diversity and the specificity of the immune response and for the adaptive aspect of the immune

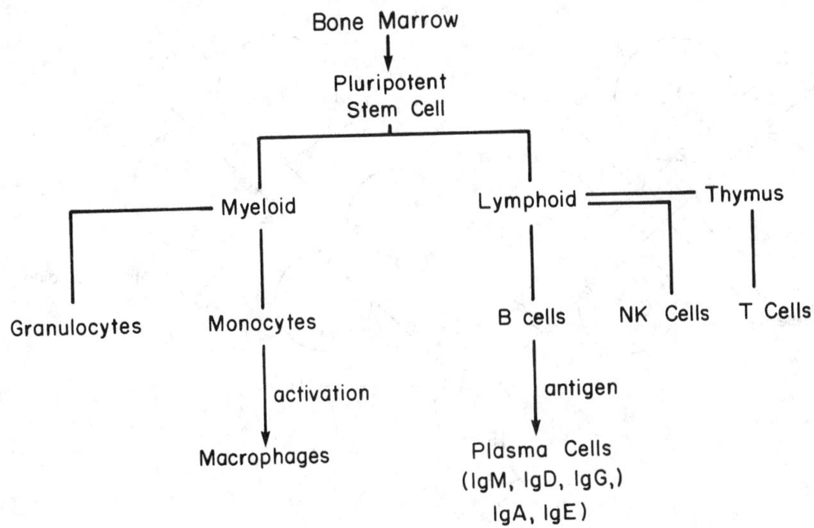

FIGURE 1.12-1 *Types of mature cells. All cells are ultimately derived from a pluripotent stem cell of bone marrow, which gives rise to myeloid or lymphoid progenitors that undergo further differentiation to mature cell types. Ig—immunoglobulin; NK—natural killer. (From A J Norin: Introduction to immunobiologic concepts. In* Depressive Disorders and Immunity, *A H Miller, editor, p 5. American Psychiatric Press, Washington,1989. Used with permission.)*

TABLE 1.12-1
Features of Natural and Specific (Acquired) Immunity

Feature	Natural Immunity	Specific (Acquired) Immunity
Physiochemical barriers	Skin, mucous membranes	Cutaneous and mucosal immune systems; antibody in mucosal secretions
Circulating molecules	Complement	Antibodies
Cells	Phagocytes (macrophages, neutrophils), natural killer cells	Lymphocytes
Soluble mediators active on other cells	Macrophage-derived cytokines; e.g., alpha and beta interferons, tumor necrosis factor	Lymphocyte-derived cytokines; e.g., gamma interferon

From A K Abbas, A H Lichtman, J S Pober: *Cellular and Molecular Immunology.* Saunders, Philadelphia, 1991. Used with permission.

system. Furthermore, T and B cells are responsible for directing the immune response against foreign targets, rather than self components. An effective specific immune response includes three conceptually separate phases; an induction phase, in which the presence of an infectious agent or antigen is detected; an activation phase, which includes the proliferation and the mobilization of the immune cells relevant to the eradication of the infectious agent; and an action or effector phase, in which the infectious agent is neutralized and eliminated.

INDUCTION PHASE Recognition of pathogens or neoplastically transformed cells is achieved through specialized receptors for antigens on the surface of B and T lymphocytes. Antigens are foreign substances that induce specific immunity and typically include molecules derived from pathogens, such as viral subunits, enzymes, and bacterial cell wall glycoproteins. The B cell antigen receptor is a membrane-bound form of immunoglobulin (Ig). A related form of immunoglobulin is secreted as antibody by mature plasma B cells. Antibodies play a central role in humoral immunity and help to kill a variety of pathogens. Each immunoglobulin or antibody molecule has two identical antigen-binding sites, and those binding sites can recognize the tertiary structure of specific proteins and other molecules, such as polysaccharides and lipids, which are important components of infectious agents (Figure 1.12-2).

The T cell antigen receptor has a single antigen-binding site. Antigen recognition by T cells takes on an added level of complexity not inherent to B cells. The T cell receptor recognizes only fragments of protein antigens. In addition, the antigen fragments must be present in association with a class of cell surface molecules called the major histocompatability (MHC) molecules (Figure 1.12-3). Virtually all nucleated cells of the body express MHC molecules on their surface. Most cells express class I MHC molecules; some cells, usually of immune system origin, also express class II MHC molecules. The induction of a T cell response depends on the ability and the effectiveness of MHC molecules to bind and present antigen. Therefore, the repertoire of MHC molecule genes that a person inherits can contribute significantly to antigen presentation and ultimately to susceptibility to infectious diseases and autoimmune disorders. T cells are MHC class-restricted—that is, T cell receptors recognize antigen only in association with one or the other class of MHC molecules. All MHC class I-restricted T cells also express an invariant surface glycoprotein, referred to as *clusters of differentiation (CD)8.* All MHC class II-restricted T cells express a different invariant surface glycoprotein, referred to as CD4. CD8 and CD4 molecules assist the binding of T cells to antigen-MHC complexes and assist in subsequent T cell activation. Most $CD8^+$ T cells are cytolytic T lymphocytes (CTLs) that have the ability to lyse cells to which they bind, whereas most $CD4^+$ T cells are helper T cells that secrete cytokines on activation. Since macrophages have the ability to engulf, degrade, and process extracellular proteins and then display the processed bits of protein in conjunction with surface class II MHC molecules, those cells play an important role in presenting antigen to $CD4^+$ T cells.

All the receptors for an antigen on a particular B or T cell are identical and unique to that cell and its descendents *(clones).* A family of lymphocytes with identical antigen receptor specificity is called a *clonal line.* Diversity in antigen recognition is derived from the vast number of different B and T cell clonal lines present in each person. Such diversity is achieved by semirandom mixing and matching of sequences of deoxyribonucleic acid (DNA) that code for the antigen-binding portion of the T cell and B cell receptors. That process of genetic diversity has been estimated to have the capacity to generate in each person more than 10^8 different receptors with functionally distinct antigenic specificity. Such high diversity makes it likely that each person possesses some clonal line of lymphocytes with an antigen receptor specificity capable of binding to a portion of any pathogen that may be encountered. Thus, the specific recognition of pathogens by the immune system entails the clonal selection of lymphocytes that are specifically responsive to the infectious agent.

ACTIVATION PHASE The binding of foreign antigens by B cells and T cells is usually not sufficient to produce cell activation; an accessory signal must also be provided. Important accessory signals are generated by a group of cytokines called *interleukins* that are secreted by T helper cells and macrophages. T helper cells and macrophages cooperate (Figure 1.12-3). Macrophages secrete interleukin-1 and other cytokines that stimulate T helper cells to secrete interferon gamma (IFN gamma), which then increases the phagocytic ability of macrophages and increases their class II MHC expression, thus improving their antigen-presenting capacity. In addition, IL-1 stimulates T cells to produce IL-2 and express IL-2 receptors on their surface. IL-2 is an important cytokine that activates multiple lymphocyte functions (Table 1.12-2).

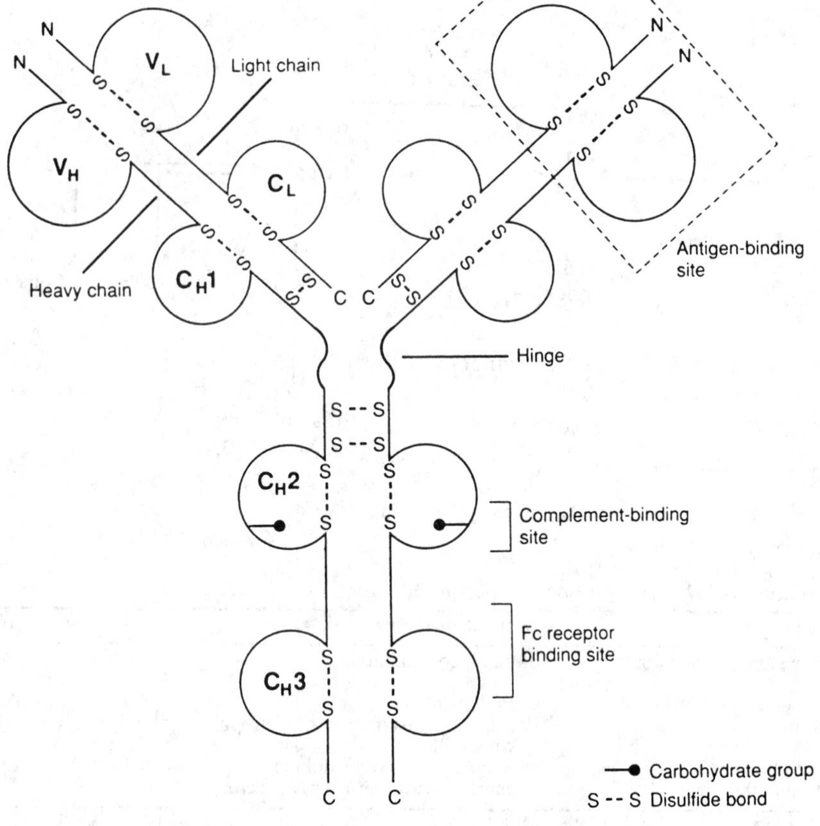

FIGURE 1.12-2 *Immunoglobulin Gr molecule. The antigen-binding sites are formed by the juxtaposition of variable (v) regions of antibody heavy chains (V_H) and antibody light chains (V_L). The locations of complement and F_C receptor-binding sites within the heavy chain constant regions are approximations. S--S refers to intrachain and interchain disulfide bonds; N and C refer to amino and carboxy termini of the polypeptide chains, respectively. (From A K Abbas, A H Lichtman, J S Pober:* Cellular and Molecular Immunology. *Saunders, Philadelphia, 1991. Used with permission.)*

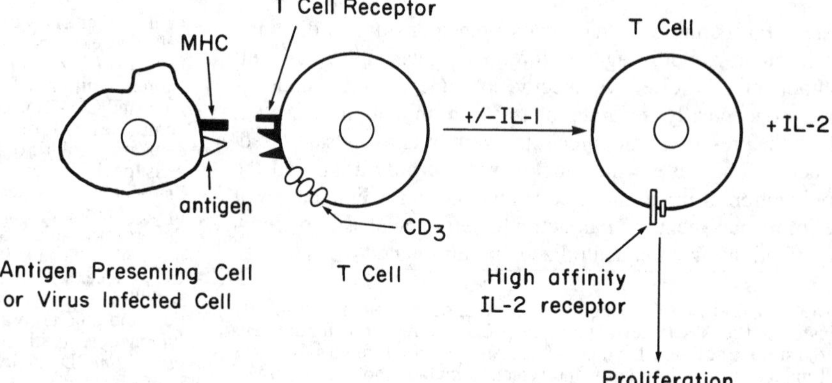

FIGURE 1.12-3 *Antigen is presented to T cells by virus-infected somatic cells or specialized antigen-presenting cells (e.g., macrophages) in association with class I or class II major histocompatability complex (MHC) gene products. The T cell receptor binds to the bimolar complex, resulting in engagement of the clusters of differentiation ($CD)_3$ complex and activation. In the presence of interleukin-1 (IL-1) (for some lymphocytes), stimulated cells then acquire high-affinity interleukin-2 (IL-2) receptors, permitting deoxyribonucleic acid (DNA) synthesis and cell proliferation on combination with IL-2. (From A J Norin: Introduction to immunobiologic concepts. In* Depressive Disorders and Immunity, *A H Miller, editor, p 9. American Psychiatric Press, Washington, 1989. Used with permission.)*

Recent evidence indicates that two subclasses of T helper cells secrete different cytokine profiles after stimulation. Those T helper (or Th) subsets have been best characterized in the mouse, in which Th1 cells secrete IL-2 and IFN gamma, resulting in CTL activation, whereas Th2 cells secrete IL-4, IL-5, and IL-6, which activate primarily B cells. Various cytokines and their effects are listed in Table 1.12-2.

After binding antigen in the presence of stimulatory cytokines, T and B lymphocytes with the appropriate binding sites are activated, leading to cell growth, division, and proliferation. Activation also results in the clonal expansion of immune cells with the identical high-affinity specificity for the foreign antigen. Some of the progeny during clonal expansion undergo further differentiation into mature effector cells, such as antibody-secreting plasma B cells, and CTLs. By contrast, some descendents of activated B cells or T cells become memory cells that are primed for activation on further stimulation by the same antigen. Reexposure to that antigen results in a secondary immune response *(acquired immunity),* which is usually more rapid and more robust than the first or primary immune response to that antigen. Memory cells may live for many years, thus providing long-lasting acquired immunity.

EFFECTOR PHASE The ultimate aims of an immune response are the neutralization and the elimination of pathogens. The principal effector mechanisms of acquired immunity are mediated by antibodies *(humoral immunity)* secreted from B cells and by cytolytic T cells *(cellular immunity).* Humoral immunity is especially effective in combating extracellular pathogens, such as bacteria and parasites; cellular immunity is effective in protecting against viral infection and, as with NK cells, may provide some protection against tumor cells.

The effector components of natural immunity are also recruited, enhanced, and directed toward specific pathogens as a result of the actions of B and T cells. For example, circulating antibodies can neutralize pathogens by binding to and coating the pathogens *(opsoniza-*

TABLE 1.12-2
Cytokines and Their Effects

Cytokines	Sources	Targets	Primary Effects
Mediators of natural immunity:			
Type I interferon (alpha IFN, beta IFN)	Monocytes, macrophages, others	All	Antiviral, antiproliferative, increased class I MHC expression
		NK cells	Activation
Tumor necrosis factor (TNF)	Monocytes, macrophages, T cells	Neutrophils	Activation (inflammation)
		Liver	Acute phase reactants
		T cells, B cells	Costimulator
		Hypothalamus	Fever
Interleukin-1 (IL-1)	Monocytes, macrophages, others	T cells, B cells	Costimulator
		Hypothalamus	Fever
Interleukin-6 (IL-6)	Monocytes, macrophages, T cells	T cells, B cells	Costimulator
		Mature B cells	Growth
Mediators of lymphocyte activation:			
Interleukin-2 (IL-2)	T cells	T cells	Growth, cytokine production
		NK cells	Growth, activation
		B cells	Growth, antibody production
Interleukin-4 (IL-4)	$CD4^+$ T cells	T cells	Growth
		B cells	Activation, isotype switching to IgE
Transforming growth factor-beta (TGF-beta)	T cells, others	T cells	Inhibit activation and proliferation
		Monocytes, macrophages	Inhibit activation
Mediators of effector cell activation:			
Interferon gamma (IFN-gamma)	T cells, NK cells	Monocytes, macrophages, NK cells	Activation
Interleukin-5 (IL-5)	T cells	Eosinophils	Activation
		B cells	Growth and activation
Mediators of immune cell growth and differentiation:			
Interleukin-3 (IL-3)	T cells	Immature progenitors	Growth and differentiation to all cell lines
Granulocyte-macrophage colony stimulating factor (G-M CSF)	T cells, monocytes, macrophages, others	Immature progenitors	Growth and differentiation to all cell lines
		Committed progenitors	Differentiation to granulocytes, monocytes, and macrophages
Macrophage CSF	Monocytes, macrophages, others	Committed progenitors	Differentiation to monocytes, macrophages
Granulocyte CSF	Monocytes, macrophages, others	Committed progenitors	Differentiation to neutrophils, eosinophils, basophils
Interleukin-7	Fibroblasts, bone marrow stromal cells	Immature progenitors	Growth and differentiation to B cells

CD—clusters of differentiation; CSF—cerebrospinal fluid; MHC—major histocompatibility complex; NK—natural killer.
Adapted from A K Abbas, A H Lichtman, J S Pober: *Cellular and Molecular Immunology.* Saunders, Philadelphia, 1991. Used with permission.

tion). Pathogens that are opsonized are made susceptible to lysis by complement factors and phagocytosis. Natural killer cells and *phagocytic cells,* such as neutrophils and macrophages, have receptors for the Fc portion of antibodies. Furthermore, complement proteins bind to and are activated by the Fc regions of some types of antibodies. Thus, antibodies can link effector cells and cytolytic proteins of natural immunity with pathogens, lending a level of specificity that is not inherent in the effector processes themselves. Although a large diversity of antigen-binding domains are present in different antibodies, the rest of the molecule is highly conserved, and there are a limited number of different types of Fc portions *(isotypes)* of the molecule (Figure 1.12-2). Since the Fc portion of the antibody is the effector portion of the molecule, antibodies with different isotypes have different effector features (Table 1.12-3).

IMMUNE SYSTEM AND DISEASE The general effectiveness of the immune system in protecting the body against pathogens has been made dramatically clear by the extensive pathology that characterizes AIDS in persons infected by the human immunodeficiency virus (HIV). HIV selectively binds to the CD4 molecule on T helper cells and thereby gains entry and inhibits T helper cell function. Since T helper cells play a critical role in facilitating all aspects of specific immunity, the incapacitation of T helper cells by HIV has catastrophic effects on the immune system. AIDS patients become susceptible to a wide spectrum of pathogens, such as protozoa *(Pneumocystis),* bacteria *(Mycobacterium tuberculosis),* fungi *(Candida),* and viruses (herpes simplex). Furthermore, AIDS patients have a high incidence of malignant tumors, especially those known to result from virally induced cellular proliferation and transformation. The nervous system is also affected in many AIDS patients, as evidenced by memory loss and other nonspecific neuropsychiatric disorders. No evidence indicates that HIV directly infects neurons; however, the infection of macrophages in neural tissues may lead to the impairment of neuronal function.

At the other end of the spectrum from immunodeficiency is autoimmunity. A number of relatively common diseases—such as type I diabetes, rheumatoid arthritis, and systemic lupus erythematosus—have in recent times been suspected of resulting from a specific autoimmune response directed against self-antigenic components. Clear genetic links to the expression of autoimmune disorders are often associated with specific types of MHC molecules. In most cases, however, a genetic background is not sufficient for the expression of disease. For example, the much greater prevalence of rheumatoid arthritis and systemic lupus erythematosus in women than in men suggests that, at

TABLE 1.12-3
Antibody Isotypes and Their Features

Properties	IgM	IgD	IgG	IgA	IgE
Human adult serum level (Ig makes up 20% of all serum protein)	0.5–2 mg/mL	0–0.4 mg/mL	8–16 mg/mL	1–4 mg/mL	10–400 μg/mL
Activates complement	++++	–	++	–	–
Crosses placenta	–	–	+	––	
Binds to macrophages, neutrophils, and NK cells	–	–	+	–	–
Binds to mast cells and basophils	–	–	–	–+	
Primary role	Primary immune response	?	Secondary immune response	Mucosal immunity	Immediate hypersensitivity (allergic response); protects against parasites

Ig—immunoglobulin; NK—natural killer.

TABLE 1.12-4
Some Defined Clusters of Differentiation (CD) Molecules and Their Known Functions

CD Designation	Main Cellular Expression	Known Functions
CD2	T cells, NK cells	Adhesion molecule, binds CD58 and sheep red blood cells
CD3	T cells	Signal transduction from T cell receptor to cytoplasm
CD4	T helper cells	Involved in MHC class II restricted antigen recognition
CD7	Some T cells	Fc receptor for IgM
CD8	Cytotoxic-suppressor T cells	Involved in MHC class I restricted antigen recognition
CD16, 32, and 64	NK cells, neutrophils, macrophages, B cells	Low-, intermediate-, and high-affinity receptors for IgG
CD21	Mature B cells	Complement factor (C3d) receptor; Epstein-Barr virus receptor
CD23	Activated B cells, macrophages	Low-affinity receptor for IgE
CD25	Activated T and B cells and macrophages	Low-affinity IL-2 receptor
CD54	Broad	Adhesion molecule (ICAM-1)
CD58	Broad	Adhesion molecule for CD2
CD71	Activated T and B cells, macrophages	Transferrin receptor

ICAM—intercellular adhesion molecules; IgG—immunoglobulin G; IgM—immunoglobulin M; IL—interleukin; MHC—major histocompatability complex; NK—natural killer.

least in some cases, there may be a hormonal component to the expression of autoimmune diseases.

The extent to which the immune system provides protection against cancer is still undetermined. Several effector mechanisms of the immune system are capable of destroying tumor cells in vitro (NK cells, CTLs, and TNF). The relatively rare occurrence of nonvirally induced tumors in immunodeficient patients suggests that the immune system plays a role primarily in protecting against tumor-inducing viruses, rather than providing widespread tumor surveillance and elimination.

METHODS USED IN STUDYING THE IMMUNE SYSTEM

In vitro assays Much of the understanding of the immune system has been derived from in vitro studies. In vitro assays may be especially useful in dissecting the direct and indirect mechanisms by which neurally controlled factors can influence immune cell function. Two of the most widely used assays in the study of neural-immune interactions are assays that assess the proliferative capacity of lymphocytes and those that determine the cytolytic capability of CTL and NK cells.

For proliferative assays, mononuclear cells, including lymphocytes, are removed from the experimental subject and are challenged in vitro with a mitogenic stimulus. Commonly used mitogenic stimuli (including concanavalin A, phytohemagglutinin, pokeweed mitogen, and lipopolysaccharide) are glycoproteins derived from plant lectins or bacterial cell walls that have been found to polyclonally stimulate lymphocyte proliferation. Proliferation is monitored by the incorporation of hydrogen 3-thymidine into the DNA of the dividing cells. The limitations of proliferative assays are their notorious interassay variability and a limited understanding of the relation between the polyclonal proliferative response to a mitogen and the clonally selective proliferative response to a specific antigen or pathogen.

NK cell assays have been widely applied to studies of neural-immune interactions. Typically, immune cells, isolated from a subject, are incubated in vitro with chromium 51-labeled target cells. Lysis of target cells results in the release of chromium 51 into the incubation medium, which is then collected and measured.

Flow cytometry The development of monoclonal antibodies against specific immune cell surface markers, such as the various CD determinants, has been useful in monitoring and sorting subclasses of immune cells (Table 1.12-4). Fluorescently tagged monoclonal antibodies and the cells to which they bind can be detected by a laser-controlled flow cytometer. Clinically, flow cytometry has important applications in monitoring the proportion of subsets of immune cells in patients' peripheral blood. For example, a diagnostic feature of the onset of AIDS is the precipitous decline in the proportion of circulating CD4-positive cells. Experimentally, flow cytometry may be useful in studying the effects of various treatments and environmental factors on the proportion of immune cell subpopulations present in the various immune compartments.

REGULATION OF THE IMMUNE RESPONSE An effective immune response requires the cooperation of many components of the immune system, often resulting in the augmentation of each component's contribution to the overall immune response. However, the simultaneous indiscriminate amplification of all aspects of the immune system would not be efficient and, in fact, could be disastrous. An overactive immune system may contribute to autoimmunity; furthermore, the inflammatory component of immune responses can be damaging if not controlled, as is seen in immune complex diseases and septic shock. Therefore, regulation of the immune response is necessary to make sure that the response is energy-efficient, focused on the infectious agent, counterbalanced in a fashion that does not cause self-damage, and reversible once the pathogen has been eliminated. The modes and the extent of immune system regulation are still poorly understood.

Probably the most important form of *intrinsic regulation* of the immune system is mediated by the various cytokines. Several examples of facilitatory effects of cytokines have been cited; however, some cytokines, such as transforming growth factor-beta, also produce potent inhibitory effects on lymphocyte activation and proliferation (Table 1.12-2). In addition, some evidence indicates that a subclass of $CD8^+$ T cells (T suppressor cells) act primarily to suppress the function of other T cells, either by secreting inhibitory cytokines or by cytolysis. The isolation of a unique subset of T cells that has a predominant suppressor action has been elusive, and the details concerning T-suppressor cells await clarification. Another important mode of intrinsic regulation may result from the production of antibodies or T cells that bind to determinants (idiotypes) in the antigen-binding domain of other antibodies or T cell antigen receptors and serve to influence further antigen-antibody interactions.

Whether there is significant *extrinsic regulation* of the immune response remains to be established. However, recent evidence of neural-immune interactions indicates that extrinsic factors of central nervous system origin may play an important role in the modulation of the immune system.

EVIDENCE OF NERVOUS SYSTEM AND IMMUNE SYSTEM INTERACTIONS

IMMUNE CELL RECEPTORS As outlined in Table 1.12-5, cells from the immune system express receptors for a wide variety of molecules that are, in part, regulated by or derived from the nervous system. Historically, the first receptor to be characterized in lymphocytes was the β-adrenergic receptor. Subsequently, receptors for the other classic neurotransmitters have been described. As in the nervous system, receptors for the neurotransmitters in immune cells are located in the cell membrane and in most cases are coupled to G proteins and associated second-messenger pathways. Nevertheless, the biochemical mechanisms for the receptor-mediated activity of the majority of the molecules listed in Table 1.12-4 has yet to be fully elucidated.

Several important concepts from research on receptors in immune cells and tissues are central to understanding the effects of neurally derived molecules on immune function. First, the expression of receptors is heterogeneous. For example, of the two types of receptors for adrenal steroids, type I (commonly referred to as mineralocorticoid receptors) and type II (referred to as glucocorticoid receptors), only the type II receptor is expressed in the thymus, whereas both type I and type II adrenal steroid receptors are expressed in the spleen. Related to heterogeneity in receptor expression in immune cells and tissues is heterogeneity in receptor density. For example, of the three subsets of T cells, the number of β-adrenergic receptors is highest for T suppressor cells, followed by T cytotoxic cells and then T helper cells.

TABLE 1.12-5
Receptors for Chemical Messengers in Cells and Tissues of the Immune System

Neurotransmitters	Neuropeptides	Steroid Hormones
β-Adrenergic	Growth hormone	Adrenal steroids, types I and II
α-Adrenergic	Prolactin	Estrogens
Dopamine	ACTH	Progesterones
Serotonin	CRH	Androgens
Acetylcholine	Substance P	
Histamine	Somatostatin	
	VIP	
	Thyroid hormone	
	Endorphins, enkephalins	
	Vasopressin	

ACTH—corticotropin; CRH—corticotropin-releasing hormone; VIP—vasoactive intestinal peptide.

Heterogeneity of both receptor expression and receptor density is relevant for understanding the sensitivities of the various immune cells and tissues to circulating hormones and is important for determining the net effect of those agents on immune function in vivo. Thus, even though β-adrenergic agents generally inhibit lymphocyte function in vitro, the increased susceptibility of T suppressor cells to the inhibitory effect (secondary to increased receptor density) may paradoxically lead to an enhancement of the immune response in vivo.

Another important concept is that an increase of circulating hormone is not necessarily associated with the activation of receptors in all immune compartments. For example, stress-related increases in glucocorticoids are more effective in activating type II adrenal steroid receptors in the peripheral blood and the thymus than in the spleen. Thus, the microenvironment of any given tissue is critical in determining hormonal or neurotransmitter influences on immune function. Taken together with the heterogeneity in receptor density and expression, the findings suggest that the influence of any given molecule on the immune system is a function of (1) the type of cell that exhibits the relevant receptor, (2) the density of the receptors on that cell, and (3) whether that cell is located in an immune compartment that allows access of the relevant molecule to the receptor under the conditions being studied.

Cross talk between receptor-associated second-messenger systems is another important biochemical mechanism by which neurally derived or regulated molecules influence the immune response (Figure 1.12-4). For example, dual signaling through the β-adrenergic and T cell receptors can lead to a synergistic rise in cyclic adenosine monophosphate (cAMP), which may alter the early events in T cell activation. Changes in those early events may then influence the transcription of multiple genes, including the genes for interleukin-2 (IL-2) and the IL-2 receptor, as well as genes for other cytokines.

IN VITRO AND IN VIVO EFFECTS Numerous chemical messengers derived from or regulated by the nervous system are capable of altering immune cell function and distribution. Table 1.12-6 provides a necessarily simplified, representative listing of selected molecules and their effects. The immunolog-

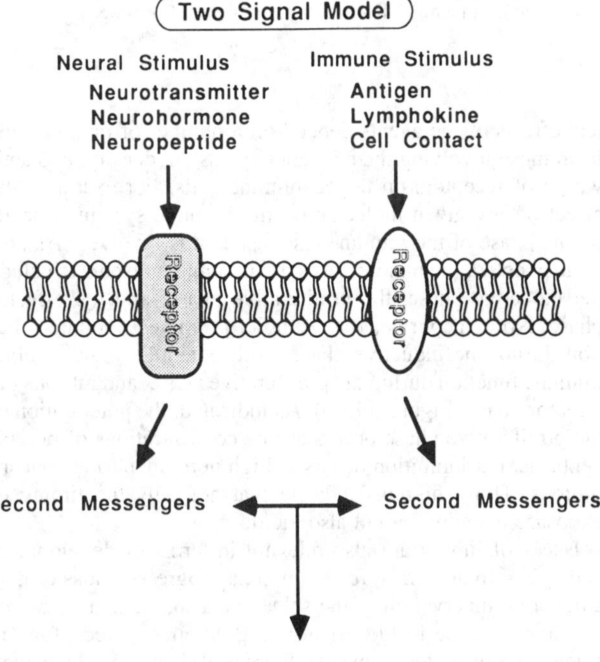

FIGURE 1.12-4 *Two-signal model of the interaction of neurally and immune-derived substances with their respective receptors on lymphocytes. The figure shows the potential cross talk between second messengers, with resulting modulation of lymphocyte function. The models assume that the lymphocytes are in G_0 of the cell cycle. (From T L Rozman, S L Carlson: Neural-immune interactions: Circuits and networks. Prog Neuro Endocrin Immunol 4: 71, 1991. Used with permission.)*

TABLE 1.12-6
Chemical Messengers and Their Immunological Effects

Chemical Messengers	Immunological Activity	
	In Vitro	In Vivo
Hormones:		
Adrenal steroids	Inhibition of IL-1, IL-2, and interferon; augmentation of IL-4 production; inhibition of NK activity, mitogen proliferation, and antigen presentation	Thymic involution, lymphopenia, monocytopenia, neutrophilia, suppression of inflammation and cell-mediated immunity
Estrogen	Inhibition of T suppressor-cell activity; increased macrophage phagocytosis and lysosomal activity	Lymphopenia; decreased mitogen responsiveness, NK activity, and macrophage phagocytosis
Progesterone	Decreased mitogen responsiveness at high concentrations	Increased skin graft survival; decreased $CD4^+$ cell numbers
Growth hormone	Enhancement of mitogen responsiveness and cytotoxic T cell activity; priming of macrophages for superoxide anion release; augmentation of neutrophil differentiation	Increased thymus size; augmentation of antibody synthesis, IL-2 production, mitogen responsiveness, and NK activity
Prolactin	Removal of PRL from culture media inhibits DNA synthesis and cell proliferation	Counteracts glucocorticoid-mediated immunosupression; PRL removal reduces NK activity and T cell proliferation and increases lethality of *Listeria* challenge
Neurotransmitters:		
Norepinephrine	Stimulation of T cell proliferation at low concentrations; high concentrations are inhibitory	Inhibition of NK cell activity and cytolytic T cell activity
Serotonin	Suppression of lymphocyte reactivity to mitogens and antigens at suprapharmacological concentrations	Suppression of humoral and cellular immune responses; enhancement of immune activity when serotonin availability is decreased
Neuropeptides:		
Endorphins	Enhancement of T cell proliferation, NK activity, cytokine production and generation of cytotoxic T cells	Mediation of immunosuppressive effects of stress on NK activity
Substance P	Enhancement of lymphocyte proliferation, monocyte chemotaxis, and monocyte production of IL-1, IL-6, and TNF; augmentation of IgA synthesis	Increased severity of adjuvant-induced arthritis; associated with hypersensitivity reactions and chronic inflammatory disorders
ACTH	Suppression of antibody production and disruption of macrophage-mediated tumoricidal activity	Activation of immunoregulatory glucocorticoids
VIP	Enhancement of monocyte chemotaxis; inhibition of Ig and IL-2 production; inhibition of NK activity and one-way MLR	Inhibition of egress of lymphocytes from sheep lymph nodes

ACTH—corticotropin; IG—immunoglobulin; IL—interleukin; MLR—mixed lymphocyte reaction; NK—natural killer; PRL—prolactin; TNF—tumor necrosis factor; VIP—vasoactive intestinal peptide.

ical effects of the agents depend on a number of factors aside from those involving the relevant expression, density, and activation of receptors on target immune cells. For example, the effect of any given molecule on the immune system depends on the phase of the immune response that is involved. As previously noted, the major phases of an immune response include the inductive phase, the proliferative phase, and the effector phase. Norepinephrine, for example, promotes immune function during the inductive phase, both potentiates and inhibits immune function during the proliferative phase, and inhibits the effector phase (Figure 1.12-5). As indicated, the potentiation of the proliferative phase occurs at low concentrations of norepinephrine, but inhibition occurs at high norepinephrine concentrations. Those findings indicate that not only the timing of exposure is important but also the dose.

Issues of timing are also relevant in terms of development and aging. In aged rats, for example, a progressive loss of noradrenergic innervation of the spleen is accompanied by a progressive increase in the density of β-adrenergic receptors on splenic lymphocytes. However, there is also an age-related dysfunction that involves impaired coupling between the β-adrenergic receptor and adenylate cyclase, indicating that noradrenergic agents may have variable, unpredictable effects on the immune function in old animals.

Related to the phase of the immune response and developmental stage of the animal is the type of immune response in terms of pathophysiology. Substances that are primarily inhibitory to immune function may promote tumor development in animals with cancer but may attenuate the development of autoimmune disease. For example, the administration of glucocorticoids accelerates the growth of tumors in mice. But glucocorticoids inhibit the development of several types of autoimmune disorders, including experimental allergic encephalitis (a model of multiple sclerosis) and streptococcal cell wall-induced polyarthritis (a model of rheumatoid arthritis).

Another important factor in determining the immunological effect of a particular molecule is its indirect effects, as well as its direct effects, on the immune system. In vitro studies provide important information on the direct effects of the various chemical messengers, but the influence of those agents in vivo may be completely different. For example, a number of in vitro studies have shown that opioid peptides are capable of enhancing natural killer (NK) cell activity. However, in vivo, opioid peptides play an important role in mediating the inhibitory effects of shock stress on NK cell activity, most likely through effects in the brain. In vivo, neurally derived molecules act against a complicated background of multiple hormones that may have synergistic or antagonist effects or both. For instance, prolactin antagonizes the effects of glucocorticoids on spleen mitogen responses in mice. Furthermore, many of the hormones and transmitters influence other bodily systems, including the cardiovascular system, which may influence the traffic of immune cells to various organs, immunological and otherwise. Changes in immunocyte distribution may ultimately have effects on cellular function.

NEURAL INNERVATION OF LYMPHOID TISSUES Historically, the identification of nerve fibers derived from the sym-

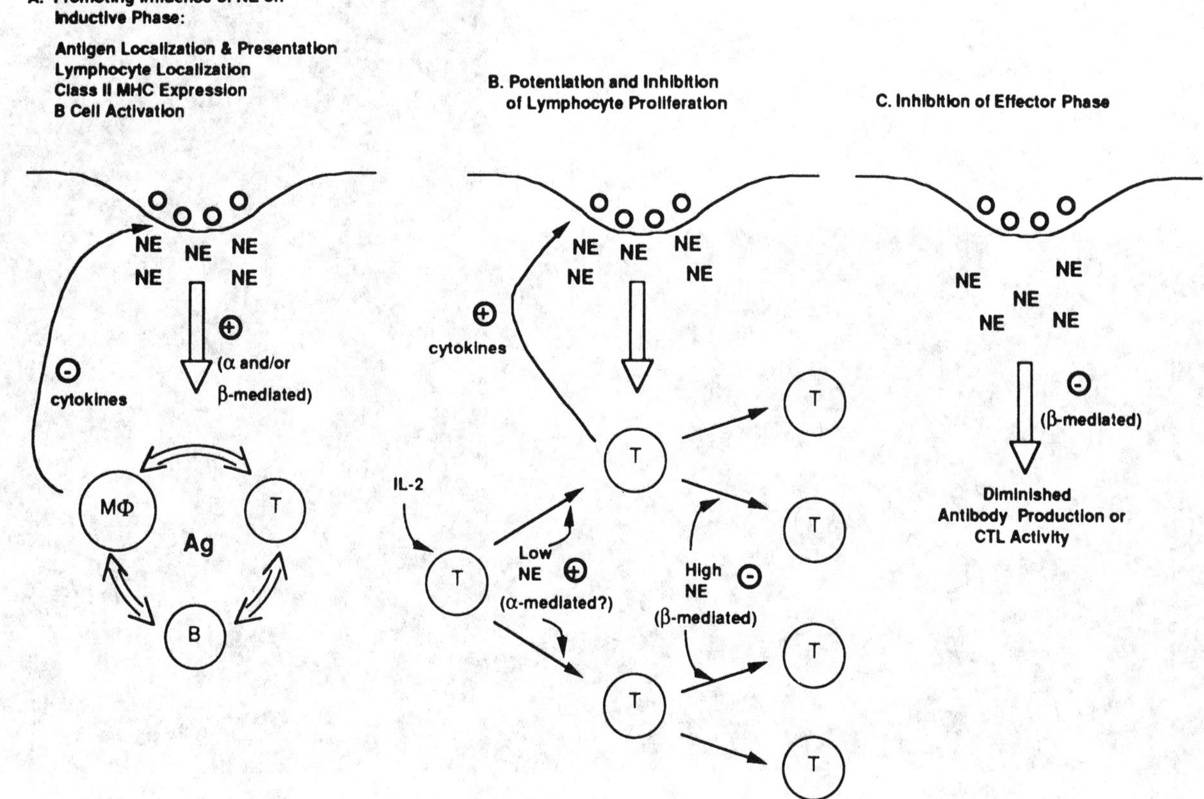

FIGURE 1.12-5 *Working model for bidirectional communication between norepinephrine (NE) and cells of the immune system. The diagram depicts the potential modulatory effects of NE during different phases of an immune response. The capacity for cellular responsiveness to NE depends on the presence of adrenoceptors, on cell type, and on the activational state. (A) In the presence of antigen, NE may have an enabling influence on lymphocyte and accessory cell function. For the proper balance between α-mediated and β-mediated effects, regulation of NE levels may be critical. (B) Low levels of NE may stimulate α-adrenoreceptors and thus potentiate lymphocyte proliferation. (B,C) With increasing NE, β-adrenoreceptor-mediated inhibition of lymphocyte proliferation and effector function may occur. The response to NE may be influenced by and may alter the production of cytokines, such as interleukin-2 (IL-2), and neuroendocrine peptides (not shown for clarity). Products of the immune system may modulate NE availability by altering release or turnover. Ag—antigen; CTL—cytolytic T lymphocyte; Mo—macrophage. (From K S Madden, S Livnat: Catecholamine action and immunologic reactivity. In* Psychoneuroimmunology, *R Ader, D L Felten, N Cohen, editors, ed 2, p 298. Academic Press, New York, 1991. Used with permission.)*

pathetic nervous system in immune tissues was one of the first indications that communication between the CNS and the immune system was possible. Sympathetic nerve fibers have been identified in organs that are responsible for the development, the education, and the function of lymphocytes. Specifically, nerve fibers are found in the bone marrow, the thymus, the spleen, and the lymph nodes. The nerves that innervate the thymus gland, for example, are derived from the vagus, phrenic, and recurrent laryngeal nerves and from the stellate and other small ganglia of the thoracic sympathetic chain. The nonmyelinated nerves that innervate the bone marrow arise from the level of the spinal cord associated with the location of the bone. The spleen obtains its sympathetic nerves from the celiac ganglion. Autonomic nervous system innervation of the lymph nodes is not as dense or as uniquely distributed as noted for the spleen and the thymus. In general, sympathetic nerve fibers enter the lymphoid tissues in association with the vascular supply. Because those nerves play an important role in vascular tone, their presence in association with the smooth muscle cells of the blood vessels is not unexpected. However, the nerve fibers travel with small blood vessels devoid of smooth muscle cells and are present in the parenchyma of the lymphoid tissue, associated not with blood vessels but with lymphocytes and other immune cells (Figure 1.12-6).

The existence of noradrenergic nerve terminals in the parenchyma of lymphoid tissues suggests that the release of norepinephrine in those areas may interact with the neurotransmitter receptors on nearby cells and ultimately influence their function.

Since catecholamines (including norepinephrine) have stimulatory effects on immune function at low concentrations and inhibitory effects at high concentrations, differential sympathetic nervous system effects on the immune response are possible, depending on local concentrations of catecholamines and the location of the immune cell relative to the point of neurotransmitter release. Chemical sympathectomy has variable effects on immune function, depending in part on the phase of the immune response studied. The reported effects of sympathectomy include suppressed antibody responses to sheep red blood cells, suppressed cytolytic T cell activity, and enhanced natural killer cell activity. Splenic sympathectomy also leads to an up-regulation of β-adrenergic receptors on lymphocytes and a decrease in suppressor lymphocyte function. Aside from the phase of the immune response, other factors that may influence the effects of nervous innervation on immune function include the animal's age, sex, and strain.

Nerves containing a variety of neuropeptides—including neuropeptide Y, substance P, vasoactive intestinal peptide, and calcitonin gene-related peptide—have also been identified in organs of the immune system. Those nerves and their distribution have not been as extensively studied as have noradrenergic nerve fibers, and their relative significance has yet to be determined.

CNS LESIONS AND CELLULAR IMMUNITY Some of the earliest studies demonstrating CNS involvement in the regulation of immune phenomena were those involving lesions in specific areas of the brain in laboratory animals. In a series of

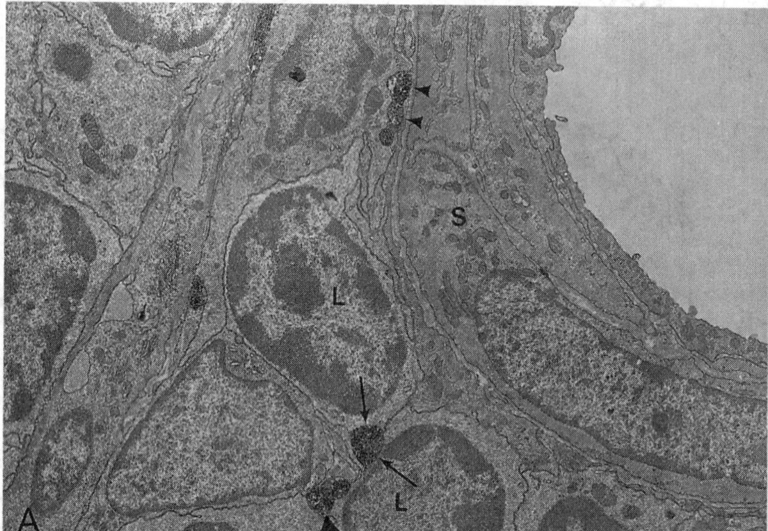

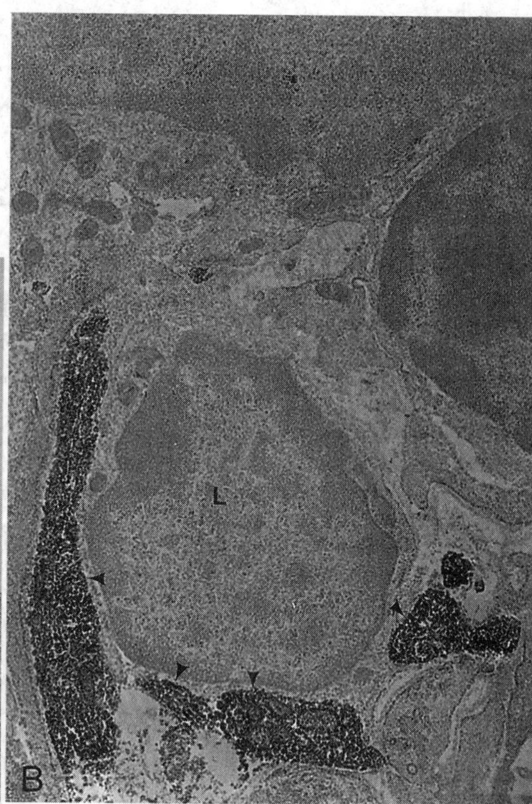

FIGURE 1.12-6 *Panel A. Tyrosine hydroxylase-immunoreactive nerve terminal (arrows) in direct contact with two lymphocytes (L), one of which has another terminal (large arrowhead) in contact with it. Terminals also contact (small arrowheads) the smooth muscle of the artery (S). Rat splenic white pulp. Transmission electron micrograph, x6250. Panel B. Tyrosine hydroxylase-immunoreactive terminals (arrowheads) circling a lymphocyte (l) and in direct contact with it for long distances in the rat splenic white pulp. Transmission electron micrograph, x3580. (From S Y Felten, D L Felten, Innervation of lymphoid tissue. In* Psychoneuroimmunology, *R Ader, D L Felten, N Cohen, editors, ed 2, p 67. Academic Press, New York, 1991. Used with permission.)*

experiments in the early 1960s, lesions of the anterior hypothalamus were found to protect guinea pigs from death by anaphylactic shock when compared with sham and control lesions. Such protection was not apparent with median and posterior hypothalamic lesions. Lesions of the anterior hypothalamus were also accompanied by decreases in thymus and spleen cell number, splenic mitogen responsiveness, antigen responsiveness, and natural killer cell activity. In contrast, bilateral electrolytic lesions of the hippocampus and the amygdala have been associated with increases in thymic and splenic mitogen responsiveness and no change in thymus and spleen cell number. Left-sided neocortical lesions have been associated with decreases in spleen T cell numbers, T cell mitogen proliferation, T cell cytotoxicity (measured in mixed lymphocyte cultures), and natural killer cell activity; those immune parameters were either unchanged or enhanced by right-sided lesions. B cell and macrophage responses were not affected by right-sided or left-sided neocortical ablations.

Some investigators have reported an increased prevalence in humans of immune disorders, especially those involving the thyroid and the gastrointestinal tract, in association with atypical cerebral dominance (left-handedness). The relation between cerebral dominance and immune dysfunction in humans lends support to the notion that lateralized alterations in CNS function may have differential effects on the immune response. However, some patients with brain tumors and head injuries have gross disturbances of in vitro lymphocyte function, and there is no evidence that the immune changes are related to the laterality of the lesion.

BEHAVIORAL CONDITIONING The notion that learning processes are capable of influencing immunological function is another example of interactions between the immune system and the nervous system. Several classical conditioning paradigms have been associated with the suppression or the enhancement of the immune response in various experimental designs. The conditioning of immunological reactivity provides further evidence that CNS events can have significant immunomodulatory effects.

Some of the first experiments on immunological conditioning were derived from the serendipitous observation that animals undergoing extinction in a taste-aversion paradigm with cyclophosphamide, an immunosuppressive agent, were noted to have unexpected mortality. In that taste-aversion paradigm, the animals are simultaneously exposed to an oral saccharin solution (the conditioned stimulus [CS]) and an intraperitoneal injection of cyclophosphamide (unconditioned stimulus [UCS]). Since the animals experience considerable physical discomfort from the cyclophosphamide injection, through the process of conditioning, they begin to associate the ill effects of cyclophosphamide with the taste of the oral saccharin solution. If given a choice, the animals avoid the saccharin solution (taste-aversion). The conditioned avoidance can be eliminated or extinguished if the saccharin is repeatedly presented in the absence of cyclophosphamide. However, it was observed that animals undergoing extinction of cyclophosphamide-induced taste-aversion unexpectedly died, leading to the speculation that the oral saccharin solution had a specific conditioned association with the immunosuppressive effects of cyclophosphamide.

Repeated exposure to the saccharin-associated conditioned immunosuppression during extinction might explain the unexpected death of animals.

To test that hypothesis, the researchers conditioned the animals with saccharin (CS) and intraperitoneal cyclophosphamide (UCS) and then immunized them with sheep red blood cells. At different times after immunization, the conditioned animals were reexposed to saccharin (CS) and examined. The conditioned animals exhibited a significant decrease in mean antibody titers to sheep red blood cells compared with the controls. Thus, the evidence demonstrated that immunosuppression of humoral immunity was occurring in response to the CS of saccharin alone.

Because the immunological effects of conditioned immunosuppression were not large, the influence of immunological conditioning on the development of a spontaneously occurring autoimmune disease in New Zealand mice was investigated. Those animals provide a standard model for the study of systemic lupus erythematosus, an autoimmune disorder that is similar to that found in humans and is fatal. Death in the New Zealand mice can be delayed by weekly injections of the cyclophosphamide. In the initial studies the animals were first conditioned with saccharin and cyclophosphamide and then divided into three groups: (1) saccharin only (CS group), (2) saccharin and cyclophosphamide (CS plus UCS group), and (3) no treatment. As shown in Figure 1.12-7, the animals given saccharin alone had a mortality rate as low as the animals receiving saccharin plus weekly injections of cyclophosphamide. Those findings again supported the notion that conditioned immunosuppression was occurring in response to saccharin alone.

The ability to condition immunosuppression with T cell-independent antigens and a graph versus host response has indicated that conditioned immunosuppression generalizes to both humoral and cell-mediated immunity. Furthermore, conditioned enhancement of natural killer cell activity in response to the CS, camphor, has been found after repeated pairing of the immunostimulant poly I:C with camphor odor. Recently, studies of conditioning of immune responses have been expanded to include demonstrations that environmental stimuli, such as those inherent in passive avoidance paradigms, can be associated with conditioned immunosuppression.

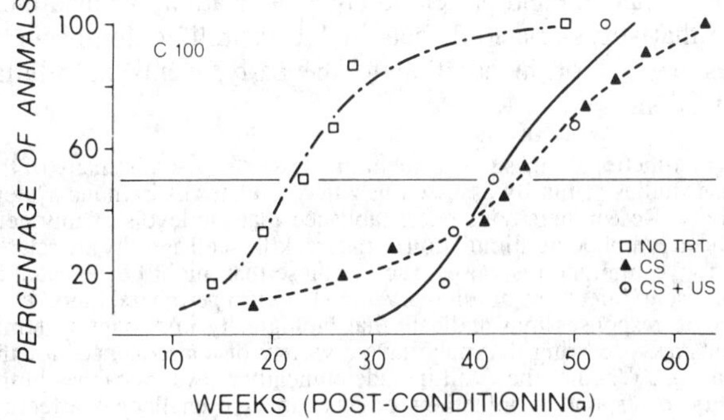

FIGURE 1.12-7 *Mortality rate in New Zealand female mice treated with saccharin and cyclophosamide (CY) weekly and then continued on a regimen of saccharin and CY (group CS + US, N = 6), continued on saccharin alone (group CS, N = 11), or deprived of both saccharin and CY (no TRT, N = 6). CS—conditioned stimulus; N—number; no TRT—no treatment; US—unconditioned stimulus. (From R Ader: Behaviorally conditioned modulation of immunity, In* Neural Modulation of Immunity, *R Guillemin, M Cohen, T Melnechuk, editors, p 63. Raven Press, New York, 1985. Used with permission.)*

STRESS AND THE IMMUNE RESPONSE Interest in the effects of stress on the immune system has grown out of a series of animal and human studies that suggest that stressful stimuli can influence the development of immune-related disorders, including infections, cancer, and autoimmune diseases. Experiments in animals in the late 1950s and the early 1960s, for example, indicated that a wide variety of stressors—including isolation, rotation, crowding, exposure to a predator, electric shock, and unprotective housing—increased morbidity or mortality to a number of conditions, including several types of tumors and infectious diseases due to both viruses and parasites. Critical variables in the effects of stress on illness in animals involved the timing of the stressor application and the type of infectious agent or tumor. For example, mice subjected to electric grid shock one to three days before the injection of Maloney murine sarcoma virus-induced tumor cells exhibited a decreased tumor size and incidence. In contrast, mice exposed to grid shock two days after tumor cell injection exhibited an increase in tumor size and number.

Fewer studies have been carried out on the relation between stress and immune-related illnesses in humans, and in general they are difficult to interpret because of the many factors that can influence both illness and illness behavior. Nevertheless, from prospective studies on upper respiratory infections verified either by physician diagnosis or by biological methods, evidence indicates that stressful life events can increase the susceptibility to infectious diseases in humans. For example, in a recent study investigators found that infection rates by five separate rhinoviruses administered intranasally were significantly greater in persons experiencing a high degree of psychological stress than in those under low stress. Prospective studies in humans on the development of cancer are mixed. Some studies have indicated a relation between depressive symptoms (presumably secondary to increased stress and inability to cope) and cancer development; others have been unable to replicate those findings. Once cancer has developed, however, data on women with metastatic breast cancer indicate that supportive group therapy may increase the time of survival by more than one year, although group therapy did not alter the mortality rates in the patients. Similar findings of increased survival have been found in patients diagnosed with malignant melanoma who were provided with a six-week structured psychiatric group intervention.

In an attempt to understand the potential mechanisms of the effect of stress on illness, researchers have focused considerable attention on the effects of stress on a variety of immune parameters in laboratory animals and humans.

Animal studies Early studies using 19 hours of tail shock showed that intense stress is capable of inhibiting mitogen-induced lymphocyte proliferation in the peripheral blood of rats. Subsequent studies have indicated that the stressor also inhibited natural killer cell activity and the production of interferon and interleukin-2 in the blood and spleen of rats. Since the early studies on tail shock, there has been an explosion of reports on the effects of many types of stress on virtually every aspect of immune function. In general, the stressors inhibit immune responses (Table 1.12-7). However, several studies using either chronic stressors or mild or brief stressors have noted an enhancement of both cellular and humoral aspects of the immune system. For example, in a study of mice exposed to 0.3, 0.8, or 1.2 milliampere of electric foot shock over a one-hour period, there was a graded enhancement of the proliferative response of T cells to the mitogen concanavalin A as the shock level increased. Proliferative assays using the B cell mito-

TABLE 1.12-7
Stress-Induced Changes in the Immune System of Rodents

Stressor	Subject	Immunological Effect
Restraint	Rat	Involution of the thymus
Restraint	Mouse	Decreased macrophage cytotoxic activity
Noise	Mouse	Decreased lymphocyte proliferation to mitogenic stimulation, reduced lymphocyte cytotoxicity; prolonged noise enhanced immune responses
Noise	Rat	Leukopenia
Isolation	Rat	Decreased lymphocyte proliferation to antigenic stimulation
Crowding	Rat	Increased lymphocyte stimulation to antigenic stimulation
Passive avoidance of learning task	Mouse	Decreased interferon production, delayed allograph rejection, decreased antibody response to challenge, increased death rate after antigenic challenge
Uncontrollable shock	Rat	Decreased natural killer cell activity, decreased interleukin-2 (IL-2) production, decreased IL-2 receptor expression
Heat stress	Mouse	Diminished delayed-type hypersensitivity

Table adapted from J M Weiss, S Sundar: Effects of stress on cellular immune responses in animals. In *Annual Review of Psychiatry,* vol 11, p 146. American Psychiatric Press, Washington, 1992. Used with permission.

gen lipopolysaccharide did not show any significant effect of the shock treatments on that measure of immune function. Differential effects of stress on various measures of the immune system have been further demonstrated in a study in which physical restraint in mice significantly depressed the cellular immune response to influenza virus infection without affecting the humoral response as measured by antiviral IgG antibody levels.

Stress-induced suppression of immune function may be related to the psychological state of the animal. One study suggested that coping is an important variable in stress effects on the immune system. Whereas phytohemagglutinin and concanavalin A stimulation of lymphocytes was suppressed in rats exposed to inescapable, uncontrollable electric shock for 80 minutes, followed by several minutes of tail shock 24 hours later, animals receiving the same total amount of shock using a yoked paradigm but able to terminate the stressor did not have decreased lymphocyte activity compared with nonstressed controls. Those findings are consistent with the hypothesis that the ability to cope with a stressor may mitigate against some of its noxious effects.

Human studies The effect of stress on measures of the immune system in humans has also attracted considerable attention. In studies on academic stress among medical students, a decrease in natural killer cell activity was found during the final examination period as compared with a preexamination baseline. Examination stress was also associated with changes in the number of T cells, mitogen responses, interferon production, and antibody titers to latent herpes viruses. Investigators have also reported decreased measures of immune function in persons exposed to chronic life stressors, such as divorce and the caretaking of Alzheimer's disease patients.

Conjugal bereavement is one of the most stressful of commonly occurring life events, and it has been associated with increased medical morbidity and mortality. One group investigated the effects of bereavement on immune measures in a prospective longitudinal study of spouses of women with advanced breast carcinoma. Lymphocyte stimulation was measured in men before and after the deaths of their wives. Lymphocyte stimulation responses to phytohemagglutinin, concanavalin A, and pokeweed mitogen were significantly lower during the first two months after bereavement compared with the prebereavement immune responses. The number of peripheral blood lymphocytes and the percentage and the absolute number of T and B cells during the prebereavement period, however, were not significantly different from those in the postbereavement period. Follow-up during the remainder of the postbereavement year revealed that lymphocyte stimulation responses had returned to prebereavement levels for the majority of the men but not all. Prebereavement mitogen responses did not differ from those of age-matched and sex-matched controls.

Immunological mechanisms Only recently have investigators begun to examine the immunological mechanisms through which stress may affect the immune system. In general, a stressor can alter immune function in two major ways. First, the stressor can lead to changes in the distribution of immune cells in any given part of the body. Since the immune response depends on the interplay of various immune cell subtypes, a redistribution of relevant cell types into or out of a particular immune compartment can directly influence the local immune response. Second, the stressor can alter the function of immune cells themselves. Studies have shown that stressors can alter a variety of cell-specific activities, including IL-2 production and the expression of the IL-2 receptor gene. In a study examining the biochemical mechanisms of stress-induced impairment of T cell mitogenesis, spleen cells isolated from rats exposed to two brief stressors (five minutes of restraint or two minutes of foot shock) exhibited a diminished response to both T cell mitogens and a combination of the phorbol ester, tetradecanoylphorbol acetate, and the calcium ionophore, ionomycin. Since stimulation with the latter two agents mimics early signals generated by mitogen surface receptor binding, including increased intracellular calcium and protein kinase C activation, the data indicate that stress-related defects in T cell proliferation occur at sites beyond or in addition to the early events in cellular activation.

The functional measures of the immune system used in many of the stress studies primarily assessed in vitro correlates of immune system activity. Researchers have not established that the levels of mitogen-induced lymphocyte stimulation or natural killer cell activity are related to in vivo immune responses, such as those that might be expected in response to infections or tumors. Altered in vitro peripheral blood lymphocyte responses may indicate that biologically important systemic events are occurring that may have a variety of consequences for the organism. Whether they will include clinically relevant changes in the ability to respond to infections or other in vivo challenges affecting health outcome remains to be determined.

For example, a great deal of attention has been directed to the notion that stress and depression may influence immunocompetence in human immunodeficiency virus (HIV)-seropositive persons, thereby serving as cofactors in the progression of HIV infection to AIDS. Several recent studies have explored the relation of psychosocial factors and the number of T cell subsets among HIV-seropositive adults. No relation was found between life stress or depression and counts of helper T (CD4) lymphocytes, suppressor T (CD8) cells, or helper-suppressor T cell ratios in a cohort of 124 HIV-seropositive homosexual men. Furthermore, the stress and depression measures were not related to advanced illness or mortality over time. Nevertheless, the virulence of HIV may

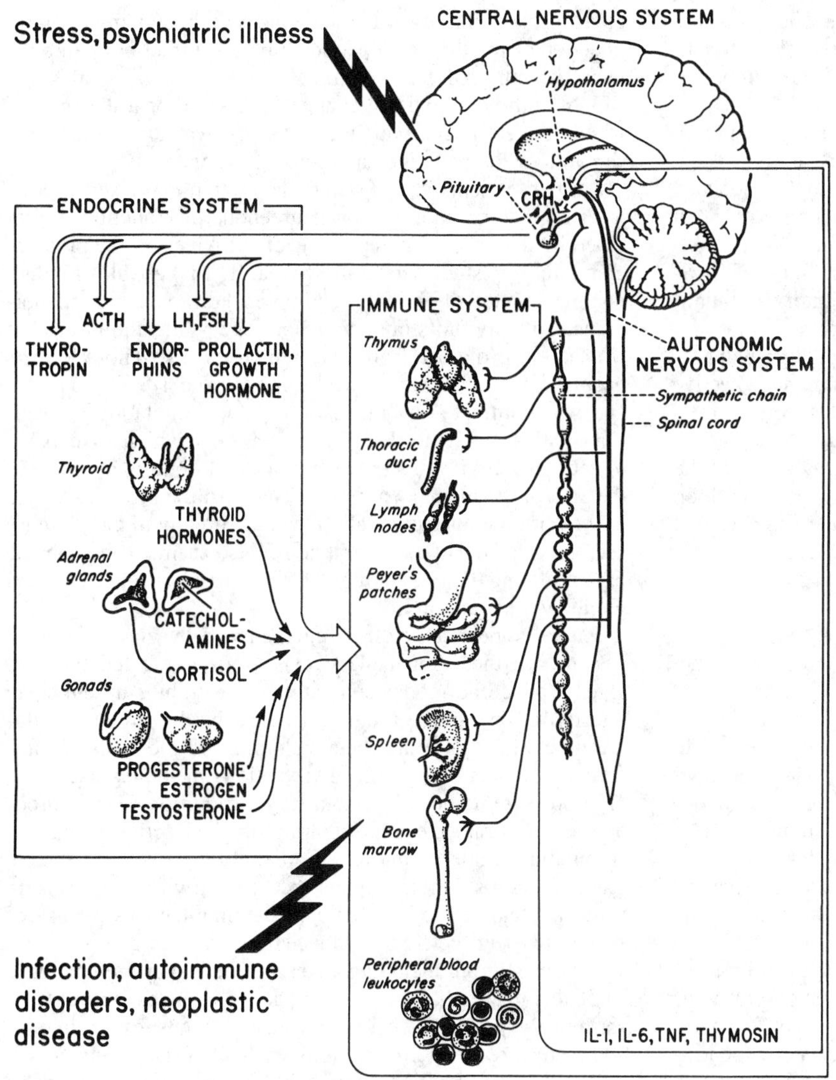

FIGURE 1.12-8 *Bidirectional communication between the central nervous system (CNS) and the immune system. The endocrine system and the autonomic nervous system are depicted as important mediators of CNS effects on the immune system. Inflammatory cytokines—including IL-1, IL-6, and tumor necrosis factor (TNF)—are shown closing the loop and interacting with the brain. ACTH—corticotropin; CRH—corticotropin-releasing hormone; FSH—follicle-stimulating hormone; IL—interleukin; LH—luteinizing hormone. (Drawn by Ellen Felten, Medical Arts Department, Mount Sinai Medical Center, New York, New York.)*

confound the psychosocial effects on immune measures. However, both those reports raise questions about the relation between, on the one hand, stress and measures of the immune system and, on the other hand, health and illness, and the reports suggest that psychosocial factors, such as stress, may not have a measurable or substantial effect on the immune system in relation to severe immunological disorders, such as AIDS.

Several recent animal studies have begun to address the issue of direct evidence of a causal relation among stress, immune alterations, and disease states. One study has found that rats exposed to an acute swimming stress exhibited decreased natural killer cell activity against a mammary tumor in vitro and an increase in tumor lung metastases when the same tumor cells were injected in vivo. In addition, investigators have shown that restraint stress in mice not only suppressed measures of the cellular immune response to a specific herpes simplex viral infection but also was associated with an increased herpes simplex virus local infection. Those two animal studies support the hypothesis that stress effects on tumors and infection are a result of stress-induced suppression of the immune system.

PUTATIVE MECHANISMS AND MEDIATORS

A number of studies have focused on the neuroendocrine mechanisms by which stress or alterations in CNS function may influence the immune response. The two systems that have received the most attention are the endocrine system, especially the hypothalamic-pituitary-adrenal (HPA) axis, and the autonomic nervous system (Figure 1.12-8). Those two systems are intimately associated with the organism's response to stress, and, as described in detail above, immune cells and tissues not only express receptors for the transmitters and hormones emanating from those systems but also receive direct innervation from autonomic nervous system fibers.

The interplay of the HPA axis and autonomic nervous system with the immune system has been the focus of numerous recent experiments. The data indicate that both the HPA axis and the autonomic nervous system have specific and selective effects on the immune system that are determined in part by which immune compartment and which immune response is examined. For example, after mild foot shock, investigators have found suppression of both splenic and peripheral blood lymphocyte responses to nonspecific T cell mitogens. Removing endogenous corticosteriods by adrenalectomy prevented the shock-induced suppression of the proliferative response of T cells in the peripheral blood. However, adrenalectomy had no effect on the stress-induced suppression of T cell proliferation in the spleen. But β-adrenergic receptor antagonism using propranolol (Inderal) and nadolol (Corgard) attenuated the shock-induced suppression of T cell proliferation in the spleen but had no effect on stressed-induced suppression of T cell mitogen responses in the peripheral blood. The findings that stress-induced changes of immune parameters in the peripheral blood are adrenal-dependent or pituitary-dependent, whereas stress effects on immune parameters in the spleen are related to catecholamine release, have been demonstrated in a number of laboratories using a variety of paradigms.

In addition to catecholamines, endorphins appear to play a role in stress effects on natural killer cell activity in the spleen. Rats subjected to a foot-shock paradigm known to be associated with opioid analgesia exhibited a decreased natural killer cell activity that was prevented by injections of the long-acting opioid antagonist naltrexone (Trexan). Much of the focus of CNS-immune interactions has emphasized the inhibitory immunological effects of neurally derived or regulated molecules, but several pituitary hormones, including prolactin and growth hormone, seem to have immune-enhancing or immunoprotective properties. For example, removal of the pituitary before stress resulted in a pronounced inhibitory effect of stress on a variety of immune parameters. Finally, the effects of cytokines on the nervous system and the endocrine system close the loop between the brain and the immune system and indicate that neural-immune interactions are bidirectional (Figure 1.12-8).

IMMUNE SYSTEM EFFECTS ON CNS AND ENDOCRINE FUNCTION

Research lending support to the idea of interactions between the immune system and the CNS includes the discovery that certain cytokines are capable of exerting profound effects on the CNS and neuroendocrine function. Acting at the level of the hypothalamus, the pituitary, and the adrenal glands, immune system products—including IL-1, IL-6, and TNF—appear to play a role in the regulation of sleep, temperature, feeding behavior, and the secretion of multiple hormones, most notably the glucocorticosteroids.

One group of investigators made electrophysiological recordings from individual neurons in the ventromedial hypothalamus at various time intervals after an antigenic challenge. The maximal increase in hypothalamic neuronal firing rate corresponded with the peak of the immune response, when presumably the release of immunological mediators is greatest. Furthermore, blood levels of glucocorticoids were noted to increase at that time of peak responsivity, whereas norepinephrine concentrations in the hypothalamus were found to be decreased. To determine whether cytokines were influencing hypothalamic norepinephrine concentrations and ultimately glucocorticoid secretion, the researchers injected supernatants from mitogen-stimulated lymphocytes into rats and measured hypothalamic norepinephrine concentrations. They saw a significant drop in norepinephrine concentrations two hours after injection. That decrease was similar to the decrease in norepinephrine seen during a normal immune response except that, as anticipated, the kinetics were much accelerated. Those studies have been repeated, using IL-1, with similar results. Thus, evidence exists that cytokines are capable of influencing the CNS and neuroendocrine function by acting at the level of the hypothalamus. Recently, IL-1 has been shown to exhibit direct stimulation of the secretion of hypothalamic CRH and, therefore, is capable of activating the neuroendocrine cascade, resulting in increased corticosteroid release. In addition, IL-1 beta and its messenger RNA have been found in nerve cell bodies and nerve fibers within the hypothalamus, the hippocampus, and other regions in human and rodent brains.

Thymic hormones, especially the thymosin peptides, have also shown the ability to stimulate the release of adrenocorticotropic hormone (ACTH), beta-endorphin, and glucocorticoids through activity at the level of the hypothalamus. Microinjection of the thymosin peptide, thymosin fraction 5, into the hypothalamus led to a significant increase in adrenal gland weight with no associated changes in thyroid or testes weight. In addition, intracerebral injections of thymosin $alpha_1$ were shown to selectively increase corticosterone levels.

Further evidence that the immune system may exert a powerful regulatory influence on neuroendocrine function is provided by data showing the effects of cytokines on the pituitary gland. In vitro studies have shown that IL-1 is capable of inducing the release of ACTH, leutinizing hormone, growth hormone, and thyroid-stimulating hormone while inhibiting the release of prolactin from rat pituitary cells. Those effects occurred at concentrations between 10^{-9} and 10^{-12} molar (M) and was eliminated by incubation of the stimulating preparations with antibody to IL-1. Brain glial cells, which are capable of secreting IL-1, are strategically located in large numbers in the area of the median eminance. That position provides access to the portal venous circulation leading directly to the pituitary secretory cells. Thymosin fraction 5 also seems to be capable of stimulating the secretion of ACTH in assays using a cultured monolayer of pituitary cells.

Finally, evidence of direct interaction between the immune system and the adrenal gland exists. Virus-infected lymphocytes produce hormones concomitantly with human leukocyte interferon. Two of the products are structurally similar to pituitary-derived ACTH and beta-endorphin on the basis of antigenicity, molecular weight, and retention time on reverse phase high-pressure liquid chromatography. In addition, the two products demonstrate the appropriate biological activity—that is, stimulating primary cultures of adrenal tumor cells to secrete glucocorticoids, binding opiate receptors in vitro, and causing analgesia and catatonia in mice. The simultaneous release of ACTH-like and beta-endorphin-like products in response to a variety of stimuli, including CRH, indicates that immunocytes (probably macrophages), like pituitary cells, are capable of transcribing the proopiomelanocortin gene, which is responsible for coding the precursor protein from which ACTH and beta-endorphin are derived. Other hormones found to be secreted by immunocytes include somatostatin, vasoactive intestinal polypeptide, thyrotropin, and prolactin. Lymphocyte production of an ACTH-like hormone suggests that immunocytes may be capable of tapping directly into the hypothalamic-pituitary-adrenal (HPA) axis at the level of the adrenal gland, giving rise to a so-called lymphoid-adrenal axis. Although controversial, the lymphoid-adrenal axis seems to be physiologically relevant, since hypophysectomized mice mount a time-dependent increase of corticosterone after innoculation with Newcastle disease virus.

RELEVANCE OF INTERACTIONS TO PSYCHIATRY

Interactions between the CNS and the immune system are relevant to psychiatry in at least three major ways. First, psychiatric conditions, which inherently involve disordered CNS function, may lead to or be associated with disordered immune function. Alterations in immune function may then predispose persons with psychiatric conditions to immune-related illnesses, including cancer, infectious disease, and autoimmune disorders. Second, disordered immune function or immune-related diseases may lead to or be associated with alterations in CNS activity. This area of inquiry is often referred to as neuroimmunology and involves the investigation of the potential causative role of infectious, paraneoplastic, and autoimmune processes in psychiatric and neurological syndromes. Third, in the context of neural-immune interactions, peripheral immunological events may serve as models of CNS events.

PSYCHIATRIC DISORDERS, IMMUNOCOMPETENCE, AND HEALTH AND ILLNESS The psychiatric disorder that has been most investigated in terms of the competence of the immune system is major depression. More than 30 studies have examined immune parameters in depression; in general, the results have been inconsistent. Although a number of investigators have reported depression-related alterations in peripheral blood immune cell numbers and decreases in peripheral blood mitogen responses and natural killer cell activity, the findings have not been reliably replicated. Therefore, alterations in the immune system do not appear to be a specific biological correlate of depression. Nevertheless, depression-related immune changes may occur in association with other variables that characterize persons with depression, such as age, sex, and symptom severity. For example, in a large study of 91 depressed patients and 91 controls, investigators found no mean differences in immune measures between the groups. However, in that study both advancing age and severity of depression were associated with decreases in CD4 cell numbers and mitogen responsiveness of peripheral blood lymphocytes in depressed patients. Moreover, two studies have reported sex differences in the immune function and depression. One study, which reported decreased NK activity in males, found no changes in females, and the other study found no changes in depressed men and increased NK activity in depressed women compared with controls.

Since depressed patients frequently exhibit alterations in cortisol secretion and since cortisol has potent immunoregulatory effects, a number of studies have examined the relation between measures of cortisol secretion and the immune response in depressed patients. As indicated in Table 1.12-8, no clear association between those variables has emerged. Reports of decreased receptors for cortisol and decreased sensitivity to the inhibitory immunological effects of glucocorticoids in vitro and in vivo on peripheral blood lymphocytes from depressed patients may explain the findings.

Epidemiological data have not supported the idea that depressive symptoms or mood disorders are associated with an increased mortality from immune-related diseases. For example, several studies have examined mortality in large numbers of patients with psychiatric disorders; in general, the results suggest that psychiatric disorders are significantly associated not with death from natural causes but, rather, with unnatural mortality, such as suicide and accidental death. Furthermore, recent reports indicate that depressive symptoms, in contrast to the results of previous studies, are not clearly associated with an increased risk of cancer morbidity and mortality. Although a prospective study on 2,018 male employees of the Western Electric Company has most often been cited to support a relation between depressive symptoms and cancer, at least three subsequent reports with larger samples have failed to find such a relation. Taken together with the inconsistent findings of immune dysfunction in depressed patients, those results indicate that persons with depression do not clearly exhibit evidence of impaired immunocompetence and are not clearly at risk for immune-related conditions. Nevertheless, the above reports primarily focused on persons free of physical illness at the time of the study, and considerable evidence suggests that persons with physical illness complicated by depression have a worse outcome than persons without depression.

TABLE 1.12-8
Neuroendocrine Function and the Immune System in Depression

Neuroendocrine Measure	Immune Measure	Results
DST	M	Suppressors = nonsuppressors
DST	E, M	Suppressors = nonsuppressors
DST	E	Lower lymphocyte number and percentage in nonsuppressors
DST	E	Suppressors = nonsuppressors
UFC	M	Hypersecretors = normosecretors, no correlation
Plasma cortisol	E	No correlation
Plasma cortisol	N	No correlation
Plasma cortisol	M	Negative correlation between cortisol and M in all subjects combined
1–4 PM plasma cortisol	N	Hypersecretors = normosecretors, no correlation

DST—dexamethasone suppression test; UFC—urinary free cortisol; M—mitogen-induced lymphocyte proliferation; E—enumeration of immune cells; N—natural killer cell activity.
Adapted from A H Miller, M Stein: The immune system and depression. In *American Psychiatric Press Review of Psychiatry,* vol 11, A Tasman, M B Riba, editors, p 191. American Psychiatric Press, Washington, 1992. Used with permission.

NEUROIMMUNOLOGY Disorders that are typically associated with the immune system, including infectious diseases and autoimmunity, can influence CNS function. Infectious agents can invade the brain and either infect cells in the nervous system directly, such as the infection of microglial and endothelial cells by HIV, or grow locally outside the brain cells, as in bacterial meningitis. Both conditions lead to an inflammatory reaction, and alterations of CNS function in those cases are a combination of the direct effects of the infectious agent on the various cell types in the nervous system and the effects of cytokines and other inflammatory products on neurons.

The idea that infectious agents can lead to psychiatric disorders has been well established. Obvious examples include the mental retardation after congenital infection with rubella or cytomegalovirus, the delirium that accompanies acute meningoencephalitis after CNS infection by herpes simplex virus type I, and the dementias caused by slow viruses, such as kuru and Creutzfeldt-Jakob disease. Several lines of evidence suggest that CNS infection by a virus may be involved in the pathogenesis of some cases of schizophrenia. The data include (1) an excess number of patient births in the late winter and early spring, suggesting possible exposure to viral infection in utero during the fall and winter peak of viral illnesses; (2) the association between exposure to viral epidemics in utero and the later development of schizophrenia; and (3) the presence of gliosis, a process known to accompany infection and inflammation, in some brain areas of schizophrenic patients. In addition, investigators have reported various alterations in immune markers in schizophrenic patients. The alterations include increased levels of interferon, decreased IL-2 production, and increased IL-2 receptors. Cerebrospinal fluid (CSF) immunoglobulins have also been increased in some studies. Although those immune findings in schizophrenic patients may indicate evidence of immune system activation secondary to infection, they may also indicate that an autoimmune process is involved in the disorder. Attempts to isolate infectious agents, especially viruses and viral DNA, from schizophrenic patients have been unsuccessful. For example, in a recent study the polymerase chain reaction was used to amplify specific viral DNA sequences for cytomegalovirus (CMV) in brain tissues from schizophrenic patients, suicide victims, and normal controls. No evidence of cytomegalovirus DNA was found in any of the tissue samples.

A second major process whereby the immune system can lead to CNS dysfunction is the development of autoantibodies to central nervous system tissue components. Several autoimmune disorders, including autoimmune disorders of the thyroid and such collagen vascular diseases as systemic lupus erythematosus, are capable of indirectly or nonspecifically altering CNS function, but only a few autoimmune conditions directly involve brain antigens. Neural cells are the target for autoantibodies in the paraneoplastic syndromes, and autoantibodies to γ-aminobutyric acid (GABA)-ergic neurons in the serum and the CSF appear to be the mechanism behind the stiff-man syndrome, a rare disorder characterized by progressive rigidity, accompanied by recurrent painful muscle spasms (Table 1.12-9).

Multiple sclerosis (MS) and acute disseminated encephalomyelitis are also believed to result from autoimmune processes. However, the hypotheses are based on the inflammatory features of pathological lesions and the presence of nonspecific immunological abnormalities in patients suffering from the disorders, rather than the isolation of specific autoantibodies to nervous system tissue. The development of an MS-like syndrome (experimental allergic encephalomyelitis) in animals injected with myelin basic protein, the major protein constituent of myelin, supports the notion that MS is an autoimmune disorder.

As previously noted, an autoimmune cause has been suspected in some patients with schizophrenia. Nevertheless, attempts to isolate autoantibodies to CNS tissue constituents in schizophrenic patients have failed to yield consistent results. Furthermore, since schizophrenia may involve various forms of CNS tissue damage, with the resultant release of brain antigens, autoantibodies to CNS tissues in those instances may be the result of CNS pathology, rather than the cause.

NEURAL-IMMUNE INTERACTIONS Mounting evidence indicates a reciprocal interaction between the CNS and the immune system, and functional alterations in the CNS may be manifest in immune cells. Therefore, immune cells may serve as useful peripheral models for CNS alterations in psychiatric disorders.

Immunocytes as models of receptor function in depression Unlike brain cells, immune cells are readily available from the peripheral blood and express receptors for hormones and transmitters that are altered in a variety of psychiatric disorders. Immune cells may, therefore, provide useful receptor models for exploring the molecular and biochemical mechanisms that may be involved in altered neuroendocrine or neurotransmitter function. For example, as previously noted, adrenal steroid receptors are expressed in immune tissues, and, after long-term exposure to glucocorticoids in rats, those receptors in immune tissues exhibit down-regulation in parallel with adrenal steroid receptors in multiple brain regions, including the hypothalamus and the hippocampus. Peripheral immune cells from depressed patients also exhibit decreased adrenal steroid receptor numbers. Whether the decreased receptor number in lymphocytes from depressed patients is secondary to hypercortisolism or a primary aspect of the depressed state is unknown. Nevertheless, the evidence of altered glucocorticoid receptor number in lymphocytes may be relevant, since abnormalities in HPA axis activity in depression are believed to be related, in part, to reduced glucocorticoid receptor responsiveness to feedback inhibition by glucocorticoids at the level of the hippocampus, the hypothalamus, and the pituitary. Evidence of altered glucocorticoid receptor number in lymphocytes from depressed patients indicates that the glucocorticoid resistance may be reflected in the readily accessible cells from the immune system. Abnormalities in lymphocyte glucocorticoid receptor expression have also been found in patients with posttraumatic stress disorder (PTSD). In constrast to patients with depression, patients with PTSD exhibit significantly higher numbers of glucocorticoid receptors than in controls: Those findings are accompanied by significantly lower concentrations of plasma cortisol in PTSD patients. Immune cells may, therefore, provide a useful receptor model for both identifying persons with HPA axis alterations and exploring the molecular mechanisms involved.

Another lymphocyte receptor that has been evaluated in the depressive disorders is the β-adrenergic receptor. In the majority of studies, β-adrenergic receptors of peripheral immune cells from depressed patients have exhibited evidence of diminished β-adrenergic responsiveness. The decreased responsivity may be the result of desensitization (diminished function, normal number) or down-regulation (diminished number) of leukocyte β-adrenergic receptors. Since postmortem brain β-adrenergic receptors from depressed patients (death by suicide) have been shown to be up-regulated (increased receptor binding), brain and lymphocyte β-adrenergic receptors appear to have an inverse relation in the depressive disorders. However, whether the decreased responsivity of immune cell β-adrenergic receptors is due to an increase in plasma catecholamines or whether a decrease in peripheral sensitivity to catecholamines leads to an increase in brain catecholamine production is unknown. Nevertheless, as with glucocorticoid receptors, immune cells may be an important tool for identifying and evaluating β-adrenergic receptor alterations in the depressive disorders.

SUGGESTED CROSS-REFERENCES

Functional neuroanatomy is discussed in Section 1.2, neurotransmitters in Sections 1.3 and 1.4, and psychoneuroendocri-

TABLE 1.12-9
Paraneoplastic Syndromes Involving the Central Nervous System

Clinical Syndrome	Identified Antigens	Associated Neoplasms
Encephalomyelitis	35-40 kd neuronal nucleoprotein	Small-cell lung carcinoma
Subacute cortical cerebellar degeneration (PCD)	34-38 kd cytoplasmic proteins in Purkinje's cells	Breast carcinoma, ovarian cancer
Opsoclonus	55 and 80 kd neuronal proteins (anti-Ri)	Breast carcinoma
Necrotizing myelopathy	52 kd protein from spinal cord tissue	Lymphoma
Cancer-associated retinopathy	23 kd retinal antigen	Small-cell lung carcinoma

kd—kilodalton; PCD—paraneoplastic cerebellar degeneration.
From I Wirguin, I Steiner, O Abramsky: Immunologically related disorders of the central nervous system. Prog Neuro Endocrin Immunol *4:* 218, 1991. Used with permission.

nology in Section 1.11. Multiple sclerosis is discussed in Section 2.6, infectious diseases in Section 2.7, and endocrine disorders in Section 2.8. Dementia is discussed in Chapter 12, Alzheimer's disease in Section 49.6a, schizophrenia in Chapter 14, mood disorders in Chapter 16, psycho-oncology in Section 26.11, and AIDS in Sections 29.2 and 29.2a. Bereavement is discussed in Section 29.6 and suicide in Section 30.1.

REFERENCES

*Abbas A K, Lichtman A H, Pober J S: *Cellular and Molecular Immunology.* Saunders, Philadelphia, 1991.

*Ader R, Felten D L, Cohen N, editors: *Psychoneuroimmunology,* ed 2. Academic Press, New York, 1991.

*Ben-Eliyahu S, Yirmiya R, Liebeskind J C, Taylor A N, Gale R P: Stress increases metastatic spread of a mammary tumor in rats: Evidence for mediation by the immune system. Brain Behav Immun *5:* 193, 1991.

Berkenbosch F, Oers J V, Del Rey A, Tilders F, Besedovsky H: Corticotropin-releasing factor-producing neurons in the rat activated by interleukin-1. Science *238:* 524, 1987.

Besedovsky H, Del Rey A, Sorkin E: The immune response evokes changes in brain noradrenergic neurons. Science *221:* 564, 1983.

Bonneau R H, Sheridan J F, Feng N, Glaser R: Stress-induced modulation of the primary cellular immune response to herpes simplex virus infection is mediated by both adrenal-dependent and independent mechanisms. J Neuroimmunol *42:* 167, 1993.

Breder C D, Dinarello C A, Saper C B: Interleukin-1 immunoreactive innervation of the human hypothalamus. Science *240:* 321, 1988.

*Cohen S, Tyrell D A J, Smith A P: Psychological stress and susceptibility to the common cold. N Engl J Med *325:* 606, 1991.

Division of Health Sciences Policy, Division of Mental Health and Behavioral Medicine, Institute of Medicine: *Behavioral Influences on the Endocrine and Immune Systems.* National Academy Press, Washington, 1989.

Evans D L, Folds J D, Pettito J M, Golden R N, Pederson C A, Corrigan M, Gilmore J H, Silva S G, Quade D, Ozer H: Circulating natural killer cell phenotypes in men and women with major depression, relation to cytotoxic activity and severity of depression. Arch Gen Psychiatry *49:* 388, 1992.

Fawzy F I, Fawzy N W, Hyun C S, Elashoff R, Guthrie D, Fahey J L, Morton D L: Malignant melanoma; effects of an early structured intervention, coping, and affective state on recurrence and survival 6 years later. Arch Gen Psychiatry *50:* 581, 1993.

Glaser R, Kennedy S, Lafuse W P, Bonneau R H, Speicher C, Hillhouse J, Kiecolt-Glaser J K: Psychological stress-induced modulation of interleukin 2 receptor gene expression and interleukin 2 production in peripheral blood leukocytes. Arch Gen Psychiatry *47:* 707, 1990.

Goetzl E J, editor: Neuromodulation of immunity and hypersensitivity. J Immunol *135* (8, Suppl): 739, 1985.

Justice A: Review of the effects of stress on cancer in laboratory animals: Importance of time of stress application and type of tumor. Psychol Bull *98:* 108, 1985.

Keller S, Schleifer S J, Liotta A S, Bond R N, Farhoody N, Stein M: Stress-induced alterations of immunity in hypophysectomized rats. Proc Natl Acad Sci U S A *85:* 9297, 1988.

Keller S E, Weiss J M, Schleifer S J, Miller N E, Stein M: Suppression of immunity by stress: Effects of a graded series of stressors on lymphocyte stimulation in the rat. Science *213:* 1397, 1981.

Miller A H, editor: *Depressive Disorders and Immunity.* American Psychiatric Press, Washington, 1989.

Perry S, Fishman B: Depression and HIV: How does one affect the other? JAMA *270:* 2609, 1993.

Riley V: Psychoneuroendocrine influences on immunocompetence and neoplasia. Science *212:* 1100, 1981.

Saphier D: Neurophysiological and endocrine consequences of immune activity. Psychoneuroendocrinology *14:* 63, 1989.

Schleifer S J, Keller S E, Camerino M, Thornton V C, Stein M: Suppression of lymphocyte stimulation following bereavement. JAMA *250:* 374, 1983.

Spiegel D, Kraemer H C, Bloom J R, Gotheil E: Effects of psychosocial treatment on survival of patients with metastatic breast cancer. Lancet *2:* 888, 1989.

*Stein M, Miller A H, Trestman R L: Depression, the immune system and health and illness. Arch Gen Psychiatry *48:* 171, 1991.

Stein M, Schiavi R C, Camerino M: Influence of brain and behavior on the immune system. Science *191:* 435, 1976.

Yehuda R, Boisoneau D, Mason J W, Giller E L: Glucocorticoid receptor number and cortisol excretion in mood, anxiety, and psychotic disorders. Biol Psychiatry *34:* 18, 1993.

1.13 CHRONOBIOLOGY

THOMAS A. WEHR, M.D.

INTRODUCTION

Chronobiology is the study of biological rhythms. Such rhythms span a spectrum of periods from the fraction-of-a-second fluctuations of the electroencephalogram to multiyear cycles in populations of predators and their prey. This section focuses on the physiology and the neurobiology of two types of biological rhythms, circadian (daily) rhythms and seasonal rhythms. Those rhythms enable the organism to anticipate and adapt to corresponding cycles in the environment.

PHYSIOLOGY

CIRCADIAN RHYTHMS Because the Earth rotates on its axis, it presents two different environments—a daytime world and a nighttime world—to the organisms that live on it. In the course of their evolution, most animals have specialized in the active engagement of only one of those two environments. Because adaptations that make animals fit for one environment are liable to make them unfit for the other, animals have also adopted ways of withdrawing from the unfavorable environment (by sleeping in secure refuges, for example) to avoid danger and to prevent the inefficient use of energy.

Thus, as the world alternates between phases of light and of darkness, animals alternate between phases of active engagement and of withdrawal. That alternation of behavioral states is not simply a passive response to the alternation of day and night. Animals possess clocklike mechanisms that automatically switch them from one state to the other in anticipation of the transitions between day and night. Those mechanisms also switch back and forth between contrasting physiological states that are geared to engagement or to withdrawal. For that reason, circadian rhythms in animals' behavior and physiology often exhibit two distinct phases, a diurnal phase and a nocturnal phase, with relatively discrete transitions between them (Figure 1.13-1). In human beings, for example, the *diurnal phase* is one of active engagement of the environment, high body temperature, and decline or cessation of the secretion of several hormones, including pineal melatonin, pituitary thyrotropin, pituitary prolactin, pituitary corticotropin, and adrenocortical steroids. Conversely, the *nocturnal phase* is one of withdrawal from the environment, rest, sleep, low body temperature, and augmentation of the secretion of the above hormones (Figure 1.13-1).

The best evidence that circadian rhythms are not simply passive responses to cyclic changes in the external environment but are generated by endogeneous processes is the fact that the rhythms persist when organisms are placed in constant conditions. In that situation the rhythms continue to oscillate but with an intrinsic period that differs slightly from 24 hours (hence the name "circadian," about daily). In human beings, for example, the period is slightly longer than 24 hours. In a normal environment the circadian system responds to external stimuli that serve as *time cues, zeitgebers,* in such a way that the period of its oscillations is adjusted to 24 hours and a characteristic *phase relationship* to the day-night cycle is maintained. Thus, in human beings, external time cues advance the phase of their

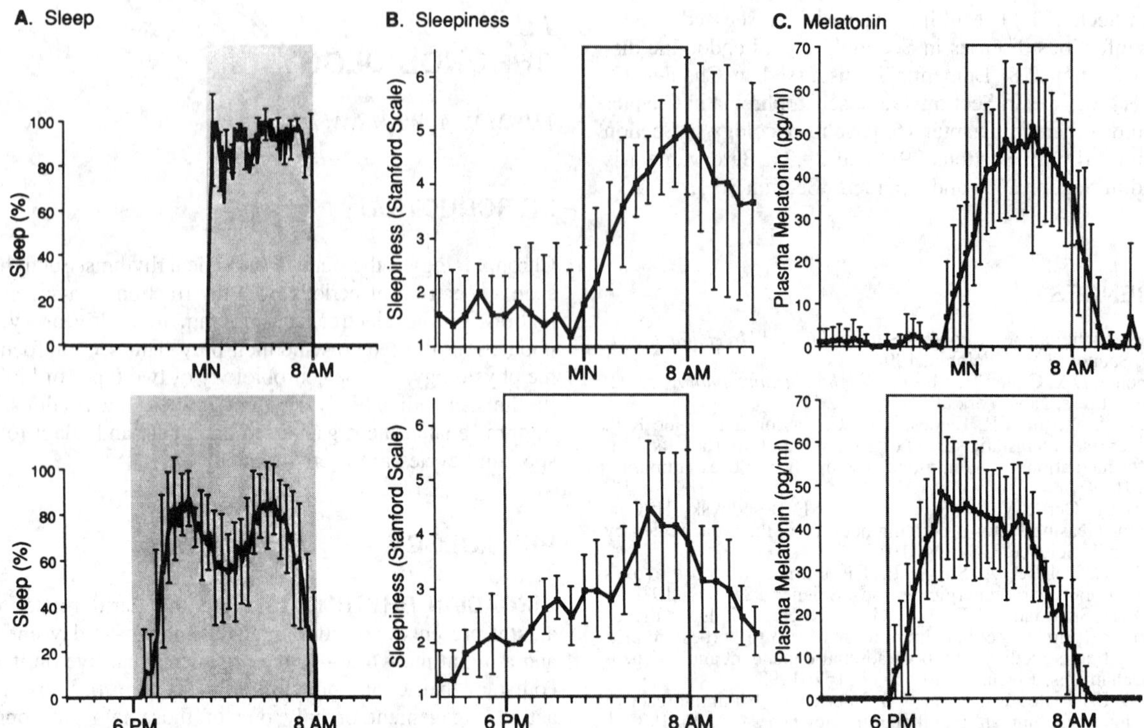

FIGURE 1.13-1 *In human beings, durations of the nightly sleep phase (A), of the nightly rising phase of sleepiness (B), and of the nightly phase of active melatonin secretion (C) all expand when the duration of night is lengthened from 8 hours (top) to 14 hours (bottom). The dark phase of each photoperiod schedule is indicated by shaded rectangles. Sleepiness and melatonin levels were measured during continuous wakefulness in constant dim light. The dark phase of the photoperiod to which the persons had been exposed in the weeks before the latter measurements is indicated by open rectangles. (From T A Wehr: The durations of human melatonin secretion and sleep respond to changes in daylength (photoperiod). J Clin Endocrinol Metab 73: 1276, 1991. Used with permission.)*

longer-than-24-hour circadian rhythms several minutes each day, so that sleep recurs every 24 hours and recurs at night. Otherwise, humans would go to sleep later and later each day and would make a full circuit around the clock.

Light, acting on the retina, is the most important stimulus for phase resetting of the circadian system. The direction and the magnitude of the phase-resetting effect of light depends on the circadian phase at which it is applied. For example, early-morning light shifts the oscillations of the circadian system to an earlier *advanced-phase position;* late-evening light shifts the oscillations to a later *delayed-phase position.* Light in the middle of the day has little or no effect. Thus, in human beings, evening light delays the time of sleep onset, but morning light advances it. The dependence of light's phase-resetting effects on the circadian phase at which it is applied can be shown quantitatively in a *phase-response curve* that indicates the magnitude and the direction of phase shifts induced by light pulses at each circadian phase (Figure 1.13-2). The phase-resetting properties of light have led to its use in the treatment of certain types of sleep and mood disorders and of jet lag.

Light-oriented rhythms and behavior-oriented rhythms Circadian rhythms in animals appear to be of two types: (1) rhythms whose phase relations to the external light-dark cycle are similar in day-active and night-active species but whose phase relations to the endogenous activity-rest cycle are opposite (Type I) and (2) rhythms whose phase relations to the external light-dark cycle are opposite in day-active and night-active species but whose phase relations to the endogenous activity-rest cycle are similar (Type II).

Type I rhythms have the same orientation to the light-dark cycle in both day-active and night-active species. They include the rhythm in the circadian system's responses to light pulses, which reaches its maximum at night (Figure 1.13-2); the rhythm in the hypothalamic suprachiasmatic nucleus's electrical multiple-unit activity and glucose utilization (Figure 1.13-3), which reaches its maximum in the daytime; the rhythm in retinal disk shedding, which reaches its maximum in the morning; the rhythm in melatonin secretion, which reaches its maximum at night (Figure 1.13-1); and the rhythm in cerebrospinal fluid arginine vasopressin secretion, which reaches its maximum in the daytime. Most of those rhythms are intimately connected with mechanisms responsible for the generation and the entrainment of circadian rhythms, and one of their most important functions appears to be the transmission of information about the timing of day and night to other parts of the organism.

Type II rhythms have the same orientation to the activity-rest cycle in both day-active and night-active species. They include the rhythm in sleep, which reaches its maximum during the rest phase (Figure 1.13-1); the rhythm in body temperature, which reaches its maximum during the activity phase; and the rhythms in pituitary thyrotropin secretion, pituitary corticotropin secretion, and adrenocortical steroid secretion, which reach their maximums during the rest phase. Those rhythms seem to be directly connected with the maintenance of internal conditions that serve active engagement of and withdrawal from the environment.

If Type I rhythms are directly connected with clock mechanisms and Type II rhythms are directly connected with the expression of behavioral rhythms that are driven by those clock mechanisms, it is likely that Type II rhythms occupy a more subordinate position than Type I rhythms in the hierarchical organization of the circadian system.

Sunrise and sunset For organisms to coordinate the timing of their diurnal and nocturnal phases with the timing of day and night, they must track and anticipate the transitions between day and night. That task is complicated by the fact that the Earth's axis of rotation is tilted, causing the interval between dawn and dusk to vary during the course of the year. Animals appear to

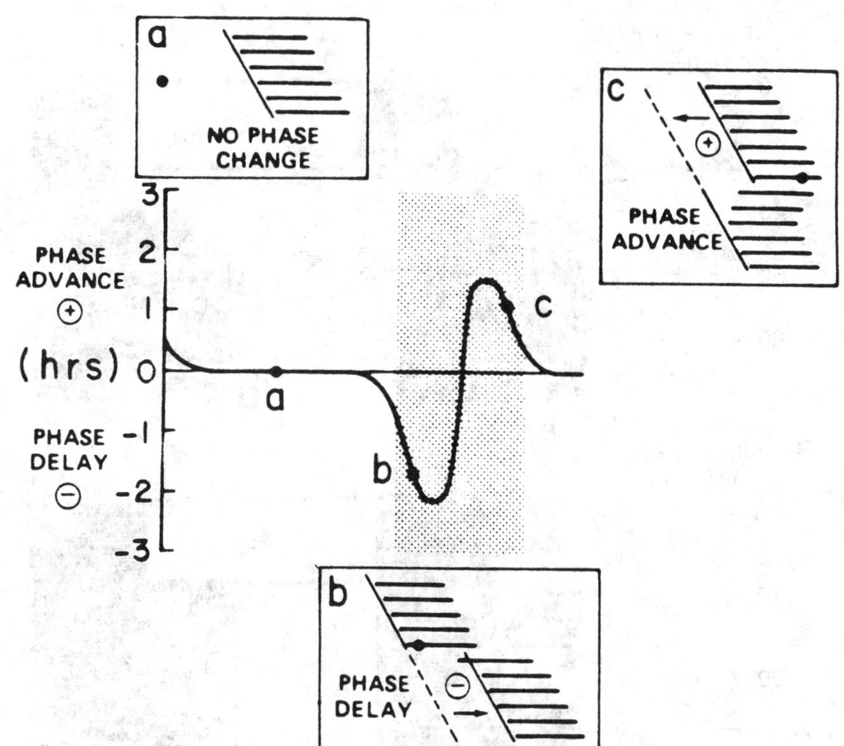

FIGURE 1.13-2 *The derivation of a phase-response curve for the phase-resetting effect of light pulses in an animal whose circadian locomotor activity rhythms are free-running in constant darkness. Light pulses result in no phase change (a), a phase delay (b), or a phase advance (c), depending on the phase of the circadian cycle at which the stimulus occurred. (From C A Czeisler, G S Richardson, R M Coleman, J C Zimmerman, M C Moore-Ede, W C Dement, E D Wertzman: Chronotherapy: Resetting the circadian clocks of patients with delayed sleep phase insomnia. Sleep 4: 1, 1981. Used with permission.)*

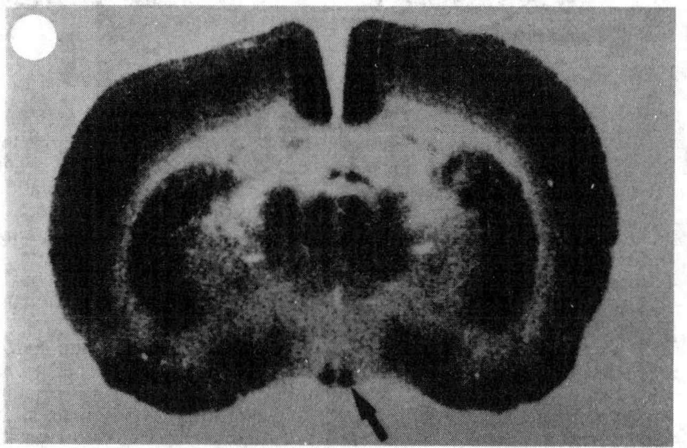

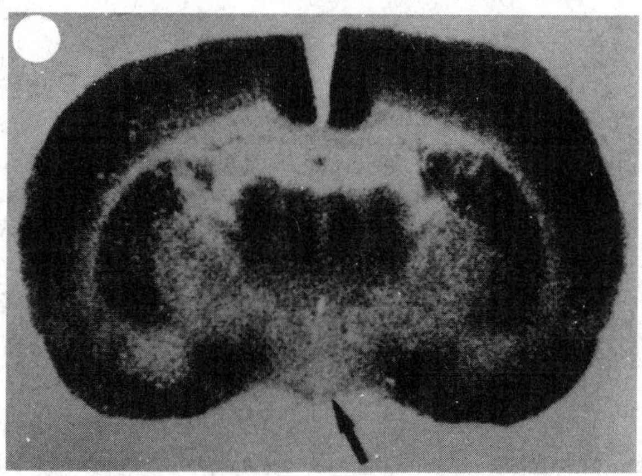

FIGURE 1.13-3 *In autoradiographs of coronal sections of rat brain, 2-deoxyglucose uptake in the suprachiasmatic nuclei of the hypothalamus (indicated by arrows) is higher during the light phase (left) than during the dark phase (right). (From W J Schwartz, C B Smith, L C Davidsen: In vivo glucose utilization of the suprachiasmatic nucleus. In* Biological Rhythms and Their Central Mechanism, *M Suda, O Hayaishi, H Nakagawa, editors, p 355. Elsevier, New York, 1979. Used with permission.)*

deal with the situation by using two separate mechanisms to track and to anticipate the times of dawn and dusk. In that way they are able to modify the durations of diurnal and nocturnal phases to match the changing durations of day and night. According to one model, that is accomplished by a circadian pacemaker that consists of two coupled oscillators. One oscillator, entrained to sunset, controls the timing of the transition from the diurnal phase to the nocturnal phase of the circadian system; a second oscillator, entrained to sunrise, controls the timing of the transition from the nocturnal phase to the diurnal phase of the circadian system. According to that model, in human beings the dusk-entrained oscillator controls the onset of sleep and the onset of nocturnal melatonin secretion, and the dawn-entrained oscillator controls the offset of sleep and the offset of nocturnal melatonin secretion. Thus, when nights become longer in winter, the sleep phase and the melatonin secretory phase become longer, too (Figure 1.13-1).

The fact that activity or sleep in animals and human beings tends to be bimodally distributed, with a peak near dusk and a peak near dawn (Figure 1.13-1 and 1.13-4), seems consistent with a two-oscillator model. The strongest support for the model comes from the phenomenon of *splitting* of activity-rest cycles: when nocturnal rodents are exposed to constant light, their activity sometimes splits into two circadian components that seem to oscillate independently (Figure 1.13-5). A phenomenon that resembles splitting has also been described in human sleep-wake cycles.

SEASONAL RHYTHMS The system of dawn-tracking and dusk-tracking circadian mechanisms that adjusts the durations of diurnal and nocturnal phases to match the durations of day and night has a second important function. The timing of dawn

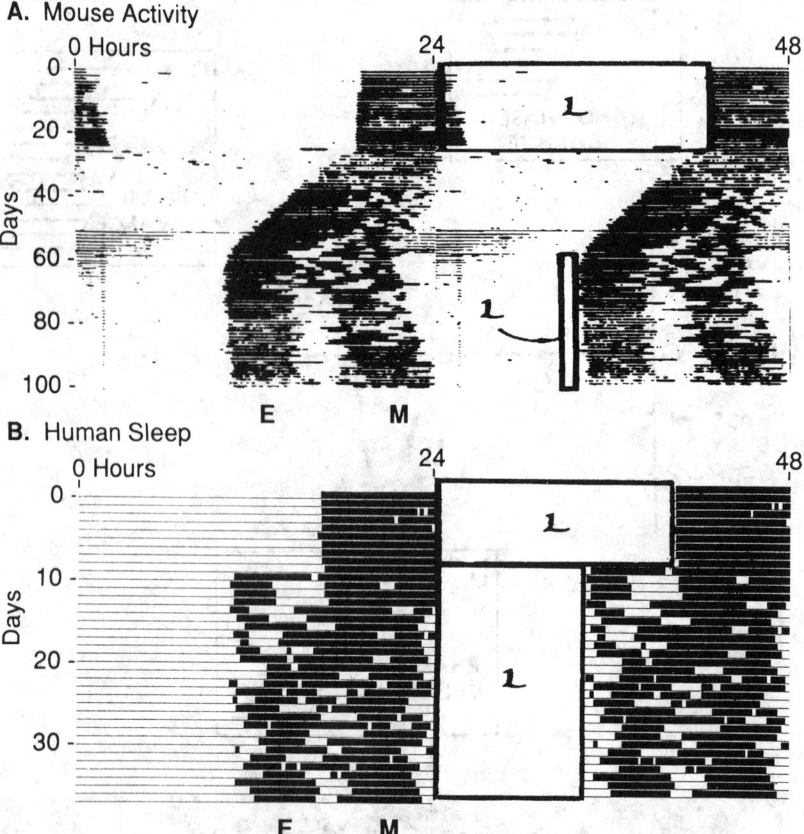

FIGURE 1.13-4 *When schedules of daily light exposures (L) were shifted from long days to short days, the nocturnal sleep phase of a human being (B) expanded and separated into an evening component (E) and a morning component (M). Shortening the photoperiod causes similar changes to occur in the activity phase of nocturnal rodents, as the record of mouse wheel-running activity (A) illustrates. Successive 24-hour intervals of data (wheel revolutions in the mouse and electroencephalographically monitored sleep in the human being) are plotted beneath one another, and the records are double-plotted over 48-hour intervals to facilitate visual inspection of the courses of the activity-rest cycles and the sleep-wake cycles. (From T A Wehr: The durations of human melatonin secretion and sleep respond to changes in daylength (photoperiod). J Clin Endocrinol Metab 73: 1276, 1991. Used with permission.)*

relative to the timing of dusk is an indicator of the time of year. Taking advantage of that fact, animals also use dawn-tracking and dusk-tracking mechanisms as a kind of annual clock. With such a clock they can anticipate conditions that will prevail at particular times of the year and can initiate responses that are likely to be adaptive. For example, animals respond to critical changes in day length *(photoperiod)* by storing energy in anticipation of seasonal scarcity of food or by conceiving offspring in anticipation of seasonal abundance of food.

Melatonin The pineal hormone *melatonin* plays an important role as a chemical mediator of the effects of seasonal changes in the photoperiod on reproduction and other functions. As mentioned previously, in some animals the duration of nocturnal melatonin secretion appears to be regulated by separate circadian processes that are synchronized with dusk and with dawn and that trigger the onset and the offset of secretion. Thus, in winter, when nights are long, the duration of nocturnal melatonin secretion is long. In summer, when nights are short, the duration of melatonin secretion is short (Figure 1.13-1). In many species those changes in the duration of melatonin secretion serve as chemical signals that convey information about the duration of night to target sites in the body that induce season-specific changes in behavior and physiology. For example, numerous experiments have shown that the effect of the photoperiod on breeding is mediated by changes in the duration of nocturnal melatonin secretion.

Elements of the reproductive system that respond to melatonin appear to possess *interval timers* that measure the duration of melatonin secretion. When the duration increases by a certain amount, winter-type reproductive responses are triggered. When the duration declines by a certain amount, summer-type responses are triggered. Further research has shown that the direction of change in the duration of melatonin secretion is also important in determining the nature of the response. Intermediate durations of melatonin secretion can elicit either summer-type responses or winter-type responses, depending on whether the duration to which an animal was previously exposed were long or short.

The exact nature of an animal's reproductive responses to photoperiod-induced changes in melatonin secretion depends on its species and the length of its gestational period. For example, short photoperiods and long melatonin durations induce breeding in sheep, but long photoperiods and short melatonin durations induce breeding in hamsters. Because the gestational period of sheep is long and the gestational period of hamsters is short, the offspring of each species tend to be born at approximately the same time of year, the late spring—a time when conditions are favorable for their survival. Thus, melatonin is generically neither progonadal nor antigonadal. Rather, it conveys information about the duration of the photoperiod, and that information is used in different ways by different animals.

Melatonin binding sites have been identified, and they are concentrated in the suprachiasmatic area of the hypothalamus and the pars tuberalis of the pituitary. It seems likely that the effects of melatonin on reproductive function are mediated, at least in part, by interval timers associated with melatonin receptors in those areas. Recently, a 420-amino acid melatonin receptor has been identified and cloned. Structural analysis revealed that the receptor protein is a newly discovered member of the guanine nucleotide binding protein-coupled receptor family. Identification of a melatonin receptor should facilitate understanding of melatonin's action at the cellular and molecular level.

By using artificial light, human beings expose themselves to an unvarying, long photoperiod that, to some extent, overrides the natural photoperiod. However, when human beings are exposed to artificial photoperiods of different lengths, some of their responses are similar to those that occur in animals. For example, when persons are transferred from conventional, summer-type photoperiods (16 hours of light and 8 hours of darkness) to winter-type photoperiods (10 hours of light and 14 hours of darkness), the distribution of human sleep becomes bimodal (Figures 1.13-1 and 1.13-4). That pattern in nocturnal sleep or activity in short photoperiods has been observed in many other animals, including insects, reptiles, birds, and mammals (Figure 1.13-4).

After a transfer to short photoperiods, the duration of nocturnal melatonin secretion increases in humans and in animals (Figure 1.13-1). Whether that change ultimately induces changes in human reproductive function, like the changes that occur in animals, is unknown. Recent reports of an association between increased melatonin secretion and suppression of reproductive function in pathological states in human beings suggest that the possibility ought to be investigated.

Unicellular algae also produce melatonin at night, and they use photoperiod-induced changes in the duration of their nocturnal production to trigger encystment, an adaptive response to conditions that prevail in winter. The fact that human beings and algae both use changes in the duration of nocturnal melatonin secretion to code for seasonal

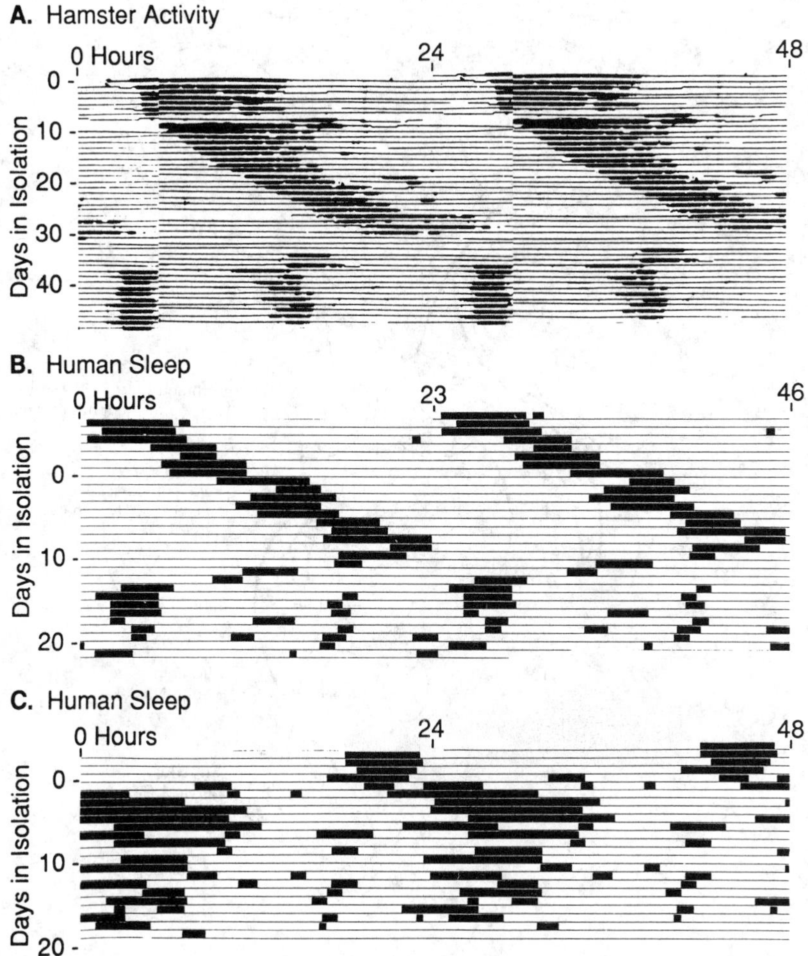

FIGURE 1.13-5 *Splitting of free-running circadian rhythms of hamster-running wheel activity (top) and electroencephalographically monitored human sleep (middle and bottom) into two components that become stably recoupled approximately 180° apart. The human data are from a hypomanic patient treated with the monoamine oxidase inhibitor clorgyline (middle) and from a drug-free bipolar disorder patient who switched from depression to mania during the course of the experiment (bottom). (From T A Wehr: In short photoperiods, human sleep is biphasic. J Sleep Res 1:* 103, *1992. Used with permission.)*

changes in the duration of the night points to an ancient evolutionary origin for the mechanism.

Circannual rhythms Certain types of seasonal rhythms in animals, such as rhythms in hibernation, persist in experimental conditions when the duration of the photoperiod and all other conditions are held constant. Apparently, those seasonal rhythms are not simply passive responses to seasonal changes in the photoperiod; they are endogenous and capable of self-sustainment. In constant conditions, their intrinsic period is slightly different from one year (hence the name ''circannual,'' about yearly). In the natural environment the circannual rhythm responds to zeitgebers in such a way that its period is adjusted to one year, and a characteristic phase relationship to the seasons is maintained. Annual changes in light, temperature, and diet have been shown to serve as zeitgebers for various types of circannual rhythms.

The behavior of hamster and sheep breeding cycles under various experimental conditions suggests that an absolute distinction does not always exist between externally driven photoperiodic seasonal rhythms and internally driven circannual rhythms. When a hamster is transferred from long days to short days, its gonads regress. However, if it is maintained in short days, its gonads spontaneously recrudesce after a number of weeks. In that situation the animal is said to have become photorefractory. From that point on, short days do not reinduce regression until the animal has again been exposed to long days. If the animal is maintained in long days, it never regresses. Thus, in constant short days the hamster cycles through a part of its annual breeding rhythm, as would occur with a circannual rhythm, but then arrests. In constant long days it arrests and does not even begin to cycle. Like hamsters, sheep become photorefractory to short days; however, unlike hamsters, they also become photorefractory to long days. As a consequence, their breeding cycle, which is normally driven by changes in the photoperiod, persists in constant conditions, like a circannual rhythm.

FEEDBACK Some outputs of the circadian system feed back onto its rhythm-generating mechanisms and modify their oscillatory behavior. For example, pharmacological studies suggest that the onset of melatonin secretion in the evening, which is triggered by the circadian system, may feed back on the system and phase advance it. That effect of melatonin may be mediated by high-affinity melatonin binding sites that are found in the suprachiasmatic nucleus (SCN) of the hypothalamus, which is the site of a circadian pacemaker. Experiments have shown that arousing stimuli—such as forced exercise, social interactions, and novel environments—when applied near the time of onset of the activity phase, phase advance circadian rhythms. That finding suggests that the daily onset of the activity phase, which is triggered by the circadian system, may also feed back on the system and phase advance it.

NEUROBIOLOGY

The circadian system consists of three elements: (1) a rhythm generator or pacemaker, (2) visual inputs to the pacemaker that mediate its entrainment to the photoperiod, and (3) efferent connections that drive and coordinate numerous physiological and behavioral output rhythms. Research over the past two decades has revealed that the retinohypothalamic-pineal axis contains

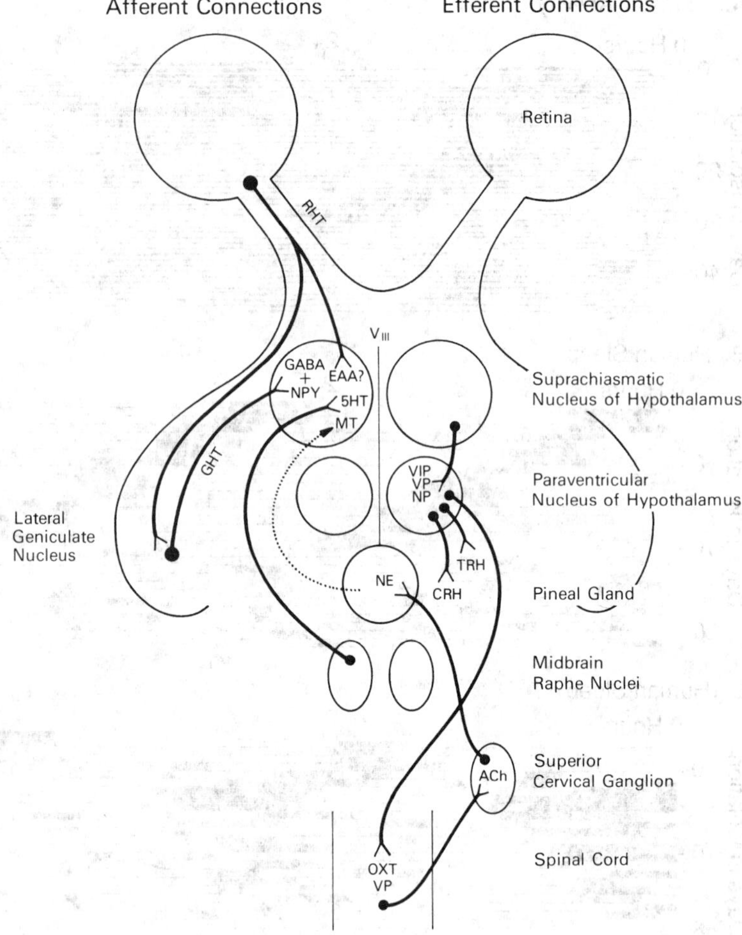

FIGURE 1.13-6 *Important pathways and neurotransmitters of the retinohypothalamic-pineal/midbrain raphe axis (schematic drawing, not to scale).* Anatomical structures: *V_{III} = third ventricle; RHT = retinohypothalamic tract; GHT = geniculohypothalamic tract.* Neurotransmitters: *EAA = excitatory amino acids; NPY = neuropeptide Y; 5HT = serotonin; VIP = vasoactive intestinal peptide; VP = vasopressin; NP = neurophysin; NE = norepinephrine.* Hormones: *MT = melatonin; CRH = corticotropin-releasing hormone; TRH = thyrotropin-releasing hormone.*

all those elements and is the core of the mammalian circadian system (Figure 1.13-6).

PACEMAKER The mammalian brain has at least two circadian pacemakers, but only one, the SCN of the hypothalamus, has been identified. (A second oscillator, which can be entrained by feeding and which survives SCN lesions, has not been localized.) The SCN consists of bilateral compact cell groups lying above the caudal third of the optic chiasm on either side of the third ventricle (Figure 1.13-3). The evidence that the SCN generates and coordinates circadian rhythms in mammals includes the following:

1. The SCN is directly innervated by the retinohypothalamic tract (RHT), a pathway that originates in the retina and is necessary and sufficient for the entrainment of circadian rhythms by light.
2. SCN lesions disrupt many types of circadian rhythms.
3. The SCN exhibits circadian rhythms in multiunit electrical activity, even when it is isolated from the rest of the brain by knife cuts that create a hypothalamic island in vivo.
4. SCN explants continue to exhibit circadian rhythms in multiunit electrical activity, vasopressin release, and metabolic activity in vitro.
5. Fetal SCN transplants restore circadian rhythmicity to animals whose circadian rhythms have been disrupted by SCN lesions.
6. When such SCN transplants are obtained from mutant donors whose circadian rhythms oscillate unusually rapidly, the recipient's circadian rhythms also oscillate unusually rapidly.

Intact SCNs have also been shown to be necessary for the expression of photoperiodic seasonal rhythms.

The SCNs of a variety of mammalian species share a number of common properties. The SCN can be divided into dorsomedial and ventrolateral subdivisions. The *dorsomedial* subdivision contains neurons exhibiting vasopressinlike and somatostatinlike immunoreactivity. Most vasopressin-containing cells and somatostatin-containing cells seem to be local circuit neurons that do not project beyond the confines of the SCN. The *ventrolateral* subdivision contains a large number of vasoactive intestinal polypeptide-immunoreactive neuronal perikarya. The majority of those cells also appear to be local-circuit neurons confined to the boundaries of the SCN, although there is a small projection to the periventricular and anterior hypothalamic area.

The normal neuroanatomical organization of the SCN is not necessary for its cells to generate circadian rhythms. Dispersed cultures of SCN cells are capable of generating circadian rhythms in vasopressin release, and transplants of those cultures are capable of restoring circadian rhythms in animals whose circadian rhythms have been disrupted by SCN lesions. Those results suggest that circadian rhythm generation in the SCN may be a property of individual cells or of small networks of cells. The fact that all successful transplants included vasoactive intestinal polypeptide-containing cells may indicate that those particular SCN cells play an important role in the generation of circadian rhythms.

Since protein-synthesis inhibitors phase shift mammalian circadian rhythms, protein synthesis may be part of the SCN's mechanism for generating those rhythms. Results of experiments with fruitflies seem to indicate that gene expression also participates in the rhythm-generating process. The existence of clock mutations in hamsters and mice raises the possibility that gene expression may play a role in rhythm generation in mammals, too. Recently, for example, a semidominant mutation, *Clock,* that lengthens the circadian period and abolishes the persistence of rhythmicity in mice has been mapped to the midportion of mouse chromosome 5, a region that is syntenic to human chromosome 4.

Circadian-rhythm generation by the SCN pacemaker is reflected in changes in multiple-unit electrical activity and metabolism, which increase in the daytime in both day-active and night-active mammals (Figure 1.13-3). Furthermore, circadian rhythms in that activity persist when knife cuts isolate tissue containing the SCN from the rest of the brain. When splitting occurs in hamsters, the pattern of glucose metabolism becomes asymmetrical in the two SCNs.

AFFERENTS TO THE SUPRACHIASMATIC NUCLEUS PACEMAKER The SCN receives three major afferents, a direct visual pathway, an indirect visual pathway, and a pathway from the raphe nuclei of the brainstem (Figure 1.13-6). All three pathways terminate on cells in the ventrolateral subdivision of the SCN, and all three pathways have been shown to affect the expression of rhythms generated by the SCN.

Direct visual pathway Entrainment of circadian rhythms in animals requires intact visual pathways. If the eyes are removed or the optic nerves cut, the circadian pacemaker expresses its own intrinsic rhythm and free runs, even in the presence of a light-dark cycle. The pathways responsible for photic entrainment are unusual in some respects. The threshold for photic effects on entrainment is rather high and resembles that of cone photoreceptors. In fact, genetic mutant mice that lack rods can be entrained perfectly normally to light-dark cycles, suggesting that cones or some novel type of photoreceptor is responsible for phase resetting by light. The photic entrainment system is also unusual in that it can integrate light over long durations. It responds optimally to pulse durations of five minutes.

The RHT—which passes from the retina along the optic nerve, exits from the optic chiasm, and enters the SCN—is both necessary and sufficient for photic entrainment of circadian rhythms. If the optic tracts, which are distal to the chiasm, are cut, entrainment is preserved.

Neurophysiological studies have shown that the SCN contains many cells whose electrical activity is modified when the retina is exposed to light. The visual fields of those cells are wide, and they code exclusively for luminance (as opposed to spatial characteristics of light that may be useful for image processing). With light stimulation, electrical activity is enhanced in some cells and suppressed in others.

Which neurotransmitters mediate RHT input to the SCN is still not certain. Currently, several lines of evidence point to excitatory amino acids. They have been found in the RHT and its terminals, and their levels are reduced by optic nerve transection. Furthermore, an *N*-methyl-D-aspartic acid (NMDA) glutamate receptor antagonist can block light-induced phase shifts in rodents.

Photic entrainment may depend on transcriptionally regulated signal transduction processes in the SCN. Light triggers production of mRNA and protein products of the proto-oncogene c-fos in the SCN. That stimulation exhibits the same circadian-phase dependence and the same photic threshold as circadian-rhythm phase-shifting effects of light, and the stimulation can be blocked with an NMDA antagonist. Light also stimulates the jun-B protooncogene family, which forms a dimer with c-fos, called AP-1, which serves as a transcription factor.

Indirect visual pathway An indirect visual pathway reaches the SCN through the lateral geniculate nucleus and the intergeniculate leaflet. That pathway is not necessary for entrainment; nevertheless, it appears to be capable of modifying the responses of the SCN circadian pacemaker to photic and nonphotic entraining stimuli. In hamsters, destruction of the intergeniculate leaflet prevents lengthening of the intrinsic period of circadian rhythms that is normally caused by constant light, reduces the magnitude of phase shifts that are induced by light pulses, and advances the time of onset of the nocturnal activity phase under conditions of entrainment to a light-dark cycle. Furthermore, electrical stimulation of the lateral geniculate nucleus causes phase shifts in circadian rhythms.

Geniculohypothalamic tract input to the SCN appears to be mediated by neuropeptide Y, which is present in cells of the tract and which is released from terminals in the SCN when the lateral geniculate nucleus is electrically stimulated. Moreover, injections of neuropeptide Y directly into the SCN produce phase shifts that resemble those produced by electrical stimulation of the lateral geniculate nucleus. In nocturnal rodents, the phase shifts produced by electrical stimulation of the lateral geniculate nucleus and by applications of neuropeptide Y to the SCN resemble phase shifts produced when dark pulses are applied against a background of constant illumination.

In human beings neuropeptide Y cell bodies do not appear to be present in the lateral geniculate nucleus. Instead, they are found within the SCN itself. That fact may indicate that in human beings the indirect visual input to the SCN is circumscribed and bypasses the lateral geniculate nucleus.

Pathway from the raphe nuclei From the serotonergic raphe nuclei, extensive projections terminate in the SCN, mainly on the vasoactive intestinal polypeptide-containing cells. Furthermore, the SCN shows a diurnal rhythm of serotonin uptake and sensitivity. In contrast to excitatory amino acids and neuropeptide Y, which are excitatory neurotransmitters, serotonin is inhibitory and suppresses spontaneous electrical activity of SCN cells.

Although lesion studies have shown that raphe input is not necessary for photic entrainment, the raphe cells do appear to influence the rhythmic behavior of the SCN pacemaker and its responses to light-dark cycles. For example, in rodents housed in constant darkness, lesioning of the raphe causes activity rhythms to disintegrate. That finding suggests that raphe input may be necessary to maintain the coherent expression of SCN rhythms.

The raphe nuclei also appear to modulate animals' responses to the photoperiod. As was described previously, animals adjust the durations of the diurnal and the nocturnal phases of their circadian systems to match the photoperiod. In rodents exposed to a fixed light-dark cycle, lesioning of the raphe nuclei causes the onset of locomotor activity to advance to an earlier time and the offset to delay to a later time, so that the duration of the nocturnal activity phase increases (as also occurs when the photoperiod is shortened). Lesion studies suggest that the effects of serotonergic input on the times of onset and offset of activity may be mediated by separate tracts—a tract from the dorsal raphe nucleus that modulates the time of activity offset and a tract from the median raphe nucleus, lateral to the other tract, that modulates the time of activity onset.

The idea that serotonergic input from the raphe nuclei modulates or reinforces the SCN circadian pacemaker's responses to the entraining light-dark cycle is also supported by observations that quipazine, a serotonin agonist, can induce phase shifts in the circadian rhythm of spontaneous electrical activity of the SCN in vitro. Since increases in serotonergic activity have been shown to be correlated with increased arousal in rats, phase shifts induced by arousing stimuli may be mediated by serotonergic input to the SCN from the raphe nuclei. The effects of serotonin on the circadian pacemaker appear to be mediated by a novel receptor, the serotonin type 7 (5-HT_7) receptor.

Other afferent connections to the SCN have been described, but their function and their physiological significance are obscure. A few dopamine-containing terminals are present in the SCN, and there are afferents from the anterior hypothalamic nucleus, ventromedial nucleus, arcuate nucleus, and paraventricular thalamic nucleus. There are also numerous commissural projections between the SCNs.

EFFERENT CONNECTIONS The SCN drives circadian rhythms in locomotor activity, food intake, water intake, sexual behavior, deep body temperature, sleep, adrenocorticotropic hormone (ACTH) secretion, prolactin secretion, melatonin secretion, and gonadotropin secretion. Presumably, the imposition of rhythms on those functions is mediated by efferent pathways from the SCN to networks that regulate those functions.

Efferent projections of the SCN are confined mainly to the hypothalamus. Besides the commissural connections, six efferent pathways to fiber terminals can be identified.

The principal efferent from the SCN is a dense plexus of fibers that terminates in the subparaventricular zone, below the posterior part of the the paraventricular nucleus. A few of those fibers continue through the paraventricular nucleus and midline thalamic nuclei and end in the paraventricular nucleus of the thalamus. Fibers from the SCN to the paraventricular nucleus and subparaventricular zone contain vasoactive intestinal polypeptide, vasopressin, and neurophysin. The hypothalamic paraventricular nucleus is a way station in the multisynaptic pathway that connects the SCN to the pineal gland and that mediates the effects of light and pacemaker activity on nocturnal melatonin secretion (Figure 1.13-6). The pathway proceeds through the intermediolateral cell column of the spinal cord and the superior cervical ganglion and terminates in noradrenergic sympathetic fibers on the pineal gland. At night the SCN triggers the release of norepinephrine, which stimulates the synthesis and the release of melatonin by the pineal gland. Lesions of the paraventricular nucleus and the superior cervical ganglion abolish the nocturnal rhythm of melatonin secretion and abolish seasonal photoperiodic reproductive rhythms. The fact that melatonin inhibits spontaneous electrical activity and glucose metabolism in the SCN suggests that the SCN modulates its own activity through a pineal neuroendocrine feedback loop.

Since the paraventricular nucleus contains cell bodies of thyrotropin-releasing hormone neurons and corticotropin-releasing hormone neurons that regulate pituitary thyroid-stimulating hormone secretion and pituitary ACTH secretion, the connections between the SCN and the paraventricular nucleus may also be the route through which the SCN pacemaker imposes daily rhythms on the secretion of thyroid-stimulating hormone and ACTH by the pituitary. Paraventricular nucleus lesions do not interfere with the expression of activity and sleep circadian rhythms.

Other pathways consist of relatively fewer fibers. One pathway runs rostrally and ends in the ventral part of the medial preoptic area. Probably through this connection the SCN imposes circadian rhythms on water intake, deep body temperature, and reproductive behavior. Another pathway runs rostrally through the medial preoptic nucleus and ends in the intermediate lateral septal nucleus. Other fibers terminate in the bed nucleus of the stria terminalis, the parataenial nucleus, the paraventricular nucleus of the thalamus, the midbrain central gray nuclei and raphe nuclei, the lateral geniculate nucleus, a zone near the arcuate nucleus, and the lateral hypothalamic area. Interruption of that last pathway by lesions of the dorsomedial nucleus interrupts the circadian control of food intake without affecting rhythms in body temperature, drinking, and locomotor activity.

Efferent projections from the SCN terminate in the intergeniculate leaflet and in the raphe nuclei, areas from which afferents to the SCN arise. Through those feedback loops, the SCN may modify its own inputs.

Parallels exist between the closely related indoles serotonin and melatonin (serotonin is a precursor of melatonin) (Figure 1.13-7). The SCN drives daily rhythms in the synthesis and the release of each indole, and each feeds back on the SCN—one acting as a neurotransmitter, the other as a hormone. Each appears to be capable of inducing phase shifts in rhythms generated by the SCN pacemaker, and each appears to play a role, as mediator or modulator, in the pacemaker's responses to seasonal changes in the photoperiod.

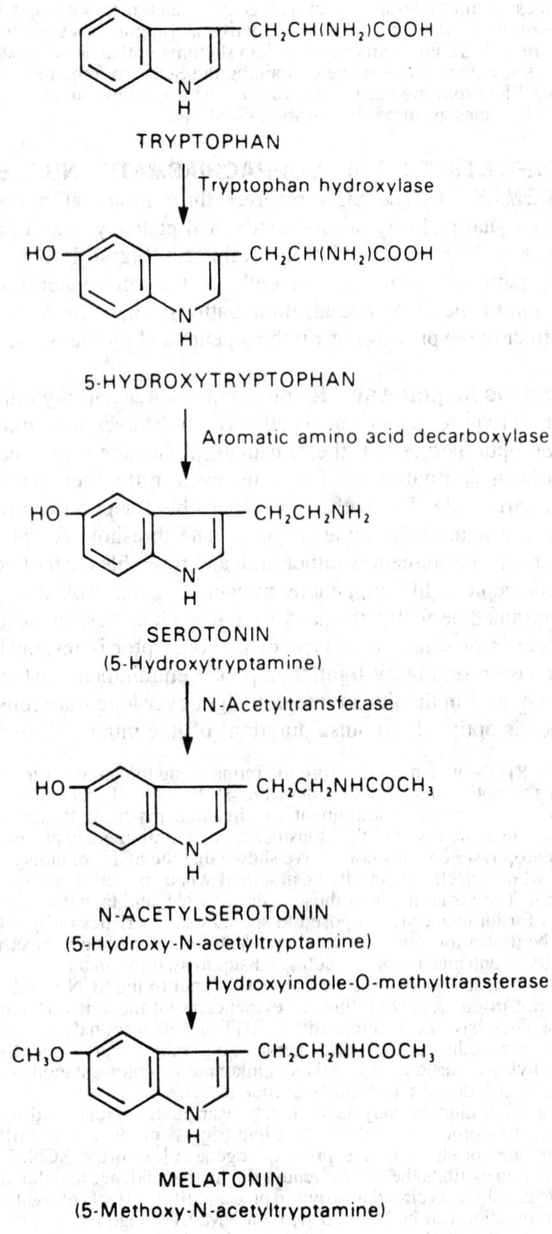

FIGURE 1.13-7 *Biosynthesis of serotonin and melatonin (From D Sugden: Melatonin biosynthesis in the mammalian pineal gland. Experientia 45: 923, 1989. Used with permission.)*

BIOLOGICAL RHYTHMS IN PSYCHIATRY

DELAYED SLEEP PHASE SYNDROME The circadian system and its substrate, the retinohypothalamic-pineal axis, may play an important role in the pathophysiology of some sleep and mood disorders. The evidence for such a role is clearest in the case of *delayed sleep phase syndrome,* a type of insomnia characterized by difficulty in falling asleep in the evening and in waking in the morning. Delayed sleep phase syndrome appears to represent a pure circadian rhythm disorder. In persons afflicted with the syndrome, sleep is entirely normal except that the timing of the sleep-wake cycle is shifted abnormally late (delayed) relative to the day-night cycle. When the syndrome sufferers attempt to go to sleep at a conventional hour, they are unable to do so. Instead, they remain awake until the early-morning hours. Then, if undisturbed, they sleep normally and wake up in the late morning or early afternoon. However, if they wish to wake up at a conventional hour, they find it difficult to do so, and they function poorly during the hours when they would otherwise have been asleep. If they habitually wake themselves at that hour (for example, to go to work), they have a chronic sleep deprivation syndrome as a complication of their delayed sleep phase syndrome. Apparently, in persons with the syndrome, the circadian pacemaker is unable to adopt a normal phase position when it entrains to the day-night cycle; instead, the pacemaker adopts an abnormally delayed phase position. Using principles derived from the human phase-response curve for light, clinical researchers have successfully treated delayed sleep phase syndrome by exposing patients to bright light in the morning, which advances their rhythms, and by shielding them from light in the evening, which delays their rhythms.

CYCLIC MOOD DISORDERS Animals use dawn-tracking and dusk-tracking components of their circadian system to lengthen or to shorten the duration of their sleep and activity phases to match seasonal changes in the duration of night and day. They also use the photoperiod-tracking mechanism to trigger dramatic seasonal changes in their behavior and physiology. For example, at one time of the year, they may become active and aggressive, seek out the environment, become interested in sex, sleep less than usual, and lose weight. At another time of the year, they may become less active, withdraw from the environment, lose interest in sex, sleep more than usual, and gain weight. All those changes are reminiscent of changes that occur in cyclic mood disorders in human beings. The parallels raise the possibility that a photoperiod-tracking mechanism in human beings underlies the changes that occur in cyclic mood disorders.

Major depressive disorder, with seasonal pattern The possible role of the circadian system and the retinohypothalamic-pineal axis has been extensively investigated in a type of major depressive disorder, with seasonal pattern, characterized by recurrent winter depression. On the basis of animal models, clinical investigators have hypothesized that winter depression is triggered by seasonal changes in the photoperiod and that the effect is mediated by photoperiod-induced changes in the duration of nocturnal melatonin secretion. Consistent with that model, exposure to light can reverse symptoms of winter depression. The light must be administered through the eyes (not the skin) to be effective, and some of the therapeutic effects of light can be reversed by administering melatonin to patients who respond to the treatment. Furthermore, the effects of morning light treatments can be mimicked by morning administration of a β-adrenergic receptor antagonist, which suppresses the terminal phase of nocturnal melatonin secretion and improves winter depression. However, other experimental evidence seems inconsistent with the model. Evening administration of a β-adrenergic receptor antagonist fails to improve winter depression, and suppression of melatonin secretion by light does not appear to be essential for its therapeutic effect. Nevertheless, some evidence shows that the antidepressant effect of light may depend on the capacity of light to shift the timing of the melatonin circadian rhythm.

Bipolar disorder Cycles of bipolar disorder (whether seasonal or nonseasonal) are often characterized by dramatic, state-dependent changes in the duration of sleep (the sleep phase shortens in mania and lengthens in depression). Those changes in sleep may play important roles in the pathogenesis of the disorder. In patients with bipolar disorder, experiments have shown that deprivation of sleep is antidepressant and can induce mania and that sleep is a depressant. Therefore, when shortening of sleep occurs in the course of bipolar disorder, it may help trigger or intensify mania. When lengthening of sleep occurs, it may help trigger or intensify depression.

In light of those observations, the mechanisms that regulate the duration of human sleep are important. As was already mentioned, the duration of human sleep is partly regulated by components of the circadian system that track dawn and dusk and adjust the duration of sleep to match the duration of night. Shifts in the relative timing of dusk-tracking and dawn-tracking mechanisms that control sleep onset and sleep offset may be responsible for cyclic changes in the duration of sleep that occur in bipolar disorder. In typical cases in which manic-depressive cycles are not synchronized with seasonal changes in the photoperiod, such shifts may be triggered by nonphotic, internal stimuli acting on the suprachiasmic nucleus circadian pacemaker. A possible source of such stimuli is the raphe serotonergic input to the pacemaker. As mentioned previously, that input can modulate the duration of nocturnal and diurnal phases defined by the pacemaker. The duration of the nocturnal cortisol-secretory phase is increased in depression (the time of the onset of the nightly increase in the rate of secretion is advanced relative to the time of the offset). That finding is consistent with the hypothesis that the duration of the nocturnal phase of the circadian system lengthens in depression and that the lengthening is responsible for the increased duration of sleep in the depressive phase of bipolar disorder. That hypothesis can be tested further by investigating whether the nocturnal melatonin-secretory phase, measured in dim light, also lengthens.

What precisely is ill in bipolar disorder has never been clear. This section has described a system centered in the retinohypothalamic-pineal axis (Figure 1.13-6) that, in animals, codes for seasonal changes in the duration of the photoperiod and orchestrates dramatic changes in sleep, activity, sexual behavior, hormones, and many other functions that are disturbed in bipolar disorder. Recent research shows that a homologous system in human beings is capable of coding for changes in the duration of the photoperiod and of orchestrating changes in sleep and melatonin. (Other functions under its control remain to be investigated.) The hypothesis that an illness in that system underlies the cycles of some forms of bipolar disorder is an attractive one that can be tested further.

SUGGESTED CROSS-REFERENCES

Sleep and the REM-non-REM sleep cycle are discussed in Section 1.9 on the basic science of sleep. The menstrual cycle and the neuroendocrine systems are discussed in Section 1.11 on psychoneuroendocrinology. Excitatory amino acids are discussed in Section 1.4 on amino acid neurotransmitters; neuropeptide Y is discussed in Section 1.5; and the serotonergic system is discussed in Section 1.3 on monoamine neurotransmitters. Sleep disorders are discussed in Chapter 23, and mood disorders are discussed in Chapter 16.

REFERENCES

Armstrong S M: Melatonin and circadian control in mammals. Experientia *45*:932, 1989.

Aronson B D, Johnson K A, Loros J J, Dunlap J C: Negative feedback defining a circadian clock: Autoregulation of the clock gene frequency. Science *263:* 1578, 1994.

Aschoff J, editor: *Handbook of Behavioral Neurobiology,* Plenum, New York, 1981.

Balzer I, Hardeland R: Photoperiodism and effects of indoleamines in a unicellular alga, Gonyaulax polyedra. Science *253:* 795, 1991.

Bartness T J, Goldman B D: Mammalian pineal melatonin: A clock for all seasons. Experientia *45:* 939, 1989.

Card J P, Moore R Y: The suprachiasmatic nucleus of the golden hamster: Immunohistochemical analysis of cell and fiber distribution. Neuroscience *13:* 415, 1984.

Ebisawa T, Karne S, Lerner M R, Reppert S M: Expression cloning of a high-affinity melatonin receptor from *Xenopus* dermal melanophores. Proc Natl Acad Sci *91:* 6133, 1994.

Glotzbach S F, Sollars P J, Pickard G E: 14C-2-deoxyglucose (2DG) uptake reveals bilateral asymmetry in the suprachiasmatic nucleus (SCN) of hamsters with split circadian activity rhythms. Neurosci Abstr *262:* 5, 1991.

Goodless-Sanchez N, Moore R Y, Morin L P: Lateral hypothalamic regulation of circadian rhythm phase. Physiol Behav *49:* 533, 1991.

Johnson R F, Smale L, Moore R Y, Morin L P: Paraventricular nucleus efferents mediating photoperiodism in male golden hamsters. Neurosci Lett *98:* 85, 1989.

Kripke D F: Critical interval hypotheses for depression. Chronobiol Int *1:* 73, 1984.

Meijer J H: Physiological basis for photic entrainment. Eur J Morphol *28:* 308, 1990.

*Meijer J H, Rietveld W J: Neurophysiology of the suprachiasmatic-circadian pacemaker in rodents. Physiol Rev *69:* 671, 1989.

Moore R Y, Card J P: Neuropeptide Y in the circadian timing system. Ann NY Acad Sci *611:* 247, 1990.

Moore R Y, Card J P: Visual pathways and the entrainment of circadian rhythms. Ann NY Acad Sci *453:* 123, 1985.

Moore-Ede M C: Physiology of the circadian timing system: Predictive versus reactive homeostasis. Am J Physiol *250:* R735, 1986.

*Moore-Ede M C, Czeisler C A, Richardson G S: Circadian timekeeping in health and disease. N Engl J Med *309:* 469, 1983.

Morgan P J, Williams L M: Central melatonin receptors: Implications for a mode of action. Experientia *45:* 955, 1989.
Morin L P, Michels K M, Smale L, Moore R Y: Serotonin regulation of circadian rhythmicity. Ann NY Acad Sci *600:* 418, 1990.
Mrsovsky N, Reebs S G, Honrado G I, Salmon P A: Behavioural entrainment of circadian rhythms. Experientia *45:* 696, 1989.
Prosser R A, Miller J D, Heller H C: A serotonin agonist phase-shifts the circadian clock in the suprachiasmatic nuclei in vitro. Brain Res *534:* 336, 1990.
Rosenwasser A M, Adler N T: Structure and function in circadian timing systems: Evidence for multiple coupled circadian oscillators. Neurosci Biobehav Rev *10:* 431, 1986.
Rusak B: The mammalian circadian system: Models and physiology. J Biol Rhythms *4:* 121, 1989.
*Rusak B, Bina K G: Neurotransmitters in the mammalian circadian system. Annu Rev Neurosci *13:* 387, 1990.
Sack R L, Lewy A J, Blood M L, Stevenson J, Keith L D: Melatonin administration to blind people: Phase advances and entrainment. J Biol Rhythms *6:* 249, 1991.
*Takahashi J S: Circadian rhythms: From gene expression to behavior. Curr Opin Neurobiol *1:* 556, 1991.
Vitaterna M H, King D P, Chang A-M, Kornhauser J M, Lowrey P L, McDonald J D, Dove W F, Pinto L H, Turek F W, Takahashi J S: Mutagenesis and mapping of a mouse gene, *Clock,* essential for circadian behavior. Science *264:* 719, 1994.
Wehr T A: The durations of human melatonin secretion and sleep respond to changes in daylength (photoperiod). J Clin Endocrinol Metab *73:* 1276, 1991.
Wehr T A: Effects of sleep and wakefulness on depression and mania. In *Sleep and Biological Rhythms.* J Montplaisir, R Godbout, editors, p 42. Oxford University Press, London, 1990.
Wehr T A, Goodwin F K, editors: *Circadian Rhythms in Psychiatry.* Boxwood Press, Pacific Grove, CA, 1983.
*Wehr T A, Moul D E, Barbato G, Giesen H A, Seidel J A, Barker C, Bender C: Conservation of photoperiod-responsive mechanisms in humans. Am J Physiol *265:* R846, 1993.
Wehr T A, Rosenthal N E: Seasonality and affective illness. Am J Psychiatry *146:* 829, 1989.
Wever R A: *The Circadian System of Man.* Springer, New York, 1979.

1.14 BASIC MOLECULAR NEUROBIOLOGY

STEVEN E. HYMAN, M.D.
ERIC J. NESTLER, M.D., Ph.D.

INTRODUCTION

The genetic blueprint of all living organisms, from bacteria to human beings, is encoded by the macromolecule deoxyribonucleic acid (DNA). DNA permits the transfer of information from generation to generation, and it contains the information required for the development of an organism in interaction with the environment. A common misconception is that the pattern of gene expression within a cell is rigidly determined during development and is a stable attribute of the cell thereafter. In fact, the expression of genes is constantly regulated in response to environmental signals. Changes in gene expression in response to physiological and pharmacological stimuli are involved in many homeostatic mechanisms and permit cells to make long-term adaptations to the environment.

Understanding the mechanisms by which environmental factors—such as life experience, drugs, infections, and injuries—affect the expression of neural genes is critical for an understanding of the pathophysiology of psychiatric disorders. Family, twin, and adoption studies make it apparent that both genetic and environmental factors play important roles in the normal development of temperament, personality, and many behavioral traits, and in the pathogenesis of major psychiatric disorders. Unlike some genetic disorders, such as Tay-Sachs disease and Huntington's disease, the major psychiatric disorders that have been investigated do not result solely from the unfolding of genetic information. Twin studies of schizophrenia, bipolar disorder, and panic disorder, for example, indicate that none of those disorders exhibits complete genetic penetrance. In other words, concordance for those disorders among monozygotic twin pairs (who have all their DNA in common) is less than 100 percent. Therefore, environmental factors must interact with the genome or its protein products to produce those illnesses.

In the coming decades an understanding of the pathogenesis of disorders such as bipolar disorder and schizophrenia is likely to be based, at least in part, on the identification of the disease genes that confer vulnerability to those disorders, combined with attempts to identify and study the environmental factors that interact with disease genes to produce the disorders. Analysis of those disorders in which inheritance of vulnerability involves a large number of genes may take a good deal longer, but the principles governing the pathogenesis of disorders are likely to be similar. Indeed, most psychiatric disorders and, for that matter, behavioral traits probably involve an interplay between a limited number of genes and specific environmental factors.

Gene-environment interactions may play a role not only in the initial expression of psychiatric disorders but also in their course. For example, some persons with mood disorders exhibit a worsening course over time, with episodes becoming progressively more frequent, more severe, and more refractory to treatment. Other disorders, such as bulimia nervosa and drug abuse, may begin as relatively controlled learned behaviors, but with repetitive experience (either binging or purging or repetitive drug administration) they become compulsive, with markedly diminished voluntary control, accompanied by dramatic effects on mood and cognition. In all those cases one can hypothesize that neurotransmitters or hormones released or otherwise affected by the disease, behavior, or drug administration produce long-term changes in neural functioning (that is, neural plasticity) that have a negative effect on the symptoms and the course of the disorder. A likely mechanism for such long-term changes is the neurotransmitter-mediated alteration of gene expression in the brain.

In the case of mood disorders, a number of hypotheses are consistent with such a model. For example, long-term exposure to high levels of glucocorticoid hormones is toxic to hippocampal neurons that are normally involved in producing counterregulatory restraints on the stress response. Because many patients with major depression have high levels of glucocorticoids, hippocampal neurons may, over time, be lost in those patients, permanently impairing the negative feedback on the neuroendocrine systems that contribute to both stress and depression. That model still lacks direct evidence in humans.

Another hypothetical approach, which is still more preliminary than the steroid toxicity model, analogizes episodes of mood disorder to kindling stimuli in an animal model of epilepsy. In the kindling model, repeated subthreshold electrical or drug stimuli are delivered to limbic structures, such as the amygdala, resulting eventually in an autonomous seizure focus. Although the models may be borne out, one need not posit such dramatic occurrences as hippocampal cell death or kindling of limbic structures to begin to hypothesize about how neurotransmitters, hormones, and drugs alter the course of a psychiatric disorder. Even normal intercellular signaling mechanisms function constantly to fine-tune levels of gene expression within the brain, permitting adaptive responses to environmental circumstances. Excessive or repetitive activation of intracellular signaling systems caused by diseases, by learned behaviors, or by drugs may drive those adaptive mechanisms in an abnormal fashion, resulting in plastic changes that may exacerbate or even produce psychiatric symptoms.

Alterations in neural gene expression may also be central to the mechanism of action of many psychotherapeutic drugs. In contrast to benzodiazepine anxiolytics, most other types of psychiatric drugs—such as antidepressants, antipsychotic drugs, and lithium (Eskalith)—work over a period of days to weeks, rather than minutes to hours. The direct, rapidly occurring effects of those drugs on neurotransmitter reuptake transporters, neurotransmitter receptors, and other components of the synaptic machinery apparently do not represent their ultimate therapeutic mechanism but, rather, are initial stimuli for slower-onset therapeutic actions. Although the regulation of gene expression begins rapidly (within minutes) in response to drugs, it can continue to produce biological effects with a time course consistent with the process progressively changing over a period of weeks.

For none of the examples cited above—pathogenesis of psychiatric disorders, course of psychiatric illnesses, and mechanism of action of psychotropic drugs—are the detailed mechanisms known. However, a great deal of molecular neurobiology is now known, permitting critical thinking about those central problems in psychiatry.

MACROMOLECULAR BUILDING BLOCKS

DNA is a double helix composed of two strands. Each strand is a linear polymer constructed of four small building blocks called nucleotides. The four nucleotides that make up DNA are the purines adenine (A) and guanine (G) and the pyrimidines cytosine (C) and thymine (T). As shown in Figure 1.14-1, the double helix is constructed of a sugar-phosphate backbone, with the nucleotide bases oriented toward the inside. On the inside of the helix, a purine (A or G), the large type of nucleotide, is always found directly opposite a small pyrimidine (T or C). In fact, the nucleotide A is always paired with T, and G is always paired with C. That situation is described by stating that A is complementary to T and that G is complementary to C. A maximum number of stabilizing hydrogen bonds form only between pairs of complementary nucleotides; any other arrangement of bases destabilizes the structure of the DNA.

The principle of complementary base pairing forms the basis of DNA replication and of the transcription of DNA into ribonucleic acid (RNA), which is the first step in gene expression. Because DNA is a linear polymer, it can serve as a template for the synthesis of other macromolecules. In either DNA replication or RNA synthesis, the double helix unwinds, and a new complementary strand of DNA or RNA is synthesized by successively incorporating complementary bases (for example, an A in the new strand across from a T in the template strand). Since the new strand contains a nucleotide sequence that is the exact complement of the sequence of the template, both strands contain the same information. In DNA replication each strand of the parent double helix can serve as a template for the synthesis of a new complementary strand, resulting in two double-helical molecules of DNA identical to the first. In RNA synthesis only one strand of the DNA serves as a template for the synthesis of a single-stranded RNA, which then dissociates from the template.

In higher (eukaryotic) organisms the DNA is contained within a specialized organelle called the *nucleus* and is organized into several discrete *chromosomes* (humans have 46) that are composed of long molecules of DNA bound by structural and regulatory proteins. Each chromosome contains multiple segments of DNA called *genes*. As a first approximation, a gene is a region of DNA that codes for the synthesis of a single protein (although RNA processing can introduce some variety into the protein products of a single gene). In addition to their coding regions, which specify the structure of proteins, genes contain regulatory regions that determine in which cells, under what circumstances, and to what extent the genes will be expressed. The human genome is thought to contain about 100,000 genes.

The structure of DNA is ideally suited for information storage and transfer, but its chemical simplicity and its relatively rigid helical structure limit the functions that DNA molecules can perform in the cell. As a result, the information contained within DNA is expressed through other molecules: RNA and proteins. RNA, like DNA, is a linear polymer of four nucleotides, but, unlike DNA, it is a nonrigid single strand, free to fold into a variety of conformations; it is, therefore, functionally more versatile than DNA. *Messenger RNA* (mRNA) functions as an intermediate between the sequence of DNA and the sequence of proteins. As in the case of DNA, mRNA carries information encoded in its linear sequence of nucleotides.

Proteins are constructed from 20 kinds of amino acids. By incorporating so many different amino acids, with their chemically diverse side chains (diverse in size, shape, hydrophobicity, and charge), proteins have much greater functional versatility than either DNA or RNA. The specific properties of proteins depend not only on the linear sequence of their amino acid building blocks (primary structure) but also on their folded,

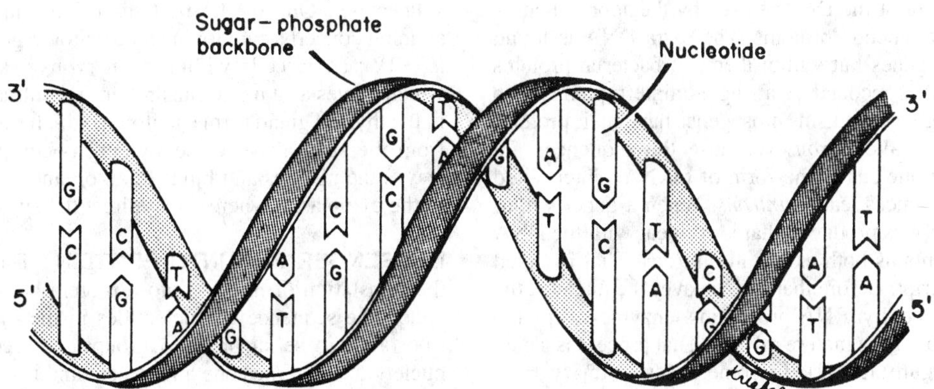

FIGURE 1.14-1 *The double helix of DNA. Two complementary strands of DNA hybridize with one another to form a double helix. The backbones of the two strands are formed by alternating sugar and phosphate groups; the nucleotide bases are found on the inside. Formation of a DNA double helix is stabilized when hydrogen bonds form between complementary bases of the two strands. (From S E Hyman, E J Nestler:* Molecular Foundations of Psychiatry, *p 4. American Psychiatric Press, Washington, 1993. Used with permission.)*

three-dimensional characteristics (secondary and tertiary structure). In addition, individual proteins (polypeptide chains) may form complexes with other proteins (quarternary structure); in such cases the individual proteins are called subunits. Proteins function in markedly different ways and serve virtually every aspect of cellular function. For example, proteins can serve as cytoskeletal and other structural components of cells and thereby determine their highly specialized shapes and control the transport of subcellular components; as enzymes, which catalyze and regulate the chemical reactions that occur within cells and thereby determine the other chemical constituents of cells; as ion channels and pumps, which regulate the flow of ions and other small molecules across cell membranes; as receptors and postreceptor signal transduction molecules that control the flow of information from the outside to the inside of cells; and even as intercellular messengers, such as hormones, growth factors, cytokines, and neuropeptides.

INFORMATION FLOW

Proteins are synthesized not directly from DNA but, rather, in two sequential processes: *transcription* of DNA into messenger RNA, which occurs in the nucleus, and *translation* of the mRNA into a protein, which occurs in the cytoplasm. Conceptually, transcription is similar to DNA replication in that one of the two strands of DNA serves as a template to produce an exact complement in terms of nucleotide sequence. However, instead of producing a second strand of nucleic acid that remains annealed to the template strand (as in DNA replication), transcription produces an RNA strand that is released from the template. That release allows the DNA of the gene to reform the double helix, and the RNA, which remains single-stranded, can be further processed and then exit the nucleus for translation. Since it is an exact complement of the gene, the mRNA produced by transcription retains all the information of the DNA sequence from which it was synthesized. The process of transcription can be subdivided into three major steps: *initiation,* mRNA chain *elongation,* and chain *termination.* In eukaryotes, the transcription of genes that encode proteins is carried out by the enzyme RNA polymerase II and associated regulatory proteins. The proteins that are involved in regulating transcription are called transcription factors.

RNA INTO MESSENGER RNA Eukaryotic cells contain far more DNA than is needed for their genes. In the human genome only about 1 percent of the DNA is used by the approximately 100,000 genes that encode proteins. The extra DNA is found not only between genes but within them. In bacteria, proteins are almost invariably encoded by a single uninterrupted stretch of DNA, but in higher organisms most genes have their protein-coding sequences, called *exons* (because the sequences are *ex*ported from the nucleus in the form of mRNA), interrupted by noncoding sequences, called *introns.* When a gene is transcribed, a long RNA is produced that is colinear with the DNA and, therefore, contains both exons and introns. That is called the primary transcript. Before that RNA leaves the nucleus, the introns are removed by RNA-processing enzymes, and the exons are joined to form a mature mRNA. That process is called *RNA splicing* (Figure 1.14-2). In some cases, primary transcripts may be spliced in alternative ways, depending on the cell type or the stage of development, to produce different mRNAs and hence different proteins. The mechanism enables more than one protein to be synthesized from a single gene and primary transcript, depending on which exons are retained or spliced out. One of the best-studied examples of alternative splicing concerns calcitonin and calcitonin gene-related peptide (CGRP): some cells within the nervous system form CGRP, which serves as a neurotransmitter; in contrast, medullary cells in the thyroid gland form calcitonin, which serves as a hormone, from the same gene. Once splicing is completed, the mRNA leaves the nucleus and binds to an organelle called a ribosome in the cytoplasm, where it can direct the synthesis of a protein.

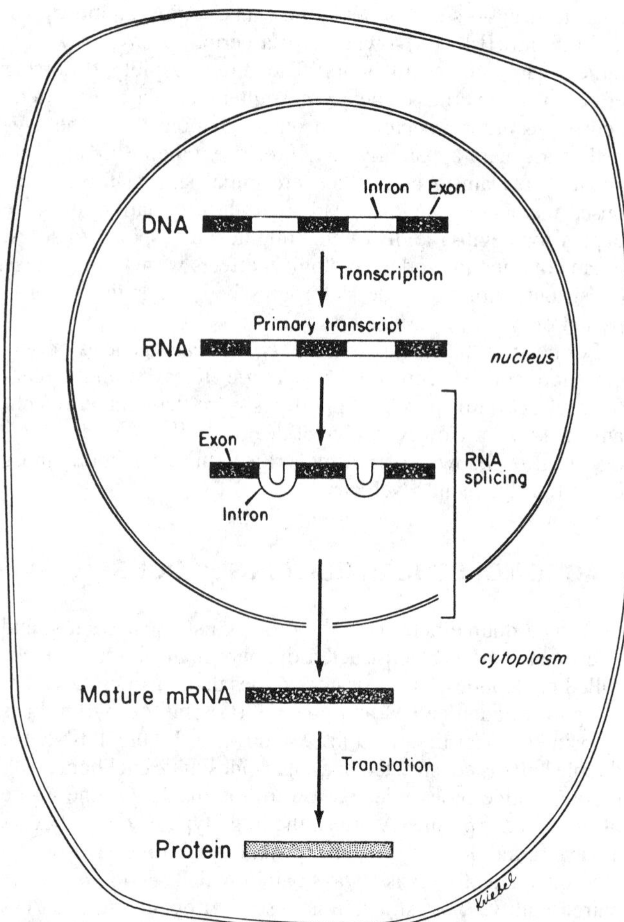

FIGURE 1.14-2 *RNA splicing. DNA contains exons, which encode polypeptides, and introns, which do not. The primary RNA transcript produced by RNA polymerase II contains both exons and introns. Before the transcript leaves the nucleus, a series of enzymes (themselves partly composed of RNA) recognize particular sequences as exon-intron boundaries and splice out the intron sequences. The mature messenger RNA (mRNA), containing only exons, is then exported from the nucleus into the cytoplasm, where it can bind to ribosomes and be translated into protein. (From S E Hyman, E J Nestler:* Molecular Foundations of Psychiatry, *p 17. American Psychiatric Press, Washington, 1993. Used with permission.)*

MESSENGER RNA INTO PROTEIN The rules governing the translation of mRNA into a protein are called the genetic code. The sequence of nucleotides in the mRNA are read on ribosomes in serial order in groups of three. Each triplet of nucleotides specifies one amino acid and is called a *codon.* The codons within an mRNA do not interact directly with the amino acids they specify; the translation of mRNA into a protein depends on the presence of adaptor RNA molecules, called transfer RNAs (tRNAs), that recognize the three bases within a codon and carry a corresponding amino acid. Transfer RNAs do that by providing a covalent attachment for a specific amino acid and a loop of RNA with a sequence complementary to a particular codon (Figure 1.14-3). The loop is called an anticodon and allows the tRNA to interact with the mRNA and to deliver its amino acid to the growing peptide chain. Each codon triplet has a corresponding tRNA species that specifies an amino acid. Ribosomes provide the structure on which tRNAs can interact (through their anticodons) with the codons of an mRNA in sequential order. The ribosome finds a specific start site on the mRNA and then moves along the mRNA molecule, translating the nucleotide sequence one codon at a time, using tRNAs to add amino acids to the growing end of the polypeptide chain. When the ribosome reaches the end of the message, both the mRNA and the newly synthesized protein are released from the ribosome, which then dissociates into individual subunits. That process is illustrated schematically in Figure 1.14-4. After and often coincident with translation, proteins are further processed: by specific cleavages to produce smaller peptides and proteins; by covalent modification, such as glycosylation, of particular amino acid residues within the protein; and by specific folding mechanisms. At that point, proteins are targeted to their proper location within the cell—for example, within the cell membrane or the membranes of particular organelles, within the cytoplasm, to other cellular locations, or to secretory pathways.

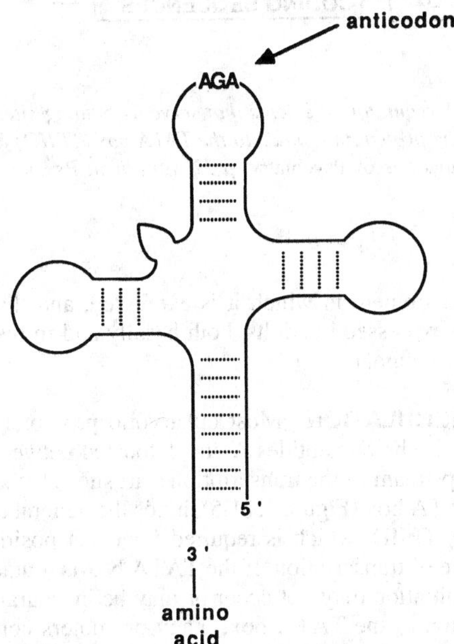

FIGURE 1.14-3 *Chemical structure of tRNA. Transfer RNA (tRNA) is a single strand of RNA that folds on itself through the apposition of complementary base pairs and the subsequent formation of hydrogen bonds, indicated by the dashed lines in the figure. One of the loops formed contains the anticodon, the sequence of three nucleotides on the tRNA that binds to the complementary codon on a messenger RNA (mRNA) molecule. For the anticodon AGA shown in the figure, the corresponding codon on the mRNA is UCU. The free 3′ end of the tRNA binds to a specific amino acid. Each tRNA, with a given anticodon, binds only one type of amino acid, determined by the genetic code. In the case shown in the figure, the amino acid is serine. (From S E Hyman, E J Nestler:* Molecular Foundations of Psychiatry, *p 19. American Psychiatric Press, 1993. Used with permission.)*

In summary, information within the genome is read out by a series of processes, each of which is highly regulated by the cell. Those processes include transcription of DNA into messenger RNA, mRNA splicing, translation of mRNA into a protein, and posttranslational modification of proteins.

REGULATION OF GENE EXPRESSION

Although many levels of regulation are important, transcription initiation appears to be the most important control point gating the flow of information out of the genome. As described above, transcription of protein-encoding genes, including genes for peptide hormones and neurotransmitters, is carried out by RNA polymerase II and associated proteins. The regulation of transcription initiation involves two critical processes, the positioning of polymerase at the correct start sites of genes and controlling the efficiency of initiations to produce the appropriate transcriptional rate for the cell. Those control functions are served by short stretches of DNA within genes, called *cis-regulatory elements* (Figure 1.14-5), that serve as specific binding sites for *transcription factors* (the proteins that regulate the rate of transcription).

Cells contain a large number of transcription factors with

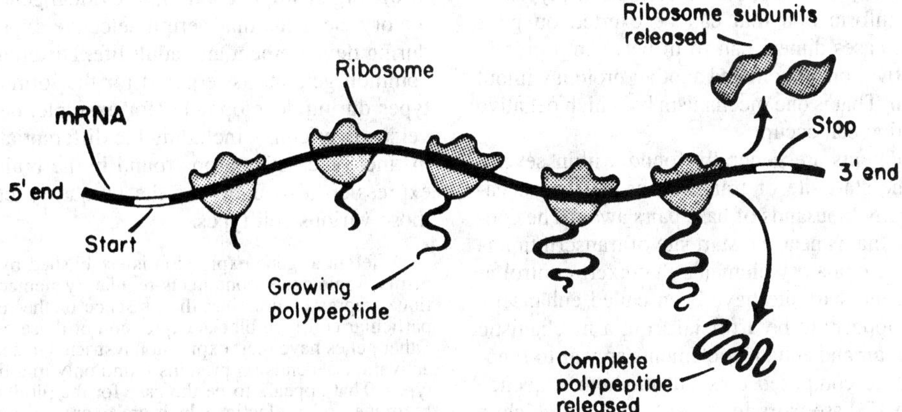

FIGURE 1.14-4 *The translation of messenger RNA (mRNA) into protein. Ribosomal subunits bind together on mature mRNAs to form actively translating ribosomes. The ribosome begins adding amino acids when it reaches a start codon on the mRNA and moves down the mRNA, one codon at a time, adding the appropriate amino acid as it is delivered by a transfer RNA (tRNA). When a stop codon is reached, the ribosome releases the polypeptide chain and dissociates from the mRNA. Each mRNA that is being actively translated has multiple ribosomes moving sequentially down its length, forming a polyribosome complex. (From S E Hyman, E J Nestler:* Molecular Foundations of Psychiatry, *p 20. American Psychiatric Press, Washington, 1993. Used with permission.)*

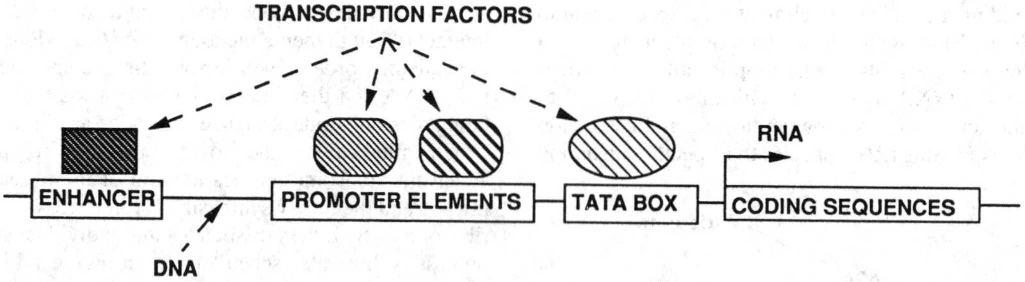

FIGURE 1.14-5 *An idealized eukaryotic promoter. The open rectangles represent DNA regulatory elements that serve as binding sites for transcription factors (stippled squares and ovals) involved in transcriptional regulation. The protein that binds to the TATA box (TFIID) determines the exact start site of transcription. (From S E Hyman, E J Nestler:* Molecular Foundations of Psychiatry, *p 12. American Psychiatric Press, Washington, 1993. Used with permission.)*

markedly different functional and structural properties. Some factors interact with many genes, others with only a small number. Transcription factors can increase or decrease the rate of expression of genes with which they interact. The ability of some transcription factors to activate or repress the expression of genes is regulated by physiological signals, such as protein phosphorylation.

Most known cis-regulatory elements are relatively short, 8 to 16 nucleotides in length. The role of those elements is to tether the appropriate transcription factors to the correct target genes but not to other genes. In an analogy with neuropharmacology, the specific DNA sequences of cis-regulatory elements act as receptors for transcription factors. The specificity of the binding site for a given transcription factor protein is determined by the particular order of bases in that short stretch of DNA. Most transcription factors contain two domains: one that recognizes and binds to the DNA sequence of a specific cis-regulatory element and another, often called the transcription-activation domain, that interacts with RNA polymerase II and associated proteins to form an active transcription complex. Many transcription factors are active only as dimers, either of identical proteins (homodimers) or of two different proteins (heterodimers). In such cases both proteins within the dimer often contribute both to the DNA binding site and to the activation domain. The ability of transcription factors to form heterodimers increases the diversity of transcription-factor complexes that can form in cells and, as a result, increases the types of specific regulatory information that can be exerted on gene expression. In some cases dimers can form between a protein with a functional activation domain and another protein without an activation domain. That is one mechanism by which negative control of transcription can occur.

Cis-regulatory elements are generally found within several hundred bases of the start site of transcription but can occasionally be found many thousands of base pairs away. The control region of a gene that is near the start site of transcription is called the promoter. Regulatory elements that exert control at some distance from the start site have been called enhancers, but that distinction appears to be artificial from a mechanistic point of view. Promoter and enhancer elements appear to function similarly; both are composed of small modular sequence elements (often 7 to 12 base pairs in length), each of which is a specific binding site for one or more transcription factors. Studies in which the elements have been removed or mutated have shown that each gene has a particular combination of cis-regulatory elements, the nature, number, and spatial arrangement of which determine the gene's unique pattern of expression, including the cell types in which it is expressed, the times during development in which it is expressed, and the level at which it is expressed in adults, both basally and in response to physiological signals.

BASAL REGULATION Most eukaryotic promoters have a region rich in the nucleotides A and T located between 25 and 30 bases upstream of the transcription start site. That sequence, called a TATA box (Figure 1.14-5), binds the general transcription factor, TFIID, which is required for exact positioning of the start site of transcription. If the TATA box is mutated, transcription initiation may not occur or may be inaccurate.

In addition to the TATA box, many promoters contain one or more cis-regulatory elements that bind transcription factors that confer a basal level of transcriptional activity on the gene. Such basal cis-regulatory elements are used by many genes. Common examples are the GC box (rich in the nucleotides G and C), which binds a transcriptional activator protein called SP1, and the CCATT box, which binds several different transcription factors. A gene that contains those types of regulatory elements is expressed constitutively (that is, at some finite level even when the cell is unstimulated), unless the gene also binds a repressor protein that prevents its expression under certain circumstances.

REGULATION DURING DEVELOPMENT Since all cells of an organism contain the same DNA (that is, a complete copy of the organism's genome), individual genes must contain regulatory elements that permit selective expression of the genes during development and adult life. Differential expression of a common genome is required for the formation of distinct cell types during development (for example, neuron versus kidney versus liver cells), including the differentiation of thousands of distinct types of neurons found in the brain. Differential gene expression also underlies the unique functional properties of those various cell types.

Differential gene expression is established by a number of mechanisms. Some genes contain cis-regulatory elements that bind transcriptional repressor proteins; the presence of the repressor proteins in a particular cell type blocks expression of those genes in that cell type. Other genes have their expression restricted to certain cell types if their activation depends on proteins found only in a limited number of cell types. That appears to be the case for the pituitary hormones, growth hormone and prolactin, which are expressed only in pituitary lactotrophs and somatotrophs because their main positive activator, a protein called Pit 1, is found only in those two cell types in the adult organism.

Mechanisms underlying the restriction of expression of genes only to appropriate cells is a complex subject that is understood in detail only in a few cases. In many cases, specificity of gene expression may be achieved through a combination of mechanisms: a given gene may contain multiple types of both repressor binding sites and activator binding sites that act in concert to determine which cells can express that gene. A major problem in developmental biology is understanding how cells come to express the particular set of activator and repressor proteins that determine which other genes are expressed in that cell.

REGULATION BY PHYSIOLOGICAL SIGNALS Many and possibly most genes contain cis-regulatory elements that confer responsiveness to physiological signals. Such cis-elements are often called response elements. Response elements work by binding transcription factors that are activated (or inhibited) by specific physiological signals, such as by second-messenger-dependent phosphorylation or hormone binding. That type of regulatory mechanism, which transduces physiological signals into changes in gene expression, is probably involved in many types of plasticity in the nervous system, including the events underlying learning and memory. Such plasticity is also likely involved in the onset and the course of psychiatric disorders and the therapeutic actions of psychotropic medications. Regulation of neural gene expression by neurotransmitters, hormones, and drugs can potentially produce long-lasting alterations in virtually all aspects of a neuron's functioning by regulating levels of neurotransmitter-synthesizing enzymes, peptide neurotransmitters, receptors, ion channels, signal transduction proteins, cytoskeletal components within the cells, and other critical neural proteins.

Steroid hormone receptors One important family of physiologically regulated DNA elements are the glucocorticoid response elements (GREs). Glucocorticoid and other steroid hormones bind to and thereby activate specific receptors within the cytoplasm of cells. The activated receptors then translocate into the nucleus, where they bind to GREs (or other steroid-hormone response elements) contained within particular genes. Such binding increases or decreases the rate at which those target genes are transcribed, depending on the precise nature and the DNA sequence context of the element. Most of the known effects of glucocorticoids, gonadal steroids, thyroid hormone, and vitamin D on cellular function are mediated by such actions on gene expression.

Neurotransmitters and second messengers Gene expression in the brain can be regulated by normal physiological processes, by experience, and by synaptically active drugs. The process is sometimes referred to as transsynaptic regulation of gene expression. The general mechanism by which synaptic signals are transduced to the genome involves the activation of intracellular second-messenger systems and their cognate protein kinases. The protein kinases then phosphorylate specific transcription factors or associated proteins, which alters their transcriptional activity. Phosphorylation of a transcription factor can alter its binding to the appropriate cis-regulatory element or, if already bound to DNA, its ability to regulate the activity of the polymerase II complex.

That schema has two major variants. One involves direct activation of a transcription factor that preexists within the neuron even under basal conditions. The other mechanism is indirect; phosphorylation activates a preexisting transcription factor that, in turn, activates the expression of genes that encode additional transcription factors. The newly synthesized factors can then activate or repress an additional set of target genes. The first mechanism occurs more rapidly than the second and partly explains the widely different time courses observed for transsynaptic regulation of gene expression. Thus, some neurotransmitter receptor-stimulated changes in gene expression occur within minutes, whereas others require many hours and depend on new protein synthesis. Both direct and indirect mechanisms are widely used by neurons to regulate their long-term responses to environmental signals.

DIRECT ACTIVATION BY CYCLIC AMP The first type of second-messenger response element to be characterized was one that conferred activation by cyclic adenosine monophosphate (cAMP) on the genes in which it was found. Similar cAMP response elements (CREs) have now been found within many neural genes. The discovery and the analysis of CREs and other response elements have depended on the ability to mutate candidate DNA sequences in vitro and then to reintroduce them into eukaryotic cells in culture. One can then observe the effects of the mutation on the activation of the gene. The process by which DNA is introduced into cultured cells is called *transfection.* Analysis of the expression of transfected genes is greatly facilitated by removing the coding sequences of the gene and replacing those sequences with those of a reporter gene, which yields an easily assayed protein product. The result is called a fusion gene. That type of analysis is schematized in Figure 1.14-6, in which the regulatory sequences of the human proenkephalin gene are shown fused to one commonly used reporter gene, bacterial chloramphenicol acetyltransferase (CAT). Other commonly used reporter genes include firefly luciferase and bacterial β-galactosidase.

Once fusion genes are constructed and transfected into tissue culture cells, the cells can be treated with neurotransmitters or drugs that activate the cAMP or other second-messenger systems. Induction of the reporter activity (for example, CAT activity) is a quantitative marker for regulation of the gene regulatory sequences being investigated. The simplest approach is to analyze progressive deletion of the regulatory sequences of the gene. Those progressive deletions eventually abolish the response to second messengers, thereby defining a region of DNA containing the response element. The identified region can then be examined in fine detail, such as by altering single bases within the region. As shown in Figure 1.14-6, the critical DNA regulatory element within the proenkephalin gene that makes the gene cAMP-responsive has the sequence TGCGTCA.

In addition, cAMP response elements have been identified in many other neural genes, including those for somatostatin, vasoactive intestinal polypeptide, tyrosine hydroxylase, and c-fos. By comparing response element sequences within many genes, one can derive an idealized consensus sequence. For CREs the consensus nucleotide sequence is TGACGTCA, and the nucleotides CGTCA are absolutely required.

The first transcription factor found to bind CREs was called CREB (for CRE binding protein). When bound to a CRE, CREB activates transcription when it is phosphorylated by cAMP-dependent protein kinase. However, the regulation of gene expression by cAMP turns out to be quite complex. At least three different forms of CREB have been cloned to date, and CREB is a member of a larger family of proteins. Moreover, members of another family of proteins, the Jun family, may bind CREs; in particular, JunD may bind to and activate the proenkephalin CRE in response to cAMP. Finally, CREB and perhaps JunD may be activated not only by cAMP through cAMP-dependent protein kinase but also by calcium entry through calcium-calmodulin-dependent protein kinases. The potential complexity of the regulation is likely to result in a great deal of flexibility and specificity in the way different types of cells respond to the environment.

INDIRECT ACTIVATION BY IMMEDIATE EARLY GENES Genes that are transcriptionally activated by synaptic activity, drugs, and growth factors are often roughly classified into two groups. Genes that are activated rapidly (within minutes), transiently, and without requiring new protein synthesis are referred to as cellular immediate early genes (IEGs). Genes that are induced or repressed more slowly (over hours) and are dependent on new protein synthesis are referred to as late-response genes. Protein products of certain IEGs may function as transcription factors that bind to DNA regulatory elements contained within late-response genes (target genes) to activate or repress them (Figure 1.14-7). In that scheme, late-response genes encode proteins involved in the differentiated functions of the cell.

The term "IEG" was used initially for viral genes that are activated immediately after infection of eukaryotic cells. Viral immediate early genes encode transcription factors that are needed to activate viral late gene expression. The terminology has been extended to cellular (non-viral) genes. However, the terminology has not been entirely successful. Cellular IEGs often encode transcription factors but not always. Many genes involved in the differentiated functions of cells, such as the cAMP-regulated genes for proenkephalin and tyrosine hydroxylase, appear to be activated rapidly and independently of new protein synthesis (by phosphorylation of CREB or JunD). Those are not generally included under the rubric of IEGs, even though a prototypical IEG, c-fos, is activated by a similar mechanism (Figure 1.14-7).

c-Fos protein is present in most neurons at barely detectable levels under resting conditions, but the expression of its gene can be induced

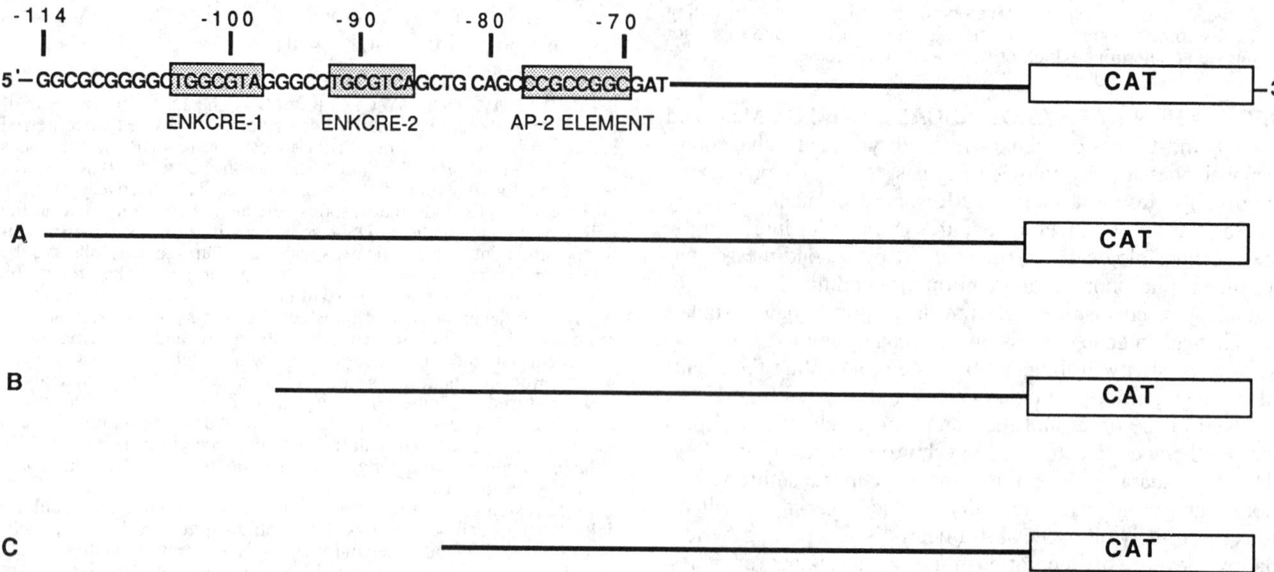

FIGURE 1.14-6 *Deletion analysis of a DNA regulatory region: the proenkephalin gene as an example. The top line shows the known DNA regulatory elements (shaded boxes) that constitute the proenkephalin enhancer. The relevant DNA sequences are shown; the rest of the regulatory region of the gene is shown as a line. The coding sequence of the gene has been replaced by a reporter gene, chloramphenicol acetyltransferase (CAT). Alterations can be made in the regulatory region of the DNA construction, and CAT expression can be assayed after transfection into eukaryotic cells. Lines A to C illustrate a deletion analysis, which is the initial approach used to analyze a promoter. Line A represents the entire enhancer sequence of the proenkephalin gene. When it is transfected and the cells are treated with cyclic adenosine monophosphate (cAMP), the gene is fully activated as measured by increased expression of CAT activity. In line B, one of the DNA regulatory elements (ENKCRE-1) has been deleted; when that construction is analyzed, the response of the gene to cAMP is diminished 10-fold. The deletion shown in line C removes a second regulatory element (ENKCRE-2) in addition to the first element. The gene is now inactive—despite a remaining element, activator protein-2 (AP-2)—which is apparently not strong enough to work on its own. The gene can now be further analyzed by mutating individual bases within the response elements. Even such small mutations can alter the ability of transcription factors to bind to their respective DNA elements. This type of analysis was used to define the boundaries of the regulatory elements in the proenkephalin gene promoter that mediate the gene's responsiveness to cAMP. The response element termed ENKCRE-2 binds the AP-1 and cAMP response element binding protein (CREB) families of transcription factors and is the critical element in cAMP-mediated signal transduction. (From S E Hyman, E J Nestler:* Molecular Foundations of Psychiatry, *p 222. American Psychiatric Press, Washington, 1993. Used with permission.)*

dramatically in response to a variety of stimuli, including neuronal depolarization. The newly synthesized c-fos mRNA is then translocated to the cytoplasm, where it is translated into new c-Fos protein. c-Fos protein, in turn, is translocated back to the nucleus, where it functions as a transcription factor. However, c-Fos protein and the protein products of the closely related IEGs—FosB, Fra-1 (fos-related antigen-1), and Fra-2—are unable by themselves to bind DNA with high affinity. The various members of the Fos family interact with members of the Jun family, a family of related transcription factors, to form heterodimers that bind DNA strongly. The Jun family includes c-Jun and JunB, which are regulated as IEGs (similar to c-fos), and JunD, which, as described above, is not regulated as an IEG in that it is constitutively expressed and regulated primarily by phosphorylation. Fos and Jun heterodimers bind to DNA at the sequence TGACTCA, the activator protein-1 (AP-1) binding site, to activate or repress transcription of the genes to which they are bound. Fos and Jun form heterodimers by juxtaposing conserved α-helical domains within each protein that contain leucines spaced seven amino acid residues apart, the so-called leucine zipper. Heterodimers can form between each of the proteins in the Fos family and the proteins of the Jun family. In addition, unlike the Fos proteins, the Jun proteins can form homodimers that bind to AP-1 sites, albeit with lower affinity than Fos and Jun heterodimers. Since many additional members of the Fos and Jun families are likely to be found, complex regulatory interactions can readily be imagined. What is the biological significance of those interactions? Different heterodimer and homodimer pairs apparently have different activator and repressor properties; for example, c-Fos and c-Jun are generally transcriptional activators; in contrast, c-Fos and JunB heterodimers and heterodimers containing FosB may function largely as repressors.

The IEGs and their protein products can be conceptualized as components of a molecular cascade that transduces signals from cell-surface receptors to the nucleus. Thus, IEGs such as c-fos have been termed third messengers in signal transduction cascades when neurotransmitters are designated as intercellular first messengers and small molecules, such as cAMP, are designated as intracellular second messengers. Alternatively, IEGs can be considered fourth messengers, with the CREB-like transcription factors (whose phosphorylation mediates the induction of c-fos and possibly some other IEGs) considered the third messengers. By either terminology, characterization of the biological actions of IEGs within particular neurons has many analogies with understanding the functions of other molecules within signal transduction cascades. Together with the direct mechanisms described above and shown in Figure 1.14-7, activation of IEG transcription factors serves to couple stimulation by drugs and neurotransmitters to activation or repression of genes involved in neuronal function. The observation that multiple IEGs, including c-fos, are activated in specific brain regions by psychotropic drugs—such as haloperidol (Haldol), cocaine, and amphetamine—has initiated many investigations of the mechanisms by which the drugs produce long-term alterations in neural functioning and, hence, behavior.

SUGGESTED CROSS-REFERENCES

Intraneural signaling pathways are discussed in Section 1.6, neurotransmitters in Sections 1.3 and 1.4, and genetics in Sections 1.15 and 1.16.

REFERENCES

Abeliovich A, Chen C, Goda Y, Silva A J, Stevens C F, Tonegawa S: Modified hippocampal long-term potentiation in PKC gamma-mutant mice. Cell *75:* 1253, 1993.

Borsook D, Konradi C, Falkowski O, Comb M, Hyman S E: Molecular mechanisms of stress-induced proenkephalin gene regulation: CREB interacts with the proenkephalin gene in the mouse hypothalamus and is phosphorylated in response to hyperosmolar stress. Mol Endocrinol *8:* 22, 1994.

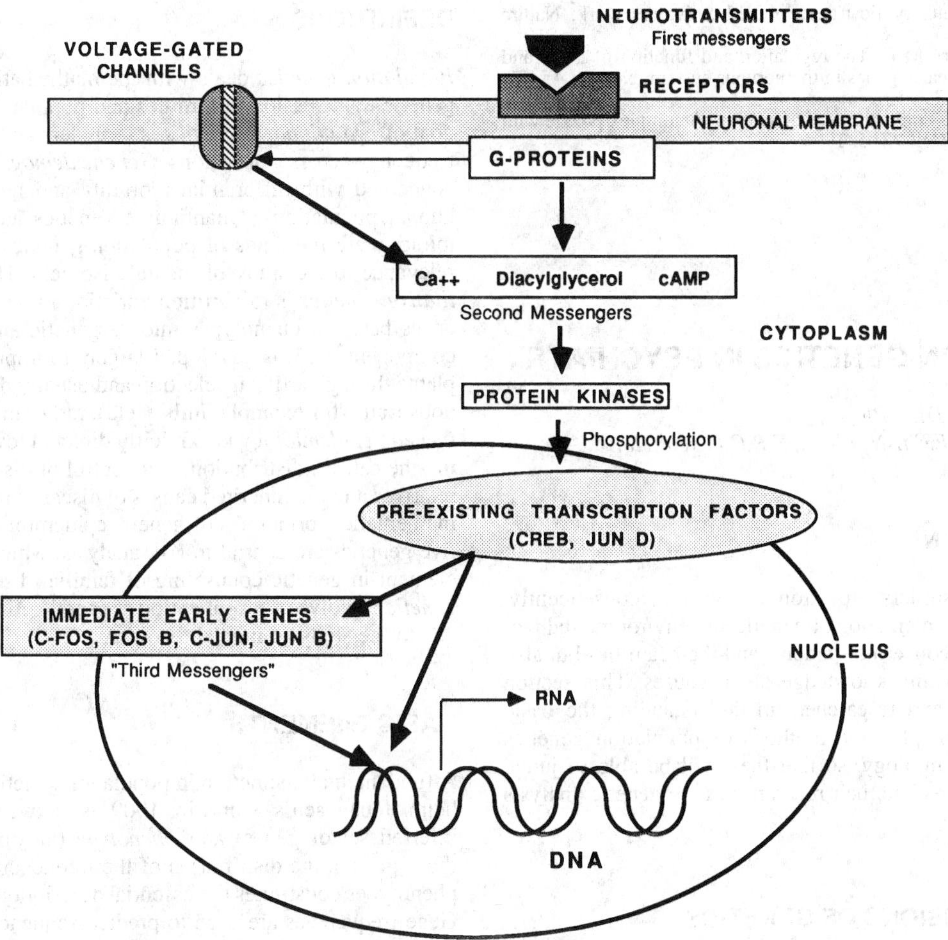

FIGURE 1.14-7 *Receptor-mediated signals being transduced to the nucleus. Neurotransmitter binding to its receptor may activate second-messenger systems, which in turn activate protein kinases. Phosphorylation of constitutively expressed transcription factors activates the transcription of both immediate early genes and other cellular genes. The protein products of immediate early genes may then activate or repress additional cellular genes. (From S E Hyman, E J Nestler:* Molecular Foundations of Psychiatry, *p 107. American Psychiatric Press, Washington, 1993. Used with permission.)*

Bouchard T J Jr, Lykken D T, McGue M, Segal N L, Tellegen A: Sources of human psychological differences: The Minnesota study of twins reared apart. Science *250:* 223, 1990.

Bourne H R, Nicoll R: Molecular machines integrate coincident synaptic signals. Cell *72* (Suppl): 65, 1993.

Comb M, Birnberg N C, Seasholtz A, Herbert E, Goodman H M: A cyclic AMP- and phorbol ester-inducible element. Nature *323:* 353, 1986.

*Comb M, Hyman S E, Goodman H M: Mechanisms of trans-synaptic regulation of gene expression. Trends Neurosci *10:* 473, 1987.

Crick F H C: The genetic code: III. Sci Am *215* (4): 55, 1978.

Dragunow M, Robertson G S, Faull R L M, Robertson H A, Jansen K: D_2 dopamine receptor antagonists induce fos and related proteins in rat striatal neurons. Neuroscience *37:* 287, 1990.

Ginty D D, Kornhauser J M, Thompson M A, Bading H, Mayo K E, Takahashi J S, Greenberg M E: Regulation of CREB phosphorylation in the suprachiasmatic nucleus by light and circadian clock. Science *260:* 238, 1993.

Gold P W, Goodwin F K, Chrousos G P: Clinical and biochemical manifestations of depression. N Engl J Med *319:* 349, 413, 1988.

Gonzalez G A, Montminy M R: Cyclic AMP stimulates somatostatin gene transcription by phosphorylation of CREB at serine 133. Cell *59:* 675, 1989.

Graybiel A M, Moratalla R, Robertson H A: Amphetamine and cocaine induce drug specific activation of the c-fos gene in striosome-matrix compartments and limbic subdivisions of the striatum. Proc Natl Acad Sci USA *87:* 6912, 1990.

Hope B, Kosofsky B, Hyman S E, Nestler E J: Regulation of IEG expression and AP-1 binding by chronic cocaine in the rat nucleus accumbens. Proc Natl Acad Sci USA *89:* 5764, 1992.

*Hyman S E, Nestler E J: *Molecular Foundations of Psychiatry.* American Psychiatric Press, Washington, 1993.

Kendler K S, Eaves L J: Models for the joint effect of genotype and environment on liability to psychiatric illness. Am J Psychiatry *143:* 279, 1986.

Konradi C, Kobierski L, Nguyen T V, Heckers S, Hyman S E: The cAMP-response-element-binding protein interacts, but Fos protein does not interact with the proenkephalin enhancer in rat striatum. Proc Natl Acad Sci USA *90:* 7005, 1993.

Li Y, Erzuraml R S, Chen C, Jhaveri S, Tonegawa S: Whisker-related neuron patterns fail to develop in the trigeminal brainstem nuclei of NMDAR1 knockout mice. Cell *76:* 427, 1994.

Maniatis T, Goodbourn S, Fischer J A: Regulation of inducible and tissue-specific gene expression. Science *236:* 1237, 1987.

Miller J C: Induction of c-fos mRNA expression in rat striatum by neuroleptic drugs. J Neurochem *54:* 1453, 1990.

*Mitchell P J, Tjian R: Transcriptional regulation in mammalian cells by sequence-specific DNA binding proteins. Science *245:* 371, 989.

Morgan J I, Cohen D R, Hempstead J L, Curran T: Mapping patterns of c-fos expression in the central nervous system after seizure. Science *237:* 192, 1987.

*Morgan J I, Curran T: Stimulus-transcription coupling in the nervous system: Involvement of the inducible proto-oncogenes fos and jun. Annu Rev Neurosci *14:* 421, 1991.

Nestler E J: Molecular mechanisms of drug addiction. J Neurosci *12:* 2439, 1992.

Nestler E J, Hope B T, Widnell K L: Drug addiction: A model for the molecular basis of neural plasticity. Neuron *11:* 995, 1993.

Nguyen T V, Kosofsky B, Birnbaum R, Cohen B M, Hyman S E: Differential expression of c-fos and zif268 in rat striatum after haloperidol, clozapine, and amphetamine. Proc Natl Acad Sci USA *89:* 4270, 1992.

Plomin R: The role of inheritance in behavior. Science *248:* 183, 1990.

*Ptashne M: How eukaryotic transcriptional activators work. Nature *335:* 683, 1988.
Sheng M, Greenberg M E: The regulation and function of c-fos and other immediate early genes in the nervous system. Neuron *4:* 477, 1990.
Tjian R, Maniatis T: Transcriptional activation: A complex puzzle with few easy pieces. Cell *77:* 5, 1994.

1.15
POPULATION GENETICS IN PSYCHIATRY

STEVEN O. MOLDIN, Ph.D.
IRVING I. GOTTESMAN, Ph.D., F.R.C.Psych.(Hon.)

INTRODUCTION

Many mental disorders are strongly familial; consequently, understanding the interaction of genetic and environmental factors is not only a concern of patients and their families but also essential to advancing knowledge about causes. This section assists clinicians and researchers in understanding the basic mathematical principles and methods of population genetics and genetic epidemiology, so that they will be able to judge new data and appreciate their relevance in the genetic analysis of mental disorders.

MAIN SUBDIVISIONS OF GENETICS

The scientific study of heredity, which began less than a century ago, gradually developed into five major disciplines, as depicted in Figure 1.15-1. *Biochemical genetics* is concerned with the biochemical reactions by which genetic determinants are replicated and produce their effects. *Developmental genetics* is concerned with the study of mutations that produce developmental abnormalities so that researchers can gain an understanding of how normal genes control growth and other developmental processes. *Molecular genetics* studies the structure and the functioning of genes at the molecular level. *Cytogenetics* deals with the chromosomes that carry those determinants. *Population genetics* may be subdivided into the partially overlapping fields of evolutionary genetics, genetic demography, quantitative genetics, and genetic epidemiology.

DEFINITIONS

Population genetics deals with the mathematical properties of genetic transmission in families and populations. The primary goal of *evolutionary genetics* is to understand changes in gene frequency across generations. *Genetic demography* is primarily concerned with differential mortality and fertility (fitness) in human populations. Quantitative genetics and genetic epidemiology are the fields of population genetics that are of most relevance to the study of mental disorders. The goal of *quantitative genetics* is to partition variation in the observed differences between phenotypes into its genetic and environmental components. It was developed largely to improve animals and plants through artifical selection and usually deals with continuous traits (for example, milk yield), rather than discrete traits. *Genetic epidemiology* is explicitly directed toward understanding the causes, distribution, and control of disease in groups of relatives and the inherited causes of disease in populations. The mathematical principles of genetic epidemiology and quantitative genetics are central to risk analysis, which is the essential element in genetic counseling of familial disease. *Psychiatric genetics* involves the application of genetic principles and methods to the study of mental disorders.

BASIC ELEMENTS

A fundamental distinction in population genetics dating to Wilhelm Johannsen's work in 1909 is between *genotype* (an inferred set of genes) and *phenotype* (an observed effect of those genes); the distribution of the frequencies of the various phenotypes constitutes the essential description of a population. Gene frequencies are used to predict frequencies of genotypes and phenotypes and vice versa under a set of assumptions that include the following: (1) From the pattern of familial inheritance, the genotypes can be distinguished unequivocally, such that the frequencies of phenotypes are the same as those of the underlying genotypes. This relationship between phenotypic and genotypic frequencies requires the related assumptions of negligible mutation rates and the occurrence of segregation of genes according to Mendel's laws: (2) There is no selection—that is, the expected number of fertile progeny from a mating that reaches maturity does not depend on the genotypes of the mates. (3) The population structure is such that all matings take place at random with respect to the genetic differences being considered in a population of infinite size. Consequently, the probability of mating between persons is in no way influenced by their genotype at a given locus.

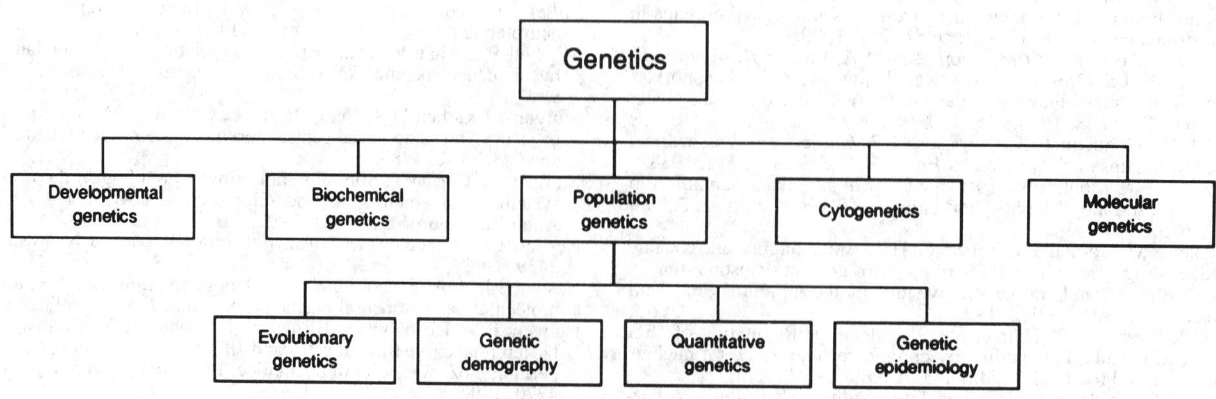

FIGURE 1.15-1 *The relationship of population genetics to the field of genetics.*

A general theorem formulated in 1908 independently by Godfrey Harold Hardy and Wilhelm Weinberg is derived from those assumptions and fits the facts well in many cases. In its simplest form the *Hardy-Weinberg law* states that, if the gene frequencies of two alternative forms of a gene *(alleles)*, A_1 and A_2, in parents are p_1 and p_2, respectively, the relative genotypic frequencies among the progeny with genotypes A_1A_1, A_1A_2, and A_2A_2 are p_1^2, $2p_1p_2$, and p_2^2, respectively. That relationship between gene frequencies and genotype frequencies is of the greatest importance because many of the deductions in quantitative and population genetics rest on it.

A basic distinction in population genetics of direct relevance for the analysis of mental disorders is that between *quantitative* and *qualitative* phenotypes. That is, do persons belong to a small number of discrete classes and differ in kind, or do they belong on a continuum and differ in degree? Disease phenotypes are qualitative—that is, persons are classified as affected or unaffected. Contemporary genetic analysis usually posits an underlying unobservable liability to affection that is continuous, with affected cases consisting of persons at an extreme end of the continuum. That is analogous to having height as the phenotype but only being able to measure tall versus nontall, rather than height in feet and inches. Quantitative phenotypes are those in which an observable continuous scale is used to measure the variable under consideration; enzyme levels and blood pressure are typical quantitative phenotypes.

A variable measured on a continuous scale has greater information content than one measured as a dichotomous variable; therefore, quantitative traits that are highly correlated with liability to an illness can make important contributions to genetic analysis. Highly specific and sensitive quantitative measures unfortunately have not been found for mental disorders, but data provided by both diagnostic interviews (determination of affected versus unaffected status) and biological-biobehavioral quantitative measures can be analyzed conjointly to identify genetic or environmental factors important in familial transmission.

GENETIC MODELS

Mathematical models are required in population genetics to represent the ways in which genes and the environment interact to form complex phenotypes transmitted within families. The most common transmission models applicable to the study of psychiatric phenotypes are presented in Table 1.15-1.

SINGLE MAJOR LOCUS MODEL The single major locus model assumes that all relevant genetic variation is due to the presence of alleles at a single locus and that environmental variation is nonfamilial. The variance in a trait attributable to a single gene can be distinguished from the variance attributable to several genes at multiple loci acting together; in that context the single gene is a *gene of large effect*. With two alleles, *A* and *a*, of respective frequencies p_1 and p_2, three genotypes are possible: *AA*, *Aa*, and *aa*. When both alleles are the same, it is a *homozygous* genotype; when two alleles are different, it is a *heterozygous* genotype. The sum of the allele frequencies totals unity, so, by definition, $p + q = 1$. If the environment is constant, such that each genotype corresponds to only one phenotype, the gene at a given locus is *completely penetrant*. The important discovery in 1993 of trinucleotide (triplet) repeats within single dominant genes helps to explain the variations in both age of onset and severity, without invoking an additional modifying locus.

Diseases transmitted through a single major locus are referred to as Mendelian diseases, as the pattern of inheritance in families follows the rules of Mendelian segregation and can usually be recognized through visual inspection of pedigrees. Genetic disorders transmitted through a single major locus are quite rare and include retinitis pigmentosa, Duchenne's muscular dystrophy, Huntington's disease, phenylketonuria, and cystic fibrosis.

Familial patterns of inheritance can be characterized by whether the disease gene is on an autosome or on a sex chromosome and by whether both alleles are required for expression (recessive disease) or only one allele is sufficient (dominant disease). The liability distributions in the general population resulting from a diallelic major locus in Hardy-Weinberg equilibrium are shown in Figure 1.15-2.

Single major locus modes of inheritance The following criteria for different single locus models of disease transmission are required: (1) *Autosomal dominant*—(a) transmission continues from generation to generation without skipping; (b) except for freshly mutated cases, every affected child has an affected parent; (c) the two sexes are affected in equal numbers; and (d) in marriages of an affected heterozygote to a normal homozygote, the probability that a child born into that family will be affected (the segregation ratio) is ½; (2) *Autosomal recessive*—(a) if the disease is rare, parents and relatives (except siblings) are usually normal; (b) all children of two affected parents are affected; (c) in marriages of two normal heterozygotes, the segregation ratio in offspring is ¼; and (d) the two sexes are affected in equal numbers. (3) *Sex-linked recessive*—(a) if the disease is rare, parents and relatives (except maternal uncles and other male relatives in the female line) are usually normal; (b) hemizygous affected men do not transmit the disease to children of either sex, but all their daughters are carriers; (c) heterozygous carrier women are normal but transmit the disease to their sons with a segregation ratio of ½, and half of the daughters are normal carriers; and (d) except for

TABLE 1.15-1
Genetic Models of Disease Transmission

	Source of Familial Resemblance		
Genetic Model	Single Major Locus	Polygenes	Common Environment
Single major locus	Yes	No	No
Multifactorial	No	Yes	Yes
Mixed	Yes	Yes	Yes

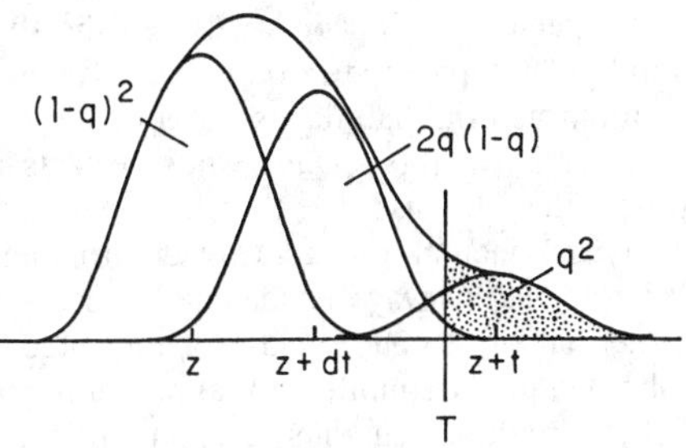

FIGURE 1.15-2 *Liability distributions resulting from a single major locus in Hardy-Weinberg equilibrium. The proportion of persons with a given genotype who are above the threshold* T *gives the penetrance of that genotype. The shaded area gives the lifetime cumulative incidence of the disease* (K_p).

mutants, every affected male child comes from a carrier mother. (4) *Sex-linked dominant*—(a) heterozygous mothers transmit to both sexes in equal frequency, with a segregation ratio of ½; (b) except for new mutants, every affected child has an affected parent; (c) if the disease is rare, the frequency is approximately twice as great in females as it is in males; and (d) hemizygous affected males transmit the trait only to daughters, the segregation ratio being 1 in daughters and 0 in sons.

The irregular patterns of inheritance of the common illnesses with genetic components—such as hypertension, coronary artery disease, diabetes, cancer, epilepsy, and mental disorders—do not meet any of the above criteria for fully penetrant single major locus transmission in most families. The concept of *incomplete penetrance* has been introduced, by which persons with identical genotypes have different phenotypes because of variability in nontransmissible environmental factors that contribute to the phenotype. The penetrance is the probability that a person with a given genotype will manifest the illness; probabilities are usually denoted by the letter *f*. The lifetime cumulative incidence or morbid risk of a disease is frequently denoted by the letters K_p. In the case of a disorder caused by a diallelic autosomal single major locus—in which the respective gene frequencies of the *A* and *a* alleles are p_1 and p_2 and the respective penetrances associated with the *AA*, *Aa*, and *aa* genotypes are f_1, f_2, and f_3—$K_p = f_1p_1^2 + 2f_2p_1p_2 + f_3p_2^2$. Current single major locus models allow for incomplete penetrance (such that one or more *f*s are not equal to zero or one) with transmission of a fully penetrant major locus contained as a submodel.

Elucidation of abnormal protein products and subsequent resolution of pathophysiology is theoretically more straightforward in the case of disease transmission through a gene of large effect than in the case of disease transmission through polygenes. However, the genetics of single major locus diseases can still be complicated, as exemplified by Huntington's disease. A dominant disease locus was linked to genetic markers on chromosome 4 in 1983, but the precise gene or biochemical abnormality was only identified in 1993.

MULTIFACTORIAL MODEL The multifactorial model assumes that all relevant genetic and environmental contributions to variation can be combined into an unobserved normally distributed variable termed *liability*. One or more threshold values are on the liability scale; affected persons are those with liability values that exceed the threshold. Familial inheritance is modeled through correlations in liability between family members, with the following assumptions: (1) relevant genes act additively and are each of small effect in relation to the total variation; (2) environmental contributions are due to many events, whose effects are additive; and (3) there may be multiple thresholds, such that persons with scores between threshold values represent mild phenotypic or spectrum cases. The genetic contribution to multifactorial liability is not a single major locus but, rather, several loci *(polygenes)* whose effects aggregate. Liability to manifest the disorder, therefore, is the cumulative effect of many risk factors (polygenic or environmental). Normal traits inherited in this way include intelligence, stature, skin color, total dermal ridge count, and probably blood pressure. Diseases inherited under a multifactorial model include hypertension, diabetes mellitus, ankylosing spondylitis, pyloric stenosis, rheumatoid arthritis, peptic ulcer, most cases of breast cancer, spina bifida, and coronary artery disease. Liability distributions in the general population for single-threshold and two-threshold multifactorial models are shown in Figure 1.15-3.

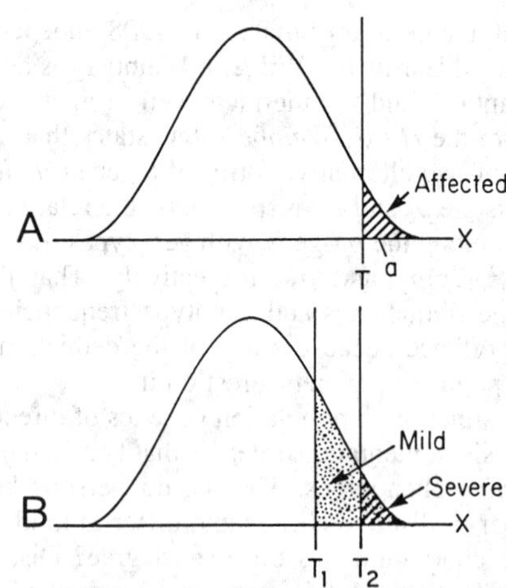

FIGURE 1.15-3 *Liability distributions with (a) a single threshold* T *and mean liability of affected persons denoted by* a *and (b) two thresholds,* T_1 *and* T_2*, used to model severity, such that persons with a liability score above* T_2 *have a core phenotype, and persons whose liability is between* T_1 *and* T_2 *have a milder form of the illness (spectrum condition). The shaded areas give the lifetime cumulative incidences of the disease* (K_p).

MIXED MODEL The mixed model is a marriage of the single major locus and the multifactorial models. An unobservable distribution of liability is determined by the effects of a major locus, a multifactorial transmissible background (polygenes or environmental factors), and residual nontransmissible environmental factors. A crucial distinction from the single major locus model is that the variation within a genotype for the major locus in the mixed model is in part familial.

The mixed model and other related formulations have a number of conceptual and practical advantages over other approaches. When generalized so that the background is multifactorial, the mixed model is the most comprehensive and realistic model, since common illnesses are likely to have both major locus and multifactorial (polygenes or common transmissible environment) causes. Since both the single major locus model and the multifactorial model are submodels, the mixed model provides a statistical advance in permitting the rigorous testing of whether a single major locus or a multifactorial component (or both) contributes to familial resemblance.

Oligogenic models Oligogenic models are extensions of the mixed model in that a small number of major loci either with or without a larger number of background polygenes contribute to disease expression. Such models also allow for interaction *(epistasis)* among loci. Oligogenic models represent the latest thinking among quantitative geneticists that a small number of loci of varying large effect that differentially contribute to disease susceptibility can be identified. Analyses of recurrence risks in first-, second-, and third-degree relatives and in monozygotic and dizygotic twins in European family studies have suggested that epistatic loci are involved in the familial transmission of schizophrenia.

RESEARCH DESIGNS

Population, family, twin, adoption, and association studies can each contribute evidence to evaluate the involvement of genetic factors in the cause of an illness. The methods have been applied extensively in the investigation of mental disorders.

POPULATION STUDIES Prevalence and incidence rates of mental and other disorders derived from community-based surveys have important scientific and health policy implications. Variations in such rates can provide clues to causes and can be used as base rates for comparative purposes in family genetic studies.

FAMILY STUDIES If genetic factors are involved in the transmission of an illness, the illness should cluster in the families of affected members at a higher rate than in appropriate control populations. However, relatives who share a number of genes also tend to share common environments, so familial clustering by itself does not necessarily implicate a genetic mechanism; culture, family environment, or infectious agents may be responsible. Family studies for mental and other disorders begin with affected persons *(probands)* selected in an unbiased way—for example, from consecutive hospital inpatient admissions. Available relatives are located and assessed for psychopathology with structured or semistructured diagnostic instruments. Countries with national health insurance and psychiatric registers can provide morbidity information across generations. Recurrence risks are expected to increase as the degree of genetic overlap between relatives increases. The closest familial relationship is that of monozygotic twins, who have all their genes in common. Dizygotic twins, full siblings, parents, and children are first-degree relatives, who share half of their genes on average. Second-degree relatives of probands—grandparents, grandchildren, uncles, aunts, nieces, nephews, and half siblings—share one fourth their genes.

A variety of factors tend to make comparisons of familial risk to mental disorders across studies difficult. Those factors include differences in sample characteristics, methods of age correction, ascertainment schemes, and diagnostic procedures. Such methodological concerns can explain how in different studies the risk for depression in first-degree relatives of depressive probands varies between 11 and 18 percent, while the risk to relatives of normal controls varies between 0.7 and 7.3 percent. Comparison of normal controls and high-risk relatives by similar case-finding and diagnostic methods are essential when interpreting mean risk estimates. Likewise, the ideal family study uses double-blind, case-controlled methods in which diagnoses of relatives are made independently of the proband's diagnosis.

TWIN STUDIES The twin method has been a popular research design to implicate or exclude genetic factors in the cause of a disease. Since monozygotic twins have identical genotypes, any dissimilarity between pair members must be due to the action of the environment, either prenatally or postnatally. Consequently, anything less than 100 percent concordance among monozygotic pairs living through the period of risk excludes genetic factors as sufficient determinants of that disease.

If genetic differences are not important for the familial clustering of a disease, no differences should be seen in the monozygotic and dizygotic concordance rates. That is the case in twin studies of diseases caused by infectious agents, such as measles. Conversely, if genes are important in causing a disease, the monozygotic concordance rate is significantly higher than the dizygotic rate. A genetic basis is the most likely explanation for the higher monozygotic concordance rate if (1) monozygotic twins are not more predisposed to having the disease and (2) monozygotic twin environments are not more alike in features that cause the disease. The twin method in psychiatry has also been useful in identifying spectrum conditions that are alternative manifestations of the disease genotype that occur in monozygotic twins discordant for the core illness.

Critics of the twin method have argued that monozygotic pairs share more similar environments than do dizygotic pairs, and that is responsible for the higher monozygotic concordance rate for mental disorders. Three ways in which environmental factors may increase the rate have been advanced: (1) monozygosity per se, (2) the effects of identification by one twin with another, and (3) the sharing of a similar ecology, with enhanced exposure to triggering events. No conclusive evidence has been advanced that those limitations have substantially biased the results of twin studies of mental disorders.

ADOPTION STUDIES Whereas monozygotic and dizygotic twin studies endeavor to hold the family environment constant to compare the resemblances between persons with the same and different genotypes, adoption studies permit the comparison of the effects of different types of rearing on groups who are assumed to be similar in their genetic predispositions. Such studies attempt to separate the effects of genes and the familial environment by capitalizing on the adoption process, in which children receive their environment from a source different from their gene source. Consequently, adoption studies provide one of the few research designs for disentangling genetic and environmental factors that contribute to the familial aggregation of a disease. The ability to draw inferences from an adoption study is strongest when the adopted children are separated from their biological parents at birth.

Potential problems of the research design are that (1) any parent-child interaction from the time of birth to the separation confounds a clear demarcation of genetic and environmental aspects and (2) the environmental circumstances of biological parents may be associated with prenatal and perinatal events relevant to the cause of the disease.

Three major designs of adoption studies have been used to study mental disorders. (1) The parent-as-proband design compares the rate of illness in the adopted offspring of ill and well persons. Support for a genetic component is indicated if the risk of illness among adopted children of ill parents is greater than the risk of illness among adopted children of well parents. (2) The adoptee-as-proband design uses ill and well adoptees as probands. Genetic factors are implicated if (a) the risk of illness in the biological relatives of ill probands is greater than that in the adoptive relatives of ill probands and (b) the risk of illness is greater in the biological relatives of ill probands than that in the biological parents of well adoptees. (3) The third design is the seldom used cross-fostering approach, which compares rates of illness in two groups of adoptees. One group have ill biological parents and are raised by well adoptive parents; the other group have well biological parents and are raised by ill adoptive parents.

A famous adoption study in psychiatry was started in the 1960s by David Rosenthal, Seymour Kety, Paul Wender, and their colleagues to study schizophrenia in Denmark. The major accomplishment of the project was to rule out some alleged environmental factors (being reared by a schizophrenic parent) as either necessary or sufficient for the development of schizophrenia in the offspring of schizophrenic parents. The data have held up remarkably well, even after probands and relatives were classified with criteria used in the third edition of *Diagostic and Statistical Manual of Mental Disorders* (DSM-III). The data also provided an opportunity to develop operational criteria for schizotypal personality disorder as a spectrum condition genetically related to the core schizophrenic phenotype, since it occurred at a higher rate in the biological realtives of adopted-away schizophrenic persons than in the adoptive relatives of schizophrenic persons and the relatives of control adoptees.

ASSOCIATION STUDIES An approach for better understanding the origin of a complex disease is to evaluate whether there is an association between genetic markers and the disease.

That is typically accomplished by studying a sample of unrelated affected persons and comparing the frequency of a particular marker phenotype in the affected group versus its frequency in a population sample or other controls through the chi-square statistic. The most widely accepted genetic explanation for a weak-to-moderate association is that there exists a disease locus linked to and in linkage disequilibrium with the marker locus. However, causal inferences based on genetic differences between cases and controls drawn from a heterogeneous population are often difficult to replicate or interpret. Such *population-based genetic association studies* are highly susceptible to the effects of the admixture of subgroups that do not randomly intermarry. Ethnic and religious groups often differ in allele frequencies at many genetic loci, and case-control matching is inadequate when the relevant variables are not known or are difficult to measure.

Association without linkage in pedigrees may be explained by one of several hypotheses: (1) population stratification or admixture, (2) epistasis or interaction among multiple genes, (3) clustered sampling of related persons, and (4) chance findings in a given sample.

The choice of a proper control group in association studies is essential to insure that an observed association is not due to population admixture. For example, if a given allele tends to occur more often in a given racial group, the control population has to be carefully matched for race. That problem was resolved by Catherine Falk and Paldo Rubenstein, by analyzing data from a sample of affected persons and their parents, assuming no differential selection between genotypes at the susceptibility locus—for example, no reduced fertility. The most appropriate control sample is the alleles at different loci received from one patient (the parental *haplotype*) not present in the affected person, which represent a random sample of haplotype pairs from the same genetic population. Under the null hypothesis of no association, each allele at the locus under investigation has an equally likely chance of being transmitted to the affected offspring. Association strategies have grown in importance as a result of negative results with linkage studies and as a result of increased density of markers covering the genome. Such family-based association tests present a viable alternative to more traditional population-based association tests as a means to detect and confirm a disease marker association.

Family-based association tests therefore distinguish between association due to linkage (with linkage disequilibrium) and association that may arise in the absence of linkage, such as that due solely to artifacts such as population stratification. In that sense, the family-based approach is a test of linkage in the classical sense and combines the advantages of a linkage study and population study without requiring ascertainment of highly multiplex families.

An efficient design for genetic studies in psychiatry may be to ascertain families and conduct a family-based association test; if association is found, pedigrees could be evaluated using all family members. Such a design would be cost-effective in that (1) new families would not need to be identified, and (2) initial pedigree ascertainment would not require multiplex pedigrees only, which are difficult to find for illnesses like schizophrenia and bipolar disorder. Independent replication would be required to establish the verisimilitude of the findings.

QUANTITATIVE METHODS

Data from the research designs described above can be analyzed by using sophisticated mathematical models and high-speed computers. The methods most typically used in the study of genetic factors are presented in Table 1.15-2.

PATH ANALYSIS Path analysis was introduced as a technique to (1) explain the interrelations among variables by analyzing their correlational structure and (2) evaluate the relative importance of varying causes influencing a certain variable. The primary goal of path analysis in genetic epidemiology is to distinguish genetic effects from transmissible environmental effects transmitted from parents to children *(cultural transmission)* that contribute to the familial aggregation of a disease. Twin and adoptive data are necessary to separate nature from nurture in path analysis. When genetic transmission is present, additive polygenic effects cannot be distinguished from single major locus effects.

Familial correlations are estimated through *maximum likelihood techniques,* statistical procedures for estimating parameters, such that the best-fitting estimates are those that maximize the probability of the observations. Comparisons of competing models are made by fitting a general model and alternative submodels. Since log likelihoods are calculated for the general model (L_1) and the submodel (L_2), then $-2(L_1-L_2)$ is approximately distributed as a chi-square with the degrees of freedom equal to the difference in the number of estimated parameters. That is the *likelihood ratio test,* the test statistic for comparing alternate models. Both qualitative (affected or unaffected status) and quantitative phenotypes may be analyzed, and examples of the results of applying path models of multifactorial transmission to analyze several traits are given in Table 1.15-3. A typical path model that has been used in the study of mental disorders is shown in Figure 1.15-4.

A useful application of complex path models was exemplified by the analysis of twin and family data from a variety of published sources for tuberculosis and schizophrenia. The results showed that the major contribution to phenotypic variance for tuberculosis came from shared family environment, rather than from genes; that result is expected for an illness caused by an infectious agent. Results from twin data alone would have been misleading in implicating a major genetic effect. In the case of schizophrenia, by contrast, the largest contribution to the variance comes from genes, with the suggestion of a modest role for the common environment.

Path analysis and complex segregation analysis both allow for adjustment to correct biases that may have occurred in the sampling

TABLE 1.15-2
Quantitative Methods of Genetic Analysis

Method	Data	Goal
Path analysis	Twin, adoption	Distinguish transmissible environment from polygenes
Complex segregation analysis	Pedigree	Distinguish a major locus from polygenes or transmissible environment
Linkage analysis	Pedigree	Establish chromosomal localization of a putative disease susceptibility major locus

TABLE 1.15-3
Genetic and Environmental Contributions to the Variance of Several Traits

Trait	Polygenes	Family Environment	Nonshared Environment
I.Q.	0.48	0.36	0.16
Personality (extroversion)	0.66	0.00	0.34
Bipolar disorder	0.86	0.07	0.07
Major depression	0.52	0.30	0.18
Dysthymia	0.08	0.54	0.38
Schizophrenia	0.63	0.29	0.08
Tuberculosis	0.06	0.62	0.32

Adapted from P McGuffin: Genetic models of madness. In *The New Genetics of Mental Illness,* P McGuffin, R Murray, editors, p 34. Butterworth-Heinemann, Boston, 1991.

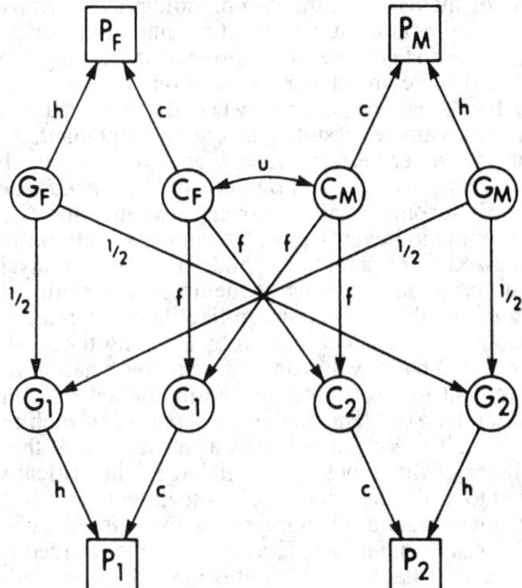

FIGURE 1.15-4 *Path model used for the transmission of schizophrenia in nuclear families.* G, C, *and* P *denote genotype, transmissible environment, and phenotype, respectively. Subscripts* F, M, 1, *and* 2 *denote father, mother, and two children respectively. The model has the following parameters: genetic heritability,* h^2*; cultural heritability,* c^2*; effect of parental environment on offspring's environment,* f*; correlation between the transmissible environments of the spouses,* u. *(From M McGue, I I Gottesman, D C Rao: The transmission of schizophrenia under a multifactorial threshold model. Am J Hum Genet 35: 1161, 1983. Used with permission.)*

procedure. For example, because mental disorders have variable ages of onset, one must make an adjustment for the fact that many of the relatives involved in the analyses have not yet lived through the full period of risk. Corrections have also been developed and implemented in path and complex segregation analysis that take into account the selection *(ascertainment)* of families through probands.

COMPLEX SEGREGATION ANALYSIS Complex segregation analysis is a powerful method for resolving a single major locus effect, but it leaves cultural inheritance confounded with additive polygenes. The unit of analysis is an entire pedigree, and the goal is to statistically assess evidence for the segregation of a major gene in the presence of other sources of familial resemblance. Inference is carried out by maximum likelihood estimation and likelihood ratio tests as described above; for example, support for a major gene is indicated when the subhypothesis of no major gene is falsified against a general alternative. Both qualitative and quantitative family data may be analyzed.

Segregation analysis is much more sensitive than path analysis to departures from distributional assumptions; consequently, when quantitative data are analyzed, a skewed distribution secondary to scaling or other measurement issues can lead to the false inference of a major gene. It is customary to use *admixture analysis* to fit mixtures of distributions to the overall distribution of quantitative data and then to remove skewness from the data through numerical transformation. That method permits conservative testing of the hypothesis of a single major locus contributing to disease inheritance.

Traditional approaches to complex segregation analysis assume the presence of multivariate normal distributions, and that assumption requires the use of complex mathematical techniques for numerical integration. Researchers have proposed different models for segregation and linkage analysis based on *logistic regression* techniques that do not require the integration of underlying multivariate normal distributions. An additional advantage of applying logistic regressive models for segregation and linkage analysis to study the inheritance of mental disorders is that covariates—such as sex, birth year, and environmental exposure—may be easily incorporated.

The application of complex segregation analysis to psychiatric family data has led to disappointing results in the sense that no single gene has been identified for any mental disorder. The inherent problems most likely are that it is difficult to resolve genetic models of disorders with complex modes of transmission when there is etiological heterogeneity and when qualitative phenotypes of indeterminate stability and validity are the only sources of information.

LINKAGE ANALYSIS Complex segregation analysis is a powerful analytic tool for identifying a major locus, but phenotypic segregation patterns alone do not provide opportunities for its identification. Linkage analysis is a statistical procedure by which pedigree data are examined to determine whether a disease phenotype is cosegregating with a genetic marker that has a known chromosomal location. Linkage analysis allows an investigator to infer that two loci (a genetic marker locus and a putative disease susceptibility locus) are located close enough together on the same chromosome that their alleles tend to be transmitted together from parent to child more frequently than would occur by random assortment. The demonstration of linkage between a putative disease susceptibility locus and one or more genetic markers thus determines on which chromosome the disease locus lies.

Genetic markers are entities known to follow a simple Mendelian mode of inheritance with an identified chromosomal location. As discussed below, at least one parent must be doubly heterozygous for that mating to be informative for linkage. Therefore, a genetic marker locus's usefulness for linkage depends on the number of alleles and the gene frequencies (its degree of *polymorphism*) in the sense that an increased polymorphism leads to an increased probability of heterozygosity.

Twenty years ago the number of available polymorphic genetic markers was severely limited to blood cell antigen loci (ABO, Rh, HLA) now known to be on chromosome 1, 6, or 9. Some of those markers were highly polymorphic, but their limited number and restricted coverage of the genome meant that even linkage studies with excellent family data had little prospect for success. However, in the late 1970s and early 1980s geneticists proposed to treat differences in the DNA sequence as allelic variants and to use them as genetic markers. Through molecular genetic techniques *restriction fragment length polymorphisms (RFLPs)* were obtained and were well suited as genetic markers in linkage analysis. RFLP markers are highly polymorphic and are available in great numbers that saturate the genome: The resulting rapid progress in molecular genetics has been a boon to human linkage analysis. A common measure of the degree of polymorphism often used is the *polymorphic information content (PIC)* value, which is defined as the probability that the marker genotype of a given offspring will allow a deduction of which of the two marker alleles of the affected parent were received. If a PIC value approaches 1, virtually all matings are informative for linkage; a PIC value of ½ means that 50 percent of matings are informative. Another common measure of the degree of polymorphism is called *heterozygosity* (H), which is the probability that a random individual is heterozygous for any two alleles at a given locus. A genetic marker's usefulness for linkage analysis is reflected in its PIC and H values; the higher the values, the greater its utility.

A classic approach in human genetics has been to search for single locus effects underlying disease transmission once a Mendelian mode of transmission has been identified and then to apply linkage analysis. Chromosomal localization through linkage analysis is the first essential step in the process of identifying, isolating, and cloning a disease susceptibility locus.

In practice, linkage analysis has been applied to the study of mental disorders in the absence of formal evidence provided by segregation analysis for a major gene effect. Recent highly publicized findings of linkage of bipolar disorder and schizophrenia to DNA polymorphisms on chromosomes 11 and 5, respectively, have not been replicated in independent samples and have not been extended in the families from whom the original reports were made. A few reports of linkage of bipolar disorder to chromosome-X markers have not been confirmed in other studies. Much controversy has been engendered by the contradictory results; possible explanations that have been advanced include genetic heterogeneity and chance. Recent large-scale family studies to delineate possible genetic mechanisms involved in the causes of schizophrenia, bipolar disorder, Alzheimer's disease, and alcoholism have been begun in cooperation with the National Institute of Mental Health (NIMH) and the National Institute of Alcohol Abuse and Alcoholism (NIAAA).

Two traditional analytical strategies are used to search for linkage in psychiatric family data: (1) apply parametric methods to analyze pedigree data and (2) examine identity-by-descent scores at a given marker locus in pairs of affected siblings (nonparametric methods).

Parametric methods The alleles at different loci received by a person from one parent are called a *haplotype*. In principle, a doubly heterozygous person—for example, *Aa, Bb*—received the *A* allele with either the *B* or *b* allele from one parent. If two loci (with alleles *A* or *a* at one locus and *B* or *b* at the other) are inherited independently of each other, a father passes the four haplotypes *AB, ab, Ab,* and *aB* to his offspring in the ratio of 1:1:1:1. If the *AB* and *ab* haplotypes look the same as the ones he received from his parents, the children receiving them are called parental types. The other two haplotypes (*Ab* and *aB*) in this case are unlike any haplotypes received by the father from the grandparents of the child and contain one allele from each grandparent (a recombination of grandparental alleles must have occurred in the father). The nonparental types (*Ab* and *aB*) are called *recombinants,* and the other two haplotypes are called *nonrecombinants.* A recombination between two genes denotes the event that two different grandparents contribute one allele at each of the two loci to a haplotype in a person, whereas a nonrecombination is said to have occurred when a haplotype in a person contains two alleles that originated from the same grandparent of that person.

When two genes are inherited independently of each other, recombinants and nonrecombinants are expected in equal proportions among the offspring. Some pairs of genes consistently deviate from the 1:1 ratio of recombinant to nonrecombinant offspring; in other words, alleles of different genes appear to be genetically coupled. That is called *genetic linkage.* The extent of genetic linkage is measured by the *recombination fraction,* which is the probability that a gamete produced by a parent is a recombinant. The recombination fraction is denoted by the Greek letter theta *(θ)*. Genes segregating independently are unlinked with $\theta = ½$, whereas linked genes are characterized by $\theta < ½$. Some pairs of genes are tightly linked, so that θ approaches 0—that is, only rarely does a recombination occur between them. The estimation of θ and tests of the hypothesis of free recombination ($\theta = ½$) versus linkage ($\theta < ½$) are the goals of linkage analysis. A mating is potentially informative for linkage between two specific genes when at least one of the parents is a double heterozygote.

Figure 1.15-5 shows in a simplified manner the chromosomal interpretation of recombination. In meiosis (cell division leading to the formation of gametes) homologous chromosomes pair up. At that point each homologous chromosome consists of two strands *(chromatids),* so that a chromosome pair consists of four strands (Figure 1.15-5, I).

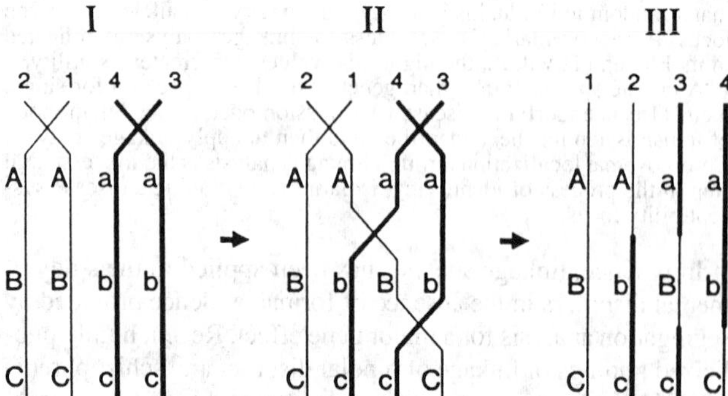

FIGURE 1.15-5 *Schematic representation of (I) a pair of homologous chromosomes, each consisting of two strands; (II) two crossovers between two homologous chromosomes during meiosis; and (III) resulting gametes with nonrecombinant (1), single recombinant (2,4), and double recombinant (3) haplotypes. (From J Ott:* Analysis of Human Genetic Linkage, *ed 2. Johns Hopkins University Press, Baltimore, 1991. Used with permission.)*

In the course of meiosis (II), the two homologous chromosomes separate from each other at most places but maintain two zones of contact *(chiasmata).* Chiasmata reflect the occurrence of *crossing over* between chromatids. In II there are two crossovers: one between the *A,a* locus and the *B,b* locus and the other between the *B,b* locus and the *C,c* locus. In III, four gametes result: 1 is a nonrecombinant, 2 is a single recombinant (crossover betwen *a* and *b* genes), 3 is a double recombinant (crossovers between *a* and *B* genes and between *B* and *c* genes), and 4 is a single recombinant (crossover between *b* and *C* genes).

Since recombination events can be recognized only on the basis of haplotypes passed from parents to children, linkage analysis requires phenotypic observations on pedigree members. Estimating θ is carried out by using the method of maximum likelihood. A relevant quantity is the likelihood ratio that is obtained by dividing the likelihood of a given family ($L(\theta)$) by its value under free recombination ($L(½)$). It is usually convenient to work not with the likelihood ratio but with its logarithm to the base 10. This is the *lod score* $Z(\theta)$, such that $Z(\theta) = \log_{10}[L(\theta)/L(½)]$. The lod score serves as a measure of the weight of the data in favor of the hypothesis of linkage. The critical value generally adhered to as the criterion for significant evidence for linkage to diseases with unambiguous phenotypes and established modes of transmission is 3 for autosomal loci. The asymptotic one-sided type I error rate associated with that value when θ is the only estimated parameter is 0.0001.

Parametic assumptions of lod score methods are as follows: (1) genetic resemblance for a disease is caused by a single major locus only and (2) no transmissible environmental effects contribute to disease inheritance.

The advantages of lod score methods for linkage analysis include the following: (1) Since it is a parametric method, it has great power to detect a true linkage. Lod score analysis, in fact, is the most powerful method to search for linkage to genetic markers, assuming that estimates of single locus inheritance parameters (gene frequencies and penetrances) are established independently through segregation analysis. (2) If affected sib-pairs are rare and etiological heterogeneity is likely, multigenerational pedigrees with affected relatives of various classes (uncles, grandparents, cousins, and so forth) can be analyzed. (3) Linkage to a particular chromosmal region can be excluded.

A consideration when applying lod score methods for linkage analysis is that the mode of inheritance is assumed to be known. When single major locus inheritance parameters (gene frequencies and penetrances) are estimated jointly with θ in linkage analysis, the critical lod score value of 3 is no longer appropriate. A further complication in the genetic investigation of mental disorders is that some abnormal conditions may or may not be related genetically to a core phenotype—for example, the relation between variants of schizoaffective disorder and schizophrenia or bipolar disorder. Several linkage analyses of mental disorders have been conducted in which the lod score was maximized over different disease definitions and different model parameters. Recent studies have shown that maximizing the lod score over many models with different disease definitions leads to an inflation of the evidence for linkage; therefore, a lod score criterion of 4 or more has been recommended in the genetic analysis of mental disorders.

Nonparametric methods Sib-pair methods have less power for detecting linkage than parametric methods and cannot be used to estimate θ, but they provide an attractive alternative to lod score methods for detecting linkage.

Essentially, the affected sib-pair method uses perturbations in the distribution of *identity-by-descent (IBD)* scores at a marker locus to detect the presence of a linked disease locus. In the absence of linkage, the probability that two siblings share neither, one, or both marker haplotypes identical by descent is independent of their disease phenotypes. Consequently, if pairs of siblings are studied because they are both affected, the distribution of their IBD scores will be ¼, ½, and ¼ for IBD = 2, 1, and 0, respectively; when a disease locus is linked to a marker locus and pairs of affected sibs are studied, there is a perturbation in the IBD score distribution at that marker locus. The distribution of marker genes shared IBD thus depends on θ between the disease susceptibility locus and the marker locus.

The specific advantages of affected sib-pair methods in the study of mental disorders are the following: (1) Specification of complex, non-Mendelian modes of transmission is not required. Concomitantly, several confounding factors that make it difficult to accurately estimate the mode of transmission in segregation analysis—for example, complex ascertainment strategies, cohort effects, sex effects, variable age of onset—do not have to be modeled. (2) Large multigenerational families with many affected persons, which are typically difficult to locate and study, are not required.

MULTIVARIATE MODELS INCORPORATIONG QUANTITATIVE TRAITS Traditional approaches in genetic epidemiology focus on the qualitative determination of disease status

TABLE 1.15-4
Tentative Quantitative Indicators of Liability to Mental Disorders

Mood Disorders	Schizophrenia	Alzheimer's Disease
Lithium erythrocyte-plasma ratio	Dopamine D_2, D_3, D_4, D_5 receptor density	Plasma membrane fluidity
TSH response to TRH	Serotonin receptor subtype variability	
Melatonin secretion	Ventricular enlargement	
Platelet imipramine binding	Hippocampus-amygdala volume	
Arecoline sensitivity	Frontal cortical activity	
Cortisol secretion	Event-related potentials	
REM sleep latency	Eye-tracking dysfunctions	
	Personality trait scores	
	Attentional-information processing deficits	

TABLE 1.15-5
Frequent Complications in the Genetic Analysis of Mental Disorders

Diagnostic error and clinical heterogeneity
Improper classification of spectrum conditions and core phenotypes
Etiologic heterogeneity
Age, sex, and cohort effects
Variable age of onset
Complex ascertainment strategies
Complex modes of disease inheritance

as the exclusive source of data for genetic analysis. That approach is problematic in the case of mental disorders, in which phenotypic assessment through structured and semistructured interviews is potentially complicated by secular trends in the prevalence of illness, inderterminate stability and validity of diagnostic assessments, and variable age of onset. Quantitative traits that cosegregate with the disease phenotype provide greater information content than do groupings of persons into affected and unaffected classes. The informativeness of pedigrees is increased, as a greater range of information is available on unaffected persons who are not yet through the risk period.

Idiopathic hemochromatosis is a clear example of the usefulness of incorporation quantitative traits in formal genetic analyses. The precise mode of inheritance of the qualitative disease phenotype was somewhat unclear, but the inclusion of a quantitative biological trait (latent capacity of transferrin) led to the discovery of a recessive gene.

Since highly sensitive, specific, and robust quantitative indicators of the liability to different mental disorders have not yet been found—for example, psychiatry has no laboratory measure that offers presumptive evidence of a given diagnosis in the way the thyroid function tests do for endocrine dysfunction—both qualitative determinations of affection status and quantitative correlated traits must be conjointly analyzed. Examples of quantitative biobehavioral traits that may index liability to different mental disorders are shown in Table 1.15-4.

Multivariate methods that incorporate both quantitative and qualitative family data have been developed and are currently being extended to allow the fitting of complex transmission models and for detecting linkage to DNA polymorphisms. The methods are implemented in multivariate segregation and linkage analysis, respectively, and will be applied in future family studies of schizophrenia and correlated traits.

FREQUENT COMPLICATIONS IN THE GENETIC ANALYSIS OF MENTAL DISORDERS

Several factors have played major roles in frustrating attempts to find single genes for mental disorders in segregation analysis and to establish linkage to DNA markers. The factors are presented in Table 1.15-5.

DIAGNOSTIC ERROR AND CLINICAL HETEROGENEITY

Without a true gold standard for the psychiatric phenotypes, all case definitions are best considered as approximations of indeterminate validity of the true disease state. A diagnostic stability model has been developed and applied to temporal assessment data. That model estimates the probability of being a true case at time 2, given a set of clinical correlates and an assessment of affection at time 1, and allows the development of an index of caseness. The method permits explicit modeling of diagnostic error and clinical heterogeneity, so further extensions, such as incorporation of quantitative information provided by biological indicators, can have powerful effects on increasing the validity of psychiatric phenotypes for segregation and linkage analysis.

ETIOLOGICAL HETEROGENEITY Although a heterogeneity test can be performed on available families, the power to detect heterogeneity is a function of the mode of transmission and the available sample size. Subtyping mental disorders on the basis of clinical characteristics may identify homogeneous and heritable entities, but the adequacy of existing approaches has generally not been demonstrated. Subtyping depression on the basis of previous episodes and an early age of onset may identify a homogeneous and heritable entity for future genetic analysis.

AGE, SEX, AND COHORT EFFECTS The establishment of the mode of inheritance requires accurate modeling of sex differences in inheritance, secular trends in illness rates (a possible cohort effect), and determination of an appropriate age correction for relatives not yet through the period of risk. *Survival analysis* techniques, including the Cox proportional hazards model, provide powerful approaches to quantify the relation between such covariates and risk of mental disorders in probands and relatives.

ASCERTAINMENT CORRECTIONS Assumptions about the pedigree sampling process must be made to accurately estimate genetic transmission parameters, as random sampling is not the way that families are identified for genetic investigations in psychiatry. Pedigrees are typically ascertained through probands, and an appropriate ascertainment correction is provided as the family is extended through a sequential sampling scheme. Another approach to ascertainment correction has been proposed that involves conditioning the likelihood of the sample on the part of the data relevant to ascertainment. Successful determination of the mode of inheritance of mental disorders will require the incorporation of such sophisticated methods for modeling complex ascertainment in segregration analysis.

TRANSMISSION UNDER MORE COMPLEX GENETIC MODELS Traditional methods in population genetics and genetic epidemiology applied to the study of mental disorders

TABLE 1.15-6
Glossary of Genetic Terms

Age-correction procedure: A statistical procedure used in genetic studies of families that takes into account the fact that different psychiatric diagnoses have different ages of onset.
Allele (allelomorph): Alternative form of a gene. There may be many alleles for a given gene, but each person possesses only two alleles for each gene, receiving one of each pair of alleles from each parent. A person with a pair of similar alleles is a homozygote; one with a dissimilar pair is a heterozygote.
Amniography: Opacification of amniotic fluid by injecting radiopaque material to visualize the fetal skeleton and soft tissues clearly.
Aneuploidy: An irregular number of chromosomes (e.g., 45, 47, or 48 chromosomes in a human being), caused by the loss or the addition of one or more chromosomes or parts of chromosomes.
Autoradiography: The process by which a radioactive label is used to identify a specific biological process or material by overlaying with X-ray film and observing exposed areas that usually appear as dots or bands.
Autosomal: Located on or transmitted by an autosome.
Autosome: A chromosome that is not a sex chromosome. A human being has 22 pairs of autosomes.
Barr body: The **sex chromatin** mass in somatic cells of the female.
Carrier: One who carries a recessive gene, either autosomal or sex-linked, together with its normal allele, but who does not show any clinically detectable effect of the gene (i.e., a heterozygote for a recessive gene).
Centimorgan: The genetic distance in which the probability of a recombination occurring is 1 percent.
Centromere: The constricted portion of the chromosome, which is the point of attachment to the equatorial plane of the mitotic or meiotic spindle.
Chromatid: A chromosome at prophase and metaphase consists of two strands attached to the centromere. Each strand is a chromatid (see Mitosis).
Chromatin: The substance in cell nuclei and chromosomes that stains intensely with basic dyes and that is composed of DNA combined with proteins. In the fixed intermitotic nucleus, chromatin usually takes the form of an irregular network of long coiled threads, which are gradually condensed into individual chromosomes as the cell undergoes division.
Chromatin-negative: Nuclei that lack the sex chromatin mass or Barr body. It is characteristic of the normal human male.
Chromatin-positive: Nuclei containing the distinctive sex chromatin mass. It is characteristic of the normal human female.
Chromosomal aberration (or **abnormality**)**:** A deviation from the normal morphology of chromosomes.
Chromosome: One of a number of small bodies, occurring in pairs, into which the chromatin material of a cell nucleus resolves itself before cell division. Chromosomes are visible only during cell division. Homologous chromosomes are the two members of one pair, one of maternal origin and one of paternal origin. Chromosomes bear the vehicles of hereditary traits, the genes. The morphological characteristics of the individual chromosomes and their total number are constant for all the somatic cells of a given species. Major chemical components are DNA, RNA, histones, and nonhistone proteins.
Chromosome number: The number of chromosomes found in the somatic cells of an individual or of a species: normally, 46 in a human being.
Clone: A colony of cells that originated from a single cell.
Concordance rate: A measure of the similarity of the presence or the absence of a disease or a specific trait in pairs of twins.
Congenital: Present at birth; not necessarily genetic.
Consanguinity: Relationship by descent from a common ancestor.
Crossing-over: The exchange of corresponding segments between maternal and paternal homologous chromosomes, occurring when maternal and paternal homologous chromosomes are paired during prophase of the first meiotic division.
Cytogenetics: The branch of genetics dealing with the cytological basis of heredity (i.e., with the study of the chromosomes).
Deoxyribonucleic acid (DNA): The primary storage molecule for genetic information. DNA consists of a long chain of nucleotides, each of which is made up of a deoxyribose (a five-carbon sugar) molecule, a phosphate group, and one of four organic bases—adenine (A), guanine (G), thymine (T), or cytosine (C). The genetic code is contained in the linear array of those organic bases. Each arrangement of three bases (e.g., ACA, GCG) specifies the incorporation of a specific amino acid into a protein molecule.
Diploid: The normal complement of chromosomes (in humans, 22 pairs of homologous chromosomes and the sex chromosomes).
Dizygotic (or **dizygous**) **twins:** Twins resulting from the simultaneous fertilization of two ova by two spermatozoa. Recurrence in families is common. (*Synonym:* Fraternal twins.)
Dominant gene: A gene that expresses its effect even when it is present on only one chromosome.
Empiric risk: The prediction of the probability that a genetic or congenital abnormality will occur in a family.
Exon: A segment of a gene that is represented in the mature messenger RNA and that codes for a portion of the structure of a protein.
Expressivity: The extent to which a trait is manifested. The kind or the degree of phenotypic expression may be slight or pronounced.
Family-risk study: Study of the occurrence of a specific disorder in the family members of an identified person, the proband, who has the specific disorder.
Gamete: A male or female reproductive cell; a spermatozoon or an ovum.
Gene: A segment of DNA that contains the coding information for a single protein molecule or a limited set of protein molecules.
Gene frequency: The relative proportion of each of two or more alleles of a particular gene in a given population. The gene frequency may be expressed as a percentage (0 to 100 percent) or as a probability (0 to 1).
Gene marker: Identified chromosomal locus for which the genomic position is known. Gene markers are used in RFLP studies.
Genetic code: The sequential order of the bases of DNA, which carry the genetic information.
Genocopy: One who shares a trait with another because they have the same gene or genes.
Genome: All the genes found in a diploid set of chromosomes.
Genotype: The full set of genes carried by a person. The term is sometimes used in a limited way to refer to the alleles present at one or more loci.
Haploid: The number of chromosomes in a normal gamete, which contains only one member of each chromosome pair; in a human being, the haploid number is 23.
Hemizygous: Having unpaired genes. Since males have only one X chromosome, they are said to be hemizygous with respect to X-linked genes.
Heritability: A measure of the relative importance of genetic information in the determination of a particular observable feature.
Hermaphrodite: One with both male and female gonadal tissue (not necessarily functional).
Heterologous: Having chromosomes or chromosomal segments that are nonhomologous (see Homologous) or nonidentical.
Heterozygote: One possessing differing alleles at a given locus on a pair of homologous chromosomes. (*Adjective:* Heterozygous.)
Homologous: Having chromosomes or chromosomal segments that are identical with respect to genetic loci and visible structure; e.g., two normal chromosome 15s. (*Noun:* Homologue.)
Homozygote: One possessing a pair of identical alleles at a given locus on a pair of homologous chromosomes. (*Adjective:* Homozygous.)
Inborn error of metabolism: A genetically determined biochemical disorder in which a specific enzyme defect produces a metabolic block that may have pathological consequences.
Incidence: The rate of new cases; e.g., the number of infants born with a condition divided by the number of live births in a given population in a period of time. (Compare with Prevalence.)
Intron: A segment of a gene that is initially transcribed but then spliced out of the messenger RNA. It is an intervening segment of DNA between two exons.
Isochromosome: A chromosome in which the arms on either side of the centromere are identical.
Karyotype: The full complement of chromosomes; the term covers the number, relative sizes, and morphology of the chromosomes.
Linkage: Genes that have their loci on the same chromosome are said to be linked. Also used to describe traits transmitted by a gene of known locus on a specific chromosome (e.g., see X-linkage).
Locus: The precise location of a gene on a chromosome. Different forms of the gene (alleles) are always found at the same locus on the chromosome.
LOD score: A measure of the probability of genetic linkage between a genetic trait and a polymorphism within a particular pedigree or series of pedigrees. The LOD score ranges from 0.0 to 0.5, with 0.5 representing no linkage.
Meiosis: Nuclear division that occurs during the formation of gametes. Two consecutive cell divisions (the first and second meiotic divisions) occur, but only one division of the chromosomes occurs. Thus, the number of chromosomes is reduced from the diploid (46) to the haploid (23) number. During meiosis, pairing of homologous chromosomes takes place, followed by chromosomal breakage and crossing-over. The end result of meiosis is four cells, each with half the number of chromosomes possessed by the original cell.

TABLE 1.15-6 (*continued*)

Mendelian: According to the genetic principles of Gregor Mendel, which included the descriptions of the heritability of dominant and recessive traits.
Metaphase: That stage of cell division (mitosis or meiosis) during which the chromosomes line up on the spindle equatorial plate.
Mitosis: A form of nuclear division in which each chromosome splits lengthwise (replicates itself); one chromatid of each chromosome passes to one daughter cell and the other chromatid to the second daughter cell. Thus, each daughter cell receives the full complement of 46 chromosomes. This type of cell division is characteristic of somatic cells and of germ cells before the onset of meiosis.
Mode of inheritance: The pattern of inheritance (e.g., dominant or recessive) of a particular allele.
Monozygotic (or **monozygous**) **twins:** Twins resulting from the division of a single zygote into two embryos after fertilization of a single ovum by a single spermatozoon. Recurrence within families is rare. (*Synonym:* Identical or one-egg twins.)
Mosaic: One with two or more cell lines differing in genotype.
Multifactorial inheritance: Inheritance of a trait governed by many genes or multiple factors. Each gene may act independently with cumulative total effect. Height, weight, and other body dimensions are determined by multifactorial inheritance.
Mutation: A permanent heritable change in the genetic material. Mutations are an important source of hereditary diversity.
Mutation rate: The frequency of detectable mutations for a genetic locus in a generation.
Northern hybridization: A research technique involving the hybridization (i.e., annealing) of complementary DNA probes to messenger RNA molecules that have been separated by gel electrophoresis and then transferred onto specialized materials (e.g., nitrocellulose membranes).
Oncogene: A gene that encodes a protein that is involved in tumor formation.
Pedigree study: A study of a family that usually includes multiple members of multiple generations. The heritability or lack of heritability of a particular trait can then be studied from one generation to the next and among members of the same generation.
Penetrance: The frequency of phenotypic expression of a dominant gene or a homozygous recessive gene. When a dominant gene produces no detectable phenotypic expression, it shows lack of penetrance.
Phenocopy: One with all the hallmarks of a particular genetic disorder but with no hereditary cause apparent in the pedigree or genome.
Phenotype: The total of all observable features of a person (including anatomical, physiological, biochemical, and psychological makeup and disease reactions, potential or actual). The phenotype is the result of interaction between the genotype and the environment. The term may also apply to the trait produced by a single gene or several genes.
Population genetics: The study of mutant genes in populations, rather than in individuals.
Prediction study: A type of family genetic study based on the prospective study of persons who are at high risk (e.g., the child of two affected parents) for the development of a specific disorder.
Prevalance: The number with a specific condition in a given population at a particular time. (Compare with Incidence.)
Proband: The person with an abnormality whose relatives are studied to determine the hereditary or genetic aspects of the trait. (*Synonyms:* Propositus [male]; proposita [female]; index case.)
Probe: A radioactive DNA or RNA sequence used to detect the presence of a complementary sequence by molecular hybridization.
Prophase: The first stage of cell division, during which the chromosomes become visible as discrete structures.
Recessive: Denoting a trait or gene expressed only in those who are homozygous (or hemizygous) for the gene concerned.
Recombination: The process by which a pair of homologous chromosomes physically exchange sections, yielding a new combination of genes.
Restriction endonucleases: A family of bacterial enzymes, each of which breaks DNA or RNA at specific base sequences. In bacteria, the enzymes restrict the entry of foreign genetic material (e.g., viruses) that would be harmful.
Restriction fragment length polymorphism (RFLP): Different-length fragments of DNA containing the same site or locus in a chromosome, as revealed by exposure of the DNA to restriction endonucleases.
Ribonucleic acid (RNA): A long chain of nucleotides that differ in two ways from the nucleotides of DNA; ribose is the sugar, instead of deoxyribose, and uracil is substituted for thymine. Several subtypes of RNA molecules are involved in the process by which the genetic information in DNA is transformed into a specific protein molecule.
Ring chromosome: A circular chromosome, resulting from breakage in both arms of a chromatid followed by fusion of the broken ends to form a ring. Varying amounts of chromosomal material are lost or deleted from both arms.
Segregation: The separation of the two alleles of a pair of allelic genes during meiosis, so that they pass to different gametes.
Sex chromatin: A chromatin mass in the nucleus of interphase cells of females. It represents a single X chromosome, which is inactive in the metabolism of the cell. Normal females have sex chromatin and, thus, are **chromatin-positive;** normal males lack it and, hence, are **chromatin-negative.** (*Synonym:* Barr body.)
Sex chromosomes: Chromosomes responsible for sex determination (XX in females; XY in males).
Sex-limited: Affecting one sex only.
Sex-linkage: Inheritance by genes on the sex chromosomes, especially on the X chromosomes.
Somatic cell: A nonreproductive cell. Somatic cells are diploid; germ cells are haploid.
Southern blot: A technique for transferring DNA fragments separated by gel electrophoresis onto nitrocellulose paper for molecular hybridization to labeled probes.
State-dependent: Denoting measures that vary with the person's particular clinical status. For example, intoxicated behavior is state-dependent on a person's being intoxicated.
Teratogen: Any agent that causes a physical defect or defects in a developing embryo or fetus.
Trait-dependent: Denoting measures that do not vary with the person's particular clinical status. For example, the genetic marker for Huntington's disease is present in an affected person both before and after the person has the symptoms of Huntington's disease.
Transcription: The molecular process by which the genetic code contained in a DNA molecule is used as a template to make a corresponding molecule of RNA.
Translation: The molecular process by which the genetic code contained in an RNA molecule is used as a template to construct a specific protein molecule.
Translocation: A change in location of genetic material, either within a chromosome or from one chromosome to another.
Trisomy: The presence of three, rather than two, chromosomes in a particular set; humans with three sex chromosomes—XXX, XXY, or XYY—are trisomic for the sex chromosomes.
X-chromosome: A sex chromosome that occurs singly in the normal male and in duplicate in the normal female.
X-linkage: Transmission of a trait by a gene on the X chromosome.
Y-chromosome: A sex chromosome that occurs singly in the normal male and is absent in the normal female.

Table adapted from R Berkow, editor: *Merck Manual,* ed 15, p 2161, Merck Sharp & Dohme Research Laboratories, Rahway, NJ, 1987. Used with permission.

have usually focused on single locus models with reduced penetrance or polygenic models with a large number of loci of equal effect. However, mental disorders are probably transmitted under oligogenic models in which a few loci of major effect either alone or with a larger number of loci of equal effect contribute to the disease. Consequently, the failure to identify the mode of inheritance of major mental disorders and to delineate single major locus effects may reflect the inadequacy of simple models and traditional analytic methods. Oligogenic models require increasingly complex methods of analysis that are currently being developed and that will be applied in the new generation of large-scale, multicenter family and genetic studies in psychiatry.

FUTURE DIRECTIONS

As an ever-increasing number of polymorphic DNA markers saturate the human genome and as progress in the construction and the completion of genetic linkage maps continues, the ability to identify genetic factors in the transmission of mental disorders will be enhanced. In addition, the following steps can be taken to facilitate the dissection of complex mental disorders into their constituent genetic and nongenetic components through the use of methods in genetic epidemiology and population genetics in future studies: (1) Diagnostic criteria and diagnostic hierarchies—for example, what conditions other than the core phenotype are considered manifestations of the affected genotype—are explicitly defined. (2) Standardized and objective methods for phenotypic assessment and analysis of genetic marker data are used. (3) New methods are developed or current methods are extended to allow for the incorporation of longitudinal or cross-sectional data in models to define caseness. That will reduce diagnostic error and clinical heterogeneity across independent samples. (4) Diagnosticians are blind to genetic marker status, and laboratory personnel are blind to diagnostic determinations. (5) All linkage analyses performed with different phenotypic definitions and different genetic models are reported to insure that proper corrections for multiple tests are made. (6) All information regarding ascertainment strategies is made explicit if genetic transmission parameters are estimated. (7) All information regarding the specification of the mode of inheritance is provided. (8) Current analytical methods are extended to allow for segregation and linkage analysis of a qualitative disease phenotype conjointly with biological quantitative data. (9) New analytical methods are further extended to allow the delineation of single genes when several major genes are involved or when there is epistasis among loci. Replication of relevant findings by independent investigators in independent samples is essential and will help establish the validity of the findings in psychiatric genetics.

SUGGESTED CROSS-REFERENCES

The principles and the methods of epidemiology are discussed in Section 5.1. Mathematical and statistical concepts useful in understanding the fundamental principles of population genetics can be found in Section 5.3. Specific findings related to the epidemiology of schizophrenia and mood disorders are presented in Scetions 14.2 and 16.2, respectively. Specific findings from the study of the genetics of schizophrenia and mood disorders are presented in Sections 14.5 and 16.4, respectively. A glossary of genetics terms is given in Table 1.15-6 on pages 152 to 153.

REFERENCES

Bonney G E: Regressive logistic models for familial disease and other binary traits. Biometrics *42*: 611, 1986.

Bouchard T J, Propping P, editors: *Twins as a Tool of Behavioral Genetics.* Wiley, Chichester, 1993.

Cavalli-Sforza L L, Bodmer W F: *The Genetics of Human Populations.* Freeman, San Francisco, 1971.

*Cloninger C R, Reich T, Suarez B K, Rice J P, Gottesman I I: The principles of genetics in relation to psychiatry. In *Handbook of Psychiatry: The Scientific Foundations of Psychiatry,* vol 5, M Shepherd, editor, p 34. Cambridge University Press, Cambridge, England, 1985.

Cloninger C R, Rice J P, Reich T: Multifactorial inheritance with cultural transmission and assortative mating: II. A general model of combined polygenic and cultural inheritance. Am J Hum Genet *31*: 176, 1979.

Crowe R R: Candidate genes in psychiatry: an epidemiological perspective. Am J Med Genet (Neuropsychiatric Genetics) *48:* 74, 1993.

Elandt-Johnson R C: *Probability Models and Statistical Methods in Genetics.* Wiley, New York, 1971.

Elston R C, Stewart J: A general model for the analysis of pedigree data. Hum Hered *21*: 523, 1971.

Falconer D S: *Introduction to Quantitative Genetics,* ed 3. Wiley, New York, 1989.

Falk C T, Rubinstein P: Haplotype relative risks: An easy reliable way to construct a proper control sample for risk calculations. Ann Hum Genet *51*: 227, 1987.

*Gershon E S, Cloninger C R: *Genetic Approaches to Mental Disorders.* American Psychiatric Press, Washington, 1994.

Goldin L R, Gershon E S: Power of the affected-sib-pair method for heterogeneous disorders. Genet Epidemiol *5*: 35, 1988.

Gottesman I I: *Schizophrenia Genesis: The Origins of Madness.* Freeman, New York, 1991.

Gottesman I I, McGuffin P, Farmer A: Clinical genetics as clues to the "real" genetics of schizophrenia. Schizophr Bull *13*: 23, 1987.

Hodge S E: Linkage analysis of "necessary" disease loci versus "susceptibility" loci. Am J Hum Genet *53:* 367, 1993.

Kendler K S: The impact of varying diagnostic thresholds on affected sib pair linkage analysis. Genet Epidemiol *5*: 407, 1988.

Kety S S, Rosenthal D, Wender P H, Schulsinger F, Jacobsen B: The biologic and adoptive families of adopted individuals who became schizophrenic: Prevalence of mental illness and other characteristics. In *The Nature of Schizophrenia: New Approaches to Research and Treatment,* L C Wynne, R L Cromwell, S. Matthysse, editors, p 25. Wiley, New York, 1978.

*Khoury M J, Beaty T H, Cohen, B H: *Fundamentals of Genetic Epidemiology.* Oxford, New York, 1993.

Kondler K S: Twin studies of psychiatric illness: Current status and future directions. Arch Gen Psychiatry *50:* 905, 1993.

Lalouel J-M, Le Mignon L, Simon M, Fauchet R, Bourel M, Rao D C, Morton N E: Genetic analysis of idiopathic hemochromatosis using both qualitative (disease status) and quantitative (serum iron) information. Am J Hum Genet, *37*: 700, 1985.

Loehlin J C: *Latent Variable Models—Introduction to Factor, Path, and Structural Analysis,* ed. 2. Erlbaum, Hillsdale, NJ, 1992.

McGue M, Gottesman I I: Genetic linkage in schizophrenia: Perspectives from genetic epidemiology. Schizophr Bull *15*: 453, 1989.

*McGuffin P, Murray R, editors: *The New Genetics of Mental Illness.* Butterworth-Heinemann, Oxford, England, 1991.

McGuffin P, Owen M, O'Donovan M, Thapar A, Gottesman I I: *Seminars in Psychiatric Genetics,* Gaskell, London, 1994.

Mendlewicz J, Hippius H, editors: *Genetic Research in Psychiatry.* Springer-Verlag, Berlin, 1992.

Moldin S O: Indicators of liability to schizophrenia: perspectives from genetic epidemiology. Schizophr Bull *20:* 169, 1994.

Moldin S O, Reich T: Genetic analysis of depression: Future directions. Clin Neurosci *1:* 139, 1993.

Moldin S O, Reich T, Rice J P: Current perspectives on the genetics of unipolar depression. Behav Genet *21*: 211, 1991.

Moldin S O, Rice J P, Van Eerdewegh P, Gottesman I I, Erlenmeyer-Kimling L: Estimation of disease risk under bivariate models of multifactorial transmission. Genet Epidemiol *7*: 371, 1990.

Morton N E: *Outline of Genetic Epidemiology.* Karger, New York, 1982.

Morton N E, Rao D C, Lalouel J-M: *Methods in Genetic Epidemiology.* Karger, New York, 1983.

Neale M C, Cardon L R: *Methodology for Genetic Studies of Twins and Families.* Kluwer Academic, Boston, 1992.

Nothen M M, Propping P, Fimmers R: Association versus linkage studies in psychosis genetics. J Med Genet *30:* 634, 1993.

Ott J: *Analysis of Human Genetic Linkage,* ed 2. Johns Hopkins University Press, Baltimore, 1991.

Plomin R, McClearn G E. editors: *Nature, Nurture, and Psychology.* American Psychological Association, Washington, 1993.

Reich T, James J W, Morris C A: The use of multiple thresholds in determining the mode of transmission of semi-continuous traits. Ann Hum Genet *36*: 163, 1972.

Rice J P, Cloninger C R, Reich T: Multifactorial inheritance with cultural transmission and assortative mating: I. Description and basic properties of the unitary models. Am J Hum Genet *30*: 618, 1978.

Rice J P, Risch N J: Genetic analysis of the affective disorders: Summary of GAW5. Genet Epidemiol *6*: 161, 1989.

Risch N J: Genetic linkage and complex diseases, with special reference to psychiatric disorders. Genet Epidemiol *7*: 3, 1990.

Risch N J: Linkage strategies for genetically complex traits: I. Multilocus models. Am J Hum Genet *46*: 222, 1990.

Risch N J: A note on multiple testing procedures in linkage analysis. Am J Hum Genet *48*: 1058, 1991.

Ross C A, McInnis M G, Margolis R L, Li S-H: Genes with triplet repeats: Candidate mediators of neuropsychiatric disorders. Trends Neurosci *16:* 254, 1993.

Sing C F, Haviland M B, Templeton A R, Zerba K E, Reilly S L: Biological complexity and strategies for finding DNA variations responsible for inter-individual variation in the risk of a common chronic disease, coronary artery disease. Ann Med *24:* 539, 1992.
Sobell J L, Heston L L, Sommer S S: Novel association approach for determining the genetic predisposition to schizophrenia: Case-control resource and testing of a candidate gene. Am J Med Genet *48:* 28, 1993.
Spielman R S, McGinnis R E, Ewens W J: Transmission test for linkage disequilibrium: The insulin gene region and insulin-dependent diabetes mellitus (IDDM). Am J Hum Genetics *52:* 506, 1993.
Suarez B K, Cox N J: Linkage analysis for psychiatric disorders: I. Basic concepts. Psychiatr Dev *3:* 218, 1983.
Suarez B K, Hampe C L, Van Eerdewegh P: Problems of replicating linkage claims in psychiatry. In *Genetic Approaches to Mental Disorders,* E S Gershon, C R Cloninger, editors, p 23. American Psychiatric Press, Washington, 1994.
Suarez B K, Rice J P, Reich T: The generalized sib pair IBD distribution: Its use in the detection of linkage. Ann Hum Genet *42*: 87, 1978.
Torrey E F, Bowler A S, Taylor E H, Gottesman I I: *Schizophrenia and Manic-Depressive Disorder: The Biologic Roots of Mental Illness as Revealed by the Landmark Study of Identical Twins.* Basic Books, New York, 1994.
Tsaung M T, Faraone S V: *The Genetics of Mood Disorders.* Johns Hopkins Press, Baltimore, 1990.
Tsuang M T, Kendler K S, Lyons M J, editors: *Genetic Issues in Psychosocial Epidemiology.* Rutgers University Press, New Brunswick, N J, 1991.
Vieland V J, Hodge S E, Greenberg D A: Adequacy of single-locus approximations for linkage analyses of oligogenic traits. Genet Epidemiol *9:* 45, 1992.
*Vogel F, Motulsky A G: *Human Genetics: Problem and Approaches,* ed 2. Springer, New York, 1986.

1.16 GENETIC LINKAGE ANALYSIS OF THE PSYCHIATRIC DISORDERS

T. CONRAD GILLIAM, Ph.D.
JAMES A. KNOWLES, M.D., Ph.D.

INTRODUCTION

Human gene mapping with polymorphic deoxyribonucleic acid (DNA) markers was born in the early 1980s. The technique relies on the earlier discoveries of a class of bacterial enzymes, the restriction endonucleases, that cleave DNA at unique recognition sites and on the invention of molecular cloning. In the early 1980s researchers predicted that abundant silent mutations in the *human genome* (all human chromosomes) could be detected as changes in the length of restriction endonuclease fragments when those mutations either altered or created a recognition site for a particular endonuclease. Using *recombinant DNA molecules* (human DNA fragments molecularly stitched together with bacterial viruses) as radioactive probes against restriction endonuclease-digested human DNA, researchers reported the first restriction fragment length polymorphisms (RFLPs) in 1981. By 1990 more than 1,900 genes and 4,500 anonymous DNA clones had been mapped to specific chromosomal locations. About half of those clones are polymorphic DNA markers that now serve as molecular signposts for mapping the human genome and for detecting disease loci.

HISTORY

The first disease to be mapped with RFLP markers was the X-chromosomal Duchenne's muscular dystrophy gene in 1982. One year later the autosomal-dominant Huntington's disease gene was mapped to the short arm of chromosome 4 by using DNA markers. In the next 10 years scores of single-locus Mendelian diseases were mapped to discrete chromosomal locations by using DNA markers and genetic linkage analysis. By 1987 DNA marker maps were reported that spanned a majority of the human genome at fairly close intervals, although a significant number of gaps between markers still existed. In recent years those maps have improved with greater representation of the genome, more densely mapped markers, and more polymorphic markers. The vast majority of disease genes lie in an interval between two closely spaced, highly polymorphic DNA markers.

Genetic linkage analysis and subsequent gene-mapping technologies have led to the isolation and the identification of a subset of the genetically mapped disease genes. Notable among them is the massive dystrophin gene, which mutates to cause not only Duchenne's muscular dystrophy but also the much milder variant, Becker type tardive muscular dystrophy. Researchers were aided in their search for the dystrophin gene by the discovery, in 1985, of a large X-chromosomal deletion from the blood sample of a young boy who suffered from Duchenne's muscular dystrophy and several other abnormalities. The identification of a gross chromosomal aberration associated with a heritable disorder has remained an important tool in gene-mapping strategies. The neurofibromatosis gene was discovered in 1989, just one year after the discovery of two chromosomal translocation events in the region of the linked DNA marker. No gross chromosomal rearrangements were found in association with the lethal autosomal-recessive cystic fibrosis gene, mapped to chromosome 7. Despite the absence of that vital clue, a combination of gene-mapping strategies (linked DNA markers, chromosome walking and jumping, identification of gene-coding sequences in the linked region, and identification of allelic association between the disease gene and the disease phenotype) led two groups to identify the cystic fibrosis transmembrane conductance regulator (CFTR) gene in 1989. The Huntington's disease gene was the first autosomal genetic disorder to be mapped by genetic linkage analysis. A decade of concerted effort by a consortium of sophisicated molecular genetic laboratories finally identified the Huntington's disease gene in 1993. Like several other prominent human heritable disorders (for example, Fragile X syndrome, spinal and bulbar spinal muscular atrophy, myotonic dystrophy, and spinocerebellar ataxia type 1), the autosomal dominant neurodegenerative disorder was shown to result from a triplet repeat sequence (CAGCAGCAG . . . and so on) immediately upstream of the disease gene, which expands from approximately 10 to 35 copies in normal persons to approximately 40 to 90 copies in persons with Huntington's disease.

Disease genes continue to be rapidly uncovered by the gene-mapping process. Some common themes are emerging in regard to the molecular basis of pathology. One of these is a common molecular mechanism (an expanding trinucleotide sequence) that may cause an increased severity of the disorder in succeeding generations. Fragile X syndrome (a leading cause of mental retardation) and myotonic dystrophy both display the phenomenon of genetic anticipation. The identification of a disease gene allows direct investigation of the normal function of the gene and study of its abnormal expression in the disease state. For example, researchers have shown that CFTR is a chloride channel protein. Mutations of the gene prevent epithelial cells from properly modulating the permeability of chloride ions, causing chronic mucus production, infection, and inflammation, which are lethal. Effective treatment of an illness based on knowledge of the gene product is much less predictable. However, early gene therapy experiments with both dystrophin and CFTR have been encouraging, with preliminary studies showing that the viral introduction of a correct copy of the gene can partially correct the phenotype in animal models. Furthermore, diagnosis has dramatically improved for the muscular dystrophies, and prenatal detection of Duchenne's muscular dystrophy, Becker type tardive muscular dystrophy, and cystic fibrosis is now possible.

In the past several years the Human Genome Project has been launched with the goal of sequencing the entire human genome in the next 15 years. This historical mission promises to unveil the approximately 50,000 human genes, the DNA sequences that regulate their expression, and, presumably, many unknown characteristics of the human genome. Although the DNA sequence alone will not explain human biology, the sequence information will usher in the next explosion of human genetic discoveries and will guide human biology and medicine for many years to come.

OVERVIEW

All mammals contain two copies of each chromosome. The individual copies are called *homologues,* and one set is inherited from the mother (maternal) and one set from the father (paternal). As the male and female germ-line cells undergo meioses, the homologues cross over or recombine to exchange genetic information. As a consequence of that *meiotic recombination,* genes that are located close together on a homologue are coinherited by the children and are referred to as *nonrecombinants.* Genes located far apart or on different chromosomes are inherited independently of one another. Those genes or *loci* (any polymorphic point on a chromosome) appear in families as recombinants and are unlinked to one another. In between are loci that are usually inherited together but that also show varying degrees of recombination. The loci appear in families more often as nonrecombinants and, thus, are *genetically linked.* Two loci that are coinherited 99 percent of the time (and recombine in 1 percent of cases) are, by definition, separated by one centimorgan (1 cM) of genetic distance. The total length of all human chromosomes (the human genome) is estimated to be 3,000 cM. Since the physical length of the human genome is estimated to be 3×10^9 base pairs, 1 cM is approximately equal to 1 million base pairs or 1 megabase of DNA. The correlation between physical distance and genetic distance varies at different locations along the chromosome.

DNA markers detect naturally occurring variations, polymorphisms, that occur fairly randomly throughout the human genome. When a DNA marker detects a variation in the DNA sequence at any point along the chromosome (a *locus*) such that the maternally and paternally inherited homologues can be distinguished, the marker is said to be *informative* for that person, and the polymorphic variants are referred to as *alleles.*

Figure 1.16-1 shows the coinheritance of a DNA marker locus and a dominantly inherited disease locus in which the father (generation II) is informative at both marker and disease loci. The mother is not informative for the disease or marker locus because she is *homozygous* (contains two identical alleles) for both the N (normal) allele and the 1 allele. Thus, all her offspring receive a 1-N from the mother, but it is impossible to determine whether that was her maternal or her paternal 1-N allele. In that case, because the paternal grandparents are also informative for the DNA marker and the grandmother is affected, the 3 allele and the D (disease) allele were inherited from the grandmother, but the 2 allele and the N allele were inherited from the grandfather. That information establishes the *phase* of the homologues in the father's DNA, as shown in the inset at top right. At this point a hypothesis is developed that the marker locus is genetically linked to the disease locus and that the phase is 3/D and 2/N. Of course, the 3 allele and the D allele could have been coinherited from the grandmother on different chromosomes (unlinked), but that is the hypothesis to be tested. When the *phase* of two alleles is known, as in this case, greater statistical evidence for or against linkage can be obtained.

To formally address whether the DNA marker locus and the disease locus are genetically linked, one must tally the ratio of *recombinants* to *nonrecombinants.* As shown in Figure 1.16-1, the 3 allele cosegregates with the D allele (or the 2 with the N) in four of five persons, suggesting that 80 percent of the offspring are nonrecombinants and 20 percent are recombinants. The last-born daughter in generation III is a recombinant. In her father's germ-line DNA a meiotic recombination has occurred at some point on the chromosome between the marker locus and the disease locus, so she inherits her father's 3 allele, together with an N allele. Alternatively, the marker and disease loci are located on different chromosomes, and, by chance, they are coinherited in four of five cases. Normally, the first offspring is used to establish the linkage hypothesis (that is, allele 2 segregates with allele N and allele 3 with allele D) and is not scored. One could estimate the *recombinant fraction* (θ) (the percent recombination between two loci) to be 20 percent or 20 cM. The validity of that conclusion depends on the likelihood that the 80-to-20 ratio of nonrecombinants to recombinants is different from the 50-to-50 ratio expected if the loci are inherited independently. The 80-to-20 ratio would certainly be significant if it were observed after scoring many children in a large number of families.

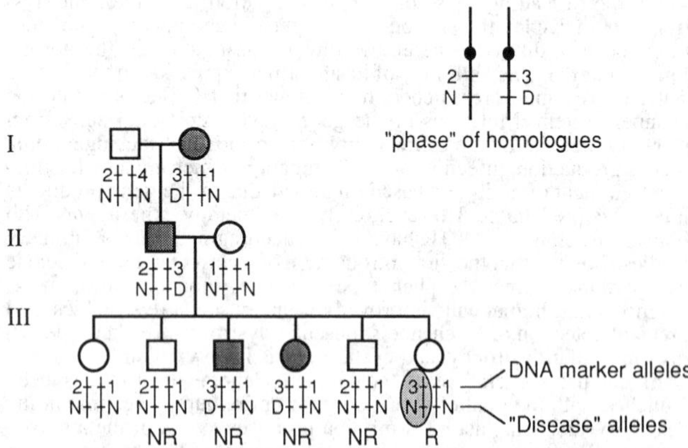

FIGURE 1.16-1 *Coinheritance of a DNA marker locus and a disease locus. This three-generational pedigree depicts the inheritance of an autosomal dominant disease. Each person displays the DNA marker alleles for their two homologues and either on N (normal) allele or a D (disease) allele corresponding to the disease locus. Shaded circles (females) and shaded squares (males) indicate affected persons. The two vertical lines below each person represent the person's homologues. In the insert (top right) the black dot on each homologue indicates the centromere. The insert shows the phase for the marker and disease alleles that can be deduced for the affected father in generation II. NR refers to those persons who show no recombination between the marker and the disease loci, and R refers to the person who displays a meiotic recombination between the DNA marker and the disease loci.*

LOD SCORE METHOD Linkage analysis calculates the relative likelihood that two loci are linked over a range of recombination fractions (θ) varying from 0 (no recombination) to 0.5 (random assortment). The likelihood ratio in the case discussed above is

$$\text{Odds ratio} = \frac{\text{likelihood of data if loci linked at } \theta = 0.2}{\text{likelihood of data if loci unlinked at } \theta = 0.5}$$

The *lod score* is the $\log_{10}$ of the odds ratio. Lod scores are convenient to use because data collected from different families can simply be added to derive the *cumulative lod score (Z).* When the phase between two loci is known, each person with cosegregation of two loci contributes a lod score of about 0.3; those with recombination between the two loci contribute about −0.2. For single-locus Mendelian disorders, positive lod scores above 3.0 are generally accepted as significant evidence for linkage, and scores below −2.0 are significant evidence against linkage. The value of θ at which Z is greatest is accepted as the best estimate of the recombination fraction and is often called the *maximum likelihood estimate.* Another example of coinheritance between a DNA marker and a dominant disease allele, together with the linkage calculations, is shown in Figure 1.16-2. The disease coinherits with the 2 allele in this family except in person III-3, who is a recombinant. A schematic diagram of a Southern blot analysis autoradiogram depicts the 6,000 base pair allele 1 and the 4,000 base pair allele 2. Of the 15 offspring of the original ancestor (I-1), only one shows a recombination. The estimated percent recombination (1 out of 14) is thus close to the 7 percent value obtained through formal analysis using the Linkage computational program. Since there is one recombination, the lod score at 0.00 (no recombination) is $-\infty$. The maximum lod score of 3.4 occurs at a point 7 cM from the disease loci. Those data can be taken as definitive evidence that the marker and disease loci are linked, since the maximum likelihood estimate exceeds 3.0.

Genetic linkage analysis begins by identifying a set of families manifesting the disease of interest. Blood samples are col-

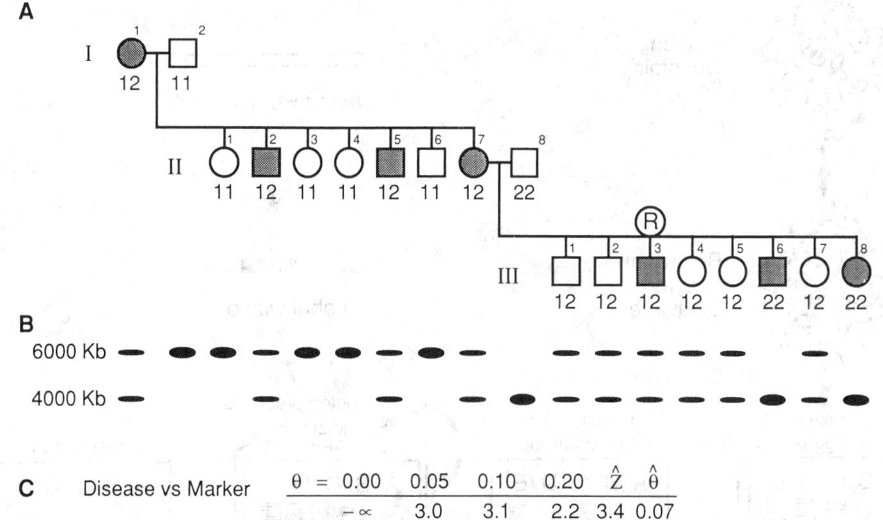

FIGURE 1.16-2 *Calculation of genetic linkage in a single pedigree. (A) A three-generational pedigree segregating a DNA marker locus and on autosomal dominant disease. Shaded circles and shaded squares indicated affected persons. The DNA marker alleles are shown below each person. III-3 shows a recombination (R) between the marker and the disease loci. (B) A schematic drawing of DNA marker alleles as they appear after Southern blot analysis and autoradiography. The larger 6,000 base pair fragment migrates slower through the agarose gel than does the 4,000 base pair fragment. Homozygotes (11 and 22) appear as darker bonds, since they are present as two copies of the identical allele (C) Linkage between the DNA marker locus and the disease locus was analyzed by using the Linkage program. θ is the recombinant fraction, the person recombination between the two loci. Thus, lod scores are calculated by sssuming 0 (no recombination), 5, 10, and 20 ercent recombination between the marker and the disease loci. The lod score is then maximized over the recombinant fractions to reveal a maximum θ at 0.07 or 7 percent recombination, with a corresponding maximum lod score Z of 3.4.*

lected from all key family members. Lymphocytes can be immortalized by viral infection to provide a renewable source of DNA for further experiments, or DNA can be isolated directly from the whole blood. Computer simulation analysis is performed to estimate the overall power of the family set to detect linkage. Once a sufficient number of samples are available to detect linkage, DNA markers are systematically tested for coinheritance with the disease phenotypes. If DNA markers are available for genes whose function implies a role in the disease pathology, those *candidate genes* may be tested first. Likewise, if candidate regions of the genome are implicated in the disease cause from cytological observations, markers from those regions may be tested first. Every step in the protocol must be carefully planned and executed, particularly for complex, non-Mendelian disorders, such as the psychiatric disorders.

DNA MARKERS

The human genome contains millions of silent mutations that human geneticists have used to map chromosomes and disease genes. If any stretch of human DNA is compared base pair by base pair between two unrelated persons, on average, one base pair in 300 will be *polymorphic*—will differ between them. The focus of human geneticists over the past 10 years has been (1) to identify increasingly larger portions of the polymorphisms and (2) to identify subsets of the mutations that are highly polymorphic throughout the population. For linkage analysis a marker must distinguish the maternal and paternal homologues (alleles) in the parents. That is, the marker must identify *heterozygous* (different) alleles, as opposed to *homozygous* (identical) alleles. When a marker is heterozygous or *informative*, one can determine which homologue was transmitted to each offspring. That is illustrated for the informative parents (I-1 and II-7) in Figure 1.16-2. Markers are often characterized by their *heterozygosity value*, which is simply the percentage of persons who will be heterozygous or informative when typed by using that marker. A major goal of human geneticists has been to find new types of polymorphisms with increasingly higher heterozygosity values.

RESTRICTION FRAGMENT LENGTH POLYMORPHISM

The first type of DNA polymorphism described was the restriction fragment length polymorphism (RFLP). That method detects only the subset of mutations that alter a specific 4-to-6 base pair sequence recognized and cleaved by a particular restriction endonuclease enzyme. The alteration may eliminate a previously existing recognition site, or it may create a new site. Either way, the mutation alters the length of the restriction fragment that can be detected by *DNA hybridization* (a kinetic process in which the DNA marker sequence recognizes and preferentially binds only to its matched or homologous sequence among the total human genome) with the DNA marker. To detect those changes in restriction (fragment) length, the investigator performs a process called a Southern blot analysis (Figure 1.16-3). Total (genomic) DNA is isolated from each person in the study and is digested to completion with a restriction endonuclease. The hundreds of thousands of DNA fragments generated are then separated on the basis of size by electrophoresis through an agarose gel. The DNA fragments are transferred (by capillary action) to a membrane for ease of handling, and radioactively labeled DNA from a particular region of the genome is allowed to find its complement on the membrane (DNA hybridization). That radioactivity can then be detected by exposure of the membrane to X-ray film. Figure 1.16-2 depicts a Southern blot analysis autoradiogram in which the marker detects restriction fragments of 6,000 base pairs and 4,000 base pairs. In generation I the affected mother is heterozygous for the marker, but the unaffected father is homozygous and uninformative. For dominant disorders only the affected parent need be informative for the marker. For diseases in which the mode of inheritance is unknown, both parents must be informative.

RFLP markers have been used to map numerous Mendelian diseases and to construct a complete genetic map of the human genome. Although several thousand RFLP markers are available, those markers have several limitations that have spurred the development of several new types of markers. First, RFLPs detect only a small fraction of all mutations. Second, RFLPs are, by definition, 2 allele systems (plus or minus the restriction site) and have limited variability in the population.

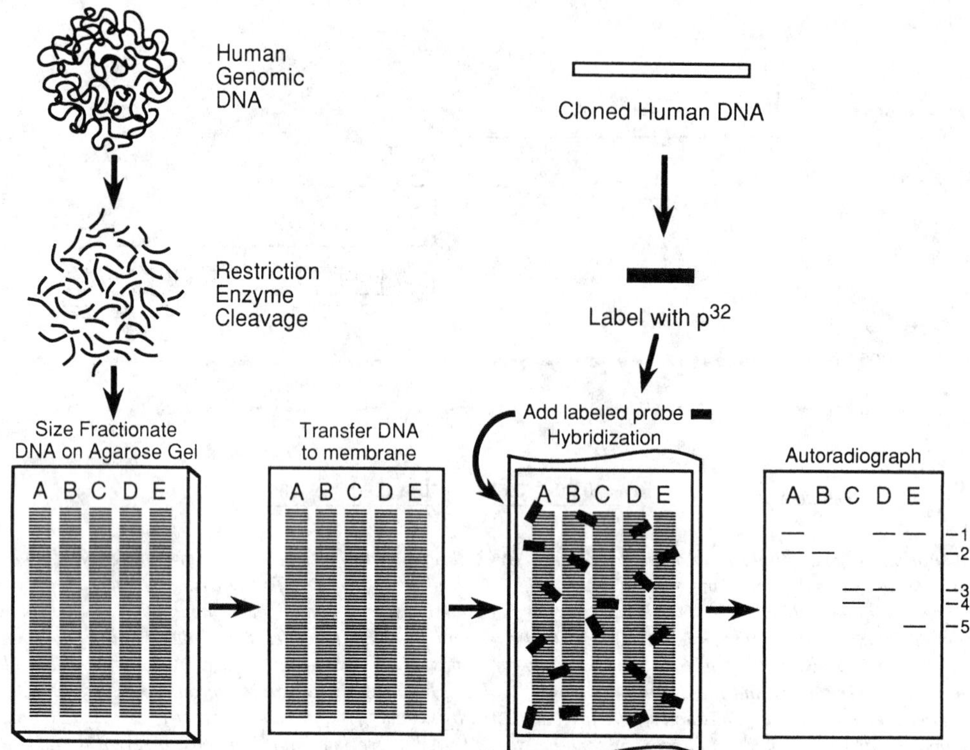

FIGURE 1.16-3 *Southern blot analysis and DNA hybridization. Human DNA is isolated from whole blood or cultured lymphocytes. The DNA is digested to completion with a restriction endonuclease, yielding hundreds of thousands of restriction fragments, which are separated by size on an agarose gel. The gel is submarined in buffer and subjected to electrophoresis; the negatively charged DNA moves through the gel twoard the positive electrode. Small restriction fragments move through the agarose pores faster than do large fragments. A-E represent individual DNA samples. The restriction fragments are transferred by capillary action to a nylon membrane, which traps the DNA fragments as an exact template of the agarose gel. The five lanes of digested DNA are now bound to the membrane, which is placed in a sandwich bag along with a radiolabeled DNA marker, a buffer, and other chemicals to enhance the DNA hybridization reaction. The radioactive marker binds to its matching DNA sequence on the membrane, marking that restriction fragment on the resultant autoradiograph. The nylon membrane is washed with a buffer and decreasing salt concentrations to release nonspecifically bound radioactivity. The membrane is dried and exposed to X-ray film overnight. The X-ray film is developed, and the resultant alleles can be read for each person. For example, this particular DNA marker detects alleles 1 and 2 in person A and alleles 3 and 4 in person C.*

At best, the alleles exist in equal frequency in the population to yield a heterozygosity value of 50 percent (half of persons are heterozygous 12, a quarter homozygous 11, and a quarter homozygous 22). If one types two markers through a family, the chance that both markers are informative and can be mapped relative to each other is, at best, 25 percent (50 percent × 50 percent). Finally, the Southern blot analysis technique is slow and labor-intensive compared with new techniques.

VARIABLE NUMBER OF TANDEM REPEATS In 1988 a second type of DNA sequence polymorphism was described, the variable number of tandem repeats (VNTR) or minisatellite markers. VNTR polymorphisms are based on the observations that naturally occurring end-to-end (tandem) repeats of DNA sequence are observed in relatively random regions along the chromosomes and that the number of repeat sequences is highly variable among persons. The tandem repeat sequences are flanked on both sides by unique-sequence DNA; cleavage of the unique sequence with the appropriate restriction endonuclease releases a DNA fragment whose length depends on the number of repeats in the tandem array. A physical analogy is a freight train with multiple identical boxcars. The boxcars represent the repeated sequences, and the engine and the caboose represent the unique-sequence DNA. The restriction fragments are detected by hybridization to DNA probes that are homologous to the unique flanking sequences, using the same Southern blot analysis method used to detect RFLP polymorphisms. Multiple alleles frequently occur at those VNTR loci (like various numbers of boxcars). Indeed, several markers have been identified that detect hundreds of alleles and are now being used for forensic fingerprinting.

Since the average heterozygosity value is 50 to 70 percent, the VNTR markers are a major improvement over RFLP markers. Unfortunately, VNTR markers do not appear to be evenly spread across the chromosomes, and they are less abundant than is ideal for mapping the entire genome. Also, VNTR markers rely on the use of Southern blot analysis and, therefore, suffer some of the same limitations as the RFLP markers.

POLYMERASE CHAIN REACTION Recently developed methods for detecting polymorphisms use the *polymerase chain reaction* (PCR), a method to selectively amplify small regions of the genome up to 10,000-fold, thus eliminating the need to perform a Southern blot analysis. The most common polymorphic DNA markers that use PCR are the *short tandem repeat* and the *microsatellite repeat* markers. Like the VNTR markers, those markers make use of naturally occurring repeated DNA sequences. The microsatellite repeat sequence is only 2, 3, or 4 nucleotides in length—typically $(CA)_n$—and the number of times that the sequence is repeated is highly variable. By cloning and sequencing a small amount of DNA on either side of the microsatellite repeat sequences, an investigator can synthesize short stretches of DNA *(oligonucleotide primers)* (20 to 30 base pairs in length) and use them to prime the PCR amplification process. The amplification products differ by two to four base pairs in size and constitute the microsatellite alleles. The products of the PCR reaction are separated by size on a polyacrylamide gel that can resolve length differences to one base pair. For a highly polymorphic microsatellite marker, two bands are observed for each person that correspond to the length of the unique flanking DNA sequence and the length of the repeated DNA sequence on the two homologues.

The rate of DNA marker typing is significantly faster for PCR-based markers than for RFLP and VNTR markers. The PCR markers are abundant, evenly spread throughout the genome, and have heterozygosity values that average 60 to 90 percent. Maps of all the human chromosomes have been constructed using only the microsatellite markers, and they have replaced the RFLP and VNTR markers for both chromosome mapping and disease gene mapping.

ANALYSIS OF PSYCHIATRIC DISORDERS

The primary assumptions underlying lod score analysis are that the traits being analyzed are the result of mutations at a single locus and that they are inherited in a predictable Mendelian pattern—that is, autosomal-dominant or autosomal-recessive or X-linked. Mendelian or monogenic inheritance is characterized by certain hallmarks. The *recurrence risk* (the risk to a first-degree relative of an affected person) in families is very high, 100 to 1,000 times the frequency in the general population. Furthermore, the risk to relatives decreases by a factor of ½ with each degree of relationship—that is, from first-degree (parent or sibling) to second-degree (grandparent or cousin) to third-degree relatives. If the risk decreases more rapidly than that, a more complex genetic model is implicated. By that definition the genetics of psychiatric disorders are complex, and that complexity makes genetic linkage analysis considerably complicated.

GENETIC BASIS The evidence that genetic factors contribute to certain psychiatric disorders is based on several lines of experimentation. The *morbidity risk* (the age-adjusted familial rate) among first-degree relatives of probands with bipolar disorder is 4 to 9 percent and about 3 to 7 percent for schizophrenia probands. The rate in the relatives of controls is 0.2 to 0.5 percent. The *relative risk* (the ratio of the risk for the patient's relatives to the risk for the relatives of normal controls) for bipolar disorder is 17 to 20, indicating a significant clustering of ill persons within families. Twin and adoption studies can be used to identify the genetic contribution within a group of families.

Familial clustering can be due to genetic or nongenetic causes. For example, table manners may show a familial cluster, but they are clearly not inherited. Because monozygotic (identical) twins share all their genes, but dizygotic (fraternal) twins share only 50 percent of their genetic component, a higher rate of concordance for illness in monozygotic twins than in dizygotic twins points to the role of genetic factors. The concordance rates for bipolar disorder (plus related mood disorder) are 80 percent in monozygotic twins and 24 percent in dizygotic twins. (In schizophrenic patients the concordance rate in monozygotic twins is slightly above 50 percent, but the rate is significantly higher than in dizygotic twins.) The *heritability estimate* (a measure of the genetic contribution to the overall familial resemblance) is 75 percent for bipolar disorder, suggesting a genetic component of large magnitude. Since 20 percent of monozygotic twins are discordant for the illness, nongenetic factors are clearly present. The population prevalences for both bipolar disorder and schizophrenia are roughly 0.5 to 1.0 percent. Since a single mutation is not likely to have survived to such a high population rate, the psychiatric disorders are probably genetically heterogeneous—that is, they have arisen from multiple mutations, some of which may not be genetically linked *(locus heterogeneity)*.

Although the evidence is compelling that genetic factors contribute to the causes of various psychiatric disorders (bipolar disorder, schizophrenia, panic disorder, Tourette's disorder, alcohol-related disorders, and others), little is known about the nature of those factors or the degree to which they contribute to illness. The inability to accurately characterize the mechanism of genetic contribution complicates conventional genetic linkage analysis.

GENETIC MODELS Current genetic and epidemiological analyses have been unsuccessful in delineating the genetic contribution (either the number of genes or the magnitude of the genetic effect) to the major psychiatric disorders. Unlike the one-to-one correspondence of genotype (DNA marker allele) and phenotype (affected status) that is characteristic of most Mendelian disorders, the relation may be weak among complex disorders. For that reason, disease genes are appropriately referred to as *susceptibility genes*. Most psychiatric genetic research to date has focused on two models: the *single major locus model* and the *multifactorial-polygenic model*. According to the single major locus model, the familial transmission of the disorder can be explained solely by a single gene that is transmitted in its normal or mutated (disease-promoting) form. Deviation from classic Mendelian inheritance is explained by reduced or *incomplete penetrance* (incomplete or lack of manifestation of the disorder in persons with the susceptibility gene) and, conversely, by *phenocopies* (affected persons who do not have the susceptibility gene). The multifactorial-polygenic model postulates the combined action of multiple genes and environmental components, each making a small additive contribution to phenotypic expression. According to the multifactorial-polygenic model, the clinical phenotype manifests when the genetic-environmental load exceeds a particular threshold. In between, the *oligogenic model* posits several but not many genes whose interaction (epistasis) is required for normal function. Mutations in one or more of the genes lead to the clinical manifestation. Unfortunately, none of those models can be excluded for schizophrenia or bipolar disorder. Schizophrenia may fit better with oligogenic models than with polygenic models, and single locus models may fit least well.

PHENOTYPIC CLASSIFICATION Another complication in the study of psychiatric genetics is ambiguity over diagnostic classification. Although recent efforts to operationalize diagnostic criteria have improved the reliability of diagnosis, it is impossible to know a priori which set of criteria will provide the best correlation between genotype and phenotype. To some extent one can define a genetic spectrum for a given disorder. A diagnosis that is genetically related to schizophrenia should occur at a high frequency among close relatives, such as monozygotic twins and first-degree relatives. That is true of unipolar depression and bipolar disorder probands and of both schizotypal and paranoid personality disorders and schizophrenia. In general, the most stringent diagnostic criteria yield the highest consensus among clinicians but provide the least power to detect linkage, since a smaller number of persons are considered affected.

Current linkage strategies often use a hierarchy of diagnostic categories. For example, a narrow classification of bipolar disorder may include bipolar and schizoaffective disorders only, but a broad classification may include those narrow classes and major depressive disorder and cyclothymic disorder. Usually, the initial classification scheme is a compromise between power to detect linkage and reliability of diagnosis. Subsequent schemes can then be tested to follow up an initial linkage finding or to reevaluate a linkage result.

BIAS AND INTERPRETATION For Mendelian disorders a maximum lod score of 3 or an odds ratio of 1,000 to 1 has traditionally been required to assert linkage. The odds that any two randomly selected loci will be genetically linked to one another *(prior probability)* in the human genome is about 2 percent. The corrected odds or *posterior odds* for linkage, given a lod score of 3, are simply the prior odds of linkage (0.02) times the odds provided by the data (1,000) or 20 to 1. That gives a posterior probability of linkage of 20 out of 21, or 95 percent, and a probability of no linkage or a false-positive probability of 5 percent. Lod score statistics for non-Mendelian diseases are not so straightforward. For the reasons cited above, linkage analysis of the psychiatric disorders requires the testing of multiple models for the mode of inheritance, the disease parameters (penetrance, phenocopies, disease allele frequency), and the diagnostic categories. The testing of multiple models leads to inflation of the resultant lod scores. To correct for the inflation, some investigators have proposed subtracting $\log_{10}t$ from the maximum lod score where t = the number of genetic or diagnostic models tested. Thus, if 10 models are used to derive a lod score of 3.0, the inflation-adjusted score is 2.0. In part because of inflationary methods, the interpretation of recent psychiatric linkage findings has been complicated; in several well-known studies, preliminary conclusions have been retracted, and other studies remain unresolved or unreplicated.

If one assumes the inheritance of dominant-susceptibility alleles, linkage analysis is most effective when the disease gene is inherited through only one side of the family *(unilateral transmission)*. That is because there is no way to distinguish persons who inherit one and not two copies of a susceptibility allele. *Bilateral transmission* (both parents affected) is a particular problem in view of locus heterogeneity, in which two different susceptibility genes segregate in the same family. Psychiatrically ill patients often mate with persons who are similarly affected, a situation referred to as *assortative mating*. That situation can increase the occurrence of bilineal transmission of susceptibility genes, which in turn confounds standard linkage analysis.

Another complication that has received much attention recently is *ascertainment bias,* in which the method of family collection is expected to bias either genetic or nongenetic contributions to illness in the families being studied. For example, the selection of families heavily loaded for illness may unwittingly select for bilineal transmission, presumably in cases in which one spouse carries an incompletely penetrant susceptibility allele. Without standard and systematized rules for family ascertainment, the comparison of individual linkage studies is complicated.

Comparison over time within societies presents unique problems also. Economic and social forces induce continued changes in society, including health and disease. *Cohort effects* and *secular trends* in rates of disorders are examples of temporal variations in the incidence or the prevalence of a disorder and are thought to reflect variations in risk factors (or exposure) over time. Such factors may include exposure to a common toxin or a shared historical event. For example, striking increases in the rates of major depression have been found in the successive decade-of-birth cohorts from 1910 to 1960 of first-degree relatives of patients with major mood disorders. Such trends are unlikely to be genetic in nature and need to be carefully documented, lest they lead to a distortion of genetic parameters, such as estimated disease allele frequency.

The psychiatric disorders present many new challenges to conventional genetic linkage analysis. To some extent, those problems will be alleviated by new methods of statistical analysis; for example, simultaneous search programs are being developed that can evaluate linkage at several loci simultaneously. Some of the complications will be offset by advances in DNA marker technology and better genetic maps and physical maps of human chromosomes. The lod score method is, however, fundamentally dependent on the correct approximation of genetic parameters, which cannot be known with certainty before linkage analysis. In general, misspecification of the mode of inheritance parameters will reduce the expected lod score and increase the estimated value of the recombination fraction.

NONPARAMETRIC STRATEGIES Methods are available to complement linkage analysis that are *nonparametric* (not dependent on assumptions regarding pattern of inheritance or penetrance) but that do retain sufficient power to detect linkage in some situations. One such strategy is the *affected-sib-pair method,* which is based on the premise that affected siblings are more likely to share identical marker alleles than would be predicted by chance when the marker and the disease locus are genetically linked. That is true regardless of the mode of inheritance, and penetrance is not an issue, since only affected persons are analyzed. Sib-pair analyses are, therefore, less prone than are other methods to produce misleading interpretations, such as false-negative findings. The major disadvantage of sib-pair analysis is that it is considerably less powerful than lod score analysis, especially in the presence of significant locus heterogeneity.

Another useful genetic strategy is the detection of *allelic association (linkage disequilibrium)* between a marker allele and the disease phenotype. A marker allele appears in association with another locus when the two loci have not been separated by meiotic recombination over a long course of history. That happens only when the two loci are extremely close together (usually separated by a tenth to several tenths of a centimorgan) and when both mutations are relatively old. Allelic association was recently used to identify the gene for cystic fibrosis and to show that alleles at the insulin gene are in linkage disequilibrium with a particular subtype (human leukocyte antigen [HLA]-D2-positive) of insulin-dependent diabetes mellitus (IDDM). That finding is of particulare interest because numerous linkage studies had failed to establish linkage between insulin and IDDM. A particular application of the association strategy is to test whether a *candidate gene* (a gene whose function implies a role in the disease pathology) harbors the susceptibility mutation.

PSYCHIATRIC GENETIC STUDIES

Despite the myriad of complications enumerated in the preceding pages, a growing number of studies portend well for the future of complex genetic linkage studies. Several studies indicate that some degree of locus heterogeneity can be tolerated by both linkage analysis and linkage disequilibrium studies. For example, Charcot-Marie-Tooth neuropathy maps to at least three different chromosomes and shows both dominant and recessive X-linked inheritance. By clinical criteria, patients with the disorder cannot be distinguished, regardless of their genetic subtype. Conversely, two widely disparate motor neuron disorders, Werdnig-Hoffmann disease and Kugelberg-Welander disease, apparently map to the identical locus on the long arm of chromosome 5 (5q). As described previously, allelic association studies identified a subtype of insulin-dependent diabetes mellitus that is tightly linked to polymorphisms in the insulin gene. In all those cases, genetic analysis overcame significant locus heterogeneity to reveal distinct genetic subtypes of illness.

Genetic linkage analysis of Alzheimer's disease is particularly relevant to the psychiatric studies. Alzheimer's disease is difficult to analyze by linkage methods because it has a late age of onset; it overlaps with nongenetic dementia, which occurs frequently in the very old; and the diagnosis can be made only postmortem. The majority of patients with Alzheimer's disease appear as sporadics with no clear family history, and Alzheimer's disease is not perceived as a genetic disorder. Despite those complexities, genetic linkage and linkage disequilibrium studies have recently made considerable inroads to the identification of genetic factors which contribute to this illness. Mutations in amyloid precursor protein, the major proteinaceous component of senile plaques, have been identified in family members affected with early-onset familial Alzheimer's disease, thereby identifying that gene as the target site for a minority of patients with the early-onset form of the illness. In 1992 strong genetic linkage evidence (cumulative lod scores over 20) identified another locus for the early-onset form of the disease on chromosome 14. By contrast to families of schizophrenic patients, a subset of early-onset Alzheimer's disease cases have been identified with a multigenerational pattern of inheritance that is consistent with a highly penetrant dominant allele. Thus, early onset was identified as a covariate that revealed a rare subtype of Alzheimer's disease with a Mendelian pattern of inheritance. In 1992 another family of Alzheimer's disease, one with typical late-onset illness, was tentatively mapped to chromosome 19. In 1993 researchers identified significant linkage disequilibrium between the ε-4 allele of apolipoprotein E on chromosome 19, and both late onset familial and sporadic Alzheimer's disease. Persons who inherited one copy of the ε-4 allele along with one copy of either the ε-2 or ε-3 allele are at roughly threefold greater risk of developing illness, while persons who inherit two copies of the ε-4 allele are at eightfold greater risk. Thus, apolipoprotein E ε-4 gene dose is a major risk factor for late-onset Alzheimer's disease, although it appears to be neither necessary nor sufficient to cause illness.

The current set of DNA markers and statistical analysis programs have proved to be adequate in the face of some daunting problems, including genetic heterogeneity, ambiguous inheritance patterns, and uncertain diagnostic classifications.

EARLY LINKAGE STUDIES The first genetic linkage studies of psychiatric disorders were conducted with conventional markers that detected protein polymorphisms. A possible linkage between schizophrenia and group-specific factor (G_c) and the immunoglobulin Gm locus was reported in 1973. Several years later there were reports of a possible linkage between both schizophrenia and bipolar disorder and the human leukocyte antigen (HLA) gene family locus. It has been proposed for nearly half a century that susceptibility to bipolar disorder is linked to the X chromosome. The lack of male-to-male transmission and an excess of affected women were observed in early family and epidemiological studies. The first evidence for X-linkage used the X-chromosome color blindness marker against two large North American families. Several laboratories later reported linkage to color blindness or the closely linked glucose 6-phosphate dehydrogenase deficiency locus. Those early findings prompted additional studies, which generally failed to replicate the original linkages. In light of the many complexities discussed here, it is not difficult to understand why independent linkage studies have largely gone unreplicated.

In the past 10 years significant advances have been made in the operationalized diagnosis of psychiatric disorders, the systematic collection of families for linkage analysis, the development of new statistical methods to analyze linkage data, and the molecular genetic analysis of pedigrees. Many of the studies performed before the mid-1980s are difficult to appraise or to compare with recent studies because of the rapid evolution of methods. A number of recent psychiatric studies have incorporated updated methodologies, several of which are summarized below, including an Amish bipolar disorder study, an X-linked bipolar disorder study, reports of schizophrenia linkage on chromosomes 5 and 22, and a study of heritable aggressive behavior.

AMISH BIPOLAR DISORDER In 1987 RFLP analysis of an Old Order Amish pedigree indicated that a dominant gene conferring a strong predisposition to bipolar disorder is located on the tip of the short arm of chromosome 11. The pedigree consisted of the extended families of six ill probands with a total of 81 persons. The Amish are an appealing population for psychiatric linkage analysis for several reasons: their large family size, clearly established paternity, geographic concentration, and social and religious prohibition of alcohol and drug abuse, which can severely complicate psychiatric diagnosis. RFLP and VNTR polymorphisms for insulin and the cellular oncogene Harvey-ras-1 (H-*ras*-1) showed relatively strong linkage to mood disorders in the pedigree. Even more convincing, the findings were robust over a wide range of penetrance values (0.55 to 0.95). Maximum likelihood analysis of the linkage data indicated that the mood disorder gene was most tightly linked to H-*ras* with a Z_{max} = 4.9.

That pioneering report also indicated that a number of clinically variant forms of bipolar disorder (bipolar I, bipolar II, major depressive disorder, schizoaffective disorder) likewise result from mutations at a single chromosome 11 locus. The indication that a simple genetic mechanism (single locus, dominant inheritance, with reduced penetrance) can account for the transmission of bipolar disorder in that extended pedigree provided a great impetus for other psychiatric studies. Unfortunately, the finding was quickly followed by reports of nonreplication and, finally, retraction. Later in the same year, two independent reports, one of North American white families of European origin and the other of three Icelandic pedigrees, failed to detect linkage with the same markers.

In 1989 the Amish study was extended by adding new DNA marker data on several members of the core pedigree, by providing updated clinical data on several recent onsets of illness in previously unaffected members, and by extending the number of persons with large lateral extensions of the original pedigree. With that new information the lod support for linkage fell dramatically. Ten persons in the core pedigree were not typed with both DNA markers in the original study. The new DNA marker typings resulted in a drop in Z_{max} from 4.08 to 2.46 for H-*ras* while insulin increased from 2.6 to 3.38. The most dramatic effect came from the updated diagnostic information on two members who became ill after the original investigation. Because they were high up in the pedigree, their change in status also affected other persons, dropping the maximum lod scores to 1.03 and 1.75 for H-*ras* and insulin, respectively. A left extension of the pedigree with six persons, two of whom were ill, dropped the scores further to 0.7 and 1.29. The right extension consisted of 31 members, four with bipolar disorder and seven with major depressive disorder. When they were analyzed separately, the extension was strongly negative. When they were added to the core pedigree, linkage could be excluded in the chromosomal region surrounding both insulin and H-*ras* loci. In 1991 another extension of the Amish families was shown to be clearly unlinked to the short arm of chromosome 11 (11 p) markers.

A key lesson learned from those pioneering psychiatric genetic studies is that researchers must be aware of the possibility that diagnosis may change with time and that follow-up studies of phenotypes are required. Nonetheless, the sophistication of the original report and the timely and thorough follow-up analyses have become the model for psychiatric genetic studies.

X-LINKED BIPOLAR DISORDER In 1987 researchers reported the linkage analysis of five large, multigenerational families heavily loaded with mood disorders from a large sample of psychiatric patients in Israel. The study included 161 adults, of whom 47 were ill with bipolar disorder or related mood disorders. Four of the five pedigrees were non-Ashkenazi (of Mediterranean or Asian origin), and one was Ashkenazi (of European origin). The pedigrees were informative for either color blindness or glucose 6-phosphate dehydrogenase deficiency, both classic phenotypic markers at Xq28 (near the telomere of the X chromosome long arm). The study provided strong evidence for the close linkage of bipolar disorder to the Xq28 markers. The maximum lod scores ranged from 7.52 to 9.17. The highest lod scores were obtained by assuming locus heterogeneity—that is, by assuming that not all the families in the study resulted from mutation at the identical locus. In the study only the non-Ashkenazi families were linked to the Xq28 markers.

A study of a Belgian population showed weaker evidence of linkage between persons with bipolar disorder and a factor IX marker located about 30 to 40 cM centromeric to the color blindness or glucose 6-phosphate dehydrogenase (G6PD) loci. On the other hand, a number of studies have failed to find linkage in the Xq27-28 chromosomal region by using either the color blindness phenotypic markers or DNA markers

A reanalysis of the Israeli bipolar pedigrees showed very little, if any, support for linkage to 13 DNA markers which map to the Xq27-28 chromosomal region. The reanalysis included the three pedigrees that demonstrated the strongest support for linkage in the 1987 study. The pedigrees were extended and new persons were analyzed, all diagnoses were updated, and DNA markers from both the color blindness locus and the G6PD locus were substituted for visual examinations and enzyme assays respectively. That reanalysis uncovered inaccuracies in the inference of genotype based on enzyme assays (G6PD deficiency) in the 1987 study, it revealed recombination events not detected by the less informative phenotypic evaluations, and it revealed new recombination events between DNA markers and the putative disease locus which resulted from changes in diagnostic status over time. The 1987 linkage study and the 1993 reanalysis yielded radically different support for linkage to bipolar disorder at chromosome Xq28. The statistical support for linkage dropped by 6 to 9 lod units in the 1993 study. The lesson from the 1993 reanalysis is that DNA markers are more informative and more reliably interpreted than their phenotypic counterparts. The more important concern for psychiatric geneticists is how such overwhelming support for linkage could be subverted by a more thorough analysis of the same core pedigrees plus additional relatives. The contribution of previously missed genetic information plus errors in the enzyme assay system would not be expected to shift the evidence significantly for, or against, support for linkage. It is most likely that some form of systematic bias went undetected, presumably in the earlier study, since the reanalysis detects significantly more of the genetic information in the three Israeli pedigrees. Genetic analysis of behavioral disorders is particularly susceptible to bias in the correlation of genotype and disease status. Diagnostic classification is exceedingly complex and prone to change over time so that there is the tendency for these studies to extend for long periods. Under those circumstances it can be very difficult to keep laboratory workers and field workers blind to phenotypic and genotypic data, respectively. Nonetheless, recent DNA marker studies of psychiatric disorders seem to have avoided the major sources of false-positive errors. The challenge for future studies will be to avoid false-negative errors, and to detect evidence for linkage in the face of numerous complicating factors.

SCHIZOPHRENIA In 1988 investigators described a family in which an extra copy of a short segment of chromosome 5 was coinherited along with schizophrenia. In the same year a British group reported genetic linkage between DNA markers from that duplicated chromosomal region and ill status in British and Icelandic families with schizophrenia and related disorders. The study consisted of five Icelandic and two English families with 39 cases of schizophrenia (including all main subtypes), five cases of related schizoid personality disorder, and 10 cases of fringe phenotypes not usually associated with schizophrenia (phobia and other anxiety disorders and major depressive disorder). Two chromosome 5 long arm (5q) RFLP-type DNA markers were coinherited with a putative dominant allele predisposing to schizophrenia and related disorders. Using relatively high penetrance values (73 to 86 percent), the investigators calculated maximum lod scores of 3.22 (for persons with schizophrenia), 4.33 (schizophrenia and schizoid personality disorder), and 6.49 (schizophrenia, schizoid personality disorder, and fringe phenotypes, including alcoholism).

It was surprising that linkage increased by a lod score of 3.3 with the inclusion of fringe phenotypes, which are not typically found at high frequency in the families of schizophrenic patients. In general, one would predict that evidence for linkage would decrease when the phenotypic definition of the illness is widened to include less certain cases, because the addition of false-positive cases in a linkage analysis can significantly lower the lod scores. When the authors considered only strictly defined cases as affected (penetrance-free model), they derived a maximum lod score of 2.45.

Using a more detailed genetic map, another group of investigators immediately reported the absence of linkage to the 5q region in a single large Swedish pedigree. Soon after, a number of studies failed to find linkage in that area, although in two studies a significant portion of the families analyzed had cases of bipolar disorder in addition to schizophrenia. Since a number of epidemiological studies have shown that the two psychiatric diseases are distinct, those studies are not easy to interpret.

By 1990 a combined analysis of all studies gave a lod score of −40 in the 5q region, indicating that only a small minority of families of schizophrenic patients could be affected by mutations in that region. A thorough analysis of the original English and Icelandic families—along with additional families, presumably from the same populations—have failed to support the linkage to schizophrenia in that region. As of this writing, evidence from the original families in support of linkage has dropped below the 3.0 mark.

Of the three psychiatric linkage studies described here, the Amish report is the most nearly complete in the sense that nearly all necessary follow-up studies have been conducted and reported. It now seems fairly certain that the original finding was spurious. The chromosome-5 studies and the X-chromosome studies require further systematic follow-up analysis.

In the past several years, most of the entire genome has been tested for linkage to schizophrenia. Genome-wide searches by some groups have failed to produce convincing evidence of linkage to schizophrenia, while other groups have reported potential linkages on chromosomes 5p and 22. On chromosome 22q12-q13.1 a lod score of 1.54 was observed using a dominant genetic model on data collected from 39 multiplex pedigrees. Maximization of the lod score by varying the parameters of the genetic model raised the lod score to 2.82. An attempt to replicate the finding by a collaborative group of researchers using an additional 217 pedigrees (256 total) found no evidence of linkage or heterogeneity in the region. However, a third group has reported a lod score of 2.09 using markers from the region and a recessive model of analysis.

Velo-cardio-facial syndrome, an autosomal dominant disorder in which persons have been noted to have an increased rate of psychotic symptoms, is located on chromosome 22 centromeric to the potential linkages described. The phenotypic connection between the two disorders is strengthened by the findings of increased frequency of epicanthal skin folds, malformed ears, and high palate, which are observed in velo-cardial-facial syndrome, in schizophrenic patients as compared with controls. That connection between velo-cardial-facial syndrome and schizophrenia is currently being investigated.

AGGRESSIVE BEHAVIOR One of the most intriguing studies in psychiatric genetics is the investigation of a large Dutch pedigree in which several males are affected with a syndrome of borderline mental retardation and abnormal regulation of aggression. Men in the pedigree have displayed impulsive aggression, arson, attempted rape, and exhibitionism. The pattern of segregation of the syndrome in the pedigree appeared X-linked, and a genetic linkage analysis localized the defect to the p11-p21 region of the chromosome. The genes for monoamine oxidases A and B are located in this region and are strong candidate genes for aggressive behavior because of their role in the degradation of serotonin, noradrenaline, and dopamine. The activity of those enzymes was tested in skin fibroblast cultures from several members of the pedigree and expression of monoamine oxidase-A (MAO-A) activity was negligible in the affected men. DNA sequence analysis revealed a single base-pair mutation causing a premature stop codon in the MAO-A gene from affected men. A linkage analysis of the clinical phenotype and the point mutation gave a maximum lod score of 3.55 with a recombination fraction of zero.

The finding of a point mutation in the MAO-A gene is consistent with data from several studies that have found low concentrations of 5-hydroxyindoleacetic acid (5-HIAA) in the cerebrospinal fluid (CSF) of persons with impulsive aggression. Presumably, premature termination of the MAO-A gene in this family prevents expression of portions of the enzyme necessary for the metabolism of the monoamines, and would lead to decreased production of 5-HIAA. The synthetic pathway of serotonin has also been investigated by using DNA polymorphisms. An association between a polymorphism in an intron of the tryptophan hydroxylase gene and CSF 5-HIAA concentration has been observed in a sample of impulsive, alcoholic, violent offenders. The polymorphism was also associated with a history of suicide attempts in a sample of impulsive and nonimpulsive violent offenders. At this time, the intronic DNA polymorphism is thought to be functionally insignificant, but it may provide a marker for a genetically linked mutation in the tryptophan hydroxylase gene.

SUGGESTED CROSS-REFERENCES

Population genetics is discussed in Section 1.15, and genetic counseling is discussed in Section 31.11. Schizophrenia is discussed in Chapter 14, mood disorders in Chapter 16, anxiety disorders in Chapter 17, and Alzheimer's disease and other dementing disorders in Section 49.6a.

REFERENCES

Barnes D M: Troubles encountered in gene linkage land. Science *243:* 313, 1989.

Baron M, Endicott J, Ott J: Genetic linkage in mental illness: Limitations and prospects. Br J Psychiatry *157:* 645, 1990.

Baron M, Freimer N F, Risch N, et al: Diminished support for linkage between manic-depressive illness and X-chromosome markers in three Israeli pedigrees. Nature Genet *3:* 49, 1993.

Baron M, Risch N, Hamburger R, Mandel B, Kushner S, Newman M, Drumer D, Belmaker R H: Genetic linkage between X-chromosome markers and bipolar affective illness. Nature *326:* 289, 1987.

Coon H, Holik J, Reimherr F: Analysis of chromosome 22 markers in nine schizophrenia pedigrees. Am J Med Genet *54:* 72, 1994.

Corder E H, Saunders A M, Strittmatter W J, Schmechel D E, Gaskell P C, Small G W, Roses A D, Haines J L, Pericak-Vance M A: Gene dose of apolipoprotein E type 4 allele and the risk of Alzheimer's disease in late onset families. Science *261:* 921, 1993.

Diehl S R, Kendler K S: Strategies for linkage studies of schizophrenia: Pedigrees, DNA markers, and statistical analyses. Schizophr Bull *3:* 403, 1989.

Donnis-Keller H, Green P, Helms C: A genetic linkage map of the human genome. Cell *51:* 319, 1987.

*Egeland J A, Gerhard D S, Pauls D L, Sussex J N, Kidd K K, Allen C R, Hostetter A M, Housman D E: Bipolar affective disorders linked to DNA markers on chromosome 11. Nature *325:* 783, 1987.

Falconer D S: The inheritance of liability to certain diseases estimated from the incidence among relatives. Ann Hum Genet *29:* 51, 1965.

Goate A, Chartier-Harlin M-C, Mullan M: Segregation of a missense mutation in the amyloid precursor protein gene with familial Alzheimer's disease. Nature *349:* 704, 1991.

Goate A M, Haynes A R, Owen M J, Farrall M, James L A, Lai L Y C, Mullan M J, Roques P, Rossor M N, Williamson R, Hardy J A: Predisposing locus for Alzheimer's disease on chromosome 21. Lancet *1:* 352, 1989.

Gottesman I I, Shields J A: A polygenic theory of schizophrenia. Proc Natl Acad Sci USA *58:* 199, 1967.

Gusella J F: Location cloning strategy for characterizing genetic defects in Huntington's disease and Alzheimer's disease. FASEB J *3:* 2036, 1989.

Huntington's Disease Collaborative Research Group: A novel gene containing a trinucleotide repeat that is expanded and unstable on Huntington's disease chromosomes. Cell *72:* 971, 1993.

Kelsoe J R, Ginns E I, Egeland J A, Gerhard D S, Goldstein A M, Bale S J, Pauls D L, Long R T, Kidd K K, Conte G, Housman D E, Paul S M: Re-evaluation of the linkage relationship between chromosome 11p loci and the gene for bipolar affective disorder in the Old Order Amish. Nature *342:* 238, 1989.

Kety S S: The significance of genetic factors in the etiology of schizophrenia: Results from the national study of adoptees in Denmark. J Psychiatr Res *4:* 423, 1987.

*Lander E S, Botstein D: Mapping complex genetic traits in humans: New methods using a complete RFLP linkage map. Cold Spring Harb Symp Quant Biol *51:* 49, 1986.

Malaspina D, Quitkin H M, Kaufmann C A: Epidemiology and genetics of neuropsychiatric disorders. In *The American Psychiatric Press Textbook of Neuropsychiatry,* ed 2, S C Yudofsky, R E Hales, editors, p 187, American Psychiatric Press, Washington, 1992.

Martin J B: Molecular genetic studies in the neuropsychiatric disorders. Trends Neurosci *12:* 130, 1989.

McKusick V A: Current trends in mapping human genes. FASEB J *5:* 12, 1990.

Mendlewicz J, Simon P, Sevy S, Charon F, Brocas H, Legros S, Vassart G: Polymorphic DNA marker on X chromosome and manic depression. Lancet *1:* 1230, 1987.

Orkin S H: Reverse genetics and human disease. Cell *47:* 845, 1986.

Ott J: *Analysis of Human Genetic Linkage.* Johns Hopkins University Press, Baltimore, 1985.

Ott J: Genetic linkage analysis under uncertain disease definition. In *Banbury Report: Genetics and Biology of Alcoholism,* vol 33, C R Cloninger, H Beglieter, editors. Cold Spring Harbor Laboratory Press, Cold Spring Harbor, NY, p 327.

Pericak-Vance M A, Bedout J L, Gaskell P C, Roses A D: Linkage studies in familial Alzheimer's disease—evidence for chromosome 19 linkage. Am J Hum Genet *48:* 1034, 1992.

Poustka A, Pohl T, Barlow D P, Zehetner G, Craig A, Michiels F, Ehrich E, Frischauf A-M, Lehrach H: Molecular approaches to mammalian genetics. Cold Spring Harb Symp Quant Biol *51:* 131, 1987.

Pulver A N, Karayiorgou M, Lasseter V K, et al: Follow-up of a report of a potential linkage for schizophrenia on chromosome 22q12-q13.1: Part 2. Am J Med Genet *54:* 44, 1994.

Pulver A N, Karayiorgou M, Wolyniec P S, et al: Sequential strategy to identify a susceptibility gene for schizophrenia: Report of potential linkage on chromosome 22q12-q13.1: Part 1. Am J Med Genet *54:* 36, 1994.

Rieder R O, Kaufmann C A: Genetics: In *The American Psychiatric Press Textbook of Psychiatry,* J A Talbott, R E Hales, S C Yudofsky, editors, p 33. American Psychiatric Press, Washington, 1988.

*Risch N: Genetic linkage and complex diseases, with special reference to psychiatric disorders. Genet Epidemiol *7:* 3, 1990.

Risch N: Genetic linkage: Interpreting lod scores. Science *255:* 803, 1992.

Saiki R H, Gelfand D H, Stoffel S: Primer-directed enzymatic amplification of DNA with a thermostable DNA polymerase. Science *239:* 487, 1988.

*Sherrington R, Brynjolfsson J, Petursson H, Potter M, Dudleston K, Barraclough B, Wasmuth J, Dobbs M, Gurling H: Localization of a susceptibility locus for schizophrenia on chromosome 5. Nature *336:* 164, 1988.

*Straub R E, Gilliam T C: Genetic linkage studies of bipolar affective disorder. In *Genome Analysis,* vol 6, *Genome Maps and Neurological Disorders,* K E Davies, S M Tilgman, editors, p 77. Cold Spring Harbor Laboratory Press, Cold Spring Harbor, NY, 1993.

Suarez B, O'Rourke D, Van Eederwegh P V: Power of the affected-sib-pair methods to detect disease susceptibility loci of small effect: An application to multiple sclerosis. Am J Hum Genet *12:* 309, 1982.

Van Broeckhoven C, Backhovens H, Cruts M, DeWinter G, Bruyland M, Crass P, Martin J-J: Mapping of a gene predisposing to early-onset Alzheimer's disease to chromosome 14q24.3. Nature Genet *2:* 335, 1992.

Weber J L: Informativeness of human $(dC\text{-}dA)_n$ $(dG\text{-}dT)_n$ polymorphisms. Genomics *7:* 524, 1990.

Weeks D E, Brzustowicz L M, Squires-Wheller E, Cornblatt B, Lehner T, Stefanovich M, Bassett A, Gilliam T C, Ott J, Erlenmeyer-Kimling L: Report of a workshop on genetic linkage studies in schizophrenia. Schizophr Bull *16:* 673, 1990.

Weissenbach J, Gyapay G, Dib C, Vignal A, Morissette J, Millasseau P, Vaysseix G, Lathrop M: A second-generation linkage map of the human genome. Nature *359:* 794, 1992.

1.17 FUTURE DIRECTIONS IN NEUROSCIENCE AND PSYCHIATRY

SOLOMON H. SNYDER, M.D.

INTRODUCTION

Much of psychiatry's future will probably be inseparable from the neurosciences. Already, the use of sophisticated drugs in psychiatry requires practitioners to keep up with the latest advances in neurosciences. Yet drugs available today are based on what was known of neurotransmitters and their receptors one or two decades ago. A generation ago the only clearly established neurotransmitters were acetylcholine and norepinephrine, although serotonin had recently been identified and was thought to be of interest. γ-Aminobutyric acid (GABA) had already been identified in the brain, but it was not widely accepted as a neurotransmitter until the mid-1960s. Next to nothing was known of the neuropeptides, and there was virtually no understanding of amino acids, such glutamate and glycine, as neurotransmitters. Today, most drugs used in psychiatry act through the neurotransmitters serotonin and the catecholamines. Drug companies are actively pursuing agents that may act through neuropeptides, such as substance P and cholecystokinin, but the lag between drug identification and clinical application indicates that most agents acting through the newest-known neurotransmitter systems will be arriving in the 21st century.

Molecular biology will affect clinical research and practice more and more. The major molecular biological tools are already being incorporated into all branches of biomedical research. People no longer speak about "doing molecular biology" and applying it to the neurosciences. Rather, molecular neuroscience is taken for granted as an integral part of the field. Similarly, when electron microscopes were first developed in the 1950s, some scientists were called "electron microscopists." Now the electron microscope is merely a machine used by many biomedial researchers without particularly specialized training.

THERAPIES BASED ON MESSENGER MOLECULES

Drugs currently used in psychiatry act on various aspects of neurotransmitter systems. For instance, amphetamines facilitate the release of the catecholamines norepinephrine and dopamine. Tricyclic antidepressants inhibit the reuptake inactivation of serotonin and norepinephrine. Opiates directly stimulate opiate receptors, which normally interact with the opiatelike peptide neurotransmitters the enkephalines. Benzodiazepines facilitate the actions of the inhibitory neurotransmitter GABA by binding to a distinct site on GABA receptors, enhancing the binding affinity of GABA for its receptor site. Antipsychotic drugs block dopamine receptors.

Those agents act through a limited number of neurotransmitter systems. Moreover, they generally lack subtype selectivity. Thus, chlorpromazine (Thorazine) blocks all dopamine receptors, but five or more dopamine receptor subtypes are now known. Clearly, one theme in the coming decades will be the development of agents that are more selective than presently used agents. Recent advances in receptor subtypes reflect what may only be the tip of the iceberg of receptor selectivity.

In the case of dopamine receptors, in the late 1970s differential drug effects established two subtypes, D_1 and D_2. The major antipsychotic actions are associated with the blockade of D_2 receptors because of the close correlation between the blockade of D_2 receptors and antipsychotic potency, whereas the blockade of D_1 receptors parallels antipsychotic actions only modestly. Thus, haloperidol (Haldol), one of the most clinically potent antipsychotic drugs, is quite potent at D_2 receptors but weak at D_1 receptors. Both D_1 and D_2 receptors are localized in the corpus striatum and in the limbic system. By blocking receptors in the corpus striatum, those drugs elicit extrapyramidal side effects, but antipsychotic actions reflect the blockade of limbic dopamine receptors. The molecular cloning of genes for dopamine receptors led to the identification of novel subtypes. For instance, D_3 and D_4 dopamine receptors are quite similar to D_2 receptors but display notable differences. Specifically, both of those new receptors are substantially more concentrated in the limbic system than in the corpus striatum. Clozapine (Clozaril), the atypical antipsychotic drug with a low incidence of extrapyramidal side effects, is 10 times more potent at D_4 than at D_2 receptors, whereas most antipsychotics are more potent at D_2 than at D_4. sites. Accordingly, the unique antipsychotic actions of clozapine and its low incidence of extrapyramidal side effects may reflect selective actions at D_4 receptors. Clearly, chemicals that specifically block D_4 receptors are likely to be more potent and safer clozapinelike agents than agents that block D_2 receptors. One can readly express cloned receptors in cell culture systems and monitor drug binding to them. Thus, from the perspective of drug development, molecular biology provides powerful tools to attain highly selective agents.

The example with dopamine receptors applies similarly to numerous other receptor systems. Multiple serotonin receptor subtypes have been cloned. Presently, the antianxiety drug buspirone (BuSpar) is the only major drug in psychiatry that acts directly on a particular serotonin receptor subtype. Serotonin is relevant to many drugs influencing neurological and psychiatric processes. Selective inhibitors of serotonin reuptake inactivation are already dominating the therapy of depression. Drugs such as sumatriptan, which stimulate serotonin 5-HT_{1D} subtype receptors, are providing a new generation of highly effective antimigraine agents. Drugs influencing 5-HT_3 serotonin receptor subtypes relieve nausea and vomiting associated with cancer chemotherapy. One serotonin receptor subtype that may become increasingly important in psychiatry is the 5-HT_2 subtype receptor. Drugs such as ritanserin, which block that type of receptor, seem to influence the negative symptoms of schizophrenia favorably. In the future, psychiatrists may selectively titrate the positive symptoms of schizophrenic patients with dopamine-antagonizing antipsychotics and the negative symptoms with serotonin 5-HT_2 antagonists. Drugs such as risperidone (Risperdal), which block D_2 and 5-HT_2 receptors, may afford such combination therapy in a single medication.

Molecular biological analysis reveals that most neurotransmitter receptors exist in a number of subtypes. For instance, the $GABA_A$ receptor, at which benzodiazepines act, comprises at least three distinct subunit proteins, designated alpha (α), beta (β), and gamma (γ). Several subtypes have been cloned for each of those subunits. Functional GABA receptors comprise various combinations of the subunit subtypes; 20 to 200 distinct GABA receptor subtypes may regulate neurotransmission. Certain drugs act differently at the various GABA-benzodiazepine receptor subunits. Some of those drugs exert varying ratios of sedative-to-antianxiety effects. Thus, one may be able to sculpt new benzodiazepinelike agents that are safer and more effective than present agents.

Drug development using glutamate receptors is particularly prominent in neurology. Glutamate is the major excitatory neurotransmitter in the brain. The *N*-methyl-D-aspartate (NMDA) subtype of glutamate receptor appears to be relevant to neurotoxicity in vascular thrombosis. After the occlusion of a cerebral artery, a large outpouring of glutamate acts on NMDA receptors to elicit neurotoxicity. Experimental drugs that block NMDA receptors greatly diminish neuronal destruction after a thrombosis, even when the drugs are given to animals after tying off an artery. In clinical application, vascular thrombosis patients will receive intravenous injections of the drugs soon after the first symptoms of stroke, analogous to the treatment of patients with myocardial infarctions by using tissue plasminogen activator. Numerous subtypes of glutamate receptors have been cloned. What types of therapeutic effects one may expect from drugs that stimulate or block other non-NMDA glutamate receptor subtypes is not yet clear. Presumably, drugs that block glutamate receptors will be similar to agents that stimulate GABA receptors. The possible therapeutic actions include the relief of anxiety, anticonvulsant effects, and sedation.

The diverse antidepressants that inhibit neurotransmitter uptake were developed long before a molecular appreciation of the uptake recognition sites. In 1991 molecular cloning was reported for GABA, norepinephrine, dopamine, and serotonin transporter proteins. Whether transporter subtypes for each neurotransmitter exist is not yet clear. The expression of those cloned transporters in cell culture systems will provide a valuable tool for developing more potent and selective uptake inhibitor drugs. Besides drugs that inhibit biogenic amine uptake, the clinical actions of drugs that inhibit GABA, glutamate, and glycine uptake would be of interest. Inhibitors of GABA uptake should potentiate GABA and elicit antianxiety, sedative, and anticonvulsant effects. Inhibitors of glutamate uptake can be expected to be stimulants, conceivably with antidepressant actions.

SECOND MESSENGERS AND NOVEL MESSENGERS

Most therapeutic agents in psychiatry act through particular neurotransmitters. Little effort has been devoted to developing drugs that act through second-messenger systems, such as the cyclic adenosine monophosphate (cAMP) and the phosphoinositide (PI) systems. One might theorize that those second messengers serve so many different neurotransmitters that agents affecting them would be too global in their actions. However, one example does not fit that generalization—namely, lithium (Eskalith). No one is certain about the molecular site of lithium's actions. However, much evidence indicates that lithium slows the PI cycle. Lithium inhibits the enzyme that converts inositol-1-phosphate to inositol, providing a damper on the PI cycle. Neurophysiological studies reveal a dampening of synaptic activity after lithium treatment, with a lessening of both excessive inhibition and excessive excitation, fitting with lithium's clinical normalizing effects. Those actions of lithium on PI turnover and related neurotransmission occur at therapeutic concentrations of about 0.5 to 1.5 mM. Since one can monitor PI turnover biochemically, it should be possible to develop nonmetallic drugs that could act like lithium but lack the side effects associated with lithium's substitution for sodium. As with neurotransmitter receptors, molecular biology has revealed heterogeneity of enzymes and receptor sites associated with second-messenger systems, so that one may achieve considerable selectivity.

Recently, atypical messenger molecules have been characterized that do not fit classical definitions of neurotransmitters and second messengers. Adenosine 5-triphosphate (ATP) has long been advanced as such a substance. ATP is stored with catecholamines in synaptic vesicles and is released with them. In primary sensory neurons ATP may be released by itself to exert excitatory effects. Adenosine, which is formed from ATP, has a modulatory action that may reflect conventional neurotransmitter effects. Adenosine, like ATP, occurs in all cells but is highly concentrated in discrete neuronal populations in the brain. Adenosine inhibits the release of most neurotransmitters. Because of the predominence of the excitatory neurotransmitter glutamate in the brain, the major actions of adenosine are probably inhibitory, caused by the blockade of glutamate release. Caffeine exerts its behavioral stimulant effects by blocking adenosine receptors. Numerous pharmaceutical investigators are exploring the potential therapeutic effects of drugs that mimic adenosine. Such agents are already known to exert anticonvulsant and sedative effects and may be therapeutic in settings such as those in which benzodiazepines are currently used. New generations of adenosine antagonists may be useful behavioral stimulants in conditions such as age-associated mental impairment, in which a mild stimulant can enhance cognitive activity.

NITRIC OXIDE The most exciting novel messenger molecule is nitric oxide (NO). NO was first discovered as a mediator of the ability of macrophages to kill tumor cells and bacteria. NO also accounts for endothelial-derived relaxing factor activity. When acetylcholine dilates blood vessels, it does so by acting on receptors on endothelial cells, triggering the production of NO, which diffuses to the adjacent smooth muscle cells to promote relaxation by stimulating cyclic guanosine monophosphate (GMP) formation. NO is formed from the amino acid arginine by the enzyme NO synthase (NOS). Immunohistochemical localizations of NOS reveal concentrations in discrete neuronal populations in the brain and in autonomic nerves throughout the body. For instance, in the myenteric plexus NOS is localized to the neurons that mediate the physiological relaxation associated with peristalsis. Arginine derivatives, such as nitroarginine, which inhibit NOS activity, block physiological neurotransmission in that system. Thus, there NO fulfills all the requirements of a neurotransmitter. In most other areas of the gastrointestinal system, smooth muscles of the pulmonary system, the urethra, the penis, and other autonomic regions, NO similarly serves like a neurotransmitter.

In the brain the NOS neurons are those that stain for reduced nicotinamide adenine dinucleotide phosphate (NADPH) diaphorase activity, which reflects NOS oxidative functions. Those neurons are uniquely resistant to ischemic damage. Ischemic damage triggers a major release of glutamate, which binds to NMDA receptors and stimulates the NOS neurons to form NO. The NO diffuses to adjacent neurons, eliciting neurotoxic effects. Thus, the neurotoxicity evoked by glutamate in primary cultures or cerebral cortical neurons is blocked potently by NOS inhibitors. Similarly, neurotoxicity occurring with vascular thrombosis in animals is blocked by NOS inhibitors. Although NO mediates the toxic effects of high concentrations of glutamate acting through NMDA receptors, it also mediates the physiological synaptic effects of glutamate through NMDA receptors in which cyclic GMP formation is stimulated. Thus, the ability of glutamate to stimulate cyclic GMP levels is blocked by inhibitors of NOS.

On the basis of the known physiology of NO, NOS inhibitors will likely have therapeutic application in treating thrombosis in a fashion similar to the use of NMDA antagonists. Numerous investigators have already shown that administration of NOS inhibitors after tying off cerebral arteries blocks thrombosis damage. No one yet knows the psychiatric effects of enhancing or decreasing NO production. NOS is concentrated in a number of limbic structures of the brain and can be anticipated to play some role in behavioral regulation.

CAUSES OF MENTAL DISORDERS

To the clinician confronted with disabled patients, new therapeutic modalities are the bottom line of the profession. Of perhaps greater intellectual exictement is the likely application of molecular neuroscience to identifying fundamental abnormalities in the major mental disorders. Restriction (fragment) length polymorphism (RFLP) markers applied to deoxyribonucleic acid (DNA) samples of patients and their close relatives have pinpointed abnormal genes in several diseases relevant to the neurosciences. One of the most dramatic examples involves the discovery of the abnormal gene in Duchenne's muscular dystrophy and dystrophin, the protein that it encodes. That discovery led rapidly to diagnoses of muscular dystrophy in utero. The molecular biological findings revealed mutliple subtypes of dystrophy abnormalities, clarifying various clinical presentations of the disease. In Huntington's disease the specific abnormal gene has recently been pinpointed, which now permits the diagnosis of persons who are likely to have Huntington's disease in the future.

What about genetic markers for schizophrenia, depression, and anxiety? RFLP research in families with high concentrations of various disturbances has led to the preliminary identification of markers linked to bipolar disorder and schizophrenia. However, most of those markers have not held up as definitive links to the diseases in large populations. Some workers argue that psychiatric disturbances are so heterogeneous that one may never find the responsible molecular abnormalities. Although the challenge in psychiatry may be more difficult than for diseases such as muscular dystrophy, the major psychiatric disturbances are probably amenable to those research approaches. Will schizophrenia or mood disorders be associated with several completely unrelated molecular abnormalities? Alternatively, as in muscular dystrophy, varying mutational patterns of a single protein could provide diverse clinical patterns. Whatever the outcome, there will probably be surprises, and major molecular insights into psychiatric disability will emerge.

SUGGESTED CROSS-REFERENCES

Sections 1.3 and 1.4 discuss neurotransmitters, Section 1.5 discusses neuropeptides, Section 1.14 discusses molecular neurobiology, and Section 1.16 discusses genetic linkage analysis.

REFERENCES

*Baronde S: The biological approach to psychiatry: History and prospects. J Neurosci *10:* 1707, 1990.

*Berridge M J, Irvine R F: Inositol phosphates and cell signalling. Nature *341:* 197, 1989.

*Bredt D S, Snyder S H: Nitric oxide: A novel neuronal messenger. Neuron *8:* 3, 1992.

Burnstock G, Satchell D G, Smythe A: A comparison of the excitatory and inhibitory effects of non-adrenergic, non-cholinergic nerve stimulation and exogenously applied ATP on a variety of smooth muscle preparations from different vertebrate species. Br J Pharmacol *46:* 234, 1991.

Doble A, Martin I: Multiple benzodiazepine receptors. Trends Pharmacol Sci *13:* 76, 1992.

Garthwaite J: Glutamate, nitric oxide and cell-cell signalling in the nervous system. Trends Neurol Sci *14:* 60, 1991.

*Hokfelt T: Neuropeptides in perspective: The last 10 years. Neuron *7:* 867, 1991.

Hyman S E, Nestler E J: *The Molecular Foundations of Psychiatry.* American Psychiatric Press, Washington, 1993.

Moncada S, Palmer R M J, Higgs E A: Nitric oxide: Physiology, pathophysiology and pharmacology. Pharmacol Rev *43:* 109, 1991.

Sibley D R, Monsma F J: Molecular biology of dopamine receptors. Trends Pharmacol Sci *13:* 61, 1992.

*Snyder S H: Adenosine as a neuromodulator. Ann Rev Neurosci *8:* 103, 1985.

CHAPTER 2 NEUROPSYCHIATRY AND BEHAVIORAL NEUROLOGY

2.1 NEUROPSYCHIATRY: CLINICAL ASSESSMENT AND APPROACH TO DIAGNOSIS

JEFFREY L. CUMMINGS, M.D.

INTRODUCTION

Neuropsychiatry is the scientific discipline concerned with the identification and management of behavioral disturbances associated with brain dysfunction. It has research, education, and patient-care dimensions. Neuropsychiatry draws on the rich traditions of biological psychiatry, behavioral neurology, psychopharmacology, and neuroscience in its quest to understand the physical basis of behavior and to apply that knowledge to patients with behavioral disturbances. No aspect of human behavior is independent of its physical underpinnings, and neuropsychiatry is a cornerstone of psychiatry. All therapeutic interventions must eventually be translated into neurological events that affect behavior.

PRINCIPLES OF NEUROPSYCHIATRY

Several generalizations are applicable to clinical practice. (1) Essentially all types of behavior observed in idiopathic psychiatric syndromes can occur in association with a neurological disorder, and neurological diseases are an important part of the differential diagnosis of behavioral disturbances. (2) The phenotypic identity of psychiatric and neurological disorders does not necessarily imply pathogenetic identity, but shared pathophysiological mechanisms underlying similar behavior are likely and provide a framework for treatment and research. (3) Diagnosis informs therapy, and a thorough diagnostic evaluation should be a part of every psychiatric assessment. (4) Deficit syndromes frequently accompany productive symptoms, and a probing mental status examination aids in the identification and the characterization of neuropsychiatric syndromes. (5) Laboratory tests and neuroimaging play important roles in confirming clinical diagnoses. (6) Late-onset disorders are likely to be related to brain diseases, but neuropsychiatric disorders are not limited to the elderly. (7) Patients with neuropsychiatric illnesses usually lack the premorbid psychiatric or personality alterations that occur in many idiopathic psychiatric disorders. (8) The presence of neuromedical illness in a patient with a behavior disturbance should lead the clinician to explore potential relations between the two. (9) Patients with neuropsychiatric illness often lack the family history of psychiatric disability common in those with idiopathic psychiatric disorders. Hereditary neuropsychiatric illnesses, such as Huntington's disease, are exceptions to that rule. (10) Pharmacotherapy relies on intervention in brain processes and is applicable in both neuropsychiatric and idiopathic psychiatric disorders. (11) Neuropsychiatric syndromes are common in patients who are elderly or who have sustained brain injuries; drug dosages usually have to be adjusted downward to avoid pharmacotoxicity.

MENTAL STATUS EXAMINATION

The key to an accurate neuropsychiatric evaluation and diagnosis is a comprehensive mental status examination. Mental status testing, augmented by the clinical history, leads to a specific diagnosis or to the generation of diagnostic hypotheses. The neurological examination, selected laboratory studies, the success of treatment interventions, and repeated evaluation over time eventually complete the diagnostic process. Effective management demands accurate diagnosis. In neuropsychiatry, the diagnostic approach has added significance, since the clinician must make an accurate behavioral assessment and identify and manage the underlying brain disorder.

The elements of a comprehensive mental status examination include observation of the dress and the spontaneous demeanor of the patient, evaluation of mood and affect, and assessment of thought form (including formal thought disorder, obsessional thinking, and perseveration) and thought content (delusions, hallucinations, preoccupations). That is followed by a structured probing of intellectual function, including tests of attention, language, memory, visuospatial and constructional abilities, calculation, abstraction, judgment, and frontal-subcortical systems tasks. Interview schedules and rating scales may be used to standardize and quantify the observations. Referral to a neuropsychologist or speech pathologist may be indicated for further testing of neuropsychological and communicative abilities. Table 2.1-1 outlines the components of the mental status examination.

In neuropsychiatric assessment, behavioral phenomena are explored and cognitive functions probed as a means of investigating brain function. Although complex behavior is a product of integrated brain activity, individual brain regions or brain systems make specialized contributions to each human capacity and have hallmark syndromes when injured. Structured neuropsychiatric assessment probes the functions of the major brain regions and synthesizes the information into a comprehensive behavioral and etiologic formulation. Cortical-subcortical, right hemisphere-left hemisphere, anterior-posterior hemispheric location, and emotional-cognitive dimensions are systematically assessed.

OBSERVATIONAL ASSESSMENT Any interaction with the patient provides an opportunity for neuropsychiatric data collection. Patients with dementia, delirium, or frontal lobe syndromes may appear disheveled and unkempt; patients with schizophrenialike illnesses or secondary mania may be eccentric or flamboyant. Patients with unilateral neglect after a lateralized brain injury may ignore objects or people in one hemiuniverse and fail to dress or groom half of the body. Signs of

TABLE 2.1-1
Components of the Mental Status Evaluation

- Observational Assessment
  - Dress (disheveled, eccentric, flamboyant, unilateral neglect)
  - Demeanor (anxious, impulsive, apathetic)
  - Social interaction (suspicious, unduly familiar, distractible, excessive dependence on spouse)
  - Affect (jocular, sad, irritable, angry, labile, perplexed)
  - Speech (mutism, stutter, dysarthria, abnormal volume, disturbed speed, aprosodia)
  - Language (fluent aphasia, nonfluent aphasia, echolalia, palilalia, coprolalia)
  - Motor behavior (compulsions, absence spells, stereotypies, movement disorders, hyperactivity, gait abnormalities)
  - Psychomotor speed (slow, rapid)
- Neuropsychiatric Interview
  - Mood (happy, sad, labile, anxious)
  - Thought form
    - Thought disorder (tangential, circumstantial, loose associations, illogicality, derailment, flight of ideas)
    - Perseverations and intrusions (abnormal persistence or recurrence of ideas or words)
    - Incoherence
  - Thought content
    - Delusions
    - Hallucinations (visual, auditory, tactile, gustatory, olfactory, somatic)
    - Obsessions (involuntary intrusive ideas)
    - Depersonalization and derealization
- Mental Status Examination
  - Alertness, arousal
  - Attention (digit span, continuous performance test)
  - Memory
    - Learning (verbal, nonverbal)
    - Recall of recently learned information
    - Recognition of recently learned information
    - Recall of remotely learned information
  - Language
    - Comprehension
    - Repetition
    - Naming
    - Reading (aloud and comprehension)
    - Writing
  - Word-list generation
  - Visuospatial and constructional skills
    - Copy figures (circle, overlapping, rectangles, cube)
    - Drawing (clock, flower)
  - Calculation
    - Addition
    - Multiplication
    - Subtraction
    - Division
  - Abstraction
    - Similarities
    - Differences
    - Idioms
    - Proverbs
  - Judgment and insight
    - Understanding of personal situation
    - Planning for future
    - Social insight questions
  - Frontal-subcortical systems tasks
    - Alternating programs
    - Reciprocal programs
    - Go-no go
    - Multiple loops
    - Set shifting
    - Response inhibition
  - Miscellaneous tests
    - Praxis
    - Prosody
    - Right-left orientation
    - Finger identification
    - Singing
    - Automatic speech (reciting the days of the week, reciting the alphabet)
    - Familiar face, environment, object, voice, sound recognition

incontinence may be evident in patients with frontal lobe syndromes or dementia. The patient's spontaneous demeanor may evidence anxiety (for example, in hyperthyroidism), impulsivity (for example, in orbitofrontal syndromes), or apathy (for example, in medial frontal lobe syndromes). Social interactions are revealing: patients with delusional disorders may be suspicious and establish poor rapport, patients with orbitofrontal dysfunction may be unduly familiar with the examiner, and patients with delirium or frontal lobe disorders may be distractible. Observing patients' interactions with their spouses is critical: patients with dementia syndromes, such as Alzheimer's disease (called dementia of the Alzheimer's type in the fourth edition of *Diagnostic and Statistical Manual of Mental Disorders* [DSM-IV]), become increasingly dependent on their spouses for information and automatically turn to them for answers during the examination. Observation of the patient's affect may provide additional information. Patients with brain dysfunction may show a variety of context-incongruent affects, including jocularity, sadness, irritability, anger, affective lability, and perplexity. Each of those affective abnormalities may have diagnostic or localizing significance. Verbal output, including speech (the mechanical aspects of communication) and language (the propositional content of communication), also provides diagnostic information. Abnormalities of speech include mutism, dysarthria, increased or decreased voice volume, stuttering, abnormal rate of speech, and disturbed speech prosody (loss of melody or inflection). Language disturbances in neuropsychiatric syndromes include aphasia (fluent or nonfluent), echolalia (echoing what the examiner says), and palilalia (repeating what the patient says). Patients with Tourette's disorder have involuntary vocalizations ranging from subtle sighs, sniffs, grunts, and barks to shouting and coprolalia (swearing). A wide variety of diagnostically important motor behaviors may be evident during the examination, including movement disorders (tremor, chorea, parkinsonism, tics, myoclonus, tremor, gait abnormalities), compulsions, stereotypies, hyperactivity, and absence spells. Alterations of the patient's posture may also be diagnostically meaningful. Patients with Parkinson's disease have a flexed posture, whereas patients with progressive supranuclear palsy have an extended posture. The clinician should note the patient's psychomotor speed. Response latencies may be prolonged, or the patient may impulsively interrupt the examiner, anticipating the question. Speech and movement may be slowed or executed with abnormal rapidity. Slowing of central processing is typical of subcortical neurological disorders, medial frontal syndromes, and depressive disorders. Patients with secondary mania or disinhibited orbitofrontal syndromes may have accelerated speech and increased motor activity.

NEUROPSYCHIATRIC INTERVIEW The neuropsychiatric interview includes evaluation of the patient's mood and affect and of thought form and thought content. Observations relevant to personality function and alterations may also be made. The interview is conducted in the same way as a conventional psychiatric assessment, but a wider variety of phenomena may be observed, and the expression of abnormalities may be modified by concomitant delirium, dementia, aphasia, or amnesia.

Disturbances of mood *Mood* is an internally experienced pervasive emotion; *affect* is the outward emotional display.

Mood disturbances are common in the course of neurological disease. Depression is the most frequent mood disturbance, occurring in patients with cerebrovascular disorders, Parkinson's disease and other movement disorders, epilepsy, and multiple sclerosis. Sadness and feelings of hopelessness, helplessness, worthlessness, and guilt should be assessed. The overall range of mood and affect may be reduced. Suicidal ideation may range from passive wishes for death to directed suicidal activities. Among neuropsychiatric illnesses, Huntington's disease and epilepsy have substantially increased suicide rates. Loss of interest in work, hobbies, or recreational activities may be marked; patients may acknowledge their fatigue and loss of energy. Associated disorders include insomnia (difficulty in falling asleep, frequent nocturnal awakenings, early morning awakening), alterations in appetite, loss of libido, and motor behavior changes (agitation, slowed movement and speech, reduced voice volume). Tearfulness and sobbing are typical changes of affect.

Euphoria, hypomania, and mania may also occur in neuropsychiatric disorders. Euphoria is most common in frontal lobe dysfunction (trauma, frontal lobe tumors, frontal lobe degenerative diseases, frontal infections) and in secondary mania. The patients may exhibit an elevated mood, undue optimism, inflated self-esteem, grandiosity, exaggerated confidence, and motoric hyperactivity. Distractibility, flight of ideas, racing thoughts, and pressured speech may be evident. Insomnia, increased appetite, and exaggerated libido may also occur.

Anxiety occurs in a variety of neuropsychiatric conditions, including metabolic encephalopathies (for example, hyperthyroidism, anoxia), toxic disorders (for example, lidocaine toxicity), and degenerative disorders (for example, Alzheimer's disease, Parkinson's disease). The patient exhibits excessive worry and apprehension, undue pessimism, and feelings of impending death or disaster. Somatic symptoms—including palpitations, tachycardia, shortness of breath, light-headedness, fleeting pains, dry mouth, nausea, diarrhea, and perspiration—are often prominent. The patient may appear tense, with furrowed brow and worried expression; tremor, tachypnea, pupillary dilation, and restless fidgeting may be observed.

Mood lability is a disorder of mood regulation observed in neuropsychiatric syndromes. Patients may shift rapidly from sadness to jocularity. Typically, patients with marked lability are irritable and vacillate from anger to apathy to euphoria. The emotional outbursts are usually short-lived. Lability is common in patients with frontal lobe dysfunction or mental retardation. In the mood lability syndromes, mood and affect are congruent (the patient feels and appears angry, sad). Lability is to be distinguished from the affective instability of pseudobulbar palsy, in which mood and affect are incongruent.

Mood and affect may be dissociated in neuropsychiatric disorders. *Pseudobulbar palsy* is a disorder of affect in which the patient's emotional expression is a gross exaggeration of the associated mood or is completely at variance with it. The patients may weep in minimally sad situations or when no appropriate stimulus is present. Alternatively, the patient may laugh when sad or when no humorous event has occurred. The abnormal pseudobulbar affect is accompanied by other evidence of loss of supranuclear control of bulbar functions, including dysarthria, dysphagia, increased gag response, increased jaw jerk and facial muscle stretch reflexes, and facial weakness with hypomimia. Congruence between mood and affect should be explored in patients with neuropsychiatric illness, and the associated signs of pseudobulbar palsy must be sought during the neurological examination. In most cases, patients with pseudobulbar palsy have bilateral lesions of the descending corticobulbar tracts. Common causes are cerebrovascular disease, multiple sclerosis, amyotrophic lateral sclerosis, traumatic brain injury, and brainstem or skull base tumors.

Disorders of thought form Formal thought disorders are less common than are delusions as a manifestation of psychosis in neuropsychiatric diseases, but classic thought disorders have been observed in the schizophreniclike illnesses accompanying epilepsy, Huntington's disease, and idiopathic basal ganglia calcification. Tangentiality, circumstantiality, loose associations, illogicality, derailment, and thought blocking may be observed. Flight of ideas occurs in secondary mania; circumstantiality is evident in some patients with temporal lobe epilepsy or alcohol-related dementia.

Perseveration, intrusions, and incoherence are disorders of the form of thought unique to neuropsychiatric conditions. *Perseveration* is the inappropriate continuation of an act or a thought after its proper context has passed. *Intrusions* are late recurrences of words or thoughts from an early context. Perseverations and intrusions are seen in aphasias, frontal lobe syndromes, and dementing illnesses. Incoherence occurs when words have no logical association. Incoherence occurs in extreme cases of psychosis but is most common in delirium and cortical dementias, such as Alzheimer's disease.

Disorders of thought content A plethora of disorders of thought content may be observed in neuropsychiatric diseases. Delusions are the principal manifestations of psychosis in neurological disorders. A *delusion* is a false belief based on incorrect inferences about external reality and firmly held in spite of evidence to the contrary. The most common types of delusions are persecutory beliefs involving the conviction of personal endangerment, theft of personal property, and entry by unwelcome strangers into one's home. Content-specific delusions, such as Capgras's syndrome, may also be observed in neurological illnesses, and the type of delusion is not helpful in distinguishing schizophrenia or other idiopathic psychotic illnesses from the delusions of neurological disease. Table 2.1-2 lists and defines the content-specific delusions that have been reported in neuromedical disorders with delusions.

TABLE 2.1-2
Content-Specific Delusions in Neuropsychiatric Disorders

Delusion	Content
Capgras	A significant other (usually a family member) has been replaced by identical-appearing imposter.
Fregoli's	A persecutor is able to assume the appearance of others.
Intermetamorphosis	Persons in the environment take on the appearance of tormentors.
Othello	The patient's spouse is unfaithful.
Parasitosis	The patient is infested with insects, worms, lice, vermin.
Lycanthropy (werewolfism)	The patient periodically turns into an animal.
Heutoscopy (the double, Doppelganger)	The patient has a twin or second self.
de Clérambault (erotomania)	The patient is secretly loved by another, usually someone of higher social or economic status.
Incubus	The patient has a demon or phantom lover.
Phantom boarder	Unwelcome guests are living in the patient's home.
Dorian Gray	Others are aging, but the patient appears to remain the same age.

Schneiderian first-rank symptoms are delusional experiences that include hearing one's thoughts spoken aloud, hearing voices arguing about oneself, hearing voices commenting on one's actions, having bodily sensations imposed from outside, attributing one's feelings to external sources, experiencing one's drive and actions as controlled from outside, having one's thoughts inserted or withdrawn from the mind, broadcasting one's thoughts, and attributing special delusional significance to one's perceptions. Although most common in schizophrenia, first-rank symptoms have been recorded in a number of neurological illnesses with schizophrenialike manifestations, including epilepsy, Huntington's disease, and idiopathic basal ganglia calcification.

Hallucinations are common manifestations of neuropsychiatric illness. *Hallucinations* are sensory perceptions occurring without appropriate external stimulation of the relevant sensory organ. Hallucinations and delusions may occur together as elements of a psychotic process, or hallucinations may be recognized by the nondelusional patient as unreal. Hallucinations by themselves are neither necessary nor sufficient evidence of psychosis. Hallucinations may occur in any sensory modality, including visual, auditory, tactile (formication), gustatory, and olfactory. Somatic hallucinations are sensory experiences involving the patient's body and internal organs. Hallucinations may be formed, well-defined, and recognizable sensations (for example, visual hallucinations of people or animals; auditory hallucinations of voices) or unformed elementary sensations (visual hallucinations of flashing lights or colors; auditory hallucinations of unrecognizable noises).

Obsessions are another type of anomalous thought content. In *obsessions* the patient experiences recurrent, intrusive thoughts, images, or impulses that are ego-dystonic and involuntary. The obsessional thoughts typically involve violent, sexual, or visceral-eliminative themes. Patients with obsessions frequently also have *compulsions*—repetitive stereotyped behaviors that are recognized as senseless but cannot be resisted. Washing and checking compulsions are the most common, although nearly any action can be ritualized and become the object of compulsive repetition.

Depersonalization and derealization are also examples of altered thought content. They refer to dissociative experiences; the patient may feel as if in a dream. *Depersonalization* is a state of altered experience in which the feeling of one's own reality is temporarily lost. There may be a loss of ability to experience emotion and disturbed perception of time. *Derealization* usually refers to the sense of unreality about one's surroundings. Neuropsychiatric disorders to be considered in the differential diagnosis of depersonalization include epilepsy, migraine, encephalitis, and systemic metabolic disorders.

MENTAL STATUS EXAMINATION Systematic probing of the patient's mental state is a crucial part of neuropsychiatric assessment. Diagnostic hypotheses generated while taking the history and conducting the neuropsychiatric interview are further refined by mental status testing. The examination should be conducted methodically and should comprehensively assess the major domains of neuropsychological function (Table 2.1-1). When possible, the examination should be quantified to facilitate comparisons among patients and documentation of changes in the patient's function over time. The patient's age, handedness, educational level, and sociocultural background may all influence the mental status examination and should be determined before initiating the evaluation. The Mini-Mental State questionnaire is a useful scale to grade cognition (see Table 9.8-11 in Section 9.8, Psychiatric Rating Scales).

Alertness and attention The patient's level of arousal and attention are evaluated by observation and testing. Levels of hypoarousal vary from drowsiness to obtundation, stupor, and coma. The *drowsy* patient is fatigued and falls asleep when unstimulated. *Obtundation* is a state of moderately reduced alertness, with slow responses and diminished interest in the environment. *Stupor* is the next most severe level of impaired consciousness. Stuporous patients must be vigorously stimulated to be aroused and engaged in questioning. Stupor returns when stimulation ceases. *Coma* is a state of unarousable unresponsiveness. Comatose patients have no psychological response to external stimulation or internal needs. Impaired arousal occurs in toxic-metabolic encephalopathies, increased intracranial pressure, severe cerebrovascular disorders, encephalitis, and traumatic brain injury. *Hyperarousal* with anxiety, autonomic hyperactivity (tachycardia, tachypnea, hyperthermia), and exaggerated startle responses may occur in metabolic disorders, particularly during withdrawal from alcohol, opiates, or sedative-hypnotic agents.

Stupor must be distinguished from akinetic mutism, locked-in syndrome, and catatonic unresponsiveness. *Akinetic mutism* is a state of silent, alert-appearing immobility. The patient's eyes are open and may follow environmental events; the patient has regular sleep-wake cycles. The patient may be completely inert or may have occasional brief movements or postural adjustments spontaneously or in response to vigorous stimulation. The disorder has occurred with large frontal lobe injuries, bilateral cingulate gyrus damage, and midbrain pathology. *Locked-in syndrome* occurs with bilateral pontine lesions that render the patient mute and paralyzed. Intellectual function, however, is not impaired, and the patient can communicate by eye movements or eye blinks (for example, blinking once for "yes" and twice for "no"). In *catatonic stupor* the patient is mute and motionless. A psychological pillow and waxy flexibility may be elicited. Brief impulsive acts may punctuate the catatonic period. Catatonia occurs in a wide variety of neurological, toxic-metabolic, and psychiatric disorders, including frontal lobe syndromes, hypoglycemia, schizophrenia, and depression.

Attention is impaired in disorders of arousal but may also be abnormal in patients who are fully alert. Delirium and acute confusional states are characterized by abnormal attention in alert patients. Two types of tests are particularly useful in detecting compromised attention: digit-span forward and continuous performance tests. The *digit-span test* is conducted by asking the patient to repeat increasingly long series of numbers said aloud by the examiner. The numbers are given at a rate of one a second in a monotone voice. A normal forward digit span is seven digits long; fewer than five digits is abnormal and indicates impaired attention. Sustained attention is evaluated by a *continuous performance test,* such as the "A" test, in which the clinician says a series of random letters at a rate of one a second. The patient is asked to signal each time the letter "A" occurs. The test continues for one minute and assesses the patient's ability to sustain concentration over time. Distractible patients make errors of omission, failing to detect one or more of the "As." Persons with normal attention perform the test perfectly. Acute confusional states and impaired attention are usually indicative of a toxic or metabolic disorder but also occur in cases of increased intracranial pressure, frontal lobe disorders, and focal lesions of the posterior right hemisphere.

Mental control tests are tasks that require intact attention but also depend on other intellectual resources. Serial subtractions, spelling words backward, reverse digit span, and reciting the days of the week or the months of the year in reverse order are examples of tests used to investigate mental control. Both the accuracy and the speed of performance are observed. Attention, language, frontal lobe functions, and calculation skills contribute to mental control abilities.

Impaired attention conditions all aspects of behavior and intellectual function. Patients who are drowsy or in acute confusional states perform badly on comprehension, repetition, drawing, and calculation tests because of their inability to sustain attention. In general, conclusions regarding a potential underlying dementia or memory disturbance cannot be drawn while the patient is in a confusional episode. Management efforts are directed to controlling the associated disorder and restoring attention; reexamination then reveals the baseline mental condition.

Memory Aspects of memory to be assessed in the course of a mental status examination include learning, recall of recently learned information, recognition, and recall of remotely learned information. Learning, recall, and recognition can be assessed in both verbal and nonverbal domains.

Inquiring about personal orientation is one means of assessing recent memory. Temporal and spatial orientation must be continuously updated, and patients with memory abnormalities may fail to learn the current day, date, or place. Orientation to self is rarely lost and has little value as a memory test.

Word-list memory tests are a common means of assessing learning, recall, and recognition. The patient is given three words to remember and then is asked to recall them three minutes later. The examiner notes how much difficulty the patient has in learning the three words initially and how many times the words must be presented before the patient can repeat all three. A few minutes later the patient is asked to remember the three words. If the patient can do so, the performance is normal. If the patient cannot remember the words, the patient is given clues (for example, the category of items to which a word belongs or a list of words containing the target and several foils) to distinguish between storage and recall deficits. Patients with encoding or storage deficits (for example, amnesia) are not aided by prompting and clues; patients with intact storage but impaired recall (for example, patients with frontal-subcortical circuit disturbances) are aided by the maneuvers. Memory performance patterns are often more readily discerned by using a 10-word list than by using a 3-word list.

Nonverbal memory can also be tested to distinguish between encoding and access impairments. The patient is asked to copy several figures (usually as part of the constructional task described below); a few minutes later the patient is asked to reproduce the drawings from memory; if the patient cannot spontaneously remember the drawings, a group of figures containing the targets and several foils is presented. Patients who cannot recognize the original drawings have a nonverbal encoding disturbance as part of an amnestic syndrome; patients who cannot recall the drawings but are able to recognize them within a group of stimuli and foils have a nonverbal memory retrieval abnormality resulting from a frontal-subcortical circuit disorder.

Remote-memory testing evaluates the patient's ability to remember events and persons of the remote past. Information is gathered on that aspect of memory while taking a history of the patient's illness by inquiring about the patient's significant life events (dates of marriage, birth dates of children) and by asking about political leaders and important historical events. Remote information is not stored in specific focal brain areas, and recall failures do not provide localizing information. The temporal profile of remote memory may be diagnostically revealing. Amnestic syndromes are characterized by a period of anterograde amnesia after the onset of the disorder (that period may continue indefinitely if the patient fails to recover or may be time-limited if memory function returns), a period of retrograde amnesia extending backward in time for a few seconds to a few years from the time of the onset of the amnesia, and intact remote recall for material beyond the period of the retrograde amnesia.

Language Language assessment includes observing the patient's spontaneous speech and testing language comprehension, repetition, naming, reading, and writing. Language-related abilities that may be evaluated include speech prosody, automatic speech, singing, and right-left orientation. Abnormalities of language are usually observed in the course of taking the history and conducting the neuropsychiatric interview, and patients with those abnormalities require the most detailed testing. When the verbal exchange has been unremarkable, testing a few difficult items in the major linguistic categories is adequate to establish normal language function.

Spontaneous speech reveals abnormalities of thought and language, and the two types of abnormalities must be carefully distinguished. Disorders of thought form and content have been discussed above. *Aphasia* is any disturbance of the linguistic aspects of verbal communication. Aphasic disturbances of spontaneous verbalization are characterized as fluent or nonfluent. *Fluent aphasias* feature normal or excessive amounts of speech, normal phrase length with complex sentence structures, preserved speech melody, no dysarthria, a paucity of information content with excessive dependence on words of indefinite reference (such as "thing" and "it"), and paraphasic errors. *Paraphasias* may involve the substitution of one phoneme for another (for example, "nook" for "book") in phonemic paraphasias, the replacement of one word with another in verbal or semantic paraphasias, or the construction of new words in neologistic paraphasias. *Nonfluent aphasias* exhibit essentially the opposite features of fluent aphasias. The patient has reduced verbal output, shortened phrase lengths or one-word replies, agrammatism with a tendency to omit the syntactic functor words (for example, "and," "but," "the"), increased articulatory effort and impaired speech initiation, reduced speech melody, and dysarthria. The patient has few or no paraphasias, and information content is relatively normal. Abnormalities of language must be distinguished from disorders of speech (dysarthria), abnormalities of inflection and melody (aprosodia), and absence of linguistic output (mutism).

Language *comprehension* is tested by asking the patient to follow verbal commands, respond to yes-or-no questions, or decipher complex linguistic constructions. The easiest commands are one-step orders involving whole-body functions, such as "Stand up" and "Turn around." Next in order of difficulty are single-step commands involving midline body parts, such as "Open your mouth," "Close your eyes," and "Stick out your tongue." Pointing to room objects and body parts assesses the next level of comprehension. Patients are asked to point to one, two, or three objects visible in the examination room (for example, "Point to the ceiling, then to the floor, then to the desk") or to one, two, or three body parts (for example, "Point to your nose, then to your shoulder, then to your knee"). Pointing to objects in an array of items laid in front of the patient is more difficult for most patients than is sequential pointing to room objects or body parts. A vertical array—such as a comb, a pen, a coin, and keys—is provided, and the patient is asked to point to several of the items in turn (for example, "Point to the keys, then to the comb, then to the pen"). Each time the test is repeated, the item order is changed. Pointing tasks may also be made more difficult by asking the patient to point to an item that is described, rather than named (for example, "Point to the entrance to the room'' or ''Point to the source of illumination''). Pointing is impossible for some patients because of paralysis or apraxia, and yes-or-no questions may be used to minimize the motor demands of the task. The questions may range from easy (for example, ''Are the lights on in this room?'') to modestly difficult (for example, ''Do you put your shoes on before your socks?''). Complex questions—such as, ''Is my wife's brother a man or a woman?'' and ''If a lion is killed by a tiger, which animal is dead?''—allow the examiner to determine if the patient can follow complex linguistic formulations. Impaired comprehension usually implies dysfunction of posterior structures of the left hemisphere. Comprehension is abnormal in many aphasic syndromes, dementia, and delirium.

Repetition is assessed by asking the patient to repeat increasingly long phrases or sentences, beginning with a single word and progressing to sentences 8 to 10 words in length (for example, ''The quick brown fox jumped over the lazy dog''). Abnormalities include omissions and paraphasic substitutions. The repetition span is typically one or two words longer than the digit span, and patients with shortened digit spans are able to repeat only brief phrases. Conversely, the digit span is a repetition test, and patients with repetition disturbances, such as several of the aphasias, have abnormal digit spans.

Assessment of *naming* involves asking the patient to name objects and parts of objects, body parts, pictures or drawings of objects, and colors. Naming is compromised systematically with the impairment of rarely used low-frequency words before commonly used high-frequency words. A thorough language examination must include the naming of both low-frequency and high-frequency words. As a rule of thumb, objects are of higher frequency than the parts of the objects (for example, ''wristwatch'' is a more common word than ''watchband'' or ''crystal,'' and ''glasses'' is a higher-frequency word than ''lens'' or ''bow''). Error types include the failure to respond, the production of paraphasic errors, and circumlocutory responses, in which the patient describes the object or its use but does not name it. Anomia occurs in aphasias, dementias, and deliria. Adequate vision must be assured before errors are ascribed to naming deficits.

Evaluation of *reading* entails the assessment of the patient's ability to read aloud and to comprehend what is read. Those two aspects of reading may be impaired independently. The most elementary assessment of reading involves asking the patient to read aloud and to point to an object whose name has been written (for example, ''nose'' or ''door''). Comprehension of complex written material is evaluated by asking the patient to read and to follow written commands (for example, ''Raise your right hand'') or to read and to fill in the blanks in incomplete written sentences (for example, ''A man who repairs cars and trucks is known as a ______________''). Again, adequate vision must be demonstrated before failures are ascribed to an alexia. Abnormalities of spontaneous speech are usually recapitulated in reading aloud, and deficits in reading comprehension typically co-occur with disturbances of comprehension of spoken language. In some cases, *alexia* (the inability to understand the meaning of written words) and *agraphia* (the loss of the ability to produce written language) may occur in patients without aphasic disturbances.

Writing may be disturbed on a mechanical basis or an aphasic basis. Mechanical agraphias occur in patients with limb paresis, limb apraxia, or movement disorders, such as tremor and chorea. Micrographia is a characteristic aspect of parkinsonism in which the patient's script becomes progressively smaller as the patient writes a sentence or extended series of numbers or letters. Aphasic agraphias accompany aphasic syndromes, and the same types of errors noted in verbal output are reproduced in written form. For example, patients with Broca's aphasia have impoverished agrammatic output, whereas patients with Wernicke's aphasia have fluent paraphasic writing. Agraphia occurs without aphasia in Gerstmann syndrome (agraphia, acalculia, right-left disorientation, finger agnosia), alexia with agraphia, and disconnection agraphia (left-handed agraphia in patients with an injury to the corpus callosum). Agraphia also occurs in dementia and is a sensitive index of the attentional deficit in delirium. *Acalculia* is the inability to perform simple arithmetic problems. *Agnosia* is the inability to recognize sensory stimuli that are adequately perceived.

Word-list generation Word-list generation tasks involve asking the patient to think of as many members of a specific category or as many words beginning with a specific letter as possible in one minute. Typically, the patient is asked to produce as many animal names as possible in one minute or is asked to think of as many words beginning with the letter ''F'' as possible in one minute (excluding numbers; proper names, like France and Frank; and repetitions of words with the same core, such as ''fix,'' ''fixed,'' ''fixing,'' and ''fixation''). Normal persons produce between 12 and 24 animal names in one minute (the mean is 18; fewer than 12 is abnormal) and between 10 and 20 words beginning with the letter ''F'' (the mean is 15; fewer than 10 is abnormal). Word-list generation is sensitive to word-finding disturbances, lexical search abnormalities associated with frontal-subcortical circuit dysfunction, and psychomotor retardation.

Visuospatial skills The visuospatial abilities include spatial attention, perception, construction, visuospatial problem solving, and visuospatial memory. Construction tasks are the most widely used screening tests of visuospatial ability. Clock drawing and copying figures of increasing complexity are useful assessment techniques. In the clock-drawing test, the patient is asked to draw a clock and to fill in the clock numbers; when that task is complete, the patient is asked to draw in the clock hands to indicate that the time is 10 minutes after 11 o'clock. Patients with poor planning skills draw a clock face that is too small to conveniently contain the required numbers or space the numbers inappropriately. Patients with unilateral neglect ignore half of the clock face. Patients with frontal-lobe disorders may have stimulus-boundedness and place one hand on the 10 and one on the 11 when attempting to set the clock for 10 minutes after 11:00.

Tests of copying begin by having the patient reproduce a relatively simple figure, such as a circle; then the patient is asked to copy two or three more challenging figures (for example, intersecting circle and triangle, overlapping pentagons, cube). Abnormalities include distortions of size, the failure to reproduce the shapes accurately, the absence of perspective, perseveration on individual elements, drawing over the stimulus figure, and unilateral neglect. Hemineglect is a valid indicator of contralateral brain injury, but other types of construction abnormalities do not have precise localizing value. An injury to the posterior aspect of the right hemisphere produces the most severe and the most enduring visuospatial deficits, but dysfunction of frontal, occipital, or parietal lobes of either hemisphere (cortical or subcortical) can adversely affect drawing abilities. Preliminary evidence suggests that the two hemispheres have complementary roles in construction abilities; the right hemisphere mediates the external configuration, and the left hemisphere mediates the internal details. Drawing disturbances are common with focal brain damage, degenerative disorders, and toxic and metabolic encephalopathies. The term ''drawing apraxia'' is avoided here; apraxia is applied to disorders characterized by an inability to do on command tasks that can be performed spontaneously. By that definition, drawing disturbances are not apraxias.

Calculation Calculation skills tested on the mental status examination include addition, multiplication, subtraction, and division. High-order mathematical skills are not assessed except in specific circumstances in which the patient's premorbid mathematical abilities are well documented. Patients are asked to perform one-digit and two-digit tasks (for example, $16 + 32$, 15×3) mentally or to address demanding problems with the aid of pencil and paper. Calculation abilities are determined by the patient's education and occupational history. Acalculias occur in aphasic syndromes in which aphasic substitutions of one digit for another lead to inaccurate answers, visuospatial disorders leading to the incorrect alignment of columns of numbers, and primary anarithmias in which basic mathematical processes are disrupted. Anarithmias occur after damage to the posterior aspect of the left hemisphere.

Abstraction Abstraction skills refer to the patient's ability to derive a general principle from a specific example. Similarities, differences, idioms, and proverbs are used to assess abstracting capacity. *Similarities* require the patient to identify the class or the category to which two items belong (for example, rose and tulip, bicycle and train, watch and ruler). *Differences* require the patient to identify the salient distinguishing feature between two similar items (for example, child and midget, lie and mistake). *Idioms* are metaphorical statements or aphorisms that require the patient to generalize to a larger meaning (for example, ''seeing eye to eye,'' ''levelheaded,'' and ''eyes peeled''). *Proverbs* are usually double metaphors that require the patient to ignore the immediate meaning and to derive a lesson or a maxim (for example, ''Don't cry over spilled milk,'' ''People who live in glass houses shouldn't throw stones,'' ''The tongue is the enemy of the neck''). A concrete response to the proverb ''People who live in glass houses shouldn't throw stones'' is, ''The glass will break.'' Success on abstraction tasks depends on the patient's level of education. In addition, the tests are not culture-fair, and proverbs from the patient's own culture must be used to make a valid assessment of abstraction abilities. Abstraction is sensitive to many types of brain dysfunction, and task failure is a nonspecific indicator of cerebral dysfunction.

Judgment and insight Assessing judgment is an important aspect of mental status testing. The assessment should be done so as to yield ecologically valid results that meaningfully relate to the patient's everyday decisions. Questions regarding patients' insight into their own conditions, their plans for the future, and their understanding of their own limitations best show their insight and judgment. Questions such as, ''What would you do if you were walking beside a lake and saw a 2-year-old child playing alone at the end of a pier?'' help explore the patient's interpersonal and social judgment. Judgment is impaired in many neurological conditions. Orbitofrontal damage produces particularly marked alterations in social judgment.

Frontal-subcortical systems tasks Frontal-subcortical systems tasks assess the integrity of a complex circuit involving the frontal cortex, the caudate nuclei, the globus pallidus, the thalamic nuclei, and the connecting white matter tracts. Frontal-subcortical functions are among the most difficult to examine either with bedside techniques or with formal neuropsychological measures. Some areas of the frontal lobe, such as the orbitofrontal cortex, produce few identifiable cognitive changes when injured but have major behavioral ramifications, with obvious disinhibition and impulsiveness. The principal abnormalities observed in patients with frontal-subcortical systems dysfunction include perseveration, motor programming deficits, apathy, poor word-list generation, impaired set maintenance, abnormal recall with preserved recognition memory, stimulus-boundedness, concrete interpretation of proverbs, imitation of the examiner's actions (imitation behavior), and impulsive responses to environmental events (utilization behavior).

Motor programming tasks sensitive to injury to the convexities of the frontal lobe and the related subcortical structures include alternating programs (Figure 2.1-1) (for example, alternating shapes or ''m''s and ''n''s are copied from a sample provided by the examiner and then extended across a page of paper), reciprocal programs (for example, the patient holds the right hand in a fist close to the face and extends the left hand, making a ring with the thumb and the first finger; then the positions are repeatedly reversed), and the go-no go test (for example, when the examiner taps under the table once, the patient taps twice; when the examiner taps twice, the patient makes no response). Another task, copying multiple-loop figures, often elicits perseveration (Figure 2.1-2). The execution of serial hand sequences is also frequently disrupted in patients with frontal-subcortical systems abnormalities. In that task, the examiner demonstrates a sequence of three hand positions (for example, fist, slap, side of hand) and asks the patient to learn and to perform the sequence. If the patient fails, the examiner asks the patient to say aloud, ''Fist, slap, side.'' If the patient cannot use verbalization to guide the hand sequence, frontal-subcortical circuit dysfunction is implicated.

Difficulty in maintaining a mental set and limitations in appropriately changing between tasks are also typical of patients with frontal-subcortical systems dysfunction. Tests to elicit those deficits include trail-making tests (for example, asking the patient to sequentially alternate between numbers and letters: 1A, 2B, 3C) and card-sorting tests (for example, the Wisconsin Card Sorting Test), in which the patient sorts cards according to a criterion—such as color, shape, or number—that

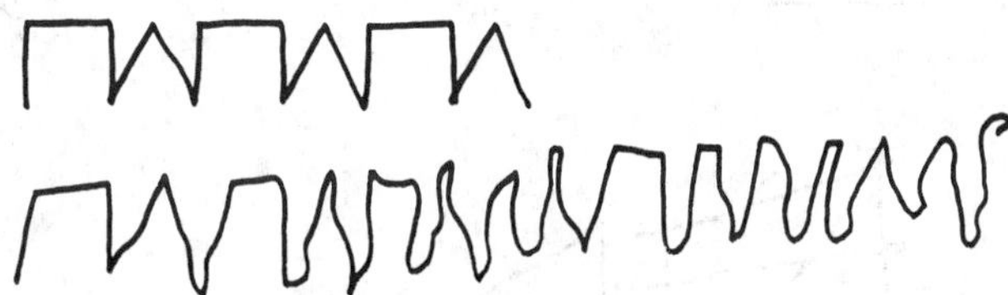

FIGURE 2.1-1 *Alternating programs. The examiner's model is above, the patient's attempt to duplicate the pattern is below. Failure to alternate between the two shapes is evident.*

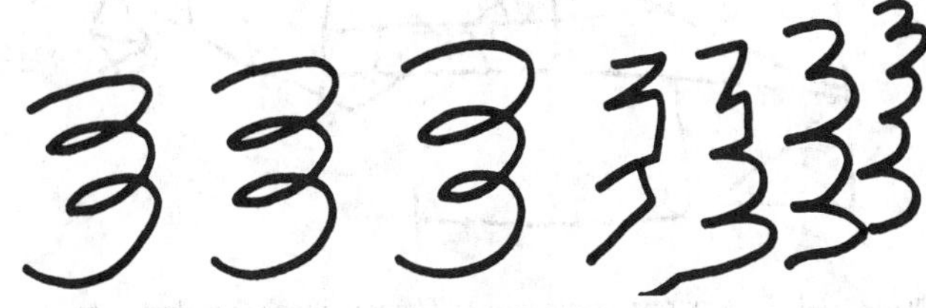

FIGURE 2.1-2 *Multiple loops. The three figures on the left were drawn by the examiner. When the patient attempted to copy the figures (right), perseveration, with the production of additional loops, was shown.*

the patient must discover and apply and that changes during the course of the testing.

Environmental dependence and poor response inhibition can be shown in patients by creating situations with competing demands. One such test, the Stroop Test, involves writing the name of a color in a different color (for example, writing the word ''blue'' in the color red) and asking the patient to ignore the color name and to read the color of the writing. Patients with frontal-subcortical systems deficits often cannot inhibit the tendency to read the word, rather than state the color.

In addition, poor abstracting abilities, stimulus-boundedness on clock-drawing tests, poor word-list generation, and adopting poor strategies when drawing complex figures (Figure 2.1-3) aid the examiner in concluding that a frontal-subcortical systems disturbance is present. Those deficits are common in patients with head trauma, frontal-lobe degenerations, frontal-lobe neoplasms, chronic multiple sclerosis, Huntington's disease, and other basal ganglia disorders, multiple subcortical infarctions, and some brain infections, such as syphilis.

Miscellaneous tests A variety of miscellaneous tests not necessarily performed with every examination may aid diagnosis or localization in specific circumstances. Testing of praxis, prosody, right-left orientation, finger identification, singing, automatic speech, and visual recognition are among those specialized tasks. *Ideomotor apraxias* are abnormalities of learned motor behavior that occur in the absence of motor, sensory, or comprehension deficits; they involve motor tasks that the patient can perform spontaneously but cannot execute on command. Apraxias of limbs and buccofacial structures may be detected.

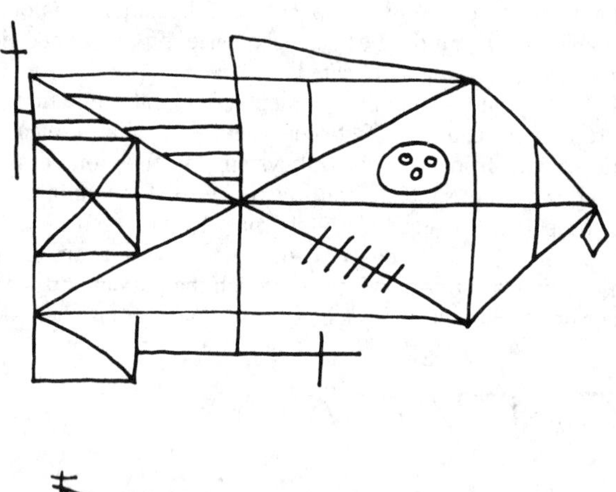

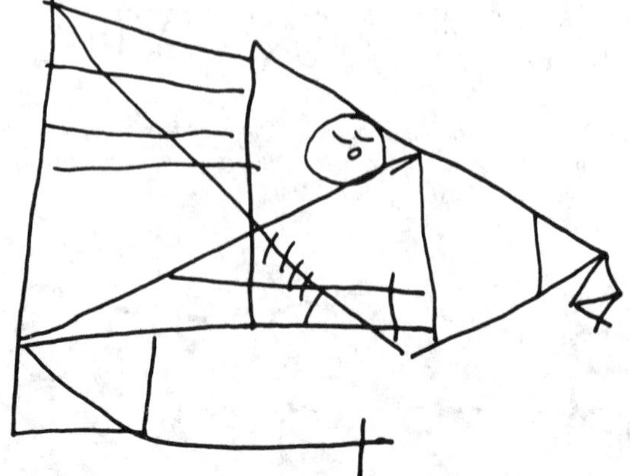

FIGURE 2.1-3 *Rey-Osterreith figure. The top figure was drawn by the examiner; the figure below is an attempt to copy the model by a patient with frontal lobe dysfunction.*

Limb commands include telling the patient to perform an action that ordinarily requires no object (for example, thumb a ride, wave good-bye) and to pantomime the use of an object (for example, throw a ball, hammer a nail). Typical oral-lingual commands include telling the patient to pretend to blow out the flame of a burning match, cough, lick the lips, and pretend to sniff a flower. Failures may involve substituting a limb for the imaginary object (for example, using a hand for the hammer, instead of pretending to hold the hammer) and, in severe cases, simply failing to perform the act adequately. Ideomotor apraxias of the type described here occur with lesions of the left hemisphere or the corpus callosum.

Aprosodies are disorders of speech melody and inflection. They assume particular importance in neuropsychiatry because prosody is the means by which emotion is communicated, and any disruption of that mechanism impairs patients' abilities to relay their emotional states. Executive aspects of prosody are tested by having the patient inflect a neutral sentence (for example, ''I'm going to the store'') to provide a variety of different meanings, such as anger, happiness, and surprise. Prosodic comprehension is assessed by having the patient guess the emotion when the examiner differentially inflects the same or a similar neutral test phrase. Executive prosody is disrupted by lesions of the right premotor cortex or the basal ganglia; receptive prosody is impaired by lesions of the posterior superior right temporal lobe (the equivalent of Wernicke's area in the right hemisphere).

Disturbances of right-left orientation and finger identification occur in conjunction with agraphia and acalculia as part of Gerstmann syndrome. *Right-left orientation* is assessed by asking the patients to point to their own body parts, using various combinations of right and left (for example, ''Point to your right shoulder''; ''With your right hand, touch your left knee''). If they perform those tasks accurately, they are asked to point to specific parts of the examiner, who is seated facing the patient. The patient is thus required to perform a mental reversal to correctly respond to the commands (for example, ''Point to my right hand''; ''Point to my left shoulder''). The examiner may make the task more difficult by crossing his or her own hands and asking the patient to touch the examiner's right or left hand, thus requiring another reversal by the patient. *Finger identification* is also tested with a hierarchy of increasingly complex tests. At the most elementary level, the patients are asked to name each finger (for example, thumb, forefinger, middle finger, ring finger, pinkie or little finger). If the patients are able to perform that task, they are asked to point to the equivalent finger of one hand while the examiner touches a finger of the other hand held out of sight above the patient's head. Another taxing test of finger identification involves having patients close their eyes and then state how many fingers are between the fingers of one hand touched by the examiner (for example, if the examiner touches the thumb and the pinkie, three fingers are between them). Gerstmann syndrome occurs with lesions of the left angular gyrus. All four components—agraphia right-left disassociation, finger agnosia, acalculia—must be present for the syndrome to have localizing significance.

Singing and automatic speech may be useful adjuncts in language assessment, particularly in a patient with limited verbal output. In some cases, patients who are mute and incapable of propositional speech are nevertheless able to sing. That occurs in extrapyramidal syndromes, such as advanced Parkinson's disease, and in patients with nonfluent aphasias. *Automatic speech* is the recitation of overlearned sequences, such as the days of the week, the months of the year, the alphabet, and memorized poems and prayers. Automatic speech, like singing, may be preserved when little other verbal output can be demonstrated. Preserved automatic speech, despite severely impaired spontaneous verbal output, is characteristic of isolation aphasia (also known as mixed transcortical aphasia) and may also occur in patients with mental retardation syndromes and advanced dementias.

Visual recognition skills may be compromised by specific lesions of the nervous system. Visual perception is intact, and naming skills are normal, but the patient cannot recognize a familiar object, place, or person. When complaints warrant, the recognition of objects, places, and faces should be tested. *Visual object agnosia* occurs with bilateral lesions of the inferior longitudinal fasciculi or the adjacent cortex of the medial occipitotemporal regions. Patients can see the objects, they have intact language skills, and they can accurately identify the objects by palpation, but they cannot identify the objects by visual means. *Prosopagnosia* is impaired recognition of familiar faces. The patient can tell that the faces are not identical but cannot recognize familiar persons, such as friends, family members, and celebrities. The patient's auditory recognition skills are intact, and the patient can distinguish among persons when they speak. Prosopagnosia can occur with lesions limited to the right posterior hemisphere, but many patients have bilateral posterior hemispheric injuries. *Environmental agnosia*—the inability to recognize familiar places, such as the patient's own home—may accompany prosopagnosia. *Phonagnosia* is the inability to recognize familiar voices, and *auditory agnosia* involves the loss of recognition of all sounds. Cerebrovascular disease is the most common cause of all types of agnosia.

NEUROLOGICAL EXAMINATION

The neurological examination consists of the assessment of the cranial nerves, the motor systems, the sensory abilities, the muscle stretch reflexes, and the primitive reflexes.

CRANIAL NERVE EXAMINATION The function of the *first cranial nerve (olfactory)* is tested by asking the patient to identify a variety of distinctive odors (for example, perfume, coffee, chocolate, soap, spices). Requiring patients to close their eyes during the testing helps make sure that olfaction per se is being assessed. The olfactory nerves, bulbs, and tracts are located on the inferior surface of the frontal lobe, where they are vulnerable to damage by contusions in the course of closed-head trauma and compression by subfrontal tumors. Olfaction is also compromised by smoking, sinusitis with rhinitis, and nasal trauma.

Examination of the *second cranial nerve (optic)* includes visual inspection of the nerve head, assessment of visual acuity, and mapping of the visual fields. The optic nerve is the only nerve directly accessible to visual inspection by the examiner. By means of ophthalmoscopy, the clinician can detect optic atrophy (a pale disk), papilledema reflecting increased intracranial pressure, and papillitis associated with optic nerve ischemia or inflammation. Macular degeneration, pigmentary retinopathy, retinal infarction, narrowing of the retinal vessels, and retinal hemorrhages or exudates may also be seen.

Visual acuity is tested with Snellen's test held 18 inches from the face; each eye is tested separately with glasses or through a pinhole to minimize visual disturbances produced by abnormalities of the shape of the optic globe (astigmatism). Acuity should be correctable to 20/20 if optic nerve function is normal. Impaired acuity after correction implies the presence of prechiasmatic optic nerve dysfunction, such as ischemic optic neuritis or inflammation associated with multiple sclerosis or other inflammatory disorder. Papilledema is associated with an enlarged blind spot but does not impair acuity.

Visual field defects are identified by covering one of the patient's eyes and comparing the patient's visual field with that of the clinician's by determining when the patient detects a stimulus (moving finger or small stimulus item) entering the visual field from the periphery. The shape of the visual field is determined by repeating that maneuver in all quadrants. Bilateral double simultaneous visual stimulation allows the detection of visual neglect; if the patient has full visual fields with monocular testing but extinguishes stimuli in one field during double simultaneous stimulation, a neglect syndrome is present. Damage to the optic nerve produces a monocular visual-field defect of the ipsilateral eye. Postchiasmatic injury between the optic chiasm and the occipital lobe usually produces a homonymous visual-field defect. Occipital injuries produce highly congruent field defects of similar size and shape in both fields; anterior lesions (for example, damage to the geniculocalcarine radiation in the temporal lobe) produce incongruent field defects. Midline tumors in the region of the optic chiasm, such as craniopharyngiomas and chromophobe adenomas, may compress the chiasm medially, producing a bitemporal visual-field defect. Hemianopsias are often associated with *release hallucinations* (formed or unformed visual hallucinations occurring in the blind field). Visual neglect occurs most often with lesions of the parietal cortex but has also been reported with frontal lobe and subcortical lesions.

Ocular motility, pupillary responses, and eyelid position are mediated by the *third, fourth, and sixth cranial nerves* (*oculomotor, trochlear, and abducens,* respectively). The rectus externus moves the eye laterally and is innervated by the abducens nerve; the superior oblique moves the eye downward when the globe is in the adducted position and is innervated by the trochlear nerve; all the remaining ocular movements, the pupillary responses, and the position of the eyelid are determined by oculomotor nerve function.

Pursuit movements are tested by having the patient follow the examiner's finger through seven positions (adduction, adducted and up, abducted and up, abducted, abducted and down, adducted and down, convergence). The patient's saccadic movements (volitional movements) are then tested by asking the patient to look to the right, left, up, and down without following a visual target. Conjugate gaze is mediated by gaze centers in the pons (lateral movements) and the midbrain (vertical movements). Brainstem lesions, extrapyramidal movement disorders, and bilateral upper motor neuron lesions may produce supranuclear gaze palsies manifested by incomplete ocular movements, hypometric (abnormally small) saccadic movements, and irregular pursuit movements. *Pupillary changes* occur in response to light stimulation and in conjunction with convergence (constriction of the pupil with near vision). The third cranial nerve is responsible for pupillary constriction through its parasympathetic branches; pupillary dilation is a function of the sympathetic nervous system. *Lid position* is determined by the balanced input from the third nerve, responsible for volitional eye opening; the seventh cranial nerve, mediating lid closure; and sympathetic input that also participates in keeping the lid open. *Pupillary abnormalities* occur with brainstem lesions, syphilis (Argyll Robertson pupil, in which the reaction to light is lost but the convergence mechanism is intact), diabetes, and compression by aneurysms and other mass lesions. *Third-nerve palsy* results in ptosis, a nonreactive pupil, and an inability to adduct, elevate, or depress the eye. *Lid retraction* may occur with lesions of the collicular plate or in parkinsonian syndromes. *Horner's syndrome* includes ptosis, pupillary constriction, and diminished sweating on the ipsilateral side of the face. It results from sympathetic paralysis caused by medullary infarcts, cervical cord lesions, pulmonary apical and mediastinal lesions, and neck trauma.

The *fifth cranial nerve (trigeminal)* innervates the muscles of mastication and is responsible for facial and corneal sensation. The fifth cranial nerve is involved in tic douloureux and other facial pain syndromes.

The *seventh cranial nerve (facial)* supplies the facial musculature, including the platysma muscles of the anterior neck, the orbicularis oris and buccinator muscles, the orbicularis oculi, and the frontalis. In addition, its branches innervate the lacrimal and salivary glands, the stapedius muscles, and the taste fibers of the anterior two thirds of the tongue.

Fibers supplying the upper facial muscles receive supranuclear input from the ipsilateral and contralateral motor cortex; fibers innervating the lower facial muscles receive only contralateral input. Peripheral nerve lesions result in ipsilateral paralysis of upper and lower face, but upper motor neuron lesions above the level of the seventh nerve nucleus produce only contralateral lower facial paresis. All human faces are asymmetrical, and facial asymmetry by itself should not be regarded as evidence of paresis; asymmetries, however, can result from weakness, and detection of asymmetries should lead to testing for evidence of muscle paresis. The facial nerve receives input from both descending pyramidal neurons, mediating volitional movements, and nonpyramidal limbic system connections, mediating emotional responses. That dual innervation results in the preservation of emotional responses in spite of paralysis of volitional facial movements in patients with pyramidal tract lesions (most evident in the syndrome of pseudobulbar palsy) and a lack of emotional facial responses with intact volitional movements in patients with lesions of the limbic system. The latter condition has been observed, for example, in patients with seizure foci arising from lesions of the temporal lobes. The facial musculature is also involved in generalized movement disorders (for example, chorea, tics, parkinsonism).

The *eighth cranial nerve (acoustic)* is responsible for hearing (*auditory* branch) and balance (*vestibular* branch). Auditory compromise is associated with deafness and can produce auditory hallucinations.

Vestibular end organ and nerve lesions produce nystagmus and vertigo and, when acute, may be associated with the experience of sudden shifts in the environment (for example, vertical inversion). Vestibular nystagmus is characterized by horizontal or combined horizontal-rotatory eye movements and is typically accompanied by vertigo and nausea. Lesions disrupting vestibular connections in the central nervous system can produce nystagmus in any direction and are usually not associated with vertiginous or nauseous sensations. Vestibular nystagmus should be distinguished from gaze-paretic nystagmus resulting from inadequate ocular deviation and occurring with paresis of cranial nerves III, IV, or VI. The quick or jerky phase of the nystagmus occurs in the direction of the weakened muscle. Nystagmus also occurs with a variety of medications, particularly anticonvulsants and sedative-hypnotics. Table 2.1-3 presents the differential diagnosis of nystagmus and related disorders of ocular movement.

TABLE 2.1-3
Types of Nystagmus and Related Ocular Movements

Pendular nystagmus (consists of sinusoidal movements of equal speed in both directions)
- Brainstem lesions
- Cerebellar lesions
- Blindness or reduced visual input
- Congenital nystagmus

Jerky nystagmus (consists of alternating slow and quick movements)
- Vestibular (labyrinth, nerve, nucleus, brainstem connections)
- Gaze-evoked
  - Gaze-paretic, associated with gaze palsy
  - Drug-induced (anticonvulsants, sedative-hypnotic agents)
  - Cerebellar disease

Special types of nystagmus
- Physiological (end-point) nystagmus
- Dissociated nystagmus (more severe in one eye than in the other)
- Rotatory nystagmus (produced by involvement of central vestibular connections)
- Seesaw nystagmus (alternating downward beating in one eye, upward beating in the other)
- Convergence-induced nystagmus
- Periodic alternating nystagmus (horizontal jerk nystagmus that periodically reverses directions)
- Downbeat nystagmus (typically associated with disorders of the craniocervical junction)
- Upbeat nystagmus (occurs with lesions of the cerebellar vermis or the brainstem)
- Rebound nystagmus (gaze-evoked nystagmus that beats in the opposite direction of the previous fixation after returning to the primary position)
- Circular, elliptic, or oblique nystagmus (usually indicative of demyelinating brainstem lesions)
- Voluntary nystagmus (very rapid conjugate horizontal oscillations)

Ocular movements to be distinguished from nystagmus
- Ocular myoclonus (pendular oscillation in concert with simultaneous palatal movements in the syndrome of palatal myoclonus)
- Ocular bobbing (rapid conjugate downward ocular jerks followed by a slow return to midposition; occurs in comatose patients with pontine lesions or metabolic encephalopathies)
- Square-wave jerks (conjugate eye movements away from [in either direction] and back to the fixation point; occur in cerebellar disease and with progressive supranuclear palsy)
- Ocular dysmetria (undershooting or overshooting of an ocular target followed by compensatory saccadic movements)
- Ocular flutter (brief, intermittent conjugate, horizontal oscillations occurring during straight-ahead fixation; occurs in same conditions as opsoclonus)
- Opsoclonus (rapid, chaotic, unpredictable conjugate eye movement [saccadomania]; occurs with cerebellar disturbances and as a remote effect of neuroblastoma and other carcinomas)
- Oculogyric crises (sustained conjugate ocular deviations; induced by antipsychotic drugs and in postencephalitic parkinsonism)

The *ninth and 10th cranial nerves* (*glossopharyngeal and vagus*, respectively) control pharyngeal and laryngeal function, taste, and the gag reflex. The glossopharyngeal nerve conveys sensory information (including taste sensation from the posterior third of the tongue); the vagus nerve is primarily responsible for the motor aspects of those structures. Dysfunction of the vagus nerve results in a hoarse voice or aphonia and dysphagia. Supranuclear lesions in the syndrome of pseudobulbar palsy produce an exaggerated gag reflex.

The *11th cranial nerve (accessory)* innervates the upper half of the trapezius muscle and the sternocleidomastoid muscle. The *12th cranial nerve (hypoglossal)* innervates the tongue. Tongue weakness is common in pseudobulbar palsy.

MOTOR SYSTEM EXAMINATION The motor system examination includes the assessment of muscle bulk, strength, and tone; tests of coordination; and the identification of movement disorders. Normal motor function depends on the functional integrity of the pyramidal motor system, the extrapyramidal nuclei, the cerebellum, the spinal cord, the peripheral nerves, the myoneural junction, and the muscles. Assessment of the motor system is particularly important in neuropsychiatry: psychiatric disturbances frequently produce associated motor system manifestations; movement disorders are often accompanied by neuropsychiatric abnormalities; and many of the agents used to treat psychiatric diseases adversely affect the motor system.

Muscle bulk, strength, and tone Muscle *bulk* is examined by visual inspection and palpation and occasionally by measurement. The dominant limbs, particularly the upper extremities, have slightly greater bulk than the nondominant extremities. Muscle wasting may occur with volitional disuse, muscle disease, and nerve or spinal disease and in generalized weight loss secondary to malnutrition, systemic illness, and advanced brain diseases.

Strength is tested by asking the patient to exert maximal power of specified muscle groups.

Strength is graded as 0, no evidence of muscle contraction; 1, muscle contraction without movement of the limb; 2, limb movement after gravity is eliminated; 3, limb movement against gravity; 4, limb movement against partial resistance; 5, normal strength. The upper and lower limbs and both proximal and distal musculature should be assessed.

Distal weakness is characteristic of peripheral neuropathies; proximal weakness is a manifestation of primary muscle disease. Weakness below a specific level of innervation occurs with spinal cord diseases (paraparesis and quadriparesis), and fatigability is most characteristic of muscle and myoneural junction disorders (for example, myasthenia gravis). Lateralized weakness (hemiparesis) is a manifestation of lesions of the contralateral brainstem or above. Pyramidal tract pathology produces a predilection pattern of weakness affecting the extensor muscles of the upper limbs and the flexor muscles of the lower limbs; that is known as a decorticate posture, and it imitates the antigravity posture of the biped. Pyramidal lesions of the pons result in flexor weakness of all limbs and consequent extensor posturing; extension of all limbs is known as the decerebrate posture, and it recapitulates the antigravity posture of the quadruped.

Muscle *tone* is evaluated by passively manipulating the patient's limbs or neck while the patient relaxes. Additional information can be garnered by asking the patient to perform motor activities with the contralateral limb while tone in the ipsilateral limb is determined (for example, the patient is asked to draw a large square in the air with one arm while the examiner is testing the tone of the other arm). Activation of tone by that maneuver (Froment's sign) is characteristic of parkinsonian-type extrapyramidal syndromes.

Hypotonia is relatively unusual in neuropsychiatric disorders. Muscle tone is decreased in muscle and peripheral nerve diseases, cerebellar syndromes, early in the course of many choreiform disorders, and in the first few days following onset of an upper motor neuron lesion. Episodic hypotonia occurs in narcolepsy and accounts for the cataplectic attacks experienced by narcoleptic patients.

Increased muscle tone (rigidity) is encountered in a variety of neuropsychiatric conditions. *Spasticity* is a form of rigidity in which the muscle is flaccid at rest and reacts with increasing tone to a slow passive stretch. In many cases the tone abruptly decreases after reaching a certain magnitude, resulting in a sudden loss of resistance (the clasped-knife phenomenon). Spasticity results from upper motor neuron lesions that result in disinhibition and hyperexcitability of the alpha and gamma motor neurons of the spinal cord. Muscle stretch reflexes are mediated through the same mechanism as spasticity and are exaggerated in spastic disorders. Parkinsonian-type extrapyramidal syndromes produce *plastic rigidity* (also known as lead-pipe rigidity) characterized by an increased resistance to passive movement that is independent of the velocity of limb movement. The rigidity is produced by a dysfunction of the nigrostriatal projection or the globus pallidus. Plastic rigidity may involve primarily the appendicular musculature (in Parkinson's disease), or it may be pronounced in the axial structures, such as the neck and the trunk (in progressive supranuclear palsy). *Cogwheel rigidity*, observed in some extrapyramidal disorders, results from the occurrence of tremor that is palpated as intermittent resistance when manipulating the limbs; it may occur with or without plastic rigidity. *Gegenhalten* (also known as paratonia) is characterized by resistance to movement; it is encountered in advanced brain diseases. It is characterized by active resistance to all limb movements. It may result from the release of primitive protective or position-holding mechanisms similar to the released motor programs responsible for grasp and suck reflexes. *Waxy flexibility* is the tone change classically associated with catatonia. The patient's limb has moderate resistance to passive movement and maintains the end position of the movement (like candle wax). *Catatonia* occurs in a variety of psychiatric, frontal lobe, extrapyramidal, and toxic-metabolic disorders.

Coordination assessment *Coordination* may be disrupted by many types of motor and sensory abnormalities but depends primarily on intact cerebellar function. Disturbances of coordination must be interpreted with caution to avoid ascribing the effects of weakness, spasticity, or sensory loss to cerebellar disease.

Tests of coordination used in the standard neurological examination include rapid alternating movements (alternating supination and pronation movements of the hand), fine finger movements (repeated apposition of the thumb and the first finger), finger-to-nose movements (the patient alternates between touching his or her own nose and the examiner's finger), heel-knee-shin maneuvers (the patient touches the knee of one leg with the heel of the other and then gently slides the heel down the shin), and rebound check tests (the clinician suddenly releases the patient's extended arms as they push upward, against the examiner's resistance; the clinician observes whether the patient can arrest the upward movement after the release). Gait, eye movement, and tremor-related observations aid in identifying a cerebellar disorder. Dysdiadochokinesia (abnormal rapidly alternating movements), ataxia, loss of rebound check, and intention tremor are characteristic cerebellar disturbances.

Gait and posture are examples of motor acts dependent on successful motor and sensory integration. Systematic gait observations should assess step initiation, stride length, step height, base width, step symmetry, path deviation, trunk stability, speed, turning, and adventitious (superfluous, hyperkinetic) movements. *Festination of gait* is increasingly fast forward movement with an inability to stop. Asking the patient to perform tandem toe-to-heel walking makes cerebellar, sensory, and vestibular disturbances of gait and balance evident. Table 2.1-4 summarizes the principal types of gait abnormalities.

Posture may be extended or flexed. In addition, sensory abnormalities, cerebellar disorders, and extrapyramidal disturbances may contribute to postural instability. Parkinson's disease and many parkinsonian syndromes produce a tendency to flexion of all limbs; progressive supranuclear palsy causes a characteristic extended posture. Postural stability is tested by asking the patient to stand with legs comfortably apart and eyes open; the examiner then stands behind the patient and pulls backward on the patient's shoulders with a short, rapid jerk. Patients with extrapyramidal disorders fall backward or must take a compensatory backward step. Sensory input to postural mechanisms can be tested by asking the patient to stand with feet together and eyes closed. Patients with sensory abnormalities from peripheral neuropathy or posterior column disease can stand with eyes open but not with eyes closed (Romberg's sign); patients with cerebellar ataxia cannot stand with feet together, whether the eyes are open or closed.

Soft signs are minor motor and sensory abnormalities that are normal in the course of early development but abnormal when present beyond childhood. They have been reported with increased frequency in a variety of psychiatric disorders, including schizophrenia and sociopathy. Soft signs lack definitive localizing significance but are indicative of subtle brain dysfunction. Table 2.1-5 lists the main soft signs elicited in the course of the neurological examination.

TABLE 2.1-4
Abnormalities of Gait

Observation	Abnormality	Cause
Step initiation	Start hesitation	Parkinsonism
Stride length	Shortened	Parkinsonism
Step height	Decreased	Parkinsonism
	Increased	Sensory abnormality
Base width	Increased	Cerebellar ataxia, chorea, sensory abnormalities
Step symmetry	Asymmetric	Pain with unilateral avoidance, hemiparesis
Path course	Deviation	Cerebellar or vestibular ataxia
Trunk stability	Unsteady	Cerebellar or vestibular disorders
Speed	Slowed	Parkinsonism
Turning	En bloc	Parkinsonism
Adventitious movements	Present	Chorea, athetosis, dyskinesia, tics, tremor, myoclonus, dystonia

TABLE 2.1-5
Neurological Soft Signs

Test	Soft Sign
Articulation	Mild dysarthria
Finger tapping	Slow, clumsy, irregular
Foot tapping	Slow, clumsy, irregular
Rapid alternating movements	Slow, clumsy, irregular
Eye closure	Cannot maintain on command
Tongue extrusion	Cannot maintain on command
Arms extended	Minor choreiform movements
Finger to nose	Jerky, clumsy
Heel to shin	Jerky, clumsy
Heel walking	Unsteady, posturing of upper limbs
Toe walking	Unsteady, posturing of upper limbs
Standing on one foot	Cannot balance
Hopping on one foot	Unsteady
Tandem walking	Unsteady
Tandem walking backward	Unsteady
Face-hand test	Distal stimulus extinguished when distal and proximal stimuli are delivered simultaneously
Two-point discrimination	Perceives two separate points only when they are more widely separated than normal
Graphesthesia	Errors
Romberg's sign	Present (cannot stand with feet together and eyes closed)

Movement assessment A wide variety of *movement disorders* may be observed in the course of the neuropsychiatric examination. Four general classes of movement disorders can be distinguished—parkinsonism, hyperkinesias, dystonia, and tremor. The first three are irregular disorders; the last is a regular hyperkinesia. Parkinsonian syndromes are characterized by rigidity and bradykinesia. Dystonic disorders produce sustained postural deviations. Hyperkinesias include chorea, dyskinesias, athetosis, tics, and myoclonus. Tremors are regularly alternating movements. Several types of movement disorders (for example, parkinsonism, dystonia, and tremor) can occur simultaneously.

Parkinsonism may be produced by degenerative disorders (Parkinson's disease, progressive supranuclear palsy), multiple small cerebrovascular events (lacunar state), metabolic disorders (hypothyroidism, hypoparathyroidism), head trauma, central nervous system (CNS) infections (Creutzfeldt-Jakob disease, human immunodeficiency [HIV] encephalopathy), CNS tumors, hydrocephalus, and drug treatment. Medications most likely to induce parkinsonism include dopamine-blocking agents, such as phenothiazines and butyrophenones. Table 2.1-6 lists the causes of parkinsonism. The parkinsonian syndrome features bradykinesia and plastic rigidity with or without a rest tremor. Manifestations of bradykinesia include a masked face, reduced spontaneous blinking, diminished spontaneous swallowing with sialorrhea, start hesitation when initiating a movement, shuffling gait (combination of reduced stride length and decreased step height), decreased arm swing when walking, en bloc turns, slowed movement, and reduced spontaneous gesturing.

Hyperkinetic movement disorders include athetosis (observed primarily in cerebral palsy), chorea (Huntington's disease, Sydenham's chorea, neuroacanthocytosis), tardive dyskinesia, myoclonic disorders (Creutzfeldt-Jakob disease, myoclonic epilepsy, hereditary myoclonus, drug-induced myoclonus), ballismus (usually occurring as hemiballismus after an infarction of the subthalamic nucleus), and tic disorders (Tourette's disorder, simple tic syndromes). In *hemiballismus* the patient manifests large-amplitude flinging movements of the arm and the leg contralateral to a lesion of the subthalamic nucleus. With time, the movements may evolve into hemichorea. *Chorea* is an irregular hyperkinesia intermediate in speed between the slow athetosis and the fast myoclonus. The choreic movements resemble normal movements and may be incorporated into semipurposeful gestures to partially obscure their occurrence. Electromyographic recordings, however, reveal that antagonistic muscles are active at inappropriate times. In Sydenham's postinfectious chorea the movements involve the distal musculature more than the proximal musculature; in Huntington's disease the proximal musculature is more affected than is the distal musculature. *Dyskinetic movements* observed in tardive dyskinesia are a special instance of chorea. *Myoclonus* is characterized by random,

TABLE 2.1-6
Causes of Parkinsonism

- Degenerative disorders
  - Parkinson's disease
  - Progressive supranuclear palsy
  - Corticobasal degeneration
  - Idiopathic basal ganglia calcification
  - Cortical Lewy body disease
  - Rigid Huntington's disease (Westphal variant)
  - Parkinsonism-dementia-amyotrophic lateral sclerosis complex of Guam
  - Wilson's disease
  - Hallervorden-Spatz disease
  - Azorean disease
  - Striatonigral degeneration
  - Olivopontocerebellar atrophy
  - Shy-Drager syndrome
  - Pallidal atrophies
- Vascular disorders
  - Lacunar state
  - Binswanger's disease
- Metabolic conditions
  - Hypothyroidism
  - Hypoparathyroidism
- Drugs and toxins
  - Antipsychotic agents and other dopamine receptor blocking agents
  - Methyl-phenyl-tetrahydropyridine (MPTP)
  - Reserpine
  - Manganese
- Traumas
  - Posttraumatic encephalopathy
  - Dementia pugilistica
- Infections
  - Creutzfeldt-Jakob disease
  - Human immunodeficiency virus (HIV) encephalopathy
  - Syphilis
  - Encephalitis lethargica
- Miscellaneous disorders
  - Hydrocephalus
  - Carbon monoxide intoxication
  - Neoplasms
  - G_{M1} gangliosidosis
  - Neuronal intranuclear inclusion disease
  - Ceroid lipofuscinosis (Kuf's disease)

TABLE 2.1-7
Principal Hyperkinetic Disorders

- Chorea
  - Huntington's disease
  - Benign hereditary chorea
  - Wilson's disease
  - Neuroacanthocytosis
  - Olivopontocerebellar atrophy
  - Azorean disease
  - Basal ganglia infarction
  - Systemic lupus erythematosus
  - Sydenham's chorea
  - Chorea gravidarum (with pregnancy)
  - Chorea induced by oral contraceptives
  - Non-Wilsonian hepatocerebral degeneration
  - Hyperthyroidism
  - Tardive dyskinesia
  - Levodopa-induced chorea
  - Anticonvulsant-induced chorea (phenytoin, phenobarbital, carbamazepine, ethosuximide)
  - Stimulant-induced chorea (amphetamines, cocaine, pemoline, methylphenidate)
- Myoclonus
  - Essential myoclonus (hereditary, sporadic)
  - Epilepsy
  - Progressive myoclonic epilepsy
  - Creutzfeldt-Jakob disease
  - Alzheimer's disease (advanced stage)
  - Subacute sclerosing panencephalitis
  - Metabolic encephalopathies (renal failure, anoxia, hepatic encephalopathy)
  - Postanoxic myoclonus
- Tics
  - Idiopathic tics
    - Transient tic disorder
    - Chronic motor tic disorder
    - Tourette's disorder
  - Secondary tics
    - Postencephalitic tics
    - Postrheumatic chorea
    - Carbon monoxide poisoning
    - Neuroacanthocytosis
    - Drug-induced (stimulants, levodopa, antipsychotics) tics

asynchronous, brief muscle jerks large enough to move a limb. *Tics* are similar to myoclonus in amplitude and duration but are stereotyped, repetitively involving the same muscles, and they are subject to partial temporary volitional suppression. Table 2.1-7 summarizes the principal hyperkinetic movement disorders. *Athetosis* is a slow, writhing hyperkinesia.

Dystonia is a movement disorder in which tonic contraction of antagonistic muscle groups leads to sustained postural abnormalities. Initially, the muscle contractions may be intermittent, giving rise to an irregular tremorlike disorder. Dystonia may be focal, involving a single body part (for example, torticollis); segmental, involving adjacent body parts (for example, torticollis plus the involvement of one shoulder); or generalized. Table 2.1-8 provides the differential diagnosis of dystonia. Idiopathic dystonias appear to have few neuropsychiatric associations; secondary dystonias occur in conjunction with many of the other hyperkinesias (including Huntington's disease and Parkinson's disease), and dystonia is a frequent side effect of treatment with antipsychotic agents. Drug-induced dystonias may be acute, occurring within a few hours of initiating treatment or increasing the drug dosage, or they may be manifestations of tardive dyskinesia.

Tremor is a more or less regular oscillation of a body part around a fixed point. Table 2.1-9 presents a classification of tremors, including rest tremors, postural tremors, and kinetic tremors. *Rest tremors* include the typical large-amplitude, low-frequency (approximately 4 to 6 Hz) tremor of Parkinson's disease and other parkinsonian states. The tremor disappears with sleep and is characterized as a tremor of alert repose, occurring when the patient is alert but inactive. Rest tremor is suppressed by volitional movement. The principal *postural tremors* include exaggerated physiological tremors and essential tremors. They are small-amplitude, high-frequency (10 to 12 Hz) tremors that are absent at rest and occur during postural maintenance and intentional activities (holding the arms outstretched in front of the body, writing).

TABLE 2.1-8
Differential Diagnosis of Dystonia

- Primary
  - Idiopathic torsion dystonia (hereditary or sporadic)
- Secondary
  - Dystonia with other movement disorders
    - Huntington's disease
    - Parkinson's disease
    - Wilson's disease
    - Idiopathic basal ganglia calcification
    - Neuroacanthocytosis
    - Azorean disease
    - Olivopontocerebellar atrophy
    - Progressive supranuclear palsy
    - Corticobasal degeneration
    - Hallervorden-Spatz disease
    - Pallidal atrophies
  - Acquired dystonias
    - Perinatal or adult anoxia
    - Kernicterus
    - Carbon monoxide intoxication
    - Postencephalitic dystonia
  - Drug-induced and toxin-induced dystonias
    - Acute antipsychotic-induced dystonia
    - Tardive dystonia
    - Levodopa-induced dystonia
    - Manganese-induced dystonia

TABLE 2.1-9
Classification of Tremors

Tremor Type	Frequency	Amplitude	Cause
Rest	4–6 Hz	Large	Parkinson's disease, antipsychotic agents
Postural			
Physiological	10–12 Hz	Small	Fatigue, anxiety, hypoglycemia, thyrotoxicosis, drugs (lithium, tricyclic agents, sympathomimetic drugs), alcohol and sedative-hypnotic withdrawal
Essential	10–12 Hz	Small	Hereditary, sporadic
Kinetic	3–5 Hz	Crescendo*	Cerebellar dysfunction from multiple sclerosis, head trauma

*Tremor amplitude increases as the target is approached.

Exaggerated physiological tremors occur with fatigue, excitement, hypoglycemia, and thyrotoxicosis and in metabolic encephalopathies and drug-induced toxic states (lithium, tricyclic agents, sympathomimetics). Essential tremors are usually inherited but may occur sporadically. Kinetic tremors are those that worsen with movement. Cerebellar intention tremors are the classic examples of kinetic tremors.

SENSORY EXAMINATION The examination of sensory function includes the assessment of primary sensory modalities mediated at the thalamic level and secondary or cortical sensation. Sensory information is projected from the peripheral receptors to the postrolandic sensory cortex by the peripheral nerves, the spinal cord, the brainstem, and the thalamus; damage at any of those levels may produce a sensory deficit. The primary modalities include light touch, pain (tested by examining the patient's ability to distinguish a sharp pin from a dull object), temperature and vibration. Vibration should be tested with a 128-Hz tuning fork. The cortical sensory modalities include joint position sense, *two-point discrimination* (ability to discriminate two closely spaced areas of stimulation from a single stimulation), *graphesthesia* (ability to identify numbers "written" on the tips of the fingers), and *stereognosis* (ability to recognize, by touch, objects placed in the hand). Double simultaneous stimulation is a sensitive and valuable means of detecting unilateral neglect. Patients are told that they will be touched in one or two areas, including the face, the dorsum of the hands, or the front of the lower legs. The patients' ability to perceive bilateral simultaneous stimuli is then systematically assessed. Patients with neglect fail to perceive stimuli on one side of the body when they are simultaneously stimulated on the other side. The primary sensory abilities (for example, light touch) must be intact to perform the test. Patients with unilateral neglect may manifest the related behavioral disorder of *anosognosia* (denial of illness).

MUSCLE STRETCH REFLEXES Muscle stretch reflexes are monosynaptic spinal cord reflexes that are modulated by descending connections. Muscle stretch reflexes are decreased in muscle, peripheral nerve, and nerve root disorders and increased in the presence of upper motor neuron lesions. Every muscle has an associated muscle stretch reflex, and the examiner chooses a small number that can routinely be examined in the screening evaluation and tests additional reflexes to explore hypotheses generated in the course of the examination. A reasonable screening examination includes the following muscle stretch reflexes: biceps, brachioradialis, triceps, finger flexors, knee jerks, and ankle jerks. Reflexes are graded as 0, absent or unobtainable; 1, decreased; 2, normal; 3, brisk with spread of the contraction response to adjacent muscles; 4, clonus. *Clonus* is the series of rhythmic reflex contractions observed when a muscle is suddenly subjected to sustained stretch. Clonus is most easily elicited at the ankles but may be observed in the knees, the wrists, and the jaw. Lateralized increased reflexes in conjunction with weakness, spasticity, and Babinski's sign constitute the upper motor neuron syndrome indicative of a contralateral lesion of the descending pyramidal system. Reflexes are diminished in the acute phase of an upper motor neuron lesion and gradually increase during the first few weeks after the injury.

PATHOLOGICAL AND PRIMITIVE REFLEXES Babinski's sign is the most important pathological reflex sought in the neurological examination. It is typically elicited by stroking the lateral aspect of the plantar surface of the foot from back to front with a semisharp object. A normal response consists of plantar flexion of the great toe; a pathological response *(Babinski's sign)* consists of dorsiflexion of the great toe with or without fanning of the other toes. It is produced by upper motor neuron lesions and is a fragment of a protective flexion reflex. In its completely developed form (observed in infants and in some patients with severe spinal cord injuries), there is a flexor synergy with flexion of the hip, the knee, and the toe, removing the foot from the noxious stimulus. Babinski's sign, like other primitive reflexes, represents the release from suprasegmental control of primitive motor programs. No equivalent reflex appears in the upper extremity, but Hoffmann's sign (thumb flexion elicited by briskly flexing the distal phalanx of the middle finger while holding the digits in a dorsiflexed position) may be used to assess hyperreflexia in the upper extremities and is frequently present in patients with upper motor neuron lesions and Babinski's signs in the lower limbs.

The *glabella tap reflex* (Myerson's sign) is often mistakenly considered a primitive reflex similar to grasp and sucking reflexes. Continued blinking with tapping of the glabellar region is associated with extrapyramidal dysfunction and is seen in Parkinson's disease and drug-induced parkinsonism. To be abnormal, the blinking must continue to occur after four or more glabella taps.

The *grasp reflex* is the involuntary gripping of objects in or near the patient's hand. Four types of grasp response have been described: (1) the simple grasp response occurs when the patient's thenar eminence is stimulated; (2) the hooking response occurs when the patient's flexed fingers are gently extended; (3) if the hooking response is marked, there is loss of voluntary relaxation, and the patient grips steadily as the examiner withdraws the patient's hand (traction grasp); (4) in patients with advanced disease, the sight of the examiner's hand or the light touch of the hand by the examiner causes the patient to move to grasp the examiner's hand (groping response or magnetic grasp). Grasp reflexes occur in patients with advanced brain disease and with lesions restricted to the medial frontal lobes. Grasp responses can be elicited in the feet, as well as in the hands.

The *sucking reflex* comprises sucking movements of the lips, the tongue, and the jaw elicited by gentle stimulation of the lips. It is related to the *snout reflex,* characterized by puckering and protrusion of the lips in response to tapping of the upper or lower lip. Like the grasp reflex, those are primitive motor programs that occur normally in infants and reappear as age-inappropriate signs in patients with frontal lobe and diffuse brain dysfunction.

The *palmomental reflex* features ipsilateral contraction of the mentalis muscle in response to stroking of the thenar eminence of the hand. The reflex can be seen in normal aged patients and may be regarded as pathological when it is unilateral or when it does not fatigue with repeated stimulation.

PHYSICAL EXAMINATION

Selected aspects of the general physical examination are particularly important in neuropsychiatric assessment. Dysmorphological features are important in the recognition of congenital and chromosomal syndromes. The manifestations of fetal alcohol syndrome, for example, may be evident in adults and include microcephaly, short palpebral fissures, maxillary hypoplasia, short nose, smooth philtrum with thin and smooth upper lip, small distal phalanges, and small fifth fingernails.

Examination of the head and the neck is essential. Patients may have enlarged heads from compensated hydrocephalus (normal men should have a head circumference of less than 58.4 cm and normal women less than 57.5 cm) or small heads from inadequate brain development. Palpation of the head may reveal evidence of a previous craniotomy not revealed or recalled by the patient. A short neck is characteristic of platybasia associated with congenital deformities of the posterior fossa (Arnold-Chiari malformation) and of basilar impression (occurring, for example, with Paget's disease of the skull) that may give rise to hydrocephalus.

The neuro-ophthalmological examination may contribute essential information in the neuropsychiatric examination. Examination of the optic nerve, the visual fields, extraocular movements, lid position, and pupillary responses were discussed above. In addition, inspection of the eyes may reveal a Kayser-Fleischer ring at the corneal limbus in Wilson's disease. Retinal inspection may reveal macular degeneration (associated with blindness and visual hallucinations) and retinal degeneration, which occurs with phenothiazines, particularly thioridazine (Mellaril), and some hereditary CNS disorders. Cataracts may be present in diabetes, hypoparathyroidism, and Wilson's disease and after treatment with chlorpromazine (Thorazine) and corticosteroids.

Cardiovascular assessment is of obvious interest in neuropsychiatry. Cardiac and carotid auscultation and blood pressure measurement are necessary in most examinations. Abdominal palpation may occasionally reveal organomegaly in neuropsychiatric illnesses, including hepatomegaly in alcoholism. Skin changes in neuropsychiatric disorders include pigment deposition after long-term treatment with chlorpromazine, small pigmented papules (angiokeratoma corporis diffusum) in Fabry's disease, and a variety of anomalies in mental retardation syndromes.

BEHAVIORAL DISTURBANCES

Behavioral disturbances with neurological disorders may be divided arbitrarily into neurobehavioral syndromes and neuropsychiatric syndromes. *Neurobehavioral syndromes* conventionally include *deficit disorders,* such as aphasia, amnesia, alexia, agraphia, aprosody, acalculia, apraxia, frontal lobe disorders, neglect, and anosognosia. Those syndromes have in common an acquired loss of function after the onset of a brain disorder. Each syndrome is characterized by the absence of an ability that the patient was previously able to exercise, and in most cases it has been possible to correlate each deficit syndrome with a specific focal injury to the cerebral cortex, deep hemispheric nuclei, or white matter tracts. Deficit disorders are anatomically determined and occur in nearly all cases in which the appropriate anatomical lesion is present.

Neuropsychiatric syndromes traditionally include *productive disorders* that closely resemble or are identical to idiopathic psychiatric illnesses. Productive syndromes include delusions, hallucinations, depression, mania, personality alterations, anxiety, obsessive-compulsive disorder, and paraphilias that occur for the first time after the onset of a brain disorder and that are secondary to acquired brain dysfunction. In some cases, productive syndromes have been associated with focal brain injury (for example, visual hallucinations in the blind hemifield after contralateral occipital injury), but in other cases the lesions may occur anywhere within a system of functionally related structures, and precise anatomical localization is less evident (for example, delusions with limbic system lesions). Productive disorders are anatomically contingent; the lesion must be in an anatomically appropriate location for the disorder to occur, but the existence of the lesion by itself is often insufficient to produce the disorder. Other characteristics that contribute to the occurrence of the disorder include the age of the patient, the patient's age at the onset of the disorder, unilateral or bilateral distribution of the brain dysfunction, genetic vulnerability to a specific behavioral disorder, gender, comorbidity, premorbid personality, environmental stress, coping skills, and social support. Table 2.1-10 summarizes the anatomical relations of deficit disorders and productive disorders.

NEUROBEHAVIORAL SYNDROMES

Aphasia *Aphasia* is characterized by the loss of language abilities produced by brain dysfunction. The most common cause of isolated aphasia is cerebrovascular disorder, but it may also occur with brain tumors, infections, and trauma and in the course of degenerative diseases, such as dementia of the Alzheimer's type.

There are eight major aphasia syndromes, each identifiable by a distinctive combination of changes of fluency, comprehension, and repetition (Table 2.1-11). *Wernicke's aphasia* has a fluent output with poor comprehension and impaired repetition. Naming is abnormal, reading comprehension is impaired, reading aloud is compromised, and writing contains errors similar to the fluent paraphasic output. *Broca's aphasia* is characterized by a terse nonfluent output, intact comprehension, and poor repetition. Reading comprehension is largely preserved, and reading aloud has the same nonfluent characteristics as spoken language. Naming and writing are impaired. *Global aphasia* is the most severe aphasic syndrome: spontaneous output is nonfluent and often severely limited, comprehension is abnormal, and repetition is disturbed. Naming, reading comprehension, reading aloud, and writing are all abnormal. *Anomic aphasia* is a mild aphasic syndrome with fluent output, preserved comprehension, and intact repetition. The principal disturbances are a word-finding deficit and abnormalities of naming. Reading aloud and writing contain the same abnormalities noted in spontaneous speech. *Conduction aphasia* resembles Wernicke's aphasia in having fluent output and impaired repetition, but comprehension is preserved. Conduction aphasia patients read with comprehension but cannot read aloud. Writing contains paraphasic errors. The typical paraphasias of conduction aphasia are phonemic substitutions, whereas patients with Wernicke's aphasia have verbal and neologistic paraphasias. *Transcortical sensory aphasia* is similar to Wernicke's aphasia (fluent output, poor comprehension) with intact repetition. Reading and writing are compromised. *Transcortical motor aphasia* has features similar to Broca's aphasia (nonfluent output, intact comprehension) with normal repetition. Reading comprehension is intact; reading aloud and writing are abnormal. *Mixed transcortical aphasia* resembles global aphasia (nonfluent, poor comprehension) but has preserved repetition.

Each of the aphasic syndromes is associated with a different region of cerebral cortical dysfunction. Wernicke's aphasia is produced by a lesion of the posterior superior left temporal gyrus (Wernicke's area). Broca's aphasia reflects pathology of the middle third of the left inferior frontal gyrus (Broca's area). Global aphasia is associated with a large left hemisphere lesion involving the anterior and posterior lateral convexity. Anomic aphasia occurs with lesions of the posterior inferior left temporal gyrus, the left angular gyrus, or the top of the left temporal lobe. Conduction aphasia is seen with disruption of the arcuate fasciculus connecting Wernicke's and Broca's areas. Transcortical sensory aphasia is caused by lesions of the posterior inferior parietal region. Transcortical motor aphasia may occur with lesions of the left medial frontal lobe or the convexity area superior to Broca's area. Mixed trans-

TABLE 2.1-10
Anatomical Relation of Deficit Disorders and Productive Disorders

Structure	Deficit Disorders	Productive Disorders
Left frontal lobe	Broca's aphasia Transcortical motor aphasia Executive aprosody Poor word-list generation Poor motor programming Motor perseveration Stimulus-bound behavior Apraxia Poor verbal memory Poor concentration	Major depressive disorder Disinhibition Apathy
Right frontal lobe	Executive aprosody Amusia Poor design fluency	Mania
Left temporoparietal region	Wernicke's aphasia Anomic aphasia Conduction aphasia Transcortical sensory aphasia Alexia with agraphia Gerstmann syndrome Acalculia Right-left disorientation Finger agnosia Construction disturbance Contralateral neglect Denial of aphasia Verbal memory loss Apraxia	Delusions Auditory hallucinations Visual hallucinations Minor depression
Right temporoparietal region	Construction disturbance Contralateral neglect Contralateral neglect Anosognosia Dressing disturbance Receptive aprosody Receptive amusia Nonverbal memory loss Environmental agnosia Receptive amusia Nonverbal memory loss Environmental agnosia	Delusions Anxiety Minor depression Visual hallucinations Mania
Left occipital	Alexia without agraphia Anomia Color agnosia Contralateral achromatopsia	Visual hallucinations
Right occipital	Contralateral achromatopsia Prosopagnosia	Visual hallucinations
Left basal ganglia	Executive aprosody Poor word-list generation Poor motor programming Motor perseveration Stimulus-bound behavior Poor verbal memory Poor concentration	Disinhibition Major depressive disorder
Right basal ganglia	Executive aprosody Poor design fluency Poor nonverbal memory Poor concentration	
Left thalamus	Poor verbal memory Anomia	Apathy
Right thalamus	Poor nonverbal memory	Mania
Corpus callosum	Apraxia Alexia without agraphia Left-hand anomia Left-hand agraphia Alien hand Right-hand construction disturbance	

cortical aphasia is produced by lesions combining the syndromes of transcortical motor aphasia and transcortical sensory aphasia or by large lesions of the anterior and posterior medial left hemisphere.

Localizing principles regarding lesion location in aphasic patients can be derived from those observations. Syndromes with impaired repetition all have lesions bordering directly on the sylvian fissure of the left hemisphere (Wernicke's, Broca's, and conduction aphasias), whereas syndromes with intact repetition (all transcortical aphasias) have lesions that spare the immediate perisylvian structures. Disorders with impaired comprehension have lesions affecting posterior hemispheric structures (behind the rolandic fissure), whereas aphasic syndromes with intact comprehension typically have lesions limited to anterior hemispheric structures. Those localization rules apply only to right-handed adults. Children often exhibit nonfluent aphasias regardless of the lesion localization in the left hemisphere. Left-handed patients may have mixed cerebral dominance, resulting in atypical aphasia syndromes after localized left-hemisphere injuries.

Causal diagnosis is aided by aphasia syndrome identification. Wernicke's aphasia and conduction aphasia are most often caused by emboli, usually arising from the heart. Transcortical aphasias arise from lesions of the vascular border zone regions and are typically seen with large-vessel diseases involving the extracranial carotid arteries. Transcortical sensory aphasia is commonly observed in the middle phases of Alzheimer's disease. Global aphasia usually occurs with thrombotic occlusion of the left middle cerebral artery.

Amnesia and memory disorders Amnesia is an inability to learn new information despite normal attention, language, and other intellectual abilities. The amnestic syndrome is typically characterized by a period of *retrograde amnesia* extending back from the time of the onset of the amnesia and encompassing from a few seconds to a few years of the patient's life. Retrograde amnesia does not include all the patient's past life, and personal identity is not forgotten. "Amnesiacs" claiming to have forgotten all personal history are usually malingering or are suffering from an idiopathic psychiatric disorder. Amnestic syndromes also have an *anterograde amnesia* that extends forward from the time of the onset of the memory disorder. Anterograde amnesia may be temporary, lasting until memory functions recover, or it may be permanent. Patients exhibiting recovery of memory function may have a concomitant shrinking of retrograde amnesia as the anterograde amnesia resolves. The memory dysfunction in amnesia is an inability to store new information for later recall. Memory for newly learned information is not aided by clues or prompting strategies. *Confabulation* is characterized by untrue responses to questions but without a deliberate attempt to mislead. The confabulated responses are often drawn from the patient's actual experiences but are produced out of context. For example, when asked about their occupations, patients may produce detailed but untrue descriptions, the details of which are taken from jobs they had 10 or 20 years previously. Confabulation is common in the acute phases of amnesia but is rare in chronically amnestic patients.

The amnestic syndrome is associated with a restricted set of lesions involving limbic structures of the medial aspect of the cerebral hemispheres. The damage producing amnesia affects the hippocampus, the fornix, the mammillary bodies, or the medial thalamic nuclei. Severe amnesia usually reflects bilateral damage, whereas unilateral injury results in relatively modest and hemisphere-specific deficits, with left-sided lesions producing verbal amnesia and right-sided pathology causing deficits in learning nonverbal and visuospatial information.

The differential diagnosis of amnesia includes pathological processes that predominantly affect the medial hemispheric limbic areas. Table 2.1-12 lists the most common causes of amnesia and the site of the associated lesion. Hippocampal injury occurs with closed-head trauma, occlusion of the basilar or posterior cerebral artery, anoxia, hypoglycemia, and herpes simplex encephalitis. The hippocampus is involved early in the course of Alzheimer's disease, and an amnestic disorder is occasionally the presenting manifestation of that degenerative disorder. The fornix can be involved by surgery, brain tumors, and the rupture of anterior cerebral artery aneurysms. Mammillary bodies are affected in the Wernicke-Korsakoff syndrome and by brain tumors. The medial thalamic nuclei are involved in Wernicke-Korsakoff syndrome, brain tumors, and some cerebrovascular disorders

TABLE 2.1-11
Characteristics of the Major Aphasia Syndromes

Aphasia Type	Fluency	Comprehension	Repetition	Naming	Reading Comprehension	Reading Aloud	Writing
Wernicke's	F	Impaired	Impaired	Impaired	Impaired	Impaired	Impaired
Anomic	F	Normal	Normal	Impaired	Normal	Normal	Impaired
Conduction	F	Normal	Impaired	Impaired	Normal	Impaired	Impaired
Transcortical sensory	F	Impaired	Normal	Impaired	Impaired	Normal	Impaired
Broca's	NF	Normal	Impaired	Impaired	Normal	Impaired	Impaired
Transcortical motor	NF	Normal	Normal	Impaired	Normal	Impaired	Impaired
Mixed transcortical	NF	Impaired	Normal	Impaired	Impaired	Impaired	Impaired
Global	NF	Impaired	Impaired	Impaired	Impaired	Impaired	Impaired

F: fluent; NF: nonfluent.

TABLE 2.1-12
Most Common Causes of Amnesia and the Associated Site of the Lesion

Syndrome	Anatomical Site of Pathology
Wernicke-Korsakoff syndrome	Mammillary bodies, medial dorsal nucleus of the thalamus
Head trauma	Hippocampus
Cerebrovascular disease (posterior cerebral artery)	Hippocampus, thalamus
Subarachnoid hemorrhage (rupture of aneurysm of anterior cerebral artery)	Fornix
Anoxia	Hippocampus
Hypoglycemia	Hippocampus
Herpes simplex encephalitis	Hippocampus
Alzheimer's disease	Hippocampus
Neoplasms	Fornix, hypothalamus, thalamus
Surgery (lobectomy)	Temporal lobe
Transient global amnesia	Hippocampal ischemia (in some cases)
Electroconvulsive therapy	Uncertain

(occlusion of the thalamoperforant branches of the posterior communicating and posterior cerebral arteries).

A few clinical signs help distinguish the amnestic disorders. The Wernicke-Korsakoff syndrome classically evolves through an acute phase of Wernicke's encephalopathy, characterized by ophthalmoplegia, ataxia, and delirium. If the responsible thiamine deficiency is not reversed, the patient progresses into the Wernicke-Korsakoff syndrome, which includes amnesia, nystagmus, and ataxia. A peripheral neuropathy is usually present, and a history of alcohol abuse is common, although any cause of thiamine deficiency (starvation, prolonged vomiting, gastric carcinoma) can produce the Wernicke-Korsakoff syndrome. Lesions of the hippocampus (for example, posterior cerebral artery occlusion, herpes encephalitis) commonly impinge on the adjacent fibers of the optic radiation and cause a superior quadrantanopsia or homonymous hemianopsia. Frontal-lobe-type behavioral disturbances commonly accompany posttraumatic amnesias because of orbitofrontal injuries occurring in conjunction with the temporal lobe damage.

Amnesia must be distinguished from several other types of memory abnormalities. *Age-associated memory impairment* (also known as benign senescent forgetfulness) occurs in the course of normal aging. It is characterized by impaired spontaneous recall, retained recognition skills, an absence of deficits in other neuropsychological domains, and an awareness of the loss of timely recall. It is not the harbinger of a dementing illness. The characteristic memory disturbance of *Alzheimer's disease* features both difficulty in learning new information and impaired remote recall. In the early phases of the disease, remotely learned information is better recalled than recently learned material. Late in the course of the illness, the patient is unable to remember both remote information and newly learned material. The memory abnormality in the *subcortical dementias,* such as Huntington's disease and Parkinson's disease, is a recall deficit with intact recognition. Patients learn and retain information but have difficulty in spontaneously retrieving it. Unlike amnestic patients, they are aided by clues, prompting strategies, and encoding enhancement techniques, such as embedding the to-be-remembered material in a story.

Frontal lobe disorders Frontal lobe disorders are among the most important syndromes in neuropsychiatry. Frontal lobe dysfunction is present in many idiopathic psychiatric diseases (depressive disorders, schizophrenia, obsessive-compulsive disorder), and frontal lobe lesions produce profound behavioral alterations. Lesions of the deep subcortical and the superficial cortical structures of the frontal lobe produce behavioral disorders; frontal systems dysfunction reflects the anatomy of the conditions with frontal-lobe-type behaviors.

Three behavioral complexes are currently recognized with frontal systems dysfunction: an orbitofrontal disinhibition syndrome, a medial frontal apathetic-akinetic syndrome, and a frontal convexity motor programming disorder (Table 2.1-13). Combinations of symptoms are the rule, rather than the exception, in most patients with frontal lobe disorders. An understanding of the symptoms of frontal lobe dysfunction is evolving, and a more definitive clinical classification is likely to be developed.

The *orbitofrontal syndrome* is the best known and most flamboyant of the frontal lobe behavioral disorders. Patients with the syndrome are disinhibited, making tactless remarks and acting on impulse. They are coarsened, lack empathy, and show little concern for the feelings of others. They fail to plan ahead and exhibit little concern about their illness or the future. Their mood is typically irritable and labile, with a fatuous euphoria. Inappropriate jocularity and an insensitive humor *(witzelsucht)* may be observed. The patient shows a lack of social restraint and an undue familiarity with strangers. Despite the marked behavioral alterations, the patient may have few or no neuropsychological deficits and may exhibit intact language, memory, and visuospatial skills. The orbitofrontal syndrome occurs with posttraumatic encephalopathy, frontal brain tumors (particularly inferior frontal meningiomas), anterior cerebral artery occlusions or aneurysm rupture, multiple sclerosis, and degenerative frontal lobe diseases, such as Pick's disease. Deficits in olfaction are common accompaniments of

TABLE 2.1-13
Principal Frontal Lobe Syndromes

Behavioral Syndrome	Location of Major Pathology	Features
Disinhibition	Orbitofrontal	Impulsiveness, loss of tact, coarseness, facetiousness
Apathy	Medial frontal	Limited motivation and initiative
Executive deficits	Frontal convexity	Perseveration, impersistence, impaired serial order behavior

the syndrome because of the proximity of the olfactory nerves, bulbs, and tracts to the orbital surface. The syndrome has been observed with inferior caudate lesions and disturbances of the orbitofrontal cortex.

The *medial frontal lobe syndrome* is also a striking behavioral disorder. The severity of the syndrome extends from *akinetic mutism* at the most severe end of the spectrum to a mild lack of motivation on the other end. Akinetic mutism occurs with bilateral medial frontal lesions and is characterized by mutism and limited spontaneous movement. Patients with the syndrome, however, appear alert, have their eyes open, exhibit ocular following movements of environmental events, eat when fed, and may move with persistent stimulation or pain. The syndrome has been reported with bilateral anterior cerebral artery occlusions, trauma, hydrocephalus, bilateral thalamic infarction, and midline tumors of the thalamus, the third ventricle, the hypothalamus, and the pituitary. Partial amelioration of the syndrome with dopaminergic agents (pergolide [Permax], bromocriptine [Parlodel]) suggests that interruption of the ascending dopaminergic fibers plays a role in the pathophysiology of the disorder. An attenuated form of the syndrome occurs with unilateral medial frontal lobe lesions. Loss of initiative, poor motivation, limited gesturing, and apathy characterize the spontaneous behavior of patients with medial frontal lesions. A variety of neurobehavioral and neuropsychological abnormalities may accompany the neuropsychiatric disorders. With left-sided lesions, patients manifest transcortical motor aphasia with little speech initiation, nonfluent output, intact comprehension, and preserved repetition. With lesions of either hemisphere, a callosal apraxia with inability to perform learned motor acts on command with the left hand may also be present. If the lesion extends posteriorly to the medial central gyrus, paresis of the contralateral leg and foot is evident.

Frontal convexity lesions produce abnormalities of sequential behavior, including perseveration (abnormal continuation of behavior), impersistence (abnormal early termination of behavior), deficits in set shifting, and disturbances of programming sequential motor acts, such as alternating programs, reciprocal programs, multiple loops, and serial hand sequences (Figures 2.1-1 and 2.1-2). Patients also have difficulty in developing strategies that facilitate the copying of complex figures (Figure 2.1-3), exhibit poor judgment, and are concrete on tests of abstraction. The patient may have no elementary neurological abnormalities. Tumors, cerebrovascular trauma, and frontal degenerations account for most cases of frontal convexity syndromes. The condition has been observed with dorsal caudate lesions, as well as frontal convexity lesions.

Depression occurs with lesions in many regions of the brain but is most common with lesions of the frontal lobe and the caudate nucleus. Within the left hemisphere, the closer the lesion is to the frontal pole, the more frequent and the more severe are the associated depressive symptoms. Depression frequently accompanies the frontal convexity syndrome.

Frontal lobe syndromes contrast with clinical disorders associated with temporal, parietal, and occipital dysfunction (Table 2.1-10). The hallmark of left temporoparietal disorders is fluent aphasia; medial left temporal lesions produce verbal amnesia. Right temporoparietal lesions produce receptive aprosody and amusia, contralateral neglect, anosognosia, and construction disturbances. Neglect and construction impairment occur with both left and right temporoparietal lesions but tend to be less severe and less enduring with left temporoparietal lesions. Medial right temporal disorders cause nonverbal amnesia, and bilateral medial temporal lesions are associated with *Klüver-Bucy syndrome* (placidity, hyperorality, hypermetamorphosis, hypersexuality, and psychic blindess). Bilateral temporoparietal lesions cause *Balint's syndrome* (ataxia of optically guided movements, inability to refixate the eyes after fixations without first closing the eyes, inability to see more than one object at a time). Left occipital lesions produce alexia and agraphia if the posterior aspect of the corpus callosum is also involved. Anomia and visual hallucinations have also been associated with left posterior dysfunction. Right and left occipital lesions cause visual hallucinations. Bilateral occipital lesions may produce either *cerebral blindness* or markedly constricted visual fields. *Anton's syndrome* is the combination of cerebral blindness and denial of blindness.

Neglect and anosognosia Unilateral *neglect* is a hemi-inattention syndrome in which the patient fails to attend to or act on stimuli in one hemiuniverse. Visual neglect is striking and easily demonstrable, but, in its fully developed form, hemisensory neglect includes all sensory modalities, including hearing and touch. Hemimotor neglect may also occur, with the patient failing to act in one hemispace. The patient with neglect ignores one half of objects when copying or drawing, may not dress or groom one-half of the body, does not see or hear persons and events occurring on one side of the body, and extinguishes (fails to perceive) stimuli on the side contralateral to the lesion when both sides of the body or the visual field are stimulated. Hemisensory neglect is more common and more enduring with lesions of the right parietal lobe or the right thalamus than with left-sided lesions, but it occurs with injury to either hemisphere. Motor neglect occurs with frontal or subcortical damage.

Anosognosia is the denial of hemiparesis that occurs in some patients with unilateral neglect. In some usages, the term has been extended to encompass all forms of denial of illness. A variety of anosognosic phenomena have been described, enlarging the syndrome to include all types of abnormal regard for the affected limbs. *Hemiasomatognosia* is neglect of one side of the body when there is no hemiparesis, and *somatophrenia* is the term denoting denial of ownership of one's paretic limbs. When limb weakness is acknowledged but minimized, the term *anosodiaphoria* is used; hatred of a weak limb is called *misoplegia*. Preoccupation and personification (for example, naming the limb) are two other variants of anosognosia.

NEUROPSYCHIATRIC SYNDROMES

Delusions *Delusions* are false beliefs held despite evidence to the contrary and occur in a variety of neurological disorders. They are most common in Alzheimer's disease, vascular dementia, Huntington's disease, temporal lobe epilepsy, and multiple sclerosis. They also occur in posttraumatic encephalopathy, Wilson's disease and other degenerative extrapyramidal disorders, and brain tumors, but they are not common in those conditions. Delusions are rare in Parkinson's disease except as a manifestation of dopamine or anticholinergic toxicity. Delusions are frequent in delirium. When delusions occur with focal lesions, the injury is usually in the left or right temporoparietal region. With left-sided lesions, delusions occur in conjunction with Wernicke's aphasia; with right-sided lesions, prominent visual hallucinations commonly accompany the delusional disorder. Together, those clinical observations indicate that delusions are most common in diseases affecting the temporal lobe cortex or the basal ganglia, particularly the caudate nucleus. Delusions are more frequent in disorders with bilateral damage than in disorders with unilateral alterations.

Several principles aid in characterizing and understanding delusions in neurological diseases. First, delusions are not reactions to declining intellectual function; the more intact the delusional patient's cognition, the more complex the delusions tend to be. Patients with dementing illnesses have simple delusions, whereas patients with single cerebrovascular events or other limited lesions exhibit complex, well-structured, and firmly held delusional beliefs. The intellect is in the service of the delusional process. Second, no specific neuropsychological correlates of delusions (for example, deficits in memory, language, visuospatial functions, and frontal lobe abilities) have been consistently identified. Third, no delusional content distinguishes neurological illnesses from such idiopathic psychotic processes as schizophrenia. Most delusions in neurological illness tend to be persecutory beliefs, but any type of delusional content can be observed (Table 2.1-2). Fourth, visual hallucinations are more common in conjunction with delusions in neurological illness than in conjunction with idiopathic psychoses. Auditory hallucinations occur with delusions in both neurological and idiopathic psychiatric disorders. Fifth, delusions are most common in diseases affecting both hemispheres, such as the degenerative disorders and vascular dementia. Sixth, when delusions follow unilateral lesions, the laterality of the damage may influence the delusion content. Schneiderian first-rank symptoms are common with left-sided lesions, and delusions of substitution, such as Capgras's syndrome, are common with right-hemisphere lesions. Seventh, delusions are not invariably linked to lesions in specific anatomical structures in the same way that a hemiparesis predictably follows a pyramidal tract lesion, and other nonanatomical factors (biochemical changes, developmental factors, environmental conditions) must participate in determining the occurrence of the delusions. Eighth, the onset of the delusions is often delayed for considerable periods after the occurrence of a brain insult. In temporal lobe epilepsy, for example, several years may elapse between the occurrence of the brain injury with the onset of the seizures and the first appearance of delusions. Ninth, the treatment of delusions in a neurological illness involves addressing both the delusions and the underlying illness. Delusions may respond to antipsychotic agents and rarely improve with anticonvulsants and other nonantipsychotic medications.

Hallucinations *Hallucinations* are sensory perceptions occurring without the appropriate stimulation of the corresponding sensory organ. Visual hallucinations are common in neurological illness. The differential diagnosis of visual hallucinations is presented in Table 2.1-14. Ocular disorders that produce total or partial blindness—enucleation, cataracts, macular degeneration, retinal diseases, and vitreous traction—are common causes of hallucinations. *Vitreous traction* produces unformed flashes of light; the other processes may produce formed or unformed hallucinations. Inflammation of the optic nerves from ischemic optic neuritis or optic nerve demyelination can cause phosphenes or unformed flashes of light.

Lesions of the midbrain produce the syndrome of *peduncular hallucinosis,* characterized by visual hallucinations typically of a formed type occurring in the evening and associated with a benign affect. A sleep disturbance is usually present. The condition rarely lasts more than a few days. Peduncular hallucinosis has been produced by midbrain cerebrovascular insults and brainstem tumors.

Lesions of the geniculocalcarine radiations produce visual field defects. Hallucinations within the field abnormality are common in the period soon after the injury occurs. Known as *release hallucinations,* they are usually formed, are not necessarily stereotyped from episode to episode, last from minutes to hours at a time, and may be modified by moving or closing the eyes.

Focal seizures may produce visual hallucinations. Occipital foci tend to produce unformed hallucinations; parietal and temporal foci produce formed hallucinations. *Ictal hallucinations* are brief and stereotyped. They may be associated with other seizure phenomena (for example, interruption of consciousness, head or eye deviation) and are generally not lateralized in the visual field. Micropsia (things look small and far away), macropsia (things look large and close), and metamorphopsia (distortions) may also occur in the course of seizures.

Hallucinations in *migraine* vary from simple light flashes to scintillating scotomata to fully formed complex visions. The classic hallucination of migraine is a fortification spectrum that looks like the jagged top of the wall of a fort or a castle. Hallucinations precede the headache and may be the dominant aspect of the migrainous attack. Micropsia and macropsia may occur in migraine, in which they are termed the Alice in Wonderland syndrome.

Narcolepsy is associated with the tetrad of sleep attacks, visual hallucinations, cataplexy (loss of muscle tone with subsequent falling), and sleep paralysis (momentary inability to move or speak on awakening from sleep). The hallucinations occur on falling asleep (hypnagogic) or on awakening (hypnopompic) and are usually terrifying in nature. Documentation of sleep-onset rapid eye movement (REM) sleep confirms the diagnosis.

Visual hallucinations are common in delirium associated with toxic and metabolic encephalopathies, in alcohol and sedative-hypnotic withdrawal, and with the ingestion of hallucinogenic agents, such as lysergic acid diethylamide (LSD), psylocibin, mescaline, and phencyclidine (PCP). Visual hallucinations occur in up to 30 percent of patients with Parkinson's disease treated with dopaminergic agents, such as levodopa, bromocriptine, and pergolide.

Visual hallucinations occur in idiopathic psychoses, including schizophrenia, depression, and mania. They are rarely the dominant type of hallucination in those circumstances. Normal people may experience visual hallucinations on falling asleep or in the course of sensory or sleep deprivation. The imaginary companions of childhood often have a visual aspect.

Hallucinations in other sensory modalities are less common than visual hallucination in neurological illnesses. *Auditory hallucinations* occur in conjunction with persecutory delusions in delusional disorders. Hallucinations may also occur with deafness, brainstem lesions, and epilepsy. *Tactile hallucinations* are reported in delirium and withdrawal (particularly opiate withdrawal) and in association with delusions of infestation. *Gustatory and olfactory hallucinations* occur in psychoses and epilepsy.

TABLE 2.1-14
Differential Diagnosis of Visual Hallucinations

Condition or Lesion Location	Cause
Ocular pathology	Enucleation Cataracts Macular degeneration Vitreous traction
Optic nerve pathology	Optic neuritis (ischemic, demyelinating)
Brainstem pathology	Peduncular hallucinosis (infarction, tumor)
Cerebral hemispheric lesions	Geniculocalcarine lesions (infarction, tumor) Epilepsy
Neurological illnesses	Migraine Narcolepsy
Medical illnesses	Delirium
Toxic disorders	Delirium Withdrawal Hallucinogens
Psychiatric disorders	Schizophrenia Mania Depression
Normal conditions	Hypnagogic hallucinations Imaginary companions of childhood Sensory deprivation Sleep deprivation

Depression Depressive symptoms are common in neurological diseases. In some cases the mood changes represent grief for a lost function, an altered role and status, and increased dependence. In many patients, however, the depression is more severe than anticipated for the functional disability and greater than that experienced by patients with nonneurological disabling diseases. In those patients, the depression is a behavioral manifestation of the brain dysfunction. Neurological diseases in which depression has been identified as a prominent abnormality include Parkinson's disease, Huntington's disease, Wilson's disease, idiopathic basal ganglia calcification, cerebrovascular disorders, multiple sclerosis, and epilepsy. Endocrine disorders, systemic illnesses, and a wide variety of medications are also capable of inducing a depressive disorder.

The diagnosis of depression in patients with neurological illness presents a difficult challenge. Many neurological diseases without mood changes produce symptoms that are characteristic of depressive episodes—diminished pleasure and interest, weight loss, insomnia, agitation, retardation, fatigue, impaired concentration—and may lead to the misdiagnosis of depression. Other neurological illnesses, such as the parkinsonian disorders, produce psychomotor slowing, bowed posture, fatigue, and impaired concentration; the presence of depression in those disorders can easily be overlooked. Experiential manifestations of depression—including feelings of sadness, worthlessness, hopelessness, and recurrent thoughts of death or suicide—are the most dependable indicators of a depressive syndrome and should be sought. Patients with dementia, however, may be unable to describe the subjective symptoms, and depression must be inferred from the associated symptoms.

A few observations pertain to most neurological disorders manifesting depression as part of their symptom complex. First, the entire spectrum of depression severity may be observed, with some patients manifesting few mood symptoms and others meeting all the criteria for a major depressive episode. Second, frontal-subcortical systems structures are the sites most often implicated in the depression syndromes. Depression syndromes may occur with lesions elsewhere in the nervous system, but they are less common and less severe. Left-sided lesions are more commonly associated with depression than are right-sided lesions. Third, preliminary evidence indicates that depressive symptoms may differ subtly in different neurological disorders. Suicide is common in Huntington's disease and epilepsy but is rare in Parkinson's disease; psychosis is common in depressed patients with epilepsy and rare in Parkinson's disease; the depression of Parkinson's disease is characterized by more anxiety and less guilt than is idiopathic depression; psychomotor retardation is more extreme in poststroke depression than in other depression syndromes. Fourth, depression in neurological diseases usually responds to treatment with psychopharmacological agents or electroconvulsive therapy.

Mania Mania (secondary mania) is much less common than depression in the course of neurological illness. Manic symptoms have been observed in Huntington's disease, Wilson's disease, idiopathic basal ganglia calcification, cerebrovascular disorders, trauma, multiple sclerosis, general paresis, viral encephalitis, and postencephalitis syndromes, frontal degenerative disorders and after a thalamotomy. A variety of medications also produce manic behavior, including steroids, triazolobenzodiazepines, dopaminergic agents, thyroid preparations, sympathomimetics, and stimulants. Antidepressants may precipitate manic episodes in depressed patients.

Structural lesions producing mania usually involve the basotemporal region, the parathalamic structures, and the inferior medial frontal lobe. When lateralized, the lesions have a marked right-sided predominance. A family history of psychiatric illness is more common in patients with secondary mania than in normal controls or in patients with secondary depression, and genetic vulnerability may facilitate the appearance of mania in the setting of brain dysfunction. The natural history of secondary mania is variable; patients may experience a single manic episode, recurrent mania, or alternating periods of depression and mania. The optimal treatment of secondary mania has not been determined. Tranquilization may be necessary in the acute phases of the manic episode; lithium (Eskalith), carbamazepine (Tegretol), clonazepam (Klonopin), and valproate (Depakene) may be used in the treatment of secondary mania; those agents may also be used prophylactically in patients who experience repeated episodes of manic behavior.

Personality alterations *Personality* is the term used for the stable patterns of behavior that include the way one relates to, perceives, and thinks about the environment and oneself. It is the least explored area of neuropsychiatry. Personality changes have been difficult to quantify for study, and personality alterations may be difficult to distinguish from the delusional and mood disorders that also occur in neurological illness. Moreover, the effects of personality vary among the neurological disorders, and few generalizations are currently possible. Table 2.1-15 summarizes the personality alterations routinely observed in specific neurological diseases and conditions.

TABLE 2.1-15
Personality Alterations in Neurological Illnesses

Neurological Disease	Personality Alteration
Alzheimer's disease	Disengagement, indifference
Frontal lobe degenerations	Disinhibition or apathy
Huntington's disease	Irritability, impulsiveness
HIV* encephalopathy	Apathy
Focal lesions	
Orbitofrontal	Irritability, impulsiveness, pseudopsychopathy
Medial frontal	Apathy, loss of motivation and initiative
Right hemisphere (childhood)	Schizoid
Right hemisphere (adult)	Alexithymia
Left hemisphere (Wernicke's area)	Suspiciousness, irritability
Bilateral temporal lobe	Placidity (component of the Klüver-Bucy syndrome)
Ventromedial hypothalamus	Rage
Temporal lobe epilepsy	Suspiciousness, Geschwind's syndrome (hyperreligiosity, circumstantiality, hypergraphia, viscosity, hyposexuality)

*HIV: human immunodeficiency virus.

Alzheimer's disease has a profound effect on personality, and the behavioral changes may predate the neuropsychological deficits. Early in the illness, patients become disengaged and indifferent, showing little concern about their own disease and little insight into the feelings of family members. Late in the course of the disease, impulsiveness and aggression are often exhibited. Patients with other dementia syndromes exhibit contrasting personality alterations. Frontal lobe degenerations, such as Pick's disease, usually produce the disinhibition, impulsiveness, and facetiousness characteristic of orbitofrontal dysfunction or the apathy suggestive of medial frontal pathology. Huntington's disease combines marked irritability with impulsiveness, sometimes leading to aggression, violence, and suicide. Many subcortical dementia syndromes (for example, Parkinson's disease, progressive supranuclear palsy, and HIV encephalopathy) cause apathy and indifference.

Focal lesions may also be associated with personality alterations. The marked personality alterations after orbitofrontal and medial frontal lesions were described above. Patients with Wernicke's aphasia are often suspicious, demanding, aggressive, and irritable. Preliminary studies of adults with right-hemisphere lesions suggest that they exhibit alexithymia, with a reserved expression of emotions and a tendency to forgo symbolic thought. Right-hemisphere damage sustained in childhood may result in a schizoid type of behavioral pattern, perhaps because the inability to perceive or to execute emotional cues limits the child's ability to engage in interpersonal relationships.

Limbic system lesions have profound effects on personality. Ventromedial hypothalamic lesions produce a syndrome of dementia, hyperphagia, and rage. Bilateral medial temporal lobe lesions produce Klüver-Bucy syndrome, characterized by placidity, hypersexuality and altered sexual behavior, visual agnosia, *hypermetamorphosis* (compulsive exploration of environmental stimuli), and hyperorality.

A controversial area of research in neuropsychiatry concerns personality changes in epilepsy. Personality inventories reveal that the most common type of personality change in epileptic patients is increased suspiciousness and paranoia. An uncommon syndrome (known as the temporal lobe epilepsy personality or Geschwind's syndrome), occurring in patients with partial complex seizures, consists of hypergraphia, circumstantiality, interpersonal viscosity, hyperreligiosity, and hyposexuality. That personality style is not unique to epilepsy but occurs with increased frequency in epileptic patients and can be the presenting manifestation of the limbic seizure disorder.

Anxiety Anxiety is a state of apprehension, tension, or uneasiness that occurs in anticipation of internal or external danger. The anxiety syndrome includes motor tension, autonomic hyperactivity, apprehensive expectation, and heightened vigilance. Anxiety occurs in a variety of neurological and medical disorders and can be precipitated by drugs. Neurological diseases causing anxiety include brain tumors (particularly in the regions of the temporal lobe and the third ventricle), trauma, cerebrovascular disorders, migraine, encephalitis, multiple sclerosis, epilepsy, Parkinson's disease, Huntington's disease and Wilson's disease. The principal medical conditions associated with anxiety include hypoxia, hypoglycemia, hyperthyroidism, Cushing's disease, and mitral valve prolapse. Medications capable of causing anxiety are amphetamines, cocaine, sympathomimetics, caffeine, organophosphate compounds, lidocaine (Xylocaine), and procaine penicillin. Withdrawal from alcohol and sedative-hypnotics is frequently accompanied by anxiety. When anxiety is associated with focal brain lesions, the pathology usually involves the right temporal lobe.

The treatment of anxiety in neurological disorders requires attention to the underlying condition, as well as to the anxiety symptoms. When pharmacological agents are indicated, conventional anxiolytics and β-receptor blocking agents are used.

Obsessive-compulsive disorder *Obsessions* are recurrent, intrusive, senseless ideas, thoughts, and images that are egodystonic and involuntary. *Compulsions* are repetitive activities carried out in response to an obsession or executed in a stereotyped and ritualized fashion. Lesions in the basal ganglia are associated with obsessive-compulsive behavior (Table 2.1-16). Conditions affecting the basal ganglia and producing obsessive-compulsive disorder include idiopathic Parkinson's disease, postencephalitic Parkinson's disease, Huntington's disease, progressive supranuclear palsy, Tourette's disorder, neuroacanthocytosis, Sydenham's chorea, carbon monoxide poisoning, neonatal hypoxia, bilateral caudate infarctions, cardiopulmonary arrest, and manganese poisoning. Obsessional thinking has also been observed in conjunction with antipsychotic-induced and postencephalitic oculogyric crises.

The treatment of obsessions and compulsions in neurological disorders entails treating the underlying disease and providing symptomatic relief for the obsessive-compulsive disorder.

Paraphilias and altered sexual drive Neurological disorders can produce paraphilic behavior and alterations in the sexual drive. Markedly diminished libido occurs with temporal lobe epilepsy, hypothalamic lesions, and right-hemisphere brain injuries. Heightened sexual drive occurs in secondary mania, in the postictal period after a seizure, after markedly improved seizure control in patients with epilepsy (for example, after temporal lobectomy or with improved anticonvulsant control of seizures), after the introduction of levodopa or other dopaminergic agents in Parkinson's disease, with diencephalic or frontal lobe lesions, with septal injury, and in Klüver-Bucy syndrome. Hypersexuality has also been induced by amphetamines, cocaine, hyperthyroidism, hypercortisolism, and androgen administration.

Paraphilias are characterized by intense sexual urges and sexually arousing fantasies, usually involving nonhuman objects or animals, the suffering or humiliation of oneself or one's partner, or children or other nonconsenting persons. Examples of paraphilias include exhibitionism, fetishism, frotteurism, pedophilia, sexual masochism, sexual sadism, transvestic fetishism, voyeurism, bestiality (zoophilia), and telephone scatologia. Paraphilic behavior has been described in association with temporal lobe epilepsy, postencephalitic states, Tourette's disorder, frontal lobe disorders, Huntington's disease, brainstem tumors, bilateral temporal injury, septal injury, and multiple sclerosis. Paraphilic behavior has occasionally occurred with dopaminergic therapy for Parkinson's disease.

TABLE 2.1-16
Neurological Disorders Associated with Obsessive-Compulsive Disorder

Parkinsonism with compulsions during on period in patients experiencing on-off swings
Postencephalitic parkinsonism
Progressive supranuclear palsy
Huntington's disease
Neuroacanthocytosis
Tourette's disorder
Sydenham's chorea
Carbon monoxide poisoning with bilateral caudate nucleus lesions
Carbon monoxide intoxication with bilateral globus pallidus injury
Bilateral caudate nucleus infarctions
Anoxic injury to the caudate and the putamen
Anoxia with bilateral globus pallidus lesions
Manganese intoxication
Acute dystonic reactions with oculogyric crises

SUGGESTED CROSS-REFERENCES

Other sections in Chapter 2 discuss the neuropsychiatric aspects of various disorders. Neuroimaging is discussed in Sections 1.10 and 2.10. Clinical assessment and diagnosis are also discussed in Chapter 9; Section 9.8 discusses psychiatric rating scales, including the Mini-Mental State examination. Cognitive disorders are discussed in Chapter 12, schizophrenia in Chapter 14, mood disorders in Chapter 16, anxiety disorders in Chapter 17, and paraphilias in Section 21.2. Biological therapies are discussed in Chapter 32.

REFERENCES

Adams R D, Victor M: *Principles of Neurology,* ed 4. McGraw-Hill, New York, 1989.

Bruton D J, Stevens R, Frith C D: Epilepsy, psychosis, and schizophrenia: Clinical and neuropathologic correlations. Neurology *44:* 34, 1994.

*Coffey E C, Cummings J L, editors: *Textbook of Geriatric Neuropsychiatry.* American Psychiatric Press, Washington, 1994.

Cummings J L: Behavioral complications of drug treatment of Parkinson's disease. J Am Geriatr Soc *39:* 708, 1991.

Cummings J L: *Clinical Neuropsychiatry.* Grune & Stratton, New York, 1985.

*Cummings J L: Depression and Parkinson's disease: A review. Am J Psychiatry *149:* 443, 1992.

Cummings J L: Frontal-subcortical circuits and human behavior. Arch Neurol *50:* 873, 1993.

*Cummings J L: The neuroanatomy of depression. J Clin Psychiatry *54* (11, Suppl): 14, 1993.

Cummings J L, Petry S, Dian L, Shapira J, Hill M A: Organic personality disorder in dementia syndrome: An inventory approach. J Neuropsychiatr Clin Neurosci *2:* 261, 1990.

Cummings J L, Victoroff J I: Noncognitive neuropsychiatric syndromes in Alzheimer's disease. Neuropsychiatr Neuropsychol Behav Neurol *3:* 140, 1990.

Cutting J: *The Right Cerebral Hemisphere and Psychiatric Disorders.* Oxford Medical, New York, 1990.

*Damasio H, Damasio A R: *Lesion Analysis in Neuropsychology.* Oxford University Press, New York, 1989.

DeJong R N: *The Neurologic Examination,* ed 4. Harper & Row, New York, 1979.

Folstein M F, Folstein S E, McHugh P R: "Mini-Mental State": A practical method for grading the cognitive state of patients for the clinician. J Psychiatr Res *12:* 189, 1975.

Glaser J S: *Neuro-ophthalmology.* Harper & Row, New York, 1978.

Irle E, Peper M, Wowra B, Kunze S: Mood changes after surgery for tumors of the cerebral cortex. Arch Neurol *51:* 164, 1994.

Jones K L: *Smith's Recognizable Patterns of Human Malformation,* ed 4. Saunders, Philadelphia, 1988.

Jorge R E, Robinson R G, Arndt S V, Forrester A W, Geisler F, Starkstein S E: Comparison between acute- and delayed-onset depression following brain injury. J Neuropsychiatry Clin Neurosci *5:* 43, 1993.

Kiernan R J, Mueller, J, Langston J W, Van Dyke C: The Neurobehavioral Cognitive Status Examination: A brief but differentiated approach to cognitive assessment. Ann Intern Med *107:* 481, 1987.

Lance, J W, McLeod J G: *A Physiological Approach to Clinical Neurology,* ed 3. Butterworth, Boston, 1981.

*Laplane D, Levasseur M, Pillon B, Dubois B, Baulac M, Mazoyer B, Tinh T, Sette G, Danze F, Baron J C: Obsessive-compulsive and other behavioural changes with bilateral basal ganglia lesions. Brain *112:* 699, 1989.

Lishman W A: *Organic Psychiatry*, ed 2. Blackwell Scientific, Boston, 1987.
Mayberg H S, Starkstein S E, Peyser C E, Dannals R F, Folstein S E: Paralimbic frontal lobe hypometabolism in depression associated with Huntington's disease. Neurology *42:* 1791, 1992.
McKeith I G, Fairburn A F, Bothwell R A, Moore P B, Ferrier I N, Thompson P, Perry R H: An evaluation of the predictive validity and inter-rater reliability of clinical diagnostic criteria for senile dementia of the Lewy body type. Neurology *44:* 872, 1994.
Miller B L, Cummings J L, McIntyre H, Ebers G, Grode M: Hypersexuality or altered sexual preference following brain injury. J Neurol Neurosurg Psychiatry *49:* 867, 1986.
Pearlman A L, Collins R C, editors: *Neurobiology of Disease*. Oxford University Press, New York, 1990.
Pillon B, Deweer B, Agid Y, Dubois B: Explicit memory in Alzheimer's, Huntington's and Parkinson's disease. Arch Neurol *50:* 374, 1993.
Plum F, Posner J B: *The Diagnosis of Stupor and Coma*, ed 3. Davis, Philadelphia, 1980.
Robinson R G, Starkstein S E: Current research in affective disorders following stroke. J Neuropsychiatry Clin Neurosci *2:* 1, 1990.
Shukla S, Cook B L, Mukherjee S, Godwin C, Miller M G: Mania following head trauma. Am J Psychiatry *144:* 93, 1987.
Simon R P, Aminoff M J, Greenberg D A: *Clinical Neurology, 1989*. Appleton & Lange, Norwalk, CT, 1989.
Squire L R, Zola-Morgan S: The medial temporal lobe memory system. Science *253:* 1380, 1991.
Starkstein S E, Mayberg H S, Bertheir M L, Fedoroff P, Price T R, Dannals R F, Wagner H N, Leiguarda R, Robinson R G: Mania after brain injury: Neuroradiological and metabolic findings. Ann Neurol *27:* 652, 1990.
Strub R L, Black F W: *The Mental Status Examination in Neurology*, ed 2. Davis, Philadelphia, 1985.
Sultzer D L, Cummings J L: Drug-induced mania: Causative agents, clinical characteristics and management. Med Toxicol Adverse Drug Exp *4:* 127, 1989.
Sultzer D L, Levin H S, Mahler M E, High W M, Cummings J L: A comparison of psychiatric symptoms in vascular dementia and Alzheimer's disease. Am J Psychiatry *150:* 1806, 1993.
Tinetti M E: Performance-oriented assessment of mobility problems in elderly patients. J Am Geriatr Soc *34:* 119, 1986.
Weiner W J, Lang A E: *Movement Disorders. A Comprehensive Survey*. Futura, Mount Kisco, NY, 1989.
Wragg R E, Jeste D V: Overview of depression and psychosis in Alzheimer's disease. Am J Psychiatry *146:* 577, 1989.

2.2 NEUROPSYCHIATRIC ASPECTS OF CEREBROVASCULAR DISEASES AND TUMORS

WILLIAM E. REICHMAN, M.D.

INTRODUCTION

The clinical study of the effects of cerebrovascular disease (commonly called stroke) on cognition, mood, and personality has yielded valuable information about the neural basis of behavior. Like cerebrovascular diseases, mass-occupying lesions, such as primary and metastatic intracranial tumors, produce direct and indirect effects on brain functions that often result in behavioral alterations. This section reviews the neurological, neurobehavioral, and psychiatric consequences of brain injury resulting from cerebral infarctions, hemorrhages, and tumors. Attention is directed to the pathogenesis of the disorders and to evaluative techniques, including neuroimaging and laboratory assessment.

CEREBROVASCULAR DISEASES

DEFINITION AND CLINICAL CHARACTERISTICS *Stroke* is a syndrome of focal cerebral dysfunction caused by a vascular event. The clinical hallmark of stroke is the sudden onset of neurological signs and symptoms. Disturbances of the cerebral circulation culminating in stroke result from thrombosis, embolism, hemorrhage, systemic hypotension, hypertension, anoxia, and disorders of the blood, such as polycythemia. The clinical features of stroke may include focal neurological deficits, such as hemiparesis, hemisensory loss, and aphasia. The sudden onset of headache, dysarthria, or ataxia may also herald the onset of a cerebrovascular event. In hemorrhagic stroke the onset is often marked by a dramatically severe headache accompanied by emesis and drowsiness. Neck stiffness and photophobia may also be noted but are not accompanied by fever, as in meningitis. Intracranial hemorrhage is generally the consequence of aneurysmal rupture; the observed clinical syndrome reflects the anatomical site of bleeding. In embolic stroke the clinical signs and symptoms develop most rapidly, as there is less time for the development of collateral circulation.

ETIOLOGY Cerebrovascular events may result from extracranial hypoperfusion, intracranial thrombosis or hemorrhage, and embolization from the heart or the large extracranial vessels. In addition to hypertensive atherosclerosis, stroke may be associated with a large number of systemic illnesses that affect perfusion and the cerebral vasculature (Table 2.2-1). Factors such as age, sex, race, and geographic setting influence the incidence and prevalence figures related to the cause of stroke. Although thrombotic stroke is uncommon before the fifth decade of life, the incidence rates of cerebral embolism and subarachnoid hemorrhage are evenly spread throughout all age groups. Specifically, the incidence of cerebral hemorrhage appears to be greatest between the ages of 40 and 60. The incidence of cerebral infarction, caused by a thrombosis or an embolism, is greatest in those aged 60 to 80 years. Although

TABLE 2.2-1
Causes of Stroke

- Atherosclerosis
- Embolism
- Saccular aneurysm or arteriovenous malformation (ruptured or unruptured)
- Arteritis
  - Infectious: meningovascular syphilis; pyogenic and tuberculous meningitis; rare infections, such as typhus, schistosomiasis, trichinosis, malaria
  - Inflammatory: connective tissue diseases, polyarteritis (Wegener's, allergic, and necrotic granulomatosis), temporal arteritis, systemic lupus erythematosus, Takayasu's disease, giant cell arteritis of the aorta
  - Cerebral thrombophlebitis: secondary to infection (ear, paranasal sinus, face), meningitis, and subdural empyema; postpartum; postoperative; cardiac failure; hematological diseases (polycythemia, sickle cell disease); and of undetermined cause
  - Hematological disorders: polycythemia, sickle cell disease, thrombotic thrombocytopenic purpura
  - Trauma to carotid artery
  - Dissecting aortic artery aneurysm
  - Systemic hypotension with arterial stenosis: secondary to sudden blood loss; myocardial infarction; Stokes-Adams syndrome; traumatic and surgical shock; sensitive carotid sinus; simple faint; severe postural hypotension
  - Complications of arteriography
  - Migraine with persistent deficit
  - Vascular occlusion with tentorial, foramen magnum, and subfalcial herniations
  - Miscellaneous conditions (postirradiation, complication of contraceptives, local dissection of middle or carotid arteries, lateral pressure of intracerebral hematoma, unexplained middle cerebral infarction in closed head injury)
  - Moyamoya disease
  - Undetermined cause, as in children and young adults—e.g., moyamoya disease

the figures derived from clinical material and autopsy studies vary, cerebral infarction caused by a thrombosis or an embolism accounts for nearly 80 percent of strokes, with the remainder resulting from intracranial hemorrhages (Table 2.2-2).

The temporal course and the duration of cerebrovascular events may vary significantly. When little or no necrosis occurs before the restoration of the blood supply and when the signs and symptoms last for 15 to 60 minutes, a *transient ischemic attack* (TIA) is diagnosed. When the residua last longer (usually in excess of 24 hours) but essentially resolve within a few weeks, a minor stroke or *reversible ischemic neurological deficit* is described. Longer-lasting deficits are said to result from *major strokes*. Slowly emerging neurological deficits of vascular cause are occasionally referred to as *strokes in evolution*.

The brain metabolism is altered after about 30 seconds of interrupted blood supply. After a full minute, neuronal functions are essentially halted. After five minutes, continued anoxia leads to a series of pathological events that result in cerebral infarction. *Cerebral infarction* denotes a region of brain within which hypoxia or ischemia has irreversibly damaged the neurons, the glial cells, and the endothelium. The clinical consequences of those events may not be permanent if the blood supply is returned soon enough.

Stroke may involve the vascular territories of the cortical vessels—such as the anterior, the middle, and the posterior cerebral arteries and their branches—or may involve subcortical vessels, such as those supplying the basal ganglia and the subcortical white matter. *Lacunar infarctions* are small subcortical strokes that are concentrated in the thalamus, the basal ganglia, the internal capsule, the brainstem, and the cerebellum. They are the most common type of infarction and result from the occlusion of perforating arteries damaged by chronic hypertension or diabetes mellitus. In *Binswanger's disease* (subcortical arteriosclerotic encephalopathy), multiple areas of demyelination associated with narrowing of the penetrating medullary arteries and arterioles are noted in the periventricular and subhemispheric white matter.

EPIDEMIOLOGY AND RISK FACTORS Cerebrovascular disease is the most common neurological disorder in adults. In the Western industrial nations, stroke is the third most frequent cause of death; the incidence is about 150 per 100,000 persons each year. In the United States alone, nearly 300,000 people are disabled, and 275,000 die from strokes each year.

In the United States the risk of stroke is twice as high in blacks as in whites, and males are at a slightly higher risk than are females (1.3 to 1). Age is the most prominent risk factor associated with stroke, along with arterial hypertension, ischemic and valvular heart disease, atrial fibrillation, and diabetes mellitus. Cigarette smoking appears to minimally increase the risk of stroke in men under the age of 65.

PROGNOSIS Overall, the mortality rate in stroke is about 30 percent and is slightly higher in the elderly than in young victims. Nearly 25 percent of patients die in the acute phase of cerebral infarction. The mortality rate for cerebral hemorrhage is higher, about 35 percent. In hemorrhagic stroke, nearly half of the patients who succumb do so within the first two days. An additional 30 percent of those mortally affected die by the end of the first week. Of those who die from cerebral thrombosis, only one third succumb within the first week. The remainder who eventually die suffer from heart failure, pulmonary embolism, or pneumonia. More than two thirds of patients who survive a stroke have at least limited ability to ambulate during recovery; 30 percent are severely disabled and need institutional-based care. The death rate from cerebrovascular disease has significantly declined over the past 25 years.

Several factors contribute to the prognosis for recovery after a stroke. In the acute phases of stroke, impaired consciousness, brainstem findings, altered respiration, bilateral features, and decorticate posturing all portend a bad prognosis. Loss of proprioception, neglect, and visual field deficits also appear to negatively influence the outcome. The location and the size of the stroke (the volume of the infarcted tissue) affect the resulting clinical state. For example, relatively small strokes in the internal capsule can result in substantially greater disability than much larger lesions located in the nondominant temporal lobes or frontal regions.

PATHOGENESIS Atherosclerosis and hypertension are the most common contributors to infarction. *Atherothrombosis* occurs when a clot develops at the site of an ulcerated plaque in a vessel wall. With enlargement of the clot, either the vessel lumen is occluded, or small emboli are shed into distal arteries. The plaques typically originate at the bifurcation of the common carotid artery into the external and internal carotid arteries and at the origins of the middle and anterior cerebral arteries.

Cerebral embolism results from the occlusion of an artery by a fragment of clotted blood, fat, air, neoplasm, bacteria, or other substance. Vasospasm may be an associated element. As a result, the surrounding neural tissue becomes ischemic. The most common emboli arise from fragments of an atherosclerotic plaque within the heart. Less frequently, the source is an intra-arterial plaque within the carotid circulation.

Intracerebral hemorrhage can result from a vessel rupture anywhere in the cerebral circulation. In hypertensive patients the most vulnerable sites for hemorrhagic stroke are microaneurysms in the intracerebral arterioles supplying the basal ganglia. Less commonly, hemorrhages occur in the cerebral lobes, the brainstem, and the cerebellum. As a consequence of an intracerebral hemorrhage, the surrounding parenchyma is compressed and displaced by an enlarging mass of blood. In nearly 90 percent of cases, blood enters the ventricular system. *Subarachnoid hemorrhage* occurs when blood leaks into the subarachnoid space, usually from a ruptured cerebral aneurysm.

MAJOR CEREBRAL STROKE SYNDROMES The onset of a stroke is typically sudden and may occur during sleep, with signs and symptoms evident on awakening. After the onset of a thromboembolic event, symptoms may continue to worsen for 24 to 48 hours. Except for infarctions of the brainstem, consciousness is usually preserved, although the patient may experience transient confusion. The specific clinical features that result from a stroke depend on its pathogenesis (thromboembolic or hemorrhagic), the size and the site of the involved cerebrovascular territory and its collateral circulation, and variations in the region supplied by a particular artery.

Middle cerebral artery occlusion Cerebral infarction in the territory of the middle cerebral artery often occurs with embolization from the anterior carotid circulation.

If the main trunk of the middle cerebral artery is occluded, the afflicted patient has eye deviation to the side of the infarction, contralateral sensory loss and weakness, global aphasia (if the occlusion is left-sided), severe visuospatial impairment (if the occlusion is right-sided), and hemianopia. Because the infarction typically involves the

TABLE 2.2-2
Incidence by Age of Cerebrovascular Lesions in Autopsy-Proved Cases

	Infarction		Hemorrhage	
Age in Years	Thrombotic (%)	Embolic (%)	Intraparenchymal (%)	Primary Subarachnoid (%)
<20	0	9	1	11
20–29	0	9	0	17
30–39	1	14	3	19
40–49	7	14	21	20
50–59	24	27	27	18
60–69	36	22	26	10
70–79	25	0	20	4
>80	7	5	2	1
Total	100%	100%	100%	100%

cerebral convexity and deep structures (such as the posterior limb of the internal capsule), the face, the arm, and the leg are often equally affected. When deep structures are spared, weakness and sensory loss are greater in the face and the arm than in the leg. When unilateral cerebral infarction occurs, maximum disability involves the extensor muscles of the arm and the flexors of the leg. If weakness is severe, muscle tone may be initially decreased. After several days or weeks, spasticity, hyperactive reflexes, and Babinski's sign are noted. When weakness is mild, clumsiness and incoordination are more evident than is the loss of strength. Infarction of the middle cerebral artery may result in disturbances in position sense and two-point discrimination. Pain and temperature sense may be impaired but are rarely completely lost. When infarction involves the prefrontal cortex, damage to the frontal eye field may result (Brodmann's area 8). Clinically, there is acute eye deviation to the side of the infarction and difficulty with volitional eye deviation (saccades) to the opposite side.

APHASIA Disturbances of language frequently arise from an infarction involving the left hemisphere. An anterior lesion of the upper division of the middle cerebral artery, in the area of the posterior third of the inferior frontal gyrus and the adjacent areas of the operculum and the insula, give rise to *Broca's aphasia.* Language output is nonfluent, effortful, and agrammatical. Speech is characterized by dysarthria and disturbances of prosody (melody, inflection, and timber). Comprehension is relatively well-preserved, but repetition and the ability to write and read aloud are impaired. Left-sided frontal lesions caused by an occlusion of branches of the middle cerebral artery that spare Broca's area may result in isolated language disturbances, such as impaired verbal fluency.

Wernicke's aphasia results from an occlusion of a branch of the middle cerebral artery supplying the posterior third of the left superior temporal gyrus and the adjacent posterior temporal and inferior parietal areas. Patients manifest a fluent verbal output with multiple paraphasic errors (word or phoneme substitutions) and impaired language comprehension and repetition. Writing, reading aloud, and reading comprehension are all affected. However, significant variability is seen in the relative severity of the loss in each of those areas. *Transcortical sensory aphasia* is similar to Wernicke's aphasia but is distinguished by the retention of repetition ability. The left temporoparieto-occipital junction region is the most common site of the corresponding lesion. Involvement of the left angular gyrus can also result in visuoconstructional disturbances, right-left disorientation, dyscalculia, and finger agnosia *(Gerstmann syndrome).*

Lesions that involve the entire territory of the left middle cerebral artery produce *global aphasia,* with impairment in nearly all aspects of language. Patients, if they can speak at all, often verbalize in a stereotyped fashion, with nonsense utterances or overlearned stock phrases. *Conduction aphasia* is an uncommon disturbance resulting from lesions of the arcuate fasciculus in the region of the left parietal operculum. Language output is fluent, with multiple phonemic paraphasic errors (for example, substitution of one sound for another), relatively intact comprehension, and disproportionately impaired repetition. Reading comprehension is intact, although reading aloud and writing are disturbed. In its pure form *anomic aphasia* results from a lesion in the left angular gyrus or adjacent posterior second temporal gyrus, but more often it is a residual disorder after recovery from Wernicke's or conduction aphasia. Anomia is the cardinal clinical feature; comprehension and repetition are preserved. Reading aloud and reading comprehension are spared. Language output is fluent, with few paraphasic substitutions.

APRAXIA Infarctions of the left hemisphere convexity, particularly in the parietal region, can cause bilateral *ideomotor apraxia.* In the disorder, patients cannot perform on command motor behaviors that can be done spontaneously, such as brushing the hair, throwing a ball, and saluting. Strokes involving the right parietal convexity may also result in difficulty in dressing *(dressing apraxia),* with excessive impairment in the ability to orient garments to particular limbs. *Buccolingual apraxia,* in which such motions as blowing out a match and sucking through a straw are disturbed, also follows left-brain injury. Anterior left-sided lesions may cause *sympathetic apraxia.* In that syndrome, there is a right hemiparesis, and the left arm is apraxic.

CONSTRUCTIONAL DISTURBANCES Impairment in the ability to copy pictures, make spontaneous drawings, or reproduce designs with matchsticks or blocks results from hemispheric lesions in a variety of locations. With stroke, lesions in the parieto-occipital and frontal regions most often result in constructional disability. Infarction in the left hemisphere results in the simplification and the omission of constituent elements in constructed pictures. Right-sided lesions produce profound disruptions of the overall construction, with a loss of perspective and severely distorted relations among the constituent parts. Stroke involving the frontal lobes, in particular the right frontal lobe, results in drawings that are perseverative, poorly planned, and excessively segmented.

NEGLECT, DENIAL, AND ANOSOGNOSIA Although not exclusively the product of right-hemispheric lesions, unilateral neglect is most frequent and most severe with acute lesions of the right parietal lobe. It less commonly results from right frontal lesions in the territory of the middle cerebral artery or from right subcortical lesions. In unilateral neglect or hemi-inattention, the patient fails to notice or to respond to tactile, visual, and auditory stimuli in half of the extrapersonal space, usually the left side. Such patients may dress or groom only one side of the body, copy only one side of a construction, or draw only one side of a clock. When the deficit is mild, neglect may be elicited only by double simultaneous stimulation, in which the stimulus (tactile, auditory, or visual) is extinguished on one side of the body. After a stroke, mild forms of neglect may persist for several months and may present an obstacle to progress in rehabilitation.

Denial of illness or *anosognosia* is most profound with right parietal lesions. However, fluent aphasic patients with posteriorly placed left-sided infarctions may also demonstrate the syndrome. The afflicted patient denies that a sensory, motor, or language deficit exists, despite objective evidence to the contrary.

EXECUTIVE FUNCTIONS Vascular lesions of the anterior branches of the middle cerebral artery supplying the lateral convexity of the frontal lobes can give rise to deficits in a group of neuropsychological domains called executive functions. Afflicted patients may show inflexibility, motor perseveration and impersistence, difficulty in programming novel motor behavior, disturbances in the ability to follow directions sequentially, and inability to vary modes of performance when given new directions. Such patients also have *stimulus boundedness,* as shown by the tendency, when asked to draw a clock with the time set at 11:10, to put one hand on the 10 (stimulus-bound) and the other on the 11.

In addition, deficits in the ability to tap rhythms and to copy alternating sequences and reciprocal commands (each time the examiner shows one finger, the patient is to show two) are noted. Frequently, the patient shows a tendency toward easy distractibility and difficulty in maintaining attention. Performance on tests that assess vigilance (continuous performance tasks) is typically impaired.

Anterior cerebral artery occlusion When infarction occurs in the territory of the anterior cerebral artery, the most common signs are referable to the paramedian frontal lobe, the caudate, and the anterior perforating substance.

The signs include weakness, sensory loss, and incoordination of the distal contralateral leg. The hand may be normal, but shoulder weakness and incontinence are occasionally noted. If the territory of the diencephalic branch (recurrent artery of Heubner) is involved, the anterior limb of the internal capsule is affected, giving rise to weakness of the face. Bilateral infarction in the territory of the anterior cerebral artery results in additional neurological impairment, including suck and grasp reflexes, diffuse rigidity *(gegenhalten),* and impaired responsiveness. One of the commonly encountered stroke syndromes of the anterior cerebral artery circulation involves an aneurysm arising from the anterior communicating artery. The specific clinical features of the aneurysm may vary, depending on the degree of ischemia to the surrounding regions. Generally, if rupture occurs, the clinical presentation is dominated by signs of subarachnoid hemorrhage, such as meningism, altered consciousness, and obstructive hydrocephalus. As a result, specific neurobehavioral sequelae are often obscured, at least during the short-term stages of the event. Personality alterations—disinhibition and impulsiveness—are common after recovery from the rupture.

APHASIA Infarction of the anterior cerebral artery in the region of the medial left frontal lobe (supplementary motor area and adjacent cingulate gyrus) results in *transcortical motor aphasia.* The distubance is often initially characterized by mutism. A nonfluent language output with relatively well-preserved repetition and reading aloud ability follows the mute period. Auditory comprehension is generally preserved, with variable reading comprehension.

AKINETIC MUTISM AND RELATED STATES Bilateral infarction of the anterior cerebral artery in the vicinity of the cingulate gyri of the medial frontal lobes results in a behavioral state in which the patient is mute and unresponsive to commands. There is most notably a lack of spontaneous motor behavior *(akinesia),* despite intact sensory-motor function.

Afflicted patients may show intermittent agitation and aimless aggressivity. The syndrome appears to be similar to *catatonia* but lacks the associated features of stereotypy, mannerisms, waxy flexibility, and catatonic posturing. In addition to medial frontal lesions, the syndrome can also be produced by damage to the brainstem reticular formation, bilateral infarction of the globus pallidus, and interruption of the medial forebrain bundle as it courses through the anterior hypothalamus to the anterior cingulate region. A related disorder is the *locked-in syndrome,* in which basilar artery occlusion with pontine infarction causes a state of motor paralysis that includes the limbs and the cranial nerves. Only the ocular movements remain, and patients communicate by blinking.

Bilateral infarction of the putamen, the caudate, or the globus pallidus can lead to extreme hypokinesis, rigidity, and mutism. That state of *extrapyramidal mutism* can also be caused by carbon monoxide poisoning. In the *apallic state of Kretschner,* near-total destruction of the mantle zone of the hemispheric convexity (pallium) results in mutism, akinesia, and unresponsiveness. The condition is the consequence of injury to associative and secondary sensory-motor areas with preservation of the primary motor strip. Muscle tone and posture are markedly affected. The causes include anoxia, carbon monoxide poisoning, and a variety of miscellaneous conditions, such as closed head injury, syphilis, and chronic viral encephalitis.

ANTERIOR CALLOSAL DISCONNECTION SYNDROME The anterior cerebral artery supplies the anterior 80 percent of the corpus callosum, resulting in callosal injury when there is infarction in the vascular supply. The stigmata of anterior callosal disruption include apraxia of the left arm, left-hand tactile anomia and agraphia, constructional disability, and impaired cross-replication of hand postures.

Posterior cerebral artery occlusion Occlusion of the posterior cerebral artery usually results from embolization and produces contralateral homonymous hemianopsia as a common sign.

Because of collateral circulation to the occipital pole by the middle cerebral artery, macular vision is generally spared. If the infarction is bilateral, the patient may have cortical blindness. Other patients may experience impaired hand-eye and gaze coordination and *metamorphopsia* (distortions of visualized objects). *Achromatopsia* is the acquired loss of vision in a quadrant, a hemifield, or the entire visual field. Unilateral infarction of a branch of the posterior cerebral artery supplying the medial occipitotemporal cortex results in contralateral hemiachromatopsia. Bilateral infarction in the region produces total color blindness. When infarction of the posterior cerebral artery is proximal, lesions may involve subcortical structures, such as the thalamus or the midbrain. Midbrain damage may result in striking eye signs, such as refractory nystagmus, oculomotor nerve palsy, internuclear ophthalmoplegia, vertical gaze paresis, lid retraction, and decreased pupillary reactivity. The pupil may also be eccentrically positioned *(corectopia).* When the midbrain peduncle is damaged, contralateral hemiparesis may result. If cerebellular outflow is interrupted above its decussation, contralateral ataxia will also occur. Damage to the reticular activating system can lead to lethargy, stupor, or coma. A stroke involving the subthalamic nucleus can result in contralateral hemiballismus.

AMNESIA Bilateral proximal posterior cerebral artery occlusion results in interrupted blood supply to the medial aspects of the medial temporal lobe, including the hippocampus. That interruption can lead to a severe and sustained organic amnestic syndrome. Although most such disorders result from bilateral infarction, a few cases of stroke-induced amnesia have been described with unilateral left-sided hippocampal damage. *Transient global amnesia* is the sudden onset of a temporary period of memory loss. Usually, an anterograde component lasts several hours, and a period of retrograde amnesia may extend back a few weeks. Patients can generally recall their own identities and recognize familiar persons, but they are amnestic for recent occurrences and new events. Afflicted patients frequently repeat the same questions and appear to be befuddled. No associated neurological signs are associated with the spells. Although not definitively understood, the disorder may result from a transient ischemic event of the vertebrobasilar circulation or the posterior cerebral circulation.

AGNOSIA Infarction within the posterior circulation can result in a variety of disturbances in recognition that occur despite intact sensory function.

In visual object agnosia there are two types of disturbances: apperceptive and associative. In *apperceptive visual agnosia* the patient retains the ability to detect light intensity, to identify color, and to appreciate movement and its direction. However, as a result of bilateral posterior cerebral artery infarction, visual perception is impaired, as the patient cannot distinguish one form from another (for example, a box from a cross) or draw presented objects. In contrast, in *associative visual agnosia,* perception is intact, but recognition is impaired. Affected patients can successfully match pictures or draw presented objects but cannot identify their meaning or their use. That type of disturbance results most commonly from bilateral medial occipitotemporal lesions that interrupt the inferior longitudinal fasciculi connecting the occipital and temporal cortices.

Bilateral medial occipital lesions or, less often, a unilateral right-sided posteromedial lesion may lead to *prosopagnosia,* the disturbed ability to recognize familar faces or different members of a particular class (for example, makes of cars). Infarction involving the medial left occipital cortex and the splenium of the corpus callosum results in *color agnosia,* the inability to correctly name a presented color or to match a color to a name. The deficit occurs despite intact color perception as assessed by a normal performance on color-matching tests. Because of callosal disruption, resulting in a disconnection of the left hemisphere (language) from the right occipital cortex (vision), the responsible infarction may also cause alexia without agraphia or aphasia.

Topographic or *environmental agnosia* can result from a unilateral right-sided occipitotemporal infarction, but it is commonly the consequence of bilateral medial occipital lesions. The impairment consists of the loss of familiarity with the surrounding environment. Patients may need to rely on verbal cues to identify their neighborhoods or their own homes.

Simultanagnosia results from bilateral cerebral infarction in the parieto-occipital watershed region between the anterior and posterior cerebral artery circulations. Patients are unable to perceive more than one element of a multifaceted stimulus. For example, if told to look at a card with a cross and a circle, the patient detects only one of the figures; if shown a complex photograph, only one portion of it is perceived. *Balint's syndrome* is the presence of simultanagnosia and associated disturbances in the ability to shift gaze at will to any new visual stimuli (*optical apraxia* or sticky fixation) and to point to a target under visual guidance *(optic ataxia).*

With bilateral posterior cerebral artery infarction resulting in cortical blindness, the patient may not recognize or admit that the visual deficit exists *(Anton's syndrome).*

Watershed infarction The watershed regions exist at the borders between the vascular territories of the major cerebral arteries. The areas are especially vulnerable to the effects of reduced cerebral perfusion resulting from cardiac arrest or blood loss. The most vulnerable watershed region is the parieto-occipital cortex, located between the territories supplied by the middle and posterior cerebral arteries. The clinical features of watershed infarction, for example, are variable. They include transcortical aphasia syndromes, proximal muscle weakness, and proximal sensory loss. Dementia may also result from infarction in those regions.

Thalamic stroke The most prominent signs and symptoms of thalamic infarction involve altered sensation.

Infarction of the ventral posterior nucleus results in contralateral loss of all sensation. Occasionally, dissociation of sensory modalities is present; pain and temperature are lost, but two-point discrimination, touch, and proprioception are retained. The syndrome consists of residual and chronic pain, which occur as sensation is restored after thalamic damage.

APHASIA Thalamic aphasia is most often the consequence of hemorrhage in the left thalamus, with accompanying pressure effects on distal cortical structures. The language disturbance consists of an initial period of mutism followed by the emergence of a fluent verbal output with paraphasia. Comprehension impairment is variable, and repetition is generally preserved. Reading comprehension is also relatively intact, although reading aloud and writing ability are compromised. The aphasia is often transient and accompanied by articulatory difficulties. Infarction of the thalamus tends to produce less striking language disturbances than those seen in hemorrhage.

Internal carotid artery occlusion The clinical manifestations of internal carotid artery thrombosis are variable.

As a result of significant collateral circulation, occlusion of the internal carotid artery may be neurologically silent. In other situations, however, occlusion may lead to catastrophic stroke involving all or the anterior two thirds of the cerebral hemispheres. Most vulnerable is the territory of the middle cerebral artery. If the anterior communicating artery is relatively small, the distribution of the anterior cerebral artery may also be affected. In some cases the posterior cerebral artery receives most of its supply from the internal carotid artery instead of the basilar artery. When that occurs, the clinical symptoms are localized to the territory of that vessel as well. If at an earlier time the other internal carotid artery was occluded, thrombosis of the remaining internal carotid artery can lead to bilateral massive cerebral infarction, resulting in coma and quadriplegia.

Multi-infarct (vascular) dementia The accumulation of multiple cerebral infarctions in the distributions of the middle, anterior, and posterior cerebral arteries results in dementia characterized by variable impairment across several domains of intellectual function. The state is accompanied by a history compatible with cerebrovascular disease and neurological signs and symptoms.

MOOD DISORDERS AND STROKE The literature describing stroke and mood disorders has been limited in part by methodological difficulties, such as imprecision in the definitions of "stroke" and "depression." In addition, the assessment of mood disturbance in stroke may be hampered by aphasic patients' impaired ability to elaborate their feelings verbally or comprehend questions about depression. Conversely, patients with right-hemisphere stroke may minimize the symptoms because of pathological denial. Diagnostic confusion may also result when neurovegetative symptoms attributed to depression are actually nonspecific somatic concomitants of stroke. Many of the relevant studies have been based on limited sample sizes and have intermittently included patients with premorbid histories of psychiatric illness or previous strokes. Given those limitations, the literature devoted to mood changes and stroke must be interpreted cautiously. Table 2.2-3 lists the neuropsychiatric syndromes associated with stroke.

Depression and stroke

PHENOMENOLOGY The period of greatest vulnerability to the occurrence of depression after cerebral infarction appears to be the two years after the onset of stroke. About 25 to 30 percent of stroke patients are depressed at the time of the initial interview.

During the poststroke period, a variety of depressed mood states have been described. Some patients have a clearly verbalized dysphoria related to diminished functional ability and accompanying loss of self-esteem. It is most often recognizable as an adjustment disorder with depressed mood. Most authors have noted that depressed feelings in reaction to perceived losses may constitute only a subset of clinical depressions associated with stroke. Evidence has been derived from the observation that the adequacy of the social supports and the degree of neurological and physical impairment does not predict the likelihood of an occurrence or the severity of the depression after stroke. Depression negatively influences poststroke recovery by slowing the speed and lowering the success rate of rehabilitation.

About 25 percent of acute stroke patients fulfill the diagnostic

TABLE 2.2-3
Neuropsychiatric Syndromes Associated with Stroke

Neuropsychiatric Syndromes	Anatomical Region
Mood disorders	
Depression	Cortical and subcortical areas, left > right,* anterior > posterior
Mania	Cortical and subcortical areas, especially orbitofrontal cortex, perithalamic regions, basal forebrain
Anxiety disorders	
Anxiety with depression	Same as for depression, cortical > subcortical (basal ganglia)
Obsessive-compulsive symptoms (with parkinsonism)	Basal ganglia
Personality alterations	
Apathetic	Medial frontal lobes; paramedian thalamus, globus pallidus
Disinhibited (pseudopsychopathic)	Orbitofrontal cortex; ventromedial caudate
Klüver-Bucy syndrome	Anteromedial temporal lobes
Psychosis	
Hallucinations	
Visual	Temporal, parietal, and occipital lobes; right > left,** more formed if anterior lesion; midbrain
Auditory	Temporal auditory cortex, pons
Delusions	Temporoparietal and subcortical areas

*Left > right; more commonly seen with left-sided lesions than with right-sided lesions
**Right > left; more commonly seen with right-sided lesions than with left-sided lesions

criteria for major depressive disorder, with symptoms consisting of depressed mood, anhedonia, loss of energy, and difficulty with concentration. Symptoms such as anorexia, diminished libido, disturbed sleep with early-morning awakening, and suicidal ideation have also been frequently noted. Several studies have reported spontaneous remission of the disorder within one or two years of the onset of the stroke.

A third depressive disturbance associated with cerebrovascular disease consists of a mild depression whose chronicity approaches that outlined in the diagnostic criteria for dysthymic disorder. The symptoms of the depression are similar qualitatively to major depressive disorder but are less severe and appear to last more than two years poststroke.

LESION LOCATION Cortical or subcortical infarctions in the left anterior hemisphere have been reported to produce a higher rate of depression than do similar-sized lesions in other cerebral locations. Within the frontal regions, the closer the proximity of the lesion to the frontal pole, the greater is the incidence of poststroke depression. Premorbid enlargement of the lateral and third ventricles (subcortical atrophy) may predispose to the occurrence of depression after stroke. Other recent neuroimaging-based analyses suggest that additional topographic factors, such as whether the infarction is in a ventral or a dorsal location, may affect which cluster of depressive symptoms are most prominent. The duration of the depressive symptoms is greater when the lesions are cortical, rather than subcortical. A recent study using single photon emission computed tomography (SPECT) in stroke patients demonstrated that the volume of the ischemic area correlated with depression scores.

PSEUDOBULBAR AFFECT The tendency to cry or laugh easily may occur with bilateral cerebral infarctions that interrupt descending corticobulbar pathways. Afflicted patients show additional signs of *pseudobulbar palsy,* such as dysarthria, dysphasia, and exaggerated gag and facial reflexes.

TREATMENT A paucity of well-controlled studies examine the role of pharmacotherapy and, to a smaller extent, nonpharmacological approaches to the treatment of poststroke depression. One randomized double-blind study of the tricyclic nortriptyline (Pamelor) in 34 poststroke depressed patients showed it to be effective, despite a dropout rate of 28 percent attributed to side effects. Few data support any particular treatment modality or combination of treatments for poststroke depression. The successful treatment of poststroke depression with serotonergic antidepressant agents, psychostimulants, and electroconvulsive therapy has been reported.

Mania and stroke Poststroke mania appears less commonly than poststroke depression and is not as thoroughly studied. The sudden onset of manic behavior has been described with unilateral cerebral infarction that is more often right-sided than left-sided. Responsible lesions have usually involved diencephalic structures (thalamus and hypothalamus) abutting the third ventricle or the adjacent regions of the basal forebrain. Lesions of the inferomedial frontal lobes may also produce mania. The psychiatric symptoms are generally indistinguishable from the manic state of bipolar disorder, although in poststroke mania there may be pathological denial of the accompanying neurological deficits. In addition, the patient may have retrograde amnesia for the period of time in which the mania was evident. In some patients the disturbed mood state resolves spontaneously in four to six weeks. In others the mania is persistent or recurrent, and treatment with lithium carbonate (Eskalith) is warranted. A family history of mood disorder increases the risk of poststroke mania, unlike poststroke depression.

ANXIETY DISORDERS AND STROKE The relation of stroke to anxiety disorders has received little exploration. One recent study found that, although major depression with significant anxiety was associated with a higher frequency of cortical lesions, major depression without anxiety was more frequently associated with subcortical (basal ganglia) infarctions.

PERSONALITY ALTERATIONS The most commonly encountered personality alterations in stroke involve damage to the frontal lobes and their connections. The majority of the syndromes result from bilateral frontal dysfunction. Damage to the lateral convexities resulting in altered demeanor is much more commonly the consequence of trauma, neoplasm, demyelinating disease, and degenerative processes than the result of stroke. The most striking abnormalities accompanying lateral convexity damage are those involving neurobehavioral deficits.

Aneurysms of the anterior communicating artery can exert mass effects or ruptures into the surrounding orbitofrontal and medial frontal regions, producing striking alterations in personality. Cerebral infarction alone rarely gives rise to the orbitofrontal syndrome but has been frequently associated with medial frontal injury. The consequences of orbitofrontal vascular damage on the personality include disinhibition, impulsivity, inappropriate jocularity, facetiousness, and euphoria. Patients are often affectively labile, show poor judgment and insight, and lack concern for others *(pseudopsychopathic).* Conversely, damage to the medial frontal systems results in a behavioral syndrome manifested by akinesia and sparse verbal output. A tendency toward confabulation can result from frontal vascular damage when memory is impaired. That tendency often arises from an anterior communicating artery aneurysm that extends into the medial basal forebrain. On questioning, patients may either offer false answers partially based on past events or invent fantastic, bizarre, or impossible experiences. *Reduplicative paramnesia* results when the patient inappropriately relocates the present environment to another location, generally one close to home. It may be seen in the setting of an acute infarction that involves the right frontal and parietal regions.

At present, no consistently efficacious agents are used to treat the personality alterations seen in frontal dysfunction. After an acute stroke, significant resolution of the symptoms often occurs spontaneously. Pharmacological treatment of the orbitofrontal syndrome has consisted of antipsychotics, benzodiazepines, carbamazepine (Tegretol), and propranolol (Inderal), all with inconsistent results. The medial frontal apathetic syndrome may, at times, improve with the use of psychostimulants. Dopaminergic agents such as bromocriptine (Parlodel) have been tried with variable results in the akinetic state resulting from medial frontal injury.

In addition to frontal injury-induced changes, temporal lobe damage may result in alterations in demeanor. Bilateral anteromedial temporal vascular damage has been associated with the *Klüver-Bucy syndrome.* The most typical features of the disorder include placidity, varied dietary behaviors, hyperphagia, sexual alterations, hyperorality, compulsive exploration of objects in the environment, and agnosia.

Personality alterations have also been described with vascular lesions affecting the ventromedial caudate (disinhibition), the paramedian thalamus (apathy), and the globus pallidus when bilaterally infarcted (apathy).

STROKE-INDUCED PSYCHOSIS

Vascular hallucinosis Visual hallucinations can result from any focal vascular hemispheric lesion within the visual pathways of the temporal, parietal, or occipital lobes. Hallucinations arising in that manner are termed *release hallucinations*. Hemispheric lesions causing those hallucinations are most commonly right-sided and may reflect the particular role of the right hemisphere in visuoperceptual processes. Often, the hallucinations are experienced within an associated visual field defect. The images seen are generally formed, vary in content, and last minutes to hours. Their character may be changed by opening or closing the eyes.

Acute infarction of the occipital lobe can cause psychedeliclike hallucinatory experiences. Patients visualize geometric forms, spirals, checkerboards, and funnels.

Palinopsia is a specific variety of release hallucination that occurs with posterior lesions of either hemisphere, preferentially with pathology on the right side. In the disorder visual images persist or recur after a stimulus is no longer present. The image often endures despite a shift in gaze. Palinopsia often begins abruptly in the setting of an infarct, a trauma, or a tumor but remits in several hours or a few days.

Cerebrovascular events involving the hemispheres less commonly cause *ictal hallucinosis* associated with seizures. The experiences are brief and more stereotyped than release phenomena. Anteriorly located ictal foci in the temporal lobes cause formed visual hallucinations. A visual field defect may not necessarily accompany them, as the visualized image most often occupies the entire field. The content of the hallucinations, when they are well-formed, is often of past events. An alteration in consciousness is often associated during or after the hallucinatory experience.

Focal vascular lesions of the midbrain produce *peduncular hallucinosis*. The characteristic visual hallucinations are typically complex images that tend to occur in the evening. Patients are frequently entertained by the phenomena and have altered sleep-wake cycles. Because of the midbrain location of the responsible lesion, concomitant brainstem findings are often found on neurological examination.

Another form of visual hallucinosis, *autoscopy* (heutoscopy), can occur in the course of a subarachnoid hemorrhage, a migraine, or other vascular events. During the experience patients see their own images. They may or may not have the associated delusion of there being a true double *(Doppelganger)*.

Auditory hallucinations may result from structural lesions of the brain (particularly tumors) in the region of the temporal auditory cortex but are rarely the consequence of vascular lesions. Temporal lobe infarctions occasionally result in *palinacousis*, in which previously experienced auditory stimuli persist or recur later. Pontine hemorrhage has also been implicated in the origin of vascular-induced auditory hallucinations.

Stroke and delusions Delusions attributed to cerebrovascular disease most often are persecutory or take the form of Schneiderian first-rank symptoms, Capgras's and related delusions, and heutoscopy (Doppelganger). In addition, stroke may lead to delusional denial of illness (anosognosia) and blindness (Anton's syndrome). Poststroke delusions typically result from thrombosis or intracerebral hemorrhage in the right and left temporoparietal regions or from subcortical and lacunar infarctions.

EVALUATION

Thrombotic infarction Within a few hours of a thrombotic infarction, ischemic areas are visualized by magnetic resonance imaging (MRI). In contrast, computed tomography (CT) may take a few days before showing such evidence. Like MRI, radionuclide scanning and positron emission tomography (PET) may show regions of ischemia before CT shows them. The most definitive neuroimaging technique for thrombotic occlusion is arteriography, in which collateral flow can also be assessed. Because the associated injection of radiopaque material in arteriography may potentialy extend an infarction, it has been largely replaced by digital subtraction angiography. That technique allows visualization of the major arteries of the neck and the brain and is generally indicated when anticoagulant or surgical therapy is being considered.

Unless a thrombotic infarction is large or has significant edema, cerebrospinal fluid (CSF) pressure is most often within normal limits. Occasionally, CSF protein is mildly elevated, and in the early stages a mild leukocytosis (3 to 8 per cubic millimeter) may be present. Much less commonly, it is followed by a transient pleocytosis of 400 to 2,000 polymorphonuclear leukocytes per cubic millimeter. When the CSF cell count remains high, that suggests an underlying inflammatory or infectious vasculitis or a nonvascular process causing strokelike signs and symptoms. In that context the serum sedimentation rate may be elevated, but that finding is nonspecific. In collagen vascular diseases, such as systemic lupus erythematosus, laboratory measures used to confirm the diagnosis or to follow the disease activity, such as anticardiolipin antibodies, may not correlate well with neurological manifestations. The clinician must establish, for each individual patient, a profile of laboratory tests that are most sensitive to collagen vascular disease activity. In thrombosis, serum cholesterol or triglycerides may be elevated, but that finding is nonspecific. A complete blood count with differential and prothrombin and partial thromboplastin times are generally performed to exclude hemopathy and coagulopathy. An electroencephalogram (EEG) may reveal focal slow-wave activity over the site of the infarction, but the finding tends to depend on lesion size.

Embolic infarction Many of the same laboratory findings occur in cerebral embolism as in thrombotic occlusion; the exceptions include hemorrhagic infarction and septic embolization.

Hemorrhage occurs in about 30 percent of embolic strokes; in a minority, blood leaks into the ventricular system, causing erythrocytes to be evident in the CSF. Hemorrhagic embolic infarction may first be evident on CT scanning after the first two days poststroke. When septic embolization occurs, the CSF may show a leukocytosis (generally up to 200 cells per cubic millimeter). Erythrocytes may also be evident, with a resultant red discoloration of the CSF. Although the glucose content of the CSF is within the normal range, the protein is generally elevated. Bacteria are most often absent, and CSF cultures are negative for the growth of microorganisms. In cerebral embolization, echocardiography is often indicated to evaluate for a cardiac embolic source.

Hemorrhagic infarction

INTRAPARENCHYMAL HEMORRHAGE CT scanning is the visualization method of choice in the evaluation of intraparenchymal bleeding. When blood extravasates into the CSF, CT becomes somewhat less valuable. CT also visualizes any accompanying features, such as hydrocephalus, shifting of intracerebral structures, and edema. After four to five weeks, CT may no longer visualize hemorrhage and is clearly inferior to MRI.

Lumbar puncture must be done with great caution to avoid temporal lobe herniation resulting from increased intracranial pressure. The CSF is often grossly bloody, with cell counts ranging from a few thousand to a million cells per cubic millimeter. Intracranial hemorrhage may also be associated with an elevated sedimentation rate, glucosuria, and a peripheral leukocytosis that is greater than that typically encountered with thrombosis. The EEG may nonspecifically show high-voltage, slow waves.

SUBARACHNOID HEMORRHAGE CT scanning detects bleeding within the parenchyma or the ventricular system. Angiography is the most sensitive technique available to reveal aneurysms. The CSF is generally under increased pressure and reveals a red discoloration. Initially, the proportion of red to white cells mirrors the peripheral circulation. In some cases, however, a CSF leukocytosis may appear within a few days. The CSF protein is usually increased, and glucose levels are diminished. Glucosuria and albuminuria are frequent. Occasionally, a peripheral leukocytosis is found. The EEG is usually of little diagnostic use.

TREATMENT The optimal treatment of stroke and associated neurological and behavioral sequelae has three phases: (1) short-term management, (2) restoration of the circulation and prophylaxis, and (3) physical therapy and rehabilitation.

Thrombotic infarction and embolism To optimize cerebral perfusion, clinicians generally keep patients in a horizontal position for the first few days after stroke onset. On ambulation, patients are encouraged to avoid standing still for extended periods. Maneuvers to maintain and increase the systemic blood pressure are instituted to optimize cerebral blood flow while coexistent anemia or hypoxia is maximally treated to enhance cerebral oxygenation. The effects of anticoagulants and vasodilators are inconsistent and somewhat unpredictable. The use of anticoagulant medication mandates that cerebral hemorrhage has been thoroughly excluded by neuroimaging. Once thrombotic infarction has been well-established, drugs such as heparin and coumadin (Warfarin) are not of use. Whether those agents have significant prophylactic value in the prevention of further thrombotic strokes is unclear, but the attendant risk of hemorrhage generally outweighs any potential benefits. However, when a cerebral embolism has occurred with a myocardial infarction, atrial fibrillation, or valvular prosthesis, the long-term use of anticoagulants is warranted. In the early phases of embolization, anticoagulant therapy is best delayed several days. The therapy may be instituted after CT scanning and lumbar-puncture tests have been performed to exclude prior hemorrhage. The risk of anticoagulant-induced hemorrhage is increased in large cerebral infarctions and when the patient is hypertensive.

A contrasting approach uses such alternative agents as aspirin, dipyridamole (Persantine), and sulfinpyrazone (Anturane), which reduce clotting by diminishing platelet adhesiveness and aggregation. Aspirin is prescribed for patients with thrombotic events for stroke prophylaxis; the efficacy of other agents is unproved. An additional approach to increasing cerebral blood flow in stroke is the use of calcium channel inhibitors, such as nimodipine (Nimotop). Those agents lessen vasoconstriction and appear to limit neuronal death. Occasionally, cerebral edema complicates stroke during the first few days. Controlled ventilation and the use of a steroidal agent, such as dexamethasone (Decadron), is indicated. Intravenous mannitol and glycerol are also used to treat the complication.

Hemorrhagic stroke The basic principles of management in thrombotic and embolic strokes are applicable in the setting of cerebral hemorrhage. In general, therapy reduces intracranial pressure by using controlled hyperventilation and such dehydrating agents as mannitol and furosemide (Lasix) and by limiting fluid intake. In the early stage of hemorrhage, before the onset of deep coma, surgical removal of the clot may be indicated, especially if the intracranial pressure cannot be adequately controlled. When hemorrhage occurs because of an aneurysmal rupture, surgical treatment may relieve signs of hydrocephalus and prevent further bleeding. Surgical procedures are often delayed until the patient's course has stabilized. The procedures consist of occluding the stem of the aneurysm to prevent rupture.

Rehabilitation Rehabilitation of the stroke patient requires physical therapy, occupational therapy, speech therapy when appropriate, and treatment of any associated psychiatric or behavioral symptoms, including appropriate psychotropic medications and supportive psychotherapy. As the physical and neuropsychiatric aspects of stroke are identified and treated, attention is directed to optimizing performance in the activities of daily living.

INTRACRANIAL TUMORS

DEFINITION Intracranial masses encompass all neoplasms that may arise from the brain parenchyma, the blood vessels, the cranial nerves, the pituitary, the meninges, and the skull. Also included are metastases from extracranial neoplasms, parasitic cysts, granulomas, and lymphomas. Brain tumors may be classified by their histopathologic type and location (Table 2.2-4). Because a wide variety of tumor types can affect the brain, significant variability is seen in growth rate, potential size, and invasive quality.

PRINCIPAL INTRACRANIAL TUMORS

Gliomas The glia, cerebral connective tissues, are the most common cell types to give rise to primary intracranial tumors. The astrocyte is the most common glial constituent cell type, and the *astrocytoma* is the most common primary intracranial tumor.

Additional but less common glial tumors are the oligodendrocytomas, the ependymomas, and the medulloblastomas. Those tumors are graded from I to IV, depending on such variables as the degree of anaplasia, the mitotic frequency, and the presence of giant cells and necrosis.

TABLE 2.2-4
Distribution of Major Brain Tumors by Age and Location

Location	Tumor Type	Percentage of All Tumors
Infancy and Adolescence (0–20 years)		
Supratentorial	Glioma of cerebral hemisphere	10–14
	Craniopharyngioma	5–13
	Ependymoma	3–5
	Choroid plexus papilloma	2–3
	Pinealoma	1.5–3
	Optic glioma	1–3.5
Infratentorial	Cerebellar	
	Astrocytoma	15–20
	Medulloblastoma	14–18
	Brainstem glioma	9–12
	Ependymoma	4–8
Middle Age (20–60 years)		
Supratentorial	Glioblastoma	25
	Meningioma	14
	Astrocytoma	13
	Metastases	10
	Pituitary tumors	5
Infratentorial	Metastases	5
	Acoustic neuroma	3
	Meningioma	1
Old Age (>60 Years)		
Supratentorial	Glioblastoma	35
	Meningioma	20
	Metastases	10
Infratentorial	Acoustic neuroma	20
	Metastases	5
	Meningioma	5

Glioblastoma multiforme (malignant astrocytoma, grades III and IV) is the most common primary brain tumor, comprising 20 percent of all intracranial tumors. The mean age of afflicted patients is 56 years. It is a particularly malignant tumor, with a tendency to attain a large size before becoming clinically evident. It usually infiltrates extensively into the surrounding brain tissue. The tumor affects primarily the cerebral hemispheres but may also be found in the brainstem, the cerebellum, and the spinal cord. About 50 percent of the tumors occupy more than one lobe or both cerebral hemispheres; extraneural metastasis is rare. Pathologically, the tumor is highly vascular and has a variegated appearance. Surrounding tissue is often significantly displaced, with distortion and displacement of the ventricles. Histological examination reveals hypercellularity, cellular pleomorphism, hyperchromatism of the nuclei, tumor giant cells, mitotic figures, and hyperplasia of the endothelial cells lining the small vessels. Thrombosis, hemorrhage, and tissue necrosis are often noted.

Lower-grade astrocytomas are somewhat less frequent and may occur almost anywhere in the brain, including the cerebrum, the cerebellum, the hypothalamus, the brainstem, the spinal cord, and the optic nerves and chiasm. When involving the cerebral hemispheres, the tumor type is most common in young adults aged 20 to 40 years. The tumor is frequently found in nonhemispheric locations in children and adolescents.

Oligodendrogliomas are rare tumors (approximately 6 percent of intracranial gliomas) found most often in the deep white matter of the frontal lobe. They are most common in young adults. *Ependymomas* arise from the cells lining the ventricles and the spinal canal. They are most commonly found in the fourth ventricle and account for about 5 percent of intracranial gliomas. Infratentorial (posterior fossa) ependymomas are frequent in early childhood; those in a supratentorial location are evenly distributed among all age groups.

Meningiomas These histologically benign tumors are second in prevalence to gliomas and arise from the arachnoidal cells of the meninges. Meningiomas may be located in the following regions: parasagittal (30 percent), convexity (30 percent), lesser wing of the sphenoid (15 percent), and subfrontal (15 percent). Additional sites include the cerebellum and the spinal canal. Unlike gliomas, meningiomas are more common in women than in men (2 to 1) and reach their highest incidence in the seventh decade. They can extend through the dura and invade and erode the cranial bones. The size that is critical for producing neurological signs and symptoms is a function of the location of the mass. In general, meningiomas are slow-growing tumors that may reach enormous size before coming to medical attention.

METASTATIC TUMORS Neoplasms of extracranial origin account for about 6 percent of intracranial tumors. Intracranial metastasis may be to the skull and the dura, the brain parenchyma, and the meninges. Any neoplasm that tends to metastasize to bone can reach the skull or the meninges. The most common tumors associated with that pattern of metastasis are carcinoma of the breast, carcinoma of the prostate, and multiple myeloma. Neoplastic cells apparently reach the cranium by a vertebrel venous plexus that courses the length of the vertebral column from the pelvis.

Metastasis to the brain parenchyma is by hematogenous spread. The most common neoplasms associated with that type of metastasis are carcinoma of the lung, carcinoma of the breast, and malignant melanoma. Additional primary tumors giving rise to intraparenchymal brain metastasis are carcinomas of the colon, the rectum, the kidneys, the gallbladder, the liver, the thyroid, the testicles, the uterus, the ovaries, and the pancreas. Some primary neoplasms are particularly likely to metastasize to the brain (75 percent of melanomas, 57 percent of testicular tumors, and 35 percent of bronchial carcinomas). When metastasis to the parenchyma occurs, the foreign tumor incites little glial reaction but significant edema. Most metastatic lesions are solid, with a subset appearing cystic or hemorrhagic.

In *meningeal carcinomatosis,* tumor cells are widely disseminated throughout the meninges and the ventricles. That pattern of metastasis is most common with tumors of the breast, the lung, and the gastrointestinal tract and with melanomas and childhood leukemia.

EPIDEMIOLOGY For intracranial disease, only stroke exceeds tumor as a cause of death. In the United States the incidence each year of all brain tumors is 46 per 100,000, and for primary tumors the incidence is 15 per 100,000. In about 20 percent of all patients with cancer, the brain, the meninges, or the skull is secondarily infiltrated by tumor at some point in the disease course. With the possible exceptions of radiation exposure and, to a smaller extent, viral infection, no risk factors are clearly established for the development of a brain tumor.

CLINICAL FEATURES The clinical features accompanying intracranial tumors reflect alterations in neural function arising from direct parenchymal invasion, mass effect on distant structures, edema, hydrocephalus, or stroke.

The symptoms produced by intracranial tumors are generally progressive. The signs and the symptoms may suddenly appear with the striking onset of a seizure or, more commonly, develop insidiously, with slowly evolving cognitive deficits, depression, and such physical complaints as headache. The features may develop over weeks to months. Unfortunately, no particular cluster of signs or symptoms is pathognomonic of an intracranial tumor.

Historically, headache, emesis, and papilledema were considered the clinical hallmarks; those findings, however, are inconstant. When the features are found in combination with other signs of increased intracranial pressure, such as unsteady gait and sphincteric incontinence, the presence of a mass lesion must be strongly suspected.

Additional symptoms often associated with the presence of an intracranial mass include altered states of consciousness, diplopia or blurred vision, vasomotor symptoms, and focal clinical signs, such as weakness, sensory abnormalities, speech and language difficulties, and visual field defects. In general, the same types of focal neurological abnormalities found in stroke may also be present with a mass lesion. In contrast to stroke, mass lesions are more apt to produce distant clinical effects on brain function because of mass effect and noncommunicating hydrocephalus. For example, when a brain tumor causes increased intracranial pressure, the focal symptoms may be accompanied by nonfocal signs, such as psychomotor retardation, lethargy, and, ultimately, obtundation or coma.

In certain settings, *false localizing signs* may develop. For example, with increased intracranial pressure, unilateral or bilateral *abducens palsy* may be noted because of stretching of the sixth cranial nerve. In addition, when intracranial pressure is sufficiently elevated, transtentorial herniation may result. If the responsible mass is unilateral and temporal, the medial temporal lobe can be displaced inferomedially through the tentorial notch, producing *uncal herniation.* As a result, falsely localizing signs may develop, such as ipsilateral ptosis and pupillary dilatation (third-nerve compression), contralateral homonymous hemianopsia (posterior cerebral artery compression), ipsilateral hemiparesis (contralateral cerebral peduncle compression), and contralateral hemiparesis with bilateral Babinski's signs (midbrain compression).

Although variable, headaches are an early symptom in about one third of patients later found to have a brain tumor. The headache that occurs with an intracerebral tumor cannot be reliably distinguished from headaches of other causes by clinical features alone. However, their nocturnal occurrence, their presence on initial awakening, and a deep, nonpulsatile quality may be distinguishing characteristics of the headache associated with a brain tumor. Headaches are not directly related to the level of intracranial pressure. When intracranial pressure is normal, a headache may result from traction or pressure on such structures as the dura, the blood vessels, and the sensory nerves.

Emesis also occurs in about one third of tumor patients and is more frequent with lesions in the posterior fossa. It may be accompanied by headache, dizziness, and vertigo. Most often, the vomiting is not directly related to meals and may occur after awakening.

Focal or generalized seizures occur in 20 to 50 percent of patients with intracranial tumors. The seizures are more commonly manifestations of masses in the cerebral hemispheres than in the posterior fossa or the brainstem. In one series of approximately 450 patients, the tumor type influenced the occurrence of seizures; they were most frequent in vascular tumors (69 percent), followed by astrocytomas (55 percent), meningiomas (41 percent), metastatic tumors (35 percent), and glioblastomas (31 percent).

Like stroke, intracranial tumors may have profound effects on intellectual function, mood, and personality. Tumors have also been implicated as causes of such psychotic symptoms as hallucinations and delusions and such dissociative phenomena as depersonalization and derealization. Brain tumors may also give rise to chronic confusional states.

Mood and personality alterations The alterations in mood and personality described under Cerebrovascular Diseases are also potential consequences of intracerebral mass lesions.

PSYCHOMOTOR (MENTAL) ASTHENIA Although apparently nonlocalizable, a relatively common behavioral manifestation of intracerebral tumors includes a symptom complex consisting of inertia, impaired insight, forgetfulness, apathy, lack of spontaneity, and irritability in the absence of a clearly depressed mood or excessive anxiety. Patients are also prone to complaints of weakness, fatigue, and dizziness. They have long latencies of responsiveness and may appear sleepy or excessively reserved. Cerebral tumors most likely to cause the syndrome are gliomas of the frontal lobes, the temporal lobes, and the corpus callosum.

DEPRESSION AND MANIA Intracranial neoplasms appear to cause depression most often when the mass is temporal. As in stroke, left-sided lesions are most often associated with depressive symptoms. Tumors may also cause depression on a less focal basis in obstructive hydrocephalus. The depressive symptoms are accompanied by the triad of dementia, gait instability, and urinary incontinence. After shunting procedures to reduce the degree of hydrocephalus, the depressed mood may improve. Right-sided mass lesions in the vicinity of the hypothalamus and the inferomedial frontal lobes have been particularly associated with mania.

PERSONALITY ALTERATIONS The effects of brain tumors on the personality include the medial frontal apathetic state and the orbitofrontal disinhibited state. Often, brain damage resulting from mass lesions creates personality alterations that represent a combination of those states. In addition to frontal personality disorders, personalities complicated by violent rage reactions have been described with neoplasms involving the hypothalamus. Tumors that bilaterally encroach on limbic structures in the vicinity of the medial temporal lobes may give rise to an excessively placid demeanor.

Psychosis

HALLUCINATIONS Mass lesions that interrupt the visual pathways may cause visual hallucinosis in the same manner as strokes. The resultant hallucinations may be release phenomena or ictal events. The disturbances are relatively uncommon with frontal lesions, but mass effects caused by tumors in that location may exert pressure on the temporal lobes or the brainstem, resulting in hallucinatory phenomena. Olfactory hallucinations commonly arise with tumors impinging on the olfactory pathways. Disruption of the amygdaloid nuclei may play a particularly important role in that type of experience. Auditory hallucinations have also been associated with central nervous system tumors. They are either formed or unformed and tend to be most closely associated with temporal lobe tumors. Temporal lobe tumors can also cause palinacousis, in which there is persistence or the late recurrence of previously experienced auditory stimuli.

DELUSIONS Temporal lobe neoplasms can cause the emergence of persecutory and Schneiderian first-rank delusions. Capgras's delusions have also been associated with brain tumors, particularly right-hemispheric lesions.

Dementia and delirium Tumors may sufficiently alter neural functions to cause dementia. Unlike other more common causes of dementia, like Alzheimer's disease and vascular dementia, mass lesions frequently cause early and enduring alterations in arousal, attention, and concentration. As a result, the dementia syndrome associated with mass lesions has characteristics of a chronic confusional state. Focal neurological signs and symptoms or evidence of increased intracranial pressure may also be present.

Extracerebral neoplasms that may be occult can rarely cause *paraneoplastic syndromes* without evidence of metastasis. Often, patients have the insidious onset of cerebellar findings—such as dysarthria, ataxia, and nystagmus—in addition to cognitive loss. The disorder is probably immune-mediated; a number of studies document the presence of anti-Purkinje's cells antibodies in the cerebrospinal fluid. Tumors that have been associated with the syndrome include carcinomas of the lung (mostly oat cell carcinomas) and the breast and Hodgkin's disease. *Limbic encephalitis* is a poorly understood paraneoplastic condition in which there are neuropathological changes, such as neuronal loss, lymphocytic proliferation, gliosis, and necrosis concentrated in the limbic areas. In addition to a chronic confusional state, patients may manifest profound amnesia, hallucinations, anxiety, and depression. There may be evidence of extralimbic involvement as well, with cerebellar or brainstem signs.

Postirradiative encephalopathy Radiation therapy for cerebral or pituitary tumors occasionally causes a delayed coagulation necrosis of the white matter and, less commonly, the brainstem. The major cause of the disorder is thought to be radiation-induced damage of the blood vessel walls, with resultant fibrinoid necrosis and thrombosis. The symptoms may first appear three months to three years after radiation treatment. Typical features include dementia, seizures, and increased intracranial pressure. CT scanning may reveal a low-density, contrast-enhancing mass that is best distinguished from a tumor by MRI.

EVALUATION The evaluation of an intracranial mass lesion involves careful neurological and medical examinations and the assessment of cognitive function, mood, and behavior. Neuroimaging, such as CT or MRI with contrast, is indicated. In addition, a chest radiograph should be ordered to exclude the possibility of metastasis from the lung. In selected mass lesions, angiography may be desired to elucidate the circulation for intended surgical exploration or to exclude the possibility of a giant aneurysm presenting as a tumor. When multiple tumors are present, a primary source for metastasis must be sought; a chest X-ray, a gastrointestinal series, an intravenous pyelogram, a barium enema, a liver scan, and a bone scan may be indicated.

DIFFERENTIAL DIAGNOSIS The diagnosis of an intracranial tumor must be strongly suspected when slowly developing and progressive focal neurological symptoms—dizziness, seizures, atypical headaches, and psychiatric symptoms—are found. The conditions that must be excluded before diagnosing a brain tumor include subdural hematoma, aneurysm, stroke, infection, demyelinative diseases, degenerative neurological diseases, hydrocephalus, and pseudotumor cerebri.

In general, a subdural hematoma is accompanied by a history of a recent head injury. However, in the case of a chronic subdural hematoma, neuroimaging may be needed to exclude the condition. Large aneurysms can present with similar signs and symptoms as tumors but are readily differentiated by CT, MRI, or angiography.

The symptoms of a stroke usually have a more abrupt clinical onset than does a tumor, although that distinction is not absolute. In addition, signs of increased intracranial pressure are much more common in tumors than in strokes, but differentiation may also rely on neuroimaging findings.

Infections of the nervous system are also usually readily distinguished from mass lesions by CT or MRI and the results of lumbar-puncture tests. In some cases, abscesses can be distinguished from neoplasms only by cerebral biopsy. Demyelinating diseases, such as multiple sclerosis, have different clinical signs than do tumors, such as a relapsing and remitting course. However, rare disorders, such as Schilder's disease, may appear with nonspecific clinical signs and a mass lesion (on neuroimaging) resembling a glioma. The diagnosis may then need to be made on the basis of a cerebral biopsy. Degenerative diseases, such as Alzheimer's disease, typically have an insidious onset and are progressive, like brain tumors. However, in Alzheimer's disease, focal neurological signs or seizures are rarely seen early in the disease course. Signs of increased intracranial pressure are also incompatible with the diagnosis. In degenerative diseases, neuroimaging also excludes the presence of a mass lesion.

Pseudotumor cerebri (benign intracranial hypertension) is particularly common in overweight female adolescents and adult women. Its cause is unknown. Symptoms of increased intracranial pressure develop over weeks to months. The clinical profile consists of headache, dizziness, blurred vision, and, occasionally, unilateral facial numbness. The patient's arousal and cognitive functioning are intact. Neurological examination reveals papilledema and, less often, abducens palsy or nystagmus on far lateral gaze. Visual loss is a rare consequence of the disorder. CT or MRI reveals a normal or constricted ventricular size, without a mass lesion.

Occasionally, *papillitis,* swelling of the optic disk despite normal intracranial pressure, is confused with papilledema. In papillitis, the patient usually has a sudden onset of impaired vision in one or both eyes, a scotoma, pain with eye movement, and tenderness on palpation of the globe. Nearly 75 percent of afflicted patients show other signs of multiple sclerosis within 15 years.

COURSE, PROGNOSIS, AND TREATMENT The course and the ultimate prognosis for a patient with an intracranial tumor are a function of its histological type, rate of growth, invasiveness, and response to treatment. In general, brain tumors of glial origin are lethal. However, some strides have been made in the development and the availability of refined microsurgical techniques, radiation therapy, and chemotherapeutic agents. In many tumor types the cerebral edema may be treated with steroids; associated symptoms, such as seizures, are treated with anticonvulsant medications.

Psychiatric and behavioral manifestations of brain tumors are judiciously treated with appropriate psychotropic medications, with special attention paid to the potential side effects, such as excessive sedation and lowered seizure threshold. Often, afflicted patients benefit from supportive psychotherapeutic techniques directed at maintaining the patient's self-esteem and sense of control over the future. Many patients need to be helped through the several stages of grieving that accompany such terminal illnesses as brain tumors.

In glioblastoma, less than 20 percent of afflicted patients survive for one year after the onset of the symptoms. After two years, only 10 percent of the patients are still alive. Unfortunately, the contemporary treatment of the tumor is largely unsuccessful. Surgery usually cannot resect the entire mass because of its infiltrative character. Survival may be increased by about five months after three to four weeks of daily radiation (up to 5,000 rads a day). Chemotherapy increases survival to a limited extent.

Less malignant astrocytomas are somewhat more amenable to surgical resection. Although data are incomplete, radiation therapy may also prolong survival. The average survival period after the onset of symptoms is five to six years. Tumors confined to the cerebellum have somewhat better survival rates (nearly eight years).

Meningiomas, if accessible, are often permanently cured by surgical resection. If resection is incomplete, however, recurrence is likely. Adjunctive radiation therapy improves the cure rates, whether or not the mass is completely resected.

SUGGESTED CROSS-REFERENCES

Functional neuroanatomy is discussed in Section 1.2, neuroimaging in Sections 1.10 and 2.10, schizophrenia in Chapter 14, mood disorders in Chapter 17, anxiety disorders in Chapter 18, and Alzheimer's disease and other dementing disorders in Section 46.6a.

REFERENCES

*Adams R D, Victor M: *Principles of Neurology,* ed 4. McGraw-Hill, New York, 1989.

Bannister R: *Brain's Clinical Neurology,* ed 6. Oxford University Press, New York, 1986.

Benson D F, Stuss D T: *The Frontal Lobes.* Raven, New York, 1986.

Castillo C S, Starkstein S E, Fedoroff J P, Price T R, Robinson R G: Generalized anxiety disorder after stroke. J Nerv Ment Dis *181:* 100, 1993.

*Catapno F, Galderisi S: Depression and cerebral stroke. J Clin Psychiatry *51:* 9, 1990.

Coffey C E, Figiel G S, Djang W T, Weiner R D: Subcortical hyperintensity on magnetic resonance imaging: A comparison of normal and depressed elderly subjects. Am J Psychiatry *147:* 187, 1990.

*Cummings J L: *Clinical Neuropsychiatry.* Grune & Stratton, New York, 1985.

Cummings J L, Mendez M F: Secondary mania with focal cerebrovascular lesions. Am J Psychiatry *141:* 1084, 1984.

Ebrahin S, Barer D, Nouri F: Affective illness after stroke. Br J Psychiatry *151:* 52, 1987.

Fedoroff J P, Starkstein S E, Parikh R M, Price T R, Robinson R G: Are depressive symptoms nonspecific in patients with acute stroke? Am J Psychaitry *148:* 1172, 1991.

Kaneyama M, Tomonaga N, Aiba T: *Cerebrovascular Disease.* Igaku-Shoin, New York, 1988.

Marsden C D, Fowler T J: *Clinical Neurology.* Raven, New York, 1989.

Marshall J, Thomas D J: Vascular disease. In *Diseases of the Nervous System,* A K Asbury, G M McKhann, W I McDonald, editors, vol 2, p 1101. Saunders, Philadelphia, 1986.

Mesulam M M: *Principles of Behavioral Neurology.* Davis, Philadelphia, 1985.

Morris P L, Robinson R G, Andrzejewski P, Samuels J, Price T R: Association of depression with 10-year poststroke mortality. Am J Psychiatry *150:* 124, 1993.

Morris P L, Robinson R G, Raphael B: Prevalence and course of depressive disorders in hospitalized stroke patients. Int J Psychiatry Med *20:* 593, 1990.

Power C, Hachinski V: Stroke in the elderly. In *Principles of Geriatric Medicine and Gerontology,* ed 2, W R Hazzard, R Andres, E L Bierman, J P Blass, editors, p 926. McGraw-Hill, New York, 1985.

Robinson R G, Lipsey J R, Rao K, Price T R: Two year longitudinal study of poststroke mood disorders: Comparison of acute onset with delayed onset depression. Am J Psychiatry *143:* 1238, 1986.

Robinson R G, Parikh R M, Lipsey J R, Starkstein S E, Price T R: Pathological laughing and crying following stroke: Validation of a measurement scale and a double-blind treatment study. Am J Psychiatry *150:* 286, 1993.

Robinson R G, Starr L B, Kubos K L, Price T R: Poststroke affective disorders. In *Cerebrovascular Disease,* M Reivich, H I Hurtig, editors, p 137. Raven, New York, 1983.

Robinson R G, Szetela B: Mood change following left hemispheric brain injury. Ann Neurol *9:* 447, 1981.

Rowland L P, editor: *Merritt's Textbook of Neurology,* ed 8. Lea & Febiger, Philadelphia, 1989.
Schwartz J A, Speed N M, Mountz J M, Gross M D, Modell J G, Kuhl D E: Tc-hexamethylpropyleneamine oxime single photon emission CT in poststroke depression. Am J Psychiatry *147:* 242, 1990.
Shapiro W R, Shapiro J R: Primary brain tumors. In *Diseases of the Nervous System,* A K Asbury, G M McKhann, W I McDonald, editors, vol 2, p 1136. Saunders, Philadelphia, 1986.
Starkstein S F, Cohen B S, Fedoroff T, Parikh R M, Price T R, Robinson R G: Relationship between anxiety disorders and depressive disorders in patients with cerebrovascular injury. Arch Gen Psychiatry *47:* 246, 1990.
Starkstein S E, Fedoroff J P, Price T R, Leiguarda R, Robinson R G: Catastrophic reaction after cerebrovascular lesions: Frequency, correlates, and validation of a scale. J Neuropsychiatry Clin Neurosci *5:* 189, 1993.
*Starkstein S E, Robinson R G, Price T R: Comparison of patients with and without poststroke major depression matched for size and location of lesion. Arch Gen Psychiatry *45:* 247, 1988.
*Stern R A, Bachman D L: Depressive symptoms following stroke. Am J Psychiatry *148:* 351, 1991.

2.3 NEUROPSYCHIATRIC ASPECTS OF EPILEPSY

MARIO F. MENDEZ, M.D., Ph.D.

INTRODUCTION

Our understanding of psychiatric disorders in epilepsy has had a turbulent history. Epileptic patients have had every possible type of behavioral abnormality attributed to them until modern times, when an opposition to any special association between epilepsy and psychiatric illness began to prevail. Only recently have we begun to decipher and to define the neuropsychiatric aspects of epilepsy. Although most epileptic patients are psychologically normal, there is an increased prevalence of psychosis, depression, borderline personality disorder, and hyposexuality among seizure patients. Evidence links both seizures and behavioral changes with the mediobasal temporal limbic region, the most common location of pathological changes in adult epilepsy.

DEFINITION

Epileptic *seizures* are sudden, involuntary behavioral events associated with either excessive or hypersynchronous electrical discharges in the brain. The seizure itself is known as the *ictus.* The *interictal period* is the period between the end of postictal abnormalities and the next ictus. *Periictal* refers to the period just before and after the ictus and is applied when there is insufficient information about when the ictus begins or ends. Epileptic seizures can be primary, secondary to a neurological condition, or reactive to a situational factor such as sleep deprivation or drug withdrawal. *Epilepsy* is the recurrent tendency to experience seizures. *Status epilepticus* is a condition of prolonged or repetitive seizures without intervening recovery.

In epilepsy, abnormal electrical discharges are caused by hyperexcitable neurons with sustained postsynaptic depolarization. Proposed mechanisms for the sustained depolarization include changes in ionic conductance, decreased γ-aminobutyric acid (GABA) inhibition of cortical excitability, and increased glutamate-mediated cortical excitation. In animals, alumina-induced membrane changes alter the ratio of intracellular-extracellular ionic concentrations and result in abnormal neuronal firing. Anticonvulsants such as phenytoin (Dilantin), carbamazepine (Tegretol), and valproate (Depakene) reduce this repetitive firing through effects on sodium channels. Ethosuximide (Zarontin) works through blockage of calcium currents. Penicillin-induced cortical injury causes seizures through decreased GABA inhibition. Barbiturates and benzodiazepines may reduce seizures by enhancing GABA-receptor current, and valproate through blockage of GABA catabolism. Kainic acid, a glutamate agonist, induces seizures through increased synaptic action at its *N*-methyl-D-aspartate (NMDA) receptors. Much work is underway on potential anticonvulsants which may work by inhibiting that excitatory receptor mechanism.

The electroencephalogram (EEG) is a surface recording of brain wave activity used in the evaluation of seizures. Basic waves include normal waking alpha waves (8 to 13 Hz), which are most prominent over the occipital region, high frequency β waves (above 13 Hz), and theta (4 to 7.5 Hz) and delta slowing (3.5 or less Hz) waves. Seizures are manifested as multiple spike of spike and wave discharges on the EEG (Figure 2.3-1). A spike is a sharp transient with a duration of 20 to 70 msec. Interictally one may see single spikes and other markers of abnormal electrical activity, often emanating from a temporal lobe.

HISTORY

In his book on epilepsy, *On the Sacred Disease,* Hippocrates (460 to 377 BC) attacked the prevailing belief that those afflicted with epilepsy were possessed by gods or goddesses. He proposed that epilepsy was a brain disease caused by the blockage by phlegm of air-carrying vessels to the brain. Despite this initial view, epilepsy was construed throughout most of human history as demonic possession or the accumulation of bad humors. Attempts at exorcism involved trephination, cautery of the back of the skull, diuretics, emetics, bloodletting, purging, sweating, and even sexual intercourse to release sperm. In the 18th century, the first scientific treatise on epilepsy since ancient times attributed seizures to masturbation. By happenstance, bromides, which were introduced to diminish libido and masturbation, proved to be the first successful anticonvulsant medication. With the development of effective anticonvulsants and the introduction of the EEG, we have come full circle to Hippocrates' belief that epilepsy is rooted in organic brain disease.

The association of epilepsy with behavioral disorders also dates to antiquity. The brain was regarded as the seat of both the falling sickness and madness, and both were related to phlegm. Unusual or abnormal behaviors were attributed to seizure patients even during their seizure-free periods. At the turn of the 19th century, Emil Kraepelin emphasized in his writings that epileptic patients possessed personality changes and a predisposition to psychosis. With the greater understanding of the physical basis of epilepsy, many clinicians sought to protect epileptic patients from the demonic stigma of their disease. In their view, psychiatric problems resulted from the psychosocial difficulties associated with seizures rather than any unique relationship of epilepsy with psychiatric illness. The present view was initiated by the definition of temporal lobe epilepsy and the concept of a physiological disturbance in the limbic or emotional brain. Again, one has come full circle back to the view of Hippocrates and the ancients that epilepsy is associated with mental illness, at least in some patients.

NOSOLOGY

The International Classification of Epileptic Seizures divides seizures into generalized and partial (Table 2.3-1). Generalized seizures have initial widespread bihemispheric involvement, and partial seizures emanate from a focus in one hemisphere. In adults, most generalized seizures are tonic-clonic seizures (grand mal seizures or convulsions) and are characterized by an abrupt loss of consciousness with tonic rigidity, followed by a synchronous, clonic release. Partial seizures are either complex partial seizures (psychomotor or temporal lobe epilepsy) or simple partial seizures, depending on whether or not there is complex symptomatology such as an alteration of consciousness or psychic symptoms (Table 2.3-2). Simple partial seizures pro-

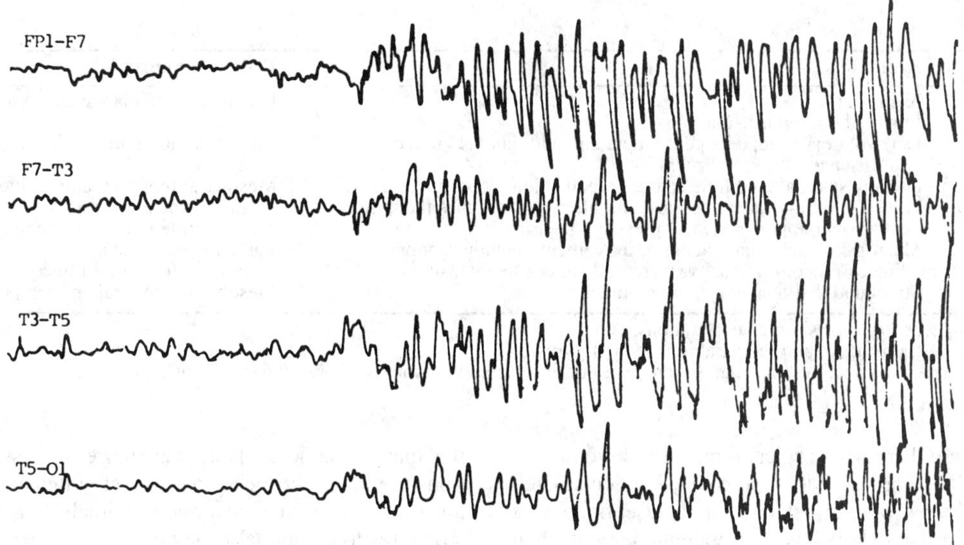

FIGURE 2.3-1 *Electroencephalogram showing right temporal spikes consistent with complex partial seizures.*

TABLE 2.3-1
The International Classification of Epileptic Seizures

I. Partial (focal, local) seizures
   A. Simple partial seizures
      Motor, somatosensory, autonomic, or mixed symptoms
   B. Complex partial seizures
      1. Begin with symptoms of simple partial seizure but progress to impairment of consciousness
      2. Begin with impairment of consciousness
      3. Involve psychic symptoms with or without impairment of consciousness
   C. Partial seizures with secondary generalization
      1. Begin with simple partial seizure
      2. Begin with complex partial seizure (including those with symptoms of simple partial seizures at onset)
II. Generalized seizures (convulsive or nonconvulsive)
   A. Absence (typical and atypical)
   B. Myoclonus
   C. Clonic
   D. Tonic
   E. Tonic-clonic
   F. Atonic-akinetic
III. Unclassified

duce isolated motor, somatosensory, autonomic, or mixed symptoms in a clear sensorium. The simple partial seizures that evolve to complex partial seizures are considered auras. Complex partial seizures are usually characterized by motionless staring combined with simple automatisms, or automatic motor activity, and they last about one minute. Complex partial seizures that evolve to generalized tonic-clonic seizures are secondarily generalized. Finally, a second form of generalized seizures, absence (petit mal) seizures, occur less commonly in adults and are characterized by brief lapses of consciousness. Absence seizures differ from complex partial seizures in being short (10 sec) and very repetitive; in lacking auras, postictal confusion, or complex automatisms; and in having characteristic 2 to 4 Hz spike and wave discharges on the EEG.

EPIDEMIOLOGY

Seizure disorders are common and usually have an early onset. Epilepsy affects 20 to 40 million people worldwide, has a prevalence of at least 0.63 percent and an annual incidence of about 0.05 percent. The overall incidence is high in the first year of life, drops to a minimum in the 30s and 40s, then increases again in later life. More than 75 percent of patients have their first seizure before age 18, and 12 to 20 percent have a familial incidence of seizures.

PSYCHOPATHOLOGY Epidemiological studies from communities, psychiatric hospitals, and epilepsy clinics have indicated a higher prevalence of psychiatric problems among epileptic patients as compared to normal controls.

About one quarter of all those with epilepsy and one half of those specifically with CPSs had psychosis, depression, anxiety, or childhood behavioral problems. The percentage of epileptic patients in psychiatric hospitals was also higher than the general prevalence of epilepsy and ranged from 4.7 percent of all inpatients in a British psychiatric hospital to 9.7 percent in a U.S. Veterans Affairs psychiatric facility. Furthermore, of patients attending epilepsy clinics, about 30 percent had a prior psychiatric hospitalization and 18 percent were on at least one psychotropic drug. Despite criticisms of selection bias, these studies constitute a broad spectrum of sources indicating greater overall psychopathology in epilepsy.

Is epilepsy associated with greater psychopathology than other disorders in similarly impaired patients? If this were so, it would suggest that the psychopathology is of biological origin rather than a less specific reaction to chronic disease. Although disputed by some investigators, several studies report more psychopathology among epileptic patients than among patients with chronic diseases that do not directly affect the brain. Furthermore, the pattern of behavioral changes in seizure patients appears specific to epilepsy. For example, on the Minnesota Multiphasic Personality Inventory (MMPI), despite a lack of difference in overall psychopathology, patients with epilepsy have higher schizophrenia scale and paranoia scale scores than patients with other neurological disabilities.

PSYCHOSIS Psychoses are the specific psychiatric disorder most clearly associated with epilepsy. The lifelong prevalence of all psychotic disorders among epileptic patients ranges from 7 to 12 percent. In a follow-up of 100 children with complex partial seizures for up to 30 years, of the 87 who survived to adulthood and did not have mental retardation, 9 (10 percent) experienced a psychotic illness. Moreover, in temporal lobec-

TABLE 2.3-2
Psychic Auras

Type	Symptoms	Probable Source
Dysphasic*	Nonfluent Impaired comprehension	Left perisylvian language areas
Dysmnestic	Déjà vu, déjà vécu, déjà pensé, déjà entendu, jamais vu, etc., prescience, illusion of memory	Mesobasal temporal,† especially on right
Cognitive	Dreamy state, altered time sense, derealization, depersonalization Forced thinking, forced actions, and altered or obscure thoughts	Mesobasal temporal and and temporal neocortex Frontal association cortex
Affective	Fear/anxiety/apprehension, depression, pleasure, unpleasure	Mesobasal temporal and temporal neocortex
Illusions‡	Macropsia, micropsia, teleopsia, movement, metamorphopsia, increased color intensity, increased stereopsis intensity	Lateral superior temporal neocortex, especially on right for visual illusions
Hallucinations‡	Structured, hallucinatory remembrances	Mesobasal temporal and temporal neocortex

*Does not include speech arrest or simple vocalizations.
†Includes hippocampus, amygdala, and the parahippocampal gyrus.
‡Includes either interpretive (size, motion, shape, stereopsis) or experiential (elements of past experience or involvement).

tomy studies, where there was surgical removal of an epileptic focus, psychosis occurred in 7 to 8 percent of patients, even long after the seizures were arrested. That represents about a two-fold or greater risk of psychosis for epileptic patients than for the general population, with a particular risk in epileptic patients with a mediobasal temporal focus.

LOCALIZATION AND LATERALITY Many studies have found an association between psychopathology and seizures emanating from mediobasal temporal lesions. Psychiatric disturbances, primarily psychotic and personality disorders, are two to three times more common in patients with complex partial seizures, most of whom have a temporal focus, than in those with GTCSs. Other studies have failed to find a difference. Nevertheless, 60 to 76 percent of epileptic adults, regardless of seizure type, have a temporal lobe focus, and many generalized tonic-clonic seizures are secondarily generalized from a temporal lobe focus without a preceding complex partial seizure. One cannot exclude the presence of mediobasal temporal limbic pathology in comparison groups with generalized tonic-clonic seizures.

Studies on the laterality of the seizure focus suggest an association of a left-sided focus with psychosis. Although conclusions derived from a surface EEG recording are open to criticism, depth recording of presurgical patients shows that twice as many patients with left temporal lesions have psychosis. Positron emission tomography (PET) scans and single photon emission computerized tomography (SPECT) scans may show predominant left temporal hypometabolism in psychotic epilepsy patients. Psychological studies also suggest a greater incidence of ideational orientation, self-criticism, and depression among epileptic patients with a left hemisphere focus. Conversely, studies have not established the proposed association of right hemisphere foci with mania and other disorders.

ETIOLOGY

Most new-onset epilepsy is idiopathic, but other frequent causes include trauma in the third and fourth decades, neoplasms in the fifth and sixth decade, and cerebrovascular disease in the elderly. Although some complex partial seizures originate from frontal or temporal neocortex and other areas, at least two thirds of complex partial seizures and generalized tonic-clonic seizures originate from the mediobasal temporal limbic structures (hippocampus, amygdala, and parahippocampal gyrus).

PSYCHOPATHOLOGY The relation among seizures, psychiatric syndromes, and the mediobasal temporal lobes implies that many behavioral changes are more than psychological reactions to the psychosocial stressors of epilepsy. Stimulation and ablation studies in humans and animals link temporal limbic structures to emotional behavior.

For example, temporal limbic stimulation in a person evokes psychic auras and automatisms, and amygdalar stimulation and ablation in animals results in either aggression or placidity. Moreover, psychotic behavior in cats occurs when their limbic structures undergo kindling (that is, the repeated application of epileptic agents in order to induce lasting behavioral changes).

There are several potential organic causes of psychiatric disturbances in epilepsy (Table 2.3-3). First, the pathology itself may be the source of both seizures and behavioral changes. Left hemisphere and temporal lobe lesions may be associated with a schizophreniform psychosis, and psychosis in epilepsy may be particularly frequent if there is specific underlying pathology or ventricular enlargement. Second, ictal or subictal epileptiform activity may promote behavioral changes by facilitating distributed neuronal connections, increasing limbic-sensory associations, or changing the overall balance between excitation and inhibition. Third, the absence of function, such as in the interictal hypometabolism observed on PET scans, may lead to depression or other interictal behavioral changes. Fourth, seizures may result in neuroendocrine or neurotransmitter changes that affect behavior, such as increased dopaminergic or inhibitory transmitters, decreased prolactin, increased testosterone, or increased endogenous opioids. Furthermore, organic factors

TABLE 2.3-3
Proposed Relationships of Psychiatric Disturbances to Epilepsy

Common neuropathology, genetics, or developmental disturbance
Ictal or subictal discharges potentiate abnormal behavior
- Kindling or facilitation of a distributed neuronal matrix
- Changes in spike frequency or inhibitory-excitatory balance
- Altered receptor sensitivity (e.g., dopamine receptors)
- Secondary epileptogenesis

Absence of function at the seizure focus
- Inhibition and hypometabolism surrounding the focus
- Release or abnormal activity of remaining neurons
- Dysfunction or down-regulation of associated areas

Neurochemical changes
- Dopamine and other neurotransmitters
- Endorphins
- Gonadotrophins

Psychodynamic factors
- Dependence, learned helplessness, low self-esteem
- Disruption of reality testing
- Weakening of defense mechanisms

Organic and psychodynamic potentiate each other
Sleep disturbance
Drug-induced factors

may be potentiated by psychodynamic factors, such as feelings of helplessness, dependency, low self-esteem, and the disruption of reality testing. In sum, the psychiatric manifestations of epilepsy are heterogeneous disorders with a multiplicity of causes.

DIAGNOSIS AND CLINICAL FEATURES

In epilepsy, the various psychiatric behaviors occur ictally, periictally, or interictally (Table 2.3-4). Depression is the most common of these psychiatric behaviors, but psychosis, borderline personality disorder, and hyposexuality are also frequent.

ICTAL FEATURES Seizure discharges can produce semipurposeful automatisms and psychic auras such as affective changes, forced thinking, derealization, and depersonalization. When these arise in isolation or persist beyond the ictus, they may present as one of the cognitive disorders. Ictal fear, which ranges from a vague apprehension to abject fright, has occurred without any other seizure manifestation, and ictal depression has extended days or longer after the seizure has passed. An inescapable, recurrent forced thought suggests psychotic or obsessive thinking, and feelings of derealization could impair reality testing. Some epileptic patients have pleasurable auras. Fyodor Dostoyevsky had "ecstatic auras," where he felt in perfect harmony with the entire universe and "would give 10 years of this life, perhaps all of it, for a few seconds of such bliss."

Cognitive disorders follow status epilepticus with simple partial seizures, complex partial seizures, or absence seizures. Recurrent or prolonged SPSs do not result in alteration of consciousness or invariable abnormalities on the EEG, and, if manifested by psychic auras, simple partial seizures may be difficult to distinguish from primary psychiatric disturbances. Status epilepticus from complex partial seizures and absence seizures result in prolonged alterations of responsiveness. With the addition of various ictal auras, CPS status can appear psychotic. Finally, recurrent EEG complexes known as periodic lateralizing epileptiform discharges may be associated with prolonged confusional behavior and focal cognitive changes.

A 68-year-old man had a left temporal-parietal hemorrhagic stroke. An initial fluent aphasia and right hemiparesis completely resolved, but he developed poststroke epilepsy. His seizures began with speech arrest and were followed by secondary generalization to generalized tonic-clonic seizures. The postictal periods lasted days due to continued left hemisphere periodic lateralizing epileptiform discharges. During these prolonged postictal periods, he was confused, placid, and had a return of his aphasia.

One year later, after achieving seizure control, the patient developed mania for the first time in his life. His mania was in a clear sensorium without a change in his neurological examination or epileptiform activity on the EEG. He did not sleep, had flight of ideas, and had grandiose ideation, including beliefs that he was a three-star general, had killed Hitler, and was now a millionaire. He exposed himself to everyone, including his daughter, and inserted pencils up his penis because he believed that he needed catheterization. His psychosis lasted for three months until he had two generalized tonic-clonic seizures. Postictally, for 10 days he remained placid, confused, and asphasic, with a right beating nystagmus and periodic lateralizing epileptiform discharges maximal in the left temporal region (Figure 2.3-2). With a new anticonvulsant medication he returned to normal with total resolution of his mania.

TABLE 2.3-4
Behavioral Disorders in Epilepsy

I. Ictal
  A. Ictal psychic symptoms
  B. Non-convulsive status: simple partial seizures, complex partial seizures, and periodic lateralizing epileptiform discharges
II. Periictal (includes preictal, postictal, and mixed ictal)
  A. Preictal prodromal symptoms: dysphoria, apprehension, etc.
  B. Postictal confusion
  C. Periictal psychosis
    1. Concomitant with increased seizure frequency
    2. Alternating psychoses
    3. Postictal psychoses
III. Interictal psychosis and personality disturbances
  A. Chronic schizophreniform psychosis
  B. Heightened significance personality characteristics
  C. Borderline personality disorder
IV. Behavioral disturbances variably related to ictus
  A. Dissociative states
  B. Mood disorders
  C. Suicide
  D. Sexuality
  E. Aggression and violence
  F. Other behaviors

PERIICTAL FEATURES Periictal behavioral changes occur before seizures (preictal), after seizures (postictal), or during intermittent seizure activity. Dysphoria, insomnia, anxiety, or build-up of tension may precede seizures or be relieved by them. The postictal period is characterized by a confusional state lasting minutes to hours or, occasionally, days. Some twilight states result from a protracted period of intermixed ictal and postictal changes.

Investigators have also described brief psychotic episodes, which may be precipitated or relieved by seizures or alternate with them, particularly in patients who have complex partial seizures with secondary GTCSs. These periictal psychotic episodes usually constitute days to weeks of agitated, hallucinatory, paranoid, and impulsive behaviors, often accompanied by sudden mood swings and suicide attempts. Some patients develop psychosis concomitant with an increase in seizure frequency or anticonvulsant withdrawal and, on control of the seizures, have resolution of the psychosis. Others develop a psychosis immediately after a flurry of seizures and may occasionally continue to display psychotic symptoms for an extended period of time. These postictal psychotic episodes are often delayed after a latency of 12 to 48 hours, during which the immediate postictal confusion may resolve. A third group of patients develop psychosis after their seizures are controlled, and the psychosis promptly resolves once the seizures recur. The terms "alternating psychosis" and "forced or paradoxical normalization" refer to a demonstrable antagonism between the periictal psychosis and the seizures or EEG discharges. The disappearance of seizures or EEG discharges may precipitate other behaviors, such as a more chronic interictal schizophrenialike psychosis.

A 33-year-old man with a 15-year history of generalized tonic-clonic seizures and a 4-year history of periictal psychotic episodes was hospitalized several times for recurrent postictal psychosis. The initial flurry of GTCS's was followed by a 24- to 48-hour latency period, and, subsequently, two to seven days of delusions, hallucinations, and disordered thought processes. He believed that people could transmit messages to him and read his thoughts, and that voices commanded him to love his neighbor. The patient claimed to read the future and to communicate with a dead grandfather who voiced dissatisfaction with things on earth. During those episodes, the patient had loose associations, euphoria, agitation, and occasional spike and waves on the EEGs. Between psychotic episodes, he was psychiatrically and neurologically normal, and his EEGs showed left temporal interictal spikes. After the postictal psychosis, the patient returned to baseline without residual changes in behavior.

INTERICTAL PSYCHOSIS Most epileptic patients with a schizophrenialike psychosis have a chronic interictal illness without known direct relations to seizure events or ictal discharges. Those patients often have an 11 to 15 year history of poorly controlled seizures, most commonly poorly controlled

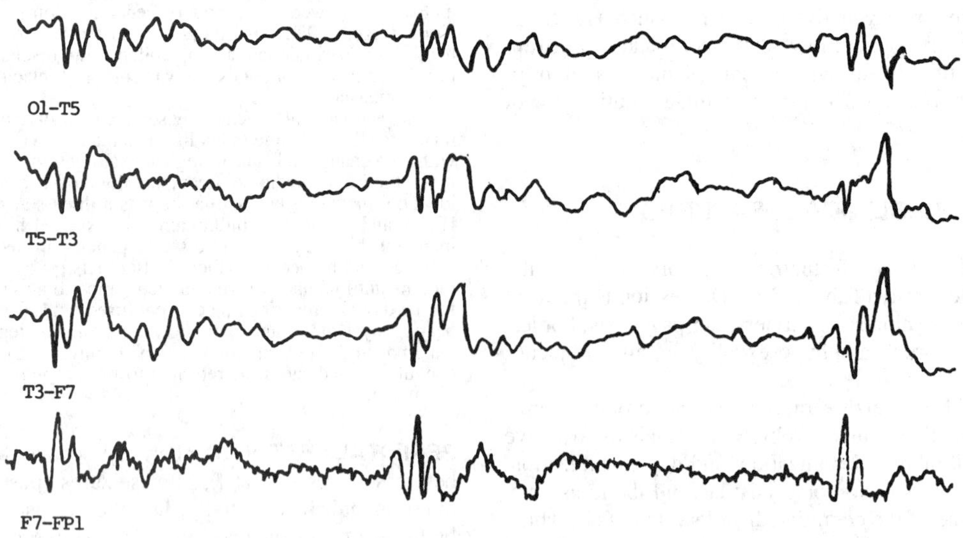

FIGURE 2.3-2 *Periodic lateralizing epileptiform discharges (PLEDs).*

complex partial seizures and auras. However, seizure control with anticonvulsants or removal of the seizure focus does not prevent the development of this psychosis, which occasionally emerges for the first time after successful seizure treatment. This disorder sometimes resembles a schizoaffective disorder with intermixed affective symptoms. In addition, there are prominent paranoid delusions, relative preserved affect, normal premorbid personality, and no family history of schizophrenia. Other reported differences with idiopathic schizophrenia are outlined in Table 2.3-5.

A 23-year-old man developed paranoid delusions after his daily complex partial seizures were controlled for the first time. His seizures dated from age 8 years and consisted of a rising epigastric sensation and facial flushing followed by a motionless stare and automatisms, often culminating in secondary generalized tonic-clonic seizures. Prior to initiating anticonvulsant therapy, the patient had no history of paranoid or psychotic behavior. Afterwards, he believed that people were sending energy to him through small concealed batteries. He felt able to work this energy off with his fluorescent watch dial and a one-armed plastic crucifix in his boot. The patient also felt that people were observing him, trying to manipulate him, and threatening him through telephone lines and telephone poles. His examination was remarkable for the degree of emotion he exhibited while relating his bizarre ideas. He had a lesion in the left anterior temporal area, probably consistent with an old calcified cyst, and left temporal spikes on the EEG. His paranoid delusions subsequently abated with antipsychotic therapy.

TABLE 2.3-5
Predisposing Factors for the Chronic Interictal Psychosis of Epilepsy

Epilepsy Characteristics:
- Complex partial seizures with secondary generalized tonic-clonic seizures
- More auras and automatisms than in nonpsychotic epilepsy patients
- Epilepsy present for 11–15 years before psychosis
- Long interval of poorly controlled seizures
- Recently diminished seizure frequency, especially of GTCSs
- Left temporal focus
- Mediobasal temporal lesions, especially tumors

Psychosis Characteristics:
- Atypical paranoid psychosis
- Psychosis alternating with seizures
- Preserved affective warmth
- Failure of personality deterioration
- Less social withdrawal than in schizophrenia
- Less systematized delusions than in schizophrenia
- More hallucinations and affective symptoms than in schizophrenia
- More religiosity than in schizophrenia
- More positive as opposed to negative symptoms
- Few Schneiderian first-rank symptoms
- Negative family history for psychosis
- Absent schizophrenogenic background

HEIGHTENED SIGNIFICANCE PERSONALITY Although there is no general epileptic personality, specific personality traits occur in a subset of patients with complex partial seizures. Some epileptic patients with a temporal limbic focus develop a sense of the heightened significance of things. Those patients are serious, humorless, overinclusive, circumstantial, tenacious, or viscous in interpersonal encounters and have an intense interest in philosophical, religious, and moral issues. They may spend a long time getting to the point, give detailed background information with multiple quotations, or write copiously about their thoughts and feelings. In addition, some of these epileptic patients experience multiple religious conversions or experiences.

A 39-year-old man developed seizures following a contusion of the left temporal region. His seizures began with stereotypical voices and spread to secondary generalized tonic-clonic seizures. He was extremely circumstantial and tangential, stressed every detail, and had difficulty getting to the point. Ironic and minor philosophical insights were fascinating to him. He wrote 30-page rambling letters to his physician, and his writings were full of metaphors and quotes. An example of his writing was as follows: ''I became overwhelmed by the sentiment of a letter composed in my head before reaching paper. The sentiment of this letter continued to expand in all dimensions until it seemed no longer connected to any specific ideal, but more to an all-pervasive color, yellow, and a smell, like burning leaves. I felt deliriously happy, but I felt in danger as well. Afterwards I got an acute attack of aphasia and could do nothing but shrug. My prior prophet voices which went away with the Dilantin were saying something profound that I needed to get down on paper. It seems as though I am a prophet and I will never have another problem for the rest of my life.''

Conclusive proof that epileptic patients with a temporal lobe foci are prone to this heightened sense of significance has remained elusive. Most of the early studies used the MMPI, a test that proved insensitive to most of the specific traits attributed to epilepsy. Studies with the Bear-Fedio Inventory, an MMPI-like instrument developed to assess those so-called epileptic traits, found that epileptic patients with temporal lobe foci were sober and humorless, dependent, circumstantial, and had strong philosophical interests. In addition, those with a left-sided focus had a more reflective ideational style and maximized their problems, while those with a right-sided focus had emotional tendencies and minimized their problems. Further investigations with the Bear-Fedio Inventory described those seizure patients as having viscosity in interactions, prominent religious interests, a pronounced sense of personal destiny, and deepened affect. However, other applications of this inventory found the same characteristics in nonepileptic patients with psychiatric disorders or with comparable physical disabilities. Although these personality characteristics do occur in some epileptic patients, they may not be specific for patients with seizure disorders.

BORDERLINE PERSONALITY DISORDER The most common personality disorder in epilepsy is borderline personality disorder. Epileptic patients frequently lack a stable character structure and may be immature and impulsive. That personality constellation partially explains the increased incidence of irritability, suicide attempts, and intermittent explosive disorder. Those with epilepsy are stigmatized, feared, and subject to difficulties in obtaining a job, driving, and maintaining a marriage. Those psychosocial difficulties, along with any associated mental retardation, contribute to the dependency, low self-esteem, and overall borderline personality traits present in many epileptic patients.

DISSOCIATIVE STATES A specific association of epilepsy with dissociative identity disorder, depersonalization disorder, possession states, fugue states, and psychogenic amnesia is intriguing but unresolved. Studies of patients with dissociative identity disorder reveal frequent EEG changes but few actual seizures. It is conceivable that temporary personality disintegration occurs in some patients as part of postictal confusion or periictal psychosis, particularly in those with a right temporal focus. Persistent alterations in the experience of self and feelings of being taken over by others may occur in patients with auras of derealization and depersonalization. In epilepsy, prolonged periods of compulsive wandering with amnesia have resulted from an admixture of ictal and postictal changes and have been termed ''poriomania.'' Finally, some patient may have periods of amnesia or lost time, possibly due to complex partial seizures without surface EEG abnormalities.

MOOD DISORDERS Depressive disorder is the most prevalent neuropsychiatric disorder in epilepsy and the main diagnosis among epileptic patients in mental hospitals. Depressive disorder is twice as common in seizure patients as in comparably disabled populations suggesting that it is more than just a psychological reaction to a disability.

There are subgroups of depression in epilepsy. Many ''depressileptics'' have a chronic interictal depression or dysthymia and frequent paranoid delusions and hallucinations emphasizing the continuum with psychotic disorders. The rare occurrence of ictal depression may not only outlast the actual ictus but may lead to suicide. Depression also occurs periictally. Episodic mood disturbances, often with agitation, suicidal behavior, and psychotic symptoms, may occur with increasing seizure activity. Several investigators also report a decrease in seizures prior to the onset of depressive symptoms ranging from prodromal dysphoria to a schizoaffective disorder. Patients with that alternating depression experience relief with a seizure, particularly a secondary generalized tonic-clonic seizure, much like the effects of electroconvulsive therapy (ECT). Finally, postictal depression is common, and, a prolonged depressive state occasionally follows complex partial seizures even when ictal experiences do not include depression.

Mood disorder due to epilepsy with manic features or with mixed features is much rarer than mood disorder due to epilepsy with depressive features or with major depressivelike features but may emerge with an increase in seizure frequency or after seizure control. Although a right temporal focus was suggested as the source of mania in epilepsy, that laterality is not established.

SUICIDE The risk of completed suicide in epileptic patients is about 4 to 5 times greater than among the nonepileptic population, and those with complex partial seizures of temporal lobe origin have a particularly high risk, up to 25 times greater than the nonepileptic population. A comparison of suicide attempts among epileptic patients and comparably handicapped nonepileptic controls has revealed that 30 percent of those with epilepsy had attempted suicide as compared with 7 percent of the controls. The increased risk of suicide continues even long after temporal lobectomy and successful control of seizures. Most suicidal behavior among epileptic patients is not directly due to reactions to the psychosocial stressors of a seizure disorder. Rather, epileptic patients are likely to attempt suicide in conjunction with borderline personality disorder behaviors and likely to complete suicide from psychosis. Contributors to successful suicides include paranoid hallucinations, agitated compunction to kill themselves, and occasional ictal command hallucinations to commit suicide.

A 26-year-old woman had her initial seizure during her first pregnancy at age 18. Her seizures included echoing sounds ''like walking in a cave,'' a motionless stare with stereotypical automatisms, postictal confusion, and occasional secondary generalized tonic-clonic seizures. Because of a variable anticonvulsant response, she underwent closed-circuit television video-EEG telemetry that documented both complex partial seizures from a right temporal focus and nonepileptic seizures. The patient, who had six children by six different men, had prominent feelings of inadequacy and isolation and was considering cutting her wrists ''just to see if anyone cared.'' Her multiple suicide attempts and threats resulted in five psychiatric hospitalizations. During one period of time, she complained of decreased menses, weight gain, stretch marks, increased appetite and sleep, and exhaustion. She insisted that she was pregnant despite six negative pregnancy tests and multiple evaluations.

SEXUALITY Epileptic patients often have a disinterest in all the usual libidinous aspects of life. They may lose erotic fantasies or dreams and may suffer from impotence or frigidity. Hyposexuality appears directly related to seizure events. Substantial improvement to the point of public hypersexuality can occur after seizures are brought under control. Moreover, prior to temporal lobectomy, most epileptic patients are hyposexual, but nearly one third of them have an increase in libido after the operation.

Other sexuality changes are rare. Individual cases of homosexuality, transvestism, fetishism, and gender dysphoria are not frequent enough to exclude a coincident association. True ictal sexual manifestations are also unusual; however, libidinous feelings, erotic sensations, sexual remembrances, and even orgasm rarely occur, primarily in women, and probably result from seizure discharges in the amygdala. In addition, ictal masturbation has occurred with absence status. A woman with erotomania proved to have incidental sexuality from sensory simple partial seizures caused by a tumor in the sensory cortex, representing her genital region.

AGGRESSION Lay people have accredited to epilepsy aggressive and violent acts and have even used that epilepsy defense in criminal proceedings. Investigators have bolstered this association with studies showing aggressive verbalizations with stimulation of the amygdala and interictal defensive rage in cats with epileptic hippocampal lesions. Furthermore, the prevalence of epilepsy among prisons has been two to four times higher than among the general population.

Yet epilepsy is not a cause of premeditated violence. Studies from both Britain and the United States have failed to find more violent crimes among epileptic prisoners compared with nonepileptic prisoners. Most directed aggression in epilepsy is associated with psychosis or intermittent explosive disorder and correlates with subnormal intelligence, low socioeconomic status, childhood behavior problems, prior head injuries, and possible orbital frontal damage. Semidirected ictally related aggression rarely occurs as an automatism or, after a delay, as a response to an unpleasant or emotional aura or periictal sensation (Table 2.3-6). More commonly, nondirected violent movements, aimless destructive behavior, or angry verbal outburst occur during the postictal confusional state when patients react violently to attempts to restrain them.

A 38-year-old man had complex partial seizures and secondary generalized tonic-clonic seizures since age 5 years. His seizures began with a sensation of buzzing in his head and turning to the right, and were associated with a left temporal focus. He also had frequent violent behavior consisting of breaking windows, destroying property, and making personal assaults. The patient actually complained of wanting to hurt others and of an urge to kill people. When he was accused of homicide, he underwent a court-ordered neuropsychiatric evaluation. He stated that he was excessively irritable, prone to lose his temper, and believed that people were talking about him and wanted to hurt him. When people walked behind him, he felt that they would stick a knife in him. His affect was normal, and his intellectual level was average. The neuropsychiatric assessment concluded that his violence resulted from a paranoid psychosis rather than from ictal aggression.

OTHER BEHAVIORAL CHANGES Other psychiatric disorders may be associated with epilepsy or epileptiform EEG activity. Among the impulse control disorders, intermittent explosive disorder is characterized by a prodromal mounting tension and irritability, postictal remorse, and increased temporal spikes on the EEG. Among the somatoform disorders, some epileptic patients have a conversion disorder, often manifested as nonepileptic seizure events. Finally, compared to the nonepileptic population, epileptic patients are subject to greater anxiety and adjustment disorders, subtle cognitive effects of seizures, and the potential behavioral effects of anticonvulsant medications.

PATHOLOGY AND LABORATORY EXAMINATION

NEURODIAGNOSTIC TESTS In addition to the routine laboratory data and toxicology screens used to exclude reactive seizures, several neurodiagnostic tests are useful in the assessment of epilepsy. The EEG is the most widely used confirmatory test for seizures; however, single EEGs are frequently normal and must be repeated, particularly with provocative maneuvers, such as sleep. Occasionally, closed-circuit television video-EEG telemetry for an extended period of time is necessary to capture seizure activity. Neuroimaging procedures such as magnetic resonance imaging can more precisely visualize a seizure focus or even mesial temporal sclerosis (Figure 2.3-3). Other tests, which are primarily of interest in research, occasionally aid in localizing the seizure focus, include quantitative EEG, SPECT, and PET scanning. PET scans may show interictal hypometabolism around the temporal seizure focus and are also useful in the presurgical assessment of medically intractable seizure patients. Neuropsychological examinations, particularly during a Wada Test, further help in localizing and lateralizing memory and language prior to surgery.

TABLE 2.3-6
Criteria for Assessing Ictal Violence in Epilepsy

1. The diagnosis of epilepsy is established by at least one specialist in epilepsy.
2. The presence of epileptic automatisms is documented by history and by closed-circuit television video-EEG telemetry.
3. The presence of violence during epileptic automatisms is verified in a videotape-recorded seizure in which ictal epileptiform patterns are also recorded on the EEG.
4. The aggressive act is characteristic of the patient's habitual seizures, as elicited by history.
5. A clinical judgment is made by the epilepsy specialist, attesting to the possibility that the aggressive act was part of a seizure.

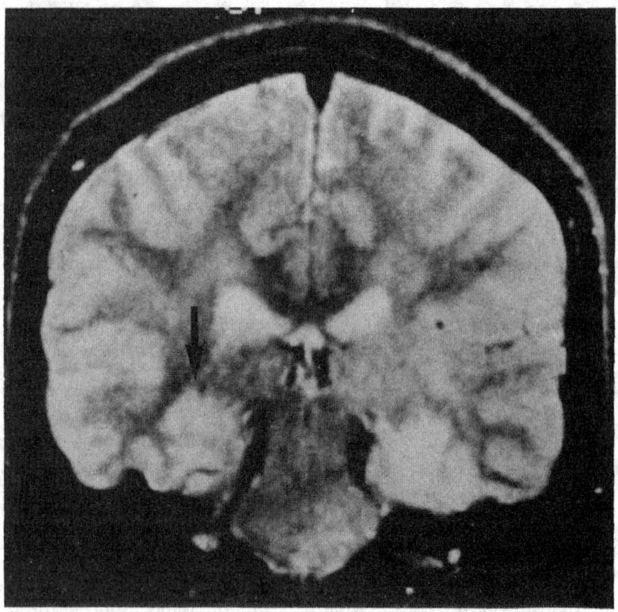

FIGURE 2.3-3 *Magnetic resonance imaging of the head showing right-sided mesial temporal sclerosis (irregular shaped area of increased signal in right hippocampal region). (Photograph courtesy of John Gates, M.D., and the Minnesota Epilepsy Group.)*

NEUROPATHOLOGY The common pathological findings in epilepsy are mediobasal temporal lobe lesions. About two thirds of epileptic adults have a temporal lobe focus and two thirds of those have mesial temporal sclerosis with pyramidal cell loss in the hippocampus. Theories about the cause of mesial temporal sclerosis include perinatal insults, dysgenesis, and kindling from reactive seizures. Another 20 to 25 percent of those with temporal lobe lesions have tumors such as hamartomas and gangliogliomas. The rest have scars from trauma and other causes or lack a distinct histological lesion.

DIFFERENTIAL DIAGNOSIS

Epileptic seizures may be particularly difficult to distinguish from two other transient behavioral events, syncope and nonepileptic seizures, or pseudoseizures. Syncope is a loss of consciousness usually with premonitory lightheadedness, autonomic reactivity, a brief atonic ictus, and little or no postictal confusion. Syncope lacks both the many characteristic features of seizures and a clear epileptiform EEG. Nonepileptic seizures, on the other hand, are involuntary, psychogenically induced spells that, by definition, mimic many epileptic behaviors. These spells are not due to malingering but usually result from conversion reactions, personality disorders, or depression.

Differentiating nonepileptic seizures can be difficult, and even epileptologists are incorrect from 20 to 30 percent of the time. Patients with nonepileptic seizures are most commonly women between the ages of 26 and 32 years with psychological stressors and poor coping skills. Many have a true seizures disorder as well, and nonepileptic seizures may result from the elaborating or highlighting of epileptic seizures. Nonepileptic seizures are characterized by a sudden collapse or by motor activity which does not fit a typical complex partial seizure or a generalized tonic-clonic seizure (Table 2.3-7). However, every epileptic behavior can occur occasionally, including tongue biting and incontinence, and nonepileptic events are especially difficult to differentiate from the atypical motor behavior of frontal lobe epilepsy. The most helpful differentiation feature may be an ictal duration of two or more minutes. In addition, nonepileptic seizures usually occur in the presence of a witness, can often be induced with injections or suggestions, and respond poorly to anticonvulsant treatment. Ultimately, the differentiation may require CCTV-EEG telemetry along with the assessment of the absence of a seizure-induced rise in serum prolactin levels.

COURSE AND PROGNOSIS

Most epileptic patients have a good prognosis. The majority of seizures can be sufficiently controlled with anticonvulsant medications so that the patient can live a productive life. Some seizures, such as absence seizures, tend to disappear by adulthood. For epileptic patients who are medically intractable, epilepsy surgery offers a good alternative (that is, temporal lobectomy or corpus callosotomy), provided the focus can be localized or lateralized. In addition, most epileptic patients will not have psychiatric disorders, and others have psychiatric difficulties only if they endure many years of poorly controlled seizures. For those with behavioral problems, anticonvulsant drugs or epilepsy surgery may relieve some symptoms, such as hyposexuality and aggression, but may not affect the emergence of others, such as psychosis and suicidal behavior.

TREATMENT

ANTICONVULSANT MEDICATIONS In the treatment of psychiatrically disturbed epileptic patients, a first consideration is the behavioral effects of anticonvulsant medications. Encephalopathic changes occur at toxic levels of all these medications. Even at therapeutic levels, barbiturates may need to be discontinued because of drug-induced depression, suicidal ideation, sedation, psychomotor slowing, and paradoxical hyperactivity in the very young and the very old. In the treatment of behaviorally disturbed seizure patients, the best drugs may be carbamazepine or valproate. Both drugs are mood stabilizers with significant antimanic and modest antidepressant effects, including some efficacy in long-term prophylaxis. Carbamazepine appears to be a more significant antimanic agent particularly with rapid-cyclers and those with dysphoria. Clonazepam (Klonopin), in addition to its anxiolytic properties, can serve as a supplement to other antimanic therapies. Both carbamazepine and ethosuximide may have value for borderline personality disorder, and carbamazepine can ameliorate some dyscontrolled, aggressive behavior. Other anticonvulsant medications do not have clearly established psychotropic properties, but much more research is still needed in this area.

PSYCHOTROPIC MEDICATIONS A second consideration is the seizure threshold lowering effect of psychotropic medications (Table 2.3-8), a problem which can occasionally reach clinical significance in poorly controlled epilepsy. Psychotropic drugs are most convulsive with rapid introduction and in high doses. Clozapine (Clozaril), for example, has induced seizures in 1 to 4.4 percent of patients, particularly when the dose was rapidly increased. When initiating psychotropic therapy, it is best to start low and go slow while monitoring anticonvulsant levels and EEGs.

DRUG INTERACTIONS A third treatment consideration is the potential for interaction of anticonvulsant and psychotropic medications (Table 2.3-9). Most commonly, an anticonvulsant drug increases the metabolism of a psychotropic drug with a consequent decrease in its therapeutic efficiency. Conversely, withdrawal of anticonvulsant drugs can precipitate rebound elevations in psychotropic levels. Moreover, the initiation of a psychotropic drug may result in competitive inhibition of anticonvulsant metabolism with elevations of anticonvulsant levels to toxicity.

SURGERY Epilepsy surgery is a fourth treatment consideration and is limited to patients with medically intractable sei-

TABLE 2.3-7
Nonepileptic Seizures: Helpful But Not Diagnostic Ictal Characteristics

Preceding ictus
- Presence of emotional precipitants and a model for seizures
- Seizures can be induced
- Seizures only occur when others are present
- Anxiety auras: palpitations, choking, dizziness, paresthesias

During ictus
- Do not fit known seizure types or seizure sequence
- Gradual onset, prolonged duration, and abrupt termination
- Sudden collapse
- Asymmetric, out-of-phase movements of arms or legs
- Pelvic thrusts, hyperarching, side-to-side head movements
- Absence of whole body rigidity, autonomic reactivity, incontinence, tongue-biting, or injury on falling, and presence of corneal reflex
- Avoidance of noxious stimuli or eye opening
- Vocalization at the start and crying, screaming, or talking
- No increase in prolactin
- Normal ictal EEG

Following ictus
- No postictal confusion
- Normal postictal EEG and no interictal spikes
- Subsequent recall of events during the ictus
- Absence of stereotypy (i.e., different from attack to attack)
- No relationship of ictal events to anticonvulsant drugs or levels

TABLE 2.3-8
Seizure Threshold Lowering Effect of Psychotropic Medications

Potential	Antipsychotic	Antidepressant	Other Psychotropic
		Proconvulsant	
High	Chlorpromazine	Buproprion	
	Clozapine	Imipramine	
		Maprotiline	
		Amitriptyline	
		Amoxapine	
		Nortriptyline	
Moderate	Most piperazines	Protriptyline	Lithium
	Thiothixene	Clomipramine	
Low	Fluphenazine	Doxepin	Ethchlorvynol
	Haloperidol	Desipramine	Glutethimide
	Loxapine	Fluoxetine	Hydroxyzine
	Molindone	Trazodone	Meprobamate
	Pimozide	Trimipramine	Methaqualone
	Thioridazine		
	Resperidone		
		Anticonvulsant	
Low	Methylphenidate	MAOIs	Oral benzodiazepines
	Detroamphetamine		
High			Barbiturates

TABLE 2.3-9
Anticonvulsant-Psychotropic Drug Effects on Blood Levels

Anticonvulsant	Indication*	Psychotropic† Effects on Anticonvulsant	Anticonvulsant Effect on Psychotropic†
Carbamazepine	SPS, CPS, GTCS	Potentially decreased	Decreased
Phenytoin	SPS, CPS, GTCS	Potentially decreased or increased, rarely toxic levels	Decreased
Phenobarbital and primidone	SPS, CPS, GTCS	Potentially decreased	Significantly decreased
Valproic acid	CPS, GTCS, absence	Potentially increased, rarely toxic levels	Potentially decreased
Ethosuximide	Absence	None known	None known
Clonazepam	Myoclonic	Potentially decreased	Potentially decreased

*Note: SPS = simple partial seizure, CPS = complex partial seizure, GTCS = generalized tonic-clonic seizure
†Antipsychotic and antidepressant drugs; lithium and the minor tranquilizers have few drug interactions with anticonvulsant drugs.

zures. The main operation involves resection of epileptogenic tissue by removal of 4 to 6 cm of the anterior temporal lobe. Over 80 percent of temporal lobectomy patients experience some reduction in their seizure frequency and over 50 percent are entirely seizure-free. Despite removal of the amygdala and most of the hippocampus, there are few postoperative behavioral effects. A few patients have an anomia or a verbal memory deficit after resection of the dominant hemisphere, and patients occasionally develop a transient postoperative depression. Others experience a reduction in preoperative depression and relief of hyposexuality, but epileptic patients may continue to develop psychosis, personality changes, and suicidal behavior even long after the temporal lobectomy.

Less common epilepsy surgeries include the resection of extratemporal lesions, the removal of the epileptogenic hemisphere, and the ligation of the corpus callosum. Corpus callosotomy, which aims to prevent the interhemispheric spread of seizures, results in a unique, transient disconnection syndrome of mutism, apathy, agnosia, apraxia of the nondominant limbs, and difficulty naming and writing with the nondominant hand.

SEIZURE MANAGEMENT In treating the neuropsychiatric disorders of epilepsy, a final consideration is altering the seizure management itself. In addition to the occasional behavior alleviated by strict seizure control, allowing seizures under carefully controlled conditions, much like ECT, relieves some cases of periictal psychosis, depression, or other behaviors.

SUGGESTED CROSS-REFERENCES

Most of the specific psychiatric syndromes associated with epilepsy are discussed in more detail in the appropriate sections devoted to them: Personality disorders are discussed in Chapter 25, mood disorders are discussed in Chapter 16, and sexual disorders are discussed in Chapter 21. The rest of the neuropsychiatric sections in Chapter 2 are also pertinent to epilepsy.

REFERENCES

Adamec R E: Does kindling model anything clinically relevant? Biol Psychiatry *27:* 249, 1990.
*Bear D, Fedio P: Quantitative analysis of interictal behavior in temporal lobe epilepsy. Arch Neurol *34:* 454, 1977.
Diehl L W: Epilepsie und suizid. Psychiatr Neurol Med Psychol *38:* 625, 1986.
Dongier S: Statistical study of clinical and electroencephalographic manifestations of 536 psychotic episodes occurring in 516 epileptics between clinical seizures. Epilepsia *1:* 117, 1959–1960.
Engel J, Ludwig B, Fetell M: Prolonged partial complex status epilepticus: EEG and behavioral observations. Neurology *28:* 863, 1978.
Ervin F, Epstein R W, King H E: Behavior of epileptic and nonepileptic patients with "temporal spikes." Arch Neurol Psychiatry *74*:488, 1955.
Falconer, M A: Reversibility by temporal-lobe resection of the behavioral abnormalities of temporal-lobe epilepsy. N Engl J Med *289:* 451, 1973.
Gates J R: Psychogenic seizures. Merritt-Putnam Quarterly *4:* 3, 1987.
Gibbs A: Ictal and non-ictal psychiatric disorders in temporal lobe epilepsy. J Nerv Ment Dis *113:* 522, 1951.
Gudmundsson G: Epilepsy in Iceland: A clinical and epidemiological investigation. Acta Neurol Scand *25* (Suppl): 1, 1966.
Heath R G: Psychosis and epilepsy: Similarities and differences in the anatomic-physiologic substrate. Adv Biol Psychiatry *8:* 106, 1982.
Koch-Weser M, Garron D C, Gilley D W, Bergen D, Bleck T P, Morrell F, Ristanovic R, Whisler W W Jr: Prevalence of psychological disorders after surgical treatment of seizures. Arch Neurol *45:* 1308, 1988.
Landolt H: Serial electroencephalographic investigations during psychotic episodes in epileptic patients and during schizophrenic attacks. In *Lectures on Epilepsy,* L de Haas, editor. Elsevier, New York, 1958.
*Lindsay J, Ounsted C, Richards P: Long-term outcome in children with temporal lobe seizures: III. Psychiatric aspects in childhood and adult life. Dev Med Child Neurol *21:* 630, 1979.
Logsdail S J, Toone B K: Post-ictal psychosis, a clinical and phenomenological description. Br J Psychiatry *152:* 246, 1988.
Mark V H, Ervin F R: *Violence and the Brain.* Harper & Row, New York, 1970.
Mathews W S, Barabas G: Suicide and epilepsy: A review of the literature. Psychosomatics *22:* 515, 1981.
*Mendez M F, Cummings J L, Benson D F: Depression in epilepsy, significance and phenomenology. Arch Neurol *43:* 766, 1986.
Mendez M F, Doss R C, Taylor J L, Salquero P: Interictal depression in epilepsy: Relationship to seizure variables. J Nerv Ment Dis *181*:444, 1993.
Mendez M F, Grau R, Doss R C, Taylor J L: Schizophrenia is epilepsy: Seizure and psychosis variables. Neurology *43:* 1073, 1993.
Mendez M F, Lanska D J, Manon-Espaillet R, Burnstine T: Causative factors for suicide attempts by overdose in epileptics. Arch Neurol *46:* 1065, 1989.
Pakalnis A, Drake M E, John K, Kellum J B: Normalizations: Acute psychosis after seizure control in seven patients. Arch Neurol *44:* 289, 1987.
Meierkord H, Will B, Fish D, Shorvon S: The clinical features and prognosis of pseudoseizures diagnosed using video-EEG telemetry. Neurology *41:* 1643, 1991.
Perez M M, Trimble M R: Epileptic psychosis:—diagnostic comparison with process schizophrenia. Br J Psychiatry *37:* 245, 1980.
Pond D A, Bidwell B H: A survey of epilepsy in 14 general practices: II. Social and psychological aspects. Epilepsia *1:* 285, 1959–1960.
Ramani V, Gumnit R J: Intensive monitoring of interictal psychosis in epilepsy. Ann Neurol *11:* 613, 1982.
Robertson M M, Trimble M R, Townsend H R A: Phenomenology of depression in epilepsy. Epilepsia *28:* 364, 1987.
Rodin E, Schmaltz S: The Bear-Fedio personality inventory and temporal lobe epilepsy. Neurology *34:* 591, 1984.
Slater E, Beard A: The schizophrenia-like psychosis of epilepsy: Psychiatric aspects. Br J Psychiatry *109:* 95, 1963.
*Smith D B, Treiman D M, Trimble M R: *Neurobehavioral Problems in Epilepsy.* Raven, New York, 1991.
*Trimble M R: *The Psychosis of Epilepsy.* Raven, New York, 1991.
Williams D: The structure of emotions reflected in epileptic experiences. Brain *79:* 29, 1956.

2.4 NEUROPSYCHIATRIC ASPECTS OF HEAD TRAUMA

DANIEL X. CAPRUSO, Ph.D.
HARVEY S. LEVIN, Ph.D.

INTRODUCTION

Deficits in cognitive functioning and social behavior are the most disabling consequences of brain trauma. Although many patients attain good physical recoveries from brain trauma, personality changes and cognitive deficits frequently bring survivors of head injury to the attention of psychiatrists. The neuropsychiatric effects of head injury include neuropathological, cognitive, and behavioral features.

HISTORY

A spectacular accident that befell Phineas Gage in 1848 resulted in the first detailed clinical report of pathological personality change after a head trauma. While Gage was working with explosives, a pointed iron rod 1.25 inches in diameter and 3.5 feet long was blasted through his left frontal lobe and temporal pole (Figure 2.4-1). Despite the severity of the trauma, Gage survived the accident for 11 years; during that time he was productively employed, albeit with frequent job changes. Gage's personality was dramatically altered by the accident. Before the accident he was described as well-balanced, honest, reliable, efficient, and capable. After the injury he was described as childish, capricious, inconsiderate, and profane and as having poor judgment. It was said that the balance between his intellectual abilities and his animal propensities had been destroyed. Friends described him as "No longer Gage."

The case of Phineas Gage received wide attention, and documentation of other cases of pathological behavior after a head injury were soon published. In 1888 Leonore Welt published the case of a man who had sustained a severe penetrating frontal fracture after plunging from a fourth-floor window. Like Gage, the patient recovered quickly, but significant changes in personality were noted after the injury. Although he was described as having been industrious and cheerful before the accident, he became aggressive, malicious, and prone to distasteful jokes after the accident. After the patient's death from a lung infection, an autopsy revealed bilateral destruction of the gyrus rectus and lesioning of the right inferior frontal gyrus. A survey of the literature revealed that in many cases of frontal lobe pathology no psychopathological sequelae were apparent. Of eight autopsied persons who showed personality change, all had lesioning of the orbital gyri.

COMPARATIVE NOSOLOGY

Several of the mental disorders in the fourth edition of *Diagnostic and Statistical Manual of Mental Disorders* (DSM-IV) are commonly observed in patients with head trauma. Those disorders are delirium, amnestic disorder, dementia, and personality change due to head trauma. A comparison of neurological-neuropsychological and DSM-IV psychiatric nosologies is seen in Table 2.4-1.

The depth and duration of impairment in consciousness are the features typically used to classify the severity of head trauma in which acceleration-deceleration is the primary traumatic force. At a minimum, a brief loss of consciousness is typically considered necessary for brain trauma to have taken place, although as discussed in the proposed DSM-IV category of postconcussional disorder, there is currently no universally accepted threshold for determining the degree and duration of altered consciousness that is minimally necessary for determining whether brain trauma has occurred. In emergency rooms and trauma centers the degree of disturbance in level of consciousness is evaluated with the Glasgow Coma Scale (GCS). GCS scores are summed ratings of the patient's best eye opening, best verbal response, and best motor response (Table 2.4-2). For those patients who do not obey commands, responding is assessed by observing the reaction to painful stimulation. As seen in Table 2.4-3, head injuries may be classified into mild, moderate, and severe categories based on initial GCS scores. Patients with GCS scores indicating mild head injury but with intracranial complications or abnormal neurological examination are placed into the moderate category despite the favorable GCS score.

Historically, the term "concussion" originated to describe head trauma patients with rapidly resolving cognitive dysfunction but without obvious resulting brain pathology. Later, the term developed an etiological meaning to describe the physical

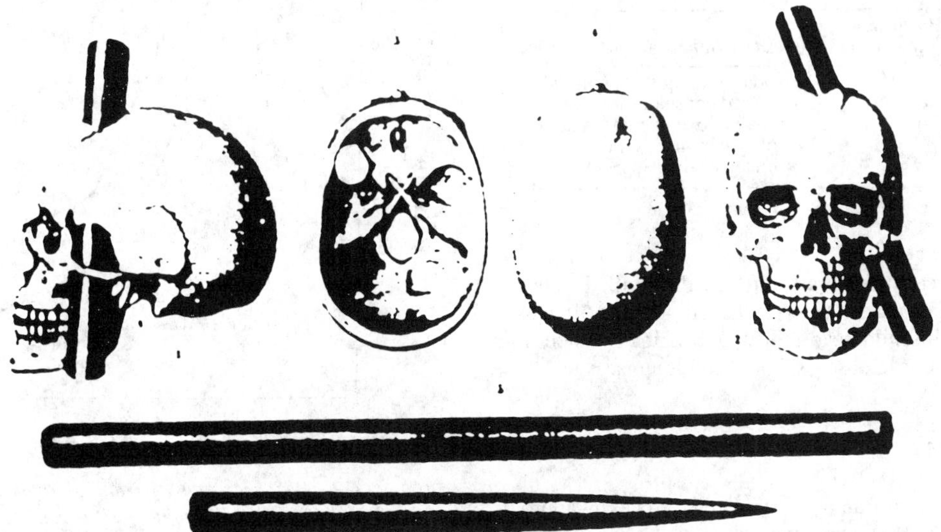

FIGURE 2.4-1 *Brain trauma sustained by Phineas Gage in 1848 as reconstructed by a surgeon who examined Gage two years after the head injury. The iron bar that was blasted through Gage's head is shown below the skull. (From H J Bigelow: Dr. Harlow's case of recovery from the passage of an iron bar through the head. Am J Med Sci* 39: *13, 1850. Used with permission.)*

TABLE 2.4-1
Comparative Nosology of Behavioral Disturbances Associated with Brain Trauma

Neurological-Neuropsychological	DSM-IV
Coma	—
Transitional phase of recovery	
Confusional state	Delirium due to head trauma
Posttraumatic amnesia	Amnestic disorder due to head trauma
Long-term phase of recovery	
Posttraumatic dementia	Dementia due to head trauma
Organic personality syndrome	Personality change due to head trauma
Pseudodepressed	Apathetic type
Pseudopsychopathic	Disinhibited or aggressive type

TABLE 2.4-2
Glasgow Coma Scale

Eye Opening	
None	1
To pain	2
To speech	3
Spontaneous	4
Motor Response	
No response	1
Extension	2
Abnormal flexion	3
Withdrawal	4
Localizes pain	5
Obeys commands	6
Verbal Response	
No response	1
Incomprehensible	2
Inappropriate	3
Confused	4
Oriented	5

Glasgow Coma Scale Score = Eye Opening + Motor Response + Verbal Response

Table adapted from B Jennett, G Teasdale: *Management of Head Injuries*. Davis, Philadelphia, 1981.

TABLE 2.4-3
Head Injury Classification

Head Injury	Glasgow Coma Score	Acute Clinical Features
Mild	13 to 15*	Headache, fatigue, dizziness
Moderate	9 to 12*	Impaired consciousness, no coma
Severe	3 to 8	Coma: no eye opening, inability to obey commands, no understandable speech

*Initial and lowest score.

translation of force to the brain through the skull. In current clinical and research usage the term "concussion" is often used synonymously with mild head injury to describe transient loss or impairment of consciousness from head trauma.

EPIDEMIOLOGY

The incidence of head trauma in the United States is approximately 200 per 100,000 population. The overall mortality rate is approximately 25 per 100,000 in the population. Men suffer head injuries at double the rate of women, and men are four times more likely than women to suffer fatal head injuries. The incidence increases with age and peaks in the 15-to-24 age range in the white population and in the 25-to-40 age range in the black population. The incidence then decreases, with another increase beginning at age 60 (Figure 2.4-2). Black urban men suffer the highest incidence of head injury. Motor vehicle accidents are the primary cause of head injuries in the United States, with falls and gunshot wounds the other leading causes.

CLINICAL FEATURES

The degree and duration of impairment in the level of consciousness are the principal clinical features in head trauma. GCS scores are typically recorded serially once the patient is brought to an emergency room or trauma center. Any deterioration in GCS scores obtained serially may indicate the development of a potentially fatal complication.

COURSE IN MILD HEAD INJURIES A mild head injury is characterized by an initial GCS score of 13 to 15, with no intracranial complication and normal neurological examination. Typically, persons suffering from mild head injuries experience a brief loss of consciousness lasting 20 minutes or less. In the emergency room or trauma center they may be alert and completely oriented, they may be slightly dazed or disoriented, or they may have a rapidly resolving transient amnestic disorder for events occurring since the injury.

There are a variety of cognitive and somatic complaints frequently reported by patients in the first weeks of recovery from mild head injury, including headaches, fatigability, dizziness,

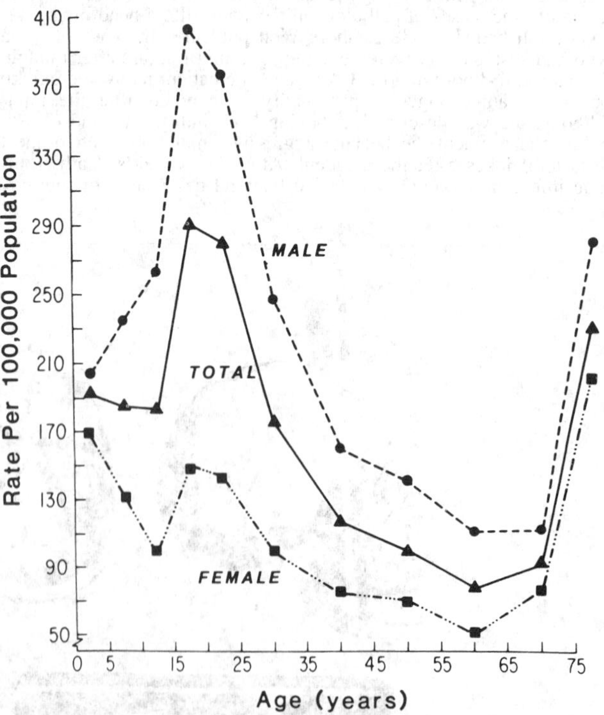

FIGURE 2.4-2 *Incidence rates of brain injury per 100,000 population in San Diego County, California, 1981. (From J F Kraus, M A Black, N Hessol, P Ley, W Rokaw, C Sullivan, S Bowers, S Knowlton, L Marshall: The indicidence of acute brain injury and serious impairment in a defined population. Am J Epidemiol 119: 186, 1984. Used with permission.)*

sleep disturbance, and memory deficit (Table 2.4-4). A number of those subjective complaints have been selected as research criteria for a proposed DSM-IV diagnostic category of postconcussional disorder. Possible etiologies of those symptoms could include a mild degree of diffuse axonal injury, focal cerebral contusions, small intracranial hematomas, labyrinth injury contributing to dizziness, focal scalp injuries contributing to headaches, and vasomotor alterations in the superficial cranial vessels possibly contributing to headaches. Nonspecific emotional reactions to trauma, hospitalization, and litigation and preexisting psychiatric disturbance, substance abuse, and such psychosocial risk factors as family and occupational problems may be contributory. Any combination of those neurological and psychiatric factors may interact to help produce postconcussion symptoms.

Multicenter studies have indicated that in the first week following mild head injury, impairment in memory and information processing speed is usually evident on psychometric testing. Within one to three months, patients with mild head injury typically recover cognitive functioning to the level of normal controls, although cognitive and somatic complaints may persist indefinitely in a minority of patients sustaining mild head injury. Again, whether those persisting sequelae reflect neurological or psychological disturbance is unclear; an interaction of neurological, psychological, and social factors may account for the long-term symptoms in some patients following mild head injury. The rate of prolonged postconcussional complaints can be as high as 15 percent in patients with mild head injury, and this figure approximates the 15 to 20 percent base rate of preexisting neuropsychiatric disorder in the population with mild head injury.

Because in most patients postconcussional symptoms represent acute and subacute phenomena that typically resolve within three months of a mild head injury, the proposed DSM-IV criterion requiring a symptom duration of three months is out of step with the clinical course observed in the majority of patients. Although an actual physical trauma may initiate the symptoms, the persistence of those symptoms far beyond the three-month limit typically seen in other patients with mild head injury makes consideration of a somatoform disorder necessary in the differential diagnosis. After careful evaluation, many patients with chronic postconcussional complaints are more appropriately diagnosed as having somatoform, mood, or anxiety disorders. Malingering in the hope of obtaining a favorable medical-legal settlement following a minor accident is also to be considered in the differential diagnosis. As the following clinical vignette will illustrate, patients attributing an often extensive list of chronic complaints to seemingly trivial incidents in which no substantial loss or alteration of consciousness took place are extremely common in neurological settings.

A 40-year-old man was referred for cognitive evaluation by a neurologist following two incidents, five months apart, that each resulted in scalp lacerations requiring stitches. A lawsuit was pending regarding the second injury. The patient denied measurable loss of consciousness, anterograde, or retrograde amnesia resulting from either incident. Computed tomography (CT) of the brain following the second injury was normal. Despite several months off from work for recovery, the patient showed a deteriorating clinical course with escalating complaints of memory loss and an extremely wide variety of somatic complaints. Despite his memory complaints, which were of an atypical nature for persons with mild head injury (for example, the patient reported that he forgot how to spell his own name), the patient scored at normal to above-normal levels on all standardized psychometric tests that were administered. For example, he recalled 12 out of 12 list items following a 30-minute delay. In contrast, his objective personality testing was grossly abnormal. Psychiatric, rather than neurological, treatment was recommended.

Empirical studies have demonstrated that repeated mild head injuries apparently have a cumulative effect in reducing information processing speed, although the mechanism of cumulative injury is not known and replication of those studies is necessary. Theoretically, repeated injuries have the effect of reducing the reserve of cerebral neuronal reserve that is used in the performance of challenging attentional tasks. Whether repeated mild head injuries sustained in boxing can cause cognitive deficits of the severity required for the diagnosis of dementia is currently a controversial issue on which no firm agreement has been reached in the research, clinical, and editorial literature. However, DSM-IV mentions dementia pugilistica as a potentially progressive condition under the rubric of dementia due to head trauma.

TABLE 2.4-4
Frequency of Postconcussional Symptoms Reported in a Three-Center Study of Mild Head Injury

Symptom	Percent Reporting (N = 155)
Headaches	71
Fatigability	56
Dizziness	50
Sleep	44
Recent memory	39
Depression	36
Anxiety	33
Appetite	31
Thinking	30
Concentration	30
Blurred vision	29
Coordination	27
Noise sensitivity	23
Patience	19
Vertigo	19

Table adapted from H S Levin, H E Gary, W M High, S Mattis, R M Ruff, H M Eisenberg, L F Marshall, K Tabaddor: Minor head injury and the postconcussional syndrome: Methodological issues in outcome studies. In *Neurobehavioral Recovery from Head Injury,* H S Levin, J Grafman, H M Eisenberg, editors, p 267. Oxford University Press, New York, 1987. Used with permission.

COURSE IN MODERATE AND SEVERE HEAD INJURIES

As indicated in Figure 2.4-3, recovery from a moderate or severe brain trauma typically involves a progression through a sequence of neurobehavioral syndromes. The initial stage for severely head-injured patients is coma. When consciousness is recovered, a period of delirium and then posttraumatic amnesia is typically seen. The retrograde component of posttraumatic amnesia is the failure to recall events occurring before the head injury. The anterograde component of posttraumatic amnesia is the failure to store and recall ongoing events occurring since the head injury. Retrograde amnesia lasts only seconds or minutes for most mild to moderate head injuries, and it is typically much shorter than the anterograde amnesia. Retrograde amnesia for intervals of more than two days is rare, although in some patients recovering from severe head injuries, retrograde amnesia for intervals as long as nine years has been reported.

The following clinical vignette illustrates a patient's evolution through a sequence of neurobehavioral syndromes from coma, through delirium due to head trauma, and transient amnestic disorder due to head trauma, to a mental status marked by normal orientation but with residual cognitive deficits on psychometric memory testing:

A 23-year-old professional woman in the physical sciences sustained a severe closed head injury when her car was destroyed in a collision with a truck. After being extracted from the vehicle, she was noted to be unresponsive and required intubation. She was admitted to the hospital with a GCS score of 3 and fixed pupils. The patient had cranio-

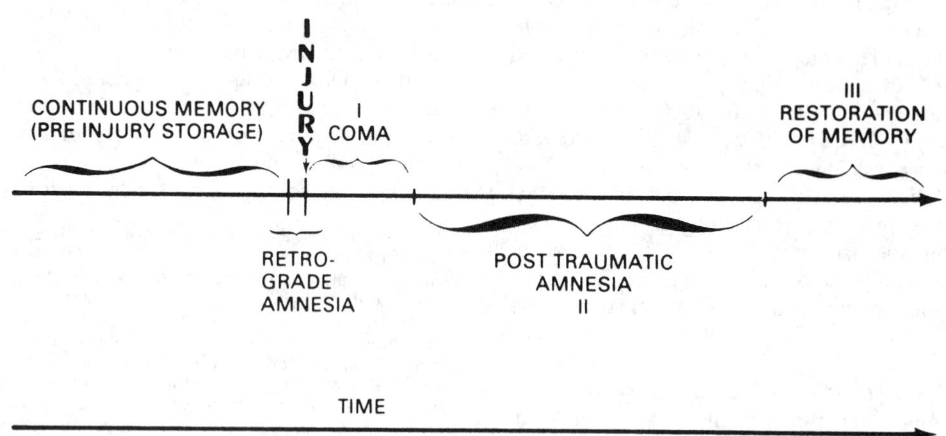

FIGURE 2.4-3 *Sequence of acute alterations in memory after a closed head injury. (From H S Levin, A L Benton, R G Grossman:* Neurobehavioral Consequences of Closed Head Injury, *p 74. Oxford University Press, New York, 1982. Used with permission.)*

tomy for extraction of a left extradural hematoma and cardiothoracic surgery for repair of a ruptured aorta. At 24 hours following admission the patient had improved to a GCS score of 14, with brisk pupillary responses. When first cognitively evaluated eight days posttrauma, the patient appeared to have mildly clouded consciousness. She was oriented to place and some personal information (for example, her date of birth), but disoriented to time and some other aspects of personal information, including her proper age, address, and occupation. She provided confabulatory answers to questions that she could not answer correctly. She as unable to learn a 12-item list and her 30-minute delayed recall was 0 out of 12 list items. Two weeks later the patient was fully alert, had normal orientation in all spheres, and was no longer confabulatory. Psychometrically, she was able to attain a full-scale intelligence quotient (I.Q.) of 134 (99th percentile), but had persisting deficits in verbal learning and memory; her 30-minute delayed recall for list items was 3 out of 12 (less than first percentile). She had no memory for events occurring several hours before the accident (retrograde amnesia) and no memory for events occurring during the initial one and a half weeks of her hospitalization (anterograde amnesia).

The pattern of memory impairment for autobiographical information observed in head-injured patients conforms to the law proposed by Theodore Hercule Ribot in 1882: the most recent memories are the most susceptible to disruption by trauma, whereas recall of remote memories is least affected (Figure 2.4-4). The resolution of retrograde amnesia also follows Ribot's law: the period of memory loss shrinks backward toward the accident, with the most remote memories being recovered first. The recovery of orientation after a head injury also tends to be sequential. The majority of patients regain orientation to personal information first, then to place, and finally to time. Few patients remain disoriented to personal information when oriented to time or place or both.

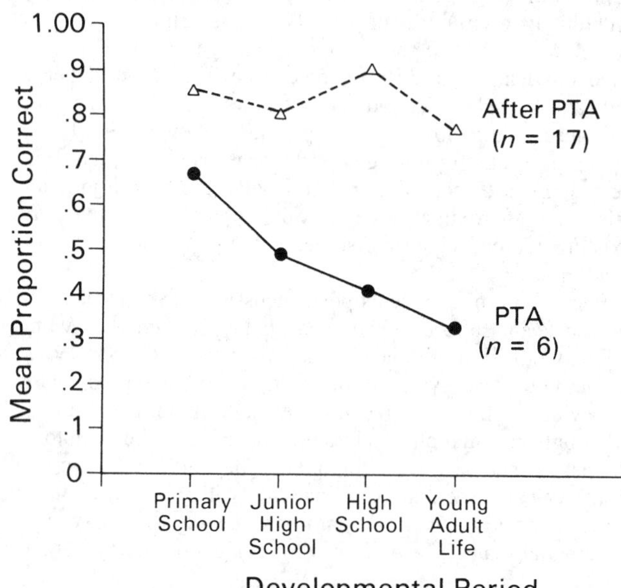

FIGURE 2.4-4 *Mean proportion of correct recall of autobiographical events plotted across developmental periods for head-injured patients during and after posttraumatic amnesia (PTA). (From H S Levin, W M High, C A Meyers, A von Laufen, M Hayden, H M Eisenberg: Impairment of remote memory after closed head injury. J Neurol Neurosurg Psychiatry* 48: *551, 1985. Used with permission.)*

DIAGNOSIS OF COGNITIVE DISORDERS DURING RECOVERY FROM HEAD TRAUMA The course of recovery from head trauma typically demands a sequence of differing DSM-IV diagnoses that are directly related to the acute pathophysiological effects of the injury followed by the evolution of various stages of recovery. For example, patients may initially be in coma, but will often evidence a delirium as they recover from unconsciousness. That delirium may resolve into a dementia, transient or chronic amnestic disorder, or essentially normal recovery. When diagnosing any DSM-IV mental disorder due to head trauma the clinician should also code head injury on Axis III.

Amnestic disorder due to head trauma Amnestic disorders varying from transient to chronic are very common in patients recovering from head traumas. Although memory deficits are typically the most severe chronic cognitive sequelae of head trauma, owing to the diffuse nature of the neuropathology of severe head injuries, most patients with gross posttraumatic memory deficits will be more appropriately diagnosed with dementia.

Dementia due to head trauma DSM-IV recognizes head trauma as a common cause of dementia. The most salient features of dementia due to head trauma are memory impairment and disturbance in executive functioning (that is, planning, organizing, sequencing, abstracting). Aphasia as a component of the dementia is uncommon, and is typically less pronounced than either the memory or executive features unless there has been a focal left hemisphere lesion, such as a hematoma. Although aphasia is not a common component of dementia due to head trauma, various nonaphasic language disturbances, such as tangential and illogical speech, are common components of posttraumatic dementia. Apraxia and agnosia, typically associated with extensive posterior cerebral damage, are rare features of dementia due to head trauma except in the most severe and globally impaired patients. As mentioned in DSM-IV, personality change is a frequent concomitant of dementia due to head trauma.

APHASIA After penetrating missile wounds, the type of aphasia manifested is related to the localization of the damage produced by the track of the projectile and resulting bone fragments. Although the relation between the classic aphasia syndromes and the localization of lesions resembles the pattern found after cerebrovascular insults, atypical aphasia syndromes commonly result from penetrating missile wounds because projectiles rarely produce the same territorial patterns of damage caused by a stroke. As in cerebrovascular disease, left-handed persons are less likely to develop aphasia than are right-handed persons after unilateral left-hemisphere wounds, but left-handed persons are more likely to develop aphasia after unilateral right-hemisphere wounds. Outcome studies conducted up to 15 years after penetrating missile wounds indicate that roughly two thirds of patients with aphasia showed good recovery.

Anomic aphasia is the most common syndrome of language disturbance after a closed head injury. The disorder is characterized by fluent speech and relatively preserved repetition and comprehension but defective naming ability. Circumlocutions and word-finding difficulties may be readily apparent on confrontation naming and in conversational speech. The second most frequent aphasic disorder after a closed head injury is *Wernicke's aphasia*. That disorder is characterized by poor language comprehension and impaired repetition in the context of fluent speech. Semantic paraphasic errors are apparent on confrontation naming (for example, saying "horse" or "ant" for a picture of an elephant) and jargon may be present.

After a severe closed head injury, the recovery of language functioning tends to be sequential. The comprehension of gestures and oral language appears first, with oral expression, reading, and writing recovering at a slower rate. Articulation and phonation are often persistently impaired. Anomia and perseveration are common sequelae of a severe closed head injury.

OUTCOME OF MODERATE TO SEVERE HEAD INJURIES

Six months is the recommended interval at which assessment of outcome should be made. The Glasgow Outcome Scale (GOS) includes death and four categories of survival: persistent vegetative state, severe disability, moderate disability, and good recovery.

Persistent vegetative state Some patients never recover consciousness from the initial brain trauma and are classified either as brain-dead or as existing in a persistent vegetative state. *Brain-dead* patients have a complete absence of both cerebral and brainstem functioning as documented by respiratory arrest and the absence of all brainstem reflexes. Those patients require mechanical respiration, and cardiac arrest typically occurs within days. Patients in a *persistent vegetative state* give no indication of cerebral cortical functioning, although a working brainstem allows vegetative functioning to continue. Although the patients have sleep-wake cycles, may visually track objects, and may move their limbs, those actions are considered spontaneous and reflexive if they have no communicative value and do not imply cognitively meaningful activity.

Of 100 patients in a persistent vegetative state in Japan, 45 percent were still alive after three years. Of the 38 patients in the sample for whom closed head injury was the cause, the mean survival time was 33 months (standard deviation, 26). Only 3 of the 100 patients became communicative.

A study of 650 severe closed head injury patients in the United States found that 14 percent were discharged in a persistent vegetative state. Of 84 vegetative patients, 40 percent regained consciousness by six months posttrauma, with an additional 11 percent regaining consciousness by one year, and an additional 6 percent regaining consciousness by three years. If a patient does not regain consciousness by one year, the prognosis is poor for improvement of the persistent vegetative state.

Severe disability Conscious but dependent is how patients with severe disability are best described, because they require supervision in the activities of daily living. Disability may derive primarily from physical or cognitive limitations. In some instances both physical and cognitive functioning remain relatively intact, but the patients are so disinhibited or apathetic that they cannot be left to their own devices. Patients who cannot care for themselves for 24-hour intervals are put in this category.

Moderate disability Patients with moderate disability are best described as independent but disabled. Although they may live independently, retain employment at a reduced level, and use public transportation, they suffer from neurobehavioral or other physical deficits that compromise their functioning when compared with their premorbid status.

Good recovery Patients who make a good recovery may have some neurological complications and may show some residual deficits on cognitive testing, but they remain physically and socially competent and are independent and capable of returning to full employment.

PREDICTING OUTCOME Survival rates after a head injury are strongly influenced by the initial (that is, postresuscitation) GCS score, initial pupillary reactivity, and age. For patients younger than 40 years with an initial GCS score no higher than 8, the mortality rate is less than 50 percent, but the mortality rate rises to 50 to 80 percent for patients more than 40 years old.

The initial and worst postresuscitation GCS score is a reliable predictor of the cognitive outcome after two years for those patients who survive a severe head injury (Table 2.4-5). Approximately two thirds of the surviving patients with a GCS score of 3 to 4 are in a persistent vegetative state or have severe cognitive deficits. One quarter of the surviving patients with a GCS score of 5 to 7 have severe cognitive deficits. Surviving patients with a GCS score of at least 8 infrequently suffer severe or permanent cognitive deficits, and only 16 percent have mild deficits on formal testing. Pupillary reactivity and lowest GCS score were more predictive of the magnitude of residual cognitive impairment than initial GCS scores. Initial GCS scores are too susceptible to mediation effects and transient changes in intracranial pressure to reflect the depth of neurological damage truly, which is more validly measured by pupillary reactivity. The duration of the posttraumatic amnesia, as measured by the Galveston Orientation and Amnesia Test, is another useful predictor of outcome. As indicated in Table 2.4-6, posttraumatic

TABLE 2.4-5
Cognitive Outcome at Two Years in Survivors of Head Injury as Predicted by Initial Glasgow Coma Scale (GCS) Score

	Initial GCS Score (in %)		
Cognitive Outcome	3–4 (N = 25)	5–7 (N = 47)	8–15 (N = 30)
Minimal or no deficit	10	34	84
Mild deficit	23	40	16
Severe deficit	60	26	—
Vegetative	7	—	—

Table adapted from A Alexandre, F Colombo, P Nertempi, A Benedetti: Cognitive outcome and early indices of severity of head injury. J Neurosurg *59:* 751, 1983. Used with permission.

TABLE 2.4-6
Duration of Posttraumatic Amnesia as a Predictor of Long-Term Outcome

	Duration of Posttraumatic Amnesia as Measured by Galveston Orientation and Amnesia Test						
Long-Term Outcome	**0–1 Day**	**4–7 Days**	**8–14 Days**	**15 Days–1 Month**	**1–2 Months**	**>2 Months**	**Total**
Good recovery	3	4	7	2	—	—	16
Moderate to severe disability	—	—	1	5	5	5	16

Table from H S Levin, V M O'Donnell, R G Grossman: The Galveston Orientation and Amnesia Test: A practical scale to assess cognition after head injury. J Nerv Ment Dis *167:* 681, 1979. Used with permission.

amnesia for more than two weeks is associated with long-term outcomes of moderate to severe disability in most patients, whereas patients with posttraumatic amnesia for less than two weeks typically have long-term outcomes of good recovery. Verbal learning performance on neuropsychological testing is the single best predictor of the ability of patients to return to work and to maintain employment after a closed head injury.

PATHOLOGY

PENETRATING MISSILE INJURY In a penetrating missile injury (usually gunshot or shrapnel) the projectile typically forces a shower of bone fragments into the brain as it perforates the skull. Further damage is caused by shock waves and the expansion of hot gases in the wake of the projectile, so that the missile leaves a trail of damage larger than its own diameter. A missile that does not retain enough velocity to exit the skull may be deflected back into the brain, or it may continue its travels along the inner surface of the skull.

Patients who retain consciousness after a penetrating missile wound have a relatively good prognosis (Phineas Gage, for example, was noted to be talking and ambulatory within minutes of his accident). However, death is the expected outcome for those in deep coma, and only 20 percent of comatose patients who react to pain are expected to live. When the destruction wrought by a penetrating missile wound is confined to focal areas of the brain, the patient typically shows a syndrome of deficits related to the functional properties of the areas destroyed by the projectile. For example, a patient with a right parietal lobe missile wound may show spatial disabilities, whereas another patient with a right temporal wound may have difficulties in discriminating faces. A substantial proportion of the existing knowledge of local brain functioning is derived from veterans with penetrating missile wounds.

CLOSED HEAD INJURY A closed head injury results from the impact of a blunt moving object on the head; it may occur when the head is rapidly accelerated (as in whiplash) or decelerated (as in a fall or a motor vehicle accident). Contusions may result under the site of impact. Laceration of the brain may also occur if there is a depressed skull fracture. Contrecoup contusions may occur remote from the site of the impact.

The structural irregularities of the temporal lobe and the irregularity of the lesser wing of the sphenoid bone underlying the frontal and temporal lobes result in the greatest amount of physical force being concentrated in the frontal and temporal regions of the brain. As a result, lesions are typically concentrated in the ventral aspects of the frontal and temporal lobes and in the temporal poles, regardless of the original site of the impact. In contrast, the smooth and regular surfaces overlying the occipital lobes result in that area's sustaining the least amount of contusion during a closed head injury (Figure 2.4-5). Contrecoup lesions may also result from cavitation. A rapid acceleration of the skull contents results in the formation of a pressure gradient, with the lowest pressure level occurring opposite the point of traumatic impact. Cavitation occurs if fluids in the brain reach a pressure level below their vapor pressure level, causing them to convert to a gaseous state and boil violently, thereby damaging the brain tissue at the point opposite the site of the impact.

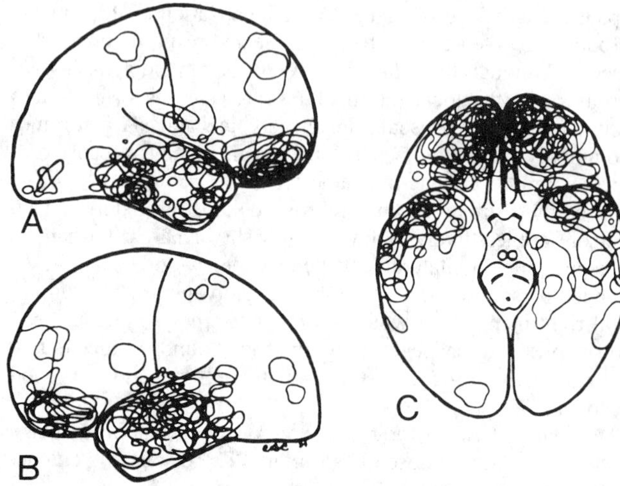

FIGURE 2.4-5 *Overlap of surface contusions of the brain in 40 consecutive cases of brain trauma. A: lateral view of the right hemisphere; B: lateral view of the left hemisphere; C: ventral view. (From C B Courville:* Pathology of the Central Nervous System, *Pacific Press, Mountain View, CA, 1937. Used with permission.)*

Although contusions and hematomas are the most gross pathological features observed after a closed head injury, diffuse damage occurs throughout the brain because of rotational acceleration or deceleration. The brain rarely suffers an impact focused on its center of gravity. Therefore, rotational forces are generated as the brain pivots around its center of gravity in response to the impact. The brain has no rigidity, and various brain components differ in mass, compliance, and elasticity. During rapid rotational acceleration or deceleration those differences in physical properties cause gray matter, white matter, and blood vessels to separate obliquely through shear strain. Axons, blood vessels, and other brain components stretch to their limits and snap, producing diffuse microscopic lesions. A centripetal sequence of damage is caused by shear strain, with the surface of the cerebrum sustaining the most damage, the diencephalon sustaining a smaller proportion of damage, and the mesencephalon sustaining the least proportion of damage. The fibers coursing from the mesencephalon to the frontal lobes typically receive a significant proportion of the damage caused by shear strain and contusion. Midsagittal magnetic resonance imaging (MRI) frequently shows corpus callosum lesions or atrophy, and neuropathological studies have shown that the callosum may sustain extensive microscopic lesioning in the absence of visible lesions on neuroimaging.

Secondary effects In addition to the primary brain damage suffered as a direct consequence of the impact, secondary effects are common in both penetrating missile injuries and closed head injuries. The most lethal secondary effect of a closed head injury is raised intracranial pressure, which can result from edema or a hematoma. Hematomas are formed by the accumulation of blood from the contusion, laceration, or rupture of blood vessels through shear strain. Hematomas may be intradural, subdural, or intracerebral. The displacement of cerebrospinal fluid can compensate for raised intracranial pressure to a certain point, but continued rises in intracranial pressure can result in herniation (Figure 2.4-6). The most common type of herniation is the displacement of the parahippocampal gyrus and the uncus downward through the tentorial hiatus. The brainstem may also be displaced downward into the posterior fossa. Respiratory arrest can result from

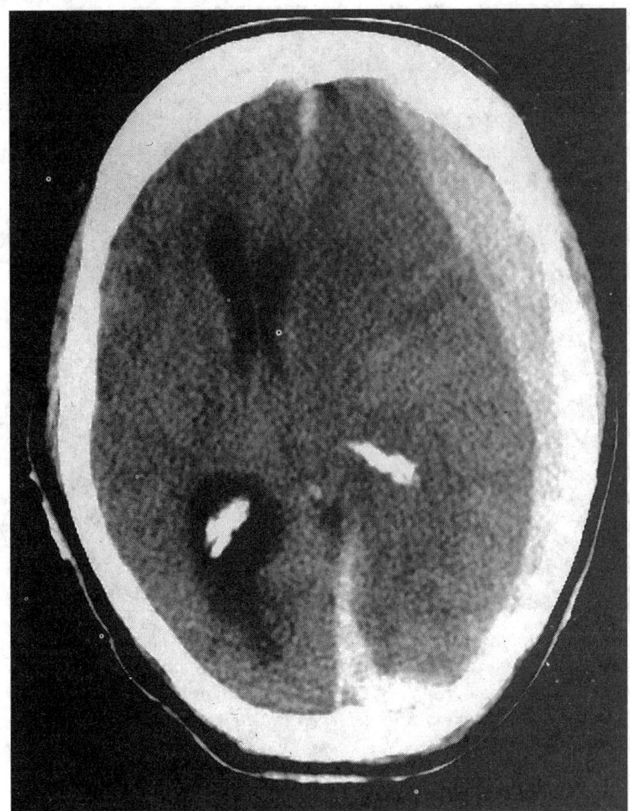

FIGURE 2.4-6 *Computed tomography (CT) scan of the brain of a 47-year-old woman who sustained a closed head injury in a fall and who had an initial Glasgow Coma Scale (GCS) score of 4. An acute subdural hematoma lines the left cerebral convexity and extends into the falx cerebri posteriorly. A massive cerebral shift across the midline is visible; it resulted in both subfalcine and uncal herniation. Three months after a craniotomy and the removal of the hematoma, the patient had recovered to the point of obeying simple commands.*

brainstem dysfunction associated with herniation. Raised intracranial pressure may also reduce cerebral blood flow and cause diffuse ischemia, although ischemia may also result from inadequate ventilation or anemia caused by blood loss. Subarachnoid hemorrhage may lead to communicating hydrocephalus.

The olfactory nerve is frequently damaged, even in minor head injuries, because of its location overlying the cribriform plate on the orbitofrontal surface of the brain. Olfactory function returns in approximately half the patients suffering anosmia. Optic nerve injuries may occur, most frequently because of damage to the optic canal. Lesions of the oculomotor nerve may occur, although unilateral dilatation of the pupil typically receives careful investigation because of the possibility of an extracerebral mass lesion. Frontal scalp lacerations frequently lesion the supraorbital branch of the trigeminal nerve. A variety of types of hearing loss are possible as a consequence of a head injury, with bilateral symmetrical sensorineural loss in the high-frequency range the most common clinical occurrence. Asymmetrical and unilateral auditory difficulties may also be seen.

Epilepsy Posttraumatic epilepsy occurs in 2 to 5 percent of patients after a closed head injury. The onset of posttraumatic epilepsy may occur within a week of the injury *(early epilepsy)* or beyond *(late epilepsy)*. Of those adults who do not have early epilepsy, only 3 percent subsequently have late epilepsy. In contrast, 30 percent of those adults with early epilepsy go on to late epilepsy. Factors increasing the risk of posttraumatic epilepsy are an acute hematoma, a depressed skull fracture, and posttraumatic amnesia for more than 24 hours. Patients with penetrating missile wounds have a higher incidence of late epilepsy than do patients with closed head injuries, particularly in the presence of torn dura or damage to multiple lobes or when the path of the missile is deep enough to reach a ventricle. Once a patient with a head injury has had even one late seizure, there is a high probability of recurrent seizures.

LABORATORY TESTS

NEUROIMAGING Radiographic examination of the head is used to identify and delineate fractures of the skull. CT and MRI allow for the detection of contusions, hematomas, and other intracranial pathologies in a noninvasive fashion (Figures 2.4-6 and 2.4-7). Focal brain lesions 15 cm^3 or larger are present in about 25 percent of initial CT scans of patients in a traumatic coma, with one intracerebral lesion present for every two extracerebral lesions.

Ventriculomegaly has proved to be a useful correlate of behavioral functioning after a closed head injury (Figure 2.4-7). Ventricular enlargement is related to a long coma and a bad outcome on neuropsychological measures, but only when the onset of the ventriculomegaly is gradual and subacute. Gradual ventricular enlargement suggests a diffuse axonal injury or ischemic hypoxia as the underlying pathological mechanism, instead of the effects of focal lesions.

Although CT is as useful as MRI in detecting rapidly expanding lesions, MRI can detect lesions in up to 85 percent of patients with mild to moderate closed head injuries and normal CT scans. Neurobehavioral functioning is correlated with total lesion volume as measured by MRI but is not correlated with lesion volume as measured by CT. Studies using MRI have proved the centripetal model of brain damage in closed head injuries by showing that the depth of the parenchymal lesion on MRI is strongly correlated with a variety of clinical and outcome factors. As the depth of the lesion increased from the cortex to the brainstem, patients showed greater impairments in the level of consciousness, longer durations of impaired consciousness, greater ventricular enlargement, and worse quality of outcome. Despite MRI's superior anatomical resolution and increased sensitivity to structural lesions, the short-term effects of closed head injuries are imaged by CT because of its greater speed, its sensitivity to hemorrhages, and the difficulty of placing patients on life-support equipment in a magnetic field.

Positron emission tomography (PET) studies of small samples of closed head injury patients have shown reductions in the metabolic rates in the anterior temporal lobe bilaterally, with intact metabolism in the posterior temporal lobes during recovery. When CT and MRI showed unilateral structural damage, PET showed reduced metabolism in the damaged temporal lobe. However, after six months, metabolism was also reduced in the structurally intact temporal lobe, suggesting that diaschisis may play a role in outcome.

NEUROCHEMICAL ANALYSIS The extreme agitation of many patients recovering from head injuries suggests some form of sympathetic hyperactivity. The somatic symptoms of increased sensitivity to noise and of photophobia also suggest that the noradrenergic system is failing to perform its presumed function of gating and regulating the perceived intensity of incoming stimuli. One study has shown that elevations in the levels of circulating catecholamines are related to GCS scores and that circulating norepinephrine levels are quadrupled and dopamine levels are tripled in patients with GCS scores of 3 to 4 when compared with normal levels (Figure 2.4-8 and Table 2.4-7). Delirious and agitated patients also have decrements in dopamine metabolites.

ELECTROENCEPHALOGRAPHY Electroencephalography (EEG) of patients in posttraumatic coma is characterized by slowing of spontaneous activity, abnormal rhythm, and reduction or abolition of the startle response to sensory stimulation. The recovery from coma is accompanied by an increasing frequency of alpha waves, spontaneous variation in rhythm, and increased responsiveness to sensory stimulation. Despite its diagnostic usefulness in patients with posttraumatic epilepsy, EEG has not proved to be a better predictor of the development of posttraumatic seizures than such clinical features as early epilepsy, acute hematoma, and depressed skull fracture. The degree of abnormality in evoked potentials is predictive of outcome and has been shown to be related to other neurological indexes of the severity of injury. However, evoked potentials are time-consuming to perform and thus are not commonly used in neurotrauma centers.

PSYCHIATRIC ASPECTS

PREMORBID PERSONALITY When compared with the general population, head-injured patients show a disproportionate degree of premorbid psychiatric disturbance and personality

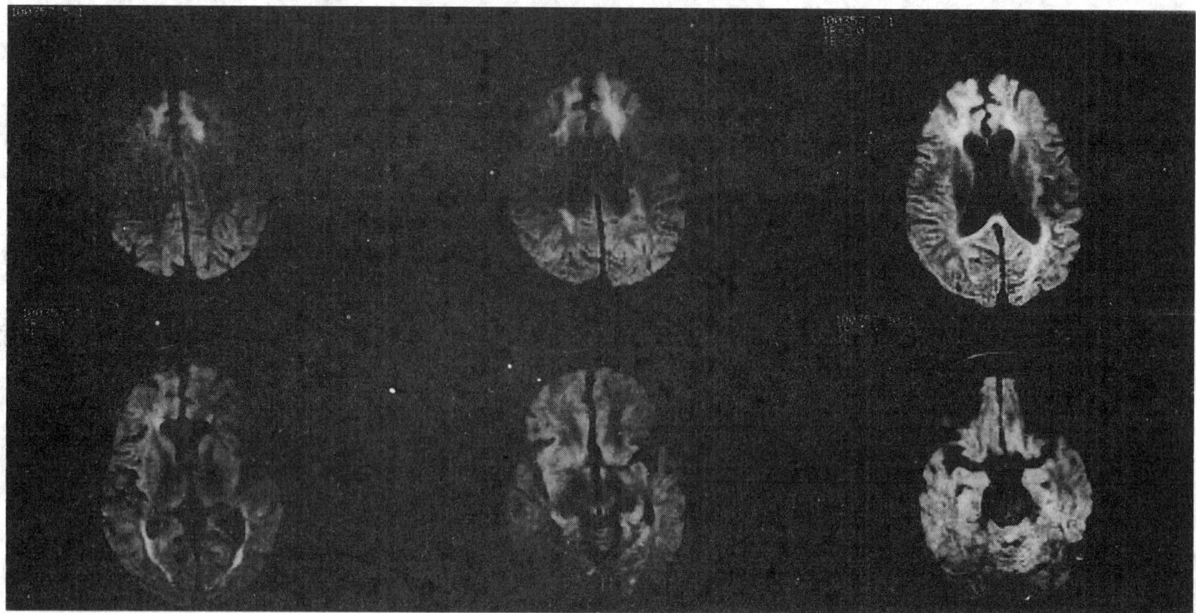

FIGURE 2.4-7 *Magnetic resonance imaging (MRI) of the brain of a 24-year-old woman five years after she sustained a severe closed head injury in a motor vehicle accident. Areas of abnormal signal intensity may be seen in the frontal lobes bilaterally and in the occipitotemporal white matter. There is prominent ventriculomegaly and widening of the sulci. Serial computed tomography (CT) scans had disclosed only diffuse injury in the patient, whereas MRI also documented the presence of focal lesions. Although the patient had achieved excellent grades in high school, after her head injury she required seven years to complete an Associate of Arts in Horticulture from a community college, a course of study that typically requires only two years.*

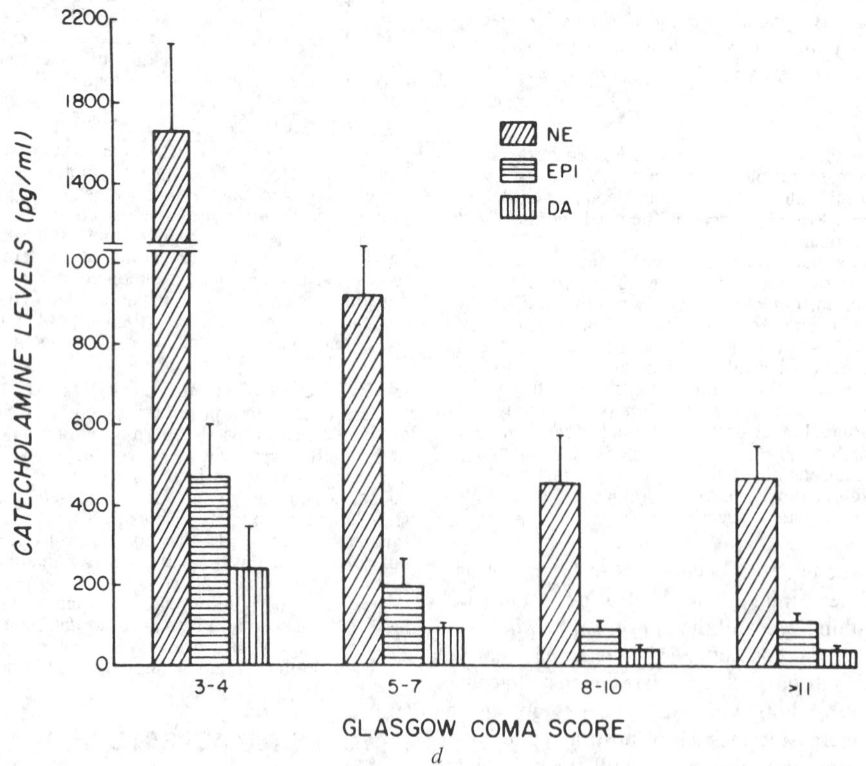

d

FIGURE 2.4-8 *Catecholamine levels within 48 hours of head injury in patients grouped by initial Glasgow Coma Scale score. (From R W Hamill, P D Woolf, J V McDonald, L A Lee, M Kelly: Catecholamines predict outcome in traumatic brain injury. Ann Neurol 21: 440, 1987. Used with permission.)*

TABLE 2.4-7
Mean Catecholamine Levels within 48 Hours of Brain Trauma*

	Glasgow Coma Score			
Catecholamine	**3–4**	**5–7**	**8–11**	**11–15**
Norephinephrine	1,687 (1,501)	919 (644)	477 (218)	463 (146)
Epinephrine	430 (621)	208 (192)	76 (38)	118 (54)
Dopamine	236 (395)	80 (42)	26 (11)	27 (9)

*Standard deviations are indicated in parentheses. Table adapted from R W Hamill, P D Woolf, J V McDonald, L A Lee, M Kelly: Catecholamines predict outcome in traumatic brain injury. Ann Neurol *21:* 440, 1987. Used with permission.

maladjustment. A recent study indicated that 56 percent of patients suffering from penetrating missile wounds or closed head injuries had indicators of severe premorbid psychopathology. Because many head injuries are alcohol-related, those suffering head injuries have a high proportion of alcoholism. Of those patients who suffered head injuries during intoxication, 75 percent had indicators of severe premorbid psychopathology. Increased premorbid incidences of hyperactive, impulsive, and antisocial personality characteristics have been noted in patients suffering from head injuries, presumably because those patients are prone to engage in risk-taking and thrill-seeking activities. Also, depressed and other emotionally pained persons are thought to be more likely than psychiatrically healthy persons to engage in such potentially self-destructive activities as driving at excessive speeds. For depressed persons, the automobile often represents an ideal vehicle for the indirect expression of suicidal impulses. Argumentative and aggressive persons are likely to suffer head injuries during altercations that may escalate to involve fists, such blunt instruments as baseball bats, and, ultimately, firearms. In fact, of those patients who had penetrating missile wounds, 88 percent had indicators of severe premorbid psychopathology, as compared with 47 percent of those suffering from closed head injuries.

Premorbid personality factors not only increase the likelihood that some persons will sustain head injuries but also interact with the neurological effects of the head injury. Some clinicians have suggested that disinhibition is the sole factor involved in pathological behavior after a head injury. In that sense, there may be no personality change after a head trauma, only the emergence of maladaptive tendencies that were present premorbidly but that were sensibly restrained during the majority of social interactions. Some researchers have suggested the concept of intolerances developing as negative symptoms after a head trauma. Head-injured patients often show a dramatic reduction in their ability to tolerate a variety of social and personal stressors.

Research with both soldiers and civilians suffering head traumas indicates that a history of psychiatric disorder in the immediate family increases the probability that a patient will suffer significant psychiatric sequelae after a head injury. Consequently, both dysfunctional family dynamics and genetic predisposition may be factors in the development of psychiatric complications after a head trauma. However, studies following identical twins, one of whom had suffered a head trauma, indicate that the rate of psychiatric disturbance is equivalent for both the control twin and the injured twin.

PSYCHOLOGICAL REACTIONS Maladaptive behavior not only may stem from physical brain damage but also may occur as a reaction to a new reality in which survivors of brain trauma are no longer capable of performing certain tasks or of behaving appropriately in certain social situations. The term ''catastrophic reaction'' has been used to describe the extreme withdrawal that may occur when neurologically impaired patients are confronted with the scope and the severity of their impairments. Some researchers have found that relatives report increased psychiatric symptoms in head-injured patients after the first six months. Presumably, psychiatric symptoms increase as the patients experience increasing frustration and failure in their attempts to resume their previous employment and social status.

AWARENESS OF DEFICITS Although some head-injured patients are painfully aware of their deficits, many head-injured patients are oblivious to their own social inappropriateness and ineffectuality. Researchers have repeatedly found that one of the most devastating behavioral sequelae of frontal lobe lesions is an inability to evaluate one's own cognitive abilities accurately. As a consequence, patients with head injuries often have unrealistic goals for the future.

A 19-year-old man with 12 years of formal education underwent neuropsychological evaluation three years after an automobile accident in which he sustained a severe closed head injury with an initial GCS score of 3. His coma lasted 3.5 weeks. The patient attained a full-scale I.Q. score of 73 (fourth percentile). His verbal and visual memory performances were markedly impaired (first percentile). The patient stated that his vocational goal was to become a stockbroker.

PSYCHOTIC SYMPTOMS Psychotic symptoms are often seen during the early recovery from a head injury, even in those patients with no previous psychiatric or substance-abuse history. In those patients psychosis is almost always a component of delirium or posttraumatic amnesia and is primarily characterized by confabulations and delusions. For example, in a series of 10 patients with posttraumatic psychosis, two women and one man expressed the delusion that they were having a baby. Paranoid ideation and reduplicative paramnesia for place were common. As opposed to the systematized delusions seen in paranoid schizophrenia, the delusions present in posttraumatic psychosis tend to be fragmented.

In some respects, patients recovering from brain traumas resemble persons suffering from schizophrenia, disorganized type. Conceptual disorganization is typically one of the most salient features apparent during an interview with a patient recovering from a brain trauma. Head-injured patients tend to be illogical, rambling, and tangential.

Preservation is often present and can be so severe that it makes a conventional mental status examination almost impossible. The patient's speech may be echolalic and palilalic. Proverb interpretation tends to be concrete or highly personalized. The following material was obtained from the mental status examination of a 45-year-old man still in posttraumatic amnesia 29 days after a motor vehicle accident in which he sustained a severe head injury and after he had an initial GCS score of 4:

Examiner: Where are you right now?
Patient: I'm right here.
Examiner: What kind of place are you in?
Patient: You're looking at it.
Examiner: What type of building is it?
Patient: An oxygen tent. [The patient was in a conventional hospital room; he was not in an oxygen tent.]
Examiner: How old are you?
Patient: You tell me. How should I know? I just got up.
Examiner: What year is it now?
Patient: 1988. [The correct answer was 1991.]
Examiner: How is your memory?
Patient: Fine, how is your memory?
Examiner: What does this saying mean: People in glass houses shouldn't throw stones.

Patient: It's logical. You don't throw stones if you live in a house made of glass. You live on a glass river.
Examiner: Can you count backward from 100 by 1? . . . What is 100 minus 1?
Patient: Zero, nothing, nothing to advance to or from. A zero point. Zero, zero, zero, one.

A CT scan of the patient's brain, conducted four days after the injury and shown in Figure 2.4-9, revealed bilateral frontal lobe pathology and a hemorrhage of the left basal ganglia. Profound personality change was also apparent in the patient, with frequent episodes of violence, inappropriate sexual flirtation, and profane speech.

Patients may present as psychotically disturbed, incoherent, or delusional even during long-term recovery. For example, a previously normal 19-year-old woman who had a good cognitive recovery six months following a severe head injury had delusions that a man repeatedly placed and ignited explosives inside her body cavities.

The following material was obtained from an interview with a 30-year-old woman two years after a severe closed head injury:

They hit me. . . . I think they like it because they keep hitting and hitting and hitting me. . . . They're behind a mask, a bloody mask. They look pretty tall.

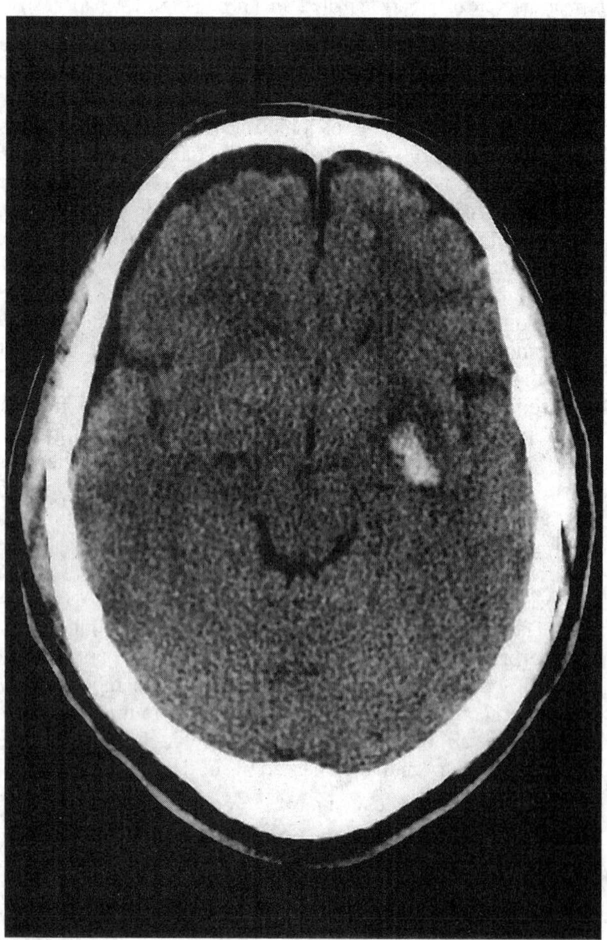

FIGURE 2.4-9 *Computed tomography (CT) scan of the brain of a 45-year-old man. The scan was obtained four days after he sustained a severe head injury in a motor vehicle accident. A hemorrhagic contusion and associated edema are apparent in the left basal ganglia and deep white matter of the left frontal lobe. Bifrontal subdural fluid collections are also apparent.*

Follow-up examination after several months of recovery in patients with posttraumatic psychosis indicates no psychiatric sequelae in a minority of patients but persisting behavioral disturbances in the remaining patients. Although some patients manifesting posttraumatic psychosis have no period of coma and have normal CT scans, the majority of patients have CT results indicating diffuse cerebral swelling and intracranial shifting secondary to hematoma.

MOOD DISORDERS Depressive or manic episodes secondary to head injury are diagnosed as mood disorder due to head trauma in DSM-IV. The development of mood disorders due to head trauma is more common in patients with previous personal or family psychiatric histories. Recent research has distinguished acute posttraumatic depression from depression developing several months to one year following the trauma. Acute posttraumatic depression is typically characterized by a higher frequency of vegetative symptoms whereas later-onset depression is characterized by a higher frequency of psychological symptoms. It has been proposed that acute posttraumatic depression is secondary to neurophysiological or neurochemical changes wrought by the head injury, whereas later-onset posttraumatic depression may be secondary to psychosocial factors and psychological reaction to the consequences of the injury. Depressive mood disorders secondary to head trauma are particularly associated with left dorsolateral frontal and left basal ganglia lesions. Prominent acute anxiety symptoms presenting in addition to depression tend to be associated with the presence of right hemisphere lesions. Those acutely anxious and depressed patients tend to have a longer course of depression than those with depressive symptoms alone. In patients with closed head injuries, mood disorder with manic features has been found in association with right hemisphere lesions, particularly with involvement of the basotemporal cortex or limbic system structures. An increased prevalence of posttraumatic epilepsy has been reported among patients with posttraumatic manic features.

The findings of depression after left-hemisphere lesions and of mania after right-hemisphere lesions have experimental correlates with unilateral lesions in the rat. In the rat, massive noradrenergic projections pass rostrally from the locus ceruleus to the neocortex in an anterior-to-posterior fashion, passing through the frontal lobes. Therefore, lesions close to the frontal poles significantly damage noradrenergic neurons before they undergo increasingly extensive arborization as they pass toward the posterior cortices. Right-hemisphere infarctions in the rat have been observed to result in hyperkinetic behavior, with no significant change in activity levels elicited by similar left-hemisphere lesions.

PERSONALITY CHANGES Clinicians and researchers have observed that there are a number of manifestations of disordered personality which may be seen following head trauma. Most commonly observed have been the *pseudodepressed personality* characterized by apathy and limited emotional reactivity and purportedly associated with lesions of the dorsomedial aspects of the frontal lobes. Using DSM-IV terminology those patients would be diagnosed with personality change due to head trauma, apathetic type. The *pseudopsychopathic personality* is characterized by disinhibition, egocentricity, and sexual inappropriateness and is reportedly associated with lesions of the orbital frontal lobes. Using DSM-IV terminology those patients would be diagnosed with personality change due to head trauma, disinhibited type, aggressive type, or combined type, depending on the predominant feature or features. Phineas Gage, for example, would have been diagnosed with personality change due to head trauma, disinhibited type.

The following clinical vignette illustrates not only the sexual disinhibition sometimes observed after a closed head injury but also the egocentricity that is one of the most pronounced features of personality change due to head trauma.

A 19-year-old woman had exhibited childish behavior and hypersexuality since an automobile accident in which she sustained a severe closed head injury and a period of coma. Two months after the accident she was informed by rehabilitation staff members that her fiancé had been killed in the accident. The patient's immediate reaction was to express her consternation that her main source of sexual gratification was gone.

The second vignette illustrates the effect personality change due to head trauma can have on vocational adjustment:

A 36-year-old woman sustained a closed head injury resulting in a combined period of coma and posttraumatic amnesia equaling one month. She returned to her work in a state developmental center following the head injury but was eventually suspended from her job because of her profane and verbally abusive interactions with residents. Also reported were memory deficits compensated for by paranoia. For example, the patient accused residents of stealing items that she herself had misplaced. The patient denied most of the incidents in question but admitted very poor frustration tolerance.

BEHAVIORAL SEQUELAE Studies have been conducted, using psychiatric rating scales, to quantify the profile of behavioral disturbance during the subacute phase of recovery from a closed head injury. The most common behavioral sequelae were found to be conceptual disorganization, inaccurate self-appraisal, poor insight, unrealistic goals, poor planning for the future, memory deficits, disorientation, expressive speech deficits, depression, blunted affect, fatigue, motor retardation, and somatic concerns. When comparing patients with mild, moderate, and severe head injuries, researchers found that the severity of the head injury was related to disordered cognition and to deficits in insight, goals, planning, and expressive speech (Figure 2.4-10). However, the extent of the somatic concerns was found to be inversely proportional to the severity of the injury, probably because of the low levels of insight and the inaccurate self-appraisals by the severely head-injured patients.

A great severity of behavioral sequelae was found in those patients who had compressed ventricles on early CT scans, indicating significant brain edema. An abnormal EEG was also related to the degree of the disturbed behavior observed during recovery. The presence of agitation—as indicated by combativeness, screaming, and other forms of sympathetic arousal—was related to severe behavioral sequelae after the acute period of agitation had subsided.

EFFECTS ON THE FAMILY Head injury results in a high incidence of psychiatric illness in the family involved, as well as in the injured patient. Family members of head-injured patients suffer deterioration in social and psychological functioning. In one study 57 percent of the relatives of head-injured patients had reached clinical levels of mental distress three months after the injury. That decrease in the mental health of family members can also be long-term and deteriorative, rather than the result of short-term distress because of the relative's head injury. Years after the head injury, up to two thirds of the parents caring for severely head-injured patients gradually lose most or all social contacts. Even siblings may stop visiting. Among those head-injured patients who were married at the time of the injury, divorce rates six years after the injury were 42 percent for patients attaining good recovery, 64 percent for those with moderate disability, and 62 percent for those with severe disability. Among those who remained married, the spouse frequently changed from a marital partner to a caretaker. Sexual contact may continue between the partners, but the uninjured partner frequently complains that sexual contact loses the empathic and sharing qualities that were present before the injury.

Family members often use defense mechanisms when confronted with the realities of a head injury. Denial is particularly common. Family members may believe that their relative will recover from a state of severe disability, despite all the evidence to the contrary. Health care professionals may be distrusted, disbelieved, and, in some instances, attacked when they are tactfully conveying a grim but realistic prognosis.

HEAD TRAUMA IN CHILDREN

After a focal lesion of the brain, the recovery of function (specifically language functioning) is often much more satisfactory in children than in adults because of the plasticity of the child's developing nervous system. Unfortunately, the same principle cannot be applied to diffuse cerebral insult. Diffuse injury to the brain, such as that produced by a closed head injury, produces more severe and longer-lasting sequelae in children than in adults.

OUTCOME As in adults, controlled empirical studies have demonstrated no lasting cognitive sequelae in children suffering mild head injuries. Memory is the cognitive function most frequently compromised in children as a result of moderate to severe head injuries. By six months to one year after the injury, children suffering moderate head injuries typically have memory performances consistent with those of normal controls, whereas children recovering from severe head injuries typically perform significantly below both the controls and children with moderate injuries. Severely head-injured children show dramatic improvement in memory functioning six months after the injury but still perform significantly below the controls and children with mild to moderate head injuries. As with adults, the rate of recovery in children seems to reach an asymptote after six months. After 12 months severely head-injured children typically show little improvement over memory performances measured after six months. Executive functioning is also impaired in children with moderate to severe head trauma, and the size of frontal lobe lesioning on MRI has been found to be associated with the extent of executive dysfunction.

Scores on I.Q. tests typically reflect 10- to 30-point decrements in full-scale I.Q. scores when compared with premorbid estimates in children recovering from severe closed head injuries. Although deficits in both verbal and performance I.Q. scores are typically seen soon after recovery from posttraumatic amnesia, verbal I.Q. scores often show steady improvement on serial testing. Persisting deficits are often observed in performance I.Q. scores and are correlated with a reduction in motor speed during simple tasks. Among academic skills, arithmetic disturbance is a frequent sequela of severe closed head injuries in children, whereas reading and spelling performances are relatively well-preserved. Reading and spelling are thought to be automatized and overlearned and are, therefore, resistant to brain injury, whereas arithmetic operations require a great degree of sustained attention and concentration.

PSYCHIATRIC ASPECTS As with adults, such premorbid behavioral features as impulsivity and hyperactivity place certain children at a high risk for sustaining head trauma. For example, retrospective examination of school records indicates a higher frequency of teacher-reported behavioral problems in

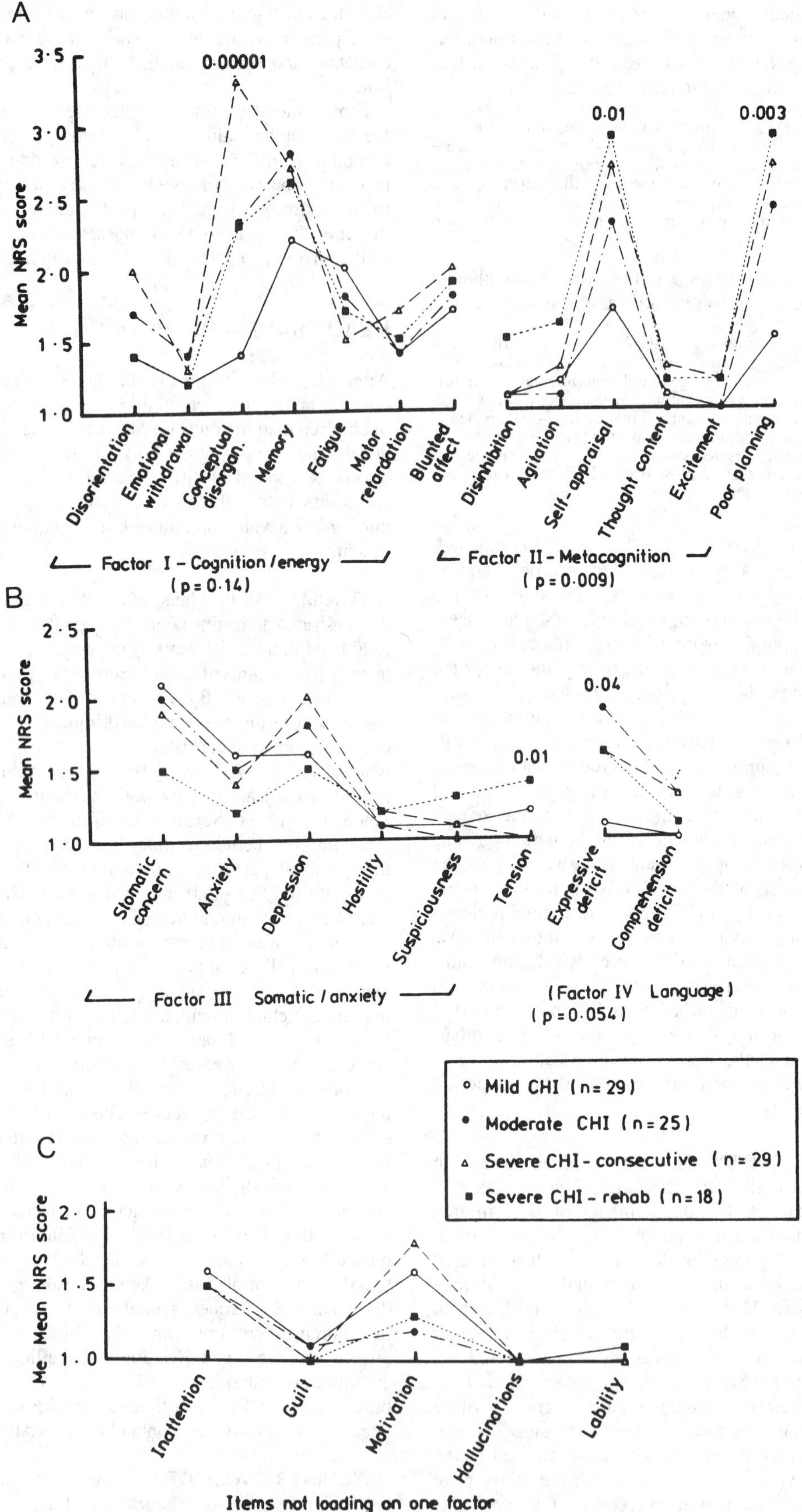

FIGURE 2.4-10 *Mean scores for 27 neurobehavioral rating scale variables plotted for four samples of head-injured patients. The variables are plotted according to their loadings on four factors. The significant main effects are indicated by probability values above the respective variables. (From H S Levin, W M High, K E Goethe, R A Sisson, J E Overall, H M Rhoades, H M Eisenberg, Z Kalisky, H E Gary: The neurobehavioural rating scale: Assessment of the behavioural sequelae of head injury by the clinician. J Neurol Neurosurg Psychiatry* 50: *188, 1987. Used with permission.)*

children suffering head trauma as compared with controls. Longitudinal studies have documented that the rate of new psychiatric disorders is directly related to the severity of head trauma in children. Children with a history of head trauma have higher rates of distractibility, poor anger control, irritability, low frustration tolerance, and aggression, when compared with children having behavioral disorders but without a history of head trauma. Children with severe head injuries have a rate of psychiatric disorders triple that of orthopedic controls two years after the injury, although behavioral problems are estimated to be at least partially due to premorbid psychiatric features in approximately one third of children with severe head trauma. After a head trauma, premorbidly maladjusted children often develop new and more severe forms of behavioral disturbance. Recovery of social and adaptive functioning in children has been found to be associated with adaptive family characteristics, such as the degree of cohesion, extent of positive interrelationships, and flexibility in the families of the recovering children.

NEUROPSYCHOLOGICAL TESTING

Neuropsychological testing provides an objective and quantified appraisal of the cognitive deficits that may accompany head trauma. During the early stages of recovery from moderate to severe head injury, assessment should focus on the presence of retrograde and anterograde amnesia. The Galveston Orientation and Amnesia Test and its pediatric analog, the Children's Orientation and Amnesia Test, are practical instruments for the measurement of posttraumatic amnesia and are useful predictors of long-term outcome.

After recovery from posttraumatic amnesia, formal and more extensive neuropsychological testing may be performed. If the test results indicate well-preserved cognitive functioning in relevant cognitive domains, a return to work or school may be feasible within one month. Areas of deficit may be identified that can then be made the focus of treatment intervention by rehabilitation professionals. Although the clinical course is typically characterized by at least a partial resolution of the cognitive deficit, the mechanism of recovery remains conjectural. The reduction of edema, the reorganization of intact brain areas into a new functional arrangement, and the development of compensatory skills through rehabilitation have been postulated to underlie clinical recovery. However, some deficits (for example, memory disturbance) may prove refractory.

The results of neuropsychological evaluations during the initial hospitalization or shortly after discharge should be interpreted cautiously as prognostic indicators of long-term functioning if the evaluation is performed less than six months after the injury. Serial assessments characterizing the early rate of recovery are more informative than a single evaluation, which may provide only a modest amount of prognostic information. The rate of recovery is conventionally considered to be relatively stable after six months, although further improvement may occur, depending on the individual patient.

Neuropsychological evaluation typically assesses the major cognitive domains of memory, attention, intellect, language, perception, and motor performance. However, evaluation of those domains must be supplemented by careful assessment of executive functioning. The *executive or frontal lobe systems* are responsible for motivating, planning, regulating, and controlling the quality of behavioral performance. *Executive deficit syndromes* are disorders in the application of intellectual abilities to specific situations in the environment. Patients with head traumas often retain impressive levels of skill and knowledge but are unable to apply those abilities in an adaptive and effective manner, as they did before the injury.

Many neuropsychological tests (such as intelligence tests) are highly structured, with explicit instructions about the tasks involved. Patients may perform well on a standard battery of neuropsychological tests but then exhibit profound deficits on tasks that are unstructured and in which patients must abstract the solution by actively planning and monitoring their own behavior. Several tests of abstract problem-solving ability and resistance to perseveration are relatively unstructured and sensitive to executive functioning. Those tests should be a standard component of the evaluation of patients with traumatic brain injuries.

REHABILITATION

Rehabilitation of brain-injured patients is a multidisciplinary endeavor primarily involving psychologists, physiatrists, speech pathologists, physical therapists, occupational therapists, and professionals from other disciplines. Behavior-modification techniques are used to eliminate or reduce the frequency of maladaptive behaviors, such as aggressiveness and social inappropriateness. Cognitive retraining focuses on finding alternative strategies to compensate for deficits in memory or executive functioning. For example, patients with memory deficits may be given training in the extensive use of memory prostheses, such as appointment books and reminder notes posted conspicuously at home or at work. Patients with executive deficits may be taught to break complex tasks down into simpler component steps before attempting them, or they may be taught to organize their behavior into highly automatized routines to overcome their inertia. In addition to the remediation of dysarthria and anomic deficits, treatment of communication disorders in head-injured patients extends to learning pragmatic skills in topic maintenance, concise delivery of an essential message, and taking balanced turns in conversation.

Traditional rehabilitation programs are confined to speech, occupational, and physical therapy. Whether supplementing those traditional programs with cognitive rehabilitation produces improved neurobehavioral outcomes is currently an issue of contention. Controlled outcome studies are needed to resolve the issue.

SUGGESTED CROSS-REFERENCES

The use of the mental status examination and the general clinical approach to neuropsychiatric disorders are discussed in Section 2.1. Delirium, dementia, and amnestic and other cognitive disorders, mental disorders due to a general medical condition, and postconcussional disorder are covered in Chapter 12. The use of neuropsychological tests in the examination of psychiatric and neurological patients is described in Sections 9.5 and 9.6. Relevant aspects of neurology are discussed in Section 1.2, and neuroimaging is described in Section 1.10.

REFERENCES

Becker D P, Povlishock J T, editors: *Central Nervous System Trauma Status Report*. National Institute of Neurological and Communicative Disorders and Stroke, Bethesda, 1985.

Ben-Yishay Y, Diller L: Cognitive remediation in traumatic brain injury: Update and issues. Arch Phys Med Rehabil *74:* 204, 1993.

Brooks N, editor: *Closed Head Injury: Psychological, Social, and Family Consequences*. Oxford University Press, New York, 1984.

*Brown S J, Fann J R, Grant I: Postconcussional disorder: Time to acknowledge a common source of neurobehavioral morbidity. J Neuropsychiatry Clin Neurosci *6:* 15, 1994.

Clifton G L, Kreutzer J S, Choi S C, Devany C W, Eisenberg H M, Foulkes M A, Jane J A, Marmarou A, Marshall L F: Relationship between Glasgow Outcome Scale and neuropsychological measures after brain injury. Neurosurgery *33:* 34, 1993.

Dikmen S, Machamer J, Temkin N: Psychosocial outcome in patients with moderate to severe head injury: 2-year follow-up. Brain Inj *7:* 113, 1993.

Fenton G, McClelland R, Montgomery A, MacFlynn G, Rutherford W: The postconcussional syndrome: social antecedents and psychological sequelae. Br J Psychiatry *162:* 493, 1993.

*Jennett B, Teasdale G: *Management of Head Injuries.* Davis, Philadelphia, 1981.

Jorge R E, Robinson R G, Arndt S V, Forrester A W, Geisler F, Starkstein S E: Comparison between acute- and delayed-onset depression following traumatic brain injury. J Neuropsychiatry Clin Neurosci *5:* 43, 1993.

Jorge R E, Robinson R G, Starkstein S E, Arndt S V: Depression and anxiety following traumatic brain injury. J Neuropsychiatry Clin Neurosci *5:* 369, 1993.

Jorge R E, Robinson R G, Starkstein S E, Arndt S V, Forrester A W, Geisler F H: Secondary mania following traumatic brain injury. Am J Psychiatry *150:* 916, 1993.

*Levin H S, Benton A L, Grossman R G: *Neurobehavioral Consequences of Closed Head Injury.* Oxford University Press, New York, 1982.

Levin H S, Culhane K A, Mendelsohn D, Lilly M A, Bruce D, Fletcher J M, Chapman S B, Harward H, Eisenberg H M: Cognition in relation to magnetic resonance imaging in head-injured children and adolescents. Arch Neurol *50:* 897, 1993.

Levin H S, Eisenberg H M, Benton A L, editors: *Frontal Lobe Function and Dysfunction.* Oxford University Press, New York, 1991.

Levin H S, Eisenberg H M, Benton A L, editors: *Mild Head Injury.* Oxford University Press, New York, 1989.

Levin H S, Grafman J, Eisenberg H M, editors: *Neurobehavioral Recovery from Head Injury.* Oxford University Press, New York, 1987.

Lezak M D, editor: *Frontiers of Clinical Neuroscience,* vol 7: *Assessment of the Behavioral Consequences of Head Trauma.* Liss, New York, 1989.

*Lishman W A: *Organic Psychiatry: The Psychological Consequences of Cerebral Disorder,* ed 2. Blackwell, London, 1987.

Michaud L J, Rivara F P, Jaffe K M, Fay G, Dailey J L: Traumatic brain injury as a risk factor for behavioral disorders in children. Arch Phys Med Rehabil *74:* 368, 1993.

Mittenberg W, DiGiulio D V, Perrin S, Bass A E: Symptoms following mild head injury: Expectation as aetiology. J Neurol Neurosurg Psychiatry *55:* 200, 1994.

Newcombe F: *Missle Wounds of the Brain.* Oxford University Press, New York, 1969.

Ommaya A K, Gennarelli T A: Cerebral concussion and traumatic unconsciousness: Correlation of experimental and clinical observations on blunt head injuries. Brain *97:* 633, 1974.

Silver J M, Hales R E, Yudofsky S C: Neuropsychiatric aspects of traumatic brain injury. In *Textbook of Neuropsychiatry,* ed 2, S C Yudofsky, R E Hales, editors, p 363. American Psychiatric Press, Washington, 1992.

*Vinken P J, Bruyn G W, Klawans H L, editors: *Handbook of Clinical Neurology,* vol 13: *Head Injury.* Elsevier Science, New York, 1990.

Wehman P, Sherron P, Kregel J, Kreutzer J, Tran S, Cifu D: Return to work for persons following severe traumatic brain injury. Supported employment outcomes after five years. Am J Phys Med Rehabil *72:* 355, 1993.

Wood R L, editor: *Neurobehavioural Sequelae of Traumatic Brain Injury.* Taylor & Francis, New York, 1990.

2.5 NEUROPSYCHIATRIC ASPECTS OF MOVEMENT DISORDERS

WILLIAM C. WIRSHING, M.D.

INTRODUCTION

Movement disorders have neurological and psychiatric manifestations. In many instances the neuroanatomical site responsible for the condition is known, in some cases the specific neurochemical defect has been identified, and, rarely, the particular genetic abnormality causing the movement disorder has been localized. Those characteristics are typical of many neurological syndromes. Conversely, those conditions are also notoriously responsive to stress, are commonly ameliorated by sleep, are prone to psychogenic embellishment, and have been associated with a wide spectrum of concomitant psychiatric ailments, including obsessive-compulsive disorder, depressive disorders, psychotic disorders, anxiety disorders, and personality alterations. That association implies common neuroanatomical control, common electrochemical deviation, or perhaps closely linked heritability.

The various neuropsychiatric syndromes that have been noted in movement disorders might conceivably be secondary or reactive to the primary neuromotor dysfunction. The disorders are, after all, socially and functionally limiting and can be fatal. If that were the case, however, the neuropsychiatric reactions of all movement-disordered patients should be indistinguishable from one another and from other progressive and handicapping illnesses (for example, rheumatoid arthritis, multiple sclerosis, and chronic myelogenous leukemia). Furthermore, no psychiatric symptoms should be apparent before the movement disorder is demonstrable. Both conditions are contrary to clinical experience. In addition, both the movement disorder and the psychiatric syndromes are somewhat amenable to pharmacological manipulations of various and sometimes different monoaminergic systems. Those findings argue against a simple psychiatric reaction to a primary illness. Table 2.5-1 summarizes the psychiatric syndromes associated with the most common movement disorders, discussed in this section, and Table 2.5-2 highlights unusual movement disorders and their neuropsychiatric correlates.

Movement disorders have traditionally been considered the motoric expressions of disorders within the basal ganglia. Those phylogenetically ancient subcortical structures are, in fact, vital in controlling and modulating movements, particularly those that are overlearned (for example, postural control, walking, and alternating movements). They have a well-documented reciprocal neuronal connection with the supplementary motor area and the motor cortex (through the thalamus) and have been implicated in virtually every known pathological movement disorder.

The cortical connectivity of the basal ganglia, though, extends well beyond the motor areas and includes virtually all cortical regions. The basal ganglia integrate, process, and modulate those wide-ranging inputs before sending the resultant responses through the thalamus to any of a number of specific cortical targets. Most generally, the basal ganglia can be seen as responsible for maintaining the present state (for example, sitting still, walking, concentrating, euthymic mood), excluding unwanted states (for example, adventitial movements, intrusive thoughts, impulsive or compulsive behaviors, depressed moods) and terminating old states and initiating new ones (for example, rising from a chair, beginning ambulation, changing the focus of mental concentration, ceasing a ruminative thought). It performs those functions in concert with many other brain structures. A perturbation anywhere in the striatothalamocorticostriatal network loop could result in a disorder in one or more of those general properties. Thus, a dopamine-blocking agent could at once cause parkinsonism through its effect on striatal-

TABLE 2.5-1
Movement Disorders and Their Associated Neuropsychiatric Aspects

Disorder	Neuropathology	Neurochemical Abberations	Associated Neuropsychiatric Syndromes	Pharmacotherapeutics
Parkinson's disease	Loss of nigrostriatal dopaminergic fibers, with resultant gliosis and intracytoplasmic inclusion bodies (Lewy bodies); other brain areas are also affected, including the pigmented nuclei of the brainstem, the globus pallidus, and the substantia innominata	Decreased dopamine in the nigrostriatal, mesolimbic, and mesocortical pathways; serotonin is also decreased, but that may be a secondary effect	Depression	Tricyclic antidepressants, lithium, MAOIs, atypical antidepressants; serotonin-specific agents may be at once more effective and better tolerated by the patient
			Neuropsychiatric deficits	None available
Huntington's disease	Marked atrophy and cell loss of the caudate and the putamen, with smaller degrees of atrophy in the globus pallidus and the thalamus; the cortex shows neuronal loss and gross atrophy in severe cases	Loss of GABA-ergic striatal outflow neurons is the most consistently demonstrated finding	Mood disturbances, predominantly depression	Tricyclic antidepressants, lithium, MAOIs, atypical antidepressants
			Psychosis	Antipsychotics and antidepressants
			Personality changes	Antipsychotics
			Neuropsychological deficits	None available
Tourette's disorder	None identified	Hypofunction of dopamine system, although no specific site has been identified	Obsessive-compulsive disorder	Serotonin-augmenting agents
			Aggressive behavior	Antipsychotics and serotonin-augmenting agents
			Hyperactivity	Stimulants may attenuate the hyperactivity but will worsen the tics

outflow neurons and anhedonia by disrupting reward learning through its effects on the neurons in the ventral striatum.

Movement disorders can be seen as the motoric manifestations of network disfunction. When the perturbation is small and specific, no other abnormalities are present. However, when the disruption is extensive, the movement disorder is but one aspect in a rich spectrum of functional disturbances. In the latter instances, the motoric abnormalities provide cleanly monitorable symptoms that can be assessed, along with modulation of mood, aggressive behaviors, obsessional thoughts, and cognitive performance. The motoric abnormalities are, in a sense, neurological reference points from which behavioral changes in response to disease courses or treatments can be gauged. This section reviews the phenomenology of movement disorders, discusses the major neurological illnesses that have movement disorders as their most salient features, and presents the neuropsychiatric aspects of those illnesses.

DEFINITION

Movement disorders may be conceptually classified into hypokinetic, characterized by slowed movement, and hyperkinetic. The disorders include such phenomena as dystonia, athetosis, chorea, tremor, tics, and myoclonus.

HYPOKINETIC SYNDROME The causes of this syndrome (also known as parkinsonism and akinetic-rigid syndrome) are many. Table 2.5-3 lists the diseases and conditions that may manifest a hypokinetic syndrome during at least part of the clinical course. Parkinson's disease is the prototypical akinetic-rigid syndrome.

The classic clinical tetrad of Parkinson's disease consists of muscular rigidity, bradykinesia, loss of righting reflexes, and resting tremor. Rigidity is manifested as muscular resistance to passive movement of the body part. It is believed to be mediated through central (basal ganglia) overactivation of the so-called long loop or transcortical reflexes.

Bradykinesia (slow movement) leads to excessively long performance or movement time during voluntary motor tasks. Clinically, it manifests as slow movement and low-amplitude-with-frequent-arrests performance on such tasks as rapid alternating movements. Some authors believe that akinesia represents the extreme end of the bradykinetic spectrum, in which volitional movement has come to a near halt and the afflicted patient is frozen in space. Others define akinesia separately and see it as a lack of spontaneous movements and an exaggerated delay in initiating movement. Generally, the patients with pronounced bradykinesia have prolonged reaction times, but those components are separated frequently enough in hypokinetic patients to suggest that they are mediated by distinct pathophysiological mechanisms.

Loss of righting reflexes relates to the patient's inability to balance properly, with resulting disequilibrium, festination, and tendency to fall.

Resting tremor is characteristic of Parkinson's disease and occurs variably in other hypokinetic disorders. It can affect any body region, but the upper extremity is generally involved most prominently. It has a regular frequency (three to six cycles per second), is usually suppressed during volitional action of the involved body part, is exacerbated by stress and anxiety, and classically involves alternating contractions of opposing muscular groups (for example, the pronators and the supinators of the forearm). Although a resting tremor is clearly a disorder of excessive movement, it is described and classified here because the tremor accompanies syndromes that are hypokinetic in overall appearance. Furthermore, it generally remits with pharmacological interventions that mitigate other components of the hypokinetic syndrome.

HYPERKINETIC SYNDROME This syndrome has more varied and complex manifestations than does the hypokinetic symptom complex. It is usually fractionated into clinically recognizable subsyndromes that range in speed from a fixed posture (dystonia) to very fast and brief adventitial movements (tics and myoclonus). Table 2.5-4 delineates the clinical characteristics of each of the subsyndromes, their respective speeds in cycles per second, their common areas of distribution, and the most common associated disease states.

PARKINSON'S DISEASE

EPIDEMIOLOGY Parkinson's disease is the most common idiopathic extrapyramidal syndrome seen in the aging population. Prevalence estimates vary between 85 and 180 per 100,000 population. The mean age of onset is 60 years, and the disease

TABLE 2.5-2
Common Neuromotor Syndromes and Their Associated Neuropsychiatric Findings

Disease Entity Alternate Nomenclature	Neuropathology	Clinical Features	Associated Neuropsychiatric Syndromes
Multiple system atrophies Olivopontocerebellar degeneration Shy-Drager syndrome Striatonigral degeneration	A combination of degenerative lesions in the pontine nuclei, the cerebellum, the inferior olivae, the pigmented nuclei, the striatum, and the spinal cord; the specific classification applied to a given patient (e.g., Shy-Drager versus striatonigral degeneration) depends on which clinical characteristics predominate	Hypokinetic (i.e., parkinsonian) features tend to be the most common, but choreas, dystonias, and, rarely, ballistic and myoclonic movements can be present; in addition, there is ataxia (cerebellar involvement) and corticobulbar and corticospinal signs (pontine and spinal involvement); other less common neurological features are cranial nerve palsies, retinal degeneration, peripheral neuropathy, autonomic dysfunction (Shy-Drager), and deafness; autosomal dominant and recessive inheritance is most common, but sporadic cases do occur; the disease is invariably progressive and ends in incapacitation and death	Cognitive functions generally remain relatively intact, but progressive intellectual decline of the cortical type does occur (cerebrocerebellar degenerations)
Progressive supranuclear palsy Steele-Richardson-Olszewski syndrome	Atrophy of the brainstem and the cerebellum dominate the gross pathology; microscopically, there is neuronal loss, gliosis, granulovacuolar degeneration, and neurofibrillary tangles (15 nm straight filaments) in the subthalamic nucleus, the nucleus basalis of Meynert, the pontine and the midbrain tegmentum, the red nucleus, the reticular formation, the globus pallidus, and a number of other midbrain nuclei	The disease generally begins in the 50s and progresses to death over a period of 10–15 years; there is vertical supranuclear ophthalmoplegia, axial rigidity (with neck-extended posturing), appendicular spasticity, pseudobulbar palsy (emotional lability, explosive coughing, dysarthria, and dysphagia), and pyramidal track findings (hyperreflexia, clonus, spasticity, and extensor plantars)	Emotional lability without major behavioral disturbances predominates the early course of the illness; later, there is a mild progressive dementia of the so-called subcortical variety that includes cognitive slowing, forgetfulness, and personality changes
Wilson's disease Hepatolenticuar degeneration	Bilateral degeneration of lenticular nuclei that ranges from discoloration to cavitation caused by excessive accumulation of copper in the CNS; destruction of white matter areas and the cerebral cortex is also occasionally seen; microscopically, neuronal loss and astrocytic degeneration are commonly seen	A parkinsonian syndrome with a generally severe tremor that exacerbates during action is commonly the presenting motoric abnormality; function is generally affected out of proportion to the apparent severity of the hypokinetic syndrome; dysarthria, dysphonia, dysphagia, and ataxia accompany the parkinsonism; dystonic and, less commonly, choreic movements are also seen in untreated cases; the neurological findings are present with hepatic disturbances (ranges from acute hepatitis to cirrhosis) and ocular changes (Kayser-Fleischer rings and sunflower cataracts); most but not all clinical manifestations improve with chelation therapy	No specific neuropsychiatric syndrome is associated with Wilson's disease, but up to 25% of patients initially present to psychiatrists for a variety of emotional reasons, ranging from simple adjustment reactions to mood disturbances to frank and occasionally unremitting psychotic states; it is not known whether any of the reported syndromes are due to the co-occurrence of illnesses, the excess deposition of CNS copper, or the reaction of the adolescent or young adult to a debilitating neurological illness
Basal ganglia calcification Fahr's disease	Calcification of CNS structures can be secondary (to parathyroid disturbances, birth anoxia, lead poisoning, tuberous sclerosis, AIDS, radiation therapy, mitochondrial diseases, and other causes) or primary; the striatum and the globus pallidus are most frequently affected, but other cerebral structures can be involved	In the idiopathic variety a parkinsonian syndrome usually manifests in the third decade of life; choreoathetoid and dystonic movements can also be present, as can seizures, ataxia, and dysarthria; the illness is progressive, with death ensuing from secondary illness	Depression, anxiety, psychosis, and cognitive decline are among the commonly reported neuropsychiatric correlates; only dementia is clearly related to the underlying neurological deterioration that accompanies the idiopathic variety; in the congenital forms of pseudohypoparathyroidism, there may also be mental retardation, but it is not due to the resultant calcification of subcortical structures

TABLE 2.5-2 (*continued*)

Hallervorden-Spatz disease	Grossly there is rust-brown discoloration of the globus pallidus, the substantia nigra, and the red and subthalamic nuclei; iron, neuromelanin, and lipofuscin constitute the pigment; gliosis, spheroids (swollen axon fragments composed of glycoprotein, lipid, and mitochondria), and neuronal loss are prominent in the internal segment of the pallidum and the substantia nigra zona reticulata and to a smaller extent in the zona compacta	The illness generally begins in childhood and is relentlessly progressive, with death ensuing on average a decade after onset; parkinsonian motor features are most common, but, when present, the tremor is more often worse during posture-maintaining procedures; dystonia and chorea can also be present at different stages of the illness; pyramidal tract signs (e.g., hyperreflexia and extensor plantar responses), dysarthria, and reduced visual acuity (secondary to retinal pigment deposition or optic atrophy) also occur	Mental retardation may be present, but mental deterioration that ranges from mild cognitive deficits to frank dementia can intervene; about 15% of the patients reported have normal mentation; other neuropsychiatric characteristics are not commonly reported
Sydenham's chorea St. Vitus dance	The neurological lesions are widespread and nonspecific; there is inflammation, neuronal degeneration, petechial hemorrhages, and vasodilation; antibodies to striatal-specific antigens have been reported to occur, but their exact significance remains obscure; like the other streptococcal-related syndromes (arthritis, carditis), Sydenham's chorea is a vanishingly rare disorder	The syndrome is almost invariably choreic, but dysarthria and hypotonia frequently occur; females predominate, and affected children are generally between 5 and 15 years old; about a third give a history of acute streptococcal infection one to six months before the symptoms; the course is time-limited and usually remits after three to six months; rarely are patients left with some permanent neurological impairment	The syndrome frequently presents with irritability, a personality change, or even an overt toxic confusional state (about one fifth of patients); like the chorea, the behavioral disturbances generally worsen over two to four weeks and then slowly abate over the ensuing three to six months; there are occasionally some residual behavioral abnormalities
Idiopathic torsion dystonia Dystonia musculorum deformans Childhood-onset dystonia	Although a disturbance of dopamine neurotransmission in the striatum of the substantia nigra has been suspected, convincing documentation is lacking	This generally progressive illness typically begins between ages 6 and 12 with a focal action dystonia of the leg; it reaches its most severe point 5 to 10 years after onset and involves virtually all body regions with fixed and deforming postures; bulbar musculature involvement results in dysphonia, dysphagia, and respiratory disturbances; in adulthood the syndrome remains static or gradually improves; about 20% of patients experience remissions lasting hours to years, but recurrence is common; it is thought to be genetically transmitted, but the exact nature of that transmission (i.e., autosomal recessive, autosomal dominant with incomplete penetrance, X-linked) is unclear	Adjustment reactions to this chronic and neurologically debilitating disease is common; there is no intellectual impairment, increased incidence of psychosis, bipolar disorder, or other behavioral syndromes
Adult-onset focal dystonias Cranial dystonia Meige's syndrome Blepharospasm-oromandibular dystonia Breughel's syndrome Spasmodic torticollis Truncal dystonia Writer's cramp and other occupational dystonias	A disturbance of dopamine neruotransmission in the striatum or the substantia nigra has been suspected in adult-onset focal dystonias; the few postmortem studies have suggested that nonspecific abnormalities (i.e., cell loss, Lewy bodies, and rare neurofibrillary tangles) are present in the nigra and other pigmented brainstem nuclei, as well as in the striatum (particularly the putamen)	The form of the syndrome depends on the body region affected; generally, the illness begins between ages 20 and 50; it is progressive over the next five years; partial, temporary remissions are common, but complete recovery rarely, if ever, occurs; emotional stress exacerbates the condition, and patients are commonly given a psychogenic diagnosis at some point during their illness course	Reactive depression is the most commonly associated neuropsychiatric symptom; cognition is unaffected, and other behavioral disturbances are uncommonly reported; some investigators report that patients are likely to have a rigid, fastidious, and repressed personality style; however, such patients may be merely unable to adapt to the neurological impairment

reaches its highest prevalence in the eighth decade. Approximately 80 percent of parkinsonian patients are in their seventh or eighth decade of life. Neither gender appears to have an enhanced risk.

ETIOLOGY Despite the passage of nearly two centuries since James Parkinson described shaking palsy in 1817, its cause remains unknown. Speculations about the cause have clustered in three areas: genetic, accelerated aging, and environmental and toxic.

For most patients with Parkinson's disease, twin studies and direct examination of the relatives of probands have failed to reveal any genetic role in the cause of the disease. Certain families, however, are at particular risk. In those high-risk pedigrees, the genetic pattern

TABLE 2.5-3
Diseases and Conditions with Hypokinetic Syndromes Associated with the Clinical Course

Idiopathic Parkinson's disease
Postencephalitic parkinsonism
- Encephalitis lethargica
- Other encephalitides

- Parkinsonism in other degenerative diseases
- Multiple-system atrophies
  - Olivopontocerebellar degeneration
  - Shy-Drager syndrome
  - Striatonigral degeneration
- Pallidal degenerations
- Progressive supranuclear palsy
- Hepatolenticular degeneration (Wilson's disease)
- Acquired hepatocerebral degeneration (e.g., secondary to alcohol-induced hepatic encephalopathy)
- Nigrospinodentatal degeneration with ophthalmoplegia (Machado-Joseph-Azorean disease)
- Alzheimer's disease
- Creutzfeldt-Jakob disease
- Cortical-basal ganglionic degeneration
- Pick's disease
- Parkinson-dementia-amyotrophic lateral sclerosis (ALS) complex of Guam
- Rigid variant of Huntington's disease (Westphal variant)
- Hallervorden-Spatz disease
- Calcification of the basal ganglia (Fahr's syndrome)
- Rare variants of other neurodegenerative and neurometabolic disorders (e.g., Gaucher's disease, G_{M1} gangliosidosis; Chédiak-Higashi syndrome; chorea-acanthocytosis syndrome (neuroacanthocytosis); neuronal intranuclear inclusion disease; familial depression, alveolar hypoventilation and parkinsonism)

- Drug- or toxin-induced parkinsonism
- Antipsychotics, antiemetics
- 1-Methyl-4-phenyl-1,2,3,6-tetrahydropyridine (MPTP)
- Manganese

- Parkinsonism caused by other known triggers
- Postanoxic
- Toxic
  - Carbon monoxide intoxication, cyanide poisoning, carbon disulphide, methanol, ethanol
- Dementia pugilistica (punchdrunk syndrome)

- Hydrocephalus (normal-pressure and high-pressure)

- Space-occupying lesions: tumors, arteriovenus malformations

- Multiple cerebral infarcts (atherosclerotic parkinsonism)

appears to be an autosomal dominant pattern with incomplete penetrance.

Cell loss within the zona compacta region of the substantia nigra (the cells that are destroyed in Parkinson's disease) occurs with age, and some authors have proposed that the disease is a consequence of accelerated aging. Arguing against such an explanation is the fact that not all very aged persons have Parkinson's disease. Furthermore, the risk rises with age until about the mid-70s, when the incidence declines significantly. Thus, age-related changes in that brain area are probably not causally related to Parkinson's disease but do contribute to disability.

Evidence in support of the environmental and toxic cause is varied and indirect. Young-onset Parkinson's disease patients are more likely to have been exposed to well water in a rural environment than were their older-onset counterparts. The Chamorro people of Guam are known to have an unusual syndrome, called Parkinson-dementia-amyotrophic lateral sclerosis-complex of Guam, that is marked by parkinsonism, muscular weakness, and dementia. Excessive consumption of the cycad nut (cycad circinalis, the seed of a palmlike plant) has been proposed as the cause of the syndrome. In primate experiments the use of β-N-methylamino-L-alanine, an amino acid derived from cycad, causes the delayed development of basal ganglia dysfunction. The intravenous use of 1-methyl-4-phenyl-1,2,3,6-tetrahydropyridine (MPTP), a toxic by-product of the clandestine synthesis of a potent meperidine analogue, causes selective destruction of nigral dopamine neurons and an irreversible parkinsonian syndrome in primates and humans. Those unusual clinical syndromes account for only a tiny fraction of those afflicted with parkinsonism. Taken together, though, the data indicate that the neuronal structures responsible for Parkinson's disease are susceptible to environmental and toxic insults and hint that such a cause underlies the common forms of the disease. Attempts to identify toxic exposure or environmental commonality in the general parkinsonian population have been uninformative to date.

CLINICAL FEATURES

Neurosomatic features In addition to the cardinal features of the hypokinetic syndrome, Parkinson's disease patients can also manifest hypomimia (masked facies), hypophonic and monotonous voice, seborrheic dermatitis, constipation, sialorrhea (secondary to decreased swallowing), dysphagia, mild orthostatic hypotension, delayed gastric emptying, decreased appetite, urinary bladder dysfunction, impotence, and episodic diaphoresis. That constellation of neurosomatic symptoms is rarely present in any one patient, and some symptoms, such as dysphagia, are late manifestations.

Neuropsychiatric features Conceptually, the neuropsychiatric concomitants of Parkinson's disease may be put into four categories: those that are unrelated to the disease (for example, preexisting bipolar disorder and schizophrenia), reactive psychiatric syndromes (for example, reactive depressive disorder), psychiatric perturbations secondary to medications (for example, levodopa hallucinosis), and parkinsonism-linked behavioral changes (for example, dementia and depression). Although such a framework has undeniable heuristic usefulness, the categorical determination may be difficult to make in individual patients.

DEPRESSION Depression is the most frequent psychiatric concomitant of Parkinson's disease, afflicting 20 to 90 percent in cross-sectional epidemiological studies. Some investigators have reported that the severity of the mood symptoms correlated with the severity of the motor disability and improved when the movement disorder was treated. Those observations led to the conclusion that parkinsonian depression is either reactive to the neurological morbidity or biologically mediated by the same neurochemical perturbations that account for the neurological symptoms.

Other investigations have indicated that depressive symptoms are unresponsive to antiparkinsonism medications and that the severity of the motor symptoms does not correlate with the depressive symptoms. Studies separating major depressive disorders from dysthymic syndromes suggest that major depressive disorder is independent of the motor manifestations and treatment and that modest depressive syndromes have a reactive profile. Some authors have suggested that the apparent investigational inconsistency is because the depression of Parkinson's disease is an organically based, heightened mood reactivity; that is, its neuropathology makes patients susceptible to responding to stress or disability with depression.

The depression of Parkinson's disease is largely indistinguishable from its nonparkinsonism counterpart. Depressed Parkinson's disease patients as a group have more somatic symptoms and less commonly report pathological guilt than do nonparkinsonism-depressed patients. Some authors have inferred that there is a natural progression to the depression of Parkinson's disease, with recent-onset patients manifesting relatively few somatic features and neither vegetative signs nor cognitive impairment. Long-duration patients with depression often show marked somatic features and both vegetative signs and cognitive impairments.

Biochemically, the cerebrolspinal fluid (CSF) of Parkinson's disease depressives has been reported to reflect hypofunction of the dopaminergic, serotonergic, adrenergic, and cholinergic systems, and all those neurotransmitters have been implicated in the cause of the mood syn-

TABLE 2.5-4
Hyperkinetic Subsyndromes

Subsyndrome	Clinical Characteristics	Speed*	Areas of Distribution	Associated Disease States
Dystonia	Sustained postures produced by continuous muscular tension; it can be spasmodic and give the appearance of being almost rhythmic in quality; the postures are generally maintained for at least 30 seconds but can become permanent if ankylosis or contractures supervene	0–1	The entire musculature with the exception of the sphincters may be affected; torticollis, anterocollis, retrocollis, blepharospasm, jaw opening or closure, tongue protrusion, lordosis, opisthotonos, hyperpronated forearm with extended elbow, flexed wrist and extended fingers, and inversion of the foot are among the common presentations	Idiopathic torsion dystonia (dystonia musculorum deformans), Wilson's disease, G_{M1} and G_{M2} gangliosidosis, Lesch/Nyhan syndrome, homocystinuria, glutaric acidemia, metachromatic leukodystrophy, methylmalonic acidemia, Hartnup disease, triosephosphate isomerase deficiency, Leigh's disease, Hallervorden-Spatz disease, neuronal ceroid lipofuscinosis, dystonic lipidosis, calcification of the basal ganglia, ataxia telangiectasia, chorea-acanthocytosis, Pelizaeus-Merzbacher disease, Huntington's disease secondary to brain injury, infection, or toxic insult, corticobasal ganglionic degeneration, dystonic amyotrophy, dystonia with neural deafness, myoclonic dystonia with nasal malformation, psychogenic, malingering
Chorea	Excessive spontaneous movements, irregularly timed, generally nonrepetitive, randomly distributed, and slow to abrupt in character	1–2	All voluntary muscles can be affected, but the face (especially the lips, jaw, and tongue) and the upper extremities are most commonly involved; in severe syndromes, the legs, back, muscles of respiration, and pelvic muscles may be involved	Huntington's disease, benign hereditary chorea, senile chorea, Wilson's disease, neuroacanthocytosia, tardive dyskinesia, basal ganglia infarct, Tourette's disorder, olivopontocerebellar atrophy secondary to medications (e.g., stimulants, antiparkinsonian agents, anticonvulsants, steroids, antihistamines), numerous metabolic disturbances, systemic lupus erythematosus, renal failure, postrheumatic chorea, and many of the hereditary diseases described under both the hypokinetic syndrome and dystonia
Ballismus	Violent, large-amplitude flinging movements of the extremities caused by contractions of the proximal limb musculature; it is virtually inseparable from chorea except that it tends to be more violent and involve the proximal musculature more extensively	1–3	The upper and lower extremities can both be affected, and the syndrome is usually unilateral (i.e., hemiballismus); in some cases the leg is affected more than the arm, but in others the opposite is true	Multiple sclerosis, cerebral trauma, levodopa-induced, oral contraceptives, exogenous estrogens, phenytoin intoxication, hyperglycemia, tuberculous meningitis, subthalamic nucleus cyst, ischemic or hemorrhagic insult of subthalamic nucleus, arteriovenous malformation, metastatic tumor
Tics	Involuntary, repetitive purposeless, usually rapid movements involving one or more muscle groups; they are transiently suppressible, preceded by a rising sense of tension that is relieved by the tic, and may be motor or phonic	2–8	Virtually all areas of the body, including the sphincters, can be affected; motor tics range from simple eye blinking, neck streching, and fist clenching to skipping, finger cracking, and echopraxia; phonic tics can be as simple as sniffing or throat clearing or as complex as panting or coprolalia	Simple tics of childhood, chronic simple or multiple motor tics, adult-onset or senile tic, Tourette's disorder, postencephalitic chorea, postrheumatic chorea, head injury, CO poisoning, cerebrovascular diseases, neuroacanthocytosis, drugs (e.g., stimulants, antiparkinsonian agents, anticonvulsants, antipsychotics [tardive Tourette's disorder]), mental retardation syndromes
Myoclonus	Brief, asynchronous, shocklike muscular jerks; most myoclonus is of the positive type that is due to inappropriate muscular contractions, but many patients also manifest lapses in posture—negative myoclonus	7–12	Any area of the body may be affected; the myoclonic jerks may occur in only one area or region (focal or segmental) or may involve multiple areas (multifocal); in extreme cases the entire musculature can be affected	Physiological (e.g., hypnic jerks, hiccough, benign infantile myoclonus while feeding), essential myoclonus (hereditary, sporadic, myoclonic ocular jerks), epileptic myoclonus (fragments of epilepsy, childhood myoclonic epilepsies, benign familial myoclonic epilepsy, Baltic myoclonus), Lafora body disease, lipidoses, ceroid lipofuscinosis, sialidosis, Ramsay Hunt's syndrome, Friedreich's ataxia, ataxia telangiectasia, Wilson's disease, idiopathic torsion dystonia, Hallervorden-Spatz disease, progressive supranuclear palsy, Huntington's disease, Parkinson's disease, corticobasal ganglionic degeneration, Creutzfeldt-Jakob disease, Alzheimer's disease, viral encephalopathies, hepatic failure, renal failure, hyponatremia, hypoglycemia, hyperglycemia, heavy metal poisoning, levodopa toxicity, tricyclic antidepressants, poststroke

*Cycles per second.

drome. Dopaminergic and serotonergic abnormalities have been the most consistently demonstrable. The neurodestructive process that devastates the dopamine neurons in the nigra and accounts for the motoric manifestations of Parkinson's disease may also affect the ascending serotonergic neurons originating in the dorsal raphe. Alternatively, destruction of the ascending mesocortical dopamine neurons (projecting from the ventral tegmental area to the orbital frontal and prefrontal cortex) may cause metabolic hypofrontality and secondary serotonergic dysfunction by disrupting the descending cortical projections to the dorsal raphe. The report that monoamine oxidase inhibitors are able to restore CSF serotonin but not dopamine to normal levels supports the suggestions that the dopamine deficit is structural and that the serotonin abnormality is secondary. The cerebral metabolism, as reflected by 2-(F^{18})-fluoro-2-deoxy-D-glucose (FDG) positron emission tomography (PET), of parkinsonism depressives reveals relative hypofunction of the inferior and orbital areas of the frontal lobes as compared with nondepressed Parkinson's disease patients.

NEUROPSYCHOLOGICAL DEFICITS Although Parkinson's original paper on shaking palsy reported that the disease was unassociated with intellectual dysfunction, an estimated 10 to 70 percent (average 30 percent) of patients manifest dementia at some point in their illness. Since only 10 percent of the non-parkinsonism population over 65 have dementia, Parkinson's disease carries a significantly increased risk of cognitive decline. The most consistently reported abnormalities on the neuropsychological tests not dependent on motor performance are on memory recall (but not recognition) and frontal systems tasks (that is, cognitive flexibility, acquisition of novel skills, selective screening of competing stimuli). In addition, *bradyphrenia,* slowed mentation, has been described. Language and visuospatial skills are relatively spared.

The conjectured cause of the cognitive decline has included enhanced concordance of Alzheimer's dementia, loss of cholinergic fibers from the nucleus basalis of Meynert, and disturbed frontal-subcortical circuits in the syndrome of subcortical dementia. The loss of norepinephrine neurons from the locus ceruleus, the toxicity of antiparkinsonism medications—particularly the anticholinergic agents—and hypofunction of the prefrontal cortex secondary to deficiency of ascending dopamine fibers may contribute to the intellectual deficiencies. The correlation between the degree of intellectual impairment and the severity of the motor dysfunction seen in many patients indirectly implicates dopamine deficiency as the common factor. Like depression, Parkinson's disease may have its intellectual impairment mediated through the disruption of the ascending mesocortical dopamine fibers resulting in prefrontal cortical hypofunction. Supporting that hypothesis is the observation that the virtually pure dopamine deficiency of MPTP-induced parkinsonism results in impairments of both frontal systems tasks and visuospatial abilities.

MISCELLANEOUS PSYCHIATRIC DISTURBANCES Some authors have said that the long-term effects of the neurological compromise in Parkinson's disease lead to a personality pattern that is progressively passive, dependent, and constricted. Early psychodynamically oriented observers even reported that certain personality styles were predisposed to Parkinson's disease. Such conceptual links between Parkinson's disease and personality function are now largely passé. However, the hypofrontality seen in some Parkinson's disease patients could possibly result in a neurologically based apathetic behavioral syndrome (amotivation, impaired initiative, flattened affect). Anxiety is common in parkinsonism both in association with depression and in nondepressed patients.

In patients with postencephalitic parkinsonism (late sequelae to encephalitis lethargica, also called von Economo's disease and epidemic encephalitis), compulsive thinking, writing, and use of words; paroxysmal paranoia, agitation, restlessness, and somatic sensations; and chronic fatigue states have been described. Those symptoms are rare in idiopathic Parkinson's disease.

Pathology Severe neuronal loss in the zona compacta of the substantia nigra, other pigmented nuclei of the brainstem, the globus pallidus, and the substantia innominata is noted in the brains of Parkinson's disease patients at autopsy. Gliosis and intracytoplasmic inclusions (Lewy bodies) are also observed. Those latter structures are acidophilic spherical inclusions with an amorphous dense core from which filaments radiate. Although not pathognomonic for Parkinson's disease, they are characteristic.

Neurochemically, the most profound abnormality is found in the nigrostriatal dopaminergic system. The dopamine metabolites homovanillic acid and dihydroxyphenylacetic acid and the activity of the enzyme tyrosine hydroxylase are all profoundly (that is, more than 70 percent) decreased in the striatum, and those changes are more pronounced in the putamen than in the caudate nuclei. Those chemical alterations parallel the motor dysfunction in life and the nerve cell loss noted at autopsy.

Other dopamine neurons (for example, mesolimbic, mesocortical) are also affected, although to a more variable degree than is the nigrostriatal system. Additional neurotransmission systems—serotonergic, noradrenergic, cholinergic, γ-aminobutyric acid (GABA)-ergic, and neuropeptide—have all had functional or structural abnormalities described. Of those secondary systems, the dorsal noradrenergic is the most consistently abnormal; its clinical expression remains unclear.

COURSE AND PROGNOSIS The course of idiopathic Parkinson's disease is progressive but at widely variable rates. In some cases the progression is so rapid that death from intercurrent infection or asphyxiation follows within a few years of diagnosis. At the other extreme, several decades may elapse before functional activities show a significant decline. Current pharmacological treatments have extended life expectancy, and the average patient now survives 15 to 20 years after diagnosis.

TREATMENT The recognition of the loss of pigmented neurons in the nigra and the reduction of dopamine concentration in the striatum of Parkinson's disease patients led to trials of levodopa replacement therapy. Dopamine itself could not be used because the molecule is highly lipophobic (that is, hydrophilic) and does not cross the blood-brain barrier. Levodopa (a dopamine precursor), however, is lipophilic and is readily taken up by brain tissue, where it is enzymatically decarboxylated by the presynaptic neuron to dopamine (Figure 2.5-1). Because 95 to 99 percent of orally ingested dopa is converted to dopamine outside the central nervous system, peripheral decarboxylation must be blocked with the concomitant use of a hydrophilic decarboxylase inhibitor (for example, carbidopa or benserazide). Combinations of levodopa and peripheral decarboxylase inhibitors (for example, Sinemet) have been remarkably successful at remediating the protean motoric manifestations of Parkinson's disease, particularly bradykinesia and rigidity.

Dopamine replacement is not a cure for Parkinson's disease; it does nothing to alter the disease's rate of progression. It is, however, an effective palliative strategy and extends life by 5 to 10 years. Levodopa requires an intact presynaptic neuron (the ones destroyed in Parkinson's disease) to be decarboxylated to dopamine (Figure 2.5-1). Agents that act directly on the postsynaptic D_2 receptor, the subtype of dopamine receptor in the striatum that modulates motor behavior, could theoretically remain effective after the efficacy of dopamine replacement wanes. Bromocriptine (Parlodel) is such an agonist, and its long duration of action makes it particularly useful in some patients. However, bromocriptine apparently requires a partially functioning presynaptic neuron for in vivo efficacy, and it works best when used in combination with levodopa preparations. Because stimulation of the D_1 receptor augments the response of simultaneous stimulation at the D_2 receptor, nearly pure D_2 agonists, like bromocriptine, could conceivably require some endogenous activity at the D_1 site to be maximally effective (Figure 2.5-1). Pergolide (Permax) and lisuride are more potent and longer-acting D_2 agonists than is bromocriptine. Although neither requires the presence of the presynaptic neuron for activity, they have not been clearly shown to be superior to

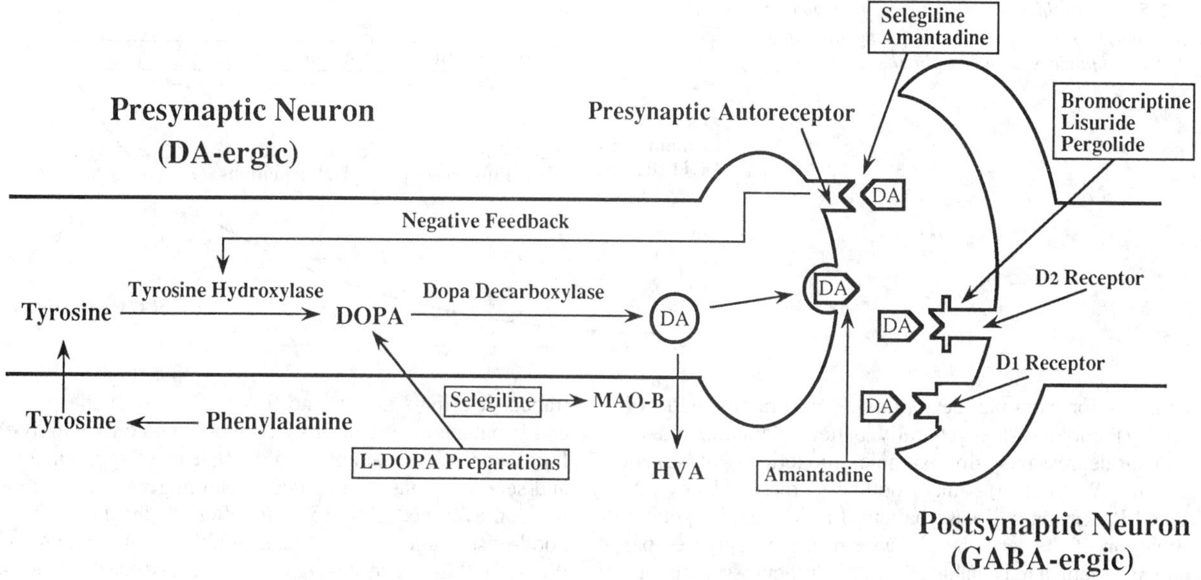

FIGURE 2.5-1 *Schematic of the intrastriatal neuronal connection between the dopaminergic presynaptic neuron, whose cell body is in the zona compacta region of the nigra, and the GABA-ergic postsynaptic neuron. The putative sites of action of the various antiparkinsonian agents are depicted.*

bromocriptine. Combined administration of carbidopa-levodopa and a dopamin-receptor agonist reduces the late consequences of long-term carbidopa-levodopa therapy, such as the on-off phenomenon.

Amantadine (Symmetrel) is a weak dopamine-agonist that works by enhancing presynaptic dopamine release and by blocking its reuptake (Figure 2.5-1). It is somewhat useful in early Parkinson's disease and may be of benefit in smoothing the motoric fluctuations that occur later with levodopa treatment. Anticholinergic agents—for example, benztropine mesylate (Cogentin), trihexyphenidyl hydrochloride (Artane), and biperiden hydrochloride (Akineton)—are also of some usefulness in early Parkinson's disease and putatively have a selective effect on resting tremor. Elderly patients and patients with dementia are particularly prone to the adverse side effects of anticholinergic agents.

Selegiline (Eldepryl) (L-deprenyl) is an irreversible and selective inhibitor of monoamine oxidase B (MAO-B) and also acts as a dopamine reuptake inhibitor. It is lipophilic, penetrates quickly into tissues, is highly (94 percent) protein-bound, reaches maximal concentrations about one hour (range 0.5 to 2 hours), is metabolized predominantly by the hepatic microsomal cytochrome P-450 system, and has a plasma half-life of about 40 hours. It effectively (more than 90 percent) inhibits platelet MAO-B at daily dosages of 10 mg and, because of its irreversible activity, maintains that inhibition for three to five days after drug discontinuation. At daily dosages of less than 20 mg, it does not cause the tyramine-induced hypertensive crises, the so-called cheese reactions, that are associated with nonselective or A-type MAO inhibitors; thus, no dietary restrictions are necessary. Although it has little short-term antiparkinsonism effect, it appears to slow the progression of the disease, possibly by slowing the elaboration of neurodestructive free radicals or by preventing the oxidative conversion of unidentified exogenous or endogenous molecules to highly neurotoxic compounds. Polypharmacy is common in Parkinson's disease. Early in their course, patients are usually treated with selegiline and carbidopa-levodopa; later they may require a complex combination of selegiline, carbidopa-levodopa, bromocriptine or pergolide, and amantadine.

Psychiatric effects of pharmacotherapy Dopamine-augmenting strategies commonly result in behavioral toxicities that limit their dose-tolerated and functional efficacy. In general, those effects are dose-related and progress in more or less predictable order (Figure 2.5-2). At first, insomnia with vivid dreams develops and is followed by visual misperceptions, nonthreatening visual hallucinations, and agitation with paranoid ideations. Auditory phenomena are infrequently reported, and patients adapt quickly to the visual illusions and hallucinations and are largely undisturbed by them. Exceptions to the progression rule occur, and confusion (that is, delirium) can develop at any time, especially if concomitant anticholinergics are used.

Treatment of behavioral syndromes Accurate phenomenological identification of the behavioral perturbation in Parkinson's disease patients is of critical importance. Patients who are described by their families as acting withdrawn, disinterested, and needing help with the activities of daily living may have experienced motoric worsening, a delirium from adjunctive anticholinergic medications, an intercurrent depression, or cognitive decline. Appropriate intervention depends entirely on the inferred cause of the behavioral change.

When it is of functionally handicapping severity, parkinsonism-associated depression should be treated with antidepressant medications or electroconvulsive therapy (ECT). The Parkinson's disease patient has altered sympathetic tone and an impaired righting reflex and is particularly prone to orthostatic hypotension and falls. Thus, the α-adrenergic-blocking properties of the antidepressants are especially troublesome. All tertiary amine tricyclic antidepressants—for example, doxepin (Adapin), amitriptyline (Elavil), and imipramine (Tofranil)—and the nonselective MAOIs—for example, tranylcypromine (Parnate), phenelzine (Nardil), isocarboxazid (Marplan)—have troublesome side-effect profiles in that population. The second-

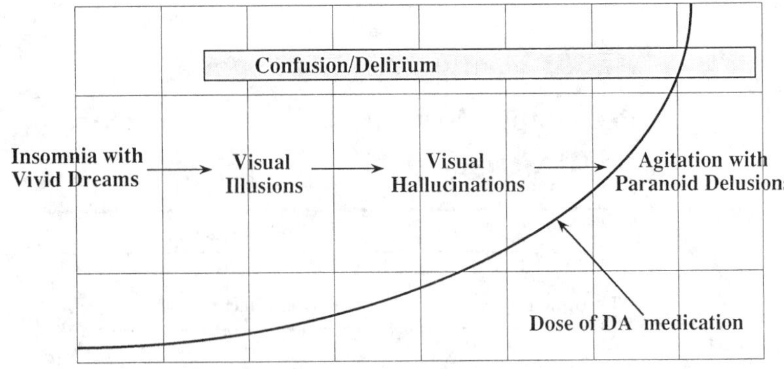

FIGURE 2.5-2 *Graphical relation between the amount of dopaminergic replacement therapy and the emergence of psychiatric side effects in the treatment of Parkinson's disease.*

ary amines—for example, desipramine (Norpramin) and nortriptyline (Pamelor)—are generally better tolerated, and the atypical antidepressants—for example, fluoxetine (Prozac) and bupropion (Wellbutrin)—may be best tolerated by the depressed Parkinson's disease patient. In view of the putative hypofunction of the serotonergic system in the depressed parkinsonism patient, a reasonable choice of antidepressant therapy is a selective inhibitor of serotonin reuptake (for example, fluoxetine or fluvoxamine). Lithium (Eskalith) has also been used with limited success in Parkinson's disease patients prone to recurrent depressions. Depressed patients intolerant of or unresponsive to pharmacotherapy are candidates for ECT. The motor symptoms, as well as the mood disorder, may improve with ECT; the motor response is usually transient.

Pharmacotherapy has been of distinctly limited usefulness in the cognitively impaired Parkinson's disease patient. Although theory has implicated (among other things) hypofunction of the extrastriatal dopamine systems in the cause of the dementing syndrome in parkinsonism, dopamine replacement does not convincingly improve cognitive performance. In fact, excessive dopamine replacement can cause a confusional syndrome that enhances the deficits. At present, the best pharmacological approach is to optimize the antiparkinsonism regimen and to avoid all medications that could potentially aggravate the cognitive deficits (for example, anticholinergics).

The psychotic disturbances that occasionally result from dopamine replacement therapy present a classic therapeutic dilemma. Attempts to decrease the dopamine replacement will worsen the motor symptoms, as will adjunctive antipsychotic agents. In some cases the clinician can adjust the dopamine-replacement regimen to provide acceptable motor function and avoid intolerable paranoia and hallucinosis. At other times, however, no such window of therapeutic opportunity exists. In those cases, adjunctive antipsychotic treatment must usually be instituted. The low-potency antipsychotics—for example, thioridazine (Mellaril)—have traditionally been used because of their low extrapyramidal syndrome liability, but concomitant α-adrenergic blockade may result in unacceptable cardiovascular effects. The atypical antipsychotic agent clozapine (Clozaril) has been used in those patients with encouraging results. It and its pharmacological successors—for example, risperidone (Risperdal) and sertindole—may be the treatment of first choice in those pharmacologically challenging patients.

HUNTINGTON'S DISEASE

ETIOLOGY AND EPIDEMIOLOGY Huntington's disease is a genetically transmitted disease that invariably follows an autosomal dominant type of heritability with 100 percent penetrance. It afflicts about 2 to 9 per 100,000 of the population, and spontaneous mutations have not been convincingly found. It has a peak onset at about 35 to 40 years of age, but childhood and senescent-onset cases occur. Huntington's disease patients live, on average, 13 to 15 years after the diagnosis, but childhood-onset patients usually succumb to complications of their illness within six to seven years. The disorder has no gender bias, but offspring whose fathers were affected are at greater than usual risk for the rigid-akinetic variant of the illness in childhood.

The gene responsible for Huntington's disease has been localized to the distal portion of the short arm of chromosome 4 by intensive linkage analyses. The mutant gene itself has recently been identified and is a variably repeated and unstable trinucleotide (CAG) sequence. This trinucleotide is repeated on the normal chromosome 11 to 34 times, but is repeated 37 to 86 times on the mutant chromosome. When the mutant gene is transmitted by the father, there is a tendency for the affected offspring to have an even longer redundant sequence. It is thought that this accounts for the clinical observation of paternal transmission resulting in a more malignant course of disease.

CLINICAL FEATURES

Neurological features Adult-onset Huntington's disease is often heralded by the development of random fidgeting. It progresses to clinically identifiable chorea over a period of years. Before the chorea is convincingly manifested, the movements of the patient may appear eccentric, manneristic, and excessive but look pathological only in retrospect. Fully developed chorea consists of excessive spontaneous movements that are irregularly timed, generally nonrepetitive, randomly distributed, and slow to abrupt in character. The chorea is usually first apparent in the face and the upper extremities but generally progresses to involve all the extremities, the trunk, and the muscles of articulation and deglutition. The chorea is exacerbated during action of the involved body part (for example, walking) and is suppressible to only a modest extent by patient effort. Gait disturbances, eye movement abnormalities, dysarthria, and dysphagia are virtually universal in the fully developed syndrome. The dysphagia involves all aspects of food intake and contributes greatly to choking and aspiration pneumonia, the proximal cause of death in many Huntington's disease patients. The differential diagnosis of chorea is given in Table 2.5-4.

About 10 percent (range 6 to 16 percent) of patients have onset before the age of 20, with less than 1 percent manifesting the disease before age 10. This juvenile-onset group have a more malignant course, and about 75 percent (range 60 to 85 percent) have an akinetic-rigid form of the illness (Westphal variant). In addition, the childhood-onset form has a high prevalence of generalized seizures (about 35 percent) and a rapidly progressive dementia. The course typically begins with behavioral disturbances, school difficulties, and mild chorea that is rapidly succeeded by parkinsonism, cognitive decline, dysarthria, and seizures. About 6 percent of adult-onset patients have the Westphal variant.

Neuropsychiatric features

DEPRESSION Between 30 and 40 percent of Huntington's disease patients have major mood disturbances, about 25 percent attempt suicide, and approximately 6 percent die by their own hands (about four times the rate in the general population). The bulk of the suicide attempts and completions occur early in the course of the illness. Depression is the most frequent mood disorder, and it commonly reaches delusional intensity, with psychomotor retardation and pathological guilt predominating. Depression may be evident several years before overt movement abnormalities are apparent. The depressive episodes can last from weeks to years and are responsive to conventional antidepressant medications.

A small fraction of patients with mood disturbances have manic episodes marked by psychomotor hyperactivity, flight of ideas, insomnia, and grandiose delusions that are indistinguishable from idiopathic bipolar disorder. The episodes usually last only weeks and are generally terminated with a return to the depressive state. They are thought to be only partially responsive to the usual thymoleptic agents, such as lithium and carbamazepine (Tegretol), and are usually treated with antipsychotic medications.

PSYCHOTIC STATES Although 10 to 30 percent of Huntington's disease patients are reported to have schizophreniclike disturbances, their psychotic syndromes are marked almost exclusively by positive psychotic experiences, especially delusions and a variety of hallucinatory experiences. Like the mood disturbance, the psychotic syndrome may develop before any demonstrable neurological changes. It usually begins with a vague but growing sense that the world has changed, with common events taking on bizarre, supernatural, or otherworldly importance. Those altered beliefs have been called delusional mood, and they tend to consume the mental life of the patient. Succeeding that modified view of reality are a series of ill-defined delusions of control, influence, persecution, or grandiosity. Patients may report, for example, that they are the targets of study by beings from another world or that family members are trying to control their thoughts. Hallucinations generally occur at that point; although they are usually auditory, they can be either visual or tactile.

Those psychotic states can last for several months and can occasionally present precipitously. They respond somewhat to both conventional antipsychotic and antidepressant treatment, but residual symptoms are frequently present.

PERSONALITY CHANGES Huntington's disease patients show two overlapping personality syndromes: apathetic and disinhibited. The apathetic syndrome is marked by slowness, disinterest in usual activities, hygienic neglect, and social avoidance. That syndrome generally accompanies the cognitive decline and is unresponsive to pharmacological interventions that typically remediate the mood disturbance. The disinhibited syndrome consists of irritability, anger outbursts, interpersonal violence, and a markedly labile and reactive mood. It can co-occur with elements of the apathetic syndrome and generally manifests in patients with both cognitive disturbance and mood disorder.

NEUROPSYCHOLOGICAL DEFICITS Relentless decline in intellectual functioning is a virtually universal finding in Huntington's disease. As in the other psychiatric syndromes, cognitive impairment may precede the motor symptoms. The intellectual decline is usually severe only after years of overt neurological abnormality.

The first symptom reported is an inability to think through routine problems with customary efficiency. The subtle meaning of language and the grasp of personal circumstances may be lost, and patients report trouble recalling information effectively. Formal testing at that point usually reveals a disturbance of both verbal and auditory memory, with a relative sparing of language and visuospatial function. The memory disturbance is not a true amnesia but an impaired efficiency of the recall of learned information. Parallel to those deficits is a progressively worsening mental apathy. It begins with disinterest in usual activities, a decline in intellectual curiosity, and diminished physical vitality. As the dementia advances, patients reach the point at which they are nearly mute, akinetic, globally disinterested, unable to recognize family members and friends, and incapable of managing their activities of daily living.

Pathology Grossly, the whole brain is abnormal, with mild to moderate atrophy of the cortex, most marked in the frontal lobes. The corpus striatum is markedly atrophic, with the adjacent lateral ventricles being correspondingly dilated. Smaller degrees of atrophy are seen in the globus pallidus and the thalamus, with the brainstem, the spinal cord, the substantia nigra, and the cerebellum being relatively spared. Microscopically, neuronal loss is apparent in the cortex (particularly layers 3 to 5) and in the caudate nucleus and the putamen, where up to 70 percent of the tissue can be lost. The medium-sized spiny neurons are most affected, with a number of morphological changes in the remaining neurons. Somewhat less neuronal destruction is seen in the ventral striatum (the nucleus accumbens) and the ventral anterior putamen.

Those pathological changes are reflected in life; cerebral computed tomography and magnetic resonance imaging reveal a concavity in the area of the caudate, instead of the usual convex bulging into the lateral ventricle. FDG PET shows hypometabolism in the caudate in Huntington's disease patients, and some investigators have found similar abnormalities in asymptomatic persons at risk for the disease.

Neurochemically, many abnormalities have been reported in brains at autopsy. The GABA-ergic system (the major outflow from the striatum) is most frequently reported to be abnormal, but levels of dopamine, acetylcholine, and the neuropeptides substance P, cholecystokinin, vasoactive intestinal polypeptide, and metenkephalin are also diminished.

COURSE AND PROGNOSIS Like Parkinson's disease, Huntington's disease is a progressive, fatal disease. It has less variability of course than does Parkinson's disease, with few patients surviving more than 20 years after the onset. Childhood-onset patients rarely survive more than 10 years. Currently available treatments have done little to affect the time to death, which is usually caused by complications of aspirations or infections that result from the patient's bed-bound status in the terminal phase of the disease.

TREATMENT Pharmacotherapy has only a modest effect in Huntington's disease. Antidopamine agents (that is, antipsychotics) are useful early in the course to reduce the chorea. High-potency antipsychotics are usually preferred—for example, haloperidol (Haldol), pimozide (Orap), fluphenazine (Prolixin)—but all types have been used. In addition to decreasing the chorea, those agents are partially useful in attenuating the irritability, paranoia, hallucinations, violent tendencies, and bizarre behaviors that sometimes accompany the disease. Anticholinergics usually exacerbate the cognitive impairments and worsen both the chorea and the dysphagia. GABA replacement strategies have been largely ineffective, as have cholinergic augmentation. The antidepressants are useful in those patients with mood disturbances and occasionally as an adjunct to antipsychotics in those patients with psychotic symptoms.

TOURETTE'S DISORDER

ETIOLOGY AND EPIDEMIOLOGY Tourette's disorder (also known as Gilles de la Tourette's syndrome) has a lifetime prevalence somewhere between 10 and 100 per 100,000 of the population. Males are afflicted more often than females, and the syndrome tends to run in families. The exact mode of inheritance is unknown, but it is most likely a type of autosomal dominant, sex-influenced, partially penetrant trait. In addition, the phenotypic heterogeneity may indicate genotypic variability. In pedigrees with abundant Tourette's disorder, obsessive-compulsive disorder and chronic motor tics are also overrepresented, giving rise to speculations that those syndromes share either closely linked heritability or a similar neuropathological substrate.

CLINICAL FEATURES

Neurological features Tourette's disorder begins in childhood or adolescence (average age 7), with simple or complex motor tics (Table 2.5-4). Those repetitive, brief, stereotyped, purposeless movements can be suppressed for varying lengths of time, are exacerbated by stress, and are lessened by relaxation and concentration. The face, the head, and the neck are most frequently involved, but the upper and lower extremities and the trunk can be affected. Patients may also show compulsive touching, self-injurious behavior, and occasionally echopraxia. The severity of the tics waxes and wanes over time, and the form of the tic may change over weeks to months (for example, eye blinking may give way to a repetitive shoulder lift). The variability becomes less pronounced in adulthood, when stable manifestations develop.

In some patients the tics seem to be dystonic or choreic in appearance (Table 2.5-4). Tics are distinct from the other two hyperkinetic syndromes in that Tourette's disorder patients describe a rising tension as the urge to tic mounts; the tension is relieved after the tic is completed. Electroencephalographically (EEG), the tics are not preceded by the premovement potential that immediately antedates volitional movements, including mimicking the tic movement. The differential diagnosis of tics is presented in Table 2.5-4.

Tourette's disorder patients also have vocal tics (Table 2.5-4) during some part of their illness. Coprolalia (the involuntary utterance of obscenities) is the most notorious of the vocal tics, but only about 50 percent of Tourette's disorder patients ever manifest it. Common vocal tics are throat clearing, grunting, and sniffing. Occasionally (15 percent), a patient presents with only vocal tics; the motor tics appear later.

In addition, Tourette's disorder patients commonly report a number of sleep disturbances, including somnambulism, frequent awakenings, and enuresis. They also have a number of soft neurological signs, excessive left-handedness, and minor EEG abnormalities. The EEG abnormalities have not been found by all investigators, and their significance in certain Tourette's disorder patients remains obscure.

Neuropsychiatric features No progressive intellectual decline is seen in Tourette's disorder. The other psychiatric concomitants have a long and still contentious history. Some reports have concluded that Tourette's disorder patients show no excessive psychopathology or cognitive impairments; other reports describe a vast array of neuropsychopathological syndromes. Included in the list are obsessive-compulsive disorder, mood disorders, attention-deficit/hyperactivity disorder, anxiety disorders, self-mutilating behavior, learning disabilities, psychotic disorders, paranoia, inappropriate sexual activity, and impulsive, aggressive, and antisocial behaviors. The exact meaning of the reported co-occurrences is unclear.

OBSESSIVE-COMPULSIVE BEHAVIOR The tic itself is reminiscent of the obsessions and the resultant rituals of obsessive-compulsive disorder. Preceding the ritual, the tic counterpart, a rising sense of tension and anxiety is relieved by the stereotyped ritualistic behavior. Like the tic, the ritual can be suppressed for a time but at a cost of escalating tension and anxiety. Behaviors similar to those seen in obsessive-compulsive disorder have been reported in 10 to nearly 90 percent of Tourette's disorder patients (average about 50 percent). The behaviors are reported in the absence of any alterations in mood. Typical examples of behaviors are checking rituals, smelling objects, avoiding certain items, repetitive rituals, excessive hand washing, arithmomania, and obsessions of doing harm to others. Furthermore, patients with severe Tourette's disorder have the most behaviors seen in obsessive-compulsive disorder. Those behaviors usually respond to serotonergic agents, behavioral therapy, or, in the most extreme cases, psychosurgery. They do not remit, as the tics do, with antipsychotic therapy.

AGGRESSIVE BEHAVIOR As in the obsessive-compulsive disorder symptoms, the co-occurrence of aggressive behavior, either toward self or others, increases with the severity of Tourette's disorder. The reported prevalence of the behaviors ranges from 5 to 50 percent. The acts of self-directed violence include compulsively picking at sores, lip biting, tongue biting, repeated eye damage (sometimes resulting in blindness), punching the body, and tooth extraction. Other-directed violence, including punching and touching others, is thought to be associated with the symptoms of forced touching and coprolalia and occasionally responds to antipsychotics or serotonergic agents.

Hyperactivity About 50 percent of children with Tourette's disorder evidence hyperactivity. Treatment with stimulants frequently exacerbates the tics and may lead to the initial recognition of the disorder.

Pathology No neuropathological abnormalities have been identified in Tourette's disorder, although the number of autopsy studies is small. Neurochemically, the most frequently reported abnormality is a decrease in dopamine turnover, as shown by low levels of CSF homovanillic acid. That finding has been interpreted to mean that Tourette's disorder patients have dopamine-receptor supersensitivity. The decrease in homovanillic acid is thought to be secondary to enhanced negative feedback from the supersensitive presynaptic autoreceptor, and the palliative effect of antipsychotics on the tics is hypothesized to be due to the blockade of an abnormally sensitive postsynaptic D_2 receptor (Figure 2.5-1). In vivo studies of dopamine-receptor sensitivities, using C^{11}-labeled 3-N-methylspiperone (a D_2-specific ligand) PET scans, have not shown any abnormalities in Tourette's disorder patients. In support of dopamine supersensitivity is the fact that 70 percent of Tourette's disorder patients have a decrease in tics with the high-potency antipsychotics, such as haloperidol and pimozide. Furthermore, dopamine-stimulating agents like methylphenidate (Ritalin), cocaine, and amphetamine generally exacerbate tics, and a tardive form of Tourette's disorder has been described after the long-term use of dopamine-blocking drugs. Serotonin and acetylcholine have also been implicated in the pathophysiology of Tourette's disorder, but pharmacological attempts to manipulate those systems have been largely unsuccessful. Because of the partial efficacy of the antiadrenergic agent clonidine (Catapres), that neurotransmission system has also been implicated. No convincing evidence for adrenergic hyperfunction has been uncovered.

COURSE AND PROGNOSIS Although Tourette's disorder is a lifelong illness, its manifestations vary in both form and severity over time. Spontaneous remissions occur in about 10 percent of patients but rarely last more than one year. The disease is not progressive but usually becomes constant in adulthood.

TREATMENT Not all cases require pharmacological intervention; antipsychotics are the mainstay of suppressive treatment of the tics seen in Tourette's disorder. The drugs neither cure nor influence the course of the disease, but they are effective in suppressing the manifestations in about 70 percent of those afflicted. Likewise, dopamine-depleting agents like reserpine (Serpasil) and tetrabenazine have shown some ability to suppress tics. Those drugs carry the same liability for the development of extrapyramidal side effects for the Tourette's disorder patient as they do for the psychotic patient. In fact, tentative evidence indicates that Tourette's disorder patients may be more sensitive than are psychotic patients.

Clonidine has also been used and is somewhat effective at suppressing tics and attenuating obsessive-compulsive behavior. Its effects may wane after a few months. Clomipramine (Anafranil) and fluoxetine successfully ameliorate obsessive-compulsive behavior in some Tourette's disorder patients. A panoply of additional compounds have been tried with limited or mixed results. The compounds include antidepressants, anxiolytics, lithium, anticonvulsants, corticosteroids, antihistamines, and megavitamins.

SUGGESTED CROSS-REFERENCES

Neuroimaging is discussed in Sections 1.10, 2.10, and 49.5c. Cognitive disorders are discussed in Chapter 12, mood disorders in Chapter 16, obsessive-compulsive disorder in Section 17.3, attention-deficit/hyperactivity disorder in Chapter 38, tic disorders in Chapter 41, and dementing disorders in the elderly in Section 49.6a. Psychotherapies are discussed in Chapter 31 and biological therapies in Chapter 32.

REFERENCES

Agid Y, Ruberg, M, Dubois B, Javoy-Agid F: Biochemical substrates of mental disturbances in Parkinson's disease. Adv Neurol *40:* 211, 1984.

Bates G P, MacDonald M E, Baxendale S, Youngman S, Lin C, Whaley W L, Wasmuth J J, Gusella J F, Lehrach H: Defined physical limits of the Huntington disease gene candidate region. Am J Hum Genet *49:* 7, 1991.

Baxter L R Jr, Schwartz J M, Bergman K S, Szuba M P, Guze B H, Mozziotta J C, Alazraki A, Selin C E, Munford P: Caudate glucose metabolic rate changes with both drug and behavior therapy for obsessive compulsive disorder. Arch Gen Psychiatry *49:* 681, 1992.

Comings D E, Comings B G: A controlled study of Tourette syndrome: IV. Obsessions, compulsions, and schizoid behaviors. Am J Hum Genet *41:* 782, 1987.

Comings D E, Comings B G: Tourette syndrome: Clinical and psychological aspects of 250 cases. Am J Hum Genet *37:* 435, 1985.

Cummings J L: Behavioral complications of drug treatment of Parkinson's disease. J Am Geriatr Soc *39:* 708, 1991.

Cummings J L: Depression and Parkinson's disease. A review. Am J Psychiatry *149:* 443, 1992.

Denny-Brown D: *Diseases of the Basal Ganglia and Subthalamic Nucleus.* Oxford University Press, New York, 1946.

Farrer L A. Suicide and attempted suicide in Huntington's disease: Implications for preclinical testing of persons at risk. Am J Med Genet *24:* 305, 1986.

*Gilles de la Tourette G: Étude sur une affection nerveuse caracterisée par le l'incoordination motrice accompagnée del'echolalie et de copralalie. Arch Neurol *9:* 19, 158, 1885.

Gusella J F, MacDonald M E, Ambrose C M, Duyao M P: Molecular genetics of Huntington's disease. Arch Neurol *50:* 1157, 1993.

Hakim A M, Mathieson G: Dementia in Parkinson's disease: A neuropathologic study. Neurology *29:* 1209, 1979.

*Huntington G: *On Chorea.* Lea & Blanchard, Philadelphia, 1872.

*Lees A J, Smith E: Cognitive deficits in the early stages of PD. Brain *106:* 257, 1983.

Marsh G G, Markham C H: Does levodopa alter depression and psychopathology in Parkinsonian patients? J Neurol Neurosurg Psychiatry *36:* 925, 1973.

Mayeux R, Stern Y, Rosen J, Leventhal J: Depression, intellectual impairment, and Parkinson disease. Neurology *31:* 645, 1981.

Mazziotta J C, Phelps M E, Pahl J J, Huang S-C, Baxter L R, Riege W H, Hoffman J M, Kuhl D E, Lanto A B, Wapenski J A, Markham C H: Reduced cerebral glucose metabolism in asymptomatic subjects at risk for Huntington's disease. N Engl J Med *316:* 357, 1987.

*Parkinson J: *An Essay on the Shaking Palsy.* Sherwood, Neely, & Jones, London, 1817.

Robertson M M, Trimble M R, Lees A J: Self-injurious behavior and the Gilles de la Tourette syndrome: A clinical study and review of the literature. Psychol Med *19:* 611, 1989.

Shapiro A K, Shapiro E, Wayne H, Clarkin J: Psychopathology of Gilles de la Tourette's syndrome. Am J Psychiatry *129:* 427, 1972.

Tatton W G, Lee R G: Evidence for abnormal long-loop reflexes in parkinsonian patients. Brain Res *100:* 671, 1975.

Taylor A, Saint-Cyr J A, Lang A E: Dementia prevalence in PD. Lancet *1:* 1037, 1985.

Tyler A, Harper P S: Attitudes of subjects at risk and their relatives toward genetics counseling in Huntington's disease. J Med Genet *20:* 179, 1983.

*Weiner W J, Lang A E: *Movement Disorders: A Comprehensive Survey.* Futura, Mount Kisco, NY, 1989.

2.6 NEUROPSYCHIATRIC ASPECTS OF MULTIPLE SCLEROSIS AND OTHER DEMYELINATING DISORDERS

PETER V. RABINS, M.D., M.P.H.
FRANCIS J. McMAHON, M.D.

INTRODUCTION

Myelin is the principal component of the proteinaceous-lipoid sheath surrounding C fibers in the central nervous system (CNS). Myelin is distributed throughout the neuraxis and is primarily responsible for the white matter seen in gross sections of the brain and with imaging techniques, such as T2-weighted magnetic resonance imaging (MRI) scans. The diseases that affect myelin and cause neuropsychiatric symptoms can have genetic, infectious, or autoimmune causes or, like multiple sclerosis, have an as yet undiscovered cause.

The demyelinating disorders account for considerable neurological and cognitive disability and often cause significant psychiatric disability as well. The psychiatric complications are sometimes an understandable or neurotic reaction to the underlying illness. Often, they are specific psychiatric disorders triggered pathophysiologically by the demyelinating disease, and are responsive to the same treatments that are effective for those disorders in the general population.

MULTIPLE SCLEROSIS

Multiple sclerosis (MS), called diffuse sclerosis in Great Britain and *sclerose en plaque* in France, is the most common demyelinating disorder. It was first described clinically by the French neurologist Jean-Martin Charcot more than 100 years ago as a disorder in which neurological symptoms are disseminated in both time and space. That is, the clinical diagnosis required at least two distinct episodes of neurological impairment and evidence on examination or history (and now radiologically) of at least two separate lesions.

MS most commonly begins between ages 20 and 40 and affects women more than men. The course is usually one of exacerbation (active symptoms) followed by remission (partial or complete resolution of the symptoms), although it may become chronically progressive in time. With repeated exacerbations the neurological deficits accumulate. In elderly patients MS may become chronically progressive early in its course. The most common symptoms are presented in Table 2.6-1.

MS becomes more prevalent with increasing distance from the equator. The risk is determined by age 15; persons who move after age 15 are at the same risk as persons residing at the latitude at which they lived before age 15.

Magnetic resonance imaging (MRI) has dramatically altered the diagnostic process. MRI often shows definite demyelinating lesions that have never been clinically manifest; it can show evidence of demyelinating lesions that are disseminated in space (multiple locations in the brain), even when no clinical evidence is available to identify multiple distinct episodes of neurological impairment. MRI findings resembling MS lesions also occur in the general population, and clinical or laboratory confirmation of the diagnosis, in addition to MRI alterations, is necessary.

Pathologically, multiple sclerosis consists of multifocal demyelination. Among the common disorders that should be considered in the differential diagnosis are vascular disease, particularly the vasculitides, meningovascular syphilis, mass lesions, and the neurodegenerative disorders.

No laboratory test is definitive for MS. A lumbar puncture may reveal monocytosis, an elevated percentage of γ-globulin, or an elevated myelin basic protein, especially during an exacerbation. Slowed visual-evoked responses provide objective definite evidence of an abnormality in the visual pathways. Since optic neuritis is a common early symptom of MS but one of which the patient may be unaware, the presence of slowed evoked response and another focal lesion strongly supports the diagnosis. Laboratory tests should be used together with the clinical and radiological findings in making a diagnosis.

TABLE 2.6-1
Presenting Symptoms in Multiple Sclerosis

	Patients	
Symptom	**Number (Total 144)**	**Percent***
Paresthesia	53	37
Gait difficulty	50	35
Weakness or incoordination of one or both lower extremities	25	17
Visual loss (retrobulbar neuritis)	22	15
Weakness or incoordination of one or both upper extremities	15	10
Diplopia	14	10
Urinary difficulty	9	6
Dysarthria	8	6
Hemiparesis	7	5
Severe fatigue	5	3
Vertigo	4	3
Impotence	4	3
Convulsion	3	2
Severe emotionality	3	2
Lhermitte's sign	2	1
Muscle cramps (legs)	2	1
Fecal incontinence	2	1
Dysphagia	1	<1
Severe movement tremor	1	<1
Hearing loss	1	<1

*Total is more than 100 percent because some patients presented with more than one major symptom.
Table from J W Swanson: Multiple sclersosis: Update in diagnosis and review of prognostic factors. Mayo Clin Proc *64:* 577, 1989. Used with permission.

ETIOLOGY The cause of MS is unknown. The epidemiology and the pathology suggest an immunological-infectious cause, but that is unproved. There is a familial predisposition but no clear genetic diathesis.

Anecdotal evidence has long suggested that stressful life events may precede the onset of MS or precipitate exacerbations. Because the cause of multiple sclerosis is unknown, the theory has remained attractive. A definite answer has been difficult to obtain for several reasons. First, determining when an exacerbation of multiple sclerosis has occurred is sometimes difficult. Symptoms can be worsened by heat or the occurrence of other medical conditions, such as a urinary tract infection, or physiological events, such as pregnancy. Many of the studies have been retrospective and subject to recall bias. Research on life events has shown that stressful events are better remembered by patients who are asked about them or who have a reason to remember. Furthermore, many neurological disorders are known to be more symptomatic during periods of emotional upset. It is sometimes difficult to distinguish between a mild worsening of symptoms related to emotional distress and the development of a mild exacerbation that then leads to emotional distress. Mood and other emotional variables worsen during MS exacerbations. Although retrospective studies find that patients can identify a precipitating stress in one half to three quarters of cases, prospective studies and studies using comparison groups of patients with other neurological illnesses have found no greater frequency of adverse life events in MS patients than in controls.

The difficulty in ascertaining when an exacerbation has occurred suggests that there is no definitive answer to the question at present. A satisfactory answer may require the development of a biological marker for exacerbation.

PSYCHIATRIC ASPECTS In his original clinical description Charcot listed three psychological symptoms as prominent features of MS: (1) "mental depression suggesting classic forms," (2) "stupid indifference," and (3) "foolish laughter without cause." Research over the past 125 years has confirmed a substantial prevalence of those symptom complexes in MS.

Disorders of emotion

DEPRESSION Reported rates of depression in MS patients vary widely, ranging from 20 to 60 percent. To determine if MS carries a specific association with depression, several studies have used medically ill comparison groups to control for the presence of medical illness. Those studies have generally found higher rates of depression in MS patients than in controls. Studies that found similar rates of depression in MS patients and patients with other neurological or medical conditions had sample sizes too small to detect a difference if it existed.

Few studies provide data to distinguish between major depression and adjustment disorder. Most find no relation between the extent of the neurological or functional impairment and depression, arguing against a reactive cause for the depression. Another finding supporting a nonreactive cause is that patients with brain lesions have higher rates of depression than do those with only spinal cord lesions, even though the spinal cord lesion patients are often more disabled than the brain lesion patients (Figure 2.6-1). Complicating the diagnosis of depression in MS are the co-occurrence of emotional lability, emotional incontinence, dementia, and euphoria. Nevertheless, the fact that antidepressant therapy and behavioral treatments improve mood more than does a placebo emplasizes the need to recognize and treat mood disorders.

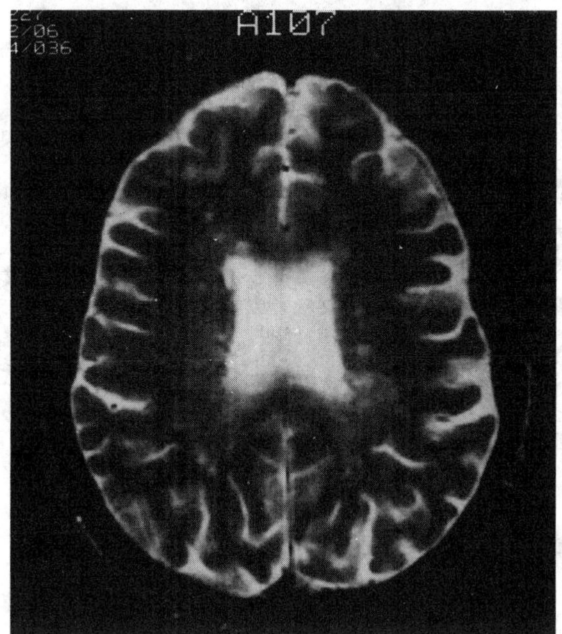

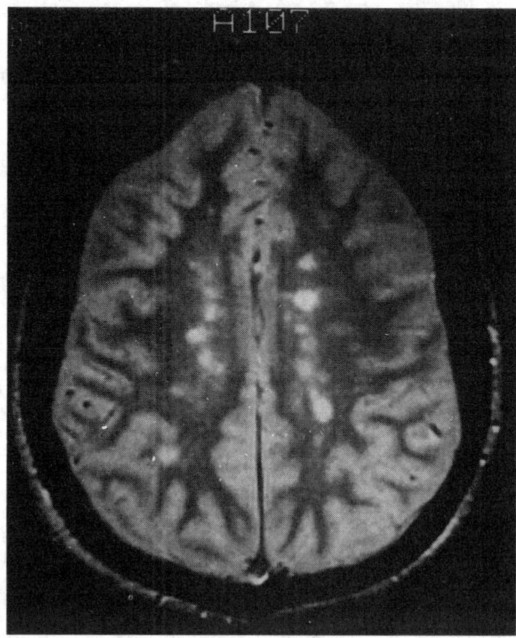

FIGURE 2.6-1 *T1 and T2 weighted-head magnetic resonance imaging (MRI) scan, showing ventricular enlargement and demyelination in a 30-year-old man with a mood disorder and multiple sclerosis (MS).*

EUPHORIA AND MANIA Euphoria is the most controversial psychological symptom in MS. A high prevalence was emphasized by the influential neurologist Samuel A. Kinnier Wilson, and mania is the one symptom often known to practitioners who have little contact with the disease. Investigators have distinguished between *elation,* a truly elevated mood, and *eutonia,* a sense of well-being that appears incongruous with the patient's physical state. The prevalence of eutonia in MS is less than 15 percent. Several pieces of evidence suggest that the lack of concern (sometimes called *la belle indifférence*) of eutonia results from frontal lobe damage or a frontal disconnection syndrome, rather than psychogenic denial or lack of awareness.

Bipolar disorder occurs in MS at rates higher than would be expected from its prevalence in the general population. One series of consecutive MS patients found a 15 percent prevalence of bipolar disorder. The patients with a history of mania were more likely than those without such a history to have left temporal lobe lesions. The association between bipolar disorder and MS is given further support by a community-based study carried out in Rochester, New York, that found more than twice the rate of bipolar disorder in MS patients compared with other persons in the community.

EMOTIONAL INCONTINENCE Emotional incontinence, also called *pathological crying and laughing,* is a disorder of the expression of emotion. Weeping or laughter comes on rapidly and is often triggered by events that have little or no sad or happy content. Emotional incontinence often occurs in patients who have evidence on neurological examination of *pseudobulbar palsy* (hyperactive jaw jerk, spastic function of cranial nerve VII, hyperactive gag reflex, difficulty in swallowing, and high-pitched, dysarthric speech). Pathological crying is more common than pathological laughing and can sometimes be mistaken for a depressive disorder. Both crying and laughter can be sources of distress and can impair social interactions.

Impairment of social and work functions The neurological impairment caused by MS ranges from mild visual difficulty to quadriparesis. In view of the frequent occurrence of MS in young persons, it is not surprising that marked disruptions of family, interpersonal, and social functioning occur. Impairment in work performance and in the activities of daily living—such as walking, dressing, and driving—can be difficult to adapt to at any age but are particularly devastating to the young adult who is just beginning to establish work and family routines and to develop mature social networks and activity patterns. The likelihood of job loss correlates with the degree of neurological and cognitive impairment. Therefore, neuropsychological assessment should be a part of the evaluation of any MS patient who is having work difficulty.

Fatigue Fatigue is a common symptom of multiple sclerosis and is distinct from depression. Most evidence suggests that it is a physiological symptom, but it can be difficult to distinguish from apathy and the anhedonia of depression. Fatigue is sometimes misinterpreted by patients and their families as resulting from a personality defect or a lack of initiative.

Unpredictability MS is among the most unpredictable of neuropsychiatric disorders. That is particularly distressing to some patients and is a common issue in individual and group psychotherapy.

Cognitive disorder Estimates of the prevalence of cognitive disorder in MS have ranged widely since MS was first described a century ago. Most recent studies report that 25 to 50 percent of patients have significant cognitive impairment and that mild impairment is even more prevalent. Several problems confound the study of cognitive impairment in MS. First, many neuropsychological tests depend on motor performance and are timed. Poor performance could, therefore, be caused by the motor disorder and the slowing caused by the neuromuscular impairment. Second, sensitive neuropsychological tests can pick up cognitive changes that are clinically irrelevant. Third, many of the studies of cognitive disorder have examined patients followed in university centers or persons from the list of the local Multiple Sclerosis Society. Those are not representative samples of MS patients who reside in the community and are probably biased toward including persons with severe disease. Each of those biases tends to increase the rate of cognitive impairment detected.

A study of 100 patients who were members of the local MS society compared their performances with those of 100 controls matched for age, gender, and education. Defining impairment as a performance worse than 95 percent of community residents, the researchers found the rate of cognitive impairment to be 43 percent. They found correlations between cognitive disorder and job failures. The clinician treating patients with MS should be careful to include cognitive disorder in the differential diagnosis of any behavioral change.

As might be expected from its predominant effect on white matter, MS has characteristics of a subcortical dementia. Memory, speed, and mental flexibility are commonly impaired, but language, praxis, and recognition are generally spared. Attempts to link specific neuropsychological deficits with specific plaque locations have been largely unsuccessful, probably because MRI is too sensitive and computed tomography (CT) scans too insensitive.

Medication-induced symptoms Several of the drugs used to treat MS can cause psychiatric symptoms. Baclofen (Lioresal) and benzodiazepines can cause delirium. Steroids can cause depression, elation, delirium, and paranoia—all psychiatric symptoms associated with MS itself. Therefore, identifying the cause of those symptoms can sometimes be accomplished by decreasing or stopping the offending drug.

Schizophrenia Case reports of coincident MS and schizophrenialike syndromes were common in the first half of the 20th century. Recent case series studies of MS patients that use structured examinations rarely turn up such cases, and there is little evidence that the two disorders occur together more than by chance. Many of the published case reports describe patients with severe neurological impairment and probable dementia who have psychotic symptoms. Since current diagnostic criteria do not allow a diagnosis of schizophrenia when a specific organic abnormality is present and since delusions and hallucinations can be seen in any brain injury, many of the case reports probably do not represent true schizophrenic illness.

Hysteria Charcot was interested in both MS and hysteria, and associations between the two conditions have been suggested for 100 years. Recent studies do not confirm a specific association, although cases of patients with MS and unexplainable physical symptoms still occur. Hysteria apparently occurs no more frequently in MS patients than in patients with other physical illnesses. Furthermore, some cases of hysteria and MS may result from silent lesions in areas affecting primarily behavior and cognition, such as the frontal lobes.

TREATMENT No specific treatment for MS exists. A variety of anti-inflammatory therapies have been tried because MS is hypothesized to have immunological, autoimmune, or chronic infectious causes. Brief courses of high-dose steroids can shorten the length of an exacerbation, but steroid therapy does not affect the long-term course, and no evidence indicates that other anti-inflammatory agents are beneficial. In one double-blind study, lithium carbonate (Eskalith) was shown to prevent the development of steroid psychosis in MS patients. Because lithium itself can induce delirium in those patients, caution should be used in prescribing it.

Treatment of psychiatric symptoms Since the range of psychiatric symptoms associated with multiple sclerosis is broad, the clinician should choose a specific treatment to treat a specific symptom. In MS patients with symptoms of major depression, tricyclic antidepressants have been shown in a double-blind study to be more effective than a placebo, whereas lithium carbonate has been shown to be effective in case reports of MS patients with manic symptoms.

Emotional incontinence also responds to antidepressant therapy. One double-blind study used amitriptyline (Elavil), but clinical experience suggests that other antidepressants are equally effective and may have fewer side effects than amitriptyline.

The wide range of functional and social disabilities dictates the appropriate use of rehabilitation therapy, job retraining, and information on aids that are available to maximize functional performance.

Individual, group, and family psychotherapy are important supports. Several studies have shown that interpersonal and cognitive therapy are more effective than nontreatment in improving the emotional state of MS patients. The practitioner using psychotherapy must have knowledge of or close working contact with professionals who understand the neurological impairments suffered by each individual patient. The goals of psychotherapy are often multiple and include such issues as helping the patient accept and adapt to limiting physical impairments, helping the patient make the changes necessary for maximal function, and helping family members understand, accept, and adapt to the changes in mood, behavior, and function that are caused by the disease.

OTHER DEMYELINATING DISORDERS

A variety of genetic diseases lead to illnesses that predominantly affect the white matter of the CNS. Most of the disorders follow a recessive inheritance and affect the production of enzymes. The production of enzymes is a multistaged synthesis. Within each enzyme cascade, one of several specific enzymes may be deficient. Much of the variation in the age of onset and the symptom presentation of each disorder results from the specific enzyme deficiency. A complete absence of the enzyme usually leads to impairment at birth or during the first years of life. Normal amounts of less active enzymes lead to onset in adolescence or young adulthood. The symptom profile often depends on age of onset. In general, the late-onset conditions are likely to manifest neuropsychiatric symptoms early in the course of the disease, and obvious neurological symptoms appear somewhat later. Because many of the disorders are rare, most reports are small case series.

Metachromatic leukodystrophy is caused by an accumulation of cerebroside sulphate in the CNS and a variety of other organs. It is due to a deficiency of arylsulfatase A, a lysosomal acid hydrolase. Schizophrenialike symptoms have been reported; in most cases the hallucinations and delusions are accompanied by a mild cognitive impairment. Disordered behavior is common in adolescent and adult patients, but no specific psychiatric syndrome is associated with this disorder.

The *gangliosidoses* are a good example of some of the general principles described above. Complete absence of the enzyme hexosaminidase A results in *Tay-Sachs* disease, a progressive neurodegenerative disorder that presents in early infancy and results in death after several years. In contrast, partial deficiency or absence of the enzymes hexosaminidase A and B results in adolescent (*Sandhoff's* disease) or early adult onset G_{M2} gangliosidosis. Many patients have symptoms of bipolar disorder, and the condition may present with mood symptoms before neurological symptoms are manifest. The mood disorder symptoms appear to respond to standard treatments, although, for theoretical reasons, antipsychotic drugs are thought to be contraindicated. Hexosaminidase A levels can be measured in leukocytes and used as a diagnostic test.

Subacute sclerosing panencephalitis is a progressive demyelinating illness that generally occurs in childhood or adolescence. It is an autoimmune disorder thought to be triggered by a measles virus infection. Behavioral disorder can be an early symptom and is a common sequela of the encephalomyelitis.

Kufs disease (neuronal ceroid lipofuscinosis) presents with progressive dementia, motor dysfunction, and facial dyskinesias. Personality changes may be the earliest symptom. No specific test is available that can diagnose all cases, but urinary dolichols are accurate in about 70 percent of cases. Different eponyms have been applied to different ages of onset. In infants it is called *Haltia-Santavuori* disease, late infantile onset disease is called *Jansky-Bielschowsky* disease, juvenile onset is called *Spielmeyer-Vogt* disease, and adult onset is called *Kufs* disease.

Several other neurodegenerative disorders can present during adolescence or early adulthood and have behavioral symptoms or personality change among the first manifestations. Included in that group are cerebrotendinous xanthomatosis, adrenoleukodystrophy, metachromatic leukodystrophy, Gaucher's type I disease, Niemann-Pick type II-C disease, Sanfilippo's syndrome (mucopolysaccharidosis type III-B), Fabry's disease (which presents with painful extremities, nonblanching purple papules, hypohidrosis, and corneal or lens opacities), and Krabbe's disease (globoid cell leukodystrophy), in which motor symptoms develop before dementia.

SUGGESTED CROSS-REFERENCES

Functional neuroanatomy is discussed in Section 1.2, neuroimaging in Sections 1.10 and 2.10, schizophrenia in Chapter 14, and mood disorders in Chapter 16.

REFERENCES

Argov Z, Navon R: Clinical and genetic variations in the syndrome of adult G_{M2} gangliosidosis resulting from hexosaminidase A deficiency. Ann Neurol *16:* 14, 1984.

Burnfield A, Burnfield P: Common psychological problems in multiple sclerosis. Br Med J *1:* 1193, 1978.

Canter A H: Direct and indirect measures of psychological deficit in multiple sclerosis: Part I. J Gen Psychol *44:* 3, 1951.

Charcot J-M: *Lectures on the Diseases of the Nervous System.* New Syndenham Society, London, 1877.

Coker S B: The diagnosis of childhood neurodegenerative disorders presenting as dementia in adults. Neurology *41:* 794, 1991.

Compston A, Scolding N, Wren D, Noble M: The pathogenesis of demyelinating disease: Insights from cell biology. Trends Neurosci *14:* 175, 1991.

Cottrell S S, Wilson S A K: The affective symptomatology of disseminated sclerosis. J Neurol Psychopathol *7:* 1, 1926.

Dalos N P, Rabins P V, Brooks B R, O'Donnell P: Disease activity and emotional state in multiple sclerosis. Ann Neurol *13:* 573, 1983.

Feigenson J S, Scheinberg L, Catalano M, Polkow L, Mantegazza P M, Feigenson W D, LaRocca N G: The cost-effectiveness of multiple sclerosis rehabilitation: A model. Neurology *31:* 1316, 1981.

Fluharty A L: The relationship of the metachromatic leukodystrophies to neuropsychiatric disorder. Mol Chem Neuropathol *13:* 81, 1990.

Foley F W, Traugott U, LaRocca N G, Smith C R, Perlman K R, Caruso L S, Scheinberg L C: A prospective study of depression and immune dysregulation in multiple sclerosis. Arch Neurol *44:* 338, 1992.

Grant I, Brown G W, Harris T, McDonald W I, Patterson T, Trimble M R: Severely threatening events and marked life difficulties preceding onset or exacerbation of multiple sclerosis. J Neurol Neurosurg Psychiatry *52:* 8, 1989.

Honer W G, Hurwitz T, Palmer M, Paty D W: Temporal lobe involvement in multiple sclerosis patients with psychiatric disorders. Arch Neurol *44:* 187, 1987.

Jambor K L: Cognitive functioning in multiple sclerosis. Br J Psychiatry *115:* 765, 1969.

Joffe R T, Lippert G P, Gray T A, Sawa G, Horvath Z: Mood disorder and multiple sclerosis. Arch Neurol *44:* 376, 1987.

Krup L B, Alvarez L A, LaRocca N G, Scheinberg L C: Fatigue in multiple sclerosis. Arch Neurol *45:* 435, 1988.

Larcombe N A, Wilson P H: An evaluation of cognitive-behaviour therapy for depression in patients with multiple sclerosis. Br J Psychiatry *145:* 366, 1984.

*Matthews W B, editor: *McAlpine's Multiple Sclerosis.* Churchill Livingstone, New York, 1991.

*McIntosh-Michaelis S A, Roberts M H, Wilkinson S M, Diamond J D, Mc Lellan D L, Martin J P, Spackman A J: The prevalence of cognitive impairment in a community survey of multiple sclerosis. Br J Clin Psychol *30:* 333, 1991.

Nisipeanu P, Korczyn A D: Psychological stress as risk factor for exacerbations in multiple sclerosis. Neurology *43:* 1311, 1993.

O'Connor P, Detsky A S, Tansey C, Kucharczyk W: Effect of diagnostic testing for multiple sclerosis on patient health perceptions. Arch Neurol *51:* 46, 1993.

Poser C M: Exacerbations, activity, and progression in multiple sclerosis. Arch Neurol *37:* 471, 1980.

Pratt R T C: An investigation of the psychiatric aspects of disseminated sclerosis. J Neurol Neurosurg Psychiatry *14:* 326, 1951.

Rabins P V, Brooks B R: Emotional disturbance in multiple sclerosis patients: Validity of the General Health Questionnaire (GHQ). Psychol Med *11:* 425, 1981.

*Rabins P V, Brooks B R, O'Donnell P, Pearlson G D, Moberg P, Jubelt B, Coyle P, Dalos N, Folstein M F: Structural brain correlates of emotional disorder in multiple sclerosis. Brain *109:* 585, 1986.

*Rao SM, editor: *Neurobehavioral Aspects of Multiple Sclerosis.* Oxford University Press, New York, 1990.

Rao S M, Leo G J, Bernardin L, Unverazgt F: Cognitive dysfunction in multiple sclerosis: I. Frequency, patterns, and prediction. Neurology *41:* 685, 1991.

Rao S M, Leo G J, Ellington L, Nauertz B S, Bernardin M S, Unverzagt F: Cognitive dysfunction in multiple sclerosis: II. Impact on employment and social functioning. Neurology *41:* 692, 1991.

Reischies F M, Baum K, Nehrig C, Schorner W: Psychopathological symptoms and magnetic resonance imaging findings in multiple sclerosis. Biol Psychiatry *33:* 676, 1993.

Ron M A, Logsdail S J: Psychiatric morbidity in multiple sclerosis: A clinical and MRI study. Psychol Med *19:* 887, 1989.

Schiffer R B, Babigan H M: Behavioral disorders in multiple sclerosis, temporal lobe epilepsy, and amyotrophic lateral sclerosis: An epidemiologic study. Arch Neurol *41:* 1067, 1984.

*Schiffer R B, Herndon R M, Rudick R A: Treatment of pathologic laughing and weeping with amitriptyline. N Engl J Med *312:* 1480, 1985.

Schubert D S P, Foliart R H: Increased depression in multiple sclerosis patients. Psychosomatics *34:* 124, 1993.

Surridge D: An investigation into some psychiatric aspects of multiple sclerosis. Br J Psychiatry *115:* 749, 1969.

Swanson J W: Multiple sclerosis: Update in diagnosis and review of prognostic factors. Mayo Clin Proc *64:* 577, 1989.

Thygesen P: *The Course of Disseminated Sclerosis: A Close-Up of 105 Attacks.* Rosenkilde and Bagger, Copenhagen, 1953.

Valleroy M L, Kraft G H: Sexual dysfunction in multiple sclerosis. Arch Phys Med Rehabil *65:* 125, 1984.

Warren S, Greenhill S, Warren K G: Emotional stress and the development of multiple sclerosis: Case-control evidence of a relationship. J Chron Dis *35:* 821, 1982.

Whitlock F A, Siskind M M: Depression as a major symptom of multiple sclerosis. J Neurol Neurosurg Psychiatry *43:* 861, 1980.

2.7
NEUROPSYCHIATRIC ASPECTS OF INFECTIOUS DISORDERS

WILFRED G. VAN GORP, Ph.D.
JEFFREY L. CUMMINGS, M.D.

INTRODUCTION

Infectious agents affecting the central nervous system (CNS) have provided some of the best-documented relations between brain dysfunction and neuropsychiatric alterations. A major impetus to the growth of neuropsychiatry can be traced to the discovery that an infection involving the nervous system (syphilis) could cause severe behavioral abnormalities and dementia (general paresis). Other infectious diseases have since been identified that cause neuropsychological and emotional abnormalities (for example, Creutzfeldt-Jakob disease, herpes encephalitis); recently, human immunodeficiency virus (HIV) infection has become a major cause of neuropsychological and neuropsychiatric morbidity. Infectious agents can produce a variety of neurobehavioral and neuropsychiatric disturbances, including amnesia, aphasia, bradyphrenia, depression, mania, psychosis, hallucinations, and dementia.

This section focuses on the neuropsychiatric syndromes produced by infectious agents affecting the CNS. Special emphasis is given to the neuropsychiatric features associated with HIV type I (HIV-1) infection, since HIV is responsible for more cases of dementia than any other infectious agent and is the cause of more cases of nontraumatic dementia in young adults than is any other condition. In addition, the sheer quantity of research that has been conducted on the neuropathology, neuropsychiatry, and neuropsychology of HIV infection allows rich insights into the relation between a brain infection and the resulting neuropsychiatric manifestations.

NOSOLOGY

Infectious agents and diseases affecting the central nervous system can be divided into six categories: slow virus infections, prion disorders, acute viral encephalitis, and bacterial, fungal, and parasitic infectious encephalopathies.

Slow virus infections characteristically progress gradually over weeks, months, or years and should be considered whenever a patient presents with a history of insidious, subacute, or chronic changes in cognitive, motor, or behavioral function. Among the slow virus infections are HIV-related disorders, subacute sclerosing panencephalitis, progressive multifocal leukoencephalopathy, progressive rubella encephalitis, and paraneoplastic limbic encephalitis.

Creutzfeldt-Jakob disease, fatal familial insomnia, and kuru are examples of prion disorders. Prions have also been called unconventional viruses because they are transmissible but have few of the characteristics of conventional viruses. Table 2.7-1 lists the common slow virus and prion diseases.

In contrast to slow virus and prion infections, acute viral infections typically produce an abrupt change in mental status. Herpes encephalitis is an example of an acute viral infection of the CNS.

Bacterial, fungal, and parasitic infectious encephalopathies include syphilis-related disorders, Whipple's disease, chronic meningitides (including tuberculosis and cryptococcosis), and opportunistic infections (such as toxoplasmosis) occurring in immunosuppressed hosts.

HIV-ASSOCIATED DEMENTIA

DEFINITIONS HIV-1 is an infectious viral agent that produces severe immunosuppression in its host. The Centers for Disease Control (CDC) uses a staging system in which HIV-1 infection is classified into one of three categories: asymptomatic infection (CDC Group A); minor symptoms including oral candidiasis, cervical dysplasia, prolonged unexplained diarrhea, and so on (CDC Group B); and AIDS defining illnesses or infections such as pneumocystis carinaii pneumonia, cytomegalovirus infection, tuberculosis, Kaposi's sarcoma or lymphoma, and so on (CDC Group C). Each category is divided into subgroup 1 if the CD4 count has always been 500 or more, subgroup 2 if the CD4 lowest count was between 200 and 499, or subgroup 3 if the CD4 count was ever less than 200.

Immune system markers commonly used in patients infected by HIV-1 are the absolute immune helper (CD4) and suppressor (CD8) cells, and their ratio (CD4:CD8). A ratio less than 0.2 indicates advanced disease and is a criterion for prophylaxis to prevent *Pneumocystis carinii* pneumonia.

A variety of terms have been used for the constellation of cognitive, motor, and behavioral changes associated with the effects of HIV-1 on the CNS, including ''subacute encephalitis,'' ''AIDS dementia complex,'' ''HIV encephalopathy,'' and ''HIV-associated cognitive-motor complex''. Although those terms refer to essentially the same symptom constellation, the term ''HIV-associated cognitive-motor complex'' is used here, since the term implies a specific set of diagnostic criteria. In adults the complex is diagnosed when neuropsychological or mental status changes are evident, along with the reduced activities of daily living. In HIV-1-associated dementia complex, the ability to work and to function independently are notably impaired, but only the most difficult or demanding activities of daily living are impaired in patients with an HIV-1-associated minor cognitive-motor complex. In children, evidence of HIV-1 infection is required (a positive HIV-antibody test)—together with evidence of the loss of developmental milestones or intellectual ability, impaired brain growth, or motor deficits (paresis, abnormal tone, pathological reflexes, ataxia, or gait disturbance)—to establish a diagnosis of HIV-associated cognitive-motor complex.

ETIOLOGY HIV-1 is the viral agent responsible for AIDS, but the pathogenesis of HIV-associated dementia complex is less well defined. HIV can be cultured from the cerebrospinal fluid and the brains of half or more of infected patients; it is found primarily in glial cells and not in the neurons. That fact has led to speculation that HIV is transmitted to the central nervous system by infected macrophages crossing the blood-brain barrier. By that route, macrophages could exert a deleterious effect on the function of nearby neurons. A neurochemical disturbance, such as increased levels of quinolinic acid, that exerts a toxic effect on the central nervous system has also been proposed. Accompanying viral agents, such as cytomegalovirus infection of the CNS, in an immunocompromised host may also contribute to the dementia.

CLINICAL FEATURES Immunocompromised patients infected with HIV are subject to a number of CNS-related disorders. Although the most common condition is the HIV-associated dementia complex, other opportunistic infections and processes may develop, including cytomegalovirus infection (in 15 to 30 percent of patients), toxoplasmosis (3 to 30 percent), cryptococcal meningitis (2 to 11 percent), progressive multifocal leukoencephalopathy (1 to 6 percent), and CNS lymphoma (1 to 5 percent).

Recent studies have found little evidence of overt neuropsychological deficits in asymptomatic persons as a group, although slow reaction times in that population have been reported in some studies. HIV-associated dementia complex occurs most often in the presence of significant immunosuppression (that is, below CD4 200 mm^3) and concurrent constitutional illness. Patients whose immune systems are compromised (with CD4 values at or below 200 mm^3 or whose CD4 values drop precipitously) are most at risk for the dementia. An HIV-related dementia is the sole presenting sign of HIV infection in a small number of patients.

Patients who exhibit HIV-associated cognitive-motor complex typically present with a constellation of cognitive, motor, and behavioral changes characteristic of a subcortical dementia. Psychomotor slowing, difficulty in concentrating, and a pattern of memory performance characterized by poor retrieval and intact recognition are often the initial features. That presentation is consistent with early involvement of the thalamus and the basal ganglia. Table 2.7-2 summarizes the pattern of cognitive strengths and weaknesses observed in HIV-1-associated dementia.

Attention Most studies have found attention, as measured by digit span and the A test, to be intact, although expanded and more taxing mental control tasks and computerized measures of sustained attention, concentration, and reaction time have found differences between seropositive and seronegative persons. Tasks requiring patients to divide their attention between two competing stimuli are affected in a subset of patients. The difficulty with sustained and divided attention may give rise to the frequent subjective complaint of many HIV-infected patients that they are less able to concentrate and often lose their train of thought.

TABLE 2.7-1
Principal Infections Producing Neuropsychiatric Disorders

Viral infections
- Slow virus infections
  - HIV encephalopathy
  - Subacute sclerosing panencephalitis
  - Progressive multifocal leukoencephalopathy
- Acute viral disorders
  - Herpes simplex encephalitis
  - Other viral encephalitides

Prion infections
- Creutzfeldt-Jakob disease
- Fatal familial insomnia
- Kuru

Chronic fungal infections
- Cryptococcosis
- Coccidioidomycosis
- Histoplasmosis
- Candida

Parasitic infections
- Malaria
- Cysticercosis
- Toxoplasmosis

Chronic bacterial infections
- Tuberculosis
- Whipple's disease
- Syphilis
- Lyme disease (borreliosis)

TABLE 2.7-2
Pattern of Cognitive Impairments in HIV-Associated Dementia Complex

Impaired	Preserved
Complex attention and reaction time	Basic attention and digit span
Performance I.Q.	Verbal I.Q. (less affected than performance I.Q.)
Recall memory	Recognition memory
Psychomotor speed	Language
Visuospatial skills (+/−)	Visuospatial skills (+/−)
Motor speed and coordination	
Mood and affect	

Language Language function in HIV-infected patients is preserved until end-stage disease is reached. Performances on tests of confrontation naming (such as the Boston Naming Test), measures of vocabulary (revised Wechsler Adult Intelligence Scale [WAIS-R] vocabulary subtest), and word list generation are normal.

Visuospatial Some studies have found HIV-infected symptomatic persons to have poor cube drawing, reproduction of a complex figure (the Rey-Osterrieth Complex Figure), and construction of blocks to match a design (block design from the WAIS-R); other studies have not observed those abnormalities. Thus, variable performance among HIV-infected persons is evident on visuospatial tasks; definite abnormalities occur in patients with advanced stages of illness.

Memory Verbal memory tasks that require learning and the recall of a series of unrelated words over a number of trials are performed more poorly by symptomatic HIV-infected persons than by seronegative controls. However, information presented in a meaningful context (prose passages) is learned and recalled as well by seropositive as by seronegative persons. The majority of studies have also found symptomatic persons to exhibit deficits on nonverbal memory tasks, particularly as the test difficulty increases. Thus, difficult memory tasks, such as learning a list of words or recalling a complex design, are impaired in HIV-infected persons, but learning and the recall of prose passages or less complex information are retained until moderate stages of dementia are reached.

Motor speed Motor involvement is a hallmark of HIV-associated dementia complex, being among the triad of features characteristic of the condition (cognitive, motor, and behavioral abnormalities). Studies specifically assessing pure motor speed have failed to find evidence of slowing in asymptomatic persons, but, as the patient becomes more symptomatic, motor speed and strength decline. Psychomotor slowing, rather than pure motor slowing, per se, is most characteristic of HIV-associated dementia complex. The greatest deficits are seen on tasks in which thought is tied to action. Nevertheless, motor slowing itself is evident in patients with advanced stages of the illness.

Psychomotor speed and speed of information processing Of all cognitive domains, psychomotor speed is the one most affected in HIV-infected symptomatic persons. Examples of such measures include the Trail Making Test, in which the person is asked to connect numbers distributed on a page from 1 to 25, in order, as fast as possible with a pencil (Trail Making Test A) or to sequentially alternate between number and letter—for example, 1-A, 2-B, 3-C, 4-D (Trail Making Test B). Trail Making Test B reveals the most consistent deficits in symptomatic persons. The other task especially sensitive to HIV-associated cognitive impairment is the digit symbol substitution task from the WAIS-R. On that task, the person is shown a series of numbers, each associated with a unique symbol. The person is then asked to match the symbols associated with a series of numbers as quickly as possible in 90 seconds. That task requires psychomotor speed, attention, and memory.

Most studies of reaction time and speed of information processing in HIV-infected persons have found symptomatic seropositive persons to perform worse than seronegative persons. In some studies, asymptomatic infected persons have performed worse than their seronegative counterparts. Although the measures may well reflect subtle cognitive changes associated with early CNS infection by the virus, the deficits are sufficiently slight that they do not significantly affect the activities of daily living.

Executive and frontal systems functions Although frontal systems deficits are often found in various subcortical dementias, they are not particularly common among HIV-infected persons. At least one study has found seropositive persons to have difficulty in getting into the set of a task, but most studies have not found differences on measures of perseveration, category and concept shifting, and abstraction. Thus, other than difficulty on a task requiring both psychomotor speed and set shifting (Trail Making Test B), most nontimed measures of frontal systems function have not shown HIV-infected persons to perform worse than seronegative controls.

Global cognitive functioning and intelligence The few studies that have examined the performance of HIV-infected patients on the Mini-Mental State Examination have not found that test to be sensitive to HIV-related cognitive impairment until the disorder is severe. In contrast, most studies have found symptomatic HIV-infected persons to have lower WAIS-R verbal, performance, and full-scale I.Q. scores than do seronegative controls.

Mood and affect Depression is a common feature in subcortical dementias, and elevated findings on various mood measures have been reported in symptomatic seropositive persons. An initial acute depressive reaction has been reported in as many as 90 percent of HIV-infected persons. Although the depression resolves in most patients, 15 to 30 percent meet the criteria for major depression at some point during the course of the illness.

The dementia syndrome of depression (pseudodementia), found in depressed elderly persons, is infrequent in young people infected with HIV. Studies comparing the neuropsychological test performances of depressed persons with AIDS with nondepressed AIDS persons have shown that the clinically depressed AIDS persons performed no worse than the nondepressed AIDS patients except on measures of pure motor speed. Those data suggest that, in nonelderly AIDS persons, cognitive function is unaffected by depression. Individual case reports have documented the dementia syndrome of depression in some young AIDS patients, but that circumstance is relatively uncommon.

Depression correlates with a patient's subjective sense of cognitive dysfunction. Several studies have compared HIV-infected patients' subjective complaints of everyday cognitive failures with their actual neuropsychological test performances. In patients without diagnosed dementia, their subjective appraisals of their cognitive functioning related more to their scores on measures of depression than to their actual neuropsychological performances. These findings indicate that a person's own report of cognitive difficulties must be combined with objective neuropsychological and affective measures before determining that a dementia is present. Otherwise, a misdiagnosis of HIV-associated dementia complex may be made when the patient is actually depressed, rather than demented.

Other psychiatric manifestations are also frequently observed in HIV-infected persons. An acute psychiatric disturbance, such as a psychosis, can also be the sole initial sign of HIV infection. In symptomatic persons, anxious mood has been reported to occur in up to 64 percent of infected persons, secondary mania in as many as 30 percent, delusional thinking in 29 percent, paranoid mentation in 23 percent, and hallucinations in 27 percent.

The cause of the psychiatric symptoms in most HIV-infected persons has not been fully determined. The psychological trauma sustained when one is given a diagnosis of a terminal illness, especially one that is tainted by social stigma, is often emotionally devastating. The predilection of HIV for subcortical and limbic structures suggests that the psychiatric features may, at least in part, have a biological underpinning.

LABORATORY EXAMINATION HIV serum status is typically determined by an enzyme-linked immunosorbent assay (ELISA) with anitbody positive results confirmed by Western blot analysis to reduce the number of false-positive findings. Less frequently, antibody status is determined by a polymerase chain-reaction technique or actual serum or cerebrospinal fluid (CSF) culture. The polymerase chain-reaction technique is far more sensitive than ELISA or the Western blot assay but is used primarily for research purposes because of the labor-intensive nature of the procedure, the skill and the equipment required, and the high number of false-positive results.

Various imaging approaches have been used to assess HIV encephalopathy. Typically, the findings of magnetic resonance imaging (MRI) and computed tomography (CT) are normal in HIV-associated minor cognitive-motor complex but show atrophy with ventricular enlargement in HIV-associated dementia complex. Patchy areas of high signal intensity in the white matter may be seen on MRI. Caution should be exercised, however, in interpreting areas of high signal intensity without clinical correlation; several studies have shown that at least one quarter of seronegative controls also have patchy areas of high signal intensity on their scans. MRI and CT are most helpful in excluding focal opportunistic infections and lesions of the central nervous system.

In contrast to MRI and CT, functional imaging approaches, such as positron emission tomography (PET) and single photon emission computed tomography (SPECT), have shown distinctive alterations. Abnormal cerebral metabolic activity (hypermetabolism) and cerebral blood flow have been consistently found in the basal ganglia and the thalamus of patients with HIV-associated mild cognitive-motor complex; widespread (cortical and subcortical) abnormalities with reduced cerebral metabolic activity and blood flow have been seen in patients with advanced dementia. Within the cortex the temporal lobes have been reported to be among the regions to first show abnormal glucose metabolism.

Like functional neuroimaging measures, electroencephalograms (EEG) may also be sensitive to early features of HIV-associated cognitive-motor complex. Theta slowing of the frontal and frontotemporal regions has been reported in up to 30 percent of patients. Reduced P300 amplitudes and increased evoked response latencies have also been described in HIV encephalopathy. Although the EEG may reveal abnormalities before cognitive changes are evident, the EEG is normal in the majority of infected patients, even when dementia is manifest.

PATHOLOGY Neuropathological abnormalities can be found in 90 percent or more of autopsied HIV-infected persons. Enlarged ventricles and cortical atrophy are present in substantial numbers of patients. Abnormalities are most striking in the subcortical white matter, where diffuse pallor is usually present. Gliosis, small foci of necrosis, microglial nodules, demyelination, and multinucleated giant cells are characteristic histopathological changes. The amygdala, the basal ganglia, the hippocampus, and the cortex (temporal and parietal lobes preferentially) are affected in a significant number of patients. Often, surprisingly little relation is found between the degree of the clinical dementia apparent and the extent of the neuropathological abnormalities.

DIFFERENTIAL DIAGNOSIS When encountering an HIV-infected patient with suspected cognitive impairment, the clinician must first determine through serum studies, lumbar puncture, and neuroimaging (MRI, CT, SPECT) if a focal or multifocal opportunistic process is present. If a focal process is implicated on imaging or neurological examination, infarctions and neoplastic processes must be assessed, including toxoplasmosis, progressive multifocal leukoencephalopathy, and lymphoma. If progressive multifocal leukoencephalopathy is suspected, a brain biopsy may be required to establish the diagnosis conclusively.

Cognitive impairment in an HIV-infected patient with no alternate cause for dementia (for example, head injury, learning disability, alcoholism) and no focal abnormalities suggests the presence of HIV-associated cognitive-motor complex. Other subcortical dementias must also be considered, including multiple sclerosis, Wilson's disease, and progressive supranuclear palsy. Neurosyphilis must be excluded if the results are positive on the Venereal Disease Research Laboratory (VDRL) test or the rapid plasma reagin (RPR) test.

Among the most common differential diagnostic challenges is the one between HIV-associated cognitive-motor complex and the dementia syndrome of depression. Although the dementia syndrome of depression occurs in only a small subset of HIV-infected patients, it must be considered if a patient is found to be clinically depressed or agitated and presents with cognitive impairment. If the clinician has any doubt, the depression should be aggressively treated and the patient reexamined after the treatment of the underlying mood disorder.

COURSE AND PROGNOSIS Early reports indicated that, once a patient evidences signs of the AIDS dementia complex, death is likely to occur within weeks to months. With increasing prophylactic measures to prevent opportunistic infections, however, patients with HIV-associated cognitive-motor impairment may live months to years after the diagnosis. Whether the course follows a steady downhill trajectory or has long plateau periods is unclear. Evidence indicates that cognitive deterioration is most apparent when precipitous declines of the CD4 count occur. Opportunistic infections of the CNS may cause death quickly. For instance, mortality associated with a diagnosis of progressive multifocal leukoencephalopathy is usually within days, weeks, or months, with only an occasional patient surviving longer than six months after the initial diagnosis.

TREATMENT Zidovudine (Retrovir), formerly called azidothymidine (AZT), has been shown to improve neuropsychological test performances in HIV-infected patients, particularly those with AIDS. Although the degree of improvement can be substantial (particularly in cognitively impaired patients), it is not known how long the benefits are sustained. High-dose AZT (that is, more than 1,200 mg a day) may result in greater cognitive improvement than does lower-dose treatment, but conclusive dose-response data are not yet available. With longer survival, memory retraining procedures may assist the affected patient in retaining as much independence as possible.

Individual opportunistic infections may benefit from specific therapy regimes.

OTHER INFECTIOUS ILLNESSES

SUBACUTE SCLEROSING PANENCEPHALITIS Subacute sclerosing panencephalitis is a rare, slow virus infection that affects approximately one person per million each year. It results from a conventional Paramyxovirus infection of the CNS.

Children and adolescents are predominantly affected, with most cases occurring before age 18. Mental status changes are commonly first apparent between ages 5 and 15. More cases occur in boys than in girls. The clinical course is relatively rapid, with death occurring within one to three years after the diagnosis; in many cases, survival is as short as three months. In rare cases, survival up to 10 years has been reported.

The dementia syndrome seen in patients with the disease consists of a constellation of cognitive, behavioral, motor, and other neurological signs. Initially, the child or adolescent may exhibit behavioral problems or acting out at school, poor grades, and distractibility and forgetfulness. Hallucinations have also been reported in the initial stage. Cognitive deterioration is apparent in the middle stage and includes reduced intelligence test scores, difficulty in reading and writing, and problems with visuospatial processing and constructions. Neurobehavioral symptoms may also be apparent, including apraxia, agnosia, and Balint's syndrome (optic ataxia, simultanagnosia, and sticky fixation). Myoclonus is common, initially involving the head and eventually affecting the trunk and the limbs. The jerking movements occur only occasionally at first; as the disease progresses, they occur regularly every 5 to 15 seconds. Generalized or focal seizures often occur in the middle stage of the illness.

In the advanced phases the cognitive manifestations are pronounced, with eventual global cognitive deterioration and mutism. In the final phase, extrapyramidal dysfunction is present, with masked face, limited spontaneous movement, and dystonic posturing. Finally, decerebrate rigidity occurs.

Laboratory analyses reveal elevated measles antibody titers and otherwise unremarkable findings on conventional serological testing. Cerebrospinal fluid studies usually find an elevated protein, with immunoglobulin G accounting for up to 60 percent of the protein concentration, and high measles antibody titers.

In addition to the clinical features described above and the presence of measles antibodies, the EEG is a key diagnostic tool, showing high-amplitude bilateral and stereotyped complexes that repeat every four to five seconds. When myoclonus is present, the complexes occur simultaneously with the myoclonic jerks.

CT studies typically reveal enlarged ventricles and cortical, cerebellar, and brainstem atrophy. MRI often shows lucent areas in the basal ganglia. As in HIV encephalopathy, PET scans often show early subcortical *hyper*metabolism followed by global cortical and subcortical *hypo*metabolism. Autopsy studies show gray and white matter microscopic abnormalities consisting of lymphocytic and plasma cell infiltrates. Neuronal loss and astrocytic and microglial hyperplasia have also been found on pathological examination. Eosinophilic inclusions are present in the cytoplasm and the nuclei of the neurons and the glial cells.

As indicated above, the clinical course usually results in rapid deterioration, with death occurring in weeks, months, or sometimes up to three years after the diagnosis. Amantadine (Symmetrel), isoprinosine, and intraventricular interferon have been associated with temporary remissions and somewhat increased life spans relative to untreated patients; no treatments reverse the disease.

CREUTZFELDT-JAKOB DISEASE Creutzfeldt-Jakob disease is a rare dementia syndrome with an incidence of approximately one case per million each year. It results from a prion infection of the CNS and manifests signs of cortical and subcortical dysfunction. Mental status changes may include aphasia, amnesia, marked visuospatial impairment, diminished executive (that is, frontal lobe-type) functions, and changes in mood and affect. The onset is often abrupt and may include fatigue, apprehension, and nonspecific influenzalike symptoms. After several weeks the dementia syndrome becomes prominent and typically progresses to death over a period of a few months. After the initial stages, myoclonus and pyramidal and extrapyramidal signs are present.

The prion protein responsible for the disease may be inherited or it may be transmitted from an infected host. The infectious prion is a self-replicating agent that commandeers the host cell machinery for reproduction. Transmission from humans to various primate species, cats, pigs, and mice has been documented, and human-to-human transmission has also been recorded. In one instance, human growth hormone harvested from infected persons was administered to children with growth failure, and several children who received the substance subsequently had Cruetzfeldt-Jakob disease. Transmission rarely occurs without direct inoculation of the agent; health care workers, spouses, sexual partners, and others who come into contact with patients exhibiting features of the disease do not have a higher rate of diagnoses than do the general population.

Conventional blood and urine studies are not helpful in the diagnosis of the disease. Although not diagnostically pathognomonic, EEG abnormalities are characteristic: a gradual slowing in the background rhythm and periodic complex discharges are seen. Both CT and MRI findings may be normal or reveal mild atrophy or sulcal enlargement; SPECT and PET findings reveal multifocal areas of decreased activity.

On microscopic inspection, the gray matter may show diffuse or multifocal cortical and subcortical neuronal loss and astrocytic hypertrophy. The cortex, the thalamus, the caudate nucleus, and the putamen show spongiform pathology with intraneuronal vacuoles.

Currently, no treatment for Creutzfeldt-Jakob disease is known.

HERPES ENCEPHALITIS Herpes encephalitis is a dramatic neuropsychiatric disorder resulting from direct viral invasion of the CNS by the herpes simplex virus. The onset is typically rapid, with an acute syndrome characterized by cognitive changes, focal neurological signs, seizures, and eventual coma. Temporal-limbic structures are usually most affected, and a variety of behavioral changes may herald the onset of the disorder. Amnesia (inability to learn) is the most common permanent neuropsychological deficit; many patients also exhibit some form of aphasia, and cognitive deficits can often be found with neuropsychological testing. Klüver-Bucy syndrome and dementia have been reported in a number of patients in the postencephalitic state after herpes encephalitis.

EEG abnormalities in the acute stage include slowing (diffuse or focal) and high-voltage sharp waves in the temporal regions. Imaging studies (CT, MRI, SPECT) often reveal structural changes or reduced blood flow in the temporal lobes and the orbitofrontal regions. Pathologically, there is an acute necrotizing encephalitis with neuronal loss and perivascular lymphocytic infiltrates. Intranuclear inclusion bodies in the neurons and the glia are characteristic.

Treatment with arabinosyladenine reduces mortality and morbidity if initiated early.

SYPHILIS An noted above, syphilitic infection showed the organic underpinnings of many neurospychiatric syndromes. General paresis (as the dementia was initially termed) was once among the most common disorders producing dementia and neuropsychiatric disorders. With penicillin treatment, however, neurosyphilis is now diagnosed only occasionally and is responsible for only a small fraction of psychiatric admissions to hospitals. Nevertheless, the panoply of cognitive, behavioral, and affective features that can appear in infected patients illustrates how an infection can produce profound neuropsychiatric disease. The various cognitive and behavioral changes that can result contribute to the reputation of syphilis as the great imitator, and the neuropsychiatric features contribute to misdiagnosis. Half or more of the patients with neurosyphilis have features of dementia. However, one quarter or more of those patients have prominent neuropsychiatric manifestations as well, including secondary mania, depression, paranoia, and psychosis. The cognitive changes include distractibility, diminished intellectual test performance, memory disturbance and confabulation, anomia, apraxia, and pseudobulbar palsy. The dementia is progressive in most untreated cases, and seizures, spasticity, diminished reflexes, and mutism occur in the final stage of the illness. Children born to infected parents may exhibit juvenile paresis, characterized by delayed developmental milestones, regressive behavior, and global cognitive impairment.

The symptoms of tertiary neurosyphilis generally become evident 10 to 20 years after the initial infection of the host by the agent *Treponema pallidum,* although the reported range from infection to symptom onset is 3 to 40 years. Ten percent of untreated but infected persons go on to teritiary neurosyphilis, but half or more have transient CNS infection.

The diagnosis of neurosyphilis presumes documented seropositive findings for syphilis (positive VDRL and serum fluorescent treponemal antibody-absorption test [FTA-ABS]), and reactive cerebrospinal fluid. Elevated cerebrospinal fluid protein, pleocytosis, and increased gamma globulin are also seen. After successful treatment, all but the FTA-ABS may revert to a nonreactive status.

Contemporary treatment of neurosyphilis involves the administration of penicillin or related antibiotics—typically, weekly injections of 2.4 million units of penicillin G benzathine (Bicillin) for three weeks or 9 million units of daily aqueous penicillin G procaine injections for 15 days. Regular monitoring of the serum and spinal fluids for the reemergence of reactivity should occur during the first year after treatment; if the results are positive for *Treponema pallidum,* treatment should be repeated. The majority of patients with neurosyphilis improve in cognition and the activities of daily living after treatment.

Cortical atrophy is the most common neuroimaging feature, with frontal and temporal lobe atrophy most prominent. Cortical cellular derangement is apparent on microscopic examination, with neuronal loss, astrocytosis, and the presence of microglial cells. Special studies are needed to show the spirochetal organisms.

CHRONIC MENINGITIDES Chronic meningitides can result from various fungal, parasitic, and chronic bacterial infections (Table 2.7-1). Although the conditions producing a chronic meningitis are typically diagnosed by findings on laboratory studies, mental status changes may be prominent features of the conditions. A slow, insidious process of cognitive and intellectual impairment is often seen, as are anergia, apathy, and lethargy. Difficulty in maintaining vigilance and concentration, together with memory difficulties, is common. Focal neurological and neuropsychological features are present if a focal lesion is part of the underlying pathology.

PROGRESSIVE MULTIFOCAL LEUKOENCEPHALOPATHY This disease results from a papovavirus infection and becomes manifest in persons with significant immunosuppression (such as secondary to HIV infection) and chronic lymphoproliferative or granulomatous conditions. Patients with progressive multifocal leukoencephalopathy typically present with an abrupt onset and focal neurological and neuropsychological signs, dependent on the site of the lesions. Aphasia, hemineglect or visual field abnormalities, striking visuospatial disturbance, and apraxia are examples of specific neuropsychological syndromes that can be seen in the condition. The disease progresses rapidly, with death occurring in two to four months in most cases, but cases with survival for 12 months or even longer have been reported. No unique diagnostic findings are seen in analyses of serum, blood, urine, and the cerebrospinal fluid; brain biopsy is the only means of making a certain diagnosis. Neuroimaging studies are helpful; multifocal areas of high signal intensity are typically seen in the white matter. CT findings also reveal nonenhancing lucent areas in the white matter. PET and SPECT studies may likewise reveal multifocal areas of reduced metabolic activity and blood flow, respectively.

Some patients may show temporary improvement when treated with cytarabine (Cytosar), but in most cases the disease is irreversible, and it is invariably rapidly progressive.

SUGGESTED CROSS-REFERENCES

Functional neuroanatomy is discussed in Section 1.2, the interactions of the immune system and the central nervous system in Section 1.12, the neuropsychological aspects of adults with HIV disorders in Section 29.2a, and the psychiatric aspects of AIDS in Section 29.2. Neuroimaging is discussed in Sections 1.10 and 2.10. The mental status examination is discussed in Sections 2.1 and 9.1. Mood disorders are discussed in Chapter 16 and the biological therapies in Chapter 32.

REFERENCES

*American Academy of Neurology AIDS Task Force: Nomenclature and research case definitions for neurologic manifestations of human immunodeficiency virus-type 1 (HIV-1) infection. Neurology *41:* 778, 1991.

Aylward E, Henderer J, McArthur J, Brettschneider P, Harris G, Barta P, Pearlson G: Reduced basal ganglia volume in HIV-1 associated dementia: Results from quantitative neuroimaging. Neurology *43:* 2099, 1993.

Baker H F, Ridley R M: The genetics and transmissibility of human spongiform encephalopathy. Neurodegeneration *1:* 3, 1992.

*Brown P, Cathala F, Castaigne P, Gajdusek D C: Creutzfeldt-Jakob disease: Clinical analysis of a consecutive series of 230 neuropathologically verified cases. Ann Neurol *20:* 597, 1986.

Butters N, Grant I, Haxby J, Judd L L, Martin A, McClelland J, Pequegnat W, Schacter D, Stover E: Assessment of AIDS-related cognitive changes: Recommendations of the NIMH workshop on neuropsychological assessment approaches. J Clin Exp Neuropsychol *12:* 963, 1990.

Centers for Disease Control: Revision of the CDC surveillance case definition for acquired immunodeficiency syndrome. MMWR *36:* 3S, 1987.

Cummings J, Benson D F: *Dementia: A Clinical Approach,* ed 2. Butterworths, Boston, 1992.

Davis L E, Schmitt J W: Clinical significance of cerebrospinal fluid tests for neurosyphilis. Ann Neurol *25:* 50, 1989.

DeCarli C, Civitello L A, Brouwers P, Pizzo P A: The prevalence of computed tomographic abnormalities of the cerebrum in 100 consecutive children symptomatic with the human immune deficiency virus. Ann Neurol *34:* 198, 1993.

Gabuzda D H, Ho D D, de la Monte S M, Hirsch M S, Rota T R, Sobel R A: Immunohistochemical identification of HTLV-III antigen in brains of patients with AIDS. Ann Neurol *20:* 289, 1986.

Gabuzda D H, Levy S R, Chiappa K H: Electroencephalography in AIDS-related complex. Clin Electroencephalogr *19:* 1, 1988.

Glass J, Wesselingh S, Selnes O, McArthur J: Clinical-neuropathologic correlation in HIV-associated dementia. Neurology *43:* 2230, 1993.

Goethe K E, Mitchell J E, Marshall D W, Brey R L, Cahill W T, Leger G D, Hoy L J, Boswell R N: Neuropsychological and neurological function of human immunodeficiency virus seropositive asymptomatic individuals. Arch Neurol *46:* 129, 1989.

Goldfarb L G, Peterson R B, Tabafon M, Brown P, LeBlanc A C, Montagna P, Cortelli P, Julien J, Vital C, Pendelbury W W, Haltia N M, Will P R, Hann J J, McKeever P E, Monari L, Schrank B, Swergold G D, Autilio-Gambetti L, Gajdusek D C, Lugaresi E, Gambetti P: Fatal familial insomnia and familial Creutzfeldt-Jakob disease: Disease phenotype determined by a DNA polymorphism. Science *258:* 806, 1992.

Grant I, Atkinson J H, Hesselink J R, Kennedy C J, Richman D D, Spector S A, McCutchan J A: Evidence for early central nervous system involvement in the acquired immunodeficiency syndrome (AIDS) and other human immunodeficiency virus (HIV) infections. Ann Intern Med *107:* 828, 1987.

Hinkin C H, Van Gorp W G, Satz P, Weisman J D, Thommes J, Buckingham S: Depressed mood and its relationship to neuropsychological test performance in HIV-1 seropositive individuals. J Clin Exp Neuropsychol *14:* 289, 1991.

Ho D D, Bredesen D E, Vinters H V, Daar E S: The acquired immunodeficiency syndrome (AIDS) dementia complex. Ann Intern Med *111:* 400, 1989.

Janssen R S, Cornblath D R, Epstein L G, McArthur J, Price R W: Human immunodeficiency virus (HIV) infection and the nervous system: Report from the American Academy of Neurology AIDS Task Force. Neurology *39:* 119, 1989.

Janssen R S, Saykin A J, Cannon L, Campbell J, Pinsky P F, Hessol N A, O'Malley P M, Lifson A R, Doll L S, Rutherford G W, Kaplan J E: Neurological and neuropsychological manifestations of HIV-1 infection: Association with AIDS-related complex but not asymptomatic HIV-1 infection. Ann Neurol *26:* 592, 1989.

Krawiecki N S, Dyken P R, Taher El G, DuRant R H, Swift A: Computed tomography of the brain in subacute sclerosing panencephalitis. Ann Neurol *15:* 489, 1984.

Krup L B, Lipton R B, Swerdlow M L, Leeds N E, Llena J: Progressive multifocal leukoencephalopathy: Clinical and radiographic features. Ann Neurol *17:* 344, 1985.

Maj M: Psychiatric aspects of HIV-1 infection and AIDS. Psychol Med *20:* 547, 1990.

Martin E, Robertson L, Sorensen D, Jagust W, Mallon K, Chirurgi A: Speed of memory scanning is not affected in early HIV-1 infection. J Clin Exp Neuropsychol *15:* 311, 1993.

McArthur J C, Becker P S, Parisi J E, Trapp B, Selnes O A, Cornblath D R, Balakrishnan J, Griffin J W, Price D: Neuropathological changes in early HIV-1 dementia. Ann Neurol *26:* 681, 1989.

*McArthur J C, Cohen B A, Selnes O A, Kumar A J, Cooper K, McArthur J H, Soucy G, Cornblath D R, Chmiel J S, Wang M, Starkey D L, Ginzburg H, Ostrow D G, Johnson R T, Phair J P, Polk B F: Low prevalence of neurological and neuropsychological abnormalities in otherwise healthy HIV-1 infected individuals: Results from the Multicenter AIDS Cohort Study. Ann Neurol *26:* 601, 1989.

McArthur J C, Hoover D, Bacellar H, Miller E, Cohen B, Becker J, Graham N, McArthur J H, Selnes O, Jacobson L: Dementia in AIDS patients: Incidence and risk factors: Multicenter AIDS Cohort Study. Neurology *43:* 2245, 1993.

Miller E N, Selnes O A, McArthur J C, Satz P, Becker J T, Cohen B A, Sheridan K, Machado A M, Van Gorp W G, Visscher B: Neuropsychological performance in HIV-1 infected homosexual men: The Multicenter AIDS Cohort Study (MACS). Neurology *40:* 197, 1990.

Navia B A, Jordan B D, Price R W: The AIDS dementia complex: I. Clinical features. Ann Neurol *19:* 517, 1986.

*Navia B A, Price R W: The acquired immunodeficiency syndrome dementia complex as the presenting or sole manifestation of human immunodeficiency virus infection. Arch Neurol *44:* 65, 1987.

Perry S, Marotta R F: AIDS dementia: A review of the literature. Alzheimer Dis Assoc Disord *1:* 221, 1987.
Prusiner S B: Prions and neurodegenerative diseases. N Engl J Med *25:* 1571, 1987.
Schmitt F A, Bigley J W, McKinnis R, Logue P E, Evans R W, Drucker J L, AZT Collaborative Working Group: Neuropsychological outcome of zidovudine (AZT) treatment of patients with AIDS and AIDS-related complex. N Engl J Med *319:* 1573, 1988.
Seilhean D, Duyckaerts C, Vazeux R, Bolgert F, Brunet P, Katlama C, Gentilini M, Hauw J: HIV-1-associated cognitive/motor complex: Absence of neuronal loss in the cerebral neorcortex. Neurology *43:* 1492, 1993.
Selnes O A, Miller E, McArthur J, Gordon B, Mu oz A, Sheridan K, Fox R, Saah A J, Multicenter AIDS Cohort Study: HIV-1 infection: No evidence of cognitive decline during the asymptomatic stages. Neurology *40:* 204, 1990.
*Serban D, Taraboulos A, DeArmond S J, Prusiner S B: Rapid detection of Creutzfeldt-Jakob disease and scrapie prion proteins. Neurology *40:* 110, 1990.
Simon R P: Neurosyphilis. Arch Neurol *42:* 606, 1985.
Van Gorp W G, Miller E N, Satz P, Visscher B: Neuropsychological performance in HIV-1 immunocompromised patients: A preliminary report. J Clin Exp Neuropsychol *11:* 763, 1989.
Van Gorp W G, Satz P, Hinkin C, Miller E N, D'Elia L F: In *Neuropsychology of Alzheimer's Disease and Other Dementias,* R W Parks, R F Zec, R S Wilson, editors, p 153. Oxford University Press, New York, 1993.

2.8 NEUROPSYCHIATRIC ASPECTS OF ENDOCRINE DISORDERS

ROBERT A. STERN, Ph.D.
ARTHUR J. PRANGE, JR., M.D.

INTRODUCTION

Endocrine disorders are among the most common medical conditions that result in neuropsychiatric symptoms (Table 2.8-1). In many situations, without appropriate laboratory data, differential diagnosis between endocrine abnormalities and idiopathic psychiatric illness or degenerative dementia is difficult, if not impossible. Many of the psychiatric and neurocognitive manifestations of the disorders are reversible if the underlying endocrine disturbance is diagnosed and treated in a timely fashion.

Among the endocrinopathies, thyroid disorders are most frequently associated with neuropsychiatric impairment. Perturbations of the hypothalamic-pituitary-thyroid (HPT) axis are cited as some of the most significant causes of reversible dementia and secondary psychiatric disturbance. This section focuses primarily on the HPT axis, including detailed descriptions of the physiology, epidemiology, causes, clinical features, laboratory examination procedures, and treatment of the major thyroid disorders. After that thorough review, brief clinical descriptions of two other endocrine systems associated with neuropsychiatric dysfunction are presented: disorders of the hypothalamic-pituitary-adrenal (HPA) axis and diabetes mellitus. Other endocrine disorders are associated with neuropsychiatric dysfunction, but the disorders discussed below are the most commonly observed and have received the most scientific study with regard to associated neuropsychiatric symptoms.

THYROID DISORDERS

Overt forms of thyroid dysfunction, such as myxedema and Graves' disease, have historically been associated with profound neuropsychiatric symptoms. In recent years, subclinical forms of thyroid disorder have also been linked to psychiatric and neurocognitive abnormalities. Differential diagnosis of primary psychiatric illness and thyroid disorder is difficult but crucial for making appropriate treatment decisions. The causal relation between thyroid dysfunction and neuropsychiatric symptoms is easily shown in patients without any personal or family history of psychiatric illness in whom the emergence of behavior change is temporally associated with alterations in thyroid hormone levels. However, differential diagnosis is more difficult when the patient has psychiatric or neurocognitive symptoms that predate the clinical manifestations and hormonal

TABLE 2.8-1
Physical and Neuropsychiatric Signs and Symptoms of Select Endocrine Disorders

Endocrine Disorder	Physical Signs and Symptoms	Neuropsychiatric Symptoms
Hyperthyroidism	Heat intolerance, tachycardia, appetite increase, weight loss, warm skin, bowel changes, hyperactive reflexes, goiter, exophthalamus (in Graves' disease)	Irritability, anxiety, emotional lability, mood may resemble agitated depression or (in elderly) apathetic depression, restlessness, distractibility, problem-solving and organization difficulties, possibly psychosis, decreased sleep
Hypothyroidism	Cold intolerance, bradycardia, weight gain, dry thickened skin, delayed reflexes, constipation	Fatigue, abulia, lethargy, depression, occasional psychosis, generalized neurocognitive impairment with mental slowing and diminished attention
Hypercortisolism (Cushing's syndrome)	Central obesity, hypertension, muscle wasting, moon facies, hirsutism, impotence or menstrual dysfunction, abdominal striae, glucose intolerance, osteoporosis	Secondary to endogenous glucocorticoids: anxiety, depression, suicidal ideation, diminished memory, spatial deficits Secondary to exogenous glucocorticoids: euphoria, irritability, pressured speech, diminished memory, psychosis
Hypocortisolism (Addison's disease)	Weakness, weight loss, fatigue, skin pigmentation, hypotension, abdominal symptoms, hypoglycemia	Apathy, depressed mood, anhedonia, negativism, occasional psychosis, global neurocognitive impairment, stupor
Hyperglycemia (diabetes mellitus)	Fatigue, polydipsia, polyuria, polyphagia, blurry vision, occasional impotence	Fatigue, lethargy, depression, global neurocognitive impairment, stupor, coma
Hypoglycemia	Weakness, sweating, tachycardia, tremulousness, tingling of lips and extremities	Acute phase: anxiety, panic, confusional state Chronic phase: depression, psychosis, changes in personality, global neurocognitive impairment

alterations of a thyroid disorder. Similarly troublesome is the presentation of neuropsychiatric symptoms in the presence of subclinical thyroid alterations that are diagnosed only by less routine laboratory tests. Many of the clinical signs and symptoms of thyroid disorders are similar to those of psychiatric illnesses, such as mood and anxiety disorders. Familiarity with the shared and unshared signs and symptoms aids in the diagnostic dilemmas.

DEFINITION

Hypothalamic-pituitary-thyroid axis The hypothalamic-pituitary-thyroid *(HPT)* axis is a homeostatically controlled system that involves both central (hypothalamus) and peripheral (pituitary and thyroid glands) tissues (Figure 2.8-1) and the secretions from those tissues (Table 2.8-2). Thyroid hormones affect virtually every organ and tissue in vertebrates. In many cases the effects are a direct result of hormonal action, but in other situations the effects are secondary to hormones with which the thyroid hormones interact. With respect to thyroid hormone effects on the brain, the relation is even more complicated because of the numerous interactions that thyroid hormones and other secretions of the HPT axis have with neurotransmitter and neuropeptide systems.

In general, the principal role of *thyroid hormones* is to govern the overall metabolic rate of the body. Metabolism is also influenced by many other variables, but its rate is generally proportional to the amount of available thyroid hormones. Not only do the hormones affect numerous sites throughout the body, but they also act at multiple sites within a given cell.

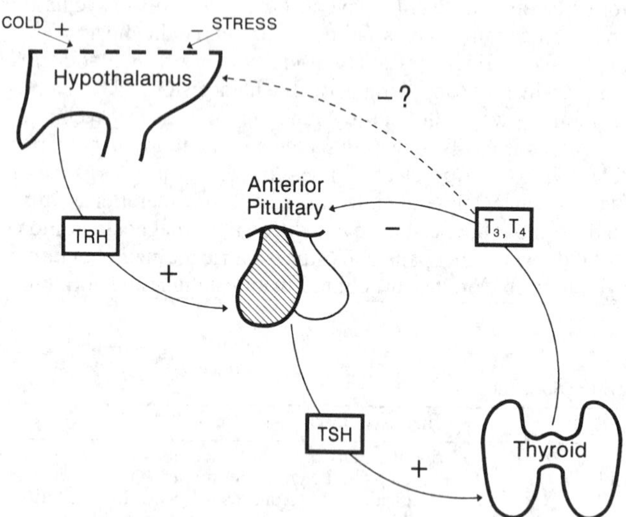

FIGURE 2.8-1 *The hypothalamic-pituitary-thyroid axis. (Prepared by Lisa Duke.)*

Thyrotropin-releasing hormone and thyroid-stimulating hormone Thyroid-releasing hormone *(TRH)* is a tripeptide that is secreted from the hypothalamus into the hypothalamic-pituitary portal venous system. The release of TRH is governed by numerous factors, including inhibition from stress and stimulation from cold. TRH is carried to the anterior pituitary, where it binds to membrane receptors on thyrotroph cells. Those cells then respond by releasing thyroid-stimulating hormone *(TSH)* into the general circulation. TSH subsequently binds to receptors on thyroid cells, inducing the production and the release of thyroid hormones.

Thyroid hormones The thyroid synthesizes and releases two hormones, tetraiodothyronine (thyroxine, T_4) and triiodothyronine (T_3), into the general circulation. Approximately 80 percent of serum T_3 is produced through the deiodination of T_4 by peripheral tissues and not through direct secretion from the thyroid. In general, T_3 is the active hormone in the periphery; T_4 must be deiodinated to T_3 to have a metabolic effect on tissues. In that respect, T_4 serves primarily as a prohormone for the active T_3. Within the circulation, T_3 and T_4 are quickly bound to three proteins: thyroxine-binding globulin (TBG), thyroxine-binding prealbumin (TBPA), and albumin. That avid binding results in less than 1 percent of T_3 and less than 0.1 percent of T_4 remaining unbound or free and, thus, active. By negative feedback, the unbound T_3 and T_4 diminish TSH and, possibly, TRH secretion.

Free-circulating thyroid hormone concentrations are carefully regulated to maintain appropriate metabolic homeostasis. When free T_3 and T_4 concentrations are out of their normal ranges (Table 2.8-3), they almost always indicate HPT axis dysfunction or systemic illness. However, in special circumstances when decreased peripheral metabolism is needed, such as in starvation and some medical illnesses, the careful homeostasis of thyroid function is shifted. In those instances T_4 is converted to an inert stereoisomer of T_3, reverse T_3 (rT_3). Although it is adaptive in those circumstances to have diminished metabolism in the periphery, the thyroid economy of the brain must remain intact. The exact mechanisms for the process are not yet fully known; two mechanisms may be involved: First, unlike other organs and tissues, the brain appears to use T_4 as its active thyroid hormone. Second, the brain tissue may be uniquely efficient in converting T_4 to T_3.

HYPERTHYROIDISM

History Caleb Parry first described hyperfunction of the thyroid in 1825, attributing the condition to traumatic fear. In 1835 Robert Graves also suggested that a patient's psychological state could play a role in the development of hyperthyroidism, linking it in particular to globus hystericus in women. That relation between psychological state and the

TABLE 2.8-2
Hormones of the Hypothalamic-Pituitary-Thyroid Axis

Hormone	Abbreviation	Primary Origin	Principal Function
Thyrotropin-releasing hormone	TRH	Hypothalamus	Stimulates synthesis and release of TSH; is also a neuromodulator, with several non-HPT-axis functions in the central nervous system (CNS)
Thyroid-stimulating hormone	TSH	Anterior pituitary	Stimulates synthesis and release of thyroid hormones
Thyroxine	T_4	Thyroid gland	Precursor of T_3; may be active hormone in brain
Triiodothyronine	T_3	Thyroid gland; deiodination of T_4 by peripheral tissues	Primary determinant of metabolism in periphery (with possible exception of brain)
Reverse triiodothyronine	rT_3	Deiodination of T_4 by peripheral tissues	Inhibits T_4 to T_3 deiodination; role in brain unknown

TABLE 2.8-3
Laboratory Tests of Hypothalamic-Pituitary-Thyroid Axis Function

Test	Measurement Technique	Approximate Range*
Total T_4	RIA	4–12 μg/dL
Total T_3	RIA	70–190 μg/dL
T_3 resin uptake (T_3U)	Resin uptake of labeled T_3	40–60% saturation
Free thyroxine index (FTI)	Calculated from total T_4 and T_3U	1.5–5.5
TSH	IRMA	0.5–3.5 μU/mL
TRH-stimulation test	TSH measured 0, 15, 30, 45 min after IV administration of 500 μg TRH	ΔTSH > 5 μU/mL

*Reference ranges vary among laboratories and specific assay kits. T_4 = thyroxine; T_3 = triiodothyronine; TSH = thyroid-stimulating hormone; TRH = thyrotropin-releasing hormone; RIA = radioimmunoassay; IRMA = immunoradiometric assay.

onset of hyperthyroidism has since received much attention. In the early 20th century Walter Cannon explored the role of environmental excitation in the onset of hyperthyroidism. In 1951 George Ham proposed a mechanism in which the breakdown of psychological adaptation leads to hyperthyroidism. To date, however, an animal model of the stress-hyperthyroid mechanism has not been successfully constructed, and empirical studies in humans have been inconclusive.

In addition to the causal role of psychological state in hyperthyroidism, the neuropsychiatric symptoms secondary to hyperthyroidism have been described historically. The reason for the historical connection between thyroid dysfunction and neuropsychiatric abnormalities is clear to any practitioner who has examined a hyperthyroid patient. As described below, many of the cardinal features of the disorder are behavioral, such as nervousness, irritability, and diminished concentration. Although the neuropsychiatric symptoms of hyperthyroidism are traditionally described in endocrinology textbooks, there has been surprisingly little objective, empirical investigation of the neuropsychiatric correlates of Graves' disease and other forms of hyperthyroidism.

Nosology *Thyrotoxicosis* is characterized by excessive amounts of circulating thyroid hormones. The term ''hyperthyroidism,'' frequently used as a synonym, is often used in a narrower sense, implying the condition resulting from the production of excessive amounts of thyroid hormones by the thyroid gland. That definition contrasts with conditions arising from the overingestion of thyroid hormone medications. *Subclinical or preclinical hyperthyroidism* is a term used when a patient has normal circulating thyroid hormone levels in the presence of a blunted to absent TSH response to exogenous TRH (that is, to a TRH-stimulation test).

Epidemiology The prevalence of hyperthyroidism in the general population is about 0.5 percent. Graves' disease is the most common cause of hyperthyroidism, accounting for more than 80 percent of cases. Toxic multinodular goiter accounts for about 10 percent of cases, and toxic adenoma accounts for 5 percent of cases. The remaining cases are caused by a variety of conditions, such as hydatidiform moles and choriocarcinomas, iodine supplementation, and pituitary resistance to the negative feedback from circulating thyroid hormones.

This section focuses on Graves' disease, since it is by far the most common cause of hyperthyroidism. Graves' disease occurs predominantly in women, with only 20 to 30 percent of the cases involving men. Although it may present at any age, the majority of cases occur during the third and fourth decades of life.

Etiology Graves' disease is an autoimmune disorder in which an antibody to the TSH receptor on the thyroid follicular cell causes stimulation of the receptor and eventually thyrotoxicosis. Although the cause of the production of the antibody, thyroid-stimulating immunoglobulin, is unclear, Graves' disease appears to be familial. The presence of antithyroid antibodies and the genetic loading for Graves' disease both militate against the purely psychogenic cause for the disorder that has been postulated since it was first described.

Clinical features The classic features of Graves' disease are goiter, weight loss in the presence of increased appetite, weakness, palpitations and arrhythmias, heat intolerance, warm moist skin, excessive perspiration, dyspnea, tremor, hyperactive reflexes, amenorrhea or impotence, insomnia, fatigue, and muscle wasting. Ophthalmic involvement includes the retraction of the upper lid secondary to increased sympathetic tone and exophthalmos, a protrusion of the eyes caused by the deposition of mucopolysaccharides within the retro-orbital space and by edema. The ophthalmic disorders of Graves' disease may either run a parallel course to Graves' disease itself or progress independently.

In patients with disease of long duration, a variety of additional signs and symptoms may occur. They include onycholysis (loosening of the nail from its bed), dermopathy of Graves' disease (pretibial orange-peel thickening), and cardiomegaly.

In contrast to the typical presentation of Graves' disease, some elderly hyperthyroid patients exhibit an atypical clinical picture. Rather than the nervous, irritable, and hyperactive presentation of young patients, elderly patients exhibit apathy and depression as their primary symptoms. Patients with *apathetic thyrotoxicosis* often do not have a goiter and may be lacking the ophthalmic signs of classic Graves' disease. Instead, the clinical profile may include fatigue, temporalis muscle wasting, proximal myopathy, and a variety of cardiac abnormalities, including heart block and atrial fibrillation.

PSYCHIATRIC FEATURES Frequently, the behavioral and psychiatric manifestations of hyperthyroidism lead patients to treatment. Too often, the symptoms result in misdiagnosis and subsequent mistreatment. The most common psychiatric complaints include emotional lability, nervousness, restlessness, irritability, fatigue, and insomnia. In general, the presentation is similar to that seen in agitated depression and in anxiety disorders. In those patients who report anxiety symptoms, the picture is usually similar to generalized anxiety disorder, although cases of social phobia and panic disorder (with and without agoraphobia) have been described. Although depressive symptoms are frequently reported, both the hyperthyroidism symptoms and the thyroxine level appear to correlate with the severity of the anxiety symptoms and not with depression.

In thyroid storm (an increasingly rare condition, probably because of early detection and treatment of hyperthyroidism), the psychiatric features may be marked and include psychosis and profound agitation. Elderly hyperthyroid patients with apathetic thyrotoxicosis appear depressed and exhibit significant psychomotor retardation. They may be indistinguishable from patients with major depressive disorder.

As in many secondary psychiatric disorders, the symptom complex of hyperthyroidism does not necessarily include actual mood state changes consistent with a primary mood or anxiety disorder. That is, the hyperthyroid patient may show several of the symptoms of anxiety or depression but may not report feeling dysphoric or anxious.

Many of the signs and symptoms of hyperthyroidism are

shared with anxiety disorders; nevertheless, each disorder also has unique symptoms (Table 2.8-4). Several of the shared signs and symptoms are most likely due to the increased nonadrenergic function directly caused by thyrotoxicosis. Some signs that are related to increased peripheral sympathetic tone are diminished when patients are given β-adrenergic antagonists (β-blockers), a common initial treatment for Graves' disease. However, many of the neuropsychiatric complaints of hyperthyroid patients are probably due to the central effects of the thyroid hormones themselves.

NEUROPSYCHOLOGICAL FEATURES Hyperthyroid patients frequently complain of a variety of neuropsychological difficulties. The most typical complaints are of poor attention, diminished concentration, and memory problems. However, only a few comprehensive, objective neuropsychological investigations of hyperthyroid patients have been reported in the literature. The results of existing studies indicate a variety of subtle deficits, including diminished concentration and memory. In addition, some studies have revealed diminished reaction times, especially on tasks requiring visual discrimination. Many of the tests on which hyperthyroid patients perform poorly involve complex visual processing, conceptualization, and the organization of spatial information. The patients may also have impairments in executive functioning and mental flexibility.

Many of the neurocognitive difficulties exhibited in hyperthyroid patients are possibly secondary to peripheral sympathetic hyperactivity (for example, poor concentration). However, just as with the psychiatric symptoms, some of the neurocognitive impairments may be due to central dysfunction, directly or indirectly caused by the disruption of the brain's thyroid economy. Several of the neuropsychological symptoms appear to be clinically consistent with prefrontal lobe dysfunction (for example, organization, conceptualization, mental flexibility). Specific functional imaging techniques capable of elucidating regional metabolic dysfunction—such as positron emission tomography (PET), single photon emission computed tomography (SPECT), and magnetic resonance imaging (MRI) spectroscopy—have not yet been used in this population. Nonetheless, electroencephalogram (EEG) and evoked potential studies, both in patients with Graves' disease and in healthy volunteers, suggest that alterations in the thyroid state have a variety of nonspecific electrophysiological effects.

On the basis of self-reports and objective measurements, most neuropsychological symptoms appear to remit after successful treatment of the hyperthyroidism. However, some of the neurocognitive deficits may be irreversible in patients with long-standing hyperthyroidism. Comprehensive, longitudinal follow-up studies have yet to be conducted.

TABLE 2.8-4
Clinical Signs and Symptoms of Hyperthyroidism and Anxiety

Hyperthyroidism Only	Anxiety Only	Hyperthyroidism and Anxiety
Goiter	Anxious or dysphoric mood	Shakiness
Exophthalmos	Fear of dying	Palpitations
Heat intolerance	Dizziness	Sweating
Warm moist skin	Unreality	Decreased sleep
Increased appetite	Chest pain	Fatigue
Weight loss	Faintness	Shortness of breath
Amenorrhea or impotence		Nervousness
Hyperactive reflexes		Irritability
Muscle wasting		Diminished concentration
Onycholysis		

Although the specific mechanisms underlying the effects of thyrotoxicosis on mental functioning are not yet known, possibilities abound. For example, one theory holds that thyroid hormones increase central β-adrenergic receptor sensitivity to norepinephrine. Another possible mechanism involves the γ-aminobutyric acid (GABA) system. Thyroid hormones have been shown to inhibit GABA uptake. That inhibition would, in turn, lead to increased GABAergic transmission and to alterations of other interrelated neurotransmitter systems (for example, dopamine).

LABORATORY EXAMINATION The initial screen for suspected hyperthyroidism should include serum T_4 levels and an estimation of the free thyroxine index (FTI), which is a product of total T_4 and T_3 resin uptake (T_3U) (Table 2.8-3). Elevation of the FTI alone, however, does not identify the cause of the specific thyrotoxic disorder. Serum T_3 is elevated in most cases of hyperthyroidism, regardless of cause, and, except in specific situations, is not necessary to make the diagnosis of hyperthyroidism. The ultrasensitive immunoradiometric assay (IRMA) techniques can measure TSH levels as low as 0.01 μU/mL and are helpful in the determination of hyperthyroidism.

The TRH-stimulation test may be useful in patients who are suspected of having hyperthyroidism but in whom the results of traditional thyroid function tests are negative or equivocal. In the TRH-stimulation test the patient is administered TRH intravenously after a baseline serum TSH level is obtained. While the patient is supine, TSH levels are then determined at set intervals. The normal, positive response is a rise of at least 5 μU/mL above the baseline. In hyperthyroid patients the response is abolished; a positive response, therefore, excludes hyperthyroidism.

To make a conclusive diagnosis, especially in those patients without overt clinical signs (for example, exophthalmos, pretibial dermopathy), the clinician should order a thyroidal radioactive iodine uptake (RAIU) test. That test involves administering a trace amount of radioactive iodine orally and subsequently determining the amount of radioactivity taken up by the thyroid, using an external detector or scan. Elevated uptake is found in Graves' disease, whereas low RAIU is seen in such conditions as subacute thyroiditis and painless thyroiditis.

Treatment Antithyroid drugs are the backbone of hyperthyroidism treatment. The thionamides, propylthiouracil (PTU) and methimazole (Tapazole), block the synthesis of thyroid hormones by inhibiting thyroperoxidase. In addition, PTU but not methimazole blocks the peripheral deiodination of T_4 to T_3. β-Adrenergic blockers are frequently prescribed as adjuvant therapy with antithyroid medications. The β-adrenergic blockers result in rapid symptomatic improvement by blocking the increased adrenergic activity associated with hyperthyroidism. Such medications also appear to reduce serum T_3 levels by diminishing T_4 to T_3 conversion.

Medications alone are frequently insufficient in the treatment of hyperthyroidism. Radioactive iodine (RAI) has become the definitive therapy for the disorder. In the procedure, I^{131} is administered, resulting in the gradual ablation of the thyroid gland, typically over a six-month period. Many nuclear medicine practitioners and endocrinologists prescribe thyroxine soon after I^{131} treatment. Others wait until the overt signs and symptoms of hypothyroidism develop before starting replacement therapy. Many patients require two or more doses of I^{131} before adequate thyroid destruction can be achieved.

Surgical ablation of the thyroid gland, most typically subtotal thyroidectomy, has been a form of treatment for more than 50 years. However, the procedure has several potential complications, such as hypoparathyroidism, laryngeal nerve palsy, and keloids. Furthermore, many patients have recurrent hyperthyroidism after surgery and require additional treatment. In general, thyroidectomy is used only if other forms of treatment are not possible, as in cases of allergy to thionamides and unwillingness to undergo I^{131} therapy.

In most cases, successful treatment of the hyperthyroidism itself is effective in reducing the neuropsychiatric symptoms.

β-Blockers in conjunction with antithyroid medications ameliorate many of the symptoms of anxiety. Adjunctive psychopharmacological treatment remains controversial. Tricyclic antidepressants are typically contraindicated and have the risk of central toxicity. Although lithium (Eskalith) has antithyroid properties of its own, it is generally avoided in Graves' disease because of the possibility of exacerbating the exophthalmos. Occasionally, antipsychotics are needed in severely agitated or psychotic patients, although haloperidol (Haldol) has been found to result in neurotoxicity and possibly the initiation of thyroid storm. Case reports have suggested that electroconvulsive therapy may be helpful in alleviating severe agitated depression symptoms in hyperthyroid patients.

Subclinical hyperthyroidism The terms "subclinical hyperthyroidism" and "preclinical hyperthyroidism" are used when patients are clinically euthyroid with normal circulating thyroid hormone levels but exhibit a blunted to absent TSH response to exogenous TRH. That finding is occasionally observed in patients who have been previously treated for Graves' disease and in patients in the early stages of hyperthyroidism. Subclinical hyperthyroidism has been associated with many of the same neuropsychiatric symptoms seen in overt hyperthyroidism, such as nervousness, tachycardia, tremor, fatigue, irritability, and diminished concentration. Blunted TSH responses have been observed in depressed patients without other thyroid abnormalities.

The neuropsychiatric symptoms seen in subclinical hyperthyroidism may be merely a reflection of mild sympathetic alterations. They may also reflect the brain's sensitivity to even mild changes in central thyroid economy. Comprehensive empirical investigation of the neuropsychiatric correlates of subclinical hyperthyroidism is needed. At this time, the issue of whether to treat patients with the disorder remains undecided.

HYPOTHYROIDISM

History William Gull first described the neuropsychiatric features of hypothyroidism in 1873, detailing a clinical picture of overall mental and physical slowing. The term "myxedema" was introduced in 1878 by William Ord, who postulated that the overall apathy, fatigue, and weariness of the patients was due to a "jelly-like" swelling of connective tissues. Ten years later, the Clinical Society of London released its classic report on myxedema. That report indicated that insanity, manifested by delusions and hallucinations, was seen in more than one third of the patients and that dementia was also observed in a significant number. Mental slowing was observed in all but 3 of 109 cases presented. Since that time, myxedema madness has been described in single case reports and in case series as embracing a variety of psychiatric symptoms, including striking personality changes, overt psychosis, and delirium.

Today, hypothyroidism remains one of the most common causes of reversible dementia and of new-onset psychiatric disturbance in the elderly. The striking and prevalent neuropsychiatric alterations associated with the endocrine disorder underscore the need for the psychiatrist to be keenly aware of differential diagnosis and treatment issues.

Nosology *Primary hypothyroidism* is typically of thyroidal origin and results in diminished circulating thyroid hormones and a lack of hormonal effects on body tissues. *Secondary hypothyroidism* results from hypopituitarism, and *tertiary hypothyroidism* results from hypothalamic dysfunction. Those two disorders can be distinguished from primary hypothyroidism by the presence of a low basal serum TSH concentration or by the lack of a TSH response to exogenous TRH.

Although the term *"myxedema"* is often used synonymously with hypothyroidism and sometimes severe hypothyroidism, it more accurately describes one aspect of the disorder—namely, the infiltration of the skin and other tissues with mucopolysaccharides, resulting in puffiness of the face, the hands, and the feet.

Overt or *grade I hypothyroidism* is the clinical condition of primary hypothyroidism with the typical signs and symptoms of hypothyroidism described below. It is associated with diminished serum thyroid hormone levels and elevated TSH (Table 2.8-5). In two grades of *subclinical hypothyroidism,* the serum thyroid hormone levels are within normal limits, and they may or may not have associated clinical symptoms (grades II and III hypothyroidism). *Grade II hypothyroidism* is defined by normal thyroid hormone levels and elevated baseline TSH. *Grade III hypothyroidism* is characterized by normal thyroid hormone and TSH levels with an elevated TSH response to exogenous TRH.

TABLE 2.8-5
Grades of Hypothyroidism

Grade	Free Thyroxine Index (FTI)	Basal TSH	Stimulated TSH*
I (overt)	↓	↑	↑
II (subclinical)	Normal	↑	↑
III (subclinical)	Normal	Normal	↑

*TSH test—TSH after administration of TRH.

Hashimoto's thyroiditis (chronic lymphocytic thyroiditis) is an autoimmune disorder that specifically affects the thyroid gland. Although the disorder may eventually lead to overt hypothyroidism and less often to hyperthyroidism, it is frequently asymptomatic, with the exception of a diffuse goiter.

Epidemiology Hypothyroidism has an overall prevalence of 0.5 to 1.0 percent, increasing to 2 to 4 percent in the elderly. Women are three to four times more likely to have hypothyroidism than are men. It occurs most commonly in the fifth and sixth decades of life. Both overt and subclinical hypothyroidism are common in rapid-cycling bipolar disorder.

Etiology Hypothyroidism has several potential causes. One of the most common causes is prior ablation of the thyroid gland, either through I^{131} therapy or by surgical resection. Another frequent cause is Hashimoto's thyroiditis, either in a symptomatic early stage or in later stages, when the chronic inflammation leads to significant thyroid dysfunction. Other potential causes include endemic iodine deficiency, the ingestion of antithyroid agents (for example, thionamides, thiocyanate), certain genetically determined thyroid hormone synthesis defects, and peripheral resistance to the effects of thyroid hormone.

Clinical features Hypothyroidism is characterized by the following signs and symptoms: reduced basal metabolic rate; dry, flaky, thickened, and cool skin; brittle, dry hair; lateral eyebrow hair loss; cold intolerance; myxedema (puffy face, hands, and feet); hoarse voice; weight gain in the presence of reduced food intake; delayed tendon reflexes; constipation; bradycardia and reduced cardiac output; hyperlipidemia; slightly elevated diastolic blood pressure; anemia (typically normocytic); and menorrhagia.

PSYCHIATRIC FEATURES The psychiatric manifestations of hypothyroidism have been observed for nearly 200 years. In fact, psychiatric symptoms may be the presenting complaint of patients with hypothyroidism. As with hyperthyroidism, differentiating the symptoms of hypothyroidism from those of a primary psychiatric disorder, such as major depressive disorder, is not an easy task (Table 2.8-6). For example, among the psychiatric symptoms of hypothyroidism are apathy, fatigue, anergia, suicidal ideation, emotional lability, overall slowing, diminished libido, delusions, increased sleep, and weight gain in the presence of decreased appetite.

Unlike hyperthyroidism, in which a specific alteration in mood state is not necessarily part of the symptom complex,

TABLE 2.8-6
Clinical Signs and Symptoms of Hypothyroidism and Depression

Hypothyroidism Only	Depression Only	Both Hypothyroidism and Depression
Cold intolerance	Weight loss	Depressed mood
Hyperlipidemia	Sleep decrease	Apathy
Brittle, dry hair	Appetite increase	Emotional lability
Eyebrow hair loss		Weight gain
Dry, thickened skin		Appetite decrease
Bradycardia		Sleep increase
Delayed reflexes		Fatigue, anergia
Myxedema		Diminished concentration
Reduced basal metabolic rate		Memory complaints
Anemia		Mental slowing
Menorrhagia		Diminished libido
Goiter		Suicidal ideation
		Delusions
		Constipation

hypothyroidism is often manifested by a dysphoric mood. That makes differential diagnosis challenging. In fact, in the elderly hypothyroid patient with complaints of dysphoria and suicidal ideation, laboratory data are essential to avoid misdiagnosis. That need has resulted in the routine practice of ordering thyroid hormone and TSH levels when patients present with depressive symptoms.

NEUROPSYCHOLOGICAL FEATURES In addition to the psychiatric symptoms described above, intellectual impairment was also part of the earliest clinical descriptions of hypothyroidism. Today, hypothyroidism should always be considered in the differential diagnosis of patients presenting with neurocognitive dysfunction. The typical presentation includes mental slowing and long response latencies, diminished concentration, and memory complaints. Surprisingly, given the prevalence of cognitive disturbance associated with hypothyroidism, few comprehensive neuropsychological investigations of large groups of hypothyroid patients have been conducted. Therefore, a specific neuropsychological profile of hypothyroid patients does not yet exist.

Some evidence indicates that in many patients the neuropsychological impairments caused by hypothyroidism may not completely remit after replacement hormone therapy. That may be due to neuronal death, associated with long-standing hypothyroidism.

The cause of the neuropsychiatric symptoms observed in hypothyroidism is unclear. Among the many hypothesized mechanisms are decreased central β-adrenergic receptor sensitivity and diminished central metabolism, the latter manifested by alterations in cerebral blood flow, glucose, or oxygenation. Although no systematic functional neuroimaging studies of hypothyroid patients have used PET or SPECT, EEG studies have shown a variety of abnormalities. Many of the studies have revealed slowing and a reduction in the amplitude of dominant rhythms. In addition, visual evoked potentials often show long average latencies and small average amplitudes.

LABORATORY EXAMINATION A typical battery of diagnostic tests for hypothyroidism includes serum T_4, FTI, and TSH (Table 2.8-3). Serum TSH assays are highly sensitive and are the best single indicators of primary hypothyroidism; a low FTI, accompanied by elevated TSH concentrations, is diagnostic of hypothyroidism. However, because transient abnormalities have been observed in psychiatric patients, it is best to repeat the test before starting treatment.

Treatment The treatment of choice in hypothyroidism is synthetic sodium levothyroxine (Synthroid), which produces stable levels of both T_3 and T_4. In the treatment of hypothyroidism, both the patient and the clinician must realize that clinical improvement may take up to three months. Serum T_4 may return to the normal range in a matter of days. However, T_3 levels may take two to four weeks to normalize, and TSH frequently takes six to eight weeks to return to the normal range.

In most cases the neuropsychiatric symptoms of hypothyroidism remit with appropriate replacement hormone therapy, leading to euthyroidism. However, some patients, especially those who initially exhibit psychosis, may have an exacerbation of the neuropsychiatric symptoms during the initial phase of replacement therapy. With careful, low-dose therapy, their symptoms usually abate. Exacerbation of symptoms, mania in particular, may be most likely in patients whose psychiatric illnesses predated their endocrine disorders. Therefore, in all patients, especially in those with previous psychiatric disorders, care should be taken when initiating thyroid hormone replacement therapy.

Frequently, adjuvant psychotropic medications may be desirable when treating hypothyroidism. That is especially true in patients who are severely psychotic or delusional and in patients whose neuropsychiatric symptoms do not completely remit with thyroid hormone therapy and the subsequent return to a euthyroid state. Unfortunately, no controlled clinical trials of the efficacy of combined thyroid hormone and psychopharmacological treatment of hypothyroidism have been conducted. On the basis of anecdotal reports, antidepressant medications typically are not effective until euthyroidism is achieved. Lithium carbonate has antithyroid properties and subsequently is generally avoided in hypothyroid patients. Carbamazepine (Tegretol) does not lead to overt hypothyroidism but has been found to lower serum T_3 and T_4 levels. Additional anecdotal evidence indicates that hypothyroidism may lead to antipsychotic-induced cardiac dysrhythmias. Benzodiazepines may be safe in those patients, but their drug metabolism may be slowed by hypothyroidism.

Until recently, practitioners sometimes prescribed thyroid hormone as a treatment for generalized fatigue, without any supportive laboratory evidence of either overt or subclinical hypothyroidism. Perhaps even more inappropriate has been the prescription of thyroid hormone for the purpose of weight loss in euthyroid patients. Both practices are not supported by empirical findings and may be dangerous.

Subclinical hypothyroidism Subclinical or marginal hypothyroidism is defined by the laboratory findings of an elevated basal serum TSH or an exaggerated TSH response to TRH in the presence of normal thyroid hormone concentrations (Table 2.8-5). The condition is highly prevalent; it is thought to be present in at least 1 out of 20 persons. In women over the age of 60, the prevalence is reported to be as high as 15 percent. Although the common somatic manifestations of overt (grade I) hypothyroidism are not present in subclinical hypothyroidism, it is apparently not completely asymptomatic from a neuropsychiatric standpoint.

Some investigations have suggested that patients with subclinical hypothyroidism exhibit anergia, malaise, and abulia and that such symptoms may remit with thyroid hormone replacement therapy. Other uncontrolled and small sample studies have suggested that patients with subclinical hypothyroidism have subtle neuropsychological deficits, such as difficulties in selective attention and new learning. Evidence also indicates that patients with subclinical hypothyroidism have an increased lifetime history of depression, as compared with euthyroid controls. Subclinical hypothyroidism has also been found to occur frequently in patients with rapid-cycling bipolar disorder. However, whether the limited empirical evidence is strong enough to warrant thyroid hormone treatment for all patients who show the laboratory findings of subclinical hypothyroidism is unclear.

ADRENAL DISORDERS

The hypothalamic-pituitary-adrenal (HPA) axis is another endocrine system that has long been associated with neuropsychiatric functioning. Like the HPT axis, the HPA axis is a homeostatically controlled system, involving both central (hypothalamus) and peripheral (pituitary and adrenal cortex) tissues (Figure 2.8-2) and the secretions from those tissues. The hypothalamus releases *corticotropin-releasing hormone (CRH),* also referred to as corticotropin-releasing factor (CRF), which is transported by the hypothalamic-pituitary portal venous system to the anterior pituitary. CRH release varies diurnally and is influenced by stress. In the anterior pituitary, CRH interacts with receptors on *corticotropin*-producing cells, stimulating adrenocorticotropic hormone (ACTH) secretion. ACTH is then released into the general circulation and is carried to the adrenal cortex, where it interacts with receptors on adrenocortical cells, thus stimulating the production and the release of the glucocorticoid *cortisol.* Completing the loop, cortisol negatively feeds back to the hypothalamic release of CRH.

The adrenal cortex produces several steroid hormones in addition to cortisol, such as the mineralocorticoid aldosterone and several estrogens and androgens. Because of its importance to neuropsychiatry, however, only cortisol and its regulatory system receive attention in this section.

Cortisol, directly and through its effects on other hormones, has many functions. In addition to being the primary stress-response hormone, cortisol maintains vascular reactivity to catecholamines; functions in the regulation of carbohydrate, protein, and lipid metabolism; and modulates peripheral blood cell counts. Although the underlying neuropathological mechanisms are not yet fully understood, alterations in cortisol levels result in pronounced neuropsychiatric disturbances.

HYPERCORTISOLISM *Cushing's syndrome* is a family of disorders, each with different causes, which share the presence of excessive cortisol levels. *Cushing's disease* is characterized by excessive pituitary release of ACTH and is typically the result of a pituitary tumor. Occasionally, Cushing's disease is caused by increased hypothalamic secretion of CRH. Autonomously functioning adrenal tumors are another cause of hypercortisolism, as are ACTH-secreting ectopic tumors. In addition to those endogenous causes of hypercortisolism, the sustained exogenous administration of glucocorticoids can also lead to Cushing's syndrome and is by far the most common cause of the condition.

One of the most frequently occurring endocrine abnormalities associated with mood disorders is hypercortisolism, *pseudo-Cushing's syndrome.* For example, patients with major depressive disorder often exhibit elevated levels of cortisol and have abnormal findings on dexamethasone-suppression tests.

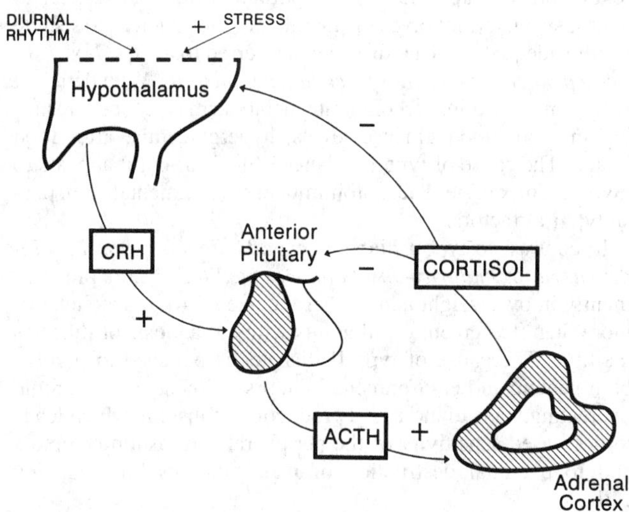

FIGURE 2.8-2 *The hypothalamic-pituitary-adrenal axis. (Prepared by Lisa Duke.)*

Clinical features Cushing's syndrome is characterized by centripetal obesity, hypertension, glucose intolerance, amenorrhea or impotence, hirsutism, purple abdominal striae, plethoric (moon) facies, proximal myopathy, osteoporosis, acne, and easy bruising. Although those signs and symptoms are recognized as the classic features of Cushing's syndrome, much variability is seen in their presentation.

PSYCHIATRIC FEATURES Psychiatric disturbance has been observed to be part of the clinical presentation of Cushing's syndrome since the earliest descriptions of the disorder. Most studies have revealed that psychiatric abnormalities occur in at least 50 percent of all Cushing's syndrome patients, with anxiety and depressed mood being the most common symptoms. Suicidal ideation, insomnia, irritability, emotional lability, and decreased libido are features often associated with the anxious depression seen in Cushing's syndrome. Although psychosis is not as common as anxiety and depression, it is seen in about 15 percent of cases.

In many patients, neuropsychiatric symptoms, such as irritability and diminished libido, may be the first presenting complaints of Cushing's syndrome, with the other physical signs and symptoms of the disorder following. The psychiatrist must be vigilant to the possibility that a differential diagnosis of even chronic psychiatric disturbance should include hypercortisolism. The dexamethasone-suppression test is often used as an initial screen for Cushing's syndrome. Since a positive result is frequently found in many patients with major depressive disorder but without endocrinopathy, additional laboratory assessment may be warranted.

Evidence suggests that the psychiatric presentation of patients with iatrogenic Cushing's syndrome (that is, it results from the administration of exogenous glucocorticoids) is different from that seen in patients with endogenously caused Cushing's syndrome. After the short-term administration of glucocorticoids, patients frequently report euphoria, hyperactivity, insomnia, increased appetite, and, occasionally, feelings of anxiety and irritability. The sense of well-being frequently leads to dependence and the abusive administration of the drugs. After the administration of glucocorticoids (at the equivalent daily dose of prednisone 40 mg) for several days, however, *steroid psychosis* may develop, but it typically remits on discontinuation of the medication.

NEUROPSYCHOLOGICAL FEATURES Few comprehensive studies of the neurocognitive correlates of Cushing's syndrome have been reported. On the basis of the limited available information, a specific profile of neuropsychological functioning does not appear to be present, but a wide variety of deficits are present. Among the deficits are difficulties in attention, concentration, memory, and spatial functioning. Although most patients with Cushing's syndrome exhibit neurocognitive abnormalities, many—perhaps up to one third—do not. Some evidence suggests that the neurocognitive dysfunction seen in Cushing's syndrome is related more to high ACTH levels than to high cortisol levels.

The few specific studies of the neuropsychological functioning associated with exogenously administered steroids suggest deficits in selective attention and memory. The memory impairment appears to involve errors of commission (that is, self-generated intrusions when recalling previously learned material), rather than errors of omission. That type of deficit is supported by electrophysiological data indicating that exogenous steroids diminish average evoked potential responses to relevant information but not to irrelevant information. In addition, some evidence indicates that the memory impairment is more intermittent in those patients than in patients with endogenous Cushing's syndrome.

The mechanisms underlying the neurocognitive deficits associated with hypercortisolism are not yet known. However, animal research links increased corticosterone levels to the damage of select hippocampal neurons, structures known to be important in both mood and memory functioning.

HYPOCORTISOLISM Hypocortisolism has three major causes. *Primary adrenocortical insufficiency* results from the destruction of the majority of the steroid-secreting tissues in the adrenal cortex. The pituitary is not impaired; therefore, diminished circulating corticosteroids result in increased ACTH. *Addison's disease,* an autoimmune disorder, accounts for 70 to 80 percent of the cases of primary adrenocortical insufficiency. Tuberculosis accounts for 10 to 20 percent of the cases, with the remaining cases caused by amyloidosis, hemochromatosis, sarcoidosis, neoplastic infiltration, adrenal hemorrhage, and previous bilateral adrenalectomy.

Secondary adrenocortical insufficiency is pituitary or hypothalamic dysfunction resulting in diminished ACTH or CRH or both, thereby reducing the adrenocortical output of glucocorticoids. The effect on mineralocorticoid production is minimal. A third cause of adrenocortical insufficiency is the *rapid withdrawal of corticosteroid medications* after long-term treatment (for example, corticosteroid-containing dermatological preparations) that had suppressed the HPA axis.

Clinical features The principal features of Addison's disease are fatigue, weakness, weight loss, hypoglycemia, and gastrointestinal symptoms. Because of the concomitant loss of mineralocorticoids in primary adrenocortical insufficiency syndromes such as Addison's disease, hypoaldosteronism also occurs. Consequently, symptoms of salt craving, sodium wasting, hypotension, hyperkalemia, hyponatremia, and metabolic acidosis are present. The increase in ACTH and melanocyte-stimulating hormone also leads to hyperpigmentation, usually localized to exposed areas (for example, knuckles, knees, scars) and around the lips.

PSYCHIATRIC FEATURES Psychiatric symptoms have been included in the clinical reports of Addison's disease since the initial description of the disorder in the mid-1850s. Although the underlying pathophysiology of Addison's disease is in some ways the opposite of Cushing's syndrome, the psychiatric profiles of the two disorders are similar. The most common psychiatric symptoms of Addison's disease are apathy, anhedonia, depressed mood, negativism, fatigue, and an overall poverty of thought; symptoms of anxiety are less common. Psychosis can occur in the acute phase of the disorder and can occasionally be as pronounced as delirium or stupor. In some cases the presenting features of Addison's disease may involve psychiatric symptoms, although those features are not as frequent as in the thyroid disorders and in Cushing's syndrome. Psychotropic medications are typically avoided in patients with Addison's disease because of the drugs' potential to exacerbate hypotensive episodes.

NEUROPSYCHOLOGICAL FEATURES The neurocognitive manifestations of Addison's disease are less well studied and documented than are the endocrine disorders previously described. Case descriptions mention impaired attention and concentration; in acute stages of the disease, generalized and severe cognitive dysfunction may occur. Some evidence suggests alterations in visual evoked potentials, including diminished amplitudes and prolonged latencies.

Although clinicians initially presumed that the neuropsychiatric symptoms associated with Addison's disease were due to diminished glucocorticoid levels, recent evidence suggests that some of the symptoms may result from the central nervous system (CNS) effects of increased ACTH or CRH.

DIABETES MELLITUS

Neurons require an appropriate amount of blood glucose for proper functioning. Disorders that result in either too much glucose (that is, *hyperglycemia*) or too little glucose (that is, *hypoglycemia*) in the CNS can, therefore, have significant neuropsychiatric ramifications. Unlike disorders of the HPT axis and the HPA axis, in which the direct or indirect effects of hormones on specific receptors in the CNS result in neuropsychiatric symptoms, disorders of glucose regulation produce their CNS effects by altering the availability of blood glucose to neuronal tissues.

The hormonal regulation of blood glucose involves two products of the pancreas, insulin and glucagon. *Insulin,* produced by the β cells of the pancreatic islets of Langerhans, lowers blood glucose levels and the levels of fatty acids and amino acids, aiding in the conversion to their respective storage forms of glycogen, triglycerides, and protein. *Glucagon,* synthesized by the α cells of the islets of Langerhans, affects similar metabolic pathways but generally in the opposite direction. The carefully balanced effects of both insulin and glucagon result in proper fuel metabolism and *normoglycemia* or euglycemia (Figure 2.8-3).

The autonomic nervous system appears to play an important role in insulin and glucagon regulation. For example, stress raises blood glucagon levels, probably through the sympathetic nervous system. Similarly, acetycholine and parasympathetic activation also increase glucagon levels.

The most frequently studied form of glucose metabolism dysregulation, perhaps the most important form with respect to neuropsychiatry, involves the inability of the pancreas to secrete insulin adequately. That disorder is referred to as *type I* or *insulin-dependent* or *juvenile-onset diabetes mellitus.* With deficient secretion of insulin, carbohydrate metabolism is reduced, resulting in high blood glucose levels, hyperglycemia, after food intake. The cause of type I diabetes is unclear, but it appears to involve a mix of genetic, autoimmune, environmental, and, possibly, viral factors.

In contrast to type I diabetes, *type II diabetes* (*non-insulin-dependent* or *maturity-onset diabetes mellitus*) occurs predominantly in overweight adults over the age of 40. It accounts for more than 90 percent of all adults with a diagnosis of diabetes mellitus. The cause of type II diabetes is believed to involve both genetic and environmental factors. In most cases, chronic overeating leads to increased production of insulin, which leads to decreased sensitivity of the peripheral cell insulin receptors and to eventual destruction of pancreatic insulin-producing cells.

CLINICAL FEATURES The onset of type I diabetes typically represents a medical emergency. Initial clinical features include

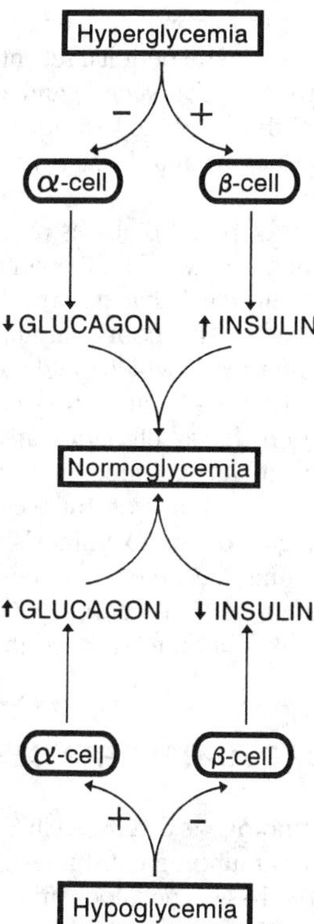

FIGURE 2.8-3 *The effects of hyperglycemia and hypoglycemia on the pancreatic secretion of insulin and glucagon. (Prepared by Lisa Duke.)*

polyuria, polydipsia, polyphagia, and rapid weight loss. Additional symptoms may include blurred vision, fatigue, nausea and vomiting, and shortness of breath. If the disease is left untreated, ketoacidosis and marked dehydration may occur and eventually lead to stupor, diabetic coma, and death. The long-term medical consequences of type I diabetes include increased risk of cerebrovascular disease, myocardial infarction, kidney disease, neuropathies, and ophthalmic disorders.

Treatment of type I diabetes involves the injection of exogenous insulin. Because of the lack of adequate endogenous metabolic control, a common and potentially dangerous result of treatment is hypoglycemia, both chronic and acute. The clinical features of hypoglycemia include weakness, sweating, tachycardia, tremulousness, and tingling of the lips and the extremities. In acute hypoglycemia, seizures, confusional state, and coma may result.

The onset of type II diabetes is more insidious than that of type I diabetes and rarely presents as a medical emergency. Although the long-term medical consequences (for example, cerebrovascular disease, myocardial infarction, neuropathies) are similar to those of type I diabetes, patients with type II diabetes do not typically experience ketoacidosis and subsequent coma.

Because of the significant effects of dysregulation of glucose metabolism on the brain, neuropsychiatric symptoms are frequently observed in both type I and type II diabetes. The brain depends on the constant availability of blood glucose to maintain proper functioning. In central thyroid hormone homeostasis the brain appears to be somewhat protected from peripheral changes in thyroid hormone availability, but the brain does not have compensatory mechanisms to protect itself from fluctuations in blood glucose levels. The body, by contrast, has robust mechanisms that respond to hypoglycemia. Among the mechanisms are the release of growth hormone and cortisol, stimulation of the sympathetic nervous system, and the secretion of epinephrine. The arousal of the autonomic nervous system (adrenergic features), along with the direct depression of the CNS (neuroglucopenic features), leads to a variety of the neuropsychiatric symptoms observed in diabetes. *Acute hypoglycemia* may result in both the adrenergic and the neuroglucopenic signs, whereas *chronic hypoglycemia* may be associated with only the neuroglucopenic features.

Psychiatric features As early as the 17th century, reports of diabetes mellitus included descriptions of accompanying depression. Since that time, depression and occasionally mania have been viewed as part of the clinical picture of diabetes, both type I and type II. Recent studies of diabetes have found a lifetime prevalence of major depressive disorder as high as 33 percent, a rate much greater than that found in most other chronic medical illnesses. Anecdotal reports associate manic symptoms and bipolar disorder with diabetes, but carefully controlled research has yet to substantiate those observations.

The cause of the major depressive disorder or depressive symptoms in diabetes is uncertain, but several possible causes exist. Among the possibilities are various psychological factors associated with having a chronic disease in general and diabetes specifically (for example, social isolation, stress, the need to maintain a strict dietary regimen, concern over and guilt surrounding dietary indiscretions). In addition, many patients with diabetes suffer from significant chronic pain secondary to diabetic neuropathy. In some of them, depressive symptoms may be a psychological reaction to pain, or pain and depression may share some underlying neuropathological mechanism. Some form of shared neuroendocrine dysfunction is another possible explanation for depression in diabetes. For example, many depressed psychiatric patients and nondepressed diabetic patients have in common an increased production of cortisol, suggesting a shared dysregulation of the HPA axis. Diabetes-induced vascular changes may produce cerebral ischemia and an associated depression.

The pharmacological treatment of mood disorders in diabetic patients poses some difficulties for the clinician. Many of the difficulties are related to the medical complications of diabetes, such as cardiovascular disease and neuropathy, and to the control of glucose metabolism itself. For example, many heterocyclic antidepressants block α-adrenergic receptors, thereby blunting the growth hormone response to hypoglycemia. There have also been reports of either increased or decreased blood glucose as a side effect of heterocyclics. Moreover, monoamine oxidase inhibitors have been associated with hyperglycemia. Electroconvulsive therapy has been observed to result in both decreases and increases of blood glucose in depressed diabetic patients.

In addition to the relation between diabetes mellitus and syndromal mood disorders, some evidence indicates that alterations in blood glucose result in specific mood state changes.

HYPERGLYCEMIA Mild or moderate hyperglycemia typically results only in fatigue. With chronic hyperglycemia, the patient often has a significant feeling of lethargy, depressed mood, and anorexia. Although uncommon, schizophreniclike symptoms may also occur in patients with long-standing chronic hyperglycemia.

HYPOGLYCEMIA Many of the psychiatric features of diabetes are caused by the autonomic arousal secondary to acute hypoglycemia. Among the symptoms are anxiety and feelings of panic, with accompanying palpitations and sweating. Acute hypoglycemia also has associated cerebral glucopenia, with accompanying headache, confusional state, and light-headedness. Chronic hypoglycemia typically does not result in autonomic arousal and its accompanying psychiatric symptoms. Rather, long-term decreases in blood glucose can cause such subtle symptoms as changes in personality characteristics, chronic depressive symptoms, and occasionally psychotic features.

Neuropsychological features Numerous investigators have studied the neuropsychological alterations associated with diabetes mellitus. There is now general agreement that diabetic patients (both type I and type II), compared with controls, exhibit a wide range of neurocognitive deficits, including impaired attention, information processing, memory, problem-solving abilities, visuoconstructional skills, and language functioning. In most studies of patients with type I diabetes, the degree of neuropsychological impairment has been strongly associated with the history of hypoglycemia (for example, the number of hypoglycemic unconsciousness events), rather than with the severity or the chronicity of the hyperglycemia. In type II diabetes, evidence suggests that many of the neurocognitive deficits are associated with or secondary to a depressed mood state.

Studies of the short-term effects of alterations in blood glucose also show that the brain is more sensitive to mild-to-moderate levels of hypoglycemia than it is to hyperglycemia.

HYPERGLYCEMIA Untreated *severe hyperglycemia* can lead to stupor and diabetic coma. In contrast, very little overt or subjective neurocognitive dysfunction appears to be directly associated with mild or even *moderate hyperglycemia* (that is, glucose concentrations of 300 mg/dL). Moderate chronic hyperglycemia is believed to be the cause of many of the vascular complications of diabetes, such as nephropathy, retinopathy, neuropathy, cardiovascular disorders, and cerebrovascular diseases (including both small and large vessels); most of those disorders have known neuropsychiatric complications. Therefore, neurocognitive dysfunction may occur as a *secondary complication* of hyperglycemia in diabetes.

Recent studies suggest that short-term increases in blood glucose may actually improve memory performance in nondiabetic animals and humans. And memory functioning may be enhanced in healthy elderly persons during periods of mild hyperglycemia, compared with periods of euglycemia. Neither the specific underlying mechanisms nor the clinical usefulness of those findings is clearly understood at this time.

HYPOGLYCEMIA Even mild drops in blood glucose levels can lead to significant alterations in neurocognitive functioning. Diabetic patients often have subjective feelings of thinking more slowly and of becoming more easily confused when their blood glucose levels are low than when the levels are normal. Objective investigations support those self-reports, indicating that diminished blood glucose in diabetic patients results in diminished attention, slowed information processing, and decreased fluency. Many of the neuropsychological features of hypoglycemia are consistent with those seen in patients with compromised function of the bilateral frontal lobes.

In addition to the effects of mild to moderate hypoglycemia, profound neuropsychological and neurological impairments result from severe drops in blood glucose levels. As the levels approach 40 mg/dL, slurred speech may become evident. Increasing overall cerebral impairment and, finally, seizures and coma occur when blood glucose levels drop to 10 to 15 mg/dL.

Type I diabetes typically presents in childhood, and the issue of developmental neuropsychological dysfunction has received a great deal of investigation. Several studies have described specific neuropsychological deficits and generalized learning and educational difficulties in both children and adolescents. Up to 25 percent of diabetic children have clinically evident cognitive dysfunction. Research indicates that the earlier in childhood the onset of diabetes, the greater are the neuropsychological impairments. One compelling explanation is that young children are more prone to experiencing hypoglycemic seizures than are older children and adolescents. The early seizure activity may subsequently lead to long-standing brain dysfunction. Therefore, in an adult with type I diabetes and neuropsychological deficits, it is difficult to distinguish among several causative factors, including long-standing developmental neuropsychological deficits, recently acquired impairment caused by chronic hypoglycemia and acute fluctuations in brain glucose availability, and the secondary effects of cerebrovascular disease, cardiovascular disease, renal failure, and ophthalmic impairment.

Ongoing treatment of type I diabetes requires the active participation of the patient. Frequently, the neurocognitive impairments in patients with type I diabetes result in limited understanding of their disease and in poor compliance with their complicated medical regimen, which includes careful insulin dosing, multistepped blood-sugar-testing procedures, and diet and caloric calculations based on anticipated physical activity. The neurocognitive deficits exhibited in the patients may appear on the surface to be mild or nonexistent because of the patient's compensatory strategies or the examiner's limited evaluation. Consequently, care must be given to obtain a detailed mental status examination or formal neuropsychological testing to assess the patient's likelihood to succeed in self-care.

SUGGESTED CROSS-REFERENCES

Psychoneuroendocrinology is discussed in Section 1.11. Neurochemical, viral, and immunological studies in schizophrenia are discussed in Section 14.4. The biochemical aspects of mood disorders are discussed in Section 16.3. Anxiety is discussed in Chapter 17. Endocrine and metabolic disorders as they relate to psychosomatic disorders are discussed in Section 26.6. Biological therapies are discussed in Chapter 32. The use of thyroid hormones to treat psychiatric disorders is discussed in Section 32.22. Children's reactions to illness are discussed in Section 47.4 and the psychiatric problems of the medically ill elderly in Section 49.6i.

REFERENCES

Braverman L E, editor: *Werner and Ingbar's The Thyroid: A Fundamental and Clinical Text,* ed 6. Lippincott, Philadelphia, 1991.

Cannon W B: *Bodily Changes in Pain, Hunger, Fear and Rage.* Macmillan, New York, 1941.

Graves R: Clinical lectures. Med Classics *5:* 35, 1940.

Gull W: On a cretinoid state supervening in adult life. Trans Clin Soc Lond *7:* 180, 1873.

Haggerty J J Jr, Stern R A, Mason G A, Beckwith J, Morey C E, Prange A J Jr: Subclinical hypothyroidism: A modifiable risk factor for depression? Am J Psychiatry *150:* 508, 1993.

Ham G, Alexander F, Carmichael H: A psychosomatic theory of thyrotoxicosis. Psychosom Med *13:* 19, 1951.

Haupt M, Kurz A: Reversibility of dementia in hypothyroidism. J Neurol *240:* 333, 1993.

*Holmes C S, editor: *Neuropsychological and Behavioral Aspects of Diabetes.* Springer, New York, 1990.

Holmes C S, editor: *Psychoneuroendocrinology: Brain, Behavior, and Hormonal Interactions,* Springer, New York, 1990.

Joffe R T, Levitt A J: Major depression and subclinical (grade 2) hypothyroidism. Psychoneuroendocrinology *17:* 215, 1992.

*Joffe R T, Levitt A J, editors: *The Thyroid Axis and Psychiatric Illness.* American Psychiatric Press, Washington, 1993.

Kathol R G, Delahunt J W: The relationship of anxiety and depression to symptoms of hyperthyroidism using operational criteria. Gen Hosp Psychiatry *8:* 23, 1986.

Loosen P T, Chambliss B, DeBold C R, Shelton R, Orth DN: Psychiatric phenomenology in Cushing's syndrome. Pharmacopsychiatry *25:* 192, 1992.

Monzani F, Del-Guerra P, Caraccio N, Pruneti C A, Pucci E, Luisi M, Baschieri L: Subclinical hypothyroidism: Neurobehavioral features and beneficial effects of *L*-thyroxine treatment. Clin Investig *71:* 367, 1993.

*Nemeroff C B, Loosen P T, editors: *Handbook of Clinical Psychoneuroendocrinology.* Guilford, New York, 1987.

Ord W M: On myxedema, a term proposed to be applied to an essential

condition in the "cretinoid" affection occasionally observed in middle-aged women. Roy Med Chir Soc Trans *61:* 57, 1878.
Osterweil D, Syndulko K, Cohen S N, Pettler-Jennings P D, Hershman J M, Cummings J L, Tourtellotte W W, Solomon D H: Cognitive function in nondemented older adults with hypothyroidism. J Am Geriatr Soc *40:* 325, 1992.
Parry C: *Collected Works,* vol 1. Underwoods, London, 1825.
Prange A J Jr, editor: *The Thyroid Axis, Drugs, and Behavior.* Raven, New York, 1974.
Ryan C M, Williams T M: Effects of insulin-dependent diabetes on learning and memory efficiency in adults. J Clin Exp Neuropsychol *15:* 685, 1993.
Schlote B, Schaaf L, Schmidt R, Pohl T, Vardarli I, Schiebeler H, Zober M A, Usadel K H: Mental and physical state in subclinical hyperthyroidism: Investigations in a normal working population. Biol Psychiatry *32:* 48, 1992.
Starkman M N, Gebarski S S, Berent S, Schteingart D E: Hippocampal formation, volume, memory dysfunction, and cortisol levels in patients with Cushing's syndrome. Biol Psychiatry *32:* 756, 1992.
Starkman M N, Schteingart D E: Neuropsychiatric manifestations of patients with Cushing's syndrome. Arch Intern Med *141:* 215, 1981.
Tallis F: Primary hypothyroidism: A case for vigilance in the psychological treatment of depression. Br J Clin Psychol *32:* 261, 1993.
Tarter R E, Van Thiel D H, Edwards K L, editors: *Medical Neuropsychology: The Impact of Disease on Behavior.* Plenum, New York, 1988.
Whelan T B, Schteingart D E, Starkman M N, Smith A: Neuropsychological deficits in Cushing's syndrome. J Nerv Ment Dis *168:* 753, 1980.
Whybrow P C, Prange A J Jr: A hypothesis of thyroid-catecholamine-receptor interaction. Arch Gen Psychiatry *38:* 106, 1981.
*Whybrow P C, Prange A J Jr, Treadway C R: Mental changes accompanying thyroid gland dysfunction. Arch Gen Psychiatry *20:* 48, 1969.
*Wilson J D, Foster D, editors: *Williams' Textbook of Endocrinology,* ed 8. Saunders, Philadelphia, 1991.
Wolkowitz O M, Reus V I, Weingartner H, Thompson K, Breier A, Doran A, Rubinow D, Pickar D: Cognitive effects of corticosteroids. Am J Psychiatry *147:* 1297, 1990.

2.9 NEUROPSYCHIATRIC ASPECTS OF HEADACHE

ELYSE J. SINGER, M.D.

INTRODUCTION

Headache (pain above the orbitomeatal line) is one of the most common and often one of the most frustrating symptoms that physicians evaluate. Diagnosis of headache is complicated by the complex anatomy and physiology of the head and the neck; by the confusing, often eponymous, nomenclature of headache syndromes; and by the many psychosocial factors that can influence pain.

HISTORY

The earliest physicians were consulted for headaches. The practice of trephining the skull to treat headache dates back as far as 3000 BC, and headaches are mentioned in the oldest medical writings. Modern descriptions of headache began in the 1800s.

A major contemporary advance came in 1962, when an ad hoc committee of the National Institutes of Health (NIH) published a headache classification system that was widely adopted by physicians. The NIH classification consisted of short descriptions of common headache types, grouped by the presumed mechanism. The NIH system lacked research diagnostic criteria, making it impossible to conduct accurate epidemiological studies. Continuing research into the pathogenesis of headache cast doubt on the accuracy of the NIH classification.

In 1988 the International Headache Society published a new classification that included research diagnostic criteria for different headaches and incorporated new hypotheses on pathophysiology. That system is part of the tenth revision of the *International Classification of Diseases and Related Health Problems* (ICD-10) and is used in this section.

EPIDEMIOLOGY

In Western societies headache occurs in more than 70 percent of the population. Women are afflicted slightly more often than men, although some headaches (for example, cluster headache) are more common in men than in women. The prevalence of headache declines after age 60. An epidemiological study using ICD-10 criteria found that, of the persons surveyed who had headache, 82 percent had tension-type headache, and 16 percent had migraine. A large United States pain study revealed that many headache sufferers—including persons with frequent, severe headaches—do not consult health care professionals. That finding suggests that data from tertiary-care referral centers may not accurately reflect the headache population, because those institutions do not attract a representative sample of persons with headache. That suggestion may be particularly relevant in studies of the personality characteristics of headache patients.

ETIOLOGY AND PATHOPHYSIOLOGY

Pain in the head can be generated by the stimulation of peripheral *nociceptors* (receptors that are preferentially sensitive to noxious or potentially tissue-damaging stimuli) or by the dysfunction of central or peripheral nervous system pathways. Pain-sensitive structures in the external head and neck include the skin, fasciae, muscles, eyes, external ears, auditory canals, the auditory apparatus, temporomandibular joints, tooth pulp, periodontia, the tongue, the mucosa of the oropharynx and the larynx and sinuses, and the periosteum of the craniofacial and upper cervical bones. Pain-sensitive intracranial structures include the great vessels of the brain, such as the venous sinuses and the large arteries; the meningeal arteries; portions of the dura proximal to the large blood vessels and cranial nerves V, VII, IX, and X and the upper three cervical nerves. The bone parenchyma, parts of the dura, most of the pia-arachnoid, the ventricular ependyma, and the choroid plexus are insensitive to pain, as is the brain parenchyma itself.

Craniofacial sensation (including the mouth, the anterior two thirds of the tongue, the supratentorial dura, and the cerebral vessels) is supplied primarily by cranial nerve V. Cranial nerve VII supplies a small area of mastoid skin, parts of the tympanic membrane and the external auditory meatus, the soft palate, and the pharynx. Cranial nerve IX supplies the posterior third of the tongue, portions of the pharynx, the soft palate, the tonsils, the eustachian tubes, and the tympanic cavity. Cranial nerve X supplies portions of the pharynx, the larynx, and the upper esophagus. The upper three cervical nerves supply the upper neck, the upper cervical vertebrae, and the occiput. Cranial nerves IX and X and the upper three cervical nerves innervate the posterior fossa, including the infratentorial dura and the blood vessels.

Exteroceptive pain sensation initiated by the stimulation of peripheral nociceptors travels centrally through the primary afferent nerve fibers (A delta or C fiber types). The cell bodies of the trigeminal primary afferent fibers are located in the trigeminal (semilunar, gasserian) ganglion in the middle cranial fossa. The central processes of those neurons (sensory root of cranial nerve V) enter the pons; those that convey pain, temperature, and soft touch descend as a group (the spinal tract of the trigeminal nucleus) to the caudal medulla and the upper cervical cord. As the spinal tract descends, it gives off fibers to the nucleus of the spinal tract of the trigeminal nerve, which parallels the downward course into the cervical cord. The central axonal processes of nociceptive V neurons synapse on second-order relay neurons in the spinal nucleus of the trigeminal nerve, which is divided into upper (pars ovalis), middle (pars interpolaris), and lowest (pars caudalis) subnuclei. The second-order neurons relay impulses to the contralateral brainstem, where they ascend in the ventral trigeminothalamic tract to synapse on neurons of the ventral posteromedial and intralaminar nuclei of the thalamus. From the thalamus, impulses are relayed to the somatosensory cortex. Considerable modulation (augmentation or suppression) of nociception can occur as sensation is processed.

Most nociceptive primary afferents carried in cranial nerves VII, IX, and X terminate in the nucleus of the solitary tract; and most nociceptive afferents from the upper three cervical nerves terminate in the dorsal horn of the spinal cord. However, a significant minority of nociceptive fibers—from cranial nerves VII, IX, and X and from the upper three cervical nerves—terminate in the trigeminal subnucleus caudalis, a part of the V spinal nucleus that is anatomically contiguous with and physiologically analogous to the dorsal horn of the spinal cord. That convergence of nociceptive input in the V subnucleus caudalis provides the anatomical substrate for widely referred pain in the head and the neck and for the substantial functional interactions between the upper cervical nerves and the cranial nerves.

About 20 percent of the primary afferent C fibers of cranial nerve V contain substance P, a peptide thought to be one of several nociceptive neurotransmitters. When activated, substance P-containing neurons fire impulses either orthodromically (centrally, to activate second-order relay neurons) or antidromically (retrograde, onto the peripheral structures supplied by the cranial nerves, such as blood vessels). Retrograde transmission of substance P, neurokinin A, and calcitonin gene-related peptide from C-fiber axons causes dilation of blood vessels, constriction of other smooth muscle cells, protein extravasation, glandular secretion, the release of histamine and serotonin from mast cells, the excitation of autonomic ganglia, and the local synthesis of prostaglandins and kinins. Similar substance P-containing neurons have been found in the geniculate ganglion of the facial nerve. The phenomena of blood vessel dilatation and protein exudation initiated by the retrograde discharge of substance P and other vasoactive neuropeptides has been called *neurogenic inflammation* and is thought to play an important role in the pathogenesis of migraine and cluster headaches.

Nociceptive stimulation also activates the brain's endogenous pain-control systems. Those systems include descending serotonergic (5-hydroxytryptamine [5-HT]) and noradrenergic (norepinephrenergic [NE]) nuclei that are thought to suppress incoming nociceptive transmission at the level of second-order neurons in the subnucleus caudalis and in the dorsal horn of the spinal cord, either by direct postsynaptic inhibition or through enkephalinergic interneurons. Derangements of central 5-HT and NE systems have been implicated in the pathogenesis of chronic pain and headache. Increased biological availability of 5-HT or NE in those pathways is a putative mechanism for the therapeutic effect of tricyclic antidepressants on chronic pain.

CLINICAL EVALUATION

Headache is a symptom, not a disease. Clinical evaluation should be directed toward the classification of the patient's headache; appropriate diagnosis is the basis for successful treatment. The most important factor in diagnosis is obtaining a thorough history. Physical examination and laboratory tests support hypotheses based on the history. The most common cause of headache misdiagnosis is failure to perform a complete history and physical examination, rather than the failure to perform enough laboratory tests. The diagnostic process begins by determining whether the headache is primary (caused by the derangement of normal physiology) or secondary to some underlying illness.

If the patient has more than one type of headache, each type should be described individually. Essential data include pain location, quality, time course, duration, age of onset, precipitating factors, ameliorating or exacerbating factors, and associated symptoms. Concurrent medical illnesses and a family history of headache should be pursued. The use of some medications or medication withdrawal may cause headache, and the patient's medication regimen should be reviewed. All patients should be asked about depression, anxiety, recent life stressors, and nonprescription drug or alcohol use. The examination should include vital signs; inspection of the tympanic membranes, the oropharynx, and the temporomandibular joint; funduscopy; range of motion in the cervical spine; palpation of the craniofacial and neck muscles; and a careful neurological examination, including mental status, cranial nerves, motor nerves, sensory nerves, coordination, and reflex function.

A computed tomography (CT) or magnetic resonance imaging (MRI) scan is often part of a headache evaluation. Neuroimaging is most likely to be productive if the patient has a new-onset headache disorder or new changes in an old headache especially after age 40 or if loss of consciousness, trauma, seizures, systemic illness that could involve the brain, fever, meningism, papilledema, or focal neurological signs are present. In most cases CT with contrast suffices. CT is less expensive, faster (making it easier to scan restless patients), and superior to MRI in the imaging of bone and fresh blood (for example, for head trauma and subarachnoid hemorrhage). CT can be used for patients with cardiac pacemakers and other magnetic devices. MRI is superior to CT in the evaluation of small lesions, vascular diseases, demyelinating diseases, cerebral infections, metabolic diseases, and posterior fossa lesions. Lumbar puncture should be preceded by neuroimaging in headache patients whenever possible to rule out mass lesions with the potential to cause herniation. Lumbar puncture is indicated to search for blood in the cerebrospinal fluid (CSF) that was missed by neuroimaging, to measure CSF pressure, and to diagnose intracranial infection or inflammation. Electrodiagnostic tests, such as electroencephalography and evoked potentials, usually add little to a headache evaluation.

MIGRAINE

Migraine is a separate ICD-10 classification, no longer included as a vascular headache, because of the debate about whether the pathophysiology is primarily neuronal or vascular. Migraines are stereotypic, recurrent phenomena that often occur in cycles. A positive family history is found in 50 to 60 percent of patients; 90 percent of migraine patients experience their first attack before age 40, often in early childhood.

Migraines afflict females more often than males.

MIGRAINE WITHOUT AURA Migraine without aura (common migraine) is characterized by headaches lasting 4 to 72 hours, with at least two of the following characteristics: unilateral location, pulsating quality, moderate to severe intensity, and aggravation by physical activity. The headache is associated with nausea, vomiting, and photophobia or phonophobia. Common but nondiagnostic associated symptoms include diarrhea, blurred vision, sensitivity to odors, lightheadedness, tenderness of the pericranial muscles and scalp and carotid arteries, flushing, pallor, and fluid retention before the attack, followed by diuresis during the attack, mood swings, and slowed thinking. Emotional stress, menses, glaring lights, physical exertion, fatigue, alcohol, hunger, head trauma, oral contraceptives, sleeplessness, and food containing vasoactive substances may trigger attacks.

MIGRAINE WITH AURA Migraine with aura (classic migraine, ophthalmic or hemiplegic migraine, migraine accompagnee, complicated migraine) is characterized by recurrent attacks of focal neurological symptoms (the aura) that can be localized to the cerebral cortex or the brainstem, usually develop over 5 to 20 minutes, last less than one hour, and are usually followed within an hour by headache, nausea, and photophobia. The headache typically lasts from 4 to 72 hours but may be completely absent.

Preceding the attack of migraine with aura, regional cerebral blood flow declines in the brain region that corresponds to the aura symptoms. Blood flow reduction usually starts posteriorly and spreads anteriorly in a nonvascular pattern and may persist for a prolonged period of time after the headache abates. The precise relation of cerebral blood flow to the aura symptoms or to the headache itself is unknown. After one to several hours, hyperemia develops in the same region. Regional cerebral blood flow changes have not been documented in migraine without aura.

Migraine with typical aura can be diagnosed when one or more of the following aura symptoms develop and completely recede, followed by the typical headache: homonymous visual disturbances (such as homonymous hemianopsia), scotomata (areas of depressed or absent vision surrounded by normal vision), photopsia (sensations of unformed flashes of light), unilateral paresthesias or numbness, unilateral weakness, aphasia, or other speech disturbance.

Migraine with prolonged aura (complicated migraine) is characterized by aura symptoms lasting from one hour to one week, without evidence of brain infarction on neuroimaging.

Basilar migraine is characterized by brainstem or bilateral occipital symptoms, such as visual changes afflicting both temporal fields and both nasal fields, dysarthria, vertigo, tinnitus, deafness, diplopia, ataxia, bilateral sensory or motor symptoms, and syncope.

Migraine aura without headache (migraine equivalent) consists of focal neurological symptoms without headache and must be differentiated from transient ischemic attacks.

OTHER MIGRAINES Other categories of migraine include *ophthalmoplegic migraine* (aura of paresis of one or more ocular cranial nerves); *retinal migraine* (monocular scotomata or amaurosis); *status migrainosus* (migraine headache lasting over 72 hours, despite treatment); and *migrainous infarction* (aura symptoms last more than three weeks and are associated with an infarction on CT scan).

PATHOPHYSIOLOGY Although no single hypothesis explains the entire pathophysiology of migraine, derangements of normal physiology have been reported, in addition to blood flow changes in migraine with aura, that may contribute to the pathophysiology of migraine. Plasma and platelet-bound 5-HT levels decrease during an attack, followed by a rise in urinary levels of 5-HT and its metabolites. Hyperaggregability of platelets in migraine patients has been reported and may be associated with the synthesis of prostaglandins and the release of 5-HT. In experimental paradigms, prostaglandin infusion is associated with the onset of migrainelike headache, nausea, dilatation of the extracranial arteries, and impaired cerebral autoregulation; some drugs that inhibit prostaglandin synthesis alleviate migraine. Some investigators postulate that trigeminal depolarization and the antidromic release of substance P onto the dura or the cranial arteries may initiate the process of neurogenic inflammation and cause headache and vascular changes. The concept of a migrainous personality has not been confirmed and has been largely discarded.

TREATMENT The treatment of migraine includes the avoidance of triggering factors, learned control over the autonomic nervous system to prevent or abort attacks, and pharmacotherapy. Infrequent attacks are treated symptomatically. Prophylaxis is recommended when attacks are frequent (more than two a month) or disabling.

Most of the effective drug therapies for migraine act at one or more subtypes of the 5-HT receptor. It is hypothesized that abortive antimigraine agents act at the 5-HT_1 receptor subtype whereas prophylactic antimigraine agents act at the 5-HT_2 and the 5-HT_{1C} receptors. Mild attacks may be relieved by rest, sleep, ice packs, or nonprescription analgesics.

Pharmacotherapy Drugs that are helpful in the treatment of migraine appear to share an affinity for 5-HT receptors. Ergotamine (Ergomar), a 5-HT_1 agonist and vasoconstrictor, alone or in combination preparation with caffeine (Cafergot, which contains 1 mg ergotamine and 100 mg caffeine), should be used immediately at the onset of an attack (for example, 1 mg of ergotamine by mouth at the onset; if necessary, that can be followed by another dose in a half hour, to a limit of 6 mg of ergotamine a day or 10 mg a week). The bioavailability of oral ergot preparations may be reduced by gastric stasis; alternative routes include sublingual tablets, rectal suppositories, and use of an ergotamine inhaler. Dihydroergotamine mesylate (D.H.E. 45) can be used to abort acute migraine attacks in adults (1 mg subcutaneously or intramuscularly every hour up to 3 mg a day or 1 mg intravenously followed by 0.5 mg to 1.0 mg to a total of 3 mg a day or 6 mg a week). Some authors recommend slightly higher doses of dihydroergotamine to break episodes of status migrainosus. Ergots are contraindicated during pregnancy and in patients with coronary artery, renal, hepatic, or peripheral vascular diseases or hyperthyroidism. Some patients become ergot-dependent and have severe rebound headaches during drug withdrawal.

Metoclopramide (Reglan), given 10 mg intravenously, may be used to relieve the nausea or the gastric stasis that accompanies migraine. Its adverse effects include restlessness and occasional movement disorders. Sumatriptan (Imitrex) is a new 5-HT_1 receptor agonist that has demonstrated efficacy in the treatment of acute migraine. The dose is 6 mg given subcutaneously by an autoinjector that allows self-administration; that dose may be repeated in one hour if the headache does not completely resolve. Patients typically begin to experience pain relief within 30 to 60 minutes. The maximal dose is 12 mg in 24 hours. Common adverse effects include local reactions, such as redness or pain at the injection site, and atypical sensations, such as tingling or burning, flushing, dizziness, or vertigo. Less common adverse effects include chest pressure or tightness, which may radiate to the neck or face, electrocardiographic changes, and arrhythmias. Up to 40 percent of all patients may experience some headache recurrence, usually at a less severe level, as the drug wears off. The drug should be avoided in persons with cardiac disorders or uncontrolled hypertension and in those who received ergot alkaloids within the preceding 24 hours. Persons at high risk for cardiac disease should take their first dose of sumatriptan under direct medical supervision, as in an emergency room.

A wide range of drugs have been used for migraine prophylaxis. β-Adrenergic blockers that do not possess intrinsic sympathomimetic activity, such as propranolol (Inderal), 40 to 320 mg a day by mouth, and metoprolol (Lopressor), 100 to 200 mg a day by mouth, act to prevent vasodilation and may also act on 5-HT receptors. Their adverse effects include fatigue, insomnia, postural hypotension, dizziness, diarrhea, weight gain, and depression. They are contraindicated during pregnancy and in patients with asthma, congestive heart failure, poorly controlled diabetes, and second- or third-degree heart block.

Tricyclic antidepressants, such as amitriptyline (Elavil), a 5-HT_2 receptor antagonist, given 10 to 150 mg a day by mouth, or nortriptyline (Pamelor), 25 to 100 mg a day by mouth, have shown efficacy in the prophylaxis of migraine, tension, and mixed headaches. Amitriptyline acts to block the reuptake of 5-HT and NE and may thus activate endogenous pain-control pathways. Tricyclics are contraindicated in patients with second- or third-degree heart block, narrow-angle glaucoma, and prostatic hypertrophy and in patients taking monoamine oxidase inhibitors (MAOIs). The adverse effects of tricyclics include dry mouth, blurred vision, constipation, sedation, orthostatic hypotension, tachyarrhythmias, and increased appetite. The antidepressant fluoxetine (Prozac), a serotonin-specific reuptake inhibitor, 20 mg a day by mouth, was reported to decrease headache scores in a small placebo-controlled clinical trial. Fluoxetine is contraindicated in persons using MAOIs concurrently or within two weeks prior to fluoxetine administration. Potential adverse side effects include allergic reactions, rash, increased anxiety, insomnia, anorexia, activation of mania or hypomania, and seizures. Fluoxetine has a prolonged half-life, is eliminated slowly, and may have significant interactions with several other psychopharmacological agents.

Calcium channel antagonists, such as verapamil (Calan), given 80 to 480 mg a day by mouth in three divided doses, may help in migraine prophylaxis. Their putative mechanisms include the prevention of cerebral hypoxia, the prevention of vasoconstriction, decreased prostaglandin synthesis, and 5-HT_2 receptor antagonism. Their adverse side effects include constipation, light-headedness, nausea, fluid retention, orthostatic hypotension, and fatigue. Verapamil is contraindicated in patients with advanced heart block, some arrhythmias, or severe left ventricular dysfunction.

In several open studies and in two placebo-controlled clinical trials, sodium valproate (Depakote), an anticonvulsant, has been reported to decrease the frequency and severity of migraine refractory to other prophylactic agents. The dosages used varied in each study, ranging approximately between 800 and 1,500 mg a day by mouth. Potential adverse effects of sodium valproate include nausea, vomiting, abdominal cramps, anorexia, weight gain, sedation, tremor, hair loss, and skin rash. Rare but potentially fatal episodes of hepatic failure have been reported in some patients. Thrombocytopenia, other coagulation abnormalities, pancreatitis, and elevated ammonia levels have also been reported. The drug is contraindicated in patients with hepatic disease, significant hepatic dysfunction, and clotting disorders and in pregnant women. Anticonvulsants and other medications may interact with sodium valproate. All patients taking this drug should be closely monitored by their physicians; however, no significant adverse side effects were reported in any of the headache subjects studied.

Naproxen (Naprosyn), a nonsteroidal antiinflammatory drug that reduces prostaglandin formation, has been reported to reduce migraine severity. The usual dose of naproxen is 250 to 1,250 mg a day by mouth. Its adverse effects include nausea, abdominal pain, fluid retention, dizziness, and tinnitus. Its long-term use can be nephrotoxic and may cause gastrointestinal bleeding. Naproxen is contraindicated in persons allergic to aspirin.

Methysergide (Sansert), given orally 2 to 8 mg a day, is a highly effective 5-HT_2 receptor antagonist and is helpful in migraine prophylaxis. Methysergide is most often given to patients who have failed other antimigraine drugs. Many patients cannot tolerate the drug because of its potent adverse effects, which may include nausea, abdominal pain, muscle cramps, peripheral vasoconstriction, pedal edema, weight gain, limb claudication, drowsiness, and mental confusion. The most serious consequences that may occur with prolonged use are pulmonary, retroperitoneal, or cardiac valvular fibrosis. Patients must go on a one-month drug holiday every five months, and physicians must monitor for fibrotic changes.

Temperature biofeedback Temperature biofeedback is the best-studied nonpharmacological technique for the control of migraine. Several studies have shown biofeedback to be superior to a placebo in migraine management, but others have not; no study has shown biofeedback to be superior to drug prophylaxis. Temperature biofeedback may be more successful in children with migraine than in adults.

CLUSTER HEADACHE

Cluster headache (ciliary or migrainous neuralgia, Horton's headache, histaminic cephalalgia, petrosal neuralgia, sphenopalatine neuralgia, vidian or Sluder's neuralgia) is a relatively uncommon headache disorder, with a prevalence of approximately 69 cases per 100,000 people. Cluster headache was previously classified as a vascular headache; however, research studies have failed to show changes in cerebral blood flow in conjunction with the attacks. Cluster headache is now classified with chronic paroxysmal hemicrania, a rare cluster headache variant. Cluster headache occurs in men five to six times more often than in women and commonly begins between age 20 and age 40. No familial pattern is present.

Cluster headaches are characterized by attacks of severe, strictly unilateral pain in the orbital, supraorbital, and temporal areas. The pain is stabbing, sharp, or constant (nonpulsatile); may radiate to the ipsilateral face and neck; and lasts from 15 minutes to three hours. Attacks occur in series, lasting weeks to months to years. The episodic form is more common (90 percent) than the chronic form (10 percent), in which periodicity is lost.

During a cluster headache attack, headaches occur from every other day up to eight times a day and are associated with at least one of the following on the painful side: conjunctival congestion, lacrimation, nasal congestion, rhinorrhea, sweating, miosis, ptosis, and eyelid edema. Nausea and vomiting are not present. Pericranial muscle tenderness, visual blurring (without other visual symptoms), and systemic autonomic changes (sweating, bradycardia, arrhythmias, hypertension) may accompany an attack. Clusters frequently occur at the same time of day or during the same season each year.

The pathophysiology of cluster headaches is unknown. Various hypotheses have been proposed to account for their unique characteristics, including dysregulation of central hypothalamic pacemakers to account for the rhythmicity of the attacks and the systemic autonomic disturbances; excessive release of histamine during the attacks; and the stimulation of trigeminal pathways to release substance P both orthodromically, giving rise to pain, and peripherally onto blood vessels, producing dilatation of the extracranial vessels, facial flushing, and nasal congestion. Low levels of CSF met-enkephalin have been reported in cluster headache patients, suggesting a defect in the endogenous pain-control system.

TREATMENT The treatment of cluster headache is almost exclusively pharmacological; behavioral therapies and acupuncture are ineffective. Individual attacks can be treated with ergotamine, preferably with an inhaler to speed absorption (one puff or 0.36 mg every five minutes, up to six puffs in 24 hours or 15 puffs a week). Dihydroergotamine mesylate, 1 mg given intravenously, has been reported to abort cluster headache attacks. Sumatriptan, 6 mg given subcutaneously, has also been reported to abort cluster headache. Recommendations for the administration and dosage of both dihydroergotamine and sumatriptan are the same as those for migraine. One-hundred-percent oxygen administered with a face mask at a flow rate of 8 to 10 liters a minute for 10 to 15 minutes can be used up to five times a day to abort attacks. Intranasal lidocaine (1 mL of Xylocaine 4 percent topical solution) has been reported to ameliorate some cluster headache attacks.

For prophylaxis, ergotamine, 1 to 2 mg by mouth or as a rectal suppository, can be taken several hours before an expected attack. A series of cluster headaches can often be aborted by a course of prednisone, 50 to 75 mg a day by mouth for one week, followed by a tapering course; the dosage may be increased if the symptoms reappear. The potential adverse effects include glucose intolerance, hypertension, weight gain, edema, and ulcers.

Lithium (Eskalith), 300 to 1,200 mg a day by mouth in divided doses, ameliorates chronic cluster headaches but may require several weeks before it is effective. Plasma levels should be kept under 1.2 mEq/L. The adverse effects include tremor, polyuria, nausea, diarrhea, ataxia, and suppression of thyroid function. Intoxication may cause hypotension, convulsions, and renal failure.

TENSION-TYPE HEADACHE

Tension-type headache (muscle-contraction headache) remains poorly understood, despite the fact that it is by far the most common headache type. Tension headaches are divided into episodic and chronic types and by the presence or the absence of pericranial muscle spasm and tenderness to palpation. Diagnosis by the ICD-10 criteria requires at least two of the following: pressing or tightening quality (nonpulsatile), mild to moderate severity, bilateral location, and lack of aggravation by physical activity. Patients do not experience vomiting or more than one of the following: photophobia, phonophobia, and nausea. Other commonly reported features are occipitonuchal or bifrontal location, a bandlike sensation around the head, and its occurrence in relation to emotional stress or anxiety.

Tension headaches are more common in women than in men and usually begin between age 20 and age 40. Although many patients with tension headaches report daily or near-daily pain, sometimes lasting years, relatively few consult physicians. Many patients have both tension-type and migraine headaches.

The pathogenesis of tension headache is unknown. Previously, sustained pericranial muscle contraction was assumed to cause ischemia and muscle pain. Recent studies show no correlation between decreased pericranial muscle blood flow and pain or tenderness. Surface electromyographic (EMG) studies have failed to consistently confirm elevated muscle activity in tension headache patients; in fact, muscle tension levels are often higher in migraine patients. Despite the role that stress, anxiety, and depression appear to play in the pathogenesis of tension headaches in many patients, no unique psychological profile is present in the person with episodic tension-type headache. Recently, attention has focused on possible central causes for tension headache. Beta-endorphin levels are decreased in the CSF; CSF, plasma, and platelet 5-HT levels are low in patients with chronic tension headaches; and amitriptyline, which increases the biological availability of 5-HT, is often effective in the prophylaxis of tension-type headaches. Those observations suggest a role for 5-HT in the pathogenesis of tension headaches.

TREATMENT Most persons with episodic tension-type headaches successfully treat themselves with rest, hot or cold packs, and nonprescription analgesics, such as aspirin, 625 mg by mouth; acetaminophen, 1,000 mg by mouth; and ibuprofen, 200 to 800 mg by mouth. Patients with frequent or disabling headaches can be treated prophylactically with amitriptyline, 25 to 150 mg a day by mouth; nortriptyline, 25 to 150 mg a day by mouth; or imipramine (Tofranil), 50 to 200 mg a day by mouth. Those drugs are especially helpful if an associated depression or sleep disorder is present. Muscle relaxants or benzodiazepines, such as diazepam (Valium), 2.5 to 10 mg by mouth three times a day, can be used for the short-term relief of episodic tension headache but may be associated with habituation, tolerance, or depression. Such drugs are not recommended for chronic pain.

Physical therapy, such as stretching exercises, with or without the use of heat or cold, and fluorimethane spray (15 percent dichlorodifluoromethane and 85 percent trichloromonofluoromethane) to reduce pain and relax muscle spasms are helpful and low-risk treatment modalities for many people with muscle spasm and tenderness. Ideally, physical treatments should be combined with some sort of behavioral intervention, such as biofeedback, Jacobsen's progressive relaxation therapy, self-hypnosis, meditation, or cognitive-behavioral therapy. EMG biofeedback has been shown to be superior to no treatment or a placebo in several controlled studies but is probably not more effective than other relaxation techniques.

POSTTRAUMATIC HEADACHE

Posttraumatic headaches occur within 14 days of a head injury or within 14 days of regaining consciousness, if consciousness has been lost. An estimated one of every 100 persons suffers from a concussion each year, and up to 50 percent of those persons experience chronic headaches that last more than two months. The pathogenesis is likely to be organic in most cases, although litigation is often suspected to be a contributing factor. Damage may occur to the brain, even in cases without a skull fracture or intracerebral hemorrhages. In closed head injuries, acceleration-deceleration forces may cause tearing or stretching of brain tissues and diffuse axonal injury. Chronic muscle spasms caused by whiplash-type injuries may also contribute to the headache.

Posttraumatic headaches can resemble migraine, tension-type, or mixed tension-migraine headaches. They may be associated with other postconcussive symptoms, such as nausea, vomiting, dizziness, vertigo, decreased concentration, and emotional lability. Patients may become anxious or depressed and require psychological treatment. Narcotics and benzodiazepines should be avoided except immediately after the injury. Posttraumatic headache resembling migraine or tension-type headache should be treated in the same way as those primary headache types. Chronic muscle spasms should be treated with physical therapy.

POST-LUMBAR-PUNCTURE AND OTHER LOW-CSF-PRESSURE HEADACHES

Post-lumbar-puncture headache is a bilateral headache that occurs within seven days of a lumbar puncture. It is worse within 15 minutes of the patient's sitting or standing upright and is relieved within 30 minutes of lying flat. Similar headaches can occur with posttraumatic, postoperative, and idiopathic CSF leaks. Post-lumbar-puncture headaches are more common in women than in men and in persons with low body mass or headache prior to lumbar puncture occur less frequently after age 70 and in persons with cerebral atrophy.

The presumed cause is persistent CSF leakage after the spinal needle is removed, with resultant loss of CSF volume and tension on the brain's pain-sensitive anchoring structures. Lowered CSF pressure may also cause intracranial venous distention and pain. Occasionally, nausea, stiff neck (caused by muscle spasm), blurred vision, photophobia, tinnitus, vertigo, diminished hearing, and postural syncope is associated with a severe headache. The pain is worsened by a cough, strain, head movement, or jugular compression. The average headache lasts less than four days but in rare cases may persist for two to three weeks.

In an extensive study the incidence of post-lumbar-puncture headache was inversely correlated with the needle gauge (diameter), suggesting that small-gauge (25 or 26) needles should be used whenever possible. Hydration, postural maneuvers, rest, and the use of an abdominal binder were relatively ineffective prophylactic measures. If a post-lumbar-puncture headache occurs, the best treatment is to keep the patient flat in bed and to use analgesics and other symptomatic therapies. Prolonged headache can be treated by the injection of sterile autologous blood into the epidural space (epidural blood patch) to seal the puncture. The potential complications of that therapy include backache and radiculitis.

HEADACHE ASSOCIATED WITH INTRACRANIAL NEOPLASM

Headaches are popularly assumed to be the most common initial symptom of brain tumors; in fact, most patients with brain tumors experience behavioral changes or seizures before headaches, unless the tumor obstructs CSF outflow and raises intracranial pressure early in its course.

Most tumor headaches start as mild, episodic, dull headaches that are present on arising from sleep and get better as the day progresses and the patient is upright. Over time, they become continuous and intense. Occasionally, tumor headache is paroxysmal in nature if the intracranial pressure suddenly rises or if there is bleeding into the tumor. Tumor headache is often associated with nausea or vomiting and is made worse by coughing, straining, and the Valsalva maneuver. Patients with such headaches should always get a contrast-enhanced MRI or CT, whether or not the neurological examination results are normal. The presumed pain mechanisms include traction on the dura or other pain-sensitive structures, increased intracranial pressure, and direct tumor compression or invasion of pain-sensitive structures.

Treatment should address the tumor itself by surgery, radiation therapy, and steroids to reduce the cerebral edema. Narcotics may increase the intracranial pressure but should not be withheld from terminally ill patients.

HEADACHE ASSOCIATED WITH SUBARACHNOID HEMORRHAGE

Subarachnoid hemorrhage is the leakage of blood into the subarachnoid space; it is usually accompanied by an acute neurological deficit. Approximately 28,000 cases a year occur in North America. The most common cause is a ruptured congenital saccular arterial aneurysm (berry aneurysm). Subarachnoid hemorrhage most frequently occurs in persons 30 to 60 years of age and is slightly more common in women than in men.

The headache characteristically begins suddenly during physical exertion, is severe and bilateral, and often radiates to the neck or the back. It may peak rapidly and taper off or linger. Up to two thirds of patients lose consciousness or have altered levels of consciousness immediately after a bleed. Associated features may include a stiff neck, elevated temperature, nausea, vomiting, photophobia, focal neurological signs, subhyaloid hemorrhage, an elevated white blood count, hypertension, and cardiac arrhythmias. Up to two thirds of patients lose consciousness or have altered levels of consciousness accompanying a subarachnoid bleed. Warning or sentinel headaches may occur before a major bleed and should trigger an immediate investigation.

Subarachnoid hemorrhage is a medical emergency. Up to 40 percent of patients die in the first 24 hours, and survivors are at risk for rebleeding and delayed ischemic complications. Suspected cases should be sent immediately for a CT scan, which is the most sensitive method of detecting recent intracranial hemorrhage. MRI may be preferable if the event is more than a week old. The scan should be followed immediately by a lumbar puncture if the scan findings are normal; subarachnoid bleeding not evident on a CT or MRI scan may be detected in the spinal fluid. Patients with evidence of hemorrhage must be hospitalized at strict bed rest and sedated if necessary to reduce their physical activity. Nimodepine (Nimotop), a calcium channel blocker, 90 to 240 mg a day by mouth in divided doses, should be given to reduce the incidence of postrupture vasospasm and ischemia. Urgent neurosurgical consultation should be obtained to decide the optimal timing of angiography and surgery.

HEADACHE ASSOCIATED WITH GIANT CELL ARTERITIS

Headache is the most common initial symptom of giant cell arteritis (temporal arteritis), an inflammatory obliterative arteritis of large and medium-sized arteries. It is closely linked with polymyalgia rheumatica, an illness characterized by pain and stiffness of the limb-girdle muscles and by inflammatory synovitis. Giant cell arteritis is more common in women than in men and typically begins between ages 50 and 85.

The headache is described as constant and boring or aching, located over the temporal region, worse at night, and increased by cold air. Associated symptoms include tenderness of the scalp and the superficial arteries, visual obscurations, malaise, anorexia, myalgias and arthralgias, and claudication of the jaw, the tongue, and the limbs. A physical examination may reveal absent arterial pulses, bruits, muscle tenderness, fever, hand swelling, joint effusions, and peripheral neuropathy. The erythrocyte sedimentation rate is usually elevated over 50 mm an hour but is occasionally normal. Diagnosis is confirmed by a biopsy of a 4- to 6-cm length of the temporal artery that shows a patchy arteritis. Inflammatory cells invade the tunica intima and tunica media and disrupt the internal elastic membrane. Thrombosis may be present.

Suspected giant cell arteritis is a medical emergency because of its potential ischemic complications, such as blindness (from ischemia of the optic nerve), cerebrovascular disorder, and myocardial infarction. Treatment with prednisone should be started empirically before a biopsy as soon as the diagnosis is suspected (40 to 80 mg a day by mouth is generally recommended, but a few patients require more). Typically, corticosteroid therapy relieves the pain within 48 hours and may prevent the loss of vision during the diagnostic evaluation. Most patients require between one and three years of steroid treatment before the disease remits.

HEADACHE FROM SUBSTANCE WITHDRAWAL

Withdrawal headaches can occur after acute substance use (for example, the morning-after hangover from alcohol) and after chronic, high-dose substance use. The headaches appear within hours after the substance is eliminated from the body and are relieved by ingesting another dose of the substance. A common example is rebound migraine, occurring within 48 hours after chronic ergotamine intake (usually 1 to 2 mg a day) is abruptly discontinued. Severe ergotamine withdrawal headaches may require inpatient detoxification and intravenous dihydroergotamine mesylate treatment. Other examples include withdrawal headaches from narcotics, barbiturates, caffeine, and nonprescription analgesics.

SUGGESTED CROSS-REFERENCES

Functional neuroanatomy is discussed in Section 1.2, neurotransmitters in Sections 1.3 and 1.4, neuroimaging in Sections 1.10 and 2.10, and the neuropsychiatric aspects of brain trauma in Section 2.4. Behavior therapy is discussed in Section 31.2, hypnosis in Section 31.3, cognitive therapy in Section 31.6, and tricyclic antidepressants in Section 32.24.

REFERENCES

Adly C, Straumanis J, Chesson A: Fluoxetine prophylaxis of migraine. Headache *32:* 101, 1992.

Anthony M, Lance J W: Plasma serotonin in patients with chronic tension headaches. J Neurol Neurosurg Psychiatry *52:* 182, 1989.

*Bonica J J: Anatomic and physiologic basis of nociception and pain. In *The Management of Pain,* ed 2, J J Bonica, J D Loesser, C R Chapman, W E Fordyce, editors, vol 1, p 28. Lea & Febiger, Philadelphia, 1990.

Bruyn G W, Lanser J B K: The post-concussional syndrome. In *Handbook of Clinical Neurology, Head Injury,* R Braakman, P J Vinken, O W Bruyn, H L Klawans, editors, vol 13, p 421. Elsevier Science, New York, 1990.

Diener H C, Dichgans J, Scholz E, Geiselhart S, Gerber W D, Bille A: Analgesic-induced chronic headache: Long-term results of withdrawal therapy. J Neurol *236:* 9, 1989.

Goadsby P J, Edvinsson L: The trigeminovascular system and migraine: studies characterizing cerebrovascular and neuropeptide changes seen in humans and cats. Ann Neurol *33:* 48, 1993.

Hardebo J E: On pain mechanisms in cluster headache. Headache *31:* 91, 1991.

*Headache Classification Committee of the International Headache Society: Classification and diagnostic criteria for headache disorders, cranial neuralgias, and facial pain. Cephalalgia *8* (7, Suppl): 1, 1988.

Hering R, Kuritsky A: Sodium valproate in the treatment of migraine: a double-blind study versus placebo. Cephalalgia *12:* 81, 1992.

Hunder G G: Giant cell (temporal) arteritis. Rheum Dis Clin North Am *16:* 399, 1990.

Jensen R, Brinck T, Olesen J: Sodium valproate has a prophylactic effect in migraine without aura: a triple-blind, placebo-controlled crossover study. Neurology *44:* 647, 1994.

Kelly R E: Post-traumatic headache. In *Handbook of Clinical Neurology: Headache,* F C Rose, P J Vinken, G W Bruyn, H L Klawans, editors, vol 4, 383, Elsevier Science, New York, 1986.

Kuntz K M, Kokman E, Stevens J C, Miller P, Offord K P, Ho M M: Post-lumbar puncture headaches: experience in 501 consecutive procedures. Neurology *42:* 1884, 1992.

Lance J W: *Mechanism and Management of Headache,* ed 4. Butterworth, Boston, 1982.

Langsmark M, Jensen K, Olesen J: Temporal muscle blood flow in chronic tension-type headache. Arch Neurol *47:* 654, 1990.

Marshall S B, Marshall L F, Vos R H, Chestnut R M: *Neuroscience Critical Care: Pathophysiology and Patient Management.* Saunders, Philadelphia, 1990.

Mathew N: *Cluster Headache.* Spectrum, New York, 1984.

Moskowitz M A: The neurobiology of vascular head pain. Ann Neurol *16:* 157, 1984.

*Moskowitz M A: Neurogenic inflammation in the pathophysiology and treatment of migraine. Neurology *43*(3, Suppl): S16, 1993.

Olesen J: Cerebral and extracranial circulatory disturbances in migraine: Pathophysiological implications. Cerebrovasc Brain Metab Rev. *3:*1, 1991.

Olesen J, Bonica J J: Headache. In *The Management of Pain,* ed 2, J J Bonica, J D Loeser, C R Chapman, W E Fordyce, editors, vol 1, p 687. Lea & Febiger, Philadelphia, 1990.

Peroutka S J: Antimigraine drug interactions with serotonin receptor subtypes in human brain. Ann Neurol *23:* 500, 1988.

Peroutka S J: Migraine. In *Principles of Drug Therapy in Neurology,* M V Johnston, R L MacDonald, A B Young, editors, p 161. Davis, Philadelphia, 1992.

Raskin N H: *Headache,* ed 2. Churchill Livingstone, New York, 1988.

Rasmussen B K, Jensen R, Olesen J: A population-based analysis of the diagnostic criteria of the International Headache Society. Cephalalgia *11:* 129, 1991.

*Sessle B J: Neural mechanisms of oral and facial pain. Otolaryngol Clin North Am *22:* 1059, 1989.

Silberstein S D: Advances in understanding the pathophysiology of headache. Neurology *42*(2, Suppl): 6, 1992.

Silberstein S D: Tension-type and chronic daily headache. Neurology *43:* 1644, 1993.

Subcutaneous Sumatriptan International Study Group: Treatment of migraine attack with sumatriptan. N Engl J Med *325:* 316, 1991.

Sumatriptan Cluster Headache Group: Treatment of acute cluster headache with sumatriptan. N Engl J Med *325:* 322, 1991.

Taylor H, editor: *The Nuprin Pain Report.* Harris, New York, 1985.

Tourtellotte W W, Henderson W G, Tucker R P, Gilland O, Walker J E, Kokman E: A randomized double-blind clinical trial comparing the 22 versus 26 gauge needle in the production of the post-lumbar puncture syndrome in normal individuals. Headache *12:* 73, 1972.

*Welch K M A: Drug therapy of migraine. N Engl J Med *329:* 1476, 1993.

2.10 NEUROIMAGING IN CLINICAL PRACTICE

BRUCE L. MILLER, M.D.
JEFFREY L. CUMMINGS, M.D.
ISMAEL MENA, M.D.
JACQUES DARCOURT, M.D.

INTRODUCTION

The past 15 years have seen an enormous increase in the imaging techniques made available to clinicians for studying the structure and function of the brain. When the earliest computed tomography (CT) scanners arrived at clinical centers in 1976 the practicing psychiatrist, for the first time, was able to obtain a high-resolution image of brain structures, something that was previously possible only at postmortem examination. The introduction of CT led to subtle modifications in the approach to psychiatric patients and now clinicians commonly use neuroimaging as part of the assessment of a variety of patients with psychiatric symptomatology. The frequent identification of structural brain injury in such patients has reinforced the concept that dysfunction in specific brain structures is the basis for psychiatric disease.

In 1983 magnetic resonance imaging (MRI) was introduced to clinical medicine. It affords substantially better resolution than CT and improved visualization of the anatomical regions that are particularly important to psychiatrists, such as the anterior temporal and basal frontal lobes. However, the role of MRI in the evaluation of psychiatric patients is still undefined and the clinician must decide whether its better resolution as compared with CT is outweighed by the additional cost and patient inconvenience.

In addition to structural brain scans tests are now available that quantify brain function and chemistry. With single photon emission computed tomography (SPECT) cerebral blood flow (CBF) is imaged with a resolution of 7 millimeters (mm) and with positron emission tomography (PET) the resolution of glucose metabolism has reached the 3-mm range. Studies of brain metabolism and neurotransmitter receptor density can now be performed with both techniques. A distinct advantage of PET and SPECT for psychiatry is that there are many conditions in which brain structure is grossly and even microscopically normal but brain function is severely disturbed. The distinction is particularly clear with the degenerative dementias in which functional and clinical disturbances often precede gross structural changes.

Finally, hydrogen 1 (^{1}H) and phosphorus 31 (^{31}P) magnetic resonance spectroscopy (MRS) can noninvasively acquire information concerning brain chemistry. ^{1}H MRS measures the concentration of glutamate, glutamine, *N*-acetylaspartate

(NAA), creatine, lactate, myoinositol, glucose, and choline-containing compounds and ^{31}P MRS determines the pH and the concentration of phosphorous-containing energy metabolites in the brain.

NEUROIMAGING TECHNIQUES

COMPUTED TOMOGRAPHY With CT an image of tissue density is obtained. Radiation is emitted from a collimated beam that rotates around the head, with the head placed between the radiation source and the scintillation counters that detect the radiation. The amount of radiation that reaches the scintillation detectors depends on the tissue density of the brain; it subsequently is translated into a black, gray, and white two-dimensional X-ray photograph. Black areas represent tissues with low attenuation, such as cerebrospinal fluid (CSF), whereas white areas represent areas of high attenuation, such as bone. Gray areas have intermediate attenuation values. The spatial resolution of a scan can be enhanced by obtaining multiple small slices. Additional information can be derived by injecting iodinated contrast material intravenously. Regions enhance if there is breakdown of the blood-brain barrier, such as in a patient who recently suffered a cerebrovascular disorder or has a brain tumor or a focal brain infection, such as bacterial abscesses. Blood vessels are also more evident with contrast dye so that arteriovenous malformations and aneurysms often can be visualized with contrast enhancement.

The technique is relatively inexpensive and changes that are detected have been carefully studied with postmortem evaluations, making it clearer to interpret abnormal findings than with MRI. However, tissue resolution with CT is inferior to that with MRI and is particularly poor in areas adjacent to bone, such as the temporal and basal frontal lobes and the brain stem.

MAGNETIC RESONANCE IMAGING MRI is a noninvasive imaging technique that uses information regarding the proton density of tissue to reconstruct an image of brain structure. The patient is placed in a static magnetic field in which all of the water-containing molecules realign in the same direction. The molecules then are subjected to a radiofrequency pulse that flips them 90 or 180 degrees. As the molecules move back toward their original direction of spin they emit an energy, which is detected by a computer, that reflects the distribution and concentration of the protons. The energy information is converted into an image of water density throughout the brain.

Three main types of scans are utilized—T_1, T_2, and the proton density scan (Figures 2.10-1A, 2.10-1B, and 2.10-1C). The T_2-weighted scans show the CSF as white and the cortex as gray, whereas the T_1-weighted scans show the CSF as dark. The proton density scan is intermediate in density. MRI demonstrates most pathological processes as areas of increased water. The T_2 scan is particularly good for detecting brain pathology, and the T_1 scan is better for defining normal anatomy. Blood flowing through arteries and veins is not detectable and appears as a dark flow void. It is now possible to obtain angiographic visualization with MRI. As with CT contrast agents that detect the breakdown of the blood-brain barrier are now available with MRI; the agent currently used is gadolinium diethylenetriaminepentaacetic acid (DTPA).

MRI has distinct advantages over CT, including better spatial resolution, which, with multiple small slices, currently is as high as 2 to 3 mm and its theoretical limits have not yet been achieved. Unlike CT, where bone limits resolution in areas critical to psychiatry such as the anterior temporal and basal frontal cortex, MRI resolves those areas well. It also is more sensitive than CT for diseases that involve white matter, such as multiple sclerosis and certain types of ischemic brain injury. In examining most psychiatric patients MRI is more informative than CT.

Its major disadvantage is that it costs three to four times more than does CT. In addition, although MRI sensitivity is high, many of the abnormalities that it detects have no clear pathological meaning. A good example is the detection of small white matter lesions in normal elderly persons that are often missed with CT.

SINGLE PHOTON EMISSION COMPUTED TOMOGRAPHY Brain SPECT is a noninvasive imaging method that detects conventional single photon emitters (technetium Tc 99m or iodine 123 [^{123}I]) that have been labeled with molecules that cross the blood-brain barrier, such as ^{99m}Tc-d,1, hexamethyl-propyleneamine-oxime (HMPAO), and ^{123}I-amphetamine. The labeled molecule is injected intravenously and the lipophilic molecules cross the blood-brain barrier. Brain uptake is proportional to cerebral perfusion, and from that information an image of the CBF is reconstructed. Xenon 133 gas, administered through inhalation, can also be utilized to measure and image cerebral perfusion (Figure 2.10-2).

SPECT instruments with single- or triple-headed rotating cameras that detect single photons are readily available in most nuclear medicine laboratories. Some centers have brain-dedicated multiring imaging devices that allow the quantification of blood flow with xenon. All SPECT imaging devices collect information in a 360 degree circle around the brain and generate a three-dimensional image that can be displayed in transaxial, coronal, and sagittal cuts 1 to 1½ centimeters thick. Resolution with brain-dedicated machines is approximately 7 to 9 mm and with single-headed cameras it is around 15 mm.

Image display can use a radiographic gray scale or be converted to a color scale. Some investigators prefer black and white images but many use color scales to maximize the information derived from an individual scan. Color images are normalized to the area of maximum uptake in the brain. A threshold of 60 percent of maximum depicts ideal specificity, whereas a threshold of 66 percent affords the best sensitivity. For the imaging technique used to generate the illustrations presented here, the threshold changes color from red to yellow; therefore, any area in the image displayed in yellow denotes 63 percent diminished blood flow. The next shift occurs at 50 percent and those regions are green (Figure 2.10-3).

For clinical purposes qualitative images supply important information but research requires quantifiable results. Those results are achieved by measuring the blood flow in small regions defined as regions of interest (ROI), which limit the area of observation. Radioactivity is measured in an ROI and is expressed in absolute numbers. The size of the ROI can be standardized, allowing the expression of results in counts per pixel. With xenon the counts represent absolute flow measurements whereas in HMPAO imaging counts must be expressed as a ratio to a normal reference ROI, such as the cerebellum, calcarine cortex, or whole brain. An ROI can be drawn manually by a knowledgeable observer or by using automated programs.

Receptor-specific binding agents labeled with ^{123}I are being utilized to study the functional capacity of muscarinic, dopaminergic, and serotonergic receptors. The approach offers the potential of localizing the chemical dysfunction associated with specific diseases at the presynaptic or postsynaptic receptor level.

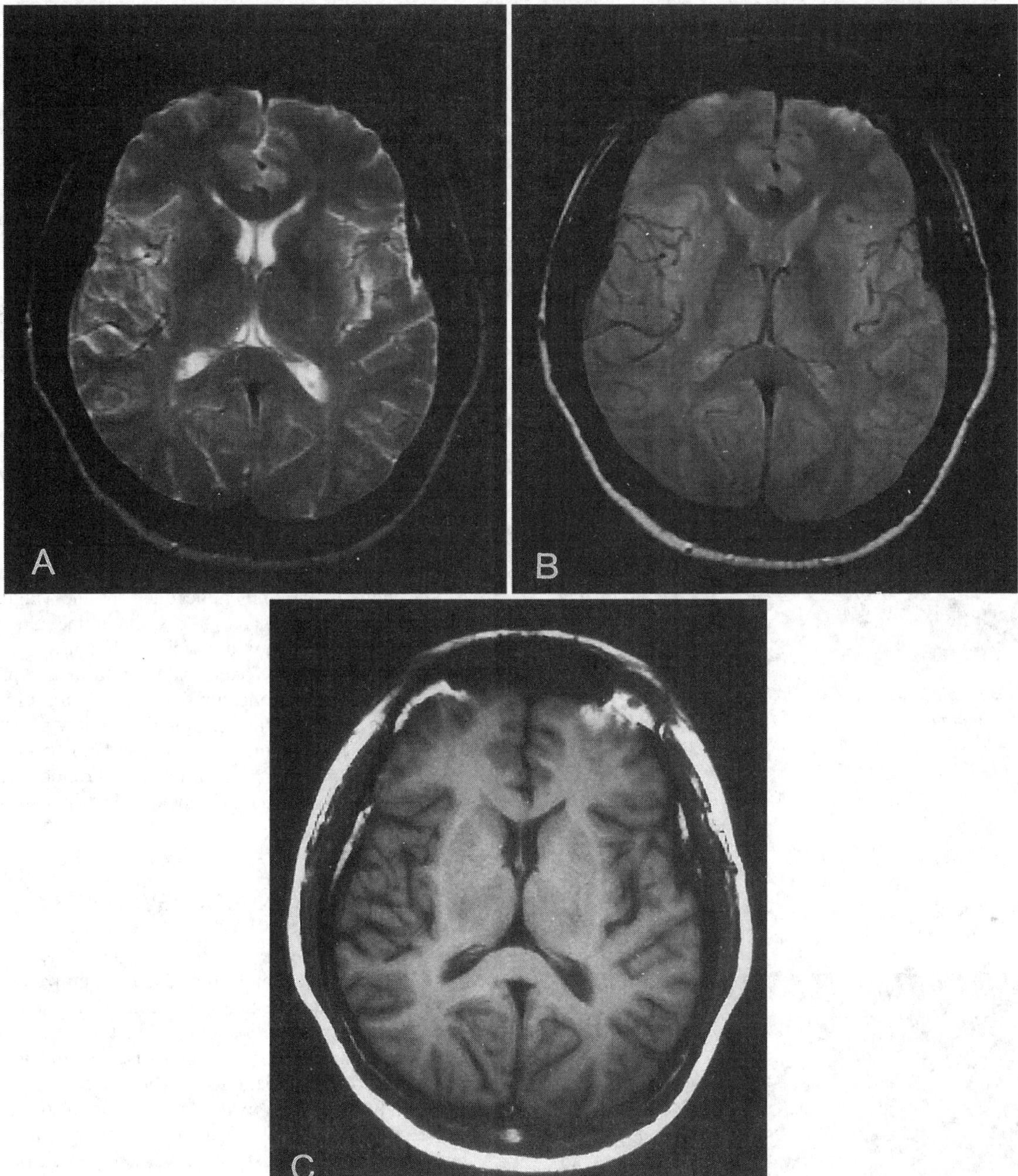

FIGURE 2.10-1 *Normal MRI of a healthy elderly man: T_2 weighted (A), intermediate (B) and T_1 weighted (C).*

POSITRON EMISSION TOMOGRAPHY PET, a noninvasive technique, uses special radionuclides that emit high-energy radiation, which is generated when isotopes collide and emit energy from one pair of gamma rays, each traveling in the opposite direction. Therefore, each radioactive event can be detected simultaneously with detectors located 180 degrees apart. The isotopes commonly employed are fluorine 18, oxygen 15 (^{15}O), and nitrogen 13. The most frequently used compound is ^{18}F deoxyglucose (FDG): brain cells with high metabolic rates will have an increased uptake of FDG and areas with decreased metabolism will exhibit diminished uptake. Nitrogen 13 is useful for the measurement of CBF and ^{15}O for oxygen utilization. Because the radionuclides have short lives they must be prepared on-site with a cyclotron. PET utilizes brain-dedicated multiring systems with resolution as low as 3 mm. Image display is similar to that of SPECT, with transaxial, coronal, and sagittal reconstructions, and results are usually expressed as a ratio of uptake as compared with a standardized zone.

PET has contributed significantly to understanding the pathophysiology of many psychiatric and neurological conditions. Initial studies imaged and measured brain blood flow and brain uptake of glucose in a variety of degenerative, vascular, and psychiatric conditions. More recently, investigators have attempted to image specific brain receptors of the dopaminergic, cholinergic, serotonergic, and opiate systems.

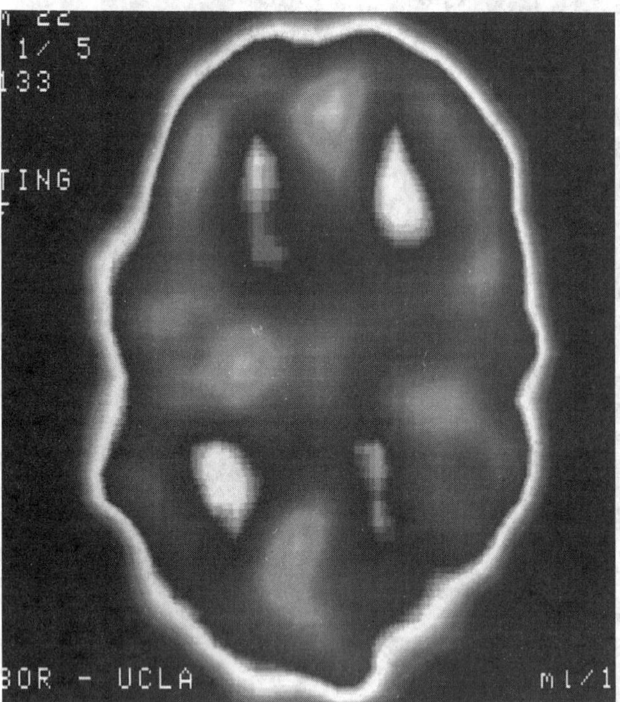

FIGURE 2.10-2 *Xenon 133 image of cerebral blood flow in a healthy elderly man. Blood flow ranges from 57 mL/100 g tissue a minute in the periventricular regions to 82 mL/100 g tissue a minute in the frontal and occipital regions. (See Color Plate 4.)*

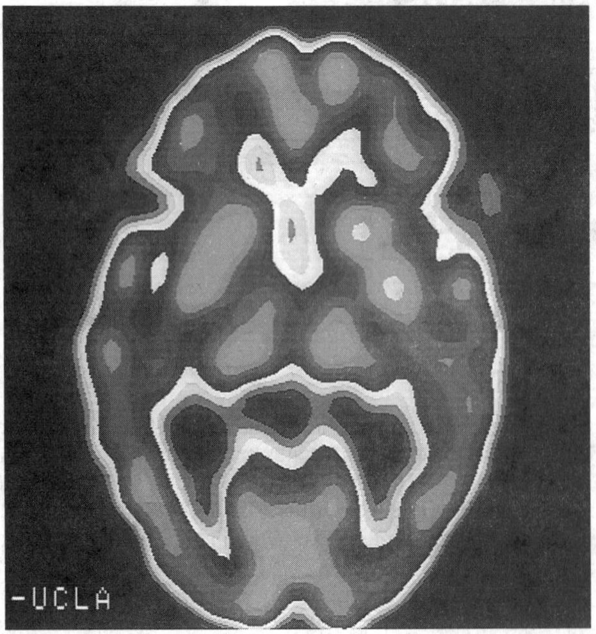

FIGURE 2.10-3 *SPECT of a normal subject using ^{99m}Tc-d,l, hexamethyl-propyleneamine-oxime (HMPAO). The color scale is set to maximum uptake with a shift to yellow at 66 percent maximum uptake and shift to green at 50 percent maximum uptake. (See Color Plate 4.)*

MAGNETIC RESONANCE SPECTROSCOPY MRI provides an image of the brain water whereas MRS determines the concentration of specific molecules. It measures molecules from atoms that contain protons and neutrons with an odd number, such as carbon 13 (^{13}C), fluorine 19 (^{19}F), sodium 23 (^{23}Na), and potassium 39 (^{39}K). The most exciting clinical advances with MRS have occurred with hydrogen 1 (^{1}H) and phosphorus 31 (^{31}P), although measurements of ^{13}C, ^{19}F, ^{23}Na, and ^{39}K spectra may lead to a better understanding of a variety of psychiatric conditions.

With MRS the chemical shift identifies the specific molecule and the height of the peak is used to determine its concentration. Generally, for a chemical to be detectable with current clinical ^{1}H and ^{31}P MRS techniques, it must reach a concentration of at least 1 millimolar; mobile water-soluble molecules are seen better than are immobilized fat-soluble compounds. Excitatory and inhibitory neurotransmitters, such as glutamate and α-aminobutyric acid (GABA), reach the millimolar concentration, but acetylcholine, dopamine, and serotonin do not.

More chemicals can be measured with ^{1}H than with ^{31}P MRS, and ^{1}H MRS allows measurements within a smaller area of interest. The main ^{1}H peaks seen are NAA, total creatine (creatine), and choline-containing molecules (choline) (Figure 2.10-4), whereas lactate, glutamate, GABA, glutamine, glucose, and myoinositol are all visible with special techniques. Spectra can be acquired from multiple voxels and the information presented as a map of metabolite concentrations with a brain resolution approaching 7 mm. Absolute quantitation is now possible.

With ^{31}P MRS the resolution is poorer and most groups report spectra using large voxels; it is used to determine pH, monoester, diester, phosphocreatine, nucleoside triphosphate, and inorganic phosphate peaks.

NEUROIMAGING IN NEUROPSYCHIATRIC DIAGNOSIS

DEMENTIAS Both CT and MRI have been utilized widely in the diagnosis of various dementing conditions and are now routinely ordered in dementia patients to exclude structural brain diseases, including tumors, cerebrovascular disorders, and hydrocephalus. In those patients in whom a treatable illness is not detected by a routine physical examination and blood studies, a CT or MRI must be performed; without such tests even the best clinician will occasionally miss a reversible or partially treatable brain disorder. The addition of CT and MRI to dementia evaluations has been an important factor in the steady decline in the misdiagnosis of Alzheimer's disease (called dementia of the Alzheimer's type in the fourth edition of *Diagnostic and Statistical Manual of Mental Disorders* [DSM-IV]) seen over the past decade.

Alzheimer's disease A progressive degenerative disease of the brain. The pathological substrate of Alzheimer's disease is bilaterally symmetrical neuronal loss associated with amyloid plaques and neurofibrillary tangles. Changes occur primarily in the temporal-parietal neocortex and hippocampus, with the frontal lobes less intensely involved and the primary motor, sensory, and visual cortex relatively spared. Subcortical structures have less pathological involvement.

The distribution of the pathology determines the clinical characteristics of Alzheimer's disease with marked losses of memory and language, visuospatial, and cognitive skills seen early in the disease as a result of dysfunction in the hippocam-

Normal Brain B

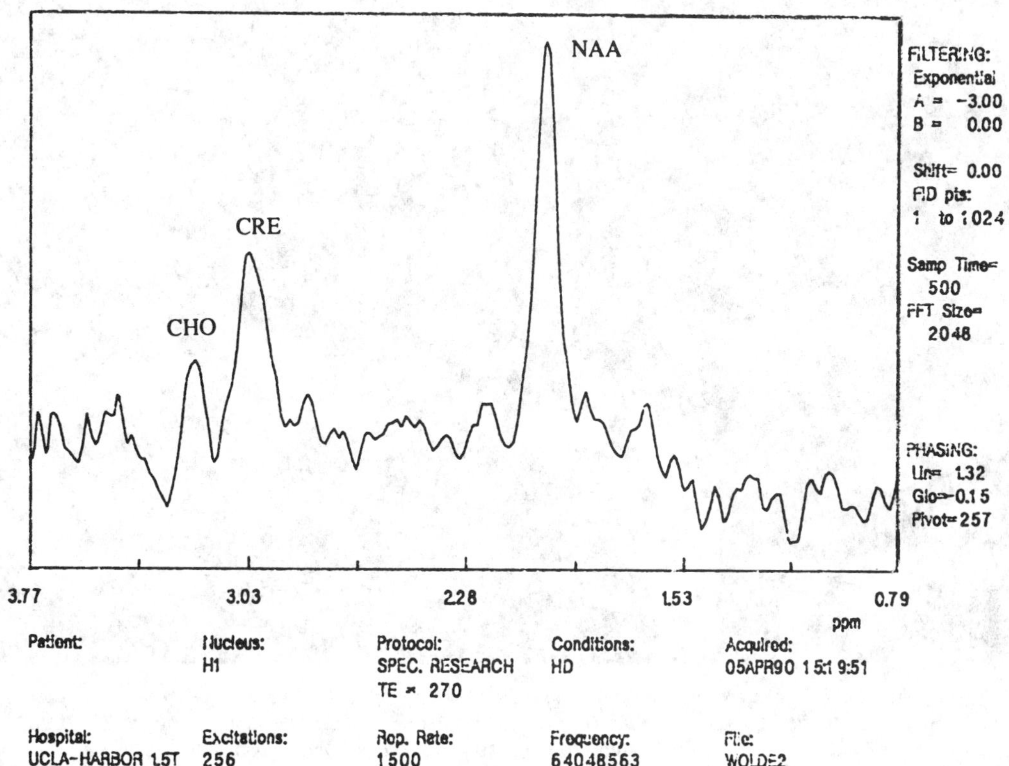

FIGURE 2.10-4 *Normal ^{1}H magnetic resonance spectrum obtained from a 27-cm voxel in the right occipital lobe. The three main peaks detected are NAA at 2.0 ppm, creatinine-phosphocreatinine at 3.0 ppm, and choline-containing compounds at 3.2 ppm.*

pus and temporal-parietal neocortex. Personality changes are variable, although social graces are often initially spared. Psychosis is common in the middle stages of the disease. Alzheimer's disease progresses slowly, with a duration from onset to death of approximately 11 years.

Either CT or MRI will demonstrate brain tumors, cerebrovascular disorders, or hydrocephalus, all of which may clinically mimic Alzheimer's disease. Patients with Alzheimer's disease exhibit a greater degree of brain atrophy than do normal elderly persons. However, many processes can cause brain atrophy; some patients with early Alzheimer's disease do not demonstrate significant atrophy and some normal elderly persons show marked brain atrophy. Thus it is not possible to confirm the diagnosis of Alzheimer's disease on the basis of an atrophic scan.

Functional imaging studies, such as PET and SPECT, show promise for improving diagnostic accuracy in Alzheimer's disease. PET reveals extensive hypometabolism of glucose in temporal-parietal neocortex in patients within the early stages of the disease (Figure 2.10-5). As the disease progresses there is more extensive hypometabolism of frontal cortices, although primary motor, sensory, and visual cortices show normal metabolism into the later stages. Similarly, in early Alzheimer's disease SPECT shows mild global decreases in CBF, with more marked decreases in the temporal-parietal cortex (Figures 2.10-6A and 2.10-6B). As Alzheimer's disease progresses the overall CBF declines further and frontal lobes show even more extensive hypoperfusion.

The changes are usually symmetrical, although some patients

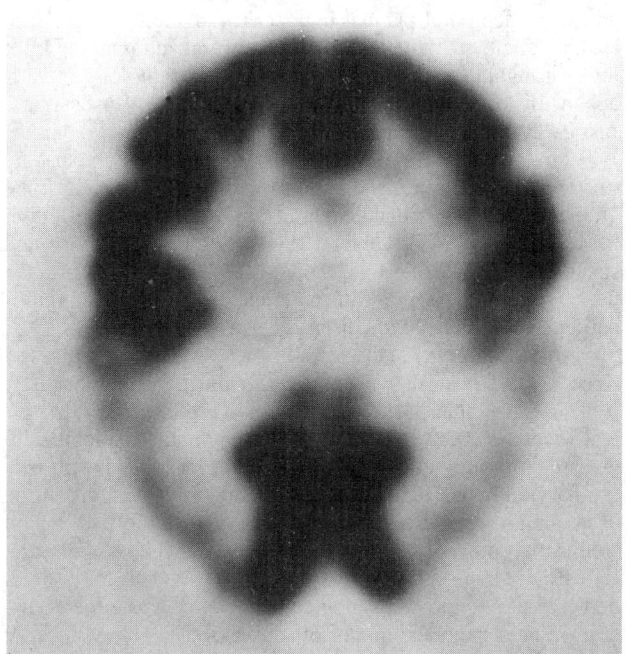

FIGURE 2.10-5 *A PET of a patient with Alzheimer's disease. It shows markedly decreased glucose uptake in the temporal-parietal cortex with normal uptake in the motor, sensory, and visual cortex.*

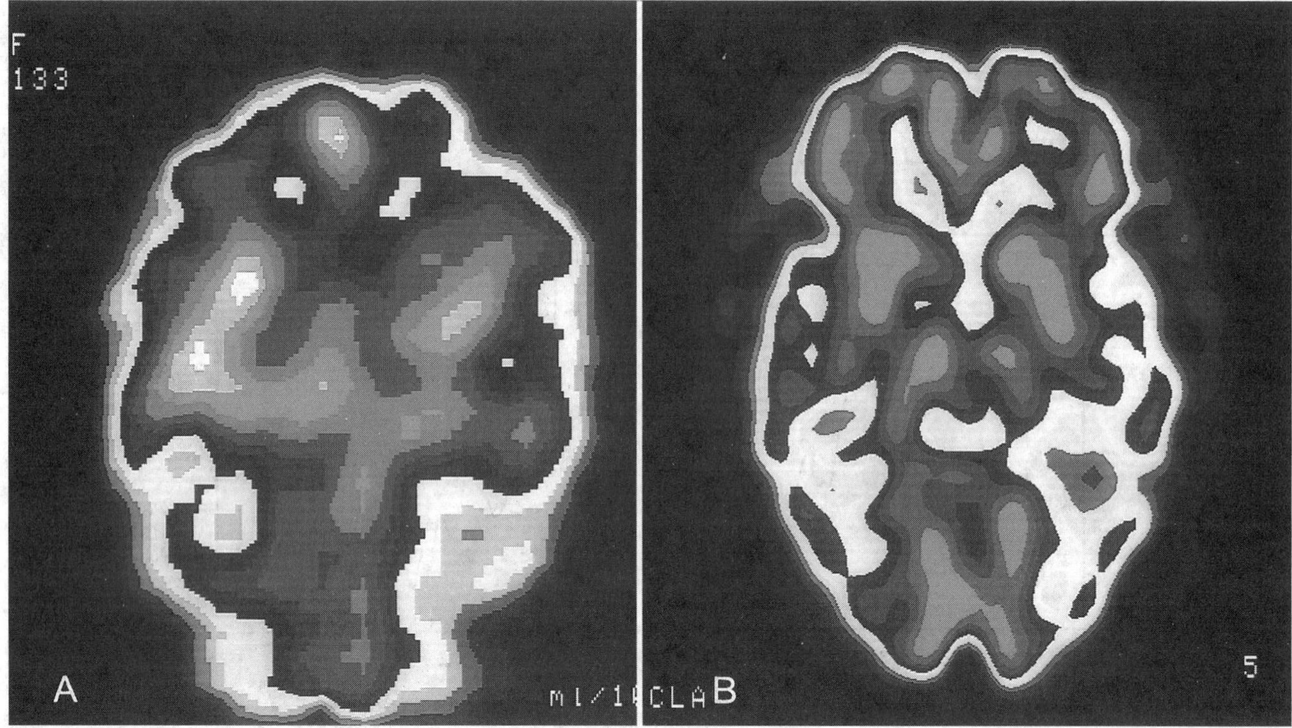

FIGURE 2.10-6 *A, Xenon 133 image of cerebral blood flow in a 69-year-old man with Alzheimer's disease. In the posterior temporal-parietal cortex blood flow is 18 to 25 mL/100 g tissue a minute whereas maximum flow occurs in the motor cortex at 46 mL/100 g tissue a minute. B, HMPAO SPECT from the patient in Figure 2.10-6A demonstrating a 50 percent reduction in blood flow in the posterior temporal-parietal cortex. (See Color Plate 4.)*

exhibit unilateral or asymmetrical temporal-parietal hypoperfusion in the early stages of the disease. In those patients the symptoms are also restricted; patients with left hemisphere hypoperfusion have more language dysfunction whereas those with right temporal-parietal hypoperfusion show more visuospatial deficits. In patients with focal clinical and imaging findings throughout the course the postmortem pathology is variable, with Alzheimer's disease, focal gliosis, Pick's disease, and Jakob-Creutzfeldt disease all reported.

Temporal-parietal hypoperfusion with SPECT is not specific to Alzheimer's disease and patients with sleep apnea, hypoxic brain injury, and vascular dementia may all demonstrate similar SPECT changes. Despite limitations in their sensitivity and specificity, SPECT and PET show great promise for improving the diagnostic capabilities of the clinician in the evaluation of patients with Alzheimer's disease.

^{31}P MRS may eventually help diagnose Alzheimer's disease. Recent work has shown increases in the phosphomonoester peak in Alzheimer's disease, and in preliminary studies ^{31}P MRS was 100 percent accurate in differentiating patients with disease from normal controls. Work with ^{1}H MRS is still preliminary, although some suggest that the NAA peak might be used to map areas of reduced neuronal concentration. In several studies myoinositol has been elevated in Alzheimer's disease. ^{1}H MRS is being used to test the hypothesis that the brain is depleted of choline-containing compounds in Alzheimer's disease. Whether the addition of other peaks such as myoinositol will help in the diagnosis is still unknown.

Pick's disease Pick's disease involves the anterior temporal and frontal lobes and spares the temporal-parietal regions. Initial symptoms often involve behavior and personality changes, with dementia symptoms occurring later. Common early symptoms include apathy and behavioral disinhibition, with some patients showing features of the Kluver-Bucy syndrome even before dementia occurs. The loss of organizational skills and of language output are often the first signs of dementia whereas there is relative sparing of mathematical and visuospatial skills.

At postmortem, atrophy and gliosis that are more prominent in the frontal and anterior temporal lobes and cytoplasmic inclusion bodies, the so-called Pick bodies, are seen. There are many patients with the clinical features of Pick's disease who at postmortem have lobar frontal and temporal atrophy and gliosis but no Pick bodies. In one series the number of patients with frontotemporal dementia with Pick bodies was only 20 percent. Patients without Pick bodies may be part of the spectrum of Pick's disease, with the presence or absence of Pick bodies a variable characteristic of the illness. It is also possible that those patients with Pick bodies represent a distinct disease process.

With frontotemporal dementia there is atrophy of the frontal and anterior temporal lobes, although for many patients CT or MRI studies are normal in the early stages. PET reveals frontal and anterior temporal hypometabolism with sparing of other brain regions in frontotemporal dementia and Pick's disease. SPECT shows marked symmetrical frontal hypoperfusion with more modest decreases in perfusion in the temporal-parietal area (Figures 2.10-7A and 2.10-7B). Those findings are seen in patients without dementia when the only manifestations of disease are behavioral alterations. As intellectual decline occurs the temporal-parietal cortex shows diminished perfusion. Like temporal-parietal hypoperfusion, frontal hypoperfusion is not specific to Pick's or frontotemporal dementia and patients with motor neuron disease, progressive supranuclear palsy, and depressive disorder have all been found to exhibit reduced per-

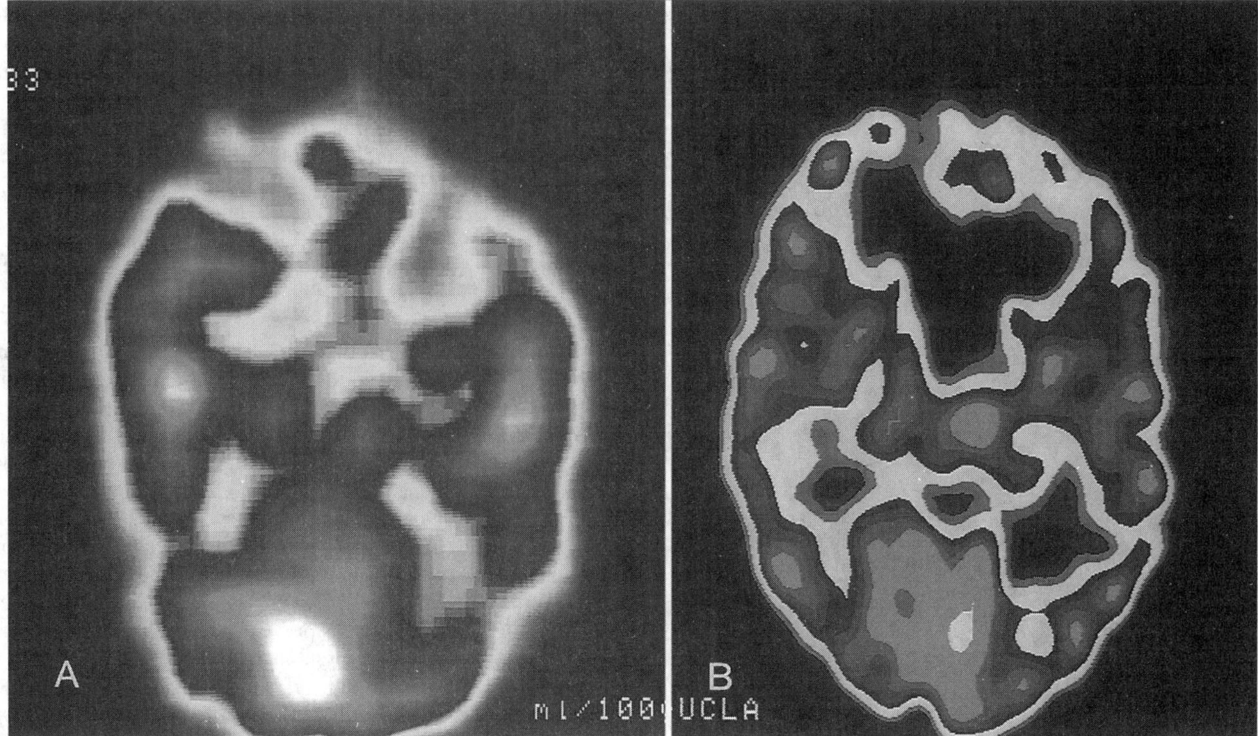

FIGURE 2.10-7 *A, Xenon 133 image of cerebral blood flow in a 52-year-old woman with a progressive frontal lobe degeneration. Blood flow ranges from 18 mL/100 g tissue a minute in the anterior frontal lobes to 74 mL/100 g tissue a minute in the occipital regions. B, HMPAO SPECT from the patient in Figure 2.10-7A demonstrating a 50 percent reduction in blood flow in the frontal regions. (See Color Plate 5.)*

fusion of the frontal lobes. Research criteria for frontotemporal dementia have been established.

Parkinson's disease and parkinsonian syndromes Patients with Parkinson's disease show progressive bradykinesia, tremor, and rigidity. Depression is common and the prevalence of dementia is higher than in age-matched controls. It is important to differentiate patients with idiopathic Parkinson's disease from those in whom parkinsonian symptoms are produced by a different disorder, particularly for those patients in whom dementia is present. Pathologically, Parkinson's disease is characterized by a greater than 90 percent loss of dopamine-containing cells in the substantia nigra and the presence of Lewy bodies in the remaining neurons. There are various possible causes for dementia in Parkinson's disease and some patients have both Parkinson's disease and Alzheimer's disease. However, recent work shows that some patients with a combination of dementia and parkinsonism have Lewy body dementia, a disorder marked by the diffuse deposition of Lewy bodies throughout the cortex. Another disease to be considered in the differential diagnosis of parkinsonism with dementia is progressive supranuclear palsy, although distinctive eye findings are usually present in patients with that condition. Shy-Drager syndrome is a parkinsonian syndrome associated with profound autonomic failure.

Structural imaging of Parkinson's disease is nondiagnostic. In parkinsonism resulting from brain infarction, CT or MRI shows multiple white matter and basal ganglia cerebrovascular disorders. Large CT lucencies or hyperintensity on MRI in the basal ganglia suggest other causes for the parkinsonian syndrome, including Wilson's disease, Hallervorden-Spatz disease, carbon-monoxide intoxication, striatonigral degeneration, Leigh's disease, or adult aminoaciduria. Atrophy of the dorsal midbrain is a feature of supranuclear palsy and olivopontocerebellar degeneration is characterized by atrophy of the medulla, pons, and cerebellum (Figure 2.10-8) with variable increases in lucency in the basal ganglia.

Calcification of the globus pallidus is common with normal aging, but calcification that spreads into the putamen, thalamus, or cerebellum requires investigation. If CT or MRI shows calcifications in globus pallidus, putamen, and cerebellar dentate nuclei (Figure 2.10-9), a search for calcium, phosphorus, or thyroid hormone abnormalities should be pursued. Polycystic lipomembranous osteodysplasia produces calcification of the basal ganglia and multiple carpal and metacarpal bone cysts. Idiopathic basal ganglia calcification is a diagnosis of exclusion, made after calcium metabolism abnormalities and the other diseases have been excluded.

MRI detects iron deposition in the basal ganglia, thalamus, red nucleus, and substantia nigra and is more sensitive to iron deposition than is CT. In adults MRI hypointensity in the globus pallidus, red nucleus, and pars reticularis of the substantia nigra are common owing to iron deposition. In the eighth and ninth decades those changes often spread to the putamen. In Parkinson's disease hypointensity in the putamen and substantia nigra decreases, but that finding is nonspecific and MRI cannot be used to diagnose Parkinson's disease.

A role for functional imaging in Parkinson's disease is uncertain and SPECT imaging of CBF and PET images of glucose metabolism are often normal in idiopathic Parkinson's disease. However, several investigators have found decreased uptake of radiolabeled compounds that bind to dopamine receptors in patients with Parkinson's disease. Supranuclear palsy shows hypoperfusion in the frontal lobes with SPECT. In some

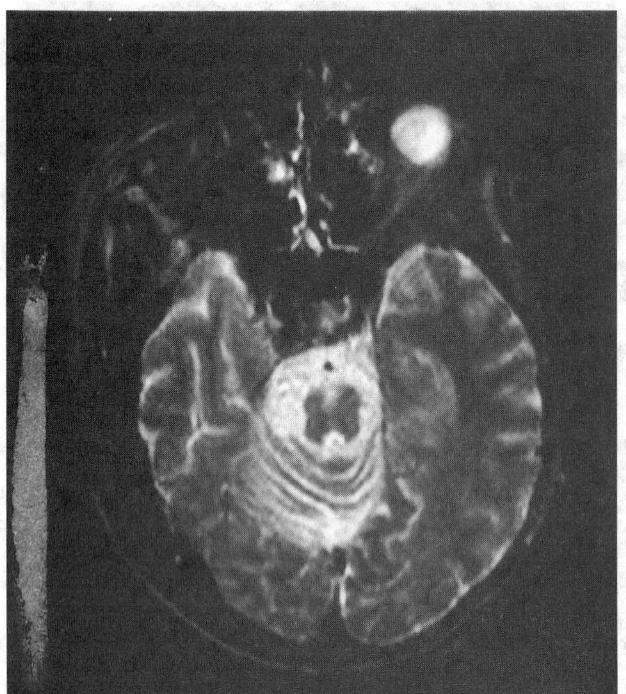

FIGURE 2.10-8 *A T_2-weighted MRI scan that shows a markedly atrophic pons.*

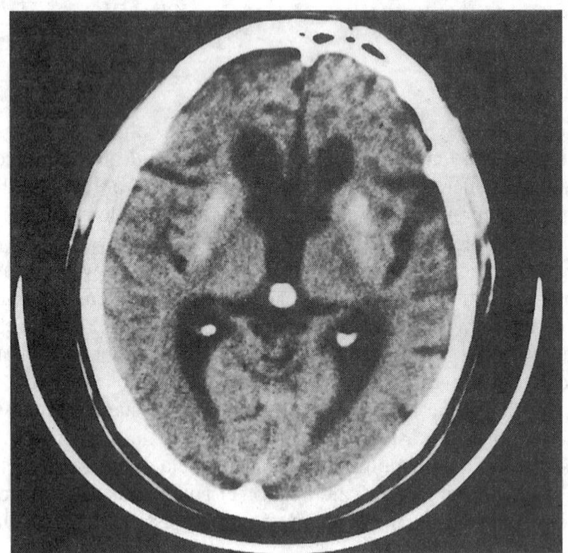

FIGURE 2.10-9 *A CT scan of a patient with progressive idiopathic basal ganglia calcification. Calcium deposition is evident in the caudate and putamen bilaterally.*

patients with dementias due to Parkinson's disease PET shows temporal-parietal hypometabolism, suggesting a combination of Alzheimer's disease and Parkinson's disease.

Huntington's disease Huntington's disease is an autosomal-dominant inherited disease characterized by a movement disorder and dementia. Psychiatric symptoms, including personality alterations, psychosis, depression, and mania, are all common in the disease. Patients typically develop symptoms during the third or fourth decade of life and survive about 11 years. On CT and MRI generalized atrophy and focal atrophy of the caudate nucleus are evident. However, those structural changes occur once the disease is clinically apparent and are not helpful for diagnosis in the early stages. Most investigators believe that even in the presymptomatic stages of Huntington's disease glucose metabolism studies with PET show caudate hypometabolism (Figure 2.10-10). Similar changes can be seen with SPECT (Figure 2.10-11). It is one of the few diseases of the nervous system where an imaging technique can detect a progressive degenerative brain disease before it is clinically apparent.

Normal-pressure hydrocephalus In normal-pressure hydrocephalus, first described in 1956, the ventricles are diffusely enlarged although CSF pressure is normal. Blockage of CSF absorption over the cerebral convexities is responsible for the dilatation of the ventricles. Although clinical symptoms are variable the classical normal-pressure hydrocephalus triad includes memory disturbance, gait apraxia, and urinary incontinence. Mental status changes can include apathy, depression, or an akinetic mute state. Vascular or degenerative dementia can mimic the clinical and imaging features of the syndrome.

No imaging technique has proved to be foolproof in defining those patients likely to respond to diversion of the CSF through a ventriculoperitoneal shunt. CT shows diffuse enlargement of the lateral, third, and fourth ventricles. Unlike Alzheimer's disease, in which the ventricles and sulci are all diffusely enlarged, the sulci should appear normal or compressed in normal-pressure hydrocephalus. MRI detects the ventricular enlargement and is useful for ruling out a fourth ventricular mass as the cause for the hydrocephalus. In patients with hydrocephalus there may

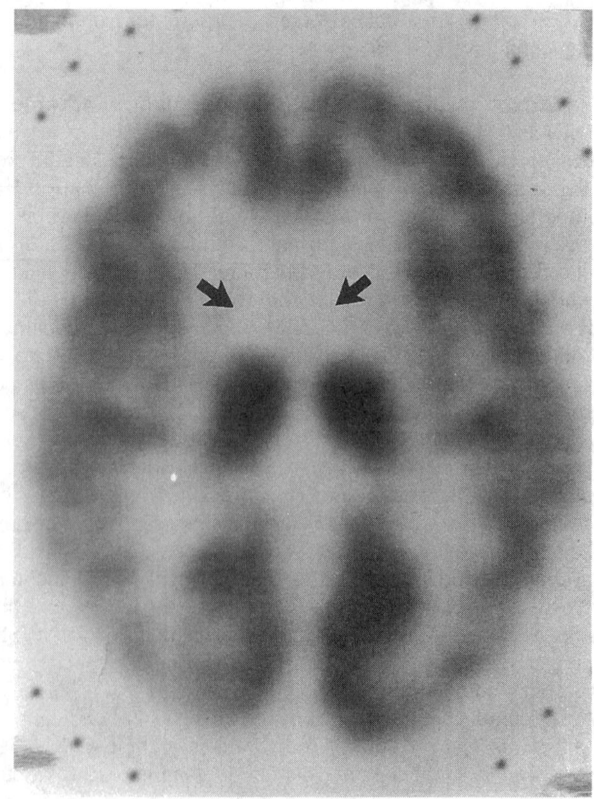

FIGURE 2.10-10 *FDG-18 PET scan of a patient with Huntington's disease that shows extensive hypometabolism of glucose in the caudate nuclei (arrows).*

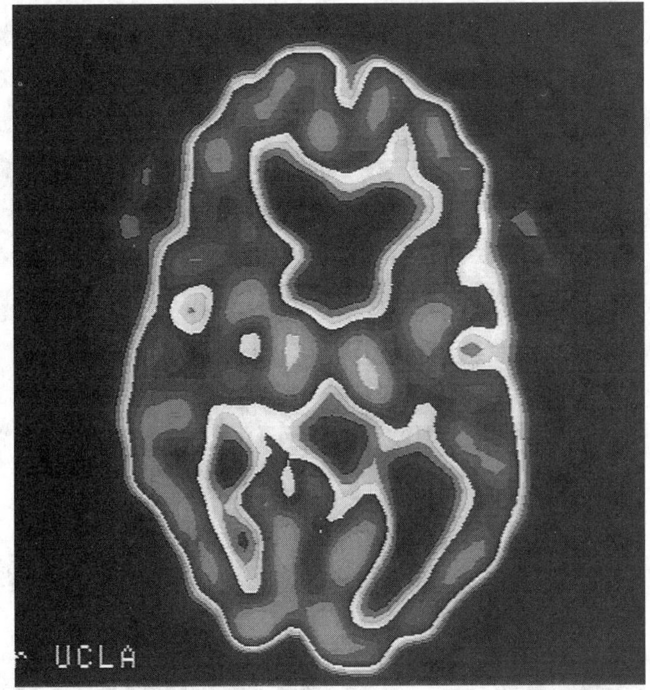

FIGURE 2.10-11 *HMPAO SPECT of a 46-year-old woman with dementia and chorea secondary to Huntington's disease. It shows marked hypoperfusion of both caudate regions. (See Color Plate 5.)*

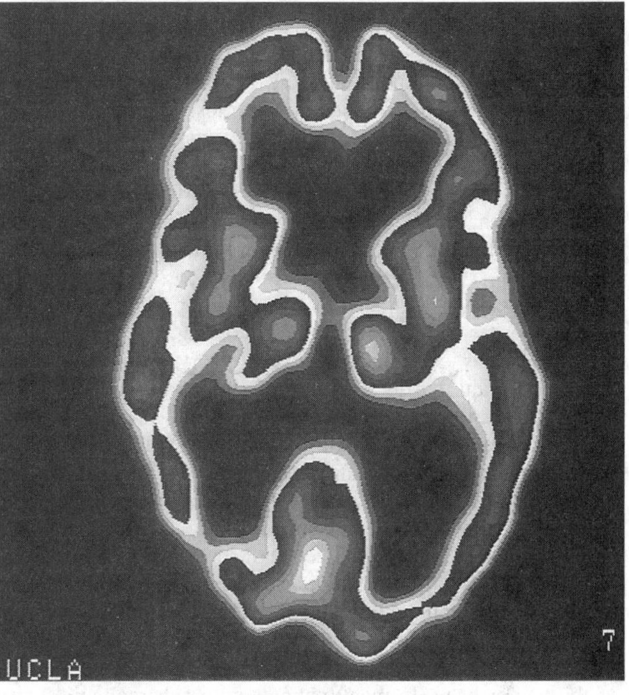

FIGURE 2.10-13 *SPECT of a patient with normal-pressure hydrocephalus that shows mild diffuse cortical and subcortical hypoperfusion. (See Color Plate 5.)*

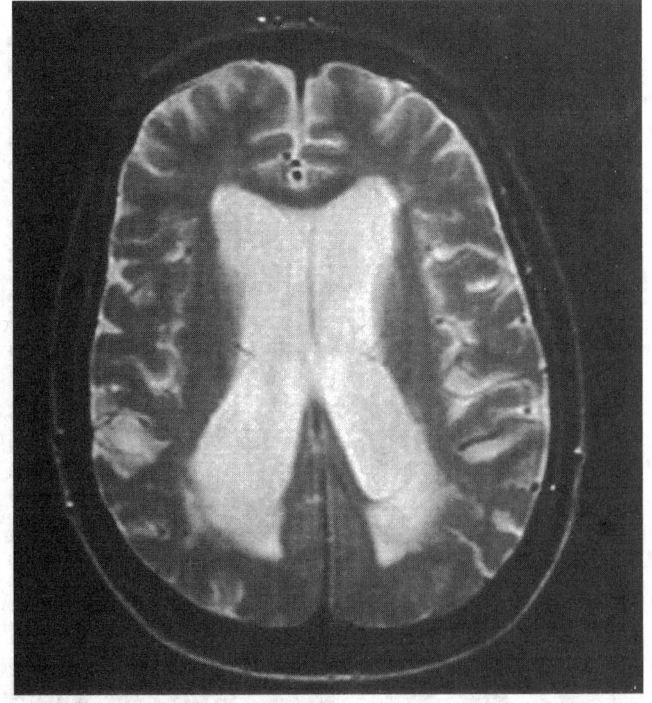

FIGURE 2.10-12 *A T_2-weighted MRI scan of a 76-year-old patient with dementia and gait apraxia secondary to normal-pressure hydrocephalus. It shows large periventricular white matter lesions and hydrocephalus. (See Color Plate 5.)*

be hyperintensities surrounding the lateral ventricles secondary to transudation of CSF into adjacent tissue (Figure 2.10-12). Many patients with vascular dementia have similar findings, however, and the presence of periventricular hyperintensity cannot reliably distinguish the two syndromes.

Nuclear medicine studies add information on selected patients. The flow of CSF can be delineated by the injection of radiolabeled albumin into the lumbar subarachnoid space. Normally the compound is absorbed into the ventricles and then percolates over the cerebral convexities. Most of the compound should be gone within 48 hours, although the radioactivity remains trapped in the ventricles and over the convexities. Unfortunately, false positives and false negatives occur with this technique.

The literature on SPECT and PET findings in normal-pressure hydrocephalus is limited. Many patients show global cerebral hypoperfusion or metabolism and do not demonstrate the Alzheimer's disease pattern of selective temporal-parietal changes (Figure 2.10-13). However, there are some patients with that pattern in whom shunting has been successful.

Jakob-Creutzfeldt disease A rapidly progressive dementia caused by infectious prion particles, its presentation is variable, although the rapid onset of dementia with extrapyramidal dysfunction and myoclonus is characteristic. CT and MRI findings are often normal or show nonspecific atrophy. PET shows multifocal patchy areas of hypometabolism.

VASCULAR DISEASE

Cerebrovascular disorder The result of an occlusion or hemorrhage from a blood vessel supplying brain tissue, the clinical syndrome depends on the type of cerebrovascular disorder and the tissue injured. The main types are thrombotic, embolic, intraparenchymal hemorrhage, and subarachnoid hemorrhage;

the vessels that supply cortex are the anterior, middle, and posterior cerebral arteries. The basal ganglia, thalamus, and capsule are supplied by small penetrating vessels coming from the anterior, middle, and posterior cerebral arteries. Neuroimaging has dramatically influenced the diagnostic approach to patients with cerebrovascular disorder.

In the setting of an acute event CT is performed to exclude brain hemorrhage. It is often normal for the first 24 to 48 hours following acute ischemic injury. Approximately 24 hours after acute ischemia nonenhanced CT reveals a loss of the junction of the gray and white matter in a wedge-shaped area at the site of the disorder and CT performed following the infusion of a dye reveals cortical enhancement secondary to breakdown of the blood-brain barrier. Within 72 hours a wedge-shaped lucency is seen, whereas the contrast scan shows enhancement of the cortical gyri at the site of infarction (Figure 2.10-14). After several months focal atrophy and a wedge-shaped cortical lucency remain. However, due to the resorption of tissue and remodeling of brain, little evidence may remain that a cerebrovascular event has occurred. Lacunar disorders in the brain stem and basal ganglia follow a similar pattern of enhancement and resorption, but brain hemorrhage is seen as an area of increased intensity with surrounding lucency secondary to edema. The hematoma is gradually resorbed, leaving a lucency at the site of the hemorrhage. In many patients with subarachnoid hemorrhage CT and MRI show blood in the subarachnoid space.

There are certain cerebrovascular syndromes in which MRI has a distinct advantage over CT. Disorders in the brain stem, basal ganglia, and subcortical white matter (Figure 2.10-15) are better resolved with MRI than with CT. Also, small arteriovenous malformations, angiomas, and capillary telangiectasias show well with MRI but are often missed with CT.

The role of SPECT in the setting of a cerebrovascular disorder has not yet been determined, although it appears that it

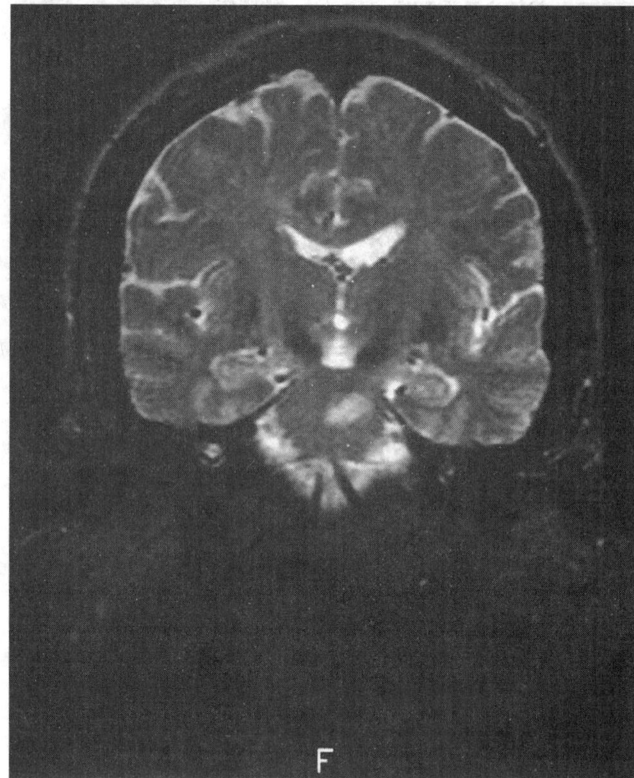

FIGURE 2.10-15 *The T_2-weighted MRI shows a small area of hyperintensity in the left pontine region in a patient with a cerebrovascular disorder.*

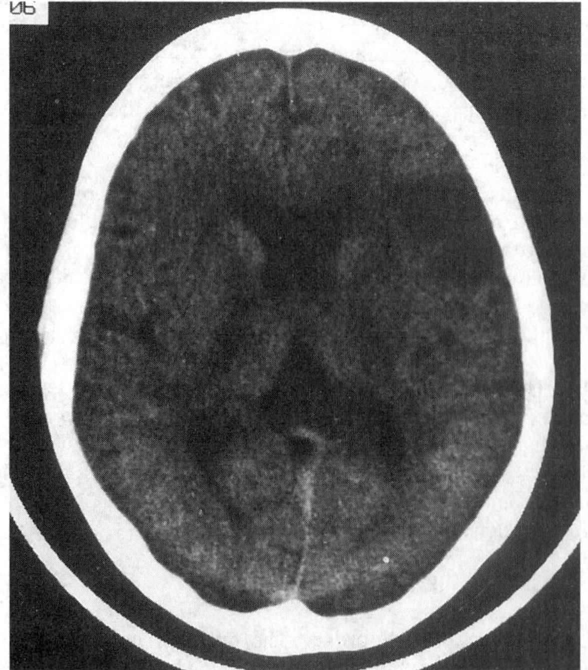

FIGURE 2.10-14 *A CT scan of an elderly woman with long-standing Broca's aphasia. It shows a wedge-shaped lucency in the left frontal region.*

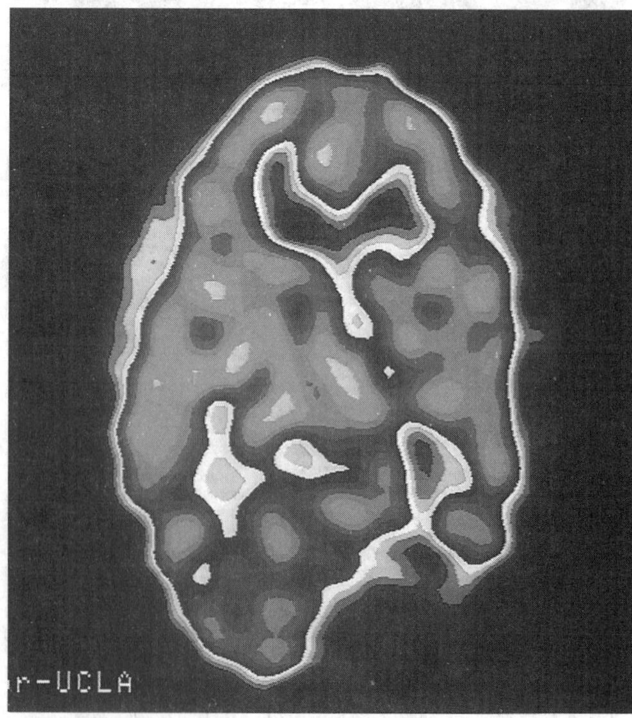

FIGURE 2.10-16 *HMPAO SPECT showing a 50 to 70 percent reduction in cerebral perfusion in the left occipital lobe in a patient with alexia without agraphia. (See Color Plate 6.)*

will eventually have value in the assessment of selected patients. In ischemic cerebrovascular disorder wedge-shaped hypoperfusion is seen within minutes of the acute insult and SPECT often exhibits a larger area of abnormality than is exhibited with structural scans (Figure 2.10-16). Those wider areas of hypoperfusion probably reflect imaging of tissue that is dysfunctional as opposed to structural imaging, which demonstrates injured tissue. Lesions that have receded on CT or MRI may persist for years with SPECT. However, SPECT cannot separate hemorrhage from ischemia and is poor at delineating ischemia in the white matter, basal ganglia, and brain stem.

PET has been utilized in cerebrovascular disorder and has the distinct advantage that it can be used to measure oxygen utilization and CBF simultaneously. In permanently infarcted tissue CBF and oxygen utilization are both decreased whereas tissue that is ischemic but not infarcted shows decreased blood flow but elevated oxygen utilization. That phenomenon occurs in the ischemic penumbra.

With acute ischemia ^{31}P MRS shows a drop in brain pH associated first with a decrease in phosphocreatine and followed by losses of adenosine triphosphate. With ^{1}H MRS NAA is seen to decrease, which probably reflects neuronal loss. Also, there is a rise in lactate secondary to a shift to anaerobic metabolism. Surprisingly, lactate may remain elevated for months in the infarcted region.

Vascular dementia The diagnosis of vascular dementia is made when a person has multiple cerebrovascular events and they cause a dementia syndrome. The Hachinski scale is a quantitative test that delineates the clinical features of vascular dementia: abrupt onset, stepwise deterioration, and focal neurological symptoms and signs. The pattern is often associated with multiple cortical infarcts and the diagnosis in patients with this form of vascular dementia is usually straightforward. However, in patients with subcortical or white matter cerebrovascular disorder the deterioration can be slowly progressive, as in Alzheimer's disease. It is important to identify patients with vascular dementia as the illness often has treatable and reversible components.

Early studies showed that the loss of a critical volume of tissue as a result of a cerebrovascular disorder (100 cubic centimeters) was always associated with a dementia whereas the occurrence of intellectual decline was more variable in patients with smaller volumes of infarcted tissue. Recent MRI studies have confirmed that patients with a cerebrovascular disorder without dementia have smaller areas of infarction than do patients with vascular dementia. Also, there may be critical regions in the cortex that must be involved to produce dementia. For example, infarction in the dominant angular gyrus causes right-left disorientation, visuospatial deficits, acalculia, agraphia, and alexia; a single lesion in that region can lead to a syndrome that mimics Alzheimer's disease. Also, MRI studies have shown that the left posterior cortex is much more likely to be affected in patients with vascular dementia than in patients with a cerebrovascular disorder without dementia.

Functional imaging shows promise for improving the diagnosis in patients with vascular dementia. SPECT reveals multifocal areas of brain hypoperfusion (Figures 2.10-17A and 2.10-17B) and with PET multifocal areas of hypometabolism are seen. With both SPECT and PET deficits that are not detectable with CT or MRI can be visualized. Recent work suggests that those techniques could be utilized to demonstrate patients with a dementia that is due to a combination of vascular dementia and Alzheimer's disease. In such patients the scans might show both temporal-parietal and multifocal perfusion deficits. Research criteria for vascular dementia were recently established.

White matter lesions in elderly persons With MRI a sizable percentage of normal elderly persons are seen to have detectable abnormalities within their white matter. Those white matter lesions increase in size with each decade, are rare in subjects under the age of 50, and are present in over 50 percent

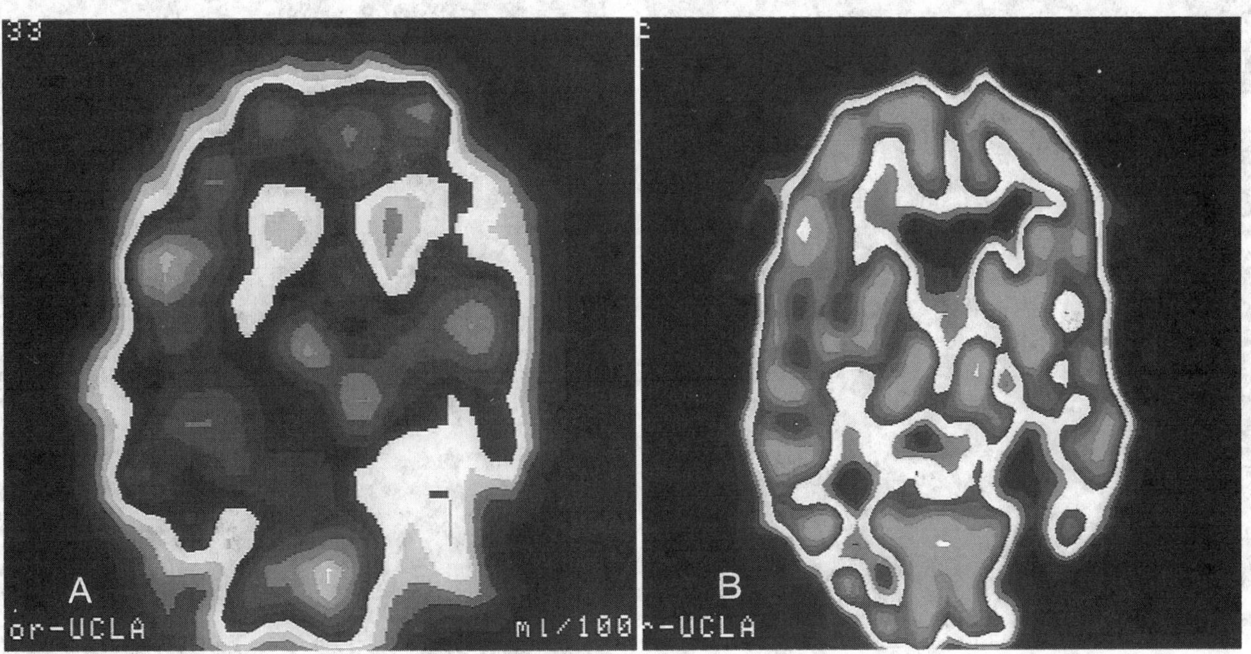

FIGURE 2.10-17A,B *Xenon 133 and HMPAO scans in a patient with vascular dementia show wedge-shaped areas of hypoperfusion in the left frontal and posterior parietal and right frontal areas. (See Color Plate 6.)*

of persons over 70. There is a high prevalence of white matter lesions in patients with hypertension and vascular dementia. The lesions have a predilection for the periventricular regions and commonly surround the lateral ventricles as a halo or appear as scattered small punctate lesions in the deep hemispheric white matter. However, about 6 percent of normal elderly have large white matter lesions (Figure 2.10-18). When the lesions are large they are usually seen with CT as white matter lucencies.

The etiology of white matter lesions is debatable; some researchers hypothesize that the lesions are benign, representing only pallor of white matter, and others state that they represent incomplete infarctions. In some cases small punctate lesions may be secondary to leakage of fluid or possibly direct pressure from hyalinized hypertensive vessels. The periventricular area is a watershed zone and may be more susceptible to ischemia in elderly persons. White matter lesions are more common in patients with vascular dementia than in normal elderly persons and in several studies of vascular dementia nearly 100 percent of the patients had large confluent white matter lesions. But it is unlikely that all of those lesions are attributable to chronic hypertension and the strongest risk factor is age. Other hypothesized risks include episodic hypotension and cerebral amyloid angiopathy.

The clinical symptoms associated with white matter lesions in elderly patients remain to be determined. Small lesions are common and a direct relationship between them and cognitive deterioration is unlikely. However, even in normal elderly persons large white matter lesions are associated with deficits on frontal systems tasks and there is a high frequency of such lesions in patients with depression and psychosis presenting for the first time late in life. In an elderly patient with large white matter lesions the clinician should look for potentially treatable cerebrovascular risk factors, such as hypertension. In one study of patients with severe hypertension the lesions disappeared following treatment. In rare elderly patients demyelinating disease or a leukodystrophy will be etiological.

Cocaine-induced cerebrovascular disorder and vasculitis Urban centers have seen an epidemic of cerebrovascular disorders in young persons who abuse cocaine. In many patients with cocaine-induced brain hemorrhage, hypertension from cocaine causes hemorrhage from occult arteriovenous malformations or aneurysms. In cocaine-precipitated ischemic cerebrovascular disorder the etiology is obscure and angiographic studies have typically been normal. In patients intoxicated with cocaine brain SPECT shows multifocal areas of hypoperfusion. Small focal areas of cortical hypoperfusion and large scalloped areas of hypoperfusion that surround the lateral ventricles are also seen (Figure 2.10-19). In PET studies multifocal areas of hypometabolism have been detected. The clinical significance of the lesions is unknown, although SPECT is probably detecting focal vasospasm in small cerebral vessels.

DEMYELINATING DISEASES AND LEUKODYSTROPHIES

Multiple sclerosis Multiple sclerosis is caused by an immunological attack on white matter. It often follows a relapsing and remitting course but in some patients it is slowly progressive. Many patients with multiple sclerosis have no psychiatric symptoms, particularly when the disease primarily affects the spinal cord. When hemispheric white matter is involved psychiatric symptoms are common. Mania and depression often occur and a small subset of patients develop psychosis. Those with large areas of demyelination usually develop a dementia. Mild CSF pleocytosis is common and oligoclonal bands are present in over 90 percent of patients. Evoked potentials may show dysfunction in areas not clinically affected, such as the optic nerve or brain stem.

Both CT and MRI can aid in the evaluation of patients with

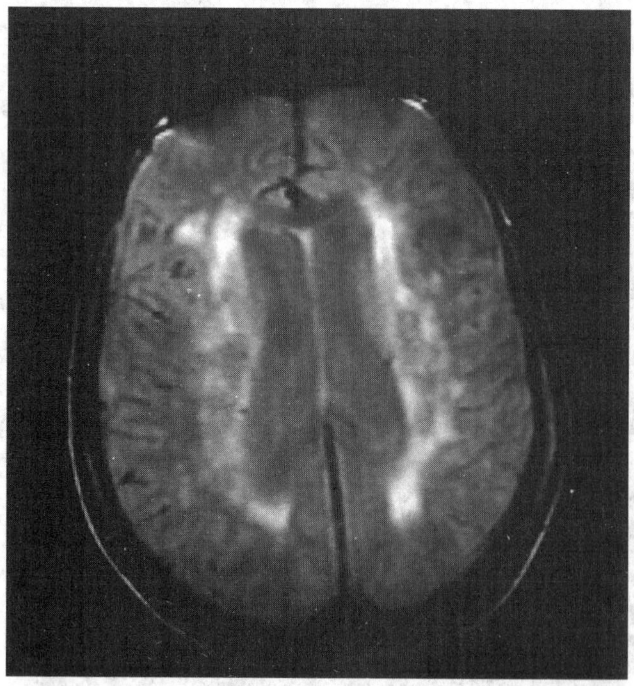

FIGURE 2.10-18 *MRI scan from a healthy elderly person with mild deficits on neuropsychological testing shows large confluent periventricular white matter lesions.*

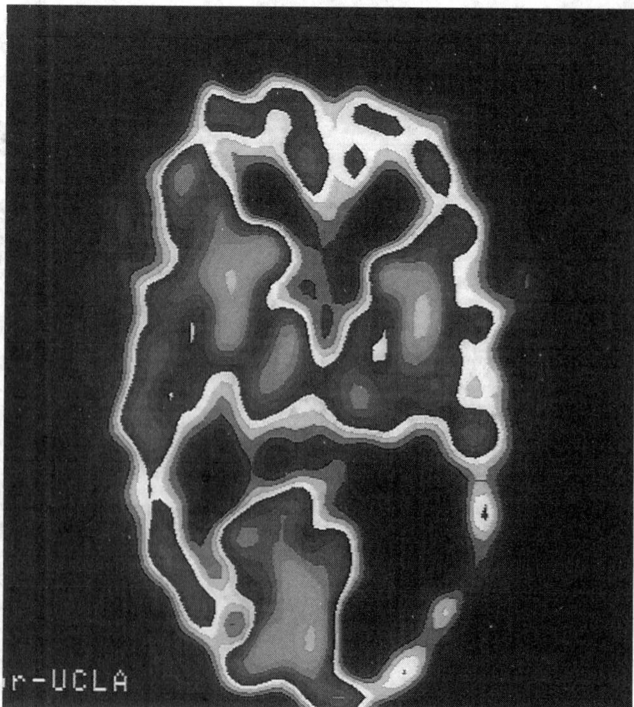

FIGURE 2.10-19 *HMPAO SPECT showing multifocal areas of hypoperfusion in a patient with chronic cocaine abuse. (See Color Plate 7.)*

multiple sclerosis. With CT both old and new large white matter lesions are seen as lucencies. Acute demyelination has a predilection for the regions surrounding the lateral ventricles and with contrast is detected as an enhancing area. MRI is more sensitive to white matter lesions than is CT and the T_2-weighted scan is excellent for showing multiple sclerosis plaques (Figure 2.10-20). MRI is also good for detecting lesions in the brain stem and spinal cord. The age of a plaque can be estimated with gadolinium, which detects the breakdown of the blood-brain barrier associated with acute inflammation. Enhancement with gadolinium lasts for as long as eight weeks following an acute attack.

Clinical studies show a strong relationship between cognition and MRI lesions, and several investigators report that the burden of white matter disease correlates with neuropsychological performance. Persons with extremely large areas of white matter lesions are often demented. Weaker relationships have been found between psychiatric symptoms and white matter lesions, although in one study the volume of temporal lobe lesions strongly correlated with psychosis.

Functional imaging has not added significantly to the clinical evaluation of patients with multiple sclerosis, although SPECT shows hypoperfusion in overlying white matter plaques and similar abnormalities have been reported with PET. However, ^{1}H MRS shows promise for differentiating between acute and chronic demyelination. Chronic multiple sclerosis lesions show decreased NAA, but with acute multiple sclerosis, NAA is often normal. Others have described increases in both lactate and lipids in patients with acute multiple sclerosis.

Leukodystrophies The leukodystrophies are rare diseases that produce degeneration of brain myelin. The most common types are adrenal and metachromatic leukodystrophy. Adrenal leukodystrophy is an X-linked demyelinating disease of the brain associated with an excess of long-chain fatty acids. It affects young boys and the history is frequently one of school failure or visual and motor disturbances that begin following normal early development. In adrenal leukodystrophy there is a predilection for temporal-occipital white matter and CT shows lucencies in those regions. MRI is able to detect the lesions in white matter prior to their visibility with CT.

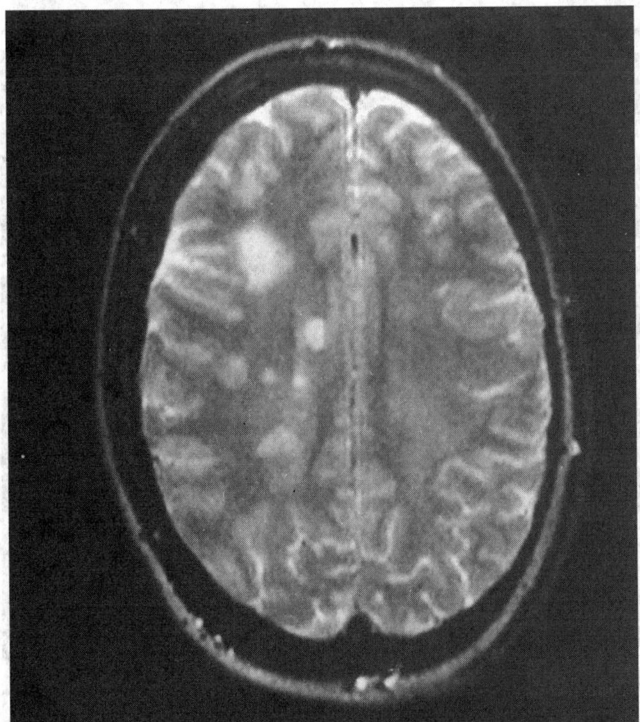

FIGURE 2.10-20 *T_2-weighted MRI showing multiple patchy white matter lesions in the right subfrontal region.*

Metachromatic leukodystrophy often presents in childhood with motor and cognitive deterioration. However, a subtype develops in adulthood, with some cases reported as late as the seventh decade. Most adult metachromatic leukodystrophy patients reported were initially diagnosed as having schizophrenia. The syndrome tends to be more diffuse or preferentially affects the frontal lobes. As with adrenal leukodystrophy, patients show white matter lucency on CT and hyperintensity on MRI. An even rarer leukodystrophy is adult Krabbe (globoid cell) leukodystrophy, which can present as a degenerative disease of adulthood. In globoid cell leukodystrophy diffuse symmetrical occipital white matter lesions, along with generalized cerebral atrophy, have been reported. Finally, there is a form of multiple sclerosis, Schilder's disease, that presents as slowly progressive dementia secondary to progressive immunologically mediated demyelination of subcortical white matter.

Rare adult neurodegenerative diseases There are a variety of diseases that typically begin in childhood but sometimes present as degenerative diseases in adults. Those rare diseases include Alexander's disease, Kuf's disease, cerebrotendinous xanthomatosis, Lafora's disease, GM_1 gangliosidosis type III, GM_2 gangliosidosis, Gaucher's disease type 1, Niemann-Pick disease type II-C, mucopolysaccharidosis type III-B, and Fabry's disease.

Two other degenerative diseases, Canavan's disease and mitochondrial encephalopathies, represent disease processes in which exciting advances in ^{1}H and ^{31}P MRS are providing additional information about diagnosis and pathogenesis. Canavan's disease causes progressive macrocephaly and motor and intellectual regression beginning during the first year of life. An enzymatic abnormality leads to the accumulation of NAA in the brain and body. MRI shows extensive white matter degeneration and ^{1}H MRS shows massive elevations of NAA, which can help confirm the diagnosis.

Mitochondrial encephalopathies are a heterogeneous group of disorders caused by mitochondrial dysfunction. Patients with those conditions typically exhibit a mixture of heart, peripheral muscle, and brain symptoms. The three main adult syndromes are Kearns-Sayre syndrome (ophthalmoplegia, ragged red fibers), MELAS (mitochondrial encephalomyopathy, lactic acidosis, and strokelike episodes), and MERRF (myoclonic epilepsy and ragged red fibers). In a few cases MRI has shown extensive white matter lesions, and with Kearns-Sayre syndrome a calcification of the basal ganglia occurs. ^{31}P MRS of muscle and brain shows abnormal phosphorus metabolism.

WERNICKE-KORSAKOFF SYNDROME In patients who are chronically deprived of thiamine (vitamin B_1) leakage of capillaries in the areas surrounding the third and sometimes fourth ventricle can occur. That condition typically arises in persons who abuse alcohol and who come into the hospital and are given an intravenous carbohydrate load without thiamine. During the acute phases of the disease (Wernicke's syndrome) patients exhibit a delirium. Ataxia, ophthalmoplegia, and peripheral neuropathy are often present. A patient who is not quickly treated with thiamine may progress to an extensive periventricular hemorrhage and die. Even with treatment some develop develop Korsakoff's syndrome. During Wernicke's syndrome the CT or MRI may be normal, although in florid cases hemorrhages surrounding the third, and perhaps the fourth, ventricle are seen. Atrophy of the mammillary bodies can sometimes be visualized on coronal MRI studies of patients with Korsakoff syndrome.

HEAD TRAUMA CT represented a significant advance for the study of head trauma, and in the setting of acute trauma made it possible to detect lesions that require acute surgical intervention, such as extradural, subdural, and intraparenchymal hematomas. Epidural hematomas appear as a unilateral area of increased density in the space between the brain and the skull. They are usually football shaped, and a shift of brain substance away from the side of the hematoma and compression of adjacent brain are seen. In contrast, acute subdural hematomas spread over the cortex and are often bilateral. Shifts of brain substance and acute hydrocephalus also occur.

Head trauma produces parenchymal or subarachnoid blood, which can lead to the development of communicating hydrocephalus. Common sites for contusions are the frontal and anterior temporal lobes. After head trauma the carotid or vertebral arteries may be injured, leading to superimposed cerebrovascular disorders. Herniation may compress the anterior or posterior cerebral arteries, producing ischemic deficits. Visualization of any of those findings on CT should elicit an emergency neurosurgical consultation. In severe brain trauma there is a loss of gray-white matter contrast, often a precursor of brain death.

Chronic head-injury patients are often seen in a psychiatric setting. Chronic subdural hematoma causes changes in attention, awareness, and mood, and should be considered in patients with those symptoms, even without focal neurological findings. Subacute subdural hematoma acquires the same density as brain and can be missed with CT, particularly if bilateral symmetrical hematomas are present. Chronic subdural hematomas acquire the density of water. Both CT and MRI detect intra- and extracerebral hematomas, although more subtle injuries can be missed. In many patients with behavioral deficits following head injury the structural image is normal. One possible explanation is that the injuries shear small white matter tracts (Strich lesions), producing alterations below the resolution of CT and MRI. In the years following a head injury there are resorption and remodeling of brain tissue and all that may remain as a remnant of an old injury is mild atrophy or even a normal CT or MRI.

However, SPECT and PET can both demonstrate functional deficits associated with remote head trauma. SPECT shows focal hypoperfusion at the site of the lesion whereas PET reveals focal hypometabolism at the site of injury. Coupe and contra-coupe lesions are also well demonstrated with SPECT (Figures 2.10-21A and 2.10-21B) and PET. As with cerebrovascular disorder areas distant from the area with structural injury show hypoperfusion or hypometabolism, suggesting that SPECT and PET detect dysfunction in neuronal systems and not just at the direct site of the injury (Figure 2.10-22). More research is required with SPECT and PET, but both techniques show promise for delineating the areas that are injured as a result of brain trauma.

TUMORS Many factors determine when and how a brain tumor will cause symptoms; some general principles apply to brain tumors in psychiatric disease. The first manifestation of a brain tumor is often a seizure and evaluation of a new onset seizure should include a contrast CT or an MRI. Tumors in certain anatomical areas are more likely to cause psychiatric symptoms. Frontal lobe meningiomas and gliomas are notorious for causing depression, behavioral disinhibition, and apathy. Occipital tumors, particularly right-sided ones, often cause visual hallucinations whereas temporal lobe masses can lead to irritability, language disturbances, and memory lapses—symptoms that can be mistaken for psychiatric diseases. In patients

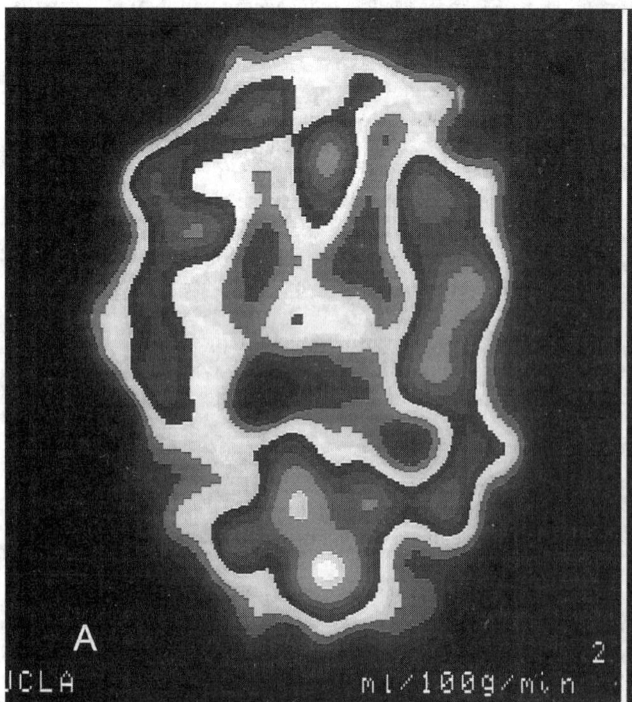

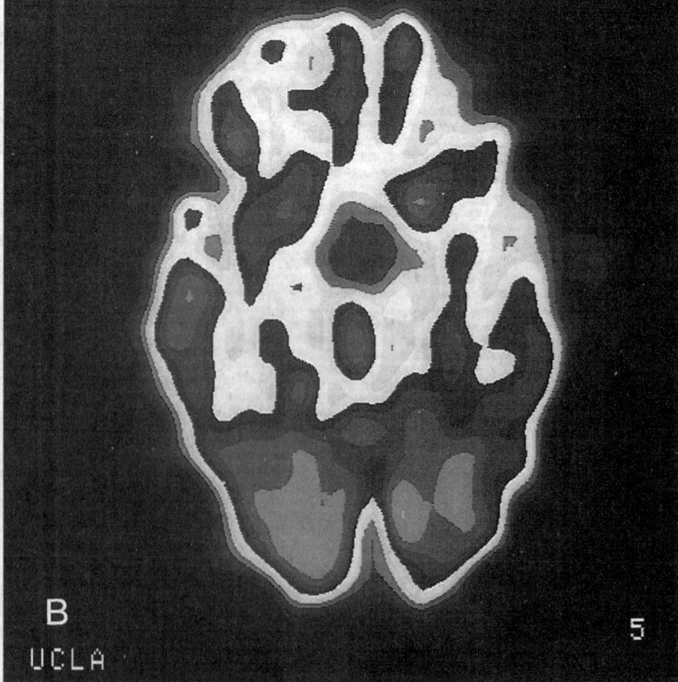

FIGURE 2.10-21A,B *Xenon 133 and HMPAO SPECT scans demonstrate bifrontal and bitemporal areas of hypoperfusion and a right posterior parietal contrecoup area of hypoperfusion. (See Color Plate 7.)*

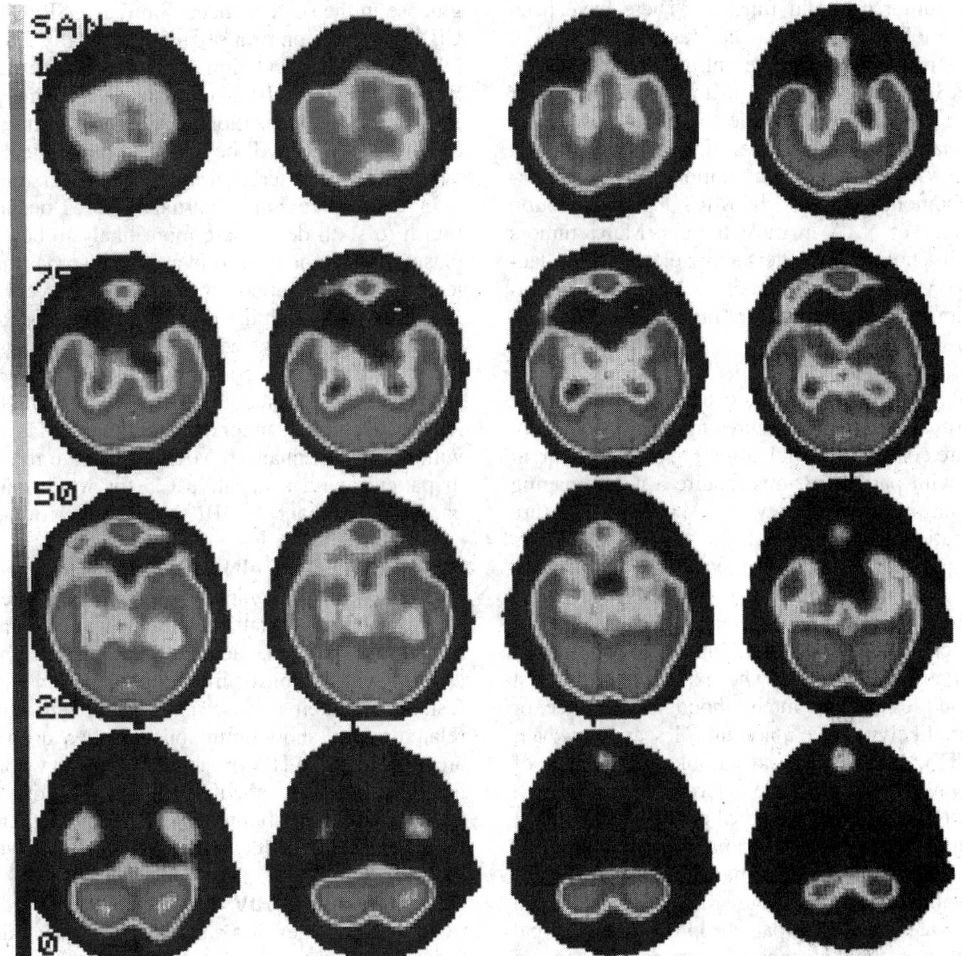

FIGURE 2.10-22 *HMPAO SPECT shows bifrontal hypoperfusion in a patient with a previous frontal leukotomy. Although only white matter fibers were cut the overlying cortex exhibits extensive hypoperfusion. (See Color Plate 8.)*

with such symptoms a contrast CT or MRI scan should be performed.

The main types of brain tumors are those of primary brain origin and those that are metastatic. Many primary brain tumors have benign characteristics and can be surgically cured. However, the most common brain tumor type, glioma, is usually fatal. Tumors are intra-axial if they are located in brain parenchyma or extra-axial if they are located outside the brain. Intra-axial brain tumors exert their effect by infiltrating and disrupting normal tissue. Extra-axial tumors compress normal brain tissue. Both intra- and extra-axial tumors cause symptoms by exerting direct pressure and by causing brain edema.

Contrast CT is a highly reliable imaging technique for suspected tumors. However, it is not as sensitive as MRI for detecting tumors in the brain stem, particularly those that lie adjacent to bone (such as cerebellopontine neurofibromas). Also, MRI is better at delineating edema and determining the true extent of tumor spread. A small percentage of tumors missed with CT are seen with gadolinium-enhanced MRI, which should be employed in selected cases.

Most primary and metastatic brain tumors appear on CT as areas of hypointensity, although a few types of metastatic tumor appear hyperintense even without contrast. Less malignant gliomas often show no or only slight enhancement with contrast whereas malignant astrocytomas often have a thick shaggy rim of surrounding enhancement. More malignant astrocytomas have a hypodense area surrounding the tumor that is due to edema. Only rarely are gliomas multicentric, so the presence of multiple enhancing lesions suggests either metastatic tumor or brain infection. Tumors often show an irregular and thick ring of enhancement whereas bacterial abscesses and cysticercal cysts have thin, symmetrical rims. Meningioma is the most common extra-axial tumor and exerts its effect by compressing adjacent brain.

In many regions of the third world, and even in some parts of the southwestern United States, the most common type of focal brain mass is cerebral cysticercosis, an infection by a parasite that invades the brain. Approximately 3 to 5 percent of the population in Mexico have cerebral cysticercosis at autopsy. With active cerebral cysticercosis the lesion appears on CT as a lucency. It is often surrounded by a rim of enhancement and in some instances the scolex of the worm can be visualized. Edema is variable and often is most intense when the larvae first invade the brain and when they die. MRI is better than CT at delineating the cyst, the scolex, and surrounding edema. Eventually the cysts calcify and those small calcifications are well visualized with CT or MRI.

SPECT, PET, and MRS are promising research tools for the study of brain tumors and infections. Both SPECT and PET have the advantage of being able to demonstrate the physiological effect of the tumor on brain function. There have been attempts to utilize PET to characterize the presence and type of tumor on the basis of the receptors present in the tumor.

^{31}P and ^{1}H MRS have been used to differentiate one tumor type from another chemically, to grade the degree of malignancy of a particular tumor, and to determine the response of a tumor to therapy. With ^{31}P MRS many tumors show an elevation of the phosphomonoester peak. ^{1}H MRS depicts depletion of the neuronal marker NAA in most tumors. Many tumors exhibit increases in choline and others show elevations of lactate or alanine. ^{1}H MRS might eventually be used to differentiate focal infections from brain tumor (Figure 2.10-23A and 2.10-23B).

EPILEPSY Epileptic seizures are caused by excessive synchronous neuronal discharge. Seizures may be generalized, involving the entire cortex, or partial, affecting only focal brain regions. Patients with partial seizures require a neuroimaging evaluation to determine the etiology and site of the seizure focus, whereas patients with generalized seizures are more likely to have idiopathic, genetic, or metabolic etiologies for the seizures.

The patient with a seizure that by electroencephalographic (EEG) or clinical characteristics is partial in origin requires, at the minimum, a brain CT. Patients who experienced the first onset of partial complex seizures in childhood, adolescence, or early adulthood are likely to have a normal CT scan. However, comprehensive EEG, MRI, PET, and pathological studies of patients with idiopathic epilepsy have determined that in such patients there are a variety of pathological processes. The most common pathological entity is hippocampal sclerosis, although focal trauma, cortical dysgenesis, gliomas, arteriovenous malformations, and hamartomas also occur. MRI in hippocampal sclerosis demonstrates hippocampal atrophy, hippocampal hyperintensity, and sometimes atrophy of the temporal lobe and dilatation of the ipsilateral temporal horn. The technique is exquisitely sensitive for detecting small gliomas, malformations, and areas of cortical dysgenesis that lead to intractable partial complex seizures.

During a focal seizure PET shows increased utilization of glucose in the seizure focus. Similarly, SPECT shows elevated CBF in the region of a seizure. Postictally PET shows glucose hypometabolism and diminished cerebral perfusion is seen with SPECT (Figure 2.10-24). In surgical studies the use of PET improves the localization of a seizure focus. It is likely that SPECT and PET will be added to the clinical armamentarium of the clinician interested in the site of seizures.

In the United States partial seizures occurring during the fourth to sixth decade are more likely to be caused by a neoplasm, trauma, or a cerebrovascular disorder than by congenital lesions, such as hippocampal sclerosis or cortical dysgenesis. In the seventh, eighth, and ninth decades vascular and degenerative brain diseases become the major etiology for focal seizures, with tumors accounting for a smaller percentage. A focal seizure in an adult should prompt a contrast CT as certain focal lesions, including tumors and infections, can be detected only with contrast. Enhanced MRI is sensitive to small tumors and in patients with a negative CT for whom suspicion is high, gadolinium-enhanced MRI should be performed.

HIV-RELATED BRAIN DISEASE The majority of patients infected with the human immunodeficiency virus (HIV) develop neuropsychiatric symptoms. Approximately 40 percent of patients with the acquired immune deficiency syndrome (AIDS) will exhibit neurological symptoms as the first manifestation of their disease, and 90 percent who die of AIDS-related causes show brain abnormalities at postmortem. There are three types of HIV-infected patients in whom neuroimaging has been utilized: patients with dementia due to HIV disease, patients with focal brain masses, and persons who are infected with HIV but have few or no AIDS-related symptoms.

Dementia due to HIV disease Patients with dementia due to HIV disease develop a slowly progressive dementia characterized by mental slowing, apathy, depression, forgetfulness, and visuospatial deficits. It eventually progresses to severe dementia and ultimately to death. Patients with the syndrome show severe generalized brain atrophy and extensive subcortical white matter changes on CT and MRI. PET studies have found hypermetabolism in the basal ganglia early, followed by

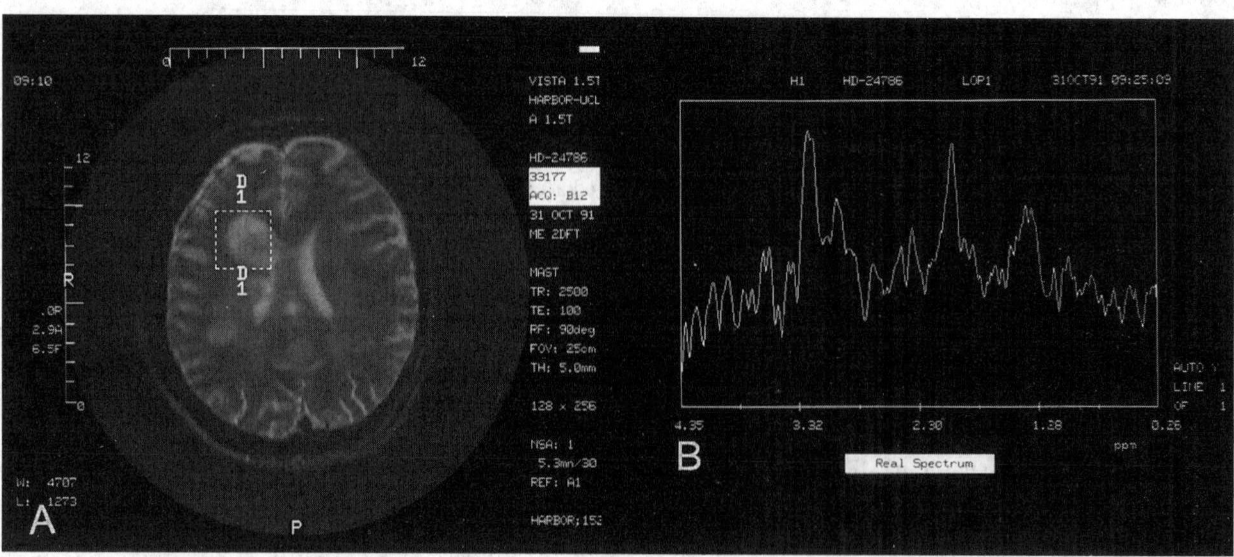

FIGURE 2.10-23 *A T_2-weighted MRI showing a large periventricular mass lesion in a patient with AIDS (A). Biopsy revealed a lymphoma. A 27-cm^3 spectrum from within the mass (B), which shows a marked loss of NAA with a large lactate peak. The largest peak is choline and the lactate-to-choline ratio is greater than 1.*

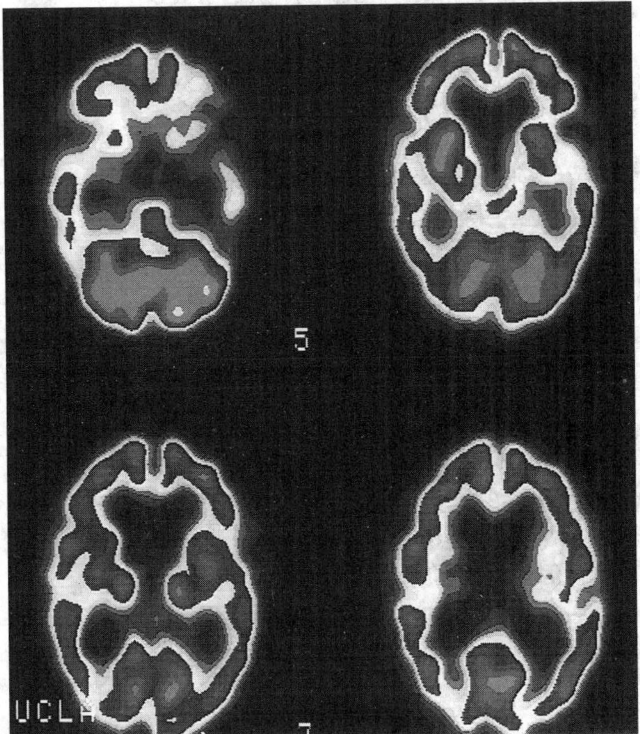

FIGURE 2.10-24 *HMPAO SPECT demonstrates severe left temporal and posterior left frontal hypoperfusion in a postictal woman with partial complex seizures. (See Color Plate 8.)*

global cortical hypometabolism in the later stages of the disease. Treatment with azidothimidine (AZT) may improve the PET abnormalities. In the few SPECT studies that have been performed multifocal areas of hypoperfusion (not unlike the pattern seen with vasculitis) are seen in some subjects; others show focal frontal or temporal hypoperfusion. Preliminary ^{31}P MRS studies suggest that there may be global brain decreases in phosphorus-containing compounds. ^{1}H MRS has shown decreases in NAA suggesting neuronal loss. Although there has been a tendency to describe dementia due to HIV disease as a homogeneous entity, it is more likely that there are many different diseases that cause dementia in AIDS patients and neuroimaging studies may be helpful in separating the different syndromes.

Focal brain masses in AIDS Focal brain infections and primary brain tumors are seen in as many as 40 percent of the patients infected with HIV. Toxoplasmosis, cryptococcomas and other fungal abscesses, and progressive multifocal leukoencephalopathy are the most common opportunistic infections, and primary brain lymphoma is the most frequent tumor. MRI is more sensitive than CT to those AIDS-related masses and may show multifocal lesions when CT shows only a single mass. Toxoplasmosis is often multifocal with a predilection for the basal ganglia, whereas progressive multifocal leukoencephalopathy primarily involves white matter. Lymphomas spread in the regions around the ventricles and are usually solitary.

Despite those general rules it is often impossible to discriminate one infection from another or an infection from a tumor on clinical or MRI findings. It may eventually be possible to use ^{1}H MRS to separate one infection from another chemically and to differentiate tumors from infections. In preliminary work tumors have shown elevations in choline whereas infections often have resulted in massive elevations of lactate.

LATE-ONSET DEPRESSIVE AND PSYCHOTIC DISORDER Imaging of patients who develop the first onset of depressive or psychotic disorder after the age of 45 has been particularly helpful. After excluding patients with clinical evidence of dementia 64 percent of patients with late-onset depressive disorder were found to have significant medical or neurological disease as compared with less than 10 percent of elderly controls. The major abnormality that accounted for the difference was the presence of large confluent white matter lesions in the depressed group (50 percent as compared with 9.7 percent of controls). A strong association also has been found between white matter lesions and depressive disorder. In the foregoing study, two of 14 patients had evidence of early degenerative dementia, two had tumors, and one had evidence of posttraumatic brain injury. SPECT studies of those patients showed a high prevalence of frontal and temporal hypoperfusion, although with SPECT the patients could not be uniformly differentiated from normal elderly controls. Similarly, another study showed that patients experiencing the first onset of psychotic disorder had a higher prevalence of structural brain disease than did elderly controls.

The studies indicate a greater degree of structural and functional brain disease in patients with late-onset psychotic or depressive disorder. Those abnormalities include large white matter lesions, cerebrovascular disorder, brain tumor, and degenerative dementias. Although functional imaging studies of those populations did not present a specific SPECT pattern, there was a higher frequency of focal brain dysfunction, which was most severe in the frontal and temporal regions. Any patient with a late-life onset of psychotic or depressive disorder requires a neuroimaging evaluation to search for structural brain injury. Ongoing neuroimaging and neuropathological studies in younger patients with psychiatric illnesses will almost certainly continue to demonstrate links between brain injury and brain dysfunction in many psychiatric conditions.

FUTURE DIRECTIONS

Neuroimaging has had a major influence on the diagnostic approach to patients with psychiatric disease and CT or MRI is now frequently utilized to study selected psychiatric patients. The discovery that some psychiatric patients have structural brain injuries that contribute to or cause their psychiatric symptoms has reemphasized the role of structural brain injury in the pathogenesis of certain psychiatric diseases.

Although CT has practically achieved its diagnostic potential, MRI resolution may continue to improve and microscopic imaging theoretically is possible. The emergence of in vivo ^{1}H and ^{31}P MRS is an exciting advance. Resolution with MRS is improving and the number of chemicals that can be reliably measured continues to rise. The techniques are relatively easy to use clinically and it is likely that, in the coming years, MRS will provide valuable information on specific psychiatric diseases.

The powerful techniques of SPECT and PET are now being used in a variety of psychiatric conditions and often show functional brain deficits when structural images are normal. They are particularly valuable in diagnosing degenerative dementias, and show promise for other psychiatric conditions as well. It is unlikely that a single pattern of hypometabolism or perfusion will be delineated with most psychiatric conditions, although SPECT and PET can help to differentiate degenerative demen-

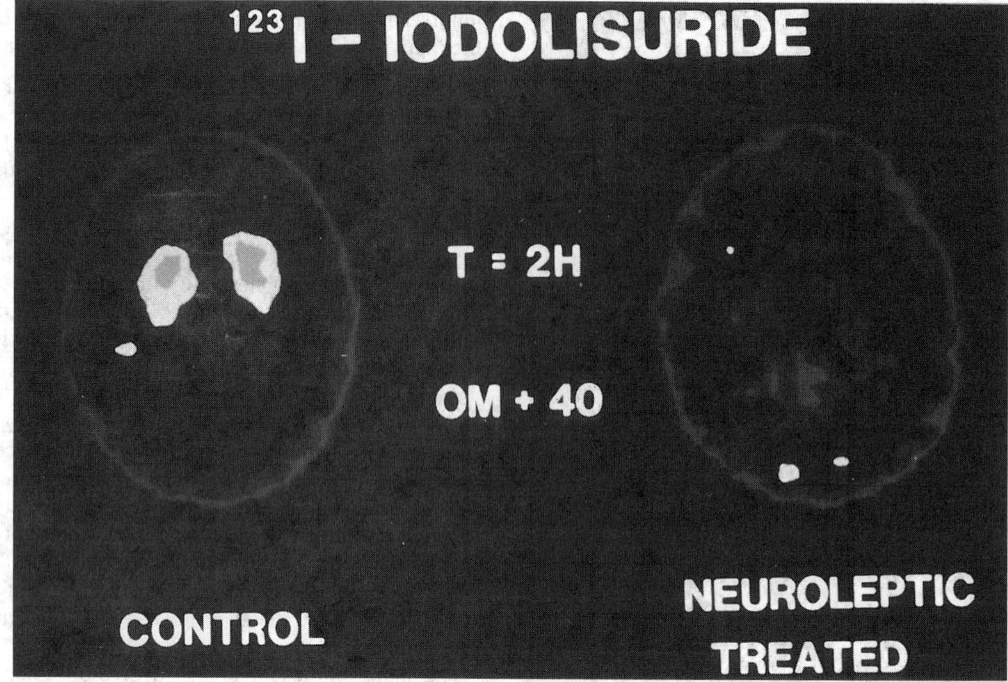

FIGURE 2.10-25 *Iodine 123-labeled lisuride SPECT. The D_2 agent shows extensive uptake in the basal ganglia which is eliminated by preloading with the dopamine antagonist haloperidol (Haldol). (See Color Plate 9.)*

tias from purely psychiatric diseases. The techniques may prove of diagnostic value in subgroups of patients with psychiatric conditions, and both are beginning to pinpoint brain regions that are dysfunctional in specific syndromes.

Future receptor labeling with PET and SPECT may help to define the site in the brain where neurochemical dysfunction is present. Receptor imaging has been extensively studied with PET, but D_2 receptor imaging with SPECT now is possible (Figure 2.10-25). An exciting use for this technique will be to assess whether drug treatment has effectively reached the receptor sites.

SUGGESTED CROSS-REFERENCES

The principles of neuroimaging are discussed in Section 1.10, the neuropsychiatric aspects of multiple sclerosis and other demyelinating disorders are discussed in Section 2.6, and medical assessment and laboratory testing are discussed in Section 9.7. The psychiatric aspects of the acquired immune deficiency syndrome are discussed in Section 29.2 and the neuropsychological and neuropsychiatric aspects of HIV infection are discussed in Section 29.2a. The use of neuroimaging in geriatric practice is discussed in Section 49.5c.

REFERENCES

Arnold D L, Matthews P M, Francis G, Antel J: Proton magnetic resonance spectroscopy of human brain in vivo in the evaluation of multiple sclerosis: Assessment of the load of disease. Magn Res Med *14:* 154, 1990.

Brun A, Englund B, Gustafson L, Passant U, Mann D M A, Neary D, Snowden J S: Clinical and neuropathological criteria for frontotemporal dementia. J Neurol Neurosurg Psychiatry *57:* 416, 1994.

Brunetti A, Berg G, Di Chiro G, Cohen R M, Yarchoan R, Pizzo P A, Broder S, Eddy J, Fulham M J, Finn R D, Larson S M: Reversal of brain metabolic abnormalities following treatment of AIDS dementia complex with 3″-azido-2′, 3′-dideoxythymidine (AZT, zidovudine): A PET-FDG study. J Nucl Med *39:* 581, 1989.

Ciricillo S, Rosenblum M: Use of CT and MR imaging to distinguish intracranial lesions and to define the need for biopsy in AIDS patients. J Neurosurg *73:* 720, 1989.

Coffey C E, Figiel G S, Djang W T: White matter hyperintensity on magnetic resonance imaging: Clinical and neuroanatomic correlates in the depressed elderly. J Neuropsychiatry Clin Neurosci *1*: 135, 1989.

Coker S B: The diagnosis of childhood neurodegenerative disorders presenting as dementia in adults. Neurology *41:* 794, 1991.

Davis P C, Hudgins P A, Peterman S B, Hoffman J C: Diagnosis of cerebral metastases: Double-dose delayed CT vs contrast-enhanced MRI. Am J Neurorad *12:* 293, 1991.

Engel J: *Seizures and Epilepsy*. Davis, Philadelphia, 1989.

Ernst T, Kreis R, Ross B D: Absolute quantitation of water and metabolites in the human brain: I: Compartments and water. J Magn Res *B102:* 1, 1993.

Grady C L, Haxby J V, Schapiro M B, Gonzalez-Aviles A, Kumar A, Ball M J, Heston L, Rapoport S I: Subgroups in dementia of the Alzheimer type identified using positron emission tomography. J Neuropsychiatry Clin Neurosci *2*: 373, 1990.

Gur R C, Gur R E, Obrist W D, Skolnick B E, Reivich M: Age and regional cerebral blood flow at rest and during cognitive activity. Arch Gen Psychiatry *44:* 617, 1987.

Lesser I M, Miller B L, Boone K B, Hill E, Mehringer C M, Wong K, Mena I: Brain injury and cognitive function in late-onset psychotic depression. J Neuropsychiatry Clin Neurosci *3*: 33, 1991.

Liu C K, Miller B L, Cummings J L, Goldberg M, Mehringer C M, Howng S L, Benson D F: A quantitative MRI study of vascular dementia. Neurology *42:* 138, 1992.

Matthews, P M, Tampieri D, Berkovic S F, Andermann F, Silver K, Chityat D, Arnold D A: Magnetic resonance imaging shows specific abnormalities in the MELAS syndrome. Neurology *41:* 1043, 1991.

*Mazziotta J C, Phelps M E, Carson R E, Kuhl D E: Tomographic mapping of human cerebral metabolism: Auditory stimulation. Neurology *32:* 921, 1982.

Meyerhoff D J, Ner Nat, MacKay S, et al: Reduced brain *N*-acetylasparate suggests neuronal loss in cognitively impaired human immunodeficiency virus-seropositive individuals: In vivo ^{1}H magnetic resonance spectroscopic imaging. Neurology *43:* 509, 1993.

Miller B L: The choline peak in ^{1}H NMR spectroscopy. NMR Biomed *5:* 1, 1991.

Miller B L, Chang L, Mena I, Boone K, Lesser I: Clinical and imaging features of right focal frontal lobe degenerations. Dementia *4*: 204, 1993.

*Miller B L, Cummings J L, Villaneuva-Meyer J, Boone K, Mena I: Frontal lobe degeneration: Clinical, neuropsychological and SPECT characteristics, Neurology *41:* 1374, 1991.

Miller B L, Lesser I M, Boone K, Hill E, Mehringer C M, Wong K: Brain lesions and cognitive function in late-life psychosis. Br J Psychiatry *158:* 76, 1991.

Miller B L, Mena I, Daly J, Giombetti R J, Goldberg M A, Lesser I M, Garrett K, Villaneuva-Meyer J, Liu C K: Temporal-parietal hypoperfusion with SPECT in conditions other than Alzheimer disease. Dementia *1*: 41, 1990.

Miller B L, Moats R, Shonk T, Ernst T, Wooley S, Ross B D: Abnormalities of cerebral myoinositol in patients with early Alzheimer disease. Radiology *187:* 334, 1993.

Neirinckx R D, Canning L R, Piper I M, Nowotnik D P, Pickett R D, Holmes R A, Volkert W A, Forster A M, Weisner P S, Marriott J A, Chaplin S B: Technetium-99m d, l-HM-PAO: A new radiopharmaceutical for SPECT imaging of regional cerebral perfusion. J Nucl Med *28:* 191, 1987.

Perry E K, Irving D, Kerwin J M, McKeith I G, Thompson P, Collerton V, Fairbairn A F, Ince P G, Morris C M, Cheng A V, Perry R H: Cholinergic transmitter and neurotrophic activities in Lewy body dementia: Similarity senile dementia of the Lewy body type: A clinically and neuropathologically distinct form of Lewy body dementia in the elderly. J Neurol Sci *95:* 119, 1990.

*Pettegrew J W, Keshavan M S, Panchalingam K, Strychor S, Kaplan D B, Tretta M G, Allen M: Alterations in brain high-energy phosphate and membrane phospholipid metabolism in first-episode, drug naive schizophrenics. Arch Gen Psychiatry *48:* 563, 1991.

Roman G C, Tatemichi T K, Erkinjuntti T, Cummings J L, Masdeu J C, Garcia J H, Amaducci L, Orgoggozo J M, Brun A, Hofman A, Moody D M, O'Brien M D, Yamaguchi T, Grafman J, Drayer B P, Bennett D A, Fisher M, Ogata J, Kokmen E, Bermejo F, Wolf P A, Gorelick P B, Bick K L, Pajeau A K, Bell M A, DeCarli C, Culebras A, Korczyn A D, Bogousslavsky J, Hartmann A, Scheinberg P: Vascular dementia: Diagnostic criteria for research studies: Report of the NINDS-AIREN International Workshop. Neurology *43:* 250, 1993.

*Ross B D, editor: Proton spectroscopy in clinical medicine. NMR Biomed: *4*: 49, 1991.

Seeman P, Niznik H B: Dopamine receptors and transporters in Parkinson's disease and schizophrenia. FASEB *4*: 237, 1990.

Sidtis J J, Gatsonis C, Price R W, et al: Zidovudine treatment of the AIDS dementia complex: Results of a placebo-controlled trial. Ann Neurol *33:* 342, 1993.

Skomer C, Stears J, Austin J: Metachromatic leukodystrophy (MLD): XV. Adult MLD with focal lesions by computed tomography. Arch Neurol *40:* 354, 1983.

*Smith F W, Besson J A, Gemmell H G, Sharp P F: The use of technetium-99m-HM-PAO in the assessment of patients with dementia and other neuropsychiatric conditions. J Cereb Blood Flow Metab *8*: 116, 1988.

Snow B J, Nygaard T G, Takahashi H, Calne D B: Human positron emission tomographic [18F]fluorodopa studies correlate with dopamine with dopamine cell counts and levels. Ann Neurol *34:* 324, 1993.

Tzika A A, Ball W S, Bigneron D B, Dunn R S, Kirks D R: Clinical proton MR spectroscopy of neurodegenerative disease in childhood. Am J Neurorad *14:* 1267, 1993.

Wolinsky J S, Narayana, P A, Fenstermacher M J: Proton magnetic resonance spectroscopy in multiple sclerosis. Neurology *40:* 38,

CHAPTER 3 CONTRIBUTIONS OF THE PSYCHOLOGICAL SCIENCES

3.1 PERCEPTION AND COGNITION

DANIEL J. SIEGEL, M.D.

INTRODUCTION

Perception and cognition are important domains of study in understanding psychopathology. In the past few years an explosion in the field of cognitive science has focused on such topics as attention, perception, memory, thinking, intelligence, information processing, schemata, and control of action. In the past the field of cognitive psychology played the major role in studying those areas. Now that field has been joined by anthropology, psycholinguistics, artificial intelligence, computer science, philosophy, and the neurosciences. The convergence of those disciplines in the 1980s brought an abundance of insights into mental processes that are relevant to the psychiatry of the 1990s.

Some basic questions addressed by cognitive science include the following: (1) How is the external world sensed and perceived? (2) How are mental representations of the external world acted on to allow higher cognitive processing, such as generalizations, deductions, and schematizations? (3) What is thinking? (4) What is imagery? (5) What are mental models? (6) What is consciousness? (7) How do emotions interact with cognition?

Although mainstream cognitive scientists generally do not discuss social cognition, emotions, and subjective experience, many leaders in the field encourage their study since they are fundamental aspects of human mental functioning.

Emotions, memories, desires, images, ideas, and thoughts emanate from the complex neural structures encased in the skull. Even the subjective experience of self-awareness can be understood as a cognitive-perceptual process that internally focuses attention on the cognitive processes of itself. Neuroanatomy reveals that the billions of cells in the brain are distributed in a complex interwoven network. Recently designed computer models of parallel distributed processes can mimic such things as perceptual recognition, decision processes, and learning. Thus psychiatrists need not postulate a mind substance that is separate in location, quality, or quantity from the functioning of the brain. Biological, psychodynamic, and social psychiatry can find a common home and language in the field of cognitive science.

BASIC CONCEPTS

COGNITIVE PSYCHOLOGY The information-processing model has been the dominant theoretical influence on research paradigms. Each of the disciplines has been able to incorporate that conceptualization into its theoretical approaches to varying degrees. A basic model (Figure 3.1-1) focuses on the flow of information between stimuli and response. That view includes taking in external stimuli (energy), filtering them into perceptual data (information), and using a short-term or working memory process in which the data are analyzed, encoded into long-term memory, and retrieved from long-term memory and returned to short-term (working) memory. Sensory input can also be encoded in some forms without passing through working memory, such as in divided-attention experiments. Representations in long-term memory are then available for further cognitive processing (generalizations, deductions, comparisons) as they are retrieved back into working memory. The retrieval process can influence the form of the representations in long-term memory. Output or action can be a verbal or a nonverbal behavioral response (bodily movement, speech, writing).

An important aspect is the direction of processing. In *bottom-up* (stimulus-driven or data-driven) processing the dominant thrust of the information flow is from external stimuli to higher processes. For example, in viewing a painting that one has never seen before, careful attention to lines, contrasts, and combinations of colors dominates the processing of the visual information. In *top-down* (conceptually driven or theory-driven) processing a dominant influence on processing is from higher cognitive functions. Thus prior knowledge, semantic classification schemes, memory for similar events, and prior exposure to similar stimuli influence the processing of perceptual data.

INFORMATION PROCESSING The term ''sensation'' refers to the initial stages of the input process. The term ''perception'' refers to the processes that identify and interpret the initial sensory image and act on its information content. Perceptual processes thus extract certain features from sensory input.

The term ''cognition'' can be used to refer to the entire range of mental processes from input to output, to just the complex functions that act directly on perceptual representations, or to representations retrieved from long-term memory. Examples of those functions include rehearsing, noting similarities, classifying, storing, and retrieving information. Other higher-order processes relate to the elaborate functions of logical deduction, schematization, and the manipulation of language

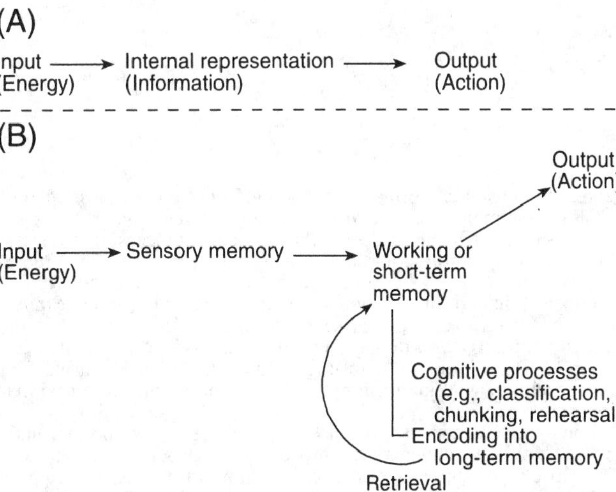

FIGURE 3.1-1 *Information-processing models. (A) Basic elements. (B) Expanded model of information flow showing some steps from input to encoding to output. Attention processes can act at any of the arrow stages and are thought to regulate the flow of information processing.*

FIGURE 3.1-2 *Act* (A) and Soar (B), two cognitive architectures that outline computational approaches to information processing. Both architectures emphasize the basic elements of input, working memory, long-term memory, and output. (Figure from A Newall, P S Rosenblum, J E Laird: Symbolic architectures for cognition. In* Foundations of Cognitive Science, *M I Posner, editor, p 93. MIT Press, Cambridge, MA, 1989. Used with permission.)*

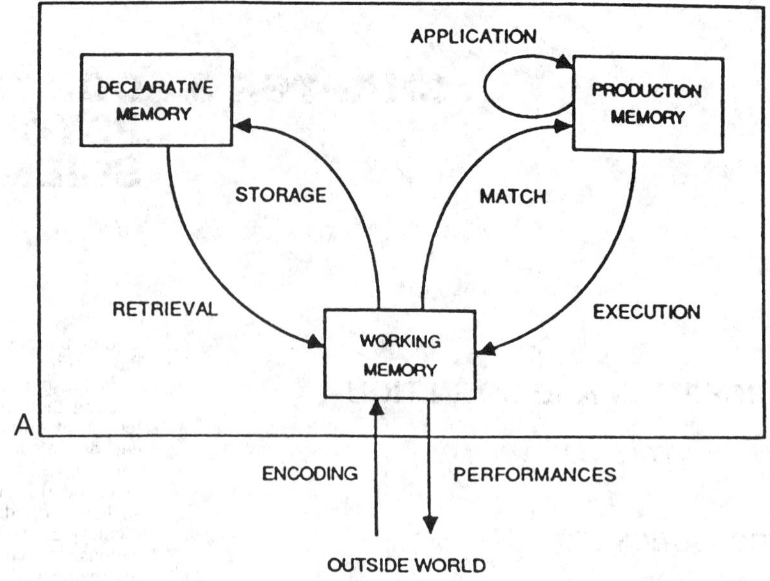

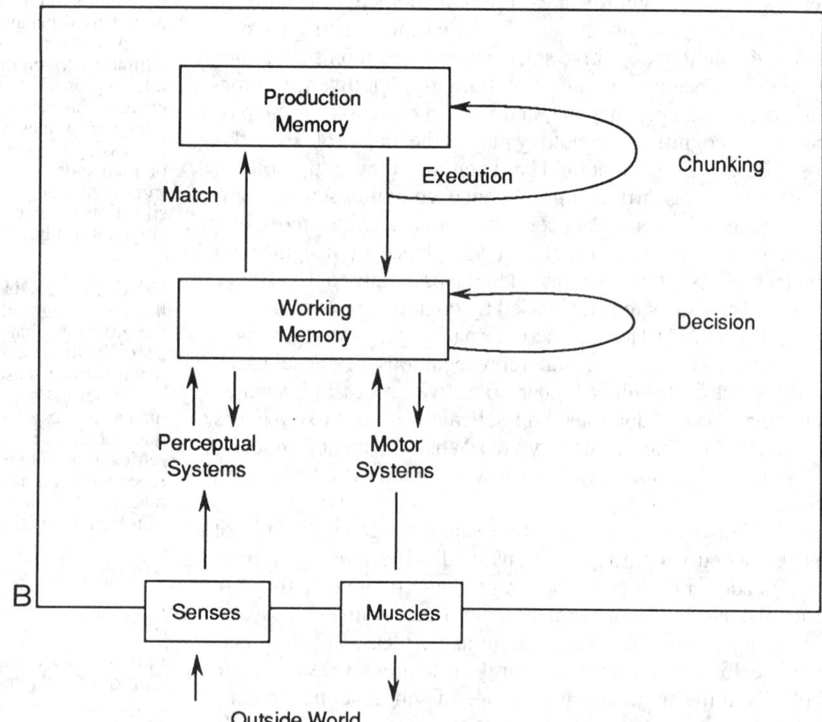

representations in the formation of speech. Those processes are part of what are commonly referred to as thinking and memory.

A basic feature of the model is that conscious processing of mental representations (information) occurs only for items in working memory. Working memory has a limited capacity in duration and volume (number of units of information stored in one period of time). Studies have found, for example, that seven plus or minus two items is the quantity capacity for working memory. Cognitive processes that can group bits of information into large chunks (chunking) can increase the capacity of working memory by making each unit more information-rich.

Long-term memory is thought to have an associative or schematic organization that influences the processes of encoding and retrieval. The retrieval of stored information in long-term memory is required for certain further processes to be carried out on those representations. Reencoding of the transformed information can lead to a modification of the originally stored data. Thus the retrieval of information and its active processing modify long-term memory stores. That may be an important principle in various models of psychotherapy.

REPRESENTATIONS, PROCESSES, AND STRUCTURES

Thoughts, ideas, images, and even emotions are manifestations of neural excitation. The media for those phenomena are patterns of neural activation that are displayed across billions of dendritic connections among complex networks distributed in parallel fashion in the brain. Thus a sensory image is a pattern of neural excitation with a characteristic activation of particular neurons. That pattern is what is meant by the term ''mental representation.'' Representations can be thought of as similar to the data of a personal computer.

Cognitive processes involve the transformation of mental representations into elaborate forms that contain complex relations to other representations. The processes can alter the form in which representations are stored and thus retrieved from long-term memory. Processes are analogous to the software programs of a personal computer and act directly on the stored data (representations).

''Cognitive structure'' is a term used to describe a highly complex function, such as working memory or schema, that seems to be a fundamental part of the information-processing system. In the computational design of cognitive architectures the structures can be thought of as the hardware of the computer. Representations (data) thus are manipulated by processes (programs) that function in the setting of cognitive structures (computer hardware). Care must be taken not to make those conceptualizations overly concrete.

COGNITIVE ARCHITECTURES The attempt to build computational models of cognitive functioning led to the development of several architectures that have been used as frameworks for computer design. Figure 3.1-2 shows the Act and Soar models. The serial or linear nature of those models derives from early computer-science notions that were based on the designers' awareness of their own sequential, logical processes. Although those computer-based models have provided important insights into computational functioning, they are seriously limited in their resemblance to human mental activity.

A new computational approach is based on the neural networks of the brain, which are distributed in parallel fashion, not in sequential order. The brain-based connectionist model for computer architecture shows remarkable similarities to human mental functioning. The parallel distributed processing model may become a relevant tool in understanding mental functioning in both health and disorder. Figure 3.1-3 provides a schematic representation of a simple network.

ATTENTION Attention is the process that controls the flow of information processing. Controversies have arisen concerning the phenomena regulating attention processes, but a practical division of attention into three components identifies specific deficits in a number of psychiatric disorders. Those features are selectivity, capacity, and sustained concentration. Various neuroanatomical and neurotransmitter systems may be responsible for the various aspects of attention function.

Early conceptualizations of attention were based on Donald Broadbent's idea of a filter that selects a limited amount of incoming stimuli to be further processed. In that view the limited capacity of attention was attributable to the inability to process the overwhelming amount of incoming stimuli. An attention bottleneck was described as occurring either early in the sensory process and thus automatically or late in the perceptual processing stage and involving such processes as identification and classification. Recent views of attention have deemphasized the idea of a filter as a cognitive structure and have fostered the development of the concept of general cognitive resource capacity, which limits the stimuli processed. Those theoretical frameworks of information processing help explain findings in various psychopathological conditions, such as schizophrenia and attention-deficit/hyperactivity disorder.

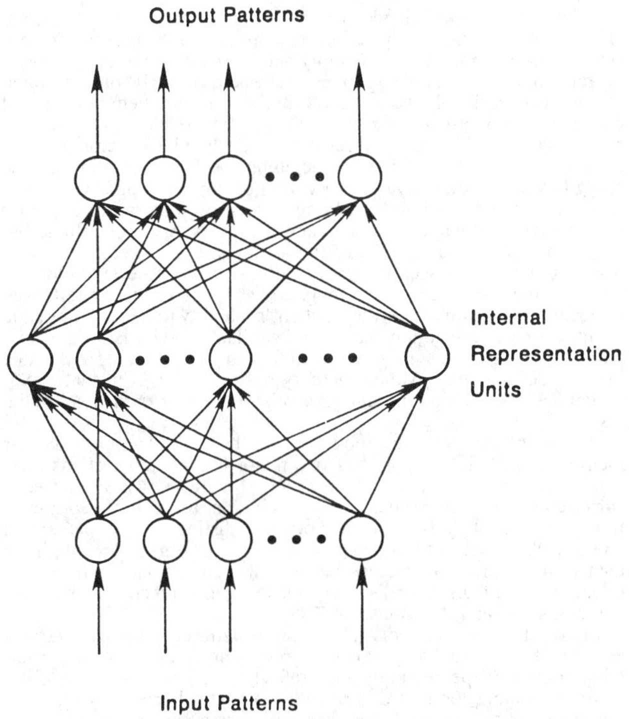

Selective attention One aspect of attention processes is that they focus a metaphorical spotlight on given external stimuli or internal mental representations or processes.

In Broadbent's conceptualization selectivity has three dimensions: (1) filtering, focusing on specific physical attributes (for example, small circles); (2) categorizing, based on stimulus class (for example, attending to letters in whatever script they are written); and (3) pigeonholing, reducing perceptual information needed to place a stimulus into a specified category. Each of those aspects acts on incoming stimuli to make a determination of fit for the sought-after characteristic. Schizophrenic patients show greater difficulty with pigeonholing than with filtering when they are symptomatic.

Another conceptualization of selective attention distinguishes between two interactive ways of processing sensory input. *Preattentive* processing (a parallel function) assesses global, holistic patterns and appears to be an early component of the perceptual process. *Focal* attention (a serial process) follows preattentive processing and involves a detailed analysis of stimuli characteristics. Focal attention can be directed at one stimulus form only and is thus limited in its capacity. Parallel (preattentive) attention processes, in contrast, do not appear to have limited capacity and can detect gestalt aspects of environmental stimuli from numerous sources. The ability to hear one's name called out by a nonattended voice in a crowded, noisy room is an example of an ongoing parallel process with the ability to detect gestalt features and extremely familiar (and thus automatically processed) stimuli.

Attention capacity The concept of processing capacity involves the idea that a given task makes a demand on a limited pool of resources. A task with a high processing load draws more resources from the finite pool than does a task with a low processing load, thus inhibiting the accessibility of resources for other simultaneous functions drawing from the same pool. Focal attention requires cognitive effort and thus has a high processing load demand. Cognitive models describing several resource pools suggest an executive process that distributes resources to various cognitive functions. Serial processes that demand processing capacity inhibit the simultaneous action of other serial high-load processes. In contrast, parallel processes have low or no processing capacity demands and can function simultaneously with numerous other functions without inhibiting them.

Optimal performance is attained with moderate levels of arousal that allow for the establishment of task goals and feedback from the performance of the task, leading to appropriate resource allocation. Low levels of arousal impair those processes and lead to inadequate resource allocation. High levels of arousal may be detrimental to the performance because of poor discrimination of stimuli and diminished efficiency of allocation, resulting in poor attention functioning. Pupillary dilation is directly proportional to the level of arousal and has been used as a measure of the degree of processing demand for specific cognitive tasks.

Sustained attention The ability to sustain attention is called vigilance and can be tested with task demands for alertness and concentration over a period of a few minutes to an hour. Usually the tests involve detection requirements for target stimuli that occur infrequently at random intervals. An example of such a test is the continuous performance test, which has been used to study various psychiatric disorders. Important aspects of the tests are derived from signal detection theory and include the factors of sensitivity and response criterion. Sensitivity is the distinguishing of target from nontarget stimuli. The response criterion is the amount of perceptual evidence required to support the decision regarding a target versus a nontarget item.

SENSATION AND PERCEPTION Sensation is the initial encoding of simple sensory data from peripheral sensory organs to sensory memory. The process rapidly analyzes basic features of the physical stimuli and transforms them into a mental representation in sensory memory. For example, in the visual system the stimulus of a vertical line activates retinal cells, producing a distribution of excitation in the visual cortex. Neural processing of that excitation pattern yields a summary analysis called an iconic image, which encodes various features of the stimulus, such as its linearity, direction, size, and color.

Output Patterns

Internal Representation Units

Input Patterns

FIGURE 3.1-3 *Multilayer connectionist network in which input patterns are recoded by internal representation units. The parallel distribution of input influences subsequent stages of representation; output patterns are derived from further parallel processing. In complex models activating and inhibiting influences, as in neural networks, contribute to the subsequent representations. (Figure from D E Rumelhart, G E Hinton, R J Williams: Learning internal representations by error propagation. In* Parallel Distributed Processing: Explorations in the Microstructure of Cognition, *J L McClelland, D E Rumelhart, editors, vol 1, p 320. MIT Press, Cambridge, MA, 1986. Used with permission.)*

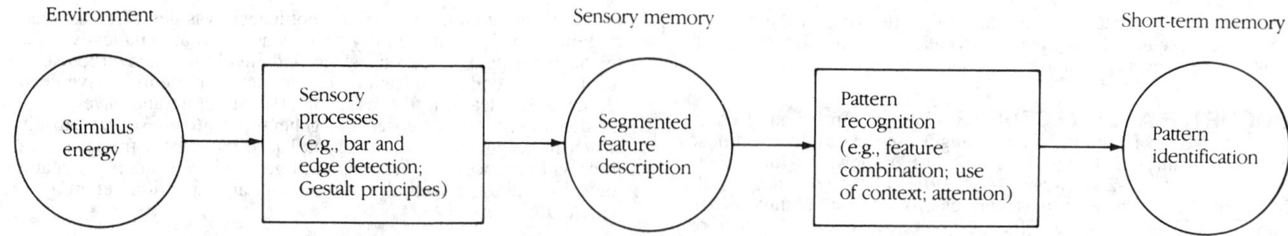

FIGURE 3.1-4 *Flow of information from the environment to its perceptual representation. The information indicated in the circles is operated on by the sensory and perceptual processes indicated in the boxes. (Figure from J R Anderson:* Cognitive Psychology and Its Implications, *ed 3, p 84. Freeman, New York, 1990. Used with permission.)*

Attention processes at the level of sensory memory act on the sensory image with higher cognitive functions (for example, classification and chunking) as it enters working memory. That set of early, lower processes is what is usually considered sensation (Figure 3.1-4). Studies of patients with schizophrenia reveal specific deficits at that stage of cognitive processing.

Perception occurs as the initial stimulus is acted on by the higher cognitive processes. This can happen with or without awareness. Numerous studies have shown that perception is processed differently if focal attention with awareness is not applied to the sensory data. The studies also show, however, that long-term memory does store representations of the nonaware perception, as demonstrated by indirect measures. Blindsight patients are an example of perception without awareness.

The perceptual systems of vision, audition, olfaction, taste, and touch all have unique aspects and have been studied to varying degrees. Vision has been the most extensively studied perceptual system, with complex research paradigms, computational models, and elegant neuroanatomical descriptions of functioning. One feature of the study of sensation and perception that is thought to apply to at least visual and auditory systems is gestalt processing. Perception appears to extract general sensory patterns from the whole of a stimulus. Those basic components are then assembled into a large picture based on pattern recognition, which is heavily influenced by top-down processing. Figure 3.1-5 is an example of how pattern contrasts can be extracted from figure-ground presentations and of how top-down processing can influence perception. What is encoded in short-term memory is the perceived stimulus, not the sensory data.

The study of imagery has a long history, with the bulk of the work focusing on visual images. Mental imagery can involve the generation, inspection, retention, and transformation of perceptual images. One finding is that the processing of mental images appears to require timing and effort similar to that required when the imaged object is perceived externally. Studies show that complex visual mental images require more time and effort to rotate mentally than do simple forms. Images in other perceptual modalities have been described but not studied to the same extent as visual images. Mental imagery is used in several forms of psychotherapy, such as hypnosis, cognitive-behavioral treatment, and guided imagery. The basic capacity of the brain to generate mental images may be an important process in the production of the hallucinations and illusions seen in several disorders.

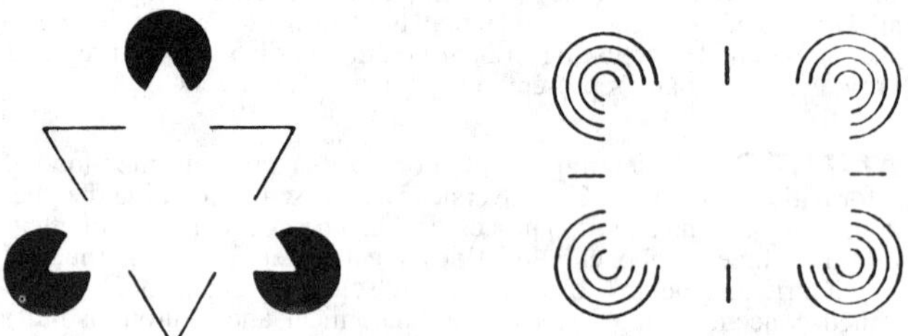

FIGURE 3.1-5 *Perception involves the registration of patterns from contours. Top-down processing influences the form of the image perceived. (Figure from E C Hildreth, S Ullman: The computational study of vision. In* Foundations of Cognitive Science, *M I Posner, editor, p 133. MIT Press, Cambridge, MA, 1989. Used with permission.)*

MEMORY Memory is generally viewed either as multiple-storage systems or as having distinct forms of processing. For example, memory has been divided into procedural, episodic, and semantic memory stores: Procedural memory stores are learned behavioral responses, episodic memory stores are autobiographical memory (recalling oneself in an episode), and semantic memory stores are knowledge representations. Memory has also been divided into procedural and declarative memory; declarative memory is accessible to verbalization. Those are examples of the dominant multiple-storage-systems models of memory function. Figure 3.1-2 is a schematic diagram of a computational cognitive architecture, using the separation of procedural (or production) memory from declarative memory.

One influential processing model describes memory as implicit or explicit. Implicit memory includes behavioral, emotional, and perceptual learning due to a past experience but not involving a sense of consciousness recollection when retrieved. Indirect measures of memory, such as priming effects and time saving for relearning a task, and learned skilled activity are ways in which implicit memory can be assessed. Priming refers to the increased likelihood and speed of retrieval of an item from memory. Implicit memories cannot be stated directly and a person may be unaware of how the memories were acquired. Explicit memory stores information that can be verbalized and assessed by means of direct measures, such as recall and recognition tasks.

Studies have revealed dissociations in the normally associated memory functions of implicit recall and explicit recall in various mental states. Explicit memory, by definition, implies that the person can consciously recall an item from memory and use language to express what is retrieved. Korsakoff's patients revealed dissociations between implicit (intact) recall and explicit (impaired) recall. Neuroanatomical correlations suggest that the hippocampus and related structures are required for the encoding and retrieval of declarative or explicit long-term memory; other structures, including the basal ganglia and the amygdala are fundamental to procedural or implicit memory. Studies of the effects of benzodiazepines on normal persons reveal a similar dissociation: normal functioning and awareness during testing, but impaired explicit recall in the setting of intact implicit recall. Similar dissociations can be seen in hypnotically induced amnesia, childhood amnesia, memory changes in aging, and cases of surgical anesthesia. In posttraumatic stress disorder a patient's inability to recall a traumatic event and yet avoid contextual stimuli similar to the initial trauma and have startle reactions to those stimuli can be explained by intact implicit but impaired explicit memory retrieval. However, that explanation needs validation through research into memory processes in the disorder.

A cognitive architecture model called the multiple-entry modular memory system is composed of two major interrelated systems, perceptual (P) and reflective (R) processes (Figure 3.1-6). Within each subsystem related component processes act on information from multiple levels. That division of memory into distinguishable perceptual and reflective systems has provided a model for organizing empirical data from a variety of studies on normal memory and with clinical populations with amnesic disorders due to a general medical condition, confabulation, and delusions.

In the retrieval of memory in that model items encoded with various degrees of perceptual and reflective processing contain profiles of relative degrees of perceptual versus reflective components for a given memory. Marcia Johnson described a function called reality monitoring, which is viewed as the process by which a person discriminates, when remembering, between information that had a perceptual source and information that was self-generated from thought, imagination, fantasy, or dreams. Research in various settings suggests that the more reflective the processing is at the time of an event, the better able a person is to distinguish the memory of that event as internally generated. Reflective processing at the time of encoding, in that model, enables the retrieval process to identify the origin of a memory.

Although the model has not yet been applied to the process that allows for discrimination between ongoing sensory input and retrieved memory, applications to the understanding of flashback phenomena, such as experienced by patients with posttraumatic stress disorder, theoretically are possible.

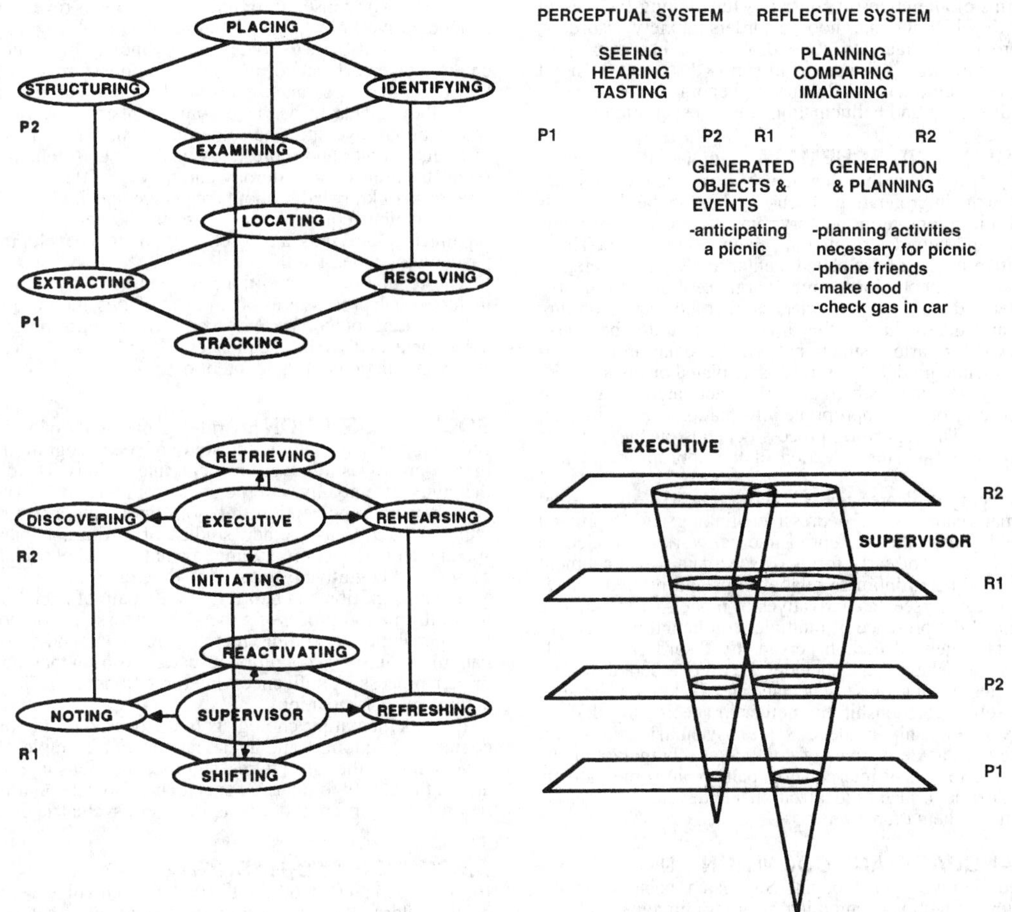

FIGURE 3.1-6 *Schematic outline of the multiple-entry modular memory system. Perceptual (P1 and P2) and reflective (R1 and R2) processes act on income data in the encoding of memory. The retrieval of memory yields a processing profile of P and R components that were present at the time of encoding. (Figure from M K Johnson: Reflection, reality monitoring and the self. In* Mental Imagery, *R G Kunzendorf, editor. Plenum, New York, 1991. Used with permission.)*

CONSCIOUSNESS AND UNCONSCIOUSNESS Consciousness has intrigued philosophers for centuries and is an active domain of study for cognitive scientists. Most mental activity is nonconscious (that is, out of awareness or not in phenomenal experience). *Phenomenal awareness* is the subjective experience of being aware or cognizant of a phenomenon. Disorders with cognitive effects thus may be out of the awareness of the patient. Experimental studies have found that information is processed differently, depending on the state of awareness of the person, and that nonaware forms of perception can directly influence a person's emotional state, thought, and behavior. Some psychiatric disturbances may be the result of primary disturbances in the cognitive process of consciousness (such as depersonalization, derealization, hallucinations, obsessive thoughts, or distorted body image). Rigorous scientific attempts to update psychodynamic theory have used cognitive science as a means of exploration. Cognitive therapy techniques that are effective in the treatment of several disorders are mediated through conscious attention to verbal communication.

Consciousness can be understood as a subjective awareness of some aspects of ongoing cognitive processing, rather than as a way station required for further processing. Awareness can be directed at sensory data from external stimuli or toward internal cognitive processes, such as memories, images, and thoughts. Conscious awareness can be described as a complex serial selective sampling of mental activity being processed in parallel form.

Another view, based on a biological assessment of brain function, is that of Gerald Edelman, which describes two forms of consciousness that derive from the resonant interactions between groups of neurons. In that model primary consciousness stems from the interaction between perceptual categorizations and conceptual categorizations. That form of consciousness, called the remembered present, is also found in higher animals and is unable to transcend momentary awareness. It is embedded in the present but is influenced by categorizations from the past. In human beings the capacity for lexical or language processing enables a secondary or higher-order consciousness to exist and stems from the resonance between those processes and conceptual categories. Higher-order consciousness frees inner experience from the prison of the present and allows for views of the past and plans for the future. Included in those forms of consciousness is a scene of the present situation in which the self is placed in a temporospatial context.

Cortically blind patients state that they cannot see visual stimuli, but they respond behaviorally as if they were fully sighted. They describe being unaware of visual perception, but they make eye and hand movements that reflect the processing of information about stimulus location, shape, orientation, and direction of motion. In information-processing terms behavioral tests reveal that blindsighted patients do sense and perceive visual stimuli but do not have conscious awareness of the perceptual process. That is an example of a dissociation of the normally associated processes of perception and consciousness or awareness of phenomena.

Misidentification syndromes are other examples of subjective, conscious experience disturbances. In prosopagnosia patients are unable consciously to access memories regarding persons familiar to them. In the Capgras syndrome patients are able to recognize a familiar person's face but feel that it is not really that person. Being certain, as in recognition, is one aspect of consciousness as a cognitive process. The pathological uncertainty in patients with obsessive-compulsive disorder theoretically can be viewed as a disturbance in that aspect of conscious functioning.

Consciousness provides a sense of continuity. Various studies find perceptual discontinuity (for example, the presence of a blind spot in the visual field, blurred peripheral vision, saccadic eye movements that displace the visual field with sudden shifts) but the subjective experience of continuity in consciousness.

Many psychiatric patients experience profound senses of discontinuity and confusion that may be related to a dysfunction in the sense-making, continuity-creating process of consciousness. Some psychiatric symptoms, including derealization and depersonalization, may be understood in terms of alterations in conscious functioning (as seen in some patients with schizophrenia, mood disorders, anxiety disorders, dissociative disorders, posttraumatic stress disorder, and some personality disorders), distorted body image (as in eating disorders or mood disorders), intrusive memories and flashback phenomena (as in posttraumatic stress disorder), and hallucinations (as in psychotic states).

MENTAL MODELS AND SCHEMATA Studies of perception and memory support the view that the mind has organizational structures that influence the interpretation of sensory data, shape the encoding of information into long-term memory, bias the retrieval of items stored in memory, and help determine the behavioral response. Those organizing cognitive functions are called mental models or schemata.

Mental models are unconscious, highly organized structural processes that are derived from past experiences, that aid in interpreting present stimuli, and that influence the direction of future behavior. Mental models exist for various situations. When a situation is appropriate for a given mental model, that model is activated or instantiated. The process, which regulates which model is activated at a given moment, helps to carry out the appropriate information processing and subsequent behavior. The regulation process depends on the accurate reading of the situation and the selection of the appropriate mental model.

Aaron Beck's theory of depression is based on the idea that mental models or schemata can produce depressive thinking and depressed moods. John Bowlby used the concept of internal working models to describe the development of early forms of schemata for attachment relationships. Difficulties in intimate relationships and related behavioral dysregulation can be seen as derivatives of models of inadequate early attachment and the presence of multiple, conflictual models.

Mardi Horowitz's view of certain personality disorders and maladaptive interpersonal behavior also includes the role of mental models or person schemata. Among those schemata are models of the self, another, and the self in relationship to another in specifically defined maladaptive role relationship models. Some psychiatric signs and symptoms can be seen as derivatives of conflictual schemata and situations. Classic descriptions of interpersonal patterns in some patients with personality disorders, such as idealization and devaluation, can be seen as maladaptive schema functions.

THOUGHT, LANGUAGE, AND COGNITION There is no universally accepted definition of thought. Suggested basic elements include propositions (functions containing meaning), images, and lexical and semantic symbols. Cognitive processes can be carried out in parallel, simultaneously, and without consciousness. Cognitive processes, such as thoughts, are often directly known only through translation into consciousness and language. As in the study of mental models clinical observation and experimental paradigms can infer the nature of thought processes only through indirect measures. Those concepts are important in interpreting what is implied by the term "thought disorder."

Thinking involves the mental representation of some aspect of the world or of the self and the manipulation of those representations. Thinking depends on both explicit memory and implicit memory for prior experiences. In addition, thought processes can be influenced by a person's emotional state and mental models. The basic components of thinking include categorization, judgment, decision making, and general problem solving. The assignment of representations of events or objects to categories is important to subsequent thought processing, because thoughts can act on the general class to which an item belongs, rather than on individual representations. That is another example of top-down processing influences.

The ability to judge the probability of uncertain events, a primary role of judgment, is a fundamental aspect of the rationality of thought. The lack of conformity of thinking to the rules of logic is one aspect of disordered thought processing. Thinking is important in choice, the decision to choose among various options. Each of those processes contributes to the goal of problem solving; data are assessed, classified, transformed, and compared on the basis of logical rules to produce a choice that solves a problem. Failures in those steps can result in limitations and distortions in normal thought processes.

Psycholinguistics is a complex domain that focuses on the cognitive process of language formation and semantic analysis. Cognitive science views language as a dominant influence on subjective experience. It is the medium that dominates human social communication and one of the major features distinguishing *Homo sapiens* from other species. In the human infant language shapes the ways in which the world is perceived, the manner in which desires are communicated and satiated, and the way in which society responds. Disorders in receptive and expressive language functions influence both the subjective experience of the world and social functioning; children with such disorders often have multiple levels of maladaptation. The ability to communicate through nonverbal language depends on social cognitive processes.

METACOGNITION Metacognition concerns processes that act on the cognitive processes themselves—thinking about thinking. The thinking can be conscious or unconscious and is revealed through either metacognitive knowledge or the regulation of cognition. Knowledge about cognition appears to develop by the age of about 6 when a child enters elementary school and takes various forms, including what is known as the appearance-reality distinction: Things may not actually be as they appear to be. Two components of that awareness are representational diversity (the same object may appear to be different to different people) and representational change (thoughts today are different from those of yesterday and may be different again tomorrow). That form of knowledge about the person-specific meaning of cognitive representation requires some sense of the person's awareness of the separateness of minds, a theoretical domain in developmental cognitive psychology called the theory of mind.

The regulation of cognition, also called metacognitive monitoring, includes such processes as planning activities, monitoring the activities, and checking outcomes. Metacognitive monitoring may involve the assessment of thinking sequences for fallacious logic, factual errors, and contradictions in the content of speech.

SOCIAL COGNITION Bridging the fields of social psychology and cognitive psychology, the study of social cognition focuses on the mental processes involved in social interactions. The domains include the study of empathy, interpersonal communication (verbal and nonverbal), person perception, relationship scripts, and group processes. Other related areas include studies of attribution bias, memory for social interactions, stereotyping, mental control of social cognitive processes, and cognitive origins of a sense of self.

Social cognition can be seen as a domain of social psychology that uses information-processing theory to assess the components of attention, perception, encoding, memory, retrieval, and schemata. A dominant theme in social cognition research has been that top-down, theory-driven processing influences interpretations of social situations and actions in such situations.

Developmental psychologists have focused on the origins of social cognitive functioning and its deviations. For example, autistic children have, among other difficulties, significant deficits in empathic capacity and in the ability to interpret social cues. Social cognitive deficits may be present in different domains in other psychiatric disorders.

DISCOURSE AND NARRATIVE Discourse is communication from one person to another; it is thought to involve a sense of intention or plan. Normal discourse follows a set of rules that ensure the coherence and effectiveness of communication: What is intended to be stated by the sender is understood by the listener or receiver. Some researchers support the idea that discourse is a cognitive function that follows the basic principles of information processing, including a schema for effective communication, and of social cognition, such as taking into account the listener's perspective.

Incoherent discourse can be noted by analyzing unlicensed violations of the primary maxims of discourse. Another technique is that of discourse analysis, which examines the ways in which discourse deviates from an assumed discourse plan. The exact method to quantify abnormalities in discourse remains controversial, but clinical impressions of incoherence remain important for assessing deficits in social communication. The deficits may be due to learned behavior, inherent cognitive abnormalities in thought or language, or deviations in social cognitive functioning. Deviations from normal discourse can be a general finding in need of further assessment. Abnormal discourse is clinically evident in psychosis, specifically in schizophrenia.

Narrative is a broad domain ranging from the literary study of fiction to the developmental psychology investigations of the origin of autobiographical accounts. From a cognitive point of view narrative is important in understanding the relations of language, memory, consciousness, mental models, self-schemata, and social cognition. Narrative can be generally defined as the way in which a person creates a verbal account of events in the world.

Autobiographical narrative begins early in life, as the capacity for language develops. Studies of early monologues find that young children are interpreting and assigning meaning to events in their world from an early age.

As with other areas in child development, debate concerns whether that aspect of cognition develops from a biological imperative (that is, the brain needs to make sense of the world, and narrative is the language output derived from that innate process) or from an internalization of social experiences (that is, families tell stories, and children practice taking the narrator role). Anthropologists who study psycholinguistic development across cultures have described a phenomenon called coconstruction, in which family members collaboratively create a story of daily events in their lives. How those family behaviors influence the child's emerging capacity to organize experiences and encode them into long-term memory to be retrieved later in the production of autobiographical narrative is a fundamental question for many disciplines in cognitive science. Specific deficits in early family experiences and in innate cognitive capacities may theoretically result in effects on the child's narrative capacity.

COGNITIVE DEVELOPMENT Developmental theories and research can be divided into several views. Stage theories (Jean Piaget, neo-Piagetian, the sociocultural school of Alexander Luria and Lev Vygotsky) describe discontinuous periods of development, with times of stability and consolidation alternating with instability and transition. Information-processing models have not been explored in as much detail with regard to child development, but the models do postulate a nonstage theory, in which the emergence of cognitive capacity is a continuous process that does not require a set of invariant sequences. Both stage and nonstage views embrace the idea that a hierarchial integration and an ongoing differentiation are fundamental aspects of cognitive development.

Another distinguishing feature is the degree to which the theories view the contributing role of innate, biological factors and the role of culturally determined social learning experiences. Do cognitive capacities emerge from a genetically determined plan (Piagetian view), or do they develop in response to experience (sociocultural view)? Developmental psychologists have found features of both views, supporting the idea of a transaction between innate factors and environmental experiences.

Psychiatric disturbances in cognition may reflect arrested patterns of normal cognition (as in mental retardation), deviant developmental pathways (for example, social cognitive functioning in persons with autistic disorder), and specific cognitive impairments (schizophrenia) that may have been present early on or only became evident as life requirements, such as school, became demanding (some cases of attention-deficit/hyperactivity disorder). Investigations into the developmental features of those disorders is a major focus of the field of developmental psychopathology.

COGNITION AND PSYCHIATRIC DISORDERS

Since the time of Emil Kraepelin and Eugen Bleuler psychiatrists have known that certain disorders include profound deficits in mental functioning, such as attention and reasoning in the case of schizophrenia. Since the 1950s researchers have attempted to determine the exact nature of such deficits. With the advances in computer technology and the technical ability to analyze stimulus presentation and response times of the order of tens of milliseconds, cognitive psychologists have been able to devise research paradigms capable of testing when such deficits are present. Those advances led to revisions in the proposed structural models of processing.

Processing research has focused on the three domains of sensation, perception, and cognition. Sensory processing studies focus on post-stimulus events up to a maximum of one second, using simple stimuli. Perceptual studies examine processing after a period of up to about five seconds after a slightly more complex stimulus. Cognitive processing experiments can examine early processing (for example, phenomena occurring within the first 30 seconds) of complex, long-term cognitive processes that can occur over minutes, hours, or days. Studies of long-term memory can examine processes that involve an indefinite post-stimuli period.

Recent attempts have been made to correlate complex cognitive findings with clinical presentations. General problems with the approach include the diversity of patients falling under the same syndrome classification. Thus schizophrenia can more appropriately be considered as the schizophrenias or schizophrenia spectrum disorder. The same may be true for other disorders, such as attention-deficit/hyperactivity disorder and major depressive disorder. An array of cognitive dysfunctions identified for certain subsets of syndromes must be interpreted in the light of the heterogeneity of some patient populations.

A related problem is the distinction between general deficits and specific deficits. Care must be taken in interpreting experimental data that show a difference in results between normal controls and a patient group. Do psychiatrically ill patients perform less well on a given paradigm because they are ill or because of a deficit specific to the disorder? The creative design of experimental tasks can help distinguish between general deficits and specific deficits. A comparison of target patient populations with matched normal persons and other psychiatric patients can help to determine disorder-specific cognitive dysfunction.

Another general issue is that of state markers versus trait markers. For example, a patient with schizophrenia may have a persistent cognitive deficit when actively psychotic (state) and also when asymptomatic (trait). Those abnormal results have been found in certain cognitive tests of attention that correlate with improvement on medications; the abnormal results are also found in nonschizophrenic first-degree relatives. Is the marker of genetic vulnerability a coincidental finding or part of the core deficit in schizophrenia? An exploration of the implications of those cognitive abnormalities for the daily life of the patient is an important application of the research findings to clinical psychiatry.

SCHIZOPHRENIA Almost a century ago Kraepelin described a primary attention deficit in his elaborate clinical description of schizophrenic patients. Numerous investigators since that time have attempted to define the nature of the cognitive deficits in schizophrenia. A general approach is that an early perceptual processing deficit leads to problems in perceptual organization. In general, information-processing models note that two things are processed: energy (in the form of external stimuli impinging on the senses) and information (a stimulus that carries a signal value based on significance derived from the prior processing of similar energy configurations). Schizophrenic patients appear to have deficits in the processing of both energy and information.

Some cognitive tasks have been identified as trait-linked markers of schizophrenic disorder: reaction time crossover, backward masking, dichotic listening, serial recall tasks, vigilance (sustained attention) tasks requiring high processing loads, and span-of-apprehension tests with large visual arrays. Deficits in those areas have been explored through thousands of cognitive studies examining various aspects of processing.

Crossover and modality shift effects Those paradigms examine the general finding that schizophrenic patients have a slower than usual response on tasks that require rapid reaction times. A stimulus is presented with varied combinations of warning signals and preparatory intervals. Schizophrenic patients show an advantage only with short preparatory intervals and long response times with regularly spaced stimuli, a pattern distinct from that of normal controls (crossover effect). In a related paradigm, when the modality of the stimulus is varied (for example, light is interspersed with tone), the latency (delay) of the response in schizophrenic patients, when compared with controls, is longer if the preceding stimulus was of a different modality. That is termed the modality shift effect, revealing a greater degree of cross-modal retardation in schizophrenic patients than in controls.

A number of theories have been proposed to explain those effects. They may be quantitative, rather than qualitative, distinctions from normal control groups. However, both the crossover and modality shift effects support the idea that schizophrenic patients are overly influenced by stimuli that occurred immediately before the effect. The information-processing stages that explain the persistence of prior stimulus effects is under investigation.

Visual backward masking, sensorimotor gating, and habituation That aspect of cognitive functioning in which rapidly presented stimuli are abnormally attended to by schizophrenic patients, as compared with normal controls has been examined. In visual backward masking a stimulus is followed by an interstimuli interval, and then a subsequent stimulus is presented. Figure 3.1-7 shows a typical masking experiment. The presentation of the secondary stimulus leads the schizophrenic patient to not report, to mask, the initial stimulus. Lengthening of the interstimulus interval beyond 500 milliseconds (ms) can lead to normalization, with no masking present. Thus the rapidity of presentation of the secondary stimulus is the factor determining whether it will influence the perception or, at least, the reporting of the initial stimulus. Some studies find that the impairment improves with treatment by medication and can be induced in nonschizophrenic patients given catecholaminergic agents. Other studies find that the impairment may be a marker of increased vulnerability to schizophrenia.

Sensorimotor gating and habituation are the processes by which stimuli become less attended to with rapidly repeated presentation. Habituation is believed to involve preattentive processing, and the visual masking requires higher cognitive functions. Schizophrenic patients show a markedly diminished capacity to habituate. One common study examines the persistent acoustic startle reflex as the person continues to blink with repetitive tones. Parallel findings are those of the studies that showed that lysergic acid diethyamide (LSD) administration and the intracerebral injection of dopaminergic agents in rats lead to similar findings, supporting the idea that excessive dopamine activity, thought to be central in schizophrenia, can induce those deficits.

In general, the diminished habituation and visual backward masking lend further cognitive support to the idea that schizophrenic patients have a markedly diminished capacity to regulate the flow of rapidly presented information, leading to an inundation by stimuli that in a normal person are gated out. The disruptive effects of the externally derived stimuli, as demonstrated in those experimental paradigms, are thought to occur also for internally generated stimuli.

Psychomotor slowing A general deficit, not specific to schizophrenia, is a generalized slowing of response rate. Cognitive science is concerned with all stages in information processing, from attention, sensation, perception, and cognition to action. Multiple neural integrative systems are involved in the processes, from stimulus to response. Numerous disorders may result in a common finding of diminished reaction time. The general nature of the deficit should not lead clinicians and researchers to ignore the importance of response rate deficits in interpreting clinical and experimental data. Attempts to assess the interdependence of input, central processing, and action are part of psychomotor studies in schizophrenic patients.

Selective attention Numerous studies have attempted to determine the nature of deficits in selective attention in schizophrenic patients. Early studies were based on the idea of a bottleneck that limits the attention processing capacity at some stage in the information flow. Those studies were based on the idea that some cognitive structure devoted to filtering is impaired. Analysis of the studies revealed consistent deficits in shadowing (the ability to repeat what the person is selectively focusing on in a dichotic condition) and in verbal recall. In general, selective attention paradigms present the person with a target stimulus and distracters to be nonattended. Findings reveal that schizophrenic patients have an impairment in their ability to avoid distracting stimuli (to filter) and to pigeonhole (to use category features to reduce stimulus qualities needed to respond). The studies found that distractibility is a core cognitive deficit, supported by its high incidence in genetically vulnerable persons, its improvement with medications, and its worsening in acutely psychotic states.

Those findings were explained by using the framework of an impaired filtering structure and pigeonholing process, but recent conceptualizations have examined a generalized impairment of the information-processing capacity in schizophrenia. The capacity model examines the way in which a pool or pools of attention capacity can be allocated across mental activities. Two components are quantity of resources available (capacity) and executive allocation policy. Other areas of deficit may involve an impaired response selection process, leading to abnormal results on tasks.

Several possibilities have been proposed to explain attention deficits in schizophrenic patients on the basis of the capacity model: (1) deautomatization of normally automatic preattentive processes, (2) disproportionate allocation of attention to schema-relevant but task-irrelevant information, (3) inability to sustain controlled processes needed to maintain attention allocation without shifting, (4) inability to shift allocation biases to correct wandering attention, and (5) disorganized response selection because of heightened arousal under distracting conditions. Studies of selective attention may begin to examine those possibilities in a capacity model, rather than in the previously explored structural framework.

Sustained attention Sustained attention, or vigilance, is required to process stimuli of long duration. The most common research paradigm in cognitive studies of sustained attention and psychopathology is the Continuous Performance Test. The test is a rapidly paced set of vigilance tasks with varied spacing and timing of target and nontarget stimuli. Continuous Performance Tests have the following features: The presentation of a

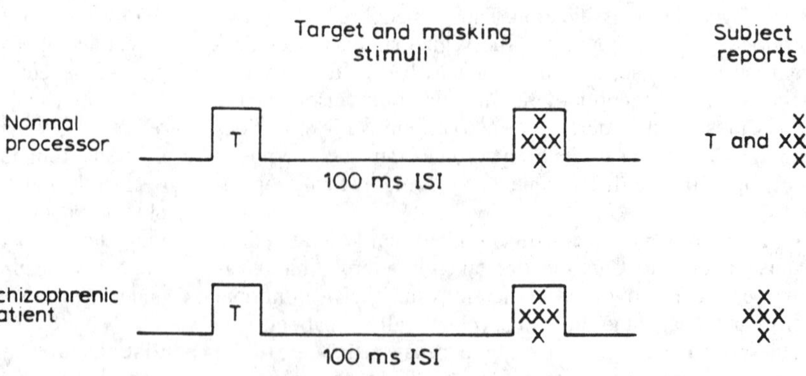

FIGURE 3.1-7 *Diagram showing the difference in the verbal reports of normal versus schizophrenic subjects presented with a single backward masking trial with a 100-ms interstimulus interval (ISI). The T represents the target stimulus and the Xs represent the masking stimulus. (Figure from D L Braff, D T Saccuzzo, M A Geyer: Information processing dysfunctions in schizophrenia: Studies of visual backward masking, sensory motor gating and habituation. In* Handbook of Schizophrenia, *vol 5,* Neuropsychology and Information Processing, *S R Steinhauer, J H Gruzelier, J Zubin, editors, p 303. Elsevier Science, New York, 1991. Used with permission.)*

random sequence of visual stimuli on a small screen (numbers or letters), a fixed stimulus pace with a rapid rate (one to two seconds), a brief stimulus exposure time (40 to 200 ms), designated stimuli or sequences of stimuli as targets, and the use of a button with which the person can respond. The processing load for a Continuous Performance Test can be varied by blurring the stimulus presented or by changing the rapidity of presentation.

Vigilance tests, such as the Continuous Performance Test, require analysis of response features on the basis of the signal detection theory. The two elements distinguished are sensitivity and the response criterion. Diminished sensitivity is a sign of decreased vigilance and results in a high miss rate (errors of omission). The response criterion can be diminished, leading to a high false-positive rate (error of commission). The analysis is important in the interpretation of results.

Schizophrenic patients appear to have a specific diminishment in sensitivity but not a lowering of the response criterion for both verbal and spatial stimuli. Various forms of the Continuous Performance Test contain variations in stimulus pace and processing load that reveal deficits in schizophrenic patients. Some forms of the test have shown vigilance deficits that are thought to be trait markers, exacerbated in symptomatic states, that improve with medications. Diminished responses on certain tests are found in only about half the schizophrenic patients studied. The impaired responses were significantly associated with specific clinical features in the patients and first-degree relatives. Test abnormalities, although present in other disorders, appear to be most robust in schizophrenia.

Positron emission tomography (PET) in schizophrenia patients performing a Continuous Performance Test found differential activation, with lower metabolic activity than in normal persons, in the prefrontal cortex bilaterally but normal or elevated activation in the occipital region, leading to a hypofrontal pattern. That finding is consistent with other findings supporting the idea of impaired frontal function in schizophrenia.

The vigilance studies using the Continuous Performance Test reveal that schizophrenic patients have a deficit in their ability to distinguish target stimuli from nontarget stimuli when the stimuli are presented as brief signals at a rapid pace. That finding is consistent with the other features of attention abnormalities revealed in other paradigms.

Language and discourse Assessments of language dysfunction in schizophrenia have focused on the basic question of whether the abnormalities in speech are reflections of a core disorder of thought or an abnormality in speech production. The search for a schizophrenic language has yielded negative conclusions. Discourse analyses of conversations with schizophrenic patients suggested that they may have significant difficulties in the maintenance of a specific topic (derailment) and in the lack of a discourse plan directing speech (disorganization).

Other investigators have argued that schizophrenic patients have impaired capacities to perceive the needs of others and may be schema driven in the direction of their speech, rather than intending to communicate effectively. One study showed that delusion-consistent material presented in the nonattended channel in a dichotic listening task leads to diminished attention to the target channel. A clinical implication of that experimental finding is the possibility that schema-driven processing during speech production may be diverting attention to internal stimuli and away from the potentially confusing social demands of conversation.

Span of apprehension Span of apprehension is an experimental paradigm that illustrates a cognitive psychological approach to the core deficit of schizophrenic patients. In the span-of-apprehension test an array of letters is displayed for a brief period (from 50 to 100 ms in most studies). One of the letters is a ''t'' or an ''f'' and the person must detect which letter is present. The number of nontarget letters is increased, and significant differences in detection are found for displays of 10 or more letters. Figure 3.1-8 provides an example of a visual display for the span-of-apprehension test.

The detection form of the test was derived after other forms had been established. The speed of presentation by a tachistoscope is too rapid for saccadic eye movements to scan the display. An analysis of the steps involved in detection can help elucidate mechanisms in attention and thus which cognitive processes may be abnormal, as assessed by the paradigm.

The first step in attention is registration into sensory image or register. For vision that is called iconic memory, and for audition it is called echoic memory. The decay rate of the sensory memory is thought to be in the range of 250 ms. Studies have shown that persons have far more items in their iconic memory than they can report. The detection for that version of the span-of-apprehension test avoids the limitation by emphasizing the search for a ''t'' or an ''f,'' rather than verbal reporting of each of the letters in iconic memory.

The iconic image of the 50-ms display is thought to have passed through the automatic portion of sensory processing and forms a representation that contains the physical features of the display itself (size, color, location of items). Persons raised to read English scan the image from left to right, top to bottom. That finding has been confirmed by assessing response rates as a function of the placement of target stimuli in the display. In the onset of top-down processing, categorical features (''Is that a 't' or an 'f'?'') are used as a schema to investigate the display in iconic memory. That stage of iconic memory scanning occurs within the first 250 ms after the display terminates and is a more central process than is the initial sensory register.

A proposed functional attention spotlight scans the iconic image. The factors affecting the scanning process are similar to those in the conscious scanning of a visual stimulus: number of letters displayed, size of print, spatial arrangement, intensity of light in the room, and the distance of the focus point from a peripheral element on the page. The serial scanning process is an element of focal attention. Parallel processing in the search involves increased aspects of assessment of figure-ground and textual segregation and is thought to be an automatic process.

Studies have shown that the sequential scanning of the attention spotlight is directly affected by increasing the complexity of certain display characteristics, leading to increased errors in detection. That is logical, since the iconic image has a limited display time and the scanning of the image may be incomplete by the time it decays from such an ultrabrief form of memory.

FINDINGS IN SCHIZOPHRENIC PATIENTS Schizophrenic patients show significantly increased errors in the span-of-apprehension test under conditions of increased complexity of display. Their scores are also worse in psychotic conditions and are improved with symptomatic improvement while taking medications. Increased errors are also found

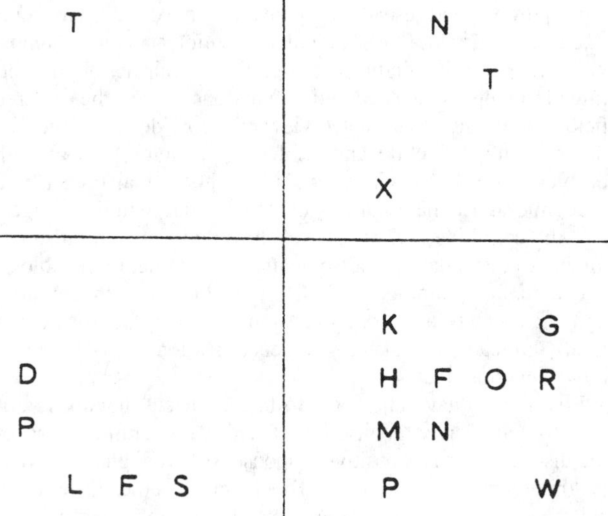

FIGURE 3.1-8 *Sample arrays used in the wide-visual-angle version of the partial report span-of-apprehension task. (Figure courtesy of Robert F Asarnow, PhD.)*

in nonschizophrenic mothers of children with schizophrenia. Thus the span-of-apprehension test is a measure of both state and trait in some cases of schizophrenia.

Only about half of the patients with the diagnosis of schizophrenia have abnormal results on span-of-apprehension tests. Those who do have abnormal results also have the clinical symptom of anergia. Other psychiatric disorders studied did not reveal those findings. Thus the abnormal results on the test appear to be specific to some forms of schizophrenia. Both short-term and long-term outcome studies have found that those patients with abnormal test results whose scores improve after receiving antipsychotics have a good clinical response to pharmacotherapy.

The span-of-apprehension test taps into some aspect of cognitive function specific to some patients with schizophrenia, their nonschizophrenic relatives, and persons at risk for developing schizophrenic symptoms. To scan the iconic image the person must (1) engage attention to the iconic register, (2) move the focus of attention, and (3) disengage the focus of attention. Impairments in performing any one of those tasks can explain the test-result abnormalities. Another cause of the deficiency may be that, with each fixation of attention, less information is processed. Thus, although the individual steps of iconic scanning may be intact, less visual information is processed and more errors occur. A third possibility is that the initiation of the attention process is delayed. That possibility is consistent with the increased reaction times revealed on numerous other tasks. The delay in the face of a rapid decay rate of sensory memory places the patients at a disadvantage when rapid responses are required. That possibility is also consistent with the other forms of attention deficit described earlier.

Another view, in contrast to the structural models described, focuses on the capacity model of attention. With a general limit on the cognitive resources available at a given moment, tasks that require an increased processing load (as in the case of time requirement or more letters on the display) diminish the resources available for other processes (such as scanning the image for the target letter and reporting the determination).

Schizophrenic patients may have a number of structural and capacity deficiencies. The hypotheses are not mutually exclusive. Further studies are needed to elucidate the nature of the cognitive state-trait marker for schizophrenic patients and persons vulnerable to the disorder.

ATTENTION-DEFICIT/HYPERACTIVITY DISORDER The change in 1980 of the terms "hyperkinetic" and "minimal brain dysfunction" to "attention-deficit disorder" in the third edition of the Diagnostic and Statistical Manual of Mental Disorders (DSM-III) and the change in 1987 to "attention-deficit hyperactivity disorder" in the revised third edition (DSM-III-R) emphasized the role that attention factors are thought to play in children, adolescents, and adults with the disorder. In the fourth edition of DSM (DSM-IV) attention-deficit/hyperactivity disorder integrates two categories from DSM-III-R: attention-deficit hyperactivity disorder and undifferentiated attention-deficit disorder. Diagnostic criteria embrace a number of forms of the syndrome, and research into the cognitive deficits have outlined a wide array of tasks in which attention capacity is abnormal. The pervasive findings of cognitive impairment in the setting of numerous intact cognitive functions has left the research field with no clearly accepted view of a core deficit in the disorder. Clinically, child and adolescent patients present with problems in school, with peers, and at home that reflect both academic and behavioral dysfunctions. Many studies suggest that the cognitive and behavioral dysfunctions in the disorder may be independent processes with different neurophysiological bases. For example, the finding that children with attention-deficit/hyperactivity disorder are impulsive may be true behaviorally but cannot be stated as a generalization about their cognitive functioning.

Researchers have attempted to find clear-cut diagnostic criteria to help clarify the disorder. There is no definitive test for the disorder, nor is a positive response to psychopharmacological intervention pathognomic. Biochemical studies have found abnormal urinary catecholamine metabolites that normalize as the patients' behavior improves when taking psychostimulants. Those findings and PET scan data suggest abnormal brain functions in patients with attention-deficit hyperactivity disorder.

What are the cognitive features of attention-deficit/hyperactivity disorder? Data from numerous studies show that the patients have dysfunctions on a variety of tasks (Table 3.1-1). Intact performance has been found on a number of memory tasks requiring verbal processes (for example, digit span, word tests, story recall) and nonverbal processes (for example recall, visual arrays, block series).

A number of theories have been elaborated to explain those differences between patients with the disorder and normal persons. Each theory has strengths, weaknesses, and varied support by the data, but each highlights the complexity of the cognitive dimensions of the disorder. In general, patients with the disorder evidence behavior that has been compared to that of patients with frontal lobe damage: deficits in the control of motor responses, in the execution of fine motor movements, and in the inhibition of ongoing response patterns. Memory tasks and basic aspects of information processing are intact, but the patients have impaired performance across modalities (auditory, visual, motor, perceptual-motor), suggesting some global deficit. The patients also appear to be unusually susceptible to boredom when the required tasks are long and repetitive.

Another view examines two proposed systems—an underactive behavioral inhibition system and an impaired behavioral reward system—to explain the behavioral problems that children with the disorder often have. A related view is that the rule-governed behavioral system is not intact; patients with the disorder appear to do especially poorly in a system with delayed or nonexistent rewards as in tasks that require sustained attention, accuracy, or task-directed activity governed by another person's direction or rules. Under those conditions the patients' poor regulation and inability to meet functional demands are revealed. A related issue is a diminished motivational drive and possibly a diminished arousal regulation system.

Yet another approach supported by research data is that the patients have metacognitive deficits. According to that perspective metacognitive processes that help plan, monitor, and regulate performance are impaired. The patient's ability to assess the task and determine strategies also has deficits. That is an example of top-down aspects of attention, with impairment of the higher cognitive processes that regulate information flow. Additional bottom-up deficiencies involve basic aspects of attention focus because of abnormalities in arousal, selectivity, and capacity.

The finding that numerous factors can influence the appearance of deficits led Virginia Douglas to the hypothesis that attention-deficit/hyperactivity disorder is a self-regulatory disorder with pervasive effects. The impairments affect each of four domains—attention, inhibition, reinforcement, and arousal—resulting in deficits in several aspects of self-regulation: (1) the organization of information processing, including planning, metacognition, executive functions, adapting appropriate cognitive sets for a given task, regulating arousal levels and alertness, and self-monitoring and self-correction; (2) the mobili-

TABLE 3.1-1
Tasks on Which Deficits Have Been Found in Attention-Deficit/Hyperactivity Disorder

Monitoring tasks and automated reaction time tasks
Deploying continuous, careful, and sustained attention to ongoing stimuli
Inhibiting responses to inappropriate stimuli
Inhibiting responses at inappropriate times
Perceptual search tasks
Conducting an organized, exhaustive, intensive, and focused search of task stimuli
Ignoring irrelevant stimuli
Inhibiting responses to irrelevant stimuli
Logical search tasks
Clarifying task demands
Generating and evaluating possible problem-solving strategies
Generating and evaluating possible solutions
Inhibiting premature, inadequate responses
Memory tasks
Processing task stimuli adequately
Generating and applying effective rehearsal strategies
Generating and applying effective retrieval strategies
Motor control and perceptual motor tasks
Guiding and controlling movement
Inhibiting inappropriate movement
Carrying out a careful perceptual analysis of complex figures
Drawing accurate reproductions of complex figures

Table from V I Douglas: Cognitive deficits in children with attention deficit disorder with hyperactivity. In *Attention Deficit Disorder: Criteria, Cognition, Intervention,* L M Bloomingdale, J A Sergeant, editors, p. 65. Pergamon, Oxford, 1988, Used with permission.

zation of attention, including the deployment and the maintenance of adequate attention; and (3) the inhibition of inappropriate responses such as withholding responses to extraneous stimuli and reinforcers. Those deficits in self-regulation imply that increased processing demands would lead to a diffusion of attention processes and to a subsequent impairment of the in-depth, coherent acquisition of knowledge and understanding.

One line of research has been based on the additive factor method, in which experimenters attempt to isolate the stage of the deficit. The model for that approach entails four stages: encoding (the identification of a stimulus), serial comparison (of the stimulus with elements related to the category in long-term memory), decision (pertaining to the category into which the stimulus is stored), and translation and response organization. Studies using evoked potentials suggest that deficits are found after the search and decision stages (the first three stages). The response preparation and execution processes appear to be impaired. Features that increase the processing load—such as speed demands, complexity of stimuli, distracters leading to divided attention, and increased duration of task—reveal different areas of deficit. That fact may explain the diversity of methods and research data supporting various theories. The variables affecting outcome include information-processing demands, the availability of alternate stimuli to which to attend, and the presence of an external regulator.

The diversity of research findings and theoretical explanations is paralleled by the clinical finding that children who are severely impaired in the classroom may have no attention problems in the confined, one-on-one setting of the psychiatrist's office. Such children may also be able to attend for indefinite periods to video games and yet be unable to follow complex conceptual information. The important principle is that cognitive dysfunction in psychopathological conditions may be task specific as a function of the nature of the cognitive impairment. The patient's clinical history and evaluation must consider potentially hidden domains of abnormal cognition.

AUTISTIC DISORDER Early descriptions of autism delineated the social functioning deficits that impair normal functioning. Autistic children were seen as having difficulties in normal emotional contact. Cognitive dysfunctions in autism were described later and were found to involve a number of areas, including abstraction, sequencing, language, and comprehension. Researchers are now focusing on the nature of the core deficit in the disorder. Issues of specificity and universality of areas of dysfunction in the disorder are important. How the cognitive domains relate to the social-affective deficits is an area of particular interest.

Seventy-five percent of the patients with autistic disorder are also mentally retarded. Mental retardation involves global cognitive and language impairments that may make it difficult to distinguish autistic disorder features. General cognitive impairments may be especially difficult to assess if language functioning is severely limited. Studies of high-functioning patients with autistic disorder have permitted various deficits to be determined.

Studies of the cognitive deficits in autistic disorder have distinguished an array of dysfunctional areas, including numerous language problems, excessive or impaired responsiveness to stimuli of various modalities, different encoding of auditory stimuli, and impairment in the ability to extract important features from incoming information. That range of deficits is thought to require the transformation of symbolic representations. In contrast, some autistic patients have relatively intact visuospatial and gestalt functions, musical abilities, and rote memory. Performances on standardized tests reveal relatively good results in object assembly and block design but poor results in comprehension.

Language deficits vary and include syntactic and phonological domains. Those findings initially suggested a left-hemisphere deficit, but other findings, including deficits in prosodic and pragmatic language functions, suggested right-hemisphere involvement as well. The findings can be interpreted as both deviations from normal language functioning and delays in language functioning. The wide array of dysfunctions in autistic disorder may be due to a number of subtypes, with characteristic deficits and possibly different brain loci of dysfunction.

Other studies have focused on the social cognition of patients with autistic disorder. They have examined the nature of the patients' emotional behavior and understanding to assess the earliest clinical descriptions of an abnormal emotional connection between autistic children and their parents. Two findings supported the initial impressions: autistic children were much less likely than usual to imitate adult vocalizations and gestures, and they showed much less sophisticated representational play with objects than did normal children. Those findings led to the suggestion that a core deficit in autistic disorder is the representation of representations (metarepresentations), leading to deficits in symbolic play and the inability to understand the mental states of others. The inability to transfer cognitive representations into language symbols may also be a related metarepresentation deficit.

A series of studies explored the relation of those possible cognitive impairments to socioemotional behavior. In contrast to clinical lore, autistic children were found to look at their parents; they had eye contact with their parents when social interactions were parentally elicited, and they revealed normal behavioral patterns of attachment. The studies did find a marked lack of social referencing (looking to parents for emotional cues in ambiguous situations) and protodeclarative gestures (pointing to objects and showing objects to familiar adults).

Three domains have been proposed to explain those findings: (1) Autistic children may not have the capacity to have a representation of another person as having ideas, perspectives, or emotions that can be shared. That proposal is consistent with a theory-of-mind hypothesis, in which the core deficit is believed to be the inability to have a sense of another's mind. (2) Autistic patients may have an impaired ability to perceive or comprehend the emotional (usually facial) signals of others. (3) The core deficit may involve either a lack of interest in others or an aversion to responding to others.

Studies have found that although autistic children do express emotions, they have less positive affects in response to their (relatively infrequent) periods of joint attention. Furthermore, they have an impairment in their responsivity to the display of strong emotion by another, whether of distress or of pleasure. Tests of high-functioning autistic patients reveal poor performance on emotion-recognition tasks, little comprehension of and empathy with depictions of social situations, and difficulty in talking about socially derived emotions such as pride and embarrassment. Autistic patients with relatively high intelligence use adaptive cognitive strategies to interpret social stimuli to compensate for impaired emotion-processing abilities.

The development of social cognition and socioemotional understanding requires complex interactions among the cognitive, perceptual, and emotional processes. A series of interactive elements essential to the development of social understanding have been proposed (Figure 3.1-9). That model describes the basic precursors of emotional responsiveness; the ability to attend to, encode, and interpret verbal and nonverbal social stimuli; the awareness of one's own and others' emotional responses; and the ability to contrast oneself with others. Out of that matrix develops the ability to understand others' views, desires, and beliefs. Accordingly, a deficit in any of those basic elements may explain the characteristic deficits observed in the social understanding of autistic persons.

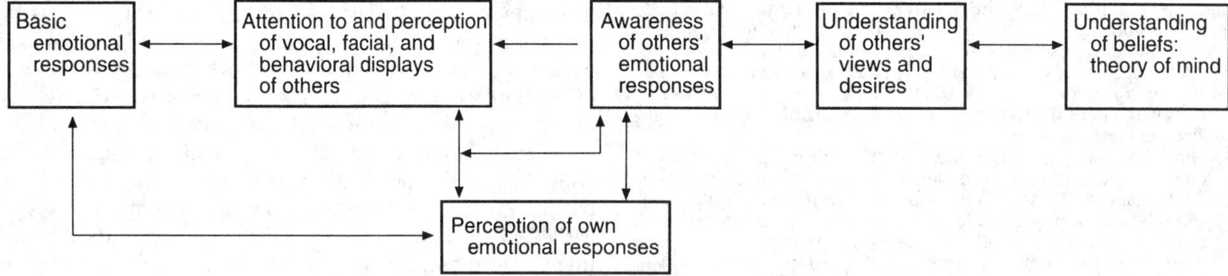

FIGURE 3.1-9 *Sigman's model for the development of socioemotional understanding. (Figure courtesy of M Sigman.)*

MOOD DISORDERS In contrast to schizophrenia, attention-deficit/hyperactivity disorder, and autistic disorder, the mood disorders do not appear to have core cognitive deficits that are diagnosis specific. Instead, cognitive abnormalities appear to be related to the degree of psychopathology and to the severity of the mood disturbance. Most studies have examined depressed patients; only a few studies have assessed cognitive functioning in patients with bipolar disorder in a manic state. In depressed patients the severity of the depression has ranged from mild depression in students to severe illness in hospitalized patients with major depressive disorders. The studies have examined primarily attention and memory for neutral and emotionally toned stimuli.

Depressive disorders Depressed patients often complain of difficulties with concentrating, learning, and remembering. Studies have documented that such patients perform poorly on tasks that require sustained attention or effortful and elaborate rehearsal. Thus controlled limited-capacity processes appear to be impaired in major depressive disorder. That limitation on access to capacity-demanding resources appears to be directly related to the severity of the depression and normalizes with remission from a depressive episode.

In contrast to patients with dementia, who have impaired semantic recall, depressed patients have intact access to long-term knowledge stores. Studies have found that although explicit memory for recently learned tasks is impaired in both depressive disorder and dementia, implicit memory (as shown by priming tasks) is intact in depression but impaired in dementia. That finding supports numerous studies showing that effort-requiring tasks are impaired in states of depression.

A dual-process model distinguishes between elaboration and activation. *Activation* makes items accessible and readily available to subsequent cognitive processes and is thought to be an automatic process fundamental to implicit memory. *Elaboration* is defined as the way in which the associative linkages are formed and strengthened between the current stimuli and other representations in memory. Elaboration occurs over an extended time and makes an item retrievable by the creation of several retrieval paths. The finding of intact implicit memory suggests that the automatic process of activation is unaffected in depression, whereas the effortful process of elaboration is impaired, thus influencing explicit memory.

Other studies of memory function reveal that depressed patients are likely to remember emotionally negative words and negative events in their lives during a depressive episode. Although studies of anxious patients have found consistent attention biases favoring attention to threat-related words, studies of attention effects in depression have yielded inconsistent results. Thus processing and recall in depressed patients appear to be more related to emotional effects on cognition than to attention biasing.

Depressed patients have also been found to have an increased response criterion; they require increased supportive data from the presented stimuli to respond in a test situation. Whether that need to be certain before responding is a psychological response to being depressed or a specific feature of the depression itself has not yet been determined. The reluctance to respond needs to be considered in interpreting research data and clinical interview findings.

The attention and memory findings have suggested several theoretical frameworks that are clinically useful. A schema theory of depression outlines a positive feedback loop in which negative self-schemata prime persons to have negative thoughts, to recall negative events in their lives, and to interpret present events with a negative bias. Whether as a cause or as a maintaining influence, those depressogenic schemata are thought to create a series of cognitive functions that produce and maintain a depressed mood.

A network theory of memory and emotion has been supported by research on depressed and nondepressed persons in which mood leads to a spreading activation of items in memory that are congruent with the mood. Thus emotion directly influences retrieval by a process of state-dependent learning and memory. Depressed patients are likely to encode items while depressed in a form that makes them readily accessible when retrieved in a depressed state. Depressed mood thus becomes an internal context cue that accesses depression-related memories.

Both the network and schemata theories of depression are consonant with research findings but do not explain all the cognitive and clinical findings in depression. They provide a framework for understanding how emotions and moods influence cognitive processing, such as memory retrieval and mental models. The conceptualization may be applicable to both transient mood states and severe mood episodes. Thus emotions in both health and illness can act as a context cue, leading to the activation of previously formed schemata for oneself and others. The activated schemata, in turn, can produce retrieval biasing and behavioral responses that can further elicit a negative emotional response. A reinforcing loop is established to support the continuation of the depressed mood and depressive cognition.

Some patients may be especially prone to marked cognitive alterations because of an emotional state that may be a fundamental part of a clinical presentation.

Bipolar disorder Patients with manic states present a spectrum of cognitive dysfunctions that appear to be related to the severity of their mood episode and that normalize with remission. The disturbances have been described clinically as rapidly paced thinking and speech, quick associations to self-generated or other-generated stimuli, grandiosity, and increased distractibility.

Formal studies of patients with bipolar disorder are technically difficult to carry out because of the patients' lack of cooperation and their restlessness and because such patients are few in number. The studies have suggested a high rate of combinatory thinking, the inclusion of loosely associated but related intrusions, and increased distractibility. The clinical impression of humor (even in the face of an underlying dysphoria) in some patients with bipolar disorder is corroborated by playful, extravagant, or flippant elaborations and intrusions in speech.

Those findings seem to indicate primarily state-dependent symptoms that improve on recovery. Thus forced-choice span-of-apprehension and backward masking tasks reveal impairments similar to those seen in actively schizophrenic patients but unlike those seen in schizophrenic patients who have persistent deficits in the remitted state. Bipolar disorder patients who are not actively ill reveal normal information processing.

POSTTRAUMATIC STRESS DISORDER Studies of posttraumatic stress disorder have extended the findings of information-processing abnormalities in anxiety disorders: attention biases toward fear-related and threat-related stimuli. Many of the studies were hampered by poorly defined clinical populations and control groups. However, some general trends, noted especially in the well-controlled paradigms, are promising and provide important insights into the psychopathological cognitive mechanisms in posttraumatic stress disorder.

Cognitive studies of patients with anxiety disorders have focused primarily on either attention or memory. Various research paradigms have been applied to assess attention bias and memory retrieval for neutral and emotionally activating stimuli. Studies find that anxious patients have an increased tendency to attend to fear-related and threat-related words. One research approach includes a dichotic listening task in which an anxious patient is more easily distracted than are controls by fear-related stimuli in the nonattended channel. That finding suggests that the patients have automatic, parallel attention processes that are primed to detect certain types of stimuli. Another approach uses the Stroop paradigm, in which words are presented in different-colored inks, and the person's task is to look at the word and state the color of the ink. Anxious patients have a significant delay in their response times for fear-related words. That finding suggests that increased attention capacity or cognitive processing is necessary when those words are perceived and the color of the ink is determined.

One theory that explains those findings is the idea of a fear network that encodes fear-related information in a memory structure that is readily accessible and able to influence cognitive, motor, and psychophysiological responses. The theoretical fear networks, which may be similar to mental models, are thought to contain three related forms of information: fear-eliciting stimulus cues, specific response patterns, and the meaning of both the cues and the responses for that particular person. In that theory patients with anxiety disorders are believed to have fear networks that are especially coherent and stable and that require few environmental cues to become activated.

Patients with posttraumatic stress disorder have been found to have attention biases toward threat-related stimuli specific to the experienced traumatic event. Many of the patients studied were combat veterans, and further work needs to establish the generalizability of those findings to other forms of posttraumatic stress disorder. The disorder is clinically characterized by both intrusive processes (memories, images, emotions, thoughts) and avoidance elements (psychic and emotional numbing, amnesia, behavioral avoidance of environmental cues resembling the initial trauma). The patients are thought to have a unique configuration of fear networks with stimulus cues (environmental stimuli), response components (cognitive, motoric, and psychophysiological), and meaning elements (for example, the moral implications of the trauma, survivor guilt, and the meaning of intentional trauma versus accidental trauma).

Some theories argue that states of excessive arousal during trauma impair attention capacity and memory encoding during the event. Emotional processing during and after the traumatic experience may also be hampered by the states of psychophysiological arousal and altered memory storage. The subsequent clinical syndrome may have some adaptive aspects; cognitive attention biases that are primed to detect fear-related stimuli may permit the early detection of threatening situations that, if not avoided, would produce incapacitating psychophysiological arousal. Automatic, nonconscious behavioral avoidance response patterns, embedded in the proposed fear networks or mental models, allow the patients to minimize excessive arousal by avoiding trauma-related situations.

The psychopathological aspects of posttraumatic stress disorder can be cognitively exemplified as follows: A combat veteran with chronic posttraumatic stress disorder may have no direct recall (impaired explicit memory) of a helicopter crash in which his best friend, who was seated next to him, was killed. Years later continued avoidance of airports, amnesia for combat, general apathy, and social withdrawal (avoidance elements)—combined with startle response, panic attacks, intrusive images, and nightmares (intrusive components)—suggest intact implicit memory for the combat trauma. The veteran is emotionally, behaviorally, and cognitively impaired.

The evaluation and treatment of patients can be greatly enhanced by an understanding of cognitive processes, including memory, and its careful application to the assessment of presenting symptoms and signs. Several areas that have interested clinicians for decades have become of great societal concern. Two topics that inspire intense controversy are the delayed recall of repressed memories of traumatic events and the suggestibility of patients influenced by clinicians, society, or friends to believe that they are the victims of childhood trauma.

Delayed recall Many scientists and clinicians believe in the cognitive capacity of patients to be unaware for years or decades of severely traumatic experiences that took place in their childhoods. Other researchers disagree and emphasize the paucity of studies of corroborated cases of childhood trauma that have been followed prospectively into adulthood with documentation of impaired access of consciousness to events presumably stored in memory.

A cognitive science view of delayed recall can examine the role of memory processes, development, and the effect of trauma on the processing of information to describe a theoretically coherent but yet-to-be-proved set of mechanisms.

A repressed memory can be thought of as originating from the active, intentional suppression of memory from consciousness. The mechanisms underlying the process then may become automatic and the contents of memory inhibited from retrieval into consciousness. The blockage may exist to avoid flooding the person's awareness with information that is associated with excessive anxiety or fear that would impair normal functioning.

In contrast, a traumatic event may be so overwhelming that normal processing may be impaired. If focal attention is divided, the nonfocally attended (traumatic) material will only be processed implicitly. Thus, in order to adapt to a traumatic event, some persons may have the capacity to focus their attention on a nonthreatening aspect of the environment or on their imagination during the trauma. That may be an underlying mechanism in a process called dissociation. Traumatic memory that has been only implicitly encoded will affect behavior and emotions and possibly will contain intrusive images and bodily sensations that are devoid of a sense of past, of self, or of something being recalled. That may, in part, explain the findings of posttraumatic stress disorder with amnesia (blocked conscious access to a memory or its origin) in the setting of avoidance behaviors, hyperarousal, intrusive images, and flashbacks.

Thus two distinct mechanisms that may explain delayed recall of childhood trauma are the concept of repressed memories and the concept of dissociated memories. A person may utilize both mechanisms for different aspects of a traumatic event. Recollection of the traumatic memory may take different forms. Repressed memories may have been processed to some degree in narrative form whereas dissociated memories probably lack that more integrative processing. The latter form thus may be experienced as nonpast and nonself, making the intrusive retrieval of dissociated memories a confusing and frightening experience.

Studies of the development of memory in children suggest

that the shared construction of narratives about experienced events is often crucial in making those events accessible to long-term retrieval. The establishment of a personal memory system appears to be a function of such memory talk in which parents discuss with children the contents of their memory. In children who have been forced to keep traumatic events a secret, as may occur with childhood abuse, the normal developmental process of narration may be blocked. That may be an additional cognitive mechanism underlying the inaccessibility of some forms of childhood trauma to consciousness in adult patients.

Suggestibility Dissociation and repression provide theoretical scientific explanations for the underlying mechanisms that may lead to delayed recall of childhood trauma, but clinicians must also be aware of other cognitive processes that influence memory. Numerous studies have demonstrated that the human mind is easily influenced. Human suggestibility can be used to the benefit or detriment of others. Suggestibility is adaptive for a social being that relies on the experiences of others to inform its knowledge of the world and thus to increase its chance for survival. Thus listening to the stories of others, reading a textbook, and being coached in athletics all require the receiver to accept data from the sender. The learner (listener) needs to trust the reliability of the teacher (teller) in order to accept the incoming information. Critical analysis of the data received is an important component of learning. The metacognitive function of assessing the accuracy or usefulness of newly acquired information may be suspended under certain conditions, including hypnosis, drug-altered states, and conditions of severe threat.

Studies of human suggestibility indicate that postevent questioning can bias the metamemory processes that help to determine the source and accuracy of a retrieved memory. The verbal and nonverbal cues given by the interviewer may influence a person to believe that aspects of an event, or an entire event, that may have never happened actually took place. A person can be convinced of the accuracy of an event despite its lack of correspondence with actual experience. Factors that may influence the biasing of interviewees include a belief in the trustworthiness and authority of the interviewer, not being aware that "I don't know" is a permissible response, repetition of a question that already has been answered, and the interviewer's beliefs as communicated through emotional tone and nonverbal gestures.

It is crucial for clinicians to be aware of human suggestibility in order to avoid iatrogenic distortions. Likewise, it is important for persons who experienced severe trauma early in life to receive informed and empathetic evaluations and treatment. There is a delicate balance between supportive neutrality and active advocacy in assessment and intervention. Awareness of those fundamental cognitive processes may help guide the clinician toward achieving that goal.

Approaches to the treatment of patients with posttraumatic stress disorder need careful evaluation but generally include the view that the impaired emotional processing of the traumatic event requires the active recollection, in explicit terms, of the details of the experience. The process of effectively treating unresolved trauma usually involves the active cognitive processing of specific memories, including emotional responses and the psychophysiological arousal at the time of the traumatic event. The provision of new cognitive information in the course of psychotherapy can, in theory, alter the configuration of the fear networks and allow previously inaccessible information to be explicitly processed and made available to consciousness for incorporation into an ongoing autobiographical narrative. Such changes may diminish the avoidant and intrusive components of the clinical syndrome of posttraumatic stress disorder and improve social, emotional, and cognitive functioning.

IMPLICATIONS FOR THE FUTURE

Cognitive science offers a breadth of conceptualizations for understanding the way in which the mind functions in health and in disease. The broad interdisciplinary field provides numerous research paradigms helpful in further elucidating the nature of psychopathology through techniques from the neurosciences to computer models of brain functioning. The cognitive understanding of emotions and consciousness may also expand psychiatry's framework for knowing about human subjective experience. The clinical tools, from medications to in-depth psychotherapy, may also find wider application as the process of psychological change is better understood.

Psychiatry, in turn, has much to offer the field of cognitive science. The long history of descriptive psychopathology and the attempt to synthesize views of the mind and the brain can provide nonclinical cognitive scientists with unique data and relevant questions. The invitation is open for psychiatry to join in the search for understanding the cognitive processes of the human mind.

SUGGESTED CROSS-REFERENCES

Piaget and emotional development are discussed in Section 3.2, memory in Section 3.5, cognitive impairment disorders in Chapter 12, schizophrenia in Chapter 14, mood disorders in Chapter 16, and anxiety disorders in Chapter 17 (particularly posttraumatic stress disorder in Section 17.4). Dissociative disorders are discussed in Chapter 20 and personality disorders in Chapter 25. Behavior therapy is discussed in Section 31.2, hypnosis in Section 31.3, and cognitive therapy in Section 31.6. Mental retardation is discussed in Chapter 35, learning disorders in Chapter 36, pervasive developmental disorder in Chapter 37, and attention-deficit/hyperactivity disorder in Chapter 38.

REFERENCES

Alba J W, Hasher L: Is memory schematic? Psychol Bull *93:* 203, 1983.

Anderson J R: *Cognitive Psychology and Its Implications,* ed 3. Freeman, New York, 1990.

Brewin C R: Cognitive change processes in psychotherapy. Psychol Rev *96:* 379, 1989.

Broadbent D E: *Decision and Stress.* Academic Press, New York, 1971.

Brothers L, Ring B: A neuroethological framework for the representation of minds. J Cognitive Neurosci *4:* 107, 1992.

Damasio A R: *Descarte's Error: Emotion, Reason and the Human Brain.* Putnam, New York, 1994.

Dennett D C: *Consciousness Explained.* Little, Brown, Boston, 1991.

Douglas V I: Cognitive deficits in children with attention deficit disorder with hyperactivity. In *Attention Deficit Disorder: Criteria, Cognition, Intervention,* L M Bloomingdale, J A Sergeant, editors, p 65. Pergamon, Oxford, 1988.

*Edelman G: *Bright Air, Brilliant Fire.* Basic Books, New York, 1992.

*Flavell J, Miller P H, Miller S A: *Cognitive Development,* ed 3. Prentice-Hall, Englewood Cliffs, NJ, 1993.

Frith U, Happe F: Autism: Beyond "theory of mind." Cognition *50:* 115, 1994.

Grice H P: Logic and conversation. In *Syntax and Semantics: III: Speech Acts,* P Cole, J L Moran, editors, p 41. Academic Press, New York, 1975.

Horowitz M J, editor: *Person Schemas and Maladaptive Interpersonal Patterns.* University of Chicago Press, Chicago, 1991.

Johnson M H, Magaro P A: Effects of mood and severity on memory processes in depression and mania. Psychol Bull *101:* 28, 1987.

Johnson M K: Reflection, reality monitoring and the self. In R G Kunzendorf, editor. *Mental Imagery,* Plenum, New York, 1991.
Johnson-Laird P N: *Mental Models: Towards a Cognitive Science of Language, Inference and Consciousness.* Harvard University Press, Cambridge, MA, 1983.
Kihlstrom J F: The cognitive unconscious. Science *237:* 1445, 1987.
Kosslyn S M: *Image and Brain: The Resolution of the Imagery Debate.* MIT Press, Cambridge, MA, 1994.
Lister R G, Weingartner H J, editors: *Perspectives on Cognitive Neuroscience.* Oxford University Press, New York, 1991.
Litz B T, Keane K M: Information processing in anxiety disorders: Application to the understanding of posttraumatic stress disorder. Clin Psychol Rev *9:* 243, 1989.
MacLeod C: Mood disorders and cognition. In *Cognitive Psychology: An International Review,* M W Eysennck, editor, p 9. Wiley, Chichester, England, 1990.
Main M: Metacognitive knowledge, metacognitive monitoring, and singular (coherent) vs. multiple (incoherent) models of attachment: Findings and directions for future research. In *Attachment Across the Life Cycle,* P Marris, J Stevenson-Hinde, C Parkes, editors. Routledge & Kegan Paul, New York, 1991.
Marcel A, Bisiach E, editors: *Consciousness in Contemporary Science.* Oxford University Press, New York, 1988.
McClelland J L, Rumelhart D E, editors: *Parallel Distributed Processing: Explorations in the Microstructure of Cognition,* vols 1 and 2. MIT Press, Cambridge, MA, 1986.
*Metcalfe J, Shimamura A P: *Metacognition: Knowing About Knowing.* MIT Press, Cambridge, MA, 1994.
Morris R G M, editor: *Parallel Distributed Processing: Implications for Psychology and Neurobiology.* Clarendon, Oxford, 1989.
Nelson K, editor: *Narratives from the Crib.* Harvard University Press, Cambridge, MA, 1989.
O'Mara S, Walsh V, editors: The cognitive neuropsychology of attention. Cogn Neuropsychol *11:* 96, 1994.
Osherson D N, Kosslyn S M, Hollerbach J M, editors: *Visual Cognition and Action: An Invitation to Cognitive Science, vol 2.* MIT Press, Cambridge, MA, 1990.
Osherson D N, Smith E E, editors: *Thinking: An Invitation to Cognitive Science, vol 3.* MIT Press, Cambridge, MA, 1990.
Pettinati H M, editor: *Hypnosis and Memory.* Guilford, New York, 1988.
*Posner M I, editor: *Foundations of Cognitive Science.* MIT Press, Cambridge, MA, 1989.
Roediger H L, Craik F I M, editors: *Varieties of Memory and Consciousness: Essays in Honor of Endel Tulving.* Erlbaum, Hillsdale, NJ, 1989.
Schacter D L, Tulving E, editors: *Memory Systems 1994.* MIT Press, Cambridge, MA, 1994.
Schneider D J: Social cognition. Ann Rev Psychol *42:* 527, 1991.
Schumacher J F, editor: *Human Suggestibility: Advances in Theory, Research and Applications.* Routledge & Kegan Paul, New York, 1991.
Siegel D J: Memory, trauma and psychotherapy: A cognitive science view. J Psychother Pract Res 4: 93, 1995.
Sigman M: What are the core deficits in autism? In *Atypical Cognitive Deficits in Developmental Disorders: Implications for Brain Function.* S H Broman, J Grafman, editors, p 139. Erlbaum, Hillsdale, NJ, 1994.
Singer J L, editor: *Repression and Dissociation: Implications for Personality Theory, Psychopathology and Health.* University of Chicago Press, Chicago, 1990.
Steinhauer S R, Gruzelier J H, Zubin J, editors: *Handbook of Schizophrenia,* vol 5: *Neuropsychology and Information Processing.* Elsevier Science, New York, 1991.
Terr L: *Unchained Memories: True Stories of Traumatic Memories, Lost and Found.* Basic Books, New York, 1994.
Watts F N, editor: *Neuropsychological Perspectives on Emotion. vol 7: Cognition and Emotion.* Erlbaum, Hillsdale, NJ, 1993.
*Yudofsy S C, Hales R H, editors: The neuropsychiatry of memory. In *Psychiatry,* vol 12, J M Oldham, M B Riba, A Tasman, editors, p 661. American Psychiatric Press, Washington, 1993.

3.2 PIAGET'S APPROACH TO INTELLECTUAL FUNCTIONING

STANLEY I. GREENSPAN, M.D.
JOHN F. CURRY, Ph.D.

INTRODUCTION

In recent studies of human learning cognitive theorists have emphasized the importance of the child's unique experiences and abilities as well as the importance of the experimental context and task. In so doing they have challenged and revised aspects of Jean Piaget's model of developmental psychology as well as a number of his specific conclusions. Yet his theory and insights remain a basic foundation for inquiries into the developmental stages of human intelligence. The following overview first introduces Piaget's basic theoretical concepts and briefly summarizes his model of the stages of intellectual development in childhood and adolescence. A discussion follows on how Piaget's model can be elaborated into a more general developmental model that includes effectual development and individual differences. The latter model is seen to have special clinical utility. Jean Piaget (1896–1980) was born in Neuchatel, Switzerland.

GENETIC EPISTEMOLOGY

Widely renowned as a child or developmental psychologist, Piaget referred to himself primarily as a genetic epistemologist. That self-designation reveals at once that Piaget's central project was not the articulation of a child psychology, as this term is generally understood, but rather an account of the progressive development of human knowledge.

On the classic question of the origins of knowledge Piaget was neither a nativist nor an empiricist; however, his position should not be considered an amorphous form of interactionism. Piaget stated in detail the nature of the interactionist position to which he ascribed. It is, in his words, a "constructivist structuralism," according to which the origin of mental structures is to be sought in the actions of the subject (the child) on objects as the subject strives to adapt to its environment. Structures are constructed within the subject as a consequence of interactions between subject and object. What Piaget judged to be innate is an intelligent functioning that makes possible the production of progressively more adequate structures of knowledge on the basis of abstraction from actions performed during the stages of development.

For example, the concept of space is a fundamental mental structure developed in the earliest period of children's lives. In earliest infancy the child is aware of not one homogeneous space but of several heterogeneous spaces, each centered on a certain part of the child's body (for example, visual space and tactile space). As children act on objects that may traverse these various spaces (for example, a rattle occupying visual, tactile, and auditory spaces) they come to coordinate these individual spaces. Eventually, actions representing displacements in space are organized mentally into the general concept of space. That concept is a structure that can be described in logico-mathematical terms.

EQUILIBRATION For Piaget the general criterion for intelligent functioning is *equilibration,* briefly defined as "a compensation for an external disturbance.'' Hans Furth described equilibration as ''the factor that internally structures the developing intelligence. It provides the self-regulation by which intelligence develops in adapting to external and internal changes.'' At every level of development the equilibration mechanism is operative in furthering adaptation, but as development proceeds toward the highest level of cognitive functioning, equilibration becomes progressively more adequate in enabling the organism to adapt to a wider range of internal and external disturbances. Piaget's notion of intelligence as adaptation is therefore essentially bound to an equilibration model of intelligent functioning.

ASSIMILATION AND ACCOMMODATION To explicate the equilibration model further it is necessary to introduce Piaget's concepts of the assimilation and accommodation processes. The biological foundation of Piaget's developmental theory is nowhere more clearly evident: those processes are considered functional invariants of all intelligent behavior. At every level of intellectual development, from infancy to adulthood, the processes are operative in the overall process of adaptation.

The assimilation-accommodation account of development stresses the interaction between organism and environment. A certain readiness is postulated as a necessary condition within the organism for change or development to take place. In Piaget's view associationism (empiricism) in psychology has committed the fallacy of crediting only half of those conditions necessary for learning with all explanatory power. A full account of human development must include not only the influence of stimuli on respondents (S → R), but also the influence of the responding organism on incoming stimuli (S ← R). Such an account is provided by Piaget's assimilation-accommodation viewpoint: ''From a biological point of view, assimilation is the integration of external elements into evolving or completed structures of an organism. In its usual connotation, the assimilation of food consists of a chemical transformation that incorporates it into the substance of the organism.''

Furth referred to assimilation as ''an inward-directed tendency of a structure to draw environmental events towards itself.'' Assimilation is the conservative side of intellectual development, assuring continuity and coherence by incorporating new aliments into existing mental structures. However, assimilation alone cannot account for growth or change within those structures.

Accommodation occurs during the developmental periods when new data cannot be wholly assimilated to the child's existing mental structures, and yet the data are not so entirely foreign to those structures that their existence can be ignored. Furth referred to accommodation as ''an organism-outward tendency of the inner structure to adapt itself to a particular environmental event.'' Read Tuddenham pointed out the variations in accommodation relative to levels of intellectual development as follows: ''At the lowest psychological level, accommodation refers to the gradual adaptation of the reflexes to new stimulus conditions—what others have called conditioning or stimulus generalization. At higher levels it refers to the coordination of thought patterns to one another and to external reality.''

Following this line of thought it can be seen in what sense intelligence is defined by Piaget in terms of equilibration. The equilibration to which he refers is not a static, balanced system, but a dynamic or mobile equilibration between assimilation and accommodation as the child responds to the environment.

STRUCTURALISM Intelligence has been discussed in terms of an equilibration process involving assimilation of aliments to structures and accommodation of structures to new, somewhat different aliments. Before the stages of intellectual development through which that process passes can be analyzed, it is necessary to understand more fully Piaget's notion of intellectual structure and to take a more fundamental look at the origins and developmental forms of the cognitive structures.

The term Piaget used for a cognitive structure is scheme *(schema)*: ''A scheme is the structure or organization of actions as they are transferred or generalized by repetition in similar or analogous circumstances.'' Schemata exist in the infant in the form of perceptual-motor behavior patterns, such as the grasping reflex. They also exist in mature intelligence, although, as Furth pointed out, schema is more commonly used to refer to an early mental structure, whereas general schemata resulting from use of higher intelligence are referred to as *operations*.

The abstraction process that leads to the formation of cognitive structures is called *reflective* or *formal abstraction*. It is an abstraction from *actions*, according to which the similarities inherent in various behavioral acts are dissociated from their particularized contexts. (See, for example, the earlier example of the rattle in space.) According to Furth and colleagues, ''More precisely, reflective abstractions are an enriching feedback into the structures of the organism from the most general coordinations of actions.''

THEORY OF STAGES

The preceding discussion of Piaget's thought has been general, designed to provide a theoretical perspective on genetic epistemology. Forming an integral part of that system is a psychology of cognition, which seeks to answer descriptively the question of how knowledge develops and changes. The genetic framework for that and the process of intellectual adaptation during the major early periods of life are provided in Piaget's theory of the stages of cognitive development.

The stages of cognitive development that Piaget and his associates delineated on the basis of research are not defined merely by the dominance of some aspect that remains present in a less dominant manner throughout development. Rather, each stage constitutes a structured whole and can be defined by reference to a set of criteria.

Concerning his stages of cognitive development, Piaget was not entirely consistent, but the only possible source of confusion in his later writings is whether the so-called preoperational period is to be considered apart from the period of concrete operations, in which it culminates. On the basis of John Flavell's 1963 study and Piaget's 1983 summary, three major periods and one subperiod of intellectual development are delineated (Table 3.2-1). Within these periods are found subdivisions, referred to as stages. The major developmental periods are as follows:

1. The sensorimotor period, which extends from birth until approximately 1½ years of age. The period is divided into six stages, which are described in general in the following discussion with reference to the development of the concept of the permanent object.
2. A period of preparation for and acquisition of concrete operations. This period is initiated by the appearance (at about age 2) of the symbolic (semiotic) function and ends with the beginning (at about age 7) of higher mental operations applied to concrete objects.
3. The period of formal operations, which begins at approximately 11 years of age. During this period, full adult intelli-

TABLE 3.2-1
Stages of Intellectual Development Postulated by Piaget

Age (years)	Period	Cognitive Developmental Characteristics
0–1½ (to 2)	Sensorimotor	Divided into six stages, characterized by (1) inborn motor and sensory reflexes (2) primary circular reaction (3) secondary circular reaction (4) use of familiar means to obtain ends (5) tertiary circular reaction and discovery through active experimentation (6) insight and object permanence
2–7	Preoperations subperiod*	Deferred imitation, symbolic play, graphic imagery (drawing), mental imagery, language
7–11	Concrete operations	Conservation of quantity, weight, volume, length, and time based on reversibility by inversion or reciprocity; operations; class inclusion and seriation
11 through end of adolescence	Formal operations	Combinatorial system, whereby variables are isolated and all possible combinations are examined; hypothetical-deductive thinking.

*This subperiod is considered by some authors to be a separate developmental period.

gence develops as the operations are extended to apply to propositional or hypothetical thinking.

SENSORIMOTOR PERIOD The sensorimotor period of intelligence is so named because construction by the child of mental schemata is in no way aided by representations, symbols, or thoughts. Rather, schemata are dependent totally on perceptions and bodily movements.

Stage 1 of sensorimotor development is marked by a relatively few organized reflexes that stand out against the background of the spontaneous general activity of the neonate. Among those early reflexes are the sucking reflex and the palmar reflex. Those primitive reflexes take on the nature of the first schema through three types of assimilation: (1) reproductive (repeating the actions); (2) generalizing (repeating the actions on new objects); and (3) recognitory (performing different varieties of the actions on different objects).

Stage 2 is that of the first habit and the primary circular reaction. The first habits develop out of the original schemata as those are applied to objects in the environment or to parts of the infant's body, but without any differentiation between means and end. In a primitive state of consciousness, the infant is aware only of action sequences, and not even aware of self. Primary circular reactions occur when by chance the infant experiences a new consequence of a motor act, and then tries to repeat the act.

In stage 3 of the sensorimotor period an initial distinction between means and end becomes apparent, but in a primitive sense. The infant repeats a particular action pattern that succeeded in achieving one end for the purpose of achieving many other (unrelated) ends. For example, a baby who succeeds in shaking a rattle by pulling a string may repeatedly pull the string in an attempt to effect other sounds or results.

In stages 4 and 5 infants use a variety of available means to obtain particular goals. The distinction between stages 4 and 5 lies in the relative creativity or newness of the means employed. Stage 4 is marked by use of already familiar means. Stage 5 is marked by a search for new means based on further differentiations of already known schemata and by the tertiary circular reaction. The latter differs from a secondary circular action in that the child no longer produces schemata that were effective in one situation to produce magically efficacious results in every situation. Instead, the child relies on exploration of the environment and means variation to test for effectiveness. Discovery is a hallmark of stage 5. For example, a child may use a stick to move an object not within reach.

Stage 6 is transitional, leading into the preoperational subperiod. In stage 6 the child becomes capable of inventing new means, not by direct actions on objects but by mental combination. Whereas discovery marked stage 5, insight is a characteristic of stage 6. For example, a child, having seen the father bang on a drawer to loosen it, may bang on a toy box to make it easier to open.

During the sensorimotor period, a number of significant concepts are developed, including the child's concepts of space, time, and causality. These categorical concepts develop in a process parallel to the sequence of the six stages outlined previously. Most important, during the sensorimotor phase, the child develops the schema of object permanence, the first major victory of *conservation* and the foundation of all future knowledge.

Schema of object permanence The knowledge that objects in the external world have an existence independent of the child's actions on them or interactions with them is a major accomplishment of the sensorimotor period. Flavell has outlined Piaget's observations and interpretations of infants' reactions to the disappearance of interesting objects, which are the foundation for the theory of development of object permanence. In stages 1 and 2, for example, a child simply continues to look at the place where the object was last seen. In stage 3 if an object such as a spoon drops to the floor, the infant will look for it (for example, by leaning over and looking at the floor). In stage 4 if an object is repeatedly hidden at point A (in sight of the child) and then hidden at point B (also in sight of the child), the child searches for it at the original, rather than the current, hiding place (that is, at A, not B). Stages 5 and 6 mark the child's increasing understanding of object permanence in that the infant is able to follow multiple displacements of the object through points in space, even if the object is hidden within another object.

PREOPERATIONAL SUBPERIOD AND SEMIOTIC FUNCTION The advent of the preoperational subperiod is marked by the appearance of what Piaget called the *semiotic function.* This new ability was defined by Piaget and Bärbel Inhelder as follows: "It consists in the ability to represent something (a signified something object, event, conceptual scheme, etc.) by means of a signifier which is differentiated and which serves only a representative purpose: language, mental image, symbolic gesture and so on."

During the sensorimotor period, a thing could be represented in a limited sense by a part of itself (for example, the mother's voice might represent the presence of the mother in the room). However, such signifiers are indices undifferentiated from their significants (the voice is part of the mother). Symbols and signs are signifiers that are differentiated from their significants. They become available to the child only with the appearance of the semiotic function, with which representational thought becomes possible. As Furth pointed out, representation has first of all an active meaning in Piaget's theory. The child becomes capable of summoning up a symbol or sign to stand for a given significant. It is essential to state that, for Piaget, representation is not of the essence of thought. It serves rather an auxiliary function.

Characteristic behavior patterns The semiotic function is heralded by five characteristic behavior patterns in evidence during the second year of life: (1) deferred imitation or imitation that starts after the disappearance of the model; (2) symbolic play or the game of pretending; (3) drawing or graphic imagery; (4) mental image, which appears as an internalized imitation and not as a function of perception; and (5) verbal evocation of events not occurring at the time. Each behavior pattern shows the origins of representational thought as the preoperational subperiod of cognitive development begins.

For Piaget the semiotic function, which serves to enlarge the children's worlds to such a great extent—liberating them from the bonds of immediate space and time and enabling them to begin to manipulate symbols and to think rather than just to act on immediately present objects—finds its roots in imitation.

IMITATION It is possible to follow the development of imitation through the same six sensorimotor stages delineated for the concept of object permanence. Piaget has done this in his volume *Play, Dreams and Imitation in Childhood.* A radically new form of imitation occurs during the second year of life: *deferred imitation.* For example, children may put on their father's hat and walk as their father does, even hours after the father has gone off to work.

For Piaget intelligence is an equilibration process in which assimilation and accommodation are in balance. Imitation, however, is behavior in which accommodation outweighs assimilation. According to Piaget, imitation is behavior in which "the subject's schemes of action are modified by the external world without his utilizing this external world." In imitation the child's cognitive structures undergo temporary change without simultaneously incorporating new aliment.

SYMBOLIC PLAY A second new behavior pattern that now appears is symbolic play. In imitation the imbalance between assimilation and accommodation is weighted in favor of accommodation; however, the opposite holds true in symbolic play, which is a lessening of the demand of the adaptive process.

Play, too, can be followed in its development through the six stages of sensorimotor intelligence, but the use of symbols in play is found only after the sensorimotor period, in the type of play characterized by games of pretending. For example, a little girl will pretend that she is asleep, that a box is her pet cat, or that she herself is a church. In each instance symbols are generated "in order to express everything in the child's life experience that cannot be formulated and assimilated by means of language alone."

According to Piaget's theory, these symbols are created by the same process of imitation that gives rise to deferred imitation at this time. In fact, Piaget views imitation as the process underlying the development of the entire semiotic function. In symbolic play, then, symbols are generated by a process in which accommodation outweighs assimilation. But instead of being used accurately (that is, to represent that from which they are derived), they are placed at the service of a process in which a liberating assimilation outweighs accommodation.

DRAWING A third behavior pattern associated with the rise of the semiotic function is drawing, or graphic imagery. Piaget sees in this activity elements of play and of imitation. In developmental terms, he considers drawing as "halfway between symbolic play and the mental image," appearing at about age 2 or 2½ years. Drawing is playful activity in the sense that it is an end in itself and is characterized by reproductive assimilation; in other words, the child enjoys producing drawings for their own sake. However, the graphic play also has accommodative elements especially as the child grows older and attempts to draw not just formless scribble, but some thing.

MENTAL IMAGE Very closely related to drawing is the mental image. Piaget viewed the genesis of mental imagery as tied to accommodation and imitation. He explicitly denies that mental images can be the product of perception; they are a construction, something the child creates. The mental image is not directly given by perceptual input; rather, it is constructed by the process of accommodation.

VERBAL EVOCATION OF EVENTS The fifth behavior pattern associated with the rise of the semiotic function has to do with language. It consists of the verbal evocation of events that are not present. Piaget gave the example of a little girl saying "Anpa, bye-bye" (Grandpa went away) while pointing to the path he had taken when he left. The parallel with deferred imitation is clear, but here the new representational ability is supported by the social system of language.

CONCRETE OPERATIONS A crucial difference between preoperational and concrete-operational thought is the presence within operative thinking of concepts of conservation. When concrete operations have been organized into a system, they enable the child to conserve, that is, "to discover what values do remain invariant . . . in the course of any given kind of change or transformation." The progressive and continual structure building that takes place in the concrete operational period is evident in the increase, with development and age, in the scope of such concepts, such as conservation of quantity, substance, and number.

Conservation of quantity The clearest sign that a child remains in the preoperational subperiod is the absence of the concept of conservation. For example, if liquid is poured from a short, wide glass into a tall, narrow one, the child in the preoperational stage thinks the amount of liquid has changed. At the level of concrete operations, however, children are no longer overwhelmed by the perceptual discrepancy between the two configurations. They begin to reason about the transformation, and their correct judgments regarding the conservation of quantity of liquid are accompanied by explanations grounded in logical properties. It is assumed that children are not aware of the logic they utilize.

When problems of conservation begin to be solved, the child passes from the preoperational subperiod into the period of concrete operations, for which the former was a long time of transition and preparation.

Conservation of substance At the age (on average) of about 7 or 8 the child can solve the conservation-of-quantity problem and can perform similar judgments of conservation when, for example, a lump of clay is transformed in shape. Between the ages of 9 and 10, the child discovers that the weight of a given object is also conserved even when its shape is transformed. However, not until approximately age 11 or 12 do children have a logical comprehension that the volume displaced by a given object is conserved even after transformation of the object's shape. Conservation entails the logical certainty that one characteristic of an object remains invariant while the object itself undergoes some type of perceived transformation.

Concept of cardinal numbers The concept of cardinal numbers also develops from an initially nonconserving to a conserving stage. Children in the preoperational subperiod can be presented with two horizontal rows of colored dots in one-to-one correspondence (that is, imaginary vertical lines could be constructed between each red dot and its corresponding blue dot). When the experimenter destroys this optical correspondence by spreading out one of the rows of dots, the child in the preoperational period thinks the larger row contains more dots. Only after conservation of cardinal number has been established as a logical necessity does the child maintain the numerical equivalence of the spread-out row. Clearly, preoperational concepts of number provide inadequate bases for arithmetic skills. It is possible that a lag in the development of number conservation could underlie certain types of arithmetic-related learning disabilities. Again, that points to the importance of children's active experience as a foundation for subsequent concept formation.

OPERATIONS Notions of conservation are the mark of well-established concrete operational thinking. It is therefore essential to discuss the meaning of *operation* in Piaget's thought. Operations, themselves, constitute essential thinking. For Piaget an operation is an action that is (1) interiorized, (2) reversible, and (3) part of an organized system of such actions.

The operations that form this system are, first, interiorized actions. In the sensorimotor period external behavior patterns gave rise through a process of abstraction to the construction of sensorimotor schemata. In similar fashion internal thinking patterns later give rise to operations. According to Furth, it is the generalizable aspects of actions, "those which can be found in any coordination of action," that enter into the construction of operations. To say that the crucial aspect of actions in this regard is their generalizability is to explain the importance of interiorization in the construction of operations. *Interiorization* refers to "the increasing dissociation of general form from particular content." In other words, the notions of generalizability and interiorization merely point out the process of abstraction that is occurring. For example, a child adds two apples and three apples to obtain five apples. In another instance a child adds seven blocks and one block to obtain eight blocks. In a third instance a child combines the category of fathers with that of mothers to obtain the category of parents. The operation abstracted from these three mental actions is that of addition or combining, without reference to the particular content of numbers, objects, or categories.

Not only must an operation be interiorized action, it must also be reversible. The action of combining (addition) is not an operation until its relationship to the action of separating (subtraction) is comprehended. To understand reversibility is to understand the third criterion of an operation, its inclusion in a system.

The reversibility essential to operatory thought may be either of two types: inversion or reciprocity. In reversibility by inversion, an action $+A$ is reversed by $-A$. For example, in the above conservation-of-quantity example, the pouring of liquid into container 2 $(+A)$ may be mentally reversed: that is, mentally poured back into container 1 $(-A)$. In reversibility by reciprocity a relation $A < B$ is reversed by a relation $B < A$. Referring again to the conservation-of-quantity example, let A stand for container 1, and B stand for container 2. The rising height of liquid in container 2 $(A < B)$ is offset by its narrower width $(B < A)$.

Corresponding to these two types of reversibility are the two major categories of concrete operations: those pertaining to classes and those pertaining to relations. In the system of operations performed on classes, reversibility is by way of inversion; in those performed on relations, it is by way of reciprocity. For example, subtraction and addition relate to inversion; comparing sticks of different sizes relates to reciprocity.

Class inclusion The concrete operation demonstrating understanding of classes is the class inclusion task. In this task a child is shown, for example, an array of pets (superordinate class) consisting of dogs and cats (subordinate classes). After counting the number of dogs, cats, and pets, the child is asked whether there are more dogs or more pets. Children in the preoperational subperiod cannot maintain in mind the superordinate class while perceiving only the subordinate classes. Thus, they fail the task frequently over a series of such arrays.

Relations The concrete operation that demonstrates an understanding of relations is seriation. Children are asked, for example, to arrange a set of rods in order of increasing size. Children in the preoperational subperiod may subgroup the rods but will have difficulty completing an entire array along the required dimension. They may understand the concept of smaller versus larger but have difficulty with comprehending the gradual nature of change.

FORMAL OPERATIONS In the third and final stage in Piaget's conception of the intellectual development in the child the logical structures of concrete operations are superseded by structures referred to as formal operations.

The relationship between the real and the possible that is characteristic of adolescent thinking represents a reversal of that relationship in the thinking of the concrete operational child. Inhelder and Piaget note that the real has priority for the younger child and that possibility is conceived of merely as a prolongation or extension of real operations, "as, for example, when, after having ordered several objects in a series, the subject knows that he could do the same with others." For the adolescent, however, the possible occupies a place of priority and the real is seen as a particular instance of it. "Henceforth, they conceive of the given facts as that sector of a set of possible transformations that has actually come about." This immediately presupposes that the adolescent can take a given empirical event (such as, "the long, thin rod bends") and categorize it within a system of possible combinations of events (for example, long rods or short rods, thin rods or thick rods, bending or not bending). Three characteristics follow from this fundamental reorientation in thought: (1) adolescent thought is hypothetical-deductive in nature; (2) it deals in propositions rather than in concrete events; and (3) it is capable of isolating variables and of examining all possible combinations of variables.

Hypothetical-deductive thought As a hypothetical-deductive form of thought, formal operational intelligence proceeds from the possible to the real. In this sense, it mirrors scientific reasoning. The implications of a propositional statement are drawn and then tested against reality. Rather than building up a proposition by induction from disparate concrete examples to a loose generalization, formal intelligence operates systematically from general statement to particular instance by means of testable hypotheses. In Flavell's words, "To try to discover the real among the possible implies that one first entertains the possible as a set of hypotheses to be successively confirmed or infirmed. Hypotheses which the facts infirm can then be discarded; those which the data confirm then go to join the reality sector."

Propositional thought When it is said that formal operations deal in propositions rather than in concrete events, an increased freedom from immediate content is implied, with a correspondingly greater intellectual mobility. At one level this freedom implies the ability to manipulate abstractions that have been tied to concrete examples or events. The adolescent, for example, can perform a transitive inference ($A < B, B < C$; therefore, $A < C$) without any empirical demonstration of referents for the terms A and B. At another level this freedom implies that, having performed a concrete operation, the adolescent can abstract the results of that operation and perform further operations on them. For example, an adolescent can perform the concrete operation of combining two liquids to observe the color of the resultant mix and then take the result of this operation and systematically relate it to results of all other combinations of available liquids.

Isolating variables and examining combinations The example that follows helps to explain the third characteristic of adolescent thought mentioned by Flavell: the isolation of variables and the examination of all possible combinations. Instead of dealing with disparate concrete experiments, hypothetical-deductive adolescents can organize their investigations into a coherent pattern *a priori,* then perform all relevant combinations of variables to test their hypotheses, in that way isolating causal factors. Piaget's theory of formal operational cognition has focused on scientific thinking. For example, the weight, speed, shape, and size of an object may all be seen to have their relative contribution to the size of a hole the object will make when hitting the ground.

Children in the preoperational substage merely describe what they see, and causal thinking is expressed in an undifferentiated form (for example, "It has to"). The child with concrete operational thinking can categorize and order the relevant variables independently but has difficulty integrating the system of all relevant variables. The adolescent, however, can generate all possible combinations of relevant variables and can proceed to a systematic test of the importance of each variable.

A complete combinatorial system makes its appearance only during the period of formal operations. Instead of focusing on empirical givens, as a child in the concrete operational stage does, the adolescent using formal operational thinking constructs a hypothetical system of which the empirical givens are members. Whereas the younger child was capable of classifying events according to various categories, such as length, width, and weight, the adolescent uses that classification as a basis on which to abstract all possible combinations of variables. Having done this, the adolescent can then test hypotheses derived from the combinatorial system. The end result of this new ability is the capacity to test the causal significance of each individual factor in succession by holding all other factors constant.

Piaget interprets the rise of formal operational thought in the context of his equilibrium model of cognitive development. Thus, he considers neurological maturation and experience of the object and interpersonal world as necessary but not sufficient conditions to explain this qualitative improvement in thinking. In essence, the equilibration explanation is as follows: During the stage of concrete operations, a number of qualitatively heterogeneous factors are constructed by the child, resulting in the achievement of conservation of the factor in question even in the face of perceptual transformations. Such factors include quantity, weight, volume, time, and length. Eventually, the child discovers that in many concrete instances the operation of these factors is interrelated. Thus, although the factors have been constructed mentally in relative isolation from one another, their presence in real objects is mixed. Through experience with both impersonal and interpersonal objects, the child's concrete operational understanding of these factors is shown to be insufficient, and a more comprehensive, more intelligent understanding is stimulated.

EGOCENTRISM

Each major period of cognitive development discussed previously is characterized by a qualitative shift toward more comprehensive and more adaptive cognitive structures. In this sense, the adolescent is more intelligent than the infant. However, each transition to a higher level of cognitive organization is initially accompanied by a lack of full differentiation between self and object. Each period has an early organizational phase that is followed by the phase of accomplishment of cognitive developmental tasks. During the early organizational phase, the child's failure to differentiate fully the self from objects is manifest in behavior reflecting stage-specific forms of egocentrism. David Elkind has summarized the process. Each developmental period has characteristic forms of egocentrism.

In the sensorimotor period egocentrism refers literally to a lack of differentiation between self and object, as perceived in the lack of object permanence. The existence of objects independent of action patterns of the self is not acknowledged. In the preoperational subperiod the capacity to engage in symbolic thinking is accompanied by initial failure to differentiate fully between symbols and their referents. That may be manifest, for example, in failure to differentiate such mental images as dreams from real objects. In the concrete operational period the capacity to engage in logical operations is accompanied by an unrealistic certainty in which probability is not appreciated and mental construction of the self (self-definition) is not differentiated from facts. Finally, at adolescence, the capacity to engage in hypothetical thinking and to understand others' points of view is accompanied by characteristic patterns of thought in which others are unrealistically presumed to be focusing on the self. As Elkind has pointed out, adolescent egocentrism is a "belief that others are preoccupied with (the adolescent's) appearance and behavior," when, in fact, the adolescent is preoccupied with these topics.

EXTENSIONS OF PIAGET'S THEORY

In his classic statement of theory and in the bulk of his scientific research, Piaget focused on the development of logico-mathematical reasoning, the operative aspects of thinking. Others, however, have extended a similar structural model to the investigation of other domains. The best known example of such an extension of Piagetian theory is probably Lawrence Kohlberg's theory of the stages of moral reasoning. Kohlberg proposed six stages in the development of moral reasoning. These begin with the moral stance of the preschool child, based on reward or punishment, and proceed through middle childhood, when moral judgment tends to be based on desire to obtain the approval of others or to uphold authority. Only with adolescence does the morality of internalized principles, such as the rights of individuals or the notion of a natural law, begin to take effect. In Kohlberg's model each major stage of moral development requires that the child attain a commensurate level of cognitive development. For example, conventional morality, which develops during middle childhood, requires concrete operational thinking, and principled morality requires formal operational thinking.

A broader area of development in which Piaget's observations have been extended has been referred to as social cognition. As noted earlier, a central construct throughout Piaget's developmental model is that of egocentricity versus decentration. In the social domain decentration has been referred to as role taking or the ability to take the perspective of others. That skill may be observed at a perceptual, a cognitive, or an affective level. Perceptual role-taking involves the ability to recognize how a perceptual array appears from the perspective of another when that perspective differs from one's own. Cognitive and affective role-taking involve analogous processes in which the thoughts and feelings of others are taken into account when they differ from one's own. Thus, role-taking is a condition necessary for the development of empathy. Kohlberg took the position that it was also a necessary condition for the development of higher levels of moral reasoning.

In general, social cognitive processes refer to role-taking and communication skills that enable children, adolescents, and adults to understand one another's thoughts and feelings. Social cognitive processes are central to the concerns of psychiatry, because deficiencies in these processes impair communication and correlate with symptomatology, and because reconstruction of social cognitive processes is a direct concern of psychosocial interventions. For example, the deficiencies in social cognition that are characteristic of aggressive, conduct disordered boys have been delineated by Kenneth Dodge, John Lochman, and others, and then identified as targets for intervention with these youngsters.

Flavell recently reviewed three decades of work in the area of perspective-taking or role-taking. After a period focused on communication skills, perspective-taking researchers concentrated on cognitive processes in which children develop knowledge of themselves and others as learners and rememberers. For example, during development children become aware of strategies for encoding bits of information that need to be recalled. Studies of such metacognition are another example of the extension of a Piagetian model to domains of practical importance to psychiatry and applied psychology. Deficiencies in metacognitive skills have been identified in youngsters with attention-deficit/hyperactivity disorder or learning disorders, and can serve as targets for psychoeducational intervention.

Recently, post-Piagetian research in perspective-taking has focused on what has been described as children's theory of mind. That pertains to children's awareness that others have cognitive processes similar to their own, or that others have an internal mental state and the ability to represent the mental states of others in their own mind. An example of a theory of mind task is the false belief task. In that task, a child is shown a popular, brand name candy box and asked what it contains. The child is then shown and told that the box does not contain candy, but instead contains a pencil. The pencil is then put back into the box, and the child asked to predict what another child would say is in the box, as well as asked to say what is actually in the box. Thus, the task involves predicting an erroneous belief in another that differs from one's own correct belief. Young children master this task at about age 4. However, children with autistic disorder, show specific deficiencies on this task, whereas children in whom language is merely delayed have no such difficulty. Thus, theory of mind may be an area of cognitive deficiency specific to autistic disorders.

NEO-PIAGETIAN RESPONSE TO CRITICISMS OF PIAGET'S THEORY Major criticisms of Piaget's theory have emanated from the Anglo-American empirical tradition and from sociocultural theorists. Empiricists have pointed to findings, including the effectiveness of training interventions in accelerating Piaget's proposed pace of cognitive development and to weak correlations among scores on tasks that purportedly measure the same underlying cognitive structure. Sociocultural theorists consider Piaget's emphasis on logicomathematical reasoning and on the isolation and manipulation of variables as a bias inherent in Western forms of thought. Cross-cultural research has shown that different tasks are mastered at different ages in different cultures. In addition to these external critics Piaget has been criticized within his own school of thought for failing to address individual differences in cognitive abilities, for failing to investigate cognitive development during adulthood, and for giving an insufficient explanation of the processes by which stage transitions occur.

Neo-Piagetian theorists, such as Juan Pascual-Leone and Robbie Case, attempt to address these criticisms while retaining the core assumptions of Piaget's theory. Instead of positing broad cognitive structures that subsume a variety of specific tasks, these theorists focus more on narrow-band structures and elaborate on the mechanisms or processes by which such structures change. In so doing they have moved neo-Piagetian theory closer to other branches of cognitive science and have delineated processes that are more readily studied in relation to biological or neurological variables.

Pascual-Leone, for example, has emphasized the role of attention in the process of structural changes. To move from a lower to a higher level cognitive structure a child must first inhibit the application of an old cognitive structure to an environmental stimulus or aliment and then coordinate a new set of schemata through mental effort. That effort involves deployment and maintenance of attention. Case, on the other hand, emphasizes the cognitive processes of problem-solving and exploration in the transition from lower to higher levels of cognitive structure. Both theorists take the view that change occurs on one or a few structures at a time and that the specific structure undergoing change will be a function of individual differences or environmental opportunities. Neo-Piagetian theory is thus less universal in its model of cognitive development and more accommodating of cultural and individual differences. Nevertheless it retains the basic Piagetian concepts of an active, developing child who is constructing cognitive structures on the basis of interaction with the external and social environment. However, even neo-Piagetian theory has not solved the key challenge of how to fully integrate emotional and intellectual development.

NEW CONCEPTS OF INTELLIGENCE: EMOTIONAL BASIS OF INTELLIGENCE

Human emotions have traditionally been viewed as somewhat separate from cognition and as a minor concern to overall development. New clinical observations by the first author and emerging findings from a number of recent studies suggest that emotions are central to cognition and may actually regulate and orchestrate cognitive capacities. They may also be critical to development of cognitive capacities. It is suggested that babies' emotional exchanges with their caregivers, rather than their ability to complete cognitive tasks, should become the primary measure of developmental and intellectual competence.

Twelve-month-old Cara sits in her mother's lap at a table, eyes locked onto the psychologist who tries to get her to follow the bean he is putting under the cup and search for it. Cara knocks over the cup. Is that little girl, as her mother fears, cognitively delayed? Does a 1-year-old child who never babbles like other children her age and violently flings food and toys away from her show signs of a significant intellectual deficit? After a battery of similarly frustrating tests, the evaluator concludes that cognitive delay is the likely diagnosis in Cara's case.

For 50 years developmental testers have expected babies to sit still in their mothers' laps, pay attention, and perform prescribed tasks while adults assess their basic intelligence. Traditional wisdom has long insisted that carefully scoring how well a tiny child fits pegs into boards, sorts cards by shape, or hunts beads under cups can reveal an accurate measure of intelligence and developmental competence. However, recent results from research and clinical practice by the first author and others suggest that that entire approach to assessing children's capacities rests on false premises and has inadvertently led to mistaken diagnoses that can stigmatize children throughout their school years.

When a second evaluator schooled in this new thinking assessed Cara, he focused on her spontaneous interactions with her caregiver. He looked at each of Cara's intentional behaviors as a sign of her emotional interests. For instance, he observed her delight in yanking her mother's nose. At the assessor's suggestion the mother permitted the tugging on her nose to continue and playfully responded, "Toot, toot." Cara smiled and pulled again. The baby was rewarded with another "Toot, toot" and a big smile from her mother. Cara soon began to copy her mother's gestures and eagerly thrust her nose towards Mom. When the mother squeezed Cara's nose, the 1-year-old girl chirped, "Mo, mo," her very first words.

Cara showed that she could initiate social interactions and comprehend their consequences. That demonstrated degree of understanding put Cara at at least the 12-month level of cognitive development. Further observation revealed an extremely energetic, active, highly physical toddler who liked to have her way and control her surroundings. With the consultant's help, Cara's mother later altered her parenting style. She learned to follow Cara's behavioral lead, enthusiastically then engaging her daughter in creative interactions while simultaneously setting firm limits. Cara's energy quickly became more focused; her babbling, richer. Before long she was saying real words and actively cooperating with her parents.

If a series of such simple, pleasurable interactions with her mother could reveal and foster Cara's language development and organizational ability, then any conception of intellect that marked her as cognitively delayed because of an inability to search for a bean has serious flaws. Those flaws are based on a long-standing mistaken belief that the intellect is superior to and supervises the passions. Clearly, as Cara's linguistic debut demonstrates, analysis of a child's early relationships and sensory and emotional experiences is a vital key to accurate assessment of intelligence and developmental competence.

Until now, however, no one has offered an explanation of how emotions give birth to intelligence. In fact, a baby's earliest feelings play a pivotal role in all later intellectual development. Unlikely as the connection between feeling-states and intelligence may seem, the emotions orchestrate a vast array of cognitive operations throughout an individual's life span. Indeed, they make possible all creative thought.

Results from four distinct lines of inquiry have recently shed new light on the importance of emotions for intelligence. In work with Arnold Sameroff the first author has found that children with four or more family emotional risk factors had 24 times the chance of scoring an I.Q. below 80 than children without those risks. Stephen Porges and the first author have shown that measurements in 8-month-old infants of a part of the brain that regulates emotions correlate with these same children's IQ scores at age 4.

The first author's work with a group of autistic children, who suffer some of the most severe thinking and language problems imaginable, has also confirmed the inextricable linkage of emotional and cognitive development. Therapeutic programs for these severely challenged children have traditionally concentrated on trying to stimulate their cognition and teach them language. However, a program based on emotional cuing (like that which revealed Cara's true abilities) proved to be more effective for a number of these children in fostering empathy, warmth, and creative thinking.

One young patient, Ashley, neither spoke nor made any response or eye contact with those around her. The 2-year-old child spent hours staring into space, rubbing persistently at the same patch of rug. Her abnormal repetition was viewed by the clinician observing her as more than just a distressing symptom of her autism. That symptom revealed an underlying interest and motivation that could be harnessed and redirected toward interacting with others. To initiate her cognitive progress the clinician had to first motivate her to communicate with the simplest of emotional gestures—a smile, or smirk, or purposeful hand movements. He suggested that her mother place her hand next to Ashley, on the favorite stretch of rug. When Ashley pushed it away, the mother gently put her hand back. Each time the child pushed, the mother's hand would return. A cat-and-mouse game ensued, and after three sessions of these rudimentary interactions, Ashley was looking, smiling, and anticipating.

From that tiny beginning, through a comprehensive therapeutic program, grew a bridge to emotional relationships and eventual verbal exchanges. For example, as therapy progressed, the therapist helped Ashley use her imagination by repeatedly initiating pretend play. He recognized that each time Ashley repeatedly flung herself on her mother, the child was deriving sensory-based simple pleasure from her behavior. He instructed the mother to whinny like a horse each time Ashley lunged at her. Soon Ashley imitated mother's sounds and then started initiating her own sounds and words. In that way the therapist helped the mother stretch a pleasant sensation for Ashley into a richer, more complex interaction. Over time mother and child pretended to be neighing horses, mooing cows, and barking dogs. Their social and emotional interchange grew increasingly complex, passing through the same series of developmental stages identified in children without difficulties. At age 7 Ashley now enjoys warm friendships, argues as well as her lawyer father, and scores in the low superior I.Q. range.

A fourth line of inquiry, microscopic clinical observations of children's thinking, further clarifies the relationships between emotion and reason by revealing two necessary elements of thinking. The first process—creating a new idea—stems from a person's ability to use his or her own emotional experience to assign meaning and significance to daily events or concepts. The second process—reflection and logical analysis—examines the newly created idea according to whatever principles of logic the person possesses, and places it in a wider frame of reference.

To understand those processes in action, the authors put a simple question to two young boys seen in therapy not long ago. When asked by the clinician, "What do you think about people who act bossy to you?" Chris replied, "Well, teachers are bosses, babysitters are bosses, policemen are bosses." That articulate 7-year-old child lacked the emotional pathways that permit creative and intuitive thought. He could provide a formal classification of different types of bosses but was incapable of making observations that relate these categories to his own life. However, 7-year-old Josh had no such difficulties. In response to the same question about bosses, he announced, "Most of the time I don't like being bossed, especially when my parents try to tell me when I can watch TV and when I have to go to sleep. I'm big enough to decide for myself. Sometimes when I'm being bad, I guess I need bossing, though. Maybe bosses are okay some of the time, and some of the time they're not." Josh finds his answer in his own, apparently generally irritating, brushes with bosses. Rather than simply listing categories or incidents, he is able to abstract a principle from the emotional core of those incidents.

How exactly did Josh's ability to think and abstract develop? A baby's experience begins with sensations like touch and sound. Each sensation, however, also gives rise to an emotion. A toy may feel interesting or boring; a voice, soothing or jarring. Even young infants react to sensations emotionally. They prefer the sound or smell of their mother, for example, to any others and by 4 months of age can react to certain persons with fear. Furthermore, contrary to long-held assumptions, basic sensations like touch and sound can be perceived differently by different people, giving rise to emotional differences.

Emotional meaning also adheres in early concepts like "big and little," "more and less," "near and far," and "now and later." "A lot" is a bit more than makes a child happy. "Near" is snuggled next to him in bed. "Later" is a frustrating stretch of waiting. For a child without an intuitive sense of "few and many," numbers have no meaning. Furthermore, a young child's experience of any sensation always occurs within the context of a relationship that gives it broader meaning. Playing with mother's hair, for example, may occasion smiles and hugs or an angry scolding.

Each sensory experience has such a dual aspect and is labeled by both its physical properties and its emotional qualities. This double coding helps the child both place the memory or experience in a catalogue of experience and retrieve or reconstruct it when needed. As the child grows, emotional reactions come to operate as a sixth sense that allows the child to recognize and understand situations.

Emotion orchestrates complex judgments as well. One of modern psychology's main enigmas is how does a child learn to discriminate among situations ("When can I yell and kick") and generalize from one to another ("Should I behave at school like I do at home?"). Consider how a child makes a seemingly simple judgment about when to say "hello." She doesn't learn a set of cognitive rules like greeting only those who live on her street or only those who wave at her. Rather, from countless specific encounters she abstracts an emotional pattern; there is a feeling of warmth and friendliness in situations that rate "hello." Her interactions create an emotional signaling system that tells her when to say hello and that it is okay to punt the football but not to kick Sarah or Charlie in the shins. That emotional signaling system, which acts like an orchestra leader for the vast array of cognitive instruments, is a quintessentially human process. No computer, for all its apparent so-called brainpower, can ever get beyond limited elements of logical analysis and think like a person. Advocates of artificial intelligence may claim that current computational capacity limits creative, humanlike thought, but the real limit is a machine's inherent inability to engage the world emotionally. No collection of microchips can ever have a child's lived emotional experience of bosses and "hello," of noses and rugs. None, therefore, can ever create the emotionally based meaning from which creative thought grows and on which it depends.

TOWARD A GENERAL DEVELOPMENTAL MODEL

The relationship of cognitive to emotional development is yet another challenge to investigators. Piaget made few contributions in this area. The diagnosis and treatment of emotional and developmental disorders in infants and young children, however, requires the clinician to take into account all facets of the child's experience. It is necessary, therefore, to have a model with which to look at how constitutional-maturational (regulatory), family, and interactive factors work together as the child progresses through each developmental phase, and each phase must be viewed from affective, as well as cognitive, perspectives.

A developmental, structuralist model has been formulated by the first author that integrates cognitive and affective development, and applies the types of structure Piaget described to a range of experience. Most important, that model also considers individual difference in terms of biology and interaction. The model can be visualized with the infant's constitutional-maturational patterns on one side and the infant's environment, including caregivers, family, community, and culture, on the other side. Both sets of factors operate through the infant-caregiver relationship, which can be pictured in the middle. Those factors and the infant-caregiver relationship, in turn, contribute to the organization of experience at each of six developmental levels (consistent with both cognitive and affective milestones), which may be pictured just beneath the infant-caregiver relationship.

What is potentially unique about this particular clinical and research model is the ability it gives the user to look at the back-and-forth influence of highly specific, verifiable constitutional-maturational factors on interactive and family patterns and vice versa, in relationship to specific developmental processes (and to relate these processes to later developmental and psychopathological disorders).

DEVELOPMENTAL LEVELS In the model are six developmental levels. Those include the infant-child's ability to accomplish the following:

1. Attend to multisensory affective experience and at the same time organize a calm, regulated state and experience pleasure.
2. Engage with and evidence affective preference and pleasure for a caregiver.
3. Initiate and respond to two-way presymbolic gestural communication.
4. Organize chains of two-way communication (opening and closing many circles of communication in a row), maintain communication across space, integrate affective polarities, and synthesize an emerging prerepresentational organization of self and other.
5. Represent (symbolize) affective experience (for example, pretend play, functional use of language). That ability calls for higher level auditory and verbal sequencing ability.
6. Create representational (symbolic) categories and gradually build conceptual bridges between these categories. That ability creates the foundation for such basic personality functions as reality testing, impulse control, self-other representational differentiation, affect labeling and discrimination, stable mood, and a sense of time and space that allows for logical planning. The ability rests not only on complex auditory and verbal processing abilities, but also on visual-spatial abstracting.

At each level, one looks at the range of emotional themes organized (for example, can the child play out [symbolize] only dependency themes and not aggressive ones; is aggression behaved out and dealt with presymbolically?). One also looks at the stability of each level. Does a minor stress lead a child to lose his ability to represent, interact, engage, or attend?

In their use in day-to-day clinical work the six developmental levels can be collapsed into four essential processes that characterize development in infants and young children. Those processes have to do with how an infant and the parents or caregivers negotiate the various phases of their early interactions. It is necessary to understand how these four processes serve as a basis for diagnosis and treatment.

A 7½-month-old infant's mother worried that, "He cries any time I try to leave him, even for a second. If I'm not standing right next to him when he is sitting on the floor, he cries and I have to pick him up. He's a tyrant. He's waking up four times at night and is a fussy eater. He eats for short bursts [breast-feeding] and then stops eating. I'm feeding him all the time."

The mother was feeling cornered, controlled, manipulated, and bossed around. Her baby was like a "fearful dictator" (therapist's term). She said, "That's the perfect way to describe him." The father was impatient with the mother; he felt that she indulged the baby too much. He was getting "fed up," because she had no time for him.

The baby was interactive and sensitive to every emotional nuance. As he came into the room, he immediately caught the clinician's eye. They exchanged smiles and motor gestures. He interacted with his parents with smiles, coos, and motor movements. Father intruded somewhat. He would roughhouse until the baby would cry, put the baby down, and then roughhouse again. Mother, in contrast, was ever so gentle, but long silences passed between her vocalizations. During her long silences, the baby would rev up, get more irritable, and start whining. There was whining with the mother and fearful crying with the father. Even before he could finish his motor gestures or vocalizations, his mother moved in and picked him up, or gave him a rattle, or spoke for him. In this way she undermined his initiative. Even while whining, however, he was interactive and contingent.

On physical examination this baby was sensitive to loud noises and to light touch on the arms, legs, abdomen, and back. He had a mild degree of low motor tone and was posturally insecure. He was not yet ready to crawl.

In terms of his mastering the first developmental challenge of shared attention and engagement, the infant's constitutional and maturational patterns did not compromise development. This was an attentive, engaged baby. But at the second developmental stage, intentional communication and assertiveness, he was a passive reactor. He was not learning to initiate two-way communication, to be assertive and take charge of his interactions. His low motor tone was compromising his ability to control his motor movements. His sensory hyperreactivity was compromising his ability to regulate sensation. He was frequently overloaded by just the basic sensations of touch and sound and he was not receiving support from his mother through the nurturing and rhythmic caretaking that would foster self-initiative.

This family required therapeutic work on a number of tasks simultaneously. The infant's special constitutional-maturational patterns were discussed. Hands-on practice helped the parents help their baby be attentive and calm. Those tasks included helping the mother to be more patient and wait for the baby to finish what he started, and how to support his initiative (for example, putting something in front of the baby while the baby was on his tummy in order to motivate him to crawl and reach); getting the mother to put more affect into her voice and to increase the rhythm and speed of her vocalizations; and getting the father to be more gentle. The parents' own feelings about the interactions were explored: the father's tough-guy background, the mother's fear of her own assertiveness, her fear of her baby being injured, and their own associated family patterns.

Gradually, the baby began to sleep through the night and became more assertive and less clinging and fearful. He also became happier. He was slow to reach his motor milestones, so an occupational therapist began to work with him and to give the parents advice on motor development and normalizing his sensory overreactivity. In four months, this infant was functioning in an age-appropriate manner with a tendency toward a cautious, but happy and assertive, approach to life's developmental challenges.

As developmental clinicians and researchers build on Piaget's findings and formulations, the developmental model will serve as a basis for understanding social and emotional development and provide a framework for clinical and educational intervention.

SUGGESTED CROSS REFERENCES

Perception and cognition are discussed in Section 3.1, learning theory in Section 3.3, aggression in Section 3.4, biology of memory in Section 3.5, and brain models of mind in Section 3.6. Chapter 38 addresses attention-deficit disorders. Chapter 36 focuses on learning disorders, motor skills disorder, and communication disorders. Feeding and eating disorders in children are the subject of Chapter 40, and mental retardation is covered in Chapter 35.

REFERENCES

Anthony E J: The system makers: Piaget and Freud. Br J Med Psychol *30:* 255, 1957.

Case R: Neo-Piagetian theories of intellectual development. In *Piaget's Theory: Prospects and Possibilities,* H Beilin, P Pufall, editors, p 61. Erlbaum, Hillsdale, NJ, 1992.

DeGangi G A, Porges S W, Sickel R Z, Greenspan S I: Four-year follow-up of a sample of regulatory disordered infants. Infants Ment Health J *14:* 4, 1993.

Elkind D: Egocentrism in adolescence. Child Dev *38:* 1025, 1967.

Elkind D: Piagetian psychology and the practice of child psychiatry. J Am Acad Child Psychiatry *21:* 45, 1982.

Flavell J: *The Developmental Psychology of Jean Piaget.* Van Nostrand, New York, 1963.

*Flavell J: Concept development. In *Carmichael's Manual of Child Psychology,* P Mussen, editor, p 983. Wiley, New York, 1970.

Flavell J: Perspectives on perspective taking. In *Piaget's Theory: Prospects and Possibilities,* H Beilin, P Pufall, editors, p 107. Erlbaum, Hillsdale, NJ, 1992.

Furth H G: Piaget and Knowledge. Prentice-Hall, Englewood Cliffs, 1969.

Furth H G, Youniss J, Ross B: Children's utilization of logical symbols: An interpretation of conceptual behavior based on Piagetian theory. Dev Psychol *3:* 36, 1970.

Greenspan S I: *Intelligence and Adaptation: An Integration of Psychoanalytic and Piagetian Developmental Psychology,* Monograph 47/48. Psychological Issues, 1979.

Greenspan S I: *The Clinical Interview of the Child.* McGraw Hill, New York, 1981.

*Greenspan S I: *The Development of the Ego: Implications for Personality Theory, Psychopathology, and the Psychotherapeutic Process.* International Universities Press, Madison, CT, 1989.

*Greenspan S I: *Infancy and Early Childhood: The Practice of Clinical Assessment and Intervention with Emotional and Developmental Challenges.* International Universities Press, Madison, CT, 1992.

Hamlett K W, Pellegrini D S, Conners C K: An investigation of executive processes in the problem-solving of attention deficit-hyperactive children. J Pediatr Psychol *12:* 227, 1987.

Inhelder B, Piaget J: *The Growth of Logical Thinking from Childhood to Adolescence.* Basic Books, New York, 1958.

Lochman J E, Dodge K: Social cognitive processes of severely violent, moderately aggressive, and nonaggressive boys. J Consult Clin Psychol *62:* 366, 1994.

Pennington B F: *Diagnosing Learning Disorders.* Guilford, New York, 1991.

*Piaget J: *The Early Growth of Logic in the Child.* Norton, New York, 1969.

Piaget J: Piaget's theory. In *Manual of Child Psychology,* P Mussen, editor, p 103. Wiley, New York, 1983.

Piaget J: *Play, Dreams and Imitation in Childhood.* Norton, New York, 1951.

Piaget J: The stages of the intellectual development of the child. Bull Menninger Clin *26:* 120, 1962.

Piaget J: *Structuralism.* Basic Books, New York, 1970.

Piaget J, Inhelder B: *The Origin of the Idea of Chance in Children.* Norton, New York, 1975.

*Piaget J, Inhelder B: *The Psychology of the Child.* Basic Books, New York, 1969.

Pinard A, Laurendeau M: Stage in Piaget's cognitive-developmental theory: Exegesis of a concept. In *Studies in Cognitive Development: Essays in Honor of Piaget,* D Elkind, J H Flavell, editors, p 121. Oxford University Press, New York, 1969.

Sameroff A, Seifer R, Barocas R, Zax M, Greenspan S I: IQ scores of 4-year-old children: Social-environmental risk factors. Pediatrics 1986.

Sternberg R J, Berg C, editors: *Intellectual Development.* Cambridge University Press, Cambridge, 1992.

Tuddenham R: Jean Piaget and the world of the child. Am Psychol *21:* 207, 1966.

Wolff P H: *The Developmental Psychologies of Jean Piaget and Psychoanalysis,* Monograph 5. Psychology Issues, 1960.

3.3 LEARNING THEORY

W. STEWART AGRAS, M.D., F.R.C.P. (C)

G. TERENCE WILSON, Ph.D.

INTRODUCTION

Learning is central to an understanding of the genesis of the psychiatric disorders and to their treatment. The basic concept of learning is that the organism acquires new behaviors as a result of experience. Much of the disordered behavior that characterizes the syndromes of interest in psychiatry is learned and maintained within a social context, particularly within the family. Psychotherapeutic treatment can be regarded as educational in nature, enabling the patient to learn adaptive coping skills and to extend personal control over problem behaviors. Therapists must have a firm grasp of the principles of modern learning theory so that they can understand and modify problem behaviors in the most effective manner.

Among the building blocks of learning theory are classical and operant conditioning. In *classical or Pavlovian conditioning* (also known as *respondent conditioning*) learning occurs when one stimulus or event comes to predict another as a function of the logical and perceptual relations between the two events. In *operant or instrumental conditioning* learning occurs as a result of the consequences of one's actions and the resultant effect on the environment. As B. F. Skinner, the father of radical behaviorism, put it, "A person does not act upon the world, the world acts upon him." Skinner, in his definition of the sphere of interest of pysychology, specifically eschewed the role of intervening variables, such as thoughts. *Social-cognitive learning theory* incorporates both the respondent and the operant models of learning. However, social learning theory acknowledges the reciprocal interaction between persons and their environments; environments determine some aspects of behavior, but persons can alter aspects of their personal environments, which in turn may alter their behavior. Cognitive processes are viewed as important factors in modulating the persons' responses to environmental events.

Psychoanalytic theory and practice developed concurrently with learning theory. A number of attempts have been made over the past half century to integrate the two theoretical approaches. For example, in 1950 John Dollard and Neal Miller reformulated many psychoanalytic concepts in terms of learning theory. One of the principal concepts underlying the theory is that fear can be understood as a drive that motivates learning, particularly the learning of inhibited responses in conflictual situations—responses that reduce fear. But such attempts at theoretical fusion have not had a lasting influence on psychoanalytic thought or therapy. Instead, behavior therapies based on various aspects of learning theory have been developed over the past quarter century, and, because of the experimental and hypothesis-testing emphasis deriving from learning theory, the therapies have become the mainstream of psychotherapy research. Nonetheless, psychoanalytic theory has raised many issues of consequence to learning theorists, and those issues will ultimately be addressed experimentally.

Recently, researchers have shown much interest in the neurophysiological and biochemical components of learning. For example, research with simple organisms—such as aplysia, a sea mollusk—has revealed that the learning of avoidance behavior alters the chemical structure of cells in the nervous system; when the avoidance is unlearned, the chemical changes are reversed. Thus, the foundation for understanding the neurochemistry of learning has been laid, and a reciprocal interaction between ongoing biological processes in the central nervous system and behavior changes resulting from environmental influences is evident.

This section lays the foundation for understanding the process of behavior change, particularly when directed toward the amelioration of disordered thought, feelings, and actions; therefore, the various behavior-change procedures deriving from the different models of learning are particularly emphasized here. Since most therapies consist of an articulated package of procedures aimed at changing behavior and then maintaining that change, the singling out of particular procedures is somewhat artificial. Nonetheless, the approach is necessary to the understanding of the role of learning in the treatment of psychiatric disorders. Four models of learning are described here: classical conditioning, two-factor conditioning theory, operant conditioning, and social-cognitive learning theory. Definitions of some of the concepts and principles used in the context of learning are given in Table 3.3-1.

CLASSICAL CONDITIONING

HISTORY The idea that learning takes place when two events occur closely together in time has a long history, stemming from association theory developed by the British school of philosophical empiricism. But it was the Russian physiologist Ivan Petrovich Pavlov and his coworkers who over many years documented the parameters of this form of learning in carefully conceived experiments. Traditional accounts of classical conditioning stated that learning occurs when an initially neutral stimulus, the *conditioned stimulus* (CS), is paired with a stimulus that naturally elicits a response, the *unconditioned stimulus* (US). The response elicited by the US is the *unconditioned response* (UR). After repeated and contiguous pairing of the two stimuli, the CS elicits the UR, which is then called the *conditioned response* (CR).

Pavlov's work was enthusiastically espoused by American psychologists, such as John B. Watson, who demonstrated that classical conditioning can give rise to phobiclike behavior in a now-classic experiment. The subject of the experiment was Albert B., who was 11 months old. Watson demonstrated that a few pairings of a loud noise (US) with the sight of a white rat (CS) led Albert to avoid not only the rat, which had not caused fear before, but also related objects, such as cotton wool and sealskin, an example of *stimulus generalization* in which stimuli similar to the original CS may elicit the CR, although usually with a weakened response. In that view of classical conditioning, a view that is still widely held by psychologists and psychiatrists, classical conditioning was a rather simple, limited, and automatic form of learning. Current thinking, however, differs substantially from that traditional account.

CURRENT VIEWS Temporal contiguity between two stimuli is neither necessary nor sufficient for classical conditioning to take place. Two classic examples illustrate the point. In the first example a rat is exposed to five pairings of a tone and an electric shock in one situation. In another situation the tone is presented 10 additional times in the absence of shock. The contiguity of tone and shock is the same in both situations, but classical conditioning occurs only in the first situation. The reason is that only in that situation does the tone predict or provide information about the US. In the other situation the US is equally likely whether or not the tone is sounded. Nor is contiguity necessary for conditioning to occur. If the presentation of the tone and the shock is arranged so that shocks never occur in the presence of the tone, the tone comes to predict the nonoccurrence of the shock, a phenomenon called *conditioned inhibition*.

In the second example two groups of animals are exposed to a compound stimulus (tone plus light) that signals a shock. One group have a history of learning in which the light predicts a shock; the other group do not. Both groups have the same contiguous exposure to the tone-light compound stimulus, but, for the group with pretraining, the tone is redundant. When both groups are tested for their conditioning to the tone, the group with pretraining with the light stimulus show significantly worse conditioning than the other group. The reason is that, despite equivalent contiguity, the tone conveys different information to the two groups.

Nor is classical conditioning necessarily a slow process dependent on repeated pairings of stimuli. Learning is often rapid and efficient. As Robert Rescorla noted:

> Pavlovian conditioning is not a stupid process by which the organism willy-nilly forms associations between any two stimuli that happen to co-occur. Rather the organism is better seen as an information seeker using logical and perceptual relations among events, along with its own preconceptions, to form a sophisticated representation of the world.

TABLE 3.3-1
Common Terms Used in Learning Theory

Aversive conditioning: A procedure in which punishment or aversive stimulation is used to reduce the frequency of a target behavior.
Avoidance learning: A form of operant learning in which an organism learns to avoid certain responses or situations.
Classical conditioning: The association of a neutral stimulus with an unconditioned stimulus such that the neutral stimulus comes to bring about a response similar to that originally elicited by the unconditioned stimulus.
Conditioned response (CR): In classical conditioning the response elicited by the conditioned stimulus.
Conditioned stimulus (CS): In classical conditioning the originally neutral stimulus that comes to be associated with the unconditioned stimulus and eventually elicits a conditioned response.
Continuous reinforcement: A schedule of reinforcement in which, every time a response is emitted, a reward is administered.
Covert reinforcement: A method of increasing behavioral frequency by using the imagination of pleasant events as a reinforcement.
Covert sensitization: A method of reducing the frequency of behavior by associating it with the imagination of unpleasant consequences.
Discrimination learning: A process in which the tendency toward stimulus generalization is counteracted and responses are made only to specific stimuli.
Experimental neurosis: An abnormal behavior pattern produced in animals through the application of classical or operant conditioning techniques.
Extinction: The reduction of frequency of a learned response as a result of the cessation of reinforcement.
Fixed-interval schedule: A reinforcement schedule in which a reward is given after a specific amount of time has passed.
Fixed-ratio schedule: A reinforcement schedule in which a reward is given after a specific number of responses have been emitted.
Habituation: A simple form of learning in which the response to a repeated stimulus lessens over time.
Higher-order conditioning: In classical conditioning the establishment of a new conditioned stimulus through association with an established conditioned stimulus.
Instrumental learning: Operant conditioning.
Law of effect: The principle that behaviors followed by pleasant consequences are strengthened and those followed by negative consequences are weakened.
Modeling: Observational learning.
Negative practice: A method for reducing the frequency of a behavior by the intense repetition of the response.
Observational learning: Learning new behaviors by observing others responding and receiving some form of consequence; vicarious learning.
Operant conditioning: A form of learning in which behavioral frequency is altered through the application of positive and negative consequences.
Partial reinforcement: A schedule of reinforcement in which rewards are not given each time a response is made, rendering a learned response highly resistant to extinction.
Primary reinforcer: A stimulus affecting a biological process (e.g., food that increases the probability of behaviors it follows).
Reinforcer: A stimulus that increases the frequency of responses it follows.
Respondent learning: Classical conditioning.
Secondary reinforcers: Stimuli that gain the power to reinforce a behavior through association with primary reinforcers.
Shaping: An operant procedure in which a desirable behavior pattern is learned by the successive reinforcement of approximations to that behavior.
Spontaneous recovery: The increase in the strength of an extinguished behavior after the passage of a period of time.
Successive approximation: See Shaping.
Unconditioned response (UR): In classical conditioning a response that occurs spontaneously to the unconditioned stimulus.
Unconditioned stimulus (US): A stimulus that, without any training, produces a specific response.
Variable-interval schedule: A reinforcement schedule in which a reward is given after varying periods of time have passed.
Variable-ratio schedule: A reinforcement schedule in which a reward is given after a varying number of responses have been emitted.

Table by Marshall P Duke, PhD, and Stephen Nowicki, Jr, PhD.

Indeed, in teaching undergraduates, I favor an analogy between animals showing Pavlovian conditioning and scientists identifying the cause of a phenomenon. If one thinks of Pavlovian conditioning as developing between a CS and a US under just those circumstances that would lead a scientist to conclude that the CS causes the US, one has a surprisingly successful heuristic for remembering the facts of what it takes to produce Pavlovian associative learning.

Classical conditioning has been viewed as either (1) an automatic process that occurs similarly in the mollusk and the human being, requiring little or no conscious processing or awareness, or (2) learning that, in humans at least, requires conscious or controlled processing and awareness of the relations between events. On the one hand, evidence indicates that classical conditioning can occur in the absence of intention to learn, without awareness, and even if it is resisted. For example, both animals and humans acquire conditioned aversions to specific smells and tastes (the CS) if they are associated with drug-induced or illness-induced nausea (the US-UR). People develop highly specific aversions to food that they may have eaten with the onset of seasickness or a gastrointestinal illness. The food becomes a conditioned stimulus for them, despite their knowledge that it did not cause their nausea. That is what happens to patients who have conditioned nausea to stimuli associated with chemotherapy. In those instances people seem to be biologically prepared to have some conditioned responses and not others. For example, nausea is readily conditioned to smell and taste but not to sight and sounds. Some phobic reactions in humans may provide other examples of prepared learning of that sort (for example, fears of animals and heights). The hypothesis is that people are biologically predisposed to learn certain fears as a result of their evolutionary past, when it was adaptive to do so. That explains the fact that people have phobias only to selected situations and objects, which presumably were once associated with threats to survival.

On the other hand, a good deal of evidence shows that awareness of a relation between events is often necessary for conditioning to occur and greatly facilitates learning. It seems reasonable to conclude that classical conditioning in humans occurs through hierarchically organized neural systems. The operation of some of those systems may predispose to automatic processing while others do not.

CLINICAL APPLICATIONS Classical conditioning has influenced the way in which clinical disorders have been conceptualized and has generated methods for their treatment. Its role in the analysis and the treatment of anxiety disorders is discussed below. Another area of application has been in the treatment of substance abuse. Cues associated with repeated alcohol and drug use come to elicit CRs. Some of the CRs are opposite in nature to the unconditioned effects of the substance. They are known as *classically conditioned compensatory reactions,* which are believed to reflect homeostatic mechanisms. That conditioning process contributes to the development of behavioral tolerance to alcohol and drugs. In alcohol-dependent or drug-dependent persons the CRs are believed to be subjectively experienced as craving or anticipatory withdrawal reactions. An alternative view is that the CSs trigger craving because they come to signal the positively rewarding consequences of alcohol or drug use. In either case it follows that cues associated with substance abuse need to be addressed in treatment. Cue-exposure treatment for alcoholic persons and drug addicts is based on the principle of extinction—the procedure of presenting the CS in the absence of the US. Doing so results in the elimination of the CR when the CS no longer predicts its occurrence. For example, alcohol-dependent patients are presented with alcohol-related cues (for example, the sight and the smell of alcohol), which reliably elicit craving, without being allowed to drink (the US). Since negative emotional states can function as CSs, cue-exposure treatment also involves the induction of relevant mood states.

Classical conditioning is no longer necessarily linked to the philosophy of behaviorism, with which it was once associated. Its concepts and methods lend themselves to current perspectives on human behavior, and they continue to play an important role in contemporary behavior therapy, which itself has become more eclectic and theoretically broader than it was during its early origins in behaviorism.

TWO-FACTOR CONDITIONING THEORY

O. H. Mowrer proposed a two-factor theory of avoidance behavior that had a major influence both on models of psychopathology and on treatment. The theory made two basic assumptions: (1) Anxiety is an acquired drive established by classical conditioning in which a neutral stimulus comes to signal an aversive or traumatic event. (2) The classically conditioned anxiety motivates escape and avoidance behavior, which is reinforced by the reduction of the underlying anxiety drive. That theory has been fruitfully applied to phobic avoidance and obsessive-compulsive behavior. In the case of compulsive hand washers, for example, it is assumed that their anxiety about dirt and contamination is a classically conditioned response that drives them to wash their hands repeatedly after touching anything believed to be contaminated. Hand washing removes the dirt and reduces the anxiety. The anxiety reduction then reinforces and maintains the hand washing.

CLINICAL APPLICATIONS More important than the models of psychopathology it generated were the treatment methods that two-factor theory spawned. The techniques of exposure and response prevention followed directly from the theory. In *exposure treatment* for phobic disorders, patients are gradually and systematically exposed to the situations they fear and avoid until the phobic reactions are extinguished. In the technique of *systematic desensitization*—pioneered by Joseph Wolpe, one of the founding fathers of behavior therapy—the exposure is to imagined representations of the feared stimuli while the patient is in a state of relaxation. That technique was thought to be an example of *reciprocal inhibition,* in which one response (anxiety) is inhibited by an opposite response (relaxation). However, it is more effective to conduct exposure to real-life situations (for example, guiding an agoraphobic patient to enter shopping malls, supermarkets, crowded buses, and other feared situations) than to imagined scenes. In *response prevention* the therapist encourages patients to persist in coping with the anxiety they experience in response to approaching a feared situation without leaving the scene. For example, compulsive hand washers resist the urge to wash their hands after exposure to a feared substance.

PROBLEMS Despite its historical significance in the field, two-factor conditioning theory has been criticized on several counts. One problem is the difficulty it encounters in explaining why phobic reactions are resistant to extinction. Classically conditioned fear reactions in laboratory animals extinguish rapidly when the US is omitted. But phobic fears persist, even though phobic persons frequently come into contact with the situations they fear (exposure to the CS) without any aversive event (the US)—by definition, the conditions for the extinction of the fear and the avoidance behavior. A second difficulty for the theory is the evidence showing that avoidance behavior is not causally mediated by fear or anxiety, whether the anxiety is defined as autonomic nervous system arousal or subjective self-report. Avoidance behavior can be eliminated without inhibiting the accompanying anxiety. Anxiety reduction may precede, accompany, or even follow changes in avoidance behavior—an impossibility if anxiety is said to cause the avoidance behavior. A more accurate conclusion is that both anxiety and avoidance behavior are correlated coeffects of some still undetermined central mediating state. Third, whereas the effectiveness of exposure treatments has been well documented, two-factor theory fares poorly in accounting for its therapeutic mechanisms. The amount of exposure should be closely correlated with the degree of change in phobic avoidance behavior, yet it is a poor predictor of such change. An alternative explanation of exposure treatment is discussed below.

OPERANT CONDITIONING

The notion that learning occurs as a consequence of action was espoused in the pioneering work of Edward Lee Thorndike, whose learning theory dominated United States psychology for the first half of this century. A typical experiment devised by Thorndike consisted of placing a hungry cat in a cage with some form of latching device that, when correctly manipulated, allowed the cat access to a second cage for a bite of food. Thorndike noted that the cat became efficient at opening the lock, a sequence of events termed *trial-and-error learning.* Thorndike hypothesized that the appropriate behaviors were strengthened by experiences of success and failure. B. F. Skinner and his colleagues, following up on Thorndike's work, made the effects of environment on behavior a central aspect of learning.

The principles and procedures of operant conditioning are the product of Skinner's philosophy of *radical behaviorism.* In that approach, overt behavior is the only acceptable target of scientific investigation. Skinner argued that subjective experience (private events) should be included in the experimental analysis of behavior, but their role has always been restricted. Thoughts and feelings are epiphenomena in operant conditioning; they cannot exert a causal influence on behavior. Strictly speaking, aside from biological determinants (and those have always been minimized), it is assumed that human behavior is exclusively a function of environmental events that are ultimately beyond personal control. Another hallmark of operant conditioning has been its emphasis on the study of the individual organism. The repeated measurement of the behavior of a person under controlled conditions is the methodological contribution of operant conditioning. Skinner rejected statistical comparisons between groups of subjects, claiming that group averages obscure what is important—namely, the behavior of individual subjects. The application of the principles and the procedures of operant conditioning to human problems is known as *applied behavior analysis.*

Aside from a set of philosophical assumptions about behavior and innovative methods for analyzing it, operant conditioning has contributed to the field of behavior change a number of influential learning principles.

POSITIVE REINFORCEMENT The best known contribution of operant conditioning to the field of behavior change is the principle of *positive reinforcement*—the process by which certain consequences of behavior raise the probability that the behavior will occur again. On the whole, positive reinforcers are viewed as pleasant (for example, food, attention, praise, money). Reinforcers that affect biological processes, such as food, may be defined as *primary reinforcers.* Such reinforcers are now rarely used with humans. Events viewed as aversive by some may be reinforcing for others. For example, the behavior of some children is reinforced by scolding, which, after all, is a form of attention. Many drugs appear to be positive reinforcers, including opioids, barbiturates, and such stimulants as amphetamine and cocaine. Animals and humans self-administer the substances, reliably discriminating between the active drug and a placebo. Complex patterns of behavior can be shaped in animals using drugs as reinforcers.

Traditional textbook descriptions state that reinforcement of a response must be immediate. But, as with classical conditioning, temporal contiguity is not necessary for learning to occur in operant conditioning. Recent research shows that the behavior of even a simple organism, such as the laboratory rat, can be controlled by the aggregate consequences of a series of reinforcements of multiple responses over time. Revision of the requirement that reinforcement be immediate if it is to control behavior greatly extends the explanatory power of operant conditioning. But the mechanism by which the organism is able to integrate reinforcing consequences over time is never specified. Critics of operant conditioning point out that the delayed effect of reinforcement contingencies must be mediated by cognitive processes.

NEGATIVE REINFORCEMENT Reinforcement increases the probability of behavior. *Negative reinforcement* is the process in which behavior leading to the removal of an aversive event strengthens that behavior. Negative reinforcers tend to be aversive events. For example, avoidance behavior, such as phobic reactions and compulsive rituals, is negatively reinforced because it forestalls actual or perceived aversive outcomes. Research shows that, when patients with anorexia nervosa are placed in a restricted hospital environment to facilitate the use of positive reinforcement for eating and gaining weight, they work (eat and gain weight) in order to get out of the aversive environment, adding negative reinforcement effects to the positive reinforcement effects.

PUNISHMENT Punishment is the presentation of an aversive stimulus contingent on the occurrence of a particular response. The removal of a positive consequence contingent on behavior, known as *time out* from reinforcement, can also be viewed as punishment. The procedure is commonly used as a means of disciplining children with behavior problems. One must distinguish punishment from negative reinforcement. Punishment decreases the probability of the behavior's occurring, whereas negative reinforcement increases the probability. One must also distinguish between the usual use of the term "punishment" and the technical use of the term given here. In the punishment paradigm the punishing event is always delivered contingent on performance and demonstrably reduces the frequency of the behavior being punished. That is considerably different from the use of the term to denote imprisonment, for example, since the prison sentence follows long after the crime and may not affect future criminal behavior. (Figure 3.3-1 summarizes the major principles of operant conditioning and the effects they have on behavior.)

RECIPROCAL INFLUENCES Since much human behavior occurs within an interpersonal context, reciprocal influences do occur. An example of the way in which such reciprocal influences may give rise to complex behavior patterns is afforded by the study of predelinquent behavior. Family studies suggest that predelinquent behavior patterns are set in motion by the excessive and inconsistent use of punishment on the part of parents. A mother may severely scold her small son, who in response may whine or have a temper tantrum. If the mother then responds by talking to the child to calm him down, the child stops whining. Thus, the child's whining punishes the mother's scolding and makes her less likely to scold in the future. The mother's attention to the child's whining reinforces that unpleasant behavior on the part of the child. Such a behavior pattern, when well established in the child, is viewed as unpleasant and aggressive by others and increases the likelihood that the child will be rejected by parents, peers, and teachers, thus initiating a complex series of events, such as poor school performance and joining a deviant peer group, which predisposes to delinquent behavior.

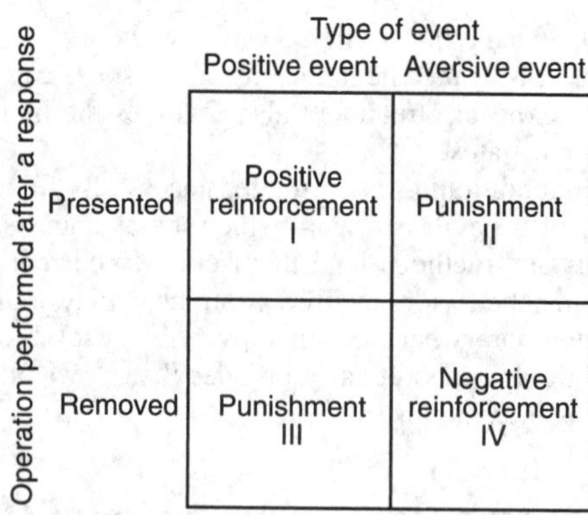

FIGURE 3.3-1 *The principal procedures of operant conditioning, depending on whether a positive or an aversive event is applied or removed after the behavior is performed. (From A E Kazdin:* Behavior Modification in Applied Settings, *ed 2. Dorsey Press, Homewood, IL, 1983. Used with permission.)*

CLINICAL APPLICATIONS Operant conditioning procedures have been applied to a wide range of problems in all age groups in psychiatry, education, rehabilitation, and medicine. In general, the procedures are most commonly used today in changing the behavior of young children, retarded persons, and institutionalized populations, such as long-term mental patients. Behavior therapists in clinical practice, particularly with adult outpatient disorders, rarely describe themselves as applied behavior analysts, and they draw on broad theoretical perspectives.

Reinforcement procedures may be used alone as applications of operant conditioning, or such procedures may be combined with others, such as extinction and punishment. However, reinforcement occurs in any form of psychotherapy, since the therapist differentially attends to the verbal behavior of the patient. Moreover, most behavior therapists today combine the use of reinforcement procedures with many other procedures derived from learning theory.

Positive reinforcement Much is known about various *schedules of reinforcement,* defined as the patterns or frequencies with which a reinforcer is delivered as a consequence of behavior. The most frequently used schedules are listed in Table 3.3-2. One of the most frequently used schedules in clinical practice is *partial reinforcement,* in which reinforcement only occasionally results from a particular behavior. Such a pattern of reinforcement maintains the behavior at full strength. Moreover, partially reinforced behavior may be particularly resistant to extinction. Since many deviant behaviors provoke attention from others, they are maintained by the social environment. Observational and experimental work, for example, has shown that hospital staff members tend to reinforce their patients' abnormal behaviors by attending to them. When the staff members learn to stop giving such attention and to attend more frequently to adaptive behaviors, patient behavior improves. Similar findings have been made in school. Teacher attention rein-

TABLE 3.3-2
Reinforcement Schedules in Operant Conditioning

Reinforcement Schedule	Example	Behavioral Effect
Fixed-ratio (FR) schedule	Reinforcement occurs after every 10 responses (10:1 ratio); 10 bar presses release a food pellet; workers are paid for every 10 items they make.	Rapid rate of response to obtain greatest number of rewards. Animal knows that next reinforcement depends on a certain number of responses being made.
Variable-ratio (VR) schedule	Variable reinforcement occurs (e.g., after the third, sixth, then second response and so on).	Generates fairly constant rate of response because probability of reinforcement at any given time remains relatively stable.
Fixed-interval (FI) schedule	Reinforcement occurs at regular intervals (e.g., every 10 minutes or every third hour).	Animal keeps track of time. Rate of responding drops to near 0 after reinforcement and then increases at about expected time of reward.
Variable-interval (VI) schedule	Reinforcement occurs after variable intervals (e.g., every three, six, and then two hours), similar to VR.	Response rate does not change between reinforcement. Animal responds at steady rate in order to get reward when it is available; common in trout fishermen, use of slot machines, checking mailbox.

forces disruptive behavior in the classroom; when such attention is withdrawn, the disruptive behavior decreases.

The most used reinforcement procedure is a *shaping paradigm,* in which a particular behavior is changed in form by reinforcing components of the final behavior sequentially. For example, in teaching a mute schizophrenic patient to talk, the first behavior to be reinforced may be simply looking at the therapist, followed by any mouthing movement, followed by any vocalization (perhaps imitating the therapist), and, finally, simple words and sentences. A *continuous reinforcement schedule* may first be used; in it reinforcement is delivered for every appropriate response. That schedule may be followed by partial reinforcement; each component behavior is first developed with continuous reinforcement and then strengthened with partial reinforcement. If speech is reinforced only in the presence of one therapist, the patient may remain mute with others, an example of *discriminative learning*. Similar behavior is seen in everyday life when a motorist stops at a red light and drives off when the light changes to green—behaviors that are highly reinforced in this society. To overcome discriminative learning, the therapist first establishes the beginnings of speech and then adds other therapists to the patient's experience to ensure generalization of the new behavior. When speech is fully developed, artificial reinforcement can be phased out, since speaking should be more reinforcing than being mute. That is also an example of *chaining* of behaviors and reinforcement, since all the initial behavioral sequences are necessary for the final behavior of talking, and a complex sequence of behaviors is gradually built up and reinforced.

Many problem behaviors seen in humans have been developed in animals by using various schedules of reinforcement. Thus, head banging, a behavior seen frequently in retarded and autistic children, has been developed in monkeys with the use of reinforcement such that the monkeys actually injure themselves. Although experiments of that kind do not prove that similar behaviors seen in humans are learned, they do call attention to the powerful effect of reinforcement in developing deviant behavior and to the fact that many behaviors are developed and maintained in that way.

Reinforcement, often given in the form of attention and praise contingent on certain behaviors, is a basic ingredient of most therapies. Skilled therapists of most persuasians use contingent verbal reinforcement, as has been shown even in nondirective psychotherapy, so that certain therapeutic themes are strengthened. Other methods used in reinforcement paradigms include tokens exchangeable for goods or activities that cannot be bought or engaged in otherwise. What is reinforcing for one person may not be for another; therefore, when reinforcement is used, the clinician must observe and measure the behavior being reinforced to make sure that it is being strengthened. The data from a clinical example of the use of token reinforcement to increase social communication is shown in Figure 3.3-2.

The patient was a 21-year-old man who was extremely withdrawn. He spent most of his time in his hospital room, rarely approaching others or initiating conversation. Skilled psychiatric nursing care had not altered his behavior. As a first step in increasing his conversational ability, reinforcement for approaching nurses was instituted. The patient was first carefully observed, and it was noted that he enjoyed listening to the radio and watching television. He was told that, for every two minutes that he talked with the nurses during three daily sessions, he would earn a token that could be exchanged for three minutes of listening to the radio or watching television and that talking was the only way in which he would earn the right to engage in those activities. The nurses, in turn, were instructed not to approach him during the sessions but to engage in conversation only if he initiated and maintained it, thus reinforcing a chain of behaviors: approaching nurses, initiating conversation, and maintaining conversational behavior. The nurses also timed the number of minutes of conversation, using a stopwatch.

As can be seen in Figure 3.3-2, the patient engaged in little conversation with the nurses during the baseline measurement period. When the token system was introduced, he began to speak with the nurses for increasing lengths of time. In the third phase of the treatment study, he was given a free supply of tokens equivalent to what he had earned in the previous phase; the tokens were no longer contingent on his behavior. Under those conditions the amount of conversation gradually declined, an example of extinction. When the original reinforcement conditions were reintroduced during the final experimental phase, his conversational ability improved. Similar procedures were used to generalize his new-found conversational ability to other staff members, eventually allowing the patient to engage successfully in a rehabilitation program.

PREMACK'S PRINCIPLE Premack's principle states that a behavior engaged in at a high frequency can be used to reinforce a lower-frequency behavior. In one experiment David Premack observed that children spent more time playing with a pinball machine than eating candy when both were freely available. When he made playing with the pinball machine contingent on eating a certain amount of candy, the amount of candy eaten by the children increased. In a therapeutic application of the principle, schizophrenic patients were observed to spend more time sitting down and doing nothing than working at a simple task in a rehabilitation center. When five minutes of sitting down was made contingent on a certain amount of work, their work output increased considerably, as did their skill acquisition.

EXTINCTION Disordered behavior is often developed and maintained by reinforcement in the form of attention from oth-

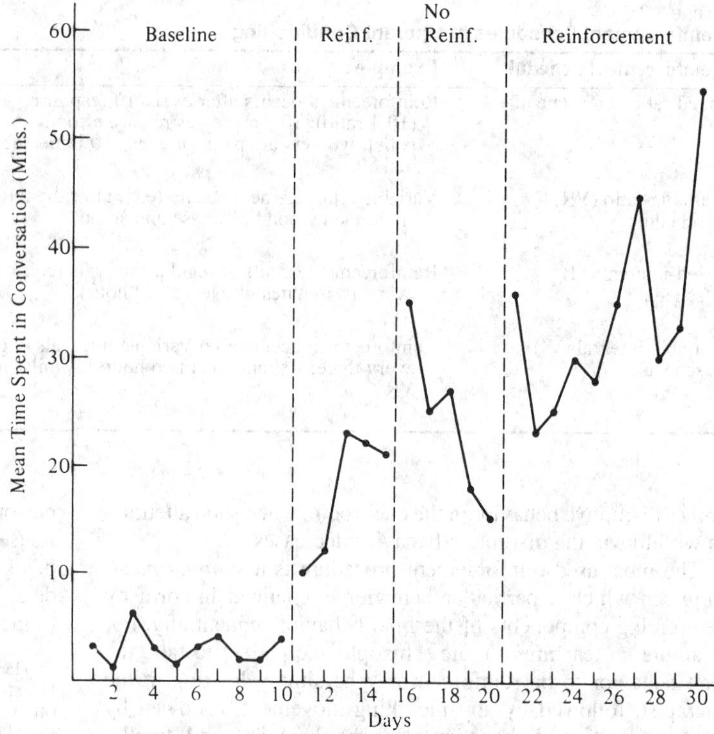

FIGURE 3.3-2 *The time spent by a withdrawn patient conversing with nurses during sequential experimental phases: baseline (measurement only), reinforcement delivered in the form of tokens, after reinforcement was withdrawn, and when reinforcement was reinstated. The effect of positive reinforcement is demonstrated by an increase in conversational time during the two phases in which tokens were delivered.*

ers. In such cases the clinician must identify the reinforcer and remove it from the patient's environment, a procedure known as *extinction.* A simple example of the use of extinction is the case of a young child who cries interminably before going to sleep. When the mother puts the child to bed, the crying begins after a few minutes, and the mother returns to find out what the problem is. She then reads to the child or engages in some other activity. When she leaves, the pattern is repeated. Clearly, maternal attention is reinforcing the crying. The treatment is to persuade the mother not to return to the child's bedroom once the child is settled for the night. However, she needs to be warned that the amount of crying may increase for two or three nights before it diminishes. That phenomenon is known as an *extinction burst;* the person exhibits more behavior in order to increase the probability of gaining positive reinforcement. When the reinforcement is not forthcoming, the behavior diminishes in frequency.

Punishment Punishment is less useful as a therapeutic procedure than either reinforcement or extinction, since it may produce unwanted side effects, such as aggressive behavior, and the possibility of inflicting physical damage is always present. For the most part, punishment is used only in situations in which the behavior to be changed threatens injury to the patient.

A clinical example of such a condition is rumination disorder, in which infants regurgitate their food mouthful by mouthful, which leads to malnutrition, dehydration, and frequently a threat to life. One treatment is to use the principle of punishment, making an unpleasant event contingent on each episode of regurgitation. In the case illustrated in Figure 3.3-3, lemon juice was used as the unpleasant event. During the baseline period before treatment, the infant ruminated between 40 and 70 percent of the time it was awake. Once the lemon juice was presented contingent on spitting up food, the frequency of rumination steadily declined. Punishment was then briefly removed, and rumination returned to the baseline levels, demonstrating the efficacy of punishment. The reintroduction of punishment eventually led to the virtual elimination of the behavior and a return to normal weight with no relapse at one-year follow-up.

The use of punishment in a clinical situation should be carefully overseen and should follow certain rules. The behavior to be addressed should have been resistant to well-thought-out behavior-change procedures involving the use of positive reinforcement. Behaviors incompatible with the problem behavior can often be reinforced and, thus, the problem eliminated. In addition, the behavior to be changed should be severely incapacitating and should threaten physical integrity (for example, the self-injurious behavior of some autistic children). Punishment procedures that themselves cause tissue damage should not be used. The behavior to be changed should be observed, measured, and recorded (as shown in Figure 3.3-3); in that way the effects of punishment can be seen, as can the amount of punishment used. Usually, effectively used punishment rapidly brings a behavior under control, and incompatible behaviors can then be built up with the use of positive reinforcement.

SOCIAL-COGNITIVE LEARNING THEORY

MODES OF LEARNING Albert Bandura, a psychologist, has integrated traditional classical and operant conditioning principles into an expansive and theoretically rich account of behavior change and psychological treatments. A primary tenet of the approach is that the influence of environmental events on the acquisition and the regulation of behavior is primarily a function of cognitive processes. The processes are based on prior experience and determine what environmental influences are attended to, how they are perceived, whether they will be remembered, and how they may affect future action.

Reinforcement is regarded not as an automatic strengthener of behavior but as a source of guidance for behavior by anticipated outcomes. By observing the consequences of behavior, the person learns what action is appropriate in what situation. By symbolic representation of anticipated future outcomes of behavior, the person helps to generate the motivation to initiate and maintain behavior. Classical conditioning and operant conditioning are viewed as sources of learning about predictive relations among events. A third mode of learning is modeling (vicarious learning). In *modeling,* learning occurs through observation alone. The person need not emit any behavior or be directly reinforced for behavior. Modeling expands the scope and the complexity of learning influences on behavior. For

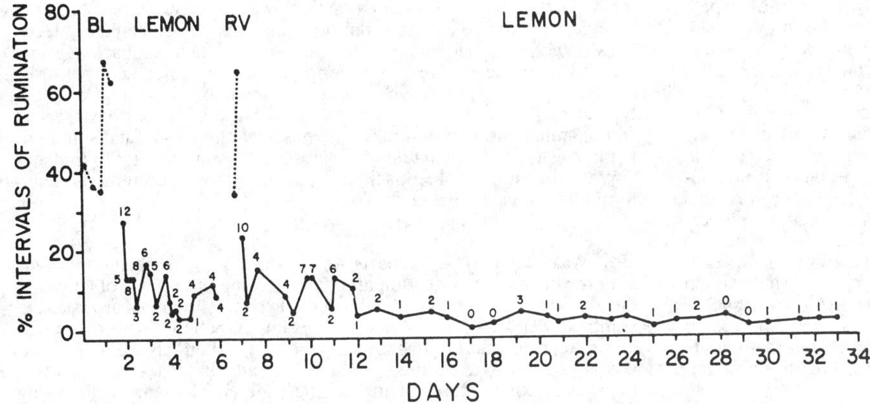

FIGURE 3.3-3 *The effect of punishment in an experiment in which lemon juice was delivered contingent on ruminative vomiting in an infant. The frequency of rumination was rapidly reduced from the baseline (BL) levels and was increased only when punishment was withdrawn during the reversal phase (RV). The number of applications of punishment (lemon juice) is shown by the number above each data point.*

example, it helps explain how phobic reactions may be acquired in the absence of any direct traumatic experience. Young monkeys acquire a severe and lasting fear of snakes after observing their wild-reared parents act fearfully in the presence of a snake. Modeling has many therapeutic applications. For example, it has prepared children for pending surgery by having them observe a film in which a child successfully copes with novel and frightening events.

The traditional emphasis on conditioning principles gave short shrift to verbal instruction as a mode of learning. The potential therapeutic effects of verbal instructions are illustrated by a study of hypertensive patients (Figure 3.3-4). All participants in the experiment were told that relaxation training would help them reduce their blood pressure. Half of the participants were also told that their blood pressure would show reductions after three sessions of relaxation training given in one morning. The other half were told that they could expect reductions only after prolonged relaxation practice. As shown in Figure 3.3-4, the groups have no difference in diastolic blood pressure readings. In systolic blood pressure, however, large and significant differences are shown; the group receiving immediate-lowering instructions showed lower blood pressure readings, but the other group did not. The mechanism underlying the effect is unknown. However, an expectancy of blood pressure lowering may be needed to induce the biochemical changes necessary to lower blood pressure. It is an example of the complex interactions that occur between environmental events, in this case the instructions given to the patient, the patient's cognitive appraisal of the instructions, and neurochemical processes. Therapists tend to neglect the effect of therapeutic instructions, but experimental work suggests that the therapist should do everything to enhance the development of realistic outcome and efficacy expectations.

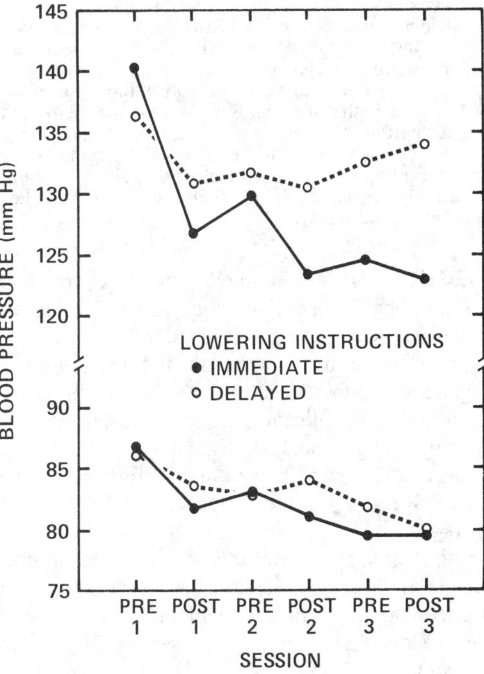

FIGURE 3.3-4 *The effects of two expectancies on systolic (top lines) and diastolic (bottom lines) blood pressures of hypertensive persons. Systolic blood pressure was markedly reduced in the group of patients told that relaxation training would lower their blood pressure after only one or two training sessions but was less reduced for those who were told to expect lowering only after prolonged training.*

SELF-EFFICACY THEORY A component of social-cognitive learning theory with ramifications for the treatment of clinical problems is self-efficacy theory. With *efficacy expectations* people are confident that they can cope effectively with a particular situation. *Outcome expectations* are defined as beliefs that particular actions will produce a certain outcome. Self-efficacy is the end product of different cognitive processes. To alter *self-efficacy,* people must actively appraise a specific experience and attribute successful coping to themselves, as opposed to some transient factor outside their control. Self-efficacy theory and cognitive-social learning theory in general draw heavily on the principles of attribution theory (a cognitive approach concerned with how people perceive the causes of behavior) from modern social psychology.

The self-efficacy theory predicts that the greater the self-efficacy (that is, the more people feel capable of predicting and controlling threatening events), the less vulnerable they are to anxiety and stress disorders in response to traumatic experiences. Research with primates supports the prediction. Infant monkeys were reared in an environment in which they either exercised control over food, water, and special treats (the masters) or received reinforcers administered automatically, independent of their behavior (the controls). Months later, the masters were significantly less fearful in response to a threatening situation than were the controls.

The theory also predicts that psychological treatments, such as exposure, are effective because they enhance self-efficacy for coping with threatening events. Behavioral performance is the most powerful means of increasing self-efficacy, but self-efficacy is also influenced by sources of information derived from vicarious learning and verbal persuasion. Numerous studies have established that exposure treatment is one of the most effective methods for eliminating phobic disorders. Exposure also produces greater increases in self-efficacy than do other methods. The greater the increase in self-efficacy, the greater the change in phobic behavior, regardless of the type of treatment. Outcome expectations (that is, self-reports of anticipated anxiety about entering a phobic situation) tend to be correlated with efficacy expectations. If the correlation with efficacy expectations is eliminated statistically, outcome expectations fail to predict outcome, suggesting that change in self-efficacy is the important variable underlying behavior change.

Critics have charged that self-efficacy is only correlated with treatment-induced changes in phobic behavior and does not cause the behavior change. Bandura, however, points to the systematic covariation of experimentally induced levels of efficacy expectations and phobic behavior as evidence of their causal nature. Self-efficacy is related to measures of fear arousal other than self-reports and behavioral performances. Increases in self-efficacy in phobic patients is associated with reductions in autonomic nervous system reactivity and neuroendocrine responses to phobic stimuli. The theory also suggests an explanation of the apparent resistance to the extinction of phobic behavior. Whether phobic reactions are eliminated by exposure to feared situations depends on the nature of the information that people derive from such experiences and not simply on the quantity of exposure. If people conclude that they can cope effectively, they cease to avoid the feared situations. But no change occurs if people conclude that they are unable to cope and, hence, experience unnerving anxiety. By strengthening phobic patients' expectations that they cannot cope, exposure may even enhance their phobic sensitivity. Treatment should be aimed at increasing the patients' sense of predictability and controllability through enhanced self-efficacy. Treatment of phobic patients along those lines produces results superior to treatment that passively exposes patients to feared stimuli without fostering coping skills, even if the length of the exposure is greater in the latter therapy.

Beyond furthering the analysis and the treatment of phobic disorders, self-efficacy has proved fruitful in the experimental analysis of a wide range of clinical problems, including pain management, the effects of stress on behavior and the immune system, and the prevention of relapse in substance abusers.

SELF-REGULATION In marked contrast to operant conditioning and radical behaviorism, social-cognitive learning theory emphasizes a capacity for self-regulation of behavior. Cognition is more than a passive conduit of external influences; it serves a generative function, allowing people to initiate thought, affect, and action to influence their circumstances, which, in turn, affect their cognition. People are neither driven inexorably by internal forces, nor are they passive reactors to environmental pressures. Rather, they are both agents and objects of external influences.

Self-control strategies have become important components of most therapeutic interventions in behavior therapy. Among the most important elements of self-regulation of behavior are goal setting and feedback, self-monitoring, self-evaluation, and self-reinforcement.

Goal setting and feedback People set both long-term and short-term goals for themselves. The setting of sequential short-term goals leads to better performance than setting a distant goal. Presumably, the reason is related to the reinforcing qualities of goal attainment, since reinforcing successive small steps is better than reinforcing the final behavior, at least until the behavior is well established. The definition of the goal is also important, since the attainment of well-specified goals is more easily recognized than is the attainment of poorly defined goals. In general, the higher the goal set, the better the performance. At the highest levels of goal setting, performance begins to decline, underlining the fact that unrealistic goals undermine performance. Goal attainment enhances self-efficacy and affects future performance.

From a therapeutic viewpoint the therapist should help the patient define and set realistic, well-specified goals that signal small steps along the way to the overall goal. In that way demoralization can be kept at bay by success. Patients must set their own goals, since self-determined goals lead to better performance than goals imposed by others. Teaching patients a problem-solving strategy that they can use in many situations is a useful aspect of most therapies.

Goal attainment is not the only indicator of improvement in performance. Behavior change itself, if observed by the patient, can provide information regarding progress toward a particular goal. The process known as *informational feedback* enhances performance in a wide variety of tasks, such as learning to shoot accurately at a target, driving an automobile, and self-regulating autonomic processes.

Removing informational feedback leads, at least temporarily, to setbacks. Information regarding therapeutic progress can be fed back to the patient in several ways. First, patients can observe their own progress when the desired behavior change is relatively linear, such as approach to a phobic object or situation. Many behaviors, however, are complex. In such cases self-monitoring the behavior can enhance feedback. In addition, patients can plot the results of such feedback in graph form to examine progress over long periods. Enhancement of information regarding progress is the central focus of biofeedback. In the typical *biofeedback* paradigm, processes that are not easily observed (for example, blood pressure, small muscle contractions, and skin temperature) are made available for inspection by amplification. With sensitive and continuous feedback, the patient has the opportunity to learn to regulate invisible behaviors.

Self-monitoring The basis of all self-control strategies is *self-monitoring,* the identification and the recording of target problems and the conditions under which they occur. Typically, patients are asked to complete daily written records. For example, patients with panic disorder track all panic attacks and record the thoughts, feelings, and actions that preceded and accompanied the attacks. The goal is to identify the proximal determinants of the problem. Patients with eating disorders monitor their pattern of binge eating and purging against a background of daily food intake. The purpose is not only to identify situations that trigger binge eating and purging but also to prove to patients that, as their eating habits return to normal, they purge less than before and do not necessarily gain weight. Continual self-monitoring provides patients with feedback of gradual progress that facilitates compliance with therapeutic prescriptions.

Self-monitoring not only provides patients with an awareness of how their behavior affects their social environment but also prompts behavior change. As patients identify specific influences on their behavior, they are able to make changes.

Self-evaluation and self-reinforcement People who adopt certain standards and monitor their performances evaluate their success or failure in achieving those standards. That self-evaluation is the basis for self-reinforcement. Performances that match or exceed the standards serve as cues for rewards, and people deny themselves rewards for substandard performance. The essence of self-reinforcement is that people make freely available rewards contingent on behavior that meets preset standards. Common clinical problems, such as depression, involve the adoption of unrealistic or perfectionistic standards or excessively harsh and judgmental self-evaluation, regardless of objective performance.

CLINICAL APPLICATIONS As a broad-based framework that emphasizes the multidimensional nature of psychological functioning, social-cognitive learning theory provides a flexible guide for therapists trying to design treatments for individual patients. Treatment programs typically combine several principles and procedures. For example, treatment for panic disorder includes systematic exposure to internal stimuli (physical sensations) that trigger panic attacks. Typical ways to elicit relevant internal cues for exposure are to have patients imagine panic-related situations, engage in shallow and rapid breathing (hyperventilation) to induce paniclike feelings, and run in place. Exposure is continued until the cues no longer evoke anxiety.

A second component of treatment is to complement exposure with relaxation training. Patients learn to use relaxation to cope with anxiety and to keep it from spiraling into a panic attack. A third component is to modify the way in which patients appraise cues that trigger panic attacks. Panic disorder patients misinterpret benign physical sensations as harbingers of some catastrophe (for example, acceleration in heart rate is construed as the onset of a heart attack). Patients are taught to identify and to modify the catastrophic thoughts by considering alternative explanations and disconfirming them through mutually agreed on behavioral tests (for example, inducing and then controlling hyperventilation without panicking). That strategy is consistent with social-cognitive theory but is drawn from the cognitive therapy of Aaron Beck. Cognitive-behavioral treatment of that type has proved highly effective in the treatment of panic disorder.

Several components are also used in the cognitive-behavioral treatment of bulimia nervosa. For example, a female patient is presented with a rationale for the treatment, which includes the idea that societal pressures lead young women to overvalue a thin body and to diet. That leads to binge eating and weight gain and ultimately to even more stringent dieting, with the formulation of various rules concerning good and bad foods. Ultimately, the cycle leads to progressive worsening of binge eating, more threatened weight gain, and purging. The patient is then given the expectation that, by making slow step-by-step changes, she can regain self-control over the pattern. In the next phase of treatment, self-monitoring is used to examine her unique feeding pattern, binge eating, and purging episodes. The therapist uses that information to plan the initial treatment approach, which involves shaping three or more meals a day, using instructions and social reinforcement in the form of approval for positive change to strengthen new behaviors. As regular meals are reestablished, forbidden foods are slowly introduced. That leads to an examination of the patient's distorted thinking about body shape and weight and the role of various foods and activities in affecting those factors. Self-monitoring may then focus on factors that lead to loss of control of eating—often interpersonal problems leading to negative affect. Problem solving is then used as a method to deal with such problems effectively. In addition, skills training in assertion may be used at this point. Finally, the therapist examines situations that may lead to lapses once the binge eating and the purging are under control, and the patient works out and practices effective ways of coping with such situations.

The social-cognitive learning approach not only represents the theoretical foundations of cognitive behavior therapy but also informs broader, eclectic approaches, such as Arnold Lazarus's multimodal therapy. It also dovetails with Aaron Beck's cognitive therapy. Cognitive therapy is something of a misnomer because it explicitly uses behavioral procedures to challenge and correct the dysfunctional cognitions presumed to cause such clinical disorders as depression. A cardinal principle of social-cognitive learning theory is that, whereas behavioral procedures are the most effective means of producing therapeutic change, they are mediated by cognitive processes.

Theories of relapse One of the major problems facing therapists of all persuasions is that of patient relapse. Some instances of relapse can be easily understood; for example, the original environmental influences reinforcing symptomatic behavior may not have altered, and the patient's behavior is brought under their control once treatment has ended. That is an example of insufficient treatment; perhaps, for example, the family should have been brought into therapy. Sometimes, however, relapse denotes an impossible situation for the therapist, who is unable to alter a noxious psychological environment.

Less is known about the process of relapse than about the acquisition of behavior. For the most part, relapse has been studied in the addictive disorders, such as alcoholism and opiate addiction, and in related disorders, such as cigarette smoking and obesity. The basic theory concerning relapse involves situations that pose a high risk for engaging in the problem behavior, situations in which the behavior has occurred at a high frequency in the past. If such a situation is coped with successfully, the person experiences an increase in self-efficacy, and that increase leads to a low probability of relapse. The assumption is that the person has been taught or has developed usable coping skills. However, a former substance abuser who is deficient in coping with the high-risk situation develops a positive expectancy regarding the beneficial effects of the substance and starts using the substance again. That practice leads to an *abstinence violation* effect, defined as the breaking of a self-imposed rule, leading to a diminished sense of self-efficacy, negative cognitions and mood, and an increased probability of relapse. Several studies have found levels of self-efficacy to be predictive of outcome.

A fair amount is known about the characteristics of high-risk situations and the determinants of relapse, particularly for alcoholism, cigarette smoking, and the eating disorders. Physiological processes underlying the withdrawal syndrome are an important factor in relapse in many addictive disorders, since abstinence from the abused substance often leads to symptoms that are alleviated by the substance. Cravings and urges may also be conditioned responses to environmental stimuli associated with the use of the substance, whether it be alcohol, cigarettes, or food. Those cravings may persist in specific circumstances for a long time, thus increasing the probability of relapse. Such a scenario may also be true for bulimic patients, who crave their regular binge food, particularly in specific stimulus circumstances (for example, when alone at home). However, symptoms of withdrawal and conditioned cravings may be responsible for only a small proportion of the instances of relapse.

Negative emotional states—such as depression, anxiety, and stress—appear to be important determinants of lapses. More than half of the relapse episodes in alcoholism, cigarette smoking, and bulimia nervosa are associated with negative moods. Since the use of substances, such as alcohol, tends to relieve a negative mood in the short term, the sequence of negative-mood onset and drinking alcohol is learned. Future occurrences of negative mood triggered by stressors then lead to drinking. Factors militating against a negative mood, such as adequate social support, tend to protect against relapse. Such support is most powerful when it comes from family or friends; however, therapeutic groups are also potential sources of support.

All treatments should contain relapse-prevention procedures. The most important element of such a program is a careful analysis of the circumstances under which lapses occur during the treatment program, including events, cognitions, and moods. Self-monitoring is combined with a problem-solving procedure to identify behaviors that are incompatible with relapse. Such behaviors are then practiced in high-risk situations and refined through experience. Among the promising techniques are extinction procedures aimed at breaking the connections between environmental cues and the cravings that promote relapse.

BIOLOGICAL BASIS OF LEARNING

The major experimental models for studying the biology of learning and memory are (1) identified neuronal pathways controlling specific behaviors in invertebrates (for example, *Hermissenda* and *Aplysia californica*), (2) cerebellar neuronal pathways controlling the rabbit nictitating membrane and eyelid response, and (3) hippocampal neurons involved in the long-term potential of behavioral sequences in vertebrates. Research conducted by Eric Kandel and his colleagues at Columbia University with *Aplysia californica* has been particularly well covered in the psychiatric literature. It is now clear that a reciprocal interaction between central nervous system biological processes and environmental influences results in the development and the modification of behaviors.

The aplysia, a sea mollusk, is a useful animal to study because of the simplicity of its nervous system as compared with that of humans. The aplysia contains about 20,000 neurons, many of them large and readily identifiable. The specific behavior studied is a defensive reflex involving the withdrawal of the snail's siphon when the animal is tactually stimulated. If the snail is touched repeatedly, it learns not to withdraw its siphon and gill, a process called *habituation*. If the snail receives a strong stimulus, such as an electric shock, it becomes *sensitized*, such that even a previously subthreshold tactile stimulation causes the animal to withdraw its gill and siphon. Furthermore, one can condition the snail classically so that it withdraws its siphon and gill to a conditioned stimulus. Habituation, sensitization, and classical conditioning of the reflex in the snail can be considered forms of learning and memory.

The neuronal anatomical and chemical bases for the learning processes have been well worked out in that animal model. Sensory neurons receiving tactile information form excitatory synapses with the gill and siphon motor neurons that cause the withdrawal activity. Habituation, sensitization, and classical conditioning all involve neurochemical changes in the sensory neuron, resulting in alterations in the amount of excitatory neurotransmitter released. The neurochemical basis of habituation is that, after repeated stimulation of the sensory neuron (for example, repeated tactile stimulation), less calcium than usual enters the presynaptic nerve terminal, resulting in less neurotransmitter being released and, thus, less activity by the motor neurons. Sensitization requires the presence of additional neurons, called *facilitator interneurons*, that synapse onto the sensory neurons. The sensitizing stimulus, such as an electric shock, causes the facilitator interneuron to release serotonin that binds to serotonin receptors on the sensory neuron. Activation of the serotonin receptors activates adenylate cyclase, producing cyclic adenosine monophosphate (cAMP), thereby activating a cAMP-dependent protein kinase, which is believed to phosphorylate an S-type potassium channel. Phosphorylation of the potassium channel results in increased calcium influx during the action potential and increased neurotransmitter release. Although classical conditioning also results in an increased amount of neurotransmitter released by the sensory neuron, the neurochemical basis is less well understood at this time but may involve additional protein kinases.

Experimental work with young aplysia has shown that the processes of habituation and sensitization develop at different times, with habituation preceding sensitization. It may be possible to identify the separate biological processes that give rise to both of the important learning phenomena.

SUGGESTED CROSS-REFERENCES

Applications of the principles and procedures discussed in this section, together with an assessment of the effectiveness of such therapeutic applications to various conditions, can be found in Section 31.2 on behavior therapy and Section 31.6 on cognitive therapy. Issues basic to learning are discussed in Chapter 1 on neural sciences and in Section 3.1 on perception and cognition. Derivations from the principles and procedures exemplified in this section are discussed in Chapter 8 on theories of personality and psychopathology derived from psychology and philosophy.

REFERENCES

Bandura A: *Principles of Behavior Modification*. Holt, Rinehart & Winston, New York, 1969.

*Bandura A: Self-efficacy: Toward a unifying theory of behavioral change. Psychol Rev *84:* 191. 1977.

Bandura A: *Social Foundations of Thought and Action: A Social Cognitive Theory*. Prentice-Hall, Englewood Cliffs, N J, 1986.

Beck A T: *Cognitive Therapy of Depression. A Treatment Manual*. Guilford, New York, 1979.

*Brownell K D, Marlatt G A, Lichenstein E, Wilson G T: Understanding and preventing relapse. Am Psychol *41:* 764, 1986.

Clark G A, Hawkins R D, Kandel E R: Cell biological perspectives on learning. In *Diseases of the Nervous System*, A K Ashury, M McKhann, W I MacDonald, editors, p 262. Saunders, Philadelphia, 1986.

Dollard J, Miller N E: *Personality and Psychotherapy*. McGraw-Hill, New York, 1950.

Fairburn C G, Agras W S, Wilson G T: The research on the treatment of bulimia nervosa: Practical and theoretical implications. In *The Biology of Feast and Famine: Relevance to Eating Disorders*, G H Anderson, S H Kennedy, editors, p 318. Academic Press, New York, 1992.

Haaga D A F, Stewart B L: Self-efficacy for recovery from a lapse after smoking cessation. J Consult Clin Psychol *60:* 24, 1992.

Hilgard E R, Bower G H: *Theories of Learning*, ed 4. Prentice-Hall, Englewood Cliffs, N J, 1975.

Kandel E R, Spencer W A: Cellular neurophysiological approaches in the study of learning. Physiol Rev *48:* 65, 1968.

*Kendall P C. Healthy thinking. Behav Ther *23:* 1, 1992.

Lazarus, A A: *Multimodal Behavior Therapy*. Springer, New York, 1976.

Mineka S, Davidson M, Cook M, Keir R: Observational conditioning of snake fear in rhesus monkeys. J Abnorm Psychol *93:* 335, 1984.

Mineka S, Gunnar M, Champoux M: Control and early socioemotional development: Infant rhesus monkeys reared in controllable versus uncontrollable environments. Child Dev *57:* 1241, 1986.

Mischel W: Toward a cognitive social learning reconceptualization of personality. Psychol Rev *80:* 252, 1973.

Mowrer O H: *Learning and Behavior*. Wiley, New York, 1960.

Pavlov I P: *Conditioned Reflexes*. Clarendon Press, London, 1927.

Poling A: *A Primer of Human Behavioral Pharmacology*. Plenum, New York, 1986.

Premack D: Reinforcement theory. In *Nebraska Symposium on Motivation*, M Jones, editor. University of Nebraska Press, Lincoln, 1965.

Rachlin H: *Introduction to Modern Behaviorism*. Freeman, New York, 1970.

*Rescorla R A: Pavlovian conditioning. It's not what you think. Am Psychol *43:* 151, 1988.

Seligman M E P: Phobias and preparedness. Behav Ther *2:* 107, 1971.

Sherman J E, Jrenby D E, Baker T B: Classical conditioning with alcohol: Acquired preferences and aversions, tolerance, and urges/craving. In *Theories on Alcoholism*, C D Chaudron, D A Wilkinson, editors, p 187. Addiction Research Foundation, Toronto, 1988.

*Skinner B F: *Science and Human Behavior*. Macmillan, New York, 1951.

Thorndike E L: *Human Learning*. Century Company, New York, 1931.

Watson J B, Rayner R: Conditioned emotional reactions. J Exp Psychol *3:* 1, 1920.

Wolpe J: *Psychotherapy by Reciprocal Inhibition*. Stanford University Press, Stanford, CA, 1958.

3.4 AGGRESSION

JOHN R. LION, M.D.

INTRODUCTION

Most clinicians have encountered an aggressive patient at some point in the course of their clinical careers. Indeed, violence spans the entire spectrum of mental disorders, commonly appearing in the behavior of patients with schizophrenia, bipolar disorder, agitated depressive states, and conduct disorder in childhood. Rages are prominent features of characterological disorders such as borderline and narcissistic personality disorders, and temper proneness and aggressive outbursts can be seen in disorders such as personality change due to a general medical condition, aggressive type, mental retardation; and intermittent explosive disorder.

Despite its ubiquity, the clinical literature concerning aggression in humans is scant compared with that describing mood disorders or thought disorders. The clinical study of violence has largely been relegated to the forensic realm, while more basic scientific inquiries into the biochemistry and neurophysiology of aggression in animals and humans have appeared mainly in the basic sciences literature. One reason for the reluctance of the psychiatric profession to involve itself in the problem of aggression is that violent behavior has always been viewed as a manifestation of badness and criminality. In contrast, psychosis or depression are clearly perceived as madness and as genuine illnesses worthy of recognition and research.

An added complexity is that of distinguishing normal from pathological aggression. A surgeon in the operating room or a basketball player on the court may be very aggressive, but in highly controlled ways. If the surgeon throws an instrument or rages at a nurse, the behavior may not be tolerated by his or her colleagues. The basketball player who incurs many fouls may be disqualified. Conversely, passive adolescents who begin to assert themselve at home and verbally fight with their parents may be showing healthy aggression. Thus, aggression is a behavior which is on a continuum, the product of sublimations. Those complexities of definition are obviously less present among animals, where aggression appears to be more simplistic. But even here, various forms of violence have been noted, such as predatory aggression in acquiring food, territorial aggression, and violence during mating.

THEORETICAL BACKGROUND

PSYCHOANALYTIC AND PSYCHODYNAMIC VIEWS

Sigmund Freud initially postulated a theory of libido in which there existed dual sexual and aggressive instincts or drives. The aggressive drives could be traced through the various oral, anal, and phallic manifestations of the sexual drive. For example, aggressive instincts in infants could be seen by oral activity, such as biting, or appear as soiling in the anal phase or as later phallic behavior; those phases were further divided into erotic and sadistic stages, depending on resolution. Sadism, then, was seen as an aggressive component of the sexual instinct. But Freud also began to recognize that impulses of cruelty could arise from sources independent of sex. Thus, years later, influenced by the war around him, he revised his entire theory of instincts and hypothesized life and death instincts, Eros and Thanatos. Aggression, or destructiveness, was still viewed as a fundamental human drive, though the forces could be diverted or modified in the service of the organism.

Non-Freudian psychoanalytic theories of aggression stressed other origins for violence. Alfred Adler saw the inferiority complex and a quest for power as responsible for destructive aggression, while Carl Jung viewed aggression as the unleashing of primordial archetypical behavior inherent in the collective unconscious. Otto Rank departed significantly from Freud by devising a theory in which birth trauma was the cause of neurosis; thus, violence sprang from early conflicts between mother and child. In the interpersonal theory of neurosis, Harry Stack Sullivan viewed aggression as resulting from parataxic distortions in interpersonal relationships. Erich Fromm, further developing social and cultural aspects of psychopathology, conceptualized benign and malignant aggression. The former was more instinctive, animalistic, and defensive, while the latter was unique to humans and could be seen in sadistic characters in history, such as Joseph Stalin. Later theoreticians, attempting to integrate Freudian views with the principles of learning observed in the laboratory, viewed aggression as an elicited drive, secondary to frustration or pain. John Dollard and colleagues proposed the frustration-aggression theory, in which the blocking of an ongoing goal-directed behavior led to the arousal of an aggressive drive and a subsequent attack on the source of the frustration.

INSTINCT THEORY Instinct views of aggression focused on innate tendencies most easily observed in animals. Konrad Lorenz, like Freud, invoked a hydraulic model to understand nature. From his observation of animals, Lorenz postulated that aggressiveness was not necessarily a reaction to any outside stimulus but a fighting instinct fed by energy continuously accumulating in neural centers. Organisms needed sources and expression for the release of that built-up aggressive energy. Most often, the release took the form of behavior adaptive for the organism. For example, fighting dispersed animals over wide areas and thus insured adequate supplies of food. Lorenz's instinct theory is somewhat difficult to grasp, particularly when extrapolated to humans from the more rudimentary forms of violence seen among mammals.

LEARNING THEORY Learning theories of aggression have tended to view violence not as innate or instinctual, but as the manifestation of experience. There are three main concepts in learning theory: acquisition of aggressive modes of behavior, instigation of aggression, and reinforcement of the behavior. An example of acquisition is the direct observation of violence in families or on television. Instigation occurs, for instance, when models of violence are allowed to exist without sanctions. People who are repeatedly exposed to combative models will be more assaultive in their interactions than those who observe nonviolent styles of conduct. Learning theory is based on the assumption that humans are not born with a full repertoire of aggressive responses but acquire them through experience. Additionally, learning theory is based on the fact that many forms of aggression in a culture, ranging from sports to crime to warfare, are positively sanctioned and shaped by the society in which those behaviors flourish.

PHYSIOLOGICAL ASPECTS

BIOCHEMISTRY IN ANIMALS AND HUMANS A variety of experimental techniques have been used to replicate animal models of aggression. Most commonly, mice and rats are subjected to either prolonged isolation, electric shock, pharmacological manipulation, or brain stimulation or lesions. Muricidal rats, which spontaneously kill mice introduced into their cages, can also be bred and subjected to those experimental procedures. Analysis of specific areas of the brain involved in the regulation of aggression in those animals, such as the olfactory bulbs, has revealed that the inhibitory neurotransmitter γ-aminobutyric acid (GABA) has a regulatory effect on violence. The potentiation of GABAergic inhibition by such drugs as valproic acid (Depakene) results in decreased aggressiveness. That effect is seen not only in muricidal rats, but in normal animals subjected to isolation or shock-induced aggression.

The role of serotonin has also been addressed in aggression research. A decrease of brain serotonin is found in the brainstems of muricidal rats and of animals made aggressive by isolation. The administration of tryptophan, a serotonin precursor, reduces or abolishes violence. Other studies indicate not only a decrease in inhibitory neurotransmitter metabolism in aggressive rats, but also an increase in metabolism of excitatory neurotransmitters, such as norepinephrine. Drugs that increase functional noradrenergic activity increase aggressiveness in animals.

Nonhuman primates have also been used to study the neurochemistry of aggression, but results have been variable. Some workers, using drugs to manipulate central nervous system (CNS) serotonin activity in vervet monkeys, have produced increased or decreased aggressiveness. Those animals with high blood serotonin and cerebrospinal fluid (CSF) 5-hydroxyindoleacetic acid (5-HIAA), a metabolite of serotonin, tend to be dominant. One methodological problem in those research efforts is to maintain colonies of highly aggressive monkeys or chimpanzees. More recent studies have been performed on free-ranging monkeys. From observations of the animals and inspection of their fight wounds, rankings were made and the chemistries blindly assayed. There was a significant negative correlation between high rankings for aggression and CSF 5-HIAA, while positive correlations were found between aggression and norepinephrine. Plasma testosterone was also studied, but no positive correlation was found.

Human studies associated with CSF neurotransmitters have looked at 5-HIAA and the norepinephrine metabolite 3-methoxy-4-hydroxyphenylglycol (MHPG). Work has focused on both suicide and externally directed violence, as they often coexist in patients who are labile and manifest aggressive dyscontrol. Many studies have shown diminished CSF 5-HIAA concentrations in impulsive and violence-prone subjects. The individual cases and small populations studied include psychopathic military personnel, children with histories of torturing animals, incarcerated murderers, suicidal patients, and persons who killed their children. Suicidal patients who use violent means show lower 5-HIAA than their less violent counterparts, and significantly higher aggression rating scores were found in patients with suicidal histories compared with those without such histories. It appears that very impulsive and aggressive patients direct their violence both inwardly and outwardly and are unable to regulate those rages. Impulsivity and disinhibition appear to be the parameters associated with lowered CSF serotonin.

NEUROANATOMY A vast literature exists linking specific brain structures to aggressive behavior in mammals and nonhuman primates. Both facilitory and inhibitory areas have been identified. For example, the hypothalamus plays a crucial role in the expression of aggression in animals, but there appear to be multiple aspects to its functions, depending on the species used for experiment and the nature of the lesions or stimulations.

Stimulation of the anterior hypothalamus causes predatory attacks in cats, while activation of the dorsomedial aspect produces aggression in which the animal ignores the presence of an available rat and attacks the experimenter. Destruction of aggression-inhibiting areas, such as the ventromedial nucleus of the hypothalamus, produces permanently aggressive cats and rats. Following cortical ablation, stimulation of the posterior lateral hypothalamus of the cat elicits the so-called sham rage, a posture of preparation for attack. Further stimulation of the posterior lateral portion of the hypothalamus shortens the latency of attack, while stimulation of the medial ventral area prolongs the latency of attack. Other areas implicated in aggression include the midline thalamus, lateral preoptic region, mammillary bodies, hippocampus, and cingulate gyrus, or frontal lobe areas.

The amygdala has been extensively studied in rodents, nonhuman primates, and humans. Bilateral lesions of the amygdala tame a variety of innately hostile and vicious animals, while irritative lesions or electrical stimulation can lead to rage outbursts. Results are not always consistent and depend on which portion of the amygdala is stimulated. In humans, reports of surgical intervention for the relief of mental or structural brain disease or epilepsy have shown that both the amygdala and other temporal lobe and limbic system structures control aggression. Limbic system tumors, infections, and blood vessel abnormalities have also been associated with violence. Although it is clear that various limbic system structures have an inhibitory or excitatory effect on aggression, the precise nature of the aggression pathway is still far from established.

HORMONES AND AGGRESSION Many studies deal with the effects of hormones on animal aggression; results reveal complex relationships. For example, the castration of postpubertal male rats diminishes spontaneous fighting, whereas testosterone therapy restores the readiness to fight. Testosterone treatment of adult male rats does not restore fighting, however, if castration is done at a neonatal age, when, presumably, there is CNS differentiation occurring. In male rhesus monkeys, plasma testosterone levels correlate positively with behavioral dominance and aggressiveness. If a single male monkey is placed with other aggressive males, he becomes submissive and shows a dramatic fall in plasma testosterone level, revealing that endogenous hormone production can be affected by behavioral variables.

The same may be true for humans. In one study of human aggression, for example, a correlation between plasma testosterone and prison violence could not be made, but testosterone levels were elevated in juvenile prisoners who had committed violent crimes against persons. In another study, a positive relationship appeared between testosterone and the aggressiveness of hockey players. But cause-and-effect is far from clearly established by these studies, and it may well be that aggressiveness stimulates the production of testosterone rather than the reverse.

Castration has been effective in the control of certain violent sex crimes in men, while the therapeutic use of estrogens and antiandrogens have been shown to reduce aggressiveness and sexual offenses. Medroxyprogesterone acetate (Provera) has been used to treat aggressive paraphiliac persons, but the reasons for its efficacy are unknown. The drug decreases testosterone secretion by the testes but also appears to act centrally on the brain, because there is no compensatory elevation of follicle-stimulating hormone (FSH) or luteinizing hormone (LH) production by the pituitary gland in response to lowered serum testosterone. Dosages of medroxyprogesterone acetate can effectively decrease erotic imagery but leave serum testosterone unchanged.

GENETICS AND AGGRESSION Genetic studies of criminality, delinquency, and antisocial behavior have shown that adult criminality, as a manifestation of antisocial personality disorders, has some genetic etiology. Studies have related adult antisocial personality disorder among adoptees to biological backgrounds of criminality or antisocial behavior. For example, one study revealed a greater incidence of antisocial personality disorder in the offspring of convicted felons than in adoptees whose mothers were not felons. Another study showed that adoptees from backgrounds of antisocial behavior were more likely to have antisocial personality disorder. In Danish studies, significant correlations were found between adoptees and their biological parents with respect to convictions for property crimes, but not for crimes of violence.

Environment also plays a major role. In studies of adolescent twins, the correlation for aggressive and antisocial behaviors was roughly the same for monozygotic twins and dizygotic twins, thus providing evidence for the effects of a common environment. However, twin studies suggest that antisocial behavior in adult life is related more to genetic factors than to environmental factors. Sex factors have also been studied, showing in one study that female criminals are more likely than other women to have criminal relatives.

On the basis of prevalence studies of the proportion of chromosomal variants found in incarcerated populations, researchers at one time suggested a link between the XYY variant and violence. However, those studies did not take into account such parameters as family background and other factors that might lead to institutionalization; consequently, the link between

XYY and violence has not been confirmed. Certain inborn errors of metabolism and syndromes of mental retardation are associated with aggression. Children with Cornelia de Lange syndrome or those with Lesch-Nyhan syndrome, for example, engage in severely self-mutilative behavior. They manifest outward aggression when attempts are made to stop the self-injurious behavior.

CURRENT PHENOMENOLOGICAL CONSIDERATIONS

The 1974 American Psychiatric Association Task Force on Clinical Aspects of the Violent Individual defined violence as an act leading to physical harm or destruction. That operational description leaves much to be desired. For example, a common clinical problem is assessing the dangerousness of a psychiatric patient. In such cases, the patient's thoughts and fantasies are often more urgent concerns than the behavior. Indeed, such patients may not have exhibited violent behavior and yet may be perceived as potentially homicidal. In contrast, a clinician may be asked to see a patient who has killed another but is at no risk for killing again at the time of the assessment. Clearly, labeling a patient violent is problematic. Verbal aggression is especially difficult to assess because it may be a function of social class and clinical status. Some patients threaten a good deal but are not aggressive in person, while others store their rages and ultimately explode in anger. How a patient handles aggressive urges requires evaluation not only of what he or she says, but also of past behavior. The clinician must ask, what is the patient's most violent act? Has he or she used a weapon? Has he or she threatened a spouse or lover? Should that person be evaluated as well? Violence involves other people, and the assessment of violence requires the clinician to move outside the realm of the patient.

DIAGNOSTIC ISSUES

DEFINITIONS In the fourth edition of the American Psychiatric Association's *Diagnostic and Statistical Manual of Mental Disorders* (DSM-IV), the disorder most intensively studied with respect to aggression is intermittent explosive disorder. The origins of the term date to concepts advanced by Karl Menninger, who viewed aggression as a severe psychic dyscontrol in which explosive outbursts of rage, usually of psychotic proportions, occurred. The second edition of DSM (DSM-II) included a disorder called the explosive personality, characterized by behavior patterns with ''gross outbursts of rage or verbal or physical aggressiveness.'' In 1970 Russell Monroe published a monograph on the episodic behavior disorders, in which he attributed aggression to brain dysfunction, such as psychomotor epilepsy. Intermittent explosive disorder was thus perceived as an ictal disorder, and it was accordingly conceptualized in the 1980 third edition of DSM (DSM-III) as a disorder of impulsive control with associated features ''suggesting an organic disturbance . . . such as nonspecific electroencephalographic (EEG) abnormalities or minor neurologic signs and symptoms thought to reflect subcortical or limbic system dysfunction.'' That view has since been challenged, leading to the current perception of intermittent explosive disorder as temper proneness without a clear organic etiology. Violence of organic etiology is identified in DSM-IV as personality change due to a general medical condition, aggressive type. Table 3.4-1 lists the various disorders in DSM-IV that include aggression or violence.

TABLE 3.4-1
DSM-IV Categories Which Include Violence and Aggression

Alcohol-related disorders
Amphetamine intoxication
Inhalant intoxication
Phencyclidine intoxication
Antisocial personality disorder
Borderline personality disorder
Dementia
Delirium
Intermittent explosive disorder
Mental retardation
Conduct disorder
Oppositional defiant disorder
Posttraumatic stress disorder
Personality change due to a general medical condition, aggressive type
Sexual sadism
Schizophrenia, paranoid type

SCIENCE, POLITICS, AND AGGRESSION Using a model of ictal, or epileptoid, aggression, Vernon Mark and Frank Ervin stated that all forms of human aggression might have their origins in underlying seizure states. That generalization led more conservative scientists and government groups to counter with statements that directed violence rarely sprang from epilepsy, although it could be seen as a manifestation of a postictal confusional state. So heated did the controversy about brain dysfunction and violence become, that the National Institute of Health placed a moratorium on federally funded psychosurgical programs, in part fearing that surgical treatments might be misused on prisoner populations. In a recent investigation of the link between aggression and seizure states, researchers concluded that directed violence is extremely rare during a seizure state. The debate over the etiological role of epilepsy and other forms of brain dysfunction and aggression continues. For the practicing clinician, it may be useful to consider an organic evaluation in the case of a paroxysmally aggressive patient. Yet the causality of most violence is far more complex and reflects social forces, psychodynamic factors, and personality.

PHARMACOLOGICAL CONSIDERATIONS Although serotonergic compounds, such as the serotonin-specific reuptake inhibitor (SSRI) group of antidepressants, might seem a logical choice in the management of aggression, they have not proved systematically effective. Eltoprazine, one of a new class of so-called serenic compounds (drugs that induce serenity), is a central serotonin receptor agonist shown to have an antiaggressive effect in animal paradigms of aggression, but clinical trials have not substantiated its effectiveness in humans. The anticonvulsants, such as carbamazepine (Tegretol), have been described as beneficial for patients with epileptoid forms of aggression. Lithium (Eskalith) has been shown in double-blind studies to reduce aggressiveness in prisoners, although the basis for its efficacy remains unclear. Antipsychotic agents are regularly employed to treat psychoses in which there is aggression, but their primary mode of action is to reduce the underlying thought disorder; by themselves, those drugs possess no antiaggressive properties. The β-adrenergic receptor antagonists, such as propranolol (Inderal), have been found empirically useful in the treatment of aggression in mentally retarded and brain-damaged patient populations. Benzodiazepines have been advocated for certain characterologically aggressive patients by reducing the anxiety and irritation that fuel reactive aggression.

Two other groups of drugs for the treatment of aggression in humans deserve mention. Isolated case reports have shown narcotics antagonists to be effective in reducing self-injurious behavior in mentally retarded patients. In one study, such patients had higher concentrations of opioid peptides in their CSF, which could account for their higher threshold to self-induced pain. Used on a wider scale, antiandrogen or progestational agents, such as medroxyprogesterone acetate, for the treatment of sexually aggressive men were found to be effective. Given parenterally in depot form, medroxyprogesterone acetate has been shown to decrease erotic imagery and arousal and to effect a corresponding decrease in paraphiliac behavior.

A variety of drugs have been implicated in the unleashing of aggression in humans. Those include CNS stimulants, such as dextroamphetamine (Dexedrine), and hallucinogens, such as phencyclidine (PCP). Marijuana is actually a pacifying agent. Heroin, likewise, is a pharmacological agent that induces quiescence, although violence is certainly used to procure it. The benzodiazepines have been implicated in so-called paradoxical rage outbursts, yet in one study of the treatment of aggressive outpatients by high dosages of benzodiazepines no disinhibition was noted.

The antidepressant fluoxetine (Prozac) has received adverse publicity for allegedly activating aggressive behavior, including violence, murder, and suicidal acts. It is unlikely, however, that any one agent produces violence. Rather, the drug may cause some disinhibition in a patient already prone to violence or suicide. Recent studies of the response of anger to fluoxetine treatment suggest that there exists a subset of depressed patients who may have greater central serotonergic dysregulation than depressed patients without that condition. Alcohol is still the most common disinhibiting agent.

VECTORS OF VIOLENCE Freud formulated that in the state of depression the organism turns its aggression toward itself. That view of depression as anger turned inward has persisted and is often offered as the explanation for impulsive acts of suicide by patients reacting to loss. But the matter appears to be more complex, and the vector of aggression may be more a function of the sum of the patient's aggression and faulty regulatory mechanisms than the simple dynamic of internalization. In one study, investigators found that severely violent patients had histories of many acts of attempted suicide, not just externally directed acts of aggression. A five-year follow-up study of 100 patients who threatened homicide found that four patients had committed suicide and three had committed homicide. A 1966 study of a group of murderers in England revealed that one third of them committed suicide after the murders. The population included two large groups: women who committed infanticide and despondent elderly patients who killed their spouses and then themselves. In the United States the suicide and murder rates are almost comparable; in 1990 the homicide rate per 100,000 population was 10.2 and the suicide rate 12.3. In Scandinavia, there is a tenfold higher rate of suicide than of homicide. Those statistics suggest that culture plays a major role in determining the vectors of aggression and may have an impact on shame and guilt.

The problem of assessing the vector of aggression is hardly an academic one for clinicians faced with a potentially violent patient. A depressed patient may choose to harm a spouse or child, while a narcissistic patient may commit suicide out of rage and humiliation. Rageful borderline disorder patients may find their own anger intolerable and take overdoses of drugs to quench the painful affect or cut themselves to relieve the tension accompanying anger. Conversely, a patient who sees no hope of salvation may decide to kill those persons considered responsible for his or her unhappiness. It is a common practice to watch new inmates in jail for the first six weeks, when suicidal risk is high.

Self-mutilation and other forms of self-injurious behavior constitute another class of inwardly turned aggression. Such behaviors as head banging are often difficult to control and require a combination of pharmacological intervention, mechanical restraint, and behavioral conditioning.

THE MEASUREMENT OF AGGRESSION A common problem is to quantify the aggressiveness of a patient or assess how violent he or she may become. Traditionally, projective tests, such as the Rorschach test or Thematic Apperception Test (TAT) have helped to address the issues. Other tests, such as the Buss-Durkee test, rely on true-false questions about violent ideation (''I seldom strike back, even if someone hits me first'': true or false) or queries about the intensity of anger. There are marked limitations to those rating scales in the evaluation of dangerousness. Assessment of risk for release from prison or hospital depends much more on subjective parameters, such as the patient's alliance or compliance with medication, than on formal tests, and the past history is still the most important determinant in the process of risk assessment. Table 3.4-2 illustrates a rating scale based on inpatient behavior. The scale quantifies verbal aggression, physical destructiveness, aggression against self, and aggression against others. Such a scale is useful in pharmacological studies.

SOCIOLOGICAL ASPECTS

AGGRESSION IN HOSPITALS AND ON MENTAL HEALTH PROFESSIONALS Assaults in psychiatric hospitals have been studied by a number of workers. One survey of assaults for a 10-year period among some 27,000 Scandinavian inpatients found eight fatalities—seven patients and one staff person. The peak incidence of assault occurred when a newly admitted male schizophrenic patient was mixed with an older, feebler patient during a temporary period of understaffing. Among other studies of patients who commit violent acts, the most common diagnoses are schizophrenia, personality disorders, cognitive disorders, and alcohol-related disorders. A history of violence remains the most important parameter in identifying the patient who is most likely to become violent during hospitalization.

The problem of institutional violence in this country has been recently reviewed. Most violence occurs within public mental hospitals where chronically psychotic patients are housed; hence the finding that schizophrenic patients are more commonly involved than others in assaultive behavior. Extrapolating on the basis of published studies, it has been estimated that there are thousands of assaults in American hospitals each year, although how many of those are fatal is not known. Nurses are most often injured, largely because they are the primary caregivers to violent patients. Most assaults occur during restraint and seclusion. The emergency room is a site of risk for mental health workers; two studies have commented on weapons found on patients seen in that location.

Assaults on mental health professionals have also been studied. One study found that 40 percent of clinicians in a university health service had been assaulted during the course of their career. Seven psychiatrists have been killed by patients in the

TABLE 3.4-2
Overt Aggression Scale

Identifying Data

Name of Patient: ______________________ Name of Rater: ______________________

Sex of Patient: ____ Male ____ Female
Date: ____ /____ /____ (mo/da/yr)
Shift: ____ Night____ Day____ Evening

No aggressive incident(s) (verbal or physical) against self, others, or objects during the shift ____

Aggressive Behavior (Check All That Apply)

Verbal Aggression

- ____ Makes loud noises, shouts angrily.
- ____ Yells mild personal insults, e.g., "You're stupid!"
- ____ Curses viciously, uses foul language in anger, makes moderate threats to others or self.
- ____ Makes clear threats of violence toward others or self ("I'm going to kill you") or requests to help to control self.

Physical Aggression Against Self

- ____ Picks or scratches skin, hits self, pulls hair (with no or minor injury only).
- ____ Bangs head, hits fist into objects, throws self onto floor or into objects (hurts self without serious injury).
- ____ Small cuts or bruises, minor burns.
- ____ Mutilates self, causes deep cuts, bites that bleed, internal injury fracture, loss of consciousness, loss of teeth.

Physical Aggression Against Objects

- ____ Slams door, scatters clothing, makes a mess.
- ____ Throws objects down, kicks furniture without breaking it, marks the wall.
- ____ Breaks objects, smashes windows.
- ____ Sets fires, throws objects dangerously.

Physical Aggression Against Other People

- ____ Makes threatening gesture, swings at people, grabs at clothes.
- ____ Strikes, kicks, pushes, pulls hair (without injury to them).
- ____ Attacks others, causing mild–moderate physical injury (bruises, sprain, welts).
- ____ Attacks others, causing severe physical injury (broken bones, deep lacerations, internal injury).

Time incident began: ____ ____ : ____ ____ a.m. / p.m.

Duration of incident: ____ ____ : ____ ____ (hours:minutes)

Intervention (Check All That Apply)

- ____ None.
- ____ Talking to patient.
- ____ Closer observation.
- ____ Holding patient.
- ____ Immediate medication given by mouth.
- ____ Immediate medication given by injection.
- ____ Isolation without seclusion (time out).
- ____ Seclusion.
- ____ Use of restraints.
- ____ Injury requires immediate medical treatment for patient.
- ____ Injury requires immediate treatment for other person.

Table from S C Yudofsky, J M Silver, W Jackson, J Endicott, D Williams: The overt aggression scale for the objective rating of verbal and physical aggression. Am J Psychiat *143:* 35, 1986. Used with permission.

past 15 years in the United States. Because 10 to 15 percent of persons admitted to psychiatric inpatient facilities have been aggressive to someone in the year prior to hospitalization, the management of aggression is an important issue. The American Psychiatric Association Task Force on Clinician Safety has published recommendations for aggression management in the workplace. Items to consider include the physical handling of patients, availability and use of proper restraint appliances, use of seclusion, training of security staff, panic alarm installation, and policies concerning the disposition of aggressive patients and the prosecution of patients who have been aggressive during hospitalization.

THE PREDICTION OF VIOLENCE AND DANGEROUSNESS The topic of prediction, of considerable interest to parole boards, judges, and clinicians, has an extensive literature. The methodological problems associated with accurate predictive statements include the definition of the term "dangerous," the problem of predicting a low base-rate event, and the problem of false positives—identifying patients as dangerous when they are not. The prediction of dangerousness has had increasing medicolegal ramifications since the 1976 Tarasoff legal decision, in which a California therapist was held responsible for determining that his patient was homicidal; in that case, the patient repeatedly threatened to kill his girlfriend and actually went on to do so. The Tarasoff duty to protect ruling set a legal precedent which forces the clinician not only to determine if a patient intends to do harm, but to take active steps to prevent it. A standard of care is evolving that mandates the clinician to assess the risk a patient poses to society. A clinician may be held liable for the incorrect determination of that risk and the failure to intervene appropriately.

Clinical risk assessment is usually based on answers to the following questions. What is the history of violence in the patient? Does he or she use alcohol or disinhibiting drugs? Does he or she own a weapon, and has he or she used it? Has the patient been violent or threatened harm to a specific person? Does the patient have poor impulse control or some other form of ego dysfunction? Does the patient form an alliance with a therapist, and is he or she compliant with medication? Subjectively, how do examiners feel about the patient?

CRIMINAL VIOLENCE AND FAMILY VIOLENCE The four crimes classified as violent by the Federal Bureau of Investigation (FBI) are homicide, armed robbery, rape, and assault. There are over 20,000 homicides in the United States every year, and those deaths are largely an urban phenomenon. Handguns are the weapons used in over half of murders, and men are three times more likely than women to be killed. In 9 out of 10 homicides, perpetrator and victim are of the same race; homicide rates among blacks are many times higher than among whites. The peak age for homicide victims is about 25 years, and alcohol is involved in 25 to 75 percent of homicides. In one study of youthful murderers on death row, many had neurological abnormalities and brain dysfunction.

Homicide often occurs in families, where domestic quarrels are a major factor. Most police departments, recognizing the risk to officers who must respond to dangerous family altercations, now give courses to personnel on safe ways to defuse arguments.

The family as the cradle of violence is now well documented. Several studies have shown that between one half and three fourths of women have experienced physical violence from their partners at some time. The terms "spouse abuse" and "wife battering" are now common, attesting to increased awareness of family abuse. The frequency of marital abuse is difficult to ascertain because so much of it goes unreported. Based on one study in Delaware of reported and nonreported serious family assaults, the incidence ranged from 26 to 7,016 in 100,000. Shame, guilt, and fear on the part of the victim still make underreporting a significant problem.

That a cycle of family violence exists is now documented. In a study of 100 battered wives, half of the batterers and a quarter of the victims had experienced a violent childhood; one third of the abused wives and one half of the abusive husbands had abused their children. The most likely perpetrators of violence are those persons who were themselves victimized as children. Without effective intervention, generations of abuse can occur. Treatment, however, is far from simple. It involves raising self-esteem in the victims, as well as helping them to understand the complex psychodynamics of victimhood.

Within families, children are hardly immune from violence. Indeed, child abuse has been known for centuries, but it was only with the 1946 publication of a syndrome of subdural hematoma and abnormal radiological changes in the long bones that the medical profession became aware of the problem. Child abuse reporting laws now exist in all states. Estimates of the number of children physically and sexually abused vary widely and run from 50,000 to 2.5 million a year. In 1989, 1,237 children were killed by their parents.

Studies of the dynamics of child abuse have revealed that abusive parents may look on the child as fulfilling some of their own unmet needs. A role reversal occurs wherein the parent views the child as hostile and unloving. Because the parent is likely to have been abused, he or she may respond to disappointment in the child with rage and physical punishment. The parents of abused children are often emotionally immature, and in one study, one half the mothers were clinically depressed.

TREATMENT OF CRIMINAL VIOLENCE AND ANTISOCIAL SYNDROMES The literature on aggressive sociopathy attests to society's limited abilities to formulate and execute effective treatment strategies for recidivist aggressive criminals. Two projects deserve mention. In Denmark, George Sturup pioneered long-term incarceration treatment programs using group and behavior therapy in an indeterminate-sentence facility. A similar program took place in the United States at Patuxent Institution in Maryland, where ''defective delinquents'' were at one time also treated during indeterminate sentences. Over the past decade the indeterminate sentence has been abolished, however, and the facility has been converted to a fixed-sentence unit where severely violent recidivists can elect to undergo intensive psychological treatment, chiefly involving group therapy. Prisoners are given progressively greater freedom within the institution and are gradually weaned from the prison into half- and quarter-way houses where they receive work and living supervision.

The effectiveness of those treatment programs is still a matter of controversy. Prisoners released into the community from indeterminate-sentence facilities have shown a lower rate of recidivism than prisoners released after the expiration of their fixed sentences; however, since they are usually kept in the institution longer than the average criminal, the effectiveness of indeterminate sentences has not been independently confirmed. Beyond those experimental programs for severely aggressive offenders, little in the way of treatment or rehabilitation goes on in the majority of prisons in the world.

Workers have commented on behavior modification paradigms in the therapy of aggressive patients, including such traditional interventions as time-out and negative and positive conditioning (privileges and tokens). A recent alternative involves the use of social constructionism for intractably violent individuals. Here, a planned disruption between patient and caretakers occurs. For example, the patient's privilege level is determined randomly rather than being tied to behavior. Under such circumstances, a pathological feedback loop is interrupted, and the patient, sensing the detachment of the clinician, stops the adverse behavior. No extensive or systematic studies of the efficacy of such therapy has been carried out.

FUTURE ISSUES FOR RESOLUTION

With the discovery of a class of serenic compounds that may have antiaggressive efficacy comes new hope of treating violence in humans. Unfortunately, the matter is complicated by phenomenological and ethical issues. The Food and Drug Administration has viewed aggression as a nonspecific behavior and has hesitated to approve the marketing of an antiaggressive drug. Consequently, clinical trials for the assessment of pharmacological efficacy have not begun in America. Society has ambivalent attitudes toward the suppression of aggression, fearing the potential political or scientific misuse of any antiaggressive agent. Since western society places a high value on self-determinism, the availability of a drug to pacify citizens is bound to evoke dismay. To some extent, similar concerns have been raised about the tranquilizers in general and benzodiazepines in particular.

Some efforts are currently under way to conceptualize aggression as a mood disorder. There are many similarities between aggression and other affective states, such as mania or depression. Psychodynamically, those affects have long been viewed as related. Aggression is often heralded by a prodromal dysphoric state, while the behavior of aggression is itself dysphoric. Aggression can be associated with depression through the established serotonergic links between externally directed violence and suicide. It can be associated with mania through the accompanying psychomotor and physiological arousal. More work in that direction needs to be done.

SUGGESTED CROSS-REFERENCES

Personality disorders are discussed in Chapter 25. Adult antisocial behavior and criminality are the subject of Section 28.3. Sexual abuse of adults is discussed in Section 29.7. Section 32.19 is devoted to the serotonin-specific reuptake inhibitors.

REFERENCES

Allen N: *Homicide: Perspectives on Prevention.* Human Sciences Press, New York, 1980.

Beck J C: *The Potentially Violent Patient and the Tarasoff Decision in Psychiatric Practice.* American Psychiatric Press, Washington, 1985.

Brown G L, Goodwin F K: Human aggression: A biological perspective. In *Unmasking the Psychopath,* W H Reid, D Dorr, J I Walker, J W Bonner, editors, p 132. Norton, New York, 1986.

Caldwell F: Applying social constructionism in the treatment of patients who are intractably aggressive. Hosp Community Psychiatry *45:* 597, 1994.

Conn L, Lion JR: Psychopharmacology of violence. Psychiatr Clin North Am *7:* 879, 1984.

Corrigan P W, Yudofsky S C, Silver J M: Pharmacological and behavioral treatments for aggressive psychiatric inpatients. Hosp Community Psychiatry *44:* 125, 1993.

Delgado-Escueta A V, Mattson R H, King L, Goldensohn E S, Spiegel H, Madsen J, Crandall P, Dreifuss F, Porter R J: The nature of aggression during epileptic seizures. N Engl J Med *305:* 711, 1981.

Dubin W, Lion J R, editors: *Clinician Safety: A Report of the American*

Psychiatric Association Task Force. American Psychiatric Press, Washington, 1993.
Eichelman B: Toward a rational pharmacotherapy for aggressive and violent behavior. Hosp Community Psychiatry *39:* 31, 1988.
Fava M, Rosenbaum J F, Pava J A, McCarthy M K, Steingard R J, Bouffides E: Anger attacks in unipolar depression, Part I: Clinical correlates and response to fluoxetine treatment. Am J Psychiatry *150:* 1158, 1993.
Favazza A R, Rosenthal R J: Diagnostic issues in self-mutilation. Hosp Community Psychiatry *44:* 134, 1993.
Fromm E: *The Anatomy of Human Destructiveness*. Holt, Rinehart and Winston, New York, 1973.
Golden R N, Gilmore J H, Corrigan M H, Ekstrom R D, Knight B T, Garbutt J C: Serotonin, suicide, and aggression: Clinical studies. J Clin Psychiatry 52 (Suppl): 61, 1991.
Herman H H, Hammock M K, Arthur-Smith A A, Egan J, Chatoor I, Werner A, Zelnick N: Naltrexone decreases self-injurious behavior. Ann Neurol *22:* 550, 1987.
Higley J D, Mehlman P T, Taub D M, Higley S B, Suomi S J, Linnoila M, Vickers D V M: Cerebrospinal fluid monoamine and adrenal correlates of aggression in free ranging rhesus monkeys. Arch Gen Psychiatry *49:* 436, 1992.
Lewis D O, Pincus J H, Bard B, Richardson E, Prichep L S, Feldman M A, Yeager C: Neuropsychiatric, psychoeducational, and family characteristics of 14 juveniles condemned to death in the United States. Am J Psychiatry *145:* 584, 1988.
Lion J R: Intermittent explosive disorder. Psychiatr Ann *22:* 64, 1992.
Lion J R: Training for battle: Thoughts on managing aggressive patients. Hosp Community Psychiatry *38:* 882, 1987.
*Lion J R, Reid W H, editors *Assaults Within Psychiatric Facilities*. Grune & Stratton, New York, 1983.
*Lystad M, editor: *Violence in the Home: Interdisciplinary Perspectives*. Brunner/Mazel, New York, 1986.
MacDonald J: Homicidal threats. Am J Psychiatry *124:* 475, 1967.
Mark V H, Ervin F R: *Violence and the Brain*. Harper & Row, New York, 1970.
Monahan J: *The Clinical Prediction of Violent Behavior*. National Institute of Mental Health, Rockville, MD, 1981.
Monahan J: Mental disorder and violent behavior. Am Psychol *47:* 511, 1992.
*Monroe R R: *Episodic Behavioral Disorders*. Harvard University Press, Cambridge, MA, 1970.
Raghoebar M, Olivier B, Rasmussen D L, Mos J, editors: Eltoprazine: A serenic compound. Drug Metab Drug Interact (Special Issue #1-2) *8:* 1, 1990.
*Ratey J, editor: *Clinical Aggression Research*. J Neuropsychiatry 3 (Suppl) 1991.
Restraint and Seclusion: Report of the American Psychiatric Association Task Force. American Psychiatric Press, Washington, 1985.
Rosenbaum J F, Fava M, Pava J A, McCarthy M K, Steingard R J, Bouffides E: Anger attacks in unipolar depression, Part 2: Neuroendocrine correlates and changes following fluoxetine treatment. Am J Psychiatry *150:* 1164, 1993.
Roy M, editor: *Battered Women: A Psychosocial Study of Domestic Violence*. Van Nostrand Reinhold, New York, 1977.
Sarles R M: Child abuse. In *Rage, Hate, Assault, and Other Forms of Violence*, D J Madden, J R Lion, editors, p 1. Spectrum, Jamaica NY, 1976.
Sturup G K: *Treating the Untreatable: Chronic Criminals at Herstedvester*. Johns Hopkins University Press, Baltimore, 1978.
*Tardiff K: *Assessment and Management of Violent Patients*. American Psychiatric Press, Washington, 1989.
Valzelli I, Morgese I, editors Aggression and Violence: A Psychobiological and Clinical Approach. Edizioni Centro Culturale E. Congressi, Saint Vincent, Milano, 1981.
Valzelli L: Psychobiology of Aggression and Violence. Raven, New York, 1981.
Virkkunen M, Kallio E, Rawlings R, Tokola R, Poland R E, Guidotti A, Nemeroff C, Bissette G, Kalogeras K, Karonen S L, Linnoila M:Personality profiles and state aggressiveness in Finnish alcoholics, violent offenders, fire setters, and healthy volunteers. Arch Gen Psychiatry *51:* 28, 1994.
West D J: *Murder Followed by Suicide*. Harvard University Press, Cambridge, MA, 1960.
Yudofsky S C, Silver J M, Jackson W, Endicott J, Williams D: The overt aggression scale for the objective rating of verbal and physical aggression. Am J Psychiatry *143:* 35, 1986.

3.5
BIOLOGY OF MEMORY

LARRY R. SQUIRE, Ph.D.
RICHARD D. McKEE, Ph.D.

The topic of memory is fundamental to the discipline of psychiatry. Personality is in part a set of habits and dispositions that develop from experience. The neuroses are largely products of learning; that is, anxieties, phobias, and predispositions are founded on specific experiences or on repeated patterns of experience. Psychotherapy itself is a process by which new behaviors are acquired through the accumulation of new experiences. Thus, memory is at the heart of psychiatry's concern with the individual, personal identity, and growth and development. Memory makes possible autobiographical recollection, it connects the present moment to what came before, and it is the basis for cultural evolution.

For the biologically trained psychiatrist, memory is of particular interest. Disorders of memory, and complaints about memory function, are common in neurological and psychiatric illness. Among patients with neurological disease, memory problems are considered to be among the most common initial complaint of higher function. Memory functions are also of special concern as side effects of certain psychiatric treatments, especially electroconvulsive therapy. Accordingly, the effective clinician needs to understand some of what is known about memory, its psychological organization and neurological foundations, and also about the varieties of memory dysfunction—how they present and what they mean. This section reviews the biology of memory and considers memory disorders from a biological perspective and describes how memory function can be evaluated in patients.

BIOLOGY OF MEMORY

MEMORY AS SYNAPTIC CHANGE Memory is a special case of the more general phenomenon of *neural plasticity*. At the level of nerve cells and synapses, the problem of memory can be illuminated by understanding the plasticity of neurons, that is, how neurons can show history-dependent behavior by responding differently as a function of recent input. In the last decade of the 19th century, researchers proposed that existing nerve cells can grow and that such growth could account for the stability of memory. Others have restated this idea since then, making explicit the hypothesis that the synapse is the critical site of plastic change. However, a number of possibilities are consistent with this general idea. The persistence of memory could in principle be based on structural alterations in the number of contacts between neurons or on structural changes in existing contacts that increase their strength. Alternatively, memory could be based on stable biochemical changes within neurons, which are not expressed as growth, but which nevertheless alter the way in which neighboring neurons communicate with one another.

During the past two decades, neurobiological studies have provided strong evidence in support of two related conclusions about the biology of memory: (1) distinct cellular and synaptic events are involved in short-lasting synaptic plasticity (which persists for seconds or minutes) and long-lasting synaptic plasticity (which may persist for days, weeks, or longer); and (2) long-term memory ultimately depends on physical growth of neural processes and on an increase in the number of synaptic connections.

One major source of information about the neurobiology of learning and memory has come from extended study of one invertebrate, the sea hare *(Aplysia californica)*. That marine mollusc is well suited for neurobiological study because the animal has a nervous system consisting of fewer than 20,000 neurons distributed among nine ganglia (Figure 3.5-1). Many of the cells are large enough to be seen by the naked eye, and they can be identified from animal to animal. In addition, the connections between the neurons can be determined, and it has been possible to work out much of the wiring diagram of simple behaviors. The *Aplysia* is capable of nonassociative learning (habituation and sensitization), and associative forms of learning, including classical conditioning and operant conditioning. The neurobiological analysis of memory has focused on the gill-withdrawal reflex (Figure 3.5-2), a defensive reflex whereby the application of tactile stimulation causes the gill and the siphon to retract. The reflex can be modified by behavioral experience. For example, the gill-withdrawal reflex is facilitated (sensitized) when tactile stimulation of the siphon is preceded by strong stimulation to the head of the animal. Under appropriate training conditions sensitization can persist for weeks.

In reduced preparations designed to investigate the cellular mechanisms underlying sensitization, it was found that short-lasting synaptic facilitation can be produced by a single application of serotonin, a transmitter released by stimuli that produce sensitization. The facilitation is based on an enhanced release of transmitter by the presynaptic neuron and is accompanied by covalent modifications of preexisting proteins. Changes lasting more than one day can be produced by several repeated applications of serotonin, distributed over a period of 1½ hours. The long-term change resembles the short-term change in several respects. For example, the long-term change occurs at the same site as the short-term change, and the long-term change, like the short-term change, is based on enhanced release of transmitter. However, in contrast to the short-term change, the long-term change is blocked by inhibitors of transcription or translation. That is, the long-term change uniquely requires the expression of genes and the synthesis of proteins. In addition, the long-term change, but not the short-term change, is accompanied by growth of the processes of the sensory neuron and by an increase in the number of synaptic connections between the sensory neuron and the motor neuron.

Less direct evidence is available about the neural basis of long-lasting memory in vertebrates. However, it is clear that behavioral manipulations can result in measurable changes in the brain's architecture. For example, rats reared in enriched environments show an increase in the number of synapses ending on individual neurons in neocortex. These changes are accompanied by numerically small but statistically reliable increases in cortical thickness, in the diameter of neuronal cell bodies, and in the number and length of dendritic branches. Thus, experience can increase the number of synapses, presumably either by forming them outright or by selectively preserving synapses from a population that is continuously being replaced. Behavioral experience can exert powerful effects on the wiring of the vertebrate brain.

Many of these same structural changes have been found in adult animals given a period of exposure to an enriched environment, and some have been found in adult animals given

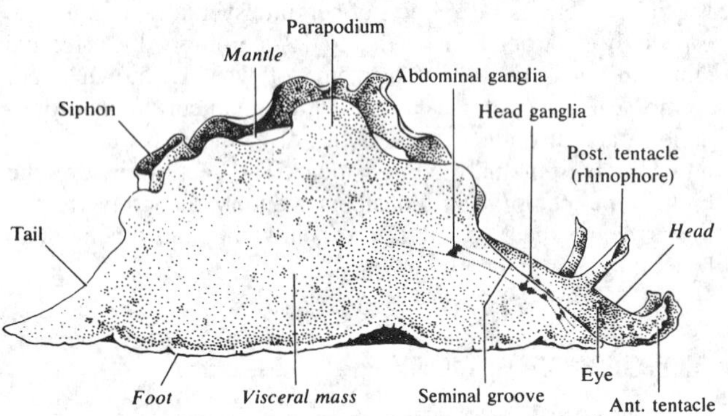

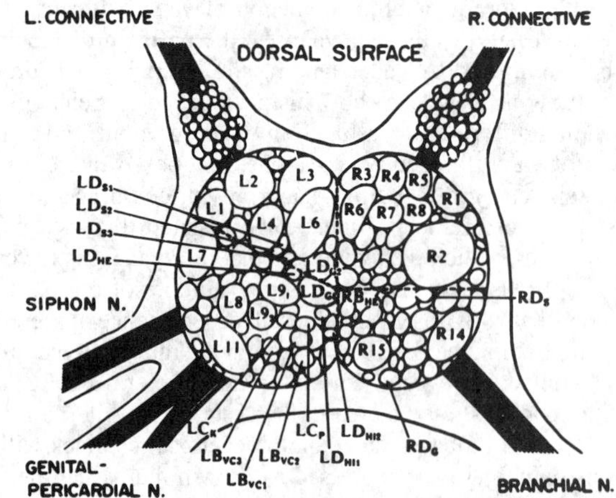

FIGURE 3.5-1 *(Top) Lateral view of the marine snail* Aplysia californica. *(Bottom) Cross-sectional view of the abdominal ganglion of* Aplysia *showing identified cells. The relative simplicity of the nervous system makes* Aplysia *a valuable organism for studying cellular and synaptic mechanisms of behavioral memory. (Top figure from E R Kandel:* Cellular Basis of Behavior. *Freeman, San Francisco, 1976. Used with permission. Bottom figure from E R Kandel: Psychotherapy and the single synapse. N Engl J Med 301: 1028, 1979. Used with permission.)*

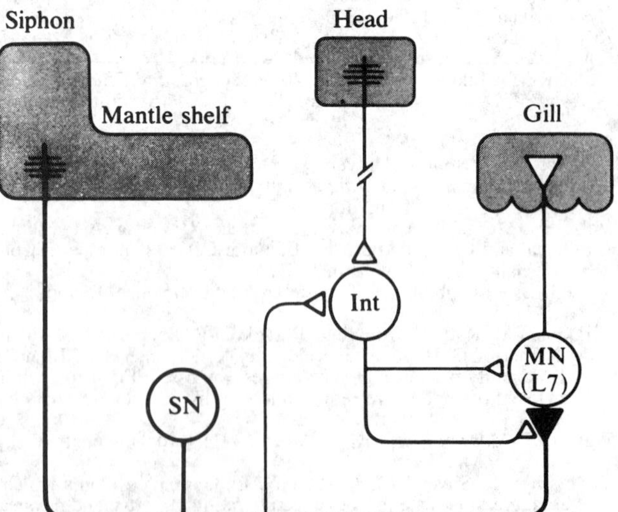

FIGURE 3.5-2 *A simplified schematic representation of the neuronal circuit underlying behavioral habituation and sensitization of the gill-withdraw reflex in* Aplysia. *The synapse between the sensory neuron (SN) and the motor neuron (MN) is an important site of habituation. Sensitization results from activation of the interneuron (Int) pathway. (Figure from E R Kandel:* Cellular Basis of Behavior. *Freeman, San Francisco, 1976. Used with permission.)*

extensive maze training. In this case, opaque contact-lens occluders were used to restrict vision to one eye, and the corpus callosum was transected to prevent information received by one cerebral hemisphere from reaching the other hemisphere. In these monocularly trained animals, increases in the size of dendritic fields of pyramidal neurons of occipital cortex were found only in the trained hemisphere. This finding rules out a number of nonspecific influences including motor activity, indirect effects of hormones, and overall level of arousal. Although more direct data are needed, it seems likely that long-term memory in vertebrates is generally based on morphological growth and change.

A potentially important cellular mechanism for memory in vertebrates is the phenomenon of long-term potentiation (LTP). LTP is a form of neural plasticity in which the response strength of a postsynaptic neuron is persistently increased following a brief burst of high-frequency stimulation. LTP has a number of properties that make it a promising memory mechanism. First, it is established quickly and then lasts for a long time. Second, it is associative; that is, it depends on the co-occurrence of postsynaptic depolarization and presynaptic activity. Third, it is synapse specific, that is, it occurs only at the potentiated synapses, not at all the synapses terminating on the target cell. Finally, LTP occurs prominently in the hippocampus, a structure in the medial temporal lobe that is importantly involved in memory function. The induction of LTP is known to be mediated postsynaptically and to involve the N-methyl-D-aspartate (NMDA) receptor, which when activated permits the influx of calcium into the cell. The mechanism of how LTP is maintained and expressed is not yet understood. Evidence has been presented in favor of a presynaptic locus of change—increased transmitter release, but evidence has also been presented favoring a postsynaptic locus—an increase in the sensitivity or number of postsynaptic receptors. Rapidly developing structural changes in the dendritic spines of the postsynaptic neuron have also been described in association with LTP. Currently, LTP is the best available mechanism for memory in vertebrates, and it merits intensive study. Although its potential role in memory is not well understood, it will be clear from what follows that LTP, at least in the hippocampus where it is most commonly studied, cannot be the mechanism for recording permanent memories. The role of the hippocampus in memory is only temporary. LTP could provide the mechanism by which the hippocampus carries out its contribution to memory, but hippocampal LTP is not a mechanism for the recording of complex experiences at the synapses where LTP occurs.

ORGANIZATION OF MEMORY Understanding the biology of memory requires more than just an understanding of the synaptic events that store memory. It is also essential to understand how and where synaptic events are organized in the brain. Many levels of analysis can be identified between synaptic change and behavioral memory, and many important questions about memory address levels of biological analysis that are intermediate to synapses and behavior.

One major issue concerns the question of where memory is stored. In the 1920s Karl Lashley carried out a series of famous experiments that were directed at this problem. Lashley recorded the number of trials that rats needed to relearn a preoperatively trained maze problem after removal of different amounts of neocortex. The deficit was proportional to the amount of cortex removed and, further, it seemed to be qualitatively similar, regardless of what region of cortex was removed. Lashley concluded that memory for the maze habit was not localized in any one part of the brain, but instead was distributed equivalently over the entire cortex. Subsequent work has led to a revision of this idea. Maze learning in rats depends on many forms of information, including visual, tactual, spatial, and olfactory information, which is processed and stored in different areas. Thus, the correlation between retention score and lesion size that Lashley observed reflects the progressive encroachment on specialized cortical areas serving the many components of cognition important to maze learning.

Other examples indicate that restricted areas of the cerebrum are involved in different kinds of memory. For example, the eyeblink-nictitating membrane response in rabbits has been used to study classical conditioning. In that paradigm repeated pairings of a tone (conditioned stimulus) and an airpuff (unconditioned stimulus) to the eye lead to a conditioned eyeblink in response to the tone. Eyeblink conditioning provides the best evidence available for the involvement of specific pathways in the storage of specific information in the vertebrate nervous system. Lesions of the deep nuclei of the cerebellum eliminate the classically conditioned response without affecting the unconditioned response, which indicates that the cerebellum contains part of the essential circuitry for the conditioned stimulus-unconditioned stimulus (CS-US) association. This finding does not mean that all the changes occurring in the animal during conditioning involve the cerebellum; it means only that some of the essential neural changes responsible for the CS-US link depend on this circuitry.

Other work has concerned how visual information is processed and stored in nonhuman primates. The cortical pathway for visual information processing (Figure 3.5-3) begins in primary visual cortex (V1 in Figure 3.5-3) and proceeds from there along parallel pathways or streams. One stream projects ven-

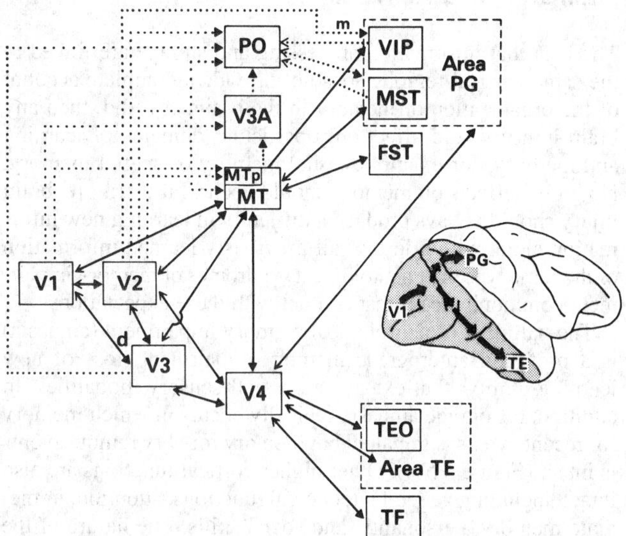

FIGURE 3.5-3 *Summary of cortical visual areas and some of their connections. There are two major routes from striate cortex (V1): One follows a ventral route into the temporal lobe via V4, and the other follows a ventral route into the parietal lobe via MT. Heavy arrowheads indicate forward projections, and light arrowheads indicate backward projections. Intermediate projections are indicated by two heavy arrowheads. The use of "d" indicates a projection that is limited to the dorsal portion of the area; "m," one that is limited to the medial portion. Other potential pathways into the parietal lobe include those carrying input from the peripheral visual field (dotted lines). (Figure from L G Ungerleider, R Desimone: Cortical connections of visual area MT in the macaque. J Comp Neurol 248: 190, 1986. Used with permission.)*

trally to the inferotemporal cortex (area TE in Figure 3.5-3) and processes information about visual pattern. Another stream projects dorsally to parietal cortex and processes information about spatial location. Electrophysiological studies in the monkey show that neurons in area TE register specific and complex features of visual stimuli, for example, particular kinds of curvature and handlike shapes. Furthermore, TE lesions impair visual learning and memory without loss of visual acuity. These findings have led to the view that, in addition to being a higher-order visual processing system, TE is a storehouse of the visual memories that result from the processing.

Memory in the nervous system is both distributed and localized. It is distributed in the sense that, as Lashley found, there is no one center where entire memories are stored. Many parts of the nervous system participate in representing a single event in memory. Memory is localized in the sense that different aspects or dimensions of memory for an event are stored at specific sites, in the same regions that are already specialized to analyze and process particular aspects or dimensions of information.

In monkeys, information stored in visual area TE may serve to identify objects, but other important components of events involving objects will be processed and stored separately (for example, spatial, temporal, tactual, or olfactory information). Viewed in this way, the problem of memory storage involves a series of related issues. First, any particular event or learning task is composed of a number of components. Second, each component engages a particular processing site. Third, each processing site stores information as an outcome of the processing that is done.

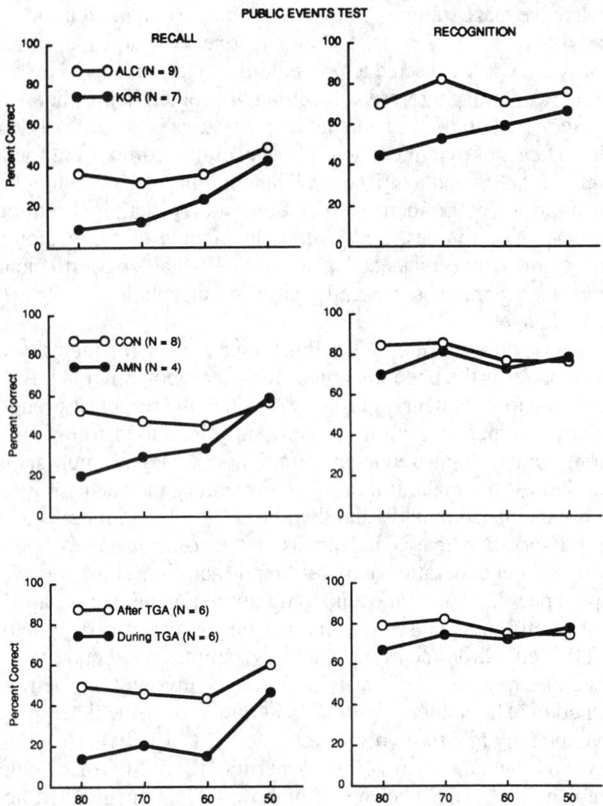

FIGURE 3.5-4 *Remote memory performance of amnesic patients with Korsakoff's syndrome (KOR), alcoholic control subjects (ALC), amnesic patients with confirmed or suspected damage to the hippocampal formation (AMN), healthy control subjects (CON), and patients with transient global amnesia (TGA). (Left) Recall of past public events that had occurred in one of the four decades from 1950 to 1985. (Right) Performance on a multiple-choice test (four alternatives) involving the same public events (Figure from M Kritchevsky, L R Squire: Transient global ischemia: Evidence for extensive, temporally graded retrograde amnesia. Neurology 39: 213, 1989. Used with permission. Also from L R Squire, F Haist, A P Shimamura: The neurology of memory: Quantitative assessment of retrograde amnesia in two groups of amnesic patients. J Neurosci 9: 828, 1989. Used with permission.)*

MEMORY AND AMNESIA

The idea that information processing and storage are linked to the same cortical regions does not provide a complete account of the organization of memory in the brain. If it did, then any brain injury would affect only particular domains of learning and memory, for example, visual memory or spatial memory. No global effects on memory should occur. Furthermore, brain injury should always produce a difficulty in learning new information along with a loss of all previously learned information of the same type. Yet neurological syndromes of memory impairment commonly occur that conflict with these expectations.

The hallmark of neurological memory impairment (amnesia) is a profound anterograde memory impairment (loss of new learning ability) that extends across all sensory modalities. In addition, retrograde amnesia typically occurs in which memory for recent events is impaired but memory for very remote events is intact (Figure 3.5-4). Other higher cortical functions are also intact, including general intellectual functions, attention, immediate memory, personality, and social skills. The nature of the memory deficit in amnesia makes the important point that the brain has separated to some extent its intellectual functions and perceptual processing functions from the ability to lay down a record of the memories that ordinarily result from this processing. The finding that anterograde amnesia can occur despite intact remote memory indicates that the brain structures damaged in amnesia are not the long-term repositories of memory. Detailed studies of human amnesic patients and animal models of amnesia have illuminated these issues considerably.

NEUROANATOMY OF AMNESIA Amnesia results from damage to either of two brain regions: the medial temporal lobe or the midline diencephalon. Early studies of one remarkable patient (H M) particularly stimulated investigation of the role of the medial temporal lobe. H M became amnesic in 1953, when he sustained a bilateral resection of the medial temporal lobe to relieve severe epilepsy. The removal included the amygdala, the anterior two thirds of the hippocampus, and underlying cortex. Following the surgery, H M's seizure condition was much improved, he had normal language, preserved intellectual functions, and a normal short-term memory (for example, digit span). However, he had a profound anterograde amnesia, together with some retrograde amnesia. In the early 1990s H M is in his late 60s and continues to participate in experimental studies.

More recently, favorable cases of amnesia have permitted more detailed analysis of the anatomy of medial temporal lobe memory functions. For example, patient R B was a 52-year old former postal worker who in 1978 developed a moderately severe anterograde amnesia (and little retrograde amnesia) following an episode of global ischemia. After his death five years later, extensive histological studies of his brain revealed a circumscribed bilateral lesion of hippocampal area CA1 (Figure 3.5-5). Only minor additional pathology was found and none

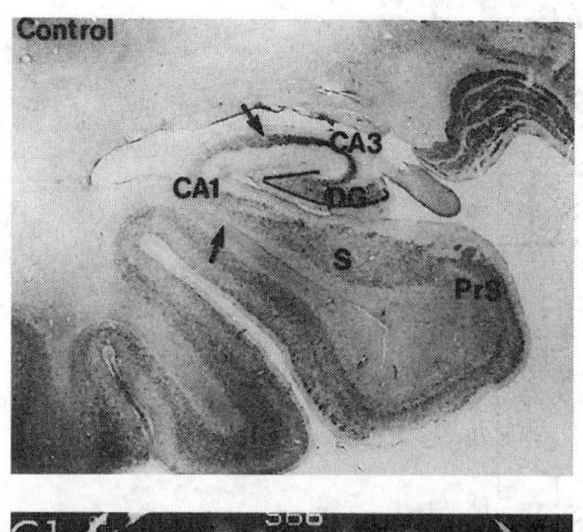

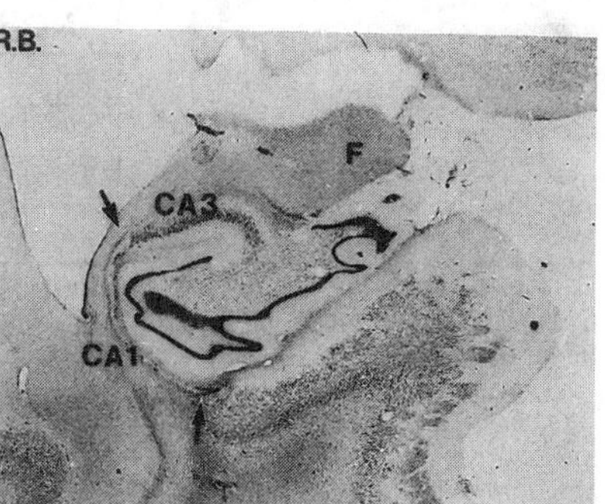

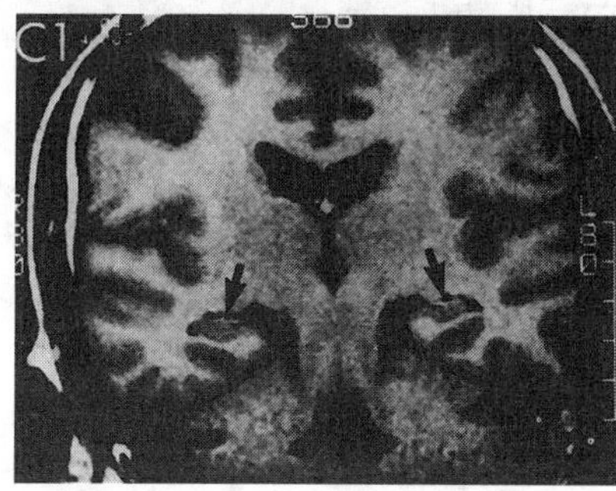

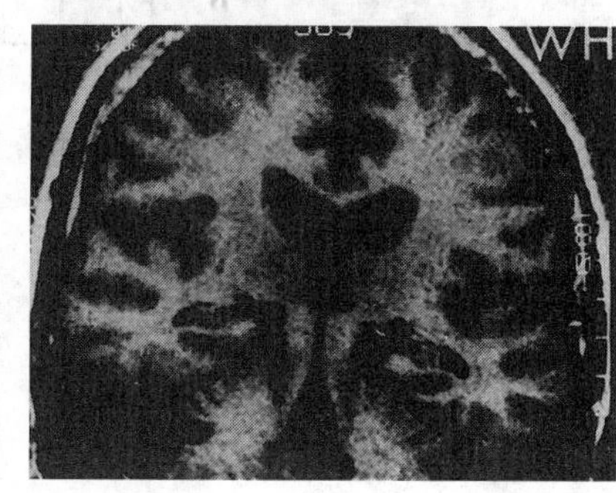

FIGURE 3.5-5 *(Top left panel) Section through the hippocampus of a normal subject. (Top right panel) Section through the hippocampus of amnesic patient R. B., showing damage to the CA1 region. (Bottom left panel) Magnetic resonance scan of a normal subject (resolution = 0.625 mm). Several anatomical features of the hippocampal formation can be distinguished. (Bottom right panel) Magnetic resonance scan of amnesic patient W. H. using the same protocol. The hippocampal formation is markedly reduced in size. The calibration bars to the right represent 5 cm in 1-cm increments. (Top panels reprinted from L R Squire: The mechanisms of memory. Science* 232: *1612, 1986. Used with permission. Bottom panels reprinted from G A Press, D G Amaral, L R Squire: Hippocampal abnormalities in amnesic patients revealed by high-resolution magnetic resonance imaging. Nature* 341: *54, 1989. Used with permission.)*

that could reasonably explain the memory impairment. More recently, improved high-resolution protocols using magnetic resonance imaging (MRI) have been able to identify pathological change in the hippocampal region of other amnesic patients. The significant finding is that even damage limited to the hippocampus itself can result in clinically significant memory impairment. Furthermore, because H M is considerably more amnesic than R B, hippocampal regions other than field CA1 or, more likely, structures in the medial temporal lobe in addition to the hippocampus, must contribute to memory functions.

The findings from human amnesia inspired the development of models of amnesia in experimental animals. Early studies with animals yielded contradictory findings that could not be easily related to memory impairment. In part, the difficulty was that human amnesia itself was poorly understood. As discussed below, memory is now appreciated to be a collection of different abilities and not a unitary mental faculty. Human amnesia affects only one kind of memory. Until researchers learned this lesson, it was unclear what parallels should be looked for in experimental animals, and it was unclear what kinds of tasks would be appropriate for modeling amnesia in experimental animals.

In the early 1980s an animal model of human amnesia was successfully developed in the nonhuman primate. Several years of systematic study subsequently identified the important structures and connections in the medial temporal lobe memory system. In those studies, monkeys with surgical damage to specific structures were trained to perform tasks that are identical to or, in some cases, analogous to tasks that are sensitive to memory impairment in humans. Monkeys with large medial temporal lobe lesions, which were intended to approximate the damage that occurred in patient H M, exhibited many features of human amnesia. For example, the impairment was multimodal (that is, it occurred in more than one sensory modality), short-term memory was intact, the deficit was enduring, skill learning was preserved, and retrograde amnesia was temporally graded. The important structures are the hippocampus and adjacent, anatomically related cortex including entorhinal, perirhinal, and parahippocampal cortices (Figure 3.5-6).

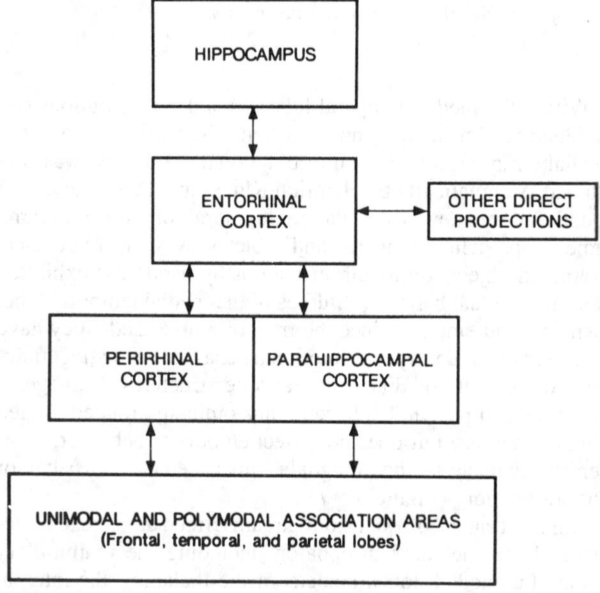

FIGURE 3.5-6 *A schematic view of the medial temporal lobe memory system. The system consists of the hippocampus and the underlying entorhinal, perirhinal, and parahippocampal cortices. The entorhinal cortex is the major source of projections to the hippocampus. Nearly two thirds of the cortical input to the entorhinal cortex originates in the adjacent perirhinal and parahippocampal cortices, which in turn receive projections from unimodal and polymodal areas in the frontal, temporal, and parietal lobes. The entorhinal cortex receives other direct inputs from orbital frontal cortex, cingulate gyrus, insular cortex, and superior temporal gyrus. All these projections are reciprocal. (Figure from L R Squire, S Zola-Morgan: Science* 253: *1380, 1991. Used with permission.)*

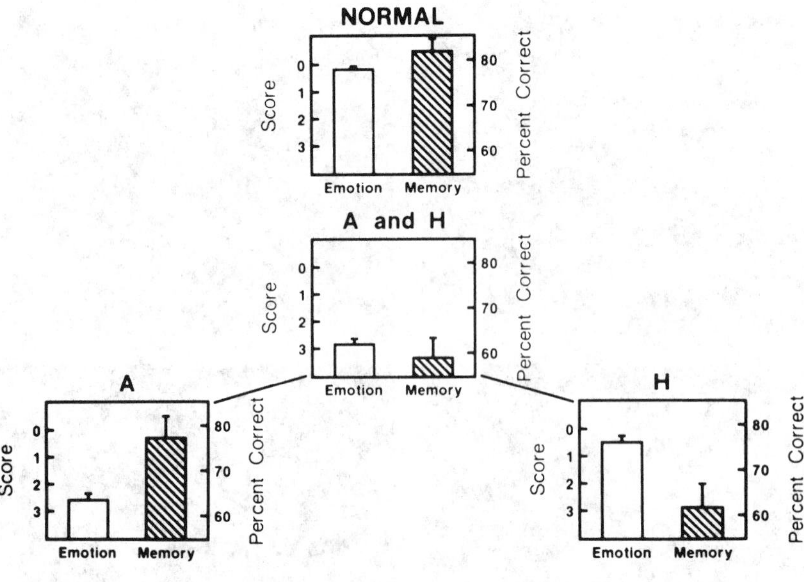

FIGURE 3.5-7 *Dissociation of emotional reactivity and memory by lesions of the amygdala and the hippocampal formation. The score for emotional reactivity was obtained by measuring the responsiveness of monkeys to seven objects that could elicit investigatory or consummatory behavior. The memory score is the score on the delayed nonmatching to sample task at a 10-minute delay. In both cases, a high score indicates normal performance. Normal (top panel) performance of 15 normal monkeys. A and H (middle panel): performance of monkeys with damage to both the hippocampal formation and the amygdala. A (lower left panel): performance of monkeys with damage to the amygdala but not the hippocampal formation. H (lower right panel): performance of monkeys with damage to the hippocampal formation and associated cortical areas, but not the amygdala. Brackets show the standard error of the mean. The figure shows that lesions of the amygdala impaired emotional reactivity, lesions of the hippocampal formation or related cortex impaired memory, and combined lesions produced both kinds of impairment. (Figure from S Zola-Morgan, L R Squire, P Alvarez, R Clower: Independence of memory functions and emotional behavior: Separate contributions of the hippocampal formation and the amygdala. Hippocampus* 1: *207, 1991. Used with permission.)*

Within the medial temporal lobe, separate contributions can be identified for memory and emotion. The participation of the medial temporal lobe region in emotional expression was first studied systematically by Heinrich Kluver and Paul Bucy, who found that monkeys with bilateral temporal lobectomy became tame, approached animals and objects without reluctance, examined objects by mouth instead of by hand, and exhibited abnormal sexual behavior. Studies of the medial temporal lobe, memory, and emotion since the time of Kluver and Bucy have indicated that memory and emotional behavior are distinct functions of separate medial temporal lobe structures. Damage to the hippocampus and adjacent, anatomically related cortex impairs memory but does not affect emotional behavior. Conversely, damage to the amygdala impairs emotional behavior but not memory (Figure 3.5-7).

Amnesia can also result from circumscribed damage to structures of the medial diencephalon, including the mammillary nuclei, the medial dorsal nucleus of the thalamus, the internal medullary lamina, and the mammillothalamic tract. Korsakoff's syndrome is the best studied example of diencephalic amnesia. However, patients with alcoholic Korsakoff's syndrome typically have frontal lobe pathology in addition to diencephalic damage, and the frontal lobe pathology produces a pattern of cognitive impairment which is dissociable from amnesia itself and which, in the case of the patient with Korsakoff's syndrome, is superimposed on severe memory impairment (Table 3.5-1).

Because medial temporal lobe and diencephalic amnesia involve damage to separate brain regions, it has been natural to suppose that the two forms of amnesia should be distinct behaviorally as well. In fact, there is as yet no compelling demonstration of qualitatively different patterns of memory impairment for medial temporal lobe and diencephalic amnesia. Although it is reasonable to expect that the brain regions damaged in these two groups should make different contributions to normal memory, each region may also be a critical component of a larger functional system. If so, it may be difficult to demonstrate a difference in the functional contribution of each region using behavioral measures.

The brain regions damaged in amnesia are not the permanent repositories of memory. Damage to the hippocampus or related structures in the medial temporal lobe produces a loss of memory for events that were acquired prior to the time that the damage occurred. Retrograde memory loss is temporally graded affecting recent memories more than remote memories (Figure

TABLE 3.5-1
Associated and Dissociated Deficits in Amnesia

Test	Amnesia	Korsakoff's syndrome	Frontal lobe damage
Delayed Recall	+	+	−
Dementia rating scale: memory index	+	+	−
Dementia rating scale initiation/perseveration index	−	+	+
Wisconsin Card-Sorting Test	−	+	+
Temporal order memory	+	++	++
Metamemory	−	+	+
Release from proactive interference	−	+	−

Pattern of cognitive impairment associated with amnesia (e.g., after medial temporal lobe damage), Korsakoff's syndrome, and frontal lobe pathology without amnesia. Korsakoff's syndrome is associated with both diencephalic lesions (which produce amnesia) and with frontal lobe pathology.
(+) Deficit; (−) no deficit; (++) disproportionately impaired relative to item memory.
Table from Squire L R, Zola-Morgan S, Cave C B, Haist F, Musen G, and Suzuki W A: Memory, organization of brain systems and cognition. *In* Cold Spring Harbor Symposia on Quantitative Biology, Vol LV. Cold Spring Harbor Laboratory Press, Plainview, NY, 1990. Used with permission.

3.5-8). This graded memory loss has been demonstrated retrospectively in studies of amnesic patients and prospectively in studies of monkeys, rats, and mice. Thus, the limbic-diencephalic structures damaged in amnesia make only a temporary contribution to memory. As time passes after learning, the contribution of these structures gradually diminishes, and a more permanent memory gradually develops, presumably in neocortex. The limbic-diencephalic structures damaged in amnesia are needed at the time of learning and during this gradual process. After sufficient time has elapsed, long-term memories are maintained and retrieved independently of limbic-diencephalic structures.

MULTIPLE MEMORY SYSTEMS

Not all kinds of memory are impaired in amnesia. The kind that is impaired has been termed *declarative* (or *explicit*) *memory*. Declarative memory includes conscious recollections of facts and events. Thus, a deficit in declarative memory presents itself

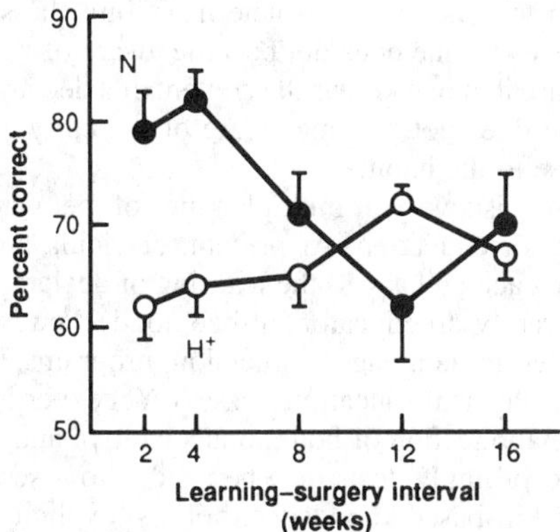

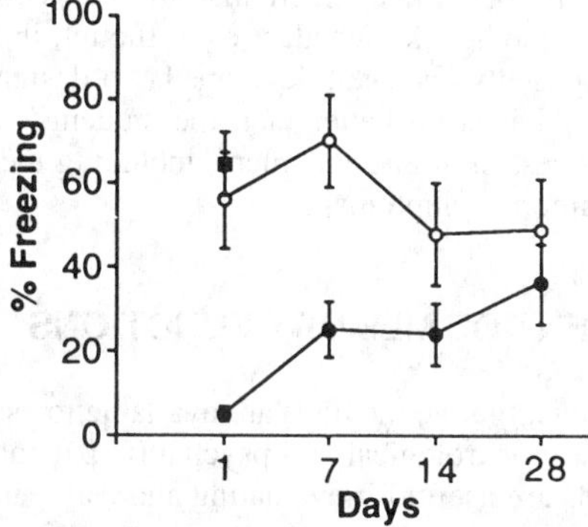

FIGURE 3.5-8 *Temporally graded retrograde amnesia following damage to the hippocampal formation in prospective studies of the monkey and rat. (Top) Retention of 100 object discrimination problems learned approximately 2, 4, 8, 12, and 16 weeks before hippocampal surgery (20 pairs per time period). Retention was assessed two weeks after surgery in monkeys with lesions (H^+) ($n = 11$) or after an equivalent interval in unoperated animals (N) ($n = 7$). Brackets show standard error of the mean. (Bottom) Freezing behavior in rats tested after fear conditioning. The hippocampus (closed circles) was removed at different times after conditioning, as shown, and testing occurred seven days after surgery. The cortical lesion group is shown by a square, the control animals by open circles. Brackets show ± standard error of the mean. (Figure from J J Kim, M S Fanselow: Modality-specific retrograde amnesia of fear. Science 256: 675, 1992. Used with permission.)*

as a global disorder that impairs memory for routes, lists, faces, melodies, objects, and other verbal and nonverbal material, regardless of the sensory modality in which the material is presented. However, many other kinds of learning and memory are preserved, specifically a heterogeneous collection of nonconscious abilities, collectively termed *nondeclarative* (or *implicit*). Nondeclarative memory includes skill learning, habit learning, conditioning, and the phenomenon of priming. Thus, amnesic patients can acquire certain perceptual, perceptuomotor, and cognitive skills as rapidly as normal subjects. For example, amnesic patients learned to read mirror-reversed text at a normal rate, they exhibited the normal facilitation in reading speed with successive (out loud) readings of normal prose, and they improved as rapidly as normal subjects at speeded reading of repeating nonwords. Amnesic patients were also able to classify novel strings of letters as rule-based or not rule-based after seeing several strings of letters that were generated by a finite-state rule system. Subjects first studied the letter strings one at a time and then were told for the first time that the letter strings could be generated by a complex set of rules. Performance on the classification test was similar in the amnesic patients and the normal subjects, despite the fact that the amnesic patients were unable to remember the previously studied items or the events of training as well as normal subjects.

Priming refers to a facilitation of the ability to detect or identify stimuli based on their recent presentation. Priming also occurs at full strength in amnesia. Thus, amnesic patients exhibit the normal tendency to complete three-letter stems (for example, MOT____) with previously encountered words (MOTEL) when they are instructed to produce the first word that comes to mind. They also exhibit priming of object names and priming of novel objects. For example, in one experiment, patients named pictures of new objects with a latency of about 1190 msec. They named pictures of previously presented objects faster than new objects (response latency = 1020 msec), even after a delay of a week. This facilitation occurred at normal levels in amnesic patients, despite the fact that the patients were markedly impaired at identifying which pictures had been presented previously. Recent positron emission tomography (PET) studies and divided visual-field studies of word-stem completion priming suggest that repetition priming occurs at early stages of perceptual processing. In the PET studies, priming of visually presented words was associated with changes in cortical sensory processing systems in right extrastriate cortex.

A tentative organization of memory systems appears in Figure 3.5-9. One memory system, which supports declarative memory, depends on medial temporal lobe and diencephalic structures. The system provides for the rapid learning of facts (semantic knowledge) and events. Nondeclarative memory depends on several different brain systems, depending on what is being acquired. Habits likely depend on connections between the neocortex and the neostriatum. The cerebellum is important for conditioning of skeletal musculature, the amygdala for emotional learning, and the neocortex for priming.

Declarative and nondeclarative memory differ in important ways. Declarative memory is phylogenetically more recent than nondeclarative memory. In addition, declarative memory is flexible and is available to conscious recollection; that is, acquired information is available to multiple response systems. Nondeclarative memory tends to be inflexible and inaccessible to awareness. Nondeclarative learning is stored as changes in the processing systems themselves, changes that are encapsulated with limited accessibility to other processing systems.

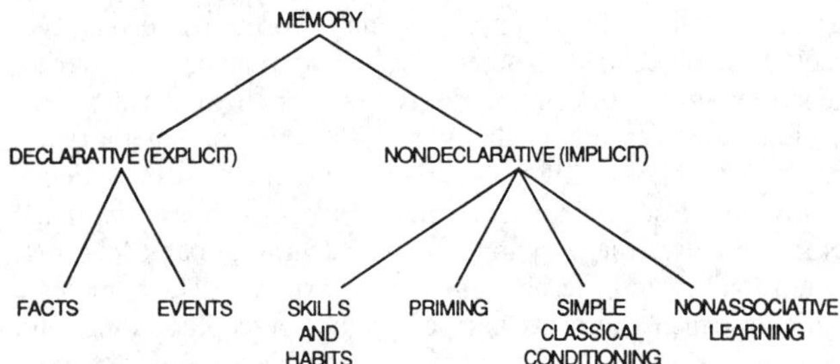

FIGURE 3.5-9 *A tentative memory taxonomy. Declarative memory refers to conscious recollections of facts and events and depends on limbic/diencephalic brain structures. Nondeclarative memory refers to a collection of abilities and is independent of these structures. In these cases performance changes as the result of experience but without affording access to the original experience or to any conscious memory content. Nonassociative learning includes habituation and sensitization. (Figure from L R Squire, S Zola-Morgan: The medial temporal lobe memory system. Science* 253: *1380, 1991. Used with permission.)*

IMPLICATIONS FOR PSYCHIATRY

Current understanding of the biology of memory has significant implications for certain traditional issues in psychiatry, for example, the problem of infantile amnesia, which is the apparent absence of conscious memory for experiences that occurred during approximately the first three years of life. Traditional views of infantile amnesia have emphasized the role of either repression (psychoanalytic theory) or retrieval failure (developmental psychology). The assumption was that adults retain memories of early events but cannot bring them into consciousness. More recently, it was suggested that nondeclarative memory capacity (for example, classical conditioning and skill learning) emerges early in infancy but that declarative memory abilities do not become available until about the third year, perhaps because the limbic-diencephalic structures essential for declarative memory are not fully developed until that time. By this view, infantile amnesia results not from the adult's failure to retrieve early memories, but from the child's failure to store them in the first place. This is an intriguing suggestion, but experiments designed to test this possibility have not supported the strong version of this idea. First, recall-like memory abilities have been demonstrated in young infants. In addition, it now appears that one of the most commonly employed tests of infant memory, the visual-paired comparison task, depends on declarative memory.

Infantile amnesia may still reflect the slow development of declarative memory. However, what likely limits its development is not the maturation of the limbic-diencephalic structures essential for declarative memory, but rather the gradual development and maturation of the neocortex. As the neocortex develops, the memories supported and stored there can become more complex. Strategies emerge for organizing incoming information, language develops, and declarative memories become more richly encoded and persistent. The existence of multiple forms of memory and the gradual maturation of neocortex suggest an alternative to traditional views of infantile amnesia. It is not necessary to suppose that memories were fully formed and that the only difficulty is in retrieval. An alternative view is that the capacity to store a viable declarative memory develops only gradually.

The existence of multiple memory systems also has implications for issues of interest to psychoanalytic theory, including the construct of the unconscious. In considering the effects of past experience, it is significant what view one takes of the nature of memory. By the traditional view, memory is a unitary faculty, and representations in memory vary mainly in strength and accessibility. In this view, material that is unconscious is below some threshold of accessibility and could potentially be made available to consciousness. In contrast, the discovery that there is more than one kind of memory has resulted in a distinction between conscious memory (declarative memory) that by its nature can be brought to mind and other kinds that are by their nature nonconscious, in the sense that the knowledge is expressed through performance without affording any conscious memory content. In this view, early experience might affect later behavior, but the manner in which the experience persists to affect behavior need not include a record of the event itself. Behavior is simply different. Thus, experience accumulates in altered dispositions, preferences, conditioned responses, habits, and skills, but these changes do not afford any actual awareness that behavior is being influenced by past experience. In this sense, the unconscious does not become conscious. Behavioral change can occur by acquiring new habits that supersede old ones, or by becoming sufficiently aware of a habit that one can to some extent isolate it or limit the stimuli that elicit it. However, one does not become aware of its content in the same sense that one knows the content of a declarative memory, and one does not become aware of the early experiences that gave rise to the habit.

Finally, the discovery of multiple kinds of memory has some significance for education. At present, curricula are designed primarily to teach and assess the learning of declarative knowledge. Only rarely do educators utilize nondeclarative memory (for example, in language immersion programs, vocational training, and physical education classes). Yet expertise in a field involves the application of both nondeclarative and declarative memory. Accordingly, tests may be needed to assess expertise and related skill-based knowledge, not just explicit knowledge of facts. It has been observed that fourth-year medical students typically perform better than practicing physicians on multiple-choice tests of medical knowledge, even though their clinical skills are supposedly less well developed. To design a test on which the physicians do better than the students, one would presumably assess skill and judgment, including the ability to see patterns among symptoms.

ASSESSMENT OF MEMORY FUNCTIONS

A variety of quantitative methods are available to assess memory functions in neurological and psychiatric patients. Quantitative methods are useful for evaluating and following patients longitudinally as well as for carrying out a one-time examination to determine the status of memory function. It is usually desirable to obtain information about the severity of memory function as well as to determine, if a memory problem is detected, whether memory is selectively affected or whether memory problems are occurring, as they do in dementia, against a background of intellectual deficits. The following section presents a rationale for evaluating memory and identifies areas of memory function that should be evaluated in any comprehensive assessment. Although there are some readily available tests, such as the Wechsler Memory Scale-Revised, which provide a useful measure of memory, most single tests assess memory rather narrowly, and even general-purpose neuropsychological batteries provide for only limited testing of memory functions. A complete assessment of memory usually involves a number of specialized tests which sample intellectual functions, new learning capacity, remote memory, and memory self-report.

INTELLECTUAL FUNCTIONS The assessment of general intellectual functions is fundamental to any neuropsychological examination. In the case of memory testing, information about intellectual functions provides both information about a patient's general test-taking ability and a way to assess the selectiveness of memory impairment. Useful tests include the Wechsler Adult Intelligence Scale-Revised, a test of object naming such as the Boston Naming Test, a rating scale to assess the possibility of global dementia, a test of word fluency, and specialized tests of frontal lobe function.

NEW LEARNING CAPACITY Memory tests are sensitive to impaired new learning ability when they adhere to either of two important principles. First, tests are sensitive to memory impairment when more information is presented than can be held in immediate memory. For example, one might ask patients to memorize a list of 10 faces, words, sentences, or digits, as 10 items is more than can be held in mind. The paired-associate learning task is an especially sensitive test of this kind. In the paired-associate task, the examiner asks the patient to learn a list of unrelated pairs of words (for example, queen-garden, officer-river) and then to respond to the first word in each pair by recalling the second word.

Second, tests are sensitive to memory impairment when a delay, filled with distraction, is interposed between the learning phase and the test phase. In that case, researchers typically ask patients to learn a small amount of information and then distract them for several minutes by conversation, to prevent rehearsal. Recollection is then assessed for the previously presented material. Memory can be tested by unaided recall of previously studied material (free recall), or by presenting a cue for the material to be remembered (cued recall), or by any of several methods for testing recognition memory. In multiple-choice tests of recognition memory, the patient tries to select previously studied items from a group of studied and unstudied items. In yes-no recognition tests, patients see both studied and unstudied items one at a time and are asked to say "yes" if the item was presented previously and "no" if it was not. These various methods for assessing recently learned material can be ranked in terms of their sensitivity for detecting memory impairment (from most sensitive to least sensitive: free recall, cued recall, yes-no recognition, multiple-choice recognition). In practice, a cued-recall test can vary widely in its sensitivity, depending on how effective a cue is provided.

VERBAL AND NONVERBAL MEMORY The specialization of the cerebral hemispheres means that left and right unilateral damage to limbic-diencephalic structures is associated with different kinds of memory problems. Accordingly, different kinds of memory tests must be used when either left or right unilateral damage is a possibility. Damage to limbic-diencephalic structures in the left cerebral hemisphere causes difficulty remembering verbal material such as word lists and stories. Damage to limbic-diencephalic structures in the right cerebral hemisphere impairs memory for faces, spatial arrangements, and other material that is typically encoded without verbal labels. For example, left medial temporal lobe damage impairs memory for both spoken and written text. Right medial temporal lobe damage impairs the learning of spatial arrays, whether the layouts are examined visually or by touch. One well-known test of nonverbal memory asks patients to copy a complex geometric figure and then, without forewarning, to reproduce it after a delay of several minutes (Figure 3.5-10).

REMOTE MEMORY Disorders of memory are frequently accompanied by retrograde amnesia, that is, memory loss for events that occurred before the amnesia began. Evaluations of retrograde memory loss should attempt to determine both the severity of the loss and the time period that it covers. Most quantitative tests of remote memory are composed of material in the public domain that can be corroborated. For example, tests have involved questions about former one-season television programs, news events, or photographs of famous persons. An advantage of these methods is that one can sample large numbers of events and can often target particular time periods. At the least, one can identify time periods before which the information could not have been learned. (Knowledge that Sarah Jane Moore tried to assassinate President Ford could not have been acquired prior to the 1970s.) However, a disadvantage is that those tests are not so useful for detecting memory loss during the weeks or months immediately prior to the onset of amnesia. The tests sample time periods rather broadly and are too coarsely grained to detect memory impairment that covers only a few months.

Autobiographical memory tests provide a potentially effective method for obtaining fine-grained information about a patient's retrograde memory. In the word-probe task, devised by Francis Galton in 1879, patients are asked to recollect specific episodes from their past in response to single word cues (for example, bird and ticket) and to date the episodes. When normal subjects take the test, the frequency of episodic recall is lawfully related to the time period from which the episode is taken. Most of the memories come from recent time periods (the past one or two months). Patients with amnesia often exhibit temporally graded retrograde amnesia, drawing few episodic memories from the recent past, but producing as many remote autobiographical memories as normal subjects (Figure 3.5-11). When the same test is repeated a few weeks later, patients tend to assign the same dates to their recollections as

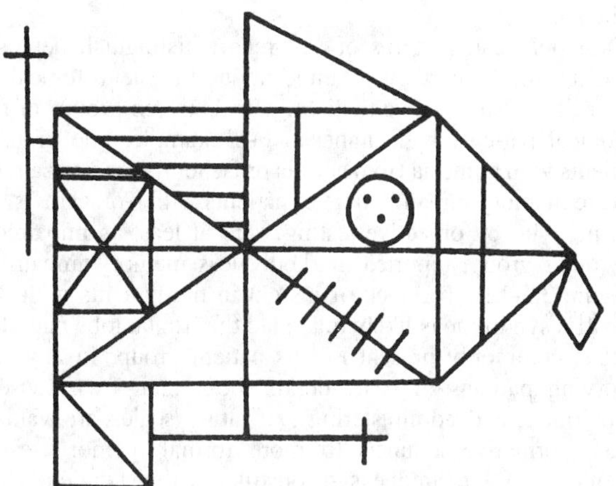

FIGURE 3.5-10 *The Rey-Osterreith figure, as used to assess delayed recall of nonverbal material. Patients are asked to copy the figure and then after a delay of several minutes, and without forewarning, patients attempt to reproduce the figure from memory. (Figure from P Osterreith: Le test de copie d'une figure complexe. Arch Psychol* 30: *206, 1944. Used with permission.)*

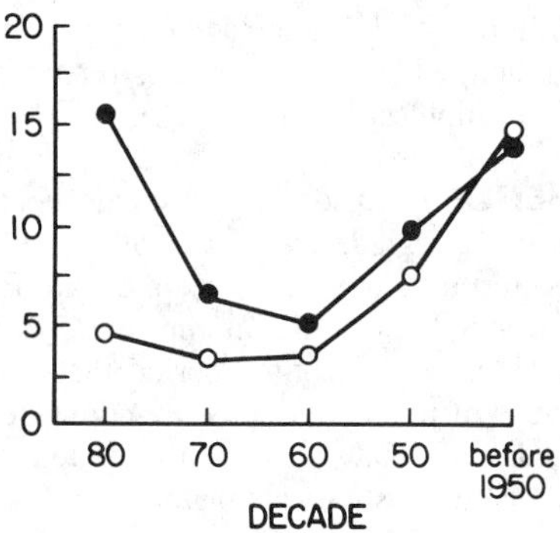

FIGURE 3.5-11 *Time periods from which five amnesic patients (filled circles) and five normal subjects (open circles) recalled well-formed autobiographical memories in response to 75 single-word cues (for example, tree, flag, window). (Figure from D MacKinnon, L R Squire: Autobiographical memory in amnesia. Psychobiology* 17: 247, 1989. *Used with permission.)*

they did during the first testing. This suggests that the recollections are not outright fabrications.

MEMORY SELF-REPORTS Patients can often supply accurate, useful descriptions of their memory problems that are extremely useful for understanding the nature of their impairment. Self-rating scales are available that yield both quantitative and qualitative information about memory impairment. As a result, it is possible to distinguish memory complaints associated with depression from memory complaints associated with amnesia (Figure 3.5-12). Depressed patients tend to rate their memory as poor in a rather undifferentiated way, endorsing equally all the different items on a self-rating form. By contrast, amnesic patients tend to endorse some items more than others; that is, there is a pattern to their memory complaints. Thus, amnesic patients do not report difficulty in remembering very remote events or in following what is being said to them, but they do report having difficulty remembering an event a few minutes after it happens. Indeed, the self-reports match rather closely the description of memory dysfunction that emerges from objective tests. Specifically, new learning capacity is affected, immediate memory is intact, and very remote memory is intact.

Not only can patterns of self-report distinguish depressed patients from patients with amnesia due to a neurological disorder, it is also possible to distinguish between groups of neurological patients with amnesia. For example, one group of patients with amnesia from anoxia or ischemia reported a rather severe memory impairment. Yet patients with Korsakoff's syndrome, who by objective testing were at least as impaired as the other group, reported markedly less memory impairment (Figure 3.5-12). The lack of insight in the patients with Korsakoff's syndrome is likely related to the frontal lobe pathology that is commonly present in this patient group. In any case, querying patients in some detail about their own sense of impairment and administering self-rating scales are valuable and informative adjuncts to more formal memory testing. Another useful technique is to construct, with the patient's help, a time line that shows the past time periods that the patient has difficulty remembering (Figure 3.5-13).

PSYCHOGENIC AMNESIA VERSUS NEUROLOGICAL AMNESIA Differentiating psychological (or dissociative) amnesia from a neurological condition is less difficult than

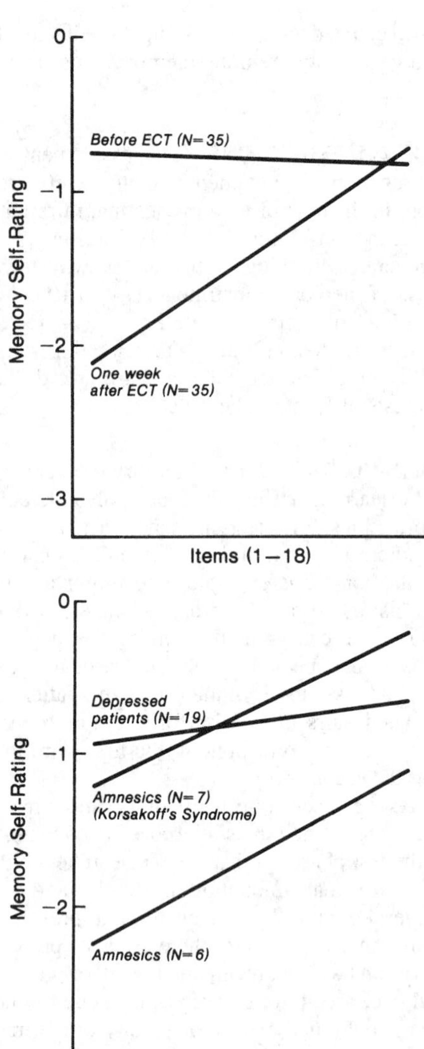

FIGURE 3.5-12 *(Top) Self-ratings of memory functions on an 18-item test, as reported by 35 psychiatric patients before a prescribed course of electroconvulsive therapy (ECT) and again one week after completion of treatment. The data are presented as best-fitting lines across the mean scores for all 18 test items. The items are ordered according to the score obtained one week after ECT. Item 1 produced the lowest score, and item 18 produced the highest score. (Bottom) Self-ratings of memory functions on the same 18-item test, as reported by depressed patients (DEP), amnesic patients with Korsakoff's syndrome (AMN-KORS), and non-Korsakoff amnesic patients (AMN). The data are presented as best-fitting lines across the mean scores for all 18 test items. The order of the items, from left to right, is the same as in the top panel. The similarity between the pattern of self-ratings reported by patients with ECT and by amnesic patients suggests that memory complaints after ECT reflect the experience of amnesia. The patients with Korsakoff's syndrome were as severely amnesic as the other amnesic patients, according to neuropsychological tests, but the patients underestimated their memory impairment. An impaired ability to self-monitor memory function has been observed in other tests of patients with Korsakoff's syndrome and is likely related to the frontal lobe atrophy that typically occurs in that group. (Figure from L R Squire, J Zouzounis: Self-ratings of memory dysfunction: Different findings in depression and amnesia. J Exp Clin Neuropsychol* 10: 722, 1988. *Used with permission.)*

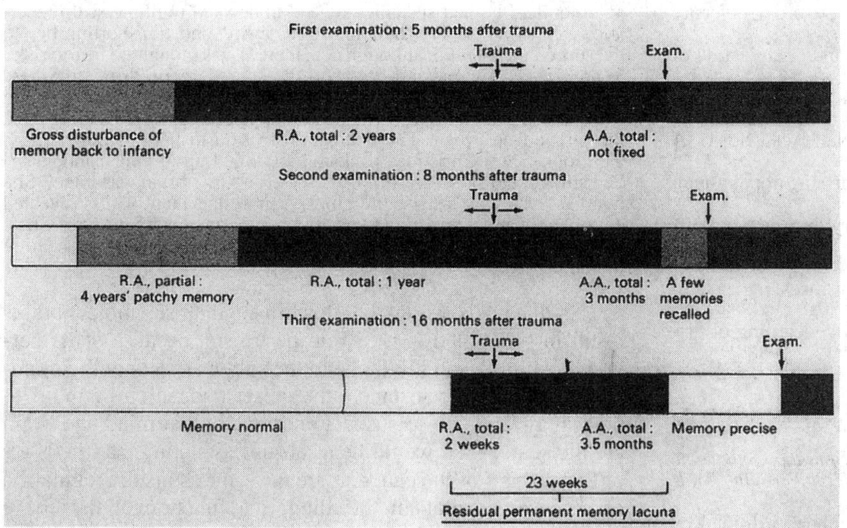

FIGURE 3.5-13 *An illustration of time periods that were difficult to remember at three different intervals after a severe head injury. (Figure from J Barbizet:* Human Memory and Its Pathology. *Freeman, San Francisco, 1970. Used with permission.)*

might be supposed. First, psychogenic amnesia is much rarer than the memory disorder that results from neurological injury or disease. Moreover, the two kinds of amnesia have markedly different characteristics. Psychogenic amnesias typically do not affect new learning capacity. Patients enter the hospital able to lay down a continuing record of daily events. By contrast, new learning problems are at the core of neurological amnesia. The main positive symptom in psychogenic amnesia is extensive and severe retrograde amnesia. Patients may be unable to recall their own name or to recollect pertinent autobiographical information from childhood. By contrast, patients with neurological amnesia never forget their name, and their remote memory for the events of childhood and adolescence is typically normal unless there is damage beyond the limbic-diencephalic brain structures associated with memory functions.

Some patients with psychogenic amnesia have circumscribed retrograde memory loss that covers a particular time period or that covers only autobiographical memories. One patient was reported to be able to answer questions about past public events but not questions about past personal events. Another patient scored close to zero on a test of famous photographs, far worse than any neurological amnesic patient would score, and was also unable to identify proper names, such as "Los Angeles" and "Pontiac." The challenge for the clinician is not in distinguishing psychogenic amnesia from neurological amnesia, but in distinguishing psychogenic amnesia from conscious malingering. Indeed, the diagnosis of psychogenic amnesia can be difficult to substantiate and may be met with skepticism by hospital staff. Often, the clinical picture remains unclear until the amnesia clears, which it sometimes does after a period of days.

SUGGESTED CROSS-REFERENCES

Functional neuroanatomy is presented in Section 1.2. Delirium, dementia, and amnestic and other cognitive disorders, including memory disorders, are discussed in Chapter 12. Dissociative disorders, including dissociative amnesia, are discussed in Chapter 20. The broad issue of neuropsychological and intellectual assessment of cognitive functions is discussed in Sections 9.5 and 9.6.

REFERENCES

Alvarez P, Squire L R: Memory consolidation and the medial temporal lobe: A simple network model. Proc Natl Acad Sci USA *91:* 7041, 1994.

Bailey C H, Chen M: Time course of structural changes at identified sensory neuron synapses during long-term sensitization in *Aplysia.* J Neurosci *9:* 1774, 1989.

Byrne J H: Cellular analysis of associative learning. Physiol Rev *67:* 329, 1987.

Greenough W T, Bailey C H: The anatomy of a memory: convergence of results across a diversity of tests. Trends Neurosci *11:* 142, 1988.

Hawkins R D, Kandel E R, Siegelbaum S A: Learning to modulate transmitter release: Themes and variations in synaptic plasticity. Annu Rev Neurosci *16:* 625, 1993.

Knowlton B J, Squire L R: The learning of categories: Parallel brain systems for item memory and category knowledge. Science *262:* 1747, 1993.

Lashley K S: *Brain Mechanisms and Intelligence: A Quantitative Study of Injuries to the Brain.* Chicago University Press, Chicago, 1929.

LeDoux J E: Emotion. In *Handbook of Physiology: The Nervous System,* V J M Brookhart, V B Mountcastle, editors. American Physiological Society, Bethesda, 1987.

Lezak M D: *Neuropsychological Assessment,* ed 2. Oxford University Press, New York, 1983.

Madison D V, Malenka R C, Nicoll R A: Mechanisms underlying long-term potentiation of synaptic transmission. Annu Rev Neurosci *14:* 379, 1991.

McKee R, Squire L R: On the development of declarative memory. *J Exp Psychol* [Learn Mem Cogn] *19:* 397, 1993.

*Mishkin M: A memory system in the monkey. In *Philos Trans R Soc Lond* [Biol] D E Broadbent, L Weiskrantz, editors, vol 298, p 85. The Royal Society, London, 1982.

Polich J, Squire L R: P300 from amnesic patients with bilateral hippocampal lesions. Electroencephalogr Clin Neurophysiol *86:* 408, 1993.

Pratt R T C: Psychogenic loss of memory. In *Amnesia,* ed 2, C W M Whitty, O L Zangwill, editors, p 104. Butterworth, London, 1977.

Press G A, Amaral D G, Squire L R: Hippocampal abnormalities in amnesic patients revealed by high-resolution magnetic resonance imaging. Nature *341:* 54, 1989.

Schacher S, Glanyman D, Baryilai A, Dash P, Grant S G N, Keller F, Mayford M, Kandel E R: Long-term facilitation in *Aplysia:* Persistent phosphorylation and structures changes. In *Cold Spring Harbor Symposia on Quantitative Biology,* vol. 55, *The Brain.* Cold Spring Harbor Laboratory Press, Plainview, NY, 1990.

Schacter D L, Chiu C Y, Ochsner K N: Implicit memory: A selective review. Annu Rev Neurosci *16:* 159, 1993.

Schacter D L, Wang P L, Tulving E, Freedman M: Functional retrograde amnesia. Neuropsychologia *20:* 523, 1982.

Scoville W B, Milner, B: Loss of recent memory after bilateral hippocampal lesions. J Neurol Neurosurg Psychiatry *20:* 1121, 1957.

*Squire L R. *Memory and Brain.* New York, Oxford University Press, 1987.

Squire L R: Memory and the hippocampus: A synthesis of findings with rats, monkeys, and humans. Psychol Rev *99:* 195, 1992.

Squire L R: The neuropsychology of memory dysfunction and its assessment. In *Neuropsychological Assessment of Neuropsychiatric*

Disorders, I Grant, K Adams, editors, p 268. Oxford University Press, New York, 1986.
*Squire L R, Knowlton B, Musen G: The structure and organization of memory. Annu Rev Psychol *44:* 453, 1993.
Squire L R, Ojemann J G, Miezin F M, Petersen S E, Videen T O, Raichle M E: Activation of the hippocampus in normal humans: A functional anatomical study of memory. Proc Natl Acad Sci USA *89:* 1837, 1992.
*Squire L R, Zola-Morgan S: The medial temporal lobe memory system. Science *253:* 1380, 1991.
Squire L R, Zouzounis J A: Self-ratings of memory dysfunction: Different findings in depression and amnesia. J Clin Exp Neuropsychol *10:* 727, 1988.
Thompson R F, Krupa D J: Organization of memory traces in the mammalian brain. Annu Rev Neurosci *17:* 519, 1994.
Thompson R F: The neural basis of basic associative learning of discrete behavioral responses. Trends Neurosci *11:* 152, 1988.
Tulving E: What is episodic memory? Curr Dir Psychol Sci *2:* 67, 1993.
*Tulving E, Schacter D L: Priming in human memory systems. Science *247:* 301, 1990.
Victor M, Adams R D, Collins G H: *The Wernicke-Korsakoff Syndrome and Related Neurological Disorders Due to Alcoholism and Malnutrition,* ed 2. Davis, Philadelphia, 1989.
Zola-Morgan S, Squire L R: The neuroanatomy of amnesia. Annu Rev Neurosci *16:* 547, 1993.
Zola-Morgan S, Squire L R: The primate hippocampal formation: Evidence for a time-limited role in memory storage. Science *250:* 288, 1990.
Zola-Morgan S, Squire L R, Amaral D G: Human amnesia and the medial temporal lobe region: Enduring memory impairment following a bilateral lesion limited to field CA1 of the hippocampus. J Neurosci *6:* 2950, 1986.

3.6
BRAIN MODELS OF MIND

KARL H. PRIBRAM, M.D.

INTRODUCTION

For two centuries brain models of mind have fascinated scientists and the lay public alike. The intense interest began with the pioneering correlations between brain pathology and characteristic personality histories of patients inaugurated by Francis J. Gall. As with every major advance in understanding the mind-brain relation, Gall's demonstrations became a popular fad in the form of phrenology, reading bumps on the skull. Today a similar fad involves the application of the findings regarding hemispheric specialization: educators and politicians alike exhort people to use their right brains, lest the human race fall forever into sinister damnation.

Brain models of mind show a remarkable coherence during the 19th and 20th centuries, despite the often acrimonious bickering regarding emphasis on this or that phenomenon to the exclusion of a comprehensive analysis. When carefully considered, each of the often opposing views captures important aspects of the issues, and reconciliation devolves on making distinctive definitions and reading the proposals in their original form with those definitions in mind.

Gilbert Ryle provided a definition of mind: mind comes from minding, paying attention. In old English *gemynd,* akin to remind, was derived from terms indicating to warn and to intend. The Sanskrit *manas* means to think.

THE MIND-BRAIN RELATION

A case-history highlights this definition. A neurosurgeon is called regarding a 14-year-old girl who had fallen out of a rapidly moving automobile. She had sustained a head injury and multiple scalp lacerations. She was several hundred miles away, and transporting her to the surgeon's hospital, although considered, was thought to be too risky to an already traumatized head. So the neurosurgeon drove to where she was bedded. Her head was swathed in bandages, through which some blood had oozed, making them appear bright red. By contrast, the girl looked green. The neurosurgeon said to her: "Hello, Cathy. You look like a Christmas package, all dolled up in your bandages." She smiled and said, "Hello, Doctor." The girl's brain was intact. She minded, even with a sense of humor. A thorough examination revealed a broken rib and a puncture to one lung, giving her a green color. Chest bandages and a brief time in an oxygen tent quickly allowed healing to commence.

The diagnosis rested on the truism that scrambled brains result in scrambled minds. But the truism, because of its pervasive validity, can blind one to the subtle aspects of the mind-brain relation. For instance, the close association of mind to brain may lead one to suspect uncritically that mind and brain are the same. That would be as absurd as stating that the islets of Langerhans of the pancreas are the same as insulin regulation of glucose metabolism. Minding is a function of the entire organism's interacting with its environment, just as glucose metabolism is a function of the organism's metabolizing environmentally derived nutrients. What is common to brain and mind is their organization, much as what is common to a computer's hardware and the various levels of programming software is the information being processed.

On the whole, people accept the special relation between brain and conscious experience but are not at all agreed on the subtleties inherent in the nature of the relation or on the consequences that the understanding of that nature may have on their understanding of themselves and their relationships to others. In that respect people have apparently come no further than the philosophers of the past two millennia.

Each of the philosophical stances toward the mind-brain relation has merit as long as it is restricted to the database that defines the stance. Thus what becomes important is the special relation between various brain processes and the variety of mental processes. On the other hand, what is ontologically neutral to the material brain and mental (psychological) processes is order, order as measured scientifically in terms of energy, entropy, and information.

With respect to the special relation between brain processes and the variety of mental processes, the ontological neutrality is expressed by showing that conscious and unconscious processes are coordinate with identifiable brain processes occurring in identifiable brain systems. That is, at some level the descriptions of brain processes and the descriptions of mental processes become homomorphic.

An example from computer science illustrates what is meant by homomorphic: One uses a computer as a word processor by typing English words and sentences. The word-processing system converts the keyboard input to binary, which is the language of the computer. Nothing in the description of English and in the description of binary machine language appears to be similar. Nevertheless, by virtue of the various transformations produced in the encoding and decoding operations of the various stages leading from typescript to binary, the information (the form within) of the typescript is preserved in the binary language of the operation of the computing machine.

In a similar fashion, little in conscious experience resembles the operations of the neural apparatus with which it has such a special relation. However, when the various transformations (the transfer functions, or the codes that intervene between experience and neural operations) are sufficiently detailed, a level of description is reached in which the transformations of experience are homomorphic with the language used by the brain. That language is the language of the operations of a microprocess taking place in synaptodendritic fields, a mathematical language similar to what describes processes in subatomic physics.

At the microprocessing level, therefore, an identity describes the relation between brain and mental processes. At remote processing levels that encompass large-event structures (assemblers, operating systems or their counterparts in computer or brain systems), pluralism and eventually (at the natural language level) dualism characterize the relation.

The special relation between brain and mental processes is thus not unitary, except in implementation at the microprocessing level. At the neuronal level and even at the neural-system level, several types of relations with psychological processes can be discerned.

First, neurochemical states of neuronal assemblies determine and are determined by states of consciousness. The field of psychoneuropharmacology is replete with evidence of relations between catechol and indole amines acting in specified brain locations to produce states of consciousness, such as wakefulness and sleep, depression and elation, and perhaps even dissociated states, such as those seen in schizophrenia. The relations between relative concentrations of blood glucose and osmolarity and hunger and thirst, between sex hormones and sexually characteristic behaviors, and between such peptides as the endorphins and the enkephalins and the experiences of pain and stress are all well documented.

Second, the relations between the sensory systems of the brain and the sensory aspects of perception, such as the contents of consciousness, have been described in detail. States of consciousness often determine contents and are often determined by them. When hungry a person tends to be aware of restaurant signs; smelling the aroma of freshly baked bread while walking past a bakery whets the appetite. The connection between states of consciousness and the contents of consciousness is mediated by a process ordinarily called *attention* (the control of sensory input), *intention* (the control of motor output), and *thought* (the control of remembering). An understanding of those processes of minding is critical to the understanding of the special relation between brain states and the contents of conscious experience.

VARIETIES OF BRAIN ORGANIZATION

LOCALIZATION AND DISTRIBUTION OF FUNCTION

Gall brought the issue of localization of function to the fore by correlating local brain pathologies with the histories of the cadavers he autopsied. Although often wrong in detail, Gall was correct in the methods he carefully detailed. He was naive in delineating the faculties of mind for which he sought localization, but the systematic classification of mental functions is still elusive despite half a century of operational behaviorism. Today it is popular to discuss the modularity of mind and component systems of the brain and to relate them, in both the clinic and in the laboratory, by crafting experimental designs and behavioral and verbal testing procedures. The use of these techniques can be traced directly to Gall's enterprise.

The excesses of phrenology brought a reaction. First, the question was raised as to which brain system brought together the various faculties into a conscious self. The unity of being, the soul, was challenged by breaking mentation into a mere collection of faculties. Furthermore, experimental evidence showed a relation between, on the one hand, impairments in complex behaviors and verbally reported experiences and, on the other hand, the amount of brain tissue destroyed, regardless of location. In the recent past Karl Lashley became the exponent of that mass-action view.

However, if one reads Lashley carefully, one finds the seeds of conciliation. In a letter to Fred Mettler, Lashley once stated his exasperation with being misinterpreted. He knew, of course, that the front of the brain does something different from the back end. The visual sensory input terminates in the occipital lobes. Electrical stimulations of the pre-Rolandic areas elicit movements and the front parts are more enigmatic in their functions. But these observations beg the issue.

What concerned Lashley was that certain selected mental functions appeared to be related to brain processes that are nonlocal. For instance, he pointed out that sensory and motor equivalences could not be accounted for even by a duplication of brain pathways:

> "Once an associated reaction has been established (e.g., a positive reaction to a visual pattern), the same reaction will be elicited by the excitation of sensory cells which were never stimulated in that way during training. Similarly, motor acts (e.g., opening a latch box) once acquired, may be executed immediately with motor organs which were not associated with the act during training."

An example of motor equivalence was reported by A. A. Ukhtomski. A dog was conditioned to raise his right hind leg at the sound of a tone. After that conditioned response was well-established, his right motor cortex (which controls the left side of the body) was exposed. Then, during the performance of the conditioned reaction, a patty of strychninized filter paper (which chemically excited the cortical tissue) was placed on the area that controls the left forepaw. Immediately, the dog switched the responding leg: He now raised his left forepaw to the conditional signal. A temporary dominant focus of excitation had been established in the cortex by the chemical stimulation. E. Roy John summarized the experiments that demonstrate such shifts in cerebral dominant foci in Figure 3.6-1 (the experiment by Lev Abramovich Zal'manson in the illustration is the one reported by Ukhtomski).

The distributed aspect of brain function becomes most evident in memory storage. Even with large deletions of brain tissue, such as those resulting from cerebrovascular diseases and resections for tumor, specific memories, or engrams, are seldom lost. When amnesias do occur they are apt to be spotty and difficult to classify. That fact suggests that memory is stored in a distributed and statistically more or less random fashion. The storage process dis-members the input, which is then re-membered when recognition and recall became necessary. The retrieval processes, in contrast to storage, are localized, at least in such systems as those that are sensory-specific. When such systems are damaged, sensory-specific and even category-specific agnosias result. Thus, with regard to memory, both distributed and localized processes can be identified, depending on which property of the process is being considered.

HIERARCHY AND HETERARCHY The fact that a temporary dominant focus in the cerebral cortex can take control of the expression of a learned behavior indicates that hierarchical control operates in the central nervous system. Equally persuasive is the evidence for control over spinal cord activity by the brainstem and the forebrain. Neuronal activity in the spinal cord displays a high rate of spontaneous impulse generation. These generators are modulated by inhibitory local circuit neurons in such a way that the resultant activity can be modeled in terms of coupled ensembles of oscillatory processes.

The ensembles of oscillators become organized by brainstem systems that consist of cholinergic and adrenergic neurons. The cholinergic set regulates the frequency of a wide range of tonic rhythmic activities, such as those involved in locomotion, respiration, cardiovascular responses, and sleep. The cholinergic system is coupled to an adrenergic set of neurons that segment the rhythmic activities into episodes. Both systems are subject to further hierarchical control by the dopaminergic system of the basal ganglia.

Clinically, the loss of hierarchical control becomes manifest

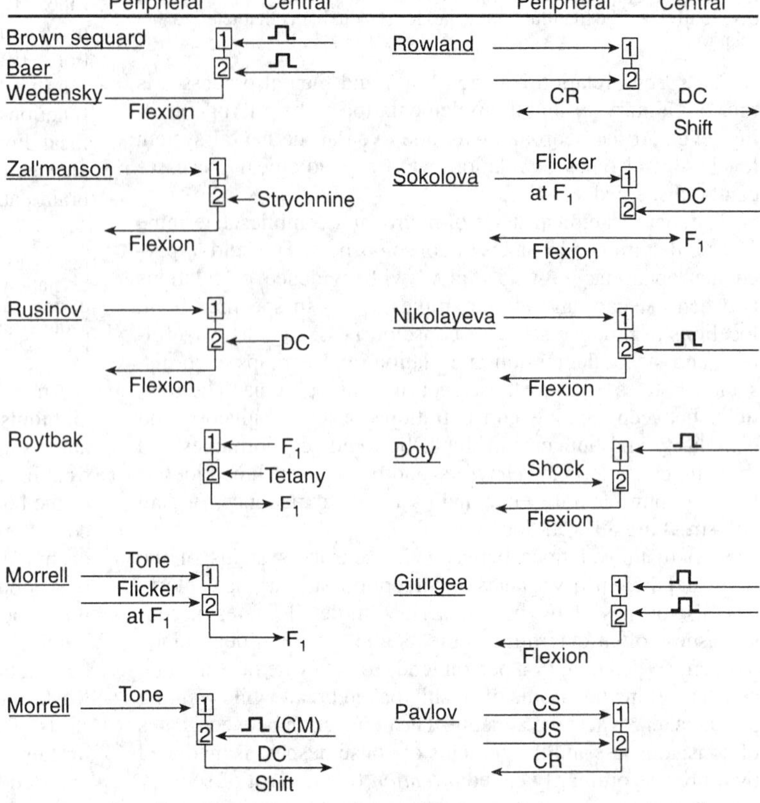

FIGURE 3.6-1 *Methods of conditioning that have been used by various investigators to establish and produce shifts in cerebral dominant foci. The example in the text refers to Zal'manson's experiment. (Figure from K Pribram:* Languages of the Brain: Experimental Paradoxes and Principles in Neuropsychology, *p 79. Random House, New York, 1971. Used with permission.)*

in an exaggeration of the normally present, almost subliminal tremors that, under extreme conditions, lead to spastic paralysis, hyperreflexia, and uncontrollable fits of oscillatory muscular spasm.

But the evidence from the experiments that showed temporary dominant foci can be viewed from another perspective: The flexibility demonstrated by the shift from one controlling locus to another shows the organization of the cortical system to be heterarchical. Any locus within the system can become dominant if sufficiently excited. Warren McCulloch used the following story to illustrate the nature of heterarchical organization.

After the 1916 battle of Jutland during World War I, in which the British navy took a beating, both the British and American navies were reorganized to change from hierarchical to heterarchical control. Battleships no longer had to await orders from a central command source to engage in defensive maneuvers.

During World War II the American fifth fleet was stationed in an only slightly dispersed mode of operation somewhere in the Pacific Ocean when it was attacked from two directions by separate air squadrons. Sightings of the attackers were made from two locations in the fleet by observers on the ships closest to one or the other of the attacking squadrons. In essence, the sailor who made the sighting became a dominant focus, and his ship and those in his proximity took off to defend against the attackers. However, since the attack came from two directions, two dominant foci were created, each commanding parts of the fleet to steam away in opposite directions. That left the ship at the center of the fleet, which housed its admiral, haplessly unprotected and, since no sightings were made by the admiral's ship, at a momentary loss as to what to do. Fortunately, both attacking squadrons were defeated and turned back without any damage accruing to the fifth fleet.

Thus, a penalty may be paid for the flexibility achieved by a heterarchical dominance, albeit temporary, over processing.

SERIAL AND PARALLEL PROCESSING Ordinarily, hierarchical control is conceived to be accomplished by way of a serial process. When control is direct, a causal connection exists between the controller and the controlled. Causality implies that the origination of the control signal precedes its effect on the system being controlled. Seriality remains when feedback loops are present. However, when feedforward operations are inserted into the process, seriality is no longer as clear-cut. In a thermostat or in homeostasis, if one lowers the temperature or the blood sugar, the sensor closes a circuit, and the effector responds: a serial process. But if one places a control dial or other bias on the process, the sensor can be adjusted in two or more ways. One can reset the thermostat's dial; thus the sensor has parallel inputs one from the dial and the other from the heat in the room. Herman von Helmholtz is credited with pointing out that voluntary processes, such as those by which people move their eyes, are constituted of such feedforwards: parallel corollary discharges to the effectors. Control can be hierarchical yet dependent on a parallel process.

Heterarchical organization, by definition, involves the potential for parallel processing. However, when control is exerted over other systems, a serial process becomes implemented. In general, the brain is composed of hierarchies of heterarchical systems.

Processing in the cerebral cortex is massively parallel. Simulations of those parallel cortical processes have been implemented on personal computers to such an extent that the endeavors have been dubbed a cottage industry.

Computer simulations of neural networks are capable of pattern recognition, language learning, and decision making that are remarkably true to life. Single-layered simulations have given way to three-layered computations, which involve an input layer, an output layer, and a hidden layer. All the elements of the network are interconnected, each element with all the others. In several such simulations the input is fed forward through the net and the output is compared with one that is desired; the difference between the actual and the desired is fed back to the net. The process is repeated until the desired output is achieved.

Variations on that theme abound, each variation being better adapted than its alternatives for a particular purpose.

Relevant to the issue of localization and nonlocal processing is the fact that information contained in the input becomes fragmented and distributed in the elements of the layers. The simulations are said to be parallel-distributed processes. That makes them akin to the optical information-processing systems, such as holography and tomography, from which they were derived.

ROLE OF BASAL BRAIN SYSTEMS IN ORGANIZING MIND

BASAL FOREBRAIN SYSTEMS William James noted that the delineation of minding—that is, consciousness—devolves on processes usually referred to as attention and intention (volition). Thought should be added. Controls on attention determine the span of sensory processing; controls on intention determine the span over which action becomes effective; and controls on thought determine the span of memories that become considered.

The neural processes in the control of attention involve three mechanisms: One mechanism deals with short phasic responses to an input (arousal-familiarization); a second mechanism relates to the organism's prolonged tonic readiness to respond selectively (activation-selection); and a third mechanism (effort-comfort) acts to coordinate the phasic (arousal) and tonic (activation) processes. Separate neural and neurochemical systems are involved in these processes: The phasic process is centered on the amygdala; the tonic process is centered on the caudate nucleus, while the coordinating system critically involves the hippocampus, a phylogenetically ancient part of the neural apparatus.

Evidence from the analysis of changes in the electrical activity of the brain evoked by brief sensory stimulation has shown that the arousal and activation systems operate on a basic process centered on the dorsal thalamus, the way station of sensory input to the cerebral cortex. Brain electrical activity evoked by sensory stimulation can be analyzed into components. Early components reflect processing by systems that directly (through the thalamus) connect sensory surfaces with cortical surfaces. Later components reflect processes initiated in the thalamocortical and related basal ganglia systems that operate downward onto the brainstem (tectal region), which influences a thalamic gate that modulates activity in the direct sensory pathways. The activity reflected in these later components constitutes activation.

The thalamic gate is, however, also regulated by input from the system centered on the amygdala, the arousal system. That system, when stimulated, produces an effect on the gate that is the opposite of the effect of the activation system.

The evidence also indicates that the coordination of phasic (arousal) and tonic (activation) attentional processes often demands effort. When attention must be paid the hippocampal system becomes involved; it influences the arousal system rostrally through frontal connections with the amygdala system and the activation system caudally through connections in the brainstem. At that juncture the relation of attention to intention—that is, to volition (will)—comes into focus. William James pointed out that a good deal of what is called voluntary effort is the maintaining of attention or the repeated returning of attention to a problem until it yields a solution.

Emotion and motivation William James apposed will to emotion and motivation (which he called *instinct*). Beginning with Walter Cannon's experimentally based critique of James and followed by Lashley's critique of Cannon, the anatomically based suggestions of James Papez, and their more current versions by Paul MacLean, brain scientists have been deeply concerned with the processes that organize emotional and motivational experience and expression. Two major discoveries have accelerated the ability to cope with the issues and have placed the early speculative accounts into perspective. One of the discoveries is the role of the reticular formation of the brainstem and its chemical systems of brain amines that regulate states of alertness and mood. Donald Lindsley proposed an activation mechanism of emotion and motivation on the basis of the initial discovery and detailed the pathways by which such activation can exert control over the brain processes. The other discovery is the system of brain tracts that, when electrically excited, results in reinforcement (that is, an increase in the probability of recurrence of the behavior that has produced the electrical brain stimulation) or deterrence (that is, a decrease in the probability that such behavior will recur).

To organize these discoveries and other data that relate brain mechanisms to emotion, one must distinguish between those data that refer to experience (feelings) and those that refer to expression and must distinguish emotion from motivation. Feelings encompass both emotional and motivational experience—emotional as affective processes and motivation as readiness. The affective processes of emotion are based on arousal, the ability to make phasic responses to input that stop the motivational processes of activation that maintain selective readiness. Feelings are based on neurochemical states (dispositions or moods) that become organized by appetitive (motivational, go) and affective (emotional, stop) processes.

James is almost universally misinterpreted as holding a peripheral theory of emotion and mind. Throughout his writings he emphasized the effects that peripheral stimuli (including those of visceral origin) exert on brain processes. Nowhere did he identify emotions with bodily processes. Emotions are always the resultant effect on brain states. However, what James failed to take into account is the role of expectations (the representational role of the organization of arousal-familiarity and activation-selection) in the organization of feelings. Those representations, or neuronal models, of prior experience entail the functions of the basal ganglia, including the amygdala.

Nonetheless, James was explicit when he discussed the nature of the input to the brain from the viscera. He pointed out two possibilities: emotions are processed by a separate brain system, or they are processed by the same systems as are perceptions. Today, both possibilities are known to play a role: parts of the frontolimbic forebrain (especially the amygdala and related systems) process visceroautonomic bodily inputs, and the results of processing are conveyed to brainstem systems that distribute to and diffusely influence the perceptual systems.

In addition, James defined the difference between emotions and motivations: Emotional processes take place primarily within the organism; motivations reach into the organism's environment. James may have overemphasized the visceral determination of emotional experience, but he did occasionally include attitudinal factors as depending on sensory feedback from the somatic musculature.

The distinction between the brain mechanisms of motivation and will were less clearly enunciated by James. He grappled with the problem and set the questions that must be answered. Clarity did not come until the late 1960s, when several theorists began to point out the difference between feedback, homeostatic motivational processes on the one hand and voluntary programs—which are feedforward, homeorrhetic processes—on the other hand. Feedback mechanisms depend on error processing and are, therefore, sensitive to perturbations. Programs, unless completely derailed, run themselves off to completion, regardless of the obstacles placed in their way.

Voluntary and involuntary behavior Clinical neurology classically distinguished the mechanisms involved in voluntary behavior from those in involuntary behavior. The distinction rests on the observation that lesions of the cerebellar hemispheres impair intentional (voluntary) behavior, but basal ganglia lesions result in disturbances of involuntary movements. Damage to the cerebellar circuits are involved in a feedforward mechanism, rather than a feedback mechanism.

The cerebellar hemispheres may operate by performing calculations in fast time—that is, extrapolate where a particular movement would end if it were to continue and send the results of such a calculation to the cerebral motor cortex, where they can be compared with the target to which the movement is directed. Experimental analysis of the functions of the motor cortex has shown that such targets are composed of images of achievement, constructed in part on the basis of past experience.

Just as the cerebellar circuit serves intentional behavior, the basal ganglia are important to involuntary processes, such as the readiness of the organism to respond selectively (activation). Lesions in the basal ganglia grossly amplify tremors at rest and markedly restrict expressions of motivational feelings. Neurological theory has long held that these disturbances are due to the lesion's interference with the normal feedback relations between the basal ganglia and the cerebral cortex. In fact, surgical removal of the motor cortex has been performed on patients with basal ganglia lesions to redress the imbalance produced by the initial lesions. Such resections have been successful in alleviating the often distressing continuing disturbances of involuntary movement that characterize basal ganglia diseases.

CEREBRAL CORTEX AND MINDING

Reflective consciousness and unconscious processes

The distinction between the systems that control intentional behavior and those that control involuntary behavior extends to the control of sensory input and the processing of memory. With regard to sensory input, the distinction between the contents of awareness and the person who is aware was delineated by Franz Brentano and called *intentional inexistence.* The dualism of a minding self and objective matter (the brain) was already present in the writings of Ernst Mach and René Descartes. Although Cartesian dualism is perhaps the first overt nontrivial expression of the issue, the duality between subject and object and some causal connection between them is inherent in language once it emerges from simple naming to predication. Eric Neumann and Julian Jaynes suggested that a change in consciousness (that is, in distinguishing an aware self from what the self is aware of) occurred somewhere between the time of the *Iliad* and the time of the *Odyssey.* That occurrence may be linked to the invention and promulgation of phonemically based writing. Prehistory was transmitted orally-aurally. Written history is visual-verbal. In an oral-aural culture a great share of reality is carried in memory and is personal; once writing becomes a ready means of recording events, they become a part of extrapersonal objective reality. The shift is especially manifest in a clearer externalization of the sources of conscience, the gods no longer speak personally to guide individual humans.

The process of ever-clearer distinctions between personal reality and extrapersonal objective reality culminates in Cartesian dualism and Brentano's intentional inexistence, which Edmund Husserl shortened to *intentionality.* That reading of the subject-object distinction is what philosophers ordinarily mean when they speak of the difference between conscious processes and unconscious processes.

Sigmund Freud had training in both medical practice and philosophy. When he emphasized the importance of unconscious processes, was he implying the medical definition or the philosophical definition? Most interpretations of Freud suggest that unconscious processes operate without awareness in the sense that they operate automatically, much as do respiratory and gastrointestinal processes in someone who is stuporous or comatose. Freud himself seems to have promulgated that view by suggesting a horizontal split between conscious, preconscious, and unconscious processes, with repression operating to push memory-motive structures into deep layers, where they no longer have access to awareness. Still, in "Project for a Scientific Psychology," memory-motive structures are neural programs located in the core portions of the brain that gain access to awareness by their connections to the cortex, which determines whether a memory-motivated wish comes to consciousness. When the neural program becomes a secondary process it comes under voluntary control, which involves reality testing and consciousness. To use language as an example, one may well know two languages but at any one time connect only one language to the cortex; thus the other language remains unconscious and voluntarily unexpressed.

The linking of reflective consciousness to the cortex is not as naive as it first appears. As recently reported cases have shown, blind-sight results when patients are subjected to unilateral removal of the visual cortex. Such patients insist that they cannot see anything in the field contralateral to their lesion, but, when tested, they can, by guessing, locate and identify large objects in their blind hemifield with remarkable accuracy. Furthermore, some patients have unilateral neglect after suffering parietal lobe lesions. Neglect patients can often get around by using their neglected limbs appropriately. A still different syndrome giving the same type of result was observed in a patient who sustained an amygdala-hippocampal resection; when he was trained in operant tasks the effects of the training persisted without decrement for years, despite protestations from the patient that he did not recognize the situation and that he remembered nothing of the training. Monkeys with such lesions have shown almost perfect retention of training after a two-year period, and the retention was better than that shown by controls. Those monkeys and the blind-sight patients are clearly conscious in the medical instrumental sense. What went wrong was their ability to reflect on their behavior and experience, an inability within the impaired sphere of clearly distinguishing personal from extrapersonal reality. They were left with impaired consciousness in the philosopher's sense: Behavior and experience were no longer intentional.

The thrust of most recent thinking by psychoanalysts and experimentalists is in the direction of interpreting the conscious-unconscious distinction in the philosophical sense. For instance, Ignacio Matte Blanco proposed that consciousness be defined by the ability to make clear distinctions, to identify alternatives. Making clear distinctions includes being able to tell personal reality from extrapersonal reality. By contrast, unconscious processes, according to Matte Blanco, are composed of infinite sets "where paradox reigns and opposites merge into sameness." When infinities are being computed the ordinary rules of logic do not hold. Thus dividing a line of infinite length results in two lines of infinite length—that is, one = two. Being deeply involved allows love and ecstacy but also suffering and anger to occur. In keeping with this, Carl Gustav Jung defined unconscious processes as those involving feelings. Bringing the wellsprings of behavior and experience to consciousness means making distinctions, providing alternatives, making choices, becoming informed in the sense of reducing uncertainty.

Unconscious processes as defined here are thus not completely submerged and unavailable to experience. Rather, unconscious processes produce feelings that are difficult to localize in time or in space and difficult to identify correctly. The unconscious processes construct the emotional dispositions and motivational context within which extrapersonal reality and personal reality are constructed. As the classic experiments of Seymore Schachter and Jerome Singer showed, feelings are to a large extent undifferentiated; people tend to know and label them according to the circumstances in which the feelings were manifested.

It is in this sense that behavior comes under the control of the unconscious processes. When people burst out in anger, they are aware that they have done so and are aware of the effects of the anger on others. They may or may not have attended the buildup of feeling before the blowup. And they may have projected the buildup onto others or introjected it from them. But they could have been aware of all that (with the guidance of a friend or a therapist) and still found themselves in uncontrolled anger. Only when the events leading to the anger become clearly separated into alternative or harmoniously related distinctions is unconscious control converted into conscious control. People with obsessions or compulsions are aware, in the instrumental sense, of their experience or behavior, and they feel awful. But they cannot, without aid, cope, that is, differentiate controls on the behavior generated by their feelings.

Cerebral dominance and the unity of consciousness As noted above, the topic of hemispheric specialization is currently fashionable not only in the behavioral neurosciences but also among the public at large. Three important discoveries fueled this interest. First, the rediscovery during the latter half of the 19th century of the fact that, in most right-handed persons, speech is controlled by the left hemisphere. That fact was already known to Hippocrates and may well have been learned by him from the Egyptians. Running from back to front, comprehension, grammar, and fluency are affected by lesions centering on the sylvian fissure. But dominance is not as complete in women as it is in men, nor is it pervasive in cultures that do not use phonemic writing.

Second, what is new in the appreciation of hemispheric specialization is the realization that the non-speech-dominant hemisphere has its own characteristic modes of processing. The left hemispheres of right-handed persons being taken over by an aural-oral dimension may have been due to the fact that the right hemisphere was used by primates to process visual-spatial relations leaving the right hand free for further manipulations. *Spatial* here means the space defined by the body in motion—egocentric and allocentric, as differentiated from occulocentric and object-centered spaces.

These specializations in processing modes refer primarily to the semantic and syntactic aspects of language. With regard to the emotional tone of language (prosody), right-sided frontal lesions result in monotone speech. Right-sided posterior lesions leave the patient unable to understand those aspects of communication that depend on intonation and emphasis (these syndromes are known as "aprosodias").

The third and most pervasive and persistent focus of interest has been a theme that also organized a debate regarding localization of function in the 19th century: the unity of consciousness. When the corpus callosum was severed in patients who had suffered severe unilateral epileptic seizures to prevent the involvement of the healthy hemisphere, testing revealed that what was sensed by the right hemisphere could be expressed only nonverbally by that hemisphere. The left, verbal, hemisphere appeared to be ignorant of what had transpired. It seemed as though consciousness had been split when the hemispheres were sundered. The assumption that there is ordinarily a unity to consciousness received support in that this unity had been ruptured.

These observations led to the conception that civilization suffers from left-brain dominance and that training for brain balance would restore balance to civilization. Of course, that is pure rot. All but the most rudimentary processing involves both hemispheres, as innumerable studies have demonstrated. Even in language, the appreciation and the expression of emotional communication involves the right hemisphere, and extreme specialization is limited to right-handed men raised in a phonemic literary environment.

Although the popular overgeneralization is to be deplored (as is the overgeneralization that led to phrenology), the original observations did renew interest in the question of whether consciousness can be divided. Sir John Eccles has argued that consciousness is tied to language, an argument also made by Freud, and that the right, speechless, hemisphere is essentially unconscious. However, the right hemisphere clearly communicates with left-handed, nonverbal instrumental responses to the input presented to it. The nonverbal hemisphere obviously has a mind of its own. But conscious minding is of two sorts: instrumental and intentional. Eccles's proposal is tenable if what is meant is intentional consciousness. Brain facts as they relate to behavior, mind, and consciousness often spring surprises on the unwary.

VARIETIES OF CONSCIOUS EXPERIENCE

OBJECTIVE CONSCIOUSNESS

Posterior cerebral convexity Surrounding the major fissures of the primate cerebral cortex lie the terminations of the sensory and motor projection systems. These systems have been labeled extrinsic because of their close ties (by way of a few synapses) with peripheral structures. The sensory surface and the muscle arrangements are mapped more or less isomorphically onto the perifissural cortical surface by way of discrete, practically parallel lines of connecting fiber tracts. When a local injury occurs within these systems, a sensory scotoma or a scotoma of action ensues. A *scotoma* is a spatially circumscribed hole in the field of interaction of the organism and the environment—for example, a blind spot, a hearing defect limited to a frequency range, or a section of the skin where tactile stimuli fail to elicit a response. Those are the systems where what Henry Head called epicritic processing takes place. The extrinsic sensory-motor projection systems are so organized that movement allows the organism to project the results of processing away from the sensory and muscular surfaces where the interactions take place and out into the world external to the organism, much as a stereo effect is obtained by adjusting the phase between the output of two speakers. Processing within the extrinsic systems constructs an objective reality for the organism.

In between the perifissural extrinsic regions of the cortex lie other regions of the cortex variously named association cortex, uncommitted cortex, and intrinsic cortex. These names reflect the fact that there is no apparent direct connection between peripheral structures and those regions of the cortex that make up most of the convexity of the cerebrum.

Corporeal reality and extracorporeal reality Lesions of parts of the intrinsic cortex of the posterior cerebral convexity result in sensory-specific agnosias in both monkeys and humans. Research on monkeys has shown that the agnosias are due not to a failure to distinguish cues from one another but a failure to make use of those distinctions in making choices among alternatives. The ability to make use of those distinctions is the essence of information processing in the sense of reducing uncertainty. The sensory-specific posterior intrinsic cortex determines the range of alternatives, the sample size that a particular informative element must address. A patient with agnosia can tell the difference between two objects but does not know what the difference means. As Charles Peirce once noted, what people mean by something and what they mean to do with it are synonymous. In short, alternatives, sample size, choice, cognition, information, and meaning are closely interwoven concepts. When agnosia is severe, it is often accompanied by what is termed neglect. The patient appears not only not to know that he does not know but to actively deny the agnosia.

Typical is a patient who repeatedly had difficulty in sitting up in bed. Her physician pointed out to her that her arm had become entangled in the bedclothes. She acknowledged that fact momentarily, only to "lose" that arm once more in a tangled environment. Part of her perception of her body, her corporeal consciousness, seemed to have been extinguished.

Such observations can readily be conceptualized in terms of an extracorporeal and corporeal *objective* reality. For a time it was thought that corporeal (egocentric) reality (personal body space) depended on the integrity of the frontal intrinsic cortex and that the posterior convexal cortex was critical to the construction of extracorporeal (allocentric) reality. That scheme was tested in experiments with monkeys and human patients and was found wanting. In fact, the corporeal-extracorporeal distinction involves the parietal cortex. Perhaps the most clear-cut example comes from studies showing that cells in the parietal cortex respond when an object is within view but only when it is also within reach. In essence, studies have been unable clearly to separate the brain locations that produce agnosia from those that produce neglect. Furthermore, the studies indicate that agnosia is related to meaning as defined by corporeal use.

In monkeys the disturbances produced by restricted lesions of the convexal intrinsic cortex are also produced by lesions of the parts of the basal ganglia (implicated in activation, selective readiness) to which those parts of the cortex project. That finding takes on special meaning from the fact that lesions of the thalamus (which controls the relaying of sensory input to the cortex) fail to produce such effects. The special connection between the posterior intrinsic (association) cortex and the basal ganglia further clarifies the intentional process that those systems make possible—the distinction between an objective egocentric corporeal self (the me) and an extracorporeal allocentric reality (the other).

NARRATIVE CONSCIOUSNESS

Frontolimbic forebrain Frontal lesions were produced for a time in an effort to relieve intractable suffering, compulsions, obsessions, and endogenous depressions. When effective in pain and depression these psychosurgical procedures portrayed in humans the now well-established functional relation between the frontal intrinsic cortex and the limbic forebrain in nonhuman primates. Furthermore, frontal lesions can lead either to perseverative, compulsive behavior or to distractibility in monkeys and in humans depending on environmental circumstance. A failure to be guided by the consequences of their behavior can account for both effects. Extreme forms of distractibility and obsession are due to a lack of sensitivity of the activation (selective readiness) process to feedback from consequences. Both the results of experiments with monkeys and clinical observations attest to the fact that those with frontal lesions—whether surgical, traumatic, or neoplastic—fail to be guided by the consequences of their behavior.

Consciousness as conduct and narrative *Consequences* are the outcomes of behavior. In the tradition of the experimental analysis of behavior, consequences are reinforcers that influence the recurrence of the behavior. Consequences are thus a series of events (Latin *ex-venire,* out-come), outcomes that guide action and thereby attain predictive value (as determined by confidence estimates). Such con-sequences—that is, sequence of events—form their own confidence levels to provide contexts that, in humans, become envisioned event-ualities.

Confidence implies familiarity. Experiments with monkeys and humans have shown that repeated arousal to an orienting stimulus habituates—that is, the orienting reaction gives way to familiarization. Familiarization is disrupted by limbic (amygdala) lesions and frontal lesions. Ordinarily, familiarization allows continued activation of selective readiness; disruption of familiarization leads to repeated distraction (orienting) and thus a failure to allow con-sequences to form. When the process of familiarization is disrupted, the outcomes-of-behaviors, events, become inconsequential. When intact, the familiarization process is segmented by orienting reactions into episodes within which confidence values can become established.

In such an episodic process the development of confidence is a function of coherences and correlations among the events being processed. When coherence and correlation span multiple episodes, the organism becomes *committed* to a course of action (a prior intention, a strategy), which then guides further action and is resistant to perturbation by particular orienting reactions (arousals). The organism is now *competent* to carry out the action (intention-in-action, tactic). Particular outcomes now guide competent performance; they no longer produce orienting reactions. In humans coherent competence provides the basis for ethical behavior. Thus in several languages the meaning of consciousness and conscience are conflated.

The cascade that characterizes episodic processing leads ultimately to considerable autonomy of the committed competence. Envisioned events are woven into coherent subjectivity, an ''I,'' whose story is a narrative, the myth by which the person lives. The narrative composes a practical guide to action in achieving (temporary) stability in the face of a staggering range of variations of events.

Consciousness is manifest (by verbal report) when familiarization is perturbed, when an episode is updated and incorporated into a larger contextual scheme (the narrative) that includes both the familiar episodes and the novel episodes. Consciousness becomes attenuated when actions and their guides cohere; the actions become skilled, graceful, and automatic.

TRANSCENDENTAL CONSCIOUSNESS The contents of consciousness are not exhaustively described by the *qualia* of feelings of familiarity and novelty that are the basis for episodic and narrative consciousness nor by those of extracorporeal allocentric and corporeal egocentric consciousness. The esoteric tradition in Western culture and the mystical traditions of the Far East are replete with instances of uncommon states that produce uncommon contents. Those states are achieved by a variety of techniques, such as meditation, yoga, and Zen. The contents of processing in such states appear to differ from ordinary feelings and perceptions. Experiences are described as oceanic, a merging of corporeal reality and extracorporeal reality, or as out-of-body—that is, corporeal reality and extracorporeal reality continue to be clearly distinguished but are experienced by still another reality, a meta-me. Or an ''I'' that becomes transparent: a throughput experiencing everything everywhere; there is no longer the segmentation into episodes; nor do events become enmeshed in a narrative structure.

All these experiences have in common a transcendental relation between ordinary experience and an encompassing organizing principle. That relation is ordinarily termed ''spiritual.'' The spiritual contents of consciousness can be accounted for by the effects of excess excitation of the frontolimbic forebrain (ordinarily involved in narrative construction) on the dendritic microprocess that characterizes cortical receptive fields in the sensory extrinsic systems (ordinarily involved in the construction of objective reality).

In addition to the gross topological correspondence between cortical receptive fields and the organization of sensory surfaces that gives rise to the overall characteristics of processing in the extrinsic systems, a microprocess that depends on the internal organization of each receptive field comes into play. The internal organization of receptive fields embodies, among other characteristics, a spectral domain: receptive fields of neurons in the extrinsic cortex are tuned to limited bandwidths of frequencies of radiant energy (vision), sound, and tactile vibration.

The most dramatic data are those that pertain to vision. The cortical neurons of the visual system are arranged, as are the other sensory systems, so as to reflect more or less isomorphically the arrangement of the receptor surfaces to which they are connected. (Thus, the homunculi that Wilder Penfield and others have mapped onto the cortical surface of the extrinsic projection systems.) However, within that gross arrangement lie the receptive fields of each of the neurons—a receptive field determined by the dendritic arborization of the neuron that makes contact with the peripheral parts of the system. Thus, the receptive field of a neuron is that part of the environment processed by the parts of the system to which the neuron is connected. Each receptive field is tuned to approximately an octave of spatial frequency. The frequency-selective microprocess thus operates in a holographiclike manner.

Processing can be conceived to function somewhat like the production of music by a piano. The sensory surface is analogous to a keyboard. The keyboard and the strings are spatially related to provide the overall organization of the process. When individual strings are activated, they resonate over a limited bandwidth of frequency. The combination of the spatial arrangement and the frequency-specific resonance of the strings makes the production of music possible.

The gross organization and the microorganization of the cortical neurons in the extrinsic systems resemble the organization of a multiplex hologram. A multiplex hologram is characterized by a Gabor elementary function, which Dennis Gabor called a quantum of information. A Gaussian envelope constrains the otherwise unlimited sinusoid described by the Fourier transform to make up the Gabor function. Experiments have shown that electrical excitation of the frontal and limbic structures relaxes the Gaussian constraints that are manifested as inhibitory surrounds or flanks in the receptive field architecture. When the relaxation of the constraint is moderate as during ordinary excitation of the frontolimbic systems of the forebrain, processing leads to narrative construction. When frontolimbic excitation becomes overwhelming, experience is determined by a totally unconstrained holographic process.

Holograms of the type involved in brain processing are composed by converting (for example, by Fourier transformation) successive sensory images (for example, frames of a movie film) into their spectral representations and patching the microrepresentations into orderly spatial arrangements that represent the original temporal order of the successive images. When such conversions are linear (as when they use the Fourier transform), they can readily be reconverted (for example, by the inverse Fourier transformation) into moving (successive) sensory images. The spectral domain is peculiar in that information (in the Gabor sense) becomes both distributed over the extent of each receptive field (each quantum) and enfolded within it. Thus sensory-image reconstruction can occur from any part of the total aggregate of receptive fields. That gives the aggregate its holographic, holistic aspect. All input becomes distributed and enfolded, including the dimensions of space and time and, therefore, causality. That apparently timeless-spaceless-causeless aspect of processing, which can be instigated by overwhelming frontolimbic excitation, is responsible for the extrasensory dimensions of experience that characterize the esoteric traditions.

Because of their enfolded property, these processes tend to swamp distinctions, such as corporeal reality and extracorporeal reality. In the esoteric traditions consciousness is not limited to that type of reality.

A related development (because it deals with the specification of an encompassing, cosmic order) has occurred in quantum physics. Over the past 50 years it has become clear that there is a limit to the accuracy with which certain measurements can be made when other measurements are being taken. The limit is expressed as an indeterminacy. Gabor, in his description of a quantum of information, showed that a similar indeterminacy describes communication, thus leading to a unit of minimum uncertainty, a limit on the maximum amount of information that can be packed for processing. As a consequence there is a convergence of the understanding of the microstructure of communication—and, therefore, of observation—and the understanding of the microstructure of matter. The need to specify the observations that lead to inferring the properties of matter has led noted physicists to write a representation of the observer into the description of the observable. Some of those physicists have noted the similarity of that specification to the esoteric descriptions of consciousness.

A revolution in Western thought is therefore in the making. The scientific tradition and the esoteric tradition have been at odds since the time of Galileo. Each new scientific discovery and the theory developed from it have, up until now, resulted in the widening of the rift between objective science and the subjective spiritual aspects of human nature. The rift reached a maximum toward the end of the 19th century: people were asked to choose between God and Charles Darwin, and Freud showed that heaven and hell reside within people, not in their relation to the natural universe. The discoveries of 20th century science do not fit that mold. For once, the recent findings of science and the spiritual experiences of humanity are consonant. That augurs well for the coming millennium. A science that comes to terms with the spiritual nature of humanity may well outstrip the technological science of the immediate past in its contribution to human welfare.

SUGGESTED CROSS-REFERENCES

Neuroanatomy is discussed in Section 1.2, electrophysiology in Sections 1.7 and 1.8, perception and cognition in Section 3.1, psychoanalysis in Section 6.1, and psychosurgery in Section 31.27.

REFERENCES

Bolster B, Pribram K H: Cortical involvement in visual scan in the monkey. Percept Psychophysics *53:* 505, 1993.

*Bracewell R N: The Fourier transform. Sci Am *260:* 86, 1989.

Cannon W B: The James-Lange theory of emotions: A critical examination and an alternative theory. Am J Psychol *39:* 106, 1927.

Efron R: *The Decline and Fall of Hemispheric Specialization.* Erlbaum, Hillsdale, NJ, 1989.

Gabor D: Theory of communication. J Inst Elect Eng *93:* 429, 1946.

James W: *Principles of Psychology.* Dover, New York, 1950.

Lashley D: The thalamus and emotion. In *The Neuropsychology of Lashley,* F A Beach, D O Hebb, C T Morgan, H W Nissen, editors, p 345. McGraw-Hill, New York, 1960.

Luria A R, Pribram K H, Homskaya E D: An experimental analysis of the behavioral disturbance produced by a left frontal arachnoidal endothelioma (meningioma). Neuropsychologia *2:* 257, 1964.

*Matte Blanco I: *The Unconscious as Infinite Sets.* Duckworth, London, 1975.

Mountcastle V B, Lynch J C, Georgopoulos A, Sakata H, Acuna C: Posterior parietal association cortex of the monkey: Command functions for operations within extrapersonal space. J Neurophysiol *38:* 871, 1975.

Neumann E: *The Origins and History of Consciousness.* Princeton University Press, Princeton, NJ, 1954.

Penfield W: Consciousness, memory and man's conditioned reflexes. In *On the Biology of Learning,* K H Pribram, editor, p 127. Harcourt, Brace & World, New York, 1969.

*Pribram K H: *Brain and Perception: Holonomy and Structure in Figural Processing.* Erlbaum, Hillsdale, NJ, 1991.

Pribram K H: How is it that sensing so much we can do so little? In *Central Processing of Sensory Input,* F O Schmitt, F L G Worden, editors, p 249. MIT Press, Cambridge, MA, 1974.

Pribram K H: *Languages of the Brain: Experimental Paradoxes and Principles in Neuropsychology.* Prentice-Hall, Englewood Cliffs, NJ, 1971.

*Pribram K H: Localization and distribution of function in the brain. In *Neuropsychology After Lashley,* J Orbach, editor, p 273. Erlbaum, Hillsdale, NJ, 1982.

Pribram K H: *Rethinking Neural Networks: Quantum Fields and Biological Data.* Erlbaum, Hillsdale, NJ, 1993.

Pribram K H: The intrinsic systems of the forebrain. In *Handbook of Physiology, Neurophysiology,* J Field, H W Magoon, V E Hall, editors, p. 1323. American Psychological Society, Washington, 1960.

Pribram K H: The isocortex. In *American Handbook of Psychiatry,* D A Hamburg, H K H Brodie, editors, vol 6. Basic Books, New York, 1974.

Pribram K H: The orienting reaction: Key to brain representational mechanisms. In *The Orienting Reflex in Humans,* H D Kimmel, editor, p 3. Erlbaum, Hillsdale, NJ, 1980.

*Pribram K H, Gill M: *Freud's "Project" Reassessed.* Basic Books, New York, 1976.

Pribram K H, McGuiness D: Attention and para-attentional processing: Event-related brain potentials as tests of a model. Ann NY Acad Sci *658:* 65, 1992.

Pribram K H, Nuwer M, Baron R: The holographic hypothesis of memory structure in brain function and perception. In *Contemporary Developments in Mathematical Psychology,* R C Atkinson, D H Krantz, R C Luce, P Suppes, editors, p 416. Freeman, San Francisco, 1974.

Pribram K H, Reitz S, McNeil M, Spevack A A: The effect of amygdalectomy on orienting and classical conditioning in monkeys. Pavlov J *14:* 203, 1979.

Rose J E, Woolsey C N: Organization of the mammalian thalamus and its relationship to the cerebral cortex. Electroencephalogr Clin Neurophysiol *1:* 391, 1949.

Ryle G: *The Concept of Mind.* Barnes & Noble, New York, 1949.

Schachter S, Singer T E: Cognitive, social and physiological determinants of emotional state. Psychol Rev *69:* 379, 1962.

Sidman M, Stoddard L T, Mohr J P: Some additional quantitative observations of immediate memory in a patient with bilateral hippocampal lesions. Neuropsychologia *6:* 245, 1968.

Stevenson I: *Telepathic Impressions: A Review and Report of Thirty-Five New Cases.* University Press of Virginia, Charlottesville, 1970.

Thatcher R W, John E R: *Functional Neuroscience.* Erlbaum, Hillsdale, NJ, 1977.

Ukhtomski A A: Concerning the condition of excitation in dominance. Novoe Refteksol Fiziol Nerv *2:* 3, 1926.

Weiskrantz L: *Blindsight: A Case Study and Implications.* Clarendon, Oxford, 1986.

Willshaw D: Holography, associative memory and inductive generalization. In *Parallel Models of Associative Memory,* G E Hinton, J A Anderson, editors, p 83. Erlbaum, Hillsdale, NJ, 1981.

CHAPTER 4 CONTRIBUTIONS OF THE SOCIOCULTURAL SCIENCES

4.1 ANTHROPOLOGY AND PSYCHIATRY

MELVIN KONNER, Ph.D., M.D.

INTRODUCTION

Traditional accounts of the relation between anthropology and psychiatry have usually been limited to cultural psychiatry: the definition of culture, interactions between it and the individual, culture-specific syndromes, and cross-cultural differences in definitions of health, illness, and healing. But those categories represent only a part of the current interface between the two fields. When the interface was first extensively explored during the 1930s and 1940s psychoanalytic theory seemed the most promising domain in psychiatry and anthropologists independently saw its potential as a powerful tool for the study of culture. The interaction between psychoanalysts or psychiatrists and anthropologists was both natural and fruitful.

It immediately became clear that cultures differ in their definitions of health, illness, and healing and also vary greatly in child-rearing patterns, social models and expectations, role opportunities, and other major variables that would be anticipated by psychodynamic theory to influence the etiology and course of psychiatric disorders. To say that these observations are still valid would be an understatement, and some of the evidence supporting them will be reviewed below. However, both anthropology and psychiatry have been transformed during the past 30 years, owing largely to the increasing importance of biology in each of those fields. The interface between them has become much more complex and thus the goal here is to reconceptualize in current terms the relation between anthropology and psychiatry. (Parenthetical notes in the text refer by number to pertinent cases at the end of this section.)

BIOLOGY, PSYCHOLOGY, AND CULTURE: HISTORICAL PERSPECTIVE

Over the past several decades psychiatry has evolved from a primarily psychological discipline to one that is biopsychological. Inevitably the transformation has been somewhat wrenching, and what is often described as eclectic psychiatry is often a not very well-integrated amalgam of psychodynamics, psychopharmacology, and behavioral and clinical pragmatism. The transformation of anthropology during the same period has been parallel in important ways. As two eminent pioneers in cultural anthropology, Alfred L. Kroeber and Margaret Mead, had recognized by the 1950s the increasing delineation of cross-cultural variety must carry with it the potential for describing the invariant features of human behavior and mental life. That proved to be a prescient observation as the description of universals of language, culture, facial expressions, parent-offspring interactions, and many other aspects of human life would soon become possible. Those universals constitute a part of what is meant by human nature, a term that must be considered again, after decades of being in disfavor, as having scientific legitimacy.

In the 19th century it was not unusual for treatises on aspects of human psychology to refer to ethnographic data. Darwin's 1872 book on facial expression cited the occurrence of certain expressions in primitive societies as evidence for their biological basis, and attempted to relate them to facial expressions in animals in an evolutionary sequence. Edward Westermarck, whose theory of incest aversion is still read and tested, appealed to ethnographic evidence to illuminate a deeper psychodynamic process he considered to be as universal as certain facial expressions. In the late 19th century it was common for prominent anthropologists to attempt to array nonindustrial societies in an evolutionary sequence of social complexity, religion, or language. And in the early years of the 20th century ethnological expeditions tested members of primitive societies for the presence of proposed perceptual universals.

Those trends, which might be seen as early efforts to characterize human nature and its origins, were greatly affected by the development of modern social and cultural anthropology and by the parallel emergence of psychoanalysis. Anthropologists on both sides of the Atlantic, despite many differences of opinion, came to share a contempt for the evolutionary sequencing of cultures, replacing it with accurate if not exhaustive descriptive characterizations of cultures as independent units. Proposed universals of human behavior or mental function were met with equal skepticism, and anthropologists still like to say, ''Not among my people, they don't,'' a kind of statement that has been called the anthropological veto.

PSYCHOANALYTIC THEORY Early generalizations by Jean Piaget and others were tested cross-culturally, but none elicited the enthusiasm for such testing that psychoanalysis did. The British social anthropologist Bronislaw Malinowski attempted to demolish the universality of the Oedipus complex by describing a separation of male authority (vested in the mother's brother) from the object of male jealousy (the biological father) in his society in the Trobriand Islands (an argument still actively debated). With the skeptical encouragement of Franz Boas, the dean of American cultural anthropology, such disciples as Margaret Mead tried to undermine certain psychoanalytic convictions by using cross-cultural comparisons but at the same time attempted to use psychoanalytic and other psychodynamic theory to explain culture.

The fundamental theorem of that school was that cultures are distinctive because of distinctive patterns of child rearing, and that a unified approach combining psychoanalysis and cultural anthropology could explain culture and elucidate laws of psychological development simultaneously. During World War II the approach reached its florescence with speculations about the national character of Russians, Japanese, Germans, and Americans, relating those speculations to unscientific observations of infant and child care. Sigmund Freud's method, difficult enough when applied to a single patient studied in a concentrated way for hundreds of hours over a period of years, was thus adopted for a completely distinct task for which it was inappropriate.

By the 1950s the approach had generated some research that to some extent delegitimized it through refinement and measurement. Both the assessment of adult psychological disposition and the objective description of child training were made quantitative, the first through projective testing and the second through direct behavior observation, with interviewing supporting both approaches. Cora Dubois and Anthony F. C. Wallace demonstrated through projective testing and interviewing that even small-scale societies with relatively homogeneous cultures do not have what might be called a basic personality (an entity corresponding to national character in large-scale societies). Individual variation in personality and character is great in every known culture, however primitive. At best there is perhaps a modal personality (from the statistical concept of mode) shared by a substantial minority of a culture's members—as shown by Wallace for two distinct Native American groups. In any case a culture must derive its distinctiveness from the particular mutual articulation of its various personality types and the opportunities it provides for their expression, rather than from fundamental tendencies shared by a majority—a sort of symphony orchestra model of culture and personality, but with the proviso that the symphony may frequently and even intrinsically be more cacaphonous than harmonious.

Research on the genetics of personality has become far more rigorous in the past decade owing to large systematic national samples in Scandinavia and Finland, multiple replications of findings on American samples, increasingly developmental emphasis, subtle consideration of environmental contributions to variance, and cross-national replications using similar instruments and comparable samples. The studies have converged on a five-factor model of personality that has proved quite robust: (1) extraversion or positive emotionality, (2) compliance or agreeableness, (3) conscientiousness or will to achieve, (4) neuroticism or negative emotionality, and (5) intellect or intelligence. The last factor may be considered as separate from personality but it is clearly an important human trait that influences psychological adaptation and psychiatric health.

The factors are derived empirically through factor analysis, not generated intuitively or theoretically. Their consistency thus is remarkable. On the basis of many new and rigorous studies (rather than dubious old ones) personality overall is seen to have a heritability of approximately 50 percent. A reasonable hypothesis, according to studies to date, would be that the five factors will prove to be present in all cultures, thus underscoring the need for the symphony-orchestra model of culture and personality. Also, different cultures can be expected to favor different loadings on the five factors and to try to shape children in a particular direction. However, it is clear that every culture must come to terms with the variety of human personalities and perhaps specifically with the five factors described. Perhaps culture is like the conductor of the orchestra, balancing and shaping the musicians' expressions of what they themselves can do.

CHILD TRAINING At the same time John Whiting and Beatrice Whiting were trying to place the cross-cultural study of child training on a scientific foundation. A 1953 study by John Whiting and Irvin Child using a large cross-cultural sample demonstrated that themes in childhood experience of interest to psychoanalysts are correlated with similar themes in religion, folklore, and other cultural expressions (which they called projective systems). They focused on a culture's traditional explanations of illness and its treatment, reasoning that those beliefs might reflect chronic, shared anxieties. Cultures rated as causing infants and children high levels of anxiety in relation to their oral needs (as through early weaning or the withholding of food as a form of punishment), for example, tended to be the same cultures that used oral themes to explain illness (as in deeming it a result of the ingestion of prohibited foods). Cultures in which child-training anxieties were high in the area of aggressive behavior tended to be those in which adults explained illness as an attack by a human sorcerer or an evil spirit.

The researchers recognized, however, that such correlations might arise from causes other than those most friendly to psychoanalysis and that childhood experience needed to be measured more rigorously. The Whitings devoted the next three decades to such measurement in a number of societies around the world and developed a model of the influence of fundamental features of society—such as ecology, economy, and vulnerability to external attack—on child-training practices, which in turn might give rise to certain consistent adult predispositions. But it was rarely possible to establish such relations beyond the level of correlations, and many cultural anthropologists became disillusioned with such theories.

CROSS-CULTURAL DIAGNOSIS A parallel development relevant to cultural psychiatry was the attempt to study systematically the incidence of psychiatric disorders cross-culturally, an approach associated with the reputation of Alexander Leighton and Jane Murphy among others. That attempt continues to be fruitful, but is beset by doubts about the cross-cultural validity of diagnostic categories. Recent attempts to rationalize nosology at the national and international levels reveal similar obstacles to cross-cultural diagnosis. Nevertheless, certain still valid conclusions emerged from such work: first, both the general category of psychological deviance and at least several distinct syndromes appear to be characteristic of all cultures for which information is available; second, some psychiatric disorders appear to be relatively or largely culture-specific; third, it is extremely difficult, if not impossible, usefully to compare the incidence or prevalence of most disorders cross-culturally, much less to draw conclusions about the etiology of alleged cross-cultural differences in prevalence.

MEDICAL ANTHROPOLOGY By the late 1950s the subdiscipline of medical anthropology had emerged and had established certain firm generalizations. The sick role, whether in relation to psychological illness or to physical illness, is seen in all cultures but carries many different meanings and expectations. The same ailment, even what is apparently the same degree of physical pain, varies greatly in designation and interpretation, to the extent that some cultures recognize diseases unrecognized as abnormalities in others and some encourage the expression of pain whereas others discourage it.

In early Christianity, which was a healing religion, suffering through illness was often simply to be borne and could bring about a state of grace. Among the !Kung San, hunter-gatherers of the Kalahari, the sick person was under attack from the spirit world and an aggressive stance against the spirits might be appropriate. A classic study of subcultural or ethnic group differences in American cities revealed that both Jewish patients and those of Italian ancestry feel free to express their pain, whereas Old Americans (white Anglo-Saxon Protestants) do not. Italians are oriented to the pain itself and express confident gratitude to the doctor when pain remits. Both Old Americans and Jews are more oriented to the prognosis, but the former are optimistic about it whereas the latter remain skeptical of the doctor.

Finally, the role and responsibility of the healer show a comparable degree of variation. The Christian physician—even the modern fundamentalist trained by Oral Roberts—joins healing to salvation. The !Kung healer enters deep trance, risking his life as his soul leaves his body (and he runs off into the bush or dives into the fire) so that he can berate the spirits on behalf of the sick person. And most physicians recognize that the more traditional members of American ethnic groups may require different bedside manners than do other patients. Such findings have usually been presumed to have even stronger implications in the realm of psychiatric illness and treatment than in other branches of medicine.

CURRENT APPROACHES The stage was now set for the transformation of anthropology that began in the 1960s. Although some cultural anthropologists drifted out of science altogether, finding their affinities with literary criticism and nonanalytic philosophy, others, along with most archeologists and many linguists, became increasingly quantitative, scientific, and biological in orientation. The four subfields of traditional American anthropology—cultural anthropology, archeology, linguistics, and biological anthropology—became reunified in an enterprise that had been moribund since the late 19th century: the characterization of human nature and its evolutionary origins. Although not every anthropologist subscribed to that purpose, it became once again a highly legitimate one, and the only one with the potential for unifying and invigorating anthropology as a whole.

The unification is advancing on seven fronts simultaneously: (1) the adoption, extension, and testing of evolutionary theory, particularly as it applies to behavior; (2) the characterization of human origins as revealed in an ever-improving fossil record; (3) the systematic description and analysis of the behavior of nonhuman primates, both to test evolutionary theory and to make inferences about the behavior of the human race's protohuman ancestors; (4) the study of contemporary and recent hunting-gathering societies with a view toward making inferences about behavior and social organization in the environment of human evolutionary adaptedness; (5) the rise of scientific archeology with its attempt to reconstruct the social worlds of past societies and relate them to the recent ones studied by cultural anthropologists; (6) the corresponding attempt by cultural anthropologists to understand ecological influences on stability and change in contemporary nonindustrial societies (for example, hunter-gatherer societies that become settled and gain access to cow's milk shorten their birth spacing, with many consequences for social structure and psychological development); and (7) the characterization of cross-cultural universals of language, nonverbal behavior, and culture, including universals of abnormal behavior and its classification and of attempts at healing.

Those approaches proceeded in parallel with the continued effort to document the extant, and steadily disappearing, variety of human cultures. Some cultural anthropologists remain aloof from that unified enterprise, but they admit to being aloof from science as a whole.

INTERPRETIVE ANTHROPOLOGY OF THE EMOTIONS The 1980s saw a marked resurgence of interest in the cross-cultural study of the emotions. However, far from being motivated by psychoanalytic or any other Western psychological theory, the new work abandoned all such theoretical bases. Its central tenet was that the ethnologist of emotions must read or experience the emotional expressions of the members of another culture without any theoretical biases or filters. By analogy with the reading of literary texts, practitioners of interpretive anthropology see their method as more respectful of their subject of study than a more conventional theory-based approach. Many literary scholars, for example, would find a psychoanalytic approach to Shakespeare irrelevant, or even destructive, to the reader's understanding of the text. Similarly, interpretive ethnographers want to engage the culture under study on its own terms and to experience it on a human level that they deem incompatible with an elaborate theoretical apparatus. To deepen the analogy, however, one must recognize that a naive approach may not be sufficient. For example, Lear's rage may seem universal in some respects but a knowledge of the culture of royalty in Shakespeare's England is surely relevant to an understanding of Lear's feelings and of the way they are expressed.

In one of the new ethnographies of the emotions, Unni Wikan's *Managing Turbulent Hearts: A Balinese Formula for Living,* the author uses the ethnographic method of thick description to set out many instances in life in Bali in which the expression of the emotions seems far different from such expression in Western culture. In particular, she delves deeply into the Balinese desire to suppress sadness and anger, showing how the culture encourages suppression and masking, not only by insisting that it is better for the suffering person, but through the more intimidating shaming tactic of citing the effect on the mental health of family, friends, and neighbors. The sufferer is repeatedly reminded that expressing sadness stirs up sadness in others and that the ultimate result is damage to the mental health of the community as a whole. Wikan also describes how the Balinese insist that the conventional Western distinction between thought and feeling can be misleading. "Stop thinking," she repeats they would say to her when they saw she was being misled in that way. "'You'll never understand what we mean if you only use your thinking!'" Just as young psychotherapists are often urged by their preceptors to use their feelings toward the patient as part of their assessment, the ethnographer was being reminded by her own study subjects to stop trying to gain an understanding of their feelings through rational thought alone. Showing the influence of her Balinese friends, Wikan makes a plea for resonance, her translation of the Balinese phrase *ngelah keneh.* It is a deep understanding between one person and another, based on what she calls "feeling-thought." It can only be achieved by not making false distinctions between thought and feeling.

Such ethnographies have been used, however, to discredit earlier, perhaps less sensitive but still valuable, ethnographic work. More relevant for psychiatry, they have been used to attack the notion that there are universal emotions. One anthropologist cited Wikan's work as disproving the hypothesis that grief is universal. Study of the work itself reveals how misleading that influence is. Wikan tells the story of a young woman who received a telegram announcing the death of her fiance. She first interpreted it as a joke but on having the news confirmed began to weep. Those who saw her responded with laughter, saying: "What's the matter with you, are you crazy [gila]?" The woman composed herself, assumed a happy expression, and smiled to passersby as she walked home.

She did take the extraordinary step of borrowing money to travel to her fiance's memorial and had herself photographed prostate on his grave. Three months later she cried openly, once.

Still, she was widely admired in her community (a testimony to the difficulty of what she did). Her remarkable composure, exceptional even in Bali, appeared to confirm the reputation Bali has among anthropologists of being the only culture in which death does not call forth tears. As the woman explained, "'I am afraid to think of it, that I might go mad, so I try to be cheerful always that I may forget my sadness.'"

But it is absurd to claim, as some anthropologists have done, that the Balinese anecdote disproves the universality of grief. There was much evidence of the young woman's grief, including at least two episodes of crying. What the Balinese case, and others like it, does show is that culture strongly shapes the expression of the emotions—which is not news to anthropology or psychiatry. As the stiff-upper-lip British superimpose calm and fortitude on grief the Balinese superimpose cheerfulness. As a clown Pagliacci must go before the audience and laugh although he is grieving. The show must go on. Those culturally mandated performances must have some influence on underlying emotions, but the claim that they disprove the universality of emotions is groundless. The distinction is vital because psychiatrists have often been misled by anthropologists' claims. Ethnography can still serve to break down ethnocentric prejudices about human mind and behavior but exaggerations of cross-cultural variation are misleading. Catherine Lutz titled her book about Ifaluk, a Polynesian island, *Unnatural Emotions,* but there are no unnatural emotions to be found in it, merely culturally guided expression of the emotions that all human beings share.

Another problem is the confusion of emotion words with the emotions themselves. Different languages label emotions in different ways. English distinguishes between liking and loving but the French say only *aimer.* That certainly does not mean that the French do not know or feel the difference. The joy felt at the suffering of a rival or an enemy is expressed in the German word *Schadenfreund,* but its mere presence in the German language does not reflect a different fundamental emotional makeup among Germans. Lutz finds it difficult to translate the Ifaluk word *fago,* which contains elements of compassion, love, sympathy, and perhaps even what Wikan would call resonance. But to conclude, as Lutz and others do, that the word means that Ifaluk feelings are fundamentally different from those of other persons is to mistake the word for the thing.

An important attempt to solve the problem is found in Karl Heider's *Landscapes of Emotion: Mapping Three Cultures of Emotion in Indonesia.* His study uses the statistical technique of multidimensional scaling to generate maps of emotion words in three different Indonesian cultures and languages: the Minangkabau language of West Sumatra, the Indonesian language spoken in the same region, and the Indonesian of Central Java. Based on similar analyses done on European cultures, Heider posits eight proposed basic pancultural emotions: sadness, anger, happiness, surprise, love, fear, disgust, contempt. Those are tested against the clusters emerging from the multidimensional scaling of Minangkabau and Indonesian emotion words. The result is a strong confirmation of the universality of sadness, anger, happiness, and surprise, and confirmation of the other four in the list with decreasing strength in the order given. Words in the Indonesian languages clearly cluster in confirmation of the first four, but for the second four, boundaries between emotions that Westerners would draw with the words love, fear, disgust, and contempt are drawn in different ways. Love loads with components of happiness in Western usage whereas in Indonesia it loads more with components of sadness. That strongly confirms the universality of certain emotions and also points to the different ways in which different cultures use emotion words. It does not prove, however, that Indonesians experience love, fear, disgust, and contempt in different ways, but only that they use different words to describe those feelings.

Most recent work on the ethnology of the emotions is less scientific than Heider's. Usually, the writings in the field make passing reference to the biological underpinnings of human mental life. For example, Lutz writes, "While the physiological aspects of emotional experience have not been considered in this work, it is important to stress again in conclusion that the biological basis of human experience, including that termed emotional, is not denied here." Similarly, Claudia Strauss, in the introduction to *Human Motives and Cultural Models,* states: "All humans have a built-in receptiveness to the form human cultures take, and all human cultures probably share some bedrock commonalities because of these coevolved features of human neurophysiology and morphology." But those, and similar works, then go on to conduct their analyses of emotions and motives as if biology were irrelevant. What if a biomedical scientist were to agree that chemistry is undeniable and then proceed to ignore it in all analyses? For some purposes—say, the Starling curve of heart function or the calculation of load on hip bones—chemistry can be temporarily ignored in favor of physics. But it is the mark of maturity of biomedical science that it now rests firmly on a foundation of chemistry and physics. The anthropology of the emotions will be similarly mature when it rests on, and fully uses, a foundation in biology and psychology.

BIOLOGICAL AND BEHAVIORAL EVOLUTION

The fossil evidence for human and protohuman evolution has accumulated steadily for more than 100 years. However, new discoveries are made each year that change the details of the picture, and during the past two decades biochemical taxonomy has further altered understanding. Many controversies remain. Thus it is clear that the chimpanzee (although perhaps the pygmy chimpanzee *Pan paniscus* rather than the common chimpanzee *Pan troglodytes*) is the human being's closest relative, but estimates of the time that the human diverged from the ape line range from 5 to 13 million years ago. It is clear that there were more than one species of hominids (protohuman forms) around two million years ago, but there may have been as few as two or as many as four. Upright posture was established before most of the evolution of the human brain took place, but the lag between the two and the role of tool using or tool making in brain evolution remains controversial.

Psychiatry probably has little to gain by closely following each argument in human paleontology. But there is much to be gained from understanding (1) the general higher primate background of human evolution; (2) the environment of human evolutionary adaptedness, that of hunting and gathering; and (3) the principles of evolutionary adaptation as applied to behavior and reproduction. Those three categories of knowledge can be described in such a way as to be relatively insensitive to future disruption by discoveries regarding the details of paleontology and evolutionary lineages.

HIGHER PRIMATE BACKGROUND All higher primates (monkeys, apes, and humans) are social animals with great learning capacity and with the mother-offspring bond at the center of social life. That bond is always prolonged, as is the anatomical and behavioral course of individual development, including each phase of the life cycle and the life span as a whole. Laboratory and field studies demonstrate the capacity for complex social cognition and social learning, up to and including the cultural transmission of social rank, tool-using techniques, and knowledge of food sources. Play, especially social play, is characteristic of all primate species, particularly during development, and is believed to provide an important opportunity for learning. As shown by Paul MacLean the higher primate emphasis on both the mother-infant bond and juvenile play represents an intensification of the pattern established by the early mammals and is essential to the understanding of the phylogeny of the limbic system and the emotions.

Primate groups generally include a core of genetically related individuals with associated nonrelatives. In most instances the core is a matrilineage, stable over the life course of individual members, but in a few species, including the common chimpanzee, the core is a patrilineage and female members are the unrelated migrants. The distribution of acts of social support and generosity is preferentially toward genetic relatives, but not exclusively so. Monkeys and apes aid nonrelatives and can usually expect reciprocal aid. Cooperation is ubiquitous, but so is competition, and one of the major purposes of cooperation is mutual defense against conspecifics. Dominance hierarchies may reduce conflict, but conflict is still frequent. Both sexes participate, but male primates generally exhibit more aggression than do female primates.

Beyond those broad generalizations great variation exists in social organization both between and within species. Gibbons and some South American monkeys are monogamous, but in most species larger group associations subsuming more temporary (although sometimes more than transient—see Case P1) associations between individual male members and individual female members of the group are the rule. Among orangutans *(Pongo pygmaeus),* despite their phylogenetic proximity to humans, the usual social groupings are a female orangutan with her offspring and (separate from those units) solitary male orangutans. The causes of that variation in higher primate social organization remain obscure, although some relevant evolutionary principles will be considered here.

Some generalizations may also be made about the nature and social context of individual development among monkeys and apes. Because the New World monkeys separated from the Old World monkeys and the apes approximately 40 million years ago, some of those generalizations do not apply to all New World monkeys. However, they do apply to all the catarrhines, a category that subsumes all Old World higher primates, including monkeys, apes, and humans. The catarrhine mother-infant complex is characterized by (1) a hemochorial placenta, with exceptionally intimate maternal and fetal circulations; (2) single birth; (3) frequent nursing, at least four times an hour; (4) late weaning, at around 25 to 30 percent of the age at first estrus or menses; (5) direct mother-infant physical contact more than 90 percent of the time in the immediate postnatal months; (6) close, frequent mother-infant proximity at least until weaning; (7) gradual transition to a multiaged play group; and (8) variable but low involvement of male adults in most species.

Interpretation of primate field studies in relation to human behavior is aided by an increasing body of laboratory data on the consequences of manipulation of early rearing conditions. Those experiments provide an epistemological link between anthropological primatology and psychiatry. Although there are important species variations it may be generally said that higher primates are sensitive to significant perturbations of the early social environment, such as isolation rearing or repeated involuntary mother-infant separation, and that those perturbations give rise to abnormalities of sexual, maternal, and aggressive behavior that in humans would be viewed as psychopathology.

In a number of species isolation rearing gives rise to stereotypical behavior, such as rocking and self-directed aggression, and mother-infant separation gives rise to symptoms usually described as protest followed by depression. Even deprivation of contact with peers during development has produced abnormal behavior in many experiments. Apparent human analogs of those causal relationships, although difficult to interpret, have encouraged the use of primate models and enhanced the interpretive value of field studies. They emphasize the extent to which the normal development of behavior in such animals has come to depend on a social matrix.

Natural variation in stable individual behavior patterns (personality) occurs in free-ranging monkey and ape groups and extends to variants that would be considered pathological in humans, such as hyperaggressive, isolative, phobic, or depressed behavior. It is rarely possible to explore the etiology of such variants. However, most cannot result from specific abnormalities of social rearing, such as are deliberately instituted in typical laboratory experiments, but are probably both genetic and environmental in etiology. Some abnormalities, such as severe depression (as in Case P2, an 8-year-old wild chimpanzee after the death of its mother) may be incompatible with survival. Others, however, such as hyperaggressiveness (as in Case P3, a female chimpanzee that, together with her daughter, systematically and repeatedly killed the infants of other female chimpanzees) may actually enhance reproductive adaptation for the abnormal individual.

HUNTING-AND-GATHERING ENVIRONMENT The foregoing generalizations probably apply to the social and psychological world of protohuman higher primate species for a period of approximately 40 million years. Against this background hominids evolved during the past few million years, culminating in the emergence of the species within the past few hundred thousand years, and finally in the appearance of modern *Homo sapiens* about 30,000 to 40,000 years ago. Although still controversial, the hypothesis arises from comparative studies of mitochondrial deoxyribonucleic acid (DNA) that everyone living today originated from a small group of persons who lived no more than 200,000 years ago—strongly arguing for the biological unity of humankind. But that would have been preceded by the completion of the evolutionary transition from apes to humans. Aside from the increase in intelligence, as indicated by increasing relative and absolute brain size as well as by the increasing complexity of stone tools, one hallmark of the transition to hominids was a greater reliance on scavenging and hunting. Monkeys and apes are largely vegetarian and the instances of meat eating are relatively infrequent.

Among the most technologically primitive humans, however, meat eating is of major importance. Most of the stone tools that have survived archeologically were used in hunting or butchering, and the demands caused by those activities have long been thought central to the emergence of human intelligence and social organization. It has been shown that the stone used sometimes had to be traded over long distances, implying unexpectedly complex social networks among human ancestors at least two million years ago. Furthermore, even chimpanzees share meat after a kill (but not plant foods) and among human hunter-gatherers the following of elaborate regulations for such sharing may be a life-and-death matter. Finally, with one noteworthy exception (the Agta of the Phillipines, where women routinely hunt) all hunting-and-gathering societies in the ethnographical record have a division of labor by sex—men do almost all of the hunting and women supply most of the plant foods. Thus some peculiarly human aspects of social life are probably attributable to the advent of hunting, but those features had to have been grafted onto an already complex social life characteristic of nonhuman higher primates.

In many hunting-and-gathering societies, plant foods gathered by women constitute most of the diet and are shared with others (although not beyond the immediate family), as they are not among nonhuman primates. Postweaning mortality is much higher in juvenile nonhuman primates than in human children, and it has been speculated that the provision of plant foods to their children by human mothers accounts for the difference. Also, the early advent of upright posture may have had more to do with the need to carry plant foods as well as infants to a base camp than with any advantage it conferred in hunting. It may be that digging sticks and carrying devices for plants or infants were the first tools invented, probably by women. Those tools, however crucial to daily life, would not have been preserved archeologically.

The psychodynamic theorist John Bowlby used the phrase "environment of evolutionary adaptedness" (EEA) to describe the hunting-and-gathering way of life. The phrase correctly implies that it was the context for which natural selection prepared human beings, and from which they departed only during the past 10,000 years, a short time in evolutionary terms. From many studies of recent and current hunting-and-gathering peoples, combined with archeological evidence of those of the distant past, it is possible to make the following generalizations about that context. (1) Social groups are usually small, ranging in size from 15 to 40 persons related through blood or marriage. (2) Groups are nomadic, moving frequently to take advantage of changing subsistence opportunities, and are flexible in composition, size, and adaptive strategies. (3) Daily life involves physical challenge, vigorous exercise, and occasional hunger, but with a usually dependable food base from a moderate work effort and with a marked division of labor by gender. (4) Diseases, mainly infectious, produce high rates of mortality, especially in infancy and early childhood, with consequent frequent experiences of loss. (5) Virtually all of life's activities are carried out in a highly social context with persons one knows well—often the same persons for different activities. (6) Privacy is limited but creative expression in the arts is frequently possible and conflicts and problems are dealt with through extensive group discussions that often include highly personal revelations. (Case H1, a woman among the !Kung San of Botswana, illustrates some of those points.)

The generalizations outlined describe the contexts in which almost all of human evolution and history have occurred, so it is often said that modern human beings are, in effect, hunter-gatherers in offices and factories. Simplistic observations about the consequences of the change are of little value. Life in such societies is not simply more or less stressful; the stresses are quite different. Social density crudely measured is neither demonstrably higher or lower, but strangers are rarely encountered and both privacy and loneliness are unusual. Bosses and teachers make no demands, but environmental exigencies make many. A thoughtful set of analyses of the differences between psychological conditions in modern society and in the kind of society in which humans spent most of their history has not yet been carried out.

Childhood experience Child care is distinctive in such societies. It includes (1) frequent breast-feeding (up to four times an hour) and late weaning (at 2 to 4 years of age); (2) close, essentially constant mother-infant contact, including extensive skin-to-skin carrying and adjacent sleeping until weaning (Figure 4.1-1); (3) prompt response to infant crying and indulgent response to other infant and child demands; (4) a gradual transition from an intense mother-infant bond to a multiaged child play group of mixed gender; (5) relatively little responsibility in the sense of chores or schooling in middle childhood, with most learning taking place through observation and play; and (6) liberal premarital sexual mores, with sex play throughout middle childhood gradually giving rise to adolescent sexuality, but with late menarche limiting the opportunities for childbearing until the late teens.

Those characteristics of the hunter-gatherer childhood extend the patterns found among nonhuman higher primates. Some of the features, such as breast-feeding and sleeping in the same room with the infant, usually in the same bed, can be generalized to all nonindustrial societies. Other characteristics, such as a high degree of premarital sexual freedom, are significantly more applicable to hunting-and-gathering societies than to agricultural or herding societies. Either way, they are characteristics of the environment of human evolutionary adaptedness, and they suggest many hypotheses (still largely untested) about the possible consequences of the departure by modern industrial societies from those patterns.

Largely because of morbidity and mortality the hunter-gatherer pattern of childhood experience is not idyllic. Frustration and loss come mainly from inadvertent features of the environment rather than from parental attitudes, but the outcome of the child-care practices in such societies is the development of mental illnesses, both major and minor. All of the societies experience some violent conflict, up to and including homicide, which in the !Kung San (Bushmen) of Botswana has been shown to exceed that in American cities, belying the common description of the group as "the harmless people." Human behaviors often considered undesirable, such as selfishness, deceit, adolescent rebellion, adultery, desertion, and child abuse, are seen in such societies (Case H1), although it is impossible to compare the rates of such behaviors with those in the West.

NEO-DARWINIAN THEORY OF BEHAVIOR Since the late 1960s a field of evolutionary study known as neo-Darwinian theory or, more commonly, sociobiology, has emerged. It has been quickly adopted by most investigators who study animal behavior under natural conditions, including ethologists and behavioral ecologists, and has also influenced many anthropologists and psychologists. Briefly summarized, the principles are as follows:

1. An organism is in essence a gene's way of making another gene. More strictly, it is a way found by thousands of genes, through short- or long-term cooperation, to make copies of themselves. As long as it is admitted that no forces other than physicochemical ones can operate in nature, continued membership in an ongoing germ plasm can be the only goal served by any given gene. To the extent that a gene influences behavior, it can only continue in the germ plasm if it maintains or enhances, through the behavior, the number of copies of itself in the gene pool of the next generation. Contrary to a frequently repeated confusion, the cohesiveness of the genome through pleiotropy and epistatic and regulatory effects has only quantitative bearing on the validity of the principle. Recent theoretical and experimental work on intragenomic conflict strongly suggests that the cohesiveness of the genome in some respects has often been exaggerated.

2. Genes increase their number by enhancing reproductive success. Enhancing survival is only one way of doing this. Where the two goals are in conflict, genes that enhance reproductive success will replace genes that enhance survival. The concept of fitness in evolutionary theory has no meaning except the relative frequency of characteristics and of the genes that influence them. It is a tautological dimension of reproductive success and has nothing necessarily in common with medical, social, athletic, or ethical definitions of fitness, all of which can be achieved without an increase, or even with a decrease, in technically defined reproductive fitness. That principle has profound implications for medicine, and for psychiatry especially. Psychiatrists attempt to

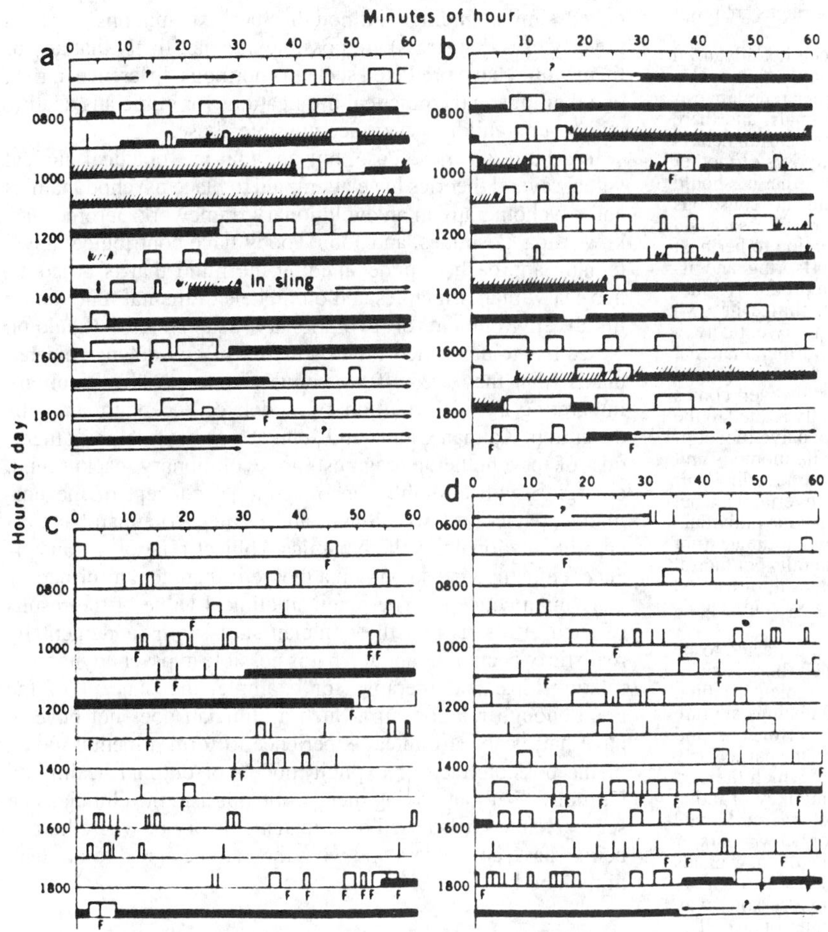

FIGURE 4.1-1 *Breast-feeding in hunter-gatherers. A day in life of each of four infants among !Kung San hunter-gatherers of northwestern Botswana in 1975: (A) a 4-day-old boy; (B) the same boy at 15 days; (C) a 12-month-old girl; (D) a 17-month-old boy. The long dark bars are sleep. The higher open bars and vertical lines are nursing bouts. (Figure from M Konner, C Worthman: Nursing frequency, gonadal function and birth spacing among !Kung hunter-gatherers. Science 207: 788, 1980. Used with permission.)*

adjust patients to a commonly understood professional standard of medical and psychological equilibrium, usually subscribed to by the patients, their families, or both. In many particulars that goal must be unrelated to the goal of enhancing reproductive fitness, for which the human organism, like all organisms, was primarily designed.

3. Fitness is properly defined as *inclusive fitness,* by which evolutionary theorists mean the tendency of genes to influence their frequency, not only through the survival and reproduction of the individual carrying them, but also through the survival and reproduction of closely related others who may be carrying the same gene through common descent. The concept was introduced by W. D. Hamilton to account, using the mathematics of evolutionary genetics, for the existence of altruism in animals, which previously seemed to be something that should be culled by the process of natural selection. Thus a newly defined subprocess of natural selection, called *kin selection,* was needed. If one twin dies to save an identical twin, then the frequency of any gene that helped predispose to that action will (all else being equal) be unaffected by the death. In general terms such genes, or any genes predisposing an individual to self-sacrifice for a relative, should be favored under conditions where $b/c > 1/r$, where b is the benefit to the recipient, c is the cost to the altruist, and r is the degree of genetic relatedness or the likelihood that any gene found in one individual is identical to the same gene found in another by common descent. That concept has been invoked to explain self-sacrifice of soldier ants for the colony, alarm calls of birds and ground squirrels, and nepotism in human beings, among many other phenomena. Other theories that have been brought to bear on the problem of altruism are reciprocal altruism and the prisoner's dilemma model of cooperation, neither of which requires that the altruist and the recipient be related. Reciprocal altruism assumes that the organism has some memory capacity and lives long enough to repay an act of generosity with a reciprocal one—preferentially directed toward the original altruist. It is difficult to make such a system resistant to the evolution of cheating, but the prisoner's dilemma model accounts for that factor by making the reciprocity simultaneous—in effect, cooperation. The game consists of a situation in which two prisoners must either cooperate or not cooperate (defect). The reward is greatest if one prisoner defects while the other cooperates. However, if the game is repeated again and again, the other prisoner will not continue to cooperate. When both defect, which will happen repeatedly, both will gain much less than they would have if both had cooperated. It is not obvious what should be done, assuming that there will be many trials, but it has been shown empirically, through computer simulation, that one successful strategy is tit for tat—doing what the other prisoner did the last time—rather than consistent defection. Changing the rules or the context, however, can result in different long-term adaptations.

4. As argued by Robert Trivers from a suggestion of Darwin's, in species with two sexes in which there is a physiological or behavioral difference in the energy invested in individual offspring, the sex that invests more will become the scarce resource over which members of the other sex will compete. Among mammals and in most birds the female sex exhibits greater investment, but direct male parental investment may be very high in some species. Species in which male parental investment is high tend to be those in which pair formation of a breeding male member with a breeding female member is long-lasting; sexual dimorphism, both morphological and behavioral, is low; male-male competition for female mates is low; and variability among male members in reproductive success is low. Such pair-bonding species, a category including 8,000 species of birds but only a minority of mammal species, may be contrasted with lek or tournament species, so called because they sometimes have annual seasonal breeding tournaments in which male members of the species compete fiercely for female members. Those species often have high sexual dimorphism for display or fighting (for example, antlers or peacock feathers); a low tendency for pair formation; low direct male parental investment in offspring; and high variability in male reproductive success. In the elephant seal *Mirounga angustirostris,* 4 percent of the male seals account for 85 percent of the copulations during the breeding season, a skewing of reproductive success that can result in a very rapid rate of evolution and accounts for the extreme sexual dimorphism in that species. Human beings are considered to be near but not at the pair-bonding end of the continuum, as indicated by the amount of sexual dimorphism, degree of direct male involvement in the care of offspring in a wide range of cultures, and the known distribution of human marriage forms. (Polygyny, in which one man marries more than one woman, is allowed or encouraged in most cultures in the anthropological record: 708 of 849, or 83 percent. The converse arrangement, polyandry, is rare: four of 849. Furthermore, a double standard of sexual

restriction is extremely common; still, most human marriages are probably monogamous, at least in intent.)

5. The neo-Darwinian model of parent-offspring conflict advanced by Trivers has implications for the nature of the family that are as profound as those arising from the theory of differential parental investment. Weaning conflict is very common among mammals, and there are equivalent phenomena among birds, even including tantrum behavior on the part of the weanling. If the evolutionary purposes of mother and offspring were isomorphic, then they should agree (that is, should have been selected to act as if they agreed, implying no conscious intent) that a given level and duration of investment are necessary and sufficient, after which the mother should turn her attention to her next potential offspring. However, even if the current offspring and its unborn sibling have the same father, the offspring's reproductive success will be twice as great if it acts selfishly to maximize its own reproductive value, as compared with that of its sibling. Eventually, a point is reached at which the offspring's need for further maternal investment is outweighed by the inclusive fitness advantage gained through the birth of a subsequent sibling. That point, however, comes later for the offspring than for the mother, who is equally related to the weanling and the potential unborn sibling. Although a naive model of the nature of the family assumes that it functions as a harmonious unit under ideal conditions, it was not so designed. Like the breeding pair the family is an association among individuals with overlapping but distinct evolutionary purposes. Its members naturally pursue individual goals that are sometimes at odds with one another's ultimate (not merely temporary) purposes, and their relations are naturally conflictful rather than harmonious. The natural conflict is not the result of friction in what should or could be a smoothly functioning system, but is intrinsic.

6. Competition among unrelated individuals can be expected to be extreme at times. Virtually all animal species for which there is sufficient evidence have been seen to exhibit extremes of violent conflict, including homicide, in the wild. The belief that human beings are rare among animal species in that they kill their own kind is erroneous, and more evidence to the contrary accumulates every year. One particularly noteworthy phenomenon is competitive infanticide, of which the paradigmatic description is that of the Hanuman langur monkey of India, *Presbytis entellus*. Langur troops consist of a core of related female monkeys and their offspring, associated for periods of a few years or less with unrelated immigrant male monkeys. Occasionally, new males monkeys arrive and challenge the resident male monkeys. If the newcomers win and take over the troop, they drive their predecessors away and proceed to kill all resident infants under 6 months of age. The mothers of those infants then come into estrus again (much sooner than they would have if the infants had survived and continued to nurse) and are impregnated by the new male monkeys. Controversy has centered over whether that is normal behavior or a response to crowding or other social stress. Such controversy misses the point that the behavior enhances the reproductive success of the new male monkeys at the expense of the old ones, and can be expected to be favored by natural selection. Similar phenomena (for example, the killing of a number of infant chimpanzees by two unrelated female chimpanzees under natural conditions) have been observed in many species.

Evolutionary psychiatry In the late 1980s and early 1990s a new subfield of psychiatry began to take shape in response to neo-Darwinian theory. Known as evolutionary or Darwinian psychiatry, its concepts and assertions range from the useful to the outrageous. The notion that phobias are the result of what once were probably adaptive fears is not surprising, nor does it contribute in any evident way to patient care, except perhaps by offering the patient an explanatory model of the phobia—but one that clinicians did not need sociobiologists to suggest to them. Sociopathy may be the result of an evolutionary adaptation for increasing reproductive success, but that does not make it any more treatable or the sociopath's victims any less wronged; the theorist may find the model satisfying, but that does not necessarily help anyone else.

Some findings generated by neo-Darwinian theory, however, have been rather unexpected and may have practical value. Martin Daly and Margo Wilson, reasoning from inclusive fitness theory, predicted that rates of child abuse would differ between stepfathers and biological fathers. Data from Canada in the 1970s and 1980s showed that the risk of death by homicide to a child under 2 years of age was 70 times greater in a household with a stepparent (usually a stepfather) than in one with two natural parents. American and English samples produced similar findings. Although other explanations (such as poverty or social stress) are possible, it is not likely that any of them would have predicted such an enormous difference in risk, one that must have practical implications for clinicians dealing with young children who face possible abuse.

In a more abstract sense, but one that has practical clinical value, several theories have attempted to place psychodynamics and psychotherapy in an evolutionary framework. Jerome Barkow, Lida Cosmides, and John Tooby have contributed a systematic approach to understanding the mind that is based on neo-Darwinian principles and on models of mental functioning in an environment of evolutionary adaptedness. Randolph Nesse has reinterpreted Freud's theory of ego defense mechanisms (that they are self-protective tactics of self-deception), integrating it with evolutionary models of deception and self-deception. Kalman Glantz and John Pierce have set their methods of psychotherapy against an evolutionary background, emerging with a slightly unconventional concept of the normative. Malcolm Owen Slavin and Daniel Kriegman have set current relational psychodynamics—object relations, transference, empathy, and so on—in a theoretical context informed by Darwinian concepts. The practical clinical value of the results of such efforts is that the clinician starts with fundamentally realistic expectations about what is possible in psychodynamics, relationships, and therapy (for example, the concept of the good-enough relationship). Such a clinician does not have to have had years of clinical experience to form a mental model of the possible tacit or explicit models of optimal health and harmony. Without risking therapeutic nihilism the clinician can set reachable goals based on a realistic theory of where human beings have come from and what they are designed to do, feel, think, and be.

Value judgments Neo-Darwinian or sociobiological theory is sometimes presumed to include value judgments. That presumption merely repeats an ancient philosophic fallacy, according to which whatever is, is right. An extension of the fallacy would hold that sickle cell anemia or thalassemia must be accepted because natural selection has maintained it through balanced polymorphism, the heterozygotes being at an advantage in malaria resistance; or that myopia should not be corrected because natural selection in favor of sharp vision has relaxed in the human population since the end of the hunting-and-gathering era. Human judgments about what is desirable are separate from any observations or explanations of what exists in nature, although they may be enhanced by taking the facts of the natural world into account.

That caution applies equally to clinical and ethical judgments. Just as those two kinds of value judgments must be kept separate from each other, so each must be separated from Darwinian fitness, and one can imagine situations in which all three types of judgments would lead to different conclusions. There is something satisfying, however, about the fact that survival and reproduction—priorities reordered by the neo-Darwinians as reproduction and survival—show a symmetry with the goals of mental health as Freud defined them: *lieben und arbeiten*, or to love and to work.

CROSS-CULTURAL CONSISTENCY AND VARIATION IN HUMAN BEHAVIOR

MODEL OF CULTURE AND PERSONALITY Figure 4.1-2 shows how the elements of human social organization and culture may articulate with the universal characteristics of the

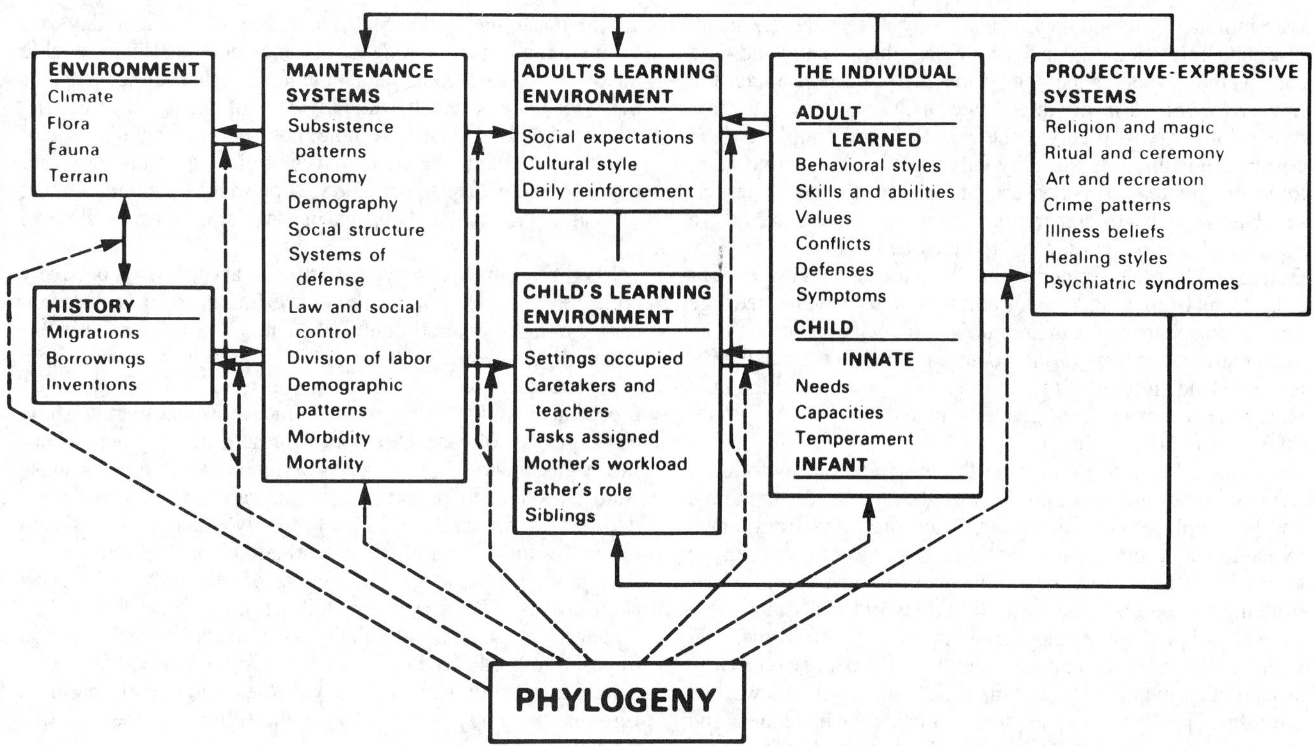

FIGURE 4.1-2 *Model of the interrelationships of child training, adult personality, and various aspects of society and culture under the influence of phylogeny. Modified from a model of John and Beatrice Whiting. (Figure from M J Konner: Evolution of human behavior development. In* Handbook of Cross-Cultural Human Development, *R H Munroe, R L Munroe, B B Whiting, editors, p 3. Garland STPM Press, New York, 1981. Used with permission.)*

human life cycle, especially the developmental phase, to produce the variation observed in the anthropological record. It is loosely based on a model developed by John and Beatrice Whiting to summarize their view of culture and personality after several decades of work in psychological anthropology.

The model carries on a tradition begun in the 1930s of assuming that (1) some aspects of society and culture are likely to determine the major features of childhood experience, (2) such childhood experience markedly influences the adult personality of the typical member of the society, and (3) some other aspects of society and culture are likely to be consequences of the typical adult personality and so of the childhood experiences. Phylogeny was not explicitly part of the Whiting model, but is added here as a result of the foregoing considerations, which will be extended and integrated with the rest of the model.

Even without the phylogenetic arrows the model is explicitly Darwinian in intent. The environment is considered primary and the society and culture as a response to the environment, much as in the longer course of evolution individual morphology and innate behavioral capacities of different species are responses to the environment. (The addition of history to the model was a relatively late development; defined as it is in terms of borrowings and inventions, it does not change the basic concept of society and culture as responses to the environment.) *Maintenance systems* are the aspects of social organization most heavily influenced by the demands of adaptation, especially subsistence ecology and defense. Those demands, according to the model, constrain the learning environment in childhood and adulthood, producing distinctive features of individual personality and behavior. Finally, *projective systems,* aspects of culture theoretically only indirectly dependent on the environment, are determined largely by the culture's particular collection of adult personalities.

Many studies in psychological anthropology have been inspired by such a model, which emerged initially from collaborations between anthropologists and psychoanalysts. Cross-cultural applications of psychoanalytic theory continue to be fruitful, as in the work of Robert LeVine *(Culture, Behavior, and Personality)* and Robert Paul *(The Tibetan Symbolic World),* both anthropologists who undertook psychoanalytic training, and in that of Robert Levy *(Tahitians),* who was a practicing psychiatrist before becoming an anthropologist. Melford Spiro's *Oedipus in the Trobriands* defends the concept of the putatively universal oedipal conflict against the old objection of Malinowski that it could not occur in a Western society in which the traditional father's role was split between the father and the mother's brother.

Most recent studies do not rely on psychoanalytic constructs, however, but on categories of behavior and child development that are easier to operationalize. Consider a cross-cultural study carried out by Whiting and Whiting in 1975 that exemplifies both the appeal and the limitations of the approach. The study used the Human Relations Area Files, one of the most important tools for quantitative research in anthropology. The files consist of nested samples of societies and cultures studied by anthropologists throughout the world, especially a core sample of 60 and a larger sample of nearly 200. Among criteria for inclusion are (1) quality of data, as indicated by training and language competence of the ethnographers, person-years of study at the field site, number of published pages, and other measures; (2) geographical and cultural representativeness of the entire known range of several thousand societies and cultures; and (3) mutual independence of influence, to maximize the likelihood that each society entered in the world sample will function as a statistically independent unit.

The Whitings analyzed a dimension they called "husband-wife intimacy,'' which they measured by three intercorrelated, independently rated dimensions: whether the husband and wife eat together, whether they sleep together, and how much the father is involved in the direct care of the children. All three dimensions vary markedly in the world cultural sample, but the covariance is high; that is, they vary together. Furthermore, all three are related to a measure of how much the society is involved in war and preparations for war. At one extreme are the typical warlike cultures of the crowded highlands of New Guinea, with collective houses in which men eat and sleep separate from women and young children, and to which teenage boys are sent to begin their training for belligerency. At the other extreme are non-warlike societies—such as the small, protected, island cultures of the south Pacific—that have high husband-wife intimacy and greater involvement of men with infants and young children.

The model is used to interpret those correlations as follows: Some societies are thrust into warfare because of demographic and geographical conditions; others are protected from attack by natural conditions. Distinct maintenance systems arise in the two types of society with consequences for child care, such as bringing teenage boys into an all-male world that trains them for war and predisposes them to avoid contact with women and young children. In the realm of adult learning being exclusively around other men reinforces a man's identification with warlike purposes. Projective systems, such as distinctive male dress and hair style, religious beliefs, and beliefs about male superiority (not directly incorporated into the study), would be seen as epiphenomena of the basic or typical male personality.

The study is appealing because fitting it to the model involves primarily commonsense assumptions about the relations within and among the various systems. However, it remains an interpretation of correlations and not an actual causal demonstration. It might be argued that in warlike societies the first event was a historical accident—say, the advent of a very belligerent leader. That person may have invented men's houses and trained boys for war, which eventually led to a state of chronic belligerency toward neighboring societies. In that model, accepted by some historians and anthropologists, ideology and individual predisposition precede fundamental environmental adaptations. The model may seem plausible in the explanation of the structure and function of a given society at a given moment, but it is difficult to argue convincingly that regularities, such as those observed in broad cross-cultural statistical analyses involving scores or even hundreds of societies, could emerge from a collection of such ideological or historical accidents.

CHILDHOOD EXPERIENCE AND ADULT PREDISPOSITION The model faced its most troubling difficulties not in the anthropological realm of the relation between maintenance systems and ideology, but in the psychological realm of the relation between childhood experience and adult predisposition. In the early 1970s the developmental psychologist Jerome Kagan became involved in research on cross-cultural psychological development. That research led him to initiate a major challenge to one of the most fundamental assumptions not only of behavioral and social science, but also of psychiatry and clinical psychology. The assumption was that childhood experiences, especially in early childhood, have different and more lasting effects on the formation of adult predispositions and abilities than do later experiences. Specifically, in studying cognition in infancy and childhood in a remote Guatemalan Indian village he and his colleagues found that lack of stimulation and substantial deficits in infancy did not entail deficits in later childhood. In the United States he found that being in day care for eight hours a day throughout infancy did not affect available measures of cognition, attachment, or other dimensions of behavior. The research and judgment of many other experimental developmental psychologists seem to challenge that assumption, fundamental to psychological anthropology and psychodynamic psychiatry, and to support the counterclaim that little if anything that happens in early life is irreversible in effect.

Psychodynamic clinicians routinely accept retrospectively collected interview data as evidence for the relation between early environment and adult personality; rigorous experimentalists do not seriously entertain such data in relation to that particular question. Some investigators of child development do prospective studies using excellent measures that seem to show consequences of early experience for later development; skeptics argue that without random assignment of subjects those studies produce mere correlations that can be readily explained without a particular causal effect of early experience. Research on the lasting effects of early deprivations or interventions, as long as they are not extreme, has generally failed to support such effects. The research includes follow-up studies of low Apgar scores, lack of stimulation in infancy, breast-feeding as opposed to bottle feeding, day care in infancy, Head Start preschool interventions, and other variables. In general, the more rigorous the study and the longer the follow-up, the less was the detectable effect.

Counterarguments are also numerous. Specific measures used in childhood or adulthood may be inappropriate, behavior under stress rather than baseline behavior may be the right outcome measure, random assignment of subjects is unethical, and so on. The fact remains that developmental psychologists, psychiatrists, and educators have failed to show that decisive lasting effects of early experience exist. They also have failed to show how such effects might operate or what they might specifically be, despite the strong beliefs of many clinicians about those relationships.

Developmental behavioral genetics Significant new insights on both sides of this controversy have come from an unexpected but increasingly valuable direction: developmental behavioral genetics. The emphasis on developmental process among behavioral geneticists is new, and in the relatively near future it may provide solutions to many old problems in the development of personality, abilities, and psychopathology. Ironically, developmental behavioral genetics may be one of the few paradigms for generating believable results regarding environmental influences, because it is the only nonexperimental paradigm that controls for gene effects and genotype-environment correlation. Recent work by Robert Plomin, David Rowe, and others has established an extraordinary fact about family influence. In rigorous twin, adoption, and family studies variance in personality, as well as in mental ability, can be statistically partitioned among various sources. The results routinely accord a large proportion of the variance to environmental influence (roughly half in a number of studies), although it remains difficult to specify the time points after conception at which the environmental influence takes place or how it is distributed among various environmental independent variables (for example, trauma, infection, psychodynamic processes, school, and peer pressure).

The extraordinary finding is that family influence in numerous studies appears to be very small. That inference follows from the fact that the portion of the variance in outcome measures (such as behavior and questionnaire results) attributable to environment is composed almost entirely of within-family variance, such as sibling differences. Identical twins reared together are routinely found to be no more similar in personality than identical twins reared in separate families, and sometimes the latter are found to be more similar. To the extent that children in different families differ in personality, the difference can be explained almost entirely by their genetic differences. Differences between nonidentical-twin siblings, however, cannot be explained by their genetic differences alone, but require environmental explanations as well.

That is an extraordinary conclusion. It seems to indicate that everything parents do to treat their children similarly (rules, religion, schooling, toys, television) does not make them more similar in personality, or more different from their counterparts in other families, than they would be on the basis of genes alone. No one understands why that is so. It could have to do with siblings' influences on one another, as in the case of identical twins reared together, who may have stronger motives to differentiate themselves from each other than do identical twins reared apart. Birth-order effects have also been explored but rigorous research shows them to be far smaller than folklore and popular psychology have claimed. More plausible is the model suggested by Sandra Scarr, a developmental psychologist and behavioral geneticist. According to Scarr, a child's genotype leads the child to seek out a particular, compatible environment, and may lead parents to provide such a tailored environment. Whatever the explanation, the challenge posed by the extremely small magnitude of measurable between-family variance poses a major challenge to the explanatory paradigms of child psychiatry, psychodynamic theory, and developmental psychology.

Animal models The only really decisive evidence concerning those processes comes from studies of animal models, which are given insufficient attention by some psychodynamic clinicians and cultural anthropologists. Animal studies using random assignment and rigorous control of other independent variables have repeatedly shown that early experience can make a lasting impression not only on behavior and psychological predisposition, but also on neural and neuroendocrine structure and function.

In the jewel fish early social experience changes the number and shape of the dendritic spines on the pyramidal neurons of the tectum. In the chick imprinting (the formation of early attachments, normally to the mother) alters neuronal structure and glucose utilization in the hyperstriatum and permanently determines the juvenile attachments the bird will make and also its adult sexual choice. Rats stimulated or handled in infancy have faster rates of growth, larger body size, and greater resistance to being killed by starvation, drowning, tumor injection, and other means. They are less fearful in strange situations, exploring more and defecating less, and they have improved learning ability as compared with controls. All those effects are believed to be related to an altered pattern of corticosterone secretion from the adrenal cortex—a pattern in which secretion is low when stress is low but rises markedly when stress is high.

Male mice raised in isolation for three weeks after weaning are much more likely to fight when paired with another male mouse than are controls raised in groups and then paired with strange male mice. Such isolation also results in altered levels, turnover, and related enzyme activities of monoamine neurotransmitters, although the precise relation of the neurochemical changes to the increased aggressiveness is not known. Rats of any age, including those at the end of the life span, can experience brain alterations in response to experiential enrichment: in the occipital region of the cerebral hemispheres the thickness and weight of the cortex, the number and size of synapses, the complexity of dendritic branching and density of dendritic spines, and the activity of choline acetyltransferase are favorably affected.

In rhesus monkeys the closure of one eye for a few days during the first six months of life will result in permanent impairment of depth perception; incoming stimuli from the two eyes are at that time in competition for sites on binocularly responsive cells in the visual cortex and removal of stimulation from one eye allows the other to take over all sites on the cells, which will then be unable to respond binocularly. In rhesus monkeys, as in several other species of monkeys and apes, isolation rearing results in a variety of permanent impairments of social and reproductive behavior; in the presence of pathological behavior, such as stereotypical rocking and self-directed aggression at baseline; and in a lower threshold for the elicitation of such pathological behaviors by amphetamine, even in monkeys that have recovered from the isolation-induced syndrome. Even short separations of a week or so in rhesus monkeys have been shown to have lasting effects on their behavior in strange situations.

TRANSFERABILITY TO HUMANS The lessons to be drawn are complex. Most of the results cannot be transferred in a simple manner to humans, yet some principles may be transferable. The fact that a variety of stimulating tactics in infancy in rats, some of which are simply stressors, have the same apparently positive effects must lead to caution in interpreting early stress effects in humans. The monocular closure experiment demonstrates that a particular distortion of input can produce permanent damage in a short time, even though closure of both eyes, a blanket deprivation, at the same age would have little permanent effect. If that could be extrapolated to human social and emotional development, it might vindicate psychodynamic thinking about early emotional trauma. The amphetamine challenge experiment shows that monkeys that have recovered behaviorally from early isolation still have neurochemical abnormalities that make them vulnerable to neuropharmacological challenge, suggesting that some psychodynamic theorists may be right in thinking that the behavioral measurements of developmental psychologists do not necessarily get at the underlying structure of the psyche.

Given the number and variety of those and related findings, and the fact that they range over the entire vertebrate phylogenetic tree, only an assumption of the most unlikely discontinuity between the nature of the human brain and behavioral development and that of animals can support the expectation that similar effects on human development will not be shown. Such effects, when properly delineated, will form the core of a new body of theory in both clinical psychodynamics and psychological anthropology. To believe that such effects exist is reasonable, but to hold strong specific beliefs about how early experience and cultural variations in child care influence adult personality, in the absence of clear evidence, can only impede the growth of knowledge about those processes.

CROSS-CULTURAL UNIVERSALS OF HUMAN BEHAVIOR, MIND, AND CULTURE Although the main enterprise of cultural anthropology in general, and of psychological anthropology in particular, has been the description and analysis of cross-cultural variation, that enterprise has always had an inevitable complement: the characterization of features of human behavior that do not vary or that vary relatively little. The concept of universals has at least five different meanings:

(1) behaviors, such as coordinated bipedal walking or smiling in social greeting, that are exhibited by all normal members of every known society; (2) behaviors that are universal within an age or sex class, such as the Moro reflex in all normal neonates or the ejaculatory motor action pattern in all postpubertal males; (3) population characteristics that apply to all populations but not to all individual members of the population, such as the sex difference in physical aggressiveness; (4) universal features of culture rather than of behavior, such as the taboos against incest and homicide, or the highly variable but always present institution of marriage, or the social construction of illness and attempts at healing; and (5) characteristics that, although unusual or even rare, are found at some low level in every population, such as homicidal violence, thought disorder, depression, suicide, and incest.

The list of characteristics in those five categories is much longer than earlier anthropologists would have predicted. (The ethologist Irenaus Eibl-Eibesfeldt has been responsible for the description of many remarkable constancies in nonverbal communication and social relationships.) The search for societies without violence, or without gender differences that go beyond reproduction, or without mental illness, or even without the ability to make and use fire has been a vain one. Although there is convincing documentation of variation in the incidence or context of expression of most human behaviors, the existence of a large core of always-present, if variable, features constitutes a demonstration of the reality of human nature and its validity as a scientific construct. It should be emphasized that those universals are fundamental to the nature of the human species in a deeper way than are the features found in human hunter-gatherers but departed from by later forms of society; the universals are found in all societies regardless of environment or subsistence ecology and thus are likely to be related to human nature in an even more intrinsic way.

Traditional cultural anthropologists have shown little or no interest in such universals, viewing them as trivial or outside their subject matter. That attitude is like being interested in the height difference between the Watusi and the Pygmies, but not in the mechanism of action of growth hormone. The elucidation of universal features of human behavior and culture is increasingly being recognized as one of the central task of the discipline, and one likely to enhance the analysis of cultural variation. Even many cultural anthropologists have attempted to delineate such universals as symbol systems and mental structures whose common underlying characteristics link widely disparate kinds of art, language, and ritual.

With regard to the model in Figure 4.1-2, the delineation of universal features of human behavior is central to the elucidation of the effects of phylogeny, shown as dotted lines in the diagram. Phylogeny is shown as directly affecting the box representing the individual, especially the innate needs, drives, and capacities. But most of its effects on the system are modeled as occurring through its influence on other arrows. Natural selection operating on ancestral organisms created not only individuals with certain needs, drives, and capacities, but also equations (if-then statements) relating the environment to the social system, the social system to the individual member, and so on. To refer again to the study of husband-wife intimacy, phylogeny appears to have provided a system in which separating men from women and small children enhances their effectiveness as warriors. It does not mean that they must be warriors or that they must be aloof from their wives, but that aloofness may increase effective belligerency, and perhaps the converse. The universal characteristic here is not only a phenotypic characteristic (aggression is more a male characteristic than a female characteristic) but also an underlying mechanism relating two sets of characteristics to each other (the male-female difference is exaggerated by gender separation and reduced by gender proximity).

Recent applications In the past decade the application of neo-Darwinian or sociobiological theory to ethnological materials has produced many findings that seem to bypass the complex questions of the relations among society, culture, and individual development. For example, societies in which young men inherit land from their mothers' brothers are more lax about the prevention of female adultery than are societies in which young men inherit from their fathers; in societies in which polygyny is allowed, wealthier men tend to have more wives; and in small-scale societies in which the adoption of children is common, it tends to follow patterns predicted by genetic relatedness. Investigators usually declare that they do not claim any direct genetic basis for those variations in human behavior, and some of the most egregious confusion about sociobiology stems from a failure to appreciate the distinction between the propositions of neo-Darwinian theory and those of traditional behavioral genetics or molecular genetics.

Even in a nonhuman species such as the redwing blackbird *Agelaius phoeneceus,* male birds singing on richer territories mate with several female birds instead of one. But the mechanism of that flexible adaptive system, known as a *facultative adaptation,* must be quite different in blackbirds than in human beings (although it would probably underestimate blackbirds to assume that in them the system is under tight genetic control). The wings of insects come from thoracic tissue, the wings of birds from forearm structures, the wings of bats from fingers, and the wings of humans from technology. Those four adaptations to the problem of flight arrive at similar functions through extremely different developmental processes. The same will prove to be true of adaptations in social behavior.

Incest Sociobiologists (and classical evolutionists and geneticists before them) predicted that incest would be avoided in most sexually reproducing species to avoid the appearance of maladaptive homozygous recessive members of the species. But adults on the verge of mating must recognize close kin. In insects and in some vertebrates such recognition depends on pheromones. In humans the unlikelihood of that mechanism has led to a search for other ontogenetic explanations. The anthropologist Arthur Wolf, motivated by considerations apart from sociobiology, has shown conclusively that in traditional China, where young girls sometimes came to live with the families of their intended spouses (also children), the resulting marriages had a much higher rate of failure and infertility than did other arranged marriages. He has further identified a sensitive period of contact for the effect to occur. Related findings emerge from studies of the marriage rate among Israeli kibbutz cohort members.

Thus the familiarity breeds contempt hypothesis of incest, first introduced by Westermarck in the last century, receives support. The implication is that human beings avoid inbreeding through a psychological mechanism that depends on cultural choice, even though the evolutionary effects may ultimately be the same as in species that rely on pheromones for their incest avoidance. In such analyses the purposes and methods of psychological anthropology and sociobiology are joined, and the study of human behavior in general is much better served than it is by debates about nature and nurture.

UNIVERSALS AND VARIATIONS IN PSYCHOSOCIAL GROWTH Freud postulated, and present-day child psychiatry continues to accept in altered and disputed forms, a universal sequence of emotional development on which the social environment of the family could be claimed to operate to produce enduring traits of emotional disposition. Beyond some very general elements (the existence of infantile sexuality, the formation of an attachment to a primary caretaker who is usually the mother, the ubiquity of conflicts and jealousies within the family) that allegedly universal sequence has never found empirical support; hence unresolvable disputes have arisen among different schools of child psychoanalysis, along with the skepticism of outsiders. Extensive cross-cultural studies of human behavioral and psychological development have not furnished evidence relevant to those particular models, but they have produced extensive evidence supporting more empirically grounded putative universals of psychosocial growth. In the absence of knowledge of neuropsychological development psychoanalytic theory postulated a libidinal theory of neural development that many question. However, the growing body of knowledge about neural and neuroendocrine development can now begin to provide an anatomical foundation for newer, more empirically grounded studies of psychosocial growth.

Among the well-established cross-cultural universals of psychosocial development, the following are the best supported, and in most cases can be plausibly related to putative underlying neural or neuroendocrine maturational events: (1) the emergence of sociality, as heralded by social smiling, during the first four months of life, in parallel with the maturation of basal ganglia and cortical motor circuits; (2) the emergence of strong attachments, as well as of fears of separation and of strangers, in the second half of the first year of life, in parallel with the maturation of the major fiber tracts of the limbic system; (3) the emergence of language during the second year and after, in parallel with the maturation of the thalamic projection to the auditory cortex among other circuits; (4) the emergence of a sex difference in physical aggressiveness in early and middle childhood, with male children on the average exceeding female children, a consequence in part of prenatal androgenization of the hypothalamus; (5) the emergence of adult sexual motivation and functioning in adolescence, in parallel with and following the maturation of the hypothalamic-pituitary-gonadal axis at puberty, against the background of the previously mentioned prenatal androgenization of the hypothalamus.

Other probable cross-cultural developmental universals, such as increased babbling in the second half of the first year and progress through the first three or perhaps four of the six stages in Lawrence Kohlberg's scheme of moral development in childhood, are neither as well established nor as plausibly related to underlying maturational events as are the five advanced here. Although their underlying neuropsychology is at an early stage of elucidation, their cross-cultural universality is well established, and in each case there is extensive experimental evidence to support the maturational nature of the process in behavioral development. They thus constitute a first approximation of the true structural basis of psychosocial development, which Freud was groping for with his theory of libidinal development in the nervous system.

The universals also constitute a firm basis for the future understanding of how variations in social experience, whether clinical or cross-cultural, act on the maturing psychosocial competence to produce potentially lasting variations. In each of the five processes mentioned cross-cultural differentiation of the maturing competence begins almost as soon as the maturation occurs. In some cases there is sufficient evidence to state provisional rules relating environment to differentiation, for example: "Infants whose smiles are favorably responded to will smile more," or, "All children will acquire languages with similar cognitive and social functions, but with whatever arbitrary semantic content is presented." In others, such as the differentiation of the strength of attachment in different cultures, it has been difficult to discern any plausible relation to the characteristics of the social and emotional world that preceded the attachment, despite the expectation of such relationships.

The more interesting developmental events are more refractory to explanation, but the acceptance and increasingly detailed and reliable description of the maturational constants underlying the variation in psychosocial growth will provide a steadily firmer place on which to stand while attempting to understand the true, and undoubtedly large, role of cultural and individual experience.

CROSS-CULTURAL PSYCHIATRY

Cross-cultural psychiatry as it has been practiced by anthropologists and psychiatrists has consisted of three closely related enterprises: (1) *psychological anthropology,* using psychodynamic theory to interpret the relation among elements of society and culture; (2) *comparative psychiatry,* using formal epidemiological or less formal observational and clinical methods to describe and analyze cross-cultural variation in the incidence or prevalence of syndromes and symptoms; and (3) *medical anthropology,* using traditional anthropological methods to elucidate cross-cultural variation in the social and cultural construction of illness from disease and in the elaboration of healing or caretaking roles and relationships.

COMPARATIVE PSYCHIATRY Comparative psychiatry has been a difficult enterprise under the best of circumstances. The fourth edition of *Diagnostic and Statistical Manual of Mental Disorders* (DSM-IV) was developed in an attempt to rationalize and reduce the wide variation in diagnostic styles found even among major medical centers in the United States. Ongoing debates prove that much disagreement still exists. The international equivalent of the manual, under the supervision of the World Health Organization, is quite different and is subject to similar controversy. Yet one often sees statements about the prevalence of psychiatric disorders in different countries and cultures that seem to presume the nonexistence or unimportance of such nosological controversy.

It is often said that the incidence of schizophrenia is roughly similar in all countries, with ½ to 1 percent incidence the figure usually cited. England and the United States alone, two English-speaking countries with excellent medical cooperation and communication, have had major differences in the definition of schizophrenia that would preclude any meaningful statement about whether the incidence of the disorder is roughly similar or very different in the two countries. And the comparison takes place under ideal conditions, relatively free of doubt about differences in the age and mortality of the populations, the likelihood of case location, the quality and integrity of hospital records, and other factors that plague the cross-cultural epidemiological study of even the best-defined diagnoses in medicine and surgery.

The implication often drawn from that purportedly constant cross-cultural incidence of schizophrenia (namely, that it supports a genetic basis for the disorder) is also misleading. Most known genetic diseases have marked population variation in their incidence that is well known to physicians and anthropologists. Various categories of evidence support some genetic hypothesis of schizophrenia defined in almost any way, but the alleged cross-cultural constancy in incidence, even if true, is not one of them. (It could, for example, merely reflect a cross-cultural constancy in the threshold for labeling a thought disorder as serious or chronic.)

CROSS-CULTURAL INCIDENCE AND PREVALENCE When the discussion turns to questions of incidence in small-scale societies, such as those most often studied by anthropologists, the size of the cohort is too small to support meaningful comparative study. Still, two generalizations about the cross-cultural incidence and prevalence of psychiatric disorders can be made, regardless of the scale of the societies under comparison.

Symptom clusters First, the major psychiatric symptoms and symptom clusters, including those at the core of the major disorders and syndromes variously defined, appear to exist in all societies. They include anxiety, mania, depression, suicidal ideation, major thought disorder, paranoia, somatization, and many other diagnoses or components of diagnoses on Axis I of DSM-IV. In addition, they include a range of normal and abnormal personality types that is suggestive of the range exhibited by the diagnoses on Axis II.

Those disorders frequently are manifest as folk illnesses, with labels that subdivide the range of symptom patterns differently than psychiatrists do. Some cultures fail to label at all, but recognize the abnormality, and even its treatability. And many give labels that are close to cross-national comparisons of Western psychiatric diagnoses. Jane Murphy's research among the Eskimo of northwest Alaska and the Yoruba of rural Nigeria provides several illustrations. Persons in both of those cultures clearly recognize a syndrome resembling schizophrenia—an idiosyncratic severe thought disorder, chronic or chronically recurring, that markedly impairs social functioning. The Eskimo call it *nuthkavihak* and the Yoruba *were* (in English, "crazy" or "insane"). Its victims are responded to with a mixture of compassion and fear, and treated with persistent attempts at decent maintenance as well as restraint. The syndrome is carefully distinguished from shamanistic thought disorder, which is believed to be voluntary, despite temporary hallucinations and delusions.

In the realm of nonpsychotic symptomatology both cultures have labeled such complaints as insomnia, night terrors, agoraphobia, anxiety, and claustrophobia, and considered them treatable by folk healers, but neither has a general label corresponding to neurosis. Each culture has a word (*kulangeta* in Eskimo, *arankan* in Yoruba) for the rare person who would be called a sociopath by psychiatrists (DSM-IV antisocial personality disorder) and each considers the condition untreatable.

Folk views of human character make quite subtle distinctions even in very simple societies. Case H2 is that of a man who, in a culture in which all men had extensive homosexual experience, was recognized as deviant in his devotion to such experience, and (although not labeled there) would perhaps merit the diagnosis of sexual disorder not otherwise specified, with persistent and marked distress about one's sexual orientation as the main symptom. Case H3 is that of a woman in Guatemala who experienced an isolated episode of what might be called a brief reactive psychosis and which received the folk label *colera*. Years later, when she was mature, she was recognized as having special powers in a positive sense, an excellent long-term resolution given her history.

Culture-bound syndromes Second, the cross-cultural distribution of some disorders is so skewed that the differences can probably be accepted even without strictly reliable epidemiological methods. Those so-called culture-bound or culture-specific syndromes should be referred to as syndromes usually found in one or more particular cultural settings. Thus the disorder may not only have a label, social construction, explanation, or even a mental content that is culturally unique (which is true of virtually every diagnosis defined by any society), but it is so bound up with its cultural meaning that it would not exist (would be something else) in the absence of the particular cultural framework.

Psychiatric tradition in Western culture includes at least two diagnoses that are probably in this category. Conversion disorder remains in the DSM-IV classification but appears to have been a much more common condition in the bourgeois society of Europe in the late 19th century than in any other cultural context, and it is likely that it was, to some extent, a specific interaction of individual predisposition with the cultural expectations of that subculture. Anorexia nervosa, in the past few decades an increasingly common disorder of middle-class adolescent and postadolescent women, appears likely to be evoked by particular cultural conditions affecting body image and self-expectation. Both disorders are or were strongly culturally constructed and subject to spread through psychocultural communication. In addition, many DSM-IV substance-use disorders have been, if not culture bound, certainly highly skewed in their patterns of subcultural distribution within society, and some have even had the quality of giving rise to transient cultural fads in self-treatment or self-stimulation.

The following are among the frequently cited syndromes believed to be characteristic of specific non-Western cultural settings: (1) *amok,* a condition among traditional Malay men in which a period of brooding is followed by an outburst of frenzied, often homicidal, violence ending in exhaustion and amnesia; (2) *pibloktoq,* a form of Arctic hysteria described among the Eskimo of northern Greenland, characterized by irritability followed by up to half an hour of wild excitement and dangerous and inappropriate behavior ending in seizures, and finally some hours of stuporous sleep ending in amnesia; (3) *latah,* an extreme startle reaction to a novel stimulus that especially affects middle-aged women in Southeast Asia, with disorganized speech and action, echolalia, and echopraxia, among other symptoms; (4) *koro,* another Southeast Asian malady consisting of extreme anxiety with the mental content of fear of involution of the genitalia and fear of death; and (5) *windigo,* a psychosis among the Algonkian Indians in which the fear of becoming a cannibal through possession by the windigo, a mythic creature, is a prominent feature of the thought disorder.

Other culturally defined syndromes seem insufficiently distinctive to merit inclusion among culture-bound syndromes, yet have a folk definition that makes it seem inadequate simply to translate them into a DSM-IV diagnosis. *Ataque de nervios,* a syndrome first described for Costa Rica but common elsewhere in Latin America (loosely translated as "attack of nerves," and perhaps related to North American symptom patterns that go by that folk label) consists of complaints of headache, insomnia, loss of appetite, fears, anger, trembling, falling, disorientation, fatigue, and despair. It is common, is considered hereditary, and legitimizes psychological complaints (allowing secondary gains) in a culture that otherwise resists them. *Susto,* a condition of general malaise and anhedonia resulting from a severe fright, is another example of a widespread Latin American folk diagnosis. In modernizing sub-Saharan Africa many male students experience what they call *brain fag* (headache, visual difficulties, agnosia, and chronic fatigue), which, despite its seemingly humorous name, causes much anguish. And in Trinidad the folk view recognizes a particularly severe form of reactive depression, *tabanka,* peculiar to men whose wives have left them; although the victim is considered ridiculous, he is also at serious risk for suicide.

In all those diagnoses—certainly the folk illnesses, but also the more distinctive culture-bound syndromes—the uniqueness can be questioned by any experienced psychiatrist, and in some cases (such as the *windigo* psychosis) the existence of the disorder is in dispute. *Ataque de nervios* has been studied in relation to disorders described in the revised third edition of DSM (DSM-III-R) by Michael Liebowitz and his colleagues at the Hispanic Anxiety Disorders Clinic of the New York State Psychiatric Institute. Patients presenting at the clinic who said that they suffered *ataque de nervios* did not differ in DSM-III-R diagnoses from those who did not give themselves this label. A variety of anxiety and depressive disorders was present in both group. But for the subgroup of *nervios* patients who were diagnosed with panic disorder (40 percent of those who used the folk label), symptom checklists showed that the patients used the folk label in reference to the same symptoms that the psychiatrists used to arrive at the diagnosis of panic disorder.

But neither *ataque de nervios* nor any other culture-bound syndrome has been sufficiently well studied to permit the assignment of a DSM-IV or other standard diagnosis, or to establish firmly the need for a new diagnosis. However, given the protean nature of human mental life in health and disease, it is not unlikely that the complex biopsychosocial dynamics of mental illness would produce some entities in some cultures that fall outside the range of DSM-IV. Premature assignment of DSM-IV diagnoses to those syndromes may prevent important discoveries about the mechanisms of psychiatric disorder. Such mechanisms may not be culturally determined. *Pibloqtoq,* for example, has been variously hypothesized to be the result of hypothermia, hypocalcemia, and hypervitaminosis A, among other proposed (including cultural) causes. Its elucidation might be prevented by the assurance that it is not unique. (Similar attitudes delayed the recognition of the causes of the New Guinea neurological disorder *kuru* and of pellagra.) Labeling theory provides a set of cultural mechanisms that attempt to explain some symptoms and syndromes as the result of learning. It is known that patients admitted to psychiatric hospitals in the United States take on characteristics that the staff members expect them to have, a response to labeling that should be even more possible in a traditional society. The existence of voodoo death alone should be sufficient evidence of the power of culturally defined symbols to produce illness, and some culture-bound syndromes and folk illnesses may be in a similar category. But it must also be noted that the great range of variation in human cultural and social life might have been expected to have produced more exotic syndromes than those few disputed entities, unless there were fundamental biological constraints on the way that the human mind and behavior break down.

MEDICAL ANTHROPOLOGY Dispute about the question of completely distinctive culture-bound syndromes misses the important point about this material. Whether or not such syndromes are homologous with the DSM-IV diagnoses, they have a distinct psychiatric reality by virtue of the cultural definitions, expectations, and responses that surround them. In that sense the most prosaic symptom or disorder in DSM-IV may become exotic when it appears in any other culture. Even medical and surgical illnesses undergo a similar transformation in non-Western cultural or subcultural settings.

The presence of an actual underlying biological disease is not at issue here, but it is clear that culture changes the meaning of the biological disease reality in ways that directly affect the physician. The differential diagnosis and treatment of a diffuse abdominal or lower back pain will be altered in cultures that have elaborate beliefs about discomfort in those anatomical areas. The differential diagnosis of ideas of reference or paranoid delusions will be even more subject to such cultural differences; moreover, the psychiatrist's role in consultation and liaison may make the circumstances of cultural expectation more critical for psychiatry than for most other fields of medicine.

Medical anthropology is a subfield of anthropology that is devoted in part to culture-bound syndromes and to non-Western concepts and systems of healing. It is not difficult to reconcile that kind of cross-cultural variation with the evolutionary perspective. Nonhuman primates have many response patterns that a psychiatrist would label abnormal in a human being (Cases P1, P2, and P3). Still, such abnormal behaviors, including prolonged grief after a loss, isolative behavior, or excessive violence, produce social effects and responses. Even illnesses and wounds are responded to by other group members with caretaking attempts.

It is hardly surprising that all human cultures have made some attempt to define abnormal conditions of body and mind and to respond to them with healing. Disease in general was probably the most important selective force operating on human ancestors during evolution, and it is inconceivable that cultural creatures with increasing intelligence should fail to try to do something about it. Although it can be argued that some of the most primitive attempts at healing may have had biological effectiveness, one does not have to go that far to conclude that the placebo effect of the mere attempt, for the patient, and the calming effect for others who might be frightened or saddened by the patient's condition would constitute an adaptive response that could enhance survival and reproduction.

Explanatory model of illness Medical anthropologists draw a distinction between disease and illness, disease being the underlying biological reality (to the extent that one exists) and illness the result of the social construction of the disease. Although it has proved difficult to introduce the specific terminology for the distinction into typical medical environments where the two terms are used interchangeably, health-care professionals will recognize the validity of the distinction. The social construction, or illness, involves a series of intersecting or nested explanatory models for the disease, held or promulgated variously by the patient, the family, the physician, other health-care personnel, and the larger culture as represented, for example, by religious authority or the law. Some medical anthropologists have argued for the addition of an Axis VI to DSM-IV on which the cultural or subcultural explanatory model offered by the patient or the patient's family would be recorded. That modification would strike most physicians who have worked in different cultures, or even with patients from different subcultures, as potentially valuable.

Among traditionally oriented persons in modern Taiwanese culture, for example, patients with syndromes that would be called anxiety neuroses routinely attempt to define their symptoms as primarily somatic, and hold a somatopsychic rather than psychosomatic explanatory model of the syndrome (Case H4). The explanation is not psychobiological but is a cruder reasoning from vaguely defined aches, pains, and pressures in particular body parts to the symptoms of psychological distress. The patient's relations with the family, not in the sense of remote, early, formative effects but of currently acting ones, are held to be strongly operative. Patients and families often also refer to the balance or loss of yin and yang to explain their symptoms and may, in addition, visit either a Taoist priest or a shaman, who provides a spiritual formulation of the disorder and undertakes to help placate the gods alleged to have caused the problem or to drive away ghosts or evil spirits. In addition, herbalists with various theories of particular illnesses sell their wares to patients. All those explanatory models may influence a patient who is attempting to get help.

In a much less complex culture, that of the !Kung San, hunter-gatherers of Botswana, a person who is ill either medically or psychiatrically will usually be viewed as being the target of some motivation (anger, capriciousness, grief) of either a god or the spirit of a dead relative. The community, consisting of a small band of relatives, responds by convening a trance dance, which is both the central religious experience of the culture and the main approach to healing. Women sit around the fire clapping and singing while men dance in a circle around them and gradually enter trances, during which their souls may separate from their bodies and which make them capable of healing. In one case of malaria (which the !Kung recognize as a separate diagnosis) in a young woman, a healer in trance traveled to the world of the spirits where he found her father, recently dead, holding her in his arms. Through vigorous argument he convinced the father that he was being selfish in taking such a young woman away from the living, and the effort was believed to have healing efficacy.

Such psychological insight is not unusual in the traditional healing systems of non-Western cultures, and as long as the patient is aware of the explanatory model, some genuine effect (corresponding to what might be called a placebo effect, bedside manner, counseling, or even psychotherapy) is not implausible. In some cases the anticipation of Western psychological theories and techniques is remarkable, as in a form of group discussion for the purpose of dream analysis found among the 17th-century Iroquois. Explanatory models in some other cultures are not so benign. Many cultures have theories of witchcraft or voodoo in which some persons are believed to put curses or hexes on others. Those theories not only serve as explanatory models of conventional illness, but have been found capable of causing distress, illness, and death in persons who believe that they are the targets of such curses. Some such cases may be coincidences, but others remain a challenge to medical science, especially to psychiatry.

Psychiatric disorders may be even more subject to spiritualistic explanation than medical or surgical disorders. In many cases not only the behavior and situation of the patient but also those of other persons involved, such as the healer or the witch, are of psychiatric interest. Healers are often respected by marginal persons in traditional societies (the !Kung are exceptional in that many can heal) and may have attained healing power through trances, hallucinations, self-starvation, substance use, or other processes that psychiatrists would consider to be in their province, and which are often of great psychological interest. Theories relating shamanism to mental illness (specifically acute schizophrenia, but the arguments would apply as well to bipolar disorders or borderline personality disorder) either individually or familially have been advanced; if true, they would help to explain the maintenance of those conditions in humans during evolution. (Among the !Kung San a young woman with a recurring thought disorder that may have been either a bipolar disorder or remitting schizophrenia was the daughter of a woman whose trance and healing powers were legendary.)

Conversely, in many societies psychiatric disorders evoke an explanatory model than labels their victims as witches who are held responsible for other's illnesses and misfortunes. (Some Soviet psychiatric practices, recognized as abuses by the World Psychiatric Association, appear to have reversed the phenomenon, giving psychiatric diagnoses to persons who are healthy according to all criteria but political cooperation.)

Those and many other examples demonstrate that explanations of illness, including culture-specific symbol systems, as well as behaviors and relations involved in healing, vary greatly across cultures in ways that are of direct concern to psychiatry. Closer attention to those variations can aid psychiatrists and other physicians in a myriad of daily tasks involving consultation, liaison, compliance, hypochondria, factitious disorders, placebo effects, abuse of the health-care system, and other problems. As for the core of disorders for which psychiatrists are directly responsible (psychoses, neuroses, substance use, personality disorders, and more acute reactive symptomatology) only a purely psychopharmacological explanation, such as is not really tenable for any disorder, could lead to the conclusion that non-Western approaches must be devoid of value. Any other currently accepted psychiatric explanatory model (psychodynamic, existential, cognitive, behaviorist, family dynamic, or community based) must lead to serious consideration of the possible effectiveness of non-Western explanatory models and their resulting treatments.

CULTURE AND MENTAL ILLNESS IN WESTERN CONTEXTS If cultural construction, labeling, and explanatory models affect the course of mental illness in non-Western societies, then they should do so in Western contexts as well. As in the case of *susto* or *pibloktoq* certain symptom patterns in Western cultures have a particular history, social place, and meaning that, if understood, greatly enhance clinical understanding. The approach does not entail the devaluing of standard psychiatric interpretations of etiology or treatment. It merely adds cultural flesh to the bare bones of neurobiological or psychodynamic explanation, giving the clinician new routes of interpersonal access through shared frameworks of cultural meaning.

Common sense suggests that suicidal ideation will have a different meaning for a Japanese person than it will for some others, because of unique Japanese cultural traditions regarding suicide and honor. But as shown by A. Alvarez, suicide has literary and religious traditions in Western culture as well, and it is likely that a clinician's ability to speak the language of those traditions will enhance his or her effectiveness with some patients. Similar historical and cultural analyses have been made by Joan Jacobs Brumberg for anorexia nervosa, by David Morris for chronic pain, by Armando Favazza for self-mutilation, by Kay Redfield Jamison for bipolar disorder in relation to creativity, by Anthony Storr for solitude, and by Ethel Spector Person for passionate romantic love. Those accounts give depth and complexity to the clinical entities, and it would be ideal if clinicians could enrich their understanding with such works of history and interpretation.

In a sometimes less sophisticated but parallel fashion, patients experience mental illness in many dimensions of life that go beyond the restrictive accounts of psychiatric nosology, even with all five axes of DSM-IV. Martin deVries has pioneered the use of pagers and systematic self-observation (the experience sampling method) to find out what patients are actually doing and feeling, in whatever environments they inhabit, throughout the day and night. Such research, inspired by methods in ethology and anthropology, gives personal meaning to a patient's clinical symptoms, course of illness, and treatment in much the way that cultural interpretation provides historical and philosophical meaning. As Arthur Kleinman has written, ''Most experienced psychiatrists learn to struggle to translate diagnostic categories into human terms so that they do not dehumanize their patients or themselves. . . . Irony, paradox, ambiguity, drama, tragedy, humor—these are the elemental conditions of humanity that should humble even master diagnosticians.''

POVERTY, RACE, AND GENDER AS MANIFESTATIONS OF CULTURE Even with ascertainment bias strongly favoring the well-to-do mentally ill, epidemiological surveys show an increased prevalence of many disorders among the poor, especially among the homeless. If stressful life events contribute to unfavorable diatheses in chronic mental conditions, then such diatheses will be more common in poverty. In addition, groups that are subject to invidious discrimination, whether poor or not, can also be expected to suffer more from mental illness than those who are able to exorcise such discrimination against them. Growing up with feelings of inferiority because of inferior social status and limited options has demonstrable negative effects on mental health. Cultural frameworks are crucial in determining patterns of poverty and discrimination. The United States, with its extreme cultural valuation of independence, tolerates more poverty than do other industrial states, which practice a more communistic version of capitalism. Many Americans label the mentally ill as sinful, responsible for their own illnesses. The American tolerance for handgun violence is another manifestation of the cultural ethos of independence, and its consequences particularly affect the poor.

Communities have shown little willingness to provide the support systems needed by those with chronic mental illnesses after hospital discharge. The result is often a downward spiral of poverty, homelessness, physical illness, and eventual hospital readmission. Since it is now clear that the chronically mentally ill are more likely to have acute crises if they lack a favorable milieu and adequate family or other social support, it should also be clear that the culture's neglect of them is extremely harmful, and not a gift of independence. Mentally ill women in poverty have the added burdens of a constant fear of sexual assault and harassment and an extreme concern for any children. Mentally ill African-Americans must often shoulder the added burden of bigotry.

The evolutionary perspective is not at odds with the recognition of those cultural forces predisposing to mental illness. On the contrary, it predicts that the privileged will use their greater resources to maintain their privilege and deceive themselves into thinking that all is well, and that the weak will suffer at their hands because of the self-deception. Yet it offers no comfort in the form of social Darwinism, a misconstrual of evolution to which Darwin never subscribed. Instead, it tends to make people more aware of the unfairness of stratified social systems and of the abuse of power and privilege. Because of the facts of evolution and every-person-for-himself/-herself mode of social life will never produce the ideal society or the kind of care for the mentally ill that a decent society must have. Thus the principles of evolution and those of cultural psychiatry point to the need for a greater sense of community to reduce those cultural forces that tend to increase the prevalence of mental illness.

CASES FROM ANTHROPOLOGICAL LITERATURE

Each of the following cases illustrates several different, usually disparate, points. The first three cases are from the nonhuman primate literature and the rest from the cross-cultural literature. Each is both a context (a different species or culture) and an individual member of that species or culture, with the context introduced before the individual member is described. Although those selected are unusual in some way against the species or cultural background, their inclusion does not necessarily imply a presumption of diagnosable psychiatric abnormality.

CASES FROM NONHUMAN PRIMATE LITERATURE

Case P1 Barbara Smut's book *Sex and Friendship in Baboons* exemplifies the complex interactionist outlook advocated here at the level of nonhuman primates. Resting on a groundwork of evolutionary theory, it recognized the extreme complexity of social behavior and its determination in the life cycle. Characteristically in the species (olive baboons, *Papio cynocephalus anubis*, a large ground-living Old World monkey considered highly relevant to human behavior), sexual relations are frequently inseparable from male-female friendships and are properly thought of as nonexclusive sexual friendships. Foreign male monkeys immigrate to troops and must form friendships with female monkeys, which may eventually become sexual, a process that can take months to a year or more.

One male monkey, whom she called Ian, was a mature (10-year-old) immigrant to her main study troop who never made the transition. He had great difficulty in establishing relationships with female monkeys. He almost always provoked alarm in them, and unlike most male monkeys his age, did not seem to know how to calm them by sitting at a distance and making friendly sounds and gestures. Instead, he pursued them, frightening them further, and even elicited screams that brought a group response that drove him from the troop. Eventually, he failed to integrate and he disappeared. (Another male monkey his age who had arrived at the same time, and who had the appropriate behavior toward female members of the troop, was by then fully absorbed into the troop.) It is not known what individual life history led to his behavioral inadequacy, which may have been genetic or environmental or both in causation. The negative impact on his reproductive success seems clear.

Case P2 Jane Goodall's studies of *Pan troglodytes*, the chimpanzee species that is the human's second closest animal relative, culminated in *The Chimpanzees of Gombe: Patterns of Behavior*. The book summarizes 25 years of study of known groups of wild chimpanzees, whose relationships are subtler and more complex than those of baboons, and details not only life histories but family histories up to three generations long. Among many other observations were the responses of 11 young chimpanzees up to 9 years of age (the approximate age of female sexual maturity) to the deaths of their mothers. Classic behavioral depression and other abnormalities were characteristic of the younger chimpanzees, most of whom did not survive, but the severity of the grief reaction was inversely proportional to age, and three of the four that were between the ages of 7 and 9 showed few effects.

The fourth, called Flint, has become famous for his extreme grief reaction. When he was 5 years old his infant sibling died, and he had resumed dependence on his mother that was extreme for his age, including riding on her back and sleeping in her nest. That dependence, which eventually became mutual, continued until her death three and a half years later, at a stage of development roughly equivalent to that of a human 12-year-old. He lingered near her body for many hours and became increasingly lethargic over the next six days. He was lost sight of for four days and when seen again was in a markedly deteriorated physical condition that worsened until his death two weeks later of autopsy-proved gastroenteritis and peritonitis. It has been speculated that psychoimmunological vulnerability induced by an abnormal grief reaction may have played a role in his death, but his dependency was definitely abnormal.

Case P3 Another chimpanzee in Goodall's study, a female chimpanzee known as Passion, was also to become well known for abnormal behavior. She was first identified in 1961 before coming into estrus and was in the study until her death of an unknown wasting disease in 1982. In 1965 she gave birth to an infant, Pom, and exhibited inefficient and indifferent maternal behavior. Pom survived and a close and lasting bond formed between the two. Beginning in 1970 Passion became increasingly isolative, spending most of her time with her own offspring, eventually three in number. In 1971 she suffered an eye injury that resulted in two weeks of monocular closure and evident pain, with a runny nose and eyes and a whitish patch on the iris. Eye healing was apparently complete but her nose continued to run for more than 10 years. Although most of their hunting is done by male chimpanzees four of seven bushbuck fawns seen to be captured were killed by female chimpanzees, two of them by Passion in 1977.

Her truly divergent behavior, however, was cannibalistic infanticide. Of six chimpanzee infants killed by adult chimpanzees three were killed by male chimpanzees in the course of attacks on the mothers, and later eaten, and three were killed systematically, with attacks on the infant only, by Passion with the cooperation of her adolescent daughter Pom. In two other cases they made unsuccessful attempts on other infants. Without their close cooperation it would have been impossible for them to overpower the infants' mothers, but Passion was clearly the leading force. The pair may have taken seven other infants in addition, unobserved. Those events took place between 1974 and 1977 and it is not known why they began or why they stopped. Pom gave birth herself in 1978 but the infant died about two years later, upon which the mutual dependency of Passion and Pom intensified. Infanticide with and without cannibalism has been observed in many species and in several other studies of chimpanzees, but it is very unusual, and Passion's devoted pursuit of it so far is unique in the literature.

CASES FROM CROSS-CULTURAL HUMAN LITERATURE

Case H1 Marjorie Shostak's *Nisa: The Life and Words of a !Kung Woman* describes the life history of an essentially normal woman among hunter-gatherers in northwestern Botswana. The outlines of the culture and child-rearing pattern fit the model described for hunter-gatherers in general. Nisa was the third child (a second died in infancy) of a then stably married couple living traditionally. She remembered her life as idyllic until weaning shortly before the birth of her younger brother, which she attended and whom she claimed to have saved from infanticide by her mother. She described intense sibling rivalry with her brother (for example, continuing attempts to nurse) and attributed her small stature and other problems to allegedly early weaning. Her father fought violently with her mother but they remained together until Nisa was in adolescence. She was married several times premenarcheally and (despite a culturally typical pattern of sex play throughout childhood) had a stormy introduction to adult sexuality, but her parents tolerated her flight from her husbands.

She remained with her fourth husband, Tashay, and eventually had four children; two of them died in infancy and early childhood, one died of illness in his youth, and a fourth was killed by her own husband shortly after marriage. Those losses, along with Tashay's death shortly after the birth of her third child in her late 20s, shaped her adulthood. She had occasional contacts with lovers both before and after his death, a habit she had not given up by the time she was interviewed at ages 50 and 55, despite two further marriages, her then-current one being quite stable. Her menopause near age 50 caused a period of sadness and self-assessment, but at 55 she had accepted her childlessness and was bringing up her younger brother's two children. She was vibrant, mildly eccentric with a bawdy sense of humor, eloquent on both her own life and the culture, open to new relationships, including the interview relationship with its probing self-exploration, and proud of having surmounted difficulty and tragedy with a willingness to go forward and a continuing joy in life.

Case H2 Gilbert Herdt's book *Guardians of the Flutes* is the best known of a series of ethnographies on cultures in a region of New Guinea (the semen belt) where male homosexuality is a universal aspect of adolescent development, and the symbolic framework involves the belief that semen must be absorbed, usually through fellation, although also in some cultures through anal intercourse, in order for a boy to become a man. Among the Sambia studied by Herdt boys engage in homosexual activity exclusively beginning at age 7 to 10 and continuing until they are married in their late teens or early 20s. They must suck the penises of postpubertal boys as often as possible until they go through puberty, after which they are fellated very frequently by younger boys. It all proceeds in an atmosphere of extreme misogyny and of hypermasculine preparations for warriorhood and hunting. At the end of the period they marry and become exclusively heterosexual husbands and fathers in almost every case—a challenge to several theories of homosexuality and an answer to the obvious Darwinian objections to such an apparently maladaptive pattern.

The psychoanalyst Robert Stoller and Herdt published an aberrant case, Kalutwo, who had married four times by his mid-30s, marriages that were infertile and perhaps unconsummated. He had been the illegitimate son of an older widow and a man married to someone else who could have taken the widow as his second wife. Stigmatized, Kalutwo was raised by his mother, who was bitter about men and had no contact with his father. He showed an unusually keen enjoyment of fellatio, had unusually strong homoerotic feelings and attachments, and committed the serious indiscretion of continuing to fellate younger boys even after he reached puberty. Although he acted tough he never displayed what were considered masculine achievements, such as suffering war injuries or undertaking acts of courage. Stoller and Herdt argue for a classic psychoanalytic provenance of homosexuality in his case, but regardless of its etiology they argue that Kalutwo would be a homosexual anywhere, independent of the culture's erotic customs, which in themselves do not produce homosexuality.

Case H3 Benjamin and, until her death, Lois Paul studied the community of San Pedro la Laguna, a small Zutuhil (Mayan Indian) village in highland Guatemala, for more than 45 years, with periodic field trips beginning in 1941. In that traditional community, which had little contact with the mainstream Ladino culture of the region or the Hispanic culture of the country, many ancient beliefs and rituals remained functional, including strong well-defined roles for shamans (men) and midwives (women), the latter being adept at spiritual as well as obstetrical pursuits.

Maria, who was 18 at the time they met her in 1941, was an attractive woman who had had two failed marriages and had a 9-month-old daughter. Her father was one of six shamans in a village of 2,000 persons and was held to be an expert on insanity, but he was also lazy, opportunistic, and given to drinking. Her mother, stable and dutiful, had lost three infants before Maria was born. Maria was somewhat sickly and was cared for attentively until the birth of two siblings in succession (at 15 months and between two and three years) displaced her. She became her father's companion for some years, but he eventually changed his attitude toward her, becoming punitive and scolding. She had an intense rivalry with her next younger sister, eventually over the same boyfriend. She was considered masculine in her competitiveness, disobedience, and general willfulness, but was nonetheless seductive, charming, and a popular dancer. She was vivacious with occasional morose lapses, witty with a flair for the gruesome, gossipy, and irresponsible. She fell in love and eloped, leaving her baby with her parents (cause for a lawsuit in that culture) but soon was fighting with her new husband.

One night he struck her and she suffered an attack of *colera,* essentially an adult temper tantrum believed to result from swelling of the heart resulting from bad blood, with symptoms of gasping and suffocation. Later that night she lapsed into a state of unconsciousness (''cold and stiff as though dead for good'' according to her husband and his father) that was so serious that the case was rejected by a shaman. She awoke spontaneously after two hours and began to wail that spirits of the dead were surrounding her and trying to take her. She was unresponsive to persons and events around her, talking only to the spirits. She was labeled *loca* (crazy) and her father was called in because of his expertise with insanity. He took her (and most of her and her husband's families) to a more powerful shaman in a neighboring village, whose advice (although spiritual) subdued many intense family conflicts and involved the kinship network in a common effort against the spirits trying to take Maria. She continued to have auditory hallucinations and delusions of persecution for about a week (with content seemingly related to her life situation, such as an insistence that she nurse the babies in the spirit world). She had one further dramatic episode during which she beat and attempted to castrate her husband, but it remitted and she was free of the symptoms thereafter. Her symptoms were defined in spiritual terms and treated as such.

She continued to have marital difficulties and eventually left the village with a fifth husband and in 1962, while in her late 30s, she complained of various physical symptoms that she attributed to bewitchment and to her powers. A shaman treating her divined that she was being called to be a midwife, a profession that made a great virtue of her eccentricities and even her ideas of reference and persecution. Her younger sister, who had always been more stable and had stayed in their home town, became a midwife at about the same time through a more conventional route, but one that also involved illness (a protracted grief reaction, with anorexia, to their mother's death) and ideas of reference, although in a milder form than Maria's. Maria, in accordance with recommended practice, avoided sex since becoming a midwife and encouraged her husband to find lovers, but in a conflict with him and one of his mistresses she became ill again, bedridden with abulia and anorexia for weeks until cured by miraculous intervention in a dream.

Case H4 Arthur Kleinman's study of traditional healing in Taipei, a large urban community in Taiwan, is one of the few such efforts to be conducted by someone trained in both psychiatry and anthropology. Intensive observations of patients with medical as well as psychiatric symptoms and syndromes were made with a focus on the various traditional attempts at healing. Mr. Chen was a 44-year-old lower-middle-class master woodworker who belonged to the ethnic subgroup Hakka within the Chinese majority. For 16 years he had complained intermittently of a feeling of pressure in his chest, general anxiety, weakness, malaise, and neck tension. He traced the problem to a time when he was in financial difficulties, lonely, and unhappy, but was not helped by visits to four Western-style physicians, who could not identify his illness, or by Chinese-style physicians, who gave him a diagnosis and an explanation and who prescribed various remedies. He believed that his illness was physical, not psychological, but he also believed a fortune-teller who told him that he had bad fate because he was being bothered by an ancestor, and that he had to find out who it was. He immediately reasoned that it was his biological mother, who had been divorced from his father when Mr. Chen was 4 years old, and whom his father had forbidden him to visit when she lay dying. He propitiated her ghost and his symptoms disappeared. He was free of them for 10 years.

Six years previously, however, they had reappeared and had waxed and waned since. They returned strongly at a time when his business was at a crucial juncture, and a series of negative tests by Western-style physicians resulted in a diagnosis of neurasthenia. Finally, he visited a shaman with whom Kleinman was working. A full mental status examination revealed marked anxiety and somatic preoccupation but no other abnormalities, with limited insight into the nature of the illness, and resulted in a diagnosis of chronic anxiety neurosis. The shaman performed several rituals but the milieu of the shrine seemed as important to the patient as the rituals, and the main thrust of the visit was that he should devote himself to the service of the god and return to the shrine frequently. After five nightly visits and much effort he entered a subjectively described trance state, threw himself around violently, and eventually collapsed, a pattern that would become habitual although more controlled. Two days after his first trance he was evaluated at home by Kleinman, who found him greatly improved both objectively and subjectively. "My overall impression was . . . that his former anxiety had been largely, and perhaps entirely, relieved." The improved state continued on periodic follow-up for two years, during which the patient became increasingly involved with the shrine, eventually becoming a leader who entered trance nightly.

Case H5 In *Saints, Scholars, and Schizophrenics,* her study of the cultural context of mental illness in a remote rural area of western Ireland, Nancy Scheper-Hughes explores the unusually high prevalence of serious mental illness in that region. She documents the relentless generations-long series of social stresses in that population, impoverished and condemned to farm very poor land; dwindling in size and losing its traditions owing to the emigration of young persons, especially women; experiencing a breakdown of respect for the elders of the community; and losing a certain degree of time-honored tolerance of, and even respect for, persons with strange visions. Those stresses occurred against the background of a culture and child-rearing pattern characterized by severe sexual repression, canings, ridicule and scapegoating of children, and both longing for and fear of intimacy. Thematic Apperception Test (TAT) and Draw-a-Person test results with psychiatric patients are consistent with her emphasis of those themes. Without denying the basic biological nature of vulnerability to schizophrenia, she argues persuasively that those sociocultural stresses account in part for the unusually high prevalence of schizophrenia and other serious mental illnesses. Two briefly described cases illustrate certain characteristic female and male themes.

Kitty was a 20-year-old woman hospitalized for the first time with a diagnosis of schizophrenia, which began during a brief period of emigration to work in a low-grade London pub. She was the second youngest in a large family with an occasionally brutal father who abused alcohol and a compulsively religious and sexually repressed mother. She became hysterical over her task of recycling leftover beer slops into fresh glasses, which she equated with the whoring behavior of her Protestant English clients, who recycled their defiled sexuality into their wives in a similar way. During her illness she was obsessed with themes of polarity, such as order-disorder, female-male, pure-impure, Catholic-Protestant, and Celt-Anglo.

Patrick was a 34-year-old farmer, fourth in a family of seven and the youngest son, who carried the diagnosis of chronic schizophrenia. His parents had imposed on him a guilty sense that he must stay and care for them in their old age, and he had remained unmarried and celibate in a dying village from which most young women had fled. In the hospital he rarely spoke. His spotty responses on the TAT described the figures as statues or as pictures of a picture. In describing his relationship to his parents he said, "I am their dead son."

Those and other cases cited by Scheper-Hughes demonstrate the power of cultural context to invest a severe thought disorder with specific content, but also may be relevant to explaining the high prevalence of severe mental illness in traditional rural western Ireland during the 1970s.

Case H6 Among the traditional Zuni, as well as among other pueblo dwellers of the American Southwest, and to some extent among Native North Americans generally, culture defined a role for men who wished to comport themselves as women (as well as for women who wanted to act as men), an institution known as *berdache*. Such persons not only were accepted and treated with dignity but were viewed as being somewhat special, even treasured members of the community. It is unlikely that more than a small number of them were born with anomalous genitalia but most knew from childhood that they wanted to assume a cross-sexual role. Their easily spotted tendencies were viewed as a different *onnane* or life road. They were typically, but not always, homosexual in adulthood, but their alliances, including marriage, were with nonberdache same-sex partners. Zuni child rearing generally emphasized nonaggressive, cooperative behavior. Physical punishment of children was rare, although religious training included some frightening elements.

The most famous berdache (*lhamana* in Zuni), We'wha, is described in a book by Will Roscoe, *The Zuni Man-Woman.* He was born in 1849 in a highly traditional community frequently subjected to raids by nearby Navajo and Apache. He was adopted into a rich and influential family; his adoptive father was a rain priest. At first he received male-typical religious training, but as his berdache tendencies became apparent he began learning domestic skills and crafts from women. He mastered and carried out advanced skills of weaving (this was the classic period of pueblo textiles), ceramics, cooking, and gardening. At the age of 30 We'wha was a matron, or supervisor, at the Zuni mission school. At that time he became friendly with Matilda Stevenson, an anthropologist, who many years later wrote that We'wha's "strong character made his word law among both the men and women . . .", and yet he "was loved by all the children, to whom he was ever kind."

For years, Stevenson had believed that We'wha was a woman. "She was perhaps the tallest person in Zuni; certainly the strongest, both mentally and physically. . . . She possessed an indomitable will and an insatiable thirst for knowledge. Her likes and dislikes were intense. She would risk anything to serve those she loved." We'wha eventually became a diplomat, visiting Washington for extended periods of lobbying for the Zuni. She died before the age of 50, of heart disease, and the anthropologist, now a close friend, was there. "The writer never before observed such attention as every member of the family showed her . . . [I]n a feeble voice she said, in English, 'Mother, I am going to the other world' . . . The family suppressed their sobs that the dying not be made sad . . . Her face was radiant in the belief that she was going to her gods."

Case H7 Anthropologist Oscar Lewis and his research team in their ethnography of very poor people defined what some have called the culture of poverty. Lewis's legacy includes thousands of pages of published observations and interviews that offer respectful, detailed, compassionate, and comprehending access to the practical and psychological worlds of the poor. In *La Vida: A Puerto Rican Family in the Culture of Poverty—San Juan and New York* he presents interlocking life-history interviews with many members of the same family, and adds observations based on days spent with each of them. Fernanda, a short, muscular, attractive San Juan woman of African descent was interviewed by a woman research assistant. She was a mother and a former prostitute.

"I am as frank as I am ugly and I don't try to hide what I am," she began. "There is nothing good about me. I have a bad temper, why should I deny it?. . . When I get into rages, it makes no difference to me whether I kill or get killed. I never feel sorry or anything." She drank heavily, threatened her husbands and boyfriends, and carried a razor blade hidden in her mouth. "I'm not afraid of anyone but God . . . I'm 40 now and I've had six husbands, and if I want, I can have six more. I wipe my ass with men." She also reported a compassionate side; she would prostitute herself to earn money for others in need. She was born in a small country town in Puerto Rico, was mistreated by her grandmother, and was sickly as a child; she specified rickets as one of her illnesses. She loved her mother but was frequently badly beaten by her. The mother was chronically ill, in pain, and raged at her.

She did not adjust well to school and was held back in the first grade because of her frequent fighting. She prided herself on being able to beat up boys. She lived for a time with her grandmother, but went back to her mother: "I had to be at my mother's side forever . . . I loved my mother dearly and I loved only her." She fell in love only once, with a boy of whom her mother disapproved, and she did not go with him. When she was between 12 and 14 years of age her stepfather frequently made sexual advances to her until the man who was to be her first husband, but whom she did not love, took her away. He later beat her severely, while she was pregnant, until her mother threw boiling water at him, causing him permanent injury. Her first child, a girl, was born when Fernanda was 15. Three more came in rapid succession. "I never did get along very well with kids and I didn't let my children be close to me. They never dared cling to me because if they did, I'd yank the hair off their scalps."

When she was 21 and her husband was in the army and away most of the time, she began prostituting herself. She netted little money, often went to jail, and eventually gave it up because she was thin and sickly. She worked in laundries and restaurants. She was to have five more husbands; to raise her children as she had been raised, with a combination of beatings and love; and to maintain a fearful temper and fierce will throughout. At the age of 40, she was living with a man to whom she was very attached and they were fairly good to each other. She was optimistic about the future, if unrealistically so: "I'm 40 years old, but I can still have 50 more babies if I want to. Other women my age have had babies, what would be so strange about my having one? I'm still young." That such a life, in such conditions, is lived with optimism and produces children who grow up to become parents themselves is a tribute to the resilience of the human spirit.

SUGGESTED CROSS-REFERENCES

Sociology and psychiatry are discussed in Section 4.2 and sociobiology in Section 4.3. Aggression is presented in Section 3.4. Atypical psychotic disorders and culture-bound psychoses are discussed in Section 15.3. Culture shock is discussed in Section 28.5 on additional conditions that may be a focus of clinical attention.

REFERENCES

Alvarez A: *The Savage God: A Study of Suicide*. Random House, New York, 1972.
*Barkow J, Cosmides L, Tooby J, editors: *The Adapted Mind*. Oxford University Press, New York, 1992.
Betzig L, Borgerhoff Mulder M, Turke P: *Human Reproductive Behavior: A Darwinian Perspective*. Cambridge University Press, New York, 1988.
Bowlby J: *Attachment and Loss* (3 vols). Hogarth Press, London, 1969–1977.
Brumberg J J: *Fasting Girls: A History of Anorexia Nervosa*. Harvard University Press, Cambridge, MA, 1988.
Csikszentmihalyi M: *Flow: The Psychology of Optimal Experience*. Harper Collins, New York, 1990.
Dahlby L C: *Geisha*. University of California Press, Berkeley, 1983.
Daly M, Wilson M: *Homicide*. Aldine de Gruyter, New York, 1988.
DeVries M, editor: *The Experience of Psychopathology: Investigating Mental Disorders in Their Natural Settings*. Cambridge University Press, New York, 1992.
Digman J M: Personality structure: Emergence of the five-factor model. Ann Rev Psychol *41:* 417, 1990.
Dunbar R I M: *Primate Social Systems*. Cornell University Press, Ithaca, NY, 1988.
Edgerton R B: *Sick Societies: Challenging the Myth of Primitive Harmony*. Free Press, New York, 1992.
Erchak G M: *The Anthropology of Self and Behavior*. Rutgers University Press, New Brunswick, NJ, 1992.
Favazza A: *Bodies Under Siege: Self-mutilation in Culture and Psychiatry*. Johns Hopkins University Press, Baltimore, 1987.
Glantz K, Pierce J: *Exiles from Eden: Psychotherapy from an Evolutionary Perspective*. Norton, New York, 1989.
Goodall J: *The Chimpanzees of Gombe: Patterns of Behavior*. Harvard University Press, Cambridge, MA, 1986.
Gregor, T: *Anxious Pleasures: The Sexual Lives of an Amazonian People*. University of Chicago Press, Chicago, 1985.
Hahn M E, Hewitt J K, Henderson N D, Benno R, editors: *Developmental Behavior Genetics: Neural, Biometrical, and Evolutionary Approaches*. Oxford University Press, New York, 1990.
*Heider K: *Landscapes of Emotion: Mapping Three Cultures of Emotion in Indonesia*. Cambridge University Press, New York, and Editions de la Maison des Sciences de l'Homme, Paris, 1991.
Jamison K R: *Touched With Fire: Manic Depressive Illness and the Artistic Temperament*. Free Press, New York, 1993.
*Kagan J: *The Nature of the Child*. Basic Books, New York, 1984.
Kenny M G, editor: *New Approaches to Culture-Bound Mental Disorders*. Soc Sci Med *21*(2): 162, 1985.
Kleinman A: *Patients and Healers in the Context of Culture*. University of California Press, Berkeley, 1980.
Kleinman A: *Rethinking Psychiatry: From Cultural Category to Personal Experience*. Collier-Macmillan, London, 1988.
Konner M: Human nature and culture: Biology and the residue of uniqueness. In *The Boundaries of Humanity: Humans, Animals, Machines*, J J Sheehan, M Sosna, editors, p 103. University of California Press, Berkeley, 1991.
*Konner M: *The Tangled Wing: Biological Constraints on the Human Spirit*. Holt, New York, 1989 (originally 1982).
Konner M: Universals of behavioral development in relation to brain myelination. In *Brain Maturation and Cognitive Development*, K R Gibson, A C Petersen, editors, p 181. Aldine-DeGruyter, New York, 1991.
Konner M: *Why the Reckless Survive, and Other Secrets of Human Nature*. Viking, New York, 1990.
Leibowitz M R, Salman E, Jusino C M, Garfinkel R, Street L, Cardenas D L, Silvestre J, Fyer A J, Carrasco J L, Davies S, Guarnaccia P, Klein D P: Ataque de nervios and panic disorder. Am J Psychiatry *151:* 6, 1994.
LeVine R: *Culture, Behavior, and Personality*. Aldine, Chicago, 1973.
Lin K-M, Kleinman A: Psychopathology and clinical course of schizophrenia: A cross-cultural perspective. Schizophr Bull *14:* 555, 1988.
Lutz C A: *Unnatural Emotions: Everyday Sentiments on a Micronesian Atoll and Their Challenge to Western Theory*. University of Chicago Press, Chicago, 1988.
MacLean P D: Brain evolution relating to family, play, and the separation call. Arch Gen Psychiatry *42:* 405, 1985.
McGuire M, Marks I, Nesse R M, Troisi A: Evolutionary biology: A basic science for psychiatry. *Acta Psychiatr Scand*, 1992.
Morris D B: *The Culture of Pain*. University of California Press, Berkeley, 1991.
Murphy J M: Psychiatric labeling in cross-cultural perspective. Science *191:* 1019, 1976.
Nesse R, Lloyd A T: The evolution of psychodynamic mechanisms. In *The Adapted Mind*, J Barkow, L Cosmides, J Tooby, editors, p 601. Oxford University Press, New York, 1992.
Paul R A: *The Tibetan Symbolic World: Psychoanalytic Explorations*. University of Chicago Press, Chicago, 1982.
Person E S: *Dreams of Love and Fateful Encounters: The Power of Romantic Passion*. Norton, New York, 1988.
Plomin R, Daniels J: Why are children in the same family so different from one another? Behav Brain Sci *10:* 1, 1994.
Roscoe W: *The Zuni Man-Woman*. University of New Mexico Press, Albuquerque, 1991.
Rosenblatt P C, Walsh R P, Jackson D A: *Grief and Mourning in Cross-Cultural Perspective*. Human Relations Area Files Press, New Haven, CT, 1976.
Rosenhan D L: On being sane in insane places. Science *179:* 250, 1973.
Rowe D C: *The Limits of Family Influence: Genes, Experience, and Behavior*. Guilford, New York, 1994.
Rubel A J, O'Nell C W, Collado-Ardon R: *Susto, A Folk Illness*. University of California Press, Berkeley, 1984.
Scheper-Hughes N: *Saints, Scholars, and Schizophrenics: Mental Illness in Rural Ireland*. University of California Press, Berkeley, 1979.
Shostak M: *Nisa: The Life and Words of a !Kung Woman*. Harvard University Press, Cambridge, MA, 1981.
*Simons R C, Hughes C C, editors: *The Culture-Bound Syndromes: Folk Illnesses of Psychiatric and Anthropological Interest*. D. Reidel, Boston, 1985.
Slavin M O, Kriegman D: *The Adaptive Design of the Human Psyche: Psychoanalysis, Evolutionary Biology, and the Therapeutic Process*. Guilford, New York, 1992.
Spindler G D, editor: *The Making of Psychological Anthropology*. University of California Press, Berkeley, 1978.
Storr A: *Solitude: A Return to the Self*. Free Press, New York, 1988.
Trivers R L: *Social Evolution*. Benjamin Cummings, Menlo Park, CA, 1985.
Whiting J W M, Whiting B B: Aloofness and intimacy between husbands and wives. Ethos *3*: 183, 1975.
Wikan U: *Managing Turbulent Hearts: A Balinese Formula for Living*. University of Chicago Press, Chicago, 1990.

4.2 SOCIOLOGY AND PSYCHIATRY

RONALD C. KESSLER, Ph.D.

INTRODUCTION

Sociology is the behavioral science that studies the organizing principles of social life, the impact of societal and world-historic forces on these principles, and the way in which these principles affect individual and organizational behavior. Sociologists presume that fundamental social forces influence individual action by determining ranges of possible behavioral choices. Sociological inquiry seeks to illuminate those social forces in order to understand the motives underlying human behavior.

Contemporary sociology is relevant to psychiatrists in a number of ways. Over the past decade, sociologists have studied the sociocultural determinants of mental health and illness, social factors in psychiatric help-seeking, attitudes toward the mentally ill, and mental health care organization. In each of these areas, an interdisciplinary body of theory and research exists, with contributions made not only by sociologists but also by psychiatrists, psychologists, and epidemiologists.

SOCIAL AND CULTURAL DETERMINANTS OF MENTAL ILLNESS

Research on social and cultural factors in psychopathology has been dominated during the past decade by an interest in the health-damaging effects of stressful life experiences.

LIFE EVENTS Although the hypothesis that stress can cause mental disorder is an old one, serious population-based research on the topic has been conducted only during the past two decades. Most of the research has used a life events inventory to measure stress and to estimate its effects. Early work was limited to case-control studies in which retrospective reports about life events were obtained from psychiatric patients and from controls. More recent work has been based on general population samples and longitudinal designs.

It is difficult to document causal effects of life events on mental illness due to the fact that an event-illness association may reflect an influence of the illness on the event rather than the converse. Job loss, divorce, and many other major life events may result from pre-existing disorders, and there is no certain way of discounting that possibility in the nonexperimental studies that are the mainstay of stress research.

Nevertheless, studies which focus on events known to be independent of prior disorder have elucidated the effects of stress. Studies of job loss due to plant closings, for example, have documented rates of clinically significant anxiety and depression among unemployed workers two to three times higher than those found among the stably employed.

Over the past decade, as social scientists have focused on adjustment to particular life crises, efforts have been made to specify the dimensions of crises that make them stressful. The differential impact of events can be explained, in part, by differences in the ways those dimensions coalesce in particular instances. For example, job loss seems to promote anxiety and depression by increasing financial strain and heightening reactivity to unrelated stresses. As a result, the most serious psychiatric outcomes associated with job loss are found among people who lack financial reserves and who experience another major crisis (for example, a child developing a life-threatening illness) during the period of unemployment. The next decade is likely to see a major expansion of research aimed at delineating the contextual features of stressful experiences that predict healthy adjustment and recovery.

Two related lines of research have also developed over the past decade. Studies of posttraumatic stress disorder following rape or combat have elaborated the lifetime impact of such stressors. That work has motivated researchers to consider the long-term effects of early life adversities (for example, parental death or family violence) in the context of a developmental perspective on psychopathology.

The other line of research has studied the effects of prior history of psychopathology on stress reactions, sometimes in conjunction with an investigation of the impact of early life adversities on emotional reactions to adult life events. That research has established that adult stresses promote clinically significant episodes of disorder primarily among persons who are already vulnerable. The implications of the finding for future research and prevention efforts have not yet been fully appreciated; it is hoped that future interventions will target those people most vulnerable to adult stresses.

CHRONIC STRESS Research on the relation between chronic stress and emotional disorder is much less well developed than work on life events. It is easier to determine that an event has occurred than to measure the existence of an ongoing stressful situation, and it is easier to make a causal interpretation about the effect of a discrete event than of a chronic stress. Consequently, many researchers have favored life event measures over chronic stress measures.

That preference does not imply that life events are more important than chronic stresses. Recent research, using community surveys, suggests that chronic stresses are more predictive of psychological disorders than are life events. More reliable procedures for measuring chronic stresses and their effects have yet to be developed.

The most developed work of that kind to date concentrates on job stress. Naturalistic studies have documented that time pressure, closeness of supervision, job insecurity, and a variety of other job stress dimensions are associated with a higher incidence of depression, anxiety, and substance abuse. Based on those results, more closely focused studies of such high-risk occupations as assembly line work and air-traffic control have been undertaken. Those studies have associated particular constellations of job conditions with emotional disability. For example, several studies have established a link between the combination of high job demands (for example, a job in which workers must rush to meet important deadlines) and low decision latitude (that is, low control over either the pace or organization of work) with both emotional disability and cardiovascular disease.

Several major corporations have agreed to carry out job redesign experiments aimed at modifying some of those health-damaging job conditions. Motivated partly by a desire to increase worker productivity, the experiments are providing an unparalleled opportunity to study the effects of chronic stress. They should yield important new knowledge about the determinants of chronic job stress and about effective strategies for changing work environments to reduce the most pernicious kinds of stress.

VULNERABILITY FACTORS Only a small minority of people who are exposed to stressful life experiences develop clinically significant emotional disorders. In fact, emerging evidence indicates that stressful encounters can sometimes promote competence. The major thrust of current research on life stress, accordingly, is to identify variables that help explain differences in stress response. Some investigators have emphasized enduring psychological characteristics such as cognitive flexibility, effective problem-solving behaviors, and interpersonal skills. Others have focused on more social resources such as social support and financial assets.

Social support The term *social support* has been widely used to refer to the mechanisms by which interpersonal relationships protect people from the deleterious effects of stress. The popularity of the term was triggered by a series of influential review papers in the mid-1970s that demonstrated a consistent relation between psychiatric disorders and such factors as marital status, geographic mobility, and social isolation. Although highly inferential in their arguments and not always clear about their definition of the concept, the papers generated a great deal of scientific interest in the possibility that social support can have health-promoting effects.

Over the intervening years, the issues and evidence have been subjected to a critical examination. Various types of social support have been identified, and distinctions have been made empirically among the effects of the various dimensions. Several different functions of social support have been identified, such as the expression of positive regard, expression of agreement with the person's beliefs or feelings, encouragement of ventilation, and provision of advice or information.

Normal population and case-control studies Most recent research has concentrated on the ability of social support to ameliorate the impact of stress on health. For example, it has been shown that the impact of life events in provoking episodes of major depressive disorder is reduced among persons who have intimate, confiding relationships with friends or relatives. In one study, nearly 40 percent of the stressed women without a confidant became depressed compared with only 4 percent of those women with access to a confidant. That result has been replicated in several community surveys and case-control studies.

Although those studies provide suggestive evidence, methodological problems obscure the results. There is virtually no way to rule out the possibility that some predisposition to depression accounts for the presumed buffering effect; persons who are so predisposed may, for reasons related to the predisposition or its personality correlates, be less likely than others to form close, confiding personal relationships.

Experimental intervention Experimental interventions have examined the effect of support on such outcomes as preoperative anxiety, recovery from surgery, and compliance with medical regimens. Support interventions have also been instituted to facilitate coping with such life crises as widowhood, rape, and job loss.

Those interventions have operationalized support in numerous ways, although all of them have involved both emotional and informational interactions with support providers. Most have been provided by health care professionals and have been modest in scope, generally using limited resources and involving a small number of sessions. In the vast majority of cases, such manipulations have been effective in fostering adjustment to life crises.

Although social support may protect against emotional disorders that can be linked to life crises, intervention experiments have not been designed to clarify the mechanisms through which that influence occurs. Furthermore, as most of the interventions were multifaceted, it is impossible to specify which aspects of support are most effective.

Clinical studies Research comparing the social networks of psychiatric patients and normal subjects shows that psychotic patients have very tight kin-based networks, and neurotic patients have loose and sparse networks, as compared with controls. Those network structures may be causally implicated, but it is equally likely that they are results of the disorders.

That causal ambiguity has been resolved to some degree by research in which the supportiveness of social networks at the time of illness onset was assessed to predict subsequent relapse. The most important work in this tradition was that of sociologist George Brown and his colleagues, who isolated a pattern of expressed emotion characterized by hostile feelings and intrusiveness on the part of the families of schizophrenic patients, which is strongly associated with poor prognosis after discharge. More recent work based on Brown's model has resulted in the design of family interventions that have been effective in altering that expressive style. When experimentally evaluated, the work has been shown to reduce relapse among first-episode schizophrenic patients. Parallel research on relapse for major depressive disorder has begun, but it lags far behind the research on schizophrenia.

Future directions The evidence suggests that social support may play an important part in protecting against both the onset and the continuation of psychopathology. A clearer understanding of those influences will require research advances in several directions. One advance would involve further specification of the components of social support, including its differential effects depending on the provider. A related issue pertains to the effects of negative social interactions. The literature clearly suggests that interactions between psychiatrically impaired individuals and their social networks are not merely unsupportive but openly conflictual. It would be useful to assess negative social exchanges as risk factors for onset and prolongation of psychiatric disorders. In the few studies that have compared positive and negative elements of social interaction, the negative elements have been uniformly more strongly related to mental health outcomes. More must be learned about the relative importance of positive and negative components as stress buffers and risk factors.

Researchers must also grapple with the consistent finding that the perception of *hypothetical* availability of crisis support—the perception that support would be available if it were requested—is the dimension of support most strongly associated with good emotional functioning in the face of severe life stress. The evidence is much less clear that actually receiving support promotes adjustment to stress. There is even evidence that some supportive behaviors backfire and make matters worse. Those miscarried helping efforts seem particularly likely to occur when help undermines the crisis victim's sense of self-control and competence.

The best current thinking on the importance of the perception of hypothetical support availability is that it leads to appraisals of the situation as manageable. The perception, in turn, appears to promote active, self-reliant coping efforts, which give the person some sense of mastery over the crisis situation. Some support interventions have been developed with that perspective in mind. Research on the victims of natural disasters, for example, shows that emotional adjustment is improved if the disaster relief team mobilizes disaster victims to participate actively in reconstructive work rather than sitting by with blankets and coffee. Future research is needed to link supportive interventions with self-help interventions, and to understand more about the capacity of support to mobilize active coping.

Prior psychopathology Important recent research has conceptualized prior history of psychopathology as a vulnerability factor. We now know that stressful events have much more powerful effects on recurrence of depression than on first onset of depression in adulthood. Prior history has also been associated with many of the psychosocial variables that are known to be vulnerability factors for depression, including sociodemographic variables such as social class and sex, social resources such as access to social support, and personality variables such as neuroticism and self-esteem. The association of prior history with all those vulnerability factors raises the question of whether the putative effects of these variables may be due, at least in part, to prior history.

GROUP DIFFERENCES IN PSYCHIATRIC DISORDER Much of the sociological research on psychopathology has been concerned with structural correlates of psychiatric illness, such as social class, sex, race, age, and urbanicity. Recent research has centered on those same associations in a way that reflects the contemporary issues.

The most obvious hypothesis to test in examining such associations is that differential exposure to stress explains group differences in mental illness. It is now clear that the hypothesis can be rejected. Although people in comparatively disadvantaged positions in society (for example, women, lower-socioeconomic status persons, nonwhites) are exposed to more stress than their advantaged counterparts, differential exposure cannot explain their higher rates of anxiety, depression, and nonspecific distress in general population samples.

Vulnerability factors have taken center stage in research on group differences. The research has shown consistently that there are group differences in vulnerability to stress which play an important part in explaining differences in rates of psychiatric disorder.

SOCIAL CLASS One of the oldest and most firmly established associations in psychiatric epidemiology is that between social class and mental illness. People in socially disadvantaged positions have higher rates of psychiatric disorder than their more advantaged counterparts, as measured by treatment statistics, nonspecific distress in community surveys, and clinically significant psychiatric disorders in epidemiological studies.

Early work on social class and psychopathology was based on the influential work of A. B. Hollingshead and F. C. Redlich, who defined social class in terms of a two-factor index that combined information on educational attainment and occupational prestige. They studied patterns of social class variation in psychiatric hospitalization and documented clearly that lower-class people both have a significantly higher probability of hospitalization and remain hospitalized longer than their middle-class counterparts. Subsequent work has used the term "social class" to describe measures as diverse as family income, occupational prestige, education, and even the Marxian concept of class that distinguishes workers from owners. The most recent descriptive work on the issue shows that it is important to discriminate among the various measures rather than to combine them as Hollingshead and Redlich did. The evidence now suggests that income (among men) and education (among women), rather than class, are the primary correlates of psychopathology. Furthermore, the effect of income is actually due to personal earnings rather than to total family income, which implies that financial adversity is not the central operating factor.

Until the early 1970s, the dominant line of thinking in the literature on class and mental illness was that lower-class people were exposed to more stressful life experiences than those of more advantaged social status, and that this differential exposure accounted for the negative relationship between class and mental illness. The view was first challenged in a study which documented that stressful life experiences have a greater capacity to provoke mental health problems in the lower class than in the middle class. Subsequent work has shown that class-linked vulnerability to stress accounts for the major part of the association between social class and depression as well as between social class and nonspecific distress.

There are several ways in which that differential vulnerability might arise. One of the most plausible is that some type of selection or "drift" of incompetent copers to the lower class might lead to the relationship between class and vulnerability. Another explanation is that one's experience as a member of a particular class leads to the development of individual differences in coping capacity as well as to differences in access to interpersonal coping resources.

Available evidence supports both hypotheses. Most of the evidence for the drift hypothesis comes from studies of major mental illnesses, primarily schizophrenia, which show that the early onset of a disorder can reduce one's changes of socioeconomic achievement, a fact that seems true primarily for people who become ill before establishing a career. Less severe disorders apparently do not interfere with socioeconomic achievement.

Evidence for the linkage of vulnerability factors and class is widespread. Lower-class people are disadvantaged in their access to supportive social relationships. Personality characteristics associated with vulnerability to stress, such as low self-esteem, fatalism, and intellectual inflexibility, are more common among lower-class people. To date, the major efforts in that area have been confined to the study of social support. One study found that lower-class people have fewer confidants than those in the middle class, which apparently increases their vulnerability to undesirable life events. The finding has been replicated in several investigations, but more work needs to be done to assess in parallel fashion the importance of coping strategies and personality characteristics. As most investigations of class and stress have focused on life events, a more serious consideration of ongoing stressful situations may lead to a better understanding of the relationship between class and psychopathology.

GENDER Community surveys show that adult women are twice as likely as men to report both extreme levels of psychiatric distress and a history of mood disorders. Two lines of research on sex differences in nonspecific distress and affective disorders can be distinguished. The first is based on indirect assessments of role-related stress. For the past decade, the dominant perspective has held that women are disadvantaged relative to men because their roles expose them to more chronic stress. Because of the difficulties in measuring chronic stress objectively, empirical analysis has used indirect assessments, based on measures of objectively defined role characteristics or constellations of multiple roles, to document the relation.

The second line of research has examined stressful events. Studies have shown a significant interaction between gender and undesirable events in predicting distress, with women appearing more vulnerable than men to the effects of stressful events. Several hypotheses have been advanced to account for female vulnerability to stress, including the argument that females are disadvantaged in access to social support, in the use of effective coping strategies, and in personality characteristics.

Although aggregate analyses of life event inventories show that women are on average more vulnerable than men, there are some events for which this is not true. Research on widows, for example, shows that women adjust to spousal death better than men. Women also adjust as well as or better than men to divorce. Furthermore, financial difficulties do not affect women as much as men.

A challenge for future research is to reconcile the discrepancy between the studies of particular life events and aggregate life event surveys. The only such attempt to date, a meta-analysis of several large-scale community surveys in which the effects of different types of events were assessed separately, found no evidence that women are more distressed than men by such major life crises as job loss, divorce, or widowhood. Their greater vulnerability was primarily associated with events that happen to people close to them—death of a loved one other than a spouse being the most commonly reported event in that regard.

The greater impact of network events on women can be interpreted in several ways. One component of the difference is probably linked to the fact that women provide more support to others than men do, creating stresses and demands that can lead to psychological impairment. Another interpretation is that women may be more empathic than men, or that they may extend their concern to a wider range of people. Those and other possibilities need to be investigated, since the role played by network events appears to account for a very substantial part of the overall gender-distress relation.

Recent survey research on the different predictors of onset and recurrence of depression shows clearly that, while women are twice as likely as men to report a recent episode of depression, there is no significant gender difference in risk of recurrence. The seeming anomaly can be explained by the fact that women are twice as likely as men to have a lifetime history of depression. Among men and women with such a history, there is no gender difference in recurrence risk. The observation means than an understanding of gender differences requires an understanding of the determinants of first onset. Analysis of gender-specific age of onset curves shows that the two-to-one female-to-male ratio of lifetime depression occurs by the mid-20s and that rates of first onset after that age are fairly similar for men and women. That means that the focus of attention in studies of gender differences in depression needs to be redirected from the midlife period, where most of the current research on gender roles is concerned, to the late adolescent and early adult periods.

RACE Much of the research on race differences in psychopathology has focused on black-white differences. Research is also increasing on the comparison of Americans of Mexican and of Anglo-Saxon heritage.

Black-white differences Although community surveys paint a consistent picture, with blacks clearly evidencing higher average levels of distress than whites, statistical control for the fact that blacks generally have lower socioeconomic levels than whites usually accounts for the race difference. That implies that minority status and the life experiences associated with it are not in themselves instrumental in creating mental health problems. It appears that minority status, although related to experiences of prejudice and discrimination, is also related to structural resources that can help protect against the adverse mental health effect of those stresses.

The stress-buffering effect of group solidarity among members of deprived groups has long been emphasized. Theoretically, the effect may stem from at least two sources: (1) the group provides cognitions that assign responsibility for their deprivation to structural conditions, thus removing any self-blame for their lack of financial achievement; and (2) the group provides emotional support that can buffer the effects of life stress in a variety of ways.

Initial attempts have been made to investigate the counterbalancing effect of group solidarity on the mental health of blacks. However, the work has been hampered by the fact that the stresses of minority status have not been measured explicitly. Only one study of race differences in exposure and response to life events has been reported in the literature, and it found both greater exposure and vulnerability to undesirable events among nonwhites. Other researchers have inferred from available data that blacks are exposed to more stresses than whites, by virtue of their disadvantaged social status, but there have been no attempts to measure those stresses explicitly.

Evidence has been presented to support indirectly the view that blacks develop cognitions which shield them from the self-esteem assaults associated with some types of stress. Specifically, the relationship between personal efficacy and self-esteem is much weaker among blacks than among whites. Perhaps a group ideology that explains low personal efficacy as a result of discrimination negates the damaging effects that feelings of low efficacy would otherwise have. More work is needed on that possibility and on extensions that would take into consideration vulnerabilities to particular types of stress situations.

Anglo-Hispanic differences Consistent evidence exists that Americans of Mexican heritage are underrepresented in treatment statistics relative to their proportions in the population. Furthermore, community surveys of Anglo-Hispanic differences in nonspecific psychological distress report mixed results, with no consistent evidence for a difference in the levels of distress experienced by members of the two groups.

The underrepresentation of persons of Mexican origin in treatment groups and the inconclusiveness of normal population surveys have been the source of much speculation. Minority scholars share the general view that Mexican-Americans have much greater mental health needs than the statistics show, and that further research should attempt to measure that need accurately and to study the determinants of underutilization.

There has been considerable research on the extent to which minority communities and family structures provide protective resources, which enhance the mental health of Hispanics. Most of the work focuses on the relation between group identification and mental health. The general view is that acculturation leads to heightened psychological distress by exposing individuals to conflicting values and alienating them from the supportive environments that traditionally ameliorated the effects of life stress. There is no systematic evidence regarding that issue or the related issue of how minority families foster identities and provide nurturant environments. Personal identity is created in the context of an early childhood environment, where a child's most significant interactions take place with people of the same race or ethnicity. Group identity, in comparison, takes place later as a result of contacts with the larger society. There is a great deal of current interest in the parallel developments of those two identities and the conditions under which they are bound. The ability to develop a deeper understanding of minority mental health hinges on unraveling those developmental processes and their implications for self-attributions, supports, and coping efforts.

AGE Most reviews of the epidemiological literature have documented inconsistency in the relation between age and screening scales of psychological distress. Recent meta-analyses have demonstrated a stable nonlinear association between age and distress, with distress elevated among young adults, then declining from the mid-20s to a stable low level, and increasing again beginning in the mid-70s. The apparent inconsistency of the age-distress relationship in earlier studies was due to the fact that surveys with younger samples found the relationship to be negative, those with older samples found it to be positive, and those with balanced age distributions found no linear relationship at all.

There is currently a great deal of interest in both ends of the nonlinear age distribution. The elevated levels of distress found in surveys of adolescents and young adults is consistent with recent evidence that first onset of many psychiatric disorders occurs during that period of the life course. Psychosocial research aimed at explaining the concentrations of mental disorder among adolescents and young adults has focused on developmental challenges associated with the transition to adulthood. Up to now, that literature has not dealt seriously with the fact that early-onset mental disorders tend to be associated with family histories of disorder, which means that genetic factors could be involved. New collaborative work between social scientists, psychiatrists, population geneticists, and psychiatric epidemiologists is now attempting to sort out the influences of genes, childhood stresses associated with having a mentally ill parent, and gene-environment interactions on early-onset disorders.

The fact that mental disorders are clustered with a larger set of problem behaviors in adolescence is intriguing. The clustering becomes much weaker during the transition to adulthood, at the same time that distress and active psychiatric problems begin to decrease. Investigation of the reasons for those changes is part of the emerging interdisciplinary area of developmental psychopathology, which is fundamentally concerned with timing and critical change points in problem behaviors over the life course, many of them linked to social and structural factors which constrain options at critical life course decision points. A number of collaborative longitudinal studies of the transition to adulthood currently under way are likely to increase our understanding of those issues over the next decade.

There is also a good deal of interest in the elevated levels of distress found among elderly people. The evidence from general population surveys shows that this increase begins in the mid-70s. The main focus of work has been on the themes of disengagement and loss; increased exposure to loss events and decreased resources for coping with them apparently conspire to promote high levels of psychological distress among the elderly. Innovative experiments designed to facilitate living situations for the elderly and for increasing opportunities to maintain a sense of purpose and control in life are being carried out in an effort to develop structural correctives which can minimize those problems.

In seeming contradiction to the evidence on increased psychological distress among the elderly, population surveys of clinically significant psychiatric disorders show that rates of depression, anxiety, alcoholism, and drug abuse all decrease among older people. There is reason to think that those decreases are due, at least in part, to methodological problems. Physical illness becomes increasingly implicated in psychiatric disorders among older people. That, in turn, leads to higher levels of diagnostic exclusions for possible organic causes and to errors in diagnosis because psychiatric problems are masked by physiological complaints. Those factors cannot explain the more puzzling fact, however, that not only current disorders but lifetime disorders are reported to be less prevalent among elderly persons. That pattern could be due to differential recall accuracy as a function of age, to selection bias (a history of psychiatric disorder predicts early death), or to the fact that the most seriously impaired elders are excluded from community samples because of institutionalization.

Another possibility, and the subject of lively debate over the past few years, is that there may have been a cohort shift in rates of psychiatric disorders, with cohorts born after World War II having higher rates of psychopathology than older cohorts. There is clear evidence consistent with that hypothesis for the increased prevalence of drug abuse and dependence among more recent cohorts. Evidence from general population surveys of distress over time are also consistent with the hypothesis. Recent replications of large-scale surveys carried out in the late 1950s and early 1960s document substantially elevated levels of distress in more recent cohorts. The reasons for those cohort changes are only now being considered.

PSYCHIATRIC HELP-SEEKING

Needs assessment surveys show that most people with serious emotional problems do not seek professional help. Informal helpers are still approached most often in times of emotional turmoil. Furthermore, a person seeking professional help is more likely to turn to a primary care physician than to a mental health specialist. That choice is partly due to the dearth of mental health specialists in some areas of the country, but other variables are also involved.

Most of our direct knowledge about those other determinants comes from general population surveys that ask respondents about emotional problems and whether they sought professional help for them. Those surveys have documented several consistent attitudinal, demographic, and system-dependent determinants of help-seeking.

Sociologists have been particularly interested in structural determinants, the strongest and most consistent of which is social class. A positive correlation between social class and help-seeking persists even though community mental health centers and other inexpensive treatment facilities have reduced the financial barriers to care. In the most recent surveys, education has emerged as a stronger predictor of help-seeking than income, which suggests that some cultural facilitating factors are more important than financial resources in accounting for the influence of social class.

Women are much more likely than men to seek mental health care, even given the higher prevalence of disorder among women. Sociological research over the past few years has made considerable progress in understanding the gender difference by showing that women are more likely than men to recognize their problems, and that recognition is the main point in the decision-making process that discriminates men and women. Once either men or women recognize a problem, they do not differ in their likelihood of obtaining professional help. The subject of why women are more likely than men to recognize their problems is currently under study.

The most recent surveys suggest that the determinants of utilization differ markedly from one community to another, suggesting that local alternatives and barriers play a major part in determining who will seek treatment. That result is likely to lead to a greater emphasis on comparative case studies of particular communities.

The most careful case studies document that the critical point in the help-seeking process is the decision that help is needed. Most people have no conception of when a personal problem is big enough to warrant professional care. As social scientists come to appreciate the importance of problem definition, more sophisticated theories about how people make sense of symptoms are being developed. Recent research suggests that people operate on the basis of "schemas" for explaining particular kinds of illnesses. Those schemas contain lay accounts of the cause, course, symptoms, and prophylaxis for various illnesses. A number of different schemas appear to exist for particular medical conditions, and characteristics of the schema held by a particular person provide important insights into his or her help-seeking and compliance habits. Although systematic research into schemas for psychiatric disorder is in its infancy, it is likely to become a major area of investigation over the next decade.

An issue of considerable current interest is the finding that persons with comorbid conditions are more likely than those with a single disorder to seek professional help for psychiatric difficulties. That result is consistent with the more general finding that likelihood of seeking help is positively associated with severity of symptoms. Persons with comorbid disorders are more severely distressed than those with only one disorder, and they very often have alcohol or drug problems superimposed on anxiety or depression. Their help-seeking patterns direct them disproportionately to community substance use programs, where underlying psychiatric problems are often overlooked and untreated.

The problems associated with comorbid diagnoses could be addressed by intervention efforts aimed at attracting psychiatrically disordered persons into treatment before they develop secondary disorders. Early interventions might be effective in preventing the onset of secondary comorbid conditions. The challenge to implementing that approach is that the motivation to seek help often occurs only in the context of the severe role impairments associated with comorbid conditions. In light of recent evidence about the early onset of primary disorders among persons who later develop comorbid conditions, effective early intervention will almost certainly require the screening of school-aged populations.

COMMUNITY RESPONSES TO THE MENTALLY ILL

ATTITUDES Attitudes about the mentally ill have been charted in public opinion surveys since the 1950s. Dislike and fear have remained high among the attitudes surveyed. Negative attitudes are pronounced among poorly educated and elderly respondents, and men consistently report more negative attitudes than do women.

The core concerns about mentally ill persons revolve around their presumed unpredictability and dangerousness. Those concerns have some basis in reality, because patients released from state psychiatric hospitals have comparatively high arrest rates. However, most crimes committed by released patients are property crimes that do not involve violence.

Intensely negative attitudes about the mentally ill may be part of a larger cluster of beliefs, attitudes, and values characterized by an absence of sympathy for people who need help, a deep-seated distrust of people and institutions who are different, and a rigid outlook on what is right and wrong. People with that orientation cannot easily be swayed by rational arguments to change their views.

Fortunately, most people have much less intense negative feelings that can be modified on the basis of experience and as they learn to make finer distinctions about kinds of mental illness and treatment. Visits to a psychotherapist, for example, have much less stigma attached than hospitalization for a mental illness. Private hospitalization seems to be less stigmatizing than public hospitalization. Drug therapies are perceived as evidence of greater disorder and so provoke more fear and distrust of the patient than do talk therapies. For a similar reason, treatment by a psychiatrist involves more negative attitudes than consultation with a psychologist, social worker, or member of the clergy.

Survey data suggest that attitudes of community members are affected by contact with the mentally ill. Survey respondents who report knowing someone with a history of mental illness are, in general, less negative than people who report no personal contact. It is difficult to sort out cause and effect here, because negative attitudes might be associated with the failure to report the mental illness of a close relative.

Family studies and studies of the reintegration of former patients into their old work roles show that contact with former coworkers and associates promotes more positive attitudes about the mentally ill. Seeing a former patient perform adequately in a normal role is particularly important in that regard. Self-disclosure by the former patient about what it was like to have a mental illness and to be hospitalized also helps to promote normalization and acceptance by reducing the aura of mystery that otherwise surrounds the illness.

Much less is known about how to change negative attitudes in the general population. Studies of the mass media show that the stereotyped depictions of former patients that commonly appear on television and in movies reinforce negative public perceptions about the mentally ill. Whether more sympathetic portrayals of mentally ill people would change those negative attitudes, or whether informational campaigns making use of the mass media could increase public knowledge about mental illness is less well understood.

That issue is attracting considerable interest because several large mass media campaigns to increase public awareness, recognition, and treatment of mental illness are currently under development. The largest campaign has been developed by the National Institute of Mental Health to increase knowledge about anxiety and depression and to encourage voluntary help-seeking for those disorders. Unfortunately, the campaigns do not include active evaluation components, so it can only be inferred which kinds of message strategies and information channels lead most effectively to attitude and behavior changes among persons with those disorders. Gauging from the experiences of health educators in campaigns aimed at other public health problems, information of that sort is vitally important to successful campaign design and implementation.

COMMUNITY REACTIONS TO SHELTERED-CARE HOMES Negative attitudes about the mentally ill are important for a number of reasons, including the fact that they inhibit help-seeking for personal problems. A subject of recent sociological attention is the organization effect of negative attitudes on attempts to establish group homes for the mentally ill.

In the extensive research on collective action, community opposition to group homes has become one of the mobilization activities studied. The research clearly indicates that middle-class neighborhoods are much more resistant than lower-class neighborhoods to having group homes in their midst. That greater resistance can be traced to effective mobilization efforts. In particular, efforts to meet and organize local opposition are accomplished more quickly in middle-class neighborhoods, where a person or a committee is more likely to be selected to act on the neighborhood's behalf and where multipronged political actions are more likely to occur.

Community attitudes also play an important part in the success of group homes in fostering readjustment among deinstitutionalized patients. Ethnographic research shows clearly that patients are aware of the accepting or rejecting attitude climates in their neighborhoods, and that that awareness influences their social functioning. The ease with which the residents of sheltered-care homes adjust to life in the community depends to a large degree on community acceptance. The conflict that can attend the creation of a home does not make a good foundation on which to build such acceptance. In general, public opinion surveys show that contact with former patients who are strangers exacerbates whatever fears and uncertainties community residents already have, particularly in cases where conflict arose about the establishment of the group home.

Those issues have been neglected in most sociological studies of community opposition to group homes, which generally concentrate on structural determinants of neighborhood mobilization and on strategies available to agencies for diffusing opposition. Research is urgently needed on what happens after the home is opened and the residents must live in the neighborhood. Because contact with a former mental patient who was known prior to hospitalization can foster positive attitude changes, especially when that person is seen performing adequately in normal roles, a challenge for the future is to create structured situations that will facilitate contact between residents of sheltered care homes and their neighbors in such a way that positive attitude changes can occur.

ORGANIZATION OF MENTAL HEALTH SERVICES

INTERORGANIZATIONAL COORDINATION Research on complex organizations is one of the liveliest areas in sociology today as a result of the enormous organizational changes in American society and the innovative work of social theorists in developing new frameworks within which to understand those changes. The mental health care delivery system has been a favorite example used by theorists to test new ideas about interorganizational linkage, because it provides unique opportunities to study a decentralized system consisting of many overlapping organizations with complex coordinating functions.

One focus has been on the continuing diminution of state mental hospitals and the impact of that downsizing on general hospitals and community-based programs. Although it is generally perceived that most of the reductions in state mental hospital systems throughout the country occurred in the 1950s and 1960s, there were decreases of up to 50 percent in the numbers of inpatients in many state mental health systems during the 1980s. The result has been an increased burden on general hospitals and a revolving door policy whereby patients are treated during periods of crisis and largely ignored between admissions.

Case studies of community responses to those changes have documented enormous coordination problems and inconsistencies in organizational rationalities. Historical analyses show that those problems result from the accumulation of many specific decisions that seemed rational from a narrow perspective when they were made but which lack any overall plan or purpose. The challenge for researchers is to combine those case studies into a comparative analysis in order to pinpoint the fundamental coordinating mechanisms that facilitate rationality in the relations among community organizations.

Researchers have attempted to trace the influences of state and national policy initiatives on community-based organizations and systems. Studies have been done, for example, on how strategic decision-making in local organizations is affected by considerations of the future actions of state and national funding agencies. The studies show that instability of state and national initiatives to develop community-based programs leads to local processes of adaptation that were not intended by the program developers. At present, comparative studies are underway to isolate characteristics of community systems that determine local responses.

There is also a great deal of interest in designing and evaluating organizational innovations that may improve the quality of care for chronically mentally ill patients, particularly those who cannot afford private care. Capitation programs (for example, HMOs in which health-care providers are reimbursed on a per-capita basis rather than on a fee-for-service basis), managed care programs, programs that mainstream the mentally ill into existing or specially created HMOs are among the organizational innovations currently under discussion. Sociologists recognize that notions of treatment success for the chronically mentally ill patient must be broadened to include fundamental quality of life issues, such as adequacy of housing, nutrition, employment, and social integration.

ORGANIZATIONAL FACTORS IN SERVICE DELIVERY Another kind of organizational research extends the work on job stress by studying the influence of organizational structure on the health, well-being, and productivity of its members. Some of the work has focused on the structural components of mental health care organizations that affect staff satisfaction with their work. A few studies have also examined the impact of organizational structure on patient outcomes. All of the work has been naturalistic rather than experimental, and comparative rather than based on case studies of individual treatment settings.

One finding is that staff satisfaction and productivity are positively associated with decision latitude. Patient functioning in long-term mental hospitals is also positively associated with the decision latitude of low-level staff. Other correlates of good patient functioning include high staff job satisfaction and high staff participation in treatment decisions. Patient functioning in acute-care inpatient settings is positively associated with an active management style; functioning of patients in community-based shelter care homes is likely to be better when the homes are small, have flexible rules, and require patients to take some responsibility for activities of daily living.

As those results suggest, there is as yet no overarching theoretical framework that integrates the specific findings into a coherent model of organizational influence on staff and patient functioning. Integrative work of that type will be facilitated by the insights being obtained from job redesign experiments in industrial settings. Similar experiments in treatment settings (for example, sheltered-care homes) are much less common, although innovative experiments are now under way to change the structures of community-based shelter care homes in an effort to reduce the problems of staff burnout and turnover. It is likely that the success of organizational redesign efforts will determine whether similar experiments are carried out in a wide range of treatment settings.

EVALUATION OF COMMUNITY MENTAL HEALTH SERVICES The development and maintenance of an effective community-based mental health care system require a cyclical process of service planning, implementation, evaluation, and feedback. The first step is usually a *needs assessment,* which identifies the mental health problems in the community and establishes priorities for the creation of services to address them. Such an assessment is vitally important to organizational success by monitoring demand for services and pinpointing needs not recognized by community residents.

The most direct way to conduct a needs assessment is by a large-scale community survey. However, such surveys are very expensive and few local service organizations can afford them, a number of innovative approaches have been devised to obtain more indirect information about needs at a lower cost. Those techniques include systematic interviews with key informants, the establishment of citizen advisory councils, the use of national statistics on need profiles in conjunction with small-area social indicators on community demographics, and extrapolation from data on demand for services to estimates about need for services.

Once programs are developed, research can also be important in evaluating effectiveness and targeting areas that need to be changed. Program effectiveness depends on at least two levels of research. The first focuses on success in attracting participants to the program; the second focuses on success in helping people with their problems. Behavioral scientists have been more active in the first research area than in the second area.

Research on success in attracting program participants emphasizes acceptability, accessibility, and awareness. Acceptability refers to how willing community residents are to use the new service. Accessibility involves the ease with which the program can be reached. Time, distance, transportation, and financial barriers are all important to consider here. Awareness relates to community knowledge that the service exists and that it is appropriate for particular needs. An understanding of local culture is required to develop programs that are sensitive to those issues. Sociological research, using ethnographic or other strategies can increase the sensitivity of program staff to local norms and customs.

Research that evaluates the effectiveness of programs is much less common for several reasons, including the substantial costs of implementing a carefully controlled study of treatment effectiveness, the high level of methodological sophistication required, and the potential threat to clinicians and program administrators of openly studying the therapeutic value of their services. Although the expertise for such work is available, that area of investigation remains underdeveloped.

SOCIAL CONTEXT OF PROFESSIONAL ACTIVITY The medical profession is undergoing enormous change, engendered by such things as diagnostic related groups (DRGs) and other new payment arrangements, shifting of care from inpatient to ambulatory settings, diversification of the medical care industry, increasingly overt competition among providers, and the growing importance of third-party payers. Those changes are part of broader societal forces that include the aging of our population and cohort shifts, that have led to massive expansion in the plant facilities of the medical care industry and a marked increase in the number of physicians in the marketplace.

Sociologists have been keenly interested in the implications of those trends for the future of medicine. One perspective holds that physician domination of the health care system is too firmly established to be shaken by the ongoing changes in social context. The legal subordination of nurses, pharmacists, and other medical care professionals to the physician is cited as a critical factor, as are the exclusive licensing powers granted to physicians as gatekeepers of the medical care system.

An opposing view is that the medical profession is in a period of declining power as a result of the resurgence of consumerism in medicine. The greater number of medical patients who suffer from chronic rather than acute conditions creates an interest group of lay people who acquire considerable technical knowledge about their own afflictions, band together in self-help groups, and sometimes challenge the professionals who care for them. The technical diversification of medical procedures and the increasingly important contributions to health care by technician-specialists who are not physicians are also thought to play a part. With changes in the organization of professional care, new systems of ownership and management have promoted competition among physicians, which inevitably brings with it increased consumer control. Finally, the dominant position of large insurers consolidates the bargaining position of consumers in a novel way. Those views are particularly relevant to psychiatrists, because the existence of auxiliary mental health specialists, such as clinical psychologists and psychiatric social workers, has no counterpart among other medical specialties.

Another perspective on the changing nature of medical practice involves the proletarianization of medical work. More and more physicians, especially psychiatrists are working as salaried employees in large, bureaucratic organizations. As those organizations institute managerial styles orchestrated by the graduates of business schools rather than of medical schools, changes in procedures for professional control will invariably occur. Formal review procedures are being applied to a wider range of professional behaviors. Within particular institutions, mechanisms are being developed to monitor and control the technical decisions of clinicians. All of those trends will result in increasing external control of the domain of professional practice.

SUGGESTED CROSS-REFERENCES

Other perspectives on sociocultural influences on psychiatry may be found in Section 4.1 on anthropology and psychiatry and in Section 4.3 on sociobiology and psychiatry.

REFERENCES

*Aiken L H, Mechanic D, editors: *Applications of Social Science to Clinical Medicine and Health Policy.* Rutgers University Press, New Brunswick, NJ, 1986.

Aseltine R H, Jr, Kessler R C: Marital disruption and depression in a community sample. J Health Soc Behav *34:* 237, 1993.

*Brown G W, Harris T, editors: *Social Origins of Depression.* Free Press, New York, 1978.

Christianson J B, Lurie N, Finch M, Moscovice I S, Hartley D: Use of community-based mental health programs by HMOs: Evidence from a medicaid demonstration. Am J Public Health *82:* 790, 1992.

Costello C G, editor: *Basic Issues in Psychopathology.* Guilford, New York, 1993.

Karasek R, editor: *Healthy Work: Stress, Productivity, and the Reconstruction of Working Life.* Basic Books, New York, 1990.

*Kendler K S, Neale M C, Heath A C, Kessler R C, Eaves L J: Life events and depressive symptoms: A twin study perspective. In *The New Genetics of Mental Illness,* P McGuffin, R Murray, editors, pp 146–164. Butterworth-Heinemann, Oxford, 1991.

Kessler R C, Foster C, Webster P S, House J S: The relationship between age and depression in two national surveys. Psychology and Aging *7:* 119, 1992.

Kessler R C, Kendler K S, Heath A, Neale M C, Eaves L J: Perceived support and adjustment to stress in a general population sample of female twins. Psychol Med *24:* 317, 1994.

Kessler R C, Magee W J: Childhood adversities and adult depression: Basic patterns of association in a U.S. national study. Psychol Med *23:*679, 1993.

Kessler R C, Magee W J: Childhood family violence and adult recurrent depression. J Health Soc Behav *35:* 13, 1994.

Kessler R C, Magee W J: The disaggregation of vulnerability to depression as a function of the determinants of onset and recurrence. In *Stress and Mental Health: Contemporary Issues and Prospects for the Future,*W R Avison, I H Gotlib, editors, p 239, Plenum, New York, 1992.

Kessler R C, McGonagle K A, Swartz M, Blazer D G, Nelson C B: Sex and depression in the National Comorbidity Survey I: Lifetime prevalence, chronicity and recurrence. J Affective Disord *29:* 85, 1993.

Kessler R C, McGonagle K A, Zhao S, Nelson C B, Hughes M, Eshleman S, Wittchen H-U, Kendler K S: Lifetime and 12-month prevalence of DSM-III-R psychiatric disorders in the United States: Results from the National Comorbidity Survey. Arch Gen Psychiatry *51:* 8, 1994.

*Kessler R C, Price R H, Wortman, C B: Social factors in psychopathology: Stress, social support, and coping processes. Annu Rev Psychol *36:* 531, 1985.

*Mechanic D. Strategies for integrating public mental health services. Hosp Community Psychiatry *42:* 797, 1991.

McHugh S, editor: *Illness Behavior: A Multidisciplinary Model.* Plenum, New York, 1986.

Regier D A, Narrow W E, Rae D S, Manderscheid R W, Locke B Z, Goodwin F K: The de Facto U.S. Mental and Addictive Disorders Service System: Epidemiologic Catchment Area prospective 1-year prevalence rates of disorders and services. Arch Gen Psychiatry *50:* 85, 1993.
Rolf J, Masten A S, Chicchetti D, Nuechterlein K H, Weintraub S, editors: *Risk and Protective Factors in the Development of Psychopathology.* Cambridge University Press, New York, 1990.
Sarason B R, Pierce G R, Sarason I R: Social support: The sense of acceptance and the role of relationships. In *Social Support: An Interactional View,* B R Sarason, I G Sarason, G R Pierce, editors, pp 97-149. Wiley, New York, 1990.
Scott W R, Black B L, editors: *The Organization of Mental Health Services.* Sage, Beverly Hills, CA, 1986.
Turner J B, Kessler R C, House J S: Factors facilitating adjustment to unemployment: Implications for intervention. Am J Community Psychol *19:* 521, 1991.

4.3
SOCIOBIOLOGY AND ITS APPLICATIONS TO PSYCHIATRY

RUSSELL GARDNER, JR., M.D.

INTRODUCTION

Sociobiology applies biology to social processes. Psychiatric illnesses can be considered subsets of those processes. The term ''sociobiology'' came into use shortly after World War II, when animal behavior research flourished, but it became popular and controversial because of Edward O. Wilson's book on social behaviors in animal life, *Sociobiology: The New Synthesis,* published in 1975. Wilson strongly emphasized evolutionary factors in his formulation but omitted psychiatry except to mention suicide in his opening sentences.

Wilson defined *sociobiology* as ''the systematic study of the biological basis of all social behavior.'' The field has been chiefly influenced by population biology, with attempts to predict behavior in groups, often focusing on the adaptive features of various traits. Inclusive fitness theory—emphasizing that kin share genes—is considered by some to be synonymous with sociobiology, but sociobiology has become much more inclusive, and Wilson's original definition is important to emphasize.

With new technologies and conceptual frameworks, natural history facets of biology are increasingly merged with biological research traditionally associated with the basic sciences of medicine. Sociobiological research on all levels has increasingly recognized the importance of evolutionary factors. Systematic comparisons of human behavior with the behavior of other animals has high importance. Sociobiology assumes that interactions between a genetically derived repertoire of behavioral propensities modified by experience result in specific organism behaviors. Data on human-nonhuman similarities and differences come from many disciplines: paleontology; morphological, behavioral, and macromolecular comparisons; and investigations of unique human characteristics, such as upright posture, brain size, suppressed evidence of ovulation, extended childhood, language, and culture.

Despite Wilson's omission, psychiatric disorders can be considered disturbances in the person's communication behaviors that cause social difficulties. That is, psychiatric symptoms—now easily considered biological, in part because they respond to pharmacological agents—are usually related to problems in the patient's interactions with people. The depressed person feels worthless with respect to other people. The manic person tries to unduly influence and control others. Schizophrenic, paranoid, and brain-diseased patients may hallucinate voices and be delusional about persecution by others, who are usually vague in specific identity but felt to be clearly hostile out-group people. Schizoid and negative symptoms refer to withdrawal from others. The agoraphobic person is fearful of other people, as in the marketplace. Moreover, all treatments—psychopharmacological treatment and family, group, and individual psychotherapy—feature social interactions.

Sociobiology has related fields. For example, *behavioral ecology* is the observation and quantitative study of animal behavior in its surroundings and is not confined to social acts; for example, an optimality theory has allowed predictions about how the nature of food supply within an animal's ecological niche resulted in particular foraging behaviors. Behavioral ecology overlaps with sociobiology because any niche includes not only predators and prey but also others of its own kind *(conspecifics). Sociophysiological* research includes studies of normal processes known to be affected by psychotropic drugs and developmental psychobiology.

Wilson publicized the core perception that human behavior is as biological as other animal behavior. He asserted that sociology, anthropology, and psychology are biological disciplines that have ignored their biological bases too much. He thought that observations of behaviors and intuitive conclusions about their explanation (which in his opinion psychology and ethology have exemplified) were insufficient; those sciences require definitive linkage to their biological roots on the one hand and rigorous study that uses strong-inference scientific procedures that operate by ruling out alternative hypotheses on the other hand. He and other animal researchers advocated the use of mathematical modeling of population and genetic mechanisms as methods in biological research. With those methods *evolution* is defined as changes in gene frequencies in a population over time according to principles outlined by Charles Darwin in the mid-19th century.

DARWIN'S MODEL FOR EVOLUTION

Darwin proposed that changes in organisms over generations occur fundamentally from the interaction of three factors: diversity in the behaving organism, natural selection of those specimens that best fit their environment, and hereditary mechanisms for passing on the traits that help survival most.

EXAMPLES Two examples illustrate Darwin's principles on a relatively short time scale: deceptive communication between species and genetic sequelae of intergroup exploitation.

Deceptive communication between species Melanism occurred in British moths over decades in the second half of the 19th century as a result of soot production in industrial cities. Bird predators found few of the black moth variants when the background coloration was also dark. The original variant, in pepper-and-salt shades that provide protective coloration when the moths rest on lichens, remained most prevalent in unpolluted areas and, from updates on the original work, were prevalent again in the urban areas as they have become less polluted than in the past. Darwin's principles are illustrated in that black variants of the moths (diversity of phenotype) survived most often with good protective coloration (natural selection) and lived to furnish progeny with genes that also determined the black coloration (hereditary factors). Evolution had occurred because the black gene frequency had increased. The same process operated in reverse when pollution became less of a factor.

Genetic sequelae of intergroup exploitation The prevalence of salt-sensitive hypertension in many African Americans has been attributed to survival in those ancestors whose kidneys had retained salt during the arduous trips from Africa to the New World over the 350 years of the African slave trade. That trait had already been selected to an extent by salt-deficient environments. Subsequently, water and salt deprivation occurred on the trip before and during the transatlantic crossing. Further, water and salt loss occurred because of vomiting secondary to seasickness and because of diarrhea caused by nonhygienic ocean travel conditions. Survivors of those conditions conveyed their salt-retaining genes (and consequent vulnerability to hypertension) to their descendants. In contrast to the reversed melanism of the moths, hypertensive people are as evolutionarily fit as others when those dying from the disease do so after they have reproduced and nurtured their children.

EVOLUTIONARY FITNESS Key to the core concept of evolutionary fitness is the fact that traits enhancing continued life are conveyed into the next generations. Various forms of the *phenotype* (the manifest behaving form of the organism) are acted on by factors that influence survival and reproduction, such as environment, health, mate choice, fecundity, and parenting. Evolutionary fitness refers less to a person's attributes (direct fitness) and more to the ability to perpetuate descendants, although the two are often correlated. Thus, a small person with surviving healthy grandchildren has demonstrated more evolutionary fitness than a large person with no descendants, even if the small person died at age 30 and the large one at 80 years.

OBJECTIONS TO EVOLUTIONARY THEORY In the 19th and early 20th centuries survival of the fittest ideas—referring to direct fitness only—resulted in the misapplication of evolutionary theory to social actions, and xenophobic attitudes were acted on. In the eugenics movement mentally ill and retarded persons were sterilized. In Adolph Hitler's Third Reich mass exterminations took place. Worries that biological theory and oversimplified, biased research will again be misapplied to rationalize negative cultural practices have led to a potent resistance to the propositions, discussion, and application of the disciplines of sociobiology and have motivated concern that its science be appropriate and responsible.

An important facet of evolutionary biology that stimulated early objections to Darwin's theory was its seeming presumption of supernatural programming. *Teleology* is a belief that nature operates with predetermined ends and is not congruent with the physicochemical processes that modern science has assumed to operate. Effective arguments in rebuttal have held that biological forms are, indeed, programmed and that the programming results from physicochemical processes. Biological forms of matter are fundamentally different from other forms for that reason. *Teleonomic processes* accurately label such programming yet remove the supernatural connotation.

Early physicists used a short estimate for the age of the Earth (20 to 40 million years) as an objection to Darwin's ideas. Subsequent geological data, however, testified to a greater age of Earth. Life originated 3.5 billion years ago, and that is considered an adequate time for evolutionary processes to have taken place.

ULTIMATE AND PROXIMATE CAUSES IN EVOLUTION

The adaptations increasing evolutionary fitness illustrated by the changed melanism of the urban moths and the salt-retaining kidneys of the slaves who survived are referred to as ultimate, distal, or *evolutionary causation,* the why of evolutionary change. Evolutionary causation is a population biology term in that groups of organisms with the trait survive better than do others because Darwin's three factors—diversity, natural selection, and inheritance—have operated in the individuals who make up the population. Individuals reflect the history of traits as reinforced in their ancestors and then actualized in themselves. Methodologically, researchers operating from that framework use the black-box approach of examining organism outputs, inputs, and external characteristics, rather than the biology within.

Proximate causation is illustrated by immediate mechanisms, the how of evolution. Proximate causes include detailed molecular factors, such as those that enhanced the production of melanin-containing cells in the moths and the biochemical changes that occurred in the slaves' kidney cells. Such factors are often investigated by biochemists and physiologists in the traditions of medical biology. Proximate causes also label immediate factors at other system levels, such as salt hunger, anxious fear, and delusions not yet fully explained by genetic and central nervous system mechanisms.

MENDELIAN GENETICS

A major problem for Darwin's theory in his time was the lack of a mechanism for inheritance. That lack was remedied by the modern synthesis of Darwin's theory and Mendelian genetics; the idea of a gene in a gene pair that is expressed *(dominant allele)* or not expressed *(recessive allele)* in a competitive manner provides the concept of inherited whole traits, rather than infinite gradations of heritable materials. Such ideas about inheritance mechanics, supported by convincing data, caused new thinking and modeling that uses organisms with short life spans, such as fruit flies and guinea pigs.

Although alleles at a gene pair are basic units with dominance and recessive effects, additive and other effects have been described with respect to their consequences on an individual's phenotype. Other non-Mendelian genetic concepts include *mosaicism,* in which somatic cells variously register a genetic variant and which is seen in fragile X syndrome. In *genomic (parental) imprinting,* the sex of the parent determines how a genetic defect is phenotypically realized. For example, deletions of chromosome 15 cause a mental retardation syndrome complicated by voracious appetite and obesity if the defect stems from the father *(Prader-Willi syndrome)* and another if from the mother *(Angelman syndrome).* The two phenotypes contrast; for example, Angelman syndrome patients exhibit more profound retardation, incessant laughter, and larger variants of mouth structure than do patients with the counterpart syndrome. In some cases of both syndromes, the phenomenon of uniparental disomy occurs; two copies of one parent's genetic material replace genes that usually stem from both parents, causing a de facto deletion from the other parent.

GENE FREQUENCY The Hardy-Weinberg equilibrium equation, which describes relative frequencies of genes in a population, provides a quantitative approach to evolution versus genetic stasis. Genetic polymorphisms can be assumed to occur as part of each individual's genetic equipment, illustrated by the genes that determine melanotic versus pepper-and-salt moths. Sexual reproduction alters gene combinations among particular individuals in a population, even though overall population gene frequencies generally stay the same (most evolution proceeds over many generations). Artificial breeding, which influenced Darwin, demonstrated that assortative mating can accelerate the effect of selection in changing gene frequencies, as in the many dog breeds. Relevant for psychiatry is the fact that behavioral and temperamental characteristics are among the variables in dogs and other domesticated animals.

In natural populations various kinds of natural selection have taken place, and genes or gene combinations have had effects on reproductive success. The black moths survived better than the pepper-and-salt moths in the era of coal pollution, and those persons with salt-retaining kidneys survived best during the transit from Africa to America. Genetic drift occurs when small isolated populations have some genetically determined characteristic at a great frequency and convey that characteristic to their descendants, heightening the frequency in them, compared with other members of the population. Some disease-producing mutations, such as those contributing to mental retardation, have become amplified in that way. Although mutations seem rare and are usually deleterious, some contribute significantly to beneficial change.

In 1953 new work was stimulated by the discovery of detailed mechanisms, the double helix of deoxyribonucleic acid (DNA) and the promulgation of the central dogma that DNA coding sequences (genes) determine ribonucleic acid (RNA) sequences, which in turn code proteins (DNA→RNA→protein). DNA now clearly connects the generations. The field of molecular biology has flourished since that discovery, with increasing information available about detailed proximate mechanisms. Structural and regulatory genes have been distinguished. *Structural genes* determine the sequence of proteins that compose the body, and *regulatory genes* determine tissue allocation and expression, timing of appearance, inhibition, and many other facets of cell function.

HOMOLOGY VERSUS CONVERGENT TRAITS Evolutionary theory called attention to historical factors in the formation of biological traits. Inherited traits shared by different species are *homologous* if the common ancestor also possessed the trait. That is true even if the present-day functioning of the trait is different in the species compared. For instance, the mouth of a human is homologous to the mouth of a worm or a fish, despite different methods of food capture and processing and such added functions as respiration and communication. A common ancestor of all three groups of animals also possessed a mouth.

In addition to historical factors, adaptation to environment has markedly shaped organisms over generations. *Convergent evolution* occurred if structures with different histories have a similar function. Thus, flight as a functional trait to exploit the ecological niche of air has convergently evolved in bats, birds, and moths. All three groups have a common ancestor—remotely in the past for the common ancestor of the insects and the vertebrates—and have characteristics in common—for example, all are multicellular and motile. To the extent that they possess common features with the common ancestor, the features are homologous. But that ancestor did not fly, so flight was a convergent trait.

New molecular techniques have detected identical nucleotide and amino acid sequences in widely divergent species. That finding has enhanced and highlighted the search for homologies versus convergences. Similar genes figure in the cellular machinery (that is, metabolism and replication) of the cells of all organisms (housekeeping genes). At the same time, what characterizes particular species are recent elaborations of those basic plans and parts.

Biological mechanisms that seem manifestly complex have solved an adaptive problem in the simplest way available to the organisms reproducing during the era in which the adaptation was initially made. Evolution has been compared to a tinkerer in that natural selection processes work only with the materials furnished, similar to someone's grandmother recycling bed sheets by making curtains from them. Insect wings that facilitate insect behavior may have evolved from lateral protuberances on ancestral insects that were initially adaptive for thermoregulatory functions.

Some comparisons stem from the less remote past. Chimpanzees and humans have such similar structural genes that their different phenotypes may be almost exclusively the consequence of regulatory genes and their products. For example, *neoteny,* the continued expression of juvenile traits into adult life, may have influenced such differences. Comparisons of adult humans and immature chimpanzees show more similarities than when adults of the two species are compared (adult humans have a face, a jaw, and a forehead that are youthful by chimpanzee standards). Playfulness is typically a characteristic of young mammals (perhaps to help them practice adult skills) but distinguishes many adult humans throughout life and may be an adaptive feature of human thinking. That morphological and behavioral youthful features fail to alter may be due to a removal of some usual regulatory gene products that ancestrally caused developmental change over an individual's life span (as in a human ancestor that resembled the adult chimpanzee more than the present-day human).

Phenomena that seem simple, including behavioral phenomena exhibited by humans, may have convoluted and complex determinants and mechanisms. Conversely, environmentally complex mechanisms that greatly change survival capabilities may have resulted from simple biochemical variations. In humans only a single amino acid substitution in hemoglobin gave rise to the sickle-cell variant adaptive in malaria-ridden Africa.

GENE-FOCUSED THEORY

That genetically determined phenotypical characteristics enhanced adaptation has been a powerful conceptual tool and provides fresh impetus to psychiatric scientists who are now not encumbered by machine similes, such as drives and hydraulics, unrelated to physiological realities. A major puzzle features unselfish behavior. Self-preservative and sexual behaviors are easily included in biologically determined contexts, such as eating and defensive maneuvers. But self-sacrificial and helping behaviors seem less obvious than those behaviors. Major segments of social insect and nude mole rat populations, for instance, do not themselves reproduce but, rather, seem to work for the good of the colony. Young human soldiers risk dying in war. What are the mechanisms through which those behaviors provide benefit? Do individuals calculate the good of the species in such sacrifices?

That they may do such calculations—a formerly popular concept called group selectionism—was challenged in an influential book, *Adaptation and Natural Selection,* by George C. Williams in 1966. His persuasive counterproposal held that adaptive behaviors must be understood not from a vague calculus that involves the good of the species but with respect to how they increase the genes held by the individual carrying them into subsequent generations. Much of Wilson's sociobiology was based on the increased scientific leverage that the model seemed to furnish. Genetic material is the fundamental unit of selection that continues to live through the generations.

To highlight a need for rigor and to underline that counterintuitive idea, proponents of the approach have used fresh metaphors, such as the selfish gene, with the body described as a survival machine in the service of its DNA. If altruism is not explained by group selection, other explanations of altruistic phenomena are necessary within the constraints of the gene-centered model, which is possible because genes and soma can be clearly differentiated. Much research has been done with those premises but not without criticism.

John Paul Scott, who has extensively investigated genetic effects on mammalian behaviors, argues that the anthropomorphic image is that of the selfish entrepreneur, a popular hero. Naive assumptions about independence of the various genes (that is, bean-bag genetics) have had to be made to allow the seemingly more rigorous science to ask questions. Scott noted that "genes do not and cannot act by themselves but only as components of an ongoing system." Many gene loci affect any phenotypic characteristic, any one locus affects many characters, any allele uniquely contributes to the phenotype, and dominance of a particular allele at a gene position varies according to the whole genotype and to the environment. However, proponents think that conceptual advances and data-based research have flourished with the oversimplification; for example, the intensity and the rate of selection for melanism in the English moths were predicted three decades before it was found to be true.

ECONOMIC METAPHOR AND GAME THEORY Researchers in animal behavior have focused on the evolutionary benefits of particular behaviors and on their evolutionary risks; for instance, when a bird displaying *parental investment* distracts a predator from its nest, it benefits to the extent that its eggs or fledglings are saved and is at risk to the extent that the predator may capture and consume it, even as the predator benefits or spends fruitless energy. Terms such as "investment," "benefits," "risks," and "spending" reflect imagery from human economics.

Game theory has extended the economic metaphor into the examination of rules of exchange, as seen with fighting behaviors in stereotyped combat known as *ritual agonistic behavior*. Contests between animals, such as between males competing for females, can be described in terms of game theory, using relatively simple formulas. In an early example, male beetles competing for females always won on the basis of size. Although size and strength are often variables for other species, too, the determinants of conflict resolution (rules) are usually complex and depend on many other factors, such as cleverness, the use of allies, delay now for challenge later, and surreptitiously impregnating estrous females. Figure 4.3-1 shows young male giraffes using their necks and heads as weapons in intrasexual competition. Such contests can be understood as components of sexual selection, described by Darwin and discussed further below.

Evolutionary strategies Examples of evolutionary strategies involve actions and reactions that are genetically programmed, including the capacity to estimate what is needed for victory and how to cut losses if defeat occurs. Those behavioral and cognitive operations are less the product of conscious considerations on the part of the acting animal than they are perceptual bias sets genetically determined in ancient neural and hormonal basic plans activated in each new generation. Such strategies describe the decision rules and behaviors of many individuals of a species that have provided sufficiently high benefit-cost ratios to have been maintained in the genetic code.

Those become *evolutionarily stable strategies* if they occur invariantly. For example, in a prototypical game of hawk-dove (representing strategies of always win or always give in), algorithms subjected to computer modeling and testing have shown that a population cannot sustain either mode of behavior as an evolutionarily stable strategy; rather, mixed and conditional strategies are likely. Peaceable cooperation also occurs. Grouping behaviors (for example, herds, flocks, and schools) assist survival. Even dinosaurs 200 million years ago seem to have displayed herd behavior that differentiated parental behavior within it; the young seem to have occupied the center of groupings, and large animals occupied the periphery.

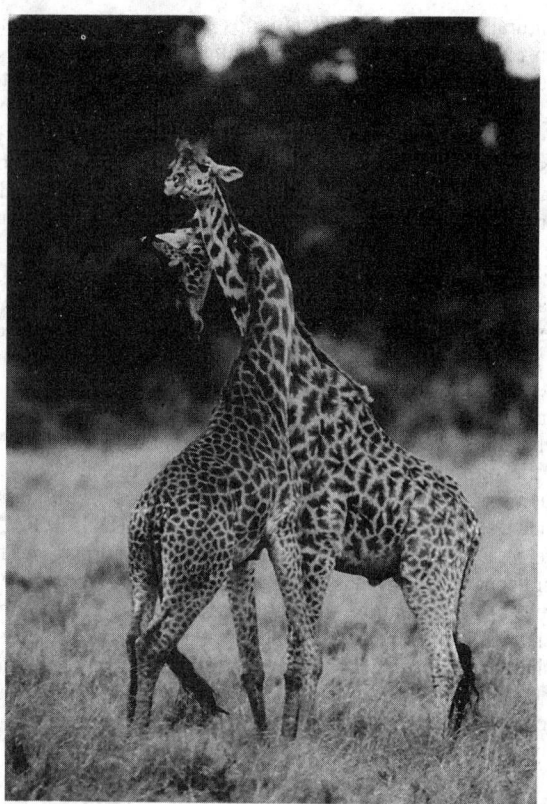

FIGURE 4.3-1 *Young male giraffes demonstrate friendly competition by necking. They are practicing intrasexual competition, using the powerful weapon that the neck and the head together have become in giraffes. They use the neck as a sling, with the skull at the end as a momentum-producing weight. The weapon is used not only against fellow males but, even more devastatingly, against other antagonists, such as predators. (Courtesy of Gregory G. Dimijian.)*

Both competitive and cooperative strategies abound in complex combinations. Population biology terms describe responses averaged over many individuals, but for some species, such as humans and other primates, diversity of conditional responses on the part of different individuals within a group or within any one individual over time is more highly adaptive than are stereotyped responses.

Reciprocal altruism *Altruism* is helpful behavior that raises the recipient's fitness while lowering the donor's fitness. An act whose benefit is reciprocated is called *reciprocal altruism*. Like lending or investing money, an unselfish behavior by a person may be expected to redound to that person's benefit—or to the benefit of kin—at a later time. Such calculations in humans are often conscious. In studies of chimpanzee politics, those primates also establish coalitions with each other and keep track of political debts.

Cheating and attempts at unfair bargaining have also been studied with computer models. After making simplifying assumptions, researchers tested numerous simple and complex algorithms and showed that a simple tit-for-tat strategy—meaning that a recipient of an honest or dishonest signal reacts in the same way the signaler acted—proved to be more effective than numerous complex strategies.

Resource-holding potential In developing equations to describe the evolution of ritual agonistic behavior, researchers have used the intervening variable of resource-holding potential to express fighting capacity or, when extrapolated to human conflict, the ability to deal successfully with various competitive exchanges. Resource-holding potential is an ability to fight for one's position or to otherwise successfully enhance it. For ritual agonistic behavior to evolve as an evolutionary strategy, each person uses knowledge about its own resource-holding potential in conjunction with that of competitors. When they are compared, the difference is conceptualized as *relative resource-holding potential*. In humans relative resource-holding potential has been correlated with self-esteem.

Individuals have developed ways to signal resource-holding potential to competitors and to decode competitors' counterpart signs of those quantities. Part of resource-holding potential is substantive, consisting of real resources like size, strength, skill, and allies—akin to real financial resources, such as gold reserves. A *ritual component* of resource-holding potential is lowered or raised by signals from others, as from allies. A *situational component* (such as being on home ground or, if human, being in the right) may add strength. In animal groupings, including humans, a *group-membership component,* deriving from affiliations, may heighten the likelihood of victory.

Two modes of group living Two modes of group living in primates have been noted, one characterized by tension and fighting *(agonic mode)* and the other by relaxation and playfulness *(hedonic mode).* In the agonic mode, subordinates pay great attention to punitively dominant alpha animals. In contrast, when a grouping is in the hedonic mode, the dominant or control (alpha) animal may be hard to distinguish. Human groupings can be similarly classified, and observers of business effectiveness have noted that companies with relaxed atmospheres have increased productivity. *Social-attention-holding power* is a variation on resource-holding potential independent of fighting that has become a factor for group-living animals with leaders. It labels the ability of an alpha person to be attractive to the group (prestige in humans). Followership behavior (counterpoint to leadership) has been described in cult formation. Hypnosis may be a social communicative (followership) state within any one person that is both helpful in therapy and pathogenic in conditions such as dissociative identity disorder.

SEXUAL SELECTION A mate choosing a sexual partner makes the choice on the basis of estimates of the other's fitness (perhaps quantified, as in resource-holding potential calculations)—that is, which potential mate would most enhance the survival of the chooser's genes in their joint offspring? Chosen examples include animals that are the ruddiest (thereby least anemic) or that have the most elaborate plumage or other showy attributes, reflecting health and resourcefulness that cause them to be chosen preferentially as mates. Such characteristics seem to be cues for the chooser of a potential mate about factors that auger well for the chooser's offspring (for example, resistance to disease and predators). Behavioral phenomena that are otherwise mysterious, such as *lekking* (male defense of a small territory to demonstrate prowess, exhibited by some birds and mammals), seem to illustrate those cues, as do male bowerbirds, who show their capability by elaborate courtship rituals and nest building. The male's efforts and their extent may figure more importantly for a choosing female than does the size of the territory or the nest's effect on the offspring.

Which sex does the choosing? In imagery borrowed from sellers' versus buyers' markets, that may be influenced by which sex has the scarce and expensive resources. Differential gamete size in plants and animals *(anisogamy)* contrasts to motile isogamy of both gametes typical of undifferentiated life forms. In complex species, sperm are easily and numerously produced, whereas the female egg—with its elaborate yolk, large size, immobility, and limited number—is much more expensive for its maker than is the sperm. The expensive egg may determine coyness in the female, frequently the chooser sex, although males of some species may prevent her making choices by keeping other males away.

Runaway positive feedback effects demonstrate sexual selection consequences, such as the peacock's tail. Competition with one's gender mates for the opposite sex may, however, become an arms race with deleterious consequences. The call of the male Túngara frog, used for attracting females, is exploited by frog-eating bats for locating the frogs as prey.

Specific methods of sexual rivalry include sperm competition at many system levels. The male damselfly, for example, has a special brush at the end of his penis that sweeps out a predecessor's sperm, so that only the last male to mate is the successful one. After mating, the male then hovers about the female to ward off competitors. In species closer to humans, many baboon and chimpanzee males mate with counterpart estrous females. The most dominant baboons, however, mate at the female's most receptive time. Chimpanzees may compete on a cellular level, so that relatively large testes have evolved to generate more sperm in each ejaculate. Few gorilla males mate per female (dominants zealously guard their females), and they have correspondingly smaller testes than do chimpanzees.

Human males have testes that are intermediate in size between chimpanzees and gorillas but have penises larger than either primate. Conjectures based on across-species comparisons have held that human males may rely on direct sperm competition to a degree intermediate between the other two primates, but the visible attribute of the penis may have more importance for human female choice. *Sexual dimorphism*—gender differences in body attributes—generally hinges on the degree to which male rivalry and female choice occurs within a species. In species in which males and females cannot be distinguished (no dimorphism), strict monogamy prevails. Such monogamy may be an evolutionary strategy to assure male parental investment.

Human female and male psychological attributes may be not only the result of childhood learning but also the outcome of male and female brains' and bodies' having differently evolved for strategic reasons. A prominent question is why women suppress evidence of ovulation (in contrast to the evident estrus of most mammals). A proposed answer is that the suppression may enhance continued male interest in them and, hence, in their children—that is, it may represent another strategy to bring about increased *parental investment* on the man's part.

KIN SELECTION AND INCLUSIVE FITNESS Behaviors that enhance the survival of genes shared by kin result in *kin selection.* William D. Hamilton's belief that close relatives share genes has had a powerful effect on sociobiology. Benefit to a relative thereby benefits one's own genes, even though the replicas that survive are carried by another person. The closer the relationship, the greater the benefit to one's own DNA. That benefit has been labeled *inclusive fitness,* the reproductive success of identical genes carried in organisms related by common descent. A formula that describes how altruistic acts may enhance inclusive fitness is $rB > C$, where B=benefit to recipient, C=cost to donor, and r=coefficient of relatedness, for example, full siblings and parent-offspring relatedness have an r of ½, half siblings and grandparent-grandchild have an r of ¼, and the r of first cousins is ⅛.

Giving up reproduction, therefore, but working to benefit one's siblings and cousins should help one's own genes, even if they reside in the bodies of others. Figure 4.3–2 shows evidence of bonding and familial investment among sibling elephants. Data collected on pied kingfishers indicate that the nonbreeding males documented as helping a breeding pair most were, in fact, offspring of a previous nesting. Distantly related males also helped somewhat.

The most effective and most efficient way to benefit one's own genes in later generations is parenting. Differential attention to offspring has been described as K and r selection strategies. In K selection, which is typical of many mammals, the parents invest energy and resources in a few offspring for lengthy periods, thereby sacrificing the production of more offspring (parental investment). In r selection, parental energy goes, instead, into the production of a large number of fertilized gametes, although fewer survive without the parental investment of the K strategy.

Despite the high relatedness possessed by parents and their children and by siblings to each other, they have conflicts of interest. Behavioral phenomena within families may have genetic determinants. In the metaphor, parents wish that all the siblings get equal shares because all have the same amount of parental genes, but each of the offspring is most interested in furthering its own personal cause. Sibling rivalry is, therefore, not surprising, nor is parental disapproval of it.

HUMAN AS HUNTER-GATHERERS Humans may have originated in the Great Rift valley of Africa. Hominid ancestors evolved upright posture sooner than they evolved increased brain size. On an evolutionary time scale, they evolved recently and quickly and then migrated worldwide, rapidly occupying

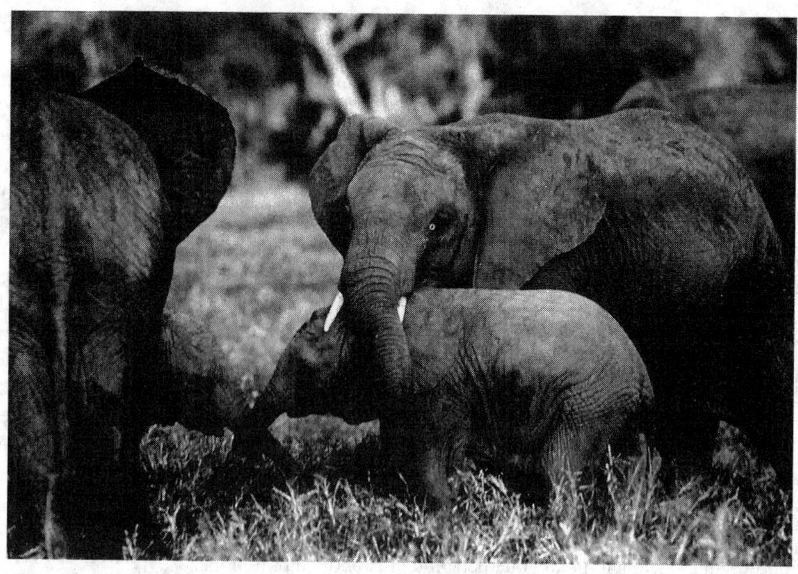

FIGURE 4.3-2 *An elephant family palpably demonstrate familial bonding (the trunk of an adolescent is draped about a little one). This illustrates kin selection and inclusive fitness. (Courtesty of Gregory G. Dimijian.)*

many and varied ecological niches. Hominids and early humans were hunters and gatherers for a much lengthier period (millions of years) than they have been agriculturalists and city dwellers (thousands of years). The rapid cultural innovation may have caused adaptations stemming from the earlier time period to be evident today and to be potentially maladaptive.

For example, the prototypical nuclear family of modern times may be a biological novelty, quite different from the large groupings typical of hunter-gatherer societies, in which many adults are in constant contact with the offspring and there is less strain on the relationship of the marital pair and their immediate offspring than in the nuclear family. Of course, civilization has developed to accommodate the needs of people, and, given varied allocations of resources, inequity may result now, as was probably true then. Critics have noted that present-day hunter-gatherers at the periphery of favorable habitats cannot be considered representative of those ancestral groups.

MEDICAL USE OF THE ADAPTATIONIST ASSUMPTION The *adaptationist assumption* (also called *selectionist thinking*) holds that a trait is adaptive unless otherwise demonstrated. Adaptationism has been hard to apply to psychiatry because, by definition, psychiatric disorders do not help but, rather, hinder survival and reproduction. Adaptationist assumptions are often used by biological scientists in hypothesis-generating phases of their research (for example, what may have been an adaptive function over evolutionary time of an attribute of the cell, the body, or a behavior), but most dispense with that part of the thought process in research reports because it bears little on the disproof or the confirmation of hypotheses in testing phases of research.

Some recent scholars, however, in defining Darwinian medicine and Darwinian psychology, have advocated the application of selectionist thinking to arenas beyond hypothesis formation, as in counseling patients. They point to adaptive features of otherwise distressing problems. For example, a high temperature (fever) helps combat disease, despite the discomfort induced. In a behavioral adaptation, reptiles without internal temperature-elevating mechanisms seek out the sun when they are infected.

Medications that overzealously treat uncomfortable side effects may reduce the benefits of the evolved adaptation. Obsessive-compulsive behaviors may have been adaptive for survival from communicable diseases. That is, neural mechanisms that enhanced hand-washing compulsions may have improved survival during epidemics of infectious disease and, hence, may be like the salt retention of the former slaves—more adaptive once than now. However, clomipramine (Anafranil), which seems to ameliorate the present-day overuse of compulsions, may be a culturally evolved (that is, drug-company-developed) interference with an evolutionarily evolved behavior that is no longer adaptive.

HOMICIDE, ABUSE, ABORTION, AND SUICIDE Inclusive fitness theory predicts that kin are less likely to suffer from aggression than are nonrelatives. For example, a male lion taking over a new pride kills cubs not fathered by himself, and infanticide of nonkin has been reported in other species. Research has shown that humans may also use such evolutionary strategies. Criminal statistics on family crimes from many countries show that homicide and abuse rates are much lower when the recipients are genetically related to the criminals than when they are not genetically related. For example, a perpetrator's spouses, stepchildren, and in-laws are 11 times more likely to die than are the children, parents, and siblings living in the same household. Moreover, epidemiological evidence shows that pregnant women and girls with available families or mates (more available parental investment) are less likely to make the decision to have an abortion than are those without families or mates.

People who are likely to complete suicides have little new to contribute to the inclusive fitness of their genes. That is, those who died were unlikely either to have had future offspring or to be able to contribute to the welfare of the offspring and other genetic relatives that they did have.

CRITIQUE OF ADAPTATIONIST APPROACHES In the title of a widely noted paper Stephen J. Gould and Richard C. Lewontin used vivid imagery, "The Spandrels of San Marco and the Panglossian Paradigm: A Critique of the Adaptationist Programme." They criticized the circular reasoning inherent in adaptationist thinking (that is, the Panglossian paradigm indicates an assumption that things are there because they were meant to be there, a folk theory counterpart to teleology). The authors argued that, although a biological feature may clearly have a purpose, that fact fails to indicate that the feature evolved to fulfill that purpose. To illustrate the concept that evolutionarily recent biological features may be useful in adaptation, Gould and Lewontin asserted that spandrels—mosaics that decorate spaces next to the curves of cathedral arches—are there not for the first purpose of structure but as add-ons, as late-arriving features with communicative functions.

Another criticism of the adaptationist approach maintains that, in contrast to the selfish-gene metaphor, those explanations of altruism, in fact, only explain variations on selfishness. However, a proximate mechanism, avidity for learning or *docility,* has been proposed as an explanation for true human altruism. Docility may be such a helpful mechanism in humans that it is adaptive for people to accept a tax of altruism—that is, to give without expectation of direct return. However, a person doing so is honored by other people. Distinctions, admiration, and reputation are intangible commodities, but honors conferred for unselfish behavior are meaningful. Docility may be an add-on proximate mechanism with evolutionary payoffs.

SOCIOPHYSIOLOGY: COMMUNICATION AND INDIVIDUAL BIOLOGY

The chief contribution of sociobiology to psychiatry is that it lays the foundations for an adequate biological basic science for the specialty. Beyond the black-box premises and deductive methods of ultimate causation advocates, research on proximate mechanisms in the individual must be done for a subset of sociobiology, labeled sociophysiology, to be an adequate basic science of psychiatry. Only recently have investigators begun to expand the population biological aspect of sociobiology to the examination of individuals, human and nonhuman, with an eye to the dimensions on which they can be compared (Table 4.3-1).

Among the studies bearing on proximate causation at different system levels, top-down and bottom-up research can be distinguished. In bottom-up research, cellular-molecular studies bear on the behaviors of whole organisms, similar to the way that a low antidepressant blood level may explain a treatment nonresponse. In top-down work, whole organism behaviors point to molecular data, as polyphagia, polydipsia, and polyuria predict hyperglycemia and hypoinsulinemia, part of the pathogenesis of diabetes mellitus. In contrast to that disease, however, most psychiatric disorders provide few molecular clues. Yet such clues to pathogenesis are a legitimate objective of sociobiological science.

EMOTION DISPLAYS AS SOCIAL REGULATORS In top-down analyses the most appropriate interpretation of organism behavior helps define the parameters at the different levels. Ordinarily, the distinction between emotions as fundamentally communication and emotions as reflections of internal states has little meaning. Observations of context-dependent displays in birds provided investigators with the view that emotions have been evolutionarily reinforced because they are interpersonal signals that organize and modulate exchanges between people.

Research on emotions in social settings shows that signals such as smiling are displays, rather than spillovers from internal

TABLE 4.3-1
Sociophysiological Model of the Individual

A B C D E **Cell**
1. Cell division and metabolism
2. Natural selection (NS) /unicellular
3. Basic housekeeping genes
4. (((((EEEE))))) E = core genes
5. All cells have common elements
6. Lesch-Nyhan mental retardation

D **Body**
1. Cell adhesion, nutrition, and maintenance
2. NS/early multicellular life stages
3. Basic genes (BG) +intercell add-ons (IA)
4. ((((DEEEED)))) D=cell specialty genes
5. Oral cells: epithelial, neural, muscular
6. Delirium from electrolyte abnormality

C **Individual**
1. Body integrity: food and security
2. NS/obligate multicellular stages
3. BG+IA+add-on genes for body integrity (BI)
4. (((CDEEEEDC))) C=food intake+protection genes
5. Biting occurs for eating and defense
6. Panic disorder, anorexia nervosa

B **Family**
1. Gene perpetuation: bonding, gamete production, direct parenting, sibling cooperation/competition
2. NS + kin selection for ↑ inclusive fitness/groups
3. BG+IA+BI+ add-on genes for familial bonding (FB)
4. ((BCDEEEEDCB)) B= genes for kin detection/bonding
5. To bond, mother and infant both laugh, using mouth2/6. Infantile autism, child abuse

A **Species**
1. Gene enhancement: selection of best mate available; parental investment; conspecific groups for feeding, defense, and reproduction; social rank hierarchies
2. NS + sexual selection for best genes/group living
3. BG+IA+BI+FB+ add-ons for mate selection + group behavior
4. (ABCDEEEEDCBA) A=genes for mate selection devices
5. Males sing (orally), and female smiles at choicest male
6. Manic patients are hypersexual + overassume control

A–E: Levels of investigation. 1. Organism functions at each level. 2. Kind of evolutionary selection/era when evolved. 3. Basic plan schemata, with new contributions at each level. 4. Speculative diagram of responsible gene/gene complexes. 5. Examples of gene-determined mouth-functions at each level. 6. Psychiatric illness from dysfunction at each level. The five levels of investigation can be related to any one of the others by top-down (e.g., A/B with C/D or E), bottom-up (e.g., E or D with A/B), or mixed approaches.

states. For example, bowlers throwing strikes or spares do not smile when alone at the time of the achievement, but they do smile a little later, when they encounter the gaze of an onlooker.

Instead of considering anger as simply a fundamental emotion variously held in check (that is, behaviors indicative of it are decoded as expressed, concealed, or displaced), clinicians should consider displays of anger as signals that the person is about to aggress in a variety of potential ways contingent on the social setting and what happens next. A person with incompletely hidden anger may be displaying not so much concealment as tentative signs of an inclination to aggress; an explosion occurring later may result from another person's reacting to the first display in a way that escalates it. Relative aspects of the interactants—such as age, rank, and relationship—may partly determine the next behavior.

Such concepts can be exemplified by clinical experience in psychiatry, as in the assessment and the treatment of potentially violent patients with many possible diagnoses (angry displays are not diagnosis-specific). Clinicians know that violence potential rises when a possible aggressor begins to speak loudly, paces, and shows an inability to hear. Reactive displays of counteraggression and loud voices heighten the probability of violence. Calming and cooperation are best attained with (1) nonthreatening distance (that is, the clinician stays outside the person's body buffer zone, which increases in a person potentially violent), (2) offers of food or drink while continuing efforts at verbal negotiation are voiced softly, and (3) a show of unambiguous but gentle potential force, as when a number of large men quietly surround the person while the clinician is quietly authoritative. Registration of other nonverbal displays during psychotherapeutic sessions similarly assist in deciphering the complex melange of patient messages.

More—not less—aggression results when a potentially violent patient is laughed at by antagonistic strangers. Laughter is an emotional signal in humans with both alienating and bonding effects. Laughter causes particular distress and potential fury in a person ridiculed, but it enhances closeness for those laughing together.

HUMAN BEHAVIOR AS ELABORATED BASIC PLANS

Animals communicate with one another on cognitive and noncognitive levels. Programmed spacings and linkages in conspecifics are exhibited; they often take the form of propensity states antedating language in communication. Strategies evolving over evolutionary time represent the contemporary action of basic biological plans that have originated early and then endured, such as eating, defense, sex, and parenting. Each may have given rise to derivative communicative states with distinctive add-on components.

Eating Eating is so significant an animal activity that it probably has not reevolved over evolutionary time, as flying obviously did, but the details vary markedly in what is eaten and how food capture and processing are accomplished. Foraging mechanisms often involve conspecific communication in ways that are highly specialized and elaborated in species-specific ways.

For example, in rats the odor caused by what a fellow rat has recently ingested has a major influence on the smeller; what the other rat ate becomes preferred food. On an evolutionary basis that preference may have evolved to avoid poison while yet exploiting most what is available—that is, a fellow rat alive enough to emit the odor may assure safety for that food.

Humans have undergone quite separate counterpart oral evolutions. For example, in contrast to other animals, humans tell stories that may serve as guides to the future actions of the hearers. Such activities are derivative, in part, of genes that program the mouth, pharyngeal, and laryngeal apparatus.

Flight-fight As is well known from flight-fight reactions, defensive behaviors also reflect basic plans. Panic and anxiety disorders may reflect unduly triggered human variants. Indeed, as mentioned above for obsessive-compulsive disorders, many psychiatric disorders may represent the activation of basic patterns of reactivity that to outside observers are inappropriate to the context; studies of their pathogenesis may eventually involve investigation of what actions are basic and what are add-on components. For example, monkeys whose ancestors evolved where snakes prey on monkeys are not born with snake aversions but instantly learn such aversions from observations of other monkeys, whereas aversion to other objects, such as flowers, are not acquired.

Sex The identification of conspecifics that are potential mates seems to have stemmed from the adaptation that sexual reproduction provided. The mixing of genes to stay ahead of mutating microorganisms may have reinforced the adaptation. Species that reproduce by parthenogenesis tend to be short-lived as distinct entities. On the proximate level of analysis, reproductive and other sexual hormones have figured in the mechanics of sexual proliferation, as they are homologous factors in many species with varied ancestries; sex hormones are the result of basic plans and are constituent basic parts. Sexual biology also involves communication (for example, testosterone causes a deep voice).

Incest taboos In work bearing on the prevention of deleterious genetic consequences from inbreeding, evidence exists for incest taboos in many species other than humans, and the taboos probably exist in humans as well, not so much as a result of the oedipal complex but antedating it in the infant's life. Familial bonding seems to preempt sexual bonding later and is based evidently on early contact, more than genetic relatedness; for example, unrelated children growing up together in a kibbutz behave as though they were siblings and show no later interest in mating. Only when familial bonding is disrupted do evidences of sexual bonding occur. Oedipal temptations probably happen only when preoedipal bonding has been disrupted.

Parenting Mammals are highly invested in their offspring. Babies are attention-getters for adults and show that genetic predispositions interact with the environment to heighten adaptation. Human neonates, for instance, seem to have a preprogrammed interest in adult facial expressions. Observers without knowledge of a specific stimulus can tell from a baby's imitative reaction whether a stimulus face was smiling or frowning.

Cries and smiles are aimed at adults, who have somatic and behavioral responsivity to such stimuli; adults' pupils enlarge and interest heightens on perceiving pictures of infants, even if the infants are unrelated to the perceiver. Men tend to display pupillary dilation once they have become parents but not before, whereas women and girls of all ages display the response. That gender difference may exemplify differential *parental investment* in the two sexes: the basic plan is there for both sexes, but the plan is more readily apparent and easily elicited in women than in men. That the response exists when unrelated infants are the stimulus shows that proximate mechanisms (similar to docility, described above) may outweigh deduced calculations of genetic relatedness (selfish genes). Such proximate mechanisms seem to allow humans to adopt unrelated offspring.

Experiments with rat mothers and infants using invasive measures impossible in humans have shown that, at each developmental stage, the mother and the pup are complexly attuned to each other, including related temperature, heart rate, and gastric secretion variables. Smell is a critical variable for a pup seeking the teat of its dam; moreover, specific constituents in the mother's milk influence the rat pup's maturation.

PRIMATE DIVERSITY AND CONSISTENCY Problems for biological research on behavior exist partly because of behavioral diversity in humans and other primates. Approximately 200 primate species occupy numerous ecological niches and do so with remarkably different social interactions, varying among and within species. For example, the longitudinal study of chimpanzee troups by Jane Goodall showed that food concentration may have caused cooperative communications to be succeeded by aggressive behaviors.

Similarly, the behavioral variability of humans is also extraordinarily diverse, resulting from individual learning, cultural traditions, and biological differences. How can evolutionarily ancient versus recent traits be distinguished phenotypically? How can one determine which behaviors and their biological mechanisms are promising for investigation? For top-down approaches, the phenomena of psychiatric disorders—which are not diverse but, rather, stereotyped—may help the basic science. Mood disorders are here described as prototypical illustrations.

Mood disorders as sustained display states In contrast to primate diversity, psychiatric disorders show communicative behavioral states with features so consistent that their defining qualities are agreed on formally by large numbers of psychiatrists. Moreover, some syndromes resemble communication propensity states seen not only in humans but also in other group-living animals. John S. Price described resemblances in human depression and in low-ranking birds, as in chicken peck orders, and has postulated that much depression may reflect a communicative state stemming from losing reactions programmed by highly conserved ritual agonistic behaviors; a loser may be signaling that it represents no threat to the victors to enhance its own survival for possible future efforts at reproduction; for the most convincing display, losers fool even themselves in the process. That theory reconceptualizes learned helplessness, a label for the same behaviors that has helped foster animal models for human depression. Viewed sociophysiologically, learned helplessness is less a learned state than an activation of the basic plan of a communication propensity embedded in the genetic code, homologous across reptiles, birds, and mammals, whose common ancestors date approximately 300 million years ago.

Manic and hypomanic states resemble alpha behavior—in humans, high-profile, charismatic leadership—but are maladaptive in their extent, timing, and choice of audience. Activity levels, communicative push, planning behaviors, lessened sleep need, increased appetites, creativity, elated happiness, and infectious good humor are also seen in high-profile human leaders.

Leads to the cellular and the molecular counterparts of both poles of mood disorders and their normal variants may be inferred from what is known preliminarily of the mechanisms of drugs used effectively in their treatment. One of the important metabolites involved is serotonin.

Social rank correlates of serotonin High social rank in vervet monkey groups correlates robustly with high blood serotonin levels, a finding also true in humans. Moreover, in subsequent bottom-up research, when drugs affecting serotonin have artificially heightened such levels in monkeys, dominance behaviors increased. Those findings relating systemic serotonin levels to behavioral states have not yet been fully integrated with other findings that connect central nervous system serotonin to behavior (lower spinal fluid levels have been associated with impulsivity, and antidepressant drugs have been associated with the blocking of serotonin uptake in synapses).

Search for gene-behavior correlations For another bottom-up approach, a promising natural experiment has shown genetic deletions to be associated with stereotyped behavioral communications. A deletion in chromosome 15 has been typically associated with a mental retardation syndrome that involves laughter. People with Angelman syndrome never learn to speak, but most laugh and smile incessantly. Genes on chromosome 15 in the nondeleted normal condition, therefore, may be regulating factors for those key communicative attributes in humans. Angelman syndrome patients also have large mouths and jaws. In Prader-Willi patients with a similar deletion on chromosome 15, small mouth structures occur, along with overeating behaviors. Perhaps basic plans for eating with more recently evolved communication nuances stem from that chromosomal region, although many other chromosomal regions also figure in the determination of such important signals and mental states.

Homosexual men have increased male homosexual kin on the maternal side only. A finding that the X chromosome displays a distinctive set of DNA markers in homosexual men stimulated a sociobiological hypothesis that explains the seeming paradox of a powerful behavioral propensity without reproductive advantage. Since the X chromosome is inherited by men from their mothers only, the distinctive DNA in homosexual persons could indicate a coding that causes heightened sexual interest in men in the developed brain of not only women but men as well. Both sexes would experience this, the theory holds, but only the women can use it for reproductive advantage. That there might be potential reproductive payoff for the genetic region stems from the fact that women have twice as many X chromosomes as men, and over the generations any one X chromosome exists twice as long in women as in men. In economic metaphor, therefore, these are *selfish genes:* The genetic material of the region sacrifices the reproductive success of men for a conjectured reproduction by the women of the kindred that outweighs the loss from the nonreproducing men ($B > ½ C$, where B = benefit and C = cost). That illustrates sociobiological reasoning based on partial data. It is not an established conclusion because yet to be demonstrated are data that the women of a homosexual person's kin share the same distinctive DNA sequences and that these are in turn correlated with a heightened female sexual interest in men and consequent increased reproduction.

IMPLICATIONS FOR PSYCHIATRY

As a specialty of medicine, psychiatry has not previously had the focus of sociophysiology as a biological basic science, although psychiatric disorders and even sexual preferences, such as homosexuality, are considered by some to be biological (no longer cultural or learned) in origin. Several decades ago and until recently, behavioral modification theories assumed that behavioral variations, adaptive and maladaptive, were the result of learning that affected an identical substrate *(tabula rasa)* in each child whose behavioral and psychological uniqueness developed later. That assumption, which emphasized developmental factors to the exclusion of other factors, has given way to the recognition that there are interactions between genetic and environmental factors, both of which need extensive definition and study within and between their respective levels of analysis. Sociobiology greatly extends that domain of work.

GENETIC DELETIONS AND COMMUNICATIVE SIGNALS Study of the pathophysiology of Alzheimer's disease (called dementia of the Alzheimer's type in the fourth edition of *Diagnostic and Statistical Manual of Mental Disorders* [DSM-IV]) has been enhanced because it resembles changes evident in Down's syndrome, in which a known genetic defect causes definable biochemical changes. Other genetically caused mental retardation syndromes can be approached as indexes of investigation, especially if the genes can be located and the behaviors are definable (for example, stereotyped) and interesting. Thus, Angelman syndrome and Prader-Willi syndrome, both often associated with a deletion on chromosome 15, feature dysregulations of a mental set (appetite) and a communicative signal (laughter), both of high interest for psychiatry. That natural experiment points to fresh studies of phenomena meaningful in psychiatry from both bottom-up and top-down perspectives. The meaning of laughter in interpersonal exchanges needs to be investigated, as do the genes on chromosome 15 missing in patients with Angelman syndrome and Prader-Willi syndrome. How does variation in each set of data affect variation in the other? Other natural experiments include the fragile X syndrome and its relation to autistic behavior, self-abusive behaviors, and the distal regions of the X chromosome.

PRACTICE IMPLICATIONS Biological psychiatry may have caused psychiatric practitioners to become less blaming, compared with what had been implicitly the case when the idea of the schizophrenogenic mother, for example, was current several decades ago. But a thoroughgoing appreciation of the pathophysiology of disorders may allow all concerned to experience them as sequelae of disease, rather than as moral turpitude, more akin to the altered personality of a patient with a brain tumor than to a despised criminal. As can be appreciated by everyday experiences with dilemmas posed by courtroom trials for aberrant behavior, the pathophysiology of troubling actions requires much study.

To learn that mania and depression, for example, may be facets of unfortunately triggered communication propensity states puts them into a different context for the practitioner, the patient, the family, and the public. It allows the psychiatrist to be more confident and more convincing than is provided by a simple assertion of a chemical imbalance inferred by empirical response to medication but without further placement in a pathophysiological framework. Indeed, when the basic plans that are activated have had biologically adaptive reasons for being, a propensity to the affliction may even be seen positively. Families of bipolar disorder patients, for example, are documented to be more successful than are others. For the moment treatment plans may be little affected—lithium (Eskalith) and carbamazepine (Tegretol) may continue to be used—but, with further study and definition of the problem, other remedies may be obvious.

An increasingly better pathophysiology for psychiatric illnesses should stem from sociobiological research on communication biases. On the one hand, that research may result from comparative studies using adaptationist thinking and population biology to learn about ultimate causes of communication. On the other hand, sociophysiological research on proximate mechanisms should produce new data from study of the DNA molecule and other proximate causes, using top-down and bottom-up methods that do not neglect or overly constrict either level of analysis. Most important, a better understanding of the mysterious processes that psychiatrists confront should render the practice of the specialty more helpful to its patients.

PSYCHOTHERAPY IMPLICATIONS Successful psychotherapy is considered by some theorists to be biological learning, causing changes that can be investigated with such tools as positron emission tomography and magnetic resonance imagery. Increasing realization that social processes are no less biological than other bodily processes will no doubt motivate such investigations in the future. To this point, however, the major emphasis of sociobiological applications has focused on adaptationist assumptions. Views of human behavior can become refocused when its characteristics are aligned with the behavior of other animals and evaluated for how its genomic history and proximate structures have caused it to enhance natural, sexual, and kin selection and evolutionary and inclusive fitness.

Selectionist thinking and Freud Several authors have surveyed ways in which selectionist thinking has helped clarify phenomena noted and preliminarily explained by Sigmund Freud. Two examples are repression and oral behavior. Repression may be a form of deceiving others by way of deceiving oneself, especially by the verbal language route. Repression, therefore, is a subtle form of combined cooperation and cheating.

Oral behavior can be understood as sucking independent of hunger that evolved when babies nursed at the breast. It may have evolved to stave off rival siblings born to the mother by inhibiting her ovulation through nipple stimulation, a physiological effect documented to last two to three years. Evidence exists from third-world countries that a child's survival is enhanced if the next baby is delayed. That finding suggests that genes that enhance impulses to suck nonnutritively help offspring survive and seems to constitute a powerful message from child to mother received on a noncognitive level. Others have speculated that the typical terrible-twos behavior of the small child evolved to divert the attention of the mother toward its own benefit and away from a younger sibling.

Relief from confusion and undue responsibility Guilty or ashamed people and those distressingly mystified and confused about their own behaviors may feel less so when counseled that they possess automatic psychological and behavioral responses that are biologically programmed and that have been perhaps inappropriately triggered. Those responses are exemplified by panic and other anxiety states conceptualized as flight-fight responses out of proportion to reality and experienced as fear without consciously appreciated reasons. Moreover, some therapists have provided conceptual schemata that reassure patients with the information that troubles may arise because humans evolved as hunter-gatherers. Since many reactions appropriate in that era of adaptation may work less well in modern times, the reactions may seem unpleasant and maladaptive, similar to out-of-control allergic reactions.

Self-esteem and resource-holding potential Self-esteem is an important concept in psychiatry generally, as mood disorders and some personality disorders are seen to have its dysregulation as a defining feature. The likely existence of ancient basic plans for communication behaviors in the context of aggression helps delineate problems of human self-esteem with methods of comparative psychology; that is, self-esteem may result from comparisons of self-prowess with the prowess of others, as in contests stemming from sexual-selection processes. Elaborations are exemplified by social-attention-holding power (for example, attractiveness for elected leaders), which often characterizes human political processes.

Resource-holding potential is a useful concept because (1) all the components of agonistic behavior can be described in terms of signals of either absolute resource-holding potential (for example, family wealth, large size, good looks) or relative resource-holding potential (for example, a person wins or loses an encounter with another, as in an athletic contest, or boosts or puts down another, as with a compliment or a sarcastic comment); (2) as an index of self-esteem, resource-holding potential can be applied not only in humans but also in animals, so that precursors of the primordial self-concept (states of having won or lost) can be studied in nonhumans; and (3) resource-holding potential and mood are closely correlated, so that an analysis of interpersonal exchanges in terms of resource-holding potential may clarify the conceptualization of mood change, including profound depression, as it may represent self-deceptive operations about the loss of self-worth. Persons who not only declare themselves worthless but also believe it are perhaps more persuasive to others experienced as threatening than if they are insincere about the message.

Specifically in psychotherapy, resource-holding potential has been used as a facilitating concept; acceptance of having lost, if one has lost, may be an important therapeutic event. Convincing displays of losing are no longer necessary, and the person can go on to other things, instead of expending or risking resource-holding potential on pursuing revenge. That variant on cognitive therapy for depression provides a comprehensive biological rationale for that form of treatment.

SUGGESTED CROSS-REFERENCES

Molecular neurobiology is discussed in Section 1.14, genetics in Sections 1.15 and 1.16, aggression in Section 3.4, and animal research in Section 5.2. Mood disorders are discussed in depth in Chapter 16, anxiety disorders in Chapter 17, and personality disorders in Chapter 25.

REFERENCES

Alexander R D: *The Biology of Moral Systems.* Aldine de Gruyter, New York, 1987.

Alcock J: *Animal Behavior.* Sinauer Press, Sunderland, Mass, 1989.

Badcock C R: *Evolution and Individual Behavior: Introduction to Human Sociobiology.* Blackwell, Cambridge, MA, 1991.

Bailey K G: *Human Paleopsychology: Applications to Aggression and Pathological Processes.* Erlbaum, Hillsdale, NJ, 1987.

Barkow J H: *Darwin, Sex and Status: Biological Approaches to Mind and Culture.* University of Toronto Press, 1989.

Bickerton D: *Language and Species.* University of Chicago Press, Chicago, 1990.

Birtchnell J: *How Humans Relate: A New Interpersonal Theory.* Praeger, Westport, CT, 1993.

Brandon R N, Burian R M, editors: *Genes, Organisms, Populations: Controversies over the Units of Selection.* MIT Press, Cambridge, MA, 1984.

Calvin W H: *The Ascent of Mind: Ice Age Climates and the Evolution of Intelligence.* Bantam, New York, 1990.

*Chance M R A, editor: *Social Fabrics of the Mind.* Erlbaum, Hillsdale, NJ, 1988.

Corballis M C: *The Lopsided Ape: Evolution of the Generative Mind.* Oxford University Press, New York, 1991.

Crick F: *What Mad Pursuit: A Personal View of Scientific Discovery.* Basic Books, New York, 1988.

Daly M, Wilson M: *Homicide.* Aldine de Gruyter, New York, 1988.

Dawkins R: *The Selfish Gene,* ed 2. Oxford University Press, New York, 1989.

deCatanzaro D: Human suicide: A biological perspective. Behav Brain Sci *3:* 265, 1980.

de Waal F: *Chimpanzee Politics: Power and Sex among Apes,* ed 2. Johns Hopkins Press, Baltimore, 1989.

Diamond J: *The Third Chimpanzee: The Evolution and Future of the Human Animal.* HarperCollins, New York, 1992.

*Donald M: *Origins of the Modern Mind: Three Stages in the Evolution of Culture and Cognition.* Harvard University Press, Cambridge, MA, 1991.

Erickson M T: Rethinking Oedipus: An evolutionary perspective of incest avoidance. Am J Psychiat *150:* 411, 1993.

Fridlund A J: Evolution and facial action in reflex, social motive, and paralanguage. Biol Psychol *32:* 3, 1991.

Fridlund A J: *Human Facial Expression: An Evolutionary View.* Academic Press, New York, 1994.

Galanter M: *Cults: Faith, Healing, and Coercion.* Oxford University Press, New York, 1989.

Gardner R: Mechanisms in manic-depressive disorder: An evolutionary model. Arch Gen Psychiatry *39:* 1436, 1982.

Gilbert P: *Human Nature and Suffering.* Erlbaum, Hillsdale, NJ, 1989.

Glantz K, Pearce J K: *Exiles from Eden: Psychotherapy from an Evolutionary Perspective.* Norton, New York, 1989.

Gould S J, Lewontin R C: The spandrels of San Marco and the Panglossian paradigm: A critique of the adaptionist programme. Proc R Soc Lond *205:* 281, 1979.

Itzkoff S W: *The Making of the Civilized Mind.* Lang, New York, 1989.

MacLean, P D: *The Triune Brain in Evolution: Role in Paleocerebral Functions.* Plenum, New York, 1990.

Magenis R E, Toth-Fejel S, Allen L J, Black M, Brown M G, Budden S, Cohen R, Friedman J M, Kalousek D, Zonana J, Lacy D, Lafranchi S, Lahe M, MacFarlane J, Williams C P S: Comparison of the 15q deletions in Prader-Willi and Angelman syndromes: Specific regions, extent of deletions, parental origin, and clinical consequences. Am J Med Genet *35:* 333, 1990.

Marks I M: *Fears, Phobias, and Rituals: Panic, Anxiety, and Their Disorders.* Oxford University Press, New York, 1987.

Masters R D: *The Nature of Politics.* Yale University Press, New Haven, CT, 1989.

Maynard Smith J: *Evolutionary Genetics.* Oxford University Press, New York, 1989.

Mayr E: *The Growth of Biological Thought: Diversity, Evolution, and Inheritance.* Harvard University Press, Cambridge, MA, 1982.

Price J S: Hypothesis: The dominance hierarchy and the evolution of mental illness. Lancet *2:* 243, 1967.

*Price J S, Sloman L, Gardner R Jr, Gilbert P, Rohde P: The social competition hypothesis of depression. Br J Psychiatry *164:* 309, 1994.

Raleigh M J, McGuire M T, Brammer G L, Pollack D B, Yuwiler A: Serotonergic mechanisms promote dominance acquisition in adult male vervet monkeys. Brain Res *559:* 181, 1991.

Reynolds V, Falgar V S E, Vine I, editors: *The Sociobiology of Ethnocentrism: Evolutionary Dimensions of Xenophobia, Discrimination, Racism and Nationalism.* University of Georgia Press, Athens, 1986.

Scott J P: *The Evolution of Social Systems.* Gordon and Breach, New York, 1989.

Shair H N, Barr G A, Hofer M A: *Developmental Psychobiology: New Methods and Changing Concepts.* Oxford University Press, New York, 1991.

Simon H A: A mechanism for social selection and successful altruism. Science *250:* 1665, 1990.

Slavin M O, Kriegman D: *The Adaptive Design of the Human Psyche: Psychoanalysis, Evolutionary Biology, and the Therapeutic Process.* Guilford, New York, 1992.

Sloman L, Gardner R, Price J: The biology of family systems and mood disorders. Fam Process *28:* 387, 1989.

*Smith C U M: Evolutionary biology and psychiatry. Br J Psychiatry *162:* 149, 1993.

Smith W J: *The Behavior of Communicating: An Ethological Approach.* Harvard University Press, Cambridge, MA, 1977.

Smuts B B, Cheney D L, Seyfarth R M, Wrangham R W, Struhsaker T T: *Primate Societies.* University of Chicago Press, Chicago, 1987.

Trivers R: *Social Evolution.* Benjamin-Cummings, Menlo Park, CA, 1985.

Wenegrat B: *Sociobiological Psychiatry: A New Conceptual Framework.* Lexington Press, Lexington, MA, 1990.

Wenegrat B: *Sociobiology and Mental Disorder: A New View.* Addison-Wesley, Menlo Park, CA, 1984.

Williams G C: *Adaptation and Natural Selection.* Princeton University Press, Princeton, NJ, 1966.

Williams G C, Nesse R M: The dawn of Darwinian medicine. Q Rev Biol *66:* 1, 1991.

*Wilson D S: Evolutionary epidemiology: Darwinian theory in the service of medicine and psychiatry. Acta Biotheoretica *41:* 205, 1993.

Wilson E O: *Sociobiology: The New Synthesis.* Harvard University Press, Cambridge, MA, 1975.

CHAPTER 5 QUANTITATIVE AND EXPERIMENTAL METHODS IN PSYCHIATRY

5.1 EPIDEMIOLOGY

DARREL A. REGIER, M.D., M.P.H.
JACK D. BURKE, JR., M.D., M.P.H.

INTRODUCTION

Psychiatric epidemiology has begun to demonstrate its value to clinicians, researchers, and policymakers. Recent findings provide new understanding of the course and co-occurrence of psychiatric disorders, measure the impairment in functioning they cause, establish a basis for policy decisions on mental health, and set a starting point for analyzing access to care and use of mental health services. Advances in epidemiological methods have created opportunities to integrate epidemiological findings with clinical research and have pushed clinical research methods to new sophistication.

Nevertheless, one principal goal in epidemiology, to find ways to lessen the occurrence of new illnesses, still eludes investigators. Progress in prevention depends on continuing evolution of methods and an even closer tie to findings in basic and clinical research on mental disorders.

DEFINITION

Mental disorder epidemiology is the quantitative study of the distribution and causes of mental disorder in human populations. The definition has several important components.

POPULATION FOCUS Population groups, rather than individuals, are the basic focus of research. Although individuals within population groups must be accurately diagnosed, the scientific questions addressed by epidemiology begin with descriptions of how mental disorders are distributed across different population subgroups.

QUANTITATIVE METHODS Because of its focus on the health status of population groups, epidemiology is often referred to as the basic science of public health. Higher than average disease rates in population groups are referred to as epidemics, from the Greek *epi* (upon) and *deme* (the people). Although there are many clinical, journalistic, and political ways of describing the impact of an illness on a population, it is the province of epidemiology to provide a quantitative assessment of the frequency with which illnesses affect different segments of the population at different points in time. Quantitative statistical methods are the means by which differences in the frequency of disorders in population groups are assessed.

CORRELATES Pathological states are not randomly distributed in the population, but rather are differentially associated with physical, biological, social, and temporal characteristics of human beings and their environment. Epidemiologists seek to discover characteristic factors that may define populations with excessively high rates of a mental disorder. That approach is used initially to narrow the range of characteristics associated with a disorder and ultimately to identify characteristic risk factors that, if altered, would interrupt a causal network producing a disorder.

SPECIAL FEATURES Despite efforts in the past 30 years, both in the United States and abroad, progress in psychiatric epidemiology has been slow because of several methodological problems that are just now being overcome.

Nosology The relative quiescence of epidemiological mental health research over the past generation may be attributed in part to limits on the state of the art in the clinical research field of nosology. The grouping of morbidity states for quantitative analysis requires that classification of disorders be explicit and reliably applied across large populations. If mixed conditions are included under one diagnostic category, risk factors associated with one of the component disorders will have their statistical association diluted and, thus, fail to be recognized by the epidemiological method.

A limiting factor in psychiatric nosology has been the heavy reliance on manifestational criteria (such as signs, symptoms, clinical course, and treatment response manifestations) as opposed to causal criteria (such as toxins, trauma, and metabolic defects). Dependence on manifestational criteria in the absence of convincing causal factors increases the likelihood that heterogeneous groups may be combined in one diagnosis. The problem is shared by the rest of clinical medicine, which attempts to move beyond a diagnosis based on symptoms such as fever to a specific etiological agent or anatomical defect. The new descriptive approach to psychiatric nosology has been an important intermediate stage that will facilitate more rigorous investigations of causal factors in clinical and epidemiological studies.

Case identification methods Without clearly defined nosological categories, it has been difficult both to define a case and to develop case-identification (diagnostic) techniques that are appropriate for large-scale population studies. Such techniques require explicit criteria if clear communication to other researchers and reliability in administration are to be feasible. In the absence of reliable assessment methods, epidemiologists have often used self-report questionnaires that assess the dimensions of psychological and psychophysiological symptoms. Cutoff scores on various symptom scales have been calibrated with symptom profiles of patients under treatment. Thus, persons in the general population could be assessed in terms of their probability of having disorders similar to those seen in clinical settings. The absence of face validity of many such questionnaires, the lack of diagnostic specificity, and the tautological assumption that mental disorders under treatment should define the full spectrum of all types of mental disorder led to clinician apathy about epidemiological survey results. Recently, however, standardized clinical interview methods have been adapted for use in epidemiological surveys—a development that has brought advances in psychiatric epidemiology.

Risk factors At a more advanced level of investigation, another difficulty has been to determine what psychosocial and biological factors are likely candidates for identifying high-risk groups for particular psychiatric disorders. Once identified, those factors must also be measured in objective ways as part of an epidemiological study.

The relative paucity of clearly defined and modifiable risk factors available for study has led to overdependence on associations with descriptive and relatively unmodifiable factors, such as age, sex, and ethnic status. Although presumably modifiable factors (such as stressful life events) have recently emerged, the multifactorial interaction between individual susceptibility and stress has not been fully explicated.

Chronic disease epidemiology paradigm Other difficulties in psychiatric epidemiology are common to the pursuit of the epidemiology of chronic medical diseases. Those difficulties primarily have to do with the time-disease relation and include incomplete information on the temporal aspects of the clinical course, uncertainty about the time at which causative factors may have affected the individual, an undefined lag time between the onset of a pathogenic influence and the occurrence of a disorder, and the absence of any generally accepted concept as to when a disorder may be considered to be eradicated in a patient with a history of the illness. Although those are not problem areas in all mental disorders, they are common to cancer, cardiovascular disease, and rheumatological disease epidemiology.

USES OF EPIDEMIOLOGY

There are three levels of epidemiological investigation. Those levels are defined according to their basic intent as follows:

1. Descriptive—studies that produce basic estimates of the rates of disorder in a general population and its subgroups.
2. Analytical—studies that explore the basis of variations in illness rates among different groups in order to identify risk factors that may contribute to the development of a disorder.
3. Experimental—studies that test the presumed association between a risk factor and a disorder and that seek to reduce the occurrence of illness by controlling the risk factor.

At each level of investigation, information is obtained that can be used to improve clinical practice and to plan public health policies. As past difficulties with nosology, case-identification techniques, risk-factor specification, and chronic disease paradigms have been addressed, it has been possible to realize more fully the seven basic applications of epidemiology identified by J. N. Morris. Those basic uses are discussed below in relation to the three stages of epidemiological inquiry—descriptive, analytical, and experimental—to demonstrate the important applications of epidemiological knowledge, even in the earliest studies at the descriptive level of investigation.

DESCRIPTIVE LEVEL

1. Community diagnosis The starting point for epidemiological research is to estimate rates of illness in a defined population. Community diagnosis provides a baseline for understanding the burden of illness in a population, the mix of disorders present, and the proportion of untreated cases in the population. Those basic rates are needed before more elaborate studies of risk factors can be undertaken, and they are important for health planners who want to know what kind of treatment services may be needed in the community, especially if untreated cases are to be brought into the health care system.

When the President's Commission on Mental Health examined mental health issues in the United States in the late 1970s, two fundamental questions that were addressed were the extent of mental illness in the population and the role of health services in providing treatment to persons with mental disorders. Because of previous difficulties in obtaining valid estimates for those figures, the figures were derived from a synthesis of information from a variety of studies. With that method it was estimated that about 15 percent of the United States population could be diagnosed as having a mental disorder in one year. More recent estimates have shown a higher rate of 22 percent in one year, which increases to 28 percent if the addictive disorders are added. However, about 15 percent of the population actually receives some mental or addictive disorder services in the course of a year.

2. Completing the clinical picture More precise rates of illness in a community can be obtained only if a standardized assessment procedure is used to ascertain the diagnostic status of the large number of persons sampled in a study. If the case ascertainment is done well, then epidemiological studies will improve clinical understanding and benefit the field of public health. The full clinical picture of a disorder can be studied by characterizing subclinical or mild cases, by studying relatives to determine the familial occurrence of the condition, and by following the progression of the illness to determine its course and prognosis. The value of that effort rests on the fundamental rule of epidemiology, which is to sample individuals from a geographically defined population without the bias that may rise if a sample is drawn only from patients seen in particular treatment settings. For example, with the new classification of schizophrenic and related disorders in the fourth edition of *Diagnostic and Statistical Manual of Mental Disorders* (DSM-IV), it is important to determine the associated features for each condition, the prognosis, and the course of the illness in longitudinal studies.

3. Identification of syndromes Similarly, it may be that some conditions occur in a population sample that have not previously been recognized in clinical populations. The opportunity to identify new syndromes in the population is provided both by representative sampling of the population and by the application of thorough, standardized assessment procedures to all individuals in a sample. One example is agoraphobia without history of panic disorder, which appears to occur more commonly in the general population than in clinical samples.

ANALYTICAL LEVEL

4. Assessing individual risks Once the basic rates of illness are established, it is possible to identify groups in the population with unusually high rates of illness. Such a comparative analysis provides a variety of hypotheses for testing to see if some characteristics of the more commonly affected group can be linked to a causal chain for the illness. An example is the finding by psychiatric epidemiologists in the 1930s that rates of schizophrenia appeared to be higher among low-income, inner-city residents. The first problem in assessing such a finding is to determine whether it reflects a potentially higher risk of developing schizophrenia among those who live in such conditions, or whether those who have schizophrenia move into such areas through downward social mobility. That question still awaits a definitive resolution.

Even if place of residence seems to be an antecedent characteristic rather than a consequence of the disorder, it is still necessary for investigators to pursue the study of possible risk factors that may underlie the apparent association between the group characteristic and the disorder. It may be that particular features of poverty, poor housing, or population density are risk factors, or that genetic, nutritional, or other familial risks are higher in people who live in such areas, or that toxic or infectious agents are the true contributors and occur more commonly in such areas.

Moving from the demonstration of higher rates in a particular group to more targeted studies of putative risk factors for individuals is an essential but difficult step in the progression of epidemiological investigations.

5. Historical study Identification of risk factors may be made easier if some historical variation can be shown. That type of evidence may help strengthen the arguments for studying one or another putative risk factor. For example, to judge from a 25-year study of one community population in Sweden, depression may be increasing and dementia may be decreasing in an industrialized Western society. Other epidemiological studies have shown that depression and drug abuse and dependency may be occurring at higher rates and with earlier onset in more recent generations.

EXPERIMENTAL LEVEL

6. Identifying causes As risk factors are demonstrated, epidemiologists can help reduce contributors to a disorder by intervening in the causal chain that links a risk factor to the occurrence of the disorder. Studies undertaken to modify a risk factor and to assess the impact of that intervention in reducing the onset of illness are the long-term goals of epidemiologists. That type of investigation promises to elucidate opportunities for the primary prevention of mental disorders by intervening to reduce the chances that high-risk individuals will develop an illness. A quantitative, population-based method of epidemiological investigation can be used to measure the impact of preventive interventions being tested. Such assessment is important both to determine the benefits of the intervention for high-risk individuals and to assess the magnitude of any unintended negative effects of the program.

7. Working of health services Although the epidemiological method is usually taken as a guide to the primary prevention of disorders, it can also be used for secondary prevention, early diagnosis, and prompt, effective treatment of persons who have already developed signs of the illness. Thus, in the broader perspective epidemiological methods can also be applied to clinical populations and to general populations in the community.

Just as epidemiological findings can assist primary prevention efforts through assessment and reduction of risk factors, so they can be used for secondary prevention. Once the prevalence of clinical disorders is determined, as has been done for depression among primary care patients, it is possible to assess the extent of early diagnosis and prompt, effective treatment. Despite the common occurrence of depressive disorders in primary care patients, recent studies in the United States and abroad have suggested that those disorders are not often diagnosed or treated.

Interventions to improve clinical practice through secondary prevention can be tested, just as primary prevention and intervention efforts are tested. Epidemiological research applied to clinical populations is known as clinical services research.

EPIDEMIOLOGICAL METHODS

Epidemiology has several important characteristics, including a population-centered research strategy that requires an adequate sampling plan. Especially in psychiatry, epidemiological research had to await advances in the nosology of mental disorders before acceptable case-identification instruments could be developed. With those prerequisites met, quantitative research in psychiatric epidemiology has become possible. The following discussion reviews sampling methods, how to evaluate the validity of case-assessment instruments, and basic measures used in estimating rates of disorder, measuring associations of risk factors with disorders, and determining the effectiveness of experimental interventions.

SAMPLING One of the most powerful features of the epidemiological method is that two desirable conditions about the sample of people under study can be met: A suitable reference population or universe can be defined, and persons in the study can be related to that defined universe in a specified way. If those conditions are satisfied, the results of the study can be generalized to the universe.

In the present discussion the universe is the hypothetical population to which study results will be generalized and the study population is the operational equivalent of the universe that will actually be studied by the investigator. For example, a universe may be all residents of a delimited area, but a study population may consist of customers of a local electric utility. The study population should be as equivalent to the specific universe as possible.

Once the study population has been defined and judged equivalent to the universe, its members can be assessed to determine their risk or illness status. All members of the study population can be assessed in a total count if money, time, and other resources are adequate. Usually, though, it is necessary to select a few representative members of the study population to form the study sample.

Sampling design The fundamental principle of sampling is to select subjects in such a way that the sample results will be representative of the entire study population and ensure equivalence to the intended universe. To ensure that the sample does represent the entire study population, the members of the study sample must be selected without bias and with a known probability of selection. The basic case is the simple random sample. All members of the study population are rostered and a sample is selected randomly.

Sample selection Consider, for example, a study population of 3,000 persons who can be listed individually. The investigator plans to examine 300 subjects, a 10 percent sample of the study population. Using a random selection procedure, such as choosing subjects by a table of random numbers, the investigator can select, on the average, one in every 10 persons to be in the study. In simple random samples, every member of the population has an equal and known probability of being selected for the sample, in this case a one in 10 chance. With large numbers chosen, random selection tends to produce a sample that in the aggregate reflects the composition of the study population. In the above example, if the distribution of females in the 3,000 population members is 60 percent, it will be roughly the same in the sample. The larger the total number of persons chosen for the sample, the more likely it is that all the characteristics in the study population will be reflected accurately in the study sample.

Sample size The drive to reproduce overall population characteristics in the sample by random selection is one reason why large sample sizes are desirable. Another reason is that estimates of rates or other statistics are more precise when a large number of persons are used as the basis for estimation.

Point estimate Study sample A, drawn by the investigator as described above, is not the only one that could be drawn from the study population. With a different starting point in the table of random numbers, a different series of 300 individuals would be selected for the study sample; this second sample can be called B. Its composition would also reflect, roughly, the characteristics of the overall population of 3,000. The proportion of females in sample B would also be about 60 percent, but it probably would not be exactly the same proportion as was calculated for sample A. If the investigator drew repeated samples and continued to calculate the proportion of females in each sample, the various sample estimates of the proportion of females in the overall population would form a range of values tending to center on the true population value of 60 percent. The estimate produced from a sample is called point estimate of the proportion of females in the study population.

Standard error Although repeated sampling of 300 individuals from a total population of 3,000 can be easily described, it is almost never feasible in a world of limited time, money, and researchers. If the first sample was drawn at random, it is possible to calculate a statistic, the standard error of the proportion, that describes how much variation exists in a large series of repeated samples, each one composed of 300 subjects, that could theoretically be selected from a given population. With the standard error, which is easily calculated using data from one sample, it is possible to calculate the range of values that allows investigators to say that they are 95 percent confident that the true proportion of females lies between those estimates. That range is known as the 95 percent confidence interval, and it is customary for investigators to report the range along with the point estimates of characteristics they have assessed in their samples. Larger numbers of individuals permit more stable point estimates, and the confidence interval is correspondingly smaller than it would be with fewer subjects in the sample.

Confidence interval uses Confidence intervals are helpful in comparing rates of illness. Suppose that in the sample of 300 subjects the investigator assessed the presence of major depressive disorder and wanted to compare rates for all high school graduates with those who have less education. The point estimates may look different—for example, 3.0 percent for graduates and 9.5 percent for nongraduates. A valid comparison requires a consideration of how rough those point estimates may be in terms of the true population-based rates of illness.

Calculating 95 percent confidence intervals helps the investigator determine if the apparent difference in rates is due to the roughness of the point estimates or to a true difference. With such a small sample the confidence intervals may be large, say 0.3 to 5.7 percent for graduates and 4.8 to 14.2 percent for nongraduates; there is an overlap, so the differences may be due to variability of point estimates associated with sampling from the population. Because the 95 percent confidence intervals are large enough to overlap, it may not be possible to say that the difference in point estimates of 3.0 percent and 9.5 percent is a real one. When confidence intervals overlap, a definitive comparison of point estimates can be made by a statistical test, such as the χ^2 test. Larger numbers of subjects in the sample lead to smaller confidence intervals around point estimates, so there is a premium placed on having enough subjects. Statistical power analysis allows investigators to plan their studies so that they can be sure of a reasonable chance of having enough subjects to support confidence intervals that are smaller than the anticipated differences in the most important rates that will be compared.

Stratified sampling In many cases simple random sampling is not useful. In the example being considered, suppose that the investigator wanted to look at subgroups—for example, college graduates—that occurred in the population much less commonly than high school graduates and nongraduates. Rather than collapsing the college graduates into a category with all who finished high school, the investigator may want to be sure that the study sample includes enough subjects who are college graduates. With the equal probability of selection entailed in simple random sampling, college graduates would only be as common in the sample as they were in study population.

A more complicated approach to sampling would be to roster the 3,000 individuals in three separate groups or strata, rather than in a single listing, and then to sample each stratum separately. The investigator could decide to have 100 subjects from each educational stratum. If the study population contained 1,500 individuals who were nongraduates, the probability of selecting any one of them for the study would be 100 ÷ 1,500, or about 0.07. If the college graduates numbered only 500, the probability of selection would be 100 ÷ 500, or 0.20.

That type of sampling is called stratified random sampling, and it requires slightly more complex statistical techniques than simple random sampling to calculate point estimates and confidence intervals for proportions. In stratified random sampling, each subject is weighted according to the selection probability; estimates can be obtained for specific strata as well as for the total study population.

Cluster sampling One problem with simple and stratified random sampling is that individuals in the study population must be listed in order to be sampled. Listing all potential subjects may be possible for small populations whose members can be identified, such as patients seen in a clinical setting, but it is usually not possible or economical for large populations, especially of community residents. An alternative is to use lists of groups or clusters of individuals. The only roster of units that can be sampled in a community may be a list of census tracts or a map of city blocks. Once a sample is chosen, all the households within the selected block can be listed, and a sample of households can be selected. After the households are chosen, individuals who live there can be entered into the study. Cluster sampling is often the only feasible method, because lists of individuals in a population cannot always be obtained, and it is more efficient than simple or stratified random sampling of individuals in enrolling a large sample. It produces less precise estimates, however, and therefore larger confidence intervals.

In studies of the total population, cluster sampling can become complicated. Clusters can be selected from several different types of strata—households and institutions, urban and rural—and some individuals, such as the elderly or children, can be sampled at higher rates. In such cases the calculation of selection probabilities and the associated efforts to produce confidence intervals and more sophisticated statistical comparisons become complex.

NOSOLOGY Before acceptable case-identification instruments can be developed in epidemiology, it is necessary to write diagnostic criteria that can be unambiguously interpreted. Once explicit diagnostic criteria for each disorder are available, it is possible to create examination protocols based on such statements. Proposed sets of explicit criteria for psychiatric diagnoses were first published in the 1970s with the St. Louis research criteria and the Research Diagnostic Criteria (RDC). In 1980 the third edition of DSM (DSM-III) adopted the approach of writing explicit criteria to use as the basis for clinical practice and for epidemiological and other research; that approach proved useful for researchers and clinicians and has been continued in DSM-IV.

CASE ASSESSMENT Information about a subject can be collected in several ways. Medical records often are used for patients seen in clinical settings; they provide essential documentation about prior course of the illness, other disorders or preexisting risks, and the type and course of the treatment provided. In some studies the diagnoses listed in the medical records are used to identify cases of rare disorders.

Records in central data banks can be important for identifying very rare disorders and for studying patterns of treatment in a defined area. Case registers are now maintained on a national basis for specific types of cancer. They provide a roster of patients with the disorder and information that can be used to test hypotheses about risk factors or other features of the illness. For more common disorders, geographically based case registers provide a longitudinal record of all persons in the population who received treatment for the disorder. For two decades a register of all patients seen in mental health treatment facilities in Monroe County, New York, has been used to describe population treatment patterns in an urban community. A similar register was also maintained through the late 1970s for the state of Maryland.

The most important source of information about a subject in the study is often the direct interview or examination of the individual. Until the late 1970s, the major obstacle in psychiatric epidemiology was the lack of an acceptable case-assessment instrument to identify persons with mental disorders that could be used in studies of the total area population.

CRITERIA FOR ASSESSMENT INSTRUMENT Several criteria must be satisfied by an assessment instrument before it can be used successfully in studies of human subjects.

Safety The assessment of subjects should not cause them harm. If risks do exist, the benefits of the study must outweigh the potential harm. Anyone participating in such a study must do so voluntarily after being informed of the nature and extent of potential risks, and must be able to withdraw at any time. Those requirements are enforced by institutional review boards for the protection of human subjects at an investigator's institution. At present, there is no reason to believe that participating in epidemiological studies that include a diagnostic psychiatric interview harms either adults or children.

Feasibility With research funds becoming more limited, it has been increasingly important to develop assessment procedures that yield adequate information about large numbers of subjects without being unduly time-consuming, burdensome for subjects, or dependent on a highly skilled examiner whose services are expensive. For population surveys that assess large samples, it has become prohibitively expensive to use highly trained mental health clinicians to perform psychiatric interviews. Alternatives were needed before such major studies could begin.

Reliability An important psychometric property of assessment instruments is reliability. *Reliability* usually refers to an instrument's capacity to give consistent results when used by different examiners or at different times.

Validity An instrument that has acceptable levels of interrater (defined below) and test-retest reliability can be assessed to determine if it is measuring what it intends to measure. That property is called *validity.*

Reliability and validity are so important that a more extensive discussion of their role in evaluating case-identification instruments is provided.

Reliability An instrument's property of yielding equivalent results when used by different examiners on the same subject is known as interrater reliability. The property of producing equivalent results when used on the same subject on different occasions is called test-retest reliability. Although those two properties are necessary, they are not sufficient for an instrument; for example, at least hypothetically a diagnostic instrument could show high interrater and test-retest reliability but could give consistently wrong results. Accuracy would be attenuated without consistency, however, so demonstration of acceptable reliability is usually required of any assessment instrument proposed for use in an epidemiological study before the study begins. Several measures of reliability are available; to a large extent, choice of the proper measure depends on the type of information the assessment instrument uses. In the simplest case, consider an interrater reliability pretest of a diagnostic interview that used two examiners to assess the presence or absence of a disorder in a series of 100 individuals. A two-way table can be used to summarize the results from the two interviewers.

Proportion of Subjects Classified by Two Raters

		Examiner A		
		Present	Absent	Total
Examiner B	Present	$a = 0.07$	$b = 0.08$	$B_1 = 0.15$
	Absent	$c = 0.11$	$d = 0.74$	$B_2 = 0.85$
		$A_1 = 0.18$	$A_2 = 0.82$	1.00

Po= proportion of agreement observed $= a + d = 0.81$.
Pc= proportion of agreement by chance $=$
$A_1 \times B_1 + A_2 \times B_2 = 0.724$.
$\kappa = (Po - Pc) / (1 - Pc) =$
$(0.81 - 0.724) / (1 - 0.724) = 0.31$.

A simple measure of agreement for dichotomous data—presence versus absence, for example—is the proportion of observed agreement, or the percentage of patients in whom the two examiners agreed that the disorder was present or absent. In the instance illustrated in the table, the results indicate 81 percent agreement; however, the measure is not recommended.

When two judgments are compared, there is some probability of agreement through chance alone, without regard to how consistent the interview may be. To adjust for the potential contribution of chance agreements, a better measure of agreement is kappa (κ). Calculation of κ as shown in the Table yields a value of 0.31. Another advantage of κ is that its confidence interval can be calculated for a determination of how stable the point estimate is of the true value of κ.

The κ statistic can be used to measure agreement between the raters at different levels of information. Judgments about any disorder considered in the interview, about just one of the specific disorders, as in the example, or about an individual item for a specific disorder can be described using κ. As the levels become broader, the reliability is likely to improve, because there are more ways to qualify as having any disorder than there are ways to qualify as having an individual symptom. An important characteristic of κ is that its value depends on how common the particular condition is in the study sample. For less common disorders with a frequency below 5 percent, the value of κ will be so low in most cases that some investigators suggest not calculating it for those conditions.

For data that are expressed as ratings on an ordinal scale, other statistical measures are appropriate, including an intraclass correlation coefficient using analysis of variance techniques. κ can also be calculated for complex situations like shifting numbers of multiple examiners and when some items are weighted in importance.

Acceptable reliability has become an expected feature of psychiatric assessment instruments, especially diagnostic interviews, because substantial research has demonstrated that routine clinical diagnoses are not reliable. The classic demonstration of that inconsistency occurred in the United States-United Kingdom Diagnostic Project, which showed that psychiatrists in New York and London used the same diagnostic terms in widely varying ways, both for their own patients and for patients interviewed on videotape and shown to both groups. That study led to the development of standardized interview schedules that were designed to reduce the most important sources of inconsistency in diagnostic assessments. Those sources of inconsistency included the following:

1. Information variance—examiners collect different types of information about patients.
2. Observation variance—examiners interpret the subject's answers and nonverbal behavior in different ways.
3. Criterion variance—examiners evaluate information about the subject according to different diagnostic rules.

The development of standardized interviews has reduced, but not eliminated, those sources of inconsistency. Two other sources of variance remain: (1) subject variance—the subject has different conditions at different times, and (2) occasion variance—the subject is in different stages of the same condition at different times, or at least reports different information about it.

Validity Reliability is assessed by comparing agreement between examiners or between examinations. Validity testing requires a demonstration that the test results are accurate, ideally by comparison with a well-known standard of truth. In a new field that uses descriptive criteria for diagnosis and that has just begun developing standardized instruments because clinical examinations have been shown to be unreliable, there is no reference standard to use as an absolute measure of truth in diagnostic assessment. In practice, the choice of an acceptable criterion instrument to use as a standard of comparison in validity testing of a new diagnostic instrument is one of the most difficult aspects of the study.

A simple validity study would involve administration of the test instrument and, independently, of the criterion instrument to each subject, with the order of administration changed randomly to be sure that one instrument does not influence the results of the other. Different statistical measures are calculated to measure validity than are used for reliability. In reliability tests, no assumptions are made that one examiner is more likely than the other to obtain the true answer, so a simple comparison of their agreement is made. In validity testing, however, the criterion instrument is assumed to produce the truth, and the measures calculated are designed to indicate how well results from the new instrument being tested match the results from the criterion instrument. A two-way table is constructed, as shown:

		Truth (Criterion Instrument Results)		
		Disorder Present	Disorder Absent	Total
New Instrument	Disorder present	$a = 35$	$b = 8$	$a + b = 43$
	Disorder absent	$c = 5$	$d = 52$	$c + d = 57$
		$a + c = 40$	$b + d = 60$	100

$$\text{Sensitivity} = \frac{a}{a+c} = \frac{35}{40} = 0.875$$

$$\text{False-negative rate} = \frac{c}{a+c} = \frac{5}{40} = 0.125$$

$$\text{Specificity} = \frac{d}{b+d} = \frac{52}{60} = 0.87$$

$$\text{False-positive rate} = \frac{b}{b+d} = \frac{8}{60} = 0.13$$

Sensitivity is a measure of the new instrument's ability to detect the true cases of disorder identified by the criterion instrument. The false-negative rate is the proportion of true cases missed by the new instrument.

Specificity is a measure of the new instrument's ability to identify the true noncases identified by the criterion instrument. The false-positive rate is most commonly measured as the proportion of true noncases mistakenly identified as cases by the new instrument.

Those measures allow basic judgments to be made about the new instrument's ability to identify cases that it is designed to identify. Higher values of sensitivity and specificity are always desirable. For a given instrument, there are trade-offs between those two values. The only way to improve both sensitivity and specificity without a trade-off is to improve the instrument itself.

Another useful measure related to validity is the proportion of apparent cases, as detected by the new instrument, that are true cases as determined by the criterion measure. That proportion is the *positive predictive value.* Of the 43 apparent cases in the example, only 35 were true cases, so the positive predictive value = 35/43 = 0.814. The positive predictive value is affected by the base rate, so it is especially difficult for diagnostic tests to achieve a high positive predictive value with rare disorders.

CRITERION VALIDITY All of the measures discussed so far are based on a type of validity known as criterion validity, because results of the test instrument are compared with results of a similar but presumably more accurate instrument. If the new instrument had been compared with a criterion that would be administered at some point in the future, the method would have been predictive criterion validity.

FACE VALIDITY Other types of validity besides use of a criterion have been described. The simplest is face validity, which refers to a judgment that the new instrument makes sense to an investigator. Standards for face validity usually are not clear; however, face validity does have some usefulness in increasing acceptability by clinicians and subjects of a new and otherwise unusual instrument.

CONTENT VALIDITY Content validity refers to a systematic examination of the new instrument by an expert to ensure that its items cover the types of information that will be needed for later interpretation and scoring of the examination. Verification of content validity is especially important for such instruments as standardized diagnostic interviews that are intended to collect information to be used with a set of explicit diagnostic criteria.

PROCEDURAL VALIDITY Procedural validity has recently been introduced to refer to tests of whether a particular type of examiner (such as nonclinician) can use the new instrument and achieve the same results as a skilled examiner (such as a research psychiatrist). Because the concept of procedural validity involves both a comparison between examiners, as in reliability testing, and a comparison with a criterion, as in criterion validity testing, investigators have reported both κ and sensitivity-specificity measures for those studies.

CONSTRUCT VALIDITY The most important concept of validity is construct validity, which refers to the demonstration that the thing being measured exists in a way that the instrument designed to measure it assumes it does. Establishing construct validity for a mental disorder is a difficult problem for research. The concept of construct validity is described later.

Ideally, safety, feasibility, reliability, and validity are examined before an instrument is used to assess subjects in an epidemiological study. In practice, the difficulty in picking a criterion instrument with its own validity already established means that only the first three properties—safety, feasibility, and reliability—can be well studied for psychiatric assessment instruments. In an effort to establish at least minimum standards for new instruments, the instruments can be assessed for content and procedural validity, and comparison with other similar instruments can be made. Although those other instruments cannot be used as legitimate criterion instruments, they can provide useful comparisons if they have met the same standards, including reliability and content validity, as the new instrument being studied.

DESCRIPTIVE STUDIES Once an appropriate sampling plan and acceptable assessment instruments are available, epidemiological investigations can begin to explore the distribution of disorders in the population. For rare disorders a total area population survey may be unrewarding, but for most psychiatric illnesses the starting point is an area survey to determine basic measures of frequency of the illness.

In epidemiological studies, which emphasize careful sampling to produce results that can be extended to the universe of interest, the results based on number of cases of a disorder are expressed not in raw numbers but in terms of population rates. In general those rates are proportions that require both a numerator, the number of cases, and a denominator, the total number in the population, including cases and noncases.

$$\text{Rate} = \frac{\text{Cases in the population}}{\text{Total population (includes cases and noncases)}}$$

The rate is therefore a proportion, a fraction that includes cases in both the numerator and the denominator. Some writers reserve the term "rate" to refer to an instantaneous change and express it using methods of calculus. To simplify that concept, the term "average rate" can be used for measures that involve rates over specified time periods.

Point prevalence Most surveys in psychiatric epidemiology have examined the prevalence of disease in the population. The term "prevalence" encompasses several types of rates but always refers to cases who have the disorder at a specified time, regardless of how long ago the disorder started. The basic measure is the point prevalence rate, which refers to the proportion of individuals in the population who have the disorder at a specified point in time. That point can be a day on the calendar, such as April 1, 1990, as in the national census, or it can be a point defined in relation to the study assessment, such as the day of interview, regardless of the calendar date.

$$\text{Point prevalence rate} = \frac{\text{Cases at } t_o}{\text{Population at } t_o}$$

Although a day is often taken as the definition of a point in time, the use of diagnostic criteria that require multiple symptoms to cluster, with a minimum duration of symptoms, has sometimes led to extension of the point measure back in time to refer to the previous week or previous month. Expanding the concept of point to include a period more than one month before the interview is not advisable because it can lead to confusion and raises methodological problems, which are discussed later in relation to lifetime prevalence.

To establish a point prevalence rate for depression, an investigator might sample the residents of a defined area, administer an assessment instrument that detects a current depressive illness at that time, and calculate the rate as the proportion of the sample with current depression. Because such a study would likely take several weeks or months to conduct, if the sample size is large, the rate would probably be based on a point that is the time of interview, rather than asking subjects to report their symptoms retrospectively from the starting date of the field survey. (Unless a simple random sample was chosen, the investigator would also need to weight the sample results to reflect the overall population figures according to an individual's probability of selection.)

Incidence In epidemiological research incidence also has a specific meaning. It refers to a rate that includes only new cases of illness that started within a clearly defined time period. The most common time period is one year; thus, the annual incidence rate is the usual rate reported. A study of incident cases is more difficult than a study of prevalent cases. A careful study of incidence requires at least two examinations of each person in the sample, at the start and again at the end of the designated time period. The initial assessment is needed to determine which members of the sample already have the disease; they are not eligible to become new cases because they already have the illness, so they are omitted from the numerator of new cases counted at the end of the study. They are also excluded from the denominator because they are not part of the population considered at risk of developing a new case of the disorder. At the start of the study the numerator is set to zero; at the end of the study those individuals who have developed the illness are counted as cases. If on the second examination the assessment instrument is unable to provide retrospective coverage of the entire time period being used, such as one year, it would be necessary to resurvey the population at risk more often than just at the end of the period.

For some disorders that are characterized by recurrent episodes it is useful to use an incidence figure that includes both first and later episodes of illness (for example, a second episode of major depressive disorder). A broader concept of total incidence includes those with a new episode of illness, regardless of whether there have been previous episodes.

An alternative way to study incidence is to conduct a single examination of subjects, as if it were the end of the time period chosen for study, and to ask them to recall their disease status at the beginning of the time period. Besides problems of recall, the simpler design has the problem of systematically omitting some categories of new cases, including the cases of persons who died during the time period and cannot be sampled and cases of persons who left the circumscribed geographical area.

The preceding description of incidence rates is the traditional one. More precise concepts of incidence have been developed that take into account change over time and the possible loss to follow-up of persons in the at-risk population. The term "incidence density" (ID) refers to an average incidence rate over the time period of interest:

$$ID = \frac{\text{Number of incident cases in one year}}{\text{Population-time (person-years of observation)}}$$

Because some members of the at-risk population sample will develop the disease and some will drop out of the study (by moving without establishing a forwarding address, or by dying from an unrelated illness), the denominator is calculated in terms of a person-time figure, such as person-years of observation, until the individual leaves the at-risk population. That calculation depends on knowing when during the year an individual develops an illness or otherwise leaves the at-risk population. If for 1,000 people being followed, 20 are lost at the end of six months, another 100 develop disease at the end of six months, and 880 are free of disease at the end of one year, the person-time figure for observation of at-risk, disease-free individuals is $(880 \times 1 \text{ year}) + (20 \times \frac{1}{2} \text{ year}) + (100 \times \frac{1}{2} \text{ year}) = 940$ person-years, and

$$ID = \frac{100 \text{ persons}}{940 \text{ person-years}} = 0.1064 \text{ per year}$$

One advantage of the more precise approach is that in stable populations the point prevalence rate can be related in a simple way to the incidence density by the equation $P = ID \times D$, where D is the average duration of illness before termination (where termination may be death from the illness or recovery, for example). In that case a stable population is one that is stable in size and in age distribution and has constant incidence and prevalence rates.

Incidence rates are more difficult to calculate and require more extensive data collection than point prevalence rates. Point prevalence rates reflect the accumulated burden of chronic cases of very long duration, however, so incidence figures based on new cases in a specified time period are more useful in analytical studies of risk factors. Point prevalence surveys are more useful for descriptive purposes, as in portraying the frequency of illness in a community population and in relating disease frequency to potential need for services.

OTHER PREVALENCE RATES Although point prevalence and annual incidence rates are the fundamental measures used for descriptive and analytical studies in epidemiology, other types of prevalence figures have also been described and have some usefulness.

Period prevalence The period prevalence rate is used to summarize the number of cases of a disorder that exist at any time during a specified time period. Its numerator includes any existing cases at the start of the period plus any new cases that develop during the time period. For a one-year period the annual period prevalence rate is approximately equal to the point prevalence rate (existing cases ÷ population at the start) plus the annual incidence rate (new cases in a year ÷ population at risk). The period prevalence rate has less value than the separate expression of its two components, point prevalence rate and annual incidence rate. It may be useful, however, for research studies in which annual treated prevalence rates are contrasted with annual true prevalence rates.

Lifetime prevalence Lifetime prevalence rate is a measure of persons considered at a point in time who have ever had the illness under study. It may be useful to describe conditions that remit but can often recur, such as major depressive disorder. There are at least three potential problems with the lifetime prevalence rate:

1. It is almost always based on subject recall, which can be inaccurate.
2. It covers persons over the full age range represented in the study population, including many who have not yet reached the age of highest risk for onset of the disorder. It is possible to report lifetime rates separately for specific age groups. That figure may be misleading for some purposes, however, if no provision is made for the fact that persons who contracted the disease at earlier ages may have experienced different death rates than those without the disease.
3. Used in a summary way, the lifetime prevalence rate does not allow for the fact that incidence rates may have changed over the years. Therefore, different age groups may have true differences in rates that are obscured by using an overall rate and by the possible differences in mortality between those with and without the disorder.

Several alternatives to the lifetime prevalence rate, as determined from a point prevalence survey, have been described. One method uses a life table approach to estimate age-specific lifetime rates based on age-specific incidence and mortality figures. For psychiatric disorders detailed age-specific information is rarely available. Another method calculates lifetime risk by including persons in a birth cohort with and without the disorder who died or otherwise left the study population before the age designated as the cutoff. The latter method can also be used to impute probable risk for those without illness who have not yet reached the cutoff age. That approach is the most useful expression of risk, rather than actual development of illness, and is especially important for genetic studies, which must include children and deceased relatives.

Treated prevalence Treated prevalence usually refers either to a point prevalence rate or to an annual period prevalence rate that is determined by counting all residents in a defined geographical population who receive treatment for a given disorder.

Administrative prevalence A more restricted form of treated prevalence has been used for studies that include, as their population denominator, registered patients at a clinical facility rather than all area residents. The form of treated prevalence in which registered patients form the denominator population has been called administrative prevalence. It does present difficulties, because the denominator is dependent on registration status, rather than being based on those who perceive the study facility as their usual source of care, and the numerator is assumed to be all treated cases in the population, although some persons may in fact seek care elsewhere.

ANALYTICAL STUDIES Measures of disease frequency allow comparisons to be made between groups within the study sample. If one group has high rates of a disorder compared with other groups, then a search for factors that led to the higher rate of disorder can be undertaken. Many studies of disease frequency have shown that women have higher rates of major depressive disorder than men. From that consistent finding, based on group comparisons, it is possible for investigators to formulate hypotheses about what factors place women at higher risk. Whether those putative risk factors are biological or psychosocial, they can next be studied in targeted investigations to see if women with the presumed risk factor have higher rates of major depressive disorder than women without the risk factor. To make comparisons among groups, and later among groups with and without suspected risk factors, investigators have several options for study design.

Cross-sectional prevalence survey One approach to examining the apparent higher frequency of major depressive disorder among women is to conduct a sample survey of the total population in an area and calculate the point prevalence rates for men and women. Those rates could be compared, and, as an example, it may be found that women have twice the point prevalence rate of men. If the investigator examined characteristics thought to be risk factors, such as the use of oral contraceptives, it would also be possible to compare the rates among women who used that medication and those who did not.

Such a design has been used for the purpose described, but it has several drawbacks. As shown in the discussion on incidence rates, the point prevalence rate is affected both by the rate at which illness develops, as reflected in the incidence rates, and by the duration of the illness after it develops. If men and women with major depressive disorder had different average durations of illness they would also have different point prevalence rates, even with identical incidence rates; it is conceivable that the point prevalence rate for women could be twice the rate for men simply because those women who developed major depressive disorder had more chronic forms and tended to accumulate in the population. A second problem with a cross-sectional design is that it may be difficult to know whether women with the suspected risk factor, use of oral contraceptives, had been using the medication before they became ill, as would be required if there were a causal chain leading to major depressive disorder.

Incidence study and relative risk To isolate the frequency of onset from the duration of a disorder once it has developed, and to assess possible risk factors accurately, studies of incidence rates are much more useful.

The fundamental measure for comparing two groups is the relative risk (RR), a form of risk ratio:

$$\text{RR} = \frac{\text{Incidence rate in group with risk factor}}{\text{Incidence rate in group without risk factor}}$$

In terms of the usual two-way table, relative risk can be expressed as follows:

Incident Series of Cases

	New Cases	Noncases
With risk factor	a	b
Without risk factor	c	d

$$\text{RR} = \frac{a}{a+b} \div \frac{c}{c+d}$$

If the relative risk is greater than 1.0, the group with the suspected risk factor does have a higher incidence rate of the disorder. In that study design, risk factor status (for example, use of oral contraceptives) could be examined at the start of the time period for all those without the disorder; those persons could be reexamined during or at the end of the period (or both) to assess both the development of illness and the continued use of the medication.

Prospective cohort study The prospective cohort study design assesses incidence rates and risk ratios. A cohort is a group formed by sampling from a single, well-specified population, such as residents of a circumscribed area. A prospective cohort study allows extension of the study findings to the universe of interest, and as a prospective study it allows determination of risk factor status in persons with the disorder who are followed to identify newly developed cases.

Case-control study For very rare disorders, or sometimes for exploratory studies of possible risk factors, a study using identified cases rather than potential cases may be used. The design is called a case-control study. It recruits cases (persons with the disorder) already diagnosed, usually by monitoring records at clinical facilities like hospitals. That method of sampling cases assumes that everyone with the disorder is likely to present for medical attention and to be accurately diagnosed. It also assumes that all relevant facilities are monitored, or else that no differences exist in persons who stay at home or use different facilities.

One problem with the case-control study is that the universe from which cases are drawn cannot be specified, at least in customary terms, such as geographical area of residence. Another problem is that a comparison group of noncases (persons without the disorder) is not easy to specify. To compensate, often a comparison group is drawn from other patients in the same facility, and a second one is drawn from community residents in the area presumably served by the hospital. It is conceivable that either one of those comparison groups could be drawn from a different universe than the hypothesized one that is reflected in the sample of cases.

In case-control studies ascertainment of possible risk factors is usually possible only by retrospective report of the subjects unless prior documentation exists, as in medical records.

ODDS RATIO Because incidence rates cannot be calculated in such a case-control design, the typical calculation of risk ratio must be altered. Instead of a relative risk, the odds ratio is calculated for case-control studies:

	Cases	Noncases
Possible risk factor present	a	b
Possible risk factor absent	c	d

$$\text{Odds ratio} = \frac{a}{b} \div \frac{c}{d} = \frac{ad}{bc}$$

BIAS Analytical studies to assess risk factors can be flawed by three types of bias:

1. Selection bias. If a study sample is not drawn properly, it may not accurately reflect the study population; also, the study population may not be equivalent to the universe of interest. In case-control studies the selection of cases may be distorted if the clinical diagnoses used to determine eligibility are not accurate.
2. Observation bias. If the assessment instruments are invalid, information about subjects will be wrong. In case-control studies examiners who know the case or noncase status of subjects can be influenced in assessing the risk factors being studied.
3. Confounding bias. In a particular study sample some other causal factors of the disorder may be related to the risk factor being studied. That effect can often be examined and some adjustments can be made during data analysis.

Those potential flaws can affect the validity of a study's findings. A second question is whether the findings considered applicable to a particular universe also apply to other possible universes. For example, does a risk factor studied in one local community have the same association to disease in other types of communities? The answer to the second question is a matter of judgment until equally valid replications are performed.

Risk factors and causality Epidemiological data demonstrate an association between risk factors and a disorder. Because an association does not indicate causality, the desire to study human illness has led epidemiologists to consider standards of evidence that may support an interpretation of a causal connection between a risk factor and a disorder.

1. Temporality. Unless the risk factor precedes the disorder, it cannot cause the disorder. Clear demonstration of the prior occurrence of a risk factor strengthens the possibility of causality.
2. Replication. Repeated, consistent demonstration of a risk factor's relation to a disorder in multiple studies strengthens the possibility that a risk factor may be causative.
3. Magnitude of association. A large risk ratio tends to support an interpretation of causality, as does demonstration of a dose-response effect.
4. Plausibility. If a possible causal mechanism can be postulated within the framework of existing knowledge, it may lend credibility to the interpretation of a causal relation; however, in new fields where knowledge is growing, that criterion may not be so relevant.
5. Specificity. If a proposed risk factor can be associated with a single disorder and no others, that association may strengthen belief in a possible causal relation. Some factors, such as adverse life events, may lead to a variety of disorders, however, so that the failure of specificity does not discredit a potential risk factor.
6. Experimental intervention. Experiments to control a risk factor may support a causal role for the factor if the occurrence of disease is reduced; however, with such an experiment, it is possible that unintended or unknown factors may have been the true responsible agents and may have been affected by the intervention.

EXPERIMENTAL STUDIES An important goal of psychiatric epidemiology is to reduce the burden of illness. Epidemiological investigations, because they entail the study of populations, are well suited to assessing the impact of broad efforts to reduce the occurrence of illness and to reduce its duration and associated disability.

Population attributable risk For primary prevention—the effort to reduce onset of a disorder in those persons at risk for developing it—a measure of the potential impact of controlling an established risk factor is derived from the attributable risk (AR), the risk difference measure based on incidence rates (IR) for persons with and without the risk factor.

$$\text{AR} = (\text{IR with risk factor}) - (\text{IR without risk factor})$$

The proportion of cases in the group with the risk factor that may be caused by that factor is the population AR:

$$\text{Population AR} = \frac{\text{IR (total population)} - \text{IR (without)}}{\text{IR (total population)}}$$

When the more precise figures of incidence density are used, that measure has been called the etiological fraction. In some instances it may be possible to demonstrate that a protective factor has caused a lower rate of illness among those persons exposed to it; then the formula is reversed to show the preventive fraction. Studies of low dental caries rates in areas with fluoridated water provide the best example. Calculation of the etiological fraction from observational studies indicates the maximum benefit likely to occur with an intervention that is designed to reduce the pathogenic effect of the risk factor. Demonstration that an intervention has been effective rests on a controlled design, with calculation of a preventive fraction based on those persons with a risk factor who received the intervention and those with the risk factor who did not receive the intervention.

Preventive applications In addition to studies that test interventions to prevent a disorder from occurring, the method described above can be used for secondary and tertiary prevention as well. Secondary prevention is aimed at reducing the prevalence of illness by reducing its duration in those who have just developed it. Factors that tend to prolong an episode of illness can be targeted in secondary prevention efforts.

Reduction of disability produced by a disorder, or tertiary prevention, can also be assessed, even if full recovery does not occur. Tertiary prevention studies use instruments that assess the severity of illness and do not simply produce a dichotomous present-absent rating. Studies with that design are commonly used in controlled clinical trials to assess the effectiveness of new therapies to reduce duration until recovery or to reduce the severity of illness in persons who do not achieve full recovery.

Primary prevention efforts are especially difficult to study because it is not clear how to choose large groups to study, how to demonstrate that they have received the intervention, and how to ensure that no other, unplanned intervention actually produced any improvement that occurred. Even if those conditions are met, it may be difficult to demonstrate that the intervention was effective for the reasons postulated and that its costs, including any unintended negative consequences, did not overwhelm any benefits that did occur.

EPIDEMIOLOGICAL METHODS IN PSYCHIATRY

Special problems have delayed progress in psychiatric epidemiology. Although the general field of epidemiology has advanced to the point of being most concerned about such issues as controlling confounding bias in risk-factor studies and developing ways to measure the impact of preventive interventions, methodological concerns in studies of mental disorders are more basic. They have centered on difficulties in applying complex sampling techniques, in developing acceptable case-assessment instruments, and in identifying potential risk factors that merit study in large-scale investigations. The most important of those problems has been the development and application of case-assessment instruments for large-scale studies.

CASE ASSESSMENT The major obstacle to valid identification of cases in large samples of nonclinical populations has been the lack of an explicit set of criteria for diagnostic classification. Researchers who had access only to earlier systems, such as the first edition of DSM (DSM-I), were forced to rely on detailed descriptions of symptom patterns that were formulated by the investigators in order to achieve a meaningful classification of cases. During the 1960s and 1970s, the effort to use detailed specifications for disorders led to more explicit statements of empirically based criteria for specific mental disorders. Until that goal was met, with the publication of the third edition of DSM (DSM-III) and DSM-IV, investigators had only a few alternatives in selecting instruments to identify cases. The most common approach was to employ a self-report questionnaire, usually with a concentration on psychophysiological symptoms, that could yield a score based on positive answers by the subject. The scores were intended to reflect the probability that a subject had a diagnosable mental disorder, with higher scores indicating a greater likelihood. In most cases a cutoff score was calculated to separate the sample into two groups, cases and noncases. (In some studies those scales and other information were also reviewed by clinicians, who attempted to form an overall judgment about the subject's psychiatric status.)

The second major effort to develop standardized assessment instruments was to produce diagnostic interview protocols with acceptable interrater reliability. The first such instrument was the Present State Examination (PSE), an interview form that concentrates mainly on psychotic conditions and that has been used in major international studies, such as the United States-United Kingdom Diagnostic Project, the International Pilot Study of Schizophrenia, and other studies of schizophrenia supported by the World Health Organization (WHO) and the National Institute of Mental Health (NIMH). The PSE is intended for use by skilled clinicians, usually psychiatrists, who have been trained in its use; after training, the interviewers are commonly expected to participate in a pretest of any investigation to demonstrate adequate levels of interrater reliability.

The ninth edition of the PSE (PSE-9) does have drawbacks. As it is limited to coverage of the one-month period prior to interview, historical information is not obtained. The very features that generate its capacity to be used reliably—an explicit glossary of psychopathological concepts to guide examiners, and a careful computer program (CATEGO) to score the interview—may not reflect the diagnostic practices of any particular school of psychiatry; the authors of PSE-CATEGO present it as a nondiagnostic classification system that is not directly tied to any existing classification scheme. Although general outlines of the complex CATEGO algorithms have been published, detailed study by others has only recently been undertaken.

The PSE was not designed to yield diagnostic labels according to an established classification system, because the lack of explicit criteria in the early 1970s made it difficult to determine unambiguous standards for a given category. Only with the advent of formally stated, sufficiently detailed criteria for a range of psychiatric diagnoses was it possible to construct interviews that attempted to perform a diagnostic assessment and assign persons to specific categories of disorder. More recently, the PSE has been updated to reflect criteria in the revised third edition of DSM (DSM-III-R) and the 10th revision of the *International Classification of Diseases and Related Health Problems* (ICD-10) as part of the WHO- and National Institutes of Health (NIH)-sponsored Schedules for Clinical Assessment in Neuropsychiatry (SCAN). A new version of the PSE (10th edition) and of CATEGO form the core of the modular SCAN examination protocol.

When the St. Louis research criteria and the RDC were formulated in the 1970s, they were accompanied by interview schedules that investigators would use to assess subjects in a study. Those instruments were the Renard Diagnostic Interview (RDI) for the St. Louis criteria and the Schedule for Affective Disorders and Schizophrenia (SADS) for the RDC. Because those schedules required skilled clinicians to spend up to three months learning them and because epidemiological studies need a large number of such high-level interviewers, they were not used much in community surveys. An important exception was the SADS Lifetime version (SADS-L), which was used in a follow-up study of 511 community residents in New Haven. That study demonstrated that the SADS-L could be used successfully in epidemiological studies of community subjects.

Stimulated by that demonstration of feasibility and usefulness, and aware that DSM-III would adopt the approach of using operationalized criteria, as in the St. Louis and RDC systems, NIMH epidemiologists sponsored development of a fully structured interview that could be used by nonclinicians to assess a large number of subjects according to DSM-III criteria. The new instrument, the NIMH Diagnostic Interview Schedule (DIS), was based on the RDI and SADS interviews and was written by authors of those two earlier interviews. Following extensive use of the DIS in the United States and many other nations, WHO and three NIH institutes agreed to sponsor international field trials of an updated and slightly modified DIS. That instrument, the Composite International Diagnostic Interview (CIDI), has the same structural characteristics of the DIS described below, with new computer scoring programs that use ICD-10 and DSM-IV diagnostic criteria. Multiple international training sites are now available to prepare research investigators for using both the CIDI and SCAN in epidemiological and clinical research settings.

STRUCTURE OF THE DIS AND CIDI To allow nonclinicians to administer the DIS and CIDI reliably, the interview contains the exact wording to be used for each question; examiners need only read the question aloud for each item being assessed. Once a question is answered positively, several types of probes are used to determine whether the item can plausibly be counted toward a psychiatric diagnosis. A severity criterion, based on the subject having told a physician or other professional about the symptom or having experienced life interference as a result of the symptom, is used to separate common and insignificant problems from clinically meaningful phenomena. If the symptom has always occurred as a result of physical illness or injury or in relation to medication, alcohol, or drugs of abuse, it is coded as being explained by those conditions and not by a psychiatric illness. Those two features are intended to ensure consistency, accuracy, and selectivity in the assessment of positive reports of symptoms. Interviewer observations are used only for behavior-related psychotic conditions, and extensive use of marginal notes and examples is encouraged to allow editors and reviewing clinicians to judge any uncertain items.

Another effort to achieve reliability and accuracy is the use of a computer program to score the information and make diagnostic assignments. The program is written in a straightforward style so that clinicians can easily interpret the scoring algorithms. Questions on the DIS have been formulated to allow criteria to be assessed for categories specified in the RDC and St. Louis systems and in DSM-III; however, only selected DSM-III categories are covered. The DIS was updated for DSM-III-R and revised for DSM-IV. The CIDI covers both ICD-10 and DSM-IV.

Unlike the PSE, which concentrates on the one-month period prior to interview, the DIS and CIDI assess the occurrence of symptoms throughout the patient's lifetime. The lifetime approach allows a diagnosis of some disorders in which symptoms accumulate to a threshold (for example, somatization disorder, antisocial personality disorder), of disorders in which the history is important in the diagnosis (schizophrenia, bipolar disorder), and of prior episodes of recurring disorders (major depressive disorder). That approach also permits estimation of age at onset for subjects in a study as well as identification of subjects with a history of multiple disorders. Once a diagnosis is established on a lifetime basis, its most recent occurrence is dated. A modification of the DIS and CIDI permits dating of the most recent experience with any positive symptoms.

Several aspects of the DIS and CIDI approach have been noted as potential weaknesses. The approach minimizes examiner observation and judgment and therefore is limited to subject self-report to a great extent. Self-reports may not be adequate for assessment of some disorders, such as schizophrenia and mania. Eliciting self-reports of symptoms on a lifetime basis means that poor recall may also affect the validity of symptom reporting; that possibility has been raised particularly for persons with previous psychotic conditions. Although many aspects of the history of an illness can be obtained, such as age at onset and symptoms during the worst episode (for recurrent illnesses), some aspects of the course cannot be determined. It is also possible that variations in training and editing procedures may result in an effective ceiling on the degree of standardization that can be achieved in multisite studies.

CHARACTERISTICS OF THE DIS AND CIDI In the large epidemiological study that it was designed to support, the DIS was shown to be a feasible and safe instrument. It has been administered to about 20,000 subjects in five parts of the United States, and the refusal and dropout rate among persons who agreed to start the DIS has been less than 1 percent. The CIDI was used in the National Comorbidity Survey to interview subjects as a random sample across the United States.

Because the RDI and SADS interviews have been demonstrated to be reliable for current and lifetime reports in a range of subjects, and because the DIS is similar to them but has more structure and is accompanied by a computer program to score information, it was decided to perform interrater reliability studies at the higher level of procedural validity. In the first test, agreement was measured between two examiners, a nonclinician and a psychiatrist. Acceptable levels of agreement were reached, and further field testing was undertaken in the context of the epidemiological studies. The CIDI has been shown to have high interrater reliability in a multinational field trial conducted in varied languages.

Criterion validity for a diagnostic interview, especially one based on a new classification system, is hard to test, because there are no other validated interviews to use. The desire to apply a routine clinical judgment by psychiatrists using the clinical methods suffers from the possible effects of information, observer, and criterion variance that led to the development of standardized interview schedules 20 years ago. One alternative is to use similar instruments that apply the same standards of evidence and use scoring procedures based on the same system of diagnostic criteria. The purpose of such studies is not to validate any single instrument but to understand better any discrepancies with the comparison instrument. Studies comparing the CIDI and SCAN, as well as other interviews like the Structured Clinical Interview for DSM, are being undertaken for that purpose.

CONSTRUCT VALIDITY Construct validity, theoretically the most important form of validity for an assessment instrument, refers to a demonstration that an instrument does measure what it intends to measure, that in fact the entity exists and can be quantified by the instrument. The psychological literature has proposed various ways to accomplish that task. In psychiatric epidemiology the question involves more than whether an instrument detects a given disorder as specified by a classification system's rules. In practice those rules cannot be applied independently of a specified, reliable assessment instrument; therefore, the construct validity of the diagnostic entities in a system of classification remains to be shown for many categories for DSM-IV.

As psychiatric nosology has advanced, ways to establish validity for a diagnostic entity have been considered. The first requirement suggested was to demonstrate that a clinical picture with characteristic features can be described for the disorder, and that the features can be used to separate the disorder from others that may resemble it. The second type of evidence can be derived from external criteria and includes biological variables, such as those that are obtained from biochemical and neuroanatomical studies; psychosocial and personality styles, including methods for coping with adverse life events; familial and genetic variables, such as patterns of transmission of the disorder in relatives; clinical course and outcome variables, such as stability of the diagnosis over time and response to treatment; epidemiological variables, such as systematic occurrence in certain groups or places; and multivariate statistical analysis to demonstrate separation from and relation with other disorders in terms of the listed variables or to examine the latent structure of the underlying category.

Ideally, such studies would be based on assessments by several different, commonly used instruments to determine which technique most capably identifies homogeneous groups of subjects with little overlap with groups having other disorders.

STUDIES OF HISTORICAL IMPORTANCE

The results of epidemiological studies are most usefully reviewed within the framework of the population studied. That framework emphasizes the primacy of the population group as the basic unit of analysis in epidemiology and illustrates that a variety of descriptive, analytical, and experimental studies may be appropriate with any population group, provided that the selection characteristics of the group are clearly defined and considered in the design. The population groups reviewed here include (1) treated populations in specialty mental health settings, (2) patients registered in general medical practice settings, (3) noninstitutionalized community populations, and (4) persons with specific mental disorders within defined populations.

The definition of the study population group frequently affects decisions on the type of mental disorder criteria used, interviewer selection, interview method, and the descriptive or analytical variables used. Although the public health framework of epidemiological surveys begins with a community population and proceeds to primary care medical practices, then to specialty mental health treated populations, the reverse order more frequently has been the rule in the development of psychiatric epidemiology. That pattern is found in the rest of medicine, where the usual progression is from clinical observation to the laboratory for more intensive study—the laboratory, in the case of epidemiology, being large population groups. The choice of treated populations arises from the relative ease of defining a treated population, the availability of highly trained personnel to conduct assessments, and the existence of extensive diagnostic and related information in the medical records.

The impetus for proceeding from specialty mental health setting surveys to primary care surveys has been to broaden the population base so that it is more representative of the total community. In so doing it is still possible to retain highly trained physicians for case identification and longitudinal medical record data analysis in order to increase the pool of information about subjects beyond the amount that could be obtained in cross-sectional studies. Selection bias may affect both the dependent variables of syndromes and diagnoses and the associated descriptive and independent risk-factor variables that may lead to better understanding of etiology. Limitations on generalization to different populations develop whenever the population base from which the disorders are drawn is narrowed to a clinical setting. Likewise, the association of causal or descriptive variables with disorders may be confounded by the tendency of some variables to be strongly associated with use of services, as patients may visit primary care practitioners or psychiatrists for reasons unrelated to a mental disorder.

With that background in mind, a few selected studies of historical importance are presented.

SPECIALTY MENTAL HEALTH SECTOR TREATED POPULATIONS

Social class and mental illness One of the most prominent specialty mental health treated prevalence surveys was reported by August De Belmont Hollingshead and Fredrick Carl Redlich in the early 1950s. By exhaustively surveying every mental health facility and private office practice psychiatrist that treated any patient in the New Haven area, the authors defined an overall mental disorder, six-month treated prevalence rate of 8 in 1,000 population in the community. The rates varied, however, by socioeconomic status. Treated prevalence rates ranged from 5 to 7 out of 1,000 in social classes I through IV to 17 out of 1,000 in the lowest social class V. Patients were assessed by clinicians using a protocol report form that was dependent on the use of unspecified clinical judgment methods and unspecified criteria for specific diagnoses. Social class was a principal descriptive variable used to stratify frequency of diagnoses and the frequency of treatment setting use (Table 5.1-1). Although careful attention was given to controlling for potential confounding variables of age, sex, and type of mental disorder, a strong association was found between higher social class, less severe disorders, and private office treatment settings. By contrast, severe disorders were concentrated in the lower social classes and in long-stay public mental hospital institutions. New cases coming into treatment settings (treated incidence) composed only one eighth of the total six-month prevalence, with a much narrower range of about 1.0 out of 1,000 population for classes I through IV to 1.4 out of 1,000 population for social class V. Incidence rates were less discrepant across the social class groups than prevalence rates, which indicates that there was a longer duration of disorders in the lower social classes (prevalence ÷ incidence = duration). That finding could be partially explained by the diagnostic distribution across social classes, which showed a gradient increase in the proportion of psychotic to neurotic disorders from class I through V.

TABLE 5.1-1
Classification of Social Class by Hollingshead and Redlich

Class	Characteristics of the Sample in New Haven, Conn.
I	Class I, the highest social class, was composed of the community's business and professional leaders. Members of this group were well educated; they frequently had a history of attending private schools and both men and women had at least some college education. They earned the highest incomes, or lived on inherited wealth, and resided in the "best" areas of New Haven.
II	This class was composed of adults who had been upwardly mobile in their lives, and had jobs as managers or lower-ranking professionals. Their incomes were comfortable, but they had little accumulated wealth. Almost all of the adults had attended college, and they attributed their success to educational attainment.
III	The men in this class held administrative or semiprofessional positions or were skilled manual workers; many of the women worked in clerical or sales positions. They had economic security with some savings; most were high school graduates.
IV	In class IV, the men were skilled and semiskilled workers, and almost all women were employed in factory, clerical, or sales positions. Adults had usually left high school before graduating. Their incomes went for living expenses, and despite efforts to save, they had little, if any, savings accumulated.
V	In the lowest social class, employable adults were unskilled and semiskilled workers with low salaries. They had no savings and faced a constant struggle to cope with financial or social crises. Few of the adults had completed the ninth grade.

The Hollingshead and Redlich study may be seen as a combined descriptive and analytical epidemiological study of the treated prevalence and incidence of mental disorders, in which the community population was examined only for social class and other demographic variables. As such it provided treatment rates and showed strong associations between social class and the frequency, severity, and treatment setting of patients with mental disorders. The absence of standardized assessment procedures in the total population made it impossible to determine if diagnoses were reliably assessed across treatment settings, if social class was associated with mental disorders or only with a treatment frequency, or if social class was related in any etiological way to the presence of mental disorders or merely concentrated more direct risk factors within that population group.

Despite its methodological limitations, the Hollingshead and Redlich study had a major impact on the collective social conscience of the day and may be seen as a classic example of the power of simple frequency and descriptive variable associations to have important administrative and health policy impacts while generating, but not testing, hypotheses about etiology. The implications of social class-determined treatment and the possibility that community characteristics might have a role in the etiology of mental disorders supported major public policy decisions in the United States to expand specialty mental health services and the community mental health center legislation.

National reporting program An additional source of treated prevalence data is available from the Mental Disorder National Reporting Program (NRP) recently transferred from NIMH to the Center for Mental Health Services in the new Substance Abuse and Mental Health Services Administration. The NRP complements the United States Public Health Service National

Health Survey, which consists of periodic health examinations and facility surveys conducted by the National Center for Health Statistics (NCHS) and other Public Health Service agencies. Components of the NRP include the annual census of state and county mental hospitals, the inventory of specialty mental health facilities, and the sample patient surveys drawn from the universe of facilities. Routine data on office-based psychiatrists are drawn from the NCHS National Ambulatory Medical Care Survey.

The annual census of state and county mental hospitals describes the age, sex, and diagnostic composition of resident patients present in those hospitals at the end of each calendar year, and admissions during the year. A comprehensive inventory of all mental health facilities records information on the staffing and organizational characteristics of the facilities and information on caseload and capacity, including number of episodes of care. Episodes are defined as residents at year's end plus all admissions during the year. Because some patients may have more than one admission in a year, the indicator is slightly inflated over annual treated prevalence rates. Finally, the sample patient surveys provide more detailed information on patient characteristics, including diagnoses, length of stay, and type of treatment received.

Besides being the major source of national service use data, the NRP has proved an invaluable source of longitudinal trend data on patients under treatment in the specialty mental health sector. For example, the decreased number of residents in state hospitals during the period of deinstitutionalization, from a high of 559,000 in 1955 to a level of 92,000 in 1990, can be documented (Figure 5.1-1). Also, the shift in care from one type of facility to another can be analyzed. In 1955 1.7 million episodes of care were delivered, of which 49 percent were inpatient episodes in state and county mental hospitals; in 1988 7.8 million episodes were delivered and only 5 percent were inpatient episodes in state and county mental hospitals, with 12 percent of care episodes delivered in general hospital psychiatric units, 5 percent in private psychiatric hospitals, 3 percent in Veterans Administration medical centers, 2 percent in other inpatient settings, and 72 percent in all outpatient psychiatric services (Figure 5.1-2).

Such data illustrate the value of treated prevalence data in describing the workings of the health care system. They also demonstrate how treated prevalence rates reflect administrative and policy decisions that affect patterns of treatment.

PRIMARY CARE SETTINGS Because primary medical care settings reflect a much broader population base than specialty settings while retaining the potential for engaging patients in treatment, many epidemiological investigations have examined mental disorders in general medical populations. Various studies in the United States have indicated that at least 70 percent of the noninstitutionalized population use general medical services over the course of a year, so general physicians are in a position to screen for mental disorders in a much larger proportion of the population than the 1 to 6 percent who may be seen in specialty mental health services in a year.

Recent studies of mental disorder in primary care patients have used contemporary diagnostic interviews to demonstrate that 15 to 30 percent of patients visiting primary care offices have a current mental disorder. However, some of the same studies suggest that few of those disorders are recognized, diagnosed, or treated by the primary care clinician. A major public health campaign has been developed by NIMH to increase the awareness, recognition, and treatment of the most common mental health condition, depression. That effort, known as Project D/ART (Depression/Awareness, Recognition, Treatment), is providing educational materials to the general public, primary care clinicians, and mental health specialists. Similar programs on panic disorders and eating disorders have been initiated.

COMMUNITY POPULATION STUDIES To overcome the problems of selection bias and unreliability of routine clinical diagnosis in treatment settings, epidemiologists rely most heavily on direct surveys of community residents. Before World War I epidemiological studies used institutional records or key informants to generate prevalence estimates of mental disorders. More recent studies have used direct interviews of community residents, with the information recorded on structured protocols by nonclinicians. Three studies conducted in the 1950s were classic investigations that attempted to generate prevalence estimates of mental disorders in accordance with one or more of the major diagnostic practices in use at the time. Two of them, conducted in Stirling County, Canada, and in midtown Manhattan, also examined specific etiological hypotheses about the causal relationship of socioenvironmental factors to the occurrence of mental disorders.

Stirling County study The study of Stirling County, directed by Alexander H. Leighton and continued by Jane Murphy, was

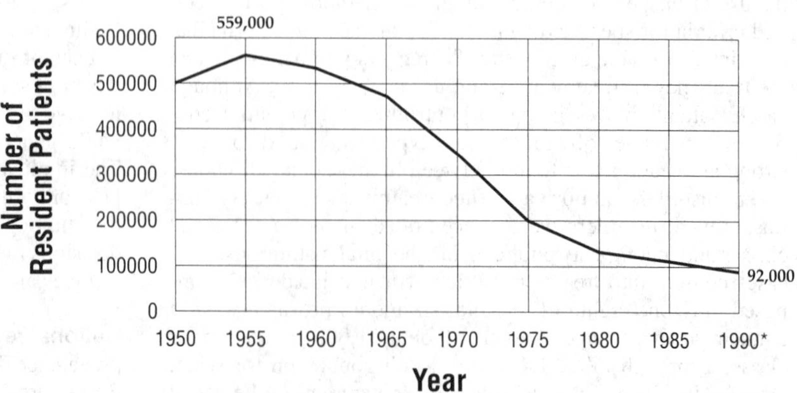

FIGURE 5.1-1 *Number of resident patients at year end in state and county hospitals.*

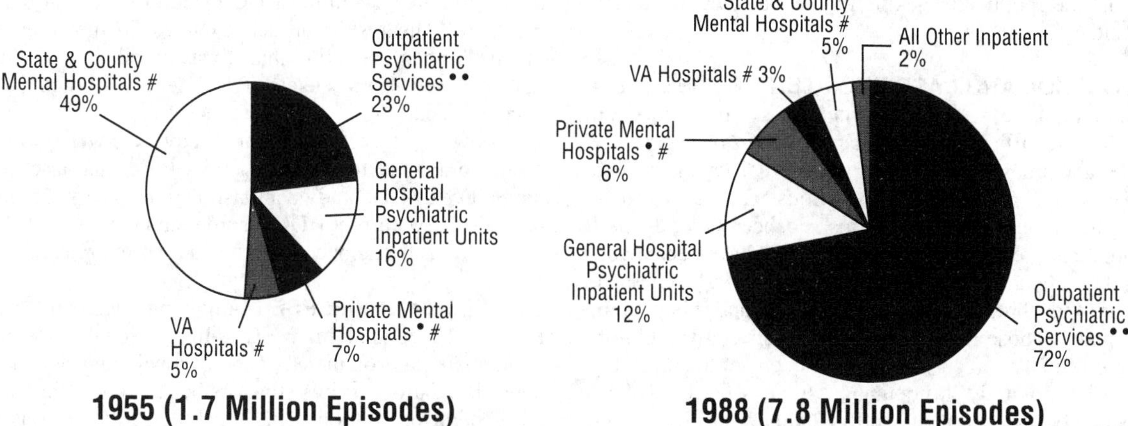

• Includes residential treatment centers for emotionally disturbed children

Inpatient services only

• • Includes free-standing outpatient services as well as those affiliated with psychiatric and general hospitals (for 1988, 6 percent of total care episodes are partial care and are included in this category. No partial care data obtained in 1955.)

FIGURE 5.1-2 *Percent distribution of inpatient and outpatient care episodes in mental health facilities, by type of facility, in the United States in 1955 and 1988. (Figure from Statistical Note 204, Table 2, 1992. DHHS Publication Number (ADM) 92-1911, U.S. Government Printing Office, Washington, 1992.)*

begun in the 1950s. Out of 20,000 residents of a rural county in Canada, 1,010 adults were sampled. Independent variables, hypothesized to be causally related to mental disorders, were cultural and community characteristics. The dependent variables were mental disorders defined in accordance with the newly developed DSM-I criteria and were rated in terms of the presence or absence of 32 detailed symptom patterns, impairment levels, and the need for psychiatric attention. Trained field-workers surveyed the population sample with a structured psychiatric interview that was clinically evaluated later by two psychiatrists. Additional information was gathered from all county general practitioners, who served as key informants for obtaining more detailed medical, psychological, and social data about each sample member.

Estimates of the lifetime prevalence of the dependent variables included rates of 57 in 100 population for all DSM-I conditions, 24 in 100 for conditions associated with significant impairment, and 20 in 100 for conditions in need of psychiatric attention; the last rate is regarded as the most clinically meaningful estimate. Higher rates of disorders were found in communities characterized by social disintegration, although the exact causal factors within the gross environmental descriptive categories could not be specified.

Midtown Manhattan study The Midtown Manhattan study of Thomas Rennie, Leo Srole, and colleagues also began in the early 1950s. From an area of midtown Manhattan that had a population of 110,000 adults, a sample of 1,660 adult residents was selected. The independent variables included various measures of stress, immigration status, social class, occupation, and marital status; the dependent variable was a measure of impairment in adult life function rated on a six-point gradient scale from none to incapacitated.

Psychologists and social workers used a structured psychiatric interview to obtain information from respondents, which was subsequently rated by two psychiatrists. The most celebrated findings were that 81.5 percent of the population had at least mild impairment from psychological symptoms and 23.4 percent had significant impairment. Although correlations were found between sociodemographic and social stress variables with levels of impairment, one of the most significant results of the study was a debate about the dependent variable measure of mental health status. If less than 20 percent of the population could be identified as mentally healthy, the clinical usefulness of mental disorder definitions was open to question. The importance of using more rigorous criteria for diagnoses was immediately apparent to other more medically oriented epidemiologists.

Baltimore study A third major study, undertaken in Baltimore, Maryland, sampled the entire noninstitutionalized population, including children. The study was a two-stage morbidity survey. The first stage consisted of household interviews by census interviewers; the second stage consisted of clinical examination of 809 subjects stratified by level of disability. General medical internists and pediatricians conducted a medical history and examination, followed by a psychiatrist's rating of all protocols with psychological symptoms or impairment related to mental disorders. Because the study was a morbidity survey conducted to identify the prevalence of individuals with chronic medical or mental disorders for purposes of improving services, no attempt was made to test etiological hypotheses. Diagnostic categories provided in the *International Statistical Classification of Diseases* (ISCD) were used for all physical and mental disorders, although no effort was made to assess the reliability or validity of assessments. A point prevalence rate of 10.9 percent was found for all ISCD mental disorders, with 1.4

percent of the population exhibiting moderate or severe impairment.

CASE-CONTROL AND CASE REGISTER STUDIES Population samples are especially important for avoiding selection bias, but they are difficult to use for rare disorders or to generate hypotheses about possible risk factors. Case registers have been maintained for rare disorders that are serious and likely to come to medical attention, such as rare forms of cancer. Over the past two decades, case registers of psychiatric cases have been maintained in the state of Maryland, in Monroe County (Rochester), New York, and abroad in Oxford, England, and Mannheim, West Germany. Those registers have been especially useful in providing information about schizophrenia, one of the most difficult disorders to study in population surveys because of its relatively rare occurrence and the difficulty of ensuring an accurate diagnosis.

Danish adoption study One of the most prominent case-control studies in psychiatric epidemiology is that of Seymour Kety and colleagues, begun in 1964. They studied a defined population of 5,483 adoptees, registered from 1924 through 1947, in the city and county of Copenhagen, Denmark. At that time the adoptees ranged from 17 to 40 years old. Of the total population, 507 were known to have some admission to a psychiatric hospital, and 33 of that group were assessed as having a diagnosis within a spectrum of schizophrenic disorders. An equal number of matched adoptees who had no history of mental hospitalization were identified for comparison.

For cases and comparison adoptees, a systematic search of available records was conducted to assess the rate of schizophrenialike conditions in biological relatives. Of the 150 biological relatives of the schizophrenic adoptees, 8.7 percent had a diagnosis of schizophrenia, compared to 1.9 percent of the 156 biological relatives of the comparison group of adoptees. The highly significant difference in those rates indicated a genetic contribution to schizophrenia in the index cases, because environmental influences had been removed through adoption. That classic study has recently been extended with an examination of adoptees throughout the rest of Denmark. At present, the genetic mechanism that increases passive susceptibility or that causes active expression of particular genes has not been identified.

Experimental epidemiology Prospective trials have been used to test the effect of treatments among identified cases, with random assignment of cases to experimental or control groups used to control for possible selection bias. Longitudinal designs allow comparisons of rates of expected outcome between the control and experimental subjects. Similar clinical trial designs are being used to test preventive interventions in high-risk populations.

CONTEMPORARY EPIDEMIOLOGICAL STUDIES

STUDIES using SADS As the SADS interview was being developed for clinical studies in the mid-1970s and was shown to be appropriate for both patients and normal controls in those studies, investigators began testing the feasibility of employing it in large population-based studies of community residents and primary care patients. In a follow-up study of 1,095 adults first studied in New Haven in 1967, Jerome Myers and Myrna Weissman conducted interviews with 511 who were still available for study in 1975–1976. They found that 15.1 percent of the sample had a definite RDC mental disorder at the time of interview. The results attracted interest in the research community by demonstrating that it was possible to conduct community-based studies using assessment instruments that produced clinically meaningful diagnoses.

Following that successful study, NIMH investigators designed a study for primary care settings that also employed the SADS-L. That study demonstrated that nearly 28 percent of patients had a current RDC disorder and that fewer than one in 10 of the cases had been recognized by primary care clinicians.

STUDIES using the PSE Following successful use of the PSE in 12 centers in WHO's International Pilot Study of Schizophrenia, conducted in both developing and developed countries, European investigators began conducting studies of the general population using the PSE as the core assessment instrument. Although the PSE by itself does not generate diagnoses, it provides information that can be related to ICD disease categories for the month preceding the examination. Among the multiple studies conducted with the PSE, five have been conducted in reasonably comparable ways and permit comparison of results for depressive and anxiety disorders (Table 5.1-2). Because those disorders typically show female predominance, whereas such disorders as alcohol abuse and dependence, which are more common among male patients, are not assessed in detail by the PSE, it is common for such studies to show that the total rate of the disorder is higher in female patients than in male patients; however, such conclusions need to be qualified according to the range of disorders covered in the study. Rates of depressive conditions in Athens and Camberwell, England were generally equivalent and higher than rates in Canberra, Australia, and Edinburgh; the highest rates by far were those reported from two Ugandan villages, and they are still unexplained. Rates of anxiety conditions among women were reported to be quite high in Athens.

An especially interesting finding was reported by investigators in Edinburgh, who incorporated ratings of RDC criteria into their interview protocol, which was built around the core items of the PSE. As shown in Table 5.1-2, the rates of the PSE-derived categories of depression and anxiety in their sample of women were roughly comparable to the rates reported from Canberra and Camberwell. However, the rates of depression and anxiety, based on information from the same interviews and evaluated according to RDC criteria, were much higher in the Edinburgh sample, compared with the rates found in the New Haven cohort follow-up study that had used the SADS interview. That finding highlights the need for greater diagnostic comparability in epidemiological investigations, particularly for international comparisons.

NIMH EPIDEMIOLOGIC CATCHMENT AREA PROGRAM The NIMH Epidemiologic Catchment Area (ECA) program grew out of a combination of scientific developments and historical events within the mental health field. An important scientific development was the emergence of operational criteria for diagnoses that produced DSM-III and culminated in DSM-IV and ICD-10. A logical extension of the use of those criteria was the construction of standardized clinical instruments to elicit information on the presence of requisite symptom patterns from research subjects in a reliable manner.

In addition to the development of operationalized diagnostic criteria and standardized instruments, the 1978 President's Commission on Mental Health demonstrated major gaps in knowledge of specific mental disorder population rates and how such disorders are treated. By synthesizing information from

TABLE 5.1-2
Rates of ICD-Equivalent Disorders from the PSE in General Population Surveys (in percent).

	Depression		Anxiety		All Disorders		
Location	Males	Females	Males	Females	Males	Females	Total
Athens	4.3	10.1	3.9	12.1	8.6	22.6	16.0
Canberra	2.6	6.7	4.1	3.0	7.0	11.0	9.0
Camberwell	4.8	9.0	1.0	4.5	6.1	14.9	10.9
Edinburgh	—	5.9	—	2.8	—	8.7	—
Uganda	17.0	21.0	2.8	4.0	23.6*	27.0*	25.3*

*Rates calculated from tabular data published by authors.

the NIMH NRP, psychiatric case registers, general practice epidemiological surveys, the Baltimore morbidity survey, and various other sources, it was possible to provide conservative estimates of overall annual prevalence rates and the health care sector in which persons with such disorders received care. Analysis of secondary epidemiological and services research data resulted in mental disorder point prevalence rate estimates of 10 out of 100 population in the United States, an annual incidence rate of 5 out of 100 population, and an annual period prevalence rate of 15 out of 100 population. Based on treated prevalence data, it was estimated that only 3.1 in 100 population were seen by any mental health specialist in the course of one year and that the majority (54 percent of the 15 in 100 population) were seen exclusively in the general medical outpatient sector.

Fundamental deficits in knowledge of specific mental disorder frequency rates, the proportion of ill persons treated and untreated, and the locus of treatment became readily apparent. The recommendation to proceed with a new wave of epidemiological and services research studies received favorable response from the NIMH leadership when the need was buttressed with evidence that the new diagnostic criteria and prototype standardized instruments could be applied for epidemiological purposes.

Methodology The NIMH ECA program was a multisite epidemiological and health services research study that assessed mental disorder prevalence, incidence, and service use rates in about 20,000 community and institutional residents. The survey used the DIS as a diagnostic assessment instrument.

The essential features of the research design included geographically defined community populations of at least 200,000 residents, from which stratified random probability samples were drawn to obtain completed interviews from approximately 3,000 adult (age 18 and over) community residents and 500 institutional residents. The five participating universities were Yale, Johns Hopkins, Washington University (St. Louis), Duke, and the University of California at Los Angeles. Several of the sites oversampled special populations, including the elderly and minority groups.

After sample selection, each subject was interviewed by a trained lay interviewer with the DIS and service utilization questions. With a longitudinal design, each site conducted at least two face-to-face interviews one year apart and one intervening telephone or face-to-face interview to assess service use and change in symptom or diagnostic status. A total of 18,571 persons were interviewed in the first wave of community sampling, and the sample extends to 20,000 when persons institutionalized in prisons, nursing homes, and mental hospitals are added. Estimates for the United States were made by first weighting each person in proportion to his or her probability of selection in the individual catchment area site, and subsequently weighting each person in proportion to his or her representation in 36 age by sex by race-ethnicity groups in the 1980 United States census of adults ages 18 and over.

The one-month community population rates for persons ages 18 and over are provided below to document the current state-of-the-art point prevalence rates using the DIS case-identification instrument. Standard errors are provided to illustrate the relative stability of those estimates of DIS-defined DSM-III disorder prevalence rates.

It is important to emphasize that the specific disorder rates allow multiple disorders for each person and do not include any exclusionary diagnoses that are allowed for by DSM-III. Although DSM-III would exclude a diagnosis of panic disorder if schizophrenia was present, the current diagnostic algorithms of the DIS do not unduplicate diagnoses based on exclusions.

Results Current one-month point prevalence rates (with standard errors in parentheses) are presented in Table 5.1-3 for the United States estimates derived from the combined data collected in all five sites. Those data, which are weighted to the 1980 United States Census noninstitutionalized population, provide a major advance in the ability to estimate national rates over what was available at the time of the President's Commission on Mental Health. In addition to providing overall prevalence rates of DIS and DSM-III disorders, it has also been possible to identify sociodemographic correlates of those disorders that identify groups having relatively high or low rates of those disorders.

Table 5.1-3 shows that 15.4 percent of the United States noninstitutionalized population can be estimated to have had one or more DIS and DSM-III disorder in the one month prior to interview. There is a small but significant difference between overall rates for male interviewees (14.0 percent) and female interviewees (16.6 percent) although those differences cease to be significant when age, marital status, race-ethnicity, and socioeconomic status variables are controlled. A summary rate of 11.5 percent, which excludes persons with only substance use disorders or severe cognitive impairment, is included to facilitate comparison with the PSE-based studies that also exclude those disorders. When those disorders are excluded, the rates for male subjects (8.2 percent) and female subjects (14.6 percent) are close to the median rate (Camberwell) of the PSE-based studies of male subjects (6.1 percent) and female subjects (14.9 percent). Those data show the importance of including alcohol and drug abuse disorders in epidemiological studies, particularly when accurate rates for men are desired. Because diagnostic exclusions were not used, it is possible for subjects to have more than one diagnosis. The sum of the rates for individual disorders is greater than the overall rate.

The addition of institutionalized persons raised the one-month rates of any disorder to 15.7 percent of the total adult population. When the one-year follow-up examinations of that cohort were analyzed, it was shown that 12.3 percent of the population developed a new or recurrent disorder in the follow-

TABLE 5.1-3
One-Month Point Prevalence Rate Estimates per 100 U.S. Community Residents for Selected DIS/DSM-III Disorders, NIMH Epidemiologic Catchment Area Program (ECA).* Data Combined from Five Sites and Weighted to 1980 Census of U.S. Population

Disorder	Rate per 100 Community Population		
	Total (N = 18,571)	Male (N = 7,618)	Female (N = 10,953)
Any DIS/DSM-III disorder covered	15.4 (0.4)†	14.0 (0.5)	16.6 (0.5)
Any disorder except severe cognitive impairment or substance use	11.5 (0.3)	8.2 (0.4)	14.6 (0.4)
Schizophrenic/schizophreniform disorders	0.7 (0.1)	0.7 (0.1)	0.7 (0.1)
Schizophrenia	0.6 (0.1)	0.6 (0.1)	0.6 (0.1)
Schizophreniform disorder	0.1 (0.1)	0.1 (0.0)	0.1 (0.0)
Affective disorders (mood disorders)	5.1 (0.2)	3.5 (0.3)	6.6 (0.3)
Manic episode	0.4 (0.1)	0.3 (0.1)	0.4 (0.1)
Major depressive episode	2.2 (0.2)	1.6 (0.2)	2.9 (0.2)
Dysthymia	3.3 (0.2)	2.2 (0.3)	4.2 (0.3)
Anxiety disorders	7.3 (0.3)	4.7 (0.3)	9.7 (0.4)
Phobia	6.2 (0.2)	3.8 (0.3)	8.4 (0.3)
Panic	0.5 (0.1)	0.3 (0.1)	0.7 (0.1)
Obsessive-compulsive disorder	1.3 (0.1)	1.1 (0.1)	1.5 (0.2)
Substance use disorders	3.8 (0.2)	6.3 (0.4)	1.6 (0.2)
Alcohol abuse, dependence	2.8 (0.2)	5.0 (0.4)	0.9 (0.1)
Drug abuse, dependence	1.3 (0.1)	1.8 (0.2)	0.7 (0.1)
Somatization disorder	0.1 (0.0)	0.0 (0.0)	0.2 (0.1)
Antisocial personality disorder	0.5 (0.1)	0.8 (0.1)	0.2 (0.1)
Cognitive impairment—severe	1.3 (0.1)	1.4 (0.1)	1.3 (0.1)

*The Epidemiologic Catchment Area Program (ECA) is a series of five epidemiological research studies performed by independent research teams in collaboration with staff of the Division of Biometry and Epidemiology (DBE) and the Division of Clinical Research (DCR) of the National Institute of Mental Health (NIMH). The NIMH principal collaborators are Darrel A. Regier, Ben Z. Locke, and Jack D. Burke, Jr.; the NIMH project officers are Carl A. Taube (1978–1985) and William Huber (1985–). The principal investigators and coinvestigators from the five sites are: Yale University, UO1 MOH 34223—Jerome K. Myers, Myrna M. Weissman, and Gary L. Tischler; Johns Hopkins University, UO1 MH 33870—Morton Kramer, Ernest Gruenberg, and Sam Shapiro; Washington University, St. Louis, UO1 MH 33883—Lee N. Robins and John Helzer; Duke University, UO1 MH 35386—Dan Blazer and Linda George; University of California, Los Angeles, UO1 MH 35865—Marvin Karno, Richard L. Hough, Javier I. Escobar, M. Audrey Burnam, and Dianne M. Timbers.
†Numbers in parentheses represent standard errors.

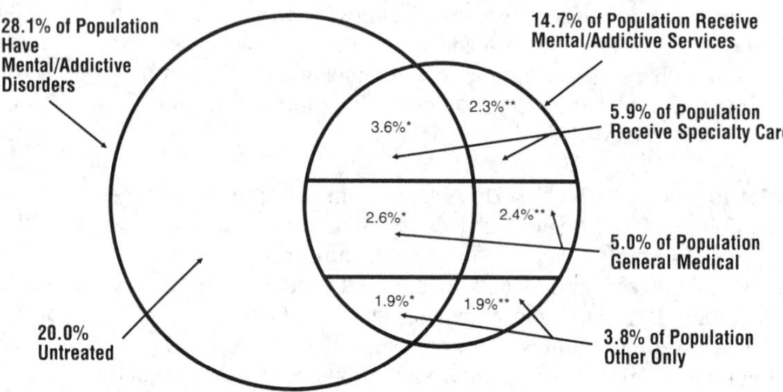

FIGURE 5.1-3 *Annual prevalence of mental-addictive disorders and services.*

ing year. In one year, 28.1 percent of the total population experienced sufficient symptoms to meet criteria for one or more mental or addictive disorders. By contrast, the earlier estimates from the President's Commission were that only 15 percent of the population would experience such a disorder in one year.

Detailed information also became available on the treated prevalence of those disorders and the proportion of the population that received any mental health treatment in one year. A total of 14.7 percent of the population reported use of some mental health services in one year for emotions, nerves, or for alcohol or drug abuse (Figure 5.1-3); 5.9 percent of the total adult population received such care from a mental health specialist and an additional 5.2 percent received such services exclusively in general medical settings. It is also possible to account for 3.4 percent of the population that used mental health services outside the above health sectors from social service agencies, the clergy, other human service professionals, self-help groups, family, or friends.

Although about 45 percent of those using mental or addictive services had symptoms that were below full diagnostic threshold, fully 80 percent of the outpatient and 95 percent of the inpatient admissions had prior life-time diagnoses and sub-threshold symptoms of severe disorders associated with significant morbidity in other analyses.

SCHIZOPHRENIA Schizophrenia was found in 0.7 percent of the population, with equal rates in men and women. The highest rates were found in the age group 25 to 44 years (1.1 percent), followed by a rate of 0.8 percent in the age group 18 to 24 years. Significantly higher rates were found in separated and divorced persons (1.5 percent) and in lower socioeconomic groups, an odds ratio of 8 was identified for the lowest socioeconomic class as compared with the highest class.

AFFECTIVE DISORDERS Affective (mood) disorders were found at an overall rate of 5.1 percent and were significantly higher in women (6.6 percent) than in men (3.5 percent). Although those rates are consistent with previous studies such as the median (Camberwell) for those using the PSE, specific biological or social factors that may account for the sex ratio discrepancy have not yet been identified. Rates were highest (6.4 percent) in the age group 25 to 44 years and lowest (2.5 percent) in the 65 and older age group. An NIH consensus conference discussed the possible need for a lower threshold for clinically significant depressive disorders in the elderly; however, no change in diagnostic criteria was introduced in DSM-IV for that age group.

Of all the sociodemographically defined groups, the separated and divorced marital status group had the highest overall level of affective disorders, 11.1 percent, compared with a rate of 4.1 percent for married subjects. Major depressive episode was found in 2.2 percent of the population, and manic episode, necessary for bipolar I disorder diagnostic criteria, was found in 0.4 percent of the population. Dysthymia, which requires a two-year duration of symptoms for DSM-III criteria, was identified only on a lifetime basis (3.3 percent) but is included in the current one-month prevalence rates because of the higher probability of patients' recalling more recent episodes and to avoid a serious underestimate of affective disorders. For example, the Camberwell group found a higher rate of total affective disorders (7.0 percent) and the same ratio of men (4.8 percent) to women (9.0 percent).

ANXIETY DISORDERS As a group, the anxiety disorders exhibited the highest overall prevalence (7.3 percent), with women (9.7 percent) having significantly higher rates than men (4.7 percent). Phobic disorders, which include simple phobias, social phobias, and agoraphobia, constituted the largest single diagnosis. Within the five sites, that disorder had the highest prevalence rates and the greatest variation between sites, ranging from 4 to 5 percent in three sites (New Haven, St. Louis, Los Angeles) to 11 percent in two sites (Baltimore, Durham). The marked discrepancy in the prevalence rates of one diagnosis led the investigators to examine whether any of the following types of bias existed: observational bias (differences in interviewer training or questionnaire construction), selection bias (differences in characteristics of subjects), or confounding bias (another factor, such as socioeconomic status, may be related to both a causal factor of phobia and the population of subjects with high rates of the disorder). Once methodological explanations have been ruled out, environmental or other variables associated with the geographically defined populations in Baltimore and Durham that are not found in the other three sites need to be examined. Of the remaining anxiety disorders, panic disorder and obsessive-compulsive disorder were also found somewhat more frequently in women; the respective rates were 0.5 percent and 1.3 percent.

SUBSTANCE USE DISORDERS Overall substance use disorders were found in 3.8 percent of the population, with markedly higher rates in men (6.3 percent) than in women (1.6 percent). Alcohol abuse or dependence rates (2.8 percent) showed a significant difference between men and women, with men having over five times the rate of women. Sex ratios of that magnitude were found in only one other disorder, antisocial personality disorder, which had a low prevalence rate and a male to female ratio of four to one. In contrast, rates of drug abuse and dependence (1.3 percent) in men were slightly more than two times higher than in women. Finding a higher male to female ratio for alcoholism in comparison to the higher female to male ratio for depression and anxiety disorders led other investigators to question whether a similar underlying biological disorder results in a differential phenotypical manifestation of depression or anxiety disorders in females and alcoholism in males because of social-role expectations. Population, genetic, and neurobiological research may eventually find measurable risk factors to test that hypothesis by case-control methods.

SOMATIZATION DISORDER The only somatoform disorder covered in the DIS is somatization disorder, which is closely related to Briquet's syndrome in the St. Louis research criteria for mental disorders. It was found almost exclusively in women (0.2 percent), which, in the absence of any cases in men, resulted in an overall population rate of 0.1 percent.

SEVERE COGNITIVE IMPAIRMENT Cognitive impairment is not a DSM-III or DSM-IV diagnosis but is determined by a score of 0 to 17 on the Mini-Mental State Examination (MMSE). A major objective of that component of the DIS is to identify subpopulations with a high probability of having mental disorders due to a general medical condition, including the dementias (such as dementia of the Alzheimer's type), delirium, or other syndromes due to a general medical condition that affects cognition. Low scores of 0 to 17 on the MMSE indicate severe cognitive impairment, scores of 18 to 23 indicate mild impairment, and scores of 24 to 30 indicate little or no impairment. To assess the range of disorders included and the sensitivity and specificity of the screening instrument for a detailed criterion assessment, detailed psychiatric and neurological examinations have been conducted on the sample of subjects with those disorders at the Baltimore site.

ANTISOCIAL PERSONALITY DISORDER Antisocial personality disorder was found predominantly in men (0.8 percent), with a rate of 0.2 percent in women and an overall population rate of 0.5 percent. It was also found predominantly in the age group under 45 years (0.8 to 0.9 percent) and was associated with a separated or divorced marital status (1.1 percent), compared with a 0.5 percent rate in married persons. Rates were higher in persons of lower socioeconomic status levels 3 and 4 (0.7 to 0.9 percent) than in persons of higher socioeconomic status levels 1 and 2 of (0.2 to 0.3 percent).

OTHER PERSONALITY DISORDERS Psychiatrists conducted additional interviews of 762 respondents at the Baltimore ECA site using a semistructured examination for DSM-III personality disorders. The prevalence rate for any personality disorder was 5.9 percent at a definite level of certainty and 9.3 percent when provisional cases were added. The most common personality disorders were histrionic (2.1 percent) and compulsive (1.7 percent). Rates were especially high in respondents who were separated or divorced (15.6 percent).

SUMMARY RATES The diagnostic algorithms for computing rates allowed for multiple diagnoses, and did not exclude diagnoses as allowed in DSM-III. Summary rates were used to present the total number of persons in the population with any one of the disorders, and were included for comparative purposes. It should be emphasized that the summary rates do not identify the total rate of mental disorder in the population, but only that proportion of persons having one of the DSM-III disorders and cognitive impairment identified by the DIS.

ONSET AND COMORBIDITY Data from the ECA are consistent with other studies that demonstrate a higher rate and earlier onset of major depressive disorder in generations born since World War II. The change happened too quickly to be attributed to genetic factors, but the underlying cause is not yet known. An effort to determine whether that finding resulted from methodological problems, namely the cross-sectional examination using a lifetime approach, as in most recent epidemiological studies, showed that many other disorders did not demonstrate such a shift. One disorder that showed a shift to earlier age at onset and higher rates in young adults was drug abuse and dependence, and its shift occurred only in the group with adolescent-onset major depressive or anxiety disorder. Earlier studies had demonstrated that a history of major depressive disorder or an anxiety disorder in adolescence or young adulthood doubled the risk of developing a subsequent drug abuse and dependence disorder. Those findings raise the possibility that early intervention to treat first episodes of major depressive and anxiety disorders, especially in adolescents, may help reduce the risk of subsequent drug abuse and dependence.

Comorbidity Results from the ECA program demonstrated that disorders tend to co-occur in some individuals more commonly than expected from their prevalence rates. Of particular importance for their high degree of overlap with mental disorders were alcohol and other substance use disorders. That finding led the three NIH institutes dealing with those conditions to sponsor a national survey of mental disorders co-occurring with alcohol and other drug use disorders.

NATIONAL COMORBIDITY SURVEY A sample of 8,098 respondents aged 18 to 55 years were interviewed from 1990 to 1992 with the CIDI, modified to reinforce the instructions to subjects to try to recall their past experiences with symptoms relevant to the disorders. The results showed much higher rates of disorders than were found in the ECA. Lifetime rates of mental disorders covered on the CIDI for all respondents were 48.0 percent, and one-year rates were 29.5 percent. For major depressive disorder, the lifetime rates were 17.1 percent for all respondents and 21.3 percent for women. One-month rates of major depressive disorder were 4.9 percent for all respondents and 5.9 percent for females.

Explanations for rates higher than those reported in earlier studies like the ECA range from issues of sampling, interview methodology, change over time, and more accurate case identification. Whether the national sample (as opposed to the five-site survey in the ECA), or the restricted age sample, or the memory cuing on the modified CIDI, or the progression of disease over a decade led to the higher rates is not yet determined, but if methodological differences can be ruled out as the explanation, the findings offer a fascinating challenge to epidemiologists, who try to interpret differences in the distribution of illness as a clue to risk factors. Results from the National Comorbidity Survey (NCS) were also consistent with studies that have suggested that major depression occurs with earlier age at onset with younger generations.

Health policy issues Data from the ECA have been used as a basis for estimating the total direct and indirect cost of mental disorders to the United States. For 1988 the costs were estimated to total $129.3 billion, including $55.4 billion for treatment costs and $57 billion in lost productivity. Assessing the costs of early mortality and lost productivity is difficult because fewer than 30 percent of persons with a psychiatric disorder in one year receive any services from mental health, primary care, or other human service providers during that year. Those results have strengthened the arguments of policymakers who want to provide equivalent coverage of mental disorders in health care benefit packages. Similarly, data on childhood and early adolescent onset of many disorders spurred efforts to improve the delivery of mental health services to children and adolescents in the early 1990s.

FUTURE EFFORTS

Although questions remain about the validity of DSM-IV diagnoses, which are based largely on manifestational rather than causal criteria, the explicit nature of the criteria renders them susceptible to empirical hypothesis testing. Removal of presumed etiological criteria from mental disorder diagnoses has actually facilitated research on the scientific veracity of etiological hypotheses. Epidemiological studies using DSM-IV criteria are expected to produce external validating criteria to assess the degree to which groups identified with specific disorders are homogeneous with regard to biological, demographic, social, and clinical course characteristics. Stability of mental disorder rates in populations with similar characteristics would support the validity of the diagnoses, whereas variations in rates may lead to additional subtyping or even etiological clues.

With improvements in nosological and case-identification tools for epidemiological research, it will be necessary to extend the application of epidemiological methods to new population groups, including those in other cultures. Further refinements in the basic tools for evaluating childhood disorders and culture-specific disorders should expand research opportunities in those understudied groups. After 15 years of effort, investigators collaborating with NIMH recently completed developmental work on the Diagnostic Interview Schedule for Children and field-tested it in four sites. A combined prevalence and services use study of children and adolescents is expected in the near future.

Once the intrinsic research base of epidemiology is more secure, it should be possible to extend the interface with other research fields, including service systems, clinical services, and clinical and neurobiological research areas. Many potential etiological or clinical service improvement risk factors emerging from those other research areas will require validation in large population studies using experimental epidemiological research designs.

The full potential of psychiatric epidemiology for public health purposes has yet to be realized. Improved understanding of the epidemiology of mental disorders should facilitate allocation of resources to mental health services, broaden the safety and effectiveness of specific treatments for persons with a mental disorder, and lead to effective prevention efforts to reduce the onset of new cases of mental disorders.

SUGGESTED CROSS-REFERENCES

Other quantitative and experimental methods in psychiatry are discussed in the other sections in Chapter 5. The classification of mental disorders is discussed in Section 11.1. Schizophrenia is the subject of Chapter 14; mood disorders are covered in Chapter 16; anxiety disorders are the focus of Chapter 17; substance-related disorders are discussed in Chapter 13; somatization disorder is discussed in Chapter 18; and personality disorders are the subject of Chapter 25.

REFERENCES

Bebbington P, Hurry J, Tennant C, Sturt E, Wing J K: Epidemiology of mental disorders in Camberwell. Psychol Med *11:* 561, 1981.

Blazer D G, Kessler R C, McGonagle K A, Swartz M S: The prevalence and distribution of major depression in a national community sample: The National Comorbidity Survey. Am J Psychiatry *151:* 979, 1994.

*Burke J D, Burke K C, Rae D S: Increased rates of drug abuse and dependence after onset of mood or anxiety disorders in adolescence. Hosp Community Psychiatry *45:* 451, 1994.

Burke K C, Burke J D, Rae D S, Regier D A: Comparing age at onset of major depression and other psychiatric disorders by birth cohorts in five U.S. community populations. Arch Gen Psychiatry *48:* 789, 1991.

Cross-National Collaborative Group: The changing rate of major depression: Cross-national comparisons. JAMA *268:* 3098, 1992.

Dean C, Surtees P G, Sashidharian S P: Comparison of research diagnostic systems in an Edinburgh community sample. Br J Psychiatry *142:* 247, 1983.

Goldstein R B, Weissman M M, Adams P B, Horwath E, Lish J D, Charney D, Woods S W, Sopbin C, Wickramaratne P J: Psychiatric disorders in relatives of probands with panic disorder and/or major depression. Arch Gen Psychiatry *51:* 383, 1994.

Gonzales J J, Magruder K M, Keith S J: Mental disorders in primary care services: An update. Public Health Rep *109:* 251, 1994.

Henderson S, Duncan-Jones P, Byrne D G, Scott R, Adcock S: Psychiatric disorder in Canberra: A standardized study of prevalence. Acta Psychiatr Scand *60:* 355, 1979.

Hollingshead A B, Redlich F C: *Social Class and Mental Illness.* Wiley, New York, 1958.

*Kahn H A, Sempos C T: *Statistical Methods in Epidemiology.* Oxford University Press, New York, 1989.

*Kessler R C, McGonagle K A, Zhao S, Nelson C B, Hughes M, Eshleman S, Witchen H U, Kendler K S: Lifetime and 12-month prevalence of DSM-III-R psychiatric disorders in the United States: Results from the National Comorbidity Survey. Arch Gen Psychiatry *51:* 8, 1994.

Kety S S, Wender P H, Jacobsen B, Ingraham L J, Jansson L, Faber B, Kinney D: Mental illness in the biological and adoptive relatives of schizophrenic adoptees: Replication of the Copenhagen study in the rest of Denmark. Arch Gen Psychiatry *51:* 442, 1994.

Kleinbaum D G, Kupper L L, Morgenstern H: *Epidemiologic Research: Principles and Quantitative Methods.* Lifetime Learning Publications, Belmont, CA, 1982.

Kramer M S: *Clinical Epidemiology and Biostatistics: A Primer for Clinical Investigators and Decision-Makers.* Springer-Verlag, Berlin, 1988.

Leighton D C, MacMillan A M, Harding H S, Macklin D B, Leighton A H: *The Character of Danger.* Basic Books, New York, 1963.

Mavreas V G, Beis A, Mouyias A, Rigoni F, Lyketsos G C: Prevalence of psychiatric disorders in Athens: A community study. Soc Psychiatry *21:* 172, 181, 1986.

Michels R, Marzuk P M: Progress in psychiatry. N Engl J Med *329:* 552, 1993.

Morris J N: *Uses of Epidemiology,* ed 2. Williams & Wilkins, Baltimore, 1964.

Orley J, Wing J K: Psychiatric disorders in two African villages. Arch Gen Psychiatry *36:* 513, 1979.

Regier D A: ECA contributions to national policy and further research. Int J Methods Psychiatr Res *4*: 73, 1994.

Regier D A, Boyd J H, Rae D S, Burke J D, Locke B Z, Myers J K, Kramer M, Robins L N, George L K, Karno M: One-month prevalence of mental disorders in the U.S.: Based on five epidemiologic catchment area (ECA) sites. Arch Gen Psychiatry *45:* 977, 1988.

*Regier D A, Narrow W E, Rae D S, Manderscheid R W, Locke B Z, Goodwin F K: The de facto U.S. mental and addictive disorders service system: Epidemiologic Catchment Area prospective one-year prevalence rates of disorders and services: Arch Gen Psychiatry *50:* 85, 1993.

*Robins L N, Regier D A, editors: *Psychiatric Disorders in America.* Free Press, New York, 1990.

Samuels J F, Nestadt G, Romanoski A J, Folstein M F, McHugh P R: DSM-III personality disorders in the community. Am J Psychiatry *151:* 1055, 1994.

Schwab-Stone M, Fallon T, Briggs M, Crowther B: Reliability of diagnostic reporting for children aged 6–11 years: A test-retest study of the Diagnostic Interview Schedule for Children-Revised. Am J Psychiatry *151:* 1048, 1994.

Weissman M M, Myers J K, Harding P S: Psychiatric disorders in a U.S. urban community: 1975–1976. Am J Psychiatry *135:* 459, 1978.

Wittchen H U, Robins L N, Cottler L B, Sartorius N, Burke J D, Regier D A: Cross-cultural feasibility, reliability, and sources of variance of the Composite International Diagnostic Interview (CIDI). Br J Psychiatry *159:* 645, 1991.

5.2
ANIMAL RESEARCH AND ITS RELEVANCE TO PSYCHIATRY

WILLIAM T. McKINNEY, M.D.

INTRODUCTION

Since the previous edition of this textbook, the field of animal research as it relates to psychiatry has continued to undergo rapid development despite the continued lack of an effective, organized effort at the federal level. Increasing attempts have been directed to conceptual clarification of the role of animal models, including their advantages and limitations in the study of human development and psychopathology, and a broader range of animal preparations with important interfaces to the basic and clinical sciences have been developed.

A theme which will be apparent throughout this section is that there is no single comprehensive animal model for any clinical syndrome. All proposed animal models have their advantages and limitations. However, there is a range of models for studying specific components or aspects of psychiatric illness, and, indeed, that is a more useful way of viewing animal models (that is, as experimental preparations developed in one species for understanding phenomena occurring in another species).

The primary focus of this section will be on presenting the rationale for the use of animals in psychiatric research and on discussing the general categories of animal models. Animal research relevant to three illustrative disorders, mood disorders, schizophrenia, and anxiety disorders will be discussed in more detail to illustrate the general conceptual points.

Obviously, one has to be cautious and scientifically accurate in cross-species reasoning. Overextended comparisons have no place in comparative psychiatry and have sometimes given the field a bad name. However, there are principles to guide attempts to learn something about the behavior or neurobiology of one species by studying another species, and they must always be respected and used.

Most psychiatric illness can be best understood by using a multivariate approach. Animal studies, where variables can be controlled rather precisely, have the potential for permitting the study of both the main effects of single variables and, especially, how they interact. Such approaches are highly relevant to a biopsychosocial view of human psychopathology.

HISTORY

Ivan Pavlov is often said to have been the originator of research relevant to animal modeling of human psychopathology in general. His use of clinical terms, as well as the experimental techniques he used, may seem foreign to most psychiatric clinicians. However, the fact that his work represented one of the first moves away from the correlational method of behavioral analysis to the experimental study of psychopathology is of central importance. As H. D. Kimmel has said:

> The significance of this change in direction may best be comprehended in relation to its two most important implications. First, the completely correlational method of behavioral analysis, which was the empirical foundation of all earlier systematic efforts to understand psychological abnormality, including everything from Hippocrates' humors and Franz Gall's prominences to the ingenious psychoanalytic theorizing of Sigmund Freud, could now be supplemented, if not altogether supplanted, by a direct experimental approach which was much less fraught with the dual dangers of loose conjecture and empirical untestability. Second, and historically of possible greater significance, the continuity of animal morphology, physiology, and behavior, already beginning to assume a position on center stage in man's philosophical thinking, received a new extensive thrust from the early Pavlovian findings since for the first time even such uniquely human phenomena as emotional breakdowns were seen to occur in subhuman animals.

Pavlov was followed by a number of other workers, and it is difficult to know what conclusions to draw about the early history of the field of experimental psychopathology research. Some have not seen it as a particularly noteworthy beginning. However, the early pioneers may have been more successful than it appears in developing certain principles that seem to be being rediscovered today. Those include the following:

1. The demonstration that psychopathology could be experimentally studied in animals as well as in the strictly correlational studies done previously in humans.
2. The demonstration of the importance of both careful behavioral observations and serendipity. Although most of the early workers did not use the more sophisticated and quantifiable behavioral scoring techniques now available, they were keen observers and literate in their descriptions.
3. The repeated proposal of an interactive model of psychopathology. The role of the temperament of the animals, along with a variety of social and neurobiological variables, was repeatedly stressed in the early literature. The concept of individual variability was part of the early work, and investigation of the sources of such variability continues to be an important area of research.
4. The development that there could be a persistent internal response, even after the inducing stimulus was no longer present, a discovery that remains a major contribution to the understanding of a number of forms of psychopathology.
5. The recognition of the importance of unpredictability and uncontrollability of which systematic investigations continue today.
6. Experimental paradigms for adaptive behavioral processes that provide the foundation on which maladaptive behavior patterns are built in the presence of altered environmental demands. Adaptive mechanisms of animals and humans are fragile and share a tenuous relationship with the environment. Either internal changes in the organism (for example, with drugs or other altered neurochemistry) or changes in the external environment (for example, separation, the imposition of uncontrollability) can lead to serious behavioral changes, which can, in turn, lead to neurobiological changes and the development of a vicious circle. The study of those interactions is becoming a cornerstone of animal modeling research in depression and other forms of psychopathology.

One of the problems in early experimental psychopathology was that clinical terms were applied far too loosely and prematurely to a set of behavioral changes induced by methods that seemed to bear only a faint resemblance to inducing conditions for human syndromes. The result was a certain amount of skepticism and cynicism about the whole field by clinicians.

The work of Harry Harlow, in particular, helped to stimulate interest by clinicians in the field of primate behavioral research. With his passing in 1981 the field of primatology lost one of its most prominent scientists.

Harlow's research with primates began in about 1930 with observations at the local zoo. He soon discovered that monkeys and apes were much smarter than rats, and that tests designed to study rodent learning did not begin to tap the primates' intellectual capabilities. It became apparent that more challenging or complex learning tasks and a better physical environment in which to test his primates were needed. Harlow addressed those two basic problems by developing the Wisconsin General Test Apparatus and a primate laboratory.

The Wisconsin General Test Apparatus brought to the study of primate learning capabilities a means by which a large number of discrete learning tests could be rapidly presented in highly standardized fashion to subject after subject. Studies of primate learning proliferated in the following years, and a battery of discrimination learning and memory tasks was developed that provided a standardized intelligence test for monkeys. Harlow then proceeded to study cortical localization of learning capabilities by lesioning different primate brain areas and noting subsequent differential patterns of deficits in their performance on the test battery.

In the late 1940s Harlow achieved a major conceptual and methodological breakthrough with his discovery of learning sets. He showed that rhesus monkeys presented with long series of six-trial, two-choice discrimination problems soon learned to achieve near-perfect performance on the second and subsequent trials of each problem. He was able to demonstrate unequivocally that the monkeys had acquired a strategy for problem solving. What the monkeys had learned was an abstract concept ("learning to learn," in his words), rather than the product of simple associative learning.

Harlow's interest in the processes underlying primate learning extended to two lines of research. The first line involved motivation. In an effort to understand the factors that influenced learning performance, he discovered major inconsistencies with classic notions of drive reduction. It was not readily apparent why monkeys should solve puzzles more effectively when motivated by mere curiosity than when driven by hunger or thirst, but they did. Convinced that drive reduction and other motivational theories then in vogue in psychology and psychiatry could not possibly account for most of a monkey's behaviors, he began to look for alternative formulations.

At about the same time, Harlow began studies of the ontogenic development of learning capabilities in rhesus monkeys. The task required both devising a new battery of age-sensitive learning tests and acquiring suitable subjects. The latter requirement led to the establishment of a captive breeding colony and a nursery suitable for the hand-rearing of large numbers of baby monkeys.

More recent work from Mortimer Mishkin's laboratory has demonstrated that an experience can enter into memory in monkeys in two ways: (1) as cognitive information stored in a cortico-limbo-thalamo-cortical system involving higher-order sensory areas of the cortex, amygdala, hippocampus and interrhinal cortex, medial thalamic nuclei, ventromedial prefrontal cortex, and basal forebrain, and (2) as a habit perhaps stored in a cortical striatal system involving sensory cortical areas, caudate, and putamen. The two systems seem to be developmentally dissociable. The system for noncognitive association (habit system) seems to develop early in infancy. By contrast, the system for cognitive association (memory system) appears to develop late in infancy, presumably because the neural circuit on which it depends has a slow ontogenetic maturation. Neonatal removal of the limbic system (that is, combined amygdalo-hippocampal removal) produces a severe memory deficit from birth onward that is accompanied by socio-emotional abnormalities that are strikingly similar to those seen in autistic children (that is, they have in common an absence of social interactions, blank facial expressions, motor stereotypies, and memory deficits). Thus, neonatal damage that leads to a severe memory disorder can have extremely serious consequences for personality and social development, in part because of the cognitive memory impairment that is present from infancy onward, but also because of the direct effect of limbic lesions on mechanisms of emotionality.

Next came the cloth- and wire-covered surrogate mothers and the entrance of primatology into clinical psychiatry. Infant rhesus monkeys reared with a choice between a wire surrogate that fed them and a cloth surrogate that did not overwhelmingly preferred the cloth "mother." Contrary to prevailing wisdom, contact comfort, as Harlow called it, was much more instrumental than feeding in bonding those infants to their surrogates. Harlow's discoveries with the surrogates sounded the end for drive reduction theory and revolutionized thinking about the socialization process in children. They also opened up the field of primate social development to serious scientific inquiry.

Eventually, Harlow shifted the major focus of his research to the study of social behavior and its development, both normal and abnormal. He developed the concept of affectional systems, the idea that social ontogeny involves the establishment of qualitatively different types of social relationships with a variety of others in the social network—parents, siblings, peers—as one grows up. At the same time, he studied the consequences of blocking the formation of different affectional systems through social isolation rearing or disrupting the attachment bonds once formed by experimental separations. Those studies clearly established the overwhelming importance of early social experiences for the development of species-normative adult social activities, including reproduction and maternal behavior.

Harlow spent his last years at Wisconsin expanding on the twin themes of normal and abnormal social behavior. Along with Margaret Harlow, he was instrumental in establishing the nuclear family living unit, in which adult male-female pairs and various offspring could live together in a laboratory but in a situation rich in stimulation compared with the more typical laboratory environment.

Harlow made a career of using rhesus monkey subjects to study human capabilities and problems not easily researched in humans themselves, and many of the fundamental concepts he developed, which were the source of considerable controversy at the time, are now fully incorporated into developmental theories.

RATIONALE FOR USING ANIMALS IN PSYCHIATRIC RESEARCH

The following reasons for including animal modeling research as part of a comprehensive psychopathology research program are illustrative rather than comprehensive. Issues concerning the development, practical use, and potential benefits of animal models are also summarized in Table 5.2-1.

1. Many critical questions about the origins of human psychopathology cannot be studied directly in humans. By using animal preparations, it is possible to control inducing conditions rather precisely and to study the behavioral and neurobiological effects on both a short-term and long-term basis. For example, in relation to depression, prospective studies examining the effects of developmental events on behavior and on neurobiology can be done much more easily in animals. The timing and exact nature of certain alterations in development can be specified, and the short- and long-term consequences studied. That aspect of modeling research is relevant to the question of developmental vulnerability based on early experiences and the mediating mechanisms of vulnerability.

A particular line of research where animal preparations have a special contribution to make is in prospective studies of the effects of developmental events on behavior and neurochemistry. The interactions between those variables can be studied in a controlled and prospective manner. Animal preparations have been developing in the past decade that make such investigations feasible and that will facilitate the movement beyond correlation and retrospective analysis to cause-and-effect studies.

2. The underlying mechanisms associated with specific behaviors and patterns of behaviors can be studied more directly in certain animal species. Animal models potentially make possible the dissection of mechanisms in a more direct way than is possible in human clinical research, and they complement ongoing efforts in human protocols. More direct, and potentially more invasive, studies of neurobiological mechanisms can be done, although such procedures need to be suited to both the species and the overall purpose of the experimental paradigm. Not all procedures are justified on ethical or economic grounds in all species. The questions have to be clear and specific, especially in proposing such studies in higher-order primates.

The time is ripe for a vigorous effort in that area. The area of experimental psychopathology in animals has become complex enough to require the involvement of multiple laboratories, much as collaborative human studies of psychopathology often involve many centers. For example, different strategies and approaches need to be employed with several species, and techniques now generally available in only one laboratory need to be applied to many of those preparations. Attention needs to be given to how to do what kinds of mechanism studies in a given species. Molecular or submolecular studies may be indicated in some preparations, but that may not be the only reasonable way to approach mechanism studies, for example, in a socially behaving species. The issues are complex but probably solvable with enough discussion and with the development of some collaborative protocols across laboratories that take advantage of complementing expertise.

3. Single variables can be evaluated in terms of their main effects and in terms of the nature of their interaction with each other. For example, the nature of the interactions among genetic, developmental, social, and biological variables can be studied in various combinations in different species. In human clinical research, multiple variables interact simultaneously, and it has been impossible to sort them out in any quantifiable way.

4. The ability to isolate specific behavior patterns in animals and to study their origins, pathophysiology, and responsiveness to treatment techniques is important. Typically, in clinical work one is dealing with a broad range of behaviors that occur together, and it is impossible to study one or two in isolation and to understand them more completely. The many examples include anhedonia, stereotypic rituals, social withdrawal, and altered learning and cognitive abilities. If one can begin to understand those and other particular aspects of psychopathological syndromes better, it might be possible to expand the understanding of situations where they typically occur together.

5. Animal models have played an important role in the preclinical evaluation of drugs. That topic, which relates to the empirical or predictive validity of animal models, will be discussed further with regard to the general kinds of animal models.

A related aspect of the use of animal models is their contribution to a better understanding of the mechanism of the action of drugs in altering specific behavior patterns. That assistance goes beyond a mere prediction of whether drugs work or do not work and relates to the behavioral effects of agents with relatively specific mechanisms of action.

6. Animal models can also be used to help understand the mechanisms of established treatment techniques. They potentially make possible the investigation of the mechanisms in terms not only of pathogenesis but also of treatment responsiveness. That is, why do some drugs work whereas others do not? What are the mechanisms of action of electroconvulsive therapy in depression? Why are certain behavioral interventions effective and others are not?

7. Animal models also permit the understanding of a specific behavior or set of behaviors in terms of the developmental and social context as well as pathophysiologically. Rather than focusing on global syndromes, one can investigate behaviors as to their origin, context, and responsiveness to certain interventions.

8. Animal modeling research, especially with primates, has led to the development of improved behavioral, ethologically based rating methods that can now be used in clinical research

TABLE 5.2-1
The Development, Practical Use, and Potential Benefits of Various Types of Animal Models

Criteria for Development	Use in Research	Benefits
Similarity of inducing conditions Similarity of behavioral syndromes Similarity of neurobiological mechanisms Similarity in response to clinically effective treatments Other criteria appropriate for the specific model	Treatment screens Study of developmental determinants Study of underlying mechanisms Study of interactions between social and biological components	New treatments Better definition of syndromes in humans Identification of at-risk persons Development of improved diagnostic tests

settings to evaluate social interactions, as between mother and infant or among peers.

In his work with animal models of depression, Paul Wilner provides additional perspective on the rationale and philosophy of using animals in psychiatric research. He makes the point that, in the case of depression, animal models have been most frequently encountered in the pharmaceutical industry, where they have been used in screening tests in the development of new antidepressants. He indicates that animal models are also being used as simulations for investigating the psychobiology of depression, and that some models have been specifically developed for that purpose. His concepts of validity include *predictive validity,* which primarily concerns the correspondence between drug actions in the model and in the clinic, *face validity,* which includes phenomenological similarities between the model and the disorder, and *construct validity,* which is a sound theoretical rationale for the model.

There are a number of approaches in developing animal models for any psychiatric disorder, and there is no such thing as a best model for any single syndrome. Animal models should be understood as basically experimental preparations that are developed in one species for the purpose of studying phenomena occurring in other species. The concern should be, and increasingly is, to develop a variety of experimental paradigms in animals to study selected aspects of human psychopathology rather than to attempt to develop a model of a given syndrome. Certain paradigms are suitable for studying certain phenomena, whereas others are more suitable for studying other aspects. The best model for depression, schizophrenia, and so on depends on what the question is.

CATEGORIES OF ANIMAL MODELS

Animal models can be divided into four categories: (1) those developed to simulate a specific sign or symptom of the human disorder (behavioral similarity models); (2) those developed to evaluate etiological theories (theory-driven models); (3) those developed with the primary purpose of studying underlying mechanisms (mechanistic models); (4) those developed to permit preclinical evaluation of treatment methods (empirical validity models). There is obvious overlap among the categories.

BEHAVIORAL SIMILARITY MODELS Behavioral similarity models are designed to simulate specific symptoms of the human disorder in animals. The primary intent is to produce a particular symptom or set of symptoms, not to evaluate any specific etiological theory or to study underlying mechanisms or treatment responsiveness. The validity is judged by how closely the model approximates the human disorder from a phenomenological standpoint.

THEORY-DRIVEN MODELS In a theory-driven model a theory drives the development of a specific experimental paradigm. It is not necessary to assume the validity of the theory in order to proceed with the research. The attempt is made to operationalize the theory and to develop experimental paradigms to evaluate the effects of such inducing conditions. The approach is sometimes criticized on the basis that the theory has not been substantiated in humans, so its use in animals is questionable. The response is that the very reason for developing the paradigm is to test or evaluate the theory. Most etiological theories of psychopathology have developed from studies of sick humans and, therefore, are retrospective. Using inducing conditions as an independent variable, one can evaluate prospectively the effects of specific conditions designed to represent certain causative theories.

MECHANISTIC MODELS The issue of the use of animals to study mechanisms is complex. For some, mechanism studies represent the only reason for developing animal models, which are evaluated by how well they lend themselves to those studies. With the increasing availability of high-technology methods for studying underlying neurobiological mechanisms, many researchers have become preoccupied with the molecular and submolecular basis of the altered behavior seen in many proposed animal models, and they consider useful only a model that permits those types of studies.

One must be careful, however, with the term "mechanisms." Mechanistic studies certainly include the application of high-technology neuroscience techniques to the study of different mechanisms in the various models, but they also include social, behavioral, and developmental mechanisms. One cannot necessarily transpose techniques of mechanism studies from rodents to monkeys or vice versa. One must study mechanisms as appropriate in a particular species and recognize that each approach has certain advantages and disadvantages. Behavior and psychopathology occur in a social and developmental context and, therefore, the continued study and monitoring of social behavior is essential. A serious challenge for researchers remains the development of noninvasive techniques for mechanism studies in socially behaving animals that will be satisfactory to basic neuroscientists as mechanism studies. Compromises between directness of neurobiological studies and sophisticated ongoing assessment of social behaviors may be necessary.

EMPIRICAL VALIDITY MODELS The best known and oldest use of animal models involves the use of animal preparation to develop and test clinically effective drugs. Basically, an ideal animal model would be one in which there are no false positives and no false negatives; that is, when a drug works in animals it is predictive of its clinical effects in humans and vice versa. Unfortunately, there is never 100 percent correspondence between the effects of a drug in an animal model and in a clinical condition, although there are a number of models with established high empirical validity. The establishment of an animal model as valid on empirical grounds (or on any other grounds) does not necessarily establish its validity on other parameters.

ILLUSTRATIVE ANIMAL MODELS

MOOD DISORDERS

Pharmacological models In one approach, drugs are administered to animals in order to reproduce some of the phenomenology of human depressive syndromes. A related approach is to use certain drugs to produce a set of changes in animals that do not necessarily resemble human depression but have high empirical validity in terms of predicting clinical drug responses. A third class of animal models is heterogeneous and, although not based on drug-induced changes, has been found useful in predicting and characterizing antidepressant activity. That type of model may have empirical validity in terms of drug screening, but in terms of induction techniques or behaviors, it bears little relationship to human depression (for example, the bulbectomized rat syndrome and kindled amygdaloid convulsions).

Among pharmacological models, the syndrome induced by reserpine (Serpasil) and related compounds has been the most widely used. Reserpine, when given to animals of various species, produces a characteristic set of behaviors, including ptosis, hypothermia, inactivity, social withdrawal, and sedation. The interest in that animal model came from the clinical observation that drugs containing reserpine were reported to induce depression in humans who took them for the treatment of hypertension. That clinical observation, at least in its initial form, has been called into question on the basis of recent evidence. It appears that humans who become depressed while taking reserpine-containing drugs have a history of depression and are presumably vulnerable in that area.

The reserpine syndrome as an animal model of depression has been reviewed extensively. In addition, a number of related compounds have been used to induce symptoms qualitatively similar to those produced by reserpine, although a number of factors are different, such as the speed of onset, duration, and central and peripheral effects. Initially, it was thought that most clinically active antidepressant drugs antagonized some or all of the symptoms induced by reserpine. In general, that is true, but there are a number of inconsistencies. The reserpine syndrome is not a unitary entity, but involves many different effects. For example, ptosis antagonism, although probably a peripheral effect, seems to characterize the greatest number of clinically effective antidepressants, including several of the newer ones, some of which are regarded as false negatives in other reserpine procedures. In evaluating the empirical validity of the model, one must be specific about which behavior is involved. Some behaviors could have high empirical validity in terms of predicting clinical drug response, although the mediating mechanism may not even be central in origin. Reserpine has so many different neurochemical effects that one cannot reason directly from such studies to possible mechanisms associated with the behaviors produced, let alone human depression.

Several other pharmacologically induced models have been developed. One is the amphetamine withdrawal model. Animals subjected to repeated amphetamine treatments, which are then stopped, evince a number of effects, including decreases in motor activity and self-stimulation behavior. Those effects have been reported to be reversed to a certain extent by amitriptyline (Elavil), imipramine (Tofranil), mianserin, and pargyline (Eutonyl), when given on an acute basis, but especially when given on a chronic basis.

Another proposed pharmacological model is clonidine (Catapres)-induced behavioral depression. Clonidine, an α-adrenergic receptor stimulant, is thought to act at presynaptic receptor sites to reduce the release of norepinephrine, resulting in hypothermia, analgesia, and marked sedation. Clonidine-induced hypoactivity has been proposed as a test for antidepressant drugs. Although it is not clear which drugs will work in that model, it may play a role in screening for antidepressants that might be inactive in other models.

Another class of procedures widely used in pharmacology involves the potentiation by antidepressants of the behavioral and other effects of amines or their precursors. Those procedures do not attempt to mimic the clinical condition, but are based on theories about the role of the amines in depression. Thus, they are designed to show how amines interact with each other and are influenced by antidepressant drugs. By such routes, important information can be obtained that may ultimately have a bearing on mechanism questions, which can be tested in more highly developed behavioral models. Examples of such procedures include the potentiation by antidepressants of the various central effects of amphetamine and yohimbine (Yocon).

Pharmacologically induced models continue to be important for screening clinically effective drugs. Thus, in evaluating them, attention should be paid primarily to their empirical or predictive validity. Each has false negatives and false positives, but by using several such tests in a battery, it may be possible to achieve an even higher degree of empirical validity.

In the case of all empirically based tests, it should be kept in mind that the mechanism by which the drug presumably acts in the animal preparation is not necessarily the same as its mechanism of action in human depression. Too many variables can intervene, and additional types of animal preparations may be necessary to assist with mechanism questions.

Separation models Disruption of attachment bonds, whether in humans or nonhumans, has been established as a very stressful event. Humans and many animal species are in their most stable condition when they have developed secure social attachment systems. Disruption of such systems almost invariably leads to the development of grief reactions and can precipitate clinical depression in some vulnerable individuals. Many developmental, social, and neurobiological variables are known to influence the reaction to separation. However, determining the influence of those variables in humans, and how they interact with one another, has been extremely difficult. Investigators have therefore turned to animal models for a more systematic study of the effects of separation.

BEHAVIORAL RESPONSES TO MATERNAL SEPARATION The earliest work on separation in animals began in the 1960s at a number of laboratories with the short-term separation of pigtail macaque infants from their mothers at the ages of 5 and 7 months, followed by reuniting them with their own or another mother. The behaviors seen following separation have been divided into two categories, labeled agitation or protest, and depression or despair.

The protest and despair response seen in many primate species after maternal separation has been compared with the responses in human children diagnosed with anaclitic depression or observed in institutions (usually hospitals or nurseries) where they were unavoidably separated from their mothers and families. The stages of response of human infants to maternal separation have been described as protest, despair, and denial (later changed to detachment). Those stages have played a key role in the development of the theory of primary separation anxiety.

As animal researchers extended the original work on the response to maternal separation, it became apparent that the response of the infants was influenced by a number of parameters, including the species, age, and social conditions.

The reaction to maternal separation in primates represents a true biobehavioral syndrome. Not only are there significant behavioral effects as described above, but there are also major neurobiological changes.

PHYSIOLOGICAL RESPONSES TO MATERNAL SEPARATION Pigtail macaque infants undergoing maternal separation have been studied using totally implanted multichannel biotelemetry systems to monitor heart rate, body temperature, and sleep physiology before, during, and after the separation. In those studies, the biological mother was usually removed from a group living situation and the infant was left in the group. Attachment bonds have been found to be as central to the development of monkeys as they are to humans, with disruption of those bonds leading to serious changes. In one study, for example, the infant's heart rate and body temperature increased significantly immediately after maternal separation. The changes were most pronounced early in separation and diminished as the separation continued. Beginning with the first night, both the heart rate and body temperature showed marked decreases from baseline levels and the behavioral patterns became more depressivelike. During reunion, both the heart rate and body temperature returned to normal, although some infants exhibited a lower heart rate well into the reunion. An increased incidence of cardiac arrhythmias as a result of maternal separation has also been reported. Significant sleep changes have included increased sleep latency, more frequent arousals, less total sleep, and a disruption of rapid eye movement (REM) sleep.

In other research, neurochemical effects were examined in rhesus monkey infants that were in the protest stage following maternal separation. Positive findings included elevated serotonin levels in the hypothalamus and significantly higher levels in the adrenal gland of all of the major enzymes involved in catecholamine syntheses. Resting levels of norepinephrine and dopamine were unchanged in any of the brain regions examined. The study measured resting levels of those substances at one point in time and thus gives no information about possible dynamic changes occurring over time. However, it provides additional confirmation of the powerful effects of disrupting the maternal attachment bond. The syndrome is neither transient nor mild.

Squirrel monkeys, when separated from their mother or from a surrogate, show a marked increase in the pituitary-adrenal response. Initially, it was reported that there was an identical physiological response whether the infant was separated from a mother or from a surrogate. The monkey mother also showed an elevated corticoid response to separation. The latter finding is interesting in that the mother's responses to infant removal have been very minimally described in most studies because investigators have been preoccupied with assessment of the infant. The mother has been typically described as acutely upset but as getting over it very quickly. The infant's corticoid response was felt to be due to the separation itself rather than to the new cage in which it was housed during the separation phase, and that finding has been supported by data from a number of studies. The presence of a familiar animal during the separation phase did not alter the corticoid response, suggesting that the disruption of the specific attachment bond between mother and infant was the main cause of the increased corticoid levels.

Physiological and behavioral changes following separation may not occur simultaneously. For example, separation from the surrogate results in a behavioral response but no corticoid response. Later work shows that infants of highly dominant mothers manifest the greatest adrenocortical response to separation, and that they may not always exhibit concomitant behavioral changes. This important research illustrates the complexity of understanding the neurobiological and behavioral changes that may accompany separation. It is important to obtain adequate baseline behavioral profiles of both the group structure and individual behavioral assessments.

Desipramine (Norpramin) has been reported to be effective in preventing the response to maternal separation in primates, and imipramine has a similar therapeutic effect on the responses to peer separation.

OTHER RESPONSES TO MATERNAL SEPARATION When infant lagur monkeys were separated from their mothers at 6 to 8 months of age, all infants showed changes in social behavior, which varied from minimal to severe and included two deaths. All infants sought substitute caretaking during the separation and adopted a major substitute caretaker. Most infants remained with the substitute even when the mother returned.

Some researchers have used distress vocalizations in various animals as an index of separation and have studied the effects of many pharmacological agents on those vocalizations. In general, the distress vocalizations are reported to be relieved by morphine and made worse by the narcotic antagonist naloxone (Narcan) when those drugs are given as single injections. A variety of opiatelike peptides have been tested, and all have been reported to be effective in decreasing distress vocalizations in separated animals when injected into the vicinity of the fourth ventricle in quite low doses. Additional maternal separation studies have been done using canine puppies, guinea pigs, and chicks. From those studies, researchers have developed the theory that brain endorphins may play a critical role in the mediation of social bonds, and that when those bonds are disrupted by separation, a syndrome much like that following narcotic withdrawal is produced.

PEER SEPARATION Rhesus monkeys and most other primate species develop strong, complex social bonds, and paradigms have been developed that involve experimental disruption of those bonds in peers of various ages, including adults. In general, the behavioral reaction to peer separation is quite similar to that following maternal separation in terms of the classic protest-despair response. Furthermore, when peer groups are formed and separations are repeated, the response is seen with each separation. Not surprisingly, a number of variables can influence the nature of the response, including age; rearing conditions; housing conditions before, during, and after each separation; and treatment with pharmacological agents. Significant individual variability can be related to a number of developmental and neurobiological variables. For example, cerebrospinal fluid (CSF) norepinephrine appears to be a trait-related marker predicting a more severe response to separations. Animals with lower CSF norepinephrine respond to separation with more huddling and self-directed behaviors than animals with higher levels. By contrast, CSF homovanillic acid (HVA) and 5-hydroxyindoleacetic acid (5-HIAA) are state-related markers that reflect the behavioral response to separation no matter how the response is obtained.

Pharmacological agents can affect the response to peer separation. Imipramine reverses the reaction to peer separation and prevents the reaction to future separations as long as the monkeys are kept on it. They return to more typical separation behavior when the drug is withdrawn. Amphetamine modifies the behavioral response to separation in a very similar manner to imipramine, but the overall effects of the two drugs on group social behavior can be distinguished. *a*-Methylparatyrosine, which blocks tyrosine hydroxylase and thereby lowers norepinephrine and dopamine levels, can exacerbate the response to peer separation at doses so low that they have no effect when the monkeys are living as a stable social group. It is only when one combines the stress of separation with low-dose *a*-methylparatyrosine that one sees other effects of the drug in that paradigm. Parachlorphenylalanine, which blocks serotonin synthesis, has no effect. Low doses of alcohol alleviate the peer separation response whereas high doses make it worse.

RESEARCH APPLICATIONS With regard to proposed depression models, the rationale for separation studies in animals is that the bulk of evidence strongly suggests social separations as risk factors that cut across types of depressions. Animal studies represent one way of studying those risk factors. Although many factors are involved in depression, separations appear to be important events for vulnerable individuals and so are worthy of additional investigation. An even more important context in which to view separation studies is as prototypes for the study of stressful events in general. With the recent advances in the knowledge of both developmental and neurobiological influences on behavior, it becomes increasingly important to have experimental paradigms in which the interactions between neurobiological factors and social risk factors can be examined. That type of animal preparation provides the opportunity to control social and developmental variables and to do prospective studies of both behavioral and neurobiological parameters. The long-term effects of early alterations can be examined in a much shorter period of time. One can obtain repeated measurements of neurobiological variables, as in the CSF, in a way that cannot be carried out in humans and in relation to specific units of behavior. One can also evaluate the effects of drugs on parameters similar to those being studied in humans, and determine what those changes mean with regard to specific social behaviors. The role that specific neurotransmitter systems play in influencing specific units of social behavior, including responses to separation, can also be clarified. Humans are fundamentally social creatures, and an understanding of the social origins of psychopathology and how they are related to neurotransmitter systems becomes possible in that kind of preparation.

Learned helplessness The animal model of learned helplessness has been extensively studied for more than 15 years. It relates closely to some important aspects of clinical depression, particularly cognitive aspects, such as a negative conception of the self, negative interpretations of one's experiences, and a negative view of the future. Those cognitive aspects are reflected in feelings of helplessness and hopelessness. Whether the phenomena are primary or secondary is a moot point for the present discussion. The point is that they occur as core aspects of depression frequently enough to be worthy of further study. Both etiological theories and therapeutic approaches have developed from that cognitive view of depression.

In the original experimental study with animals, dogs were placed in one of three situations. In the first situation, they were put in harnesses and subjected to electric shock that they could terminate by touching a panel. Not surprisingly, they learned to escape the shock rather quickly. In the second situation, the dogs were prepared as in the preceding situation, but when the shock was given, they were unable to terminate it. Finally, to control for the effect of the shock itself, dogs were put in harnesses but were not shocked at all. In phase 2 of the study, dogs were given electric shock while unharnessed in a shuttle box. Normally, dogs have no difficulty learning to avoid the shock by going to the other side of the box, which proved to be true for the dogs that had been exposed to escapable shock while in the harness. However, the dogs that had been exposed to inescapable shock failed to learn that they could escape from the electric shock in phase 2 by jumping over a barrier that separated the two sides of the shuttle box. They were described as being initially agitated in reaction to the shock but, rather than to run around frantically until they discovered that they could escape the shock by crossing the barrier, they would sit or lie down, quietly whining—that is, they acted as if they were helpless and incapable of escaping. The interpretation was that something had happened during the earlier experience to make them unable to cope with the present situation, and that that something was the inescapable shock. One explanation was that they had learned during their initial experience that outcomes were not contingent on their behavior. No matter what they did, it did no good; they learned to be helpless.

In an attempt to reverse this state, attempts were made to retrain the dogs by trying to coax them across the barrier. That strategy was very difficult, and ultimately it was found that the only effective way was to drag the dogs across the barrier forcibly and thus to terminate the shock. It took many efforts before most of the dogs could learn that response and do it by themselves when placed in the shuttle box.

Recent studies suggest cortisol may be specifically elevated in helpless animals. One study found that animals showing deficits in escape performance have norepinephrine depletions, specifically in the locus ceruleus, and the researchers have used an antagonist to manipulate that system. They suggest that the α_2-receptor system is involved. That has been confirmed in mice by other studies on the effects of serotonin and acetylcholine. Other investigators have suggested specific alterations in the hippocampal β-receptors that occur with the development of helpless behaviors. They suggest that those changes are reversed by antidepressant drug treatments, and that 5-hydroxytryptamine (5-HT) appears to regulate β-receptor levels in the hippocampus. Along with lesion studies implicating the fornix and septal regions in the behavioral alterations, that study points to the septal-hippocampal pathway as an important site for 5-HT regulation of norepinephrine function. The latter group has been successful in selective breeding for learned helplessness through several generations. That use of the learned helplessness model is leading to some detailed hypotheses about the neurological regulation of affect is improving the understanding of human mood disorders.

RESEARCH APPLICATIONS The literature on learned helplessness is enormous and, as in the case of separation models, controversial. However, one set of recent findings merits closer scrutiny and illustrates clearly how experimental paradigms in animals can be used to investigate the interrelations between behavioral events and neurobiology, an interface critical to understanding human psychopathology. Again, as in the separation models, one does not have to agree with the validity of the model itself to appreciate the value of that kind of work in a spectrum of research approaches aimed at understanding specific aspects of human depression.

Severe, inescapable trauma, for example, has been found to produce a deficiency in central noradrenergic activity, namely, depletion of locus ceruleus norepinephrine levels. However, studies have shown that if the subjects were able to control the noxious experiences, they did not develop the noradrenergic deficiency and were able to respond quite efficiently. When the drop in noradrenergic activity was prevented by treatment with drugs, the learned helplessness phenomenon did not occur. Unfortunately, those kinds of data have sometimes been cited as evidence that the concept of learned helplessness is not valid.

A major finding, by contrast, has shown that a state that is clearly induced behaviorally is associated with major changes in certain neurobiological systems, and that if those changes can be prevented, one can prevent the behavioral state, which results from certain well-described behavioral manipulations, or reverse it once developed. It would be interesting to learn if behavioral reversal of the syndrome leads to reversal of the biological changes, or if reversal of the biological changes alone (once the syndrome is set in motion) will reverse the behavioral aspects. Investigators know that in human depression not all of the significant behavioral and cognitive changes are necessarily reversed with drugs, which presumably alleviate whatever underlying biological alterations may be present. One sometimes has to deal directly with the altered cognitions and behaviors, as well as the underlying neurochemistry. The evidence of a complex interplay between a cognitive-behavioral state and neurobiology clearly warrants further investigation.

Other ongoing work in learned helplessness mainly relates to that interface between the behavioral state and neurochemical substrates. Several such substrates may prove to be important, and it will be critical to ascertain their interaction with behavioral variables.

Chronic stress models In chronic stress paradigms rats are subjected to a chronic stress regimen that is designed to be unpredictable with regard to the stimulus properties of the stress, as well as the time of stress delivery. Stressors are administered every one to two days over a period of 21 days at various points in the circadian cycle. Stressors include switching of cage mates, removal from double housing to single housing for 24 hours, 30 minutes of scrambled unpredictable foot shock, 46 hours of food deprivation, 46 hours of water deprivation, a cold water swim, shaker stress, and tail pinch. After 21 days, when the rats are tested in an open field test situation, they do not exhibit normal open field activity or the usual response to an acute stress. The decreased exploratory behaviors can be reversed by a variety of drugs, including monoamine oxidase inhibitors (MAOIs) and tricyclic antidepressants, as well as by electroconvulsive therapy (ECT). Amphetamine and scopolamine are ineffective. Thus, the model appears to have good pharmacological specificity and is one in which studies of the neurobiological substrates could readily be done. That approach emphasizes the combined influence of chronicity and unpredictability in producing the behavioral alterations.

Changes in dominance in hierarchy Another proposed model reflects the importance of dominance in the relationships of many nonhuman primates. It has been postulated that changes in the stability of the dominance arrangement cause behavioral alterations. It is hypothesized that the behavior that occurs in association with gaining higher dominance ranking may be elation, and with falls in one's position in the hierarchy, depression. Depression, in that theory, is postulated to be adaptive as it prevents the descending animal from fighting back. It has been reasoned that, if this is so, one could try to induce depression by altering the dominance hierarchy in some nonhuman primates. The theory rests on limited data since the evidence for particular behavior patterns occurring in association with specific changes in the hierarchy is fragmentary. Dominance hierarchies are not easy to manipulate. However, recent work concerning dominance and serotonin metabolism will be interesting to follow. The work is not concerned primarily with animal models of depression, but it does involve manipulation of the dominance hierarchy, careful behavioral observations, and study of the serotonin system.

Intracranial self-stimulation models Another proposed animal model of depression is the reward-reduction model using self-stimulating animals. The involvement of catecholamines in the mediation of intracranial self-stimulation (ICSS) has been well established, although there is controversy about their relative importance. In general, agents that enhance the effects of catecholamines tend to increase ICSS responding, whereas those that impair catecholamine actions tend to depress ICSS response rates. However, the actions of tricyclics in the model appear anomalous as they do not enhance ICSS responding despite their well-documented antidepressant action and their effects on catecholamine systems. Those drugs tend to decrease the rate of responding and to raise the reward threshold. Attempts have been made to find an animal model in which tricyclics potentiate ICSS responding. One such model has been suggested, in which reinforcement requires increasing effort. In those progressive fixed-ratio schedules, responding typically drops gradually to zero. Antidepressants have been reported actually to enhance responding. However, efforts to replicate the work have been unsuccessful. Rats that had electrodes chronically implanted in the medial forebrain bundle were trained in progressively increasing fixed ratio schedules. Two tricyclic antidepressants (imipramine and protriptyline [Vivactil]) were given, but neither resulted in response enhancement. Thus, additional work is indicated to evaluate more fully the reward-reduction model involving ICSS as an animal model of depression. It is worth pursuing, however, in view of the important finding that anhedonia is a key feature in many cases of severe depression. It would be valuable to have an animal model in which the mechanism and pharmacology of that sign could be studied.

Conditioned motionlessness The proposed model involves pairing a buzzer (conditioned stimulus) with a tetrabenazine injection (unconditioned stimulus) for at least 11 trials. Following conditioning, some rats exhibited motionlessness after the presentation of the buzzer alone. Imipramine attenuated the conditioned motionlessness. Subsequent neurochemical studies of those rat preparations supported the conclusion that the motionlessness observed was associated with an excess of functional serotonin at the synaptic cleft. Motionlessness after tetrabenazine is not blocked by imipramine. When the conditioned response is reversed by imipramine, however, the biochemical data resemble those for control subjects.

Behavioral despair The model involves the use of a test based on the observation that when rats or mice are forced to swim in a restricted space from which they cannot escape, they eventually cease their attempts to escape and become immobile. It has been suggested that the characteristic behavioral immobility reflects a state of despair in the rats or mice. The immobility is reduced by most clinically active antidepressants, as well as by nonpharmacological treatments such as ECT, REM sleep deprivation, or exposure to an enriched environment. The effects can be seen after acute administration, but more marked effects are seen after repeated treatments with lower doses. The drug effects do not appear to be caused by increased motor activity as the doses used generally decrease motor activity. Antidepressants seem to prolong the escape-directed behavior observed at the beginning of a test session, whereas psychostimulants or anticholinergics cause a generalized behavioral stimulation. Those potential false positives can be distinguished from the effects of true antidepressants. However, as with all models, there are both false positives and false negatives. False-positive results have been reported with antihistamines, subconvulsant doses of convulsants, and some neuropeptides. False negatives have been found with clomipramine (Anafranil) in rats and salbutamol in rats and mice.

The model was developed mainly for drug screening and thus must be evaluated in terms of its empirical validity, which seems at least as good as that of most drug-screening models. At a theoretical level, its relationship with learned helplessness or uncontrollability models needs to be clarified. Mechanism studies remain to be done. Recent years have seen a major expansion in the number of behavioral paradigms that have been proposed as animal models of depression.

Other considerations of animal models of mood disorders Because it is ethically unacceptable to use human subjects to conduct manipulative experimental hypothesis testing research on major depressive disorder, investigators interested in the depressive disorders have turned to observation of models with humans and to interactive models with animals. The models based on limbic dysfunction could be used to explore specific neurosubstrates of depression. In that context, the rat with limbic dysfunction induced by olfactory bulbectomy is felt to fulfill best the requirements for a model of depression. Discovery of a genetic strain of animals that show comparable behavioral and neurovegetative deficits and similar selected drug responses to those seen in depressed patients, would help to advance the field and increase the understanding of the neurobiology of the limbic system.

Comparatively little work has been done to develop animal models of bipolar mood disorders, and that is an area of great need. Most work has involved the antagonism by lithium (Eskalith) of drug-induced states in animals and man. Table 5.2-2 summarizes those studies. Some of the newer thinking is represented by an evolutionary model of manic depressive disorder, the essence of which is that manic and depressive behaviors are evidence of triggered fundamental alpha (α) and omega (ω) states of social rank and not by themselves pathological.

SCHIZOPHRENIA Is it possible to produce an animal model for schizophrenia? Several authors have suggested standards that should be satisfied if a particular preparation is to qualify as an adequate animal model. Those criteria have been mostly drug-related; for instance, clinically effective antipsychotic drugs should reverse the abnormal behaviors, and clinically ineffective drugs should not.

There should be no argument about the need for animal models of psychiatric diseases, in general, and for schizophrenia, in particular. Although significant progress is being made in clinical research on schizophrenia, the development and use of suitable animal preparations could facilitate many kinds of studies that, for ethical and practical reasons, are impossible to do in humans.

There are no animal analogues for many of the core signs and symptoms of schizophrenia. Clinicians and animal researchers need to pay careful attention to ways of making schizophrenic signs and symptoms operational, possibly through a more ethological analysis of human schizophrenia than has so far been done. If different types of human schizophrenia could be analyzed ethologically, the same, or a similar, system could then be applied to the development of animal models, and analogues for specific behaviors might then become more feasible. There also needs to be a major conceptual shift away from the idea that one can develop an animal model of schizophrenia. It is more realistic to develop animal preparations for studying specific aspects of schizophrenia and to understand better some fundamental issues. Figure 5.2-1 summarizes some of the existing animal models of schizophrenia along with some future approaches.

TABLE 5.2-2
Antagonism by Lithium of Drug-Induced States of Animals and Humans

State	Lithium Effect: Humans	Lithium Effect: Animals
Amphetamine (low dose) Hyperactivity, activation	Blocked	Reduced
Amphetamine (high dose) Stereotypical behavior	Unchanged or prolonged	—
Morphine Excitement, euphoria	Reduced or unchanged	Unchanged
DMA plus tetrabenazine Hyperactivity	Reduced or unchanged	—
L-Dopa Hyperactivity, hypomania	—	Possibly reduced
Ethanol High	—	Unchanged
MAO-inhibitor Hyperactivity	Enhanced	—

Drug-related animal models

AMPHETAMINE MODEL The amphetamine model has attracted a considerable amount of attention in connection with schizophrenia and hyperactivity, because amphetamine psychosis in humans can closely mimic paranoid schizophrenia.

Do the data indicate, as some investigators have suggested, that animals become schizophrenic when they are given amphetamine? Clearly, the paranoid delusions have no direct measurable analogue in the animal model, although inferences have been made from certain behaviors. Some investigators have reported that animals are hypervigilant when given amphetamine, as shown by their increased alertness and visual attention to other animals in their environment. Subordinate rats actively withdraw from social interactions, retreat to strategically defensible positions in their environment, and remain hypervigilant. Some have theorized that that behavior may be a manifestation of paranoia.

When given to rats, cats, and monkeys, amphetamine produces stereotypical behaviors, and many researchers find that fact particularly intriguing. It should be remembered that stereotypical behavior is not included in any list of major human schizophrenic symptoms, and, thus, a model is being proposed based mainly on a behavior that is nonspecific and nondiscriminating for schizophrenia. However, from the standpoint of empirical validity, drugs that have antipsychotic properties in humans block the amphetamine-induced stereotypical behavior

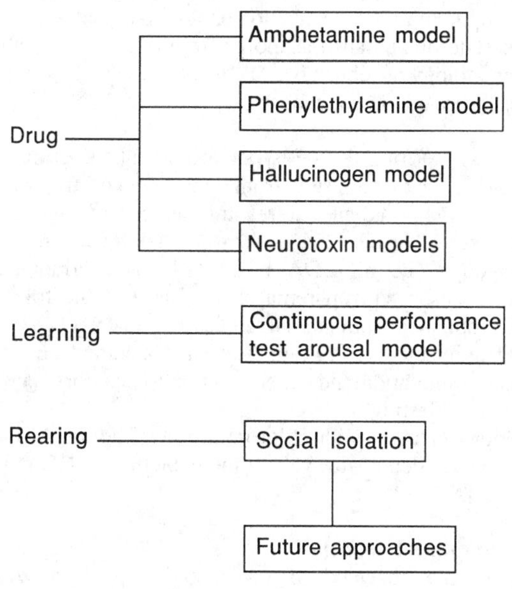

FIGURE 5.2-1 *Existing animal models of schizophrenia and future approaches.*

in both animals and humans. That finding has been related to the possible dopaminergic mechanisms in schizophrenia on the assumption that amphetamine-induced stereotypical behavior in animals is mediated by increased dopamine turnover.

Some investigators have tried to separate the stereotypical behavior from the increased locomotor activity produced by amphetamine by relating the behavior to the release of striatal dopamine, which is significantly increased with repeated amphetamine administration. By contrast, the increased locomotor activity is thought to be mediated by norepinephrine. Tolerance develops in locomotor activity with repeated doses of amphetamine, but not to the effects on stereotypical behaviors. That kind of approach attempts to distinguish the different types of amphetamine-induced behavioral alterations in animals and to elucidate the neurochemical mechanisms that may be involved.

Other researchers have examined the effects of amphetamine on a variety of behaviors in rats and have focused on locomotor activity and stereotypy. A progressive augmentation of both behaviors with repeated drug administration has been reported. The duration of stereotypy was not necessarily increased, but the onset of stereotypy was. Those data were interpreted to mean that long-term amphetamine administration tended to produce increased preservation of progressively more focused and restricted behaviors. A similar phenomenon has been reported in rhesus monkeys.

PHENYLETHYLAMINE MODEL Another proposed drug-induced model of schizophrenia involves phenylethylamine (PEA), a neuroamine that is an endogenous component of mammalian brain and is most highly concentrated in the limbic system of the human brain. That drug produces stereotypies that closely resemble those produced by amphetamine.

HALLUCINOGEN MODEL Many animal experiments using hallucinogenic agents have been very productive in promoting the understanding of the behavioral pharmacology of those compounds, but they have not provided convincing animal models of schizophrenia. As the phenomenology of hallucinogenic-induced states in humans was more carefully compared with the symptomatology of schizophrenia, the proposed behavioral isomorphism became less persuasive.

NEUROTOXIN MODELS One hypothesis about the etiology of schizophrenia is that it results from impairment of the structural integrity of the noradrenergic reward mechanism, and that the impairment is chronic and at least partially irreversible. 6-Hydroxydopamine (6-OHDA) is said to be the aberrant metabolite that causes schizophrenia on the basis of the following evidence obtained from animal studies:

1. When injected into certain brain sites in animals, 6-OHDA decreases stimulation and other rewarded behaviors, and that effect is long-lasting.

2. Prior treatment with chlorpromazine (Thorazine) blocks the behavioral deficits as well as the depletion of NE induced by 6-OHDA.

Nondrug animal models

AROUSAL It has been postulated that patients with schizophrenia operate at excessive arousal levels and that impaired attention resulting from hyperarousal constitutes a major deficit. By training rats on an operant task thought to be analogous to a test of attention (the Continuous Performance Test) used to study schizophrenic patients, attempts have been made to produce an animal model for the attentional deficit. Low levels of electrical stimulation to the reticular formation in rats cause the animals to make errors similar to those made by schizophrenic patients. In general, those drugs with antipsychotic properties are most effective in reversing the deficit.

PRIMATE SOCIAL ISOLATION Isolation seems to share some components with schizophrenia, as illustrated in Figure 5.2-2, but one should be extremely cautious about such linkages until further studies have been done.

There are two potentially productive approaches toward creating animal models of schizophrenia. The ethological approach would focus on a specific behavioral analysis of schizophrenia. Those data could, in turn, provide the foundation for comparisons with other species. The second approach would involve creative operational paradigms for animals based on the present level of analysis of human schizophrenia and move away from attempts to develop global models of the disorder.

Another proposed animal model of schizophrenia relates to the concept of sensorimotor gating. The background comes from reports of oversensitivity to sensory stimulation in schizophrenic patients that theoretically correlates with stimulus overload and leads to cognitive fragmentation. There have been experimental paradigms using cortical event-related potentials and the prepulse inhibition of startle responses which show that schizophrenic patients have impaired central nervous system inhibition (sensorimotor gating). Animal model studies have shown that sensorimotor gating failure similar to that seen in schizophrenic patients can be reproduced. The time course of the observed schizophrenic and animal model deficits is compatible with a temporal map of monoaminergic neuron functions. The workers make the point that studies of sensorimotor gating would allow investigators to comment on the spatial and temporal mapping of neurons, trait and state deficits, and vulnerability factors in a schizophrenic spectrum of disorders. That approach, where one is studying sensorimotor gating research in schizophrenic patients and related animal model experiments, should permit one to understand the functional significance of neurotransmitter abnormalities and the relationship of those abnormalities to cognitive disturbances seen in schizophrenia.

ANXIETY DISORDERS It is well known to clinicians that anxiety can be either a symptom or a specific syndrome. The literature on animal models is often very confusing in that regard. In some work, anxiety seems to be used synonymously with neuroses; in other paradigms, what is being studied seems more akin to fear or to certain kinds of learning behavior. In any case, it is important to keep in mind the core features of the human syndrome.

In the case of anxiety, proposed models must be evaluated according to how they behaviorally resemble human anxiety and how they conform to treatment responsiveness criteria. Neither in itself is completely satisfactory, but investigators do not know enough about the etiology, pathogenesis, or mechanisms of human anxiety to use them as validating criteria for animal models. Some of the proposed animal models of anxiety may help to clarify those issues.

Most approaches to animal modeling of anxiety use variations of operant conditioning paradigms, and validity is evaluated on an empirical basis—that is, how well do clinically effective antianxiety agents work in the paradigms and how specific is the response? A number of the approaches have high empirical validity. Although they may not bear any relationship to the etiology or pathogenesis of human anxiety, they may still have merit in the context of that aspect of animal modeling. The

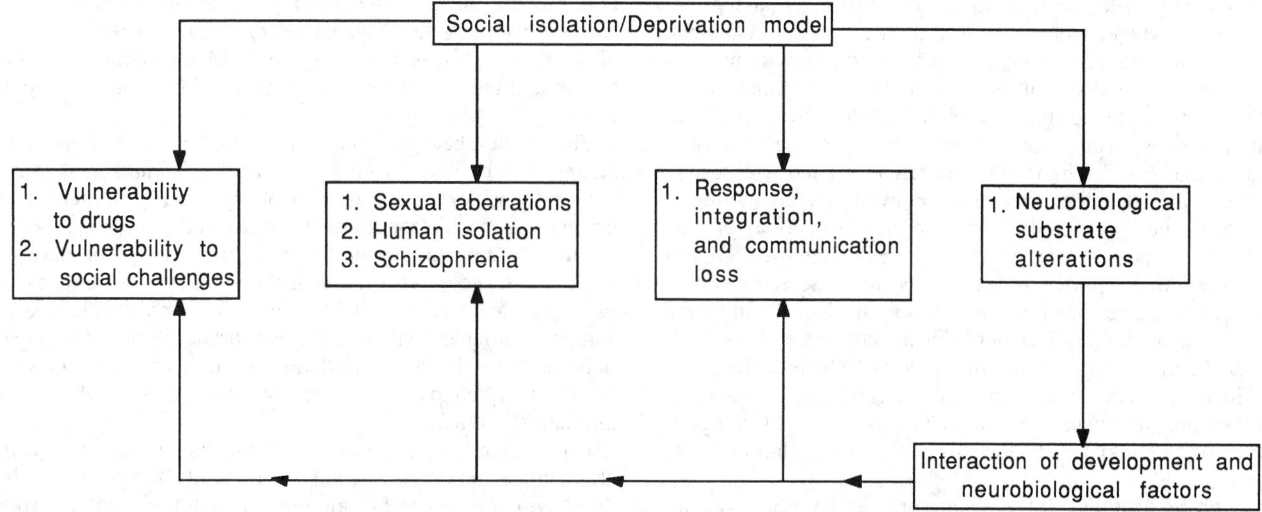

FIGURE 5.2-2 *Applications of the social isolation-deprivation model of human psychopathology.*

assessment of behavior is of vital importance in the development of any animal model, and anxiety is no exception. One cannot talk to animals; thus, what defining characteristics of human anxiety (symptom or syndrome) should researchers attempt to measure in animals? The inducing conditions for many forms of human anxiety are unknown, and so it is impossible to use those conditions as criteria. Also, not enough is known about its mechanisms to use anxiety as a criterion.

Operant conditioning paradigms The basic strategy is to use operant techniques to elicit a behavior with a high frequency of occurrence. After the response is well established, the behavior is suppressed by punishing it when it occurs. The analogy to fear is the conditioned association between the behavior and the punishment. Potential antianxiety drugs are evaluated according to their ability to restore responding to what it was at presuppression levels.

The Geller Conflict Test, one of the best known of such tests, is widely used in screening for potential antianxiety drugs. In the original Geller paradigm, rats were trained on a multiple variable interval (VI) two-minute continuous reinforcement (CR) schedule for milk reinforcement; that is, there was a two-component operant behavior schedule. In the VI portion, signaled by one stimulus, bar pressing was reinforced at variable intervals, with the mean interval being two minutes. In the CR portion, signaled by a different stimulus, every bar pressing was reinforced. When foot shock was given concurrently with the positive reinforcement, response rates were suppressed.

Drug-induced increases in the rate of punished responding are interpreted as an index of antianxiety activity, while decreases in unpunished responding are interpreted as indicating depressant activity. In other words, the type of behavior that originally occurs frequently, but is subsequently suppressed by certain manipulations is highly sensitive to the benzodiazepines and meprobamate (Miltown) but not to chlorpromazine. In general, the test, along with many modifications of it, identifies clinically active anxiolytic agents, predicts their clinical potency, and is generally insensitive to stimulant, antipsychotic, antidepressant, or analgesic drugs. It seems to work in different species and to be relatively independent of the schedules of positive reinforcement or punishment. Thus, the operant conflict approach has high empirical validity in terms of predicting clinical drug responsiveness.

The model, involving conflict behavior, has been used to evaluate several biochemical hypotheses concerning the mechanism of action for the antianxiety, or the so-called emotional analgesic, properties of benzodiazepines. With the increasing interest in the possible neurobiological substrates of anxiety, the availability of a paradigm in which the mechanism of drug action can be explored simultaneously with measures of operant behavior is necessary for future research. Over the past few years, with the identification of benzodiazepine receptor sites, evidence has begun to accumulate that those receptors may mediate the therapeutic effects of such drugs. The relationship of those receptor sites for benzodiazepines to the understanding of the neurobiological mechanisms of anxiety states is complex and remains an active area of investigation. The involvement of various neurotransmitter systems with those receptor sites is important to understand, and the continuing development of experimental systems in which the complex interrelationships can be studied would be helpful. A number of theories, especially with regard to the γ-aminobutyric acid (GABA) and the serotonin systems, purport to explain the effects of the anxiolytic drugs. However, anxiety has many different components, and different neurotransmitters may be involved with each. For example, the muscle relaxant or anticonvulsant properties may be neurochemically mediated in one way, but the anxiolytic effects as revealed in conflict paradigms may be mediated by other neurotransmitters. It is important to have careful behavioral descriptions available along with the specific neurochemical technology.

Alteration of locus ceruleus function The locus ceruleus is a brain structure with a very high density of norepinephrine-containing neurons and numerous projections to other brain regions. Various techniques to alter its function provide one way to learn more about the function of one noradrenergic system in the brain. The system has been studied in the cat, macaque monkey, and squirrel monkey with such techniques as electrical stimulation, ablation, and pharmacological probes. Significant species differences are found in the catecholamine-containing cells in the brain stem, in addition to significant variations in behaviors. Cross-species reasoning from such studies is difficult, but a recent set of studies in nonhuman primates may be particularly relevant to animal models of anxiety.

Increasing locus ceruleus function, whether by electrical

stimulation or with drugs, led to an increase in threat-associated behaviors, whereas decreasing it reduced those behaviors. Those behavioral effects are said to be consistent with the critical role of the locus ceruleus in mediating anxiety and fear.

It has been argued that the behavioral measures associated with the locus ceruleus function in primates are the same ones that change with environmental stimuli associated with fear in humans, and that they are lessened by diazepam (Valium). However, the approach does not permit a distinction between fear as a response to an externally threatening situation and anxiety, which typically is less related to a specific environmental precipitant. The problem arises in much of the literature on animal modeling of anxiety, where the terms "anxiety," "fear," and "learning" are often used interchangeably.

The general conclusion is that the locus ceruleus is essential, though not sufficient, for the behavioral and physiological expression of anxiety. The locus is likened to an alarm system.

Studies of *Aplysia* It has been proposed that not only anxiety as a general state, but several specific subcategories of anxiety, can be modeled in the sea snail, *Aplysia*. It is contended that the molecular basis of anxiety can be studied in that type of animal preparation because of its relatively simple nervous system. The approach has attracted interest because it offers the possibility of more direct approaches to studying the cellular mechanisms of behavior. Behavior in such a preparation has a very different meaning from that in some of the previous models. It is not social behavior, and it is closest to a variant of conditioning paradigms that has been used for some time in the animal modeling field. In *Aplysia,* classically conditioned fear has been said to model anticipatory anxiety, and what is called long-term sensitization to model chronic anxiety.

Many workers have speculated about the relationship of aversive conditioning paradigms in animals to human anxiety. The situation in which the conditioned stimulus serves as a cue for the occurrence of the unconditioned stimulus and various behavioral changes take place, presumably in anticipation of that stimulus, has been likened by investigators to anticipatory or signaled anxiety. In the sea snail, for example, exposure to the extract of shrimp elicits the withdrawal and reflex responses. The term "chronic anxiety of long-term sensitization" has been widely used to describe the state when there is repeated exposure to the unconditioned stimulus alone without any cueing or prior exposure to the conditioned stimulus. Researchers have speculated about the role of the unpredictability of uncontrollability as a factor in mediating that response.

Social manipulations The initial stage of reaction to separation, historically labeled the agitation or protest stage, has been more recently conceptualized in an anxiety context. The first phase is characterized by the infant's being very active behaviorally. Such infants have marked activation of the pituitary adrenal system and an increase in the enzymes involved in catecholamine synthesis. Those findings and others support the view of separation as a very powerful event from both behavioral and neurobiological standpoints, and they are consistent with a large body of literature regarding the behavioral and biological effects of a variety of stressors. To what extent the initial stage of reaction responds to anxiolytic pharmacological agents and how specific the response may be are not known.

Phobias and other anxiety disorders Fear is an emotion produced by present or impending danger. The cause is apparent. Anxiety, on the other hand, is an emotion of which the cause is vague or less understandable. Fear can lead to one's either freezing up or becoming mute. Much literature reports the same thing (for example, rats freezing up in an open field) as being caused by stress.

The relation between conditioning models and theories, and anxiety and phobia models in animals has a number of shortcomings when extended to human phobias. Many animal experiments that assume conditioned fear, as well as avoidance conditioned by trauma, are models of human phobic (or anxiety) reactions. Although it is true that such induction techniques do produce fear of relatively specific stimuli and enable one to study the variables that are important for the learning about fear in humans, rarely can the initiation of a human phobia (or anxiety) be ascribed to a definable event (that is, a definable unconditioned stimulus).

It is contended that research on animals has little to impart about human anxiety, which exists internally and symbolically, often without observable motor or autonomic concomitants. Anxiety is difficult to define. Some investigators feel that Pavlovian or Skinnerian conditioning paradigms are useless for modeling human phobias (anxieties). Human phobias and anxiety just do not fit into conditioning language or paradigms. It has been argued that conditioning language makes assumptions about etiology and treatment that are not borne out in practice, and that the terminology is difficult to apply to clinical events.

One approach to the study of phobias involved the development of two lines of pointer dogs. One line was bred for fearfulness and lack of friendliness toward people and the other for the opposite characteristics. The basic hypothesis was that inheritance would largely determine many behavioral characteristics of the dog, including susceptibility to breakdown under acute and chronic stress. Through the process of selection and inbreeding, it was possible to establish the two lines of dogs and to study their behavior on a number of parameters. Throughout 10 generations, about 80 percent of each litter were similar in temperament to the parents. The phobic line of dogs was extremely timid, avoided humans, and showed decreased exploratory activity. They showed an excessive startle response, and had a slower heart rate and an increased incidence of atrioventricular heart block. Even the dogs with the most severe disturbance could learn operant conditioning bar pressing, but it was necessary to facilitate that process with benzodiazepines—the most efficacious drugs. Both amphetamine and cocaine disrupted the behavioral responses of genetically nervous dogs to a far greater extent than the stable dogs.

There has been some recent work relevant to developing animal models of generalized anxiety disorder and panic disorder. That work should help to clarify the possible roles of neurotransmitter systems as well as to alter developmental experiences and how those two might be related in the etiology of those widespread and disabling illnesses. Those studies involve use of lactate to induce acute endogenous distress in nonhuman primates. Since lactate has been reported to induce panic disorder in humans, if it also does so in animals, then it may be possible to do studies more directed at the mechanisms of those disorders. Additional animal models for anxiety have been reported in the context of the increasingly complex serotonergic receptor systems. There has also been animal work relevant to other ethologically based animal models of anxiety disorder, including generalized anxiety and panic disorders, phobic disorders, obsessive-compulsive disorder and posttraumatic stress disorder.

PSYCHIATRY AND ETHOLOGY

Several authors have suggested that work in the biological science of ethology might be useful in psychiatry. John Bowlby has been taking an ethological approach to psychiatry for many years and as early as 1957 suggested that such an approach might be useful in psychiatric research. Other authors who have written about the interface between ethology and psychiatry generally approached the topic by defining ethology, presenting its vocabulary, describing its methodology, and suggesting conceptual and specific applications of ethological findings to psychiatry. Nevertheless, ethological methods and research findings have had little impact on psychiatry, although it would seem that ethology does have much to contribute to psychiatry, and psychiatry to ethology. The failure of that collaboration to materialize to the extent it should have appears to be the result mostly of artifactual factors, rather than of an intrinsic incompatibility between ethological and psychiatric approaches.

The roots of ethology lie in the natural science of biology, in particular, zoology. The principal philosophical tenet is a naturalistic one, that is, that studies of behavior should take place in natural settings. Its origin in biology and the emphasis on the study of behavior in context have led to ethology's being largely an observational, nonexperimental science. Several authors have contrasted that characteristic with the field of comparative psychology, which has different historical origins and emphases. Research in ethology has at times seemed indistinguishable from that in comparative psychology, as ethologists have used various techniques, from studying naturally occurring phenomena, to introducing experimental factors into a natural setting, to actually working in a laboratory. Researchers usually consider those occasional excursions into the laboratory as attempts to refine mechanisms of behavior, always cognizant of the fact that the behavior evolves in a natural setting.

A glossary of some key ethological terms is provided in Table 5.2-3.

It has been suggested that psychiatric research and practice might benefit from the careful observational techniques ethologists employ in describing both specific behavioral patterns and the context in which the behaviors occur. Those techniques would be applicable to both nonverbal and verbal behavior, as well as to the communicative aspects of each. A more general methodological issue relates to the use of the scientific method in research. In particular, it has been stressed that the ambiguity in the interpretation of findings in psychiatric research could be reduced by a greater use of operational definitions of behavior. One example is the definition of attachment behavior as any behavior that results in an increased proximity between two (or more) members of a species, rather than its being defined in more global terms that make inferences about the internal states of the individuals involved.

Another aspect of ethology that has been stressed in previous approaches to the interface between psychiatry and ethology is the phylogenetic origins of behavior. Ethologists are involved in the comparative study of behavior and derive hypotheses based on phylogenetic assumptions. In the same way that hypotheses are derived in the comparative study of anatomy, behavior can also be studied using the comparative method. The underlying assumption is that the behavioral patterns being studied have evolved as a result of mutation and natural selection in the same way as anatomical systems.

The more recent use of cybernetics, both control theory and information theory, in the understanding of behavioral systems in ethology has been paralleled to some extent in psychiatry. Therefore, the cybernetic approach may be a useful theoretical bridge between the two fields.

One area frequently cited with regard to the application of ethological methodology and theory to psychiatry has been that of attachment systems. The research on separation and on the relationship between separation and depression is a corollary of the work on attachment systems. Another area commonly suggested where ethological research might be useful in psychiatry is that of aggression, particularly in the study of hierarchical and territorial behavior.

TABLE 5.2-3
Selected Glossary of Ethological Terms

Term	Definition
Action-specific energy	Energy associated with the innate releasing mechanism and specific to a particular behavior pattern, which builds up if the releasing stimulus is not present to activate the behavior pattern, and conversely is depleted by repetition
Aggression	Intraspecific conflict manifested by physical attack or social signaling
Appetitive behavior	Phase of behavior involving the active seeking of sign stimuli and thought to be driven by action-specific energy accumulating through inactivity of the specific behavior pattern
Consummatory response	Phase of behavior whereby the energy driving the appetitive phase is released. Involves the perception of sign stimuli, the activation of the innate releasing mechanism (IRM), and the performance of the fixed action pattern (FAP)
Critical period	The time during which imprinting must occur, usually shortly after birth or early in life. Also, "sensitive period."
Displacement activity	A set of behavior patterns occurring alongside an unrelated set of behavior patterns. Originally, irrelevant movements from one behavioral system occurring in the presence of powerful but thwarted drive from another behavior system.
Ethology	The biological study of behavior. From the Greek *ethos,* meaning custom, usage, manner, habit. The modern usage is attributed to Oskar Heinroth, Konrad Lorenz' teacher
Fixed action pattern (FAP)	A genetically determined behavior pattern which is initiated by stimuli particular to the pattern and which consists of species-specific stereotyped movements
Imprinting	A specialized form of learning occurring early in life and often influencing behavior later in life. The exposure to the stimulus situation must occur during a particular period, the critical period, and the exposure can be of short duration and without obvious reward. The learning is particularly resistant to change
Innate	Genetically determined behavior patterns, in theory not influenced by experience
Innate releasing mechanism (IRM)	Sensory mechanism selectively responsive to specific external stimuli and responsible for triggering the stereotyped motor response
Instinct	A developmental process resulting in species-typical behavior
Redirection activity	The venting of one drive from two or more incompatible, but simultaneously activated, drives on some third animal or object
Ritualization	Process of a behavior pattern being incorporated through evolution into a primary signaling function, frequently with exaggeration and embellishment of some of the movements

A natural relation between psychiatry and ethology results from their parallel positions within their respective broader disciplines. The medical sciences are based principally on the biological sciences. Psychiatry is the area within medicine most concerned with the study of behavior, and ethology has an analogous position in biology. However, ethology is still not commonly taught or used in training programs in psychiatry or child psychiatry in the United States. Nikko Tinbergen has delineated three conditions that have contributed to the relative lack of communication between psychiatrists and ethologists.

The first condition is communication difficulties that arise because of differences in scientific language. The second is the obvious differences in the education of students in the two disciplines. The third is the likelihood that the people who study ethology as graduate students are different from those who enter medical school and subsequently train in psychiatry. But even if the people themselves are not particularly different, the stereotypes and the expectations of them by others can inhibit communication between psychiatrists and ethologists.

In 1973, the Nobel prize in medicine was awarded to three ethologists: Karl von Frisch, Konrad Lorenz, and Nikko Tinbergen. That occasion highlighted the importance of ethology for medicine and its special relevance for psychiatry in a manner not dissimilar to the relation between molecular biology and medicine. The contributions of those three ethologists that are particularly relevant to psychiatry are summarized below.

KARL VON FRISCH Von Frisch, who was born in 1886, conducted studies on changes of color in fish and demonstrated that fish were capable of learning to distinguish among several colors and that their sense of color was fairly congruent with that of human beings. He later went on to study the color vision of bees.

Von Frisch's subsequent research was almost entirely concerned with the behavior of bees, and he is most widely known for his analyses of how they communicate with each other—that is, their language, or what is known as their dances. His description of the complex behavior of bees has prompted an investigation of information systems of other animal species.

KONRAD LORENZ Born in 1903, Lorenz is known for his studies of animals, mainly birds, which he allowed to remain free but trained so that they would not be disturbed by his presence. Lorenz was a systematic observer who brilliantly described behavioral traits exhibited by animals. Many of his conclusions have been verified in experimental studies by himself and by other researchers. His interest focused from the beginning on instinctive actions, meaning certain movements performed in a proscribed manner and provoked by certain key stimuli. Those forms of behavior are now called fixed motor patterns. Lorenz showed that, in several animal species, when a fixed motor pattern has been provoked it proceeds automatically. It seems to be genetically programmed and, once started, is not affected by the environment. Fixed motor patterns presumably develop as a result of evolution, through the pressure of selection. Lorenz studied those patterns in several species, including jackdaws, ducks, and geese.

According to Lorenz, fixed motor patterns are provoked by stimuli specific to each pattern, which are called key stimuli. Those stimuli can be assumed to correspond to a particular organization of the central nervous system, originally called das angeborene auslosende Schema, and later, at Tinbergen's suggestion, as the innate releasing mechanism (IRM). The mechanism is assumed to react to key stimuli by prompting or releasing corresponding fixed motor patterns. Lorenz has emphasized that not only instinctive actions but all kinds of learning have their basis in the genetically programmed equipment of the individual.

Lorenz is perhaps best known by psychiatrists for his studies of imprinting. During a certain short period of development, a young animal is highly sensitive to a certain type of stimulus that then, but not at other times, provokes a specific behavior pattern. Lorenz described how newly hatched goslings are programmed to follow a moving object, whereupon they rapidly become imprinted to follow it and possibly similar objects. Typically, the mother is the first moving object the young sees, but should it see something else first, the gosling will follow it. For instance, a gosling imprinted by Lorenz followed him and refused to follow a goose. Imprinting is an extremely important concept for psychiatrists to understand in their effort to link early developmental experiences with later behaviors.

Lorenz also studied the forms of behavior that function as sign stimuli (that is, as social releasers) in communications between individuals of the same species. Many of the signals have the character of fixed motor patterns in that they appear automatically and provoke equally automatic reaction in other members of the species.

Lorenz is also well known for his interest in problems of aggression. He has written about the practical function of aggression, such as the defense of their territory by fish and birds. Aggression among members of the same species is common, but Lorenz has pointed out that, in normal conditions, it seldom leads to killing, or even to serious injury. Although the animals attack one another, a certain balance appears between tendencies to fight and flight, with the tendency to fight being strongest in the center of the territory and the tendency to flight strongest at a distance from the center.

In many of his works Lorenz has tried to draw conclusions from his ethological studies of animals that can also be applied to human problems. Many of his suggestions are by now well-known and provocative. The postulation of a primary need for aggression in humans, cultivated by the pressure of selection, is a primary example. That need might have served a practical purpose at an earlier time when human beings lived in small groups that had to defend themselves from other groups. Competition with neighboring groups became the most important factor of selection. However, Lorenz has pointed out how that need has survived the advent of weapons that can be used not merely to kill individuals but to wipe out all human beings.

NIKKO TINBERGEN Tinbergen, who was born in 1907, conducted a series of experiments to analyze various aspects of animal behavior. He also was successful in quantifying behavior and in obtaining measures of the power or strength of different stimuli in eliciting specific behavior. Tinbergen's first studies were of the digger wasp, *Philantus*. He determined that those insects dig individual nests, where they deposit captured bees to nourish their larvae. He was also able to show that they find their way back to their nests with the aid of various landmarks. Above all, they rely on their visual sense and learn the landmarks by means of an endogenously programmed aerial circuit.

Tinbergen's well-known studies of the various key stimuli that can provoke fixed motor patterns and of how they work together have been very valuable. Different stimuli can provoke the same motor pattern with different degrees of intensity. Particularly elegant is his analysis of the properties of the beak of the herring gull, which encourages its young to solicit food. For example, where the beak is narrow and yellow underneath, there is a contrasting red patch against which the young birds peck.

By using dummies of different shapes and colors, and with different degrees of contrast, he was able to measure the different degrees of force with which the stimuli prompted the young to peck.

Tinbergen's discovery of so-called displacement activities represents another key contribution. Those activities have been studied mainly in birds. For example, in a conflict situation, when the need for fight and the need for flight are of roughly equal strength, birds sometimes do neither. Rather, they display behavior that appears to be irrelevant to the situation. For example, a herring gull defending its territory can start to pick grass. Displacement activities of that kind vary according to the situation and the species concerned. It is well known that human beings can engage in displacement activities when under stress.

In one of his later works, Tinbergen, together with his wife, studied early childhood autism. They began by observing the behavior of autistic and normal children when they meet strangers, employing the techniques used in observing animal behavior. In particular, they observed the conflict that arises in animals between fear and the need for contact and noted that it can lead to behavior that is similar to that of autistic children. They hypothesized that in certain specially predisposed children, fear can greatly predominate and can be provoked by stimuli that normally have a positive social value for most children. That innovative approach to studying infantile autism has opened up new avenues of inquiry. Although their conclusions about preventive measures and treatment must be considered tentative, the methodology illustrates another way in which ethology and clinical psychiatry can relate to each other.

CONSIDERATIONS FOR FUTURE STUDY Aspects of the interaction between psychiatry and ethology can be broadened in a number of ways.

This first aspect is methodology. Recent years have seen a beginning in the study of child behavior by ethological techniques similar to those used during the past quarter of a century in the study of primate behavior and involving operational definitions of specific behaviors and the careful observation and recording of their occurrence.

The second aspect is the relative differences in interest in normal and abnormal behavior. The focus in medicine and psychiatry tends to be on the abnormal, whereas ethologists generally study the parameters of normal behavior for a given species. In a general sense, ethologists and psychiatrists are both interested in differences in adaptation—the ethologist in species differences as related to varying ecological niches, and the psychiatrist in intraspecies differences in response to varying life situations. There has been a growing awareness in recent years of deficiencies in the objective understanding of normal human development, and more interaction with ethology could be useful in improving that situation.

The third issue that an interaction with ethology will force psychiatry to confront is that of the uniqueness of the human species. In psychiatry, it is often assumed that humans are so different from other species that the study of those species is of little use in understanding human behavior. Although a phylogenetic point of view is acknowledged in human anatomy and physiology, it is certainly not emphasized in psychiatry.

The fourth aspect to be considered is the size of the behavioral units of interest to each area. Historically, ethologists have been interested in thoroughly studying the specifics of behavior to the point of a microscopic dissection, and recently, at the other extreme, through a more global approach. Psychiatry has been more interested in the behavior that takes place between these two extremes; that is, psychiatrists are not concerned about specific measurements of facial expression or difficulties in adaptation human beings are confronting today, but with the general behavior of individuals, families, and groups. Exceptions to the generalization include behavior modification at the more specific end of the spectrum and general systems theory at the more global end.

Inasmuch as ethology is a biological science, one might expect that the area of biological psychiatry is where the integration with ethology is most likely to occur. However, with the exception of the use of certain animal models for the understanding of the mechanism of action of a few psychopharmacological agents, biological psychiatrists have been among the least interested in the rich findings of that particular area of biology. Rather, biological psychiatry has tended to be quite reductionistic with its use of animal models. There is a growing body of literature on the effect of psychopharmacological agents in various species, but without much consideration of such factors as the phylogenetic status of the animal, its prior experience, and the effect of these agents on the animal in a natural setting.

A school of thought within psychiatry that has interesting parallels with an ethological perspective is that of psychoanalysis. The libidinous and aggressive drives about which Sigmund Freud and others have written could be viewed as analogous to some of the behavioral states studied in ethology. Much of the ethological literature has dealt with courtship and mating behavior, as well as aggression, whether expressed in hierarchical behavior or in territoriality. Much of Tinbergen's work dealt with the problem of achieving reproductive success when tendencies for courtship and tendencies of aggression occur simultaneously between prospective mates. Bowlby has articulated the natural relationship between psychoanalytic and ethological thought, and his work demonstrates the usefulness of doing so. It both has increased knowledge of the specific components of attachment behavior and broadened the understanding of their existence.

Ethology seeks to understand behavior within an evolutionary or comparative framework and to use descriptive assessment techniques. There has been some interest in applying those ethological descriptive techniques for assessing social behaviors to psychiatric patients. For example, do patients with different types of psychiatric disorders show differences in their nonverbal social behaviors? Do those changes reflect the underlying illness, or do they represent some key feature of the disorder? The use of some of the methods developed by ethologists would permit more definitive and, potentially, specific characterization of disorders along those lines. Conventional psychiatric rating scales used in clinical research studies focus on individual behaviors, whereas the supplementation with ethologically based scales would permit the assessment of a broader range of key aspects of a person's functioning. For example, one study presents data to show that flight and impaired sociability are significant features of the nonverbal behavior of depressed persons. Furthermore, that study and others suggest that while deficits in sociability and flight may cut across several diagnostic groups, there are significant differences in the usage and temporal sequencing of the constituent elements that go into those behavior constellations. For example, in depression, the study documented a reduction of the input and output of socially meaningful information. That, in turn, further isolates the person from others. Are such phenomena secondary to the illness (that is, state related), or are there traits that would characterize the baseline behaviors of persons prone to develop such disorders? Those are questions parallel to the ones being asked in biological psychiatry, where state-trait discussions are very common and where there is great interest in trait markers. The other concept that is important here is the integration of data in man and animals using related rating scales and units of measurement.

SUGGESTED CROSS-REFERENCES

Section 1.4 is a discussion of amino acid neurotransmitters. Section 1.7 covers basic electrophysiology. Learning theory is the subject of Section 3.3. Normal child development is covered in Section 33.2. Chapter 14 focuses on schizophrenia, Chapter 16 covers mood disorders, and sleep disorders are reviewed in Chapter 23. Biological therapies are the subject of Chapter 32.

REFERENCES

Anisman H, Zacharko R M: Behav Brain Sci *5:* 89, 1982.

Bachevalier J, Mishkin M: An early and late developing system for learning and retention in infant monkeys. Behav Brain Res *20:* 249, 1986.

Braff D L: Information processing and attention dysfunctions in schizophrenia. Schizophr Bull *19:* 233, 1993.

Braff D L, Geyer M A: Sensorimotor gaiting and schizophrenia. Human and animal studies. Arch Gen Psychiatry *47:* 181, 1990.

Dixon A K, Fisch H U, Huber C, Walser A. Ethological studies in animals and man, their use in psychiatry. Pharmacopsychiatry *22:* 44, 1989.

*Gardner R: Mechanisms in manic-depressive disorder: An evolutionary model. Arch Gen Psychiatry *39:* 1436, 1982.

Ginsberg S D, Hof P R, McKinney, W T, Morrison J H: Quantitative analysis of tuberoinfundibular tyrosine hydroxylase- and corticotropin-releasing factor-immunoreactive neurons in monkeys raised with differential rearing conditions. Exp Neurol *120:* 95, 1993.

Harris J C: Experimental animal modeling of depression and anxiety. Psychiatr Clin North Am *12:* 815, 1989.

*Henn F A, Johnson A, Edwards E, Anderson P: Melancholia in rodents: Neurobiology and pharmacology. Pharmacol Psychopharmacol Bull *21:* 443, 1985.

Kanner M: *The Tangled Wing.* Harper & Row, New York, 1982.

Kornetsky C, Markowitz R: Animal models and schizophrenia. In *Model Systems in Biological Psychiatry,* D Ingle, H Shein, editors. MIT Press, Cambridge, MA, 1975.

Kraemer G W: Causes and changes in brain norepinephrine systems and later effects in response to social stressors in rhesus monkeys: The cascade hypothesis. In *Antidepressants and Receptor Function,* CIBA Foundation Symposium, nos. 126 and 127. Wiley, New York, 1986.

Kraemer G W, Ebert M H, Schmidt D E, McKinney W T: A longitudinal study of the effect of different social rearing conditions on cerebrospinal fluid norepinephrine and biogenic amine metabolites in rhesus monkeys. Neuropsychopharmacology *2:* 175, 1989.

*Kraemer G W, Ebert M H, Schmidt D E, McKinney W T: Strangers in a strange land: A psychobiological study of infant monkeys before and after separation from real or inanimate mothers. Child Dev *62:* 548, 1991.

Li T K, Lumeng L, Doolittle D P: Selective breeding for alcohol preference and associated responses. Behav Gen *23:* 163, 1993.

Lister R G: Ethologically-based animal models of anxiety disorders. Pharmacol Ther *46:* 321, 1990.

Marks I: Phobias and obsessions: Clinical phenomena in search of a laboratory model. In *Psychopathology: Experimental Models.* J Maser, M Seligman, editors. Freeman, San Francisco, 1977.

Matthyse S, Haber S: Animal models of schizophrenia. In *Model Systems in Biological Psychiatry,* D I Ingle, H Shein, editors. MIT Press, Cambridge, MA, 1975.

McGuire M T, Marks I, Nesse R M, Troisi A: Evolutionary biology: A basic science for psychiatry? *Acta Psychiatrica Scand, 86:* 89, 1992.

McKinney, W T: Animal models of schizophrenic disorders. In *Schizophrenia: Scientific Progress.* S C Schulz, C A Tamminga, editors, p 141. Oxford University Press, New York, 1989.

McKinney, W T: Basis of development of animal models in psychiatry: An overview. In *Animal Models of Depression.* G F Koob, C L Ehlers, D J Kupfer, editors, p 3. Birkhauser, Basel, 1989.

*McKinney W T: *Models of Mental Disorders.* Plenum, New York, 1988.

Mishkin M, Appenzeller T: The anatomy of memory. Sci Amer *256:* 80, 1987.

Mishkin M, Malamut B, Bachevalier J: Memories and habits: Two neural systems. In *Neurobiology of Learning and Memory,* G Lynch, J L McGaugh, N M Weinberger, editors, p 65. Guilford, New York, 1984.

Pavlov I P: *Lectures on Conditioned Reflexes.* International Publishers, New York, 1928.

Porsolt R D: Pharmacological models of depression. In *The Origins of Depression: Current Concepts and Approaches,* J Angst, editor. Springer-Verlag, Berlin, 1983.

Post R M, Weiss R B: Sensitization, kindling and anticonvulsants in mania. J Clin Psychiat *50* (Suppl): 45, 1989.

Redmond E A: Alterations in the function of the nucleus locus coerulus: A possible model for studies of anxiety. In *Animal Models in Psychiatry and Neurology,* I Hanin, E Usdin, editors. Pergamon, New York, 1977.

Reeke G N Jr, Sporns O: Behaviorally based modeling and computational approaches to neuroscience. Annu Rev Neurosci *16:* 597, 1993.

Richardson J S: Animal models of depression reflect changing views on the essence and etiology of depressive disorders in humans. Prog Neuropsychopharmacol Biol Psychiatry *15:* 199, 1990.

Siegel S J, Ginsberg S D, Hof P R, Foote S L, Young W G, Kraemer G W, McKinney W T, Morrison J H: Effects of social deprivation in prepubescent rhesus monkeys: Immunohistochemical analysis of the neurofilament protein triplet in the hippocampal formation. Brain Res *619:* 299, 1993.

Snyder S: Amphetamine psychosis: A model schizophrenia mediated by catecholamines. Am J Psychiatry *130:* 161, 1973.

Sunderland G, Friedman S, Rosenblum L A: Imipramine and alprazolam treatment of lactate induced acute endogenous distress in nonhuman primates. Am J Psychiatry *146:* 1044, 1989.

Swerdlow N R, Braff D L, Taaid N, Geyer M A: Assessing the validity of an animal model of deficient sensorimotor gating in schizophrenic patients. Arch Gen Psychiatry *51:* 139, 1994.

Weiss J M, Goodman P: Neurochemical mechanisms underlying stress-induced depression. In *Stress and Coping,* P McCabe, N Schneiderman, editors, vol 1. Erlbaum, Hillsdale, NJ, 1984.

*Wilner P: The validity of animal models of depression. Psychopharmacology *83:* 1, 1984.

Yehuda R, Antelman S M: Criteria for rationally evaluating animal models of posttraumatic stress disorder. Biol Psychiatry *33:* 479, 1993.

5.3 STATISTICS AND EXPERIMENTAL DESIGN

ROBERT M. KAPLAN, Ph.D.
IGOR GRANT, M.D.

INTRODUCTION

Descriptive statistics are used to organize, summarize, and describe observations. They might include summaries of symptom checklist scores for a selected group of neurotic patients, a summary of neuroendocrine data for a group of schizophrenic patients, or a descriptive summary of the correlation between watching television violence and behaving aggressively. *Inferential statistics* are required for drawing general conclusions about probabilities on the basis of a sample. They have many uses. Statistical inference might be used, for example, to make statements about the eating habits of Americans on the basis of study of a small fraction of the American people, or to decide whether to attribute differences between two groups to chance or to nonchance factors.

DESCRIPTIVE STATISTICS

Descriptive statistics are used to summarize observations and to place those observations within context. The most common descriptive statistics include measures of central tendency and measures of variability.

MEASURES OF CENTRAL TENDENCY There are three commonly used measures of central tendency: the mean, the median, and the mode. The *mean* is the arithmetic average, the *median* is the point representing the 50th percentile in the distribution, and the *mode* is the most common score. Sometimes those measures are all the same. On other occasions, the mean, the median, and the mode can be different.

The mean, median, and mode will be the same when the distribution of scores is normal. The *normal distribution,* shown in Figure 5.3-1, is a theoretical distribution of scores that is symmetrical. Under most circumstances, the mean, median, and mode will not be exactly the same. The mode is most likely to misrepresent the underlying distribution and is rarely used in statistical analysis. Investigators typically choose between the mean and the median as a measure of central tendency. The major consideration is how much weight should be given to extreme scores. The mean takes into account each score in the distribution; the median finds only the halfway point.

Table 5.3-1 shows how the mean and median can have very different values. The table lists weights of two groups of college women. There are five women in each group, but four of them are in both groups (Sally, Sue, Leslie, and Dana). The fifth member in group 1 is Allison and in group 2 is Bertha. Allison and Bertha have very different weights. As the example shows, the median is exactly the same in the two groups. However, the estimation of the mean is affected by the addition of the extreme case. Because it best represents all subjects and because of its desirable mathematical properties, the mean is typically favored in statistical analysis.

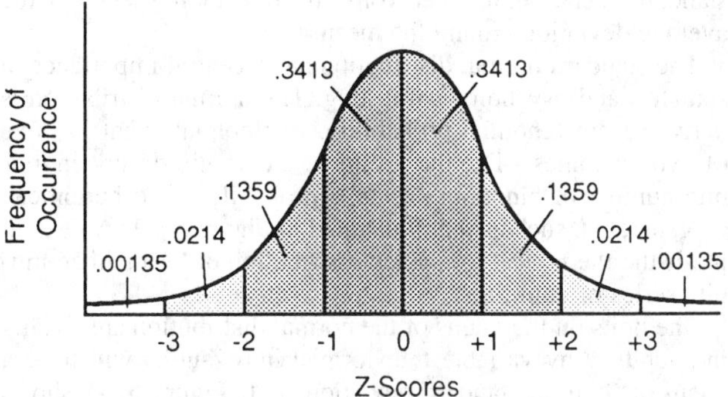

FIGURE 5.3-1 *The normal distribution and areas under the normal curve for Z-scores from −3 to +3.*

TABLE 5.3-1
Mean and Median for Weights (in Pounds) of Two Groups of College Women

Group 1		Group 2	
Woman	**Weight**	**Woman**	**Weight**
Sally	95	Sally	95
Sue	100	Sue	100
Leslie	105	Leslie	105
Dana	110	Dana	110
Allison	115	Bertha	275
Mean ($\bar{X}$) = 105		Mean ($\bar{X}$) = 137	
Median (Md) = 105		Median (Md) = 105	

The median also has some advantages. In particular, the median disregards outlier cases, whereas the mean moves further in the direction of the outliers. Thus, the median is often used when the investigator does not want scores in the extreme of the distribution to have a strong impact. The median is also valuable for summarizing data for a measure that might be insensitive toward the higher ranges of the scale. For instance, a very easy test may have a ceiling effect (that is, it is too easy to measure the true ability of the best students). Thus, if some scores stack up at the extreme, the median may be more accurate than the mean. If the high scores were not bounded by the highest obtainable score, the mean might actually be higher.

As noted, the mean, median, and mode are exactly the same in a normal distribution. However, not all distributions of scores have a normal or bell-shaped appearance. The highest point in a distribution of scores is called the *modal peak.* A distribution with the modal peak off to one side or the other is described as *skewed.* The word "skew" literally means slanted.

The direction of skew is determined by the location of the tail or flat area of the distribution. The skew is positive when the tail goes off to the right of the distribution. Negative skew occurs when the tail or low point is on the left side of the distribution. Figure 5.3-2 illustrates the normal distribution, a distribution that has positive skewness, and one that has negative skewness.

The mode is the most frequent score in the distribution. In a skewed distribution, the mode remains at the peak. The mean and the median shift away from the mode in the direction of the skewness. The mean moves furthest in the direction of the skewness, and the median typically falls between the mean and the mode. The relative positions of the mean, median, and mode in normal and skewed distributions are shown in the illustration.

MEASURES OF VARIABILITY Measures of central tendency, such as the mean and median, are used to summarize information. They are important because they provide information about the average score in the distribution. Knowing the average score, however, does not provide all of the information required to describe a group of scores. Measures of variability are also required. The simplest method of describing variability is the *range*—the difference between the highest score and lowest score. Another statistic, known as the *interquartile range,* describes the interval of scores bounded by the 25th and 75th percentile ranks. In other words, the interquartile range is bounded by the range of scores that represent the middle 50 percent of the distribution.

In contrast to ranges, which are used only infrequently in statistical analysis, the variance and standard deviation are used commonly. To understand the characteristic of a distribution of scores, some estimation of deviation around the mean is important. Because the mean is the average score in a distribution, the sum of the deviations around the mean will always equal zero. However, the squared deviations around the mean can yield a meaningful index. The *variance* is the sum of the squared deviations around the mean divided by the number of cases. It is described by the formula:

$$\sigma^2 = \Sigma\frac{(X_i - \bar{X})^2}{N}$$

where σ^2 is the variance, Σ means sum, X_i is the score of the ith case, $\bar{X}$ is the mean for the population, and N is the number of cases.

The variance is a very useful statistic and is commonly

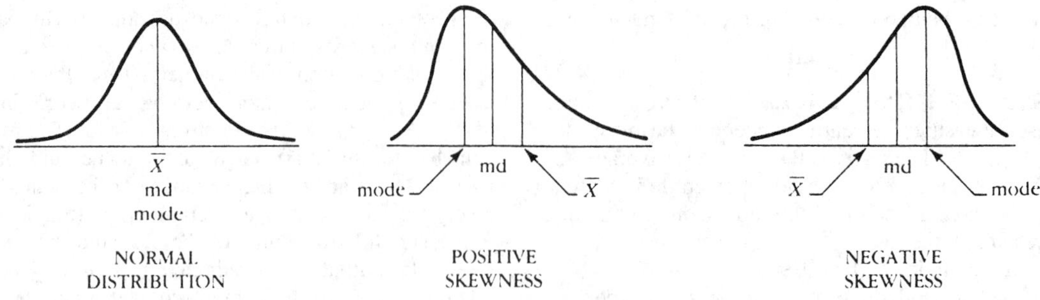

FIGURE 5.3-2 *Examples of normal distribution, positive skewness, and negative skewness.*

employed in data analysis. However, as its calculation requires finding the squared deviations around the mean rather than the simple deviations around the mean, the result will always be in squared units. Taking the square root of the variance puts the units back into their original metric. The square root of the variance is known as the *standard deviation,* which is an approximation of the average deviation around the mean.

SAMPLES AND POPULATIONS The methods discussed so far describe populations. The *population* is the entire collection of a set of objects, people, events, and so on in a particular context. In other words, population refers to the collection of all items on which statements will be based. Examples are all schizophrenic patients in a particular hospital or all depressed persons in a community.

In statistics, means and standard deviations for populations are typically estimated from observations taken from samples. A *sample* is a subset of observations selected from the population. It may be unusual for an investigator to describe only patients with schizophrenia in a particular hospital, and it is unlikely that an investigator will measure every depressed person in a community. More frequently, statements are made about populations on the basis of samples. The mean of a population can be estimated on the basis of a random and unbiased sample of individuals from a community. The formulas for estimating the standard deviations for samples differ slightly from those that are used for populations. The denominator in the radical $N - 1$ is used for sample statistics instead of N, which is used for population statistics. Thus, the definitional formula for the standard deviation of a sample is

$$S = \sqrt{\frac{\Sigma(X_i - \bar{X})^2}{N - 1}}$$

The computational formula for a sample standard deviation is

$$S = \sqrt{\frac{\Sigma X^2 - \frac{(\Sigma X)^2}{N}}{N - 1}}$$

The computational formula does not require the calculation of each deviation from the mean. Instead, it uses the sum of the squared scores and the square of the summed scores, which can be easily obtained using spreadsheet programs for microcomputers.

STANDARDIZED SCORES

The meanings of means and standard deviations are not independent of context. For example, if the mean of a set of scores is 57.6, it still does not convey all the information necessary for an interpretation. Other metrics are designed for more direct interpretation. The Z-score is a transformation into standardized units that are easier to interpret. It is the difference between the score and the mean, divided by the standard deviation.

$$Z = \frac{X - \bar{X}}{S}$$

In other words, a Z-score is the deviation of a score, X, from the mean, $\bar{X}$, expressed in standard deviation units. If a score is equal to the mean, its Z-score is zero. Consider the example of a score of 4 taken from a sample with a mean of 5.75 and a standard deviation of 2.11. The Z-score would be

$$Z = \frac{4 - 5.75}{2.11} = \frac{-1.75}{2.11} = -0.83$$

That means that the observed score (4) is 0.83 standard deviation below the average score or that the score is below the mean but its difference from the mean is slightly less than one standard deviation. In other words, the deviation is less than the average deviation around the mean.

The standard normal distribution has a central importance in statistics and psychological testing. The normal distribution is derived from binomial probability. A binomial event has one of two outcomes—like the results of a coin flip. Using an infinite number of binomial events, a probability distribution can be generated, such as that illustrated in Figure 5.3-1. An example is the theoretical frequency distribution of heads in an infinite series of coin flips.

The units on the x-axis of the normal distribution are usually in Z-units. Any variable transformed into Z-units will have a mean of 0 and a standard deviation of 1. Figure 5.3-1 shows the areas under the normal curve associated with those Z-units. For example, 34.13 percent or 0.3413 of the cases fall between the mean and one standard deviation above the mean. Since 50 percent of the cases fall below the mean, we can conclude that if a score is one standard deviation above the mean it will be in the 84th percentile rank ($50 + 34.13 = 84.13$). A score that is one standard deviation below the mean will be in the 16th percentile ($50 - 34.13 = 15.87$).

Translation of Z-scores into percentile ranks is accomplished by using a table for the standard normal distribution. Certain Z-scores are of particular interest in statistics and psychological testing. The Z-score 1.96 represents the 97.5th percentile in a distribution, whereas -1.96 represents the 2.5th percentile. A Z-score less than -1.96 or greater than $+1.96$ falls outside of a 95 percent interval bounding the mean of the Z-distribution. Some statistical definitions of abnormality view those defined deviations as cutoff points. Thus a person who is more than

1.96 Z-scores from the mean on some attribute might be regarded as abnormal.

McCALL'S T There are a variety of other systems by which raw scores can be transformed to give them more intuitive meaning. One system was established in 1939 by W. A. McCall, who originally intended to develop a system to derive equal units of mental quantities. McCall suggested that a random sample of 12-year-olds be tested and that the distribution of their scores be obtained. Then percentile equivalents were to be assigned to each raw score, showing the percentile rank in the group for the persons obtaining that raw score. After that had been done, the mean of the distribution would be set at 50, to correspond to the 50th percentile. In McCall's system the standard deviation was set at 10.

In effect, McCall's system is exactly the same as that of standardized scores (Z-scores), except that the mean in McCall's system is 50 rather than 0 and the standard deviation is 10 rather than 1. Indeed, a Z-score can be transformed to a T-score by applying a linear transformation.

$$T = 10\,Z + 50$$

The T-score system is commonly used in psychological tests. For example, the Minnesota Multiphasic Personality Inventory (MMPI) uses McCall's system. Thus a score of 60 on any subscale is one standard deviation above the mean. A score of 60 places an individual in approximately the 85th percentile relative to the standardization sample. A score of 70 or above is more than two standard deviations above the mean, and might thus be considered unusual in relation to the normative population.

CONFIDENCE INTERVALS In most statistical inference problems, the sample mean is used to estimate the population mean. Each sample mean is considered to be an unbiased estimate of the population mean. Although the sample mean is unlikely to be exactly the same as the population mean, repeated random samples will form a sampling distribution of sample means. The mean of the sampling distribution is an unbiased estimate of the population mean. However, because taking repeated random samples from the population is difficult and expensive, it is necessary to estimate the population mean based on a single sample.

Because sample means are distributed normally around the population mean, the sample mean is probably near the population value, but it may be an overestimate or an underestimate of the population mean. Statistical inference is used to estimate the probability that the population mean falls within some defined interval. The first step in creating that interval is to find the standard error of the mean, which is the standard deviation divided by the square root of the sample size. Using information about the standard error of the mean, it is possible to put a single observation of a mean into context.

The ranges that are likely to capture the population mean are called *confidence intervals*. The confidence interval is defined as a range of values with a specified probability of including the population mean, and is typically associated with a certain probability level. For example, the 95 percent confidence interval has a 95 percent chance of including the population mean. A 99 percent confidence interval is expected to capture the true mean in 99 of every 100 cases. The confidence limits are defined as the values for points that bound the confidence interval.

Creating a confidence interval requires a mean ($\overline{X}$), a standard error of the mean ($S_{\overline{X}}$) and the Z-value associated with the interval (Z_α). It is calculated with the formula:

$$CI = \overline{X} \pm Z_\alpha\, S_{\overline{X}}$$

Consider the 95 percent confidence interval. It is obtained by taking the mean plus or minus the standard error of the mean multiplied by the Z-score for the 95 percent interval, or 1.96.

If smaller sample sizes are involved, it may be advisable to use another sampling distribution instead of the standard normal distribution. For example, it is common to use the t-distribution to create confidence intervals for smaller samples.

t-TESTS In experimental sciences, comparisons between groups are very common. Usually, one group is the treatment, or experimental, group and the other group is the untreated, or control, group. If patients are randomly assigned to those two groups, it is assumed that they differ only by chance before treatment. Measurements are taken after the treatment to determine whether the groups differ. The statistician's task is to determine whether any observed differences between the groups after treatment should be attributed to chance or to the treatment. The t-test is commonly used for that purpose. There are several types of t-tests, which are summarized in Table 5.3-2. The table also shows the formulas used to calculate the t-values.

Most statistical tests have a common logic. All of the procedures are based on a ratio of observed differences to expected differences. The top half of the ratio is the observation. For the t-test the numerator is usually the observed difference between means. The denominator of the ratio is the standard error for that same observation. It is an estimate of the extent to which the means could be expected to differ by chance alone. The standard error of the mean is the standard deviation of the sampling distribution. It is an approximation of the average deviation that could be expected in estimating the population mean from a sample.

Consider the t-test for differences between independent

TABLE 5.3-2
Types of t-Tests

1. Comparison of a sample mean with a hypothetical population mean.
2. Comparison between two scores in the same group of individuals.
3. Comparison between observations made on two independent groups.

Formulas:

1. $t = \dfrac{\overline{X}_1 - \mu}{S_{\overline{X}}}$

where $\overline{X}_1$ is the sample mean, μ is the hypothetical population mean, and $S_{\overline{X}}$ is the standard error of the sample mean.

2. $t = \dfrac{\overline{D}}{\dfrac{S_D}{\sqrt{N_1}}}$

where $\overline{D}$ is the mean of the differences between pairs of observations, S_D is the standard deviation of the difference scores, N is the number of pairs, and $\dfrac{S_D}{\sqrt{N_1}}$ is the standard error of differences, defined as:

$$\sqrt{\frac{N\Sigma D^2 - (\Sigma D)^2}{N - 1}}$$

3. $t = \dfrac{\overline{X}_1 - \overline{X}_2}{S_{\overline{X}_1} - \overline{X}_2}$

where $\overline{X}_1$ is the mean of sample 1, $\overline{X}_2$ is the mean of sample 2, and $S_{\overline{x}_1} - \overline{x}_2$ is the standard error of the difference between means.

means. For that test, the numerator is the observed difference between those independent means. The bottom half of the equation is the standard error of the differences between means. In other words, the observed differences between means are divided by an approximation of the average deviation that could be expected as a result of sampling error. If the ratios are large, then the numerator—the observed deviation—is greater than would be expected by chance. If the ratio is small, then the numerator, or difference between groups, is equal to or less than what might be expected by chance. The rationale is quite similar for other types of t-tests. For example, the t-test on paired observations compares the deviations of pairs (numerator) against the standard error for those deviations (denominator).

ANALYSIS OF VARIANCE (ANOVA) Psychiatric and psychological studies often require comparison of the means of more than two groups (for example, a comparison of the depression scores of persons in three groups: mood disorder, schizophrenia, and nonpatient controls). The t-tests are suitable only for two-sample problems. When there are three or more samples, and the data from each sample are thought to be distributed normally, analysis of variance (ANOVA) may be used.

Mathematically, it can be shown that if two or more samples are drawn from the same population, then the variances (S^2) of the several samples will all be estimates of the population variance (σ^2). Furthermore, the ratio of the variances derived from two samples of the same population will form a distribution called the F-distribution. The shape of the F-distribution depends on the size of each sample (or, more accurately, on $N - 1$ for each sample, which represents the degrees of freedom [df] associated with each sample; df $= N - 1$ because once the mean is known and all but the very last observation is specified, then the very last observation must be invariant).

When two or more samples are being compared, two sources of variance must be considered. As an example of a three-sample problem, investigators may wish to compare the depression scores of patients with mood disorders (X_m) with those of schizophrenic patients (X_s) and with controls (X_c). The task is to evaluate the hypothesis (null hypothesis) that the patients with mood disorders, the schizophrenic patients, and the controls have been sampled from the same population with respect to depression scores. That population will have a mean depression score X. The mean scores for the three groups will probably not be exactly the same (even if they come from the same population), but they will vary around X. That is called *between groups variance* and is calculated in the ANOVA procedure.

The between groups variance provides an estimate of the difference between group means. How can it be determined whether that variability is meaningful or random? To index between groups variance, an independent estimate of variability is used. Within each of the groups the variability of individual scores around their own group mean provides an estimate of how depression scores are expected to vary by chance. When aggregated across groups, the variance of individual scores around their group means becomes an estimate of error, or *within groups variance*. The F-ratio then becomes a fraction in which the numerator is the between groups variance estimate and the denominator is the within groups variance estimate. The larger the F-ratio, the more likely it is that we can reject the null hypothesis, namely, that the mood-disordered, schizophrenic, and control subjects came from the same population with respect to depression scores. Critical values of F, for various degrees of freedom at desired levels of significance, can be obtained from standard F-tables.

In much psychiatric research, subjects will actually be classified in several different ways, giving rise to a two-factor model, a three-factor, and so on. For example, in the analysis of depression scores the subjects might be divided not only by diagnostic classification (mood disorders, schizophrenia, control normals), but also by sex, giving three-by-two factorial design (three diagnoses by two sexes). F-ratios can then be computed for each of the two *main effects* (that is, diagnosis and sex). A main effect is a statistical difference that is independent of the influence of other variables. It is thus possible to determine whether there are significant differences in depression among diagnostic groups and also between men and women. The factorial design allows us to make each of those assessments independently. Typically, studies are designed so that those independant variables are orthogonal, or uncorrelated.

Where two or more factors or classifications are being considered, an *interaction* may occur. Interactions are joint effects of two or more variables. For example, female patients with mood disorders may have higher depression scores than female schizophrenic patients or controls, but the differences between the diagnostic groups may be smaller for men. That effect might be even greater than would be expected when taking into account the independent contributions of diagnosis and sex. Such a systematic variation in depression scores as a function both of sex and diagnosis is an interaction, or a difference of differences. The difference in depression scores attributable to diagnostic groupings is larger for female than for male patients. Once again, an F-ratio can be computed for the interaction effect.

Table 5.3-3 illustrates the results of a two-way ANOVA. Beck Depression Inventory scores were obtained for 10 patients with mood disorder, 10 patients with schizophrenia, and 10 controls. Half of the subjects in each group were women. A glance at the raw scores suggests that there were differences between patients and controls and between men and women. Are those differences greater than would be expected by chance (defined as occurring less than 5 percent of the time due to chance if the null hypothesis is true)? The ANOVA computation indicates that the F-ratio for the diagnosis effect ($F_{2/24} = 100.79$, $p <$

TABLE 5.3-3
Summary of Two-by-Three ANOVA for Sex by Diagnostic Group

Data	Controls ($N = 10$)	Schizophrenic Patients ($N = 10$)	Mood Disorder Patients ($N = 10$)
Men ($N = 15$)	2	8	11
	4	9	9
	3	8	16
	1	7	12
	2	6	10
Women ($N = 15$)	4	12	20
	4	11	16
	2	9	18
	3	11	16
	6	13	22

ANOVA Summary Table*

Source	MS	df	F	p
Diagnosis main effect	354.433	2	100.787	<.001
Sex main effect	116.033	1	32.995	<.001
Interaction	18.433	2	5.242	<.02
Error	3.52	24		

*MS = mean square, df = degrees of freedom, F is the F-ratio, and p is the probability level.

.001) is greater than the table value of F (5.61) at the .01 significance level for 2 and 24 df. Thus there is a diagnosis main effect. Similarly, for gender, the F-ratio exceeds the tabled value for 1 and 24 df at the .01 level (table value = 7.82). Finally, the F associated with the interaction is also larger than the tabled .05 level (3.40) for 2 and 24 df, demonstrating a systematic influence of the combination of sex and diagnosis on Beck scores (that is, women with mood disorders had significantly higher Beck scores than would be predicted from considering diagnosis and sex alone).

CHI-SQUARE

The methods used to estimate population parameters such as the mean and the standard deviation are *parametric*. Using them requires that assumptions be made about population characteristics. For example, one assumption is that the variable under study is normally distributed within the population from which the sample is drawn. Although violations of that assumption have relatively little impact on a statistical test for most applications in basic statistics, there are circumstances in which substantial bias will be introduced. To address the problem, there is another family of statistical procedures that do not make assumptions about population distributions. They are called *nonparametric,* or distribution-free, techniques. Many research workers prefer nonparametric methods because they rest on fewer assumptions. Those techniques are also appropriate to the analysis of data that do not have continuous numerical properties, for example, data that exist as categories, ordinal data (for example, clinical ratings of severity on a six-point scale), or ranked data.

The most commonly used nonparametric test for categorical data is the chi-square. The chi-square statistic is used to evaluate the relative frequency or proportion of events in a population that fall into well-defined categories. For each category, there is an expected frequency that is obtained from knowledge of the population or from some other theoretical perspective. There is also an observed frequency for each category, which is obtained from observations made by the investigator. The chi-square statistic expresses the discrepancy between the observed and the expected frequency. The formula for chi-square is

$$\chi^2 = \Sigma \frac{(O - E)^2}{E}$$

where O is the observed frequency and E is the expected frequency.

An example of a situation in which chi-square is used is in evaluating the association between sex and diagnosis of major depressive disorder. The investigator would consider whether each man and each woman in a sample did or did not carry the diagnosis. Under the null hypothesis, the expected frequency for major depressive disorder would be assumed to be equal for men and women. The chi-square test would be used to evaluate the two-by-two table.

There are also nonparametric alternatives to problems that suggest the possibility of using a t-test or ANOVA, but where the properties of the data render application of parametric statistics inappropriate. For a two-sample experiment the Mann-Whitney U test may be preferable to the t-test, whereas, for problems involving three or more samples, the Kruskal-Wallis procedure can replace the ANOVA. Both of those nonparametric methods involve transformation of the data into ranks.

TYPES OF ERRORS

When the null hypothesis is rejected, the observed differences between groups are deemed to be improbable by chance alone. For example, if drug A is compared with a placebo for its effects on depression and the null hypothesis is rejected, the investigator concludes that the observed differences are most likely not explainable simply by sampling error. The key word is *probable.* When offering that conclusion, the investigator has the odds on his or her side. However, what are the chances that the conclusion is incorrect?

In statistical inference there is no way to say with certainty that rejection or retention of the null hypothesis was correct. There are two types of potential errors: *type I errors* and *type II errors.*

TYPE I ERROR Type I errors occur when the null hypothesis is rejected but should have been retained. That might happen when a researcher decides that two means are different. He or she might conclude that the treatment works or that the groups are not sampled from the same population, whereas, in reality, the observed differences are attributable only to sampling error. In a conservative scientific setting, type I errors rarely should be made. There is a great disadvantage to advocating treatments that really do not work. Because of the desire to avoid type I errors, statistical models have been created so that the investigator has control over the probability of a type I error, denoted by the Greek letter alpha (α). At the .05 significance or alpha level, a type I error is expected to occur in 5 percent of all cases. At the .01 level, it may occur in 1 percent of all cases. Thus, at the .05 alpha level, one type I error is expected to be made in every 20 independent tests. At the .01 alpha level, one type I error is expected to be made in every 100 independent tests.

TYPE II ERROR The motivation to avoid a type I error might increase the probability of making a type II error, in which the null hypothesis is retained when it was actually wrong. For example, an investigator may reach the conclusion that a treatment does not work when it is actually efficacious. The probability of a type II error is symbolized by the Greek letter beta (β). Table 5.3-4 shows four possible outcomes broken down in a 2 × 2 table. In the left column we have the decisions the researcher made about the null hypothesis. The hypothesis (H_o) can be rejected or retained. Across the top of the table is the actual situation. Hypothetically that is the decision that should have been made. In teaching, it often referred to as God's model, implying that there is a correct decision that could have been made but it is beyond the human capacity to know what it was.

The upper-left box shows that the null hypothesis is rejected

TABLE 5.3-4
Four Possible Outcomes of Decisions Concerning the Null Hypothesis

		"God's Model" What Actually Is True	
		H_0 is True *It should have been retained*	H_0 is False *It should have been rejected*
Researcher's Decision	Reject H_0	Type I error $p = \alpha$	Correct decision $p = 1 - \beta$ (also called the power of the test)
	Retain H_0	Correct decision $p = 1 - \alpha$	Type II error $p = \beta$

even though it is true. That is a type I error. It will occur with a probability (p) of alpha (α), or the significance level for the test. For example, at the .05 alpha level, the probability of a type I error is 5 in 100. The bottom right box in the table shows the decision not to reject the null hypothesis, which in reality was false. That is a type II error with the probability of beta (β).

Not all decisions are incorrect. The table also shows two boxes where the researcher made the correct decision. The lower left box shows the decision to retain the null hypothesis, which was in fact true. That is a correct decision, which occurs with a probability of $1 - \alpha$. Finally, the upper right box shows the decision to reject the null hypothesis, which was in fact false. That is a correct decision with a probability of $1 - \beta$, a probability often referred to as the power of the test.

Statistical power There are several maneuvers that increase control over the probability of different types of errors and correct decisions. One type of correct decision is the probability of correctly rejecting the null hypothesis. *Power* is defined as the probability of rejecting the null hypothesis when, in the real world, it should have been rejected. Ultimately, the statistical evaluation will be more meaningful if it has high power, especially when the null hypothesis is retained. Retaining the null hypothesis with high power gives the investigator more confidence in stating that differences between groups were nonsignificant. One factor that affects the power is the sample size. As the sample size increases, power increases. The larger the sample, the greater is the probability that a correct decision will be made as to whether to reject or retain the null hypothesis.

Another factor that influences power is the *significance level.* As alpha or significance increases, the power increases. For instance, if the .05 level is selected rather than the .01 level, there will be a greater chance of rejecting the null hypothesis. However, there will also be a higher probability of a type I error. Reducing the chances of a type I error entails reducing the chances of correctly identifying the real difference (power). Thus the safest way to affect power without affecting the probability of a type I error is to increase the sample size.

The third factor affecting power is *effect size.* The larger the true differences between two groups, the greater is the power. Experiments that attempt to detect a very strong effect, such as the impact of a very potent treatment, might have substantial power even with small sample sizes. The detection of subtle effects may require very large samples in order to achieve reasonable statistical power.

Not all statistical tests have equal power. The probability of correctly rejecting the null hypothesis is higher with some statistical methods than with others. Nonparametric statistics are typically less powerful than parametric statistics, for example.

CORRELATION

Clinicians and researchers are often interested not so much in how samples might differ, but in how variables that represent characteristics of some particular sample or population are related to each other. For example, one might wish to know the relationship between an oral dose of haloperidol (Haldol) and plasma level, between rapid eye movement (REM) latency and Beck depression scores, or between the volume of the third ventricle and degree of amnesia. Figure 5.3-3 displays results from a clinical study in which plasma haloperidol was determined one hour after each of 10 single oral doses of the drug. The distribution of points in the scatter plot suggests that the

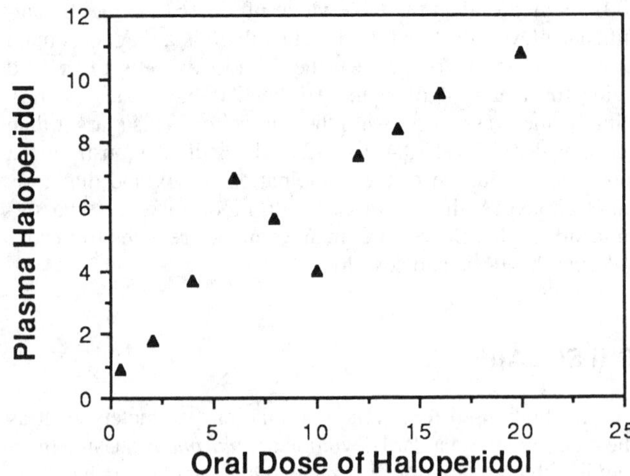

FIGURE 5.3-3 *Hypothetical relationship between oral dose of haloperidol and plasma concentration of haloperidol. The linear relationship accounts for 86 percent of the variance.*

data could be modeled in terms of a straight line, called a *regression line.* The question is, how well can plasma levels be predicted from oral dose? In statistical terms, how much of the total variation in plasma haloperidol is attributable to the oral dose, and how much can be explained by other factors (for example, age, diet, or body mass)?

The regression line that expresses the relationship between plasma haloperidol (Y) and oral dose (X) can be expressed by the equation: $Y' = a + bX$, where Y' is the predicted value of plasma haloperidol taken from the regression line, a is the intercept of the line on the y-axis, and b is the slope of the regression line.

Once the regression line has been fitted to the data, the next question is, what is the strength of the linear relationship between plasma haloperidol and oral dose? The strength of the association is expressed as the ratio of the variance in y that is attributable to its relationship to x divided by the total variance in the model. That ratio has been designated r^2. In Figure 5.3-3 the r^2 was computed as .86. That means that 86 percent of the total variation in plasma haloperidol can be attributed to its relationship to the oral dose, and that 14 percent of the variation is the result of unexplained factors, such as measurement error or characteristics of subjects.

Customarily, the strength of the linear relationship between two variables is actually reported as the correlation coefficient (product moment correlation, Pearson's r, or simply r). The correlation coefficient is the regression coefficient when both X and Y variables are expressed in standardized or Z-units. The regression coefficient allows a translation between X and Y in natural units. It is the amount of expected change in Y for each unit change in X. For example, the equation $Y = 3.25 + .5X$ suggests that each unit change in X is expected to correspond with a 0.5 change in Y. The value 3.25 is the intercept, the value of Y when X is 0. The correlation coefficient is also the square root of r^2. In the above example, $r = .93$. To determine whether a product moment correlation falls outside the bounds of chance, one can compute a t-statistic using a standard formula that takes into account the number of degrees of freedom. In the case of a correlation between two variables, the degree of freedom equals $n - 2$, where n is the number of pairs. In the above example, t was computed as 7.13, which exceeds $t =$ 2.90, the critical value of $\alpha = .05$ for 8 df. Thus it can be concluded that the r is significantly larger than would be expected by chance. The formulas for the correlation coefficient and the evaluation of statistical significance using the t-test are

$$r = \frac{N\Sigma XY - (\Sigma X)(\Sigma Y)}{[N\Sigma X^2 - (\Sigma X)^2][N\Sigma Y^2 - (\Sigma Y)^2]}$$

$$t = r\sqrt{\frac{N-2}{1-r^2}}$$

where N is the number of cases and X and Y are scores on measured variables.

Cautions in interpreting the correlation coefficient Several issues need to be borne in mind in interpreting the correlation coefficient. First, it is important to inspect the data that are being modeled. For example, the linear correlation between plasma concentration of an antidepressant and score on a symptom checklist is low in Figure 5.3-4. That is not because the variables are unrelated, however. The data are best modeled as a U-shaped function, rather than as a straight line.

Correlation coefficients can be biased by a single extreme value, as is illustrated in Figures 5.3-5 and 5.3-6. Figure 5.3-5 shows the correlation between scores on an inventory of life events and a self-rated depression checklist. As shown, there is only a very weak correlation between the scores ($r = -.11$). Figure 5.3-6 displays the same relationship with the addition of a single outlier. That one case had many life events and a high depression score. With the addition of that one extreme point, the correlation rises to .97. The example illustrates the sensitivity of correlational methods to extreme scores. Investigators should inspect their data to avoid spurious high correlations caused by outliers.

Figure 5.3-7 illustrates another problem with interpreting the meaning of the correlation. Here data collected from two samples were pooled, and a product moment correlation was computed. Inspection of the scatter plot shows that the apparent linear relationship is explained by the fact that the two samples differed in their mean scores for memory errors and third ventricle width (that is, the samples came from different populations), but that within each sample there was no relationship between the two variables.

The range of variability in data will also determine the size of the correlation coefficient. For example, if the range of variability is very restricted (that is, there is not much "play" in the scores), then the observed value of Pearson's r will be constrained near 0. The level of r at which a significant value is attained also depends on the size of the sample. In extremely large samples (for example, hundreds or thousands of subjects), even tiny values of r (for example, $r = 0.1$) may be statistically significant but have little practical meaning.

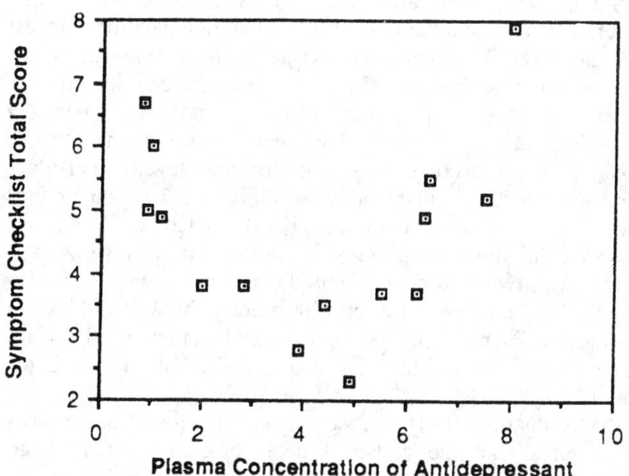

FIGURE 5.3-4 *The systematic U-shaped relationship between plasma concentration of antidepressant and scores on a symptom checklist is not detected by Pearson product moment correlational methods, which are designed to describe linear relationships.*

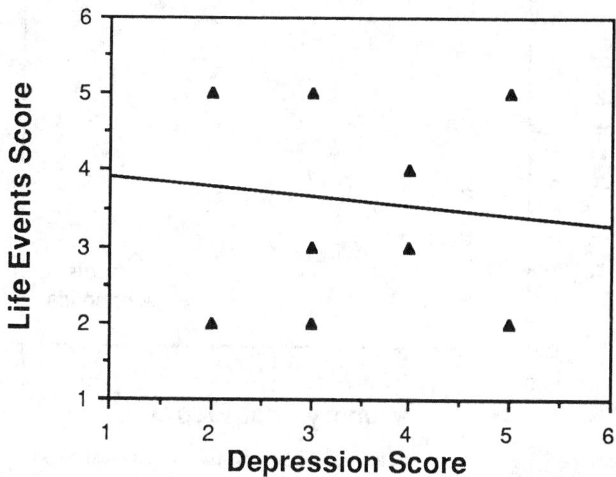

FIGURE 5.3-5 *Scatter plot of depression and life events scores.*

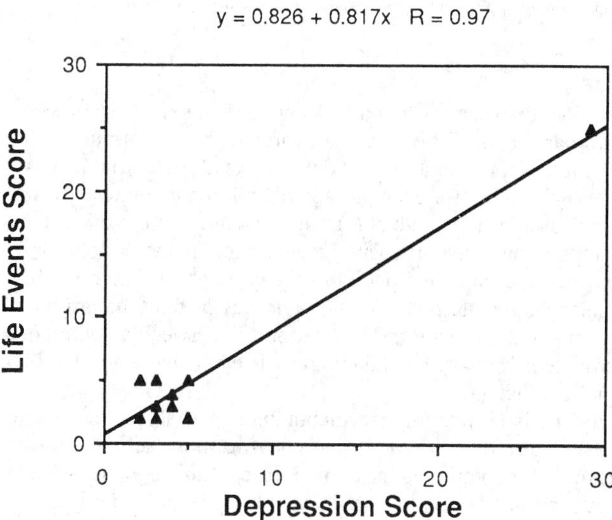

FIGURE 5.3-6 *The same data as in Figure 5.3-5 with the addition of one outlier. A single outlier can have a significant effect on estimates of linear correlation.*

Correlation when variables are not continuous In the discussion above, it was assumed that the two variables being correlated, X and Y, were both continuous. Correlations can also be computed even if one or both variables are not continuous. The distinction must be drawn between dichotomous variables that are "true," such as male versus female sex, and those that have been artificially divided to form dichotomies, for example, the division of a continuous test score into normal and abnormal categories. The types of correlation coefficients used to find the

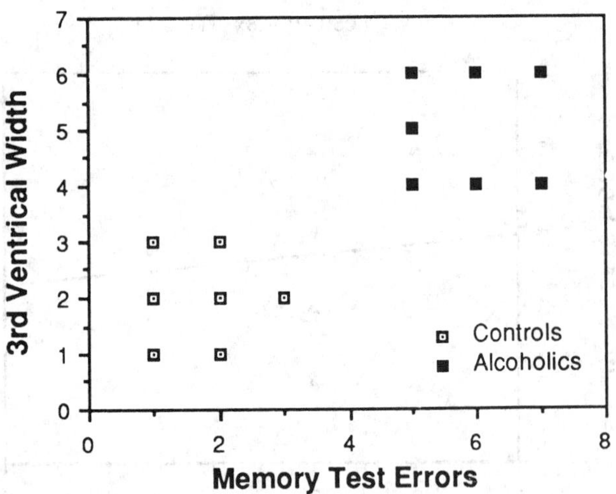

FIGURE 5.3-7 *Example of ecological correlation, which must be interpreted with caution. The correlation between memory and third ventricle width is low within both alcoholic-patient and control groups. However, after merging both groups, a significant correlation appears. The fact that the correlation from the pooled samples is significant does not demonstrate a true association between ventricle width and memory.*

relation between dichotomous and continuous variables are summarized in Table 5.3-5. If variable Y is continuous (for example, scores on a manual dexterity test), but variable X is a true dichotomy (for example, sex of children being tested), and if one assigns the value of 0 to one sex and 1 to the other, then computation of the product moment correlation will yield a special statistic called the point biserial correlation. The point biserial r can be interpreted in the same way as the standard product moment correlation. The relationship between a continuous variable and an artificial dichotomy is evaluated using the biserial coefficient.

If one is correlating two dichotomous variables, and one at least is true dichotomous, then entering those scores into the formula for computing the correlation coefficient yields another statistic called the phi coefficient (ϕ). The phi coefficient is related to the more commonly known chi-square. In fact, it can be shown that $\chi^2 = N\phi^2$, where N is the number of cases.

The significance of phi can be determined by computing $N\phi^2$ and referring to a chi-square table with one degree of freedom. When both variables are artificial dichotomous, another coefficient known as the tetrachoric r is used.

Rank order correlation Sometimes observations are made to which it is difficult to assign precise values. For example, a clinician might wish to relate the amount of belligerence exhibited by drug-abusing patients to the strength of their phencyclidine abuse habit. The notion of belligerence may be difficult to quantify, although it might be possible to rank the patients from most to least belligerent. Similarly, the notion of strength of drug abuse habit may be difficult to quantify, but it may be possible to order the subjects from heaviest to lightest user. A rank order correlation coefficient called Spearman's rho, can then be computed. By computing a Z-value, using formulas that can be found in standard texts, it is possible to evaluate the significance of rho for the particular sample size. It should be noted that Spearman's rho may be preferred over the product moment correlation when the variables being related have distributional properties that depart significantly from normality. For example, the distribution of grams of alcohol consumption

TABLE 5.3-5
Appropriate Correlation Coefficients for Relations Between Dichotomous and Continuous Variables*

Variable Y	Variable X		
	Continuous	Artificial dichotomous	True dichotomous
Continuous	Pearson r	Biserial r	Point biserial r
Artificial dichotomous	Biserial r	Tetrachoric r	Phi
True dichotomous	Point biserial r	Phi	Phi

*The entries in the table suggest which type of correlation coefficient is appropriate given the characteristics of the two variables. For example, if variable Y is continuous and variable X is true dichotomous, the point biserial correlation will be used.

among those who regularly drink has a strongly positive skew. Rank correlation methods may be preferred in studies of alcohol use because of that nonnormal distribution.

MULTIVARIATE ANALYSIS

Multivariate analysis considers the relationship between combinations of three or more variables. For example, the prediction of the number of psychiatric readmissions of schizophrenic patients from the linear combination of age, premorbid adjustment, presenting symptoms, and treatment history would be a problem for multivariate analysis. The field of multivariate analysis is a technical one, requiring an understanding of linear and matrix algebra. A schematic representation of the techniques involved may help to place them in context, while showing the basic similarity of approaches that might appear to be quite different.

Fundamentally, multivariate techniques involve the manipulation of matrix data (that is, data organized in columns and rows). The data in columns are termed variables and those in rows are called observations. More specifically, multivariate analyses operate on matrix columns.

Figures 5.3-8A–E illustrate how the family of multivariate analysis techniques is related. Figure 5.3-8A represents multiple regression, where variable Y is being predicted from a linear combination (L_x) of variables X_1, X_2, and X_3. In Figure 5.3-8B, there are two predictors (X_1, X_2) and two outcome (dependent) variables (Y_1, Y_2). That illustrates the basis of canonical correlation—finding the relationship of the linear combinations of two or more predictors (L_x) and two or more outcomes (L_y) simultaneously. In Figure 5.3-8C, there is one outcome (Y), but instead of being continuous, it has discrete levels. That illustrates linear discriminant analysis. In Figure 5.3-8D the predictors X_1 and X_2 are dichotomous, but the outcomes Y_1, Y_2, and Y_3 are continuous. That represents multivariate analysis of variance, with two factors and multiple outcome variables. In Figure 5.3-8E only the relationships among the X variables are being considered, and new linear combinations of them are expressed as the factors Lx_1 and Lx_2. That illustrates factor analysis.

What distinguishes those techniques is the model being specified rather than the statistical theory or computational detail that underlies them. The various methods differ in the number and kind of predictor variables they use. They are similar in that they all transform groups of variables into linear combinations, or weighted composites of the original variables. The weighting system combines the variables to achieve some goal.

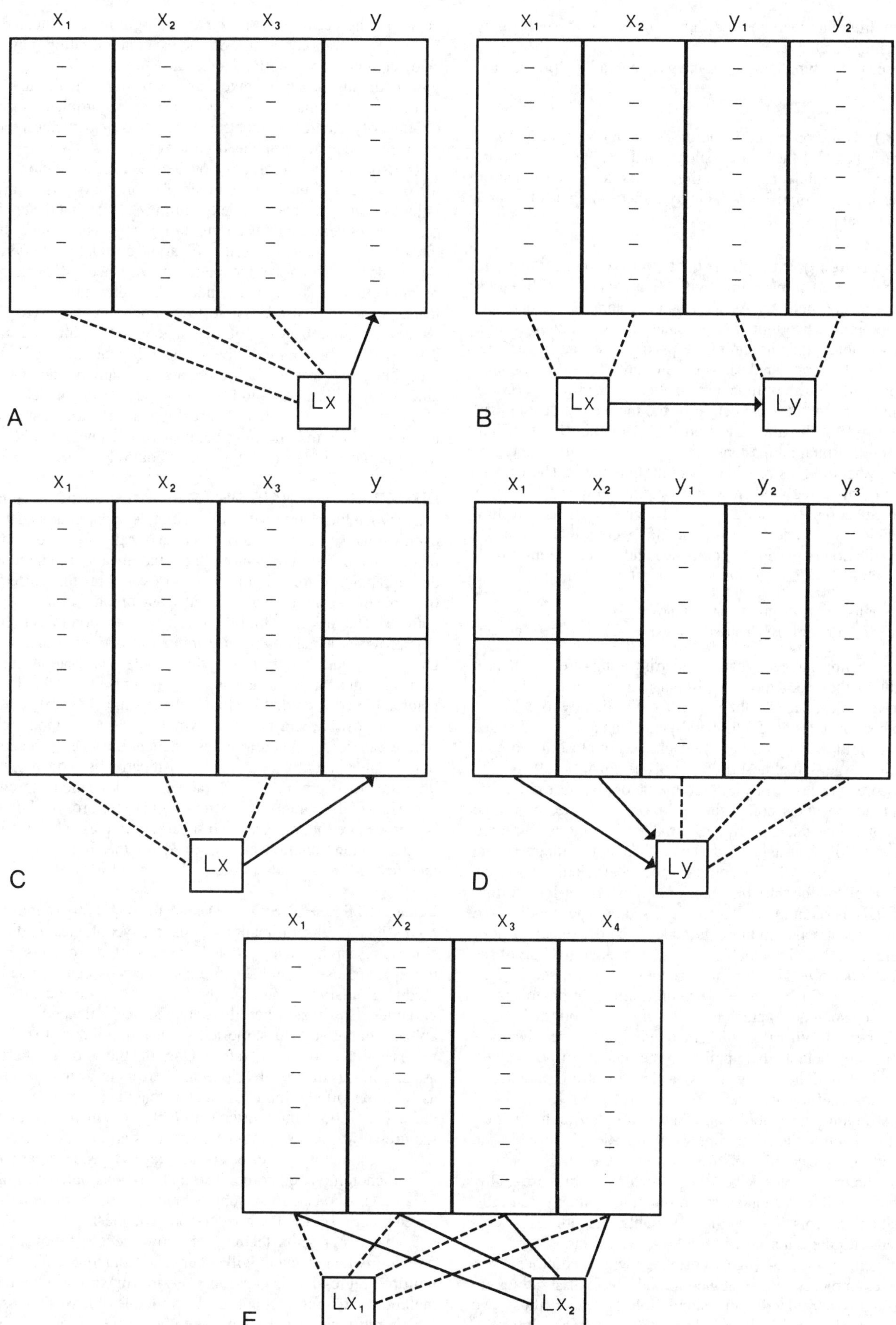

FIGURE 5.3-8 *Schematic representations of multivariate models. (Figure modified from J P Van de Geer:* Introduction to Multivariate Statistics for the Social Sciences. *Freeman, San Francisco, 1971.)*

The multivariate techniques differ according to the goals they are trying to achieve.

A linear combination of variables is generally expressed as:

$$Y' = a + b_1X_1 + b_2X_2 + b_3X_3 + \cdots + b_kX_k$$

where Y' is the predicted value of Y, a is a constant, X_1 to X_k are variables and there are k such variables, and b_1 to b_k are regression coefficients. The entire right side of the equation creates a new composite variable by transforming a set of predictor variables.

Example using multiple regression Variables that are important in a combination will be associated with larger regression coefficients. As an example, suppose researchers want to predict the number of psychiatric hospitalizations from three variables: income, rating by psychiatrists, and age. That type of multivariate analysis is called multiple regression, and its goal is to find the linear combination of the three variables that provides the best prediction of the number of hospitalization episodes. The aim is to find the correlation between the criterion (hospital admissions) and some composite of the predictors (income plus psychiatrist rating plus age). The combination of the three predictors, however, is not just the sum of the three scores. Instead, a computer algorithm is used to find a specific way of adding the predictors together that will make the correlation between the composite and the criterion as high as possible. A weighted composite might be:

Admissions = .3 (Z-scores for income)
+ .6 (Z-scores of psychiatrist ratings) + .03 (Z-scores for age)

The example suggests that psychiatrist ratings are given more weight in the prediction of hospital admissions than are the other variables, because the rating is multiplied by .6, whereas the other variables are multiplied by much smaller coefficients. Age is multiplied by only .03, which is very close to no contribution. Age will almost drop out of the equation.

Z-scores are used for the three predictors because the coefficients in the linear composite will be greatly affected by the range of values taken on by the variables. Income is measured on a scale of thousands of dollars, whereas the range in age might be 15 to 70. To compare the coefficients with one another, all of the variables must be transformed into similar units. That is accomplished by using Z-scores. The standardized coefficients attached to those variable Z-scores are called β, or β weights. When the variables are not expressed in Z-units, the coefficients or weights for the variables are expressed in their natural units. For example, in finding an equation to use in estimating someone's predicted level of success on the basis of certain personal characteristics, there would be some advantage to using coefficients that applied to the untransformed values. When that is done, the weights in the model are called raw regression coefficients (sometimes called "*b*'s").

Interpreting regression coefficients can be difficult. In addition to reflecting the relation between a particular variable and the criterion, the coefficients are affected by the relations among the predictor variables. When the predictor variables are highly correlated with one another, it is difficult to evaluate their individual coefficients. Two predictor variables that are highly correlated with the criterion will not both receive large regression coefficients if they are highly correlated with each other.

For example, suppose that income and psychiatrist ratings are both highly correlated with readmission. However, those two predictors also are highly correlated with each other. In effect, they seem to be measures of the same thing (which should not be surprising because the psychiatrist might include income in his or her overall appraisal). So the psychiatrist rating may get a lower regression coefficient because some of its predictive power already has been taken into consideration through its association with income. That is known as the problem of multicolinearity. Regression coefficients are most easily interpreted when the predictor variables do not overlap.

The strength of the association between the predictors and the outcome is expressed, as in simple correlation, as a correlation coefficient, usually called multiple R. Note that the uppercase R is conventionally used in multiple regression rather than the lowercase r typically used in bivariate correlation. Squaring R provides an estimate of the amount of variance in Y explained by predictors X. There are methods for determining the significance of R. It is also possible to compute an "adjusted R," which takes numbers of subjects and variables into account. That is desirable because the replicability of the regression model becomes less likely if there are too many predictor variables in relation to the number of subjects from which such observations derive. Generally speaking, as the ratio of subjects to variables begins dropping below 10 to 1, one's confidence in the replicability of the regression should decrease.

DISCRIMINANT ANALYSIS Multiple regression is appropriate when the criterion outcome variable is continuous. However, in many cases the criterion is a set of categories. For example, a researcher might want to know the linear combination of demographic, historical, and symptom variables that differentiate positive-symptom and negative-symptom schizophrenic patients. The task is to find the linear combination of variables that provides a maximum discrimination between categories. One appropriate way to model that problem is to apply linear discriminant analysis. The technique attempts to find that linear combination of predictors that achieves the best separation between positive and negative symptom cases. A model chi-square can be computed to assess the significance of the solution. If an apparently successful classification is achieved, it is important to determine the generalizability of the model through one of several techniques and cross-validation. Cross-validation is a procedure that requires two separate samples. The discriminant function equation is developed for the first sample and then tested for accuracy in the second sample.

LOGISTIC REGRESSION Despite the popularity of multiple regression and discriminant analysis in psychological and psychiatric research, those models have presented problems. Both multiple regression and discriminant analysis can be used to predict a binary outcome on the basis of several independent variables. However, when the outcome or the dependent variable has only two values, the statistical assumptions of multiple regression are often violated. One of the most important assumptions is that the distribution of errors is normal. Another assumption, often difficult to meet, is that the independent variables will follow multivariate normality. Logistic regression requires fewer assumptions and provides an excellent alternative for estimating the effect of several independent variables on a dichotomous outcome. The dichotomous outcome might be a diagnostic category (schizophrenic–not schizophrenic) or a treatment response (responder-nonresponder).

Logistic regression techniques allow the estimation of the probability that an event will occur. The technique differs from multiple regression because it uses the maximum-likelihood method. Linear regression uses the principle of least squares, in which regression coefficients are the result of the smallest squared distances between observed and predicted values. The maximum-likelihood method uses a rule that the coefficients are based on the most likely result. Logistic regression also allows the characterization of nonlinear relationships.

The interpretation of logistic regression coefficients is different from that for multiple regression coefficients. In regression analysis the coefficient gives the amount of change in the dependent variable for each unit change in the independent variable. Coefficients in logistic regression describe the odds of an event's occurring. The odds are the probability of an event divided by the probability of no event. Coefficients in logistic regression offer the log-odds or the logarithm-of-the-odds ratio.

LOG-LINEAR MODELS Essentially, chi-square is a test of nonindependence, but it does not provide estimates of the relationship between variables. The chi-square test becomes very complicated if more than two variables are in the analysis. Log-linear analysis allows the construction of systematic models to evaluate the relationship between categorical variables. Complex models can be constructed, and specific significance tests can be ordered. Tests for hierarchical relationships can also be evaluated. For instance, the relationship between employment status and alcohol abuse can be evaluated separately with those persons with and those without a diagnosis of mood disorder.

FACTOR ANALYSIS Discriminant analysis and multiple regression analysis are techniques that find linear combinations of variables that maximize the prediction of some criterion. Factor analysis is used to study the interrelationships among a set of variables without reference to a criterion. It might best be thought of as a data-reduction technique. With responses to a large number of items or a larg? number of tests, it is often desirable to reduce the information into more manageable chunks. The task in correlation is to find the best fitting line through the points created by a two-dimensional scatter diagram. As more variables are added in multivariate analysis, the number of dimensions increases. For example, a three-dimensional plot is shown in Figure 5.3-9. Scatter diagrams for more than three dimensions can only be imagined.

In factor analysis a matrix of correlations between every variable and every other variable is created. Then the linear combinations of the variables that describe as many of the interrelations between the variables as possible are obtained. Those linear combinations of the variables are called principal components, and the goal in creating them is to describe as much of the association between the variables as possible. As many principal components as there are variables can be obtained. However, each principal component is extracted according to

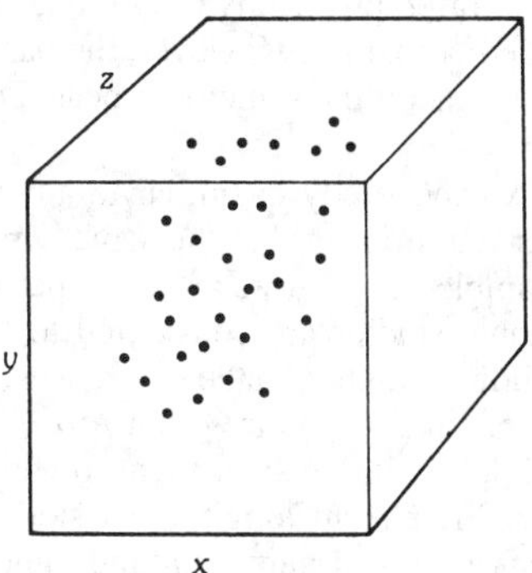

FIGURE 5.3-9 *Three-dimensional scatter plot represented as a box. In addition to the* X- *and* Y-*axes, points must be located with respect to a third,* Z-*axis.*

mathematical rules that make it independent, or uncorrelated with all of the other principal components. The first component will be the most successful in describing the variation among the variables, and each succeeding component will be somewhat less successful. Typically, only a few components that account for larger proportions of the variation are extracted for further study.

Once the linear combinations or principal components have been found, the correlations between the original items and the factors are obtained. Those correlations are called factor loadings. The expression "item 7 loaded highly on factor I" means that there was a high correlation between item 7 and the first principal component. By examining which variables load highly on each factor, the factors come to be interpreted and named.

Factor analysis is a complex and technical method, and there are many options the user must consider. For example, investigators frequently use methods that help them get a clearer picture of the meaning of the components by transforming the variables in a way that pushes the factor loadings toward the high or the low extreme. Those transformation methods involve rotating the axes in the space created by the factor. These transformations have been labeled methods of rotation. Such rotation methods can improve the scientific utility of the factor solution. There are several options for methods of rotation, and there are other options concerning the characteristics of the matrix that is originally entered into the analysis.

SURVIVAL ANALYSIS Survival analysis evaluates the timing of events. In biomedical research survival analysis is typically used to evaluate life expectancy. However, a whole series of time-dependent questions can be evaluated using survival analysis techniques (for example, age of onset of psychological illness, time to relapse for those in treatment, or the timing of developmental milestones, such as first word spoken, age of initiation of smoking, or age at marriage). Virtually any time-dependent variable can be analyzed, such as duration of marriage or duration of employment.

Survival analysis requires the construction of a follow-up life table. Building the table requires a defined starting point, for example, birth, date of initiation of therapy, or date of diagnosis. Next, a follow-up interval, such as a year, is defined. The central focus of survival analysis is the time until a defined event occurs. For each time interval, survival analysis calculates the probability that the event has occurred.

Survival analysis allows comparisons between different defined groups. For example, smokers with coaddictions might be compared with those who use tobacco only. For each of these groups, a hazard rate is created. A *hazard rate* is defined as the estimated probability that a person who has not experienced an event at the beginning of an interval will experience that event during the interval.

An example of survival analysis in psychiatric research is provided in studies of alcoholism.

> Alcoholic persons had previously been reported to experience excess mortality, which meant that greater proportions died at a given age as compared with nonalcoholic persons. The alcoholic persons who achieved long-term sobriety had improved mortality as compared with relapsed alcoholic persons. The investigators wished to compare the mortality of the two groups of alcoholic persons with that of nonalcoholic persons. Figure 5.3-10 illustrates the results. The starting point for the analysis was date of entry into the study. The follow-up period ranged from 1 to 11 years. The number of deaths in each group is plotted as a function of time. Cumulatively, 19 of 101 relapsed alcoholic subjects died, compared with 4 of 98 continuously abstinent alcoholic subjects and 1 of 92 nonalcoholic controls. The 99 percent confidence intervals were 9.64 to 33.38 for the relapsers, 0.67 to 12.59 for

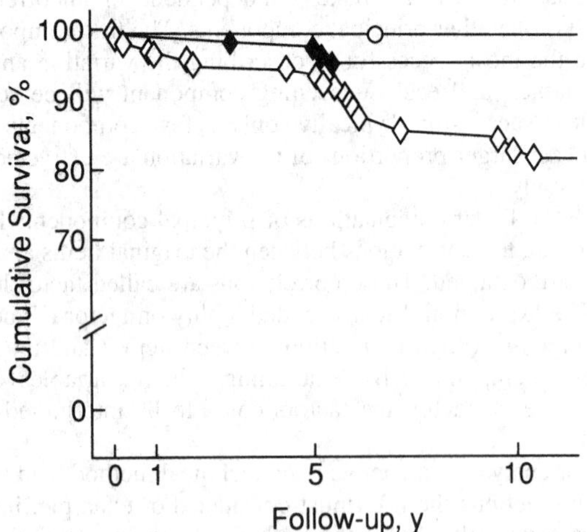

FIGURE 5.3-10 *Life table survival experience for all subjects. Open diamonds (◇) represent expired relapsed alcoholic subjects* (N = 19/101)*; solid diamonds (◆) represent expired abstinent alcoholic subjects* (N = 4/98)*; circles (○) represent expired nonalcoholic controls* (N = 1/92)*.*

the abstainers, and 0.01 to 7.43 for the nonalcoholic subjects. The confidence interval for relapsers does not overlap with that of the nonalcoholic subjects, so there was 99 percent confidence that the two groups did not differ by chance.

Survival analysis has many attractive features. For example, it allows the use of time-varying covariates, which means that the influence of a covariate may be different at different points in time. The effects of depression on substance use, for example, may be stronger at some ages than at others. Survival analysis allows the modeling of some of those relationships. In the example with alcoholic subjects, factors such as relapse, lifetime alcohol use, neuropsychological status, and personality measures were considered, but relapse was found to be the only significant predictor. These techniques have received relatively little attention in the psychiatric literature.

COMPUTATIONALLY INTENSIVE METHODS

Most classic measures of statistical analysis were developed between 1920 and 1950, but a major advance in statistical computing came with the widespread availability of high-speed computers. Within the past decade a whole range of new statistical methods has been introduced. These methodologies require literally millions of calculations. Sometimes they are used to resolve difficult mathematical problems. For instance, it is easy to estimate the mean and the standard deviation for a group of scores. However, investigators often want to study other estimators, such as the trimmed mean, which is defined as the average of the middle 50 percent of the data. Estimating the standard deviation for that trimmed mean can be difficult. Computationally intensive methodologies, such as the bootstrap technique, use random samples from the original data to provide those estimates.

Computationally intensive methodologies have provided a whole new range of options for estimating functional relationships between variables and for building complex decision trees.

EPIDEMIOLOGICAL MEASURES

A variety of epidemiological measures are commonly used in psychiatric research. Epidemiological studies typically focus on outcomes expressed as morbidity and mortality. Morbidity rates are divided into two major types: incidence and prevalence. Incidence refers to the rate at which new cases are occurring, and is defined as the number of new cases that arise in a specific population within a defined time interval. The incidence rate typically is expressed per 1,000 in the population. Conceptually, it is

$$\text{Incidence rate per 1,000} = \frac{\text{New cases per unit of time}}{\text{Persons exposed or at risk per unit time} \times 1{,}000}$$

Prevalence rates describe the number of diagnosed cases at a particular point in time.

$$\text{Prevalence rate per 1,000} = \frac{\text{Cases at specific time point}}{\text{Persons in population at specific time point} \times 1{,}000}$$

Prevalence rate is equal to the incidence rate times the duration of the disease. For example, if the average duration of dementia is five years and its incidence is 3 per 1,000 each year, the prevalence would be 15 per 1,000. Epidemiologists often make the distinction between point prevalence and period prevalence. Point prevalence refers to the number of cases at a defined time period, such as the year 1995. Period prevalence is relevant to a time interval. Period prevalence begins with an estimate of prevalence at the beginning of some time period and includes all new cases accumulated until the end of that defined period.

RESEARCH DESIGNS

Virtually all research designs common to clinical and experimental research are used in psychiatry and behavioral sciences.

OBSERVATIONAL STUDIES

Observational studies do not attempt to manipulate variables in a systematic fashion. Instead, inferences are made on the basis of an ongoing series of observations. Some of the most common observational studies include the cohort study, the panel study, and the case-control study.

Cohort study In a cohort study, groups of those who share some common characteristics are followed over time. Those studies, which are often prospective, resample the same populations on repeated occasions. However, the participants in the study may not be exactly the same on repeated observations.

Panel study A panel study is similar to a cohort study, but it has the stricter requirement that the same persons who were in the original sample be followed at each repeated assessment.

Cohort and panel studies are considered to be *longitudinal* designs. Longitudinal studies make inferences about changes over the course of time. They are often *prospective* and have the advantage of documenting antecedents of new cases. *Cross-sectional studies* differ from longitudinal studies in that they examine different groups of persons at the same point in time. To make inferences about drug use in college, for example, the cross-sectional method would require the sampling of each current class. Then first-year students could be compared with sophomores, juniors, and seniors. They would not be members of the same class or birth cohort.

Case-control study A case-control study compares a group of persons diagnosed with a particular disease (cases) with one or more groups that have not been given the same diagnosis. Case-control studies are typically retrospective because they make inferences about events that have caused currently diagnosed cases.

Observational studies do not exercise control over variables, as is common in experiments. To compensate, investigators often use correlational and multivariate statistical techniques. Variables that are uncontrolled through the experimental design are often matched or controlled using statistical methods.

EXPERIMENTAL STUDIES In contrast to observational studies, in which important variables are not controlled, experimental studies typically involve the systematic manipulation of variables. Mental illnesses have a natural history, and in most instances their course fluctuates considerably without treatment. One of the difficulties in determining the effects of an intervention is that it may occur at a time of crisis. For example, patients with mood disorder might seek psychiatric care on days when they are most depressed. If the exacerbation of the illness is self-limiting (as in the case of mood disorders), the patient's condition will spontaneously improve. A control group can help sort out the effect of treatment from other factors. A group receiving the intervention under study is compared with the control group to determine whether there are differences attributable to the intervention.

It is widely accepted among medical and biobehavioral scientists that a control or comparison group is required to establish causal inference. In some cases investigators are willing to accept quasi-experimental data in which an *ad hoc* control is used, or where there is a stable baseline of observations prior to an intervention. However, several authors have argued that an experiment characterized by a single observation, an intervention, and a second observation is virtually impossible to interpret from a causal perspective.

For experiments using control groups, random assignment to treatment and control conditions is very desirable. Simply stated, randomized clinical trials remove several sources of bias.

The value of randomized clinical trials has been emphasized in a series of review articles. In 1982, Harvey Sacks, Thomas Chalmers, and Henry Smith reviewed six therapies for which approximately equal numbers of randomized clinical trials and nonrandomized trials had been reported in the literature. They found that 79 percent of the studies in which patients were not randomly assigned to groups reported that the therapy was better than the control regimen. The same therapies were found to be effective in only 20 percent of the studies in which patients had been randomly assigned to the treatment or control condition. In a related review Chalmers and his colleagues analyzed 145 papers, which were divided into three categories: those in which the randomization process was blinded, those in which the randomization was unblinded, and those in which assignment to treatment or control was by a nonrandom process. Review of those studies suggested that there was a systematic relationship between the rigor of the experimental design and the probability of finding a treatment benefit. There was a significant treatment benefit in 58 percent of the studies in which the subjects were not randomly assigned. The same benefit was observed in 24 percent of the unblinded randomized studies and in approximately 9 percent of the blinded randomized studies.

There are many sources of bias in studies that do not use control groups, and the end result is frequently an overestimate of the effects of the therapy under study. Those biases are reduced in experimental studies, but the rigor of the experimental design is systematically related to the chances of finding a treatment benefit. Valid scientific inferences must be built on a solid experimental foundation.

ISSUES IN RESEARCH STUDIES

RELIABILITY ATTENUATES RELATIONSHIPS Reliability is the extent to which the test or measure is free of measurement error. Measurement error is the discrepancy between an observed score and the true value for a particular attribute. Under most circumstances the error is assumed to be random and independent of the true score. Reliability is estimated in a variety of ways. If the measure is supposed to be stable over the course of time, such as a personality trait, reliability can be assessed by examining the correlation between scores on the same test for the same subjects when the test is administered at two points in time. Other forms of reliability consider the internal consistency of a test. For example, a measure designed to tap depression may be composed of many items, each of which is an independent assessment of the general depressive attribute. A test is more reliable if responses to those independent items are correlated with one another. Measures of internal consistency, including the Kuder-Richardson 20 and coefficient alpha, are typically correlationlike indexes with ranges from 0 to 1.0. The nearer the reliability coefficient is to 1.0, the higher is the reliability of the test.

The definition of an acceptable level of reliability depends on the purpose of the test. It has been suggested that reliability estimates in the range of 0.70 to 0.80 are high enough for most purposes in basic research. In many research studies the investigator needs only an approximate estimate of whether two variables are correlated. If the result looks promising, it may then be worth the extra time and effort to make the research instruments more reliable. Increasing the reliability beyond 0.90 may increase expense and burden in the respondents. In clinical settings high reliability is extremely important. When tests are used to make important decisions about individual patients, it is essential that classification error be minimized. Thus a test with a reliability of 0.9 might not be good enough.

A number of procedures are available to increase the reliability of a test. For example, increasing the number of items tends to increase the reliability of a measure. A prophecy formula is available that permits the estimation of the specific number of items that need to be added in order to achieve a defined level of reliability. A second strategy is to factor analyze the items. Thus homogeneous subsets of items can be obtained. Selection of items from these homogeneous subsets increases the reliability of the test.

The effect of low reliability on correlations has been well documented in the psychometric literature. Observed correlations between two variables are attenuated when either or both variables are measured with error. The expected observed correlation between two variables measured with error is defined as the true correlation times the square root of the product of their reliabilities or

$$r = tr\sqrt{r_{11}r_{22}}$$

where r is the expected observed correlation, tr is the expected true correlation, r_{11} is the reliability of the first measure, and r_{22} is the reliability of the second measure.

Consider the example of the association between a measure of life stress and a measure of social support. The Schedule of Recent Experiences (SRE) has an observed reliability of 0.55. The Arizona Social Support Interview Schedule has an observed reliability of 0.52. Suppose that the true correlation between these measures was a substantial 0.50. Because each measure contains measurement error, the observed correlation between the two measures would be 0.27. In a study with 50 participants ($r = 0.27, p > 0.05$) the investigator would fail to find a significant correlation between those two variables, even though there is indeed a substantial association.

MULTIPLE COMPARISONS It is common in psychiatric research to use multiple outcome measures. Investigators believe they are beneficial because psychiatric outcomes are complex and a multitude of measures are required to capture them. The use of multiple measures, however, creates other statistical biases. When multiple comparisons are made, the probability of finding at least one difference by chance increases. At the .05 significance level, one significant difference is expected for each 20 independent tests (or 5 percent of all comparisons). Thus, a certain number of significant differences between groups are expected by chance alone. Multiple-comparisons problems occur under two circumstances. First, they may be common when the investigator is comparing multiple groups on the same outcome measure. The number of possible comparisons is equal to

$$j(j-1)/2$$

where j is the number of groups.

For example, with six groups, the number of comparisons would be 15. That difficulty is avoided by using such methods as ANOVA, with appropriate follow-up tests such as the Neuman-Keuls test.

The problem of multiple outcome measures is more difficult. The probability of finding at least one significant difference by chance is defined as:

$$\text{Probability of one or more type I errors} = 1 - (1 - \alpha)^C$$

where C is the number of tests

As the number of tests increases, the investigator can expect to find more spurious results. For example, the probability of finding at least one spurious statistical difference in five contrasts is 0.23. For 10 contrasts, the probability is 0.40, whereas for 20 tests the probability is 0.64. In other words, the chances of drawing the wrong conclusion about the null hypothesis can become quite high when multiple comparisons are performed.

There are several remedies for that situation. In order to avoid false conclusions, some investigators adjust the significance level to be more conservative. That is the basis for the Bonferroni inequality, a common procedure for correcting for multiple comparisons. According to the procedure, if α was originally set at 0.05 but 10 comparisons were performed, the adjusted would be $\alpha/N = 0.005$, where N is the number of comparisons. However, such adjustments may be problematic because some of them are so conservative that the null hypothesis is rarely rejected (that is, a type II error may be introduced). Another approach is to use multivariate techniques that take multiple comparisons into consideration or to reduce the data set to a smaller number of manageable dimensions. For example, if 20 neuropsychological tests were administered to 200 subjects, factor analysis might be used to reduce the neuropsychological domain to three or four factors.

SAMPLE SIZE ISSUES Generally speaking, there are fewer biases in studies with large sample sizes than in studies with small sample sizes. However, a large sample size does not necessarily ensure that conclusions will be meaningful, and many studies with small sample sizes have appropriate internal validity. For studies attempting to estimate prevalence or incidence rates, representativeness is more important than sample size.

In a famous case the *Literary Digest* attempted to forecast the outcome of the 1936 presidential election in which the nominees were Roosevelt (the Democrat) and Landon (the Republican). The magazine drew its sample from its readers, from automobile registrations, and from telephone directories. In 1936 all of those sources overrepresented the wealthy, and most of the subjects were Republicans. The poll showed that Landon would win by a landslide. Roosevelt won by one of the greatest margins in American history. Thus, survey results are of little value if the sample is not random. There was no problem with the sample size in the *Literary Digest* poll; it was very large. In contrast, election day polls using as few as 2,000 respondents to represent all of the voters in the United States have repeatedly been shown to be very accurate. Relatively small samples can be of great value if they are drawn in a random and representative fashion.

Most statistical tests take sample size into consideration. Thus, the probability of rejecting the null hypothesis by chance when the sample size is 10 is 0.05 if the 0.05 alpha level is used, and it is also 0.05 at the 0.05 level for a sample size of 10,000. In other words, there is an inherent correction for sample size. It is commonly asserted that studies that reject the null hypothesis but have a small sample size are of little value. However, obtaining a significant difference with a small sample size often requires that the experimental effect be significantly stronger than obtaining the effect at the same alpha level with a larger sample. Thus demonstrating treatment efficacy with a sample size of 10 per group might require that the treatment effect account for 30 percent or more of the variance in the outcome variable. Obtaining the same significance level with a large sample size (say 300 per group) might require that only 1 percent or 2 percent of the variance be accounted for.

POWER ANALYSIS AND SAMPLE SIZE PLANNING Statistical power defines the probability that a statistical test will produce a significant result. In most research studies the investigator evaluates the null hypothesis—the hypothesis of insufficient evidence for the hypothesis of interest. Typically, the researcher prefers to reject the null hypothesis in favor of the alternative that he or she hopes to support.

When statistical tests are nonsignificant, the investigator is typically unable to conclude that the null hypothesis is correct. Significant treatment effects can be missed because the experiment does not have sufficient power. For example, if too few subjects are in the study or if there is substantial variability, a potentially beneficial treatment might be overlooked.

To avoid making these type II errors, sample size planning is required. That typically requires a power calculation. Formulas for power calculations are available for most types of statistical tests.

A common formula for an experiment that compares two groups is

$$N = \frac{2s^2(Z_\alpha + Z_\beta)^2}{\Delta^2}$$

where s is the standard deviation of the outcome, Z_α is the Z-score associated with the probability of a type I error, Z_β is the Z-score associated with the power of the test, and Δ is the expected differences between the experimental and control groups.

An investigator wants to study changes in neuropsychological functioning following the administration of a β-blocker medication. Patients will be randomly assigned to use the drug or to take a placebo. The neuropsychological test expresses outcomes in *T*-scores (mean = 50, standard deviation = 10), and the drug is expected to reduce performance in comparison with placebo by about five points. The investigator needs to estimate how many patients would be required to have a 90 percent chance of detecting a difference with the probability of a type I error set at 0.05.

The *Z*-score for the 0.05 significance level is 1.96 (Z_α) and that for a power of 0.90 (Z_β) is 1.28. The following calculations are made:

$$N = \frac{2(10)^2(1.96 + 1.28)^2}{5^2} = \frac{200(3.24)^2}{5^2} = \frac{2{,}100}{25} = 84$$

Thus the experiment would require 84 subjects, or 42 in each of the two groups.

SELECTIVE BIASES A variety of biases are common to psychiatric research.

Selective attrition Many studies involve follow-up of patients. However, patients may be available for follow-up on a selective basis. For example, it has been demonstrated that in treatment studies those who are available for follow-up are not a representative sample of the original population. It is common for those available for follow-up to be among those who succeeded in the treatment program. That can be a particular problem in studies where the loss to follow-up is different for treatment and control subjects.

Detection bias A common problem in studies of the etiology of a disease is that those with the diagnosis may be examined in a different way than those who have not already been so labeled. If at all possible, it is valuable to blind the observers.

EX POST FACTO DESIGN PROBLEMS One of the most common designs in biomedical research is the case-control study. In the research methodology literature, that is known as the *ex post facto* design. In such analyses the investigator already knows that the groups being compared differ in some respect. Typically, persons who have a diagnosed disorder are compared with a matched group of persons who have not been placed in the same diagnostic category. The matching occurs for a limited number of variables, and the investigator attempts to determine whether the two groups differ on various previous or current exposures to causal factors. The case-control study is also known as the case-referent study or the case-comparison study design. An example of that design is a comparison between patients with a diagnosis of paranoid schizophrenia (cases) with persons without schizophrenia (controls). Prior histories for the two groups might be compared.

In contrast to true experiments, the case-control or *ex post facto* method has many deficiencies. The investigator clearly knows that the two groups differ on at least one variable. The observation that the groups differ on other variables implies relatively little about causation. In effect, those designs represent parallel correlational studies.

Often in case-control studies an investigator matches patients on a particular variable or uses the variable as a covariate or covariable. If the matching variable or covariate fails to change the difference between the cases and controls, it is assumed that the variable does not explain the underlying basis of the condition. However, there are many rival explanations for the failure of covariables to explain an observed relation. One important explanation is that the covariates were measured with error or that the match was imperfect. To the extent that those problems occur, the effect of adjustment will be greatly attenuated. Thus the fact that a covariable does not have an effect does not necessarily mean that the covariable is unimportant in the observed relationship.

COMPUTER APPLICATIONS The availability of computer software has greatly facilitated the execution of most statistical techniques. The many statistical packages run on different types of platforms or computer configurations. There are three main classes of platforms: mainframe, workstation, and microcomputer. Mainframe computers are now used less frequently for data analysis because many complex analyses can be achieved on less expensive workstations and microcomputers. The two most common types of microcomputers are IBM-compatible and Apple-Macintosh. Intensive computer software is now available for each of them. For general data analysis the Statistical Package for the Social Sciences (SPSS, distributed by SPSS, Inc., Chicago, Illinois), the BMDP series (distributed by BMDP Statistical Software, Los Angeles, California), and the Statistical Analysis System (SAS, distributed by the SAS Institute of Cary, North Carolina) are recommended. They are general-purpose statistical packages that perform essentially all of the analyses common to biomedical research. In addition, a variety of newer packages have emerged. SYSTAT runs on both IBM-compatible and Macintosh systems and performs most of the analyses utilized in biomedical research. The popular SAS program has been redeveloped for Macintosh systems and is sold under the name JMP. Other commonly used programs include Stata, which is excellent for the IBM-compatible computers. It is distributed by the Computing Resource Center of Los Angeles. The developers of Stata publish a regular newsletter providing updates, which makes the package very attractive. StatView is a general-purpose program for the Macintosh computer distributed by Abacus Concepts of Berkeley, California. Newer versions include an additional program called Super ANOVA, which is an excellent set of analysis-of-variance routines. StatView is user-friendly and also has superb graphics. For users interested in epidemiological analyses, Epilog, which is distributed by Epi Center Software of Pasadena, California, is recommended. Epilog is a relatively low-cost program that runs on IBM-compatible platforms. It is particularly valuable for rate calculations, analysis of disease clustering patterns, and survival analysis.

Historically, a major concern of data analyzers was that each analysis program required its own data format. A recent software advance helps alleviate that problem. A program called DBMS/Copy allows the user to move files among a number of spreadsheets, databases, and commonly used statistical packages. It uses a form of artificial intelligence to create a directory of information about the data. With that directory, it can reformat the data so they can be used in most of the commonly available programs. DBMS/Copy is now distributed by SPSS, Inc. A summary of some available computer programs is offered in Table 5.3-6.

Computer software programs that create easy access to highly sophisticated statistical methodologies represent both opportunities and dangers. On the positive side, no serious researcher need be concerned that he or she will not be able to use precisely the statistical technique that best suits his or her purpose, and do so with the kind of speed and economy that was inconceivable just two decades ago. The danger is that some investigators may be tempted to employ after-the-fact statistical manipulations to salvage a study that was flawed at the start, or to extract significant findings through use of progressively more sophisticated multivariate techniques. Such *ex post facto* ransacking of databases does not advance knowledge. Progress in psychi-

TABLE 5.3-6
Summary of Common Statistical Software

Program	Distributor	Platform	Special Features
SPSS*	SPSS, Inc.	Mainframe, IBM, Mac	All purpose, advanced and basic
BMPD†	BMD Statistical Systems	Mainframe, IBM	All purpose, advanced and basic
SAS‡	SAS Institute	Mainframe, IBM	All purpose, advanced and basic
SYSTAT§	SYSTAT, Inc	IBM, Mac	Most routines available, includes multidimensional scaling, excellent graphics
Stata	Computing Resource Center	IBM	Basic statistics, graphics and data management
StatView	Abacus Concepts	Mac	Excellent for ANOVA and graphics
Epilog Plus	Epicenter Software	IBM	Superb simple program for epidemiology, survival analysis

*SPSS Statistical Program for the Social Sciences
†BMDP Biomedical Computing Programs Series D
‡SAS Statistical Analysis System
§SYSTAT The System for Statistics

TABLE 5.3-7
Glossary of Statistical Terms

analysis of variance: A set of statistical procedures designed to compare two or more groups of observations.

canonical correlation: A multivariate technique for simultaneously finding the relation of linear combinations of two or more predictors and two or more outcomes.

chi-square: A set of statistical procedures used to evaluate the relative frequency or proportion of events in a population that fall into well-defined categories.

confidence interval: An interval that is likely to capture the population mean with a specified level of confidence. For the 95 percent confidence interval, the chances are estimated to be 95 in 100 that the true mean falls within that interval.

correlation: A statistical index of the relation between variables. The most common correlation coefficient is the Pearson product moment correlation, an index of bivariate association that varies between −1.0 and 1.0.

dependent variable: The phenomenon of interest in a research study, often called the outcome variable.

descriptive statistics: Methods used to summarize, organize, and describe observations. Examples include the mean, standard deviation, and variance.

discriminant analysis: A multivariate method for finding the relation between a single discrete outcome and a linear combination of two or more predictors.

factor analysis: A data-reduction technique used to reduce a large number of variables to a smaller number of linear combinations of variables.

incidence rate: The rate at which new cases of a disease or a condition are occurring. The incidence rate per 1,000 persons in the population is the number of new cases that occur within a defined unit of time, divided by the persons exposed or at risk during the same time unit, multiplied by 1,000.

independent variable: A variable studied in relation to an outcome of dependent variables. In experiments the independent variable is controlled by the experimenter.

inferential statistics: Methods used for drawing general conclusions about probabilities on the basis of a sample.

logistic regression: A multivariate method for estimating the effect of several independent variables on a dichotomous outcome. The method requires fewer assumptions than discriminant analysis or multiple regression.

log-linear analysis: Methods that allow the construction of systematic models to evaluate the relation between categorical variables. Complex models can be constructed and specific significance tests can be ordered. Tests for hierarchical relationships can also be evaluated.

McCall's T: A specialized standard score with a mean of 50 and a standard deviation of 10.

multiple regression: A form of multivariate analysis in which a scaled variable is correlated with a linear combination of independent or predictor variables.

multivariate analysis: Methods for considering the relationship of three or more variables. Multivariate methods include multiple regression, discriminant analysis, canonical correlation, and factor analysis.

multivariate analysis of variance: A multivariate technique that uses an analysis-of-variance design but includes a dependent variable that is a linear combination of variables.

nonparametric statistics: Statistical methods that do not require restrictive assumptions about population distributions.

null hypothesis: The hypothesis that observed differences or variation in scores can be attributed to random sources. When the null hypothesis is rejected, observed differences between groups are deemed to be improbable by chance alone.

population: The entire collection of a set of objects and so on having the same definition.

power: The probability of rejecting the null hypothesis when, in the real world, it should have been rejected. Power is the probability of identifying a true difference.

power analysis: Analytical methods for estimating the sample size required to detect statistical effects of defined size for variables with known variances.

prevalence rate: The number of diagnosed cases of a disease or a condition. Point prevalence is the number of cases at a particular point in time. The point prevalence rate per 1,000 is defined as the cases at a specific point in time, divided by the number of persons in the population at a specific point in time, multiplied by 1,000. Period prevalence is the number of cases occurring during a specified period of time.

probability: A quantitative statement of the likelihood that an event will occur. A probability of 0 means that the event is certain not to occur; a probability of 1.0 means the event will occur with certainty.

random variable: A variable for which the variation is determined by chance.

sample: A subset of observations selected from a population.

standard deviation: The square root of the variance. The standard deviation gives an estimate of the average deviation around the mean.

standardized or Z-score: The deviation of a score from its group mean expressed in standard deviation units.

survival analysis: Methods for evaluating the timing of events. The methods can be used to evaluate life expectancy, age of onset of psychological illness, time to relapse for those in treatment, or the timing of developmental milestones, such as first word, age of initiation of smoking, age at marriage, and any other time-dependent variable.

***t*-test:** A statistical procedure designed to compare two sets of observations.

type I error: The error that occurs when the null hypothesis is rejected when it should have been retained.

type II error: The error that occurs when the null hypothesis is retained when it should have been rejected.

variance: An estimate of variability. The sum of the squared deviations around the mean, divided by the number of cases.

atry will depend increasingly on careful crafting of hypotheses, experimental design, and appropriate statistical modeling.

Brief definitions of commonly used statistical terms are given in Table 5.3-7.

SUGGESTED CROSS-REFERENCES

Section 5.1 discusses epidemiology. Section 5.2 discusses the methods used in animal research and its relevance to psychiatry.

REFERENCES

Bullock K D, Reed R J, Grant I: Reduced mortality risk in alcoholics who achieve long-term abstinence. JAMA *267:* 668, 1992.

Chalmers T C, Celano P, Sacks H, Smith H: Bias in treatment assignment in controlled clinical trials. N Engl J Med *309:* 1358, 1983.

Cohen J: *Statistical Power Analysis for the Behavioral Sciences.* Erlbaum, Hillsdale, NJ, 1988.

Cohen J, Cohen P: *Applied Multiple Regression/Correlation Analysis for the Behavioral Sciences.* Erlbaum, Hillsdale, NJ, 1983.

*Cook T D, Campbell D G: *Quasi-experimentation: Design and Analysis Issues for Field Studies.* Rand-McNally, Chicago, 1979.

Daniel W W: *Applied Nonparametric Statistics,* ed 2. PWS-Kent, Boston, 1990.

Darlington R B, Carlson P M: *Behavioral Statistics: Logic and Methods.* Free Press, New York, 1987.

Dawson-Saunders B, Trapp R G: *Basic and Clinical Biostatistics,* ed 2. Appleton & Lange, Norwalk, CT, 1994.

Edwards L K, editor: *Applied Analysis of Variance in Behavioral Science.* (*Statistics: Textbooks and Monographs,* vol 137). Marcel Dekker, New York, 1993.

*Efron B, Tibshirani R: Statistical data analysis in the computer age. Science *253:* 390, 1991.

Glantz S A: *Primer of Biostatistics,* ed 3. McGraw-Hill, New York, 1992.

Gottman J M, Rushe R H: The analysis of change: Issues, fallacies, and new ideas. J Consult Clin Psychol *61:* 907, 1993.

*Ingelfinger J A, Mosteller F, Thibodeau L A, Ware J H: *Biostatistics in Clinical Medicine,* ed 3. McGraw-Hill, New York, 1994.

Jessor R, Jessor L J: *Problem Behavior in Psychosocial Development.* Academic Press, New York, 1977.

Kaplan R M: *Basic Statistics for the Behavioral Sciences.* Allyn & Bacon, Newton, MA, 1987.

Kaplan R M, Sacuzzo D P: *Psychological Testing: Principles, Applications, and Issues,* ed 3. Brooks/Cole, Monterey, CA, 1993.

Keppel G: *Design and Analysis.* Prentice-Hall, Englewood Cliffs, NJ, 1991.

Keren G, Lewis C: *A Handbook for Data Analysis in the Behavioral Sciences: Statistical Issues.* Erlbaum, Hillsdale, NJ, 1993.

Keselman H J, Keselman J C: Analysis of repeated measurements. In *Applied Analysis of Variance in Behavioral Science,* vol 137 of *Statistics: Textbooks and Monographs,* Lynne K Edwards, editor, p 105. Marcel Dekker, New York, 1993.

Maxwell S E, Delaney H D: *Designing Experiments and Analyzing Data. A Model Comparison Approach.* Wadsworth, Belmont, CA, 1990.

McCall R: *Fundamental Statistics for Psychology,* ed 5. Harcourt Brace Jovanovich, New York, 1990.

*Sacks H, Chalmers D C, Smith H: Randomized versus historical controls for clinical trials. Am J Med *72:* 233, 1982.

Siegel S, Castellan J Jr: *Nonparametric Statistics for the Behavioral Sciences,* ed 2. McGraw-Hill, New York, 1988.

Smith M B, Glass G D: *Research and Evaluation in Education and the Social Sciences.* Prentice-Hall, Englewood Cliffs, NJ, 1987.

*Tabachnick B G, Fidell L S: *Using Multivariate Statistics,* ed 2. Harper & Row, New York, 1989.

Van de Geer J P: *Introduction to Multivariate Analysis for the Social Sciences.* Freeman, San Francisco, 1971.

Winer B J: *Statistical Principles in Experimental Design.* McGraw-Hill, New York, 1971.

CHAPTER 6 THEORIES OF PERSONALITY AND PSYCHOPATHOLOGY: PSYCHOANALYSIS

6.1 PSYCHOANALYSIS

GLEN O. GABBARD, M.D.

INTRODUCTION

Contemporary psychiatrists are blessed with an impressive array of treatments in their therapeutic armamentarium. Among these highly effective therapeutic tools are electroconvulsive therapy, highly specific pharmacotherapeutic agents, sophisticated protocols for behavioral desensitization, hypnosis, family and marital psychotherapies, group psychotherapy, individual psychotherapy, and psychoanalysis. On the basis of a thoroughgoing understanding of the patient, clinicians must determine which modality to prescribe. Not all patients take medication as prescribed, nor do all patients carry through on prescribed behavioral exercises. Only a systematic understanding of the patient's personality can explain this noncompliance.

When it comes to unraveling the mysteries of the human mind, no body of knowledge approaches that of psychoanalytic theory. Although the basic contributions of Sigmund Freud, the founder of psychoanalysis, have undergone considerable revision since their development 100 years ago, several of Freud's fundamental hypotheses regarding the workings of the mind remain central to psychiatric practice today.

PSYCHIC DETERMINISM Freud discerned that such diverse aspects of human experience as symptoms of psychiatric disorders, vocational choices, dreams, selection of marital partners, and slips of the tongue all had meaning. Behavior, thoughts, feelings, and symptoms are the final common pathways of unconscious processes. The concept of overdetermination—the notion that several intrapsychic factors operate simultaneously to create a specific symptom, thought, or behavior—is still a pivotal construct in contemporary psychoanalytic thinking. For example, a young woman may choose to be a surgeon because of the confluence of several unconscious determinants: (1) she is seeking to win the approval of her father, who is also a surgeon; (2) she wishes to outdo her mother, who is a homemaker; (3) she is channeling aggressive wishes into a socially acceptable and productive activity; and (4) she wishes to repair the damage she feels she did to her younger siblings while growing up.

Biological factors also influence symptoms and behavior. Hallucinations and suicidal wishes, for example, may be the end product of aberrations of brain chemistry. However, the meanings given to those phenomena are still psychically determined on the basis of the psychological makeup of the individual patient.

THE UNCONSCIOUS As implied by the principle of psychic determinism, the construct of the unconscious mind is also a central feature of psychoanalytic thinking. In his clinical work with hysterical patients, Freud noted that long-forgotten memories reemerged in the process of the treatment. That discovery led him to conclude that the human mind has a form of censorship that deems certain memories, thoughts, and feelings unacceptable. The material is *repressed*—that is, buried in the unconscious—and the person is no longer consciously aware of the phenomena that have undergone repression.

Freud observed that parapraxes, slips of the tongue, provided concrete evidence of the role of the unconscious in everyday life. The eruption of a repressed thought or feeling when one word is substituted for another often reveals an unacceptable unconscious wish. One woman meant to say she was "a Protestant" and instead blurted out "a prostitute."

Freud's work with his patients' dreams provided another avenue of confirmation that his model of the unconscious was valid. The manifest or overt content of dreams often deals with material that would be entirely unacceptable in waking life. Moreover, Freud was able to demonstrate that a repressed childhood wish is almost always a motivating force that generates the content of the dream.

PAST IS PROLOGUE The psychoanalytic viewpoint stresses the crucial role of childhood development in the shaping of the adult. All major psychoanalytic schools of thought view developmental successes and failures as central to the evolution of adult character and highly influential in the pathogenesis of adult psychiatric disorders. Pathogenetic factors may include both actual trauma and subtle and repetitive forms of interaction that occur between children and their parents and between children and their siblings.

Freud's theory of childhood development was particularly remarkable in that he was able to delineate psychosexual stages. Freud postulated the existence of sexual energy, which he termed *libido,* as an organizer of developmental stages. As psychoanalysis evolved, greater emphasis came to be placed on the interpersonal context in which the libidinal transitions took place. Specific patterns of *object relations,* by which Freud meant relationships with significant figures in one's life, are formed during childhood and repeated again and again in adult life. Similarly, one's sense of self is forged in this smithy of interactions with others during those formative years.

Although this section is devoted to psychoanalysis proper as both a theory and a treatment, the basic tenets enumerated here are useful in a variety of nonanalytic settings in clinical psychiatry. The data of psychoanalysis originated in the method of free association, whereby patients say whatever comes to mind without attempting to censor unacceptable thoughts. However, the theory of human behavior that grew out of those data harbors the potential to enrich and extend the practice of psychiatry.

HISTORY

The history of psychoanalysis is inextricably linked to the life of Sigmund Freud. He was born on May 6, 1856, in Freiburg, a small town in Moravia, which has since become a part of Czechoslovakia. When Freud was 4 years old, his father, a Jewish wool merchant, moved the family to Vienna. He grew up there, was educated there, and practiced there almost his entire life. In 1938 Freud fled the Nazis by moving to England, where he died the next year (Figures 6.1-1 through 6.1-10).

FREUD'S CAREER

Freud was first and foremost an empirical scientist. He was convinced that the key to unlocking the secret of mental processes was to be found in the study of brain physiology. The dominant approach to human physiology in Europe during Freud's formative years was the Hermann Helmholtz school of physiology. According to the deterministic principles of that school, physiological and mental processes resulted from causal laws and sequences that could ultimately be reduced to the tenets of physics, such as the principles of inertia and conservation of energy. Freud was also influenced by the theories of Charles Darwin, which were much discussed in scientific circles in his day.

Coexisting with Freud's tendency to embrace scientific empiricism was his lifelong fascination with literature, particularly the writings of Johann Wolfgang von Goethe and William Shakespeare. Freud had a deep appreciation and respect for the word as a result of being raised in the Jewish tradition. Through his immersion in literature and religion, Freud became familiar with the complexities of the human psyche and the roles of symbolism and meaning in understanding human nature. Freud's thinking always displayed a romantic element, and it was no accident that he was ultimately awarded the Goethe Prize for literature.

Medical training

Freud's experience in medical school laid the foundation for his subsequent scientific orientation. It was during those years that he was exposed to the ideas of Darwin and Helmholtz. The intellectual currency of the day was scientific empiricism; an emphasis on measurement and observation was replacing the mysticism and romanticism that had pervaded scientific thought in central Europe in the first part of the 19th century.

During his medical school years, Freud was profoundly influenced by two mentors, Ernst Brücke and Theodore Meynert. Those two figures—along with Sigmund Exner, who worked in Brücke's laboratory—dominated the physiological research in Europe during that era. Freud also worked in Brücke's laboratory and viewed Brücke in particular as a role model whose integrity and scientific discipline Freud strove to emulate.

Brücke, Meynert, and Exner all endorsed the idea that the nervous system operates through the transmission of quantitatively variable excitations from afferent to efferent nerve endings. Because the chemical basis of neural conduction was poorly understood, Brücke assumed that conduction is electrical in nature. Central to Brücke's thinking was the notion that the mind and the body are organized along principles of psychophysical parallelism. The reflex arc was his model of neural functioning. In other words, no spontaneous central activity exists in the nervous system; it merely functions as a passive instrument that remains quiescent until stimulated by exogenous energies. The end result of the stimulus is the reduction of incoming irritation to a minimum. That physiology of force and energies, drawing heavily from the doctrine of conservation of energy, was to have a far-reaching effect on Freud's own thinking.

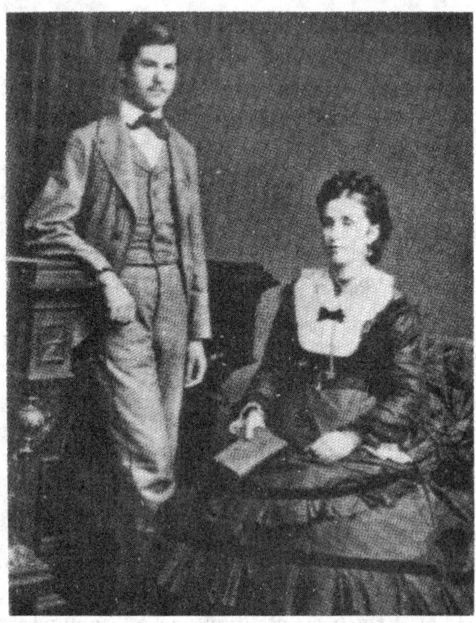

FIGURE 6.1-2 *Sigmund Freud and his mother in 1872. (Courtesy of Austrian Information Service, New York.)*

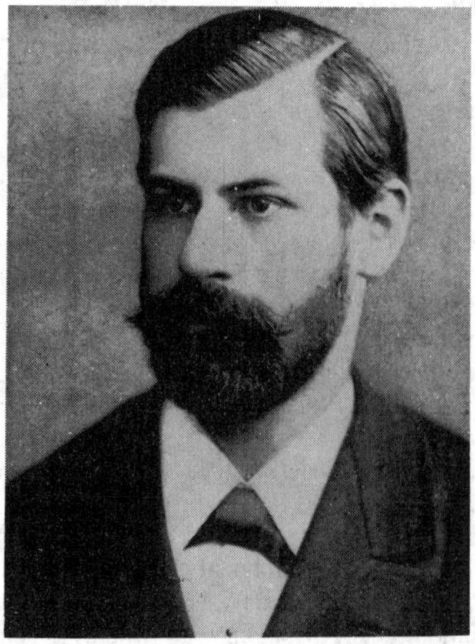

FIGURE 6.1-1 *Sigmund Freud as a young man. (Courtesy of Austrian Information Service, New York.)*

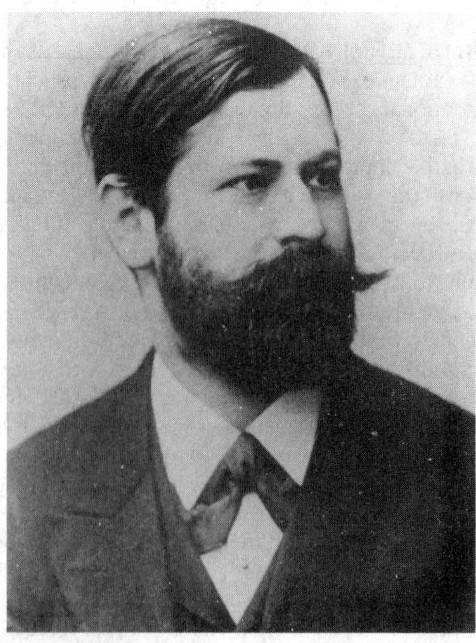

FIGURE 6.1-3 *Sigmund Freud in 1891 at age 35. (Courtesy of Menninger Foundation Archives, Topeka, Kansas.)*

Medical career After graduation from medical school, Freud continued to work in Brücke's laboratory for a year. There Freud developed his overriding scientific ambition to apply the principles of Helmholtz and Brücke to the nervous system. He was convinced that both psychopathological manifestations and normal mental functioning could ultimately be explained in terms of the forces and energies that regulate the nervous system.

Freud's research was interrupted when he realized that laboratory work could not generate sufficient income to support a family. He had fallen in love with Martha Bernays, and he was forced to enter medical practice to provide an adequate standard of living for his new bride. In 1882 he began work as a general physician in the Vienna General Hospital. After a stint in the surgical service, he served in Theodore Meynert's psychiatric clinic. Although Freud had some reservations about Meynert's clinical competence, his study of Meynert's amentia (acute hallucinatory psychosis) had a lasting effect on him and contributed to the concept of wish fulfillment, which later became a crucial part of Freud's theory of the unconscious.

Neurological career Freud's exposure to neuroanatomy and neuropathology under the charismatic leadership of Meynert led him to choose neurology as a specialty. In 1885 he received a grant that allowed him to study for 19 weeks at the Salpêtrière in Paris. There his career was powerfully shaped by the great French neurologist, Jean-Martin Charcot (Figure 6.1-5).

Under Charcot's influence, Freud became fascinated with the problem of hysteria. Whereas most neurologists did not take hysterical phenomena seriously, Charcot viewed them as worthy of careful study. He viewed them as related to a congenital degeneration of the brain, but he placed considerable emphasis on the role of hypnosis in the treatment of hysterical disorders. When Freud observed the precipitation of hysterical manifestations through the use of hypnotic suggestion, he began entertaining the possibility that hysteria has a psychological origin.

When Freud returned to Vienna in 1886, he was determined to pursue his dual interests in hypnosis and neurology. Hungering for more knowledge about the clinical applications of hypnosis, he journeyed to Nancy, France, to study with Ambroise-Auguste Liébault, who was attempting to remove neurotic symptoms through hypnotic suggestions. Liébault's associate, Hippolyte Bernheim, was also studying the characteristics of suggestibility and noted that it was present in patients with neurotic disorders other than hysteria. Freud's observations of the therapeutic uses of hypnosis used by Bernheim and Liébault convinced

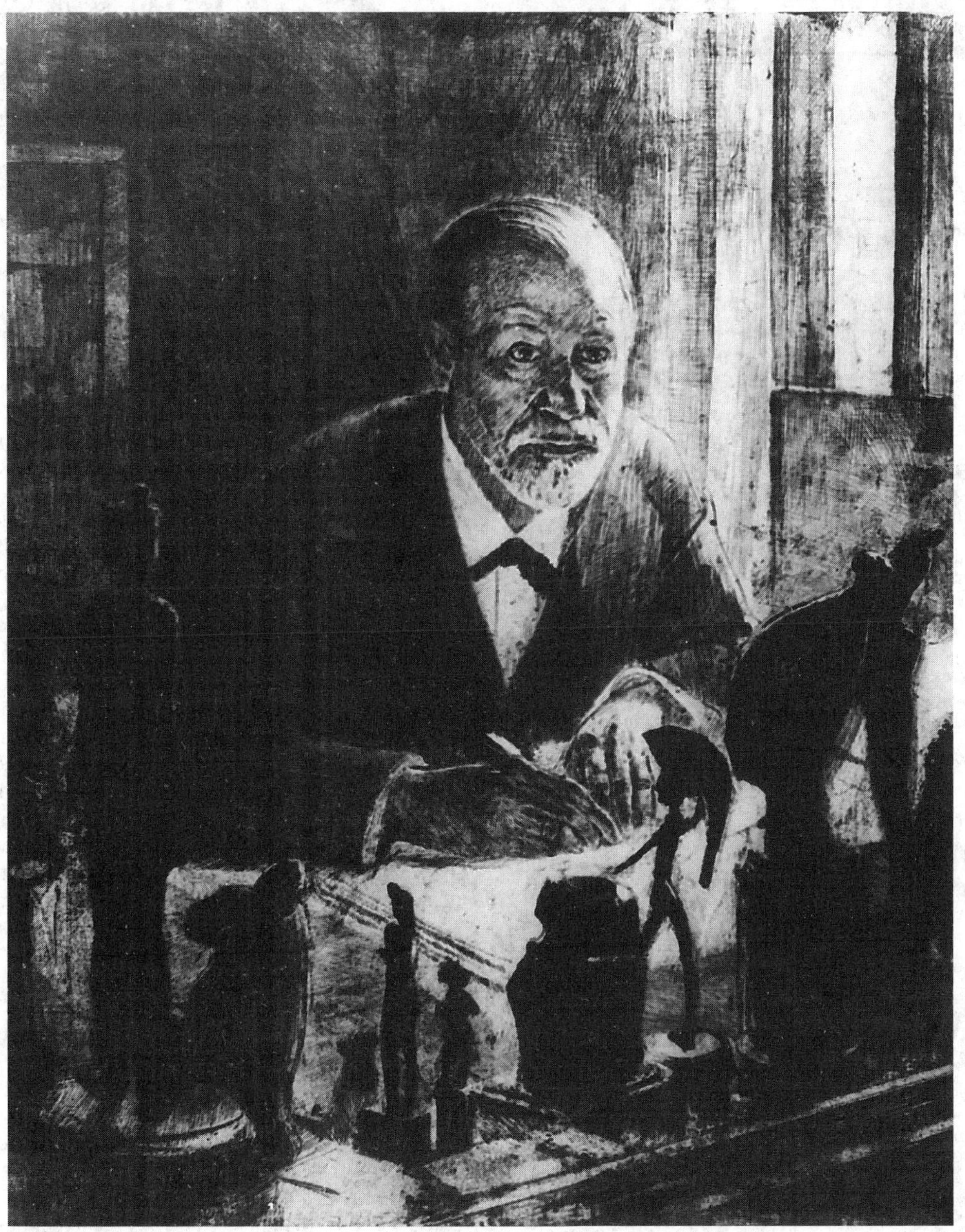

FIGURE 6.1-4 *Sigmund Freud in his Vienna office. (Etching by Max Pollak. Courtesy of Menninger Foundation Archives, Topeka, Kansas.)*

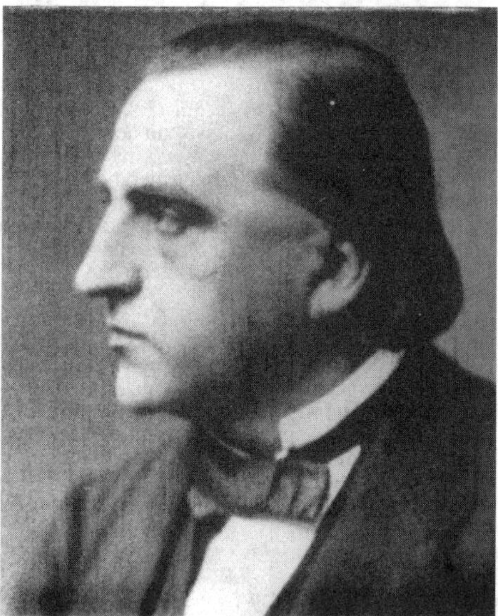

FIGURE 6.1-5 *Jean-Martin Charcot. (Courtesy of the New York Academy of Medicine.)*

him that powerful unconscious forces were involved in human motivation and behavior. He also learned that physicians themselves may play significant roles as instruments of psychotherapeutic change.

Freud's first major neurological work appeared in 1891. Entitled *Aphasia*, it offered a functional explanation that accounted for variants of aphasic disorders in terms of disruptions of the radiating associative pathways. That same year with Oscar Rie, a pediatrician, he was coauthor of a major work on unilateral paralysis in children. Two years later he wrote a massive monograph on children's paralysis that received major acclaim.

Project for a Scientific Psychology The period between 1895 and 1897 represented a turning point in Freud's career. Intent on anchoring psychology to neurophysiology, Freud struggled to apply the principles of the Helmholtz school to the workings of the mind. The result was his pivotal work, *Project for a Scientific Psychology*. Freud was disgusted with what he had written and wanted it destroyed. It was finally published posthumously because of the recognition that it had a far-reaching influence on Freud's subsequent ideas.

Freud's explanation of the mechanisms of the nervous system revolved around the principles of neuronic inertia, which asserted that neurons tend to divest themselves of Q, the quantity of excitation. Pain can be related to an excess of nervous excitation, and pleasure can be viewed as the end result of the discharge of that excitation. At the root of the theory was a model of the nervous system as a passive recipient of stimulation from external forces and a concept of motivation in terms of tension or drive reduction.

Influenced by the principle of conservation of energy, Helmholtz had insisted that the sum of forces must remain constant in any isolated system. Freud elaborated on that principle of constancy in his *Project* by developing the idea that mental processes constantly strive for equilibrium or homeostasis. In 1893 Freud formulated the principle as follows: "If a person experiences a psychical impression, something in his nervous system, which we will for the moment call the sum of excitation, is increased. Now in every individual there exists a tendency to diminish this sum of excitation once more, in order to preserve his health." This principle of constancy served as the economic foundation for Freud's theory of instincts.

Although many of Freud's ideas in his *Project* have been confirmed by more sophisticated neuropsychological studies, he was unable to forge the grand synthesis between the psychological and the neurological to which he had aspired. Nonetheless, in a number of his other works, "Preliminary Communication" (1893) and *Studies on Hysteria* (1895), the notions of the discharge of affect and cerebral excitation clearly derive from ideas generated in *Project for a Scientific Psychology*. Moreover, the model of the mind set forth in Freud's magnum opus, *The Interpretation of Dreams* (1900), also had clear roots in his *Project*. Finally, his understanding of the pleasure-unpleasure principle was profoundly influenced by the basic theorems of his *Project*. As late as 1920, in *Beyond the Pleasure Principle*, the derivatives are clearly in evidence.

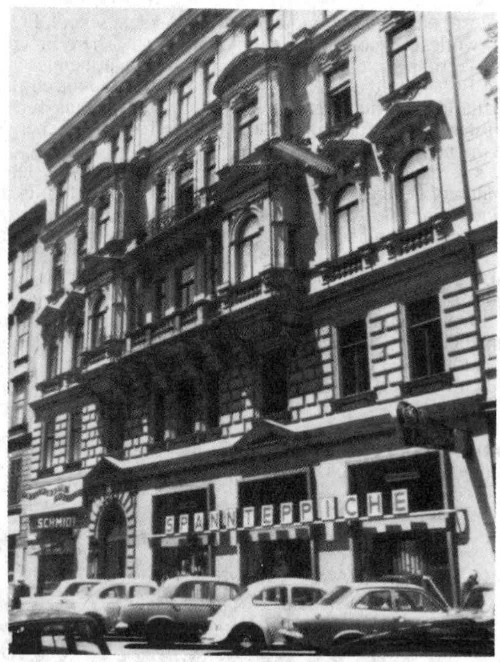

FIGURE 6.1-6 *Berggasse 19, the building in which Freud had his offices. It now houses the Freud Museum. (Courtesy of Austrian Information Service, New York.)*

EVOLUTION OF PSYCHOANALYSIS

During the decade from 1887 to 1897, Freud's interests in clinical neurology gradually waned. His collaboration with Josef Breuer, a distinguished older colleague with whom he had worked at Brücke's institute of physiology, led him into the nether regions of the unconscious mind, a subject that attracted his interest away from neurology and toward the evolution of psychoanalysis. As the two clinicians struggled together to understand the mysteries of hysteria, they gave birth to psychoanalysis as a therapeutic technique, as a scientific discipline, and as a method of investigation.

COLLABORATION WITH BREUER: THE CASE OF ANNA O. AND *STUDIES ON HYSTERIA* The body of theory, knowledge, and technique that is now referred to as psychoanalysis had its origins in one typical case treated by Breuer. The patient, Bertha Pappenheim, consulted Breuer in December 1880 and continued in treatment with him until June 1882. Referred to by Breuer as "Anna O.," she was an intelligent and attractive woman of 21 years who presented a plethora of hysterical symptoms in association with her father's fatal illness. The symptoms included serious disturbances of sight and speech, inability to ingest food, paralysis of three extremities with contractures and anesthesias, and a nervous cough. She also manifested two distinct states of consciousness: one a relatively normal young woman, the other a troublesome and naughty child. Breuer observed that the shift between the two discrete personalities seemed to be induced by some form of autohypnosis, and he was able to bring about the transition by placing Anna O. in a hypnotic state.

Breuer knew that Anna had been very attached to her father and had nursed him alongside her mother while he was on his death bed. During her altered states of consciousness, Anna could recall vivid fantasies and powerful feelings she had experienced as her father lay dying. Breuer was astonished to note that his patient's recollection of the affect-laden circumstances

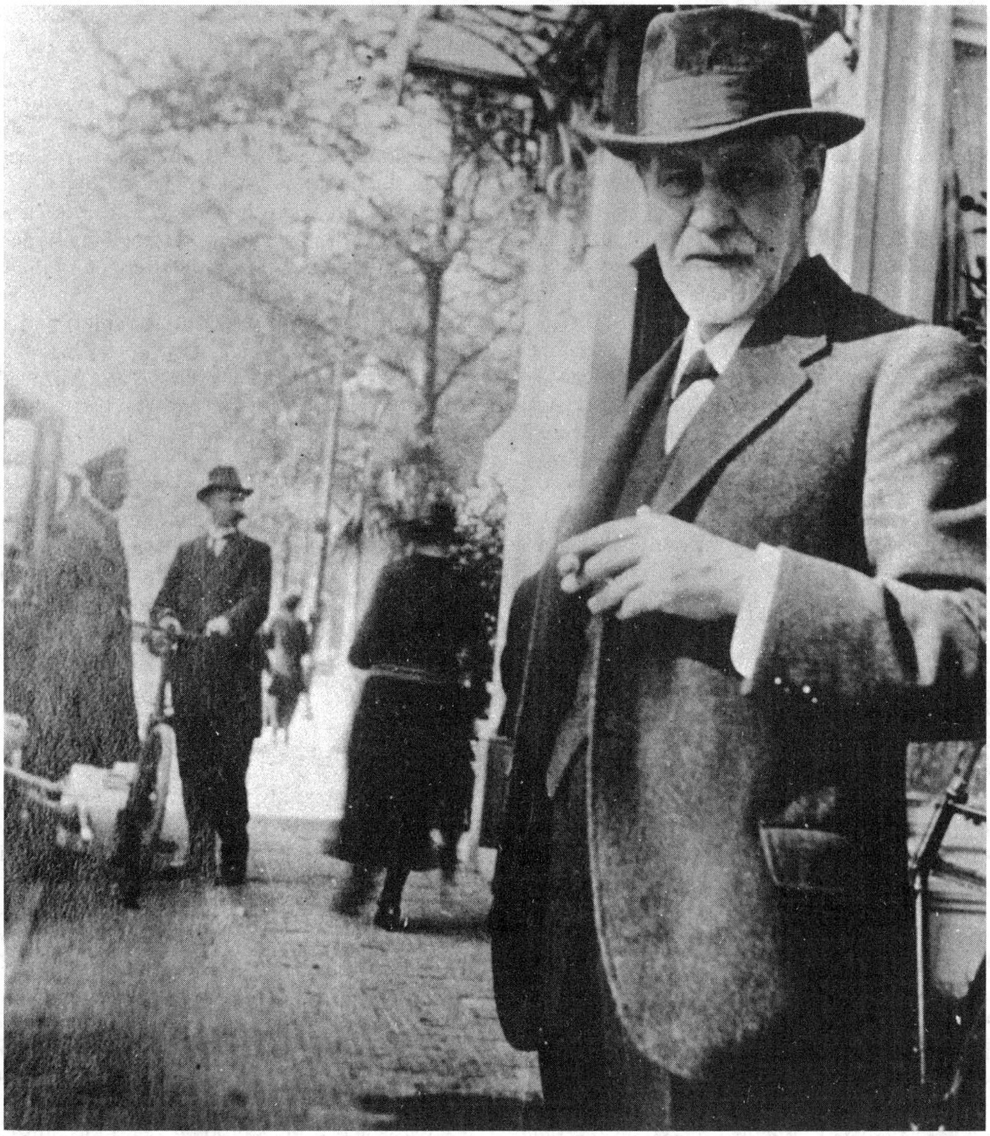

FIGURE 6.1-7 *Sigmund Freud on a street in Vienna. (Courtesy of Menninger Foundation Archives, Topeka, Kansas.)*

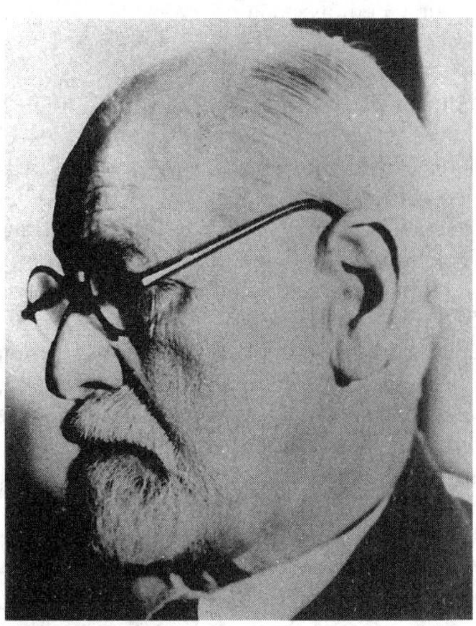

FIGURE 6.1-8 *Sigmund Freud in 1938. (Courtesy of Menninger Foundation Archives, Topeka, Kansas.)*

during which her symptoms first appeared led those same symptoms to disappear. Anna O. dubbed this process the "talking cure." She was so taken by it that she continued to discuss one symptom after another. For example, she remembered sitting at her father's side while her mother was absent and having a fantasy or daydream about a snake. In her vision the snake was about to bite her father. She tried to ward off the snake, but her arm had gone to sleep as a result of having been draped over the back of her chair. The paralysis remained until she was able to recall the scene under hypnosis and regain use of her arm.

Breuer became enchanted with his extraordinary patient. He spent so much time with her that his wife grew jealous and resentful. Frightened by the sexual connotations of his wife's complaints, he abruptly terminated the treatment of Anna O. Several hours after that termination, he was called to Anna's bedside in the midst of a crisis. He found her in an agitated state in the throes of hysterical childbirth. Although he had been unaware of any sexual feelings toward him, the phantom pregnancy (pseudocyesis) reflected Anna O.'s intense erotic longings for Breuer. He calmed his patient down by inducing a hypnotic trance, and in a state of extreme agitation he arranged for an immediate departure to Venice with his wife for a second honeymoon.

Although Breuer found the whole experience with Anna O. to be highly disconcerting, Freud was intrigued by the power of unconscious memories and suppressed affects to produce hysterical symptoms. Breuer was reluctant to publish his account, but Freud insisted that he write it up from memory some 13 or 14 years after it had occurred. The collaboration of Breuer and Freud resulted in the publication of "Preliminary Communication" in 1893. In that document they articulated the causal linkage between psychic traumata and hysterical symptoms.

In 1895, with the publication of *Studies on Hysteria,* Breuer and Freud presented a much more sophisticated clinical and theoretical treatise on the pathogenesis and treatment of hysterical symptoms. The hysterical patient suffers from "reminiscences," according to Freud. In other words, a repressed incompatible idea is the source of the symptomatic manifestations. The patient had experienced a childhood trauma that stirred up overwhelming feelings of an intensely unpleasant nature. The traumatic experience represented an incompatible idea to the patient and was, therefore, intentionally dissociated or repressed from consciousness. The nervous excitation associated with the incompatible idea was transformed or converted into somatic channels that produced hysterical symptoms. As a result, all that was left in conscious awareness was a mnemonic symbol that was only remotely connected with the traumatic event, often through disguised links. Freud thought that, if the memory of the traumatic experience could be brought back into the patient's conscious awareness, along with the strangulated affect associated with it, the symptoms would disappear as the affect was discharged.

EVOLUTION OF FREUD'S TECHNIQUE

Use of hypnosis Although Freud had used hypnosis since he opened his practice in 1887, he had initially used the technique simply as a means to remove symptoms through suggestion. When he encountered disappointing results, he shifted to the *cathartic method* as a result of Breuer's account of Anna O. In 1889 Frau Emmy von N. consulted Freud for treatment of a variety of hysterical complaints, including anesthesia and pain in her leg, an ovarian neuralgia, deliriums, hallucinations, phobias, and abulias. For the first time Freud used Breuer's cathartic method, attempting to remove the woman's symptoms through a process of recovering and verbalizing suppressed feelings with which they were associated. The method came to be known as *abreaction.*

Freud soon became dissatisfied with the abreactive approach when he observed that the therapeutic benefits lasted only as long as the patient maintained contact with the physician. The personal relationship with the physician appeared to have greater therapeutic importance than the specific hypnotic technique. His understanding of the doctor-patient relationship was expanded by an incident in which one of his patients awoke from a hypnotic trance and threw her arms around Freud's neck. Experiences such as those, coupled with Breuer's report of Anna O., led Freud to realize that the patient's attachment to the physician had an erotic component. However, instead of fleeing in panic from such developments, as Breuer had done, Freud investigated them as he did any other phenomena encountered in treatment. Those early encounters led Freud to discover *transference,* a concept that was to become a cornerstone of psychoanalytic theory and technique. Transference refers to the displacement onto the analyst of thoughts, feelings, and behavior originally associated with significant figures from the past.

Freud's discovery of transference contributed to his abandonment of hypnosis. In his view, hypnosis concealed aspects of the transference, so that they could not be investigated as part of the process. He also felt that hypnosis encouraged the patient to please the hypnotist, instead of learning about the origins and the meanings of symptoms. Freud also observed that many patients were simply refractory to hypnosis.

Concentration method and development of free association One of the patients who was particularly resistant to the hypnotic abreactive technique was Elizabeth von R. Freud evolved his method of concentration as a way of dealing with the refractory nature of that patient. He remembered that Bernheim had asserted that all forgotten memories could be recalled consciously if the physician asked appropriate leading questions and urged the patient to remember.

Freud asked his patient to lie down on a couch and to close her eyes. He asked her to concentrate on a particular symptom and to recall any memories that might assist in understanding the origin of the symptom. Freud would then press his hand on the patient's forehead and reassure her that she would indeed recall relevant memories when he questioned her about them.

Much to Freud's credit, he allowed himself to learn from his patients. Elizabeth von R., for example, responded to the concentration method by telling Freud, "I could have told you that the first time, but I didn't think it was what you wanted." Freud then modified his technique by informing patients to simply ignore all censorship. When Elizabeth von R. reproached him for interrupting her flow of thoughts with his questions, Freud modified his technique again by reducing the frequency of his questions so as not to interfere with the natural flow of the patient's associations.

By the late 1890s Freud had come to realize that the concentration technique was more an impediment than a facilitator. He abandoned the procedures of directing the patient's attention, placing pressure on the forehead, directing the patient to close her eyes, and asking probing questions. Instead, he had the patient lie on the couch and say whatever came to her mind, the method of *free association,* which remains a central part of psychoanalytic technique today.

REPRESSION AND RESISTANCE In addition to Freud's discovery of transference, two other seminal psychoanalytic concepts—resistance and repression—grew out of his clinical investigations of hysterical patients in the 1890s. In the evolution of his technique from hypnosis to the concentration method to free association, Freud noted that certain patients *resisted* the therapeutic technique. Some could not be hypnotized. Others were unable to recall memories of causative significance. Still others encountered a mental block when they attempted to free-associate. Freud discerned that a stubborn refusal to cooperate was not at the root of the resistance. Many of his patients who were genuinely distressed by their symptoms were also the most resistant to the therapeutic techniques. Freud concluded that active forces in the patient's unconscious mind were excluding unpleasant thoughts or memories from conscious awareness. He referred to that active force as *repression.*

Freud's studies of hysterical symptoms convinced him that repression was a pivotal force in the process of symptom formation. He described the mechanism in the following manner:

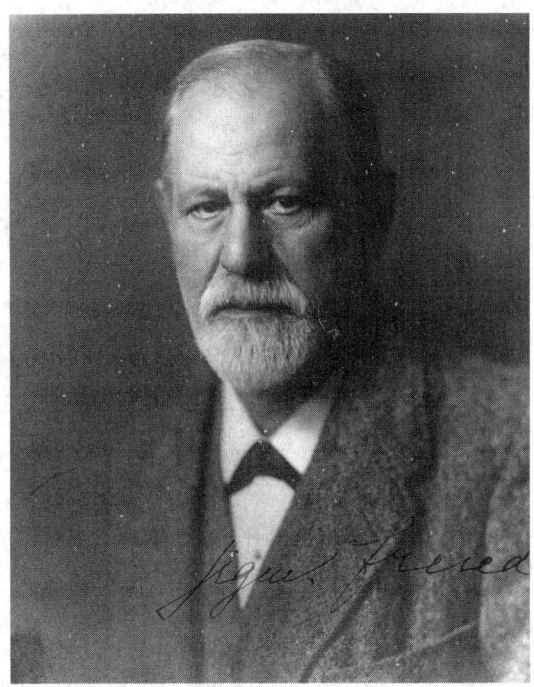

FIGURE 6.1-9 *Sigmund Freud in 1920. (Courtesy of Menninger Foundation Archives, Topeka, Kansas.)*

A traumatic experience or a series of experiences, usually of a sexual nature, that had occurred in childhood had been forgotten or repressed because of its painful or unacceptable nature, but the excitement associated with the incident was not extinguished, and traces persist in the unconscious in the form of repressed memories. The memories may remain without pathogenic effect until a contemporary event, such as a disturbing love affair, revives them. The so far successful repression fails at that point, leading the patient to experience what Freud referred to as *the return of the repressed.* The original sexual excitement is revived and comes to the surface in the form of a neurotic symptom.

On the basis of his understanding of repression, Freud postulated that symptoms arise from a compromise between a repressed impulse and the countervailing forces of repression. In cases of hysteria, Freud believed that impulses that were unacceptable and therefore repressed were diverted into somatic pathways, resulting in such symptoms as paralysis, blindness, and disturbances of sensation. He speculated that similar mechanisms are involved in the development of paranoid ideation and obsessive-compulsive symptoms. The main thrust of treatment then was to assist patients in the retrieval of repressed memories of sexual experiences so that the excitations attached to them could emerge into conscious awareness and be discharged through verbalization.

THEORY OF INFANTILE SEXUALITY Freud's treatment of hysterics during the early years of the 1890s convinced him that childhood sexual seduction plays a major role in causing the neuroses. Many of his patients reported such seductions by nursemaids, fathers, and caretakers, and Freud believed that repressed memories of actual sexual traumata created neurotic symptoms.

In the latter half of the 1890s, he began to reconsider those views and ultimately made a dramatic shift in his thinking. Fantasies of sexual seduction by parental figures began to displace actual seduction as the pivotal pathogenetic factor in the neuroses. Although the reasons for the shift are not entirely clear, several reasons have been suggested: (1) Working from the hypothesis that childhood sexual seduction is the cause of neurosis, Freud had been unable to bring a single analytic case to an entirely successful conclusion. (2) He had always been skeptical about the reports of perverse acts by fathers, and the frequency of hysteria made it difficult for him to believe that so many sexually abusive fathers could exist in the Vienna of his day. (3) Some of the reports from his patients sounded so fantastic that it became difficult for Freud to distinguish the difference between truth and fiction in such accounts. Emma Eckstein, for example, reported a "memory" of encountering the devil and being tortured by him as he inserted needles into her fingers. Many other patients recounted stories of torture and possession linked to witchcraft. (4) In both his self-analysis and further clinical investigations, Freud became convinced of the importance of internal psychological processes and the role of fantasy in distorting reality to conform to wishes.

Although Freud's subsequent writings indicate that he never entirely abandoned his belief that actual sexual seductions by parents took place, by the late 1890s he had clearly moved to a position of stressing childhood sexual fantasies as the core of the neuroses. By adopting a psychodynamic theory of infantile sexuality in which the child's psychosexual life occupies center stage, psychoanalysis had taken a new direction, coming into its own as a depth psychology. The child was no longer portrayed as an innocent victim of wicked adults but was seen as a sexual being with powerful fantasies and wishes. By the waning years of the 19th century, Freud had completed his self-analysis, proposed a dynamic theory of infantile sexuality, developed the technique of free association, postulated the origins and the pathogenesis of the neuroses, and designed a theory of the mind that included the unconscious as its centerpiece. Psychoanalysis as it is known today was clearly recognizable at that point, and as the 20th century approached, Freud was immersed in perhaps his most monumental work, *The Interpretation of Dreams.*

THE INTERPRETATION OF DREAMS

SIGNIFICANCE OF DREAMS Freud became aware of the significance of dreams when he noted that patients frequently reported their dreams in the process of free association. Through their further associations to the dream content, he learned that the dreams were definitely meaningful, even though that meaning was often hidden or disguised. Most of all, Freud was struck by the intimate connection between dream content and unconscious memories or fantasies that were long repressed. That observation led Freud to declare that the interpretation of dreams was the royal road to the understanding of the unconscious.

Freud's self-analysis also contributed to his appreciation of the significance of dreams. One of his principal methods in conducting his own analysis was to rely on dreams and his associative exploration of those dreams. Indeed, Freud used many of his own dreams as illustrative examples in *The Interpretation of Dreams,* which appeared in 1900. Considered by many to be Freud's greatest work, the book still informs clinical psychoanalytic work with dreams today. In his magnum opus Freud put forth the notion that a dream is the disguised fulfillment of an unconscious childhood wish that is otherwise not readily accessible to conscious awareness in waking life.

In attempting to characterize the psychology of dreaming, Freud laid the foundations for ego psychology. He suggested that unconscious childhood wishes can be transformed into disguised conscious manifestations only if a censor exists in the mind. The censor, acting in the service of the ego, functions to preserve sleep. By disguising disturbing thoughts and feelings, the censor makes sure that the dreamer's sleep will not be disturbed. Moreover, early forms of defense mechanisms in the ego were delineated by Freud's investigation of the different methods of disguise used by the ego—for example, displacement, condensation, and symbolic representation. Freud also drew beginning parallels between the dream mechanisms and the pathological thoughts of psychotic patients in the waking state.

ANALYSIS OF DREAM CONTENT The dream, as it is recalled by the dreamer, is the result of the unconscious mental activity that occurs during sleep. Freud believed that dreaming is simply the conscious experience of thoughts during sleep. Contemporary research has revealed that the cognitive activity of sleep actually has considerable variation. The dreaming activity described by Freud is probably more or less restricted to the stage 1 rapid eye movement (REM) periods of the sleep-dream cycle; those periods occur approximately every 90 minutes during the night. The thoughts that occur in non-REM sleep periods tend to be more logically organized, briefer, and more realistic.

Freud distinguished between two layers of dream content. The *manifest dream* refers to the content as it is recalled by the dreamer, including the affect and sensory experiences accompanying the dream and any commentaries on the dream that occur within the dream. The unconscious thoughts and wishes that threaten to awaken the dreamer constitute the *latent* content. Freud referred to the unconscious mental operations by which the latent dream content is transformed into the manifest dream as the *dream work*. Freud's technique of dream interpretation was based on free association, in which the patient would say whatever came to mind in response to aspects of the dream. Through that approach the manifest content of the dream would gradually give way to the underlying latent content in which the unconscious meaning of the dream is contained.

Freud initially believed that internal or external stimuli initiate dreaming. Modern dream research has demonstrated that endogenous patterns of activation in the central nervous system associated with particular phases of sleep are responsible for the onset of dreaming activity. A more contemporary understanding of what Freud viewed as initiating stimuli are that such phenomena are simply incorporated into dream content and influence the material in the dream to that extent.

Nocturnal sensory stimuli A variety of sensory impressions—including hunger, pain, thirst, and urinary urgency—may influence dream content. For example, a man whose thirst is beginning to interfere with his sleep may dream that he has risen from bed, gone to the bathroom, drunk a glass of water, and returned to bed as a way of safeguarding the continuity of sleep. Freud's view of dreaming as the guardian of sleep is still considered a valid function of dreaming, but recent research suggests that the function of dreams is considerably more complex in that the preservation of sleep is only one of many functions.

Day residues Freud discerned that an important influence on the dream thoughts is the residues of feelings, ideas, and thoughts associated with experiences of the preceding day. The final form of the manifest content of the dream is shaped by those day residues, as well as by sensory stimuli. Seemingly innocuous or unimportant elements from the day residues may be used as the vehicle for the disguised expression of unconscious drives and wishes of an erotic or aggressive nature. Hence, events of the preceding day may effectively conceal the infantile impulse at the core of the dream.

Repressed infantile drives Following the dictum that a dream represents the disguised fulfillment of an unconscious childhood wish, Freud understood the driving forces behind dream activity as impulses or wishes from the earliest years of life. Those repressed wishes, usually sexual or aggressive and stemming from oedipal and preoedipal levels of development, are melded with day residues and nocturnal stimuli to produce the end result. Despite some challenges from discoveries of recent sleep research, Freud's observations continue to have clinical utility.

Dreams by young children are particularly unique because they show little distinction between infantile and current conflicts. In general, the dreams of young children are less disguised than the dreams of older persons and show much less distinction between manifest and latent dream content because of the relative immaturity of the defensive operations of the child's ego.

DREAM WORK As just noted, the dream work comprises several processes that transform latent dream content into manifest dream content. The theory of the nature of dream work, which Freud first put forth in *The Interpretation of Dreams,* became the fundamental description of the operation of unconscious processes. The mechanisms that Freud elaborated from his study of dreams proved to have broad applications to neurotic symptom formation and to a general psychology of the mind.

Dream formation The basic problem of dream formation is to determine how the latent dream content represents itself through the manifest dream. In Freud's view the state of sleep leads to a relaxation of repression. With the repressive forces weakened, unconscious impulses and wishes are allowed to press for gratification and discharge. Since an outlet in motor expression is blocked by the sleep state, those repressed wishes and impulses have to find means of representation through mechanisms of thought and fantasy. Both elements of day residues and nocturnal stimuli are appropriated to express those latent wishes or impulses in the manifest dream.

The unconscious wishes and impulses that emanate from childhood are repressed because they are painful or unacceptable. Although repression is relaxed during sleep, Freud postulated that a dream censor is still actively involved in resisting the discharge of those impulses and disguising their true nature. The dream censor serves to attach impulses and wishes to neutral or innocent images from the residues of the dreamer's current psychological experience. Trivial or insignificant images from the dreamer's day residues are presumably linked on the basis of some resemblance that allows connections to be established. To enable those neutral images to surface in the dream, the dream work uses a set of disguised mechanisms that include condensation, displacement, symbolic representation, and secondary revision.

Condensation In condensation several unconscious impulses, wishes, or feelings can be combined and attached to one manifest dream image. For example, a composite character may appear in the dream that has the name of one person in the dreamer's life, a beard like another person, and a musical instrument that reflects a third person. The feelings associated with those three persons may be disguised in the resulting amalgam and may become apparent only through analysis of the various dream elements. The converse of condensation, diffusion, can also occur in a dream when a single latent wish or impulse is distributed through multiple representations in the manifest content.

Displacement In displacement the energy or intensity associated with one object is diverted to a substitute object that is associatively related but more acceptable to the dreamer's ego. Murderous wishes toward one's mother, for example, may be redirected toward a neutral or insignificant figure in one's life. In that manner the dream censor has displaced affective energy in such a way that the dreamer's sleep can continue undisturbed.

A special instance of displacement, projection, involves the attribution of the dreamer's own unacceptable impulses or wishes to another character in the dream. For example, a dreamer who finds homosexual impulses unacceptable may attribute them to his analyst in the dream. In some cases different aspects of the dreamer are represented in several characters in the dream.

Symbolic representation Freud noted that the dreamer would often represent ideas or objects that were highly charged by using innocent images that were in some way connected with the idea or object being represented. In that manner an abstract concept or a complex set of feelings toward a person could be symbolized by a simple, concrete, or sensory image. Freud noted that symbols have unconscious meanings that can be discerned through the patient's associations to the symbol. However, he also believed that certain symbols have universal meanings—for example, a flower as a symbol for female genitalia, a snake as a symbol for the penis.

Secondary revision The mechanisms of condensation, displacement, and symbolic representation are characteristic of a type of thinking that Freud referred to as *primary process.* That primitive mode of cognitive activity is characterized by illogical, bizarre, and absurd images that seem incoherent. Freud believed that a more mature and reasonable aspect of the ego is at work during the dream to organize some of those primitive aspects of the dream into a more coherent form. He called that process *secondary revision;* in it intellectual processes of a more mature nature make the dream somewhat more rational. The process is related to more mature activity characteristic of waking life, which Freud termed *secondary process.*

TYPICAL DREAMS For the most part Freud believed that the underlying meaning of a dream reveals itself only through a proper analysis of the dreamer's associations. However, just as he made exceptions to certain universal symbols, he also thought that certain dreams are universal in their meaning, and he referred to them as *typical dreams.*

Anxiety dreams Freud's dream theory preceded his development of a comprehensive theory of the ego. Hence, his understanding of dreams stressed the importance of discharging drives or wishes through the hallucinatory contents of the dream. He viewed such mechanisms as condensation, displacement, symbolic representation, projection, and secondary revision primarily as facilitating the discharge of latent impulses, rather than protecting the dreamer from anxiety and pain. Freud understood anxiety dreams as reflecting a failure in the protective function of the dream work mechanisms. In other words, the repressed impulses succeed in working their way into the manifest content in a more or less recognizable manner. The ego reacts to the emergence of the threatening content with intense anxiety; the dreamer often experiences severe distress or may even partially awaken.

Punishment dreams Dreams in which the dreamer experiences punishment represented a special challenge for Freud because they appear to represent an exception to his wish-fulfillment theory of dreams. He came to understand such dreams as reflective of a compromise between the repressed wish and the repressing agency or conscience. In the punishment dream the ego anticipates condemnation by the dreamer's conscience if the latent unacceptable impulses are allowed direct expression in the manifest dream content. Hence, the wish for punishment by the patient's conscience is satisfied by giving expression to punishment fantasies. In that formulation Freud anticipated the concept of the superego and the interplay between the ego and the superego, which he did not elaborate into the structural model for some 20 years.

TOPOGRAPHIC MODEL OF THE MIND

The publication of *The Interpretation of Dreams* in 1900 heralded the arrival of Freud's topographic model of the mind. That model divides the mind into three regions: the conscious system, the preconscious system, and the unconscious system, each of which has its own unique characteristics. That theory of the psyche embraces four central assumptions. The first assumption is the notion of psychological determinism derived from Freud's Helmholtzian background. The second assumption is the existence of unconscious psychological processes. The third assumption postulates that neurotic symptoms are related to unconscious psychological conflicts and forces. Finally, the topographic theory assumes that some psychological energies originated in instinctual drives.

THE CONSCIOUS The conscious system in the topographic model is characterized as the part of the mind in which perceptions coming from the outside world or from within the body or mind are brought into awareness. Consciousness is viewed as a subjective phenomenon whose content can be communicated only by means of language or behavior. Freud assumed that consciousness employs a form of neutralized psychic energy that he referred to as *attention cathexis.* In other words, one is aware of a particular idea or feeling as a result of the investment of a discrete amount of psychic energy in that particular idea or feeling. Up until 1923 Freud viewed the conscious mind as in control of motor activity as well. Freud devoted little of his own energies to the conscious system, so it is relatively undeveloped in his theory of the mind, as compared with the unconscious.

THE PRECONSCIOUS The preconscious system comprises those mental events, processes, and contents that are capable of being brought into conscious awareness by the act of focusing attention. Although most people are not consciously aware of the appearance of their first-grade teachers, they can ordinarily bring that image to mind by the deliberate focusing of attention on the memory. Conceptually, the preconscious interfaces with both the unconscious region and the conscious region of the mind. To reach conscious awareness, the contents of the unconscious must become linked with words and thus become preconscious. The preconscious also maintains the repressive barrier and censors unacceptable wishes and desires. Unlike the unconscious, which is characterized by primary process thinking, the preconscious is characterized by secondary process thinking and the delay of drive discharge.

THE UNCONSCIOUS The unconscious system is a dynamic one. In other words, the mental contents and processes of the unconscious are kept out of conscious awareness through the force of censorship or repression. The repressive force, sometimes referred to as *countercathexis,* manifests itself as the resistance to remembering. The essence of the unconscious can be captured in five key features:

1. The unconscious is closely related to instinctual drives. In Freud's theory of development, instincts were then thought to consist of sexual and self-preservative drives, and the unconscious was thought to contain primarily the mental representations and derivatives of the sexual instinct.
2. The content of the unconscious is limited to wishes seeking fulfillment. Those wishes provide the motivation for dream and neurotic symptom formation. That view is now considered reductionistic.
3. The unconscious system is characterized by primary process thinking, which has as its principal aim the facilitation of wish fulfillment and instinctual discharge. Primary process thinking is governed by the pleasure principle and, therefore, disregards logical connections, has no conception of time, represents wishes as fulfillments, permits contradictions to exist simultaneously, and denies the existence of negatives. The primary process is also characterized by extreme mobility of drive cathexis, meaning that the investment of psychic energy can shift from object to object without opposition. The mental mechanisms of displacement, condensation, and symbolic representation, discussed as part of the dream work, are part of the primary process as well. That form of thinking is also associated with creativity and with severe mental illness.
4. Memories in the unconscious have been divorced from their connection with verbal symbols. Hence, when words are reapplied to for-

gotten memory traits, as in psychoanalytic treatment, the verbal recathexis allows the memories to reach consciousness again.

5. The contents of the unconscious can become conscious only by passing through the preconscious, where censors are overpowered, allowing the elements to enter into consciousness.

DYNAMICS OF MENTAL FUNCTIONING

Freud conceptualized the psychic apparatus in the context of the topographic model as a kind of reflex arc. The arc consists of a series of segments arranged consecutively, with the perceptual or sensory system at one end and the motor system at the other. The memory and association systems were conceived of as occupying the segments between the two extremes. Perceptions are thus modified and stored in the form of memories, and the mental energy associated with unconscious ideas seeks discharge through thought or motor activity. Hence, the normal pathway of discharge in the waking state is from the perceptual to the motor end. Freud suggested that the flow of psychic energy can be reversed in sleep, moving from the motor to the perceptual end. That reversal of the normal flow of energy, which he called *topographic regression,* is the basis for the appearance of childhood images in dreams and the presence of hallucinations in psychoses.

When Freud subsequently abandoned the reflex arc model of the mind, he nevertheless retained the concept of regression as a key component to his theory. In neurosis, for example, the patient is thought to revert to earlier modes of instinctual discharge or to earlier levels of fixation. That form of regression is termed *libidinal* or *instinctual* regression.

FRAMEWORK OF PSYCHOANALYTIC THEORY

After the development of the topographic model, Freud turned his attention to the complexities of instinct theory. The *source* of the instinct refers to the part of the body from which it arises, to the somatic process that gives rise to stimuli that are represented in mental life as emotions, or to drive representations. The *impetus* or pressure refers to the amount of force or energy created by the instinctual stimulus. The *aim* refers to the action-directed gratification of the instinct. And the *object* is the target or recipient of the action-directed gratification and may be a person or a thing.

INSTINCT OR DRIVE THEORY

Freud was determined to anchor his psychological theory in biology. That choice led to terminological and conceptual difficulties when Freud used terms derived from biology to denote psychological constructs. Instinct, for example, refers to a pattern of species-specific behavior that is genetically derived and, therefore, more or less independent of learning. Used primarily by students of animal behavior, the word "instinct" applies to such phenomena as migration, nesting, and maternal behavior.

Ethological studies have increasingly demonstrated that instinctual patterns are modified through experiential learning. The effects of adaptation on instinctually derived patterns have made Freud's instinctual theory problematic. Confusion also surrounds the translation of the German word *Trieb* into English; it does not have an unequivocal correlate. Freud was referring to powerful, imperative strivings, such as self-preservation and sexuality. Hence, *Trieb* has been translated as "drive," "instinct," and "instinctual drive."

Confounding matters further is the fact that Freud himself shifted his view of instinct theory over time. His clearest definition appeared in his 1915 paper "Instincts and Their Vicissitudes," in which he referred to an instinct as "a concept on the frontier between the mental and the somatic, as the psychical representative of the stimuli originating from within the organism and reaching the mind, as a measure of the demands made upon the mind for work in consequence with its connections with the body." The ambiguity inherent in this concept on the borderland between the biological and the psychological has led to considerable debate about whether the mental representation aspect of the term and the physiological component should be integrated or separated.

Although "drive" may have been closer than "instinct" to Freud's meaning, he preferred not to translate *Trieb* in that manner because behavior theorists of his time had already appropriated the term "drive." In contemporary usage, "drive" and "instinct" are often used interchangeably.

CLASSIFICATION OF INSTINCTS Freud's instinct theory grew out of clinical observations. The sexual drive, for example, appeared to be central to the pathogenesis of hysteria. Hence, Freud was primarily preoccupied with the sexual drive during the 1890s and into the early 20th century. Although he originally postulated a self-preservative instinct in the 1890s, he did not elaborate it until some 20 years later. As psychoanalytic theory continued to evolve, his theorizing about the role of instincts became more and more abstract and divorced from clinical data.

Libido Freud defined *libido* as "that force by which the sexual instinct is represented in the mind." The association of libido with sexuality is somewhat misleading in that Freud's intent was to encompass the general notion of pleasure, as well as sexuality, including both the physiological underpinnings and the mental representations. The linkage of genital sexuality with libido was viewed as the end result of a course of development in which libidinal expression takes a variety of forms, as is elaborated in the discussion of libidinal zones later in this section.

Ego instincts From 1905 on, Freud maintained a dual-instinct theory subsuming sexual instincts and ego instincts connected with self-preservation. Until 1914, with the publication of "On Narcissism," Freud had paid little attention to ego instincts. In that communication Freud invested ego instinct with libido for the first time. He postulated an ego libido and an object libido. Freud thus viewed narcissistic investment as an essentially libidinal instinct and called the remaining nonsexual components the ego instincts. In that rather confusing model Freud suggested that the clash between libido and ego instincts may produce symptoms of neurosis. At that point ego instincts connoted both the drives of self-preservation, such as hunger and thirst, and early aspects of the superego or conscience.

Aggression When psychoanalysts today discuss the dual-instinct theory, they are generally referring to libido and aggression. However, Freud originally conceptualized aggression as a component of the sexual instincts in the form of sadism. As he became aware that sadism has nonsexual aspects to it, he made finer gradations, enabling him to categorize aggression and hate as part of the ego instincts and to categorize the libidinal aspects of sadism as components of the sexual instincts. With that differentiation, the impulse to attack in order to defend oneself can be seen as aggression associated with the ego instincts, and sadism can be regarded as a fusion of sexual and aggressive instincts.

Freud ran into much greater difficulty when he attempted to explain self-destructive behavior with his newly developed taxonomy of

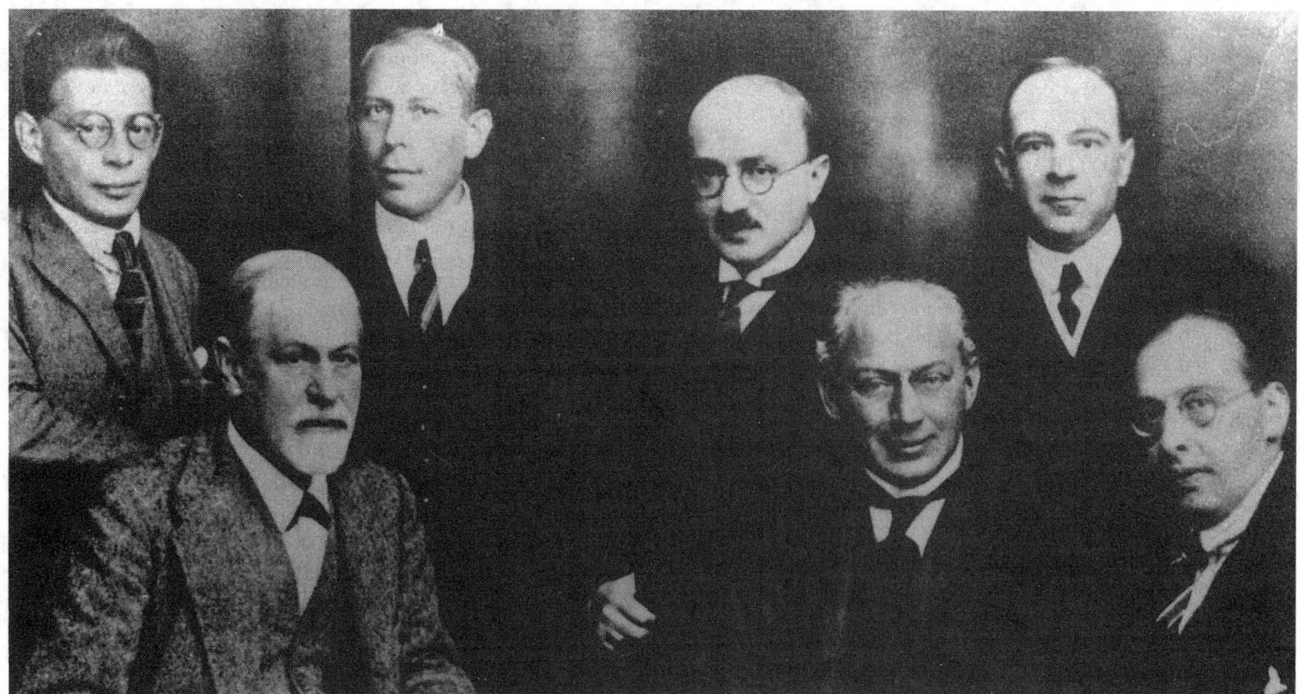

FIGURE 6.1-10 *Freud and his disciples in 1922. From left to right: Otto Rank, Sigmund Freud, Karl Abraham, Max Eitingon, Sandor Ferenczi, Ernest Jones, and Hans Sachs. (Courtesy of Menninger Foundation Archives, Topeka, Kansas.)*

instincts. How, for example, could he view the self-mutilation of masochistic patients as part of the ego instincts of self-preservation? Finally, to account for the clinical data he was observing, in 1923 he was compelled to conceive of aggression as a separate instinct in its own right. The source of that instinct, according to Freud, is largely in skeletal muscles, and the aim of the aggressive instincts is destruction. He also noted that aggression in response to the frustration of libido is secondary, rather than primary.

Life and death instincts Before the designation of aggression as a separate instinct, Freud, in 1920, subsumed the ego instincts under a broader category of life instincts. Life instincts were juxtaposed with death instincts, and the two were referred to as *Eros* and *Thanatos* in *Beyond the Pleasure Principle.* The life and death instincts were regarded as forces underlying the sexual and aggressive instincts. Although Freud could not provide clinical data that directly verified the death instinct, he thought it could be inferred by observing the *repetition compulsion,* the tendency of persons to repeat past traumatic behavior. Freud felt that the dominant force in biological organisms had to be the death instinct. He viewed it as a tendency of all organisms and their component selves to return to an inanimate state. Here again, Freud was linking psychology to principles of hard science—specifically, the notions of entropy and constancy from physics.

In contrast to the death instinct, Eros, the life instinct, refers to the tendency of particles to reunite or bind to one another. That counterpoint to entropy leads to organization and greater unities of systems. Sexual reproduction is the most obvious example. The death and life instincts are directly analogous to catabolism and anabolism. In modern psychoanalytic thinking the death instinct has been largely discounted except by followers of Melanie Klein. The prevalent view today is that the dual instincts of sexuality and aggression are sufficient to explain most clinical phenomena.

PLEASURE AND REALITY As noted in the discussion of Freud's *Project,* the constancy principle, the tendency of an organism to maintain a particular state or equilibrium, was one of the cornerstones for the evolution of psychoanalytic theory. Freud's notion of the death instinct was clearly linked to the constancy principle and was also associated with what he termed the *Nirvana principle,* which postulates that an organism strives to discharge internal tension and to seek a state of rest. In 1911 Freud further elaborated the nature of the human organism's need to maintain a state of equilibrium when he described two basic tenets of mental functioning, the pleasure principle and the reality principle.

Freud essentially recast the primary process and secondary process dichotomy into the pleasure and reality principles, thus taking an important step toward solidifying the notion of the ego. Both principles, in Freud's view, are aspects of ego functioning. The *pleasure principle* is defined as an inborn tendency of the organism to avoid pain and to seek pleasure through the discharge of tension. The *reality principle,* on the other hand, is considered a learned function, closely related to the maturation of the ego, that modifies the pleasure principle and requires the delay or postponement of immediate gratification.

INFANTILE SEXUALITY

In 1905 Freud published *Three Essays on the Theory of Sexuality.* He regarded that work as second only to *The Interpretation of Dreams* in importance. Contrary to popular belief, Freud's ideas did not create much of an uproar among the scientific community or even among the public. The Vienna of his day was exposed to a great deal of popular literature that openly discussed an array of sexual problems. However, Freud's notion that children are influenced by sexual drives has made it difficult for some people to accept psychoanalysis throughout its 100-year history.

Freud's book was significant because it set forth three major tenets of psychoanalytic theory. First of all, Freud broadened the definition of sexuality to include forms of pleasure that transcend genital sexuality. Second, Freud established a developmental theory of childhood sexuality that delineated the vicissitudes of erotic activity from birth through puberty. Third, he forged a conceptual linkage between neuroses and perversions.

PSYCHOSEXUAL DEVELOPMENT

Freud's ideas about psychosexual developmental stages and libidinal zones have worked their way into popular culture. It is commonplace to hear someone who is greedy or voracious referred to as "oral." Persons who are withholding and stubborn may be regarded as "anal." The popular usage reflects the fact that Freud's identification of psychosexual stages also laid the groundwork for the subsequent psychoanalytic theory of character.

The earliest manifestations of infantile sexuality, in Freud's view, are basically nonsexual. They are associated with such bodily functions as feeding and bowel and bladder control. As the libidinal energy shifts from the oral zone to the anal zone to the phallic zone, each stage of development is thought to build on and to subsume the accomplishments of the preceding stage. The oral stage occupies the first 12 to 18 months of life. The anal stage picks up where the oral stage leaves off and extends to approximately 36 months of age. The phallic stage is usually associated with the period of time between ages 3 and 5.

Throughout each of the psychosexual stages, specific erotogenic zones, when stimulated, give rise to erotic pleasure. During the oral stage the infant derives pleasure from nursing, in addition to satisfying the physiological need to assuage hunger. Karl Abraham, a disciple of Freud, divided the oral period into a sucking phase and a biting phase, thus incorporating aspects of aggression and sadism into the notion of sexual pleasure. Similarly, Abraham divided the anal stage into an anal-sadistic phase and an anal-erotic phase.

The phallic stage is initially focused on urination as the source of erotic activity. That urethral phase was briefly noted by Freud but was elaborated on by a number of later writers. During the urethral phase the primary eroticism is pleasure in urination and a secondary urethral retention pleasure. One may see derivatives of that phase in paraphilic activities involving sexual excitement associated with urinating on others or being urinated on by others.

Freud suggested that phallic erotic activity in boys is a preliminary stage leading to adult genital activity. Whereas the penis remains the principle sexual organ throughout male psychosexual development, Freud postulated that the female has two principal erotogenic zones, the vagina and the clitoris. He thought that the clitoris is the chief erotogenic focus during the infantile genital period but that erotic primacy shifts to the vagina after puberty. Studies of human sexuality have subsequently questioned the validity of that distinction.

VICISSITUDES *Three Essays on the Theory of Sexuality* also discusses the vicissitudes of libido, by which Freud meant the different paths that the instinct can take within the sexual life of the person. Although in normal adult functioning sexual activity is dominated by the genital zone, pregenital libidinal zones continue to play a role, specifically during foreplay. Kissing, for example, constitutes a pleasurable stimulation of the oral zone, and stimulation of the anus may also accompany foreplay or be part of lovemaking. In healthy adults who have attained mature genital potency, the sexual act culminates in the pleasure of orgasm.

Freud conceptualized infantile sexuality as *polymorphously perverse*—that is, composed of partial or component instincts that allow sexual excitation to occur from multiple sources. For example, oral and anal stimulation involves such component instincts as pleasure in watching *(scoptophilia),* pleasure in showing *(exhibitionism),* and pleasure in cruelty *(sadism).* Those component instincts emerge as pairs of opposites. Scoptophilia and exhibitionism are instinctual pairs, as are sadism and masochism. Freud thought that all those components are combined into a unity at puberty under the primacy of the genital zone. Unacceptable components are either repressed or confined to foreplay. If the libido becomes irrevocably attached to one of the pregenital erotogenic zones or if a part instinct predominates, the result may be a perversion in which the normal act of intercourse is replaced by some other activity, such as fetishism or voyeurism. Freud termed the persistent attachment of the libido to a particular phase of genital development a *fixation.*

NEUROSIS AND PERVERSION In studying perversions, Freud noted that perverse fantasies are ubiquitous in the human unconscious. He thought that neurosis is the negative of perversion. In other words, whereas persons with perversions express their fantasies and impulses in action, neurotic persons repress similar fantasies and impulses, which manifest themselves only as neurotic symptoms. Although that conceptualization continues to be valid in some cases, it perhaps oversimplifies the pathogenesis of perversions. Freud's formulation, for example, cannot explain why a part instinct in one person is repressed and transformed into a neurotic symptom whereas in another it is expressed overtly as a perversion. More theoretical sophistication was required to explain those individual differences.

OBJECT RELATIONS IN CLASSICAL THEORY

Although Freud's thinking is usually associated with drive theory and ego psychology, he also evolved his own version of object relations theory. He always held that early experiences with parenting figures have profound influences on subsequent development. He believed that adult relationships are later editions of childhood relationships. However, in Freud's opinion, the development of object relations is intimately connected with the sexual drive. Infants, in his view, have limited awareness of the mothering figure. Their main focus is on internal states of tension and relaxation. Hence, their longing for the object is, in fact, a longing for drive discharge or tension release. The object is viewed as a vehicle to satisfy drive pressures. As a result of that perspective on the infant's world, Freud's developmental line of object relations is intimately interwoven with psychosexual stages of development.

ORAL STAGE In the earliest months of life, the infant experiences hunger and frustration in the absence of the breast and the need-satisfying discharge of tension when the breast is present. Tension and hunger force the recognition and acceptance of persons in the outside world. In Freud's view, then, the first psychological awareness of an object arises from the intense physiological need for a familiar experience that provides gratification and relieves tension.

The mother's responsiveness to the child is critical in laying the foundations for the most rudimentary and essential basis for the subsequent development of object relations and the capacity for entering the world of human beings. She becomes the first love object for the infant in that she is recognized as the source of gratification of hunger and the provider of the erotogenic pleasure that the infant obtains from sucking. If a warm, trusting, and affectionate relationship has been established between mother and child during the first few months of life, the stage is set for the development of trusting and affectionate relationships with others throughout life.

Conversely, when the early mother-infant bond and the feeding experience are disturbed, the groundwork is established for subsequent problems in the area of object relations. If the mother is unavailable during the early sucking phase of the oral stage, frustration may be so intense that the infant grows up with intense longings to be nurtured and taken care of by others. If the fixation occurs during the biting phase of the oral stage, the child may be plagued with oral aggressive tendencies throughout life. Those impulses may be manifested in a voracious appetite or in a tendency to make biting comments about others that is destructive to relationships.

ANAL STAGE After infants pass through the oral stage during the first 18 months of life, they enter the anal stage, which lasts from about 18 to 36 months of age. One striking difference is that in the anal stage the child is much less passive than in the oral stage. Moreover, the demands of toilet training during the anal period lead to a struggle of wills between mother and child. The erotization of the anal stage involves both the pleasurable sense of excretion and, later, the erotic stimulation of the anal mucosa through the retention of feces.

Freud noted the connection between anal and sadistic drives. Initially, the object of anal-sadistic activity is the feces, and pinching off is regarded as a sadistic act. As the anal stage progresses, the sadism becomes more interpersonal in nature. In the developing struggles over toilet training, the child learns to exercise power over the parents by either giving up or retaining the feces. The sense of power over the environment that comes with sphincter control represents another sadistic element.

Before toilet training, elimination and pleasurable retention are essentially autoerotic because they do not require the presence or the assistance of an outside object. The act of defecation during that early period is imbued with a sense of omnipotence as a result. The feces become libidinized because they represent pleasure. Later, the child develops an ambivalent view of feces as body contents that are both external and internal. In other words, the child regards the feces as both "me" and "not me." On the one hand, the feces are loved and retained or reinternalized; on the other hand, they are hated and pinched off.

The ambivalence associated with the anal stage may also be transferred to objects in the external environment. The stimulation associated with having the anal area cleansed may lead to strong erotic feelings toward the mother. Later, battles over toilet training lead to aggressive and hateful feelings toward parental figures. Freud suggested that obsessive-compulsive persons had regressed to the anal stage of development. The ambivalence associated with the feces in conjunction with the parental control led those persons to become compulsively neat, rigid, domineering, and pedantic. Freud also described them as intensely ambivalent, tormented by simultaneous feelings of love and hate and by simultaneous wishes both to control and retain the object and to expel and destroy it.

URETHRAL STAGE Although Freud did not discuss the urethral psychosexual stage in any depth, some clinicians think it has particular relevance to issues of performance and control. The urethral stage is generally viewed as transitional between the anal and the phallic psychosexual stages. Pleasure in urination is referred to as urethral erotism, and urethral functioning may be associated with sadistic urges carried over from the anal stage. Competitiveness and ambition are often viewed as compensation for the shame associated with loss of urethral control.

PHALLIC STAGE Around the age of 3 the child enters the phallic stage, in which the penis or the clitoris is the primary erotogenic zone. The phallic stage of psychosexual development heralds the arrival of the oedipal level of development, in which relationships become more complicated than they were in the past. The emphasis is on triangular or three-person relationships, instead of dyadic or two-person relationships. The phallic stage is also characterized by greater tolerance of ambivalence and the ability to withstand frustration in the absence of significant objects because of the ability to maintain an internal representation of the absent object.

Another major contrast between the pregenital psychosexual stages of development and the phallic stage is the nature of the child's libidinal activity. In the oral and anal stages, such activity is, for the most part, autoerotic in that the child's sexual impulses are directed toward the child's own body. Pleasure is still derived from one's own body in the phallic phase, but that period of development is also characterized by the fundamental task of finding a love object that will establish later patterns of object choice in adult life.

Oedipus complex The period of life between ages 3 and 5 is known as the oedipal stage of psychosexual development because the culmination of infantile sexuality—the *Oedipus complex*—occurs at that time. Freud discovered this crucial cornerstone of psychological development during his own self-analysis and in his clinical work with patients in which fantasies of incest with the parent of the opposite sex emerged with regularity in association with feelings of jealousy and murderous rage toward the parent of the same sex. Drawing an analogy between such fantasies and the Greek myth of Oedipus, who unknowingly killed his father and married his mother, Freud termed the intrapsychic constellation the Oedipus complex.

The oedipal phase of development is of central importance in the pathogenesis of neuroses and many anxiety disorders. Oedipal issues are also prominent in the psychodynamics of character neuroses and high-level personality disorders, such as hysterical personality and obsessive-compulsive personality. The Oedipus complex presents a developmental challenge for the child, and the resolution of the child's dilemma differs according to the child's gender.

RESOLUTION FOR BOYS The first love object of the male child is his mother. Unlike the little girl, the little boy does not need to shift his affection to another parent at the beginning the oedipal phase. The male child essentially falls in love with his mother. He wishes to be at the center of her world, to sleep with her, to caress her, and to have all her attention. It becomes apparent that such plans are interfered with by the relationship of his mother and father. As a result, he begins to view his father as a rival and develops murderous wishes toward him. Those thoughts create a predicament for the little boy because he also loves his father. Murderous wishes produce guilt. They also produce fear of retaliation, accompanied by anxiety about that impending retaliation.

Freud repeatedly noted that the chief source of the boy's anxiety in the Oedipus complex is that the father will retaliate by removing the child's penis. The male child's investment in keeping his genitals intact supersedes his sexual wishes for his mother, and he renounces those wishes as a result. Freud termed the renunciation of oedipal strivings secondary to castration anxiety the *castration complex*. Hence, the Oedipus complex in boys is resolved by the castration complex. The male child identifies with his father and decides to find a woman *like* his mother so that he can become *like* his father. That resolution is often referred to as *identification with the aggressor*. One aspect of the male resolution of the Oedipus complex is that the retaliatory father is internalized to form the superego, which Freud regarded as heir to the Oedipus complex.

Freud viewed bisexuality as a fundamental aspect of the unconscious. Loving feelings for the father coexist with the view of him as a rival who must be murdered. At times, the mother is regarded as interfering with the father-son relationship, and the male child has murderous wishes about his mother. Freud referred to that constellation as the *negative Oedipus complex,* which he considered a universal aspect of psychosexual development.

RESOLUTION FOR GIRLS Freud was frank throughout his writings about his difficulty in understanding psychological development in girls. He often dealt with that difficulty by assuming that female development occurs along lines that are essentially analogous to male development. In attempting to explain the resolution of the Oedipus complex in little girls (called the Electra complex), Freud noted that, although the Oedipus complex in male children is resolved by the castration complex, in female children it is promulgated by an awareness of their "castrated" state. Freud believed that little girls feel like little boys during the preoedipal psychosexual stages until the age of 3, when the girls discover the existence of the penis. He postulated that the discovery leads to feelings of inferiority and narcissistic injury and to penis envy. The little girl then blames her mother for bringing her into the world less well equipped than her male counterparts and turns to her father as her love object. The wish to have a baby with her father then replaces her wish for a penis.

The discovery of the little girl's "genital inferiority," according to Freud, leads to one of three outcomes: (1) a defiant hypermasculinity, (2) a neurotic cessation of all sexuality, or (3) normal feminity, entailing the renunciation of clitoral sexuality. Whereas the fear of castration leads to the resolution of the little boy's Oedipus complex, fear of losing the mother's love leads the little girl to a satisfactory resolution of the Electra complex. When the female child realizes that her mother disapproves of her wishes toward her father, she decides to renounce her oedipal strivings to maintain her bond with her mother.

Freud's view of female development has undergone significant revision by modern psychoanalytic authors. It is now known that the sense of being female is present long before the onset of the phallic-oedipal stage of development. Child observational research suggests that both sexes become aware of anatomical genital differences at approximately 16 to 18 months of age. Also, studies of persons with chromosomal anomalies and ambiguous genitalia have persuasively demonstrated that the primary source of femaleness is not the nature of the genitalia but the parents' conviction about the nature of the child's gender. Moreover, penis envy is no longer regarded as a bedrock phenomenon that defies further understanding and analysis. Contemporary psychoanalytic writers regard penis envy as only one aspect of the development of feminine identity, not the origin of it. They point out that following a strictly Freudian model of development may lead a clinician to help a female patient regard herself as a genitally inferior form of male. The mysterious nature of the little girl's genitalia may provoke anxiety independent of their differences from the genitals of little boys, and those anxieties can be fruitfully explored in psychoanalysis.

SIGNIFICANCE OF THE OEDIPUS COMPLEX Freud viewed the Oedipus complex, along with its successful or unsuccessful resolution, as the nucleus for the pathogenesis of adult neurosis. He also thought that personality, fixations, object choices, and identifications are significantly influenced by the oedipal phase of development. Incestuous oedipal feelings reemerge in both sexes at puberty, and one of the tasks of adolescence is to withdraw libidinal urges from parental figures and direct them toward more suitable love objects.

LATENCY STAGE This stage of development begins with the resolution of the Oedipus complex (discussed above) around the age of 5 or 6 and ends with the onset of puberty, somewhere between 11 and 13 years of age. The name "latency" derives from the fact that the sexual drive is relatively quiescent during those years. The inactivity of the sexual drive can be explained by the institution of the superego as the heir to the Oedipus complex. The control of instinctual impulses by the superego allows for further integration and consolidation of sex-role identity in sex roles. The latency stage of development is also associated with the development of a sense of industry and a capacity for mastery that enhances autonomous functioning.

GENITAL STAGE This stage of psychosexual development corresponds with the adolescent phase that begins with the onset of puberty and ends with the achievement of young adulthood. Most clinicians who work with adolescents think it is useful to subdivide the period into preadolescent, early adolescent, middle adolescent, and late adolescent subphases. The most striking influence on this period of development is the physiological maturation of hormonal systems that results in an intensification of drives, particularly sexual drives. This rather extended psychosexual stage of development, without a doubt one of the most challenging in the life cycle, requires the development of psychological mastery over drive pressures. In addition, a key developmental task associated with the genital stage is the establishment of mature object relations and genital sexuality with an appropriate partner. A major aspect of that achievement is the psychological separation from one's own parents and the establishment of an independent life-style.

Freud's stages of psychosexual development are discussed in Table 6.1-1.

CONCEPT OF NARCISSISM

The first systematic discussion of narcissism in Freud's work was published in 1914. Freud was dissatisfied with the paper and wrote to Karl Abraham, "The narcissism was a difficult labor and bears all the marks of a corresponding deformation." Nevertheless, Freud's thinking about narcissism led him to important modifications in his understanding of libido and instinct theory in general.

THEORETICAL BASIS According to the Greek myth, Narcissus was a young man who fell in love with his own reflection in the water of a pool and drowned in his attempt to embrace the beloved image. Freud used the term *narcissism* to describe situations in which a person's libido is invested in the ego itself, rather than in other people. That conceptualization of narcissism presented Freud with vexing problems for his instinct theory. It essentially violated his distinction between libidinal instincts and ego or self-preservative instincts. Freud's understanding of narcissism led him to use the term to describe a wide array of psychiatric disorders, very much in contrast to the contemporary usage of the term to describe a specific kind of personality disorder. For example, in 1908 Freud noted that in cases of schizophrenia (which was then known as dementia precox), the person's libido is withdrawn from objects and turned inward. He believed that the withdrawal of libidinal attachment to objects accounted for the loss of reality testing in psychotic patients. Grandiosity and omnipotence in such patients reflected excessive libidinal investment in the ego.

Freud did not limit his use of narcissism to psychoses. In states of physical illness and hypochondriasis, he observed that libidinal investment is frequently withdrawn from external objects and from outside activities and interests. Similarly, he suggested that, in normal sleep, libido is withdrawn and reinvested in the sleeper's own body. Homosexuality, which Freud regarded as a perversion, he understood as an instance of a narcissistic form of object choice, one in which a person falls in love with an idealized version of himself or herself projected onto another person. He also found narcissistic manifestations

TABLE 6.1-1
Stages of Psychosexual Development

	Oral Stage		
Definition	The earliest stage of development in which the infant's needs, perceptions, and modes of expression are primarily centered in the mouth, lips, tongue, and other organs related to the oral zone.	Objectives	To establish a trusting dependence on nursing and sustaining objects, to establish comfortable expression and gratification of oral libidinal needs without excessive conflict or ambivalence from oral sadistic wishes.
Description	The oral zone maintains its dominant role in the organization of the psyche through approximately the first 18 months of life. Oral sensations include thirst, hunger, pleasurable tactile stimulations evoked by the nipple or its substitute, sensations related to swallowing, and satiation. Oral drives consist of two separate components: libidinal and aggressive. States of oral tension lead to a seeking for oral gratification, typified by quiescence at the end of nursing. The oral triad consists of the wish to eat, to sleep, and to reach that relaxation that occurs at the end of sucking just before the onset of sleep. Libidinal needs (oral erotism) are thought to predominate in the early parts of the oral phase, whereas they are mixed with more aggressive components later (oral sadism). Oral aggression may express itself in biting, chewing, spitting, or crying. Oral aggression is connected with primitive wishes and fantasies of biting, devouring, and destroying.	Pathological traits	Excessive oral gratifications or deprivation can result in libidinal fixations that contribute to pathological traits. Such traits can include excessive optimism, narcissism, pessimism (often seen in depressive states), and demandingness. Oral characters are often excessively dependent and require others to give to them and to look after them. Such persons want to be fed but may be exceptionally giving to elicit a return of being given to. Oral characters are often extremely dependent on objects for the maintenance of their self-esteem. Envy and jealousy are often associated with oral traits.
		Character traits	Successful resolution of the oral phase provides a basis in character structure for capacities to give to and receive from others without excessive dependence or envy and a capacity to rely on others with a sense of trust, as well as with a sense of self-reliance and self-trust.
	Anal Stage		
Definition	The stage of psychosexual development that is prompted by maturation of neuromuscular control over sphincters, particularly the anal sphincters, thus permitting more voluntary control over retention or expulsion of feces.	Objectives	The anal period is essentially a period of striving for independence and separation from the dependence on and control of the parent. The objectives of sphincter control without overcontrol (fecal retention) or loss of control (messing) are matched by the child's attempts to achieve autonomy and independence without excessive shame or self-doubt from loss of control.
Description	This period, which extends roughly from 1 to 3 years of age, is marked by a recognizable intensification of aggressive drives mixed with libidinal components and in sadistic impulses. Acquisition of voluntary sphincter control is associated with an increasing shift from passivity to activity. The conflicts over anal control and the struggle with the parent over retaining or expelling feces in toilet training give rise to increased ambivalence, together with a struggle over separation, individuation, and independence. Anal erotism refers to the sexual pleasure in anal functioning, both in retaining the precious feces and in presenting them as a precious gift to the parent. Anal sadism refers to the expression of aggressive wishes connected with discharging feces as powerful and destructive weapons. These wishes are often displayed in such children's fantasies as bombing and explosions.	Pathological traits	Maladaptive character traits, often apparently inconsistent, are derived from anal erotism and the defenses against it. Orderliness, obstinancy, stubbornness, willfulness, frugality, and parsimony are features of the anal character derived from a fixation on anal functions. When defenses against anal traits are less effective, the anal character reveals traits of heightened ambivalence, lack of tidiness, messiness, defiance, rage, and sadomasochistic tendencies. Anal characteristics and defenses are most typically seen in obsessive-compulsive neuroses.
		Character traits	Successful resolution of the anal phase provides the basis for the development of personal autonomy, a capacity for independence and personal initiative without guilt, a capacity for self-determining behavior without a sense of shame or self-doubt, a lack of ambivalence and a capacity for willing cooperation without either excessive willfulness or sense of self-diminution or defeat.
	Urethral Stage		
Definition	This stage was not explicitly treated by Freud but is envisioned as a transitional stage between the anal and the phallic stages of development. It shares some of the characteristics of the preceding anal stage and some from the subsequent phallic stage.	Objectives	Issues of control and urethral performance and loss of control. It is not clear whether or to what extent the objectives of urethral functioning differ from those of the anal period.
Description	The characteristics of the urethral stage are often subsumed under those of the phallic stage. Urethral erotism, however, is used to refer to the pleasure in urination, as well as the pleasure in urethral retention analogous to anal retention. Similar issues of performance and control are related to urethral functioning. Urethral functioning may also be invested with a sadistic quality, often reflecting the persistence of anal sadistic urges. Loss of urethral control, as in enuresis, may frequently have regressive significance that reactivates anal conflicts.	Pathological traits	The predominant urethral trait is that of competitiveness and ambition, probably related to the compensation for shame due to loss of urethral control. In control this may be the start for the development of penis envy, related to the feminine sense of shame and inadequacy in being unable to match the male urethral performance. This is also related to issues of control and shaming.
		Character traits	Besides the healthy effects analogous to those from the anal period, urethral competence provides a sense of pride and self-competence derived from performance. Urethral performance is an area in which the small boy

TABLE 6.1-1 (*continued*)

	Urethral Stage (*continued*)		
		Character traits	can imitate and match his father's more adult performance. The resolution of urethral conflicts sets the stage for budding gender identity and subsequent identifications.
	Phallic Stage		
Definition	The phallic stage of sexual development begins sometime during the third year of life and continues until approximately the end of the fifth year.	Pathological traits	The derivation of pathological traits from the phallic-oedipal involvement are sufficiently complex and subject to such a variety of modifications that it encompasses nearly the whole of neurotic development. The issues, however, focus on castration in males and on penis envy in females. The other important focus of developmental distortions in this period derives from the patterns of identification that are developed out of the resolution of the oedipal complex. The influence of castration anxiety and penis envy, the defenses against both, and the patterns of identification that emerge from the phallic phase are the primary determinants of the development of human character. They also subsume and integrate the residues of previous psychosexual stages, so that fixations or conflicts that derive from any of the preceding stages can contaminate and modify the oedipal resolution.
Description	The phallic phase is characterized by a primary focus of sexual interests, stimulation, and excitement in the genital area. The penis becomes the organ of principal interest to children of both sexes, with the lack of a penis in the female being considered as evidence of castration. The phallic phase is associated with an increase in genital masturbation accompanied by predominantly unconscious fantasies of sexual involvement with the opposite-sex parent. The threat of castration and its related castration anxiety arise in connection with guilt over masturbation and oedipal wishes. During this phase the oedipal involvement and conflict are established and consolidated.		
Objectives	The objective of this phase is to focus erotic interest in the genital area and genital functions. This focusing lays the foundation for gender identity and serves to integrate the residues of previous stages of psychosexual development into a predominantly genital-sexual orientation. The establishing of the oedipal situation is essential for the furtherance of subsequent identifications that will serve as the basis for important and enduring dimensions of character organization.	Character traits	The phallic stage provides the foundations for an emerging sense of sexual identity, a sense of curiosity without embarrassment, initiative without guilt, as well as a sense of mastery not only over objects and persons in the environment but also over internal processes and impulses. The resolution of the oedipal conflict at the end of the phallic period gives rise to powerful internal resources for regulation of drive impulses and their direction to constructive ends. This internal source of regulation is the superego, and it is based on identifications derived from primarily parental figures.
	Latency Stage		
Definition	The stage of relative quiescence or inactivity of the sexual drive during the period from the resolution of the Oedipus complex until pubescence (from about 5–6 years until about 11–13 years).	Pathological traits	The danger in the latency period can arise either from a lack of development of inner controls or an excess of them. The lack of control can lead to a failure of the child to sufficiently sublimate energies in the interests of learning and development of skills; an excess of inner control, however, can lead to premature closure of personality development and the precocious elaboration of obsessive character traits.
Description	The institution of the superego at the close of the oedipal period and the further maturation of ego functions allow for a considerably greater degree of control of instinctual impulses. Sexual interests during this period are generally thought to be quiescent. This is a period of primarily homosexual affiliations for both boys and girls, as well as a sublimation of libidinal and aggressive energies into energetic learning and play activities, exploring the environment, and becoming more proficient in dealing with the world of things and persons around them. It is a period for the development of important skills. The relative strength of regulatory elements often gives rise to patterns of behavior that are somewhat obsessive and hypercontrolling.	Character traits	The latency period has frequently been regarded as a period of relatively unimportant inactivity in the developmental schema. Recently, great respect has been gained for the developmental processes that take place in this period. Important consolidations and additions are made to the basic postoedipal identifications. It is a period of integrating and consolidating previous attainments in psychosexual development and establishing decisive patterns of adaptive functioning. The child can develop a sense of industry and a capacity for mastery of objects and concepts that allows autonomous function and with a sense of initiative without running the risk of failure or defeat or a sense of inferiority. These important attainments need to be further integrated, ultimately as the essential basis for a mature adult life of satisfaction in work and love.
Objectives	The primary objective in this period is the further integration of oedipal identifications and a consolidation of sex-role identity and sex roles. The relative quiescence and control of instinctual impulses allow for the development of ego apparatuses and mastery skills. Further identificatory components may be added to the oedipal ones on the basis of broadening contacts with other significant figures outside the family, such as teachers, coaches, and other adults.		
	Genital Stage		
Definition	The genital or adolescent phase of psychosexual development extends from the onset of puberty from ages 11–13 until the person reaches young adulthood. In current thinking, there is a	Pathological traits	The pathological deviations due to a failure to achieve successful resolution of this stage of development are multiple and complex. Defects can arise from the whole spectrum of

Genital Stage (*continued*)			
	tendency to subdivide this stage into preadolescent, early adolescent, middle adolescent, late adolescent, and even postadolescent periods.		psychosexual residues, since the developmental task of the adolescent period is in a sense a partial reopening and reworking and reintegrating of all those aspects of development. Previous unsuccessful resolutions and fixations in various phases or aspects of psychosexual development will produce pathological defects in the emerging adult personality. A more specific defect from a failure to resolve adoelscent issues has been described by Erikson as identity diffusion.
Description	The physiological maturation of systems of genital (sexual) functioning and attendant hormonal systems leads to an intensification of drives, particularly libidinal drives. This produces a regression in personality organization, which reopens conflicts of previous stages of psychosexual development and provides the opportunity for a reresolution of these conflicts in the context of achieving a mature sexual and adult identity.	Character traits	The successful resolution and reintegration of previous psychosexual stages in the adolescent, fully genital phase sets the stage normally for a fully mature personality with a capacity for full and satisfying genital potency and a self-integrated and consistent sense of identity. Such a person has reached a satisfying capacity for self-realization and meaningful participation in the areas of work and love and in the creative and productive application to satisfying and meaningful goals and values. Only in the last few years has the presumed relationship between psychosexual genitality and maturity of personality functioning been put in question.
Objectives	The primary objectives of this period are the ultimate separation from dependence on and attachment to the parents and the establishment of mature, nonincestuous object relations. Related to this are the achievement of a mature sense of personal identity and acceptance and the integration of a set of adult roles and functions that permit new adaptive integrations with social expectations and cultural values.		

Table adapted from W. W. Meissner in *Comprehensive Textbook of Psychiatry, fourth edition.* Adapted by Glen O. Gabbard, M.D.

in the beliefs and myths of primitive people, especially those involving the ability to influence external events through the magical omnipotence of their own thought processes. In the course of normal development, children also exhibit a belief in their own omnipotence.

NARCISSISM AND OBJECT RELATIONS According to Freud, the infant is born into a state of primary narcissism in which the libido is stored in the ego. He viewed the neonate as completely narcissistic, with the entire libidinal investment in physiological needs and their satisfaction. He referred to that self-investment as *ego libido.*

The infantile state of self-absorption changes only gradually, according to Freud, with the dawning awareness that a separate person—the mothering figure—is responsible for the gratification of the infant's needs. That realization leads to the gradual withdrawal of the libido from the self and the redirection toward the external object. Hence, the development of object relations in the infant parallels the shift from primary narcissism to object attachment. The libidinal investment in the object is referred to as *object libido.*

If the developing child suffers rebuffs or trauma from the caretaking figure, object libido may be withdawn and reinvested in the ego. Freud called this regressive development *secondary narcissism.*

One of the confusing aspects of Freud's conceptualization of narcissism is that his usage of the term varied according to context. At times, he discussed narcissism as a perversion in which persons use their own bodies or body parts as objects of sexual arousal. At other times, he used the term to describe a developmental phase, as in the state of primary narcissism, when there is no differentiation of self and other and when autoeroticism predominates. That usage is particularly problematic because narcissism operates at all stages of psychosexual development, from the deprivation of oral needs during the earliest months of infancy to the losing out to a rival during the oedipal phase. In still other instances, Freud used the word "narcissism" to refer to a particular type of object choice. He distinguished love objects who are chosen "according to the narcissistic type," in which case the object resembles the subject's idealized or fantasied self-image, from objects chosen according to the "anaclitic type," in which case the love object resembles a caretaking figure from early in life. And Freud occasionally used the word "narcissism" interchangeably and synonymously with "self-esteem."

Freud's developmental view of narcissism and object relations has caused considerable controversy in the field. Part of the difficulty stems from the fact that a certain amount of narcissistic libido is necessary for healthy self-regard. Freud's maturational model implies that, in the course of healthy development, one should outgrow investment in oneself and devote one's libidinal energies primarily to others. Others have noted that Freud's model implies that investment of the libido in a love object results in depletion of libidinal investment in oneself. That conceptualization does not explain how it is that persons are likely to feel the greatest sense of self-esteem when they are in love. And Freud's model does not lend itself well to the differentiation between normal narcissism and pathological narcissism. Subsequent psychoanalytic theorists, discussed later in this section, have dealt with some of those difficulties.

EGO PSYCHOLOGY

Although Freud had used the construct of the ego throughout the evolution of psychoanalytic theory, ego psychology as it is known today really began with the publication of *The Ego and the Id* in 1923. That landmark publication also represented a transition in Freud's thinking from the topographic model of the mind to the tripartite structural model of ego, id, and superego. He had repeatedly observed that not all unconscious processes can be relegated to the instinctual life of the person. Elements of the conscience, as well as functions of the ego, are clearly unconscious as well. From 1923 to 1937 Freud developed both his theory of ego psychology and his later theory of anxiety. After his death, such psychoanalytic contributors as Heinz Hartmann, Ernst Kris, David Rapaport, and Erik Erikson continued the general thrust within psychoanalysis away from the instinctual life toward a greater emphasis on ego functioning and development and toward social and cultural perspectives.

EARLY CONCEPTS OF THE EGO Freud's concept of the ego was ill-defined and imprecise during the formative years of psychoanalysis. He used the term to refer to the dominant place of the person's conscious thoughts and values, as opposed to the domain of repressed impulses and wishes. The ego's primary function is defensive, which at that time denoted repression. Impulses and wishes, primarily of a sexual nature, are barred from conscious awareness because of the counterforce provided by the ego. In the early years of the 1890s, Freud viewed the memories of sexual trauma as the main source of the defensive response. Those memories arouse unpleasant affect, which leads to repression, which in turn causes a damming up of energy that produces anxiety. That formulation, however, produces a contradiction in the nature of the ego's function. On the one hand, the ego reduces tension and avoids unpleasant affects through repression; on the other hand, the process of repression *produces* anxiety, which is an equally unpleasant affect. When Freud shifted in 1897 from his emphasis on actual seduction to the role of childhood fantasy, he also suspended his thinking about the function of the ego.

During the ensuing years, Freud devoted much of his attention to the instinctual drives and their vicissitudes. His studies led him back to consideration of the ego. In his 1915 work "Instincts and Their Vicissitudes," Freud noted that the sexual instinct is subjected to repression, sublimation, turning on oneself, and reversal into its opposite (a sadistic impulse transformed into a masochistic one). Those vicissitudes came to be understood as defense mechanisms of the ego.

Topographic theory failed to provide Freud with all the answers he needed to explain the functioning of the mind. For example, since neither the preconscious nor the ego instincts can be viewed as solely responsible for regression or censorship, how can repression be explained? Freud tried to explain repression by postulating that certain ideas remain in the unconscious as a result of libidinal withdrawal. He suggested that the withdrawal is a repetitive process of countercathexis that operates on an unconscious basis. He eventually assigned that function to the ego.

FREUD'S EGO PSYCHOLOGY Freud's first comprehensive theory of the ego appeared in *The Ego and the Id.* There, although the ego is primarily organized around the perceptual conscious system, it also includes the structures responsible for *unconscious* defenses and resistance in the clinical setting. The ego is regarded as the agency that organizes mental processes and functions. It is one of three major functional subdivisions of the mental apparatus—one that responds in a mostly passive way to pressures from the other two, the id and the superego. The ego has its origins in the id, in Freud's view, and is later depicted by him as a helpless rider on the id's horse, going in whichever direction the id dictates. The ego also responds to reality influences.

In 1926 Freud introduced the notion of signal anxiety in *Inhibitions, Symptoms and Anxiety.* There the ego is no longer viewed as a passive servant of the id. Signal anxiety is seen as an autonomous function of the ego that initiates defensive maneuvers in response to the threatened emergence of unacceptable wishes and impulses from the unconscious.

The concept of the ego was further expanded to include adaptation as a result of Freud's continued elaboration of the reality principle. Adaptation enables the ego to control instinctual drives when real danger prompts those drives into action. Intrinsic to the maturation of the ego is the substitution of the reality principle for the pleasure principle. In addition to reducing tension from the id, the reality principle gauges the limitations, requirements, and possibilities of the environment with an eye to attaining greater pleasure in the future. By the last decade of his life, Freud viewed the ego as the executive organ of the psyche, a powerful regulatory force for the integration and control of impulses, and as an agent of adaptation in relation to reality. In 1937 Freud made it clear that the ego evolves independently of the id.

STRUCTURE OF THE PSYCHIC APPARATUS

Contemporary psychoanalytic ego psychology is based on Freud's structural theory, which divides the psychic apparatus into the id, the ego, and the superego (Figure 6.1-11). The id encompasses the mental representations of the instinctual drives and some but not all the contents of the unconscious system in Freud's topographic theory. The id operates according to primary process and to the dictates of the pleasure principle. The ego occupies the position between the drives and the demands of the outer world. It evaluates, perceives, coordinates, and integrates perceptions in the service of taming the intensity of drives. The ego attempts to achieve optimal gratification of instinctual strivings while maintaining good relations with the superego and with external reality. The superego assists the ego in the regulation of tensions arising from the id. It encompasses internalized moral values, prohibitions, and standards of parental figures.

ID Freud referred to the id as "the dark inaccessible part of our personality. . . . We approach the id with analogies: we call it a chaos, a cauldron full of seething excitation." Freud borrowed the term from Georg Groddeck, a psychoanalytically informed internist, who coined the term "id" to mean all that was ego-alien. It was viewed as a reservoir of the unorganized instinctual drives. Operating under the domination of the primary process, the id lacks the capacity to delay or modify the instinctual drives with which the infant is born. The id should not, however, be viewed as synonymous with the unconscious because both the ego and the superego have unconscious components.

EGO The ego spans all three topographic dimensions of conscious, preconscious, and unconscious. Logical and abstract thinking and verbal expression are associated with conscious

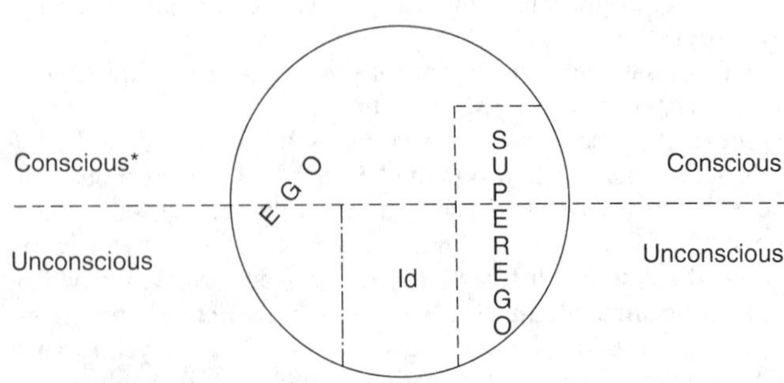

FIGURE 6.1-11 *Freud's structural model. (From G O Gabbard:* Psycyodynamic Psychiatry in Clinical Practice, *p 21. American Psychiatric Press, Washington, 1990. Used with permission.)*

and preconscious functions of the ego. Defense mechanisms reside in the unconscious domain of the ego. The most comprehensive definition of the ego can be found in Freud's *An Outline of Psycho-Analysis,* which he wrote in 1938:

Here are the principal characteristics of the ego. In consequence of the pre-established connection between sense and perception and muscular action, the ego has voluntary movement at its command. It has the task of self-preservation. As regards *external* events, it performs that task by becoming aware of stimuli, by storing up experiences about them (in the memory), by avoiding excessively strong stimuli (through flight), by dealing with moderate stimuli (through adaptation) and finally by learning to bring about expedient changes in the external world to its own advantage (through activity). As regards *internal* events, in relation to the id, it performs that task by gaining control over the demands of the instincts, by deciding whether they are to be allowed satisfaction, by postponing that satisfaction to times and circumstances favorable in the external world or by suppressing their excitations entirely. It is guided in its activity by consideration of the tension produced by stimuli, whether these tensions are present in it or introduced into it.

In essence, then, the ego controls motility, perception, contact with reality, and, through the mechanisms of defense available to it, the delay and modulation of drive expression.

Origins of the ego In Freud's view, the neonate has no ego to speak of, and the coherent system of functions now associated with the concept is regarded as an outgrowth of the id. Specifically, the ego arises out of the modification of the id created by the demands of the external world. The ego forms in tandem with the increasing influence of external reality on the infant, gradually replacing the pleasure principle with the reality principle. The role of conflict, first between the id and the outside world and later between the id and the ego, Freud viewed as central to ego development.

Later contributors to ego psychology—such as Hartmann, Kris, and Loewenstein—made significant modifications to the theory of ego development. Hartmann, in particular, stressed the adaptational aspects of the ego. In his view, one can delineate a line of ego development that is independent of instinctual drives. He postulated the existence of primary autonomous ego functions that do not have their origins in the id. Those functions include perception, motility, memory, and intelligence; all are present from birth and therefore determined, at least in part, by genetic factors. In that expanded view of the ego, the origins of both the ego and the id were thought to be in a common undifferentiated matrix present at birth. That shift toward the primacy of the ego was instrumental in the movement within psychoanalytic theory away from drive theory and toward a greater focus on the complexities of the ego.

Functions of the ego Although Freud periodically used the term "ego" to mean self, the concept is best viewed as a structure within the personality. It is an agency or an organization of functions that have in common the task of mediating between the instincts and the outside world. Ego psychologists have identified a set of basic ego functions that characterize the ego. The following descriptions reflect the activities that are generally regarded as basic and fundamental to the operation of the ego:

1. CONTROL AND REGULATION OF INSTINCTUAL DRIVES The development of the capacity to delay or postpone drive discharge, like the capacity to test reality, is closely related to the progression in early childhood from the pleasure principle to the reality principle. That capacity is also an essential aspect of the ego's role as mediator between the id and the outside world. Part of the infant's socialization to the external world is the acquisition of language and secondary process or logical thinking, both of which assist in the control of instinctual drives. The capacity to think in a logical and abstract manner allows for the representation of drives in fantasy, which may circumvent the need to discharge them in action.

The ego's capacity to regulate thinking and to control drive discharge is intimately connected with its defensive functioning. One example of the linkage between control of drives and defensive functioning can be seen in the ego's use of signal affects. Affect states such as guilt, anxiety, shame, and depression serve as signals of the potential breakthrough of threatening impulses from the unconscious. Those signals then act to mobilize defenses in the ego to prevent the breakthrough. That function of the ego is also instrumental in building a capacity to tolerate pain, anxiety, and frustration within manageable limits.

2. JUDGMENT A closely related ego function is judgment, which involves the ability to anticipate the consequences of one's actions. As with the control and regulation of instinctual drives, judgment develops in parallel with the growth of secondary process thinking. The ability to think logically allows for an assessment of how one's contemplated behavior may affect others. The consequences to oneself can also be ascertained through the use of secondary process thinking. The ego function of judgment may assist regulatory aspects of the ego in the avoidance of impulse discharge. Both those ego functions are commonly impaired in impulsive personality disorders.

3. RELATION TO REALITY The mediation between the internal world and external reality is a crucial function of the ego. The relationship with the outside world can be divided into three aspects: the sense of reality, reality testing, and adaptation to reality. The sense of reality develops in concert with the infant's dawning awareness of bodily sensations. The ability to distinguish what is outside the body from what is inside is an essential aspect of the sense of reality, and disturbances of body boundaries, such as depersonalization, reflect impairment in that ego function.

Reality testing is an ego function of paramount importance in that it differentiates psychotic persons from nonpsychotic persons. Reality testing refers to the capacity to distinguish internal fantasy from external reality. That function of the ego gradually develops in parallel with the increasing dominion of the reality principle over the pleasure principle.

The third aspect, adaptation to reality, involves the ability to use one's resources to develop effective responses to changing circumstances on the basis of previous experiences with reality. One may perceive reality accurately but not use one's full resources to make an informed judgment about the necessary response. In that sense, adaptation is closely linked to the concept of mastery with respect to both control of drives and accomplishment of external tasks. Adaptation to reality is also intimately connected with defensive functions of the ego. One commonly calls on a variety of defensive maneuvers to master situations that may produce anxiety or other affects. To deal with overwhelming trauma, for example, one may use temporary denial to get through the crisis.

4. OBJECT RELATIONSHIPS The significance of object relationships in normal psychological development and in psychiatric disorders was not fully appreciated until relatively late in the evolution of classical psychoanalysis. The capacity to form mutually satisfying relationships is in part related to patterns of internalization stemming from early interactions with parents and other significant figures. That ability is also a fundamental function of the ego in that satisfying relatedness depends on the ability to integrate positive and negative aspects of others and oneself and to maintain an internal sense of others, even in their absence. Similarly, mastery of drive derivatives is crucial to the achievement of satisfying relationships.

5. SYNTHETIC FUNCTION OF THE EGO First described by Herman Nunberg in 1931, the synthetic function refers to the ego's capacity to integrate diverse elements into an overall unity. Different aspects of oneself and others, for example, are synthesized into a consistent representation that endures over time. The function also involves organizing, coordinating, and generalizing or simplifying large amounts of data.

6. PRIMARY AUTONOMOUS EGO FUNCTIONS A direct outgrowth of the work of Hartmann, the primary autonomous functions refer to rudimentary apparatuses that are present at birth and that develop independently of intrapsychic conflict between drives and defenses, provided that what Hartmann referred to as an *average expectable environment* is available to the infant. As noted previously, those functions include perception, learning, intelligence, intuition, language, thinking, comprehension, and motility. In the course of development, some of those conflict-free aspects of the ego may eventually become involved in conflict if they encounter opposing forces.

7. SECONDARY AUTONOMOUS EGO FUNCTIONS Hartmann originally used the concept of the conflict-free sphere of ego functioning to identify areas of primary autonomy. However, that area may be enlarged by functions that originally arise in the service of defense against drives but subsequently become independent of them. Those functions are referred to as *secondary autonomous ego functions.* For example, a child may develop caretaking functions as a reaction formation against murderous wishes during the first few years of life. Later, the defensive functions of the style may be neutralized or deinstinctualized when the child grows up to be a social worker and cares for the homeless. That neutralization, leading to desexualization of

libidinal drives or deaggressivization of aggressive drives, provides the ego with independent energies that were formerly used to deal with drive pressures.

8. DEFENSIVE FUNCTIONS OF THE EGO Freud acknowledged the existence of several defense mechanisms, but his writings focused predominantly on repression, which he regarded as the queen of the defenses. In many of his contributions, defense and repression are used almost synonymously. Repression provides a barrier against the direct expression of impulses and wishes from the unconscious. With the ascent of the structural model, Freud shifted the function of defense to the ego. However, defense mechanisms could not be systematically studied until after 1926, when Freud formulated his theory of signal anxiety and the mobilization of defenses in response to danger signals.

The first comprehensive study of defense mechanisms was written not by Sigmund Freud but by his daughter Anna in her landmark 1936 work, *The Ego and the Mechanisms of Defense*. Anna Freud (Figure 6.1-12) expanded her father's work by providing detailed descriptions of a number of individual defense mechanisms, including regression, reaction formation, undoing, introjection, identification, projection, turning against the self, reversal, and sublimation. She pointed out that everyone uses a characteristic repertoire of defense mechanisms that are intimately related to that person's character. She also insisted that the ego should be the focus of psychoanalytic treatment, in addition to the uncovering of repressed drive derivatives. Her famous observation that "there is depth in the surface" reflected her appreciation of the complexity of the defensive aspects of the ego.

Evolution of defense mechanisms In the course of development, defenses emerge as a reflection of the ego's attempts to mediate between the pressures of the id, on the one hand, and the demands of external reality, on the other hand. At each phase of psychosexual development, then, the specific drive components evoke specific ego defenses. For example, defense mechanisms like introjection and projection are seen in concert with the development of oral incorporative impulses; reaction formations such as shame and disgust develop in response to anal impulses and pleasures. Pregenital defense mechanisms may persist into adult life, lending an infantile cast to the adult personality. In the course of normal development, mechanisms like repression and intellectualization supersede immature defenses.

The defense mechanisms most commonly used by a person to deal with unpleasant situations or distressing internal affective states constitute a significant component of that person's character. Obsessive-compulsive character traits, such as excessive orderliness and miserliness, may initially develop in response to instinctual drives, but they are subsequently divorced from them as they take a central role in the person's overall functioning, even in conflict-free situations. The defenses may be adaptive and healthy, as well as pathological; in normal functioning they are critical to the preservation of psychological well-being.

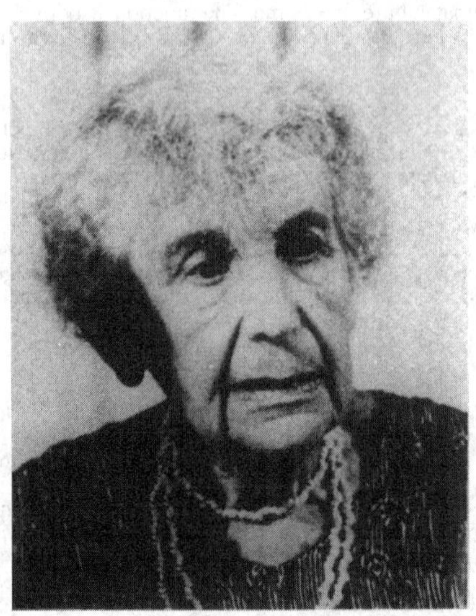

FIGURE 6.1-12 *Anna Freud. (Courtesy of UPI/Bettman Newsphotos.)*

In psychopathological states, one may see various alterations of normal defensive functioning. In hysterical and obsessive-compulsive persons, for example, one sees hypertrophied development of particular defenses, as though the dangers from infantile impulses were just as threatening in adulthood as they were in childhood. Exaggerated repression is characteristically associated with hysterical patients; such defenses as reaction formation, undoing, isolation of affect, and intellectualization are associated with obsessive-compulsive patients. Persons who are fixated at the oral psychosexual stage may rely on such defense mechanisms as denial and projection. The failure of defenses may lead to a breakthrough of direct drive expression with obvious regression in the ego's control of thought and affect, a condition most clearly manifested in the schizophrenias.

Classification of defenses The defenses of the ego can be classified in a variety of ways. Psychoanalysts themselves disagree as to the best taxonomy, and most acknowledge that any one classification is inadequate in its capacity to take into account all the relevant factors. Defense mechanisms can be categorized according to the psychosexual stage with which they are associated, but that system does not address the fact that some defense mechanisms (such as regression) are used in every developmental stage.

Other systems assign defenses according to the nature of the psychopathology with which they are associated. According to that taxonomy, hysterical defenses include conversion, repression, somatization, and dissociation. Freud himself classified defenses according to severity of psychopathology. Denial, distortion, and projection, he believed, are defense mechanisms associated with psychosis. The neurotic defense mechanisms include repression, isolation, undoing, displacement, and reaction formation. He considered mature defenses to be sublimation, altruism, humor, and suppression. A classification that draws both on the level of psychopathology and on developmental maturity is provided in Table 6.1-2, along with definitions of commonly recognized defense mechanisms.

Although analysts disagree as to the total number of defense mechanisms, most agree with Freud's assessment that defense mechanisms must possess the following properties: (1) they manage instinct, drive, and affect,; (2) they are unconscious; (3) they are discrete; (4) they are dynamic and reversible; and (5) they can be adaptive, as well as pathological.

SUPEREGO The third component of the tripartite structural model is the superego. The superego establishes and maintains the person's moral conscience on the basis of a complex system of ideals and values internalized from one's parents. As noted previously, Freud viewed the superego as the heir to the Oedipus complex; it is, therefore, influenced by the resolution of oedipal conflict. It conducts an ongoing scrutiny of the behavior, thoughts, and feelings of the person; makes comparisons with expected standards; and offers approval or disapproval. Criticisms and reproaches lead to a variety of painful feelings; praises and rewards raise the person's self-esteem. Those activities occur unconsciously to a large extent, reflecting the clinical observation that self-criticism operates as much outside conscious awareness as aggressive and sexual drive derivatives do.

The idea of the superego first appeared in 1896 with Freud's *Further Remarks on the Neuro-Psychoses of Defence*, in which

TABLE 6.1-2
Classification of Defense Mechanisms

Narcissistic Defenses*			
Denial	Avoiding the awareness of some painful aspect of reality by negating sensory data. Although repression defends against affects and drive derivatives, denial abolishes external reality. Denial may be used in both normal and pathological states.	Projection	Perceiving and reacting to unacceptable inner impulses and their derivatives as though they were outside the self. On a psychotic level, this defense mechanism takes the form of frank delusions about external reality (usually persecutory) and includes both perception of one's own feelings in another and subsequent acting on the perception (psychotic paranoid delusions). The impulses may derive from the id or the superego (hallucinated recriminations) but may undergo transformation in the process. Thus, according to Freud's analysis of paranoid projections, homosexual libidinal impulses are transformed into hatred and then projected onto the object of the unacceptable homosexual impulse.
Distortion	Grossly reshaping external reality to suit inner needs (including unrealistic megalomanic beliefs, hallucinations, wishfulfilling delusions) and using sustained feelings of delusional superiority or entitlement.		
Immature Defenses			
Acting out	Expressing an unconscious wish or impulse through action to avoid being conscious of an accompanying affect. The unconscious fantasy is lived out impulsively in behavior, thereby gratifying the impulse, rather than the prohibition against it. Acting out involves chronically giving in to an impulse to avoid the tension that would result from the postponement of expression.	Passive-aggressive behavior	Expressing aggression toward others indirectly through passivity, masochism, and turning against the self. Manifestations of passive-aggressive behavior include failures, procrastination, and illnesses that affect others more than oneself.
Blocking	Temporarily or transiently inhibiting thinking. Affects and impulses may also be involved. Blocking closely resembles repression but differs in that tension arises when the impulse, affect, or thought is inhibited.	Projection	Attributing one's own feelings and wishes to another person because of intolerable inner feelings or painful affects. Characteristically present in psychotic states, especially paranoid syndromes, projection is also widely used under normal conditions. In psychoses, projection takes the form of frank delusions about external reality, usually persecutory in nature, and includes the perception of one's own feelings toward another and subsequent acting on that perception.
Hypochondriasis	Exaggerating or overemphasizing an illness for the purpose of evasion and regression. Reproach arising from bereavement, loneliness, or unacceptable aggressive impulses toward others is transformed into self-reproach and complaints of pain, somatic illness, and neurasthenia. In hypochondriasis, responsibility can be avoided, guilt may be circumvented, and instinctual impulses are warded off. Because hypochondriacal introjects are ego-alien, the afflicted person experiences dysphoria and a sense of affliction.	Regression	Attempting to return to an earlier libidinal phase of functioning to avoid the tension and conflict evoked at the present level of development. It reflects the basic tendency to gain instinctual gratification at a less-developed period. Regression is a normal phenomenon as well, as a certain amount of regression is essential for relaxation, sleep, and orgasm in sexual intercourse. Regression is also considered an essential concomitant of the creative process.
Introjection	Internalizing the qualities of an object. Although vital to development, introjection also serves specific defensive functions. When used as a defense, it can obliterate the distinction between the subject and the object. Through the introjection of a loved object, the painful awareness of separateness or the threat of loss may be avoided. Introjection of a feared object serves to avoid anxiety when the aggressive characteristics of the object are internalized, thus placing the aggression under one's own control. A classic example is identification with the aggressor. An identification with the victim may also take place, whereby the self-punitive qualities of the object are taken over and established within one's self as a symptom or character trait.	Schizoid fantasy	Indulging in autistic retreat in order to resolve conflict and to obtain gratification. Interpersonal intimacy is avoided, and eccentricity serves to repel others. The person does not fully believe in the fantasies and does not insist on acting them out.
		Somatization	Converting psychic derivatives into bodily symptoms and tending to react with somatic manifestations, rather than psychic manifestations. In desomatization, infantile somatic responses are replaced by thought and affect; in resomatization, the person regresses to earlier somatic forms in the face of unresolved conflicts.
Neurotic Defenses			
Controlling	Attempting to manage or regulate events or objects in the environment to minimize anxiety and to resolve inner conflicts.	Dissociation	Temporarily but drastically modifing a person's character or one's sense of personal identity to avoid emotional distress. Fugue states and hysterical conversion reactions are common manifestations of dissociation. Dissociation may also be found in counterphobic behavior, multiple personality disorder, and the use of pharmacological highs or religious joy.
Displacement	Shifting an emotion or drive cathexis from one idea or object to another that resembles the original in some aspect or quality. Displacement permits the symbolic representation of the original idea or object by one that is less highly cathected or evokes less distress.		

TABLE 6.1-2 (*continued*)

Neurotic Defenses (*continued*)			
Externalization	Tending to perceive in the external world and in external objects elements of one's own personality, including instinctual impulses, conflicts, moods, attitudes, and styles of thinking. Externalization is a more general term than projection.	Reaction formation	Transforming an unacceptable impulse into its opposite. Reaction formation is characteristic of obsessional neurosis, but it may occur in other forms of neuroses as well. If this mechanism is frequently used at any early stage of ego development, it can become a permanent character trait, as in an obsessional character.
Inhibition	Consciously limiting or renouncing some ego functions, alone or in combination, to evade anxiety arising out of conflict with instinctual impulses, the superego, or environmental forces or figures.	Repression	Expelling or withholding from consciousness an idea or feeling. Primary repression refers to the curbing of ideas and feelings before they have attained consciousness; secondary repression excludes from awareness what was once experienced at a conscious level. The repressed is not really forgotten in that symbolic behavior may be present. This defense differs from suppression by effecting conscious inhibition of impulses to the point of losing and not just postponing cherished goals. Conscious perception of instincts and feelings is blocked in repression.
Intellectualization	Excessively using intellectual processes to avoid affective expression or experience. Undue emphasis is focused on the inanimate in order to avoid intimacy with people, attention is paid to external reality to avoid the expression of inner feelings, and stress is excessively placed on irrelevant details to avoid perceiving the whole. Intellectualization is closely allied to rationalization.	Sexualization	Endowing an object or function with sexual significance that it did not previously have or possessed to a smaller degree in order to ward off anxieties associated with prohibited impulses or their derivatives.
Isolation	Splitting or separating an idea from the affect that accompanies it but is repressed. Social isolation refers to the absence of object relationships.		
Rationalization	Offering rational explanations in an attempt to justify attitudes, beliefs, or behavior that may otherwise be unacceptable. Such underlying motives are usually instinctually determined.		
Mature Defenses			
Altruism	Using constructive and instinctually gratifying service to others to undergo a vicarious experience. It includes benign and constructive reaction formation. Altruism is distinguished from altruistic surrender, in which a surrender of direct gratification or of instinctual needs takes place in favor of fulfilling the needs of others to the detriment of the self, and the satisfaction can only be enjoyed vicariously through introjection.	Humor	Using comedy to overtly express feelings and thoughts without personal discomfort or immobilization and without producing an unpleasant effect on others. It allows the person to tolerate and yet focus on what is too terrible to be borne; it is different from wit, a form of displacement that involves distraction from the affective issue.
Anticipation	Realistically anticipating or planning for future inner discomfort. The mechanism is goal-directed and implies careful planning or worrying and premature but realistic affective anticipation of dire and potentially dreadful outcomes.	Sublimation	Achieving impulse gratification and the retention of goals but altering a socially objectionable aim or object to a socially acceptable one. Sublimation allows instincts to be channeled, rather than blocked or diverted. Feelings are acknowledged, modified, and directed toward a significant object or goal, and modest instinctual satisfaction occurs.
Asceticism	Eliminating the pleasurable effects of experiences. There is a moral element in assigning values to specific pleasures. Gratification is derived from renunciation, and asceticism is directed against all base pleasures perceived consciously.	Suppression	Consciously or semiconsciously postponing attention to a conscious impulse or conflict. Issues may be deliberately cut off, but they are not avoided. Discomfort is acknowledged but minimized.

*The categorization of these defenses as narcissistic is controversial. Many psychoanalysts would subsume them under "Immature Defenses."
Table adapted from G E Vaillant: *Adaptation to Life,* Little, Brown, Boston, 1977; E Semrad: The operation of ego defenses in object loss. In *The Loss of Loved Ones,* D M Moriarity, editor. Charles C Thomas, Springfield, IL. 1967; and G L Bibring, T F Dwyer, D S Huntington, A A Valenstein: A study of the psychological process in pregnancy and of the earliest mother-child relationship: Methodological considerations. *Psychoanal Stud Child 16:* 25, 1961. Adapted by Glen O. Gabbard, M.D.

he described "self-reproaches which have reemerged in transmuted form and ... relate to some sexual act that was performed with pleasure in childhood." In early discussions of dreams, Freud commented on the activities of a self-criticizing agency that censors the entry of unacceptable ideas into consciousness because the ideas are morally offensive. In his 1914 paper "On Narcissism," Freud spoke of a special self-critical agency and of a hypothetical state of narcissistic perfection originating in children's idealized views of themselves. As that idealized version of self is tarnished through the slings and arrows of development, the child attempts to recover the lost narcissism by creating an ego-ideal. Having postulated that construct, Freud needed to create a special agency whose function it was to be sure that the person's behavior and thoughts measure up to the expectations of the ego-ideal. The construct of the superego, then, grew out of the need for monitoring and preserving the ego-ideal.

Ego-ideal The distinction between the superego and the ego-ideal has always been ambiguous. The most common usage today is to refer to the ego-ideal as an agency that *prescribes* what one should do and to refer to the superego as an agency of moral conscience that *proscribes*—that is, dictates what one should *not* do. Freud, however, did not always make that distinction. In 1921 he referred to the self-critical agency responsible for guilt and self-reproaches in melancholia and depression as the ego-ideal. In *The Ego and the Id* two years later, he assigned both the conscience and the ego-ideal to the superego. Today most analysts conceptualize the ego-ideal as comprising a set of functions contained within the structure of the superego.

The ego-ideal is best conceptualized as an amalgam of internalized representations. The ideal object, stemming from internal images of an admired and omnipotent parent, is one such representation. The ideal self, based on fantasies of a self-image that would result in maximal parental approval, is another representation contained within the concept. Representations of actions that should be done to attain an ideal relationship with significant figures in one's life are also involved.

The ego-ideal becomes an internal standard of what one should be. In this regard it is intimately connected with the affect of shame, which is a response to an internal perception that one has not lived up to one's ego-ideal. Although guilt is a closely related affect, it is generally regarded as a response to the transgressions of superego prohibitions, particularly sexual or aggressive wishes toward others.

Origins of the superego As described earlier, the superego is a relatively mature structure resulting from the resolution of the Oedipus complex. In the case of the little boy, his love for his mother engenders murderous wishes toward his father. His observation of the genital differences between males and females leads him to fear that his oedipal wishes will be punished with castration. Under the influence of the perceived threat from his father, the little boy renounces his incestuous longings for his mother and identifies with his father. That resolution involves the installation of the parental moral values as the superego structure.

In the case of the little girl, she renounces oedipal strivings for her father because she realizes that a victory over her mother would result in the loss of her mother's love. Freud initially postulated that little girls grow up with less moral conviction and character as a result of the absence of the castration threat. That view is no longer held by contemporary psychoanalysts. Recent empirical studies suggest that moral developmental differences between boys and girls do exist but along different lines. Boys tend to place high moral value on achievement and fair play; girls are more likely to develop a moral code based on affiliation and relatedness to others.

Evolution of the superego Primitive superego precursors are formed early in life from the internalization of frightening and aggressive perceptions of parental figures. In some cases those perceptions are based on real behaviors of the figures; in other cases the perceptions are influenced by distortions deriving from fantasies by the child and from projections of the child's rage and sadism onto external objects. As a child matures and resolves the Oedipus complex, identifications with both parents become integrated to form an intricate and well-rounded internal object representation within the ego that interacts with the other contents of the ego as a superego. The parental identification is further reinforced by the child's struggles to repress unacceptable sexual and aggressive wishes and by the child's identification with the parents' superegos.

The ego originates to a large extent through interactions with the external world. The superego, however, is much more closely related to the id in its origins. It emerges from a powerful struggle with the drive pressures emanating from the id and is, therefore, more internal in its origins than is the ego. The identifications constituting the superego continue to undergo modification as role models and authority figures in one's life become incorporated into a set of internal standards, values, aspirations, and ideals.

As the oedipal phase of psychosexual development is resolved, the child moves into the stage known as *latency*. That stage, ranging from age 5 or 6 until the onset of puberty, is a period of relative quiescence, when the pressures from instinctual drives are more or less under control. Punishments and restrictions previously imposed by the parents are now firmly ensconced in the superego, which judges and guides behavior even in the absence of external authorities.

With the onset of puberty and the entry into adolescence, sexual and aggressive drives resurge. The superego is undermined as abandoned incestuous strivings are rekindled. The well-known phenomenon of adolescent rebellion can be understood as both an instinctual mutiny against the prohibitions of the superego and an attempt to take flight from the forbidden impulses toward parents arising from the hormonal changes of puberty. A major developmental task of adolescence is to modify the superego from a rigid and overly punitive structure to one that allows and sanctions an adult sexual object choice.

THEORY OF ANXIETY

The development of Freud's understanding of anxiety is of fundamental importance to the theory and the practice of psychoanalysis. His clinical observations in the 1890s led him to regard anxiety as the result of "dammed-up libido." In other words, a physiological increase in sexual tension leads to a corresponding increase in libido, the mental representation of that physiological event. The normal outlet for such tension is, in Freud's view, sexual intercourse. However, abnormal sexual practices, such as abstinence and coitus interruptus, prevent tension release and result in *actual neuroses.* Those conditions of heightened anxiety related to libidinal blockage include neurasthenia, hypochondriasis, and anxiety neuroses, all of which Freud regarded as having a biological basis.

Freud differentiated the actual neuroses from the *psychoneuroses*—hysteria, phobias, and obsessional neuroses. He understood those conditions and the anxiety associated with them to be primarliy related to psychological factors, rather than physiological factors. Intrapsychic conflict is responsible for anxiety in psychoneuroses, and Freud observed that the resulting anxiety is less intense and dramatic than what he observed in actual neuroses.

Freud's early theory of anxiety cannot account for objective anxiety related to the threat of real danger that is unrelated to accumulated sexual tensions. That gap in Freud's theory led him to expand his conceptual framework of the pathogenesis of anxiety to include self-preservation and the adaptive function of anxiety.

ANXIETY AS A SIGNAL With the publication of *Inhibitions, Symptoms and Anxiety* in 1926, Freud created a new theory of anxiety that reflects the ascendence of the structural model over its topographic predecessor. Accordingly, the role of instinctual drives and physiological pressures is of less importance in that theory. Instead, the new theory accounts for both real external anxiety and neurotic internal anxiety as a response to a danger situation.

Freud identified two types of anxiety-provoking situations. One situation involves overwhelming instinctual stimulation, the prototype of which is the experience of birth. In situations of that variety, the excessive amount of drive pressure penetrates the protective barriers of the ego, producing a state of helplessness and trauma. The second and more common situation involves anxiety that develops in *anticipation* of dangers, rather than as the result of those dangers. That warning to the organism, known as *signal anxiety,* operates at an unconscious level and serves to mobilize the ego's resources to avert the danger. Either external or internal sources of danger may produce such a signal that leads the ego to marshal specific defense mechanisms to guard against or to reduce the degree of instinctual excitation.

Freud's new theory of anxiety explains neurotic symptoms as a partial failure of the ego to cope with distressing stimuli. The drive derivatives associated with danger have not been adequately contained by the defense mechanisms used by the ego. In phobias, for example, Freud explained the fear of an external threat (such as dogs or snakes) as an externalization of an internal danger. In psychotic conditions the breakdown of ego-defensive functioning is so thoroughgoing that associated distortions of ego functioning take place in an effort to accommodate the idiosyncratic distortions of the external world perceived by the patient.

Although Freud focused much more of his attention on signal anxiety in the latter part of his career than in his early career, he always maintained that physiologically based actual neuroses exist alongside the psychoneuroses. Freud's differentiation of two forms of anxiety—one biologically mediated and the other psychologically generated—proved to be remarkably prophetic. That distinction parallels what we now view as panic disorder and generalized anxiety disorder. Panic disorder may be mediated by stimulation of the locus ceruleus, the largest noradrenergic nucleus of the brain. Dysregulation of the γ-aminobutyric acid system seems to trigger that form of anxiety; psychological factors, unrelated to the locus ceruleus, appear to trigger a milder form of anticipatory or generalized anxiety. It has been postulated that an underlying neural structure may lead to a diathesis for the more severe form of anxiety and that the absence of such a neural structure leads to a milder form of expression, signal or anticipatory anxiety.

DEVELOPMENTAL HIERARCHY OF ANXIETY Freud realized that each stage of psychological development contains a characteristic danger situation involving phase-specific issues. Hence, a developmental hierarchy of anxiety can be constructed based on the specific fears associated with each stage. The earliest danger situation is a fear of disintegration or annihilation, often associated with concerns involving fusion with an external object. As one matures to the recognition of the mothering figure as a separate person, separation anxiety or fear of the loss of the object becomes more prominent.

During the oedipal psychosexual stage, the girl child is most concerned about losing the love of the most important figure in her life, her mother. The male child is primarily anxious about bodily injury or castration. After the resolution of the oedipal conflict, a more mature form of anxiety occurs, often termed *superego anxiety*. That latency-age concern involves the fear that internalized parental representations, contained in the superego, will cease to love the child or will angrily punish the child. The symptoms of anxiety may have determinants from several of those developmental stages. A major task for the psychoanalytic clinician treating anxiety is to understand the particular danger situations and their associated developmental phases that have contributed to the anxiety of a particular patient in a particular situation.

IMPLICATIONS OF THEORY Freud's theory of signal anxiety heralded a decisive shift in his formulation of the ego. Before the introduction of the structural theory in 1923, Freud regarded the ego as a passive, weak, and fragile agency that responds to the bidding of the instinctual drives from the id and the punitive demands of the superego. In his revision of his anxiety theory, however, the ego is an executive agency that exerts control over the forces of the id. Anxiety appearing before repression is operative, and the ego is endowed with sufficient autonomy to exercise certain functions on its own.

The conceptualization of anxiety as a signal also has important clinical implications. Anxiety should not be viewed simply as a pathological symptom to be removed. A healthy ego must develop the capacity to use anxiety signals to mobilize ego resources in efforts at mastery and control. Indeed, psychoanalysts view a person's capacity to tolerate anxiety as a significant sign of ego integration and psychological health.

PSYCHOANALYTIC CONCEPT OF CHARACTER

Although the term ''character'' has moralistic meanings in popular usage, in psychoanalysis, *character* refers to the enduring patterns of functioning typical of a person. Others know a person's character by that person's habitual way of behaving, feeling, speaking, and thinking. A variety of theoretical underpinnings have been proposed to explain character formation. As previously noted, Freud linked certain character traits with certain psychosexual stages. For example, persons who are developmentally fixated at the anal stage are likely to manifest orderliness, obstinacy, and miserliness. In a classic paper on anal eroticism and character, Freud concluded that permanent character traits represent ''unchanged prolongation of the original instincts, or sublimation of those instincts, or reaction formation against them.''

Freud was faced with a challenge in differentiating neurotic symptoms from character traits. He suggested that neurotic symptoms represent a ''return of the repressed,'' reflecting his formulation that the failure to repress drive derivatives leads to neurotic symptom formation. In contrast, he postulated that character traits are the end result of the *successful* use of repression and other defenses, particularly reaction formation and sublimation. Freud's development of the structural model allowed him to expand his understanding of character formation further by including identification as a defense. He observed that a person may be able to relinquish an object attachment only by a process of identification, in which the lost object is firmly established inside the ego. Through a series of identifications, children develop their own characters. The formation of the superego is a related identificatory process that also contributes to the end result of a unique character structure.

Karl Abraham delineated character traits linked to oral, anal, and genital eroticism and, in so doing, advanced Freud's rudimentary ideas to a much more sophisticated and detailed description of character. Wilhelm Reich also made significant contributions by identifying the close relationship between resistance to psychoanalytic treatment and the nature of the patient's character traits. Reich's observations about character resistance remain useful today in the work of contemporary psychoanalytic clinicians.

CURRENT CONCEPTS OF CHARACTER Today the concept of character and that of personality are used interchangeably, particularly in discussions concerning Axis II personality disorders and traits. Psychoanalytic interest has expanded beyond specific character traits to a broadened understanding of character as a series of compromise formations between instinctual wishes and opposing defenses, on the one hand, and constellations of internal representations of self and others, on the other hand. Increasing evidence from studies of twins and other research indicate that genetic and constitutional factors play key roles in the development of character. The unique stamp of personality of any one person appears to be the final common pathway of a complex mixture of innate biological predispositions and environmental-psychological factors. For example, recent research suggests that shyness involves an inherited diathesis that requires particular environmental circumstances to attain phenotypic manifestations.

Discussions of character lead directly to related concepts of self, ego, and identity—all of which have developed varied meanings in contemporary psychoanalytic usage. The following discussion of object relations theory attempts to explicate those terms in more detail.

OBJECT RELATIONS THEORY

The ego-psychological approach to psychoanalysis, often referred to as the classical view, is one of three major theoretical frameworks that are widely used by modern psychoanalytic clinicians. The other two theoretical schools, object relations theory and self psychology, are both emblematic of a trend within psychoanalysis away from an emphasis on drives and defenses and toward an increasing interest in relationships. Self psychology, which is discussed later in this section, derives from the interpersonal tradition established by Harry Stack Sullivan but most eloquently formulated and elaborated by Heinz Kohut and his followers. Object relations theory originated in the work of Melanie Klein and members of the British school, including D. W. Winnicott and W. R. D. Fairbairn.

BASIC CONCEPTS The ego-psychological perspective conceptualizes drives as primary and object relations as secondary. In that model the infant is motivated by the wish to discharge tension under the pressure of instinctual drives. By contrast, object relations theory stresses the fact that all drives emerge in the context of a mother-infant relationship; therefore, object seeking must be considered a motivation equal to or of even greater importance than drive discharge.

Freud made many references to the importance of internalized objects. For example, in his 1923 landmark work on the structural model, *The Ego and the Id,* he noted that "the character of the ego is a precipitant of abandoned object-cathexes and . . . contains the history of these object choices." In other words, he firmly believed that a person's ego results from identification with such external objects as parental figures. Similarly, the superego and the ego-ideal are conceptualized as internalizations of aspects of one's parents.

Freud laid the groundwork for a theory of object relations within the framework of the structural model, but his followers began to notice certain limitations of the model. For example, it became increasingly apparent that the id is not simply an amorphous cauldron of explosive drives. Aggressive and sexual wishes are connected with fantasies and meanings organized around relationships. Similarly, the view of the ego as subservient to an internal critical agency called the superego is seen as having limited clinical usefulness. The superego has both loving and critical aspects to it, and the complexity of its interaction with the ego can most usefully be conceptualized as an internal object relationship. Conceptualizing an object relationship strictly in terms of its cathexis with drive energy does not do justice to the full range of needs and affects associated with relationships. Such wishes and needs as affirmation, safety, reassurance, and self-esteem are not easily subsumed under the dual-instinct theory.

In strict terms, object relations theory is not an interpersonal model of psychoanalysis. It is a theory of unconscious internal object relations involving the transformation of interpersonal relationships into internalized structures. As infants grow and develop, they internalize an experience of a self in relationship to an other. The feeding experience is perhaps the best prototype of the process. While a hungry infant is screaming for its mother, a template of unpleasant experience is laid down in its brain, involving an experience of the self as greedy, demanding, and angry and an experience of an object (the mother) as frustrating, unavailable, and inattentive. That self-object constellation is also accompanied by powerful affects.

When the mother finally feeds the baby, the self-object-affect unit is transformed into a positive experience of the self, a positive view of the object as nurturant and attentive, and a positive affective experience of pleasure and satiation. At around 16 months of age, the infant's cognitive and perceptual apparatuses have sufficiently developed so that those two experiences are internalized as two opposing sets of self-object-affect units.

That examination of the feeding experience illustrates a basic tenet of object relations theory—namely, that object relations always involve an interaction between a self and an object associated with an affect. Internalized representations of self and object do not occur in isolation. A second point of crucial importance is that the structures laid down by the child are significantly determined by the child's fantasy life. For example, the mother who is not responding to her child's demands to be fed may in actuality be a perfectly competent mother who is simply occupied with other siblings. However, the infant's fantasies may involve a mother who is evil, rejecting, and abandoning, so that the internal structure laid down by the child may include such distorted characteristics. Freud was clearly aware of that phenomenon when he noted in 1940, "It is a remarkable thing that the super-ego often displays a severity for which no model has been provided by the real parents." Hence, a one-to-one correlation may not exist between the real external object and the internalized object.

Object relations theory also views motivation differently from Freudian ego-psychological theory. For example, the infant transforms its mother into an internal soothing presence as a way of dealing with its fear of losing its mother. In that manner both the external mother and the internalized version of the mother represent safety and an enhanced sense of well-being for the child, independent of drive discharge. Internalizing bad or negative aspects of the mother is more complex and involves the fantasy of gaining control over the bad object by capturing it within oneself, developing mastery through repetitive traumatic experiences with the object, yearning to transform the bad object into a good object, and needing to hang on to the bad object because it is preferable to no object at all.

The development of the self-object units in the child's internal world reflects the operation of two distinct internalization mechanisms. *Introjection* involves the taking in of an object that continues to exist as an other, an internal presence that may be experienced as a soothing companion or a critical parent, as in the case of the superego. Introjects, then, continue to be experienced as *objects,* rather than as parts of the child's self. *Identification,* in contrast, involves a modification of the self on the basis of the internalization of a significant external figure who is used as a model. That assimilation process in identification leads to the child's experience of those parental qualities as part of the self, rather than as a foreign body, as in the case of introjection. Identification with an introject may also take place over the course of development.

Whereas ego psychology regards conflict as struggles between wishes and defenses or between intrapsychic agencies, such as the id and the superego, object relations theory views conflict quite differently. Unconscious conflict is perceived as a struggle between different self-object-affect units striving for center stage in the psyche. The notion of character is also conceptualized in a different manner. Instead of the ego-psychological view that the end result of instinctual drives and specific defensive operations deals with those drives, character is viewed as heavily influenced by the predominant constellations of self-representations and object representations deriving from introjections and identifications.

HISTORICAL EVOLUTION Object relations theory as a separate school of psychoanalytic thought originated in the United Kingdom. The British Psychoanalytic Society is divided into three segments as a result of disagreements that took place before and during World War II. Those three discrete groups, still in existence today, include the A group, followers of Melanie Klein; the B group, followers of Anna Freud; and the independent group, who are often referred to as the middle groupers. The third group—consisting of such notable clinicians as D. W. Winnicott, W. R. D. Fairbairn, Harry Guntrip, Michael Balint, Margaret Little, and John D. Sutherland—are responsible for the theory of object relations as it is known today. They formed the British school of object relations out of a wish to avoid taking sides with either the Kleinians or the Anna Freudians. However, they owe a substantial debt to Melanie Klein, who is generally acknowledged to be the pivotal figure in the shift from classical theory to object relations theory.

Melanie Klein Heavily influenced by Freud, Melanie Klein evolved a theory of internal object relations that was intimately linked to drives. She arrived in England in 1926, having emigrated from Budapest and Berlin. Her unique perspective largely grew out of her psychoanalytic work with children, in which she became impressed with the role of unconscious intrapsychic fantasy. She believed that a fear of annihilation associated with Freud's death instinct was a key factor in the first few months of the infant's life. She postulated that the ego undergoes a splitting process to deal with that terror; derivatives of the death instinct—such as aggression, hatred, sadism, and all other forms of "badness"—are disavowed and projected into the mother.

Klein viewed projection and introjection as the primary defensive operations at that stage of life. After projecting the death-instinct derivatives into the mother, the infant begins to suffer from persecutory anxiety, in which the infant lives in dread of an invasive attack from the mother. In that terrifying fantasy, the "bad mother" created by the infant's projections gets inside the infant (that is, the "bad mother" is reintrojected) and destroys the remaining "goodness" (that is, libidinal derivatives) that were originally protected by the splitting and projection of the "badness."

That persecutory anxiety characterized what Klein called the *paranoid-schizoid position,* the infant's mode of organizing experience in which all aspects of the infant and the mother are split into good and bad elements. Klein thought that external and internal objects cannot be clearly distinguished because the actual figures in the external world are heavily colored by the infant's projections and ensuing perceptions are distorted. She conceptualized oscillating cycles of introjection and projection to keep bad aspects of the self separated from good aspects of the self and to keep the bad aspects of objects separated from the good aspects. In that manner the child can prevent good, loving aspects of its experience from being destroyed by bad, hateful aspects of experience. In the second half of the first year of life, according to Klein's developmental timetable, the child's part-object world (that is, a world containing an "all-bad" mother and an "all-good" mother) begins to change. The child becomes aware that the hateful, rejecting mother and the loving, nurturing mother are simply aspects of the same person. As those disparate views are integrated, the infant becomes concerned that it may have harmed or destroyed its mother through its hostile and sadistic fantasies directed toward her. At that developmental point the child has arrived at the *depressive position,* in which the mother is viewed ambivalently as having both positive and negative aspects and as being the target of a mixture of loving and hateful feelings.

In contrast to the paranoid-schizoid position, in which the primary concern of the infant is external attack, in the depressive position the infant's primary concern is that it may harm love objects, particularly the mother. The possibility of losing the good object through sadistic and aggressive impulses produces guilt feelings in the child. Anxiety about loss of the love object through one's own destructiveness is known as *depressive anxiety.* To deal with guilt feelings, the child engages in a process of *reparation,* in which efforts are made to assure that love prevails over hate and that damage done through one's own destructiveness is repaired through loving behavior. Because the maternal object is recognized as a whole object in the depressive position, Klein postulated that the Oedipus complex begins in the second half of the first year, and she recast the whole oedipal constellation as an effort to resolve depressive anxieties and guilt through reparation.

Kleinian theory has been criticized for its significant shortcomings. One of its primary difficulties is the assumption that an infant in its first year of life possesses a highly sophisticated capacity for abstract and conceptual thinking. The infant's perceptual-cognitive development is actually too rudimentary when that young to be capable of elaborating the sophisticated fantasies that Klein postulates. Hence, her developmental timetable, which compresses preoedipal and oedipal phases into the first year, is no longer tenable.

Klein's emphasis on envy and greed have considerable clinical utility, but her view that such states, as well as aspects of sadism and aggression, derive from the death instinct has fallen out of favor. Klein has also been criticized for relying too heavily on fantasy and thereby discounting the role of actual environmental trauma on children and the influence of real parental objects on the child's development. Post-Kleinian theorists have suggested that the paranoid-schizoid and depressive positions are not developmental phases that are outgrown but, rather, two modes of generating experience that continue in a dialectic with one another throughout adult life. Viewed from that perspective, Klein's formulations have a great deal of clinical value, particularly in the treatment of highly disturbed patients.

Independent group The British analysts who constitute the middle group had several key features in common. First, like Klein, they were involved in the psychoanalytic treatment of patients who were more severely disturbed than the classical neurotic patient. As a consequence of that particular clinical experience, they tended to focus on preoedipal development and dyadic object relations, rather than the triangular oedipal constellation. Also, they counterbalanced Klein's focus on intrapsychic fantasy with detailed attention to the actual environment provided by the mothering figure in the earliest months of life. The group was also intensely interested in a theory of *deficit*—that is, a theory that encompassed the effects of insufficient maternal nurturance on the developing child and that conceptualized certain forms of psychopathology as involving the absence of or an insufficiently developed intrapsychic structure, rather than interagency conflict. Each of the leading figures of the British school of object relations theory made unique contributions.

W. R. D. FAIRBAIRN Although heavily influenced by Klein, Fairbairn (Figure 6.1-13) reversed her focus on the role of fantasy in the infant's creation of its objects. He saw the causes of his patients' difficulties in their mothers' failure to provide appropriate nurturance, rather than in the frustration of drives. He thought that infants have a basic need for a kind of love and acceptance from the mother that assures the infants that they are persons in their own right. In that regard he conceptualized the need for the recognition of personhood as primary and the physiological needs related to the drives as secondary. He did not deny the existence of libido and aggression but thought that they are fundamentally object-seeking, rather than pleasure-seeking.

Although Klein stressed that fantasy is the earliest and most basic activity of the infantile mind, Fairbairn regarded fantasy as substitutive, rather than primary. The welfare of the developing child lies fundamentally in the experience of the mother's acceptance of it, and internal objects are elaborated only in compensation for unsatisfactory relationships with real external objects.

Fairbairn is particularly known for his insight into the primacy of the schizoid condition. He suggested that, when the mothering figure fails to fulfill the baby's basic needs, the infant splits the object and the ego into various components, leading to a schizoid state. Hence, in contrast to classical theory, the Fairbairn theory views the ego as whole

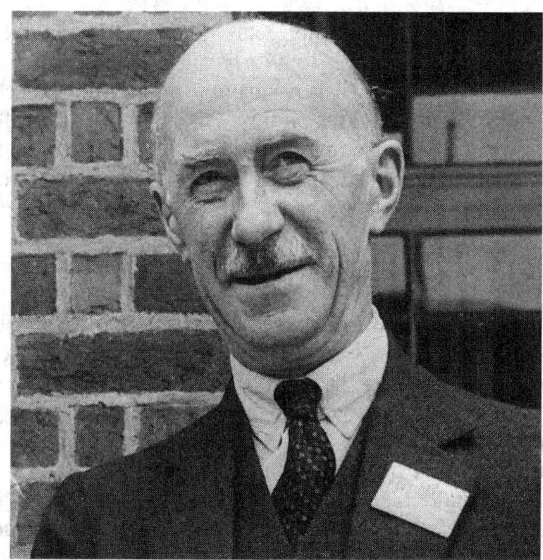

FIGURE 6.1-13 *W. R. D. Fairbairn. (Courtesy of John D. Sutherland, Edinburgh, Scotland.)*

at birth, only to become split as it encounters unfavorable experiences with early mothering figures. In the Fairbairn model, libidinal object-seeking is primary, and aggression occurs as a natural defensive reaction to the frustration of the libidinal drive.

D. W. WINNICOTT Of all the middle groupers, Winnicott is probably the best known. Like Fairbairn, he was a Kleinian revisionist who gave greater credence to the role of external reality in development. He was particularly interested in the creation of a *holding environment* by the mother that made it ultimately possible for the child to develop awareness as a separate person. In Winnicott's view the mother plays a key role in bringing the world to the child and in offering empathic anticipations of the infant's needs. The mother provides a fundamentally crucial relationship that enables the nascent self of the infant to emerge. Trained as a pediatrician, Winnicott gave primary attention to the mother-infant dyad. Little of importance was written about the father in Winnicott's work.

Winnicott coined the term *good-enough mothering* to designate a mothering figure who is able to provide an optimal amount of comfort and constancy for the infant, so that the infant can proceed along normal developmental lines. Such a mother tunes in to the infant and meets the child's omnipotent needs without challenging them and offers her support according to the infant's own timetable, rather than imposing herself on the child as a consequence of her own needs. She also lets the infant separate at the appropriate time and allows for an optimal disillusionment of the child's omnipotence.

Winnicott was also responsible for the concept of the *transitional object,* the infant's not-me possession, usually a treasured blanket or toy. The object, often suffused with the mother's scent, enables the child to separate emotionally from the mother without undue anxiety. The transitional object preserves the illusion of the comforting maternal object, even in her absence. Winnicott described *transitional phenomena* as objects, sounds, sights, and smells that exist in an intermediate realm that has elements both of external reality and of the child's own subjectivity. Art, religious experience, and creativity may well derive from that sphere of experience.

Winnicott's distinction between the *true self* and the *false self* is widely used in clinical discussions. The true self refers to the inherited potential that constitutes the kernel of the child. The true self is the child's authentic being that will emerge if a good-enough mothering experience with an appropriate holding environment is offered. The false self is a facade constructed by the child in reaction to a self-involved mother who insists on certain responses from her child. The false self may develop to protect the true self by complying with the maternal demands.

Winnicott's conceptual framework of the mother-infant relationship led to a form of psychoanalytic treatment that radically departed from the classical approach. He thought that the analyst must provide the appropriate facilitating environment that was missing during the patient's early development. Only then can the true self, which was frozen in a state of developmental arrest, continue its growth and overtake the false self constructed by the patient. Like Fairbairn, Winnicott thought that psychopathology results from the mother's failures, rather than from interagency conflict or intrapsychic fantasy. His own technique took on a unique character in that he advocated a prolonged holding period before making interpretive interventions.

MICHAEL BALINT Balint thought that the search for the primary love object underlies virtually all psychological phenomena. The infant wishes to be loved totally and unconditionally, and, if the mother is not forthcoming with appropriate nurturance, the child devotes its life to a search for the love that was missed in childhood. Balint described the feeling in many patients that something is missing as *the basic fault.* Like Fairbairn and Winnicott, Balint understood that deficit in internal structure to be the result of maternal failures. He viewed all psychological motivations as stemming from that failure to receive adequate maternal love.

Unlike Fairbairn, Balint did not entirely abandon drive theory. He suggested that libido, for example, is both pleasure-seeking and object-seeking. He also worked with primitively organized patients, and, like Winnicott, he felt that certain aspects of psychoanalytic treatment occur at a more profound level than verbal explanatory interpretations. Although some material involving genital psychosexual stages of development can be interpreted from an intrapsychic conflict perspective, Balint believed, certain preverbal phenomena are reexperienced in analysis, and the relationship itself is decisive in dealing with that realm of experience.

MIXED MODELS When object relations theory began to cross the Atlantic and to influence North American thinkers, attempts were made to integrate American ego-psychological concepts with the object relations perspectives of Klein and members of the British school. Two prominent contributors to that mixed-model approach are Edith Jacobson and Otto Kernberg. The melding of ego psychology and object relations theory typical of their work has led Jacobson and Kernberg, as well as those influenced by them, to be categorized as American object relations theorists.

Edith Jacobson In contrast to members of the British school, Jacobson understood the infant's disappointment with the maternal object to be not necessarily related to actual failure by the mother. In Jacobson's view, disappointment is always related to a specific, drive-determined demand, rather than to a global striving for contact or engagement. She viewed the infant's experience of pleasure or unpleasure as the core of the early mother-infant relationship. Satisfactory experiences lead to the formation of good or gratifying images, whereas unsatisfactory experiences create bad or frustrating images. Normal and pathological development are based on the evolution of these self-images and object images. As far as Jacobson was concerned, the concept of fixation refers to modes of object relatedness, rather than modes of gratification.

Jacobson believed that the structural model and an emphasis on object relations are not fundamentally incompatible. She thought that the ego and self-images and object images exert a reciprocal influence on one another's development. The ego, as it matures, integrates early pleasure-unpleasure experiences into partial primitive images of the self and the object. Subsequent events continue to be divided into either gratifying or frustrating experiences.

By the second year of life, with further maturation of the ego, the child is able to distinguish specific features of the love object and to entertain the notion of being like the admired object, rather than of becoming the object. If conditions are favorable, selective identification, the tendency to be like the object, gradually replaces the tendency to regress into merger fantasies. Eventually, competition with peers and the same-sex parent contributes to stable ego identification and the establishment of an ego-ideal. Jacobson viewed the ego-ideal as a fusion between ideal self-images and ideal object images that partially compensate for the lost fantasies of merger.

For Jacobson the superego develops in three phases. The early superego consists of archaic, sadistic images formed on the basis of introjective and projective processes. The second phase involves the fusion of ideal self-images and ideal object images into the entity of the ego-ideal. The third and final stage involves the internalization of realistic parental demands, values, and prohibitions.

Otto Kernberg Perhaps the most influential of the American object relations theorists, Otto Kernberg was substantially influenced by both Melanie Klein and Edith Jacobson. Much of his theory was derived from his clinical work with patients suffering from borderline personality disorder (discussed later). In brief, Kernberg places great emphasis on the splitting of the ego and the elaboration of good and bad self-configurations and object configurations. Although he continues to use the structural model, he views the id as composed of self-images, object images, and their associated affects. Drives appear only to manifest themselves in the context of internalization of interpersonal experience. Good and bad self-relationships and object relationships become associated, respectively, with libido and aggression. Not only do object relations constitute the building blocks of structure, but they are also the building blocks of drives. Goodness and badness in relational experiences precede drive cathexis. In other words, the dual instincts of libido and aggression arise from object-directed affective states of love and hate.

The influence of Klein on Kernberg is apparent in his view of infantile development as moving from splitting toward integration. Idealized or good images of self and object are gradually integrated with devalued or bad self-images and object images, leading to ambivalent, whole-object configurations of self and other. That integration leads to feelings of guilt, concern, and mourning, much as Melanie Klein described the process. Kernberg's view of the superego follows Jacobson's model in delineating three layers based on the three developmental phases of Jacobson.

The principal features of the major object relations theorists are summarized in Table 6.1-3.

DEFENSE MECHANISMS IN OBJECT RELATIONS THEORY Although the clinical work of ego psychologists has focused primarily on neurotic defense mechanisms, the object relations theorists have traditionally worked with more disturbed patients. That clinical perspective has delineated a set of primitive defense mechanisms characteristic of severe personality disorders and psychoses that are in common usage by object relations theorists.

Splitting Although Freud described splitting of the ego in his discussions of fetishism, Melanie Klein was the first analyst to recognize the universal importance of splitting in early development. It can be defined as an unconscious process that actively separates contradictory self-representations, contradictory object representations, or contradictory feelings from one another. Splitting is crucial for emotional survival because it allows the infant to separate the negative views of the mother as a rejecting, unavailable figure from the positive views of the nurturing, feeding mother, so that the feeding experience itself is not contaminated by the terrifying anxieties about the ''bad mother.'' Splitting helps the developing child separate love from hate, pleasure from unpleasure, good from bad, and positively colored experience from its negative counterparts. Splitting may also be viewed as a basic mode of ordering experience into separate compartments on the basis of the fear that all that is good will be destroyed by all that is bad unless the good and the bad are kept separate. Splitting is secondarily elaborated into a psychological defense.

Kernberg has been instrumental in making the defense of splitting clinically relevant to the diagnostic understanding and treatment of severe personality disorders. He has identified four common clinical manifestations of splitting: (1) the coexistence of contradictory and alternating self-representations that cause the patient to look quite different from day to day, (2) the division of persons in the environment into an idealized or all-good group and a devalued or all-bad group, (3) selective problems with impulse control, and (4) the expression of behaviors and attitudes that alternate and are contradictory but are regarded by the patient with lack of concern and bland denial. Although Kernberg has cited splitting as the key defensive operation in borderline patients, it may also be found in psychotic patients and those with neurotic or higher-level personality disorders.

Projective identification Splitting works hand in hand with the second defense mechanism, projective identification, which is an unconscious three-step process by which object representations or self-representations are disavowed and attributed to someone else. The three steps involve the following:

1. The patient unconsciously projects an object representation or self-representation into the clinician.

2. The clinician unconsciously identifies with what is projected and begins to behave or feel like the patient's projected object representation or self-representation in response to interpersonal pressure exerted by the patient's behavior. That step in the phenomenon has been referred to as projective counteridentification.

3. The clinician psychologically processes the projected contents, which are, therefore, modified to some extent before finally returning to the patient through reintrojection. When

TABLE 6.1-3
Object Relations Theorists

	Klein	Winnicott	Fairbairn	Balint	Jacobson	Kernberg
Theoretical school	A Group	Independent or middle group	Independent or middle group	Independent or middle group	American mixed model	American mixed model
Emphasis on drives vs. environmental failures	Drives	Environmental failures	Environmental failures	Environmental failures	Both important	Both important
Emphasis on conflict vs. deficit	Conflict	Deficit	Deficit and conflict	Deficit	Conflict	Conflict
Major contributions	Paranoid-schizoid position Depressive position Seminal roles of splitting, envy, greed, and reparation	Need for holding environment Transitional objects and relatedness Good-enough mothering True self-false self	Need for recognition of personhood by mother is primary; drives and fantasy are secondary Primacy of the schizoid condition Ego is whole at birth and splits in reaction to unfavorable mothering experiences	Search for love object is primary Basic fault Emphasis on preverbal development	Disappointment related to drive-determined demand Integrated structural model and emphasis on object relations Three phases of superego development	Drives appear in context of self-object-affect units Object relations are building blocks of structure Delineated borderline personality organization Formulated concept of pathological narcissism

those modified projected contents are returned to the patient, there is a corresponding modification of the patient's internal object relatedness.

Whereas that definition is geared to the treatment situation, a similar pattern occurs in nonclinical settings, although the processing and the modification of the third step are likely to be far less extensive when the target of the projective identification is not a clinician.

Projective identification as defined in that three-step model can be viewed as both an intrapsychic defense mechanism and an interpersonal process. Splitting and projective identification work in tandem to separate good and bad elements from one another. For example, a woman who has introjected a physically abusive parent may use projective identification to keep the internal bad object representation outside herself, so that she can control it. Her behavior may coerce treaters to assume the role of the abusive parent and to struggle with feelings of anger and hatred toward her. The treater's feeling of being controlled or bullied into assuming a specific role vis-à-vis the patient is a hallmark of projective identification. Although Melanie Klein originated the concept of projective identification, Wilfred Bion elaborated it to encompass a developmental situation in which the infant projects unacceptable aspects of itself into the mother, who serves as a container for the infant's projections before returning them in a modified form.

Projective identification is a controversial term, and some authors have limited its use to describe an intrapsychic defense that may or may not result in a complementary response from the clinician. In that model the identification process is regarded as occurring within the patient, rather than within the clinician who is the target of the projection. By maintaining the empathic bond or identification with the projected contents, the patient can maintain a fantasy of complete control over the target of the projection and over the projected material itself.

The distinction between projection and projective identification is also somewhat controversial. However, if one assumes that the three-step model involves both an intrapsychic defense and an interpersonal process, projective identification requires a transformation of the target of the projection. Projection does not require such a transformation. Paranoid patients, for example, may assume that people who are walking up and down the street are members of the Central Intelligence Agency, but that projection of malevolence does not alter the feelings or the behaviors of those people.

Primitive idealization and devaluation Primitive idealization and devaluation also occur in concert with splitting. External objects are viewed as either all good or all bad as a way of preventing the destruction of the loving aspects of others and of the self by their hateful counterparts. Hence, by attributing omnipotence and perfection to certain figures in the environment, a patient may bask in the reflected glory of the object and defend against feelings of contempt and envy toward the object. Similarly, by devaluating another person as thoroughly worthless, the patient may defend against painful feelings of envy and inferiority.

CONCEPT OF THE SELF Whereas ego psychologists concentrated their efforts on the ego, object relations theorists have sought to clarify the role of the self in psychoanalytic theory. The confusion between the self and the ego goes back to Freud's ambiguous usage of *Ich,* which James Strachey translated as ''ego'' in *Standard Edition of the Complete Psychological Works of Sigmund Freud.* Freud used the term to connote both the person and the intrapsychic agency within the person. In other words, a term that can be literally translated from the German as ''I'' was used interchangeably to refer both to subjective self-experience and to a collection of organizing functions within the psyche. However, the self-experience meaning gradually became lost in the increasingly preferred usage of ''ego'' as an impersonal executive organ of the psyche.

Hartmann attempted to distinguish the two meanings of *Ich* by defining the interactional context. The self interacts with objects, and the ego interacts with the id and the superego. That clarification was useful because it stresses the fact that the self evolves in relational configurations to objects. Hence, one's experience of oneself is discontinuous in that the nature of the self varies with the nature of the object to which it is relating. In that regard the person's self embodies the history of many internalized relationships. The concept of the self should then refer to a multiplicity of points of view from which one experiences, observes, and feels. Everyone behaves differently from others and has a different sense of internal experience, depending on the figure with whom the person is relating.

Despite the presence of that array of selves responding to diverse environmental contexts, a person has some sense of continuity over time. The sum of the component selves is regarded as one's *identity,* a term defined by Erik Erikson as a conscious sense of inner solidarity that endures over time.

If one considers a sentence such as, ''I think about myself,'' one becomes aware that the self is used to describe both an object of reflection and an experiential consciousness that is doing the thinking. That distinction has been the source of another major controversy surrounding the self—namely, whether the word ''self'' should be used to refer to an intrapsychic representation, conscious or unconscious, or to an initiator of action in its own right. Ego-psychological thinkers have traditionally viewed the self as representational, but members of the British school have preferred a concept that includes subjective experience or personal agency. Kernberg has suggested that there is room for both the self-as-agency view and the self-as-representation perspective. The self-as-agency is embedded in the ego and may be conceptualized as the end result of the integration of a myriad of self-representation.

Contemporary psychoanalytic theory has been enhanced by conceptualizing the self as a content of the ego. The ego is useful for understanding and dealing with drive-defense conflicts, character, and compromise formations, but the self offers a subjective side to the ego that is relevant to such issues as narcissism, identity, self-other differentiation, and internal object relations. Moreover, the notion of self is important in clinical work with primitively organized patients who use such defenses as splitting and projective identification. Kohut's view of the self as a primary, supraordinate entity implying motivational status is discussed under the heading ''Self Psychology.''

INFANT OBSERVATION STUDIES Recent interest in object relations theory has been bolstered by the findings of infant observation studies conducted by Margaret Mahler (Figure 6.1-14) and her colleagues. Those investigations focused on both normal and abnormal mother-infant pairs during the first three years of life. The investigations were specifically designed to study the manner in which a child achieves an intrapsychic sense of separateness from its mother. As a result of the research, three developmental phases in mother-infant object relations have been widely accepted.

An *autistic* phase occurs during the first two months of life, during which the infant spends most of its day in a half-sleeping, half-waking state, more concerned about physiological matters than relatedness. From 2 to 6 months of age, the infant enters the phase of *symbiosis,* a term Mahler used to describe an undifferentiated state of fusion between infant and mother. The onset of that phase is heralded by the infant's smile response and the baby's dawning awareness of a dimly perceived source of need satisfaction in its environment, although that maternal source is viewed as within the orbit of an omnipotent dual unity.

Most of Mahler's research focused on the third phase of the development of object relations, which she termed *separation-individuation.* That period extends from around 6 months to 36 months of age and involves the infant's psychological birth as a separate person apart from the mother. Observational data indicated that the third phase can be divided into four subphases. The first subphase, *differentiation,* occurs between 6 and 10 months of age and is linked to the child's awareness that the mother is a separate person. That awareness often results in the child's attachment to a transitional object, as described by Winnicott, to substitute for the mother when she is not available.

The second subphase, which Mahler termed *practicing,* occurs between the ages of 10 and 16 months and is characterized by elated investment in the child's newfound autonomy that results from acquiring locomotor skills. The toddlers explore their environment as though their mothers were no longer important, only to return for periodic refueling through physical contact.

The third subphase of separation-individuation, known as *rapprochement,* occurs between 16 and 24 months of age. In contrast to the toddler's relative obliviousness of the mother's presence during the previous subphase, in rapprochement the toddler shows a marked increase in its awareness of vulnerability to separations from its mother. Children at that age demonstrate a seemingly constant concern about the actual location of their mothers and display a wish for their mothers to be involved in sharing new experiences. A great need for maternal love can also be observed during the third subphase. Rapprochement is crucial in the development of object relations in which the child uses splitting of self-representations and object representations. The toddler's anger at its mother is viewed as dangerous because of the risk that the anger will destroy the positive internal representation of the mother, and the absence of the child's mother during the third subphase leads to a predominance of bad self-representations and object representations, which may be quite frightening to the child.

The fourth subphase of separation-individuation is marked by the beginnings of object constancy and the consolidation of the child as a separate person. The period corresponds to the third year of the child's life and involves the integration of the good and bad aspects of both self-representations and object representations. Moreover, the major accomplishment of the fourth subphase is the development of *object constancy,* by which the mother becomes introjected as an integrative whole object that is felt as a soothing internal presence. Because an internal image of the mother is sustained during periods of separation, the child no longer feels threatened by the comings and goings of the mother.

The empirical data gathered by Mahler and her colleagues demonstrate the crucial importance of object-seeking in the course of development. Clinicians have shown that the concepts of separation-individuation, object constancy, and, particularly, the rapprochement subphase have considerable applicability in the understanding of primitively organized patients, such as those with borderline personality disorders. The implications of that research on the understanding of pathogenesis is discussed under the heading "Psychoanalytic Psychopathology."

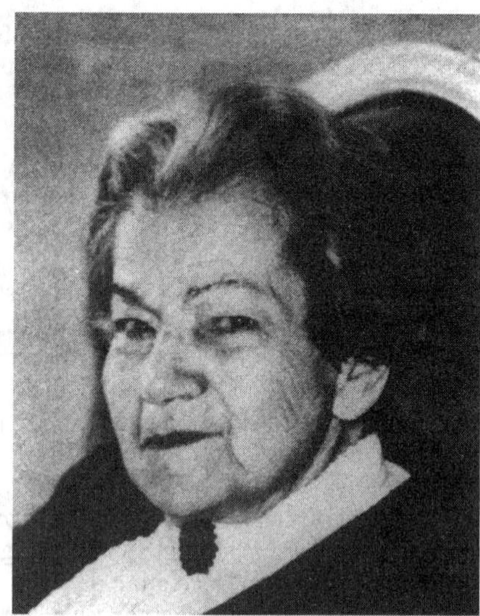

FIGURE 6.1-14 *Margaret S. Mahler, M.D. (Courtesy of Margaret S. Mahler, M.D.)*

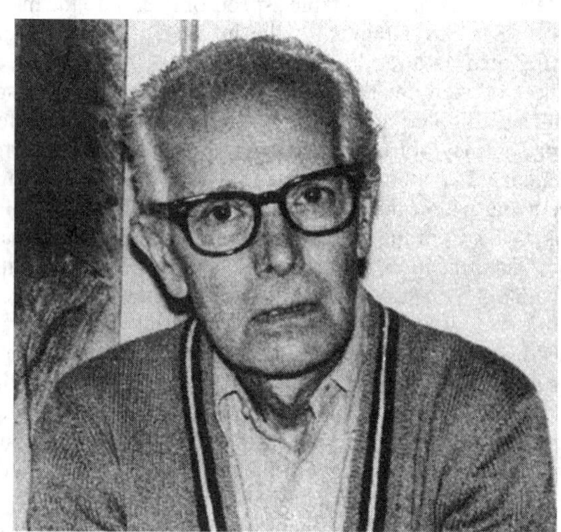

FIGURE 6.1-15 *Heinz Kohut. (Courtesy of AP/Wide World Photos.)*

SELF PSYCHOLOGY

The third major theoretical school in modern psychoanalysis is self psychology. (The other two schools are ego psychology and object relations theory, discussed above.) Derived from the work of Heinz Kohut (Figure 6.1-15), the self psychology model of the mind regards the person as needing particular kinds of responses from others in the environment to develop and maintain a sense of self-esteem and well-being. Although object relations theory and self psychology have some similarities, object relations theory stresses the importance of internalized relationships between self-representations and object representations, and self psychology focuses on the role of actual external relationships in creating self-cohesion and self-esteem. In that regard, self psychology can be viewed as a derivative of the Sullivanian interpersonal tradition, given the fact that it is essentially a self-object or two-person psychology.

Kohut's self psychology departs from classical ego psychology in a number of ways. Defects or deficits, rather than conflicts, take center stage in self psychology. Faulty structures are viewed as responsible for faulty functioning, and the emphasis is on infantile needs, rather than repressed wishes and drives. Hence, the analyst's therapeutic goals involve understanding those needs and partially meeting them in the treatment, rather than frustrating infantile wishes that must ultimately be renounced. Building the psychic structure and repairing self-defects are seen as more important than the resolution of conflict.

KOHUT'S DOUBLE-AXIS THEORY Self psychology evolved out of psychoanalytic work with narcissistically disturbed patients. In treating those patients, Kohut noted that ego psychology based on the structural model lacks sufficient explanatory power with those patients. Instead of having discrete neurotic symptoms, those narcissistic patients had vague complaints related to disappointing patterns in relationships and a hypersensitivity to slights from others.

Kohut thought that a new theory was required to provide a conceptual framework for the analytic treatment of such patients. His theory evolved directly from clinical observations, specifically the tendency of his patients to form one of two kinds of transference: the mirror transference and the idealizing transference. The mirror-transference patients seem in desperate need of the analyst's approval and will do whatever is necessary to gain that affirmation or validation from the analyst. Those patients often appear to be performing or showing off to obtain the analyst's admiration. Kohut viewed the mirror transference as a revival of an infantile situation in which the child shows off to capture the gleam in the mother's eye that makes the child feel confirmed and validated. Kohut referred to that developmental arrest as the *grandiose-exhibitionistic self,* a term he used nonpejoratively to describe a normal developmental phase in which the child's self-worth is dependent on empathic mirroring responses from the mothering figure. Without that empathy, children cannot maintain their sense of self-cohesion or wholeness, and their sense of self fragments. That sense of fragmentation of the self can be experienced along a continuum from mild anxiety or distress to full-blown panic associated with feelings of disintegration. Those children who are not provided with adequate maternal empathy are regarded as developmentally frozen and doomed to go through life seeking mirroring responses from others.

In the idealizing transference the patient regards the analyst as a perfect and omniscient parent who meets all the patient's needs. The patient may show little interest in insight or understanding in such cases because the patient's primary wish is to bask in the reflected glory of the idealized analyst. Kohut viewed that transference manifestation as similar to the developmental arrest in which the child has not been provided with a parental model worthy of idealization. As a result, the analyst is needed to perform the function that was missing in childhood.

Kohut's observations led him to postulate a double-axis theory that takes into account both narcissistic needs and object love. Kohut was impressed that narcissistic needs are never outgrown but, rather, persist throughout life in parallel development with the person's needs for object love. On the basis of that perspective, he postulated a separate axis for narcissistic development that exists alongside the classical line of development leading to object love, as depicted in Figure 6.1-16. In that model the self begins as a set of fragments that gradually achieve cohesiveness if the child's phase-appropriate developmental needs are greeted with maternal empathy.

At some point in development, a point that Kohut left unspecified, children are threatened by losing the blissful perfection of the mother-infant bond and resort to one of two strategies to recapture the perfection. In one scenario the perfection is assigned to a grandiose self within the infant, in which case the adult manifestation in the psychoanalytic setting is the mirror transference. In the other scenario the infant assigns perfection to an idealized parental imago, in which case the idealizing transference appears in the analytic setting. In the course of normal development, the grandiose self evolves into healthy ambitions, and the idealized parent imago is eventually internalized as a structure akin to Freud's ego-ideal or superego—that is, a set of values and ideals that lead to moral conduct. If, however, the child's developmental needs for mirroring or idealization or both are met with maternal failures of empathy, a developmental arrest occurs at the point of the grandiose self or the idealized parental image. Those two poles of self-development Kohut termed the *bipolar self.*

Inherent in Kohut's double-axis theory is an accepting view of narcissistic needs. He thought that Freud's model of the progression from primary narcissism to object love as an expectation in the normal maturational process contains a moralizing, pejorative tone toward narcissism. In other words, Freud's view suggests that narcissism should be outgrown and that the mature adult should be primarily devoted to the needs and concerns of others. Kohut regarded that attitude as hypocritical; after all, everyone has narcissistic needs that are crucial to one's sense of personal happiness and fulfillment. Indeed, one of Kohut's major contributions was his insistence that, in addition to the dual drives of sexuality and aggression, needs for self-esteem

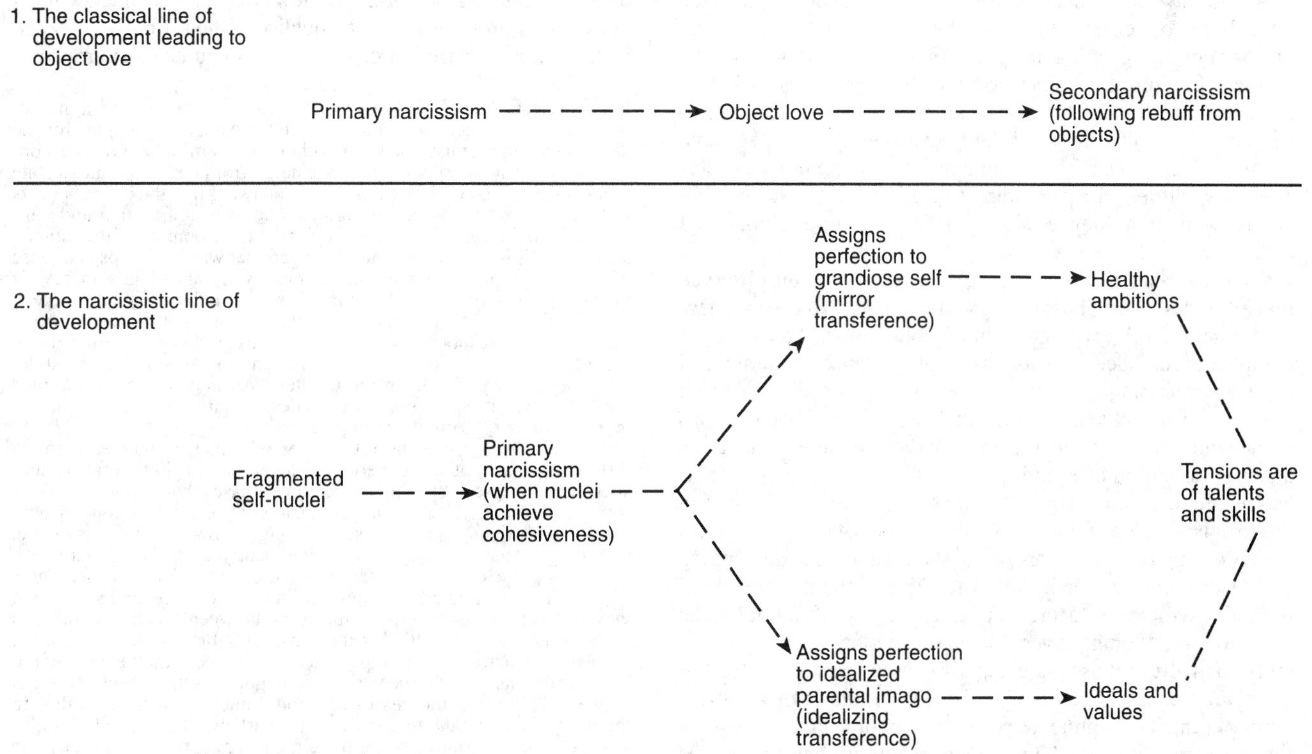

1. The classical line of development leading to object love

Primary narcissism ------→ Object love ------→ Secondary narcissism (following rebuff from objects)

2. The narcissistic line of development

Fragmented self-nuclei ---→ Primary narcissism (when nuclei achieve cohesiveness)

Assigns perfection to grandiose self (mirror transference) ---→ Healthy ambitions

Tensions are of talents and skills

Assigns perfection to idealized parental imago (idealizing transference) ---→ Ideals and values

FIGURE 6.1-16 *Kohut's double axis theory (1971). (From G O Gabbard:* Psychodynamic Psychiatry in Clinical Practice, *p 39. American Psychiatric Press, Washington, 1990. Used with permission.)*

also occupy a place of central importance in the psyche. Self psychology, then, provides a conceptual framework for the analyst that advocates empathy for the patient's narcissistic needs, instead of viewing them as immature and contemptible. Another implication of the double-axis model is that the development of a cohesive sense of self may in and of itself be a legitimate goal for psychoanalytic treatment, regardless of the patient's capacity for object love.

SELFOBJECT CONCEPT Throughout the evolution of self psychology, Kohut struggled with the extent to which his new theory would depart radically from the classical model in which he had been trained. He initially tried to incorporate drive theory by suggesting that narcissistically disturbed patients invest objects with a special form of narcissistic libido. However, as his theory evolved, he eventually found that mixed models were unsatisfying to him, so he made a complete break from classical theory. He also thought that his theoretical formulations were no longer limited to narcissistic personality disorders. He greatly expanded the scope of self psychology to include all forms of psychopathology.

Within that broadened view, the term "selfobject" became a central tenet of his theory. *Selfobjects* are viewed as fundamental needs of all persons that are required for normal development. Selfobjects may best be conceptualized as functions (such as mirroring, validating, soothing, idealizing, and affirming), rather than actual persons. As the term "selfobject" implies, other people are not viewed as separate objects with their own centers of autonomy and their own distinct needs. Rather, they are viewed as present only to gratify the needs of the nascent self. Kohut believed that selfobjects are necessary for emotional survival in the same way that oxygen in the atmosphere is needed for physical survival. Throughout life all persons are dependent on others to maintain their sense of self-esteem and well-being.

At the time of his death in 1981, Kohut had conceptualized a third area of selfobject needs, which he termed the *twinship* or *alter ego*. Originating in a childhood wish to merge with the mothering figure, this dimension of selfobject needs makes its appearance in the transference in the form of a wish or need to be exactly like the analyst. Infantile antecedents of that transference development can be found in such commonplace occurrences as a little girl's pretending to feed her doll as her mother is busy nursing a younger sibling. Hence, Kohut's bipolar self became a *tripolar self*.

As a result of that expansion of the theory, Kohut observed that all forms of psychopathology can be traced to disturbances of the self-selfobject relationship in childhood. The Oedipus complex is regarded as secondary in importance in the light of the self-psychological view that all psychiatric disorders are based on distortions of the self, weakness of the self, or defects in the structure of the self. Oedipal conflicts involving castration anxiety, inhibition of aggression, and other neurotic symptoms are regarded as breakdown products of preoedipal failures in the provision of selfobject needs. An adequate self-selfobject matrix during the early years of life should allow the developing child to weather the oedipal constellation without residuals of neurotic symptoms. Moreover, most forms of pathological behavior—including perversions, binge eating, sexual promiscuity, and drug abuse—are regarded as efforts to restore or maintain a cohesive sense of self under the threat of fragmentation. In that conceptual model, disintegration anxiety, involving the concern that the failure of adequate selfobject responses from persons in the environment will lead to fragmentation of the self, becomes the fundamental fear leading to emergency attempts to restore harmony to the self through pathological behaviors.

Despite the central importance of the self in Kohut's theory, Kohut himself never offered a simple definition of the self. He seemed to think that an overarching structure of such fundamental importance defied definition. If one follows the development of his theory from the late 1960s to the time of his death in 1981, however, his view of the self appears to have undergone a transformation from that of a self-representation to a supraordinate center of initiative and experience that was regarded as the main motivating agency in the primary constellation of the psyche. In that regard the self in Kohut's self psychology is both an experiential self and a center of initiative that establishes and repairs self-esteem. Hence, even self psychology cannot escape the dialectic of self as simultaneously subject and object. That theoretical perspective can also be characterized by a marked de-emphasis on the ego and its functions and a corresponding increase in the importance of conscious subjective experience. Also, in the light of the minimization of the role of drives and defenses, aggression is viewed as a secondary reaction to selfobject failures, rather than as an instinctual drive of a primary or innate nature.

Although Kohut was always vague about the developmental timetable appropriate to his theory, certain implications can be drawn. First, Kohut believed that a psychological connection to a mothering figure is present from birth, an idea in stark contrast to Mahler's autistic phase. The infant, in Kohut's view, is born into a self-selfobject bond that is much closer to Mahler's concept of the symbiotic phase. Second, Kohut's emphasis on the lifelong need for appropriate selfobjects suggests that psychological separation is a myth. He regarded Mahler's object relations view, which revolves around the notion that the child moves in the direction of autonomy from supportive caretakers, as containing a moralistic stance. Kohut's notion of lifelong dependence on selfobjects places him in opposition to Mahler's developmental framework. His view was that dependency itself does not diminish; instead, the quality of the selfobjects needed by the self moves from archaic to more mature and appropriate.

INFANT OBSERVATION DATA Recent infant research, particularly that of Daniel Stern, has provided considerable support for the developmental premises of self psychology. Stern's observations convinced him that the infant does not emerge from the womb into a state of autistic self-absorption. From the first days of life, the infant appears to be aware of the mothering figure. Moreover, affirmation and validation from the caretaker is crucial for the development of the infant's sense of self. In that regard Stern stressed that what develops is a sense of self-with-other, and the role of fantasy, as in Klein's theory, is viewed as of only minimal significance. The infant primarily experiences reality, in Stern's view, and relates to the real presence of the mother, whose responses allow the infant to grow. Stern believed that the infant is an adept observer of reality and that it is the older toddler who uses fantasy and distortion to alter what is perceived. He argued that secondary process thought precedes primary process thought and is the bedrock of normal development.

Stern delineated five discrete senses of self. He regarded them as different domains of self-experience, rather than as phases that are subsequently eclipsed by the succeeding phase. Each domain, once formed, remains for the entire life span and operates in concert with the other coexisting senses of self. During the first two months of life, an emergent self appears; it is predominantly a bodily self based on physiological needs. A core sense of self emerges from 2 to 6 months of age; it is associated with greater interpersonal relatedness. Stern viewed the third sense of self, appearing between 7 and 9 months, as a major advance. He called it the sense of subjective self because it involves the matching of intrapsychic states between mother and infant. The fourth sense of self, the verbal or categorical sense of self, emerges between 15 and 18 months of age and coincides with the ability to think symbolically and to communicate verbally. The arrival of a fifth sense of self, a narrative sense of self, appears between 3 and 5 years of age. Stern believed that the fifth sense of self, the historical view of the self, is the one encountered when patients present their life stories in the analytic setting.

Stern identified four essential features of the sense of self: agency, coherence, affectivity, and continuity (or historicity). He also noted that such fundamental issues as attachment, trust, and security transcend phase specificity and are issues for the entire life span. He also questioned the notion of symbiotic merger postulated by Mahler as occurring in the first six months of life. In Stern's view, such wishes for and fears of union are the product of a much more mature mind, one that is capable of thinking abstractly about such concepts as fusion and merger. A central tenet of Stern's work is that the infant develops as a result of sensitive affective attunement by the mothering figure. Kohut and other self psychologists argue that the same kind of empathic resonance is necessary in the analytic situation to repair the patient's self-defects.

PSYCHOANALYTIC PSYCHOPATHOLOGY

In an age in which neuroscience research has made giant strides in the understanding of many Axis I disorders, psychoanalytic theory still has much to contribute to the overall understanding of causes and pathogenesis,. Although biological factors play major roles in such illnesses as schizophrenia and mood disorders, environmental and psychological stressors are influential in triggering the underlying biological diathesis. Moreover, the clinical management of Axis I disorders is greatly enhanced by a psychoanalytically based understanding of the personality factors that contribute to the illness. In the following survey of the psychoanalytic contributions to the understanding of psychiatric disorders, the emphasis is on psychological and environmental factors. However, whenever appropriate, the interaction between those factors and biological determinants of the illness is pointed out.

SCHIZOPHRENIA Freud thought that patients with psychotic disorders are not amenable to psychoanalytic treatment, so he did not accumulate the kind of clinical experience with psychoses that he did with neuroses. Nevertheless, he attempted to place psychotic disorders in a psychodynamic conceptual framework. Freud thought that the sine qua non of schizophrenia is the withdrawal of object cathexis, by which he meant that schizophrenic patients detach themselves from any libidinal or emotional investment in external objects or their intrapsychic representations. He regarded schizophrenia as a regression from object love to an autoerotic stage of development in which one does not have to deal with the frustrations and conflicts encountered in interpersonal relationships.

Freud's decathexis theory underwent revision after the structural model had been developed. In his revised view of schizophrenia, he contrasted neurosis and psychosis on the basis of the nature of the conflict involved. He regarded neurosis as a conflict between the ego and the id, but in psychosis the conflict occurs between the ego and the external world; reality is remodeled to conform to the patient's internal distortions. Even after that substantial revision, Freud continued to write about withdrawal of object cathexis and used that concept to assert that patients suffering from schizophrenia cannot form transference attachments to treaters.

Subsequent psychoanalytic writers have demonstrated that schizophrenic patients do develop transference, although it is qualitatively different from the variety seen in the psychoanalytic treatment of neurotic patients. Harry Stack Sullivan and Frieda Fromm-Reichmann, who spent their professional careers involved in the psychoanalytic treatment of psychotic patients, regarded schizophrenia as arising from early interpersonal difficulties in the child-parent relationship that required understanding and repair in the context of a therapeutic relationship. In their view, faulty mothering led to anxiety and distrust of others, causing persons with schizophrenia to withdraw from interpersonal relatedness.

One controversy in the psychoanalytic literature involves whether or not the conflict theory used to explain neuroses is sufficient to explain schizophrenia as well. Jacob Arlow and Charles Brenner believed that psychosis can be explained by the same compromise-formation model that is applied to neuroses and that the two conditions may differ quantitatively, but qualitatively they are fundamentally alike. Arlow and Brenner conceptualized the quantitative differences as schizophrenia's involving greater disturbances of ego and superego functioning, more severe regression, and more intense conflicts revolving around aggression. They regarded schizophrenic symptoms, such as delusions and hallucinations, as compromise formations developed in response to conflict, much in the same way that neurotic symptoms are developed. Similarly, Arlow and Brenner viewed the withdrawal of object cathexis that Freud emphasized as simply a defensive retreat from conflict.

Biological research on schizophrenia has identified primary difficulties with information processing and attention in schizophrenia; both difficulties are improved by antipsychotic medication. Indeed, most schizophrenic patients experience themselves as being bombarded by a variety of external and internal stimuli. Approaching the illness from a deficit model, James Grotstein suggested that the schizophrenic inability to screen out incoming stimuli is the fundamental problem in the illness of schizophrenia. The defective stimulus barrier makes it extremely difficult for patients with schizophrenia to deal with the chaotic feelings within, so unacceptable impulses and affects are projectively disavowed and placed in the mothering figure. Conflict then arises in the mother-child relationship, and the conflict is reenacted in the transference with a clinician.

MOOD DISORDERS Biological factors play major roles in the causes and pathogenesis of mood disorders. A vast literature on genetic transmission and neurotransmitter changes attests to that fact. Nevertheless, research suggests that intrapsychic and environmental stressors are involved in the onset of major depressive episodes in the majority of cases. It is useful in the light of that perspective to separate cause from pathogenesis. Environmental factors, such as the loss of a loved one, and intrapsychic factors, such as falling short of internal standards, may be crucial causative determinants of a particular depressive episode. The ensuing response to those environmental and intrapsychic triggers, however, occurs at the level of brain chemistry. Hence, the cause may well be intrapsychic, but the pathogenesis is neurochemical.

Depression Freud originally understood depression as internally directed anger. In his view the self-reproaches and the loss of self-esteem commonly experienced by depressed patients are directed not at the self but, rather, at an introject. He noted that in some cases the only way the ego can give up an object is to introject it, so the anger directed at the ambivalently held object takes on the clinical manifestations of depression. After his development of the structural model, he expanded his understanding of depression to include a harsh superego that punishes the person for harboring destructive wishes toward parental figures and other loved ones.

Melanie Klein suggested that depression is linked to a reactivation of the depressive position; depressed patients are convinced that they have destroyed their internal good objects because of their own aggression and greed. As a result, they feel persecuted by internal bad objects while longing for the lost love objects.

Contemporary psychoanalytic contributors have downplayed the role of aggression in the development of depression. They are likely to view depression as a disturbance of self-esteem in the context of interpersonal relationships. A consistent observation is that depressed patients feel that they have not lived up to internal standards of conduct. The depressed patient's awareness of the disparity between their actual performance and those high internalized expectations leads them to feel helpless and powerless. Often, their internal expectations involve eliciting a certain kind of response from important persons in the environment. Depressed persons often live their entire lives for others, rather than for themselves. Depression may begin when they feel hopeless about their life plans because they realize that their efforts have been wasted in living for someone else.

From an object relations perspective, many depressed patients unconsciously experience themselves to be at the mercy of a tormenting internal object that is unrelenting in its persecution of them. In cases of psychosis, that primitive forerunner of the superego may actually be hallucinated as a voice that is unrelentingly critical. From the self-psychological point of view, depression is related to a sense of despair about ever getting one's selfobject needs met by people in the environment.

Mania Follow-up research on patients with bipolar disorders has demonstrated that psychological issues frequently precipitate manic episodes. Psychoanalytic exploration of psychological factors contributing to mania has consistently revealed underlying depressive themes. Manic episodes serve a defensive function so that the patient does not get in touch with the painful affects associated with the undercurrent of depression. A euphoric disposition may serve to deny any aggression or destructiveness toward others. Manic episodes frequently occur in response to significant losses as a way of denying the grief associated with the losses. Melanie Klein noted that manic defenses have several functions: to deny that one is dependent on love objects, to disavow the presence of bad internal objects, and to restore and rescue lost love objects.

ANXIETY DISORDERS AND NEUROSES The evolution of Freud's theory of the neuroses has been extensively covered in preceding parts of this section. Freud's famous psychoneurotic cases are summarized in Table 6.1-4. In brief, his early view included a heavy emphasis on the traumatic consequences of childhood seduction and on the physiological buildup of libido. As Freud shifted to a model based on psychic conflict, he viewed neurotic symptoms as reflecting the breakthrough of infantile sexual impulses in response to failures of repression. With the advent of the structural model, Freud understood neurotic symptoms to be compromise formations between unconscious wishes and defenses against those wishes produced as a result of conflict between intrapsychic agencies. That view was further refined in 1926, when anxiety became understood as a signal of the presence of danger in the unconscious that mobilized ego defense mechanisms to bolster repression. The relabeling of neuroses as anxiety disorders in the last three editions of the American Psychiatric Association's *Diagnostic and Statistical Manual of Mental Disorders* (DSM-III, DSM-III-R, DSM-IV) has led to an unfortunate tendency for clinicians to think about anxiety as an *illness* to be eliminated with pharmacological intervention, rather than as an overdetermined *symptom* of unconscious conflict that requires understanding.

Panic disorder As noted earlier in this section, recent biological research has borne out Freud's early observations that there are two forms of anxiety, one involving a purely psychological cause and the other more clearly related to an underlying neurophysiological substrate. Psychological anxiety is now regarded as a milder form of anticipatory or signal anxiety, and neurophysiological anxiety takes the form of panic disorder. Many patients who experience episodes of panic feel that the attacks come out of the blue and are, therefore, psychologically contentless. Nevertheless, psychodynamic investigations of those attacks find that many of them have psychological meaning. The experience of them as coming out of the blue may only reflect the fact that the psychological triggers are unconscious. A number of studies have demonstrated a close link between separation anxiety and panic disorder. In addition, as many as 43 percent of all panic-disordered patients show improvement after taking a placebo; that finding suggests that the interpersonal involvement with a physician who is concerned about the symptoms may ameliorate certain psychological factors involved in the onset of panic attacks.

One of the clearest examples of psychologically precipitated panic attacks can be found in patients who have not attained object constancy, as described in Mahler's developmental scheme. Patients with borderline personality disorder are often psychologically arrested before that developmental achievement and cannot internalize a soothing image of the therapist at times of distress. That incapacity may precipitate panic attacks that have all the physiological symptoms of the disorder, accompanied by the thought that the therapist has died or abandoned them. At such times a brief telephone conversation with the therapist reassures them that they have not been abandoned and immediately quiets the panic attack. Such clinical instances illustrate how psychodynamic factors may trigger neurotransmitter disturbances and how psychotherapeutic interventions may calm those disturbances.

Phobias The classical psychodynamic understanding of phobias is based on the mobilization of ego defense mechanisms in response to signal anxiety. An unacceptable aggressive or sexual thought begins to enter conscious awareness, and the phobic person worries about the possibility of retaliatory punishment for such thoughts. The result is the activation of signal anxiety, which enlists the ego's help in deploying three defense mechanisms—displacement, projection, and avoidance—that work in concert. The unconscious impulse is displaced and projected outward onto a neutral stimulus, such as a dog or an elevator, which is then avoided.

Obsessive-compulsive disorder Freud regarded obsessive-compulsive neurosis as reflecting a defensive retreat from the presence of oedipal conflicts in response to the threat of castration anxiety. In Freud's model obsessive-compulsive patients regress to the preceding psychosexual stage, the anal stage, because they feel relatively safe from the threats associated with the oedipal constellation. That regression leads to an unraveling of the smooth fusion between the sexual and the aggressive drives, so that obsessive-compulsive neurotic patients suffer from intense ambivalence. The patients often feel paralyzed with doubt and indecision because of the simultaneous presence of hateful and loving feelings. To defend against aggressive and sexual impulses that are experienced as on the verge of being out of control, obsessive-compulsive patients use reaction formation, intellectualization, isolation, and undoing.

Recent research suggests that the psychodynamic explanation is only partially explanatory. Because patients with obsessive-compulsive disorder have smaller caudate nucleus volumes than do healthy controls and have almost no placebo responses in

TABLE 6.1-4
Classical Psychoneurotic Reactions[a]

	Conversion Reaction (Dora)	Phobic Reaction (Hans)	Obsessive-Compulsive Reaction (Rat Man)	Mixed Psychoneurotic Reaction (Wolf Man)
Family history	Striking family history of psychiatric and physical illness	Both parents treated for neurotic conflict but not severe	No family history of mental illness	Striking family history of psychiatric and physical illness
Symptoms	Enuresis and masturbation 6–8 yrs. Onset of neurosis at 8. Migraine, nervous cough, and hoarseness at 12. Aphonia at 16. "Appendicitis" at 16. Convulsions at 16. Facial neuralgia at 19. Change of personality at 8 from "wild creature" to quiet child	Compulsive questions at 3–3½ yrs. in regard to sex difference. Jealous reaction to sibling birth at 3½. Overt castration threat. Overt masturbation at 3½. Overeating and constipation at 4–5. Phobic reaction at 4–5. Attack of flu at 5 worsens phobia. Tonsillectomy at 5 worsens phobia	Naughty period at 3–4 yrs. Marked timidity after a beating by father at 4. Recognizing people by their smells as a child ("Renifleur"). Precocious ego development. Onset of obsessive ideas at 6–7	Tractable and quiet up to 3¼ yrs. "Naughty" period at 3¼–4 yrs. Phobias at 4–5 with nightmares. Obsessional reaction at 6–7 (pious ceremonials). Disappearance of neuroses at 8
Causes	Seduction by older man. Father's illness. Father's affair	Seductive care by mother. Sibling birth at 3½	Seduction by governess at 4. Death of sibling at 4. Beating by father at 4	Seduction by older sister at 3¼. Mother's illness. Conflict between maid and governess

[a]Adapted from S. Freud and from E. J. Anthony in *Comprehensive Textbook of Psychiatry, first edition.* Adapted by Glen O. Gabbard, M.D.

controlled medication trials, biological factors appear to play major roles in causing the disorder. However, even biologically based disorders have psychological meanings, and the elucidation of those meanings may be instrumental in the clinical management of those patients.

Posttraumatic stress disorder Freud originally placed great importance on trauma in the development of neurosis. Contemporary psychodynamic understanding of anxiety states reflects a rediscovery of the pivotal role of actual environmental trauma in many patients suffering from severe anxiety. Posttraumatic stress disorder became a legitimate diagnostic entity in the official nomenclature as a result of the substantial evidence accumulated regarding the severe and disabling effects of trauma on Vietnam War veterans and on victims of incest, sexual abuse, and rape. One contribution of psychoanalytic thinking has been to understand the meaning of the environmental stressor to a particular patient. Different persons respond differently to the same stressor. Seemingly minor stressors can produce major symptoms in one person, but overwhelming trauma may have no effect on another person.

Modern studies on the effects of psychic trauma in childhood have shown that an arrest of affective development occurs in response to such trauma. However, trauma in adulthood tends to produce a regression in affective development. The end result is that trauma victims are unable to use affects as signals. A kind of psychic numbing occurs because any intense emotion is internally regarded as a threat that the original trauma is returning. Consequently, affects are somatized, and many patients who have experienced trauma have psychosomatic illnesses accompanied by an inability to identify emotional states, a condition known as alexithymia. Associated with those developments, patients with posttraumatic stress disorder are often incapable of soothing themselves, so that they are in a permanent state of hyperarousal.

Many patients who experience childhood sexual abuse learn to dissociate under the duress of the trauma. They thus convince themselves that the trauma is happening to someone else who has a different name and a different identity. In that manner multiple personality disorder, which many view as a form of chronic posttraumatic stress disorder, develops.

Generalized anxiety disorder Patients with generalized anxiety disorder may experience mild symptoms of autonomic discharge but nothing comparable to the experience of patients with panic disorder. Anxiety in cases of generalized anxiety disorder is a signal of an unconscious danger or threat to the person. The psychodynamic meaning of the signal can be discerned only by a careful evaluation of the source of the patient's fear. As noted earlier in this section, anxiety stems from various developmental levels, each of which has its own characteristic fear. If anxiety stems from oedipal conflicts, a male patient may fear castration or physical harm in response to forbidden wishes or thoughts. Preoedipal concerns may lead to separation anxiety in which patients fear that an important loved one is about to abandon them. At higher developmental levels patients may suffer from superego anxiety, in which case the concern is that they are not living up to the internalized ideals and standards of their parents.

PARAPHILIAS The classical view of the origin of the paraphilias or perversions is that they serve the function of denying castration. For example, a male exhibitionist may display his genitals in public as a way of reassuring himself that he has not been castrated. Freud noted that perversions are complex and multilayered, observing that passive and active counterparts of perverse activity ordinarily coexist in the same person.For example, sadists have a flip side that is masochistic, and exhibitionists are unconsciously voyeuristic.

From a self-psychological perspective, paraphilias are regarded as desperate responses to the absence of appropriately empathic selfobjects. Perverse sexual activity may restore a sense of cohesiveness to the self in the paraphilic patient. Similarly, sexual acting out during a psychoanalytic process may relate to empathic failures in the analyst.

Contemporary views of the paraphilias have stressed the role of object relatedness in their cause and pathogenesis. Robert Stoller has noted that the essence of perverse sexual activity is the conversion of a passively experienced trauma into an adult act of triumph and mastery. For example, if parents dress a little boy as a girl, he may seek to master his humiliating childhood traumas by becoming a transvestite as an adult. Joyce McDougall has viewed deviant sexual behavior as resulting from unconscious scripts stemming from a complicated set of identifications and counteridentifications with the erotic desires and conflicts of one's parents. She has also noted a fear of self-disintegration involved with much perverse activity, so that certain deviant sexual practices may be experienced as medicating the internal fear of dissolving into nothingness.

ANOREXIA NERVOSA Patients with anorexia nervosa typically lack a sense of autonomy and selfhood. Many patients with the disorder experience their bodies as somehow under the control of their parents.

Self-starvation may be an effort to gain validation as a unique and special person. Only through acts of extraordinary self-discipline can the anorexic patient develop a sense of autonomy and selfhood.

Psychoanalytic clinicians who treat patients with anorexia nervosa generally agree that those young patients have been unable to separate psychologically from their mothers. The body may be perceived as if it were inhabited by an introject of an intrusive and unempathic mother. Starvation may have the unconscious meaning of arresting the growth of that intrusive internal object and thereby destroying it. Often, a projective identification process is involved in the interactions between the patient and the patient's family. Many anorexic patients feel that oral desires are greedy and unacceptable, so that those desires are projectively disavowed. Parents respond to the refusal to eat by becoming frantic about whether the patient is actually eating. The patient can then view the parents as the ones who have unacceptable desires and projectively disavow them. Others are voracious and ruled by desire but not the patient.

BULIMIA NERVOSA Patients suffering from bulimia nervosa lack the superego control and ego strength of their counterparts with anorexia nervosa. The bulimic patients' difficulty in controlling impulses is often manifested by chemical dependency and self-destructive sexual relationships, in addition to the binge eating and purging that are hallmarks of the disorder. Many bulimic patients have histories of difficulty in separating from caretakers manifested by the absence of traditional objects during their early childhood years. Some clinicians have observed that bulimic patients use their own bodies as transitional objects. The struggle for separation from the maternal figure is played out in the ambivalence toward food; eating may represent a wish to fuse with the caretaker, and regurgitating unconsciously expresses a wish for separation.

Psychodynamic treatment of patients with bulimia nervosa has revealed a tendency to concretize introjective and projective defense mechanisms. In a manner analogous to splitting, food is divided into two categories: those items that are nutritious and those that are unhealthy. Food that is designated as good may be ingested and retained within because it unconsciously symbolizes good introjects. But junk food is unconsciously associated with bad introjects and is, therefore, expelled through vomiting, with the unconscious fantasy that all destructiveness, hate, and badness are being evacuated. Patients may temporarily feel good after vomiting because of the fantasized evacuation, but the associated feeling of being all good is short-lived because it is based on an unstable combination of splitting and projection.

PERSONALITY DISORDERS Axis II in DSM-IV consists of personality disorders, an area of psychopathology in which psychoanalytic thinking makes perhaps its most significant contribution to contemporary psychiatry. Personality disorders are long-standing modes of thinking, feeling, and relating to others that are deeply ingrained within the patient. The major features of personality disorders are often *ego-syntonic,* meaning that they are not subjectively experienced by the patient as foreign or distressing in the way neurotic symptoms are. However, personality disorders do create problems for those who must relate to the patient. In many cases those with Axis II disorders do not even seek treatment until the interpersonal and social consequences of their character traits create so much concern that they feel the need to change.

Persons who suffer from personality disorders have generally resolved intrapsychic conflict through the formation of stable defensive patterns that result in severe inhibitions in work and play or that allow for partial gratification of instinctual wishes under certain conditions. The term "character neurosis" is used to describe higher-level personality disorders, such as those of a predominantly obsessive-compulsive or hysterical nature. In those conditions, discrete neurotic symptoms are absent, but certain defensive patterns and cognitive styles pervade the entire personality. Some lower-level personality disorders, such as borderline and antisocial conditions, may involve deficit, as well as certain conflict, and may manifest themselves in certain characteristic ego weaknesses, particularly in the areas of frustration tolerance, drive regulation, object relations, and affective control.

Paranoid personality disorder Persons suffering from paranoid personality disorder have rigid, pervasive cognitive styles involving suspiciousness, hypervigilance, inability to trust or confide in others, pathological jealousy, and a proneness to be easily slighted. Their intrapsychic world is organized along the lines of the paranoid-schizoid position described by Melanie Klein. Splitting, projection, and projective identification are the typical defense mechanisms by which those patients separate out all badness, hatred, and aggression within themselves and deposit it projectively into others. As a result, those patients maintain a stable equilibrium but live with persecutory anxiety connected to the constant threat of attack or mistreatment by others. Moreover, because of their defensive style, the patients must be hypervigilant at all times and attempt to control others, so that the perceived threat is kept at bay. Low self-esteem and feelings of inferiority and weakness are at the core of paranoia, and the grandiosity often seen in the patients is a compensatory defense to deal with the pain caused by those unacceptable feelings.

Schizoid and schizotypal personality disorders Persons with schizoid and schizotypal personality disorders are often considered misfits who seem to avoid other people. Outwardly, they may appear to prefer isolation to relatedness and show little conflict over their solitary existence. However, psychodynamic treatment of them has demonstrated that their apparent lack of concern for their mode of adjustment may mask considerable confusion and deepening longings for relatedness. From a psychoanalytic perspective, the term "schizoid" refers to a splitting or fragmentation of the self into a myriad of self-representations that produce a sense of identity diffusion. The patients' absence of conviction about who they are and what they want may cause schizoid persons to feel paralyzed and to withdraw from attempting interpersonal relatedness. Many have also experienced thoroughgoing frustration as children regarding their ability to get their emotional needs met by others, so they attempt to be self-sufficient to avoid the pain of repeated rejections and of disappointments in others. They may feel that their neediness is so voracious that it would destroy others or drain them of all they have to give. Alternatively, they may fear that they will be consumed or smothered by those from whom they seek emotional sustenance. Hence, many feel caught in a schizoid compromise in which they adjust to a solitary existence as a way of dealing with the twin fears of driving others away by their neediness and of being consumed by the demands of others.

Borderline personality disorder Although the borderline concept has been around for many years, the work of Otto Kernberg from his ego psychological-object relations perspective in the 1960s provided the first comprehensive psychodynamic understanding of the condition. He used the term "borderline personality organization" to describe a cluster of characteristics typical of a group of patients who appear to have a mixture of both neurotic and psychotic symptoms. Kernberg's structural analysis of that level of ego organization include the following four elements:

1. Nonspecific manifestations of ego weakness, including poor anxiety tolerance, poor impulse control, and poorly developed subliminatory channels
2. A shift toward primary process thinking, particularly under the pressure of strong affects or in unstructured situations, such as projective psychological testing
3. A pattern of specific defensive operations, including splitting, projective identification, primitive idealization, denial, omnipotence, and devaluation
4. Pathological internalized object relations based on split-

ting, so that representations of self and others are alternatingly all good or all bad.

Although Kernberg's psychodynamic conceptualization applies to most patients with borderline personality disorder, it was developed as a level of *ego organization* that also encompasses other personality disorders. Kernberg subsumed narcissistic, schizoid, antisocial, paranoid, and lower-level histrionic (infantile) personality disorders under the umbrella of borderline personality organization.

Kernberg also linked the cause and the pathogenesis of borderline personality disorder to a specific developmental arrest during the rapprochement subphase delineated by Mahler and her colleagues. Because those patients can distinguish self from object, Kernberg thought that they had fully traversed the symbiotic phase but had not been able to successfully negotiate separation-individuation. In Kernberg's view, something goes wrong during the rapprochement subphase of development, so that borderline patients never get over the fear that maternal figures will abandon them. He postulated that either a disturbance in the mother's emotional availability or an inborn excess of aggression in the child (or perhaps a combination of both) results in the developmental arrest. As a consequence, the children grow up with chronic anxiety about being abandoned by significant people in their lives. Similarly, they are never able to integrate positive and negative aspects of self-representations and object representations and to internalize well-rounded and complex internal images of the mother to provide object constancy.

Gerald Adler, by contrast, has approached borderline personality disorder from a deficit or insufficiency model that is influenced by self-psychological theories. He understood the borderline patient to be one who grew up in an environment where selfobject needs were not satisfied. Hence, the patients continue to search for selfobjects as adults because they have not developed a holding-soothing introject. Whereas Kernberg viewed the borderline patient as suffering from a predominance of hostile introjects, Adler regarded those same patients as suffering from an absence of introjects, so that they are prone to fragmentations of the self when others do not provide selfobject functions for them. Adler referred to that fear of self-disintegration as *annihilation panic.*

Narcissistic personality disorder The two major psychodynamic theories of narcissistic personality disorder are those of Kohut and Kernberg. Kohut's theory of the cause and pathogenesis was discussed under the heading of "Self Psychology." In brief, Kohut's view is that narcissistic patients are developmentally arrested because of parental failures of empathy in response to the child's phase-appropriate needs for idealization, mirroring, and twinship experiences. Those children then grow up treating others as though they exist only to gratify their narcissistic needs. Persons who are expected to fill selfobject functions for narcissistic persons are usually alienated by the self-centered nature of the relationship and reject the narcissistically disordered person. Hence, a patient with narcissistic personality disorder goes through life suffering repeated fragmentations of the self in response to the failure of others to fulfill those selfobject needs.

Kernberg offered a different psychodynamic formulation of narcissistic personality disorder. He saw a person with the disorder as essentially similar to a person with borderline personality disorder in that they both operate from the same level of personality organization. The corresponding defensive operations and pathological internal object relations are also present. Kernberg differentiated a narcissistic patient from a borderline patient on the basis of the presence in the narcissistic patient of an integrated but pathologically grandiose self. He conceptualized the grandiose self as being a defensive structure in narcissistic personality disorder that denies dependency on others. Kernberg saw the grandiose self as a fusion of the real self, the ideal object, and the ideal self. In other words, a narcissistic patient maintains an illusion of self-sufficiency through the grandiose self-image.

Kernberg further differentiated narcissistic personality disorder from borderline personality disorder by the presence of higher-level ego functioning in the narcissistic personality disorder. Narcissistic patients, then, look much the same from day to day because their self-representation is more continuous than the alternating self-representations of the patient with borderline personality disorder.

Kohut discussed the libidinal and selfojbect needs of narcissistic patients, but Kernberg stressed the underlying envy and aggression in patients with narcissistic personality disorder. Because of excessive aggression from either constitutional or environmental sources, narcissistic patients are seen as suffering from chronic intense envy that leads them to destroy and spoil the positive aspects of others whom they envy. Kohut thought that envy does not play a central role in causing narcissistic personality disorder and that aggression is secondary to narcissistic injury, rather than primary, as Kernberg argued. Although Kohut postulated that idealization, commonly seen in narcissistic patients, is a normal developmental need, Kernberg conceptualized idealization as defensive against underlying contempt, rage, and envy.

Antisocial personality disorder Of all the Axis II conditions, antisocial personality disorder is the one most clearly linked to biological underpinnings. Twin studies suggest that genetic factors are influential, neuropsychological testing demonstrates the presence of organically based cognitive impairment, and measures of autonomic indicators suggest that antisocial patients are autonomically hyporeactive. The normal attachment process of the infant to the mother may be compromised by those innate constitutional factors. In addition, patients with antisocial personality disorder frequently report a history of abuse or neglect by parental figures. Some authors believe that antisocial personality disorder is psychodynamically related to narcissistic personality disorder. Therefore, a pathological grandiose self is often a key feature of persons with antisocial tendencies. However, such patients differ from narcissistic patients in the nature of the parental introject. Typically, antisocial persons have internalized a cruel, malevolent parental figure, instead of the ideal object that is internalized by those with narcissistic personality disorder.

Because persons with antisocial personality disorder do not experience a loving maternal figure in the early months of life, they never develop basic trust in others. Moreover, the antisocial person never really becomes sensitive to other people as separate persons with needs and feelings of their own. Those major impairments in the internalization process result in a person with no moral conscience. The only trace of superego development may be the presence of sadistic superego precursors. The only value system, if one can call it that, in patients with antisocial personality disorder is the exercise of power and destructiveness over others. Every relationship is approached as an opportunity for exploitation and cruelty. The absence of superego development in those patients makes them extraordinarily difficult or impossible to treat.

Histrionic personality disorder Histrionic personality disorder is best conceptualized as a continuum between a lower-level orally fixated histrionic patient on one end and a higher-level hysterical patient with a phallic fixation on the other end. In the case of a female patient at the lower end of the continuum, she typically turns to her father for maternal nurturance that she feels she did not receive from her mother. She learns that dramatic affective displays are required to capture the attention of her father and other men. Genital sexual relations may be characterized by primitive oral neediness. She then discovers that sexual behavior is rarely satisfying because she is searching for a maternal breast and is receiving a penis instead, an unconscious fantasy known as the *breast-penis equation.*

At the higher end of the continuum, a hysterical female patient has typically been more successful in receiving maternal nurturance than was the female patient at the lower end. However, the hysterical woman is unable to relinquish her libidinal attachment to her father and grows up with an incompletely resolved oedipal situation. She idealizes her father as a man who has no equal. She finds herself in triangular relationships throughout her life, in rivalrous situations with other women for the affections of a man who may be forbidden or unattainable. The hysterical woman frequently chooses romantic partners who are already married or otherwise inappropriate as a way of assuring herself that she will not have to give up her attachment to her father. Because repression is a primary defense used by a patient with hysterical personality disorder, the attachment is often entirely unconscious, and only through psychoanalysis or psychotherapy does she become aware of her tendency to repeat the oedipal drama throughout her adult life.

Although hysterical personality disorder is commonly associated with women, male patients may also meet the diagnostic criteria. The dynamics of such cases is remarkably similar to those found in female patients. The histrionic male patient turns to his father for maternal nurturance. In the absence of an emotionally available father, the boy child may either show a hypermasculine flight from concerns about feminine identification with the mother or show a passive effeminate identity in direct identification with his mother. At the higher end of the continuum, the male patient with hysterical personality disorder remains attached to his mother in an incompletely resolved oedipal situation, much like his female counterpart. He may find that the women he meets are disappointing because they never measure up to his mother, or he may choose a celibate or isolated life-style to maintain his unconscious attachment to his mother.

Obsessive-compulsive personality disorder The early papers on the obsessive-compulsive character emphasize regression to an anal fixation in response to castration anxiety encountered in the oedipal phase. The anal traits associated with the character pattern include parsimony, excessive orderliness, and stubbornness. Much like patients with symptomatic obsessive-compulsive neurosis, anal characters were viewed as victims of a harsh superego that is prone to be punitive in response to sexual and aggressive wishes.

As psychoanalytic theory has shifted more and more in the direction of the vicissitudes of object relations, the literature on obsessive-compulsive personality disorder has focused less on anal character traits and more on difficulties in self-esteem, management of dependency and anger, cognitive style, and problems with intimacy. Self-doubt is a common trait of obsessive-compulsive patients, and psychoanalytic treatment frequently reveals the entrenched conviction that they were not loved or valued by their parents. Intense anger directed at the parents and dependent longings are frequently defended against through reaction formation and isolation of affect.

Obsessive-compulsive patients also reveal perfectionistic strivings that are designed to transcend such unacceptable feelings as rage and dependency. They often feel that, if they could just do enough, they will finally win the parental approval that they missed in childhood. Intimacy presents a risk to obsessive-compulsive patients because they fear that their dependent yearnings and angry resentment will be triggered and then get out of control. Most patients with obsessive-compulsive personality disorder prefer work to the unpredictable intimacy of personal relationships. Spouses and significant others often complain that their obsessive-compulsive loved ones are too controlling and lack spontaneity in marriage and other close relationships.

Avoidant personality disorder Although it has been controversial because of its overlap with other personality disorders, avoidant personality disorder can be linked to the psychoanalytic tradition of identifying character neuroses that evolved from studying symptomatic neuroses. Just as obsessive-compulsive personality disorder is regarded as a characterological form of obsessive-compulsive neurosis, avoidant personality disorder can be viewed as a characterological version of phobic neurosis. Persons with avoidant personality disorder are extremely shy and fear social situations in which they may experience humiliation or embarrassment. Although social phobias involve specific situations, the threat in avoidant personality disorder is far more generalized.

The defensive posture of shyness or avoidance typically protects against anticipated rejection, failure, humiliation, and embarrassment. Shame is often a key affective experience for patients with avoidant personality disorder. Psychodynamic exploration reveals that close relationships and social situations are avoided because of the fear that personal inadequacies will be obvious to everyone. Avoidant patients feel that they can never measure up to their own internal standard of performance. Hence, they experience a form of stage fright in interpersonal situations. Some research suggests a genetic-constitutional basis for shyness, but environmental experiences of ridicule or rejection seem to be necessary to produce the full characterological manifestations of avoidant personality disorder.

Dependent personality disorder Persons with dependent personality disorder often reveal family backgrounds characterized by overinvolved parents. Messages are given to the children that autonomy within the family is potentially dangerous. Loyalty to and dependency on the family are rewarded. Classical psychoanalytic explanations involving oral-stage fixation are no longer viewed as pertinent to the pathogenesis of dependent personality disorder because the stage specificity of that hypothesis is a dubious proposition. Persons who are extremely dependent have generally experienced parental messages about the dangers of separation throughout the entirety of childhood, a pervasive pattern that is not linked to one particular stage of development. Psychodynamic exploration of patients with dependent personality disorder has also shown that dependency may mask considerable hostility and aggression.

PSYCHOANALYTIC TREATMENT

INDICATIONS AND ANALYZABILITY The determination of which patients are suitable for psychoanalysis has undergone an evolution that parallels the historical changes in theory and technique. The original indications for psychoanalytic treatment were relatively straightforward—only those patients suffering from symptomatic neuroses of a hysterical, obsessive-compulsive, or phobic nature were suitable for psychoanalytic treatment. Freud also believed that, as patients age, their lack of psychological malleability makes them less amenable to psychoanalysis. Hence, only young patients, generally those in their 20s and 30s, were viewed as ideal candidates for analysis.

Those rather narrow indications are now considered limiting, if not archaic. Few patients present to clinicians with complaints of discrete neurotic symptoms, as they did in Freud's day. Manifestations of pervasive character pathology, such as difficulties in a patient's ability to love and to work, are likely to be the presenting complaints today. The changes in the conditions that patients bring to psychoanalysis have been mirrored in the advances in technique that are based on developments in self psychology and object relations theory. It is now common to refer to the *widening scope* of psychoanalytic treatment in the context of the expanded indications for such treatment.

Moreover, the age restrictions advocated by Freud have largely been discounted, as an increasing amount of research and clinical data attest to the malleability of middle-aged and elderly patients. Adult developmental studies indicate that significant changes in defenses, internal object relations, and self-representations occur throughout the adult life cycle. It is now common for analysts to treat patients in their 50s, 60s, and even 70s.

Conditions considered amenable to analysis today include, in addition to the symptomatic neuroses, certain anxiety disorders, higher-level personality disorders (such as the obsessive-compulsive and hysterical character neuroses), most patients with narcissistic personality disorder, and patients at the upper end of the spectrum of borderline personality disorder who have the necessary ego strength and motivation to tolerate the procedure.

The preceding list of indications for psychoanalysis is incomplete, however, without also taking into consideration generalized criteria for analyzability that apply regardless of the diagnosis. Significant suffering must be present, so that the patient is motivated to make the sacrifices of time and financial resources that are required for psychoanalysis. Also, patients who enter analysis must have a genuine wish to understand themselves, rather than a desperate hunger for symptomatic relief. They must be able to withstand the frustration, anxiety, and other strong affects that emerge in analysis without fleeing or acting out their feelings in a self-destructive manner. Other ego functions that must be intact, in addition to the ability to delay impulses and control affects, are reality testing and self-object differentiation. Without reasonably good ego functioning in those areas, a stable, workable transference will not be established.

The presence of reasonably mature superego development is also necessary for a patient to be analyzable. Patients who are pathological liars, who are morally corrupt, or who commit criminal acts are rarely suitable for psychoanalytic treatment. At least average, if not superior, intelligence is required for analytic work, as is a well-developed capacity to verbalize internal experiences. The patient must have some capacity to regress in the service of the ego but also an ability to reinstitute defenses by the end of the session.

One other important criterion of analyzability is a form of thinking that is usually referred to as *psychological mindedness*. Patients who possess the trait have the ability to think abstractly and symbolically about the unconscious meanings of their behavior. They have a tendency to look inward for explanations about things that happen to them, rather than to externalize responsiblity for events in their lives. They also possess the ability to think in terms of analogy—that is, something that happens in outside relationships is analogous to similar developments in the transference relationship to the analyst.

The psychoanalyst must also take into account certain external life situations in determining a patient's suitability for analysis. It is generally better not to begin analysis in the midst of a major upheaval or life crisis, such as a job loss or a divorce. Sufficient stability in one's work situation is necessary to assure that a patient will be in the same geographical location for a period of several years. Serious physical illness may interfere with the patient's ability to invest in a long-term treatment process. The patient must have enough financial resources so that analytic treatment does not present an unbearable economic hardship. The final decision must take into account those external life factors, in addition to a careful psychodynamic evaluation of the patient's ability to use psychoanalysis productively, based on the previously noted criteria.

A 1994 survey of 580 analytic patients suggested that psychoanalysis is often used when previous treatments have not been entirely successful. That survey found that 82 percent of the patients currently in psychoanalysis had undergone other forms of psychotherapy in the past. The mean age at the beginning of the analysis in the sample was 36.2 years, and 59 percent of the patients were female. Of the 580 patients, 71.4 percent had at least one personality disorder diagnosis. Of the Axis I diagnoses, a mood disorder was the most common, and anxiety disorder was the second most common diagnosis. A significant number of the patients, 27 percent of the total, had been sexually abused or assaulted. High levels of sexual dysfunction, 43.4 percent of the total, were also found in the group.

ANALYTIC PROCESS In formal psychoanalysis the process is conducted four or five times a week in sessions that last either 45 or 50 minutes. The patient usually reclines on a couch while the analyst sits behind the couch out of the patient's view. The patient is invited to say whatever comes to mind without censoring it or passing judgment on it. That technique, known as *free association,* promotes a useful regression in the patient that encourages attunement to internal processes and the establishment of a transference attachment to the analyst. In addition to the process of free association, the patient is expected to mobilize basic ego resources to make connections between the associations that emerge and to gain mastery through insight. In that regard, the patient works in a collaborative process with the analyst, rather than taking a passive position in which the analyst does all the work.

When Freud shifted from the use of hypnosis and suggestion to the technique of free association, his goal was to bring repressed material into conscious awareness, so that the patient gains insight through an understanding of how dynamically repressed childhood events contributed to the symptoms experienced as an adult. Freud noted that the regression produced by the analytic setting allows for the reemergence of infantile conflicts in the form of a *transference neurosis,* in which all the feelings and fantasies involved in the oedipal constellation of childhood are reactivated in the relationship with the analyst.

Psychoanalysis as a therapeutic procedure, then, was originally based on the notion of uncovering and reconstructing the analysand's past through the re-creation of that past in the transference neurosis with the analyst. However, the understanding of the analytic process has undergone considerable expansion as a result of increasing interest in the analyst's role in the analytic relationship. The reexperience or reenactment of the past is now viewed as influenced by the current analyst-patient relationship and the contributions of the analyst to that relationship. Hence, the meaning of analytic data in a particular hour is gleaned not exclusively from the historical past of the patient but also from the interplay between patient and analyst in the present. The past is influenced by the present, just as the present is influenced by the past in the analytic setting.

Phases of the analytic process The analytic process has traditionally been divided into three phases, although the gradations are acknowledged to be somewhat arbitrary and, to some extent, overlapping. The first or opening phase involves the patient's establishment of a therapeutic alliance with the analyst. That alliance involves the development of trust and a willingness to work collaboratively with the analyst in the pursuit of understanding. The second or middle phase is characterized by the appearance of a transference neurosis, which is then systematically analyzed and worked through in the analyst-patient relationship. The issues that arise in the middle phase generally stem from the oedipal conflicts but also include preoedipal and postoedipal issues to varying degrees. The third or termination phase of analysis requires the patient to mourn and give up infantile attachments to parental figures at the same time that the loss of the analyst as a real person is being mourned. Autonomy, independence, and the development of the capacity for continuing self-analysis are also prominent issues during the termination phase. Analysts do not typically view an analysis as finished or complete nowadays. All analyses end with a certain degree of unfinished business that the analysand continues to analyze by identifying with the analyst's role and by continuing the process of self-analysis.

PRINCIPLES OF TECHNIQUE Freud established the basis of psychoanalytic technique when he designated the *fundamental rule:* the patient must agree to be completely honest with the analyst. That rule is applied in clinical practice through the technique of free association. The free-associative process induces the necessary regression and passive dependence required to establish and work through the transference neurosis, and it provides content for the analytic work itself. Although free association is the cornerstone of psychoanalytic technique, several guiding principles anchor the analyst's conceptualization of what is happening in the process, what needs to be said, and what should be left unsaid until further work is accomplished.

Resistance One of Freud's greatest insights into the human psyche was that most people, no matter how extensive their suffering, do not wish to change. Powerful internal forces oppose the analyst's efforts to produce insight and to promote new modes of adaptation. Indeed, those internal forces, which Freud termed *resistance,* were crucial in the evolution of psychoanalytic technique. Hypnosis and abreaction did not produce lasting change, Freud learned, because forces of resistance tenaciously cling to the neurotic compromise formation. In one of his 1912 papers on technique, Freud observed that "the resistance accompanies the treatment step by step. Every single association, every act of the person under treatment must reckon with the resistance and represents a compromise between the forces that are striving toward recovery and the opposing ones."

Resistance is ubiquitous in psychoanalysis. It may be viewed as the analyst's daily bread-and-butter work. It pervades every aspect of the patient's behavior and associations and may take a variety of forms, including falling asleep during sessions; forgetting the analyst's insights; withholding important thoughts and feelings from the analyst; demanding symptom relief, instead of understanding, from the analyst; falling silent during the sessions; failing to pay the bill; and even free-associating in such a literal manner that none of the material is connected or used constructively to produce understanding.

Although resistances may be either conscious or unconscious, resistance to the analytic process automatically arises as soon as one is invited to free-associate. The exercise of a patient's willpower is often insufficient to overcome those powerful forces. Neither should the analyst approach resistances with the intent of overcoming them. Analysts approach resistances with the idea that they must be analyzed. Through the patient's associations to them and the analyst's observations of the setting in which they occur, resistances are investigated with the idea of learning more about their structures, their sources, and the specific affects with which they are associated. Moreover, the form that a patient's resistances take provides a gold mine of information about that particular patient's characteristic defense operations. Resistance may be conceptualized as the manifestation of the patient's typical defense mechanisms in the analytic setting. Another way of making the distinction is to say that defenses, which operate intrapsychically, are translated into resistances, which appear interpersonally, when the patient enters an analytic relationship with the analyst.

Resistances take many forms. One particular subgroup of special importance is *transference resistance.* That resistance involves fantasies, thoughts, feelings, and wishes that directly involve the analyst. Loving or sexual wishes directed toward the analyst, for example, may serve the function of avoiding the analytic task of developing insight. Transference resistance may also take the form of defending against the awareness of feelings toward the analyst. Also, one set of transference feelings or wishes may defend against awareness of another, more disturbing set. Transference itself may be regarded as a resistance when it interrupts the process of the analysis, and the systematic analytic working through of intense feelings constitutes a good deal of psychoanalytic treatment.

Resistance tends to change in character during the course of an analysis. In the opening phase, resistance may take the form of avoiding a meaningful attachment or relationship with the analyst. In the middle phase, it may involve intense and irrational feelings toward the analyst. In the termination phase, resistance may manifest itself as a return of symptoms that were present at the beginning of the analysis or a reluctance to give up the passive and dependent regressed relationship with the analyst.

Analyses that are conducted from a self-psychological perspective approach resistance in a manner radically different from the classical ego-psychological model described here. As a consequence of the deemphasis on the ego and its defense mechanisms in self psychology, the role of those defenses as they emerge in the analysis is also minimized. The view of the analytic process is not one of an inexorable unraveling of defenses. Rather, the analyst attempts to emphathize with the core subjective experience of the patient in the interest of reactivating growth in the domain of the self. From that standpoint, both defenses and resistances are reviewed as healthy intrapsychic activities that safeguard and preserve the integrity of the self. Kohut preferred to speak of the defensiveness of patients, rather than their resistances, and he stressed that defensive attitudes are both psychologically valuable and adaptive.

Object relations theory provides yet another perspective on resistance. Particular self-object-affect units within the patient gain prominence for compelling intrapsychic reasons, and the patient only reluctantly gives up those object relations paradigms in the interest of developing new forms of object relatedness. The patient's internal object relations are repeated in the analytic setting with the hope that they will be altered in some manner in the context of a new relationship. At the same time, however, relinquishing internal objects and their corresponding self-representations involves feelings of loss and grief. Those feelings are often defended against through a strong propensity in the patient to cling tenaciously to familiar self-object-affect units.

Transference *Transference* is the term that refers to the displacement onto the analyst of attitudes and feelings originally experienced in relationships with people from the past. Transference patterns appear automatically and unconsciously in the analytic relationship. Analysands suddenly find that they are reacting to the analyst with intense feelings that are inappropriate, at least in part, to the current situation. Patients unconsciously reenact a past relationship, instead of remembering and verbalizing it. Transference is not unique to the analytic setting. Every significant relationship in adult life is a new edition of the original attachments of childhood. The chief difference between transference in the analytic setting and transference in extra-analytic relationships is that transference is analyzed in the analytic setting.

Freud encouraged analysts to be opaque to their patients, much like a tabula rasa on which the patients can impose their stored object representations of past relationships. In that classical model of transference, an infantile relationship from the past is brought into the present without contamination or contribution from the analyst. In the contemporary view, transference is regarded as a mixture of the new relationship with the analyst and a reenactment of a past relationship with a significant childhood figure. Also, in the contemporary perspective the analyst is regarded as an active participant in the therapeutic relationship. In the current conceptual framework, the analyst's personal characteristics exert a powerful influence on the specific shape and intensity of the patient's transference. The notion of opacity is considered a myth, and the analyst's real characteristics must be taken into account when the analyst formulates therapeutic interventions.

In the classical view the transference neurosis is the distinct and pivotal entity that develops in the middle phase of the analysis as a consequence of the replication of the childhood neurosis. The patient's attachment to the analyst is so intense that emotional satisfaction from the analyst becomes more important than the original therapeutic goals. From the contemporary perspective of transference, object relations ideas are regarded as more significant than drive-derived aims aroused by the analytic regression. The term "transference neurosis" is seen as lacking specific meaning or utility in the analytic setting; the term is replaced by references to all transference responses as shifting self-representations and object representations that are influenced by the analyst-analysand relationship.

Therapeutic alliance The controversial term *therapeutic alliance,* used interchangeably with *working alliance,* refers to the conscious aspect of the relationship between the analyst and the patient involving the collaborative pursuit of common therapeutic goals. In the therapeutic alliance the patient identifies with the general aims and strategies of psychoanalytic treatment and cooperates with the analyst in the search for understanding and insight. To form such an alliance, the patient must have the ability to split the ego into a functioning component that is involved in free-associating and an observing component that is identified with the analyst's task of analyzing.

Freud originally delineated three types of transference: an excessively positive or erotic transference, a negative transference, and an unobjectionable positive transference. He described the third type of transference as an aspect of a healthy and mature doctor-patient relationship and the vehicle of success in psychoanalytic treatment. In other words, the unobjectionable positive transference differs from the other two forms of transference in that it facilitates the analytic process, but the other two serve as resistances to the process. Freud's conceptualization was a forerunner of the idea of therapeutic alliance, although he conceptualized unobjectinable positive transference as an aspect of transference, rather than as an entity distinct from transference.

The term "unobjectionable positive transference" is controversial today because of the implication that the patient reacts to a real relationship in a conscious and rational way, free from transference contaminations. Some analysts argue that the repetition in analysis of childhood attitudes—such as cooperativeness, reliance, and trust—may have considerable positive value but are, nevertheless, transference repetitions and should be regarded as such. The analyst runs the risk of failing to analyze the childhood origins of collaboration with the analyst if the collaboration is regarded as a therapeutic alliance that occurs outside the transference.

Countertransference Freud originally used the term *countertransference* to refer to unconscious conflicts from the analyst's past that were displaced onto the patient. In other words, he regarded the countertransference as the analyst's transference to the patient. Freud viewed it as an interference with the analyst's optimal functioning, and he issued an injunction that the analyst "shall recognize this counter-transference in himself and overcome it." That conceptualization of countertransference is now known as the *narrow* or classical view.

The term "countertransference" has undergone considerable revision in the past few decades; a *broad* or modernist view is now in wide use among analysts to connote the analyst's total emotional reaction to the patient. That shift was fueled by Klein, Winnicott, and Kernberg—all of whom viewed countertransference reactions, particularly in work with seriously disturbed patients, as stemming more from the patient than from the analyst. In other words, through projective identification the analyst begins to feel powerful affects that are associated with the patient's internal self-representations and object representations. Winnicott referred to one variant of such phenomena as *objective hate* to reflect the fact that certain patients cause everyone to hate them; therefore, the analyst's feelings do not reflect specific unconscious conflicts from the analyst's past.

Another implication of the broadened conceptualization of countertransference introduced by the object relations theorists is that the analyst's feelings provide important information about the analysand's internal world. Moreover, by reacting to the patient in a role-responsive manner, the analyst gains greater understanding about the typical problems that occur in the patient's other relationships. Hence, countertransference is regarded not as an obstacle to the analyst's functioning but as an indispensable aid to the analyst's ability to understand and to intervene effectively with the patient.

The most widely held view of countertransference today is that it is a joint creation involving contributions both from the analyst's past and from the patient's internal world. One of the analyst's principal tasks is to engage in a continuing process of self-scrutiny in which the two components are distinguished and understood.

Interpretation *Interpretation* is the analyst's ultimate therapeutic instrument in psychoanalysis. It involves an explanatory statement by the analyst that links a symptom, thought, feeling, or behavior to its unconscious meaning. It is the vehicle by which the analyst delivers understanding to the patient. In the ideal situation, interpretation is designed to make the patient consciously aware of unconscious material that is close to the surface of consciousness.

Genetic interpretations are statements that connect thoughts, conflicts, and feelings in the present with their childhood antecedents. The analyst reconstructs the patient's past on the basis of memories, dreams, free associations, and transference distortions to shed light on how the present situation is a repetition of the past.

Transference interpretations are often viewed as the analyst's central mutative activity. Such interventions explain to the patient how the distortions in the analytic relationship are reenactments of past significant relationships. The historical conceptualization of transference interpretation generally involves genetic reconstructions. But the contemporary view de-emphasizes reconstruction and helps the patient see how current wishes and expectations in the analytic setting are influenced by the past. Moreover, the analyst interprets with the patient as a collaborator in understanding the current interpersonal situation with the analyst in the context of past relationships.

Transference interpretation has two broad categories. The first involves explanations of resistance to the resolution of the transference. The explanations may involve genetic elements or may focus on the here-and-now situation. An example of a genetic interpretation is: "You do not want to give up your erotic attachment to me because you hope that it will lead to getting a response from me that you never received from your father." An example of a here-and-now interpretation is: "You do not want to give up your erotic attachment to me because you have the fantasy that you can control me with your sexual demands." The second category of transference interpretation involves explications of resistance to the awareness of transference. An example is: "I wonder if your sudden need to launch into an extramarital affair is related to the development of sexual feelings for me that you cannot yet acknowledge."

A single interpretation does not resolve either transference or resistance in one fell swoop. The analyst's initiation of an interpretive strategy marks the beginning of a prolonged process that Freud referred to as *working through.* Freud commented that "one must allow the patient time to become more conversant with his resistance with which he has now become acquainted, to work through it, to overcome it, by continuing, in defiance of it, the analytic work according to the fundamental rule of analysis." Similar transference and resistance themes are encountered in a variety of different situations, and the repetitive interpretation process each time those familiar patterns emerge eventually leads to mastery and insight.

From an ego-psychological perspective, working through is necessary because of the tenacity of ego defenses. For the patient to relinquish those defenses and allow the warded-off drive components to enter conscious awareness, a single demonstration of the impulse-defense configuration is not sufficient. Repeated confrontations of the defensive strategies are necessary in a variety of situations to accomplish a major shift in the intrapsychic relationships of ego, superego, and id.

Object relations theorists and self psychologists view the working-through process somewhat differently. Proponents of the British school, such as Fairbairn and Winnicott, stress that the analytic setting provides a new object for the patient. Working through involves attaching to the new object, internalizing the new object relationship, and relinquishing the old internal object relations units as the new relationship takes center stage in the patient's psyche. Self psychologists do not conceptualize the working-through process as involving resolution of intrapsychic conflict. Instead, they regard it as the resumption of previously arrested developmental processes. The patient's relationship with the analyst in the present reactivates that frozen development so that selfobject transferences can evolve. Through the repetitive examination of self-selfobject disruptions in the transference, the patient gradually internalizes the empathic interactions with the analyst to repair defects in the self.

Neutrality Freud used the term "neutrality" in different ways throughout his writings. The most widely accepted contemporary meaning is a nonjudgmental stance regarding the patient's feelings, wishes, and behaviors. That idea is in keeping with Anna Freud's understanding of neutrality, which was based on the structural model—that is, the analyst remains equidistant from the id, the ego, the superego, and the demands of external reality. By maintaining a neutral position, the analyst eventually helps patients become aware that their own critical attitudes are being attributed to the analyst.

Neutrality is occasionally misunderstood to suggest that analysts should remain cold and aloof. Concern, empathy, and emotional warmth are all part of effective analytic work, and a cold, rejecting attitude in the analyst may become an aspect of the real relationship in the present that is incorporated into the patient's transference experiences. The influence of object relations theory on psychoanalytic technique has redefined the analyst's role as one involving participation in the process. When analysts allow themselves to respond in a disciplined yet spontaneous manner to the patient's projections, they find that their role-responsive reactions to the patient's projective identification process provide useful information and an empathic sense of the patient's internal world.

GOALS AND THERAPEUTIC ACTION It is customary in most of medicine to speak of cure as a treatment goal, but one must be considerably more cautious in discussing the outcome of psychoanalysis. A key aspect of the analyst's neutral position is to avoid therapeutic zeal. The analyst's task is to analyze, interpret, and provide understanding. The patient's task is to decide how much and in what direction to change. When analysts start to have a specific therapeutic agenda for their patients, they are at risk of creating a situation in which the patient changes to please the analyst, a re-creation of a common parent-child situation. Hence, the goals of analysis emanate as much from the patient as from the analyst.

The goals of psychoanalysis are intimately linked to conceptualizations of the therapeutic action of psychoanalytic treatment and are, therefore, a source of controversy in the field. When Freud first began treating hysterical patients in the 1890s, the therapeutic action of psychoanalysis was simple and straightforward: through abreaction the analysis helps the patient work through the release of dammed-up affects. Previously repressed fantasies, memories, and feelings are brought into conscious awareness. After Freud developed the structural model, abreaction became of less significance, and he regarded the therapeutic action of psychoanalysis as involving a redistribution of the interrelationships among the three intrapsychic agencies. In Freud's words, "Where id was, there ego shall be."

Freud always thought that transference work is crucial to effecting change in the patient. However, James Strachey in 1934 most clearly articulated an understanding of how transference interpretation produces change in psychoanalysis. Strachey believed that a harsh superego is at the core of most neuroses and that modification of the superego through interpretation is the essential therapeutic action of psychoanalysis. Strachey identified a vicious cycle that takes place in analysis in which the patient's id impulses and harsh superego are transferred to the analyst. The analyst is then experienced as a dangerous and frightening object. Seeing the analyst as a threat produces further destructive impulses toward the analyst; those impulses are then projected in the service of creating an even more hostile object.

That vicious cycle is broken, in Strachey's view, through mutative transference interpretations. After interpretation of the transferred id impulses to the analyst, patients become aware that their hostile impulses are directed toward internal parental objects, rather than real objects in the present, such as the analyst. As those interpretations are repeated in the context of the process of working through, patients realize the discrepancy between their own perceptions of the analyst and the real nature of the analyst. The analyst then becomes a much less frightening object, and the superego is correspondingly modified.

Mechanisms of change and analytic goals vary according to one's theoretical perspective. Analysts working within the framework of the British school of object relations theory believe that an analysis must do more than alter interrelationships between intrapsychic structures. They stress the need for change in mental representations of self and object and in the affective linkage between those representations. They believe that such changes are brought about partly through interpretation but also through the analytic relationship itself. Through the provision of a holding environment, the analyst's persistent curiosity and interest in the internal experience of the patient, and the analyst's ability to endure attacks or seductions from the patient, a new emotional experience is provided for internalization.

Proponents of the British school emphasize the process of containment in producing change. Through projective identification, the analyst becomes a container of the patient's self-representations and object representations, often in association with powerful affective states. Before those projected contents are returned to the patient by the process of reintrojection, the analyst psychologically processes and thereby modifies the patient's representations. For example, if a patient projects an abusive internal object representation into the analyst, the analyst resists becoming abusive toward the patient and, instead, attempts to process and understand the projected contents. When the patient reintrojects the abusive internal object representation, it has been modified by the analyst's containment process. The modified object representation then modifies the corresponding internal self-representation. In other words, a new mode of object relatedness has been internalized through the process of projective identification and containment.

Object relations theory views the patient as developmentally frozen. The experience of the analyst as a new object allows the patient to resume development and to experience previously thwarted relational and emotional capacities of a positive nature. Some analysts have compared it to a reparenting model in which the analyst conveys acceptance and validation of the patient's uniqueness and autonomy.

Self psychology views the goal of psychoanalytic treatment as the strengthening of a weakened self so that it can move from a dependence on archaic selfobject experiences to a position of greater self-cohesion that allows for reliance on mature selfobjects. Kohut asserted that the goal was accomplished by the laying down of psychic structure through optimal frustration and transmuting internalizations. He noted that failures of empathy are unavoidable in analysis, and the systematic interpretation and understanding of those empathic failures provide optimal frustration and the gradual internalization of the analyst as a new object. The essential curative aspect of the analytic process, however, is the establishment of empathic attunement between the self and the selfobject on a mature level. The experience of empathy allows the patient to overcome enslavement to archaic selfobjects in the service of maintaining self-cohesion.

Regardless of which theoretical school the analyst embraces, patients at the termination of a successfully conducted analysis feel certain predictable changes. They often have a sense of being freed up from previously mystifying internal constrictions. They may feel more creative and productive, so that they are able to pursue work and leisure-time activities with more enthusiasm. They are also likely to experience a much greater sense of mastery over their internal states. Greater tolerance of anxiety, for example, allows them to use that disturbing affect as a signal to reflect on what internal and external circumstances are causing concern and thereby to understand the source of the anxiety. Most patients at the end of analysis also experience a much expanded capacity to love others without contamination by conflicted relationships from the past. Through identification with the analyst, patients have internalized a self-analytic process that can be used to understand and master new situations as they arise throughout the life cycle.

A synthesis of the various developmental theorists—among whom are Margaret Mahler, John Bowlby, Sigmund Freud, Erik Erikson, Jean Piaget, and Daniel Stern—is provided in Table 6.1-5.

Some of the material in this section was derived from the chapter by William W. Meissner, S.J., M.D., "Classical Psychoanalysis," which appeared in the fourth edition of *Comprehensive Textbook of Psychiatry,* and from the section by Normund Wong, M.D., "Classical Psychoanalysis," which appeared in the fifth edition of *Comprehensive Textbook of Psychiatry.*

PSYCHOANALYTIC THINKING IN CONTEMPORARY PSYCHIATRY

This section focuses on formal psychoanalysis for the most part, but psychoanalytic or psychodynamic thinking is relevant to the practice of general psychiatry. Psychodynamic and biological approaches often work synergistically in treatment settings. Despite the either-or polarization of the biological and psychodynamic orientations in some quarters, psychodynamic psychiatry is not inherently antibiological, and an integrated approach has much to offer.

For psychiatry to avoid the twin pitfalls of becoming either mindless or brainless, clinicians must acknowledge the complex relations between neurophysiological and psychosocial factors in the cause and the pathogenesis of psychiatric disorders. To say that a chemical imbalance, for example, is the cause of a disorder is reductionistic. Neurophysiological or biochemical, processes in the brain are mediating mechanisms, rather than causal agents. The subjective meaning of the information perceived from the environment sets the biological processes in motion.

The interface between psychological trauma and brain functioning has been amply documented in primate research. Squirrel monkeys who are removed from their mothers undergo dramatic physiological changes, some of which become permanent if the separations are repeated. Among the physiological changes produced by early separation are persistently elevated plasma cortisol, lasting alterations in the sensitivity of noradrenergic receptors, permanent changes in the sensitivity and the number of brain opiate receptors, changes in adrenal gland catecholamine-synthesizing enzymes, and changes in hypothalamic serotonin secretion. Moreover, the psychoanalytic idea that environmental insults may cause varying degrees of psychological damage, depending on the specific developmental phase during which they occur, receives some support from the primate research. In one series of experiments, isolating infant monkeys from their mothers resulted in a more serious effect if the separation occurred at 90 days than if it occurred at either 60 or 120 days; perhaps the difference is related to a link between certain forms of bonding behavior and myelinization of the nervous system.

The brain is not a static structure. It is remarkably plastic and undergoes functional and structural changes almost daily. At the most fundamental level, psychotherapy must work by altering brain activity. Psychiatric disorders with strong biological

TABLE 6.1-5
A Synthesis of Developmental Theorists

Age (Years)	Margaret Mahler	John Bowlby	Sigmund Freud	Erik Erikson	Jean Piaget	Daniel Stern
0–1	Normal autistic phase (birth to 8 weeks) · State of half-sleep, half-wake · Major task of phase is to achieve homeostatic equilibrium with the environment Normal symbiotic phase (8 weeks to 6 months) · Dim awareness of caretaker, but infant still functions as if he or she and caretaker were in state of undifferentiation or fusion · Social smile characteristic (2–4 months) The subphases of separation-individuation proper First subphase: differentiation (6–10 months) · Process of hatching from autistic shell (i.e., developing more alert sensorium that reflects cognitive and neurological maturation) · Beginning of comparative scanning (i.e., comparing what is and what is not mother)	Phase I (birth to 8–12 weeks) · Infant's ability to discriminate one person from another is limited to olfactory and auditory stimuli · To any person in infant's vicinity, infant will: –orient to that person –have tracking movements of the eyes –grasp and reach –smile –babble –stop crying on hearing voice or seeing face · These behaviors, by influencing the adult's behavior, are likely to increase time the baby is in proximity to mother (adult) Phase II (8–12 weeks to 6 months or much later, according to circumstances) · Continuation of phase I activities but more marked in relation to mother more specifically	Oral phase (birth to 18 months) · Major site of tension and gratification is the mouth, lips, tongue –includes biting and sucking activities	Basic trust vs. basic mistrust (oral sensory) (birth to about 18 months) · Social mistrust demonstrated by ease of feeding, depth of sleep, bowel relaxation · Depends on consistency and sameness of experience provided by caretaker · Second 6-months' teething and biting moves infant "from getting to taking" · Weaning leads to "nostalgia for lost paradise" · If basic trust is strong, child maintains hopeful attitude	Sensorimotor phase (birth to 2 years) · Intelligence rests mainly on actions and movements coordinated under *schemata*. (Schema is a pattern of behavior in response to a particular environmental stimulus.) · Environment is mastered through *assimilation* and *accommodation*. (Assimilation is the incorporation of new environmental stimuli. Accommodation is the modification of behavior to adapt to new stimuli.) · *Object permanence* is achieved by age 2 years. Object still exists in mind if disappears from view: search for hidden object · Reversibility in action begins	Emergent self (birth to 2 months) · A bodily self based on physiological needs Core sense of self (appears between 2 and 6 months) · Associated with greater interpersonal relatedness Sense of subjective self (appears between 7 and 9 months) · A major advance involving the matching of intrapsychic states between mother and infant
1–2	· Characteristic anxiety: stranger anxiety, which involves curiosity and fear (most prevalent around 8 months) Second subphase: practicing (10–16 months) · Beginning of this phase marked by upright locomotion—child has new perspective and also mood of elation · Mother used as home base · Characteristic anxiety: separation anxiety Third subphase: rapprochement (16–24 months) · Infant now a toddler—more aware of physical separateness, which dampens mood of elation · Child tries to bridge gap between self and mother—concretely seen as bringing objects to mother	Phase III (6–7 months and continues throughout second and into third year) · Attachment to mother figure evident · Following departing mother · Greeting her on her return · Using her as base from which to explore · Waning of friendly, undifferentiated responses to others · Treating strangers with caution, alarm, withdrawal	Anal phase (18–36 months) · Anus and surrounding area are major source of interest · Acquisition of voluntary sphincter control (toilet training)	Autonomy vs. shame and doubt (muscular-anal) (about 18 months–3 years) · Biologically includes learning to walk, feed self, talk · Muscular maturation sets stage for holding on and letting go · Need for outer control, firmness of caretaker before development of autonomy · *Shame* occurs when child is overtly self-conscious because of negative exposure · *Self-doubt* can evolve if parents overly shame child (e.g., about elimination)		Verbal or categorical sense of self (appears between 15 and 18 months) · Coincides with the ability to think symbolically and communicate verbally

	· Mother's efforts to help toddler often not perceived as helpful, temper tantrums typical · Characteristic event: rapprochement crisis; wanting to be soothed by mother and yet not being able to accept her help · Symbol of rapprochement: child standing on threshold of door not knowing which way to turn in helpless frustration · Resolution of crisis occurs as child's skills improve and child is able to get gratification from doing things					
2–3	Fourth subphase: consolidation and object constancy (24–36 months) · Child better able to cope with mother's absence and to engage substitutes · Child can begin to feel comfortable with mother's absences by knowing she will return · Gradual internalization of image of mother as reliable and stable · Through increasing verbal skills and better sense of time, child can tolerate delay and endure separations	Phase IV (from 24 months) · Mother figure seen as independent · Object seen as persistent in time and space · More complex relationship with mother develops–partnership between mother and child develops, in which child acquires insight into mother's feelings and motives · Child observes mother's behavior and what influences it			Preoperational phase (2–7) years) · Appearance of *symbolic* functions, associated with language acquisition. · *Egocentrism:* child understands everything exclusively from own perspective · Thinking is illogical and magical · Nonreversible thinking with absence of conservation –*Animism:* belief that inanimate objects are alive (i.e., have feelings and intentions) –*Immanent justice:* belief that punishment for bad deeds is inevitable	
3–4 4–5			Phallic-oedipal phase (3–5 years) · Genital focus of interest, stimulation, and excitement · Penis is organ of interest for both sexes · Genital masturbation common · Intense preoccupation with *castration anxiety* (fear of genital loss or injury) · *Penis envy* (discontent with one's own genitals and wish to possess genitals of male) seen in girls in this phase · *Oedipus complex* universal: child wishes to have sex with and marry parent of opposite sex and simultaneously be rid of parent of same sex	Initiative vs. guilt (locomotor genital) (3–5 years) · *Initiative* arises in relation to tasks for the sake of activity, both motor and intellectual · *Guilt* may arise over goals contemplated (especially aggressive) · Desire to mimic adult world; involvement in oedipal struggle leads to resolution through social role identification · Sibling rivalry frequent		Narrative sense of self (appears between ages 3 and 5) · The historical view of the self encountered when patients present their life stories in treatment

TABLE 6.1-5 (*continued*)

Age (Years)	Margaret Mahler	John Bowlby	Sigmund Freud	Erik Erikson	Jean Piaget	Daniel Stern
5–6			Latency phase (from 5–6 years to 11–13 years) · State of relative quiescence of sexual drive with resolution of oedipal complex · Sexual drives channeled into more socially appropriate aims (i.e., schoolwork and sports)			
6–11			· Formation of *superego:* one of three psychic structures in mind that is responsible for moral and ethical development, including conscience · (Other two psychic structures are *ego,* which is a group of functions mediating between the drives and the external environment, and the *id,* repository of sexual and aggressive drives · The id is there at birth, and the ego develops gradually from rudimentary structure present at birth)	Industry vs. inferiority (latency) (5–13 years) · Child is busy building, creating, accomplishing · Receives systematic instruction and fundamentals of technology · Danger of sense of inadequacy and inferiority if child despairs of his tools, skills, and status among peers · Socially decisive age	Concrete (operational) phase (7–11 years) · Emergence of logical (cause-effect) thinking, including reversibility and ability to sequence and serialize · Understanding of part and whole relationships and classifications · Child able to take other's point of view · Conservation of number, length, weight, and volume	
11+			Genital phase (from 11–13 years) · Final stage of psychosexual development—begins with puberty and the biological capacity for orgasm but involves the capacity for true intimacy	Identity vs. role diffusion (13 years through end of adolescence) · Struggle to develop *ego identity* (sense of inner sameness and continuity) · Preoccupation with appearance, hero worship, ideology · *Group identity* (peers) develops · Danger of *role confusion,* doubts about sexual and vocational identity · *Psychosocial moratorium,* stage between morality learned by the child and the ethics to be developed by the adult	Formal (abstract) phase (11 years through end of adolescence) · Hypothetical-deductive reasoning, not only on basis of objects but also on basis of hypotheses or of propositions · Capable of thinking about one's thoughts · Combinative structures emerge, permitting flexible grouping of elements in a system · Ability to use two systems of reference simultaneously · Ability to grasp concept of probabilities	

Table by Sylvia Karasu, M.D., and Richard Oberfield, M.D. Adapted by Glen O. Gabbard, M.D.

underpinnings are not devoid of meaning. Illnesses are elaborated psychologically by patients who suffer from them, and clinicians must incorporate questions of meaning into an overall diagnostic understanding and treatment plan.

Clinical illustration A 29-year-old single man with a 10-year history of obsessive-compulsive disorder was admitted to a psychiatric hospital. He had been housebound for the preceding eight years because his obsessional thoughts and compulsive rituals had become incapacitating. The patient's mother had retired from her career so that she could be at home with the patient and accommodate his demands for cleanliness.

The patient lived in constant fear of contamination. Specifically, he worried that he might have semen on his hands that would impregnate women. He washed his hands compulsively to make sure that his fears would not come to fruition. He demanded that his mother be with him virtually every hour of the day. She did not enter the shower with him, nor did she sleep with him, but she helped him dress because he feared his clothes would become contaminated with germs if he touched them. The patient insisted on a complex 58-step ritual when his mother prepared his meals. If she made a small deviation from the ritual, he insisted that she throw out all the food she had prepared and start from scratch. She had wasted thousands of dollars each year in her efforts to conform to the rituals demanded by her son. The patient ordered his father to stay away from the house, lest the father bring in germs from the outside world. The father complied by staying in a separate part of the house, where he rarely had contact with his son.

The patient's early childhood had been basically unremarkable from a developmental perspective, but he did recall a vivid and frightening event when he was 5 years old. He remembered seeing his mother crying out for him to rescue her after his father had grabbed her by the breasts. He remembered trying to stop his father but could not succeed in getting him away from his mother.

By the time the patient had turned 19, he had been severely compromised by obsessive-compulsive symptoms and had been to many psychiatrists. Each time, he refused to return after one appointment. One psychiatrist had managed to obtain the patient's agreement to take clomipramine (Anafranil). However, the patient refused to take the medication after the first dose produced ill-defined side effects.

The patient was finally admitted to a hospital because he was completely incapacitated by his symptoms. On admission, his hospital psychiatrist asked him why he was seeking treatment. The patient responded, "I'm determined to be dependent—I mean, independent." The doctor noted that he initially had said "dependent" and asked, "Is there perhaps a part of you that would like to be dependent?" The patient replied, "You mean on my mother?" The psychiatrist responded that he was sure the patient would know better than he. The patient then thought about his situation momentarily and observed, "Well, she does take pretty good care of me." He went on to say that his mother also made him nervous when she dressed him. The patient speculated that "there was something sexual about that."

After a week of hospitalization, the patient became less anxious and less controlled by his symptoms. He was able to touch doorknobs without fearing that he would contract germs, and he could even touch magazines that others had read. He also spent less time washing his hands than he had before admission to the hospital. Those improvements occurred without the assistance of clomipramine or other medication. The patient said he was less anxious because he was away from his mother and did not need to worry about the sexual aspects of her dressing him.

Psychodynamic-biological interface The interface between the psychodynamic and the biological is illustrated by the above clinical vignette. Obsessive-compulsive disorder is a condition that is biologically based to a large extent. Patients with the disorder have a smaller caudate nucleus volume than do healthy control persons. Monozygotic twins have a higher rate of concordance for the disorder than do their dizygotic counterparts. Also, patients with obsessive-compulsive disorder manifest virtually no response to a placebo.

Nevertheless, in the case of the above patient, the obsessive-compulsive symptoms were rich in psychological meaning. The patient's symptoms reflected the psychoanalytic concept known as *compromise formation:* they contained both the direct expression of an underlying wish and a defense against that wish. The patient's obsessional thoughts and compulsive rituals defended against his sexual wishes for his mother by causing him to spend every waking moment in hand washing rituals and other activities. However, these symbolic rituals also produced a situation in which his mother showered attention on him, even to the point of dressing him, while his father stayed in another part of the house. For all practical purposes the patient had created a symbolic oedipal victory; he had successfully stolen his mother away from his father. His resistance to taking clomipramine can be understood as a refusal to give up his triumphant position with his mother. His oedipal victory also created guilt and anxiety, which led to increased reliance on the rituals and obsessions. The hospitalization removed him from the anxiety-producing situation at home; therefore, his symptoms were not necessary to deal with his anxiety.

An analogy from a common elementary school demonstration is useful in explicating the relation between the biological and the psychodynamic. If iron filings are placed on a sheet of paper with a magnet underneath, the filings line up in formation on the surface and follow the movement of the magnet as it glides beneath the paper. Similarly, psychodynamic themes often appropriate the powerful magnetlike biological forces in the brain for their own purpsoes. The obsessive-compulsive patient's unconscious wishes and his defenses against them appropriated the neurophysiologically driven obsessive-compulsive symptoms and used them as a vehicle for the expression of his wishes and defenses.

Noncompliance Noncompliance with pharmacotherapeutic regimens is an everyday problem in contemporary psychiatry. The psychodynamic concepts of resistance and transference may be extraordinarily useful in understanding noncompliance. In the case of the obsessive-compulsive patient above, the psychoanalytically informed understanding of his resistance to taking medication was essential to his successful treatment, which ultimately involved medication and therapeutic work with the family. The patient's slip of the tongue made him aware for the first time that any improvement in his symptoms would threaten his privileged position with his mother.

The psychodynamic understanding of the patient's obsessive-compulsive symptoms illustrates an important distinction within dynamic psychiatry, namely, the difference between causation and meaning. The obsessive-compulsive symptoms may be caused by biological forces, but they are imbued with meaning by the unconscious of the patient. Similarly, only one fourth of persons who witness a traumatic event develop symptoms of posttraumatic stress disorder. Although there may be genetic vulnerability in some cases, one can also speculate that particular forms of trauma have specific unconscious meanings to certain persons that may contribute to their becoming symptomatic.

PANIC DISORDER In other anxiety disorders, such as panic disorder, the psychodynamic and biological approaches can best be integrated by differentiating pathogenesis from cause. The pathogenesis of panic disorder appears to involve dysregulation of γ-aminobutyric acid (GABA) in the locus ceruleus. The neurophysiological underpinnings of panic disorder are further substantiated by other findings, including a higher incidence of panic disorder in panic patients' families than in control families, a higher rate of concordance in monozygotic twins than in dizygotic twins, and the induction of panic attacks by sodium lactate infusion in patients suffering from panic disorder.

As persuasive as those research findings are regarding the biological dimensions of panic disorder, they say little about what causes the condition. To determine what triggers an episode of panic, clinicians must think psychodynamically. Psychoanalytically oriented interviews have been successful in identifying psychological stressors that precede the onset of panic attacks, even when the patients themselves have not recognized the stressors. There is also a high correlation between maternal separation in early childhood and the subsequent development of panic disorder. Patients with panic disorder have a high incidence of stressful life events, particularly loss, in the months preceding the onset of panic whem compared with control persons. Moreover, patients with panic disorder tend to experience greater distress about events in their lives than do controls. In other words, stressors have greater than usual psychological meaning to persons who then experience panic episodes.

A psychological variable appears to mediate between external events and neurophysiological mechanisms that ultimately produce panic episodes. Psychological treatments can alter the neurophysiology of panic disorder. Patients who have panic induced by sodium lactate infusion can no longer have panic induced after they receive effective treatment of panic disorder with cognitive psychotherapy. Findings such as those indicate that psychological interventions targeted at the mind influence physiological processes located in the brain. The richness and the complexity of human functioning cannot be reduced to molecular genetics and neurotransmitters. To understand the causes of psychiatric disorders, clinicians must factor in psychological meaning. What is crucial to cause and pathogenesis is also crucial to informed treatment planning. Mind and brain are inseparable.

SUGGESTED CROSS-REFERENCES

The psychoanalytic perspective is relevant to virtually every chapter of this book. Of particular interest are the discussion of Erik Erikson in Section 6.2, other psychodynamic schools in Chapter 7, approaches derived from psychology and philosophy in Chapter 8, psychodynamic to neurodynamic theories and individual psychotherapy of schizophrenia in Sections 14.6 and 14.10, psychodynamic etiology and psychological treatments of mood disorders in Sections 16.5 and 16.8, anxiety disorders in Chapter 17, personality disorders in Chapter 25, psychoanalysis and psychoanalytic psychotherapy in Section 31.1, evaluation of psychotherapy in Section 31.10, and psychotherapy with the elderly in Section 49.7a.

REFERENCES

Abend S A: Countertransference and psychoanalytic technique. Psychoanal Q *58:* 374, 1989.

Balint M: *The Basic Fault: The Therapeutic Aspects of Regression.* Brunner/Mazel, New York, 1979.

Brenner C: *The Mind in Conflict.* International Universities Press, New York, 1982.

Cooper A M: Changes in psychoanalytic ideas: Transference interpretation. J Am Psychoanal Assoc *35:* 77, 1987.

Doidge N, Simon B, Gillies L A, Ruskin R: Characteristics of psychoanalytic patients under a nationalized plan: DSM-III-R diagnoses, previous treatment, and childhood trauma. *Am J Psychiatry 151:* 586, 1994.

Eagle M: The concepts of need and wish in self psychology. Psychoanal Psychol *7:* 71, 1990.

Fairbairn W R D: *Psychoanalytic Studies of the Personality.* Routledge & Kegan Paul, London, 1952.

*Freud A: *The Ego and the Mechanisms of Defense* (1936). In *The Writings of Anna Freud,* vol 2, ed 2. International Universities Press, New York, 1966.

*Freud S: *Standard Edition of the Complete Psychological Works of Sigmund Freud.* Hogarth Press, London, 1953–1966.

Friedman L: How and why do patients become more objective? Sterba compared with Strachey. Psychoanal Q *61:* 1, 1992.

Gabbard G O: *Psychodynamic Psychiatry in Clinical Practice: The DSM-IV Edition.* American Psychiatric Press, Washington, 1994.

Gabbard G O: Psychodynamic psychiatry in the ''decade of the brain.'' Am J Psychiatry *149:* 991, 1992.

Gill M: *Analysis of Transference,* vol 1, *Theory and Technique.* International Universities Press, New York, 1982.

Goldberg A: Farewell to the objective analyst. Int J Psychoanal *75:* 21, 1994.

*Greenson R R: *The Technique and Practice of Psychoanalysis,* vol 1. International Universities Press, New York, 1967.

Hartmann H: *Essays on Ego Psychology: Selected Problems in Psychoanalytic Theory.* International Universities Press, New York, 1964.

Hoffman I Z: Dialectical thinking and therapeutic action in the psychoanalytic process. Psychoanal O *63:* 187, 1994.

Holzman P S, Aronson G: Psychoanalysis and its neighboring sciences: paradigms and opportunities. J Am Psychoanal Assoc *40:* 63, 1992.

Jacobson E: *The Self and the Object World.* International Universities Press, New York, 1964.

Jacobson J G: Signal affects and our psychoanalytic confusion of tongues. J Am Psychoanal Assoc *42:* 15, 1994.

Kernberg O F: *Borderline Conditions and Pathological Narcissism.* Aronson, New York, 1975.

Kernberg O F: The current status of psychoanalysis. J Am Psychoanal Assoc *41:* 45, 1993.

Klein M: *Envy and Gratitude and Other Works, 1946–1963.* Free Press, New York, 1975.

*Kohon G: *The British School of Psychoanalysis: The Independent Tradition.* Yale University Press, New Haven, 1986.

Kohut H: *The Analysis of the Self: A Systematic Approach to the Psychoanalytic Treatment of Narcissistic Personality Disorder.* International Universities Press, New York, 1971.

*Kohut H: *How Does Analysis Cure?* University of Chicago Press, Chicago, 1984.

Kohut H: *The Restoration of the Self.* International Universities Press, New York, 1977.

Mitchell S A: Contemporary perspectives on self: Toward an integration. Psychoanal Dial *1:* 121, 1991.

Ogden T H: The concept of internal object relations. Int J Psychoanal *64:* 227, 1983.

Ogden T H : *Subjects of Analysis.* Aronson, Northvale, NJ, 1994.

Parsons M: The refinding of theory in clinical practice. Int J Psychoanal *73:* 103, 1992.

Renik O: Analytic interaction: conceptualizing technique in light of the analyst's irreducible subjectivity. Psychoanal O *62:* 553, 1993.

Sandler J: On internal object relations. J Am Psychoanal Assoc *38:* 859, 1990.

Scharff J S: *Projective and Introjective Identification and the Use of the Therapist's Self.* Aronson, Northvale, NJ, 1992.

Simon B: In search of psychoanalytic technique: Perspectives from on the couch and from behind the couch. J Am Psychoanal Assoc *41:* 1051, 1993.

Stern D N: *The Interpersonal World of the Infant: A View from Psychoanalysis and Developmental Psychology.* Basic Books, New York, 1985.

Tyson P: Theories of female psychology. J Am Psychoanal Assoc *42:* 447, 1994.

Van der Kolk B A: *Psychological Trauma.* American Psychiatric Press, Washington, 1987.

Wakefield J C: Freud and the intentionality of affect. Psychoanal Psychol *9:* 1, 1992.

Winnicott D W: *The Maturational Process and the Facilitating Environment: Studies in the Theory of Emotional Development.* Hogarth Press, London, 1965.

Winnicott D W: *Playing and Reality.* Basic Books, New York, 1971.

6.2
ERIK H. ERIKSON

PETER M. NEWTON, Ph.D.
DORIAN S. NEWTON, Ph.D.

INTRODUCTION

Erik Erikson was a lay psychoanalyst whose book *Childhood and Society* expanded the understanding of psychological growth, conflict, and pathology by describing stages in the development of the ego throughout the life cycle. His other famous works include *Young Man Luther, Gandhi's Truth,* and countless articles, many of which have been collected into anthologies. In his psychological biographies of the great religious leaders, Erikson demonstrated the interrelations between individual psychodynamics and development on the one hand and social structure and history on the other hand without reduction to any single level of explanation. His unparalleled success in doing so extended the influence of his thinking far beyond the boundaries of the clinical disciplines to include the social sciences, the humanities, and the arts. Reviewing his biography of Martin Luther, the English poet W. H. Auden described Erikson as "that happy exception, a psychoanalyst who knows the difference between a biography and a case history."

Erikson's students, many of whom are now leaders in their own disciplines and carrying out Erikson's work in highly distinctive ways, have been inspired by his generative concern for human life and the social institutions on which it depends and by the originality and brilliance of his scholarship. Analysts and psychotherapists who had the good fortune to be supervised by Erikson regard him as a singularly gifted clinician. There, then, was the promise of psychoanalysis fully realized—a clinician, a developmental theorist, and a humanist integrated within one coherent identity, unfolding across a long, creatively productive life.

This section illustrates Erikson's key concepts by applying them to his own life and work, primarily during youth and middle age. Erikson's concepts are italicized. The reader will encounter other terms, not italicized, but clearly derived from a theory of adult development, such as, "the life structure," the developmental phase of "becoming one's own man," and "the mid-life transition." Those terms come from Erikson's student, Daniel Levinson, who, building on his teacher's work, was a leading psychosocial theorist of the life cycle.

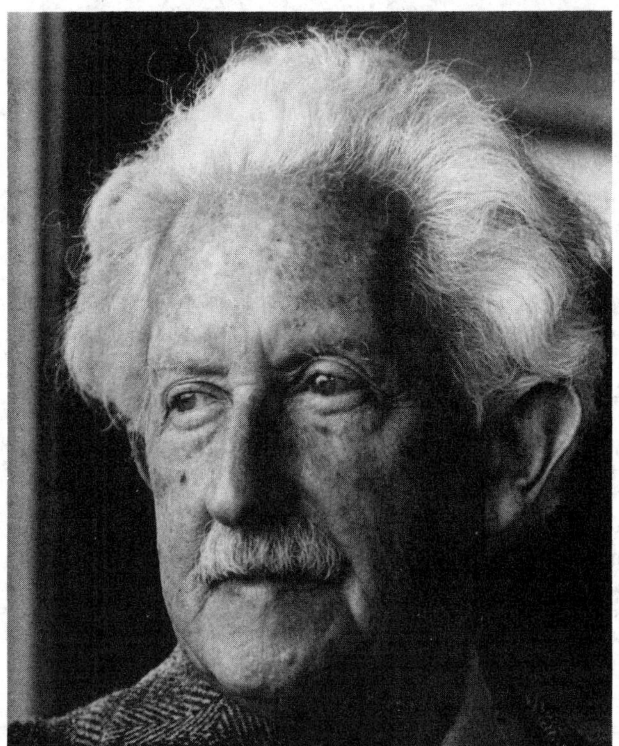

FIGURE 6.2-1 *Erik Erikson.*

LIFE AND WORK

Erik Homburger Erikson was born on June 15, 1902, in Karlsruhe, Germany, an old capital of a Lutheran principality (Figure 6.2-1). Erikson died in 1994. His father was Protestant and his mother Jewish. The parents, both Danish, had separated before his birth; his mother was visiting friends in Germany when the baby was born. She stayed in Karlsruhe and, a few years later, married her child's pediatrician, a well-to-do Jewish doctor named Theodor Homburger, in whose house young Erik grew up. That was the formative occasion of what became his lifelong pattern of getting himself adopted by kind men. During an alienated adolescence, the tall, blond boy found himself regarded as a gentile in his father's Jewish milieu and as a Jew at school. He remembered his mother as sad, bookish, and artistic; his adoptive father as professionally respected; and both as loving.

Erikson attended the Humanistische Gymnasium in Karlsruhe, where he studied Greek, Latin, philosophy, literature, and science; by 18 he had the educational attainments of an American college graduate and a far stronger base. His primary interest was in art; impatient with formal study and possessed by a restlessness he never lost, Erikson chose not to go to a university, preferring to travel about the countryside reading, drawing, and making wood carvings. Back home after a year, he tried formal art study, first in Karlsruhe and then in Munich with some success but in neither case with decisive commitment.

At about 21 Erikson went to live in Florence, where he continued his art studies informally. There he enjoyed the friendship of his old gymnasium chum Peter Blos, a writer, who later became a famous American child psychoanalyst. That sort of wandering about was not uncommon among German youth of the period, so Erikson was permitted, as his biographer Robert Coles sagely wrote, "to go through his own years of discontent and confusion without being especially singled out and thereby forced to defend behavior often best granted the limits of its own momentum." Erikson was having what he would later term a *psychosocial moratorium;* in so doing, he was also mitigating the asperities of an *identity crisis.*

BECOMING A CHILD PSYCHOANALYST By 24 or 25 Erikson's transition to early adulthood was over. Back in Karlsruhe, he was ready to make art teaching the occupational component of his first adult life structure. Peter Blos invited him to become the other faculty member in a progressive grammar school in Vienna, where Blos was teaching language and science. The year was 1927. Sigmund Freud was 71, and his last child, Anna, an educator and psychoanalyst, had started a psychoanalytically enlightened school for children with an American friend, Dorothy Burlingham. Erikson joined Blos and later recalled with ironic warmth Blos's determination to turn the feckless youth into some semblance of a disciplined worker: "To make a teacher of me . . . the highly disciplined Peter first had to teach me to keep regular work hours, a task which was initiated every morning, no matter what time of year, by a cold shower, then the preferred shock treatment for identity confusion."

Before long, Erikson found himself not only a teacher of children but also an analysand at the Vienna Psychoanalytic Institute—what is now called a candidate—in treatment with Anna Freud. Any sort of psychoanalytic approach to treating or educating children was then a radical idea. Both educationally and clinically, the Freuds constituted a sufficiently deviant group that Erikson was able to find a place in it. There was in 1927 a *configurational affinity* between his personal history and the history of psychoanalysis as a profession. But what was a fledgling artist without a university education to do among those high-powered theorists and intellectuals at the Vienna Psychoanalytic Institute?

Erikson recalled this epiphanic exchange with his analyst: "When I declared once more that I could not see a place for my artistic inclinations in such high intellectual endeavors, she said quietly: 'You might help to make them see.'" Dreams had been Freud's royal road to the unconscious; observing children's play would be Erikson's path to the understanding of the ego and its development. Looking back, Erikson thought that it was Anna Freud's simple mandate that enabled him to succeed in combining the artistic and the theoretical in *Childhood and Society.*

Erikson remained in Vienna for six years, until 1933. In those years between 25 and 31, he continued as a novice adult to develop the skills and meanings of the occupational component of his life structure. He turned his artist's eye from the observation of nature to the analysis of children; he learned about psychoanalysis by studying children's play and his own free associations as a patient, and he learned fundamental clinical skills in the supervised treatment of others. He formed mentor relationships with Anna Freud and Heinz Hartmann and a more distant admiring-inspirational relationship with Anna Freud's sick and aging but still productive father.

During his own late adulthood, Sigmund Freud had moved beyond clinical preoccupations to problems of the ego, society, and history in works such as *Beyond the Pleasure Principle* (written at age 64), *Group Psychology and the Analysis of the Ego* (at 65), and *The Ego and the Id* (at 66); during Erikson's years in Vienna, Freud was working on *The Future of an Illusion* (at 71) and *Civilization and Its Discontents* (at 73). It appears that Erikson identified with both Freuds, internalizing them as mentors, and that they provided him with a strong, inner basis for a lifetime of both psychoanalytic treatment and psychosocial research.

Equally important, during those years Erikson succeeded in committing himself to what was the other central component of his life structure. In Vienna he met his wife, Joan Serson, an American woman with a masters degree in sociology who had a special interest in modern dance and psychoanalysis. They married, and Serson joined the faculty of Burlingham's school as an English teacher. Serson's unusual combination of interests and skills—education, psychoanalysis, and sociology, coupled with her ability as a writer—gave Erikson a skilled coworker for a lifetime of intellectual work. Several articles are coauthored, Joan Erikson helped with most of the others, and the endowed chair at Harvard that was named after Erikson carries both their first names.

With the birth of their sons, Kai and Jon, Erikson had by 31 become a husband, a father, and a child psychoanalyst. He had come a long way from the aimless youth of his early 20s. His first adult life structure was fully formed, and he was productively engaged in the stage of ego development that he later characterized by the polarity *intimacy versus isolation*. He continued to work on that ego stage, but the life structure that Erikson had begun to build at 25 changed.

EMIGRATING TO AMERICA By 1933 the Fascist menace in Europe was growing. When Erikson graduated that year from the Vienna Psychoanalytic Institute, the Eriksons prepared to leave. They considered repatriating to Denmark but encountered sufficient annoying difficulties to allow them to rationalize a real emigration. Home for Erikson was always a fortuitously adoptive one, and so he allowed chance, in the form of a serendipitous meeting with Freud's disciple Hanns Sachs, to settle his future. Sachs enthusiastically invited him to come to the United States. In 1933 the Eriksons moved to Boston, and at 31 he became the city's first child psychoanalyst and a member of the faculty of the Harvard Medical School. With a new home and a new profession as a professor, Erikson was, in his age-30 transition, revising the life structure that he had created in his mid-20s. At Harvard University, Erikson joined the group of personality researchers working under the leadership of Henry Murray at the Harvard Psychological Clinic.

Murray's book *Explorations in Personality: A Clinical and Experimental Study of Fifty Men of College Age* was published in 1938. It is one of the integrative masterpieces in American psychology—experimental and biographical, psychological and sociological, Freudian and Jungian, developmental and diagnostic—and it provided a luminous example of how to study persons in their origins and in their purposes. Murray's example was helpful when Erikson later turned his hand to the biographical study of Sigmund Freud, Martin Luther, and Mohandas Gandhi.

Listed on the title page of Murray's book, among other research associates, is "Erik Homburger." The next year, at age 37, during a developmental phase that Levinson calls "becoming one's own man," Homburger renamed himself Erikson, retaining Homburger as his middle name. With characteristically bold creativity, Erikson had solved the problem of his paternity by adopting himself.

PSYCHOANALYTIC ANTHROPOLOGY In 1936 Erikson hit the road again, this time to the Institute of Human Relations in the department of psychiatry at Yale University. The interdisciplinary work of the institute shaped Erikson's interest, begun at the Harvard Psychological Clinic, in cross-cultural research, and in 1938 he joined a colleague on a research expedition to the Sioux Indians in South Dakota. On the Pine Ridge reservation he observed children and child-rearing practices and interviewed adults, resulting in his paper "Observations on Sioux Education," published in 1939. In that same year the Eriksons moved to California, where he joined the faculty of the University of California at Berkeley. There he settled down and remained for a decade, the longest period in one place since his preadulthood years in Karlsruhe. That was the culminating period of his early adulthood, a time to realize the promise and reap the rewards of youth. At Berkeley he became his own man, visible first in the outward signs of changing his name and later in refusing to sign the university's anti-Communist loyalty oath. Most important, during those 10 years, from 37 to 47, Erikson wrote his masterwork, *Childhood and Society,* and began his career as a biographer.

At Berkeley Erikson initially continued his cross-cultural research, this time with the Yurok Indians of northern California. He also lent his research skills to the war effort in articles on submarine habitation and the interrogation of prisoners of war. He also continued his research, begun at Burlingham's experimental school, on children's play. But at 40, entering his mid-life transition, something new appeared. Erikson was becoming more biographical and more interested in the adult years of the life cycle. Like other successfully developing people, he found a way to pursue his development through the strictures of exigent reality. World War II was under way, and he was deeply concerned about it. After his initial narrowly framed attempts at scholarly patriotism, he began writing his first psychobiographical essays on Adolf Hitler and the psychosocial dynamics of his appeal to young Germans. "Hitler's Imagery and German Youth" was published in 1942.

MID-LIFE TRANSITION The primary developmental task at mid-life is to terminate the existing life structure and initiate a new one suitable for middle age. *Childhood and Society* was the creative product of Erikson's developmental efforts during his mid-life transition. He had intended it to be a contribution to the psychiatric education of clinicians from various disciplines, but the book outgrew its author's intentions and found its way into every corner of the academy and beyond.

Erikson began work on the book when he was 42 and largely completed work on it by 46. *Childhood and Society,* published in 1950, is at once a product of early research, a prospectus of what was to come, and an initial integration of both. He presented clinical cases in which individual psychodynamics, society, and history are interwoven with a skill not seen before or since; analyses of children's play and development in various cultures; a theoretical sketch of the entire human life cycle; pieces on the problem of identity; and biographical essays on Hitler and the Russian writer Maxim Gorky.

As in Karl Abraham's and Sigmund Freud's psychosexual stages, Erikson's point of view is developmental, and most of his stages in ego development occur in childhood and adolescence. Unlike the Abraham-Freud conception, Erikson's stages are *psychosocial,* describing crucial steps in the maturing ego's relations with the social world, rather than a biological unfolding of neurophysiological capacities for excitation. And, whereas Freud's developmental theory falls back on itself after adolescence, Erikson's continues with characterizations of developmental tasks during youth, middle age, and old age.

Erikson's emphasis, like Freud's, is both cross-cultural and universal. Erikson's eight stages are ineluctable parts of the human life cycle, yet each person goes through them in distinct ways that are determined by culture, concrete circumstance, and personality. With *Childhood and Society* Erikson became and remained an *ego psychologist,* furthering the work of his analyst-mentor, Anna Freud, who in 1936 had written ego psychology's basic theoretical treatise, *The Ego and the Mechanisms of Defense.*

Erikson's conceptualization of psychosocial development took as its model the *epigenetic principle* of organismic growth in utero. In Erikson's view, psychosocial growth occurs in phases, with individual aspects of development proceeding according to a prefigured timetable. Each phase has its own time of quiescence and critical ascendancy, and each is dependent on the proper development of the other phases in the proper sequence. Work on any particular phase, Erikson saw, is never complete, and old developmental conflicts can be activated by critical life events.

EIGHT STAGES OF THE LIFE CYCLE Erikson's conception of the eight stages of ego development across the life cycle is the centerpiece of his life's work (Table 6.2-1). He elaborated it throughout his later work and inspired numerous Eriksonian studies of ego development. The eight stages represent points along a continuum of development in which physical, cognitive, instinctual, and sexual changes combine to trigger an internal crisis, whose resolution results in either psychosocial regression or growth and the development of specific virtues. In *Insight and Responsibility* Erikson defined *virtue* as "inherent strength," as in the active quality of a medicine or a liquor. He wrote in *Identity: Youth and Crisis* that *crisis* refers not to a "threat of catastrophe, but to a turning point, a crucial period of increased vulnerability and heightened potential, and therefore, the ontogenetic source of generational strength and maladjustment."

Trust versus mistrust (birth to about 18 months) In *Identity: Youth and Crisis* Erikson noted that the infant "lives through and loves with" its mouth. Indeed, the mouth forms the basis of its first *mode* or pattern of behavior—that of incorporation. At that stage the infant is taking the world in through its mouth, eyes, ears, and sense of touch. It is learning a cultural modality that Erikson termed *"to get"*—that is, to receive what is offered and elicit what is desired. As the infant's teeth develop and it discovers the pleasure of biting, it enters the second oral stage, the *active-incorporative* mode. The infant is no longer passively receptive to stimuli; it reaches out for sensation and grasps at its surroundings. The social modality shifts to that of *taking* and *holding on* to things. Because even under optimal circumstances the infant encounters frustration and some degree of deprivation, it also develops a basic sense of mistrust. Some measure of the sense of mistrust is an indispensable part of the person's adaptive capacity. However, if the caretaker is sufficiently attuned to the infant's needs and provides for them in a consistent, timely manner, trust predominates and *hope* as a virtue crystallizes. The mother's responses are influenced in part by the child's behavior, and the infant must control its urge to bite and chew, lest it drive her away. In *Identity: Youth and Crisis* Erikson commented, "The general state of trust . . . implies not only that one has learned to rely on the sameness and continuity of the outer providers but also that one may trust oneself and the capacity of one's own organs to cope with urges."

In keeping with his emphasis on the epigenetic character of psychosocial change, Erikson conceived of many forms of psychopathology as examples of what he termed *aggravated development crisis*—development that, having gone awry at one point, affects subsequent psychosocial change. A person who, as a result of severe disturbances in the earliest dyadic relationships, fails to develop a basic sense of trust or the virtue of hope may be predisposed, as an adult, to the profound withdrawal and regression characteristic of schizophrenia. Erikson hypothesized that the depressed patient's experience of being empty and of being no good is an outgrowth of a developmental derailment, so that oral pessimism predominates. Addictions may also be traced to the mode of oral incorporation.

Autonomy versus shame and doubt (about 18 months to about 3 years) In its development of speech and of sphincter and muscular control, the toddler experiments with conflicting impulses to hold on and to let go, and it experiences the first stirrings of the virtue that Erikson termed *will.* Much depends on the amount and the type of outer control exercised by adults over the child. Control that is exerted too rigidly or too early defeats the toddler's attempts to develop its own internal controls, and regression or false progression results. Parental control that fails to protect the toddler from the consequences of its own lack of self-control or judgment can be equally disastrous to the child's development of a healthy sense of autonomy. Erikson asserted in *Identity: Youth and Crisis:* "This stage, therefore, becomes decisive for the ratio between loving good will and hateful self-insistence, between cooperation and willfulness, and between self-expression and compulsive self-restraint or meek compliance."

Doubt and shame predominate when the child has failed to achieve a sense of self-control and free will. Yet in many ways the child cannot progress beyond the gains achieved by its parents. In *Identity: Youth and Crisis* Erikson wrote, "no matter what we do in detail, the child will primarily feel what it is we live by as loving, co-operative, and firm beings, and what makes us hateful, anxious, and divided in ourselves."

TABLE 6.2-1
Erikson's Psychosocial Stages

Psychosocial Stage	Associated Virtue	Related Forms of Psychopathology	Positive and Negative Forerunners of Identity Formation	Enduring Aspects of Identity Formation
Trust versus mistrust (birth–about 18 months)	Hope	Psychosis Addictions Depression	Mutual recognition versus autistic isolation	Temporal perspective versus time confusion
Autonomy versus shame and doubt (about 18 months–about 3 years)	Will	Paranoia Obsessions Compulsions Impulsivity	Will to be oneself versus self-doubt	Self-certainty versus self-consciousness
Initiative versus guilt (about 3 years–about 5 years)	Purpose	Conversion disorder Phobia Psychosomatic symptoms Inhibition	Anticipation of roles versus role inhibition	Role experimentation versus role fixation
Industry versus inferiority (about 5 years–about 13 years)	Competence	Creative inhibition Inertia	Task identification versus sense of futility	Apprenticeship versus work paralysis
Identity versus identity confusion (about 13 years–about 21 years)	Fidelity	Delinquent behavior Gender identity disorders Psychotic episodes		Identity versus identity confusion
Intimacy versus isolation (about 21 years–about 40 years)	Love	Schizoid personality disorder Distantiation Racism		Sexual polarization versus bisexual confusion
Generativity versus stagnation (about 40 years–about 60 years)	Care	Mid-life crisis Premature invalidism		Leadership and followership versus abdication of responsibility
Integrity versus despair (about 60 years–death)	Wisdom	Extreme alienation Despair		Ideological commitment versus confusion of values

This chart adapts and extends those found in E Erikson: *Insight and Responsibility,* p 186. Norton, New York, 1964; and E Erikson: *Identity: Youth and Crisis,* p 94. Norton, New York, 1968.

For the person who becomes fixated at the transition between the development of hope and autonomous will, the residue of mistrust, combined with the lack of a sense of self-determination, may surface years later in the paranoid conviction that others are trying to control him or her. The perfectionism, inflexibility, and stinginess of the person with an obsessive-compulsive personality disorder is rooted, according to Erikson, in the person's original struggles with conflicting tendencies to hold on and to let go. The ruminative and ritualistic behavior of the person who suffers from an obsessive-compulsive disorder is an outcome of the triumph of doubt over autonomy and the subsequent development of a *precocious conscience.*

Initiative versus guilt (about 3 years to about 5 years) The child's increasing mastery of its locomotor and language skills serves to expand participation in the outside world and to stimulate omnipotent fantasies of wider exploration and conquest. The youngster's mode of participation now is *intrusive* and its social modality that of *being on the make.* The intrusiveness is manifested in the child's fervent curiosity and genital preoccupations, competitiveness, and physical aggression. The Oedipus complex is in ascendance as the child competes with the same-sex parent for the fantasied possession of the other parent. In *Identity: Youth and Crisis* Erikson wrote that "[j]ealousy and rivalry . . . now come to a climax in a final contest for a favored position with one of the parents: the inevitable and necessary failure leads to guilt and anxiety."

The child's guilt and anxiety are assuaged through repression of the forbidden wishes, and it develops a conscience to regulate its initiative. This *conscience*—the faculty of self-observation and self-punishment—is an internalized version of parental and societal authority. At that stage the conscience is relatively primitive, harsh, and uncompromising; however, it constitutes the foundation for the subsequent development of morality. Having renounced its oedipal ambitions, the child begins to look outside the family for arenas in which it can compete with less conflict and guilt. The stage highlights the child's expanding initiative and forms the basis for the subsequent development of realistic ambition and the virtue of *purpose.*

When the person has inadequately resolved the conflict between initiative and guilt, the conflict may be played out later in the guise of a conversion disorder, inhibition, or phobia. The person who overcompensates for the conflict by driving himself or herself too hard may undergo such stress as to produce psychosomatic symptoms.

Industry versus inferiority (about 5 years to about 13 years) The child has now entered latency and has discovered the pleasures of production. It has developed industry by learning new skills and takes pride in the things made. Erikson wrote in *Childhood and Society* that the child's "ego boundaries include his tools and skills: the work principle . . . teaches him the pleasure of work completion by steady attention and persevering diligence." As the child works, it identifies with its teachers and imagines itself in various occupational roles.

If the child is unprepared for that stage of psychosocial development, either through insufficient resolution of previous stages or by current interference, the child may despair of ever amounting to much and may develop a sense of inferiority and inadequacy. Society, in the form of teachers and other role models, becomes crucially important in the child's ability to overcome that sense of inferiority and to achieve the virtue known as *competence.* In *Identity: Youth and Crisis* Erikson wrote: "[T]his is socially a most decisive stage. Since industry involves doing things beside and with others, a first sense of division of labor and of differential opportunity—that is, a sense of the technological ethos of a culture—develops at this time."

The pathological outcome of a poorly navigated stage is less well defined in industry versus inferiority than in previous stages, but it may concern the emergence of a slavish immersion into the world of production, so that creativity is stifled and identity is subsumed under the worker's role.

Identity versus identity confusion (about 13 years to about 21 years) With the onset of puberty and its myriad social and physiological changes, the adolescent becomes preoccupied with the question of identity. Erikson noted in *Childhood and Society* that youth are now "primarily concerned with what they appear to be in the eyes of others as compared to what they feel they are, and with the question of how to connect the roles and skills cultivated earlier with the occupational prototypes of the day." Childhood roles and fantasies are no longer appropriate, yet the adolescent is far from equipped to become an adult. In *Childhood and Society* Erikson wrote that the integration that occurs in the formation of ego identity encompasses far more than the summation of childhood identifications. "It is the accrued experience of the ego's ability to integrate these identifications with the vicissitudes of the libido, with the aptitudes developed out of endowment, and with the opportunities offered in social roles."

The formation of cliques and the intolerance of individual differences are ways in which the young person attempts to ward off a sense of identity loss. Falling in love—a process by which the adolescent clarifies a sense of identity by projecting a diffused self-image onto the partner and seeing it gradually assume a distinctive shape—and an overidentification with idealized figures are means by which adolescents seek to define themselves more clearly. With the attainment of a clearer identity, the youth develops the virtue of *fidelity,* a faithfulness not only to the nascent self-definition but to an ideology that provides a version of self-in-world. As Erik Erikson, Joan Erikson, and Helen Kinnik wrote in *Vital Involvement in Old Age:* "[F]idelity is the ability to sustain loyalties freely pledged in spite of the inevitable contradictions of value systems. It is the cornerstone of identity and receives inspiration from confirming ideologies and affirming companionships."

Identity confusion ensues when the person has been unable to formulate a sense of identity and belonging. Erikson holds that delinquency, gender identity disorders, and psychotic episodes can result from such confusion.

Intimacy versus isolation (about 21 years to about 40 years) Freud's famous response to the question of what a normal person should be able to do well—*"Lieben und arbeiten"* (to love and to work)—is one that Erikson often cited in his discussion of this psychosocial stage, and it underlines the importance he placed on the virtue of *love* within a balanced identity. Erikson asserted in *Identity: Youth and Crisis* that Freud's use of the term "love" referred to "the generosity of intimacy as well as genital love; when he said love and work, he meant a general work productiveness which would not preoccupy the individual to the extent that he might lose his right or capacity to be a sexual and a loving being."

The person who cannot tolerate the fear of ego loss arising out of experiences of self-abandonment (for example, sexual orgasm, moments of intensity in friendships, aggression, inspiration, and intuition) is apt to become deeply isolated and self-absorbed. *Distantiation,* an awkward term coined by Erikson in *Identity: Youth and Crisis* to mean "the readiness to repudiate, isolate, and, if necessary, destroy those forces and people whose essence seems dangerous to one's own," is the pathological outcome of conflicts surrounding intimacy and forms the basis for various forms of prejudice, persecution, and psychopathy.

Erikson's separation of the psychosocial task of achieving identity from that of achieving intimacy and his assertion that substantial progress on the former task must precede development on the latter task have engendered much criticism and debate. Critics have argued that Erikson's emphasis on separation and occupationally based identity formation fails to take into account the importance, for women, of continued attachment and the formation of an identity based on relationships.

Generativity versus stagnation (about 40 years to about 60 years) Erikson asserted in *Identity: Youth and Crisis* that "[g]enerativity . . . is primarily the concern for establishing and guiding the next generation." The term *generativity* applies not so much to rearing and teaching one's offspring as to a protective concern for all the generations and for social institutions. Having previously achieved the capacity to form intimate relationships, the person now broadens that investment of ego and libidinal energy to include groups, organizations, and society. *Care* is the virtue that coalesces at this stage. Erikson underlined the importance to the mature person of feeling needed; through generative behavior, the person is able to pass on knowledge and skills while obtaining a measure of satisfaction in having achieved a role with senior authority and responsibility in the tribe.

When persons are unable to develop true generativity, they may settle for pseudoengagement in occupational roles; or they may restrict their focus to the technical aspects of their roles, at which they may have become highly skilled, eschewing larger responsibility for their organization or profession. That failure of generativity can lead to profound personal stagnation, masked by a variety of escapisms, such as alcohol and drug abuse and sexual and other infidelities. Mid-life crisis or *premature invalidism* (physical and psychological) may occur. In that case, pathology appears not only in middle-aged persons but also in the organizations that depend on them for leadership. Thus, the person's failure to develop at mid-life can lead to sick and withered or destructive organizations that spread the effects of failed generativity throughout society. Examples of such failures have become so common as to constitute a defining feature of modernity.

Integrity versus despair (about 60 years to death) In *Identity: Youth and Crisis* Erikson defined integrity as "the acceptance of one's one and only life cycle and of the people who have become significant to it as something that had to be and that, by necessity, permitted of no substitutions." From the vantage point of this stage of psychosocial development, persons relinquish the wish that important people in their lives had been different and are able to love in a more meaningful way—one that reflects an acceptance of responsibility for one's own life. The person in possession of the virtue of *wisdom* and a sense of *integrity* has room to tolerate the proximity of death and to achieve what Erikson termed in *Identity: Youth and Crisis* a "detached yet active concern with life."

When the attempt to attain integrity has failed, the person may become deeply disgusted with the external world, contemptuous of both persons and institutions. Erikson wrote in

Identity: Youth and Crisis that such disgust masks a fear of death and a sense of despair that "time is short, too short for the attempt to start another life and to try out alternate roads to integrity."

Implications for therapists Erikson's belief that psychosocial development continues throughout the life cycle led him to caution psychotherapists against a theoretical reductionism in which symptomatic behavior is viewed as the result of a traumatic past and in which insufficient attention is paid to contemporary conflicts in the ego's relations with the world. A psychotherapy informed by Eriksonian principles emphasizes not only interpretations based on reconstruction but also an analysis of the patient's struggles with current developmental tasks. When patients' resolutions of previous psychosocial stages have been so faulty as to seriously compromise their adult development, they have the opportunity to rework early development through the relationship with the therapist. For example, the psychotherapeutic treatment of the person who suffers a schizophrenic break in young adulthood initially revolves around the painstaking establishment of a sense of basic trust between the patient and the therapist. However, the treatment eventually has to consider contemporary obstacles to building a sense of identity in work and intimacy in relations with others.

Psychotherapy is an intervention—sometimes an entire chapter—in the ongoing biography of the patient. The treatment uses new energies to redirect the patient, whose psychosocial development has been blocked. By dint of temperament, education, and conscientious self-analysis, the therapist is prepared to identify and to promote a variety of directions that subsequent development may take, avoiding a countertransference rigidity that could further inhibit the patient's growth. As Erikson noted in *Identity: Youth and Crisis,* the object of psychotherapy is not to head off future conflict but to assist the patient in emerging from each crisis "with an increased sense of inner unity, with an increase of good judgment, and an increase in the capacity 'to do well' according to his own standards and to the standards of those who are significant to him."

BECOMING A BIOGRAPHER OF YOUTH In 1949, as *Childhood and Society* was going to press, Erikson's stand on the University of California loyalty oath had rendered his position at the university untenable. News of his availability spread east, and other institutions vied to capitalize on the university's mistake. Erikson was well known at the Menninger Clinic in Topeka, Kansas, where he had lectured, so when Robert Knight left the clinic to become the director of the Austen Riggs Center in Stockbridge, Massachusets, he took Erikson with him. The Austen Riggs Center was devoted to psychoanalytic research and to the treatment of severely disturbed adolescents and young adults. Erikson had been happily adopted once again.

Erikson stayed at Austen Riggs from 1950 to 1960, from age 48 to 58, when he returned to the faculty at Harvard University. During those years, Erikson completed the transition to biographer, forming more fully the approach foreshadowed in his incomplete essays on Hitler, Gorky, and George Bernard Shaw. The transition was not easy; Coles describes that time as constituting a second "identity crisis." The authors say that, having completed the mid-life transition and having left the era of early adulthood, Erikson faced the difficult developmental task in his late 40s and early 50s of forming and revising a life structure for middle age. He had been a clinician and a theorist of youth. He was now old enough to enact the program promised in *Childhood and Society* and to become a biographer and theorist of the whole life cycle. But before he wrote *Young Man Luther,* he once again returned to Freud and the origins of his own professional identity. The way to the future was through the past.

In his early 50s, Erikson wrote three biographical essays on Freud: "The Dream Specimen of Psychoanalysis," "Freud's 'The Origins of Psychoanalysis,'" and "The First Psychoanalyst." Those essays all concern themselves with the crisis Freud suffered during his own mid-life transition, as he struggled to leave neuropathology and to define a new professional identity as a psychoanalyst. Strengthened by that reexamination of Freud's successful transition (and perhaps having reassured himself of Freud's blessing), Erikson began writing one of the genuine masterworks of psychoanalysis, *Young Man Luther.*

As always, Erikson's clinical work and observations enriched his theorizing about the life cycle. He acknowledged his debt to Austen Riggs and the Western Psychiatric Institute at the University of Pittsburgh in his preface to *Young Man Luther.* His work there had allowed him to "study the afflictions of young patients as variations on one theme, namely, a *life crisis,* aggravated in patients, yet in some form normal for all youth. I could identify those acute *life tasks* that would bring young people to a state of tension in which some would become patients."

But he would neither make Martin Luther a patient nor reify the psychopathology of the young people who were his patients. Instead, he asserted that comparisons between Martin Luther and his patients were "not restricted to psychiatric diagnosis . . . but . . . oriented toward those moments when young patients, like young beings anywhere, prove resourceful and insightful beyond all professional and personal expectation. *We will concentrate on the powers of recovery inherent in the young ego.*" [Italics added.]

Working with the young Riggs patients helped Erikson hone his understanding of identity formation. As he later put it in "The Problem of Ego Identity," "From a genetic point of view, . . . the process of identity formation emerges as . . . a configuration which is gradually established by successive ego syntheses and re-syntheses throughout childhood. It is a configuration gradually integrating *constitutional givens, idiosyncratic libidinal needs, favored capacities, significant identifications, effective defenses, successful sublimations, and consistent roles.*"

Those "ego syntheses and re-syntheses" were about to receive great attention as he attempted his biography of Luther. But to do that work, Erikson the biographer had to move further away from his own professional origins as a child psychoanalyst. He had criticized psychoanalysis for its *originology,* which he defined as the belief that something has been explained by making an analogy to its earliest manifestations. Yet his own conception of the life cycle, with most of its stages occurring within the preadult era, left him still heavily rooted in childhood. In his study of Luther he was trying to understand a life, not just a personality; from that perspective, childhood and adolescence had to be introductory, rather than the story itself.

Seeing that a child-centered view was not adequate for the tasks of biography, Erikson deftly, without either formally changing the imbalance in his theory or neglecting childhood determinants, devoted the greatest attention to an explication of development in the adult years. So successful was he in interrelating Luther's adult problems with those of his early development that *Young Man Luther* provided the seminal inspiration for the next generation of life-cycle investigators. Some of those investigators formally redressed in their own theories the originological bias vestigial in Erikson's theory.

In Luther's early or mid-20s, according to some of his contemporaries, the young monk had fallen to the floor of the choir of his monastery in a fit and shouted, *"Ich bin's nit!"* or *"Non Sum!"*—"It isn't me," or "I am not." Erikson's task as a psychological biographer was to explain how Luther got from the identity crisis of his 20s to nailing his 95 theses to the door of the church in Wittenberg at 32. Yet *Young Man Luther* is also, as it is subtitled, a study in psychoanalysis and history. Since it is not a psychoanalysis of history, some nonreductionist connecting concepts between the person and the collectivity were needed. One of Erikson's connecting concepts was *ideology,* which he defined as "an unconscious tendency underlying religious and scientific as well as political thought: the tendency at a given time to make facts amenable to ideas, and ideas to facts, in order to create a world image convincing enough to support the collective and the individual sense of identity."

Luther had personal and even psychiatric problems, but, in his defiance of Catholic orthodoxy, he created a new religious ideology that not only supported his own identity but the identities of emerging generations of Europeans as well. *"Ich bin's nit,"* expressed the young monk's identity crisis, as he found himself "fatally overcommitted" to what he was not—a young man authentically embarking on a future as an orthodox Catholic priest. "In some periods of history," Erikson concluded in his preface, "and in some phases of his life cycle, man needs . . . a new ideological orientation as surely and as sorely as he must have air and food." As such a man, Luther commanded Erikson's "sympathy and empathy" as he "faced the problems of human *existence* in the most forward terms of his era."

The reception of the book cemented Erikson's reputation, initially won by *Childhood and Society* and now international, as the leader in original, humane thought about psychological development. In no other biography have the dynamics of individual conflict and development been so seamlessly interwoven with those of society and history. With *Young Man Luther,* in his late 50s, Erikson ascended from the first rank of developmental psychoanalysts to that of a cultural seer and international *Gehlehrte.*

BECOMING A BIOGRAPHER OF MIDDLE AGE As Erikson moved through the transition from middle age to old age, he abandoned clinical work with patients to turn his attention fully to the study of the life cycle and the survival of the species. His emphasis, emergent in *Young Man Luther* and implicit in all his earlier work, was on the ego virtues that permit a person to live in a constructively critical relation with the social institutions of the time. Earlier, Erikson had described the stages in the development of the ego across the life cycle. In 1964 he wrote more about the ego virtues in *Insight and Responsibility.* He was getting ready, amid the American moral and political crises of the mid-1960s, to embark on his last major work, a study of the great moral leader Mohandas Gandhi. In the end he dedicated it to Martin Luther King, Jr.

Young Man Luther had been a story of personal choice and historical change wrought by a young man establishing and revising a first adult life structure. Erikson, in his mid-60s, had gained sufficient perspective on the life cycle to analyze a case of decisive crisis and change in a man who was going through a mid-life transition and solving it by creating a vital life structure for middle age. Gandhi did that, as he himself put it, by realizing "his vocation in life," leading *satyagraha* (truth force) campaigns in his nation, in his family, and in his own soul. Gandhi was entering the stage of the life cycle in which Erikson's ego polarity of *generativity versus stagnation* becomes active; from his developmental work on that polarity, Gandhi was earning the ego virtue of *care.*

Erikson saw that Gandhi, like Luther, was both a leader and a *religious actualist.* As a leader, he succeeded in articulating inner concerns in a way that struck a collective chord. Self-rule and home rule were inextricably combined in Gandhi's program. He would have endorsed in his own terms, Erikson believed, Luther's assertions, "Christ comes today; God's way is what makes us move; we must always be reborn, renewed, regenerated; to do enough means nothing else than always to begin again."

Gandhi had begun and successfully completed his political novitiate as an Oxford-trained barrister in South Africa during his 20s and 30s. By his late 30s, he had developed passive resistance as a political strategy to defeat the Black Act, a law that required all Indians in the Transvaal to register with the government and to carry identification papers on their persons. At 40 he staked out his claim for leadership in his Indian Home Rule Manifesto, and during the next few years of his mid-life transition he developed the device of the *satyagraha* campaign, culminating in the great march of striking mine workers in South Africa when he was 44.

When Gandhi returned to India in 1915, at 45, he did so, Erikson wrote, "like a man who knew the nature and the extent of India's calamity and that of his own fundamental mission." As a mature, middle-aged man, he was, in Erikson's view, a person who has determined what "he does and does not *care for*" as well as "what he *will* and *can* take *care of.* He takes as his baseline what he irreducibly *is* and reaches out for what only he can, and therefore, *must do.*"

What Gandhi had to do was lead a labor strike at the mill in Ahmedabad and the next year, at 50, a national strike for independence from Great Britain. "At the time of the Ahmedabad strike," Erikson wrote, "Gandhi was forty-eight years old. . . . That the very next year he emerged as the father of his country only lends greater importance to the fact that the middle span of life is under the dominance of the universal human need and strength which I have come to subsume under the term *generativity.*" Erikson refers here not merely to the generativity that a parent at 20 or 30 may feel for a child. That point is important because Erikson's concept of generativity in often mistakenly taken to apply to the child-rearing work of young adults. He is describing the protective concern for the generations and their retarding-facilitating social institutions, which is the special, though not sole, province of the middle-aged.

In the early 1970s Erikson returned to the San Francisco Bay area to live and begin again. The Eriksons returned to Cambridge, Massachusetts, some 10 years later. In 1981 the Eriksons and psychologist Helen Kivnik undertook an intensive study of 29 octogenarian parents of children whose lives had been meticulously scrutinized in the guidance study begun in 1928 at the Institute of Human Development at the University of California at Berkeley. Their book, *Vital Involvement in Old Age,* described in rich detail the ways in which the fundamental polarities of the eight stages must be reworked and reintegrated in late life. The joint reflections on old age contained in the book are at once an effort to elucidate the psychosocial process of vital involvement and an attempt by Erikson to extend his observations to the outer limits of the life cycle.

SUGGESTED CROSS-REFERENCES

Sigmund Freud's ideas are discussed most fully in Section 6.1. Other theories of personality and psychopathology are discussed in Chapters 7 and 8. Schizophrenia is discussed in Chapter 14, mood disorders in Chapter 16, personality disorders in Chapter 25, and psychosomatic disorders in Chapter 26. Normal child development and adolescent development are discussed in Sections 33.2 and 33.3, respectively; adulthood is discussed in Chapter 48, normal human sexuality in Section 21.1, and normal aging in Section 49.4. Psychoanalysis and psychoanalytic psychotherapy are discussed in Section 31.1.

REFERENCES

Auden W H: Greatness finding itself. In *Forewords and Afterwords,* E Mendelson, editor, p 79. Vintage, New York, 1974.

Bailey W T: Psychological development in men: Generativity and involvement with young children. Psychol Rep *71:* 929, 1992.

Butz M R: The fractal nature of the development of the self. Psychol Rep *71:* 1043, 1992.

*Coles R: *Erik H. Erikson: The Growth of His Work.* Little, Brown, Boston, 1970.

Cote J E: Foundations of a psychoanalytic social psychology: Neo-Eriksonian propositions regarding the relationship between psychic structure and cultural institutions. Dev Rev *13:* 31, 1993.

*Erikson E: *Childhood and Society.* Norton, New York, 1950.

Erikson E: The dream specimen of psychoanalysis. J Am Psychoanal Assoc *2:* 5, 1954.

Erikson E: The first psychoanalyst. Yale Rev *46:* 40, 1956.

Erikson E: Freud's "The Origins of Psychoanalysis." Int J Psychoanal *36:* 1, 1955.

*Erikson E: *Gandhi's Truth.* Norton, New York, 1969.

Erikson E: Hitler's imagery and German youth. Psychiatry *5:* 475, 1942.

Erikson E: *Identity and the Life Cycle.* Norton, New York, 1980.

Erikson E: *Identity: Youth and Crisis.* Norton, New York, 1968.

Erikson E: *Insight and Responsibility.* Norton, New York, 1964.

Erikson E: *Life History and the Historical Moment.* Norton, New York, 1975.

Erikson E: Observations on Sioux education, J Psychol *7:* 101, 1939.

Erikson E: The problem of ego identity. Psychol Issues *1:* 379, 1959.

*Erikson E: *Young Man Luther.* Norton, New York, 1962.

Erikson E, Erikson J, Kivnik H: *Vital Involvement in Old Age.* Norton, New York, 1986.

Evans R: *Dialogue with Erik Erikson.* Harper & Row, New York, 1967.

Freud A: *The Ego and the Mechanisms of Defense.* International Universities Press, New York, 1966.

Freud S: Beyond the pleasure principle. In *Standard Edition of the Complete Psychological Works of Sigmund Freud,* vol 18, p 7. Hogarth Press, London, 1955.

Freud S: Civilization and its discontents. In *Standard Edition of the Complete Psychological Works of Sigmund Freud,* vol 21, p 64. Hogarth Press, London, 1961.

Freud S: The ego and the id. In *Standard Edition of the Complete Psychological Works of Sigmund Freud,* vol 19, p 19. Hogarth Press, London, 1961.

Freud S: The future of an illusion. In *Standard Edition of the Complete Psychological Works of Sigmund Freud,* vol 21, p 5. Hogarth Press, London, 1961.

Freud S: Group psychology and the analysis of the ego. In *Standard Edition of the Complete Psychological Works of Sigmund Freud,* vol 18, p 69. Hogarth Press, London, 1955.

Gilligan C: Woman's place in man's life cycle. Harv Educ Rev *49:* 431, 1979.

Howenstine R, Silberstein L, Newton D, Newton P: Revitalizing the life structure: An adult developmental approach to psychodynamic psychotherapy. Psychiatry *55:* 194, 1992.

*Levinson D: *The Seasons of a Man's Life.* Knopf, New York, 1978.

McAdams D P, de St Aubin E, Logan R L: Generativity among young, midlife, and older adults. Psychol Aging *8:* 221, 1993.

Murray H: *Explorations in Personality: A Clinical and Experimental Study of 50 Men of College Age.* Oxford University Press, New York, 1938.

Newton P: Freud's mid-life crisis and the birth of psychoanalysis. Psychoanal Psychol *9:* 22, 1992.

Newton P: Samuel Johnson's breakdown and recovery in middle-age: A lifespan developmental approach to mental illness and its cure. Int J Psychoanal *11:* 93, 1984.

Newton P: Science and humanism in the biographical study of lives. Contemp Psychiatry *7:* 77, 1988.

Newton P, Levinson D: Crises in adult development. In *Outpatient Psychiatry,* A Lazare, editor. Williams & Wilkins, Baltimore, 1979.

O'Connell A N: The relationship between life style and identity synthesis and resynthesis in traditional, neotraditional, and nontraditional women. J Pers *44:* 675, 1976.

Peterson B E, Stewart A J: Generativity and social motives in young adults. J Pers Soc Psychol *65:* 186, 1993.

Roker D, Banks M H: Adolescent identity and school type. Br J Psychol *84:* 297, 1993.

Schein S, editor: *Erik Erikson: A Way of Looking at Things.* Norton, New York, 1987.

Vondracek F W: The construct of identity and its use in career theory and research. Career Dev Q *41:* 130, 1992.

CHAPTER 7 THEORIES OF PERSONALITY AND PSYCHOPATHOLOGY: OTHER PSYCHODYNAMIC SCHOOLS

MYRON F. WEINER, M.D.
PAUL C. MOHL, M.D.

INTRODUCTION

The subject of this chapter is the work of Adolf Meyer, Alfred Adler, Carl Gustav Jung, Sandor Rado, Melanie Klein, Otto Rank, Karen Horney, Franz Alexander, Harry Stack Sullivan, Wilhelm Reich, Erich Fromm, Jules H. Masserman, and Eric Berne.

Although the 13 men and women presented in this chapter made their contributions in the early and middle years of this century, they are worlds apart from present-day psychiatry. Theirs was a simpler world, more subject to capture in overarching theories of the mind. None of them doubted that mind has a physical basis, but they were not burdened by having to explain the relationship of mental phenomena to neurotransmitter systems or changes in cerebral metabolism. Because of that, they were able to stand back from the physical organism and view humans as psychological entities.

Their lack of technology and their inability to assess brain function directly forced them to learn about their patients psychologically, thus blurring the distinction between diagnostic entities and emphasizing the common elements of different psychopathologies. Carl Gustav Jung stated that, with each new patient, he had to abandon all theory and listen afresh. Contrast that statement with the current trend to diagnose and treat by manual. Present-day psychiatrists are not more scientific in their approach because they have formulated criteria and created manuals. The scientific method involves observation, hypothesis formation, hypothesis testing, and coming to conclusions. All the theorists considered in this chapter were scientists in that sense. The proof of their theories is that they fit the observations. Their major flaw is that, with the exception of Meyer and Masserman, they overexplained mental phenomena in psychological terms.

This chapter addresses the contributions of the 13 theorists to the current view of normal personality development, psychopathology, and the treatment of both mental illnesses and the minor emotional disorders. Their greatest contribution is their effort to make mental and emotional disturbances understandable as psychological phenomena. They were able to do so in large measure because of their involvement with psychoanalysis, whose basic credo is that mental and emotional symptoms are potentially understandable in psychological terms.

All except Adolf Meyer had experience with or trained in psychoanalysis. Alfred Adler, Carl Gustav Jung, Otto Rank, Wilhelm Reich, Sandor Rado, and Franz Alexander had strong personal involvements with Sigmund Freud. Jung was Freud's first heir apparent. To Alexander, Freud wrote in 1926, "all of us [in psychoanalysis] count on you as one of our strongest hopes for the future." Except for Klein, Rank, and Fromm, all were physicians. All had unique, strong personalities. Many had schools of therapy develop around them; the schools were partly of their own devising and partly based on the needs of their followers to establish a credo. The best-known schools are Jung's analytic psychology, Adler's individual psychology, and Berne's transactional analysis. Theories of personality development and psychopathology and the treatment methods were confirmed by consensus among their followers. The theories developed and the treatment techniques based on those theories are widely divergent.

The divergence of those theories and techniques and their success as explanations and treatments suggest that each is useful in some contexts and that none is applicable in every context. In attempting to use any of the theories or techniques, one must ask what theory or technique is useful with what patient under what circumstances and in the hands of what therapist, instead of attempting to force all patients into one theoretical conceptualization or one treatment modality.

ADOLF MEYER

Adolf Meyer (1866–1950) emigrated to the United States after having trained as a neuropathologist in Europe (Figure 7-1). Not interested in metapsychology, he espoused a commonsense psychobiological method for the study of mental disorder, emphasizing the interrelationship of symptoms and individual psychological and biological functions. His approach to the study of personality was biographical. Despite his biological orientation, he supported the psychotherapeutic treatment of schizophrenia. He attempted to bring psychiatric patients and their treatment out of isolated state hospitals and into communities, and he was also a strong advocate of social action for mental health. His career began as a clinically oriented state hospital pathologist and culminated in the presidency of the American Psychiatric Association and a 32-year tenure as chairman of the psychiatry department at Johns Hopkins University. His major social contribution was helping to found the National Committee on Mental Hygiene.

PSYCHOBIOLOGY Meyer strongly opposed Emil Kraepelin's view of mental illness as having a predetermined course. Instead, he proposed a dynamic point of view. He held that habitual reaction patterns made persons susceptible to specific types of breakdown. Meyer used biographical study to understand each person's reaction patterns. He observed reaction patterns, attempted to predict the conditions under which they might occur, and tested and validated methods for their modification. He acknowledged the contributions of Freud and Jung but thought they were too narrow. A thoroughgoing pragmatist, he preferred common sense to metapsychological constructs as the means to understand and deal with psychopathology.

Meyer believed that, through a basic tendency toward integration, multiple biological, social, and psychological forces

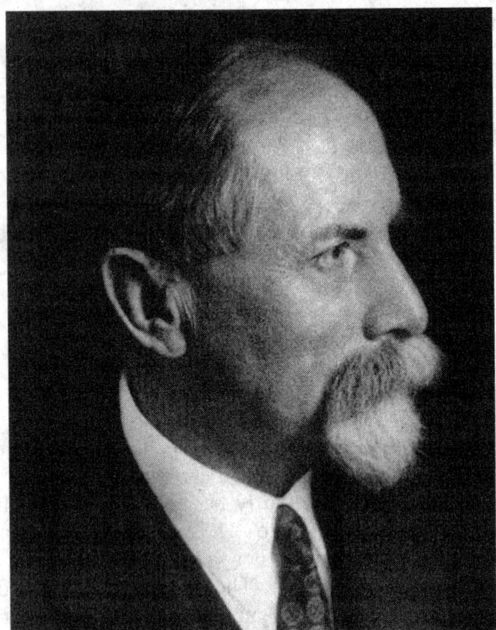

FIGURE 7-1 *Adolph Meyer. (Courtesy of New York Academy of Medicine.)*

contribute to personality development. The vulnerable person uses poorly planned, ill-adapted means. Meyer saw in the biographical approach a practical guide for eliciting information about personality development, for organizing the information, and for checking and reevaluating information obtained under different circumstances. His clinical examination assessed each patient's life history; physical, neurological, genetic, and social status; and the relation between those factors and personality factors. A diagnosis and an individual treatment plan were based on that assessment.

TREATMENT The aim of his psychobiological therapy was to help patients make the best possible adaptation to changing environmental circumstances. It began with the development of a collaborative relationship. Out of the collaborative relationship came distributive analysis, an examination of the factors in patients' lives that contributed to their adjustment or lack of adjustment, and concluded with distributive synthesis, helping patients understand themselves and thereby develop better coping skills. The first step in distributive analysis is the patient's own exposition of the presenting problem. The patient's assets and liabilities are then determined by eliciting the patient's life history in terms of the memories immediately available and later fleshed out by reconstructing past experiences.

The cooperation of the healthy aspect of the patient's personality is needed, and treatment is initiated by focusing on the patient's assets. Therapy involves psychological, chemical, physical, and environmental measures as needed. In severe cases, attention is paid first to the patients' sleep habits, nutrition, and daily routines, which must be normalized before any psychological work can be done. Patients are helped to describe their difficulties in detail. The therapist elicits patients' complaints or worries and asks what eases or worsens their complaints or worries and what significance they attach to their symptoms and concerns. In doing that, the therapist attempts to use the patients' own language and concepts to communicate suggestions and advice.

Meyer did not concern himself with the Freudian unconscious but, instead, focused on the patient's functioning in reality. Both present-day and long-term adaptive patterns were considered. Therapeutic sessions proceeded from immediate, obvious problems in the present to longer-term issues and historical data. With guidance, patients investigated their personality problems, ascertained the origin of their conflicts, and worked to develop more useful behavior patterns, the latter termed ''habit training.'' When unhealthy adaptive patterns were modified, proper adjustment and personal satisfaction resulted.

ALFRED ADLER

Alfred Adler (1870–1937) was born in Vienna and spent most of his life there (Figure 7-2). A general physician, he became one of the original four members of Freud's circle in 1902. Adler never accepted the primacy of the libido theory, the sexual origin of neurosis, or the importance of infantile wishes. In 1911 he resigned as president of the Vienna Psychoanalytic Society and continued the development of his own socially conscious theory of development. His personality theory posited a striving for self-esteem and attempting to overcome a sense of inferiority. He equated psychological health with constructive social consciousness. He developed a system that he called individual psychology, which is still vigorous in many countries. His major social contribution was the establishment of child guidance centers in Vienna that served as a model for the rest of the world.

PERSONALITY THEORY If Adolf Meyer's system were captured in a phrase, that phrase would be ''common sense.'' Adler's system may be described in a word as *Menschenkenntnis,* the concrete, practical knowledge of humankind. In contrast to Freud and his emphasis on unconscious intrapsychic conflict, Adler saw persons as unique, unified biological entities, all of whose psychological processes fit and justify an individual lifestyle *(Lebensstil).* In addition to that principle of unity, Adler postulated a principle of dynamism—that every person is future-directed and moves toward a goal. Once the goal is established, the psychic apparatus shapes itself toward the attainment of that goal. Life goals are chosen and are thus subject to change; such changes require the modification of memories,

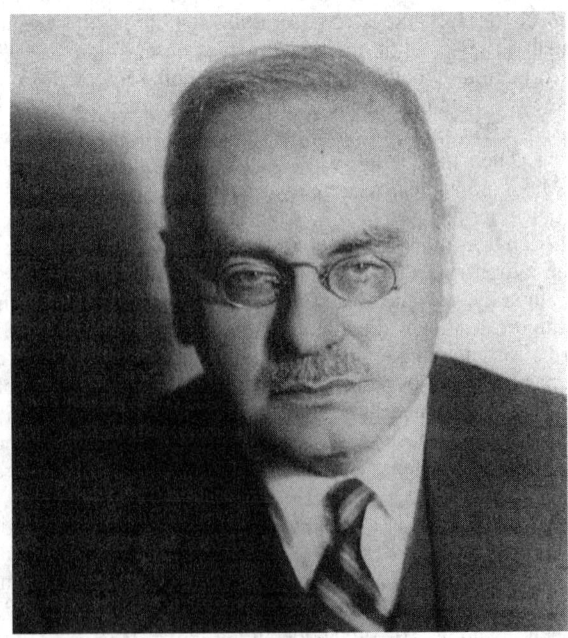

FIGURE 7-2 *Alfred Adler. (Courtesy of Alexandra Adler and James Moore.)*

dreams, and perceptions to fit the accomplishment of that goal. Adler also emphasized the interface between persons and their social environment and emphasized action in the real world over fantasy. Community-mindedness, acceptance of the need to conform to the legitimate demands of society, is an important precept, but Adler also indicated that a dialectic occurs between persons and their interpersonal environment, each constantly reacting to and shaping the other.

Normal personality and adaptation The cornerstone of Adler's personality theory is the concept of moving from a sense of inferiority to a sense of mastery. Early in life, everyone has a sense of inferiority resulting from realistic comparison with adults' size and abilities. Moving from that sense of inferiority to a sense of adequacy is the important motivational motif in life. Thus, the ideal person strives for superiority and does so through high social interest and activity; the emotionally handicapped person continues to feel inferior and reinforces that position through lack of striving and social interest.

Many obstacles may block the development of self-esteem and social interest. Prominent among them are poorly developed or inferior organs or systems (such as poor eyesight and poor eye-hand coordination), childhood diseases, pampering, and neglect. Physical handicaps and childhood diseases may promote self-centeredness and loss of social interest. Another factor contributing to personality development is birth order. First-born children, after they have lost their position of only child, tend to not share. They become conservative. Second children favor change and become social activists. Youngest children feel secure because they have never been displaced.

THEORY OF PSYCHOPATHOLOGY Emotional disorders result from mistaken life-styles, which are subject to change by will and by self-understanding. Persons subject to emotional disorders have false ideas about themselves and the world and inappropriate goals that lead them away from constructive social interests. Those with a pampered life-style, for example, expect and demand from others, avoid responsibility, and blame others for their failures but, because their well-being depends on pressing others into service, feel incompetent and insecure. If life poses no challenge, a mistaken life-style may have no consequences. When a mistaken life-style is ineffective, symptoms develop. Those symptoms protect self-esteem while helping the person avoid dealing realistically with the problem being confronted. The difference between minor and major mental disorders is that those with minor disorders maintain social interest but are blocked from life goals by symptoms but those with major mental disorders lose social interest and retreat to their own worlds.

PSYCHOTHERAPY Because Adler's theory emphasized the harmony of the psychic apparatus and the dysharmony of mistaken life-styles with the demands of the real world, he focused on blocks to living productively in the real world and not on exploring unconscious conflicts. His aim was to point out mistaken self-views and mistaken views of the world and then, by mobilizing will, to make the needed changes, including a change in life goal.

Therapeutic process Starting with three sessions a week and tapering off to once a week, the therapist establishes a positive relationship with patients and, in the context of that relationship, leads patients to an awareness of their life-styles and reorients and reeducates them. Instead of striving for goals of no social value that falsely raise self-esteem, the patients are pushed to work toward ameliorating their real situations. Having become aware of the obstacles they have placed in their own paths and of the discouragement caused by those self-defeating behaviors, the patients are helped to develop constructive interests in themselves and others. As they become less self-engaged, they find themselves better accepted by others, which reinforces their constructive efforts. Persons who have dedicated themselves to symbolically defeating others (he has a better job than I, but I am better than he because I would not prostitute myself to the system by working long hours) learn to cooperate and advance toward useful goals (I am now willing to work for what I want and to risk failure). Any endeavor in which patients can develop real competence is encouraged, whether social, work, artistic, or musical.

Patients are encouraged to remove the concrete obstacles to their developing a useful life-style; slow readers are encouraged to get reading instruction, and persons who wear glasses but are self-conscious about their appearance are encouraged to get contact lenses. Early recollections, birth order, dreams, daydreams, and present-day interactions are all used to help patients see the inappropriateness or falseness of their ideas and life goals. Actual life events or memories of events are less important than the patients' reactions to those events or memories. Because memories are likely to be retrospective falsifications that justify an erroneous life-style, the therapist need not ascertain their truth or falseness. Nor need the therapist look for latent content in dreams; they are merely expressions of present-day concerns. Nor need the therapist's interpretations be correct. They need only help patients build a useful conception of themselves and the world.

Several of Adler's techniques now enjoy wide popularity. They include reframing and paradoxical communication. *Reframing* is viewing data from a different point of view. Indecision, for example, is reframed from being a product of mixed feelings to a wish to maintain the status quo. Failure to act keeps everything the same, which is the self-fulfilling prophecy of the discouraged person. After the reframing statement, the therapist pushes patients to act constructively. *Paradoxical communication* is instructing patients to do the opposite of what the therapist wishes them to do. In dealing with an indecisive person, for example, the therapist may caution against doing anything rash. Adler also paid attention to the effects of his patients on their environment and recognized that persons do much to create their own interpersonal worlds. In response to complaints about being treated unfairly by others, Adler would ask patients how they dealt with the persons about whom they complained. Above all, Adler treated his patients as rational and as able to learn productive ways of living.

CARL GUSTAV JUNG

Carl Gustav Jung (1875–1961) was a lifelong resident of Switzerland (Figure 7-3). He trained in psychiatry under Eugen Bleuler at the Burgholzli Mental Hospital in Zurich. He was strongly involved with Freud and the psychoanalytic movement from 1906 to 1914, when he resigned as president of the International Psychoanalytic Association. After a "creative illness" that lasted from 1914 to 1918, Jung emerged as an advocate of active introspection as the means to intrapsychic change. Although he rejected Freud's notion of libido as sexual energy and the Oedipus complex as a universal developmental stage, he believed not only in the unconscious mind but in a shared collective unconscious. In his own typology an intuitive introvert, Jung was not interested in the practical aspects of living in the world. His focus was on individuation through becoming aware of the unconscious. Jung founded a school of psychotherapy and psychology that he named *analytic psychology*.

PERSONALITY THEORY Jung developed an elaborate metapsychology. His construct of the psychic apparatus differed from the Freudian topology of ego, superego, id, and ego-ideal, diagramed for the sake of comparison in Figure 7-4. Figure 7-5 presents Jung's view of the psychic apparatus. Below an outer rim of consciousness is the personal unconscious, containing the complexes. Contained within the personal unconscious and connected to the complexes are the archetypes, the elements of the self, which in turn connects to the surface of the personality as the ego.

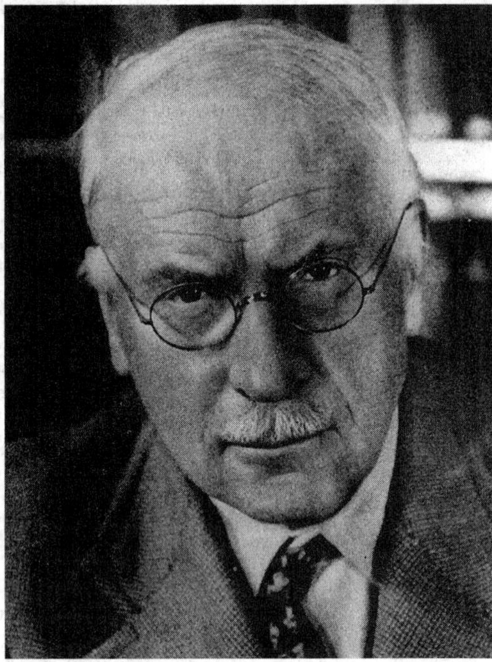

FIGURE 7-3 *Carl Gustav Jung. (Courtesy of Routledge and Kegan Paul, Ltd.)*

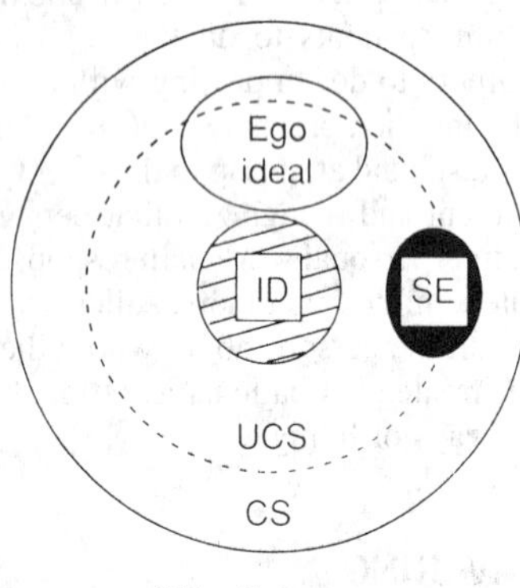

FIGURE 7-4 *The Freudian topology of the psychic apparatus.*

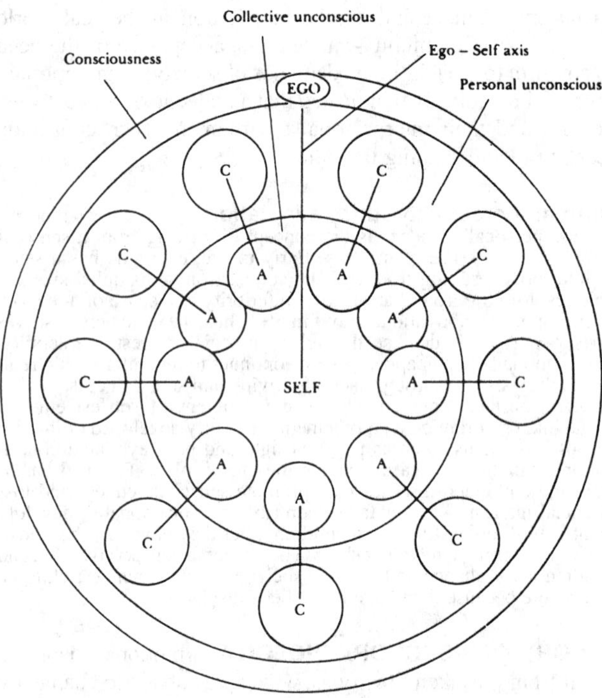

FIGURE 7-5 *The Jungian psychic apparatus. (From A Stevens:* On Jung, *p 29. Routledge, London, 1990. Used with permission.)*

Complexes Complexes are groups of unconscious ideas associated with particular emotionally toned events or experiences. Jung inferred them from his early word-association studies when he noted that certain words provoke intense reactions or produce less reaction than expected. Complexes are built around hard-wired psychic structures known as archetyes, which are explained below. Complexes are also reinforced by environmental events and by selective attention or inattention and are thus self-perpetuating. They are endowed with psychic energy from their affective tone—positive, negative, mild, or strong. The more intense the complex, the greater the emotion, imagery, and tendency to action. Complexes are often stimulated by interactions with others. A father complex can be stimulated by a person who symbolizes a father (such as an older friend) or by a stimulus, such as music or art, that evokes father memories. The complex, formerly dormant in the unconscious, comes to the fore and tends to dominate consciousness and to displace other complexes, which then sink into unconsciousness. Father-related emotions, images, memories, and ideas come to awareness and are expressed during this period, called "lowering of consciousness." As the father-related external stimuli diminish, so may the father complex, including what was thought, felt, and expressed during its ascendancy.

Some complexes are conscious, well developed, and ego-syntonic; others are less conscious, poorly developed, and ego-alien. The latter are projected into the environment, especially by the immature psyches of children; from that process, projective and introjective processes evolve. One person may introject and identify with a complex being projected by another person. Thus, therapists may become psychologically infected by their patients. One may also project a complex that is not integrated into oneself onto another person and then develop a relationship with that projected complex. One can envision an interpersonal environment charged with projected complexes potentially available for introjection, thus offering endless potential for psychic mutation in an interpersonal field.

Another important aspect of complexes is their bipolarity. Each complex has a positive pole and a negative pole, such as good father and bad father or rewarding father and punishing father. One pole of a complex can be projected onto another person, who in turns acts on it in a relationship. In that way the theory of complexes is a theory of interpersonal relationships as well as intrapsychic relationships.

In Jungian theory the ego is also a complex. It serves the same function as the Freudian ego, controlling conscious life and bridging the intrapsychic world and the external world. The other complexes that make up the psyche may align with or oppose the ego. For example, emotionally charged primitive complexes have a great tendency to become autonomous and may behave like partial personalities that oppose or control the ego. Those personalities appear as images in dreams, as hallucinations, and as separate personalities in cases of multiple personality disorder. They also appear in seances when mediums bring forth so-called personalities from the dead. For Jung, that phenomenon also explained animism and states of possession.

Archetypes Complexes are connected to structures embedded deeply in the psychic apparatus, the archetypes (Figure 7-5). Complexes, the superficial aspect of the complex-archetype continuum, are related to events, feelings, and memories from individual lives. They are the means by which archetypes express themselves in the personal psyche. Archetypes are inherited capacities to initiate and carry out behaviors typical of all human beings, regardless of race or culture, such as nurturing and accepting nurturance, becoming aggressive, and dealing with aggression by others. Those predispositions are analogous to the organization of the cerebral cortex into the anlage for perception of visual or auditory stimuli that becomes the capacity to see and hear but that specifically requires stimulation for its development. Just as vision cannot develop without visual input during physiologically critical stages, so archetypes require interactional stimulation for their elaboration into complexes. Thus, the human infant's psyche is not amorphous energy awaiting organization by the environment. It is, instead, a complex and organized set of potentials whose fulfillment and expression depend on the appropriate environmental stimuli. There are as many archetypes as there are prototypical human situations.

The mother complex-archetype illustrates the interrelation of complex and archetype. The mother complex is based on experiences with mothers or mother surrogates—their attitudes, personalities, and relationship to the person. The mother archetype is found in dreams or fantasies, often as a huge woman or an animal with many breasts. The motif of a many-breasted animal, found in many cultures, is that of unlimited nurturance.

Unconscious In contrast to Freud's unconscious (Figure 7-4), the Jungian unconscious has two layers, the more superficial layer being the personal unconscious and the deeper layer being the collective unconscious. The complexes exist in the personal unconscious, the archetypes in the collective unconscious or objective psyche. The *personal unconscious* is the equivalent of the Freudian unconscious, a repository of what has been repressed. The *collective unconscious* is the residue of what has been learned in humankind's evolution and ancestral past, much as human deoxyribonucleic acid (DNA) is an aggregate of the past. In that portion of the psyche reside the instincts, the potential for creativity, and the spiritual heritage.

The psyche, like all other living systems, attempts to stay in balance. Jung's term for homeostasis in the relation of conscious to unconscious life was the "law of compensation." For any conscious attitude or experience that is overly intense, there is an unconscious compensation. A person experiencing neglect may fantasy or dream of a huge, many-breasted mother. When interpreting dreams, Jung would ask himself for what conscious attitude the dream compensated.

Symbols Although Jung accepted certain symbols as universal, he suggested that, in dealing with patients, the therapist should view symbols as expressions of content not yet consciously recognized or conceptually formulated. A tall, cylindrical object may symbolize a penis, but it may equally well stand for creativity or healing. Symbols are often attempts to unite images from the collective unconscious with the personal unconscious and to strike a balance between the two. A tall, cylindrical object that symbolizes a penis in the personal unconscious may symbolize the phallic principle of creativity or fertility in the collective unconscious.

Personality structure At the center of the conscious personality is the complex called the *ego*. Several universal complexes attend the ego. The *persona* (named after the mask worn by ancient Greek actors), the public personality, mediates between the ego and the real world. The *shadow*, a reverse image of the persona, contains those traits unacceptable to the persona, whether they are positive or negative. A brave persona, for example, has its fearful shadow. The archetype of the shadow is the enemy or feared intruder. The *anima* is the deposit of all the experiences of woman in a man's psychic heritage; the *animus* is the deposit of all the experiences of man in a woman's psychic heritage. The anima or animus connects the ego to the inner world of the psyche and is projected onto others in day-to-day or intimate relationships. When connected with the shadow, a man, for example, may see the attributes of woman as undesirable and may experience guilt when encountering such qualities in himself.

SELF The self is the archetype of the ego; it is the innate potential for wholeness, an unconscious ordering principle directing overall psychic life that gives rise to the ego, which compromises with and is partly shaped by external reality. In Jungian metapsychology, the unconscious gives rise to integration, order, and individuation. The self appears from the unconscious in dreams, fantasies, and altered states of consciousness to give direction. In the first half of life, the ego attempts to identify with the self and to appropriate the power of the self in the service of the ego's growth and differentiation. During that time the ego may become inflated with an unrealistic sense of power—the arrogance of youth. If cut off from the self, the ego may be alienated and depressed.

INDIVIDUATION In the second half of life, the ego begins to attend more to the self than to the conscious realm of life. Jung called that developmental process "individuation," the drive for a person both to become unique and to fulfill the spiritual propensities common to all humanity. Often, the process requires withdrawing from earlier identities and conventional definitions of success and seeking new paths. The change often has the paradoxical effect of leading to broader and more mature relationships and to greater creativity.

Psychological types Jung's theory of psychological types has three axes (Figure 7-6). The *extraversion-introversion* polarity concerns object relatedness. Extraverts are oriented to others and to the world of consciousness. Their energy flows outward first, then inward. Introverts are oriented to their inner worlds, their energy flowing first inward and then to outer reality. Introverts may, therefore, be seen as selfish and unadaptable because they attend first to their inner worlds and then determine how the outer world can fit them.

The *sensation-intuition* polarity has to do with perception. The perceptive type that Jung called sensation-oriented is stimulus-bound and attuned to the specifics of here-and-now reality. The intuitive type blurs the details but apprehends the overall picture. The sensation type comes to understand a situation by assembling the details; the intuitive type grasps the overall situation before attempting to assimilate its parts. The sensation type sees the trees first; the intuitive type sees the forest first.

The polarity of *thinking* and *feeling* deals with information processing and judgment. In the thinking mode, data are evaluated according to logical principle. Feeling, at the opposite pole, involves making judgments through nonlogical processes having to do with values and

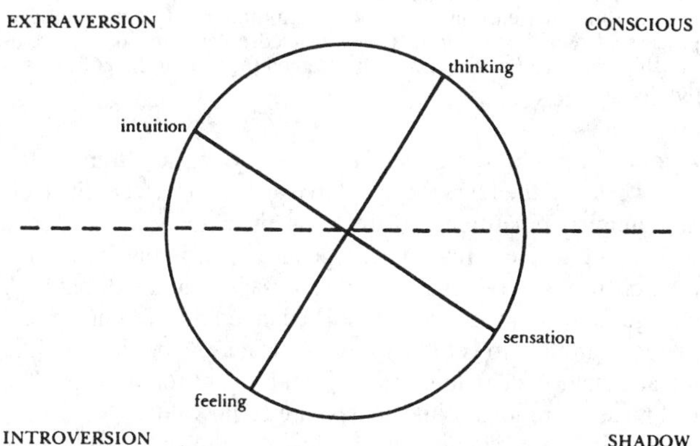

FIGURE 7-6 *The three personality axes: extraversion-introversion, thinking-feeling, and intuition-sensation. (From A Stevens:* On Jung. *Routledge, London, 1990. Used with permission.)*

understanding relations. In social relationships, the thinking type deals with people according to their social rank and the tradition of etiquette; a feeling type deals with others in terms of their present social relationship or perceived emotional state.

The three axes indicated in Figure 7-6 type each person. Sensation ascertains that something exists. Thinking tells what it is. Feeling attributes value to it. Through intuition, its possibilities can be ascertained. An extraverted-sensation-thinking type is oriented to the real world, tends to perceive details, and organizes them into a logical structure. An introverted-intuition-feeling type is self-oriented, grasps situations as a whole, and is sensitive to their emotional implications.

Everyone's psyche contains all the types. But each person has a superior set of functions, types that are evolved from early life and that are shaped strongly by constitutional factors. In the second half of life, adults who continue the process of individuation attempt to integrate or broaden and deepen their understanding of their inferior functions. Thinking types become more aware of feelings; sensation types allow themselves to rely more on intuition.

PSYCHOPATHOLOGY Jung defined *neurosis* as a dissociation of the personality as the result of complexes. When another complex becomes incompatible with the ego complex, a person experiences anxiety. To contain the anxiety, the person splits off the incompatible complex from the ego and moves unconsciously against the ego or other complexes identified with the ego. That splitting enables the person to live out the two incompatible complexes, one more ego-identified and the other more ego-alien. The ego-alien complex is often experienced as being inflicted by the outer world ("I am being mistreated," rather than "I have inner conflict"). The splitting is particularly evident in conversion and dissociative disorders and is an especially good explanation of the phenomenon of multiple personalities. Within the psyche, ego or part personalities or complexes operate along with shadow personalities antithetical to them. In addition, the anima or animus and the archetypal images of the self attempt to integrate and to control the chaos. The various personalities that appear in multiple personality disorder are manifestations of the complexes and the self.

Extraverts tend to develop conversion symptoms or to become antisocial. Introverts become dysthymic, anxious, and obsessional. The symptoms are often related to the attempted emergence of inferior functions. Viewed in that way, pathological conditions may contain within them the struggle toward wholeness or health; inferior functions attempt to become integrated, instead of dissociated from consciousness. The integration of the inferior functions often requires emotionally painful rearrangements of conscious thoughts, attitudes, and life-style.

The attempted expression of inferior functions need not result in psychopathology. Persons with highly developed thinking functions may find themselves wishing to experience life more fully and may involve themselves in highly emotional extramarital relationships. On exploration, one may find unresolved loss of a mothering person with resultant inability early in life to achieve intimacy with a woman. The process of reaching for intimacy is enacted outside the marital relationship because the wife has been assigned the role of the cold, abandoning mother.

Application Jung suggested that therapy begin with four visits a week and then be spaced out to one or two a week. Present-day Jungian practitioners work with their analysands once a week, face-to-face. Jung placed great emphasis on the human relationship between analyst and analysand and noted that both change in the course of analysis. He defined transference as the patient's attempt to get into psychological rapport with the doctor and held that, without rapport and object relationship, the technical operations of the analyst are of no value.

With its emphasis on reintegration, symbolism, and dreams, Jungian analysis seems well suited to help educated persons deal with developmental problems of mid-life. Having achieved a professional identity, material success, and a firm family role, they often begin to ask, "What is the real me?" "What is most meaningful to me?" and "What is my relationship to humankind and human history?" Such persons, often given strongly to self-criticism in the service of self-improvement, may be relieved to find themselves described as trying to become fully themselves, instead of being mentally disordered.

SANDOR RADO

Hungarian-born and Hungarian-trained in psychiatry, Sandor Rado (1890–1972) emigrated to the United States in 1931 after having helped to organize the Hungarian Psychoanalytic Society and having been a member of the Berlin Psychoanalytic Institute (Figure 7-7). In 1945 at Columbia University he directed the first psychoanalytic institute within a university medical school. He thought that learning and cultural and parental influences were of greater importance than instinctual factors as causes of emotional and behavior disorders but felt strongly that an underlying genetically determined biochemical abnormality was present in schizophrenia.

ADAPTATIONAL PSYCHODYNAMICS Rado viewed the psychic apparatus as an organ of adaptation. Effective adaptation is psychological health. Psychological illness or maladaptive behavior is a failure of the adaptive mechanism. The hierarchical levels of human mental integration are hedonic, emotional, emotional thought, and unemotional thought. Those levels parallel the phylogenetic and ontogenetic evolution of the brain and the gradually increasing influence of the neocortex over the more primitive parts of the brain. The hedonic level is the realm of pain and pleasure. Pain signals impending damage and causes flight. Pleasure indicates benefit and elicits clinging or moving toward. Persistent pain has the secondary effect of reducing self-esteem through a sense of failure; pleasure has the secondary effect of enhancing self-esteem through a sense of success. The emotional level of psychic integration consists of the emergency emotions, such as fear and rage, and the tender or welfare emotions, such as love and pride. The emergency emotions are responses to real or anticipated pain and result in flight or fight. The welfare emotions are responses to actual or anticipated pleasure or benefit and prepare the organism to

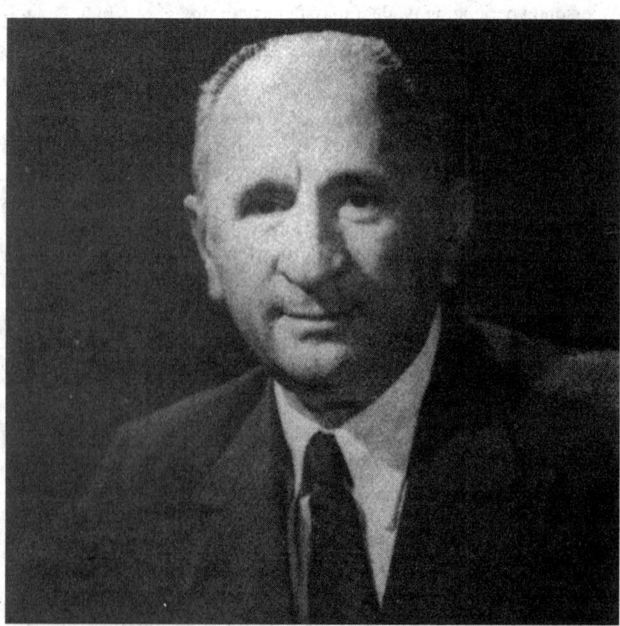

FIGURE 7-7 *Sandor Rado. (Courtesy of New York Academy of Medicine.)*

embrace the pleasurable stimulus. Rado's observation that ordinary human mental activity is primarily at the hedonic and emotional levels was borne out by George Vaillant's later studies that followed a group of successful college undergraduates into their middle years.

Emotional thought justifies and reinforces the emotions from which it springs and is not reality-based. It corresponds to Freud's primary process. Examples of emotional thought include dreams, fantasies, delusions, and the hallucinations of functional psychiatric illness. Rational or unemotional thought operates on Freud's reality principle, making it possible to delay action and gratification, to forgo present pleasure for future gain, and to control emotional responses. Rado concluded that ordinary adults exert much effort to combat emotional thinking and that the emergency emotions are far stronger than the welfare emotions.

Conscience Conscience is the part of the mature psychic apparatus, operating unconsciously, that rewards good behavior, thereby raising self-esteem, and punishes bad behavior by guilt, thus lowering self-esteem. Conscience facilitates cooperation with others and reduces destructive forms of competition. Although conscience stimulates adaptive behavior, it also produces pathological behavior.

Conscience development is based on the dependent child's wish and need to remain in its parents' good graces. Initially, the child projects its own omnipotent feelings onto the parents. Believing that parents see and know all causes the child to fear punishment that it feels is unescapable. A child who misbehaves experiences guilty fear, which has the positive effect of stimulating expiatory behavior. The child admits wrongdoing and accepts punishment to restore the parents' positive feelings. That action relieves the painful guilty fear and restores self-esteem. Pain-dependent or masochistic behavior is a form of expiatory behavior based on guilty fear. The fear motivates the person to seek punishment in advance, which may permit satisfaction of a formerly proscribed desire. Although Rado did not provide a complete explanation of masochistic behavior, he did provide an important link in its understanding.

Both discipline and conscience formation are complicated by the buildup of rage that occurs when the child obeys or submits to its parents. The rage, which is repressed, constantly seeks discharge and presents a potentially serious problem to both the person and society.

Concept of self Rado substituted the term ''action-self'' for ego. A child's first or primordial concept of self is that of an omnipotent, magical being. When children discover that their actual powers are limited, they repress their magical notions. On the way to developing a more realistic concept of self, children delegate their omnipotence and magical powers to their parents, whom they suppose will use those powers for the children's benefit. Rado conceived of the organism's appreciating itself as a ''proven provider of pleasure.'' That emotional appreciation of self is the basis of self-esteem or pride.

TREATMENT According to Rado, psychological health is a predominance of welfare emotions in a reasonably independent, self-reliant person. Such a person creates a self-reinforcing interpersonal field by stimulating pleasurable feelings in others. The emergency responses are still active but are released nondestructively through various types of play or constructive activity and through dreaming.

The aim of psychotherapy is to increase the influence of the welfare emotions on behavior and to reduce the influence of the emergency emotions. The therapist encourages patients to relinquish the dependency that both causes and results from maladaptive behavior and to become reasonably self-reliant. The past is explored in therapy primarily to increase understanding of the present, rather than to reconstruct the past. Rado focused more on examining patients' present-day behavior than on the recovery and analysis of memories and the development of insight based on those reconstructions. He educated patients directly, instead of developing and analyzing the transference, as was done in classical analysis.

MELANIE KLEIN

A lay analyst educated in Germany, Melanie Klein (1882–1960) developed a school of psychoanalysis in England (Figure 7-8). She was an object relations theorist who developed a theory of psychosexual development and psychopathology based on intrapsychic and interpersonal events presumed to occur during the first year of life. Her theory of psychopathology, based on observation of children's free play, was that excessive innate aggression or the psychic reaction to aggression was the cause of severe emotional disturbances, such as the psychotic disorders. She attempted to deal with the intrapsychic forces with classical analytic technique and early interpretation of unconscious impulses. Like Anna Freud, she was a pioneer in child analysis, but, unlike Anna Freud, she excluded parents from the treatment because she believed that the fundamental problem was intrapsychic. Klein's major contributions are in her emphasis on the importance of early object relations, the demonstration of superego function early in psychic development, her description of the primitive defenses characteristic of borderline personality disorder and psychosis, and her use of children's play as a medium for interpretation.

PERSONALITY THEORY Melanie Klein agreed with Sigmund Freud that aggression and libido are the two basic instincts. She also agreed with Freud that the aggressive instinct is an extension of the death instinct and libido an extension of the life instinct. Klein differed from Freud in the assumption that the ego exists at birth. She believed that the death instinct is translated after birth into oral sadism, which, projected outward, gives rise to fantasies of a bad, destructive, devouring breast. Both aggression and libido are expressed from birth on by unconscious fantasies. Klein differentiated envy, greed, and jealousy as manifestations of the aggressive instinct. *Envy* is the angry feeling that someone else has and enjoys something desirable; the envious response is to take it away or spoil it. Oral

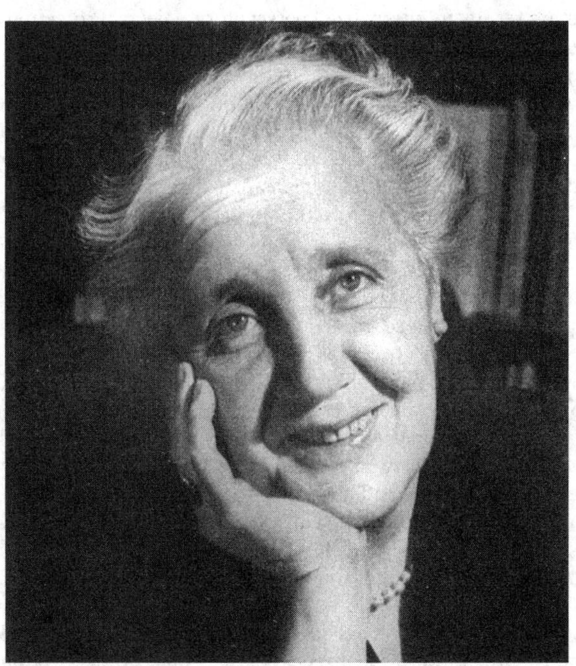

FIGURE 7-8 *Melanie Klein. (Courtesy of Melanie Klein and Douglas Glass.)*

envy, for example, results from the fantasy that the frustrating breast withholds deliberately. It leads to efforts to spoil the frustrating breast and make it less desirable. That primary envy gives rise to other forms of envy, including penis envy. At a more mature level, envy is directed toward others' creativity and frustrates the development of personal creativity because of the fear of envy projected onto others. *Greed* is the manifestation of human insatiability; its aim is destructive taking in of the desired object. *Jealousy* is fear of losing what one has. It develops from triangular relationships, as in the oedipal situation; the third person is hated because that person's receiving love or attention potentially diminishes the availability of libidinal supplies. Although the death instinct is largely projected as paranoid fears, part of it fuses with libido, giving rise to masochistic tendencies.

From the time of birth, the ego attempts to preserve a view of itself as only a source of pleasure and positive feelings; tension and displeasure are projected onto objects that are then seen as persecutory. The infant is grateful when it is physically or emotionally satiated. That gratitude, the earliest manifestation of the life instinct, is the basis of love and of generosity. Libido is invested in objects such as the breast. The gratifying breast is then introjected as the basis for a sense of the self as good. Projection of the good inner object on newly experienced objects is the basis of trust, which makes learning and the accumulation of knowledge possible.

Theory of the ego The ego both experiences and defends itself against anxiety. It develops and maintains object relations and has integrative and synthetic functions. Anxiety is the ego's response to the death instinct. It is reinforced by the separation of birth and by frustrated bodily needs, such as hunger. At first the fear of persecutory objects, anxiety later becomes the fear of introjected bad objects that are the origin of primitive superego anxiety. Fears of being devoured at the oral stage of development become anal-stage fears of being controlled and poisoned and oedipal fears of castration.

The primary means of ego growth and ego defense are *projection* and *introjection,* which integrate the ego and neutralize the death instinct. Projection of inner tensions and awareness of painful external stimuli result in paranoid fears. Their introjection results in internalized persecutory objects. Projection of pleasurable states gives rise to trust. Introjection of positive experiences makes it possible to develop good internal objects that are the basis for ego growth. Before objects in the environment, such as the mother, are recognized as such, certain aspects, such as the breast, are treated as objects. Thus, a transitional stage in object relations is part-object relations.

Unpleasant experiences and emotions associated with external and introjected objects are dissociated from pleasant experiences and emotions through a process of splitting. As the child matures, splitting diminishes, the synthesis of good and bad aspects of objects occurs, and ambivalent relationships become possible. Part-object relations characterize the earliest stage of development, the paranoid-schizoid position; whole object relations characterize the depressive position. The eventual synthesis of good and bad part-objects enables ego growth and the integration of reality. If aggression predominates over libido, idealization occurs, and splitting is reinforced. Reinforcement of splitting may interfere with accurate perception and may result in the eventual denial of reality.

Idealization is a defensive operation that preserves all-good internal and external objects, thus satisfying fantasies of unlimited gratification, such as an inexhaustible breast to protect against frustration. Idealized external objects also protect against persecutory objects. Flight toward an idealized inner good object may protect the person from reality but may do so at the cost of impaired reality testing and may give rise to exalted or messianic psychotic states.

Projective identification, the prototype of all projective mechanisms, projects split-off parts of an internal object onto another person and is used mainly to expel bad inner objects and bad parts of the self. The person onto whom the projection of sadistic impulses is made becomes seen as a persecutor who must be controlled. Attempts to control the perceived persecutor then become a vehicle for the acting out of sadism against the imagined persecutor. Although Klein agreed that environmental factors may play a role in stimulating excessive aggression, she emphasized as the cause of emotional disturbance the inborn strength of aggression, coupled with the ego's excessive anxiety formation and low anxiety tolerance.

Paranoid-schizoid and depressive positions The term "position" was preferred by Klein over "stage" because it emphasizes the effect of the child's point of view on its object relations. The paranoid-schizoid position and the depressive position occur in the first and second half, respectively, of the first year of life. They also recur at various times in life as defensive constellations and are involved in conflicts related to all psychosexual levels.

The paranoid-schizoid position is characterized by splitting, idealization, denial, projective identification, part-object relations, and a basic concern or persecutory anxiety about survival of the self. The persecutory fears are projected oral-sadistic and anal-sadistic impulses. If they are not overintense, the paranoid-schizoid position gives way in the second six months of life to the depressive position. If, however, innate aggression is overly strong and if bad introjects predominate, secondary splitting of the bad introjects may lead to projection onto many external objects, resulting in many external persecutors. Splitting may persist and fragment affective experiences, leading to depersonalization or affective shallowness. It may also interfere with accurate perception and lead to the denial of reality.

In the depressive position, libido predominates over aggression, the infant recognizes that its mother both gratifies and frustrates, and it becomes aware of its own aggression directed toward her. Recognition of its mother as a whole person makes the child vulnerable to loss, especially loss caused by the child's aggression. The mechanism of idealization evolves during the depressive period into idealization of the good object (mother) as a defense against the child's aggression toward her and its accompanying guilt. That sort of idealization leads to an overdependence on others. The bad aspects of needed persons are denied, leading to an impoverishment of both reality experience and reality testing. The depressive position also mobilizes manic defenses, whose main characteristic is the denial of painful psychic realities. Ambivalent feelings and dependence on others are denied; objects are omnipotently controlled and treated with contempt, so that their loss does not give rise to pain or guilt.

SUPEREGO THEORY The Kleinian superego functions like the classical Freudian superego. It places value on behavior, and it punishes or prohibits behavior it holds to be wrong or bad. Klein held that superego development begins during the depressive position; excessive superego pressure causes regression to the paranoid-schizoid position. The superego develops from split-off, projected bad objects, experienced as persecutory, that are later introjected. Guilt is the reaction to the sadistic urges attributed to those introjects that become part of the self. In the depressive period, objects are introjected into both the ego and the superego. The ego takes in those objects with which it can identify positively. The superego takes in the demanding, prohibitive aspects of those objects. The normal predominance of love over hate in the depressive position results in the internalization of mainly good objects into the superego. Those good objects neutralize the bad inner objects, but even under ideal circumstances predominantly good superego objects are contaminated by the bad objects. The superego, therefore, has persecuting (derived from persecutory introjects) and demanding (derived from the demanding aspects of idealized good parents) qualities. Through guilt or concern over the loss of parental love, the superego protects its introjected good objects. The more idealized the good objects contained in the superego, the more perfectionistic are the superego's demands. The idealization of good inner objects usually leads to good behavior and to restitution for bad behavior.

EARLY STAGES OF THE OEDIPUS COMPLEX The early stages of the Oedipus complex begin during the depressive position. Klein assumed an inborn knowledge of the genitals of both sexes, with oral and genital fantasies influential from birth onward. The wish for oral dependency on the mother is displaced onto the father. Longing for the good breast becomes a wish for the father's penis. The bad breast is also displaced to the bad penis. The predominance in boys of a good image of the father's penis fosters the development of the positive Oedipus complex; trust in a good father and endowment of the mother with a good penis initiates a positive Oedipus complex in girls. When aggression predominates, the oedipal boy sees the father as a dangerous potential castrator. Castration fear is, in fact, fear of the projected oral-sadistic desire to destroy the father's penis. That fear makes identification with the father difficult and predisposes to sexual inhibition and fear of women. Guilt over aggression toward the father reinforces repression of the Oedipus complex.

Good oral experiences in girls results in the expectation of a good penis; that expectation is based on the experience of a good breast. Excessive aggression in girls may give rise to unconscious fantasies of robbing the mother of the father's love, penis, and babies and may stimulate fears of maternal retaliation. In girls, the oral and genital desires for the father's penis combine, with penis envy developing as a derivative of earlier breast envy. Thus, penis envy derives from oral sadism and is not a primary envy of male genitals or a primary aspect of female sexuality.

As splitting decreases during the first year of life, the child becomes aware that the good and bad external objects are actually one. Infants then recognize their aggression toward the good object and also recognize the good aspects of persons whom they have attacked for being bad. That recognition undercuts the mechanism of projection. In addition, children become aware of their own bad internal parts and, in contrast to the fear of external harm encountered in the paranoid-schizoid position, the primary fear in the depressive position is of harming the good internal and external objects—hence, the need for the superego.

The primary emotional task of the depressive position is to deal with the ego's fear of losing the good internal and external objects. The corresponding emotional reactions are anxiety and guilt. Preservation of good objects becomes more important than preserving the ego itself. Internalized bad objects that were formerly projected make up the primary ego, which attacks the ego with guilt feelings. The bad objects within the superego, as noted above, may contaminate the good internal superego objects that have become incorporated into the superego because of their demands for certain types of behavior (I will love you if you do well at your chores; I will accept you only if you work hard).

WORKING-THROUGH MECHANISMS Normally, the mechanisms of reparation, increased reality testing, acceptance of ambivalence, gratitude, and mourning enable the child to work through the depressive period. Reparation, the antecedent of sublimation, is a healthy effort to reduce guilt over having attacked the good object by trying to repair the damage, expressing love and gratitude and thus preserving it. The child cries, rushes to its mother, throws its arms around her, and says, "I'm sorry."

Increased reality testing results from decreased splitting and the growing capacity to evaluate whole objects and the total self. Introjected objects are seen as whole and alive, instead of as autonomous fragments. Through being loved, children come to see themselves and their inner objects as good. Growing awareness of loving and hating the same person brings about the capacity to experience and tolerate ambivalence, optimally with a preponderance of love over hate. Klein believed that mourning normally reactivates the guilt of the depressive position, the difference being that during weaning in the depressive position the real, good mother is still present and helps the infant reconstitute and consolidate good internal objects.

PSYCHOPATHOLOGY Many types of severe psychopathology are attributed to fixation at one of the two Kleinian positions. Fixation in the paranoid-schizoid position leads to a number of psychotic disorders. Psychotic disorders in general deny reality, use projection extensively, and engage in splitting. Escape into an idealized inner object leads to autistic exalted states; generalized splitting and reintrojection of multiple, fragmented objects leads to confusional states. Predominant fear of external persecutors is the hallmark of delusional disorder; projection of persecutors onto one's own body results in hypochondriasis. Persons with schizoid personality disorder are emotionally shallow and intolerant of guilt, tend to experience others as hostile, and withdraw from object relations.

From fixation at the depressive position comes pathological mourning (depression) or excessive development of manic defenses. Pathological mourning results from the fantasied destruction by sadistic attack of good internal and external objects. The bad internal objects that remain function as a primitive sadistic superego, evoking excessive guilt and stimulating the feeling that all good objects are dead and the world is without love. The sadistic superego is cruel, demands perfection, and opposes the instincts. Attempts are made to idealize external objects as a means of self-preservation; thus, any reproaches are made against the self, instead of others. Suicide may embody the notion that the good external object can be preserved only by destroying the bad self.

Hypomanic and manic syndromes are brought about by a predominance of manic defenses, including omnipotence, identification with the superego, introjection, manic triumph, and manic idealization. Omnipotence results from identification with an idealized good object and denial of the rest of reality. Identification with a sadistic superego allows external objects to be treated with contempt. Introjection is manifested as object hunger, with denial of danger to and from the objects; manic triumph is manifested by a sense of having conquered the world; and manic idealization is manifested by fantasies of fusion with God.

TECHNIQUE Klein believed that all anxiety-producing situations, including the analytic hour, reactivate paranoid-schizoid and depressive position anxieties. The primitive defenses and fears are interpreted from the first session onward as deeply as possible and involve both transference (you wish to annihilate me) and nontransference (you wished to eliminate your mother's bad breast) material. The same technique is used with all patients, focusing on unconscious fantasies that represent the content and the defensive operations at the most primitive levels of the mind. The technique was used even with children less than 6 years of age, using their free play as the basis for interpretation in 50-minute sessions five days a week. To Klein a child's free play was analogous to an adult's free associations. Her views opposed those of Anna Freud, the other leading child analyst of the day, who held that analysis of a prelatency child's Oedipus complex is not possible, as it may interfere with parental relationships; that child analysis is largely an educational experience for the child; that a transference neurosis cannot be effected, because of the parents' activity in the child's daily life; and that the analyst should make every effort to gain a child's confidence. Klein held that a transference neurosis can be effected and then resolved by interpretation. Rather than attempting to gain favor with the child, Klein immediately interpreted negative transferences (you want to be rid of me) and found that doing so relieved anxiety, rather than intensifying it.

Kleinian therapists are interested in treating patients in whom primitive conflicts and defenses predominate. They do so by assuming a strictly interpretive stance, interpreting both negative and positive aspects of the transference but especially emphasizing the negative aspects.

OTTO RANK

Otto Rank (1884–1939) was a 21-year-old student when he met Sigmund Freud. Rank went on to earn a doctorate in psychology and eventually to become Freud's peer. He saw each person as an artist whose ultimate task is the creation of an individual personality. To Rank the neurotic is an *artiste manqué,* a person whose strong creative urge is stultified by the negative use of will (Figure 7-9).

RANKIAN DIALECTIC The basis for his break with Freud was Rank's view that the birth trauma is more important than the oedipal conflict. According to Rank, the physical and psychological experiences of birth give rise to a primal anxiety that is dealt with by primal repression. The crucial intrapsychic conflict that occurs at all developmental phases is the conflict between maintaining the primal bliss of attachment and experiencing the excitement and fear associated with separation.

Union stands in contrast to separation; likeness stands in contrast to difference. Union-separation and likeness-difference are polarities held in tension. In adulthood, movement toward another person is possible only if one knows who one is, which can come about only through having experienced separation. Movement toward autonomy is possible only after the person has established the sense of belonging and self-worth that derive from the experience of belonging.

Moving toward union or separation is not an innate biological process. It is, instead, an act of will. In moving toward and engaging with another, all persons experience their need to belong. Moving away from others allows persons to experience their uniqueness. Maturity is in a sense the triumph of will over the forces—guilt, death-fear, and life-fear—that inhibit movement both toward and away from others.

Rank saw guilt as the price to be paid for any act of will. Moving toward union causes guilt over being needy; moving away causes the guilt of abandoning another person. Death-fear is the fear of losing identity by fusing with another person. The weaker one's personal identity is, the stronger is the death-fear. Life-fear, by contrast, is fear of losing all ties in the process of becoming separate. Every person experiences the cycle of movement from union to separation and back again as part of the life process. The movement takes place at various levels—family, societal, artistic, and spiritual. At each level there is one or more movements toward union and rebirth. Each person, for example, usually yields to a love experience in which personal differences are set aside to experience unity with another, to experience self-worth, and to be relieved of the sense of difference. The yielding to another ends when the will asserts its separateness and a new affirmation of individuality occurs.

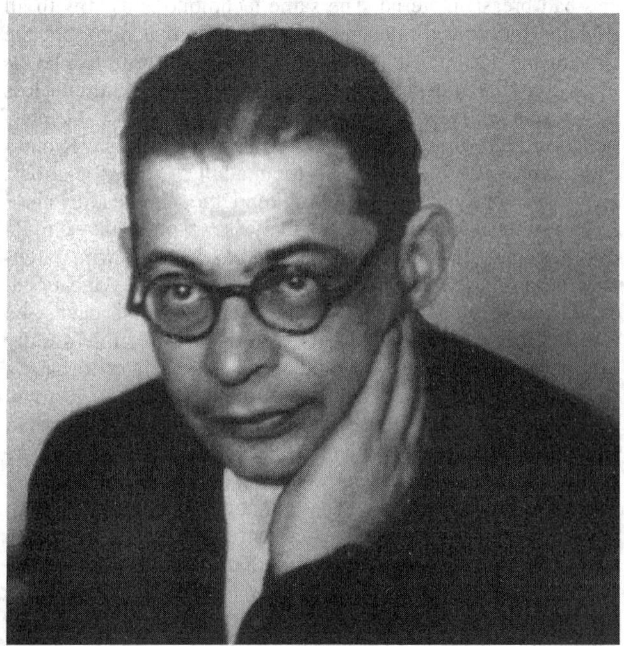

FIGURE 7-9 *Otto Rank. (Courtesy of New York Academy of Medicine.)*

Will, the prime mover in the Rankian dialectic, is an irreducible creative force. It is not solely an agency for the expression of Freudian sexual or aggressive impulses; nor is it a will to power in the Adlerian sense. The beginning of will is in the child's "no," an assertion of what it will not do. In maturation, will becomes a positive force. Neurotic persons, however, deny their will because of guilt over what they will. They deal with that guilt by using such defense mechanisms as projection and rationalization. Viewed from that perspective, neurotic persons are strong-willed and cannot acknowledge what they will or even that they will. As a result, they cannot use their will constructively in the service of their greatest potential artistic creations, their own personalities.

TREATMENT Rankian psychotherapy is a here-and-now interaction with the therapist that mobilizes the patient's will and results in a rebirth experience. The treatment, which is time-limited, focuses on the relationship with the therapist. In the therapist-patient relationship are reenacted earlier life struggles, especially struggles involving intimacy. After patients are strengthened through the therapist's acceptance, they begin a process of negative will assertion that is seen as resistance in classical analysis. Rank regarded negative will assertion as indicative of growth and supported it. Once able to provide self-affirmation on their own, patients free themselves of the therapist and begin to individuate. They overcome the life-fear by living up to their fullest potential.

Therapy is not aimed at reconstructing personal history. It is a struggle in the here and now between the therapist as a representative of transference objects and reality. The aim of the therapy is to free the patient's will.

The therapeutic process parallels the process of personality growth. At first, the therapeutic relationship recapitulates prototypical early relationships. The first rebirth experience for patients is claiming their own individual personalities and their uniqueness as human beings. The second phase is their discovery of the physical universe and their likeness to it. Later, they claim their distinctness as creators of themselves. With the emergence of the self, patients unite with ideological, philosophical, and spiritual reality and experience the final birth of the ideal person, a self-fulfilled person who no longer needs to create to justify his or her existence.

KAREN HORNEY

Physician-psychoanalyst Karen Horney (1885–1952) emphasized the preeminence of social and cultural influences on psychosexual development, focused her attention on the differing psychologies of men and women, and explored the vicissitudes of marital relationships (Figure 7-10). Her view that the repression and the sublimation of biological drives are not the primary determinants of personality development led to her removal as an instructor in the New York Psychoanalytic Institute and her founding in 1941 of the American Psychoanalytic Institute.

PERSONALITY THEORY Horney held that personality development results from the interaction of biological and psychosocial forces that are unique for each person. As the core of each personality is an enduring *real self.* Equivalent partly to the Freudian ego and partly to Eric Berne's child ego state, the real self combines choice, will, responsibility, identity, spontaneity, and aliveness. A natural unfolding process of *self-realization* leads to the development of human potential in three basic directions—toward others, to express love and trust; against others, to express healthy opposition; and away from others toward self-sufficiency.

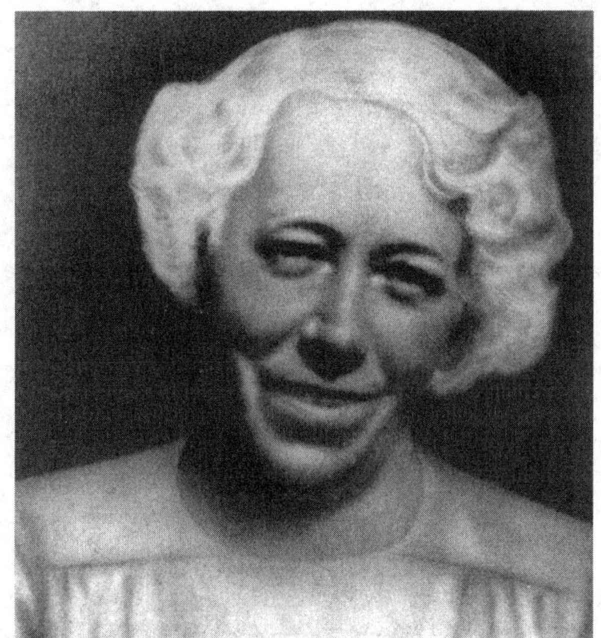

FIGURE 7-10 *Karen Horney. (Courtesy of New York Academy of Medicine.)*

Although conditions during childhood may block psychological development, healthy growth is always possible if the internal blockages are removed. Children whose family situations lead them to feel endangered concentrate on psychological survival and may do so by developing stereotyped coping mechanisms.

Horney thought that the attributes of passivity and suffering were not biologically specific to women, as taught by the analysts of her day, and that male and female personalities are, in fact, culturally determined.

THEORY OF NEUROSIS Horney defined neurosis in both intrapsychic and interpersonal terms. She noted that her patients complained not of the symptomatic neuroses, such as phobias and compulsions, but of unhappiness, blockage and lack of fulfillment in their work, and inability to establish or maintain relationships. She saw those patients as having complex systems of self-perpetuating defensive patterns against basic anxiety that began in early childhood—character neuroses.

Safety seeking Children move psychologically in three directions to relieve their anxiety, to make life safe and predictable, and to achieve satisfaction. They seek affection and approval, or they become hostile, or they withdraw. Children eventually use the coping strategy that best meets their needs, but, if only one basic strategy is used, children become limited in their coping repertoire and their experience of themselves and their world. Their sense of safety is tenuous because they have danger from within from suppressed or repressed feelings and impulses. If unfavorable environmental conditions continue, their conflicting feelings are driven into the unconscious, and such children are left with a sense of discomfort, anxiety, and apprehension and an insecure sense of self. At that juncture, their point of reference is externalized, patterns of behavior rigidify, and increasing blockages to growth develop. Horney designated those complex, relatively fixed attitudes toward self and others as neurotic trends.

CHARACTER TYPES Horney's three main character types are based on the predominant mode of relating to others. The *compliant, self-effacing type* results from the defensive operation of clinging to others. Such persons try to curry the favor of others, subordinate themselves to others, and are reluctant to disagree for fear of losing favor. The *aggressive, expansive type* results from moving against others and places heavy reliance on power and mastery as a means to achieve security. The *detached, resigned type* results from moving away from others to avoid both dependency and conflict. They are very private persons who, while refusing to compete openly, see themselves as rising above others.

SUPPLEMENTAL MEANS TO RELIEVE INNER TENSION The overdevelopment of one of the three basic interpersonal styles suppresses the two others. In a manner analogous to Jung's complexes, the repressed impulses continue to be active and to produce conflict. An artificial harmony is achieved by the use of such mental mechanisms as blind spots, compartmentalization, rationalization, and coping techniques such as excessive self-control, arbitrariness, elusiveness, cynicism, and externalization.

Idealized image During their teen years, future neurotic persons create a fantasied ideal image that, if achieved, promises to end their painful feelings and provide self-fulfillment. The idealized image counterbalances the alienation from their core selves that developing neurotic persons undergo because the survival techniques they adopted earlier force them to override their genuine wishes, feelings, and thoughts. The idealized image covers all the contradictions, conceals the defensive nature of their behavior, and restores a sense of wholeness. Energy formerly available for self-realization is used in efforts to become like the idealized image. For example, a person who has adopted the strategy of moving toward others and is consequently dependent on others for affection and approval experiences the fear of reasonable self-assertion as saintly humility and consideration of others.

Because the ideal self is imaginary, neurotic persons are readily bruised by confrontation with reality, and they work excessively hard to prove that they are, in fact, their ideal selves. Doing so results in a type of perfectionism that insists on flawless excellence in which "I should" replaces "I want" or "I need." It also results in the neurotic ambition to be first and in a strong drive for revenge on those perceived to have interfered with their becoming their ideal selves.

Claims, shoulds, and self-hatred Despite their frequent self-disparagement, neurotic persons expect to be treated as though they were their ideal selves. Those claims to special treatment, when frustrated, produce anger, righteous indignation, and resentment.

The "shoulds," self-imposed demands that they live up to their idealized selves, are irrational and unrelated to the realities of daily life. The "shoulds" are projected, are experienced as demands made by others, and are also demanded of others. Doing so results in the neurotic person's being critical of others and sensitive to criticism.

Self-hatred results when the threat arises that neurotic persons may be unable to achieve their idealized selves. If support were not needed for the idealized self, the claims, "shoulds," and self-hatred would not be such important parts of the psychic apparatus.

Neurotic pride and the pride system Glorifying aspects of the idealized self, *neurotic pride,* substitutes for healthy self-confidence. Thus, when their pride is injured by others, neurotic persons become enraged and seek to avenge their injury and to conceal their self-deception by achieving a vindictive victory over the offending person. Together with supporting claims and shoulds, neurotic pride and self-hatred form a defensive network or *pride system* that protects the idealized self. Any attempt to reduce elements of the pride system is experienced as an attack on the person. Despite the armoring of their defensive network, neurotic persons are not at peace because they are in inner conflict with the forces that protect them. The conflict between the pride system and the forces driving toward healthy self-realization is the *central inner conflict.*

Conflict also exists within the pride system itself. Neurotic pride and claims are associated with the glorified idealized image; self-hatred and shoulds are associated with the unacceptable aspects of self. When attempts are made to satisfy both forces simultaneously, conflict arises. Attempts to avoid those conflicts involve further alienation from the real self.

Alienation Alienation from self is one of the most serious consequences of neurotic development. Alienation results from the combination of repeated denial of external reality and the repression of genuine thoughts, feelings, and impulses. As the process of alienation continues, neurotic persons lose touch with the core of their being and can no longer determine or act on what is right for them. Their feelings may range from uncertainty and confusion to inner deadness and emptiness.

ANALYTIC TREATMENT Horney did not regard adult neurotic persons as recapitulating childhood experiences and, thus, did not focus on the recovery of childhood memories. She dealt, instead, with the self-perpetuating neurotic process. She stressed the importance of dreams in analysis and, later, the exploration of the patient-analyst relationship. She was one of the earliest analysts to recognize and make constructive use of her own feelings toward patients. To Horney, psychoanalysis is a cooperative venture that enables patients to free themselves from their neurotic structures and to mobilize themselves toward self-realization. The analyst's responsibility is to assist in liberating patients from *blockages,* the forces that impede healthy growth.

Early in therapy, during the *disillusioning process,* the two types of blockages are identified and examined. The first group of safety-oriented blockages, the *protective blockages,* help avoid the anxiety caused by self-awareness. The protective blockages include silence, lateness, depreciating the analyst, the use of drugs, and even the use of self-accusation to avoid further exploration.

Positive-value blockages reinforce the patients' satisfaction with themselves and support their idealized selves. In the disillusioning process, the analyst identifies both types of blockages, exposing the protective blockages before exposing the blockages that defend the idealized image. Analyzing the positive-value blockages first would arouse too much fear.

Qualities of the analyst The analyst's qualities, later described by Carl Rogers as therapist-offered conditions, include maturity, belief in constructive conflict resolution, and the ability to communicate hope and respect. The analyst listens, clarifies, provides directions, and suggests alternative resolutions to conflicts. Horney emphasized the need for the analyst to help move patients out of their alienation and suggested that therapists be flexible, tailoring their interventions to the patients' needs at the moment. She did not emphasize using the couch or a fixed number of sessions each week.

Therapeutic process Horney believed that fundamental attitudinal changes are the best means to change self-defeating, self-alienating behaviors. She created a setting in which patients were able to assess themselves as persons free to discover and choose personal values that fit with their real selves. That type of reorientation begins after the disillusioning phase of treatment. As patients begin to question their present values and their idealizing process abates, they are enabled to revise their values and to develop more flexible values consonant with their inner selves. Dreams are used in all phases of treatment to bring patients into better contact with their real selves. As unconscious attempts to solve conflicts, dreams can show constructive forces at work that are not yet discernible in the patients' conscious thoughts and behavior.

As patients mobilize their constructive forces, they experience the struggle between the pride system and the real self. In the process they experience uncertainty, psychic pain, and self-hatred. As the central conflict is resolved successfully, patients move into the final phase of treatment, the discovery and use of their real inner selves.

FRANZ ALEXANDER

Franz Alexander (1891–1964) was one of the second generation of psychoanalysts (Figure 7-11). He was born in Budapest and attended its medical school, graduating in 1912. He conducted research in bacteriology at the Institute for Experimental Pathology until World War

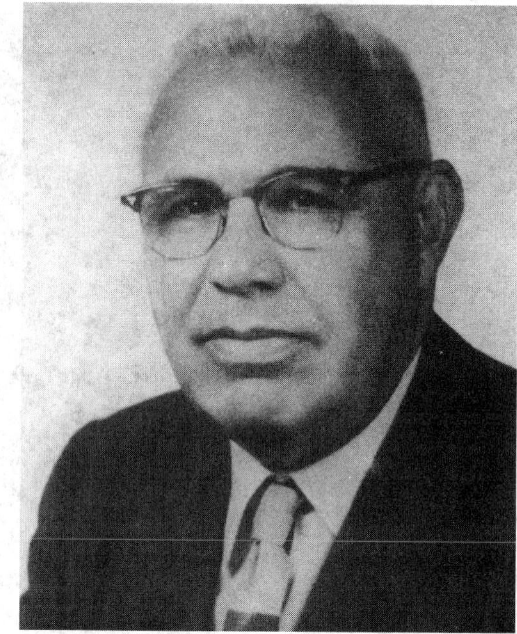

FIGURE 7-11 *Franz Alexander. (Courtesy of Franz Alexander.)*

I, when he practiced clinical microbiology on the Italian front, primarily combating malaria. After the war he joined the department of psychiatry at the University of Budapest Medical School as a brain researcher. That research led to an encounter with Freud's work, and in 1919 he became the first student in the Berlin Psychoanalytic Institute. In 1930 he became a visiting professor of psychoanalysis at the University of Chicago and in 1932 founded the Chicago Psychoanalytic Institute. He established the institute independent of the psychoanalytic societies, leading the Chicago institute to be one of the most creative sources of psychoanalytic thought. During the same time he began his interest in psychosomatic illnesses, helping to found the journal *Psychosomatic Medicine.* A guiding principle of his work was to make psychoanalysis an integral part of medicine.

In 1946 Alexander became professor of psychoanalysis at the University of Southern California, where he continued his work on psychosomatic medicine and became interested in the interface of learning theory, the psychophysiology of stress, and psychoanalysis.

THEORY OF PERSONALITY Alexander did not develop a unique overarching theory of personality. His contribution was his application of psychoanalytic thought to pathophysiological processes. He laid the groundwork for the burgeoning fields of psychosomatic medicine, behavioral medicine, and psychophysiology. He created the basis for the biopsychosocial model and studied the mind and the body at a time when American psychiatry, despite Freud's original ideas, had become purely psychological in its orientation. In studying and treating many patients with serious physical illnesses, he was also forced to consider creative modifications of therapeutic techniques.

Alexander and his group began by intensively studying, by means of clinical interviews, patients who had one of seven illnesses that had been identified by general practitioners as regularly having strong psychological components. Out of those clinical studies emerged the specificity hypothesis. The *specificity hypothesis* proposed that certain illnesses are the products of complex interactions of specific constitutional predispositions, specific unconscious conflicts, and specific types of stressors that activate such conflicts. Alexander and his group then tested those hypotheses in a series of clinical studies of patient populations. The independent variable was usually the ability of skilled clinicians to predict a patient's illness from disguised case reports. The model Alexander proposed remains the fundamental psychosomatic conceptualization; a variety of illness situations are now studied by controlling for genetic influences while measuring and modifying intrapsychic conflict and external stressors.

In the area of psychotherapy, Alexander was one of many who sought to shorten the analytic process. He hypothesized that intellectual insight is not the central curative factor in therapy. Rather, he emphasized the role of corrective emotional experience. That emphasis led him to experiment with variations in technique that may facilitate such experiences. That controversial stand nearly ruptured his relations with the psychoanalytic movement.

THEORY OF PSYCHOPATHOLOGY The seven diseases that Alexander studied were peptic ulcer disease, ulcerative colitis, essential hypertension, rheumatoid arthritis, bronchial asthma, neurodermatitis, and Graves' disease. Alexander and his group identified what they believed to be the single, specific core conflict that, in interaction with constitutional predispositions and a particular stressor, activates the disease.

The core conflict identified in *peptic ulcer disease* is hyperindependence as a defense against unacceptable dependency needs. The stressor that results in an acute attack is any situation that demands that the afflicted person openly acknowledge dependency needs or ask that they be met. Ordinarily, such patients use dominance and control to intimidate others into meeting their dependency needs. Alexander was the first to describe the "little boy" business executive prone to peptic ulcers. The groundwork was laid for John J. Brady's executive monkey experiments. That particular illness model has received more confirmatory evidence than any of the others; in a study of army inductees, psychological profiles described by Alexander, in combination with measurements of serum pepsinogen, were extraordinarily successful in predicting the development of duodenal ulcers.

Alexander's theory of *ulcerative colitis* also implicates dependency conflicts; however, rage at unmet needs is seen as the defining feature. The rage provokes guilt and the urge to make restitution to the object of anger by gifts of achievement and success. The model here is clearly the angry child seeking to placate a parent by means of performance. The precipitating event for reactivation of the illness is the perception that the efforts at placation will be unsuccessful. Alexander claimed that the perception results in excess parasympathetic activity leading to diarrhea. In Alexander's own study, skilled internists and psychiatrists reviewed case descriptions in which each patient had one of the seven identified psychosomatic illnesses and then predicted which illness each patient had; the physicians correctly identified more than half of the ulcerative colitis patients from their dynamics alone—a result well beyond chance. However, most clinicians now regard George Engel's object-relations-based formulation to be the more accurate.

Alexander's hypothesis about *essential hypertension* focuses on inhibited anger and suspiciousness in an outwardly compliant, cooperative person. A hypertensive patient often goes for long periods with blood pressure under good control and then, seemingly inexplicably, experiences dramatic rises in blood pressure. Alexander attributed those episodes to incidents when the chronic anger is exacerbated and intense defenses must be used, causing chronic sympathetic, fight-flight activation. Several psychophysiological studies have suggested that the idea has some accuracy, at least in terms of short-term changes in the blood pressure of a subset of hypertensive patients. Labile hypertensive patients appear to fit the model best.

The proposed specific conflict for *rheumatoid arthritis* postulates conflicts over rebellion against overprotective parents. A compromise formation in which the conflict is discharged through physical activity, especially sports, works for a time, but the anger is eventually expressed in self-sacrifice designed to control others. Failure of the pattern results in increased ambivalent tension, directly expressed by muscular contractions that lead to joint degeneration. A remarkable amount of confirmatory evidence for this constellation appeared in a series of psychological test studies; however, more recent research has failed to replicate much of those results and has implicated more general stress issues, life changes, and psychoneuroimmunological mechanisms.

Alexander proposed that the wheeze of *bronchial asthma* represents a symbolic cry. The specific conflict, according to him, is the wish for protection versus the fear of envelopment. That conflict leads to sensitization to separation issues, which become the events that provoke the suppressed cry of the asthma attack. In recent years it has become clear that the population with asthma is far more heterogeneous both psychologically and physiologically (in terms of vulnerability to allergens) than was recognized in Alexander's time. The role of a vicious physiological-psychological cycle in which asthma stimulates panic, which in turn triggers pathological pulmonary psychophysiological responses, has been a focus of recent research.

Although the role of conflicts in *neurodermatitis* remains widely accepted by clinicians, the specific conflict proposed by Alexander, that early deprivation leads to wishes for closeness that are opposed by a fear of it, is no longer accepted. Finally, *Graves' disease* is no longer widely accepted as a psychosomatic illness. Alexander's hypothesis was that premature responsibility leads to a martyrlike denial of dependency.

TREATMENT The specificity hypothesis led Alexander to focus his psychotherapeutic efforts in a way that other analysts of his time did not. He reasoned that, if he could help patients resolve their core conflicts without necessarily addressing other parts of the personality structure, the medical illness would improve. Indeed, he published numerous case studies suggesting just that kind of success. In addition, he was among the first to question the value of intellectual insight as the curative agent in psychotherapy. He proposed that a *corrective emotional experience* is the central agent of change. A corrective emotional experience involves disconfirmation within the transference relationship of previous assumptions and projections.

Alexander felt justified in introducing a variety of techniques that would, initially, induce and heighten the emotional experience of the transference and, subsequently, challenge the underlying unconscious assumptions. Those techniques included manipulating the frequency and the length of sessions, making direct suggestions about the patient's life, self-conscious alteration of the therapist's behavior according to the patient's conflict, and behavior therapy techniques. In many ways those techniques were the most controversial aspects of Alexander's work. Serious questions about the validity of his suppositions and the ethics of his manipulative stance were raised. He was impatient with the slow, methodical process of convincing his colleagues; his intellectual energy led him to embark on ever newer experiments while other analysts were still struggling to digest his previous suggestions. Yet, today, few quarrel with the concept that emotional learning is at least as important as intellectual insight in psychotherapeutic success. Alexander's efforts to modify and shorten the analytic process are closer to the norm in psychiatric practice than is classical analysis.

Ironically, although Alexander's therapeutic innovations seem prescient today, his specificity hypothesis, which was in his time far less controversial, seems simplistic, naive, and forced. He did not have available the sense of how complicated illness causation truly is. The dominant model then was infectious diseases—one organism, one illness. In addition, the complexity of social phenomena and stressors was unknown in his time. Yet he was the one who first postulated a multicausal etiology for disease—a specific constitutional defect, a specific conflict, and a specific stressor. He was also the first to study mind-body interactions in a systematic way. Thus, Alexander himself laid the basis on which his own formulations seem limited today.

HARRY STACK SULLIVAN

Harry Stack Sullivan (1892–1949) is generally acknowledged as the most original and distinctive American-born theorist in dynamic psychiatry (Figure 7-12). Most American psychiatrists make significant use of concepts and approaches that he developed. For many years the primary theoretical dispute within dynamic psychiatry circles was between the classical Freudians and the Sullivanians or interpersonal psychoanalysts. When psychiatrists use the term "parataxic distortion," apply the concept of self-esteem, consider the importance of preadolescent peer groups in development, or view a patient's behavior as an interpersonal manipulation, they are applying knowledge that Sullivan's ideas and observations supplied.

Sullivan graduated from medical school in Chicago in 1917. From 1921 to 1930 he was in the Washington, D.C., area, working with schizophrenic patients at St. Elizabeth's and then Sheppard and Enoch Pratt hospitals. He developed a reputation as a remarkable clinician with an uncanny ability to communicate with floridly psychotic patients, and he initiated the first of what are now called therapeutic communities. Later, he entered private practice in New York and eventually returned to the Washington area, where he was involved in clinical, consulting, and teaching activities. In the 1920s and 1930s he

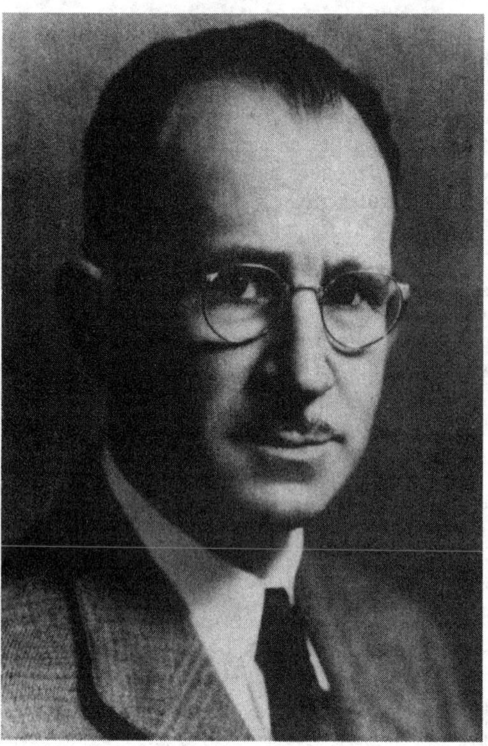

FIGURE 7-12 *Harry Stack Sullivan. (Courtesy of Dr. Otto Will.)*

wrote a number of papers on schizophrenia, later collected in *Schizophrenia as a Human Process.* His other books were compiled by his students from his lectures; most were published posthumously. That process accounts for some of the density and seeming disorganization of his written work.

PERSONALITY THEORY Sullivan rejected the Kraepelinian dogma of his day that dominated psychiatric thinking about schizophrenia. He would read passages of patient speech that Emil Kraepelin had presented as an example of how schizophrenic speech made no sense, and Sullivan would bring forth its meaning. He turned initially to Freud but reacted to him as he had to Kraepelin, rejecting an increasingly rigid and dogmatic structure. Sullivan developed his own working theory of personality, psychopathology, and therapy.

Sullivan was concerned that language can be misleading. He was wary of self-reifying conceptualizations that lead to rigid theories. He tried to emphasize the psychiatrist as participant-observer in the clinical situation. By emphasizing that aspect of the psychiatrist's role, he sought to keep observations as objective as possible, although he recognized the difficulty that presented in dealing with private emotional experiences. What can be observed is the social interaction of patients; thus, Sullivan defined personality as the "relatively enduring pattern of interpersonal relations which characterize a human life." His focus at the outset was quite apart from the intrapsychic emphasis of psychoanalysis. By approaching psychopathology in that way, he necessarily created a field theory, rather than a structural theory. Temporal and interactive processes became the hallmark. Sullivan defined a *dynamism* as "the relatively enduring pattern of energy transformations"—that is, recurrent interpersonal behavior patterns.

Sullivan's theory is fundamentally a theory of needs and anxiety. The needs are the needs for satisfaction and the needs for security. Anxiety occurs when fundamental needs are in danger of not being met; anxiety is the primary motivator of human behavior. Needs for satisfaction include physical needs—such as air, water, food, and warmth—and emotional needs, especially for human contact and for expressing one's talents and capacities. Because the infant is utterly unable to meet its own needs, interpersonal relationships become the central concern from the beginning. Decades before Margaret Mahler wrote of a symbiotic stage in infant development, Sullivan spoke of the "empathic linkage" between caretaker and infant, and he described the complicated interaction of infants' communicating tension and anxiety, arousing anxiety in the caretaker and leading to tender responses to the infant's needs. Failure to meet those needs results in loneliness and anxiety.

Sullivan defined security as the absence of anxiety. Needs for security include the need to avoid, prevent, or reduce anxiety. Since no mother is perfect, anxiety is inevitable and becomes the primary driver in personality development. The *self-system* or *self-dynamism* was defined by Sullivan as the dynamism that is responsible for avoiding or reducing anxiety. Sullivan equated the self-identity-ego with the person's developed patterns for avoiding the discomforts that arise from the failure of others to meet one's fundamental needs. The self-system exists, like all else, purely within an interpersonal framework. The self-system develops a set of mechanisms, called security operations, that reduce anxiety.

Security operations function within Sullivan's theory much as defense mechanisms do within psychoanalytic theory. However, the specific security operations were defined interpersonally, and Sullivan tried to link them closely to actual observations or experiences. Some security operations bear the same labels and definitions as Anna Freud's mechanisms of defense, but Sullivan is best known for three contributions that bear his distinct stamp: apathy, somnolent detachment, and selective inattention. Those security operations were drawn from observing the way infants and young children react to painful interactions, such as scolding, with their parents.

The self-system accrues from ever-evolving interpersonal experiences—for example, fulfillment of needs for satisfaction as a result of the empathic linkage with the mother. The most difficult experiences are not necessarily those involving failure to meet the child's needs but the child's sensing of the caretaker's anxiety in the process of responding to those needs. The caretaker's anxiety arouses anxiety in the child, promotes the need to establish a sense of security, and leads to the evolution of the self-system and the development of security operations. The self-system is divided into three parts—good me, bad me, and not me. The *good me* is a set of images, experiences, and behaviors associated with an unanxious, tender, empathic, and approving and accepting response from the environment. The *bad me* comes to be associated with ideas, actions, and perceptions that provoke anxiety and disapproval from caretakers. Some situations, however, provoke such intense anxiety that they are entirely disavowed and disowned; they become part of the *not me*. Eventually, the empathic linkage becomes unnecessary, and the self-system operates autonomously within the person, developing ever more subtle and complex ways to manage the person's anxiety.

DEVELOPMENTAL THEORIES

Cognitive development Sullivan postulated three developmental cognitive modes of experience whose degree of persistence into adulthood is important in understanding psychopathology. (1) The *prototaxic mode,* characteristic of infancy and early childhood, involves a series of disconnected brief states experienced as totalities with no temporal relationship. In later life, mystical experiences and schizophrenic fusion represent persistent prototaxic experiences. (2) *Parataxic experience* begins early in childhood as the self-system begins its independent functioning. It, too, involves a series of momentary experiences; however, they are recorded in sequence and with apparent connection to one another. They may be given symbolic meanings, but rules of logic are absent, and coincidence plays a major role in how the world is perceived. The self-system uses parataxic experience to seek effective anxiety-reducing behaviors and to repeat them, seeking sameness and predictability. Sullivan used the mode to explain transference, slips of the tongue, and paranoid ideation. (3) The *syntaxic mode* of experiencing is based on the development of language and consensual validation. *Consensual validation* is the acceptance of the shared perceptions of others as a basis for defining objective reality. The world and the self are perceived within rules of logic, temporal sequencing, external validity, and internal consistency. Thinking about oneself and others becomes testable and modifiable on the basis of rigorous analysis of experiences in a variety of different situations. Maturity may be defined as extensive predominance of the syntaxic mode of experiencing.

Social development Social development is based to some extent on those evolving cognitive modes. However, disturbed interpersonal relationships may cause the primitive ways of experiencing the world to persist. Social development is characterized by the satisfaction needs that predominate and the interpersonal sphere in which the satisfaction needs and their resulting security needs are fulfilled. Each stage is also characterized by the primary zone of interaction—bodily areas through which the person channels needs, anxiety, and relief. Sullivan's theory bears a superficial parallel to Freud's genetic theory; however, for Sullivan the role of the zones was far less important than in psychoanalytic libido theory.

Infancy, from birth to the onset of language, is characterized by the primary need for bodily contact and tenderness. The prototaxic mode predominates, and the primary zones of interaction are oral and, to some extent, anal. To the extent that needs are fulfilled with a minimum of anxiety, the infant experiences euphoria and a sense of well-being. To the extent that some anxiety is commonly present in the caretakers, apathy and somnolent detachment are regularly used security operations, persisting into adult life as a basic detached and passive stance. If anxiety and inconsistency are severe, intense experiences of dread persist, presenting in later life as the eerie, uncanny, bizarrely disruptive internal states seen in schizophrenic patients.

Childhood, which begins with the onset of usable language, continues until the beginning of school and is characterized by the child's focus on the parents as the other from whom praise and acceptance are sought. The primary mode of experience shifts to the parataxic, and the most common zone of interaction is anal. The child needs an approving adult audience. That need leads to a variety of areas of learning—of language, behavior, and self-control. It can also be observed in a variety of trial-and-error efforts by the child to find what pleases. Gratification leads to an expansive self-system with many facets of life associated with the good me and positive self-esteem. Moderate anxiety leads to chronic anxiety, uncertainty, and insecurity. Extreme anxiety results in giving up known successful behavior in favor of self-defeating patterns that fulfill what has come to be expected by others.

The juvenile era covers ages 5 to 8 years. The shift to the syntaxic cognitive mode begins, and the interpersonal focus spreads to the peer group and to outside authority figures. The opportunity exists for peers and teachers to approve and accept behavior previously inhibited within the family—for example, talking "dirty" with one's friends. Interpersonal cooperation, competition, play, and compromise become the gratifying experiences. Juveniles learn to negotiate their own needs with a legitimate social concern without sacrificing self-esteem in the process. The risks of excessive anxiety are either too great a need to control and dominate social situations or internalization of restrictive, prejudicial social attitudes.

Preadolescence, ages 8 to 12, marks the child's movement from peer-group cooperation and competition based on rules to genuine intimacy with a chum. Sullivan saw the phase as a particularly important stage in which the give-and-take with the special friend can repair and undo distortions caused by excessive anxiety at earlier stages. The child truly moves outside the family for the first time and engages in a free give-and-take with another person unfettered by the same family dynamics. The major shift toward syntaxic thinking takes place, although some distortions may persist into adolescence. A capacity for attachment, love, and collaboration emerge or fail to develop in the face of excessive anxiety. Although sexual exploration may be a part of the chum relationship, Sullivan did not see sexuality as a central element in preadolescence.

Adolescence, beginning at puberty, has in its early stage similar concerns as preadolescence, with the important exception that lust is added to the interpersonal equation. The same needs for a special sharing relationship persist but shift to the opposite gender for their outlet, leading to a major opportunity for learning or severe anxiety. As the person faces culturally defined stereotyping, many new opportunities for social experimentation may lead to the consolidation of self-esteem or to self-ridicule. The struggle to integrate lust with intimacy is accomplished by painful trial and error. If the integration is completed with the self-system relatively intact, the later years of adolescence become an opportunity to expand the syntaxic mode to such areas as a consensual view of interpersonal relations, values and ideals, career decisions, and social concerns.

THEORY OF PSYCHOPATHOLOGY Sullivan abhorred diagnostic labeling as unhelpful, overly restrictive, dehumanizing, and used primarily to impress patients or colleagues. Perhaps his most famous quotation was, in discussing persons with schizophrenia, "We are much more simply human than otherwise." He sought to understand the fundamental human process going on within his patients, especially his sickest ones. He saw psychopathology as resulting from excessive anxiety that arrests development of the self-system and, thereby, limits both opportunities for interpersonal satisfaction and available security operations. He viewed psychiatric patients as struggling to maintain their self-esteem with limited means. To understand them, one has to gauge the developmental phase at which they are operating and grasp the interpersonal needs they are expressing.

Sullivan thought that several factors affect the form that the disturbances take. The level of anxiety at a particular developmental stage can lay the groundwork for a developmental arrest. Basic cognitive capacity may play a role in the choice of security operations relied on or retained. The degree of success achieved interpersonally, combined with whatever capacities are used, affects later success. The chance occurrence of stresses encountered during life is also a factor. Sullivan thought that, at least in theory, anyone may become schizophrenic, even persons with relatively successful developmental histories, should their chosen defenses fail dramatically and their life stresses mount in the extreme. However, schizophrenic patients are likely to be highly vulnerable along all four dimensions: developmental level, cognitive capacity, interpersonal achievement, and stress exposure; others with greater developmental strengths may become obsessive, hysteroid, schizoid, or paranoid.

INTERPERSONAL PSYCHOTHERAPY Sullivan emphasized that the psychiatrist is a participant-observer in all interactions with patients. He thought about the nuances and the opportunities involved in that unique situation. When the psychiatrist interacts actively with patients, verbal and nonverbal expressions of recurrent interpersonal patterns become apparent. Those observations then inform the therapist's further behavior, thus creating the opportunity for change. The process occurs over seconds and over months and years as the psychotherapy unfolds. Sullivan saw that perspective as an antidote to what he perceived as the wrongheaded emphasis on objective neutrality embodied by the blank-screen model of psychotherapist behavior. He argued that parataxic distortions emerge in all interactions, not only in the classical analytic situation.

Sullivan saw therapy as elucidating the patient's interpersonal patterns, exploring their usefulness in the service of the patient's needs, and considering alternative and more favorable possibilities. He emphasized the patient's experiencing of the distortions, the needs, the patterns, and the potential changes within the ongoing interaction with the therapist. He saw great power in the very entanglement of the therapist with the patient and recognized the ability of a skilled therapist to manage the interpersonal process to reveal patterns and to shape the patient's emotional experience. Yet he constantly emphasized and respected the ultimate autonomy of his patients, who could still, in the end, choose not to reshape their approach to the world.

Sullivan divided therapy into four distinct stages: inception, reconnaissance, detailed inquiry, and termination. *Inception* involves the very beginning, often only a part of the first interview, during which the contract and the roles are stipulated. *Reconnaissance* may go on for as many as 15 sessions, during which the therapist identifies the patient's recurring patterns and assesses their adaptive and maladaptive qualities. The *detailed inquiry* is a lengthy process of exploring the patient's thoughts, feelings, and memories and of evaluating and reevaluating data from earlier stages, seeking to recognize, clarify, and change persistent parataxic distortions. The recurrent patterns are discussed within the context of the patient's developmental history, needs, anxieties, failures, and successes. There is often much ongoing interchange between patient and psychiatrist as feelings and perceptions are validated or questioned within the context of mutual emotional interchange in each session. *Termination* is a product of the evolving contract and understanding between the patient and the therapist and may reflect either extensive or limited goals. Sullivan emphasized the constant reassessing of goals by the therapist and the power of the ongoing negotiation and renegotiation of the therapeutic contract to reveal and change parataxic distortions. The ultimate goals of psychotherapy are to achieve as much experiencing within the syntaxic mode as possible and to broaden the repertoire of the self-system. To the extent that those goals are achieved, patients are able to become responsible for their ongoing growth through subsequent interpersonal interactions.

WILHELM REICH

Wilhelm Reich (1897–1957) was one of Freud's most controversial followers; his late years were marred by mental illness (Figure 7-13). Reich fixed on and elaborated Freud's early but later discarded view that neurosis results from the damming up of sexual energy. Reich held that blockage of normal orgasm can lead to partial conversion of sexual energy into aggression, but that residual tension manifests in the form of characteristic physical tensions that reflect the underlying character armor of each person.

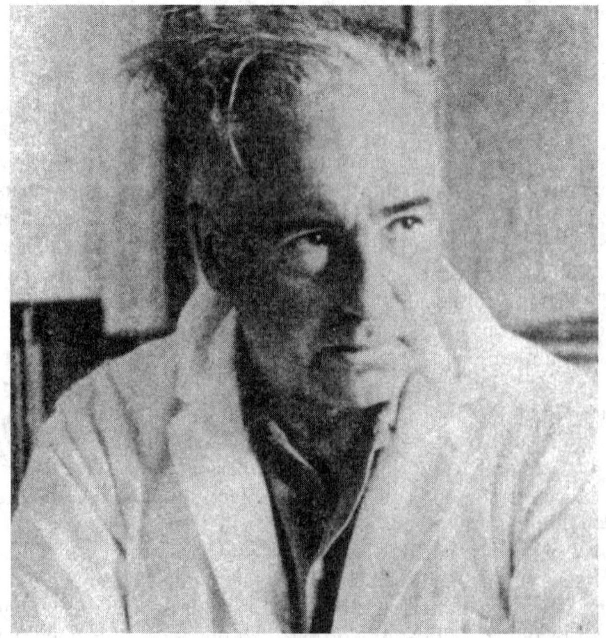

FIGURE 7-13 *Wilhelm Reich. (Courtesy of New York Academy of Medicine.)*

PERSONALITY THEORY Reich did not disagree with Freud's ideas concerning personality development, including the character types based on fixation at specific levels of psychosexual maturation. Reich went on to elaborate the interpersonal and physical behavior of those personality types. The specific behavioral traits constitute a *character armor* that defends against internal and external dangers. The traits are involuntary, repetitive, ego-syntonic behaviors that prevent the emergence of repressed impulses. For instance, the trait of ingratiation frequently defends against hostile impulses, just as the traits of hostility and self-assertion may defend against wishes to be dependent and passive. The traits are manifested physically in the voluntary musculature as characteristic postures (clenched jaw or fist, rigid or bowed back) or in stiffness or fluidity of movement.

Hysterical character The hysterical character has the least body armoring and, hence, the most lability of function. Body movements tend to be soft, rolling, and sexually suggestive. The persons of this type are superficial, excitable, flighty, fearful, highly suggestible, and easily disappointed. Their armor helps defend against easy sexual arousability by flushing out potential sexual stimuli in the environment and then reacting to them with anger.

Compulsive character Persons of this type are tense and restrained, walk stiffly, and sit rigidly. They are overconcerned about orderliness, tend to ruminate, and are indecisive and distrusting. They experience a blockage between their thoughts and their feelings. Because they have little access to their feelings, they have little ability to prioritize their actions, to make decisions, and to sense others' reactions to them. Compulsive characters avoid the expression of repressed impulses by rigid overcontrol. Therefore, trivial changes in routines are threatening to them.

Phallic-narcissistic character Phallic-narcissistic persons appear cold, reserved, and prickly. They are outspoken and provocative and seek positions of power. Frustrated at the genital-exhibitionist stage of development, the men are identified with the penis, and the women are identified with the fantasy of having a penis. The men have strong erective potency but little capacity for intimacy. The women actively dominate men.

Masochistic character Masochistic persons suffer, complain, and damage and self-depreciate themselves in ways that provoke and torture others. Reich differed with the classic analytic interpretation that masochists enjoy suffering. He thought the opposite—that pleasure is painful for the masochist because of an enormous need but excessive guilt and, therefore, low tolerance for love or pleasure. Suffering allows the masochist to indulge in a certain amount of self-gratification. Sexual intercourse can be enjoyed, for example, if the partner is inconsiderate or if the intercourse is accompanied by the fantasy of rape.

TREATMENT Reich's major contribution was in the realm of treatment. He was the first to recognize the need to deal with character resistances before attempting to recover repressed material through free association. He analyzed patients' character armor—their characteristic behaviors (including tone of voice, posture, and physical movements)—in the analytic setting before proceeding to an analysis of the unconscious. Reich worked face-to-face with patients and sought to relax their character armor by physical manipulation. That type of therapy, called *vegetotherapy* by Reich, is still practiced by Reich's followers as *bioenergetics*.

ERICH FROMM

Psychoanalyst Erich Fromm (1900–1980) was often thought of as the archetypical neo-Freudian; he was the leader among those who believe that culture and social setting influence a person's dynamics as much as the instincts do (Figure 7-14). Neither physician nor biologist, Fromm, a native German, received his doctorate in philosophy, sociology, and psychology from the University of Heidelberg in 1922. There he was exposed to the Marxist emphasis on the way history shapes societies and the way societies, in turn, shape persons according to economic needs. He was trained as a psychoanalyst at the Berlin Psychoanalytic Institute and then founded, with Frieda Fromm-Reichmann, the Frankfurt Psychoanalytic Institute. In 1933 he emigrated to the United States and in 1949 moved to Mexico City to found an institute. In 1974 he moved to Switzerland, where he died in 1980. As much a social critic as a personality theorist, he was later claimed by the existential and humanistic psychoanalysts. Fromm's intellectual agenda was the integration of Freud's theory of a dynamic unconscious with Marx's theory of history and social criticism.

PERSONALITY THEORY For Fromm, two central facts dominate human behavior: the inevitability of separateness and the historical and social moment into which each person is born. He argued that every person struggles to recapture the state of blissful union that existed prenatally. From the moment the baby begins to recognize itself as a separate human being, a titanic struggle begins, pitting the desperate anxiety of loneliness against the urge to fully express and actualize oneself and ultimately to transcend the self. Most persons find the loneliness too painful to bear, and they suppress their striving for *individuation* (the process of becoming a fully autonomous, separate person) in the service of maintaining the illusion of connectedness. They are socialized by their parents into the roles defined by the society into which they are born. Fromm actually used the term ''symbiosis'' years before Margaret Mahler used it for the universal human yearning for fusion, safety, and security.

Facing aloneness and choosing individuation leads to freedom and a productive life. However, true freedom is terrifying for many persons, who, instead, construct a series of illusions that engender a feeling of safety and security. They create a pseudoself, think pseudothoughts, and experience pseudofeelings in support of those illusions, thereby cutting themselves off from the fullness of their own inner lives. Fromm saw Freud's theory as a special case of his own more general ideas. The illusions of Victorian society involved the sublimation of sexuality and aggression in the service of social respectability. Social respectability, in turn, provided the illusion of acceptance and security.

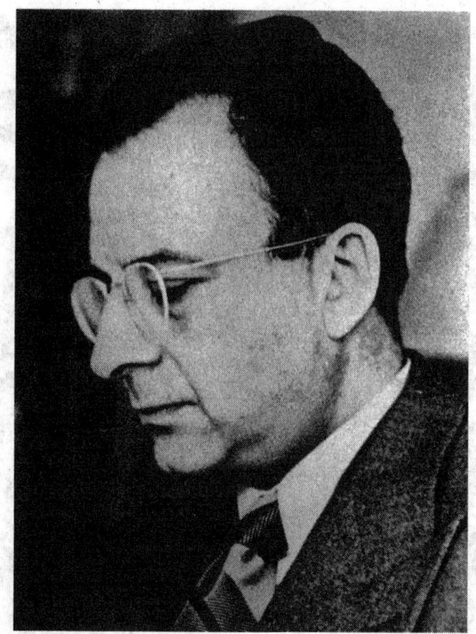

FIGURE 7-14 *Erich Fromm. (Courtesy of Erich Fromm.)*

In other places at other times, different solutions are offered. Early in World War II, shortly after his escape from Nazi Germany, Fromm wrote about the willingness of people to give up their own freedom to serve an authoritarian society. In the 1950s he wrote of the pursuit of material things in the service of postwar productivity, leading to self-satisfied conformity. Fromm's most direct application of Marxism was in his hypothesis that individual development parallels historical development: humankind frees itself from symbiosis with nature and embarks on a unique path, evolving inevitably toward the Marxist millennium—the ending of history in the universally humane society. But Fromm departed from Marxists who saw revolution as the only healthy response to an inevitably repressive society. He believed that, even within an imperfect culture, persons can face their terror, give up their pseudoselves and pseudothoughts, and choose to become themselves—encountering others who have made similar choices with love and mutuality. Before one can achieve that end, Fromm said, four basic human needs must be met: relatedness, transcendence, identity, and a frame of orientation. *Relatedness* refers to the need to feel connected to other humans. *Transcendence* refers to rising above basic instincts. *Identity* indicates the need to feel accepted yet unique. Emphasis on the need for a *frame of orientation* led Fromm, late in his career, on an exploration of the constructive and destructive roles religion may play.

THEORY OF PSYCHOPATHOLOGY As a social philosopher and critic, Fromm did not develop a systematic theory of psychopathology. He did identify three major mechanisms of retreat from individuation. Some persons, he said, seek an authoritarian solution, trying to live through someone or something external to themselves, relying on that for their sense of adequacy. Others become destructive, attacking anything that confronts them with their separateness and aloneness. Most persons develop a conformist attitude, warding off the anxiety of experiencing their own intentionality by accepting socially offered thoughts, roles, and attitudes.

Those mechanisms result in four unproductive orientations or characters typical of 20th-century society: receptive, exploitative, hoarding, and marketing. One sees, here, Fromm's economic perspective on available social roles. The *receptive character* often appears to be cooperative and open; however, the primary agenda is to establish a passive relationship with a leader who solves problems magically. *Exploitative characters* are likewise interested in filling themselves up from the outside; however, they aggressively manipulate and usurp whatever reduces their terror. *Hoarders* collect, store, and close in on themselves, often being cold and aloof in their efforts to feel secure. And *marketers* treat themselves as plastic commodities to be manipulated as needed to achieve externally validated success.

TREATMENT Fromm wrote nothing on the practice of psychotherapy; therefore, what is known is derived from anecdotal reports by those who studied with him or were treated by him. They report his emphasis on a tender and empathic inquiry into the self-deceptions and illusions created by patients in their efforts to ward off the anxiety of separateness and to maintain some sense of connectedness to significant others. He placed great emphasis on the tendency of unloved children to identify intensely with parental values to capture the magical safety the parents seem to offer. At a time when most psychoanalysts were preoccupied with detailed examinations of the instincts and defenses, Fromm contributed a sense of the range and the richness of inner experience that underlies superficial adaptation. He contributed the sense that a new authenticity can be found by those willing to confront the truth about themselves with all its terror of aloneness.

JULES H. MASSERMAN

Jules H. Masserman (1905–) studied psychobiology with Adolf Meyer and psychoanalysis with Franz Alexander. Masserman's biodynamic approach integrated the biological and dynamic aspects of all behavior. His experimental studies with animals led him to believe that all behavior is rooted in striving for individual and species survival. Each person's adaptive patterns result from a unique combination of genetic inheritance, maturational processes, and life experiences (Figure 7-15).

PSYCHOLOGICAL THEORY Masserman described three basic (*Ur-*) defenses against psychological disorganization and traumatization: belief in physical invulnerability, belief that other humans are potential friends and helpers, and belief in a higher celestial order. Those defenses lead humans to strive for physical survival, social belonging, and cosmic identity. When one of those three areas is threatened, physiological dysfunction, social maladaptation, and existential suffering result.

ANIMAL INVESTIGATIONS Masserman showed that pathological behavior can be induced by an apparatus that causes feeding-related stresses in monkeys, cats, and dogs. He called the process *neurotigenesis* and thought that the resolution of the animals' symptoms parallels the process of spontaneous recovery and of psychotherapy in humans. Some animals retest formerly frustrating feeding situations and work through their inhibited or other behavior in a manner similar to human reexploration and mastery of psychic traumas. Many animals respond to therapeutic measures. For example, a hungry animal can be slowly pushed toward food until its feeding and other inhibitions are overcome by hunger. A fearful animal often improves when placed with peers that are unafraid of the feeding situation, as do humans in response to positive group influences. In a few animals the increased conflicts between attraction and aversion cause agitation and panic. A "neurotic" animal can also be retrained by gentle steps. First, the animal is fed from the trainer's hand. Then it is urged to take food in the experimental apparatus. Later, the animal opens the feeding box with the trainer nearby. Finally, the animal works the formerly traumatizing switch and feeds itself without urging.

In human psychotherapy the patient seeks help from a therapist who uses the transference expectation of being helped. The therapist patiently and wisely reassures, guides, and supports the patient in reexamining conflicting wishes, in recognizing misinterpretations of reality, and in exploring new ways of living until the patient is sufficiently successful and confident to proceed without formal therapy.

TREATMENT The biodynamic approach uses a flexible schedule of therapeutic sessions that fits the patient's needs and resources. It is a meld of specific guidance, drugs, physical treatment, and attention to the patient's physical, social, and attitudinal problems in the here and now. History is probed only to the extent needed to clarify outmoded but continuing early patterns of behavior. Joint sessions with family, friends, employers, and others are used to help clarify and improve the patient's interactions. The criterion for success in therapy is positive behavioral change. Masserman describes the essence of psychiatric treatment as rapport, relief, review, reorientation, rehabilitation, resocialization, and recycling.

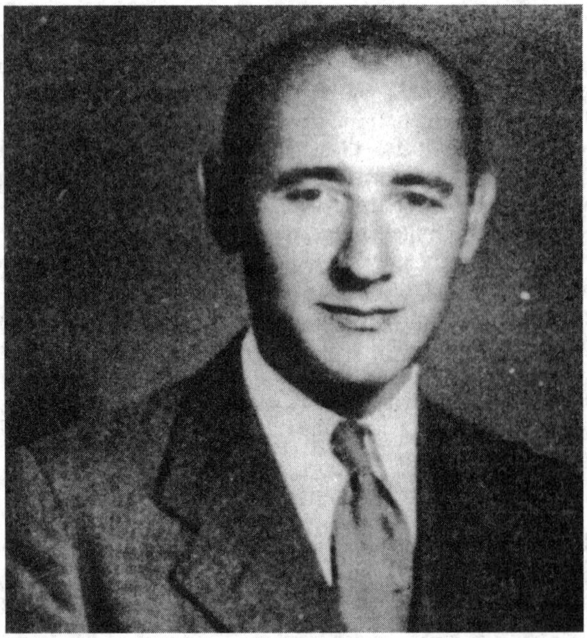

FIGURE 7-15 *Jules H. Masserman. (Courtesy of New York Academy of Medicine.)*

ERIC BERNE

Eric Berne (1910–1970) was an American original in both style and substance (Figure 7-16). He worked in the San Francisco area most of his career. He broke with psychoanalysis in the mid-1950s but never became antianalytic, as did many of his followers. Like many others, he felt the need to develop treatments briefer than those then offered. A group gathered around him and came to be known as the San Francisco transactional analysis (TA) seminars. Through weekly discussions of clinical cases and of social and political issues, Berne gradually refined his theory. He was wry and provocative in his approach to human behavior. His approach contributed to what is now called pop psychology, although its popularity and faddishness has long since faded. Few clinicians now call themselves TA therapists. Nonetheless, Berne's ideas remain useful in grasping hidden agendas in human interactions.

PERSONALITY THEORY For Berne, the primary motivator of all human behavior is the need for *strokes*—attention, recognition, and response by others. Early in life, survival depends on adequate physical contact, stimulation, and nurturance. That need remains strong, but it later becomes symbolic and interpersonal. Children rapidly learn what works within their families and practice it extensively. That observation led to one of Berne's more widely quoted statements, "Negative strokes are better than no strokes at all." People evolve ways of interacting with their world to obtain regular strokes in whatever way they can and in whatever way they have been taught to define a stroke. For example, sympathy in response to chronic depression may provide such powerful stroking that the depression cannot be given up. So great is the need for regular stroking that blatantly destructive actions persist in the face of insight, recognition, and enduring psychological or physical pain. Like Alfred Adler and Harry Stack Sullivan, Berne said that hidden

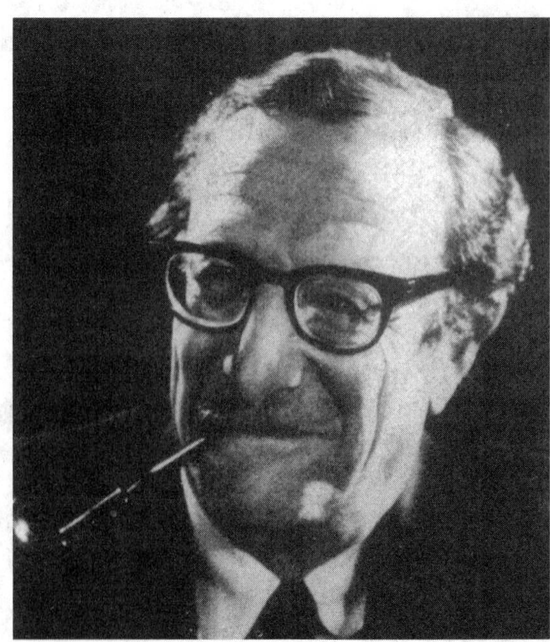

FIGURE 7-16 *Eric Berne. (Courtesy of Grove Press.)*

social needs motivate human behavior to the extent that, with rare exceptions, an interpersonal hidden agenda is present in all human activity. For Berne the unit of observation was the transaction, the short-term process of persons interacting with each other. He spent much energy analyzing transactions to discover patients' definitions of strokes and their preferred mechanism for obtaining them. He noted that most persons engage in predictable, stereotyped, repetitive transactions. The content may vary from situation to situation, but the form tends to be rigid. He called those transactions *games,* and his best-seller, *Games People Play,* captured the imagination of the American public in 1964. Some games are harmless; some are socially encouraged; many have destructive elements or, at least, limit opportunities for more gratifying relationships (intimacy); and some are highly destructive. A common socially accepted game is cocktail-party flirtation, which is ordinarily pleasant and harmless but—depending on the intensity, frequency, and seriousness with which it is played—may result in the inability to experience intimacy, in disrupted marriages, or even in physical harm.

Berne divided the human psyche into three primary parts—Child, Parent, and Adult—with two of those parts further subdivided (Figure 7-17). He called those parts ego states. An *ego state* consists of characteristic body language, voice qualities, verbal productions, and affective experiences. The Child ego state represents the persistence of childlike experiences and expressions in all persons. It is divided into three parts: the Natural Child, the ego state in which the spontaneity, joy, and intuitive perceptiveness of young children persists in all adults; the Adapted Child, the part that is compliant and cooperative; and the Rebellious Child, the repository of that part of each person prone to fight authority, challenge accepted wisdom, and struggle for autonomy. The Parent ego state is the residue of internalized parental messages and injunctions. It is divided into two parts, the Critical Parent and the Nurturing Parent. The Critical Parent bears some resemblance to Freud's superego, embodying rules, values, instruction, criticism, and restrictions. The Nurturing Parent is the internalization of positive caring experiences, the memory of loving interactions. The Adult ego state is a purely rational, data-processing element that is objective, calculating, decision making, and probability estimating.

Mental health is the flexible availability of all ego states, with no one predominating. Excess Critical Parent produces guilt and depression, but insufficient Critical Parent produces sociopathy. Excess Nurturing Parent produces a narcissistic laziness, but insufficient Nurturing Parent causes an inability to soothe oneself and maintain self-esteem.

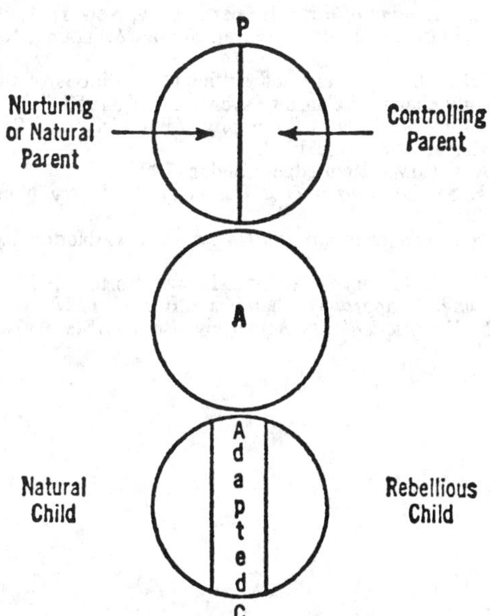

FIGURE 7-17 *Eric Berne's descriptive model of the personality. (Figure from E Berne:* What Do You Say After You Say Hello?, *p 13. Random House, New York, 1972.)*

Excess Adult results in a cold and overly rational person, but insufficient Adult leaves the person unable to balance the various internal forces in life. Too much Natural Child may result in irresponsibility, but not enough Natural Child depletes the ability to experience joy in living. Overabundance of Rebellious Child causes self-destructive battles with no constructive purpose; however, insufficient Rebellious Child may result in an overly conformist stance. Excess Adapted Child prevents appropriate autonomy striving, but insufficient Adapted Child prevents participation in group or hierarchical efforts.

Berne placed great emphasis on the child's ability to intuit parental messages and instructions, especially those communicated nonverbally and unconsciously. In that fashion the growing child may encode a conscious verbal instruction in the Critical Parent (be strong, be perfect, be smart) while internalizing a more powerful, unconscious message in the Child (do not grow up, do not leave me, do not surpass me). Usually, a model for carrying out the instruction is preserved in the Adult (be passive, drink alcohol, run around with women, act crazy). Together, the messages make a *script.* Berne emphasized the active role of the child in searching for the messages and in accepting them. That activity was crucial for him because it emphasizes the person's role in deciding to follow the script, even though the messages may have been accepted at a very young age. Scripts come in all varieties, ranging from the successful to the utterly self-destructive. For Berne the business of human living involves carrying out one's script according to the transactions learned as a child. The entire basis for psychological change lies in the person's capacity, having once accepted the script, to change his or her mind. Otherwise, the person carries out the script throughout life.

THEORY OF PSYCHOPATHOLOGY Berne's understanding of psychopathology is based on the adaptiveness of a person's games and script and the person's capacity for adaptive use of all ego states. Because Berne wrote at a time when American psychiatry rejected phenomenological diagnosis, it is difficult to map his notions of psychopathology onto the fourth edition of *Diagnostic and Statistical Manual of Mental Disorders* (DSM-IV). But he did describe numerous clinical situations and histories that are familiar to all psychiatrists, and he analyzed them according to their scripts. He was impressed with the role of fantasy and fairy tales in children's development and often asked patients what their favorite stories were as children. He then searched for the hidden identifications and messages within the story to help discern the patient's script. Insofar as he developed a nosology, it lay in the scripts encouraged by culturally sanctioned fairy tales. For example, Cinderella is a story about a young girl waiting to be rescued by a fairy godmother or charming prince and unwilling to assert herself against unjust authority. Little Red Riding Hood is a story about a girl who likes to chat with "wolves" and who gets in trouble trying to please everybody. Men, he found, identified with the wolf or Prince Charming and were unable to regard women as real persons.

Berne developed and catalogued a separate nosology of games. Examples include cocktail-party flirtation (Rapo I), which concludes when the man and the woman, having experienced the gratification of feeling attractive and attracted, part, seeking other persons to attract. Rapo II usually ends with a line like, "What kind of girl do you think I am." Rapo III ends with a painful, destructive love affair.

Another game is Why Don't You . . . Yes, But. In its mild, sociable form one person presents a problem, successfully enlisting the advice of many others; but for every proffered solution a ready explanation of why it will not work is given. The stroke or payoff is the attention and the feeling of superiority achieved by defeating others. The second-degree version of the game produces a chronic, helpless depression; the third-degree version may lead to the back wards of a state hospital.

There was no rigid mapping between games and scripts, and Berne never claimed that either was exhaustive. They were intended as clinical examples to guide the psychotherapist's thinking in evaluating each patient, who presented unique script and transactional issues. Patients were assessed according to the "straightness" of their transactions (were there hidden communications and invitations emanating from different ego states?), the adaptiveness of their scripts, and the predominant ego state and its effects. Thus, Berne might describe a compulsive person as having too much Critical Parent or a histrionic person as having too much Natural Child. In the end he saw his catalogues and any nosology as poor substitutes for the careful, clinical study of each patient.

TREATMENT Having been trained in psychoanalysis, Berne used many psychoanalytic techniques. But he applied them in unique ways. Much of his clinical work was done in groups, with the therapist being very active in confronting and interpreting the interpersonal behavior of the patients. He placed great emphasis on the initial contract with the patient and on the setting of clear, concrete goals. He encouraged therapists to inquire early on in therapy, "How will we know when our work is finished?" If a clear and specific answer was not forthcoming, he would inform the patient that therapy had not yet begun. The focus was then on the patient's difficulty in defining a recognizable end point for the work. Berne's approach was heavily informed by the psychoanalytic concept of resistance but was applied in an unusual manner. Berne examined any treatment goal defined by a patient for evidence that it was a way to continue playing games or pursuing scripts more effectively, rather than giving them up entirely.

Like Sullivan, Berne regarded the ongoing interaction between patient and therapist as the key ingredient in psychotherapy. The therapist's job is to interact actively with the patient; recognize the ego states, games, and scripts being enacted; counter them, using confrontation, interpretation, and various other interpersonal maneuvers designed to thwart the enactment; and confront the patient with a choice and an opportunity to relate in a different manner. He emphasized simple, direct statements, using everyday words to stimulate affective experience and interaction. Interactions often began with his inquiry, "What do you want to work on today?" Observers sometimes described his work as individual therapy within a group context; a dialogue would ensue, with the other patients as silent observers who often resonated emotionally to the interaction.

Berne emphasized individual responsibility for one's life and experience, which he felt had been obscured by the emphasis on historical exploration and explanation. He constantly communicated to patients the opportunity for choosing to continue or to discontinue the patterns and habits encouraged as a child. He also demonstrated to patients the invitations they offer to others to behave in various ways, thus creating their own interpersonal reality. Health lies in the potency experienced by recognizing one's options for deciding what invitations to offer to others and which to accept from others, even though they may be communicated unconsciously and nonverbally.

SUGGESTED CROSS-REFERENCES

Many sections of this textbook refer to the theorists described above. Some are included in Section 50.1 on the history of psychiatry. Others are referred to Section 6.1 on psychoanalysis, Chapter 8 on theories of personality and psychopathology: schools derived from philosophy and psychology, and Section 26.1 on the history and current theoretical concepts in psychosomatic medicine.

REFERENCES

Adler A: *The Individual Psychology of Alfred Adler: A Systematic Presentation in Selections from His Writings,* H L Ansbacher, R R Ansbacher, editors. Basic Books, New York, 1956.

Adler A: *Problems of Neurosis: A Book of Case Histories,* P Mairet, editor. Harper & Row, New York, 1964.

Alexander, F: *Psychosomatic Medicine.* Norton, New York, 1950.

Alexander F, French T, Pollock G H: *Psychosomatic Specificity.* University of Chicago Press, Chicago, 1968.

*Berne E: *Games People Play.* Grove Press, New York, 1964.

Berne E: *What Do You Say After You Say Hello? The Psychology of Human Destiny.* Bantam, New York, 1972.

Fromm E: *Escape from Freedom.* Avon, New York, 1965.

Gabbard G O: *Psychodynamic Psychiatry in Clinical Practice.* American Psychiatric Press, Washington, 1994.

Greenberg J R, Mitchell S A: *Object Relations in Psychoanalytic Theory.* Harvard University Press, Cambridge, MA, 1983.

*Grosskurth P: *Melanie Klein: Her World and Her Work.* Harvard University Press, Cambridge, MA, 1987.

Hamilton N G: A critical review of object relations theory. Am J Psychiatry *146:* 1552, 1988.

Horney K: *Neurosis and Human Growth.* Norton, New York, 1950.

*Horney K: *The Neurotic Personality of Our Time.* Norton, New York, 1937.

Jung C G: *Analytical Psychology: Its Theory and Practice.* Random House, New York, 1968.

Jung C G: *The Practice of Psychotherapy,* ed. 2. Princeton University Press, Princeton, NJ, 1966.

Jung C G: *Two Essays on Analytic Psychology.* Princeton University Press, Princeton, NJ, 1966.

Klein M: Mourning and its relation to manic-depressive states. In *Contributions to Psycho-Analysis,* 1921–1945, M Klein, editor. Hogarth Press, London, 1948.

Klein M: Notes on some schizoid mechanisms. In *Developments in Psycho-Analysis,* M Klein, P Heimann, S Isaacs, J Riviere, editors. Hogarth Press, London, 1952.

*Lieberman E J: *Acts of Will: The Life and Work of Otto Rank,* Free Press, New York, 1985.

Masserman J H: *Theories and Therapies of Dynamic Psychiatry.* Science House, New York, 1973.

McGuire W, editor: *Analytical Psychology: Notes of the Seminar Given in 1925 by C G Jung.* Princeton University Press, Princeton, 1989.

Meyer A: *Collected Papers of Adolf Meyer,* 4 vols. Johns Hopkins University Press, Baltimore, 1948–1952.

Meyer A: *Psychobiology: A Science of Man.* Charles C Thomas, Springfield, IL, 1957.

Mullahy P: *Psychoanalysis and Interpersonal Psychiatry: The Contributions of Harry Stack Sullivan.* Science House, New York, 1970.

Quinn S: *A Mind of Her Own: The Life of Karen Horney.* Addison-Wesley, Reading, MA, 1988.

Rado S: *Psychoanalysis of Behavior,* 2 vols. Grune & Stratton, New York, 1956, 1962.

Rank O: *The Trauma of Birth.* Harper & Row, New York, 1973.

Reich W: *Character Analysis.* Farrar, Strauss & Young, New York, 1949.

Rogers C R: The necessary and sufficient conditions of therapeutic personality change. J Consult Psychol *21:* 95, 1957.

Sharaf M: *Fury on Earth: A Biography of Wilhelm Reich.* St. Martin's Press/Marek, New York, 1983.

*Stevens A: *On Jung.* Routledge, London, 1990.

Sullivan H S: *The Interpersonal Theory of Psychiatry.* Norton, New York, 1953.

Sullivan H S: *Schizophrenia as a Human Process.* Norton, New York, 1962.

Vaillant G: *Adaptation to Life.* Little Brown, Boston, 1977.

Wehr F: *Jung: A Biography.* Shambbala, Boston, 1987.

Weiner M F: *Practical Psychotherapy.* Brunner/Mazel, New York, 1986.

CHAPTER 8 THEORIES OF PERSONALITY AND PSYCHOPATHOLOGY: APPROACHES DERIVED FROM PHILOSOPHY AND PSYCHOLOGY

PAUL T. COSTA, Jr., Ph.D.
ROBERT R. McCRAE, Ph.D.

INTRODUCTION

Personality psychologists have defined their subject matter in many ways, so that no single definition is possible. Some see personality as a repertoire of learned behaviors, some as a set of traits, some as a structure that organizes and integrates experience and action. But most concur that personality psychology deals with the person at a global level, describing characteristics that are pervasive and enduring and form a central part of the person's identity. To know someone's personality is to know what he or she is really like.

Descriptions of personality tend to emphasize either universal characteristics of human nature or important aspects of individual differences among people, although those two are often related. Thus, Plato and later Sigmund Freud saw human nature in terms of conflict between reason, passion, and appetite. Plato regarded them as universal elements of personality that together determine the flow of behavior. But people differ: some have strong appetites, and some have disciplined reason; those differences account for the varieties of human character. Personality theories may be defined as accounts of how people differ in their ways of being human.

Individual differences can be measured, and personality psychology as a science relies heavily on the measurement of such characteristics as anxiety, sociability, and curiosity to test theories of the nature and the development of personality. Individual differences are also central to an understanding of psychopathology, and many theories of personality have been formulated to explain variations in psychological adjustment.

This chapter selectively reviews theories of personality derived from philosophy and scientific psychology, their relations to psychopathology, and their implications for psychotherapy, with a particular emphasis on the systematic consideration of individual differences. Traditionally, personality theories have been grouped into major schools: psychoanalytic, behavioral, humanistic, and trait psychologies. Because psychoanalytic theories are covered in other chapters in this textbook, only the other schools are discussed here. In many respects those groupings are artificial: a personality theorist like Henry Murray may be regarded as a psychoanalyst or as a humanist or as a trait psychologist. Nevertheless, each of the schools has enough common themes to justify treating them together in so brief an overview as this.

PHILOSOPHICAL VIEWS

The recognition of individual differences is probably as old as human culture, but differences in personality were long confounded with differences in status, class, or caste. Persons from a high status were assumed to be superior human beings—more sensitive, honorable, and wise than other humans. They were endowed with those characteristics by education or by bloodline or—in the view of Indian philosophy—by moral behavior in a previous life.

PLATO The first major account of personality in Western thought was provided by Plato. In *The Republic* he made extended comparisons between the constitutions of different states and the constitution of the soul. Just as every state must have peasants, artisans, soldiers, and rulers, so each person has appetites (for food, sex, and so on), passions (for honor and advancement), and reason. The relative strength of those three characteristics determines character and fitness for a particular place in society. Intelligent and thoughtful people ought to rule, and passionate people should be chosen to defend the state; dull and spiritless persons, lacking reason and passion, should be given the menial chores of agriculture and industry.

Plato assumed that those psychological characteristics were, like physical strength and musical talent, largely inborn, but he regarded them as properties of the individual, not the person's social status. Although he assumed that high-status citizens normally bear children of the greatest potential, he specifically acknowledged that exceptions exist; in his ideal state children of the lower classes would be promoted, and those of the higher classes would be demoted on the basis of their own merits. Here personality would be the basis of the social order, not vice versa. His most radical extension of that idea was to argue that women should be given social equality and allowed to become soldiers and rulers if they possessed the necessary mental and physical qualifications.

One of the recurring questions in personality theory has been the relative importance of nature versus nurture. Trait psychologists, particularly those interested in the study of temperament, have frequently pointed to innate differences in personality, whereas behaviorists and psychoanalysts have laid great stress on the formative influences of the environment and early childhood experiences. Ready as he was to acknowledge the importance of inborn potential, Plato was also keenly aware of the influence of education. Much of *The Republic* is devoted to his views on the effects of physical exercise, mental instruction, and poetry and music on the development of personality. Present-day concerns about the influences of television and rock music on children follow in that tradition.

Like most philosophers, Plato was more concerned with understanding virtue and vice than psychopathology, but, because he considered vice to be the result of weak or corrupted nature rather than free but evil choice, his discussions of character can be viewed as early descriptions of what may now be viewed as personality disorders. Just as states have better and worse forms of government, so people have better and worse configurations of reason, passion, and appetite. Plato described five personality types, corresponding to five forms of government. The ideal of mental health, corresponding to government by wise rulers, is one in which reason holds in check both passions and appetites. The arrogant and ambitious types have an excess of passion or pride; the avaricious type has an excess of appetite. However, in those types reason still retains some authority; for example, avaricious persons can control most of their appetites in order to indulge their desire for money. In the self-indulgent type, appetites are undisciplined; and in the debauched type (corresponding to a government by a despot) reason is completely disregarded, and a clearly psychopathological state is reached: As Plato wrote: "Thus, when nature or habit or both have combined the traits of drunkenness, lust, and lunacy, then you have the perfect specimen of the despotic man."

ARISTOTLE Plato's vivid but rough typology was succeeded by Aristotle's detailed analysis of human character in *Nicomachean Ethics.* Courage, temperance, generosity, pride, ambition, irascibility, friendliness, boastfulness, and shame were all defined and distinguished. Aristotle attributed pathological variations on those traits to innate defects or to disease processes: "Among all the excesses of foolishness, cowardice, intemperance and irritability some are bestial, some diseased. If, e.g., someone's natural character makes him afraid of everything, even the noise of a mouse, he is a coward with a bestial sort of cowardice." Aristotle considered variation within the normal range the result of training and habit and thus subject to praise or blame.

Aristotle's basic moral precept is the golden mean: He argued that extreme standing on either end of a trait dimension should be avoided. Thus, both stinginess and extravagance are vices, whereas generosity is a virtue; similarly, vanity and humility represent excessive or insufficient self-esteem. That conception continues to influence some modern notions of psychopathology, in which marked deviation from the norm in either direction is considered pathological. Persons excessively concerned with social attention may be regarded as having a histrionic personality disorder; those insufficiently concerned with social attachments may have a schizoid disorder.

Aristotle carried conceptual analysis to a level that has seldom been surpassed—distinguishing, for example, between the superficially similar qualities of temperance and self-control: Persons are temperate if they have healthy and moderate impulses that require little control, whereas persons have self-control only if they have immoderate appetites that are nevertheless held in check. Such considerations allowed Aristotle to form rational taxonomies of traits that anticipate the empirical taxonomies proposed by 20th-century factor analysts.

KANT AND SCHOPENHAUER The last great period of the Western philosophical tradition begun by Plato and Aristotle was inaugurated at the end of the 18th century by Immanuel Kant, whose critical philosophy forms a transition between purely rational approaches to human nature and the empirical sciences that followed. One of Kant's last works, *Anthropology from a Pragmatic Point of View,* considered both natural and moral variations in character and reintroduced the Roman physician Galen's taxonomy of choleric, phlegmatic, sanguine, and melancholic types to modern psychology.

Sciences are usually distinguished from philosophy by their reliance on empirical data, but one should not imagine that philosophers made no use of experience. On the contrary, like many of the clinicians who offered psychological theories of personality, philosophers based their ideas heavily on their observations of human nature. A striking instance is provided by Arthur Schopenhauer, a 19th-century follower of Kant whose dark view of the world as a place of purposeless striving had an extraordinary influence on the early personality theorists, including Sigmund Freud and Carl Gustav Jung.

One of the central beliefs of Western thought has been that human happiness or misery is the result of external conditions, what is now called quality of life. But Schopenhauer's acute observations, reported in *The World as Will and Representation,* led him to propose "the paradoxical but not absurd hypothesis that in every individual the measure of pain essential to him has been determined once and for all by his nature. . . . His suffering and well-being would not be determined at all from without, but only by . . . what is called his temperament."

In support of that view, Schopenhauer noted that wealth and power do not make people happy, "for we come across at least as many cheerful faces among the poor as among the rich." He also argued that the effects of great misfortunes or successes are short-lived and that, for the most part, evaluations of the external causes of a state of mind are illusory attributions:

> We often see our pain result only from a definite external [cause] and . . . believe that, if only this were removed, the greatest contentment would necessarily ensue. But this is a delusion. . . . [The pain] would appear in the form of a hundred little annoyances and worries over things that we now entirely overlook.

Recent scientific research on psychological well-being has confirmed that account in every detail: well-being is chiefly a function of enduring personality dispositions; wealth, social class, and other markers of the objective quality of life are virtually unrelated to subjective happiness; and processes of adaptation quickly return persons to their own characteristic baseline of happiness after favorable or unfavorable life events. Schopenhauer's observation is also consistent with recent evidence on the heritability and lifelong stability of many mental disorders.

And yet reason and insight are not enough. On the basis of his own experience and the examples of history, Schopenhauer also concluded that "man inherits his moral nature, his character, his inclinations, his heart from the father, but the degree, quality, and tendency of his intelligence from the mother"—a conclusion flatly contradicted by the findings of modern behavioral genetics. Psychology broke from philosophy over precisely that need to seek empirical verification of hypotheses, but psychology carried with it concepts and insights accumulated over two millennia of profound thought about human nature.

BEHAVIORAL AND SOCIAL LEARNING APPROACHES

THEORIES OF PERSONALITY Behaviorism as a school of psychology grew up in reaction to the prevailing mentalistic model, in which introspection was used to determine the contents and the operations of consciousness. John B. Watson proposed that a scientific psychology should confine itself to an examination of observable behavior and explain all human conduct in terms of stimuli and learned responses. Ivan Pavlov's experiments with conditioned responses offered hope that such a science could be successful, and theorists such as Clark L. Hull provided elaborate mathematical models of learning.

Radical behaviorism Certainly the most influential behaviorist and perhaps the most influential psychologist of the 20th century was B. F. Skinner. Skinner's basic concept was *operant conditioning,* in which behaviors are a function of the organism's history of reinforcement. The observation that animals can be taught tricks by giving them rewards and punishments is nothing new. But behaviorists like Skinner refined and systematized that idea, using elegant experimental designs to tease apart the effects of the amount and the schedule of reinforcements, the use of positive and negative rewards, and the difficulty of the discriminations required. Behaviors could be shaped, maintained, or eliminated by the judicious use of those principles.

Skinner was a radical behaviorist, a purist who denied not only the scientific value but even the existence of mind. Further, he avoided any neurological or psychophysiological theorizing, preferring to study the empty organism. Individual differences were ignored in understanding basic phenomena and were explained in persons as the result of different histories of reinforcement. Even differences between species were neglected: Skinner thought that the pigeon provided an adequate model for the study of learning in all organisms; he and his followers were, in fact, able to replicate many of their animal findings in human beings. Much of Skinner's success can be attributed to his single-minded pursuit of a highly circumscribed set of variables.

Skinner's view of personality was, predictably, a reductionistic one. As he stated in *About Behaviorism,* "a self or personality is at best a repertoire of behavior imparted by an organized set of contingencies. The behavior a young person acquires in the bosom of his family composes one self; the behavior he acquires in, say, the armed services composes another." That position is rejected both by humanistic psychologists, who attribute more choice and control to the person than does Skinner, and by trait psychologists, who see consistencies of behavior that appear to transcend the consistencies of the reinforcing environment. Many personality psychologists have argued that controlled laboratory experimentation is a poor basis for theories of personality, because persons play a large role in selecting and shaping their own environments. Skinner's radical behaviorism was rejected or modified by many later learning theorists, who acknowledged the power of conditioning but also recognized differences among species and among individuals within a species.

Social learning theory One of the most distinctive features of human organisms is their use of speech, which makes possible both elaborate thinking and complex social interactions. In recent decades, learning theorists have increasingly emphasized social and cognitive processes. Among the most important learning theorists have been Julian Rotter and Albert Bandura, both of whom have offered versions of social learning theory.

Rotter's theory proposes that human behavior is guided not only by the actual history of reinforcement but also by plans, goals, and expectations of success. Persons will perform a behavior if they believe it is likely to lead to a valued goal, based on their past experiences in general and in similar situations. Persons with a history of success are likely to have a generalized expectation that they can control their lives; they are described as having an *internal locus of control.* At the opposite extreme are those whose prior efforts have been generally unsuccessful; they come to believe that rewards and punishments are a matter of luck or the arbitrary decisions of powerful others. Such persons are said to have an *external locus of control.* Locus of control has been one of the most popular variables in personality research, one that is used in numerous studies that generally support Rotter's theory.

Bandura's version of social learning theory also acknowledges the importance of internal cognitive processes. Persons learn not only on the basis of their own experience but also through vicarious reinforcement from observations of others. Bandura's demonstration of modeling effects in experiments conducted in the 1960s gave scientific legitimacy to the social learning perspective.

Both Rotter's and Bandura's are general theories of behavior, not specifically theories of personality. But personality for them is something more than a collection of learned behaviors. The total pattern of experience leads to a generalized expectation of reinforcement or to a general sense of self-efficacy that can be considered the central individual difference variable. People are characterized primarily on the basis of their beliefs in their own ability to control their lives, because those beliefs powerfully determine the effort they make to adapt to their surroundings.

Social-cognitive approaches to personality are among the most influential for current research in personality. The approaches focus on people's understandings of themselves and how those self-appraisals shape goals, plans, and behaviors. Because of the approaches' origins in social learning theory, they tend to emphasize the role of the environment, pointing out that a person's sense of self varies from setting to setting. Because of the approaches' ties to social theory, they usually explain personality in terms of the effects of social interactions. For example. Hazel Markus has suggested that a person has a number of *possible selves:* conceptions of what one is or could be, which result from the messages that significant others provide. For such theorists, concern has moved beyond the social learning of specific behaviors to the learning of entire identities.

THEORIES OF PSYCHOPATHOLOGY Psychoanalytic theories of personality grew out of attempts to understand psychopathology; thus, psychoanalysis and psychopathology have intimate connections. By contrast, behavioral approaches have focused on the general principles by which behavior is acquired and maintained; psychopathology, where it is considered at all, is usually treated as an area of application. Learning theories have had much more influence on methods of psychotherapy than on theories of psychopathology itself.

Behavioral approaches may suggest two classes of explanations for psychopathology: psychopathology may be related to the mechanisms of learning themselves, or it may be considered the result of learning behaviors that are maladaptive or socially unacceptable.

In the 1950s Hans Eysenck, a psychologist who has figured prominently in both the learning and the trait schools of personality, proposed that individual differences in the dimension of introversion-extroversion determine the ease with which persons can acquire conditioned responses, which in turn determines the form of psychopathology to which they are prone. Very introverted persons, he proposed, are easily conditioned and thus acquire many inhibitions. They are predisposed to depressive, anxious, and obsessive-compulsive disorders. By contrast, extreme extroverts are resistant to conditioning and are predisposed to hysterical and psychopathic disorders. (In later versions of Eysenck's theory, psychopathic disorders are grouped with psychotic disorders and are linked to a different dimension of personality, psychoticism.)

Most behaviorists have viewed the laws of learning as universal processes and considered psychopathology to be the result of normal learning processes. In the 1920s Irena Shenger-Krestounika taught a dog to discriminate between a circle and an ellipse as a cue for food. When the ellipse was made increasingly circular, the dog's ability to discriminate between them was taxed, and the dog began to struggle, squeal, and bite. Pavlov dubbed that behavior an "experimental neurosis" and proposed that human neuroses have parallel causes.

Probably the most famous attempt to explain psychopathology in learning theory terms was provided by John Dollard and Neal Miller. Dollard, an anthropologist, and Miller, an experimental psychologist, shared an interest in psychoanalysis. Their goal was to translate psychoanalytic concepts into the testable terminology of learning theory, as in the central psychoanalytic notion of *repression*. Sexual behaviors in the child may be punished by parents, and the child may learn to associate the behaviors with pain. By stimulus generalization, even the thought of the behaviors elicits anxiety, and cognitive processes that block those thoughts lessen anxiety and thus are reinforced. Eventually, the thoughts are effectively barred from consciousness.

Many behaviorists who did not share Dollard and Miller's enthusiasm for psychoanalysis followed their lead in attempting to explain psychopathology in terms of learning principles. Phobias, in particular, were easily explained as conditioned responses reinforced by avoidant behavior. Similarly, compulsions can be understood as a kind of self-reinforcing behavior: each time the compulsive act is performed, the anxiety associated with not performing the act is reduced, increasing the probability that the behavior will be repeated.

Social learning theorists have also noted the self-perpetuating nature of some maladaptive behavior. Persons who lack a strong sense of self-efficacy in social situations may avoid those situations. As a consequence, they fail to learn the social skills that would enhance their self-confidence. Self-defeating behaviors, which may appear irrational from an outside perspective, are often understandable in terms of the dynamics of learning.

APPLICATION OF THEORY TO THERAPY Behaviorists have a rather rudimentary view of personality, seeing it as an assemblage of learned behaviors. They also tend to see psychopathology in superficial terms. Psychological maladjustment is considered the result of learned behaviors that are called symptoms, but they are not symptomatic of any underlying disorder. Curing the symptoms cures the disorder. At worst, that position is naive and simplistic, equating the patient's presenting problem with the real source of difficulty. At best, however, it focuses attention on a specific problem that can be concretely addressed.

Many techniques for behavior modification have been used with considerable success in treating symptoms of psychopathology. Joseph Wolpe developed *systematic desensitization* as a treatment for phobias. Patients were instructed to relax and were then presented with increasingly vivid cues of the phobic object. Eventually, they were able to face the object itself without anxiety. A more dramatic technique is *implosive therapy,* in which the patient is confronted directly with the feared object (for example, a room full of snakes) without an opportunity to escape. Because the object itself is harmless and because avoidant behavior cannot be performed and is, therefore, not reinforced, the phobic reaction is swiftly extinguished.

Therapeutic interventions may be based on eliminating the reinforcements that sustain behavior, on punishments for unwanted behaviors, and on modeling or shaping of more desirable behaviors. Any variable known to affect the acquisition or the extinction of behaviors may provide an opportunity for behavior change, and behavioral techniques have been applied to physiological responses, as well as to voluntary behaviors, through biofeedback.

Behavior therapies have been used extensively in treating phobias, in controlling addictive behavior, in reducing the self-destructive behavior of autistic children, and in improving classroom discipline. For the behaviorist, the distinction between psychopathology and bad behavior is generally unimportant. Behavior therapies are most effective when the problem can be clearly traced to a particular set of behaviors or conditioned responses; they are much less effective in dealing with vague complaints of confusion and distress, although those are frequently the problems that the patient presents to the clinician.

HUMANISTIC APPROACHES

THEORIES OF PERSONALITY Psychoanalysis and behaviorism are mechanistic theories that trace human behavior and experience to the gratification of instinctual impulses or to the acquisition of learned responses. Many of the most influential personality theorists of this century have defined themselves in terms of their opposition to those two approaches. Although they vary widely in terms of their explanations of personality, humanistic approaches share a positive evaluation of human nature and emphasize their unique and distinctively human aspects. Personality both produces and reflects organization, rationality, consistency, future orientation, planfulness, self-expression, cognitive complexity, and adaptability. Human reason and freedom of will, the capacity for growth and change, the need for love and self-transcendence are prized by most humanistic theorists.

Social learning theories may be seen as a humanized form of behaviorism, because they recognize the role of complex symbolization and language in human learning. In a similar way many now-classic humanistic theories were intended as modifications of psychoanalysis. Indeed, the first major psychoanalytic revisionist was Carl Gustav Jung, who argued that human beings have spiritual needs, as well as sexual needs. Henry Murray also made major modifications to psychoanalysis in his view of personality. For example, Murray credited the mature ego with much more autonomy than Freud granted it, and he argued that the person's sense of morality is not fixed by the superego instilled in childhood but can continue to develop into more rational and altruistic forms than those developed by the child. Erich Fromm and Karen Horney minimized the instinctual origin of personality development and suggested that culture plays a large role in shaping the person. Erik Erikson proposed stages of psychosocial development to parallel Freud's psychosexual development, emphasizing such distinctly human characteristics as identity, intimacy, and generativity. Erikson also theorized that personality development continues throughout the life span, giving encouragement to research on aging and personality.

Allport Although Gordan Allport is usually classified as a trait psychologist, he was clearly a humanist in his general orientations to theorizing. For him human behavior is proactive, reflecting internal, self-initiating characteristics more than situational forces. In his view human personality possesses psychological coherence and both momentary (cross-sectional) and long-term (longitudinal) organization. Allport considered personality functioning to be characteristically rational—organized and influenced by such conscious characteristics as long-range goals, plans of action, and philosophies of life.

Perhaps the most salient and controversial feature of Allport's approach was the extreme emphasis he put on the uniqueness of the individual personality. Allport viewed the major task of *personology* (personality psychology) as the understanding and the prediction of the individual case. To grasp the real personality, one must assess personal dispositions, and doing so requires intensive study of a person's past, present, and anticipated future functioning through the use of such techniques as the case history and a content analysis of personal documents. In *Becoming: Basic Considerations for a Psychology of Personality,* Allport championed the view that concepts and laws must be developed to fit the individual case, creating the terms "idiographic" and "morphogenic" to symbolize his conviction that "each person is an idiom unto himself, an apparent violation of the syntax of the species."

Allport was deeply concerned with identifying personality functions, which he discussed under the concept of the *proprium,* the superordinate concept in his system. Propriate functioning not only organizes and integrates actions and experience but also provides the impetus to psychological growth. Allport described the functions of the proprium as *sense of body, self-identity, self-esteem, self-extension, rational coping, self-image,* and *propriate striving.* Those propriate functions are vital to personality; while they are ongoing, they are by no means considered unchanging. Allport theorized that the propriate functions are modified throughout life, predominantly in the direction of greater differentiation and integration or growth. The development of selfhood—away from the undifferentiated, opportunistic functioning of infancy and early childhood toward propriate functioning and striving—is part of human nature for Allport. Persons guide or direct their lives by attempting to fulfill their sense of self or proprium. Development continues into adulthood, with increasing signs of maturity and personal life-style.

Maslow Abraham Maslow interpreted personality in motivational terms. The person's whole life—his or her perceptions, values, strivings, and goals—is focused on the satisfaction of a set of needs, and the needs themselves are arranged in a universal hierarchy. Maslow's needs serve an organizing and integrating role in life and are not to be understood as a simple and invariant set of responses to environmental pressures. They organize and create action possibilities and external reality.

At the lowest level of the motivational hierarchy are physiological needs for food, water, sex, and sleep. The second level consists of safety needs—needs for protection and security. The third level consists of needs for love and belongingness. The fourth level consists of needs for self-respect and esteem from others. Above those needs lie the highest needs—for beauty, truth, justice, and *self-actualization,* the development of one's full potential as a unique human being.

People live at the lowest level of motivation that is troublesome for them. For example, if needs for food and shelter are not routinely met, they become the overriding concern in life: the hungry person risks danger and social ostracism to find food. Those who have always been well-fed, however, learn to take the satisfaction of physiological needs for granted, and their attention is dominated by higher needs. Instead of examining specific behaviors and their reinforcements, Maslow's theory concerns the long-term satisfaction of broad classes of needs and thus gives a broad depiction of the person.

Maslow's theory explains individual differences in terms of the levels of motivation, but, unlike trait theories, it does not assume that those differences are necessarily stable characteristics of the person. Instead, the differences reflect different life histories and life courses. In Maslow's view anyone with a history of routinely gratified physiological, safety, and belongingness needs operates on the esteem or higher levels of motivation, but precarious life circumstances can cause the person to regress to a lower level of motivation.

Maslow devoted much of his writing to a characterization of higher needs, including self-actualization, a drive to fulfill one's unique potentials. He believed that personality psychology had become obsessed with psychopathology and thought that a corrective emphasis on positive mental health was needed. His biographical studies of such exemplary persons as Eleanor Roosevelt and Abraham Lincoln suggested a number of distinctive characteristics of self-actualizers, including an accurate perception of reality, creativity, a need for privacy, and the frequent experience of mystical or peak experiences. As an exception to his general theory of motivation, Maslow also noted that such persons often skip the low levels and proceed directly to self-actualization. The most creative artists and musicians never seemed to care about poverty or the lack of social acceptance.

Kelly One of the most unconventional theories of personality was offered by George Kelly. It is in some respects a purely cognitive approach but one with few ties to traditional learning theory. Instead of seeing human beings as organisms that are conditioned by their environment, Kelly argued that they should be seen as scientists trying to make sense of their world. In *The Psychology of Personal Constructs* he stated the fundamental postulate of his theory: "A person's processes are psychologically channelized by the ways in which he anticipates events."

The basic unit for understanding personality is the *personal construct,* a schema for classifying and interpreting experiences. For example, a person may construe other people in terms of the contrast strong versus weak. Each new acquaintance is categorized as either a strong person or a weak person, and subsequent interactions with that person are guided by the original construal. In the course of experience, it is probably necessary to reclassify as weak some persons initially thought to be strong and vice versa; more important, some people may act in ways that are neither strong nor weak, leading the construer to develop new constructs (say, friendly versus hostile) that are useful in predicting other people's behavior.

Kelly elaborated a set of 11 corollaries to his fundamental postulate to provide a formal theory of personality. He explained individual differences by noting that "persons differ from each other in their construal of events." He noted that personal constructs are organized into a coherent structure, with some constructs subordinate to others; he also specified, however, that persons may from time to time use constructs that are mutually inconsistent. His choice corollary states that persons select the alternative in a dichotomy (for example, strong) that promises to best help anticipate events, and the experience corollary states that construct systems evolve as the result of experience.

That rather abstract and bloodless theory is made relevant to psychopathology by Kelly's ingenious reconstruals of some basic emotional reactions. He defined *anxiety* as the awareness that one's construct system is inadequate for construing important events. *Guilt* is the recognition that one's behavior is inconsistent with the ways in which one construes oneself. *Hostility* is the attempt to force experience to fit one's existing constructs. Such definitions are remote from both common sense and clinical notions of anxiety, guilt, and hostility, but, precisely for that reason, they offer the prospect of novel ways of treating those problems.

Rogers Carl Rogers is probably the most influential humanistic personality theorist. He articulated a formal theory of personality, pioneered a major school of therapy (client-centered therapy), and encouraged rigorous research on his theory and therapy. Rogers held that all organisms tend toward their own actualization—that mental health and personal growth are the natural condition of humankind. Psychopathology is a defensive distortion of that actualization process, and psychotherapy consists of creating conditions in which defense is unnecessary. Given those conditions, patients (or *clients,* as Rogers called them) essentially cure themselves.

The theoretical basis of Rogers's approach is phenomenological. That is, Rogers emphasized that everyone experiences the world differently and that the only world anyone knows or can know is the world of his or her own experience. Objective reality is of secondary importance to the person's perception of reality. Within that phenomenal world the most important object is the *self,* the person as he or she appears to himself or herself. (Other theorists use the terms "self-concept" and "self-image" to describe the phenomenon.)

Under ideal conditions, people's needs, desires, and goals emerge naturally as part of self-actualization and are recognized as part of the self; people are fully open to experience. In real life, however, one person's needs and desires often conflict with those of others; in particular, children find themselves in conflict with their parents, who withhold love when the child (from their perspective) misbehaves. Because love is essential, children internalize those *conditions of worth* and believe that they are good and worthwhile persons only when the self is consistent with the ideals imposed by significant others. To maintain their sense of worth, they may distort their experience; doing so leads to anxiety and to self-defeating behavior.

In some respects Rogers's theory is much like Freud's: Both see psychopathology as the result of defensive distortions and see the ideal state as one in which persons can accept conflicts and deal with them rationally. Rogers is a humanistic theorist because he assumes that human nature is essentially good and defenses ultimately unnecessary. For Freud the impulses of the id are eternally primitive and selfish, and their full actualization would be socially catastrophic.

THEORIES OF PSYCHOPATHOLOGY In general, humanistic theories of personality stress the positive aspects of human nature and discuss maladjustment in terms of failures of and blocks to the full growth and development of the person. Both Rogers and Kelly formulated their theories in the context of counseling students—persons who presumably had relatively minor maladjustments and considerable personality strengths. The applicability of humanistic theories to patients suffering from schizophrenia or dementia is certainly questionable, but the theories have had a profound effect on routine clinical practice, in which clearly diagnosable psychiatric disorders seldom account for all the patient's problems in living.

Humanistic psychologists differ tremendously in their views of the origins of maladjustment. Rogers pointed to internalized conditions of worth acquired chiefly during childhood. Erich Fromm, who was influenced by Karl Marx, blamed society as a whole for instilling in persons nonproductive orientations, such as hoarding and marketing orientations. Kelly said little about the origins of maladjustment but thought its essence is an ineffective construct system too rigid to be corrected by experience.

Other personality theorists, such as Rollo May, have been influenced by existential philosophy and have argued that the essential characteristic of human nature is freedom. Freedom, however, implies responsibility, and what Fromm called the attempted ''escape from freedom'' often leads to psychopathology. In that view people are the ultimate source of their own problems. The debate about responsibility and mental illness continues today, perhaps most conspicuously in questions about whether alcoholism should be considered a disease or a failure of self-discipline.

APPLICATION OF THEORY TO THERAPY Some humanistic theories of personality—for example, Allport's—have had little influence on psychotherapy; others, like Rogers's theory, have been tremendously influential. For decades the dominant form of therapy was psychoanalysis, a process that may require years and in which treatment is focused on dreams, childhood memories, and the ongoing relation with the therapist (the transference), rather than on the patient's immediate problems. Many of the standard techniques of contemporary counseling, clinical psychology, and psychiatry rest on a different set of assumptions about human nature that are made scientifically respectable by the work of humanistic psychologists.

Brief psychotherapies often consist of opportunities for patients to express their feelings and rethink their problems in a supportive atmosphere. The therapist may provide advice and guidance or, at least, offer new ways in which patients can think about their problems. (Many psychiatrists use that general approach as an adjunct to medication, even in the treatment of serious mental disorders.) The brief psychotherapy process implicitly assumes that people, even those requiring psychotherapy, are basically rational and are able, with some help, to solve their own problems; it also assumes that, given the right conditions, they will move toward mental health: patients are seen as scientists and self-actualizers.

The humanistic emphasis on freedom and responsibility has often clashed with the psychiatric tradition of regarding mental disorders as diseases. Labeling patients as ''schizophrenics'' or ''phobics'' is held by some to be dehumanizing, and critics like Thomas Szasz have argued that mental disorders are social and ethical judgments, not matters of medical fact. Of course, abundant evidence indicates that some mental disorders have a biological basis, but the criticisms of humanistic psychologists make the point that the disorder occurs in a human being who in many respects may be like any other person. Behaviors, experiences, and relationships may be normal or abnormal, but people are not normal or abnormal.

TRAIT AND FACTOR MODELS

Individual differences are peripheral concerns in many social learning and humanistic theories of personality; they are the central focus of trait theories. The study of variations in human character and temperament goes back at least to Theophrastus, a Greek philosopher whose *Characters* depicted 30 different types. For example, he described the morose type as follows:

> A malignant temper sometimes vents itself chiefly in ferocity of language. The man whose tongue is thus at war with all the world, cannot reply to the simplest inquiry except by some such rejoinder as—'Trouble not me with your questions:' nor will he return a civil salutation. . . . He has no pardon for those who may unwittingly shove or jostle him, or tread upon his toe. . . . He will neither wait for, nor stay with anyone long: nor will he sing, or recite verses, or dance in company. It is a man of this spirit who dares to live without offering supplications to heaven.

THEORIES OF PERSONALITY The scientific study of individual differences in personality can be traced to Sir Francis Galton in England, who laid the foundations of psychometrics, and to G. Heymans in the Netherlands, who undertook the first large-scale study of rated personality traits. The first major trait theorist in the United States was Gordon Allport, whose 1937 book, *Personality: A Psychological Interpretation,* spelled out the basic issues in trait psychology. Allport defined a *trait* as ''a neuropsychic structure having the capacity to render many stimuli functionally equivalent, and to initiate and guide equivalent (meaningfully consistent) forms of adaptive and expressive behavior.'' In that view something in the brains of morose persons makes them see even simple questions or greetings as personal affronts, and their sullen attitude is expressed in a variety of social situations.

> Allport believed that traits are concrete features of persons that uniquely describe them and that may be understood by a case study of a single person. A contrasting view is that traits are dimensions of individual difference that can be discovered only by comparing and contrasting different persons; people are then described in terms of their standing on a set of common traits. The two definitions are closely related; people who are more anxious than 99 percent of the population presumably have a neuropsychic structure that makes them anxious.

Characteristics of traits Although many different trait theories have been proposed, there is general agreement on several key features of traits: (1) Traits are tendencies to show consistent patterns of thoughts, feelings, and actions. Behaviors that are specific to a single setting or situation may better be considered habits than traits; some evidence of cross-situational consistency is necessary to infer a trait. But concrete instances of behavior have many determinants, including learned habits, aroused needs, social contexts, role requirements, and the influence of many different and potentially conflicting traits, so the influence of a specific trait on any particular behavior may be modest. Usually, only by viewing behavior across many situations can a consistent pattern be detected. (2) Traits are relatively enduring features that characterize the person. In that respect they are distinguished from transient moods or episodes of mental disorder that affect the person. The fact that traits are relatively enduring does not mean that they cannot change; traits are not immutable, even if they are durable. (3) Traits are continuously distributed, usually approximating a normal or bell curve. Although it is convenient to speak about introverts and extroverts, in fact, most persons are ambiverts, showing some of the characteristics of introverts and some of the characteristics of extroverts. With the possible exception of masculinity-femininity, there is no consistent evidence of discrete personality *types*.

Those characteristics of traits may also be used to describe abilities, needs, values, and attitudes, and trait theorists show considerable disagreement on how broadly the term "personality trait" should be construed. Allport distinguished adaptive and expressive traits, and J. P. Guilford contrasted temperamental, motivational, and ability traits. Perhaps the most common convention is to distinguish personality traits proper from ability traits and from physical characteristics. Spatial ability and physical attractiveness are not considered personality traits, whereas consistent and enduring nervousness, enthusiasm, open-mindedness, affability, and carefulness are.

From time to time controversy has surrounded the reality of traits, fueled by the fact that human beings easily and readily ascribe traits to others on the basis of little or no information, with correspondingly limited accuracy. Those personality ascriptions may be triggered by stereotypes of age or physical appearance or may be idiosyncratic. Demonstrations of that fact in laboratory experiments by social psychologists, together with the relatively loose cross-situational consistency of most traits, led a generation of psychologists in the 1970s to conclude that traits are cognitive fictions. Subsequent work—particularly demonstrations that judges who know the person well agree with each other and with the self-reports of the person about his or her standing on a variety of traits—restored faith in the consensual validity of traits. But the controversy does make the crucial points that some trait ascriptions are more accurate than others and that first impressions may be misleading. Psychiatrists ought not to assume that their clinical judgments of a patient's personality are correct; validated personality questionnaires and rating forms completed by knowledgeable others may be needed to portray and understand personality accurately.

Personality structure and factor analysis The most important differences among trait theorists are in the specific traits they have conceptualized and measured. Jung identified introversion and extroversion as basic personality variables; Bandura emphasized self-efficacy; Rogers was concerned with openness to experience. Over the years literally thousands of scales have been developed to measure traits that psychologists considered important in understanding personality. As early as 1936 Allport pointed to another source for identifying personality traits: the natural language. In a monograph he published with Henry Odbert, Allport listed some 18,000 terms extracted from an unabridged dictionary that can be used to describe people; some of them are mere evaluations (for example, "swell," "awful"), but he regarded about 4,000 as legitimate trait terms.

The problem for trait psychologists was how to choose a manageable set of traits from among the many possible constructs. Trait terms are highly redundant—for example, "anxious," "worrying," "nervous," "apprehensive," and "fearful" reflect similar, if not identical, characteristics—so what was needed was a procedure for identifying major groups of traits that covary. Factor analysis, a statistical technique that reduces the complexity of a set of correlations among variables, was first used in personality research by J. P. Guilford and has remained one of its basic tools. The factors or dimensions identified in the process correspond to groups of closely related traits; the set of basic dimensions identified by the factor analysis constitutes a model of the structure of personality traits.

Raymond Cattell developed one of the first and most influential factor models. He reasoned that, in the course of cultural evolution, any personality trait important in human social interaction would have been noticed and named; the 4,000 trait terms identified by Allport and Odbert were thus assumed to represent an exhaustive listing of personality characteristics (that assumption has become known as the *lexical hypothesis*). Cattell grouped synonyms and near synonyms together to obtain a set of 35 personality variables, and he asked respondents to rate acquaintances on each of those sets of terms. He intercorrelated the ratings and factored the correlations, identifying 12 factors. Together with four more factors found in research using self-report questionnaires, those became the basis for the 16 Personality Factor Questionnaire (16 PF), a self-report instrument that has been widely used in personality research and clinical psychology for more than 30 years.

Originally, theorists hoped that factor analysis would provide an objective solution to the question of personality structure, but for many years factor analysts agreed on little. Eysenck believed that Cattell's model was unreplicable and needlessly complex. Eysenck proposed a simple two-dimensional model that identifies extroversion-introversion (E) and neuroticism-emotional stability (N) as superfactors and showed that, if the scales of the 16 PF are themselves factored, the two largest factors resemble his E and N. He and his wife, Sybil Eysenck, developed a series of instruments to measure those factors (and later a third superfactor called "psychoticism"); the instruments have been widely used, particularly in Great Britain. Eysenck's stature as a learning theorist and a critic of psychoanalysis contributed to the importance of those dimensions in psychiatric contexts.

The five-factor model Eysenck's two factors were widely replicated, but they seemed to omit many important characteristics, such as curiosity, aggression, and achievement striving. An alternative solution was offered in 1961 by two U.S. Air Force psychologists, Ernest Tupes and Raymond Christal. They began with the 35 clusters of traits identified by Cattell and obtained ratings on those clusters in eight samples. They found that a five-factor solution fit the data in all eight samples. Two of the factors resembled Eysenck's E and N, but three other factors were new.

A small group of lexical researchers, including Warren Norman and Lewis R. Goldberg, continued to study personality structure as represented by natural language trait adjectives; after 20 years they came to the conclusion that the five-factor structure proposed by Tupes and Christal was essentially correct. Renewed interest in that model showed that the five factors can be recovered in analyses of self-reports, as well as ratings; in ratings of children, college students, and elderly adults; and in several languages, including non-Indo-European languages, like Chinese. The factors appeared in analyses of trait adjectives, descriptive phrases, and questionnaire scales. Contemporary five-factor theorists differ somewhat in their conceptualizations of the factors and, consequently, give them somewhat different labels. The terms "neuroticism" (N), "extroversion" (E), "openness to experience" (O), "agreeableness" (A), and "conscientiousness" (C) are used here. The five factors and some of the traits that define them are listed in Table 8-1.

Many psychologists were skeptical of the lexical hypothesis that led to the five-factor model. Those critics believed that personality theory and clinical experience would lead to the identification of important traits for which no lay terms existed, and they continued to offer alternative models. Isabel Myers and Katharine Briggs operationalized Jung's psychological functions in the Myers-Briggs Type Indicator, which classifies persons in terms of the dichotomies introversion versus

TABLE 8-1
Examples of Adjectives, California Q-Sort Items, and Revised NEO Personality Inventory Facet Scales Defining the Five Factors

	Definers		
Factor Name	**Adjectives**	**Q-Sort Items**	**Facet Scales**
Neuroticism (N)	Anxious	Thin-skinned	Anxiety
	Self-pitying	Brittle ego defenses	Angry hostility
	Tense	Self-defeating	Depression
	Touchy	Basically anxious	Self-consciousness
	Unstable	Concerned with adequacy	Impulsiveness
	Worrying	Fluctuating moods	Vulnerability
Extroversion (E)	Active	Talkative	Warmth
	Assertive	Skilled in play, humor	Gregariousness
	Energetic	Rapid personal tempo	Assertiveness
	Enthusiastic	Facially, gesturally expressive	Activity
	Outgoing	Behaves assertively	Excitement seeking
	Talkative	Gregarious	Positive emotions
Openness (O)	Artistic	Wide range of interests	Fantasy
	Curious	Introspective	Aesthetics
	Imaginative	Unusual thought processes	Feelings
	Insightful	Values intellectual matters	Actions
	Original	Judges in unconventional terms	Ideas
	Wide interests	Aesthetically reactive	Values
Agreeableness (A)	Appreciative	Not critical, skeptical	Trust
	Forgiving	Behaves in giving way	Straightforwardness
	Generous	Sympathetic, considerate	Altruism
	Kind	Arouses liking	Compliance
	Sympathetic	Warm, compassionate	Modesty
	Trusting	Basically trustful	Tender-mindedness
Conscientiousness (C)	Efficient	Dependable, responsible	Competence
	Organized	Productive	Order
	Planful	Able to delay gratification	Dutifulness
	Reliable	Not self-indulgent	Achievement striving
	Responsible	Behaves ethically	Self-discipline
	Thorough	Has high aspiration level	Deliberation

Adapted from R R McCrae, O P John: An introduction to the five-factor model and its applications. J Pers *60:* 175, 1992.

extroversion, intuition versus sensing, thinking versus feeling, and judging versus perceiving. Timothy Leary argued that the traits that influence social interactions are better represented in a circular order than as a set of factors, and many instruments have been developed to measure that model.

A particularly important system was suggested by Theodore Millon, who was interested in personality traits associated with psychiatric disorders. His reviews of clinical literature led to a theory of personality and psychopathology that specifies 11 personality disorders as extreme variants of normal traits. For example, the histrionic personality disorder is supposed to be related to the trait of gregariousness; the schizoid personality disorder is related to the trait of detachment. Millon's theory had a profound effect on the formulation of Axis II in the third edition of *Diagnostic and Statistical Journal of Mental Disorders* (DSM-III) and in subsequent editions. His instrument, the Millon Clinical Multiaxial Inventory, has been widely used by psychiatrists and clinical psychologists.

The fact that trait theories of personality are usually tied to assessment inventories makes it relatively easy to make empirical comparisons, and in the past decade researchers in several countries have undertaken the task of relating trait models. Those researchers share a growing consensus that virtually all the traits measured by theory-based personality questionnaires—including those derived from psychodynamic, behavioral, and humanistic theories—are related to one or more of the five factors of Tupes and Christal. However, instruments vary in comprehensiveness. For example, the four scales of the Myers-Briggs Type Indicator correspond to four of the five factors, whereas measures of the interpersonal circle represent only two factors (extroversion and agreeableness). Table 8-2 lists some scales empirically linked to each of the five factors. At the broadest level the problem of personality structure appears to have been resolved: personality consists of five basic factors.

That statement does not mean that personality can be exhaustively described by standing on five dimensions. Most trait psychologists adopt hierarchical models of trait structure. They assume that the broadest factors are composed of specific traits, which are defined by discrete behaviors. In the Revised NEO Personality Inventory (NEO-PI-R), for example, six specific traits or facets are measured for each of the five factors or domains of personality. The facet scales are listed in Table 8-1; the hierarchical organization is illustrated in Figure 8-1. Assessment on the level of specific facets provides a detailed and personalized portrait of the individual person.

Heritability and stability of personality traits Psychoanalytic, learning, and humanistic theories have usually offered causal explanations for individual differences. Thus, differences in self-efficacy are supposed to be caused by different histories of success in pursuing goals; variations in openness to experience may be the result of differences in the conditions of worth imposed by parents. The factor analysts who scoured the dictionary for trait terms usually bypassed that issue, being content to describe the personality differences they found in adults. In principle, some traits may be inherited, some instilled by parents, some learned from experience; whatever their origin, they can be measured and used to predict important life criteria.

Until recently theorists generally assumed that personality is shaped primarily by a variety of environmental influences, including parental love and discipline, social and economic opportunities, and life experiences through childhood and adolescence. Surprisingly, that assumption has rarely been tested: little prospective longitudinal research has documented links between early childhood experiences and subsequent adult personality. A different research design, using the techniques of behavior genetics, can answer those questions by comparing personality measures in adults with degrees of genetic and environmental similarity. For example, similarity between identical twins reared apart can be attributed to genetic influences, whereas similarity between adopted siblings reared together must be due to environmental influences.

In the past 20 years behavior genetics studies using many samples,

TABLE 8-2
Some Scales Empirically Related to Each of the Five Factors

	Factor				
Instrument	**N**	**E**	**O**	**A**	**C**
Hogan Personality Inventory	Low adjustment	Sociability	Intellectance	Likability	Prudence
California Psychological Inventory	Low well-being	Sociability	Achievement via independence	Femininity	Norm-favoring
Multidimensional Personality Questionnaire	Stress reaction	Social closeness	Absorption	Low aggression	Control
Adjective Check List	Low ideal self	Self-confidence	Creative personality	Low critical parent	Military leadership
Minnesota Multiphasic Personality Inventory (MMPI)	Psychasthenia	Low social introversion			
MMPI Personality Disorder Scales	Borderline	Histrionic	Schizotypal	Low paranoid	Compulsive
Guilford-Zimmerman Temperament Survey	Low objectivity	Ascendance	Thoughtfulness		Restraint
Myers-Briggs Type Indicator		Extroversion	Intuition	Feeling	Judging
Personality Research Form		Exhibition	Sentience	Nurturance	Order
Interpersonal Adjective Scales		Dominance		Love	

Adapted from R R McCrae, O P John: An introduction to the five-factor model and its applications. J Pers *60:* 175, 1992.

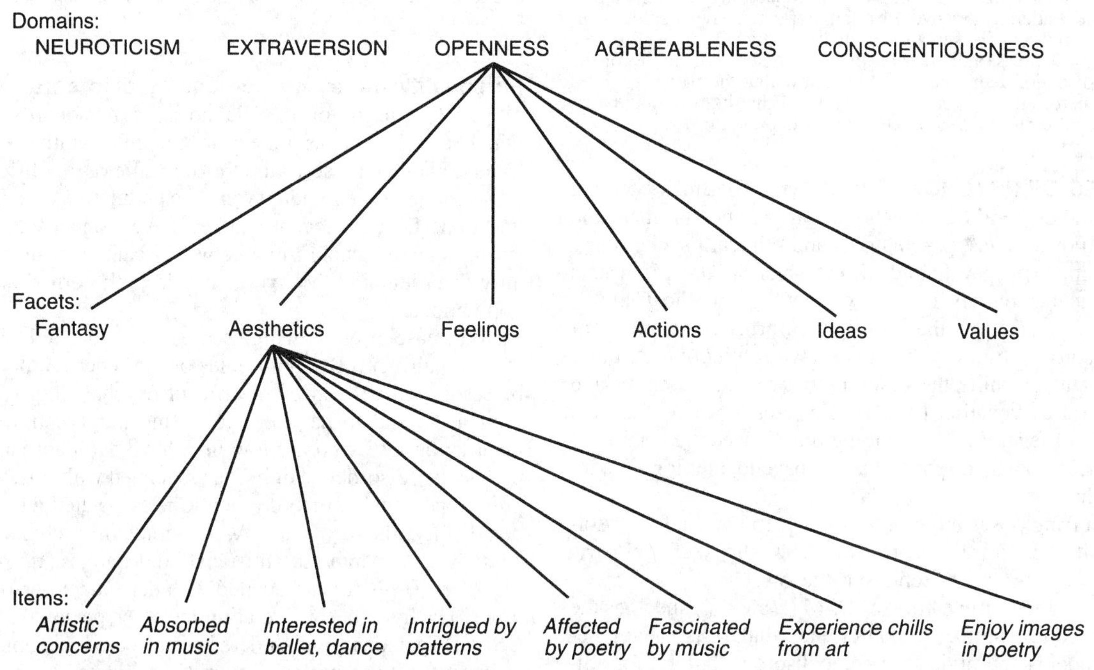

FIGURE 8-1 *An example of hierarchical organization in the revised NEO Personality Inventory: Domains, facets of openness, and items measuring openness to aesthetics.*

personality measures, and methods of data analysis have converged on the surprising conclusion that personality traits are to a considerable extent heritable and to a considerable extent caused by unknown and idiosyncratic factors but that they are hardly attributable to shared environmental causes at all. Socioeconomic status, family diet, religious training, parental modeling, and all the other influences that children growing up in the same household normally share seem to have little or no influence on adult personality. That conclusion applies most clearly to the dimensions of N and E, which have been the objects of the greatest amount of research, but seems also to hold for O, A, and C. That dramatic and counterintuitive finding will doubtless reshape theories of personality. As Sandra Scarr commented, "Psychology [currently] has no adequate theories to account for individual variation in behavior because our theories address the wrong sources of variation." Future theories will give a prominent place to genetic influences, and developmental psychology may become concerned with explaining how heritable traits come to be expressed in different family and social settings.

Research at the other end of the life span has also turned up surprising findings. Trait psychologists have always assumed that traits represent relatively enduring patterns of behavior, but most psychologists have also assumed that traits are modified by life experiences. Jung postulated that the process of individuation requires each person to express all his or her potentials, and thus the young introvert normally becomes an extrovert in old age and vice versa. Lay stereotypes of aging hold that, as they age, people become cranky, conservative, and depressed. Gerontologists have rebutted those myths of aging, arguing that old age is likely to bring maturity, wisdom, or detachment. Theories of adult development, popularized in Gail Sheehy's best-selling *Passages,* suggest that personality changes in stages and, in particular, that men and perhaps women go through a midlife crisis in their 30s or 40s.

In sharp contrast to all those theories are the findings from a number of independent longitudinal studies of personality in adulthood. Those studies present a clear picture of the predominant stability of the full range of personality traits. That is, the average levels of most traits neither increase nor decline much with age, and persons tend to maintain the same rank order. The 30-year-old who is outgoing, curious, and hardworking is likely to become an outgoing, curious, and hardworking 80-year-old. That conclusion has been supported by studies using both self-reports and ratings of all five factors of personality, and the conclusion appears to apply to both men and women. Both systematic and idiosyncratic changes in personality do appear between age 20 and age 30, although the decade still shows considerable continuity; and dementing disorders in old age often result in dramatic changes in personality. But normal life experience seems to have little effect on personality after age 30.

Few data on the long-term effects of psychopathology on personality are available. Patients in recovery from major depressive disorder generally score high on measures of N, and that may be a result of the experience of depression. However, the few prospective studies of the first onset of major depression typically show that the patients scored high on N before the first episode, suggesting that high N may be an enduring feature of people prone to clinical depression.

THEORIES OF PSYCHOPATHOLOGY The links between psychopathology and trait psychology are at once intimate and complex. For decades, psychiatrists and clinical psychologists have administered psychological tests such as the Minnesota Multiphasic Personality Inventory (MMPI) and the Cattell's measure of personality, the 16 PF, to inform the diagnosis of mental disorders; trait psychologists have routinely used those same tests to examine the relations between personality and such criteria as vocational preference, creative potential, and coping with life stress. The dividing line between normal variations in personality dispositions and psychopathology is frequently unclear.

That blurring poses more of a problem to psychiatric nosology than it does to trait theories of personality. A psychiatric diagnosis is supposed to represent the presence of a discrete disorder, and the fourth edition of DSM (DSM-IV) specifies the criteria that must be met to confer each diagnosis. That categorical model is appropriate for some disorders but not for others. It may be difficult to separate social phobia, for example, from extreme shyness and self-consciousness or to separate schizoid personality disorder from marked introversion. That difficulty is entirely consistent with trait models of personality, which regard individual differences as continuously distributed variables.

Neuroticism and psychopathology One theory of psychopathology is that some psychiatric disorders reflect extreme standing on personality traits, particularly those related to N. Among the traits that covary in normal populations to define the N factor are predispositions to experience long-term levels of negative affects, such as fear, anger, shame, and sadness. Persons with high standing on those traits may qualify for a diagnosis of generalized anxiety disorder, borderline personality disorder, social phobia, or dysthymic disorder.

Neuroticism may also be considered a risk factor for psychiatric disorders that are not themselves traitlike. Several recent studies have found that persons scoring high on measures of N are at increased risk of subsequently receiving a diagnosis of major depressive disorder. Poor control of urges and impulses and excessive concern with physical functioning are also characteristics associated with N, and persons high in N may be predisposed to eating disorders and hypochondriasis. Neuroticism is, in essence, a generalized disposition to experience psychological distress, and persons seeking psychiatric treatment are almost always distressed. Therefore, virtually all clinical populations, from drug abusers to schizophrenic patients, score high on measures of N.

Historically, the term "neurosis" or "psychoneurosis" was coined to identify psychiatric disorders of functional origin that were closely related to anxiety and its control. It survived in DSM-III-R in many secondary labels (dysthymia, for example, was also called "depressive neurosis"). Many personality psychologists object to the term "neuroticism" as a label for a dimension of normal personality because of its suggestion of psychopathology. Many psychiatrists object to the term because it appears to be tied to an outdated psychiatric nosology. But the term serves a useful purpose: it is a reminder to clinicians that patients with a wide variety of diagnoses share many features related to chronic psychological distress, and it is a reminder to personality psychologists that the difference between normal functioning and abnormal functioning is often only one of degree. The cliché that all people are more or less neurotic has some scientific basis.

Personality traits and personality disorders Axis II of DSM-IV is used for the diagnosis of personality disorders, which are defined as inflexible and maladaptive personality traits. Whether those traits are the same as or different from those encountered in nonpsychiatric populations is a reasonable question. Several recent studies have concurred in finding strong and replicable links between scales measuring personality disorders and the five factors in both normal and clinical populations.

In the case of N, only high scores are associated with psychiatric impairment. But both poles of the other factors appear to be associated with specific forms of psychopathology. Persons high in E tend to have histrionic and narcissistic personality disorders; those who are low in E have avoidant and schizoid personality disorders. High C is associated with obsessive-compulsive personality disorder; low C is associated with antisocial personality disorder. Low A, antagonism, is characteristic of persons with paranoid, antisocial, and narcissistic personality disorders. High A is associated with dependent personality disorder. The hypothesized relations between personality traits and DSM-IV personality disorders are presented in Table 8-3.

Just how those personality traits are related to the disorders is a matter of current controversy. Are normal personality traits that are carried to an extreme inherently maladaptive, or do those traits merely predispose persons to the disorders under certain circumstances? Some research has also called into question the meaningfulness of the syndromes recognized by DSM-IV; the symptoms used to define the disorders, when separately assessed, do not covary in ways that match the DSM-IV syndromes. Instead, the symptom clusters that do emerge are interpretable in terms of the five-factor model. As a result of such evidence, proposals have been made to replace the current categorical model by dimensional models that relate problems in adjustment to standing on the basic dimensions of personality. That appears to be a logical extension of trait theories of psychopathology.

TABLE 8–3
Hypothesized Relations Between DSM-IV Personality Disorders and Five-Factor Model Personality Traits

	Personality Disorder									
Personality Trait	**PAR**	**SZD**	**SZT**	**ATS**	**BDL**	**HST**	**NAR**	**AVD**	**DEP**	**OBC**
Neuroticism:										
Anxiety	h		h	h	H			H	H	
Hostility	H	L		H	H	H	H			h
Depression			h	h	H		h	h	H	h
Self-consciousness		L	H			H	H	H	h	h
Impulsiveness				H	H					
Vulnerability			h		H	h		H	H	
Extroversion:										
Warmth	l	L	L	l		H		L		L
Gregariousness	l	L	L	l		H		L		
Assertiveness									L	H
Activity						h		L		
Excitement seeking				H		h		L		
Positive emotions	l	L				H				l
Openness:										
Fantasy			H			h	H			
Aesthetics	l									
Feelings	l	L	L			H				L
Actions						h		L		
Ideas			H			l				
Values			h							L
Agreeableness:										
Trust	L		L			h				
Straightforwardness	L			L		l	l			
Altruism				L		L	L		H	L
Compliance	L	h		L	L				H	L
Modesty	l						L		H	
Tender-mindedness	l			L			L			
Conscientiousness:										
Competence	h					l				
Order										H
Dutifulness				L						H
Achievement striving		l			L				L	H
Self-discipline				L		L				
Deliberation				L						H

Note. H, L = high, low, based on DSM-IV diagnostic criteria; h, l = high, low, based on associated features provided in DSM-IV. PAR = paranoid, SZD = schizoid, SZT = schizotypal, ATS = antisocial, BDL = borderline, HST = histrionic, NAR = narcissistic, AVD = avoidant, DEP = dependent, and OBC = obsessive-compulsive.
Adapted from P T Costa Jr, T A Widiger, editors: *Personality Disorders and the Five-Factor Model of Personality.* American Psychological Association, Washington, 1994.

APPLICATION OF THEORY TO THERAPY Psychodynamic, behavioral, and humanistic theories all specify the causal mechanisms by which psychopathology is created and maintained and thus imply points of intervention. If maladjustment is caused by rigidly internalized conditions of worth, unconditional positive regard in the therapeutic setting may provide a cure; if the problem is a learned behavior, altering reinforcements may extinguish it. Trait models typically offer no causal or developmental explanations and, thus, may seem to have no implications for psychotherapy. In fact, they have many implications.

Recent evidence on the substantial heritability of most personality traits clearly indicates that Allport was right: traits do have some underlying neuropsychic structure. Research on the psychophysiology of traits is a topic of growing interest and parallels the extensive work done on the neurophysiological basis of many forms of psychopathology. In that broad sense psychopharmacological approaches to psychotherapy are, in principle, consistent with trait theories of personality: if personality traits and disorders reflect brain processes, drugs that affect the brain may offer useful instruments for psychotherapy. In practice, there is still much to learn. For example, persons with dysthymic disorder, who score high on measures of trait depression, often do not respond to antidepressant medication.

Personality assessment Historically, the chief role of trait psychology in psychotherapy has been in diagnosis and assessment. A number of self-report measures, such as the MMPI and the Millon Clinical Multiaxial Inventory, were designed specifically to measure psychopathology and include primarily items that tap psychiatric symptoms. They can be regarded as measuring psychopathological traits and states (although they are often used in college and volunteer samples as measures of personality per se). The instruments are chiefly of value as aids to psychodiagnosis. General personality questionnaires—including the 16 PF, the Guilford-Zimmerman Temperament Survey, and the Edwards Personal Preference Schedule—have also been used for decades in clinical psychology and psychiatry as part of a complete psychological assessment. Several measures of the five-factor model have recently appeared, including the Hogan Personality Inventory and the NEO Personality Inventory, and clinicians have shown considerable interest in the five-factor model. The primary advantage of that model is its comprehensiveness. By assessing traits from all five dimensions, the clinician can efficiently obtain a full portrait of the patient.

Personality psychologists and psychometricians have devoted years to the development of self-report inventories, and the usefulness of that approach to assessment is beyond doubt. Self-reports, however, are by no means infallible. Patients may not understand their own personalities or may deliberately misrepresent themselves. Concerns about defensiveness and socially desirable responses have led to the use of projective tests, the development of special validity scales to detect and correct for distorted responses, and reliance on the clinical judgment of the psychiatrist. Each of those possible solutions introduces problems of its own, however, and most clinicians rely on multiple sources of information.

One source of information that has been underused in clinical settings is informant ratings. Research in the past decade has confirmed the idea that ratings on standardized instruments by significant others, usually spouses or parents, can provide reliable and valid assessments of personality. Those findings appear to hold for clinical populations, as well as for volunteer samples. Personality ratings may be particularly valuable when patients are incapacitated or are strongly motivated to present an overly favorable or unfavorable picture of themselves.

Uses of trait profiles Traits are enduring and stable features of the patient's behavior and experience, so assessing a broad range of traits gives the clinician a sense of what the person is like, which can be useful for many purposes beyond the formulation of a diagnosis. A complete personality profile can point to the patient's strengths, as well as weaknesses; can help predict the course of therapy; and can aid in the selection of an optimal mode of treatment.

Humanistic theories of personality stress human potentials for altruism, creativity, and commitment, and they argue that psychotherapy must use those assets. Trait theorists qualify that stance: they believe that some people are altruistic, creative, or committed but that others are not. Assessing traits allows the clinician to identify and capitalize on the particular strengths that characterize each patient.

A patient's standing on trait dimensions can also give clues to the probable course of therapy. Patients who are low on agreeableness are distrustful and uncooperative, and forming a therapeutic alliance with them may be difficult; by contrast, patients who are extremely high on A may be excessively compliant and become dependent on the therapist. Conscientiousness involves commitment and self-discipline. Patients high in C will probably adhere to the treatment recommendations and work hard to solve their problems; those low in C are less persistent and dedicated, and the therapist may have to work to motivate them.

A few controlled studies and a good deal of clinical experience suggest that personality traits influence the effectiveness of various kinds of treatment interventions. Interpersonal therapies, in which patients are required to speak a great deal about themselves, appear to be most effective for extroverts; pharmacological management may be superior for introverts. Similarly, patients who are high in openness to experience benefit from such techniques as guided imagery, whereas those who are low in that trait prefer biofeedback. Ideally, the choice of therapies should be guided not only by the nature of the disorder but also by the enduring characteristics of the patient.

Psychotherapy and personality change If psychopathology is an expression or an outcome of personality traits and if, as longitudinal studies show, personality traits change little over time, how can psychotherapy be effective? The pessimistic answer is that it cannot. Many psychiatric disorders are lifelong or recurrent, and treatment consists of management, rather than cure. Those who have the best prognosis for recovery are those who are initially the least impaired. In those cases the disorder may be a transient adjustment reaction in patients who have relatively healthy personality traits. Patients very high in N and low in A and C may be poor candidates for psychotherapy.

But so pessimistic a conclusion is unwarranted. Longitudinal studies show that people change little in the course of normal experience, but the studies do not rule out the possibility that direct interventions will make changes. Psychotherapy will probably not make dramatic and lasting changes in basic personality traits, but modest improvements may be enough to allow the patient to function effectively in daily life. Interventions may be particularly effective in early adulthood, when traits are not yet fully developed. Even without changing personality, therapy may help patients adapt to their own natures. The chronically anxious person may learn techniques of relaxation; the disagreeable person may learn social skills that improve interpersonal relationships.

In some sense most forms of psychotherapy are learning experiences. Psychoanalysts promote insight into unconscious conflicts; behaviorists help their clients understand the contingencies that reinforce troubling behavior; humanistic psychologists encourage patients to discover their true potential. Trait psychology can also be a source of insight. All human beings are in some respects alike, and learning that one is not alone in one's suffering is often comforting. But in other respects, people are different from one another, and learning that fact can also be a therapeutic experience. Helping patients understand their own enduring dispositions can prepare them for some of the problems they face in life.

SUGGESTED CROSS-REFERENCES

The psychodynamic perspectives on personality and psychopathology are treated extensively in Chapter 6 on psychoanalysis and in Chapter 7 on other psychodynamic schools. Chapter 25 discusses personality disorders. Chapter 9 on diagnosis and psychiatry deals with issues of assessment; Section 9.4 on personality assessment is particularly relevant. Section 3.3 on learning theory provides technical background for the discussion of behavioral approaches to personality, and Chapter 31 on psychotherapies—particularly Section 31.2 on behavior therapy, Section 31.8 on client-centered psychotherapy, Section 31.6 on cognitive therapy, and Section 31.9 on brief psychotherapy—gives details about the application of theories of personality to therapeutic processes. A different view of adult development is explained in Chapter 48 on adulthood.

REFERENCES

Allport G W: *Becoming: Basic Considerations for a Psychology of Personality.* Yale University Press, New Haven, 1955.

Allport G W: *Personality: A Psychological Interpretation.* Holt, New York, 1937.

Aristotle: *Nicomachean Ethics.* Hackett, Indianapolis, 1985.

Bandura A: *Social Learning Theory.* Prentice-Hall, Englewood Cliffs, NJ, 1977.

Clarkin J F, Hull J W, Cantor J, Sanderson C: Borderline personality disorder and personality traits: A comparison of SCID-II BPD and NEO-PI. Psychol Assess *5:* 472, 1993.

Costa P T Jr, McCrae R R: Influence of extraversion and neuroticism on subjective well-being: Happy and unhappy people. J Pers Soc Psychol *38:* 668, 1980.

Costa P T Jr, McCrae R R: Normal personality assessment in clinical practice: The NEO Personality Inventory. Psychol Assess *4:* 5, 1992.

Costa P T Jr, McCrae R R: Personality disorders and the five-factor model of personality. J Pers Disord *4:* 362, 1990.

Costa P T Jr, McCrae R R: Personality stability and its implications for clinical psychology. Clin Psychol Rev *6:* 407, 1986.

Costa P T, Jr, Widiger T A, editors: *Personality Disorders and the Five-Factor Model of Personality.* American Psychological Association, Washington, 1994.

Digman J M: Personality structure: Emergence of the five-factor model. Annu Rev Psychol *41:* 417, 1990.

Dollard J, Miller N E: *Personality and Psychotherapy: An Analysis in Terms of Learning, Thinking, and Culture.* McGraw-Hill, New York, 1950.

Duke M P, Nowicki S Jr: Theories of personality and psychopathology: Schools derived from psychology and philosphy. In *Comprehensive Textbook of Psychiatry,* ed 5, H I Kaplan, B J Sadock, editors, p 432. Williams & Wilkins, Baltimore, 1989.

Eysenck H J, Eysenck M: *Personality and Individual Differences.* Plenum, London, 1985.

Halverson C F, Kohnstamm G A, Martin R P, editors: *The Developing Structure of Temperament and Personality from Infancy to Adulthood.* Erlbaum, Hillsdale, NJ, 1994.
Heatherton T, Weinberger J, editors: *Can Personality Change?* American Psychological Association, Washington, 1994.
John O P: The ''big five'' factor taxonomy: Dimensions of personality in the natural language and in questionnaires. In *Handbook of Personality Theory and Research,* L Pervin, editor, p 66. Guilford, New York, 1990.
Kelly G A: *The Psychology of Personal Constructs.* Norton, New York, 1955.
*Maddi S R, Costa P T Jr: *Humanism in Personology: Allport, Maslow and Murray.* Aldine, Chicago, 1972.
Maslow A H: *Motivation and Personality.* Harper & Row, New York, 1954.
McCrae R R: Consensual validation of personality traits: Evidence from self-reports and ratings. J Pers Soc Psychol *43:* 293, 1982.
*McCrae R R, Costa P T Jr: *Personality in Adulthood.* Guilford, New York, 1990.
McCrae R R, John O P: An introduction to the five-factor model and its applications. J Pers *60:* 175, 1992.
*Miller T: The psychotherapeutic utility of the five-factor model of personality: A clinician's experience. J Pers Assess *57:* 415, 1991.
Mutén E: Self-reports, spouse ratings, and psychophysiological assessment in a behavioral medicine program: An application of the five-factor model. J Pers Assess *57:* 449, 1991.
Ozer D J, Reise S P: Personality assessment. Annu Rev Psychol *45:* 357, 1994.
Pervin L A: A critical analysis of current trait theory. Psychol Inquiry *5:* 103, 1994.
*Phares E J: *Introduction to Personality.* Merrill, Columbus, OH, 1984.
Plato: *The Republic.* Oxford University Press, London, 1941.
Plomin R, McClearn G E, editors: *Nature, Nurture, and Psychology.* American Psychological Association, Washington, 1993.
Rogers C R: *On Becoming a Person: A Therapist's View of Psychotherapy.* Houghton Mifflin, Boston, 1961.
Scarr S: Distinctive environments depend on genotypes. Brain Behav Sci *10:* 38, 1987.
Schopenhauer A: *The World as Will and Representation,* ed 3. Dover, New York, 1969.
Skinner B F: *About Behaviorism.* Knopf, New York, 1974.
Strack S, Lorr M: *Differentiating Normal and Abnormal Personality.* Springer, New York, 1994.
Theophrastus: *The Characters.* Taylor, London, 1824.
Watson D, Clark L A, editors: Special issue on personality and psychopathology. J Abnorm Psychol *130:* 1, 1994.
Widiger T A: The *DSM-III-R* categorical personality disorder diagnoses: A critique and an alternative. Psychol Inquiry *4:* 75, 1993.
*Widiger T A, Trull T J: Personality and psychopathology: An application of the five-factor model. J Pers *60:* 363, 1992.
Wiggins J A, Pincus A L: Conceptions of personality disorders and dimensions of personality. J Consult Clin Psychol *1:* 305, 1989.

CHAPTER 9 DIAGNOSIS AND PSYCHIATRY: EXAMINATION OF THE PSYCHIATRIC PATIENT

9.1 THE PSYCHIATRIC INTERVIEW, HISTORY, AND MENTAL STATUS EXAMINATION

GORDON D. STRAUSS, M.D.

INTRODUCTION

Interviewing is of central importance in medicine and psychiatry. It is not only *a* core skill in all of medical practice, it is arguably *the* core skill in clinical psychiatry. In most of medicine a verbal exchange (the interview) precedes and informs a physical examination, a practice that is reflected both in our professional language and in the way medical records are kept by reference to the history and the physical examination. In psychiatry the separation is less absolute, and frequently there is no point at which the interview ends and the examination begins.

Virtually all transactions in clinical psychiatry occur within the context of an interview. That is true for diagnosis and initial evaluation, whether the process occurs in an emergency room, on a ward in a psychiatric hospital, in an outpatient office setting, or on the medical or surgical wards of a general hospital. Similarly, virtually all psychiatric treatment of individuals happens in an interview setting as well. That may seem obvious for the spectrum of psychotherapies, but it is no less true for pharmacotherapy. Whether it is the prescribing process or the ongoing monitoring of medication benefits and side effects, the psychiatrist is engaged in an interpersonal exchange which at its heart is an interview.

All interviews have some structure or form; there is no such thing as an unstructured interview. There is, however, a continuum of interviews which are more or less structured. More importantly, interviews may be well or poorly structured. As a minimum, the time available provides a structuring framework for every interview. Similarly, the task or purpose of the interview helps give a functional structure as well.

The interviewer should always have in mind a structure in the form of a schema or scenario for how the interview ideally will proceed, including a rationale for when to speak and when to keep silent and a sense of what the goals of the interaction are. The latter may be as unstructured as following the patient's lead and being attuned to the developing transference; at the other extreme is sufficient structure to obtain a history of the present illness and past psychiatric history and do a complete mental status examination within 30 minutes.

While the concept of the completely unstructured interview is a fiction, there is a meaningful distinction between interviews that are *freeform* and those that are *standardized.* Freeform interviews are tailored by the clinician, even if he or she follows a consistent and invariant interview pattern. Standardized interviews are either fully structured or semistructured and specify to varying degrees the content, order, and wording of the interview. Their reliability and validity can usually be specified. Initially, standardized interviews were developed for research purposes.

STANDARDIZED INTERVIEWS

Three prominent examples of standardized interviews are the Schedule for Affective Disorders and Schizophrenia (SADS), the Diagnostic Interview Schedule (DIS), and the Present State Examination (PSE).

The SADS is a semistructured interview designed by researchers at Columbia University for use by interviewers with clinical experience. The SADS was designed to evaluate the symptoms of disorders as defined by the Research Diagnostic Criteria (RDC), a set of diagnostic criteria which preceded and contributed to the development of the third edition of *Diagnostic and Statistical Manual of Mental Disorders* (DSM-III). A SADS interview takes a minimum of one hour (but may take up to three hours) and yields information for making both current and lifetime psychiatric diagnoses. The SADS presumes that interviewers have had clinical experience, including making judgments about manifest psychopathology.

By contrast, the DIS is a fully structured diagnostic interview developed at the National Institute of Mental Health (NIMH) for interviews conducted by nonclinicians. A DIS interviewer reads each item exactly as worded in the interview booklet. Unlike semistructured standardized interviews, the DIS allows no clinical exploration of a patient's response. Diagnoses based on a DIS interview are generated by computer.

The PSE is a clinical interview developed in England at the Maudsley Hospital. The PSE focuses on symptomatology and functioning in the month before the interview. It combines fixed structured questions with an opportunity for interviewers to follow up with questions of their own in determining whether the occurrence of the symptom warrants a positive rating. The PSE requires approximately one hour to administer and, like the DIS, leads to a computer-generated diagnosis; the diagnosis is based on the International Classification of Diseases (ICD) system rather than the *Diagnostic and Statistical Manual of Mental Disorders* (now in its fourth edition as DSM-IV).

When DSM-III was revised, a new semistructured clinical interview was introduced, tailored specifically to the revised DSM-III (DSM-III-R). The Structured Clinical Interview for DSM-III-R (SCID) was designed by many of the same people who worked on the SADS. The goals of the SCID were to produce an instrument that required less training time than the SADS, took less time to administer and code, and, once the information was collected, made the diagnostic process simpler than with the SADS. Like the SADS and the PSE, the SCID was designed to be administered by a clinician familiar with the diagnostic criteria used in the DSM-III-R. A DSM-IV version of the SCID is in preparation. The SCID was designed to be used by clinicians as well as researchers. A clinician could use either the entire SCID as part of a diagnostic assessment or sections from the SCID as a supplement to the clinician's usual interview. The SCID has two parts, one for Axis I disorders and another for Axis II personality disorders. At the start of a SCID interview, the interviewer obtains an overview of the present illness, chief complaint, and past episodes of major psychopathology before systematically asking about specific symptoms. The interview schedule itself has many questions which are open-ended so that patients have an opportunity to describe symptoms in their own words. An attempt was made to design the SCID so that the sequence of questions approximates the differential diagnostic process used by an experienced clinician. At the conclusion of the interview, which takes from 60 to 90 minutes for the part of the SCID covering Axis I diagnoses, the interviewer also completes the Global Assessment of Functioning (GAF) scale, the fifth Axis on DSM-IV.

Since the advent of DSM-III, DSM-III-R, and DSM-IV, there has been concern that the art and skill of interviewing are on the decline. Examiners for the American Board of Psychiatry and Neurology's oral examinations see too many practitioners who act as though a series of questions based on DSM-IV criteria constitute a clinical interview.

INITIAL DIAGNOSTIC INTERVIEW

Although the initial diagnostic or assessment process can extend over several days or even weeks, there can be only one first interview. Circumstances often dictate that the assessment is not completed in a single interview: some patients have long, complicated histories; there may be a need for external corroborating information; and, particularly in outpatient settings, the time available for a single interview may be limited. However, it is frequently useful for the diagnostic process to be extended over several sessions since there is informational value in seeing a patient at different points in time. The clinician ought to have an objective assessment of the stability and persistence of symptoms in addition to the patient's subjective report. Nevertheless, a single interview often encompasses a great deal of material.

It is not unusual for a first interview to be scheduled for 45 to 90 minutes. Any less time will almost certainly require the patient to return unless there are special circumstances, such as an emergency room setting, that dictate a shorter interview. Thirty minutes is the standard length for the American Board of Psychiatry and Neurology oral examination interview.

CONDUCTING THE INTERVIEW Within the context of a diagnostic assessment there are four goals for any interview: (1) establish a relationship, (2) obtain information, (3) assess psychopathology, and (4) provide feedback. There is considerable overlap among the first three.

Establish a relationship Interviewing is by nature an interpersonal process. The quality of the information which the patient reveals to the interviewer is a function of the trust and trustworthiness which the patient experiences with the interviewer. Patients will not reveal the personal, intimate, and diagnostically important details of their experience to someone they do not trust. Rapport with the interviewer is the manifestation of that trust and the evidence that a trusting relationship has been established.

A number of elements in the psychiatrist's approach to the patient contribute to the development or maintenance of a trusting relationship. One element is a demeanor of respect for the patient regardless of appearance or socioeconomic status. Another element is *compassion* for the patient's suffering and distress. Unconditional positive regard (also referred to as warmth) has been shown repeatedly to be a key element in successful therapeutic relationships. It is a stance of interest, concern, even curiosity, untainted by the flavor of judgmental evaluation. Genuineness is another of the key elements for the interviewer who wishes to establish rapport with the patient. Interviewer genuineness is a mixture of spontaneity, consistency, and authenticity. As with respect, compassion, and warmth, the patient is likely to experience the interviewer's genuineness as directly responsive to his or her personhood and behavior.

Several interview techniques contribute to establishing a good relationship, especially if done early in the interview. One of the most potent techniques is to seek out, pursue, and respond to the patient's emotions and emotionally charged areas of concern. (Failure to do this is perhaps the single most common weakness seen in candidates at the oral certifying examinations given by the American Board of Psychiatry and Neurology.) At the most basic level what is involved is a process of observation: the interviewer observes the patient's nonverbal behavior, listens for the explicit and inferable distress and emotional pain, and then responds to it. Even in such elementary techniques as simple labeling (for example, "You looked tearful just now as you spoke about your mother") is a form of empathy. To recognize, respond to, and empathize with emotion is to show compassion, warmth, and genuineness.

Another technique for enhancing rapport is to listen attentively. That means minimizing interruptions of the patient, particularly in the first 5 to 10 minutes of an interview. During that phase, it is particularly useful to follow the patient's lead. When questions and probes are needed, they should be used to clarify intended meaning, not to redirect the patient. While avoiding unnecessary interruptions, the interviewer should not pretend to understand a story that is confusing or unclear. Such pretense undermines genuineness.

Taking notes is one way for the interviewer to attend to the patient's narrative without interrupting, and to keep track of ambiguities, inconsistencies, or other confusing aspects of the patient's history, which may require review and clarification. Some form of documentation of the interview and examination will need to be made as a part of good record keeping and for medicolegal reasons, whether or not the interviewer takes notes during the session. Many psychiatrists, even if they take notes during the several sessions of an evaluation, discontinue and then make only occasional intrasession notes (for example, changes in medication, dreams, and changes in appointments). As long as the interviewer can take notes without failing to listen attentively and to maintain eye contact with the patient, the technique can be used without major risk. If note taking begins to inhibit rapport, it should be discontinued.

Less experienced interviewers are sometimes concerned that showing confusion or perplexity at something the patient says will undermine their authority. Somewhat paradoxically, just the opposite is likely unless an interviewer's questions reflect a lapse in attention or concentration (and even then most patients are remarkably forgiving unless such lapses are repeated). The physician's authority is established more by the questions asked than by advice or answers given, particularly in a diagnostic interview setting. It is by knowing which questions to ask that the interviewer demonstrates professional expertise.

The appearance and arrangement of the space where the initial interview takes place may influence the interaction. The space should be quiet, with privacy assured for the patient's confidences, and without telephones ringing, beepers sounding, or other intrusions. Chairs of roughly the same height and comfort (so as not to reify perceived differences of stature or importance) should be arranged so that the patient can choose spontaneously to sit closer to or farther from the psychiatrist. It is best if direct eye contact can be maintained easily without being enforced. The room should be arranged without physical barriers (such as a desk) between the interviewer and patient; those create distance both literally and psychologically. Fortunately, it is possible to establish rapport and begin a therapeutic relationship in space which is far from the ideal. Emergency rooms and general hospital bedrooms (or even psychiatric hospitals and clinics) may lack some or nearly all of the optimal conditions. Any setting in which the interviewer can give focused attention to the thoughts and emotions of the patient can suffice.

Obtain information Although obtaining information is the most obvious goal of all interviewing, in psychiatry the interviewer is seeking both factual and emotional information. There are general principles for obtaining information of both a factual and emotional nature and well-researched specific techniques for obtaining information of each type. The most general finding is that open-ended questions (see below) will elicit a greater volume of talk from patients than any other type of inquiry. Questions by interviewers that echo the last few words or concluding thought of the patient are also effective. Another general principle is that interview style is less important than the experience which the interviewer brings: Experienced interviewers obtain a better quality of factual information by more quickly recognizing the importance of what they are told and by a selective and efficient use of probing questions to elicit additional detail.

Several types of questions are useful in virtually all interviews:

1. *Open-ended questions:* Invite an extended narrative reply (for example, ''What do *you* mean when you say you are depressed?'' or ''How did this problem develop?'').
2. *Closed-ended questions:* Invite either a yes or no response or a short answer (for example, ''Have you lost weight in the past month?'' or ''When was your last drink?'').
3. *Echo questions:* Invite the patient to go on speaking by repeating some part of what the patient said (for example, Patient: ''I'm afraid she'll leave me because of money.'' Interviewer: ''Because of money?'').

Closed-ended questions are used for the sake of efficiency and to give the patient more structure. Those goals can go awry with certain types of closed-ended questions, two of which can be especially problematic:

1. Double questions: Pose two or more questions in the same inquiry (for example, ''Have you had problems with eating and sleeping?'').
2. Multiple-choice questions: Pose a number of alternative answers, which force the patient to give an answer that may fail to cover the range of possibilities (for example, ''Do you have nightmares during the week or just on weekends?'').

OBTAINING FACTUAL INFORMATION In obtaining factual information (events in the history, dates of developmental milestones, and so on), both open-ended and closed-ended questions are of value, and each type has advantages and disadvantages. The overwhelming advantage to open-ended questions is that they yield more information. They encourage patients to speak at greater length and in doing so they facilitate the task of establishing a relationship. The principal drawback of open-ended questions is that they may not produce focused responses; late in an interview open-ended questions may be a most inefficient way to check details or review systems. At that time closed-ended questions may be most useful. Closed-ended questions tend to narrow the focus and are useful both as a follow-up to open-ended questions and also as a way to structure the interview for patients whose thoughts wander or who are markedly circumstantial or tangential. Virtually every diagnostic interview will make use of closed-ended questions, but they are more likely to present a problem early in the interview, because they may give the patient the feeling of being interrogated.

Two other questioning techniques are effective in obtaining factual information: *checks* and *probes*. Checks, or echo questions, are often used in conjunction with open-ended questions and have a similar effect: they invite and successfully elicit narrative responses. Probes are requests for specific detail or examples. Probes may be used effectively in conjunction with both open- and closed-ended questions.

Clinical tradition and experimental research reveal that an effective strategy for obtaining factual information has two elements. First, an active questioning style (that is, one that introduces topics as the interview proceeds) yields more detailed and clinically relevant information than interview styles that are nondirective or which rely upon the patient spontaneously to raise all of the important issues. The other element in an effective strategy is the movement from a pattern of open-ended questions with checks early in the interview to more closed-ended questions and more probes later on.

OBTAINING INFORMATION ABOUT FEELINGS AND EMOTIONS Open-ended questions are far more effective than closed-ended questions in eliciting feelings and emotionally charged material, in part because such questions lead to more talk in general, which leads to more expression of emotional material. However, there are specific interventions that can be particularly effective, especially for less experienced interviewers. The simplest of them is a direct request for feelings (for example, ''How did you feel?''). Another technique is the direct request for emotionally laden personal information, including the mental health of immediate family members, family violence, criminal behavior, tension or discord between parents, parental self-criticism, or abusive sexual behavior within the family.

To a degree an interviewer is working at cross purposes when both seeking factual information and trying to get the patient to express feelings and emotions. However, it is possible to integrate the process of establishing rapport (which inevitably involves the interviewer with the patient's emotions) and the goal of obtaining information. The solution is to load the interview with open-ended questions at the outset along with direct requests for emotions and feelings. If the interviewer does that and uses each opportunity to recognize and respond empathically to the emotions and feelings expressed (or implied) by the patient, the process will facilitate establishing rapport as well as the free flow of information of both a factual and affective nature. Once a foundation of trust and rapport have been established, the interviewer can use more closed-ended questions and specific probes as the interview proceeds. It is not true, however, that open-ended questions are used only at the beginning of the interview and closed-ended questions only at the end. Closed-ended probes will often be useful in clarifying the extent of symptoms early in an interview, and open-ended questions will be useful every time the interviewer touches on a new area of the social or developmental history.

Assessing psychopathology Every diagnostic interview includes an assessment of the patient's psychopathology (or lack thereof), including not only the formal mental status testing which may be conducted but also the inferences and conclusions which an interviewer draws as the interview is conducted. The interviewer has access to a great deal of information through observation and through interacting with the patient. Appearance, psychomotor behavior, and, to some extent, emotional state are available through visual inspection during the interview. Through interactions with the patient, the interviewer can further assess psychomotor behavior, speech, emotional state (particularly connectedness), judgment, attention, concentration, intelligence, and sometimes sensorium and memory.

Although some aspects of thinking, perception, mood, and insight may be evident from the interactional behavior of the patient, those elements along with judgment, sensorium, concentration, and memory frequently require formal testing in order to describe adequately the patient's mental state.

Provide feedback There is usually an implied or explicit question posed by the patient at the conclusion of the initial interview. The question the patient would like to pose is, "Well, Doctor, what do you think?" A fuller expression of the question would include some or all of the following: "What's wrong with me? Am I crazy? Do I need to be in a hospital or on medication? Can I go home? Will you see me again? Is there any hope?"

Although giving definitive answers is often not possible at the conclusion of the first interview, it is important to recognize these concerns which virtually all patients have. Even in the first of a series of interviews in an ongoing diagnostic or treatment assessment, it may be useful to communicate an awareness of those concerns, through a statement, such as, "You may be wondering what I think about what you've told me," or "Let's talk about where we go from here." For many patients that will reinforce their sense of being understood and cared for. Even the final moments of the interview can thus be used to deepen rapport and strengthen the relationship between patient and interviewer.

CONTENT OF THE INTERVIEW As Table 9.1-1 indicates, the basic elements for a complete psychiatric history include the identifying and demographic data, chief complaint, history of present illness, past psychiatric history, past medical history, marital history or current relationships, and a detailed developmental history. While any interview can be expanded or collapsed according to the time available, it is possible to touch on all of these areas and conduct a mental status examination in an interview of 30 minutes. However, even though 30 minutes may be the average length for interviews conducted in emergency settings and is the outer limit in the board-certifying oral examinations, it is not optimal for a careful, thoughtful, and thorough diagnostic interview.

While the topics covered in the outline in Table 9.1-1 define the content of the initial diagnostic interview, they do not necessarily reflect the order in which the interview should be conducted. For example, it is rarely useful to begin the interview of a hospitalized patient with a review of demographic data. With almost all patients the development of rapport will be better served by beginning with an inquiry about the chief complaint, what brought the patient to the hospital, or what is of greatest concern at the moment. The general principle is that the clinician should make the interview responsive to the patient; the process should be as spontaneous and creative as possible. It is also important to distinguish between the content of the interview as conducted and the content of the interview as reported by the clinician in writing or verbally.

Chief complaint The clinician will usually elicit the chief complaint by beginning the interview with why the patient has come to the hospital or what has caused the patient to seek treatment. Every effort should be made to remember the patient's exact words; it is traditional to state the chief complaint in the write-up of the psychiatric history as a verbatim quote. More to the point, the first words that patients speak about their condition are extremely revealing, often indicating a great deal about their expectations of the psychiatrist as well as about their psychopathology.

TABLE 9.1-1
Outline of Psychiatric History

- I. Identifying and demographic data
  - A. Name, address, phone number
  - B. Age, ethnic group, gender, marital status, and occupation
  - C. Religion
- II. Chief complaint
- III. History of the present illness
  - A. Precipitants
  - B. Onset, course, duration
  - C. Symptoms and signs
  - D. Effects of/on environment
    - 1. Family
    - 2. Job
    - 3. Friends and relationships
  - E. Psychiatric review of systems
- IV. Past psychiatric history
  - A. Similar episodes
  - B. Other psychiatric illnesses
  - C. Treatment history
    - 1. Hospitalizations (dates/ages, durations, treatments rendered)
    - 2. Outpatient treatment
  - D. Family history of psychiatric illness
- V. Medical history
  - A. Concurrent medical problems
  - B. Current medications
  - C. Past medical history
  - D. Allergies
  - E. Medical review of systems (including use of alcohol or drugs)
- VI. Marital history or current relationships
  - A. If married: description and history of marriage and relationship with spouse
    - 1. If divorced or remarried: reasons for divorce and length of prior marriage
    - 2. If children: ages and quality of relationship with patient
  - B. If not married: quantity and quality of emotionally important relationships
- VII. Developmental history
  - A. Early childhood (preschool)
    - 1. Parents
      - a. Relationship of each to patient
      - b. Relationship of parents to each other
      - c. Parents' socioeconomic status
    - 2. Siblings
    - 3. Extended families
    - 4. Developmental milestones
    - 5. Earliest memories
  - B. School-age childhood
    - 1. Friends
    - 2. Schooling
    - 3. Key life events
  - C. Adolescence
    - 1. Puberty
    - 2. Psychosexual history
    - 3. School performance
    - 4. Dating and peer relationships
    - 5. Early experiences with alcohol, drugs
  - D. Early adulthood
    - 1. Education
    - 2. Work
    - 3. Military
    - 4. Social relations
    - 5. Recreational, avocational pursuits
    - 6. Goals
  - E. Midlife and older adulthood
    - 1. Career developments, changes
    - 2. Losses
    - 3. Aging

History of the present illness Using open-ended questions along with judiciously timed probes and checks, the interviewer elicits the history of the present illness by inviting the patient to give a narrative description of the course and chronology of his or her symptoms. How did the patient's difficulties begin? Was the onset sudden or gradual? What precipitants can be identified, and do they reflect changes in the biological, emotional, or social milieu of the patient? The information gathered here should allow the clinician not only to describe what has been happening to the patient but also to address why it is happening at this point in his or her life. In further exploring the present illness the interviewer should consider the patient's family, work setting, and friends and relationships, not only how they are affected by the patient's illness but also how they may have contributed to it. Although information germane to the present illness may emerge throughout the interview, the part devoted to the present illness should include a psychiatric review of systems so that pertinent positive and negative signs or symptoms can be evaluated.

Past psychiatric history Unless this is a first onset of psychiatric illness, there may be previous episodes with similar symptoms. If so, questions about the present illness may shade imperceptibly into an inquiry about the past psychiatric history. All previous psychiatric illnesses, whether similar to the present illness or not, should be asked about, and a careful history of the treatment for each should be obtained. Such an inquiry should focus on previous hospitalizations, with attention to the patient's age, the duration of stay, and the treatments received while in the hospital. An inquiry should also be made about periods of outpatient treatment. The patient's description of previous episodes of hospitalization or outpatient treatment may be particularly revealing of insight, and motivation for and compliance with treatment. Asking about the patient's family histories of psychiatric illness often puts the patient's own past history into a useful context, and helps to elucidate the patient's genetic vulnerability to psychiatric illness.

Medical history A psychiatric history and assessment should include a thorough investigation of the patient's medical history, not only because psychiatry is a medical specialty but also because many psychiatric patients have untreated or even undiagnosed medical problems. In addition to making a routine inquiry about past medical conditions, it is important to inquire about concurrent medical problems and about all medications, both prescribed and over-the-counter, which the patient is already taking. A general medical review of systems should be done, with particular attention to such neurological signs and symptoms as headache, seizures, head trauma, loss of consciousness, changes in vision, and episodes of disorientation or confusion. A thorough inquiry about the use of alcohol and drugs should be part of every psychiatric assessment. It is also important to inquire about a history of exposure (through transfusion, drug use, or sexual behavior) to or testing positive for the human immunodeficiency virus (HIV).

The inquiry about drugs and alcohol deserves special emphasis because physicians often fail to ask at all or too readily accept glib or vague denials or minimizations about substance use, especially alcohol. Questions such as "How much do you drink?" or "How often do you have a drink?" are more useful than "Do you drink?" If the patient is asked whether he or she drinks and says no, it is useful to follow up immediately with a question such as, "Not at all or just not much?" Asking about the preferred beverage (even the brand) and the frequency in which it is ingested is useful. Because such an inquiry may elicit defensiveness or denial, the interviewer must maintain a nonjudgmental demeanor.

Marital history or current relationships An essential part of every psychiatric assessment is the marital history and an exploration of the patient's current relationships. If the patient is married, the interviewer should elicit a qualitative description and a history of the marriage and the current relationship with the patient's spouse. If the patient is divorced or remarried, questions should be asked about the reasons for the divorce, the length of prior marriages, and the quality of the relationship with former partners. If the patient has children, their number, ages, and the quality of the patient's relationship with each should be determined. If the patient is not married, the interviewer should ask about the quality and quantity of emotionally important relationships (friends, coworkers, business associates, and so on). Besides providing a fuller picture of the patient, that area of inquiry is important for two other reasons. Diagnostically, the quality of relationships with friends, family, or other emotional intimates may be one of the most important sources of information contributing to the evaluation of Axis II (personality) psychopathology. Prognostically, the quality and nature of relatedness to the important individuals in the patient's life may help in assessing the patient's suitability for psychotherapeutic interventions.

Developmental history—early childhood through adolescence The patient's developmental history is an essential part of every first interview. The length of time devoted to it and the amount of detail that it can cover will vary according to the circumstances of the interview and assessment. If the initial interview is brief or is conducted in an emergency setting, the developmental history may do no more than hit the high points of early childhood, adolescence, education, work, and other life interests. If more time is available, or if the diagnostic assessment can be spread out over several sessions, a much more detailed history should be taken.

While elements in the developmental history may be obtained at various points during the initial interview, there is an intrinsic logic to inquiring about and tracing development chronologically. The developmental history may be extended back before the patient's birth: whether the patient's parents were legally married at the time of conception and birth, the existence of complications during the pregnancy, and the nature of the delivery may all be germane. A number of milestones during infancy are usually included, such as whether the patient was fed by breast or bottle, the age and ease of weaning, and some indication about early language and physical coordination. Most important, and often far more accessible if the patient is the only informant, is information about the parents and other members of the family, including the relationship of each parent both to the patient and to the other parent, the socioeconomic status of the patient's family, and the parental family origins. Asking about earliest memories may be quite evocative and may also reveal striking patterns of amnesia for early childhood. The other essential elements for childhood until adolescence are friends, family relations, schooling, and memorable life events.

In considering adolescent development it is important to try to date the onset of puberty. For women the age of menarche is a useful marker and is frequently an emotionally powerful life experience. For men it may be useful to inquire about when axillary and pubic hair began to appear or when voice changes occurred. Masturbation is a less reliable marker for the onset of puberty, but should be included when asking about the development of sexuality. A complete psychosexual history is not limited to adolescence, but the convergence of physiological and psychological sexual development in that period makes it an easy place to begin talking about this topic (unless the patient is an adolescent). In addition to exploring masturbatory practices (including those which precede puberty), early sexual experiences, homoerotic impulses or experiences, and the existence of fetishes or other paraphilias, the interviewer should also ask about sexual dysfunctions, including disorders of desire, arousal, or orgasm. Finally, a developmental history should not be considered complete without a sensitive but forthright exploration of sexual and physical abuse.

School performance during the teenage years reveals a great deal about psychological and social development. That is frequently the context in which to ask about dating and peer relationships. The exploration of adolescent development should also include questions about the patient's earliest experiences with alcohol and drugs.

Adult development It is now well established that development continues throughout adult life. In early adulthood the central issues are education, work, social relations, recreational and avocational pursuits, and life goals. In each of those areas there are several key points. With regard to education the issues are the amount (for example, high school, college or technical school, graduate or professional school) and quality of performance. The amount of education correlates highly with the nature of the patient's work or career, but inquiry should also be made about the duration of jobs held, satisfaction with work or career, and the quality of relationships, particularly with authority figures. If the patient served in the military, it is useful to know when and for how long, whether the patient saw combat, and the rank achieved at time of discharge.

For patients at midlife or in older adulthood there are additional developmental issues, including the relationships with growing or adult children, later career developments or retirement, aging, and losses (friends, spouse, or children).

MENTAL STATUS EXAMINATION

In oral and written presentations, a report of the patient's mental status is separate from the patient's history even though much of both may have come from the same interview. Here psychiatry follows the practice of medicine, where, although the internist may observe the unmistakable signs of congestive heart failure or chronic obstructive pulmonary disease during an interview, the results of the physical examination will be reported separately. The elements of mental status include appearance, psychomotor behavior, speech, thinking and perception, emotional state (which includes mood and affect), insight and judgment, intelligence, sensorium, attention and concentration, and memory.

Insofar as a portion of the interview is devoted to formal testing of mental status, it is often marked by a sentence or two signaling a shift from history taking to a different sort of process. The transition is easily handled with a phrase, such as, "Now I'd like to ask you a series of questions which will help me further evaluate your thinking, concentration, memory, and mood." The interviewer should avoid demeaning the interview process by saying, "Now I'm going to ask you some questions which don't have anything to do with you," or "These questions may seem silly, but please bear with me." The pejorative cast that puts on the proceedings may be minor, but it is quite unnecessary and may subtly undermine some of the rapport previously established.

APPEARANCE The patient's appearance should be considered in two ways: the overall gestalt and the particulars of grooming, hygiene, dress, and posture. In considering the overall gestalt, the interviewer should allow conscious awareness of the impression the patient makes: tasteful, garish, tailored, casual, sloppy, disheveled, meticulous, imposing, seductive, meek, and so on. Sometimes the most striking thing about the patient is age or youthfulness, particularly if the appearance goes against stated age; at other times it is the absence of anything distinctive about the appearance at all. Over the course of the interview the interviewer should take the opportunity to become consciously aware of the individual elements in the patient's appearance. Is the hair combed or brushed; is it clean? Is makeup worn, and if so is it skillfully applied? Is the patient's attire consistent with the time of day and season? Are the clothes clean and laundered, or do they look worn, rumpled, or soiled? Does the clothing combine wildly incongruous features? Is there anything striking about the patient's posture?

PSYCHOMOTOR BEHAVIOR Psychomotor behavior includes all nonverbal behavior by the patient during the interview. While psychomotor activity can be classified as increased or decreased, it is best actually to describe the patient's behavior. For example, to note that the patient "has increased psychomotor activity with agitation" is helpful, but a clearer picture is created if the patient is further described as "constantly tapping her foot, wringing her hands, and sighing deeply." Increased levels of psychomotor activity are frequently seen in states of anxiety, euphoria or elevated moods, psychoses, or confusional states due to delirium or dementia. Frequently, increased psychomotor activity in chronic psychiatric patients is partially iatrogenic, a combined manifestation of anxiety and extrapyramidal side effects of antipsychotic medication. The patient with decreased psychomotor activity will often move (and speak) slowly, with decreased gesturing and a general lack of spontaneity. Such patients, commonly described as having *psychomotor retardation,* may, in extreme situations, be mute, immobile, and virtually unresponsive.

A striking form of psychomotor activity is *catatonia.* In catatonic excitement, restlessness, agitation, and hyperactivity reach extremes. At the other end of the spectrum, catatonic posturing may be difficult to distinguish from the psychomotor retardation of severe depression. However, it is more likely that there will be repetitive odd or bizarre movements or mannerisms. Other striking forms of psychomotor activity frequently seen in psychotic conditions include tentative back and forth movements that never reach a goal (appearing very much like a behaviorally concrete form of ambivalence), *echopraxia* (the copying of the examiner's movements or posture), *catalepsy* (holding an awkward position or posture for long periods of time), and *waxy flexibility* (partial passive resistance to movement which gives way in a waxlike fashion combined with the willingness to maintain a limb extended or bent in an odd way).

SPEECH The interviewer should observe and note the patient's rate and rhythm of speech, its quantity and loudness, its grammar and syntax, and anything notable about vocabulary and choice of words. From the quality of speech the interviewer will make inferences about the processes of thinking and cognitive organization.

The interviewer should note whether the patient's speech is clear, coherent, and to the point, or whether it has any of the following properties: *Circumstantiality* is noted when the patient takes a circuitous, unnecessarily detailed path in answering the question. *Tangentiality* occurs when the patient, in attempting to answer the question, becomes side-tracked through a chain of readily understandable associations but never gets back to the point of the question. *Dysprosody* is the loss of the normal rhythm or melody of speech. *Pressured speech* refers to verbal productions which are continuous, frequently rapid, and difficult to interrupt. *Blocking* (sometimes called thought blocking) refers to an interruption of speech in mid-sentence, followed by a silence lasting from seconds to minutes; the patient eventually indicates an inability to complete (or at times even to recall) the intended thought. *Neologisms* are words created by the patient but used as if they had a specific and consensually validated meaning.

There is a spectrum of speech that is confusing, incoherent, or difficult to follow. Verbal expressions which are vague, rambling, and somewhat disconnected reflect *derailment* (metaphorically, the thoughts have left the track). In *loosening of associations* the conventional connections (associations) between expressed thoughts are reduced or lost. An utterly incoherent jumble of speech is termed *word salad*. Extremely rapid speech which changes abruptly from idea to idea (but which can often be understood if the interviewer can keep up with the patient) reflects *flight of ideas*. Speech in which the associations between thoughts are based on sounds (rhymes, homonyms, and so on) is described as *clanging*. *Echolalia* is the immediate repetition of another's words or phrases. Answers that are totally unrelated to the questions asked are *non sequiturs,* while the repetition of particular phrases or words without relevance to the question is termed *perseveration*.

THINKING AND PERCEPTION Here the nature and content of thought are considered. The concerns are the presence of thoughts which suggest the patient may be a danger to self or others, thinking which reflects impaired reality testing, and evidence of perceptual disturbances.

Every initial diagnostic interview should include an explicit inquiry about *suicidal ideation*. Handled with sensitivity and tact, there is no risk to such an inquiry. (A patient without suicidal ideation will find such a question unremarkable, nonthreatening, and perhaps irrelevant; as such it will have little or no impact.) However, the value, both to the interviewer and to the patient, of a forthright and nonjudgmental inquiry when suicidal ideation is present cannot be overstated. Such an approach may give the patient permission to reveal a subjectively terrible and terrifying secret, which may be a great relief to the patient and at the same time may alert the interviewer to levels of distress and dangerousness not previously appreciated. The interviewer should not hesitate to ask about homicidal ideation as well.

Summarizing thought content should begin with the patient's worries, anxieties, or preoccupations. The interviewer should note *ruminations* (mood-congruent ideas, which are mulled over repeatedly), *obsessions* (intrusive and unwanted ideas which occur repeatedly and are frequently accompanied by stereotyped repetitive and ritualized behaviors referred to as *compulsions*), or *phobias* (sources of unrealistic fears that the patient will go to great lengths to avoid).

The interviewer should note the presence of delusions or other thought processes which suggest impaired reality testing. Thinking which reflects a preference for an inner, idiosyncratic, or personalized reality over consensually validated external reality is referred to as *autistic* (or *dereistic*). *Delusions* are fixed false beliefs which fall outside the patient's social, cultural, or religious background. While it is not helpful to challenge a patient's delusional ideas, it is often quite valuable to ask the patient how he or she knows the delusional idea is true. Engaging the patient in such an inquiry may further reveal the breadth and depth of the psychotic process, and it may also lead the patient to reveal the presence of hallucinations. *Paranoid delusions* include delusions of persecution, grandiosity, self-reference, and religiosity, in all of which the individual has the experience of being singled out. Another type of delusion is *delusions of passivity,* which include ideas of thought broadcasting, thought withdrawal, and thought insertion, as well as the insertion of feelings, impulses, somatic sensations, and outside force or will. A *delusional perception* combines a real perception with a delusional idea about its meaning (for example, "When the doctor rubbed his nose, it meant I should go masturbate").

Paranoid delusions and delusions of passivity can usually be distinguished from those which have a more depressive cast. Sometimes that is relatively easy, as when delusions reflect the overall depressive cognition and emphasize worthlessness, badness, or inner rot. Delusions which are part of a psychotic depression may seem at first to be of a paranoid and persecutory nature. However, gentle inquiry will often reveal that what first appeared to be persecution is in fact being experienced as *punishment,* retribution for some evil deed which the patient believes he or she has committed.

An *overvalued idea* should be distinguished from a delusion. Like delusions, overvalued ideas are not open to change or correction by logical argument, but they are not as far beyond the pale of consensual reality. Unshakable biases or prejudices are examples of overvalued ideas.

Perceptions may be disturbed to varying degrees. *Depersonalization* is the subjective sense of being unreal, unfamiliar, or alien to oneself. *Derealization* is a similar subjective sense that one's environment is somehow changed, unreal, or strange. *Illusions* occur when a genuine sensory perception is misconstrued (for example, a blanket on a sofa in a poorly lit room is seen as a body). *Hallucinations* are sensory perceptions occurring without external stimuli. Although they may occur in any sensory modality, auditory and visual hallucinations are the most common type. The presence of auditory hallucinations should prompt further inquiry into the nature and content of hallucinations; *command hallucinations,* especially in the presence of suicidal or homicidal ideation, should always be noted. Although they usually reflect the presence of a severe disturbance, hallucinations are not pathognomonic of any psychiatric condition; they may be seen in psychosis, toxic and metabolic delirium, dissociative states, and even nonpathologically in acute grief. Hallucinations occurring while falling asleep are referred to as *hypnogogic,* while those occurring during the process of awakening are *hypnopompic*.

EMOTIONAL STATE This category includes an assessment of the patient's mood and affect. Those terms are often a source of confusion, in part because there is inconsistency and overlap in the definitions given by different experts. In colloquial usage, even among mental health professionals, the words "mood" and "affect" are often used interchangeably. (For example, professionals use the phrase "affective disorders" as a synonym for "mood disorders.") The definitions of mood and affect which follow maintain an internally consistent differentiation.

Mood *Mood* refers to the patient's predominant emotions. Mood has both a subjective (the patient's own assessment) and an objective (observed or described by others) component. The patient's mood, whether subjective or objective, is best described by terms that define emotional states. Typical examples include calm, happy, sad, anxious, depressed, elated, euphoric, tense, hostile, mad or angry, apathetic, serious, and ebullient.

Any mood can be further characterized in terms of its stability, reactivity, and duration. *Stability* refers to the consistency of the mood, particularly within the course of a day; some depressions, for example, have an unvarying quality while others, every bit as severe, may have a diurnal variation in which the depression lifts slightly as the day goes on. *Reactivity* refers to whether or not a particular mood changes in response to external events or circumstances. *Duration* refers to the persistence of a mood measured in days, weeks, or even years. Duration is often of diagnostic importance. For example, depressed mood must persist for two weeks or more in major depressive disorder, while the depression or dysphoria that characterize dysthymic disorder must last two years or longer.

Affect *Affect* refers to the expression and expressivity of the patient's emotions. While a patient's mood (that is, the predominant emotion) can be captured in one or two words, over the course of a 45- to 90-minute interview, the patient may experience and give expression to a number of emotions. It is the capacity or limitation of a patient to vary emotional expression in concert with thought content during the interview that is meant by affect. Affect is described in terms of (1) *range* (full, constricted); (2) *change pattern* (fluid, monotonic, labile); (3) *appropriateness* (affect is inappropriate if incongruent with thought content or if grossly at variance with what would be expected based on the patient's age and social standing); and (4) *intensity of expression* (flat or blunted if emotional expression is virtually absent or markedly reduced). Another element of the patient's affect is *relatedness,* the patient's capacity to connect with the interviewer interpersonally.

INTELLIGENCE In most clinical interviews, intelligence is inferred rather than tested specifically. The two most common ways to do this are through assessing the patient's vocabulary and ability to interpret proverbs. Over the course of the interview it should be possible to assess the sophistication of the words and usage by which the patient expresses thoughts. Vocabulary is strongly correlated with level of education; the interviewer should not lose sight of the fact that though education and intelligence are frequently highly correlated, a very intelligent person from an educationally deprived background may have a limited vocabulary and an unsophisticated use of language. In those instances, proverb interpretation may be of particular utility. The capacity to abstract a general meaning from the literal imagery of a proverb draws upon intelligence which doesn't require schooling. Poor or concrete interpretations of common proverbs suggest either a cultural block or low intelligence. Contrary to earlier beliefs, concrete proverb interpretation is not indicative of any disorder. For example, patients with schizophrenia produce proverb interpretations that are not as unusual for their concreteness as for their idiosyncratically personalized and bizarre quality.

INSIGHT AND JUDGMENT *Insight* refers both to a patient's self-awareness that there is a problem or an illness and to the nondelusional understanding of the cause or meaning. When both components of insight are present, correct and experienced emotionally and cognitively, insight (combined with motivation) can be an important element in behavioral change. Insight can be described as partial or superficial (when the problem is recognized but not its meaning or cause), intellectual (cognitive understanding without practical application), or incorrect (for example, a nonpsychotic patient who attributes his or her problems to other people's hostility when in fact the patient provokes an angry or hostile response).

By definition, insight is lacking in patients with acute psychosis. However, absent or low levels of insight are also seen frequently in a number of nonpsychotic conditions, especially in personality disorders. *Anosognosia,* literally, the denial of illness, is most often used in relation to lesions of the nondominant cerebral hemisphere, especially the parietal lobe; patients with those lesions may ignore or deny hemiplegias or blindness. Psychogenic anosognosia is seen in patients who have experienced extreme trauma or catastrophic events, and it may be part of a stress response syndrome. *La belle indifférence* is a bland indifference to a physical defect or disability. That cavalier attitude toward serious symptoms has traditionally been seen as a lack of insight, but it can also be viewed as an instance of inappropriate affect.

Judgment refers to the ability to select appropriate goals and to find or use socially acceptable and appropriate means to reach them. It is more important to assess the ability to exercise judgment in the patient's life than with regard to a contrived situation, such as fire in a theater or finding a stamped, addressed letter on the street. The interviewer can assess a more relevant aspect of judgment by asking the patient questions, such as "What are your plans?" or "What will it take for you to achieve your goals?"

SENSORIUM Sensorium refers to level of awareness and includes orientation. Level of awareness or consciousness ranges from coma and stupor through drowsiness to being alert to hypervigilance. *Clouding of consciousness* is a state of reduced wakefulness or awareness in which the patient is distractible, is startled by minor stimuli, and may misjudge sensory, especially visual, input. That state may progress to an *acute confusional state,* in which the attention span is shortened, stimuli are consistently misinterpreted, and the patient has difficulty following instructions.

There are four spheres of *orientation:* person, place, time, and circumstance or social context. Partial or complete disorientation to time is the most common. The elements of orientation to time include day, date, month, year, and season. Significant errors with regard to month and year are clinically most meaningful. Disorientation usually follows a predictable order: time before place, and disorientation to person last. Disorientation to person, while rare, signifies a serious mental disorder.

ATTENTION AND CONCENTRATION *Attention* is the ability to focus perception on an outside or inside stimulus. A simple test of attention is digit recall. The interviewer presents the patient with a series of single-digit numbers, presented at one-second intervals, and asks the patient to repeat them. Most persons can recall a 7-digit number (the equivalent of a telephone number) forward and 5 to 7 digits in reverse.

Concentration refers to sustained attention to an internal thought process. The serial 7s test is an excellent test of concentration: the patient is asked to subtract 7 from 100 and to continue to subtract 7 from the result serially. Another test of concentration is to have the patient spell a five-letter word forward and then spell the word backwards.

MEMORY It is useful to test several elements of *memory:* Immediate retention and recall, recent memory, and remote memory. *Recall* can be assessed by giving the patient a string of digits or a list of three words or phrases and asking that they be repeated back to the interviewer. That can be turned into a test of *recent memory* by asking the patient to repeat the list again in five minutes; the fraction of three objects that are recalled after five minutes is a conventional screening measure of recent memory. *Remote memory* can be assessed by asking patients about verifiable historical events, such as where they were born, where they went to high school or college, and their social security number.

Formal tests of memory are sometimes omitted when the rest of the clinical interview suggests intact cognitive functioning. However, since impaired memory function is often a sensitive indicator of a variety of cognitive disorders, tests of memory should not be omitted when any of the following factors are known or suspected: acute or chronic intoxication with alcohol or other intoxicants; head injury; acute or chronic physical illness, especially endocrinopathies or other conditions known to affect the central nervous system; ingestion of medications; and age greater than 50 years.

A sample report of a psychiatric history and mental status examination is given in Table 9.1-2.

TECHNIQUES WITH CERTAIN PATIENTS

The manner in which an interview is conducted—the specific techniques and structure—varies according to the interview setting, its purpose, and the patient's diagnosis. Patients with dif-

TABLE 9.1-2
Sample Report of Psychiatric History and Mental Status Examination

Identifying Data

This is the first psychiatric admission for this 28-year-old single Roman Catholic white native of [a middle eastern country], a graduate student in chemistry, referred from the student health service because of fears that the police are going to arrest him. The sources of information about the patient include the patient himself, who appears to be reliable, the patient's roommate, and the patient's supervising professor.

Chief Complaint

"I feel that the police can arrest me at any time and that I will be deported and not be able to complete my degree. Other people are avoiding me and giving me signs that they know about this."

History of Present Illness

The patient states that he was well and under no mental stress until approximately two years ago when he began to look out through his apartment window into an adjacent apartment where one or more women could be seen in various stages of undress. When this occurred, the patient would frequently masturbate. This process went on for a period of over a year, although from nine to eleven months, while he was going with a girlfriend, he discontinued this behavior completely. The behavior began again sometime after he broke up with his girlfriend, and over time he began to feel increasingly guilty and became convinced that his behavior had been reported to the police. Last summer, on a vacation flight home to see his family, he felt he was being followed and observed by "security agents." He states that his father can verify this.

Since returning to graduate school this past fall, he has been living in a different apartment with a new roommate, a medical student. He says that he feels that people at school and on the street know what he has done and they talk about him. He says he can frequently hear people talking about him. During the past few weeks prior to admission, his fears of arrest and subsequent deportation have grown in intensity.

On the morning of the day prior to admission he was brought to the emergency room by his roommate because he had not slept and, at approximately 4:30 AM, woke his roommate up saying he was convinced the police were coming to arrest him. He was seen by me in the emergency room, assessed as having a paranoid delusional system, and was referred to the student health service. Student health offered hospitalization to him, which he refused; instead, he agreed to return for outpatient care. On the morning of admission he was seen briefly at student health and referred to the hospital for admission because of marked anxiety and fearfulness about his imminent arrest.

He denies a major sleep disorder, saying only that he has mild difficulty in falling asleep. He admits to decreased appetite for two to three months, but denies significant change in weight and says there has been no change in his bowel habits. He denies hallucinations, but describes hearing others talk about him in a way which suggests the possibility of auditory hallucinations. He denies any recent drug use.

Past Psychiatric History

The patient denies any history of psychiatric illnesses in himself or in any other member of his family.

Past Medical History

The patient has been in generally good health and is without other symptoms. His immunizations and vaccinations are complete. He reports the usual childhood diseases without major sequelae or complications. He denies any major adult medical illnesses. He states that he has had no operations and that he has no allergies. He reports that he has never sustained serious injuries or trauma. On review of systems, the patient denies any somatic complaints.

Current medications: For one day prior to admission the patient had been given thioridazine (Mellaril), 50 mg four times a day, at student health.

Family History

The patient's father is in his late 60s or early 70s and works in the civil service of his country's government. He is described by the patient as being a very stern and rather moralistic man who did not openly display love and affection, but whose concern would always be felt if there was any kind of personal or family stress or crisis. The patient's mother is approximately age 50 and is the second wife of the patient's father. She is described as being a very warm, generous, and rather permissive person. It is clear that the patient felt that his mother would be his ally in the family. The patient is the sixth child born to his father, but the first child in his father's second marriage. Among his older half siblings, four of the five are still living. One older sister died of cancer of the uterus approximately five years ago. Another of his still living older sisters has breast cancer, and the youngest of his older brothers is reported to have bilateral choreoathetosis. None of the patient's younger siblings have any significant medical or psychiatric history.

Developmental History

The patient was born and reared in the capital city of a middle eastern country. He reports having grown up in a close family network and having felt warmth and affection from his mother and a clear expectation of his own success from his father. The patient was an excellent student in school, always at the top of his class, and did his undergraduate study in Beirut, Lebanon. The patient grew up having numerous friends and was not socially isolated in school or college. He has been a graduate student in the United States for approximately 3½ years. He successfully completed his oral exams last spring (it is perhaps notable that while the patient played down his success in the oral exams, his professor has stated that he passed them with flying colors and made one of the outstanding oral exams in the department). The patient has lived with one or more male roommates while in graduate school in off-campus apartments. Three or four months into his first year, he met and was going with a nurse for approximately one year. Their relationship included what he describes as mutually satisfactory sexual relations. The relationship ended apparently because she was interested in marriage and the patient was not. The patient has had no subsequent lasting relationships with women. He has made no attempt to involve himself in any foreign student social clubs or organizations, and his social acquaintances appear to be limited to colleagues in his department or friends of his roommate. He smokes 2 to 2½ packs of cigarettes per day. He denies alcohol consumption other than a rare social drink. He denies recent drug use, but admits to using stimulants while an undergraduate when under academic pressure. The patient does not appear to be inhibited sexually; however, he does have considerable guilt about his masturbatory activity when he was observing the women through his apartment window. He does recognize the normality of masturbation. He denies any homosexual experiences, but recognizes occasional feelings of attraction to members of the same sex.

Mental Status Examination

The patient was comfortably dressed but unshaven, appearing nervous with a mild tremor. His speech was clear with a foreign accent. He spoke with a regular rate and rhythm. His speech content was organized and his answers to questions were generally relevant. His thoughts were without loose associations but with fixed and unshakable delusions of impending arrest, disgrace, and deportation. Ideas of reference were present, but generally the patient was without grandiosity or religious preoccupations. He denies hallucinations as well as undue somatic concerns. His mood was primarily anxious although he was also somewhat depressed both subjectively and objectively. He displayed a full range of affect with some lability (he nearly broke into tears at one point), but he was able to laugh appropriately. He was fully oriented and displayed an intelligence that was well above average. Although he appeared somewhat distracted, he was able to do all routine tests of memory and concentration (serial 7s, simple calculations, recalling three objects in five minutes) without error. His insight was a mixed picture: He is increasingly aware of the need for help, but believes firmly in his delusional thought content. His judgment was distinctly impaired.

---

ferent psychiatric diagnoses differ in their capacities to participate in an interview, and they present different challenges to an interviewer. Suggestions about interviewing depressed and suicidal patients and delusional patients are provided because they are seen so frequently, while techniques for interviewing violent patients are offered because such patients present unusual difficulties.

DEPRESSED AND POTENTIALLY SUICIDAL PATIENTS

Depressed patients are often unable spontaneously to provide an adequate account of their illness because of such factors as psychomotor retardation and hopelessness. The interviewer must be prepared to ask a depressed patient very specifically about history and symptoms which the patient may not initially volunteer.

One of the most difficult aspects of dealing with depressed patients is experiencing their hopelessness. Many severely depressed patients believe their current feeling will continue indefinitely and that there is no hope. A reasonable approach is for the interviewer to communicate an awareness of how badly the patient feels, that help is certainly possible, but that it is understandable at this point for the patient not to believe that he or she can be helped. It can be a relief to a depressed patient for a psychiatrist to state that his or her depression is treatable but that it may take time for the treatment to work. Rather than convey a false reassurance (which may make depressed patients feel worse), that message conveys the psychiatrist's commitment to understanding the patient and to finding the best treatment.

The potential for suicide is of special concern when interviewing depressed patients, even in the absence of apparent suicidal risk. A suicide note, a family history of suicide, and particularly a prior suicide attempt all place the patient in a high-risk category. If the interviewer decides the patient is in imminent risk for suicidal behavior, the patient should be hospitalized or otherwise protected in a psychiatrically supervised setting. The situation where the patient does not require hospitalization but has some degree of suicidal ideation is often more challenging. Under those circumstances the interviewer should explore the patient's life situation and problems in sufficient detail to be able to help the patient see new options or choices; that will tend to counter the constricted view of the world and of the future which contributes to the hopelessness of depressed cognition.

DELUSIONAL PATIENTS As stated earlier, a patient's delusion should not be challenged directly. A delusion may be thought of as a defensive and self-protecting (though maladaptive) strategy against psychotic anxiety, lowered self-esteem, or confusion. Insisting that the delusional belief is not true or possible is only likely to increase the patient's anxiety, often with the predictable result that the threatened patient asserts the belief more strongly. More importantly, the patient feels attacked by the interviewer. A more helpful approach is to indicate that the interviewer understands that the patient believes the delusion to be true, but that the interviewer does not hold the same belief.

The approach to working with a delusional patient is like that used for overtly paranoid patients (most of whom are delusional). Direct eye contact should be intermittent rather than prolonged, and the interviewer should adopt a stance (and if possible a physical relation to the patient) to the side of the patient, in a position to view things from the patient's perspective. Showing respect and demonstrating a cognitive understanding is often more useful than a profound emotional empathy which a delusional and paranoid patient may find unnerving or intrusive.

VIOLENT PATIENTS Psychiatrists frequently encounter violent patients in a hospital setting, as, for example, when the police bring a patient to the emergency room. Since the patient is often in some type of physical restraints (for example, handcuffs), the psychiatrist must establish whether it is safe to remove them. It may be necessary to medicate the patient before attempts at interviewing can begin if reality testing is grossly impaired. If reality testing is not severely impaired, the interviewer should ask the patient directly whether it is safe to remove the restraints, giving expression to overt concern for the safety of the patient and others in the immediate area. Many interviewers opt to leave restraints on the patient until some history has been obtained and some rapport established. If the patient says or does anything that indicates that the removal of restraints is leading to increased agitation, the decision to remove them should be reassessed immediately.

With or without restraints, the interview of a violent patient should not be done alone: There should always be at least one other person present, in certain circumstances a police officer or a security guard. In an emergency setting with a violent or assaultive patient, physical safety overrides the usual priority given to privacy or strict confidentiality. Other safety measures include leaving open the interview room door and sitting so that the interviewer can exit unimpeded if necessary. A calm, nonthreatening tone of voice should be used, because many violent patients are frightened and cover that with bravado, threats, or violence. While the interviewer should be firm but nonhostile in stating that violent acts will not be tolerated, confrontation with a violent patient is to be avoided.

Once safety issues have been addressed, the principal challenge in interviewing patients who are threatening, assaultive, or potentially violent is to maintain a therapeutic stance of inquiry, concern, curiosity, and respect. Angry, violent, threatening behavior tends to elicit a predictable range of emotions: fear, anger, hatred, disgust, and aversion. It is essential not to react personally to the provocations of violent patients.

Questions that need to be asked of violent patients include those pertaining to previous acts of violence: how often; under what conditions; has the damage been to property only or also to persons; and were drugs or alcohol involved? Corroboration of the history from family, friends, and police is essential.

SUGGESTED CROSS-REFERENCES

Section 9.3 deals with the typical signs and symptoms of psychiatric illness, Section 9.5 deals with neuropsychological and intellectual assessment of adults, and Section 9.8 deals with psychiatric rating scales. Similarly, Chapter 10, on the clinical manifestations of psychiatric disorders, is an essential correlate to interviewing and examining the patient. More specialized focus is provided in Section 2.1, which deals with the clinical assessment and approach to diagnosis in neuropsychiatry. Section 3.1 on perception and cognition and Section 3.5 on the biology of memory will amplify points made in this section. Section 30.1 includes more detailed information on suicide, and Section 30.2 includes information on other psychiatric emergencies. Additional relevant information is found in Chapter 44, which deals with mood disorders and suicide in children and adolescents. Taking a developmental history implies familiarity with the aspects of normal and abnormal development; readers may find the following sections of special interest: Section 6.2 deals with Erik H. Erikson and his ideas about child and adult development; Chapter 33 deals extensively with normal development in children and adolescents; adult development is covered at great length in Chapter 48; and normal aging is the focus of Section 49.4.

REFERENCES

Bremner J D, Steinberg M, Southwick S M, Johnson D R, Charney D S: Use of the structured clinical interview for DSM-IV dissociative disorders for systematic assessment of dissociative symptoms in posttraumatic stress disorder. Am J Psychiatry *150:* 1011, 1993.

*Cox A, Hopkinson K, Rutter M: Psychiatric interviewing techniques II. Naturalistic study: Eliciting factual information. Br J Psychiatry *138:* 283, 1981.

Cox A, Holbrook D, Rutter M: Psychiatric interviewing techniques VI. Experimental study: Eliciting feelings. Br J Psychiatry *139:*144, 1981.

*Cox A, Rutter M, Holbrook D: Psychiatric interviewing techniques V. Experimental study: Eliciting factual information. Br J Psychiatry *139:* 29, 1981.

Creed F, Guthrie E: Techniques for interviewing the somatising patient. Br J Psychiatry *162:* 467, 1993.

Departments of Psychiatry and Child Psychiatry, The Institute of Psychiatry and Maudsley Hospital: *Psychiatric Examination,* ed 2. Oxford University Press, New York, 1987.
Dunner D G: Diagnostic assessment. Psychiatr Clin North Am *16*:431, 1993.
*Hassin D S, Skodol A E: Standardized diagnostic interviews for psychiatric research. In *The Instruments of Psychiatric Research,* C Thompson, editor. Wiley, New York, 1989.
Hersen M, Turner S M, editors: *Diagnostic Interviewing.* Plenum, New York, 1985.
Hodges K: Structured interviews for assessing children. J Child Psychol Psychiatry *34:* 49, 1993.
*Hopkinson K, Cox A, Rutter M: Psychiatric interviewing techniques III. Naturalistic study: Eliciting feelings. Br J Psychiatry *138:* 406, 1981.
Kendler K S, Silberg J L, Neale M C, Kessler R C, Heath A C, Eaves L J: The family history method: Whose psychiatric history is measured? Am J Psychiatry *148:* 1501, 1991.
Loewenstein R J: An office mental status examination for complex chronic dissociative symptoms and multiple personality disorder. Psychiatr Clin North Am *14:* 567, 1991.
Miller W R, Rollnick S: *Motivational Interviewing.* Guilford, New York, 1991.
Mitrushina M, Satz P: Reliability and validity of the mini-mental state exam in neurologically intact elderly. J Clin Psychol *47:* 537, 1991.
Othmer E, Othmer S C: *The Clinical Interview Using DSM-III-R.* American Psychiatric Press, Washington, 1989.
Ovsiew F: Bedside neuropsychiatry: Eliciting the clinical phenomena of neuropsychiatric illness. In *Textbook of Neuropsychiatry,* ed 2, S C Yudofsky, R E Hales, editors, p 89. American Psychiatric Press, Washington, 1992.
Rutter M, Cox A: Psychiatric interviewing techniques: I. Methods and measures. Br J Psychiatry *138:* 273, 1981.
Shea S C: *Psychiatric Interviewing: The Art of Understanding.* Saunders, Philadelphia, 1988.
Spitzer R L, Williams J B W, Gibbon M, First M B: *Users Guide for the Structured Clinical Interview for DSM-III-R.* American Psychiatric Press, Washington, 1990.
Steinberg M: The Structured Clinical Interview for DSM-IV Dissociative Disorders. American Psychiatric Press, Washington, 1993.
Stoller R J: Psychiatry's mind-brain dialectic, or the Mona Lisa has no eyebrows. In *Observing the Erotic Imagination,* R J Stoller. Yale University Press, New Haven, CT, 1986.
*Strupp H, Binder J L: The therapist's stance. In *Psychotherapy in a New Key: A Guide to Time-Limited Dynamic Psychotherapy,* H Strupp, J L Binder. Basic Books, New York, 1984.
Yager J: Specific components of bedside manner in the general hospital psychiatric consultation: 12 concrete suggestions. Psychosomatics *30:* 209, 1989.

9.2 PSYCHIATRIC REPORT

HAROLD I. KAPLAN, M.D.
BENJAMIN J. SADOCK, M.D.

When the psychiatrist has completed a comprehensive psychiatric history and mental status examination, the information obtained is written up and organized into the psychiatric report. The report follows the outline of the standard psychiatric history and mental status examination. In the psychiatric report the examiner addresses the critical questions of further diagnostic studies that must be performed, adds a summary of both positive and negative findings, makes a tentative multiaxial diagnosis, gives a prognosis, gives a psychodynamic formulation, and provides a set of management recommendations.

The following summary represents an outline the clinician or student may use in writing a psychiatric report.

I. Psychiatric history

A. *Preliminary identification:* name, age, marital status, sex, occupation, language if other than English, race, nationality, and religion insofar as they are pertinent; previous admissions to a hospital for the same or different conditions; person or persons with whom the patient lives

B. *Chief complaint:* exactly why the patient came to the psychiatrist, preferably in the patient's own words; if that information does not come from the patient, note who supplied it

C. *Personal identification:* brief, nontechnical description of the patient's appearance and behavior as a novelist might write it

D. *History of present illness:* chronological background and development of the symptoms or behavioral changes culminating in the patient's seeking assistance; describe precipitating stress, if present, at the time of onset; personality when well; how illness has affected the patient's life activities and personal relations—changes in personality, memory, speech; psychophysiological symptoms—nature and details of dysfunction; location, intensity, fluctuation; relationship between physical and psychic symptoms; extent to which the illness serves some additional purpose for the patient when dealing with stress—secondary gain; whether anxieties are generalized and nonspecific (free-floating) or specifically related to particular situations, activities, or objects; how anxieties are handled—avoidance of feared situation, use of drugs or other activities for distraction

E. *Previous illnesses*
   1. Emotional or mental disturbances: extent of symptoms and incapacity, type of treatment, names of hospitals, length of illness, effect of treatment, compliance
   2. Psychosomatic disorders: hay fever, rheumatoid arthritis, ulcerative colitis, asthma, hyperthyroidism, gastrointestinal upsets, recurrent colds, skin conditions
   3. Medical conditions: follow the customary medical review of systems, if necessary; syphilis, alcohol or substance use; at risk for acquired immune deficiency syndrome (AIDS)
   4. Neurological disorders: history of craniocerebral trauma, convulsions, or tumors

F. *Past personal history:* history (anamnesis) of the patient's life from infancy to the present to the extent that it can be recalled; gaps in history as spontaneously related by the patient; emotions associated with those life periods—painful, stressful, conflictual
   1. Prenatal history: nature of mother's pregnancy and delivery: length of pregnancy, spontaneity and normality of delivery, birth trauma, whether patient was planned for and wanted, birth defects
   2. Early childhood (through age 3)
      a. Feeding habits: breast-fed or bottle-fed, eating problems
      b. Early development: walking, talking, and teething; language development, motor development, signs of unmet needs, sleep pattern, object constancy, stranger anxiety, maternal deprivation, separation anxiety, other caretakers in home

c. Toilet training: age, attitude of parents, feelings about it
d. Symptoms of behavior problems: thumb-sucking, temper tantrums, tics, head-bumping, rocking, night terrors, fears, bed-wetting or bed-soiling, nail-biting, masturbation
e. Personality as a child: shy, restless, overactive, withdrawn, persistent, outgoing, timid, athletic, friendly, patterns of play
f. Early or recurrent dreams or fantasies

3. Middle childhood (3 to 11): early school history—feelings about going to school, early adjustment, gender identification, conscience development, punishment, peer relations, nightmares, phobias, bed-wetting, fire setting, cruelty to animals
4. Later childhood (puberty through adolescence)
   a. Social relationships: attitudes toward siblings and playmates, number and closeness of friends, leader or follower, social popularity, participation in group or gang activities, idealized figures; patterns of aggression, passivity, anxiety, antisocial behavior
   b. School history: how far the patient progressed, adjustment to school relationships with teachers (teacher's pet versus rebellious), favorite studies or interests, particular abilities or assets, extracurricular activities, sports, hobbies, relation of problems or symptoms to any school period
   c. Cognitive and motor development: learning to read and other intellectual and motor skills, minimal cerebral dysfunctions, learning disorders—their management and effects on the child
   d. Adolescent emotional or physical problems: nightmares, phobias, bed-wetting, running away, delinquency, smoking, alcohol or substance use, anorexia nervosa, bulimia nervosa, weight problems, feelings of inferiority
5. Psychosexual history (childhood through adolescence)
   a. Early curiosity, infantile masturbation, sex play
   b. Acquisition of sexual knowledge, attitude of parents toward sex, sexual abuse
   c. Onset of puberty, feelings about it, kind of preparation, feelings about menstruation, development of secondary sexual characteristics
   d. Adolescent sexual activity: crushes, parties, dating, petting, masturbation, nocturnal emissions, and attitudes toward them
   e. Attitudes toward opposite sex: timid, shy, aggressive, need to impress, seductive, sexual conquests, anxiety
   f. Sexual practices: sexual problems, heterosexual and homosexual experiences, paraphilias, promiscuity, orientation preferences
6. Religious background: strict, liberal, mixed (possible conflicts), relation of background to current religious practices
7. Adulthood
   a. Occupational history: choice of occupation, training, ambitions, conflicts; relations with authority, peers, and subordinates; number of jobs and duration; changes in job status; current job and feelings about it
   b. Social activity: whether patient has friends, is withdrawn, or is socializing well; kind of social, intellectual, and physical interests; relationship with same-sex and opposite-sex persons; depth, duration, and quality of human relationships
   c. Adult sexuality
      i. Premarital and extramarital sexual relationships
      ii. Marital history: common-law marriages, legal marriages, description of courtship and role played by each partner, age at marriage, family planning and contraception, names and ages of children, attitudes toward raising children, problems of any family members, housing difficulties if important to the marriage, sexual adjustment, areas of agreement and disagreement, management of money, role of in-laws
      iii. Sexual symptoms: anorgasmia, impotence, premature ejaculation, lack of desire
      iv. Attitudes toward pregnancy and having children; contraceptive practices and feelings about them
      v. Sexual practices: paraphilias, such as sadism, fetishes, voyeurism; attitudes toward fellatio, cunnilingus, and coital techniques; frequency
   d. Military history: general adjustment, combat, injuries, referral to psychiatrists, veteran status, disciplinary action

G. *Family history:* elicited from patient and from someone else because quite different descriptions may be given of the same persons and events; ethnic, national, and religious traditions; other persons in the home: descriptions of them—personality and intelligence—and what has become of them since the patient's childhood; descriptions of different households lived in; present relationships between patient and others in the family; role of illness in the family; history of mental illness and treatment

H. *Current social situation:* where patient lives—neighborhood and particular residence of the patient; whether home is crowded; privacy of family members from each other and from other families; sources of family income and difficulties in obtaining it; public assistance, if any, and attitudes toward it; whether patient will lose job or apartment by remaining in the hospital; person who is caring for the children

I. *Dreams, fantasies, and value systems*
   1. Dreams: prominent ones, if patient will tell them; nightmares
   2. Fantasies: recurrent, favorite, or unshakable daydreams; hypnagogic phenomena
   3. Value systems: whether children are seen as a burden or a joy; whether work is seen as a necessary evil, an avoidable chore, or an opportunity; concepts of right and wrong

II. Mental status: sum total of the examiner's observations and impressions derived from the initial interviews

A. General description

1. Appearance: body type, posture, bearing, clothes, grooming, hair, nails; healthy, sickly, angry, frightened, apathetic, perplexed, contemptuous, ill at ease, poised, old looking, young looking, effeminate, masculine; signs of anxiety—moist hands, perspiring forehead, restlessness, tense posture, strained voice, wide eyes; shift in level of anxiety during interview or abrupt changes of topic
2. Behavior and psychomotor activity: gait, mannerisms, tics, gestures, twitches, stereotypes, picking, touching examiner, echopraxia, clumsy, agile, limp, rigid, retarded, hyperactive, agitated, combative, waxy
3. Speech: rapid, slow, pressured, hesitant, emotional, monotonous, loud, whispered, slurred, mumbled, stuttering, echolalia, intensity, pitch, ease, spontaneity, productivity, manner, reaction time, vocabulary
4. Attitude toward examiner: cooperative, attentive, interested, frank, seductive, defensive, hostile, playful, ingratiating, evasive, guarded, level of rapport

B. Mood, feelings, and affect

1. Mood (a pervasive and sustained emotion that colors the person's perception of the world): how the patient says he or she feels; depth, intensity, duration, and fluctuations of mood—depressed, despairing, irritable, anxious, terrified, angry, expansive, euphoric, empty, guilty, awed, futile, self-contemptuous
2. Affective expression: how examiner evaluates patient's affects—broad, restricted, depressed, blunted or flat, shallow, anhedonic, labile, constricted, fearful, anxious, guilty; amount and range of expression; difficulty in initiating, sustaining, or terminating an emotional response
3. Appropriateness: whether the emotional expression is appropriate to the thought content, the culture, and the setting of the examination; note examples of inappropriate emotional expression

C. Perceptual disturbances

1. Hallucinations and illusions: whether patient hears voices or sees visions; content, sensory system involvement, circumstances of the occurrence; hypnagogic or hypnopompic hallucinations
2. Depersonalization and derealization: extreme feelings of detachment from self or from the environment

D. Thought process

1. Stream of thought: quotations from patient
   a. Productivity: overabundance of ideas, paucity of ideas, flight of ideas, rapid thinking, slow thinking, hesitant thinking; whether patient speaks spontaneously or only when questions are asked
   b. Continuity of thought: note whether patient's replies really answer questions; are goal directed and relevant or irrelevant; there is a lack of cause-and-effect relation in patient's explanations, statements are illogical, tangential, rambling, evasive, perseverative; there is blocking or distractibility
   c. Language impairments: impairments that reflect disordered mentation, such as incoherent or incomprehensible speech (word salad), clang associations, neologisms
2. Content of thought
   a. Preoccupations: about the illness, environmental problems; obsessions, compulsions, phobias; plans, intentions, recurrent ideas about suicide, homicide; hypochondriacal symptoms, specific antisocial urges; specific questions should always be asked about suicidal ideation
   b. Thought disturbances
      i. Delusions: content of any delusional system, its organization, the patient's convictions as to its validity, how it affects patient's life; somatic delusions—isolated or associated with pervasive suspiciousness; mood-congruent delusions—in keeping with a depressed or elated mood; mood-incongruent delusions—not in keeping with the patient's mood; bizarre delusions, such as thoughts of being controlled by external forces or thoughts being broadcast out loud
      ii. Ideas of reference and ideas of influence: how ideas began, their content, and the meaning the patient attributes to them
      iii. Abstract thinking: disturbances in concept formation; manner in which the patient conceptualizes or handles ideas; similarities, differences, absurdities, meanings of simple proverbs, such as, "A rolling stone gathers no moss"; answers may be concrete (giving specific examples to illustrate the meaning) or overly abstract (giving generalized explanations); appropriateness of answers should be noted

E. Sensorium and cognition

1. Consciousness: clouding, somnolence, stupor, coma, lethargy, alertness, fugue state
2. Orientation
   a. Time: note whether patient identifies the day correctly; can approximate date, time of day; if in a hospital, knows how long he or she has been there; behaves as though he or she is oriented to the present
   b. Place: note whether patient knows where he or she is
   c. Person: note whether patient knows who the examiner is and the roles or names of the persons with whom he or she is in contact
3. Concentration: ask patient to subtract 7 from 100 and keep subtracting sevens; if patient cannot subtract sevens, whether easier tasks can be accomplished—4 times 9, 5 times 4; whether anxiety or some disturbance of mood or consciousness seems to be responsible for difficulty
4. Memory: impairment, efforts made to cope with impairment—denial, confabulation, catastrophic reaction, circumstantiality used to con-

ceal deficit; whether the process of registration, retention, or recollection of material is involved

a. Remote memory: childhood data, important events known to have occurred when the patient was younger or free of illness, personal matters, neutral material
b. Recent past memory: the past few months
c. Recent memory: the past few days, recall of what was done yesterday, the day before; of what was eaten for breakfast, lunch, dinner
d. Immediate retention and recall: ability to repeat six figures after examiner dictates them—first forward, then backward, then after a few minutes' interruption; other test questions; whether same questions, if repeated, called forth different answers at different times; digit span measures; other mental functions, such as anxiety level and concentration
e. Effect of defect on patient: mechanisms patient has developed to cope with defect

5. Information and intelligence: patient's level of formal education and self-education: estimate of the patient's intellectual capability and whether patient is capable of functioning at the level of basic endowment; counting, calculation; general knowledge; questions that have some relevance to the patient's educational and cultural background

F. *Judgment*

1. Social judgment: subtle manifestations of behavior that are harmful to the patient and contrary to acceptable behavior in the culture; whether the patient understands the likely outcome of his or her behavior and is influenced by this understanding; examples of impairment
2. Test judgment: patient's prediction of what he or she would do in imaginary situations; for instance, what patient would do if he or she found a stamped, addressed letter in the street

G. *Insight:* degree of awareness and understanding the patient has that he or she is ill

1. Complete denial of illness
2. Slight awareness of being sick and needing help but denying it at the same time
3. Awareness of being sick but blaming it on others, on external factors, or on medical versus psychological factors
4. Awareness that illness is due to something unknown in patient
5. Intellectual insight: admission that patient is ill and that symptoms or failures in social adjustment are due to patient's own particular irrational feelings or disturbances without applying that knowledge to future experiences
6. True emotional insight: emotional awareness of the motives and feelings within patient and the important people in his or her life

H. *Reliability:* estimate of examiner's impression of patient's veracity or ability to report the situation accurately

III. Further diagnostic studies

A. *Physical examination*
B. *Additional psychiatric diagnostic interviews*
C. *Interviews with family members, friends, or neighbors by social worker*
D. *Other tests as indicated:* electroencephalogram, computed tomography scan, magnetic resonance imaging, tests of other medical conditions, reading comprehension and writing tests, tests for aphasia, projective psychological tests, dexamethasone-suppression test, 24-hour urine test for heavy-metal intoxication, illegal substances (for example, cocaine, heroin)

IV. Summary of positive and negative findings: mental symptoms, laboratory findings, psychological test results, if available; drugs patient has been taking, including dosage and duration of intake

V. Diagnosis: diagnostic classification according to the fourth edition of the American Psychiatric Association's *Diagnostic and Statistical Manual of Mental Disorders* (DSM-IV)—nomenclature, classification number, diagnoses to be ruled out; DSM-IV uses a multiaxial classification scheme consisting of five axes, each of which should be covered in the diagnosis

A. *Axis I:* consists of clinical disorders (for example, mood disorders, schizophrenia, generalized anxiety disorder) and other conditions that may be a focus of clinical attention (for example, medication-induced movement disorders, identity problem)
B. *Axis II:* consists of personality disorders and mental retardation
C. *Axis III:* consists of general medical condition or physical illness (for example, epilepsy, gastrointestinal disease)
D. *Axis IV:* refers to psychosocial and environmental stressors (for example, problems related to the social environment, occupational problems, housing problems)
E. *Axis V:* refers to the global assessment of functioning (GAF) scale by which the clinician judges the patient's overall level of functioning during a particular period (for example, the patient's level of functioning at the time of the evaluation or the patient's highest level of functioning for at least a few months during the past year). Functioning is conceptualized as a composite of three major areas: social functioning, occupational functioning, and psychological functioning (see Section 11.1)

VI. Prognosis: opinion as to the probable future course, extent, and outcome of the disorder; good and bad prognostic factors; specific goals of therapy

VII. Psychodynamic formulation: causes of the patient's psychodynamic breakdown—influences in the patient's life that contributed to present disorder; environmental, genetic, and personality factors relevant to determining patient's symptoms; primary and secondary gains; outline of the major defense mechanisms used by the patient

VIII. Treatment plan: modalities of treatment recommended, role of medication, inpatient or outpatient treatment, frequency of sessions, probable duration of therapy; type of psychotherapy: individual, group, or family therapy; symptoms or problems to be treated (*Note:* If either the patient or family members are unwilling to accept the recommendations for treatment and the clinician thinks that the refusal of the recommendations may have serious consequences, the patient [or the parent or guardian] should sign a statement to the effect that the recommended treatment was refused)

SUGGESTED CROSS-REFERENCES

A detailed discussion of DSM-IV's multiaxial system appears in Section 11.1 on the classification of mental disorders. The psychiatric interview, history, and mental status examination are discussed in Section 9.1. Medical assessment and laboratory testing are discussed in Section 9.7. The psychotherapies are presented in Chapter 31 and the biological therapies in Chapter 32.

REFERENCES

*American Psychiatric Association: *Diagnostic and Statistical Manual of Mental Disorders,* ed 4. American Psychiatric Association, Washington, 1994.

Baker N J, Berry S L, Adler L E: Family diagnoses missed on a clinical inpatient service. Am J Psychiatry *144:* 630, 1987.

Corty E, Lehman A F, Myers C P: Influence of psychoactive substance use on the reliability of psychiatric diagnosis. J Consult Clin Psychol *61:* 165, 1993.

Keller M B, Manschreck T C: The bedside mental status examination: Reliability and validity. Compr Psychiatry *22:* 500, 1981.

Kerns L L: Falsifications in the psychiatric history: A differential diagnosis. Psychiatry *49:* 13, 1986.

Kosten T A, Rounsaville B J: Sensitivity of psychiatric diagnosis based on the best estimate procedure. Am J Psychiatry *149:* 1225, 1992.

*Lewis N D C: *Outlines for Psychiatric Examinations,* ed 3. New York State Department of Mental Hygiene, Albany, 1943.

*MacKinnon R A, Michels R: *The Psychiatric Interview in Clinical Practice.* Saunders, New York, 1971.

Ryback R: *The Problem-Oriented Record in Psychiatry and Mental Health Care.* Grune & Stratton, New York, 1974.

Shea S C, Mezzich J E: Contemporary psychiatric interviewing: New directions for training. Psychiatry *51:* 385, 1988.

Stevenson I: *The Psychiatric Examination.* Little, Brown, Boston, 1969.

*Stoudemire A, editor: *Clinical Psychiatry for Medical Students,* ed 2. Lippincott, Philadelphia, 1994.

Strub R L, Black F W: *The Mental Status Examination in Neurology,* ed 2. Davis, Philadelphia, 1985.

Westermeyer J, Wahmenholm K: Assessing the victimized psychiatric patient. Hosp Community Psychiatry *40:* 245, 1989.

Wittchen H U, Burke J D, Semler G, Pfister H, VonCranach M, Zaudig M: Recall and dating of psychiatric symptoms: Test-retest reliability of time-related symptom questions in a standardized psychiatric interview. Arch Gen Psychiatry *46:* 437, 1989.

*Zarin D A, Earls F: Diagnostic decision making in psychiatry. Am J Psychiatry *150:* 197, 1993.

9.3 TYPICAL SIGNS AND SYMPTOMS OF PSYCHIATRIC ILLNESS

HAROLD I. KAPLAN, M.D.
BENJAMIN J. SADOCK, M.D.

INTRODUCTION

Psychiatry is concerned with phenomenology and the study of mental phenomena. Psychiatrists must learn to be masters of precise observation and evocative description, and the learning of those skills involves the learning of a new language. Part of the language in psychiatry involves the recognition and definition of behavioral and emotional signs and symptoms. *Signs* are objective findings observed by the clinician (for example, constricted affect and psychomotor retardation); *symptoms* are subjective experiences described by the patient (for example, depressed mood and decreased energy). A *syndrome* is a group of signs and symptoms that occur together as a recognizable condition that may be less specific than a clear-cut disorder or disease. Most psychiatric conditions are, in fact, syndromes. Becoming an expert in recognizing specific signs and symptoms allows the clinician to communicate understandably with other clinicians, accurately make a diagnosis, effectively manage treatment, reliably predict a prognosis, and thoroughly explore pathophysiology, causes, and psychodynamic issues.

The outline that follows gives a comprehensive list of signs and symptoms, each with a precise definition or description. Most psychiatric signs and symptoms have their roots in essentially normal behavior and represent various points on the spectrum of behavior from normal to pathological.

Table 9.3-1 lists in alphabetical order the mental phenomena and the signs and symptoms of psychiatric illness discussed in here. The numbers and letters in the right-hand column refer to the place in the chapter where each term is defined.

I. **Consciousness:** state of awareness

Apperception: perception modified by one's own emotions and thoughts. Sensorium: state of cognitive functioning of the special senses (sometimes used as a synonym for consciousness). Disturbances of consciousness are most often associated with brain pathology.

A. *Disturbances of consciousness*
1. Disorientation: disturbance of orientation in time, place, or person
2. Clouding of consciousness: incomplete clear-mindedness with disturbances in perception and attitudes
3. Stupor: lack of reaction to and unawareness of surroundings
4. Delirium: bewildered, restless, confused, disoriented reaction associated with fear and hallucinations
5. Coma: profound degree of unconsciousness
6. Coma vigil: coma in which the patient appears to be asleep but ready to be aroused (also known as akinetic mutism)
7. Twilight state: disturbed consciousness with hallucinations
8. Dreamlike state: often used as a synonym for complex partial seizure or psychomotor epilepsy
9. Somnolence: abnormal drowsiness

B. *Disturbances of attention:* attention is the amount of effort exerted in focusing on certain portions of an experience; ability to sustain a focus on one activity; ability to concentrate
1. Distractibility: inability to concentrate attention; attention drawn to unimportant or irrelevant external stimuli
2. Selective inattention: blocking out only those things that generate anxiety
3. Hypervigilance: excessive attention and focus on all internal and external stimuli, usually secondary to delusional or paranoid states
4. Trance: focused attention and altered consciousness, usually seen in hypnosis, dissociative disorders, and ecstatic religious experiences

TABLE 9.3-1

Index to Signs and Symptoms of Psychiatric Illness. (This table lists in alphabetical order the mental phenomena and the signs and symptoms of psychiatric illness discussed here. The numbers and letters in the right-hand column refer to the place in the section where each item is defined.)

Abreaction	II, C, 9
Abulia	III, 15
Acalculia	VIII, B, 1
Acrophobia	IV, C, 11c
Acting out	III, 14
Adiadochokinesia	VI, B, 8
Affect	II, A
Aggression	III, 13
Agitation	II, C, 4
Agnosia	VI, B
Agoraphobia	IV, C, 11d
Agraphia	VIII, B, 2
Ailurophobia	IV, C, 11f
Akathisia	III, 10e
Akinetic mutism	I, A, 6
Alexia	VIII, B, 3
Alexithymia	II, B, 12
Algophobia	IV, C, 11e
Ambivalence	II, C, 8
Amnesia	VII, A, 1
Amnestic aphasia	V, B, 3
Anhedonia	II, B, 10
Anomia	V, B, 3
Anorexia	II, D, 1
Anosognosia	VI, B, 1
Anterograde amnesia	VII, A, 1a
Anxiety	II, C, 1
Apathy	II, C, 7
Aphasic disturbances	V, B
Apperception	I
Appropriate affect	II, A, 1
Apraxia	VI, B, 6
Astereognosis	VI, B, 4
Ataxia	III, 10g
Attention	I, B
Auditory hallucination	VI, A, 1c
Autistic thinking	IV, A, 7
Automatic judgment	X, B
Automatic obedience	III, 8
Automatism	III, 7
Autotopagnosia	VI, B, 2
Bizarre delusion	IV, C, 3a
Blocking	IV, B, 15
Blunted affect	II, A, 3
Broca's aphasia	V, B, 1
Catalepsy	III, 2a
Cataplexy	III, 4
Catatonia	III, 2
Catatonic excitement	III, 2b
Catatonic posturing	III, 2e
Catatonic rigidity	III, 2d
Catatonic stupor	III, 2c
Cenesthesic hallucination	VI, A, 2, h
Cerea flexibilitas (waxy flexibility)	III, 2f
Circumstantiality	IV, B, 3
Clang association	IV, B, 14
Claustrophobia	IV, C, 11i
Clérambault-Kandinsky complex	IV, C, 3l
Clouding of consciousness	I, A, 2
Cluttering	V, A, 10
Coma	I, A, 5
Coma vigil	I, A, 6
Command automatism	III, 8
Compulsion	IV, C, 9; III, 10f
Conation	III
Concrete thinking	VIII, D
Condensation	IV, B, 9
Confabulation	VII, A, 2c
Consciousness	I
Constipation	II, D, 7
Constricted affect	II, A, 4
Conversion phenomena	VI, C
Coprolalia	IV, C, 10
Déjà entendu	VII, A, 2e
Déjà pensé	VII, A, 2f
Déjà vu	VII, A, 2d
Delirium	I, A, 4
Delirium tremens	VI, A, 11
Delusion	IV, C, 3
Delusional jealousy	IV, C, 3k
Delusion of control	IV, C, 3j
Delusion of grandeur	IV, C, 3h, ii
Delusion of infidelity	IV, C, 3k
Delusion of persecution	IV, C, 3h, i
Delusion of poverty	IV, C, 3f
Delusion of reference	IV, C, 3h, iii
Delusion of self-accusation	IV, C, 3i
Dementia	VIII, B
Dementia syndrome of depression	VIII, C
Depersonalization	VI, C, 4
Depression	II, B, 9
Derailment	IV, B, 12
Derealization	VI, C, 5
Dereism	IV, A, 6
Diminished libido	II, D, 6
Dipsomania	III, 10f, i
Disorientation	I, A, 1
Dissociative identity disorder	V1, C, 7
Distractibility	I, B, 1
Disturbances associated with cognitive disorder	VI, B
Disturbances associated with conversion and dissociative phenomena	VI, C
Disturbances in content of thought	IV, C
Disturbances in form of thinking	IV, A
Disturbances in speech	V, A
Disturbances in suggestibility	I, C
Disturbances of attention	I, B
Disturbances of consciousness	I, A
Disturbances of memory	VII, A
Diurnal variation	II, D, 5
Dreamlike state	I, A, 8
Dysarthria	V, A, 7
Dyscalculia	VII, B, 1
Dysgraphia	VIII, B, 2
Dysphoric mood	II, B, 1
Dysprosody	V, A, 6
Echolalia	IV, B, 8
Echopraxia	III, 1
Ecstasy	II, B, 8
Egomania	IV, C, 5
Eidetic image	VII, A, 4
Elevated mood	II, B, 6
Emotion	II
Erotomania	IV, C, 3l
Erythrophobia	IV, C, 11g
Euphoria	II, B, 7
Euthymic mood	II, B, 2
Excessively loud or soft speech	V, A, 8
Expansive mood	II, B, 3
Expressive aphasia	V, B, 1
Fausse reconnaissance	VII, A, 2a
Fear	II, C, 3
Flat affect	II, A, 5
Flight of ideas	IV, B, 13
Fluent aphasia	V, B, 2
Folie à deux (folie à trois)	I, C, 1
Formal thought disorder	IV, A, 4
Formication	VI, A, 1g
Free-floating anxiety	II, C, 2
Freudian slip	IV
Fugue	VI, C, 6
Global aphasia	V, B, 6
Glossolalia	IV, B, 16
Grief	II, B, 11
Guilt	II, C, 11
Gustatory hallucination	VI, A, 1f
Hallucination	VI, A, 1
Hallucinosis	VI, A, 11
Haptic hallucination	VI, A, 1g
Hyperactivity (hyperkinesis)	III, 10b
Hypermnesia	VII, A, 3
Hyperphagia	II, D, 2
Hypersomnia	II, D, 4
Hypervigilance	I, B, 3
Hypnagogic hallucination	VI, A, 1a
Hypnopompic hallucination	VI, A, 1b
Hypnosis	I, C, 2
Hypoactivity (hypokinesis)	III, 11

TABLE 9.3-1 *(continued)*

Hypochondria	IV, C, 7	Posturing	III, 2e
Hysterical anesthesia	VI, C, 1	Poverty of content of speech	V, A, 5
Idea of reference	IV, C, 3h, iii	Poverty of speech	V, A, 3
Illogical thinking	IV, A, 5	Preoccupation of thought	IV, C, 4
Illusion	VI, A, 2	Pressure of speech	V, A, 1
Immediate memory	VII, B, 1	Primary process thinking	IV, A, 9
Impaired insight	IX, C	Prosopagnosia	VI, B, 5
Impaired judgment	X, C	Pseudodementia	VIII, C
Inappropriate affect	II, A, 2	Pseudologia phantastica	IV, C, 3m
Incoherence	IV, B, 5	Psychomotor agitation	III, 10a
Increased libido	II, D, 6	Psychosis	IV, A, 2
Initial insomnia	II, D, 3a	Reality testing	IV, A, 3
Insight	IX	Recent memory	VII, B, 2
Insomnia	II, D, 3	Recent past memory	VII, B, 3
Intellectual insight	IX, A	Receptive aphasia	V, B, 2
Intelligence	VIII	Remote memory	VII, B, 4
Irrelevant answer	IV, B, 10	Repression	VII, A, 6
Irritable mood	II, B, 4	Restricted affect	II, A, 4
Jamais vu	VII, A, 2g	Retrograde amnesia	VII, A, 1b
Jargon aphasia	V, B, 5	Retrospective falsification	VII, A, 2b
Kleptomania	III, 10f, ii	Rigidity	III, 2d
		Ritual	III, 10f, vi
Labile affect	II, A, 6	Rumination	IV, C, 8
Labile mood	II, B, 5	Satyriasis	III, 10f, iv
Lethologica	VII, A, 7	Screen memory	VII, A, 5
Lilliputian hallucination	VI, A, 1i	Selective inattention	I, B, 2
Logorrhea	V, A, 2	Sensorium	I
Loosening of associations	IV, B, 11	Sensory aphasia	V, B, 2
Macropsia	VI, C, 2	Shame	II, C, 10
Magical thinking	IV, A, 8	Simultagnosia	VI, B, 7
Mannerism	III, 6	Sleepwalking	III, 10d
Memory	VII	Social phobia	IV, C, 11b
Mental disorder	IV, A, 1	Somatic delusion	IV, C, 3g
Mental retardation	VIII, A	Somatic hallucination	VI, A, 1h
Micropsia	VI, C, 3	Somatopagnosia	VI, B, 2
Middle insomnia	II, D, 3b	Somnambulism	III, 10d
Mimicry	III, 12	Somnolence	I, A, 9
Monomania	IV, C, 6	Speaking in tongues	IV, B, 16
Mood	II, B	Specific disturbances in form of thought	IV, B
Mood-congruent delusion	IV, C, 3c	Specific phobia	IV, C, 11a
Mood-congruent hallucination	VI, A, 1j	Stereotypy	III, 5
Mood-incongruent delusion	IV, C, 3d	Stupor	I, A, 3; III, 2c
Mood-incongruent hallucination	VI, A, 1k	Stuttering	V, A, 9
Mood swings	II, B, 5	Synesthesia	VI, A, 1m
Motor aphasia	V, B, 1	Syntactical aphasia	V, B, 4
Motor behavior (conation)	III	Systematized delusion	IV, C, 3b
Mourning	II, B, 11	Tactile (haptic) hallucination	VI, A, 1g
Multiple personality	VI, C, 7	Tangentiality	IV, B, 4
Munchausen syndrome	IV, C, 3m	Tension	II, C, 5
Mutism	III, 9	Terminal insomnia	II, D, 3c
Negativism	III, 3	Thinking	IV
Neologism	IV, B, 1	Thought broadcasting	IV, C, 3j, iii
Neurosis	IV, A, 2	Thought control	IV, C, 3j, iv
Nihilistic delusion	IV, C, 3e	Thought deprivation	IV, B, 15
Noesis	IV, C, 12	Thought insertion	IV, C, 3j, ii
Nominal aphasia	V, B, 3	Thought withdrawal	IV, C, 3j, i
Nonfluent aphasia	V, B, 1	Tic	III, 10c
Nymphomania	III, 10f, iii	Trailing phenomenon	VI, A, 1n
Obsession	IV, C, 8	Trance	I, B, 4
Olfactory hallucination	VI, A, 1e	Trend of thought	IV, C, 4
Overactivity	III, 10	Trichotillomania	III, 10f, v
Overvalued idea	IV, C, 2	True insight	IX, B
Panic	II, C, 6	Twilight state	I, A, 7
Panphobia	IV, C, 11h	*Unio mystica*	IV, C, 13
Paramnesia	VII, A, 2	Vegetative signs	II, D
Paranoid delusions	IV, C, 3h	Verbigeration	IV, B, 7
Paranoid ideation	IV, C, 3h	Visual agnosia	VI, B, 3
Parapraxis	IV	Visual hallucination	VI, A, 1d
Pathological jealousy	IV, C, 3k	Volubility	V, A, 2
Perception	VI	Waxy flexibility	III, 2f
Persecutory delusion	IV, C, 3h, i	Wernicke's aphasia	V, B, 2
Perseveration	IV, B, 6	Word salad	IV, B, 2
Phantom limb	VI, A, 1g	Xenophobia	IV, C, 11j
Phobia	IV, C, 11	Zoophobia	IV, C, 11k
Physiological disturbances associated with mood	II, D		
Polyphagia	III, 10h		

C. *Disturbances in suggestibility:* compliant and uncritical response to an idea or influence
   1. *Folie à deux* (or *folie à trois*): communicated emotional illness between two (or three) persons
   2. Hypnosis: artificially induced modification of consciousness characterized by a heightened suggestibility

II. Emotion: a complex feeling state with psychic, somatic, and behavioral components that is related to affect and mood

A. *Affect:* observed expression of emotion; may be inconsistent with patient's description of emotion
   1. Appropriate affect: condition in which the emotional tone is in harmony with the accompanying idea, thought, or speech; also further described as broad or full affect, in which a full range of emotions is appropriately expressed
   2. Inappropriate affect: disharmony between the emotional feeling tone and the idea, thought, or speech accompanying it
   3. Blunted affect: a disturbance in affect that is manifest by a severe reduction in the intensity of externalized feeling tone
   4. Restricted or constricted affect: reduction in intensity of feeling tone less severe than blunted affect but clearly reduced
   5. Flat affect: absence or near absence of any signs of affective expression; voice monotonous, face immobile
   6. Labile affect: rapid and abrupt changes in emotional feeling tone, unrelated to external stimuli

B. *Mood:* a pervasive and sustained emotion, subjectively experienced and reported by the patient and observed by others; examples include depression, elation, anger
   1. Dysphoric mood: an unpleasant mood
   2. Euthymic mood: normal range of mood, implying absence of depressed or elevated mood
   3. Expansive mood: expression of one's feelings without restraint, frequently with an overestimation of one's significance or importance
   4. Irritable mood: easily annoyed and provoked to anger
   5. Mood swings (labile mood): oscillations between euphoria and depression or anxiety
   6. Elevated mood: air of confidence and enjoyment; a mood more cheerful than usual
   7. Euphoria: intense elation with feelings of grandeur
   8. Ecstasy: feeling of intense rapture
   9. Depression: psychopathological feeling of sadness
   10. Anhedonia: loss of interest in and withdrawal from all regular and pleasurable activities, often associated with depression
   11. Grief or mourning: sadness appropriate to a real loss
   12. Alexithymia: inability or difficulty in describing or being aware of one's emotions or moods

C. *Other emotions*
   1. Anxiety: feeling of apprehension caused by anticipation of danger, which may be internal or external
   2. Free-floating anxiety: pervasive, unfocused fear not attached to any idea
   3. Fear: anxiety caused by consciously recognized and realistic danger
   4. Agitation: severe anxiety associated with motor restlessness
   5. Tension: increased motor and psychological activity that is unpleasant
   6. Panic: acute, episodic, intense attack of anxiety associated with overwhelming feelings of dread and autonomic discharge
   7. Apathy: dulled emotional tone associated with detachment or indifference
   8. Ambivalence: coexistence of two opposing impulses toward the same thing in the same person at the same time
   9. Abreaction: emotional release or discharge after recalling a painful experience
   10. Shame: failure to live up to self-expectations
   11. Guilt: emotion secondary to doing what is perceived as wrong

D. *Physiological disturbances associated with mood:* signs of somatic (usually autonomic) dysfunction of the person, most often associated with depression (also called vegetative signs)
   1. Anorexia: loss of or decrease in appetite
   2. Hyperphagia: increase in appetite and intake of food
   3. Insomnia: lack of or diminished ability to sleep
      a. Initial: difficulty in falling asleep
      b. Middle: difficulty in sleeping through the night without waking up and difficulty in going back to sleep
      c. Terminal: early morning awakening
   4. Hypersomnia: excessive sleeping
   5. Diurnal variation: mood is regularly worst in the morning, immediately after awakening, and improves as the day progresses
   6. Diminished libido: decreased sexual interest, drive, and performance (increased libido is often associated with manic states)
   7. Constipation: inability or difficulty in defecating

III. Motor behavior (conation): the aspect of the psyche that includes impulses, motivations, wishes, drives, instincts, and cravings, as expressed by a person's behavior or motor activity
   1. Echopraxia: pathological imitation of movements of one person by another
   2. Catatonia: motor anomalies in nonorganic disorders (as opposed to disturbances of consciousness and motor activity secondary to organic pathology)
      a. Catalepsy: general term for an immobile position that is constantly maintained
      b. Catatonic excitement: agitated, purposeless motor activity, uninfluenced by external stimuli
      c. Catatonic stupor: markedly slowed motor activity, often to a point of immobility and seeming unawareness of surroundings
      d. Catatonic rigidity: voluntary assumption of a rigid posture, held against all efforts to be moved
      e. Catatonic posturing: voluntary assumption

of an inappropriate or bizarre posture, generally maintained for long periods

f. *Cerea flexibilitas* (waxy flexibility): the person can be molded into a position that is then maintained; when the examiner moves the person's limb, the limb feels as if it were made of wax

3. Negativism: motiveless resistance to all attempts to be moved or to all instructions
4. Cataplexy: temporary loss of muscle tone and weakness precipitated by a variety of emotional states
5. Stereotypy: repetitive fixed pattern of physical action or speech
6. Mannerism: ingrained, habitual involuntary movement
7. Automatism: automatic performance of an act or acts generally representative of unconscious symbolic activity
8. Command automatism: automatic following of suggestions (also called automatic obedience)
9. Mutism: voicelessness without structural abnormalities
10. Overactivity
    a. Psychomotor agitation: excessive motor and cognitive overactivity, usually nonproductive and in response to inner tension
    b. Hyperactivity (hyperkinesis): restless, aggressive, destructive activity, often associated with some underlying brain pathology
    c. Tic: involuntary, spasmodic motor movement
    d. Sleepwalking (somnambulism): motor activity during sleep
    e. Akathisia: subjective feeling of muscular tension secondary to antipsychotic or other medication, which can cause restlessness, pacing, repeated sitting and standing; can be mistaken for psychotic agitation
    f. Compulsion: uncontrollable impulse to perform an act repetitively
        i. Dipsomania: compulsion to drink alcohol
        ii. Kleptomania: compulsion to steal
        iii. Nymphomania: excessive and compulsive need for coitus in a woman
        iv. Satyriasis: excessive and compulsive need for coitus in a man
        v. Trichotillomania: compulsion to pull out one's hair
        vi. Ritual: automatic activity, compulsive in nature, anxiety reducing in origin
    g. Ataxia: failure of muscle coordination; irregularity of muscle action
    h. Polyphagia: pathological overeating
11. Hypoactivity (hypokinesis): decreased motor and cognitive activity, as in psychomotor retardation; visible slowing of thought, speech, and movements
12. Mimicry: simple, imitative motor activity of childhood
13. Aggression: forceful goal-directed action that may be verbal or physical; the motor counterpart of the affect of rage, anger, or hostility
14. Acting out: direct expression of an unconscious wish or impulse in action; unconscious fantasy is lived out impulsively in behavior
15. Abulia: reduced impulse to act and think, associated with indifference about consequences of action; association with neurological deficit

IV. Thinking: goal-directed flow of ideas, symbols, and associations initiated by a problem or a task and leading toward a reality-oriented conclusion; when a logical sequence occurs, thinking is normal; parapraxis (unconsciously motivated lapse from logic is also called Freudian slip) considered part of normal thinking

A. General disturbances in form or process of thinking

1. Mental disorder: clinically significant behavioral or psychological syndrome, associated with distress or disability, not just an expected response to a particular event or limited to relations between the person and society
2. Psychosis: inability to distinguish reality from fantasy; impaired reality testing, with the creation of a new reality (as opposed to neurosis: mental disorder in which reality testing is intact, behavior may not violate gross social norms, relatively enduring or recurrent without treatment)
3. Reality testing: the objective evaluation and judgment of the world outside the self
4. Formal thought disorder: disturbance in the form of thought, instead of the content of thought; thinking characterized by loosened associations, neologisms, and illogical constructs; thought process is disordered and the person is defined as psychotic
5. Illogical thinking: thinking containing erroneous conclusions or internal contradictions; it is psychopathological only when it is marked and when not caused by cultural values or intellectual deficit
6. Dereism: mental activity not concordant with logic or experience
7. Autistic thinking: preoccupation with inner, private world; term used somewhat synonymously with dereism
8. Magical thinking: a form of dereistic thought; thinking that is similar to that of the preoperational phase in children (Jean Piaget), in which thoughts, words, or actions assume power (for example, they can cause or prevent events)
9. Primary process thinking: general term for thinking that is dereistic, illogical, magical; normally found in dreams, abnormally in psychosis

B. Specific disturbances in form of thought

1. Neologism: new word created by the patient, often by combining syllables of other words, for idiosyncratic psychological reasons
2. Word salad: incoherent mixture of words and phrases
3. Circumstantiality: indirect speech that is delayed in reaching the point but eventually gets from original point to desired goal; characterized by an overinclusion of details and parenthetical remarks

4. Tangentiality: inability to have goal-directed associations of thought; patient never gets from desired point to desired goal
5. Incoherence: thought that, generally, is not understandable; running together of thoughts or words with no logical or grammatical connection, resulting in disorganization
6. Perseveration: persisting response to a prior stimulus after a new stimulus has been presented, often associated with cognitive disorders
7. Verbigeration: meaningless repetition of specific words or phrases
8. Echolalia: psychopathological repeating of words or phrases of one person by another; tends to be repetitive and persistent, may be spoken with mocking or staccato intonation
9. Condensation: fusion of various concepts into one
10. Irrelevant answer: answer that is not in harmony with question asked (patient appears to ignore or not attend to question)
11. Loosening of associations: flow of thought in which ideas shift from one subject to another in completely unrelated way; when severe, speech may be incoherent
12. Derailment: gradual or sudden deviation in train of thought without blocking; sometimes used synonymously with loosening of associations
13. Flight of ideas: rapid, continuous verbalizations or plays on words produce constant shifting from one idea to another; the ideas tend to be connected, and in the less severe form a listener may be able to follow them
14. Clang association: association of words similar in sound but not in meaning; words have no logical connection, may include rhyming and punning
15. Blocking: abrupt interruption in train of thinking before a thought or idea is finished; after a brief pause, the person indicates no recall of what was being said or was going to be said (also known as thought deprivation)
16. Glossolalia: the expression of a revelatory message through unintelligible words (also known as speaking in tongues); not considered a disturbance in thought if associated with practices of specific Pentecostal religions

C. *Specific disturbances in content of thought*

1. Poverty of content: thought that gives little information because of vagueness, empty repetitions, or obscure phrases
2. Overvalued idea: unreasonable, sustained false belief maintained less firmly than a delusion
3. Delusion: false belief, based on incorrect inference about external reality, not consistent with patient's intelligence and cultural background, that cannot be corrected by reasoning
   a. Bizarre delusion: an absurd, totally implausible, strange false belief (for example, invaders from space have implanted electrodes in the patient's brain)
   b. Systematized delusion: false belief or beliefs united by a single event or theme (for example, patient is being persecuted by the CIA, the FBI, the Mafia, or the boss)
   c. Mood-congruent delusion: delusion with mood-appropriate content (for example, a depressed patient believes that he or she is responsible for the destruction of the world)
   d. Mood-incongruent delusion: delusion with content that has no association to mood or is mood-neutral (for example, a depressed patient has delusions of thought control or thought broadcasting)
   e. Nihilistic delusion: false feeling that self, others, or the world is nonexistent or ending
   f. Delusion of poverty: false belief that one is bereft or will be deprived of all material possessions
   g. Somatic delusion: false belief involving functioning of one's body (for example, belief that one's brain is rotting or melting)
   h. Paranoid delusions: includes persecutory delusions and delusions of reference, control, and grandeur (distinguished from paranoid ideation, which is suspiciousness of less than delusional proportions)
      i. Delusion of persecution: false belief that one is being harassed, cheated, or persecuted; often found in litigious patients who have a pathological tendency to take legal action because of imagined mistreatment
      ii. Delusion of grandeur: exaggerated conception of one's importance, power, or identity
      iii. Delusion of reference: false belief that the behavior of others refers to oneself; that events, objects, or others have a particular and unusual significance, usually of a negative nature; derived from idea of reference, in which one falsely feels that one is being talked about by others (for example, belief that persons on television or radio are talking to or about the patient)
   i. Delusion of self-accusation: false feeling of remorse and guilt
   j. Delusion of control: false feeling that one's will, thoughts, or feelings are being controlled by external forces
      i. Thought withdrawal: delusion that one's thoughts are being removed from one's mind by other persons or forces
      ii. Thought insertion: delusion that thoughts are being implanted in one's mind by other persons or forces
      iii. Thought broadcasting: delusion that one's thoughts can be heard by others, as though they were being broadcast into the air
      iv. Thought control: delusion that one's thoughts are being controlled by other persons or forces
   k. Delusion of infidelity (delusional jeal-

ousy): false belief derived from pathological jealousy that one's lover is unfaithful

l. Erotomania: delusional belief, more common in women than in men, that someone is deeply in love with the patient (also known as Clérambault-Kandinsky complex)

m. Pseudologia phantastica: a type of lying, in which the person appears to believe in the reality of his or her fantasies and acts on them; associated with Munchausen syndrome, repeated feigning of illness

4. Trend or preoccupation of thought: centering of thought content on a particular idea, associated with a strong affective tone, such as a paranoid trend or a suicidal or homicidal preoccupation
5. Egomania: pathological self-preoccupation
6. Monomania: preoccupation with a single object
7. Hypochondria: exaggerated concern about one's health that is based not on real organic pathology but rather on unrealistic interpretations of physical signs or sensations as abnormal
8. Obsession: pathological persistence of an irresistible thought or feeling that cannot be eliminated from consciousness by logical effort, which is associated with anxiety (also termed rumination)
9. Compulsion: pathological need to act on an impulse that, if resisted, produces anxiety; repetitive behavior in response to an obsession or performed according to certain rules, with no true end in itself other than to prevent something from occurring in the future
10. Coprolalia: compulsive utterance of obscene words
11. Phobia: persistent, irrational, exaggerated, and invariably pathological dread of some specific type of stimulus or situation; results in a compelling desire to avoid the feared stimulus
    a. Specific phobia: circumscribed dread of a discrete object or situation (for example, dread of spiders or snakes)
    b. Social phobia: dread of public humiliation, as in fear of public speaking, performing, or eating in public
    c. Acrophobia: dread of high places
    d. Agoraphobia: dread of open places
    e. Algophobia: dread of pain
    f. Ailurophobia: dread of cats
    g. Erythrophobia: dread of red (refers to a fear of blushing)
    h. Panphobia: dread of everything
    i. Claustrophobia: dread of closed places
    j. Xenophobia: dread of strangers
    k. Zoophobia: dread of animals
12. Noesis: a revelation in which immense illumination occurs in association with a sense that one has been chosen to lead and command
13. *Unio mystica:* an oceanic feeling, one of mystic unity with an infinite power; not considered a disturbance in thought content if congruent with patient's religious or cultural milieu

V. Speech: ideas, thoughts, feelings as expressed through language; communication through the use of words and language

A. Disturbances in speech

1. Pressure of speech: rapid speech that is increased in amount and difficult to interrupt
2. Volubility (logorrhea): copious, coherent, logical speech
3. Poverty of speech: restriction in the amount of speech used; replies may be monosyllabic
4. Nonspontaneous speech: verbal responses given only when asked or spoken to directly; no self-initiation of speech
5. Poverty of content of speech: speech that is adequate in amount but conveys little information because of vagueness, emptiness, or stereotyped phrases
6. Dysprosody: loss of normal speech melody (called prosody)
7. Dysarthria: difficulty in articulation, not in word finding or in grammar
8. Excessively loud or soft speech: loss of modulation of normal speech volume; may reflect a variety of pathological conditions ranging from psychosis to depression to deafness
9. Stuttering: frequent repetition or prolongation of a sound or syllable, leading to markedly impaired speech fluency
10. Cluttering: erratic and dysrhythmic speech, consisting of rapid and jerky spurts

B. Aphasic disturbances: disturbances in language output

1. Motor aphasia: disturbance of speech caused by a cognitive disorder in which understanding remains but ability to speak is grossly impaired; speech is halting, laborious, and inaccurate (also known as Broca's nonfluent, and expressive aphasia)
2. Sensory aphasia: organic loss of ability to comprehend the meaning of words; speech is fluid and spontaneous but incoherent and nonsensical (also known as Wernicke's, fluent, and receptive aphasia)
3. Nominal aphasia: difficulty in finding correct name for an object (also termed anomia and amnestic aphasia)
4. Syntactical aphasia: inability to arrange words in proper sequence
5. Jargon aphasia: words produced are totally neologistic; nonsense words repeated with various intonations and inflections
6. Global aphasia: combination of a grossly nonfluent aphasia and a severe fluent aphasia

VI. Perception: process of transferring physical stimulation into psychological information; mental process by which sensory stimuli are brought to awareness

A. Disturbances of perception

1. Hallucination: false sensory perception not associated with real external stimuli; there may or may not be a delusional interpretation of the hallucinatory experience
    a. Hypnagogic hallucination: false sensory perception occurring while falling asleep; generally considered a nonpathological phenomenon

b. Hypnopompic hallucination: false perception occurring while awakening from sleep; generally considered nonpathological
c. Auditory hallucination: false perception of sound, usually voices but also other noises, such as music; most common hallucination in psychiatric disorders
d. Visual hallucination: false perception involving sight consisting of both formed images (for example, persons) and unformed images (for example, flashes of light); most common in medically determined disorders
e. Olfactory hallucination: false perception of smell; most common in medical disorders
f. Gustatory hallucination: false perception of taste, such as unpleasant taste caused by an uncinate seizure; most common in medical disorders
g. Tactile (haptic) hallucination: false perception of touch or surface sensation, as from an amputated limb (phantom limb), crawling sensation on or under the skin (formication)
h. Somatic hallucination: false sensation of things occurring in or to the body, most often visceral in origin (also known as cenesthesic hallucination)
i. Lilliputian hallucination: false perception in which objects are seen as reduced in size (also termed micropsia)
j. Mood-congruent hallucination: hallucination in which the content is consistent with either a depressed or a manic mood (for example, a depressed patient hears voices saying that the patient is a bad person; a manic patient hears voices saying that the patient is of inflated worth, power, and knowledge)
k. Mood-incongruent hallucination: hallucination in which the content is not consistent with either depressed or manic mood (for example, in depression hallucinations not involving such themes as guilt, deserved punishment, or inadequacy; in mania hallucinations not involving such themes as inflated worth or power)
l. Hallucinosis: hallucinations, most often auditory, that are associated with chronic alcohol abuse and that occur within a clear sensorium, as opposed to delirium tremens (DTs), hallucinations that occur in the context of a clouded sensorium
m. Synesthesia: sensation or hallucination caused by another sensation (for example, an auditory sensation is accompanied by or triggers a visual sensation; a sound is experienced as being seen or a visual experience is heard)
n. Trailing phenomenon: perceptual abnormality associated with hallucinogenic drugs in which moving objects are seen as a series of discrete and discontinuous images

2. Illusion: misperception or misinterpretation of real external sensory stimuli

B. Disturbances associated with cognitive disorder: agnosia—an inability to recognize and interpret the significance of sensory impressions

1. Anosognosia (ignorance of illness): inability to recognize a neurological deficit as occurring to oneself
2. Somatopagnosia (ignorance of the body): inability to recognize a body part as one's own (also called autopagnosia)
3. Visual agnosia: inability to recognize objects or persons
4. Astereognosis: inability to recognize objects by touch
5. Prosopagnosia: inability to recognize faces
6. Apraxia: inability to carry out specific tasks
7. Simultagnosia: inability to comprehend more than one element of a visual scene at a time or to integrate the parts into a whole
8. Adiadochokinesia: inability to perform rapid alternating movements.

C. Disturbances associated with conversion and dissociative phenomena: somatization of repressed material or the development of physical symptoms and distortions involving the voluntary muscles or special sense organs; not under voluntary control and not explained by any physical disorder

1. Hysterical anesthesia: loss of sensory modalities resulting from emotional conflicts
2. Macropsia: state in which objects seem larger than they are
3. Micropsia: state in which objects seem smaller than they are (both macropsia and micropsia can also be associated with clear organic conditions, such as complex partial seizures)
4. Depersonalization: a subjective sense of being unreal, strange, or unfamiliar to oneself
5. Derealization: a subjective sense that the environment is strange or unreal; a feeling of changed reality
6. Fugue: taking on a new identity with amnesia for the old identity; often involves travel or wandering to new environments
7. Multiple personality: one person who appears at different times to be two or more entirely different personalities and characters (called dissociative identity disorder in the fourth edition of *Diagnostic and Statistical Manual of Mental Disorders* [DSM-IV])

VII. Memory: function by which information stored in the brain is later recalled to consciousness

A. Disturbances of memory

1. Amnesia: partial or total inability to recall past experiences; may be organic or emotional in origin
   a. Anterograde: amnesia for events occurring after a point in time
   b. Retrograde: amnesia prior to a point in time
2. Paramnesia: falsification of memory by distortion of recall
   a. *Fausse reconnaissance:* false recognition

b. Retrospective falsification: memory becomes unintentionally (unconsciously) distorted by being filtered through patient's present emotional, cognitive, and experiential state
c. Confabulation: unconscious filling of gaps in memory by imagined or untrue experiences that patient believes but that have no basis in fact; most often associated with organic pathology
d. *Déjà vu:* illusion of visual recognition in which a new situation is incorrectly regarded as a repetition of a previous memory
e. *Déjà entendu:* illusion of auditory recognition
f. *Déjà pensé:* illusion that a new thought is recognized as a thought previously felt or expressed
g. *Jamais vu:* false feeling of unfamiliarity with a real situation one has experienced

3. Hypermnesia: exaggerated degree of retention and recall
4. Eidetic image: visual memory of almost hallucinatory vividness
5. Screen memory: a consciously tolerable memory covering for a painful memory
6. Repression: a defense mechanism characterized by unconscious forgetting of unacceptable ideas or impulses
7. Lethologica: temporary inability to remember a name or a proper noun

B. *Levels of memory*
1. Immediate: reproduction or recall of perceived material within seconds to minutes
2. Recent: recall of events over past few days
3. Recent past: recall of events over past few months
4. Remote: recall of events in distant past

VIII. **Intelligence:** the ability to understand, recall, mobilize, and constructively integrate previous learning in meeting new situations

A. *Mental retardation:* lack of intelligence to a degree in which there is interference with social and vocational performance: mild (intelligence quotient [I.Q.] of 50 or 55 to approximately 70), moderate (I.Q. of 35 or 40 to 50 or 55), severe (I.Q. of 20 or 25 to 35 or 40), or profound (I.Q. below 20 or 25); obsolete terms are idiot (mental age less than 3 years), imbecile (mental age of 3 to 7 years), and moron (mental age of about 8)
B. *Dementia:* organic and global deterioration of intellectual functioning without clouding of consciousness
1. Dyscalculia (acalculia): loss of ability to do calculations not caused by anxiety or impairment in concentration
2. Dysgraphia (agraphia): loss of ability to write in cursive style; loss of word structure
3. Alexia: loss of a previously possessed reading facility; not explained by defective visual acuity

C. *Pseudodementia:* clinical features resembling a dementia not caused by an organic condition; most often caused by depression (dementia syndrome of depression)
D. *Concrete thinking:* literal thinking; limited use of metaphor without understanding of nuances of meaning; one-dimensional thought
E. *Abstract thinking:* ability to appreciate nuances of meaning; multidimensional thinking with ability to use metaphors and hypotheses appropriately

IX. **Insight:** ability of the patient to understand the true cause and meaning of a situation (such as a set of symptoms)

A. *Intellectual insight:* understanding of the objective reality of a set of circumstances without the ability to apply the understanding in any useful way to master the situation
B. *True insight:* understanding of the objective reality of a situation, coupled with the motivation and the emotional impetus to master the situation
C. *Impaired insight:* diminished ability to understand the objective reality of a situation

X. **Judgment:** ability to assess a situation correctly and to act appropriately within that situation

A. *Critical judgment:* ability to assess, discern, and choose among various options in a situation
B. *Automatic judgment:* reflex performance of an action
C. *Impaired judgment:* diminished ability to understand a situation correctly and to act appropriately

SUGGESTED CROSS-REFERENCES

Perception and cognition are discussed in Section 3.1. The biology of memory is discussed in Section 3.5. Psychiatric rating scales appear in Section 9.8 on psychiatric rating scales and Section 11.1 on classification of mental disorders. Cognitive disorders are discussed in Chapter 12, schizophrenia and other psychotic disorders in Chapters 14 and 15, mood disorders in Chapter 16, anxiety disorders in Chapter 17, somatoform disorders in Chapter 18, and dissociative disorders in Chapter 20. Mental retardation is discussed in Chapter 35; learning disorders, motor skills disorder, and communication disorders in Chapter 36; and sensory impairment in the elderly in Section 49.6h.

REFERENCES

*Andreasen N C: The clinical assessment of thought, language, and communication disorders: I. The definition of terms and evaluation of their reliability. Arch Gen Psychiatry *36:* 1315, 1979.

Bender M D: *Disorders of Perception.* Charles C Thomas, Springfield, IL, 1952.

Bensen D F, Blumer D, editors: *Psychiatric Aspects of Neurological Disease,* vol 2. Grune & Stratton, Orlando, 1982.

*Bleuler E: *Dementia Praecox: The Group of Schizophrenias.* International Universities Press, New York, 1950.

Campbell R J: *Psychiatric Dictionary,* ed 6. Oxford University Press, New York, 1989.

Cassano G B, Perugi G, Musetti L, Akiskal H S: The nature of depression presenting concomitantly with panic disorder. Compr Psychiatry *30:* 473, 1989.

*Cavenar J O, Brodie H K M: *Signs and Symptoms in Psychiatry.* Lippincott, Philadelphia, 1983.

Fenichel O: *Psychoanalytic Theory of Neuroses.* Norton, New York, 1945.

Frances A J, Hales R E: *Annual Review,* vol 5. American Psychiatric Press, Washington, 1986.

Geschwind N: Aphasia. N Engl J Med *284:* 654, 1971.

Hellerstein D, Frosch W, Koenigsberg H W: The clinical significance of command hallucinations. Am J Psychiatry *144:* 219, 1987.

Sadler J Z, Hulgus Y F: Clinical problem solving and the biopsychosocial model. Am J Psychiatry *149:* 1315, 1992.
*Spitzer R L, Skodol A E, Williams J B W: *Case Book: Diagnostic and Statistical Manual of Mental Disorders.* American Psychiatric Association, Washington, 1988.
*Stoudemire A, editor: *Clinical Psychiatry for Medical Students,* ed 2. Lippincott, Philadelphia, 1994.

9.4 PERSONALITY ASSESSMENT OF ADULTS AND CHILDREN

ROBERT W. BUTLER, Ph.D.
PAUL SATZ, Ph.D.

INTRODUCTION

Central to all fields of science is the concept of measurement. Accurate measurement is a necessary prerequisite for the prediction and the understanding of natural phenomena. In fields of research such as physics and biology, measurement devices are relatively sophisticated and allow for the precise and exact quantification of many processes. That sophistication in accurate measurement is due, in large part, to the fact that those sciences frequently deal with tangible phenomena and variables that are often directly observable. Personality and psychological processes, by contrast, are generally described by constructs that are not directly observable. The fact that personality comprises constructs renders the measurement and evaluation process difficult and challenging. Psychometric personality evaluation techniques have become increasingly sophisticated in attempting to quantify human behavior accurately.

PERSONALITY

The definitions of personality are numerous, but most descriptions of personality characteristics contain commonalities. *Personality* is generally conceptualized as being composed of traits, which are dispositions or tendencies for the person to behave and respond to others in a relatively consistent fashion. The emergence of trait behaviors is likely to be influenced by situational factors, leading to state-related personality characteristics. Thus, personality refers to behavior that is more or less invariant across situations and to behavior that is relatively situation-specific. When personality is conceptualized in that global fashion, assessment encompasses normal human tendencies, such as empathy and hostility, and psychopathological behavior, such as depression and anxiety. A comprehensive personality evaluation also typically assesses the presence of severe psychopathology, such as symptoms of schizophrenia and bipolar disorder. Although those disorders are probably not under the domain of personality in the strictest sense, they clearly influence the manner in which patients interact with others and express themselves.

MEASUREMENT

One cannot directly observe and measure such traits as altruism, social introversion, dysphoria, generalized fearfulness, and sadism. Those are constructs that therapists have labeled in order to describe patterns of behavior. Similarly, state-dependent, relatively transient constellations of behavior—such as depression, euphoria, and anger—are also not directly measurable. A psychological evaluation of personality aims to quantify those constructs in a meaningful manner. That goal is accomplished by identifying specific aspects of the cognitive, behavioral, and emotional constructs that reliably measure personality traits and states with an acceptable degree of validity. Relevant specific aspects of a personality construct can include individual thoughts, discrete behaviors, informant impressions, physiological responses, and even subjective perceptions. For example, the psychological measurement of anger may include having the patient respond to such statements as, "Other people upset me frequently—true or false," observing the patient for hostile or aggressive behavior, asking relatives questions about the patient's argumentativeness, recording autonomic arousal, and asking the patient to respond to unstructured stimuli, such as inkblots. In actuality, a combination of the above procedures typically occurs, and the psychologist looks for a convergence of agreement across modalities.

A psychological evaluation of personality involves more than a clinical interview. Patients are administered psychometric instruments that are designed to quantify personality characteristics. Acceptable psychometric instruments must be embodied with adequate reliability and validity. *Reliability* refers to consistency of measurement across time (provided the personality functions remain stable), and *validity* pertains to accuracy in the identification of a personality construct. A psychometrically sound assessment of personality provides data on not only the possible presence of a personality constellation but also the intensity or the degree to which the behaviors are present.

Psychological assessments of personality can be useful not only during the diagnostic evaluation but also as a barometer of change during therapeutic endeavors. A thorough and competent personality evaluation targets maladaptive traits and behaviors and also elicits data on the patient's strengths and positive attributes. Personality testing can serve as a useful benchmark against which the clinician's judgment can be compared. Although psychometric instruments are not a gold standard for the identification of personality factors, they often provide a relatively independent source of data that the clinician can use effectively in developing and testing hypotheses about the patient.

Psychiatric and psychological assessment and diagnosis have no independent criteria for the definitive identification of a behavior or a constellation of behaviors. Thus, if a patient presents with a confusing and convoluted clinical picture or interview, formal psychological assessment is likely to reveal the presence of confusing and convoluted symptoms and behaviors. That fact does not diminish the usefulness of a personality assessment. A thorough evaluation can often suggest hypotheses that are pertinent to causative and prognostic considerations. Nevertheless, psychiatry and psychology remain relatively inexact sciences, and their measurement tools are correspondingly crude. A major goal is the continual refinement of existing assessment tools and the development of new methods for the accurate measurement and quantification of behavior.

THEORETICAL FOUNDATIONS

The manner in which one measures personality is dictated, in large part, by how one conceptualizes personality and its development. In any discussion of personality assessment, it is essential that certain issues in the study of personality theory be considered.

STATE VERSUS TRAIT Anxiety as a *trait* implies that it is a relatively enduring behavior pattern across time, perhaps waxing and waning, depending on environmental conditions at the time of the assessment. Another approach to personality assessment involves the direct sampling of an occurring behavior without inferring the presence of a construct, such as a psychological trait. For example, the *state* or interactive behavioral approach to personality assessment tends to deemphasize the existence and the assessment of chronic characterological anxiety and is involved in identifying the situational demand characteristics that elicit anxious behavior on the part of the patient. Enduring characteristics do not receive detailed attention unless chronic, identifiable behavioral triggers are present.

NOMOTHETIC VERSUS IDIOGRAPHIC A *nomothetic* approach to personality emphasizes the need to have a reference point with which a person is compared. Psychological normality is viewed with a lens that considers the person in relation to the human species in general. If the majority of the population report some degree of anxiety during public speaking, that level of anxiety becomes the reference criterion for whether speech anxiety is a potential problem or abnormal behavior. An *idiographic* approach to personality, in contrast, places much less emphasis on normative groups. Whereas the nomothetic approach holds that, before making a statement on whether anxiety in a person is disabling, one needs to know how anxious the average person is, the idiographic approach is largely concerned with the fact that anxiety has been reported or observed on an individual basis. The anxiety is then examined in relation to how it affects the person's functioning psychologically, symptomatically, and interpersonally.

DYNAMIC VERSUS EMPIRICAL The *dynamic* approach to personality emphasizes the importance of underlying causative agents that determine the nature of observable behaviors. Analytical theories of personality embody that approach and typically place little significance on specific symptomatic behavior per se but, rather, consider symptoms in relation to the nature of the person's personality structure. Constructs that are remote and often unobservable become necessary for the explanation of human behavior.

The *empirical* approach to personality deemphasizes underlying constructs, such as ego functions and object relations, that mediate behavior. Instead, the empirical approach views current behavior as a function of past learning and situational determinants. The properties of reward and punishment take on explanatory roles, and directly observable behavior is given primary importance in understanding the structure of personality.

METHODOLOGICAL ISSUES

Traditionally, psychological personality assessment has been conducted by self-report, but that technique is not the only way to sample human behavior. One may obtain information from other informants, directly observe behavior, or observe behavior in contrived situations. In an ideal situation one assesses personality by all the above modalities; however, such a comprehensive assessment is rarely possible because of time and financial constraints. If it were possible, an assumption would probably be made regarding intermethod agreement; that is, the person's behavior would be expected to be consistent across assessment modalities. Although that type of agreement is desirable in most assessment situations, its absence does not necessarily represent a methodological problem in personality assessment. Any measurement of personality is colored by the patient's reactions to the assessment method and to the assessor. Often, that type of information can provide valuable information. In general, it is best to assess a facet of personality by at least two methods to maximize the likelihood of valid information.

Personality is rarely viewed as a unitary concept; rather, it has dimensions. One must determine what the dimensions are and how many are to be assessed. There is no simplistic answer or heuristic approach to the issue. Typically, the dimensions assessed are dictated by the specific question being asked or by the clinician's need to reduce the amount of data to be accumulated and digested. Also entering into the decision are incremental validity studies. Beyond a certain point, additional psychological testing may impair the global accuracy of the assessment. Parsimony in rating personality along various factors and dimensions may be preferable.

RESPONSE SETS Response sets are individual attitudes or styles in responding to personality questionnaires. For the most part, the sets appear to be problems with objective inventories; however, they are also potential sources of error with projective and behavioral assessment techniques. A *socially desirable* response set is indicative of patients who attempt to present themselves in an overly favorable light. *Faking bad* is the opposite response set; that is, patients attempt to present a more dismal outlook than is the actual case. Some of the well-constructed objective personality measures, such as the Minnesota Multiphasic Personality Inventory (MMPI) and the California Personality Inventory (CPI), have built-in scales designed to detect the presence of those types of response sets. Other troublesome response sets involve a tendency to *yea-say* or acquiesce to questions and a tendency to *nay-say* or respond in a negativistic manner. Again, a well-constructed assessment device controls for those potential problems by the careful wording of questions and the balancing of scoring properties.

One way to deal with response sets and to obtain as realistic and accurate a description of the patient as possible is by concealment of the true nature of the assessment. That approach, however, raises ethical issues that cannot be ignored. As a general rule, human dignity and the basic rights of the patient cannot be compromised. Although the specific nature of the concealment may be appropriately defended, the patient needs to be informed regarding the process of deception if it is involved. Patients always have the right to refuse to respond to questions or stimuli that they find objectionable. However, the evaluator must be aware of the refusal.

INDIVIDUAL VERSUS GROUP SETTING Psychological methods of personality assessment are most frequently administered in an individual setting, as opposed to a group setting. Some methods of assessment, particularly the objective paper-and-pencil questionnaires, lend themselves well to group administration, and the technique is permissible. Other methods, such as the projective Rorschach technique, are never administered in a group setting by a competent psychologist. In general, the decision to administer personality assessment techniques in a group or individual setting rests with the assessor. Any thorough assessment of personality functioning includes a clinical interview with the patient on an individual basis. Thus, if a group format is used, it needs to be supplemented with individual patient contact.

ADULT PERSONALITY ASSESSMENT

One's theory of personality plays a substantial role in the assessment devices selected and used. If a clinician or a researcher believes that human behavior is state-dependent and a function of prior learning that interacts with the present environment, *behavioral* personality assessment—using checklists, rating scales, self-reports, and other such techniques—is likely to be used to the exclusion of projective or objective methods. If one believes that personality comprises traits that interact with the environment and if a nomothetic orientation is preferred, *objective* personality assessment is appropriate. If a dynamic, idiographic orientation to personality theory is held, *projective* assessment is the method of choice. Table 9.4-1 provides a summary of the relation between theory and method in psychological personality assessment.

OBJECTIVE PERSONALITY ASSESSMENT The objective orientation to personality assessment is characterized by a reliance on structured, standardized measurement devices, typically self-reports. *Structured* refers to the tendency toward straightforward test stimuli, such as direct questions regarding the persons' opinions of themselves, and unambiguous instructions regarding completion of the test. *Standardization* refers to the tendency for test administration and scoring to be invariant across time and examiners. The objective approach to personality assessment is strongly nomothetic, and most tests of that nature are norm-referenced. In a *norm-referenced* test the patient's responses to various questions are typically quantified, summed, and compared to a reference group of normal—that is, nonpsychiatric—persons. The degree to which the patient deviates from the mean of the criterion reference group is noted and interpreted.

Objective personality tests can be used to measure state or trait behaviors. The tests have a clear empirical bias and are not typically used to formulate dynamic interpretations of personality structure. Proponents of objective personality assessment generally place considerable emphasis on the psychometric qualities of their assessment tools. Effort is expended to make sure that the tests possess adequate *reliability* (consistency of scores across time) and *validity* (actual measurement of the proposed construct)—characteristics deemed essential for all psychological tests.

The development of objective personality measures most frequently follows one of three general approaches. *Rational development* involves the use of confirmatory test items or questions based on personality theory. Specifically, the test developer constructs items or questions that are designed directly to assess aspects of personality that have been predicted to exist by theoretical constructs. The Millon Clinical Multiaxial Inventory (MCMI), the Edwards Personal Preference Schedule (EPPS), and the Eysenck Personality Questionnaire (EPQ) are examples of tests that have been developed by using that approach.

Empirical development involves contrasting groups of persons to find the items that successfully identify the construct in question. The approach is largely atheoretical. The MMPI and the CPI are examples of empirically derived personality tests.

The *factor analytic* approach uses advanced statistical methods, which are applied to large groups of test items to reduce them to homogeneous, internally consistent scales or subgroups. The approach is largely a mixture of empirical and theoretical thinking. The initial item pool is typically selected on the basis of some theoretical notion of personality; however, the statistical procedures define the resultant measurement scales. The scales themselves are typically labeled only after inspection of the various test items that have been shown to be highly intercorrelated. The Comrey Personality Scales (CPS) and the 16 Personality Factor Questionnaire (16 PF) exemplify the factor analytic approach to test construction.

The differences in test construction approach are important to the professional who requests a personality evaluation of a patient, particularly in regard to the referral question. For example, if knowledge regarding a patient's degree of depression is requested without concern for qualitative theoretical issues, an empirically derived test, such as the MMPI, is satisfactory. However, if the physician desires not only information on the severity of depression but also the extent to which the patient's cognitive status is characterized by depression, a rationally developed test, such as the Beck Depression Inventory (BDI), is appropriate.

A note of caution needs to be raised regarding factor analytically developed objective personality tests. As mentioned above, the constructs that the tests purport to measure are generally defined and named by inspection of the test items that make up the scales. The definitions and labels are provided by the test developer. The test consumer may or may not agree with the test constructor. Although the problem may occur with any personality test, it is most frequently an issue with the factor analytically derived instruments. In any event, it behooves the consumer of psychological personality evaluations to have at least a basic familiarity with the specific measurement tools that form the basis of the assessment. This familiarity will result in increased comfort with the information provided, and the consumer will be assured of receiving the type of information requested.

TABLE 9.4-1
Relation Between Theory and Method in Personality Assessment

Theoretical Orientation	Theoretical Approach	Preferred Method
Cognitive-behavioral	Idiographic State Empirical	Behavioral
Eclectic	Nomothetic State or trait Empirical	Objective
Psychodynamic	Idiographic Trait Dynamic	Projective

Minnesota Multiphasic Personality Inventory (MMPI) The MMPI is a 566-item, paper-and-pencil personality questionnaire. It was developed in the early 1940s, and items were selected by using an empirical approach to test construction. Subsets of the inventory items are used in the scoring of 3 validity scales, 10 clinical scales, and 4 special scales. The scales are described in detail in Table 9.4-2. A revised version of the MMPI, the MMPI-2, was published in 1989. The MMPI-2 was a major undertaking that included updating the subject-response booklet, adding several validity and personality scales, and collecting current normative data.

The original intent of the MMPI was as an aid to clinical diagnosis, hence the diagnostic labels on the clinical scales. Items for the scales were selected by comparing relatively discrete groups of diagnosed patients with nonpsychiatric persons (most frequently, patients' relatives and visitors to the hospital). The items that successfully differentiated the clinical groups from other diagnostic groups and normal persons were selected for the various scales. As a product of that empirical construction, the scale items can be grouped into obvious (those items with *high face validity*) and subtle (those items with rather *low face validity*) categories. The presence of both high and low face validity items in a personality test results in a potentially useful method of assessing the possibility of malingering, embellishment of symptoms, and denial. *Face validity* is the degree to which the test taker believes

TABLE 9.4-2
MMPI Validity and Clinical Scales

Validity

L: Lie scale A nonempirically derived social desirability scale. Items tend to reflect behaviors that are considered socially desirable but rarely practiced. The score can suggest defensiveness, illiteracy, psychosis, or personality processes, depending on various factors.

F: Infrequency scale Measures a tendency to endorse selected items that are statistically rare responses (less than 10 percent of the original normal sample). Useful in identifying illiteracy, malingering, panic, confusion, psychosis, and personality processes.

K: Suppressor scale It is used to adjust mathematically certain clinical scales in order to decrease false-positives and false-negatives. The scale is also useful in determining overall test-taking attitude and is an indication of personality variables.

Clinical

1: Hypochondriasis This scale reflects somatic concerns and preoccupation with bodily functioning. Interpretation needs to take into account such factors as age and actual health status. As with all MMPI scales, interpretation is furthered by looking at its relation with other scales.

2: Depression Scores on this scale tend to be reflective of depression as a mood disorder or neurotic depression. The fact that the scale is sensitive to situational variables suggests that it may be a good index of state personality status.

3: Hysteria Items on this scale involve the identification of classical histrionic symptoms, including the presence of physical symptoms coupled with indifference, denial, repression, and inhibition. The scale does not necessarily measure other more popularly conceived traits, such as lability and melodramatic attitude.

4: Psychopathic deviance This scale was developed to assess the amorality and asociality aspects of psychopathy rather than the criminal or antisocial. Its meaning depends on other scale configurations. The scale provides good information on the quality of interpersonal relationships.

5: Masculinity-femininity Although it was originally developed to identify homosexuality, the scale is rarely used for that purpose, although it does provide information on gender identity. The scale reflects a variety of personality and interest areas, such as dependency, sensitivity, intellectuality, and tendencies toward introspection.

6: Paranoia Developed by the empirical identification of classic paranoid persons, the scale assesses vigilance, sensitivity, delusional thought, distrust, and suspicion. Except for the paranoid areas, the members of the original criterion group were considered functional in their lives.

7: Psychasthenia A diverse scale designed to measure anxiety and obsessive-compulsive traits. Endorsed items can reflect fear, obsessive-compulsive symptoms, interpersonal hostility, tension, specific phobias, and impaired concentration.

8: Schizophrenia Reflects the acute positive symptoms of psychotic breaks with reality, rather than the chronic negative symptoms. The scale also assesses alienation, impaired self-identity, and isolation.

9: Hypomania Measures the classic symptoms of mania, including elated and unstable mood, psychomotor excitement, and flight of ideas. It also appears to reflect narcissistic personality traits. In general, the scale provides information on the degree of drivenness of the person's personality characteristics. It has a strong age component.

0: Social introversion Provides information on social withdrawal, shyness, leadership, talkativeness, levels of gregariousness, and, to a smaller degree, self-concept and neurotic tendencies. It is more two-dimensional and bipolar (introversion versus extroversion) than the other scales.

Special

A: Anxiety The first general factor extracted from factor analytic studies on the MMPI. It is thought to reflect a generalized endorsement of psychopathology.

R: Repression The second factor that is found on factor analytic studies of the MMPI. It can be conceptualized as measuring the tendency to engage in denial.

ES: Ego strength Provides an index of how functional the patient may be in terms of work and other social areas, regardless of level of psychopathology.

MAC: McAndrews alcoholism scale Estimates degree of addiction proneness, especially with alcohol and opiates. Especially sensitive to daily substance abuse, rather than episodic abuse.

Table produced with the assistance of Alex Caldwell, PhD.

that the question is measuring what the test developer intended. Thus, obvious items on the depression scale clearly assess aspects of depression, whereas subtle items generally appear to have little relation to what people believe depression entails. Subtle versus obvious item analyses were originally thought to be useful, but several recent studies have indicated that the distinction may not be clinically valid.

Numerous additional scales have been developed from the MMPI items—some using the empirical approach, others using rational and factor analytic approaches. Many of the special scales are considered experimental in nature because too little research-based evidence documents their reliability and validity. A sample of MMPI results is shown in Table 9.4-3.

Although the MMPI was initially viewed as a diagnostic aid (for example, a patient with a major depressive disorder would show an elevation on the depression scale), the advantages of a configural approach to interpretation quickly became apparent. The *configural* approach, which involves interpretations based on the patterning of the entire profile, has become the preferred method and has increased the effectiveness of the MMPI as a personality measurement device. Various researchers have identified numerous personality correlates of different MMPI scale configurations, frequently using the two highest scales as the basis for core interpretive statements. Actuarial research of that nature also serves as the basis for computerized interpretative services. Those services, although not a substitute for a compehensive personality evaluation, can assist the clinician in hypothesis formulation. Computerized services are especially useful when the MMPI is to be interpreted by a person knowledgeable in all aspects of the MMPI and the nature of the development of the computerized program. Blind use of the services by professionals not trained in the use of the MMPI is clearly inappropriate and perhaps even unethical.

TABLE 9.4-3
MMPI Results of a Male Patient with an Antisocial Personality Disorder

Validity Scales		***T* Score (mean = 50, standard deviation = 10)**
L		40
F		66
K		68
	Clinical Scales	***T*-Score (*K*-corrected as appropriate)**
1	(Hypochondriasis)	44
2	(Depression)	51
3	(Hysteria)	62
4	(Psychopathic deviance)	87
5	(Masculinity-femininity)	43
6	(Paranoia)	53
7	(Psychasthenia)	48
8	(Schizophrenia)	63
9	(Hypomania)	78
0	(Social introversion)	40
A	(Anxiety)	40
R	(Repression)	63
ES	(Ego strength)	65
MAC	(Alcoholism)	82

STRENGTHS The fact that the MMPI is the most widely used and researched psychological personality measurement device is undoubtedly one of its major strengths. Several hundred research papers on the MMPI appear in the literature each year, and it has been extensively used in cross-cultural clinical and research applications. The huge body of literature generated has resulted in a catalog of MMPI correlates on a wide variety of clinical cases, providing descriptive, predictive, diagnostic, and prognostic information.

Another strength of the MMPI is its atheoretical nature, a characteristic that probably increases its usefulness over a broad spectrum. The presence of validity scales designed to assess test-taking attitude, in addition to clinical and personality information, is a distinct advantage that the MMPI maintains over many other personality assessment tools.

WEAKNESSES Critics of the MMPI point to the outdated normative data on which interpretive statements are still being based. The MMPI-2 addresses that criticism, but the revision has not had unconditional acceptance. The normative cohort for the MMPI-2 is characterized by a relatively high degree of educational attainment and falls at the upper end of the socioeconomic status scale. When profiles are plotted against both the MMPI and the MMPI-2 normative data, significant differences in scale elevation and code type can occur. As a result, some claim that the accumulated clinical research on the MMPI is not directly transferable to the MMPI-2. Transition from the MMPI to the MMPI-2 has not been smooth, and many psychologists continue to use the MMPI for the reasons listed above. Considerable research will have to be amassed before a determination of the clinical and personality correlates of MMPI-2 results. At this time, the MMPI-2 should probably be used only with persons who closely approximate the characteristics of the normative cohort.

The MMPI and the MMPI-2 are lengthy, and patients often complain about the time required to complete the questionnaire. Several abbreviated versions of the MMPI have been developed to decrease administration time. Those versions are generally considered unsatisfactory because of the resultant compromises in reliability and validity.

Patients also complain about some of the personal questions in the MMPI. The personal nature of some questions is less likely to be a problem with the MMPI-2, since the test developers revised the inventory items to reduce the offensive content. In general, careful and sensitive administration techniques offset patient compliance problems.

Millon Clinical Multiaxial Inventory (MCMI) The MCMI is a 175-item, true-false, paper-and-pencil personality inventory developed by Theodore Millon and his coworkers in the late 1970s. The test allows for scoring and interpretation on 11 scales, which represent personality disorders from the third edition of the American Psychiatric Association's *Diagnostic and Statistical Manual of Mental Disorders* (DSM-III). The questionnaire also contains a brief validity scale and nine scales designed to assess transient, Axis I symptom disorders, which the test authors claim are generally of a less enduring nature than behavior measured with the personality scales. The scales are described in detail in Table 9.4-4.

The MCMI was revised in 1987, and the new version is the MCMI-II. Item content was reevaluated for the MCMI-II, and new validity scales were added. Normative data were enhanced by the addition of clinical samples, and the MCMI-II is compatible with the revised edition of DSM-III (DSM-III-R) but not necessarily with the fourth edition (DSM-IV).

Unlike the MMPI, which was empirically derived and is relatively atheoretical, the MCMI is based on Millon's theory of personality and psychopathology. Test items were developed by Millon and his coworkers for the purpose of making sure that the MCMI measures theory-derived variables. The inventory was also constructed to assist in arriving at DSM-III and DSM-III-R diagnoses.

Since the MCMI represents a relatively new method for assessing personality traits, relatively little published research is available beyond the initial validation studies. That state of affairs, however, is rapidly changing, and the Millon scales have been accumulating a healthy research foundation over the past few years.

The inventory embodies a number of potential advantages, such as its brevity, theoretical underpinnings, and concordance with the terminology in DMS-III and in DSM-III-R in the case of the MCMI-II. Unfortunately, some of its potential advantages may turn out to be disadvantages. The test is likely to be useful only if Millon's theories continue to receive support. The MCMI scales use a base rate scoring system, rather than interval-based severity scales. Thus, increasing values on the MCMI or the MCMI-II scale do not indicate that a personality disorder or set of behaviors is present to a severe degree. Rather, high scores on MCMI scales indicate an increased probability that the clinical entity is present. Base rate scores have advantages and limitations. They are of particular value if the goal is a binary diagnostic decision. The scores are difficult to manipulate mathematically, however, making statistical analyses problematic. Furthermore, statements regarding the degree of severity are not possible and revisions in psychiatric nomenclature pose a problem. Although minimal changes in personality diagnosis are reflected in DSM-IV, two new personality disorders were presented for research purposes in DSM-III-R, and they are not currently assessed by the MCMI. The MCMI-II does have scales designed to identify those proposed personality types. Thus, the usefulness of MCMI versions is, in part, dependent on the stability of diagnostic terminology and nosology. The Millon inventories will require continual updating and revision so as to not become outdated. For a standardized personality test, that is an expensive and time-consuming process. The inventory's primary usefulness at this time seems to involve the identification and the description of personality disorders and related symptom constellations.

The MCMI is undergoing constant revision, with attention directed to its increased usefulness at clinical levels. The authors and the publishers of the MCMI and the MCMI-II regularly sponsor seminars and symposia on the inventories and should be given credit for stimulating research efforts. Until recently, only computerized interpretative reports were available. Now, however, hand-scoring keys are available for individual use. Unfortunately, hand scoring has only recently become an option with the MCMI-II; before its availability, inventory protocols were mailed for computerized scoring and interpretation. In all likelihood, the lack of hand scoring has undermined research efforts at establishing the clinical correlates and usefulness of the MCMI and the MCMI-II. Certainly, they are instruments that deserve close scrutiny, inasmuch as their future as personality measurement devices appears bright. For now, interpretation needs to be tempered by their recent and continued development and, therefore, the lack of extensive

TABLE 9.4-4
MCMI Clinical Scales

Personality Disorders (Axis II)

Scale 1: Schizoid Assesses the probability (as do the other scales of the MCMI) that a person meets DMS-III diagnostic criteria for schizoid personality disorder. Symptoms include indifference, insensitivity, affect deficit, and apathy.

Scale 2: Avoidant Includes the measurement of characteristics of dysphoria, alienation, aversion to interpersonal behavior, and hypersensitivity.

Scale 3: Dependent Assesses trait characteristics of docility, submissiveness, initiation difficulties, poor self-image, and naivete.

Scale 4: Histrionic Assesses lability of affect, sociability, seductiveness, immaturity, inability to delay immediate need gratification, and a dissociative cognitive style.

Scale 5: Narcissistic Measures the presence of inflated self-image, exploitiveness, expansive thinking, imperturbability, and deficits in social conscience.

Scale 6: Antisocial (aggressive) High scores suggest hostile affect, vindictiveness, power-oriented life-style, malevolence, poor impulse control, and an inability to benefit from punishment.

Scale 7: Compulsive Key trait characteristics of a high score include restrained affect, conscientiousness, adherence to social conventions, conforming, cognitive constriction, and behavioral rigidity.

Scale 8: Passive-aggressive Prominent personality traits include labile affect, contrariness, disillusionment, interpersonal ambivalence, and a discontented self-image.

Scale S: Schizotypal Assesses for the presence of social detachment, eccentricity, nondelusional autistic thinking, depersonalization, emptiness, emotional flatness, and anxious wariness.

Scale C: Borderline The salient characteristics of those scoring high on this scale are intense moodiness, dysregulated activation, self-destructive behavior, dependency anxiety, and ambivalence between thought-affect and action.

Scale P: Paranoid This scale measures the enduring traits of vigilant mistrust, distorted thought, criticalness, and provocative interpersonal behavior.

Clinical Syndromes (Axis I)

Scale A: Anxiety A high score suggests apprehension, phobias, tension, indecision, and psychophysiological symptoms.

Scale H: Somatoform Assesses the degree to which psychological conflict is likely to be channeled physically and overall preoccupation with health.

Scale N: Hypomanic Measures the presence of unstable mood, restlessness, overactivity, pressured speech, impulsiveness, irritability, and other manic behaviors.

Scale D: Dysthymia An elevation on this scale is likely to suggest despondency, guilt, discouragement, futility, and other symptoms of depression. The scale does not necessarily reflect extreme severity and, instead, implies preserved ego strength.

Scale B: Alcohol abuse This scale provides a probability index for the presence or history of alcoholism.

Scale T: Drug abuse This scale extends Scale B to include substance abuse in general and also implies poor impulse control and unconventionality.

Scale SS: Psychotic thinking A high score on this scale suggests disorganized-regressed behavior, hallucinatory experiences, delusions, and inappropriate affect.

Scale CC: Psychotic depression A high score suggests the presence of a severe depression that is usually of incapacitating proportions.

Scale PP: Psychotic delusions Elevations indicate that the person is suffering from delusions, usually persecutory or grandiose in nature. Accompanying belligerency is common.

Table produced with the assistance and persmission of Theodore Millon, PhD.

supportive research. Two sample MCMI profiles with interpretative comments are presented in Table 9.4-5.

Other methods Of all the techniques used in the psychological assessment of personality, objective questionnaires are probably the most prolific. The body of research supporting the validity of the questionnaires is considerably less than that found with the MMPI. However, the MMPI is not necessarily a more appropriate measure in all cases. Many objective personality inventories have a limited but sound foundation on which reliable and valid estimates of personality processes can be formulated.

16 PERSONALITY FACTOR QUESTIONNAIRE (16 PF) The 16 PF is a factor analytically developed inventory that rates personality on 16 dimensions, including dominant, impulsive, warm, insecure, and self-disciplined. Those factors were derived from data analyses, using numerous self-reports, ratings, and performance tests. In a sense the developmental procedure for the questionnaire involved proposing a theory of personality (16 pervasive dimensions) that originated from factor analytic studies, as opposed to the common procedure of conceptualizing a theory of personality and then developing a test to validate the theory.

The 16 PF comes in numerous forms and has been the subject of a wide range of research on its usefulness with different nonclinical populations. On the surface that thoroughness appears to be an advantage; in reality, however, the data generated are extremely extensive—hence, somewhat confusing—and a high degree of sophistication is required for accurate application and interpretation.

The dimensions assessed by the 16 PF are thought to represent basic psychological processes and not necessarily elements of psychopathology. For that reason, it is most often used in describing personality attributes of normal persons in nonclinical settings, such as counseling centers, and for research projects with students. Outside of those persons who have an active interest in the theory behind it, the 16 PF inventory does not have a high degree of support or widespread use.

CALIFORNIA PERSONALITY INVENTORY (CPI) The CPI is an MMPI-type personality inventory designed for use in counseling situations, as opposed to use with clinical, pathological populations. The CPI was recently revised and updated. The inventory was developed by empirical means, much the same way the MMPI was developed, and it rates personality on 16 principal dimensions, such as sociability, tolerance, and intellectual efficiency. The CPI has generated a strong body of research and is quite widely used in counseling settings, such as university clinics. Its usefulness may also extend to less severe psychopathology, such as patients with adjustment disorders and life crises.

JACKSON PERSONALITY INVENTORY (JPI) The JPI is an example of psychometric sophistication in objective personality inventory construction. The test was developed to minimize overlap among the 15 dimensions of personality that it measures (for example, anxiety, conformity, risk taking, and social avoidedness). Test construction also minimizes possible contamination from social desirability and other response sets. Although the JPI embodies features that reflect some recent advances in objective test development, its clinical usefulness remains relatively unexplored. Because test construction and normative data are based on college students, the JPI's applicability outside that population can be seriously questioned. In addition, narrative data for the JPI are becoming dated, and the questionnaire is in need of revision.

PERSONALITY ASSESSMENT INVENTORY (PAI) Published in 1991, the PAI is a 344-item objective personality questionnaire that allows patients to respond to items on Likert-type scales. These scales measure the person's response on a continuous, rather than dichotomous, dimension. The majority of personality inventories have a forced-choice, true-false format, but the PAI allows for four gradients of endorsement. As a result, the PAI may be more sensitive to the intensity of behavioral expression and to changes in personality functioning over time.

The PAI is hand-scoreable and shares some similarities with the MMPI. Its four validity scales evaluate response sets and the patient's approach to the questionnaire. Scoring is available for 11 clinical (pathological) scales, 2 interpersonal scales, and 5 treatment scales. The treatment scales are designed to evaluate aspects of personality that are directly relevant to psychotherapy, such as suicidal ideation, aggressive acting out, and motivation for change.

The PAI was designed to reflect DSM-III-R diagnostic criteria, not necessarily DSM-IV. Virtually none of the psychological measures available at the time of this writing, however, use DSM-IV as a measure of criterion validity.

The PAI appears to be one of the few objective personality questionnaires that simultaneously evaluate both normal personality and

TABLE 9.4-5
Sample MCMI Profiles with Psychologist's Interpretations

1. 24-year-old white woman

MCMI	Base Rate Score
Scale 1: Schizoid (asocial)	18
Scale 2: Avoidant	30
Scale 3: Dependent (submissive)	46
Scale 4: Histrionic (gregarious)	97
Scale 5: Narcissistic	71
Scale 6: Antisocial (aggressive)	70
Scale 7: Compulsive (conforming)	20
Scale 8: Passive-aggressive (negativistic)	88
Scale S: Schizotypal (schizoid)	43
Scale C: Borderline (cycloid)	85
Scale P: Paranoid	70
Scale A: Anxiety	99
Scale H: Somatoform	89
Scale N: Hypomanic	85
Scale D: Dysthymic	86
Scale B: Alcohol abuse	85
Scale T: Drug abuse	81
Scale SS: Psychotic thinking	45
Scale CC: Psychotic depression	65
Scale PP: Psychotic delusions	15

Psychologist's Interpretation
This profile is valid and reflects significant elevations on several personality disorder dimensions and on most clinical scales. The patient is likely to manifest intense endogenous mood states that are poorly regulated. Ambivalence with associated anxiety is extremely likely, and the patient may have a history of chronic suicide attempts or other self-mutilating behavior. This woman can be expected to behave in a labile, immature fashion and have a poor ability to tolerate frustration or delays in immediate need gratification. Depression, anxiety, and substance abuse are likely to be present, clinically significant, and of a chronic nature.

Diagnostic Impression: Borderline personality disorder or mixed personality disorder with borderline, histrionic, and passive-agressive features. The probability of associated Axis I diagnoses is high.

2. 33-year-old Hispanic woman

MCMI	Base Rate Score
Scale 1: Schizoid (asocial)	52
Scale 2: Avoidant	81
Scale 3: Dependent (submissive)	115
Scale 4: Histrionic (gregarious)	30
Scale 5: Narcissistic	14
Scale 6: Antisocial (aggressive)	7
Scale 7: Compulsive (conforming)	65
Scale 8: Passive-aggressive (negativistic)	50
Scale S: Schizotypal (schizoid)	54
Scale C: Borderline (cycloid)	52
Scale P: Paranoid	26
Scale A: Anxiety	74
Scale H: Somatoform	67
Scale N: Hypomanic	0
Scale D: Dysthymic	79
Scale B: Alcohol abuse	10
Scale T: Drug abuse	0
Scale SS: Psychotic thinking	60
Scale CC: Psychotic depression	64
Scale PP: Psychotic delusions	30

Psychologist's Interpretation
This is a valid profile that is indicative of the presence of a personality disorder. This patient is likely to be chracteristically passive, docile, noncompetitive, and avoidant. Social anxiety can be expected, and a high degree of submissiveness to others may be present. Her dependency may be self-defeating, and initiation abilities and self-assertion are probably virtually absent. She may describe her life as empty, one of isolation, distrust, and rejection. The patient may also complain of chronic anxiety, dysphoria, and somatic problems that frequently do not have a discernible organic basis. Substance abuse is not likely to be a problem area.

Diagnostic Impression: Dependent personality disorder or mixed personality disorder with dependent and avoidant features.

TABLE 9.4-6
Objective Measures of Personality

Name	Description	Strengths	Weaknesses
Minnesota Multiphasic Personality Inventory (MMPI)	566 items; true-false; self-report format; 17 primary scales (numerous special scales)	Provides wide range of data on numerous personality variables; strong research base	Tends to emphasize major psychopathology. In need of revision with current normative data
Minnesota Multiphasic Personality Inventory-2 (MMPI-2)	567 items; true-false; self-report format	Current revision of the MMPI that has updated the response booklet; revised scaling methods and new validity scores; new normative data	Preliminary data indicate that the MMPI-2 and the MMPI can provide discrepant results. Normative sample biased toward upper socioeconomic status. No normative data for adolescents
Millon Clinical Multiaxial Inventory (MCMI)	175 items; true-false; self-report format; 20 primary scales	Brief administration time; corresponds well with DSM-III diagnostic classifications	In need of more validation research. No information on disorder severity. Needs revision for DSM-IV
Millon Clinical Multiaxial Inventory-II (MCMI-II)	175 items; true-false; self-report format; 25 scales	Brief administration time; corresponds well with DSM-III-R	High degree of item overlap in various scales. No information on disorder or trait severity
16 Personality Factor Questionnaire (16 PF)	True-false; self-report format; 16 personality dimensions	Sophisticated psychometric instrument with considerable research conducted on nonclinical populations	Limited usefulness with clinical populations
Personality Assessment Inventory (PAI)	344 items; Likert-type format; self-report; 22 scales	Includes measures of psychopathology, personality dimensions, validity scales, and specific concerns to psychotherapeutic treatment	The inventory is new and has not yet generated a supportive research base
California Personality Inventory (CPI)	True-false; self-report format; 17 scales	Well-accepted method of assessing patients who do not present with major psychopathology	Limited usefulness with clinical populations
Jackson Personality Inventory (JPI)	True-false; self-report format; 15 personality scales	Constructed in accord with sophisticated psychometric techniques; controls for response sets	Unproved usefulness in clinical settings
Edwards Personal Preference Schedule (EPPS)	Forced choice; self-report format	Follows Murray's theory of personology; accounts for social desirability	Not widely used clinically because of restricted nature of information obtained
Beck Depression Inventory (BDI)	Self-report on Likert-type format; measures depression	Follows Beck's theory of depression; widely used	Assesses mood and thought well but inadequate on neurovegetative symptoms
State-Trait Anxiety Inventory (STAI)	Self-report on Likert-type format; measures anxiety	Allows for differentiation of state and trait anxiety; well researched	STAI items are transparent
Psychological Screening Inventory (PSI)	103 items; true-false; self-report format	Yields 4 scores, which can be used as screening measures on the possibility of a need for psychological help	The scales are short and have correspondingly low reliability
Eysenck Personality Questionnaire (EPQ)	True-false; self-report format	Useful as a screening device; test has a theoretical basis with research support	Scales are short, and items are transparent as to purpose; not recommended for other than a screening device
Adjective Checklist (ACL)	True-false; self-report or informant report	Can be used for self-rating or other rating	Scores rarely correlate highly with conventional personality inventories
Comrey Personality Scales (CPS)	True-false; self-report format; 8 scales	Factor analytic techniques used with a high degree of sophistication in test construction	Not widely used; factor analytic interpretation problems
Tennessee Self-Concept Scale (TSCS)	100 items; true-false; self-report format; 14 scales	Brief administration time yields considerable information	Brevity is also a disadvantage, lowering reliability and validity; useful as a screening device only

psychopathological functions. The PAI's recent publication, however, indicates that further research will be necessary to establish its clinical usefulness.

Current status Objective personality assessment is particularly useful if one is interested in the nomothetic basis of personality attributes—that is, in how the patient compares with others on the dimensions. Objective assessment devices are also well suited for statements regarding the intensity of behaviors and the degree to which personality factors are present. The psychometric characteristics of those measures make them well suited for empirical research; hence, in contrast to projective tests, they are more appropriate instruments for such questions as, "Which form of medication or psychotherapy is most likely to benefit this patient?"

The most widely used objective measure of personality, the MMPI, has long been in need of revision, especially in regard to normative data. Unfortunately, the recent revision, the MMPI-2, does not appear to be interchangeable with the MMPI, and the new revision has met some resistance. The large amount of work that went into the development of the MMPI-2 may have been only a prelude to further research efforts on its clinical validation.

Objective assessment has been criticized by some for its reliance on normative samples. The key issue is determining an appropriate normative group. A frequently voiced recommendation is for test users to collect normative data representative of their local populations. Although that suggestion offers a partial solution to the problem, it is usually logistically and practically unfeasible to collect that type of extensive data.

Some of the popular objective techniques are summarized in Table 9.4-6.

An area of objective personality assessment that has begun to generate interest involves the estimation of premorbid personality characteristics in persons who have suffered a significant change in their level of functioning, such as an insult to the brain. Brain damage, especially those injuries that involve the frontal lobes, is often associated with alterations in mood, behavior, and personality. Disruptions in brain function can attenuate or potentiate premorbid personality characteristics or result in the emergence of previously unexhibited behavioral tendencies. Those alterations in personality can occur after closed-head trauma, cerebrovascular accidents, and tumors and also over the course of dementing illnesses.

An inventory specifically designed to assess changes in personality has recently been published, the *Neuropsychology Behavior and Affect Profile* (NBAP). The NBAP uses informant ratings on both premorbid characteristics and current behavioral status. It attempts to quantify personality change over a relatively discrete period of time. As more researchers address that methodologically difficult topic, continued refinement can be expected in the ability to document premorbid functioning when the patient is encountered after a significant change in status. The NBAP is a welcome step in that direction.

PROJECTIVE PERSONALITY ASSESSMENT The projective approach to personality assessment is defined by the use of relatively unstructured, often ambiguous test stimuli. A basic assumption is that, when confronted with a vague stimulus and required to respond to it in some manner, people cannot help but reveal information about themselves—not only in the way in which or the process by which the ambiguity is confronted but also in the content of their responses.

Test stimuli but not necessarily scoring and interpretation are typically standardized. For example, the Rorschach inkblot technique, probably the most widely used projective method, currently has six systems by which the test can be scored and interpreted. Although the approaches overlap to some degree, the variations range from a strong psychoanalytic orientation to an empirical, perceptual-cognitive approach. The net result is that one can never be sure what type of interpretation is being used when one requests an evaluation that includes projective tests. Furthermore, many scoring and interpretative approaches to projective personality assessment devices have weak empirical research foundations.

The projective approach is essentially idiographic in nature, and the tests are not usually interpreted by comparing a person's responses to a set of criterion-referenced normative data. Typically, interpretation is based on a theory of human behavior and personality, and it is assumed that people have certain needs, characteristics, defenses, and other qualities that will become apparent through the testing process. Projective assessment also tends toward a dynamic bias; a frequent assumption is that patients will project information about their need status onto the stimuli and that those projections will be symbolic of internal dynamics. Those dynamics are usually interpreted on the basis of analytical or interpersonal-environment theories of human behavior. The emphasis on personality theory and dynamics tends to focus projective assessment onto the trait aspects of human behavior; however, state variables and evidence for psychopathology can be elucidated.

With some exceptions the classic projective approach to personality assessment has tended to eschew firm adherence to measurement psychometrics. The unstructured nature of the test stimuli has been postulated to render empirical reliability and validity research difficult. Fortunately, that situation has changed somewhat over time because of the current emphasis on scientific methods in personality assessment. Nevertheless, the idiographic nature of projective methods tends to make them less psychometrically sophisticated than the objective measures of personality.

Rorschach test The Rorschach technique of projective assessment consists of 10 plates with inkblots printed on them; one of the plates is shown in Figure 9.4-1. The technique was introduced by Hermann Rorschach in 1921 and had been extensively studied by a number of psychologists by the 1950s. Interest in the technique has waxed and waned over the years, never reaching the zenith it achieved during the initial period of development.

There are essentially six major schools of administration, scoring, and interpretation of the Rorschach technique. Despite differences, the various approaches have some commonalities. Typically, administration is characterized by a brief, nondirective orientation to the task. The plates are presented to the patient one at a time, and the patient's percepts are recorded verbatim. Interaction with the assessor is kept to a minimum. On completion of that phase, the cards are reexamined, one

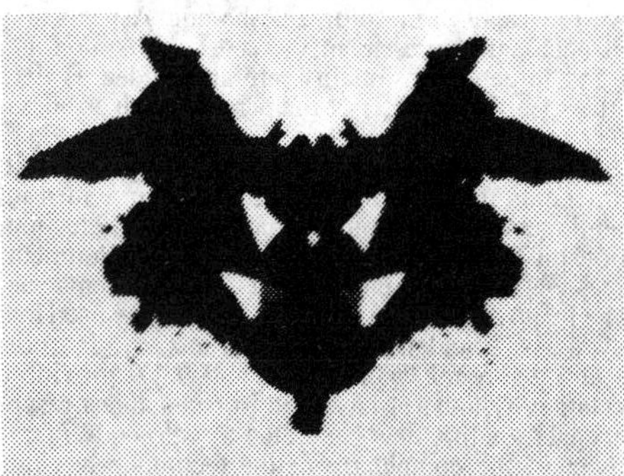

FIGURE 9.4-1 *Plate I of the Rorschach test. (From Hans Huber Medical Publisher, Berne. Used with permission.)*

TABLE 9.4-7
Personality Dimensions Assessed with Sample Rorschach Perceptions

Coping Styles

Animal movement. A response involving the kinesthetic movement of an animal. *Significance:* The number of animal movement responses are believed to be associated with the person's drive level.

Inanimate movement. A response involving movement of an inanimate object. *Significance:* The presence of this determinant suggests elevated stress levels and feelings of being out of control.

Texture. A response in which the shading features of the blot are described as tactual. *Significance:* The number of texture responses are thought to be related to the degree of need for emotional closeness.

Achromatic color. A response based on the black, gray, and white characteristics of the blot. *Significance:* This determinant suggests constraint of emotional expression.

Shading. A response based on the dark and light characteristics of the blot, without references to texture or depth. *Significance:* Suggests feelings of helplessness and loss of control.

Vista. Depth or dimensionality based on the blot's shading features. *Significance:* This determinant suggests a painfully negative self-evaluation and is most commonly found in the records of seriously depressed or suicidal patients.

Perceptual-Cognitive Operations

Distorted form. Each response is scored for goodness of fit—the appropriateness or inappropriateness of the response to the stimulus. *Significance:* This is an index of perceptual distortion. A high percentage of inaccurate perceptions (20 percent and above) can be reflective of impaired reality testing.

Whole-blot responses: detail responses. The ratio of responses based on the whole blot to responses in which a detail of the blot is used. *Significance:* This is a measure of the cognitive effort used in producing responses.

Affective Responsivity

Pure color. A chromatic color response without form characteristics. *Significance:* This determinant suggests a tendency for uncontrolled emotional discharge.

Color-shading blend. A chromatic color response with shading determinants. *Significance:* Color-shading blends are indicative of distress and occur most frequently in the records of depressed persons.

Interpersonal Attitudes

Whole human. The percept of a whole human form. *Significance:* Interpersonal interest and human relatedness are believed to be associated with the number of human responses in a protocol.

Aggressive movement. The percept of aggressive actions. *Significance:* Elevations in aggressive content indicate hostile attitudes toward others and the environment.

Self-Image

Egocentricity index. The number of pair and reflection responses in the protocol. *Significance:* This is a measure of a person's degree of self-focus.

Morbid content. Description of a percept as dead, broken, or ruined *or* attribution of dysphoric characteristics or feelings to a percept. *Significance:* An elevation of morbid responses is suggestive of a negative self-image.

Characteristics of Ideation

Human movement. A response involving kinesthetic movement of a human figure. *Significance:* The production of this type of response is thought to require the use of fantasy and intellectual resources. At least one human movement response is expected in the record of a psychologically healthy person. The form quality or form appropriateness of the human movement response is an important measure of ideational processes. The presence of a thought disorder is suggested when two or more human movement responses involve the distorted use of form.

Inappropriate combinations. These responses involve unrealistic combinations between perceived images. An inappropriate combination can consist of an implausible relation between objects (fabulized combination), an implausible merging of separate percepts into one object (incongruous combination), or an unrealistic condensation of images onto a discrete blot area (contamination). *Significance:* An elevation of these inappropriate combinations suggests a thought disturbance.

Table produced with the assistance of Ia Rorsman, PhD.

at a time, with directive questioning by the examiner to allow for an accurate coding of the responses. Although each school of Rorschach technique has its adherents, the Exner system appears to be the most widely accepted at this time. John Exner has attempted to condense the most salient and valid aspects of several other Rorschach systems into a comprehensive compilation. The Exner system is one of the few Rorschach schools to emphasize empirical research, as opposed to clinical lore. Table 9.4-7 contains examples of coding procedures and interpretation hypotheses based on the Exner system.

Although scoring systems vary, the patient's responses are typically coded under three general categories: location, determinants, and content. *Location* is the portion of the blot used. *Determinants* are those aspects of the blot that are salient to the patient's percepts. Determinants include the use of form, color, and shading. Aspects of the percept that are not necessarily present in the actual blot, such as perceived movement and three-dimensionality, are also coded as determinants. *Content* is the specific character of the percept, such as human, animal, or nature.

Interpretation is a complex and time-consuming process. Rorschach method proponents maintain that the technique provides information on the patient's level of functioning, maturity, reality testing, interpersonal relationship style, ability to organize the environment and marshal resources, balance of activity and passivity, and emotional responsiveness. The Rorschach technique is also frequently used in the assessment of psychosis, suicidality, depression, anxiety, and other clinical syndromes and disorders. Tables 9.4-8 and 9.4-9 provide diagnostic and interpretative hypotheses based on Rorschach test responses.

The Rorschach method has generated a wide body of research literature; however, the complexity of the technique has hindered the development of a comprehensive, cohesive data base. That problem has been addressed in recent years through increased efforts toward uniformity in scoring, interpretation, and scientific validation. A recent meta-analytic study compared the diagnostic validity of the MMPI with the Rorschach; neither method appeared to be superior, and both the projective and the objective assessment techniques had acceptable validity. Although the psychometric properties of the Rorschach test remain limited, the procedure is gaining power as coding systems become more specific and as researchers devote more attention to the empirical validation of Rorschach constructs.

The fact that most people enjoy having the Rorschach test administered to them is a strength of the method. The ambiguity of the stimuli and the unstructured administration can provide valuable information on how a patient copes with those types of situations. Interpretative validity may be improved by frequent use of the technique and increased clinical experience.

Thematic Apperception Test (TAT) The TAT, developed by Henry Murray, consists of 20 cards with pictures on them, some of which are age- and gender-specific. The pictures vary in content; most contain one or more characters, with different degrees of ambiguity. The patient is asked to construct a story that has a beginning, a middle, and an ending on the basis of the stimulus card. Rarely are all 20 cards administered. Typically, a number of stimulus cards are selected to pull for certain material. The basic assumption is that the person will project his or her personality into the story. Information is obtained regarding the patient's beliefs, needs, traits, attitudes, and motives—in general, a broad spectrum of behavior and cognition.

Administration of the TAT is straightforward, and, as with the Rorschach method, most patients find the task relatively nonthreatening and even enjoyable. Scoring of the TAT is by no means standardized, and numerous methods exist. Most scoring systems involve rating need

TABLE 9.4-8
Psychologist's Interpretation of Sample Responses to Rorschach Stimuli by a Depressed Female Patient

Card I. This looks like a dead leaf. (Inquiry: It is black. . . . It has the shape of a leaf, but it is ripped around the edges.)

Card VI. The top part looks like a moth with the wings destroyed. (Inquiry: It looks like the wings have been eaten out. It's not solid.)

Card VII. I see a lot of islands. A map of islands. (Inquiry: It looks almost like a photograph because of the shades of gray. That gives it a three-dimensional look. Mountains and valleys.)

Card IX. This looks like a bell. The shape is right. Looks like a rusted bell. (Inquiry: It is cracked here. Also, the gradation in the color looks like rust. I think of the Liberty Bell.)

Background: These responses are from the protocol of a 30-year-old woman with a diagnosis of major depressive disorder and treated on an outpatient basis. Her clinical picture consisted of depressed mood, feelings of guilt and worthlessness, significant weight gain, and a diminished ability to work and concentrate.

Interpretation: The above sample responses are representative of this woman's protocol. The dead leaf in card I, the moth with destroyed wings in card II, and the cracked and rusted bell in card IX are all examples of *morbid content,* suggesting a pessimistic and dysphoric view of the outside world and reflective of a negative self-image. The description of *achromatic color* (black) in card I is one of the many responses of this type presented by this patient. An elevation of achromatic color responses is common among depressed people and is believed to be associated with constraint of emotional expression. In addition, this patient produced a number of *vista* responses similar to the image produced to card VII. Vista responses are unusual in the records of normal persons and are believed to reflect painful self-inspection. Finally, the dysphoric outlook on life, harsh self-image, and constrained emotional outlet seem combined with a fair amount of cognitive confusion, as indicated by a number of responses with *color-shading blends,* as in card IX.

Table produced with the assistance of Ia Rorsman, PhD.

states or levels, following from Murray's theory of personality. Murray believed that personality is effectively described by analyzing a person's most powerful needs, such as achievement, affiliation, dominance, and play in relation to environmental press—that is, attributes of environmental stimuli that either facilitate or impede the efforts of a person to reach a specified goal. Although scoring systems exist, the typical process of interpretation is impressionistic and informal. In general, particular attention is directed at recurrent themes that may provide evidence of mood state, conflict, and the quality of interpersonal relationships.

The TAT was developed as an assessment device designed to measure trait behavior. Research, however, has tended to indicate the opposite. The TAT appears to be more sensitive to state-dependent variables than to traits. TAT use has tended to decline over the years, probably because of the relatively lengthy time required for administration and interpretation. Nevertheless, a significant number of clinicians adhere to thematic test analysis and for them the TAT is the method of choice.

Sentence completion test The sentence completion method is perhaps the least vague and the most structured projective personality assessment technique. Patients are presented with the first few words or stem of a sentence and are asked to complete it as they feel it best describes themselves. It is essentially an open-ended self-report inventory, and most items have an obvious pull in terms of the type of information being sought. For that reason, patients who choose to be less than open may produce uninformative protocols, above and beyond the fact that they are resistant to the task. In a similar fashion, sentence completion tasks are susceptible to malingering and response sets.

The numerous published versions of the incomplete sentence method vary in their degree of ambiguity and orientation. With one exception, Julian Rotter's *Incomplete Sentence Blank,* scoring for the various incomplete sentence tests is poorly standardized, and interpretation is based solely on clinical intuition. With a cooperative patient, however, considerable information can be gleaned on both state and trait personality variables.

A patient's sentence completion protocol often provides valuable additional information because, typically, patients write out their responses. A brief review of the protocol can assist the clinician in formulating hypotheses regarding written language development, the presence or the absence of academic difficulties, and evidence of early

TABLE 9.4-9
Psychologist's Interpretation of Sample Responses to Rorschach Stimuli by a Schizophrenic Male Patient

Card II. Two chickens talking to each other. (Inquiry: Heads. . . . Here are the open mouths. Talking. Red heads.)

Card III. Two women cooking. They have penises. (Inquiry: Here are the heads, their breasts, penises. . . . Women with penises.)

Card VII. Pink rats crawling up a mountain.

Card IX. This looks like a bush . . . and a face. . . . Bush face. (Inquiry: It is green, and here is the nose and the eye.)

Card X. This looks like a man being X-rayed. (Inquiry: You can see all the intestines and part of the spine. These look like his lungs, or it could be his coat. . . . I guess he has his coat on.)

Background: These responses are samples from a record of a 20-year-old male inpatient with a diagnosis of schizophrenia, undifferentiated type, subchronic with acute exacerbation. The patient was hospitalized with bizarre delusions and auditory hallucinations. At the time of the testing, these symptoms had subsided, and he presented a clinical picture with unusual perceptual experiences, various odd beliefs, and ideas of reference.

Interpretation: This patient's record was marked by a high percentage of *distorted form responses.* Many of his percept descriptions only fitted the blot arbitrarily, and several responses appeared forced on the contours of the used blot area (e.g., card X). A high percentage of distorted form responses is indicative of impaired reality testing. The record also suggests the presence of thought disorder, as reflected by several instances of *inappropriate combinations.* An incongruous combination, a mild indicator of thought disturbance, was scored twice (card III and card VII). In card III the separate blot images merged in an unrealistic fashion, creating the image of women with penises. Incongruity is further evidenced by an implausible fusion of color and form in the response to card VII. The image of two chickens talking to each other (card II) and the simultaneous impression of the inside and the outside of a body (card X) are examples of the unrealistic relations (fabulized combinations) that are often evidenced in the Rorschach records of schizophrenic patients. Although both incongruous combinations and fabulized combinations occur in normal protocols, they are rare, and the response to card IX represents a serious disorganization of thought and perceptual experiences. This merger of impressions into a single blot area (called contamination) is almost exclusively found in the records of psychotic patients. In sum, the Rorschach suggests that this is a man whose relation to the outside world is limited by misinterpretations, inaccurate perceptions, and confused and disorganized thought processes. The inappropriate combinations in the protocol suggest difficulties in reality testing and in separating various ideas, thoughts, and images.

Table produced with the assistance of Ia Rorsman, PhD.

TABLE 9.4-10
Sentence Completion Test Stimuli

I often wish ____________________

When I was young ____________________

It makes me angry when ____________________

My mother ____________________

Most people ____________________

learning disabilities. Like most projective measures, the sentence completion test can elicit symptoms of a psychotic thought process.

Examples of sentence completion test stimuli are presented in Table 9.4-10.

Other methods Similar in technique to the Rorschach method is the *Holtzman Inkblot Technique* (HIT), which was developed to rectify some of the psychometric difficulties found with the Rorschach test. The HIT consists of 45 inkblot plates (two sets permit alternate-form assessment, if desired), and the patient provides only one response to each card. The procedure ensures consistency in total responses to the HIT across patients, a condition that is rarely obtained with the Rorschach test. Although an interesting concept, the HIT is not widely used, and research documenting its validity with clinical populations has been limited. Rorschach and HIT scoring and interpretation methods do not appear to be directly comparable, a shortcoming that has probably hindered research progress and the clinical usefulness of the HIT.

Figure drawings have long been used as projective personality assessment devices. A basic assumption is that, in drawing a figure, such as a person or a house, the patient will introject interpersonal, intrapsychic, and familial conflicts onto the drawing. Perhaps the most widely used figure drawing technique is the *Draw-a-Person* procedure. Patients are presented with a blank sheet of paper and are instructed to draw a picture of a person. The projective hypothesis implies that patients will symbolically introject their own personality characteristics onto the drawing. Scoring procedures are available for estimating intelligence; however, they are generally used only with mentally retarded persons or with children. Manuals are also available that present guidelines for dynamic and analytically oriented interpretations of personality style and functioning. The technique has some degree of intuitive attractiveness, and on a case study basis one can find some valid profile interpretations. On the whole, however, the technique has little research to support most interpretative claims.

A similar technique is the *House-Tree-Person* (HTP) procedure. In addition to drawing a person, the patient is asked to draw a house and a tree. Some believe that those additional drawings, compared with just figure drawings, provide a fuller, more complete clinical picture and additional information on the patient's self-image, interpersonal relationships, and family dynamics. Little empirical research supports those claims.

A variant of figure drawing is figure copying, usually done with the *Bender-Gestalt* cards as stimuli. Some clinicians have developed elaborate rules and interpretative strategies for inferring a patient's personality characteristics on the basis of the Bender-Gestalt reproductions. The technique never developed a broad base of use or support, and currently its practice is limited. A lack of empirical support for many of the interpretative claims contributes to the infrequent use of figure reproduction as a projective assessment technique.

Current status The psychological measurement of personality by projective techniques has a long and rich history. Until recently, many of the interpretive schemata have relied on clinical lore, rather than sound empirical investigation. That situation is changing, especially in the Rorschach technique. Researchers and clinicians who advocate a scientific approach to personality assessment, however, have tended to eschew projective techniques in favor of behavioral and objective methods, which are quantifiable, face and content valid, and conducive to sound psychometric principles. Although the trend may have created a decrease in projective use, the techniques are by no means obsolete. Many practitioners firmly adhere to projective assessment, and that situation is unlikely to change in the near future.

A summary of the most widely used projective techniques is presented in Table 9.4-11.

BEHAVIORAL PERSONALITY ASSESSMENT The behavioral assessment of personality is a relatively recent outgrowth of a neobehavioral movement in clinical psychology. The movement has emphasized the use of scientific methods in addressing clinical problems. Growing dissatisfaction with traditional personality assessment techniques is also characteristic of the neobehavioral movement. The traditional testing of personality involves the measurement of theoretical constructs, which are then used to predict overt behavior. Objective personality assessment, for example, frequently measures such constructs as anxiety, sociability, and narcissism. The projective approach to assessment also purports to quantify such concepts as ego strength and neurotic dysfunction. Behavioral assessment, however, favors the direct measurement of criterion behaviors within specific situations. The behavioral assessment of ego strength, for example, involves measuring such behaviors as amount of time spent in productive work, rather than ego strength per se. Adherents to the behavioral approach point out that behavioral procedures are parsimonious, consistent with empirical evidence, and conducive to direct empirical testing. The basic rationale appears to rest on findings that the best predictors of future behavior in a given situation are past behaviors in the same type of situation. Behavioral assessment techniques are varied and include such methods as direct observation, self-monitoring, psychophysiological measurement, interviews, questionnaires, and critical-event sampling.

General approach The behavioral assessment of personality tends to be a highly structured process in which the assessor informs the patient of the purpose of the testing, what information is requested, and how it will be sought. Ambiguity is avoided unless the criterion behaviors to be measured involve the manner in which the patient copes with an unstructured situation. A behavioral approach to the assessment of a patient's response to an ambiguous situation is similar to the comments on behavior that a Rorschach test assessor may make regarding

TABLE 9.4-11
Projective Measures of Personality

Name	Description	Strengths	Weaknesses
Rorschach test	10 stimulus cards of inkblots, some colored, others achromatic	Most widely used projective device and certainly the best researched; considerable interpretative data available	Some Rorschach interpretive systems, have unproved validity.
Thematic Apperception Test (TAT)	20 stimulus cards depicting a number of scenes of varying ambiguity	A widely used method that, in the hands of a well-trained person, provides valuable information	No generally accepted scoring system results in poor consistency in interpretation; time-consuming administration
Sentence completion test	A number of different devices available, all sharing the same format with more similarities than differences	Brief administration time; can be a useful adjunct to clinical interviews if supplied beforehand	Stimuli are obvious as to intent and subject to easy falsification
Holtzman Inkblot Technique (HIT)	Two parallel forms of inkblot cards with 45 cards per form	Only one response is allowed per card, making research less troublesome	Not widely accepted and rarely used; not directly comparable to Rorschach interpretative strategies
Figure drawing	Typically human forms but can involve houses or other forms	Quick administration	Interpretative strategies have typically been unsupported by research
Make-a-Picture Story (MAPS)	Similar to TAT; however, stimuli can be manipulated by the patient	Provides idiographic personality information through thematic analysis	Minimal research support; not widely used

a patient's responses when confronted with the ambiguous Rorschach stimuli (for example, the patient requested information regarding rules, became anxious, or refused to cooperate). The assessor quantifies the responses and other similar behaviors to obtain an index of coping. The behavioral approach tends to be idiographic in nature.

Behavioral assessment is goal-directed. Rather than attempting to describe a patient in terms of dynamics, defense mechanisms, traits, or diagnosis, the assessor is interested in problem behaviors that require treatment (for example, reduction in the frequency or the strength of a target behavior). If a patient presents with an anxiety disorder, the behavioral assessor is not necessarily concerned with the dynamics, the diagnosis, or the degree of anxiety in comparison with the rest of a population. Behavioral assessment focuses on measurable target behaviors that represent the discomfort the patient is experiencing, be it increased perspiration, escape-avoidance behaviors, subjective distress, or increases in heart rate and blood pressure. The assessor determines which stimuli appear to elicit those responses, places the patient in an actual or analogous situation, and measures the responses. In selecting target or criterion behaviors to measure, the assessor considers such issues as frequency, intensity, duration, centrality to the patient's functional life, subjective distress, values, and potential risk and destructiveness of the behaviors.

The behavioral assessment process is geared toward effective empirical intervention, perhaps more so than any other method of personality assessment. The process appears to be a function of the behavioral emphasis on determining which stimuli or variables elicit the target behaviors and of the close relationship between behavioral assessment and behavior therapy. The identification of variables and stimuli that elicit the target behaviors has been labeled the most important purpose of any psychological assessment, particularly when the assessment is to have a direct effect on treatment. Behavioral assessment is frequently serial in nature and is conducted periodically throughout a treatment program to objectively document therapy effectiveness. The assessment tends to be a reciprocal feedback process in which modifications of assessment or treatment or both depend on the results of measurement.

Behavioral assessment has a strict empirical orientation and emphasizes state-dependent behaviors. Although it is not entirely atheoretical in nature (the recognition of inferential concepts, such as cognition, has become the rule with behavior therapists, rather than the exception), the method does avoid measuring personality constructs that require an additional level of inference that may not necessarily increase treatment effectiveness from a behavioral viewpoint.

The above comments tend to portray the behavioral assessor and the behavior therapist as cold, unfeeling scientists who rarely interact with their patients on a level other than that of an aloof observer. That misconception is a common one because of the historical aspects of the technique and the reliance on scientific methods. On the contrary, behaviorists typically bring the same degree of warmth, empathy, and concern into assessment and treatment settings as any other health professionals, regardless of orientation.

Interviews The interview is perhaps the most common and the most frequently used assessment technique. Almost any assessment of personality begins with or includes a clinical interview in some form. The behavioral approach to interviews involves the use of structured and semistructured formats designed to maximize the information regarding overt behavior, behavior-environment interactions, quantifiable information, and potential causative factors. Many clinicians, researchers, and diagnosticians have adopted the techniques, at times without being aware of the behavioral background and orientation that form the foundation for structured and semistructured interviews.

BRIEF PSYCHIATRIC RATING SCALE (BPRS) The BPRS is an 18-dimension rating scale that is completed after the assessor conducts a semistructured interview with the patient. Each dimension represents a domain of behavior and psychiatric symptoms—such as anxiety, hostility, affect, guilt, and orientation—that is rated on a seven-point Likert scale from "not present" to "extremely severe." Several of the domains tend not to be directly observable behaviors, but the manner in which they are assessed is sufficiently structured to qualify as a behavioral assessment. The BPRS is a brief, rather easily learned technique and provides a quantitative score that reflects global pathology. While it is possible to compute subscores from the BPRS, those variables appear to be less reliable and valid than the global score. The BPRS is useful in providing a crude barometer of a patient's overall benefit from treatment and as a dependent variable in many research protocols, particularly psychopharmacology outcome studies. On the negative side, the BPRS does not provide much information on specific behaviors because many divergent symptom complexes are covered.

HAMILTON RATING SCALE FOR DEPRESSION (HAM-D) This widely used scale is also scored on the basis of a semistructured interview. The patient is rated on depression-related symptoms, including psychomotor retardation, insomnia, mood, and insight. Several forms with different numbers of symptom ratings exist, leading to some confusion at times as to what exactly has been assessed. The combined score correlates highly with the degree of depression severity. The rating scale is effective in monitoring a depressed state over time and is useful as an index of treatment effectiveness. A weakness of the Hamilton scale is its overemphasis on biological, neurovegetative, and psychotic depressive symptoms. If used, it probably should be paired with an additional assessment device that focuses on the mood, affective, and cognitive changes known to accompany major depression.

SCHEDULE FOR AFFECTIVE DISORDERS AND SCHIZOPHRENIA (SADS) The SADS is a structured interview that has been well received by diagnosticians and researchers. Its primary purpose appears to be as a diagnostic tool. Scores on nondiagnostic symptom complexes can be obtained, however, and the SADS has been used as an index of behavioral severity. An excerpt from the SADS is reprinted in Table 9.4-12.

The SADS interview process is highly structured for both the assessor and the assessee, and it is a valuable diagnostic adjunct for a wide variety of purposes. Its use significantly improves diagnostic reliability, and it can be a useful index of behavioral change. Although the full SADS interview is time-consuming, a condensed form, the SADS-C, measures only current psychopathology. After an initial complete evaluation, using the SADS-C significantly reduces the time required if repeat assessment is desirable.

The SADS, like many other structured and semistructured interview techniques, tends to focus on the presence of pathology and not necessarily on the patient's strengths. That emphasis does not mean that the SADS embodies an inherent weakness. Rather, for a balanced assessment, both strengths and pathology need to be measured.

GLOBAL ASSESSMENT SCALE (GAS) The GAS, developed by the authors of the SADS scales, balances patient attributes. The GAS provides a quantified index of overall current health and illness that allows for evaluations that reflect positive attributes. It is typically scored after a semistructured interview. The global nature of the rating does not allow for the assessment of discrete behaviors.

Questionnaires The questionnaire is not the exclusive domain of behavioral assessment; in fact, it is well represented by objective personality assessment. However, when the goal of a questionnaire is the measurement of overt, observable behaviors, the questionnaire becomes an instrument of the behavioral assessor.

A large number of focused questionnaires have been developed for behavioral assessment purposes. The questionnaires address many diverse target behaviors, such as social skills deficits, anger, marital functioning, obsessive-compulsive behaviors, sexual functioning, ingestive disorders, fears and phobias, and menstrual dysfunction. With few exceptions, the questionnaires developed for behavioral assessment purposes lack psychometric sophistication. Despite those shortcomings, questionnaires are quickly administered and can be useful as long as one is aware of the particular instrument's psychometric limitations.

One widely used self-report questionnaire that meets the criteria of a behavioral assessment device is the *Symptom Checklist-90-Revised* (SCL-90-R). The SCL-90-R is a 90-item checklist on which the respondent indicates the degree of distress being experienced on a wide range of symptoms. The checklist can be scored to provide a unitary index of global pathology or to provide quantitative measures on nine factors, which include somatization, interpersonal sensitivity, hostility, paranoid ideation, and psychoticism. However, the validity of the various SCL-90-R subscales may change, depending on the nature of the population sampled. For that reason, many psychologists recommend that only the global score be used unless the clinician or the researcher is aware of the normative properties for a specified patient. The effectiveness of the SCL-90-R in accurately documenting change has been demonstrated in a number of clinical and research settings, and it is generally considered one of the best standardized behavioral assessment questionnaires.

Observation Observation is perhaps the assessment method most in keeping with the purpose and the orientation of behavioral assessment. Observation as an assessment technique can be naturalistic or analogue in nature. *Naturalistic observation* involves observing the patient's behavior in real-life settings and recording the data on target behaviors. If possible, more than one observer is used, and behavior is recorded independently in order to verify interrater reliability. Because the process can be time-consuming and costly, time sampling is often used. *Time sampling* typically involves identifying 15- or 30-minute segments of time and observing only during those periods, rather than continuously throughout the day.

TABLE 9.4-12
Excerpt from the Schedule for Affective Disorders and Schizophrenia

HALLUCINATIONS

Hallucinations are perceptions in the absence of identifiable external stimulation. For the purpose of this assessment, hallucinations are recorded here only if they occurred when the subject was fully awake, and neither febrile nor under the influence of alcohol or some drug. Hallucinations should not be confused with illusions, in which an external stimulus is misperceived, or normal thought processes which are exceptionally vivid. Always get the subject to describe the perception in detail. A rating of "suspected" indicates that the rater suspects, but is not certain, that the subject has experienced the particular kind of hallucination noted, as for example, when it is not clear if the subject is describing an illusion rather than a true hallucination. If the hallucination occurred in the setting of a "religious experience," inquire to determine if this is an expected perception that is idiosyncratic to the subject.

If there is no evidence from the case record, informants, or from your interview to suggest hallucinations, ask the following questions and any others from the section on hallucinations which you think are appropriate.

Has there been anything unusual about the way things looked, or sounded, or smelled?

Have you heard voices or other things that weren't there or that other people couldn't hear, or seen things that were not there?

☐ If there is still no evidence to suggest hallucinations, check here and skip to Bizarre Behavior, page 32.

Experienced auditory hallucinations of voices, noises, music, etc. (Do not include if limited to hearing name being called.)	0 1 2 3	No information Absent Suspected or likely Definite
The (sounds, voices) that you said you heard, did you hear them outside your head, through your ears, or did they come from inside your head? *Could you hear what the voice was saying?* *(Did it talk about you or repeat your thoughts?)* *Did you hear anything else? What about noises?*		
Auditory hallucinations in which a voice keeps up a running commentary on the subject's behaviors or thoughts as they occur.	0 1 2 3	No information Absent Suspected or likely Definite
Did the voice describe or comment on what you were doing or thinking?		
Auditory hallucinations in which 2 or more voices converse with each other.	0 1 2 3	No information Absent Suspected or likely Definite
Did you hear 2 or more voices talking with each other?		
Nonaffective verbal hallucinations spoken to the subject. A voice or voices are heard by the subject speaking directly to him, the content of which is unrelated to depressed or elated mood (although he may be depressed or elated at the time). Rate absent if limited to voices saying only 1 or 2 words. Examples: A woman heard voices telling her that she was having a baby and should go to the hospital. A man heard a voice telling him he was being watched by his neighbors for signs of perversion.	0 1 2 3	No information Absent Suspected or likely Definite

Table reproduced with the permission of Robert Spitzer, MD, and Jean Endicott, PhD.

Analogue observation techniques follow the same general model as naturalistic observation; however, the environment is contrived, rather than real. Whenever observation occurs with the patient's awareness, behavior can be expected to be altered. Any subsequent alteration in behavior that is reactive to the observation decreases the probability that a true sample of naturally occurring behavior has been obtained. With analogue observations patient awareness is even more of a problem because the observation technique itself is directly apparent to the patient. Despite those problems, analogue observation techniques are probably used more frequently than are naturalistic techniques because of time and cost factors. In addition, naturalistic observation is difficult to carry out logistically with target behaviors that need to be observed in outpatient settings.

A commonly used form of analogue observation is *role playing.* Role playing has been used extensively in the area of social skills training, and its effectiveness as both an assessment tool and a treatment method is promising. Typically, with the aid of assistants, an analogue situation is acted out, with the patient playing a central role. The situation is constructed to elicit certain target behaviors. Role playing as a form of assessment is likely to be expanded into other areas if the results continue to support its reliability and validity.

Self-monitoring Self-monitoring engages patients in recording data regarding their own target behaviors. If a patient is cooperative and a reliable informant, the deceptively simple technique can provide much valuable information, particularly when the target behavior is one that occurs with a low frequency, making observation techniques difficult. Self-monitoring is less expensive and less time-consuming than observation methods. However, just as a person's behavior is altered simply by knowing that he or she is being observed, changes can be expected when patients are asked to observe themselves.

Psychophysiological measurement In addition to assessing overt and covert behavioral characteristics and responses to stimuli, physiological responding can provide other important information. Physiological responding may be different from behavioral observations, and often the physiological information is needed for a thorough assessment, particularly with stress-related disorders. Some of the frequently used modalities of physiological assessment include heart rate, blood pressure, galvanic skin resistance, muscle tension, and peripheral body temperature.

In general, the psychophysiological modality used depends on the target behavior in question (for example, anxiety and pulse rate, headache and muscle tension). Psychophysiological recordings can be useful with patients who complain subjectively of disorders, such as anxiety, but show few outward behavioral symptoms and are unable to identify discrete precipitating stimuli. In addition to being useful during the initial assessment, psychophysiological recordings have treatment applications, especially as an index of therapy effectiveness.

Psychophysiological assessment is not without its drawbacks, most prominently its cost and logistical concerns. Those drawbacks are mitigated by the new, less expensive compact recording devices. Nevertheless, psychophysiological recording and monitoring equipment does tend to be expensive, bulky, and in need of frequent calibration.

Current status Behavioral personality assessment is gaining rapid acceptance, particularly among adherents to behavioral, empirical, state-oriented interventions. It is readily applicable to treatment monitoring, a decided advantage given the current emphasis on psychotherapy treatment effectiveness.

The weaknesses of behavioral assessment include its relatively recent development and, in some instances, a lack of adequate attention to the psychometric principles of reliability and validity. More important, the fact that the behavioral approach to personality measurement is atheoretical may cause disinterest among many clinicians and researchers, particularly those with a dynamic orientation. Indeed, some maintain that behavioral formulations and personality theory are contradictory terms.

Although an atheoretical approach is contrary to the scientific method, the techniques of behavioral assessment appear to be useful, regardless of orientation. For example, a psychiatrist with a dynamic orientation may wish to conduct a research project on therapy outcome. The psychiatrist may be interested in projective techniques as dependent variables. The psychiatrist may also want to use dependent variables that directly measure observable symptoms and that have readily established

TABLE 9.4-13
Behavioral Measures of Personality

Name	Description	Strengths	Weaknesses
Brief Psychiatric Rating Scale (BPRS)	Semistructured interview	Quick administration and established reliability and validity	Provides only a global pathology index
Hamilton Rating Scale for Depression (HAM-D)	Semistructured interview	Quick administration and established reliability and validity	Overemphasis on biological and neurovegetative symptoms of depression
Schedule for Affective Disorders and Schizophrenia (SADS)	Structured interview	Two versions are available, thereby allowing for relatively brief repeated assessments; increased diagnostic efficacy	The lifetime form is lengthy; some training is required for administration
Global Assessment Scale (GAS)	Rating from observation and report	Quick and easily administered index of overall functioning, which takes into account both strengths and weaknesses	The index is somewhat oversimplified
Present Status Examination (PSE)	Structured interview	Assesses a wide variety of symptoms	Somewhat lengthy, and training is required for accurate administration
Symptom Checklist-90-Revised (SCL-90-R)	Questionnaire	Brief yet reliable and valid; provides a global index of dysfunction in addition to subscores	Strict focus on pathology without adequate assessment of strengths
Direct observation	In vivo, naturalistic observation	Actually samples behaviors in question in the most direct manner possible	Expensive and time-consuming process; observation itself may alter behavior
Analogue observation	Role playing with observation	Decreases cost and time restraints of direct observation	Observation process may alter behavior
Self-monitoring	Patient records data on behaviors in question	Inexpensive method, which has been shown to be beneficial	Patient compliance is essential; self-monitoring in and of itself may alter the behavior
Psychophysiological recording	EEG, heart rate, GSR, and muscular electrical activity are most common modalities	Objective measures that provide additional information and require minimal patient compliance	Expensive technology requiring considerable upkeep

reliability and validity. Behavioral assessment offers a clear advantage over traditional projective measures for those purposes. Although orientation and theory do dictate one's approach to a large degree, one should not become blinded by theory.

A summary of various behavioral methods in personality assessment is found in Table 9.4-13.

CHILD PERSONALITY ASSESSMENT

The assessment of personality with children and adolescents raises a number of issues and methodological problems unique to those populations. Although the general approaches to personality measurement—objective, projective, behavioral—do not necessarily change, in many instances one needs to exercise caution in drawing inferences from the information obtained. For example, the dynamics behind a child's production of a percept on the Rorschach test are probably different from the dynamics involved with an adult perception.

CHILD DEVELOPMENT The interpretation of test results in child personality assessment needs to take the developmental process into consideration. However, some theoretical orientations place a greater than usual emphasis on the influences that development has on personality. For example, in the dynamic and analytical theories of personality and hence in the projective methods of personality assessment, the first few years of life are generally considered the most important for the formation of the personality. Also, developmental stages continue through adolescence. A prolonged developmental process suggests that the significance of a child's projective assessment protocol may change drastically, depending on theoretical personality development constructs. In addition, cognitive development plays a major role in accounting for changes in children's perceptions, independent of personality. Children's Rorschach test perceptions change as a function of cognitive maturity throughout the developmental span. A knowledge of those changes is essential for valid and reliable interpretations. For example, although it is normal for a child's Rorschach protocol to contain an abundance of animal content, the meaning of the animal percepts takes on new significance if the same percentage is seen in an older adolescent or an adult.

Language and academic development are also important, particularly with self-report and interview techniques. Making sure that the patient can read adequately when personality questionnaires are used is important at any age, but children's reading abilities vary dramatically as a function of grade level and age. Hence, one needs to exercise care in the administration of children's inventories. In general, children are less likely or less able than are adults to use language as a means of expression and for coping with stress and inner conflicts. Methods for eliciting valid information from a child are frequently different from those used with adults. Specific training in those areas is essential before the clinician conducts comprehensive personality assessments with children.

Language skills, insight, judgment, and moral reasoning are all less developed in the child than in the adult. For those reasons, children are likely either to deny or to maximize their problems. The child frequently lacks the advanced abilities of introspection and abstract thought. Hence, it is extremely difficult for children to evaluate their own behavior objectively—a herculean task for most adults—and to compare and contrast their own situation with what may be considered normative.

INFORMANTS In assessing aspects of personality development and status with children, clinicians should generally use their parents or caretakers as a primary source of information. With children, a thorough assessment of familial dynamics is essential. The effects of parenting and familial issues are clearly pertinent while the child is in the home. Any assessment of child personality, regardless of orientation, must directly address the structural and interactive aspects of the children with their parents and with their families in general. By the time the parents decide to seek professional help, they may no longer be objective in their observations of the child. Thus, there is an inherent problem with objective personality assessment approaches—namely, that the questionnaires are typically completed by adults. School relationships also provide valuable information on the child's personality, much in the same way that the work environment is an important source of behavioral information with adults.

Although reliance on informant reporting in child personality assessment can provide elucidating information on familial, adult, and peer interrelationships, the complexity of the evaluation also increases. Judgments on the descriptive characteristics of child and adolescent behavior vary as a function of who the informant is, the nature of the situation, and the target behaviors. In general, parents, teachers, and the child are all reliable and valid reporters of behavior. The accuracy of the report depends not only on the informant and the situation but also on the recency of the behavior and the specificity of the question.

SPECIAL NEEDS Not only does the clinician need a strong background in general clinical assessment, but additional training in developmental psychology and child psychopathology is essential. As a general rule, children are less able than are adults to inhibit impulses, and they have less ability to maintain attention and concentration in the absence of new and interesting stimuli. Those factors can have a negative effect on the validity of an evaluation if the assessor is not adequately prepared or is insensitive to the specific concerns inherent in evaluating children.

As many clinicians attest, parents often bring in children without having fully explained to them the purpose of the visit. That lack of communication often creates unnecessary confusion, anxiety, and lack of trust in the child, rendering the assessment process especially difficult. Furthermore, if the examiner does not adequately explain the purpose of the evaluation so that the child is able to comprehend it, the child's orientation toward the personality assessment may be compromised.

The basic approaches to personality assessment with children can be grouped into three major orientations—objective, projective, and behavioral—in much the same way as with adults. A major difference in child evaluations compared with adult evaluations is in objective assessment and, to a smaller degree, behavioral assessment. In those two assessment modalities, significant others are used as informants more frequently than is patient self-report. The use of reporting by others has necessitated the development of innovative psychometric methods.

In objective assessment, for example, new instruments are incorporating validity indexes specifically designed to account for the use of informants, rather than the patients themselves (for example, Personality Inventory for Children). In addition, multivariate psychometric techniques have been applied to present a representative but parsimonious taxonomy of childhood psychopathology that accounts for informant reporting (for example, Child Behavior Checklist).

Advances in behavioral assessment with children have generally mirrored those used in adult assessment. One area that behavioral assessment techniques with children have emphasized is the importance of developmental change. Child and adolescent personality assessment occurs during periods of rapid anatomical, physiological, and environmental change. The child or adolescent is less globally stable than is the typical adult, and measurement devices need to compensate for those factors. The relatively brief and situation-specific nature of behavioral assessment methods are well adapted for the fluidity of the growing years. The area of projective assessment with children, however, has tended to remain somewhat static.

OBJECTIVE PERSONALITY ASSESSMENT

CHILD BEHAVIOR CHECKLIST (CBC) The CBC is a formalized rating scale that, although similar to behavioral assessment techniques, embodies a number of sophisticated psychometric qualities that qualify it as an objective method. The CBC was constructed on the basis of a multivariate taxonomic paradigm, yielding a typology of child psychopathology that avoids both diagnostic overlap and forced choices between multiple categories. Specifically, children receive scores that indicate the degree to which they are similar to criterion groups and dissimilar from normative groups on all symptom clusters. The taxonomy itself is highly efficient.

The CBC is filled out by a knowedgeable informant who rates the child's behavior in each of a wide variety of areas (118 items), using a three-point scale: "never" a problem, "sometimes" a problem, and "frequently" a problem. The items are summated into nine scales, including schizoid, depressed, hyperactive, and delinquent. The various scales load onto two general factors, internalizing and externalizing. A sample protocol is presented in Table 9.4-14. The CBC scales are available for both boys and girls between the ages of 4 and 16 years. The CBC contains additional questions and items that are designed to measure social adjustment and interpersonal skills.

The CBC has a number of strengths. It is quickly filled out, and wording is easily understood; thus, it is useful for a wide variety of parents, teachers, and significant others. It possesses satisfactory reliability. The CBC is one of the most widely used measures of adjustment in research on child psychopathology. The rating scale can be scored according to three separate sets of norms within each sex (ages 4 to 5, 6 to 11, and 12 to 16).

Less information on profile interpretation is available with the CBC than with other questionnaires. Largely for that reason, some consider the CBC a screening instrument, at least until more specific, detailed interpretative strategies are developed.

Because the CBC is filled out by a knowledgeable significant other, there is a potential for error, attributable to the respondent's relationship with the child. To obtain as true a picture of the child's behavior and personality as possible, the clinician should have as many different

TABLE 9.4-14
Child Behavior Checklist Profile, Revised Edition (CBC), of a 9-Year-Old Boy with a Diagnosis of Attention-Deficit/Hyperactivity Disorder

Social Competence	*T* Score (mean = 50, standard deviation = 10)
Activities	40
Socialization	54
School involvement	43
Internalizing	
Schizoid-anxious	68
Depressed	68
Uncommunicative	63
Obsessive-compulsive	71
Somatic complaints	67
Withdrawal	76
Externalizing	
Hyperactive	85
Aggressive	67
Delinquent	67

raters as possible (for example, mother, father, and teacher) complete the CBC. In such cases one can determine the degree of convergence or divergence among the significant caretakers in the child's life. Convergence in that sense also provides evidence of reliability, whereas divergence may provide estimates of error in reliability or of misperceptions in how the parents or the caretakers see the child. That information can be particularly useful in treatment planning.

Personality Inventory for Children-Revised Format (PIC) The PIC is another example of a behavioral rating scale that was closely modeled after adult objective personality inventories. The full PIC contains 420 behavioral and personality descriptors that sum onto a number of dimensions, including withdrawal, anxiety, depression, social skills, and delinquency. The completion of all the items in the revised format also allows for the scoring of factor scores, validity scales, and critical items. Shortened forms of the PIC, although sacrificing some information and psychometric stabilty, tend to make the assessment process more manageable than is the original form. The PIC was constructed by using a variety of psychometric techniques, such as empirical keying and rational development, in much the same way as the MMPI's clinical, validity, and experimental scales were constructed. The PIC is appropriately used with children and adolescents between the ages of 6 and 16 years.

A prominent strength of the instrument is the inclusion of validity scales, which are designed to provide information on the possible presence of a response bias on the part of an informant. Although the feature is an advantage, one needs to keep in mind that, even with the validity scales, the PIC information is based on a rating by another person. Specifically, one is not looking at a child's self-perception but at another person's perceptions of the child. Those perceptions are colored to an unknown extent by the relationship between the child and the rater. In that sense the validity scales do not eliminate the problem but put some limits on the degree of acceptability of the error variance.

TABLE 9.4-15
Personality Inventory for Children—Revised (PIC) Profile for a 14-Year-Old Boy with a Diagnosis of Major Depressive Disorder

	T Score (mean = 50, standard deviation = 10)
Factor score I	48
Factor score II	88
Factor score III	53
Factor score IV	51
Lie	38
Frequency	71
Defensiveness	56
Adjustment	74
Achievement	53
Intellectual screening	37
Development	54
Somatic concern	52
Depression	78
Family relations	75
Delinquency	55
Withdrawal	88
Anxiety	57
Psychosis	80
Hyperactivity	36
Social skills	70

Psychologist's Interpretation

The profile is valid, and the patient's parent responded to the inventory in an open and honest fashion. The patient's profile is reflective of a significant psychological disturbance that is not likely to be accompanied by cognitive dysfunction or developmental delays. He can be expected to be significantly depressed at this time. Associated symptoms may include moodiness, pessimism, low energy level, anhedonia, serious attitude, a poor self-concept, and noncommunicativeness. This patient is likely to be socially isolative and withdrawn and to have few friends. He may be shy, passive, conforming, and generally unresponsive to his environment. The possibility of suicidal ideation should be investigated. There may be a moderate degree of disruption in family cohesiveness at this time.

Diagnostic Impression

Major depressive disorder. The possibility of dysthymic disorder should be investigated.

The PIC also contains an index of family cohesiveness, and that measure can assist in the interpretation of potential informant bias.

The PIC has been criticized for its imbalance between an extensive test construction literature and a relative dearth of validity and interpretative research. Unlike the MMPI, the PIC is not yet accompanied by well-documented actuarial manuals that provide extensive data on code types, personality characteristics, coping styles, familial relationships, diagnostic considerations, and treatment recommendations. That is somewhat surprising, as the PIC is probably the most extensive and psychometrically sound child personality questionnaire available. The PIC is best thought of as an experimental personality inventory at this time. It holds considerable promise as an objective assessment device; however, interpretative statements need to be tempered because of the lack of an adequate data base.

A sample profile of the PIC is shown in Table 9.4-15.

Millon Adolescent Personality Inventory (MAPI) The MAPI is a 150-item, true-false format questionnaire designed for adolescents ages 13 through 18 years. The inventory yields 22 scales that include measures of personality style, self-esteem, rapport, school functioning, impulse control, and validity indexes. The MAPI is one of the few personality inventories that was specifically developed for adolescents, and that fact is undoubtedly one of the measure's strengths. Adolescence is typically accompanied by unique stressors and adaptive challenges, such as emerging independence, peer adjustment, and societal expectations. The MAPI provides quantitative data that are directly pertinent to those issues. Hand scoring is not available for the MAPI; the assessor must use a mail order computerized scoring service. That is an inconvenience for many researchers and clinicians, increases the cost of using the MAPI, and tends to discourage research efforts with the inventory. These are likely to be the primary reasons for the less than common use of the MAPI.

Minnesota Multiphasic Personality Inventory Adolescent norms have been published for the MMPI. Also available are case history data on a number of adolescent MMPI profiles. However, use of the MMPI with adolescents remains rather restricted because of the limited amount of research on the MMPI with that population. Thus, interpretative hypotheses with adolescents rest on much less firm ground than those involving adult patients.

Minnesota Multiphasic Personality Inventory-Adolescent (MMPI-A) The MMPI-A is a 478-item revision of the MMPI specifically designed for adolescents ages 14 through 18. Like the MMPI and the MMPI-2, the MMPI-A is a self-report, objective measure of personality and psychopathology. It contains validity scales, clinical scales, and a large number of specialty subscales. Unique to the MMPI-A are content scales measuring areas of adjustment and personality that are especially salient for adolescents, such as immaturity, alienation, anger, school problems, social discomfort, family problems, aspirations, and self-esteem.

Like its adult counterparts, the MMPI-A has excellent psychometric properties and features, and yields a large amount and variety of clinically relevant information. A relatively new personality inventory, the MMPI-A is generating considerable interest; research and interpretative studies have begun to appear in the literature.

Hand scoring the MMPI-A is somewhat of a herculean task, and computer scoring is available only on a mail-in basis. Those drawbacks are offset by the fact that the MMPI-A represents state-of-the-art excellence in personality inventory design and construction. Its publication represents a recognition on the part of psychologists that adolescence is associated with unique characteristics and challenges for personality assessment.

Other methods A self-report version of the PIC, the *Personality Inventory for Youth (PIY),* is currently under development. When it becomes available, concurrent use of the PIC and the PIY may provide an excellent window on how both the child and the parent feel about the child's personality and psychological status.

The *Parenting Scale,* while not a direct measure of child behavior, has clear relevance for the assessment of child personality. Completed by the parent, the scale yields scores on three dimensions of parenting behavior: laxness, overreactivity, and verbosity. The scale provides a useful way of assessing interactions between relatively specific parenting behaviors and the child's behavioral and psychological reactions to those styles of parenting.

The *Children's Depression Inventory (CDI)* is a brief self-report measure of depression for children that was designed to be similar to the widely used Beck Depression Inventory. In addition to a global score for depression, the CDI includes subscales which measure mood, self-esteem, anhedonia, ineffectiveness, and interpersonal problems. Viewing the child's response to individual items is also encouraged in the interpretative process. While limited in range, the CDI provides a large amount of self-report information in a very brief time. Its use is suitable for children and adolescents ages 7 through 17.

PROJECTIVE PERSONALITY ASSESSMENT The Rorschach technique can be used with adolescents and older children, but it is rarely used with young children. The clinician interpreting a Rorschach protocol from a child or an adolescent must be knowledgeable about developmental norms for the various Rorschach responses. What is considered a pathological response in an adult may be a typical or nondeviant response in a child or an adolescent.

Children's Apperception Test (CAT) The CAT consists of 10 cards that depict animal figures in a number of settings. The cards present various scenarios designed to elicit relatively specific information. For example, one of the cards is a scene at a dinner table, and another shows a young child sleeping in a room that somewhat ambiguously shows another bed, presumably a parent's bed. The CAT has a definite psychodynamic orientation and is most appropriately used for personality assessment in which a dynamic interpretation of the child's personality is desired. The method is administered and interpreted in much the same way as the TAT. Although the CAT is dynamic in its orientation, it can also elicit considerable information concerning familial relationships, which are important in child personality assessment. Published research on validity and interpretation is available, but the test has not been extensively researched or widely used on a clinical basis.

Play therapy Play therapy techniques can be used with children to observe behavior and to make inferences regarding personality structure. Although the process is similar to the behavioral assessment procedure of analogue observation, its use is closely connected with clinicians and researchers who have a dynamic background and are prone to view the child's interaction with various play therapy stimuli as projective in nature.

Typically, the clinician presents the child with various dolls designed to represent the child and parental and sibling figures. The clinician observes the child's behavior in play with the dolls and often asks the child to make up a story, using the dolls as characters. The clinician records the story on the assumption that the child will project internal and family dynamics into the story.

Empirical research on play therapy assessment techniques is somewhat sparse; however, the procedure is widely used by dynamically oriented clinicians.

Blacky Pictures (BP) The BP consist of a set of cards that depict dog figures in various settings and scenarios. They are intended to elicit intrapsychic conflict information from adults and adolescents, but they can also be used with children. The BP were developed to provide data congruent with Freudian theory.

The pictures represent such psychoanalytic conflict arenas as castration anxiety and oedipal conflicts. The clinician asks a structured set of questions after presenting a stimulus cared.

The BP are rarely used, and many researchers and clinicians consider them no more than a curiosity. Nevertheless, it may be beneficial for psychoanalytically oriented professionals to investigate the potential usefulness of the BP.

BEHAVIORAL PERSONALITY ASSESSMENT The theory, the rationale, and the techniques of child behavioral assessment are basically identical to those for adults. In addition to the emphasis that behavioral assessment places on empirical validation, methods used with children must be particularly sensitive to the developmental process. At young ages, self-report and self-monitoring are rarely used, and other ratings and behavioral observations are more appropriate. As the child becomes more mature, a greater range of techniques are available. A multimethod approach is advocated to obtain as much information as possible, given time considerations and other practical restraints.

The behavioral assessment of personality with children incorporates several implicit assumptions regarding the causes of psychological disorders in childhood. A behavioral perspective maintains that personality has multiple determinants and that the primacy of the determinants varies with children. A priori assumptions regarding causative factors are avoided, and the assessor pays attention to the likelihood of feedback and feed-forward systems. All variables are potentially relevant, and in that sense behavioral assessment follows an ecological model.

Behavior Problem Checklist (BPC) The BPC is a relatively popular behavioral rating scale for children and adolescents. It consists of 55 items that are rated on a three-point severity scale. Scores are obtained on four dimensions: conduct, personality, immaturity, and socialized delinquency. Although the BPC does a respectable job of providing a brief screening on psychopathology, it does not provide much information on the child's strengths or areas of competence.

Louisville Fear Survey (LFS) The LFS is a rating scale composed of 81 items designed to assess a wide variety of fear and anxiety behaviors. The LFS is useful with many young children because fear syndromes and disorders, such as school phobia, are common during childhood.

Conner's scales The *Conner's Hyperactivity Rating Scale* was developed as a quantitative means of assessing hyperactivity in children. The original measure was designed to be completed by teachers and is a brief rating scale that is both reliable and valid. Continued scale development has culminated in the *Conner's Rating Scales* (CRS), which include short and long forms for both a teacher version and a parent version. The expanded rating scales not only provide an index of hyperactivity but also assess conduct disorder, anxiety, passivity, obsessional behavior, and asocial tendencies. The CRS are quickly filled out and easily scored. They are widely used and are appropriate for monitoring a child's progress over the course of therapeutic endeavors.

Self-report scales A number of self-report assessment scales have been developed for children and adolescents, including scales for measuring anxiety, socialization, depression, fear, coping, and anger. If used with caution, the techniques can be helpful, especially when combined with observation or other ratings or preferably both. Within behavioral assessment, self-report measures have tended to be underused. There is a long-standing bias against self-reports because they frequently do not directly assess the behaviors in question. That bias is changing as clinicians recognize that self-reports reveal behaviors worthy of attention.

Structured diagnostic interviews Structured diagnostic interviews have been adapted for use with children and adolescents. One commonly used diagnostic tool is the *Schedule for Affective Disorders and Schizophrenia for School-Aged Children* (K-SADS), a revision of the adult SADS. The use of structured diagnostic interviews with children is a relatively new area that is generating considerable interest. At this time the interviews are undergoing updating in response to the high degree of revision in childhood psychiatric diagnostic nomenclature that has occurred over the past 10 years.

CURRENT STATUS The assessment of personality with children and adolescents is an area that has broadened in recent years. Advances are evident in the behavioral assessment areas and in the psychometric sophistication of the inventories using an informant or other-report format. The increased psychometric sophistication has resulted in test instruments that provide data closely approximating the reliability and the validity of data found with adult objective assessment techniques.

A recent proposal recommends that childhood assessment cover five axes: parental perceptions, teacher perceptions, cognitive measures, physical conditions, and the clinician's assessment. That multiaxial approach results in an assessment that maximizes the information regarding the child's strengths and weaknesses, as well as the convergence and divergence in the perceptions of caretakers. It allows for the use of multimodal assessment devices and can incorporate objective, behavioral, and even projective methods.

INTEGRATIVE PERSONALITY ASSESSMENT

Many clinicians and researchers take a functional, pragmatic approach to personality assessment. That integrative or eclectic approach is simply the administration of a variety of assessment devices from more than one orientation. For example, both objective and projective personality instruments are frequently administered to the same patient, with the examiner then integrating the results of the two approaches. The examiner inspects the protocols for similar themes and discrepancies during the interpretative process.

The value of the multimodal approach lies in the rich clinical picture that is typically obtained. If interpretive conclusions are verified across modalities, their validity is strengthened. If discrepant results are obtained, an explanation is sought. Is the patient confused or malingering? Is one of the tests providing invalid information and, if so, why? Or is there some degree of truth in both sets of results? In any event, one generates hypotheses regarding the cause of the discrepant results and seeks out data to support or refute the hypotheses.

Incremental validity is an important issue in integrative personality assessment. Incremental validity involves the degree to which additional measures of personality functioning either increase or decrease the validity of the psychologist's interpretative statements. Increasing information beyond a certain critical point not only fails to increase assessment validity but may even have detrimental effects on the evaluation. The effect appears to be more of a serious problem with clinical judgment than with actuarial systems of interpretation. Actuarial systems use mathematical formulas in which one is able to state with some degree of certainty how much margin of error may be present on an interpretative statement. In constructing the formula, one knows exactly when to stop including information because the error margin begins to increase. In many instances the mathematical accuracy appears to be superior to judgments and impressions made on the basis of clinical experience. For those reasons the interpreter of psychological personality tests needs to exercise caution in drawing summary conclusions on the basis of an integrative assessment.

Integrative assessment can and frequently does provide a broad range of information useful for clinicians of varied orientation. Hence, it maximizes the report's usefulness, particularly in clinics where the patient may be seen by more than one team member. Integrative assessment also allows for the conceptualization of the patient on more than a unitary level.

FUTURE DIRECTIONS

Psychometric purity—defined as well-established reliability and validity not only for objective devices but also for projective and behavioral assessment methods—is receiving continued emphasis, as are environmental and situational determinants of behavior. Although these approaches have resulted in a decrease in intrapsychic, analytic-type assessment, those methods are not obsolete. Regardless of the approach, continued emphasis on meaningful and directly observable interpretations is likely.

The field of personality assessment has continued to emphasize the importance of individual patients and their views of their own psychological status. At times, diagnostic categorization is ignored. Some will always hold that diagnosis in the mental health fields is inappropriate, reductionistic, and even harmful to the patient. That position is not likely to become mainstream; it reflects those who advocate a radical idiographic approach to personality assessment. Diagnosis remains an integral part of a thorough psychological assessment, and it does not preclude attention to individual needs, integrity, wants, and desires. Diagnosis should be a design for action; within such a model, a diagnosis is more than a label; it provides the impetus for broad-spectrum treatment planning.

Psychiatry has been experiencing a growing recognition of the importance of the biological determinants of human behavior. The biological emphasis is influencing personality researchers. A unified biopsychosocial theory of personality has been proposed that has direct relevance for the assessment of both normal and abnormal personality characteristics. The most comprehensive and well-articulated proposal to date hypothesizes three independent dimensions of personality: novelty seeking, harm avoidance, and reward dependence. Those three dimensions are presumed to have a genetic inheritance that varies in a normally distributed fashion. Interactions between the dimensions are thought to be responsible for a wide range of phenotypical behavioral constellations, including diagnosable personality disorders.

A structured interview assessment system, the *Tridimensional Interview of Personality Style* (TIPS), is used to obtain Likert ratings on personality dimensions and their interactions. Modifications in behavior that occur in response to environmental conditions and factors are viewed as important, potentially adaptive or maladaptive processes. Biopsychosocial approaches can be expected to have major effects on personality assessment. The TIPS is likely to be the first in a series of efforts to integrate biological and biologically determined variables into a comprehensive personality assessment system. As sophisticated brain function measurement systems, such as positron emission tomography and quantified electroencephalographic analysis, become more refined, those measures may further broaden and improve assessment abilities.

Behavioral assessment has continued to grow in popularity. As behavioral assessment continues to incorporate cognitive factors and pays attention to dynamic social interactions, its usefulness is likely to expand. Personality assessment that provides a barometer of the patient's symptom changes is becoming more and more important, particularly in view of the recent focus on treatment accountability. The fact that behavioral assessment techniques are well suited for those purposes may contribute to their increased use and development.

The traditional integrative psychological battery of objective and projective measures remains the mainstay in clinical psychology. That situation is probably not going to change in the near future; traditional methods will likely be supplemented with behavioral and other methods, rather than replaced by them. However, many of the traditional assessment devices, such as the MMPI and the Rorschach technique, have remained unchanged for many years or have only recently been updated. Continued efforts to update normative data, to make contemporary changes, and to reestablish reliability and validity in those traditional measures can be expected.

Finally, personality assessment with children is growing by leaps and bounds. As test developers continue to take into account the problems unique to childhood assessment, methods are likely to improve and become more innovative. An example is the multiaxial system of assessment, which systematizes an integrative assessment paradigm for children. Such innovations in child assessment will undoubtedly have a beneficial effect on personality assessment methods with adults.

SUGGESTED CROSS-REFERENCES

Chapter 8 discusses the theories of personality and psychopathology derived from psychology and philosophy. Section 9.1 discusses the psychiatric interview, history, and mental status examination. Section 9.5 discusses neuropsychological aspects of adults, and Section 9.6 discusses pediatric neuropsychology. Section 9.8 discusses psychiatric rating scales and includes a copy of the BPRS. Personality disorders are discussed in Chapter 25. The psychiatric examination of infants, children, and adolescents is discussed in Chapter 34.

REFERENCES

*Achenbach T M: *Assessment and Taxonomy of Child and Adolescent Psychopathology.* Sage, Beverly Hills, CA, 1985.

Achenbach T M, McConaughy S H, Howell C T: Child/adolescent behavioral and emotional problems: Implications of cross-informant correlations for situational specificity. Psychol Bull *101:* 213, 1987.

Anastasi A: *Psychological Testing,* ed 6. Macmillan, New York, 1988.

Archer R P, Krishnamurthy R: A review of MMPI and Rorschach interrelationships in adult samples. J Pers Assess *61:* 277, 1993.

Arnold D S, O'Leary S G, Wolff L S, Acker M M: The parenting scale: A measure of dysfunctional parenting in discipline situations. Psychol Assess *5:* 137, 1993.

Bellack A S, Hersen M, editors: *Behavioral Assessment: A Practical Handbook,* ed 3. Pergamon, New York, 1988.

Butcher J N, Williams C L, Graham J R, Archer R P, Tellegen A, Ben-Porath Y S, Kaemmer B: MMPI-A: *Minnesota Multiphasic Personality Inventory–Adolescent.* University of Minnesota Press, Minneapolis, 1992.

Chick D, Sheaffer C I, Goggin W C, Sison G F: The relationship between MCMI personality scales and clinician-generated DSM-III-R personality disorder diagnoses. J Pers Assess *61:* 264, 1993.

Cloninger C R: A systemic method for clinical description and classification of personality variants. Arch Gen Psychiatry, *44:* 573, 1987.

*Cronbach L J: *Essentials of Psychological Testing,* ed 4. Harper & Row, New York, 1984.

Dahlstrom W G, Welsch G, Dahlstrom L: *An MMPI Handbook,* vol 1: *Clinical Interpretation.* University of Minnesota Press, Minneapolis, 1972.

Edwards D W, Morrison T L, Weissman H N: The MMPI and MMPI-2 in an outpatient sample: Comparisons of code types, validity scales, and clinical scales. J Pers Assess *61:* 1, 1993.

Exner J E: *The Rorschach: A Comprehensive System.* Wiley, New York, 1974.

Fischer J, Corcoran K: *Measures for Clinical Practice: A Sourcebook,* ed 2, vol 1: *Couples, Families and Children.* Free Press, New York, 1994.

Fischer J, Corcoran K: *Measures for Clinical Practice: A Sourcebook,* ed 2, vol 2: *Adults.* Free Press, New York, 1994.

Goldfried M R, Kent R N: Personality assessment: A comparison of methodological and theoretical assumptions. Psychol Bull *77:* 409, 1972.

Goldfried M R, Stricker G, Weiner I: *Rorschach Handbook of Clinical and Research Applications.* Prentice-Hall, Englewood Cliffs, NJ, 1971.

*Goldstein G, Hersen M, editors: *Handbook of Psychological Assessment.* Pergamon, New York, 1990.

Graham J R: *Assessing Personality and Psychopathology.* Oxford University Press, New York, 1990.

Holt R R: *Assessing Personality.* Harcourt Brace Jovanovich, Orlando, 1971.

Iancono W G: Psychophysiological assessment of psychopathology. J Consult Clin Psychol *3:* 309, 1991.

Jackson D N: The dynamics of structured personality tests. Psychol Rev *78:* 229, 1971.

Korchin S J, Schuldberg D: The future of clinical assessment. Am Psychol *36:* 1147, 1981.

Lachar D, Gdowski C L: *Actuarial Assessment of Child and Adolescent Personality: An Interpretative Guide for the Personality Inventory for Children Profile.* Western Psychological Services, Los Angeles, 1979.

Lachar D, Gruber C P: Development of the Personality Inventory for Youth: A self-report companion to the Personality Inventory for Children. J Pers Assess *61:* 81, 1993.

Lambert M J, Christensen E R, DeJulio S S, editors: *The Assessment of Psychotherapy Outcome.* Wiley, New York, 1983.

Mash E J, Terdal L G, editors: *Behavioral Assessment of Childhood Disorders.* Guilford, New York, 1988.

McCann J R: Convergent and discriminant validity of the MCMI-II and MMPI personality disorder scales. Psych Assessment *3:* 9, 1991.

Meehl P E: *Psychodiagnosis: Selected Papers.* Norton, New York, 1977.

Millon T: The MCMI provides a good assessment of DSM-III disorders: The MCMI-II will prove even better. J Pers Assess *49:* 379, 1985.

*Mischel W: *Personality and Assessment.* Wiley, New York, 1968.

*Mitchell V J, editor: *The Ninth Mental Measurements Yearbook.* University of Nebraska Press, Lincoln, 1985.

Rapaport J, Conners C K, Reatig N, editors: Rating scales and assessment instruments for use in pediatric psychopharmacology research. Psychopharmacol Bull *21:* 1, 1985.

Shneidman E S, Joel W, Little K B, editors: *Thematic Test Analysis.* Grune & Stratton, Orlando, 1951.

Spitzer R L, Endicott J: *Schedule for Affective Disorders and Schizophrenia: Technical Report.* New York State Psychiatric Institute, New York, 1972.

Sundberg N D: *Assessment of Persons.* Prentice-Hall, Englewood Cliffs, NJ, 1977.

Swensen C H: Empirical evaluations of human figure drawings. Psychol Bull *20:* 20, 1986.

Watson D, Clark L A, Harkness A R: Structures of personality and their relevance to psychopathology. J Abnorm Psychol *103:* 18, 1994.

Wiggins J S: *Personality and Prediction: Principles of Personality Assessment.* Addison-Wesley, Reading, MA, 1973.

Wolman B, editor: *Handbook of Clinical Diagnosis of Mental Disorders.* Plenum, New York, 1978.

Zubin J, Eron L, Schumer F, editors: *An Experimental Approach to Projective Techniques.* Wiley, New York, 1965.

9.5 NEUROPSYCHOLOGICAL AND INTELLECTUAL ASSESSMENT OF ADULTS

HARVEY S. LEVIN, Ph.D.
VICKI M. SOUKUP, Ph.D.
ARTHUR L. BENTON, Ph.D.
JACK M. FLETCHER, Ph.D.
PAUL SATZ, Ph.D.

INTRODUCTION

Neuropsychological assessment uses experimental and clinical psychology methods to analyze cognitive and behavioral disturbances resulting from injury, disease, or abnormal brain development. Used both in clinical evaluation and research, those procedures refine and extend aspects of the neurological examination. The same behavioral and mental capacities (for example, memory, language functions, orientation) that are evaluated in neurological examinations can be evaluated more precisely and objectively through neuropsychological assessment. Neuropsychological tests are standardized and yield quantifiable, reproducible results, using scores that can be compared to those of normal persons of similar age and demographic background as the person being tested.

Clinical neuropsychology was founded during a time when individual differences in ability and brain-behavior relationships (particularly with respect to cerebral localization of higher functions) were being studied. The contributions of Paul Broca and Carl Wernicke to the clinicopathological correlation between aphasia and lesions in the left hemisphere were succeeded by studies of apraxia, memory disorder, visuospatial deficit, and cognitive impairment related to frontal lobe injury. Controversies surrounding the issue of cerebral localization of higher function led to an interest in developing techniques to evaluate specific neurobehavioral deficits. In reaction, numerous universities set up experimental psychology laboratories in the late 19th century, and pioneering studies flourished. Sir Francis Galton's measurement of individual differences in motor, cognitive, and sensory capacities late in the century and the development of Alfred Binet and Theodore Simon's standardized tests for evaluating intelligence at the turn of the century anticipated the emergence of clinical neuropsychology. The demand to evaluate brain injuries for sequelae during World Wars I and II provided further encouragement for neuropsychological testing.

Until recently, it was difficult to extrapolate to psychiatric disorders those neuropsychological methods that had been developed in studies of patients with localized lesions. Demonstrating the morphological, neurophysiological and neurochemical features of those conditions that could be related to behavioral findings was a major obstacle. Advances in neuroimaging, neuropharmacology, and neurophysiology have augmented the opportunities to characterize cerebral abnormalities in psychiatric disorders and to investigate their relation to neuropsychological impairment.

PURPOSES OF THE NEUROPSYCHOLOGICAL EXAMINATION

The major role of neuropsychological test procedures is to provide an accurate and unbiased estimate of various aspects of a patient's behavioral capacity. The results can contribute to differential diagnosis and serve as both a guide to clinical management and a baseline for monitoring changes in clinical status. The indications for neuropsychological assessment are as follows:

1. To identify the presence and nature of early or mild disturbances of cognitive function in patients in whom other neurodiagnostic studies and mental status examinations have yielded equivocal findings.
2. To aid in the differentiation of depressive disorders or other causes of behavioral impairment from brain disease. The psychiatrist presented with complaints of memory impairment or slowness in thinking in a patient who is depressed or paranoid may be unsure of the possible contribution of neurological changes to the clinical picture. Indications for neuropsychological testing may be particularly evident when the findings of the neurological examination and ancillary procedures are either negative or equivocal. The differential diagnosis of incipient dementia from depression is a case in point, particularly when computed tomography (CT) fails to yield definitive results.
3. To evaluate the deficits and preserved functions in patients with neurological disease or injury to assist in planning for rehabilitation, including recommendations for speech therapy, visual neglect, and cognitive retraining. Serial assessment in nonprogressive conditions, such as head injury, documents the patient's rate of recovery and potential for returning to work.
4. To assess the neurotoxic effects of alcohol and drug abuse, including improvement and residual deficits after detoxification. Chronic alcohol abuse can result in cognitive and memory defects which resolve to a varying degree depending on the duration of abstinence.
5. To evaluate the effects of surgical intervention for epilepsy, cerebrovascular disease, and hydrocephalus. Drug therapy for neurological and psychiatric disorders can also be monitored by neuropsychological procedures. Serial administration of parallel forms of memory tests has been employed to investigate the effects of cholinergic agents and other drugs on dementia of the Alzheimer's type.
6. To evaluate school problems and developmental delay in order to differentiate between mental subnormality, emotional disturbance, and specific learning disability.
7. To provide objective data for research; neuropsychological tests are particularly useful in psychiatric investigations involving behavioral variables.

TEST BATTERIES VERSUS FLEXIBLE STRATEGY

Strategies of neuropsychological assessment may be categorized as *fixed battery* (that is, administration of a comprehensive, invariant series of tests), or as *flexible*, or "adjustive" (that is, selection of tests according to the reason for referral, pertinent clinical data, indications of deficits observed during an interview [for example, hesitancy in speech], the patient's ability to cooperate, and the results of preliminary tests which may suggest the presence of specific deficits).

Either strategy can provide a profile of abilities (that is, intellectual, linguistic, mnemonic, perceptuomotor) and, in practice, many neuropsychologists integrate complete test batteries or selected components with other procedures. While acknowledging the potential usefulness of both fixed battery and flexible strategies in neuropsychological consultation in psychiatry and neurology, the authors maintain that the examiner should be trained to conceptualize the neuroanatomical and the neurobehavioral implications of the diagnostic entities under consideration. The neuropsychologist should be capable of interpreting patterns of test scores in view of principles of lateralization and localization of cerebral function and to take account of factors which adversely affect performance (for example, fatigue, adverse drug effects, cultural deprivation, anxiety, rumination, and depression) that may mimic the neuropsychological impairment found in patients with demonstrable cerebral lesions. Clinical exigencies related to unusual neurobehavioral syndromes or extenuating circumstances may require an experimental approach to the individual patient which deviates from a standard battery.

PROCESS APPROACH The process approach to neuropsychological assessment is based on the principle that defective performance on multifactorial tasks may be obtained by patients with different neuroanatomical lesion sites. People can arrive at solutions by distinctly different processes, reflecting the activity of different structures in the central nervous system (CNS). The process approach maintains that careful monitoring of the patient's behaviors during problem solving can provide more useful information than limiting the data obtained to scores based on right versus wrong answers. By isolating and testing the various factors assumed to underlie task performance, differential diagnosis is facilitated and a better understanding of the underlying problems of a given patient emerges. The process approach considers a variety of patient variables in conjunction with the demands of a task, the nature of the stimulus parameters, and the modality of input and output. The focus on the strategies, or process, that the patient employs to compensate for cognitive problems can be informative for therapeutic interventions in rehabilitation settings and can aid differential diagnosis in psychiatric-related concerns.

Although the Wechsler Adult Intelligence Scale (WAIS) is the most widely employed test battery, it is used primarily to evaluate intellectual level and is supplemented by other tests that measure specific abilities. Consequently, this review of neuropsychological tests is organized according to function; components of batteries are included with their respective functions.

INTELLECTUAL FUNCTIONS

DEVELOPMENT OF INTELLECTUAL ASSESSMENT TECHNIQUES To assess individual differences in mental ability in school children and to identify more accurately students with mental retardation, the French psychologist Alfred Binet and the physician Theodore Simon developed a scale in 1905 which they standardized on 100 school children and on a sample of inmates from an institution for the retarded. The 30 items comprising the 1905 scale of intelligence were arranged in ascending order of difficulty. In a 1908 revision Binet and Simon introduced the concept of mental age (M.A.), which they estimated from performance on test items that could be passed by a majority of children at each age level. In 1912 William Stern introduced the intelligence quotient (I.Q.) as a quantitative index of a child's mental age (M.A.) relative to chronological age (C.A.). The ratio I.Q. was computed so that, for example, a 10 year old with an I.Q. of 100 could answer as many items correctly as the average 10 year old. An I.Q. above 100 implied that the child responded correctly to items which were typically answered correctly by older children. A child whose ceiling score corresponded to items which were usually answered correctly by younger children obtained an I.Q. below 100.

The ratio I.Q. was incorporated into the 1916 revision of the Binet-Simon scale by Lewis Terman of Stanford University. Terman expanded the scale and standardized it on a sample of approximately 1,000 children and 400 adults who were selected as a cross section of the American population. The Stanford-Binet scale was widely adopted for applications in education and psychiatry. Although Terman retained the ratio I.Q. in his 1937 revision of the Stanford-Binet scale, developmental studies revealed that standard deviations of obtained I.Q.s varied with age and were inconsistent with the underlying assumption that mental age is directly proportional to chronological age across the age span. The ratio I.Q. could no longer be regarded as equivalent from one age to another.

David Wechsler, an American psychologist, employed statistical criteria rather than mental age in his 1939 Wechsler-Bellevue I scale. By assigning the same I.Q. score of 100 to the different mean raw scores obtained on the same I.Q. test by various age groups, and by using a standard deviation of 15 I.Q. points, it was possible directly to compare I.Q. scores across various ages and to evaluate intra-individual changes over time. Wechsler's influence was reflected in the 1960 revision of the Stanford-Binet Intelligence Scale, which substituted the deviation I.Q. (mean = 100, standard deviation = 16) for the ratio I.Q. based on mental age.

Both Binet and Terman had incorporated heterogeneous items into a single scale. As chief clinical psychologist at the Bellevue Hospital in New York City, Wechsler had extensive experience with non-English-speaking patients, for whom the heavily verbal Stanford-Binet was ill-suited. To address the language problem, the Wechsler-Bellevue scale included both a verbal scale and a relatively nonverbal performance scale, each of which consisted of five subtests. The Wechsler-Bellevue yielded a Verbal I.Q., a Performance I.Q., and a Full Scale I.Q. for people between 10 and 60 years old, which could be compared with the distribution of scores obtained in persons of similar age.

The Wechsler-Bellevue I scale was revised in 1946 and replaced in 1955 by the WAIS, which retained the deviation I.Q. The WAIS (revised in 1981 as the WAIS-R) and the Wechsler Intelligence Scale for Children-3rd Revision (WISC-III) are the most widely used tests for assessment of cognitive functioning. Although the Wechsler scales were not originally designed to assess cognitive impairment associated with cerebral disease, they have the advantage of standardization on large normative populations, and they yield highly reliable results when the findings of different examiners are compared. These test batteries have also been translated for use with Spanish-speaking patients.

DISTRIBUTION AND CORRELATES OF I.Q. SCORES

Standardization of the Wechsler scales over a wide age range of normal subjects permits conversion of raw scores to standardized scores that yield a mean I.Q. of 100, with a standard deviation of 15 (Figure 9.5-1). Accordingly, 68 percent of the population have I.Q.s (85–115) within one standard deviation of the mean, and 95 percent of the population have I.Q.s (70–130) within two standard deviations of the mean. As depicted in Figure 9.5-1, the average (or normal) range is defined by an I.Q. of 90 to 110, while I.Q. scores of at least 120 are considered superior.

In their reports, psychologists frequently use percentiles to clarify the interpretation of I.Q. scores (note in Figure 9.5-1). A WAIS I.Q. of 100 corresponds to the 50th percentile, an I.Q. of 110 is at the 75th percentile, and a 90 I.Q. falls at the 25th percentile. Accordingly, an individual with a measured I.Q. of 80 has performed on a level which is exceeded by 91 of every 100 adults of comparable age (that is, the 9th percentile). In contrast, a measured I.Q. score of 119 implies that fewer than 10 out of 100 persons would perform at a higher level on the WAIS.

The American Association on Mental Deficiency defines mental retardation by an I.Q. less than 70, which corresponds to the lowest 2.2 percent of the population (Figure 9.5-1). Consequently, about 2 out of every 100 persons have an I.Q. score consistent with mental deficiency ranging from mild to severe.

Clinical interpretation of measured intelligence necessitates concurrent assessment of the person's adaptive behaviors as reflected by performance of everyday and social activities. Psychologists often obtain information from the patient (parent or guardian in the case of a child or institutionalized person) concerning performance of roles in the home, at school, and in the workplace to interpret how intellectual capacities are used. For example, the Vineland Scale of Social Maturity, which is based on information obtained from a relative (usually a parent), is a standardized scale which provides an age-equivalent level of performance in such areas as communication and social relationships. The psychologist can ascertain whether performance

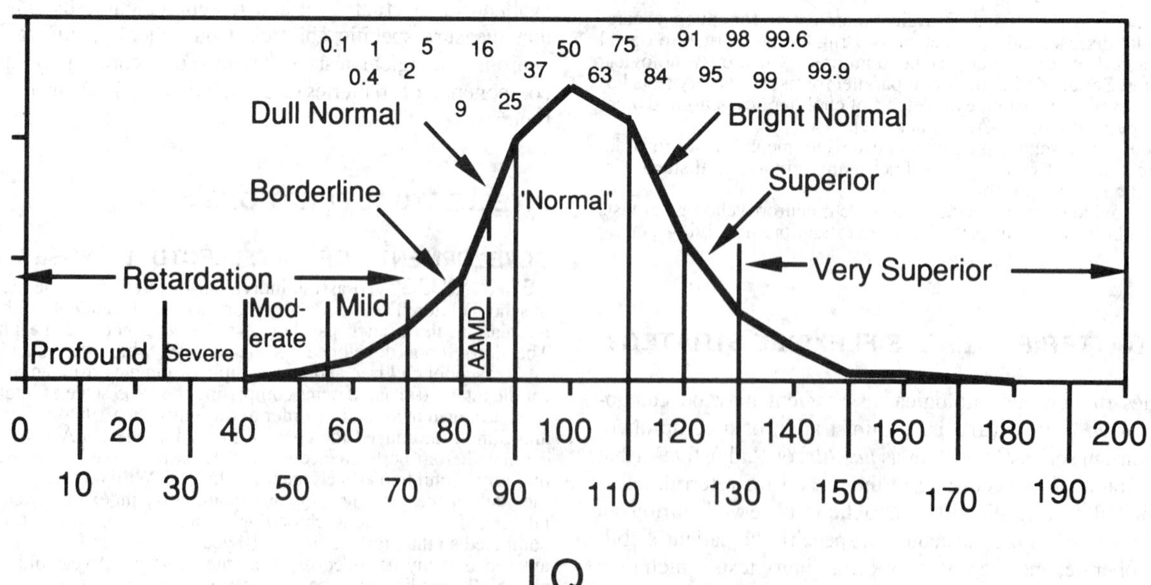

FIGURE 9.5-1 *The distribution of Wechsler Adult Intelligence Scale I.Q. categories. (Adapted from J D Matarazzo:* Wechsler's Measurement and Appraisal of Adult Intelligence, *ed 5, p 124. Oxford University Press, New York, 1972. Used with permission.)*

TABLE 9.5-1
Exemplars or Validity Coefficients of I.Q.

Exemplars	r*
IQ with Adaptive Behavior Measure	
IQ × mental retardation	0.90
IQ × educational attainment (in years)	0.70
IQ × academic success (grade point)	0.50
IQ × occupational attainment	0.50
IQ × socioeconomic status	0.40
IQ × success on the job	0.20
Related Variables	
IQ × independently judged prestige of one's occupation	0.95
IQ × parents' educational attainment	0.50

*r represents correlation
Table from J D Matarazzo: *Wechsler's Measurement and Appraisal of Adult Intelligence,* ed 5. Williams & Wilkins, Baltimore, 1972. Used with permission.

of various roles is commensurate with the estimate of intellectual capacity which is reflected by the I.Q. score.

The importance of integrating information obtained from the clinical history and the evaluation of adaptive behavior with the results of intellectual assessment is reflected by the correlation coefficients of I.Q. with various criteria of educational and occupational attainment (Table 9.5-1). Although the validity coefficient for mental retardation is high, intellectual assessment demonstrating an extreme deviation in I.Q. is required for this diagnosis. Similarly, the impressive correlation between I.Q. and the ratings assigned by a panel of judges for the prestige of various occupations encompasses extremes (for example, from ditch digger to physician). In contrast, Table 9.5-1 shows relatively modest correlations between I.Q. score and job success (4 percent of the variance accounted for) or socioeconomic status (16 percent of the variance). Given the narrower range of intellectual functioning within occupations, it is clear that noncognitive variables such as motivation, personality, and employment opportunity are contributory.

RELIABILITY OF I.Q. SCORES Test-retest reliability (stability) in adults tends to be high for the Stanford-Binet and the Wechsler I.Q. scales. Reliability coefficients typically reach the .85 to .90 range. Retesting individuals 18 years and older rarely reveals marked changes in I.Q. which exceed the measurement error of the test. However, the test-retest reliability is somewhat lower over periods of several years. Caution about extrapolating from an I.Q. score obtained several years previously is especially warranted when the initial assessment was made during childhood because marked changes in I.Q. are more common in the pediatric age range.

On the average, the reliability coefficient for the WAIS is approximately .89 for Verbal I.Q., .85 for Performance I.Q., and .90 for Full Scale I.Q. In 1981, Wechsler reported that the reliability coefficients for the WAIS-R were .95, .94, and .89 for the Full Scale, Verbal Scale, and Performance Scale I.Q.s, respectively, in one sample; and .96, .97, and .90 in a second sample over a two- to seven-week retest interval.

CLINICAL INTERPRETATION OF VERBAL, PERFORMANCE, AND FULL SCALE I.Q.s The WAIS and WAIS-R comprise two major scales—Verbal and Performance. Subtests of the Verbal Scale include Information (range of general information), Comprehension (practical reasoning and interpretation of proverbs), Similarities (abstraction and verbalization of the properties common to objects), Arithmetic (calculation of problems presented aurally), Digit Span (repetition and reversal of series of numbers given vocally by the examiner), and Vocabulary (definition of words). The Performance Scale includes Digit Symbol (a timed visuomotor coding test), Picture Completion (identification of details missing in line drawings of familiar objects and living things), Picture Arrangement (sequential arrangement of cartoon drawings to depict a theme), Block Design (timed construction using mosaic blocks of designs conforming to pictures presented on cards), and Object Assembly (timed construction of puzzles).

The Verbal Scale largely reflects retention of previously acquired (and frequently overlearned) factual information. The Performance Scale emphasizes visuospatial capacity and visuomotor speed on relatively novel problems. Neurologically normal but culturally disadvantaged persons may obtain a relatively low Verbal I.Q. (for example, because of a limited range of information and vocabulary), while highly educated and widely read persons often have a particularly high Verbal I.Q. The Performance Scale is less dependent on formal education but appears to be more sensitive to normal aging. The discrepancy between Verbal I.Q. and Performance I.Q. is generally less than 15 points.

A correction for age is introduced into the calculation of both the Verbal Scale and the Performance Scale I.Q.s on the basis of the score distributions of normal subjects at different ages. Age-corrected standard scores are also available for each subtest, thereby facilitating intraindividual comparison of abilities. For example, the cognitive efficiency of a 70-year-old patient is evaluated in terms of Verbal, Performance, and Full Scale I.Q. scores which are corrected for age and by a profile of age-corrected standard scores on the subtests. Consequently, dementia is suspected when the Verbal I.Q. or the Performance I.Q. is significantly below expectation in view of the patient's estimated premorbid ability.

From a clinical standpoint, the Full Scale I.Q. derived from the WAIS-R (or its predecessors, the Wechsler-Bellevue and WAIS) is a moderately useful index of general intellectual impairment associated with cerebral disease, provided that other explanations (for example, depression, deficient motivation) for defective scores can be excluded. The Performance Scale I.Q. is about equal to the Full Scale I.Q. as a reliable predictor of the presence of cerebral damage.

Disproportionate impairment on the Verbal Scale is primarily associated with left hemisphere damage (assuming the patient is right-handed) when aphasic disorder is present, but this disparity is unimpressive in nonaphasic cases. Specific impairment on the Performance Scale occurs in patients with right hemisphere (particularly posterior) lesions whose relatively intact language and normal Verbal I.Q. often contrast with marked impairment of visuoconstructive ability (for example, block construction), neglect of the left visual field, and difficulty in visual guidance of movement. However, exceptions to the correspondence between the direction of the Verbal-Performance discrepancy and lateralization of brain injury are not rare, and additional testing is often necessary.

Parietal lobe lesions in either hemisphere can compromise visuospatial ability (especially on constructional tasks), and subtle right-sided hemiparesis can slow coding speed and thus lower the Performance I.Q. in a patient with left hemisphere disease. For reasons that are not entirely clear, conditions that produce diffuse cerebral disturbance or multifocal lesions (for example, closed head injury, dementia of the Alzheimer's type) frequently result in lower Performance I.Q. as compared to Verbal I.Q.

A striking Verbal-Performance disparity is illustrated by the WAIS results recorded about 18 months following the onset of dementia of the Alzheimer's type in a 58-year-old physician. He obtained a Verbal I.Q. of 100 (corresponding to the population mean but considerably below the estimated premorbid level) as compared to a Performance I.Q. of 66 (more than two standard deviations below the population mean). This wide Verbal-Performance discrepancy, which reflected the patient's complete failure to assemble even the simplest block design, was essentially unchanged when he was retested 12 and 16 months later. Manifestations of the patient's visuospatial impairment included topographic disorientation (for example, he would become lost while driving) and a subjective report of visual disturbance.

However, exceptions to this pattern, such as receptive language deficit during the early stage of dementia of the Alzheimer's type, have been documented. Positron emission tomography in patients with presumptive Alzheimer's disease and in normal subjects has disclosed that asymmetry in hemispheric metabolism corresponds differentially to specific cognitive functions; that is, left hemisphere metabolism was related to verbal skills, while right hemisphere metabolism was related to visuospatial ability.

A physical handicap, neurological deficit, abnormal behavior, or cultural differences may necessitate modification of standard testing procedures or substitution of other cognitive tests. Tests such as the Leiter Scale and Raven's Progressive Matrices (for deaf patients or patients with auditory agnosia), or the Peabody Picture Vocabulary Test (for patients unable or unwilling to speak or to cooperate with the WAIS) circumvent these limitations. Failure to recognize factors other than cognitive impairment that limit performance on specific standardized tests of intelligence may result in a spurious inference of subnormality or dementia.

EXECUTIVE FUNCTIONS

Decades ago, Kurt Goldstein emphasized that, regardless of specific intellectual defects, patients with cerebral disease are likely to show cognitive impairment of a general nature that he designated as "loss of the abstract attitude." He characterized the deficit as a loss of the capacity to reason abstractly and a lack of flexibility in problem solving or in adapting to changed situations. Goldstein particularly implicated frontal lobe disease in producing these deficits. Although later research failed to support that localization of lesion associated with impaired abstract reasoning, the role of frontal lobe pathology in compromising the use of feedback to guide behavior and to solve problems has gained wide acceptance.

TESTS OF EXECUTIVE FUNCTIONS Investigators have operationalized the capacity for concept formation primarily in respect to sorting tests. The first clinical application was the *color form sorting test,* in which the patient is presented with a random array of forms (square, circle, triangle) of different colors (blue, yellow, green, red) and asked to "put those together that belong together." The crucial feature of performance that is evaluated is whether or not the patient is able to sort the forms according to a clear principle, that is, by shape or color. If the patient succeeds, the forms are once again presented in a random array, and the patient is asked to "sort them in another way," interest being focused on whether or not the patient's approach is sufficiently flexible to shift the sorting strategy. That particular color form sorting test has proved in practice to be a relatively simple task that identifies only gross impairment in reasoning and problem solving.

Wisconsin Card Sorting Test The Wisconsin Card Sorting Test has proved to be more informative than earlier tests for assessing abstract reasoning and flexibility in problem solving. Stimulus cards differing in color, form, and number are presented to the patient for sorting into groups according to a principle preestablished by the examiner. As the patient sorts the cards, he or she is told whether the responses are correct or incorrect. The number of trials required to achieve 10 consecutive correct responses is recorded. When (or if) the patient has mastered the task, the examiner once again changes the principle of sorting, and the number of trials required to achieve correct sorting is recorded. The procedure is repeated a number of times, and measures of the capacity for abstract thinking (that is, the number of trials required to achieve a solution) and of flexibility in problem solving (that is, perseverative errors on successive sorting) are derived from the patient's performance. Two abbreviated versions of the Wisconsin Card Sorting Test are available: One version uses only the initial 64 of the 128 cards; the other version is reduced in length and ambiguity to enhance receptivity among elderly patients.

Figure 9.5-2 illustrates the sensitivity of the Wisconsin Card Sorting Test. It depicts the short form protocol of a 28-year-old mechanic who had sustained a midline frontal depressed fracture and left frontal subdural hematoma after a tire which he was repairing blew up. When the patient was tested 16 months after the injury, he had an excessive number of both perseverative and nonperseverative errors. Note his tendency to persist in a response strategy after the examiner has requested him to shift to a new principle of card sorting.

Patients who have undergone frontal lobe excisions for amelioration of epilepsy exhibit a more impressive deficit on the Wisconsin Card Sorting Test than do patients with posterior surgical lesions. The basis for their failure appears to be an excessive perseverative tendency (that is, rigidity in approach) rather than defective abstract reasoning per se. Researchers have shown that chronic schizophrenic patients exhibit impaired performance on the Wisconsin Card Sorting Test which is related to reduced cerebral blood flow in their frontal lobes, while differences in other cortical regions are less impressive. The hypofrontal pattern in the schizophrenic patients was specific to the Wisconsin Card Sorting Test; their cerebral blood flow was comparable to the control group values during performance of other tasks.

Early studies suggested that patients with frontal lobe damage may perform more poorly on the Wisconsin Card Sorting Test than do patients with focal nonfrontal damage. However, recent evidence based on neuroanatomical analyses of lesion location indicates that impaired performance is not specific to frontal lobe lesions and that patients with known frontal damage do not consistently show deficits on the task. No reliable correspondence has been found between performance on the Wisconsin Card Sorting Test and the site of lesion within the frontal region (for example, orbital versus dorsolateral pathology), thus indicating the need for caution in the use of the Wisconsin Card Sorting Test as a measure of frontal lobe damage.

Category Test of the Halstead-Reitan Battery The Category Test requires the patient to solve novel problems by selecting a relevant dimension, such as color or shape, in response to stimuli that are presented in a visual display. A booklet version has also been developed. Comparisons between the Booklet Category Test and the Wisconsin Card Sorting Test have shown that the two measures are not equivalent, and that selective impairment on the Booklet Category Test may reflect difficulties in processing novel or perceptually complex information.

Shipley Abstractions Test A self-administered paper and pencil measure of conceptual thinking, the Shipley Abstractions Test requires the patient to complete logical sequences. Correct responses to the Abstraction portion of the test demand a grasp of the underlying principles. Because performance on a test of that type is related to educational background, an accompanying vocabulary test is also given to the patient, and a comparison is made between performances on the two tests. A low abstraction score in relation to vocabulary level is interpreted as reflecting impairment in conceptual thinking.

Other tests Interpretation of proverbs is often included in the mental status examination.

The organizational aspects of problem solving are assessed by *maze tests.* Maze tests demand both temporal and spatial integration of behavior, while bringing into play such personal characteristics as planfulness and impulsivity. They have been found fairly effective in identifying patients with cerebral disease. However, the idea that a deficit on that type of task is specific to frontal lobe damage has not proved to be accurate. Patients with postrolandic lesions in the right hemisphere are likely to perform as poorly as those with frontal lesions.

SCORING SHEET FOR CARD-SORTING TEST – SHORT FORM

Card Number	Sorting Category	Errors	Card Number	Sorting Category	Errors
1	F		25	N	
2	N	X NP	26	N	
3	F		27	F	X NP
4	N	X NP	28	F	X P
5	N	X P	29	F	X P
6	F		30	F	X P
7	N	X NP	31	N	
8	N	X P	32	N	
9	N	X P	33	N	
10	N	X P	34	N	
11	N	X P	35	N	
12	F		36	N	
13	N	X NP	37	F	X NP
14	N	X P	38	N	X NP
15	N	X P	39	F	X NP
16	N	X P	40	F	X P
17	F		41	N	X NP
18	N	X NP	42	N	X P
19	F		43	N	X P
20	F		44	N	X P
21	F		45	N	X P
22	F		46	N	X P
23	F		47	F	X NP
24	F		48	F	X P

SORTING CATEGORY
C = Color
F = Form
N = Number

ERROR TYPE
NP = Nonperseverative
P = Perseverative
U = Unique

ERRORS

Cards used 36-48	48
Number of categories 0-6	2
Perseverative errors 0-48	18
Nonperseverative errors 0-48	11
Unique errors 0-48	00
Total number errors 0-48	29

FIGURE 9.5-2 *Modified card sorting protocol of a 28-year-old man who had sustained a left frontal subdural hematoma associated with a severe closed head injury (Glasgow Coma Scale score = 5) 18 months previously. The patient's task was to sort the cards correctly according to the initial principle (for example, form) for six consecutive cards and then to shift to a new sorting principle at the request of the examiner. Numerous perseverative errors (for example, continuing to sort according to the previous principle after the examiner has requested that he shift to a new strategy) are present. Although the patient sorted according to form initially, he failed to follow through with consecutive responses until trials 19 to 24. Correct sorting was limited to the categories form and number and color was omitted.*

MEMORY

TYPES OF MEMORY It is customary to distinguish between two types of memory: *immediate* or *short-term memory* (STM), which persists for up to 30 seconds (for example, forward digit span) and has a capacity limited to about seven plus or minus two chunks (or alternatives) of information; *long-term memory* (LTM), which involves the consolidation of the supraspan information into a relatively permanent store that is subsequently retrievable. *Remote memory* refers to retention of information about events in the distant past (that is, months or years ago). *Recent memory* (that is, retention of experience over hours or days) is usually evaluated by informal procedures concerning orientation or the patient's environment (for example, a breakfast menu).

Whether remote memory and recent memory are parts of a temporal continuum of long-term memory or are distinct types of memory is still debated. There is considerable evidence that long-term memory and remote memory are both biologically distinguishable and clinically dissociable from STM. Memory theorists have recently distinguished between *episodic memory* (for example, recalling a telephone message in a specific spatiotemporal context) and *semantic memory,* that is, overlearned information that becomes part of a knowledge base (for example, recalling the first president of the United States).

Immediate memory is often preserved in amnestic patients who are unable to learn and retain information beyond the limits of their forward digit span. Consequently, the finding of a normal digit span does not exclude the possibility of a memory deficit. Conversely, investigation of depressed patients has disclosed that they tend to exhibit disproportionate impairment of short-term memory relative to long-term memory. This dissociation presumably reflects the disruptive effects of rumination on attention as opposed to amnestic disorder.

In one study, patients hospitalized for depression also exhibited difficulty in encoding material as reflected by their underutilization of clustering related words and their failure to organize a word list as compared to normal controls. When information was presented in an organized or structured form, recall performance by depressed patients was normal. It was postulated that hypoarousal or disrupted activation mitigated the use of these active encoding strategies by depressed patients.

To explain the relatively preserved retention of motor skills in amnestic patients, investigators have proposed that procedural memory (knowing how) can be dissociated from declarative memory (knowing what), both in performance and in neural substrate. Investigators have shown that procedural memory is relatively preserved after electroconvulsive therapy (ECT) and in patients with dementia of the Alzheimer's type. The usefulness of these concepts for routine clinical memory testing remains an open question.

MEMORY TESTS Visual short-term memory is evaluated by having the patient draw designs after they have been removed from view (Figure 9.5-3). By comparing the accuracy of the patient's reproductions from memory to the results of copying a parallel form held in view, the examiner can determine whether or not nonmnemonic factors contribute to the patient's apparent memory failure. *Memory for designs tests* are more sensitive than immediate recall of digits as behavioral measures of brain damage, probably because the task of copying complex designs from memory makes demands on the perception of spatial relations and on visuographic skill as well as on attention

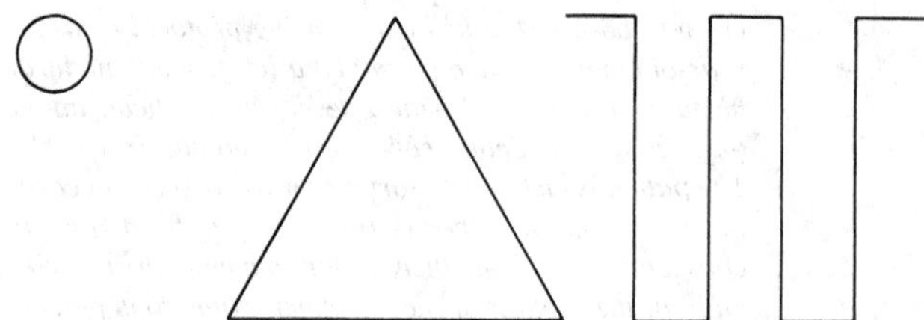

FIGURE 9.5-3 *Item from the Benton Visual Retention Test. The most frequent testing condition involves presenting each geometric figure for 10 seconds, after which the patient attempts to draw it from memory. (Figure from A B Sivan:* Benton Visual Retention Test: Clinical and Experimental Applications, *ed 5, p 23. Psychological Corporation, New York, 1992. Used with permission.)*

and immediate retention. Consequently, a patient's reproductions may be defective for one or more reasons.

Reproduction of designs from STM was one of three neuropsychological tests selected and cross-validated by a discriminant analysis of patients with dementia of the Alzheimer's type versus normal elderly people. Recent research has also shown that short-term visual memory on the Benton Visual Retention Test is impaired in schizophrenic patients with negative symptoms (that is, flat affect, asocial, inattentive) as compared to patients with only positive symptoms (for example, delusions, hallucinations).

Wechsler Memory Scale The Wechsler Memory Scale, modified in 1987 as the Wechsler Memory Scale-Revised (WMS-R), is the most widely used memory test battery for adults. The instrument comprises eight brief subtests of short-term learning and memory (involving paragraphs, paired associates, digit span, mental control, design reproduction, and figural recognition) and four subtests of long-term retention of verbal and figural material. Test items are preceded by a series of mental status questions to assess personal information and orientation. Two major composite scores are derived, yielding a general memory index and an attention-concentration index. The general memory index can be partitioned to provide composite scores for verbal and visual memory. Although factor analytic evidence does not support the distinction between verbal and visual memory, comparisons between subscores may be useful for patients with certain kinds of neurological dysfunction. The WMS-R does not assess all possible memory functions, such as biographical or procedural memory (that is, memory for learned skills), but it has the advantages of extensive normative data for people between 16 and 74 years of age, explicit scoring criteria for enhanced reliability, and transformation of scores (that is, with means and standard deviations of 100 and 15, respectively) to permit direct comparisons with WAIS-R I.Q.s.

The memory for paragraphs and mental control subtests were recently found to be among the most efficient neuropsychological measures in differentiating patients with mild senile dementia of the Alzheimer's type from normal subjects. However, many examiners and investigators prefer to employ specific tests of long-term memory that elucidate the component processes and strategies rather than to use the Wechsler Memory Scale.

Digit-learning tests A procedure that has been used occasionally in clinical and investigative work is assessment of a patient's capacity to learn a series of digits that is longer (supraspan) than his or her immediate span. The procedure provides a direct measure of learning and of long-term retention in contrast to digit span, which reflects immediate recall.

Instances have been reported of a marked disparity in performance in learning a series of digits just longer than the span. Many patients with brain disease have an unremarkable digit span (for example, six or seven digits) but are unable to learn an eight- or nine-digit span in 10 trials. Comparing forward digit span and the learning of a lengthy series of digits in patients with either known or presumed hippocampal dysfunction and in normal subjects, investigators found that there was no significant difference in digit span performance but that there was a significant difference in serial digit learning. In another study, the digit-learning procedure was used to investigate performance differences between older normal subjects and amnestic patients. The normal subjects performed unremarkably while the amnestic patients showed gross impairments. Administration of the anticholinergic drug scopolamine (Dramamine) has been found to produce a transient impairment of supraspan performance in young subjects, but it has a negligible effect on their digit span. Normative data have been published on a digit-learning task that has been standardized for clinical use.

Selective reminding tests Other verbal techniques to evaluate long-term memory include recall of word lists and recognition of words that are presented repeatedly. In a modified form of the usual recall procedure (presenting the complete list on each trial), the examiner selectively presents only those words that the patient has failed to recall on the preceding trial, that is, selective reminding.

Investigators have employed parallel forms of the selective reminding test to assess the effects of cholinergic (and other) medications on the memory deficit of patients with dementia of the Alzheimer's type. Figure 9.5-4 compares the retrieval from long-term memory in three Alzheimer's patients tested under conditions of baseline, lecithin alone, and the combination of physostigmine (Antilirium, Eserine) and lecithin. Long-term memory retrieval improved to within the range of age-matched controls under the combined physostigmine-lecithin condition.

Recent research has shown that schizophrenic patients with positive symptoms exhibited a more severe verbal memory deficit on the selec-

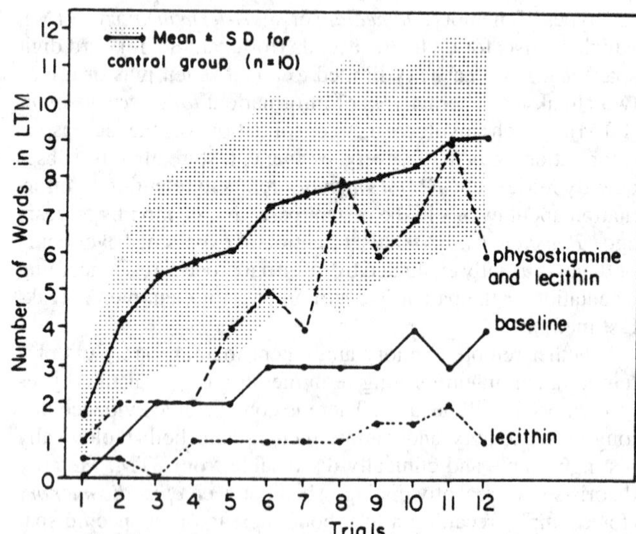

FIGURE 9.5-4 *Median number of words retrieved from long-term memory storage by three patients with dementia of the Alzheimer's type tested under conditions of baseline (no medication), subcutaneous injection of physostigmine combined with lecithin, and subcutaneous injection of a noncentrally active anticholinergic (placebo) drug combined with lecithin (indicated as lecithin in lower portion of graph). Parallel forms of the selective reminding test were employed in titration of the physostigmine dosage which preceded this randomized crossover trial. (Figure from B H Peters, H S Levin: Effects of physostigmine and lecithin on memory in Alzheimer's disease.* Ann Neurol 6: *219, 1979. Used with permission.)*

tive reminding test as compared to schizophrenic patients with primarily negative symptoms. In contrast, the direction of the group difference was opposite on a test of visual retention. Parallel forms of the selective reminding test are available for repeated assessment of memory.

Tests of verbal long-term memory The California Verbal Learning Test provides an opportunity to compare long-term memory under conditions of high and low interference. Effects of interference on verbal long-term memory have also been studied using the Rey Auditory Verbal Learning Test, whereas the relative involvement of short-term memory versus long-term memory in the Brown-Peterson distractor technique (that is, counting backwards before recall) has been debated.

Verbal long-term memory procedures facilitate the investigation of aiding recall by providing phonemic or semantic cues. Normative tables of word frequency and concreteness are available to develop parallel forms, but their equivalence must be tested directly. Specific or disproportionate impairment of verbal long-term memory accompanied by relatively preserved visuospatial long-term memory is characteristic of unilateral left hemisphere lesions.

In addition to helping detect deficits indicative of cerebral disease and evaluating the efficacy of treatment, interpretation of memory test findings based on normative data can be reassuring to patients complaining of forgetfulness, which may stem from diminished concentration, rumination, and mild depression. That fact is illustrated by the selective reminding protocol of a 41-year-old programmer who was referred for neuropsychological assessment by a neurologist because of her one-year history of memory problems and diminished work efficiency. The patient retrieved all 12 of the words by trial 7 (total consistent retrieval from long-term storage summed across 12 trials was 119 versus a mean of 113.4 and a standard deviation of 23.3 for normal adults of similar age). She correctly recalled all 12 of the words after a 30-minute delay. A detailed social history and personality assessment revealed that the patient frequently ruminated about marital problems and was mildly depressed, but that she had been reluctant to seek psychiatric treatment. The memory test findings not only reassured the patient but convinced her of the necessity for therapeutic intervention.

Tests of nonverbal memory Visuospatial material has generally been employed to test nonverbal memory using both recall and recognition procedures. The stimuli of these predominantly research tests have included faces, random designs, sequences of tapping an array of blocks, and pictures of objects. Specific impairment of visuospatial memory with relative sparing of verbal long-term memory is consistent with right hemisphere pathology.

Evaluation of long-term memory over long intervals (for example, days) is usually impractical in clinical testing. Some researchers found that patients with alcoholic Korsakoff's syndrome could recognize pictures presented a week earlier provided that the initial exposure duration far exceeded that given to normal subjects. More recent research has confirmed this normal rate of forgetting in Korsakoff's syndrome patients and in a patient with penetrating injury of the left dorsomedial nucleus of the thalamus, provided that the input duration was sufficiently long to compensate for their deficient initial learning. In contrast, this recognition procedure has disclosed rapid decay of memory in a patient with bilateral hippocampal lesions and in depressed patients following ECT. These distinctive forgetting functions have provided preliminary support for the differentiation of diencephalic type of amnesia (for example, Korsakoff's syndrome) from temporal lobe amnesia (for example, bilateral hippocampal lesions).

Tests of remote memory Retention of information from the remote past has been studied by testing recognition or recall of news events, titles of previously broadcast television shows, and photographs of persons who were prominent during a specific year or decade. These procedures have disclosed deficits in the remote memory of patients with Korsakoff's syndrome, of patients with amnestic disorders of other etiologies, and of depressed patients given ECT (a reversible deficit). However, those tests require pilot testing of normal subjects before widespread adoption because the assumption of previous exposure to the material may not be valid.

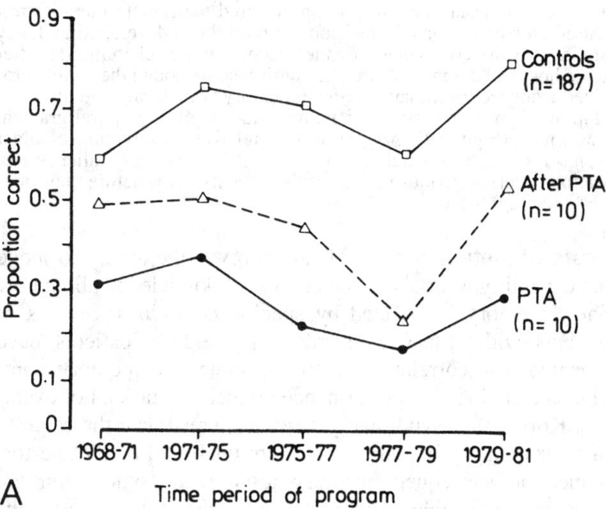

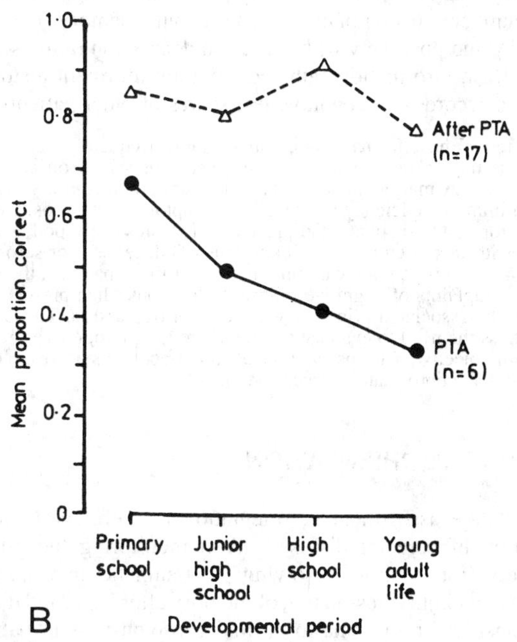

FIGURE 9.5-5 *A. Mean proportion of correct recognition of television program titles plotted against the time period of broadcast by patients with closed head injuries tested after resolution of posttraumatic amnesia (PTA) and by patients studied during PTA. Normal control subjects were studied for comparison.*
B. Mean proportion of correct recall of autobiographical information plotted against developmental periods for patients with head injuries in PTA and after PTA. The information was verified through interviews with a relative. (Figure from H S Levin, W M High, C A Meyers, A Von Laufen, M E Hayden, H M Eisenberg: Impairment of remote memory after closed head injury. J Neurol Neurosurg Psychiatry 48: *556, 1985. Used with permission.)*

In one study, remote memory impairment exhibited by Korsakoff's syndrome patients was shown to be characterized by a temporal gradient in which retention was relatively spared for the oldest information. Whether this finding reflects a progressive impairment of acquiring new information or retrograde memory loss is uncertain. In contrast, patients with dementia typically exhibit defective remote memory without a temporal gradient.

To investigate further the clinical observation of shrinking retrograde amnesia in closed head injured patients recovering from posttraumatic amnesia, the authors administered the remote memory test (based on recognition of television program titles) developed by Larry Squire and his colleagues to patients undergoing rehabilitation after acute hospitalization for closed head injuries. Although the results provided evidence for impaired remote memory both during and after resolution of posttraumatic amnesia, no evidence of a temporal gradient was found (Figure 9.5-5A). However, relative preservation of older memories was demonstrated on a recall test for personally salient information covering various periods of the patients' lives before their injuries (Figure 9.5-5B).

Tests of metamemory Metamemory is the ability to judge the capability of one's own memory and knowledge about how one's memory is affected by specific conditions. Studies of patients with amnestic disorders and elderly patients have revealed low correlations between subjective memory complaints and objective performance on memory tasks. For example, Korsakoff's syndrome patients underestimate the severity of their memory impairment and are unable to predict performance on subsequent memory tests, while other amnestic patients are capable of accurate and consistent memory self-ratings and prediction performance. Among normal elderly people, affective state is more closely related to self-ratings of memory than is objective memory performance. On the whole, the number of complaints made about memory correlate strongly and positively with scores on depression rating scales. In contrast, information gathered from an informant history is in close accord with cognitive test scores of older patients.

Depressed hospital patients complain more frequently of memory problems than patients with dementia; yet their scores on cognitive testing are only marginally lower than those of normal controls. Among human immunodeficiency virus (HIV) asymptomatic seropositive and HIV seronegative patients, the presence of depressive mood is associated with increased cognitive complaints, independent of serostatus or actual neuropsychological impairment. For those patients, the number of complaints of cognitive failures is low, but when present, they seem to be associated primarily with level of depression. Those findings stress the need to evaluate a patient's report of cognitive difficulties with objective neuropsychological and affective measures in order to formulate appropriate intervention tactics.

TEMPORAL ORIENTATION

Quantitative assessment of orientation is useful both in the detection of cerebral disease and in monitoring the rate of recovery (for example, resolving posttraumatic amnesia after closed head injury, restoration of memory after ECT, and during the transition from coma to normal consciousness in patients with metabolic, toxic, or vascular disorders). Using the schedule of questions shown in Table 9.5-2, for which data on control patients were obtained, defective performance was found in nearly one fourth of a group of patients with cerebral disease. Temporal disorientation was more common in patients with bilateral lesions (39 percent) as compared to groups with left hemisphere lesions (20 percent, excluding aphasic patients) or right hemisphere lesions (7 percent). In comparison with quantitative assessment, errors in the clinical judgment of orientation are generally of the false-negative type (that is, depicting a mildly disoriented patient as oriented times three). Temporal orientation is rather vulnerable to the influence of cerebral disease, and an objective assessment procedure can disclose a degree of disorientation that is rarely detected by the impressionistic methods typical of the routine clinical examination.

TABLE 9.5-2
Temporal Orientation Test

Questions
1. What is today's date? (The patient is required to give the day, month, and year.)
2. What day of the week is it?
3. What time is it now? (The examiner makes sure that the patient cannot look at a watch or clock.)

Scoring
A. Day of week: 1 point off for each day removed from the correct day
B. Day of month: 1 point off for each day removed from the correct day
C. Month: 5 points off for each month removed from the correct month
D. Year: 10 points off for each year removed from the correct year
E. Time of day: 1 point off for each 30 minutes removed from the correct time

Table from A L Benton, A B Sivan, K deS Hamsher, N R Varney, O Spreen: *Contributions to Neuropsychological Assessment: A Clinical Manual,* ed 2. Oxford University Press, New York, 1994. Used with permission.

ATTENTION AND VIGILANCE

Attention deficit can contribute to impaired performance on various neuropsychological tests, particularly learning and memory tasks. Attention is generally viewed as multidimensional, including selectivity, coherence (limiting the number of stimuli attended to), sustained monitoring of the environment (vigilance), and the capacity to shift attention. Impaired attention may be disproportionately affected in conditions such as closed head injury, metabolic and toxic disorders, epilepsy, and schizophrenia. Subcortical lesions may also lower the level of activation and diminish sustained attention. It has been suggested that the right parietal region integrates the various modalities of input and coordinates attention. Consistent with this view is the report that infarctions in the distribution of the right middle cerebral artery frequently cause a confusional state.

In view of the vulnerability of attention and concentration in cases of cerebral disease or of injury, it is remarkable that no battery of tests is generally available to assess various types of attention. Psychologists often use tests that were designed for other purposes. Integration of clinical observations with test data is essential to appreciate the salient features of attention deficit (for example, distractibility). Attention and information processing can be evaluated by a number of widely employed clinical procedures—for example, the Arithmetic, Digit Symbol (coding), and Digit Span subtests of the WAIS, WISC, the mental control section of the Wechsler Memory Scale, the Reitan Trail Making Test, and cancellation tests, in which the patient marks only designated letters (targets) interspersed with other letters (nontarget or distractor items) in lengthy sequences.

The Continuous Performance Test, an experimental task which involves rapid identification of a target and withholding responses to distractor stimuli, permits analysis of both the accuracy and latency of response. The Continuous Performance Test, which is one of the few tests designed to assess attention, has been widely employed in psychopharmacological research and in studies of attentional deficit in schizophrenic patients. An adjustive version of the Continuous Performance Test has been developed in which a microcomputer changes the rate of presentation according to the patient's performance. The shortest interstimulus interval at which responding is still accurate is the primary performance measure.

INFORMATION PROCESSING TASKS

Measures of information processing rate, which include the Paced Auditory Serial Addition Test and the serial subtraction of 7s, are derived from cognitive models of limited-capacity, effortful processes. Slowing of information processing may contrast with relatively preserved performance on untimed tests (for example, memory recall) or on tasks which require relatively low effort, such as attending to frequency of presentation.

Impaired serial addition is a frequent consequence of closed head injury and may be present for several weeks, even after an apparently mild injury. Although normal persons often make one or two errors on serial 7s, the inability to complete serial subtraction or making more than five errors is generally confined to patients with cerebral disease. Experimental investigations have employed vigilance tasks, in which a subject responds to the presence of an unpredictable recurring stimulus while ignoring other stimuli. Choice reaction time, that is, response to a button or key corresponding to a specific imperative stimulus which varies across trials, provides a measure of selective attention which can be compared to simple reaction time, that is, responding to the same button or key during each trial when an invariant stimulus comes on. The microcomputer permits convenient administration of these experimental tests, which were formerly tedious to administer.

Attention and vigilance tests are particularly useful in assessing patients who wish to return to an occupation in which reduced efficiency or impaired alertness would pose a safety hazard.

LANGUAGE FUNCTIONS

Clinical assessment of language and ideomotor praxis (that is, symbolic buccofacial and limb movements to exhibit gestures and to demonstrate the use of imagined or real objects) may yield findings suggestive of the locus of lesion without the aid of detailed testing. Demonstration of subtle language deficit, comparison of performance in different modalities (for example, visual versus tactile naming), and serial evaluation of recovery from aphasia are facilitated, however, by standardized, quantitative procedures. Standardized aphasia test batteries provide profiles of percentile scores of functions such as verbal fluency (retrieval of words beginning with a designated letter), repetition, naming, and receptive ability (Table 9.5-3). Writing and reading are usually also assessed. Language batteries, which permit intraindividual comparison and identify problems to be remediated in speech therapy, include the Boston Diagnostic Aphasia Battery, the Multilingual Aphasia Examination, the Neurosensory Center Comprehensive Examination for Aphasia, and the Western Aphasia Battery.

Language tests frequently disclose defects in word finding, naming, and the comprehension of complex commands that are not appreciated in patients without obvious aphasia. For example, verbal fluency has been reported to be one of a triad of neuropsychological tests which efficiently discriminate patients with dementia from normal controls. Several batteries provide correction for age, sex, and educational level, factors that are difficult to weigh in a brief clinical examination.

TABLE 9.5-3
Percentile Rank Scores of Four Aphasic Patients on Selected Tests of the Multilingual Aphasia Examination*

	Type of Aphasia			
Test	Broca's†	Wernicke's‡	Amnestic§	Conduction§
Visual naming	20	4	50	89
Sentence repetition	24	3	98	45
Word association	6	2	76	64
Oral comprehension	70	0	90	90
Reading comprehension	64	64	83	83

*Percentile rank scores based on the distribution of scores of a reference group of aphasic patients.
†Note the dissociation between levels of expression and comprehension in this patient.
‡Note the relative sparing of reading ability in this patient.
§Note the contrasting patterns of levels of naming and repetition in these patients.

Verbal fluency, or the ability to produce spontaneous speech without undue word finding difficulty, has been shown to be sensitive to the effects of left frontal and anterior bilateral hemisphere dysfunction. Measures of verbal fluency are used to detect subtle language problems that may arise, for example, in early dementia. Performance is typically evaluated by tabulating the number of words the patient produces within a restricted category (such as animals, first names, or words beginning with a certain letter) and time limit. Recent comparisons among fluency measures suggest that category fluency tasks (for example, animals, fruits, and vegetables) are superior to letter fluency tests in distinguishing dementia patients from normal elderly controls.

Language tests can also be useful in differential diagnosis of psychiatric disorders in patients with neurological complaints. A 49-year-old executive was referred for neuropsychological assessment because of a history of stammering speech and dysnomia which were episodic and associated with headaches. History of hypertension and a reported family history of Alzheimer's disease raised concern, as did the possibility of an epileptic basis for the patient's complaints. Although the patient initially had difficulty in naming line drawings on the Multilingual Aphasia Examination and his speech was occasionally halting, this appeared to be a manifestation of anxiety rather than aphasic disorder. Consistent with this interpretation, the patient achieved nearly a perfect performance on the Boston Naming Test administered later in the examination. This highly variable naming ability cast doubt on the likelihood of a left hemisphere abnormality to account for the patient's speech problems. The patient's electroencephalogram revealed no evidence of abnormal cerebral activity during an episode of halting speech.

Boston Naming Test The Boston Naming Test is a standardized procedure for naming pictures of objects that is graded in difficulty and available in parallel forms. Administration of the test has disclosed that anomic disturbance is frequently present in patients with dementia of the Alzheimer's type. The presence of dysnomia may be useful in discriminating cognitive abnormalities secondary to dementia from cognitive dysfunction associated with depression. Four equivalent abbreviated (15-item) versions of the Boston Naming Test have been developed for use in serial assessment protocols.

Boston Diagnostic Aphasia Examination The Boston Diagnostic Aphasia Examination includes a speech rating scale that is useful for comparing to test scores and a brief schedule of items for assessing ideomotor praxis. Spelling to dictation is tested by oral response, writing, and using block letters as part of the Multilingual Aphasia Examination.

Token Test The Token Test has proved a sensitive technique for detecting impairment in language comprehension, even in patients without clinically evident aphasic disorders. This test consists of oral commands of different levels of complexity to manipulate tokens that vary in shape, color, and size. The commands employ familiar words only, and the difficulty level is determined by the semantic content of the command (for example, "Put the small red circle on the large black square"). The Token Test can demonstrate impairment in verbal understanding not only in patients with clinically evident receptive aphasia, but also in patients with lesions of the left hemisphere who are not apparently aphasic on a mental status examination. In contrast, patients with lesions confined to the right hemisphere perform on a normal level (provided that the tokens are placed in the right visual field to mitigate neglect of the left visual field). Thus the test brings to light a latent or minimal aphasia in at least some ostensibly nonaphasic patients with disease of the hemisphere dominant for language.

Interpretation of receptive language performance on the Token Test is facilitated by concurrently examining verbal memory, the presence of visual (object and color) agnosia or neglect, and auditory screening to differentiate a receptive language deficit from failure secondary to memory or perceptual or sensory impairment. Axial commands not involving visual search and manipulation of objects (for example, "Look up," "Do birds fly?") are also useful to avoid misinterpretation of the Token Test and to determine the aspects of language comprehension that are preserved.

Test selection In practice, the examiner may select those subtests of an aphasia battery that are most relevant to the referral question. Modification of standard test administration and use of neurolinguistic tasks are also frequently necessary to examine the presence of a hemispheric disconnection syndrome (for example, writing and tactile letter identification with the nonpreferred hand) and to distinguish modality-specific anomia (for example, visual-verbal disconnection) from agnosia. Impairment of verbal learning and memory, which is a frequent residual of aphasia, should be investigated in follow-up examinations. Qualitative features (for example, clang associations) of nonaphasic, disturbed language in chronic schizophrenia can be useful in differentiating those patients from patients with left hemisphere structural lesions.

AFFECTIVE EXPRESSION AND PROCESSING IN RELATION TO HEMISPHERIC LATERALIZATION OF LESION

Review of the clinical literature on emotional manifestations of cerebral disease has revealed that pathological laughing, inappropriate euphoria, and mania are closely related to right hemisphere lesions, particularly involving the posterior region. In contrast, pathological crying is more strongly associated with left hemisphere disease. However, the relationship of lateralization and localization of brain infarct to poststroke depression has been inconsistent in recent studies. Bilateral lesions have been implicated in labile transitions from one emotional state to another.

Experimental studies on the evocation and identification of emotion in speech have disclosed that patients with right hemisphere lesions who exhibit visual neglect are frequently impaired in the expression and processing of affect. A double dissociation emerged whereby those patients performed above the level of patients with left hemisphere damage on tasks involving the semantic content of the same sentences. A serial study was conducted of a woman who sustained extensive right hemisphere injury in a motor vehicle accident 10 years earlier at the age of 26. Tape recordings of her speech showed, in contrast to well-preserved linguistic abilities, minimal variation in affect and prosody under conditions when she was asked to inject specific affective tones while reciting emotionally neutral sentences. Moreover, she had a corresponding deficit in identification of the affect expressed in tape recorded sentences. Impoverished affect was also evident in the patient's facial expression, whereas she exhibited appropriate social behavior. Similar differences between patients with left and right hemisphere damage have been reported for processing affective material presented visually. An implication of these studies for clinical practice is the possibility that right hemisphere disease should be considered in a differential diagnosis of patients exhibiting inappropriate or impoverished affect.

VISUOPERCEPTIVE CAPACITY

Many tests designed to disclose behavioral deficits associated with cerebral disease involve the processing and interpretation of visual information by the patient. For the most part, this emphasis on vision has been merely a matter of convenience, with the primary interest being the assessment of cognitive processes presumed to be independent of sensory modality. At times, however, the focus of interest may be on the status of higher level (essentially nonverbal) visual function, as contrasted to audition or somesthesis. These visual tasks are of a diverse nature; some assess complex visual discrimination; some assess the capacity to integrate visual information into meaningful percepts; others assess the ability to differentiate between figure and background; and still others require a search process necessary to select the design that matches a model or sample.

VISUAL FORM DISCRIMINATION The visual form discrimination test is used to establish the preservation of basic visual discrimination in patients who exhibit gross deficits on more complex tests. In giving visuocognitive tests, it is important to rule out defective visual acuity as a possible determinant of failing performance.

COMPLEX VISUAL DISCRIMINATION Although the inability to recognize familiar faces (prosopagnosia) is an uncommon disorder, defective discrimination of unfamiliar faces is a frequent finding in patients with right hemisphere or bilateral lesions. The Facial Recognition Test, in which the patient is required to identify a photograph of a face presented in a front view when it is included in various displays (for example, side view or front view with shadows) produces a high frequency of failure in patients with posterior right hemisphere lesions. Performance is generally intact in patients with left hemisphere lesions (provided that receptive language is not seriously limited) and in relatively acute schizophrenic patients. The percentage of cases with impaired performance in patients with focal lesions is shown in Table 9.5-4. Similar testing procedures (using complex stimuli other than faces) have also disclosed deficits in patients with unilateral right hemisphere damage.

COLOR DISCRIMINATION Determination of a patient's capacity for color perception is useful for both clinical and research purposes. The Ishihara and Dvorine plates involve identification of embedded numbers or lines that differ in hue from the background. An achromatic condition obtained by presenting black and white photocopies is a useful control to isolate the defect in color perception. The Farnsworth-Munsell Test involves sorting hues according to saturation. This lengthy test is not feasible for use with patients exhibiting severe cognitive

TABLE 9.5-4
Facial Recognition: Relative Frequency of Defective Performance in Patients with Focal Lesions

Group	Number of Subjects	Defect (%)
Normal subjects	286	3.5
Right anterior	23	26
Right posterior	36	53
Left anterior nonaphasic	15	0
Left posterior nonaphasic	14	0
Left anterior, aphasic without comprehension defect	5	0
Left posterior, aphasic without comprehension defect	8	0
Left anterior, aphasic with comprehension defect	17	29
Left posterior, aphasic with comprehension defect	27	44

Table from A L Benton, A B Sivan, K deS Hamsher, N R Varney, O Spreen: *Contributions to Neuropsychological Assessment: A Clinical Manual,* ed 2. Oxford University Press, New York, 1994. Used with permission.

deficit. Finally, color object matching requires the patient to select the characteristic color of a familiar object, such as a banana. These tests permit a distinction to be drawn between color agnosia and visual-verbal disconnection (for example, secondary to an infarction of the left posterior cerebral artery involving the splenium).

VISUOSPATIAL TESTS

Impairment in spatial thinking, as reflected in defective localization of objects in space, misjudgment of distance and direction, and defective geographic orientation, has long been regarded as a specific sign of disease of the right hemisphere. Numerous tests have been devised to probe for that type of deficit. One such test, the Judgment of Line Orientation Test, has been found to demonstrate failing performance in an impressive proportion of patients with right hemisphere disease. The test requires matching the slope of visually presented lines or pairs of lines. As depicted in Figure 9.5-6, the patient points to or verbally identifies the lines of the display that correspond to the angular orientation of each pair of lines. As with facial recognition, patients with right hemisphere lesions are frequently defective in visuospatial tests, while patients with left hemisphere disease perform within the normal range.

HIDDEN FIGURE AND FIGURE-GROUND TESTS The capacity to discriminate figure from background under conditions of stimulus competition is typically assessed by hidden, embedded, or mixed figure tests. Examples of the stimuli employed in hidden figure tests are shown in Figure 9.5-7. Performance on that type of task is determined by factors that transcend the visual modality, as indicated by researchers who found that defective figure-background discrimination is shown by patients with and without visual field defects and with lesions in any region of either cerebral hemisphere. However, impairment in performance was closely associated with aphasic disorder.

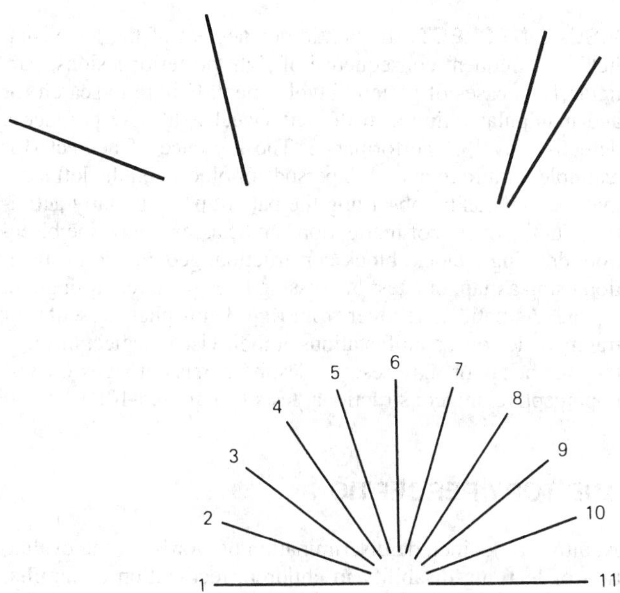

FIGURE 9.5-6 *Double-line stimuli which are matched to the multiple choice card below on the Judgment of Line Orientation Test. (Figure from A L Benton, A B Sivan, K deS Hamsher, N R Varney, O Spreen:* Contributions to Neuropsychological Assessment. A Clinical Manual, *ed 2. Oxford University Press, New York, 1994. Used with permission.)*

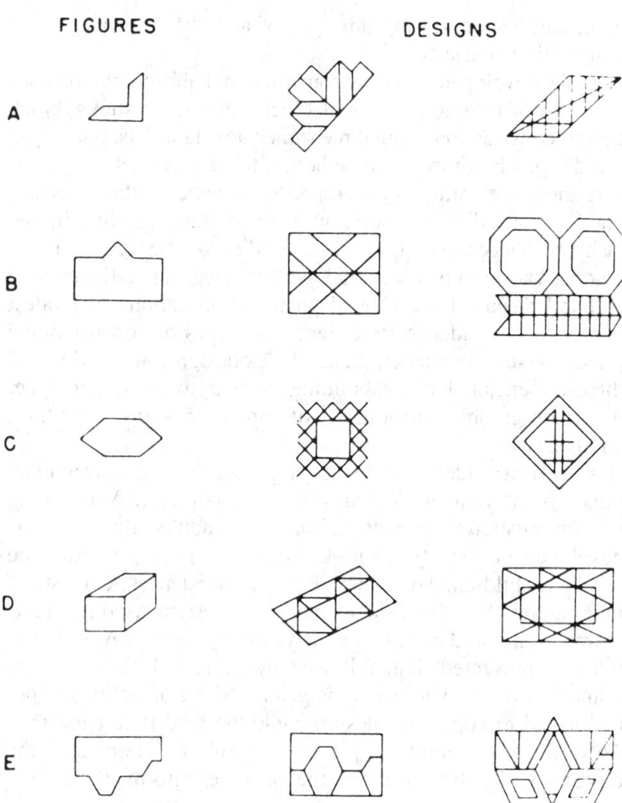

FIGURE 9.5-7 *Sample items from a hidden figures test. (Figure from M D Lezak:* Neuropsychological Assessment, p 363. *Oxford University Press, New York, 1983. Used with permission.)*

VISUAL MATRICES Raven's Progressive Matrices require the patient to select from a multiple choice pictorial display the stimulus that would complete a design in which a portion is omitted. The difficulty of the discrimination increases over trials in this lengthy test. A briefer, less difficult version (Colour Matrices) is especially useful for patients who are unable to complete the standard test, which can require 30 to 45 minutes. Impaired performance is associated with poor visuoconstructive ability and with posterior lesions of either hemisphere, but receptive language deficit may be contributory in patients with dominant hemisphere damage.

Raven's Progressive Matrices have also been employed to estimate intellectual level. In view of the modest correlation of performance with the WAIS I.Q., this practice is justified only in patients unable to take the WAIS, as in cases of bilateral motor weakness or non-English speakers. Estimates of WAIS-R Full Scale I.Q. have been reported for psychiatric patients using Matrices scores. Correlations range from 0.74 to 0.84, with predictions most accurate when age, educational level, and race are considered.

CONSTRUCTIONAL PRAXIS Constructional praxis refers to the assembly or articulation of parts to make a single entity or object. It entails a combinatory or organizing activity in which the relations among the component parts of the spatial entity must be appreciated if their synthesis is to be achieved correctly. Neurologists usually regard impairment in constructional praxis as a specific disability rather than simply as an expression of generalized mental defect. However, visuospatial and visuoconstructive deficits are frequently prominent during the early stages of dementia of the Alzheimer's type. Assessment of verbal skills and concept formation is necessary to exclude global mental deficit. Defective constructional performance is encountered fairly often in patients with cerebral disease, and tests assessing this type of activity merit a place in diagnostic batteries.

Tasks developed to assess constructional ability include construction of mosaic patterns of blocks, arranging sticks, block design construction using three-dimensional models, and copying designs by drawing. Whether all those tasks actually measure the same ability is uncertain. Some patients show considerable intra-individual variation in performance, failing in one task but succeeding in another. Studies of the interrelations among various constructional performances in patients with cerebral disease have yielded positive correlations of modest degree, with evidence for at least two types of constructional praxis. Assembling tasks, such as block design construction and three-dimensional block building, appear to form one type, while the graphic performance of copying designs constitutes another type.

The most widely employed graphic test of constructional praxis is the Bender (Visual Motor) Gestalt Test. Appropriate for administration to both children and adults, this test was developed in 1938 by Lauretta Bender to assess maturational levels in children. The material for the Bender test consists of nine figures (Figure 9.5-8) adapted from designs used by Wertheimer in his studies of Gestalt psychology. Design A in Figure 9.5-8 is presented first, followed by designs 1 through 8 in numerical order. The patient is given a sheet of unlined paper and asked to copy each design while the card is left in view. To evaluate the ability to plan the spatial arrangement of the designs on the sheet of paper, the examiner informs the patient that nine designs will be presented. There is no time limit. Availability of normative data, including a manual developed in 1963, facilitates the interpretation of this measure of visuoconstructive ability.

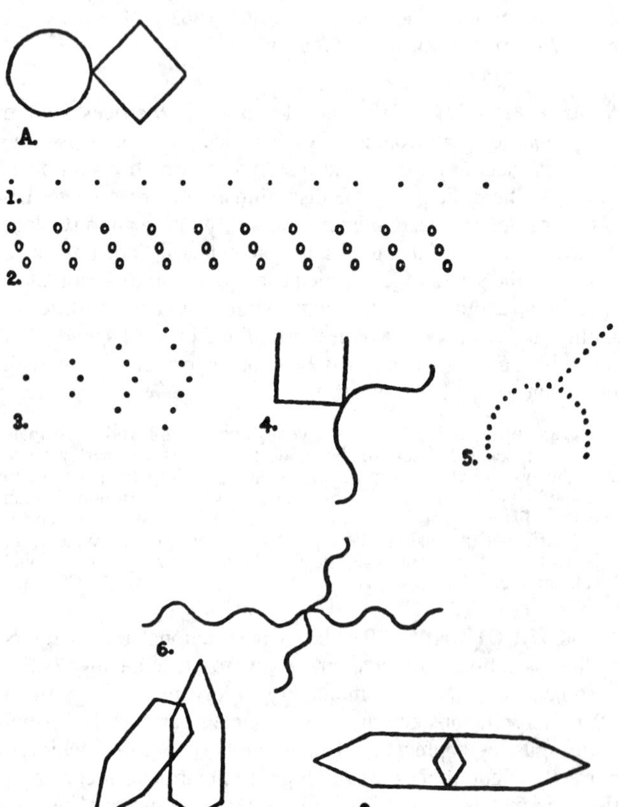

FIGURE 9.5-8 *Designs comprising the Bender (Visual Motor) Gestalt test. (Figure from L Bender:* A Visual Motor Gestalt Test and Its Clinical Use, p 4. *American Orthopsychiatric Association, New York, 1938. Used with permission.)*

Maturational changes in visuoconstructive ability are reflected in Figure 9.5-9, which depicts the percentage of children who produced the level of response depicted or better. Instances in which correct production of the design occurred are denoted by a blank box. For example, 95 percent of 11-year-old children correctly copy Designs A, 1, and 4. Note that adults typically copy all figures correctly with the exception of Design 1.

Clinicians often test the patient's reproduction of the Bender designs from memory after an interval of 45 to 60 seconds. Although this procedure can be useful in revealing a memory problem which would be undetected by the copying condition, it is advisable to confirm any suspicion of a memory deficit by administering procedures which are specifically designed for this purpose and have adequate normative data for evaluating retention.

Impairment in constructional performance is one of the most prominent deficits in patients with right hemisphere lesions. Visuoconstructive deficit is most commonly present in patients with posterior lesions, but right frontal lesion sites have also been reported in affected cases. As noted for visuoperceptive deficit, impaired constructional performance by patients with left hemisphere damage is usually associated with aphasia. Consequently, a relatively specific visuoconstructive deficit in a nonaphasic patient is consistent with a nondominant hemisphere lesion. Qualitatively distinct errors in constructional performance have also been implicated in right versus left hemisphere damage. Two types of errors in constructing block designs from three-dimensional models are primarily (if not exclusively) found in patients with documented cerebral disease. These errors include the closing-in phenomena, which refers to the patient utilizing part of the model to be copied in making his or her construction (Figure 9.5-10A). Partial or total failure to build the left half of the construction is indicative of unilateral spatial inattention or neglect associated with right hemisphere disease (Figure 9.5-10B). In contrast, global impairment of both visuospatial and verbal abilities is associated with bilateral or diffuse cerebral disease.

VISUAL NEGLECT Inattention or neglect of the left visual field is a frequent consequence of right posterior lesions, particularly in cases of parietal involvement. Failure to search for and manipulate stimuli in the left visual field may produce a defective level of performance. The presence of neglect (for example, failure to attend to persons or objects on the left side) may be obvious by observing the patient perform daily activities, but the degree of inattention can be assessed by line bisection, drawing a clock, block construction, geographic localization using a map, or a test of crossing lines scattered throughout a page. As patients recover from right hemisphere vascular or traumatic lesions, manifestations of their visual neglect in spontaneous behavior may resolve despite persistent signs on visuoperceptive and constructional tests (Figure 9.5-10B).

AUDITORY PERCEPTION

Auditory tasks include discrimination of words for the evaluation of learning disability in children, recognition of familiar nonverbal sounds to assess auditory agnosia, and appreciation of rhythm and tonal memory on the Seashore Test. Specific impairment of judgment of rhythm and tonal memory has been associated with right temporal lobe lesions.

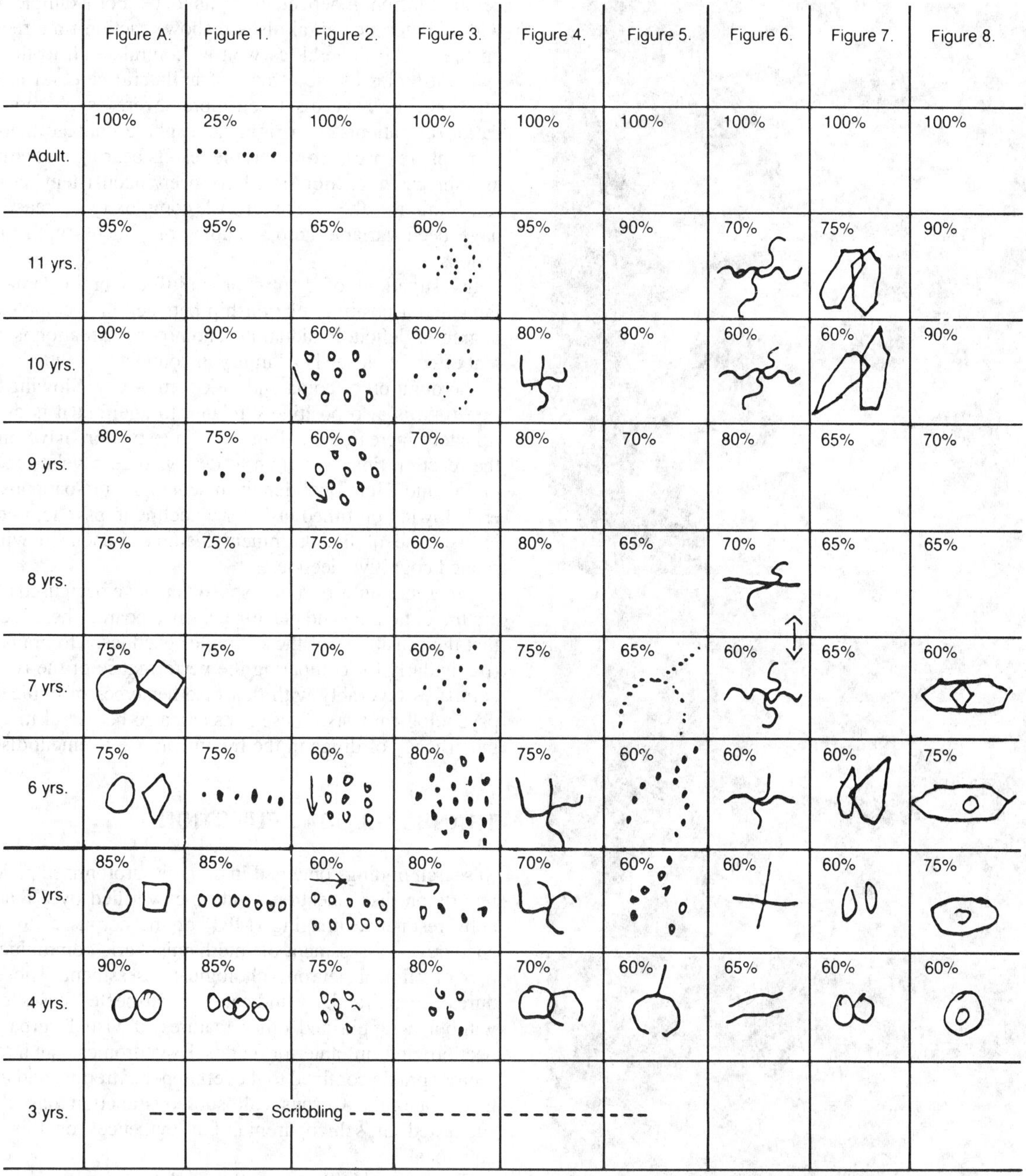

	Figure A.	Figure 1.	Figure 2.	Figure 3.	Figure 4.	Figure 5.	Figure 6.	Figure 7.	Figure 8.
Adult.	100%	25%	100%	100%	100%	100%	100%	100%	100%
11 yrs.	95%	95%	65%	60%	95%	90%	70%	75%	90%
10 yrs.	90%	90%	60%	60%	80%	80%	60%	60%	90%
9 yrs.	80%	75%	60%	70%	80%	70%	80%	65%	70%
8 yrs.	75%	75%	75%	60%	80%	65%	70%	65%	65%
7 yrs.	75%	75%	70%	60%	75%	65%	60%	65%	60%
6 yrs.	75%	75%	60%	80%	75%	60%	60%	60%	75%
5 yrs.	85%	85%	60%	80%	70%	60%	60%	60%	75%
4 yrs.	90%	85%	75%	80%	70%	60%	65%	60%	60%
3 yrs.	Scribbling								

FIGURE 9.5-9 *Percentage of children who could produce the level of response shown or better in copying the figures on the Bender (Visual Motor) Gestalt Test. Note the progressive maturational changes as reflected by increased ability to accurately reproduce the designs. (Figure from L Bender:* A Visual Motor Gestalt Test and Its Clinical Use, p 5. *American Orthopsychiatric Association, New York, 1938. Used with permission.)*

SOMATOSENSORY PERCEPTION

Somatosensory perception can be assessed by the Tactual Performance Test, which involves assembly of a form board in the absence of vision. The Tactual Performance Test is one of the most sensitive tests comprising the Halstead Reitan Battery. Tactile thresholds in patients with lesions involving parietal cortex may be assessed by stimulation with filaments of graded thickness. Tactile form perception can be evaluated by presenting a series of textured geometric designs to each hand in the absence of visual cues and asking the patient to identify the corresponding design presented in a multiple choice visual format. Protocols for localization of single and double simultaneous tactual stimulation of the fingers and right-left discrimination have been developed to detect cerebral disease, particularly of the parietal lobes.

PSYCHOMOTOR FUNCTIONS

A salient neurobehavioral effect of cerebral disease is slowness both in initiating behavior and in responding to external stimuli. In one study, for example, 40 percent of a group of brain-damaged patients were retarded in either simple reaction time (for

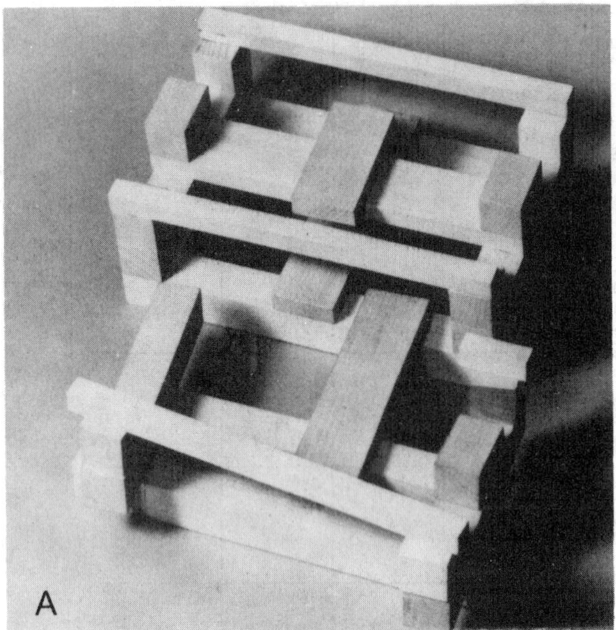

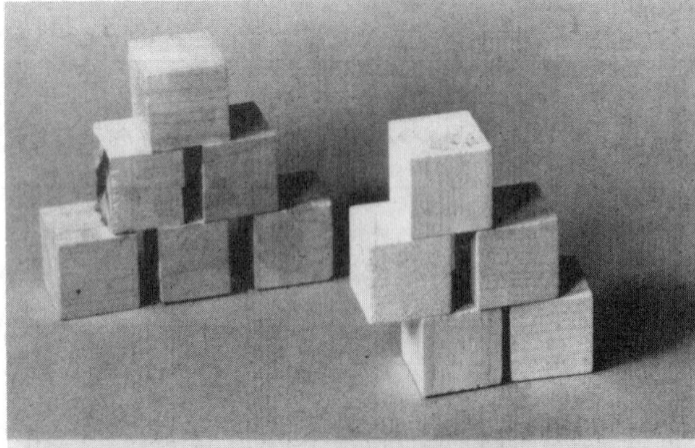

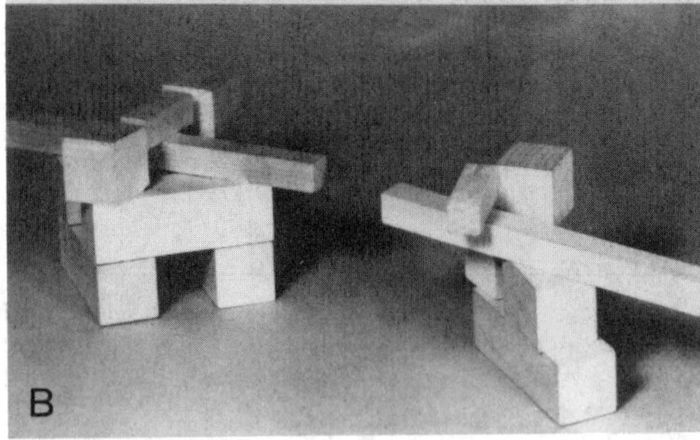

FIGURE 9.5-10 *Examples of "closing-in" error (A) and neglect of left side (B) on the three-dimensional constructional praxis test. (Figure from A L Benton, A B Sivan, K deS Hamsher, N R Varney, O Spreen:* Contributions to Neuropsychological Assessment, *ed 2,* p 121. *Oxford University Press, New York, 1983. Used with permission.)*

example, pushing the same button or key to the onset of the same stimulus each trial) or choice reaction time (for example, pushing the button or key corresponding to the onset of one of several randomly selected lights). Significant retardation is defined here as a response speed exceeded by 95 percent of control patients. Moreover, retardation in reaction time appears to reflect the presence (and possibly the size) of a cerebral lesion, independent of its locus. For example, patients with unilateral cerebral disease show reaction time retardation on the side ipsilateral, as well as contralateral, to the side of lesion. Studies of the effects of unilateral cerebral lesions on reaction time have disclosed more severe psychomotor retardation in patients with right hemisphere damage than in left hemisphere cases. However, the results bearing on hemispheric asymmetry in reaction time have been inconsistent across studies. Similarly, the effects of task complexity on reaction time have been variable across studies of patients with unilateral lesions.

Investigations of diffuse or multifocal brain damage have indicated a positive relationship between task complexity and degree of deficit. Residual psychomotor retardation is a persistent effect of closed head injury in young adults which is related to the duration of coma and task complexity. Slowing of reaction time is also positively related to age, but it is disproportionately increased by dementia. Investigators have employed the reaction time paradigm to demonstrate psychomotor retardation and attentional deficit in schizophrenic patients. A general slowing on timed tasks or a decline in psychomotor speed is also one of the prominent features associated with HIV-related cognitive decline.

Other measures of motor speed that have been used clinically are finger tapping and placing pegs in a board. There is evidence that the sensitivity of these simple speed tasks to brain damage (particularly for comparing the performance of the two hands) compares favorably with that of other types of clinical neuropsychological tests. These tests can also be useful in assessing the efficacy of drugs in the treatment of movement disorders.

TRANSCALLOSAL FUNCTION

Research findings obtained in commissurotomized patients and reports on disconnection syndromes verified by CT and magnetic resonance imaging (MRI) of the corpus callosum have encouraged assessment of interhemispheric communication as part of clinical neuropsychological assessment. Those procedures are particularly indicated in suspected cases of alexia without agraphia and other features of visual verbal disconnection and in anterior callosal syndromes, such as ideomotor apraxia confined to the left upper extremity and unilateral tactile anomia. Corpus callosum dysfunction has also been suggested in schizophrenia, but evidence for this view is equivocal.

Figure 9.5-11 illustrates the modalities and tasks employed to study the effects of commissurotomy. Similar procedures have also been used to evaluate patients with alexia without agraphia arising from occlusion of the left posterior cerebral artery or surgical division of the splenium. As depicted in Figure 9.5-11, naming objects explored by the left hand without the aid of vision and duplication of hand gestures (shown to the ipsilateral visual field or passively formed by the examiner) by the contralateral hand depend on the integrity of the anterior callosal pathways.

Tachistoscopic presentation of visual information to each visual field is employed to evaluate the capacities of the contralateral hemisphere for processing linguistic and emotive information in commissurotomized patients. Dichotic listening (that is, simultaneous presentation of competing auditory input to the two ears) may disclose markedly reduced monitoring of verbal information presented to the left ear when the corpus callosum is interrupted. This technique has been used to investigate the efficiency of right hemisphere functioning before and after treatment for depression, an illness which has been linked

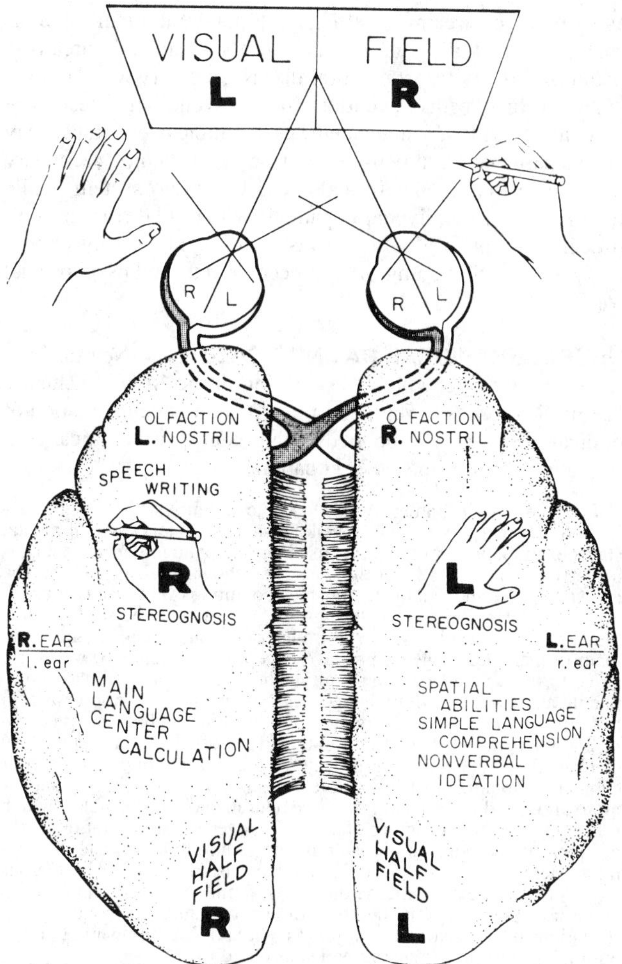

FIGURE 9.5-11 *Effects of commissurotomy on separation of neurological functions. This illustration is based on cortical lesion data and the results of studies of split-brain patients. (Figure from R W Sperry: Lateral specialization in the surgically separated hemispheres. In* Hemispheric Specialization and Interaction, *B Miller, editor. p 72. MIT Press, Cambridge, 1975. Used with permission.)*

to nondominant hemisphere dysfunction. The assessment of callosal functioning by neurobehavioral methods has recently been extended to diverse problems, including traumatic injury to the corpus callosum, interhemispheric communication in psychiatric disorder, and agenesis of the callosum.

NEUROPSYCHOLOGICAL TEST BATTERIES

HALSTEAD-REITAN BATTERY The basic battery in its present form consists of the following five tests:

1. *Category Test.* A test of abstract reasoning and hypothesis testing, in which the subject has to discover through trial and error the correct principle (for example, number, spatial position) embodied in successive presentations of pictorial stimuli. The correct principle is changed across seven subtests.
2. *Tactual Performance Test.* The subject is required to place the variously shaped blocks of the Seguin-Goddard Form Board without the aid of vision. Time taken to place the blocks is the critical response measure. An incidental test of retention follows in which the subject is required to draw the board from memory. The number of blocks correctly drawn is the memory response measure. A spatial localization measure is derived from the accuracy of drawing the relative positions of the blocks from memory. The Tactual Performance Test is presumed to assess several abilities, including motor speed, use of tactile and kinesthetic cues, learning, and incidental memory (no forewarning is given that the drawing test follows).
3. *Rhythm Test.* Adapted from Seashore's Test of Musical Talent, the Rhythm Test requires the subject to judge whether two auditory rhythmic patterns (30 pairs) are the same or different. The Rhythm Test is interpreted as a measure of nonverbal auditory perception, attention, and sustained concentration.
4. *Speech Sounds Perception Test.* The subject is required to identify spoken nonsense syllables from four visually presented alternatives. This test assesses auditory-verbal perception, attention, and concentration.
5. *Finger Oscillation.* The subject taps a mechanical counter at maximum speed for 10 seconds per trial with the index finger of each hand. Absolute motor speed and right-left asymmetries are measured.

Scoring The Halstead-Reitan Battery yields seven scores from which an Impairment Index is derived by adding the number of defective scores (based on normative data) and dividing by seven. Additions to this core examination include the Trail Making Test, which measures the time required to draw a line between scattered circles in an alphabetic (Trail A) or an alphanumeric (Trail B) sequence; various modifications of the Aphasia Screening Test of Halstead and Wepman, a somatosensory examination including finger gnosis, graphesthesia, stereognosis, and double simultaneous stimulation; and a measure of grip strength using a dynamometer. The Wechsler Memory Scale or other memory tests are also commonly administered because the Halstead-Reitan Battery is limited in this respect to an incidental recall trial on the Tactual Performance Test.

The Halstead-Reitan Battery has the advantage of providing a uniform profile of scores that must be weighed against the considerable time required for administration. Although the results adequately differentiate brain-damaged from neurologically intact persons, the differential diagnosis of psychiatric versus neurological disorder is unimpressive. Specifically, schizophrenic patients tend to perform above the level of subacutely brain-damaged patients but no differently from chronic brain-damaged groups. Moreover, the pattern of deficits on the HRB is similar in brain-damaged and schizophrenic patients. It should be noted that similar conclusions have emerged when other tests have been subjected to studies attempting to discriminate schizophrenic patients from patients with confirmed brain damage. In point of fact, neuropsychological tests are more useful for neurobehavioral investigations of schizophrenia than in routine differential diagnosis. The brief tests of sensory and motor function on the HRB appear to contribute to the assessment of lateralization of lesion, but the degree to which other components contribute information beyond the WAIS results is uncertain.

LURIA'S NEUROPSYCHOLOGICAL INVESTIGATION

Anna-Lise Christensen has developed a set of materials comprising a text, manual of instructions, and test cards that represent the techniques employed by Alexander Luria and his conceptualization of cortical functions. The procedures have been reorganized into 10 sections according to specific functions (for example, motor, sensory, visual, language skill). Items are also derived from standardized tests such as Kohs blocks and hidden figures used by Luria and from the mental status examination (for example, digit span, serial sevens).

The complex motor tasks developed by Luria are particularly innovative and are least redundant with other neuropsychological tests. The motor tests include commands requiring the patient to make a hand response that is the alternate of the examiner's hand movement (for example, "Tap once when the examiner taps twice"); a "go-no-go" discrimination (for example, "Squeeze the examiner's hand at the word red; do nothing at the word green"); alternating commands (for example, "Raise the right hand in response to one signal, the left hand to two signals"). This test battery has other unique features, including detailed assessment of arithmetic and short-term memory for hand postures.

Christensen's adaptation of Luria's methods is a potentially useful adjunct to the clinical neuropsychological examination, particularly in respect to motor integration. Although many of the tests are not sufficiently difficult to detect subtle deficit, they can be used with severely impaired patients. Insufficient normative data and omission of tests of functions such as verbal memory discourage total reliance on this battery.

LURIA-NEBRASKA NEUROPSYCHOLOGICAL BATTERY The Luria-Nebraska battery incorporates the items and the categories in Christensen's manual. These scales include: motor, rhythm, tactile (cutaneous and kinesthetic), visual (spatial), receptive and expressive speech, writing, reading, arithmetic, mnestic, and intellectual. An additional pathognomonic scale consists of the items drawn from the other scales found to be maximally sensitive to brain dysfunction. Right and left hemisphere scales, reflecting items that measure unilateral sensorimotor function, are included. In practice, a profile of transformed standard scores (after correction for age and education) is used to interpret the patient's performance.

The adaptation and modification of a portion of the techniques employed by Luria (as compiled by Christensen) and standardization for clinical use have raised methodological questions.

BRIEF COGNITIVE TESTS

In response to pressure for rapid cognitive evaluation, or screening, and increased awareness of the age-related prevalence of dementia, there has been a proliferation of brief tests (10 to 30 minutes) that purportedly provide an estimate of intellectual level. Many of the procedures are designed to assess cognition in normal elderly subjects or to provide a measure of the severity of dementia in the presenium or senile periods. The Mini-Mental State and the Mattis Dementia Rating Scale yield a single score as an index of cognitive impairment and include assessment of verbal, visuospatial, and mnemonic functions. Those measures are useful for monitoring the course of moderate to severe dementia in patients who might not be otherwise testable. However, the brief cognitive tests lack the age-based standardization across their various subtests and range of difficulty necessary for the initial evaluation of older persons suspected of an incipient dementia. The claims of a strong correlation between scores on brief cognitive tests and on the WAIS (or WAIS-R) are based primarily on patients exhibiting obvious deterioration or on studies with insufficient sample sizes. Moreover, excessive false-positive errors have been reported for elderly persons with low levels of education, while false-negative errors may occur in detection of right hemisphere pathology. Provided that the clinician is aware of the limitations of these procedures, they can serve as useful screening tests. Recognition of the limitations associated with global measures of cognitive decline has led to the development of multi-dimensional instruments for cognitive screening.

RATING SCALES

Qualitative features of patients' behavior during neuropsychological testing and an interview can provide clinically useful information with respect to differential diagnosis and serial assessment of treatment efficacy. Behavioral manifestations such as distractibility, inaccurate self-appraisal, and unrealistic planning, which reflect cerebral disease or injury, can be difficult to evaluate with conventional neuropsychological tests. The structure provided by many neuropsychological techniques may enable patients to compensate for behavioral changes secondary to focal lesions in the frontal lobes or limbic system, while findings may be equivocal in patients with mild diffuse or multifocal cerebral insult. In contrast, such patients may exhibit maladaptive functioning in their occupational and psychosocial roles.

NEUROBEHAVIORAL RATING SCALE The Neurobehavioral Rating Scale, which is a revision of the Brief Psychiatric Rating Scale, was developed to facilitate the documentation of clinical observations obtained during neuropsychological testing, interviewing, and other situations.

In a study of 101 patients with closed head injuries of varying severity and chronicity who were given a structured interview and mental status examination, investigators used a principal components analysis to derive four factors from the 27 scales shown in Table 9.5-5. The investigators found that the factors metacognition (the capacity for self-evaluation of abilities, monitoring and regulating impulses, and formulating realistic plans), cognition-energy (conceptual organization, memory), and language (expressive, receptive, articulation) were sensitive to the severity of brain injury. The fourth factor, somatic complaints-anxiety, tended to be equally or even more impressive in patients who had sustained relatively mild injuries. Follow-up neurobehavioral data based on ratings obtained at least six months postinjury confirmed that the most severely injured patients exhibited greater conceptual disorganization, inaccurate self-insight, diminished initiative-motivation, and poor planning. These neurobehavioral sequelae, which reflected difficulty in interpretation of proverbs, perseveration, difficulty in filtering tangential material, and failure to appreciate the cognitive defects resulting from injury, have been shown in numerous studies to impose an immense burden on family members and to result in chronic disability. Whether the profile of qualitative behavioral manifestations of traumatic brain injury is distinctive as compared to other etiologies of brain damage remains unsettled.

Global staging scales, such as the Global Deterioration Scale (GDS) and the Clinical Dementia Rating, provide an index of the severity of symptoms in Alzheimer's-associated dementia. Although both measures are similar in describing the middle stages of dementia, the Global Deterioration Scale provides better differentiation in the normal to early impairment range and better delineation in the most severe range.

FUNCTIONAL ASSESSMENT

In keeping with trends toward integration of cognitive measures and behavioral competency in everyday living, a variety of scales have been developed for characterizing the level of everyday functioning. Current criteria require evidence of functional impairment in social and occupational domains as a prerequisite to a diagnosis of dementia. Further, a decline in functional abilities has practical implications for caregiving assistance and decisions about institutionalization. These measures surveyed typically rely on informant reports and serve to augment dementia-related diagnostic decisions. Table 9.5-6 provides a summary of the functional domains tapped by the various instruments.

BLESSED DEMENTIA SCALE The Blessed Dementia Scale (BDS) is a 22-item behavioral rating scale that was originally introduced to quantify the cognitive and behavioral symptoms of dementia. Ratings are based on information obtained from family members concerning the person's functioning over the

TABLE 9.5-5
Neurobehavioral Rating Scale

DIRECTIONS: *Place an X in the appropriate box to represent the level of severity of each symptom.*	Not Present	Very Mild	Mild	Moderate	Mod. Severe	Severe	Extremely Severe
1. INATTENTION/REDUCED ALERTNESS—fails to sustain attention, easily distracted, fails to notice aspects of environment, difficulty directing attention, decreased alertness.	□	□	□	□	□	□	□
2. SOMATIC CONCERN—volunteers complaints or elaborates about somatic symptoms (e.g., headache, dizziness, blurred vision) and about physical health in general.	□	□	□	□	□	□	□
3. DISORIENTATION—confusion or lack of proper association for person, place, or time.							
4. ANXIETY—worry, fear, overconcern for present or future.	□	□	□	□	□	□	□
5. EXPRESSIVE DEFICIT—word-finding disturbance, anomia, pauses in speech, effortful and agrammatic speech, circumlocution.	□	□	□	□	□	□	□
6. EMOTIONAL WITHDRAWAL—lack of spontaneous interaction, isolation, deficiency in relating to others.	□	□	□	□	□	□	□
7. CONCEPTUAL DISORGANIZATION—thought processes confused, disconnected, disorganized, disrupted; tangential social communication; perserverative.	□	□	□	□	□	□	□
8. DISINHIBITION—socially inappropriate comments and/or actions, including aggressive/sexual content, or inappropriate to the situation, outbursts of temper.	□	□	□	□	□	□	□
9. GUILT FEELINGS—self-blame, shame, remorse for past behavior.	□	□	□	□	□	□	□
10. MEMORY DEFICIT—difficulty learning new information, rapidly forgets recent events although immediate recall (forward digit span) may be intact.	□	□	□	□	□	□	□
11. AGITATION—motor manifestations of overactivation (e.g., kicking, arm flailing, picking, roaming, restlessness, talkativeness).	□	□	□	□	□	□	□
12. INACCURATE INSIGHT AND SELF-APPRAISAL—poor insight, exaggerated self-opinion, overrates level of ability and underrates personality change in comparison with evaluation by clinicians and family.	□	□	□	□	□	□	□
13. DEPRESSIVE MOOD—sorrow, sadness, despondency, pessimism.	□	□	□	□	□	□	□
14. HOSTILITY/UNCOOPERATIVENESS—animosity, irritability, belligerence, disdain for others, defiance of authority.	□	□	□	□	□	□	□
15. DECREASED INITIATIVE/MOTIVATION—lacks normal initiative in work or leisure, fails to persist in tasks, is reluctant to accept new challenges.	□	□	□	□	□	□	□
16. SUSPICIOUSNESS—mistrust, belief that others harbor malicious or discriminatory intent.	□	□	□	□	□	□	□
17. FATIGABILITY—rapidly fatigues on challenging cognitive tasks or complex activities, lethargic.	□	□	□	□	□	□	□
18. HALLUCINATORY BEHAVIOR—perceptions without normal external stimulus correspondence.	□	□	□	□	□	□	□
19. MOTOR RETARDATION—slowed movements or speech (excluding primary weakness).	□	□	□	□	□	□	□
20. UNUSUAL THOUGHT CONTENT—unusual, odd, strange, bizarre thought content.	□	□	□	□	□	□	□
21. BLUNTED AFFECT—reduced emotional tone, reduction in normal intensity of feelings, flatness.	□	□	□	□	□	□	□
22. EXCITEMENT—heightened emotional tone, increased reactivity.	□	□	□	□	□	□	□
23. POOR PLANNING—unrealistic goals, poorly formulated plans for the future, disregards prerequisites (e.g., training), fails to take disability into account.	□	□	□	□	□	□	□
24. LABILITY OF MOOD—sudden change in mood which is disproportionate to the situation.	□	□	□	□	□	□	□
25. TENSION—postural and facial expression of heightened tension, without the necessity of excessive activity involving the limbs or trunk.	□	□	□	□	□	□	□
26. COMPREHENSION DEFICIT—difficulty in understanding oral instructions on single or multistage commands.	□	□	□	□	□	□	□
27. SPEECH ARTICULATION DEFECT—misarticulation, slurring or substitution of sounds which affect intelligibility (rating is independent of linguistic content).	□	□	□	□	□	□	□

Table from H S Levin, W M High Jr, K E Goethe, R A Sisson, J E Overall, H M Rhoades, H M Eisenberg, Z Kalisky, H E Gary Jr: The neurobehavioral rating scale: Assessment of the behavioral sequelae of head injury by the clinician. J Neurol Neurosurg Psychiatry *50:* 183, 1987. Used with permission.

TABLE 9.5-6
Measures for Assessment of Functional Capacity

Measures	Assessment Domains
Blessed Dementia Scale (BDS)	Everyday activities (8 items) Self-care (3) Personality (11)
Instrumental Activities of Daily Living (IADL)	Telephone use Shopping Food preparation Housekeeping Transportation Medication responsibility Handling of finances
Functional Rating Scale for Symptoms of Dementia	Eating; Dressing; Hygiene; Grooming; Continence; Verbal communication; Memory (names, events); Alertness; Confusion; Spatial orientation; Facial recognition; Emotionality; Social responsiveness; Sleep patterns
Direct Assessment of Functional Status (DAFS)	Time orientation (16 pts) Communication (14) Transportation (13) Financial skills (21) Shopping (16) Eating (10) Dressing/grooming (14)
Present Functioning Questionnaire (PFQ)	Personality (14 items) Everyday tasks (12) Language (9) Memory (14) Self-care (14)

BDS from G Blessed, B E Tomlinson, M Roth: The association between quantitative measures of dementia and of senile change in the cerebral gray matter of elderly subjects. Br J Psychiatry 114: 797, 1968. IADL from M P Lawton, E M Brody: Assessment of Older People: Self Maintaining and Instrumental Activities of Daily Living. Gerontologist *9:* 179, 1969. Functional Rating Scale for Symptoms of Dementia from J T Hutton, R L Dippelm, R B Loewenson, J A Mortimer, B L Christians: Predictors of Nursing Home Placement of Patients with Alzheimer's Disease. Tex Med *81:* 40, 1985. DAFS from D A Loewenstein, E Amigo, R Duara, A Guterman, D Hurwitz, N Berkowitz, F Wilkie, G Weinberg, B Black, B Gittelman, C Eisdorfer: A new scale for the assessment of the functional status in Alzheimer's disease and related disorders. J Gerontology *44:* 114, 1989. PFQ from D Crockett, H Tuokko, W Koch, R Parks: The assessment of everyday functioning using the Present Functioning Questionnaire and the Functional Rating Scale in elderly samples. Clin Gerontologist 8: 3, 1989.

preceding six months. The Blessed Dementia Scale is one of the few measures of severity of dementia which has been validated with neuropathological findings (for example, senile plaques) on autopsy.

INSTRUMENTAL ACTIVITIES OF DAILY LIVING In response to the need for a systematic approach to residential placement decisions, the Instrumental Activities of Daily Living (IADL) evaluates an individual's ability to perform eight complex behaviors associated with independent living. Available in an observer-rated version and a self-rated version, the measure can be used by a variety of personnel and fosters objective judgment in planning for appropriate services. A recent large-scale survey of community-dwelling elderly found that four Instrumental Activities of Daily Living items (telephone use, transportation, medication responsibility, and handling of finances) were associated with cognitive impairment, independent of age, sex, and education, suggesting that the accuracy of dementia diagnosis among poorly educated individuals can be improved with assessment of functional decline.

FUNCTIONAL RATING SCALE FOR SYMPTOMS OF DEMENTIA The Functional Scale was developed to evaluate behavioral disturbances in patients with dementia of the Alzheimer's type and to assist physicians in making individualized recommendations for nursing home placement. The measure contains 14 problem areas which are rated from 0 to 3, with higher scores indicating greater disability. Validation subjects were observed longitudinally over a span of 18 to 36 months. Scores exceeding 21 were associated with nursing home placement in six months to one year, particularly if disabilities involved incontinence, speech incoherence, and grooming deficits. In view of the small validation sample, the use of caution is advised in strict adherence to reported cut-off scores.

PRESENT FUNCTIONING QUESTIONNAIRE Using a checklist format, the Present Functioning Questionnaire (PFQ) was constructed after reviewing the literature associated with problems of everyday living. The measure provides a convenient, comprehensive, and reliable means of assessing the signs and symptoms associated with dementing disorders, and it has been found to be sensitive to differences among normal elderly subjects as compared to elderly subjects with suspected malignant memory disorders.

DIRECT ASSESSMENT OF FUNCTIONAL STATUS To circumvent the reporter bias concerns associated with family report, the Direct Assessment of Functional Status (DAFS) provides a standardized procedure for in vivo evaluation of behavioral competency. The scale can be administered in an outpatient setting, and it serves as a reliable means for evaluating the effects of pharmacological interventions. Strong correlations observed with the Blessed Dementia Scale suggest that the Direct Assessment of Functional Status is sensitive to changes in cognitive and functional status over time. Patients with mild to moderate dementia of the Alzheimer's type exhibited considerable impairment across different domains relative to normal or depressed controls.

Clinical tests and experimental tasks developed by neuropsychologists have contributed immensely to recent behavioral studies of neurological and psychiatric disorders. In clinical practice, the usefulness of neuropsychological testing depends, to a great extent, on the examiner's knowledge of the disorder in question and on both the sensitivity and the specificity of the individual measures and test batteries. Although different strategies of neuropsychological testing can often provide the psychiatrist with information pertinent to diagnosis and clinical management, the amount of information gained generally reflects the training and experience of the neuropsychologist. Positive neuropsychological findings in psychiatric patients can frequently be explained on a basis other than acquired cerebral lesions, whereas negative results hardly rule out a structural brain abnormality. Further research is needed to elucidate diagnostic implications of neuropsychological findings in psychiatric patients.

SUGGESTED CROSS-REFERENCES

The neuropsychological and intellectual assessment of children is discussed in Section 9.6. Section 9.4 addresses personality assessment. The biology of memory is discussed in Section 3.5. Attention-deficit disorders are discussed in Chapter 38. Communication disorders are the subject of Section 36.4.

REFERENCES

Anderson S W, Damasio H, Jones R D, Tranel D: Wisconsin Card Sorting Test performance as a measure of frontal lobe damage. J Clin Exp Neuropsychol *13:* 909, 1991.

Bender L: *A Visual Motor Gestalt Test and Its Clinical Use.* American Orthopsychiatric Association, New York, 1938.

Benton A L: Clinical neuropsychology: 1969–1990. J Clin Exp Neuropsychol *14:* 407, 1992.

*Benton A L: Neuropsychological assessment. Annu Rev Psychol *45:* 1, 1994.

Benton A L: Reaction time in brain disease: Some reflections. Cortex *22:* 129, 1986.

Benton A L, Sivan A B, Hamsher K deS, Varney N R, Spreen O: *Contributions to Neuropsychological Assessment,* ed 2. Oxford University Press, New York, 1994.

Berman K F, Zec R F, Weinberger D R: Physiologic dysfunction of dorsolateral prefrontal cortex in schizophrenia. II. Role of neuroleptic treatment, attention and mental effort. Arch Gen Psychiatry *43*:126, 1986.

Bryson G J, Silverstein M L, Nathan A, Stephen L: Differential rate of neuropsychological dysfunction in psychiatric disorders: Comparison between the Halstead-Reitan and Luria-Nebraska batteries. Percept Mot Skills *76:* 305, 1993.

Buschke H: Selective reminding for analysis of memory and learning. J Verb Learn Verb Behav *12:* 543, 1973.

Chouinard M J, Braun, C M-J: A Meta-analysis of the relative sensitivity of neuropsychological screening tests. J Clin Exp Neuropsychol *15:* 591, 1993.

Christensen A-L: *Luria's Neuropsychological Investigation,* ed 2. Ejnar Munksgaards Vorlag, Copenhagen, 1979.

Cohen N J, Squire L R: Preserved learning and retention of pattern-analysis skill in amnesia: Dissociation of knowing how and knowing that. Science *210:* 207, 1980.

Crossen J R, Wiens A N: Comparison of the Auditory-Verbal Learning Test (AVLT) and California Verbal Learning Test (CVLT) in a sample of normal subjects. J Clin Exp Neuropsychol *16:* 190, 1994.

Drachman D A, Leavitt J: Human memory and the cholinergic system. Arch Neurol *30:* 113, 1974.

Eslinger P J, Damasio A R, Benton A L, Van Allen M: Neuropsychologic detection of abnormal mental decline in older persons. JAMA *253*:670, 1985.

Gazzaniga M S: Right hemisphere language following brain bisection: A 20-year perspective. Am Psychol *38:* 525, 1983.

Goldberg T E, Hyde T M, Kleinman J E, Weinberger D R: Course of schizophrenia: Neuropsychological evidence for a static encephalopathy. Schizophr Bull *19:* 797, 1993.

Golden C J, Hammeke T A, Purisch A D: Diagnostic validity of a standardized neuropsychological battery derived from Luria's neuropsychological tests. J Consult Clin Psychol *46:* 125, 1978.

Grant D A, Berg E A: A behavioral analysis of degree of reinforcement and ease of shifting to new responses in a Weigl-type card-sorting problem. J Exp Psychol *38:* 404, 1948.

Heaton R K, Baade L E, Johnson K L: Neuropsychological test results associated with psychiatric disorders in adults. Psychol Bull *85:* 141, 1978.

*Heilman K M, Valenstein E, editors: *Clinical Neuropsychology,* ed 5. Oxford University Press, New York, 1993.

Kempen J M, Kritchevsky M, Feldman S T: Effect of visual impairment on neuropsychological test performance. J Clin Exp Neuro psychol *16:* 223, 1994.

Koppitz E M: *The Bender Gestalt Test for Young Children.* Grune & Stratton, New York, 1983.

Lachner G, Engel R R: Differentiation of dementia and depression by memory tests. J Nerv Ment Dis *182:* 34, 1994.

Levin H S, High W M Jr, Goethe K E, Sisson R A, Overall J E, Rhoades H M, Eisenberg H M, Kalisky Z, Gary H E Jr: The neurobehavioral rating scale: Assessment of the behavioral sequelae of head injury by the clinician. J Neurol Neurosurg Psychiatry *50:* 183, 1987.

Levin H S, High W M Jr, Meyers C A, Von Laufen A, Hayden M E, Eisenberg, H M: Impairment of remote memory after closed head injury. J Neurol Neurosurg Psychiatry *48:* 556, 1985.

Lezak M D: *Neuropsychological Assessment,* ed 2. Oxford University Press, New York, 1983.

Matarazzo J D: Wechsler's Measurement and Appraisal of Adult Intelligence, ed 5. Williams & Wilkins, Baltimore, 1972.

Meador K J, Moore E E, Nichols M E, Abney O L, Taylor H S, Zamrini E Y, Loring D W: The role of cholinergic systems in visuospatial processing and memory. J Clin Exp Neuropsychol *15:* 832, 1993.

Mesulam M M: A cortical network for directed attention and unilateral neglect. Ann Neurol *10:* 309, 1981.

Milner B: Effects of different brain lesions on card sorting. Arch Neurol *9:* 90, 1963.

Nelson A, Fogel B S, Faust D: Bedside cognitive screening instruments: A critical assessment. J Nerv Ment Dis *174:* 73, 1986.

Peters B H, Levin H S: Effects of physostigmine and lecithin on memory in Alzheimer disease. Ann Neurol *6:* 219, 1979.

Prigatano G P, Redner J E: Uses and abuses of neuropsychological testing in behavioral neurology. Neurol Clin *11:* 219, 1993.

Reitan R M: Theoretical and methodological bases of the Halstead-Reitan Neuropsychological Test Battery. In *Neuropsychological Assessment of Neuropsychiatric Disorders,* I Grant, K M Adams, editors, p 3. Oxford University Press, New York, 1986.

Sackeim H A, Greenberg M S, Weiman A L, Gur R C, Hungerbuhler J P, Geschwind N: Hemispheric asymmetry in the expression of positive and negative emotions. Neurologic evidence. Arch Neurol *39:* 210, 1982.

Schmidt R, Freidl W, Fazekas F, Reinhart B, Grieshofer P, Koch M, Eber B, Schumacher M, Polmin K, Lechner H: The Mattis Dementia Rating Scale: Normative data from 1,001 healthy volunteers. Neurology *44:* 964, 1994.

Sivan A B: *The Benton Visual Retention Test,* ed 5. Psychological Corporation, New York, 1992.

Sperry R W: Lateral specialization in the surgically separated hemispheres. In *Hemispheric Specialization and Interaction,* B Milner, editor. MIT Press, Cambridge, MA 1975.

*Stern Y: Neuropsychological evaluation of the HIV patient. Psychiatr Clin North Am *17:* 125, 1994.

Sternberg D E, Jarvik M E: Memory functions in depression. Improvement with antidepressant medication. Arch Gen Psychiatry *33:* 219, 1976.

*Storandt M, Botwinick J, Danziger W L, Berg L, Hughes C P: Psychometric differentiation of mild senile dementia of the Alzheimer type. Arch Neurol *41:* 497, 1984.

Thorndike R L, Hagen E P, Sattler J M: *Stanford-Binet Intelligence Scale: Technical Manual,* ed 4. Riverside Publishing, Chicago, 1986.

*Van Zomeren A H, Brouwer W H: Clinical Neuropsychology of Attention. Oxford University Press, New York, 1994.

Wechsler D: *WAIS-R Manual.* Psychological Corporation, New York, 1981.

Weingartner H, Cohen R M, Murphy D L, Martello J, Gerdt C: Cognitive processes in depression. Arch Gen Psychiatry *38:* 42, 1981.

Wexler B E: Cerebral laterality and psychiatry: A review of the literature. Am J Psychiatry *137:* 3, 1980.

9.6
NEUROPSYCHOLOGICAL AND INTELLECTUAL ASSESSMENT OF CHILDREN

JACK M. FLETCHER, Ph.D.
H. GERRY TAYLOR, Ph.D.
HARVEY S. LEVIN, Ph.D.
PAUL SATZ, Ph.D.

INTRODUCTION

The neuropsychological assessment of children is of growing interest to practitioners in several disciplines involved in the evaluation and treatment of children. Neuropsychological assessments have applicability to children with learning and attentional disorders, brain injuries, and behavioral problems and to a variety of diagnostic and treatment issues. As a component of the assessment of children, neuropsychological methods provide considerable information on the cognitive functioning of children and the relations of cognitive deficits to brain function and behavior. A recent study by the second author suggested that the use of neuropsychological procedures rested on two primary assumptions about validity: (1) neurological validity, or the assumption that test results are related to the integrity of the central nervous system (CNS), and (2) psychological validity, or the assumption that test results are related to meaningful components of the child's everyday functioning, such as learning abilities in school.

The validity of those two assumptions has acquired considerable support in the past few years. There is clear evidence that neuropsychological procedures are sensitive to variations in the status of the CNS. The evidence dates back to studies reported in the 1950s and early 1960s by Ralph Reitan and Arthur Benton that provided part of the foundation for the study of brain-behavior relations in children through neuropsychological approaches. Neuropsychological procedures are also of value in assessing ecologically important issues in the development of normal and handicapped children, particularly in relation to school and family functioning.

The value of neuropsychological assessment has been strengthened by the presence of different approaches to evaluating the child. Some approaches, for example, emphasize the value of neuropsychological assessment in the differential diagnosis of disorders that are functional or due to a general medical condition. That kind of approach is apparent in applications to child psychiatry and in the evaluation of behaviorally impaired children. Other approaches emphasize the value of neuropsychological assessments for determining cognitive impairments and strengths in an individual child, with remedial plans often emerging from the evaluations. Such approaches include treatment as a major goal of the assessment. Other approaches use neuropsychological assessment for lesion localization and treatment planning, such as the surgical treatment of children with intractable epilepsy. All of the approaches may use different tests and other methods for assessment.

Regardless of the approach or method used, the common view emphasizes the process of evaluating individual children. Neuropsychological assessment usually entails the administration and interpretation of a set of psychometric tests that measure a broad range of specific cognitive abilities and behavioral capacities necessary for school, community, and family functioning. The procedures have neurological and psychological validity. They are interpreted according to the psychometric properties of the tests and within the context of the child's performance (for example, school expectations, motivational and emotional factors). The assessment generally leads to a remedial plan that addresses the habilitation of the child in cognitive, behavioral, and contextual perspectives. There is considerable variability in how those goals are achieved, but all assessments are completed with some form of intervention as the end point of evaluation.

PURPOSES OF NEUROPSYCHOLOGICAL ASSESSMENT

Neuropsychological procedures have been applied to a broad range of childhood problems, including various neurological disorders (such as head injury, hydrocephalus, and epilepsy), learning and attentional disorders, and behavioral and emotional disorders. Regardless of the presenting disorder, the major questions usually concern possible cognitive impairments and their influence on school performance and behavior. Neuropsychologists also complete assessments to assist with decisions concerning the extent to which brain status or a particular neurological disorder contributes to the presenting problem, particularly as part of the evaluation of children for surgical and other medical interventions. Even in those evaluations, the focus is on identifying and measuring cognitive strengths and weaknesses as the basis for developing an intervention plan. As such, the purposes of neuropsychological assessment often overlap with those of other assessment-oriented disciplines, such as education. What distinguishes child neuropsychology from other assessment disciplines is the emphasis on a broad range of cognitive functions and an interest in the brain-related bases of behavior.

REFERRAL QUESTIONS

A variety of questions may lead to referral of a child for neuropsychological evaluation. The most common reason for referral is poor school performance, and the issues usually addressed involve the degree to which the child's academic performance is related to a learning disability or brain insult as opposed to other factors in the child's environment (for example, family problems or the school curriculum). Other reasons for referral are behavioral problems at home and in school. The question in those cases is the degree to which cognitive dysfunctions contribute to the behavioral problems. In addition to traditional psychological treatments, it may be necessary to remediate the cognitive problem and to adjust the psychological intervention according to the child's capacity for processing information. Finally, children may be referred for neuropsychological testing to localize actual brain pathology, as in the case of intractable epilepsy. The different questions addressed by neuropsychological testing may be considered simultaneously in evaluating the child, but the selection and order of procedures may vary, depending on the chief purpose of the assessment.

Referrals come from many sources, including parents, school personnel, psychiatrists, neurologists, and other health care providers. On referral the parents are informed of the nature and purpose of the evaluation. For children, early involvement of the family is critical. If the family is not centrally included in the evaluation, it is difficult to identify relevant variables (for example, parenting skills, marital dissatisfaction, sociodemographic factors) that may be contributing to the child's difficulties. In addition, any interventions must be tailored to the family's ability to respond. There is little point in recommending services that the family cannot afford or is opposed to because of poor previous experiences.

If a referral is made because of questions that are beyond the neuropsychologist's expertise, the referral questions should be discussed and clarified. For example, children sometimes are referred by educators who are concerned that a distractible child may have a seizure disorder. That issue cannot be resolved with a neuropsychological evaluation, and the evaluation should be completed only if there is a question about attention, learning, or behavior. The question of seizure disorder should be referred to a pediatric neurologist for evaluation. For more general questions, such as whether a child with a severe behavioral disorder but no evidence of overt neurological disease has a brain-related disorder, the concerns and observations that led to the referral should be discussed. In such cases the neuropsychologist seeks to determine the extent to which constitutional and environmental factors may be contributing to the presenting disorder. Neuropsychologists rarely make specific statements concerning the etiology or pathology of a disorder solely on the basis of psychometric procedures. In addition, the question is often trivial, inasmuch as the answer rarely has known treatment consequences in the behavioral domain.

The primary responsibility of the child neuropsychologist is to identify the cognitive and behavioral correlates (and consequences) of emotional, learning, and neurological disorders.

The results should be translated into a remedial plan for allied professionals (for example, physicians) and others who may implement intervention (for example, educators and parents). One advantage of an emphasis on cognitive processes is the focus on behavior and the de-emphasis on neurologizing about children. Terms such as "organic brain syndrome" or "minimal brain injury" are generally empty, with little implication for intervention. Nonetheless, such concepts are frequently proposed as the basis for referral, particularly when the etiology of the problem is not known. In accepting such referrals the neuropsychologist must establish that the assessment is an ability-oriented evaluation designed to help formulate the problem and determine specific approaches to intervention. Information may be derived that contributes to an understanding of etiology, but that information must be evaluated in conjunction with diagnostic information from other sources. Neuropsychology offers a careful analysis of ability structure and the many factors influencing the child's behavior but does not establish (in isolation) physical diagnosis or etiology.

CLASSIFICATION ISSUES AND NEUROPSYCHOLOGICAL INFERENCE

To explicate the critical issue of inference in neuropsychological evaluation, consider referrals that simply ask for an assessment of the presence or absence of a brain-related disorder. In adults the primary manifestations of many neurological diseases are behavioral (for example, memory loss in dementia). That is less true in children, in whom relations between behavior and neurological disease are less well known and possibly more indirect than in adults. Unfortunately, despite that problem, determining whether a child has a brain-related disorder is often made on the basis of behavioral signs.

The tendency to infer brain dysfunction in children solely on the basis of behavioral signs has a long history in psychology, child psychiatry, and neurology. Recently, the conceptual framework underlying that way of thinking about childhood disorders, particularly disorders in which evidence of neurological disease is lacking, has been widely criticized. The criticism is specifically applicable to common learning, attentional, and behavioral disorders in which brain injury is excluded by history and current presentation (for example, attention-deficit/hyperactivity disorder, developmental reading disorder).

The notion that certain childhood learning and behavioral disorders are brain-related is a viable hypothesis. For example, various forms of brain injury produce changes in a child's ability to learn as well as in patterns of behavior. Where problems have arisen is in the tendency to view behavioral signs as necessarily indicating underlying brain dysfunction.

HISTORY The history of such thinking can be represented as the concept of cerebral dysfunction. In the early 1900s Sir George F. Still attributed certain cases of impulsive behavior to an unobservable brain disorder. It was thought that when environmental causes could be ruled out as contributory, the children with the behavioral pattern must have had a brain dysfunction that was simply not measurable. Similarly, the organic psychiatrists Eugen Kahn and Louis Cohen argued in the 1930s that certain cases of impulsive, acting-out behavior represented brain-related disorders. The patients they observed had histories of head injury, measles encephalitis, or other neurological disorders from which physical recovery was sufficient to eliminate classic neurological signs of brain damage (for example, hemiparesis). Kahn and Cohen argued that the history supported the presence of a distinct brain damage syndrome that could not be explained by existing explanations of behavior that identified only environmental causes.

The Straussian movement, popular in the 1940s and 1950s, had the greatest contemporary influence on the concept of cerebral dysfunction. On the basis of observations of mentally retarded children, Alfred Strauss and associates argued that children who displayed impulsive, hyperactive behavior had minimal brain injury. The diagnostic category was subsequently expanded to include children with achievement deficiencies. Strauss and his colleagues contended that the pattern of behavior itself was sufficient evidence for the diagnosis of minimal brain injury, even in the absence of evidence or a history of brain injury. In the 1960s various federal task forces adopted Strauss's concept of minimal brain injury, modifying it somewhat and erecting definitions of minimal brain dysfunction and a corresponding achievement-oriented definition of specific learning disability. The validity of many of the disorders subsumed under specific learning disability was widely disputed at the time and continues to be controversial.

CEREBRAL DYSFUNCTION AND DIFFERENTIAL DIAGNOSIS The tendency to ascribe behavioral problems to cerebral dysfunction and the definitions of disorders that proceeded from that attribution have been widely criticized. The concept of cerebral dysfunction makes the following assumptions: (1) Brain injury produces unitary forms of behavioral disorder; (2) There is a continuum of brain injury, and thus, if serious forms of injury result in death or intellectual retardation, mild forms result in learning and behavioral problems; (3) There is an isomorphic relation between behavior and brain processes, such that certain behavioral signs are direct indicants of brain dysfunction. Each of those assumptions is likely incorrect and certainly misleading, with numerous logical fallacies as well as a general absence of empirical evidence supporting either the hypothesis of unitary forms of behavior disorders or a continuum of brain injury. The concept of minimal brain dysfunction is now widely disregarded and does not appear in major neurological and psychiatric classifications, such as the fourth edition of *Diagnostic and Statistical Manual of Mental Disorders* (DSM-IV).

The concepts of cerebral dysfunction and differential diagnosis pervade both observational and test-based assessments of children. Because there is no evidence for unitary patterns of behavior attributable to brain injury, overactivity and inattentiveness in a child are not direct evidence of a brain-related etiology. Similarly, the presence of paraclassical or soft neurological signs on physical examination has not been established as a reliable indicator of a biological basis for a disorder. Indeed, studies comparing learning-impaired and attentionally impaired children with conduct-disordered children on soft signs and electroencephalogram (EEG) findings have yielded null results.

In a sense, the goal of those types of studies is to infer the status of the child's CNS. Such inferences require a set of empirically validated behavior-brain relations, which have been better developed for many adult disorders. Those relations, however, can only be established when independent assessments of the child's behavior and CNS status have been made. When such correlations are established, they pertain only to that patient population and cannot be extrapolated to other populations. For example, brain-injured children may exhibit certain patterns of test responses. Observing a similar pattern in a child with no demonstrable injury to the brain does not validate an inference of the same type of injury. The pattern only indicates that the hypothesis is viable. Behavior in children is too variable and complex, and current understanding of the CNS and its relation to children's behavior is not sufficient, to permit such loose reasoning.

TREATMENT IMPLICATIONS Given these problems, it is not surprising that many contemporary approaches to child neuropsychological assessment have moved away from differential diagnosis toward an emphasis on treatment. The emphasis is not so much on deciding whether the problem is brain-related, which is a relatively straightforward decision. Rather, the emphasis is on detailed assessment of the ability structure of the child. From that assessment decisions are made concerning prognosis and remediation. With that approach a broad range of childhood disorders can be valuably served, ranging from various forms of brain injury to learning and behavioral problems in children without brain injury.

Many neuropsychologists are now engaged in systematic studies of children, particularly children with learning and attentional disorders, brain injuries, and various emotional disorders. Within those large groups specific neuropsychological patterns can be defined that have treatment and prognostic implications and that enhance understanding of the CNS basis for some of the patterns. It is increasingly possible to identify characteristic forms of cognitive disability, which often overlap across groups. By studying the relation of those profiles to variables describing the pathology of the disorders, clinicians are achieving a greater understanding of brain-behavior relations in children. However, clinical neuropsychological assessment of children continues to focus on ability strengths and weaknesses, with an emphasis on treatment.

Within the framework of ability identification, child neuropsychological assessment is a method for defining and remediating cognitive adaptational problems in children. In that respect assessment departs from the traditional use of psychometric testing for differential diagnosis. For example, the Bender Visual-Motor Gestalt Test, a visual-motor copying test for children, is frequently scored according to whether errors are indicators of emotional or neurological disorders. Using neuropsychological tests for that type of differential diagnosis assumes that (1) disorders of childhood can be easily categorized as organic (due to a general medical condition) or functional and (2) specific treatment recommendations stem from the independent diagnoses. Neither assumption is correct. The behavioral manifestations of brain disease are diverse and not easily separated into two simple groups. Moreover, treatment depends on the consequences of the disorder, not on an etiological distinction. Regardless of whether a particular disorder is organic or functional, all children with adaptational problems benefit from a careful assessment of abilities, with treatment planning following that assessment independently of diagnosis. For example, some emotionally disturbed children have difficulty learning in school. Even if the problems stem primarily from the emotional area, an assessment of school-related abilities may be useful in improving the child's response to instruction. A child who is stronger in visual-spatial skills with significant impairment of central language abilities may benefit from an approach to reading instruction that de-emphasizes phonetic decoding of words in favor of a sight-based approach. Such an approach may help reduce frustration and improve motivation. Similarly, most brain-injured children require careful instruction-oriented evaluations for school planning. However, if the child also presents with a conduct disorder, a behavioral program addressing the problem behavior may be useful. Treatment plans can be developed from assessment results for both brain-damaged and emotionally disturbed children. The need is not for a differential diagnosis but for a careful assessment of adaptive strengths and weaknesses.

APPROACHES TO NEUROPSYCHOLOGICAL ASSESSMENT

Specific methods for the neuropsychological assessment of children vary across settings and practitioners. Some neuropsychologists prefer using modified versions of standard neuropsychological batteries, such as the Halstead-Reitan Neuropsychological Battery. Neuropsychologists have systematically applied such tests to many children with learning disabilities, brain injuries, and emotional problems. Specific interpretative relations across disorders, along with remedial plans, have emerged from such applications. Other neuropsychologists focus on traditional intellectual, language, and perceptual tests and use them as the basis for assessment. The goal is to identify syndromes and develop intervention plans.

Another approach focuses on measuring specific cognitive skills. Traditional instruments are employed, but the examiners also use measures of cognitive skills drawn directly from the experimental literature on normal child development. For example, measures of phonological awareness may be used to assess reading difficulties in children because of extensive evidence that phonological processes are highly related to reading proficiency. With head-injured children, various memory tests sensitive to the effects of head injury are employed. In other applications language tests derived from contemporary psycholinguistic theories of the organization and development of language are used to assess learning-disabled and brain-injured children.

Most practitioners combine the above approaches in assessing children, for each approach contributes to the expanding knowledge base on the neurobehavioral correlates of various childhood disorders. Although different practitioners may use different specific tests, the principles, goals, and methods of interpretation in each approach are quite similar. First, psychometric tests are administered to help define the nature of the problem (for example, intellectual, learning, attentional, language, or motor disability). Second, in each approach other measures of cognitive skills correlated with the disorder are administered. For example, children with reading problems often have difficulty with language skills. In such cases an attempt is made to define the exact nature of any language deficiencies in the context of other cognitive skills. Third, environmental variables that might impinge on the child's performance on the tests and on habilitation potential are assessed. A child who is inattentive, unmotivated, or easily frustrated may not display his or her true potential on psychometric tests. Cultural variables are well-known influences on intelligence tests and have similar effects on other cognitive tasks. For remediation, family resources may limit options in terms of various available services. Fourth, results of the three levels of analysis are compared with historical and current medical data to establish relations to the child's ability structure and CNS integrity. Fifth, a remedial plan is developed on the basis of the results of the assessment. The remedial plan typically highlights areas for intervention, provides methods for remediation, and identifies potential modes of intervention (such as special education).

ASSESSMENT MODEL Figure 9.6-1 provides a schematic overview, developed by the first and second author, of the various levels of analysis that are common to the neuropsychological assessment of children. The model divides the assessment process into four components:

1. A description of the problem characterizing the child's apparent inability to meet age-appropriate expectations for performance in some settings (that is, manifest disability).
2. Assessment of the child's traits that influence the manifest disability. Those traits may be cognitive or psychosocial in nature and are often closely related.
3. Evaluation of environmental variables—social, cultural, familial, and contextual—that are directly related to the child's psychosocial traits.

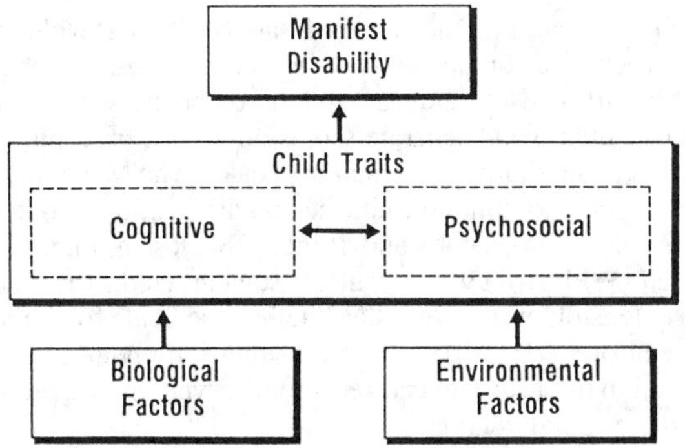

FIGURE 9.6-1 *Model for the neuropsychological assessment of children developed by Taylor and Fletcher. (Figure from H G Taylor, J M Fletcher: Neuropsychological assessment of children. In* Handbook of Psychological Assessment, *ed 2, G Goldstein, M Herson, editors, p 211. Wiley, New York, 1990. Used with permission.)*

4. Evaluation of biological variables, which can be related to CNS integrity, genetics, and medical history, that influence the cognitive traits of the child.

The four components detailed above and in Figure 9.6-1 can be represented as three levels of analysis. At the first level the neuropsychologist attempts to understand the relation between the presenting problems (manifest disabilities) and a set of core cognitive and psychosocial traits. At the second level of analysis the influence of cognitive and psychosocial factors on each other and on the manifest disabilities is considered. Children do not develop cognitive skills in isolation from environmental and internal variables, such as attitude and motivation. At the third level attempts are made to understand how various environmental and biological (CNS) variables influence the child's cognitive and psychological traits.

An important question is the degree to which the influence of biological and environmental variables is apparent in the child's ability structure. In terms of the question of whether the manifest disability is brain-related, the analysis begins at the level of behavior and proceeds to a more biological level, but always in the context of environmental variables that moderate the relation of biological and cognitive domains. The purpose is to understand the relation of the four components at behavioral and biological levels of analysis, not to make simplistic inferences concerning CNS status.

DEVELOPING A REMEDIAL PLAN Byron Rourke and colleagues have outlined a seven-step approach to developing and implementing a remedial intervention plan (Figure 9.6-2). In the first step the clinician considers the interaction of the child's ability structure and variables related to brain status, representing the product of the evaluation process outlined in Figure 9.6-1. In step 1 results of the neuropsychological assessment are formulated and decisions as to the impact of brain status on adaptive function are made. That relation is hardly direct and must be evaluated on a case-by-case basis.

In step 2 immediate and long-term demands of the environment are considered. Those demands, which include such elements as the school environment, academic expectations, and projected changes in demands as the child ages, are major considerations in the implementation of an intervention plan. They vary with age and stage of treatment, and therefore the treatment plan must be individualized and flexible.

In steps 3 and 4 the clinician attempts to develop hypotheses about prognosis (step 3) and the ideal short- and long-term treatment plan (step 4). That part of the plan should be written so that the results of any intervention can be evaluated against hypothesized outcomes and goals. In step 5 the clinician considers the availability of treatment resources, including interventions and family variables (for example, finances, child-rearing facility) that influence the family's capacity to participate in the developing habilitation plan. Along with the variables reviewed in step 2, step 5 represents what was described in Figure 9.6-1 as variables that influence the covariance of ability structure, biological variables, and the child's disability. In step 6 the most realistic remedial plan is formulated and implemented based on what is ideal (step 4) and possible (steps 2 and 5). Step 7 addresses the need to follow the child's progress with repeated assessments and modifications of the treatment plan.

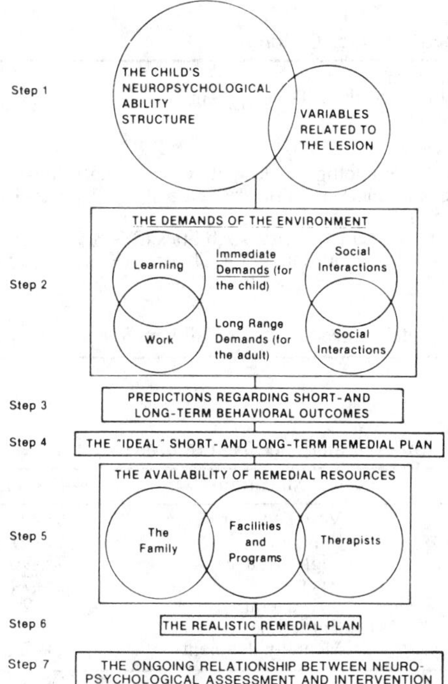

FIGURE 9.6-2 *Model for treatment plans in the neuropsychological assessment of children developed by Rourke and colleagues. (Figure from B P Rourke, J Fisk, J D Strang:* Neuropsychological Assessment of Children: A Treatment-Oriented Approach. *Guilford, New York, 1986. Used with permission.)*

Rourke's approach highlights the major considerations in clinical neuropsychological practice with children. Assessment instruments and interpretations may vary, but that is a relatively minor consideration so long as the two assumptions of neuropsychological basic reliability and validity evaluations outlined earlier are met. The approach allows the clinician to move beyond assessment to develop a specific plan for treating the child. The treatment plan may involve other disciplines and resources, but it stems from the assessment.

TESTING PROCEDURES The specific instruments used by child neuropsychologists vary across settings but commonly measure intelligence, adaptive behavior, academic achievement, behavioral adjustment, and various cognitive and motor skills.

Intelligence tests Table 9.6-1 summarizes some of the major tests used to assess intelligence in children. Each of the tests includes different scales that typically yield composite

TABLE 9.6-1
Intelligence Tests for Children

Infancy–2.5 years
- Bayley Infant Scale of Development
- Cattell Infant Scale

2.5–6 years
- Stanford-Binet intelligence test, 4th edition (2.5 years–adult)
- Wechsler Preschool and Primary Scale of Intelligence-Revised (WPPSI-R) (4–6.5 years)
- McCarthy Scales of Children's Abilities (2.5–8.5 years)
- Kaufman Assessment Battery for Children (K-ABC) (2.5–12.5 years)

6–16 years
- Wechsler Intelligence Scales for Children, 3rd edition (WISC-III)

TABLE 9.6-2
Classification of Intelligence Test Scores

I.Q.	Classification	Percentile Rank
>129	Very superior	98–99
120–129	Superior	91–97
110–119	High average	75–90
90–109	Average	25–74
80–89	Low average	9–24
70–79	Borderline	3–8
<70	Mentally deficient	1–2

scores addressing verbal and nonverbal performance skills. The scales in turn are composed of various subtests that vary in the nature and demand of the actual tasks. All of the tasks yield an overall composite I.Q., with separate scores for verbal, performance, and other subtest combinations. The tests have national standardizations across age cohorts and yield statistically derived scores that permit an estimate of the child's rank in the population. In general, scores of 100 are considered average, with scores below 70 representing the lowest 2.2 percent of the population. Children scoring below 70 are often candidates for the diagnosis of mental retardation, provided that they also show comparable decrements in adaptive behavior and social functioning. Table 9.6-2 presents a classification of I.Q. test scores as they are used to designate intellectual levels in children.

The specific tests vary with respect to constituent subtests, type of national standardization, and the underlying concept of intelligence. For example, previous versions of the Stanford-Binet Intelligence Scale, one of the earliest measures of intelligence, yielded only a single composite I.Q. score and were frequently criticized for inadequate standardizations. The Stanford-Binet Intelligence Scale was redesigned and reformatted to yield a composite I.Q. score as well as scores on four separate scales (verbal reasoning, abstract-visual reasoning, quantitative reasoning, short-term memory). Although the format and standardization are superior to earlier versions of the test, the present version has numerous psychometric problems that limit its use, particularly with younger and lower-functioning children.

The Kaufman Assessment Battery for Children (K-ABC) conceptualizes intelligence according to a model of cognitive processing that distinguishes simultaneous and sequential processing skills. Subtests are designed according to whether the task requires the child to process information along one or the other of those two dimensions. An overall score and composite scores for simultaneous and sequential processing subtests are provided. Recently, screening versions of the K-ABC have been developed that appear to have good validity.

The McCarthy Scales of Children's Abilities is a more traditional test that, like the Bayley Infant Scale of Development, yields a separate composite score for fine and gross motor skills. The McCarthy also yields an overall composite score (general cognitive index) and separate scores on verbal, perceptual-performance, quantitative, and memory scales. The McCarthy generally appeals to children, but the standardization is outdated. The Wechsler Preschool and Primary Scales of Intelligence-Revised (WPPSI-R) was recently restandardized. It is a downward extension of the Wechsler Intelligence Scale for Children, third edition (WISC-III). The recent revision updates the standardization of the test and corrects some psychometric problems with the original version.

For children over 6, the most widely used intelligence measure has been the Wechsler Intelligence Scale for Children-Revised (WISC-R). The WISC-R has been restandardized as the WISC-III, representing a revision in items, scale content, and an updated normative sample. Both versions have in common 12 subtests (Table 9.6-3), with the WISC-III adding a symbol search subtest. Four of the subtests compose the verbal comprehension scale and four compose the perceptual-organization scale. In addition, the WISC-III permits scores for a freedom from distractibility scale (digit span and arithmetic) and a processing speed scale (coding and symbol search). The verbal comprehension subtests consist of measures of general information, oral arithmetic, abstract reasoning, and vocabulary. The perceptual-organization subtests consist of measures of constructional skills (block building, puzzle assembly), visual search, and other tests. In addition to the four scales, a composite full scale I.Q. score is obtained. Mazes is a supplemental subtest that is not used to compute I.Q. scores. The different subtests and their measurement characteristics are listed in Table 9.6-3.

Tests of intelligence have many advantages. Comparisons between the child's performance on subtests requiring primarily verbal and primarily performance skills may indicate processing deficits in those areas. Because I.Q. tests measure several abilities and are well standardized, they can be used to estimate a child's general range of mental functioning. Finally, in conjunction with assessments of adaptive behavior, standardized I.Q. test results are of value in supporting placement recommendations and in surveying areas in which the child's skills may be relatively intact. However, I.Q. tests also have limitations, particularly when used by insufficiently trained practitioners or for purposes for which they were not designed.

TABLE 9.6-3
Subtests of the WISC-III

Subtest	Scale*	Operation
Information	VC	Retrieval of basic facts
Comprehension	VC	Answer questions about social situations
Arithmetic	FD	Oral arithmetic
Similarities	VC	Abstract reasoning
Vocabulary	VC	Oral vocabulary
Digit span	FD	Forward and backward digit repetition
Picture completion	PO	Recognition of missing elements
Picture arrangement	PO	Rearrange pictures depicting social situations
Block design	PO	Block construction
Object assembly	PO	Puzzle construction
Coding	PS	Incidental motor learning
Mazes	—	Completion of mazes
Symbol search	PS	Speeded visual search

*VC = verbal comprehension, PO = perceptual organization, FD = freedom from distractibility, PS = processing speed.

USES OF I.Q. TESTS, ADAPTIVE BEHAVIOR SCALES, ACADEMIC ACHIEVEMENT TESTS, AND BEHAVIOR RATING SCALES

Mental retardation The definition and classification of mental retardation used in DSM-IV correspond closely to criteria developed by the American Association for Mental Deficiency. Establishing the presence of mental retardation requires scores below the third percentile of the population scores (that is, scores less than 70) on measures of intelligence and adaptive behavior. Criteria for the diagnosis are usually legally mandated. Because of the influence of cultural factors on I.Q. scores, the need for a systematic assessment of the child's socialization, communication skills, and overall capacity for everyday functioning cannot be overemphasized. To illustrate, consider a major tool for assessing adaptive behavior, the Vineland Adaptive Behavior Scales. The Vineland can be used for early infancy through adulthood. It has national standardization and yields scores distributed like those of the K-ABC and WISC-III (100 denotes average, with units of 15 as the standard deviation). The Vineland is collected through a nondirective interview of parents or primary caretakers of the child. Four domains are addressed and scored: communication, daily living, socialization, and motor. Each of those domains includes a variety of age-appropriate items that represent behaviors or skills the child may or may not habitually demonstrate. From information obtained during the interview the examiner completes the items and obtains standardized scores for each domain and for the child's overall level of adaptive behavior. The reliability and the validity of the Vineland have been well supported.

Learning disorders DSM-IV defines learning disorders involving reading, mathematics, and written expression. The conceptual framework for DSM-IV definitions parallels current legislation requiring discrepancies between measured I.Q. and academic achievement (one to two standard deviations) relative to chronological age to establish the presence of a learning disorder. It is important to recognize that the language in DSM-IV deviates from common parlance for disabilities in academic skills, which are usually described as learning disabilities.

Table 9.6-4 lists three of the many measures of academic achievement that are commonly used in evaluating children with learning problems. Each of the tests measures basic skills in reading, spelling, writing, and mathematics, but the tests vary in how those skills are assessed. The Wide-Range Achievement Test-Revised (WRAT-R) consists of three subtests involving word identification, written spelling of single words, and computational arithmetic. The Peabody Individual Achievement Test-Revised (PIAT-R) and the Woodcock-Johnson-Psycho-Educational Test Battery-Revised (WJR) have similar tests of word identification. However, the PIAT-R measures arithmetic and spelling skills through a multiple-choice format that does not require writing. It has a separate measure of written language. The WJR has measures of computational and mental arithmetic and of written language. It also measures grammar and punctuation skills and content areas, such as social science, social studies, and humanities. Both the PIAT-R and WJR measure comprehension in reading. The PIAT-R uses a multiple-choice format in which the child silently reads a sentence and then selects from four pictures the one representing the meaning of the sentence. For the WJR, the child silently reads a sentence or passage with a missing word. Comprehension is measured by the child's ability to supply the missing word.

TABLE 9.6-4
Tests of Academic Achievement

1. Wide-Range Achievement Test-Revised (WRAT-R)
2. Peabody Individual Achievement Test-Revised (PIAT-R)
3. Woodcock-Johnson Psycho-Educational Test Battery-Revised (WJR)

Academic skills can be evaluated in a variety of ways, and detection of a learning disability often depends on the type of measure used to assess academic proficiency. For example, reading disorders in children are most commonly manifested by problems in decoding words. Comprehension problems can accompany decoding difficulties. However, children may also perform poorly on comprehension tasks for a variety of reasons not related to a reading disorder, such as lack of motivation or poor memory. It is critical to assess decoding skills for real and nonsense words in evaluating reading problems in children. Mathematics disorder often involves problems with paper-and-pencil computations. If arithmetic proficiency is assessed only by the PIAT-R, which does not require paper-and-pencil computations, an important disability may be overlooked.

There are many problems with definitions of learning disorders based on discrepancies in I.Q. and achievement as mandated by law and embedded in DSM-IV. The problems generally stem from the absence of well-accepted definitions of those disorders. Research has shown that criteria based on I.Q. and achievement discrepancies are arbitrary and do not provide a valid subclassification of children with learning disabilities. There is little evidence that children with academic problems who meet DSM-IV criteria are different from nonmentally retarded children with similar levels of academic achievement who do not show discrepancies relative to I.Q. (slow learners). The notion of specific disabilities is also widely questioned, because isolated areas of proficiency are generally rare. Many children who receive DSM-IV diagnoses of learning disorders will be placed in the learning disorder not otherwise specified category. It may have been better to indicate mixed disorders as in the DSM-IV communication disorders.

The problems in using I.Q.-achievement discrepancies for the diagnosis of learning disability stem in part from the limitations of I.Q. tests, which were not designed to diagnose learning disabilities. Intelligence tests cannot be viewed as a pure measure of learning potential. Performance on I.Q. tests reflects past learning history and genetic endowment. In terms of discrepancies between I.Q. scores and academic achievement, it should be noted that the same basic deficiencies that determine academic problems may also affect I.Q. scores. That problem challenges the frequent practice of defining learning disabilities as an I.Q.-achievement discrepancy. Similarly, the statistical limitations of computing discrepancies between moderately correlated I.Q. and achievement tests have received too little attention. Whenever discrepancy scores are computed between two correlated tests, on the average the selection of an extreme score will be associated with regression to the mean on the other test.

Another shortcoming is that I.Q. tests do not survey all possible areas of competency. The WISC-III, for example, fails to measure many aspects of social adaptation, nonverbal problem-solving, and information-processing skills. Correlations between many neuropsychological tests and academic achievement remain robust, even when the effects of I.Q. are extracted from the correlations. Further, I.Q. tests were designed to predict learning or achievement outside of the test situation, rather than to measure distinct processing skills. For that reason it is difficult to draw conclusions regarding basic skills from performance on I.Q. tests. Individual subtests often measure combinations of skills that provide few clues to component mental abilities. Finally, intelligence test results have not always been

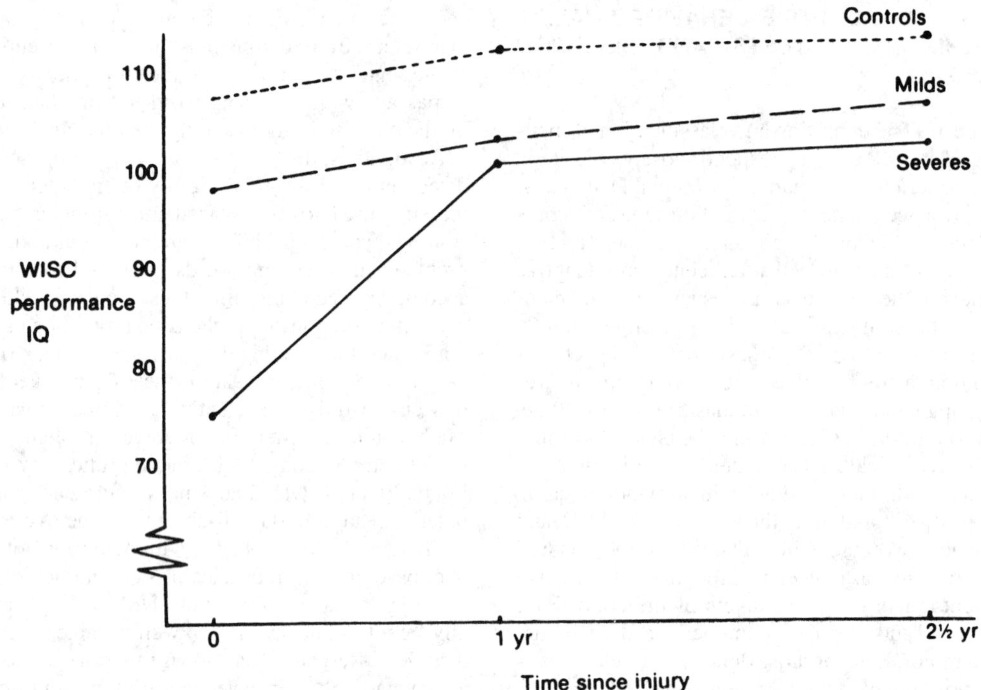

FIGURE 9.6-3 *Changes over time in the verbal and performance I.Q. scores from the Wechsler Intelligence Scale for Children-Revised in children with mild and severe head injuries and in orthopedic control patients. (Figure from O Chadwick, M Rutter, D Brown, D Shaffer, M Traub: A prospective study of children with head injuries: II. Cognitive sequelae. Psychol Med* 11: *49, 1991. Used with permission.)*

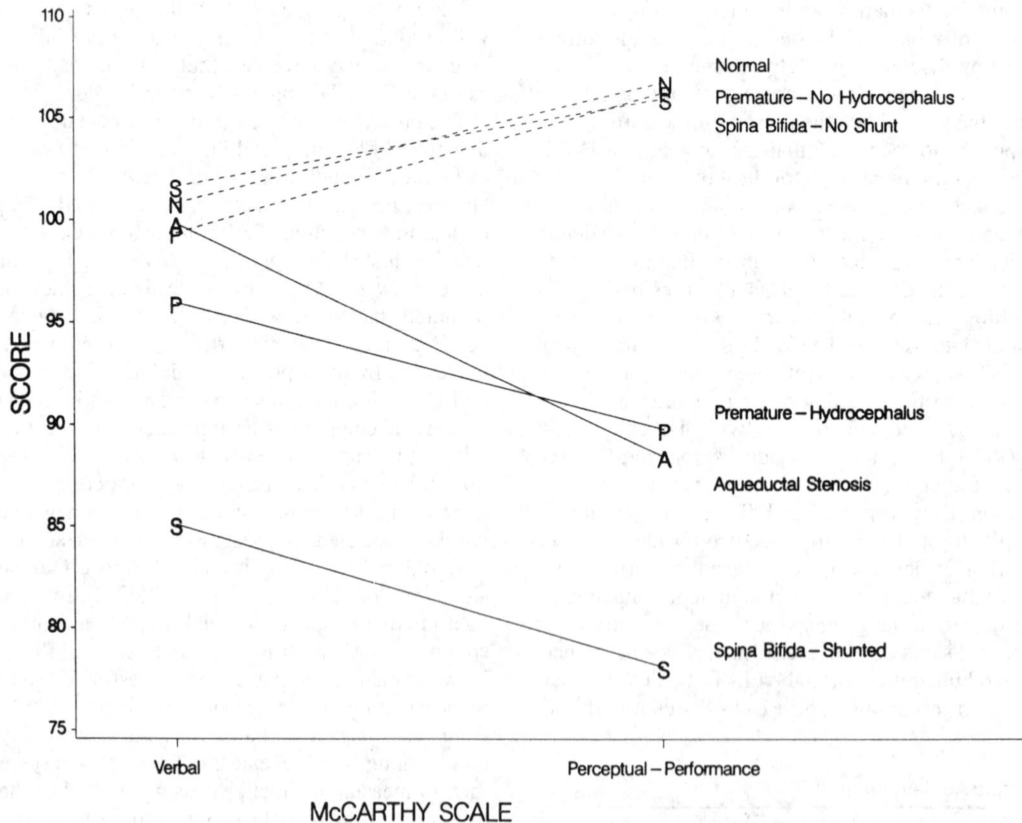

FIGURE 9.6-4 *Performance on the verbal and perceptual-performance scales of the McCarthy Scales of Children's Abilities by three groups of children with early hydrocephalus and by comparison groups.*

found useful for determining the treatment or remedial approach that is most likely to be successful for a given child. There is no reason to believe that educational strategies beneficial to children with lower I.Q. scores are any different from strategies that would be recommended for children with average or above-average I.Q. scores. Although the results of I.Q. tests can be useful in the assessment of children, they may be of relatively limited value and must be interpreted with caution. The use of I.Q.-achievement discrepancies as the sole criterion for diagnosing learning disorders is especially suspect.

Attention-deficit disorders Neuropsychological assessment can be useful for children with attention-deficit/hyperactivity disorder (ADHD). However, psychometric procedures are not diagnostic of ADHD. Attention-deficit disorders are best diagnosed through a careful history and the use of structured clinical interviews and dimensionally based rating scales. Most neuropsychologists obtain behavior ratings in addition to the psychometric tests. When possible, those ratings are obtained at home from parents and at school from the teacher.

Behavior ratings are important for ADHD because performance on cognitive tests and observations of the child in the office are not adequate for the diagnosis of ADHD. The rating scales commonly used by neuropsychologists are the Child Behavior Checklist and the Personality Inventory for Children-Revised. Psychometric testing is used to evaluate other problems (such as learning disabilities) that commonly coexist with ADHD and to facilitate planning. A baseline evaluation of attentional skills is often useful in evaluating response to pharmacological interventions in children with ADHD who do not seem to respond to stimulants.

Brain-injured children Intelligence tests should not be used to diagnose brain damage in children. Intelligence tests are sensitive to the effects of brain injury, but no uniform patterns of performance that would provide adequate criteria for the presence or absence of brain damage have been identified. The limitations of intelligence tests for learning-disabled children also apply to children with brain injury. Unfortunately, the presence of brain injury and disruption of cognitive and motor abilities is sometimes not sufficient for placement of children in special education. Eligibility guidelines often follow guidelines designed for children with learning disorders. Consequently, I.Q. tests may be required if placement recommendations are to be accepted by an educational institution. Unfortunately, tests such as the WISC-III are frequently overemphasized in the evaluation of brain-injured children and may lead to inappropriate decisions concerning placement in special education classes and concerning the effects of brain injury on the child's capacity for adaptive functioning. I.Q. scores may be reduced by the effect of the injury on cognitive skills. Despite the reduction, I.Q. tests are not sensitive to all manifestations of the brain injury, providing an incomplete assessment of the child. The WISC-III, for example, provides a limited and largely indirect assessment of memory and attentional skills, which are frequently impaired in head-injured children. Consequently, the use of I.Q. tests in brain-injured children is often unfair and prevents their entry into necessary special education classes. Indeed, children with head injury often show a decrement in I.Q. scores after injury, with subsequent recovery (Figure 9.6-3). However, recovery of adaptive behavior and memory skills often lags. If the child is evaluated shortly after injury, the I.Q. scores will be reduced and the discrepancy will not be established. Basic academic skills in reading and spelling often are not immediately affected by head injury. Reading problems may emerge several years after injury, reflecting the cumulative effects of subtle learning deficiencies. Thus, I.Q. tests may be useful with brain-injured children, but the results may provide a limited view of the child and can interfere with treatment if misused.

There are numerous studies of intellectual development and recovery in brain-injured children. For example, children with head injury often show good recovery of WISC-R verbal I.Q. scores but slower recovery of performance I.Q. scores (Figure 9.6-3). Three groups of children with congenital hydrocephalus (spina bifida-shunted, prematurity-hydrocephalus, aqueductal stenosis) showed better development on the McCarthy verbal score than on the perceptual-performance score (Figure 9.6-4). There is relatively little decrement in I.Q. scores in many cases of infectious disease. In general, those findings seem to reflect injury to the cerebral white matter in children with CNS insults,

TABLE 9.6-5
Modified Version of the Halstead-Reitan Neuropsychological Test Battery for Children Used by Rourke (Figure 9.6-2)

I. Tactile-perceptual
   A. Reitan-Klove Tactile-Perceptual and Tactile-Forms Recognition Test
      1. Tactile imperception and suppression
      2. Finger agnosia
      3. Fingertip Number-Writing Perception (9–15 years), Fingertip Symbol-Writing Recognition (5–8 years)
      4. Coin Recognition (9–15 years), Tactile-Forms Recognition (5–8 years)
II. Visual-perceptual
   A. Reitan-Klove Visual-Perceptual Tests
   B. Target Test
   C. Constructional dyspraxia items, Halstead-Wepman Aphasia Screening Test
   D. WISC picture completion, picture arrangement, block design, object assembly subtests
   E. Trail Making Test for Children, part A (9–15 years)
   F. Color Form Test (5–8 years)
   G. Progressive Figures
   H. Individual performance tests (5–8 years)
      1. Matching Figures
      2. Star Drawing
      3. Matching Vs
      4. Concentric Squares Drawing
III. Auditory-perceptual and language-related
   A. Reitan-Klove Auditory-Perceptual Test
   B. Seashore Rhythm Test (9–15 years)
   C. Auditory Closure Test
   D. Auditory Analysis Test
   E. Peabody Picture Vocabulary Test
   F. Speech-sounds Perception Test
   G. Sentence Memory Test
   H. Verbal Test
      1. WISC information, comprehension, similarities, vocabulary, digit span subtests
      2. Aphasoid items, Aphasia Screening Test
IV. Problem solving, concept formation, reasoning
   A. Halstead Category Test
   B. Children's Word-Finding Test
   C. WISC arithmetic subtest
   D. Matching Pictures Test (5–8 years)
V. Motor and psychomotor
   A. Reitan-Klove Lateral Dominance Examination
   B. Dynamometer
   C. Finger Tapping Test
   D. Foot Tapping Test
   E. Klove-Matthews Motor Steadiness Battery
      1. Maze Coordination Test
      2. Static Steadiness Test
      3. Grooved Pegboard Test
VI. Other
   A. Underlining Test
   B. WISC coding subtest
   C. Tactual Performance Test
   D. Trail Making Test for Children, part B (9–15 years)

which seems more related to performance I.Q. scores. However, studies of abrupt unilateral lesions (for example, vascular anomaly) in children tend to show more disruptions of verbal I.Q.

NEUROPSYCHOLOGICAL TESTS Two approaches to neuropsychological assessment were presented in Figures 9.6-1 and 9.6-2. A third approach recently put forward by Bruce Pennington is outlined in Figure 9.6-5. That approach classifies cognitive functions in relation to disorders that are primarily characterized by impairments in cognitive function and to the area of the brain hypothesized to mediate the cognitive function. Relative to DSM-IV, primary disorders of reading versus mathematics are thought to be subserved by areas of the left and right hemispheres, respectively. The chart also considers ADHD, pervasive developmental disorder, and one manifestation of brain injury in children (memory loss).

The tests used to implement each of the three approaches to neuropsychological assessment vary, but each approach attempts to measure a variety of skills representing critical cognitive and somatosensory-motor skills. To illustrate, Tables 9.6-5, 9.6-6, and 9.6-7 list some of the major tests used to implement the approaches modeled in Figures 9.6-2, 9.6-1, and 9.6-5, respectively. A brief description of measurement characteristics is provided here; more specific descriptions may be obtained from the primary sources.

The tests are grouped into major areas in the tables. For the approach shown in Figure 9.6-2, tests of tactile-perceptual, visual-perceptual, language, problem solving, motor, and other skills are listed in Table 9.6-5. For the approach shown in Figure 9.6-1, the tests listed in Table 9.6-6 test language, visual-perceptual, somatosensory (tactile), and motoric skills. Table 9.6-5 also includes measures of problem solving and concept formation, whereas Table 9.6-6 emphasizes memory, learning, and

TABLE 9.6-7
Neuropsychological Assessment Procedures for Evaluation of Cognitive Skills Used by Pennington (Figure 9.6-5)

I. Language
1. Boston Naming Test
2. Goldman-Fristoe-Woodcock Auditory Discrimination Test
3. Pig Latin (phoneme segmentation)
4. Speech Sounds Perception
5. Aphasia Screening Test
6. Word Fluency

II. Spatial cognition
1. Developmental Test of Visual-Motor Integration
2. Children's Embedded Figures Test
3. Constructional dyspraxia items, Aphasia Screening Test
4. Tactual Performance Test

III. Motor
1. Finger Tapping Test
2. Grooved Pegboard
3. Hand Dynamometry

IV. Sensory-perceptual
1. Modified Reitan-Klove Tactile-Perceptual Test

V. Memory
1. Story recall
2. Figure recall
3. Verbal Selective Reminding Test

VI. Social cognition
1. Childhood Autism Rating Scale
2. Theory of other minds
3. Imitation
4. Emotional perception

VII. Executive functions
1. Wisconsin Card Sorting Test
2. Tower of Hanoi
3. Matching Familiar Figures Test
4. Continuous Performance Test
5. Contingency Naming Test
6. Categories Test
7. Trail Making Test

TABLE 9.6-6
Neuropsychological Assessment Procedures for Evaluation of Cognitive Skills Used by Fletcher (Figure 9.6-1)

Construct	Test	Operation
I. Language	A. Word Fluency (WF)	Retrieval of words to letters
	B. Rapid Automatized Naming (RAN)	Naming of common pictured items
	C. Auditory Analysis Test (ATT)	Breaking words into phonological segments
	D. Token Test (TT)	Comprehension of sentences
	E. Peabody Picture Vocabulary Test-Revised (PPVT-R)	Comprehension of single words
	F. Boston Naming Test (BNT)	Confrontation naming
II. Visual-spatial and constructional	A. Developmental Test of Visual-Motor Integration (VMI)	Copying of geometric figures
	B. Judgment of Line Orientation (JLO)	Matching lines in two-dimensional space
	C. Test of Visual-Perceptual Skills (TVPS)	Battery of perceptual tests
III. Somatosensory	A. Tactile Figure Test (TFT)	Lateralized haptic processing of sandpaper figures
IV. Motor	A. Finger Tapping (FT)	Lateralized fine motor speed: tapping key
	B. Grooved Pegboard (GP)	Lateralized fine motor speed and dexterity: peg insertion
V. Memory and learning	A. Wide-Range Assessment of Memory-Story Recall (SR)	Memory for passages
	B. Design Recall (DR)	Memory for geometric figures
	C. Continuous Recognition Memory Test (CRM)	Recognition of previously presented pictures
	D. Verbal Selective Reminding (VSR)	Word list learning
	E. Nonverbal Selective Reminding (NVSR)	Memory for dot locations
VI. Attention	A. Continuous Performance Test (CPT)	Selection of target stimuli from sequentially presented stream of stimuli
	B. Verbal Cancellation Test (VCT)	Identification of letter targets in random array of letters
VII. Executive functions	A. Wisconsin Card Sorting Test (WCST)	Problem solving and attention shifts

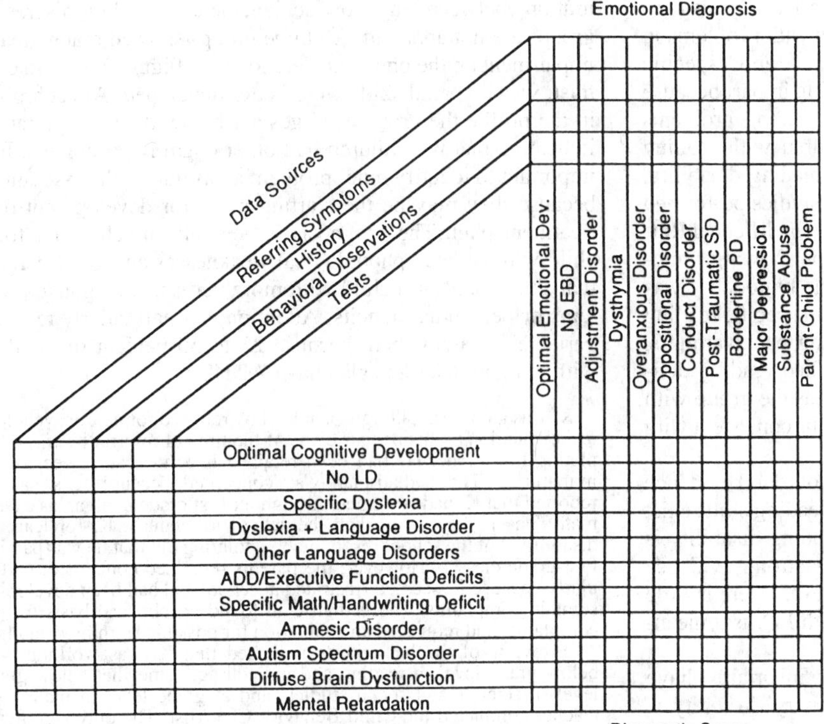

FIGURE 9.6-5 *Framework for differentiated diagnosis used for the neuropsychological assessment of children developed by Pennington. (Figure from B F Pennington:* Diagnosing Learning Disorders: A Neuropsychological Framework. *Guilford, New York, 1991. Used with permission.)*

attentional skills. Table 9.6-5 has some tasks with memory components (Tactual Performance Test) and attentional skills (Underlining Test) in an "other" category, so there is additional overlap. Memory, attention, and executive function tasks are listed in Table 9.6-7. Some tests are used in all three approaches, but the commonality is the attempt to measure a broad range of abilities and the nature of the constructs identified as important in assessment.

The tests in Tables 9.6-5 through 9.6-7 have normative information so that they can be administered to persons of different ages. However, the actual tests used with children and adults may differ in the level of difficulty. It is not assumed that the measurement characteristics and usefulness of the tests are the same for children and adults. It is misleading to simply take tests developed for adults and apply them to children (or the elderly) without considering task difficulty and differences in measurement characteristics.

The interpretations of the tests vary, depending on the nature of the assessment question and the child's presenting problem. Specific tests may be added or deleted, depending on the presenting problem and the results of the assessment. Tests are generally selected to measure abilities identified as an important correlates of school functioning, adaptive behavior, and known lesions.

There are other approaches to the neuropsychological assessment of children. Barbara Wilson has described neuropsychological assessments for infants and preschoolers. Because of the difficulties in assessing very young children, flexibility in the selection of tests is necessary. Normative information is critical for the assessment of young children. Consequently, Wilson uses a variety of standard instruments, some of which were listed in Table 9.6-1. Subtests from the instrument that measure specific processes are often picked. Whenever possible, multiple indicators of the same skill are selected to improve the reliability of the assessment, a common problem in the assessment of preschool-aged children.

Jane Holmes-Bernstein and Deborah Waber have developed a systematic approach to developmental neuropsychological assessment. It is based on a model that emphasizes both the neurological and psychological aspects of assessment. For the neurological component, assessments are designed according to a hypothetical model in which the CNS is conceptualized along three primary axes: anterior-posterior, left-right, and cortical-subcortical. Behavior is construed as a function of the dynamic interaction among those axes within the environment in which the child develops. The psychological component addresses various cognitive structures, developmental timetables, and the environmental context in which children develop. Holmes-Bernstein and Waber's approach emphasizes the qualitative assessment of behavior exhibited by children in the evaluation. Specific procedures are designed to assess the possibility of alternative strategies and approaches to an area that is particularly difficult for the child. The intervention components emphasize compensatory models, with particular emphasis on problem-solving skills that the child might bring to bear in an area of difficulty. The assessment instruments are similar to those described by the first two authors, Pennington and Rourke, but greater emphasis is placed on problem-solving processes and other more qualitative components of the child's performance. In particular, tests are chosen to address questions that arise during the evaluation, and there is no emphasis on a fixed evaluation battery. All of the approaches discussed in this section are useful, and the diversity has enriched and cross-fertilized the assessment area.

ASSESSMENT OF SPECIFIC CLINICAL POPULATIONS

The assessments outlined in Tables 9.6-5 through 9.6-7 can be applied to a broad range of clinical disorders. Applications with case examples are summarized below for children with verbal learning disabilities, nonverbal learning disabilities, head injury, and spina bifida and hydrocephalus.

VERBAL LEARNING DISABILITIES A variety of misleading terms have been used to describe children with problems in reading. The most common terms are "dyslexia" and "specific reading disability." Those terms are misleading in part because they imply that subgroups of children with reading problems exist that are somehow different from children with reading problems not reflecting dyslexia or specific reading disability. The impetus for the classification came from studies performed on the Isle of Wight and subsequently reported by Michael Rutter in the early 1980s that were interpreted as showing bimodality in the distribution of reading skills. The bimodality was represented as two groups of children, one with specific reading retardation and the other with general reading backwardness. The group with specific reading retardation had reading deficiencies that were discrepant with I.Q., whereas the group with general reading backwardness had reading skills consistent with I.Q.

More recent epidemiological studies have not found evidence of bimodality and have generally shown that reading skills exist on a continuum. That does not mean that reading disability is not biologically based. In particular, there is strong evidence for the heritability of reading disorders. However, there is little evidence that discrepancy or concordance with I.Q. is a meaningful way to classify reading disability.

Children with reading disabilities almost invariably have some form of language deficiency. The primary difficulty is inability to master decoding skills, that is, to recognize and identify single words. That deficit is most apparent when the child is asked to pronounce pseudowords (Figure 9.6-6), which are specifically assessed on the word attack subtest of the WJR. Underlying that deficiency are problems with the development of phonological awareness skills that allow the child to be aware of and to process the internal structures of words. That skill can be assessed with a variety of procedures. Figure 9.6-7 presents the Auditory Analysis Test, which requires the child to determine what word remains when a segment is deleted. Because of the phonological language deficits, spelling is also impaired. If the decoding problems are severe, reading comprehension and writing abilities are also impaired.

Reading disabilities are not solely problems with phonological language. Often language skills are more pervasively impaired, with particular problems with vocabulary and naming skills. In addition, problems with motor, perceptual, and attentional skills may be present. Figure 9.6-8 shows profiles of three groups of children across nine cognitive dimensions measured for a study of definitional variability in reading disabilities. The three groups include two defined as discrepant at different levels of severity (Rutter's specific reading retardation group) and a low achievement group that was poor in reading, average in intelligence, but not discrepant (general reading backwardness group). The profile configuration is similar in all three groups, differing only in relative severity. Differences in profile configuration between the low-achievement and I.Q.-discrepant groups are not apparent. All three groups showed much greater impairment on the phoneme deletion test (Figure 9.6-8). In contrast, visual-spatial skills were better developed. At each point in the profile the group averages are below the average range, indicating that the children had other cognitive problems. It is important to identify other problem areas during the assessment because they may be the starting point for development of a treatment plan. The prognosis is generally much better for a child with isolated phonological weaknesses and good perceptual skills than for a child with more pervasive language problems or perceptual deficits. Attention is a particularly relevant variable for assessment because 25 to 50 percent of children with reading disorders also have ADHD.

NAT

IB

HUDNED

MAFREATSUN

FIGURE 9.6-6 *Example of pseudowords that dyslexic children have difficulty identifying.*

K. was an 8-year-old right-handed boy referred for neuropsychological evaluation by his pediatrician. At the time of referral K. was completing first grade. He had been retained in kindergarten because of immaturity. The pediatrician was concerned because K.'s parents reported that K. had struggled throughout first grade in all areas except math. The parents had asked the school to evaluate K. for learning disability, but the school responded by pointing out that he was passing first-grade classes. However, the parents remained concerned, particularly because K. seemed frustrated at school and had been developing somatic complaints. The pediatrician found no physical basis for the complaints and requested an evaluation for possible learning disability.

A review of teacher reports indicated that K. was working well below grade level in reading and in spelling, somewhat below grade level in science and social studies, and at grade level in math. The teacher completed the Child Behavior Checklist. The only significant elevation was on the Attention Problems scale. Similar elevations were apparent on the parent version of the same checklist, except for a slight elevation on the anxious-depressed dimension.

Tests of academic achievement showed low scores on measures of word identification, word attack, passage comprehension, and written spelling. Average performance was apparent on a test of computational arithmetic. Because patterns of that sort are commonly associated with phonological language deficiencies, the neuropsychological test results were examined with that hypothesis in mind. In general, K. demonstrated poor performance on measures of phonological awareness, word retrieval, naming, and verbal short-term memory. Strengths were apparent on motor and perceptual skills. No intellectual problems were apparent, for both verbal and performance I.Q. scores were in the average range.

Discussion The evaluation elicited clear evidence of language-based impairments consistent with a reading disorder. In addition, there was evidence of ADHD in the parent and teacher reports and in the child's history elicited from the parents. There was evidence of the development of secondary emotional symptoms, reflecting the degree to which school was a frustrating experience.

Treatment The treatment plan devised for K. had three components. First, the child needed to be treated for ADHD with stimulant medication and environmental modifications at home and at school. Treatment of the attentional disorder was important to ensure that K. would maximally respond to instruction. The treatment program formulated for K. was one that would be standard for any child with ADHD and involved the use of stimulant medication, structured classrooms, and additional structure and consistency at home. Because there was no evidence of aggressive behavior or other behavioral problems, a systematic behavior modification program was not necessary. The second component concerned the school. K. met eligibility criteria for special education placement in reading and language arts, which was requested by the parents and arranged through a formal meeting by the school. The neuropsychologists provided a detailed treatment plan identifying specific reading programs that would be useful. The treatment plan emphasized multisensory teaching techniques to take advantage of K.'s well-developed perceptual skills to treat internal structures of words through sight recognition of morphemes and rhyming. The third component had to do with some of the secondary consequences of the learning problem, such as the somatic complaints. That component was handled primarily by an appropriate plan for the school-based problem, which was expected to relieve much of the child's concerns. The parents were educated about what to expect in the future, and plans for systematic follow-up were provided.

NONVERBAL LEARNING DISABILITIES Rourke's syndrome, the syndrome of nonverbal learning disabilities in children, is well understood but often not recognized. Although there have been many studies of children with reading prob-

Auditory Analysis Test

Name____Date____________________

School______________________________Grade______Teacher________________

Birthdate____________________

A. cow(boy)
B. (tooth)brush

1. birth(day)	21. (sh)rug
2. (car)pet	22. g(l)ow
3. bel(t)	23. cr(e)ate
4. (m)an	24. (st)rain
5. (b)lock	25. s(m)ell
6. to(ne)	26. Es(ki)mo
7. (s)our	27. de(s)k
8. (p)ray	28. Ger(ma)ny
9. stea(k)	29. st(r)eam
10. (l)end	30. auto(mo)bile
11. (s)mile	31. re(pro)duce
12. plea(se)	32. s(m)ack
13. (g)ate	33. phi(lo)sophy
14. (c)lip	34. s(k)in
15. ti(me)	35. lo(ca)tion
16. (sc)old	36. cont(in)ent
17. (b)reak	37. s(w)ing
18. ro(de)	38. car(pen)ter
19. (w)ill	39. c(l)utter
20. (t)rail	40. off(er)ing

FIGURE 9.6-7 *The auditory analysis test, a measure of phonological awareness. (Figure from J Rosner, P Simon: The auditory analysis test. J Learning Disabilities 4: 83, 1971. Used with permission.)*

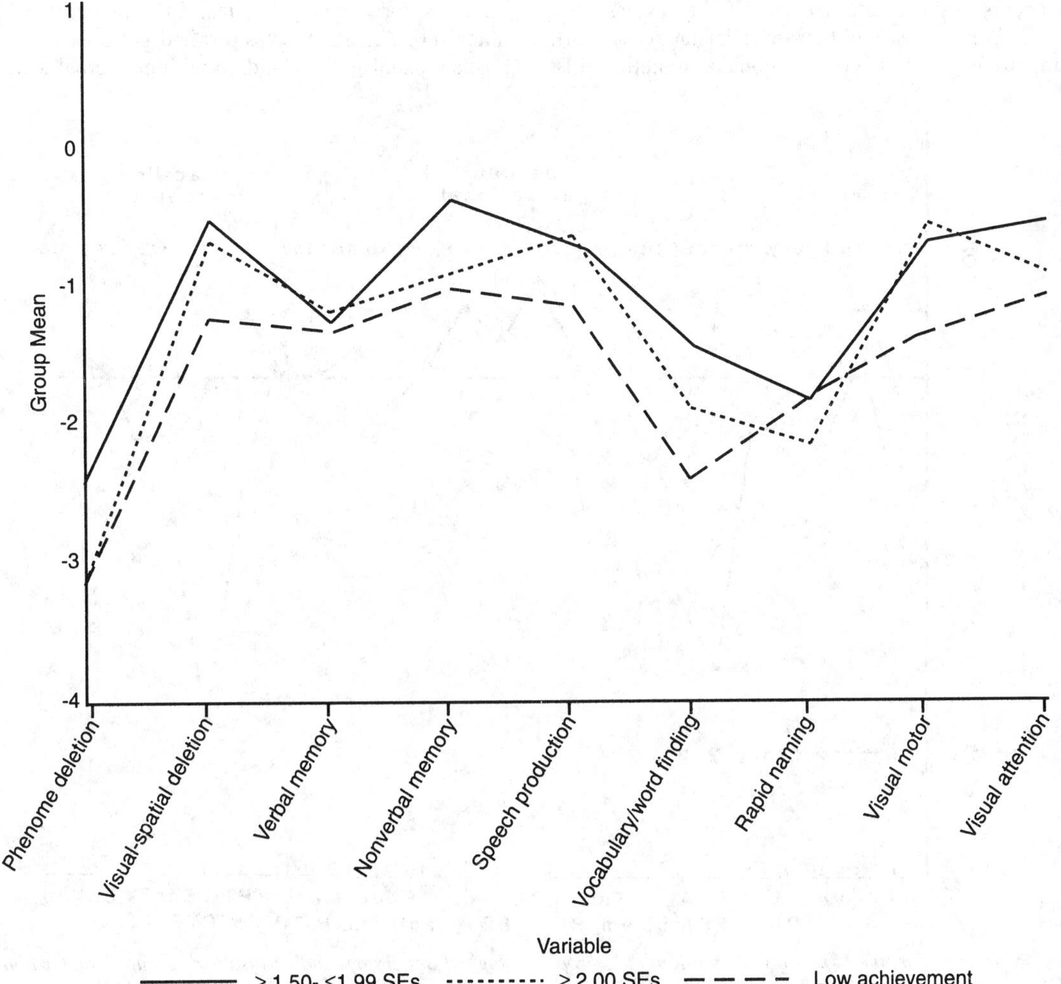

FIGURE 9.6-8 *Profile of performance in nine cognitive domains by three groups of children with reading disabilities.*

lems, relatively little research has been conducted on children who experience difficulty mastering arithmetic skills. The lack of research is surprising because a fairly large proportion of school-aged children—about 6 percent—have difficulties with arithmetic. In fact, there may be more arithmetic-disabled children than reading-disabled children (about 4 percent). The difference probably reflects the fact that most children with reading problems also have problems with arithmetic. Moreover, although the incidence of arithmetic impairment for any reason (including attention) without reading impairment is high, the incidence of reading impairment without arithmetic impairment is probably lower.

Nonverbal learning disabilities extend beyond problems with arithmetic and are not simply DSM-IV mathematics disorders. There are many types of arithmetic disabilities in children. For example, children who have motivational deficiencies may have poor grades in arithmetic. However, they often do well on standardized tests of arithmetic achievement and present with little impairment in neuropsychological or information-processing skills. Children with reading problems often have difficulty with arithmetic. Those children, whose reading problems may be related to language-processing difficulties, have special difficulty with word problems. They also forget number facts and procedures necessary for the successful execution of mechanical or computational arithmetic—errors that may reflect problems with verbal memory and the child's more general language-based learning disability.

Of special interest are children whose primary learning impairment occurs in computational arithmetic as assessed by the WRAT-R or WJR. Those children are characterized, in part, by severe impairment of basic computational arithmetic skills. However, in contrast to reading-disabled children who also show arithmetic deficits, they have excellent decoding skills with good abilities in word recognition and spelling. They often have a nonverbal learning disability, but such disabilities extend beyond math. Those disabilities were described by Pennington as a right hemisphere learning disability. In contrast to children with verbal learning disabilities, which are rarely seen in children with acquired brain injury, patterns of cognitive strengths and weaknesses characteristic of a nonverbal learning disability can be seen in children with brain injury or developmental disorders of learning.

Nonverbal learning disabilities are characterized by problems in (1) computational arithmetic and writing, (2) social competence, and (3) nonverbal cognitive skills. Errors in computational arithmetic reflect poor spatial organization, procedural errors, inattention to visual detail, and graphomotor problems. Writing is often poor, although thematic maturity may be at grade-appropriate levels. The assessment of computational arithmetic and writing abilities is typically completed with achievement tests, such as the WRAT-R, and represents an assessment of manifest disabilities (that is, problems with school achievement).

Social competency problems are often apparent in the development of social skills, particularly in unfamiliar or unstructured interpersonal situations. Anecdotal clinical descriptions include a poor understanding of other people's feelings and difficulty inferring emotions from behavior. Such problems may not reflect any particular problem with the children's capacity for empathy but instead may stem from difficulties interpreting facial expressions and gestures secondary to poor visual-spatial skills. Children with nonverbal learning disabili-

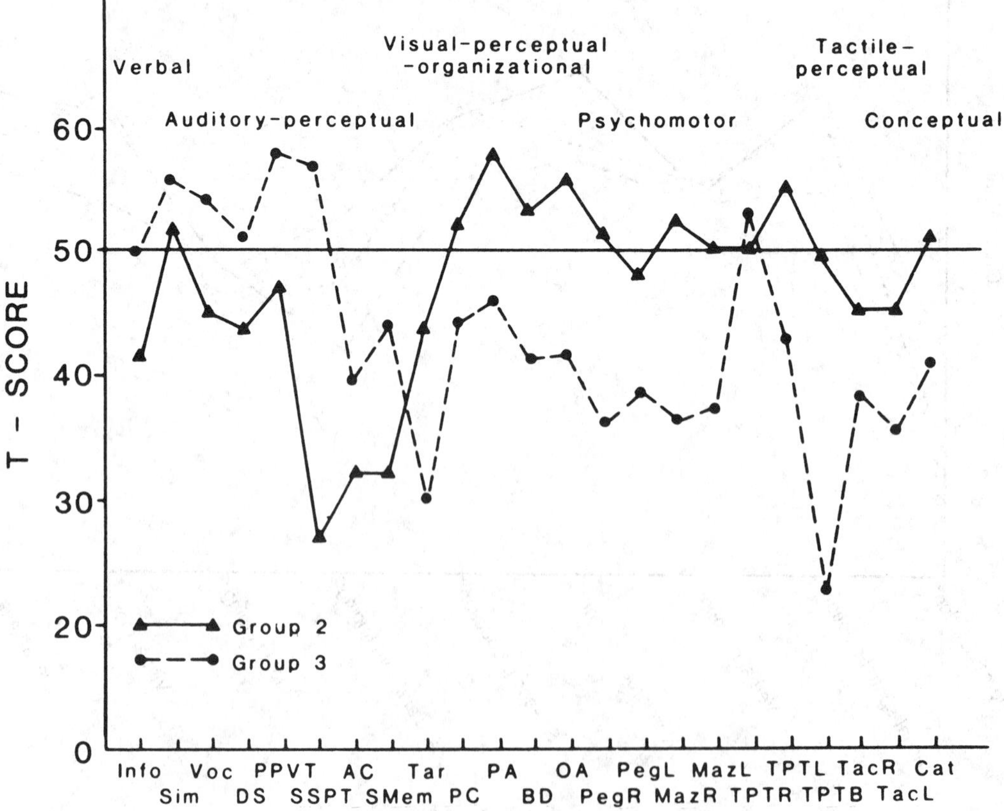

FIGURE 9.6-9 *Performance on the Modified Halstead-Reitan Neuropsychological Battery by reading-disabled (group 2) and arithmetic-disabled (group 3) children. (Figure from B P Rourke, J Fisk, J D Strang:* Neuropsychological Assessment of Children, *Guilford. New York, 1986. Used with permission.)*

ties also display body postures and facial expressions incongruent with their affect, and sometimes they show a poor understanding of appropriate interpersonal boundaries. They often talk excessively, a characteristic that reflects their well-developed automatic language skills. Although their vocabulary may be highly developed, language content sometimes seems empty, irrelevant, and tangential. They rely heavily on their verbal skills in interpersonal and learning situations and may underattend to nonverbal cues.

More generally, children with nonverbal learning disabilities seem poorly organized and unfocused. They are sometimes described as inattentive and distractible, but that behavior may reflect their poor organizational skills and reduced capacity for self-directed behavior rather than ADHD. Children with nonverbal learning difficulties often have problems initiating activities, particularly if the task is perceived as difficult, and they elicit considerable structure and direction from external figures (teachers, parents) through their verbal skills. The social component of the disability is not well understood but is important because it is a direct consequence of the information-processing disability. In other words, the nature of the cognitive problem leads to predictable problems with social competence and interpersonal behavior. That type of social problem contrasts with the reduced self-esteem, frustration, and low achievement motivation often associated with reading disabilities as secondary or indirect consequences of the effects of repeated failure. Assessment of the social component involves assessing the manifest disability and the psychosocial variables that influence adaptation to school and home. Interviews, personality tests, and behavior ratings are frequently employed and help distinguish the children with nonverbal learning disabilities from those with primary problems in attention or psychological adjustment.

In addition to problems with computational arithmetic and social competency, children with nonverbal learning disabilities exhibit characteristic difficulties on neuropsychological tasks. That pattern helps differentiate those children from reading-disabled children. Figure 9.6-9 shows the performance of groups of 9- to 14-year-old reading-disabled (group 2) and arithmetic-disabled (group 3) children on selected measures used by Rourke (Table 9.6-5). The scores have been converted into standard scores with a mean of 50 and a standard deviation of 10. A comparison of the group averages in the six areas measured by the tests shows that reading-disabled children (group 2) had significant difficulty on measures of verbal and auditory-perceptual skills but approximately average scores in other ability domains. In contrast, arithmetic-disabled children (group 3) performed at age level on verbal and auditory-perceptual tasks but displayed significant impairment on measures of visual-perceptual, psychomotor, tactile-perceptual, and conceptual abilities. By definition, children with nonverbal learning disabilities have difficulty on nonverbal processing tasks, including bilateral psychomotor and somatosensory deficits, which tend to be more apparent when the nondominant hand is tested. They may also have difficulties on tasks using novel or unfamiliar material or that require the development and application of problem-solving strategies in an unfamiliar task, even when the material to be processed can be verbally coded.

If the same groups of children had been examined using the procedures outlined in Table 9.6-6, similar patterns would have emerged. The reading-disabled children would have displayed problems on language-related tasks, including verbal memory skills. The arithmetic-disabled children would have had primary difficulties on tasks involving visual-spatial and constructional skills, somatosensory skills, motor skills, and nonverbal memory. Figure 9.6-10 compares the performance of reading- and arithmetic-disabled groups on selective reminding tasks for verbal and nonverbal material. The verbal task, shown in Figure 9.6-11, involved learning a list of animal names; the nonverbal task involved memory for dot locations (Figure 9.6-12). Two scores are provided for each task, representing long-term storage and consistent long-term retrieval. As shown in Figure 9.6-10, the reading-disabled children had difficulty on the verbal task (particularly with consistent long-term retrieval), whereas the arithmetic-disabled children had difficulty with both long-term storage and consistent long-term retrieval on the nonverbal task.

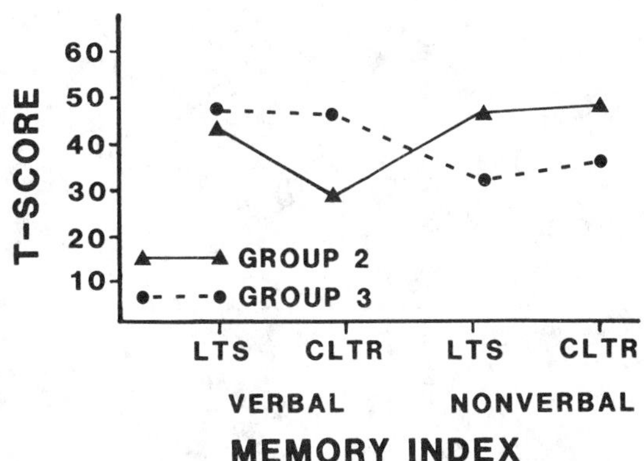

FIGURE 9.6-10 *Performance on verbal and nonverbal selective reminding tests by reading-disabled (group 2) and arithmetic-disabled (group 3) children. LTS = long-term storage, CLTR = consistent long-term retrieval.*

NAME Control ♀ DATE: 2-79
AGE 9 EDUC: 3

SELECTIVE REMINDING FOR CHILDREN ≤ 12 y.o.

	1	2	3	4	5	6	7	8
Dog		1	2	2	3	2	2	2
Fox	1	6	1	1	2	1	1	1
Horse		5	10	9	10	3	3	3
Lion		2	8	10	1	12	8	12
Elephant	3	10	6	3	8	11	7	7
Bear	4	12	9	6	7	9	9	4
Rat	2	11		5	9	10	10	9
Raccoon		3	3	8	11	8	12	6
Goat		4		4		6	11	8
Squirrel	7	8	7		4	5	5	10
Beaver	5	9	4		5	4	6	5
Turtle	6	7	5	7	6	7	4	11
Total Recall	7	12	10	10	11	12	12	12
LTR	7	11	10	9	11	12	12	12
STR	0	1	0	1	0	0	0	0
LTS	7	11	11	11	11	12	12	12
CLTR	4	8	8	9	11	12	12	12
Random LTR	3	3	2	0	0	0	0	0
Presentations	12	5	0	2	2	1	0	0

FIGURE 9.6-11 *Verbal selective reminding test for children.*

P. was a 15-year-old, right hemidecorticate girl. Pregnancy and delivery were normal, and developmental milestones were reached

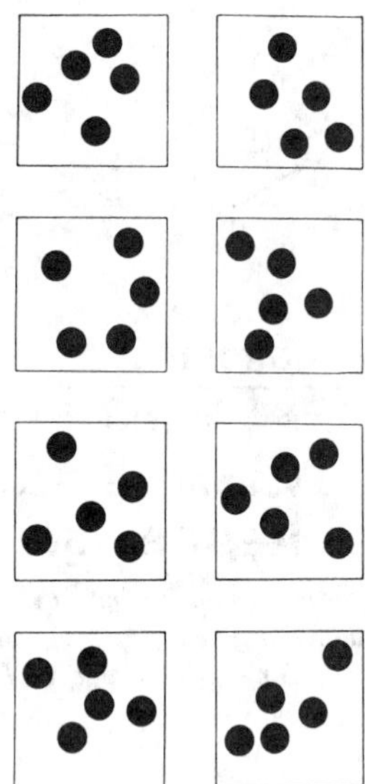

FIGURE 9.6-12 *Nonverbal selective reminding test.*

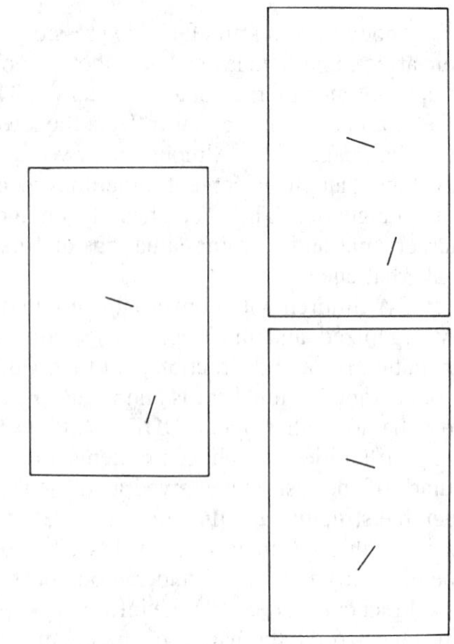

FIGURE 9.6-13 *Modified version of the judgment of line orientation test.*

early. However, at age 3½ years, P. contracted a viral encephalitis that resulted in intractable seizures. She did not respond to anticonvulsants and was in status epilepticus periodically for several months. At age 4 P. underwent surgical ablation of the right hemisphere for seizure control. The surgery resulted in complete seizure control but left P. with a left hemiparesis.

P. was referred by a child psychiatrist who was working with her on some behavioral problems. Specifically, P. came to the psychiatrist's attention because of several acting-out episodes, including frequent angry outbursts and responses that showed poor judgment. For example, after one altercation with her family, P. hopped on a bicycle and pedaled several miles to the freeway; she was found riding along a freeway feeder road. Although P. had been enrolled in a number of school environments and placed in resource classes for learning problems, the psychiatrist was concerned because P. had not undergone systematic evaluation for several years. The psychiatrist was also concerned about the demands and expectations apparent in P.'s current school environment. She was in regular middle school classes with no curriculum modifications. Consequently, the purpose of the evaluation was to determine P.'s neuropsychological functioning and to help evaluate the basis for the behavioral difficulties.

Neuropsychological results The results of the evaluation were consistent with a right hemispherectomy. Clear lateralizing deficits were apparent on measures of language and visual-spatial skills. For example, on verbal (Figure 9.6-11) and nonverbal (Figure 9.6-12) selective reminding tasks, P.'s performance was at age-appropriate levels on the verbal task but extremely impaired on the nonverbal task. Severe spatial processing problems were apparent. Figure 9.6-13 shows a modified version of Benton's judgment of line orientation test. The test requires the child to identify which orientation of lines on the bottom matches the top stimuli. P.'s score was below the first percentile for her age. It is noteworthy that although P. was hemiparetic on the left, motor and sensory functions were intact in the right hand. That would suggest good integrity of the isolated left hemisphere, which was probably reflected in her well-developed word recognition and written spelling skills. However, arithmetic abilities were poor. Comprehension skills in reading were also weak. P. was an excellent speller who used a phonetic strategy. She demonstrated problems on problem-solving tasks and had more general difficulties understanding cause and effect relationships in academic and social interpersonal situations. There was no evidence of formal psychopathology: Neither parent nor teacher ratings indicated significant problems with attention, anxiety, or depression. However, concerns were expressed about her development of social skills and her general absence of friends and social relationships.

Discussion Nonverbal learning disabilities can occur in children with and without acquired brain insults. The case of P. is interesting because it demonstrates the prototypical pattern described by Rourke for nonverbal learning disability and by Pennington for right hemisphere learning disability: P. had problems with nonverbal processing skills, executive functions, mechanical arithmetic, and social competency.

The intervention activities entailed consultation with the parents and psychiatrists, at which time the test results were presented and an alternative explanation of P.'s behavioral problems was discussed. The consequences of the right hemispherectomy were explained, with elaboration of the implications for school and personal functioning. Because of that information, psychotherapy for P. shifted from a psychodynamic model to a model recognizing the interaction of cognitive deficits with social competency. The psychiatrist altered the approach from an insight-oriented psychodynamic approach to one based on developing problem-solving skills, verbal rehearsal, and development of appropriate rules for interpersonal behavior. P. was placed on a waiting list for a special school for learning-disabled children. Because the school had a long waiting list, a meeting was held with public school personnel. Modifications of curriculum were arranged, particularly in terms of need for instruction in arithmetic. Because of the problems with reading comprehension, P. was placed with a speech-language therapist who specialized in children with learning disabilities. P. showed an immediate response to the curriculum modifications and to the tutorial intervention. Her parents thought that the tutorial intervention was more effective than psychotherapy and terminated their relationship with the psychiatrist. However, they maintained consultation arrangements around training for social skills. P. entered a regular high school with improvements in her adjustment, problem-solving skills, and interpersonal skills.

Treatment For children with nonverbal learning disabilities, the treatment plan should address the three components of the disability: educational, cognitive, and social. Didactic, compensatory approaches are generally emphasized. Intervention should not attempt directly to remediate the child's processing deficits. Such attempts may improve the deficient skill but may not generalize to the academic or behavioral deficit. Instead, remediation should address the specific academic and behavioral problems manifested in the classroom or adaptive functioning area (for example, peer relations) with an approach that emphasizes the child's strengths and helps develop compensatory mechanisms.

There are three guiding principles for treating children with nonverbal learning disabilities. First, interventions should be as verbal as possible. In completing arithmetic problems, verbal rules and routines should be emphasized. Children should rehearse steps verbally as they work arithmetic problems. Similarly, social competence skills can be improved if the behaviors are taught verbally, emphasizing repetition and rehearsal. The children will learn appropriate social behaviors less effectively if time-based contingent maneuvers are used (for example, time-out) or if training is done through a sequential contingent reward system. However, if appropriate social behavior is taught through language as a set of rules, the children have a better chance of developing appropriate social behavior. Because they often talk excessively, it may be helpful to encourage silent rehearsal and subvocalization.

Second, highly concrete and systematic teaching methods should be used. A parts-to-whole method, in which different activities (educational or behavioral) are broken into a set of component steps leading up to a sequence of activities, should be maximally effective. The children should not be expected to break down new activities into their components. Rather, the components and necessary strategies and techniques should be presented to them and taught verbally, with rehearsal and repetition. The children should not be expected to work independently, without structure and without external guidance, or the experience will be frustrating.

Third, children with nonverbal learning disabilities have significant organizational problems. They often do not understand how to approach a problem, particularly if it is unfamiliar, and may seem confused, unattentive, or unmotivated. Those difficulties do not always stem from attentional deficits; rather, they reflect intentional deficits secondary to the more general problems with organization, which may lead to difficulties in initiating new behavior. In more extreme cases such behavior can be misinterpreted as conduct problems and lead to excessive punishment that merely frustrates the child and exacerbates confusion and task avoidance. It is often tempting in such instances to remove structure from the child in an attempt to reduce dependency and increase responsibility. Such an approach is the opposite of what is needed by children with nonverbal learning disabilities. Structure should be enhanced, not reduced. The children may seem dependent when in fact they are attempting to elicit structure, which is a highly adaptive behavior. Hence, clinicians, educators, and parents should be aware of the difficulties the children have in organizing themselves and in initiating new behavior and should be prepared to provide organization and structure when needed.

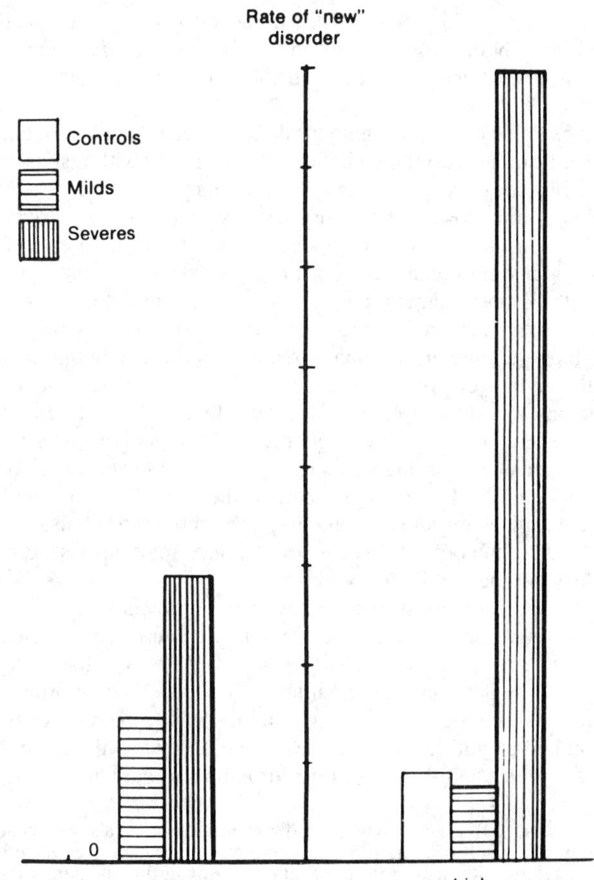

FIGURE 9.6-14 *Changes in the frequency of psychiatric disorders after mild and severe traumatic brain injury and in orthopedic control patients relative to psychological adversity. (Figure from Rutter M, Chadwick O, Shaffer D: Head injury. In* Developmental Neuropsychiatry, *M Rutter, editor, p 83. Guilford, New York, 1983. Used with permission.)*

TRAUMATIC BRAIN INJURY Neuropsychologists are commonly asked to evaluate children who have sustained traumatic brain injuries. Manifest disabilities typically involve difficulties with learning at school, accompanied by behavior problems at home or school, or both. Cognitive deficits vary with individual children. The most frequent deficits occur on (1) performance-based intelligence tests, (2) speeded motor tasks (for example, rate of finger tapping), (3) subtle aspects of language (for example, naming), and (4) memory and attention (selective reminding tasks). Psychosocial and environmental variables include the availability of rehabilitation resources in the school and community, the child's response to the injury (for example, depression), and the family's finances and capacity for dealing with an injured child. Biological variables include the nature and pathophysiological reaction of the CNS.

Memory and attentional deficits are the most frequent long-term sequelae of traumatic brain injury in children. The management and habilitation of a brain-injured child typically requires an interdisciplinary team. The plan must be revised frequently as the child recovers and the pattern of neuropsychological strengths and weaknesses changes. Behavioral changes are varied and common after head injury and must be dealt with on a case-by-case basis.

In addition to injury severity, it is important to assess the home environment before and after the injury in relation to the emergence of behavioral problems. Figure 9.6-14 shows the number of patients with mild and severe head injuries who developed a psychiatric disorder after traumatic brain injury in one study. Patients were grouped according to low or high psychosocial adversity in the home environment, with such items as divorce and financial problems representing high adversity. The incidence of subsequent behavioral problems in patients with severe brain injury was threefold higher in those who recovered in high-adversity environments. Thus, assessment of psychological and environmental variables is an important component of neuropsychological assessment.

Evaluation of biological indexes is critical in neuropsychological assessment of head injury. An evaluation of injury data should include an analysis of the nature and impact of the injury (that is, the etiology). The single most important variable is severity of the injury as assessed by depth of coma, length of posttraumatic amnesia, or duration of unconsciousness. Primary pathophysiological effects of head trauma include both multifocal, generalized injury caused by stretching of axonal fibers and the more specific mass effects of contusional injury. A host of potential secondary pathophysiological effects require careful evaluation. Head injury is associated with multiple complications, including hypoxia, increased intracranial pressure, and shock, all of which should be managed by the neurosurgeon during the acute phase of recovery. An evaluation of the child's condition includes a review of clinical neurological status, the duration of posttraumatic amnesia, and coma duration. Serial review of recovery in the intensive care unit and cerebral imaging procedures help elucidate the influence of secondary effects and late CNS changes (for example, atrophy and degeneration of white matter) that occur with head injury and potentially influence behavior.

The value of reviewing injury data has been demonstrated in several studies correlating indices of head injury with results on specific measures of cognitive development obtained after injury. From those studies injury severity appears to be the overriding correlate of recovery. Variables related to injury severity—including coma duration, indices of depth of coma, and length of posttraumatic amnesia—are most consistently associated with outcome. Longer periods of coma are associated with poorer outcomes. Brainstem abnormalities, including oculomotor and oculocephalic signs, are associated with poorer outcome on global ratings of recovery that focus on mortality and general quality of life. Higher levels of intracranial pressure are associated with higher mortality rates and lower scores on global ratings of outcome in some studies. The locus of injury as determined by cerebral tomography has not been consistently related to outcome. However, focal injury may have specific effects on the child's recovery.

For several reasons, then, clinicians need to consider neurological sources of variation in completing neuropsychological assessments of children, particularly if there is actual CNS injury. The presence of brain injury is generally known prior to referral. The task of the neuropsychologist is to establish behavioral and cognitive consequences of the injury and the relation of the injury and the recovery environment to outcome.

M. was a 14-year-old right-handed boy who sustained a severe head injury as a result of a high-speed motor vehicle accident. He was initially referred for neuropsychological evaluation during the admission hospitalization and subsequently was seen annually for several years. The initial referral sought information on the need for rehabilitation, the extent to which various cognitive skills were impaired by the head injury, and M.'s capacity for returning to independent functioning. Follow-up referrals were sought to clarify the basis for emerging school and behavioral problems.

Although substantial impairment was apparent shortly after the injury, by one year after injury M. had recovered considerably. At one-year follow-up M.'s overall performance was characterized by impulsive, inattentive behavior with poor planning and organizational skills. Memory for spatial material was at age-appropriate levels, but deficiencies in encoding and retrieving verbal information persisted. Language functions were generally intact except for mild difficulties in word retrieval and naming. Motor and perceptual skills were intact but had been markedly impaired on previous evaluations. Academically, word recognition and spelling abilities had improved, but arithmetic computations remained well below age-appropriate levels. In general, overall achievement was suppressed relative to premorbid levels, for M. had been in an accelerated program and functioning above the 80th percentile in all areas. Scores on domains of adaptive behavior were poor. Parent reports on the Vineland Adaptive Behavior Scales revealed continued concerns about attention, social judgment, and school achievement. No formal psychopathology was apparent.

The difficulties with verbal memory and computational arithmetic persisted on subsequent examinations. Attentional skills remained poor. Problems with social judgment, planning, and organization became prominent in M.'s adaptational style. Psychosocial factors were particularly pertinent and included an accelerated school placement prior to the accident. When M. was able to return to school, he and his family insisted on returning to the previous program, which was inappropriate. M.'s overall adaptation to the injury was characterized by attempts to deny the consequences of the injury, with resulting feelings of fatigue, failure, and poor self-esteem. Although the family had the resources to provide a variety of services, M. was not moved from the accelerated program until more than one year after the injury, and then was placed in a lower track of a tiered academic system. Legal action on M.'s behalf resulted in a large settlement. By age 18 he had dropped out of school, and the funds were almost depleted. On the most recent examination M. was receiving counseling and planned to attend college in a program adapted to the needs of persons with learning handicaps.

Discussion Biological factors were clearly important in M.'s case. There was a severe head injury, with initial neurological examination indicating an absence of eye opening and other oculovestibular signs consistent with a significant insult to the brainstem. The Glasgow Coma Scale scores were below 8 for eight days after injury. M. was unable to follow commands until about 15 days after the injury. Results of neuroimaging studies performed on the day of admission were within normal limits, but a follow-up computed tomography performed 12 days after injury indicated moderate ventricular atrophy. Magnetic resonance imaging performed three years after injury showed atrophy and residual changes in both frontal lobes.

Environmental factors included the child's high level of premorbid functioning and general denial by the child and family of the significance of the injury. The family resisted attempts to adjust M.'s academic program to his ability to function and had considerable difficulty adjusting to the changes M. experienced as a consequence of the injury. They were not able to place needed limits on his behavior, resulting in a period of reckless, out-of-control behavior. M. squandered a settlement that could have been used to facilitate his adjustment to adult life. The changes in adaptive functioning associated with traumatic brain injury can be seen in Figure 9.6-15, which shows declines in the overall score on the Vineland Adaptive Behavior Scales characteristic of severe versus less severe traumatic brain injury.

Treatment The treatment of brain-injured children varies according to injury severity and stage of recovery. In the acute state critical care management, often in an intensive care unit, is vital for preventing further injury to the CNS. The advent of helicopter ambulance services and trauma centers has helped reduce morbidity and mortality in brain-injured children. When the severely injured child emerges from coma, in-hospital services, particularly speech, occupational, and physical therapy, are important. When the child emerges from posttraumatic amnesia, neuropsychological evaluations are helpful for identifying areas requiring intervention and for planning reentry to community and school. Only a minority of children need (or can obtain) intensive rehabilitative services, which are usually viewed as the responsibility of the school. However, specific services may be required, such as occupational, physical, and speech therapy. Other cognitive and behavioral problems may remain and pose longer-term obstacles to habilitation. Useful methods of intervention in such cases entail services that can be provided at school and at home because of the importance of the child's reentering the community. For brain injury of any

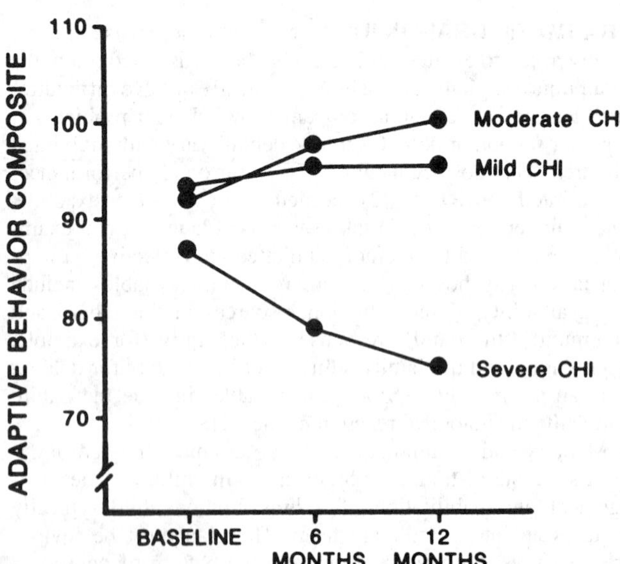

FIGURE 9.6-15 *Changes in the Vineland Adaptive Behavior Scale composite score during the first year of recovery in children with mild, moderate, and severe closed head injury (CHI). (Figure from J M Fletcher, L Ewing-Cobbs, M E Miner, H S Levin, H M Eisenberg: Behavioral changes after head injury in children. J Consult Clin Psychol 58: 93, 1990. Used with permission.)*

severity, the family must be educated about appropriate expectations for the child and for long-term progress.

HYDROCEPHALUS Another common complication of brain injury that may lead to referral for neuropsychological assessment is hydrocephalus. Hydrocephalus is generally caused by other disorders. For example, head injury and infectious diseases often lead to an increase in ventricular pressure and subsequent ventricular dilation. A variety of medical problems can lead to congenital hydrocephalus. Three principal etiologies of early hydrocephalus are aqueductal stenosis, spina bifida, and prematurity. All three conditions are also associated with other congenital neuropathological anomalies that influence development. Children with aqueductal stenosis have hydrocephalus and abnormalities of the corpus callosum, including partial agenesis. Spina bifida is a defect in neural tube closure representing a broad range of CNS changes, including spinal cord defects and multiple brain anomalies. The brain anomalies include Arnold-Chiari malformation and corpus callosum defects. Finally, some premature infants develop hydrocephalus secondary to intraventricular hemorrhage. Specific neurological deficits depend on the laterality and severity of the hemorrhage and on other complications of prematurity, such as respiratory distress.

Congenital forms of hydrocephalus have generally been associated with selective reductions in nonverbal processing skills. Most children who develop hydrocephalus early in development are not mentally deficient. However, children with early hydrocephalus often show discrepancies in the development of language versus nonverbal processing skills (Figure 9.6-4). Problems with perceptual matching, visual-motor processing, attention, and problem-solving skills are common. In addition, many hydrocephalic children experience difficulties learning arithmetic and writing. In contrast, many language skills develop normally. There may be difficulties with the pragmatic component of language, but language skills are generally preserved relative to nonlanguage skills. Sometimes children with congenital hydrocephalus experience other complications that lead to more general reductions in cognitive skills.

Neuropsychological assessment of children with hydrocephalus is important because the children can present with multiple deficits related to hydrocephalus and associated medical complications. In addition there is a tendency to view the disorder as primarily orthopedic, particularly in children with spina bifida. In such cases it is important to discriminate the components of the disorder that are related to brain function. Finally, children with early hydrocephalus have extensive medical histories and often require numerous interventions, such as shunting. Other medical problems, such as problems with bladder and bowel control, are prevalent. Some children also have cerebral palsy. Consequently, the parents may feel stressed. The assessment of children with hydrocephalus is similar to that outlined for children with right hemisphere learning disabilities and head injury.

V. was a 12-year-old right-handed boy referred for neuropsychological assessment by a neurosurgeon because of the mother's many complaints about how her child was being treated at school. V. was labeled an orthopedically handicapped child. He was in regular classes in school but was allowed to go to a support classroom if he requested special assistance. The teacher reports indicated concerns about attention and organizational skills and numerous complaints about his behavior. In particular, V. was described as lazy, unmotivated, and occasionally oppositional. Parent reports also indicated concerns about attention. On the teacher version of the Child Behavior Checklist there were significant elevations on social problems and attention and a secondary elevation on aggression. Parent ratings were elevated only on social problems and attention.

V. had a complicated medical history. He was born with a myelomeningocele that was repaired at birth. A shunt was placed during the first month of life for hydrocephalus. Subsequently, several revisions were performed to lengthen the tubing, and a period of significant obstruction required shunt replacement at age 3 years. The spinal lesion was at level T4. V. was partially ambulatory (with braces) but had problems with bowel and bladder control.

On neuropsychological testing V.'s scores were much lower on the performance I.Q. measure of the WISC-R than on the verbal I.Q. measure, consistent with the data shown in Figure 9.6-4. His strengths were in areas involving language, including phonological analysis, vocabulary, and reading. Computational arithmetic and written spelling skills were poorly developed relative to decoding skills. Memory, attention, and executive function skills were below age-appropriate levels.

Treatment The treatment plan addressed a number of issues. The first issue was the use of stimulant medication to address the attentional deficiencies observed in the evaluation. Because V.'s language skills were well developed, the verbal short-term deficits might have reflected deficient attention as opposed to actual memory deficiencies. The recommendation for stimulant medication was discussed with V.'s pediatrician, and V. was given a trial dose of 15 mg of methylphenidate (Ritalin) calculated at a therapeutic range of 0.6 mg per kg. An evaluation of short-term memory and attention skills while the medication was in effect indicated significant improvement, particularly in short-term memory. Subsequent teacher reports confirmed the efficacy of the intervention.

The second treatment issue addressed involved modifying the educational plan. Excessive demands were being placed on V. to structure his own behavior. For example, he was expected to indicate when he needed to go to content mastery instruction for assistance. Under the modified plan V. was monitored and simply instructed to go to content mastery under certain situations. Those situations included timed tests, essays, and other materials making greater demands on his attention and organizational skills. Other modifications primarily required his teachers to keep lesson plans and assignment notebooks with him. Another student wrote his assignments for him. The amount of written work required was reduced, because V. was being penalized for writing problems. Many of his outspoken behaviors were related to inability to complete written work as rapidly as required. Counseling was arranged through the school in an attempt to teach social skills in a didactic fashion. Occupational therapy was instituted with the goal of teaching keyboarding skills, and V. continued to receive physical therapy.

EMOTIONALLY DISTURBED CHILDREN Children who have primary problems with emotional functioning often have difficulty with cognitive and motor skills. Those difficulties may contribute to difficulties in implementing a treatment plan. Neuropsychological tests can be useful for establishing the extent to which a particular behavioral problem reflects emotional or cognitive factors, or both. The evaluations are conducted in much the same way as with any other child, but with more emphasis on the assessment of emotional problems. School-related difficulties with learning are dealt with in the same manner as for children with primary learning disabilities, with accommodations according to the emotional factors operant in the case (that is, psychosocial variables).

It is not always recognized that cognitive problems can contribute to the implementation of a psychotherapeutic program. In other words, children with language or visual-spatial processing deficits may have difficulty adapting to certain components of the treatment plan. Tables 9.6-8 and 9.6-9 outline a series of clinical management tools developed at a residential treatment center for children with significant emotional disturbances (Southwest Neurobehavioral Institute, San Antonio, Texas). The recommendations stemmed from an interdisciplinary assessment of children that included a neuropsychological evaluation. As the tables indicate, children's participation in social or educational milieus and procedures for setting limits on behavior and specific aspects of therapy were modified, depending on the presence of basic competency deficits in language or visual-spatial skills.

The clinical management tools in Tables 9.6-8 and 9.6-9 each begin with a set of behavioral manifestations. That portion of the tool translates the consequences of cognitive deficits into

TABLE 9.6-8
Clinical Management Tool for Language-Processing Deficits

I. Behavioral manifestations
  A. Receptive (listening) problem
    1. Does not seem to understand what is being said.
    2. Does not respond appropriately to verbal commands. Behavior doesn't match command.
    3. Child looks distractible when being given verbal commands.
    4. Child seems to forget what has been said to him or her (does not understand).
    5. Child asks many questions in order to understand.
  B. Expressive (talking) problem
    1. Poor language usage. Speaks in one-word or short sentences.
    2. Does not use language to describe affects or experiences. Has trouble telling about feelings and needs.
    3. Has difficulty communicating needs.
    4. Stammers because of word retrieval problems. Uses gestures or jargon instead.
    5. Uses incomplete sentences so that listener has to fill in material.
    6. Uses disorganized speech, talks in circles.
    7. Speech is hard to understand because of articulation problems.
II. Management techniques and approaches
  A. Receptive problem
    1. Get the child's attention (use eye contact, call name).
    2. Speak clearly and slowly.
    3. Speak in short statements.
    4. Repeat if necessary, leaving one word blank for child to fill in.
    5. Have child repeat what was said to ensure understanding.
    6. Provide list of things to be done. Child checks off each item on completion.
    7. If child cannot read, use pictures.
    8. Provide running commentary of what child or you are doing.
  B. Expressive problem
    1. Listen to what child is saying rather than how child is saying it, then confirm what you thought child said.
    2. Include the child in group activities but do not force participation.
    3. If child's communication is unclear, ask for different word or gestures.
    4. Provide child with verbal response, leaving a word to fill in.
  C. Handling time-outs (receptive and expressive)
    1. Use visual cues to warn child that a time-out is imminent.
    2. Avoid why questions. Instead, verbalize briefly what you think the child is feeling. Focus on the child's emotions and feelings. Use facial expressions and gestures.
    3. Before time-out is over and when child is calm, briefly review what caused time-out.
    4. When time-out is over, let child communicate perception or feelings nonverbally by drawing pictures, using play equipment, modeling with clay, or through drama.

everyday behavioral terminology. Because a number of staff members work with the child, jargon is avoided in favor of descriptions of potential problems. The descriptions do not fit every child but represent protypical cases. The staff is trained to observe the child using the results of the assessment and to develop specific descriptions for each case.

The second part of each management tool provides examples of program modifications that may prove useful for a given child. The modifications apply to the milieu and influence the setting of limits and discipline for various behavioral problems. Psychotherapeutic procedures may also be modified, depending on the nature of the problem. Classroom management (and instructional techniques) could also be modified after the results of the neuropsychological assessment are obtained.

The goal of an assessment is to develop habilitative plans for children, regardless of the diagnosis or presenting problem. In the cases of head injury, hydrocephalus, and emotional disturbance, the existence of CNS injury or severe emotional disorders is known prior to the evaluation. The neuropsychological evaluation helps establish the nature of the problem and the contribution of central processing deficiencies, behavioral and environmental factors, and CNS status. Simplistic causal statements are avoided in favor of a broader formulation of the nature of the child's problem. Through that formulation, a habilitative plan is developed and coordinated with other disciplines. Questions concerning brain status are addressed, but only in the context of other evaluative technologies, the child's history, and current presentation. Neuropsychological testing is a component of the assessment. A complete evaluation of the child also requires a broader focus by skilled practitioners in other disciplines, with a major emphasis on using the assessment to treat the child's disorder. Such an approach makes the best use of testing data and most fully benefits the child.

TABLE 9.6-9
Clinical Management Tool for Visual-Spatial Processing Deficits

Behavioral Manifestations
1. Difficulty understanding cause-and-effect relations. (Children have poor ability to develop insight and to learn from experience.)
2. Difficulty organizing and modulating behavioral responses to a broad range of environmental events and expectations.
3. Difficulty initiating activity, planning approach to tasks, and carrying out intentions. (Children are frequently seen as having problems attending—as lazy, disorganized, and poorly motivated.)
4. Difficulty interpreting social situations:
   a. Interpreting impact of their behavior on other people.
   b. Understanding gestures, social cues, spatial boundaries. (Children often appear undersocialized and unempathic.)
5. Difficulty conceptualizing passage of time. (Children may be seen as oppositional.)
6. Difficulty responding well to lengthy time-out procedures.
7. Difficulty orienting to place. (Children have a poor sense of direction and can get lost.)
8. Tendency to be concrete despite potential to develop more abstract abilities using language.
9. Difficulty recalling visually perceived information. (Children do not learn well by watching others.)
10. Tendency in some children to be tactually defensive and to become disorganized or fearful when touched.
11. Greater ease in processing information verbally.
12. Difficulty understanding or learning from novel experiences.

Management Techniques and Approaches
1. Encourage children to talk about experiences to others and to themselves.
2. Engage them in a verbal dialogue in which child is asked to elaborate on what is said or to fill in missing parts of dialogue or story.
3. Structure the environment to assist them in organizing time and procedures.
4. Post a written daily schedule with provision for checking off activities as completed.
5. Use procedure charts for more complicated activities.
6. Label drawers and shelves to assist the child in organizing living spaces.
7. Establish clear-cut behavioral expectations and consequences for misbehavior. Verbally explain cause-and-effect sequence after consequences have been administered.
8. Facilitate adaptation to changes in the environment by preparing the child beforehand.
9. When possible, rehearse new situations prior to actual participation.
10. Facilitate an awareness of time concepts by making references to familiar events or by using a timer or clock.
11. Consider alternative disciplinary procedures. For example, having the child write 50 times: "I will not ______." Or, if writing skills are poor, the child may record on a tape: "I will not ______."
12. When going to new places, accompany the child and talk about landmarks that will aid in finding the way. Children will need multiple tours.
13. Children frequently need to be told what is happening in social situations and need more specific directions concerning how to respond.
14. Consider structured social skills training.
15. If the child appears uncomfortable when touched, de-emphasize touching and hugging. Express feelings verbally.

SUGGESTED CROSS-REFERENCES

Supplemental approaches to testing are described in different chapters of the book. Section 9.5 describes the neuropsychological and intellectual assessment of adults. Sections 9.4 and 9.8 describe the use of psychological tests and psychiatric rating scales for behavioral problems and emotional difficulties in children. Information relevant to the syndromes discussed in this section may be found in Section 2.4 on neuropsychiatric aspects of head trauma, Section 36.2 on learning disorders, Chapter 37 on pervasive developmental disorders, Chapter 38 on attention-deficit disorders, and Section 46.3 on pharmacotherapy.

REFERENCES

Baron I S, Fennel E, Voeller K: *Pediatric Neuropsychology in the Medical Setting.* Oxford, New York, 1995.

Benton A L: Behavioral indices of brain injury in school children. Child Dev *33:* 199, 1962.

Bernstein J H, Waber D P: Developmental neuropsychological assessment: The systemic approach. In *Neuropsychology,* A A Boulton, G B Baker, M Hiscock, editors. Humana, Clifton, NJ, 1990.

*Broman S H, Grafman J, editors: *Atypical Cognitive Deficits in Developmental Disorders.* Lawrence Erlbaum, Hillsdale, NJ, 1993.

Broman S H, Michel M: *Traumatic Head Injury in Children.* Oxford, New York, 1995.

Dennis M, Barnes M: Developmental aspects of neuropsychology: Childhood. In *Handbook of Perception and Cognition,* vol 15, *Neuropsychology,* D Zaidel, editor. Academic Press, New York, 1994.

Dennis M: Neuropsychological assessment: New facts and new concepts. In *Behavioral Assessment of Childhood Disorders,* vol 5, J Call, R Cohen, S Harrison, L Stone, editors, p 146. Basic Books, New York, 1985.

Fletcher J M: Neuropsychological assessment of brain-injured children. In *Behavioral Assessment of Childhood Disorders,* ed 2, L Terdal, E Mash, editors. Guilford, New York, 1988.

Fletcher J M, Ewing-Cobbs L, Miner M E, Levin H S, Eisenberg H M: Behavioral changes after head injury in children. J Consult Clin Psychol *58:* 93, 1990.

Fletcher J M, Levin H S, Butler I J: Neurobehavioral effects of brain injury in children. In *Handbook of Pediatric Psychology,* M Roberts, editor. Guilford, New York, 1995.

*Fletcher J M, Shaywitz S E, Shankweiler D P, Katz L, Liberman I Y, Fowler A, Francis D J, Stuebing K K, Shaywitz B A: Cognitive profiles of reading disability: Comparisons of discrepancy and low achievement definitions. J Educ Psychol *85:* 1, 1993.

Fletcher J M, Taylor H G: Neuropsychological approaches to children: Towards a developmental neuropsychology. J Clin Exp Neuropsychol *7:* 24, 1984.

Kahn E, Cohen L H: Organic driveness: A brain stem syndrome and experience. NEJ Med *210:* 748, 1934.

Kaufman A: *Intelligent Testing with the WISC-R.* Academic Press, New York, 1979.

Matarazzo J D: Psychological assessment of intelligence. In *Comprehensive Textbook of Psychiatry,* ed 4, vol 2, H I Kaplan, B J Sadock, editors, p 5. Williams & Wilkins, Baltimore, 1985.

Lyon G R, editor: *Frames of Reference for the Assessment of Learning Disabilities.* Paul H Brookes, Baltimore, 1994.

*Pennington B F: *Diagnosing Learning Disorders: A Neuropsychological Framework.* Guilford, New York, 1991.

Reitan R M, Wolfson D: *Neuropsychological Assessment of Older Children.* Neuropsychology Press, Tucson, 1992.

*Rourke B P: *Nonverbal Learning Disabilities: The Syndrome and the Model.* Guilford, New York, 1989.

Rourke B P, editor: *Nonverbal Learning Disabilities: Manifestations in Neurological Disease, Disorder, and Dysfunction.* Guilford, New York, 1995.

Rourke B P, Bakker B J, Fisk J L, Strang J D: *Child Neuropsychology: An Introduction to Theory, Research, and Clinical Practice.* Guilford, New York, 1983.

Rourke B P, Fisk J, Strang J D: *Neuropsychological Assessment of Children: A Treatment-Oriented Approach.* Guilford, New York, 1986.

Rourke B P, Fuerst D: *Learning Disabilities and Psychosocial Functioning.* Guilford, New York, 1991.

Rutter M: Psychological sequelae of brain damage in children. Am J Psychiatry *138:* 1533, 1981.

Rutter M: Syndromes attributed to "minimal brain dysfunction" in childhood. Am J Psychiatry *139:* 21, 1982.

Sattler J M: *Assessment of Children's Intelligence and Special Abilities,* ed 2. Allyn & Bacon, Boston, 1982.

Satz P, Fletcher J M: Minimal brain dysfunctions: An appraisal of research concepts and methods. In *Handbook of Minimal Brain Dysfunctions: A Critical Review,* H E Rie, E D Rie, editors, p 669. Wiley, New York, 1980.

Sparrow S S, Fletcher J M, Cicchetti D V: Psychological assessment of children. In *Psychiatry,* vol 2, J O Cavenar, editor, chap 21. Lippincott, Philadelphia, 1985.

Stanovich K, Siegel L S: Phenotypic performance profile of children with reading disabilities: A regression-based test of the phonological-core variable-difference model. J Educ Psychol *86:* 24, 1994.

Strauss A A, Lehtinen L E: *Psychopathology and Education of the Brain-Injured Child.* Grune & Stratton, New York, 1947.

*Taylor H G: Learning disabilities. In *Behavioral Treatment of Childhood Disorders,* E J Mash, R A Barkley, editors, p 347. Guilford, New York, 1989.

Taylor H G: Neuropsychological testing: Relevance for assessing children with learning disabilities. J Consult Clin Psychol *56:* 795, 1989.

Taylor H G, Fletcher J M: Neuropsychological assessment of children. In *Handbook of Psychological Assessment,* ed 2, G Goldstein, M Hersen, editors, p 211. Wiley, New York, 1995.

Taylor H G, Schatschneider C: Child neuropsychological assessment: A test of basic assumptions. Clin Neuropsychologist *3:* 259, 1992.

Wilson B: Neuropsychological assessment of preschool children. In *Handbook of Clinical Neuropsychology,* vol 2, S Filskov, T J Boll, editors. Wiley, New York, 1986.

Yvilsaker M, editor: *Head Injury Rehabilitation: Children and Adults.* College Hill Press, San Diego, 1985.

9.7 MEDICAL ASSESSMENT AND LABORATORY TESTING IN PSYCHIATRY

RICHARD B. ROSSE, M.D.
LYNN H. DEUTSCH, D.O.
STEPHEN I. DEUTSCH, M.D., Ph.D.

INTRODUCTION

Psychiatrists are increasingly expected to perform medical evaluations designed to detect potential medical problems underlying a psychiatric presentation. The psychiatric manifestations (for example, hallucinations, delusions) of a particular medical disorder are usually not specific to that medical condition alone, so the clinician needs to entertain a list of organic possibilities for the patient's psychiatric symptoms. Table 9.7-1 outlines a list of medical conditions that may present with psychiatric symptoms. Each of those diagnostic possibilities may argue for a different set of laboratory or diagnostic tests. The discovery of an organic cause for a psychiatric presentation can have profound treatment implications for directing the therapy away from mere symptomatic treatment and toward an appropriate therapeutic intervention for the underlying medical problem.

A relevant medical history, a review of systems, and a physical examination are essential for the selection of appropriate laboratory and diagnostic tests. Unfortunately, it is often difficult to get a reliable medical history and review of systems from certain neuropsychiatric patients (for example, patients with dementia or delirium, patients who are psychotic and agitated, or patients who are depressed and uncommunicative). In such patients the clinician is often forced to rely on various objective measures—including the physical examination, a mental status examination, and selected laboratory and diagnostic tests—for clues suggestive of underlying medical or neurological conditions. Using the nomenclature in the fourth edition of *Diagnostic and Statistical Manual of Mental Disorders* (DSM-IV), the psychiatrist needs to be attentive to possible Axis III diagnoses of physical illnesses in patients. A criterion for many of the functional disorders listed in DSM-IV is that the patient's condition is not attributable to a known organic factor.

The laboratory has become increasingly important for the

TABLE 9.7-1
Some Medical Disorders That May Present with Neuropsychiatric Symptoms

Neurological
- Cerebrovascular disorders (hemorrhage, infarction)
- Head trauma (concussion, posttraumatic hematoma)
- Epilepsy (especially complex partial seizures)
- Narcolepsy
- Brain neoplasms (primary or metastatic)
- Normal pressure hydrocephalus
- Parkinson's disease
- Multiple sclerosis
- Huntington's disease
- Alzheimer's disease
- Metachromatic leukodystrophy
- Migraine

Endocrine
- Hypothyroidism
- Hyperthyroidism
- Hypoadrenalism
- Hyperadrenalism
- Hypoparathyroidism
- Hyperparathyroidism
- Hypoglycemia
- Hyperglycemia
- Diabetes mellitus
- Panhypopituitarism
- Pheochromocytoma
- Gonadotrophic hormonal disturbances

Metabolic and systemic
- Fluid and electrolyte disturbances (e.g., Syndrome of Inappropriate Antidiuretic Hormone Secretion [SIADH])
- Hepatic encephalopathy
- Uremia
- Porphyria
- Hepatolenticular degeneration (Wilson's disease)
- Hypoxemia (chronic pulmonary disease)
- Hypotension
- Hypertensive encephalopathy

Toxic
- Intoxication or withdrawal associated with drug or alcohol abuse
- Side effects of prescribed and over-the-counter medications
- Environmental toxins (volatile hydrocarbons, heavy metals, carbon monoxide, organophosphates)

Nutritional
- Vitamin B_{12} deficiency (pernicious anemia)
- Nicotinic acid deficiency (pellagra)
- Folate deficiency (megaloblastic anemia)
- Thiamine deficiency (Wernicke-Korsakoff syndrome)
- Trace metal deficiency (zinc, magnesium)
- Nonspecific malnutrition and dehydration

Infectious
- Acquired immune deficiency syndrome (AIDS)
- Neurosyphilis
- Viral meningitides and encephalitides (e.g., herpes simplex)
- Brain abscess
- Viral hepatitis
- Infectious mononucleosis
- Tuberculosis
- Systemic bacterial infections (especially pneumonia) and viremia

Autoimmune
- Systemic lupus erythematosus

Neoplastic
- Central nervous system primary and metastatic tumors
- Endocrine tumors
- Pancreatic carcinoma
- Paraneoplastic syndromes

Table adapted from Darrell G Kirch, MD.

safe and maximally effective use of certain psychotropic medications. Laboratory testing may be used to obtain baseline functioning of the patient's cardiac or renal status before initiating medication, to confirm treatment compliance, to monitor therapeutic blood levels, and to detect clinically unrecognized toxicity. The specific tests depend on the patient's age and medical condition and the particular organ systems affected by the psychotropic agent. The laboratory is also essential in the assessment and management of patients with substance use disorders.

MEDICAL HISTORY AND PHYSICAL EXAMINATION

A medical history and a review of systems are especially important in the initial evaluation and the evaluation of patients with new physical complaints. The traditional parameters of the medical history start with the patient's current physical complaints, the history of their onset, and current medications, including over-the-counter medications, vitamins, and home remedies. The medical history should also include an assessment of the patient's past overall health; an investigation into past injuries (such as motor vehicle accidents, head trauma, and periods of unconsciousness); surgeries; occupational and toxic exposures; illicit drug use; alcohol, tobacco, and caffeine use; previous hospitalizations for medical reasons; and allergies to medication. A review of systems may elicit symptoms suggestive of underlying medical disease. Many psychiatrists think that the therapeutic alliance is strengthened by the process of doing a medical evaluation, including a physical examination. However, psychiatric practitioners must use their judgment in determining who will perform the medical evaluation of particular patients, especially those with paranoia and sexual concerns. A chaperone should be used when appropriate during a physical examination. The deferral of a physical examination should be for as short a period of time as possible.

LABORATORY TESTING

Some clinicians and researchers support a frugal, selective approach to ordering screening tests for psychiatric patients. They provide data suggesting that few important organic causes of psychiatric dysfunction are detected by extensive screening in physically healthy psychiatric patients. However, proponents of extensive and nonselective testing strategies provide literature supporting the claim that medical problems with important treatment implications for the psychiatric patient are missed by selective screening. Although disagreement continues regarding exactly which and how many tests to perform in evaluating psychiatric patients, the relevance and the meaning of the results for a patient should be clear to the physician ordering the tests.

CHOOSING THE TESTS A patient's history and physical examination typically dictate which tests should be ordered. For instance, a young college student with a history of drug use may need an illicit drug use screen, and a patient with risk factors for acquired immune deficiency syndrome (AIDS) may need testing for human immunodeficiency virus (HIV). Tests can also be ordered to help rule out possible organic causes or contributors to the psychiatric presentation. For example, a young adult with a first psychotic episode may need a computed tomographic (CT) scan of the head to rule out possible intracranial pathology. Diagnostic tests can often serve a therapeutic function by reassuring the patient and the family that other serious medical problems are not present.

A test that is ordered should have some pretest probability of abnormal results, and the abnormality should be meaningful in the context of the patient's psychiatric or medical condition. Table 9.7-2 lists some diagnostic tests used in the evaluation of a wide range of psychiatric patients. Table 9.7-3 lists numerous psychiatric indications for diagnostic tests.

FOLLOW-UP TESTS Follow-up laboratory testing is needed whenever a significant abnormality has been found. Additional

TABLE 9.7-2
Laboratory Diagnostic Tests of Potential Relevance to the Psychiatric Patient

Hematology
- Complete blood count (CBC)*
- Sedimentation rate
- Prothrombin time, partial thromboplastin time

Chemistry
- Serum electrolytes*
- Blood glucose*
- Blood urea nitrogen (BUN)*
- Serum creatinine*
- Serum calcium*
- Serum phosphorus
- Serum magnesium
- Total protein
- Serum protein electrophoresis
- Serum albumin
- Liver enzymes
- Creatine phosphokinase (CPK)
- Alkaline phosphatase
- Blood ammonia nitrogen (plasma ammonia)
- Serum bilirubin
- Thyroid function tests
  - Thyroxine (T_4)*
  - Triiodothyronine (T_3)
  - Thyroid-stimulating hormone (TSH)
- Serum B_{12} and folate
- Plasma cortisol levels
- Blood alcohol
- Drug screen (or specific illicit drug level)
- Medication blood levels
- Erythrocyte uroporphyrinogen-1-synthetase
- Serum copper and ceruloplasmin
- Serum amylase
- Serum lipase

Serology
- Screening test for syphilis (VDRL or RPR)*
- Human immunodeficiency virus (HIV) serology
- Hepatitis screens
- LE cell preparation
- Serum antinuclear antibodies (ANA)
- Lupus anticoagulant
- Anticardiolipin antibodies (ACA)
- Antithyroid antibodies

Urine tests
- Urinalysis
- Urine screens for illicit drug use*
- Urinary uroporphyrins, porphobilinogen, and Δ-aminolevulinic acid
- Urinary catecholamines
- Urine copper and ceruloplasmin, heavy metals
- Urine myoglobulin

Stool tests
- Occult blood
- Tests for suspected laxative abuse

Radiological procedures
- Chest X-ray
- Skull X-ray
- Computed tomography (CT) of the brain
- Magnetic resonance imaging (MRI) of the brain

Other procedures
- Lumbar puncture
- Electrocardiogram (ECG)
- Electroencephalogram (EEG) and other electrophysiologic studies (e.g., brainstem evoked potential)
- Polysomnography
- Pulse oximetry
- Arterial blood gases
- Pregnancy tests in potentially childbearing women
- Dexamethasone-suppression test (DST)
- Thyrotropin-releasing hormone stimulation test (TRHST)
- Tuberculosis tests
- Blood lead levels
- Genetic testing

*Although no complete consensus exists as to which tests should be included in a routine screening battery for a psychiatric patient, these tests may be included in such a screen.

tests may help determine the cause or the seriousness of the abnormality, or a repeat of the original test may determine the reproducibility of its result. One caveat: Extensive testing may increase the chances of irrelevant and clinically insignificant abnormal results, leading to further unnecessary, expensive, and perhaps dangerous follow-up tests. Often, consultations with medical colleagues in the relevant subspecialty are necessary to guide the psychiatrist in the most appropriate use of follow-up tests.

SENSITIVITY, SPECIFICITY, AND PREDICTIVE VALUE

Sensitivity is the proportion of persons with a positive test result who have the disease out of all the persons affected with the disease. Sensitivity reflects the ability of an abnormal test result to correctly identify persons who have the disease. The more false negatives a test has, the lower is its sensitivity. *Specificity* is the proportion of negative test results among a population of persons who do not have the disease. The more false positives a test has, the lower is the test's specificity. *Predictive value* is either positive or negative. A positive predictive value is the probability of a person's having the disease, given a positive test result. A negative predictive value is the probability of a person's not having the disease, given a negative test result. Table 9.7-4 provides the formulas for sensitivity, specificity, and predictive values.

Laboratory and diagnostic tests do not have absolute sensitivities, specificities, and predictive values. Furthermore, different laboratories use different cutoff values to determine whether a result is normal or abnormal. In general, normal laboratory values for healthy persons are often described as those that fall within two standard deviations of the mean of a normal population. However, few laboratory values fall within a true Gaussian distribution. Varying cutoff values changes the sensitivity and the specificity of a test. Changes in cutoff values that increase the sensitivity of a test typically decrease its specificity and vice versa. Moreover, the predictive value of a test varies with the prevalence of the disorder in the population being studied. Hence, tests with high sensitivity can be of little value in screening if the prevalence of the disorder in the population being screened is very low. Patients with many signs, symptoms, and risk factors for a particular disease increase the predictive value of a positive test result suggestive of the disease. Patients with few signs, symptoms, and risk factors for a particular disease are less likely to belong to a population afflicted with the disease; thus, the predictive value of a negative test result is increased in such patients. Therefore, the clinician must integrate all aspects of the patient's presentation—history, review of systems, physical examination, other test results—and understand the particular test's sensitivity, specificity, and predictive values when interpreting the significance of a laboratory result.

In a hypothetical example, out of a population of 100 patients with schizophrenia, 85 are found to have abnormal smooth-pursuit eye movement, and 15 are found to have scores that fall into a previously defined normal range for smooth-pursuit performance (that is, 85 are true positives, and 15 are false negatives for schizophrenia). Hence, the sensitivity of the measure in schizophrenia is 85 percent (85/85 + 15 = 85 percent). In a population of 100 controls without schizophrenia, 20 are found to have abnormal smooth-pursuit scores (that is, 80 are true negatives, and 20 are false positives). Hence, the specificity of the measure is 80 percent (80/80 + 20 = 80 percent). The predictive value of a positive test result in all those patients studied is 81 percent (85/85 + 20 = 81 percent). The predictive value of a negative test result is 84 percent (80/80 + 15 = 84 percent). If the population had had more schizophrenic patients than controls included in the analysis, the predictive value of a positive test result would have increased; with more controls, the predictive value of a negative test result would have increased.

TABLE 9.7-3
Psychiatric Indications for Diagnostic Tests

Test	Major Psychiatric Indications	Comments
Acid phosphatase	Cognitive/medical workup	Increased in prostate cancer, benign prostatic hypertrophy, excessive platelet destruction, bone disease
Adrenocorticotropic hormone (ACTH)	Cognitive/medical workup	Increased in steroid abuse; may be increased in seizures, psychoses, Cushing's disease, and in response to stress Decreased in Addison's disease
Alanine aminotransferase (ALT) (formerly called serum glutamic-pyruvic transaminase [SGPT])	Cognitive/medical workup	Increased in hepatitis, cirrhosis, liver metastases Decreased in pyridoxine (vitamin B_6) deficiency
Albumin	Cognitive/medical workup	Increased in dehydration Decreased in malnutrition, hepatic failure, burns, multiple myeloma, carcinomas
Aldolase	Eating disorders Schizophrenia	Increased in patients who abuse ipecac (e.g., bulimic patients), some patients with schizophrenia
Alkaline phosphatase	Cognitive/medical workup Use of psychotropic medications	Increased in Paget's disease, hyperparathyroidism, hepatic disease, hepatic metastases, heart failure, phenothiazine use Decreased in pernicious anemia (Vitamin B_{12} deficiency)
Ammonia, serum	Cognitive/medical workup	Increased in hepatic encephalopathy, liver failure, Reye's syndrome; also increases with GI hemorrhage and severe congestive heart failure
Amylase, serum	Eating disorders	May be increased in bulimia nervosa
Antinuclear antibodies	Cognitive/medical workup	Found in systemic lupus erythematosus (SLE) and drug-induced lupus (e.g., secondary to phenothiazines, anticonvulsants); SLE can be associated with delirium, psychosis, mood disorder
Aspartate aminotransferase (AST) (formerly SGOT)	Cognitive/medical workup	Increased in heart failure, hepatic disease, pancreatitis, eclampsia, cerebral damage, alcoholism Decreased in pyridoxine (vitamin B_6) deficiency and terminal stages of liver disease
Bicarbonate, serum	Panic disorder Eating disorders	Decreased in hyperventilation syndrome, panic disorder, anabolic steroid abuse May be elevated in patients with bulimia nervosa, in laxative abuse, in psychogenic vomiting
Bilirubin	Cognitive/medical workup	Increased in hepatic disease
Blood urea nitrogen (BUN)	Delirium Use of psychotropic medications	Elevated in renal disease, dehydration Elevations associated with lethargy, delirium If elevated, can increase toxic potential of psychiatric medications, especially lithium and amantadine (Symmetrel)
Bromide, serum	Dementia Psychosis	Bromide intoxication can cause psychosis, hallucinations, delirium Part of dementia workup, especially when serum chloride is elevated
Caffeine level, serum	Anxiety/panic disorder	Evaluation of patients with suspected caffeinism
Calcium (Ca), serum	Cognitive/medical workup Mood disorders Psychosis Eating disorders	Increased in hyperparathyroidism, bone metastases Increase associated with delirium, depression, psychosis Decreased in hypoparathyroidism, renal failure Decrease associated with depression, irritability, delirium, chronic laxative abuse
Carotid ultrasound	Dementia	Occasionally included in dementia workup, especially to rule out multi-infarct dementia Primary value is in search for possible infarct causes
Catecholamines, urinary and plasma	Panic attacks Anxiety	Elevated in pheochromocytoma
Cerebrospinal fluid (CSF)	Cognitive/medical workup	Increased protein and cells in infection, positive VDRL in neurosyphilis, bloody CSF in hemorrhagic conditions
Ceruloplasmin, serum; copper, serum	Cognitive/medical workup	Low in Wilson's disease (hepatolenticular disease)
Chloride (Cl), serum	Eating disorders Panic disorder	Decreased in patients with bulimia and psychogenic vomiting Mild elevation in hyperventilation syndrome, panic disorder
Cholecystokinin (CCK)	Eating disorders	Compared with controls, blunted in bulimic patients after eating meal (may normalize after treatment with antidepressants)
CO_2 inhalation; sodium bicarbonate infusion	Anxiety/panic attacks	Panic attacks produced in subgroup of patients
Coombs' test, direct and indirect	Hemolytic anemias secondary to psychotropic medications	Evaluation of drug-induced hemolytic anemias, such as those secondary to chlorpromazine, phenytoin, levodopa, and methyldopa
Copper, urine	Cognitive/medical workup	Elevated in Wilson's disease
Cortisol (hydrocortisone)	Cognitive/medical workup Mood disorders	Excessive level may indicate Cushing's disease associated with anxiety, depression, and a variety of other conditions
Creatine phosphokinase (CPK)	Use of antipsychotics Use of restraints Substance abuse	Increased in neuroleptic malignant syndrome, intramuscular injection, rhabdomyolysis (secondary to substance abuse), patients in restraints, patients experiencing dystonic reactions; asymptomatic elevations seen with use of antipsychotics
Creatinine, serum	Cognitive/medical workup	Elevated in renal disease (see BUN)
Dopamine (DA) (L-dopa stimulation of dopamine)	Depression	Inhibits prolactin Test used to assess functional integrity of dopaminergic system, which is impaired in Parkinson's disease, depression
Doppler ultrasound	Impotence Cognitive/medical workup	Carotid occlusion, transient ischemic attack (TIA), reduced penile blood flow in impotence
Echocardiogram	Panic disorder	10–40% of patients with panic disorder show mitral valve prolapse
Electroencephalogram (EEG)	Cognitive/medical workup	Seizures, brain death, lesions; shortened REM latency in depression High-voltage activity in stupor; low-voltage fast activity in excitement; in functional nonorganic cases (e.g., dissociative states), alpha activity is present in the background, which responds to auditory and visual stimuli Biphasic or triphasic slow bursts seen in dementia of Creutzfeldt-Jakob disease

TABLE 9.7-3 (*continued*)

Test	Major Psychiatric Indications	Comments
Epstein-Barr virus (EBV); cytomeglovirus (CMV)	Cognitive/medical workup Anxiety Mood disorders	Part of herpes virus group EBV is causative agent for infectious mononucleosis, which can present with depression, fatigue, and personality change CMV can produce anxiety, confusion, mood disorders EBV may be associated with chronic mononucleosislike syndrome associated with chronic depression and fatigue
Erythrocyte sedimentation rate (ESR)	Cognitive/medical workup	An increase in ESR represents a nonspecific test of infectious, inflammatory, autoimmune, or malignant disease; sometimes recommended in the evaluation of anorexia nervosa
Estrogen	Mood disorder	Decreased in menopausal depression and premenstrual syndrome; variable changes in anxiety
Ferritin, serum	Cognitive/medical workup	Most sensitive test for iron deficiency
Folate (folic acid), serum	Alcohol abuse Use of specific medications	Usually measured with vitamin B_{12} deficiencies associated with psychosis, paranoia, fatigue, agitation, dementia, delirium Associated with alcoholism, use of phenytoin, oral contraceptives, estrogen
Follicle-stimulating hormone (FSH)	Depression	High normal in anorexia nervosa, higher values in postmenopausal women; low levels in patients with panhypopituitarism
Glucose, fasting blood (FBS)	Panic attacks Anxiety Delirium Depression	Very high FBS associated with delirium Very low FBS associated with delirium, agitation, panic attacks, anxiety, depression
Glutamyl transaminase, serum	Alcohol abuse Cognitive/medical workup	Increase in alcohol abuse, cirrhosis, liver disease
Gonadotropin-releasing hormone (GnRH)	Depression Anxiety Schizophrenia	Decrease in schizophrenia; increase in anorexia; variable in depression, anxiety
Growth hormone (GH)	Depression Schizophrenia	Blunted GH responses to insulin-induced hypoglycemia in depressed patients; increased GH responses to dopamine agonist challenge in schizophrenic patients; increased in some cases of anorexia
Hematocrit (Hct); hemoglobin (Hb)	Cognitive/medical workup	Assessment of anemia (anemia may be associated with depression and psychosis)
Hepatitis A viral antigen (HAAg)	Mood disorders Cognitive/medical workup	Less severe, better prognosis than hepatitis B; may present with anorexia, depression
Hepatitis B surface antigen (HBsAg); hepatitis Bc antigen (HBcAg)	Mood disorders Cognitive/medical workup	Active hepatitis B infection indicates greater degree of infectivity and of progression to chronic liver disease May present with depression
Holter monitor	Panic disorder	Evaluation of panic-disordered patients with palpitations and other cardiac symptoms
Human immunodeficiency virus (HIV)	Cognitive/medical workup	CNS involvement; AIDS dementia, organic personality disorder, organic mood disorder, acute psychosis
17-Hydroxycorticosteroid	Depression	Deviations detect hyperadrenocorticalism, which can be associated with major depression Increased in steroid abuse
5-Hydroxyindoleacetic acid (5-HIAA)	Depression Suicide Violence	Decrease in CSF in aggressive or violent patients with suicidal or homicidal impulses May be indicator of decreased impulse control and predictor of suicide
Iron, serum	Cognitive/medical workup	Iron-deficiency anemia
Lactate dehydrogenase (LDH)	Cognitive/medical workup	Increased in myocardial infarction, pulmonary infarction, hepatic disease, renal infarction, seizures, cerebral damage, megaloblastic (pernicious) anemia, factitious elevations secondary to rough handling of blood specimen tube
Lupus anticoagulant (LA)	Use of phenothiazines	An antiphospholipid antibody, which has been described in some patients using phenothiazines, especially chlorpromazine; often associated with elevated PTT; associated with anticardiolipin antibodies
Lupus erythematosus (LE) test	Depression Psychosis Delirium Dementia	Positive test associated with systemic LE, which may present with various psychiatric disturbances, such as psychosis, depression, delirium, dementia; also tested for with antinuclear antibody (ANA) and antiDNA antibody tests
Luteinizing hormone (LH)	Depression	Low in patients with panhypopituitarism; decrease associated with depression
Magnesium, serum	Alcohol abuse Cognitive/medical workup	Decreased in alcoholism; low levels associated with agitation, delirium, seizures
MAO, platelet	Depression	Low in depression; has been used to monitor MAOI therapy
MCV (mean corpuscular volume) (average volume of a red blood cell)	Alcohol abuse	Elevated in alcoholism and vitamin B_{12} and folate deficiency
Melatonin	Seasonal affective disorder	Produced by light and pineal gland and decreased in seasonal affective disorder
Metal (heavy) intoxication (serum or urinary)	Cognitive/medical workup	Lead—apathy, irritability, anorexia, confusion Mercury—psychosis, fatigue, apathy, decreased memory, emotional lability, ''mad hatter'' Manganese—manganese madness, Parkinson-like syndrome Aluminum—dementia Arsenic—fatigue, blackouts, hair loss
3-Methoxy-4-hydroxyphenylglycol (MHPG)	Depression Anxiety	Most useful in research; decreases in urine may indicate decreases centrally; may predict response to certain antidepressants

(*continued*)

TABLE 9.7-3 (*continued*)

Test	Major Psychiatric Indications	Comments
Myoglobin, urine	Phenothiazine use Substance abuse Use of restraints	Increased in neuroleptic malignant syndrome; in PCP, cocaine, or lysergic acid diethylamide (LSD) intoxication; and in patients in restraints
Nicotine	Anxiety Nicotine addiction	Anxiety, smoking
Nocturnal penile tumescence	Impotence	Quantification of penile circumference changes, penile rigidity, frequency of penile tumescence Evaluation of erectile function during sleep Erections associated with rapid eye movement (REM) sleep Helpful in differentiation between organic and functional causes of impotence
Parathyroid (parathormone) hormone	Anxiety Cognitive/medical workup	Low level causes hypocalcemia and anxiety Dysregulation associated with wide variety of organic mental disorders
Partial thromboplastin time (PTT)	Treatment with antipsychotics, heparin	Monitor anticoagulant therapy; increased in presence of lupus anticoagulant and anticardiolipin antibodies
Phosphorus, serum	Cognitive/medical workup Panic disorder	Increased in renal failure, diabetic acidosis, hypoparathyroidism, hypervitamin D; decreased in cirrhosis, hypokalemia, hyperparathyroidism, panic attacks, hyperventilation syndrome
Platelet count	Use of psychotropic medications	Decreased by certain psychotropic medications (carbamazepine, clozapine, phenothiazines)
Porphobilinogen (PBG)	Cognitive/medical workup	Increased in acute porphyria
Porphyria-synthesizing enzyme	Psychosis Cognitive/medical workup	Acute neuropsychiatric disorder can occur in acute porphyria attack, which may be precipitated by barbiturates, imipramine
Potassium (K), serum	Cognitive/medical workup Eating disorders	Increased in hyperkalemic acidosis; increase is associated with anxiety in cardiac arrhythmia Decreased in cirrhosis, metabolic alkalosis, laxative abuse, diuretic abuse; decrease is common in bulimic patients and in psychogenic vomiting, anabolic steroid abuse
Prolactin, serum	Use of antipsychotic medications Cocaine use Pseudoseizures	Antipsychotics, by decreasing dopamine, increase prolactin synthesis and release, especially in women Elevated prolactin levels may be seen secondary to cocaine withdrawal Lack of prolactin rise after seizure suggests pseudoseizure
Protein, total serum	Cognitive/medical workup Use of psychotropic medications	Increased in multiple myeloma, myxedema, lupus Decreased in cirrhosis, malnutrition, overhydration Low serum protein can result in greater sensitivity to conventional doses of protein-bound medications (lithium is not protein-bound)
Prothrombin time (PT)	Cognitive/medical workup	Elevated in significant liver damage (cirrhosis)
Reticulocyte count (estimate of red blood cell production in bone marrow)	Cognitive/medical workup Use of carbamazepine	Low in megaloblastic or iron deficiency anemia and anemia of chronic disease Must be monitored in patient taking carbamazepine
Salicylate, serum	Organic hallucinosis Suicide attempts	Toxic levels may be seen in suicide attempts; may also cause organic hallucinosis with high levels
Sodium (Na), serum	Cognitive/medical workup Use of lithium	Decreased with water intoxication; SIADH Decreased in hypoadrenalism, myxedema, congestive heart failure, diarrhea, polydipsia, use of carbamazepine, anabolic steroids Low levels associated with greater sensitivity to conventional dose of lithium
Testosterone, serum	Impotence Inhibited sexual desire	Increase in anabolic steroid abuse May be decreased in organic workup of impotence Decrease may be seen with inhibited sexual desire Follow-up of sex offenders treated with medroxyprogesterone Decreased with medroxyprogesterone treatment
Thyroid function tests	Cognitive/medical workup Depression	Detection of hypothyroidism or hyperthyroidism Abnormalities can be associated with depression, anxiety, psychosis, dementia, delirium, lithium treatment
Urinalysis	Cognitive/medical workup Pretreatment workup of lithium Drug screening	Provides clues to cause of various cognitive disorders (assessing general appearance, pH, specific gravity, bilirubin, glucose, blood, ketones, protein, etc.); specific gravity may be affected by lithium
Urinary creatinine	Cognitive/medical workup Substance abuse Lithium use	Increased in renal failure, dehydration Part of pretreatment workup for lithium; sometimes used in follow-up evaluations of patients treated with lithium
Venereal Disease Research Laboratory (VDRL)	Syphilis	Positive (high titers) in secondary syphilis (may be positive or negative in primary syphilis); RPR test also used Low titers (or negative) in tertiary syphilis
Vitamin A, serum	Depression Delirium	Hypervitaminosis A is associated with a variety of mental status changes, headache
Vitamin B_{12}, serum	Cognitive/medical workup Dementia Mood disorder	Part of workup of megaloblastic anemia and dementia B_{12} deficiency associated with psychosis, paranoia, fatigue, agitation, dementia, delirium Often associated with chronic alcohol abuse
White blood cell (WBC)	Use of psychotropic medications	Leukopenia and agranulocytosis associated with certain psychotropic medications, such as phenothiazines, carbamazepine, clozapine Leukocytosis associated with lithium and neuroleptic malignant syndrome

TABLE 9.7-4
Sensitivity, Specificity, and Predictive Value

Sensitivity (probability of a positive test result in one who has the disorder)

$$\text{Sensitivity} = \frac{\text{true positives}}{\text{true positives} + \text{false negatives}} \times 100\%$$

Specificity (probability of a negative test result in one who does not have the disorder)

$$\text{Specificity} = \frac{\text{true negatives}}{\text{true negatives} + \text{false positives}} \times 100\%$$

Predictive value of a positive test result (percentage of all positive test results that are true positives)

$$\text{Predictive value} = \frac{\text{true positives}}{\text{true positives} + \text{false positives}} \times 100\%$$

Predictive value of a negative test result (percentage of all negative test results that are true negatives)

$$\text{Predictive value} = \frac{\text{true negatives}}{\text{true negatives} + \text{false negatives}} \times 100\%$$

Table by Darrell G. Kirch, M.D.

SPECIAL POPULATIONS

GERIATRIC PATIENTS Geriatric patients are more likely than are other patient groups to have at least one chronic disease or disability. Therefore, the diagnostic assessment of a geriatric patient requires a rigorous search for organic factors that may be related to the presenting psychiatric illness. Screening laboratory tests are considered especially important in the psychiatric evaluation of a geriatric patient with a recent onset of psychiatric symptoms, a change in behavior, or symptoms resistant to therapy. The specific set of screening tests is typically determined by the patient's history and clinical presentation, but one study of psychogeriatric patients found the following five tests to be most useful in identifying illness: midstream urine, chest X-ray, B_{12}, electrocardiogram (ECG), and blood urea nitrogen (BUN).

Urinary tract infection Urinary tract infection, a common medical problem in elderly patients, can present with mental status changes, abdominal pain, nausea, and vomiting, instead of the classic symptoms of dysuria and frequency of micturition. Geriatric patients may not become febrile in the presence of serious infections. Urinalysis usually reveals bacteria, enteric rods, and pyuria, but those findings may be absent in the geriatric patient. Urine culture and sensitivity should follow for a definitive diagnosis. Men with urinary tract infection unrelated to catheterization and women with recurrent urinary tract infection should be referred to a urologist.

Anemia Anemia is an abnormality found in more than 30 percent of geriatric outpatients. The elderly anemic patient may present with confusion, apathy, or behavioral changes, whereas younger patients display the classic signs of pallor, weakness, and fatigue. Anemia should be vigorously treated in the elderly, as symptoms may improve with only a small change in the hemoglobin. A laboratory workup for anemia should begin with a complete blood count (CBC) with differential white blood count, platelet count, reticulocyte count, and peripheral smear. On the basis of those studies, the anemia can usually be classified as microcytic, macrocytic, or normocytic.

In the elderly the anemia may present as a combination of several pathological processes. Additional laboratory tests in the workup of a microcytic anemia include a serum iron level, total iron-binding capacity (TIBC), serum ferritin, and stool examination for occult blood. The presence of chronic disease in elderly patients may lead to a normal TIBC result and mask the typical laboratory findings of low iron and elevated TIBC. Therefore, in the presence of low serum ferritin and negative stool results for occult blood, colonoscopy may be indicated to identify the source of the blood loss. Macrocytic anemia may be secondary to vitamin B_{12} or folate deficiency. Red cell folate levels are more accurate reflections of folate than are serum folate levels but may not be available in all laboratories. Pernicious anemia is the most frequent cause of vitamin B_{12} deficiency in elderly patients and may present with such psychiatric symptoms as delirium, hallucinations, personality changes, delusions, depression, and mania. A neurologic examination may reveal paresthesias and abnormal proprioception. The neuropsychiatric symptoms may occur before the hematological changes, making anemia an important diagnostic consideration in any elderly patient with psychiatric symptoms. Certain clinical features—fatigue, shortness of breath, worsening angina pectoris, and peripheral edema—are common in patients with histories of heart failure and atherosclerotic heart disease. Mental status changes of confusion, depression, agitation, and apathy may occur in elderly anemic patients with no previous psychiatric histories. Dizziness is a common complaint in elderly patients, and pallor may be detected in the mucosa of the oral cavity and the conjunctiva.

Thyroid disease Thyroid disease is common among elderly persons and often presents with an atypical picture. Nonspecific symptoms—such as fatigue, constipation, and changes in functional ability—are associated with thyroid disease. Elderly patients with hyperthyroidism may present with typical symptoms (heat intolerance, weight loss, tremor, palpitations, and atrial fibrillation) or with apathetic hyperthyroidism (manifested by anorexia, weight loss, and fatigue). Hypothyroidism in the elderly may present with symptoms of lassitude, constipation, cold intolerance, fatigue, and cognitive impairment. Those symptoms may be attributed to depression or degenerative dementia. Myxedema coma is a medical emergency that occurs primarily in patients over age 50.

The laboratory screening for thyroid disease may include tests for thyroxine (T_4); triiodothyronine (T_3), T_3 resin uptake (T_3 RU), and thyroid-stimulating hormone (TSH). The free thyroxine index (FTI) corrects for protein binding, providing an accurate reflection of hormone production. Laboratory testing in hyperthyroidism reveals an elevated T_4 and FTI and very low TSH. A new TSH test allows for the distinction between euthyroid and hyperthyroid levels of TSH and has been recommended as a single screening test of thyroid function. Laboratory testing in hypothyroidism reveals a low T_4 and FTI and elevated TSH. A common pattern of abnormal thyroid test results seen in the elderly is subclinical or compensated hypothyroidism characterized by elevated TSH and normal T_4 and FTI. In patients with TSH levels greater than 20 μU/mL or with thyroid microsomal antibodies, progression to overt hypothyroidism is more likely.

Hearing and visual loss More than 25 percent of patients 65 years and older have hearing impairments that can lead to social isolation, depression, and confusion. The hearing impairment, usually in the high-frequency range, may interfere with conversation, and the psychiatrist needs to consider the impairment in the diagnostic process. The workup for hearing impairment includes an otoscopic examination of the external ear for impaction of cerumen. If the ear is clear, the patient can be screened with a hand-held audioscope or can be referred to an audiologist.

Visual impairment is present in 15 percent of persons 65 and older and twice that in patients over age 85. Cataracts and macular degeneration account for the majority of those cases, but glaucoma and diabetic retinopathy are other important causes of visual impairment. Screening tests of visual acuity include a visual acuity chart and a reading card for near vision. If the 20/40 line on the chart cannot be read with eyeglasses, a pinhole in a card can be used to increase visual acuity. If that maneuver is not helpful, immediate referral is necessary to rule out the presence of serious eye disease.

Dementia The cognitive disorder most closely associated with increasing age is dementia. All geriatric patients presenting to a psychiatrist should be screened with a brief cognitive screening examination, such as the Mini-Mental State Examination (MMSE) or the Short Portable Mental Status Questionnaire. If cognitive deficits are new and not accounted for by education, a laboratory workup for the reversible causes of dementia is indicated. The National Institutes of Health Consensus Development Conference statement on the differential diagnosis of dementing diseases recommends careful screening for a patient with a new onset of dementia in an attempt to identify the treatable causes of dementia. The conference stated that "the best diagnostic test is a careful history and physical and mental status examination by a physician with a knowledge of and an interest in dementia and dementing disease." The conference report went on:

> The laboratory tests that are used should be individualized based on the history and physical and mental status examination. Overtesting

may expose the patient to discomfort, inconvenience, excess cost, and the likelihood of false positive tests that may lead to additional unnecessary testing. Undertesting also has hazards; for example, in elderly persons, medical diseases may have nonspecific presentations such as dementia.

Although there is some consensus regarding the usefulness of a CBC, chemistry laboratory panel, and thyroid function tests for the screening evaluation of a demented patient, some argue against the routine inclusion of tests for syphilis and for B_{12} and folate levels. A supplemental test battery recommended by the conference includes computed tomography (CT), an electroencephalogram (EEG), magnetic resonance imaging (MRI), and lumbar puncture only as indicated.

SELF-ABUSERS Various diagnostic assessments can be useful in the evaluation of the patient who engages in either deliberate or unintentional self-injurious behavior. Clues to such behavior include wrist and arm lacerations and scars; the presence of open wounds, bruises, burns, or abrasions; and evidence of swelling or deformity secondary to injury. Self-damaging behavior may even cause skull deformities. Blood toxicology tests are important for the evaluation of the patient who has overdosed on prescribed or abused drugs. The degree of organ involvement in the overdose can be assessed by the appropriate diagnostic tests. For instance, in the case of a tricyclic antidepressant overdose, an electrocardiogram is needed to assess the degree of cardiac toxicity; in an acetaminophen overdose, liver function tests are important; and in an aspirin overdose, serum electrolyte determinations are needed to assess the anion gap. Deformity in a region of the body requires X-ray evaluation of that body area. Usually, consultations with medical or surgical specialists are necessary to resolve issues related to self-inflicted injuries in psychiatric patients.

RESTRAINED PATIENTS Some patients are restrained to prevent them from inflicting harm on themselves or others. Because such patients cannot attend to their own needs, they must be carefully monitored. The assessment of those patients includes the frequent monitoring of vital signs, signs of dehydration (for example, dry mouth, loss of skin turgor), and evidence of edema, swelling, or abrasions related to improper restraint techniques. Agitated patients may need to have their urine checked for evidence of myoglobinuria secondary to muscle breakdown. For patients in whom the cause of the agitated behavior is unclear, organic causes may be revealed by serum and urine toxicology screens, serum blood screens for evidence of infection or electrolyte disturbance, and computed tomography scans when a cerebrovascular disorder is suspected. Lumbar puncture and analysis of the cerebrospinal fluid (CSF) are necessary in a patient with signs of meningeal irritation or other clinical findings suggestive of infection (for example, meningitis) or vasculitis.

PSYCHIATRIC PATIENTS WITH WEIGHT LOSS Dramatic weight loss may be caused by a variety of psychiatric disturbances, including anorexia nervosa, depression, severe psychosis, catatonia, and in the context of serious alcohol or substance use disorders). A laboratory assessment is needed to determine the patient's degree of malnutrition and starvation. The monitoring of vital signs, including orthostatic blood pressure changes, is important. Frequently ordered tests include a complete blood count to determine the degree of anemia, although hemoconcentration may give an artificially elevated result before rehydration; serum electrolytes, especially potassium and blood urea nitrogen; and a urinalysis (the specific gravity is high in a dehydrated patient). Other tests that may be ordered include serum iron studies and serum total protein and albumin tests. Tests to detect other cachexia-inducing conditions, such as HIV infection or malignancy, may also be indicated.

In anorexia nervosa the recommended test batteries often include an erythrocyte sedimentation rate (ESR). The ESR is usually low in patients with anorexia nervosa and, hence, is somewhat useful in the differential diagnosis of that condition. An electrocardiogram is important to assess the effects of low potassium and starvation on the heart. Some have recommended computed tomography (CT) to rule out the presence of brain tumors. Endocrine status is frequently evaluated with tests of thyroid function and of other pituitary hormones. Stool and urine tests for laxative abuse may also be useful for some patients. Bone X-rays that reveal reduced bone densities can be useful in further assessing the physical effects of the patient's eating disorder.

SUBSTANCE ABUSERS Laboratory tests are useful in detecting substances of abuse and in evaluating the physical effects that the substance use is having on the patient's body. Often, the laboratory detection of abused substances and certain diagnostic test abnormalities related to the substance abuse (for example, abnormal liver function test results in alcohol-abusing patients) can be used therapeutically to confront the denial of a patient with a substance use disorder and to help engage the patient in treatment.

TABLE 9.7-5
Drugs of Abuse That Can Be Tested in Urine

Drug	Length of Time Detected in Urine
Alcohol	7–12 hours
Amphetamine	48 hours
Barbiturate	24 hours (short-acting) 3 weeks (long-acting)
Benzodiazepine	3 days
Cocaine	6–8 hours (metabolites 2–4 days)
Codeine	48 hours
Heroin	36–72 hours
Marijuana	3 days to 4 weeks (depending on use)
Methadone	3 days
Methaqualone	7 days
Morphine	48–72 hours
Phencyclidine (PCP)	8 days
Propoxyphene	6–48 hours

The most commonly used specimen for the detection of drugs of abuse is urine, although toxicological analyses can also be performed on blood specimens. The period of time that drugs can be detected in blood specimens is typically shorter than the length of time that drugs can be detected in urine specimens. However, the length of time that a particular drug of abuse can be detected in the urine is variable, depending on the specific drug, how long it was used, the amount of the substance used, and concomitant medical problems (for example, liver and kidney diseases). Nevertheless, Table 9.7-5 lists some common drugs of abuse that can be detected in urine specimens, along with typical lengths of time after recent use that the substances can be detected. Other specimens that have been studied to detect substance abuse include saliva and hair samples. A commercially available test measures alcohol in saliva. Equipment for the detection of recently ingested alcohol in a person's exhaled breath is commonly used in certain treatment and law-enforcement settings. The measurement of drugs of abuse in hair samples would permit detection and possible quantification of illicit substances used over a long period of time (days to weeks), but, because of various technical limitations, hair analyses of drugs of abuse remain largely a research tool at this time.

The most common method to detect substances of abuse in the potentially substance-abusing patient involves the use of a screening test and, in the case of a positive result, a more sensitive, confirmatory test (for example, enzyme-multiplied immunoassay technique [EMIT] followed up by gas chromatography-mass spectrometry [GC-MS]). GC-MS may be the most sensitive and reliable test for substances of abuse, but it is also the most expensive. Therefore, not all laboratories use GC-MS as the follow-up test. Other commonly used tests include thin-layer chromatography (TLC) and radioimmunoassay. Many laboratories do not report a positive result for a specimen unless the substance has been detected in the specimen by at least two different testing strategies. At times, the clinician needs to consult the laboratory for the best way of detecting the potential abuse of such substances as anabolic steroids and chemical solvents.

The clinician should not be sanguine that the routine drug or toxicology screen will test for all possible substances of abuse. Clinicians should check with their respective laboratories to understand which drugs are tested for by the routine drug screen that they have ordered. These routine screens might not be sensitive enough to detect such drugs as marijuana, phencyclidine (PCP), lysergic acid diethylamide (LSD), or 3,4-methylenedioxymethamphetamine (MDMA). Clinicians should also be familiar with the illicit drug use trends in their area. For instance, there have been recent reports of increases in marijuana, PCP, LSD, and MDMA use in certain localities. Only by the clinicians' knowledge about which drugs are detected by the routine drug screens they use and an understanding of the drugs being used in their area will clinicians be best able to use laboratory tests to detect substances abused by their patients.

Collection The implementation of a urine drug-testing program must first resolve issues surrounding collection. In clinical settings engaged in the treatment of known substance abusers, direct observation of urination can prevent adulteration of the specimen. In the workplace, direct observation may not be necessary, although several precautions must be observed. Ideally, the collection room should contain only a toilet whose water has been dyed; there should be no water faucets, cups, or containers. Persons entering the collection room should do so without packages or coats. The temperature of the specimen should be noted immediately after collection, and the container should be closed and sealed. The temperature of the sample should be within 2°C of the body temperature immediately after collection. Moreover, the specific gravity of the urine can be checked to detect dilution of the specimen with water. The specimens should be transported to the laboratory in tamperproof or locked boxes. A record of the signatures of all persons with access to the sample from the moment of collection should be maintained.

Results Some patients do not have positive results on urine toxicology screens when they are, indeed, abusing illicit substances; for example, they may have tampered with the specimens. Blood specimens are more difficult to tamper with and blood tests may be used for highly suspicious cases. In addition, the physical examination can provide clues to the abuse of a particular substance—needle tracks in intravenous (IV) substance users and nasal mucosal inflammation, bleeding, or septal perforation in intranasal cocaine abusers. Opioid intoxication is associated with pinpoint pupils and possibly respiratory depression; opioid withdrawal is associated with piloerection, tremor, yawning, dilated pupils, and diaphoresis. With PCP intoxication, absent corneal reflexes, alterations in sensation, hypertension, prominent nystagmus, ataxias, and catalepsy (posturing) can be found.

Initial false-negative test results do not lead to confirmatory testing. Thus, some drug abusers aim to evade detection on initial immunoassay screening tests. Benzalkonium chloride (an antimicrobial preservative contained in commercial ophthalmic solutions) causes false-negative results in enzyme immunoassay for marijuana and cocaine. Ibuprofen (Motrin), a nonsteroidal anti-inflammatory agent, can cause a false-negative result in GC-MS confirmatory testing of marijuana metabolites because of the consumption of the derivatizing agent used in the gas chromatographic procedure. Fluorescein dye in the urine interferes with the fluorescent polarization immunoassays used to screen for the presence of barbiturates and benzodiazepines in the urine. (Ibuprofen can render the fluorescent polarization immunoassay falsely positive for barbiturates and benzodiazepines.)

Several automated commercial analyzers can detect illicit substances in the urine as part of an initial screen. Two of the most widely used analyzers are the ADx (Abbott Laboratories) and the EMIT (Syntex); those analyzers use fluorescence polarization immunoassay and homogeneous enzyme immunoassay technologies, respectively. Detection cutoff values for parent drug and metabolites have been established by the National Institute of Drug Abuse. For example, values above 50 μg/L for marijuana and its metabolites and above 300 μg/L for cocaine and its major metabolite (on initial screen, but 150 μg/L for the confirmatory test) are required for a positive result. In all instances of a positive result, confirmatory testing, usually with GC-MS, is mandatory.

Cocaine use The initial urine screen to detect cocaine use involves the measurement of benzoylecgonine, a cocaine metabolite, in urine by either radioimmunoassay or enzyme immunoassay. (However, the parent compound cocaine is rapidly metabolized and is unlikely to be found in urine specimens unless cocaine use is quite recent.) Those tests can usually detect the cocaine metabolite between two and four days after drug use. Thioridazine (Mellaril) and tropane alkaloids can give false-positive results with the radioimmunoassay procedure. A positive result requires confirmation. GC-MS can detect levels of the benzoylecgonine metabolite that are below 100 ng/mL. Moreover, cocaine metabolites may be detected with GC-MS for as long as seven days after a cocaine binge.

Anabolic steroid abuse Abuse of anabolic-androgenic steroids, synthetic derivatives of testosterone, has extended beyond athletes seeking to enhance their performance to include male high school seniors seeking to enhance their physical appearance. In one study as many as 6.6 percent of the male high school seniors admitted to the use of anabolic steroids. The steroids have several legitimate and approved indications (for example, male hypogonadism and breast cancer); however, their abuse can be associated with serious morbidity, including mood disorders due to a general medical condition, psychoses, aggression, hypertension, atherogenesis, and testicular atrophy. A withdrawal syndrome associated with anabolic steroid abuse is characterized by hyperadrenergic symptoms and craving. Steroid abusers are at risk of receiving wrongly labeled preparations or veterinary preparations; dosages may be as much as 100-fold higher than the recommended therapeutic dosages. Also, intramuscular administration and the sharing of needles place the users at increased risk for HIV infection. Clinicians must maintain a high index of suspicion with respect to anabolic steroid abuse, as abuse is often denied, and the users do not recognize their addiction.

As with all substance-abuse disorders, urine testing may be necessary to confirm the diagnosis and monitor abstinence in anabolic steroid abusers. In the face of psychiatric symptoms (emotional lability, suicidality), physical signs and symptoms (acne, needle tracks in large muscles, testicular atrophy, prostatic hypertrophy), and laboratory abnormalities (increased total cholesterol), urine testing is advisable. Only a few laboratories are suitable for the urine testing, as they must screen at least 40 different steroid compounds. Morever, clinical interpretation of the results is necessary. Some exogenously administered steroids (for example, oxandrolone and stanozolol [Winstrol]) that are not metabolized to testosterone can suppress the hypothalamic-pituitary-gonadal axis and lower the levels of testosterone without altering the ratio of testosterone to epitestosterone (that is, 1 to 2.5/1). Exogenous steroids that are metabolized to testosterone and are excreted as testosterone can elevate the testosterone-to-epitestosterone ratio in excess of 6 to 1. As with all substance-abusing patients, precautions must be taken to prevent the adulteration of the urine, and samples ideally should be collected without advanced notification of the patient.

Alcohol-related disorders In patients with alcohol-related disorders, the intensity of their liver enzyme elevations (for example, γ-glutamyl transaminase [GGT], aspartate aminotransferase [AST, previously known as SGOT], alanine aminotransferase [ALT, previously known as SGPT], and other abnormal liver function tests, such as reduced serum total protein and albumin and prolonged prothrombin time) reflects the degree of liver damage in the patients. Those laboratory abnormalities can also be used to confront denial in the alcohol-abusing patient. Patients with severe alcohol-related hepatic damage may no longer be able to generate liver enzyme elevations, despite advanced liver disease. A patient with alcohol-induced hepatitis typically has a large, smooth liver; those with advanced cases have ascites, signs of portal hypertension, and even delirium related to liver failure (for example, with asterixis, liver flap). Long-term heavy alcohol use can also be associated with testicular atrophy, spider angioma, gynecomastia, and ataxia. The alcohol-abusing patient should also be assessed for possible head trauma (for example, subdural hematomas); a CT scan and a skull X-ray may be needed in cases of suspected skull injury (for example, deformity, penetrating injury).

Patients with alcohol use disorders should have a CBC to evaluate them for anemia (classically megaloblastic but can be mixed megaloblastic and microcytic). Serum levels of magnesium, electrolytes, blood urea nitrogen (BUN), and creatinine are also important.

Patients with signs and symptoms of alcohol withdrawal (for example, elevated blood pressure and pulse, tremor [six to eight counts per second]) typically have rapidly decreasing or undetectable blood alcohol levels. Alcohol withdrawal delirium is a medical emergency requiring careful attention to the patient's medical needs. Negative test results for alcohol in a patient with a history of alcohol abuse is not inconsistent with an ensuing medical emergency related to alcohol withdrawal.

Intravenous substance use A number of substances of abuse (heroin, cocaine, amphetamines) are delivered by the addict through the IV route. The needles have often been used by other addicts and have been inadequately sterilized before use. The needles can be infected with viral agents capable of causing hepatitis and AIDS.

HEPATITIS TESTING All forms of viral hepatitis have been associated with the addict's life-style. Only hepatitis B, C, and D are transmitted by the intravenous route. Hepatitis A is transmitted by the fecal-oral route but has been associated with the poor sanitary conditions that addicts (and not necessarily only IV substance abusers) are exposed to. Serum hepatitis panels for antigens and antibodies associated with hepatitis-causing viruses are indicated in patients at high risk for those hepatitides or with evidence of hepatic damage (for example, jaundice, elevated liver enzymes, elevated serum bilirubin, prolonged serum coagulation test results, and urobilinogen on urinalysis).

HIV TESTING The spread of HIV among the IV drug-abusing population is a major health care disaster. Such patients are driven by their addiction to engage in high-risk behaviors that expose them to the virus. When HIV testing is ordered, it usually involves the performance of the enzyme-linked immunosorbent assay (ELISA), with Western blot analysis as the follow-up confirmatory test. False-positive results in a high-risk population are rare. Patients undergoing HIV testing need to have appropriate counseling before and after the test. HIV brain infection can result in a myriad of neuropsychiatric manifestations, including dementia and psychosis.

MEDICAL CONDITIONS IN PSYCHIATRY

Multiple medical conditions can present with psychiatric symptoms (Table 9.7-1).

THYROID DISORDERS Both hypothyroidism and hyperthyroidism can be associated with a variety of neuropsychiatric symptoms. When routine screening tests for psychiatric patients are advocated, some degree of thyroid testing is usually included in the laboratory screening battery. Thyroid tests to evaluate a patient's thyroid status include those for T_4, T_3, TSH, T_3RU, free T_4, and FTI (sometimes referred to as T_7 or T_{12}). Other thyroid tests include those for antithyroglobulin antibodies and antithyroid microsomal antibodies and the thyrotropin-releasing hormone (TRH) stimulation test. Patients with a goiter, exophthalmus, evidence of a hypermetabolic state, a history or symptoms suggestive of thyroid disease (for example, heat or cold intolerance), or risk factors for thyroid problems (such as a history of neck or chest irradiation, thyroid surgery, iodine-131 [I^{131}] treatment, or lithium treatment) should have some type of laboratory thyroid evaluation (typically serum T_4, T_3, and TSH determinations). Patients with a serum calcium decrease and a phosphorus increase in the context of a normal alkaline phosphatase and who may show Chvostek's or Trousseau's sign should have blood parathormone level determinations.

The thyroid gland can be inspected by observing the lower half of the neck in the anterior triangles and noting the presence of an ascending mass as the patient swallows. Next, the gland can be palpated from behind or in front. Palpation of the gland from behind involves standing behind the patient and exploring the region behind the sternocleidomastoid muscles. The thyroid isthmus can be palpated on the anterior aspect of the tracheal rings. Next, the lower and upper poles of the lateral lobes are palpated. To relax the patient's neck muscles, the physician should shift the inclination of the patient's head and instruct the patient to swallow. If the thyroid gland undergoes hyperplasia and a goiter is palpated, a thyroid bruit may be auscultated from accelerated blood flow. A small diffuse goiter may be present before the menstrual period, during pregnancy, or throughout the menstrual cycle in female patients 12 to 20 years old. A goiter can also be present with thyrotoxicosis. In addition to thyroid enlargement, palpation also reveals nodules and tenderness.

ADRENAL DISEASES Adrenal diseases can be associated with a wide variety of psychiatric symptoms, including depression, anxiety, and psychosis. Low plasma cortisol is associated with Addison's disease (adrenal insufficiency); elevated blood cortisol levels are seen in Cushing's disease. Evidence of hypercortisolism can also be detected in the urine; in some patients with major depression, urinary cortisol levels approach or are in the range associated with Cushing's disease. Some researchers have proposed elevated urinary 17-hydroxycorticosteroid levels as a marker of potential suicidality. Patients with major depression can have alterations in the normal diurnal variation of plasma cortisol levels (measurable with the diurnal cortisol test) and a decreased suppression of serum cortisol by the exogenous administration of dexamethasone (measurable with the dexamethasone-suppression test). Patients with a history or a physical examination suggestive of pheochromocytoma may need a battery of tests, including a 24-hour urine test for the measurement of catecholamines and metabolites (such as metanephrine and vanillylmandelic acid [VMA]), tests for plasma levels of catecholamines, a CT scan of the abdomen, and nuclear medicine scans with iodine-131-labeled metaiodobenzyl guanidine to locate potential catecholamine-secreting tumors.

PERNICIOUS ANEMIA Pernicious anemia, caused by vitamin B_{12} deficiency, can be a confusing term for some psychiatrists, as the neuropsychiatric symptoms associated with vitamin B_{12} deficiency (such as dementia, depression, and psychosis) are not always associated with megaloblastic anemia or other classic laboratory findings typically connected with pernicious anemia (for example, abnormal Schilling test results). Elevated serum homocysteine and methylmalonic acid levels in patients with vitamin B_{12} deficiency may identify those patients whose neuropsychiatric manifestations may respond to parenteral vitamin B_{12} therapy. Serum folate levels are usually measured with B_{12} levels, as folate deficiency can result in a similar constellation of neuropsychiatric impairments. In patients with pernicious anemia, folate therapy without vitamin B_{12} can result in a normalization of the hematological abnormalities but progression of the neuropsychiatric manifestations of the disease.

ACUTE INTERMITTENT PORPHYRIA Acute intermittent porphyria can be associated with psychiatric symptoms (psychosis), although the other classic physical manifestations (abdominal pain, neuropathy, autonomic dysfunction) are not always present. During acute attacks there is typically an elevation of uroporphyrin, urine porphobilinogen (PBG), and Δ-aminolevulinic acid (ALA) levels in the urine. Elevations of those substances are much less common during asymptomatic periods. Diminished erythrocyte uroporphyrinogen-I-synthetase can be seen during both symptomatic and asymptomatic periods of the illness.

WILSON'S DISEASE Wilson's disease is an autosomal recessive disorder of copper metabolism that typically becomes symptomatic (movement disorders, psychosis, personality changes) in the second or third decade of life. There is an elevation of urine copper after a 24-hour collection, decreased serum copper, and low serum ceruloplasmin. The physician must monitor for laboratory abnormalities related to copper deposition in the liver or the kidneys. Kayser-Fleischer rings adjacent to the cornea can be seen during a slitlamp examination.

SYPHILIS In its advanced stages associated with central nervous system (CNS) invovlement, syphilis has classically been related to a wide variety of neuropsychiatric complications, including psychosis and dementia. The serum Venereal Disease Research Laboratories (VDRL) test and the rapid plasma reagin (RPR) test are the most common screening tests for syphilis. Positive results are followed up with fluorescent treponemal antibody-absorption (FTA-ABS) tests. The test that is diagnostic of tertiary (CNS) syphilis is the cerebrospinal fluid (CSF) VDRL. A positive result is typically associated with other CSF findings, such as elevated CSF protein and white blood cell counts. However, late neurosyphilis might not be associated with a positive CSF VDRL, lymphocytosis, or protein elevation. Only a CSF FTA-ABS test may be positive.

SYSTEMIC LUPUS ERYTHEMATOSUS Systemic lupus erythematosus (SLE), a rare clinical condition, can be associated with a number of psychiatric manifestations, including psychosis, delirium, depression, and dementia. The clinician must recognize the neuropsychiatric complications of SLE, as the organic treatment of the psychiatric complications requires proper treatment of the SLE-associated cerebritis (for example, steroid therapy). Laboratory tests for SLE include the LE cell preparation (phenothiazines can cause false-positive results in the test) and tests for serum antinuclear and anti-deoxyribonucleic acid (DNA) antibodies. Lupus anticoagulant (LA) and serum anticardiolipin antibodies (ACA) have been described in patients with SLE and in rare patients treated with antipsychotics. Although the presence of LA and ACA are associated with a lengthening of serum coagulation test results, such as the partial thromboplastin time and prothrombin time, it is clinically associated with an increased incidence of thrombotic events, such as stroke.

ENVIRONMENTAL CONTAMINATION Some environmental toxins have potential neuropsychiatric manifestations. Of greatest relevance is heavy metal exposure. Lead poisoning resulting in lead encephalopathy is a problem that affects both children and adults. Other heavy metals that can result in neuropsychiatric symptoms include mercury and manganese. Exposure to various solvents can also result in neuropsychiatric symptoms (for example, solvent encephalopathy or painter's syndrome).

MONITORING PSYCHOTROPIC MEDICATIONS

ANTIDEPRESSANTS There are no standardized recommendations for the evaluation of a patient about to begin taking an antidepressant medication. The clinician must have a clear understanding of the potential adverse reactions to the antidepressant and an understanding of the patient's medical condition and physiological vulnerabilities. For instance, liver enzyme tests may be ordered for a patient with a past history of liver disease, as antidepressants are metabolized by the liver; liver disease, as evidenced by elevated liver enzymes, may suggest extra caution when using antidepressants and also suggest the need for periodic follow-up tests of liver function to assess the effects of the antidepressant on liver functioning. Women of childbearing age may need a pregnancy test so that the use of an antidepressant is fully informed; the aim is to expose the fetus to as few medications as possible, even those medications that are not clearly teratogenic. Patients with a history of cardiac disease who are about to start treatment with a tricyclic antidepressant should have a baseline ECG. Tricyclic antidepressants can affect intracardiac conduction and lengthen the PR, QT, and QRS intervals; patients with baseline abnormalities of those measures may need periodic follow-up ECGs. Serious and fatal arrhythmias can result from lack of attention to these antidepressant-related ECG changes. Baseline or follow-up ECG abnormalities may suggest that the clinician choose an antidepressant less associated with alterations in ECG parameters. Tricyclic antidepressant-induced changes in cardiac conduction may be especially troublesome in elderly patients; those with preexisting cardiac conditions; those receiving type I antiarrhythmic agents, such as quinidine (Duraquin) and lidocaine (Xylocaine); those taking digoxin (Lanoxin) or other cardiac glycosides that affect AV node conduction; and those with low serum potassium or magnesium.

Therapeutic blood levels The American Psychiatric Association (APA) Task Force on Laboratory Tests in Psychiatry has recommended that blood levels of certain tricyclic antidepressants be determined in certain situations. Such situations include those in which patients show questionable compliance with their medication, patients with a poor response while taking a typical antidepressant dosage for a reasonable period of time, patients with side effects at very low dosages, and the elderly and patients with medical problems where it is important to use as low a potentially therapeutic level of the drug as possible. Wide variations in blood levels of patients taking standard doses of tricyclics (for example, between 100 and 300 mg a day) presumably reflect differences in absorption and metabolism. Blood level monitoring has also been advocated for patients who need to obtain a potentially therapeutic blood level as rapidly as possible because of their clinical conditions (for example, when the patient is severely suicidal). The APA task force recognized therapeutic levels for imipramine (Tofranil) (plasma imipramine plus desmethylimipramine levels should exceed 200 ng/mL), nortriptyline (Aventyl) (a therapeutic window between 50 and 150 ng/mL in which plasma levels above or below this range tend to be associated with a less beneficial response), and desipramine (Norpramin) (therapeutic levels are described as exceeding 125 ng/mL). Clinicians should check their laboratories for slight variances in those therapeutic levels.

Therapeutic blood levels for other antidepressants have been less clearly established but are sometimes obtained to assess compliance, poor response to a conventional antidepressant dosage, side effects experienced at low dosages of the antidepressant, and possible toxic ranges, as in overdose.

In the medical assessment of patients taking tricyclic antidepressants, the clinician should be alert to the potential for the development of clinically significant orthostatic hypotension. If clinical symptoms develop while the patient is standing, a switch to a different antidepressant associated with less orthostatic hypotension may be indicated. Tachycardia associated with the anticholinergic antidepressants is rarely a serious problem. Weight gain can be associated with many of the antidepressants, including tricyclics and monoamine oxidase inhibitors (MAOIs), and should be monitored in patients who appear to be vulnerable to weight gain. Men with prostatic hypertrophy and patients with fecal impaction or constipation are at some risk from the anticholinergic side effects of the tricyclics. Priapism has been rarely associated with the antidepressant trazodone (Desyrel), and the appearance of such priapism typically represents a medical emergency.

Monitoring of children Major depressive disorder can be recognized in childhood by using unmodified adult criteria; according to one report, about 30 to 60 percent of outpatients in child psychiatry fulfill unmodified criteria for the disorder. The disabling effect of chronic untreated prepubertal depression in children has stimulated interest in the development of effective pharmacotherapies. Diagnostic testing, including monitoring of plasma tricyclic antidepressant levels, has proved useful in that effort. Weight-corrected oral dosing of tricyclics in children has not been shown to reliably predict plasma levels in individual patients. Limitations to the upward adjustment of tricyclic dosage include the severity of the nuisance side effects and the significant ECG and cardiovascular changes (heart rate > 130/min; PR interval > 0.18 sec; QRS width > 30 percent above baseline; and blood pressure > 140/90 mm Hg). ECG monitoring is an important laboratory tool for assessing compliance.

A significant relation has been shown between clinical response and maintenance plasma levels of some tricyclics. For instance, for the tricyclic imipramine, the authors of one study recommended a therapeutic blood level discriminating cutoff value of 150 ng/mL. In another study, with the tricyclic nortriptyline, plasma levels between 60 and 100 ng/mL were associated with a positive clinical response in prepubertal depressed children. However, more study is necessary to determine meaningful therapeutic blood levels for antidepressants in children.

LITHIUM Although lithium is clearly effective in the treatment of bipolar disorder, its therapeutic and toxic blood levels are very close to one another, and in some patients the two levels seem to overlap. In addition, lithium has effects on a number of organ systems. Lithium therapy is associated with a benign elevation of the white blood cell (WBC) count, which can rise to about 15,000 cells/mm^3. That WBC elevation can sometimes be mistaken for signs of infection or be wrongly attributed to lithium in cases of infection. Lithium can also have adverse effects on electrolyte balance (especially in patients taking thiazide diuretics), thyroid function, the kidneys, and the heart.

Common lithium pretreatment tests include serum electrolytes, blood urea nitrogen (BUN), serum creatinine, urinalysis, thyroid function tests (for example, TSH, T_4, T_3RU) and an ECG. In patients with histories suggestive of possible kidney problems, a 24-hour urine test for creatinine and protein clearance is recommended; some clinicians routinely order the test in patients about to begin lithium therapy. Some have argued that antithyroid antibody testing is helpful in assessing the potential of lithium-induced hypothyroidism. Because of the potential cardiac teratogenicity of lithium, a pregnancy test in women of childbearing age should be ordered. Periodic follow-up of serum BUN, creatinine, thyroid function tests, ECG, and 24-hour urine tests for creatinine and protein clearance are recommended, with the frequency and the exact makeup of the follow-up testing battery dictated by the patient's medical condition.

Suggested therapeutic blood levels for the lithium ion in acute mania range from 0.8 to 1.5 mEq/L, although a range where potential toxicity may be manifest is 1.2 to 1.5 mEq/L (a warning range in which the risk of developing toxicity rises rapidly). Recommended maintenance therapeutic blood levels of lithium are typically around 0.6 to 0.9 mEq/L. Lithium levels for therapeutic blood level monitoring are drawn as close to 12 hours after the last dose of lithium as possible. Steady-state levels in patients without renal dysfunction are reached in about five to eight days after the initiation of lithium treatment or after a dosage change. Patients with evidence suggestive of lithium toxicity should have a level drawn immediately; they may need close medical attention, including hemodialysis when the lithium levels exceed 2 to 4 mEq/L, especially in patients in poor medical condition with poor lithium excretion.

ANTIPSYCHOTICS Except for the antipsychotic clozapine (Clozaril), no clear pretreatment and follow-up laboratory and diagnostic evaluation strategy exists, and no specific therapeutic blood levels for antipsychotics have emerged, although some suggested therapeutic blood levels for several antipsychotic agents exist in the psychiatric literature. However, blood levels can be useful in determining medication noncompliance and in identifying treatment-refractory patients who are rapid metabolizers of the agent being used.

Clinicians need to be aware of the potential toxicities of the antipsychotic agents they use and need to order laboratory and diagnostic tests accordingly. For instance, clinicians using clozapine need to be aware of its potential to cause fatal agranulocytosis and seizures (those risks exist with all the antipsychotics, albeit to a smaller extent). Fever and sore throat (from granulocytopenia), and petechiae and ecchymosis (from thrombocytopenia) may be signs of toxicity in patients taking antipsychotics. Agranulocytosis occurs in about 1 percent of clozapine-treated patients who have been receiving the agent for a year. At this time, there are no ways of predicting in whom the potentially fatal adverse event will develop.

One laboratory test that is being studied as a potential predictor of clozapine-induced agranulocytosis is human lymphocyte antigen (HLA) typing. (A combination of three alleles—B38, DR4, and DQW3—has been reported to predict which patients are at risk for agranulocytosis.) Patients with a reduced WBC, leukopenia, and agranulocytosis have been managed as described in Table 9.7-6. If during treatment with clozapine the WBC falls below 3,500/mm^3 or there is a significant decrease from a higher WBC baseline that does not fall below 3,500 or the presence of immature white cell forms is detected, the clinician should immediately obtain a repeat WBC with differential white blood count. At WBCs below 2,000/mm^3 and granulocyte counts below 1,000/mm^3, bone marrow studies are recommended. Because of the increased incidence of seizures associated with clozapine, it is perhaps prudent that a normal EEG be obtained before increasing the dosage of clozapine beyond 600 mg a day (although, according to some reports, an abnormal EEG may predict a therapeutic response to clozapine).

Other potential adverse effects of antipsychotic medication include melanism from phenothiazines (especially chlorpromazine), abnormal lactation, and gynecomastia. The clinician should establish the childbearing status of at-risk women before starting to use an antipsychotic medication.

Serious cardiac arrhythmias have been reported as associated with antipsychotic use (for example, thioridazine); patients with preexisting cardiac disorder may need ECG follow-up when antipsychotics are used. Significant orthostatic hypotension can be associated with some of the antipsychotic agents. In addition, patients with concomitant hepatic or renal disease require periodic monitoring of those organ systems with periodic physical examinations, liver function tests, and tests for BUN and creatinine.

Neuroleptic malignant syndrome The diagnosis and follow-up of this potentially fatal adverse reaction to antipsychotic medications can be assisted by the laboratory. Neuroleptic malignant syndrome typically consists of varying degrees of hyperpyrexia, autonomic instability (for example, pulse rate greater than 100), severe extrapyramidal dysfunction (95 percent with lead-pipe rigidity), and delirium. Laboratory abnormalities often include creatine phosphokinase (CPK) and WBC elevations, myoglobinuria, and occasional liver enzyme elevations. Patients with neuroleptic malignant syndrome are at risk for serious medical complications, including renal failure, pneumonia, respiratory arrest, and cardiovascular collapse. Laboratory and diagnostic testing for those conditions should be ordered as indicated.

ANTICONVULSANTS Therapeutic blood levels for carbamazepine (Tegretol) have not been clearly established when it is used for the treatment of psychiatric disorders. However, therapeutic blood levels for psychiatric conditions corresponding to the typical anticonvulsant blood levels have been proposed for the anticonvulsant valproic acid (Depakene, Depakote).

Carbamazepine has been associated with aplastic anemia in up to 1 in 10,000 patients treated with the agent, although recent data put the severe hematological side effect rate at 1 in 125,000. However, decreases in the WBC count are common in patients taking the medication. In addition, a benign drop in the red blood cells (RBCs) may occur within the first week of treatment; the count reverts to normal without stopping the drug. Recommendations for the discontinuation of carbamazepine treatment have included WBC counts of less than 3,000/mm^3, erythrocyte counts of less than 4.0×10^6/mm^3, hemoglobin counts of less than 11 mg/dL, platelet counts of less than 100,000/mm^3, and reticulocyte counts of less than 0.3 percent. A proposed timetable for laboratory monitoring of patients on carbamazepine is outlined in Table 9.7-7. Carbamazepine can also have tricycliclike effects on the ECG.

With the anticonvulsant valproic acid, laboratory testing is usually focused on follow-up tests designed to assess its potential liver toxicity, although mild elevations of liver enzymes are common. Elevated blood ammonia levels in the absence of other liver function abnormalities have been reported in patients taking valproic acid. Serious adverse reactions that have been reported during valproic acid therapy include hepatitis, liver failure, hematological abnormalities (for example, decreased platelets, bone marrow suppression), and acute hemorrhagic pancreatitis.

Carbamazepine and valproic acid are potentially teratogenic; pretreatment pregnancy testing is advised in women of childbearing age. Carbamazepine induces liver enzymes that increase carbamazepine's

TABLE 9.7-6
Clinical Management of Reduced White Blood Cell (WBC) Count, Leukopenia, and Agranulocytosis in Patients Taking Carbamazepine

Problem Phase	WBC Findings	Clinical Findings	Treatment Plan
Reduced WBC	WBC count reveals a significant drop (even if WBC count is still in normal range). "Significant drop" = (1) drop of more than 3,000 cells from prior test or (2) three or more consecutive drops in WBC counts	No symptoms of infection	1. Monitor patient closely 2. Institute twice-weekly CBC tests with differentials if deemed appropriate by attending physician 3. Clozapine therapy may continue
Mild leukopenia	WBC = 3,000–3,500	Patient may or may not show clinical symptoms, such as lethargy, fever, sore throat, weakness	1. Monitor patient closely 2. Institute a minimum of twice-weekly CBC tests with differentials 3. Clozapine therapy may continue
Leukopenia or granulocytopenia	WBC = 2,000–3,000 or granulocytes = 1,000–1,500	Patient may or may not show clinical symptoms, such as fever, sore throat, lethargy, weakness	1. Interrupt clozapine at once 2. Institute daily CBC tests with differentials 3. Increase surveillance, consider hospitalization 4. Clozapine therapy may be reinstituted after normalization of WBC
Agranulocytosis (uncomplicated)	WBC count less than 2,000 or granulocytes less than 1,000	The patient may or may not show clinical symptoms, such as fever, sore throat, lethargy, weakness	1. Discontinue clozapine at once 2. Place patient in protective isolation in a medical unit with modern facilities 3. Consider a bone marrow specimen to determine if progenitor cells are being suppressed 4. Monitor patient every 2 days until WBC and differential counts return to normal (about 2 weeks) 5. Avoid use of concomitant medications with bone marrow-suppressing potential
Agranulocytosis (with complications)	WBC count less than 2,000 or granulocytes less than 1,000	Definite evidence of infection, such as fever, sore throat, lethargy, weakness, malaise, skin ulcerations, etc.	6. Consult with hematologist or other specialist to determine appropriate antibiotic regimen 7. Start appropriate therapy; monitor closely
Recovery	WBC count more than 4,000 and granulocytes more than 2,000	No symptoms of infection	1. Once-weekly CBC with differential counts for 4 consecutive normal values 2. Clozapine must not be restarted

Table reprinted with permission of Sandoz Pharmaceuticals Corporation. Table from A MacKinnon, S C Yudofsky: *Principles of the Psychiatric Evaluation,* p 118. Lippincott, Philadelphia, 1991. Used with permission.

TABLE 9.7-7
Laboratory Monitoring of Patients Taking Carbamazepine

Test	Frequency
1. Complete blood count	Before treatment and every two weeks for the first two months of treatment; thereafter, once every three months
2. Platelet count and reticulocyte count	Before treatment and yearly
3. Serum electrolytes	Before treatment and yearly
4. Electrocardiogram	Before treatment and yearly
5. AST, ALT, LDH, alkaline phosphatase	Before treatment and every month for the first two months of treatment; thereafter, every three months
6. Pregnancy test for women of childbearing age	Before treatment and as frequently as monthly in noncompliant patients

Table from A MacKinnon, S C Yudofsky: *Principles of the Psychiatric Evaluation,* p 108. Lippincott, Philadelphia, 1991. Used with permission.

metabolism and lower its blood levels during the initial two or three weeks of its use; valproic acid is not associated with a similar metabolic increase. Carbamazepine has been reported to reduce haloperidol (Haldol) blood levels, with clinical deterioration of the patient. Carbamazepine has also been associated with lowering serum sodium levels, potentially progressing to hyponatremia and even water intoxication. Occasional dermatological adverse effects associated with the anticonvulsants include a rash with carbamazepine and alopecia with valproic acid.

BRAIN IMAGING

COMPUTED TOMOGRAPHY Most physicians agree that psychiatric patients with neurological abnormalities or past histories suggestive of brain insults (for example, focal neurological findings, abnormal EEGs, head trauma, seizures, delirium) should have a diagnostic CT scan of the head. Other physicians have proposed more liberal recommendations for obtaining CT scans in psychiatric patients. They would include CT scans as part of the workup of psychiatric patients who show confusion, dementia, delirium, movement disorders, anorexia nervosa, or prolonged catatonia or who are in a first episode of psychosis. Moreover, those physicians also recommend a CT scan in patients over the age of 50 who show a personality change or have a first episode of a mood disorder.

The use of a contrast agent in CT scanning increases its diagnostic yield. Under normal conditions the contrast agent does not cross the blood-brain barrier and enter the brain. However, in certain pathological conditions (for example, tumor and cerebrovascular disorder), the contrast agent enters the brain, providing visualization of lesions that may have been undetected. It has been recommended that for most psychiatric patients a CT scan can be performed without the use of a contrast agent, thereby minimizing the risk and the cost of the CT procedure. A contrast agent is recommended when clear signs and symptoms suggest an underlying neurological disorder that would be better visualized with a contrast agent or when a lesion is suggested on the noncontrast scan. The decision to use a contrast agent can frequently be assisted by consultation with neurologists or radiologists.

MAGNETIC RESONANCE IMAGING Magnetic resonance imaging (MRI) visualizes brain structures with remarkable clarity and offers better resolution of brain structures than does CT. The indications for using MRI in a psychiatric patient are similar to those outlined above for CT scans. However, MRI is perhaps superior to CT scans when the suspected CNS disease process includes a white matter demyelinating disease (such as multiple sclerosis), a nonmeningeal neoplasm, vascular malformation, a degenerative disease such as Huntington's disease, or a seizure. The MRI technique is also useful in patients unable to tolerate iodine-based contrast materials and intravenous procedures that may be needed during a CT scan. In addition, an MRI can be used to clarify ambiguous CT scan findings. CT is thought to be more sensitive to detecting acute subarachnoid hemorrhage than is MRI.

The MRI technique is typically contraindicated in patients with pacemakers or aneurysm clips, in pregnant women, and in patients with potentially magnetic foreign bodies. A CT scan is often recommended over an MRI when the suspected disease process involves the pituitary gland, calcified brain lesions, meningeal tumors, and acute parenchymal infarction or hemorrhage.

A variety of anxiety reactions can occur during MRI scanning (for example, claustrophobia). Some patients must be carefully screened before scanning and must be prepared for the experience, perhaps with friends and family members on hand, with prescanning behavioral desensitization, and consideration of premedication (for example, with a short-acting anxiolytic).

ELECTROPHYSIOLOGY

ELECTROENCEPHALOGRAM In patients with some likelihood of an organic CNS diathesis, an electroencephalogram (EEG) is frequently indicated. A normal result frequently reassures the clinician, the patient, and the family that an organic CNS abnormality is not present, but the clinician should realize that a single normal result does not rule out an organic cause or a seizure disorder. If a seizure disorder is strongly suspected in a patient, sampling errors can be corrected by repeat EEGs or a 24-hour ambulatory recording (often accompanied by video recordings of the patient's behavior to further document potential seizure activity). EEG recordings of sleep-deprived patients further increase the likelihood of unmasking clinically significant latent abnormal EEG activity. Some clinicians use nasopharyngeal leads to increase the diagnostic yield of the EEG in psychiatric patients. However, the nasopharyngeal leads are usually uncomfortable for the patient and interfere with the patient's falling asleep during the recording of the EEG, so they can decrease the usefulness of the EEG, as it is during sleep that latent abnormal EEG activity is often uncovered. A diagnosis of a seizure disorder is typically made on clinical grounds and is not entirely dependent on abnormal EEG findings. EEG monitoring is used by some clinicians and researchers during the administration of electroconvulsive therapy (ECT). Such EEG monitoring assures the clinician that a fully therapeutic seizure has been induced.

POLYSOMNOGRAPHY Polysomnography is used in the evaluation of various sleep disorders (for example, insomnia, sleep apnea, parasomnias, narcolepsy, male erectile disorder). Polysomnography involves the assessment of multiple physiological parameters while the patient sleeps or attempts to sleep; the parameters include EEG, electrooculogram (EOG), electromyogram (EMG), ECG, blood oxygen saturation, blood pressure, respiratory effort, and body temperature. A daytime polysomnographic evaluation called the multiple sleep latency test is used in the evaluation of narcolepsy.

EVOKED POTENTIAL Evoked potential testing can be used in the differentiation of certain organic versus functional complaints (for example, the visual evoked potential can be used to evaluate hysterical blindness). Other forms of evoked potential studies include the somatosensory evoked potential, the brainstem auditory evoked potential, and the auditory evoked potential. Evoked potentials are sometimes referred to as evoked responses. When neuropsychiatric symptoms of unclear etiology are present, certain evoked potential findings may be useful for detecting possible underlying neurological dysfunction (for example, evoked potential findings can suggest underlying demyelinating disorders, such as multiple sclerosis).

GENETIC TESTING

Clinical chromosome analysis usually takes place during a prenatal analysis of genetic disorders. Possible clinical indications for ordering a cytogenetic analysis in a psychiatric patient not in a gynecologic or obstetric setting may include congenital anomalies or nonspecific mental retardation. If a patient has cytogenetic analysis performed for some reason (for example, as part of the workup in cases of infertility, habitual abortion, amenorrhea, and ambiguous external genitalia), attention needs to be paid to the potential adverse psychological effects of the result on the patient and the family. Cytogenetic testing can provide some basis for genetic counseling.

AMOBARBITAL INTERVIEW

An amobarbital (Amytal) interview is a useful aid in differentiating certain functional versus organic conditions. For instance, in certain stuporous schizophrenic or depressed patients, amobarbital may make the patient more verbal and less guarded. A patient whose stuporous state is secondary to a neuromedical condition (for example, brain tumor, cerebrovascular disorder) is often reported to become more confused, with clear deterioration on cognitive examination, after receiving amobarbital. The interview involves the slow intravenous infusion of sodium amobarbital, with careful attention to avoid oversedation and respiratory depression.

NEW CLINICAL AND RESEARCH TOOLS

BIOLOGIC MARKERS There has been a great deal of interest in finding neurophysiologic markers of psychiatric disorders. Those biologic markers would be laboratory or other diagnostic tests for psychiatric disorders that are currently viewed as functional or idiopathic and for which no clear neuropathophysiologic lesions have yet been found. Besides being useful in helping researchers understand the pathophysiology of psychiatric disturbance, such markers might provide diagnostic tests for the practicing psychiatrist. Biologic markers could assist in (1) making accurate psychiatric diagnoses; (2) identifying persons at risk for a psychiatric disorder so that, for example, preventive steps could be implemented; (3) assessing a patient's prognosis and assisting in treatment planning; and (4) predicting which organic treatments have the greatest likelihood of therapeutic success for a particular patient. Proposed biologic markers encompass a wide range of procedures, some of which are listed in Table 9.7-8. Difficulties that have arisen for many of the proposed markers include problems with sensitivity, specificity, reliability, and contamination from artifactual influences (for example, concurrent medical illnesses, medication effects, and normal individual variation). Currently, because of those and other problems, such as certain technological hurdles, none of the markers is clearly established as useful for routine clinical practice.

Brain-imaging techniques An exciting area of biologic marker work involves several brain-imaging techniques that have become available to neuropsychiatrists. The tests provide measures of brain structure and function. Psychiatrists are now increasingly better able to image the structure and function of the brain.

ELECTROENCEPHALOGRAPHY In the computerized tomographic mapping of electrophysiological data, a computer is used to amass and process large quantities of EEG and evoked potential data from a patient. The computer analyzes the data in various ways and graphically presents the data as two-dimensional, typically color-coded maps of brain electrical activity. The technology has not yet evolved a fully agreed on niche in the diagnostic assessment of an idiopathic psychiatric disorder.

Nevertheless, some preliminary research has suggested that the computerized tomographic mapping of EEG and evoked potential data may provide some biologic markers for such psychiatric conditions as schizophrenia. For instance, somatosensory evoked potential topographic maps for schizophrenic patients reportedly have greater left temporoparietal activity than right hemispheric activity; those findings are consistent with hypotheses suggesting left temporoparietal hyperactivity, left hemispheric dysfunction, or interhemispheric imbalances in patients with schizophrenia. The P300 form of evoked potential has been reported to be attenuated in patients with schizophrenia; it has been suggested that patients with more negative symptoms of schizophrenia might have the greatest decreases in P300 amplitude.

The computerized EEG may also help in the development of the

TABLE 9.7-8
Some Biologic Markers Under Investigation

Brain-imaging techniques
- Computerized topographic mapping of electrophysiologic data
- Computed tomography (CT)
- Regional cerebral blood flow (rCBF)
- Magnetic resonance imaging (MRI—structural and functional)
- Positron emission tomography (PET)
- Single photon emission computed tomography (SPECT)
- Magnetic resonance spectroscopy (MRS)
- Magnetoencephalography (MEG)

Electrophysiologic markers
- Electroencephalography (EEG)
- Sleep EEG
- Polysomnography
- Evoked potentials (EPs)
- Electrodermal activity (EDA)
- Electroretinogram (ERG)
- Facial electromyography

Biochemical markers
- Catecholamines and catecholamine metabolites (e.g., dopamine, homovanillic acid, dihydroxyphenylacetic acid, norepinephrine, 3-methoxy-4-hydroxyphenylglycol)
- Indoleamines and indoleamine metabolites (serotonin, 5-hydroxy-indoleacetic acid)
- Other neurotransmitters and neuroregulators (acetylcholine, histamine, amino acids, melatonin, prostaglandins, opioid peptides, neuropeptides, such as neuropeptide Y, somatostatin)
- Enzymes (dopamine-β-hydroxylase, monoamine oxidase, tyrosine hydroxylase, catechol-*O*-methyltransferase, adenyl cyclase, guanyl cyclase, nitric oxide sythase)
- Receptor densities and affinities on peripheral blood and tissue elements
- Ion transport across membranes of peripheral blood elements

Psychoimmunological markers
- Immunoglobulin levels
- Lymphocyte responses (e.g., to mitogen stimulation)
- Lymphokine, cytokine, interleukin, interferon measures
- Viral serologies
- Alz-50 (monoclonal antibody directed against an antigen present in Alzheimer's disease)
- Anticardiolipin antibodies (ACA)

Neuroendocrine markers
- Dexamethasone-suppression test (DST)
- Thyrotropin-releasing hormone stimulation test (TRHST)
- Provocative challenges to growth hormone (GH)

Provocative tests for anxiety disorders
- Lactate infusion test
- CO_2 challenge test

Psychotropic medication evaluation
- Determination of therapeutic blood levels, including metabolite blood levels
- Antipsychotic medication-induced biochemical changes (e.g., pHVA)
- Antipsychotic blood activity measures (e.g., radioreceptor assay)
- Platelet MAO inhibition in patients taking MAOIs
- Lithium levels in saliva

Oculomotor measures
- Smooth-pursuit eye movement (SPEM)
- Saccadic eye movements
- Antisaccadic eye movements
- Visual fixation
- Pupillometry

Genetic markers
- HLA histocompatibility antigens
- Gene mapping
- Restriction fragment length polymorphisms (RFLPs)

Table adapted from Darrell G Kirch, MD.

EEG as a functional measure of the therapeutic activity of various psychotropics (pharmaco-EEG). The attempt is to find electrophysiologic markers of therapeutic drug activity; the technique would then help clinicians choose the best medication for a particular patient and perhaps help in titrating the best dosage of the drug. Unfortunately, inconsistencies have appeared in the literature. For instance, not all studies have found the typical antipsychotic profile for antipsychotic medications—that is, a "shift to the left of the EEG spectrum," with increases in slow frequencies and a decrease in fast frequencies. According to some reports, antipsychotic medications appear to partially normalize computerized electrophysiologic evoked potential topography in schizophrenic patients, suggesting that topographic evoked potential mapping may have some future role to play in the analysis of the effect of antipsychotics in schizophrenia.

SLEEP EEG (POLYSOMNOGRAPHY) One important biologic marker uses EEG during the sleeping state (sleep EEG). Polysomnographic findings of relevance to psychiatry include reports of decreased latency to the onset of rapid eye movement (REM) sleep (with an overall increase in the percentage of REM sleep) in patients with major depressive disorder. Neuromedical conditions giving rise to pseudodepressive presentations are typically associated with decreased REM sleep (for example, patients with dementia usually have increased amounts of non-REM sleep). In schizophrenia decreased slow-wave sleep and increased sleep latency and sleep fragmentation have been reported, especially during relapse. Computerized analysis of the sleep EEG, with the generation of topographic maps of sleep EEG activity, is also available.

COMPUTED TOMOGRAPHY Researchers continue to study possible useful subcategories of psychiatric diagnoses that could be based on computed tomography (CT) findings. Some patients with schizophrenia and enlarged ventricles may be more treatment-resistant to currently available antipsychotic agents. However, no evidence supports making functional psychiatric diagnoses based on CT scan abnormalities. The CT is commonly used by clinicians to rule out organic brain lesions, and investigators continue to use the CT to identify structural brain abnormalities in patients with idiopathic psychiatric disturbances. However, such CT scan studies are increasingly being replaced by the MRI technique because of MRI's better resolution of brain structures.

MAGNETIC RESONANCE IMAGING Various neuropsychiatric studies using the MRI technique have reported that schizophrenic patients have smaller frontal lobes, cerebrums, craniums, and hippocampi but larger lenticular nuclei than do normal controls. Differences in the symmetries of various brain structures have also been noted between schizophrenic patients and normal controls. The usefulness of the many different scanning modes in psychiatric patients has yet to be fully evaluated.

FUNCTIONAL MRI Although traditional MRI provides anatomic images of the brain, a functional MRI technique is currently under development which might ultimately provide the neuropsychiatric researcher and clinician images of brain activity that rival the clarity of MRI anatomical images. Functional MRI imaging can be directly correlated to high-resolution, three-dimensional anatomical MR images. Thus, the boundaries of activation and nonactivation can be determined precisely. For instance, using this technique, photic stimulation of human volunteers was shown to cause a localized increase in blood volume in the anatomically defined primary visual cortex. Techniques are under development for measuring increased levels of oxygenation in activated brain tissues; these techniques are based on the fact that changes in hemoglobin oxygenation affect hemoglobin's magnetic properties. The development of blood oxygenation level dependent (BOLD) MRI should obviate the need for administration of a paramagnetic pharmaceutical contrast agent to obtain a functional MR image.

MAGNETIC RESONANCE SPECTROSCOPY Magnetic resonance spectroscopy is related to MRI but uses more powerful magnets to evaluate certain aspects of brain function and metabolism. Information about brain phospholipid, carbohydrate, protein, amino acid, and high-energy phosphate metabolism; brain intracellular pH; and lithium and fluorinated psychopharmacological agents can be obtained by the technique. For instance, using phosphorus-31 nuclear magnetic resonance (P^{31} NMR) spectroscopy, researchers have studied the metabolism of brain high-energy phosphate and membrane phospholipids in the dorsal prefrontal cortex of drug-naive patients with schizophrenia. They found significant differences between the patients and controls, with dorsal prefrontal cortex hypoactivity in patients suggested by decreased adenosine triphosphate and inorganic orthophosphate levels. Alterations in membrane phospholipid metabolism were suggested by lower levels of phosphomonoesters and higher levels of phosphodiesters compared with the controls. Those and other preliminary findings suggest that magnetic resonance spectroscopy will be an exciting new neuropsychiatric research tool.

POSITRON EMISSION TOMOGRAPHY Positron emission tomography (PET) directly visualizes both cortical and subcortical brain functioning. Depending on the type of positron-emitting isotope used, different aspects of brain functioning can be evaluated, including brain glucose metabolism, cerebral blood flow, brain oxygen use, and some specific brain neurotransmitter receptor functions. PET findings have included abnormalities of the anteroposterior gradient of glucose utilization and higher subcortical/cortical glucose metabolism ratios in patients with schizophrenia compared with normal controls. PET findings in schizophrenia, bipolar disorder, substance use disorders, obsessive-compulsive disorder, and panic disorders are largely preliminary and have not always been replicated. PET remains a research tool available at only a few research centers.

SINGLE PHOTON EMISSION COMPUTED TOMOGRAPHY Single photon emission computed tomography (SPECT) has become a useful clinical and research tool. Like PET, SPECT can visualize both cortical and subcortical brain activity. Depending on the radioisotope used, different aspects of brain function can be studied, such as brain blood flow or brain receptor binding (for example, dopamine receptors). SPECT has proved to be a valuable technique for the assessment of regional cerebral blood flow in neuropsychiatric disorders. The development of SPECT for that purpose resulted from the introduction of lipophilic radiopharmaceuticals, especially N-isopropyl-p-(I^{123}) iodoamphetamine ([I^{123}] inosine monophosphate [IMP]) and (Tc^{99m}) hexamethylpropyleneamine oxime ([Tc^{99m}] HM-PAO). Those radiopharmaceuticals readily cross the blood-brain barrier, and their initial uptake into or extraction by the brain is high and dependent on blood flow. With respect to (I^{123}) IMP, there is a high first-pass extraction by the brain and retention by high-capacity, nonspecific binding sites. Optimal scans with (I^{123}) IMP should be performed about 20 minutes after injection. With Tc^{99m} HM-PAO, brain concentrations remain stable for hours, permitting scanning hours after tracer injections. Currently, perfusion studies with SPECT are described in terms of relative cerebral blood flow; that is, measurements are normalized to a structure (for example, the cerebellum), or comparisons are made between symmetrical structures on the lesioned versus the nonlesioned side. Inhalation of Xe^{133} can also be used in SPECT to obtain brain images and to measure regional cerebral blood flow. However, the technique lacks good spatial resolution and cannot be used to detect lesions in the base of the skull because of Xe^{133} gas in the paranasal sinuses.

SPECT imaging can be done with the patient at rest and in conjunction with certain activation procedures. Activation might involve the use of a cognitive challenge task such as the Wisconsin Card Sorting Test, or after pharmacological challenge with such agents as procaine (Novocain) or acetazolamide (Diamox).

A recent SPECT study used (Tc^{99m}) HM-PAO to show a relative increase in regional cerebral blood flow to the medial-frontal cortex bilaterally in patients with obsessive-compulsive disorder. The medial-frontal cortex, an area enclosed by six-degree samples of the cortical circumference on each side of the frontal midline, contained counts from the prefrontal cortex and the anterior cingulate. The finding of increased blood flow to the medial-frontal cortex of the patients is consistent with early PET findings of increased metabolism in the prefrontal cortex and the anterior cingulate. However, the increased blood flow was not correlated with the severity of the patients' obsessions or compulsions.

Patients with panic disorder have a relative deficit in frontal lobe blood flow after yohimbine (Yocon) challenge. In patients with seizure disorders, an ictal SPECT may show an area of hypermetabolism at the seizures focus, and an interictal scan may show an area of hypometabolism. Tc^{99m} HM-PAO can be injected into a patient during an ictus and imaged hours later. Such a scan might be useful in the evaluation of pseudoseizure. SPECT scan of patients with vascular dementia classically have a Swiss cheese pattern of perfusion deficits.

Other investigators using SPECT and (Tc^{99m}) HM-PAO as the imaging agent have uncovered brain perfusion abnormalities in cocaine abusers. Specifically, the investigators found focal defects in the inferior parietal cortex, the temporal cortex, the anterofrontal cortex, and the basal ganglia. In another study SPECT perfusion scans showed neurovascular abnormalities and early changes in cerebral perfusion in asymptomatic cocaine abusers. Moreover, the degree of substance abuse seemed to correlate with the severity of the abnormalities found by SPECT.

Perfusion studies with SPECT may serve an important role in the diagnostic evaluation of patients with early dementia of the Alzheimer's type. For example, in one SPECT study using I^{123} IMP, the scans of patients with Alzheimer's disease were distinguished from those of normal persons with 88 percent sensitivity (test result abnormal-disease positive) and 87 percent specificity (test result normal-disease negative). Of note was a sensitivity of 80 percent in patients whose disease was classified as mild. Patients with abnormal scan findings showed bilateral temporoparietal hypoperfusion. Moreover, perfusion defects often extended to the frontal lobes. Thus, SPECT may have a role in the evaluation of early Alzheimer's disease and the prospective evaluation of patients in medication protocols.

SPECT may also be used to image the distribution of neurotransmitter receptors in vivo. For instance, the distribution of the radiolabeled iodinated derivative of 3-quinuclidinyl benzilate (I^{123} QNB), a high-affinity muscarinic receptor antagonist, was studied in patients with primary degenerative dementia. A reduction in the relative distribution of I^{123} QNB was observed bilaterally in the posterior temporal cortex of the patients with Alzheimer's disease, compared with the controls. Cortical irregularities were seen in other areas of some of the demented patients, including focal defects of the inferior parietal cortex and the frontal cortex. The data suggest that a reduction in the binding of I^{123} QNB to a subpopulation of muscarinic receptors (perhaps the M1 receptor) occurs in at least some patients with Alzheimer's disease. Other studies suggest that SPECT may have a role in the early diagnosis and management of HIV encephalopathy.

The existence of hypofrontality (that is, diminished functional activity of the prefrontal cortex) is hypothesized in patients with schizophrenia, especially those with prominent negative symptoms. However, diminished perfusion to the frontal lobes in patients with schizophrenia has not been consistently observed. In one SPECT study using I^{123} IMP, patients with schizophrenia showed a significantly decreased perfusion in the left temporal cortex and increased perfusion in the right temporal cortex, especially the right inferior temporal pole. No significant differences in the frontal regions were seen between patients and controls. The failure to find differences between schizophrenic patients and controls in frontal lobe activity may be a function of the paradigm. In that study, patients were injected with a radiolabeled tracer and told to relax. Perhaps a perfusion defect in the frontal lobes in patients with schizophrenia must be elicited. That could be accomplished with a cognitive task (for example, the Wisconsin Card Sorting Test) whose performance engages the frontal cortex (for example, functional brain imaging with cognitive activation).

MAGNETOENCEPHALOGRAPHY In contrast to the conventional and computed EEG and evoked potential methods of recording electrophysiologic data, which gather largely cortical brain activity, magnetoencephalography (MEG) detects the magnetic fields associated with the electrical activity in both cortical and deep brain tissues. MEG is noninvasive and exposes the patient to no harmful radiation. The technology is still in its infancy and is available in only a few research centers.

REGIONAL CEREBRAL BLOOD FLOW In this nuclear medicine technique a metabolically inert radioactive substance is introduced into the body, the substance is carried to the brain by the blood, and radiation emanating from the brain is picked up by detectors surrounding the skull. The technique can delineate blood flow in cortical structures. Decreased blood flow to certain frontal regions of the brain have been reported in patients with schizophrenia.

Other neurophysiological markers

EYE MOVEMENT DEFICITS In up to 85 percent of patients with schizophrenia, a deficit in smooth-pursuit eye movement has been described. The deficit may be a biologic marker of schizophrenia. An antisaccade eye movement deficit has been described in patients with various neuropsychiatric impairments, including patients with frontal cortical and basal ganglia lesions, schizophrenia, and obsessive-compulsive disorder. The antisaccade deficit typically seen in such patients includes a decreased ability to inhibit reflexive glances toward stimuli that they are instructed to look away from. Eye movement deficits can be measured in a number of ways, including electro-oculography and infrared scleral reflectance techniques.

ELECTRORETINOGRAM The electroretinogram (ERG) measures electrical changes produced in the retina by flashes of light. ERG amplitudes are reduced in such diseases as retinitis pigmentosa and myotonic dystrophy and during the prodromes for those disorders. Decreased ERG amplitude has been reported in cases of thioridazine toxicity. In neuropsychiatric conditions, ERG amplitude reductions (specifically B-wave amplitude) have been described in many autistic patients and in patients with various types of dementia, such as Alzheimer's disease and Creutzfeldt-Jakob disease.

ELECTRODERMAL ACTIVITY The electrodermal activities that can be measured include skin conductance response, tonic skin conductive level, and skin conductance orienting response. Possible electrodermal activity markers have been reported in schizophrenia and depression. Decreased habituation of skin conductance response has been proposed as a possible correlate of suicidal behavior.

Endocrine stimulation techniques

DEXAMETHASONE-SUPPRESSION TEST Reseachers hoped that this laboratory test would be of clinical usefulness in the management of psychiatric patients. Endocrinologists use a version of the test in the evaluation of Cushing's disease, and research psychiatrists found the test to be a possible marker of major depressive illness. Researchers hoped that the test would be useful in assisting with psychiatric differential diagnosis (for example, differentiating dementia from the pseudodementia of depression and differentiating schizoaffective disorder from schizophrenia) and in predicting treatment response and suicidal potential. Many of the research findings have proved interesting, but consensus does not exist to support the routine clinical use of the test.

A common version of the test as used by psychiatrists involves the administration of a 1 mg dose of dexamethasone at 11 PM with a serum cortisol level determination before dexamethasone administration (to assess baseline cortisol levels) and other serum cortisol determinations at various points over the next 24 hours (typically at 8 AM, 4 PM, and 11 PM). The findings are considered abnormal if the serum cortisol levels after dexamethasone administration exceed about 5 μg/dL. However, the reliability of many commercial assays at about the 5 μg/dL cutoff value is questionable, so plasma cortisol levels between 4 and 7 μg/dL should be interpreted cautiously. Many other limitations on the routine use of the test have emerged, including significant potential artifactual contamination from concomitant medical conditions (such as diabetes mellitus) and medications (such as carbamazepine) and the possibility that the test results direct the clinician's attention away from other more important clinical issues. If the dexamethasone-suppression test is used, the psychiatrist should be attentive to the possible causes of false-positive or negative results outlined in Table 9.7-9.

However, some researchers and clinicians continue to argue that there is a role for the dexamethasone-suppression test in the management of depressed patients. For instance, studies have shown that a group of depressed patients who continue to show nonsuppression after apparent successful treatment for their depression are at greater risk of relapse, readmission to a hospital, and suicide than are those whose responses were normalized. When the treatment involves ECT, the clinical response after ECT has been associated with an increase in plasma dexamethasone levels; plasma cortisol levels were not related to the clinical outcome. Nevertheless, a negative result on the dexamethasone-suppression test appears to be much less informative than a positive result. If the test is used in the treatment of a patient, it should always be in the context of the patient's overall clinical condition.

THYROTROPIN-RELEASING HORMONE STIMULATION TEST Endocrinologists routinely use a version of this test in the evaluation of hypothyroidism. The hypothyroid patient has an augmented response of TSH to an intravenous injection of thyrotropin-releasing hormone (TRH). The test has also been proposed to grade different degrees of hypothyroidism. Grade 1 hypothyroidism is obvious on clinical and biochemical grounds; grade 2 hypothyroidism is less obvious, with no clear clinical features, but TSH is elevated; and grade 3 hypothyroidism has normal baseline TSH and other thyroid hormone values, but the TRH stimulation test results are abnormal. Cases of depression that are really grade 3 hypothyroidism may be missed if only the conventional serum thyroid hormone assays are used. A blunted TRH stimulation test result has been proposed as a biologic marker of major depression, with diagnostic and prognostic usefulness. A blunted result has been reported in up to 30 percent of depressed patients but does not appear to be specific for major depression; blunted results have been reported in patients with alcohol-related disorders, panic disorder, bulimia nervosa, and borderline personality disorder.

TABLE 9.7-9
Causes of False-Positive or Negative Results on the Dexamethasone-Suppression Test (DST)

False Positives	False Negatives
Cushing's syndrome	Addison's disease
Weight loss or malnutrition	Hypopituitarism
Obesity	Slow dexamethasone metabolism
Bulimia nervosa	Drugs
Pregnancy	Synthetic corticosteroids
Alcohol abuse and withdrawal	Indomethacin
Anorexia nervosa	High doses of benzodiazepines
Temporal lobe epilepsy	High doses of cyproheptadine
Dementia	
Diabetes mellitus	
Infection	
Trauma	
Recent surgery	
Advanced age	
Fever	
Carcinoma	
Renal or cardiac failure	
Renovascular hypertension	
Cerebrovascular disorder	
Antipsychotic withdrawal	
Tricyclic withdrawal	
Drugs	
High doses of estrogens	
Narcotics	
Sedative-hypnotics	
Anticonvulsants	

Table adapted from Darrell G Kirch, MD.

PROVOCATIVE TESTS OF PANIC DISORDER These tests challenge patients with carbon dioxide inhalation, IV lactate infusions, or IV infusions of such substances as caffeine, isoproterenol, β-carboline, flumazenil (Mazicon)—all of which can induce panic attacks in patients so predisposed (but less so in persons without a history of panic disorder). Lactate infusion is the most extensively studied provocative test for panic disorder, and up to 72 percent of panic disorder patients have been reported to experience a panic attack after the IV infusion of sodium lactate. Anxiogenic responses to lactate or fenfluramine (Pondimin) provocation have been described as greater in patients with high panic attack frequencies. In patients with posttraumatic stress disorder, IV infusions of lactate can trigger flashbacks of the traumatic event, at times with dramatic affective displays in response to the flashback.

Panic attacks precipitated by IV lactate infusion can be inhibited by tricyclic antidepressants and alprazolam (Xanax), psychopharmacological agents of demonstrated efficacy in the treatment of panic disorder. Simple hyperventilation procedures can also precipitate panic attacks in patients so predisposed, although hyperventilation appears to be a less potent stimulus of panic attacks than are IV infusions of lactate. However, hyperventilation procedures should be used with caution because of their ability to trigger seizures.

At this time, provocative tests are more useful as research tools to study various paroxysmal anxiety disorders than they are as diagnostic tests, although some clinician-researchers have advocated their clinical use. Responses to challenge tests for anxiety disorders may lead to useful subtyping paradigms for those disorders. However, the specificity of lactate infusions for panic disorder is unclear, as patients with primary depressive disorder and secondary panic attacks have similar rates of lactate-induced panic attacks as those patients with primary panic disorder.

Biochemical markers From blood, cerebrospinal fluid, and urine samples, one can obtain many potential biochemical markers, including neurotransmitter substances and their metabolites—dopamine, homovanillic acid (HVA), norepinephrine and its metabolite 3-methoxy-4-hydroxyphenylglycol, and serotonin (5-hydroxytryptamine [5-HT]) and its metabolite 5-hydroxy indoleacetic acid (5-HIAA)—and potentially relevant amino acids, such as tryptophan, tyrosine, glycine, and glutamate. Studies involving most of those markers and many other proposed markers have often yielded mixed results.

PLASMA HOMOVANILLIC ACID The measurement of homovanillic acid in plasma (pHVA), a major acidic metabolite of dopamine, may reflect changes in the activity of dopamine in the brain. The measurement of pHVA may have practical clinical applications in the identification of schizophrenic patients responsive to antipsychotic medications. Although most of the HVA in plasma derives from peripheral sources, some data support its use as an index of central nervous system activity. Clinical studies have found a good correlation between HVA levels in plasma and in the CSF subsequent to the inhibition of peripheral monoamine oxidase activity and the diminution of the peripheral contribution to pHVA by debrisoquin. Whereas pHVA levels in schizophrenic patients are changed by fluphenazine (Prolixin), a centrally active dopamine antagonist, the levels were insensitive to domperidone, a peripherally acting antagonist. Consistent with previous reports, a recent study suggests that responders to antipsychotics are characterized by antipsychotic-induced reductions in pHVA.

The data also suggest that the dopamine systems of some nonresponders may react differently to the antagonistic actions of antipsychotic medication than do the dopamine systems of responders. The time-dependent decreases in pHVA in treatment responders suggest that the ability to dampen presynaptic dopaminergic activity is related to the therapeutic efficacy of the antipsychotic medications. That time-dependent effect may account for the passage of weeks before maximal therapeutic effects are seen.

Clinical studies suggest that high baseline values of pHVA in schizophrenic patients may be a predictor of treatment responsiveness. Moreover, a positive association between the level of pHVA and the severity of the psychotic symptoms in drug-free schizophrenic patients has been reported. The results of several clinical trials suggest that responders to antipsychotics show higher baseline levels of pHVA and a treatment-induced reduction in levels of the metabolite compared with nonresponders.

The widespread clinical application of pHVA measurements may have relevance to treatment selection. For example, patients who do not show a reduction in pHVA after five weeks of treatment with adequate dosages of a conventional antipsychotic medication may be candidates for atypical antipsychotics or nondopaminergic interventions.

3-METHOXY-4-HYDROXYPHENYLGLYCOL When measured in 24-hour urine collections, 3-methoxy-4-hydroxyphenylglycol (MHPG) has been reported to be lower in bipolar disorder patients than in unipolar depressed patients. Low urine MHPG may predict imipramine response in depressed patients, but is probably not a useful predictor of response for other antidepressants. High urinary MHPG levels have also recently been associated with depressed patients who are more likely than depressed patients with more normal urinary MHPG levels to show the cognitive features of learned helplessness.

Low CSF MHPG (along with decreased 24-hour urinary norepinephrine-epinephrine ratios) has been used as a measure of a possible decrease in noradrenergic activity, possibly reflecting an increased predisposition to suicidal behavior.

5-HYDROXYINDOLEACETIC ACID Associations have been seen between low CSF 5-HIAA and suicidal behavior, aggression, poor impulse control and impulsive suicidal acts, disturbed behavior in childhood, violent suicide attempts, and depression in patients with diagnoses including major depression, schizophrenia, alcoholism, and adjustment disorder. 5-HIAA may not have nosological specificity; it may mark troublesome behaviors across a wide variety of psychiatric diagnoses. There have also been reports of associations between elevated CSF 5-HIAA concentrations and anxious, obsessional, and inhibited behaviors.

TRYPTOPHAN Low levels of total and free serum tryptophan have been reported in patients with major depressive disorder. The decrease in serum tryptophan does not appear to be related to the weight loss often seen in depressed patients. Special diets low in the amino acid tryptophan designed to significantly lower serum tryptophan have been shown to precipitate depression in patients so predisposed.

SERINE In psychotic patients the activity of the enzyme serine hydroxymethyltransferase has been reported to be deficient. The folate-dependent enzyme catalyzes the interconversion of serine and glycine. A deficiency in the activity of the enzyme may account for the high serine levels found in some psychotic patients. The plasma glycine levels in psychotic patients and normal controls have not been found to be significantly different.

Genetic testing Currently, no functional (idiopathic) psychiatric disorder is clearly and definitively associated with a specific chromosome or gene location or abnormality; however, work in the area is intense and may lead to the development of valuable diagnostic tools for certain psychiatric disorders. For instance, using new molecular biology techniques, some studies suggest that the Al allele of the dopamine type 2 (D_2) receptor is associated with alcoholism, Tourette's disorder, attention-deficit/hyperactivity disorder, autism, and posttraumatic stress disorder. Those studies also suggest that the presence of the mutant allele is not the primary cause of those disorders but seems to act as a modifying gene in the disorders. However, those findings have not been consistently replicated. In addition, different polymorphic forms of the D_4 receptor have also recently been identified. The D_4 receptor is of interest because the antipsychotic clozapine has a greater affinity for the D_4 receptor than for D_2 and D_3 receptors. One important question is whether a predisposition to psychotic illness is related to the presence of specific subtypes of the dopamine receptor.

For those disorders caused by a known single gene defect, the possibility exists that DNA oligonucleotide probes (about 20 nucleotides) can be synthesized to hybridize with the mutant gene under conditions of high stringency in which only perfectly matched complementary strands form stable helices. As neuropsychiatric disorders caused by single gene defects are identified, those probes will be used to identify affected heterozygous carriers and fetuses. In the procedure, DNA may be extracted from peripheral blood leukocytes or fetal cells, digested with restriction nucleases, and separated according to size by the Southern blot technique. The Southern blot procedure involves the migration of digested DNA fragments according to size in an agarose gel. The oligonucleotide probes are then used to identify mutant genes. When the mutant gene product is not known, the assessment of carrier status may still be possible if unique patterns of DNA fragments after the digestion of the cellular DNA by restriction nucleases are linked to those neuropsychiatric disorders under consideration. Thus, anonymous segments of DNA may serve as genetic markers of neuropsychiatric disorders.

Other findings in the field of molecular biology include the identification of a locus for familial Alzheimer's disease on chromosome 21; the locus appears to be near but not identical to the one encoding the amyloid precursor protein. Abnormalities in the proteolytic digestion of the amyloid precursor protein leading to the deposition of a split product in the beta-pleated sheet configuration have been implicated in the pathogenesis of Alzheimer's disease. The fragile X chromosome has been associated with some cases of infantile autism and pervasive developmental disorder; some investigators have suggested an association between female fragile X carriers and schizophrenic spectrum diagnoses and chronic mood disorders. However, those and other potential genetic markers of psychiatric disease remain only research tools at this time.

The effort to identify genes responsible for specific diseases is sponsored by the federal government's human genome project, involving the mapping of the entire human genome, which is composed of more than 100,000 genes. The mapping of the human genome should enhance the clinician's ability to diagnose all forms of neuropsychiatric diseases and should result in new conceptualizations of psychiatric disorders. The project may lead to better preventive and therapeutic measures for those disorders. However, a host of ethical issues must be resolved before those advances in molecular genetics are clinically applied to neuropsychiatric disorders.

SUGGESTED CROSS-REFERENCES

Assessment is also discussed in Section 2.1, the rest of Chapter 9, Chapter 33 on child psychiatry, and Section 49.5 on geriatric psychiatry. Neuroimaging is discussed in Sections 1.10, 2.10, and 49.5c. Substance-related disorders are discussed in Chapter 13, schizophrenia in Chapter 14, mood disorders in Chapter 16, and anxiety disorders in Chapter 17. Endocrine and metabolic disorders are discussed in Section 26.6. Psychotherapies are discussed in Chapter 31 and biological therapies in Chapter 32. Alzheimer's disease is discussed in Section 49.6a.

REFERENCES

American Psychiatric Association Task Force on the Use of Laboratory Tests in Psychiatry: The dexamethasone suppression test: An overview of its current status in psychiatry. Am J Psychiatry *144:* 1253, 1987.

*American Psychiatric Association Task Force on the Use of Laboratory Tests in Psychiatry: Tricyclic antidepressant-blood level measurements and clinical outcome: An APA Task Force Report. Am J Psychiatry *145:* 155, 1985.

Ananth J, Gamal R, Miller M, Wohl M, et al: Is the routine CT head scan justified for psychiatric patients? A prospective study. J Psychiatry Neurosci *18:* 69, 1993.

Brower K J, Catlin D H, Blow F C, Eliopulos G A, Beresford T P: Clinical assessment and urine testing for anabolic-androgenic steroid abuse and dependence. Am J Drug Alcohol Abuse *17:* 161, 1991.

Comings D E, Comings B G, Muhleman D, Dietz G, Shahbahrami B, Tast D, Knell E, Kcosis P, Baumgarten R, Kovacs B W, Levy D L, Smith M, Borison R L, Evans D, Klein D N, MacMurray J, Tosk J M, Sverd J, Gysin R, Flanagan S D: The dopamine D_2 receptor locus as a modifying gene in neuropsychiatric disorders. JAMA *266:* 1793, 1991.

Davidson M, Kahn R S, Knott P, Kaminsky R, Cooper M, DuMont K, Apter S, Davis K L: Effects of neuroleptic treatment on symptoms of schizophrenia and plasma homovanillic acid concentrations. Arch Gen Psychiatry *48:* 910, 1991.

*DeGowin R L: *DeGowin and DeGowin's Bedside Diagnostic Examination,* ed 5. Macmillan, New York, 1987.

D'Ercole A, Skodol A E, Struening E, Curtis J, Millman J: Diagnosis of physical illness in psychiatric patients using Axis III and a standardized medical history. Hosp Community Psychiatry *42:* 395, 1991.

Dolan J G, Mushlin A I: Routine laboratory testing for medical disorders in psychiatric inpatients. Arch Intern Med *145:* 2085, 1985.

Ellenhorn M J, Barceloux D G: *Medical Toxicology: Diagnosis and Treatment of Human Poisoning.* Elsevier, New York, 1988.

Galderisi S, Mucci A, Gregorio M R, Bucci P, Maj M, Kemali D: C-EEG brain mapping in DSM-III schizophrenics after acute and chronic haloperidol treatment. Eur Neuropsychopharmacol *1:* 51, 1990.

Galletly C A, Field C D, Prior M: Urine drug screening of patients admitted to a state psychiatric hospital. Hosp Community Psychiatry *44:* 587, 1993.

Garvey M, DeRubeis R J, Hollon S D, Evans M D, Tuason V B: Does 24-h urinary MHPG predict treatment response to antidepressants? Association between imipramine response and low MHPG. J Affective Dis *20:* 181, 1990.

Geller B, Cooper T B, McCombs H G, Graham D, Wells J: Double-blind, placebo-controlled study of nortriptyline in depressed children

using a "fixed plasma level" design. Psychopharmacol Bull *25:* 101, 1989.
Ghaziuddin M, Tsai L Y, Ghaziuddin N, Eilers L, et al: Utility of the head computerized tomography scan in child and adolescent psychiatry. J Am Acad Child Adolesc Psychiatry *32:* 123, 1993.
Gunther W, Baghai T, Naber D, Spatz R, et al: EEG alterations and seizures during treatment with clozapine: A retrospective study of 283 patients. Pharmacopsychiatry *26:* 69, 1993.
Hoeksema H L, de Bock G H: The value of laboratory tests for the screening and recognition of alcohol abuse in primary care patients. J Fam Pract *37:* 231, 1993.
Hoffman R S, Koran L M: Detecting physical illness in patients with mental disorders. Psychosomatics *25:* 654, 1984.
Jefferson J W, Greist J H, Ackerman D C: *Lithium Encyclopedia for Clinical Practice.* American Psychiatric Press, Washington, 1983.
Johnson K A, Holman B L, Rosen T J, Nagel J S, English R J, Growdon J H: Iofetamine I^{123} single photon emission computed tomography is accurate in the diagnosis of Alzheimer's disease. Arch Intern Med *150:* 752, 1990.
Jones P B, Owen M J, Lewis S W, Murray R M: A case-control study of family history and cerebral cortical abnormalities in schizophrenia. Acta Psychiatrica Scandinavica *87:* 6, 1993.
Keshavan M S, Kapur S, Pettegrew J W: Magnetic resonance spectroscopy in psychiatry: Potential, pitfalls, and promise. Am J Psychiatry *148:* 976, 1991.
Keshavan M S, Tandon R: Editorial: Sleep abnormalities in schizophrenia: pathophysiological significance. Psychol Med *23:* 831, 1993.
Kirch D G: Medical assessment and laboratory testing in psychiatry. In *Comprehensive Textbook of Psychiatry,* ed 5, H I Kaplan, B J Sadock, editors, p 525. Williams & Wilkins, Baltimore, 1989.
Kolman P B: Predicting the results of routine laboratory tests in elderly psychiatric patients admitted to hospital. J Clin Psychiatry *46:* 532, 1985.
Lindenbaum J, Healton E B, Savage D G: Neuropsychiatric disorders caused by cobalamin deficiency in the absence of anemia or macrocytosis. N Engl J Med *318:* 1720, 1988.
Linnoila M, Virkkunen M, Scheinin M, Nuutila A, Rimon R, Goodwin F K: Low cerebrospinal fluid 5-hydroxyindolacetic acid concentration differentiates impulsive from nonimpulsive violent behavior. Life Sci *33:* 2609, 1983.
Liu G, Sobering G, Duyn J, Moonen C T W: A functional MRI technique combining principles of echo-shifting with a train of observations (PRESTO). Magn Res Med *30:* 764, 1993.
Loosen P T, Prange A J: The serum thyrotropin response to thyrotropin releasing hormone in psychotic patients: A review. Am J Psychiatry *139:* 405, 1982.
*National Institutes of Health Consensus Development Panel: Differential diagnosis of dementing disease. National Institutes of Health Consensus Development Conference Statement *6:* 1, 1987.
Osterloh J D, Becker C E: Chemical dependency and drug testing in the workplace. West J Med *152:* 506, 1990.
Perry J C, Jacobs D: Overview: Clinical applications of the Amytal interview in psychiatric emergency settings. Am J Psychiatry *139:*552, 1982.
Puig-Antich J, Perel J M, Lupatkin W, Chambers W J, Tabrizi M A, King J, Goetz R, Davies M, Stiller R L: Imipramine in prepubertal major depressive disorders. Arch Gen Psychiatry *44:* 81, 1987.
Raj A, Sheehan D V: Medical evaluation of panic attacks. J Clin Psychiatry *48:* 309, 1987.
*Rosse R B, Giese A A, Deutsch S I, Morihisa J M: *A Concise Guide to Laboratory and Diagnostic Testing in Psychiatry.* American Psychiatric Press, Washington, 1989.
Shagass C, Roemer R: Evoked potential topography in unmedicated and medicated schizophrenic patients. Int J Psychophysiol *10:* 213, 1991.
Spurrell M T, Creed F H: Lymphocyte response in depressed patients and subjects anticipating bereavement. Br J Psychiatry *162:* 60, 1993.
Stahl S M: Peripheral models for the study of neurotransmitter receptors in man. Psychopharmacol Bull *21:* 663, 1985.
van Praag H M, Kahn R S, Asnis G M, Wetzler S, Brown S L, Bleich A, Korn M L: Denosologization of biological psychiatry or the specificity of 5-HT disturbances in psychiatric disorders. J Affective Disord *13:* 1, 1987.
Van Tol H H M, Wu Caren M, Guan H C, Ohara K, Bunzow J R, Civelli O, Kennedy J, Seeman P, Niznik H B, Jovanovic V: Multiple dopamine D_4 receptor variants in the human population. Nature *358:* 149, 1992.
Verebey K: Diagnostic laboratory: screening for drug abuse. In *Substance Abuse: A Comprehensive Textbook,* ed 2, J H Lowinson, P Ruiz, R B Millman, J G Langrod, editors, pp 425–436. Williams & Wilkins, Baltimore, 1992.
*Weinberger D R: Brain disease and psychiatric illness: When should a psychiatrist order a CT scan? Am J Psychiatry *141:* 1521, 1984.
Weinberger D R, Gibson R, Coppola R, Jones D W, Molchan S, Sunderland T, Berman K F, Reba R C: The distribution of cerebral muscarinic acetylcholine receptors in vivo in patients with dementia: A controlled study with ^{123}IQNB and single photon emission computed tomography. Arch Neurol *48:* 169, 1991.
Wilens T E, Biederman J, Spencer T, Geist D E: A retrospective study of serum levels and electrocardiographic effects of nortriptyline in children and adolescents. J Am Acad Adolesc Psychiatry *32:* 270, 1993.

9.8 PSYCHIATRIC RATING SCALES

STEPHEN R. MARDER, M.D.

Every science develops methods for measuring and characterizing its phenomena. In comparison with most fields of medicine psychiatry is at a disadvantage because the clinical manifestations of psychiatric disorders cannot be measured using physiological and biological parameters, such as blood pressure or bacteria in urine. As a result the field has resorted to the use of rating scales that are designed to translate clinical phenomena into objective and usually quantitative information. The information conveyed by a rating scale can be used to arrive at a diagnosis, to document the clinical state of a person at a point in time, or to supplement the information about a patient that is provided by a clinical examination. Such uses of rating scales can be important for both clinical care and research, although they are probably used more often for the latter purpose.

EVALUATING RATING SCALES

The clinician or researcher who has decided to use a rating scale is forced to choose among hundreds of different instruments, each with its own advantages and disadvantages. In making a selection among the instruments that propose to fulfill a particular function it is important that certain properties of the scale be considered. Those properties—usually published in the scientific literature or available from the author of the scale—will define the care with which the instrument was developed and its ability to fulfill its function.

RELIABILITY The reliability of a scale is a measure of its ability to convey consistent and reproducible information. It can be characterized in a number of different ways. Interrater reliability, which is commonly used as a measure for observer-rated scales, measures the degree to which different raters will give the same score to a subject. Typically, two or more persons will be asked to evaluate the same subject. A statistic is calculated that reflects the amount of agreement among the raters. Test-retest reliability is used as a measure for scales that theoretically are consistent over time. The scale is administered on two separate occasions and the agreement of the scores is measured. Internal consistency reliability (previously measured as split half reliability) is used for scales that have a number of items that are supposed to measure the same clinical feature. In that case reliability is a measure of whether the items in the scale are measuring the same thing.

When a scale is a continuous measure of a particular dimension, such as intelligence quotient (IQ) or severity of depression, reliabilities are usually expressed in terms of correlation coefficients. The reliability of a scale is usually represented as a coefficient or r, which is a number from 0 to 1 where 0.0 indicates that the scale is incapable of distinguishing one case from another consistently and 1.0 indicates that a person's scores are perfectly consistent. Other scales, such as diagnostic instruments, focus on whether a subject can be placed in a particular category. The most popular coefficient for indicating reliability in categorical assignments is kappa (κ), which adjusts for the fact that a certain amount of agreement will occur purely by chance. For continuous scales reliability coefficients above 0.85 are usually considered good. That level of reliability is probably necessary for clinical decisions. Kappa values above 0.75 are considered excellent and values below 0.4 are poor.

VALIDITY The validity of an instrument is the degree to which it actually measures what it is supposed to measure. The value of a scale to a clinician or a researcher most likely will be determined by its validity. Although a scale cannot be valid without reliability, the mere fact that it is reliable does not assure its validity. For example, a scale may have a scoring system that has relatively easy rules, such as rating a clinical phenomenon on the basis of eye color. In that case reliability will be high but the scale will fail to measure the phenomenon it claims to measure. Because such clinical dimensions as anxiety and depression are difficult to quantify and there are no pathognomonic symptoms that characterize most psychiatric diagnoses, the criteria for validity are difficult to find. As a result those persons evaluating the scales may report on different types of validity. Criterion validity is the amount of agreement between the instrument's score and a selected external set of criteria. For a scale of depression, for example, the external criterion could be the global rating of depression given by well-accepted experts. Similarly, depression scores should be higher for acutely admitted inpatients as compared with depressed patients living in the community. Concurrent validity is a measure of the agreement of the instrument with an already established instrument that purports to test the same phenomenon. For example, a new scale for measuring extrapyramidal side effects can be compared with an accepted scale, such as the Simpson-Angus Scale. Content validity is the degree to which the items in a scale are drawn from the proper domain of content. Face validity describes the degree to which the instrument appears to measure what it claims to measure. Predictive validity is the degree to which a scale provides information that is related to a particular outcome.

Psychiatric rating scales have important similarities to psychological tests. The distinction between the two is not always clear and sometimes is not relevant. Moreover, such tests as the Minnesota Multiphasic Personality Inventory (MMPI) and the Hopkins Symptom Checklist (SCL-90) have been used for both purposes. This section focuses on psychiatric rating scales as instruments that monitor clinical signs and symptoms of psychiatric illnesses. For the most part they do not require normative data or interpretation by a psychologist.

SELF-RATING VERSUS OBSERVER SCALES

Most of the scales described here are completed by an observer, either professional or nonprofessional. Self-rating scales, however, have an important role in the evaluation of psychopathology. First, they are economical in that they require less staff time, which makes them useful for screening or for epidemiological studies. In addition, they frequently contain more items than do observer scales and so can also screen for items that may be seen relatively infrequently. Self-rating scales also may be advantageous in rating subtle internal subjective states.

Such scales, however, have important disadvantages as well. For example, their reliability is difficult to evaluate. Patients with severe psychopathology may be unable to complete the scales. A number of studies comparing self-rating and observer scales have found a relatively low concordance rate. Patients may be reasonably accurate at scoring the presence or absence of a symptom but find it difficult to score its severity. Moreover, patients with poor insight may not be aware that they are symptomatic.

HOPKINS SYMPTOM CHECKLIST 90R (SCL-90) The SCL-90 is used to evaluate a broad range of psychopathology for patients with different disorders. It consists of 90 items and can usually be completed in less than 30 minutes. Shorter versions of the scale have also been developed, including an SCL-71, an SCL-64, and an SCL-58. The scoring system for the SCL-90 includes nine symptom scales (somatization, obsessive-compulsive behavior, interpersonal sensitivity, depression, anxiety, hostility, phobic anxiety, paranoid ideation, and psychoticism) and three global indexes. The focus is on the subject's current state. Each item is rated on a scale of 1 to 4 according to its frequency. The scale has been used in a large number of treatment studies, usually of schizophrenia or mood disorders. Its validity has been well documented.

GENERAL HEALTH QUESTIONNAIRE (GHQ) The instrument is widely used to screen populations for the presence of psychiatric illness. Two forms of the GHQ are available: the GHQ-12, which requires only two minutes to complete, and the GHQ-60, which requires 10 to 12 minutes. For each item the subject is asked whether a particular symptom or behavior occurred during the previous few weeks. The number of positive items yields a total GHQ score. A number of validity studies indicate that the total is a reasonably sensitive and specific indicator of psychopathology.

PROFILE OF MOOD STATES (POMS) Originally developed for studying neurotic patients, POMS is occasionally used to monitor mood and anxiety in a broad range of clinical trials. The subject rates adjectives along a four-point scale of intensity. The scale yields scores in tension, anger, depression, vigor, and fatigue.

DIAGNOSTIC SCALES

The development of diagnostic interviews (Table 9.8-1) was inspired by concerns regarding the apparent unreliability of psychiatric diagnoses. The problem was highlighted in the 1970s by the US-UK Diagnostic Project, which observed that United States and British psychiatrists had different conceptions of depression and schizophrenia. The difference in diagnostic criteria could be particularly serious for international studies.

PRESENT STATE EXAMINATION, NINTH EDITION (PSE-9) The PSE was developed for the purpose of standardizing diagnostic processes for international studies. Earlier versions were used in both the United States-United Kingdom project and the World Health Organization's International Pilot Study of Schizophrenia. The semistructured interview focuses on signs and symptoms at the time of the interview and symptoms during the prior month. Only symptoms that are reported by the subject to have been present within the past month are rated. Other case material may guide the questioning but cannot be

TABLE 9.8-1
Diagnostic Instruments

Instrument	Diagnostic Function	Rater	Reference
Present State Examination (PSE-9)	Psychopathology	Professional	Wing 1974
Structured Clinical Interview for DSM-III-R* (SCID)	DSM-III-R diagnosis	Professional	Spitzer 1987
Diagnostic Interview Schedule (DIS)	Diagnosis for epidemiological studies	Nonprofessional	Robins 1981
Schedule for Affective Disorder and Schizophrenia (SADS)	RDC Diagnosis	Professional	Endicott & Spitzer 1978
Composite International Diagnostic Interview (CIDI)	DSM-III-R or ICD-10 diagnosis	Nonprofessional	Robins 1988
Schedules for Clinical Assessment in Neuropsychiatry (SCAN)	DSM-III-R or ICD-10 diagnosis	Professional	Wing 1990

*A new version of SCID is being field tested for DSM-IV.

Endicott J, Spitzer R L: A diagnostic interview: the Schedule for Affective Disorders and Schizophrenia. Arch Gen Psychiatry *35:* 837, 1978. Robins L N, Wing J, Wittchen H U, et al: The Composite International Diagnostic Interview: An epidemiologic instrument suitable for use in conjunction with different diagnostic systems and in different cultures. Arch Gen Psychiatry *45:* 1069, 1988. Robins L N, Helzer J E, Croughan J, et al: National Institute for Mental Health Diagnostic Interview Schedule: Its history, characteristics, and validity. Arch Gen Psychiatry *38:* 381, 1981. Spitzer R L, Williams J B W, Gibbon M: *Instruction Manual for the Structured Clinical Interview for DSM-III-R* (SCID, 4/1/87 revision). New York State Psychiatric Institute, New York, 1987. Wing J K, Cooper J E, Sartorius N: *The Description and Classification of Psychiatric Symptoms: An Instruction Manual for the PSE and CATEGO System.* Cambridge University Press, 1974. Wing J K et al: SCAN: Schedules for Clinical Assessment in Neuropsychiatry. Arch Gen Psychiatry *47:* 589, 1990.

used for rating. The strength of the instrument lies in the richness of the information it provides about psychotic symptoms. The 140 items in the scale provide an opportunity for a thorough inventory of psychopathology. For example, more than 15 types of delusions are described and can be rated in the interview. Raters are provided with a glossary of definitions that gives detailed descriptions and criteria for rating each symptom. Also, the questions included were carefully designed to elicit psychopathology. As a result it can provide an excellent teaching device for trainees who are learning interviewing skills. It should be pointed out, however, that the PSE is not strictly a diagnostic scale but is a system for reliably documenting psychopathology.

A computer program called CATEGO organizes data collected from the PSE and can output the data into certain syndromes and to diagnoses in the ninth revision of the *International Classification of Diseases and Related Health Problems* (ICD-9). The PSE does not systematically collect historical information, however, and so is unable to provide all of the relevant information that can be used for diagnoses made according to such criteria as listed in the fourth edition of *Diagnostic and Statistical Manual of Mental Disorders* (DSM-IV) and the Research Diagnostic Criteria (RDC). A syndrome checklist is available for collecting data from outside sources, such as medical records or input from other informants. A Present State Examination Change Rating Scale has now been developed that is more sensitive to changes in psychopathology that might take place during treatment studies.

STRUCTURED CLINICAL INTERVIEW FOR AXIS I DSM-IV DISORDERS (SCID) A revised version of the Structured Clinical Interview for DSM-IV was still undergoing field trials at the time of publication. The instrument is a clinician-administered semistructured interview for making the major Axis I diagnoses according to the fourth edition of DSM (DSM-IV). After an overview that focuses on the patient's main psychiatric problems the interview moves to modules that cover mania, psychosis, depression, substance abuse disorders, anxiety disorders, posttraumatic stress disorders, somatization disorders, eating disorders, and adjustment disorders.

The instrument is useful for clinicians because it guides the interviewer through the criteria for the most important Axis I disorders. The interviewer can limit the interview to the modules that are relevant to a particular patient. Researchers can also limit the interview to the diagnostic categories that are important for a particular study.

The SCID for DSM-III-R was extensively tested in multisite studies in the United States and elsewhere. Interrater reliability has been good. In an international study test-retest reliabilities for lifetime diagnoses were above 0.6 for patient samples but were low for nonpatients.

SCHEDULE FOR AFFECTIVE DISORDERS AND SCHIZOPHRENIA (SADS) The SADS scale was developed by Jean Endicott and Robert Spitzer with the primary goal of differentiating schizophrenia from mood disorders. The scale uses RDC, which are similar to the revised third edition of DSM (DSM-III-R) but include fewer disorders. SADS resembles PSE in the use of the semistructured interview. An open-ended question begins the interview and further questions are clustered in a sensible manner. The interviewer has the latitude to alter the sequence of questions. Other sources of information, such as medical records and information from relatives, can supplement the patient's self-report. Part I of the SADS rates symptoms during two periods, the week before the interview and the one-week period during the past year when the symptoms were at their worst. Part II focuses on the past history and treatment history.

DIAGNOSTIC INTERVIEW SCHEDULE (DIS) The DIS was developed by the National Institute of Mental Health (NIMH) for use in large-scale epidemiological studies. Because it permits interviewers without any training in psychology or psychiatry to collect the information that can be used for the diagnosis of nearly all major psychiatric illnesses according to DSM-III-R, Feighner criteria, and RDC, the interview provides considerably more structure for the rater than do such instruments as the PSE, SADS, or SCID. A skilled interviewer can complete the scale in 45 to 75 minutes. In contrast to a semistructured interview, the completely structured interview leaves little room for the interviewer to modify the questions or to probe for clarification. The validity of the DIS has been reasonably well demonstrated in studies in which the diagnosis by a lay interviewer was compared with that by a psychiatrist using either the DIS or a more traditional clinical assessment.

COMPOSITE INTERNATIONAL DIAGNOSTIC INTERVIEW (CIDI) Developed for international and cross-cultural epidemiological studies, it has a significant number of questions from the DIS, but also includes PSE items, as well as DIS questions modified to improve cross-national interpretation. The scale allows investigators to diagnose patients using DSM-III-R or the tenth revision of ICD (ICD-10). It is designed for administration by lay interviewers and can be scored by a computer.

SCHEDULES FOR CLINICAL ASSESSMENT IN NEUROPSYCHIATRY (SCAN) Like CIDI, SCAN was developed by the World Health Organization. Although still undergoing field trials it has the potential to become an influential scale. SCAN consists of the latest version of the Present State Examination (PSE-10) as well as other elements that make it a more complete diagnostic instrument than PSE-9. Depending on the situation the rater may decide to rate the patient's present state, the present episode, or the "lifetime ever." SCAN also includes an Item Group Checklist, which contains psychopathology items that can be rated from such sources as medical records or another informant, and a Clinical Information Schedule, which contains summary items on intellectual level, personality disorders, social disablement, and clinical diagnosis. Data from all of these schedules may be coded and analyzed by CATEGO-5, a computer program that can categorize patients according to a number of disorders in ICD-10 or DSM-III-R and can also provide an axial formulation.

TABLE 9.8-2
Depression Scales

Instrument	Rater	Reference
Hamilton Rating Scale for Depression (HAM-D)	Professional	Hamilton 1960
Montgomery-Asberg Depression Rating Scale (MADRS)	Professional	Montgomery & Asberg 1979
Bech-Rafaelsen Melancholia Rating Scale (BRMS)	Professional	Bech & Rafaelsen 1980
Clinical Interview for Depression	Professional	Paykel 1985
Zung Self-Rating Depression Scale (SDS)	Self	Zung 1965
Beck Depression Inventory (BDI)	Self	Beck et al 1961

Bech P, Rafaelsen O J: The use of rating scales exemplified by a comparison of the Hamilton and the Bech-Rafaelsen Melancholia Scale. Acta Psychiatr Scand (*285,* Suppl): 128, 1980. Beck A T, Ward C H, Mendelson M, et al: An inventory for measuring depression. Arch Gen Psychiatry *4:* 561, 1961. Hamilton M: Rating scale for depression. J Neurol Neurosurg Psychiatry *23:* 56, 1960. Montgomery S A, Asberg M: New depression scale designed to be sensitive to change. Br J Psychiatry *134:* 382, 1979. Paykel E S: Clinical Interview for Depression: development, reliability and validity. J Affect Disord *9:* 85, 1985. Zung W W K: A self-rating depression scale. Arch Gen Psychiatry *12:* 63, 1965.

DEPRESSION SCALES

Depression can either be a mood state or the primary manifestation of a mood disorder. As a mood state depression is experienced by persons who do not have a psychiatric illness, as well as by those who have non-mood disorders, such as schizophrenia or organic disorders. Such scales as the Hamilton Rating Scale for Depression are most appropriate for mood disorders since they focus on somatic symptoms that may not be prominent in other illnesses (Table 9.8-2).

HAMILTON RATING SCALE FOR DEPRESSION (HAM-D) (Table 9.8-3) As the most widely used scale in treatment studies of depression, the instrument remains the standard against which other scales in this area are evaluated. It was developed for patients with depressive disorders and is viewed by some as not suitable for other patients or normal persons. The HAM-D has 17 to 21 items, depending on the version, that are rated according to intensity and frequency within the past few days. The ratings are based on an interview plus information from other sources. The scale should be utilized only by experienced clinicians as it requires skill both in interviewing depressed patients and in evaluating symptoms. It does not have standardized questions but depends on the skills of the interviewer to collect the information and to make rating decisions. A Structured Interview Guide for the HAM-D that was recently developed to standardize the probes of the interviewer has the advantage of improving the reliability of the individual items without adding significantly to the time it takes to administer the scale.

The HAM-D emphasizes the somatic manifestations of depression, which makes it particularly sensitive to changes experienced by patients who are severely ill, and has probably led to its widespread use in antidepressant drug trials. Most studies report the data as the total score on the basis of 17 of the 21 items. The HAM-D has been criticized for not including a number of important symptoms of depressive disorder, including hypersomnia and increases in weight and appetite.

As a result of its popularity the HAM-D has been the most widely studied instrument for depression. Its validity has been demonstrated in a number of studies in which its ratings were compared in groups of patients with different severities of illness and in studies where ratings were compared with global severity. The interrater reliability of the scale has been consistently high across a number of studies.

MONTGOMERY-ASBERG DEPRESSION RATING SCALE (MADRS) A widely used scale that was designed specifically to be sensitive to changes over time, it is frequently employed in trials of antidepressant drugs. The scale differs from the HAM-D in that it does not include somatic or psychomotor symptoms. However, it does measure some of the most important symptoms of a depressive disorder, such as sadness, inner tension, reduced sleep, lassitude, pessimism, and suicidal thoughts. Because all of the items are core symptoms of depression it has high face validity. In addition, its validity has been demonstrated by its high correlations with the HAM-D.

BECH-RAFAELSEN MELANCHOLIA RATING SCALE (BRMS) The scale was developed after an evaluation of items from the HAM-D. It has 11 items that are rated on a five-point scale. It has the advantage of specific severity anchor points to guide raters.

CLINICAL INTERVIEW FOR DEPRESSION A 36-item scale that includes both depression and anxiety, it features a semistructured interview and anchor points, which probably contribute to its relatively high interrater reliability. Although the scale takes somewhat longer to complete than does the HAM-D, the variety of items and its sensitivity to change make it a useful scale for some studies.

ZUNG SELF-RATING DEPRESSION SCALE (SDS) The scale contains 20 items that are rated according to their frequency of occurrence. Therefore, a symptom that is not severe or bothersome but occurs frequently would receive a high rating. The scale's sensitivity to change has been challenged, suggesting that it may not be well suited to antidepressant drug

TABLE 9.8-3
Hamilton Rating Scale for Depression

Clinic No. ________ Date ________ Rating No. ________ Code Number ________
Sex ____ Age ____ Patient's Name ________
Patient's Address ________ Tel ________

Item	Range	Score
1. Depressed mood	0–4	
2. Guilt	0–4	
3. Suicide	0–4	
4. Insomnia initial	0–2	
5. Insomnia middle	0–2	
6. Insomnia delayed	0–2	
7. Work and interest	0–4	
8. Retardation		
9. Agitation	0–4	
10. Anxiety (psychic)	0–4	
11. Anxiety (somatic)	0–4	
12. Somatic gastrointestinal	0–2	
13. Somatic general	0–2	
14. Genital	0–2	
15. Hypochondriasis	0–2	
16. Insight	0–4	
17. Loss of weight	0–2	
	Total Score	
Diurnal variation (M.A.E.)	0–2	
Depersonalization	0–4	
Paranoid symptoms	0–4	
Obsessional symptoms	0–4	

Table from Hamilton M: *Personal communication to the editors.* Feb. 1988. Used with permission.

The scale is designed to measure the severity of illness of patients already diagnosed as suffering from depressive illness. It is obviously not a diagnostic instrument because that requires much more information (e.g., previous history, family history, precipitating factors).

As far as possible, the scale should be used in the manner of a clinical interview. The first time the interview should be conducted in a relaxed, free, and easy manner, giving the patients time to unburden themselves and giving them the opportunity to speak of their problems and ask whatever questions they wish. It may then be necessary to obtain further information by asking them questions. At subsequent assessments, the interview can be briefer and more to the point.

An observer rating scale is not a checklist in which each item is strictly defined. The raters must have sufficient clinical experience and judgment to be able to interpret the patients' statements and reticences about some symptoms, and to compare them with other patients. They should use all sources of information (e.g., from relatives and nurses).

The scale consists of 17 items, the scores on which are summed to give a total score. There are four other items, one of which (diurnal variation) is excluded on the grounds that it is not an additional burden on the patient. The last three are excluded from the total score because they occur infrequently, although information on them may be useful for other purposes.

The method of assessment is simple. For some symptoms it is difficult to elicit such information as will permit of full quantification. If present, score 2; if absent, score 0; and if doubtful or trivial, score 1. For those symptoms where more detailed information can be obtained, the score of 2 is expanded into 2 for mild, 3 for moderate, and 4 for severe. In case of difficulty, the raters should use their judgment as clinicians.

trials. However, it may be an efficient tool for screening clinical populations for depression.

BECK DEPRESSION INVENTORY (BDI) The BDI is probably the most commonly used self-rating scale for depression. Subjects are asked to rate 21 items from 0 to 3 according to how they feel at the present time. Each of the different scores contains a one-sentence description to guide the rater. For example, one item has the following statements: (0) "I don't feel disappointed in myself." (1) "I am disappointed in myself." (2) "I am disgusted with myself." (3) "I hate myself." In contrast to the HAM-D the scale focuses on the cognitive symptoms of depression, such as pessimism and diminished self-esteem. A number of studies have found that the BDI correlates reasonably well with both the HAM-D and global ratings by psychiatrists. In addition, the scale is sensitive to change and so is useful in clinical drug trials.

SCHIZOPHRENIA SCALES

Because schizophrenia affects different dimensions of functioning, researchers and clinicians who study the illness will frequently use a number of scales (Table 9.8-4) to monitor different domains, such as positive symptoms, negative or deficit symptoms, social and vocational adjustment, and neurological side effects. Each of those areas may be affected by changes in clinical condition, and, not infrequently, improvement in one area may be accompanied by improvement or worsening in another.

BRIEF PSYCHIATRIC RATING SCALE (BPRS) Originally developed by John Overall and Donald Gorham in 1963, the scale has been modified by them and others over the years. It is by far the most widely used rating scale for treatment studies in schizophrenia, and it is uncommon to find a recent trial involving antipsychotic medications that does not use it. The original BPRS was developed following a factor analysis of the In-patient Multidimensional Psychiatric Scale (IMPS), which had been developed by Maurice Lorr and C. James Klett. It was a more lengthy instrument and was viewed by some as too cumbersome for routine use. Most forms of the BPRS consist of 16 to 24 items, each of which is rated on a scale of from 1 to 7; some forms of the scale are scored from 0 to 6. The items encompass psychosis, depression, and anxiety symptoms, although the psychosis items are most prominent. BPRS ratings should be made by an experienced clinician as the scale lacks a standardized assessment procedure. Recent modifications, including a Hillside version with anchor points and an expanded MHCRC version from the University of California at Los Angeles (UCLA), have attempted to increase reliability by adding anchor points (Table 9.8-5).

TABLE 9.8-4
Schizophrenia Scales

Instrument	Function	Rater	Reference
Brief Psychiatric Rating Scale (BPRS)	Symptoms and signs	Professional	Overall & Gorham 1962
Manchester Scale	Symptoms and signs	Professional	Krawiecka et al 1977
Positive and Negative Symptom Scale (PANSS)	Symptoms and signs	Professional	Kay et al 1987
Scale for the Assessment of Positive Symptoms (SAPS)	Positive symptoms	Professional	Andreasen 1982
Scale for the Assessment of Negative Symptoms (SANS)	Negative symptoms	Professional	Andreasen 1982
Schedule for the Deficit Syndrome	Deficit symptoms	Professional	Kirkpatrick et al 1989
Nurses' Observation Scale for Inpatient Evaluation (NOSIE)	Ward observation	Nurses	Honigfield & Klett 1965

Andreasen NC: Negative symptoms in schizophrenia: Definition and reliability. Arch Gen Psychiatry *39:* 784, 1982. Honigfeld G, Klett C J: The Nurses' Observation Scale for Inpatient Evaluation. Psychol Rep *21:* 65, 1965. Kay S R, Fiszbein A, Opler L A: The Positive and Negative Syndrome Scale (PANSS) for schizophrenia. Schizophr Bull *13:* 261, 1987. Kirkpatrick B et al: The Schedule for the Deficit Syndrome: An instrument for the research in schizophrenia. Psychiatry Res *30:* 119, 1989. Krawiecka M et al: A standardized psychiatric assessment scale for rating chronic psychotic patients. Acta Psychiatr Scand *55:* 299, 1977. Overall J E, Gorham D R: The Brief Psychiatric Rating Scale. Psychol Rep *10:* 799, 1962.

TABLE 9.8-5
Brief Psychiatric Rating Scale

<table>
<tr><td colspan="2">DEPARTMENT OF HEALTH AND HUMAN SERVICES
PUBLIC HEALTH SERVICE
Alcohol, Drug Abuse, and Mental Health Administration
NIMH Treatment Strategies in Schizophrenia Society</td><td colspan="4">PATIENT NUMBER __ __ __ __   DATA GROUP bprs   EVALUATION DATE __ __ __ __ __ __ M M D D Y Y</td></tr>
<tr><td colspan="2">BRIEF PSYCHIATRIC RATING SCALE - Anchored</td><td colspan="4">PATIENT NAME</td></tr>
<tr><td colspan="2">Overall and Gorham</td><td colspan="4">RATER NAME</td></tr>
<tr><td>RATER NUMBER</td><td colspan="5">EVALUATION TYPE (Circle)</td></tr>
<tr><td>__ __ __</td><td colspan="2">1 Baseline
2
3 4-week minor</td><td>4 Start double-blind
5 Major evaluation
6 Other</td><td>7 Start open meds
8 During open meds
9 Stop open meds</td><td>10 Early terminiation
11 Study completion</td></tr>
</table>

Introduce all questions with "During the past week have you . . ."

*1. **SOMATIC CONCERN:** Degree of concern over present bodily health. Rate the degree to which physical health is perceived as a problem by the patient, whether complaints have a realistic basis or not. Do not rate mere reporting of somatic symptoms. Rate only concern for (or worrying about) physical problems (real or imagined). **Rate on the basis of reported (i.e., subjective) information pertaining to the past week.**
1 = Not reported
2 = Very Mild: occasionally is somewhat concerned about body, symptoms, or physical illness
3 = Mild: occasionally is moderately concerned, or often is somewhat concerned
4 = Moderate: occasionally is very concerned, or often is moderately concerned
5 = Moderately Severe: often is very concerned
6 = Severe: is very concerned most of the time
7 = Very Severe: is very concerned nearly all of the time
9 = Cannot be assessed adequately because of severe formal thought disorder, uncooperativeness, or marked evasiveness/guardedness; or Not assessed

*2. **ANXIETY:** Worry, fear, or overconcern for present or future. **Rate solely on the basis of verbal report of patient's own subjective experiences pertaining to the past week.** Do not infer anxiety from physical signs or from neurotic defense mechanisms. Do not rate if restricted to somatic concern.
1 = Not reported
2 = Very Mild: occasionally feels somewhat anxious
3 = Mild: occasionally feels moderately anxious, or often feels somewhat anxious
4 = Moderate: occasionally feels very anxious, or often feels moderately anxious
5 = Moderately Severe: often feels very anxious
6 = Severe: feels very anxious most of the time
7 = Very Severe: feels very anxious nearly all of the time
9 = Cannot be assessed adequately because of severe formal thought disorder, uncooperativeness, or marked evasiveness/guardedness; or Not assessed

3. **EMOTIONAL WITHDRAWAL:** Deficiency in relating to the interviewer and to the interview situation. Overt manifestations of this deficiency include poor/absence of eye contact, failure to orient oneself physically toward the interviewer, and a general lack of involvement or engagement in the interview. Distinguish from BLUNTED AFFECT, in which deficits in facial expression, body gesture, and voice pattern are scored. **Rate on the basis of observations made during the interview.**
1 = Not observed
2 = Very Mild: e.g., occasionally exhibits poor eye contact
3 = Mild: e.g., as above, but more frequent
4 = Moderate: e.g., exhibits little eye contact, but still seems engaged in the interview and is appropriately responsive to all questions
5 = Moderately Severe: e.g., stares at floor or orients self away from interviewer, but still seems moderately engaged
6 = Severe: e.g., as above, but more persistent or pervasive
7 = Very Severe: e.g., appears "spacey" or "out of it" (total absence of emotional relatedness), and is disproportionately uninvolved or unengaged in the interview (DO NOT SCORE IF EXPLAINED BY DISORIENTATION.)

4. **CONCEPTUAL DISORGANIZATION:** Degree of speech incomprehensibility. Include any type of formal thought disorder (e.g., loose associations, incoherence, flight of ideas, neologisms). DO NOT include mere circumstantiality or pressured speech, even if marked. DO NOT rate on the basis of the patient's subjective impressions (e.g., "my thoughts are racing. I can't hold a thought," "my thinking gets all mixed up"). **Rate ONLY on the basis of observations made during the interview.**
1 = Not observed
2 = Very Mild: e.g., somewhat vague, but of doubtful clinical significance

TABLE 9.8-5 (*continued*)

3 = Mild: e.g., frequently vague, but the interview is able to progress smoothly; occasional loosening of associations
4 = Moderate: e.g., occasional irrelevant statements, infrequent use of neologisms, or moderate loosening of associations.
5 = Moderately Severe: as above, but more frequent
6 = Severe: formal thought disorder is present for most of the interview, and the interview is severely strained
7 = Very Severe: very little coherent information can be obtained

5. **GUILT FEELINGS:** Overconcern or remorse for past behavior. **Rate on the basis of the patient's subjective experiences of guilt as evidenced by verbal report pertaining to the past week.** Do not infer guilt feelings from depression, anxiety or neurotic defenses.
1 = Not reported
2 = Very Mild: occasionally feels somewhat guilty
3 = Mild: occasionally feels moderately guilty, or often feels somewhat guilty
4 = Moderate: occasionally feels very guilty, or often feels moderately guilty
5 = Moderately Severe: often feels very guilty
6 = Severe: feels very guilty most of the time, or encapsulated delusion of guilt
7 = Very Severe: agonizing constant feelings of guilt, or pervasive delusion(s) of guilt
9 = Cannot be assessed adequately because of severe formal thought disorder, uncooperativeness, or marked evasiveness/guardedness; or Not assessed

6. **TENSION: Rate motor restlessness (agitation) observed during the interview.** DO NOT rate on the basis of subjective experiences reported by the patient. Disregard suspected pathogenesis (e.g., tardive dyskinesia).
1 = Not observed
2 = Very Mild: e.g., occasionally fidgets
3 = Mild: e.g., frequently fidgets
4 = Moderate: e.g., constantly fidgets, or frequently fidgets, wrings hands and pulls clothing
5 = Moderately Severe: e.g., constantly fidgets, wrings hands and pulls clothing
6 = Severe: e.g., cannot remain seated (i.e., must pace)
7 = Very Severe: e.g., paces in a frantic manner

7. **MANNERISMS AND POSTURING:** Unusual and unnatural motor behavior. **Rate only abnormality of movements.** Do not rate simple heightened motor activity here. Consider frequency, duration, and degree of bizarreness. Disregard suspected pathogenesis.
1 = Not observed
2 = Very Mild: odd behavior but of doubtful clinical significance, e.g., occasional unprompted smiling, infrequent lip movements
3 = Mild: strange behavior but not obviously bizarre, e.g., infrequent head-tilting (side to side) in a rhythmic fashion, intermittent abnormal finger movements
4 = Moderate: e.g., assumes unnatural position for a brief period of time, infrequent tongue protrusions, rocking, facial grimacing
5 = Moderately Severe: e.g., assumes and maintains unnatural position throughout interview, unusual movements in several body areas
6 = Severe: as above, but more frequent, intense, or pervasive
7 = Very Severe: e.g., bizarre posturing throughout most of the interview, continuous abnormal movements in several body areas

*8. **GRANDIOSITY:** Inflated self-esteem (self-confidence), or inflated appraisal of one's talents, powers, abilities, accomplishments, knowledge, importance, or identity. Do not score mere grandiose *quality* of claims (e.g., "I'm the worst sinner in the world," "The entire country is trying to kill me") unless the guilt/persecution is related to some special, exaggerated attributes of the individual. Also, *the patient* must claim exaggerated attributes: e.g., if patient denies talents, powers, etc., even if he or she states that *others* indicate that he/she has these attributes, this item should not be scored. **Rate on the basis of reported (i.e., subjective) information pertaining to the past week.**
1 = Not reported
2 = Very Mild: e.g., is more confident than most people, but of only possible clinical significance
3 = Mild: e.g., definitely inflated self-esteem or exaggerates talents somewhat out of proportion to the circumstances
4 = Moderate: e.g., inflated self-esteem clearly out of proportion to the circumstances, or suspected grandiose delusion(s)
5 = Moderately Severe: e.g., a single (definite) encapsulated grandiose delusion, or multiple (definite) fragmentary grandiose delusions
6 = Severe: e.g., a single (definite) grandiose delusion/delusional system, or multiple (definite) grandiose delusions that the patient seems preoccupied with
7 = Very Severe: e.g., as above, but nearly all conversation is directed towards the patient's grandiose delusion(s)
9 = Cannot be assessed adequately because of severe formal thought disorder, uncooperativeness, or marked evasiveness/guardedness; or Not assessed

*9. **DEPRESSIVE MOOD:** Subjective report of feeling depressed, blue, "down in the dumps," etc. Rate only degree of reported depression. Do not rate on the basis of inferences concerning depression based upon general retardation and somatic complaints. **Rate on the basis of reported (i.e., subjective) information pertaining to the past week.**
1 = Not reported
2 = Very Mild: occasionally feels somewhat depressed
3 = Mild: occasionally feels moderately depressed, or often feels somewhat depressed
4 = Moderate: occasionally feels very depressed, or often feels moderately depressed
5 = Moderately Severe: often feels very depressed
6 = Severe: feels very depressed most of the time
7 = Very Severe: feels very depressed nearly all of the time
9 = Cannot be assessed adequately because of severe formal thought disorder, uncooperativeness, or marked evasiveness/guardedness; or Not assessed

*10. **HOSTILITY:** Animosity, contempt, belligerence, disdain for other people outside the interview situation. **Rate solely on the basis of the verbal report of feelings and actions of the patient toward others during the past week.** Do not infer hostility from neurotic defenses, anxiety or somatic complaints.
1 = Not reported
2 = Very Mild: occasionally feels somewhat angry
3 = Mild: often feels somewhat angry, or occasionally feels moderately angry
4 = Moderate: occasionally feels very angry, or often feels moderately angry
5 = Moderately Severe: often feels very angry
6 = Severe: has acted on his anger by becoming verbally or physically abusive on one or two occasions
7 = Very Severe: has acted on his anger on several occasions
9 = Cannot be assessed adequately because of severe formal thought disorder, uncooperativeness, or marked evasiveness/guardedness; or Not assessed

*11. **SUSPICIOUSNESS:** Belief (delusional or otherwise) that others have now, or have had in the past, malicious or discriminatory intent toward the patient. On the basis of verbal report, rate only those suspicions which are currently held whether they concern past or present circumstances. **Rate on the basis of reported (i.e., subjective) information pertaining to the past week.**
1 = Not reported
2 = Very Mild: rare instances of distrustfulness which may or may not be warranted by the situation
3 = Mild: occasional instances of suspiciousness that are definitely not warranted by the situation
4 = Moderate: more frequent suspiciousness, or transient ideas of reference
5 = Moderately Severe: pervasive suspiciousness, frequent ideas of reference, or an encapsulated delusion

(*continued*)

TABLE 9.8-5 (*continued*)

6 = Severe: definite, delusion(s) of reference or persecution that is (are) not wholly pervasive (e.g., an encapsulated delusion)
7 = Very Severe: as above, but more widespread, frequent, or intense
9 = Cannot be assessed adequately because of severe formal thought disorder, uncooperativeness, or marked evasiveness/guardedness; or Not assessed

*12. **HALLUCINATORY BEHAVIOR:** Perceptions (in any sensory modality) in the absence of an identifiable external stimulus. **Rate only those experienced that have occurred during the last week.** DO NOT rate "voices in my head," or "visions in my mind" unless the patient can differentiate between these experiences and his or her thoughts.
1 = Not reported
2 = Very Mild: suspected hallucinations only
3 = Mild: definite hallucinations, but insignificant, infrequent, or transient (e.g., occasional formless visual hallucinations, a voice calling the patient's name)
4 = Moderate: as above, but more frequent or extensive (e.g., frequently sees the devil's face, two voices carry on lengthy conversations)
5 = Moderately Severe: hallucinations are experienced nearly every day, or are a source of extreme distress
6 = Severe: as above, and has had a moderate impact on the patient's behavior (e.g., concentration difficulties leading to impaired work functioning)
7 = Very Severe: as above, and has had a severe impact (e.g., attempts suicide in response to command hallucinations)
9 = Cannot be assessed adequately because of severe formal thought disorder, uncooperativeness, or marked evasiveness/guardedness; or Not assessed

13. **MOTOR RETARDATION:** Reduction in energy level evidenced in slowed movements. **Rate on the basis of observed behavior of the patient only.** Do not rate on the basis of the patient's subjective impression of his or her own energy level.
1 = Not observed
2 = Very Mild and of doubtful clinical significance
3 = Mild: e.g., conversation is somewhat retarded, movements somewhat slowed
4 = Moderate: e.g., conversation is noticeably retarded but not strained
5 = Moderately Severe: e.g., conversation is strained, moves very slowly
6 = Severe: e.g., conversation is difficult to maintain, hardly moves at all
7 = Very Severe: e.g., conversation is almost impossible, does not move at all throughout the interview

14. **UNCOOPERATIVENESS:** Evidence of resistance, unfriendliness, resentment, and lack of readiness to cooperate with the interviewer. **Rate only on the basis of the patient's attitude and responses to the interviewer and the interview situation.** Do not rate on the basis of reported resentment or uncooperativeness outside the interview situation.
1 = Not observed
2 = Very Mild: e.g., does not seem motivated
3 = Mild: e.g., seems evasive in certain areas
4 = Moderate: e.g., monosyllabic, fails to elaborate spontaneously, somewhat unfriendly
5 = Moderately Severe: e.g., expresses resentment and is unfriendly throughout the interview
6 = Severe: e.g., refuses to answer a number of questions
7 = Very Severe: e.g., refuses to answer most questions

15. **UNUSUAL THOUGHT CONTENT:** Severity of delusions of any type—consider conviction, and effect on actions. Assume full conviction if patient has acted on his or her beliefs. **Rate on the basis of reported (i.e., subjective) information pertaining to past week.**
1 = Not reported
2 = Very Mild: delusion(s) suspected or likely
3 = Mild: at times, patient questions his or her belief(s) (partial delusion)
4 = Moderate: full delusional conviction, but delusion(s) has little or no influence on behavior
5 = Moderately Severe: full delusional conviction, but delusion(s) has only occasional impact on behavior
6 = Severe: delusion(s) has significant effect, e.g., neglects responsibilities because of preoccupation with belief that he/she is God
7 = Very Severe: delusion(s) has major impact, e.g., stops eating because believes food is poisoned
9 = Cannot be assessed adequately because of severe formal thought disorder, uncooperativeness, or marked evasiveness/guardedness; or Not assessed

16. **BLUNTED AFFECT:** Diminished affective responsivity, as characterized by deficits in facial expression, body gesture, and voice pattern. Distinguish from EMOTIONAL WITHDRAWAL, in which the focus is on interpersonal impairment rather than affect. Consider degree and consistency of impairment. **Rate based on observations made during interview.**
1 = Not observed
2 = Very Mild: e.g., occasionally seems indifferent to material that is usually accompanied by some show of emotion
3 = Mild: e.g., somewhat diminished facial expression, *or* somewhat monotonous voice *or* somewhat restricted gestures
4 = Moderate: e.g., as above, but more intense, prolonged, or frequent
5 = Moderately Severe: e.g., flattening of affect, including at least *two* of the three features: severe lack of facial expression, monotonous voice, or restricted body gestures
6 = Severe: e.g., profound flattening of affect
7 = Very Severe: e.g., totally monotonous voice, *and* total lack of expressive gestures throughout the evaluation

17. **EXCITEMENT:** Heightened emotional tone, including irritability and expansiveness (hypomanic affect). Do not infer affect from statements of grandiose delusions. **Rate based on observations made during interview.**
1 = Not observed
2 = Very Mild and of doubtful clinical significance
3 = Mild: e.g., irritable or expansive at times
4 = Moderate: e.g., frequently irritable or expansive
5 = Moderately Severe: e.g., constantly irritable or expansive; or, at times, enraged or euphoric
6 = Severe: e.g., enraged or euphoric throughout most of the interview.
7 = Very Severe: e.g., as above, but to such a degree that the interview must be terminated prematurely

18. **DISORIENTATION:** Confusion or lack of proper association for person, place or time. **Rate based on observations made during interview.**
1 = Not observed
2 = Very Mild: e.g., seems somewhat confused
3 = Mild: e.g., indicated 1982 when, in fact, it is 1983
4 = Moderate: e.g., indicates 1978
5 = Moderately Severe: e.g., is unsure where he/she is
6 = Severe: e.g., has no idea where he/she is
7 = Very Severe: e.g., does not know who he/she is
9 = Cannot be assessed adequately because of severe formal thought disorder, uncooperativeness, or marked evasiveness/guardedness; or Not assessed

TABLE 9.8-5 (*continued*)

19. **SEVERITY OF ILLNESS:** Considering your total clinical experience with this patient population, how mentally ill is the patient at this time?
    1 = Normal, not at all ill
    2 = Borderline mentally ill
    3 = Mildly ill
    4 = Moderately ill
    5 = Markedly ill
    6 = Severely ill
    7 = Among the most severely ill patients
20. **GLOBAL IMPROVEMENT:** Rate total improvement whether or not, in your judgment, it is due to treatment.
    At *baseline* assessment, mark "Not assessed" for item 20.
    For assessments *up to the start of double-blind* medication, rate Global Improvement compared to *baseline*.
    For assessments *following the start of double-blind* medication, rate Global Improvement compared to the *start of double-blind*.
    1 = Very much improved
    2 = Much improved
    3 = Minimally improved
    4 = No change
    5 = Minimally worse
    6 = Much worse
    7 = Very much worse
    9 = Not assessed

*Ratings based primarily upon verbal report.

Ratings on the BPRS are often expressed as the sum of all the items. However, the BPRS total includes such a variety of items that it is hard to interpret the dimension of psychopathology that is responsible for any changes. An alternative is to score subjects on the four BPRS factors that were developed by the developers of the instrument (Table 9.8-6).

The popularity of the scale is probably related to a number of factors: It is brief and usually requires only 15 to 30 minutes to complete. It captures the type of psychopathology that is affected by drug treatments and is sensitive to the changes that occur in treatment studies. And perhaps most important, it is familiar to most schizophrenia researchers, who are comfortable with the scale and can use it to assist them in discussing psychopathology with their colleagues. The BPRS also has limitations. Without anchor points the definitions of the items can be vague and subject to different interpretations. For example, the only item describing thought process disorder is "conceptual disorganization," which may not accurately capture that type of psychopathology.

Even with those disadvantages careful training of raters can result in high interrater reliabilities. Moreover, the validity of the scale has been demonstrated over a large number of treatment trials.

TABLE 9.8-6
Factors from the Brief Psychiatric Rating Scale

1. Thinking disturbance
   Conceptual disorganization
   Hallucinatory behavior
   Unusual thought content
2. Hostile suspiciousness
   Hostility
   Suspiciousness
   Uncooperativeness
3. Withdrawal retardation
   Emotional withdrawal
   Motor retardation
   Blunted affect
4. Anxious depression
   Anxiety
   Guilt
   Depression

MANCHESTER SCALE Also known as the Krawiecka scale, it is a relatively brief scale that is frequently used by European investigators for assessing outcome in acute treatment trials and for assessing chronic psychotic patients. It consists of eight items that are rated on the basis of replies to questions and clinical observations. Training tapes and a manual are available. Although the instrument has the advantage of brevity it is limited in the domains of psychopathology it monitors.

POSITIVE AND NEGATIVE SYMPTOM SCALE (PANSS) The scale was developed by Stanley Kay to broaden the coverage of the BPRS. It includes sections on positive symptoms, negative symptoms, and general psychopathology. All of the BPRS items are in the PANSS but the actual anchor points and definitions are slightly different. The item definitions are carefully documented in a manual and excellent training tapes are available. The scale has gained acceptance in a number of antipsychotic drug trials because of its attention to negative symptoms. Its only disadvantage in comparison with the BPRS is that it requires considerably more time to complete. Excellent interrater and test-retest reliabilities have been demonstrated with the instrument. In addition, it has been carefully validated against other instruments.

SCALE FOR THE ASSESSMENT OF POSITIVE SYMPTOMS (SAPS) The SAPS was developed by Nancy Andreasen and reflects her interest in describing psychopathology. The groups of symptoms that are rated include hallucinations, delusions, bizarre behavior, and positive formal thought disorder. Among the strengths of the SAPS is an emphasis on the evaluation of formal thought disorder, an area that is weak in such scales as the BPRS, which has a single item for conceptual disorganization. The scale provides rich definitions to characterize each scale point. It should be rated by an expert interviewer as it requires careful questioning.

SCALE FOR THE ASSESSMENT OF NEGATIVE SYMPTOMS (SANS) This scale, also developed by Nancy Andreasen, was the first to be introduced as a means of rating a broad range of negative symptoms and has become the standard against which others are compared. It includes five groups of symptoms: alogia, affective flattening, avolition-apathy, anhedonia-asociality, and attention. Each group of symptoms has several different items and a global score, which is rated 0 to 5. A manual describes the symptoms and provides anchor points. Raters should be clinically trained, as scoring is based on clinical observation as well as on reports from ward staff and family members.

SCHEDULE FOR THE DEFICIT SYNDROME William Carpenter and his collaborators developed the scale as a means of categorizing schizophrenic patients as either deficit or nondeficit subtypes. The deficit syndrome is different from other subtypes that are characterized by a prominence of negative symptoms in that some negative symptoms, such as emotional withdrawal, can be secondary to a worsening of such psychotic symptoms as suspiciousness. Carpenter focuses on deficit symptoms that endure even when the patient is in remission. Because deficit symptoms are considered independently from positive symptoms, patients may fulfill the criteria for deficit syndrome and still have severe psychotic symptoms. The schedule consists of six negative symptoms (restricted affect, diminished emotional range, poverty of speech, curbing of interests, diminished sense of purpose, and diminished social drive) and a global severity score that is rated on a scale of 0 to 4. The schedule also contains a global deficit-nondeficit categorization. The criteria for the deficit syndrome require a score of 2 or greater on two of the six symptoms. A manual for the scale gives guidelines for the interview. Studies by Carpenter and his coworkers indicate that the schedule has good interrater reliability. Studies of neuropsychological assessment and eye-tracking impairment support the validity of the deficit syndrome construct.

NURSES' OBSERVATION SCALE FOR INPATIENT EVALUATION (NOSIE) The scale rates 80 behaviors seen on inpatient units according to their frequency. Although NOSIE could apply to patients with a number of illnesses associated with abnormal behavior, the items are most applicable to schizophrenia. The scale is frequently used for antipsychotic drug trials because it is probably more sensitive to many severely disordered behavioral patterns than is the BPRS.

ANXIETY SCALES

Rating instruments have been developed to quantify the amount of normal anxiety and to measure the severity of pathological anxiety states, such as obsessional behavior, panic disorder, and phobic behaviors. In addition, normal anxiety can be a symptom associated with normal life or it can be a state that occurs in other psychiatric illnesses, such as depression and schizophrenia. Therefore, the selection of a method for assessing anxiety should take into account the patient's diagnosis. A scale that measures general anxiety may not be useful for monitoring panic disorder. And an instrument such as the BPRS may provide sufficient information about anxiety for some studies (Table 9.8-7).

ANXIETY DISORDERS INTERVIEW SCALE, REVISED (ADIS-R) The ADIS-R is a revision of the ADIS that was adapted for DSM-III-R. A semistructured interview that focuses on the diagnosis of anxiety disorders, it is a useful tool for arriving at a DSM-III-R diagnosis of anxiety disorder and in the process ruling out other illnesses. An advantage of the ADIS-R is that it provides rich information about symptoms of anxiety disorders, such as panic, generalized anxiety, and phobic avoidance, and documents the disability the patient suffers from these symptoms. The schedule includes both the Hamilton Rating Scale for Anxiety (HAM-A) and the HAM-D. The scale has demonstrated excellent reliability for simple phobia, social phobia, and obsessive-compulsive disorder, and relatively poor reliability for generalized anxiety disorder (GAD). The reliability problems for GAD may be resolved when the instrument is revised for DSM-IV.

SCHEDULE FOR AFFECTIVE DISORDERS AND SCHIZOPHRENIA—LIFETIME ANXIETY (SADS-LA) A modification of the Schedule for Affective Disorders and Schizophrenia, Lifetime version (SADS-L) designed for use in studies that focus on the lifetime occurrence of anxiety symptoms and disorders, it includes more information about a variety of anxiety symptoms, including panic attacks, phobias, fears, and avoidant behaviors. The instrument can categorize patients into nearly all anxiety disorder categories in the RDC or DSM-III-R. A life chart is prepared for each patient that includes a chronology of the patient's symptoms. The instrument has shown good to excellent reliability for diagnosing generalized anxiety disorder, social phobia, panic disorder, agoraphobia, and obsessive-compulsive disorder.

HAMILTON RATING SCALE FOR ANXIETY (HAM-A) (Table 9.8-8) The most widely used scale for measuring anxi-

TABLE 9.8-7
Anxiety Scales

Instrument	Function	Rater	Reference
Anxiety Disorders Interview Scale, Revised (ADIS-R)	Diagnosis of anxiety	Professional	DiNardo et al 1982
Schedule for Affective Disorders and Schizophrenia—Lifetime Anxiety (SADS-LA)	Lifetime occurrence of anxiety	Professional	Manuzza et al 1986
Hamilton Rating Scale for Anxiety (HAM-A)	General anxiety	Professional	Hamilton 1959
State-Trait Anxiety Inventory (STAI)	State versus trait anxiety	Self	Spielberger et al 1983
Fear Questionnaire	Phobia	Self	Marks & Mathews 1979
Leyton Obsessional Inventory (LOI)	Obsessive-compulsive symptoms	Self	Cooper 1970
Acute Panic Inventory (API)	Panic attacks	Professional	Liebowitz et al 1984
UCLA 4-D Anxiety Scale	Comprehensive anxiety	Self	Bystritsky et al 1990

Bystritsky A et al: Development of a multidimensional scale of anxiety. J Anx Disord *4:* 99, 1990. Cooper J: The Leyton Obsessional Inventory. Psychol Med *1:* 48, 1970. DiNardo P A, O'Brien G T, Barlow D H, et al: *The Anxiety Disorders Interview Schedule.* Center for Stress and Anxiety Disorders, Albany, NY, 1982. Hamilton M: The assessment of anxiety states by rating. Br J Med Psychol *32:* 50, 1959. Liebowitz M R et al: Lactate provocation of panic attacks: I. Clinical and behavioral findings. Arch Gen Psychiatry *41:* 764, 1984. Manuzza S, Fyer A, Klein D, Endicott J: Schedule for Affective Disorders and Schizophrenia—Lifetime Version modified for the study of anxiety disorders (SADS-LA): Rationale and conceptual development. J Psychiatr Res *20:* 317, 1986. Marks I M, Mathews A M: Brief standard self-rating for phobic patients. Behav Res Ther *17:* 263, 1979. Spielberger C D et al: *Manual for the State-Trait Anxiety Inventory.* Consultant Psychologist Press, Palo Alto, CA, 1983.

TABLE 9.8-8
Hamilton Anxiety Rating Scale

Instructions: This checklist is to assist the physician or psychiatrist in evaluating each patient as to his degree of anxiety and pathological condition. Please fill in the appropriate rating:

NONE = 0 MILD = 1 MODERATE = 2 SEVERE = 3 SEVERE, GROSSLY DISABLING = 4

Item		Rating	Item		Rating
Anxious mood	Worries, anticipation of the worst, fearful anticipation, irritability	____	Somatic (sensory)	Tinnitus, blurring of vision, hot and cold flushes, feelings of weakness, picking sensation	____
Tension	Feelings of tension, fatigability, startle response, moved to tears easily, trembling, feelings of restlessness, inability to relax	____	Cardiovascular symptoms	Tachycardia, palpitations, pain in chest, throbbing of vessels, fainting feelings, missing beat	____
Fears	Of dark, of strangers, of being left alone, of animals, of traffic, of crowds	____	Respiratory symptoms	Pressure or constriction in chest, choking feelings, sighing, dyspnea	____
Insomnia	Difficulty in falling asleep, broken sleep, unsatisfying sleep and fatigue on waking, dreams, nightmares, night-terrors	____	Gastrointestinal symptoms	Difficulty in swallowing, wind, abdominal pain, burning sensations, abdominal fullness, nausea, vomiting, borborygmi, looseness of bowels, loss of weight, constipation	____
Intellectual (cognitive)	Difficulty in concentration, poor memory	____	Genitourinary symptoms	Frequency of micturition, urgency of micturition, amenorrhea, menorrhagia, development of frigidity, premature ejaculation, loss of libido, impotence	____
Depressed mood	Loss of interest, lack of pleasure in hobbies, depression, early waking, diurnal swing	____	Autonomic symptoms	Dry mouth, flushing, pallor, tendency to sweat, giddiness, tension headache, raising of hair	____
Somatic (muscular)	Pains and aches, twitching, stiffness, myoclonic jerks, grinding of teeth, unsteady voice, increased muscular tone	____	Behavior at interview	Fidgeting, restlessness or pacing, tremor of hands, furrowed brow, strained face, sighing or rapid respiration, facial pallor, swallowing, belching, brisk tendon jerks, dilated pupils, exophthalmos	____
ADDITIONAL COMMENTS:					
Investigator's signature:					

Table from M Hamilton: The assessment of anxiety states by rating. Br J Med Psychol *32:* 50, 1959. Used with permission.

ety, the HAM-A was developed to rate anxiety for patients with anxiety syndromes and not for measuring generalized anxiety in other psychiatric and medical illnesses. The scale has 14 items, which are rated according to their severity. It resembles the HAM-D in its bias toward somatic experiences. Raters should be trained clinicians as it is based on open clinical interviews rather than on interviews that are programmed. The HAM-A has been thoroughly evaluated and has been found to have reasonable reliability and validity.

STATE-TRAIT ANXIETY INVENTORY (STAI) The STAI is a brief self-report measure that differentiates between state anxiety, which may be experienced in specific situations, and trait anxiety, which describes the anxiety experienced by the patient when there is no particular stress. The state questions inquire about how the patient feels at that particular moment and the trait questions ask how the patient generally feels.

FEAR QUESTIONNAIRE A self-rating instrument that is used primarily for studying phobias, one part asks subjects to rate their phobic behaviors associated with a variety of situations and a second part asks them to rate anxiety, depression, and global distress caused by a phobia. The scale yields a score for total phobia, as well for agoraphobia, blood-injury phobia, and social phobia.

YALE-BROWN OBSESSIVE COMPULSIVE SCALE (Y-BOCS) The Y-BOCS is probably the most widely used scale for rating the severity of symptoms of obsessive-compulsive disorder. It consists of a 10-item scale that is rated by clinicians, as well as a symptom checklist. Studies by the scale's developers indicate that interrater reliability is excellent for all 20 items and for the total. Utilization of the Y-BOCS in drug trials has shown it to be a sensitive instrument for measuring changes in the severity of obsessive-compulsive symptoms.

LEYTON OBSESSIONAL INVENTORY (LOI) The LOI is one of the more widely used scales for measuring obsessive-compulsive symptoms.

ACUTE PANIC INVENTORY (API) It measures the characteristics and severity of panic attacks. An advantage of the scale is its ability to discriminate panic from other anxiety symptoms.

UCLA 4-D ANXIETY SCALE The recently developed self-rating instrument was designed to be more comprehensive than other scales by including measures of the emotional, physiological, cognitive, and behavioral dimensions of anxiety. The scale consists of 40 items that ask how much the subject was bothered by certain experiences during the past week. Items are rated on a five-point scale from "not at all" to "extremely." Early studies indicate that the scale correlates well with the Zung scale.

SCALES FOR MEASURING MANIA

MANIC STATE RATING SCALE (MSRS) The MSRS, an observer-rated scale, consists of 26 items that are rated from 0 to 5 on the basis of both frequency and intensity. The items focus on behaviors that would typically be observed on an inpatient unit, such as "moves from one place to the other" or "is careless about dress and grooming." Thus it is best suited for use by trained nurses. Eleven of the items focus on elation-grandiosity and paranoid-destructiveness. The descriptions of the items are straightforward but there are no anchor points for scoring severity. However, the scale has been found to be both reliable and valid. Its main disadvantage is its length.

BECH-RAFAELSEN MANIA SCALE The instrument consists of 11 items that are rated on a five-point scale. The severity ratings have well-described anchor points, which probably accounts for the instrument's high reliability. Its developers recommend its use in conjunction with the HAM-D.

YOUNG MANIA RATING SCALE (Y-MRS) The scale has 11 items, which are rated after a clinical interview. Four items—irritability, speech rate and amount, content of thought, and disruptive-aggressive behavior—are given extra weight in the total by being scored from 0 to 8, whereas the other items are scored from 0 to 4. Clearly described anchor points are included for all of the items. High interrater reliability has been reported and the scale's validity has been demonstrated by correlations with other instruments. Moreover, predictive validity is indicated by a correlation between Y-MRS scores and the length of hospitalization.

A listing of scales for measuring mania are presented in Table 9.8-9.

SCALES FOR MEASURING COGNITIVE IMPAIRMENT

The assessment of cognitive impairment can be valuable as part of a diagnostic evaluation differentiating organic and functional disorders to determine the effects of treatment or the course of an illness (Table 9.8-10). In some circumstances neuropsychological testing is more sensitive than rating scales for docu-

TABLE 9.8-9
Mania Scales

Instrument	Rater	Reference
Manic State Rating Scale (MSRS)	Professional	Beigel et al 1971
Bech-Rafaelsen Mania Scale	Professional	Bech et al 1979
Young Mania Rating Scale (Y-MRS)	Professional	Young et al 1978

Beigel A, Murphy D, Bunney W: The Manic State Rating Scale: Scale construction, reliability, and validity. Arch Gen Psychiatry *25:* 256, 1971. Bech P, Bolwig T G, Kramp P, et al: The Bech-Rafaelsen Mania Scale and the Hamilton Depression Scale: Evaluation of homogeneity and inter-observer reliability. Acta Psychiatr Scand *59:* 420, 1979. Young R C, Biggs V T, Ziegler V E, et al: A rating scale for mania: Reliability, validity, and sensitivity. Br J Psychiatry *133:* 429, 1978.

TABLE 9.8-10
Dementia Scales

Instrument	Function	Reference
Blessed Dementia Scale (BDS)	Alzheimer's disease	Blessed et al 1968
Mini-Mental State Examination (MMSE)	Cognitive impairment	Folstein et al 1975
Sandoz Clinical Assessment—Geriatric (SCAG)	Drug trials in elderly	Shader et al 1974
Global Deterioration Scale (GDS)	Severity in dementia	Reisberg et al 1982
Brief Cognitive Rating Scale (BCRS)	Severity of cognitive impairment	Reisberg et al 1982
Alzheimer's Disease Assessment Scale (ADAS)	Alzheimer's disease	Rosen et al 1984
Structured Clinical Interview for the Diagnosis of Dementia of the Alzheimer Type, Multi-infarct Dementia, and Dementias of Other Aetiology (SIDAM)	Diagnosis of dementia	Zaudig et al 1991
Consortium to Establish a Registry for Alzheimer's Disease (CERAD)	Alzheimer's disease	Morris et al 1989

Blessed G, Tomlinson B E, Roth M: The association between quantitative measures of dementia and of senile changes in the cerebral gray matter of elderly subjects. Br J Psychiatry *114:* 797, 1968. Folstein M F, Folstein S E, McHugh P R: "Mini-mental state." A practical method for grading the cognitive state of patients for the clinician. J Psychiatr Res *12:* 189, 1975. Morris J C, Heyman A, Mohs R C, et al: The Consortium to Establish a Registry for Alzheimer's Disease (CERAD): Part I, Clinical and neuropsychological assessment of Alzheimer's disease. Neurology *39:* 1159, 1989. Reisberg B, Ferris S H, De Leon M J, et al: The Global Deterioration Scale (GDS) for assessment of primary degenerative dementia. Am J Psychiatry *139:* 1136, 1982. Rosen et al: A new rating scale for Alzheimer's disease. Am J Psychiatry *141:* 1356, 1984. Shader R I, Harmatz J S, Salzman C: A new scale for clinical assessment in geriatric populations: Sandoz Clinical Assessment—Geriatric (SCAG). J Am Geriatr Soc *22:* 107, 1974. Zaudig M, Mittelhammer J, Hiller W, et al: SIDAM—A structured interview for the diagnosis of dementia of the Alzheimer type, multi-infarct dementia, and dementias of other aetiology according to ICD-10 and DSM-III-R. Psychol Med *21:* 225, 1991.

menting mild cognitive impairment. An important limitation of rating scales is that they are influenced by intelligence, educational level, and literacy, and thus some persons who have some cognitive deterioration as compared with baseline will score in the unimpaired range.

In evaluating elderly patients other Axis I illnesses, particularly mood disorders, will frequently be part of the differential diagnosis. Therefore, such scales as the HAM-D and the BPRS may be included in pharmacological trials in those patients.

BLESSED DEMENTIA SCALE (BDS) The instrument—developed in 1968—consists of 50 items that assess such domains as orientation, recent and remote memory, and the ability of the patient to carry out the activities of daily living. It has been among the most widely used scales for diagnosing dementia of the Alzheimer's type. Frequently the scale is divided into two instruments, the Memory and Information Test and the Dementia Rating Scale. The original validation studies found that scores from the scale correlated with the number of senile plaques found at autopsy. Other studies have found that scores on the Blessed correlate with the levels of brain choline acetyltransferase in Alzheimer's disease. Although the scale has usually been used to diagnose dementia of the Alzheimer's type, it was not developed to distinguish that disease from vascular dementia.

MINI-MENTAL STATE EXAMINATION (MMSE) (Table 9.8-11) The MMSE, also known as the Folstein Scale, has become the most widely used instrument for monitoring cognitive impairment for both research and clinical populations. The examination is highly structured and so can be administered and scored by nonclinicians. The first of two sections asks questions about orientation, memory, and attention. The second section tests the ability to name objects, follow verbal and written commands, write a sentence, and copy a complex polygon. A simple scoring system is provided on the examination form. Advantages of the instrument include its brevity (it requires only 5 to 10 minutes to administer and score), its demonstrated reliability and validity, and its acceptance by the field. Whereas the Blessed Scale focuses on memory and orientation, the MMSE assesses a range of deficits. The well-standardized administration and scoring permit clinicians who are familiar with the instrument to communicate about the degree of impairment in individual patients. Reliability studies indicate that the MMSE has high interrater reliability (0.82 or better) and test-retest reliability (0.89 or better). Its validity has been demonstrated by studies in which MMSE scores were correlated with scores on the WAIS and computed tomography studies of the brain.

SANDOZ CLINICAL ASSESSMENT—GERIATRIC (SCAG) A commonly used rating scale for drug trials in elderly patients, the instrument consists of 18 items that evaluate behavioral disorders (uncooperativeness, unsociability), mood states (depression, irritability), and cognitive functions (confusion, alertness, memory impairment). The broad range of items makes it useful for evaluating the effects of treatment on different types of psychopathology, such as anxiety, depression, and confusion. Thus one group of investigators has categorized the 18 items into four orthogonal factors: agitation irritability, mood depression, cognitive dysfunction, and withdrawal. Some important symptoms, however, such as sleep disturbance, hallucinations, and suspiciousness, are not rated by the SCAG. Ratings should be made by a trained clinician based on observations of the patient.

TABLE 9.8-11
Mini-Mental State Examination

Orientation (Score 1 point for correct response)
1. What is the year?
2. What is the season?
3. What is the date?
4. What is the day of the week?
5. What is the month?
6. Where are we? building or hospital?
7. Where are we? floor?
8. Where are we? town or city?
9. Where are we? county?
10. Where are we? state?

Registration (Score 1 point for each object identified correctly, maximum is 3 points)
11. Name three objects at about one each second. Ask the patient to repeat them. If the patient misses an object, repeat them until all three are learned.

Attention and calculation (Score 1 point for each correct answer up to maximum of 5 points)
12. Subtract 7's from 100 until 65 (or, as an alternative, spell "world" backwards).

Recall (Score 1 point for each correct answer, maximum of 3)
13. Ask for names of three objects learned in question 11.

Language
14. Point to a pencil and a watch. Ask the patient to name each object. Score 1 point for each correct answer, maximum of 2 points.
15. Have the patient repeat "No ifs, ands, or buts." Score one point if correct.
16. Have the patient follow a three-stage command: "(1) Take the paper in your right hand. (2) Fold the paper in half. (3) Put the paper on the floor." Score 1 point for each command done correctly, maximum of 3 points.
17. Write the following in large letters: "CLOSE YOUR EYES." Ask the patient to read the command and perform the task. Score 1 point if correct.
18. Ask the patient to write a sentence of his or her own choice. Score 1 point if the sentence has a subject, an object, and a verb.
19. Draw the design printed below. Ask the patient to copy the design. Score 1 point if all sides and angles are preserved and if the intersecting sides form a quadrangle.

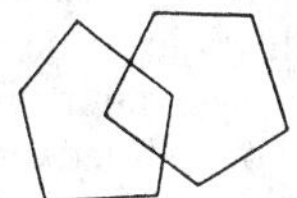

Table from Folstein M F, Folstein S E, McHugh P R: "Mini-mental state." A practical method for grading the cognitive state of patients for the clinician. J Psychiatr Res *12:* 189, 1975. Used with permission.

Studies indicate that the SCAG has excellent reliability and validity.

GLOBAL DETERIORATION SCALE (GDS) The GDS was developed by Barry Reisberg to grade the severity of dementia regardless of its etiology, largely on the basis of the amount of memory deficit. It is a seven-point scale on which 1 represents no cognitive decline and 7 represents very severe cognitive decline. The different points are clearly described according to the degree of deficit in such areas as remote and recent memory, mathematical manipulation, orientation, and ability to complete different tasks. The scale has good face and predictive validity.

BRIEF COGNITIVE RATING SCALE (BCRS) The scale assesses the magnitude of cognitive impairment in five areas: (1) concentration and cognitive ability, (2) recent memory, (3) past memory, (4) orientation, and (5) functioning and self-care. Each area is graded on a seven-point scale with anchor points describing each score.

ALZHEIMER'S DISEASE ASSESSMENT SCALE (ADAS) Developed to rate a broad range of Alzheimer's disease patients who have mild to severe dementia, the scale consists of 21 items that measure cognitive function, memory, concentration, mood, psychosis, and a number of behaviors. The ADAS includes both performance tests and ratings of the patient's behavior. The examination requires approximately 45 minutes to complete, and thus it represents a compromise between brief scales that are unable to map multiple aspects of cognitive function and scales that are too lengthy for clinical trials. Evaluations by the developers of the instrument indicate that it has high interrater and test-retest reliability. Its validity is supported by its ability to discriminate patients with Alzheimer's disease from normal elderly subjects.

STRUCTURED CLINICAL INTERVIEW FOR THE DIAGNOSIS OF DEMENTIA OF THE ALZHEIMER'S TYPE, MULTI-INFARCT DEMENTIA, AND DEMENTIAS OF OTHER AETIOLOGY (SIDAM) An instrument for diagnosing dementias according to DSM-III-R and ICD-10, it features a structured clinical interview, as well as a number of tests, including the MMSE, and items that can be collected from other informants. Although it provides a substantial amount of information, it usually can be completed in less than 30 minutes. The SIDAM also affords a means for grading the severity of cognitive impairment. Initial studies indicate good test-retest reliability and good validity when compared with diagnoses by experts.

CONSORTIUM TO ESTABLISH A REGISTRY FOR ALZHEIMER'S DISEASE (CERAD) CERAD is a consortium of investigators who have agreed on a common battery of assessments for Alzheimer's disease for both clinical use and postmortem evaluation. The clinical battery was designed to provide clinicians with sufficient information to make a confident diagnosis of Alzheimer's disease. It contains semistructured interviews with the patient and an informant; physical, neurological, and laboratory examinations; a depression scale; and a medical history. Two modified forms of the Blessed Scale and the MMSE are part of the battery, as well as a neuropsychological battery including tests of verbal fluency, word list memory, constructional praxis, and word list recognition. CERAD has developed an instruction manual that describes the administration of the tests.

The investigators administered the tests to 354 Alzheimer's disease patients and 278 elderly controls at 16 university medical centers. Both interrater and test-retest reliability varied on the instrument, although in most cases they were at acceptable levels. In addition, the battery was able to discriminate the patients from the controls.

SCALES FOR MEASURING CHILDHOOD PSYCHOPATHOLOGY

CHILDREN'S DEPRESSION INVENTORY (CDI) Probably the most widely used instrument for monitoring depression in children, it is a 27-item self-report questionnaire that is administered to 7- to 17-year-olds. Each item includes three statements with increasing severity. Evaluations of the instrument indicate good test-retest reliability.

DIAGNOSTIC INTERVIEW SCHEDULE FOR CHILDREN, REVISED (DISC-R) The scale can generate DSM-III-R diagnoses for children from 6 to 18 years old. It consists of separate interview formats for children and their parents. The interview with the child requires about 40 to 60 minutes whereas that with the parent takes 60 to 70 minutes. Both interviews can be administered by lay interviewers after going through a training program. The scale has undergone extensive testing. Both interrater and test-retest reliability are high. Validity has been confirmed by the scale's ability to discriminate between psychiatric and pediatric referrals.

DIAGNOSTIC INTERVIEW FOR CHILDREN AND ADOLESCENTS (DICA) The scale is a structured clinical interview for children aged 6 or older. It can be administered to either parents or children and requires only about 45 minutes to complete. Studies suggest that the scale has good test-retest reliability.

SCHEDULE FOR AFFECTIVE DISORDERS AND SCHIZOPHRENIA FOR SCHOOL-AGE CHILDREN (KIDDIE-SADS) It is one of the most widely used diagnostic interviews for children 6 to 17 years of age. Although the scale has been used by lay interviewers, it requires some expertise and familiarity with research criteria. The Kiddie-SADS recommends interviewing a parent first, followed by an interview with the child. The interviewer then combines impressions from both interviews on a single form. The scale has demonstrated varying reliability depending on the diagnostic categories that are being considered.

CHILD BEHAVIOR CHECKLIST (CBCL) The scale was developed by Thomas M. Achenbach to evaluate pathological behaviors and social competence in children from 4 to 16 years old. Forms are available for teachers, parents, and children. It is among the most widely used scales for both clinical use and research. The scale requires 15 to 30 minutes to complete and the time frame for rating is usually the past six months. The scale has been administered in large population surveys and thus there are substantial normative data available on the scale items. It has shown excellent test-retest reliability as well as interparent agreement. Its validity has been demonstrated in studies where scores were related to other measures of psychopathology.

KIDDIE-PANSS A childhood version of the Positive and Negative Symptom Scale (PANSS) that was developed for assessing severely disturbed children and adolescents, it is based on recent findings indicating that children with psychotic symptoms parallel adults in demonstrating both positive and negative symptoms. The instrument consists of a prepatient interview with a primary caregiver as well as a patient interview. The interviewer is guided through structured play activities for children from 6 to 10 years of age in order to gather additional information. The scale demonstrates good interrater reliability as well as the ability to differentiate patients with and without schizophrenia.

SCALES FOR ASSESSING PERSONALITY DISORDERS

The diagnosis of personality disorders has been plagued by poor reliability resulting from a number of factors, including the subjective quality of the diagnostic criteria, the frequently unreliable information obtained from patients, and the tendency of patients to meet the criteria for more than one category. Thus, rating scales for personality disorders have focused on improving diagnostic reliability.

DIAGNOSTIC INTERVIEW FOR BORDERLINES The instrument focuses on social adaptation, impulse and action patterns, affects, psychosis, and interpersonal relationships. The interviewer bases the scoring on the patient's replies to questions as well as on behaviors during the interview. The scale, which has been used in a number of studies, has demonstrated good reliability and the ability to discriminate between borderline disorder and other disorders.

STRUCTURED INTERVIEW FOR DSM-III-R PERSONALITY (SIDP-R) The SIDP-R combines information from the patient, informants, and other sources, including medical records, to make any of the DSM-III-R diagnoses. It consists of 160 questions that are related to DSM-III-R criteria, and requires approximately 60 minutes for interviewing the patient and 30 minutes for the informant.

STRUCTURED CLINICAL INTERVIEW FOR DSM-III-R PERSONALITY DISORDERS (SCID-II) The patient is first administered the SCID-I to evaluate whether or not an Axis I illness is present, which is followed by a self-rating instrument that asks the patient to respond "yes" or "no" to a number of screening questions. The interview then focuses on the responses of the patient to clarify whether the criteria for personality diagnoses are met. The instrument is being revised for DSM-IV.

PERSONALITY DISORDER EXAMINATION (PDE) A lengthy semistructured interview designed to diagnose DSM-III-R personality disorders, it consists of 359 items and requires one to two hours to complete. Items are rated on a three-point scale as to whether the item is absent, is clinically significant, or is of doubtful significance. An advantage of the scale is that the richness of information derived from the interview tends to reduce the need for the assessor to make judgments.

INTERNATIONAL PERSONALITY DISORDER EXAMINATION (IPDE) The instrument is a modification of the PDE that is compatible with the ICD-10, DSM-III-R, and DSM-IV. In a large international field trial the IPDE demonstrated reasonable interrater reliability and clinician acceptance. It is likely to be particularly useful in international studies.

SCALES FOR ASSESSING ALCOHOLISM AND SUBSTANCE ABUSE

CAGE QUESTIONNAIRE A brief and straightforward instrument that has been widely used as a screening device, CAGE is an acronym derived from the following four questions.

1. Have you ever felt you ought to *c*ut down on your drinking?
2. Have people *a*nnoyed you by criticizing your drinking?
3. Have you ever felt bad or *g*uilty about your drinking?
4. Have you ever had a drink first thing in the morning to steady your nerves or to get rid of a hangover (*e*ye opener)?

John Ewing, the scale's developer, found that answering Yes to at least two of these questions was a strong indicator for alcohol abuse by men. Although the instrument is less discriminating in outpatient than in inpatient populations, it remains useful because it is so brief and simple to administer.

MICHIGAN ALCOHOLISM SCREENING TEST (MAST) A widely used screening instrument for identifying alcohol use disorders and alcohol-related disabilities, it consists of 25 true or false questions that can be administered as a questionnaire or during an interview. Studies have supported the validity of the instrument. Briefer versions of the MAST have been developed that appear to be as valid as the original.

DRUG ABUSE SCREENING TEST (DAST) The test is a screening instrument for identifying patients with problems related to drug abuse. The 28 true or false questions are similar to those in the MAST. Studies indicate that the DAST is able to discriminate patients who seek drug abuse treatment from those who seek treatment for alcohol use disorders.

ADDICTION SEVERITY INDEX (ASI) The instrument provides an indication of the severity of problems in six domains: drug and alcohol abuse, medical, psychological, legal, family and social, and employment and support. It consists of an interview that usually requires less than an hour. As it can be administered reliably by trained technicians, it is a useful scale in both clinical and research settings. Studies indicate that the ASI is a valid instrument that can be used in treatment planning.

SCALES FOR MEASURING SOCIAL FUNCTIONING

Clinicians or researchers who are studying the outcome of an illness or the overall effects of a treatment will commonly use measures of social functioning. Because psychiatric illnesses can be associated with a range of social functioning from normal to complete dependency, a useful scale should span that entire range. Such scales as the Global Assessment Scale and the Global Assessment of Functioning Scale characterize social functioning with a single rating. However, it is not uncommon for a person to function well in one area, as in social relations, but poorly in another, such as vocational adjustment. That fact is important to note as social functioning is rated on Axis V of DSM-IV and is given a single global rating. The rating may not be sufficient for a psychosocial or pharmacological trial that may be focused on a particular social deficit.

GLOBAL ASSESSMENT OF FUNCTIONING (GAF) SCALE (see Table 11.1-7) The instrument, which is used for rating Axis V of DSM-IV, is a revision of the Global Assessment Scale (GAS) developed by Jean Endicott and colleagues. The GAS has been used in many clinical settings, as well as in numerous research studies, and clearly has face validity. The GAF scale has slightly different anchor points and eliminates subjects with superior functioning. The rater collects information on psychological, social, and occupational functioning and assigns patients a number from 1 to 100, with the higher number representing no symptoms and normal functioning. The anchor points instruct the rater to consider both the symptoms and the impairment in functioning. Two ratings are made—one for current functioning and one for the highest functioning in the past year.

The scale was designed to combine the effects of symptoms and social functioning, which is a limitation if the investigator or clinician is interested in separating those two domains.

SOCIAL ADJUSTMENT SCALE—II (SAS-II) The scale assesses social functioning during the four weeks preceding the interview. Subjects are rated on subscales that evaluate work role, household role, parental role, extended family role, conjugal and nonconjugal sexual roles, romantic involvement, social and leisure activities, and personal well-being. In addition, global ratings are developed for a number of items. An important advantage of the instrument is the completeness with which it covers the domains of social functioning. Conversely, there are relatively few items to assess the functioning of severely deteriorated patients. For example, the scale does not monitor changes in patients who perform volunteer work or participate in sheltered workshops. Similarly, it is poorly suited for monitoring changes in severely disabled patients who have only minimal social contacts.

SCALES FOR MEASURING DRUG SIDE EFFECTS

SYSTEMATIC ASSESSMENT FOR TREATMENT EMERGENT EFFECTS (SAFTEE) The instrument is useful for the systematic recording of side effects in drug trials. The investigator may choose either a general inquiry form, which asks open-ended questions about the health problems of the subject, or a systematic inquiry form, which asks questions about different systems. The scale has a number of advantages, including a format for recording a broad range of side effects, well-defined time intervals, and a computer-based data-entry program.

SIMPSON-ANGUS PARKINSONISM SCALE One of the most commonly used scales for measuring extrapyramidal side effects of antipsychotic drugs, it has undergone a number of revisions and is currently available in a shorter form. The scale is heavily focused on parkinsonism in contrast to akathisia.

ABNORMAL INVOLUNTARY MOVEMENT SCALE (AIMS) (Table 9.8-12) It is the most commonly used scale for measuring late-appearing movement disorders, especially tardive dyskinesia. Abnormal movements of different body areas (head, trunk, extremities) are rated on a five-point scale. The AIMS contains a reasonably detailed description of the method for examining patients to ascertain abnormal movements. The author recommends the use of the AIMS or a similar instrument for the routine evaluation of patients being treated with antipsychotic medications. For example, performing an AIMS test and recording the results in the medical record once every three to six months is a reasonable strategy for screening patients for tardive dyskinesia.

BARNES AKATHISIA SCALE A commonly used scale for measuring akathisia in patients who are receiving antipsychotic drugs, it includes diagnostic criteria for pseudoakathisia and mild, moderate, and severe akathisia. The scale rates both observed movements and the subjective experience of restlessness. The developer has reported reasonably good interrater reliability for the instrument.

TABLE 9.8-12
Abnormal Involuntary Movement Scale (AIMS) Examination Procedure

Patient identification: ____________________ Date ________
Rated by: ____________________

Either before or after completing the examination procedure, observe the patient unobtrusively at rest (e.g., in waiting room).

The chair to be used in this examination should be a hard, firm one without arms.

After observing the patient, he or she may be rated on a scale of 0 (none), 1 (minimal), 2 (mild), 3 (moderate), and 4 (severe) according to the severity of symptoms.

Ask the patient whether there is anything in his/her mouth (i.e., gum, candy, etc.) and if there is to remove it.

Ask patient about the current condition of his/her teeth. Ask patient if he/she wears dentures. Do teeth or dentures bother patient now?

Ask patient whether he/she notices any movement in mouth, face, hands, or feet. If yes, ask to describe and to what extent they currently bother patient or interfere with his/her activities.

Rating	Procedure
0 1 2 3 4	Have patient sit in chair with hands on knees, legs slightly apart, and feet flat on floor. (Look at entire body for movements while in this position.)
0 1 2 3 4	Ask patient to sit with hands hanging unsupported. If male, between legs, if female and wearing a dress, hanging over knees. (Observe hands and other body areas.)
0 1 2 3 4	Ask patient to open mouth. (Observe tongue at rest within mouth.) Do this twice.
0 1 2 3 4	Ask patient to protrude tongue. (Observe abnormalities of tongue movement.) Do this twice.
0 1 2 3 4	Ask the patient to tap thumb, with each finger, as rapidly as possible for 10–15 seconds; separately with right hand, then with left hand. (Observe facial and leg movements.)
0 1 2 3 4	Flex and extend patient's left and right arms. (One at a time.)
0 1 2 3 4	Ask patient to stand up. (Observe in profile. Observe all body areas again, hips included.)
0 1 2 3 4	*Ask patient to extend both arms outstretched in front with palms down. (Observe trunk, legs, and mouth.)
0 1 2 3 4	*Have patient walk a few paces, turn and walk back to chair. (Observe hands and gait.) Do this twice.

*Activated movements.

SUGGESTED CROSS-REFERENCES

The process of obtaining clinical information is discussed in Sections 9.1 and 9.3. Diagnosis in psychiatry and the current classification systems are discussed in Chapter 11. The psychiatric syndromes themselves, as well as the typical signs and symptoms, are discussed in Chapters 14 (schizophrenia), Chapter 16 (mood disorders), Chapter 17 (anxiety disorders), Chapter 25 (personality disorders), and Chapter 34 (psychiatric examination of the infant, child, and adolescent). More detailed information on psychological evaluations and the role of the clinical psychologist in evaluating psychiatric illness is included in Sections 9.4, 9.5, and 9.6.

REFERENCES

Bech P, Allerup P, Maier W, Albus M, Lavori P, Ayuso J L: The Hamilton scales and the Hopkins Symptom Checklist (SCL-90). A cross-national validity study in patients with panic disorders. Br J Psychiatry *160:* 206, 1992.

Blessed G, Black S E, Butler T, Kay D W: The diagnosis of dementia in the elderly. A comparison of CAMCOG (the cognitive section of CAMDEX), the AGECAT program, DSM-III, the Mini-Mental State Examination and some short rating scales. Br J Psychiatry *159:* 193, 1991.

Blessed G, Tomlinson B E, Roth M: The association betewen quantitative measures of dementia and of senile changes in the cerebral gray matter of elderly subjects. Br J Psychiatry *114:* 797, 1968.

Canning E H, Kelleher K: Performance of screening tools for mental health problems in chronically ill children. Arch Pediatr Adolesc Med *148:* 272, 1994.

Derogatis L R: *SCL-90: Administration, Scoring, and Procedures Manual for the Revised Version.* Clinical Psychometrics Research Unit, Baltimore, 1977.

Di Nardo P A, Moras K, Barlow D H, Rapee R M, Brown T A: Reliability of DSM-III-R Anxiety Disorders Interview Schedule—Revised (ADIS-R). Arch Gen Psychiatry *50:* 251, 1993.

Fenton W S, McGlashan T H: Testing systems for assessment of negative symptoms in schizophrenia. Arch Gen Psychiatry *49:* 179, 1992.

Fields J H, Grochowski S, Lindenmayer J P, Kay S R, Grosz D, Hyman R B, Alexander G: Assessing positive and negative symptoms in children and adolescents. Am J Psychiatry *151:* 249, 1994.

*Folstein M F, Folstein S E, McHugh P R: ''Mini-mental state'': A practical method for grading the cognitive state of patients for the clinician. J Psychiatr Res *12:* 189, 1975.

Goodman W, Price L, Rasmussen S: The Yale-Brown Obsessive-compulsive scale. II. Validity. Arch Gen Psychiatry *46:* 1012, 1989.

Gur R E, Mozley P D, Resnick S M, Levick S, Erwin R, Saykin A J, Gur R C: Relations among clinical scales in schizophrenia. Am J Psychiatry *148:* 472, 1991.

Lewis S J, Harder D W: A comparison of four measures to diagnose DSM-III-R borderline personality disorder in outpatients. J Nerv Ment Dis *179:* 329, 1991.

*Hamilton M: The assessment of anxiety states by rating. Br J Med Psychol *32:* 50, 1959.

*Hamilton M: A rating scale for depression. J Neurol Neurosurg Psychiatry *23:* 56, 1960.

Loranger A W, Sartorius N, Andreoli A, Berger P, Buckheim P, Channabasavanna S M, Coid B, Dahl A, Diekstra R F, Ferguson B: The international personality disorder examination: The World Health Organization/Alcohol, Drug Abuse and Mental Health Administration international pilot study of personality disorders. Arch Gen Psychiatry *51:* 215, 1994.

Morris J C, Heyman A, Mohs R C, Hughs J P, van Belle G, Fillenbaum G, Mellits E D, Clark C: The Consortium to Establish a Registry for Alzheimer's Disease (CERAD): Part I, Clinical and neuropsychological assessment of Alzheimer's disease. Neurology *39:* 1159, 1989.

*Oldham J M, Skodol A E, Kellman H D, Hyler S E, Rosnick L, Davies M: Diagnosis of DSM-III-R personality disorders by two structured interviews: Patterns of comorbidity. Am J Psychiatry *149:* 213, 1992.

Overall J, Gorham D: Brief Psychiatric Rating Scale. Psychol Rep *10:* 799, 1962.

Shaffer D, Schwab-Stone M, Fisher P, Cohen P, Piacentini J, Davies M, Conners C K, Regier D: The Diagnostic Interview Schedule for Children—Revised version (DISC-R): I. Preparation, field testing, interrater reliability, and acceptability. J Am Acad Child Adolesc Psychiatry *32:* 643, 1993.

Shear M K, Maser J D: Standardized assessment for panic disorder research: A conference report. Arch Gen Psychiatry *51:* 346, 1994.

Spitzer R L, Williams J B, Gibbon M, First M B: The Structured Clinical Interview for DSM-III-R (SCID). I: History, rationale, and description. Arch Gen Psychiatry *49:* 624, 1992.

Thompson C (editor): *The Instruments of Psychiatric Research* Wiley, New York, 1989.

Wetzler S (editor): *Measuring Mental Illness: Psychometric Assessment for Clinicians.* American Psychiatric Press, Washington, 1989.

Wing J K, Cooper J E, Sartorius N: *The Measurement and Classification of Psychiatric Symptoms.* Cambridge University Press, New York, 1974.

Wyatt R J: *Practical Psychiatric Practice.* American Psychiatric Press, Washington, 1994.

*Zaudig M, Mittelhammer J, Hiller W, Pauls A, Thora C, Morinigo A, Mombour W: SIDAM—A structured interview for the diagnosis of dementia of the Alzheimer type, multi-infarct dementia and dementias of other aetiology according to ICD-10 and DSM-III-R. Psychol Med *21:* 225, 1991.

Zimmerman M: Diagnosing personality disorders: A review of issues and research methods. Arch Gen Psychiatry *51:* 225, 1994.

CHAPTER 10 CLINICAL MANIFESTATIONS OF PSYCHIATRIC DISORDERS

JOEL YAGER, M.D.
MICHAEL J. GITLIN, M.D.

INTRODUCTION

Like medical disorders, psychiatric disorders express themselves in characteristic alterations in a variety of dimensions. The elicitation of subjective complaints and clinical symptoms and the observation of clinical signs of psychiatric disorders can appropriately be compared to the classic history and physical examination of medicine. In many other ways, however, psychiatric disorders stand in contrast to medical disorders. First, in comparison with medical disorders, psychiatric disorders cannot be understood without a thorough evaluation and comprehension of the broad context of the patient's complaints. For example, depressive symptoms can be evaluated and understood only in relation to the patient's interpersonal world, work role, and family life. Second, the nature and the expression of psychiatric signs and symptoms are profoundly altered by the patient's strengths, coping capacities, and psychological defenses, with the clinical picture ultimately representing a balance between psychopathology and psychological strengths. Overall, though, the most important distinction between medical and psychiatric psychopathology is psychiatry's greater reliance on internal states and subjective experiences that are, at best, difficult to describe. Trying to delineate the character and the quality of many psychiatric symptoms is often better accomplished by poets and novelists than by clinicians. Even with familiar and comprehensible feelings, it is simultaneously important and difficult to describe inner states.

A 38-year-old woman tried to explain to an evaluating psychiatrist the difference between the fatigue she experienced when she was hypothyroid and the feeling she experienced when, in a euthyroid state, she had symptoms characteristic of an atypical depression, with hypersomnia and profound fatigue. After struggling with adjectives and descriptions such as "Everything now is a mental and physical effort" and "I'm exhausted by even thinking of doing anything other than lying in bed," she felt she was not making her point adequately. After a short time, she burst into tears, exclaiming, "You'd understand if you were inside me," and refused to attempt further descriptions.

The reliance on subjective descriptions makes psychiatric symptoms inherently less reliable than quantifiable data such as blood pressure. Much of the research in psychiatric diagnosis over the past 20 years has concerned itself with increasing the reliability of observer-rated clinical symptoms. In many ways the research has had the desired effect; both clinicians and trained research personnel can, with the help of a structured interview, come to reasonable agreement on what symptoms a patient is experiencing and whether the patient meets the criteria for, say, a major depressive episode. However, the cost of that reliability has, in some instances, been the narrowing of the field of clinical vision as clinical phenomena are excluded. Although recognized by clinicians, some clinical phenomena are inherently difficult to ascertain in a structured interview. In addition, the quest for reliability can lead one only so far in describing phenomena for which few precise words are available.

Because of those observational, empathic, and semantic difficulties and because of the trends in medical practice toward rapid diagnoses and quick interventions, less attention seems to be paid to a careful description of the patient's signs and symptoms today than in years past. Nevertheless, an intensive clinical focus on a thorough description of psychopathology is important for the following reasons: (1) Important diagnostic distinctions are made on the basis of the phenomena elicited. The diagnosis made theoretically suggests a treatment course and a prognosis. For example, a psychiatrist must accurately distinguish between antipsychotic-induced akathisia and the anxiety symptoms related to psychotic thinking. On the basis of the diagnostic decision reached, opposite therapeutic strategies may be developed. (2) Clinicians' interest in the details of a patient's internal experiences helps them make some sense of what is often frightening and incomprehensible. (3) The clinician's demonstration of knowledge regarding the psychopathology diminishes the patient's sense of isolation that is characteristic of many disorders and fosters the growth of a therapeutic alliance, increasing the likelihood of treatment adherence.

PREDISPOSING VULNERABILITIES AND STRESSORS

GENETIC FACTORS Genetic vulnerabilities play a prominent role in the expression of such disorders as schizophrenia, alcohol abuse and dependence, and bipolar disorder. What is now virtually unknown is the nature of the vulnerability inherited, whether described at a neuronal level (such as a defect in the dopamine regulatory system in the mesolimbic tract), a psychophysiological level (exaggerated arousal responses to stimuli), or a psychological level (blunted responses to rewards or a weak superego).

INTRAUTERINE FACTORS The fetal alcohol syndrome is an example of how the development of children may be harmed by a noxious intrauterine environment. That syndrome also shows how genetic vulnerability for a disorder (as in a mother) may also provoke environmentally caused damage (that is, damage within the uterine environment). Other constitutionally facilitated, early development problems likely to increase subsequent psychiatric morbidity include speech and language difficulties and attention-deficit disorders. Those problems may presage the development of various adult psychiatric disorders and personality problems. Deafness, affecting as it does a major portion of the perceptual apparatus, is also associated with a high prevalence of psychiatric disturbance.

CONSTITUTIONAL FACTORS Considerable research shows that by birth or shortly afterward infants differ widely in temperament—in spontaneous activity levels; the intensity and the duration of reactions to external stimuli; the regularity or irregularity of certain biological rhythms, such as sleep; tendencies to approach or withdraw from new stimuli; the speed and the degree of adaptation; attention span and distractibility; the persistence of behavior; and qualities of mood. On the basis of such early behaviors, children may be described as having easy or difficult temperaments, being quick or slow to warm up. Temperament, however, is not immutable. There are discontinuities over time, and the development of temperament and its lasting effects on personality development are, at least in part, a function of the goodness of fit with a child's family. Nevertheless, temperamental qualities correlate somewhat with behavioral problems, at least through early childhood.

Aside from temperament, other persistent normal variations in personality development seem to be constitutionally related and may influence subsequent resilience or vulnerability. Traits such as introversion, extroversion, and neuroticism appear to be relatively enduring and stable personality dimensions. Subtypes of intelligence—such as those related to conceptual, mathematical, musical, kinesthetic, and interpersonal abilities—have been postulated as having separate genetic determinants and patterns of development. The type A and type B personality patterns, hardy and resilient personalities, and high-strung, sensitive, fussy, irritable, and pessimistic characteristics have all been described as generally lifelong qualities that originate in early childhood.

PHYSIOLOGICAL STRESSORS Physiological vulnerability may result from long-standing problems or from newly acquired problems. The metabolic, toxic, infectious, and other causes of physical illness produce increased vulnerability to psychiatric disturbance. Studies have shown that psychiatric services are used more by those are physically ill than by the healthy, and a higher than expected prevalence of physical disease is found among the psychiatrically impaired. In one study of 658 patients seen consecutively in a community mental health center, 9.1 percent had medical problems that were thought to have induced the psychiatric disturbance, and 28 percent of them were patients initially classified as suffering from a psychosis of psychiatric origin.

Human immunodeficiency virus (HIV) infection leading to seropositivity and acquired immune deficiency syndrome (AIDS) vividly illustrates the multiple and complex ways in which stressors can lead to psychiatric disturbances. Psychiatric symptoms in patients with those physical disorders may represent changes that are the direct effects of the virus on the central nervous system (CNS); the virus produces changes in cognition, personality, and mood—expectable psychological adjustments in response to an overwhelming life-threatening disorder—or the psychological stress of the viral illness may provoke the emergence of latent or quiescent primary psychiatric problems.

ENVIRONMENTAL STRESSORS There is a complex relation between the development of psychiatric symptoms and the occurrence of various life events, particularly threatening, unpredictable, and uncontrollable negative events. In general, such undesirable life events predispose a person to psychiatric symptoms, especially if the person already has a psychiatric disorder. Catastrophic events, such as incarceration in a concentration camp, cause enduring psychiatric disturbances in a high percentage of survivors, although individual responses vary widely. The stress-related consequences of combat also vary widely; some heavily exposed veterans have long-lasting posttraumatic stress disorder, but others have few persistent symptoms. Bereavement, divorce, and major physical injuries affect some people profoundly and others hardly at all in the long run. During development, certain stressors are most traumatic in critical periods. For example, the loss of a parent by a young child is likely to be more traumatic and to have more profound and longer-lasting effects that the loss of a parent by an adult.

The combined effects of negative life events and poor social supports are important in the pathogenesis of at least some psychiatric disturbances. One British study found that women who are depressed are likely to have lost a parent at an early age, to be relatively housebound with three or more children, and to lack a good confiding relationship with a spouse or other confidant. In that study, biological vulnerability to depression seemed less important than the accumulation of negative life circumstances in the development of the disorder. Persons who are ordinarily competent in all role functions may fall apart completely when a supportive spouse who has bolstered them and taken care of many of their needs suddenly dies. Patients with a depressive episode have often experienced uncontrollable actual and threatened losses, such as the death of a spouse in the year before the onset of the depression. Nevertheless, not all psychiatric disturbances are attributable to easily identified negative life events; indeed, some negative life events that at first glance appear to precede the onset of a serious psychiatric disturbance may, in fact, occur only after the onset of the disturbance. For example, someone who attributes the onset of depression to having been fired from a job several months previously may already have been functioning suboptimally at that time and have been fired as a consequence of a depression-induced decline in role functioning.

Some environmental features can counter the effects of environmental stressors and protect against breakdowns. Stable families, other social supports, and good financial circumstances offer some protection. Research has shown that persons with psychiatric disturbances have fewer social supports than do normal controls. That paucity of support may be due to friends' and relatives' withdrawal from deviant behaviors or to the disturbed person's withdrawal from deleterious family and social relationships. In contrast, physically ill persons have more social supports than do others, perhaps reflecting their ability to recruit help in times of need. Of course, the quality, as well as the quantity, of social supports is important. As has been shown in schizophrenia and mood disorders, for example, negative relationships, even in close families, may have deleterious effects both in initiating and in sustaining psychiatric disturbance.

The negative effects of a physiological or environmental stressor are closely related to its personal meaning. For example, the amputation of a cancerous breast is likely to be more distressing for a woman whose self-esteem is threatened by her physical disfigurement than to one whose self-confidence is secure.

CHARACTERISTICS OF PSYCHIATRIC SIGNS AND SYMPTOMS

Signs and symptoms form the two major categories of clinical phenomena. Classically, especially for most medical disorders, the distinction between the two is clear. Patients complain of symptoms—chest pain, headache, tingling sensations in the left leg. By their nature, *symptoms* are disturbances noted by patients that are not necessarily directly observable by another person. *Signs* are those abnormalities directly observed by an examiner, including those disturbances spontaneously observed in the course of meeting with a patient and those elicited through a physical examination.

Although the same demarcation between subjective symptoms and observable signs may be made in describing psychiatric phenomena, the line between the two is often blurred. For instance, many phenomena often considered to be symptoms of a psychiatric disorder may not be regarded as complaints by patients. A feeling of harmony with the universe may be a manifestation of a psychotic disorder, yet the patient may vigorously dispute that the experience is a symptom of any psychopathological condition. In addition, psychiatrists often consider auditory hallucinations as signs of a psychotic disorder, even though the hallucinations are subjective, internal experiences and, therefore, classically noted as symptoms. Further complicating the distinction is the tradition of inferring many psychological mechanisms—such as the classic mechanisms of defense, which are not themselves directly observable—from the presence of certain signs and symptoms.

Signs and symptoms are said to be present when the limits of normal variability are surpassed. For those qualities that can hypothetically be plotted on a continuum, those limits constitute a boundary beyond which the experience is defined as pathological and may involve the number of hours of sleep, the intensity of anger, and the extent of mood lability. Abnormalities may manifest as alterations in amplitude (such as excesses or deficits), duration, intensity, timing, and modifiability of physiological events, perceptions, emotions, thoughts, and motor activities. For other experiences the distinction between normal and abnormal is qualitative, not quantitative. In mainstream American culture, for instance, any experience of thoughts being broadcast out loud is considered pathological. For all signs and symptoms, however, exactly what constitutes normal varies from culture to culture and from context to context. A behavior or subjective experience that is defined as symptomatic in one context may be perfectly acceptable and within normal bounds in another context.

Within cultures but not across cultures, most behaviors evident in interpersonal interactions are carefully regulated by tight sets of rules and controls and are constrained by reasonably well-defined sets of expectations and acceptable limits. When observable behaviors deviate even slightly from the acceptable limits, that is quickly sensed by lay persons, as well as by professionals; because deviance is often perceived as threat, observers usually notice the deviance readily. Deviations in amplitude, duration, and intensity can occur in facial expressions, gestures, postures, vocalizations, language, and other expressions of emotion and thought. A small increase in the rate of speech, an intrusion into one person's conversation by another who does not allow proper pauses, a gesture that comes just a bit too close to a face, an excessively rigid or distant stance, or a gaze that is too staring or too avoidant—each signals social insensitivity and alerts the observer to deviant behavior.

RELIABILITY PROBLEMS Among the core difficulties in psychiatric evaluation is the fact that multiple observers may note different symptoms or may interpret signs differently when interviewing the same patient. Those discrepanices may be due to (1) differences in the observers' understanding of the symptoms or signs in question, (2) differences in information imparted by the patient, and (3) differences in interpreting the patient's responses to general presentation or questions within the interview. Those three types of reliability problems are called *criterion variance, information variance,* and *observation bias.*

Although research studies show that interrater reliability can be achieved for most symptoms of Axis I disorders, that may not hold true for personality disorders or for some specific symptoms. Furthermore, the demonstration of interrater reliability means only that consistent results may be obtained in optimal circumstances and may not reflect common clinical practice at all. To illustrate, a recent study showed the poor reliability among a diverse group of psychiatrists in distinguishing between bizarre and nonbizarre delusion, a central concept in diagnosing schizophrenia in the revised third edition of *Diagnostic and Statistical Manual of Mental Disorders* (DSM-III-R). In part because of the unreliability of that distinction, the importance of bizarre delusions is deemphasized in the diagnostic criteria for schizophrenia in the fourth edition of DSM (DSM-IV).

Even when simply responding to direct questions about symptoms, patients may respond differently, depending on how the questions are asked, their personal sense of trust or safety, whether they have answered those questions before, the amount of cuing that may signal the desired response, their fatigue, and a host of other variables.

Beyond the elicitation of symptoms and the notation of clear abnormalities in physical appearance and mental status, most clinicians still rely heavily on their own subjective responses to patients as part of a diagnostic assessment. Unfortunately, those clinical inferences, whether accurate or not, are often based on nonconscious assumptions, comparisons with other patients not well remembered, or distortions of the clinician's own personal experiences. When used correctly, intuitions can be identified and described clearly; simple trust based on faith is not sufficient. Thus, a clinician's sense that a patient is angry and potentially violent may result from the patient's subtle but verifiable body language and tone of voice, or it may be a countertransference distortion that is not prompted by signs from the patient.

When clinicians' subjective responses are used in a sloppy or inappropriate manner, contextual and cultural considerations are often ignored. Appropriateness depends heavily on context, and what is proper in a given context may be highly subjective. Appropriate behavior or dress in California may be inappropriate in Boston. A low intensity of emotional expression leading to a clinical description of constricted affect may reflect cultural norms or a psychopathological state.

NONSPECIFIC NATURE OF SIGNS AND SYMPTOMS

Until psychiatry discovers reliable diagnostic tests to define clinical syndromes, the field will continue to construct diagnostic categories based on the clustering of signs and symptoms within specific time frames. With that type of nosology, the presence of pathognomonic signs and symptoms—those characteristics that are specific for the disorder in question and that are seen only in that disorder and in no others—at least allows some diagnostic certainty. Unfortunately, no such symptoms exist; all psychiatric symptoms must be regarded as nonspecific—seen in a few and, more likely, many disorders. Depressed mood, for example, is seen in a multitude of disorders in a wide variety of diagnostic groups, including major depressive disorder, schizophrenia, some personality disorders, and mood disorder due to a general medical condition. Even Kurt Schneider's first-rank symptoms of schizophrenia are nonspecific in their diagnostic meaning; they are seen with some frequency in otherwise classic depressive and bipolar disorders.

In general medicine, symptoms not recognized as part of a clearly defined syndrome are described as being of unknown origin. Thus, a fever not associated with a disorder known to elevate temperature, such as pneumonia, is described as a fever of unknown origin. In view of the nonspecific nature of psychiatric symptoms, it seems wise to use similar appellations—such as hallucinations of unknown origin and depressed mood of unknown origin—for symptoms that cannot be clearly documented as part of a larger well-described syndrome.

Even though individual signs and symptoms may be organized into syndromes and disorders, they often have courses of their own. In the appearance or the resolution of a disorder, certain associated signs and symptoms may appear early and persist after all the other signs and symptoms have waned. In some cases certain signs and symptoms commonly associated with a given disorder may fail to appear. Each sign and symptom may have its own pattern and variability of response to treatment. In the treatment of schizophrenia, for example, some patients experience a rapid resolution of hallucinations but have persistent delusions without any other thinking disorder, whereas other patients have no residual hallucinations or delusions but still have a prominent thinking disorder. At present, no theory or approach consistently explains the dissociation of symptoms within a recognized disorder.

SYMPTOM CATEGORIES Symptoms have been categorized in a variety of ways: state versus trait, primary versus secondary, and form versus content. The state-versus-trait distinction refers to whether the symptom is an enduring characteristic of the person. Personality characteristics have *traitlike qualities,* but symptoms seen as part of a symptom-based Axis I disorder are typically *state-associated symptoms.* Some symptoms characteristic of symptom-based disorders can also be enduring traits. A person who, since childhood, has worried a great deal, tended toward catastrophic thinking, and been subjectively nervous in many environmental circumstances may be described as having trait anxiety. However, if the symptoms of anxiety are present only during a specific time, such as over a nine-month period in conjunction with a full depressive disorder, they are best described as state-related symptoms. It is unwise to infer the presence of enduring trait characteristics, such as personality traits, during the acute stages of a psychiatric disorder with dramatic state characteristics. The diagnosis of dependent personality traits based on an acutely depressed patient's behavior is often incorrect. Similarly, manipulative behavior in the midst of a hypomanic or manic episode should not be considered evidence of an enduring manipulative trait unless the behavior is also evident when the mania has clearly resolved.

Distinctions between primary and secondary symptoms have been hampered by varying definitions of those terms. The distinction may refer to causality, temporal sequence, or inability to reduce the symptoms to a clearly understood origin. Basing the distinction between *primary* and *secondary* on *causality* implies that cause and effect are understood. In attention-deficit hyperactivity disorder, for instance, the attention deficit is thought to be primary, and the hyperactivity is thought to be secondary, caused by the inability to attend. Patients with severe dependent personality traits and chronic demoralization only after many incapacitating psychotic mood episodes may be described as having a primary mood disorder and a secondary personality disorder. Conceptual models of psychopathology in which signs and symptoms are seen as restitutive, ineffective attempts to cope with an underlying problem use a primary-secondary model. For example, Eugen Bleuler viewed thought disorder as a primary symptom in schizophrenia and viewed hallucinations and delusions as secondary symptoms, formed to help the patient cope with the chaos of the primary symptoms. Those models must be viewed only as hypothetical constructs and used with great caution, since, in the vast majority of clinical phenomena, little evidence indicates that one symptom is more primary than another.

Temporal sequence is regularly used as the basis for deciding the primacy of certain symptoms, behaviors, and disorders when substance abuse occurs in conjunction with depression or anxiety. Unfortunately, establishing temporal sequence with any certainty is typically difficult, and its usefulness in establishing appropriate treatment plans is uncertain.

Those symptoms that cannot be further understood as being due to *underlying conditions* have been described as primary. Thus, the experiences of hallucinating and having delusional ideas may be regarded as primary, and the delusional content—such as paranoid ideation involving powerful punitive male strangers that is linked with early fears of a sadistic father—may be considered secondary.

CONTEXT Signs and symptoms are not necessarily static entities; they may vary in intensity or even in their existence, depending on the context. The depressed mood in a melancholic depression may persist in all situations, but the depressed mood in a mild depression may vanish completely during certain situations, including the psychiatric interview, only to reappear at another time. Symptoms that occur only in specific settings or with certain internal states are referred to as *state-dependent.* For example, some hallucinations or memories may be present only during drug or alcohol intoxication; in some patients, hives erupt as a psychophysiological response only during states of anger. Interpersonal context is also important. Some persons become violent only when involved in sadomasochistic relationships or in certain group settings, such as adolescent gangs. In gangs, social pressures for conformity and expectations of aggressive behavior may provoke or release pathological behaviors that may otherwise never be expressed by gang members individually.

NEED FOR A COMPREHENSIVE PERSPECTIVE A psychiatric disorder may be characterized by disturbances involving a wide variety of areas in the patient's life, including the biological, psychological, behavioral, interpersonal, and social spheres. Figure 10-1 illustrates some of the issues associated with each of those dimensions. In practice, common psychiatric syndromes often manifest in each of those dimensions (Table 10-1). Viewing the patient from many perspectives, referred to as the biopsychosocial model (similar to the multiaxial approach of DSM-IV), reminds clinicians to consider psychopathology and its effects on a patient's life in the broadest possible manner. Table 10-2 lists some clinical hypotheses commonly used by clinicians as they link collections of signs and symptoms into syndromes and consider the treatment options that logically follow.

Because the amount of information gathered in a thorough assessment of a psychiatric disorder is potentially overwhelming, the clinician often tends to limit the fields of vision and to appreciate only part of the available information; the clinician's theoretical orientation and other personal and cultural factors also limit what is perceived. Research has shown that clinicians tend to perceive primarily the signs and symptoms that are most in accord with their theoretical points of view and with the tools they have available to treat psychiatric disorders, a phenomenon known as *concept-driven perception.* The theoretical biases of clinicians seem to be related both to the microcultures of their training programs and to their own personality traits. Such differences may lead one clinician to see a major mood disorder, to be treated with medication, where another sees a pervasive personality disorder with dysthymia, to be treated with psychotherapy; the two use different technical terms to label roughly the same phenomena. A psychodynamic psychiatrist may see psychomotor retardation where a neuropsychiatrist sees bradykinesia; a psychodynamicist may see depressed affect and muted speech where a neuropsychiatrist sees masklike facies and aprosody; a psychodynamicist may see ruminative thought where a neuropsychiatrist sees forced thinking; a psychodynamicist may see a grimace where a neuropsychiatrist sees a tic. Words themselves help shape the concepts of reality, so the consequences of using those different labels for similar phenomena may be significant. Figure 10-2 illustrates concept-driven perception, in which each clinician who adheres to a prominent contemporary point of view perceives only some of

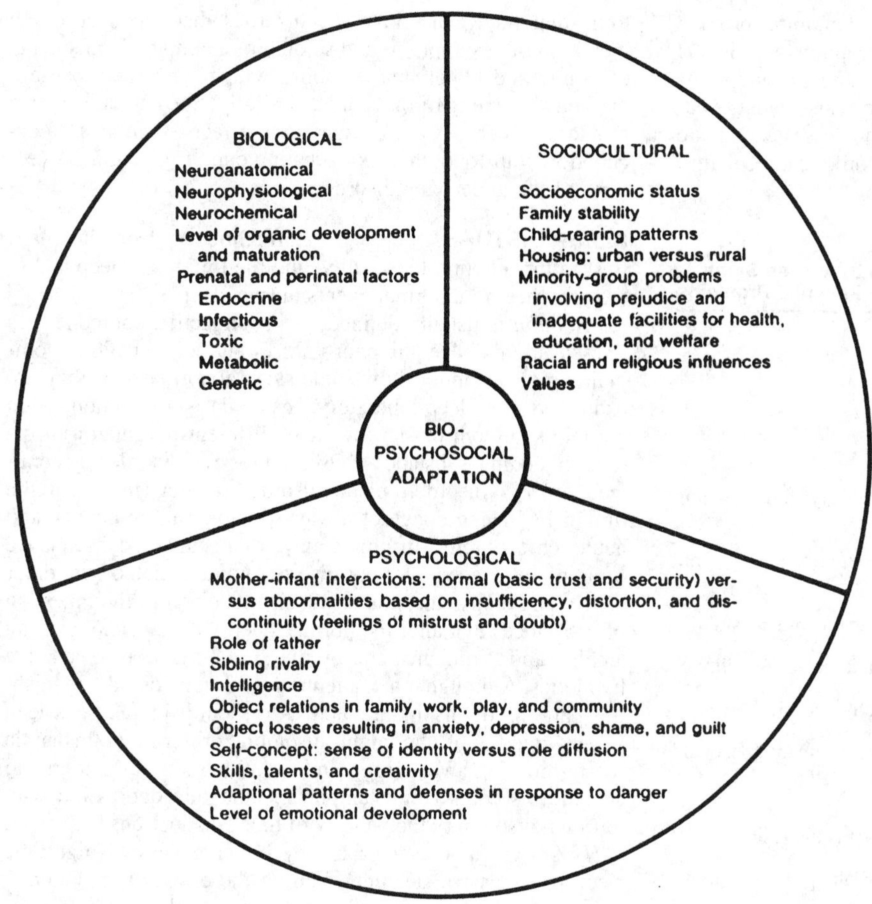

FIGURE 10-1 *Biological, psychological, and social forces interact and affect the psychiatric health of a person. (Modified after J B Richmond, S L Lustman: Total health: A conceptual visual aid. J Med Educ 29: 23, 1954. Used with permission.)*

TABLE 10-1
Biopsychosocial Features in an Illustrative Syndrome of Depression

Biological	Psychological	Behavioral	Interpersonal and Social
Current vegetative symptoms Anorexia Weight loss Constipation Impotence Sleep disturbance Diurnal variation in mood Diminished libido *Laboratory* Postive dexamethasone-suppression test Decreased REM latency *History* Seasonal variation in syndrome Similar syndrome in identical twin Treatment with antihypertensives	*Current* Depressed mood Apathy Guilt Low self-esteem Hopelessness Suicidal thoughts Delusions of having sinned Slow thinking *History* Early death of father Repeated defeats in business, school Lifelong crotchety temperament	Paucity of movement Occasional agitation Drinks more alcohol than usual Buys a pistol Irritable and withdrawn Elicits sympathy from children Elicits criticism and hostility from spouse Refuses medication	Stops working Avoids family Has burdensome financial problems Recent death of friend Disengages from major role functions as spouse, parent, member of community Shuns caretakers and interested members of community Faces pending litigation Has responsibility for aging mother

the potentially available phenomena related to a psychiatric disorder. Although there is overlap, each observer also perceives information not appreciated by the others. At the same time, all the observers may miss some information that may be highly relevant in diagnosing or treating the disorder. Clinicians 100 years from now will, no doubt, be able to detect and understand the significance of signs and symptoms not appreciated by anyone today.

For all those reasons—the intermittent nature of many psychiatric signs and symptoms, the potential unreliability of patients in reporting symptoms, differing interpretations of elicited information and observations, and subjective theoretically driven biases that influence the clinician's perception of signs and symptoms—complete assessment of a psychiatric patient requires consultation with family, friends, coworkers, and other professional observers to supplement the history and to provide observation of the patient over time.

SOMATIC MANIFESTATIONS OF PSYCHIATRIC DISORDERS

Most psychiatric disorders and virtually all Axis I, symptom-based disorders are characterized by disturbances in at least some basic physiological functions. Although frequently nonspecific in nature, the somatic signs and symptoms provide markers as to the amount of biological disruption seen in the disorders that cause them. Furthermore, the somatic symptoms not only reflect the underlying disorder but can also cause exacerbations of the disorder. If untreated, the processes can create destructive feedback loops in which the disorder causes symptoms that then exacerbate the disorder that then causes an increase in the symptoms and so on. For example, the insomnia of manic and hypomanic episodes will, if untreated, cause a marked worsening of the mania; similarly, the weight loss seen in anorexia nervosa causes starvation effects, such as a preoccupation with food, thus exacerbating one of the hallmark features of the underlying disorder.

TABLE 10-2
Common Current Clinical Hypotheses Used to Assess Signs and Symptoms: Ways of Understanding the Patient's Problems

Biologically derived hypotheses
1. As an organic mental disorder
2. As a mood disorder
3. As a nonaffective functional psychosis
4. In relation to the abuse of drugs or alcohol
5. As a disorder other than those listed in 1 through 4, above

Psychodynamically derived hypotheses
1. As being related to personality style
2. As being related to a precipitating event and its dynamic meaning
3. As a manifestation of unresolved grief
4. As a developmental crisis
5. As being related to ego functioning and related psychodynamic issues

Socioculturally derived hypotheses
1. As resulting from the nature and the social effects of stressful life events
2. As being related to the extent, the nature, and the accessibility of social support
3. As being related to definitions of and responses to breakdown in the sociocultural grouping
4. As being related to the patient's motivation, treatment goals, and the dynamics of the entry process to help seeking
5. As social communication

Behaviorally derived hypotheses
1. As disordered thinking, feeling, or acting that is the result of specific antecedent events
2. As disordered thinking, feeling, or acting resulting from reinforcing consequences of the behaviors
3. As disordered thinking, feeling, or acting in response to sociocultural and biological events
4. As a deficit of behaviors (rather than as disordered behaviors) in the areas of thinking, feeling, and acting
5. By an analysis of areas of effective functioning

Table adapted from A Lazare: Hypothesis testing in the clinical interview. In *Outpatient Psychiatry: Diagnosis and Treatment,* A Lazare, editor, p 131. Williams & Wilkins, Baltimore, 1979. Used with permission.

SLEEP DISTURBANCES Abnormalities of sleep may manifest in the amount, the quality, and the timing of sleep and in the presence of abnormal events during sleep.

Insomnia is usually defined by its subjective component as the sensation of sleeping poorly. Most but not all patients complaining of insomnia show some sleep abnormality if they are examined in a sleep laboratory. Insomnia is a common, often chronic symptom or sign of many different psychiatric disorders, including substance abuse, depressive disorder, generalized anxiety disorder, panic disorder, mania (in which the diminished sleep does not always provoke a complaint), and acute schizophrenia. Insomnia may also occur as a consequence of aging or as a symptom or disorder not associated with other psychopathology. Insomnia may also result from the ingestion of substances that alter the normal sleep-wake cycle, including alcohol and stimulants, and by the discontinuation of sedative hypnotics. Although much attention is often paid to distinguishing patterns of insomnia, such as difficulty in falling asleep versus middle of the night insomnia or terminal insomnia (early-morning awakening), and to linking specific patterns to specific disorders (for example, melancholic depression with terminal insomnia), the validity of those distinctions is unclear.

Hypersomnia, characterized by either excessive nighttime sleep or excessive sleepiness during the day, is less common than insomnia. However, hypersomnia may also reflect a number of pathological states. Some depressed patients, especially those with a history of mania or hypomania, may exhibit hypersomnia. Hypersomnia may also be seen during stimulant withdrawal, during the excessive use of sedatives or tranquilizers, and in conjunction with a variety of medical disorders. In *narcolepsy* the patient had sudden attacks of irresistible sleepiness, a symptom that may be part of a broad syndrome that includes

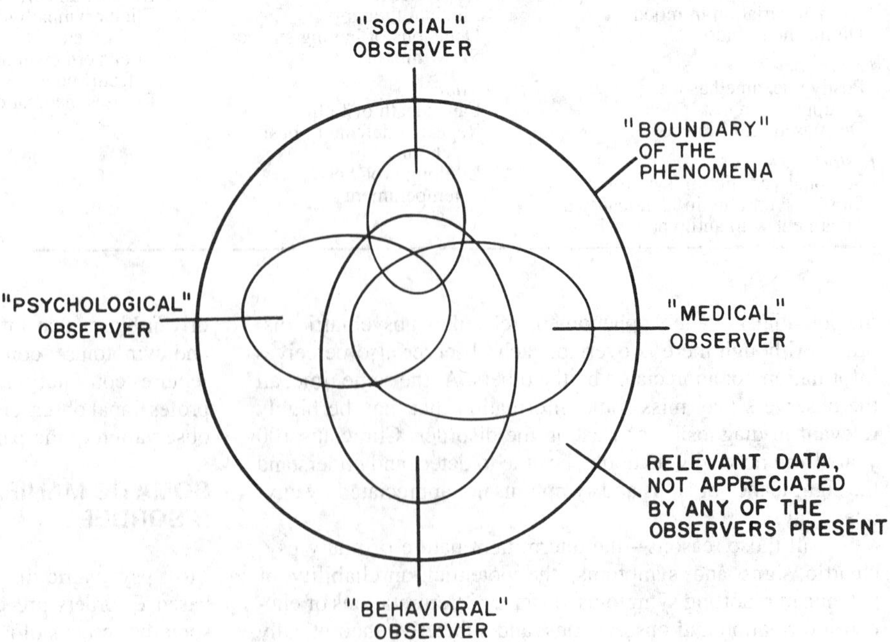

FIGURE 10-2 *Clinical data processed by four observers with different theoretical orientations. (From J Yager: Psychiatric eclecticism: A cognitive view. Am J Psychiatry* 134: *736, 1977. Copyright 1977, American Psychiatric Association. Used with permission.)*

cataplexy (sudden attacks of generalized muscle weakness, leading to physical collapse in the presence of alert consciousness), *sleep paralysis* (waking from sleep with a sensation of being totally paralyzed that may persist for minutes), and *hypnagogic hallucinations* (vivid visual hallucinations that occur at the point of falling asleep). Narcoleptic attacks are often precipitated by unusual states of arousal (for example, cataplexy may immediately follow unrestrained laughter or orgasm). Daytime sleepiness may reflect *sleep apnea.* In that disorder, typically middle-aged patients have periods of severe snoring, often first reported by their bed partners, and periods when breathing stops. The condition results from soft-palate abnormalities that cause intermittent airway obstruction throughout the night; patients wake repeatedly to find themselves gasping for air. Associated daytime fatigue is common in sleep apnea. Periodic hypersomnia also occurs in the *Kleine-Levin syndrome,* a condition typically affecting young men, in which periods of sleepiness alternate with confusional states, ravenous hunger, and protracted sexual activity. Intervals of days, weeks, or months may pass between episodes. *Sleep drunkenness* is characterized by excessive sleep and great difficulty in awakening completely, with confusion and motor incoordination experienced soon after rising. Excessive daytime sleepiness may also occur secondary to abnormalities in the brain stem, the hypothalamus, or the thalamus.

Somnambulism (sleepwalking) and *sleep terror disorder* (night terror) are two sleep disorders characterized, respectively, by aimless wandering with incomplete arousal and by acute anxiety and physiological arousal without awakening. Although both disorders typically begin in childhood, sleepwalking may be be initially precipitated by some psychotropic medications.

An obese 35-year-old woman, who was attempting to diet, experienced sleepwalking episodes in the middle of the night. Her roommate observed her go to the refrigerator and eat whatever was available, including raw flour and uncooked grains. The patient was sound asleep during those episodes. Her mother reported a history of sleepwalking since early childhood.

Sensory symptoms during sleep, typically described by patients as peculiar feelings in their legs that cause an irresistible need to move around, are characteristic of *restless legs syndrome.* The motor abnormality of repetitive myoclonic jerking of the legs, awakening both patients and their partners, is known as *nocturnal myoclonus.*

APPETITE AND WEIGHT DISTURBANCES Aside from the anorexia of medical illnesses, especially in their late stages, *loss of appetite* is most commonly seen in depressive disorders, grief, and primary anorexia nervosa and is also commonly seen in conjunction with significant anxiety. Anorexia is often accompanied by changes in taste (for example, foods begin to taste different, bitter, or flat or have an unpleasant aroma). *Hyperphagia* (increased appetite) occurs in some depressed patients, both those with and those without a history of mania or hypomania, and in binge-eating episodes characteristic of bulimic syndromes. Increased appetite may be seen, albeit rarely, in some hypothalamic disorders and in bilateral temporal lobe dysfunction, such as the Klüver-Bucy syndrome, in which it occurs in association with emotional placidity, hypersexuality, hyperorality, and other symptoms.

ENERGY DISTURBANCES Normal energy levels vary considerably among people. Some persons fatigue easily and are perceived by themselves and others as having weak constitutions; others appear to have almost boundless energy and little need for sleep.

Fatigue is a common nonspecific symptom that occurs in both medical and psychiatric disorders. It is also frequently seen as an unexplained complaint in primary care practices; in one study 24 percent of patients complaining of fatigue received no medical or psychiatric diagnosis. Historically, fatigue not caused by another disorder, typically in association with ''nervousness,'' has been labeled asthenia, neurocirculatory asthenia, neurasthenia, and psychasthenia. Many fatigued patients, having been labeled depressed or neurotic by their physicians, are referred to psychiatrists after routine workups have ruled out anemia, hypothyroidism, sleep apnea, and other frequent somatic causes.

Recently, those patients with primary complaints of tiredness have most commonly been given the diagnosis of *chronic fatigue syndrome* (previously and incorrectly labeled Epstein-Barr viral syndrome), a disorder characterized by fatigue lasting months to years, typically beginning soon after a viral syndrome. In addition to the fatigue, the syndrome is characterized by myalgias and cognitive changes, such as forgetfulness and poor concentration. Controversy continues about the extent to which cases of chronic fatigue syndrome represent discrete postviral diagnostic syndromes, mislabeled cases of depression, or modern versions of psychasthenia.

DISTURBANCES IN SEXUAL DRIVE As with energy, the normal range of sexual drives is great. Some persons are naturally lusty, whereas others have limited sexual desire. Diminished sexual drive with impotence or decreased libido is seen in a wide variety of neurological, metabolic, and other somatic syndromes. Among neurological disorders, complex partial seizures are commonly associated with hyposexuality, occurring in 50 percent of patients. Psychiatric disorders known for diminished sexual drive include depressive disorders, schizophrenia, substance abuse disorders, and marital conflict. Diminished libido, impotence, and anorgasmia are also common sequelae of many pharmaceuticals, including psychotropic medications.

Increased sexual activity may be seen in some neurological drug-induced, and psychiatric disorders. Manic patients frequently exhibit hypersexual interests and behaviors to an unusual degree compared with their euthymic interests and behaviors. Hypersexuality is occasionally seen in conjunction with epileptic syndromes and in patients who have suffered diencephalic injuries.

Altered sexuality—including fetishes, sadomasochism, and pedophilia—may occur as isolated psychiatric syndromes. In persons whose previous sexual behaviors were within the bounds of social propriety for their groups, inappropiate sexual behaviors may signal early brain disease or psychosis.

APPEARANCE The effects of general physical appearance and body language are suggested by the fact that clinicians often formulate an initial psychiatric diagnosis within 30 seconds of seeing a patient. Although about half of those initial impressions prove to be incorrect, the remainder are validated by psychiatric histories and mental status examinations, revealing just how much information is communicated by appearance and body language.

Among the physical disorders that may be relevant to psychiatric conditions are acromegaly, Cushing's disease, Down's syndrome, systemic lupus erythematosus, fetal alcohol syndrome, Klinefelter's syndrome, and Wilson's disease, to name a few. The general appearance of the skin may suggest the presence of occult psychiatric problems. The general condition and flush of the skin may reveal hypervascularity and ruddiness suggestive of alcoholism, abscesses indicative of hypodermic needle abuse, tattoos indicative of certain group affiliations, and weathering and wasting indicative of self-neglect and malnutrition. Healed scars on the wrists and arms suggest a pattern of self-mutilation from depression or personality disturbance or both. Patchy baldness, especially in conjunction with torn or infected cuticles, indicates trichotillomania, a syndrome of compulsive hair pulling. Psychophysiological symptoms reflecting psychiatric disturbance include urticarial reactions and neurodermatitis, the latter resulting, in part, from self-excoriation, destructive scratching secondary to compulsions and unrelenting sensations of discomfort. The patient's odor may reveal lack of self-care, alcoholism, diabetic ketosis, or other conditions that have psychiatric manifestations.

Examination of the head and the neck may reveal exophthalmos or puffy eyelids suggesting thyroid disease, marked pupillary dilation with anxiety or stimulant abuse, miosis with narcotic abuse, abnormal pupillary pigments in Wilson's disease, salivary gland enlargement in bulimia nervosa, or necrosis of the nasal septum in cocaine abuse. Frequent sighing is a common respiratory sign in depression. Simple sighing must be distinguished from respiratory dyskinesia in psychotic patients who have been treated with antipsychotics. Respiratory dyskinesia may occur as an acute dyskinesia caused by antipsychotic medication, or it may be a late manifestion and component of tardive dyskinesia.

DISTURBANCES IN THINKING

NORMAL THINKING *Thinking* refers to the ideational components of mental activity—processes used to imagine, appraise, evaluate, forecast, plan, create, and will. Most thought involves complex algorithms that are currently not reproducible using the formal logical rules typical of computer simulations of thought. Studying or observing the process of thinking is difficult. Most of what is known about thinking derives from the study of language as the product of (and, therefore, a reflection of) thought. Yet, a great deal of thinking takes place preverbally and in modes other than those of ordinary language. Thinking occurs in images, music, kinesthetic sensations, and symbols other than linguistic ones. Attempts to transmit preverbal and nonverbal thought using only the narrow dimensions of words are often frustrating and unsatisfactory. Creative artists have considerable difficulty in describing the inner states of tension and inchoate awareness from which ideas are distilled.

Ordinary thought is far from logical. The stream of thought is intruded on, and attention is easily distracted. Conversation is marked by recurring asides, interruptions, delays, and loss of ideas. Decisions are often made on the basis of few cues and inadequate evidence: people jump to conclusions. Beliefs are zealously held that are not supported by evidence. Thinking in stereotypes is more common than thinking in logical categories. From an evolutionary perspective, thinking in stereotypes and by approximation has probably been more adaptive than thinking in strictly defined categories. The human tendency to think in stereotypes, rather than categories, accounts for clinicians' tendencies to make diagnoses by approximation and intuition and to feel less than comfortable using formal lists of criteria found in statistical manuals, such as DSM-IV.

Characteristic styles of thinking can be described while recognizing the mixture of styles found in most persons. A cognitive style attains pathological status only when it so dominates a person's repertoire that it interferes with adaptive responses to the normal variety of life events. An *obsessional* style of thinking is marked by attention to detail and great vigilance concerning the possible implications of a particular thought. It may take the form of preoccupation with strict adherence to established rules, values, or beliefs. An obsessional style may be highly adaptive in certain jobs and professions, such as librarians and computer programmers, that require meticulous detail-oriented behavior. However, excessively rigid obsessionality may be maladaptive, such as when a person rigidly adheres to rules even when such adherence is self-destructive and shortsighted for all concerned. A *hysterical* style of thinking is characterized by global, diffuse, impressionistic, emotionally laden evaluations of situations with a lack of attention to details and nuances. The style is poorly adaptive to detail-oriented work but may be useful in the arts and in certain sales positions.

Types of thinking Because of the different ways in which both normal and abnormal thinking expresses itself, differences that are apparent to even a casual observer, a number of authors have attempted to subtype thinking types, dividing thinking into the extent to which logical versus nonlogical thought is used. One common categorical system is Freud's division of thought into primary process and secondary process.

PRIMARY PROCESS Primary process thinking is the primitive type; it is used classically in dreams, but it is also prominent in young children and in psychotic states. Primary process thinking disregards logic, permits contradictions to exist simultaneously, disregards the linear notion of time, and is dominated by wish and fantasy. It uses symbol, metaphor, imagery, condensation, displacement, and concretism in its organization, creating the jumbled and incoherent style of thinking characteristic of dreams. Primary process thinking represents what has been metaphorically called right-brain thinking, which is associated with visual images and creative thought.

SECONDARY PROCESS Secondary process thinking is characterized by logic. In contrast to primary process thinking, the secondary process uses linear notions of time, clearly delineated abstract categories, and deductive rules of logic. The abilities to think abstractly and to think in detail about future plans are characteristic of secondary process thinking. Normal secondary process thinking is also characterized by predictability, coherence, and redundancy. In interpersonal communication, words, vocal inflections, and gestures that provide important contextual cues create a sense of overall coherence to the communication. Ideas follow one another in a sequence that is understandable to the listener.

OTHER TYPES OF THINKING A non-Freudian typology of thought divides thinking into three types: fantasy thinking, imaginative thinking, and rational or conceptual thinking. *Fantasy thinking* allows the person to escape from or to deny reality; it can be seen in both normal and pathological thinking. Everyone occasionally uses fantasy thinking when daydreaming. Slips of the tongue may also be construed as a form of fantasy in which, for a moment, the speaker denies the unpleasant reality and substitutes a different image. Some dissociative and psychotic phenomena illustrate the most pathological manifestations of fantasy thinking. *Imaginative thinking* merges fantasy and memory to generate plans for the present or the future. *Rational or conceptual thinking* uses logic primarily to solve problems.

SHIFTING TYPES OF THINKING Regardless of how one categorizes thought, people can consciously shift from linear-secondary process-rational thought to fantasy-primary process-nonlogical thought, as in the free-associative method used in psychoanalysis. During free association the patient willfully surrenders the controls that maintain secondary process thinking and switches to the less controlled modes of primary process thinking in which thoughts are loosely associated by emotional associations or are based on noncentral, concrete, coincidental, loosely similar, or trivial aspects of a thought. In addition, the fact that increases in primary process thinking can be induced in normal persons under experimental conditions and in fatigued persons suggests that more primitive thought processes, such as those seen in psychosis, may be release phenomena; that is, nonlinear or psychotic thinking may indicate the functional absence of those overriding control systems that ordinarily sift, evaluate, and regulate the form and the flow of thought before it reaches consciousness.

FLOW AND FORM DISTURBANCES Because the underlying processes that govern thought are not understood, current systems for classifying thought abnormalities are primarily descriptive. Conventional classification separates form and flow from the content of thought. Yet, many types of abnormal thinking include both form and content abnormalities. Although delusions are usually classified as thought content disturbances, they are also marked by form abnormalities, such as rigidity and imperviousness of thought.

Formal thought disorder typically refers to marked abnormalities in the form and flow of thought, but some clinicians use the term broadly to include any psychotic cognitive sign or symptom. Clinicians differ as to whether or not to classify delusions and hallucinations among the types of formal thought disorder.

As with other basic aspects of human functioning, such as energy and sexuality, the flow and the form of thought vary considerably. For some people, thinking appears to be effortless—rapid and productive, exhibiting linear and goal-directed thoughts and creativity, with digressions and occasional leaps but always controlled and comprehensible. Others experience thinking as a difficult exercise—a slow, painstaking process with low output compared with others or with scattered thinking, difficulty in staying on a topic or finishing a single thought. Of course, most people experience their own thinking as mixtures of those extremes.

Disturbances in the flow and the form of thought can be divided into those reflecting its rate, continuity, control, and complexity.

Rate Thinking can be unusually slow or accelerated. *Slowed or retarded thought*—for example, the slow thinking noted in depression—is typically goal-directed but characterized by little initiative or planning. Answers to direct questions may show a long latency of response. Patients experiencing retarded thought often describe feeling that even simple thought requires monumental effort, as if molasses were cluttering their thinking. *Thought blocking,* seen in schizophrenia, is experienced as a snapping off or a sudden break in a train of thought, as if a wall suddenly came down, interrupting thinking (and speaking) in midsentence. To an outside observer, thought blocking may appear identical to *thought wihdrawal,* a disturbance in the control of thought in which the patient feels as if some alien force had intentionally withdrawn the thoughts from consciousness. The patient's further description and explanation of the inner experience are necessary to distinguish the two symptoms.

Accelerated rates of thinking, typically accompanied by fast talking, can be seen as a normal variant. Rapid rates of speech, influenced heavily by cultural and situational factors, only sometimes reflect truly rapid thought. For example, New Yorkers, who characteristically speak more quickly than people from some other cities, may not actually think at a faster rate. Similarly, auctioneers speak with an astonishing rapidity, likely reflecting a learned psychomotor skill. *Pressure of speech*—speech that is rapid, excessive, and typically loud—is characteristic of mania and hypomania, stimulant intoxication, and occasionally anxiety. *Flight of ideas* occurs when the flow of thought increases until the train of thought switches direction frequently and rapidly. The associative links between conceptual topics during flight of ideas are comprehensible to the listener, although not without considerable effort. Listening to a flight of ideas that is not overwhelmingly fast can be both a dizzying and an enjoyable experience for the listener, as exemplified by the successful performance style of certain contemporary comedians, notably Robin Williams.

Continuity Disturbances in the continuity of thought may take several forms. In *circumstantiality* the flow of thought includes many digressive associations, often including a great deal of unnecessary detail. A transcript of circumstantial thought and speech is notable for the multiple commas, subclauses, and parenthetic asides. Nonetheless, in circumstantial thought the speaker eventually returns to the initially intended point without prompting from the listener.

In contrast, in *tangentiality* the person wanders away from the intended point, moving further and further away, never returning to the original idea. If asked, the person may not even remember the original point. The person who talks past the point (*Vorbeireden,* a form of tangentiality) never quite gets to the central idea. Tangentiality is a mild form of *derailment,* in which there is a breakdown in associations. *Loose associations* exemplify severe derailment, in which the flow of ideas is no longer comprehensible to the listener, since the individual thoughts seem to have no logical relation to one another. According to some theoreticians, loose associations are a hallmark feature of schizophrenia. In extreme cases the phrases and even individual words are incomprehensible, and syntax—the rules of grammar by which phrases are organized into sentences and words into phrases—may be disrupted. *Word salad* is the stringing together of words that seem to have no logical association, and *verbigeration* is the disappearance of understandable speech, which is replaced by strings of incoherent utterances.

Clang association is a sequence of thoughts stimulated by the sound of a preceding word. For example, a manic patient said, "I'll kill with a drill or a pill—God, I'm ill—what swill." In *echolalia* the patient repeats a sentence just uttered by the examiner. Repetition of only the last uttered word or phrase is called *palilalia,* a symptom found most often in chronic schizophrenia.

Perseveration and stereotypy are two other associative abnormalities in which the flow of thought and speech appears to get stuck. In *perseveration* a sentence or a phrase is repeated, sometimes several times over, after it is no longer relevant. Perseveration is commonly seen in delirium and other organic mental syndromes. *Stereotypy* is the constant repetition of a phrase or a behavior in many different settings, irrespective of context.

Schizophrenic patients sometimes describe *crowding of thought,* an experience in which thoughts are concentrated and compressed in their heads. The thoughts are rapid and confused and not under the patient's control. The experience seems to combine some features of flight of ideas with the disjointedness of derailment.

Control Disturbances in the control of thought include primarily delusional passivity experiences and obsessional thinking. In *delusional thought passivity* patients experience their own thoughts as being under the control of other forces. Some of Schneider's first-rank symptoms of schizophrenia are thought-passivity symptoms. Thought passivity may take several forms: in *thought insertion* thoughts are experienced as having been placed within the patient's mind from the outside; in *thought withdrawal* thoughts are whisked out of the mind; in *thought broadcasting* patients experience their thoughts as escaping their minds to be heard by others. Those experiences are often combined with specific delusions of control, seemingly to explain the passivity experiences.

During his first schizophrenic episode, a 21-year-old man maintained, with utter conviction, that his thoughts were not his own and that his mind was like a freeway in which thoughts seemed to come and go quickly, without any control on his part. Initially, he would not answer any questions, explaining at a later date that, since he was sure his questioners could hear all his thoughts, he interpreted their questions as redundant and mocking. Still later, he had the unshakable delusion that his thoughts were being controlled by Satan as a test of his ultimate worthiness.

Obsessional thinking is stereotyped, repetitive, persistent thinking that is recognized as one's own thoughts. In contrast to patients with delusional thought passivity, obsessional patients do not experience their thoughts as being controlled by outside forces. Nonetheless, the patients experience only partial control over the obsessional thoughts. They can, with great effort, stop thinking the obsessional thoughts but cannot prevent them from recurring. Characteristic of obsessions are the subjective experience of compulsion, the resistance to it, and the preservation of insight. As bizarre as some obsessions are, patients know that the thoughts are irrational and are their own. At times, obsessions are pervasive enough to dominate the patient's consciousness. Obsessions may be simple, such as a sequence of words, or elaborate, such as enumerating the possible consequences of a past behavior and elaborating a cascading sequence of typically catastrophic events.

A 32-year-old woman with a mild viral syndrome picked up a carton of milk in the supermarket and then returned it to its shelf, deciding not to buy it. Over the next few days, she spent increasing amounts of time thinking about that act. She could not stop herself from thinking that the mother of a young child picked up the same container, contracted the patient's virus, and gave it to her child, who may then have gotten ill and died as a result of a fulminant infection. Despite knowing how extremely unlikely that sequence of events was, the woman could not step replaying the scenario in her mind.

Obsessional thoughts are usually seen in conjunction with compulsive behaviors, rituals linked to the obsessions that are typically constructed to undo the effects of the thoughts. Compulsive behaviors are discussed further below.

Complexity The most prominent disturbance of thinking complexity is that related to impaired capacity to think abstractly. Abstract thinking is the ability to assume a mental set, to keep simultaneously in mind all the aspects of a complex situation, to move from feature to feature as indicated by the situation, and to abstract common properties. Normal persons vary greatly in their abilities to engage in abstract thinking; geniuses in mathematics and theoretical physics leave most mortals far behind. *Concrete thinking* is a disturbance in the ability to form abstract concepts, generally illustrated by literal-mindedness and the inability to abstract the commonality of members of a group—for example, the fact that a flea and a tree are similar in that they are both living things. Concrete thinkers seem unable to free themselves from the literal or superficial meanings of words. Concrete thinking can be seen in persons with low intelligence, organic mental disorders, and schizophrenia. Schizophrenic patients may also exhibit highly selective disturbances of abstraction.

DISTURBANCES IN THOUGHT CONTENT The normal content of thought—the buzzing, booming stream of consciousness that constitutes the stuff of everyday life—is composed of awareness, concerns, beliefs, preoccupations, wishes, and fantasies occurring with various degrees of clarity, vividness, differentiation, imagination, and strength. Normal thought is often illogical, containing many beliefs and prejudices that, although they clearly contradict one another, are nevertheless held with passion and conviction.

Belief systems are the scaffolding of thought, chains of impressions and expectations around which plans and behaviors are organized. Belief systems may be attitudinal, setting general expectations and biases about the world that inform how incoming information is processed; examples are optimism, pessimism, and paranoia. Some beliefs are effervescent and fleeting; others are pervasive, tenacious, and influential. Some beliefs are unique and private; others are shared by another person, a family, or a society.

Imaginative fantasy is an important component of normal thought, starting in earliest childhood. The vivid, eidetic imaginations of young children can produce vivid fantasies in which children become fully immersed, almost as if in hypnotic states. During latency many children create imaginary companions as playmates. In later years such imaginative thinking may be the essence of the creative reverie. Artists, writers, and creative scientists retain access to those forms of thinking more readily than do others. Meditative states of mind may facilitate the emergence of imaginative insights. Such thinking may also occur in dreams. Intrusive reveries are normal and common components in the usual adult stream of consciousness. During periods of specific deprivations, such as starvation, elaborate wish-fulfilling daydreams frequently occur.

Contents in the stream of thought that are consistent with a sense of self, compatible with the person's self-image, are called *ego-syntonic*. Other thoughts that appear just as naturally may be at variance with a person's central values and may seem *ego-alien* or *ego-dystonic*. An ego-dystonic impulse to kill someone, inconsistent with one's predominant value systems, may generate a counteractive ego-syntonic thought, such as, "You really don't mean it."

Abnormal beliefs and convictions form the core of thought content disturbances. In intensity of conviction, distorted beliefs range on a continuum from overvalued ideas to the intense, unshakable belief that is characteristic of fixed delusions. Abnormal beliefs and delusions are, in most circumstances, diagnostically nonspecific. Delusions are commonly seen in mania, depression, schizoaffective disorder, dementia, substance-abuse-related syndromes, schizophrenia, and delusional disorders.

Overvalued ideas are unreasonable and sustained abnormal beliefs that are held beyond the bounds of reason. Patients with overvalued ideas have little or no insight into the fact that their ideas are unlikely to be valid; however, the ideas themselves are not as patently unbelievable as most delusions. The distorted body images of body dysmorphic disorder exemplify overvalued ideas. Morbid jealousy, in which someone is preoccupied with a spouse's possible infidelity, may constitute an overvalued idea if the person dwells on scanty shreds of potential evidence, constantly looking for clues, in the absence of clear information that an extramarital affair occurred.

Ideas of reference are false personalized interpretations of actual events: persons believe that occurrences or remarks refer specifically to them when, in fact, they do not. Some authors consider ideas of reference to be less firmly held beliefs than are delusions.

A psychotic young man enlisted in the army immediately after seeing a billboard poster of Uncle Sam pointing his finger toward him, saying, "Uncle Sam wants you." The man was convinced that Uncle Sam was directing his recruiting plea directly and solely toward him, and he felt compelled to oblige.

Delusions *Delusions* are fixed, false beliefs that are strongly held and immutable in the face of refuting evidence and that are not consonant with the person's education and social and cultural background. Delusionsal thoughts can be understood or evaluated only with at least some knowledge of patients' interpersonal worlds, such as their involvements with religious or political groups. One of the mind's primary functions is to generate beliefs, including myths and meaning systems. Those beliefs provide the person with a sense of personal and group identity and with ways of understanding reality. They are most noticeable when shared untestable beliefs form the basis for group cohesion, as in religions and cults. Some groups adhere to their cherished beliefs despite the abundance of plausible contrary evidence; for example, some fundamentalist sects take the biblical creation story literally. In the face of contrary evidence or grave personal threat, persons often cling to their primary beliefs as matters of faith—that is, as alternative, nonrefutable bases for understanding. The strong faith with which religious, political, and nationalistic convictions are held, even at the cost of death, shows the power that untestable beliefs can have on behavior.

Subjectively, delusions are indistinguishable from everyday beliefs. Therefore, the subjective experience of being delusional is no different from the subjective experience of believing that the earth is round or that one's spouse is the same person one married on their wedding day. Because of the identical experiences of delusions and consensually held beliefs, it is impossible to argue a patient out of a delusional belief.

The content of delusions is highly influenced by culture. Whereas centuries ago delusions of persecution often concerned persecution by the devil and had religious connotations, persecutory delusions today more often take on political and social perspectives.

An 18-year-old man went to an emergency room with the belief that he was controlled by a computer on board an Enterprise-like starship, an elaboration from the television series *Star Trek*. He was convinced that all his thoughts, actions, and feelings were being programmed on board the starship, which was located light years away and, therefore, could never be detected by anyone else.

An electrical engineer felt that his brain was actually that of a robot, a fancy piece of equipment. He drew up blueprints illustrating just how the mechanism worked through detailed circuitry. The fact that no such equipment was visible on X-rays of his head in no way dissuaded him, because he knew that the wiring was much too fine to be detected by mere X-rays. The patient's delusion appeared, disappeared, and reappeared, depending on how much he complied with treatment. The psychosis responded well to antipsychotic medications. During remissions he functioned well, except for an isolated life-style, and totally denied the existence of the delusional beliefs, saying that the whole thing was a bad dream. When he stopped taking his medications, the full-blown delusional system returned, identical from one episode to the next. The sequence resembled a repetitive dream or what would be expected if the delusion were a state-dependent belief.

TYPES OF DELUSIONS Although delusions are diagnostically nonspecific, some specific types of delusions are more prevalent in one disorder than in another. For example, although delusions of control and delusional percepts were listed by Schneider as first-rank symptoms of schizophrenia, those delusions are also seen, albeit less frequently, in psychotic mood disorders. Similarly, classic mood-congruent delusions—with grandiose themes seen in mania and delusions of poverty characteristic of depression—may also be seen in schizophrenia.

Table 10-3 lists some characteristics by which delusions have been classified. *Simple delusions* contain relatively few elements, whereas *complex delusions* may contain extensive elaborations of people, spirits, motives, and situations.

A man with chronic schizophrenia revealed the simple delusion that his ultimate mission in life was to raise the dead to herald the coming of a New Age. He denied ever seeing signs in his environment that referred to that mission, nor did he have auditory hallucinations telling him about it. The delusion persisted as an isolated psychotic symptom during long quiescent phases of his disorder and was also seen during his schizophrenic exacerbations, at which times the patient also had many other complicated and bizarre psychotic ideas. During the chronic phases of his disorder, the patient worked at low-level jobs and had a few ongoing but superficial relationships. The patient's behavior in no way revealed the presence of his delusion.

Systematized delusions are usually restricted to well-delineated areas and are ordinarily associated with a clear sensorium and an absence of hallucinations. They are often isolated from other aspects of behavior. In contrast, *nonsystematized delusions* usually extend into many areas of life, and new data—new people and situations—are constantly incorporated to further support the presence of the delusion. The patient usually has concurrent mental confusion, hallucinations, and some affective lability. Whereas the patient with a closed systematized delusional system may go through life relatively unperturbed, the patient with a nonsystematized delusion frequently has poor social functioning and often behaves in response to the delusional beliefs.

An agitated inpatient was convinced that the Federal Bureau of Investigation (FBI) was following and attacking him. Although he gradually accepted the good intentions of the ward staff members, at one point he became upset, and the ward staff members had to restrain him. He suddenly turned and with a frightened start said, "Ah, now I realize that you're all part of the FBI."

Complete delusions are those held utterly without doubt. In contrast, *partial delusions* are those in which the patient entertains doubts about the delusional beliefs. Such doubts may be seen during the slow development of a delusion, as the delusion is gradually given up, or intermittently throughout its course.

A young man with schizophrenia, a college dropout who could work only part-time at low-level jobs and who lived with his high-achieving family, believed he was the Messiah. When his psychosis exacerbated, he was fully convinced that his struggles and lack of occupational success were merely God's tests until the patient's true identity would be revealed. As he improved from an episode, he would, if asked, say that he was God's chosen but, when questioned further, would admit the slight possibility that he was wrong. On reaching his best clinical state, he would muse on the possibility that he was the Messiah but state that he was not sure. With every new exacerbation of the disorder, the partially held belief again became a complete delusion.

Delusions have also been divided into primary and secondary forms. Unfortunately, authors have used those terms in a variety of ways, so the distinctions are confused in the literature. According to one definition, *primary delusions* are those that are not further understandable in terms of the patient's context, such as culture or mood. In that framework a mood-congruent psychotic delusion with themes of worthlessness or guilt is a considered a *secondary delusion*. According to a different definition, primary delusion refers to and is synonymous with *autochthonous delusion*, a delusion that takes form in an instant, without identifiable preceding events, as if full awareness suddenly burst forth in an unexpected flash of insight, like a bolt from the blue. Those delusions may be elaborate.

A 17-year-old boy, characteristically an isolated loner, came to the dinner table one evening and announced that he had to leave home and climb Mount Everest in order to save the world. That knowledge came to him instantaneously, in a moment of sudden illumination. He denied that anything in particular had been troubling him beforehand, and his family had observed no recent changes in his behavior. He had never before had any interest in mountain climbing or altruistic pursuits.

Aside from the autochthonous types, three other types of delusions have been described as primary. *Delusion percept* refers to the experience of interpreting a normal perception with a delusional meaning, one that has enormous personal significance to the patient. If, in the example of the authochthonous delusion given above, the need to climb Mount Everest had occurred in response to seeing a picture of a mountain in the newspaper, the experience would represent a delusional percept. *Delusional atmosphere* or *delusional mood* is a state of perplexity, a sense that something uncanny or odd is going on that involves the patient but in unspecified ways. Ordinary events may take on heightened significance; the delusional interpretations are fleeting, but the uncanny feeling stays. Typically, after a period of time, full-blown delusions develop, replacing the delusional mood. *Delusional memory* is the memory of an event that is clearly delusional. For example, a patient "remembered" that his fourth-grade teacher slipped lysergic acid diethylamide (LSD) into his apple juice; that memory served to explain his psychotic disorder.

Patients vary considerably in the extent to which they take action in response to delusional thoughts. Just as patients can experience delusions of their thoughts being controlled (thought passivity), they may similarly experience their feelings, behaviors, and will as controlled by outside forces. Those *delusions of control* (or passivity experiences) occasionally (but uncommonly) result in dramatic self-destructive or aggressive behavior, as illustrated by the murderer who called himself Son of Sam. That psychotic killer murdered a series of people in New York and claimed that he was the powerless agent of a force that required him to commit the acts. Some patients may take bold and occasionally destructive actions on their own initiative in efforts to protect themselves or others from delusionally anticipated events.

Table 10-4 lists some classic types of delusions. Although less common than those involving paranoia, grandiosity, and influence, delusions of misidentification are prominently

TABLE 10-3
Characteristics of Delusions

Simple versus complex
Complete versus partial
Systematized versus nonsystematized
Primary (autochthonous) versus secondary
How they affect behavior

TABLE 10-4
Some Classic Types of Delusions

Delusions of persecution
Delusions of grandeur
Delusions of influence
Delusion of having sinned
Nihilistic delusions
Somatic delusions
Delusion of doubles *(Doppelgänger)*
Delusional jealousy (Othello syndrome)
Delusional mood
Delusional perception
Delusional memory
Delusions of erotic attachment (Clérambault's syndrome)
Delusions of replacement of significant others (Capgras's syndrome)
Delusions of disguise (Frégoli's phenomenon)
Shared delusions (folie à deux, folie à trois, folie à famille)

reported because of their inherently intriguing nature. In *Capgras's syndrome* the patient believes that someone close has been replaced by an exact double. In *Frégoli's phenomenon* strangers are identified as familiar persons in the patient's life. In the *delusion of doubles,* patients believe that another person has been physically transformed into themselves.

A 29-year-old woman with schizophrenia repeatedly accused her psychiatrist of switching people in her life. During one week she was convinced that he switched her college professor with an identical-looking double; the next week she was sure that her boyfriend had been switched. The psychiatrist's motive, according to the patient, was to mock and confuse her. Whenever the multiple Capgras's phenomena became too overwhelming, the patient changed her psychiatrist, whereupon the same delusions recurred with the new one.

Delusions are seen not only in isolated persons but also in couples *(folie à deux)* and in families *(folie en famille).* Many psychiatrists consider group delusions to be present in some cults as well, but exactly where the cutoff points occur between delusions and other zealous beliefs held by large, traditional, and well-organized religious and political groups is arguable.

DISTURBANCES OF JUDGMENT

Judgment involves a complex and diverse group of mental functions that includes analytic thinking, social and ethical action tendencies, and depth of understanding or insight. *Analytic thinking* includes the capacity to discriminate and to weigh the pros and cons of potential alternative actions. *Social and ethical action tendencies* are closely related to cultures and upbringing. The evidence for genetic factors in antisocial personality disorder (which is defined primarily by judgments that lead to criminal behaviors) points to the additional role of constitutional factors. *Insight* may reflect intelligence, learning, and cognitive style.

Impairments of judgment occur in many psychiatric disturbances. Anxiety states, intoxications, fatigue, and even group pressures may cause temporary impairments of judgment in otherwise normal persons. Organic brain damage and psychotic disorders may chronically impair any aspect of judgment in any person, regardless of premorbid character. Poor role models and deviant social backgrounds may lead to social and ethical action tendencies quite different from those of the examiner. Thus, someone raised in a criminal environment may have superb analytic judgment and self-awareness, which are, however, put to illegal use.

Judgment may be impaired in one dimension and spared in others. Persons may retain sound ethical judgment when their analytic capacities fail or may retain excellent analytic abilities for nonpersonal matters while lacking insight into personal situations or behaviors. Some persons who can provide socially appropriate responses to traditional mental status examination questions about what one would do in a movie theater if fire broke out or what one would do with a stamped and sealed addressed envelope found in the street may at the same time be incapable of accurately assessing crucial clinical issues related to their capacity to provide informed consent, such as the pros and cons of receiving a medication or electroconvulsive therapy, or to have insight into their own states of health or illness. The apocryphal story about the delusional patient able to accurately evaluate and fix a broken-down car that had stymied the mechanics, ending with the patient's declaring, ''I may be crazy, but I'm not stupid,'' indicates the selective nature of poor judgment within psychiatric disorders. Judgments about personal situations relevant to adaptation are clearly the most important to evaluate.

The term ''insight,'' usually in the context of self-awareness, has been used in a variety of ways. Basic *insight* refers to a superficial awareness of one's situation—for example, that one is ill. A deeper level of insight is operating when the patient has an intellectual appreciation of what is going on—for example, ''I have hallucinations and delusions, and my doctors have told me that I have schizophrenia and must take medication.'' Still deeper levels of insight reflect more complete cognitive and emotional appreciation of a situation—for example: ''I realize that I have schizophrenia, that it impairs my judgment and social function at times, and that I will have to take medications if I am to minimize my symptoms and try to make the most of my life. I feel profoundly disappointed about this affliction, because it prevents me from achieving some of the goals I've always wished for. Nevertheless, I have do my best to get over my disappointment and hurt feelings so that I can get whatever I can out of life.''

DISTURBANCES OF CONSCIOUSNESS

Consciousness can be defined as awareness of the self and the environment. If it were not for consciousness, biological organisms could probably be understood, more or less, as self-regulating automata, perhaps ultimately as elegant computers or robots. However, consciousness—as an emergent property of complex biological nervous systems, as a poorly understood property of an even more mysterious and complex universe, or as a property understandable only in religious and spiritual terms—remains unexplained and, at least from a scientific point of view, as yet unexplainable.

The term ''consciousness'' can be considered from both qualitative (such as the experiences of altered states) and quantitative viewpoints. Qualitatively, consciousness does not seem to be an all-or-none phenomenon. Even with that division, however, consciousness is far too complex to be easily categorized. In pathological states, remarkable properties of consciousness are seen—for example, coconsciousness and multiple consciousness, indicating its nonunitary nature.

Experiments involving patients with commissurotomies of the corpus callosum have shown the existence of two virtually separate systems of consciousness that seem to operate side by side. For example, when in the course of a dull experiment the picture of a nude woman was flashed only to the right brain (the left visual field) of a commissurotomized patient, the patient verbally denied being aware of anything unusual but started to squirm and blush, remarking, ''Oh, you have some machine!'' Similarly, when a cup was presented to the right brain only, the patient denied seeing anything but was able with the left hand to pick out the cup from an assortment of objects. That literal splitting of verbal awareness from visual-spatial awareness in the brain produces behavior that is at least superficially similar to that of patients who deny being consciously upset by an event but who have visceral responses. Although the formulation is simplistic, the separate consciousness for logical-verbal awareness and for spatial-visual awareness demonstrated in split-brain experiments may be crude analogues for highly differentiated and discrete types of awarenesses and modes of information processing. Furthermore, the fact that there are separate and to some extent competing modes of consciousness may increase the likelihood of psychological distress, because the two modes of consciousness are capable of yielding internally conflicting views of reality.

PSYCHOLOGICAL AND PHYSIOLOGICAL FACTORS In ordinary states of alert consciousness, persons are able to deploy adequate amounts of attention to their surroundings and to reflective thought. Normal persons vary enormously in their ability to pay attention in different settings without being distracted; individual variations may reflect differences of temperamental and cognitive styles.

A sense of increased consciousness—with heightened alertness, awareness, and thinking—may be experienced in states of high arousal for threat. Increased consciousness may also be seen in conjunction with certain emotional states, such as falling in love, and in certain situations, such as an athlete's playing in a championship game and an actor's performing in a play. Yet, alertness-arousal and awareness as two components of consciousness may be altered in opposite directions. For example, anxiety and other states of excessive emotional stimulation can simultaneously produce intense alertness-arousal and distractibility with reduced attention span. By contrast, illness and fatigue diminish the sense of alertness and attentiveness, thereby diminishing consciousness.

Consciousness involves, among other things, the experience

of a continuous environment in time and space and of a sense of self. The experience of time and its passage may be altered by shifts in the level of awareness and by emotional states, such as boredom, concentration, pain, and discomfort. The experience of time and space may be altered by hypnosis, marijuana, and psychedelic drugs.

DISTURBANCES IN LEVEL OF CONSCIOUSNESS *Levels of consciousness* (that is, alertness, awareness, and attentiveness) may be pathologically increased or decreased. Both types of change are diagnostically nonspecific and can occur in many different disorders. When pathological levels of arousal are mild, as in hypomania and after small amounts of psychostimulants are ingested, the subjective experience is typically positive, with intense alertness, prolonged concentrating ability, and hyperesthesia, in which perceptual phenomena are heightened—colors are brighter, and sounds are sharper than usual. With further increases in arousal and consciousness—as seen in mania, severe intoxications with amphetamines and cocaine, and catatonic excitement—attention fragments, heightened alertness transforms into paranoia, and the hyperesthesia becomes unpleasant.

Diminished levels of consciousness can be described on a continuum. *Clouding of consciousness* is marked by diminished awareness of sensory cues and diminished attentiveness to the environment and to the self. Secondary process thinking is most notably compromised, and primary process thinking emerges into consciousness. The level of consciousness may fluctuate rapidly in relation to the internal physiological state or to the degree of external stimulation. In alterations of consciousness, confusion may occur, with disorientation to time, place, or person. The patient is usually highly distractible and unable to pay attention to a single stimulus.

Torpor is a condition in which the patient is drowsy, falls asleep easily, and shows a narrowed range of perception and slowed thinking. *Stupor* is a state of diminished consciousness in which the patient remains mute and still, although the eyes are open and may follow external objects. In the most extreme impairment of consciousness, *coma,* the patient shows no evidence of mental activity at all. The patient appears to be functioning on a decorticate or decerebrate level. In *akinetic mutism* or *coma vigil,* patients with profound brainstem lesions appear to be awake with their eyes open, but, in fact, they show no evidence of consciousness.

Delirium, the acute confusional state, is usually characterized by a relatively abrupt onset and a short duration of clouded, reduced, and fragmented attention; impaired memory and learning; perceptual and cognitive abnormalities, such as hallucinations and delusions; disrupted sleep; and other autonomic dysfunctions. The level of consciousness may be consistently diminished, or it may fluctuate. The electroencephalogram (EEG) usually shows diffuse slowing. Typical motor abnormalities include an increase in general restlessness, fine and coarse tremors, and myoclonic jerks. Autonomic disturbances commonly include tachycardia, fever, elevated blood pressure, diaphoresis, and pupillary dilatation. The causes of delirium are legion, including such systemic medical disorders as metabolic imbalances and infections; intracranial disorders caused by traumatic, structural, and electrical causes; drug intoxications; and withdrawal states.

ALTERED STATES OF CONSCIOUSNESS Consciousness may also be qualitatively changed with the production of altered states. Drugs, such as scopolomine, with strong central anticholinergic properties; some seizures; and, on occasion, other conditions associated with delirium can induce *twilight states,* dreamlike states of wakeful consciousness in which attention is poor, a mixture of primary and secondary process thinking appears, and patients fade in and out of alertness. Dreamlike experiences intrude into the stream of conversation. Emotional outbursts or violent acts may occur during twilight states.

Mystical states of consciousness may occur in normal and pathological conditions. Intense meditation and peak or epiphanic experiences, reported by more than 10 percent of normal persons in community surveys, may produce a sense that the self dissolves or expands, that the self fuses mystically with the cosmos, that time stops, and that universal meaning becomes clear. Those perceptions may be accompanied by a sense of rejuvenation and renewed personal identity, ineffability, intense emotionality, and concurrent perceptual changes. Such experiences do not ordinarily last more than a few minutes. Many people have reached those states through the use of psychedelic agents, such as mescaline and LSD.

Hypnosis Although hypnosis lacks a consensually accepted definition, its hallmarks are selective attention, suggestibility, and dissociation. Most but not all persons can be hypnotized to some degree, and up to 90 percent of persons are capable of achieving a light trance, with 10 to 20 percent capable of entering a deep trance and exhibiting remarkable hypnotic phenomena. Hypnosis occurs when a person is in a state of heightened, not diminished, attention. EEG studies have shown hypnotized persons to be fully awake and alert. The heightened concentration probably accounts for the unusual levels of sensory and motor performance often seen under hypnosis and self-hypnosis.

Hypnotic phenomena include hypnotic anesthesia, sustained motor behaviors and acts of strength ordinarily beyond the person's capacity, and distortions of memory (both hypermnesia and amnesia). Several phenomena that reveal the multiple nature of consciousness—for example, coconsciousness—are also demonstrable. Experiments have shown that—even when a person in a deep trance has achieved profound hypnotic anesthesia and can, for example, keep a hand submerged in ice water for longer periods of time than usual—part of the hypnotized person's consciousness continues to register exactly how painful the experience actually is and can signal the researcher about the pain—for example, by finger movements—without the person's having any conscious awareness or disturbance. That phenomenon, called the hidden observer, has also been seen in postsurgical patients who, in a hypnotic trance after surgery, are able to recall conversations in the operating room that occurred while they were under general anesthesia. Dissociative and psychosomatic phenomena have also been induced with hypnosis. Posthypnotic suggestion, for example, can prompt persons to carry out complex actions, without any hint that they are doing so, because of previous hypnotic instructions. It has been suggested, not entirely facetiously, that many normal daily activities are conducted in a trancelike posthypnotic state; although those activities are attributed to conscious intention, they may, in fact, be carried out because of previous suggestion. Urticaria (hives) can be hypnotically induced and made to disappear. When plantar warts have been successfully treated with hypnosis, hypnotically induced diminished blood supply to their bases has been demonstrated. Yoga masters can exert remarkable control over basic bodily functions through self-hypnosis. As yet, little is known of the full extent to which heightened concentration may influence physiological regulation.

SUGGESTIBILITY Pathological suggestibility is seen in several clinical conditions. Automatic obedience has been described in *echolalia* (the automatic repetition of a sentence or a phrase just uttered by another person), *echopraxia* (the automatic mimicking of a movement performed by another person), and *waxy flexibility* (maintaining for a prolonged period of time a posture in which one is placed), symptoms common in catatonic states. In situations of group delusions and sometimes in cults, passive persons adopt the delusional beliefs of strong persons. In epidemic hysteria, as beautifully described among young women at the Salem witch trials in Arthur Miller's *The Crucible,* distorted and even delusional perceptions and beliefs may sweep over a group that has been highly aroused by a charismatic leader.

DISSOCIATIVE PHENOMENA *Dissociation* is the splitting off from one another of what are ordinarily closely connected behaviors, thoughts, or feelings. *Dissociative states* are those in which disturbances or alterations in the normally integrated functions of identity, memory, and consciousness appear; the states include trances, fugues, blackouts, multiple personalities, and dissociative frenzies. Although dissociative states are ordinarily thought to be functional in nature, they occur regularly with a variety of neurological disorders, particularly those with partial complex seizures. In one series one third of the patients with complex partial seizures had dissociative phenomena, including multiple personality. In those patients the dissociative phenomena were related not to the seizure activity but to interictal alterations.

As occurs in *posthypnotic amnesia* (that is, a phenomenon in which a person cannot recall events or instructions that occurred during hypnosis), elaborate activity can occur in dissociative states, and the person has no memory for what transpired during the trance state. That amnesia is functional in nature and can be reversed by hypnosis or drug–facilitated disinhibition—for example, with amobarbital (Amytal) infusion. In many of the functional dissociative states, amnestic episodes may occur for years or decades before the patient seeks medical or psychiatric attention. *Blackouts* are periods of amnesia in alcoholism or other intoxications or after a head trauma. An alcoholic blackout period may last for hours or days, after which the person has no recollection of what transpired, although other observers attest to the fact that, during the blackout, the person carried out many complicated behaviors. Memory of the blackout is lost to the predominant consciousness, but reintoxication may awaken memories of what happened during the previous blackout, indicating that memories registered during the blackout may be state-dependent.

Psychogenic fugue is characterized by sudden, unexpected travel away from customary locales, with the assumption of a new identity and amnesia for the person's past. By definition, psychogenic fugue cannot be due to a neurological disorder. In comparison, the discontinuity of experience in *psychogenic amnesia* is typically more circumscribed and does not involve assuming an entirely new identity. The dissociated memories and affects often reveal themselves in disguised form, such as nightmares, intrusive visual images, and conversion symptoms. Typically, psychogenic amnesia follows major catastrophic events—such as traumatic, gruesome combat—or less momentous events that a person prefers to forget, in order to preserve self-esteem, by denying some shameful, immoral, or illegal activity.

A 22-year-old soldier returning from Vietnam claimed to have no memory of his last month in combat. He had been assigned to a squad conducting a long-range patrol; only three of eight soldiers returned alive. Through repeated amobarbital interviews conducted in a supportive setting, gradually and with much emotion he recalled that his squad had been ambushed, that early in the firefight he had killed two or three 12- or 13-year-old Vietnamese boys who were in the attacking group, and that at a certain point he turned and ran away, leaving one or two of his wounded buddies behind, pleading with him to help.

Automatic behavior *Automatic behaviors* are complicated activities, such as writing and speaking, carried on during supposed trance states without awareness of what one is doing. Case records describe many long and creative works presumably produced by persons in states of automatic behavior. For example, *Course in Miracles*—a complicated, esoteric, widely read quasipsychological Christian spiritual tract—is said to have been written by a Jewish psychology professor from New York who perceived that she was ordered in a trance state one day to take down the book in dictation. On occasion, automatic behaviors have resulted in intellectual or artistic achievements of a quality far above the previously demonstrated capacities of the person. In one famous case an undistinguished piano teacher in the Midwest started falling into trances and wrote entire symphonies in the manner of major 18th- and 19th-century composers—works of artistic invention that were far beyond her usual talents and what anyone imagined she could produce. Although suspicion of fraud surrounds some of the reports, enough cases have been sufficiently well documented to substantiate the existence of automatic phenomena.

Dissociative identity disorder *Dissociative identity disorder* (formerly called multiple personality disorder) is a chronic, dissociative state in which two or more separate, ongoing identities or personalities alternate in consciousness. It usually occurs in persons who, as young children, were severely and repeatedly brutalized. The number of identities is variable, with some reported cases of 26 or more identities. The development of dissociated alter identities is thought to be a last-ditch psychological defense against an inescapable and unbearable traumatic situation. The identities may be of different ages and even of different sexes. Typically, the presenting identity is a dysphoric, anxious, constricted character who may suffer headaches and periods of blackout or amnesia and who is not aware of the other identities. A second identity is commonly vivacious and uninhibited. Other common identities are children, those who claim to know about all the others, and a depressed identity.

Ganser's syndrome The hallmark of *Ganser's syndrome* is that the patient responds to questions by giving approximate or patently ridiculous answers. For example, in answer to the question "What sound does a dog make?" the patient answers, "Moo." Additional features of the syndrome include alterations in consciousness, hallucinations (or pseudohallucinations), conversion phenomena, and amnesia for the episode during which the symptoms were manifest. It is generally thought to be a dissociative state, although organic features may contribute to the syndrome.

Depersonalization and derealization *Depersonalization* is an alteration in the experience and the awareness of self, leading to feelings of being unreal, of being detached from one's own body, of feeling like an automaton; it is often accompanied by a complaint of lacking all feelings and sensory experiences. *Derealization*—denoting similar changes in awareness of the external world, instead of the self—often accompanies depersonalization. Transient episodes of depersonalization and derealization occur frequently in normal persons, particularly in states of fatigue, sleep deprivation, and during acute distressing situations, such as bereavement and learning of a terminal diagnosis. Pervasive depersonalization states are typically unpleasant, ego-dystonic, and difficult to describe, especially since they are not accompanied by psychotic thinking. Those experiencing depersonalization often assume it is the harbinger of true psychosis and frequently fear that they are going crazy. Because of that fear, patients often endure depersonalization experiences for long periods before describing them to a mental health professional. Depersonalization is also characterized by frequent internal, inaudible dialogues between the participating self and the observing self but with full awareness that both parties are the same person (a feature that distinguishes depersonalization from hallucinations). Mild sensory distortions but not hallucinations are commonly associated with the experience. Depersonalization is seen in a variety of neurological and psychiatric disorders and is common in complex partial seizures. It may occur in the context of depression, anxiety disorders, and certain personality disorders, or it may occur as an entity by itself.

A 37-year-old man with a history of early childhood deprivation and chronic anxiety and dysphoria described a long and pervasive feeling of unreality. He described looking in a mirror and wondering why he looked so normal, since he felt so estranged from his body and his life. Although he was not anhedonic, the feeling of distance kept him from feeling truly alive. His relationships suffered because he constantly experienced an inner voice commenting on what was happening when he was with others. He worried continually that he was going crazy and that he would lose control of his behavior because he felt disconnected from it. Nonetheless, he always behaved appropriately, never lost control, and showed no signs of psychosis. Neurological evaluation revealed normal brain function, and extensive psychological testing found no evidence of psychotic thinking but did show significant symptoms of depression and anxiety.

DISTURBANCES OF THE SELF As the most basic level the key components of self-awareness are the *reality* and the *integrity* of the self (that I am one person), the *continuity* of self (that I am the same person now that I was in the past and that I will be in the future), the *boundaries* of self (that I can distinguish between myself and the rest of the world as not-self), and the *activity* of self (that it is *I* who is thinking, doing, feeling). Additional components of a sense of self include body image and various self-evaluations, including self-esteem and ego-ideal (ideal self). *Body image* is a person's mental representation of his or her own body. *Self-esteem* is thought to reflect how one measures up to the desired self-image. To the extent that what one sees in oneself approximates what one would like to be, self-esteem is positive. *Ego-ideals* are fantasies of the optimum person one could ever wish to be. Any of those qualities may be disturbed in psychiatric disorders.

Disturbances of the basic elements of self-awareness are seen in a variety of disorders. *Discontinuity* phenomena are characteristic of dissociative states, such as psychogenic amnesias and psychogenic fugue. *Depersonalization* reflects a mild disturbance in the awareness of self as the agent of activity. More severe disturbance is characteristic of the psychotic passivity phenomena seen in schizophrenia. *Boundary disturbances* may be considered characteristic of all psychotic states, regardless of diagnosis.

Disorders of self-integrity are characteristic of both multiple personality disorder and severe borderline personality disorder, in which a person's self-concept and the expression of that concept to others are erratic, leading to a sense of unstable identity. The *as-if personality* typically adopts characteristics of those who are particularly important to the person or characteristics that the person believes would at the moment please them. In adopting those characteristics, the as-if personality does not appear to be acting but experiences and manifests the assumed traits in a genuine and enduring manner, at least for a while. A change in relationships and situations usually prompts the as-if personality to discard previously held traits summarily and to assume new ones that better fit in with the new circumstances. Woody Allen's movie *Zelig* provides a caricature of the phenomenon.

Patients with pseudologia phantastica and the imposter syndrome show extreme examples of inconsistency in the sense of self. In *pseudologia phantastica* the patient compulsively spins out webs of lies, ordinarily self-aggrandizing ones. In the *imposter syndrome* such fantasies are acted out by liars and imposters, who seem to wish fervently that the fantasies they portray were their reality, as if they cannot accept themselves and would be overwhelmingly ashamed to be known for who they actually are. The imposter compulsively adopts the identities of others and may, for example, show up properly attired at diplomatic functions and society galas and interact with the other guests under an assumed identity. Some famous imposters have repeatedly insinuated themselves into inner circles of high society and government.

Body image may be realistic or distorted. Those persons who were overweight as children often persist in thinking of themselves as fat during their entire adult lives. Emaciated patients with anorexia nervosa may perceive themselves to be fat. Since a great deal of self-esteem is tied up in body image, many persons spend considerable effort in attempts to perfect their bodies and in attending to its adornment. *Phantom limb* phenomena are hallucinations of lost body parts. Those phenomena may result from the brain's persistent sensory expectations of stimulatory input from the missing parts, just as neural supersensitivity states follow drug withdrawals and denervations.

Transsexualism is a syndrome characterized by the feeling that one was born into a body of the wrong sex and marked by the desire from an early age to be a person of the opposite sex. Male-to-female transsexualism is reported more often than female-to-male transsexualism. Psychodynamic and biological theories have been advanced to explain the unusual phenomena.

Negative self-esteem is characteristic of depressive disorders, many personality disorders, and situational failures. Superficially inflated self-esteem is seen in mania and hypomania and, in a fluctuating manner, in narcissistic and other personality disorders.

Although some persons regard the ego-ideal as unattainable and are content to live as imperfect human beings, others strive to approximate the ideal. When that goal transcends into a demand or a driven insistence to become one's perfect self, the person is likely to be chronically dysphoric and to have poor self-esteem, since the task of becoming the ideal is doomed to failure.

Disorders of will Central to the sense of self is the concept of will or volition. Since an exact definition of will and its specific manifestations have been among the central issues debated in philosophy and religion for millennia, even the bare outlines of the debate are impossible to set down here. Psychologically, will is linked to the concept of intentionality. Will has been described as the mental agency that transforms awareness and knowledge into action, as the bridge between desire and act. For persons to manifest normal will, they must be aware and must feel desires, and those desires must arise from within themselves. Concepts related to will that may become the focus of clinical attention when disturbed include motivation and decision making—that is, the capacity to make choices.

Pathologically *heightened will,* seen primarily in manic states, is characterized by excessively intense desires and an overly facile capacity to make decisions, with complex questions being decided in an instant. With heightened psychological energy, the person can start new courses of action with astonishing rapidity. A close look at those symptoms, however, reveals that the presumably heightened will, in fact, shares much in common with decreased will, in that the intense desires and quick decisions do not reflect enduring desires or thoughtful decisions as much as they do impulsiveness, which can be considered an escape from true willing and decision making.

A *diminished sense of will* can be seen in a variety of Axis I and Axis II disorders. In schizophrenia one type of volitional disturbance is manifested by passivity phenomena, which may affect thoughts, feelings, and behaviors. Schizophrenia is also characterized by certain core components of the disorder, described as negative or deficit symptoms. The symptoms characteristic of deficient willing include lack of drive, a blunted capacity for feelings, impersistence at tasks, and a general inner flatness. Depressed patients also describe volitional disturbances, as in their general apathy and anhedonia, with decreased attention to people and activities that were previously interesting and pleasurable to them. Motivation decreases for both simple and complex activities in depressions.

A severely depressed man described how he sat in a chair all day long. In explaining why he did not get up even to make a cup of coffee (which he acknowledged he would enjoy), he answered: "You can't imagine the effort it would take to get up. I just can't be bothered with it."

In obsessive-compulsive disorder both the obsessive thoughts and the compulsive rituals are experienced as ego-dystonic and not consonant with the patient's conscious desires and will. Similarly, although patients with anorexia nervosa initially have the conscious experience of willing and controlling their intake of food, during the course of the disorder the sense of willfulness is replaced by one of passivity, of being subjugated by obsessional thoughts and compulsive behaviors that assume control of the eating behavior.

A woman with anorexia nervosa felt as if she were under the watchful eye of harsh, critical beings. Whenever she transgressed by eating more than she felt they would allow her on a given day, ordinarily 200 or 300 calories, she had the irresistible urge to harm herself by taking handfuls of laxatives. She felt that, if she refused to take the laxatives to eliminate excess calories and to punish her transgression with severe abdominal cramps and diarrhea, she would go crazy.

The disturbances of volition that are common in personality disorders are common complaints of patients presenting for psychotherapy. Persons with dependent personality disorder are characterized by difficulties in making decisions by themselves and often engage in courses of action contrary to their own desires. Similarly, persons with passive-aggressive personality disorder obscure their own desires by being excessively involved in the demands made by others. Their courses of action do not reflect their own decisions so much as the thwarting of others' desires. Persons with obsessive-compulsive personality disorder use inflexible rules, thereby precluding courses of action based on independent evaluation, desires, and decisions. In other situations they are indecisive, sometimes making impulsive decisions at the last minute when forced to decide.

Many patients seek treatment because of self-designated disturbances of willing: they do not know what they want. Often, that lack of will masks a fear of wanting and its attendant consequences. The symptom may reflect a number of other problems—for example, the fear of making a mistake and the fear of others' being angry or abandoning them if their wishes are known.

Disturbances of orientation Orientation is the person's awareness of time, place, and person. Accurate orientation requires the integrity of attention, perception, memory, and ideation. Impairments occur primarily in organic mental disorders, such as structural and toxic metabolic brain abnormalities, and occasionally in dissociative states.

Normal persons vary tremendously in their attention to the details of *time* and in the extent to which their bodies automatically keep time. Some persons have reliable built-in clocks by which they can awaken themselves at precise times or gauge the passage of time with uncanny accuracy, even in the absence of external cues—in a psychotherapy session, for example. Others have difficulty in making judgments about time and may be pathologically late or may habitually schedule more activities than can ever be accomplished in the time available. Benign disorientation to time is common. After a few days in a hosptial bed, most persons do not know exactly what the day or date is because they are not attending to or receiving their usual cues.

Pathological time disorientation can be mild or severe, with inaccuracies of estimation ranging from days to years. The dates reported by disoriented persons may have personal significance, such as those of important births, marriages, and deaths.

Because spatial cues are generally more available and obvious than temporal cues, disorientation to *place* often signifies a greater degree of cognitive impairment than disorientation to time and, therefore, rarely occurs in the absence of time disorientation. Disoriented persons may know, more or less, the type of place they are in without knowing the specific place; patients may recognize that they are in *a* hospital without being able to name *the* hospital.

A 42-year-old alcoholic man in delirium tremens, examined in a California hospital in the 1980s, was asked the date and where he was. He replied: "I'm standing on a street corner in Kansas City in 1966 minding my own business. Why don't you mind yours!"

Disorientation to *person,* a lack of awareness of one's own identity, is usually seen only in advanced dementias, such as primary degenerative dementia of the Alzheimer's type, and in dissociative states. In organically induced postconcussion amnesia, transient global amnesia, and psychogenic fugue states, knowledge of one's own identity may disappear, and a person may remain unidentified for an indefinite period until the memory for self returns.

DISTURBANCES OF MEMORY

Memory is not a unitary phenomenon. Capacities to remember vary for the different senses and perceptions. One person may have a prodigious musical memory, with the capacity to remember and reproduce whole musical pieces after one hearing, but be incapable of remembering names or telephone numbers. Exceptionally detailed verbal memories have been associated with obsessional cognitive styles. When persons with extraordinary memories complain of memory loss, ordinary memory tests may be inadequate to detect their deficits, as their relative memory loss may have reduced their capacities to a point within the range of most normal people.

Memory functions are divided into three stages: registration, retention, and recall. *Registration* or acquisition is the capacity to add new material to memory. The material may be sensory, perceptual, or conceptual and may come from the environment or from within the person. For new material to be acquired, the person must attend to the information presented, it must then be registered through the appropriate sensory channels, and it must then be processed or cortically organized. Thus, for new visual information to be acquired, the visual senses (eyes, optic nerves) and the occipital cortex must function normally. *Retention* is the ability to hold memories in storage. Many neurons are thought to be involved in the storage of a specific memory, and reverberating circuits are thought to be formed in which memory traces are held by means of changes in proteins or synaptic connectivity or both. *Recall* is the capacity to return previously stored memories to consciousness.

Newly registered material is transferred incrementally from immediate memory to short-term memory to long-term memory. Immediate memory lasts for 15 to 20 seconds, short-term or recent memory for several minutes to two days (the time involved in new learning and its early consolidation), and long-term or remote memory for longer periods of time. Different physiological processes mediate each stage of memory. Processes that affect immediate or short-term memory often spare long-term memory. The process by which memories are transferred from short-term to long-term stores is unknown.

Disturbances in memory occur through the interruption of registration, retention, or recall.

DISTURBANCES IN REGISTRATION Registration and short-term memory retention are usually impaired in disorders that affect vigilance and attention, such as head trauma, delirium, intoxications, psychosis, spontaneous or induced seizures, anxiety, depression, and fatigue. A variety of other metabolic and structural brain disturbances can also affect short-term memory, particularly lesions affecting the mamillary bodies, the hippocampus, the fornix, and closely associated areas. Patients with impaired attention and concentration who have immediate recall may not be able to retain or recollect those items from short-term memory.

DISTURBANCES IN RETENTION The retention of memories is impaired in posttraumatic amnesia and in a number of cognitive disorders, such as dementia of the Alzheimer's type and Wernicke-Korsakoff syndrome. The latter, which ordinarily results from the chronic thiamine deficiency seen in alcoholism, is associated with pathological alterations in the mamillary bodies and the thalamus.

DISTURBANCES IN RECALL Disturbances in recall can occur even when memories have been registered and are in storage. At times, failure to recall may signify that the memory traces themselves have disappeared and are no longer retrievable. However, difficulties in recall can occur separately, as in the everyday event of forgetting the name of a person or object, only to spontaneously remember it hours or days later. In normal forgetting, remote events are less well remembered than recent ones, and important events are most vividly retained in memory. Under usual conditions, forgotten events can be recalled with prompting, associative memories, or other forms of stimulation, such as hypnosis. State-dependent memories are recall failures, which are reversed by reinstituting the context in which the memory was originally formed. A classic example occurs in alcohol-dependent persons who are unable to recall experiences that happened when they were intoxicated until their next episodes of intoxication, at which time the memories are recalled easily. Recall may also be dependent on mood states, such as mania.

During his most recent manic episode, a 48-year-old man with bipolar disorder had intense grandiose, psychotic ideas. He was convinced that he could control the traffic in Los Angeles by driving on certain freeways at specified times, willing others to leave the road. At night he would drive on mountain roads, seriously considering physically pushing other cars off the road. After the manic episode ended and during the depressive episode that immediately followed, he could recall virtually no details of his previous thought content while he was manic. Later, when euthymic, he remembered only a few hazy images. A year later the beginning of a new hypomanic period was heralded by the patient's spontaneously remembering and describing in great detail the psychotic plans of the previous episode.

Amnesia is defined in a variety of ways. Overall, it is a syndrome in which short-term memory and long-term memory are impaired within a state of normal consciousness. Thus, memory disturbances in delirium should, strictly speaking, not be considered amnestic syndromes. Amnesias may be anterograde or retrograde. *Anterograde amnesia* is the inability to register or learn new information (and, therefore, to form new memories) from the onset of an illness or a trauma and for some time thereafter; it follows head trauma, states of cerebral physiological imbalance, and drug intoxication. Patients who receive electroconvulsive therapy (ECT) frequently have anterograde amnesia during the course of the treatments; the amnesia gradually fades after some weeks. *Retrograde amnesia* is an impairment in recalling memories that were established before a traumatic event. The amnesia extends backward in time for variable periods. As memory is regained, the most remote memories usually return first. A patient originally amnestic for the three-month period before an accident may ultimately be left with amnesia for events only a day or an hour just before the accident. In organically caused retrograde amnesias, remote memories are usually intact, but amnesia exists for recent events. By contrast, in *psychogenic* (functional) *amnesia* the time periods of forgotten events may be spotty or selective.

Hypermnesia, characterized by unusually detailed and vivid memories, may occur in gifted persons, in association with obsessive-compulsive and paranoid personality traits, and in hypnotic trances. Although many forgotten memories can be recalled in a hypnotic trance, retrospective falsification and distortion may also occur under hypnosis. (Memories recalled under hypnosis are usually not accepted as evidence in court.) Retrospective falsification of memory is called *paramnesia,* also known as *fausse reconnaissance.* In *confabulation,* another common form of paramnesia, the patient fills in memory gaps with inaccurate information. The responses given to questions by patients who confabulate may reflect past experiences or bizarre, fantastic stories—for example, stories involving spaceships and alien creatures. Confabulation correlates poorly with memory deficit and is thought to reflect frontal lobe dysfunction and a failure of self-monitoring. Confabulation is prominent in certain alcohol amnestic syndromes, such as Wernicke-Korsakoff syndrome, and in disorders of the mamillary bodies, the thalamus, and the frontal lobes.

A 40-year-old chronically alcoholic man, whose memory on the mental status examination was markedly impaired, frantically demanded to be released from the hospital, saying that his wife had just been in an automobile accident and that he had to rush to another hospital to see her. He said it with sincere conviction and appropriate fearful concern; for the patient, at least, the story was real. In fact, his wife had been dead for 15 years. The patient told the same story over and over again, always with evident conviction, in spite of the fact that staff members confronted him with the reality that his wife had been dead for years. The patient was never influenced by their assertions, since he could not register new memories. Although his past memory was patchy as best, he could repeatedly recall the story of his wife's emergency.

Déjà vu is the sense that one has seen or experienced what is transpiring for the first time; it is a false impression that the current stream of consciousness has previously been recorded in memory. Related phenomena are *déjà entendu,* a sense that one has previously heard what is actually being heard for the first time, and *déjà pensé,* a feeling that one has at an earlier time known or understood what is being thought for the first time. Experiences of *jamais vu, jamais entendu,* and *jamais pensé* involve feelings that one has never seen, heard, or thought (respectively) things that, in fact, one has. Those phenomena are all common in everyday life but may increase in states of fatigue and intoxication and in association with complex partial seizures and other psychopathological states.

Dementia *Dementia* is a syndrome of acquired intellectual impairment in which impairment of short-term memory and long-term memory is the essential feature, with associated impairments of abstract thinking and judgment, personality changes, and other cortical disturbances. The symptoms always involve more than one sphere of function. In the late stages, demented patients may become helpless, too confused to use a stove, and incapable of remembering the names of close relatives; they may wander into dangerous situations, oblivious of their surroundings. Dementia may be caused by a variety of pathogenic processes; some are reversible, such as hypothyroidism and subdural hematoma, but others are irreversible, such as dementia of the Alzheimer's type and vascular dementia. Although DSM-IV excludes depression as a possible cause of dementia, preferring to call the characteristic cognitive disturbances pseudodementia, many neuropsychiatrists think that profound cognitive dysfunction meeting the criteria for dementia associated with depression should properly be labeled a dementia syndrome.

DISTURBANCES IN PERCEPTION

Normal perception first requires that the person be capable of receiving information as sensations. The data must then be organized to make them meaningful and comprehensible, such as by distinguishing figure from ground or focusing attention selectively on some part of the sensory field. The organized entities are called percepts. All the sense organs contribute to organized perceptions; in states of sensory deficit—such as blindness, deafness, and anesthesia—perception is impaired, but perception is still possible because people generally perceive information about an object through several sensory modalities concurrently.

The intensity of sensation and perception is affected by vigilance and attention. Highly focused attention, as in intense concentration and hypnosis, may result in unusually acute sensations and perceptions—hyperesthesia, hyperacusis, and extraordinary visual acuity. Focused attention may also result in the failure to sense or to perceive. Deep anesthesia and negative hallucinations induced by hypnosis are simply induced failures to perceive what exists in the world.

Humans usually operate in an average expectable environment, an environment in which certain types and levels of sensory input are expected and for which the nervous system is primed. Excessive or inadequate stimulation in any sensory modality and levels of input that are extraordinarily intense can provoke distorted perceptions in most normal people. For example, total sensory deprivation produced in controlled artificial environments may elicit visual and auditory illusions and hallucinations.

The full effect of perceptions depends to a considerable extent on how they are experienced and filtered through the person's memories, emotions, and fantasies. Perceptions are colored by past experiences, associated memories, and concurrent social inputs. For example, how a person visually perceives the city of New York, as either current perceptions or as perceptual memory, depends, in part, on the person's feelings, experiences, and beliefs about the city. Some who have never been there and who know it primarily as a city of tall buildings may selectively perceive skyscrapers; other who previously lived there and disliked it may perceive (or retain a perceptual memory of) a dirty, crowded city of scowling faces.

The intensity of perceptions depends on variable individual sensitivities, mood, level of anxiety, and substance use. Depressed patients often describe colors that look faded, a sense that the world looks washed out or gray, even though their capacity to recognize and distinguish specific colors is unchanged. Similarly, mania is often characterized by heightened or intense perceptions, called *hyperesthesia.* When extreme, intense perceptions are uncomfortable. Hyperesthesia is also seen during benzodiazepine withdrawal and hallucinogen use and occasionally as part of an epileptic aura.

Stimulation of one sensory modality sometimes evokes perceptual distortions in another. Marijuana and mescaline intoxication, for example, have been associated with *synesthesia,* an experience in which sensory modalities seem fused. Synesthesia is also a normal experience for many people. Music may be experienced visually, the sound fusing with visual illusions; a tactile sensation may be experienced as a color—for example, a hot surface may feel red.

ILLUSIONS Perceptual distortions in the estimation of size, shape, and spatial relations are common even in the absence of psychiatric disorders, especially when someone is fatigued or excessively aroused. *Illusions* are misinterpretations of real sensory stimuli, as when a child in a dark bedroom sees monsters emanating from shadows on the walls or hears ghosts in the sounds of the wind. *Pareidolias* are playful and whimsical voluntary illusions that can be seen when one looks at ambiguously defined or evanescent images, such as clouds, flames in a fireplace, and patterns of sand or water. Both the onset and the termination of those perceptions are entirely voluntary. *Trailing,* another visual illusion, is the perception that an object moving steadily in space is followed by temporally distinct afterimages of itself. The effect is that of a series of stroboscopic photos. The phenomenon may occur with fatigue and is typically experienced in marijuana and mescaline intoxication.

HALLUCINATIONS Hallucinations are perceptions that occur in the absence of corresponding sensory stimuli. Phenomenologically, hallucinations are indistinguishable from normal perceptions. The hallucinated voice of the devil does not sound any more peculiar than the voice of the psychiatrist asking about the hallucination. Hallucinations are related to normal perceptions in the same way that delusions and beliefs are related to each other—they are *subjectively* identical. The only manner in which hallucinations differ from true perceptions is that hallucinations are often felt to be private, that others may not be able to see or hear the perceptions. The internal explanation is typically delusional.

Hallucinations can affect any sensory system, and they sometimes occur in several concurrently. When perception is altered, illusions and hallucinations and often delusions as well are frequently experienced together. In some studies 90 percent of patients with hallucinations also have delusions, and about 35 percent of patients with delusions also have hallucinations. About 20 percent of patients have mixed sensory hallucinations (mostly auditory and visual) that may accompany functional and organic conditions. A given external stimulus may evoke different perceptual distortions in different persons.

Three scientists floated in sensory-deprivation tanks for long periods of time. One experienced a few illusions and no hallucinations; the second had many illusions and a few faint auditory and visual hallucinations; and the third had vivid, dramatic, and complex visual and auditory hallucinations.

Hallucinations are experienced by many normal people under unusual conditions. Between 10 and 27 percent of the general population have experienced memorable hallucinations, most often visual hallucinations. *Hypnagogic* and *hypnopompic* hallucinations are common, predominantly visual hallucinations that occur during the moments immediately before falling asleep and during the transition from sleep to wakefulness, respectively. Hypnagogic and hypnopompic hallucinations both occur in normal persons and are also characteristic symptoms of narcolepsy. In acute bereavement up to 50 percent of grieving spouses have reported hallucinating the voice or the presence of the deceased; after amputations, phantom limb hallucinations are common. Those observations suggest a supersensitivity deprivation hypothesis that may explain such hallucinations and associated ones: when deprived of important and anticipated perceptual stimuli, the mental apparatus may overinterpret any sensory stimulation as evidence of the presence of the needed objects.

A perceptual release theory suggests that hallucinations emerge from the combined presence of intense states of internal arousal and of diminished sensory input (including poor attention and poor capacity to sort out relevant input from irrelevant input). Diminished input from the environment (as in sensory deprivation) and reduced capacity to attend to and take in the input (as in delirious states) heighten the likelihood that internal sensations, images, and thoughts will be interpreted as originating in the outside environment.

Hallucinations vary according to sensory modality, the degree of complexity of the hallucinated experience, and the degree to which the hallucination influences the person's behavior.

Auditory hallucinations Auditory hallucinations range in complexity from hearing unstructured sounds, such as whirring noises and muffled whispers, to hearing ongoing multiperson discussions about the patient. The simple auditory hallucinations are commonly associated with organic psychoses, such as delirium, complex partial seizures, and toxic and metabolic encephalopathies. Deafness can produce hallucinations consisting of noises or of formed music. Auditory hallucinations are classically associated with schizophrenia (seen in 60 to 90 percent of patients), but they are also frequently seen in psychotic mood disorders. Twenty percent of manic patients and almost 10 percent of depressed patients experience auditory hallucinations.

Three types of auditory hallucinations are classified as first-rank symptoms of schizophrenia (which, however, are also seen, albeit in smaller proportions, in depression and mania): (1) audible thoughts described as hallucinated voices that speak aloud what the patient is thinking; (2) voices that give a running commentary on the patient's actions; and (3) two or more voices arguing with each other, often about the patient, who is referred to in the third person.

A 21-year-old schizophrenic man heard an endless dialogue by three voices. The audible intensity waxed and waned over hours and days, but the dialogue never ceased for more than a few minutes at a time. The patient identified one voice as his angel, who spoke kindly of him, often warned him of things he had to do, and complimented him after the successful completion of tasks. A second voice was harsh and derisive in its comments, degrading the patient and caustically mocking him for what he had done. When those two voices argued with each other (which they frequently did) about the patient's merits as a person or about whether he had performed some task correctly, a third voice, a female voice, mediated the disputes.

Auditory hallucinations are frequently mood-neutral, but patients with mood disorders characteristically hear voices consistent with their moods. In major depressive disorder the voices may be unrelievedly critical and sadistic; in mania the voices often refer to the patient's specialness.

A 51-year-old Jewish man with bipolar disorder had characteristic auditory hallucinations in each of his many episodes of mania and depression. When depressed, he heard Hitler's voice saying: "All the Jews should die. I'm coming to get you. . . . I'll throw you in the ovens." When manic, the patient heard an unidentified voice encouraging him to write more poetry, since he had the most brilliant, creative mind since Shakespeare.

In *command hallucinations* the patient is ordered by voices to do things. In many instances the commands are benign reminders about everyday tasks: "Pick up your shoes" and "Clean off the table." However, the voices may also be frightening or dangerous, as they may command acts of violence toward the self or others, such as, "Jump off the roof; you're not worth anything" and "Pick up the knife, and kill your mother." Those voices vary in insistence and persistence, and patients differ in their capacities to ignore the commands. Patients with marked passivity may be helpless in the face of command hallucinations and may feel impelled to carry out the orders. Even though one recent study did not find command hallucinations to be associated with a high risk of harm to the patient or others, the presence of command hallucinations and the patient's ability to resist must be assessed carefully.

A young man with schizophrenia heard an insistent voice repeatedly telling him to stop his antipsychotic medication. After resisting the command for many weeks, the patient felt that he could no longer fight the voice, and he discontinued treatment. Two months later, he was hospitalized involuntarily; he had lost 20 pounds and was in a dehydrated state and near cardiovascular collapse. He later said that, once the medication was stopped, the voice further insisted that he should stop eating and drinking in order to be pure.

Visual hallucinations Visual hallucinations occur in a wide variety of neurological and psychiatric disorders, including toxic disturbances, drug withdrawal syndromes, focal CNS lesions, migraine, blindness, schizophrenia, and psychotic mood disorders. Although visual hallucinations are generally assumed to reflect organic disorders, one quarter to one half of all schizophrenic patients have them, often but not always in conjunction with auditory hallucinations.

Visual hallucinations range from simple and elemental, in which hallucinations consist of flashes of light or geometric figures, to elaborate visions, such as a flock of angels.

A terrified 37-year-old man in acute delirium tremens glanced agitatedly about the room. He pointed out the window and said: "My God, the Spanish armada is on the lawn. They're about to attack." He experienced the hallucination as real, and it persisted intermittently for three days before abating. Subsequently, the patient had no memory of the experience.

In some religious subcultures visual hallucinations are experienced as normal. In one fundamentalist Pentecostal church, worshipers dance themselves into a frenzy, and, without using any drugs, several participants have shared visions of the Virgin Mary at the altar.

Other types of hallucinations *Autoscopic* hallucinations are hallucinations of one's own physical self. Such hallucinations may stimulate the delusion that one has a double *(Doppelgänger)*. Reports of near-death out-of-body experiences, in which persons see themselves rising to the ceiling and looking down at themselves in a hospital bed, may be autoscopic hallucinations. In *Lilliputian* hallucinations, the person sees figures in reduced size, like midgets or dwarfs. Those hallucinations may be related to the perceptual distortions of *macropsia* and *micropsia*—respectively, the perception of objects as bigger or smaller than they actually are.

Haptic hallucinations involve touch. Simple haptic hallucinations, such as the feeling that bugs are crawling over one's skin *(formication)*, are common in alcohol withdrawal syndromes and in cocaine intoxication. When unkempt and physically neglectful patients complain of those sensations, they may be due to the presence of real physical stimuli, such as lice. Some tactile hallucinations—having intercourse with God, for example—are highly suggestive of schizophrenia but may also occur in tertiary syphilis and other conditions and may be stimulated by local genital irritation. *Olfactory* and *gustatory* hallucinations—involving smell and taste, respectively—have most often been associated with organic brain diseases, particularly with the uncinate fits of complex partial seizures. Olfactory hallucinations may also be seen in major depression, typically as odors of decay, rotting, and death.

The term "pseudohallucination" has been used in two ways. First, *pseudohallucination* refers to perceptions experienced as coming from within the mind—that is, not at the boundary or outside the mind. According to that definition, loud voices that are alien, ascribed to other beings, but that the patient knows are actually within the mind, rather than out in space, are pseudohallucinations. The term has also been used to describe hallucinatory experiences whose validity the patient doubts. A better term for that phenomenon is *partial hallucination*, analogous to partial delusion.

Functional hallucinations occur only in connection with a specific external perception—for example, in the presence of a sound (such as running water), a color, or a particular place. However, unlike illusions, the hallucinated sounds are not elaborations of the perception; they are simply triggered only in that specific context.

A patient with schizophrenia described returning repeatedly to a running brook near his parents' country home. When in the presence of the brook, he heard the voice of God calling out to him. He decided that it was his "holy place." He denied hearing hallucinations in any other setting.

Ictal hallucinations, occurring as part of seizure activity, are typically brief, lasting only seconds to minutes, and stereotyped. They may be simple images, such as flashes of light, or elaborate ones, such as visual recollections of past experiences. While the hallucinations are being experienced, the patient ordinarily experiences altered consciousness or a twilight sleep.

Migrainous hallucinations are reported by about 50 percent of patients with migraine. Most are simple visual hallucinations of geometric patterns, but fully formed visual hallucinations, sometimes with micropsia and macropsia, may also occur. The complex has been called the Alice in Wonderland syndrome, after Lewis Carroll's descriptions of the world in *Through the Looking-Glass,* which mirrored some of his own migrainous experiences. The phenomena closely resemble visual hallucinations induced by psychedelic drugs, such as mescaline.

A *flashback* is an intense visual reexperience of highly charged past events, which are often replays of hallucinations. They are typically associated with the heavy use of hallucinogens such as LSD and mescaline and often occur months after the last drug ingestion. The images may be simple or complex geometric patterns, or they may consist of previously experienced elaborate drug-induced hallucinatons. Flashback phenomena may be state-dependent. For example, visual hallucinations initially experienced with hallucinogens are likely to be subsequently experienced as flashbacks when the person is smoking marijuana. In posttraumatic stress disorder some complex intrusive flashbacklike images may attain hallucinatory vividness. Images often include horrifying memories of traumatic events that force themselves repeatedly into consciousness until they are acknowledged and worked through.

A 20-year-old man ingested LSD at least 10 times over a six-month period. In contrast to his previous experiences, his last LSD trip was frightening and dysphoric. During it he could not rid himself of illusions and hallucinations of snakes on the ground and the walls of his apartment. Two months later, while smoking marijuana for the first time since the bad LSD experience, he had a repeat performance of the snake hallucinations. He had previously smoked marijuana on many occasions without perceptual distortions. Because of the flashback experience, the patient stopped smoking marijuana entirely. Over the next few months he experienced a few brief hallucinations of the snakes, following which the perceptual distortions ceased.

Hallucinosis is a state of active hallucination in a patient who is alert and well-oriented. The condition is seen most often in alcoholic withdrawal, but it may also occur during acute intoxications and other drug-mediated states.

A 30-year-old woman being treated for depression with a monoamine oxidase inhibitor snorted cocaine at a party. For the next three days she described vivid hallucinatory experiences while in an alert state. She managed to drive her car throughout that time, although with some difficulty. In her psychiatrist's office she alternated between relating coherently to the psychiatrist and responding to her dreamlike complex visual and auditory hallucinations.

BODY IMAGE DISTORTIONS Body image, a function of self-awareness and consciousness, has perceptual and ideational components. Therefore, distortions of the body image may reflect primarily perceptual distortions or combinations of disturbed perception and appraisal.

Body-image disturbances can occur as normal responses to abrupt changes in the body (such as after an amputation), in brain disease, and in psychiatric disorders. Phantom-limb phenomena are classic body-image problems in which an amputated limb is still felt to be present. The sensation may diminish gradually over time; the phantom limb feels as though it were receding into the stump.

Agnosias, lack of awareness of body parts, may accompany brain damage, most often of the nondominant parietal lobe. Patients with obvious deficits may deny that any deficit exists *(anosognosia),* or the denial may be limited to half of the body *(hemiagnosia),* usually the left side. In *hemidepersonalization,* a less common disorder *(hemisomatognosia),* patients feel that one of their limbs is missing—again, usually on the left side. Distortions in body image in which a limb feels too heavy or weightless—termed *hyperschemazia* and *hyposchemazia,* respectively—can occur as a consequence of some neurological conditions, such as infarction of the parietal lobe. In duplication phenomena, patients feel as though part or all of them has doubled (for example, a patient has two heads or two bodies). Those rare phenomena may occur in schizophrenia, complex partial seizures, and migraine.

In *dysmorphophobia* patients distort and dislike the shape of a particular body part. The symptom is misnamed, since it contains no true phobic component, such as fear or avoidant behavior. Fine lines separate perceptual distortions and realistic but unhappy appraisals of the body, given the high social value placed on physical appearance. Dysmorphophobia is seen in some personality disorders and as an isolated disorder in which it constitutes the dominant symptom. In some ways dysmorphophobia resembles an overvalued idea. Patients may have dysmorphophobia in relation to any body part; common concerns are hair, breasts, the shape of the nose, and the shape of the entire body. For some patients, changing the body part, as in rhinoplasty for those who do not like their noses, seems to effect a lasting positive change in body image; the patients become happier with themselves and feel more attractive for years or lifetimes. When the dysmorphophobia is severe, multiple plastic surgeries may result, with the patient dissatisfied after each one. At times, the condition forms part of a large, pervasive syndrome, such as anorexia nervosa.

A 27-year-old woman with a history of borderline personality disorder, anorexia nervosa, and bulimia nervosa often became acutely suicidal after visits to her hairdresser. Whenever the hairdresser cut off a fraction of an inch more hair than she believed was proper, the patient suddenly felt that her hair was so short that she became ugly, and she believed that everyone else could see her ugliness as well. She felt too ashamed to be seen in public and would hide out in her bedroom for days or weeks until she felt presentable again.

Hypochondriacal complaints also combine perceptual and ideational distortions. Selective hypervigilance to bodily sensations may result in a high likelihood of perceptions of unpleasant and potentially pathological body experiences among the worried well, hypochondriacal populations, patients with somatization disorder (Briquet's syndrome), and some patients with panic disorder.

Body-image distortions may, at times, by severe or bizarre. Some psychotic patients with either schizophrenia or depression have somatic delusions. In depression it often expresses itself as a delusion that part or all of the body is rotting or is filled with cancer. Some culture-bound syndromes in non-Western cultures express themselves with body-image distortions, such as koro, in which the person fears that his penis is shrinking into his abdomen.

DISTURBANCES OF MOOD

Defining, describing, understanding, and categorizing feelings has long been among the most important tasks in psychiatry and, simultaneously, among the most difficult. The language of feelings is filled with terms that seem to have mostly idiosyncratic meanings as patients, phenomenologists, and psychiatrists all struggle to describe inner sensations and to correlate them with external behavior. Even to define such basic terms as "mood," "affect," "emotion," and "feelings" is difficult. The most common convention, which is used here, defines *mood* as a sustained or prevailing feeling tone or range of tones experienced by a person. *Affect* is the moment-to-moment feeling state, sometimes rapidly shifting in response to a variety of situations and objects, that the clinician can observe. *Emotions* have been defined as moods and affects that are connected to specific ideas or to the physical concomitants of moods and affects. *Feelings* are the most poorly defined of all, leading Karl Jaspers to describe them as everything for which there is no other name. In common parlance and often professionally as well, the words are sometimes used interchangeably. The term "mood disorders," adopted for DSM-III-R and DSM-IV, replaced DSM-III's "affective disorders" to describe the same group of psychiatric syndromes.

Moods, affects, and emotions can be described by a number of important qualities: intensity (shallow to deep), range (broad to narrow or flat), stability (rigid to labile), reactivity to external events (none to much), periodicity (periodic to aperiodic), congruence with thought content (congruent or appropriate to incongruent), speed of resolution (rapid to slow), and viscosity (evanescent to persistent). The lifelong predominant mood is one component of temperament. A person may be described, for example, as having a calm, buoyant, irritable, depressive, anxious, or sensitive temperament.

Moods, affects, and emotions serve as internal and external signal systems. They signal the state of the person to others and often elicit necessary help and support from the environment. A baby's face communicates its state of need, tension, or contentment, thereby recruiting appropriate maternal interventions. As adults, much of the most important interpersonal communication is transmitted nonverbally through cues that signal the observer about the communicator's mood. A sullen or even slightly scowling face powerfully alters the meaning of even the most positive verbal message, leading a listener to perceive a message of anger, regardless of the spoken words. Moods also serve as important ways of influencing others. The infectious quality of moods has been demonstrated in numerous studies. A cheerful mood toward others influences their moods toward cheerfulness and, in turn, promotes positive feelings toward the person and the situation.

Internally, moods, affects, and emotions let people know how well or how poorly they are doing, allowing them to gauge the distance between actual self-appraisal and desired self-expectations. For example, if persons desire to master an important goal and feel that they have a reasonably good chance of doing so, their emotional state in relation to the goal is pleasant. If something intervenes to assure that they never achieve the goal, so that there is an insurmountable gap between their desires and the likelihood of success, they may feel hopeless. In addition to serving as signal systems, emotional states of nonspecific tension, arousal, or anger usually imply that some activity is necessary to secure their discharge or release.

Emotional states and their expression are regulated by both biological and cultural influences. Biologically, in addition to constitutional contributions to emotional temperament, emotions are affected by periodic shifts and by drive-related processes. For example, emotional lability occurs premenstrually in some women, with varying periodicity in cyclothymic persons and in relation to such need states as hunger, sleepiness, and sexual frustration. Physiological disinhibition in the expression of emotions may result from intoxication or from brain injury, as in frontal lobe disturbances that result in emotional lability or emotional incontinence. Emotional shifts have also been related to environment-related physiological influences, such as seasonal changes in light.

Cultural regulation is significant in the expression of emotion. Although the facial expressions for basic emotions are similar in all cultures studied, the range and the style of emotional expression in relation to specific events varies greatly from culture to culture and from family to family. Some cultures and families are stiff-lipped and inhibit the open expression of emotion; others encourage emotional display. Marked differences exist among cultures in the emotional expression of acute grief, fear, pain, and affection.

DEPRESSION The term "depression" has been used variously to describe an emotional state, a syndrome, and a group of specific disorders. When seen as part of a syndrome or disorder, *depression* has autonomic, visceral, emotional, perceptual, cognitive, and behavior manifestations, as illustrated in Table 10-1. As a nonpathological, ubiquitous mood state lasting hours to days and sometimes longer, feelings of depression are synonymous with feeling sad, blue, down in the dumps, unhappy, and miserable. A depressed mood is common and appropriate after a disappointment or a loss. For most people, innate psychological resilience, alternative coping options, and supportive social networks help alleviate those brief depressive states and prevent them from becoming chronic. Some persons suffer from a chronically depressed mood, tend to view the world as a difficult place filled with obstacles and burdens, see themselves as victimized, and lack hope for the future. The extent to which constitutional, developmental, and ongoing aversive life events contribute to that pervasive stance is unknown. Persons who in early life were deprived and traumatized may be less resilient and more prone to chronic depressive features than are others. Repeated failures and the effects of unrelenting, uncontrollable, and unpredictable negative life events may set the stage for learned helplessness in humans, just as they do in animals. A subset of chronically depressed persons may suffer from a temperamental, biologically driven depression, often seen in conjunction with strong genetic loading for severe mood disorders.

Some depressive states are normal and common reactions to major unwelcome and undesirable life events. Normal *bereavement* is the best example. In bereavement, dealing with a major loss—such as the death of a parent, a spouse, or a child—persons experience sadness, pining, and yearning but do not ordinarily have the feelings of guilt, unworthiness, and self-reproach that characterize depressive disorders. Feelings of helplessness and hopelessness may be temporarily present in bereavement, but the feelings ordinarily pass with time. In uncomplicated cases the process of bereavement takes three to six months in the acute phase and up to a year for complete resolution. Bereaved persons are more likely to feel physically ill and to seek general health care than are other persons, and elderly widowers are more liable to die than are age-matched nonbereaved controls. *Pathological grief reactions,* bereavements that last more than a year, may be seen when the surviving spouse was excessively dependent on the deceased and is unable to obtain emotional and financial support elsewhere or when the survivor is unable to grieve fully because of markedly ambivalent feelings toward the deceased. *Impacted grief* is present when the initial grief response is inadequate because of the overwhelming nature of the loss or when the bereaved is unable to assimilate the loss because of developmental immaturity. The inadequate expression of grief in incomplete bereavement is thought to be pathogenic in many subsequent psychiatric disorders. For example, impulsive acting out among adolescents who have lost a parent is often assumed to be due to unresolved grief.

A variety of medical disorders may cause depressive syndromes. Most common are endocrine abnormalities, such as hypothyroidism and hypercalcemia, and CNS disorders, such as cerebrovascular disease and Parkinson's disease. Depressions are more common after cerebral diseases affecting left anterior lesions than after diseases in other locations. Medications—especially antihypertensive agents affecting adrenergic tone, such as reserpine (Serpasil) and β-blockers—may also trigger depressions. The importance of a genetic diathesis in iatrogenic depressions is not yet known. However, depressive syndromes and disorders in general are unquestionably familial and are likely to have genetic contributions, especially in depressions associated with bipolar disorder.

Severe depression The severe depressive disorders, such as *major depressive disorder,* are characterized by a depressed or apathetic mood in conjunction with a group of somatic or vegetative symptoms. Convulsive crying does not always accompany depression; in fact, many depressive syndromes are marked by tearless apathy, irritability, or anger. The *vegetative symptoms* include appetite and sleep disturbances—both of which may be increased, sleeping up to 20 hours daily or gaining 20 pounds in a month, or decreased, with marked weight loss and sleeping only a few hours a night, often seen in conjunction with early-morning awakening. Loss of libido and constipation are also common. In *major depressive episodes* with melancholia, the patient's mood may become autonomous—that is, it may be impervious to environmental stimuli, even transiently. Other melancholic features are diurnal variation, with the mood typically worse in the morning than in the rest of the day, and prominent psychomotor retardation or restless agitation and pacing. Unrelenting morbid obsessions, *ruminations,* are typically seen in melancholia; a morbid set of thoughts may be continuously experienced, like an endlessly replaying tape. Psychotic features—typically with such depressive themes as guilt, punishment, and decay—may also be seen in the most severe depressions.

A 62-year-old melancholic man was constantly plagued by the thought that he was a terrible man and that the FBI would shortly be coming to arrest him. He paced agitatedly for hours, expecting every knock at the door or ring of the telephone to be the one announcing the FBI.

Cognitive features Cognitive features of depression are prominent. Characterizing the exact nature of the memory impairment by using standardized tests has been difficult. The cognitive tasks requiring sustained effort and elaborate cognitive processing may be more disrupted in depression than are those tasks that can be accomplished almost automatically. In geriatric populations the effect of depression on cognition may be so profound as to produce a true dementia syndrome, often called *pseudodementia* (a misnomer, since the dementia is real but reversible). Profound cognitive disturbances, seen commonly in severe depressive disorders, include ruminations and feelings of worthlessness, helplessness, and hopelessness—the expectations that no one and nothing can help or is likely to help now or in the future.

Suicide Suicidal phenomena are of particular concern. Suicide is common in severe depressive disorders; 15 percent of untreated patients with depressive disorders end their lives in suicide. Depressed patients constitute the largest diagnostic group of all completed suicides. By no means, however, is suicide specific to depression. Substance abuse disorders, schizophrenia, and personality disorders are also characterized by high rates of suicide. Patients with depression with comorbid alcohol abuse may be at particularly high risk for suicide.

Suicidal persons differ in the seriousness of their intent, the precision of their planning, and the likelihood of success. In the assessment of suicide potential, the psychiatrist should examine the patient in detail regarding fantasies, perturbation (the degree of emotional upset), the strength of the impulse to act suicidally, and the lethality of the plan. Vague fantasies or wishes to be dead (''I'd be better off dead'') are less lethal than a plan to drive a car off a cliff or to use a loaded pistol when the patient has a need to quickly resolve a feeling of profound distress. Since the decision to commit suicide provides the demoralized victim with a way to regain some measure of control over events, the very act of making the decision and formulating a suicide plan may relieve anxiety and depression. For that reason, a sudden, seemingly inexplicable improvement in mood in a severely depressed person should be regarded with suspicion and should be investigated. Suicidal persons are also known to give away belongings and to make final estate plans before carrying out a suicide. Such activities in a depressed person should arouse concern.

Although consistent, useful, validated predictors of suicide do not exist, some demographic features are associated with a high risk. Those features include being white, male, old, and alone. In the psychiatric history the single most important factor is that of past suicide attempts. Among clinical signs, hopelessness, anhedonia, and severe anxiety may indicate increased suicide risk. Physical illness in association with other risk factors, such as depression, may place a patient at a high risk. Genetic predisposition toward suicidal behavior cuts across diagnostic lines and may play a role in suicide risk. A tendency toward impulsive behavior may correlate with certain measures of CNS neurotransmitter metabolites, such as low levels of 5-hydroxyindoleacetic acid (5-HIAA), the major metabolite of serotonin.

Suicidal gestures are common among impulsive depressed and self-hating persons, for whom they serve as cries for help that may enlist desired social support. Because of the association of such gestures with an increased risk for completed suicide, they should not be taken lightly. Nonsuicidal self-destructive behaviors, such as self-mutilations and repeated unnecessary risk taking, are also common in depressive syndromes and in personality disorders. Subintentional suicide may result when suicidal gestures go awry or when reckless behavior, such as taking unnecessary risks in combat or driving while drunk, prove fatal.

Other depressive phenomena *Anaclitic depression* is a psychoanalytic term referring to a helpless and withdrawn response, like that of an infant to the loss of a caretaker, that follows initial responses of protest and intense crying. With continued deprivation, the infant enters the phase of despair, becomes morose, ceases crying, and appears to feel hopeless. Some waste away and die. Anaclitic depression in later life is a helpless and withdrawn state, often seen in highly dependent persons who seem to fall apart after losing their major sources of support. *Existential depressions* result when persons no longer find meaning in their activities and lose their sense of purpose. The loss of a sense of meaning may occur in primary depressions or in response to major disappointments and unfortunate life situations.

ELATED MOODS Elated moods include euphoria, elation, exaltation, and ecstasy. They are marked by feelings of well-being, expansiveness, optimism, capability, pleasure, and grace. Such moods are normally experienced when life is going well, when long-sought-after goals are achieved, and in states of love, religious fervor, and spiritual transcendence. Peak experiences and experiences of mystic fusion are often accompanied by feelings of exaltation and ecstasy. Sexual pleasure and some chemically mediated states of altered consciousness may also induce the feelings.

Abnormal elated moods are seen primarily as part of manic states. When subtle, as in *hypomania,* the mood can be ebullient and brimming with self-confidence but with occasional irritability. Other characteristic symptoms of hypomania are increased energy, decreased need for sleep, rapidly flowing thoughts, excessive talking, inflated self-esteem with a demanding nature toward others, and diminished judgment. *Mania* is a more extreme state in which judgment and sleep are impaired to the point of marked functional disruption. As the mania exacerbates, irritability and anger increase, alternating rapidly with a brittle expansiveness. Cognition becomes increasingly disorganized. Psychotic symptoms, usually involving themes of grandiosity and specialness, occur in 50 percent or more of manic patients. With increasing escalation of the manic state, thinking becomes fragmented, psychotic symptoms are prominent, and the syndrome may appear indistinguishable from acute schizophrenia. Those three manic states—hypomania, mania, and the psychotic, fragmented manic state—are often referred to as stage I, II, and III mania, respectively.

Manic states occur in bipolar disorders and cyclothymic disorder and as a secondary mania caused by a variety of physical and toxic conditions. Secondary manias may follow specific cerebral insults, accompany systemic disorders, or occur after the ingestion of some drugs, including amphetamines, antidepressants, bromocriptine (Parlodel), decongestants, isoniazid (Cotinozin), and corticosteroids, to name but a few. Mania is the second most common neuropsychiatric disturbance induced by steroids, occurring in 30 to 35 percent of patients who have steroid-induced behavioral disorders. Up to 12 percent of patients treated with levodopa (Dopar) and bromocriptine for parkinsonism later have mania. Right hemispheric brain lesions are specifically associated with secondary mania.

ANXIETY Like depression, the term "anxiety" covers a number of different entities—a normal transient feeling, often with adaptive properties; a symptom seen in a wide variety of disorders; and a group of disorders in which anxiety as a symptom forms a dominant element. As a transient, disagreeable emotional state, anxiety may be adaptive, signaling anticipated or impending threat. In contrast to *fear,* the emotional state that exists when a source of threat is precise and well-known, anxiety occurs when the threat is not well-defined.

Patients find it difficult to describe the feeling of anxiety accurately; at its core, however, *anxiety* is characterized by intense negative affect, associated with an undefined threat to one's physical or psychological self. Subjectively, patients use words such as tense, panicky, terrified, jittery, nervous, wound-up, apprehensive, and worried in trying to delineate the sensation.

Aside from the subjective feelings, anxiety is characterized by somatic, cognitive, behavioral, and perceptual symptoms. The somatic symptoms of anxiety are legion and often dominate the subjective symptoms; a partial list includes twitching, tremors, hot and cold flashes, sweating, palpitations, chest tightness, difficulty in swallowing, nausea, diarrhea, dry mouth, and decreased libido. Cognitively, anxiety is characterized by hypervigilance, poor concentration, subjective confusion, fears of losing control or of going crazy, and catastrophic thinking. Characteristic behavioral symptoms include fearful expressions, withdrawal, irritability, immobility, and hyperventilation. Perceptual disturbances—such as depersonalization, derealization, and hyperesthesia (especially hyperacusis)—are also common symptoms.

Anxiety may be divided into state versus trait and situational versus free-floating characteristics. *Trait anxiety* is a lifelong pattern of anxiety as a temperament feature. Persons with trait anxiety are generally jittery, skittish, hypersensitive to stimuli, and psychophysiologically more reactive than are others. In contrast to trait anxiety, *state anxiety* refers to acute situationally bound episodes of anxiety that do not persist beyond the provoking situation. *Free-floating anxiety* is a condition of persistently anxious mood in which the cause of the emotion is unknown and many diverse thoughts and events seem to trigger and compound the anxiety. In contrast, anxiety may be *situational,* seen only in relation to specific situations or objects, as in phobias.

Anxiety symptoms can result from numerous physical conditions and from other psychiatric disorders. Many endocrine, autoimmune, metabolic, and toxic disorders are known to generate anxiety. The psychiatrist must differentiate the response of the patient to an underlying condition (that is, secondary anxiety) from symptoms generated by the primary disorder itself. Anxiety symptoms are common in patients with psychoses, organic mental disorders, depression, and psychoactive substance use disorders, as well as in the specific anxiety disorders. In patients with schizophrenia, anxiety must be differentiated from akathisia, a common and often overlooked syndrome of subjective restlessness, anxiety, and agitation resulting from antipsychotic medication. The coexistence of anxiety symptoms and depression in major depression is substantial; anxiety symptoms, such as anxious mood and irritability, are seen in the majority of depressed patients. In addition, half to two thirds of patients with panic disorder experience a major depressive episode over a lifetime. Drug effects—from acute use, side effects, or as part of withdrawal phenomena—are also common causes of anxiety. Many patients with severe anxiety ingest and become dependent on anxiolytic drugs—including benzodiazepines, other sedatives, and alcohol—for symptom relief. During attempts to discontinue those substances and sometimes during their ongoing use, confusing mixtures of anxiety, medication effects, and withdrawal symptoms may occur.

All symptoms characteristic of drug-related anxiety also exist in anxiety disorders. However, perceptual disturbances, such as depersonalization and hyperesthesia, may be more common in sedative-hypnotic withdrawal syndromes than in primary anxiety disorders.

Despite the general observation that anxious patients have increased startle responses, specific and consistent differences have not been found in the physiological hyperreactivity of anxiety disorder patients versus controls. In part, that nonspecificity reflects individual differences in reactivity among the patients; one person may respond to a stimulus with increased pulse and blood pressure, while another may show changes in the opposite direction. Similarly, although panic patients but not controls tend to experience panic attacks in response to sodium lactate infusion, other biological measures, especially those reflecting the catecholamine system and thought to reflect central noradrenergic activity, have failed to elucidate the biological underpinnings of anxiety. Despite the lack of consistent findings, a great deal of evidence suggests the presence of biological abnormalities as part of anxiety disorders.

Causes From a psychological point of view, anxiety frequently signals conflict between opposing desires, wishes, or beliefs on the one hand and major disequilibriums generated by negative life events on the other hand. *Role strains,* conflicts between the major social roles that form a person's identity—spouse, parent, child, wage earner, professional, community member—are common sources of anxiety. The more important the conflict and the less obvious the resolution, the greater is the associated anxiety. For example, anxiety symptoms may emerge for the first time when a person is confronted with an unavoidable unhappy choice, such as sustaining a marriage or accepting a career advancement that requires a major move that is unacceptable to the spouse. At times, those conflicts may escape conscious awareness: the person may feel anxious but not know why. Anxiety syndromes frequently result from a combination of several factors. A person in a job conflict facing an important deadline may try to alleviate the initial anxiety symptoms by overwork, then ingest caffeine or amphetamines as stimulants to keep going, then become physically exhausted and fatigued, and ultimately use alcohol excessively—each of those elements contributing separately to an anxiety state.

Certain life situations are developmentally associated with anxiety. *Stranger anxiety* develops when an infant 6 to 8 months old begins to recognize the difference between its mother and others. When a child first goes to school, mild anxiety symptoms are common; if the anxiety is excessive, school phobia may result. During adult life, anxiety often centers on issues of mastery and accomplishment in both personal life and work life. *Performance anxiety* or *stage fright* is a specific type of pathological anxiety in which anxiety escalates to episodes of panic when public performance is required. In the elderly the deterioration of the body may engender anxiety about helplessness and death anxiety.

Irritability Irritability is an unpleasant feeling state in which the person feels an inner dis-ease and discomfort. It may exist purely as a feeling state or be behaviorally associated with reduced control over temper. Irritable persons often lash out at others, usually verbally but sometimes physically. In contrast to anger, irritability does not lessen after an outburst. It is diagnostically nonspecific, seen in a variety of anxiety and mood disorders and as a lifelong temperamental quality, demonstrable from birth.

Panic *Panic attack* is a circumscribed episode of severe state anxiety lasting minutes to hours, with symptoms escalating in a crescendo pattern. Subjectively, panic is characterized by feelings of utter terror; fears that one will die, go crazy, or lose control; and many of the somatic symptoms of anxiety mentioned above, sometimes accompanied by severe chest pains, marked shortness of breath, and exhausting fatigue. Individual isolated panic attacks may be common in the general population, with up to 30 percent of the population experiencing at least one attack each year. Panic attacks may be seen more regularly and, typically, more severely as part of panic disorder or in association with other anxiety disorders. Patients with other psychiatric disorders may experience limited-symptom panic attacks in which the episodes are characterized by less intense anxiety and by fewer and milder physical symptoms, such as isolated paresthesia or difficulty in breathing. Those limited-symptom attacks may be aborted panic episodes that are not further exacerbated by secondary psychological reactions to the initial symptoms.

A 24-year-old woman was sitting in a crowded restaurant with friends when, without being conscious of any particular worries, she began to feel pressure in her chest, difficulty in breathing, and dizziness. Within minutes the symptoms escalated, and she insisted on being taken to an emergency room, where no cause for the symptoms was discovered. Over the next month she had six similar episodes, although none was as bad as the first one.

Although American psychiatry has segregated panic attacks from other forms of anxiety, assuming categorical phenomenological and biological differences, the distinction is far from universally accepted. Some psychiatrists view panic as simply an extreme form of anxiety, to be understood as part of a continuum of intensity.

Phobias Phobias are irrational fears. In an effort to reduce the intense anxiety attached to the phobic object or situation, patients do their best to avoid the feared stimuli. Thus, phobias consist of both the fear and the avoidance component. The fear itself may include all the symptoms of extreme anxiety, akin to panic. In *simple phobias* persistent, irrational fears are provoked by specific stimuli. Phobias may develop to almost any object or situation. Table 10-5 lists some phobias. Common simple phobias include fears of dirt, excrement, snakes, spiders, heights, and blood.

Behavioral, psychodynamic, and biological theories have all been advanced as causes of phobias. Some well-known phobias, such as fear of animals, may result either from early traumatic events (developing along the paradigm of classic Pavlovian conditioning) or from displacements of early psychodynamic conflicts. Genetic influences may also play a role in the development of some simple phobias; for example, some persons with blood-injury phobias, which strongly cluster among biological relatives, may be genetically predisposed by vagal responses to certain stimuli. Animal models also indicate possible biological vulnerability; some monkeys that have never been exposed to snakes become panicky when placed in the presence of a snake. Since such fear responses obviously have adaptive value, some human phobic responses may also represent exaggerations of adaptive behaviors shaped by evolutionary biology.

TABLE 10-5
Specific Phobias

Acrophobia	Fear of heights
Agoraphobia	Fear of open spaces
Amathophobia	Fear of dust
Apiphobia	Fear of bees
Astrapophobia	Fear of lightning
Blennophobia	Fear of slime
Claustrophobia	Fear of enclosed spaces
Cynophobia	Fear of dogs
Decidophobia	Fear of making decisions
Electrophobia	Fear of electricity
Eremophobia	Fear of being alone
Gamophobia	Fear of marriage
Gatophobia	Fear of cats
Gephyrophobia	Fear of crossing bridges
Gynophobia	Fear of women
Hydrophobia	Fear of water
Kakorraphiophobia	Fear of failure
Katagelophobia	Fear of ridicule
Keraunophobia	Fear of thunder
Musophobia	Fear of mice
Nyctophobia	Fear of night
Ochlophobia	Fear of crowds
Odynophobia	Fear of pain
Ophidiophobia	Fear of snakes
Pnigerophobia	Fear of smothering
Pyrophobia	Fear of fire
Scholionophobia	Fear of school
Sciophobia	Fear of shadows
Spheksophobia	Fear of wasps
Technophobia	Fear of technology
Thalassophobia	Fear of the ocean
Triskaidekaphobia	Fear of the number 13
Tropophobia	Fear of moving or making changes

Complex phobias, more elaborate than simple phobias, involve fears related to broad situations. *Agoraphobia,* the best-known, is a fear of open spaces. The predominant current formulation suggests that agoraphobia is a secondary reaction to panic attacks. In that view, persons who have become terrified of having panic attacks in social and public settings retreat to their own homes, hoping to reduce the likelihood of panic attacks by avoiding places where they were once triggered and where they may feel exposed and embarrassed. In *social phobia,* patients become overwhelmingly anxious and fear situations in which they may be observed. In the limited type only a few specific situations—such as speaking in public and urinating in a public lavatory—evoke the fear. In the general type the fear of social situations is so broad-based that it globally hampers the person's interpersonal life.

AGGRESSION, HOSTILITY, IMPULSIVENESS, AND VIOLENCE The spectrum of aggressive emotions and their behavioral manifestations is characterized by heightened vigilance in response to a sense of threat and an enhanced readiness to attack, often in response to a perceived threat. In some aggressive states, physiological tone is heightened in preparation for fight. Assertiveness, the adaptive aspect of those emotions, includes sensing that something needs to be done and feeling willing and competent to take constructive action. The manner and the extent to which aggressive emotions can be expressed varies from society to society and situation to situation. The emotions are among the most carefully regulated because of their potential destructiveness.

Individual differences in the tendency toward experiencing and expressing anger and violence are biological, developmental, and cultural in origin. Some infants are irritable from birth. Subtle birth injuries and brain anoxia may increase the susceptibility of some persons to be violent. Furthermore, studies of EEG patterns in violent persons show increased abnormalities, especially in those with histories of repeated violence and violence with little or no obvious motive. Soft neurological signs are also seen in violent criminals. Biochemically, low cerebrospinal fluid 5-HIAA has been associated with a variety of impulsive behaviors, such as violent crimes, recurrent fire setting, and violent suicide attempts.

The pathological childhood triad of bed-wetting past the age of 6 years, setting fires, and torturing animals is associated with subsequent violent behavior in adults. Interpersonally, studies show that violence-prone persons require more personal space around their physical person than do others. Violent persons feel threatened when approached too closely, particularly from the rear.

Psychological and social contributions are also strong. Violence in families breeds violence, and battered children grow up to be battering adults. Cultural norms for the expression of violence differ considerably. In some socioeconomic and ethnic groups, violent gangs organize the energies of many adolescent youth. For some, violent behavior is an adolescent socialization pattern that is necessary to prove one's manhood. Like other social organizations, violent gangs have detailed rules that inhibit the expression of violence. Some unpredictable and unsocialized violent persons, loners, are too violent to be contained even in gangs.

Aggressive or violent behavior is diagnostically nonspecific. In schizophrenia it is seen as a consequence of paranoid delusions, in response to command auditory hallucinations, and secondary to passivity experiences. Manic patients and those in mixed mood states may be violent, often in response to minimal provocation. Violent behavior is common in patients with antisocial and borderline personality disorders; those with borderline personality disorder often direct the violence against themselves, as well as others. Violent behavior is also common in epilepsy, although rarely during ictal periods; as a release phenomenon in frontal lobe syndromes; and in substance abuse syndromes, particularly with such sedatives as alcohol, which act as disinhibitors, and such stimulants as amphetamines and cocaine, which increase irritability, aggressiveness, and paranoia.

External stimuli and situations may provoke impulsive violence. Alcohol is perhaps the most common disinhibitor of violence. Intrafamilial violence, the most common setting for homicide, is frequently related to alcohol intoxication. In the syndrome of *episodic dyscontrol,* explosively violent behavioral episodes typically erupt after a person has had some alcohol, a phenomenon known as *pathological intoxication.* In the often ferocious and destructive outbursts the person may confront or provoke any potential target for violence, even total strangers, but girlfriends, wives, and parents are the frequent victims. Patients with episodic dyscontrol commonly have histories of violent sexual behavior, including rape, and, often while intoxicated, of speeding and reckless driving in automobiles, sometimes chasing down, stopping, and attacking other motorists who they feel "get in their way."

A 35-year-old man who had been jailed repeatedly for assaultive behavior appeared in an emergency room, intoxicated. He was edgy and threatening, trying to provoke staff members into a fight, and asserting that he had previously injured several policemen and security guards in similar situations. His wife confirmed the history. Ushered into a seclusion room and sedated, he pounded on the walls, bruising his hands, until he fell asleep. The next morning he was sheepish and apologetic, saying that he could hardly remember the events of the previous night.

A 35-year-old schizoid man, who had been battered as a child, avoided intimacy with people, fearing that he would be unable to relate well. He bought two dogs, hoping to teach himself to be socialized. To his horror he found that he became jealous when one dog paid attention to the other dog, rather than to him, and he sadistically beat the dog, realizing all the time that he was repeating the pattern of his father's abuse toward him. While beating the dog, he would imagine feeling the same sadistic rage that his father must have felt toward him.

Temper tantrums Immature persons with persistent personality problems may fail to develop mechanisms to inhibit the temper tantrums they displayed as children. Particularly if childhood tantrums produced the desired result, learned tantrum behaviors may persist into adult life. Although the persons may be extremely pleasant and sociable when things are going well, they often lack the capacity to tolerate frustration and are easily provoked by threats to self-esteem and self-image and by not having their own way. In those situations they may act like bullies and lose their tempers easily—glaring, snarling, yelling, shouting, intimidating, pouting, sulking, and sometimes being physically violent.

Displaced rage When circumstances prevent the expression of rage directly against those persons or institutions provoking frustration, other outlets for aggression are often found. Acts of violence that are either calculated or wanton may result. Cruelty to animals and fire setting may persist as adult forms of destructive behavior. Rape—an act of control, intimidation, terror, and humiliation—may also serve to displace frustrations that cannot be expressed more adaptively.

Sadism Sadism may occur with or without explicit sexual gratification. Calculated cruelty conducted seemingly without anger or emotional arousal may reflect the inadequate development of social morality or individual conscience, as in the conduct of torturers and some cold-blooded murderers. In some societies and under specific circumstances at certain times in history, such activity has been socially sanctioned, indicating that at least some people have few inborn inhibitions against cruelty or violence.

Self-mutilation For a variety of reasons and as part of a number of disorders, patients may commit acts of violence against themselves. Psychotic patients may enucleate their eyes, castrate themselves, or perform other self-destructive acts short of actual suicide that have apparent symbolic import. Patients with borderline personality disorder may cut themselves repeatedly with broken glass or razor blades on the arms, legs, breasts, or other parts of the body or may burn themselves with cigarettes. In explaining the behavior, patients typically deny suicidal ideation but describe the need to feel external pain as a mirror to their internal suffering, as a tension-releasing mechanism, or as a way to increase their sense of being alive, often replacing a dissociativelike numbness.

A 38-year-old woman with borderline personality disorder and a past history of anorexia nervosa and bulimia began to cut herself repeatedly on her arms after termination of her psychotherapy when her therapist moved to another city. The behavior began with superficial cuts over many weeks and escalated to deep incisions that required sutures in emergency rooms at least twice weekly. The cutting episodes occurred only at night, when the patient was alone. She described her escalating feelings of tension at those times; the tension was unrelieved by talking to her new therapist or by medication but diminished dramatically when she saw the cuts on her arms and the blood dripping.

Trichotillomania is a syndrome of compulsive hair pulling, resulting in bald patches. It is often associated with other self-mutilatory behavior, such as picking the face, nails, or cuticles to the point of infections and bleeding. Some evidence indicates that trichotillomania is related to obsessive-compulsive disorder.

Children with Lesch-Nyhan syndrome, a developmental disability syndrome caused by a congenital metabolic abnormality, bite and pick at themselves so compulsively that they do themselves great harm; they must be routinely restrained. Occasionally, patients with Tourette's disorder display compulsive self-harming behavior.

OTHER DISTURBANCES OF FEELINGS Diminished levels of affective intensity are seen in anxiety disorders, mood disorders, and schizophrenia. A mild flattening of emotion with a blunting of ability to feel joy is common in dysthymia. Some patients with narcissistic and borderline personality disorders complain of inner emptiness and pervasive boredom and ennui without displaying diminished affect in interviews. Similarly, patients with prominent depersonalization describe numbed emotions. Pathological levels of *blunt* or *flattened affect,* indicating markedly diminished affective expression in relation to specific thought content, is seen in chronic schizophrenia, some organic mental syndromes, and severe depressive disorders. Although the term ''blunted affect'' is not classically used to describe the affective flatness of severe depression, it is not always easy to distinguish between schizophrenic and depressive flatness on phenomenological grounds. *Anhedonia,* the lack of pleasurable feelings from activities that ordinarily provide pleasure, is also seen as part of severe depressive disorders and schizophrenia. Chronically psychotic patients often exhibit emotional deterioration in which affective experience and expression is entirely unrelated to thought content.

Inappropriate affect is incongruency of affective expression and thought content. The patient may display loud and raucous laughter or giggling in relation to bland or sad thoughts or may show grief without apparent reason. Inappropriate affect sometimes signifies that the thoughts have private meanings for the patient; the emotional experiences might make sense to an observer if the private meanings were understood. Inappropriate affect must be distinguished from affective expressions that are appropriate in a subculture or ethnic group but that are unfamiliar to the observer and from defensive affect, such as the nervous laughter used to alleviate tension or to ward off crying.

Affective lability is characterized by rapid shifts in affect, often within seconds or minutes. It is commonly seen during hypomanic states, premenstrual syndrome (called premenstrual dysphoric disorder in DSM-IV), postpartum blues, and some personality disorders.

Alexithymia is difficulty in identifying and describing feelings and distinguishing between feelings and physical sensations. Persons who manifest alexithymia often have constricted imaginative capacities. When distressed, the patients are simply aware of not feeling well and usually complain of somatic symptoms, leading to frustrating interactions with their primary care physicians, who cannot find physical causes for the presenting physical complaints. From one perspective, alexithymia is a means of communicating affective distress through somatic language.

DISTURBANCES IN MOTOR ASPECTS OF BEHAVIOR

Motor behavior is normally finely coordinated, purposeful, and adaptive, and necessary activities are usually carried out efficiently. In psychiatric disturbances, motor abnormalities can involve generalized overactivity or underactivity or can manifest in a wide range of specific disorders of movement.

OVERACTIVITY *Restlessness* and *agitation* are diffuse increases in body movement, usually expressed as fidgeting, rapid and rhythmic leg or hand tapping, and jerky start-and-stop movements of the entire body, accompanied by inner tension. Restlessness accompanies psychiatric conditions of high emotional arousal or confusion—such as toxic states, deliriums, mania, agitated depressive disorders, and anxiety disorders—and many medical disorders, such as hyperthyroidism. In some depressive states, agitation is often accompanied by pacing and hand wringing.

Generalized overactivity, in which patients seem to have increased physical energy, is distinguished from agitation by the lack of inner tension and by purposeful movements in generalized overactivity. It is commonly seen in mania, hypomania, anorexia nervosa, and attention-deficit hyperactivity disorder.

In *catatonic excitement,* a form of catatonic behavior less commonly seen now than in the pre-antipsychotic era, the patient exhibits disorganized hyperactive behavior, including frantic jumping, thrashing of limbs, and seemingly senseless menacing or attacking behavior. Such excitement is seen in mania, periodic catatonia, catatonic forms of schizophrenia, and such culture-bound syndromes as *amok. Confusional excitement* is a state of restlessness and generalized purposeless activity seen in ictal states, some acute intoxications, and deliriums.

DECREASED MOTOR ACTIVITY Global reductions in motor activity (motor retardation) are seen in a variety of physical disorders—such as hypothyroidism, Addison's disease, and other fatiguing illnesses—and some organic mental disorders, schizophrenias, and depressive disorders. Poverty of movement (*akinesia* or, more properly, *hypokinesia*) occurs in schizophrenia and as a side effect of antipsychotic medication. Changes in the voice frequently accompany the reduced motor activities in schizophrenia and depression, with loss of normal inflection replaced by monotonous tone and prolonged speech latency. In stuporous states, patients remain immobile, although their eyes are open and they are apparently awake.

Conversion reactions are functional, nonphysiological, psychogenic impairments in sensory or motor functions. Common motor forms include paralysis and paresis of various types, including limb paralyses, ataxias, and aphonias. In *globus hystericus* the patient is unable to swallow. Sensory conversion reactions include blindness, deafness, anesthesia, and analgesia.

Mutism may result from a variety of peripheral muscle and CNS conditions and from functional disorders. Psychiatric disorders in which mutism is seen include major depressive disorder, catatonic states, conversion disorder, and the elective mutism occasionally seen in acute adjustment disorders and some personality disorders.

MOTOR DISTURBANCES Many motor disturbances are seen in psychiatric disorders. Some form part of the core somatic symptoms of the disorders; some are characteristic of disorders that, by their nature, form the borderlands of true neuropsychiatric disorders (such as Tourette's disorder); and others are acute or chronic medication side effects.

Tremor *Tremors,* involuntary oscillating movements of the limbs or the head, may occur at rest or with movement. *Physiological tremors,* which are minimal at rest and increased with activity, are characterized by small amplitude and high frequency. They are characteristic of anxiety, fatigue, and toxic or metabolic disorders, such as caffeinism and hyperthyroidism, and are commonly seen in patients taking lithium and stimulating antidepressants. Coarse tremors with large amplitude and low frequency are seen in Parkinson's disease and cerebellar disease. *Asterixis* is a large-amplitude flapping tremor of the hands seen in hepatic disease.

Parkinsonism Parkinsonian symptoms and signs may be seen in psychiatric disorders, particularly in patients taking antipsychotic medications. The symptoms include akinesias with a marked decrease in normally spontaneous fidgety movements, a stiff gait with diminished arm swing, pill-rolling nonintention tremors (which seem to be less common in drug-induced parkinsonism than in the idiopathic type), expressionless soft and monotonous speech, micrographic handwriting, and cogwheel rigidity.

Dystonic movements Although dystonic movements are seen as part of many neurological disorders, in psychiatric patients they are almost always secondary to antipsychotic use. The dystonic reaction consists of intermittent or sustained muscle spasms, typically of the head or the neck. Common varieties include tongue spasms causing dysarthria, torticollis (neck spasm), and oculogyric crisis, characterized by a forced upward gaze. Less commonly, opisthotonos (spasm of the spinal muscle, leading to an arched posture) is seen. Those reactions are most common in young men and are typically seen soon after they begin or increase the dosage of an antipsychotic medication.

Akathisia Akathisia is a syndrome of motor restlessness seen almost exclusively in the context of antipsychotic medication use. It generally has both subjective and motor components. Subjectively, patients describe muscle tension, difficulty in finding a comfortable body position, and inability to stop moving; they feel as though they were jumping out of their skin. Objectively, the classic sign of akathisia is rocking from foot to foot while standing. When seated, patients frequently cross and uncross their legs and often arise during the interview to pace. Sleep may be disturbed because of physical discomfort. When the subjective components of akathisia are prominent, they may be difficult to distinguish from anxiety because of the primary disorder (typically, schizophrenia). Rarely, the restlessness becomes sufficiently uncomfortable to provoke acts of violence. Some authors describe *pseudoakathisia,* characterized solely by the presence of objective signs of akathisia with the subjective denial of feelings of restlessness.

A 24-year-old hospitalized schizophrenic man was given haloperidol (Haldol) 10 mg daily for a relapse of his disorder. Two days after beginning the medication, he became increasingly agitated—pacing around the ward, muttering to himself, sitting for a few moments, then arising again. It was impossible to conduct an interview, in part because he would not stand in one place. He was assessed as showing an escalation of his psychosis, and the antipsychotic dosage was doubled. Within the next few days, the patient became even more agitated but was able to tell staff members that he was convinced that a motor inside him would not stop running. (Whether the motor was metaphorical or delusional was unclear.) One of the ward psychiatrists suspected akathisia, lowered the antipsychotic dosage, and prescribed anticholingeric and β-blocking medication to combat the akathisia. Within two days the patient became far more relaxed, less restless, and less psychotic.

Tardive dyskinesia Tardive dyskinesia is a movement disorder that occurs only during the use of antipsychotic medication; occasionally the disorder appears after many months of taking the medication; more commonly it appears after years. The abnormal movements may persist with or without continued medication use or may disappear or diminish over time. The dyskinetic movements occur at rest and can usually be temporarily suppressed volitionally or by purposeful action, distraction, or sleep. The movements are varied. In the most common type, which affects the mouth and the lips, tongue thrusting, chewing movements, lip smacking, and eye blinking are seen. Another common type is characterized by choreoathetoid movements, such as writhing finger motions. In the less common but more severe truncal dyskinesias, the torso moves in thrusting motions, and respiratory dyskinesia is characterized by irregular, grunting breathing patterns. Other tardive (late) syndromes are tardive akathisia and tardive dystonia, in which the abnormal movements emerge late in treatment or when medication is discontinued.

Neuroleptic malignant syndrome Neuroleptic malignant syndrome, a potentially fatal complication of antipsychotic medication, is characterized by muscle rigidity, fever, diaphoresis, delirium, mutism, and blood pressure abnormalities. Some authors believe that the syndrome is the most severe end of a spectrum of disorders that starts with antipsychotic-induced parkinsonism, progresses to extrapyramidal syndrome with fever, and ends with fulminant neuroleptic malignant syndrome.

Rabbit syndrome This uncommon drug-induced extrapyramidal syndrome is often misdiagnosed as tardive dyskinesia. It most closely resembles a limited expression of a parkinsonian tremor. Patients make rapid chewing movements similar to those made by rabbits; the movements are ordinarily faster and more regular than the orofacial tic of tardive dyskinesia. The tongue is spared.

Blepharospasm Blepharospasm is a rapid and violent repetitive, spasmodic movement of the eyelids. The movements are often a side effect of antipsychotic or other medication but are also common in a variety of neurological disorders, including Meige's disease and Tourette's disorder.

Tics Tics are rapid, repetitive, often spasmodic, jerklike involuntary movements that serve no apparent purpose. The person may try to disguise or hide the tic in a seemingly purposive movement, and the movement may ultimately become shaped into a mannerism. Tics are the central features in tic disorders, are associated with other disorders, and are a consequence of stimulant use.

Tourette's disorder is characterized by a chronic, shifting array of motor and vocal tics. The vocal tics may include grunts, coughs, clicks, and sniffs; the motor tics may include eye blinking, tongue protrusions, facial grimacing, hopping, and twitches. Complex tics merge into complex compulsive behaviors, such as squatting, deep-knee bends, and retracing steps. *Coprolalia,* characterized by sudden verbal outbursts of obscenities, occurs in fewer than a third of Tourette's disorder patients. In mental coprolalia obscene words or phrases suddenly intrude into consciousness in an ego-dystonic manner. Obsessive-compulsive symptoms and attention-deficit symptoms are also common in Tourette's disorder.

Serotonin syndrome Serotonin syndrome, a disorder associated with excessive serotonin, is typically caused by the combination of two or more medications with serotonin-enhancing properties. It is characterized by restlessness, myoclonus, hyperreflexia, diaphoresis, shivering, tremor, and mental status changes, such as confusion.

Motor disturbances of schizophrenia Many of the abnormal movements ascribed to tardive dyskinesia and other antipsychotic-induced dystonic and choreoathetoid conditions had been described in chronically psychotic patients before the introduction of antipsychotic medications. In one series of 100 patients, the large majority of whom were classified as schizophrenic, a review of medical records before 1955 revealed that abnormal purposive movements were found in 83 percent, mannerisms and tics in 42 percent, and gait abnormalities in 10 percent. Those findings suggest that many patients with schizophrenia have neurological symptoms *not* caused by medications and that severe psychiatric disorders may have a neurological component. Other studies have reported similar findings.

Catatonia covers a broad group of movement abnormalities characteristically found in psychotic disorders. Although usually associated with schizophrenia, catatonic features are commonly found in other disorders, such as mania, depression, many neurological disorders (especially those involving the basal ganglia, the limbic system, the diencephalon, and the frontal lobes), systemic metabolic disorders, toxic drug states, and periodic catatonia. Catatonic stupor and excitement have already been noted.

Stereotypies are repetitious, seemingly non-goal-directed, complex, organized gestures or postures that are thought to have private meanings for the patient. Examples include continuously crossing oneself, blessing others, waving repeatedly in a stylized manner, and making profane gestures. The stereotypical behaviors commonly seen in autistic children (constant spinning and rocking) may provide soothing, steady sensory input that helps the patients reduce the disturbance they experience from the usual unpredictable and uncontrollable stimulation in the environment. *Bizarre posturing* is also a manifestation of a catatonic syndrome. One chronic schizophrenic patient characteristically stood for hours on one leg, like a crane, with his arms in the air. In *echopraxia* the patient imitates the examiner's movements, as if in mimicry. Some catatonic patients exhibit *waxy flexibility,* maintaining unusual postures into which they are placed for prolonged periods of time. *Negativism* may take the form of refusing to behave in a prescribed manner or of resisting passive movement.

Other motor disturbances *Gait disturbances* in patients with psychiatric disorders include a variety of neurogenic gaits consistent with brain disease, intoxications, and medication side effects. The disturbances include the festinating gait of parkinsonism, the spastic and ataxic gaits of neurological diseases and psychiatric medications, the waddling and reeling gaits associated with intoxications, and the hysterical nonphysiological gait disturbances seen in astasia-abasia, a form of conversion disorder. Gait mannerisms include clowning, prancing, and military and effeminate gaits.

Bruxism, chronic teeth gnashing, may occur involuntarily during tension states or as an isolated occurrence during stage 4 sleep, in which it has sometimes been associated with benzodiazepine or alcohol use. In severe cases serious damage to the dental enamel and temporomandibular joint pain may occur.

Myoclonus, characterized by focal muscle jerking, can be caused in psychiatric patients by certain medications, such as serotonin-reuptake-blocker antidepressants and monoamine oxidase (MAO) inhibitors. Myoclonic jerks may be difficult to distinguish from tics, but the tics often involve larger muscle groups and are more highly organized motor patterns than monoclonus. Myoclonus may be seen at rest but is more obvious during motor activity.

SEIZURELIKE BEHAVIORS In addition to the generalized, petit mal, and complex partial seizures seen in psychiatric patients, a number of nonepileptic seizurelike behaviors must be distinguished. *Breath-holding spells* usually occur in small children, who hold their breaths during moments of oppositional rage and faint as a result. The children may display associated jerking or twitching motor movements. That generally innocuous phenomenon is ordinarily impulsive and tantrumlike. *Temper tantrums* in young children may look like seizures, especially to the uninformed observer. The children may lie on the floor, screaming and kicking, and fail to respond to the environment. *Conversion seizures* must be differentiated from genuine epileptic seizures. Those *pseudoseizures* are nonphysiological. Patients do not have abnormal reflexes or incontinence. However, because so many conversion seizures occur in patients who have genuine epilepsy and who know a good deal about the condition, the differential diagnosis is sometimes difficult.

COMPULSIVE BEHAVIORS Compulsive behaviors may occur in relation to everyday activities—such as gambling, sexual conquest, shopping, and watching television—or in relation to substances, such as alcohol, cocaine, narcotics, and food. Other compulsions involve reckless risk-taking behaviors that provide stimulation and dispel dysphoric moods. Sexual compulsive perversions, such as exhibitionism and sadomasochism, may serve similar purposes. Compulsions are seen in a variety of psychotic and nonpsychotic psychiatric disorders. The cravings that underlie compulsive behaviors are strong motivating forces, and the compulsive behaviors serve to regulate emotions. As-yet-unknown similarities may underlie all compulsive and addictive mechanisms.

In obsessive-compulsive disorder the compulsions are ritualized, repetitive behavior that are performed with the goal of neutralizing and undoing obsessional thoughts. Although performed to decrease anxiety, the rituals, which are excessive compared with the fears, are never more than trivially and transiently successful. Hand-washing compulsions and compulsions to make certain that gas jets and faucets have been turned off, to be sure that doors are locked, to perform religious gestures, to count objects, and to place objects in a prescribed order are among the common compulsions.

LANGUAGE DISORDERS

Communication difficulties may be due to disorders of thinking, as previously described; abnormal speech patterns in mood disorders and schizophrenia; primary speech-fluency disorders, such as stuttering and stammering; disorders of the articulation and speech apparatus; and CNS disturbances involved in hearing and speech generation (aphasias).

Manic patients typically exhibit pressured speech, in which the speed of the stream of words is accelerated. If the disorder is severe, the speech may be garbled, imprecise, and difficult to understand. Patients with psychomotor retardation depression may speak slowly and monotonously and have a long speech latency in response to questions. Schizophrenic patients may be difficult to understand because of their disorder or because of the dysarthric effect of antipsychotic medication.

SPEECH-FLUENCY DISORDERS Stuttering and stammering (ordinarily synonymous) are disturbances in the rhythm and the fluency of speech because of blocking, convulsive repetition, or prolongation of sounds. The disorder affects males two to three times as often as females, and there is a high rate of familial transmission.

APHASIAS *Aphasias,* impairments of language produced by brain dysfunction, are ordinarily described as being fluent and nonfluent. In *fluent aphasias,* which generally reflect dysfunction in the left temporal and parietal areas, patients have a normal or even elevated verbal output, sometimes with logorrhea, but they ignore the social conventions of conversation. They produce many well-articulated phrases with normal prosody but with little informational content. The fluent aphasias are further divided according to the extent of the patient's comprehension and the patient's ability to repeat what an examiner says. The principal fluent aphasias are Wernicke's aphasia, conduction aphasia, anomic aphasia, and transcortical sensory aphasia.

Nonfluent aphasias are characterized by slow and poor verbal output, difficulty with spontaneous speech, the omission of grammatical connecting words, and poor prosody. Patients may produce one-word replies or short phrases. Brain lesions that cause nonfluent aphasias tend to occur in the anterior left hemisphere. The principal nonfluent aphasias are Broca's aphasia, transcortical motor aphasia, global aphasia, and the mixed transcortical aphasias.

DISTURBANCES IN INTERPERSONAL RELATIONSHIPS

Normal interpersonal relationships include relationships with parents, children, spouses, lovers, siblings, extended-family members, friends, comrades, coworkers, and members of the larger community. Those relationships ordinarily help provide for the satisfaction of basic drives, for affiliative needs, and for finding purpose and meaning in life. Through stable and satisfying relationships, human needs are met to have intimacy (including love, sex, and affection), to be cared for and nurtured, to provide care, to learn, to play, to relax, to dominate, and to be productive through mutual effort. Interpersonal relationships are carefully regulated by means of interpersonal signs and signals. Those communication patterns and relationships follow rules that are usually predictable, consistent, and lawful from moment to moment and over extended periods. The extent to which deviance from those patterns is tolerated in a given relationship varies from behavior to behavior, relationship to relationship, family to family, and culture to culture.

Disturbances in interpersonal relationships may be viewed as characteristics attributable to a single person or as characteristics of an interpersonal system. Individual disturbances are considered to be undesirable or maladaptive personality traits. When those traits are present to a significant extent and interfere with social functioning or cause distress, they may constitute a personality disorder. Disturbances of interpersonal relationships are also described at a systems level (for example, as dyadic and family patterns of system disturbance). However, those disturbances have not been characterized as well as have individual patterns.

INDIVIDUAL FACTORS In addition to conveying meaning through spoken words, people communicate much information through nonlexical vocalization (the music of the voice), nonverbal gestures, posture, and other aspects of appearance. A great deal of social interaction and communication is initiated, sustained, and modified by those modes of communication. The clinician's rapid diagnostic impressions rely heavily on those aspects of communication. Many clues to personality traits are immediately evident in nonverbal patterns, which must be supplemented with historical information.

Body odor Unlike members of many other cultures, Americans tend to be fastidious about body odor, bathing frequently and using a variety of scents and deodorants. A strong body odor may reflect cultural differences, a deliberate choice not to bathe, some psychiatric disorders characterized by inattention to grooming and personal hygiene, or anosmia. Strong perfume scents may reflect cultural styles and desires to be attractive.

A 34-year-old schizophrenic man had participated in an extensive social skills training group for two years, after which he bathed regularly. For the next few years the most reliable sign of an impending relapse was a marked increase in his body odor, caused by a lack of bathing, which became powerfully evident during his clinic appointments.

Clothing The type, state, and condition of clothing say much about a person's socioeconomic group, self-care and grooming, and personality. Tight, revealing clothes on a woman may signal exhibitionistic or histrionic traits; rumpled, neglected, dirty clothes may be evidence of the self-neglect that often attends cognitive impairment caused by organic or functional disorders or chronic substance abuse. Unusual articles of clothing may be emblems of subgroup affiliation or have special personal meaning, as in some psychoses and perversions. Clothing may represent a way of saying, ''I'm safe and bland,'' or a way of signaling countercultural affiliations or a personal sense of weirdness. Clothes can say, ''Stay away'' or ''Approach at your own risk.''

Skin adornment Tattoos, unusual haircuts, and scars may reveal subculture affiliation, drug use, and batterings. Highly developed muscles may reveal positive athleticism or narcissistic overinvolvement with physical attributes.

Body language Posture, gesture, and eye contact vary interculturally and interpersonally. Proxemics—posture, distancing, the use of space, touching, eye contact, voice loudness, thermal radiation, and olfaction—reveals how body language communicates psychiatrically pertinent information and quantitates the information that clinicians use intuitively all the time. At least initially, most observers are strongly swayed by body signals, and patients who wish to mislead examiners can do so by skillful misrepresentation. Clinicians often find their first impressions to be wrong, which is why they must always perform the prescribed examinations and take a detailed history.

The manner in which limbs are positioned and moved, the extent to which posture and gaze are directed or averted, and the way in which one person's body language responds to another's, regardless of the content of the ongoing verbal communication, are all highly informative. Videotape analyses of individual and family therapy sessions have shown quasi-courtship behavior—flirtatious advances, preenings, and seductive body movements—being initiated and responded to by patients and therapists who were all unaware of those body movements and who were all the while engaged in the conversation of the therapy session, which dealt with something entirely different.

Posture can convey information about ethnicity. People of northern and western European origin tend to maintain a larger personal space or physical distance from one another than do those of Mediterranean origin. Middle Easterners feel comfortable very close to one another, nearly nose-to-nose in conversation. Dominance, fear, anxiety, and the desire for intimacy are all communicated through the use of space. Irritable persons insist on maintaining personal space; dependent persons and those seeking intimacy may overstep the comfort boundary of others.

Habitual gestures may reveal personality traits and aspects of self-identity: frequent preening, patting or stroking of the hair, and examining the fingernails reveal narcissism; playing with the wedding ring reveals marital conflict; spasmodic clutching of the chest reveals hypochondriasis; repeated removal of eyeglasses and nose wiping reveal denial; and an open upper-torso body language—broad inviting, seductive gestures—but closed lower-body signals—tightly crossed or closed legs—reveal a histrionic personality trait in women.

Studies of gaze have shown extroverts to gaze more directly and more often at others than do introverts. In one study, schizophrenic patients gazed directly at an examiner only 65 percent as much as normal controls did; patients with depressive disorders gazed 73 percent as much as normal controls. The schizophrenic patients also used shorter glances (2.1 seconds) than did depressed patients (3.4 seconds) or controls (3.9 seconds). Autistic patients spend only about 4 percent of the time gazing at another person in a room, compared with 65 percent for controls.

Averted gaze may be culturally conditioned. In some societies a direct gaze is considered rude or sexually forward.

A 15-year-old devout Puerto Rican girl being interviewed by a psychiatric resident kept her body turned 90 degrees from his, refused to face him, and, except for occasional side glances, stared continuously at the floor throughout the interview. The resident initially interpreted that presentation as withdrawn and avoidant behavior, but he quickly saw that with many other people on the ward the patient was direct, friendly, and open. For that patient, who had been raised in a strict home in the Puerto Rican countryside and who had only recently come to New York, staring directly into the resident's eyes for long periods of time would have been both socially inappropriate, because of their differences in social standing, and a brazen sexual signal.

Personality traits and disorders Personality, variably defined, is the characteristic pattern of a person's attitudes, behaviors, beliefs, feelings, thoughts, and values—the sum total of a person's emotional, cognitive, and interpersonal characteristics. Personality traits are simply the prominent features of someone's personality and do not imply psychopathology. Aspects of personality are present from early on in life, and personality traits are relatively stable from adolescence onward, consistent across different environments, and recognizable by friends and acquaintances. The term ''personality disorder'' should be reserved for those consistent patterns of thought, feeling, and behavior that are inflexible and consistently maladaptive. More than almost any other construct in psychopathology, personality disturbances manifest themselves primarily in interpersonal contexts. In that way, personality disorders can be viewed as interpersonal behavior disorders.

The determinants of personality are multiple, varied, and, to a great extent, not understood. Nonetheless, personality is composed of a combination of biological and learned characteristics—of temperament (genetic or constitutional) factors and character factors, which are learned attributes presumably originating in early life experiences.

The dimensional approach to personality pathology characterizes persons along a continuum of traits; the categorical approach attempts to define a clear demarcation between having a disorder and not having one. For example, a recently proposed personality typology characterizes personality types dimensionally along three dimensions presumed to be strongly influenced genetically: (1) *harm avoidance,* (2) *novelty seeking,* and (3) *reward dependence.* In that formulation high scores on the three dimensions characterize (1) inhibition and pessimism, (2) impulsive and exploratory behavior, and (3) dependence and sentimentality. Depending on a person's score on all three dimensions, the personality type can be described. For example, antisocial personalities are characterized by high novelty seeking, low harm avoidance, and low reward dependence; dependent personalities score low on novelty seeking, high on harm avoidance, and high on reward dependence. DSM-IV, by contrast, uses a categorical approach; yet both the large overlap among the personality disorders and the clustering of the many personality disorders into three broad clusters imply a lack of clear boundaries to the currently defined categories. The three DSM-IV clusters describe odd or eccentric types (cluster A); dramatic, emotional, and erratic types (cluster B); and anxious and fearful types (cluster C).

The odd or eccentric group includes paranoid, schizoid, and schizotypal personality disorders. Patients with those personality disorders have the core traits of being interpersonally distant and emotionally constricted. Paranoid personalities are quick to feel slighted and jealous, carry grudges, and expect to be exploited and harmed by others. Schizoid personalities lack friendships or close relationships with others and are indifferent to praise or criticism by others. Schizotypal personalities display odd beliefs, engage in odd and eccentric gestures and practices, and exhibit odd speech.

The dramatic, emotional, and erratic group includes borderline, histrionic, narcissistic, and antisocial personality disorders. Patients with those personality disorders characteristically have chaotic lives, emotions, and relationships. Borderline personalities are impulsive, unpredictable, angry, temperamental, unstable in relationships, compulsively interpersonal, and self-damaging with regard to sex, money, and substance use. Histrionic personalities are attention seeking, exhibitionistic, seductive, and self-indulgent; exhibit exaggerated expressions of emotions; and are overconcerned with physical appearance. Narcissistic personalities tend to be hypersensitive to criticism, exploitative of others, and egocentric, with an inflated sense of self-importance; feel entitled to special treatment; and demand constant attention. Antisocial personalities are described almost exclusively in behavioral terms, rather than affective or relational terms. They are truant; they lie, steal, start fights, and break rules; they are unable to sustain work or school; and they shirk everyday responsibilities.

The anxious and fearful group includes avoidant, dependent, and obsessive-compulsive personality disorders. Patients with those disorders are characterized by constricting behaviors that serve to limit risks. For example, avoidant persons avoid relationships, dependent persons avoid being responsible for decisions, and obsessive-compulsive persons use rigid rules that preclude new behaviors. Avoidant personalities are hypersensitive to rejection and are reluctant to enter close relationships, in spite of strong desires for affection. Dependent personalities show excessive reliance on others to make major life decisions, stay trapped in abusive relationships for fear of being alone, have difficulty in initiating projects on their own, and constantly seek reassurance and praise. Obsessive-compulsive personalities exhibit restricted expressions of warmth, tenderness, and generosity and also exhibit stubbornness, with a need to be right and to control decisions; indecisive at times, they often use overly rigid applications of rules and morals to the point of being inflexible.

A characteristic personality disturbance commonly seen with frontal lobe damage is referred to as organic personality disorder in the tenth revision of the *International Classification of Diseases and Related Health Problems* (ICD-10) and personality change due to a general medical condition in DSM-IV. Its features include irritability, inappropriate jocularity with euphoria, inappropriate socially disinhibited behavior, and impulsiveness. Other patients, with damage to different areas of the frontal lobe, exhibit apathy and indifference.

INTERPERSONAL SYSTEMS Couples and families have been studied as systems in their own right, and numerous qualities of those systems have been identified as being clinically important. Yet no universally accepted set of guidelines has emerged for the psychological assessment of couples and families that parallels those generally used for individuals. Similarly, a single generally accepted typology of family psychopathology or interactional types has yet to be established.

Families normally provide the settings in which development and socialization take place, communication and emotional expression are learned, assumptions and expectations about the world at large are formed, one's sense of personal safety or vulnerability is established, and validation or negation of personal values, strivings, and worth occurs. Characteristics of couples and families that have received the most attention include the rules of communication, such as those governing the directness or indirectness with which disagreement and conflict are addressed; the manner (organized or chaotic) in which communications are conducted; taboo topics and secrets about which no one can openly communicate; the nature and the degree of emotional expression, including affection and anger; the cohesiveness, loyalty, and compatibility of the members; the nature of the members' shared identities, on the one hand, and their autonomous development and separateness, on the other; the extent to which the members treat one another respectfully or take one another for granted and use one another; the distribution of power and decision making among the members; the maintenance of generational boundaries (for example, the age-appropriate performance of life roles); and the members' orientation, concurrence, and disagreement about important values involving moral, religious, intellectual, cultural, financial, occupational, and child-rearing issues and about aspirations, health practices, leisure activities, and other belief systems.

Despite the lack of an accepted system for describing disturbances in family systems, some common patterns have been identified. Studies of marital patterns have shown that mating is not random. Persons with certain personality styles tend preferentially to marry spouses with complementary styles. Many imbalanced relationships in which one partner largely dominates the other may remain stable for years (*skewed* relationships). Some couples have chronically unstable relationships and constant overt conflict (*schismatic* relationships).

A characteristic family environment, called *high expressed emotion*, defines a relapse-prone environment in which one person has schizophrenia, bipolar disorder, anorexia nervosa, and possibly major depressive disorder. The key element or elements of high expressed emotion that correlates best with relapse has yet to be determined. At present, the interactional pattern includes the two characteristics of intense personal criticism and emotional overinvolvement with the identified patient. Instead of activity-based criticisms—"I don't like it when you leave your clothes on the floor"—high expressed emotion is characterized by ad hominem and globally demeaning comments—"You are a rotten and lazy kid." Aspects of overinvolvement can be measured by quantifying the number of hours of face-to-face contact and by such behaviors as relatives' categorically asserting how the patient feels without ever bothering to ask the patient. The observed relationships between high expressed emotion and increased rates of psychopathological relapse do not necessarily imply any causal relationship; they may simply reflect associations between an interactional pattern and relapse that may derive from the stressful effects of the patient's psychopathology on the family system as much as from the reverse sequence.

Couple and family system difficulties are most likely to erupt during predictable stressful events in the normal family life cycle, such as during the newlywed period; pregnancy and childbearing; difficult or contentious child-rearing periods; difficulties with parents, in-laws, and other extended family members; insurmountable and unanticipated financial or career problems; a serious illness or the death of a child or relative; the children's adolescence; the departure of children from the home; infidelity; and separation.

Pathological games Some disturbed couple and family systems play *pathological games*—repeated interactions with predictable interpersonal sequences and undesirable outcomes. Such systems may have chronic but patterned instability, with problem-maintaining feedback loops—sequences that have been called pathological games without end. Ongoing three-party-system pathological games *(perverse triangles)* may constantly generate tension but have few tension-releasing mechanisms; they function only temporarily and ineffectively and do not adequately resolve the underlying problems.

In response to a sullen and provocative teenager, one father was typically hostile, highly critical, and blaming (generating high negative expressed emotion). Whenever it seemed that physical violence was likely to erupt, the mother habitually rushed in to temporarily defuse the situation, soothing both parties and rescuing them from a further escalation of hostilities. Then, intentionally or unintentionally, in the very act of defusing or shortly thereafter, the mother always managed to do or say something that was certain to restart the buildup of tension between the father and the teenager, assuring that another round of angry confrontation would occur.

Scapegoating is another form of perverse triangulation; conflict between two people, frequently spouses, is avoided by means of recriminations or overconcern directed toward a third party, frequently a child. Pathological family coalitions and alliances may be established, cutting across the generations or excluding certain members of the family from important issues, leaving them to feel isolated and abandoned. Pathological *enmeshment,* often manifested in excessive overinvolvement of a parent with a child, may signal inadequacies in the primary marital bond.

Abnormal illness behavior Abnormal illness behavior (dysnosognosia) is a persistently pathological mode of experiencing, evaluating, and responding to one's own health status, despite a health professional's lucid and accurate appraisal of the situation and the management options. The behaviors can be considered interpersonal disorders between health care professionals and patients. Central to all the behaviors is the adoption of the sick role by the patient, who then engages in characteristic interactions with health care providers that leave both the provider and the patient dissatisfied. Patients with abnormal illness behavior typically seek repeated medical evaluations from a multitude of physicians, often undergoing a series of expensive laboratory tests. At times, the level of complaints provokes unnecessary invasive laboratory examinations or surgeries that place the patient at genuine medical risk.

Abnormal illness behavior may be unconscious or conscious. In unconscious abnormal illness behavior the patient believes that the symptoms reflect some genuine illness. The behavior may occur in somatization disorder (in which multiple symptoms and organ systems are affected), conversion disorder, somatoform pain disorder (in which no cause for the subjective level of pain can be found), and hypochondriasis (in which the primary fear is of having a serious disorder). Abnormal illness behavior in which patients act sick when they are fully aware that they are not sick include malingering (feigned illness in which external incentives, usually financial, are the motivating factors) and factitious disorders with physical or psychological symptoms (Munchausen syndrome). In *Munchausen syndrome,* patients repeatedly and compulsively present themselves for medical care with feigned or self-induced illness. The self-induced conditions may be so serious that they ultimately cause death; some patients inject themselves with feces to bring on systemic infections that will warrant hospitalization and intensive care. When the self-induced nature of the illnesses is discovered, medical staff members often become outraged at the patients. The patients rarely accept or cooperate with psychiatric care, so few have been adequately studied. Most do not appear to be psychotic but seem to have a disturbance in personality structure.

Life pattern disturbances Optimal patterns of self-expression, self-realization, and self-fulfillment require the proper development of the capacities to work, love, and play. Those patterns are acted out in the family, the school, the workplace, friendship networks, and the larger community. In each of those settings, persons adopt various social roles, through which their own activities develop and through which they define relationships to others with whom they are involved. Life pattern disturbances may occur in a single role or in multiple roles; in a single setting, such as work, or in several settings. Specific psychological conflicts may inhibit adequate performance in one of those areas. For example, in *success neurosis* a person who is conflicted about outdoing a parent or a sibling is unable to succeed professionally because unrealistic fears of retribution generate overwhelming anxiety and inhibit performance. Or chronic inability to control the expression of aggression may disrupt a career.

A 35-year-old man with an extremely ambitious, successful father had never been self-supporting, despite a variety of career starts, intelligence, and excellent, almost charismatic, interpersonal skills. With each new career he initially rose quickly, but, just before the step that would define him as a success in his field, some insurmountable problem inevitably interrupted his path. Once, it was an unexplained illness; another time, he fought with a boss; still another time, he took an unapproved vacation at a time vital for the business.

Inhibitions in interpersonal relationships—for example, shyness and fear of intimacy or sex—may set up lifelong patterns of unhappiness. Similarly, unrealistic perfectionism may prevent the establishment of satisfying long-term relationships.

An attractive, successful 32-year-old woman reported having a long string of admiring suitors and a series of intimate sexual relationships since the age of 17. Although several of the suitors to whom she was strongly attracted had proposed marriage, she felt unable to commit herself, never sufficiently in love with any of them and hoping that she would someday meet Mr. Perfect.

Life pattern disturbances sometimes result from multiple concurrent *role strains.* They occur when the person is faced with simultaneous, excessive, and conflicting demands to fulfill the duties and the obligations of work, family, and community. Demands and expectations from many sources produce the chronic overcommitment and time pressures typical of professional families that often generate chronic disturbance and dissatisfaction punctuated by intermittent crises.

A young, ambitious, devoted, and successful professional woman, the mother of two small children, found herself in repeated crisis situations at times when the demands of her job, parents, marriage, and children converged. She often had to juggle many commitments—writing reports for work, helping her children with important school projects, meeting her husband's needs for intimacy, and taking care of her ailing parents. Those circumstances resulted in frequent experiences of overwhelming tension, anxiety, panic, headache, and abdominal cramps. Nevertheless, she was chronically unable to set effective limits on the role demands in any one of those areas; she was reluctant to relinquish responsibility and had difficulty in delegating some of her responsibilities to others.

A 40-year-old physician in a successful general practice also had many business ventures in which he invested a great deal of the money he had earned from property development. The ventures frequently entangled him in legal disputes. He spent 12 to 14 hours in his medical office each day seeing patients, completed his charting and paperwork on weekends, and snatched odd moments to conduct complicated business transactions with his attorney. He was snappy and irritable with his family and expected them to be at his beck and call, seeing how "self-sacrificing" he was on their behalf. Reducing his practice, taking on an associate, and limiting his business activities were all unacceptable to him.

From an early age some persons are guided toward success or defeat by deeply ingrained attitudes and assumptions about themselves. Some persons believe themselves destined to become heroes and successes, and their activities fulfill that assumption. Others see themselves as destined to be victims and failures, perhaps repeating family patterns or fulfilling the preverse expectations of other family members; such expectations may be powerful self-fulfilling prophecies.

A 32-year-old woman had a series of relationships in which she ultimately was abused, always emotionally and often physically and sexually. Despite her conscious intent to find a caring man with whom she could have a less abusive relationship, the pattern repeated itself. Her mother had been chronically beaten by her abusive father. She recalled that her mother warned her repeatedly, "A woman's role is to give in to her husband and put up with the crap as best we can."

Life pattern disturbances may also take the form of a counterculture life-style. Dissatisfied or unsuccessful with conventional activities or feeling stymied or frustrated by various family and career failures, a person may drop out, change social role definitions and class, join a cult, or engage in other forms of social deviance, such as gang affiliations, criminality, the welfare culture, and malingering to avoid working. Career requirements—frequent geographic moves or enforced marital separations—may force life pattern disturbances on families. Certain careers and work settings carry heavy social pressures for alcohol and drug use or marital infidelity. Some families accommodate to prolonged separation but later find the demands of continuous marital intimacy and togetherness to be difficult.

A Navy couple had accommodated to the husband's long career pattern of six months at sea and six months at home. When the husband retired from the Navy, the couple experienced increasing marital conflict. Both the husband and the wife ascribed the difficulties to having lost their long periods of time apart from one another, time they had learned to enjoy, during which they had explored their own interests, developed separate relationships, and defused marital tensions.

FUTURE PROSPECTS

Like psychiatric diagnostic classifications, fashions among psychiatric signs and symptoms change; those described above must be taken in historical perspective. Characteristics once given prominence, such as the bony protuberances of the skull studied by phrenologists a century ago, are no longer accorded much importance, whereas only in the past few decades have newly described clinical phenomena, such as family-expressed emotion and alexithymia, been appreciated. Because of the shifts in what is considered relevant and because of the current dominance of biological research, it would be easy to assume that the nuances of clinical, descriptive psychopathology are mostly of historical interest. Yet some have expressed valid concerns that, as medicine and psychiatry become technologically sophisticated, both fields are in danger of losing sight of the patient as the center of concern. As long as the ultimate goals of clinical psychiatry are to help patients feel better and function better, attending to patients' subjective complaints with a firm knowledge of clinical descriptors will continue to be vital aspects of a psychiatrist's skills. Patients must feel the psychiatrist's interest in, concern with, and understanding of what frightens and ails them. Only by being curious about and aware of signs and symptoms can psychiatrists cement the types of therapeutic relationships that will allow them to maximally help their patients.

SUGGESTED CROSS-REFERENCES

The psychiatric interview, history, and mental status examination are discussed in Section 9.1. Additional definitions of typical signs and symptoms of psychiatric illness are included in Section 9.3. Perception and cognition are discussed in Section 3.1, memory in Section 3.5, and classification of mental disorders in Section 11.1. The mental disorders mentioned in this chapter are discussed in depth in many parts of this textbook: delirium and dementia in Chapter 12, substance-related disorders in Chapter 13, schizophrenia in Chapter 14, delusional disorders in Section 15.2, mood disorders in Chapter 16, anxiety disorders in Chapter 17, somatoform disorders in Chapter 18, dissociative disorders in Chapter 20, sexual disorders in Chapter 21, sleep disorders in Chapter 23, factitious disorders in Chapter 19, psychosomatic disorders in Chapter 26, and personality disorders in Chapter 25. Bereavement is discussed in Section 29.6, malingering in Section 28.2, and suicide in Section 30.1.

REFERENCES

Assad G: *Hallucinations in Clinical Psychiatry.* Brunner/Mazel, New York, 1990.

Banov M D, Kulick A R, Oepen G, Pope H G: A new identity for misidentification syndromes. Compr Psychiatry *34:* 414, 1993.

Benegal V, Hingorani S, Khanna S: Idiopathic catatonia: Validity of the concept. Psychopathology *26:* 41, 1993.

Berne E: *Transactional Analysis: Psychotherapy.* Castle, New York, 1961.

Berrios G E, Chen E Y: Recognizing psychiatric symptoms: Relevance to the diagnostic process. Br J Psychiatry *163:* 308, 1993.

Bleuler E: *Dementia Praecox: The Group of Schizophrenias.* International Universities Press, New York, 1950.

Buchanan A: Acting on delusion: A review. Psychol Med *23:* 123, 1993.

Carlson E V, Rosser-Hogan R: Cross-cultural response to trauma: A study of traumatic experiences and posttraumatic symptoms in Cambodian refugees. J Traumatic Stress *7:* 43, 1994.

Chess S, Thomas A: *Origins and Evolution of Behavior Disorders: From Infancy to Early Adult Life.* Brunner/Mazel, New York, 1984.

Cloninger R C: A systematic method for clinical description and classification of personality variants. Arch Gen Psychiatry *44:* 573, 1987.

*Cummings J L: *Clinical Neuropsychiatry.* Grune & Stratton, New York, 1985.

de Figueiredo J M: Depression and demoralization: Phenomenologic differences and research perspectives. Compr Psychiatry *34:* 308, 1993.

Fava M, Rosenbaum J F, Pava J A, McCarthy M K, Steingard R J, Bouffides E: Anger attacks in unipolar depression. Part I: Clinical correlates and response to fluoxetine treatment. Am J Psychiatry *150:* 1158, 1993.

Flaum M, Arndt S, Andreasen N C: The reliability of ''bizarre'' delusions. Compr Psychiatry *32:* 59, 1991.

Fricchione G, Sedler M J, Shukla S: Aprosodias in eight schizophrenic patients. Am J Psychiatry *143:* 1457, 1986.

*Goodwin F K, Jamison K R: *Manic-Depressive Illness.* Oxford University Press, New York, 1990.

*Hale R E, Yodofsky S C, editors: *Textbook of Neuropsychiatry,* ed 2. American Psychiatric Press, Washington, 1992.

Hall R C W, Devaul R A, Stickney S K, Poplin M K, Faillace L A: Physical illness presenting as psychiatric disease. Arch Gen Psychiatry *35:* 1315, 1978.

Hellerstein D, Frosch W, Koenigsberg H W: The clinical significance of command hallucinations. Am J Psychiatry *144:* 219, 1987.

Hilgard E R: *Divided Consciousness: Multiple Controls in Human Thought and Action.* Wiley, New York, 1977.

Hoffart A, Martinsen E W: Coping strategies in major depressed, agoraphoric and comorbid in-patients: A longitudinal study. Br J Med Psychol 66 (pt 2): 143, 1993.

Hoffman L: *Foundations of Family Therapy.* Basic Books, New York, 1981.

Howard R, Ford R: From the jumping Frenchmen of Maine to posttraumatic stress disorder: The startle response in neuropsychiatry. Psychol Med *22:* 695, 1992.

*Jaspers K: *General Psychopathology.* University of Chicago Press, Chicago, 1963.

Koenigsberg H W, Handley R: Expressed emotion: From predictive index to clinical construct. Am J Psychiatry *143:* 1361, 1986.

Larson J A: New perspectives on Type A behavior: A psychiatric point of view. Int J Psychiatry Med *23:* 231, 1993.

Lazare A, editor: *Outpatient Psychiatry: Diagnosis and Treatment,* ed 2. Williams & Wilkins, Baltimore, 1989.

Lyness J M, Caine E D, Conwell Y, King D A, Cox C: Depressive symptoms, medical illness, and functional status in depressed psychiatric inpatients. Am J Psychiatry *150:* 910, 1993.

Mumford D B: Somatization: A transcultural perspective. Int Rev Psychiatry *5:* 231, 1993.

Perry W, Braff D L: Information-processing deficits and thought disorder in schizophrenia. Am J Psychiatry *151:* 363, 1994.

Pilowksy I: The concept of abnormal illness behavior. Psychosomatics *31:* 207, 1990.

Rapaport D, editor: *Organization and Pathology of Thought.* Columbia University Press, New York, 1951.

Rogers D: The motor disorders of severe psychiatric illness: A conflict of paradigms. Br J Psychiatry *147:* 221, 1985.

Rogler L H: Culturally sensitizing psychiatric diagnosis: A framework for research. J Nerv Ment Dis *181:* 401, 1993.

Sachdev P, Loneragan C: The present status of akathisia. J Nerv Ment Dis *179:* 381, 1911.

Schneider K: *Clinical Psychopathology.* Grune & Stratton, New York, *1959.*

Shapiro D: *Neurotic Styles.* Basic Books, New York, 1965.

Sims A, editor: Delusions and awareness of reality. Br J Psychiatry *159* (Suppl 14): 22, 1991.

*Sims A: *Symptoms in the Mind: An Introduction to Descriptive Psychophathology.* Bailliere Tindall, London, 1988.

Snaith P. Anhedonia: A neglected symptom of psychopathology. Psychol Med *23:* 957, 1993.

Spiegel D, editor: Dissociative disorders. In *Review of Psychiatry,* A Tasman, S M Goldfinger, editors, vol 10, p 143. American Psychiatric Press, Washington, 1991.
Taylor C B, Arnow B: *The Nature and Treatment of Anxiety Disorders.* Free Press, New York, 1988.
Virkkunen M, DeJong J, Bartko J, Goodwin F, Linnoila M: Relationship of psychobiological variables to recidivism in violent offenders and impulsive fire setters. Arch Gen Psychiatry *46:* 600, 1989.
Winchel R M, Stanley M: Self-injurious behavior: A review of the behavior and biology of self-mutilation. Am J Psychiatry *148:* 306, 1991.
Yalom I: *Existential Psychotherapy.* Basic Books, New York, 1980.

CHAPTER 11 CLASSIFICATION OF MENTAL DISORDERS

11.1 CLASSIFICATION OF MENTAL DISORDERS

BENJAMIN J. SADOCK, M.D.
HAROLD I. KAPLAN, M.D.

INTRODUCTION

The fourth edition of *Diagnostic and Statistical Manual of Mental Disorders* (DSM-IV), published in 1994, is the latest and most up-to-date classification of mental disorders (Table 11.1-1). DSM-IV is used by mental health professionals of all disciplines and is cited for insurance reimbursement, disability deliberations, and forensic matters.

The fourth edition correlates with the 10th revision of the World Health Organization's (WHO's) *International Classification of Diseases and Related Health Problems* (ICD-10), developed in 1992. Diagnostic systems used in the United States must be compatible with ICD to ensure uniform reporting of national and international health statistics. In addition, Medicare requires that billing codes for reimbursement follow ICD.

In 1952 the American Psychiatric Association's Committee on Nomenclature and Statistics published the first edition of DSM (DSM-I). Four editions have been published since then: the second edition (DSM-II), published in 1968; the third edition (DSM-III), published in 1980; the revised third edition (DSM-III-R), published in 1987; and DSM-IV.

Although many psychiatrists have been critical of the many versions of DSM that have appeared since the first edition, DSM-IV is the official nomenclature. All terminology used in this textbook conforms to DSM-IV nomenclature.

INTERNATIONAL CLASSIFICATION OF DISEASES

ICD-10 is the official classification system used in Europe. All the categories used in DSM-IV are found in ICD-10, but not all ICD-10 categories are in DSM-IV. According to DSM-IV:

> The tenth revision of the *International Statistical Classification of Diseases and Related Health Problems* (ICD-10), developed by WHO, was published in 1992, but will probably not come into official use in the United States until the late 1990s. Those preparing ICD-10 and DSM-IV have worked closely to coordinate their efforts, resulting in much mutual influence. ICD-10 consists of an official coding system and other related clinical and research documents and instruments. The codes and terms provided in DSM-IV are fully compatible with both ICD-9-CM and ICD-10. . . . The clinical and research drafts of ICD-10 were thoroughly reviewed by the DSM-IV Work Groups and suggested important topics for DSM-IV literature reviews and data reanalyses. Draft versions of the ICD-10 Diagnostic Criteria for Research were included as alternatives to be compared with DSM-III, DSM-III-R and suggested DSM-IV criteria sets in the DSM-IV field trials. The many consultations between the developers of DSM-IV and ICD-10 (which were facilitated by NIMH [National Institute of Mental Health], NIDA [National Institute of Drug Abuse], and NIAAA [National Institute on Alcohol Abuse and Alcoholism]) were enormously useful in increasing the congruence and reducing meaningless differences in wording between the two systems.

In the United States, ICD-10 codes may be used on insurance forms and other documents requiring diagnoses. The codes in DSM-IV are fully compatible with ICD-10; however, some terms and diagnostic categories used in ICD-10 are not used in DSM-IV. ICD is discussed extensively in Section 11.2.

BASIC FEATURES OF DSM-IV

The approach to DSM-IV, as in DSM-III-R, is atheoretical with regard to causes. Thus, DSM-IV attempts to describe what the manifestations of the mental disorders are; only rarely does it attempt to account for how the disturbances come about. The definitions of the disorders usually consist of descriptions of the clinical features.

Specified diagnostic criteria are provided for each mental disorder. Those criteria include a list of features that must be present for the diagnosis to be made. The use of specific criteria increases the reliability of the diagnostic process among clinicians.

DSM-IV also systematically describes each disorder in terms of its associated features: specific age-, culture-, and gender-related features; prevalence, incidence, and risk; course; complications; predisposing factors; familial pattern; and differential diagnosis. In some instances, when many of the specific disorders share common features, that information is included in the introduction to the entire section. Laboratory findings and associated physical examination signs and symptoms are described when relevant. DSM-IV does not purport to be a textbook. No mention is made of theories of causes, management, or treatment, nor are the controversial issues surrounding a particular diagnostic category discussed.

DSM-IV provides explicit rules to be used when the information is insufficient (diagnosis to be deferred or provisional) or the patient's clinical presentation and history do not meet the full criteria of a prototypical category (an atypical, residual, or not otherwise specified [NOS] type within the general category).

MULTIAXIAL EVALUATION DSM-IV is a multiaxial system that evaluates the patient along several variables and contains five axes. Axis I and Axis II comprise the entire classification of mental disorders—17 major classifications (Table 11.1-2) and more than 300 specific disorders. In many instances the patient has a disorder on both axes. For example, a patient may have major depressive disorder noted on Axis I and obsessive-compulsive personality disorder on Axis II.

Axis I Axis I consists of clinical disorders and other conditions that may be a focus of clinical attention (Table 11.1-3).

TABLE 11.1-1
DSM-IV Classification

NOS = Not Otherwise Specified.

An x appearing in a diagnostic code indicates that a specific code number is required.

An ellipsis (. . .) is used in the names of certain disorders to indicate that the name of a specific mental disorder or general medical condition should be inserted when recording the name (e.g., 293.0 Delirium Due to Hypothyroidism).

If criteria are currently met, one of the following severity specifiers may be noted after the diagnosis:
Mild
Moderate
Severe

If criteria are no longer met, one of the following specifiers may be noted:
In Partial Remission
In Full Remission
Prior History

Disorders Usually First Diagnosed in Infancy, Childhood, or Adolescence

MENTAL RETARDATION
Note: *These are coded on Axis II.*
317 Mild Mental Retardation
318.0 Moderate Mental Retardation
318.1 Severe Mental Retardation
318.2 Profound Mental Retardation
319 Mental Retardation, Severity Unspecified

LEARNING DISORDERS
315.00 Reading Disorder
315.1 Mathematics Disorder
315.2 Disorder of Written Expression
315.9 Learning Disorder NOS

MOTOR SKILLS DISORDER
315.4 Developmental Coordination Disorder

COMMUNICATION DISORDERS
315.31 Expressive Language Disorder
315.31 Mixed Receptive-Expressive Language Disorder
315.39 Phonological Disorder
307.0 Stuttering
307.9 Communication Disorder NOS

PERVASIVE DEVELOPMENTAL DISORDERS
299.00 Autistic Disorder
299.80 Rett's Disorder
299.10 Childhood Disintegrative Disorder
299.80 Asperger's Disorder
299.80 Pervasive Developmental Disorder NOS

ATTENTION-DEFICIT AND DISRUPTIVE BEHAVIOR DISORDERS
314.xx Attention-Deficit/Hyperactivity Disorder
.01 Combined Type
.00 Predominantly Inattentive Type
.01 Predominantly Hyperactive-Impulsive Type
314.9 Attention-Deficit/Hyperactivity Disorder NOS
312.8 Conduct Disorder
Specify type: Childhood Onset Type Adolescent Onset Type
313.81 Oppositional Defiant Disorder
312.9 Disruptive Behavior Disorder NOS

FEEDING AND EATING DISORDERS OF INFANCY OR EARLY CHILDHOOD
307.52 Pica
307.53 Rumination Disorder
307.59 Feeding Disorder of Infancy or Early Childhood

TIC DISORDERS
307.23 Tourette's Disorder
307.22 Chronic Motor or Vocal Tic Disorder
307.21 Transient Tic Disorder
Specify if: Single Episode/Recurrent
307.20 Tic Disorder NOS

ELIMINATION DISORDERS
—.– Encopresis
787.6 With Constipation and Overflow Incontinence
307.7 Without Constipation and Overflow Incontinence
307.6 Enuresis (Not Due to a General Medical Condition)
Specify type: Nocturnal Only/Diurnal Only/Nocturnal and Diurnal

OTHER DISORDERS OF INFANCY, CHILDHOOD, OR ADOLESCENCE
309.21 Separation Anxiety Disorder
Specify if: Early Onset
313.23 Selective Mutism
313.89 Reactive Attachment Disorder of Infancy or Early Childhood
Specify type: Inhibited Type/Disinhibited Type
307.3 Stereotypic Movement Disorder
Specify if: With Self-Injurious Behavior
313.9 Disorder of Infancy, Childhood, or Adolescence NOS

Delirium, Dementia, and Amnestic and Other Cognitive Disorders

DELIRIUM
293.0 Delirium Due to . . . *[Indicate the General Medical Condition]*
—.– Substance Intoxication Delirium *(refer to Substance-Related Disorders for substance-specific codes)*
—.– Substance Withdrawal Delirium *(refer to Substance-Related Disorders for substance-specific codes)*
—.– Delirium Due to Multiple Etiologies *(code each of the specific etiologies)*
780.09 Delirium NOS

DEMENTIA
290.xx Dementia of the Alzheimer's Type, With Early Onset *(also code 331.0 Alzheimer's disease on Axis III)*
.10 Uncomplicated
.11 With Delirium
.12 With Delusions
.13 With Depressed Mood
Specify if: With Behavioral Disturbance
290.xx Dementia of the Alzheimer's Type, With Late Onset *(also code 331.0 Alzheimer's disease on Axis III)*
.0 Uncomplicated
.3 With Delirium
.20 With Delusions
.21 With Depressed Mood
Specify if: With Behavioral Disturbance
290.xx Vascular Dementia
.40 Uncomplicated
.41 With Delirium
.42 With Delusions
.43 With Depressed Mood
Specify if: With Behavioral Disturbance
294.9 Dementia Due to HIV Disease *(also code 043.1 HIV infection affecting central nervous system on Axis III)*
294.1 Dementia Due to Head Trauma *(also code 854.00 head injury on Axis III)*
294.1 Dementia Due to Parkinson's Disease *(also code 332.0 Parkinson's disease on Axis III)*
294.1 Dementia Due to Huntington's Disease *(also code 333.4 Huntington's disease on Axis III)*
290.10 Dementia Due to Pick's Disease *(also code 331.1 Pick's disease on Axis III)*
290.10 Dementia Due to Creutzfeldt-Jakob Disease *(also code 046.1 Creutzfeldt-Jakob disease on Axis III)*
294.1 Dementia Due to . . . *[Indicate the General Medical Condition not listed above] (also code the general medical condition on Axis III)*
—.– Substance-Induced Persisting Dementia *(refer to Substance-Related Disorders for substance-specific codes)*
—.– Dementia Due to Multiple Etiologies *(code each of the specific etiologies)*
294.8 Dementia NOS

AMNESTIC DISORDERS
294.0 Amnestic Disorder Due to . . . *[Indicate the General Medical Condition]*
Specify if: Transient/Chronic
—.– Substance-Induced Persisting Amnestic Disorder *(refer to Substance-Related Disorders for substance-specific codes)*
294.8 Amnestic Disorder NOS

OTHER COGNITIVE DISORDERS
294.9 Cognitive Disorder NOS

Mental Disorders Due to a General Medical Condition Not Elsewhere Classified
293.89 Catatonic Disorder Due to . . . *[Indicate the General Medical Condition]*
310.1 Personality Change Due to . . . *[Indicate the General Medical Condition]*
Specify type: Labile Type/Disinhibited Type/Aggressive Type/Apathetic Type/Paranoid Type/Other Type/Combined Type/Unspecified Type
293.9 Mental Disorder NOS Due to . . . *[Indicate the General Medical Condition]*

TABLE 11.1-1 *(continued)*

Substance-Related Disorders

[a]*The following specifiers may be applied to Substance Dependence:*
With Physiological Dependence/Without Physiological Dependence
Early Full Remission/Early Partial Remission
Sustained Full Remission/Sustained Partial Remission
On Agonist Therapy/In a Controlled Environment

The following specifiers apply to Substance-Induced Disorders as noted:
[I]With Onset During Intoxication/[W]With Onset During Withdrawal

ALCOHOL-RELATED DISORDERS

Alcohol Use Disorders
303.90 Alcohol Dependence[a]
305.00 Alcohol Abuse

Alcohol-Induced Disorders
303.00 Alcohol Intoxication
291.8 Alcohol Withdrawal
Specify if: With Perceptual Disturbances
291.0 Alcohol Intoxication Delirium
291.0 Alcohol Withdrawal Delirium
291.2 Alcohol-Induced Persisting Dementia
291.1 Alcohol-Induced Persisting Amnestic Disorder
291.x Alcohol-Induced Psychotic Disorder
.5 With Delusions[I,W]
.3 With Hallucinations[I,W]
291.8 Alcohol-Induced Mood Disorder[I,W]
291.8 Alcohol-Induced Anxiety Disorder[I,W]
291.8 Alcohol-Induced Sexual Dysfunction[I]
291.8 Alcohol-Induced Sleep Disorder[I,W]
291.9 Alcohol-Related Disorder NOS

AMPHETAMINE (OR AMPHETAMINE-LIKE)–RELATED DISORDERS

Amphetamine Use Disorders
304.40 Amphetamine Dependence[a]
305.70 Amphetamine Abuse

Amphetamine-Induced Disorders
292.89 Amphetamine Intoxication
Specify if: With Perceptual Disturbances
292.0 Amphetamine Withdrawal
292.81 Amphetamine Intoxication Delirium
292.xx Amphetamine-Induced Psychotic Disorder
.11 With Delusions[I]
.12 With Hallucinations[I]
292.84 Amphetamine-Induced Mood Disorder[I,W]
292.89 Amphetamine-Induced Anxiety Disorder[I]
292.89 Amphetamine-Induced Sexual Dysfunction[I]
292.89 Amphetamine-Induced Sleep Disorder[I,W]
292.9 Amphetamine-Related Disorder NOS

CAFFEINE-RELATED DISORDERS

Caffeine-Induced Disorders
305.90 Caffeine Intoxication
292.89 Caffeine-Induced Anxiety Disorder[I]
292.89 Caffeine-Induced Sleep Disorder[I]
292.9 Caffeine-Related Disorder NOS

CANNABIS-RELATED DISORDERS

Cannabis Use Disorders
304.30 Cannabis Dependence[a]
305.20 Cannabis Abuse

Cannabis-Induced Disorders
292.89 Cannabis Intoxication
Specify if: With Perceptual Disturbances
292.81 Cannabis Intoxication Delirium
292.xx Cannabis-Induced Psychotic Disorder
.11 With Delusions[I]
.12 With Hallucinations[I]
292.89 Cannabis-Induced Anxiety Disorder[I]
292.9 Cannabis-Related Disorder NOS

COCAINE-RELATED DISORDERS

Cocaine Use Disorders
304.20 Cocaine Dependence[a]
305.60 Cocaine Abuse

Cocaine-Induced Disorders
292.89 Cocaine Intoxication
Specify if: With Perceptual Disturbances
292.0 Cocaine Withdrawal
292.81 Cocaine Intoxication Delirium
292.xx Cocaine-Induced Psychotic Disorder
.11 With Delusions[I]
.12 With Hallucinations[I]
292.84 Cocaine-Induced Mood Disorder[I,W]
292.89 Cocaine-Induced Anxiety Disorder[I,W]
292.89 Cocaine-Induced Sexual Dysfunction[I]
292.89 Cocaine-Induced Sleep Disorder[I,W]
292.9 Cocaine-Related Disorder NOS

HALLUCINOGEN-RELATED DISORDERS

Hallucinogen Use Disorders
304.50 Hallucinogen Dependence[a]
305.30 Hallucinogen Abuse

Hallucinogen-Induced Disorders
292.89 Hallucinogen Intoxication
292.89 Hallucinogen Persisting Perception Disorder (Flashbacks)
292.81 Hallucinogen Intoxication Delirium
292.xx Hallucinogen-Induced Psychotic Disorder
.11 With Delusions[I]
.12 With Hallucinations[I]
292.84 Hallucinogen-Induced Mood Disorder[I]
292.89 Hallucinogen-Induced Anxiety Disorder[I]
292.9 Hallucinogen-Related Disorder NOS

INHALANT-RELATED DISORDERS

Inhalant Use Disorders
304.60 Inhalant Dependence[a]
305.90 Inhalant Abuse

Inhalant-Induced Disorders
292.89 Inhalant Intoxication
292.81 Inhalant Intoxication Delirium
292.82 Inhalant-Induced Persisting Dementia
292.xx Inhalant-Induced Psychotic Disorder
.11 With Delusions[I]
.12 With Hallucinations[I]
292.84 Inhalant-Induced Mood Disorder[I]
292.89 Inhalant-Induced Anxiety Disorder[I]
292.9 Inhalant-Related Disorder NOS

NICOTINE-RELATED DISORDERS

Nicotine Use Disorder
305.10 Nicotine Dependence[a]

Nicotine-Induced Disorder
292.0 Nicotine Withdrawal
292.9 Nicotine-Related Disorder NOS

OPIOID-RELATED DISORDERS

Opioid Use Disorders
304.00 Opioid Dependence[a]
305.50 Opioid Abuse

Opioid-Induced Disorders
292.89 Opioid Intoxication
Specify if: With Perceptual Disturbances
292.0 Opioid Withdrawal
292.81 Opioid Intoxication Delirium
292.xx Opioid-Induced Psychotic Disorder
.11 With Delusions[I]
.12 With Hallucinations[I]
292.84 Opioid-Induced Mood Disorder[I]
292.89 Opioid-Induced Sexual Dysfunction[I]
292.89 Opioid-Induced Sleep Disorder[I,W]
292.9 Opioid-Related Disorder NOS

PHENCYCLIDINE (OR PHENCYCLIDINE-LIKE)–RELATED DISORDERS

Phencyclidine Use Disorders
304.90 Phencyclidine Dependence[a]
305.90 Phencyclidine Abuse

Phencyclidine-Induced Disorders
292.89 Phencyclidine Intoxication
Specify if: With Perceptual Disturbances
292.81 Phencyclidine Intoxication Delirium
292.xx Phencyclidine-Induced Psychotic Disorder
.11 With Delusions[I]
.12 With Hallucinations[I]
292.84 Phencyclidine-Induced Mood Disorder[I]
292.89 Phencyclidine-Induced Anxiety Disorder[I]
292.9 Phencyclidine-Related Disorder NOS

(continued)

TABLE 11.1-1 (*continued*)

SEDATIVE-, HYPNOTIC-, OR ANXIOLYTIC-RELATED DISORDERS

Sedative, Hypnotic, or Anxiolytic Use Disorders

304.10 Sedative, Hypnotic, or Anxiolytic Dependence[a]
305.40 Sedative, Hypnotic, or Anxiolytic Abuse

Sedative-, Hypnotic-, or Anxiolytic-Induced Disorders

292.89 Sedative, Hypnotic, or Anxiolytic Intoxication
292.0 Sedative, Hypnotic, or Anxiolytic Withdrawal
Specify if: With Perceptual Disturbances
292.81 Sedative, Hypnotic, or Anxiolytic Intoxication Delirium
292.81 Sedative, Hypnotic, or Anxiolytic Withdrawal Delirium
292.82 Sedative-, Hypnotic-, or Anxiolytic-Induced Persisting Dementia
292.83 Sedative-, Hypnotic-, or Anxiolytic-Induced Persisting Amnestic Disorder
292.xx Sedative-, Hypnotic-, or Anxiolytic-Induced Psychotic Disorder
.11 With Delusions[I,W]
.12 With Hallucinations[I,W]
292.84 Sedative-, Hypnotic-, or Anxiolytic-Induced Mood Disorder[I,W]
292.89 Sedative-, Hypnotic-, or Anxiolytic-Induced Anxiety Disorder[W]
292.89 Sedative-, Hypnotic-, or Anxiolytic-Induced Sexual Dysfunction[I]
292.89 Sedative-, Hypnotic-, or Anxiolytic-Induced Sleep Disorder[I,W]
292.9 Sedative-, Hypnotic-, or Anxiolytic-Related Disorder NOS

POLYSUBSTANCE-RELATED DISORDER

304.80 Polysubstance Dependence[a]

OTHER (OR UNKNOWN) SUBSTANCE-RELATED DISORDERS

Other (or Unknown) Substance Use Disorders

304.90 Other (or Unknown) Substance Dependence[a]
305.90 Other (or Unknown) Substance Abuse

Other (or Unknown) Substance-Induced Disorders

292.89 Other (or Unknown) Substance Intoxication
Specify if: With Perceptual Disturbances
292.0 Other (or Unknown) Substance Withdrawal
Specify if: With Perceptual Disturbances
292.81 Other (or Unknown) Substance-Induced Delirium
292.82 Other (or Unknown) Substance-Induced Persisting Dementia
292.83 Other (or Unknown) Substance-Induced Persisting Amnestic Disorder
292.xx Other (or Unknown) Substance-Induced Psychotic Disorder
.11 With Delusions[I,W]
.12 With Hallucinations[I,W]
292.84 Other (or Unknown) Substance-Induced Mood Disorder[I,W]
292.89 Other (or Unknown) Substance-Induced Anxiety Disorder[I,W]
292.89 Other (or Unknown) Substance-Induced Sexual Dysfunction[I]
292.89 Other (or Unknown) Substance-Induced Sleep Disorder[I,W]
292.9 Other (or Unknown) Substance-Related Disorder NOS

Schizophrenia and Other Psychotic Disorders

295.xx Schizophrenia

The following Classification of Longitudinal Course applies to all subtypes of Schizophrenia:
Episodic With Interepisode Residual Symptoms (*specify if*: With Prominent Negative Symptoms)/Episodic With No Interepisode Residual Symptoms/Continuous (*specify if*: With Prominent Negative Symptoms)
Single Episode In Partial Remission (*specify if*: With Prominent Negative Symptoms)/Single Episode In Full Remission
Other or Unspecified Pattern

.30 Paranoid Type
.10 Disorganized Type
.20 Catatonic Type
.90 Undifferentiated Type
.60 Residual Type

295.40 Schizophreniform Disorder
Specify if: Without Good Prognostic Features/With Good Prognostic Features
295.70 Schizoaffective Disorder
Specify type: Bipolar Type/Depressive Type
297.1 Delusional Disorder
Specify type: Erotomanic Type/Grandiose Type/Jealous Type/Persecutory Type/Somatic Type/Mixed Type/Unspecified Type
298.8 Brief Psychotic Disorder
Specify if: With Marked Stressor(s)/Without Marked Stressor(s)/With Postpartum Onset
297.3 Shared Psychotic Disorder
293.xx Psychotic Disorder Due to . . . *[Indicate the General Medical Condition]*
.81 With Delusions
.82 With Hallucinations
Substance-Induced Psychotic Disorder *(refer to Substance-Related Disorders for substance-specific codes)*
Specify if: With Onset During Intoxication/With Onset During Withdrawal
298.9 Psychotic Disorder NOS

Mood Disorders

Code current state of Major Depressive Disorder or Bipolar I Disorder in fifth digit:
1 = Mild
2 = Moderate
3 = Severe Without Psychotic Features
4 = Severe With Psychotic Features
Specify: Mood-Congruent Psychotic Features/Mood-Incongruent Psychotic Features
5 = In Partial Remission
6 = In Full Remission
0 = Unspecified

The following specifiers apply (for current or most recent episode) to Mood Disorders as noted:
[a]Severity/Psychotic/Remission Specifiers/[b]Chronic/[c]With Catatonic Features/[d]With Melancholic Features/[e]With Atypical Features/[f]With Postpartum Onset

The following specifiers apply to Mood Disorders as noted:
[g]With or Without Full Interepisode Recovery/[h]With Seasonal Pattern/[i]With Rapid Cycling

DEPRESSIVE DISORDERS

296.xx Major Depressive Disorder
.2x Single Episode[a,b,c,d,e,f]
.3x Recurrent[a,b,c,d,e,f,g,h]
300.4 Dysthymic Disorder
Specify if: Early Onset/Late Onset
Specify: With Atypical Features
311 Depressive Disorder NOS

BIPOLAR DISORDERS

296.xx Bipolar I Disorder
.0x Single Manic Episode[a,e,f]
Specify if: Mixed
.40 Most Recent Episode Hypomanic[g,h,i]
.4x Most Recent Episode Manic[a,c,f,g,h,i]
.6x Most Recent Episode Mixed[a,c,f,g,h,i]
.5x Most Recent Episode Depressed[a,b,c,d,e,f,g,h,i]
.7 Most Recent Episode Unspecified[g,h,i]
296.89 Bipolar II Disorder[a,b,c,d,e,f,g,h,i]
Specify (current or most recent episode): Hypomanic/Depressed
301.13 Cyclothymic Disorder
296.80 Bipolar Disorder NOS

293.83 Mood Disorder Due to . . . *[Indicate the General Medical Condition]*
Specify type: With Depressive Features/With Major Depressive-Like Episode/With Manic Features/With Mixed Features
—.— Substance-Induced Mood Disorder *(refer to Substance-Related Disorders for substance-specific codes)*
Specify type: With Depressive Features/With Manic Features/With Mixed Features
Specify if: With Onset During Intoxication/With Onset During Withdrawal

296.90 Mood Disorder NOS

Anxiety Disorders

300.01 Panic Disorder Without Agoraphobia
300.21 Panic Disorder With Agoraphobia
300.22 Agoraphobia Without History of Panic Disorder
300.29 Specific Phobia
Specify type: Animal Type/Natural Environment Type/Blood-Injection-Injury Type/Situational Type/Other Type

TABLE 11.1-1 (*continued*)

300.23 Social Phobia
Specify if: Generalized
300.3 Obsessive-Compulsive Disorder
Specify if: With Poor Insight
309.81 Posttraumatic Stress Disorder
Specify if: Acute/Chronic
Specify if: With Delayed Onset
308.3 Acute Stress Disorder
300.02 Generalized Anxiety Disorder
293.89 Anxiety Disorder Due to . . . *[Indicate the General Medical Condition]*
Specify if: With Generalized Anxiety/With Panic Attacks/With Obsessive-Compulsive Symptoms
—.– Substance-Induced Anxiety Disorder *(refer to Substance-Related Disorders for substance-specific codes)*
Specify if: With Generalized Anxiety/With Panic Attacks With Obsessive-Compulsive Symptoms/With Phobic Symptoms
Specify if: With Onset During Intoxication/With Onset During Withdrawal
300.00 Anxiety Disorder NOS

Somatoform Disorders
300.81 Somatization Disorder
300.81 Undifferentiated Somatoform Disorder
300.11 Conversion Disorder
Specify type: With Motor Symptom or Deficit/With Sensory Symptom or Deficit/With Seizures or Convulsions/With Mixed Presentation
307.xx Pain Disorder
.80 Associated With Psychological Factors
.89 Associated With Both Psychological Factors and a General Medical Condition
Specify if: Acute/Chronic
300.7 Hypochondriasis
Specify if: With Poor Insight
300.7 Body Dysmorphic Disorder
300.81 Somatoform Disorder NOS

Factitious Disorders
300.xx Factitious Disorder
.16 With Predominantly Psychological Signs and Symptoms
.19 With Predominantly Physical Signs and Symptoms
.19 With Combined Psychological and Physical Signs and Symptoms
300.19 Factitious Disorder NOS

Dissociative Disorders
300.12 Dissociative Amnesia
300.13 Dissociative Fugue
300.14 Dissociative Identity Disorder
300.6 Depersonalization Disorder
300.15 Dissociative Disorder NOS

Sexual and Gender Identity Disorders

SEXUAL DYSFUNCTIONS
The following specifiers apply to all primary Sexual Dysfunctions:
Lifelong Type/Acquired Type
Generalized Type/Situational Type
Due to Psychological Factors/Due to Combined Factors

Sexual Desire Disorders
302.71 Hypoactive Sexual Desire Disorder
302.79 Sexual Aversion Disorder

Sexual Arousal Disorders
302.72 Female Sexual Arousal Disorder
302.72 Male Erectile Disorder

Orgasmic Disorders
302.73 Female Orgasmic Disorder
302.74 Male Orgasmic Disorder
302.75 Premature Ejaculation

Sexual Pain Disorders
302.76 Dyspareunia (Not Due to a General Medical Condition)
306.51 Vaginismus (Not Due to a General Medical Condition)

Sexual Dysfunction Due to a General Medical Condition
625.8 Female Hypoactive Sexual Desire Disorder Due to . . . *[Indicate the General Medical Condition]*
608.89 Male Hypoactive Sexual Desire Disorder Due to . . . *[Indicate the General Medical Condition]*
607.84 Male Erectile Disorder Due to . . . *[Indicate the General Medical Condition]*
625.0 Female Dyspareunia Due to . . . *[Indicate the General Medical Condition]*
608.89 Male Dyspareunia Due to . . . *[Indicate the General Medical Condition]*
625.8 Other Female Sexual Dysfunction Due to . . . *[Indicate the General Medical Condition]*
608.89 Other Male Sexual Dysfunction Due to . . . *[Indicate the General Medical Condition]*

—.– Substance-Induced Sexual Dysfunction *(refer to Substance-Related Disorders for substance-specific codes)*
Specify if: With Impaired Desire/With Impaired Arousal/With Impaired Orgasm/With Sexual Pain
Specify if: With Onset During Intoxication

302.70 Sexual Dysfunction NOS

PARAPHILIAS
302.4 Exhibitionism
302.81 Fetishism
302.89 Frotteurism
302.2 Pedophilia
Specify if: Sexually Attracted to Males/Sexually Attracted to Females/Sexually Attracted to Both
Specify if: Limited to Incest
Specify type: Exclusive Type/Nonexclusive Type
302.83 Sexual Masochism
302.84 Sexual Sadism
302.3 Transvestic Fetishism
Specify if: With Gender Dysphoria
302.82 Voyeurism
302.9 Paraphilia NOS

GENDER IDENTITY DISORDERS
302.xx Gender Identity Disorder
.6 in Children
.85 in Adolescents or Adults
Specify if: Sexually Attracted to Males/Sexually Attracted to Females/Sexually Attracted to Both/Sexually Attracted to Neither
302.6 Gender Identity Disorder NOS

302.9 Sexual Disorder NOS

Eating Disorders
307.1 Anorexia Nervosa
Specify type: Restricting Type; Binge-Eating/Purging Type
307.51 Bulimia Nervosa
Specify type: Purging Type/Nonpurging Type
307.50 Eating Disorder NOS

Sleep Disorders

PRIMARY SLEEP DISORDERS

Dyssomnias
307.42 Primary Insomnia
307.44 Primary Hypersomnia
Specify if: Recurrent
347 Narcolepsy
780.59 Breathing-Related Sleep Disorder
307.45 Circadian Rhythm Sleep Disorder
Specify type: Delayed Sleep Phase Type/Jet Lag Type/Shift Work Type/Unspecified Type
307.47 Dyssomnia NOS

Parasomnias
307.47 Nightmare Disorder
307.46 Sleep Terror Disorder
307.46 Sleepwalking Disorder
307.47 Parasomnia NOS

SLEEP DISORDERS RELATED TO ANOTHER MENTAL DISORDER
307.42 Insomnia Related to . . . *[Indicate the Axis I or Axis II Disorder]*
307.44 Hypersomnia Related to . . . *[Indicate the Axis I or Axis II Disorder]*

OTHER SLEEP DISORDERS
780.xx Sleep Disorder Due to . . . *[Indicate the General Medical Condition]*
.52 Insomnia Type
.54 Hypersomnia Type
.59 Parasomnia Type
.59 Mixed Type
—.– Substance-Induced Sleep Disorder *(refer to Substance-Related Disorders for substance-specific codes)*
Specify type: Insomnia Type/Hypersomnia Type/Parasomnia Type/Mixed Type
Specify if: With Onset During Intoxication/With Onset During Withdrawal

(continued)

TABLE 11.1-1 *(continued)*

Impulse-Control Disorders Not Elsewhere Classified
312.34 Intermittent Explosive Disorder
312.32 Kleptomania
312.33 Pyromania
312.31 Pathological Gambling
312.39 Trichotillomania
312.30 Impulse-Control Disorder NOS

Adjustment Disorders
309.xx Adjustment Disorder
.0 With Depressed Mood
.24 With Anxiety
.28 With Mixed Anxiety and Depressed Mood
.3 With Disturbance of Conduct
.4 With Mixed Disturbance of Emotions and Conduct
.9 Unspecified
Specify if: Acute Chronic

Personality Disorders

Note: *These are coded on Axis II.*
301.0 Paranoid Personality Disorder
301.20 Schizoid Personality Disorder
301.22 Schizotypal Personality Disorder
301.7 Antisocial Personality Disorder
301.83 Borderline Personality Disorder
301.50 Histrionic Personality Disorder
301.81 Narcissistic Personality Disorder
301.82 Avoidant Personality Disorder
301.6 Dependent Personality Disorder
301.4 Obsessive-Compulsive Personality Disorder
301.9 Personality Disorder NOS

Other Conditions That May Be a Focus of Clinical Attention

PSYCHOLOGICAL FACTORS AFFECTING MEDICAL CONDITION
316 . . . *[Specified Psychological Factor] Affecting . . . [Indicate the General Medical Condition] Choose name based on nature of factors:*
Mental Disorder Affecting Medical Condition
Psychological Symptoms Affecting Medical Condition
Personality Traits or Coping Style Affecting Medical Condition
Maladaptive Health Behaviors Affecting Medical Condition
Stress-Related Physiological Response Affecting Medical Condition
Other or Unspecified Psychological Factors Affecting Medical Condition

MEDICATION-INDUCED MOVEMENT DISORDERS
332.1 Neuroleptic-Induced Parkinsonism
333.92 Neuroleptic Malignant Syndrome
333.7 Neuroleptic-Induced Acute Dystonia
333.99 Neuroleptic-Induced Acute Akathisia
333.82 Neuroleptic-Induced Tardive Dyskinesia
333.1 Medication-Induced Postural Tremor
333.90 Medication-Induced Movement Disorder NOS

OTHER MEDICATION-INDUCED DISORDER
995.2 Adverse Effects of Medication NOS

RELATIONAL PROBLEMS
V61.9 Relational Problem Related to a Mental Disorder or General Medical Condition
V61.20 Parent-Child Relational Problem
V61.1 Partner Relational Problem
V61.8 Sibling Relational Problem
V62.81 Relational Problem NOS

PROBLEMS RELATED TO ABUSE OR NEGLECT
V61.21 Physical Abuse of Child *(code 995.5 if focus of attention is on victim)*
V61.21 Sexual Abuse of Child *(code 995.5 if focus of attention is on victim)*
V61.21 Neglect of Child *(code 995.5 if focus of attention is on victim)*
V61.1 Physical Abuse of Adult *(code 995.81 if focus of attention is on victim)*
V61.1 Sexual Abuse of Adult *(code 995.81 if focus of attention is on victim)*

ADDITIONAL CONDITIONS THAT MAY BE A FOCUS OF CLINICAL ATTENTION
V15.81 Noncompliance With Treatment
V65.2 Malingering
V71.01 Adult Antisocial Behavior
V71.02 Child or Adolescent Antisocial Behavior
V62.89 Borderline Intellectual Functioning
Note: *This is coded on Axis II.*
780.9 Age-Related Cognitive Decline
V62.82 Bereavement
V62.3 Academic Problem
V62.2 Occupational Problem
313.82 Identity Problem
V62.89 Religious or Spiritual Problem
V62.4 Acculturation Problem
V62.89 Phase of Life Problem

Additional Codes
300.9 Unspecified Mental Disorder (nonpsychotic)
V71.09 No Diagnosis or Condition on Axis I
799.9 Diagnosis or Condition Deferred on Axis I
V71.09 No Diagnosis on Axis II
799.9 Diagnosis Deferred on Axis II

Multiaxial System
Axis I Clinical Disorders
Other Conditions That May Be a Focus of Clinical Attention
Axis II Personality Disorders
Mental Retardation
Axis III General Medical Conditions
Axis IV Psychosocial and Environmental Problems
Axis V Global Assessment of Functioning

Table from DSM-IV, *Diagnostic and Statistical Manual of Mental Disorders,* ed 4. Copyright American Psychiatric Association, Washington, 1994. Used with permission.

Axis II Axis II consists of personality disorders and mental retardation (Table 11.1-4). The habitual use of a particular defense mechanism can be indicated on Axis II.

Axis III Axis III lists any physical disorder or general medical condition that is present in addition to the mental disorder. The physical condition may be causative (for example, kidney failure causing delirium), the result of a mental disorder (for example, alcohol gastritis secondary to alcohol dependence), or unrelated to the mental disorder. When a medical condition is causative or causally related to a mental disorder, a mental disorder due to a general condition is listed on Axis I and the general medical condition is listed on both Axis I and Axis III. In DSM-IV's example—a case in which hypothyroidism is a direct cause of major depressive disorder—the designation on Axis I is mood disorder due to hypothyroidism with depressive features, and hypothyroidism is listed again on Axis III (Table 11.1-5).

TABLE 11.1-2
Classes or Groups of Conditions in DSM-IV

Disorders usually first diagnosed in infancy, childhood, or adolescence
Delirium, dementia, and amnestic and other cognitive disorders
Mental disorders due to a general medical condition not elsewhere classified
Substance-related disorders
Schizophrenia and other psychotic disorders
Mood disorders
Anxiety disorders
Somatoform disorders
Factitious disorders
Dissociative disorders
Sexual and gender identity disorders
Eating disorders
Sleep disorders
Impulse-control disorders not elsewhere classified
Adjustment disorders
Personality disorders
Other conditions that may be a focus of clinical attention

TABLE 11.1-3
Axis I: Clinical Disorders and Other Conditions That May Be a Focus of Clinical Attention

Disorders usually first diagnosed in infancy, childhood, or adolescence (excluding mental retardation, which is diagnosed on Axis II)
Delirium, dementia, and amnestic and other cognitive disorders
Mental disorders due to a general medical condition
Substance-related disorders
Schizophrenia and other psychotic disorders
Mood disorders
Anxiety disorders
Somatoform disorders
Factitious disorders
Dissociative disorders
Sexual and gender identity disorders
Eating disorders
Sleep disorders
Impulse-control disorders not elsewhere classified
Adjustment disorders
Other conditions that may be a focus of clinical attention

TABLE 11.1-4
Axis II: Personality Disorders and Mental Retardation

Paranoid personality disorder
Schizoid personality disorder
Schizotypal personality disorder
Antisocial personality disorder
Borderline personality disorder
Histrionic personality disorder
Narcissistic personality disorder
Avoidant personality disorder
Dependent personality disorder
Obsessive-compulsive personality disorder
Personality disorder not otherwise specified
Mental retardation

TABLE 11.1-5
Axis III: ICD-9-CM General Medical Conditions

Infectious and parasitic disease (001–139)
Neoplasms (140–239)
Endocrine, nutritional, and metabolic diseases and immunity disorders (240–279)
Diseases of the blood and blood-forming organs (280–289)
Diseases of the nervous system and sense organs (320–389)
Diseases of the circulatory system (390–459)
Diseases of the respiratory system (460–519)
Diseases of the digestive system (520–579)
Diseases of the genitourinary system (580–629)
Complications of pregnancy, childbirth, and the puerperium (630–676)
Diseases of the skin and subcutaneous tissue (680–709)
Diseases of the musculoskeletal system and connective tissue (710–739)
Congenital anomalies (740–759)
Certain conditions originating in the perinatal period (760–779)
Symptoms, signs, and ill-defined conditions (780–799)
Injury and poisoning (800–999)

Axis IV Axis IV is used to code the psychosocial and environmental problems that significantly contribute to the development or the exacerbation of the current disorder (Table 11.1-6).

The evaluation of stressors is based on the clinician's assessment of the stress that an average person with similar socio-cultural values and circumstances would experience from the psychosocial stressors. That judgment considers the amount of change in the person's life caused by the stressor, the degree to which the event is desired and under the person's control, and the number of stressors. Stressors may be positive (for example, a job promotion) or negative (for example, the loss of a loved one). Information about stressors may be important in formulating a treatment plan that includes attempts to remove the psychosocial stressors or to help the patient cope with them.

TABLE 11.1-6
Axis IV: Psychosocial and Environmental Problems

Problems with primary support group
Problems related to the social environment
Educational problems
Occupational problems
Housing problems
Economic problems
Problems with access to health care services
Problems related to interaction with the legal system/crime
Other psychosocial and environmental problems

Axis V Axis V is the Global Assessment of Functioning (GAF) scale with which the clinician judges the patient's overall level of functioning during a particular time period (for example, the patient's level of functioning at the time of the evaluation or the patient's highest level of functioning for at least a few months during the past year). Functioning is conceptualized as a composite of three major areas: social functioning, occupational functioning, and psychological functioning. The GAF scale, based on a continuum of mental health and mental illness, is a 100-point scale, 100 representing the highest level of functioning in all areas (Table 11.1-7).

Patients who had a high level of functioning before an episode of illness generally have a better prognosis than those who had a low level of functioning.

Multiaxial evaluation report form Table 11.1-8 shows the DSM-IV multiaxial evaluation report form. Examples of how to record the results of a DSM-IV multiaxial evaluation are given in Table 11.1-9.

NONAXIAL FORMAT DSM-IV also allows clinicians who do not wish to use the multiaxial format to list the diagnoses serially, with the principal diagnosis listed first (Table 11.1-10).

SEVERITY OF DISORDER Depending on the clinical picture, the presence or the absence of signs and symptoms, and their intensity, the severity of a disorder may be mild, moderate, or severe, and the disorder may be in partial remission or in full remission. The following guidelines are used by DSM-IV:

Mild Few, if any, symptoms in excess of those required to make the diagnosis are present, and symptoms result in no more than minor impairment in social or occupational functioning.

Moderate Symptoms or functional impairment between "mild" and "severe" are present.

Severe Many symptoms in excess of those required to make the diagnosis, or several symptoms that are particularly severe, are present, or the symptoms result in marked impairment in social or occupational functioning.

TABLE 11.1-7
Global Assessment of Functioning (GAF) Scale*

Consider psychological, social, and occupational functioning on a hypothetical continuum of mental health-illness. Do not include impairment in functioning due to physical (or environmental) limitations.

Code	(Note: Use intermediate codes when appropriate, e.g., 45, 68, 72.)
100 91	Superior functioning in a wide range of activities, life's problems never seem to get out of hand, is sought out by others because of his or her many positive qualities. No symptoms.
90 81	Absent or minimal symptoms (e.g., mild anxiety before an exam), good functioning in all areas, interested and involved in a wide range of activities, socially effective, generally satisfied with life, no more than everyday problems or concerns (e.g., an occasional argument with family members).
80 71	If symptoms are present, they are transient and expectable reactions to psychosocial stressors (e.g., difficulty concentrating after family argument); no more than slight impairment in social, occupational, or school functioning (e.g., temporarily falling behind in schoolwork).
70 61	Some mild symptoms (e.g., depressed mood and mild insomnia) OR some difficulty in social, occupational, or school functioning (e.g., occasional truancy, or theft within the household), but generally functioning pretty well, has some meaningful interpersonal relationships.
60 51	Moderate symptoms (e.g., flat affect and circumstantial speech, occasional panic attacks) OR moderate difficulty in social, occupational, or school functioning (e.g., few friends, conflicts with peers or coworkers).
50 41	Serious symptoms (e.g., suicidal ideation, severe obsessional rituals, frequent shoplifting) OR any serious impairment in social, occupational, or school functioning (e.g., no friends, unable to keep a job).
40 31	Some impairment in reality testing or communication (e.g., speech is at times illogical, obscure, or irrelevant) OR major impairment in several areas, such as work or school, family relations, judgment, thinking, or mood (e.g., depressed man avoids friends, neglects family, and is unable to work; child frequently beats up younger children, is defiant at home, and is failing at school).
30 21	Behavior is considerably influenced by delusions or hallucinations OR serious impairment in communication or judgment (e.g., sometimes incoherent, acts grossly inappropriately, suicidal preoccupation) OR inability to function in almost all areas (e.g., stays in bed all day; no job, home, or friends).
20 11	Some danger of hurting self or others (e.g., suicide attempts without clear expectation of death, frequently violent, manic excitement) OR occasionally fails to maintain minimal personal hygiene (e.g., smears feces) OR gross impairment in communication (e.g., largely incoherent or mute).
10 1	Persistent danger of severely hurting self or others (e.g., recurrent violence) OR persistent inability to maintain minimal personal hygiene OR serious suicidal act with clear expectation of death.
0	Inadequate information.

*The GAF scale is a revision of the GAS (J Endicott, R L Spitzer, J L Fleiss, J Cohen: The Global Assessment Scale: A procedure for measuring overall severity of psychiatric disturbance. Arch Gen Psychiatry *33:* 766, 1976) and CGAS (D Shaffer, M S Gould, J Brasic, P Ambrosini, P Fisher, H Bird, S Aluwahlia: Children's Global Assessment Scale (CGAS). Arch Gen Psychiatry *40:* 1228, 1983). They are revisions of the Global Scale of the Health-Sickness Rating Scale (L Luborsky: Clinicians' judgments of mental health. Arch Gen Psychiatry *7:* 407, 1962).

Table from DSM-IV, *Diagnostic and Statistical Manual of Mental Disorders,* ed 4. Copyright American Psychiatric Association, Washington, 1994. Used with permission.

TABLE 11.1-8
Multiaxial Evaluation Report Form

The following form is offered as one possibility for reporting multiaxial evaluations. In some settings this form may be used exactly as is; in other settings the form may be adapted to satisfy special needs.

AXIS I: Clinical Disorders
Other Conditions That May Be a Focus of Clinical Attention

Diagnostic code	DSM-IV name
___ . ___	______________
___ . ___	______________
___ . ___	______________

AXIS II: Personality Disorders
Mental Retardation

Diagnostic code	DSM-IV name
___ . ___	______________
___ . ___	______________

AXIS III: General Medical Conditions

ICD-9-CM code	ICD-9-CM name
___ . ___	______________
___ . ___	______________
___ . ___	______________

AXIS IV: Psychosocial and Environmental Problems

Check:
- ☐ Problems with primary support group
  Specify: ______________
- ☐ Problems related to the social environment
  Specify: ______________
- ☐ Educational problems
  Specify: ______________
- ☐ Occupational problems
  Specify: ______________
- ☐ Housing problems
  Specify: ______________
- ☐ Economic problems
  Specify: ______________
- ☐ Problems with access to health care services
  Specify: ______________
- ☐ Problems related to interaction with the legal system/crime
  Specify: ______________
- ☐ Other psychosocial and environmental problems
  Specify: ______________

AXIS V: Global Assessment of Functioning Scale
Score: ___ Time frame: ______________

Table from DSM-IV, *Diagnostic and Statistical Manual of Mental Disorders,* ed 4. Copyright American Psychiatric Association, Washington, 1994. Used with permission.

In partial remission The full criteria for the disorder were previously met, but currently only some of the symptoms or signs of the disorder remain.

In full remission There are no longer any symptoms or signs of the disorder but it is still clinically relevant to note the disorder. . . . The differentiation of in full remission from recovered requires consideration of many factors, including the characteristic course of the disorder, the length of time since the last period of disturbance, the total duration of the disturbance, and the need for continued evaluation or prophylactic treatment.

MULTIPLE DIAGNOSIS When a patient has more than one Axis I disorder, the principal diagnosis is indicated by listing it first. According to DSM-IV:

> The remaining disorders are listed in order of focus of attention and treatment. When a person has both an Axis I and an Axis II diagnosis, the principal diagnosis or the reason for visit will be assumed to be on Axis I unless the Axis II diagnosis is followed by the qualifying phrase "(Principal diagnosis)" or "(Reason for visit)."

DSM-IV also states:

> When more than one diagnosis for an individual is given in an inpatient setting, the *principal diagnosis* is the condition established after

TABLE 11.1-9
Examples of How to Record the Results of a DSM-IV Multiaxial Evaluation

Example 1:		
Axis I	296.23	Major depressive disorder, single episode, severe without psychotic features
	305.00	Alcohol abuse
Axis II	301.6	Dependent personality disorder
		Frequent use of denial
Axis III		None
Axis IV		Threat of job loss
Axis V	GAF = 35	(current)
Example 2:		
Axis I	300.4	Dysthymic disorder
	315.00	Reading disorder
Axis II	V71.09	No diagnosis
Axis III	382.9	Otitis media, recurrent
Axis IV		Victim of child neglect
Axis V	GAF = 53	(current)
Example 3:		
Axis I	293.83	Mood disorder due to hypothyroidism, with depressive features
Axis II	V71.09	No diagnosis, histrionic personality features
Axis III	244.9	Hypothyroidism
	365.23	Chronic angle-closure glaucoma
Axis IV		None
Axis V	GAF = 45	(on admission)
	GAF = 65	(at discharge)
Example 4:		
Axis I	V61.1	Partner relational problem
Axis II	V71.09	No diagnosis
Axis III		None
Axis IV		Unemployment
Axis V	GAF = 83	(highest level past year)

Table from DSM-IV, *Diagnostic and Statistical Manual of Mental Disorders,* ed 4. Copyright American Psychiatric Association, Washington, 1994. Used with permission.

TABLE 11.1-10
Nonaxial Format

Clinicians who do not wish to use the multiaxial format may simply list the appropriate diagnoses. Those choosing this option should follow the general rule of recording as many coexisting mental disorders, general medical conditions, and other factors that are relevant to the care and treatment of the individual. The principal diagnosis or the reason for visit should be listed first.

The examples below illustrate the reporting of diagnoses in a format that does not use the multiaxial system.

Example 1:	
296.23	Major depressive disorder, single episode, severe without psychotic features
305.00	Alcohol abuse
301.6	Dependent personality disorder
	Frequent use of denial
Example 2:	
300.4	Dysthymic disorder
315.00	Reading disorder
382.9	Otitis media, recurrent
Example 3:	
293.83	Mood disorder due to hypothyroidism, with depressive features
244.9	Hypothyroidism
365.23	Chronic angle-closure glaucoma
	Histrionic personality features
Example 4:	
V61.1	Partner relational problem

Table from DSM-IV, *Diagnostic and Statistical Manual of Mental Disorders,* ed 4. Copyright American Psychiatric Association, Washington, 1994. Used with permission.

study to be chiefly responsible for occasioning the admission of the individual. When more than one diagnosis is given for an individual in an outpatient setting, the *reason for visit* is the condition that is chiefly responsible for the ambulatory care medical services received during the visit. In most cases, the principal diagnosis or the reason for visit is also the main focus of attention or treatment. It is often difficult (and somewhat arbitrary) to determine which diagnosis is the principal diagnosis or the reason for visit, especially in situations of "dual diagnosis" (a substance-related diagnosis like Amphetamine Dependence accompanied by a non-substance-related diagnosis like Schizophrenia). For example, it may be unclear which diagnosis should be considered "principal" for an individual hospitalized with both Schizophrenia and Amphetamine Intoxication, because each condition may have contributed equally to the need for admission and treatment.

PROVISIONAL DIAGNOSIS According to DSM-IV:

The modifier *provisional* can be used when there is a strong presumption that the full criteria will ultimately be met for a disorder, but not enough information is available to make a firm diagnosis. The clinician can indicate the diagnostic uncertainty by writing "(Provisional)" following the diagnosis. For example, the individual appears to have a Major Depressive Disorder, but is unable to give an adequate history to establish that the full criteria are met. Another use of the term *provisional* is for those situations in which differential diagnosis depends exclusively on the duration of illness. For example, a diagnosis of Schizophreniform Disorder requires a duration of less than 6 months and can only be given provisionally if assigned before remission has occurred.

PRIOR HISTORY According to DSM-IV:

For some purposes, it may be useful to note a history of the criteria having been met for a disorder even when the individual is considered to be recovered from it. Such past diagnoses of mental disorder would be indicated by using the specifier Prior History (e.g., Separation Anxiety Disorder, Prior History, for an individual with a history of Separation Anxiety Disorder who has no current disorder or who currently meets criteria for Panic Disorder).

NOT OTHERWISE SPECIFIED CATEGORIES According to DSM-IV, "not otherwise specified" categories are used as follows:

Because of the diversity of clinical presentations, it is impossible for the diagnostic nomenclature to cover every possible situation. For this reason, each diagnostic class has at least one Not Otherwise Specified (NOS) category and some classes have several NOS categories. There are four situations in which an NOS diagnosis may be appropriate:

- The presentation conforms to the general guidelines for a mental disorder in the diagnostic class, but the symptomatic picture does not meet the criteria for any of the specific disorders. This would occur either when the symptoms are below the diagnostic threshold for one of the specific disorders or when there is an atypical or mixed presentation.
- The presentation conforms to a symptom pattern that has not been included in the DSM-IV classification but that causes clinically significant distress or impairment. Research criteria for some of these symptom patterns have been included in Appendix B ("Criteria Sets and Axes Provided for Further Study"), in which case a page reference to the suggested research criteria set in Appendix B is provided.
- There is uncertainty about etiology (i.e., whether the disorder is due to a general medical condition, is substance induced, or is primary).
- There is insufficient opportunity for complete data collection (e.g., in emergency situations) or inconsistent or contradictory information, but there is enough information to place it within a particular diagnostic class (e.g., the clinician determines that the individual has psychotic symptoms but does not have enough information to diagnose a specific Psychotic Disorder).

FREQUENTLY USED CRITERIA Frequently used criteria, according to DSM-IV, are as follows:

Criteria used to exclude other diagnoses and to suggest differential diagnoses Most of the criteria sets used in DSM-IV include exclusion criteria to establish boundaries between disorders and to clarify differential diagnoses. The wordings of the exclusion criteria reflect the various types of relations between disorders:

- **"Criteria have never been met for . . ."** This exclusion criterion is used to define a lifetime hierarchy between disorders. For example, a diagnosis of Major Depressive Disorder can no longer be given once a Manic Episode has occurred and must be changed to a diagnosis of Bipolar I Disorder.
- **"Criteria are not met for . . ."** This exclusion criterion is used to establish a hierarchy between disorders (or subtypes) defined cross-sectionally. For example, the specifier With Melancholic Features takes precedence over With Atypical Features for describing the current Major Depressive Episode.
- **"does not occur exclusively during the course of . . ."** This exclusion criterion prevents a disorder from being diagnosed when its symptom presentation occurs only during the course of another disorder. For example, dementia is not diagnosed separately if it occurs only during delirium; Conversion Disorder is not diagnosed separately if it occurs only during Somatization Disorder; Bulimia Nervosa is not diagnosed separately if it occurs only during Anorexia Nervosa. This exclusion criterion is typically used in situations in which the symptoms of one disorder are associated features or a subset of the symptoms of the preempting disorder. The clinician should consider periods of partial remission as part of the "course of another disorder." It should be noted that the excluded diagnosis can be given at times when it occurs independently (e.g., when the excluding disorder is in full remission).
- **"not due to the direct physiological effects of a substance (e.g., a drug of abuse, a medication) or a general medical condition."** This exclusion criterion is used to indicate that a substance-induced and general medical etiology must be considered and ruled out before the disorder can be diagnosed (e.g., Major Depressive Disorder can be diagnosed only after etiologies based on substance use and a general medical condition have been ruled out).
- **"not better accounted for by . . ."** This exclusion criterion is used to indicate that the disorders mentioned in the criterion must be considered in the differential diagnosis of the presenting psychopathology and that, in boundary cases, clinical judgment will be necessary to determine which disorder provides the most appropriate diagnosis. In such cases, the "Differential Diagnosis" section of the text for the disorders should be consulted for guidance.

The general convention in DSM-IV is to allow multiple diagnoses to be assigned for those presentations that meet criteria for more than one DSM-IV disorder. There are three situations in which the above-mentioned exclusion criteria help to establish a diagnostic hierarchy (and thus prevent multiple diagnoses) or to highlight differential diagnostic considerations (and thus discourage multiple diagnoses):

- When a Mental Disorder Due to a General Medical Condition or a Substance-Induced Disorder is responsible for the symptoms, it preempts the diagnosis of the corresponding primary disorder with the same symptoms (e.g., Cocaine-Induced Mood Disorder preempts Major Depressive Disorder). In such cases, an exclusion criterion containing the phrase "not due to the direct effects of . . ." is included in the criteria set for the primary disorder.
- When a more pervasive disorder (e.g., Schizophrenia) has among its defining symptoms (or associated symptoms) what are the defining symptoms of a less pervasive disorder (e.g., Dysthymic Disorder), one of the following three exclusion criteria appears in the criteria set for the less pervasive disorder, indicating that only the more pervasive disorder is diagnosed: "Criteria have never been met for . . .", "Criteria are not met for . . .", "does not occur exclusively during the course of. . . ."
- When there are particularly difficult differential diagnostic boundaries, the phrase "not better accounted for by . . ." is included to indicate that clinical judgment is necessary to determine which diagnosis is most appropriate. For example, Panic Disorder With Agoraphobia includes the criterion "not better accounted for by Social Phobia" and Social Phobia includes the criterion "not better accounted for by Panic Disorder With Agoraphobia" in recognition of the fact that this is a particularly difficult boundary to draw. In some cases, both diagnoses might be appropriate.

Criteria for substance-induced disorders It is often difficult to determine whether presenting symptomatology is substance induced, that is, the direct physiological consequence of Substance Intoxication or Withdrawal, medication use, or toxin exposure. In an effort to provide some assistance in making this determination, the two criteria listed below have been added to each of the Substance-Induced Disorders. These criteria are intended to provide general guidelines, but at the same time allow for clinical judgment in determining whether or not the presenting symptoms are best accounted for by the direct physiological effects of the substance.

- There is evidence from the history, physical examination, or laboratory findings of either (1) or (2):
  (1) the symptoms developed during, or within a month of, Substance Intoxication or Withdrawal.
  (2) medication use is etiologically related to the disturbance.
- The disturbance is not better accounted for by a disorder that is not substance induced. Evidence that the symptoms are better accounted for by a disorder that is not substance induced might include the following: the symptoms precede the onset of the substance use (or medication use); the symptoms persist for a substantial period of time (e.g., about a month) after the cessation of acute withdrawal or severe intoxication, or are substantially in excess of what would be expected given the type, duration, or amount of the substance used; or there is other evidence that suggests the existence of an independent non-substance-induced disorder (e.g., a history of recurrent non-substance-related episodes).

Criteria for a mental disorder due to a general medical condition The criterion listed below is necessary to establish the etiological requirement for each of the Mental Disorders Due to a General Medical Condition (e.g., Mood Disorder Due to Hypothyroidism). . . .

There is evidence from the history, physical examination, or laboratory findings that the disturbance is the direct physiological consequence of a general medical condition.

Definition of mental disorder According to DSM-IV:

[E]ach of the mental disorders is conceptualized as a clinically significant behavioral or psychological syndrome or pattern that occurs in an individual and that is associated with present distress (e.g., a painful symptom) or disability (i.e., impairment in one or more important areas of functioning) or with a significantly increased risk of suffering death, pain, disability, or an important loss of freedom. In addition, this syndrome or pattern must not be merely an expectable and culturally sanctioned response to a particular event, for example, the death of a loved one. Whatever its original cause, it must currently be considered a manifestation of a behavioral, psychological, or biological dysfunction in the individual. Neither deviant behavior (e.g., political, religious, or sexual), nor conflicts that are primarily between the individual and society are mental disorders unless the deviance or conflict is a symptom of a dysfunction in the individual, as described above. . . .

DISTINCTION BETWEEN MENTAL DISORDER AND GENERAL MEDICAL CONDITION The terms *mental disorder* and *general medical condition* are used throughout this manual. The term *mental disorder* is explained above. The term *general medical condition* is used merely as a convenient shorthand to refer to conditions and disorders that are listed outside the "Mental and Behavioural Disorders" chapter of ICD. It should be recognized that these are merely terms of convenience and should not be taken to imply that there is any fundamental distinction between mental disorders and general medical conditions, that mental disorders are unrelated to physical or biological factors or processes, or that general medical conditions are unrelated to behavioral or psychosocial factors or processes.

Organization The DSM-IV organizational plan is described as follows:

The first section is devoted to "Disorders Usually First Diagnosed in Infancy, Childhood, or Adolescence." This division of the Classification according to age at presentation is for convenience only and is not absolute. Although disorders in this section are usually first evident in childhood and adolescence, some individuals diagnosed with disorders located in this section (e.g., Attention-Deficit/Hyperactivity Disorder) may not present for clinical attention until adulthood. In addition, it is not uncommon for the age at onset for many disorders placed in other sections to be during childhood or adolescence (e.g., Major Depressive Disorder, Schizophrenia, Generalized Anxiety Disorder). Clinicians who work primarily with children and adolescents should therefore be familiar with the entire manual, and those who work primarily with adults should also be familiar with this section.

The next three sections—"Delirium, Dementia, and Amnestic and Other Cognitive Disorders"; "Mental Disorders Due to a General Medical Condition"; and "Substance-Related Disorders"—were grouped together in DSM-III-R under the single heading of "Organic Mental Syndromes and Disorders." . . . As in DSM-III-R, these sections are placed before the remaining disorders in the manual because of their priority in differential diagnosis (e.g., substance-related causes of depressed mood must be ruled out before making a diagnosis of Major Depressive Disorder). To facilitate differential diagnosis, complete lists of Mental Disorders Due to a General Medical Condition and Substance-Related Disorders appear in these sections, whereas the text and criteria for these disorders are placed in the diagnostic sections with disorders with which they share phenomenology. For example, the text and criteria for Substance-Induced Mood Disorder and Mood Disorder Due to a General Medical Condition are included in the Mood Disorders section.

The organizing principle for all the remaining sections (except for Adjustment Disorders) is to group disorders based on their shared phenomenological features in order to facilitate differential diagnosis. The "Adjustment Disorders" section is organized differently in that these disorders are grouped based on their common etiology (e.g., maladaptive reaction to a stressor). Therefore, the Adjustment Disorders include a variety of heterogeneous clinical presentations (e.g., Adjustment Disorder With Depressed Mood, Adjustment Disorder With Anxiety, Adjustment Disorder With Disturbance of Conduct).

Finally, DSM-IV includes a section for Other Conditions That May be a Focus of Clinical Attention.

PSYCHOSIS AND NEUROSIS

Psychosis Although the traditional meaning of the term "psychotic" emphasized loss of reality testing and impairment of mental functioning—manifested by delusions, hallucinations, confusion, and impaired memory—two other meanings have evolved during the past 50 years. In the most common psychiatric use of the term, "psychotic" became synonymous with severe impairment of social and personal functioning characterized by social withdrawal and inability to perform the usual household and occupational roles. The other use of the term specifies the degree of ego regression as the criterion for psychotic illness. As a consequence of those multiple meanings, the term has lost its precision in current clinical and research practice.

According to the glossary of the American Psychiatric Association, the term "psychotic" means grossly impaired in reality testing. The term may be used to describe the behavior of a person at a given time or a mental disorder in which at some time during its course all persons with the disorder have grossly impaired reality testing. With gross impairment in reality testing, persons incorrectly evaluate the accuracy of their perceptions and thoughts and make incorrect inferences about external reality, even in the face of contrary evidence. The term "psychotic" does not apply to minor distortions of reality that involve matters of relative judgment. For example, depressed persons who underestimate their achievements are not described as psychotic, whereas those who believe that they have caused natural catastrophes are so described.

Direct evidence of psychotic behavior is the presence of either delusions or hallucinations without insight into their pathological nature. The term "psychotic" is sometimes appropriate when behavior is so grossly disorganized that a reasonable inference can be made that reality testing is disturbed. Examples include markedly incoherent speech without apparent awareness by the person that the speech is not understandable and the agitated, inattentive, and disoriented behavior seen in alcohol intoxication delirium. A person with a nonpsychotic mental disorder may exhibit psychotic behavior, although rarely. For example, a person with obsessive-compulsive disorder may at times come to believe in the reality of the danger of being contaminated by shaking hands with strangers. In DSM-IV the psychotic disorders include pervasive developmental disorders, schizophrenia, schizophreniform disorder, schizoaffective disorder, delusional disorder, brief psychotic disorder, shared psychotic disorder, psychotic disorder due to a general medical condition, substance-induced psychotic disorder, and psychotic disorder not otherwise specified. In addition, some severe mood disorders have psychotic features.

Neurosis A neurosis is a chronic or recurrent nonpsychotic disorder, characterized mainly by anxiety, that is experienced or expressed directly or is altered through defense mechanisms; it appears as a symptom, such as an obsession, a compulsion, a phobia, or a sexual dysfunction. Although not used in DSM-IV, the term "neurosis" is still found in the literature and in ICD-10. In DSM-III a neurotic disorder was defined as follows:

> A mental disorder in which the predominant disturbance is a symptom or group of symptoms that is distressing to the individual and is recognized by him or her as unacceptable and alien (ego-dystonic); reality testing is grossly intact. Behavior does not actively violate gross social norms (though it may be quite disabling). The disturbance is relatively enduring or recurrent without treatment, and is not limited to a transitory reaction to stressors. There is no demonstrable organic etiology or factor.

In DSM-IV no overall diagnostic class is called neuroses; however, many clinicians consider the following diagnostic categories neuroses: anxiety disorders, somatoform disorders, dissociative disorders, sexual disorders, and dysthymic disorder. The term "neuroses" encompasses a broad range of disorders with various signs and symptoms. As such, it has lost any degree of precision except to signify that the person's gross reality testing and personality organization are intact. However, a neurosis can be and usually is sufficient to impair the person's functioning in a number of areas. The authors believe that the term is useful in contemporary psychiatry and should be retained, especially since it is retained in ICD-10.

ICD-10 In ICD-10 a class called neurotic, stress-related, and somatoform disorders encompasses the following: phobic anxiety disorders, other anxiety disorders (including panic disorder, generalized anxiety disorder, and mixed anxiety and depressive disorder), obsessive-compulsive disorder, adjustment disorders, dissociative (conversion) disorders, and somatoform disorders. In addition, ICD-10 includes neurasthenia as a neurotic disorder characterized by mental and physical fatigability, a sense of general instability, irritability, anhedonia, and sleep disturbances. Many of the cases so diagnosed outside the United States fit the descriptions of anxiety disorders and depressive disorders and are diagnosed as such by American psychiatrists.

CHANGES FROM DSM-III-R The term "organic mental disorders" was eliminated from DSM-IV, because it incorrectly implied that other mental disorders do not have a biological component.

An appendix was added to DSM-IV to reflect the influence of culture and ethnicity on psychiatric assessment and diagnosis. That appendix describes culturally specific symptom patterns, preferred idioms for describing distress, and prevalence when such information is available. It also provides the clinician with guidance on how the clinical presentation may be influenced by the patient's cultural setting.

Multiple personality disorder was renamed "dissociative identity disorder" to highlight the failure of integration that is its central feature.

In DSM-III-R, self-defeating personality disorder was a proposed diagnostic category needing further study; after extensive debate the category was removed from DSM-IV's appendix.

A diagnostic criterion for panic disorder without agoraphobia and panic disorder with agoraphobia now emphasizes worry about the implications of the panic attack or the behavior changes, rather than the frequency of the attacks.

Appendix H in DSM-IV lists the corresponding ICD-10 codes for DSM-IV disorders.

A summary of the major changes in DSM-IV are listed in Table 11.1-11.

TABLE 11.1-11
Changes in DSM-IV from DSM-III-R

Axis I: Now includes pervasive developmental disorders, learning disorders, motor skills disorders, and communications disorders (they were coded on Axis II in DSM-III-R).

Axis II: Now contains only personality disorders and mental retardation.

Axis IV: Now used to report psychosocial and environmental problems (rather than severity of stressors).

Learning Disorders: This term replaces the older ''academic skills disorders,'' and the diagnosis is now permitted in the presence of a neurological condition or a sensory deficit.

Autistic Disorder: Age at onset before 3 years is required; individual criteria have been reduced from 16 to 12 to increase clinical utility.

Rett Disorder, Childhood Disintegrative Disorder, Asperger Disorder: These disorders have been described as separate entities within the pervasive developmental disorders in order to reduce their inappropriate inclusion in autistic disorder or as pervasive developmental disorder not otherwise specified.

Attention-Deficit/Hyperactivity Disorder: Includes attention-deficit disorder both with and without hyperactivity (as one disorder with different predominating symptom patterns: inattentive, hyperactive-impulsive, or combined). Symptoms must occur in two or more situations (school, work, home).

Conduct Disorder: Staying out at night and intimidating others are added as inclusion items to make the definition more representative of females with conduct disorder. Differentiation of subtypes based on age at onset reflects the data that show earlier age at onset confers a worse prognosis and is more likely to be associated with aggressive behavior and with adult antisocial personality disorder.

Feeding and Eating Disorders of Infancy and Childhood: The name reflects the placement of anorexia nervosa and bulimia nervosa in a separate eating disorders section.

Tic Disorders: Required age at onset has been reduced from 21 years to 18 years.

Communication Disorders: Includes both the language and speech disorders and the speech disorders not elsewhere classified of DSM-III-R.

Mixed Receptive-Expressive Language Disorder: Replaces developmental receptive language disorder, since research data indicate that receptive language problems do not occur without accompanying expressive difficulties.

Phonological Disorder: Replaces the older articulation disorder.

Delirium, Dementia, Amnestic and Other Cognitive Disorders: Replace what were previously called organic mental disorders.

Mental Disorders Due to a General Medical Condition: Includes a new category, catatonic disorder, because it is a frequent explanation for catatonic symptoms. Personality change due to a general medical condition (previously called organic personality disorder) now specifies subtypes: labile, disinhibited, aggressive, apathetic, and paranoid.

Substance-Related Disorders: Includes both the psychoactive substance use disorders and the psychoactive substance-induced organic mental disorders of DSM-III-R.

Substance Dependence: Subtypes for physiological dependence have been added that allow recognition of tolerance and withdrawal. Expanded course modifiers take into account differences between early and sustained remission, partial and full remission, and whether the patient has been on agonist therapy or in a controlled environment.

Substance Abuse: Is more clearly defined and not merely a residual category.

Alcohol Intoxication: Includes idiosyncratic intoxication because of lack of evidence that it was a distinct entity.

Schizophrenia and Other Psychotic Disorders: Brings together schizophrenia, delusional disorder, and psychotic disorders not elsewhere classified.

Schizophrenia: The required duration of active phase symptoms is increased to one month. The separate list of prodromal and residual phase symptoms has been eliminated.

Schizoaffective Disorder: Emphasis is on an uninterrupted episode of illness rather than the lifetime pattern of symptoms.

Brief Psychotic Disorder: Expands the older brief reactive psychosis to include all psychotic disturbances lasting less than one month that are not related to a mood disorder, a general medical condition, or a substance-induced disorder.

Psychotic Disorder Due to a General Medical Condition, Substance-Induced Psychotic Disorder: These disorders are included in the psychotic disorders section to facilitate differential diagnosis. Delusional disorder and hallucinosis are combined into a single psychotic disorder.

Manic Episode: The requirement of one week's duration has been reinstated. Manic episodes precipitated by antidepressant treatment are diagnosed as substance-induced rather than bipolar.

Hypomanic Episode: Is defined in a criteria set that is separate from manic episode.

Bipolar Disorders: Have been divided into bipolar I and bipolar II (at least one major depressive episode and at least one hypomanic episode but no history of manic episodes).

Mood Disorder Due to a General Medical Condition, Substance-Induced Mood Disorder: These disorders have been placed within the mood disorders section to facilitate differential diagnosis.

Major Depressive Episodes: New subtypes include with atypical features (e.g., mood reactivity, reverse vegetative symptoms, sensitivity to rejection—all of which may have implications for treatment selection); with catatonic features (reflecting evidence that many catatonic presentations are associated with mood disorders); with rapid cycling (bipolar disorder with four or more full mood episodes in 12 months, which has implications for prognosis and treatment selection); with postpartum onset (reflecting evidence that such onset may have implications for prognosis and treatment selection).

Panic Disorder Without Agoraphobia: The threshold for panic disorder has been raised, requiring recurrent unexpected panic attacks accompanied by a month or more of persistent concern about having additional attacks.

Specific Phobia: Replaces simple phobia.

Social Phobia: Includes the earlier avoidant disorder of childhood.

Posttraumatic Stress Disorder: Requires that the subject have experienced, witnessed, or been confronted with an event or events that involve actual or threatened death or serious injury, or a threat to the physical integrity of oneself or others. The previous requirement, that the stress be outside the range of normal human experience, was both unreliable and inaccurate.

Acute Stress Disorder: Acute reactions to extreme stress that last no more than a month

Generalized Anxiety Disorder: Subsumes overanxious disorder of childhood.

Anxiety Disorder Due to a General Medical Condition, Substance-Induced Anxiety Disorder: These disorders are included in the anxiety disorders section to facilitate differential diagnosis.

Somatization Disorder: The list of diagnostic items has been condensed and divided into four groups related to pain, gastrointestinal symptoms, sexual symptoms, and pseudoneurological symptoms.

Conversion Disorder: Requires the presenting problem to be a symptom or deficit that affects either voluntary motor or sensory functioning. Motor, sensory, seizure, and mixed subtypes provide increased specificity. Problems reflecting a change in functioning (e.g., pseudocyesis) are classified as somatoform disorder not otherwise specified.

Pain Disorder: Replaces the earlier somatoform pain disorder and includes pain disorder associated with psychological factors and pain disorder associated with both psychological factors and a general medical condition.

Dissociative Amnesia: Replaces psychogenic amnesia.

Dissociative Fugue: Replaces psychogenic fugue. Assumption of a new identity is no longer required, because confusion about personal identity has been found to be the predominant symptom.

Dissociative Identity Disorder: Replaces multiple personality disorder. The requirement of inability to recall important personal information has been reinstated.

Female Orgasmic Disorder, Male Orgasmic Disorder: Replace inhibited female orgasm and inhibited male orgasm.

Sexual Dysfunction Due to a General Medical Condition, Substance-Induced Sexual Dysfunction: Included to facilitate differential diagnosis.

Gender Identity Disorder: Subsumes gender identity disorder of childhood, gender identity disorder of adolescence or adulthood, and transsexualism. The disorder is placed within the group of sexual and gender identity disorders because it most often presents in adulthood.

TABLE 11.1-11 (*continued*)

Eating Disorders: A new section, recognizing that these disorders often emerge after childhood or adolescence.

Anorexia Nervosa: Binge eating and purging that occur exclusively during anorexia nervosa stay here and are no longer given a separate diagnosis of bulimia nervosa.

Sleep Disorders: The disorders are grouped by presumed etiology rather than by presenting symptoms, and the section is now compatible with the International Classification of Sleep Disorders.

Circadian Rhythm Sleep Disorders: Replace sleep-wake schedule disorder. Subtyping (delayed sleep phase, jet lag, shift work) reflects clinical usage.

Personality Disorders: Passive-aggressive personality disorder is no longer recognized.

Other Conditions That May Be a Focus of Clinical Attention: Replaces the former conditions not attributable to a mental disorder. The category has been broadened to include medication-induced movement disorders, problems related to abuse or neglect, relational problems, religious or spiritual problems, acculturation problems, and problems with cognitive decline associated with aging.

Table by Robert J Campbell, MD. Used with permission.

NEW AND CONTROVERSIAL CATEGORIES Proposed new categories that were considered controversial or for which there was insufficient information to warrant inclusion in DSM-IV were placed in Appendix B, ''Criteria Sets and Axes Provided for Further Study.'' Not all psychiatrists agree that those categories are discrete psychological disorders. Moreover, psychiatrists do not agree on the essential diagnostic features. Each category requires systematic research to determine whether it will eventually be included in the official nomenclature. Nevertheless, clinicians should be familiar with the conditions, some of which are already included in ICD-10.

In addition to the categories listed below, DSM-IV includes a list of defense mechanisms that can be added to the principal diagnosis if the clinician chooses.

Postconcussional disorder This disorder is discussed in Chapter 12. In ICD-10 it is referred to as postconcussional syndrome, which occurs after a head trauma that is usually sufficiently severe to result in loss of consciousness. The symptoms include headache, dizziness (usually lacking the features of true vertigo), fatigue, irritability, difficulty in concentrating and performing mental tasks, memory impairment, insomnia, and reduced tolerance for stress, emotional excitement, and alcohol.

Mild neurocognitive disorder This condition is discussed in Chapter 12.

Caffeine withdrawal This disorder is covered in Section 13.4.

Postpsychotic depressive disorder of schizophrenia This disorder is discussed in Section 16.6. In ICD-10, post-schizophrenic depression is described as follows:

> A depressive episode, which may be prolonged, arising in the aftermath of a schizophrenic illness. Some schizophrenic symptoms must still be present but no longer dominate the clinical picture. These persisting schizophrenic symptoms may be ''positive'' or ''negative,'' though the latter are more common. It is uncertain, and immaterial to the diagnosis, to what extent the depressive symptoms have merely been uncovered by the resolution of earlier psychotic symptoms (rather than being a new development) or are an intrinsic part of schizophrenia rather than a psychological reaction to it. They are rarely sufficiently severe or extensive to meet criteria for a severe depressive episode, and it is often difficult to decide which of the patient's symptoms are due to depression and which to neuroleptic medication or to the impaired volition and affective flattening of schizophrenia itself. This depressive disorder is associated with an increased risk of suicide.

Simple deteriorative disorder This disorder is covered in Section 14.7. In ICD-10 it is described as an uncommon disorder characterized by oddities of conduct, an inability to meet the demands of society, blunting of affect, loss of volition, and social impoverishment. Delusions and hallucinations are not evident.

Minor depressive disorder, recurrent brief depressive disorder, and premenstrual dysphoric disorder Minor depressive disorder and recurrent brief depressive disorder are covered in Section 16.6. Premenstrual dysphoric disorder is covered in Section 29.5. Minor depressive disorder is associated with comparatively mild symptoms, such as worry and overconcern with minor autonomic symptoms (for example, tremor and palpitations). Most cases never come to medical or psychiatric attention. In ICD-10, recurrent brief depressive disorder is characterized by recurrent episodes of depression, each of which lasts less than two weeks (typically two to three days) and each of which ends with complete recovery.

Mixed anxiety-depressive disorder This disorder is covered in Section 17.5. Mixed anxiety and depressive disorder is listed in ICD-10, where it is described as encompassing symptoms of both anxiety and depression, neither of which predominates.

Factitious disorder by proxy This disorder is discussed in Chapter 19. It is also known as Munchausen syndrome by proxy. In the disorder, parents feign illness in their children.

Dissociative trance disorder The dissociative disorders are discussed in Chapter 20. ICD-10 lists trance and possession disorders, in which the patient experiences a temporary loss of both the sense of personal identity and full awareness of the surroundings. The disorders are involuntary or unwanted. In some cases the patient acts as if taken over by another personality, spirit, or force.

Binge-eating disorder This disorder is a variant of bulimia nervosa, which is discussed in Chapter 22. It consists of recurrent episodes of binge eating without the compensatory behavior, such as self-induced vomiting and laxative abuse.

Depressive personality disorder and passive-aggressive personality disorder These personality disorders are classified in the not otherwise specified (NOS) category of personality disorders. Chapter 25 describes each disorder.

Medication-induced movement disorders These disorders are caused by the adverse effects of medication. They include (1) parkinsonism, (2) neuroleptic malignant syndrome, (3) acute dystonia, (4) acute akathisia, (5) tardive dyskinesia, (6) postural tremor, and (7) movement disorder NOS. They are discussed in Section 32.2.

CULTURE-BOUND SYNDROMES An appendix of culturally related syndromes includes the name for each condition, the culture in which it was first described, a brief description of its psychopathology, and a list of possibly related DSM-IV categories. Section 15.3 discusses culture-bound syndromes.

The implication of culture and its relation to diagnosis is set forth in DSM-IV as follows:

> Diagnostic assessment can be especially challenging when a clinician from one ethnic or cultural group uses the DSM-IV Classification to evaluate an individual from a different ethnic or cultural group. A clinician who is unfamiliar with the nuances of an individual's cultural frame of reference may incorrectly judge as psychopathology those normal variations in behavior, belief, or experience that are particular to the individual's culture. For example, certain religious practices or beliefs (e.g., hearing or seeing a deceased relative during bereavement) may be misdiagnosed as manifestations of a Psychotic Disorder. Applying Personality Disorder criteria across cultural settings may be especially difficult because of the wide cultural variation in concepts of self, styles of communication, and coping mechanisms.

GUIDELINES

Cautionary statement

Cautionary statement The American Psychiatric Association has issued a cautionary statement concerning the proper use and interpretation of the diagnostic categories in DSM-IV. It reads as follows:

> The specified diagnostic criteria for each mental disorder are offered as guidelines for making diagnoses, because it has been demonstrated that the use of such criteria enhances agreement among clinicians and investigators. The proper use of these criteria requires specialized clinical training that provides both a body of knowledge and clinical skills.
>
> These diagnostic criteria and the DSM-IV Classification of mental disorders reflect a consensus of current formulations of evolving knowledge in our field. They do not encompass, however, all the conditions for which people may be treated or appropriate topics for research efforts.
>
> The purpose of DSM-IV is to provide clear descriptions of diagnostic categories in order to enable clinicians and investigators to diagnose, communicate about, study, and treat people with various mental disorders. It is to be understood that inclusion here, for clinical and research purposes, of a diagnostic category such as Pathological Gambling or Pedophilia does not imply that the condition meets legal or other nonmedical criteria for what constitutes mental disease, mental disorder, or mental disability. The clinical and scientific considerations involved in categorization of these conditions as mental disorders may not be wholly relevant to legal judgments, for example, that take into account such issues as individual responsibility, disability determination, and competency.

Caveats DSM-IV describes specific caveats regarding its use:

> LIMITATIONS OF THE CATEGORICAL APPROACH DSM-IV is a categorical classification that divides mental disorders into types based on criteria sets with defining features. This naming of categories is the traditional method of organizing and transmitting information in everyday life and has been the fundamental approach used in all systems of medical diagnosis. A categorical approach to classification works best when all members of a diagnostic class are homogeneous, when there are clear boundaries between classes, and when the different classes are mutually exclusive. Nonetheless, the limitations of the categorical classification system must be recognized.
>
> In DSM-IV, there is no assumption that each category of mental disorder is a completely discrete entity with absolute boundaries dividing it from other mental disorders or from no mental disorder. There is also no assumption that all individuals described as having the same mental disorder are alike in all important ways. The clinician using DSM-IV should therefore consider that individuals sharing a diagnosis are likely to be heterogeneous even in regard to the defining features of the diagnosis and that boundary cases will be difficult to diagnose in any but a probabilistic fashion. This outlook allows greater flexibility in the use of the system, encourages more specific attention to boundary cases, and emphasizes the need to capture additional clinical information that goes beyond diagnosis. In recognition of the heterogeneity of clinical presentations, DSM-IV often includes polythetic criteria sets, in which the individual need only present with a subset of items from a longer list (e.g., the diagnosis of Borderline Personality Disorder requires only five out of nine items).
>
> It was suggested that the DSM-IV Classification be organized following a dimensional model rather than the categorical model used in DSM-III-R. A dimensional system classifies clinical presentations based on quantification of attributes rather than the assignment to categories and works best in describing phenomena that are distributed continuously and that do not have clear boundaries. Although dimensional systems increase reliability and communicate more clinical information (because they report clinical attributes that might be subthreshold in a categorical system), they also have serious limitations and thus far have been less useful than categorical systems in clinical practice and in stimulating research. Numerical dimensional descriptions are much less familiar and vivid than are the categorical names for mental disorders. Moreover, there is as yet no agreement on the choice of the optimal dimensions to be used for classification purposes. Nonetheless, it is possible that the increasing research on, and familiarity with, dimensional systems may eventually result in their greater acceptance both as a method of conveying clinical information and as a research tool.
>
> USE OF CLINICAL JUDGMENT DSM-IV is a classification of mental disorders that was developed for use in clinical, educational, and research settings. The diagnostic categories, criteria, and textual descriptions are meant to be employed by individuals with appropriate clinical training and experience in diagnosis. It is important that DSM-IV not be applied mechanically by untrained individuals. The specific diagnostic criteria included in DSM-IV are meant to serve as guidelines to be informed by clinical judgment and are not meant to be used in a cookbook fashion. For example, the exercise of clinical judgment may justify giving a certain diagnosis to an individual even though the clinical presentation falls just short of meeting the full criteria for the diagnosis as long as the symptoms that are present are persistent and severe. On the other hand, lack of familiarity with DSM-IV or excessively flexible and idiosyncratic application of DSM-IV criteria or conventions substantially reduces its utility as a common language for communication.
>
> USE OF DSM-IV IN FORENSIC SETTINGS When the DSM-IV categories, criteria, and textual descriptions are employed for forensic purposes, there are significant risks that diagnostic information will be misused or misunderstood. These dangers arise because of the imperfect fit between the questions of ultimate concern to the law and the information contained in a clinical diagnosis. In most situations, the clinical diagnosis of a DSM-IV mental disorder is not sufficient to establish the existence for legal purposes of a "mental disorder," "mental disability," "mental disease," or "mental defect." In determining whether an individual meets a specified legal standard (e.g., for competence, criminal responsibility, or disability), additional information is usually required beyond that contained in the DSM-IV diagnosis. This might include information about the individual's functional impairments and how these impairments affect the particular abilities in question. It is precisely because impairments, abilities, and disabilities vary widely within each diagnostic category that assignment of a particular diagnosis does not imply a specific level of impairment or disability.
>
> Nonclinical decision makers should also be cautioned that a diagnosis does not carry any necessary implications regarding the causes of the individual's mental disorder or its associated impairments. Inclusion of a disorder in the Classification (as in medicine generally) does not require that there be knowledge about its etiology. Moreover, the fact that an individual's presentation meets the criteria for a DSM-IV diagnosis does not carry any necessary implication regarding the individual's degree of control over the behaviors that may be associated with the disorder. Even when diminished control over one's behavior is a feature of the disorder, having the diagnosis in itself does not demonstrate that a particular individual is (or was) unable to control his or her behavior at a particular time.
>
> It must be noted that DSM-IV reflects a consensus about the classification and diagnosis of mental disorders derived at the time of its initial publication. New knowledge generated by research or clinical experience will undoubtedly lead to an increased understanding of the disorders included in DSM-IV, to the identification of new disorders, and to the removal of some disorders in future classifications. The text and criteria sets included in DSM-IV will require reconsideration in light of evolving new information.
>
> The use of DSM-IV in forensic settings should be informed by an awareness of the risks discussed above. When used appropriately, diagnoses and diagnostic information can assist decision makers in their determinations. For example, when the presence of a mental disorder is the predicate for a subsequent legal determination (e.g., involuntary civil commitment), the use of an established system of diagnosis enhances the value and reliability of the determination. By providing a compendium based upon a review of the pertinent clinical and research literature, DSM-IV may facilitate the legal decision-makers' understanding of the relevant characteristics of mental disorders. The literature related to diagnoses also serves as a check on ungrounded speculation about mental disorders and about the functioning of a particular individual. Finally, diagnostic information regarding longitudinal course may improve decision-making when the legal issue concerns an individual's mental functioning at a past or future point in time.

DECISION TREES Decision trees, also known as algorithms, are diagrammatic tracks that organize the clinician's thinking so that all differential diagnoses are considered and ruled in or out, resulting in a presumptive diagnosis. Beginning with specific signs or symptoms, the psychiatrist follows the positive or negative track down the tree (by answering "yes" or "no") until a point in the tree with no outgoing branches (known as a leaf) is found. That point is the final diagnosis. Figure 11.1-1 is an example of a decision tree for psychotic disorders. DSM-IV includes an appendix of diagnostic decision trees.

PSYCHIATRIC RATING SCALES USED IN DSM-IV

Psychiatric rating scales, also called rating instruments, provide a way to quantify aspects of a patient's psyche, behavior, and relationships with individuals and society. The measurement of pathology in those areas of a person's life may initially seem to be much less straightforward than the measurement of pathology—hypertension, for example—seen by other medical specialists. Nevertheless, many psychiatric rating scales are able to measure carefully chosen features of well-formulated concepts. Psychiatric rating scales are discussed extensively in Section 9.8.

Rating scales can be specific or comprehensive, and they can measure both internally experienced variables (for example, mood) and externally observable variables (for example, behavior). Specific scales measure discrete thoughts, moods, or behaviors, such as obsessive thoughts and temper tantrums; comprehensive scales measure broad abstractions, such as depression and anxiety.

Rating scales form an integral part of DSM-IV. The rating scales used are broad and measure the overall severity of the patient's illness.

GAF SCALE Axis V in DSM-IV uses the Global Assessment of Functioning (GAF) scale (Table 11.1-7). That axis is used for reporting the clinician's judgment of the patient's overall level of functioning. The information is used to decide on a treatment plan and later to measure the plan's effect.

SOCIAL AND OCCUPATIONAL FUNCTIONING ASSESSMENT SCALE (SOFAS) This scale can be used to track the patient's progress in social and occupational areas. It is independent of the psychiatric diagnosis and of the severity of the patient's psychological symptoms. It is described in DSM-IV as follows:

> The SOFAS is a new scale that differs from the Global Assessment of Functioning (GAF) scale in that it focuses exclusively on the individual's level of social and occupational functioning and is not directly influenced by the overall severity of the individual's psychological symptoms. Also in contrast to the GAF Scale, any impairment in social and occupational functioning that is due to general medical conditions is considered in making the SOFAS rating. The SOFAS is usually used to rate functioning for the current period (i.e., the level of functioning at the time of the evaluation). The SOFAS may also be used to rate functioning for other time periods. For example, for some purposes it may be useful to evaluate functioning for the past year (i.e., the highest level of functioning for at least a few months during the past year).

The SOFAS appears in Table 11.1-12.

TABLE 11.1-12
Social and Occupational Functioning Assessment Scale (SOFAS)*

Consider social and occupational functioning on a continuum from excellent functioning to grossly impaired functioning. Include impairments in functioning due to physical limitations, as well as those due to mental impairments. To be counted, impairment must be a direct consequence of mental and physical health problems; the effects of lack of opportunity and other environmental limitations are not to be considered.

Code	(Note: Use intermediate codes when appropriate, e.g., 45, 68, 72.)
100–91	Superior functioning in a wide range of activities.
90–81	Good functioning in all areas, occupationally and socially effective.
80–71	No more than a slight impairment in social, occupational, or school functioning (e.g., infrequent interpersonal conflict, temporarily falling behind in schoolwork).
70–61	Some difficulty in social, occupational, or school functioning, but generally functioning well, has some meaningful interpersonal relationships.
60–51	Moderate difficulty in social, occupational, or school functioning (e.g., few friends, conflicts with peers or coworkers).
50–41	Serious impairment in social, occupational, or school functioning (e.g., no friends, unable to keep a job).
40–31	Major impairment in several areas, such as work or school, family relations (e.g., depressed man avoids friends, neglects family, and is unable to work; child frequently beats up younger children, is defiant at home, and is failing at school).
30–21	Inability to function in almost all areas (e.g., stays in bed all day; no job, home, or friends).
20–11	Occasionally fails to maintain minimal personal hygiene; unable to function independently.
10–1	Persistent inability to maintain minimal personal hygiene. Unable to function without harming self or others or without considerable external support (e.g., nursing care and supervision).
0	Inadequate information.

*The rating of overall psychological functioning on a scale of 0–100 was operationalized by Luborsky in the Health-Sickness Rating Scale. (Luborsky L: Clinicians' judgments of mental health. Arch Gen Psychiatry 407, *7:* 1962). Spitzer and colleagues developed a revision of the Health-Sickness Rating Scale called the Global Assessment Scale (GAS) (Endicott J, Spitzer RL, Fleiss JL, et al: The Global Assessment Scale: A procedure for measuring overall severity of psychiatric disturbance. Arch Gen Psychiatry *33:* 766, 1976). The SOFAS is derived from the GAS and its development is described in Goldman HH, Skodol AE, Lave TR: Revising Axis V for DSM-IV: A review of measures of social functioning. Am J Psychiatry *149:* 1148, 1992.

Table from DSM-IV, *Diagnostic and Statistical Manual of Mental Disorders,* ed 4. Copyright American Psychiatric Association, Washington, 1994. Used with permission.

GLOBAL ASSESSMENT OF RELATIONAL FUNCTIONING (GARF) This scale is listed in DSM-IV to track the relations between persons using such terms as satisfactory, unsatisfactory, dysfunctional, contact, and attachment, among others. An explanation of how to use the scale is provided in DSM-IV (Table 11.1-13).

DEFENSIVE FUNCTIONING SCALE This scale lists commonly accepted defense mechanisms (also referred to as coping styles in DSM-IV) that are used to protect a person from anxiety. The major defenses are listed in alphabetical order (Table 11.1-14). A glossary of specific defense mechanisms is provided in DSM-IV (Table 11.1-15). The manual also attempts to describe the individual defense mechanisms in a classificatory table (Table 11.1-16).

FIGURE 11.1-1 *Differential diagnosis of psychotic disorders. (Figure from DSM-IV,* Diagnostic and Statistical Manual of Mental Disorders, *ed 4. Copyright American Psychiatric Association, Washington, 1994. Used with permission.)*

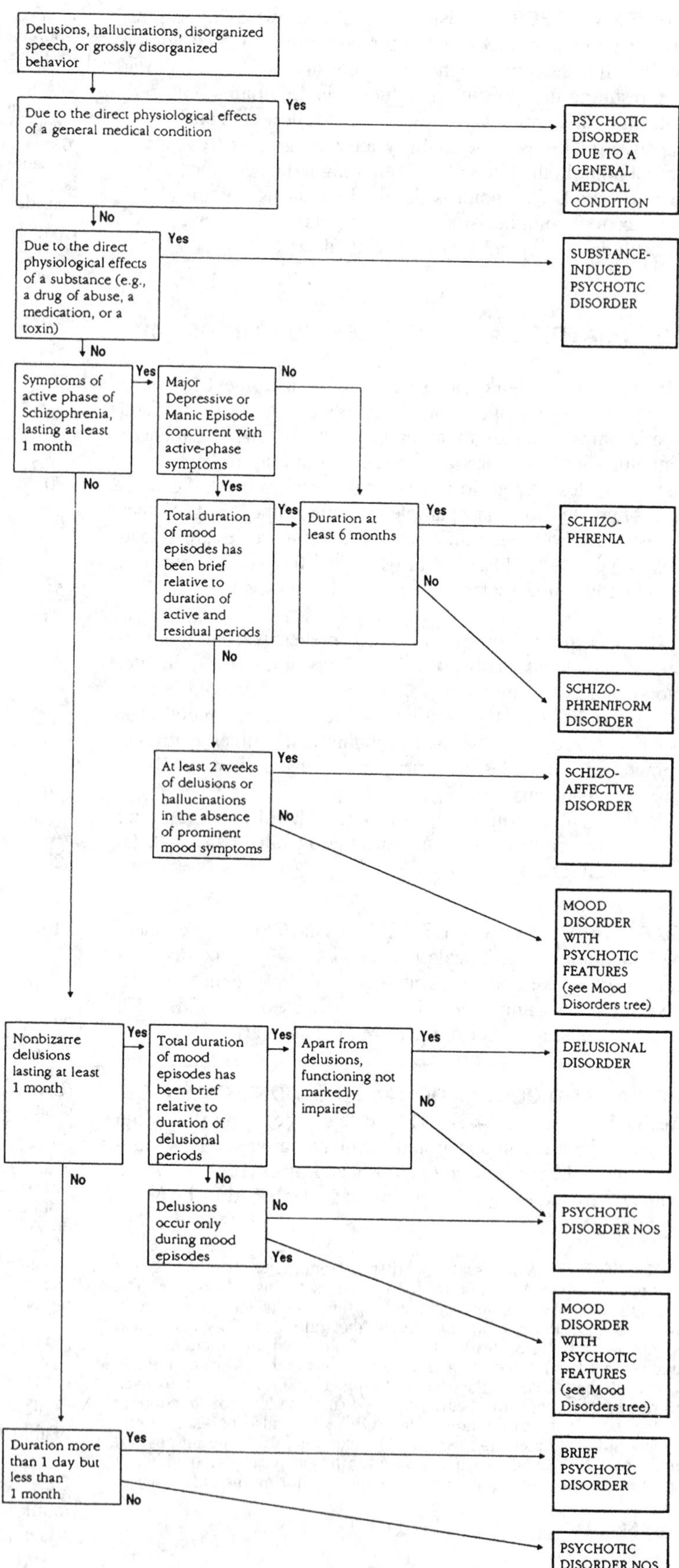

TABLE 11.1-13
Global Assessment of Relational Functioning (GARF) Scale

Instructions: The GARF scale can be used to indicate an overall judgment of the functioning of a family or other ongoing relationship on a hypothetical continuum ranging from competent, optimal relational functioning to a disrupted, dysfunctional relationship. It is analogous to Axis V (Global Assessment of Functioning scale) provided for individuals in DSM-IV. The GARF scale permits the clinician to rate the degree to which a family or other ongoing relational unit meets the affective or instrumental needs of its members in the following areas:

A. Problem solving—skills in negotiating goals, rules, and routines; adaptability to stress; communication skills; ability to resolve conflict
B. Organization—maintenance of interpersonal roles and subsystem boundaries; hierarchical functioning; coalitions and distribution of power, control, and responsibility
C. Emotional climate—tone and range of feelings; quality of caring, empathy, involvement, and attachment/commitment; sharing of values; mutual affective responsiveness, respect, and regard; quality of sexual functioning

In most instances, the GARF scale should be used to rate functioning during the current period (i.e., the level of relational functioning at the time of the evaluation). In some settings, the GARF scale may also be used to rate functioning for other time periods (i.e., the highest level of relational functioning for at least a few months during the past year).

Note: Use specific, intermediate codes when possible, for example, 45, 68, 72. If detailed information is not adequate to make specific ratings, use midpoints of the five ranges, that is, 90, 70, 50, 30, or 10.

81–100 Overall: Relational unit is functioning satisfactorily from self-report of participants and from perspectives of observers.

Agreed-on patterns or routines exist that help meet the usual needs of each family/couple member; there is flexibility for change in response to unusual demands or events; and occasional conflicts and stressful transitions are resolved through problem-solving communication and negotiation.

There is a shared understanding and agreement about roles and appropriate tasks, decision making is established for each functional area, and there is recognition of the unique characteristics and merit of each subsystem (e.g., parents-spouses, siblings, and individuals).

There is a situationally appropriate, optimistic atmosphere in the family; a wide range of feelings is freely expressed and managed within the family; and there is a general atmosphere of warmth, caring, and sharing of values among all family members. Sexual relations of adult members are satisfactory.

61–80 Overall: Functioning of relational unit is somewhat unsatisfactory. Over a period of time, many but not all difficulties are resolved without complaints.

Daily routines are present but there is some pain and difficulty in responding to the unusual. Some conflicts remain unresolved, but do not disrupt family functioning.

Decision making is usually competent, but efforts at control of one another quite often are greater than necessary or are ineffective. Individuals and relationships are clearly demarcated but sometimes a specific subsystem is depreciated or scapegoated.

A range of feeling is expressed, but instances of emotional blocking or tension are evident. Warmth and caring are present but are marred by a family member's irritability and frustrations. Sexual activity of adult members may be reduced or problematic.

41–60 Overall: Relational unit has occasional times of satisfying and competent functioning together, but clearly dysfunctional, unsatisfying relationships tend to predominate.

Communication is frequently inhibited by unresolved conflicts that often interfere with daily routines; there is significant difficulty in adapting to family stress and transitional change.

Decision making is only intermittently competent and effective; either excessive rigidity or significant lack of structure is evident at these times. Individual needs are quite often submerged by a partner or coalition.

Pain or ineffective anger or emotional deadness interfere with family enjoyment. Although there is some warmth and support for members, it is usually unequally distributed. Troublesome sexual difficulties between adults are often present.

21–40 Overall: Relational unit is obviously and seriously dysfunctional; forms and time periods of satisfactory relating are rare.

Family/couple routines do not meet the needs of members; they are grimly adhered to or blithely ignored. Life cycle changes, such as departures or entries into the relational unit, generate painful conflict and obviously frustrating failures of problem solving.

Decision making is tyrannical or quite ineffective. The unique characteristics of individuals are unappreciated or ignored by either rigid or confusingly fluid coalitions.

There are infrequent periods of enjoyment of life together; frequent distancing or open hostility reflect significant conflicts that remain unresolved and quite painful. Sexual dysfunction among adult members is commonplace.

1–20 Overall: Relational unit has become too dysfunctional to retain continuity of contact and attachment.

Family/couple routines are negligible (e.g., no mealtime, sleeping, or waking schedule); family members often do not know where others are or when they will be in or out; there is a little effective communication among family members.

Family/couple members are not organized in such a way that personal or generational responsibilities are recognized. Boundaries of relational unit as a whole and subsystems cannot be identified or agreed on. Family members are physically endangered or injured or sexually attacked.

Despair and cynicism are pervasive; there is little attention to the emotional needs of others; there is almost no sense of attachment, commitment, or concern about one another's welfare.

0 Inadequate information.

Table from DSM-IV, *Diagnostic and Statistical Manual of Mental Disorders,* ed 4. Copyright American Psychiatric Association, Washington, 1994. Used with permission.

TABLE 11.1-14
Recording Form: Defensive Functioning Scale

A. **Current defenses or coping styles:** List in order, beginning with most prominent defenses or coping styles.
1. ______
2. ______
3. ______
4. ______
5. ______
6. ______
7. ______

B. **Predominant current defense level:** ______

Table from DSM-IV, *Diagnostic and Statistical Manual of Mental Disorders,* ed 4. Copyright American Psychiatric Association, Washington, 1994. Used with permission.

CRITIQUE OF DSM-IV

DSM-IV has laudable goals, as do all the DSMs that have made the 1980s and 1990s a nosological revolution. They have modernized a diagnostic system and updated and integrated the many advances in psychiatry and psychopharmacology as they relate to nomenclature. Toward that end they have been successful; however, certain criticisms of DSM-IV have been made by psychiatrists in the United States and abroad.

In 1988 the American Psychiatric Association announced its decision to revise DSM-III-R, which had been published the previous year; initially, DSM-IV was scheduled to appear in 1992, but publication was delayed until 1994. Many believed its publication was premature. They believed there would be insufficient time to accumulate a sufficient number of research projects to provide an adequate data base on which to develop DSM-IV. Objections were raised by psychiatric residents who complained that they entered residency training learning one set

TABLE 11.1-15
Glossary of Specific Defense Mechanisms and Coping Styles

acting out The individual deals with emotional conflict or internal or external stressors by actions rather than reflections or feelings. This definition is broader than the original concept of the acting out of transference feelings or wishes during psychotherapy and is intended to include behavior arising both within and outside the transference relationship. Defensive acting out is not synonymous with "bad behavior" because it requires evidence that the behavior is related to emotional conflicts.

affiliation The individual deals with emotional conflict or internal or external stressors by turning to others for help or support. This involves sharing problems with others but does not imply trying to make someone else responsible for them.

altruism The individual deals with emotional conflict or internal or external stressors by dedication to meeting the needs of others. Unlike the self-sacrifice sometimes characteristic of reaction formation, the individual receives gratification either vicariously or from the response of others.

anticipation The individual deals with emotional conflict or internal or external stressors by experiencing emotional reactions in advance of, or anticipating consequences of, possible future events and considering realistic, alternative responses or solutions.

autistic fantasy The individual deals with emotional conflict or internal or external stressors by excessive daydreaming as a substitute for human relationships, more effective action, or problem solving.

denial The individual deals with emotional conflict or internal or external stressors by refusing to acknowledge some painful aspect of external reality or subjective experience that would be apparent to others. The term "psychotic denial" is used when there is gross impairment in reality testing.

devaluation The individual deals with emotional conflict or internal or external stressors by attributing exaggerated negative qualities to self or others.

displacement The individual deals with emotional conflict or internal or external stressors by transferring a feeling about, or a response to, one object onto another (usually less threatening) substitute object.

dissociation The individual deals with emotional conflict or internal or external stressors with a breakdown in the usually integrated functions of consciousness, memory, perception of self or the environment, or sensory-motor behavior.

help-rejecting complaining The individual deals with emotional conflict or internal or external stressors by complaining or making repetitious requests for help that disguise covert feelings of hostility or reproach toward others, which are then expressed by rejecting the suggestions, advice, or help that others offer. The complaints or requests may involve physical or psychological symptoms or life problems.

humor The individual deals with emotional conflict or external stressors by emphasizing the amusing or ironic aspects of the conflict or stressor.

idealization The individual deals with emotional conflict or internal or external stressors by attributing exaggerated positive qualities to others.

intellectualization The individual deals with emotional conflict or internal or external stressors by the excessive use of abstract thinking or the making of generalizations to control or minimize disturbing feelings.

isolation of affect The individual deals with emotional conflict or internal or external stressors by the separation of ideas from the feelings originally associated with them. The individual loses touch with the feelings associated with a given idea (e.g., a traumatic event) while remaining aware of the cognitive elements of it (e.g., descriptive details).

omnipotence The individual deals with emotional conflict or internal or external stressors by feeling or acting as if he or she possesses special powers or abilities and is superior to others.

passive aggression The individual deals with emotional conflict or internal or external stressors by indirectly and unassertively expressing aggression toward others. There is a facade of overt compliance masking covert resistance, resentment, or hostility. Passive aggression often occurs in response to demands for independent action or performance or the lack of gratification of dependent wishes but may be adaptive for individuals in subordinate positions who have no other way to express assertiveness more overtly.

projection The individual deals with emotional conflict or internal or external stressors by falsely attributing to another his or her own unacceptable feelings, impulses, or thoughts.

projective identification As in projection, the individual deals with emotional conflict or internal or external stressors by falsely attributing to another his or her own unacceptable feelings, impulses, or thoughts. Unlike simple projection, the individual does not fully disavow what is projected. Instead, the individual remains aware of his or her own affects or impulses but misattributes them as justifiable reactions to the other person. Not infrequently, the individual induces the very feelings in others that were first mistakenly believed to be there, making it difficult to clarify who did what to whom first.

rationalization The individual deals with emotional conflict or internal or external stressors by concealing the true motivations for his or her own thoughts, actions, or feelings through the elaboration of reassuring or self-serving but incorrect explanations.

reaction formation The individual deals with emotional conflict or internal or external stressors by substituting behavior, thoughts, or feelings that are diametrically opposed to his or her own unacceptable thoughts or feelings (this usually occurs in conjunction with their repression).

repression The individual deals with emotional conflict or internal or external stressors by expelling disturbing wishes, thoughts, or experiences from conscious awareness. The feeling component may remain conscious, detached from its associated ideas.

self-assertion The individual deals with emotional conflict or stressors by expressing his or her feelings and thoughts directly in a way that is not coercive or manipulative.

self-observation The individual deals with emotional conflict or stressors by reflecting on his or her own thoughts, feelings, motivation, and behavior, and responding appropriately.

splitting The individual deals with emotional conflict or internal or external stressors by compartmentalizing opposite affect states and failing to integrate the positive and negative qualities of the self or others into cohesive images. Because ambivalent affects cannot be experienced simultaneously, more balanced views and expectations of self or others are excluded from emotional awareness. Self and object images tend to alternate between polar opposites: exclusively loving, powerful, worthy, nurturant, and kind—or exclusively bad, hateful, angry, destructive, rejecting, or worthless.

sublimation The individual deals with emotional conflict or internal or external stressors by channeling potentially maladaptive feelings or impulses into socially acceptable behavior (e.g., contact sports to channel angry impulses).

suppression The individual deals with emotional conflict or internal or external stressors by intentionally avoiding thinking about disturbing problems, wishes, feelings, or experiences.

undoing The individual deals with emotional conflict or internal or external stressors by words or behavior designed to negate or to make amends symbolically for unacceptable thoughts, feelings, or actions.

Table from DSM-IV, *Diagnostic and Statistical Manual of Mental Disorders,* ed 4. Copyright American Psychiatric Association, Washington, 1994. Used with permission.

of criteria and finished just in time to learn another. Clinicians were resistant to changes in the criteria in which they were trained. Patients reported that they would be confused when their diagnoses were changed because of a different diagnostic system being used. As early as 1988 Mark Zimmerman suggested in *Archives of General Psychiatry* that the publication of DSM-IV should be delayed, and he questioned whether the changes in DSM-IV would improve the practice of psychiatry in a substantial way. He wrote:

> Resistance to adopting a new official nomenclature is understandable if a new DSM is to be published every half dozen years or so. It is ironic that one of the original primary goals of the movement to operationalize psychiatric diagnostic concepts i.e., to facilitate communication among clinicians and researchers has been, in part, undermined by the proliferation of criteria sets.

TABLE 11.1-16
Defense Levels and Individual Defense Mechanisms

High adaptive level This level of defensive functioning results in optimal adaptation in the handling of stressors. These defenses usually maximize gratification and allow the conscious awareness of feelings, ideas, and their consequences. They also promote an optimum balance among conflicting motives. Examples of defenses at this level are
- anticipation
- affiliation
- altruism
- humor
- self-assertion
- self-observation
- sublimation
- suppression

Mental inhibitions (compromise formation) level Defensive functioning at this level keeps potentially threatening ideas, feelings, memories, wishes, or fears out of awareness. Examples are
- displacement
- dissociation
- intellectualization
- isolation of affect
- reaction formation
- repression
- undoing

Minor image-distorting level This level is characterized by distortions in the image of the self, body, or others that may be employed to regulate self-esteem. Examples are
- devaluation
- idealization
- omnipotence

Disavowal level This level is characterized by keeping unpleasant or unacceptable stressors, impulses, ideas, affects, or responsibility out of awareness with or without a misattribution of these to external causes. Examples are
- denial
- projection
- rationalization

Major image-distorting level This level is characterized by gross distortion or misattribution of the image of self or others. Examples are
- autistic fantasy
- projective identification
- splitting of self-image or image of others

Action level This level is characterized by defensive functioning that deals with internal or external stressors by action or withdrawal. Examples are
- acting out
- apathetic withdrawal
- help-rejecting complaining
- passive aggression

Level of defensive dysregulation This level is characterized by failure of defensive regulation to contain the individual's reaction to stressors, leading to a pronounced break with objective reality. Examples are
- delusional projection
- psychotic denial
- psychotic distortion

Table from DSM-IV, *Diagnostic and Statistical Manual of Mental Disorders,* ed 4. Copyright American Psychiatric Association, Washington, 1994. Used with permission.

DSM-IV was eventually published in May 1994, two years behind schedule.

The criticism of a lack of replicated research data on which to base DSM-IV was addressed in the Introduction to the manual, which states that the Task Force on DSM-IV conducted a three stage-empirical process prior to publication. The stages were:

1. Literature reviews, conducted to provide comprehensive and unbiased information on which to base DSM-IV diagnostic criteria. DSM-IV notes, however, that for some issues insufficient data were available, and in those cases existing data were reanalyzed.

2. Data reanalysis that consisted of "analyses of relevant unpublished data sets" of criteria included in DSM-III-R. According to the DSM-IV Task Force, that approach made it possible for work groups to "question several criteria sets that were then tested in the DSM-IV field trials."

3. Field trials that compared DSM-III, DSM-III-R, and ICD-10 and proposed DSM-IV criteria sets. The field trials collected information on the reliability and performance characteristics of each criteria set as a whole and on specific items within each criteria set. Twelve field trials were conducted at more than 70 sites, evaluating more than 6,000 subjects. Whether that number is a large enough data base on which to base a revision is open to question. Some psychiatrists believe that insufficient time has elapsed between revisions of DSM to allow replicated research on which to base DSM-IV.

RELATION TO ICD-10 DSM-IV was published under the auspices of the American Psychiatric Association with the mandate that it be coordinated with the development of ICD-10, a publication of the World Health Organization. Each diagnosis in DSM-IV was to have a corresponding diagnosis in ICD-10. However, the language used to describe each disorder often differs significantly in the two publications. For example, neurasthenia appears in ICD-10 but is not found in DSM-IV.

DSM-IV has been criticized for including too much detail in comparison with ICD-10 and for being oriented toward researchers, not clinicians. ICD-10 presents guidelines for making diagnoses and avoids the rigid research-oriented criteria that made previous editions of DSM difficult to use in everyday psychiatric practice. ICD-10 recognizes the skills of well-trained psychiatrists to fully utilize clinical material when arriving at a diagnosis. It is considerably more user-friendly than DSM-IV.

REFERENDUM In May 1994 the American Psychiatric Association placed a referendum on its general ballot to determine the views of its membership on postponing publication of DSM-IV until 1997 and adopting instead ICD-10 as the official nomenclature of American psychiatry. In support of that position a group of psychiatrists distributed a position statement in which they claimed that (1) physicians and insurance companies use the ICD-10 classification; (2) the United States has a treaty obligation to adopt the diagnostic system used throughout the rest of the world—that is, ICD-10 (DSM-IV attempts to overcome this objection by attaching ICD-10 code numbers to the DSM-IV diagnoses); and (3) there has been an insufficient amount of time between the frequent revisions of DSM to allow for replicated research upon which to base DSM-IV. See Figure 11.1-2 for the position statement supporting the referendum. The referendum was defeated by the membership of the American Psychiatric Association; however, the fact that it was on the ballot indicated the apparent dissatisfaction that many psychiatrists have about DSM and its frequent revisions.

Some criticisms of DSM-IV are leveled at the way DSM-IV was developed. In particular, the American Psychological Association and other organizations comprised of nonpsychiatric mental health professionals, such as social workers and psychiatric nurses, have had little, if any, input into the final product. Nevertheless, those professional groups are required by law to adhere to the manual.

Robert Spitzer, M.D., special adviser to the DSM-IV Task Force, is among those critical of the process involved in the preparation of DSM-IV. In an interview with Dr. Spitzer in

DSM-IV or *ICD-10*

To qualify as folly for this purpose, the policy adopted must meet three criteria: It must have been perceived as counter-productive in its own time, not merely by hindsight. . . . Secondly a feasibly alternative course of action must have been available. To remove the problem from personality, a third criterion must be that the policy in question should be that of a group, not an individual. . . .

Barbara W. Tuchman, *The March of Folly* (1984)

In a few days you will receive this year's APA ballot. In addition to being asked to vote for officers of the APA you will have an opportunity to vote for or against the proposed DSM-IV. The choice of a diagnostic system to be used by psychiatrists throughout the United States is too important a matter to be decided by an APA committee, dominated by researchers. Through a petition drive, we have required the APA to hold a referendum of the total membership to decide which diagnostic system will become the official one in this country. The choice is between the hastily prepared DSM-IV, and the system that will be used throughout the rest of the world, the International Classification of Diseases, Tenth Edition, ICD-10.

ICD-10 was prepared for clinicians not researchers. It presents guidelines for making diagnoses and avoids the rigid research oriented criteria that have made DSM-III-R, so difficult to use in everyday clinical practice.

ICD-10 does not insult the intelligence of clinicians. It recognizes your skills, as a well trained psychiatrist, to fully utilize clinical material when arriving at a diagnosis. To show you the difference between DSM-IV's proposed criteria, and the guidelines of ICD-10, here are excerpts showing how the two systems present the Post Concussion Syndrome:

DSM-IV

A A history of head trauma that includes at least two of the following:
1. Loss of consciousness for at least 5 minutes.
2. Posttraumatic amnesia for at least 12 hours.
3. Onset of seizures within 6 months.

B Difficulties in concentration and in learning or memory, and at least three of the following:
1. Easy fatiguability.
2. Insomnia.
3. Headache.
4. Vertigo or dizziness.
5. Irritability or aggression upon little or no provocation. . . .

ICD-10

The syndrome occurs following head trauma (usually sufficiently severe to result in loss of consciousness and includes a number of disparate symptoms such as headache, dizziness (usually lacking the features of true vertigo), fatigue, irritability, difficulty in concentrating and performing mental tasks, impairment of memory, insomnia, and reduced tolerance to stress, emotional excitement, or alcohol. . . .

You now see why we believe that ICD-10 and its patient oriented guidelines are more appropriate in clinical work than DSM-IV with its inflexible criteria. The choice of internationally adopted guidelines over arbitrary research criteria, is in the best interests of both patients and psychiatrists. Your style of thinking about patients is probably much more similar to the one demonstrated in ICD-10 than that found in the proposed DSM-IV.

In addition to the problem with the criteria for the various disorders, there are many other reasons why DSM-IV should be rejected and ICD-10 be adopted. Among those reasons are:

- Psychiatrists throughout the world, and non-psychiatric physicians in the United States presently use the International Classification of diseases (ICD-9-CM) to diagnose psychiatric disorders. In 1993, they will adopt ICD-10;
- MEDICARE and most insurance companies will soon require that all diagnoses be recorded using ICD-10.
- There has been an insufficient amount of time between revisions of the DSM to allow for replicated research upon which to base DSM-IV;
- The need to validate DSM-IV will reduce resources available to study the pathophysiology and treatment of psychiatric disorders;
- With psychiatrists throughout the world with the exception of the United States using ICD-10, international cooperation in research will be seriously hampered;
- The United States has a treaty obligation to adopt a diagnostic system that is congruent with the system used throughout the rest of the world. The American Psychiatric Association can best discharge that obligation by adopting ICD-10 as the official diagnostic system for this country. Some consider the APA's plan to revise DSM-III-R as DSM-IV and to attach ICD-10 code numbers to the various diagnoses as verging on fraud;
- If the APA believes that DSM-IV should be published to explain or elaborate upon ICD-10, publication should be postponed until 1997. By that time the strengths and weaknesses of ICD-10 will be clear.

When your APA ballot arrives in a few days, be sure to vote for the immediate adoption of ICD-10 and the postponement of DSM-IV until 1997.

FIGURE 11.1-2 *Position paper supporting the use of ICD-10. (Figure courtesy of Ivan Goldberg, M.D. Used with permission.)*

Clinical Psychiatry News (May 1994), the following was reported:

> While Dr. Spitzer is pleased in many ways with the new manual, he believes that the greater autonomy granted individual work groups in some cases produced serious flaws. In the DSM-III and DSM-III-R process, the task force chairman actually chaired each work group, "so there was much more centralized control," said Dr. Spitzer, who chaired the task forces that wrote DSM-III and -III-R. "Some DSM-IV chairpeople were chosen because of distinguished careers in research, but this didn't mean they were very good at nosology. Unfortunately, some were not." As a result, there are now several diagnostic categories "that can't be supported with data."

TERMINOLOGY DSM-IV has omitted certain terms even though they are retained in ICD-10.

DSM-IV eliminated the diagnosis of organic mental disorder in an attempt to indicate that all mental disorders may have a biological basis or medical etiology. The diagnosis of organic mental disorder (OMD) is now called delirium, dementia, amnestic and other cognitive disorders in DSM-IV. ICD-10, however, retains the diagnostic category of organic mental disorders.

Neurasthenia is omitted from DSM-IV but is retained in ICD-10. Although a significant number of patients diagnosed with neurasthenia can also be classified with a depressive or anxiety disorder, there are many cases that cannot, and ICD-10 reflects that fact.

DSM-IV added the diagnosis of bipolar II disorder to refer to bipolar disorder with hypomanic episodes. The need for the terms "bipolar I" and "bipolar II" to replace the terms "bipolar disorder, current episode depression/manic" and "bipolar disorder, current episode hypomanic," respectively, is questionable because the latter terms are commonly used in the United States and are appropriately descriptive. Bipolar I and bipolar II are research terms with which most clinicians are not familiar. Those terms are not used in ICD-10.

DSM-IV eschews the term "psychogenic." Nevertheless, it still appears in ICD-10 to refer to the fact that life events or difficulties play an important role in the genesis of many psychiatric disorders. Similarly, DSM-IV has eliminated the term "neurosis," which is used in ICD-10. The authors regard both as useful terms that should be retained.

PROPRIETARY RIGHTS AND PERMISSIONS An interesting footnote in DSM-IV is the following statement: "DSM and DSM-IV are trademarks of the American Psychiatric Association. Use of these terms is prohibited without permission of the American Psychiatric Association." What this statement means is not clear. A different—and less ambiguous—approach is taken by ICD-10, which states the following:

> The World Health Organization welcomes requests for permission to reproduce or translate its publications, in part or in full. Applications and enquiries should be addressed to the Office of Publications, World Health Organization, Geneva, Switzerland, which will be glad to provide the latest information on any changes made to the text, plans for new editions, and reprints and translations already available.

STATISTICAL MANUAL OR TEXTBOOK? The DSMs have been published since 1952. They are designed to provide a system whereby psychiatric illnesses can be classified into appropriate nosological categories. As knowledge has increased, the DSM nomenclature has expanded. In addition to setting forth the criteria on which a diagnosis was to be based, DSM has added other information, such as epidemiology and differential diagnosis. Because major categories that are present in textbooks are missing from DSM, it is not and has never claimed to be a textbook; nevertheless, it is used as a text by some groups, including insurance companies, that believe it to be a comprehensive source about mental illness. DSM is authorized, but in the authors' view it is not authoritative.

TO REVISE OR NOT TO REVISE Karl Menninger in his book *The Vital Balance* described the many pitfalls, fallacies, and sources of error implicit in what he called the "irrepressible work of classification" and "the urge to classify." Among those were changes in names of mental illnesses and the fact that classification existed more for statistical purposes than for enhancing knowledge of symptoms, diagnoses, and treatment. He suggested that defining new syndromes and reordering them was "a veritable addiction of psychiatrists." In addition, the grouping of signs and symptoms may be influenced by social traditions, prevalent customs or philosophies, and unconscious determinants, such as the classifier's view of the world. Over 30 years ago, Menninger anticipated the structure of the mathematical device currently in use in DSM-IV. He wrote: "If the patient has, let us say, five symptoms, one can look up each of these symptoms and find which disease is so characterized under all five headings. Then, *voila!* the diagnosis!" Menninger suggested that the trend toward tabulating disease states was antithetical to understanding the person experiencing the illness and resulted in a deemphasis on the compassionate approach toward the patient that is the hallmark of psychiatry. That mathematical approach is reflected in the algorithms and decision trees used in DSM-IV and in the various computer programs that record signs and symptoms to provide a diagnosis.

Nosology and psychiatric classification are in a state of flux, and group consensus influences the process. The authors support Zimmerman's view that revisions to DSM should follow a "restrained, sober and deliberate pace." In their book, *The Selling of DSM,* Stuart Kirk and Herb Kutchins supported that position. They stated:

> First, none of the revisions are stimulated by clinical practitioners demanding a new classification system. Second, the writing of each revision has become more time consuming, elaborate, and politically complex. Third, the numerous changes made with each revision are justified explicitly or implicitly as improving the scientific credibility of the classification system, although the scientific basis for them is often questionable. Finally, the process of revision inevitably begins by attacking the current system, even when it has only recently been adopted, and ends by claiming the superiority of the new one.

With others, the authors believe that the publication of the various editions of DSM has been one of the most important developments in psychiatry in the past 50 years. The *Comprehensive Textbook of Psychiatry* has always relied on DSM as the template for deriving the table of contents and for organizing psychopathology. At the same time, the editors have encouraged contributors to the textbook to provide critiques of DSM and to suggest changes as they see fit. The reader will find many of those critiques throughout the book.

SUGGESTED CROSS-REFERENCES

The psychiatric report is discussed in Section 9.2, typical signs and symptoms in Section 9.3, neuropsychological assessment in Sections 9.5 and 9.6, clinical manifestations of psychiatric disorders in Chapter 10, and international perspectives on psychiatric diagnosis in Section 11.2.

REFERENCES

*American Psychiatric Association: *Diagnostic and Statistical Manual of Mental Disorders,* ed 4. American Psychiatric Association, Washington, 1994.

Berrios G E, Hauser R: The early development of Kraepelin's ideas on classification: A conceptual history. Psychol Med *18:* 813, 1988.
Bryant K J, Rounsaville B, Spitzer R L, Williams J B: Reliability of dual diagnosis: Substance dependence and psychiatric disorders. J Nerv Ment Dis *180:* 251, 1992.
*Frances A: An introduction to DSM-IV. Hosp Community Psychiatry *41:* 49, 1990.
Fyer A J, Mannuzza S, Endicott J: Differential diagnosis and assessment of anxiety: Recent developments. In *Psychopharmacology: The Third Generation of Progress,* H Y Meltzer, editor, p 326. Raven, New York, 1987.
Hughes J R, O'Hara M W, Rehm L P: Measurement of depression in clinical trials: An overview. J Clin Psychiatry *43:* 85, 1982.
Kendell R E: *The Role of Diagnosis in Psychiatry.* Blackwell, Oxford, 1975.
*Kirk S A, Kutchins H: *The Selling of DSM.* Aldine de Gruyter, New York, 1992.
Levine J, Ban T A: Assessment methods in clinical trials. In *Psychopharmacology: The Third Generation of Progress,* H Y Meltzer, editor, p 118. Raven, New York, 1987.
Menninger K: *The Vital Balance.* Viking, New York, 1963.
Mezzich J E: International experience with DSM-III. J Nerv Ment Dis *173:* 12, 1985.
Raskin A, Jarvik L S: *Psychiatric Symptoms and Cognitive Loss in the Elderly.* Wiley, New York, 1979.
*Strauss J S: A comprehensive approach to psychiatric diagnosis. Am J Psychiatry *132:* 1193, 1975.
Wilson M: DSM-III and the transformation of American psychiatry: A history. Am J Psychiatry *150:* 399, 1993.
World Health Organization: *The ICD-10 Classification of Mental and Behavioural Disorders: Clinical Descriptions and Diagnostic Guidelines.* World Health Organization, Geneva, 1992.
Zarin D A, Earls F: Diagnostic decision making in psychiatry. Am J Psychiatry *150:* 197, 1993.
*Zimmerman M: Is DSM-IV needed at all? Am J Psychiatry *147:* 974, 1990.
Zimmerman M, Coryell W, Black D: Variability in the application of contemporary diagnostic criteria: Endogenous depression as an example. Am J Psychiatry *147:* 1173, 1990.

11.2 INTERNATIONAL PERSPECTIVES ON PSYCHIATRIC DIAGNOSIS

JUAN E. MEZZICH, M.D., Ph.D.

INTRODUCTION

Diagnostic systems are offsprings of their time and context, both in regard to conceptualizations of illness and of the patient's whole clinical condition as well as concerning the organization and presentation of diagnostic information considered pertinent to clinical care, education, and research. An adequate understanding of the development of diagnostic concepts and instruments requires both a historical perspective and consideration of the international framework in which such concepts were formulated. This secton outlines major methodological developments in psychiatric diagnosis, the principles and organization of the 10th revision of the *International Classification of Diseases and Related Health Problems* (ICD-10), and the evolution of systems to harmonize the need for universal communication with the recognition of the importance of cultural diversity and the personal experience of the patient.

KEY METHODOLOGICAL DEVELOPMENTS

The most important methodological developments for psychiatric diagnosis, as collated from international surveys, are organized around two major themes: precise psychopathological description and comprehensive diagnostic formulation.

PRECISE PSYCHOPATHOLOGICAL DESCRIPTION The historical roots of systematized psychopathological description can be found in 19th-century France when symptoms were first used as units of analysis of abnormal behavior. Current concepts of psychiatric nosology can be traced back to the end of the 19th century, highlighted by Valentin Magnan's notion of clinical evolution in France and Emil Kraepelin's dichotomy of the major psychoses in Germany. Other significant contributions to the nosology of severe mental disorders of recent impact on psychiatric classification are the German description of cycloid psychoses, the Scandinavian concept of psychogenic psychosis, and the French delineation of *bouffée délirant.* In more recent times, psychopathologists from Asia, Africa, and Latin America have offered informative reports on acute transient psychoses and somatically and psychologically textured characterizations of the neuroses.

The manifestations of mental disorders constitute the focus of the so-called phenomenological description of psychopathology. That approach has encouraged careful observation of clinical presentations, particularly symptom profiles, while minimizing etiological inferences. Many questions remain regarding the organization of standard nosologies, for example, the number of major classes of mental disorders, the arrangement of subclasses, and the hierarchical relationships among diagnostic categories. Furthermore, etiopathogenic perspectives—from genetics, to psychodynamics, to general systems—may in the future contribute enriched and more valid formulations of mental disorders.

Explicit or operational diagnostic criteria, a mainstay of modern diagnostic methodology, were persuasively proposed by the British psychiatrist Edward Stengel as a step to deal with the widespread confusion in classification documented in his international survey, commissioned by the World Health Organization (WHO). The actual development of operational criteria was pioneered, chronologically, by José Horwitz and Juan Marconi in Latin America, Peter Berner in Austria, and John Feighner and associates in the United States. Operationalized diagnostic criteria probably represent the most conspicuous response to the need for clarity in psychiatry, and are regarded as essential for its progress as a scientific discipline. On the other hand, the limitations of using the criteria sets include the arbitrariness often involved in setting thresholds between cases and noncases, the cumbersomeness of their use in daily practice, and the burden they impose on meaning and usage across cultures. An approach that promises to enhance categorical definition by accommodating graded typicality and inexact boundaries involves the use of the prototypical categorization model. This is connected to mathematical *fuzzy set theory,* and its use is being explored on particularly problematic areas of psychopathology.

COMPREHENSIVE DIAGNOSTIC FORMULATION The idea of a more thorough and penetrating representation of a patient's condition has emerged predominantly under the generic term of the multiaxial approach. That model attempts to portray the complexity of the clinical condition through the systematic and separate assessment and formulation of highly informative aspects or domains. Standardized measurements, either typologies or dimensional scales, have been proposed with which to appraise each domain.

The purpose of the first multiaxial schemas in both psychiatry and general medicine was to articulate key components of an

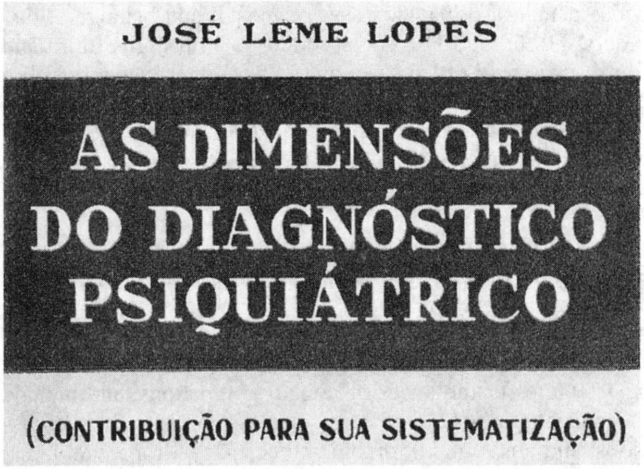

JOSÉ LEME LOPES

AS DIMENSÕES DO DIAGNÓSTICO PSIQUIÁTRICO

(CONTRIBUIÇÃO PARA SUA SISTEMATIZAÇÃO)

FIGURE 11.2-1 *Book cover of José Leme Lopes' multiaxial opus; published in 1954.*

illness. The pioneers of the field, independently proposing a methodical and almost graphical assessment of syndromes and etiology, were Erik Essen-Möller in Sweden, Maurice Lecomte and associates in France, Tadeusz Bilikiewicz in Poland, and José Leme Lopes in Brazil (Figure 11.2-1).

The first multiaxial schema in general medicine appeared to have been the Systematized Nomenclature of Pathology, which accommodated axes on topography, morphology, etiology, and symptoms. One of the latest is the International Classification of Diseases for Oncology (ICD-O), which is based on neoplastic topography and morphology (including tumor behavior and differentiation).

A more recent and far-reaching purpose of the multiaxial model is to furnish a biopsychosocial description of the patient's entire clinical condition. This encompasses not only pathologies (mental and nonmental), but also psychosocial environmental factors and the consequences of illness on the individual's functioning and quality of life. The work of John Strauss, Michael Rutter, and associates in psychiatry and of Alvin Feinstein, J. S. House, and associates in general medicine are pertinent to this objective.

Among the challenges for the further development of the multiaxial model are the need for greater simplicity and ease of use as well as the empirical appraisal of its reliability and validity across the world.

The first national diagnostic system to incorporate a multiaxial approach was the Swedish classification of mental disorders, which was based on the previously referred proposals by Essen-Möller and Snorre Wohlfahrt. More recently, the key methodological developments outlined previously (phenomenological description, explicit diagnostic criteria, and multiaxial formulation) have structured the third and fourth editions of the American Psychiatric Association's (APA) Diagnostic and Statistical Manual of Mental Disorders (DSM-III and DSM-IV), as well as the ICD-10.

ICD-10

ROOTS OF THE INTERNATIONAL CLASSIFICATION

The inspirational roots of the ICD can be found in the taxonomic work of the Swedish biologist Carolus Linnaeus in the 18th century. In *Genera Plantarum* he stated: "All the real knowledge which we possess depends on methods by which we distinguish the similar from the dissimilar . . . We ought therefore by attentive and diligent observation to determine the limits of the genera, since they cannot be determined *a priori*. This is the great work, the important labor, for should the genera be confused, all would be confusion." Linnaeus stimulated scholars from all walks of life. For example, Francois Boissier de Sauvages and William Cullen developed formidable nosologies encompassing thousands of species of disease, organized into classes, orders, and genera.

More concretely, the first International Statistical Congress held in Brussels in 1853 commissioned the Englishman William Farr and the Italian Marc d'Espine to prepare a "uniform nomenclature of causes of death applicable to all countries" as a way to obtain comparable health status information across the world. The proposals that ensued were based primarily on either topographical or etiological principles. Accommodating both, Jacques Bertillón of Paris prepared the First International Classification of Causes of Death, adopted at the International Statistical Congress of 1893.

Since then there have been revisions of the ICD approximately every 10 years. The WHO, created in 1948, assumed from its inception the preparation of these revisions as a constitutional responsibility. The sixth revision contained a critical expansion of the scope of the international classification by covering morbidity in addition to mortality. Correspondingly, psychiatric illness appeared for the first time in the classification with one category: mental illness and deficiency. The ninth revision had as one of its innovations the presentation of a glossary for the capsular definition of mental disorders. While modest in informational detail, this glossary signified recognition by the WHO that the intricacy of mental problems required more than the labels employed in all other chapters of the ICD.

PRINCIPLES OF THE 10TH REVISION The preparation of the 10th revision of the ICD started in 1979, the same year in which the ninth revision was put into effect. The developmental process involved the participation of the eight Collaborating Centers for the Classification of Diseases, specialty divisions (such as Mental Health) at both the headquarters and regional offices of WHO, nongovernmental organizations such as the World Psychiatric Association (WPA), and a miscellaneous panel of interested groups and individuals, all working under the coordination of the WHO Unit on the Development of Epidemiological and Health Statistical Services.

The first highlight of ICD-10 is its expanded scope, as denoted by its title. That continues the trend that started with causes of death, then added morbidity, and more recently is incorporating problems such as disabilities and factors that influence health status, recognizing that amplified information is needed to deal effectively with the complex issues of health care and health promotion.

ICD-10 uses an alphanumeric code composed of a letter followed by several digits. That arrangement more than doubles the number of available categories. Splitting, rather than lumping, of categories has marked the progression of ICD revisions, which has increased the need for categorical slots. The first four characters of the code are internationally official. The fifth- and sixth-character fields are available for regional and special purpose adaptations. That mechanism maintains international communication while accommodating local diversity.

Also innovative is the concept of family of disease and health-related classifications. At the core of the family are the 21 main chapters coded at the official three-character and four-character levels and the short tabulation lists of causes of death and morbidity. Peripherically located are the following classi-

TABLE 11.2-1
List of Core Chapters of ICD-10

Chapter	Title
I	Certain infectious and parasitic diseases
II	Neoplasms
III	Diseases of the blood and blood-forming organs and certain disorders involving the immune mechanism
IV	Endocrine, nutritional, and metabolic diseases
V	Mental and behavioral disorders
VI	Diseases of the nervous system
VII	Diseases of the eye and adnexa
VIII	Diseases of the ear and mastoid process
IX	Diseases of the circulatory system
X	Diseases of the respiratory system
XI	Diseases of the digestive system
XII	Diseases of the skin and subcutaneous tissue
XIII	Diseases of the musculoskeletal system and connective tissue
XIV	Diseases of the genitourinary system
XV	Pregnancy, childbirth, and the puerperium
XVI	Certain conditions originating in the perinatal period
XVII	Congenital malformations, deformations, and chromosomal abnormalities
XVIII	Symptoms, signs, and abnormal clinical and laboratory findings not elsewhere classified
XIX	Injury, poisoning, and certain other consequences of external causes
XX	External causes of morbidity and mortality
XXI	Factors influencing health status and contact with health services

fications: (1) specialty-based adaptations (for example, for oncology) where the chief difference from the core classification lies in the further extension of the ICD codes; (2) classifications for primary care and general medical practice, characterized by the condensation of categories and emphasis on less precise diagnostic terminology and immediate therapeutic utility; and (3) classifications of information outside the core ICD, such as disabilities and medical procedures. Also part of the family is the International Nomenclature of Diseases, which encompasses a list of recommended names for all diseases as well as their definitions. In contrast to the concept of nomenclature, a classification, in the words of the ICD pioneer William Farr, "groups diseases that have considerable affinity or that are liable to be confounded with each other, and therefore is likely to facilitate the deduction of general principles."

The basic forms of human illness and related conditions constitute the 21 chapters at the core of ICD-10 (Table 11.2-1).

Newly independent chapters now structure the enlarged lists of disorders of the nervous system (chapter VI), eye and adnexa (chapter VII), and ear and mastoid process (chapter VIII). The expanded chapter on neoplasms covers one full letter and shares another with blood disorders, which encompasses immunological conditions such as human immunodeficiency virus infections. Also noteworthy is that the classification of neoplasms is multiaxial (that is, one axis denotes topography and another morphology, histological type, and tumor invasiveness and differentiation).

CLASSIFICATION OF MENTAL DISORDERS In chapter V of ICD-10, on mental and behavioral disorders, all conditions are coded with the letter F (Table 11.2-2). The employment of the sixth letter of the Gregorian alphabet to denote chapter V is explained by the assignment of two letters to conditions in the chapter I, on infectious and parasitic diseases, which is lengthy.

The first digit (second character) of the chapter V diagnostic codes denotes 10 major classes of mental and behavioral disorders: F0 through F9. The second and third digits (third and fourth characters) identify progressively finer categories. For example, the code F30.2 sequentially denotes the mental chapter, mood disorders class, manic episode, and the presence of psychotic symptoms (Table 11.2-2). In this way, 1,000 four-character mental disorder categorical slots are available in ICD-10.

F0—Organic, including symptomatic, mental disorders This class is jointly characterized by having as its etiological base physical disorders or conditions involving or leading to brain damage or dysfunction. The first cluster have as prominent features disturbances of cognitive functions, and include the dementias (Alzheimer's, vascular, associated with other diseases, and unspecified), organic amnestic syndrome and delirium not induced by psychoactive substances. The second cluster has as its most conspicuous manifestations alterations in the areas of perception (hallucinations), thought (delusions), mood (depressed or manic), various emotional domains (such as anxiety and dissociation), and personality.

F1—Mental and behavioral disorders due to psychoactive substance use In contrast to earlier classifications, this class subsumes all mental disorders related to psychoactive substance use, from patterns of dependence and harmful use to various organic brain syndromes induced by substances. The diagnostic process and coding starts with the identification of the substance involved (that is, alcohol, opioids, cannabinoids, sedatives or hypnotics, cocaine, other stimulants, hallucinogens, tobacco, volatile solvents, and other substances and combinations). Identified next is the involved clinical condition, as follows: acute intoxication, harmful use (previously known as abuse and characterized by a pattern of use causing damage to physical or mental health), dependence syndrome, withdrawal state (with or without delirium), psychotic disorder, amnesic syndrome, residual and late-onset psychotic disorder, and other and unspecified mental disorders.

F2—Schizophrenia, schizotypal, and delusional disorders This class has schizophrenia as its centerpiece, a disorder characterized by fundamental and distinctive distortions of thinking and perception as well as by inappropriate or blunted affect. The remaining categories of nonorganic, nonaffective psychoses are considered as somewhat related, phenomenologically or genetically, to schizophrenia. Particularly interesting is the cluster of acute and transient psychotic disorders, which encompasses a heterogeneous set of acute-onset and relatively short-lived psychoses (polymorphic with or without schizophrenic symptoms, acute schizophrenialike, and others) reportedly frequent in industrially developing countries (where most of the world population lives).

F3—Mood (affective) disorders The fundamental disturbance in this class is a change in mood or affect, usually involving depression or elation, often accompanied by a change in level of activity. Included here are manic episode, bipolar affective disorder (characterized by recurrent episodes involving both depression and elation), depressive episode, recurrent depressive disorder, persistent mood disorder (cyclothymia, dysthymia), and other and unspecified mood disorders.

F4—Neurotic, stress-related, and somatoform disorders This grouping is based on a historical concept of neurosis, the presumption of a substantial role played by psychological cau-

TABLE 11.2-2
ICD-10 Classification of Mental Disorders

F00–F09
Organic, including symptomatic, mental disorders

F00 Dementia in Alzheimer's disease
  F00.0 Dementia in Alzheimer's disease with early onset
  F00.1 Dementia in Alzheimer's disease with late onset
  F00.2 Dementia in Alzheimer's disease, atypical or mixed type
  F00.9 Dementia in Alzheimer's disease, unspecified

F01 Vascular dementia
  F01.0 Vascular dementia of acute onset
  F01.1 Multi-infarct dementia
  F01.2 Subcortical vascular dementia
  F01.3 Mixed cortical and subcortical vascular dementia
  F01.8 Other vascular dementia
  F01.9 Vascular dementia, unspecified

F02 Dementia in other diseases classified elsewhere
  F02.0 Dementia in Pick's disease
  F02.1 Dementia in Creutzfeldt-Jakob disease
  F02.2 Dementia in Huntington's disease
  F02.3 Dementia in Parkinson's disease
  F02.4 Dementia in human immunodeficiency virus [HIV] disease
  F02.8 Dementia in other specified diseases classified elsewhere

F03 Unspecified dementia

A fifth character may be added to specify dementia in F00-F03, as follows:
  .x 0 Without additional symptoms
  .x 1 Other symptoms, predominantly delusional
  .x 2 Other symptoms, predominantly hallucinatory
  .x 3 Other symptoms, predominantly depressive
  .x 4 Other mixed symptoms

F04 Organic amnesic syndrome, not induced by alcohol and other psychoactive substances

F05 Delirium, not induced by alcohol and other psychoactive substances
  F05.0 Delirium, not superimposed on dementia, so described
  F05.1 Delirium, superimposed on dementia
  F05.8 Other delirium
  F05.9 Delirium, unspecified

F06 Other mental disorders due to brain damage and dysfunction and to physical disease
  F06.0 Organic hallucinosis
  F06.1 Organic catatonic disorder
  F06.2 Organic delusional [schizophrenialike] disorder
  F06.3 Organic mood [affective] disorders
    .30 Organic manic disorder
    .31 Organic bipolar disorder
    .32 Organic depressive disorder
    .33 Organic mixed affective disorder
  F06.4 Organic anxiety disorder
  F06.5 Organic dissociative disorder
  F06.6 Organic emotionally labile [asthenic] disorder
  F06.7 Mild cognitive disorder
  F06.8 Other specified mental disorders due to brain damage and dysfunction and to physical disease
  F06.9 Unspecified mental disorder due to brain damage and dysfunction and to physical disease

F07 Personality and behavioural disorders due to brain disease, damage and dysfunction
  F07.0 Organic personality disorder
  F07.1 Postencephalitic syndrome
  F07.2 Postconcussional syndrome
  F07.8 Other organic personality and behavioural disorders due to brain disease, damage and dysfunction
  F07.9 Unspecified organic personality and behavioural disorder due to brain disease, damage and dysfunction

F09 Unspecified organic or symptomatic mental disorder

F10–F19
Mental and behavioural disorders due to psychoactive substance use

F10. Mental and behavioural disorders due to use of alcohol

F11. Mental and behavioural disorders due to use of opioids

F12. Mental and behavioural disorders due to use of Cannabinoids

F13. Mental and behavioural disorders due to use of sedatives or hypnotics

F14. Mental and behavioural disorders due to use of cocaine

F15. Mental and behavioural disorders due to use of other stimulants, including caffeine

F16. Mental and behavioural disorders due to use of hallucinogens

F17. Mental and behavioural disorders due to use of tobacco

F18. Mental and behavioural disorders due to use of volatile solvents

F19. Mental and behavioural disorders due to multiple drug use and use of other psychoactive substances

Four- and five-character categories may be used to specify the clinical conditions, as follows:
  F1x.0 Acute intoxication
    .00 Uncomplicated
    .01 With trauma or other bodily injury
    .02 With other medical complications
    .03 With delirium
    .04 With perceptual distortions
    .05 With coma
    .06 With convulsions
    .07 Pathological intoxication

  F1x.1 Harmful use

  F1x.2 Dependence syndrome
    .20 Currently abstinent
    .21 Currently abstinent, but in a protected environment
    .22 Currently on a clinically supervised maintenance or replacement regime [controlled dependence]
    .23 Currently abstinent, but receiving treatment with aversive or blocking drugs
    .24 Currently using the substance [active dependence]
    .25 Continuous use
    .26 Episodic use [dipsomania]

  F1x.3 Withdrawal state
    .30 Uncomplicated
    .31 Convulsions

  F1x.4 Withdrawal state with delirium
    .40 Without convulsions
    .41 With convulsions

  F1x.5 Psychotic disorder
    .50 Schizophrenia-like
    .51 Predominantly delusional
    .52 Predominantly hallucinatory
    .53 Predominantly polymorphic
    .54 Predominantly depressive symptoms
    .55 Predominantly manic symptoms
    .56 Mixed

  F1x.6 Amnesic syndrome

  F1x.7 Residual and late-onset psychotic disorder
    .70 Flashbacks
    .71 Personality or behaviour disorder
    .72 Residual affective disorder
    .73 Dementia
    .74 Other persisting cognitive impairment
    .75 Late-onset psychotic disorder

  F1x.8 Other mental and behavioural disorders

  F1x.9 Unspecified mental and behavioural disorder

F20–F29
Schizophrenia, schizotypal, and delusional disorders

F20 Schizophrenia
  F20.0 Paranoid schizophrenia
  F20.1 Hebephrenic schizophrenia
  F20.2 Catatonic schizophrenia
  F20.3 Undifferentiated schizophrenia
  F20.4 Post-schizophrenic depression
  F20.5 Residual schizophrenia
  F20.6 Simple schizophrenia
  F20.8 Other schizophrenia
  F20.9 Schizophrenia, unspecified

A fifth character may be used to classify course:
  .x 0 Continuous
  .x 1 Episodic with progressive deficit
  .x 2 Episodic with stable deficit
  .x 3 Episodic remittent
  .x 4 Incomplete remission
  .x 5 Complete remission
  .x 8 Other
  .x 9 Period of observation less than one year

(continued)

TABLE 11.2-2 (*continued*)

F21 Schizotypal disorder
F22 Persistent delusional disorders
  F22.0 Delusional disorder
  F22.8 Other persistent delusional disorders
  F22.9 Persistent delusional disorder, unspecified

F23 Acute and transient psychotic disorders
  F23.0 Acute polymorphic psychotic disorder without symptoms of schizophrenia
  F23.1 Acute polymorphic psychotic disorder with symptoms of schizophrenia
  F23.2 Acute schizophrenialike psychotic disorder
  F23.3 Other acute predominantly delusional psychotic disorders
  F23.8 Other acute transient psychotic disorders
  F23.9 Acute and transient psychotic disorders unspecified

A fifth character may be used to identify the presence or absence of associated acute stress:
  .x 0 Without associated acute stress
  .x 1 With associated acute stress

F24 Induced delusional disorder

F25 Schizoaffective disorders
  F25.0 Schizoaffective disorder, manic type
  F25.1 Schizoaffective disorder, depressive type
  F25.2 Schizoaffective disorder, mixed type
  F25.8 Other schizoaffective disorders
  F25.9 Schizoaffective disorder, unspecified

F28 Other nonorganic psychotic disorders

F29 Unspecified nonorganic psychosis

F30–F39
Mood [affective] disorders

F30 Manic episode
  F30.0 Hypomania
  F30.1 Mania without psychotic symptoms
  F30.2 Mania with psychotic symptoms
  F30.8 Other manic episodes
  F30.9 Manic episode, unspecified

F31 Bipolar affective disorder
  F31.0 Bipolar affective disorder, current episode hypomanic
  F31.1 Bipolar affective disorder, current episode manic without psychotic symptoms
  F31.2 Bipolar affective disorder, current episode manic with psychotic symptoms
  F31.3 Bipolar affective disorder, current episode mild or moderate depression
    .30 Without somatic symptoms
    .31 With somatic symptoms
  F31.4 Bipolar affective disorder, current episode severe depression without psychotic symptoms
  F31.5 Bipolar affective disorder, current episode severe depression with psychotic symptoms
  F31.6 Bipolar affective disorder, current episode mixed
  F31.7 Bipolar affective disorder, currently in remission
  F31.8 Other bipolar affective disorders
  F31.9 Bipolar affective disorder, unspecified

F32 Depressive episode
  F32.0 Mild depressive episode
    .00 Without somatic symptoms
    .01 With somatic symptoms
  F32.1 Moderate depressive episode
    .10 Without somatic symptoms
    .11 With somatic symptoms
  F32.2 Severe depressive episode without psychotic symptoms
  F32.3 Severe depressive episode with psychotic symptoms
  F32.8 Other depressive episodes
  F32.9 Depressive episode, unspecified
F33 Recurrent depressive disorder
  F33.0 Recurrent depressive disorder, current episode mild
    .00 Without somatic symptoms
    .00 With somatic symptoms
  F33.1 Recurrent depressive disorder, current episode moderate
    .10 Without somatic symptoms
    .11 With somatic symptoms
  F33.2 Recurrent depressive disorder, current episode severe without psychotic symptoms
  F33.3 Recurrent depressive disorder, current episode severe with psychotic symptoms
  F33.4 Recurrent depressive disorder, currently in remission
  F33.8 Other recurrent depressive disorders
  F33.9 Recurrent depressive disorder, unspecified

F34 Persistent mood [affective] disorders
  F34.0 Cyclothymia
  F34.1 Dysthymia
  F34.8 Other persistent mood [affective] disorders
  F34.9 Persistent mood [affective] disorder, unspecified

F38 Other mood [affective] disorders
  F38.0 Other single mood [affective] disorders
    .00 Mixed affective episode
  F38.1 Other recurrent mood [affective] disorders
    .10 Recurrent brief depressive disorder
  F38.8 Other specified mood [affective] disorders

F39 Unspecified mood [affective] disorder

F40–F48
Neurotic stress-related and somatoform disorders

F40 Phobic anxiety disorders
  F40.0 Agoraphobia
    .00 Without panic disorder
    .01 With panic disorder
  F40.1 Social phobias
  F40.2 Specific (isolated) phobias
  F40.8 Other phobic anxiety disorders
  F40.9 Phobic anxiety disorder, unspecified
F41 Other anxiety disorders
  F41.0 Panic disorder [episodic paroxysmal anxiety]
  F41.1 Generalized anxiety disorder
  F41.2 Mixed anxiety and depressive disorder
  F41.3 Other mixed anxiety disorders
  F41.8 Other specified anxiety disorders
  F41.9 Anxiety disorder, unspecified

F42 Obsessive-compulsive disorder
  F42.0 Predominantly obsessional thoughts or ruminations
  F42.1 Predominantly compulsive acts [obsessional rituals]
  F42.2 Mixed obsessional thoughts and acts
  F42.8 Other obsessive-compulsive disorders
  F42.9 Obsessive-compulsive disorder, unspecified

F43 Reaction to severe stress, and adjustment disorders
  F43.0 Acute stress reaction
  F43.1 Post-traumatic stress disorder
  F43.2 Adjustment disorders
    .20 Brief depressive reaction
    .21 Prolonged depressive reaction
    .22 Mixed anxiety and depressive reaction
    .23 With predominant disturbance of other emotions
    .24 With predominant disturbance of conduct
    .25 With mixed disturbance of emotions and conduct
    .28 With other specified predominant symptoms
  F43.8 Other reactions to severe stress
  F43.9 Reaction to severe stress, unspecified

F44 Dissociative [conversion] disorders
  F44.0 Dissociative amnesia
  F44.1 Dissociative fugue
  F44.2 Dissociative stupor
  F44.3 Trance and possession disorders
  F44.4 Dissociative motor disorders
  F44.5 Dissociative convulsions
  F44.6 Dissociative anaesthesia and sensory loss
  F44.7 Mixed dissociative [conversion] disorders
  F44.8 Other dissociative [conversion] disorders
    .80 Ganser's syndrome
    .81 Multiple personality disorder
    .82 Transient dissociative [conversion] disorders occurring in childhood and adolescence
    .88 Other specified dissociative [conversion] disorders
  F44.9 Dissociative [conversion] disorder, unspecified

F45 Somatoform disorders
  F45.0 Somatization disorder
  F45.1 Undifferentiated somatoform disorder
  F45.2 Hypochondriacal disorder
  F45.3 Somatoform autonomic dysfunction
    .30 Heart and cardiovascular system
    .31 Upper gastrointestinal tract
    .32 Lower gastrointestinal tract
    .33 Respiratory system
    .34 Genitourinary system
    .38 Other organ or system

TABLE 11.2-2 (*continued*)

F45.4 Persistent somatoform pain disorder
F45.8 Other somatoform disorders
F45.9 Somatoform disorder, unspecified
F48 Other neurotic disorders
F48.0 Neurasthenia
F48.1 Depersonalization-derealization syndrome
F48.8 Other specified neurotic disorders
F48.9 Neurotic disorder, unspecified

F50–F59
Behavioural syndromes associated with physiological disturbances and physical factors

F50 Eating disorders
F50.0 Anorexia nervosa
F50.1 Atypical anorexia nervosa
F50.2 Bulimia nervosa
F50.3 Atypical bulimia nervosa
F50.4 Overeating associated with other psychological disturbances
F50.5 Vomiting associated with other psychological disturbances
F50.8 Other eating disorders
F50.9 Eating disorder, unspecified

F51 Nonorganic sleep disorders
F51.0 Nonorganic insomnia
F51.1 Nonorganic hypersomnia
F51.2 Nonorganic disorder of the sleep-wake schedule
F51.3 Sleepwalking [somnambulism]
F51.4 Sleep terrors [night terrors]
F51.5 Nightmares
F51.8 Other nonorganic sleep disorders
F51.9 Nonorganic sleep disorder, unspecified

F52 Sexual dysfunction, not caused by organic disorder or disease
F52.0 Lack or loss of sexual desire
F52.1 Sexual aversion and lack of sexual enjoyment
.10 Sexual aversion
.11 Lack of sexual enjoyment
F52.2 Failure of genital response
F52.3 Orgasmic dysfunction
F52.4 Premature ejaculation
F52.5 Nonorganic vaginismus
F52.6 Nonorganic dyspareunia
F52.7 Excessive sexual drive
F52.8 Other sexual dysfunction, not caused by organic disorders or disease
F52.9 Unspecified sexual dysfunction, not caused by organic disorder or disease

F53 Mental and behavioural disorders associated with the puerperium, not elsewhere classified
F53.0 Mild mental and behavioural disorders associated with the puerperium, not elsewhere classified
F53.1 Severe mental and behavioural disorders associated with the puerperium, not elsewhere classified
F53.8 Other mental and behavioural disorders associated with the puerperium, not elsewhere classified
F53.9 Puerperal mental disorder, unspecified

F54 Psychological and behavioural factors associated with disorders or diseases classified elsewhere

F55 Abuse of non-dependence-producing substances
F55.0 Antidepressants
F55.1 Laxatives
F55.2 Analgesics
F55.3 Antacids
F55.4 Vitamins
F55.5 Steroids or hormones
F55.6 Specific herbal or folk remedies
F55.8 Other substances that do not produce dependence
F55.9 Unspecified

F59 Unspecified behavioural syndromes associated with physiological disturbances and physical factors

F60–F69
Disorders of adult personality and behaviour

F60 Specific personality disorders
F60.0 Paranoid personality disorder
F60.1 Schizoid personality disorder
F60.2 Dissocial personality disorder
F60.3 Emotionally unstable personality disorder
.30 Impulsive type
.31 Borderline type
F60.4 Histrionic personality disorder
F60.5 Anankastic personality disorder
F60.6 Anxious [avoidant] personality disorder
F60.7 Dependent personality disorder
F60.8 Other specific personality disorders
F60.9 Personality disorder, unspecified
F61 Mixed and other personality disorders
F61.0 Mixed personality disorders
F61.1 Troublesome personality changes

F62 Enduring personality changes, not attributable to brain damage and disease
F62.0 Enduring personality change after catastrophic experience
F62.1 Enduring personality change after psychiatric illness
F62.8 Other enduring personality changes
F62.9 Enduring personality change, unspecified

F63 Habit and impulse disorders
F63.0 Pathological gambling
F63.1 Pathological fire-setting [pyromania]
F63.2 Pathological stealing [kleptomania]
F63.3 Trichotillomania
F63.8 Other habit and impulse disorders
F63.9 Habit and impulse disorder, unspecified

F64 Gender identity disorders
F64.0 Transsexualism
F64.1 Dual-role transvestism
F64.2 Gender identity disorder of childhood
F64.8 Other gender identity disorders
F64.9 Gender identity disorder, unspecified

F65 Disorders of sexual preference
F65.0 Fetishism
F65.1 Fetishistic transvestism
F65.2 Exhibitionism
F65.3 Voyeurism
F65.4 Paedophilia
F65.5 Sadomasochism
F65.6 Multiple disorders of sexual preference
F65.8 Other disorders of sexual preference
F65.9 Disorder of sexual preference, unspecified

F66 Psychological and behavioural disorders associated with sexual development and orientation
F66.0 Sexual maturation disorder
F66.1 Egodystonic sexual orientation
F66.2 Sexual relationship disorder
F66.8 Other psychosexual development disorders
F66.9 Psychosexual development disorder, unspecified

A fifth character may be used to indicate association with:
.x 0 Heterosexuality
.x 1 Homosexuality
.x 2 Bisexuality
.x 8 Other, including prepubertal

F68 Other disorders of adult personality and behaviour
F68.0 Elaboration of physical symptoms for psychological reasons
F68.1 Intentional production or feigning of symptoms or disabilities, either physical or psychological [factitious disorder]
F68.8 Other specified disorders of adult personality and behaviour

F69 Unspecified disorder of adult personality and behaviour

F70–F79
Mental retardation

F70 Mild mental retardation

F71 Moderate mental retardation

F72 Severe mental retardation

F73 Profound mental retardation

F78 Other mental retardation

F79 Unspecified mental retardation

A fourth character may be used to specify the extent of associated behavioral impairment:
F7x.0 No, or minimal, impairment of behaviour
F7x.1 Significant impairment of behaviour requiring attention or treatment
F7x.8 Other impairments of behaviour
F7x.9 Without mention of impairment of behaviour

(continued)

TABLE 11.2-2 (*continued*)

F80–F89
Disorders of psychological development

F80 Specific developmental disorders of speech and language
F80.0 Specific speech articulation disorder
F80.1 Expressive language disorder
F80.2 Receptive language disorder
F80.3 Acquired aphasia with epilepsy [Landau-Kleffner syndrome]
F80.8 Other developmental disorders of speech and language
F80.9 Developmental disorder of speech and language, unspecified

F81 Specific developmental disorders of scholastic skills
F81.0 Specific reading disorder
F81.1 Specific spelling disorder
F81.2 Specific disorder of arithmetical skills
F81.3 Mixed disorder of scholastic skills
F81.8 Other developmental disorders of scholastic skills
F81.9 Developmental disorder of scholastic skills, unspecified

F82 Specific developmental disorder of motor function

F83 Mixed specific developmental disorders

F84 Pervasive developmental disorders
F84.0 Childhood autism
F84.1 Atypical autism
F84.2 Rett's syndrome
F84.3 Other childhood disintegrative disorder
F84.4 Overactive disorder associated with mental retardation and stereotyped movements
F84.5 Asperger's syndrome
F84.8 Other pervasive developmental disorders
F84.9 Pervasive developmental disorder, unspecified

F88 Other disorders of psychological development

F89 Unspecified disorder of psychological development

F90–F98
Behavioural and emotional disorders with onset usually occurring in childhood and adolescence

F90 Hyperkinetic disorders
F90.0 Disturbance of activity and attention
F90.1 Hyperkinetic conduct disorder
F90.8 Other hyperkinetic disorders
F90.9 Hyperkinetic disorder, unspecified

F91 Conduct disorders
F91.0 Conduct disorder confined to the family context
F91.1 Unsocialized conduct disorder
F91.2 Socialized conduct disorder
F91.3 Oppositional defiant disorder
F91.8 Other conduct disorders
F91.9 Conduct disorder, unspecified

F92 Mixed disorders of conduct and emotions
F92.0 Depressive conduct disorder
F92.8 Other mixed disorders of conduct and emotions
F92.9 Mixed disorders of conduct and emotions, unspecified

F93 Emotional disorders with onset specific to childhood
F93.0 Separation anxiety disorder of childhood
F93.1 Phobic anxiety disorder of childhood
F93.2 Social anxiety disorder of childhood
F93.3 Sibling rivalry disorder
F93.8 Other childhood emotional disorders
F93.9 Childhood emotional disorder, unspecified

F94 Disorders of social functioning with onset specific to childhood and adolescence
F94.0 Elective mutism
F94.1 Reactive attachment disorder of childhood
F94.2 Disinhibited attachment disorder of childhood
F94.8 Other childhood disorders of social functioning
F94.9 Childhood disorders of social functioning, unspecified

F95 Tic disorders
F95.0 Transient tic disorder
F95.1 Chronic motor or vocal tic disorder
F95.2 Combined vocal and multiple motor tic disorder [de la Tourette's syndrome]
F95.8 Other tic disorders
F95.9 Tic disorder, unspecified

F98 Other behavioural and emotional disorders with onset usually occurring in childhood and adolescence
F98.0 Nonorganic enuresis
F98.1 Nonorganic encopresis
F98.2 Feeding disorder of infancy and childhood
F98.3 Pica of infancy and childhood
F98.4 Stereotyped movement disorders
F98.5 Stuttering [stammering]
F98.6 Cluttering
F98.8 Other specified behavioural and emotional disorders with onset usually occurring in childhood and adolescence
F98.9 Unspecified behavioural and emotional disorders with onset usually occurring in childhood and adolescence

F99 Mental disorder, not otherwise specified

Table from World Health Organization: *The ICD-10 Classification of Mental and Behavioural Disorders: Clinical Descriptions and Diagnostic Guidelines.* World Health Organization, Geneva, 1992. Used with permission.

sation, and that mixtures of symptoms are common, particularly in less severe forms often seen in primary care. Included in this block are phobic anxiety and other anxiety disorders, obsessive-compulsive disorder, reactions to severe stress and adjustment disorders, dissociative and conversion disorders, somatoform disorders, and other neurotic disorders (such as neurasthenia and depersonalization-derealization syndrome).

F5—Behavioral syndromes associated with physiological disturbances and physical factors Included here are eating disorders, nonorganic sleep disorders, and sexual dysfunctions, mental disorders associated with the puerperium and not elsewhere classified, psychological factors influencing physical disorders, and abuse of nondependence-producing substances (for example, antidepressants, hormones, analgesics, and folk remedies).

F6—Disorders of adult personality and behavior This class includes clinical conditions and behavioral patterns that tend to be persistent, and the expression of an individual's characteristic life-style and mode of relating to oneself and others. The main subclass involves personality disorders, which are deeply ingrained and enduring behavior patterns, manifesting themselves as inflexible responses to a broad range of personal and social situations. An innovative category is that of enduring personality change, not developmental nor attributable to brain damage or disease, and usually emerging after catastrophic experiences or another psychiatric illness. The broad class also includes impulse, gender identity, sexual preference, and sexual development and orientation disorders.

F7—Mental retardation This condition, one of the oldest in the history of psychiatric classifications, involves arrested or incomplete mental development, characterized by impairment of cognitive, language, motor, and social skills evidenced during the person's formative period and contributing to the overall level of intelligence. Its subcategories correspond to various levels of severity: mild, moderate, severe, and profound mental retardation. Extent of behavioral impairment is additionally coded.

F8—Disorders of psychological development These conditions are characterized, as a class, by the following attributes: onset during infancy or childhood, impairment or delay of functions connected to the maturation of the central nervous system, and a steady course unlike the remissions and relapses usual in many mental disorders. The functions affected most frequently include language, visuospatial skills, and motor coordination. A major subclass encompasses a variety of specific developmental disorders, classified by the abilities involved: speech and language, scholastic skills, and motor function. The other major subclass corresponds to pervasive developmental disorders, many of which are most saliently characterized by deviance rather than delay in development, but always involving some degree of delay. Most conspicuous here are childhood and atypical autism as well as Rett's syndrome and other childhood disintegrative disorders.

F9—Behavioral and emotional disorders with onset usually occurring in childhood and adolescence This complex class complements F7 and F8 as child-onset disorders. Included first are hyperkinetic disorders characterized by early onset, overactive and poorly modulated behavior associated with marked inattention and lack of persistent task involvement, and pervasiveness over situations and time. Conduct disorders are defined by a repetitive and persistent pattern of dissocial, aggressive, or defiant behavior. Also included in this class are emotional, social-functioning, tic, and other disorders usually starting in childhood or adolescence.

The full ICD-10 classification of mental disorders has three presentations corresponding to various degrees of definitional detail, aimed at serving different purposes and uses, as follows:

1. An abbreviated glossary containing the principal features of each disorder, for the use of statistical coders and medical librarians, published within the ICD-10 general volume.
2. Clinical descriptions and diagnostic guidelines, containing widely accepted characterizations of an intermediate level of specificity, intended for regular patient care and broad clinical studies.
3. Diagnostic criteria for research, characterized by more precise and rigorous definitions.

MULTIAXIAL PRESENTATION Within the broad international anchorage of multiaxial diagnosis, the WHO advanced some important initiatives. One was the Multiaxial Classification of Child Psychiatric Disorders, first designed in 1969 and revised several times since then. Another was the Triaxial Classification of Health Problems for Primary Care, which contained axes on physical, psychopathological, and social problems.

Building on these precedents, the WHO Mental Health Division started in the late 1980s the development of a Multiaxial Presentation of ICD-10. The conceptual bases of this development included a critical analysis of over 20 published multiaxial proposals originating in 11 countries spanning three continents, which revealed important commonalities in the clinical domains covered. A second developmental principle was simplicity in the multiaxial schema in order to enhance the prospects of its effective use across the world. The third principle was to base the instruments for axial assessment on components of the ICD-10 family of classifications, which had benefited from wide international consultations and field trials.

The Multiaxial Presentation of ICD-10 is composed of three axes: I. Clinical Diagnoses; II. Disablements; and III. Contextual Factors. The number of axes is lower than the four or five most often included in published multiaxial schemas and constitutes a condensation of those axes most frequently included in multiaxial proposals published in the international literature, which affords a measure of content validity to the schema. The value of the simplicity of the schema is enhanced by its potential for generalization beyond psychiatric practice. Information on clinical pathology, disablements, and contextual factors appears to be relevant to all health care.

Axis I. Clinical diagnoses This axis accommodates both mental and nonmental (general medical) disorders, making the point that there is a fundamental commonality among all illnesses. All significant disorders identifiable in a given individual are to be listed and coded according to chapters I through XX (the disease chapters) in the core classification of ICD-10 (Table 11.2-1).

Axis II. Disablements This axis appraises the consequences of illness in terms of impairment in the performance of basic social roles. The assessment instrument constitutes a shortened version of the WHO Disability Assessment Scale, the structure of which was condensed into four dimensions or areas. These follow (1) personal care, (2) occupational functioning (as remunerated worker, student, or homemaker), (3) functioning with family (assessing both the regularity and quality of interactions with relatives and household members), and (4) broad social behaviors (interaction with other individuals and the community at large, and leisure activities).

Axis III. Contextual factors This axis attempts to portray the context of illness in terms of several ecological domains. These include problems related to the family or primary support group, general social environment, education, employment, housing and economic circumstances, legal issues, family history of illness, and personal life management and life-style. Assessment involves the identification of problematic broad categories and the recording of specific factors. This structure is based on ICD-10 chapter XXI.

OTHER MENTAL HEALTH DEVELOPMENTS Several additional initiatives have been undertaken by the WHO to extend the usability and reach of ICD-10 within the spirit of a family of classifications. Those include a primary care version of the ICD-10 Classification of Mental Disorders, a revision of the International Classification of Impairments, Disabilities, and Handicaps, a WHO Quality of Life Instrument, and a Sociocultural Lexicon.

Primary health care version A simple, brief classification arrangement compatible with and translatable into the ICD-10 standard classification of mental disorders and linked with managements aids has been prepared for use by primary care practitioners (Table 11.2-3). The short list of categories was selected principally on the basis of importance to public health and availability of effective and acceptable management. The centerpiece of the package is a set of pocket-sized flipcards, one for each selected category. One side of the flipcard exhibits assessment information, such as presenting complaints, diagnostic features, and differential diagnosis. The other side displays management guidelines, such as essential information for patient and family, specific counseling to the patient and family, medication, and specialist consultation. Additional elements of the package involve flow charts, symptom indices, and a computerized version.

Revision of the international classification of impairments, disabilities, and handicaps Recognizing the need for the systematic appraisal of disablements, WHO published

TABLE 11.2-3
International Classification of Diseases Primary Health Care Categories

F00*	Dementia
F05	Delirium
F10	Alcohol use disorders
F11*	Drug use disorders
F17.1	Tobacco use
F20*	Chronic psychotic disorders
F23*	Acute psychotic disorders
F31	Bipolar disorder
F32*	Depression
F40*	Phobic disorders
F41.0	Panic disorder
F41.1	Generalized anxiety
F41.2	Mixed anxiety and depression
F43*	Adjustment disorder
F44*	Dissociative disorder (conversion hysteria)
F45	Unexplained somatic complaints
F48.0	Neurasthenia
F50*	Eating disorders
F51*	Sleep problems
F52	Sexual disorders
F70	Mental retardation
F90	Hyperkinetic (attention deficit) disorder
F91	Conduct disorder
F98.0	Enuresis

*More than one ICD-10 code is included.

in 1980 the first edition of the International Classification of Impairments, Disabilities, and Handicaps. Problems perceived in its conceptualization and definitions limited its use and has recently led to revision efforts. Its three constitutive elements are being redefined in regard to areas such as mental health; sensorial, visceral, locomotion, and disfigurement facets; and in attention to such uses as clinical care, research, management, and policy development. An emerging concept is that handicap arises out of an interaction between (1) impairment and disability and (2) the environment where the individual lives, the resources available, and the social and cultural setting.

WHO quality of life instrument Justifying the expanded scope of ICD-10 is the need for comprehensive health assessment, which should include not only physical and psychopathological problems, functioning or disabilities, and psychosocial environmental problems, but also quality of life. The latter is being conceptualized holistically, with an emphasis on positive aspects of health (rather than on pathology or problems) as well as on the subjective perspectives of the individual. A formidable empirical effort is being mounted by WHO to develop a Quality of Life Instrument through a worldwide network of collaborators. The domains selected include the following: I. Physical; II. Psychological; III. Level of independence; IV. Social relationships; V. Environment; and VI. Spirituality, religion, and personal beliefs. Each domain is operationalized through a number of facets and assessment questions, an approach that poses substantive cultural and translation challenges.

Sociocultural lexicon for psychiatry This document intends to facilitate the use of ICD-10 across languages and cultures. The main body of the lexicon includes introductory concepts on the interface between anthropology and psychopathology, followed by a large number of culture-related psychiatric terms and their definitions.

NATIONAL ADAPTATIONS The chaotic situation documented by Stengel in 1959 in terms of the existence of multiple independent psychiatric classifications across the world has substantially changed in recent times, particularly through the development of the ICD-10 Classification of Mental and Behavioral Disorders. ICD-10 is being accepted by most countries and by the WPA as a genuine international standard, not only for statistical reporting but also for clinical care and research. Emerging now is the need to harmonize international communication with recognition of cultural diversity and of specific local requirements. As expression of this perception, several national adaptations, versions, and annotations of ICD-10 are being developed and published, of which the following are examples.

Fourth edition of diagnostic and statistical manual of mental disorders (DSM-IV) The APA published in 1980 an innovative third edition of its diagnostic manual (DSM-III) characterized by a phenomenological emphasis in the conceptualization and organization of mental disorders, the use of explicit diagnostic criteria, and a multiaxial formulation. It acquired wide international visibility and significantly influenced the field of psychiatric classification. After preparations for ICD-10 were started by WHO, the APA initiated the development of DSM-IV, attempting this time to keep close to the international standard (which was already incorporating much of the methodological features advanced by DSM-III). Perhaps the principal attribute of DSM-IV is the scholarly emphasis of its development, based on critical reviews of the literature, reanalyses of existing data bases, and the conduction of focused field trials.

Second edition of Chinese classification of mental disorders (CCMD-II) Classification of illness has a long and rich tradition in China. In consideration of perceived changes in disease patterns associated with growing urbanization in the country, the impact of DSM-III, and the development of ICD-10, the Neuropsychiatric Branch of the Chinese Medical Association appointed in 1986 a task force to prepare a revision of the Chinese Classification of Mental Disorders. The key principle adopted was to keep close to ICD-10 while trying to maintain the Chinese traditional nosological approach. Most of the resulting categories are similar to those in ICD-10. One of the differences involves keeping the concept and term of ''neuroses'' in the Chinese classification, which subsumes the concepts of hysteria (including dissociative and conversion forms), neurasthenia, and many others. Another differential Chinese feature is the category of psychogenic disorders, which comprises induced psychosis, reactive mental disorders, and mental disorders closely related to culture. The latter is particularly interesting and includes *koro* (an episode of sudden and intense anxiety about the penis or vulva receding into the body and causing death) and *mental disorder induced by excessive Eastern gymnastic exercise,* which is regularly practiced in China (Figure 11.2-2).

Japanese clinical modification of ICD-10 Modern Japanese psychiatry constitutes a blend of traditional roots and external influences. Native concepts are exemplified by those on atypical psychosis from the Kyoto school and neurosis theories propounded by Masatake Morita and illustrated by *taijin kyofusho,* a culture-bound social phobia. European influences, particularly German, became conspicuous after the Meiji Reformation in 1868. American psychiatry reached Japan after World II, first in terms of psychodynamic concepts and more recently through the descriptive interest stimulated by DSM-III. In 1988 the Ministry of Health and Welfare appointed a committee to develop diagnostic criteria for mental disorders, which would constitute the Japanese Clinical Modification of ICD-10. Extensive field trials with ICD-10 documented both a reasonable reliability for the international standard (better than for the

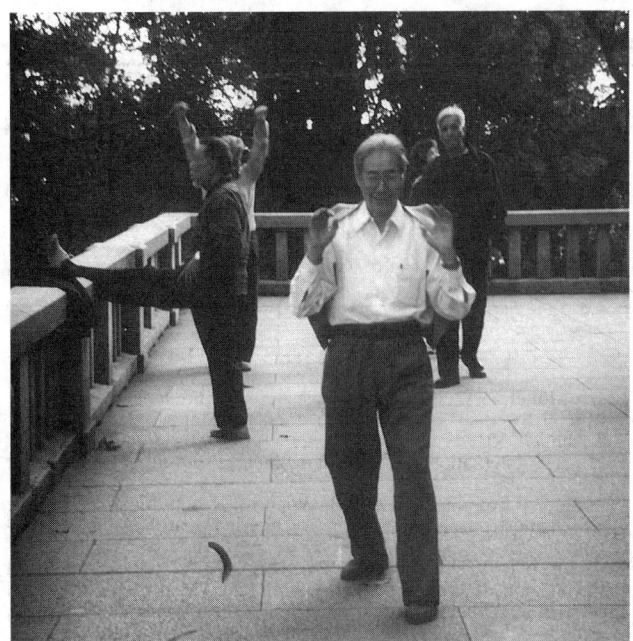

FIGURE 11.2-2 *Senior citizens practicing folk exercises in Guangdong, China.*

traditional classifications) and several problems in the applicability of ICD-10 to Japanese reality. Differential features of the Japanese Clinical Modification include the preference for the concept of atypical psychosis (reflecting Kyoto school teachings) instead of that of brief psychotic disorder, and maintenance of broad categories for neuroses and milieu reactions (in such a way that only after these are identified or diagnosed is attention given to their subtypes or specific forms).

The third Cuban glossary of psychiatry The third edition of the *Glosario Cubano de Psiquiatría* (GC-3) is inscribed within a serial enterprise to adapt the International Classification of Mental Disorders to national reality. The principle guiding these endeavors seems to have been a critical openness to international developments, examined within the framework of the local culture and the national paths for social development. The methodology employed for the preparation of the Glossaries involved national and provincial seminars dealing with conceptual issues on diagnostic assessment and practical problems arising from clinical exercises. The vast majority of the psychiatrists distributed throughout the country are listed as participants in these consultations and exercises, along with representatives of general practitioners, clinical psychologists, and social workers. The Havana Psychiatric Hospital and the Ministry of Health played key logistic roles throughout the various editions. The first Cuban Glossary (GC-1) was completed in 1971 and contained 69 adaptations of ICD-8. The second Glossary (GC-2) was published in 1983 and within its 394 pages presented 92 adaptations of ICD-9 along with rich historical information. The third Glossary (GC-3) constitutes the national adaptation of ICD-10, including its multiaxial schema, and is scheduled for presentation at national and international forums towards the end of 1994.

FUTURE PERSPECTIVES

As pointed out by the eminent historian and philosopher of science Pedro Laín Entralgo, diagnosis, more than labeling the problems suffered by a patient (diagnosis of nosological entity) or distinguishing one illness from another (differential diagnosis), consists in understanding thoroughly what happens in the mind and body of the patient who presents for care. An exploration of opportunities and models for achieving a more thorough and comprehensive diagnosis can be enhanced by employing a historical perspective (Figure 11.2-3).

The longitudinal evolution of diagnostic systems can be seen as unfolding on two parallel lines. One is represented by a synthetic, bold, and abstract Platonic conceptualization of a disease entity as a sufficient descriptor of a patient's clinical condition. The other involves an analytical, textured, and experiential Aristotelian viewpoint as well as an empathetic Hippocratic approach. The ontogeny of comprehensive diagnosis can be understood further, following Nietzschean insights on drama, as the point of convergence between an idealized and rationalistic Apollonian tradition striving for simplicity, order, and clarity, and a Dionysian tradition, vitalistic and affective.

The first tradition has articulated mainstream taxonomic endeavors in psychiatry and medicine, such as the various editions of the International Classification of Diseases and recent attempts to describe disorders more clearly and precisely. The second can be illustrated by biographical approaches, such as Adolph Meyer's dictum that an ordered presentation of the facts is a real diagnosis, and the Hippocratic prescription to keep close to the patient. Those historical lines help one to understand and substantiate an emerging model for comprehensive diagnosis. The model involves combining standardized or nomothetic diagnostic ratings with a personalized or idiographic formulation. The standardized component encompasses both nosological (illness classification) determinations and multiaxial appraisals (using categorical and dimensional scales to focus on key aspects of the patient's condition). The idiographic component covers the patient's perspectives, biographically considered, on illness manifestations, course, and explanatory models; treatment expectations; and quality of life.

The validity of psychiatric diagnosis (that is, its usefulness, particularly for clinical care) may be advanced by a comprehensive model. Standardized nosological and multiaxial ratings facilitate communication among clinicians within and across settings and allow sharing and utilizing international experience on effective treatments for specific problems and levels of dysfunction. Idiographic formulations allow a greater understanding of the patient, engaging him or her more actively in the treatment process, which, as shown by empirical studies, can enhance the outcome of care.

The components of a comprehensive diagnostic model, such as psychiatric classification, multiaxial assessment, and idiographic formulation, are displayed in Table 11.2-4 in terms of their presence in ICD-10 and DSM-IV. Concerning the structural classification of mental disorders, ICD-10 groups all into 10 major classes, consistent with its decimal statistical organi-

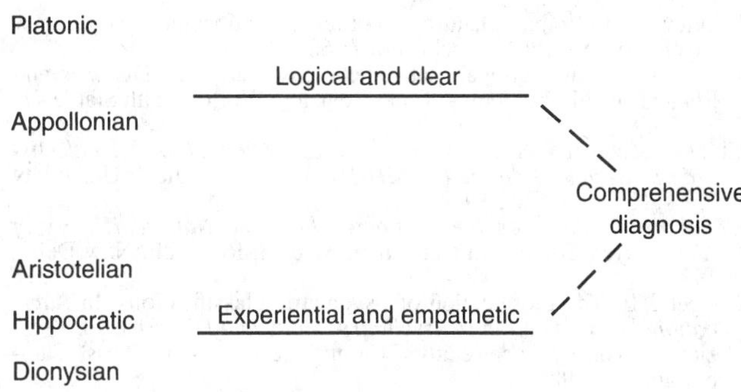

FIGURE 11.2-3 *Evolution of diagnostic systems.*

TABLE 11.2-4
Presence of Components of a Comprehensive Diagnosis Model in New Psychiatric Diagnostic Systems

Model Components	ICD-10	DSM-IV
Psychiatric classification	10 major classes	17 major classes
Multiaxial assessment	I. Clinical diagnoses	I. Mental disorders and conditions II. Personality disorders and mental retardation III. General medical conditions
	II. Disabilities III. Contextual factors	IV. Psychosocial and environmental problems V. Global functioning
Idiographic formulation	International guidelines for cultural formulation Comprehensive diagnostic assessment	

zation. With few exceptions (such as neurasthenia), the same list of disorders is grouped into 17 major classes in DSM-IV, largely following the hierarchical organization inaugurated in DSM-III.

Regarding multiaxial assessment, the almost archetypical commonalities discernible across the large number of multiaxial proposals published to date finds expression in the telescoped correspondence between the ICD-10 and DSM-IV multiaxial schemas. Besides detailed differences in the content and structure of corresponding axes, the only fundamental difference at the higher axial level involves the incorporation into one axis in ICD-10 of all the mental and nonmental disorders, which are divided into three axes in DSM-IV.

With respect to idiographic statements, the cultural formulation included in the appendix of DSM-IV constitutes one of the innovations of this diagnostic manual. It calls for a narrative summary covering the cultural framework of the individual's identity, psychiatric illness, psychosocial environment and functioning, and patient-clinician relationship. Connected to ICD-10, the International Guidelines for Comprehensive Diagnostic Assessment being prepared by the WPA contains an idiographic formulation that would include clinician's explanatory models and the patient's personal perspectives on illness and care.

SUGGESTED CROSS-REFERENCES

The classification of mental disorders is discussed in Section 11.1.

REFERENCES

Badley E M: An introduction to the concepts and classifications of the International Classification of Impairments, Disabilities, and Handicaps. Disability Rehabil *15:* 161, 1993.

Berner P: Der Lebensabend der Paranoiker. Wien Z Nervenheilkd *27:* 115, 1969.

*Berrios G E: The history of descriptive psychopathology. In *Psychiatric Epidemiology: Assessment Concepts and Methods,* J E Mezzich, M R Jorge, I M Salloum, editors. Johns Hopkins University Press, Baltimore, 1994.

Bilikiewicz T: Proba ukladu nozograficzegno etioepigenetycznego w psychiatrii. Neurol Neurochir Pol *1:* 68, 1951.

Brämer G R: International Statistical Classification of Diseases and Related Health Problems—Tenth Revision. World Health Stat Q *41:* 32, 1988.

Chinese Medical Association: *Chinese Classification of Mental Disorders, Second Edition (CCMD-II).* Human Medical University Press, Hunan, China, 1989.

Collaborative Study on the Phenomenology and Natural History of Acute Psychosis. Indian Council of Medical Research, New Delhi, 1989.

Cooper J E: The presentation of psychiatric classifications. In *International Classification in Psychiatry: Unity and Diversity,* J E Mezzich, M von Cranach, editors. Cambridge University Press, Cambridge, UK, 1988.

Essen-Möller E, Wohlfahrt S: Suggestions for the amendment of the official Swedish classification of mental disorders. Acta Psychiatr Scand *47:* 551, 1947.

Fabrega H: International systems of diagnosis in psychiatry. J Ner Ment Dis *182:* 256, 1994.

Feighner J P, Robins E, Guze S B, Woodruff R A, Winokur G, Muñoz R: Diagnostic criteria for use in psychiatric research. Arch Gen Psychiatry *26:* 57, 1972.

Feinstein A R: ICD, POR, and DRG: Unsolved scientific problems in the nosology of clinical medicine. Arch Intern Med *148:* 2269, 1988.

Frances A J, Widiger T A, Pincus H A: The development of DSM-IV. Arch Gen Psychiatry *46:* 373, 1989.

Fujinawa A: Overview of Japanese experiences on diagnostic classification: Past and present of the classification of mental disorders in Japan. In *Psychiatric Diagnosis: A World Perspective,* J E Mezzich, Y Honda, M C Kastrup, editors, Springer-Verlag, New York, 1994.

Horwitz J, Marconi J: El problema de las definiciones en el campo de la salud mental. Definiciones aplicables en estudios epidemiológicos. Bol Of Sanit Panam *60:* 300, 1966.

House J S, Landis K R, Umberson D: Social relationships and health. Science *241:* 540, 1988.

Huttenlocher J, Hedges L V: Combining graded categories: Membership and typicality. Psychol Rev *101:* 157, 1994.

Kastrup M C: Psychosocial domains in comprehensive diagnostic models. In *International Review of Psychiatry,* J-A Costa e Silva, C C Nadelson, editors. American Psychiatric Press, Washington, 1993.

Kleinman A: *Rethinking Psychiatry: From Cultural Category to Personal Experience.* Free Press, New York, 1988.

Kraepelin E: *Psychiatrie,* ed 5. Barth, Leipzig, 1896.

Laín Entralgo P: *El Diagnóstico Médico: Historia y Teoría.* Salvat, Barcelona, 1982.

Lecomte M, Damey A, Delage E, Marty P: Essai d'une statistique synoptique de médicine psychiatrique. Tech Hospitaliers *18:* 5, 1947.

Leme Lopes J: *As Dimensões do Diagnóstico Psiquiátrico.* Agir, Rio de Janeiro, 1954.

Leonhard K: *Afteilung der Endogenen Psychosen.* Akademie, Berlin, 1957.

Magnan V, Serieux P: *Le Délire Chronique á Evolution Systématique.* Gauthier Villars/Georges Masson, Paris, 1893.

*Mezzich J E, Honda Y, Kastrup M C, editors: *Psychiatric Diagnosis: A World Perspective.* Springer-Verlag, New York, 1994.

Mezzich J E, Kleinman A, Fabrega H, Parron D: *Culture and Psychiatric Diagnosis.* American Psychiatric Press, Washington, 1995.

Mezzich J E: On developing a psychiatric multiaxial schema for ICD-10. Br J Psychiatry *152:* 38, 1988.

Mezzich J E: The World Psychiatric Association and the development of ICD-10. In *Psychiatry: A World Perspective,* C Stefanis, A D Rabavilas, C R Soldatos, editors. Excerpta Medica, Amsterdam, 1990.

Ojesjo L: Psychiatric classification and diagnosis: Some guidelines. Nord Psykiatr Tidsskr *32:* 239, 1978.

Orley J, Kuyken W: *International Quality of Life Assessment.* Springer-Verlag, Heidelberg, 1994.

Otero A: *Adaptación Cultural Del Esquema Multiaxial De La CIE-10 A Través De Ejes Complementarios.* Hospital Psiquiatrico de la Habana, La Habana, Cuba, 1994.

Percy C, van Holten V, Muir C: *International Classification of Diseases for Oncology (ICD-0).* World Health Organization, Geneva, 1990.

Pull C, Chaillet G: The nosological views of French-speaking psychiatry. In *Psychiatric Diagnosis: A World Perspective,* J E Mezzich, Y Honda, M C Kastrup, editors. Springer-Verlag, New York, 1994.

Rutter M, Shaffer D, Shepherd M: *A Multiaxial Classification of Child Psychiatric Disorders.* World Health Organization, Geneva, 1975.

Sartorius N: International perspectives of psychiatric classification. Br J Psychiatry *152:* 9, 1988.

*Sartorius N, Kaelber C T, Cooper J E, Roper M T: Progress towards achieving a common language in psychiatry: Results from the field trials of the clinical guidelines accompanying the WHO Classification of Mental and Behavioral Disorders in ICD-10. Arch Gen Psychiatry *50:* 115, 1993.

Seguín C A: The concept of disease. Psychosom Med *8*: 252, 1946.

Spitzer R L, Williams J B W, Skodol A E: DSM-III: The major achievements and an overview. Am J Psychiatry *137:* 151, 1980.

Stengel E: Classification of Mental Disorders. Bull WHO *21:* 601, 1959.

Strauss J S: A comprehensive approach to psychiatric diagnosis. Am J Psychiatry *132:* 1193, 1975.

*Strauss J S: The person—key to understanding mental illness: Towards a new dynamic psychiatry, III. Br J Psychiatry *161:* 19, 1992.

Systematized Nomenclature of Pathology. College of American Pathologists, Chicago, 1965.

Üstün T B, Goldberg D A, Sartorius N: ICD-10: Classifying primary care mental disorders. Proceedings of the 146th Annual Meeting of the American Psychiatric Association, May 22-27, 1993.

*World Health Organization: *The ICD-10 Classification of Mental and Behavioral Disorders. Clinical Descriptions and Diagnostic Guidelines.* WHO, Geneva, 1992.

Wig N N, Setyonegoro K, Shen Y C, Sell H: Problems of psychiatric diagnosis and classification in the Third World. In WHO/ADAMHA: *Mental Disorders, Alcohol- and Drug-Related Problems.* Excerpta Medica, Amsterdam, 1985.

Wimmer A: Psykogene Sindssygdomsformer. In *St. Hans Hospital 1816-1915,* A Wimmer, editor, G.E.C. Gads Forlag, Copenhagen, 1916.

CHAPTER 12 DELIRIUM, DEMENTIA, AND AMNESTIC AND OTHER COGNITIVE DISORDERS AND MENTAL DISORDERS DUE TO A GENERAL MEDICAL CONDITION

ERIC D. CAINE, M.D.
HILLEL GROSSMAN, M.D.
JEFFREY M. LYNESS, M.D.

INTRODUCTION

A major conceptual transition is under way in the way clinicians and researchers view the relation between mental disorders and brain function. For much of the past century, psychiatry was trapped in an either-or dilemma—either a disease was viewed as a symptomatic manifestation of structural cerebral or systemic pathology (organic), or it was considered psychological or emotional in nature (functional).

At the same time, clinicians recognized that there are no behaviors that do not involve the brain, and that the transmission of culturally derived processes from individual to individual is influenced by each person's central nervous system (CNS). Behaviors defined by some cultures as abnormal may be mediated by normal neurophysiology; in contrast, patients with damaged brains may develop compensatory strategies reflective of CNS plasticity to ameliorate the effects of disordered neural systems. The same behavior (for example, suicide) may reflect normal or abnormal physiology. For many diseases, the CNS develops normally but acquires its dysfunction later in life, while others may reflect aberrant wiring or connections while functioning in a neurochemically or neurophysiologically normal fashion. Despite such complexity, clinicians often depended on a single criterion for defining organic disorders—either the detection of a structural lesion or, less often, the diagnosis of a known disease process. Such an approach is no longer satisfactory.

Diagnostic decisions have depended largely on available technology. For more than a century, gross postmortem examination and microscopic histopathologic examination were the primary tools. Working in a tradition of clinical-pathological correlation, psychiatrists, neurologists, and others used a dichotomous approach to both diagnosis and classification—that is, a lesion was either present or absent. That approach proved heuristically limiting and became increasingly unrewarding. The advent of new technologies has undermined the pseudocertainty of earlier years. Many patients with functional syndromes are found to have CNS abnormalities when studied with magnetic resonance imaging (MRI), positron emission tomography (PET), or single photon emission computed tomography (SPECT). Should these syndromes be reclassified as organic? Most would argue that such changes would be premature, as the pathophysiological significance of newer findings remains obscure. Such arguments are also pertinent to the entire question of organic versus functional.

The fourth edition of *Diagnostic and Statistical Manual of Mental Disorders* (DSM-IV) proposes a new approach to those questions. The terminology of organic and functional has been abandoned. When a psychopathological syndrome is known to be a symptomatic manifestation of a systemic medical or cerebral disorder, it is designated as "due to . . ." *(secondary),* with a designation of the specific disease process. When it is considered to be an idiopathic psychiatric disturbance, it is designated *primary.* A clinician should follow a careful process of case reasoning before settling on the primary or secondary status of a disorder. To appropriately diagnose a patient as having an idiopathic (that is, primary) condition, the clinician must necessarily exclude all definable, potentially etiological disease processes.

The clinician must exercise equal caution before diagnosing a disorder as secondary or symptomatic. To date there are no widely accepted guidelines for establishing probable causal relations between psychopathological conditions and detected cerebral abnormalities. Traditionally, such assignment of probable causality has been left to clinical judgment. DSM-IV outlines such guidelines; they have the effect of encouraging the clinician to undertake a thorough evaluation and to postulate causal connections conservatively.

DEFINITION

The primary-secondary classification, like similar classifications, reflects the thinking of its time. The change in terminology in DSM-IV from "organic" to "due to . . ." is more than cosmetic, as it captures the conceptual shift away from structure and lesion and toward active disease process and etiology. The broad group of cognitive disorders includes dementia, delirium, amnestic disorder, and other syndromes in which disordered cognition caused by known (or presumed) disease entities is the central characteristic feature (Table 12-1). Specific secondary syndromes are scattered through the nosology, classified along with other phenomenologically similar clinical conditions (for example, mood disorders due to general medical conditions are grouped among the mood disturbances). Such groupings are intended to foster differential diagnostic consideration; the changes in DSM-IV are intended to enhance rigorous clinical reasoning. Use of more specific designations (for example, mood disorder due to thyroid deficiency, with major depressivelike episode) strengthens diagnostic specificity when contrasted to the previously used organic mood disorder and lays the foundation for more meaningful comparative research.

Throughout this chapter, the term *neuropsychiatry* is used in

TABLE 12-1
Cognitive Disorders and Psychiatric Disorders Due to General Medical Conditions

Cognitive disorders
- Delirium
- Dementia
- Amnestic disorder
- Postconcussional
- Cognitive disorders not otherwise specified (including mild neurocognitive disorder)

Psychiatric disorders due to general medical conditions (secondary disorders)
- Psychotic
- Catatonic
- Mood
- Anxiety
- Behavioral change
- Sleep
- Sexual

Condition not attributable to a mental disorder that is a focus of attention or treatment (R code)

Age-related cognitive decline

reference to the field of medicine that considers the brain bases of mental disorders. In the United Kingdom, that field is sometimes called organic psychiatry. At one time, nearly all of psychiatry was neuropsychiatry; at another time, few would have chosen that label. This chapter reinforces the view that considering the brain substrates of behavior necessarily forces clinicians and researchers also to recognize the experiential, psychological, social, and cultural aspects of the patients and problems they encounter.

HISTORY

The development of neuropsychiatry and the growth of general psychiatry coincided with competition and ultimately cooperation between public psychiatric asylums (now called hospitals or centers) and clinical practice in universities and private offices. Different ideologies or dogmas developed, depending on whether the clinician was seeing principally institutionalized psychotic patients, for whom there was little hope for improvement or recovery, or ambulatory neurotic patients, whose apparent psychological accessibility gave rise to therapeutic optimism. Additionally, psychiatrists in the asylums (often called alienists) had different needs than the nerve doctors or neurointernists who saw the walking wounded in their offices.

Table 12-2 presents a brief categorization of historical periods in neuropsychiatry. It is probably not presumptuous to state that Wilhelm Griesinger (1817–1868) created neuropsychiatry with the publication of his book in 1845, crafted after practicing two years in one of the leading German asylums, in Winenthal. Griesinger, an advocate of physiological medicine, attempted to steer German medical practice away from both the romantic and somatic schools that existed at that time. He asserted that psychiatry was part of medicine. Griesinger is known for stating that "psychological diseases are diseases of the brain"; as well, he advocated knowing one's patients well, understanding their life course, and appreciating how their mental disease affected their overall functioning. He advanced a specific notion of the ego that attempted to explain all disease under a single conceptual view based on a gradual pathological erosion of ego integrity. He supported the idea of careful neuropathological observation, although he never pursued such work in the later fashion of Theodor H. Meynert or Karl Wernicke.

Despite Griesinger's attempted integration, many of his notions now seem simplistic or misleading, especially the idea that all mental illnesses reflected one basic pathological process that could be divided into stages. The first of Griesinger's disease stages involved an assault on the ego by the basic disease, although no frank pathological disruption was apparent. In the second and third stages, ego disintegration was completed and permanent brain changes took place. Griesinger believed that therapeutic intervention would be successful only during the first stage.

Griesinger and his contemporaries made no particular distinction between psychiatric and neurological problems, and patients with progressive neurological diseases were seen in asylums like Winenthal. He proposed joint psychiatry and neurology clinics, and founded one in Berlin in 1861. Most important, he catalyzed the development of

TABLE 12-2
Historical Periods in Neuropsychiatry

1845–1865	Griesinger—Integration I
1865–1900	Neuropathological and descriptive psychiatry
1900–1930	Gradual transition I
1930–1950	Ferment
1950–1965	Psychodynamic era (United States)
1965–present	Gradual transition II
The future	Integration II

university neuropsychiatry, in contrast to the asylum psychiatry that was prevalent in his day, and thus provided the means for developing academic, research-based approaches to questions that had largely been outside rigorous medical scrutiny.

Theodor H. Meynert (1833–1893), the next major player on the neuropsychiatric scene, steered away from Griesinger's integrative center toward an extreme of neuropathological determinism. Meynert's 1874 book, titled *Psychiatry: Diseases of the Forebrain,* largely dealt with neuroanatomy. He is probably best remembered for his histopathological studies and has deservedly been called a pioneer of neuropsychiatric pathophysiology. Meynert also consolidated within universities what proved to be both a sterile theoretical position and a form of clinical psychiatry that had little benefit for either patients in the asylum or the walking wounded. Meynert and his intellectual colleagues, perhaps unwittingly, placed neuropsychiatry in a position where it would decline. It was presumptuous to believe that all clinically significant behavioral disturbances had a demonstrable cerebral substrate, especially given available laboratory techniques. Such work took place in a context of minimal understanding of the basic aspects of neuronal or regional cerebral functioning. It was ironic, perhaps, that the driving investigative force, a search for pathologically defined brain abnormalities, was to become a basis for undoing the field. Psychiatry in general and neuropsychiatry in particular have been plagued by a sense of intellectual exclusivity—the either-or dilemma—in their intellectual conceptions. That sense of exclusivity, and the related tendency to decry integrative (multidetermined) theoretical approaches, may have reflected the ultimate conceptual complexity of the research and clinical tasks that have confronted those who would understand the cerebral bases of behavior and mental disorders: It would be paraphrased, "the brain we are studying is more complex than the brain that is studying it".

Beyond the limitations of neuropsychiatry two fundamentally different paths emerged. The first was exemplified by the work of Emil Kraepelin (1856–1926). Although Kraepelin supported the neuropathological work of Alois Alzheimer, he spent considerable effort developing a rigorous clinical classification of psychiatric disorders, particularly those observed in asylum settings. The classification was largely atheoretical, based as it was on form and course. Kraepelin perhaps hoped that clinical description and classification would ultimately lead to pathological correlation, a hope that has yet to be realized fully. The second path was developed by nerve doctors, neurointernists who saw their patients in offices or on the wards of neurological hospitals. Jean Martin Charcot (1825–1893) and Sigmund Freud (1856–1939) were notable among those practitioners. The idea of looking at an individual's development in the context of early life experience did not originate with Freud (Griesinger had advocated it as well), but Freud pushed farthest the notion of defining the meaning of particular behaviors in terms of real and imagined life events.

The different paths blazed by Freud, Kraepelin, and Meynert coexisted during the early decades of the 20th century, with no one route of investigation clearly predominant. Clinical-pathological correlation had its greatest triumphs with the recognition of the causes of general paresis and pellagra. But the large asylums remained full, and there were no specific therapies for clinicians to use.

In the United States, by contrast, the period of 1930–1950 was a time of great ferment and change, with an examination of new ideas and therapies. Shortly before World War II, clinicians experimented with a variety of somatic interventions and opined about the cerebral bases of the major psychiatric disorders. New treatments, including barbiturate coma, insulin shock, and the convulsive therapies, were developed. In this context, clinicians undertook what seemed a logical step to many—ablative neurosurgical intervention, ultimately dubbed "psychosurgery." Although it was based on poorly substantiated notions of cerebral functions and how they went awry in the major psychiatric disorders, frontal lobotomy spread rapidly in the United States following World War II, fueled by a desire to empty large state mental hospitals and reduce public expenditures for patients with chronic mental disorders. Psychosurgery offered the prospect of instituting a definitive medical procedure that either cured or markedly improved previously intractable syndromes. Psychosurgery and its practitioners failed to fulfill their promises, and neuropsychiatry eventually became a term of opprobrium. By the mid-1950s, brain-oriented views of behavior were widely considered to offer few clinically or theoretically fruitful insights, and brain-oriented psychiatrists were seen as useless or even clinically harmful to those they treated.

Juxtaposed with the 1930s' plunge into organic psychiatry and its therapies was the growth of psychoanalysis, sparked by revolutionary theories brought from Europe by analysts fleeing Adolf Hitler. Young neuropsychiatrists, neurologists, and neuroscientists proved a receptive audience for those ideas, as they discovered far greater explanatory power in the notions of Freud than in those of Charles Sherrington and the doctrine of nerve transmission. Enthusiasts found analytic insights filling unmet needs: Freud's theories and techniques supplied both tools for data collection through the free-associative interview and a coherent system to organize these findings. Of more importance, it directed specific interventions and provided the physician with something to do beyond watching impaired patients remain unchanged or become progressively symptomatic and disabled.

Stanley Cobb (1887–1968), a major figure of that era, was among the leaders in attempting to integrate psychiatry and neurology. Cobb trained in neuropathology and taught the basic neuropathology course at Harvard Medical School for several generations. A student of Adolf Meyer, he espoused a dynamic life course view. Although he maintained an appreciation for neuropathology, he moved away from a primary interest in cerebral circulation to a consideration of psychiatric disorders during the late 1920s and the 1930s. Cobb developed a conceptual pyramid as an integrative device to illustrate his views, purposefully leaving a gray, uncharted zone between pathology and clinical psychiatry. Despite subsequent advances in neuroscience, the uncharted zone seems no less opaque now than 50 years ago, when Cobb first published the conceptual pyramid in his textbooks.

The years immediately after World War II were a time of rapid change, away from neuropathology-based psychiatry and toward psychodynamic and psychoanalytic psychiatry. The growth of psychiatry departments and medical schools was spurred by federal initiative, as was the deinstitutionalization of the seriously ill. Economic motives contributed to the latter, but more important was the sense that a therapeutic triumph might be at hand. That sense was associated with the optimism brought back following World War II by psychiatrists and psychiatrists-to-be (often physicians from other disciplines who were assigned out of need to wartime psychiatry services), coupled with the hope for the successful use of psychoanalysis in a wide variety of disorders and the development, during the 1950s, of a more specific psychopharmacology. Notably, the latter did not reflect a greater degree of neuroscientific understanding; rather, serendipity and clinical acumen served as guiding beacons. Later developments of new agents did result from attempts at pharmacological modeling. Indeed, more recent understandings of CNS function were catalyzed by having specific agents that could reliably alter brain activity.

Formal psychiatric classification and nomenclature evolved during the post-World War II era. Prior to the adoption of the first edition of DSM (DSM-I), in 1952, psychiatric hospitals used the *Statistical Manual for the Use of Hospitals for Mental Disease,* first published under a slightly different title in 1918. Nearly all the categories in the *Statistical Manual* were used for classifying patients with brain-related mental disturbances. As noted in DSM, that approach proved suitable for only about 10 percent of the cases seen by the Armed Forces during World War II. In contrast to the *Statistical Manual,* DSM outlined two broad categories, one for disorders caused by or associated with impairment of brain tissue function (divided into acute and chronic), and the second for those of psychogenic origin without clearly defined physical cause or structural change in the brain. The brain disorder section classified conditions by duration and defined etiology (for example, infection, intoxication, and tumor) with no attention to clinical phenomena, while the psychogenic section began the move toward a more clinically specific categorization. For the latter, difficulties adjusting to internal and external stresses were the key pathogenic factors. Thus, a psychological theory officially supplanted the dominant brain view of earlier classification manuals. Despite the change in dominant explanatory theory, DSM maintained and further codified the same either-or philosophy set forth by the earlier post-Griesinger neuropsychiatrists.

A similar stance was taken in the second edition of DSM (DSM-II), with a separation of organic brain syndromes from psychoses not attributed to physical conditions listed previously. Brain syndromes were said to result from diffuse impairment of brain tissue and to be manifested by the following symptoms: impairment of orientation, memory, all intellectual functions (for example, comprehension and calculation), and judgment, as well as lability and shallowness of affect. The organic brain syndromes were divided into psychotic and nonpsychotic conditions, the former also including senile and presenile dementia, depending solely on the severity of functional impairment. Beyond that crude separation, there were no specifying clinical features; further classification depended on defining an etiology. Acute and chronic were indicated as diagnostic subcodes.

Psychodynamic psychiatry was not successful in treating the more seriously impaired residents of the state hospitals, and often was found wanting among ambulatory populations. Competing approaches sprang up that claimed similar or greater effectiveness. Overall, it has been difficult to definitively demonstrate treatment success when using psychotherapeutic modalities, although recent efforts at treatment evaluation have proved both more enlightening and more promising. A neurochemically oriented biological psychiatry took hold and became preeminent in the research laboratory, if not always in the clinic setting. However, there has been no successful jump from synapse to behavior, integrating our understanding anew. This dearth of explanation has made a fertile soil for the emergence of neuropsychiatry again.

COMPARATIVE NOSOLOGY

DSM-III AND DSM-III-R The third edition of DSM (DSM-III), published in 1980, and the 1987 revised third edition (DSM-III-R) moved to discard the theoretical underpinnings based on stress-related psychological reactions and emphasized phenomenology as part of an innovative multiaxial system of classification. Nonetheless, it maintained the organic versus nonorganic dichotomy. Organic mental disorders were clearer in their clinical typology, with a greater array of subtypes and causes, related either to Axis III physical disorders or conditions or to use of psychoactive substances. Importantly, categories for mood, personality, anxiety, and hallucinatory and delusional disorders were added. Those changes were made in an effort to increase recognition of clinical variations, but they lacked sufficient descriptive detail to allow reliable comparisons with idiopathic Axis I syndromes. Unfortunately, DSM-III, like DSM-I and DSM-II, provided no guidelines or discussion on how researchers and clinicians were to consider the question of causal connection between systemic medical or cerebral diseases and secondary psychiatric manifestations. Thus, there has been no consideration of the clinical reliability of the organic designation, let alone its validity.

SCIENTIFIC DEVELOPMENTS For more than two decades, another period of transition has been under way, one characterized by the absence of a dominant theoretical view within psychiatry. Scientific developments outside the field have profoundly shifted the direction of psychiatric thought. Those influences have come largely from behavioral neurology, clinical neuropsychology, and basic laboratory neuroscience. Challenged by the rehabilitative needs of many patients returning from World War II with focal cerebral lesions, a small number of neurologists and quantitative psychologists began to study the effects of those injuries, just as psychiatrists were shifting their attention away from cerebral processes. That work quickly expanded to include patients with vascular lesions. By the late 1960s, behavioral neurologists and clinical neuropsychologists were recognized specialists, although few in number, and a growing literature examined the intellectual and behavioral consequences of specific regional cerebral lesions. Those writings stimulated a modern resurgence of the clinical-pathological correlative tradition first developed during the late 1800s. For more than a decade, psychiatric researchers have drawn increasingly from the lessons of focal lesion models.

Simultaneously, basic laboratory neuroscience burgeoned, with important findings reported at a fast pace in recent years. Researchers have moved from a focus on synapses and neurons to subneuronal molecular biological processes. Investigative techniques have changed extremely quickly, facilitating the detection of variations in complex neurobiological systems while at the same time outstripping the ability to define normal and abnormal.

Even as psychiatric researchers have studied focal lesion syndromes with greater enthusiasm, the shortcomings of those models have become more apparent. Most important, they involve cerebral substrates distinctly different from those of the major idiopathic psychiatric syndromes. Whereas strokes reflect vascular anatomy, major psychopathology is probably based on dysfunction in interacting, widespread neurochemical systems. Many clinical psychiatric disorders reflect long-term (perhaps developmental) abnormalities that affect psychological growth and interpersonal events across the life course. Focal cerebral lesions, on the other hand, are acquired later in life in the context of a developmentally intact CNS. Thus, analogies must be drawn with caution.

Psychiatric researchers face another, more daunting obstacle when considering the brain bases of mental disorders. For the past two decades, many have chosen to compare specific diagnoses with putative CNS alterations. The exclusive use of categorical diagnoses, while beneficial for enhancing clinical rigor, has yet to prove a rewarding method when applied to diagnosis-brain correlative research paradigms. Although empirically defined clinical syndromes form the bedrock of modern psychopharmacology, they may not be amenable to fundamental neurobiological characterization.

The historic lessons of neuropsychiatry include a realization that a defined or unified etiology may be associated with a striking diversity of clinical presentation (for example, general paresis and Huntington's disease). Conversely, specific syndromes are often the manifestation of heterogeneous etiologies. Here again, maintenance of a rigid either-or view will likely prove disappointing. Rather, future researchers will be required to understand how experiences in the midst of normal development permanently change the brain. Too often, neuropsychiatry has viewed the universe along the trajectory of brain to behavior. It will be just as important to understand it from behavior to brain, and back again.

DSM-IV The change in terminology in DSM-IV from "organic" to "due to" represents more than a simple cosmetic transition. Rather, it emphasizes the need to define etiology, not site or structure. The term *organic,* as utilized for many years, pointed to defined pathological lesions and was contrasted with *functional* or physiological abnormalities that could not be detected by existing laboratory procedures. In the absence of sensitive and specific diagnostic laboratory tests, descriptive laboratory technology was often misapplied, giving a false impression of diagnostic validity. Similarly, the presence of a definable abnormality was considered sufficient to establish an organic diagnosis, even though no standards were available for setting a threshold of evidence or data needed to attribute the cause of a symptom to an observed lesion.

DSM-IV takes a conservative approach to the problem. Establishing a secondary diagnosis should, whenever feasible, follow a chain of reasoning that etiologically connects a psychopathological syndrome with a systemic medical or primary cerebral disorder. The coexistence of Axis I and Axis III diagnoses in an individual case is not sufficient to infer a causal relationship, even when an apparent association or correlation is present. To more confidently determine whether an association is causal, the clinician should attempt to define the strength (relative risk), consistency of form, specificity, coherence of association, and temporal relation of clinical manifestations to the proposed disease process. (Defining each attribute may not be feasible for all disorders or in every case, but it does provide stronger ground for advancing an etiological link.) When insufficient data are available to establish a causal relation, it is preferable to provide unlinked Axis I and Axis III diagnoses.

DIAGNOSIS

Thorough clinical evaluation forms the basis for diagnosing secondary disorders. Beyond a detailed personal history and mental status examination, the clinician often must depend on supplementary laboratory evaluation, including such procedures as cerebral imaging, neuropsychological testing, and electroencephalography. Four steps form the basis for establishing a secondary (due to . . .) diagnosis with greater confidence: (1) definition of the specific psychopathological syndrome, (2) delineation of other manifestations of the primary disorder, (3) demonstration of active cerebral or systemic disease, and (4) demonstration of an elevated prevalence between the proposed etiological disorder and the described psychopathological picture. Those steps may not always occur sequentially, as both syndrome and disease may be recognized.

DEFINITION OF THE SPECIFIC PSYCHOPATHOLOGICAL SYNDROME It is essential to describe the clinical disorder as precisely as possible. Subtyping should be undertaken when feasible, particularly with the specification of target symptoms for treatment. Use of broader or not otherwise specified (NOS) terminology is available for less phenomenologically specific cases. Ideally, the clinician seeks to establish etiological relationships between definable disease processes and specific clinical presentations. The multiple presentations of general paresis, however, underscore that one pathogenic agent may cause multiple syndromic forms.

Patients with many secondary psychiatric disturbances present with symptoms that are atypical of primary (idiopathic) psychiatric disorders. Other clinical features, such as older age at onset, may serve to raise the index of suspicion. Syndrome definition involves severity as well as form. Severity implies a continuum, and the application of a diagnosis implies that the disorder has exceeded a threshold of severity. For example, although behavioral changes often arise following a cerebral lesion, a categorical diagnosis is not warranted when symptoms have not had a measurable impact on a person's functional integrity. Researchers may wish to study mildly symptomatic phenomena, but clinicians typically reserve diagnoses for conditions that cause substantially disordered behaviors, those interfering with the patient's daily life and personal well-being.

DELINEATION OF OTHER MANIFESTATIONS OF THE PRIMARY DISORDER Secondary psychopathological syndromes rarely occur alone but typically keep company with other symptoms and signs of the primary systemic or cerebral disorder. Thus, it is essential to define those cognitive, neuropsychological, peripheral, or other clinically ascertained manifestations of the disease process. For example, human immunodeficiency virus (HIV)-induced manic symptoms typically are accompanied by signs of testable cognitive impairment, whereas depression due to Huntington's disease can be diagnosed with confidence only in the setting of a defined movement disorder. Identifying co-occurring manifestation provides an overall clinical context for more confidently establishing a secondary diagnosis.

DEMONSTRATION OF ACTIVE CEREBRAL OR SYSTEMIC DISEASE The clinician should seek nonbehavioral confirmation of the primary disease process. Such confirmation typically involves laboratory testing, including the full array of medical diagnostic procedures. One must be cautious, however, in the interpretation of many tests. An example is the use of cerebral imaging in psychiatric patients. Detection of a structural abnormality on computed tomography (CT) or MRI is not equivalent to demonstrating active cerebral disease, as such imaging studies provide static (nonphysiological, nonfunctional) information in most applications. Much remains unknown regarding the link between MRI findings, definable cerebral pathology, and specific pathophysiologies or diseases.

DEMONSTRATION OF AN ELEVATED PREVALENCE RATE (ASSOCIATION) BETWEEN THE PROPOSED ETIOLOGICAL DISORDER AND THE DESCRIBED PATHOLOGICAL PICTURE That guideline cannot always be fulfilled, but argues for utilizing data-based conclusions that can be applied to clinical practice. Simply recording that a change in behavior occurs after the emergence of a particular cerebral disorder, for example, is insufficient proof. A specific syndrome should occur with a prevalence in association with an etiological disorder that is above the base rate in the general population.

Many clinicians recommend as the principal criterion for establishing causality the demonstration of a close temporal association of onset and course of the primary disorder and the secondary psychiatric syndrome. Although frequently useful, the criterion of a close temporal association is not always applicable. For example, symptomatic psychosis due to epilepsy may gradually emerge 10 to 15 years after the onset of seizures. Conversely, psychiatric symptoms and signs may be the first clues to a systemic or cerebral disease, and detection of the primary pathological process may follow the emergence of psychiatric symptoms by months or longer. Many secondary psychiatric conditions also may persist after the primary disease process has resolved; examples are the secondary conditions consequent on thyroid deficiency, chronic alcohol use, or long-term exposure to neurotoxic compounds. Secondary syndromes may remit quickly, slowly, or incompletely, depending on the specific disease and whether lasting cerebral changes are present. As well, secondary syndromes may be amenable to symptomatic treatment even while the primary disorder remains without a cure.

Ultimately, the clinician must make an informed judgment as to whether the psychiatric condition is primary or secondary. Prevalence data, for example, reflect group trends, whereas the clinician seeks to make a decision regarding an individual. Two approaches are available. The clinical decision is relatively uncomplicated if a previously demonstrated elevated prevalence links a specific syndrome with a specific etiology, in the presence of additional supporting clinical features and consistent laboratory tests. Probabilistic reasoning in such cases leads to the conclusion that there is a cause-and-effect relation. A temporal association, when meaningfully present, further confirms the connection.

When a clinical research data base is less well established, however, it becomes even more critical to document rigorous clinical reasoning, in effect demonstrating how the detected historical, clinical, and laboratory features are not consistent with what is known about idiopathic psychiatric conditions. Again, establishing the causal connection should reflect the clinician's effort to undertake conscientious probabilistic case reasoning. Attribution of a secondary designation implies a link that is "more probable than not": In other words, the authors recommend a standard that exceeds 50 percent, although it may be feasible to achieve absolute certainty. Such a standard does not require that the systemic medical or primary cerebral disease be the sole factor contributing to symptom expression; rather, "due to . . ." connotes a predominant pathogenic role. When causal probability is considered less certain (that is, possible but not probable), the clinician should not define a syndrome as secondary in nature.

Diagnostic decisions based on incomplete data will be inevitable, and thoughtful clinical judgment remains the abiding rule. "Due to . . ." should be used conservatively; attribution of cause invites a careful consideration of those factors that contribute to disease formation. When doubt remains, the provision of a primary (idiopathic) psychiatric diagnosis will best serve the interests of the patient and avoid the premature closure of clinical evaluation.

NEUROPSYCHIATRIC ASSESSMENT Neuropsychiatric assessment follows the principles of all comprehensive clinical evaluations: It is based on thorough acquisition of the current and past medical history, family history, developmental and social history, and a review of personal habits. The neuropsychiatric clinician seeks to integrate the data on unique individual development, the signs and symptoms of disease, and an understanding of behavior-brain relationships into a meaningful appraisal of functional integrity.

Clinical reasoning should entail a time-oriented view with the clinician noting how the patient has progressed or failed to develop across his or her life course. The temporal perspective is buttressed by an understanding of normative development as well as by an appreciation of the natural history of disease processes. In particular, the clinician should be mindful of the unique characteristics of primary cerebral disorders, whether inborn, acquired early in life, or of later onset. Fundamental to neuropsychiatric evaluation, diagnosis, and prognosis is an understanding of disease evolution at both psychological and neurobiological levels of analysis. Frequently, the clinician must tolerate the uncertainty of not knowing (in an absolute sense) the mechanisms by which brain diseases cause behavioral problems; the clinician is then left with the task of developing practical and effective solutions to problems that may not have specific scientific answers. Despite having a recognized pathological basis, most neuropsychiatric disorders do not have specific cures and continue to require empirical, symptomatic treatment approaches.

As noted earlier in the historical review, clinicians repeatedly face a dual dilemma. Etiological specificity often is related to variable clinical expression (for example, general paresis and Huntington's disease). There is no biological law such as "one pathogen, one clinical presentation." Clinical variability is the rule rather than the exception. Conversely, there are relatively few final common pathways for the expression of a wide variety of disease processes. Those pathways include (1) alterations in arousal, attention, and concentration; (2) alterations in affective state, including both the expression of emotion and the feeling of mood; (3) alterations in perception, including distinctions between ideational and physical or internal and external; (4) alterations in intellectual function (such as memory, language, or the organization of thought processes); (5) alterations in personality; and (6) alterations in motor function. Thus, behavioral abnormalities tend to be nonspecific, and despite substantial evidence from behavioral neurology that focal lesions may lead to distinctive patterns of intellectual deficit, there are insufficient data to confidently support such assertions for major psychopathological syndromes. Moreover, idiopathic or primary psychiatric disorders may mimic symptomatic psychopathological conditions that are secondary to specific systemic medical or cerebral disease processes, and vice versa. Confounding the situation, there has been insufficient research to establish how often cerebral lesions lead to discrete psychopathological syndromes or specifically how any defined psychopathological disorder is related to a particular localized cerebral abnormality.

Thus, the clinician must use an empirical method, based on careful clinical reasoning, that allows the development of a preliminary diagnosis and an initial treatment plan. The clinician should specify in advance what possible therapeutic benefits might be derived and should understand how the natural history of the disorder will unfold if proposed treatment options prove ineffective. As well, the clinician should be ready to undertake further evaluation if an unanticipated outcome arises. By establishing a future- or outcome-oriented clinical perspective, the clinician can reduce the degree of uncertainty and establish a structural approach for systematically and self-critically scrutinizing treatment interventions.

Neuropsychiatric case reasoning The approach to neuropsychiatric case reasoning required for such formulation and planning entails blending the disparate traditions that developed in psychiatry in the past century. It draws from Meynert, as well as from the behavioral neurologists of recent decades, an appreciation of brain-behavior and behavior-brain relations, with an attempt to understand laws of the CNS. Such a method, through lesion location and an appreciation of probabilistic generalities about brain function and neuropathology, in effect argues that all nervous systems are created equal. It benefits from a thoroughly documented array of case studies that seek to define the specific behavioral expression of focal cerebral lesions. It suffers from the facts that nervous systems are not identical and that personal circumstances powerfully influence the expression of disease. Nonetheless, it has taught clinicians much about what to assess and expect when dealing with disordered brain function.

The second approach to case reasoning is derived from the Kraepelinian tradition that continues to be expressed in DSM-IV. That method argues for the precise elaboration of symptoms and signs, the definition of specific syndromes, the identification of target symptoms amenable to therapeutic intervention, and the use of diagnoses for prognostic purposes. The strengths of such an approach lie in the rigorous case definition based on thorough observation and data collection, with the derived ability to generalize from one case to another. Shortcomings, akin to the problems with lesion localization, include the substantial degree of variability that exists within the boundaries of stereotypic diagnostic descriptions and the difficult-to-quantify influences of personal life circumstances.

The third method of case reasoning is derived from dynamic psychiatry and recognizes the individual as having unique personal and developmental attributes that are expressed throughout the course of life. The clinician using this method of case reasoning seeks to understand meaning as well as event and to appreciate disease process in the patient's broader social and cultural context. The neuropsychiatric clinician must view illness in all its complexity.

The different modes of case reasoning are brought together for clinical purposes through understanding how psychological meaning, symptoms and disease process, and socially defined aspects of illness each affects the patient's ability to function autonomously. Although function is not a direct measure of pathology or disease process, assessing how each person has undertaken specific developmentally important tasks is useful for appraising the interaction of those factors. Depending on the individual case, it may be possible to more clearly state which method of case reasoning is most utilitarian or effective, both for developing a treatment plan and for understanding aspects of prognosis. Ultimately, the clinician is as much interested in the patient's return to prior functional integrity as in symptom remission. Treatment success cannot be proclaimed, for example, in the resolution of psychotic symptoms associated with epilepsy if the patient continues to be socially withdrawn or isolated and no longer capable of independent living.

Aging Age and its relation to the expression of illness must be recognized as a changing backdrop for all neuropsychiatric disorders. Age may be used as a convenient indicator for locating the patient in an evolving biological, psychological, and social matrix; a consideration of aging effects cannot await the last stages of the assessment, at which point aging is viewed solely as a factor modifying disease expression. Rather, thoughtful understanding of the aging-related context of a patient's illness is essential to obtaining the fullest view of the relevant life factors contributing to disordered behavior.

Data acquisition The patient's history is an essential feature of neuropsychiatric evaluation, as it provides the clinician the opportunity to develop the equivalent of a serial mental status examination across the patient's life course and to identify target symptoms that may respond to treatment. The clinician seeks to discern when the patient functioned autonomously and effectively, if ever, and to define those personal, social, psychological, symptomatic, and medical factors related to primary disease that contributed to a decline in function or to failure of normal development. Indeed, the history provides the opportunity to view the unfolding or evolution of signs and symptoms. The clinician strives to develop a variety of corollary information sources when assessing the patient's history so that the most complete view of the illness may be obtained. Corollary information sources may be particularly important for evaluating the history of patients who lack the cognitive capacity to effectively relate their own life stories, and they are especially important for understanding the social and cultural context of specific symptoms.

During the history taking, the clinician seeks to elicit the functional anatomy of an illness. Subtle cognitive disorders, fluctuating symptom pictures, and progressing disease processes may be effectively tracked in a detailed rendition of changes in the patient's daily routine involving such factors as self-care, job responsibilities, and work habits; meal preparation; shopping and personal support; interactions with friends; hobbies and sports; reading interests; religious, social, and recreational activities; or ability to maintain personal finances. Understanding the fabric of life for each patient provides an invaluable source of data regarding many of the final common behavioral pathways cited previously, including attention and concentration, intellectual abilities, personality, and motor skills, and more typical symptomatic psychiatric features such as mood state and perception. The examiner seeks to find the particular pursuits that the patient has identified as most important or central to his or her life-style and attempts to discern how those pursuits have been affected by the emerging clinical condition. Such a method provides the opportunity to appraise both the impact of the illness and the patient-specific settings for monitoring the effects of future therapies.

Mental status examination Following a thorough history acquisition, the neuropsychiatrist's primary tool is the assessment of mental state. Formal mental status examination fell into disrepute when descriptive psychiatry was seen as irrelevant to the effective implementation of dynamically oriented psychotherapies. Its value is now undisputed. Like the physical examination, the mental status examination is a means of surveying predetermined functions and abilities to allow a definition of personal strengths and weaknesses. It entails a repeatable, structured view of symptoms and signs; uniformity of approach assists in the reliable definition of findings and promotes effective communication between clinicians. It also establishes the basis for future comparison, essential for documenting therapeutic effectiveness, and it allows comparisons between different patients, with a generalization of findings from one to another. Table 12-3 lists the components of a comprehensive neuropsychiatric mental status examination.

GENERAL DESCRIPTION Several specific points are worthy of mention. Often, teachers and texts place the so-called sensorium as one of the last items for reporting when describing the mental status examination; the term is too broad, but consideration of arousal and responsiveness to the environment should be one of the first domains of assessment. If the patient has a significant disorder of attention or arousal, other aspects of the examination may be invalid. Together, attention and comprehension are the pillars of the mental status examination. Problems of arousal and inability to comprehend the fundamental aspects of the examination tend either to invalidate many findings or to warrant caution in their interpretation.

TABLE 12-3
Neuropsychiatric Mental Status Examination

A. **General Description**
   1. General appearance, dress, sensory aids (glasses, hearing aid)
   2. Level of consciousness and arousal
   3. Attention to environment
   4. Posture (standing and seated)
   5. Gait
   6. Movements of limbs, trunk, and face (spontaneous, resting, and after instruction)
   7. General demeanor (including evidence of responses to internal stimuli)
   8. Response to examiner (eye contact, cooperation, ability to focus on interview process)
   9. Native or primary language

B. **Language and Speech**
   1. Comprehension (words, sentences, simple and complex commands, and concepts)
   2. Output (spontaneity, rate, fluency, melody or prosody, volume, coherence, vocabulary, paraphasic errors, complexity of usage)
   3. Repetition
   4. Other aspects
      a. Object naming
      b. Color naming
      c. Body part identification
      d. Ideomotor praxis to command

C. **Thought**
   1. Form (coherence and connectedness)
   2. Content
      a. Ideational (preoccupations, overvalued ideas, delusions)
      b. Perceptual (hallucinations)

D. **Mood and Affect**
   1. Internal mood state (spontaneous and elicited; sense of humor)
   2. Future outlook
   3. Suicidal ideas and plans
   4. Demonstrated emotional status (congruence with mood)

E. **Insight and Judgment**
   1. Insight
      a. Self-appraisal and self-esteem
      b. Understanding of current circumstances
      c. Ability to describe personal psychological and physical status
   2. Judgment
      a. Appraisal of major social relationships
      b. Understanding of personal roles and responsibilities

F. **Cognition**
   1. Memory
      a. Spontaneous (as evidenced during interview)
      b. Tested (incidental, immediate repetition, delayed recall, cued recall, recognition; verbal, nonverbal; explicit, implicit)
   2. Visuospatial skills
   3. Constructional ability
   4. Mathematics
   5. Reading
   6. Writing
   7. Fine sensory function (stereognosis, graphesthesia, two-point discrimination)
   8. Finger gnosis
   9. Right-left orientation
   10. "Executive functions"
   11. Abstraction

LANGUAGE AND SPEECH The clinician may use language function, particularly when assessing output, to estimate the patient's level of education and intelligence. It is essential, whenever possible, to estimate the patient's premorbid intellectual abilities. Definition of educational attainment during acquisition of the history aids in this process, but further appraisal during mental status assessment is valuable. One must be most careful, however, when using this method, as low educational attainment, a different language or cultural background, or acquired brain damage may confound any estimation.

THOUGHT Assessment of thought processes involves appraising both form and content. Thought form relates closely to language; for example, the clinician must distinguish between fluent aphasia or other disorders of word output and formal thought disorders related to psychosis (such as tangential responses or derailment). There are no ideational or perceptual manifestations that exclusively reflect neuropsychiatric disorders. While some investigators have emphasized that olfactory hallucinations, for example, indicate brain disease specifically, such assertions have not been supported by well-designed epidemiological studies. Moreover, while the major primary psychiatric disorders have no known etiologies, there is no doubt that they involve abnormalities of brain functioning that result in the widest array of symptoms.

MOOD AND AFFECT When assessing affective and mood state, the examiner should appraise the congruence between expressed mood and demonstrated emotion. Patients with cerebral lesions occasionally demonstrate pseudobulbar affect or affective incontinence. The signs of pseudobulbar affect often include affective overshoot or disconnected affect, in which the patient responds to an appropriate stimulus but the expression is exaggerated or the emotional expression is unrelated to any defined mood. Although such behaviors can be observed in patients with idiopathic or primary psychiatric disorders, careful observation over an extended period often demonstrates that they are distinguishable from behaviors encountered in patients with mood disorders.

INSIGHT AND JUDGMENT Insight denotes looking in while judgment reflects looking out. Both entail processes of appraisal or assessment, of one's own state of mind, one's motivations and actions, or one's relationships to others. Discussing the events leading to a clinical evaluation and comparing the patient's version with data gleaned from key informants (family, friends, other clinicians) provide an opportunity defining the congruity of the patient's understanding with that of others. Comparing examination-derived findings with the patient's insight (self-appraisal of mental state) serves as a direct or first-hand assessment.

COGNITION When testing cognitive functions the clinician should evaluate memory, visuospatial and constructional abilities, and reading, writing, and mathematical abilities. Abstraction ability is also valuable to assess, although a patient's performance on tasks, such as proverb interpretation, may be difficult to evaluate when abnormal. Proverb interpretation may be a useful bedside projective test in some patients, but the specific interpretation may be due to a variety of factors, such as poor education, low intelligence, and failure to understand the concept of proverbs, as well as a broad array of primary and secondary psychopathological disturbances. Although testing similarities are also education-sensitive, similarities may be more easily understood by patients.

A variety of standardized assessments have been developed in recent decades to assist with mental status evaluation. These include psychopathological rating scales that depend on self-report as well as examiner administration and brief evaluations of cognitive function that have proved helpful in examining individuals with developing cerebral diseases. Clinicians who use brief evaluations, however, must be cautious when interpreting their findings, which are subject to both false-negative and false-positive errors. For example, many tests use single cutoff points as thresholds for establishing abnormality. However, patients with focal lesions who experience discrete intellectual impairments may remain within the normal range of performance. Patients with idiopathic psychiatric disorders, such as major depressive disorder, may perform at abnormal levels on standardized cognitive protocols, inviting unwary clinicians to diagnose them as having dementia. Such assessments may also be susceptible to systematic differences among the elderly, and nearly all are sensitive to lower educational level. Bedside cognitive tests, because they are tools for screening a large number of persons, tend to be least helpful at the extremes, either when appraising highly intelligent individuals who are suffering intellectual declines but remain above the top rung of the test or when testing those who show substantial cognitive decline. The latter may continue to have residual intellectual abilities, some of which may prove helpful for maintenance care, but tests may prove insensitive to assessing those abilities.

TABLE 12-4
Screening Laboratory Tests

General Tests
Complete blood cell count
Erythrocyte sedimentation rate
Electrolytes
Glucose
Blood urea nitrogen and serum creatinine
Liver function tests
Serum calcium and phosphorus
Thyroid function tests
Serum protein
Levels of all drugs
Urinalysis
Pregnancy test for women of childbearing age
Electrocardiography
Ancillary Laboratory Tests
Blood
Blood cultures
Rapid plasma reagin test
HIV testing (ELISA and Western blot)
Serum heavy metals
Serum copper
Ceruloplasmin
Serum B_{12}, RBC folate levels
Urine
Culture
Toxicology
Heavy metal screen
Electrography
Electroencephalography
Evoked potentials
Polysomnography
Nocturnal penile tumescence
Cerebrospinal fluid
Glucose, protein
Cell count
Cultures (bacterial, viral, fungal)
Cryptococcal antigen
Venereal Disease Research Laboratories assay
Radiography
Computed tomography
Magnetic resonance imaging
Positron emission tomography
Single photon emission computed tomography

PATHOLOGY AND LABORATORY EXAMINATION

Like all medical tests, psychiatric evaluations such as the mental status examination must be interpreted in the overall context of thorough clinical and laboratory assessment. Psychiatric and neuropsychiatric patients require careful physical examination, especially when there are issues involving etiologically related or comorbid medical conditions. When consulting internists and other medical specialists, the clinician must ask specific questions in order to focus the differential diagnostic process and use the consultation most effectively. In particular, most systemic medical or primary cerebral diseases that lead to psychopathological disturbances also manifest with a variety of peripheral or central abnormalities. Assignment of a patient's behavioral disturbance to a symptomatic or secondary status reflects, in part, the definition of other nonbehavioral manifestations of the primary disease.

An important element in the description of secondary psychiatric disorders is the use of laboratory assessment procedures to further define the characteristics of the systemic medical or cerebral process that is etiologically related to the psychiatric symptoms in question. That requires that psychiatrists understand the range of disorders that can lead to behavioral abnormalities. A screening laboratory evaluation is sought initially and may be followed by a variety of ancillary tests to increase the diagnostic specificity. Table 12-4 lists such procedures.

A clinician requesting specific laboratory tests should be led by informed clinical suspicion as well as by an appreciation of the relative costs and benefits of each test. With the exception of low-cost screening procedures, few tests should be requested without a clearly defined rationale. Different approaches are taken for inpatients versus outpatients and for those with regular medical care versus those who have none. Repetition of recently performed tests is often without value.

ELECTROENCEPHALOGRAPHY Electroencephalography (EEG) is an easily accessible, noninvasive test of brain dysfunction that has a high sensitivity in many disorders but relatively low specificity. Beyond its recognized uses in epilepsy, EEG's greatest utility is in detecting altered electrical rhythms associated with mild delirium, space-occupying lesions, and continuing complex partial seizures where the patient remains conscious though behaviorally impaired. As well, EEG is sensitive to metabolic and toxic states, often showing a diffuse slowing of brain activity. Focal slowing, when present, may be indicative of a variety of etiologies, such as space-occupying lesions (tumors, cerebral abscesses) or subdural hematomas. However, a superficial EEG (one that is recorded through the skull) is often insufficient for source localization and may prove insensitive to a variety of abnormal processes, necessitating nasopharyngeal recording to better define abnormalities generated by the temporal lobes or direct cortical (surface) recording to localize seizure foci. The EEG changes with aging, with a general reduction in alpha wave activity, and with increases in the relative amounts of theta and delta wave activity. Early in the course of disorders such as Alzheimer's disease (called dementia of the Alzheimer's type in DSM-IV), the standard EEG usually remains normal and therefore is often unrevealing. As part of sleep polysomnography, recent studies have suggested that the EEG may aid in the future in the distinction between elderly subjects with major depressive disorder associated with cognitive impairment and those with a primary neurodegenerative process underlying their dementia.

COMPUTED TOMOGRAPHY AND MAGNETIC RESONANCE IMAGING CT scanning and MRI have proved to be powerful neuropsychiatric research tools. Recent developments in MRI allow the direct measurement of structures such as the thalamus, basal ganglia, hippocampus, and amygdala, as well as temporal and apical areas of the brain and the structures of the posterior fossa. MRI has largely replaced CT as the most utilitarian and cost-effective method of imaging in neuropsychiatry. Patients with acute cerebral hemorrhages or hematomas must continue to be assessed using CT, but these patients present infrequently in psychiatric settings. MRI better discriminates the interface between gray and white matter and is useful in detecting a variety of white matter lesions in the periventricular and subcortical regions. The pathophysiological significance of such findings, designated by such terms as "rims," "caps," "unidentified bright objects," and "leukoaraiosis," remains to be defined. Such abnormalities are detected in younger patients with multiple sclerosis or HIV infection and in older patients with hypertension, vascular dementia, or Alzheimer's disease. However, their prevalence is also increased in healthy, aging individuals who have no defined disease processes. At present, those types of findings should be viewed in the same light as one would consider atrophic changes, namely, they are detected in a highly sensitive fashion but are usually nonspecific or nondiagnostic in meaning. White matter hyperintensities are more extensive and more frequent in individuals with disease, particularly those with disorders involving cognitive dysfunction, but they are too variable to contribute to the diagnosis or prognosis in an individual case. Like CT, the greatest utility of MRI when used in the evaluation of patients with dementia arises from what it may exclude (tumors, vascular disease) rather than what it can demonstrate specifically.

Because of MRI's ability to delineate brain anatomy and its sensitivity to white matter changes, these guidelines remain utilitarian when modified appropriately. Indications for ordering MRI in psychiatric patients include (1) delirium or dementia of unknown etiology; (2) a first episode of psychosis of unknown etiology; (3) a movement disorder of unknown etiology; (4) the initial evaluation of anorexia nervosa; (5) prolonged catatonia; (6) the initial onset of a major mood disorder or personality change after age 50 years; (7) the presence of unanticipated behavioral, intellectual, or functional decline in an already diagnosed psychiatric patient in whom the clinician would normally expect long-term stability or, at worst, a relapsing-remitting course with a return to baseline between episodes; and (8) the presence of any new behavioral or intellectual disorder in a patient infected with HIV.

Imaging studies have been overused in the periodic monitoring or reassessment of patients with suspected dementia of the Alzheimer's type in whom earlier examinations showed characteristic cerebral changes. Unless one suspects a missed diagnosis of normal pressure hydrocephalus, or perhaps failure to detect microinfarctions on CT when such a finding on MRI might have ruled out Alzheimer's disease, repeated scans are not warranted.

Occasional patients may become agitated in the MRI tube; premedication with a benzodiazepine can minimize the problem. The magnetic field prohibits use of MRI in patients with pacemakers or metal implants, including metallic surgical clips, although many patients now receive MRI-compatible clips at surgery.

POSITRON EMISSION TOMOGRAPHY AND SINGLE PHOTON EMISSION COMPUTED TOMOGRAPHY Physiologically based techniques for imaging the brain, such as PET and SPECT, involve the injection of radioactively labeled, naturally occurring compounds or a radiopharmaceutical, with subsequent demonstration of cerebral blood flow or the incorporation of the labeled compounds into specific metabolic pathways. Such imaging methods have shown promise in studying the neurochemical and physiological bases of a variety of neuropsychiatric disorders. However, the cost of PET currently precludes its use as a routine diagnostic procedure, and there are insufficient data to project its ultimate utility for routine clinical evaluation. SPECT can be performed more readily and at less expense, but whether it will have specific diagnostic utility in general psychiatry remains to be determined.

NEUROPSYCHOLOGICAL TESTING Neuropsychological testing provides a standardized, quantitative, reproducible evaluation of a patient's cognitive abilities. Such procedures may be useful for both initial evaluation and periodic assessment. Tests are available that assess abilities across the broad array of cognitive domains, and many offer comparative normative groups or adjusted scores based on normative samples. The clinician seeking neuropsychological consultation should understand enough about the strengths and weaknesses of selected procedures to benefit fully from the results obtained. For example, many tests do not have appropriate aging-related norms (because they have been used primarily in young and middle-aged adults who are better educated) and therefore are less utilitarian when used in children or the elderly. In general, clinicians should understand that a variety of distinct, competing neuropsychological schools of thought have developed different views regarding methods of individual evaluation, use of the tests, and interpretation of the data. Because neuropsychological evaluation is evolving rapidly and provides a remarkable array of tools for assaying disordered behavior, sophistication in the use and interpretation of those tests will benefit the clinician.

ETIOLOGY AND DIFFERENTIAL DIAGNOSIS

FACTORS AFFECTING DISEASE PRESENTATION Neuropsychiatric evaluation and diagnosis are based on a fundamental understanding of the mechanisms by which pathobiological processes, both systemic and cerebral, express themselves through altered CNS function. The factors that influence symptom expression can be approached from several perspectives.

The first perspective relates to what might be called mode of action. Systemic disorders typically express themselves indirectly, through as yet undefined centrally active substances, defined endocrine disruptions, or fundamental metabolic alterations. Their effects tend to be generalized but often include delirium, dementia, or mood disturbance. In contrast, selective destruction of specific brain regions is more frequently associated with decrements in discrete cognitive tasks or behaviors. One must be cautious with such generalizations, however, as focal lesions in key brain regions (such as those involving brain stem structures) may cause delirious states. Moreover, the clinician may encounter substantial variability in the range of behavioral abnormalities caused by specific focal damage.

A second perspective relies on knowing the natural history of particular pathological processes. Diseases tend to progress or unfold in characteristic fashions, thus allowing for continuing differential diagnostic consideration over time. As well, meaningful prognosis depends on a thorough appreciation of natural history.

A third perspective derives from recognizing the timing of an insult within a neurodevelopmental framework, where the long-term impact of any process or event will depend in part on the compensatory or recovery capacities of the brain. Such capacities change as part of the aging process (indeed, they may be fundamental to aging), but much remains unknown.

A final perspective has to do with the types of cells and regions damaged by specific diseases. Degenerative disorders (Huntington's disease, Parkinson's disease) often lead to destruction of neurochemical systems. Hypoperfusion or pulmonary insufficiency both cause hypoxia, which in turn affects regions with especially vulnerable cell populations (such as the hippocampus) or regions near the ends of vascular trees (the so-called watershed zones, including many brain association areas). Lesions due to ischemic and hemorrhagic cerebrovascular disease reflect vascular anatomy rather than the pathoanatomy associated with degeneration of functionally significant neurochemical systems. Brain toxins may act through binding to specific neurochemical receptors, causing differential damage in direct proportion to regional variations in receptor concentration. Knowledge of the cell populations and anatomical regions affected, when integrated with the other perspectives, assists in understanding or anticipating the full effects of the primary disorder.

A variety of disorders can lead to behavioral abnormalities. They can be subsumed under the following broad categories: trauma, tumor, infection, immune and autoimmune disorders, cardiovascular disease, congenital and hereditary conditions, physiological disorders, primary psychiatric disorders, metabolic disorders, demyelinating disorders, degenerative diseases, substance-induced disorders and disorders due to toxins, and malingering. This chapter does not discuss malingering.

TRAUMA Head trauma leading to brain injury is a possible etiology for all the disorders covered in this chapter, including delirium, dementia, and amnestic disorder, as well as all of the secondary psychiatric syndromes. Traumatic brain injury is largely a disease of modernity, with the majority of injuries due to motor vehicle accidents, gunshot wounds, or occupational mishaps. Estimates point to an annual incidence of 400 to 600 cases per 100,000 population, but such figures must be viewed with caution in light of variable definitions at the less severe (mild) end of the injury spectrum.

Pathophysiology Head trauma can cause brain injury through multiple mechanisms, both direct and indirect. Table 12-5 lists the factors that contribute to brain injury after head trauma. The clinician must recognize that brain injury from head trauma often results in pathology in areas beyond the site of direct impact. In addition, certain areas of the brain are more susceptible to injury regardless of the site of impact. Those areas include the orbitofrontal and frontal pole convexities as well as the anterior temporal lobes, which lie close to bony skull prominences. Rotational and horizontal movements can produce shearing in areas of the brain that are relatively immobile, such as central white matter fiber pathways. Shearing forces can produce diffuse and extensive damage, again unrelated to the actual site of impact. Thus, frontal, subcortical, and limbic structures are especially vulnerable to traumatic head injury. That may explain both the diversity of neuropsychiatric sequelae and the occurrence, at times, of disproportionate disruptions in personality, behavior, and affect when cognitive and motor functions are largely spared. Penetrating head injuries or injuries in which the head has not been able to rotate or move may spare patients from the extensive injuries associated with indirect effects, despite significant direct damage. Bullet or penetrating missile injuries, however, may disrupt neuronal function beyond the site of impact through the effects of high-frequency vibratory waves.

TABLE 12-5
Pathophysiological Mechanisms of Brain Injury After Head Trauma

Direct Effects
Contusion underlying point of trauma (coup)
Contusion linearly opposite point of trauma (contracoup)
Compression from overlying depressed skull fracture
Compression from overlying hematoma
Indirect Effects
Diffuse impact damage
Widespread damage in cerebral white matter
Discrete lesions in corpus callosum
Discrete lesions in rostral brain stem
Common cortical contusions independent of direction of impact
Orbitofrontal
Anterior temporal
Frontopolar
Secondary cerebral processes
Cerebral edema
Increased intracranial pressure with central herniation (Duret's hemorrhages)
Increased intracranial pressure with uncal herniation and posterior cerebral artery entrapment (medial occipital infarction)
Multifocal ischemic changes
Contributing secondary systemic processes
Shock (blood loss, ruptured viscera, sepsis, etc.) with hypotension
Pulmonary failure with anoxia
Long bone fracture with fat emboli

Table adapted from M P Alexander: Traumatic brain injury. In *Psychiatric Aspects of Neurologic Disease,* vol II, D F Benson, D Blumer, editors, p 219. Grune & Stratton, New York, 1982.

Psychiatric symptoms *Delirium* is the acute manifestation of all head injuries that are likely to produce long-lasting sequelae. In severe head injury there is an initial loss of consciousness (coma), followed by gradual recovery, with the delirium taking the form of progressive stages of semiwakefulness, distractibility and confusion, and finally a stable level of consciousness. The entire process may be brief or may take hours to weeks. In milder injuries there may be a brief absence of consciousness, such as momentary dazing, passing out, or transient confusion. A brief lapse of consciousness occurring after head trauma is defined as *concussion.* Significant impairment can arise from even a mild concussion, in the form of a postconcussional disorder, discussed below.

Cognitive disorders are frequent after traumatic brain injuries. Global impairment may be seen after extensive head injury or prolonged coma, although those deficits may improve dramatically in the months following injury. Dementia, or a persistence of global cognitive impairment, is less common, reflecting the high mortality associated with more severe injuries. When dementia is seen, it is usually associated with hemiparesis, aphasia, or other indicators of severe and extensive injury.

Persisting dementia with gradually progressive deficits may be associated with multiple recurrent head traumas. The condition has been termed "chronic traumatic encephalopathy," and has been noted to occur after even minor multiple head traumas. Dementia pugilistica, or boxer's dementia, is an example. Onset usually occurs at the end of a boxer's career after many bouts but chronologically earlier than the onset of the degenerative dementias. A subcortical pattern of dementia (discussed later under degenerative diseases) is typically present, with prominent parkinsonian features as well as dense memory impairment. Neuropathological studies have demonstrated global atrophy with specific involvement of the midbrain and mesial temporal lobe, presumably reflecting both direct and indirect effects of multiple injuries. Plaques and tangles are often noted, but the pathophysiological mechanism remains unknown.

Memory disturbance is nearly always present with any trauma severe enough to cause a concussion (see discussion under amnestic disorders). *Posttraumatic amnesia* occurs invariably after concussive brain injury and refers to the inability to register new memory. The duration of posttraumatic amnesia, which may be very brief, is a significant indicator of severity but can be assessed only after the patient has regained a stable level of consciousness. *Retrograde amnesia* is inability to recall events prior to the injury. It can be assessed by asking patients about their last memories before the injury. Retrograde amnesia generally shrinks with recovery, whereas a postinjury memory deficit tends to remain constant; patients do not recover memories from the period of posttraumatic amnesia. Additionally, patients may suffer persisting impairment of new learning and recall (an amnestic disorder) as a result of permanent pathological changes incurred as a result of the traumatic event. Persisting specific deficits in the context of overall robust recovery can be disabling and frustrating for the patient, who appears normal to others though still impaired cognitively and functionally. Depending on the specific nature of any deficits, these patients would be diagnosed according to DSM-IV as having cognitive disorder not otherwise specified or amnestic disorder due to traumatic brain injury.

Postconcussional disorder is a disabling cluster of symptoms of uncertain pathophysiology. It emerges within hours to days (at most, a few weeks) of a mild head injury and is characterized by headache, dizziness, fatigue, poor concentration and mild memory impairment, problems sleeping, irritability, anxiety, and often significant problems with mood regulation or frank clinical depression. Diminished spontaneity, apparent apathy, and other personality changes are noted also. The cluster of symptoms is remarkably consistent from patient to patient. Table 12-6 presents the proposed research diagnostic criteria for postconcussional disorder that are included in DSM-IV. Although occasional individuals develop posttraumatic migraine, patients with postconcussional disorder more commonly describe symptoms reminiscent of muscle tension headaches arising frontally or posteriorly and occasionally involving temporal regions as well. Some report tenderness persisting at the site of impact, but that is less frequent and its pathophysiological basis is unknown. The syndrome is usually self-limited and improves in the 5 to 10 weeks after injury. However, major depression in the context of postconcussional disorder may not remit unless specific antidepressant treatment is initiated. Postconcussional symptoms that persist beyond 10 weeks should raise suspicions of additional brain pathology, such as an undetected subdural hematoma or a chronic cognitive impairment syndrome. A thorough evaluation is warranted. Postconcussional headaches can persist and prove disabling, and patients may benefit from the judicious use of analgesics as well as antidepressants. Secondary mood disorders are commonly seen with severe injury, although they may be more common after minor injury as part of the postconcussional syndrome. All forms of psychotic symptoms that are seen in idiopathic schizophrenia can be seen after traumatic injury. They are most common in the immediate delirious period but can persist once a stable level of consciousness has been obtained.

TABLE 12-6
Research Criteria for Postconcussional Disorder

A. A history of head trauma that has caused significant cerebral concussion.
Note: The manifestations of concussion include loss of consciousness, posttraumatic amnesia, and, less commonly, posttraumatic onset of seizures. The specific method of defining this criterion needs to be established by further research.

B. Evidence from neuropsychological testing or quantified cognitive assessment of difficulty in attention (concentrating, shifting focus of attention, performing simultaneous cognitive tasks) or memory (learning or recalling information).

C. Three (or more) of the following occur shortly after the trauma and last at least three months:
(1) becoming fatigued easily
(2) disordered sleep
(3) headache
(4) vertigo or dizziness
(5) irritability or aggression on little or no provocation
(6) anxiety, depression, or affective lability
(7) changes in personality (e.g., social or sexual inappropriateness)
(8) apathy or lack of spontaneity

D. The symptoms in criteria B and C have their onset following head trauma or else represent a substantial worsening of preexisting symptoms.

E. The disturbance causes significant impairment in social or occupational functioning and represents a significant decline from a previous level of functioning. In school-age children, the impairment may be manifested by a significant worsening in school or academic performance dating from the trauma.

F. The symptoms do not meet criteria for dementia due to head trauma and are not better accounted for by another mental disorder (e.g., amnestic disorder due to head trauma, personality change due to head trauma).

Table from DSM-IV, *Diagnostic and Statistical Manual of Mental Disorders,* ed 4. Copyright American Psychiatric Association, Washington, 1994. Used with permission.

Personality change due to a general medical condition is a frequent concomitant of traumatic brain injury, owing to the vulnerability of the frontal lobes and the important role those structures play in the expression of personality. Two personality syndromes have been described with frontal lobe injury: the orbitofrontal syndrome, characterized by disinhibition, explosiveness, and jocularity; and the frontopolar syndrome, characterized by apathy, behavioral inertia, and indifference. Patients may appear indifferent to their incapacities or may confabulate regarding their injury and hospitalization. Less marked personality changes, such as irritability and a so-called short fuse, are common, especially as part of the postconcussional syndrome.

Adjustment disorders can occur at any point once a stable level of consciousness has been attained. Patient and family must adjust to loss of capacity, increased irritability and fatigue, a possible change in family roles, absence from work, financial constraints, and legal entanglements. As in all adverse circumstances, premorbid personality heavily influences the patient's adaptive capacities. Unfortunately, clinicians have at times seen the presence of an adjustment disorder or a prior history of maladaptive personality functioning as a reason to conclude that patients are not suffering from behavioral or cognitive impairments arising from brain injury. The evaluation and treatment of head trauma require clinical flexibility to address the broadest range of symptoms and syndromes.

Course and prognosis The course of recovery from post-traumatic syndromes depends on the severity of the initial injury and the location of damage. The duration of coma and of post-traumatic amnesia may be useful prognostic indicators. Dramatic improvements can occur within days and continue for up to six months. Overall recovery may continue up to 24 months, with motoric and physical improvement often preceding behavioral and cognitive restoration. Less frequently, recovery continues beyond two years after injury. The neurobiological mechanisms leading to recovery are unknown.

Treatment There are no specific treatments for the cognitive abnormalities associated with head trauma. Life-sustaining and life-supportive acute therapies may be needed initially, and the psychopathological conditions resulting from head trauma may warrant symptomatic therapies. Despite a boom in institutions and companies offering cognitive rehabilitation, it remains unproved scientifically whether those methods significantly augment natural recovery processes.

TUMOR Intracranial tumors, whether of primary CNS or metastatic origin, can cause behavioral disturbances by directly affecting brain function. They may do so by destroying or compressing brain parenchyma (from mass effect or edema), through obstructive hydrocephalus, or by disrupting brain vasculature. The nature of the ensuing behavioral disturbance depends on factors already discussed, such as time course and injury location.

Extracranial nonbrain neoplasms may indirectly alter brain function, causing psychiatric symptoms, by any of several pathways. The cancer may disturb one or more organ systems known to affect brain function. As examples, lung cancer may cause hypoxemia, or metastatic prostate carcinoma may lead to obstructive uropathy with consequent renal failure. Paraneoplastic syndromes may lead to metabolic abnormalities (for example, hypercalcemia) commonly associated with behavioral changes. Intriguingly, cancer may cause psychiatric symptoms without any known metabolic or other organ system disturbance; a commonly cited example is the onset of a major depressive disorder as the first clinical manifestation of occult pancreatic carcinoma. The mechanisms of such phenomena are unknown, although it has been speculated that blood-borne humoral factors secreted by the tumor are active centrally.

INFECTION Infections can produce any of the range of cognitive impairments or secondary syndromes, either acutely or chronically. Acute infectious processes involving the CNS often produce delirium as a component of fulminant deterioration. Chronic psychopathology can result either from a chronic infectious process, such as neurosyphilis or Creutzfeldt-Jakob disease, or from persisting structural brain damage incurred as a result of an acute infection, as in chronic sequelae of herpes simplex encephalitis.

Syphilis Syphilis is a chronic infection resulting from inoculation with the spirochete *Treponema pallidum.* It is transmitted through sexual contact. Primary syphilis is a local disease manifested by a lesion at the site of inoculation, usually the penis, vagina, or mouth, within two to three weeks after inoculation. Secondary syphilis, manifested by a recurrent rash occurring anywhere on the body but especially on the palms and soles, has its onset six weeks to six months after initial exposure. After the rash resolves, syphilis may enter a latent stage that lasts two to 10 years after inoculation. Serology remains positive throughout the latent stage. Tertiary syphilis may involve skin, bone, and the aorta, as well as the CNS. Neurosyphilis can occur five to 35 years after the initial inoculation. Neurosyphilis is divided into four stages: (1) an asymptomatic stage, without symptoms but with abnormal cerebrospinal fluid (CSF); (2) meningovascular syphilis, characterized by headache, nuchal rigidity, irritability, and, at times, delirium; (3) tabes dorsalis, with signs of posterior column degeneration, such as ataxia (due to loss of proprioception resulting in a slapping or high-stepping gait and trophic joint changes, Charcot's joints), areflexia, paraesthesias (described as lightning pains and typically involving the extremities), incontinence, impotence, and abnormal pupillary findings (the classical Argyll Robertson pupil, which accommodates but does not respond to direct light response); and (4) general paresis, also known as general paralysis of the insane or dementia paralytica, the classic neuropsychiatric disorder of tertiary syphilis.

General paresis has great significance for the history of psychiatry, as it was one of the first instances in which severe behavioral and cognitive disturbances could be attributed directly to an etiologically definable brain disease. General paresis can present as almost any form of psychiatric disturbance or dementia syndrome. The classically described grandiose presentation has become rare, while depressive presentations have become more common. Often a general change in personality is the initial presentation, with apathy, lability, and coarsening of behavior. Dementia is of a mixed pattern, with prominent impairment of memory, language, and judgment, as well as loss of initiative and psychomotor slowing. Neuropathologically the brain demonstrates diffuse degeneration with marked lymphocytic infiltration throughout.

Creutzfeldt-Jakob disease Creutzfeldt-Jakob disease, also known as Jakob-Creutzfeldt disease, depending on which of the early 20th-century reports is given precedence, is a viral infection that causes a rapidly progressive cortical-pattern dementia. The age at onset is usually in the sixth or seventh decade, although onset can occur at any age. The incidence is 1 in 1,000,000. The clinical symptoms vary with progression of the illness and depend on the regions of the brain that become involved. Patients may present initially with nonspecific symptoms, including lethargy, depression, and fatigue. Within weeks, however, more fulminant symptoms develop, including progressive cortical pattern dementia, myoclonus, and pyramidal and extrapyramidal signs. Although blood, CSF, and imaging studies are unremarkable, the EEG can demonstrate a characteristic pattern of diffuse symmetric rhythmic slow waves. A presentation with rapid deterioration, myoclonus, and the characteristic EEG pattern should raise suspicion of Creutzfeldt-Jakob disease. The definitive diagnosis is made by postmortem microscopic examination, which demonstrates spongiform neural degeneration and gliosis throughout the cortical and subcortical gray matter. White matter tracts are usually spared. Creutzfeldt-Jakob disease is caused by a slow virus or viral particle that can incubate for decades before the emergence of clinical symptoms and subsequent rapid progression. Reported routes of transmission include invasive body contacts, such as direct tissue transplantation (for example, corneal transplants) or hormonal extracts (for example, human growth hormone, before synthetic supplies were developed). Familial patterns have been reported as well, suggesting that there may be genetic susceptibility to infection. No antiviral agents have been shown to be definitively effective in retarding or slowing disease progress, although amantadine (Symmetrel) has been reported occasionally to have had some success. Death usually ensues within six months to two years of onset.

Viral encephalitis Viral encephalitis varies in severity, depending on the specific etiological agents. Mild disease is more common with mumps, and enteroviral infections can be limited to headache and malaise. Severe disease is characteristic of infections such as rabies and herpes simplex. Herpes simplex encephalitis is the most common of the severe nonepidemic encephalitides. It is of interest to neuropsychiatry because of the preferential involvement of the orbitofrontal and medial-temporal regions of the brain. A typical presentation consists of severe encephalitis of rapid onset, high fever, headache, nuchal rigidity, focal neurological signs, and delirium. Rarely, a sudden, transient psychosis may herald the onset. Occasionally the onset is more insidious, with the clinical picture at presentation limited to personality change or memory impairment. Necrosis of the frontal and temporal lobes can occur rapidly. Mortality is high, approximately 70 percent. Whenever herpetic encephalitis is suspected, a definitive diagnosis should be made as rapidly as possible by brain biopsy, with the subsequent urgent initiation of antiviral therapy. Survivors may sustain deficits related to temporal and frontal lobe damage, including a dense amnesia disproportionate to the degree of other intellectual impairment; hallucinations in all spheres, including olfactory and gustatory; components of a Klüver-Bucy syndrome; partial complex seizures; aphasia; and anosmia.

Human immunodeficiency virus Human immunodeficiency virus type 1 (HIV-1) has created a late 20th-century epidemic parallel in severity and pervasiveness to the scourges of bygone eras. Acquired immune deficiency syndrome (AIDS), the later stages of HIV infection, has been recognized for more than a decade. In recent years its neuropsychiatric manifestations have become a focal point for diagnosis and therapy, as patients live longer through the use of partially effective antiviral therapies and a variety of second-line medications employed for treating opportunistic infections. The following discussion focuses on neuropsychiatric phenomena that appear to result from HIV-1 action in the brain.

Clinicians began to recognize the variety of neuropsychiatric manifestations of HIV during the mid-1980s. Most prominent were major mood disturbances (major depressive, dysthymic, and bipolar disorders) and a characteristic progressive cognitive impairment that was labeled the AIDS dementia complex (ADC). In addition, patients developed psychoses, at times with a schizophrenic presentation, as well as alterations of personality. Intertwined with syndromes that were thought to be direct results of primary HIV infection of the CNS or secondary complications from other infections or tumors were a variety of adjustment and mood disturbances, reflecting responses to a progressive, inevitably terminal disease.

The psychopathological manifestations of HIV cover the waterfront of major symptom clusters, as well as ADC and delirium. Clinicians have used empirical treatments, many with substantial symptomatic response. Intervention with antiviral therapies also has shown beneficial behavioral effects, especially when CSF indices of CNS infective activity have suggested that the primary disease has increased in its activity. However, there have been few carefully conducted therapeutic trials to establish the overall efficacy of any symptomatic psychopharmacotherapy.

ADC is characterized predominately by a subcortical presentation (see discussion under Degenerative Diseases), with prominent psychomotor slowing and difficulties with concentration and memory. Early associated motor deficits include ataxia, leg weakness, tremor, and loss of fine motor coordination. Patients commonly become apathetic or withdrawn. The course is steadily progressive, at times punctuated by abrupt acceleration. Like other dementing disorders, ADC progresses to a late stage characterized by severe dementia, mutism, incontinence, paraplegia, and, for some, myoclonus.

During the latter part of the 1980s, controversy developed regarding the temporal sequence for the emergence of cognitive abnormalities versus other symptoms reflecting the advance of HIV infection to full-blown AIDS. There is no dispute that ADC may be the predominant feature of AIDS for some patients, but there is uncertainty regarding the presence of cognitive abnormalities in patients who are both clinically asymptomatic and without laboratory evidence of encroaching immune suppression. Many patients with HIV develop a mild (minor) cognitive disorder that has many of the same features of ADC but is neither as severe cognitively nor as impairing functionally. Recently, an American Academy of Neurology AIDS Task Force developed a set of standard nomenclature for neurological manifestations of HIV-1 infection, including both cognitive and peripheral neurological findings.

In autopsy series, 75 to 90 percent of brains of patients dying with HIV infection show neuropathological alterations. In addition to changes due to secondary or opportunistic infections, there is widespread subcortical white matter pathology with relative sparing of cortical structures. Those diffuse, noninflammatory changes are now subsumed under the term "HIV leukoencephalopathy." Microscopic examination also reveals foamy macrophages and multinucleated giant cells invading both white matter and subcortical nuclei, particularly basal ganglia structures. Such focal inflammatory findings are characterized as HIV encephalitis. As well, there may be pathology in the spinal cord associated with paraparesis, particularly vacuolar myelopathy. Insofar as many other patients have significant cognitive deficits in the context of relatively little pathological alterations, it is clear why investigators have encountered difficulty when attempting strict clinical-pathological correlation.

The mechanism by which HIV causes its functional effects remains unknown. Current data point to (1) both neurons and supporting cellular structures, through the actions of the virus itself or from its coat proteins (such as gp120); (2) the undesirable effects of activated immune components (such as activated macrophages); and (3) possible excitatory neurotoxic effects of endogenous neurotransmitters that have been dumped into surrounding interstitial fluids (for example, quinolinic acid affecting glutamate receptor subtypes, leading to the toxic accumulation of intracellular calcium).

The diagnosis of HIV-related neuropsychiatric syndromes requires a high index of suspicion and a sensitivity to possible demographic risk factors, including homosexual behavior, sexual promiscuity, intravenous substance abuse, and sexual relations with high-risk partners. In addition, there is a gradual movement of the HIV virus into the broader heterosexual population. Psychopathological changes may precede frankly defined cognitive abnormalities. The clinician also must be alert to early, subtle intellectual decline: The patient may remain within the normal range on standard neuropsychological tests but performs at a level lower than was attained previously. In addition to neuropsychological assessment, neuroimaging may demonstrate abnormalities in subcortical periventricular and deep white matter.

ADC has become a major target in pharmacotherapeutic trials to cure or ameliorate the effects of HIV infection. Preventing its emergence or prolonging the time it takes to appear have become possible end points for some studies. Others are considering ADC as a direct target for intervention. Future antiviral pharmacotherapies may be targeted specifically to the brain to eradicate any possible reservoirs of HIV, in a fashion similar to the use of irradiation or antitumor agents in children with leukemia.

IMMUNE AND AUTOIMMUNE DISORDERS Three broadly defined pathophysiological mechanisms involving the immune system can be associated with neuropsychiatric disorders. (1) Hypofunction of the immune system may contribute to infectious diseases and possibly to neoplastic illnesses. (2) Definite or putative autoimmune diseases may cause behavioral disturbances by affecting the function of organ systems in a way that compromises brain activity (for example, the hyperthyroidism of Graves' disease or hepatic failure from primary biliary cirrhosis). Autoimmune illnesses may also affect brain function more directly by causing cerebral ischemia due to vasculitis or by direct CNS parenchymal inflammation. Some primary neurological diseases may involve autoimmune pathophysiology; an example is multiple sclerosis.

A major example of an autoimmune disorder involving the CNS is systemic lupus erythematosus (SLE). Often it is considered in the differential diagnosis of new-onset psychopathological syndromes. Although the etiology of SLE is not known, evidence implicates immunological mechanisms in its pathogenesis. Numerous organ systems may be involved. SLE may affect brain function (and thereby produce psychiatric symptoms) indirectly, through such mechanisms as fever, renal failure, or pulmonary disease. In a minority of patients it may cause pathology directly, most likely from vasculitis affecting cerebral vessels. Patients with CNS disease may experience seizures, transverse myelopathies, or behavioral abnormalities, including delirium, psychotic syndromes, and affective lability. Clinicians evaluating patients with psychiatric symptoms of recent onset (particularly women in their second through fifth decades of life) should carefully consider the medical history, review of systems, physical examination findings, and routine laboratory screens, looking for evidence of systemic organ system involvement. The erythrocyte sedimentation rate, while nonspecific, is substantially elevated during acute CNS lupus and provides a useful screen. More specific laboratory tests (for example, antinuclear antibody assay and antibodies to double-stranded deoxyribonucleic acid [DNA]) may be pursued when indicated. Neuroimaging scans may show cerebral infarctions but are often normal early in the disease. Glucocorticoids are the mainstay of treatment for acute CNS SLE. Psychotropic medications may be needed to treat specific behavioral symptoms (for example, antipsychotics for severe agitation during delirium).

CARDIOVASCULAR DISEASE Because the extremely high metabolic activity of the brain is obligatorily aerobic, the brain is exquisitely sensitive to relatively minor perturbations in blood flow. Thus, alterations in cardiac function ranging from grossly obvious (cardiogenic shock) to relatively subtle (compensated congestive heart failure, chronic low-output states) often manifest with CNS dysfunction. The consequent psychiatric phenomenology may vary due to largely unknown factors, but delirium, dementia, and depressive episodes are especially common. Perfusion failure, depending on its cause, may lead to insidious, gradual changes or dramatic decrements in function. Transient profound drops in blood pressure, typically associated with major cardiac events (including surgery), may lead to mental status alterations that are difficult to pinpoint initially. Clinicians are faced with distinguishing soon-to-remit symptoms, such as postoperative delirium arising from metabolic imbalances, from subtle persisting intellectual and behavioral alterations caused by hypofusion leading to cell death.

Intrinsic cardiac illness, such as mural thrombus or valvular disease, may also be a source of embolic cerebral infarction. Cardiovascular disease may also lead to brain dysfunction by serving as a risk factor for cerebrovascular disease. Identified risk factors for stroke include hypertension, diabetes mellitus, cigarette smoking, atrial fibrillation, left ventricular hypertrophy, and coronary artery disease.

Cerebrovascular disease of any etiology and pathophysiology—thrombotic, embolic, or hemorrhagic—will affect brain function. Psychiatric symptoms may develop either acutely (presumably in relation to abrupt neuronal losses and dysregulation) or gradually (perhaps in relation to cumulative infarcted brain tissue and to longer-term adaptations of neurochemical systems). Table 12-7 presents an overview of the variety of cerebrovascular events.

Recent data undercut the long-held notion that vascular disease due to a vascular etiology always progresses in stair-step fashion, as some have described for the course of vascular dementia. Rather, progression appears to vary in rate and form, depending both on the type of vasculature affected (large versus small vessels) and on basic pathobiology (perfusion insufficiency versus occlusive disease).

It is important to recognize that psychiatric phenomena may manifest without other clinical evidence of a neurological event. For example, patients with right parietal infarction have presented with delirium but no other neurological symptoms or signs. Alternatively, an infarction in the distribution of the left middle cerebral artery may cause Wernicke's aphasia, characterized by fluent paraphasic or jargon-filled speech, poor comprehension and repetition, and suspicious or aggressive behavioral responses. No other signs of cerebral disease may be evident, and such patients have been misdiagnosed as having paranoid schizophrenia. It is also important to understand that pathology does not specify phenomenology. For example, patients with multiple infarcts on MRI are often labeled as having vascular dementia; however, multiple infarctions may manifest with dementia, with other behavioral syndromes (mood disorder, psychosis, anxiety, personality change), or with no definable neuropsychiatric syndrome.

TABLE 12-7
Types of Cerebrovascular Events

Thrombotic
Most commonly related to atherosclerotic stenosis or occlusion of cerebral vessels
May or may not be preceded by warning transient ischemic attacks (TIAs)
Onset may be gradual, stuttering, or acute
Produces ischemic infarction

Embolic
Emboli may arise from cardiac (thrombus, valve vegetation, atheromatous plaque) or carotid (thrombus) origin
Onset is typically rapid without warning TIAs
Produces ischemic, hemorrhagic, or mixed infarction

Hemorrhagic
Extradural—typically from trauma to middle meningeal artery
Subdural—from rupture of bridging veins
Subarachnoid—from ruptured saccular aneurysms (e.g., in circle of Willis)
Intracerebral—types include hypertensive, ruptured arteriovenous malformations; other contributors include hemorrhagic diatheses, vasculitis, bleeding into cerebral tumors, and septic emboli
Onset is typically rapid with further progression, without prior warning

Lacunar
Refers to occlusion of small perforating arteries, producing deep, small (2–15 mm) cavitary infarcts called *lacunes*
Associated with hypertension and atherosclerosis
Onset may be rapid, followed by partial or complete recovery, but accumulated multiple lacunes may produce secondary psychiatric syndromes

CONGENITAL AND HEREDITARY CONDITIONS Patients with congenital and hereditary conditions often present for psychiatric evaluation because of the frequency of associated behavioral disturbances. Congenital and hereditary conditions are of great significance in the understanding of brain-behavior relationships, for they are often seen in biologically homogeneous populations with relatively specific behavioral and neuropsychiatric syndromes. Congenital conditions are caused either by genetic abnormalities affecting autosomes, sex chromosomes, or single genes or by fetal insults during the pre-, peri-, or immediate postnatal periods. Table 12-8 lists several developmental and hereditary disorders with significant neuropsychiatric manifestations. In DSM-IV, those conditions are classified according to the age at which symptoms manifest, what symptoms are present, and whether the symptoms are progressive or static.

Down's syndrome Down's syndrome results in static phenotypic abnormalities, including characteristic facies and mental retardation, and has been associated with a progressive decline in functioning beginning in the third or fourth decade

TABLE 12-8
Examples of Developmental and Hereditary Disorders with Neuropsychiatric Manifestations

Syndrome	Etiology	Onset of Manifestations	Neuropsychiatric Findings
Down's syndrome	Trisomy of chromosome 21	Lifelong	Dysmorphic facies; moderate to severe mental retardation, dementia in fourth to fifth decades of life
Fragile X syndrome	X chromosome heteromorphism	Lifelong	Males: dysmorphic facies, autism, moderate to severe mental retardation, macroorchidism; females: mild mental retardation hyperactivity, affective disorder, developmental Gerstmann syndrome
Prader-Willi syndrome	Partial deletion of chromosome 15	Lifelong	Hyperphagia; lability; obesity; mild to moderate mental retardation
Learning disorder of the right hemisphere	Pre-, peri-, or postnatal insult versus genetic	Emerges in childhood	Normal intelligence but marked verbal/performance discrepancy; pathological shyness; difficulty with perception and appreciation of affect
Acute intermittent porphyria	Autosomal dominant with incomplete penetrance	Emerges after puberty, usually in third decade	Intermittent attacks with abdominal pain, polyneuropathy, seizures and delirium
Metachromatic leukodystrophy	Autosomal recessive deficiency of enzyme arylsulfatase A	Juvenile and adult forms	Personality change; auditory hallucinations; paranoid and grandiose delusions early; dementia and neurological deterioration later
Adrenoleukodystrophy	X-linked recessive	Juvenile and adult forms	Delusions and hallucinations; Addison's disease
Olivopontocerebellar degeneration (OPCA)	Autosomal dominant	Juvenile and adult forms	Subcortical dementia
Huntington's disease	Autosomal dominant; chromosome 4 linkage	Juvenile and adult forms; adult more common	Subcortical dementia; major depressive disorder, bipolar disorder

of life. Alzheimerlike pathological changes are frequently detected at autopsy, even in patients who did not exhibit functional decline before death.

Fragile X syndrome Fragile X syndrome is the second most common cause of mental retardation in men and one of the few known causes of the autism syndrome. Female heterozygotes also manifest significant psychiatric pathology, including mood disorders, difficulties with behavioral control, and a neuropsychological profile of dyscalculia, right-left disorientation, and constructional dyspraxia similar to the Gerstmann syndrome, described in patients with acquired lesions in the dominant parietal lobe. Learning disorders usually become obvious when the child begins school.

Huntington's disease Huntington's disease, also known as Huntington's chorea, has been the focus of intensive neuropsychiatric, genetic, and pharmacological research during the past two decades. First described by George Huntington on Long Island in 1872, the disorder has received intense scrutiny, and its site on chromosome 4 has been determined. The disorder is related to an unstable trinucleotide repeat, associated with more than 40 copies of the specific sequence. Onset typically occurs in middle life, usually between ages 25 and 50 years. The juvenile form, with onset occurring during adolescence, is somewhat different phenomenologically, with a greater degree of dystonia early in the disease process and a faster rate of disease progression. Huntington's disease is not diagnosed formally until the typical movements appear, although both psychiatric and neuropsychological manifestations may precede the emergence of motor abnormalities.

The psychopathology associated with Huntington's disease has a wide range of manifestations, commonly including affective presentations (typically depression, but mania as well); psychoses, often with a schizophrenic appearance; personality changes; and anxiety disorders. Some individuals, however, may proceed through the entire course of the illness with no evident psychopathology. Often the psychopathology is most florid during the early and middle stages of the disease, but as the characteristic subcortical dementia proceeds (see discussion under degenerative diseases), patients begin to emit less behavior and thus appear less symptomatic. The suicide rate is higher in patients with Huntington's disease than in the general population but suicidal ideation may be difficult to detect, as patients tend to be less spontaneous and forthcoming as a result of the cognitive difficulties associated with the disorder. Interviewers must take an active or probing approach; patients who quickly pass off inquiries when presented with open-ended questions may provide more information when queried with specifically structured interview methods.

The cognitive disorder of Huntington's disease is more consistent in its presentation than the psychopathological picture, although it, too, evolves over the course of the disorder. Patients usually experience mild memory difficulties, and the first symptoms may be subtle problems with organizing, planning, and sequencing. Spontaneity and verbal elaboration may be diminished relatively early, although that appears to be somewhat more variable in its time of onset. As the disease progresses, psychomotor slowing progresses relatively rapidly, with concomitant difficulty with complex tasks, while recall of old knowledge and factual information remains less affected. Unlike patients with dementia of the Alzheimer's type, many patients with Huntington's disease remain insightful long into the course of their disease. Thus, their mood disturbances and potential suicidality may be tied, in part, to a clear realization of their situation. Indeed, even as patients respond to standard antidepressant therapy with enhanced sleep, energy, appetite, and improved overall mood state, they may remain realistically pessimistic about their long-term situation.

Patients with Huntington's disease begin to develop an apathetic appearance as the disease progresses. Early in the course, they continue to show interest and responsiveness when presented with structured situations in which they can take part; frank apathy and disinterest develop later and persist even in the context of prompted or structured assistance. Although some degree of verbal learning impairment is an early feature of the dementia, it is more prominent later in the disease course. Similarly, subtle visuospatial processing problems may occur early but do not become prominent until later.

Just as the cognitive disturbance of Huntington's disease

evolves slowly, so, too, there is a gradual change in the associated movement disorder. In most affected adults the movement disorder is typically choreiform at the outset but becomes more dystonic and bradykinetic as the disease progresses. Toward the end of the disease course, patients are bedridden, mute, and overcome by a severe dystonic state.

The pathology and neurobiology of Huntington's disease have been studied intensively in recent years. The striatum bears the brunt of the pathology, with interruption of crucial corticostriatothalamocortical relays. Although there are no immediate, reciprocal corticostriatal connections, that multineuronal pathway similarly modulates motor function, cognition, and, apparently, mood. Recent theories suggest abnormal function of excitatory neurotransmitters, most apparently acting on glutamate receptors, that serve as endogenous neurotoxins. Although efforts have been made to use symptomatic pharmacological treatments for both the psychiatric and motor symptoms, more recent pharmacotherapeutic trials have aimed at preventing progression of the disease by employing potential glutamate receptor blockers. Such efforts have provided models for similar therapeutic approaches to Parkinson's disease and Alzheimer's disease.

The mood disorders associated with Huntington's disease have proved amenable to symptomatic treatments. Standard doses of antidepressant medications may be needed, although patients often respond sensitively to rapid changes in medication and experience unwanted side effects. Electroconvulsive therapy (ECT) has been beneficial for severe major depressive symptoms, especially in high-risk suicidal patients. The schizophrenialike presentations of Huntington's disease appear less responsive to antipsychotic therapy than phenomenologically similar idiopathic disturbances. Patients with Huntington's disease-related anxiety disorders have shown sufficient benefit from available medication regimens to warrant empirical trials. Psychotherapy, usually with the patient and family treated together, may lead to substantial therapeutic gains. Clinician commitment to the long haul may prove especially reassuring and stabilizing.

Huntington's disease, like other hereditary neuropsychiatric disorders, illustrates the need for all psychiatric evaluations to include a careful documentation of family history. Patients with Huntington's disease may present with mood or psychotic disturbances and no apparent abnormal involuntary movements and may be treated symptomatically with pharmacotherapeutic agents, only to evince later the characteristic motor disorder. Ignorance of the family history has led some to misinterpret that progression as evidence of tardive dyskinesia. The patient may remain incorrectly diagnosed until cognitive impairment becomes unmistakable. In the meantime, patients and families have lost the opportunity to clarify their life plans and develop support for future needs. Psychiatrists must remain vigilant in taking the family history whenever evaluating a new patient.

Other conditions Learning disorders involving left hemisphere functions such as reading, writing, or mathematics are well known clinically. A learning disorder of the right hemisphere has been described that is characterized by intact linguistic and academic skills; left-sided soft (nonlocalizing) neurological signs; and profound impairments in functions dependent on the right hemisphere, including visuospatial skills, modulation of affect, and the paralinguistic aspects of communication. The etiology of the learning disorder is unknown, although a retrospective history of pre- or perinatal insults is common, as is a family history of similar impairments. Acute intermittent porphyria is a hereditary disorder that is intermittent. In between episodic attacks, most patients maintain normal development. The leukodystrophies and degenerative hereditary disorders listed in Table 12-8 can produce symptoms during childhood or not until adulthood. Development until the appearance of symptoms is normal. Note, however, in each of those disorders psychiatric symptomatology can precede other evidence of the disease process and lead to an erroneous diagnosis of an idiopathic psychiatric disorder.

PHYSIOLOGICAL DISORDERS EPILEPSY Epilepsy is the prototype of a physiological disease process that manifests with psychiatric symptoms. It has long held the interest of neuropsychiatry and has been studied intensively, if not always fruitfully. The complexities of defining brain-behavior relationships in epilepsy merit extended discussion.

Definition Epilepsy is defined as a condition of recurrent seizures due to CNS disease or dysfunction. Seizures are behavioral alterations of abrupt onset and termination that are associated with sudden electrical discharges of the brain. Although the essential paroxysmal form remains constant and in fact defines a seizure, the content of the behavioral disturbance can vary widely. Seizures can be generally classified into two broad categories, generalized and focal. In generalized seizures the electrical abnormality usually originates from subcortical structures (primarily the brainstem) and then spreads simultaneously to all areas of the cortex. Loss of consciousness is invariable, and the seizure phenomenology is symmetrical and bilateral. Focal seizures originate from a specific brain locality, usually the temporal lobe. The abnormal electrical discharge may remain at the site of origin, proceed gradually to adjacent areas, or spread to include the entire cortex (secondary generalization). The clinical phenomenology of a focal seizure depends on the site from which that seizure originates and may be unilateral and restricted to a particular muscle group, sensation, affect, and so on. The epilepsies are classified based on the type of seizure and the inferred anatomical substrate (Table 12-9). Seizure type and phenomenology are usually constant within the course of a particular patient's disorder. The stereotyped presentation is a major feature of evaluation, diagnosis, and assessment of treatment efficacy.

Clinical features Seizures can proceed in stages and may include a prodrome, aura, ictus, and a postictal period. Psychopathology may manifest during any of these stages as well as during the interictal (between-seizure) period (Figure 12-1). A prodrome can be seen in generalized epilepsy, although it is more common in focal epilepsy, particularly temporal lobe epilepsy. A prodrome may consist of irritability, apprehension, sul-

TABLE 12–9
Classification of the Epilepsies

Primary generalized epilepsy
Tonic-clonic (grand mal)
Absence (petit mal)
Myoclonic
Other
Partial (focal) epilepsy
Simple (elementary) symptomatology
Focal motor
Focal sensory
Vegetative
Mixed
Complex symptomatology
Partial complex (psychomotor)
Secondary generalized
Unclassifiable

Prodrome ⟶ Aura/ictus (seizure) ⟶ Postictal ⟶ Interictal ⟶ Prodrome...

FIGURE 12-1 *Progression of phases in epileptic seizure disorders.*

lenness, or a sense of discomfort or disease that builds up gradually over hours to days before a seizure. The prodromal state remits abruptly with the onset of the seizure. The pathophysiological basis for the prodromal state is unknown.

Auras are focal seizures or the initial focal onset of a seizure and are associated with definable abnormal electrical discharges. Auras are abrupt in onset, last for seconds to minutes, may progress to a generalized seizure, or may terminate as the seizure ends. The type of clinical phenomenon depends on the site of origin and can include motor, sensory, autonomic, perceptual, cognitive, and affective abnormalities. Table 12-10 lists a number of common clinical manifestations of auras or focal seizures based on anatomical site of origin. The auras accompanying seizures originating in the temporal lobe are the most varied. In general, auras may comprise a variety of symptoms and may have unique, individual-specific features, such as the crying out of a particular phrase in a particular language. Despite the great variety of auras, in any individual auras tend to be stereotyped and consistent from seizure to seizure.

The ictus, or epileptic attack, may be generalized or focal. Primary generalized tonic-clonic epilepsy (grand mal epilepsy) is characterized by a behavioral arrest or sudden loss of consciousness. That is followed by tonic extension of the upper and lower extremities, then clonic, rhythmic jerking of the extremities. The jerking gradually decreases in frequency, leading to muscle flaccidity. The total duration of the ictus is usually two to five minutes. Associated features may include urinary and bowel incontinence, sweating, and tachycardia. Generalized absence or petit mal epilepsy is characterized by brief lapses of consciousness lasting 3 to 30 seconds. There are no associated tonic-clonic movements, nor is there loss of postural tone. There may be a slight rhythmical twitching of the mouth. Seizures can occur numerous times during the day. Absence seizures are common and occur primarily in children ages 4 to 12 years. In both types of generalized epilepsies there is amnesia for the epileptic event. Myoclonic epilepsy is characterized by nonrhythmic, brief jerks of the limbs, trunk, and head. Myoclonic jerks are asynchronous, with body parts jerking at different times and in different sequences, and there is no loss of consciousness. Myoclonic epilepsy is frequently of familial etiology, although it may be associated with brain injury or systemic disease that affects brain function, such as chronic renal disease or hepatic insufficiency.

Partial or focal seizures are distinguished by their localized site of origin. The symptomatology can be simple (elementary) or complex, with the latter characterized by some degree of impairment of consciousness. Partial seizures with elementary symptomatology include focal motor symptoms, focal sensory symptoms, autonomic symptoms, or mixed symptomatology; consciousness is retained throughout the episode, although the seizure discharges can spread to other areas of the brain (jacksonian march) and can also develop into a generalized seizure (secondary generalization). The postictal period may be characterized by a residual focal deficit, such as motor weakness (Todd's paralysis) or dysphasia. Secondary generalization may occur rapidly, giving the false impression of an immediate generalized seizure; videotaped monitoring with simultaneous EEG may be necessary for differentiation.

Partial complex seizures, also known as psychomotor seizures, temporal lobe seizures, or temporal-limbic seizures, are perhaps of greatest interest to psychiatry. The great majority of partial complex seizures originates in the temporal lobes, but the frontal lobes and other sites have also been recorded as seizure foci. The range of presenting symptomatology varies from patient to patient and may include a broad spectrum of disturbances in behavior, cognition, and affect. Auras are frequent in partial complex seizures, representing the focal onset, and it may be difficult to distinguish the aura from the ictus. Table 12-10 includes some common presentations for temporal lobe auras. They are generally associated with clouding of consciousness but retention of posture and muscle tone. The patient may exhibit simple or complex movements, such as pulling on clothing, buttoning or unbuttoning clothing, purposeless hand movements, and fumbling with objects, or may continue with the behavior initiated prior to the seizure, such as closing a window. There may be staring, lip smacking, and wandering. The actual ictus cannot be distinguished from the aura.

Psychiatrists should be familiar with the range of symptomatology associated with partial complex or temporal lobe epilepsy, as that disorder is an important diagnostic consideration in adult patients presenting with the new onset of behavioral

TABLE 12-10
Neuropsychiatric Manifestations (in the Aura and Ictus) of Focal Epilepsy

- Sensory
  - Headache
  - Focal pain
  - Paresthesia
- Motor
  - Nystagmus
  - Head turning
  - Scanning
  - Posturing
  - Stuttering
- Autonomic
  - Facial flushing
  - Hot flashes
  - Pallor
  - Dizziness
  - Chest pain
  - Tinnitus
- Perceptual
  - Micropsia, macropsia
  - Heightened auditory acuity
  - Derealization, depersonalization
  - Déjà vu, jamais vu
  - Hallucinations (visual, auditory, olfactory, gustatory, and tactile)
- Cognitive
  - Transient dysphasia
  - Speech automatisms
  - Subjective confusion
  - Obsessional thinking
  - Thought blocking
  - Distortion of time sense
- Affective
  - Fear
  - Anxiety
  - Sadness
  - Embarrassment
  - Placidity
  - Guilt
  - Anger
  - Joy
  - Elation
- Other
  - Genital sensations
  - Sexual behaviors

disturbances. In light of the protean possible manifestations of partial complex epilepsy, the physician must keep in mind that there is a general consistency to the form of partial complex seizures: They have a definite and observable onset and termination; they are always associated with impairment in consciousness, such as confusion or inability to perform cognitive tasks; and they are relatively stereotyped for an individual from episode to episode.

The postictal period may also be characterized by severe disturbances of behavior. Primary generalized tonic-clonic seizures are usually followed by a period of sleep, sometimes headache, and nausea. Focal or partial seizures may have residual focal deficits of varying duration. In partial complex seizures, recovery of consciousness may lag behind recovery of motor function. Frequently automatic behavior, such as repetitive mouth movements, arm movements, and pacing, can be observed. As the postictal period is essentially a delirious state, confusion and cognitive impairment remain. Any disturbance of mood is possible, including anger, lovingness, and the epileptic furor (random, typically nondirected displays of violence and property destruction). The postictal period usually lasts only minutes, although it may last hours to days.

Course Epilepsy has an annual incidence of approximately 20 to 50 new cases per 100,000 population. The prevalence is 0.2 to 1.0 percent. The majority of cases of epilepsy in patients older than 15 years are of the partial or focal type. Only approximately 25 percent of adolescents or adults over the age of 15 years with seizures have generalized epilepsy. Seizures with onset in childhood are more commonly generalized, particularly absence, seizures. Primary generalized tonic-clonic seizures usually occur for the first time before the age of 35 years, although they can occur at any age; absence seizures usually first manifest between the ages of 4 and 12 years. Focal seizures also have their onset commonly before the age of 20 years.

The natural history of seizure disorders has not been defined clearly. Up to one third of all seizures may remit spontaneously without treatment. Absence seizures are generally outgrown by the age of 20 years, although many patients do develop another form of generalized epilepsy as adults.

The etiological considerations for seizures vary with the age at onset. Early-onset epilepsy is usually a concomitant of genetic factors or an insult to the developing neural system in utero or in childhood. The latter can include trauma, infections, or toxic exposures. For seizures starting in adulthood, the etiological considerations include alcohol or drug withdrawal, trauma, infection, and tumors. The tumors are the primary causes of seizure disorders during the middle adult years. Cerebrovascular disease is the most common etiology among the elderly.

Psychopathology Psychopathology, namely disturbances in behavior, cognition, perception, or mood, can occur at any point in the seizure process. The prodrome may be characterized by a sense of irritability or apprehension. Families often report that they know when a relative is due to have a seizure on the basis of a change in temperament or disposition. Auras may include a variety of psychopathology, including dissociative experiences, hallucinations in all spheres, derealization, depersonalization, and disturbances of mood or affect. The disturbances of mood, such as a subjective sense of fear, anxiety, or depression, can be distinguished from normal expressions of the same emotion in that generally they are more crude, stereotyped, and brief emotional states. Joy, elation, or euphoria is less common. Ictal states can manifest striking changes in behavior that, again, are likely to be coarse and disorganized. The list of ictal manifestations in Table 12-10 includes a variety of hallucinations and dissociative experiences, as well as sudden and unpredictable shifts in mood. Other sensory or psychic experiences can occur out of their usual context (a classic case is reported of a woman who had spontaneous orgasms in church). The postictal state is a delirium that can display the full range of disturbances in level of arousal, ranging from stupor to hypervigilance. Partial seizures may be followed by a milder delirium that is detectable only from disorganization in behavior or difficulty with simple cognitive tasks such as registration and repetition. The issue of interictal psychopathology has been much studied and debated and will be discussed further below. In general, the psychiatric symptomatology associated with the prodrome, aura, ictus, and postictal state is remarkably broad—one may see virtually any thought, feeling, movement, or perception that the brain can produce. The clinician must be attentive to the form and course of these symptoms whenever considering epilepsy as a possible etiological explanation for abnormal behavior.

VIOLENCE AND AGGRESSION The issue of violence or aggression as a neuropsychiatric manifestation of an ictus has provoked much controversy. In the legal arena, epilepsy is occasionally invoked as a defense to mitigate culpability for a violent or even murderous act. Irritability or agitation can be a component of the prodrome, the aura and ictus can encompass angry affect and striking out, and the postictal state can manifest with fear and confusion with intact motor function. Although that might suggest the possibility of violent acts as a component of seizures, there is limited potential for such actions. Automatic acts of violence during epileptic seizures are short-lived, fragmentary, undirected, and most often occur in response to actions (such as attempts at restraint) that provoke or irritate the seizing individual. Examples include spitting, swearing, and striking out in a flailing fashion. For violence to be considered as a manifestation of epilepsy, it must conform to the known temporal sequence and symptomatology of a seizure; namely, there must be a clear onset and termination, together with other clinical signs (for example, confusion, incontinence, and impairment of consciousness) and stereotypy. A special 1981 epilepsy task force of the National Institute of Neurological and Communicative Disorders and Stroke (NINCDS), after studying videotapes of selected violent patients with epilepsy, recommended criteria to determine if a particular act of violence is ictal: (1) a clear diagnosis of epilepsy; (2) documented, preferably on videotape, automatisms; (3) documented aggression during the automatisms that corresponds to an EEG-proved ictus; (4) demonstration that the aggressive act is characteristic of the patient's usual seizure form; and (5) clinical consensus that the act was related to the actual seizure.

People with epilepsy have long been thought to display psychopathology during the interictal period as well. Epilepsy was thought to be a subtype or complication of insanity, and so was included in most psychiatric nosologies of the past two centuries. Epileptic patients typically were housed in asylums for the insane. In 1791 Philippe Pinel included among his recommendations for asylums the suggestion that other patients be shielded from epileptics because of their "almost always incurable" status and his sense that "few objects are found to inspire so much horror and repugnance . . . than the sight of epileptic fits." Griesinger stated that "a very great number of epileptics are in a state of chronic mental disease even during the intervals between the attacks." Interictal psychopathology can be grouped into psychotic disorders, mood disorders, personality abnormalities, cognitive disorders, and secondary repercussions.

PSYCHOTIC DISORDERS Jean Etienne Esquirol, in his 1845 description of female institutionalized epileptic patients, reported frequent psychotic symptoms, including hallucinations in all spheres: "They have hallucinations most varied . . . they think they see luminous bodies by which they fear they might be embraced . . . they smell odors the most fetid . . . they hear sounds like the bursting of a thunderbolt, the roll of drums, the clash of arms in the din of combat." Karl Jaspers, in *General Psychopathology*, classified epilepsy as one of the three major psychoses, along with schizophrenia and manic-depressive illness. He defined "genuine epilepsy" as "convulsive disorders which are not due to any known somatic process." Numerous studies have evaluated psychosis among epileptic patients. Unfortunately, most have been hampered by the lack of clear or standardized definitions for the symptoms being investigated. In addition, many studies have not distinguished between psychosis occurring in the context of the ictus, the prodrome, or the postictal state, and many have not indicated whether such symptoms were detected specifically during periods of interictal electrical stability. Few studies have discriminated between symptoms occurring in clear consciousness versus those occurring coincident with impaired consciousness.

Nonetheless, clinicians generally encounter a higher incidence of psychosis among epileptic patients, particularly those with temporal lobe foci, than in the general population. Some studies have specifically referred to paranoid ideation, delusions, ideas of reference, visual hallucinations, and first-rank auditory hallucinations as being common. Eliot Slater and A. W. Beard in 1963 identified an atypical schizophrenia, characterized by visual and auditory hallucinations, ideas of reference, and persecutory delusions, occurring in the context of preservation of affect and a level of social adaptation better than that of comparably psychotic schizophrenic patients. They further noted that the psychotic symptoms did not occur until many years after the onset of seizures (a mean of 14 years) and then occurred with an apparent periodicity. The occurrence of the psychotic episodes was unrelated both to the frequency of seizures and to measured anticonvulsant efficacy.

Although the true incidence or prevalence of psychotic disorders in epileptic patients is unknown, there is general consensus that the psychotic disorder seen in epilepsy is distinct in form from idiopathic psychiatric diseases and is characterized by the features described by Slater and Beard. Other associated findings may include an association between psychosis and left hemispheric seizure focus (especially in the temporal lobe), female sex, sinistrality, or tissue abnormality (alien tissue, such as hamartomas or focal dysplasia, is more commonly found at autopsy or after surgical excision in the psychotic patients). Those psychotic disturbances have been referred to as the schizophrenialike psychosis of epilepsy or the interictal psychosis of epilepsy. Standard antipsychotic medications are beneficial symptomatically but not as efficacious as in idiopathic psychotic disorders. Some studies have noted marked improvement in the psychotic symptoms with improved seizure control following either pharmacotherapy or surgical excision of the seizure focus. A smaller number of studies have reported an increase in psychotic symptoms occurring with improved seizure control, prompting a theory of antagonism between psychotic symptoms and seizure control.

The observation of a consistent psychotic disorder of increased prevalence in epileptic patients has led to an intense search for the underlying mechanism in the hope of describing a more general explanation for psychotic processes. Three hypothetical mechanisms for interictal psychoses have been advanced. The first hypothesis suggests that the schizophrenialike illness in epilepsy is epileptic in origin or related to abnormal electrical brain discharges. Kindling, an experimental animal model for the spread of epileptic foci, has been suggested as a paradigm for the development of psychosis in epilepsy. Chronic stimulation of the brain in animals can lower the electrical threshold for the development of electrical or clinical seizures. Over time, abnormal discharges develop at previously subthreshold levels of stimulation or even spontaneously. Abnormal behaviors associated with these experimentally induced brain discharges can also persist, even after stimulation has ceased and there are no motoric convulsions. It has been suggested that human kindling occurs at various brain foci, particularly the temporolimbic structures, resulting in psychotic and behavioral disturbances that may manifest only after years of seizure activity.

A second hypothesis for the development of interictal psychosis focuses on a proposed antagonistic relationship between seizure frequency (or, more accurately, EEG abnormality) and psychotic symptoms: *forced normalization* is the putative process by which a psychosis of sudden onset can manifest with the achievement of seizure control and associated with a normal cortical EEG. Studies of forced normalization have primarily involved case reports, and findings have been difficult to replicate. Clinical treatment regimens based on the antagonism theory, such as allowing episodic seizures or performing electroconvulsive therapy on psychotic epileptic patients, have proved ineffective, further weakening that proposal.

A third hypothesis to explain interictal psychosis suggests that it may not be related specifically to abnormal electrical activity but may instead reflect a common brain dysfunction that causes both epilepsy and psychosis. That hypothesis stresses the dysfunctional or broken brain inferred in epilepsy and regards the psychotic disorder as yet another symptomatic manifestation. Recent quantitative brain imaging studies in epileptic patients with psychotic disorders have not revealed consistent structural abnormalities within that patient group. However, specific symptom correlations have been reported, among them an increased frequency of temporal lobe structural abnormalities in epileptic patients with auditory hallucinations. Similar findings associating specific psychotic symptoms with defined cerebral abnormalities have also been reported in other psychiatric populations (for example, schizophrenia). Further symptom-based research utilizing imaging and physiologically sensitive techniques may better delineate the brain regions where dysfunction can lead to particular psychotic symptoms.

MOOD DISORDERS Affective changes can occur as part of the seizure prodrome, aura, ictus, or postictal state. Irritability is a common prodromal manifestation. Temporal lobe auras may be accompanied by mood abnormalities, most commonly fear and anxiety, although a depressive affect is possible and, more rarely, elation or euphoria. Descriptions of postictal sadness are common. All of those affective changes are generally brief, lasting minutes to hours. They differ both from normally experienced vacillations in mood, in that they occur independent of any particular context, and from the pervasive and enduring affective changes found in primary mood disorders.

Mood disorders in the interictal period have not been studied as comprehensively as psychotic or personality disorders. Many authors have noted that epileptic patients have a strong tendency to endorse items of sadness and anxiety on self-report inventories. Few studies have used clinical examinations or standardized interviews to determine the presence of mood disorders such as major depressive disorder or bipolar disorder. One study of epileptic patients diagnosed with major depressive disorder found that at least half of the patients had family histories of mood disorder and that no clear relation existed between severity of depression and seizure type, seizure frequency, seizure focus, or age at seizure onset. Although definitive studies of the incidence and prevalence of clinically defined mood disorders in epilepsy are needed, there is less support overall (compared with psychosis) for an elevated prevalence of mood disorders in epileptic patient populations. Many patients do express persisting dysphoria, perhaps reflecting the dissatisfaction and maladjustment associated with a chronic disease.

Regardless of the etiology of the dysphoria or dissatisfaction in epileptic patients, there is an increased prevalence of suicide attempts and completed suicides. The incidence of suicide in patients with epilepsy is fivefold greater than in the general population. In patients with temporal lobe epilepsy the incidence of suicide increases to 25 times that of the general population, but the underlying psychopathology remains to be defined.

PERSONALITY CHANGE There has been a long-standing misperception that an epileptic personality is distinguishable and common. Esquirol noted in his studies of 385 female epileptic patients that "only one fifth were free from intellectual derangement, but nearly all of these were irritable, peculiar, and easily enraged." Griesinger commented on the "dominant, suspicious, discontented, misanthropic perversion of sentiment . . . observed in many epileptics." Eugen Bleuler spoke of the "epileptic excess of emotion . . . easily aroused, remarkably persistent . . . difficulty in abandoning any particular thought . . . fixation to a single theme . . . precise attention to detail." Jaspers described "viscosity, slowing down, explosiveness and dementia" as characteristic of epileptic patients. Those characterizations were frequently based on chronically institutionalized patient populations representing a selection of the most severely impaired patients, in whom the effects of brain injury (especially related to repeated seizures, status epilepticus, and recurrent hypoxia), deprivations of institutionalization, and toxic treatments undoubtedly confounded clinical observation. More recent attempts at detecting a recognizable, diagnosable personality disorder in community samples of epileptic patients resulted neither in the description of a discrete personality syndrome nor in a higher prevalence of known personality disorders.

Because standard personality inventories have not uncovered specific abnormalities in epileptic populations, some researchers have focused on particular traits or behaviors. An interictal behavior syndrome of temporal lobe epilepsy has been described that encompasses four traits or behaviors: (1) altered sexuality, usually a decreased interest in sexual matters but at times involving hypersexuality or deviant sexual interests; (2) hyperreligiosity, described as an unusually deepened interest in moral affairs and matters of global importance, with vivid case descriptions of multiple religious conversions and intrusive polemicizing; (3) hypergraphia, with patients maintaining voluminous writings, including journals, essays, and novels; and (4) viscosity or stickiness, a characteristic described for more than a century, including a preoccupation with detail, digressive or overly inclusive speech, and resulting impairments in social discourse.

Although the literature supporting such a personality syndrome is rich with clinical case histories, systematic study to define such a syndrome has been difficult to replicate. Investigators using an 18-point inventory of those behaviors found they could not distinguish epileptic patients from other psychiatric populations or patients with temporal lobe from those with generalized epilepsy. Thus, the bulk of data suggests that the clinical complex of overinclusiveness in speech, interpersonal action, and writing; alteration of sexuality; and intensified emotion and cognition (hypercosmiscity) is rare and not specific for temporal lobe epilepsy. However, isolated features of this cluster may be more common among patients with temporal lobe epilepsy. When the entire picture is encountered clinically in the absence of a readily apparent seizure disorder, the clinician may wish to pursue a more intensive evaluation if the patient fails to respond to standard psychiatric therapies.

COGNITIVE DISORDERS An early view of epilepsy considered it a degenerative disorder with a progressive deterioration in cognition, similar to that seen in the degenerative dementias. Modern prospective studies, however, have disproved this belief and have demonstrated no progressive decline in cognitive skills in a general population of epileptic patients. A subpopulation of epileptic patients does demonstrate a lower I.Q. spread than the normal distribution. That likely results from a combination of factors, including the original brain damage or dysfunction responsible for the epilepsy, occasional disruption attributable to the seizure disorder, and drug effects. Numerous anticonvulsants, including ethosuximide (zarontin), phenytoin (Dilantin), phenobarbital, and carbamazepine (Tegretol), have been demonstrated to lower performance on tasks of concentration, memory, and motor speed. (The last is least impaired.) Epileptic dementia, while certainly uncommon, has been described in patients with defined CNS lesions or uncontrolled seizures. It probably reflects the cumulative effect of frequent seizure-induced hypoxic episodes and perhaps toxicity from long-standing treatment with high dosages of anticonvulsants. Phenytoin, in particular, has been demonstrated to cause cerebellar degeneration with chronic use.

BEHAVIORAL AND SECONDARY REPERCUSSIONS Despite a less glamorous research appeal, the more compelling and clinically demanding aspects of interictal function may be the behavioral, interpersonal, and social problems arising from irritability, agitation, or aggression. There are no well-defined, systematic, or tested approaches to treating those behavioral difficulties when they arise. It was long believed that maladaptive behavior, particularly aggressive behavior, as characterized by physical assaultiveness, destructiveness, and self-injury, was more common in epileptic patients. Recent methodologically rigorous studies, however, demonstrated that maladaptive behavior does not correlate with the presence of epilepsy when epileptic populations are compared with appropriately matched controls. Maladaptive behavior is, however, related to the overall extent of brain damage, in both epileptic and nonepileptic populations. That important point cannot be overemphasized: Epilepsy is a florid manifestation of a physiologically abnormal brain, and in most instances, the fundamental CNS dysfunction that causes seizures also causes associated neuropsychiatric abnormalities.

Especially among severely afflicted epileptic patients, obstacles to effective social functioning and personal autonomy pose the greatest therapeutic challenges for clinicians and families. Epileptic patients may not receive adequate education, as seizures may interfere with daily school attendance. Patients may be restricted from many occupations owing to employers' fears of patients sustaining injury in the workplace. Limitations on driving can markedly diminish the independent functioning of an epileptic patient. Many epileptic patients are compelled to remain dependent on family, even into adulthood.

PSEUDOSEIZURES Pseudoseizures simulate the motor behavior of true seizures but do not involve abnormal electrical discharges. Pseudoseizures can be distinguished from true seizures by the form of the seizure and by the lack of the usual associated features. The form does not fit the known patterns for epileptic attacks and can consist of random flailing about. Furthermore, the form can be variable from seizure to seizure, lacking the stereotypy typical of true seizures. Incontinence and tongue biting are rare. There is minimal confusion at the conclusion of the episode, and no abnormalities are detected on neurological examination. EEG can be helpful in distinguishing pseudoseizures, especially if one can be obtained during an event and then studied for evidence of electrical discharges that would correspond with the motor behavior. An EEG obtained after a true seizure should demonstrate areas of slowing that would not be seen after a pseudoseizure. Serum prolactin levels increase markedly immediately after a seizure and can be helpful in distinguishing true seizures from pseudoseizures. Video EEG telemetry is the definitive means of determining whether an observed seizure is epileptic in origin or a pseudoseizure.

Pseudoseizures are more likely in patients who suppress emotion or express emotion through somatic means. Pseudoseizures are conversion disorders in which the patient does not have conscious volitional control of the behavior; rarely are pseudoseizures the result of faking or malingering. Pseudoseizures often occur in patients who have true epileptic disorders, confounding the diagnosis. W. Alwyn Lishman has aptly noted that the diagnostic error of interpreting epilepsy as pseudoseizures is probably much more common than the obverse and far more detrimental to the patient's well-being. The diagnosis of pseudoseizures rests not on the presence of any particular personality traits or identifiable psychosocial stressors, but rather on the form of the seizure, associated features, and EEG confirmation.

PRIMARY PSYCHIATRIC DISORDERS The presence of intellectual deficits, whether identified with bedside procedures or on standardized neuropsychological tests, does not automatically warrant the diagnosis of a cognitive impairment disorder. Neuropsychological abnormalities occur frequently in many patient populations. Once neglected or considered epiphenomena of more central emotional disturbances, cognitive processing deficits are now known to be key components of clinical disorders such as major depressive disorder (especially in the elderly), acute and chronic schizophrenia, chronic alcohol dependence, and perhaps obsessive-compulsive disorder. Cognitive impairment disorders, such as dementia or delirium, or secondary psychiatric syndromes are all caused by specific disease processes; vigilant diagnostic evaluation usually leads to detection of a primary systemic or cerebral disturbance.

Difficulties may arise when the etiological disturbance is presumed but cannot be proved, as in the case of Alzheimer's disease, where the definite diagnosis must await postmortem brain examination. When a patient has both a major depressive syndrome and clinical findings consistent with incipient dementia of the Alzheimer's type, it may not be possible to determine immediately the fundamental disturbance being evaluated. Such confusing situations typically arise with the near simultaneous onset of both symptom clusters or in patients who have experienced major depressive disorder previously. They call for careful definition of symptoms, initiation of therapy for all potentially treatable conditions, and serial monitoring of the patient's responses. Documentation of the longer-term course also assists in disentangling and recognizing separately contributing disease processes.

Despite careful observation and follow-up evaluation, the clinician may remain uncertain whether a syndrome is idiopathic or secondary to other detected diseases. In such instances, it is preferable to diagnose a primary psychiatric condition on Axis I, define all systemic or cerebral conditions on Axis III, and thereafter maintain a high order of vigilance while monitoring the course of the disorder longitudinally. It is important to note questions or uncertainties in the medical record for later scrutiny, for that practice avoids premature diagnostic closure.

Clinicians must also guard against willingness to provide a psychiatric diagnosis when specialists from other medical disciplines have ruled out specific disease processes after laboratory tests have been unrevealing. The failure to define an organic disease does not warrant a functional diagnosis by default. As emphasized in DSM-III and now DSM-IV, specific clinical signs, symptoms, and course are needed to establish the presence of a primary psychiatric disorder.

METABOLIC DISORDERS Because most systemic medical conditions can directly or indirectly affect brain function, any list of illnesses that may cause a secondary psychiatric syndrome or cognitive disorder must be incomplete. Table 12-11 lists some frequently described potential etiologies, arranged by admittedly arbitrary categories.

The precise pathophysiological mechanisms by which the disease process alters brain function are poorly understood in most cases. More than one process may be involved. For example, a patient with acute myelogenous leukemia may have altered brain function due to the neoplastic process itself, anemia (with decreased oxygen delivery to the brain), brain hemorrhages (due to thrombocytopenia), and infections.

Secondary psychiatric syndromes may be the first, most prominent, or only clinical phenomena to call attention to the underlying condition (for example, depression due to occult pancreatic carcinoma and cognitive deficits due to vitamin B_{12} deficiency even in the absence of other neurological or hematological signs). Secondary behavioral changes may also be due

TABLE 12-11
Metabolic and Other Systemic Disturbances

Endocrine
- Hypo- or hyperthyroidism
- Hypo- or hyperparathyroidism
- Sex hormones—too little, too much, or cycle-related
- Hypo- or hypercortisolemia
- Pheochromocytoma
- Diabetes mellitus
- Carcinoid syndrome

Pulmonary
- Hypoxemia
- Hypercarbia
- Infections (pneumonia, bronchiectasis, abscess)
- Restrictive lung diseases
- Obstructive lung diseases
- Tumors

Hematologic
- Anemia
- Polycythemia
- Neoplasms

Hepatic
- Liver failure due to any etiology

Renal
- Renal failure due to any etiology
- Infections
- Neoplasms

Nutrition
- Marasmus
- Kwashiorkor
- Vitamin deficiencies (thiamine, niacin, B_{12}, folate)
- Dehydration

Miscellaneous
- Hypo- and hyperelectrolyte disturbances (especially sodium, potassium, phosphate, calcium, magnesium)
- Hypo- and hyperglycemia
- Acidemia
- Alkalemia
- Porphyria

to multiple etiologies, of which any one alone might or might not be sufficient to produce the psychiatric disturbance (for example, delirium due to mild anemia, mild hyponatremia, and marginal hypoxemia). The rate of change may also be important with certain etiologies. For example, a sudden drop in serum sodium to 125 mEq/L is more likely to produce behavioral changes than a chronic hyponatremia of 125 mEq/L.

Etiologies particularly identified with specific psychiatric syndromes are discussed below under each syndrome. However, most etiologies can produce more than one syndrome (for example, hypothyroidism is most often associated with a depressive state but may also cause mania, delirium, or dementia). How a specific etiology causes varied behavioral changes presumably depends on both trait-dependent and state-dependent brain diatheses that largely are not understood.

DEMYELINATING DISORDERS With regard to secondary psychiatric syndromes, multiple sclerosis (MS) is the most important demyelinating disorder. Although MS may cause delirium, dementia, and nonaffective psychoses, mood disturbances have been described frequently. Isolated, persistent euphoria has long been noted and is thought to be physiologically related to demyelinated lesions in the limbic system, frontal lobes, and basal ganglia. Emotional incontinence, also termed pathological laughing or weeping, is a state of labile affective expression that is apparently disconnected from underlying mood. Although pathophysiological mechanisms remain uncertain, it is speculated that interruption of pathways between the telencephalon and lower regions is responsible.

Depressive syndromes are especially prevalent in MS. Most studies have focused on major depressive disorder or have not used specific diagnostic criteria; therefore, little is known about minor or other subsyndromal depressions. Some data suggest that depressive syndromes can be caused directly by the demyelinating process in specific CNS regions; for example, patients with cerebral disease have higher rates of depression than patients with spinal MS. However, there is also evidence implicating psychological and social factors in the pathogenesis of depression in MS patients, and it is likely that many depressive syndromes seen in these patients are not secondary or specifically symptomatic of cerebral disease.

Bipolar syndromes are less well studied, although they appear to be more prevalent in MS populations than in the general population. Whether bipolar syndromes in MS patients represent true secondary bipolar disorders, mania induced by treatments with corticosteroids, or manifestations of a shared genetic diathesis is not known.

Other demyelinating disorders include variants of acute encephalomyelitis (including postinfectious encephalomyelitis and acute posttraumatic demyelinization). Those disorders generally manifest initially with coma or delirium, and survivors may have lasting cognitive and behavioral disturbances.

The treatment of psychiatric syndromes in demyelinating disorders, as for most secondary syndromes, is empirical and based on target symptoms (for example, antipsychotic agents for psychosis). Studies suggest that antidepressant medications, when used in conjunction with supportive psychotherapy, are helpful in patients with MS. Tricyclic antidepressants, and possibly other classes of antidepressants, reduce MS-associated emotional incontinence even in the absence of a full depressive syndrome.

DEGENERATIVE DISEASES Degenerative disease processes involve deterioration of brain function resulting in the loss of previously attained capacities. Some degree of CNS degeneration occurs as part of the aging process and is reflected in alterations in gross brain structure; neuronal cell number, morphology, and function; and neurotransmitter synthesis, metabolism, and function. The degeneration manifests clinically with psychometrically definable cognitive declines, particularly in secondary or long-term memory, speed of mental processing, visuospatial processing, divided attention, and cognitive flexibility. A range of decrements is associated with normal aging, and clinicians and investigators are developing neuropsychological procedures that distinguish such normative processes from those associated with degenerative diseases. Indeed, DSM-IV includes age-related cognitive decline (Section 49.4c) as a clinical condition that may be a focus for clinical attention although it is not a mental disorder. That allows physicians to explain to concerned healthy patients that their aging-associated decrements in cognitive processing are distinctive from incipient dementia. (Other similar conditions include problems, such as borderline mental functioning or bereavement.)

Nonetheless, the border between normative cognitive changes and incipient dementia is ill-defined. Patients who present with acquired deficits below the normal range are at higher risk statistically of developing progressive problems. However, cross-sectional cognitive tests cannot reveal time of onset, and in some individuals test results are always below normal. Conversely, people with above average intellectual abilities may experience cognitive decline without exhibiting objective deficits, for their performance remains within normal limits despite obvious functional impairments.

Degenerative CNS diseases can produce disturbances in cognition, mood, behavior, personality, and motor and perceptual function. In recent years investigators have more clearly defined that the major degenerative diseases (whether hereditary or idiopathic) reflect deterioration in specific or discrete neurochemical systems, where there is as well a regional specificity that reflects the location of both cell bodies and their ultimate terminal zones. Such diseases are best considered neurochemical system diseases. Their general pattern is one of insidious onset with a gradual progression of deficits. Dementia is the most common syndromic presentation and worsens as a reflection of the chronic progressive process; it ultimately reflects widespread CNS disease. Secondary mood, psychotic, and personality syndromes are also seen but are more likely to manifest earlier in the course, when the degeneration may be more localized.

Cortical and subcortical dementia Degenerative CNS diseases can be distinguished clinically from one another by the relative impairment and sparing of various cognitive and behavioral functions. Two basic clinical patterns of dementia have been characterized clinically, cortical and subcortical. The cortical pattern of dementia is characterized by impairments in memory (primarily a storage and recall deficit) and gnostic-practic abilities (primarily involving language, visuospatial abilities, calculation, and motor praxis). Executive functions such as organization, judgment, abstraction, and insight are similarly affected. Fine and gross motor movements are generally preserved until later in the disease course. Personality often remains intact or displays subtle variations, with patients becoming more passive or less spontaneous, or becoming coarse and crude in their interactions. With disease progression the changes in personality become more common and pronounced. Affective expression is generally preserved, although again a coarsening may be noted in the form of emotional lability. Early in the disease, patients frequently discern and express dismay about their intellectual decline.

The subcortical pattern is characterized by a generalized slowing of mental processing. Specific cognitive skills, such as calculation, naming, or copying are less affected initially, in contrast to their early decline in the cortical degenerative processes. Verbal and visual memory impairment may be present early in the course, although such impairment more often takes the form of forgetfulness or a failure of retrieval that is initially amenable to prompting, in contrast to the more severe recall deficits in cortical dementia. Patients also show deficits in learning new motor movements or complex psychomotor procedures. Planning and organizational skills are disrupted. Abnormal movements are common and manifest as a slowing and awkwardness in normal movement or as the intrusion of such extraneous movements as chorea or tremor. In contrast to the early impairment of language function in cortical disease, language is relatively spared, although the motor production of speech may be abnormal. The personality change is often marked, with striking patterns of apathy, inertia, and diminished spontaneity. Mood disorders, including major depressive disorder and mania, occur frequently. The presenting symptoms in subcortical degenerative processes may be those of a personality change or a mood disorder at a time when cognitive impairment or motor dysfunction is not yet obvious. In the cortical processes, by contrast, the presenting symptoms more often reflect cognitive impairment, particularly memory and language dysfunction. As the dementia (and, presumably, the degenerative process) progresses, the clinical presentations of cortical and subcortical diseases become nearly indistinguishable from one another.

The term ''subcortical dementia'' was first used to describe the cognitive and behavioral deficits seen in patients with Huntington's disease. A similar clinical pattern was soon described for other subcortical diseases, such as progressive supranuclear palsy and Parkinson's disease. Although the term was initially used in reference to a clinical picture that could be localized to the subcortex, subcortical dementia is now considered a pseudoanatomical designation. It is clear from imaging and neuropathological studies that cortical dementia (for example, Alzheimer's disease) is not restricted pathologically to the cortex; major affected cholinergic fiber pathways are subcortical in origin. Subcortical diseases similarly affect regions outside the subcortex, especially the frontal lobes, because of the brain's robust frontal-subcortical connections. Moreover, failure of subcortical nuclei that directly receive cortical efferent pathways can lead to clinical symptoms whose cerebral level of origin cannot be differentiated. Nonetheless, the cortical-subcortical distinction has been of clinical utility in defining patterns of cognitive, behavioral, mood, personality, and motor impairment, especially in the early stages of the degenerative disease process.

ALZHEIMER'S DISEASE Alzheimer's disease is the prototype of a cortical degenerative disease. Alois Alzheimer's original description in 1906 detailed most of the familiar clinical and neuropathological features. Of note, his patient suffered from paranoia in addition to cognitive decline. Currently, the diagnosis of Alzheimer's disease requires neuropathological confirmation, and the diagnosis of dementia of the Alzheimer's type is used clinically for cases identified antemortem. Age at onset is earlier in patients with a family history of Alzheimer's disease. Despite some data to suggest distinctive age-related clinical patterns, no phenomenological separation between early-onset and late-onset cases has been found consistently enough for age to substitute for detailed clinical description; however, early-onset Alzheimer's disease may have a more rapidly progressive course. A major component of the presenting symptoms is usually subjective complaints of memory difficulty, language impairment (''I can't find the word''), and dyspraxia (for example, difficulty driving). Diagnosis at that juncture is primarily based on exclusion of other possible etiologies for dementia. No features of the physical examination or laboratory evaluation are pathognomonic for dementia of the Alzheimer's type. Some studies have apparently discriminated patients with dementia of the Alzheimer's type from patients with dementia of other etiologies and from normal controls by using techniques such as EEG, MRI, and SPECT. Those studies have been difficult to replicate consistently, and at present, brain imaging studies are best used to exclude other identifiable etiologies. Indeed, available technological diagnostic methods have not proved more sensitive and specific than astute clinical evaluation in comparisons of patients with dementia of the Alzheimer's type and healthy control subjects. PET holds promise but currently is too costly for clinical diagnostic use.

A variety of diagnostic criteria sets have been developed for dementia of the Alzheimer's type and Alzheimer's disease. Clinical criteria have been verified prospectively in autopsy studies and have been found to be highly specific, although only moderately sensitive. Implementation of the criteria requires extensive evaluation, including an informant-based history, neurological examination, neuropsychological testing, and laboratory and neuroimaging data.

Alzheimer's disease is characterized pathologically by neurofibrillary tangles, neuritic (amyloid) plaques, and granulovacuolar degeneration. Although plaques and tangles may be detected in the brains of the nondemented elderly, they are more numerous in patients with dementia. In recent years investigators have attempted to circumvent the qualitative overlap in symptoms by developing stricter quantitative, age-adjusted pathological criteria for Alzheimer's disease. A definitive diagnosis ultimately requires both the characteristic dementia in life and the characteristic pathology after death. Occasionally, in patients with apparent dementia of the Alzheimer's type the expected pathology is not found at autopsy; conversely, autopsy studies of neurologically intact elderly samples reveal cases of Alzheimerlike pathology in the absence of clinical signs of dementia during life.

During recent years substantial effort has been devoted to the study of the pathobiology of Alzheimer's disease. Major efforts of fundamental neuroscientists have focused on the molecular biology of dementia of the Alzheimer's type, with the identification of at least two chromosomal loci associated with familial cases; the degeneration of central neurochemical systems, especially basal forebrain structures related to acetylcholine-mediated neurotransmission; factors associated with the formation of plaques and tangles; and exogenous (for example, infectious and toxic) processes that may contribute to the development of sporadic cases. Molecular biologists have sought to understand the formation of the abnormal amounts of amyloid that constitute the cerebral plaques characteristic of the disease. While amyloid itself is a normal brain product, some suggest that excessive amounts may be neurotoxic, perhaps disrupting mechanisms that maintain normal intracellular potassium levels, whereas others see amyloid accumulations solely as a disease byproduct. Attention has recently turned to amyloid precursor protein and the intriguing possibility of regulating amyloid production pharmacologically. The recent discovery of an association between apolipoprotein E4, controlled by a gene located on chromosome 19, and late-onset cases suggests further avenues for investigating risk factors and pathogenetic mechanisms. Taken together, those recent findings point to a heterogeneous array of pathobiological processes contributing to the final clinical and histological picture known as Alzheimer's disease: The postmortem and antemortem presentations may be relatively generalized (that is, nonspecific) outcomes of widely divergent etiologies.

The natural course of dementia of the Alzheimer's type, as of all the degenerative disorders, is exacerbation and progression of clinical symptomatology. Brain degeneration as measured by in vivo imaging techniques such as MRI has not been found to correlate closely with the state of clinical disease. The final common clinical picture of Alzheimer's disease is of a bedridden patient, wholly dependent on others for all basic functions, even turning in bed. Nutrition can often be provided only by nasogastric or gastrointestinal tubes. Death usually results from aspiration or from infectious processes associated with prolonged recumbency.

PARKINSON'S DISEASE Parkinson's disease, described by James Parkinson in 1817, is a prototype of a subcortical degenerative disease. Parkinson's disease is idiopathic and must be distinguished from parkinsonian syndromes that arise from a variety of etiologies.

Parkinson's disease is the result of the degeneration of subcortical structures, primarily the substantia nigra but also the globus pallidus, putamen, and caudate. Cells containing dopamine are predominantly affected, although serotonergic and other systems are disrupted as well. Just as the appellation "cortical pattern" is pseudoanatomical, so in subcortical Parkinson's disease there can be significant degeneration of cortical structures. The parkinsonian syndrome manifests with structural damage that reflects the underlying process or insult. Drug-related parkinsonism presumably involves only a dysfunction of the basal ganglia structures, without any obvious pathoanatomical abnormality. The typical age at onset of Parkinson's disease is between 50 and 60 years but may vary widely, with onset sometimes occurring one to two decades earlier. The clinical course is chronic and progressive, with severe disability attained after approximately 10 years. A smaller proportion of patients have a more rapidly progressive disease, and a yet smaller group has a slowly progressive disorder in which deterioration plateaus or remains minimal for two to three decades.

In general, subcortical diseases are thought to impinge on the three Ms—movement, mentation, and mood. In Parkinson's disease all three of those areas are affected, although not always uniformly. The movement abnormalities are characterized by the triad of tremor, rigidity, and bradykinesia. The tremor and rigidity can be unilateral or bilateral. Bradykinesia is manifested by slowness in the initiation and execution of movement. The typical presentation, with a masklike facies, minimal blink, and monotonic speech, is a concomitant of the rigidity and slowness of movement. Other prominent characteristics include postural changes such as chin-to-chest flexion and gait abnormalities. The gait is characteristically slow and shuffling, and the patient has difficulty turning (en bloc turning) and trouble initiating and stopping walking. Seborrhea, sialorrhea, excessive fatigue, and constipation are also common.

Mentation or cognition in Parkinson's disease is an area of controversy. Most patients complain of slowed thinking, called bradyphrenia by some. In general, approximately 20 to 30 percent of patients with Parkinson's disease are found to be demented, with the likelihood greater in those with late-onset disease (after age 70 years). Approximately 40 percent of nondemented patients with Parkinson's disease, however, demonstrate some neuropsychological impairment in most studies. The impairments are primarily in visuospatial capacities, as measured by copying, tracing, and tracking tasks, and in the shifting of cognitive sets, as measured by the Wisconsin Card Sorting Test or the Stroop Test. Such deficits have been noted in the absence of cognitive-based functional decline or other evidence of cognitive impairment. Controversy has emerged over whether those two patterns represent a single continuum of dementia integral to the process of Parkinson's disease or are two separate processes indicative of two distinct diseases. Neuropathologically, cases intermediate between Parkinson's disease and Alzheimer's disease exist, with the characteristic microscopic features of the latter and Lewy bodies in the substantia nigra suggesting the former. There is no clear line of division as yet between a process resembling dementia of the Alzheimer's type on which abnormal parkinsonian movements are superimposed and a clinical presentation of Parkinson's disease in which the patient slowly develops a global progressive dementia.

Mood disorders have been frequently reported in association with Parkinson's disease. Depression is the most common; mania is virtually unreported. The mean frequency of depression is approximately 40 percent, with a reported range of 4 to 70 percent. No relation has been demonstrated between the frequency and severity of depression and the patient's current age, the age at onset of symptoms of Parkinson's disease, the duration of those symptoms, the severity of motor signs, or the response to medication. No relation has been demonstrated among mood, rigidity, bradykinesia, or tremor. Although depression has been found more commonly in patients with Parkinson's disease who display prominent gait and postural changes, the relation between mood and the severity of the disability is limited. There may be some association between depression and laterality of disease, for patients with left brain disease appear to have a higher frequency of depression than patients with right brain disease. That pattern suggests that the mood disturbance is a primary manifestation of brain deterioration and not a reactive psychological response to chronic illness and disability. Although the evidence relating lateralization to a higher frequency of depression is preliminary, it does recall data regarding poststroke depression and its putative relationship to left hemisphere localization but not to the extent of disability. The phenomenology of depression in Parkinson's disease is similar to that of idiopathic major depressive disorder, for it includes subjective dysphoria, pessimism, irritability, and suicidality, but perhaps less self-disparagement and self-blame. Some patients present with anxiety or panic attacks. Of note, anergia, psychomotor retardation, and early morning awakening are three symptoms that have been found to be nonspecific for depressive disorder in those patients, as they overlap considerably with the manifestations found in nondepressed patients with Parkinson's disease. Some data support the view that the depression of Parkinson's disease is associated specifically with decreased CNS serotonin levels. The on-off syndrome, in which patients experience severe fluctuations in mobility ranging from normal movement to a frozen state, has also been associated with changes in mood. On-off phenomena usually occur after years of chronic treatment with levodopa (Larodopa, Dopar) and can manifest as a between-dosage effect or randomly throughout the day. Many studies have reported changes in mood coincident with changes in motoric function, namely, subjective and objective dysphoria in the off period and, less frequently, abnormal elation and euphoria during the on period.

Psychosis as a concomitant of Parkinson's disease has been reported primarily in the context of mood disorders or as a consequence of treatment. There are no reports of a specific personality change characteristic of Parkinson's disease except for the apparent apathy and lack of initiative that are often subsumed under bradykinesia and bradyphrenia.

The pharmacological treatment of Parkinson's disease addresses mood and movement, as there is no known regimen for the improvement of cognition. For movement dysfunction dopamine precursors, such as levodopa or levodopa-carbidopa (Sinemet), are a mainstay of treatment. Gait, posture, rigidity, and akinesia are generally more responsive to levodopa than is tremor. Anticholinergic agents and the dopamine agonists (bromocriptine [Parlodel] and pergolide [Permax]) are second-line agents. Recently, a monoamine oxidase (MAO) B inhibitor, selegiline (Eldepryl), was demonstrated to apparently slow the progression of motor dysfunction, although in the low doses used it did not have significant antidepressant efficacy. Its effects on the development of cognitive impairment are unknown. All symptomatic antiparkinsonian agents can cause delirium, a common iatrogenic concomitant of the disease. Levodopa has also been reported to cause visual hallucinations in some patients, even in the absence of delirium. Surgical treatments—stereotactic lesioning of the thalamus or globus pallidus—were used in the past to alleviate the motoric dysfunction of Parkinson's disease. Although that approach has largely been replaced by pharmacological treatment, newer more precise operative procedures have been developed in the past few years. Transplantation of fetal neural tissue into the caudate of the adrenal medulla also has been attempted, but no data from well-controlled studies are available regarding the effects of the procedure on mood and mentation. Recent findings suggest that fetal tissue transplantation may dramatically alleviate severe motor symptoms. Many differences exist in surgical protocols and transplantation methods, underscoring the highly experimental nature of those procedures.

Treatment of the mood disorder associated with Parkinson's disease involves the same agents that have proved valuable in treating idiopathic major depressive order. Antidepressants from all categories have proved efficacious. ECT is of value for treating both the mood component and the motor dysfunction; dramatic improvement in all aspects of movement has been demonstrated on standardized neurological examinations. Several studies have reported sustained improvement in motor function for as long as six months after treatment; however, most detected a short-lived improvement of days to weeks. ECT is recommended for patients with Parkinson's disease and the on-off syndrome, particularly when there are significant mood changes associated.

In summary, Parkinson's disease is a prototypical subcortical pattern degenerative disease. The overlap of clinical phenomena between a basal ganglia disease, such as Parkinson's disease, and major depressive disorder can be striking. Both are characterized by qualitatively similar impairments in the realms of movement, mentation, and mood. Differing terminologies have arisen to describe similar signs and symptoms in each. Psychomotor slowing or retardation, terms used to encompass both the motoric and cognitive slowing seen in depression, are quite similar to the bradykinesia and bradyphrenia described early in the course of Parkinson's disease. A recent study that used a nonmotor measure of bradyphrenia demonstrated close correlations between cognitive slowing and severity of the mood disorder in both depressed patients with Parkinson's disease and patients with idiopathic major depressive disorder, suggesting a close phenomenological relation between the bradyphrenia of Parkinson's disease and so-called psychomotor slowing. It underscored the idea that basal ganglia disorders are fertile ground for research and insight into the neurobiological bases of idiopathic mood disorders.

SUBSTANCE-INDUCED DISORDERS Pharmacological compounds are potent and frequent causes of psychopathology. That effect, especially when caused by environmental and occupational neurotoxins, has been little studied; more attention has been paid to peripheral or motor effects than to the less easily quantified behavioral alterations. Although alcohol-induced neuropsychiatric syndromes have long been known, the CNS consequences of abuse of recreational drugs received attention only in recent decades, in part because of societal disapproval of recreational drug use, disinterest among investigators, and the inherent difficulty of separating drug effects from confounding person effects.

Broadly speaking, there are four classes of chemically induced psychopathology: (1) that due to environmental contamination, both natural (for example, venoms and poisonous foods) and human-made (gasoline contamination of well water); (2) that due to occupational exposure; (3) that due to recreational use, abuse, or dependence on substances causing transient or lasting CNS toxic effects; and (4) the iatrogenic complications of prescribed or over-the-counter medications. Compounds must be considered from the perspectives of (1) acute or immediate effects (for example, behavioral symptoms of acute intoxication), (2) longer-term responses to persistent exposure, and (3) lasting consequences that persist after the cessation of any direct pharmacological action. The last may be especially complex because of the extremely prolonged retention (months to years) of some compounds within the body.

When considering the possibility of drug- or toxin-induced

psychopathology, the clinician must undertake a careful chain of reasoning, akin to deciding on any secondary diagnosis but differing in several respects. Initially, the clinician must ascertain whether an exposure occurred and at what level. For example, an industrial hygienist may have been exposed in a possible occupational incident. Next, it is critical to understand the toxicity of a substance (especially as it might relate to different chemical forms), its mode of action (when known), its effects in various animal species, and its clinical manifestations. Typically, those issues are within the realm of toxicologists. Subsequently, the clinician seeks to define the systemic clinical manifestations of the exposure in the particular patient. Although behavioral changes may be the only exposure-related findings, more often there is a variety of consistent symptoms, signs, and laboratory findings that together make a coherent clinical picture. It is within that larger context that the clinician views any presumptively related psychopathology.

Ideally, one would like to know the neuropsychiatric effects of all CNS toxic compounds. In the absence of such information, the clinician must describe symptoms and signs in detail and compare them with available data. The clinician defines the temporal course of exposure and assesses how the emergence of specific psychiatric manifestations relates to known actions of the compounds in question. Simultaneously, the clinician must consider the form of the disorder and establish whether it suggests a pathological CNS process or is more consistent with primary (idiopathic) psychopathology. The clinician must decide whether the syndrome in question might reflect other unrelated disease processes as well. Any measurable clinical and laboratory manifestations of CNS disease should be identified. Although no single measurement equates with proof, taken together such measurements offer the possibility of establishing a diagnosis with a high degree of clinical certainty.

The array of environmental and occupational compounds to which people may be exposed is large. Except for patients exposed to recreational and iatrogenic agents, until recently, most psychiatrists did not treat patients with toxic exposures. That is changing rapidly as a result of late 20th-century technology and increasing societal awareness. It behooves the clinician to remember that toxic exposures are used by some patients to explain a pantheon of personal ills, many of a psychiatric nature. It is neither appropriate to treat those complaints lightly nor clinically sound to accept such pathogenic explanations without firm clinical support.

Recreational drugs may be used or abused intentionally to cause dose-dependent behavioral changes, including anxiolysis with nicotine, intoxication with alcohol or marijuana, or psychosis with mescaline. There may be additional unwanted psychiatric phenomena with drug intoxication. Unwanted secondary syndromes commonly described include anxiety and insomnia due to caffeine; paranoid psychosis with cocaine; mood alterations (dysphoria, anxiety, euphoria) accompanying the perceptual disturbances induced by hallucinogenic substances; agitated (often violent) psychotic states with phencyclidine (PCP); and depressive symptoms and seemingly paradoxical disinhibition of aggressive impulses with sedative-hypnotics. However, there may be considerable variability, and therefore lack of specificity, in syndromic association with particular substances. Also, many substances in sufficient doses can cause delirium, which may itself have associated psychiatric symptoms ranging from mood disturbance to psychosis.

Withdrawal syndromes are also commonly encountered with drugs of abuse and tend to be characteristic of the class of drug. Withdrawal from nicotine may produce anxiety or irritability; withdrawal from stimulants produces a hypersomnic dysphoric crash; and withdrawal from opiates produces a well-described state that includes malaise, anxiety and irritability, drug craving, insomnia, psychomotor agitation, anorexia, and a variety of physical symptoms (for example, diarrhea, piloerection, mydriasis, hypertension, and tachycardia). Delirium often follows withdrawal from alcohol and sedative-hypnotic medications but is not a component of other drug withdrawal syndromes (for example, opiate-related).

Numerous medications have been implicated in causing psychiatric phenomena. Prescription drugs and over-the-counter preparations may cause physiologically induced behavioral changes, either through intoxication (which may involve usage at therapeutic or supratherapeutic levels) or withdrawal. As with other causes of secondary psychiatric disorders, combinations of medications and medical illnesses may cause behavioral changes even when each medication or illness alone does not.

Among prescribed medications, psychotropic drugs are designed to effect behavioral changes. Unwanted psychiatric syndromes, such as antipsychotic-induced depressive syndromes or the delirium of lithium toxicity, occur often. Countless medications have been implicated in secondary psychiatric syndromes; it is rare indeed for a medication to be listed in the *Physicians' Desk Reference* without an accompanying description of some potential neuropsychiatric side effect. However, that information must be interpreted with caution. Behavioral side effects are also noted with placebos; therefore, distinguishing physiological from psychological symptoms may be difficult. Psychiatric symptoms may also reflect the clinical manifestations of the primary illness being treated (for example, delirium in a patient receiving a new parenteral antibiotic may be due to the antibiotic or the targeted infection). Finally, numerous other factors may complicate the process of establishing the etiological significance of a particular medication. For example, β-adrenergic-blocking antihypertensives have been postulated for many years to cause depressive syndromes, yet a recent large study, carefully controlled for patient demographics, medical illness, medications, and other factors, was unable to find a significant independent association between β-blockers and depression. Despite these caveats, many medications clearly can cause secondary psychiatric syndromes.

COGNITIVE DISORDERS

DELIRIUM *Delirium,* a transient disorder of brain function manifested by global cognitive impairment and other behavioral phenomena, is a common disease state that has been described for centuries. Nevertheless, it is frequently missed or misdiagnosed, with the potential for substantial attendant morbidity and mortality. Recognition and appropriate evaluation and treatment of delirium should be an imperative, not just for psychiatrists but for all physicians.

DEFINITION DSM-IV includes delirium under cognitive disorders. Delirium is a syndrome, with core features of impairment of consciousness with attentional deficit, other cognitive alterations, and a relatively rapid onset of the disorder with a characteristically fluctuating course. Frequently there are other associated clinical phenomena, which may appear more prominent to the uneducated observer than the core features.

HISTORY Physicians have long recognized states of altered behavior, including changes in level of consciousness, of acute onset that were associated with fever, poisons, or other medical or neurological diseases. There are references to such presentations in the writings of

Hippocrates and in much subsequent Greco-Roman literature. Descriptions of the syndrome similar to modern definitions appear from the late Middle Ages through the 18th century. The history, however, is obscured by an etymological web that to this day impedes communication and education about the disorder. Numerous terms have been used to describe the syndrome of delirium, including phrenitis, frenzy, and febrile insanity; conversely, the term delirium has also been applied to other psychiatric states that led to insanity.

By the 19th century emphasis was placed on disordered consciousness as the hallmark of delirium. The phrase "clouding of consciousness" dates to that time and is still used in many quarters today despite lack of clarity as to what it means. Similarly, the term "confusion" was used frequently, despite the lack of a specific relation to delirium.

The work of George Engel and John Romano in the 1940s, summarized by them in publications from the 1950s, indicated that attentional and other cognitive disturbances were best viewed as the core features of the syndrome and that the state was associated with acute brain failure, as demonstrated by slowing on the EEG. Subsequent work on the pathophysiology of delirium has been relatively scant. Zbigniew Jerzy Lipowski, beginning in the 1960s and continuing to the present, has been instrumental in raising clinical and research awareness of delirium, defining the syndrome according to strict criteria and popularizing (especially in the psychiatric community) the use of the term "delirium." Recent years have seen alterations in diagnostic criteria, as evidenced by the removal of associated clinical features such as psychomotor changes from the required criteria. There has also been increasing study of epidemiology, clinical course, and risk factors for onset or poor outcome.

Unfortunately, etymological confusion remains. Numerous synonyms remain in common use, especially in nonpsychiatric medical fields; some of them are encephalopathy, acute confusional state, and acute organic brain syndrome. Some neurologists maintain a distinction between delirium, which they reserve to describe extremely agitated delirious states with frank thought process disorganization, perceptual disturbances, and autonomic hyperactivity, and acute confusional states, which they use to describe all other, often less severe delirious states. Most psychiatrists, and many other workers in the field, believe that such distinctions are premature at best (due to lack of evidence of differing etiologies or pathophysiologies between the two) and misleading at worst, obscuring the commonality of core clinical features, potential etiologies, and management approaches.

EPIDEMIOLOGY There have been relatively few studies of the incidence and prevalence of delirium. Little is known about the epidemiology of delirium in community or other nonpatient, noninstitutionalized populations. An estimated 10 to 15 percent of general medical inpatients are delirious at any given time, and studies indicate that as many as 30 to 50 percent of acutely ill geriatric patients become delirious at some point during their hospital stay. Rates of delirium in psychiatric and nursing home populations are not well established but are clearly substantial. Risk factors for the development of delirium include increased severity of physical illness, older age, and baseline cognitive impairment (for example, due to dementia).

Delirium is frequently unrecognized by treating physicians. Because of its wide array of associated symptoms, it may be detected but misdiagnosed as depression, schizophrenia, or other psychiatric disorder. Delirium is a frequent cause for psychiatric consultation in the general hospital but often is not recognized as such by the referring physician.

ETIOLOGY The syndrome of delirium reflects brain dysfunction that is almost always due to identifiable systemic or cerebral disease or to drug intoxication or withdrawal. A partial list of frequently encountered etiologies is given in Table 12-12. Often delirium is due to multiple simultaneous etiologies, each one of which may or may not be enough to cause delirium by itself. On rare occasions a syndrome nearly indistinguishable from delirium may manifest as part of the course of another Axis I disorder such as bipolar disorder, as discussed below.

DIAGNOSIS AND CLINICAL FEATURES The syndrome of delirium is almost always caused by one or more systemic or cerebral derangements that affect brain function. DSM-IV gives separate diagnostic criteria for delirium due to a general medical condition (Table 12-13) for delirium related to systemic medical conditions or primary cerebral conditions, substance intoxication delirium (Table 12-14), substance withdrawal delirium (Table 12-15), delirium due to multiple etiologies (Table 12-16), and delirium not otherwise specified (Table 12-17) for a delirium of unknown etiology or due to causes not listed previously, such as sensory deprivation). However, the core syndrome is the same, regardless of etiology.

The core features of delirium include altered consciousness, such as decreased level of consciousness; altered attention, which may include diminished ability to focus, sustain, or shift attention; impairment in other realms of cognitive function, which may manifest as disorientation (especially to time and space) and decreased memory; relatively rapid onset (usually hours to days); brief duration (usually days to weeks); and often

TABLE 12-12
Etiologies of Delirium

Drug intoxication
- Anticholinergics
- Lithium
- Antiarrhythmics (e.g., lidocaine)
- H_2-receptor blockers
- Sedative-hypnotics
- Alcohol

Drug withdrawal
- Alcohol
- Sedative-hypnotics

Tumor
- Primary cerebral

Trauma
- Cerebral contusion (as an example)
- Subdural hematoma

Infection
- Cerebral (e.g., meningitis, encephalitis, HIV, syphilis)
- Systemic (e.g., sepsis, urinary tract infection, pneumonia)

Cardiovascular
- Cerebrovascular (e.g., infarcts, hemorrhage, vasculitis)
- Cardiovascular (e.g., low-output states, congestive heart failure, shock)

Physiological or metabolic
- Hypoxemia, electrolyte disturbances, renal or hepatic failure, hypo- or hyperglycemia, postictal states (as examples)
- Endocrine
  - Thyroid or glucocorticoid disturbances (as examples)
- Nutritional
  - Thiamine or vitamin B_{12} deficiency, pellagra (as examples)

TABLE 12-13
Diagnostic Criteria for Delirium due to a General Medical Condition

A. Disturbance of consciousness (i.e., reduced clarity of awareness of the environment) with reduced ability to focus, sustain, or shift attention.
B. A change in cognition (such as memory deficit, disorientation, language disturbance) or the development of a perceptual disturbance that is not better accounted for by a preexisting, established, or evolving dementia.
C. The disturbance develops over a short period of time (usually hours to days) and tends to fluctuate during the course of the day.
D. There is evidence from the history, physical examination, or laboratory findings that the disturbance is caused by the direct physiological consequences of a general medical condition.

Coding note: If delirium is superimposed on a preexisting dementia of the Alzheimer's type or vascular dementia, indicate the delirium by coding the appropriate subtype of the dementia, e.g., dementia of the Alzheimer's type, with late onset, with delirium.
Coding note: Include the name of the general medical condition on Axis I, e.g., delirium due to hepatic encephalopathy; also code the general medical condition on Axis III.

TABLE 12-14
Diagnostic Criteria for Substance Intoxication Delirium

A. Disturbance of consciousness (i.e., reduced clarity of awareness of the environment) with reduced ability to focus, sustain, or shift attention.
B. A change in cognition (such as memory deficit, disorientation, language disturbance) or the development of a perceptual disturbance that is not better accounted for by a preexisting, established, or evolving dementia.
C. The disturbance develops over a short period of time (usually hours to days) and tends to fluctuate during the course of the day.
D. There is evidence from the history, physical examination, or laboratory findings of either (1) or (2):
   (1) the symptoms in criteria A and B developed during substance intoxication
   (2) medication use is etiologically related to the disturbance.*

   Note: This diagnosis should be made instead of a diagnosis of substance intoxication only when the cognitive symptoms are in excess of those usually associated with the intoxication syndrome and when the symptoms are sufficiently severe to warrant independent clinical attention.

   *Note: The diagnosis should be recorded as substance-induced delirium if related to medication use.

Code (Specific substance) intoxication delirium: (Alcohol; amphetamine [or amphetamine-like substance]; cannabis; cocaine; hallucinogen; inhalant; opioid; phencyclidine [or phencyclidine-like substance]; sedative, hypnotic, or anxiolytic; other [or unknown] substance [e.g., cimetidine, digitalis, benztropine])

Table from DSM-IV, *Diagnostic and Statistical Manual of Mental Disorders,* ed 4. Copyright American Psychiatric Association, Washington, 1994. Used with permission.

TABLE 12-15
Diagnostic Criteria for Substance Withdrawal Delirium

A. Disturbance of consciousness (i.e., reduced clarity of awareness of the environment) with reduced ability to focus, sustain, or shift attention.
B. A change in cognition (such as memory deficit, disorientation, language disturbance) or the development of a perceptual disturbance that is not better accounted for by a preexisting, established, or evolving dementia.
C. The disturbance develops over a short period of time (usually hours to days) and tends to fluctuate during the course of the day.
D. There is evidence from the history, physical examination, or laboratory findings that the symptoms in criteria A and B developed during, or shortly after, a withdrawal syndrome.

Note: This diagnosis should be made instead of a diagnosis of substance withdrawal only when the cognitive symptoms are in excess of those usually associated with the withdrawal syndrome and when the symptoms are sufficiently severe to warrant independent clinical attention.

Code (Specific substance) withdrawal delirium: (Alcohol; sedative, hypnotic, or anxiolytic; other [or unknown] substance)

Table from DSM-IV, *Diagnostic and Statistical Manual of Mental Disorders,* ed 4. Copyright American Psychiatric Association, Washington, 1994. Used with permission.

marked, unpredictable fluctuations in severity and other clinical manifestations during the course of the day, sometimes worse at night (sundowning), which may range from periods of lucidity to quite severe cognitive impairment and disorganization.

Associated clinical features are often present and may be prominent. They may include disorganization of thought processes (ranging from mild tangentiality to frank incoherence), perceptual disturbances such as illusions and hallucinations, psychomotor hyperactivity and hypoactivity, disruption of the sleep-wake cycle (often manifested as fragmented sleep at night, with or without daytime drowsiness), mood alterations (from subtle irritability to obvious dysphoria, anxiety, or even euphoria), and other manifestations of altered neurological function (for example, autonomic hyperactivity or instability, myoclonic jerking, and dysarthria). The EEG usually shows diffuse slowing of background activity, although patients with delirium due to alcohol or sedative-hypnotic withdrawal have low-voltage fast activity.

TABLE 12-16
Diagnostic Criteria for Delirium due to Multiple Etiologies

A. Disturbance of consciousness (i.e., reduced clarity of awareness of the environment) with reduced ability to focus, sustain, or shift attention.
B. A change in cognition (such as memory deficit, disorientation, language disturbance) or the development of a perceptual disturbance that is not better accounted for by a preexisting, established, or evolving dementia.
C. The disturbance develops over a short period of time (usually hours to days) and tends to fluctuate during the course of the day.
D. There is evidence from the history, physical examination, or laboratory findings that the delirium has more than one etiology (e.g., more than one etiological general medical condition, a general medical condition plus substance intoxication, or medication side effect).

Coding note: Use multiple codes reflecting specific delirium and specific etiologies, e.g., delirium due to viral encephalitis, alcohol withdrawal delirium.

Table from DSM-IV, *Diagnostic and Statistical Manual of Mental Disorders,* ed 4. Copyright American Psychiatric Association, Washington, 1994. Used with permission.

TABLE 12-17
Diagnostic Criteria for Delirium Not Otherwise Specified

This category should be used to diagnose a delirium that does not meet criteria for any of the specific types of delirium described in this section.

Examples include

1. A clinical presentation of delirium that is suspected to be due to a general medical condition or substance use but for which there is insufficient evidence to establish a specific etiology
2. Delirium due to causes not listed in this section (e.g., sensory deprivation)

Table from DSM-IV, *Diagnostic and Statistical Manual of Mental Disorders,* ed 4. Copyright American Psychiatric Association, Washington, 1994. Used with permission.

The key to diagnosing delirium is to maintain a heightened suspicion for the syndrome whenever a patient experiences a relatively rapid change in or the new onset of any psychiatric symptom or sign. Once the diagnosis is suspected, the history (usually obtained from informants such as family, nursing staff, and prior treaters) and mental status examination can elucidate the cognitive disturbances at the core of the syndrome and uncover associated clinical phenomena that may affect management or suggest the etiology.

The presence of delirium should prompt careful investigation for contributing etiologies. Delirium may be the first, most prominent, or only clinical manifestation of the new onset of a medical condition or the worsening of a previously diagnosed illness. A careful medical history (including medication and drug history), physical examination, and neurological examination must be undertaken, and various laboratory tests, neuroimaging procedures, lumbar puncture, and EEG may be useful. In searching for an etiology, physicians should remember that relatively minor abnormalities (for example, a mild anemia plus slight hyponatremia plus slight hypercalcemia) may additively produce delirium even if each abnormality alone would not normally do so. Sometimes the search for an etiology does not yield a clear cause of the delirium; the patient still has the syndrome of delirium, however, and vigilance for clinical contributing factors must be maintained. Physicians should avoid the common mistake of believing delirium to be ruled out by the lack of obvious etiology, thereby proving that the behavioral disturbance is functional in origin. EEG may be helpful in such cases by demonstrating diffuse brain dysfunction, although that in itself does not demonstrate etiology.

Current understanding of the pathophysiology of delirium is limited. Dysfunction of the reticular activating system has been speculated, given its role in arousal. There is evidence for hypofunction of cholinergic systems, particularly in the basal forebrain and pons. There is some evidence for dysfunction of several other neurochemical systems, including noradrenergic, γ-aminobutyric acid (GABA)ergic, and serotonergic; more undoubtedly await investigation. Earlier speculation about globally decreased cerebral metabolism has not been confirmed, but also has not been carefully studied in delirium despite the availability of techniques such as PET and SPECT. Even more obscure is the pathophysiological link between specific systemic conditions and delirium. The classic model of such a link is anticholinergic drug toxicity, which has been presumed to cause delirium as a direct consequence of hypoactivity of cholinergic systems. Some recent work has demonstrated increased GABAergic transmission, putatively due to increased concentrations of endogenous benzodiazepinelike substances, in patients with delirium and fulminant liver failure.

DIFFERENTIAL DIAGNOSIS Much attention has been given to differentiating delirium from dementia. Usually that distinction can be easily made by noting temporal factors (course of onset and progression of the disturbance) and by recognizing that level of consciousness and attention are affected prominently and early in delirium. Dementia by definition does not involve an alteration of consciousness, although attentional dysfunction develops as the syndrome progresses in severity. However, delirium is often superimposed on a preexisting dementia. If the history is unknown and mental status examination results are lacking in a patient with severe dementia, it can be difficult to tell if there is a new delirium, or if the delirium has resolved and the patient is back to baseline (which may, in fact, be a new baseline reflecting deterioration from a previous level of function). In such cases it is prudent to approach the patient with the presumption that the patient has delirium and with attendant careful clinical evaluation.

Although thought process disorganization, perceptual disturbances, or mood symptoms may lead the uninitiated to diagnose idiopathic psychiatric illness, the constellation of altered level of consciousness, prominent attentional and other cognitive deficits, and temporal course usually makes the differentiation of delirium from mood, psychotic, and anxiety disorders straightforward. The previous psychiatric history can be helpful, but the clinician must use care in interpreting it because patients with chronic psychiatric illness are also at risk for developing delirium due to medications, drug abuse, or other conditions. Rarely, patients with other Axis I illnesses (particularly the schizophrenias and bipolar disorders) may develop flagrantly disorganized, incoherent states with obvious attentional impairment and inability for the examiner to test other cognitive functions. (When found in the course of bipolar disorder, that state has been incorrectly called manic delirium.) Such states cannot be reliably distinguished phenomenologically from delirium due to the more usual medical causes, and they warrant the same thorough search for contributing etiologies accorded other deliria.

COURSE AND PROGNOSIS By most definitions, although not by DSM-IV criteria, delirium is a transient condition. For most patients the syndrome resolves within days to a few weeks. However, in sicker populations the mortality associated with delirium is high in the short term (acute hospitalization) and increases with several-month follow-up. It is not clear if increased mortality is independently associated with delirium or if it can be accounted for by known medical pathology. In some patients an apparently new dementia becomes evident on resolution of the delirium; the dementia may not have been present, or may have been present but unrecognized, prior to the delirium.

TREATMENT The primary treatment of delirium is to identify and ameliorate any causal or contributing medical conditions. As part of that effort, the dosages of all sedatives and other CNS-active medications should be minimized as much as possible. (The exception is delirium due to sedative-hypnotic or alcohol withdrawal, in which treatment of the underlying problem requires the administration of a cross-tolerant agent such as a benzodiazepine.) Delirious patients may need extra supportive physical care; maintenance of basic functions such as food and fluid intake is crucial to rapid recovery. Keeping the patient in an environment that is quiet and free of unnecessary stimulation may help reduce agitation. Frequent cues to orientation may also be helpful. Supportive contacts with the patient, family, and sometimes staff members are necessary to reassure the patient that the new, often frightening behavioral state reflects physical illness and that the patient is not going crazy. Attention may need to be paid to the patient's legal capacity to participate in informed clinical care decisions.

The patient with a quiet, hypoactive delirium needs no specific pharmacotherapy. However, many delirious patients show persistent or intermittent psychomotor agitation that may interfere with nursing care or necessary tests and procedures. Control of the agitation is essential to prevent inadvertent self-damage and allow appropriate evaluation and treatment. Physical restraints may be used transiently when necessary. If sedation is desired, the drug of choice is a high-potency antipsychotic in relatively low doses (for example, haloperidol [Haldol], 0.5 to 1 mg orally or parenterally, up to several mg a day). Low-potency agents, benzodiazepines, and other sedatives (antihistamines, barbiturates) should generally be avoided because they will likely worsen the delirious state. At times of severe, life-threatening agitation (for example, a patient in the intensive care unit is removing the endotracheal tube, arterial lines, and so forth), sedation at nearly any cost becomes necessary, and combinations of antipsychotics, benzodiazepines, and opioids have been used, as have neuromuscular-blocking agents, such as pancuronium (Pavulon) (use of the latter depends on the availability of adequate ventilatory support).

There have been case reports of improvement in or remission of delirious states due to intractable medical illnesses with ECT. Although ECT may rarely be advised by a consultant with expertise in the procedure, routine consideration of ECT for delirium is not advised.

DEMENTIA Interest in the study and care of patients with dementia has increased, coincident with the proportional increase of the elderly in the population. Although dementing disorders are defined by their multiple cognitive deficits, patients can present with the full array of psychiatric symptoms. And although dementia is most often associated with progressive processes, it does not, by itself, denote a deteriorating course. Thus, the clinician must seek any curable or treatable causes of dementia whenever it is recognized clinically, before irreversible CNS changes supervene.

DEFINITION Dementia is a diminution in cognition in the setting of a stable level of consciousness. Dementia denotes a decrement of two or more intellectual functions, in contrast to focal or specific impairments such as amnestic disorder or aphasia. The persistent and stable nature of the impairment distinguishes dementia from the altered consciousness and fluctuating deficits of delirium. Dementia must also be distinguished from long-standing mental subnormality, as the former represents an acquired loss of or decline in prior intellectual and functional capacities.

HISTORY The term "dementia" has long been understood as describing an acquired cognitive and behavioral decline associated with brain disease. Esquirol, in his classic, early 19th-century nosological work, *Mental Maladies: A Treatise on Insanity,* provided perhaps the first modern definition of dementia: "A cerebral affection usually chronic . . . and characterized by a weakening of the sensibility, understanding, and will." In his study of over 300 patients, Esquirol described the noncognitive symptoms of dementia, reporting hallucinations, delusions, aggressive behavior, and motoric abnormalities in many of the patients. Interestingly, however, he included among the etiologies for dementia not only aging, head trauma, syphilis, and alcohol abuse, but also conditions such as "menstrual disorders, . . . onanism, . . . disappointed affections, . . . [and] political shocks." Later investigators described neuropathological correlations for the dementia syndromes, firmly establishing the relation between brain disease and dementia. Contemporary interest has focused again on an etiological basis for the observed pathological and pathophysiological abnormalities and on risk factors, preventative measures, and specific treatments for dementia.

COMPARATIVE NOSOLOGY In DSM-III and DSM-III-R, dementia was listed as both a syndrome and a disorder. The development of specific criteria for the symptom constellation was a major departure from all previous nosologies. It proved to be a major conceptual advance for both clinical practice and research. The dementia syndrome was one of the possible presentations of psychoactive substance-induced organic mental conditions and of organic mental conditions associated with Axis III physical disorders. Dementia was also listed as a group of specific disorders, including primary degenerative dementia of the Alzheimer's type, multiinfarct dementia, dementia associated with alcoholism, and dementia not otherwise specified. A severity scale of mild, moderate, or severe was provided. DSM-IV eliminates the distinction between dementia as a syndrome and dementia as a disorder. Instead, it delineates those dementing disorders that are related to specific systemic medical or cerebral conditions (for example, dementia of the Alzheimer's type and vascular dementia). DSM-IV criteria emphasize the defining features of dementia, namely the multiple deficits that represent a decline from a previously attained level of functioning, and incorporate specific information for distinguishing the etiological subcategories from each other, relying on course of the disease, the presence or absence of focal neurological signs and symptoms, laboratory evidence of neurological damage, a history of significant substance abuse, or other evidence of a contributing medical condition. Dementia of the Alzheimer's type is, in the end, a diagnosis of exclusion, requiring that other potentially etiological CNS or systemic medical conditions be ruled out.

Beyond DSM-IV, there are alternative, conceptually overlapping systems for diagnosing dementia. The *International Classification of Diseases and Related Health Problems* (ICD) is a listing of all medical diseases, including mental disorders, that by international treaty agreement forms the basis for all nosological data recording. The 10th revision of ICD (ICD-10) includes four dementia categories: (1) dementia in Alzheimer's disease; (2) vascular dementia; (3) dementia in diseases classified elsewhere in the ICD (for example, dementia due to Pick's disease, Huntington's disease, Parkinson's disease, Creutzfeldt-Jakob disease); and (4) unspecified dementia. Although the blue book of the ICD system (*The ICD-10 Classification of Mental and Behavioral Disorders: Clinical descriptions and diagnostic guidelines*) does not specify criteria for the diagnosis of the diseases listed, the appended glossary or green book (*The ICD-Classification of Mental and Behavioral Disorders: Diagnostic criteria for research*) provides clinical and research criteria for each category of dementia.

Another set of research criteria for the diagnosis of dementia of the Alzheimer's type, established by the NINCDS and the Alzheimer's Disease and Related Disorders Association (ADRDA, now the Alzheimer's Association), has become known as the NINCDS-ADRDA criteria. Several studies have shown that a diagnosis of probable dementia of the Alzheimer's type according to NINCDS-ADRDA criteria selects patients similar to those diagnosed using DSM-III criteria. Depending on the case series, both criteria sets have been capable of identifying cases of Alzheimer's disease confirmed postmortem with a 70 to 90 percent specificity. The DSM-IV criteria share many features for the diagnosis of probable dementia of the Alzheimer's type but go beyond them to more clearly define important behavioral subtypes, akin to ICD-10, that may help guide symptomatic treatment interventions.

EPIDEMIOLOGY The prevalence of dementia rises exponentially with age. The estimated prevalence of moderate to severe dementia in a population aged 65 years or older is consistently reported at approximately 5 percent. Within that age group, the exponential curve is pronounced, so that the prevalence in the subgroup aged 65 to 69 years is 1.5 to 2 percent; in the subgroup aged 75 to 79 years, 5.5 to 6.5 percent; and in the subgroup aged 85 to 89 years, 20 to 22 percent. Dementia of the Alzheimer's type is the most common dementing disorder in clinical and neuropathological prevalence studies reported from North America, Scandinavia, and Europe. Prevalence studies from Russia and Japan show vascular dementia to be more common in those countries. It remains unclear whether those apparent clinical differences reflect true etiological distinctions or inconsistent uses of diagnostic criteria. Dementia of the Alzheimer's type becomes more common with increasing age; among persons older than 75 years, the risk is six times greater than the risk for vascular dementia. There is a suggestion of higher rates of dementia of the Alzheimer's type in females and higher rates of vascular dementia in males. In geriatric psychiatric patient samples, dementia of the Alzheimer's type is a much more common etiology (50 to 70 percent) than vascular dementia (15 to 25 percent).

Studies of the incidence of dementia have been plagued by widely differing methodology and results. Again, there is an exponential increase in incidence with age, though some reports have noted a leveling off starting around age 75 years.

ETIOLOGY Table 12-18 lists common etiologies of dementia and includes the broad systemic and cerebral disease categories noted previously in this chapter. Alzheimer's disease, the most common type of degenerative dementia, was discussed in an earlier section. Huntington's disease and Parkinson's disease were also discussed earlier in the chapter as paradigmatic examples of subcortical degenerative processes, with clinical and neuropathological descriptions separating them from cortical dementias. There may be clinical and neuropathological overlap between Alzheimer's disease and Parkinson's disease, especially among older patients. The significance of that finding remains unknown.

Frontal lobe degeneration In recent years, several authors have sought to distinguish dementias of the frontal lobe from other disorders. The uncertain status of dementias of the frontal lobe as distinct clinical and neuropathological entities has not yet warranted their formal inclusion in DSM-IV or ICD-10. They are described as cortical dementias that are found in as many as 10 to 20 percent of cases in some neuropathological series. Age at onset is apparently between 50 and 60 years for the majority, but the reported range is broad—20 to 80 years. The early clinical features of frontal lobe dementias are typified by damage to the frontal lobes and include prominent changes in personality and behavior. The personality changes include disinhibition, social misconduct, and lack of insight; those changes progress to apathy, mutism, and repetitive behaviors. A variant of the Klüver-Bucy syndrome, a condition originally described in monkeys that had undergone surgical ablation of the temporal lobes, is also described in the early stages of frontal lobe dementias and is characterized by combinations of disrupted eating behavior, hyperorality, mood disturbances, and sensory agnosias. Language, praxis, and gnosis are relatively

TABLE 12-18
Etiologies of Dementia

Tumor
- Primary cerebral*
- Metastatic*

Trauma
- Hematomas*
- Posttraumatic dementia*

Infection (chronic)
- Syphilis*
- Creutzfeldt-Jakob disease†
- AIDS dementia complex‡

Cardiac/vascular
- Single infarction*
- Multiple infarction†
- Large infarction
- Lacunar infarction
- Binswanger's disease (subcortical arteriosclerotic encephalopathies)
- Hemodynamic type*

Congenital/hereditary
- Huntington's disease‡
- Metachromatic leukodystrophy‡

Primary psychiatric
- Pseudodementia‡

Physiological
- Epilepsy*
- Normal pressure hydrocephalus*

Metabolic
- Vitamin deficiencies*
- Chronic metabolic disturbances*
- Chronic anoxic states*
- Chronic endocrinopathies*

Degenerative dementias
- Alzheimer's disease†
- Pick's disease (dementias of frontal lobe type)†
- Parkinson's disease*
- Progressive supranuclear palsy‡
- Idiopathic cerebral ferrocalcinosis (Fahr's disease)‡
- Wilson's disease*

Demyelinating
- Multiple sclerosis‡

Drugs and toxins
- Alcohol*
- Heavy metals*
- Carbon monoxide poisoning*
- Medications*
- Irradiation*

*Variable or mixed pattern.
†Predominantly cortical pattern.
‡Predominantly subcortical pattern.

spared early in the disease course, in contrast to dementia of the Alzheimer's type. However, dementias of the frontal lobe are described as progressive conditions that may in some cases involve memory as well as other cognitive functions. To date no studies have attempted to prospectively discriminate dementia of frontal lobe origin from dementia of the Alzheimer's type, with subsequent neuropathological confirmation to determine clinical diagnostic accuracy.

Neuropsychological testing in patients suspected of having dementia of frontal lobe origin may demonstrate disproportionate impairment in tasks related to frontal lobe function, such as deficiency in abstract thinking, attentional shifting, or set formation. Structural neuroimaging, such as CT or MRI, may reveal prominent atrophy of the frontal lobe, especially early in the disease process. Functional neuroimaging may prove more reliable for distinguishing dementia of frontal lobe origin from dementia of the Alzheimer's type. Regional cerebral blood flow studies using radioactively labeled xenon and SPECT studies have demonstrated disproportionate decreases in blood flow, radio tracer uptake, and glucose metabolism in the frontal lobes in patients with suspected or autopsy-confirmed frontal lobe dementia.

Presently, the definitive diagnosis of any degenerative dementia rests on postmortem neuropathological examination. Only one type of frontal lobe dementia, Pick's disease, is associated with distinctive histopathological abnormalities that allow for certain diagnosis. Swollen neurons known as Pick cells and intraneuronal inclusions known as Pick bodies define the disorder neuropathologically. Demyelination and gliosis of the frontal lobe white matter may also be found. Other frontal lobe dementias have been referred to as dementia of the frontal lobe type or frontal lobe degeneration of non-Alzheimer's type. They have been distinguished from Alzheimer's disease by their marked gross morphological involvement of frontal and anterior temporal lobes, with relative sparing of the postcentral and temporoparietal areas mostly affected in Alzheimer's disease, and by the absence of amyloid plaques and neurofibrillary tangles microscopically. The lack of positive neuropathological inclusion criteria leaves many of these clinical conditions as disease entities of uncertain status, defined histopathologically by the absence of specific features. Whenever the hallmark findings of Alzheimer's disease are present, that diagnosis has been applied, irrespective of prior clinical findings. Thus, there are no data available to determine how many clinically diagnosed cases of frontal lobe dementia have been recast as Alzheimer's disease after death.

Of the potentially multiple forms of dementia associated with progressive frontal lobe dysfunction, then, only one type can be distinguished from Alzheimer's disease neuropathologically; the others show no defining postmortem signs. They may also be difficult to distinguish clinically in life. In the early stages of disease, the predominance of behavioral and personality disturbance, the presence of primitive reflexes, and neuropsychological and neuroimaging evidence of disproportionate frontal lobe involvement can help with a more confident premortem diagnosis of frontal lobe dementia. It has been assumed by some authors that there are many variants of dementia of frontal lobe origin that cannot be distinguished from each other clinically. At present, only Pick's disease has definitive neuropathological features.

Subcortical degeneration Huntington's disease and Parkinson's disease were discussed earlier as examples of degenerative disorders with a subcortical pattern of deficits. *Progressive supranuclear palsy,* first described in 1964, is a degenerative disease involving the brainstem, cerebellum, and basal ganglia. The presenting history is usually notable for a gait disturbance, particularly spontaneous toppling. The clinical examination is notable for supranuclear paralysis of extraocular movements, particularly in the vertical plane. Dysarthria and dystonic rigidity of the neck and trunk are also common. Onset is usually after age 50 years, with progressive muscular rigidity. Neuropathology is notable for cell loss and gliosis of various nuclei in the brainstem, basal ganglia, and cerebellum, with striking preservation of the cortex. Progressive supranuclear palsy and Huntington's disease were the two disorders to which the label "subcortical dementia" was originally attached. In progressive supranuclear palsy a marked slowing of cognitive processes, apathy, and lack of initiative have been described, associated with relative sparing of language, memory, and praxis. *Fahr's disease* involves idiopathic calcification of the basal ganglia. A subcortical dementia with a parkinsonian syndrome has been described. (Mild basal ganglia calcification is frequently observed incidentally on neuroimaging studies. The clinical significance of that finding is unknown.) Basal ganglia calcification can also be seen in patients with disorders of calcium metabolism, with the expected patterns of subcortical dementia and movement disorder.

Vascular etiologies *Cerebrovascular diseases* together comprise the second most common cause of dementia. That category of dementia was referred to in the past as arteriosclerotic dementia, reflecting the belief that vascular insufficiency was responsible for the cognitive degeneration. That has now been supplanted by the belief that tissue damage or infarction underlies the vascular dementias. Cerebral infarction can be the result of a number of processes, of which thromboembolism from a large vessel plaque or cardiothrombus is the most common. Anoxia due to cardiac arrest, hypotension, anemia, or sleep apnea can also produce ischemia and infarction. Cerebral hemorrhage related to hypertension or an arteriovenous malformation accounts for approximately 15 percent of cerebrovascular disease.

The clinical characteristics of a vascular dementia depend on the area of infarction. As such, there is a wide variability in the possible presenting features of a vascular dementia. Single infarctions may result in the discrete loss of one particular function (for example, language) without dementia per se. However, some strategically located infarctions can affect more than one domain of cognitive function and mimic the clinical picture of a global dementia. An example is the angular gyrus syndrome that can occur with large posterior lesions in the dominant hemisphere. It has been characterized as manifesting with alexia with agraphia, aphasia, constructional disturbances, and Gerstmann syndrome (acalculia, agraphia, right-left disorientation, and finger agnosia). Although the findings are similar to those of dementia of the Alzheimer's type, angular gyrus syndrome can be distinguished by its abrupt onset, the presence of focal neurological, EEG, and imaging abnormalities, and preservation of memory and ideomotor praxis.

Vascular dementia is more commonly associated with multiple infarctions. The infarctions may take the form of numerous large infarctions accompanied by widespread cognitive and motor deficits. Tiny, deep infarctions, known as *lacunes,* result from disease of the small arteries that usually involves subcortical structures, such as the basal ganglia, thalamus, and internal capsule. The neurological and cognitive deficits may resolve quickly after each of the small strokes; however, the deficits may accumulate, leading to a persisting functional and intellectual decline. In the past, a stepwise pattern of deterioration was described for that type of vascular dementia, but it was dropped from the DSM-IV criteria, as no specific pattern of deterioration has been reliably demonstrated for vascular dementias. Similarly, the description of patchy deficits has been deleted, in light of the marked variability in presentation of vascular dementia, depending on the type of vasculature and the site and extent of infarction.

Binswanger's disease (subcortical arteriosclerotic encephalopathy) is characterized by microinfarctions of the white matter with sparing of the cortex. It was originally believed to be a rare form of dementia that could be diagnosed only at autopsy. With the advent of sophisticated neuroimaging techniques such as CT and MRI and the common observation of white matter hyperintensities, there is renewed interest in the disease. Binswanger's disease produces a subcortical pattern of dementia, as the neuropathology is restricted to white matter. However, the mere presence of white matter hyperintensities on MRI is not adequate for diagnosis, as those areas may represent small infarctions, focal demyelination, or simply dilated perivascular spaces. Some studies have found no postmortem pathological correlate to white matter hyperintensities detected on MRI in vivo. Recently, criteria have been proposed for the diagnosis of Binswanger's disease that include clinical and neuropsychological confirmation of dementia, the presence of vascular risk factors, evidence of focal cerebrovascular disease, evidence of subcortical dysfunction, and bilateral white matter abnormalities greater than 2×2 mm in size on CT or T_2-weighted MRI scans.

Vascular dementia of the hemodynamic type is a classification that has been used to refer to cognitive impairments that arise secondary to hypotensive episodes, such as those due to cardiac dysrhythmias or hypotension. They may overlap phenomenologically with other conditions that result from chronic hypoxia.

Dementia due to tumor, trauma, infection, and hereditary diseases has been touched on previously. Among others, *Wilson's disease* or hepatolenticular degeneration is an inherited disorder involving abnormal metabolism of copper. Copper accumulates in both the liver and the CNS, particularly in the striatum, caudate, and putamen. Onset usually occurs during childhood or adolescence, although it may be delayed until middle age. Personality change and behavioral disturbance are the most common neuropsychiatric manifestations (and frequently the presenting symptoms of the disease), but cognitive impairment may also be present. The latter takes the form of a subcortical dementia, with psychomotor slowing and loss of initiative, in the presence of relatively spared language functions, memory, and praxis. Motor symptoms are prominent in a parkinsonian pattern and include rigidity, tremor, and, at times, athetosis. The diagnosis is confirmed by assay of serum copper levels and urinary copper excretion. Treatment with chelating agents—dimercaprol (British Anti-Lewisite [BAL]) in the past and penicillamine (Cuprimine) more recently—can retard the progression of the disease and, in some instances, result in improvement in clinical features. Neuropsychiatric symptoms are treated symptomatically.

Other causes Primary psychiatric disorders can present with cognitive impairment. The term pseudodementia has been used to describe cognitive deficits that can be seen in the presence of idiopathic psychiatric illness, especially major depressive disorder. The deficits are usually subcortical in nature, involving attention, speed of mental processing, memory retrieval, and verbal fluency and elaboration. Patients may register new material but have difficulty with spontaneous recall that typically improves when they are presented with recognition cues. Pseudodementia was originally thought to be simply another expression of the depressed patient's lack of energy and unwillingness to attend to tasks. More recently, it has become clear that the deficits of pseudodementia represent fundamental cognitive deficits related to the same brain dysfunction that is responsible for the depressive symptoms. Dementia syndrome of depression is one current term that is synonymous with pseudodementia and may more accurately reflect the nature of the pathobiological process. Recent studies have indicated that it may have a poorer prognosis, especially in the elderly, and several investigators have described a persistent mild anomia in the same patient population.

Schizophrenia was viewed at first as a disorder in which cognitive impairment was a prominent feature (dementia precox). Negative symptoms such as paucity of speech, poverty of ideas, blunting of affect, and functional deterioration contributed to that perception. Contemporary studies have demonstrated consistent cognitive deficits in certain subgroups of schizophrenic patients, primarily involving neuropsychological tasks thought to be sensitive to frontal lobe function. However, it is unclear whether those deficits are acquired over the course of the illness or represent cognitive skills that have never developed, consistent with the neurodevelopmental hypothesis of schizophrenia.

Dementia in epilepsy was discussed earlier. *Normal pressure hydrocephalus* is an idiopathic disorder caused by partial obstruction to the flow of cerebrospinal fluid (CSF) into the subarachnoid space. Onset typically occurs after age 60 years. The pathophysiology is thought to be related to disruption of neural function, either through stretching of periventricular fibers or through disruption of the pressure differential between the ventricular and subdural spaces, compromising neuronal function by altering cerebral blood flow. The classic clinical triad of dementia, incontinence, and gait disturbance is not present uniformly in all patients with normal pressure hydrocephalus, especially early in the course, although it nearly always emerges if the condition goes unrecognized or untreated. The diagnosis is based on clinical findings, neuroimaging evidence of ventricular dilation in the absence of sulcal widening, and normal cerebrospinal fluid pressure measurements on lumbar puncture. The dementia can be of a subcortical or cortical pattern and may at times be reversed with cerebrospinal fluid shunt surgery. Specific indicators of a positive outcome remain to be established, although identification of the etiology and a short disease course favor improvement in the dementia. Rarely, case reports have documented marked improvements up to four years after the onset of progressive dementia.

Drug-related and toxin-related dementias were discussed earlier. *Irradiation-induced dementia* is an iatrogenic concomitant of cranial radiation treatment that has been reported with greater frequency as the posttreatment survival time for patients with intracranial tumors has lengthened. Although transient cognitive deficits can be observed coincident with treatment or soon after treatment, a progressive irreversible dementia can begin 6 to 24 months after the termination of treatment. White matter is particularly sensitive to the deleterious effects of irradiation, and the dementia is predominantly subcortical in nature, reflecting the preferential white matter degeneration. The pathophysiology has been hypothesized to involve arteriolar leakage and localized edema.

TABLE 12-19
Diagnostic Criteria for Dementia of the Alzheimer's Type

A. The development of multiple cognitive deficits manifested by both
  (1) memory impairment (impaired ability to learn new information and to recall previously learned information)
  (2) one (or more) of the following cognitive disturbances:
    (a) aphasia (language disturbance)
    (b) apraxia (impaired ability to carry out motor activities despite intact motor function)
    (c) agnosia (failure to recognize or identify objects despite intact sensory function)
    (d) disturbance in executive functioning (i.e., planning, organizing, sequencing, abstracting)
B. The cognitive deficits in criteria A1 and A2 each cause significant impairment in social or occupational functioning and represent a significant decline from a previous level of functioning.
C. The course is characterized by gradual onset and continuing cognitive decline.
D. The cognitive deficits in criteria A1 and A2 are not due to any of the following:
  (1) other central nervous system conditions that cause progressive deficits in memory and cognition (e.g., cerebrovascular disease, Parkinson's disease, Huntington's disease, subdural hematoma, normal-pressure hydrocephalus, brain tumor)
  (2) systemic conditions that are known to cause dementia (e.g., hypothyroidism, vitamin B_{12} or folic acid deficiency, niacin deficiency, hypercalcemia, neurosyphilis, HIV infection)
  (3) substance-induced conditions
E. The deficits do not occur exclusively during the course of a delirium.
F. The disturbance is not better accounted for by another Axis I disorder (e.g., major depressive disorder, schizophrenia).

Code based on type of onset and predominant features:
With early onset: if onset is at age 65 years or below
With delirium: if delirium is superimposed on the dementia
With delusions: if delusions are the predominant feature
With depressed mood: if depressed mood (including presentations that meet full symptom criteria for a major depressive episode) is the predominant feature. A separate diagnosis of mood disorder due to a general medical condition is not given.
Uncomplicated: if none of the above predominates in the current clinical presentation
With late onset: if onset is after age 65 years
With delirium: if delirium is superimposed on the dementia
With delusions: if delusions are the predominant feature
With depressed mood: if depressed mood (including presentations that meet full symptom criteria for a major depressive episode) is the predominant feature. A separate diagnosis of mood disorder due to a general medical condition is not given.
Uncomplicated: if none of the above predominates in the current clinical presentation

Specify if:
With behavioral disturbance

Coding note: Also code Alzheimer's disease on Axis III.

DIAGNOSIS AND CLINICAL FEATURES

DSM-IV DSM-IV has eliminated the general syndrome of dementia that was included in DSM-III-R. The dementia diagnoses in DSM-IV are dementia of the Alzheimer's type (Table 12-19), vascular dementia (Table 12-20), dementia due to other general medical conditions (Table 12-21), substance-induced persisting dementia (Table 12-22), dementia due to multiple etiologies (Table 12-23), and dementia not otherwise specified (Table 12-24).

TABLE 12-20
Diagnostic Criteria for Vascular Dementia

A. The development of multiple cognitive deficits manifested by both
  (1) memory impairment (impaired ability to learn new information or to recall previously learned information)
  (2) one (or more) of the following cognitive disturbances:
    (a) aphasia (language disturbance)
    (b) apraxia (impaired ability to carry out motor activities despite intact motor function)
    (c) agnosia (failure to recognize or identify objects despite intact sensory function)
    (d) disturbance in executive functioning (i.e., planning, organizing, sequencing, abstracting)
B. The cognitive deficits in criteria A1 and A2 each cause significant impairment in social or occupational functioning and represent a significant decline from a previous level of functioning.
C. Focal neurological signs and symptoms (e.g., exaggeration of deep tendon reflexes, extensor plantar response, pseudobulbar palsy, gait abnormalities, weakness of an extremity) or laboratory evidence indicative of cerebrovascular disease (e.g., multiple infarctions involving cortex and underlying white matter) that are judged to be etiologically related to the disturbance.
D. The deficits do not occur exclusively during the course of a delirium.

Code based on predominant features:
With delirium: if delirium is superimposed on the dementia
With delusions: if delusions are the predominant feature
With depressed mood: if depressed mood (including presentations that meet full symptom criteria for a major depressive episode) is the predominant feature. A separate diagnosis of mood disorder due to a general medical condition is not given.
Uncomplicated: if none of the above predominates in the current clinical presentation

Specify if:
With behavioral disturbance

Coding note: Also code cerebrovascular condition on Axis III.

TABLE 12-21
Diagnostic Criteria for Dementia due to Other General Medical Conditions

A. The development of multiple cognitive deficits manifested by both
  (1) memory impairment (impaired ability to learn new information or to recall previously learned information)
  (2) one (or more) of the following cognitive disturbances:
    (a) aphasia (language disturbance)
    (b) apraxia (impaired ability to carry out motor activities despite intact motor function)
    (c) agnosia (failure to recognize or identify objects despite intact sensory function)
    (d) disturbance in executive functioning (i.e., planning, organizing, sequencing, abstracting)
B. The cognitive deficits in criteria A1 and A2 each cause significant impairment in social or occupational functioning and represent a significant decline from a previous level of functioning.
C. There is evidence from the history, physical examination, or laboratory findings that the disturbance is the direct physiological consequence of one of the general medical conditions listed below.
D. The deficits do not occur exclusively during the course of a delirium.

Dementia due to HIV Disease
Coding note: Also code HIV infection affecting central nervous system on Axis III.

Dementia due to Head Trauma
Coding note: Also code head injury on Axis III.

Dementia due to Parkinson's Disease
Coding note: Also code Parkinson's disease on Axis III.

Dementia due to Huntington's Disease
Coding note: Also code Huntington's disease on Axis III.

Dementia due to Pick's Disease
Coding note: Also code Pick's disease on Axis III.

Dementia due to Creutzfeldt-Jakob Disease
Coding note: Also code Creutzfeldt-Jakob disease on Axis III.

Dementia due to . . . *[indicate the general medical condition not listed above]*
For example, normal-pressure hydrocephalus, hypothyroidism, brain tumor, vitamin B_{12} deficiency, intracranial radiation
Coding note: Also code the general medical condition on Axis III.

TABLE 12-22
Diagnostic Criteria for Substance-Induced Persisting Dementia

A. The development of multiple cognitive deficits manifested by both
  (1) memory impairment (impaired ability to learn new information or to recall previously learned information)
  (2) one (or more) of the following cognitive disturbances:
    (a) aphasia (language disturbance)
    (b) apraxia (impaired ability to carry out motor activities despite intact motor function)
    (c) agnosia (failure to recognize or identify objects despite intact sensory function)
    (d) disturbance in executive functioning (i.e., planning, organizing, sequencing, abstracting)
B. The cognitive deficits in criteria A1 and A2 each cause significant impairment in social or occupational functioning and represent a significant decline from a previous level of functioning.
C. The deficits do not occur exclusively during the course of a delirium and persist beyond the usual duration of substance intoxication or withdrawal.
D. There is evidence from the history, physical examination, or laboratory findings that the deficits are etiologically related to the persisting effects of substance use (e.g., a drug of abuse, a medication).

Code (Specific substance)-induced persisting dementia: (Alcohol; inhalant; sedative, hypnotic, or anxiolytic; other [or unknown] substance)

TABLE 12-23
Diagnostic Criteria for Dementia due to Multiple Etiologies

A. The development of multiple cognitive deficits manifested by both
  (1) memory impairment (impaired ability to learn new information or to recall previously learned information)
  (2) one (or more) of the following cognitive disturbances:
    (a) aphasia (language disturbance)
    (b) apraxia (impaired ability to carry out motor activities despite intact motor function)
    (c) agnosia (failure to recognize or identify objects despite intact sensory function)
    (d) disturbance in executive functioning (i.e., planning, organizing, sequencing, abstracting)
B. The cognitive deficits in criteria A1 and A2 each cause significant impairment in social or occupational functioning and represent a significant decline from a previous level of functioning.
C. There is evidence from the history, physical examination, or laboratory findings that the disturbance has more than one etiology (e.g., head trauma plus chronic alcohol use, dementia of the Alzheimer's type with the subsequent development of vascular dementia).
D. The deficits do not occur exclusively during the course of a delirium.

Coding note: Use multiple codes based on specific dementias and specific etiologies, e.g., dementia of the Alzheimer's type, with late onset, uncomplicated; vascular dementia, uncomplicated.

TABLE 12-24
Diagnostic Criteria for Dementia Not Otherwise Specified

This category should be used to diagnose a dementia that does not meet criteria for any of the specific types described in this section.
An example is a clinical presentation of dementia for which there is insufficient evidence to establish a specific etiology.

Dementia of the Alzheimer's type The DSM-IV diagnostic criteria for dementia of the Alzheimer's type emphasize the presence of memory impairment and the associated presence of at least one other symptom of cognitive decline (aphasia, apraxia, agnosia, or abnormal executive functioning). The diagnostic criteria also require a continuing and gradual decline in functioning, impairment in social or occupational functioning, and the exclusion of other causes of dementia. DSM-IV suggests that the age of onset be characterized as early (at age 65 or below) or late (after age 65) and that a predominant behavioral symptom be coded with the diagnosis, if appropriate.

Vascular dementia The general symptoms of vascular dementia are the same as those for dementia of the Alzheimer's type, but the diagnosis of vascular dementia requires the presence of either clinical or laboratory evidence supportive of a vascular cause of the dementia.

Dementia due to other general medical conditions DSM-IV lists six specific causes of dementia that can be coded directly: HIV disease, head trauma, Parkinson's disease, Huntington's disease, Pick's disease, and Creutzfeldt-Jakob disease. A seventh category allows the clinician to specify other nonpsychiatric medical conditions associated with dementia.

Substance-induced persisting dementia The primary reason that this DSM-IV category is listed with both the dementias and the substance-related disorders is to facilitate the clinician's thinking regarding differential diagnosis. The specific substances that

DSM-IV cross-references are alcohol; inhalant; sedative, hypnotic, or anxiolytic; and other or unknown substances.

Clinical diagnosis and evaluation The first step in the diagnosis of dementia is to establish that the cognitive deficits have occurred in a patient with a stable level of consciousness, without fluctuation or waxing and waning. It must also be demonstrated that the patient has multiple deficits rather than a focal disturbance such as that seen in amnestic disorder or primary progressive aphasia (the insidious onset of a slowly progressive language disturbance with relatively preserved memory, reasoning, judgment, and comportment). Once the basic criteria for the diagnosis of dementia have been met, the task is to differentiate which etiology is responsible by using the standard means of history, clinical examination, and laboratory evaluation.

For dementia of the Alzheimer's type, a family history of the dementia is probably the most important risk factor after advanced age. A family history of Down's syndrome or of hematological malignancies, such as leukemia, myelolymphoma, or Hodgkin's disease, is also associated with an increased risk for Alzheimer's disease. There is some evidence for a familial predisposition to vascular dementia, but it has not been demonstrated as clearly as for dementia of the Alzheimer's type. The family history is of greatest significance in the heredity dementias, such as Huntington's disease, which is transmitted via a single autosomal dominant gene with nearly 100 percent penetrance. A history of a parent or grandparent with a movement disorder and dementia should alert the clinician to that diagnostic possibility. Huntington's disease does not skip generations, although family members may have died from other causes prior to the emergence of definable symptoms. A familial pattern has been established for Wilson's disease, with a presumptive autosomal recessive gene responsible for abnormal copper metabolism. Metachromatic leukodystrophy similarly is inherited in a recessive pattern with incomplete penetrance.

Degenerative dementias as a group do not have well-established risk factors other than old age and familial patterns. For dementia of the Alzheimer's type, other risk factors identified tentatively in recent years include female gender, a past history of head trauma, and lower education. Vascular dementias are highly associated with the risk factors for cerebrovascular disease. Those factors include hypertension (especially with systolic pressures greater than 160 mmHg), cardiac disease, transient ischemic attacks, diabetes mellitus, carotid bruits, and sickle cell disease. Obesity, a sedentary life-style, tobacco use, alcohol consumption, and elevated serum cholesterol and lipid levels are less well-established risk factors for cerebrovascular disease.

A history of severe head trauma or multiple traumas over a period of time (such as in boxers) should raise the suspicion of dementia related to brain trauma. Although severe head trauma earlier in life increases the risk of dementia of the Alzheimer's type, its mechanism of action is unknown. A history of an untreated or partially treated sexually transmitted disease should raise the suspicion for neurosyphilis. The presence of risk factors for HIV infection, namely homosexuality, multiple sexual partners, and intravenous drug use, similarly increase the risk for ADC. Patients with chronic medical illnesses, especially if poorly controlled, such as epilepsy, renal failure, or hepatic cirrhosis, are also at greater risk for developing dementias. A history of occupational exposure to heavy metals or other toxins should be obtained as part of any evaluation for dementia.

PATHOLOGY AND LABORATORY EXAMINATION A general physical examination is a routine component of the workup for dementia. It may reveal evidence of systemic disease causing brain dysfunction, such as an enlarged liver and hepatic encephalopathy, or it may demonstrate systemic disease related to particular CNS processes. The detection of Kaposi's sarcoma, for example, should alert the clinician to the probable presence of AIDS and the associated possibility of ADC. Focal neurological findings, such as asymmetrical hyperreflexia or weakness, are seen more often in vascular than in degenerative diseases. Frontal release signs and primitive reflexes, while suggesting pathology in the frontal lobe, are present in many disorders and often point to a greater extent of progression.

Laboratory evaluation can assist in definitive identification of the etiological agent. The range of possible etiologies of dementia mandates selective use of laboratory tests. The evaluation should follow informed clinical suspicion, based on the history and physical and mental status examination results. Table 12-4 lists a number of laboratory tests useful in evaluating specific diseases presenting as dementia.

DIFFERENTIAL DIAGNOSIS The first step in the diagnosis of dementia is to exclude delirium. Delirium can mimic every possible psychiatric disorder and symptom. It is most common in the same populations in which dementia is most common, namely the elderly and the brain-injured. It can be distinguished from dementia by its cardinal feature, disturbance of consciousness. Level of consciousness or arousal must be determined to be stable before a diagnosis of dementia can be made with confidence. Dementia must also be distinguished from focal or specific cognitive impairments, such as those seen in aphasic or amnestic patients. Mood disorders can present with cognitive symptoms, particularly in the dementia of depression or pseudodementia. A history of a mood disorder or a current disturbance in neurovegetative function should alert the clinician to the possibility of a major depressive disorder.

COURSE AND PROGNOSIS The course and prognosis of a dementia syndrome vary with its etiology. Dementia does not in itself imply a progressive deterioration, although many of the pathobiological processes underlying dementia are degenerative, and there is no known means of altering the progressive clinical deterioration. The rate of progression may vary within families or from individual to individual. Occasionally, progression can be halted or slowed in the vascular dementias if contributing risk factors for further vascular events can be reduced. Some dementias, such as those related to endocrine or metabolic processes or drug intoxications, may resolve entirely with the treatment or with removal of the basic disorder. However, a long-standing cerebral insult often leads to chronic clinical deficits that persist even when the insult has been removed. Dementias related to tumor and infection usually follow a similar pattern.

Age at onset is an important feature of any illness. Alzheimer's disease is the most common etiology of dementia in the United States. Onset usually occurs after age 60 years and the prevalence increases exponentially with each successive decade, although cases have been reported in patients as young as 30 years. Familial forms of dementia of the Alzheimer's type appear to have an earlier age at onset. Vascular dementia, the second most common etiology of dementia, is associated with an earlier age at onset overall. Dementia secondary to other medical conditions usually arises only after the disease has progressed for some time. That observation is true of the dementias associated with infectious, physiological, metabolic, and toxic processes. The age at onset of Huntington's disease is usually between 30 and 50 years, but onset may occur earlier or later.

The dementias can be distinguished to some extent by their course, especially earlier in the disease process. Degenerative dementias are insidious in onset and gradually progressive. Despite the clinical rule of a steadily progressive course in dementia of the Alzheimer's type, some individuals may reach a several-year plateau in the overall functional impairment before progression resumes and continues on to death. Vascular dementias may follow a stepwise pattern, in which new deficits appear abruptly and associated with new vascular events, but the vascular dementias also often have an insidious onset and a slow but steadily progressive course. Dementias related to infection are usually acute, although syphilis and cryptococcal meningitis can have an indolent course. Metabolic dementias may begin rapidly or slowly, depending on the underlying systemic disease; correction of the basic deficiency or disturbance may result in improvement, although the cognitive deficits often persist. Drug- or toxin-related dementias may improve once the insult has been discontinued, although radiation-induced dementia is an exception: It first manifests many months after radiation exposure has ceased, and a progressive course ensues.

TREATMENT The first step in the treatment of dementia is verification of the diagnosis. Accurate diagnosis is imperative, for the progression may be halted or even reversed if appropriate therapy is provided. Preventative measures are important, particularly in vascular dementia. Such measures might include changes in diet, exercise, and control of diabetes and hypertension. Pharmacological agents might include antihypertensives, anticoagulants, or antiplatelet agents. Blood pressure control should aim for the higher end of the normal range, as that has been demonstrated to improve cognitive function in patients with vascular dementia. Blood pressures below the normal range have been demonstrated to result in further impairment of cognitive function in the demented patient. The choice of antihypertensive agent can be significant in that β-blockers have been associated with exaggeration of cognitive impairment. Angiotensin-converting enzyme (ACE) inhibitors and diuretics have not been linked to the exaggeration of cognitive impairment and are thought to lower blood pressure without affecting cerebral blood flow (cerebral blood flow is presumed to correlate with cognitive function). Surgical removal of carotid plaques may prevent subsequent vascular events in carefully selected patients.

For the degenerative dementias, no direct therapies have been demonstrated conclusively to reverse or retard the fundamental pathophysiological processes. The search for such an agent has been exhaustive and fraught with frustration. Such studies are constructed on a growing foundation of knowledge regarding brain neurochemistry and the derangements found in dementia. Numerous neurotransmitters, including acetylcholine, dopamine, norepinephrine, GABA, and serotonin, and several neuropeptides, including somatostatin and substance P, are decreased in dementia. Alzheimer's disease has been studied the most extensively, but similar decreases in neurotransmitters have been found in Huntington's disease, dementia due to chronic alcohol-related disorders, vascular dementia, Parkinson's disease, and, to a far more limited extent, in normal aging. Multiple neuropharmacological strategies have been devised in the hope of replenishing the deficient neurotransmitters. Replacement therapy for acetylcholine has been the most common and widely publicized strategy. Efforts at replenishment have included the use of acetylcholine precursors (for example, choline and lecithin), cholinergic agonists (for example, pilocarpine and arecoline), and cholinesterase inhibitors. Treatment with physostigmine (Antilirium, Eserine), a short-acting cholinesterase inhibitor, has consistently resulted in small but statistically significant improvements in memory in patients with dementia of the Alzheimer's type and in healthy control subjects during brief-duration infusion studies. A cholinergic agonist, tetrahydroaminoacridine or tacrine (tetrahydroaminoacridine, THA) (Cognex), became the focus of public debate after a 1986 study reported alleged marked improvements in 16 patients with dementia of the Alzheimer's type. That study, however, was criticized for substantial methodological limitations and was not replicated in several subsequent attempts. Two multicenter studies of varying design were published in late 1992. One study, with an enriched population, aimed to maximize detection of beneficial effect, but found only marginal improvement and no overall evidence of clinically meaningful change. The second reported statistically significant but still modest improvements in cognition. Recently, the Food and Drug Administration approved the use of tacrine as a therapeutic agent for dementia of the Alzheimer's type. Clinicians must be aware of both its limited demonstrated benefit and its hepatotoxic potential.

Many researchers have concluded that the notion of a single or selective neurotransmitter defect for any specific dementing illness is simplistic and that future research efforts should be directed toward neuronal protection and regeneration. Selegiline (Eldepryl, Deprenyl) an MAOB inhibitor, has apparently slowed the progression of Parkinson's disease, presumably by limiting endogenous generation of destructive oxidative products. Similar antioxidant treatments are being used experimentally with other dementias, including Huntington's disease and vascular dementia. Naloxone (Narcan), an opiate antagonist, is thought to have possible application in vascular dementia based on animal studies in which it was demonstrated to decrease the sequelae of cerebral ischemia. Nerve growth factor is being studied as a means of promoting neural regeneration or sprouting.

The absence of curative therapies does not preclude efforts to ameliorate disturbing clinical problems. Symptomatic measures are the rule for behavioral management of most dementia syndromes. Programs that emphasize a high degree of regularity and consistency in daily schedule and environment can mitigate the risk of development of catastrophic reactions or explosive outbursts. All pharmacological agents that are used for the idiopathic psychiatric disorders can be used in demented patients, though usually at dosages one half to two thirds lower. Antidepressants and ECT are safe and effective for significant depressive symptoms. The use of antipsychotics should be restricted to patients with defined psychotic symptoms, as demented patients are more susceptible to the parkinsonian side effects inherent in these agents. Benzodiazepines may be used briefly and judiciously for emergency sedation but otherwise should be avoided, as they can produce delirium and tend to further compromise residual cognitive capacities. Lithium carbonate (Eskalith), centrally active β-adrenergic blockers, carbamazepine, and valproic acid (Depakene, Depakote) have been used empirically in the treatment of affective lability and aggressive outbursts. Empirical management therapies should be used in conjunction with environmental modifications. Individual psychotherapy may have benefit for patients in the early stages of dementia, especially to assist them in coping with their losses. The positive effects of a therapeutic relationship can still be felt at later stages when patients have more severe cognitive deficits. Family education and support are vital components of any treatment approach, as all members benefit from extensive knowledge about course and prognosis, as well as needing assistance when assuming new roles in their relationships with the patient.

AMNESTIC DISORDERS The inclusion of amnestic disorders in the psychiatric nosology reflects the classification's roots as a manual for state hospital or asylum patients. The number of individuals given amnestic diagnoses due to nutritional deficiency, often related to chronic alcohol dependence, has declined. In contrast, traumatic causes have increased dramatically during recent decades.

DEFINITION The essential feature of amnestic disorders is the acquired impaired ability to learn and recall new information, coupled variably with the inability to recall previously learned knowledge or past events. The impairment must be sufficiently severe to compromise personal, social, or occupational functioning. The diagnosis is not made if the memory impairment exists in the context of reduced ability to maintain and shift attention, as encountered in delirium, or in association with significant functional problems due to the compromise of multiple intellectual abilities, as seen in dementia. Amnestic disorders are secondary syndromes caused by systemic medical or primary cerebral diseases, substance use disorders, or medication side effects, as evidenced by findings from clinical history, physical examination, or laboratory examination.

HISTORY AND COMPARATIVE NOSOLOGY Although amnestic disorder has been long described, its specific recognition has been relatively recent. It was most clearly elaborated by Sergei Korsakoff and was included among the alcoholic psychoses in DSM-I and DSM-II, as well as in earlier editions of the *Statistical Manual.* In DSM-I it was classified under chronic brain syndrome associated with intoxication. Understanding that psychosis was the term used to denote more severe disturbances of mental status, the authors of DSM-I stated: "The latter [severe alcohol-related brain damage] may manifest itself by the type of chronic delirium formerly diagnosed as Korsakoff's psychosis." Specific discussion of the amnestic syndromes was absent. As with DSM-I, DSM-II provided little clinical description of amnestic disorders, although a slightly longer definition was presented in the text.

DSM-III and DSM-III-R, in contrast, did provide an in-depth discussion and more specific diagnostic criteria. However, both volumes failed to underscore the essential quality of amnestic disorder as characterized by a specific cognitive deficit in the realm of memory, while dementia syndromes were reflective of multiple failures, including both memory and other impaired intellectual abilities. DSM-III and DSM-III-R required "demonstrable evidence of impairment in both short- and long-term memory," whereas the key feature of the disorder is an inability to learn and later recall new information. In addition, neither DSM-III nor DSM-III-R provided for the separation of transient from persistent amnesia.

EPIDEMIOLOGY Data are not available for estimating the point or lifetime prevalence, incidence, or lifetime risk of persistent amnestic disorder. One recent study indicated that transient global amnesia may have an incidence of 5.2 cases per 100,000 population per year. There are no specific data available on age at onset or culture- or sex-related aspects beyond those relating to the genesis of primary etiological disease processes. For example, transient global amnesia typically occurs after age 50 years.

ETIOLOGY Amnestic disorder often occurs as the result of pathological processes that cause damage to specific diencephalic and middle temporal lobe structures (for example, mammillary bodies, the hippocampus). The pathology is commonly bilateral, but deficits may arise from unilateral lesions. Pathogenic processes include closed-head trauma and penetrating missile wounds, focal tumors, surgical intervention, encephalitis due to infection from herpes simplex virus, infarction of the territory of the posterior cerebral artery, and hypoxia. A common cause of amnestic disorder is the chronic use of alcohol and associated thiamine deficiency.

Transient amnestic disorder, when encountered as a transient global amnesia, is typically associated with cerebrovascular disease and pathology in the vertebrobasilar system. Transient amnesia may also arise from episodic physiological or metabolic disorders, such as acute intoxications or seizures.

DIAGNOSIS AND CLINICAL FEATURES

Diagnosis In DSM-IV the differentiation between amnestic syndrome and amnestic disorder used in DSM-III-R has been eliminated. For the diagnosis of amnestic disorder, DSM-IV requires the "development of memory impairment as manifested by impairment in the ability to learn new information or the inability to recall previously learned information," and the "memory disturbance causes significant impairment in social or occupational functioning." A diagnosis of amnestic disorder due to a general medical condition (Table 12-25) is made when there is evidence of a causatively relevant specific medical condition (including physical trauma). DSM-IV further categorizes the diagnosis as being transient or chronic. A diagnosis of substance-induced persisting amnestic disorder is made when there is evidence that the symptoms are causatively related to the use of a substance (Table 12-26). DSM-IV refers the clinician to specific diagnoses within substance-related disorders: alcohol-induced persisting amnestic dis-

TABLE 12-25
Diagnostic Criteria for Amnestic Disorder due to a General Medical Condition

A. The development of memory impairment as manifested by impairment in the ability to learn new information or the inability to recall previously learned information.
B. The memory disturbance causes significant impairment in social or occupational functioning and represents a significant decline from a previous level of functioning.
C. The memory disturbance does not occur exclusively during the course of a delirium or a dementia.
D. There is evidence from the history, physical examination, or laboratory findings that the disturbance is the direct physiological consequence of a general medical condition (including physical trauma).

Specify if:
Transient: if memory impairment lasts for one month or less
Chronic: if memory impairment lasts for more than one month
Coding note: Include the name of the general medical condition on Axis I, e.g., amnestic disorder due to head trauma; also code the general medical condition on Axis III.

TABLE 12-26
Diagnostic Criteria for Substance-Induced Persisting Amnestic Disorder

A. The development of memory impairment as manifested by impairment in the ability to learn new information or the inability to recall previously learned information.
B. The memory disturbance causes significant impairment in social or occupational functioning and represents a significant decline from a previous level of functioning.
C. The memory disturbance does not occur exclusively during the course of a delirium or a dementia and persists beyond the usual duration of substance intoxication or withdrawal.
D. There is evidence from the history, physical examination, or laboratory findings that the memory disturbance is etiologically related to the persisting effects of substance use (e.g., a drug of abuse, a medication).

Code: (Specific substance)-induced persisting amnestic disorder: (Alcohol; sedative, hypnotic, or anxiolytic; other [or unknown] substance)

order; sedative, hypnotic, or anxiolytic-induced persisting amnestic disorder; and other (or unknown) substance-induced persisting amnestic disorder. DSM-IV also provides for the diagnosis of amnestic disorder not otherwise specified (Table 12-27).

Clinical features The inability to learn and recall new information, the cardinal feature of the disorder, is most apparent on spontaneous, unstructured recall tasks but is also evident on tasks that provide recall cues or recognition paradigms where the stimulus is presented again, often among mnemonically equivalent distractor items. Depending on lesion localization, deficits may be predominantly related to verbal or visual stimuli. (Studies have demonstrated repeatedly that individuals with amnestic disorder may learn how to perform novel procedures that are not mediated verbally, such as motoric tasks, even though they later fail to recall having undertaken those learning experiences.)

Problems remembering previously learned materials are present variably among amnestic patients. For example, a patient who suffered traumatic brain damage and who continues to exhibit deficits in new learning may remember events up to a time shortly before the injury. In some cases the interval of preinjury recall impairment may diminish as the patient recovers (shrinking retrograde amnesia), where inaccessible memories from several years before the injury are gradually produced and the extent of the amnesia diminishes in the context of clinical improvement. Recall deficits due to other etiologies may involve memory for knowledge and events gained over many years' duration.

For some forms of amnestic disorder, events from the remote past may be better remembered than more recent events. However, such a gradient of recall is not present uniformly among individuals with amnestic disorders. Typically, the ability to immediately repeat a sequential string of information (for example, a digit span) is not impaired in amnestic disorder; when such impairment is evident, it suggests the presence of attentional dysfunction that may be indicative of delirium.

Amnestic disorders may be transient, lasting for several hours to a few days, as in transient global amnesia, or persistent, lasting at least one month. In the context of a newly developed but unresolved memory impairment, the term "provisional" should be added to a diagnosis of transient amnesia.

Transient global amnesia is a form of transient amnestic disorder associated with episodes that are characterized by a dense, transitory inability to learn new information (that is, to form sustained memories), with a variable (ultimately shrinking on recovery) inability to recall events that occurred during the duration of the disturbance. The episode is followed by restoration to a completely intact cognitive state. There are no data to suggest that the memory impairment is associated with disturbed or abnormal behavior beyond the mild confusion or perplexity that may be manifest during the episode.

Depending on the etiology of the disorder, the onset of amnesia may be sudden or gradual. Head trauma, vascular events, or specific types of neurotoxic exposure (for example, carbon monoxide poisoning) may lead to acute mental status changes. Prolonged substance abuse, chronic neurotoxic exposure, or sustained nutritional deficiency exemplify conditions that may lead to an insidious memory decline, eventually causing a clinically definable cognitive impairment.

Amnestic disorder may develop as a result of alcohol dependence, associated with dietary and vitamin deficiency. Alternatively, it may be the primary clinical deficit arising from traumatic head injury and may present as the major feature of a postconcussional state. When memory dysfunction exceeds other features of a postconcussional syndrome, it is preferable to diagnose the condition as amnestic disorder due to head trauma.

Although persons with amnestic disorders may manifest other features of the primary systemic or cerebral disease that cause the development of the memory impairment, disordered mental status may be the sole presenting feature. Thus, in a blandly confabulating person, a clinician may misconstrue a person's history unless other corroborating persons are available. When amnestic disorder is the result of alcohol dependence and vitamin deficiency, other neurological complications of alcohol ingestion and malnutrition, such as peripheral neuropathy and cerebellar ataxia, may be observed.

PATHOLOGY AND LABORATORY EXAMINATION Laboratory findings diagnostic of the disorder may be obtained using quantitative neuropsychological testing. Standardized tests also are available to assess recall of well-known historical events or public figures, to characterize the nature of an individual's inability to remember previously learned information. Performance on such tests varies among individuals with amnestic disorder. Subtle deficits in other cognitive functions may be noted in individuals with amnestic disorder. However, memory deficits constitute the predominant feature of the mental status examination and account largely for any functional deficits.

Magnetic resonance imaging and computed tomography No specific or diagnostic features are detectable on imaging studies such as MRI or CT. However, damage of middle-temporal lobe structures is common and may be reflected in enlargement of third ventricle or temporal horns or in structural atrophy detected on MRI.

DIFFERENTIAL DIAGNOSIS The central feature of amnestic disorder is inability to learn and recall new information, in the context of variable difficulties recalling previously learned factual knowledge. Less efficient memory is a component of normatively defined age-related cognitive decline but is neither functionally impairing nor below the statistically normal range when assessed with quantitative procedures. Amnestic patients uniformly show significant abnormalities on cognitive or neuropsychological tests. Disordered memory is also a feature of delirium and dementia. When memory dysfunction occurs in the context of impaired consciousness, with reduced ability to focus, sustain, or shift attention, delirium predominates. The coexistence of memory impairment and multiple cognitive deficits (for example, aphasia, apraxis, agnosis, and disturbance in executive functioning) warrants the diagnosis of dementia. Confabulation is a mental status finding encountered in patients with dementia as well as amnesia.

Amnestic disorder may emerge from an evolving clinical picture that includes confusion and disorientation, occasionally with attentional problems that suggest delirium. For example,

TABLE 12-27
Diagnostic Criteria for Amnestic Disorder Not Otherwise Specified

This category should be used to diagnose an amnestic disorder that does not meet criteria for any of the specific types described in this section.

An example is a clinical presentation of amnesia for which there is insufficient evidence to establish a specific etiology (i.e., dissociative, substance-induced, or due to a general medical condition).

Table from DSM-IV, *Diagnostic and Statistical Manual of Mental Disorders,* ed 4. Copyright American Psychiatric Association, Washington, 1994. Used with permission.

classically described Korsakoff's syndrome due to thiamine deficiency has been associated most often with the delirium of Wernicke's encephalopathy. The latter typically clears quickly with appropriate treatment. Confabulation may be noted during the early stages of the disease process and is often indicated by the recitation of imaginary events to fill gaps in memory, but that sign tends to disappear with time. Profound amnesia typically is associated with disorientation to place and time but rarely to person. Disorientation to self may be encountered in patients with severe dementing disturbances characterized by multiple cognitive deficits but is atypical of pure amnestic disorder. Many patients with severe amnestic disorder lack insight into their deficits, and they explicitly deny its presence despite evidence to the contrary. The lack of insight may contribute to accusations or agitation in rare instances. More commonly, apathy, lack of initiative, emotional blandness, or other changes suggestive of altered personality function may be encountered. Individuals may be superficially friendly or agreeable, but they frequently have a shallow or diminished range of affective expression. Patients with transient global amnesia most often appear bewildered or befuddled. Although they have been described participating in complex activity or conversations in the course of an episode, that is a much less common presentation.

Occasionally, patients may demonstrate intact abilities to learn new information associated with profound memory loss for a circumscribed period of time. That pattern occurs in the setting of a discrete (time-limited) process that temporarily interferes with the patient's ability to establish new memories. Such processes include acute intoxication, transient delirium or encephalopathy (for example, a seizure), or some other transient disruption of cerebral functioning (for example, a transient ischemic attack). Such transient amnestic episodes must be defined clinically in the context of the primary disease processes; failure to establish a primary systemic or cerebral etiology suggests a psychogenic origin when that symptom pattern is encountered.

Dissociative amnesia typically does not involve deficits in learning and recalling new information; rather, patients present with a circumscribed inability to recall previously learned information while they continue to function normally in the present. Patients with resolved transient amnesia (for example, transient global amnesia) may have a superficially similar history retrospectively. They manifest failure of recall for matters or events that occurred during the discrete episode in question. Thorough clinical investigations of patients with amnestic disorder typically reveal a primary cerebral or systemic medical condition that is etiologically related to the genesis of the mental status abnormality. During an episode, patients with transient amnesia generally have a confused or bewildered demeanor and exhibit marked difficulty with new learning tasks. Episodes of psychogenic amnesia end abruptly, typically associated with an expressed awareness of having no memories for the time period of the amnestic or fugue state. In contrast, the retrograde memory defect of transient global amnesia gradually shortens as the patient recovers; when recovery is complete, the memory gap spans only the period of the episode.

COURSE Although the mode of onset is typically abrupt, data suggest that individuals with alcohol-induced amnestic disorder may develop deficits insidiously over many years as a result of repeated toxic and nutritional insults before the emergence of a final, dramatically impairing episode of illness apparently related to thiamine deficiency. Transient amnesia due to a cerebrovascular etiology may be recurrent, with episodes lasting from several hours to several days. Amnestic disorders due to head trauma, for example, may last variable amounts of time, with the greatest deficit apparent immediately after injury and improvement occurring during the ensuing two years (further improvement beyond 24 months has been noted, but less commonly). Full recovery may occur, although severe injuries are typically characterized by residual deficits. Disorders due to destruction of middle-temporal lobe structures, such as infarction, encephalitis, surgical ablation, or malnutrition in the context of alcohol dependence, may cause densely persisting impairments.

TREATMENT Whenever a primary systemic or cerebral disorder is causally tied to the amnestic syndrome, initial treatment (with thiamine, antiviral medication, aspirin) must be directed toward the underlying pathological process. Presently there are no known, definitively effective treatments for amnestic disorder that are specifically aimed at reversing apparent memory deficits. A variety of pharmacotherapeutic trials have been to no avail. Recently, centers for cognitive rehabilitation have been established whose rehabilitation-oriented therapeutic milieu is intended to promote recovery from brain injury, especially from traumatic causes. Despite the high cost of extended care at these sites, which provide both long-term institutional and daytime services, no data have been developed to define therapeutic effectiveness for the heterogeneous groups of patients who participate in such tasks as memory retraining. Persons with amnestic disturbances worthy of diagnosis experience major impediments in their social and vocational functioning. They may require supervised living situations to ensure appropriate feeding and care.

OTHER COGNITIVE DISORDERS Disorders such as dementia and amnesia are specific categorical designations that are intended to define disease states. However, intellectual functioning can also be viewed from a dimensional perspective, ranging from optimal to grossly deficient. Dementia represents an abnormal decline from a previous level of attainment; mental retardation reflects the failure to develop adequate intellectual function.

Within that broad framework multiple domains of intellect are recognized that involve a wide variety of brain-related cognitive processes. The determination of normal and abnormal usually is made by comparing a person's performance on a variety of neuropsychological tests with predetermined normative standards. Ideally, the clinician would like lifelong (that is, premorbid) serial cognitive testing to aid with diagnosis; occasionally, school, military, or vocational records provide an acceptable alternative. Usually one must compare a patient's results against published norms. Those norms may vary in quality, and the clinician should be aware whenever possible of factors such as the education, sex distribution, socioeconomic status, and age distribution of normative samples.

COGNITIVE DISORDER NOT OTHERWISE SPECIFIED DSM-IV includes a new diagnostic category, cognitive disorder not otherwise specified, to deal with patients whose clinical presentation does not conform to a diagnosis of delirium, dementia, or amnesia. The designation is useful for patients with mild deficits in cognitive functioning that result from conditions such as head trauma, chronic alcohol dependence, or HIV infection. In the recovering alcoholic, for example, or the patient with a significant but resolving posttraumatic amnesia, intellectual abnormalities may be detectable objectively and noted subjectively, although they may be only minimally impairing functionally. Those deficits may disappear over time or remain as subtle residua. HIV infection may cause a mild decline in cognition; current research has demonstrated such decrements repeatedly. Of note, the performance of many patients has remained within the normal range even as the test scores have decreased significantly. The diagnostic criteria for cognitive disorder not otherwise specified appear in Table 12-28.

Mild neurocognitive disorder To define those conditions with greater specificity, the World Health Organization developed the ICD-10 diagnostic category of mild cognitive disorder. A similar DSM-IV construct (mild neurocognitive disorder) is included in an appendix as an example of cognitive disorder not otherwise specified. Table 12-29 lists the DSM-IV research criteria for mild neurocognitive disorder. To date no results of investigations using these criteria have been published; thus, the interface between amnestic disorders or dementing disorders and mild neurocognitive disorder has not been defined.

TABLE 12-28
Diagnostic Criteria for Cognitive Disorder Not Otherwise Specified

This category is for disorders that are characterized by cognitive dysfunction presumed to be due to the direct physiological effect of a general medical condition that do not meet criteria for any of the specific deliriums, dementias, or amnestic disorders listed in this section and that are not better classified as delirium not otherwise specified, dementia not otherwise specified, or amnestic disorder not otherwise specified. For cognitive dysfunction due to a specific or unknown substance, the specific substance-related disorder not otherwise specified category should be used.

Examples include

1. Mild neurocognitive disorder: impairment in cognitive functioning as evidenced by neuropsychological testing or quantified clinical assessment, accompanied by objective evidence of a systemic general medical condition or central nervous system dysfunction (Table 12-2 for suggested research criteria)
2. Postconcussional disorder: following a head trauma, impairment in memory or attention with associated symptoms (see Table 12-6 for suggested research criteria)

TABLE 12-29
Research Criteria for Mild Neurocognitive Disorder

A. The presence of two (or more) of the following impairments in cognitive functioning, lasting most of the time for a period of at least two weeks (as reported by the individual or a reliable informant):
   (1) memory impairment as identified by a reduced ability to learn or recall information
   (2) disturbance in executive functioning (i.e., planning, organizing, sequencing, abstracting)
   (3) disturbance in attention or speed of information processing
   (4) impairment in perceptual-motor abilities
   (5) impairment in language (e.g., comprehension, word finding)
B. There is objective evidence from physical examination or laboratory findings (including neuroimaging techniques) of a neurological or general medical condition that is judged to be etiologically related to the cognitive disturbance.
C. There is evidence from neuropsychological testing or quantified cognitive assessment of an abnormality or decline in performance.
D. The cognitive deficits cause marked distress or impairment in social, occupational, or other important areas of functioning and represent a decline from a previous level of functioning.
E. The cognitive disturbance does not meet criteria for a delirium, a dementia, or an amnestic disorder and is not better accounted for by another mental disorder (e.g., a substance-related disorder, major depressive disorder).

In addition to conditions such as HIV infection, head trauma, or alcohol dependence, mild cognitive decline with neuropsychological performance below the level of age-matched peers may be encountered as an early sign of a progressive degenerative disease. The use of cognitive disorder not otherwise specified as a diagnosis can serve to describe provisionally a patient who, for example, the physician suspects will develop a more malignant dementia of the Alzheimer's type and in whom a definitive diagnosis is premature owing to the relative mildness of the symptoms and an associated lack of clarity regarding clinical course. The not otherwise specified label demands maximum clinical scrutiny and vigilance when employed in that fashion.

OTHER COGNITIVE CONDITIONS Clinical investigators and geriatric psychiatrists have recently joined cognitive psychologists in studying aging-related cognitive decrements involving such functions as spontaneous verbal memory, cognitive flexibility and abstracting ability, visuospatial processing, divided attention, speed of mental processing, and naming. Aging-related decrements in those functions do not relate to any specific or defined neuropathology, although they may reflect underlying neurobiological deterioration. Of note, objective documentation of individual decline in test performance may be impossible. Although experimental comparisons of groups of healthy older subjects with comparably educated younger groups show consistent changes with aging, there are no data to suggest that the overall decline is a harbinger of disease.

Many persons with normal (that is, normatively defined) aging-related intellectual decrements seek clinical evaluation for forgetfulness, especially out of fear that they may be developing Alzheimer's disease. Their complaints often include inability to recall names or words spontaneously, absent-mindedness, the need to use reminder lists, or subtle problems with concentration. Careful interviewing typically reveals mild anxiety about minor intellectual problems, the use of effective compensatory mental strategies, and intact personal and social functioning, with little evidence of definable interference from perceived cognitive inadequacies in their daily lives. The absence of significant functional decline, together with performance within the normative (that is, based on similarly aged samples) range on neuropsychological testing, in the context of an unrevealing general medical evaluation points to aging-associated cognitive alterations.

Because of ample data on the phenomenon and clinicians' need to provide concerned patients with an understandable terminology to define their perceived difficulties, DSM-IV groups age-related cognitive decline among those conditions not attributable to a mental disorder that are a focus of attention or treatment. A variety of other common problems are included in that class, among them borderline intellectual functioning, academic problems, adult antisocial behavior, and marital problems.

Figure 12-2 presents schematically in a dimensional perspective the relations between increasing age and cognitive performance, depicting changes in the normative range, mild cognitive impairment, and dementia. The aging-related decline in normative performance underscores the difficulty of establishing an absolute standard of cognitive deficit that is indicative of impairment due to a categorical disease process. The figure also suggests that there will always be patients detected in the range of mild impairment. As long as there are few (or no) pathobiologically exact laboratory tests to determine with certainty specific cognitive impairment disorders, thoughtful clinical judgment will remain a central part of the diagnostic process.

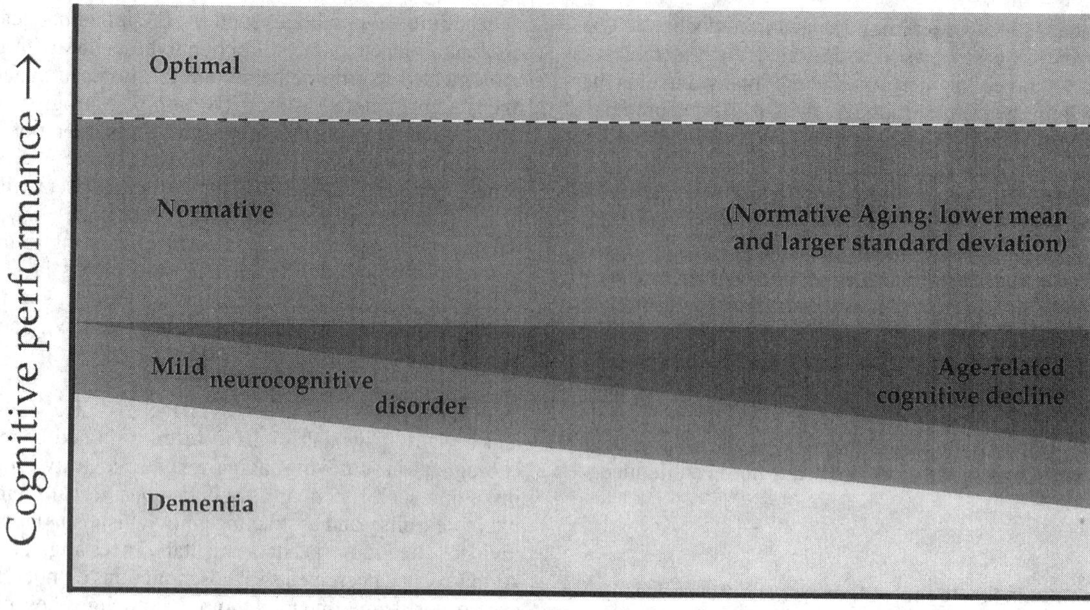

FIGURE 12-2 *Aging-associated changes in ranges of cognitive performance.*

MENTAL DISORDERS DUE TO A GENERAL MEDICAL CONDITION

DSM-IV has taken a different approach to categorizing the mental disorders due to a general medical condition than did DSM-III-R. In DSM-III-R the disorders were classified under the broader category of organic mental disorders. In DSM-IV each mental disorder due to a general medical condition is classified within the category that most resembles its symptoms (Table 12-30). For example, the diagnosis psychotic disorder due to a general medical condition is found in the DSM-IV section on schizophrenia and other psychotic disorders. The symptom-based organization of DSM-IV is meant to facilitate clinical decision making regarding the differential diagnosis of symptoms. For example, the clinician who is evaluating a patient with depression can refer to the DSM-IV section on mood disorders and find mood disorder due to a general medical condition as one of the diagnoses. That diagnosis should help clarify the importance of considering the possibility of a mental disorder due to a general medical condition for almost all psychiatric presentations.

MOOD DISORDER DUE TO A GENERAL MEDICAL CONDITION Secondary mood syndromes are characterized by a prominent mood alteration that is thought to be the direct physiological effect of a specific medical illness or agent. Those disorders are often difficult to define and have not been extensively researched; therefore, only limited information can be provided.

Definition The DSM-IV diagnostic criteria for mood disorder due to a general medical condition is found in Section 16.6. The key feature is prominent, persistent, distressing, or functionally impairing depressed mood (anhedonia) or elevated, expansive, or irritable mood, judged to be caused by either an Axis III condition or by substance intoxication or withdrawal. Cognitive impairment is not the predominant clinical feature; otherwise, the mood disturbance would be viewed as part of delirium, dementia, or other cognitive deficit disorder. The diagnostician is asked to specify if the mood syndrome is manic, depressed, or mixed, and if criteria for a fully symptomatic major depressive or manic syndromic are fulfilled.

TABLE 12-30
Mental Disorders due to a General Medical Condition

DSM-IV Category	Mental Disorders due to a General Medical Condition
Delirium, dementia, amnestic, and other cognitive disorders	Delirium due to a general medical condition Dementia due to other general medical conditions Amnestic disorder due to a general medical condition
Schizophrenia and other psychotic disorders	Psychotic disorder due to a general medical condition
Mood disorders	Mood disorder due to a general medical condition
Anxiety disorders	Anxiety disorder due to a general medical condition
Sexual disorders	Sexual dysfunction due to a general medical condition
Sleep disorders	Sleep disorder due to a general medical condition
Mental disorders due to a general medical condition not elsewhere classified	Catatonic disorder due to a general medical condition Personality change due to a general medical condition Mental disorder not otherwise specified due to a general medical condition

History and Comparative Nosology Mood disturbances secondary to medical conditions have long been described, but attention was rarely paid to the presence or absence of coexisting intellectual deficits. DSM-III introduced the term and the formal concept of organic affective syndrome, which required both mood alteration and two associated symptoms (as found in primary affective illnesses) to be present and thought due to specific medical etiologies. DSM-III-R eliminated the requirement for associated symptoms. DSM-IV marks the first explicit diagnostic criteria to denote whether or not the disturbance meets full major depressive or manic syndromic criteria. There has been much disagreement in the literature about primary depressive disorders and whether minor depressive disorders exist and how best to define them. Similar arguments might apply to lesser depressive syndromes of secondary origin. Terminology aside, there has been little research in the area of secondary mood disorders; what data exist are hampered by differing (or absent) operationalization of what constitutes sufficient evidence for defining causality.

Epidemiology There are no clear data on which to base statements of incidence or prevalence of secondary mood disorders in any clinical or community population. It is clear that depressive symptoms and a wide array of systemic and primary cerebral conditions coexist to a far higher degree than can be explained by chance. Unfortunately, establishing a causal relation between depressive symptoms and a specific medical entity is difficult; therefore, the percentage of those coexisting symptoms that can be called secondary remains unknown. Further, many reported studies did not assess a range of syndromic criteria (that is, major versus minor depression), and many simply quantified depressive symptoms by using rating scales without determining if the symptoms attained a threshold level of clinical significance. One noteworthy point is that depression in the medically ill appears to be equally prevalent by sex, or possibly slightly higher in men than in women. That disparity, when compared with the preponderance of females with primary depressive disorders, is often cited as an indicator of the importance of viewing secondary mood disturbances separately.

Rates of mood disorder in the medically ill have been carefully described in several neurological diseases. For example, at least one research group has documented high rates of criteria-defined major and minor depressive syndromes in patients shortly after cerebrovascular accidents. Correlation of stroke lesion location and size with presence (and possibly with type) of depressive syndrome suggests the role of direct disruption of brain physiology as a causal mechanism. Also, the presence or severity of depression does not correlate highly with physical impairment due to hemiparesis, for example, and may be higher than rates found in patients with similar levels of overall disability due to nonneurological conditions, suggesting that depression in neurological patients is not simply a psychological reaction to illness and disability. Similarly, less extensive descriptions of increased rates of depressive symptoms and syndromes have been reported for populations with Parkinson's disease, Huntington's disease, HIV infection (with presumed direct CNS involvement), and multiple sclerosis.

Determination of the secondary or symptomatic nature of those mood syndromes is problematic. It is further complicated by the fact that at least some of the patients with the neurological illnesses listed above had substantial cognitive impairment. Although DSM-IV attempts to address these issues directly, uncertainties remain. For example, if a patient with Huntington's disease has dementia and a depressive syndrome, the clinician might choose the diagnosis of dementia due to Huntington's disease with depressed mood. However, early in the disease process a syndromically depressed Huntington's patient with few cognitive impairments would warrant a diagnosis of mood disorder due to Huntington's disease with major depressive episode. As the intellectual impairment progresses, does the clinician abandon one diagnosis for another or add a second Axis I diagnosis of dementia? Such borderline situations are expected to generate uncertainty, which can be ameliorated by careful documentation of one's clinical reasoning.

Secondary mania appears to be much less prevalent in most neurological illnesses, with the exceptions of multiple sclerosis and possibly Huntington's disease. Case reports abound of putative secondary mania due to a variety of other causes, but the prevalence is not known.

Finally, patients with secondary mood syndromes may have increased rates of prior mood disorders and higher rates of family history of mood disorder. Therefore, secondary syndromes may reflect an interaction between a precipitating agent or illness and the patient's diathesis toward mood pathology.

Etiology The list of potential etiologies for both depressive and manic syndromes is long. Table 12-31 lists some of the etiologies most commonly considered.

Diagnosis and clinical features The depressive or manic symptoms found in secondary mood disorders are phenomenologically similar to those found in primary (idiopathic) mood disorders. It is not known if certain symptoms occur more commonly in the secondary disorders; presumably the prevalence may vary depending on the specific etiology of the secondary disorder. For example, anxiety has been described as prominent in major depressive syndromes seen in patients with Parkinson's disease; however, no studies have compared depressed patients with Parkinson's disease with similarly aged patients experiencing idiopathic major depressive disorder.

Associated clinical phenomena may include other manifestations of the cause of the secondary mood disorder, such as soft neurological signs or contributing cognitive impairment; indeed, those findings are used to support the assessment of the mood symptoms as secondary in origin.

There are no specific tests to confirm the diagnosis of a secondary mood disorder. In addition, little is known about how neurobiological abnormalities seen in idiopathic mood disorders differ from secondary syndromes. Moreover, despite recent interest in secondary mood disorders, there is still little definitive understanding of the neuroanatomical substrate of those disorders. Physical (including neurological) examination and specific laboratory tests or procedures may be crucial to establishing the presence of the primary disease state.

Differential diagnosis There are two broad domains of differential diagnosis to consider when establishing the presence

TABLE 12-31
Etiologies of Secondary Mood Disorders

Drug intoxication
- Alcohol or sedative-hypnotics (as examples)
- Antipsychotics
- Antidepressants
- Metoclopramide, H_2-receptor blockers
- Antihypertensives (especially centrally acting agents, e.g., methyldopa, clonidine, reserpine)
- Sex steroids (e.g., oral contraceptives, anabolic steroids)
- Glucocorticoids
- Levodopa
- Bromocriptine

Drug withdrawal
- Nicotine, caffeine, alcohol or sedative-hypnotics, cocaine, amphetamines

Tumor
- Primary cerebral
- Systemic neoplasm

Trauma
- Cerebral contusion
- Subdural hematoma

Infection
- Cerebral (e.g., meningitis, encephalitis, HIV, syphilis)
- Systemic (e.g., sepsis, urinary tract infection, pneumonia)

Cardiac and vascular
- Cerebrovascular (e.g., infarcts, hemorrhage, vasculitis)
- Cardiovascular (e.g., low-output states, congestive heart failure, shock)

Physiological or metabolic
- Hypoxemia, electrolyte disturbances, renal or hepatic failure, hypo- or hyperglycemia, postictal states
- **Endocrine**
  - Thyroid or glucocorticoid disturbances
- **Nutritional**
  - Vitamin B_{12}, (?)folate, deficiency

Demyelinating
- Multiple sclerosis

Neurodegenerative
- Parkinson's disease, Huntington's disease

of a secondary mood disorder. The first is phenomenological: Does the patient have clinically significant manic or depressive symptoms in the absence of evidence of a predominating cognitive deficit? That assessment requires attention to symptoms and function in the history and mental status examination. As part of the process, the clinician is also establishing whether there is a clearly defined mood syndrome sufficient to warrant an empirical treatment trial with antidepressants.

The second domain is etiological: Does the patient have an Axis III condition or a state of substance intoxication or withdrawal that is causing the mood disturbance? Establishing the presence of the relevant condition depends on standard psychiatric and medical-neurological assessments. Establishing the causal relation to the mood disorder may be difficult.

Course and prognosis Although the literature on the course of clearly defined secondary mood disorders is scant, substantial work has demonstrated that all depressive conditions that are comorbid with general medical illnesses or substance-related disorders have poorer prognoses than those that have no demonstrated associations, whether measured by means of symptomatic expression, functional disability, or mortality. It is therefore likely that secondary depressive illness is most often a chronic disease that is sometimes characterized by periods of remission followed by recurrences and sometimes by continuous illness. The prognosis varies, depending on the etiological disease state; depression secondary to a readily treatable disease (for example, hypothyroidism) has a better outcome than depression associated with a terminal, essentially untreatable condition (for example, metastatic pancreatic carcinoma). Little is known about the relation of specific depressive syndromes to outcome even within a specific etiological group. For example, there have been attempts to distinguish outcome in poststroke patients based on the presence of minor or major depressive syndromes; that work has had little replication by other investigator groups, and in any case the results may not generalize to depression secondary to other conditions. There is even less information available on the course of secondary mania, although many case reports suggest it is chronic and refractory to treatment.

Treatment Treatment response has received limited study. Standard antidepressants (for example, tricyclic antidepressants, monoamine oxidase inhibitors (MAOIs), and ECT are effective in many depressed patients with medical and neurological illnesses or substance use disorders. However, the utility of studies of antidepressants has been limited by the scant clinical definition of study patients in many publications; a designation of organic mood disorder, depressed, provides little information on specific target symptoms and their response. The efficacy of newer somatic agents (for example, serotonin-specific reuptake inhibitors, bupropion [Wellbutrin]) and of psychotherapeutic approaches has received little systematic study. A comparison of response to specific treatment modalities in syndromically similar primary and secondary mood disorders has not been done. However, the comorbid pathology found in secondary syndromes may limit treatment trials, either because of contraindications or because of increased susceptibility to side effects.

Given the severely limited data, the clinician treating a patient with a secondary mood disorder must rely on the following general guidelines. The underlying etiology or etiologies should be treated as effectively as possible. Persisting manic or major depressive syndromes will likely require somatic therapies; standard treatment approaches as used for the corresponding primary mood disorder should be employed, although the risk of toxic effects may require more gradual dosage increases. At a minimum, psychotherapy should focus on psychoeducational issues (in particular, the concept of a secondary behavioral disturbance may be new or difficult for many patients and families) and support. More specific intrapsychic, interpersonal, and family issues are addressed as indicated. Approaches to subsyndromal secondary mood disorders are even less well established, but clinically significant disturbances warrant empirical trials of the same treatments used in fully syndromic patients.

PSYCHOTIC DISORDER DUE TO A GENERAL MEDICAL CONDITION Psychosis has been a term of inconsistent definition, used in recent years to refer exclusively to symptoms of a striking nature, such as hallucinations and delusions, but in the past to severe affective syndrome (for example, psychotic versus neurotic depression); to cognitive symptoms, such as confusion, disorientation, or altered memory (such as Korsakoff's psychosis); or as a means of describing the severity of any psychiatric symptom (''of psychotic proportions''). DSM-III-R in its appended glossary defined psychosis as ''gross impairment in reality testing and the creation of a new reality.'' Hallucinations, delusions, bizarre behavior, and incoherent speech were considered direct evidence of psychosis. Psychotic symptoms have been recognized as nonspecific, as they can be seen in any of the major psychiatric illnesses, such as dementia, schizophrenia, or bipolar disorder, as well as in many systemic medical or cerebral disorders.

Definition The DSM-IV diagnostic criteria for psychotic disorder due to a general medical condition appear in Section 15.3. In order to establish the diagnosis, the clinician first must exclude syndromes in which psychotic symptoms may be present in association with cognitive impairment (for example, delirium and dementia of the Alzheimer's type) but not the defining feature, and the clinician must determine with confidence the causal link. In turn, secondary psychotic disorders must be excluded before a diagnosis of a primary (idiopathic) psychotic disorder is entertained.

History Psychotic symptoms, including delusions, hallucinations, incoherent speech or formal thought disorder, and bizarre behavior, have been recognized for centuries. In medical prehistory, they were perceived in a theological light as evidence of demonic possession or punishment for a moral failing. For Thomas Sydenham in the 18th century, at the threshold of the modern brain disease model, psychosis was sometimes attributed to a bodily dysfunction, either systemic or related specifically to the CNS. However, tension has persisted among clinicians for much of the past two centuries as to whether psychotic symptoms reflected the manifestations of a dysfunctional brain or were volitional or psychological reactions to life circumstances. Reports of secondary psychosis have abounded for centuries and have contributed to an understanding of those behaviors as specific symptoms of brain disease. Many descriptions, however, have had limited use because of vagaries in the definition of psychosis and the lack of any uniform means for establishing a correlation between psychotic symptoms and the associated systemic or cerebral medical condition under study.

Recently, three types of investigations have emerged for the study of secondary syndromes, including secondary psychosis. One type of study compares psychopathological symptoms in patient groups with and without known primary medical conditions. That comparison has been done strictly on a retrospective basis for secondary psychosis, with only one available prospective study of secondary delusional disorders. Another type of investigation has examined patient groups with known CNS disease, such as cerebrovascular disorder or Huntington's disease, with a careful description of any associated psychopathology. The third investigative track has selected patients with known psychopathology, such as hallucinations in schizophrenia, and sought evidence to correlate symptoms with CNS dysfunction using a variety of measures (for example, neuroimaging of the temporal lobe). The secondary psychotic disorders are a window through which insights into the neurobiological basis for psychotic processes may be obtained.

Comparative nosology Secondary psychotic syndromes were categorized in DSM-II as psychoses associated with organic brain syndromes. The syndromes included in that category were the dementias, deliria, and psychoses associated with other cerebral and systemic conditions. Entry into the category depended on cognitive symptoms, such as disturbances of orientation, memory, and judgment, and lability of affect. The term "psychosis" continued to be used for the sake of historic continuity, with the acknowledgment that "many patients for whom these diagnoses are clinically justified are not in fact psychotic." DSM-III improved on the nosology by establishing the general rubric of organic brain syndromes, with six specific syndromes, including organic hallucinosis and organic delusional syndrome. In DSM-IV, psychotic disorder due to . . . (with its available subtypes) has been moved out of the organic group to the phenomenological cluster to which it is related. That shift underscores the need for differential diagnosis, the clinical importance of defining etiology whenever possible, and the idea that primary psychopathology is idiopathic—that is, without known cause.

Epidemiology The incidence and prevalence of secondary psychotic disorders in the general population are unknown. The prevalence of psychotic symptoms is increased in selected clinical populations, such as nursing home residents with dementia of the Alzheimer's type, but it is unclear how to extrapolate those findings to other patient groups.

Etiology Virtually any cerebral or systemic disease that affects brain function can produce psychotic symptoms. Table 12-18 lists examples within each of the broad categories of diseases that can produce dementia; each of those diseases is also capable of producing psychotic symptoms, both in the presence and in the absence of cognitive impairment. Degenerative disorders, such as Alzheimer's disease or Huntington's disease, may present initially with new-onset psychosis, with minimal evidence of cognitive impairment at the earliest stages.

Diagnosis and clinical features To establish the diagnosis of a secondary psychotic syndrome, the clinician first determines that the patient is not delirious, as evidenced by a stable level of consciousness. A careful mental status assessment is conducted to exclude significant cognitive impairments, such as those encountered in dementia or amnestic disorder. The next step is to search for systemic or cerebral diseases that might be causally related to the psychosis. Psychotic symptomatology per se is not helpful in distinguishing a secondary from a primary (idiopathic) etiology.

Comparative studies have not demonstrated any distinguishing phenomenological features in secondary psychosis or any difference in frequency or severity of the psychosis when compared to idiopathic psychosis. Olfactory and auditory hallucinations, although claimed anecdotally to suggest a secondary or symptomatic etiology, have proved unreliable. Some studies have suggested that exclusively positive psychotic symptoms, in the absence of negative symptoms and personality change, reflect a secondary etiology. That suggestion has not been tested prospectively. Age at onset is a factor that should alert clinicians to the possible emergence of a secondary psychotic disorder, reflecting both the age-related increased prevalence of diseases affecting brain function and the natural history of primary psychotic syndromes, with their markedly diminished incidence after ages 40 to 45 years.

All patients who present with the new onset of psychotic symptoms should undergo a thorough clinical evaluation emphasizing personal medical history, family medical history, and medical review of systems. A systematic physical and neurological examination should be performed. (The examiner should bear in mind, however, that nonlocalizing, soft neurological signs and a variety of dyskinesias can be present in idiopathic schizophrenia, even in the drug-naïve patient.) The authors recommend a neuroimaging evaluation with MRI for any new-onset psychosis, irrespective of patient age.

The detection of a systemic or cerebral abnormality does not automatically lead to the determination of secondary psychosis. As emphasized earlier in this chapter, establishing a secondary status requires thoughtful clinical reasoning.

Differential diagnosis The differential diagnosis involves first establishing that the symptoms and signs encountered are in fact psychotic, according to the more specific modern definition. Confabulation may be mistaken for delusions. *Confabulation* is the spontaneous or prompted production of inconsistent and fabricated statements, often in response to questions or environmental stimuli. Although memory impairment is present in those who confabulate, the more salient cognitive deficit involves an inability to suppress or self-analyze the automatic fabrications and responses. Confabulation differs from delusions in that the fabricated beliefs are quite transient and varying. A behavioral response to the confabulated belief is usually absent. The presence of confabulation is also suggestive of brain disease, often involving the anterior temporal lobe (memory impairment) and the frontal lobes (loss of self-analysis). *Perceptual disturbances* that result in illusions or other misinterpretations of environmental stimuli must be distinguished from hallucinations, which are experienced as true perceptual experiences but without an actual stimulus. *Agnosias,* or deficit syndromes, such as prosopagnosia, topographic agnosia, or phonagnosia (inability to recognize familiar faces, places, or sounds, respectively), can occur in the context of intact peripheral perception and can be mistaken for both delusional beliefs as well as hallucinations. It is important to distinguish those deficit syndromes and to recognize that they point to parietal lobe dysfunctions that are not associated with other psychotic symptoms.

The phenomenology or type of psychotic symptom does not help distinguish idiopathic from secondary etiologies. However, once the suspicion of a secondary etiology has arisen, the specific psychotic presentation may suggest a particular brain region or direction for further investigation. Table 12-32 lists a number of specific psychotic symptoms that have been consistently associated with disease in particular brain regions. *First-rank symptoms,* originally described by Kurt Schneider as pathognomonic symptoms of schizophrenia, are now accepted as nonspecific psychotic symptoms occurring in all psychotic disorders. Although nonspecific for diagnosis, they have been associated with abnormalities in the left temporal lobe. Complex delusions have been associated with lesions in subcortical regions. Simple persecutory ideas are more common than complex or systematized delusions in patients with significant cognitive deficits. Patients apparently require a variety of intact intellectual abilities (and, presumably, underlying brain substrate) in order to produce psychotic symptoms of greater complexity. *Anton syndrome* refers to denial of blindness, classically described in patients with acquired cortical blindness arising from bilateral occipital cortex damage. More recently, it has been described in patients with peripheral optic neuropathy, suggesting that the syndrome may be a variant of the other denial-of-deficit syndromes, such as anosognosia. *Misidentification syndromes* have been described primarily in idiopathic

TABLE 12-32
Psychotic Symptoms Associated with Abnormality of Specific Brain Regions

Symptoms	Site	Laterality
First-rank symptoms	Temporal lobe	Dominant hemisphere
Thoughts spoken aloud		
Voices commenting		
Third-person voices arguing		
Made actions		
Made feelings		
Thought withdrawal		
Thought diffusion		
Delusional perception		
Complex delusions	Subcortical or limbic	
Anton syndrome	Occipital lobe, optic tract	Bilateral
Anosognosia	Parietal lobe	Nondominant hemisphere
Misidentification syndromes	Parietal, temporal, frontal lobes	Nondominant hemisphere, bilateral
Capgras syndrome		
Reduplicative paramnesia		
Fregoli syndrome		
Intermetamorphosis syndrome		

psychotic disorders, although recent studies have pointed to nondominant parietal and frontal lesions as the basis for many. One recent neuropsychological theory proposes that the right hemisphere plays a role in the appreciation of the individuality or uniqueness of people, places, and objects and that lesions in the right hemisphere can result in delusions of misidentification.

Course and prognosis The course and prognosis of secondary psychotic syndromes depend on their etiology. Vivid psychotic symptoms arising from head trauma may improve dramatically during recovery. Delusions associated with degenerative diseases may diminish as the disease worsens, for the capacity to generate those more complex cognitions is gradually lost. Some secondary psychotic disorders improve with treatment of the underlying disorder, such as the interictal psychosis of epilepsy, which often improves with the pharmacological or surgical control of seizures. Psychotic disorders secondary to infectious disease may not improve, despite eradication of the infectious organism, because of irreversible tissue damage sustained during the acute infection.

Treatment The principles of treatment for a secondary psychotic disorder are similar to those for any secondary neuropsychiatric disorder, namely, rapid identification of the etiological agent and treatment of the underlying cause. Antipsychotics afford empirical symptomatic treatment for the psychotic symptoms, although secondary psychotic disorders often prove more refractory than idiopathic disorders to such treatment. Patients with primary systemic or cerebral diseases frequently are more vulnerable to the untoward side effects of antipsychotics. To date, there has been insufficient use of nonneuroleptic antipsychotics, such as clozapine (Leponex), to judge their utility with these conditions.

ANXIETY DISORDER DUE TO A GENERAL MEDICAL CONDITION Secondary anxiety syndromes are characterized by prominent anxiety symptoms that are thought to be the direct physiological effect of a specific physical illness or agent. Those disorders have received even less careful scrutiny than secondary mood disorders; therefore, the qualifications made in the section above apply equally or more so to the following discussion.

Definition The DSM-IV diagnostic criteria for anxiety disorder due to a general medical condition is found in Section 17.5. The key feature is the presence of prominent anxiety symptoms, which may include generalized anxiety, panic attacks, obsessions, compulsions, or phobias and which are judged to be caused by either an Axis III condition or by substance intoxication or withdrawal. In addition, the anxiety symptoms are not thought to be better explained by another mental disorder (for example, the anxiety that can be seen in delirium or adjustment disorder with anxious mood). The diagnostician is asked to specify if the anxiety syndrome includes generalized anxiety, panic attacks, obsessive-compulsive symptoms, or phobias.

History and comparative nosology For centuries clinicians have described anxiety symptoms as prominent features in a variety of conditions; for most of the 20th century many of those descriptions focused on patients with endocrinopathies, neurological illnesses, mitral valve prolapse, and substance-related states. The formal concept of any organic mental disorder other than cognitive disorders was introduced by DSM-III; however, organic anxiety disorder was not presented as a distinct entity until DSM-III-R. DSM-III-R limited the diagnosis to either generalized anxiety or panic attacks; DSM-IV broadens the possible related phenomena to include obsessions and compulsions.

Secondary anxiety syndromes have received little study. There are numerous descriptions of anxiety symptoms associated with medical illness or substance-related states, but the operationalization of "secondariness" is generally absent. Further, most studies have included patients with generalized anxiety or panic symptoms; reports of secondary obsessive-compulsive phenomena are few.

Epidemiology The prevalence of anxiety symptoms is high in general medical patients and in patients with many of the specific medical illnesses that are putative potential etiologies for secondary anxiety syndromes. However, the incidence and prevalence of secondary anxiety disorders, obtained from well-operationalized criteria for syndromic and etiological diagnosis, are not known. Similarly, rates of prior anxiety disturbances or of a family history for anxiety disorders are not known.

Etiology The list of potential etiologies for anxiety syndromes is long, with nearly complete overlap with the potential etiologies for mood syndromes. Etiologies most commonly described in anxiety syndromes include substance-related states (intoxication with caffeine, cocaine, amphetamines, and other sympathomimetic agents; withdrawal from nicotine, sedative-hypnotics, and alcohol), endocrinopathies (especially pheochromocytoma, hyperthyroidism, hypercortisolemic states, and hyperparathyroidism), metabolic derangements (for example, hypoxemia, hypercalcemia, and hypoglycemia), and neurological disorders (including vascular, trauma, and degenerative). Many of those conditions are either inherently transient or easily remediable. Whether that reflects the pathophysiology of secondary anxiety or is an artifact of reporting (for example, anxiety with subacute onset and complete resolution after removal of a pheochromocytoma is more likely to be reported as an example of anxiety due to a medical illness than is chronic anxiety in the context of chronic obstructive pulmonary disease) is not known. Much attention has been paid to the association of panic attacks and mitral valve prolapse. The nature of that association is unknown, and therefore the diagnosis of panic attacks secondary to mitral valve prolapse currently is premature. Interestingly, several recent reports have sought to tie obsessive-compulsive symptoms to the development of pathology in the basal ganglia.

Diagnosis and clinical features The symptoms found in secondary anxiety disorders are by definition phenomenologically similar to those found in the corresponding primary anxiety disorder (for example, panic attacks and obsessions). It is not known if certain symptoms are found more commonly in the secondary variety; presumably the rate of co-occurrence may vary, depending on the specific etiology of the secondary disorder.

As with all secondary syndromes, associated clinical phenomena may include other manifestations of the cause of the secondary anxiety disorder, such as soft neurological signs or subtle cognitive impairment (which may have been used to support the assessment of the anxiety symptoms as being secondary in origin).

There are no specific tests to confirm the diagnosis of secondary anxiety disorder, and little is known about how neurobiological abnormalities seen in primary anxiety disorders differ in secondary syndromes. Physical (including neurological) examination and specific laboratory tests or procedures may be necessary to establish the presence of the etiological disease state.

Differential diagnosis As for other secondary disorders, two broad domains of differential diagnosis must be considered to establish the presence of a secondary anxiety disorder. The first is phenomenological: Does the patient have clinically significant anxiety, panic attacks, obsessions, or compulsions, along with an absence of evidence for another primary or secondary psychiatric syndrome? The second is etiological: Does the patient have an Axis III condition, or a state of substance intoxication or withdrawal, that is causing the phenomenology? As ever, establishing the causal relationship may be difficult.

Course and prognosis Little information is available on the course of secondary anxiety disorders. The outcome presumably depends on the specific etiology; thus, anxiety due to hyperthyroidism may well remit with treatment of the hyperthyroid state, whereas anxiety due to cardiomyopathy with a low-output state may run a more chronic course.

Treatment Well-designed treatment studies of carefully described patients with secondary anxiety disorders are lacking. Aside from treating the etiology, clinicians have found benzodiazepines to be helpful in decreasing anxiety symptoms; supportive psychotherapy (including psychoeducational issues focusing on the diagnosis and prognosis) may also be useful. The efficacy of other, more specific therapies in secondary syndromes (for example, antidepressants for panic attacks, serotonin-specific reuptake inhibitors for obsessive-compulsive symptoms, behavior therapy for simple phobias) is unknown.

SLEEP DISORDER DUE TO A GENERAL MEDICAL CONDITION Sleep disorders can result from a diversity of causes, among them stressful life circumstances, crossing time zones, pulmonary or laryngeal structural abnormalities, systemic diseases (for example, renal failure), or primary cerebral pathology. However, many sleep disorders, such as narcolepsy, sleep terrors, and enuresis, are idiopathic and occur without known systemic or central abnormalities. The epidemiology of secondary sleep disorders has not been studied systematically.

Definition and diagnosis Sleep disorders can manifest in four ways: by an excess of sleep (hypersomnia), by a deficiency of sleep (insomnia), by abnormal behavior or activity during sleep (parasomnia), and by a disturbance in the timing of sleep (circadian rhythm sleep disorders). The DSM-IV diagnostic criteria for sleep disorder due to a general medical condition is found in Chapter 23. Primary sleep disorders occur unrelated to any other medical or psychiatric illness. The DSM-IV nosology is deliberately simple and nondetailed. The patient is assigned to broad categories based on presenting symptoms and the etiological consideration of primary versus secondary disorder. The *International Classification of Sleep Disorder* is a more comprehensive and detailed nosology that requires the usage of polysomnography for many of the diagnoses.

Etiology and differential diagnosis Table 12-33 lists a number of conditions in which a disturbance of sleep has been frequently and characteristically described, allowing conditions to be designated as causes of secondary sleep disorder. *Parkinsonism,* related to either idiopathic Parkinson's disease, medications, or head trauma, frequently results in a secondary sleep disorder. As many as 75 percent of patients with Parkinson's disease complain of sleep disturbance, usually frequent awakenings during sleep. The difficulty maintaining sleep can have a number of causes. Sleep is fragmented owing to the brain degeneration that disrupts the neurophysiological and neurochemical pathways of sleep. In addition, the symptoms of Parkinson's disease can disrupt sleep. Although tremor is diminished during sleep, muscular rigidity is increased and can prevent the patient from turning or finding a comfortable position, resulting in arousal and awakening. Medications used to treat Parkinson's disease can disrupt sleep. Levodopa preparations frequently cause disruptive dreams and nightmares and may also increase nocturnal myoclonus, repetitive, brief leg jerks that awaken the patient and fragment sleep. Levodopa can be stimulating and may prevent the initiation of sleep if taken close to bedtime.

Dementia due to degenerative disease can impinge on sleep in a manner similar to parkinsonism, with the degeneration of pathways vital for normal sleep. *Sundowning,* or the emergence of severely disruptive behavior, such as agitation and paranoia,

TABLE 12-33
Medical Conditions Commonly Associated with a Secondary Sleep Disorder

Condition	Sleep Symptoms
Parkinsonism	Frequent awakenings, disturbance of circadian rhythms
Dementia	Sundowning, frequent awakenings
Epilepsy	Difficulty initiating sleep, frequent awakenings, parasomnias
Cerebrovascular disease	Difficulty initiating sleep, frequent awakenings
Huntington's disease	Frequent awakening
Kleine-Levin syndrome	Hypersomnia
Uremia	Restless legs, nocturnal myoclonus

at night, associated with inability to maintain sleep, is a major management issue in the home care of patients with dementia. The pathophysiology is unknown at present, although some have speculated that sundowning is a nocturnal delirium secondary to degeneration of the suprachiasmatic nucleus. Alternatively, sundowning is viewed as a disruption of circadian rhythms, rapid eye movement (REM) parasomnias, or simply postawakening confusion during which the demented patient is unable to distinguish between dreams and current reality. Dementia of the Alzheimer's type is accompanied by an exaggeration of the sleep changes associated with normal aging, with a decrease in total sleep time as well as in slow wave and REM sleep. The sleep disturbances worsen as the disease progresses.

Epilepsy can be a true sleep disorder. Most seizure disorders are activated by sleep or arousal from sleep. Both local and generalized epilepsy can occur during sleep, resulting in difficulties maintaining sleep. Seizures may manifest as parasomnias, such as night terrors, sleepwalking, or head banging, although most parasomnias are not related to epilepsy.

Cerebrovascular disorders can impinge on the initiation and maintenance of sleep. No specific lesions have been consistently correlated with a particular sleep disturbance, although brainstem lesions in general are apt to disrupt sleep architecture.

In *Huntington's disease* patients experience frequent awakenings and decreased total sleep time, a pattern common to many subcortical dementia syndromes. With the progression of the disease the movement disorder may manifest during sleep, further disrupting sleep.

Chronic renal failure, anemia, and *diabetes mellitus* can cause nocturnal myoclonus and the *restless legs syndrome*. The latter is characterized by the experience of deep pains in the lower calf, prompting the patient to keep the legs in constant motion and impinging severely on the ability to initiate sleep.

Kleine-Levin syndrome is a rare disorder characterized by hypersomnia, compulsive eating, sexual disinhibition, personality change, and psychosis. There is a 3 to 1 male to female predominance, with onset of symptoms typically occurring in adolescence. Hypersomnia is marked and is the most consistent feature. Compulsive eating and sexual disinhibition, such as public masturbation or propositioning of strangers, complete the syndrome. Incomplete or atypical variants are more common than the full syndrome. Irritability is frequent, and hallucinations or affective symptoms may be present. Symptoms last hours to weeks and are cyclical, with a full return to baseline on many occasions. Symptoms recur in a varying frequency of one to several months. The syndrome can be proceeded by flu-like symptoms or head trauma, although the precise etiology and pathophysiology are unknown. Presumably, there is hypothalamic system dysfunction with the manifest disturbances in sleep, eating, and sexual behavior. In most patients the episodes decrease in frequency and eventually disappear entirely.

Treatment The diagnosis of a secondary sleep disorder hinges on the identification of an active disease process known to exert the observed effect on sleep. Treatment first addresses the underlying neurological or medical disease. Symptomatic treatments focus on behavior modifications, such as improvement of sleep hygiene. Pharmacological options may also be used, such as benzodiazepines for restless legs syndrome or nocturnal myoclonus, stimulants for hypersomnia, and tricyclic antidepressants for manipulation of REM sleep.

SEXUAL DYSFUNCTION DUE TO A GENERAL MEDICAL CONDITION The DSM-IV diagnostic criteria for syndromes characterized by sexual dysfunction thought to be physiologically caused by a general medical condition are found in Section 21.1a. Specific subtypes listed are hypoactive sexual desire disorder, male erectile disorder, and dyspareunia; the remaining disorders are subsumed under sex-specific other categories.

History and comparative nosology Numerous medical conditions, medications, and drugs of abuse can affect sexual desire and performance. However, despite the attention psychiatry has given to presumed psychologically mediated sexual dysfunction, the role of physiological diseases was downplayed in earlier psychiatric diagnostic systems. DSM-III listed only functional sexual dysfunctions. DSM-III-R allowed sexual dysfunctions to be classified as psychogenic only or as due to both biogenic and psychogenic causes, but required purely biogenic syndromes to be coded on Axis III. The inclusion of secondary sexual disorders as Axis I diagnoses in DSM-IV is consistent with that edition's inclusive approach to behavioral syndromes.

Epidemiology Although surveys have repeatedly demonstrated a high prevalence of sexual dysfunctions in the general population, valid data on secondary dysfunctions are lacking. Similarly, certain medications may be associated with specific rates of sexual symptoms, but the percentage of patients with truly secondary syndromes is not known.

Etiology Potential etiologies of sexual dysfunctions are listed in Table 12-34. The type of sexual dysfunction is affected by the etiology, but specificity is rare; that is, a given etiology may manifest as one (or more than one) of several syndromes. General categories include medications and drugs of abuse, local disease processes that affect the primary or secondary sexual organs, and systemic illnesses that affect sexual organs via neurological, vascular, or endocrinological routes.

Diagnosis and clinical features The clinical features of the sexual dysfunction resemble those of the various primary dys-

TABLE 12-34
Etiologies of Secondary Sexual Dysfunctions

Medications
- Cardiac drugs, antihypertensives (e.g., reserpine, β-blockers, clonidine, α-methyldopa, diuretics)
- H_2-receptor blockers
- Carbonic anhydrase inhibitors
- Anticholinergics
- Anticonvulsants (e.g., carbamazepine, phenytoin, primidone)
- Antipsychotics
- Antidepressants (e.g., tricyclics, monoamine oxidase inhibitors, trazodone, fluoxetine)
- Sedative-hypnotics

Drugs of abuse
- Alcohol
- Opiates
- Stimulants
- Cannabis
- Sedative-hypnotics

Local disease processes that affect primary or secondary sexual organs
- Congenital anomalies or malformations
- Trauma
- Tumor
- Infection
- Postsurgical or postirradiation local neurological and vascular pathology

Systemic disease processes
- Neurological
  - Central nervous system (e.g., strokes, multiple sclerosis)
  - Peripheral nervous system (e.g., peripheral neuropathy)
- Vascular
  - Atherosclerosis, vasculitis (as examples)
- Endocrine
  - Diabetes mellitus, alterations in function of thyroid, adrenal cortex, gonadotropins, gonadal hormones (as examples)

functions discussed elsewhere in this textbook. There may be additional findings due to the underlying disease process. For example, in male erectile disorder due to diabetic autonomic neuropathy, the patient may have symptoms of bowel and bladder autonomic dysfunction (as well as evidence of diabetes mellitus itself).

Differential diagnosis Phenomenology determines the syndromic diagnosis (for example, erectile dysfunction versus orgasmic disorder). Medical history, physical examination, and relevant laboratory testing are required to demonstrate the presence of physical conditions potentially etiological for the sexual dysfunction. However, presence alone does not establish an etiological link. Clinical judgment is necessary and is based on temporal association, assessment of potentially contributory psychosocial factors (or more gross psychopathology), and other factors; the determination of secondary status is often difficult. One exception to that difficulty is male erectile dysfunction. Patients with secondary erectile dysfunction are unable to sustain erections under any circumstances, whereas those with primary (that is, psychogenic) disorders may give a history of variable erectile ability, depending on environment, partner, or other circumstances. If in doubt, a nocturnal penile tumescence study may be helpful, as only males with secondary erectile dysfunction will fail to demonstrate tumescence during sleep.

Course and prognosis The course and prognosis of secondary sexual dysfunctions vary widely, depending on the etiology. Drug-induced syndromes generally remit with discontinuation (or dosage reduction) of the offending agent. Endocrine-based dysfunctions also generally improve with restoration of normal physiology. By contrast, dysfunctions due to neurological disease may run protracted, even progressive, courses.

Treatment The treatment approach similarly varies widely, depending on the etiology. When reversal of the underlying cause is not possible, supportive and behaviorally oriented psychotherapy with the patient (and perhaps the partner) may minimize distress and increase sexual satisfaction (for example, by developing sexual interactions that are not limited by the specific dysfunction). Support groups for people with specific types of dysfunction are available. Other symptom-based treatments may be used in certain conditions; for example, yohimbine (Yocon) administration or surgical implantation of a penile prosthesis may be used in the treatment of male erectile dysfunction.

MENTAL DISORDERS DUE TO A GENERAL MEDICAL CONDITION NOT ELSEWHERE CLASSIFIED

DSM-IV has three additional diagnostic categories for clinical presentations of mental disorders due to a general medical condition that do not meet the diagnostic criteria for specific diagnoses. The first of the diagnoses is catatonic disorder due to a general medical condition (Table 12-35). The second diagnosis is personality change due to a general medical condition (Table 12-36). The third diagnosis is mental disorder not otherwise specified due to a general medical condition (Table 12-37).

Personality change due to a general medical condition

Personality refers to the constellation of enduring traits and behavioral style that essentially defines the person. Personality develops through adolescence and achieves a degree of stability in early adulthood. Both biological disposition as well as environmental factors influence the development of personality. In adults, behavioral style can be described in terms of interests, activities, pleasures, social relations, predominant mood and temperament, standards, usual outlook on life, range of coping

TABLE 12-35
Diagnostic Criteria for Catatonic Disorder due to a General Medical Condition

A. The presence of catatonia as manifested by motoric immobility, excessive motor activity (that is apparently purposeless and not influenced by external stimuli), extreme negativism or mutism, peculiarities of voluntary movement, or echolalia or echopraxia.
B. There is evidence from the history, physical examination, or laboratory findings that the disturbance is the direct physiological consequence of a general medical condition.
C. The disturbance is not better accounted for by another mental disorder (e.g., a manic episode).
D. The disturbance does not occur exclusively during the course of a delirium.

Coding note: Include the name of the general medical condition on Axis I, e.g., catatonic disorder due to hepatic encephalopathy; also code the general medical condition on Axis III.

Table from DSM-IV, *Diagnostic and Statistical Manual of Mental Disorders,* ed 4. Copyright American Psychiatric Association, Washington, 1994. Used with permission.

TABLE 12-36
Diagnostic Criteria for Personality Change due to a General Medical Condition

A. A persistent personality disturbance that represents a change from the individual's previous characteristic personality pattern. (In children, the disturbance involves a marked deviation from normal development or a significant change in the child's usual behavior patterns lasting at least one year.)
B. There is evidence from the history, physical examination, or laboratory findings that the disturbance is the direct physiological consequence of a general medical condition.
C. The disturbance is not better accounted for by another mental disorder (including other mental disorders due to a general medical condition).
D. The disturbance does not occur exclusively during the course of a delirium and does not meet criteria for a dementia.
E. The disturbance causes clinically significant distress or impairment in social, occupational, or other important areas of functioning.

Specify **type:**
- **Labile type:** if the predominant feature is affective lability
- **Disinhibited type:** if the predominant feature is poor impulse control as evidenced by sexual indiscretions, etc.
- **Aggressive type:** if the predominant feature is aggressive behavior
- **Apathetic type:** if the predominant feature is marked apathy and indifference
- **Paranoid type:** if the predominant feature is suspiciousness or paranoid ideation
- **Other type:** if the predominant feature is not one of the above, e.g., personality change associated with a seizure disorder
- **Combined type:** if more than one feature predominates in the clinical picture
- **Unspecified type**

Coding note: Include the name of the general medical condition on Axis I, e.g., personality change due to temporal lobe epilepsy; also code the general medical condition on Axis III.

Table from DSM-IV, *Diagnostic and Statistical Manual of Mental Disorders,* ed 4. Copyright American Psychiatric Association, Washington, 1994. Used with permission.

TABLE 12-37
Diagnostic Criteria for Mental Disorder Not Otherwise Specified due to a General Medical Condition

This residual category should be used for situations in which it has been established that the disturbance is caused by the direct physiological effects of a general medical condition, but the criteria are not met for a specific mental disorder due to a general medical condition (e.g., dissociative symptoms due to complex partial seizures).

Coding note: Include the name of the general medical condition on Axis I, e.g., mental disorder not otherwise specified due to HIV disease; also code the general medical condition on Axis III.

Table from DSM-IV, *Diagnostic and Statistical Manual of Mental Disorders,* ed 4. Copyright American Psychiatric Association, Washington, 1994. Used with permission.

mechanisms, and so forth. There is a robust theoretical and clinical literature delineating specific traits, such as self-consciousness, impulsivity, gregariousness, excitement-seeking, openness, and so forth, along dimensions or continua. Standardized measures are available to determine where along the spectrum for each trait a particular patient lies. That provides a personality profile that can be considered relative to standardized norms. The process is quite similar to the dimensional perspective used to assess intelligence and the determination of an I.Q.

The past concept of organic personality syndrome focused on identifying a generic category of particular traits and behaviors associated with brain injury or dysfunction. This conceptual approach has been maintained in DSM-IV, although it sought to base its classification of personality changes solely upon consistently reported behavioral alterations. Suggestions to classify disorders upon anatomical localization (such as frontal lobe syndrome) were rejected. To date there has been little theoretical work attempting to integrate the dimensional perspectives used in the description of normal personality with the categorical approach used in the study of CNS disease and related personality disturbances.

DEFINITION The DSM-IV diagnostic criteria for personality change due to a general medical condition are listed in Table 12-36. Personality change means that the person's fundamental means of interacting and behaving have been altered; that is, traits that had been regular and consistent over a lifetime have changed. Personality change must be distinguished from the transient disturbances of behavior that frequently occur in reaction to environmental circumstances. When a true personality change occurs in adulthood, the clinician should always suspect brain injury or insult.

HISTORY The impact of brain insults on personality has long been recognized. John M. Harlow's description of personality change in Phineas Gage, who sustained a penetrating head injury, remains the classic description: "He is fitful, irreverent, indulging at times in the grossest profanity (which was not previously his custom), manifesting but little deference for his fellows, impatient of restraint or advice when it conflicts with his desires, at times pertinaciously obstinate, yet capricious and vacillating, devising many plans of future operation, which are no sooner arranged than they are abandoned in turn for others appearing more feasible. A child in his intellectual capacity and manifestations, he has the animal passions of a strong man. . . . In this regard his mind was radically changed, so decidedly that his friends and acquaintances said he was 'no longer Gage.' "

The frequency of association between brain injury and personality change prompted a search for a generic personality disorder applicable to all brain injury, as well as brain locale-specific or disease-specific personality disorders. An example of the former is the organic personality disorder found in the earlier versions of DSM. Organic personality disorder was defined as a persistent disturbance of personality due to a specific organic factor involving affective instability, recurrent aggression or rage, impaired social judgment, apathy and indifference, or suspiciousness or paranoid ideation. The interictal personality disorder of temporal lobe epilepsy, characterized by hyperreligiosity, overinclusive speech and behavior, and sexual deviance, was originally presented as a disease-specific personality disorder that was thought to be of high validity. Subsequent studies did not find these traits specific for temporal lobe epilepsy or any other epilepsy. Attempts at defining locale-specific personality disorder have been hampered by difficulties in finding naturalistic human lesions that are indeed localized: Strokes, head trauma, and degenerative diseases, for example, rarely are confined to neat anatomical lobar boundaries.

Nonetheless, the most fruitful approach to delineating personality change disorders has come from the study of frontal lobe injury, where consistent and well-defined traits and behaviors have been associated with particular areas of brain injury. At least two distinct but overlapping secondary personality changes have been identified after injury to the orbitofrontal and frontal convexity areas. Frontal lobe dysfunction may play a key role in all personality and behavioral disturbances, as there are vast networks of neural connections between specific areas of the frontal lobe and various limbic and subcortical structures. A similarly complex neuropsychological system suggests that the frontal lobe (more specifically, the prefrontal cortex) modulates many of the basic cognitive, linguistic, attentional, and perceptual processes that originate in other brain areas. Injury to the frontal lobes results in dysfunction in how basic cognitive functions, such as language or memory, are expressed.

COMPARATIVE NOSOLOGY DSM-I included a category of acute and chronic brain syndromes, defined as disorders due to a diffuse impairment of brain tissue function from any cause. DSM-II provided basic symptoms for a generic organic brain syndrome, such as impairments in orientation, memory, calculation, learning, and judgment, and lability and shallowness of affect. Although there was no specific category for secondary personality change, it would have been included in the nonpsychotic organic brain syndromes. DSM-III eliminated the unitary organic mental syndrome and allowed for a variety of organic syndromes in which an organic factor was judged etiologically related. Organic personality syndrome, nonetheless, required at least one of four specific characteristics, including lability, impulsivity, apathy, or suspiciousness. DSM-III-R added recurrent aggression to the list of criteria.

The limitations of the nosology are clear. Personality encompasses a broad range of traits and behaviors not limited to those specified in the organic personality disorder category. The disturbance of personality is identified not from the presence of any particular behavior or trait, but rather from a change from premorbid personality. DSM-IV has dropped the category of organic personality disorder and replaced it with personality change due to a general medical condition. The specific phenomenological criteria were dropped in favor of a general persistent personality disturbance that represents a change from the individual's previous characteristic personality pattern. Subtypes based on the particular phenomenology evident include labile type, disinhibited type, aggressive type, paranoid type, apathetic type, other type, combined type, and unspecified type.

EPIDEMIOLOGY The epidemiological difficulties in ascertaining cases of secondary personality changes are clear: No one particular behavior or trait is diagnostic. Rather, a change in a patient's personality structure must be documented. Such documentation often requires recourse to an external informant, as patients with personality change are frequently unreliable self-informants. The overinclusive range of personality traits enumerated in previous editions of DSM allowed researchers to pick and choose traits; in addition, the means of measuring them were not consistent from study to study. As a result, reliable incidence and prevalence figures for secondary personality change are not available. Specific personality trait changes for particular brain diseases—for example, passive and self-centered behaviors in dementia of the Alzheimer's type—have been reported; the studies reporting those results, however, have not been replicated, and it remains uncertain how the findings should be applied to other disorders.

ETIOLOGY The range of etiologies of secondary personality change is vast and diverse and may involve any of the basic pathological processes described in the previous section. Diseases that preferentially affect the frontal lobes or subcortical structures are more likely to manifest with prominent personality change. Head trauma is a common cause. Strokes involving the anterior communicating or middle cerebral arteries selectively damage frontal lobe structures, often resulting in personality change. The anterior communicating artery is also a common site for aneurysms, which can result in secondary personality change. Frontal lobe tumors, such as meningiomas and gliomas, can grow to considerable size before coming to medical attention, as they may be neurologically silent (that is, without focal signs). Degenerative disorders affecting the frontal lobes can present with personality change long before cognitive symptoms are evident. Among progressive dementia syndromes, especially those with a subcortical pattern of degeneration, such as ADC, Huntington's disease, or progressive supranuclear palsy, significant personality disturbance manifests often. Multiple sclerosis can impinge on the personality, reflecting subcortical white matter degeneration. Exposures to toxins with a predilection for white matter, such as irradiation, may also produce significant personality change disproportionate to the cognitive or motor impairment.

DIAGNOSIS AND CLINICAL FEATURES The diagnosis of a secondary personality change rests entirely on the history. A clear and detailed description of the patient's premorbid personality must be obtained. That history usually is collected from an external informant who knew the patient at baseline as well as currently. The first task in evaluating the history is to determine whether a change in personality indeed has occurred or whether the current disruptive behaviors represent long-standing traits that have been exacerbated by a change in circumstance. In addition, delirium must be ruled out.

Once a diagnosis of a personality change has been established, the search for an etiological agent ensues. An insidious and progressive course is suggestive of a degenerative process or a neoplasm. An abrupt onset of personality change is more suggestive of a vascular event or trauma. Risk factors for HIV infection should raise the suspicion of ADC or neurosyphilis. A complete history of toxic exposures, including alcohol and recreational drug use, environmental or occupational toxin exposures, and medications, should be obtained. The search for a causative agent can be aided by the presence of other evidence of brain dysfunction, such as motor abnormalities and cognitive impairment.

The particular form of a personality change may be helpful in determining the locus of injury or brain dysfunction, although much research remains to be done. The prefrontal cortex is often implicated in secondary personality change disorders. Two frontal lobe personality syndromes have been described, correlating with injury to the orbitofrontal and dorsolateral frontal cortical regions. Table 12-38 outlines the behavioral and personality changes associated with each. The anatomical designations for those syndromes may be misleading, as frontal regions form rich neuronal networks with subcortical and limbic structures. Subcortical dementia also is characterized by significant personality deteriorations, such as apathy, aspontaneity, and slowing. Patients with multiple sclerosis sometimes present with a euphoric personality, probably reflecting disruption of the orbitofrontal subcortical network.

Global degenerative processes, such as dementia of the Alzheimer's type, involve significant personality change that has been less well characterized. In general, there is a coarsening of the personality with loss of subtlety and finesse. An exacerbation of premorbid traits is possible, with a suspicious patient becoming paranoid or a flamboyant patient becoming histrionic. Agitation or aggression is a common concomitant of brain disease. When they occur in a patient with a premorbid history of violence and a short temper, it may be difficult to determine if a secondary personality change has occurred, even when CNS dysfunction is evident.

Laboratory evaluation for secondary personality change is the same as for other secondary disorders. The most important element is informed clinical suspicion regarding specific disease processes.

DIFFERENTIAL DIAGNOSIS Secondary personality change must be differentiated from adjustment disorders occurring, for example, in response to environmental stressors or major medical disorders. Apathetic and amotivational symptoms in patients with dorsolateral frontal lesions may be mistaken for major depressive disorder. The former can be distinguished by a lack of pervasive dysphoria, intact neurovegetative function, and the absence of self-disparagement and hopelessness. Euphoria and disinhibition with the orbitofrontal syndrome may be ascribed to mania. The orbitofrontal syndrome, however, does not display heightened motor activity, excessive energy, and disrupted sleep. Neither does it follow the cyclical course of bipolar disorder but, rather, produces a persistent and consistent clinical picture.

COURSE AND PROGNOSIS The course of and prognosis for secondary personality syndromes depend on the course of the etiological systemic or cerebral disorder. Personality change secondary to mass lesions or hydrocephalus can improve dramatically with surgery, chemotherapy, or radiation therapy. However, each of those treatments may result in a different personality change syndrome. Personality change secondary to head trauma may improve slowly and gradually over the course of months or years, although residual disturbances may remain. Personality change due to degenerative processes can be most disruptive early in the disease process when the patient retains a measure of volition and control of motor capacities. Ironically, management of such patients may ease as the disease progresses, when the personality evolves into greater apathy, unresponsiveness, and akinesia. Personality change associated with epilepsy can improve dramatically with seizure control by pharmacotherapy or surgery.

TREATMENT Treatment for secondary personality syndromes is first directed toward correcting the underlying etiology. Symptomatic treatments as a group have been marginally effective at best. Lithium carbonate, carbamazepine, and valproic acid have been used for the control of affective lability and impulsivity. Aggression or explosiveness may be treated with lithium, anticonvulsants, or a combination of lithium and an anticonvulsant. Centrally active β-adrenergic blockers, such as propranolol (Inderal), have some efficacy as well. Antipsychotics are no more effective in the dampening of aggression than the previously mentioned agents, induce greater discomfort, and introduce the risk of tardive dyskinesia. Apathy and inertia have occasionally improved with psychostimulants. Because cognition and verbal skills may be preserved in patients with secondary personality changes, they may be candidates for psychotherapy. Families should be involved in the therapy process, with a focus on education and understanding the origins of the patient's inappropriate behaviors and coarsening. Issues such as competency, disability, and advocacy are frequently of clinical concern in those patients in light of the unpredictable and pervasive behavior change.

TABLE 12-38
Frontal Lobe Personality Change Syndromes

Orbitofrontal	Frontopolar
Disinhibition	Apathy
Inappropriate jocularity	Indifference
Affective lability	Psychomotor slowing
Impulsivity	Inaction

FUTURE DIRECTIONS

Cognitive and secondary psychiatric disorders, neuropsychiatric syndromes in which specific systemic and cerebral diseases manifest themselves through a relatively small number of common behavioral pathways, pose a daunting challenge for the clinician. Effectively evaluating, diagnosing, and treating those conditions requires rigor of thought and willingness to accept uncertainty, even as one proceeds with active therapeutic measures.

Psychiatry is moving away from the misleading dichotomy of organic and functional toward an approach that considers etiology. Diagnostic designations, such as primary and secondary, reflect both the conceptual framework of the science and specific information about discrete disorders. The clear, etiologically based designation of cognitive and secondary psychiatric syndromes highlights that most of the conditions that clinicians encounter are idiopathic, without known cause. Acknowledging that is essential for progress.

SUGGESTED CROSS-REFERENCES

A discussion of psychiatric clinical manifestations of specific neurological and systemic disorders appears in Chapter 2 on neuropsychiatry and behavioral neurology. Neuropsychological and intellectual assessment of adults is presented in Section 9.5, assessment of children in Section 9.6, and medical assessment and laboratory testing in Section 9.7. Discussions of substance-related disorders appear in Chapter 13, schizophrenia in Chapter 14, psychotic disorders in Chapter 15, anxiety disorders in Chapter 17, factitious disorders in Chapter 19, dissociative disorders (including dissociative amnesia) in Chapter 20, sexual dysfunctions in Section 21.1a on normal human sexuality and sexual dysfunctions, sleep disorders in Chapter 23, and personality disorders in Chapter 25. Psychiatry and medicine is presented in Section 29.1, psychiatric aspects of AIDS in adults in Section 29.2, and neuropsychological and neuropsychiatric aspects of HIV infection in adults in 29.2a. Physiological aspects of normal aging (including age-related cognitive decline) is discussed in Section 49.4c, and Alzheimer's disease and other dementing disorders of late life are discussed in Section 49.6a.

REFERENCES

Alexander M P: Traumatic brain injury. In *Psychiatric Aspects of Neurologic Disease,* vol II, D Benson, D Blumer, editors, p 219. Grune & Stratton, New York, 1982.

American Academy of Neurology: *Nomenclature and Research Case Definitions for Neurologic Manifestations of Human Immunodeficiency Virus–Type 1 (HIV-1) Infection.* Neurology *41:* 778, 1991.

*Bradford Hill A: The environment and disease: Association or causation? Proc R Soc Med *58:* 295, 1965.

Caine E D, Joynt R J: Neuropsychiatry . . . again. Arch Neurol *43:* 325, 1986.

Cummings J L: *Clinical Neuropsychiatry.* Grune & Stratton, New York, 1985.

Damasio H, Grabowski T, Frank R, Galaburda A M, Damasio A R: The return of Phineas Gage: Clues about the brain from the skull of a famous patient. Science *264:* 1102, 1994.

Etcheberrigaray R, Ito E, Kim C S, Alkon D L: Soluble β-amyloid induction of Alzheimer's phenotype for human fibroblast K^+ channels. Science *264:* 276, 1994.

Evans A S: Causation and disease: A chronological journey. Am J Epidemiol *108:* 249, 1975.

*Grant I, Adams K: *Neuropsychological Assessment of Neuropsychiatric Disorders.* Oxford University Press, New York, 1986.

Harlow J M: Recovery after severe injury to the head. Publ Mass Media Soc *2:* 327, 1868.

Huntington's Disease Collaborative Research Group: A novel gene containing a trinucleotide repeat that is expanded and unstable on Huntington's disease chromosomes. Cell *72:* 971, 1993.

Jaspers K: *General Psychopathology.* J Hoenig, M W Hamilton, translators. University of Chicago Press, Chicago, 1963.

*Jorm A F: *The Epidemiology of Alzheimer's Disease and Related Disorders.* Chapman & Hall, London, 1990.

Joseph A B, Young R R, editors: *Movement Disorders in Neurology and Neuropsychiatry.* Blackwell Scientific, Boston, 1992.

Krauthammer C, Klerman G L: Secondary mania. Arch Gen Psychiatry *35:* 1333, 1978.

*Lipowski Z J: *Delirium—Acute Confusional States,* ed 2. Oxford University Press, New York, 1990.

Liptzin B, Levkoff S E, Gottlieb G L, Johnson J C: Delirium. J Neuropsychiatry Clin Neurosci *5:* 154, 1993.

*Lishman W A: *Organic Psychiatry: The Psychological Consequences of Cerebral Disorder,* ed 2. Blackwell Scientific, London, 1987.

Marx O M: Nineteenth-century medical psychology. Isis *61:* 355, 1970.

Miller N E, Lipowski Z J, Lebowitz B D, editors: *Delirium: Advances in Research and Clinical Practice.* Int Psychogeriatr *3* (2), 1991.

Minden S L, Schiffer R B: Affective disorders in multiple sclerosis: Review and recommendations for clinical research. Arch Neurol *47:* 98, 1990.

O'Donoghue J L, editor: *Neurotoxicity of Industrial and Commercial Chemicals.* CRC Press, Boca Raton, FL, 1985.

Popkin M K: "Secondary" and drug-induced mood, anxiety, psychotic, catatonic, and personality syndromes: A review of the literature. J Neuropsychiatry Clin Neurosci *4:* 369, 1992.

Reynolds E H: Structure and function in neurology and psychiatry. Br J Psychiatry *157:* 481, 1990.

Robinson R G, Starkstein S E: Current research in affective disorders following stroke. J Neuropsychiatry Clin Neurosci *2:* 1, 1990.

Slater E, Beard A W: The schizophrenia-like psychoses of epilepsy. i. Psychiatric aspects. Br J Psychiatry *109:* 95, 1963.

Tucker G J, Caine E D, Popkin M K: Delirium, dementia, and amnestic and other cognitive disorders. In *DSM-IV Sourcebook,* vol 1, pp 185–337. T A Widiger, A J Frances, H A Pincus, M B First, R Ross, W Davis, editors. American Psychiatric Association, Washington, 1994.

White B V: *Stanley Cobb: A Builder of the Modern Neurosciences.* Francis A. Countway Library of Medicine, Boston, 1984.

Zegans L S, Coates T J, editors: *Psychiatric Manifestations of HIV Disease,* vol 17 (1). Saunders, Philadelphia, 1994.

CHAPTER 13 SUBSTANCE-RELATED DISORDERS

13.1 INTRODUCTION AND OVERVIEW

JEROME H. JAFFE, M.D.

INTRODUCTION

Substance use and dependence are viewed with concern by the world community. Wars have been fought over drug trafficking, and treaties have been signed aimed at controlling the production and distribution of opioids, cocaine, cannabis, and a wide range of synthetic psychoactive drugs. Most nations are signatories to two major treaties, and two permanent international bodies exist to decide which new drugs should be included under the treaty provisions. The control of illicit traffic in psychoactive drugs is often an agenda item at economic summit meetings of the world's most powerful nations. In addition, although no treaties exist to control alcohol and tobacco, actions and statements by the World Health Organization (WHO) reflect the grave concern of the world's medical community about the increasing use of tobacco in developing countries and about the impact of alcoholism on health and productivity throughout the world.

The annual economic cost of alcohol and drug abuse in the United States in 1985 was an estimated $114 billion. That estimate included the cost of acquired immune deficiency syndrome (AIDS) among drug abusers (which has since escalated), but not the cost associated with tobacco use. Whether society views substance use primarily as a moral problem or a legal problem, when it creates difficulties for the user or ceases to be entirely volitional, it becomes a concern for all the helping professions, including psychiatry.

GENERAL ORGANIZATION OF DSM-IV In the fourth edition of *Diagnostic and Statistical Manual of Mental Disorders* (DSM-IV) the substance-related disorders now include two broad categories: substance use disorders (substance dependence and substance abuse), and a diverse grouping of substance-induced disorders (such as substance intoxication, substance withdrawal, substance-induced psychotic disorders, and substance-induced mood disorders).

Thus, the topic of substance-related disorders goes beyond substance dependence and abuse and closely related problems to include a wide variety of adverse reactions not only to drugs of abuse, but also to medications and toxins. The medications associated with substance-induced disorders range from anesthetics to over-the-counter medications and include such diverse drug categories as anticholinergics, antidepressives, anticonvulsants, antimicrobials, antihypertensives, corticosteroids, antiparkinsonian agents, chemotherapeutic agents, nonsteroidal anti-inflammatory agents, and disulfiram (Antabuse). In addition, several categories of substance-induced disorders can be induced by a wide range of nonmedicinal toxic materials, ranging from heavy metals and industrial solvents to insecticides and household cleaning agents.

In the section dealing with substance dependence and substance abuse DSM-IV presents descriptions of the clinical phenomena associated with the use of the following 11 designated classes of pharmacological agents: alcohol; amphetamines or similarly acting agents; caffeine; cannabis; cocaine; hallucinogens; inhalants; nicotine; opioids; phencyclidine (PCP) or similar agents; and sedatives, hypnotics, and anxiolytics. In addition, DSM-IV includes a 12th, a residual category for a variety of agents, such as anabolic steroids and nitrous oxide, that are not included in the 11 designated classes.

DSM-IV has also changed the grouping and placement of substance-related disorders in the broad array of psychiatric disorders. Thus, the diagnostic criteria for substance dependence, abuse, intoxication, and withdrawal syndromes are grouped together in a section titled "Substance-Related Disorders," whereas the other substance-related disorders (for example, substance-induced mood disorders and substance-induced delusional disorders) are distributed in the sections covering the disorders that they most closely resemble phenomenologically (Table 13.1-1).

DEFINITION AND DIAGNOSIS

SUBSTANCE DEPENDENCE The revised third edition of DSM (DSM-III-R) and DSM-IV formulations for abuse and dependence closely follow the concepts and terminology developed in 1980 by an International Working Group sponsored by the Alcohol, Drug Abuse, and Mental Health Administration (ADAMHA) and WHO. That group defined dependence as follows:

> A syndrome manifested by a behavioral pattern in which the use of a given psychoactive drug, or class of drugs, is given a much higher priority than other behaviors that once had higher value. The term "syndrome" is taken to mean no more than a clustering of phenomena so that not all the components need always be present or not always present with the same intensity. . . . The dependence syndrome is not absolute, but is a quantitative phenomenon that exists in different degrees. The intensity of the syndrome is measured by the behaviors that are elicited in relation to using the drug and by the other behaviors that are secondary to drug use. . . . No sharp cut-off point can be identified for distinguishing drug dependence from non-dependent but recurrent drug use. At the extreme, the dependence syndrome is associated with "compulsive drug-using behavior."

That central notion is continued in DSM-IV, which states:

> The essential feature of dependence is a cluster of cognitive, behavioral, and physiological symptoms indicating that the individual continues substance use despite significant substance-related problems.

The DSM-IV criteria for substance dependence are presented in Table 13.1-2. DSM-IV uses seven criteria to describe a generic concept of dependence that applies across all 11 classes of pharmacological agents.

TABLE 13.1-1
Substance-Induced Mental Disorders Included Elsewhere in the Textbook

Substance-induced disorders cause a variety of symptoms that are characteristic of other mental disorders. To facilitate differential diagnosis, the text and criteria for these other substance-induced disorders are included in the sections of the textbook with disorders with which they share phenomenology:

Substance-induced delirium (see Chapter 12) is included in the ''Delirium, Dementia, and Amnestic and Other Cognitive Disorders'' section.

Substance-induced persisting dementia (see Chapter 12) is included in the ''Delirium, Dementia, and Amnestic and Other Cognitive Disorders'' section.

Substance-induced persisting amnestic disorder (see Chapter 12) is included in the ''Delirium, Dementia, and Amnestic and Other Cognitive Disorders'' section.

Substance-induced psychotic disorder (see Section 15.3) is included in the ''Schizophrenia and Other Psychotic Disorders'' section. (In DSM-III-R these disorders were classified as organic hallucinosis and organic delusional disorder.)

Substance-induced mood disorder (see Section 16.6) is included in the ''Mood Disorders'' section.

Substance-induced anxiety disorder (see Section 17.5) is included in the ''Anxiety Disorders'' section.

Substance-induced sexual dysfunction (see Section 21.1a) is included in the ''Sexual and Gender Identity Disorders'' section.

Substance-induced sleep disorder (see Chapter 23) is included in the ''Sleep Disorders'' section.

In addition, **Hallucinogen persisting perception disorder (flashbacks)** (see Section 13.7) is included under Hallucinogen-Related Disorder.

Table adapted from DSM-IV, *Diagnostic and Statistical Manual of Mental Disorders,* ed 4. Copyright American Psychiatric Association, Washington, 1994. Used with permission.

Like DSM-III-R, DSM-IV continues to employ a polythetic syndrome definition, in which no particular one of the seven criteria is required so long as three or more are present. However, in deference to those who believe that the presence of physiological dependence implies a distinctly different disorder, or at least a more severe form of the disorder, in DSM-IV the clinician is asked to specify whether physiological dependence (evidence of criterion 1, tolerance, or criterion 2, withdrawal) is present or absent.

In addition to requiring the clustering of three criteria in a 12-month period, DSM-IV includes a few other qualifications. It states specifically that the diagnosis of dependence can be applied to every class of substances except caffeine. That point is admittedly controversial and some workers believe that, based on the same DSM-IV generic criteria, caffeine produces a distinct form of dependence, although it is relatively benign for most persons.

Some persons use several categories of drugs and are clearly drug dependent, according to the generic criteria, but sometimes it is not possible to ascertain whether they are dependent on any one specific class of drugs. In DSM-IV, when at least three groups of substances are involved, the condition is called polysubstance dependence (Table 13.1-3). DSM-IV also makes provision for classifying substance-related disorders that cannot be classified in any of the previous categories (for example, nitrous oxide, anticholinergics, anabolic-androgenic steroids) or for an initial diagnosis in cases of dependence or abuse in which the specific substance is not known. The diagnostic criteria for other (or unknown) substance-related disorders are listed in Table 13.1-4.

Patterns of remission and course specifiers With DSM-III-R it was possible to supplement the informational value of a substance dependence diagnosis by indicating to what degree the disorder was in remission (for example, partial remission or full remission). DSM-IV expands on the theme of remission by providing six distinct modifying terms that can be appended to a diagnosis of substance dependence (Table 13.1-5). All of those course specifiers require that after a period of active dependence, there should be a period of at least 1 month during which no criteria of dependence are present. If a patient has not met any criteria for dependence for at least 1 month but for less than 12 months, the course specifier to use would be *early full remission.* If the period during which no criteria of dependence are met exceeds 12 months, the specifier of *sustained full remission* can be used. If the full criteria for dependence or abuse have not been met for less than a year but one or more criteria have been present, *early partial remission* may be used. If the period exceeds 12 months, sustained partial remission may be

TABLE 13.1-2
Diagnostic Criteria for Substance Dependence

A maladaptive pattern of substance use, leading to clinically significant impairment or distress, as manifested by three (or more) of the following, occurring at any time in the same 12-month period:

(1) tolerance, as defined by either of the following:
 (a) a need for markedly increased amounts of the substance to achieve intoxication or desired effect
 (b) markedly diminished effect with continued use of the same amount of the substance
(2) withdrawal, as manifested by either of the following:
 (a) the characteristic withdrawal syndrome for the substance (refer to criteria A and B of the criteria sets for withdrawal from the specific substances)
 (b) the same (or a closely related) substance is taken to relieve or avoid withdrawal symptoms
(3) the substance is often taken in larger amounts or over a longer period than was intended
(4) there is a persistent desire or unsuccessful efforts to cut down or control substance use
(5) a great deal of time is spent in activities necessary to obtain the substance (e.g., visiting multiple doctors or driving long distances), use the substance (e.g., chain-smoking), or recover from its effects
(6) important social, occupational, or recreational activities are given up or reduced because of substance use
(7) the substance use is continued despite knowledge of having a persistent or recurrent physical or psychological problem that is likely to have been caused or exacerbated by the substance (e.g., current cocaine use despite recognition of cocaine-induced depression, or continued drinking despite recognition that an ulcer was made worse by alcohol consumption)

Specify if:
With physiological dependence: evidence of tolerance or withdrawal (i.e., either item 1 or 2 is present)
Without physiological dependence: no evidence of tolerance or withdrawal (i.e., neither item 1 nor 2 is present)

Course specifiers:
Early full remission
Early partial remission
Sustained full remission
Sustained partial remission
On agonist therapy
In a controlled environment

Table from DSM-IV, *Diagnostic and Statistical Manual of Mental Disorders,* ed 4. Copyright American Psychiatric Association, Washington, 1994. Used with permission.

TABLE 13.1-3
Diagnostic Criteria for Polysubstance Dependence

This diagnosis is reserved for behavior during the same 12-month period in which the person was repeatedly using at least three groups of substances (not including caffeine and nicotine), but no single substance predominated. Further, during this period, the dependence criteria were met for substances as a group but not for any specific substance.

Table from DSM-IV, *Diagnostic and Statistical Manual of Mental Disorders,* ed 4. Copyright American Psychiatric Association, Washington, 1994. Used with permission.

TABLE 13.1-4
Diagnostic Criteria for Other (or Unknown) Substance-Related Disorders

The other (or unknown) substance-related disorders category is for classifying substance-related disorders associated with substances not listed above. Examples of these substances, which are described in more detail below, include anabolic steroids, nitrite inhalants ("poppers"), nitrous oxide, over-the-counter and prescription medications not otherwise covered by the 11 categories (e.g., cortisol, antihistamines, benztropine), and other substances that have psychoactive effects. In addition, this category may be used when the specific substance is unknown (e.g., an intoxication after taking a bottle of unlabeled pills).

Anabolic steroids sometimes produce an initial sense of enhanced well-being (or even euphoria), which is replaced after repeated use by lack of energy, irritability, and other forms of dysphoria. Continued use of these substances may lead to more severe symptoms (e.g., depressive symptomatology) and general medical conditions (liver disease).

Nitrite inhalants ("poppers"—forms of amyl, butyl, and isobutyl nitrite) produce an intoxication that is characterized by a feeling of fullness in the head, mild euphoria, a change in the perception of time, relaxation of smooth muscles, and a possible increase in sexual feelings. In addition to possible compulsive use, these substances carry dangers of potential impairment of immune functioning, irritation of the respiratory system, a decrease in the oxygen-carrying capacity of the blood, and a toxic reaction that can include vomiting, severe headache, hypotension, and dizziness.

Nitrous oxide ("laughing gas") causes rapid onset of an intoxication that is characterized by light-headedness and a floating sensation that clears in a matter of minutes after administration is stopped. There are reports of temporary but clinically relevant confusion and reversible paranoid states when nitrous oxide is used regularly.

Other substances that are capable of producing mild intoxications include **catnip,** which can produce states similar to those observed with marijuana and which in high doses is reported to result in LSD-type perceptions; **betel nut,** which is chewed in many cultures to produce a mild euphoria and floating sensation; and **kava** (a substance derived from the South Pacific pepper plant), which produces sedation, incoordination, weight loss, mild forms of hepatitis, and lung abnormalities. In addition, individuals can develop dependence and impairment through repeated self-administration of **over-the-counter** and **prescription drugs,** including **cortisol, antiparkinsonian agents** that have anticholinergic properties, and **antihistamines.**

Texts and criteria sets have already been provided to define the generic aspects of substance dependence, substance abuse, substance intoxication, and substance withdrawal that are applicable across classes of substances. The other (or unknown) substance-induced disorders are described in the sections of the manual with disorders with which they share phenomenology (e.g., other [or unknown] substance-induced mood disorder is included in the "mood disorders" section). Listed below are the other (or unknown) substance use disorders and the other (or unknown) substance-induced disorders.

Other (or unknown) substance use disorders
- **Other (or unknown) substance dependence**
- **Other (or unknown) substance abuse**

Other (or unknown) substance-induced disorders
- **Other (or unknown) substance intoxication**
  Specify if: With perceptual disturbances
- **Other (or unknown) substance withdrawal**
  Specify if: With perceptual disturbances
- **Other (or unknown) substance-induced delirium**
- **Other (or unknown) substance-induced persisting dementia**
- **Other (or unknown) substance-induced persisting amnestic disorder**
- **Other (or unknown) substance-induced psychotic disorder, with delusions**
  Specify if: With onset during intoxication/with onset during withdrawal
- **Other (or unknown) substance-induced psychotic disorder, with hallucinations**
  Specify if: With onset during intoxication/with onset during withdrawal
- **Other (or unknown) substance-induced mood disorder**
  Specify if: With onset during intoxication/with onset during withdrawal
- **Other (or unknown) substance-induced anxiety disorder**
  Specify if: With onset during intoxication/with onset during withdrawal
- **Other (or unknown) substance-induced sexual dysfunction**
  Specify if: With onset during intoxication
- **Other (or unknown) substance-induced sleep disorder**
  Specify if: With onset during intoxication/with onset during withdrawal

Other (or unknown) substance-related disorder not otherwise specified

Table from DSM-IV, *Diagnostic and Statistical Manual of Mental Disorders,* ed 4. Copyright American Psychiatric Association, Washington, 1994. Used with permission.

used. Two additional remission specifiers should be used when appropriate: "on agonist therapy (includes partial agonists)" and "in a controlled environment" can be used. Several factors, such as duration of remission and duration of period of dependence, must be considered in deciding that a person has fully recovered and no longer warrants a diagnosis of dependence.

SUBSTANCE ABUSE In DSM-IV the essential features of substance abuse are as follows:

> A maladaptive pattern of substance use manifested by recurrent and significant adverse consequences related to the repeated use of substances. . . . These problems must occur recurrently during the same 12-month period. . . . [T]he criteria for Substance Abuse do not include tolerance, withdrawal, or a pattern of compulsive use and instead include only the harmful consequences of repeated use. A diagnosis of Substance Abuse is preempted by the diagnosis of Substance Dependence if the individual's pattern of substance use has ever met the criteria for Dependence for that class of substances.

The DSM-IV criteria for substance abuse are shown in Table 13.1-6.

SUBSTANCE WITHDRAWAL Substance withdrawal, as used in DSM-IV, is a diagnostic term rather than a technical term. Thus minor symptoms that technically are due to cessation of substance use (for example, the coffee drinker's early morning precoffee lethargy or minor headache) would not by themselves fulfill the criteria for substance withdrawal, unless they were accompanied by a maladaptive behavior change and caused some clinically significant distress or impairment in social, occupational, or other important areas of functioning. DSM-IV does not recognize withdrawal from caffeine, cannabis, or PCP, although some observers believe that specific signs and symptoms can be observed when those agents are abruptly discontinued after a period of heavy use.

Withdrawal is commonly, but not invariably, associated with substance dependence. The signs and symptoms of withdrawal vary with the specific class of drug. In general, the severity of withdrawal is related to the amount of substance used and the duration and patterns of use. Withdrawal is seen not only when substance use is stopped but also when reduced use of a substance or a change in metabolism results in lower tissue levels. The DSM-IV generic criteria for substance withdrawal are shown in Table 13.1-7.

SUBSTANCE INTOXICATION Substance intoxication is defined more narrowly in DSM-IV than it might be in a pharmacology text. A variety of substances may produce unwanted physiological or psychological effects that could be construed as substance intoxication effects (for example, excessive sleepiness for an antihistamine), but unless the symptoms are associated with maladaptive behavior, the effects would not constitute substance-induced intoxication as defined in DSM-IV. Furthermore, whether a behavioral effect is maladaptive depends on the social and environmental context in which it occurs. A dose of ethanol (the amount of alcohol) that makes a person unusually sociable, a bit garrulous, and a little uncoordinated at a family celebration might not be maladaptive drinking behavior; the same behavior at a formal business meeting might be.

The DSM-IV general criteria for substance intoxication are shown in Table 13.1-8.

SUBSTANCE-INDUCED DISORDERS In addition to dependence, abuse, intoxication, and withdrawal, the use of certain psychoactive drugs can induce syndromes that were once called organic mental disorders. To avoid implying that other

TABLE 13.1-5
Diagnostic Criteria for Course Specifiers for Substance Dependence

Six course specifiers are available for substance dependence. The four remission specifiers can be applied only after none of the criteria for substance dependence or substance abuse have been present for at least one month. The definition of these four types of remission is based on the interval of time that has elapsed since the cessation of dependence (early versus sustained remission) and whether there is continued presence of one or more of the items included in the criteria sets for dependence or abuse (partial versus full remission). Because the first 12 months following dependence is a time of particularly high risk for relapse, this period is designated early remission. After 12 months of early remission have passed without relapse to dependence, the person enters into sustained remission. For both early remission and sustained remission, a further designation of full is given if no criteria for dependence or abuse have been met during the period of remission; a designation of partial is given if at least one of the criteria for dependence or abuse has been met, intermittently or continuously, during the period of remission. The differentiation of sustained full remission from recovered (no current substance use disorder) requires consideration of the length of time since the last period of disturbance, the total duration of the disturbance, and the need for continued evaluation. If, after a period of remission or recovery, the individual again becomes dependent, the application of the early remission specifier requires that there again be at least 1 month in which no criteria for dependence or abuse are met. Two additional specifiers have been provided: on agonist therapy and in a controlled environment. For an individual to qualify for early remission after cessation of agonist therapy or release from a controlled environment, there must be a one-month period in which none of the criteria for dependence or abuse are met.

The following remission specifiers can be applied only after no criteria for dependence or abuse have been met for at least one month. Note that these specifiers do not apply if the individual is on agonist therapy or in a controlled environment (see below).

Early full remission. This specifier is used if, for at least 1 month, but for less than 12 months, no criteria for dependence or abuse have been met.

Dependence — 1 month — 0–11 months

Early partial remission. This specifier is used if, for at least 1 month, but less than 12 months, one or more criteria for dependence or abuse have been met (but the full criteria for dependence have not been met).

Dependence — 1 month — 0–11 months

Sustained full remission. This specifier is used if none of the criteria for dependence or abuse have been met at any time during a period of 12 months or longer.

Dependence — 1 month — 11+ months

Sustained partial remission. This specifier is used if full criteria for dependence have not been met for a period of 12 months or longer; however, one or more criteria for dependence or abuse have been met.

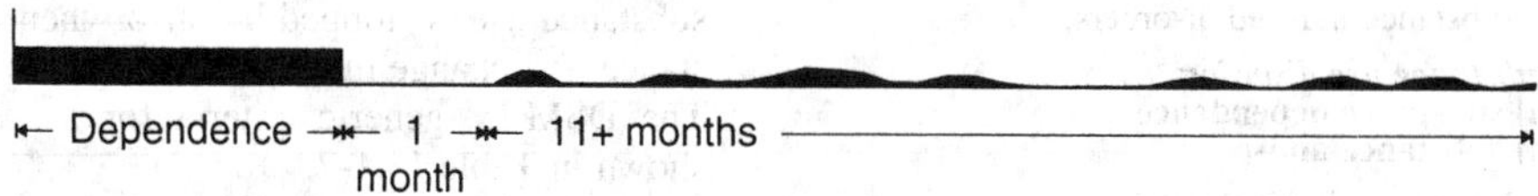

The following specifiers apply if the individual is on agonist therapy or in a controlled environment:

On agonist therapy. This specifier is used if the individual is on a prescribed agonist medication, and no criteria for dependence or abuse have been met for that class of medication for at least the past month (except tolerance to, or withdrawal from, the agonist). This category also applies to those being treated for dependence using a partial agonist or an agonist/antagonist.

In a controlled environment. This specifier is used if the individual is in an environment where access to alcohol and controlled substances is restricted, and no criteria for dependence or abuse have been met for at least the past month. Examples of these environments are closely supervised and substance-free jails, therapeutic communities, or locked hospital units.

Table from DSM-IV, *Diagnostic and Statistical Manual of Mental Disorders,* ed 4. Copyright American Psychiatric Association, Washington, 1994. Used with permission.

psychiatric disorders do not have an organic basis, DSM-IV designates those syndromes as substance-induced disorders and recognizes the following categories: substance intoxication, substance withdrawal, substance-induced withdrawal delirium, substance-induced intoxication delirium, substance-induced persisting dementia, substance-induced persisting amnestic disorder, substance-induced mood disorder, substance-induced anxiety disorder, substance-induced psychotic disorder, substance-induced sexual dysfunction, and substance-induced sleep disorder.

In recording a diagnosis of a substance-related disorder, the clinician should indicate the specific agent causing the disorder, when it is known, rather than the broad drug category: that is, substance-induced intoxication, pentobarbital (Nembutal) rather than substance-induced intoxication, sedative-hypnotics. However, the diagnostic code should be selected from the list of classes of substances provided in sets of criteria for the substance-induced disorder being recorded. For each of the substance-induced disorders (other than intoxication and withdrawal), the clinician is asked further to specify whether the onset was during intoxication or during withdrawal. Thus, a specific substance-induced disorder would have a three-part name delineating (1) the specific substance, (2) the context (whether the disorder occurred during intoxication or during

TABLE 13.1-6
Diagnostic Criteria for Substance Abuse

A. A maladaptive pattern of substance use leading to clinically significant impairment or distress, as manifested by one (or more) of the following, occurring within a 12-month period:
   (1) recurrent substance use resulting in a failure to fulfill major role obligations at work, school, or home (e.g., repeated absences or poor work performance related to substance use; substance-related absences, suspensions, or expulsions from school; neglect of children or household)
   (2) recurrent substance use in situations in which it is physically hazardous (e.g., driving an automobile or operating a machine when impaired by substance use)
   (3) recurrent substance-related legal problems (e.g., arrests for substance-related disorderly conduct)
   (4) continued substance use despite having persistent or recurrent social or interpersonal problems caused or exacerbated by the effects of the substance (e.g., arguments with spouse about consequences of intoxication, physical fights)
B. The symptoms have never met the criteria for substance dependence for this class of substance.

Table from DSM-IV, *Diagnostic and Statistical Manual of Mental Disorders,* ed 4. Copyright American Psychiatric Association, Washington, 1994. Used with permission.

TABLE 13.1-7
Diagnostic Criteria for Substance Withdrawal

A. The development of a substance-specific syndrome due to the cessation of (or reduction in) substance use that has been heavy and prolonged.
B. The substance-specific syndrome causes clinically significant distress or impairment in social, occupational, or other important areas of functioning.
C. The symptoms are not due to a general medical condition and are not better accounted for by another mental disorder.

Table from DSM-IV, *Diagnostic and Statistical Manual of Mental Disorders,* ed 4. Copyright American Psychiatric Association, Washington, 1994. Used with permission.

TABLE 13.1-8
Diagnostic Criteria for Substance Intoxication

A. The development of a reversible substance-specific syndrome due to recent ingestion of (or exposure to) a substance. **Note:** Different substances may produce similar or identical syndromes.
B. Clinically significant maladaptive behavioral or psychological changes that are due to the effect of the substance on the central nervous system (e.g., belligerence, mood lability, cognitive impairment, impaired judgment, impaired social or occupational functioning) and develop during or shortly after use of the substance.
C. The symptoms are not due to a general medical condition and are not better accounted for by another mental disorder.

Table from DSM-IV, *Diagnostic and Statistical Manual of Mental Disorders,* ed 4. Copyright American Psychiatric Association, Washington, 1994. Used with permission.

withdrawal or occurs or persists beyond those stages), and (3) the phenomenological presentation (for example, diazepam [Valium]-induced anxiety disorder with onset during withdrawal).

Table 13.1-9 shows the various disorders induced by the major categories of substances recognized by DSM-IV and indicates which disorders are seen during intoxication and during withdrawal. Although they are not included specifically in the table, anabolic-adrenergic steroids can also induce psychotic mood, anxiety, and sleep and sexual disorders, and their withdrawal can also be associated with mood and sleep disorders.

EVOLVING TERMINOLOGY The terminology used to describe the substance-related disorders has been repeatedly revised as concepts about the nature of drug-using behavior have evolved. In 1964 a WHO Expert Committee on Addiction Producing Drugs recommended substituting the term "drug dependence" for both of the previously used terms, "addiction" and "habituation." The meaning of dependence was to be defined separately for each variety of drug, but no operational criteria were provided. In the 1980 third edition of DSM (DSM-III) drug use disorders were divided into two major categories, drug abuse and drug dependence, and specific criteria for diagnosis were given. In DSM-III-R, adopted in 1987, the two categories were retained, but the diagnostic criteria were modified. Further revisions were made for DSM-IV, which adopted the terms "substance abuse" and "substance dependence," probably to eliminate the use of the more cumbersome term "alcohol and drug dependence including tobacco."

In much of the world literature on drug dependence, the term "dependence" is used to convey two distinct ideas: (1) a behavioral syndrome and (2) physical or physiological dependence. *Physiological dependence* can be defined as alterations in neural systems that are manifested by tolerance and the appearance of withdrawal phenomena when a chronically administered drug is discontinued or displaced from its receptor. Because the dual use of the word causes confusion, the 1980 ADAMHA-WHO working group recommended restricting the term "dependence" to describe the behavioral syndrome and substituting the term "neuroadaptation" for physical dependence. Such a substitution would have emphasized several points. First, the continued use of many drugs, including tricyclic antidepressants and β-adrenergic receptor antagonists, causes neuroadaptive changes followed by withdrawal phenomena, but not by drug-seeking behavior, on their discontinuation. Second, neuroadaptive changes begin with the first dose of an opioid or sedative drug, and, therefore, such changes in and of themselves are not a sufficient cause or definition of drug dependence as a behavioral syndrome.

In DSM-IV the neuroadaptive changes are referred to as physiological dependence, withdrawal, and tolerance, but the conceptual framework corresponds to that of the ADAMHA-WHO working group in that the drug-induced physiological alterations alone are not sufficient grounds for the diagnosis of drug dependence.

Why use "addiction"? The words "addict" and "addiction" often have pejorative connotations; they are also frequently trivialized and used to refer to ordinary activities, such as running and solving crossword puzzles. However, the term "addiction" continues to have the core connotation of decreased control, and some chapters in this textbook have retained such terms as "opioid addict" because they are less awkward to use than "severely opioid-dependent person" when referring to persons who are dependent on drugs to a severe degree. Here the word "dependent," unmodified, is used to mean behaviorally dependent. The term "physiological dependence" or "physical dependence" is used to refer to the physiological changes that result in withdrawal symptoms when drugs are discontinued.

COMPARATIVE NOSOLOGY

DSM-IV shares with DSM-III-R and the 10th revision of the *International Classification of Diseases and Related Health Problems* (ICD-10) the notion of a generic concept of dependence. Despite some changes in wording, the syndromes and criteria for dependence in DSM-III-R and DSM-IV are similar. DSM-IV appears to lay greater stress on tolerance and physiological dependence by requiring the clinician to specify whether tolerance and withdrawal are present; however, in practice, even requiring those criteria would not reduce substantially the number of cases meeting the criteria for dependence with most drug categories, with the exception of hallucinogens, a class of drugs for which DSM-IV does not list physiological dependence as a criterion. DSM-IV and ICD-10 employ similar concepts (the dependence syndrome varying in degree of severity), and there is generally a high level of agreement between them for making a diagnosis of dependence, although the descriptions of the criteria for determining the presence and severity of the syndrome differ. They both require three elements of the syndrome to have been present in a 12-month period.

The DSM-IV categorization of drug classes differs somewhat from the one used by ICD-10, which, constrained by a new alphanumeric system, employs only nine categories by including caffeine with amphetaminelike stimulants and PCP with other psychoactive agents.

TABLE 13.1-9
Diagnoses Associated with Class of Substances

	Dependence	Abuse	Intoxication	Withdrawal	Intoxication Delirium	Withdrawal Delirium	Dementia	Amnestic Disorder	Psychotic Disorders	Mood Disorders	Anxiety Disorders	Sexual Dysfunctions	Sleep Disorders
Alcohol	X	X	X	X	I	W	P	P	I/W	I/W	I/W	I	I/W
Amphetamines	X	X	X	X	I				I	I/W	I	I	I/W
Caffeine			X								I		I
Cannabis	X	X	X		I				I		I		
Cocaine	X	X	X	X	I				I	I/W	I/W	I	I/W
Hallucinogens	X	X	X		I				I*	I	I		
Inhalants	X	X	X		I		P		I	I	I		
Nicotine	X			X									
Opioids	X	X	X	X	I				I	I		I	I/W
Phencyclidine	X	X	X		I				I	I	I		
Sedatives, hypnotics, or anxiolytics	X	X	X	X	I	W	P	P	I/W	I/W	W	I	I/W
Polysubstance	X												
Other	X	X	X	X	I	W	P	P	I/W	I/W	I/W	I	I/W

*also Hallucinogen persisting perception disorder (flashbacks).

Note: X, I, W, I/W, or P indicates that the category is recognized in DSM-IV. In addition, I indicates that the specifier "with onset during intoxication" may be noted for the category (except for intoxication delirium); W indicates that the specifier "with onset during withdrawal" may be noted for the category (except for withdrawal delirium); and I/W indicates that either "with onset during intoxication" or "with onset during withdrawal" may be noted for the category. P indicates that the disorder is "persisting."

Table from DSM-IV, *Diagnostic and Statistical Manual of Mental Disorders,* ed 4. Copyright American Psychiatric Association, Washington, 1994. Used with permission.

Another difference among DSM-III-R, DSM-IV, and ICD-10 relates to the diagnosis of substance abuse. Whereas DSM-III-R required the presence of only one of two general criteria, DSM-IV requires one of four. Nevertheless, the agreement between DSM-III-R and DSM-IV is high for both substance dependence and abuse. However, with regard to what DSM-IV refers to as substance abuse, there is a major difference between DSM-IV and ICD-10. ICD-10 does not use the term "abuse." Instead, it includes a category of *harmful use,* which is substantially different from the DSM-IV concept of abuse. The concept of harmful use is limited to mental and physical health (for example, hepatitis and overdose), and specifically excludes social impairment, stating: "The fact that a pattern of use of a particular substance is disapproved of . . . or may have led to socially negative consequences such as arrest or marital arguments is not in itself evidence of harmful use."

The word "abuse" is also commonly used in ways that differ significantly from the definitions developed for use in DSM-IV. In popular and legislative contexts drug abuse is used to mean any use of an illicit substance or any nonprescribed use of a drug intended as a medicine, as well as the harmful or excessive use of legally available substances, such as alcohol and tobacco.

DSM-III-R described three levels of severity of dependence (mild, moderate, severe) in its section on drug dependence. DSM-IV retains the notion of severity but applies it to several disorders and describes it in its introduction. DSM-IV includes several more ways than DSM-III-R to describe patterns of remission from dependence and abuse.

Other perspectives Although the criteria for diagnosis in DSM-IV are not precisely those in DSM-III-R or ICD-10, the differences are not likely to lead to profoundly different kinds of clinical decisions because all of the sets of criteria were developed from what is essentially a biopsychosocial model of substance dependence. In such a model multiple factors—genetic, psychological, sociological, and pharmacological—contribute to the observed clinical syndromes. Such seeming unanimity about the nature of drug dependence should not obscure the existence of dissenting perspectives, which take several forms. In one the biopsychosocial model is accused of giving too much weight to biological factors and too little recognition to the notion of human will and responsibility, of medicalizing deviant behavior for the benefit of treatment professionals, and of creating universal exculpation for all those who fail to live up to reasonable societal expectations. But some professionals have implicitly criticized the same biopsychosocial model as not giving sufficient weight to the ideas that substance dependence is a specific primary disease (that is, not a symptom of other psychiatric difficulties), that those who develop the disease have no control over their intake of certain substances, that denial of the presence of a problem is a major characteristic of the disease, and that the disease is always progressive and can be managed only by lifelong and total abstinence from the particular substance.

Concepts about substance dependence can be arrayed along several dimensions that are not entirely independent or orthogonal: broad versus narrow, disease versus learned behavior, and social versus medical. The narrow concept of substance dependence accepts as disorders those maladaptive behaviors associated primarily, if not exclusively, with the ingestion of substances generally accepted as pharmacological agents. Compulsive eating, gambling, running, hair pulling, and repetitive excessive sexual activities are not included among the dependence disorders, although those problems may share certain features that resemble a decreased ability to choose and are sometimes ameliorated by participation in support groups founded on principles similar to those of Alcoholics Anonymous (AA). A broad approach would create a superclass of disorders that would include a number of such behaviors not involving pharmacological agents.

At the disease end of the disease-versus-behavioral syndrome dimension is a belief that dependence is not a learned behavior that can be modified or ameliorated with relearning but represents a primary disorder that is caused by an interaction between a substance and a person with some genetic vulnerability and that only total abstinence can arrest the progression of the disease. The medical-versus-social dimension typically describes a range of views on how best to respond to problems with substances, rather than differences about the essential nature of the problems. The medical model puts greater emphasis on issues of assessment—treatment, planning, and record keeping—and sometimes on treatment that can be rendered only by those with professional training (not necessarily physicians). The social model emphasizes the importance of social supports and the role of integrating the person with a problem into a network of recovering persons who can offer continuing support. The assessment and recording of progress and outcome as generally practiced by credentialed professionals is minimized.

HISTORY

The most commonly abused drugs have been in use for hundreds, if not thousands, of years. For example, opium has been used for medicinal purposes for at least 3,500 years, references to cannabis (marijuana) as a medicinal can be found in ancient Chinese herbals, and wine is mentioned frequently in the Bible. The indigenous people of the western hemisphere were smoking tobacco and chewing coca leaves generations before the arrival of the Spaniards. Some of the problems caused by alcohol and other drugs, such as drunkenness, are described in the Bible and in the writings of the ancient Greeks and Romans. As new and more concentrated forms of drugs were discovered or invented, or new routes of administering them were developed, new problems relating to their use emerged. For instance, the introduction of cheap gin into England in the 18th century led to alcohol-related problems that were considered more serious than those associated with beer and wine. And, although opium smoking was a major problem in Asia in the 18th and 19th centuries, the most active opioid alkaloid in opium, morphine, was not isolated until 1806. It was not commonly used by injection until the late 19th century, and the intravenous use of morphine and heroin did not begin to spread until the early part of the 20th century. Although native Americans smoked tobacco, not until the 19th century, when new methods of curing tobacco leaves to produce a mild smoking tobacco and cigarettes were introduced, did the practice of inhaling tobacco smoke deep into the lungs become common. Cigarette smoking became popular by the early decades of the 20th century.

MEDICALIZATION OF EXCESSIVE DRUG USE In 1810 Benjamin Rush, who is often credited as being the first American physician to suggest that the excessive use of alcohol was a disease rather than exclusively a moral defect, proposed the establishment of a sober house; in 1835 Samuel Woodward, a pioneer in the establishment of asylums for the insane, advocated similar asylums for inebriates. Contemporaneous with those early moves to involve medicine in dealing with excessive alcohol use was the emergence of the temperance movement and of the Washingtonians—groups of reformed drunkards concerned with helping others to adopt and maintain sobriety. In the process the Washingtonians developed many of the principles of self-help that were to be rediscovered by AA almost a century later.

When the ideas of voluntarism and self-help, as exemplified by Washingtonian Societies, failed to eliminate the problem of drunkenness, physicians began to debate more seriously the idea of coerced treatment in inebriate asylums supported by public funds. In 1870 advocates of the approach established the American Association for the Cure of Inebriates (AACI), dedicated to setting up hospitals for such persons, conducting research, and teaching medical students and physicians how to treat inebriety. At first those physicians who believed in a more spiritual, voluntary approach to the problem (neo-Washingtonians) were part of the AACI, but gradually the more somatically oriented factions, which advocated medically supervised asylums (and compulsory treatment when needed), gained ascendancy. Furthermore, the focus of concern was no longer limited to those who abused alcohol. Thomas Crothers, the secretary of AACI, saw inebriate asylums as places to treat all those who used any variety of intoxicant or narcotic to excess. However, very few publicly supported inebriate asylums ever opened.

EARLY ATTITUDES In the closing years of the 19th century there was growing concern about excessive and inappropriate drug use, including the use of alcohol and tobacco as well as opiates and cocaine.

First isolated from the coca leaf in 1860, cocaine came into widespread use in 1885 when pharmaceutical companies began to sell it in the United States and Europe. In 1884 Sigmund Freud had published a review of the potential therapeutic uses of cocaine. Some medical authorities in the United States shared his enthusiasm, and cocaine was recommended by the Hay Fever Association as a remedy for that malady. Within a few years, however, it was recognized that cocaine had the capacity to induce toxic psychosis, as well as to gain control over behavior, and that long-term opiate use had dependence-inducing effects. Nevertheless, in the United States, until the beginning of the 20th century, both the opium alkaloids and cocaine were still to be found in patent medicines that were sold over the counter for a wide variety of indications, and their labeling often did not reveal their contents.

Although the achievement of long-term cure of morphinism was reported to be exceedingly difficult, until the turn of the 20th century neither the public nor the medical profession saw the habitual user of opium or morphine as invariably suffering from a moral deficit. Those who had developed the morphine habit represented the entire socioeconomic spectrum, with women outnumbering men by about two to one. Various political and literary figures were known to use opiates but to lead otherwise productive and exemplary lives. However, it was also true that cocaine use and the morphine habit were common among gamblers, petty thieves, prostitutes, and other disreputable members of society. Also, persons with emotional problems and those who had formerly used alcohol to excess were probably overrepresented among opium users, since it was not unusual at the time for physicians to prescribe opiates to control emotional problems and alcoholism.

The problem of treating in the same institution drug users who had antisocial tendencies and those who led more conventional lives was as vexing to early advocates of medical treatment as it is to present-day practitioners. Many proponents of inebriate asylums did not want to take responsibility for persons who had frequent or serious encounters with the police because it was thought that such persons would make it impossible to create an atmosphere conducive to recovery. Partly to cope with the problem, even some of the proponents of a disease model of inebriety maintained the distinction between "inebriety the disease" and "intemperance the vice."

EARLY EFFORTS TOWARD CONTROL: EVOLUTION OF THE CRIMINAL MODEL By the late 1890s the public and the medical community were no longer indifferent to drug use and habituation. In 1893 the Anti-Saloon League was founded, reinvigorating a temperance movement that advocated the total prohibition of alcohol. Medical texts in England, Europe, and the United States contained descriptions of morphinism, theories of its causation, and recommendations for withdrawal and postwithdrawal treatment. Some texts also described problems of cocainism. Medical authorities in the United States cautioned against overly liberal prescribing of cocaine and opiates by physicians and expressed great concern about the presence of those drugs in unlabeled proprietary over-the-counter medicines. State laws were passed aimed at controlling the sale of opiates and cocaine, especially in patent medicines. In 1900 the cocaine in Coca-Cola was replaced by caffeine.

Partly to support the efforts of the Chinese government to control opium use in China, representatives of the United States government led the movement to negotiate an international treaty to control traffic in opium, cocaine, and related drugs. The first such treaty was signed at The Hague in 1912. Negotiators from the United States were also interested in the international control of cannabis but could not get other nations to view the substance as sufficiently problematic to warrant it. (Such control was achieved in 1925 at the Second Geneva Convention.) The Hague Convention required the signatories to pass domestic legislation controlling opiates and cocaine. The Harrison Act of 1914, the first federal legislation to regulate opiates and cocaine, was designed to restrict access to opiates and cocaine to doctors, dentists, pharmacists, and legitimate importers and manufacturers and brought the United States into compliance with the convention.

State regulations concerning the sale of opiates and cocaine, the introduction of aspirin and the barbiturates, and the Pure Food and Drug Act of 1906, which required the labeling of patent medicines, were already having an impact on the use of opiates in medicine when the Harrison Act was passed in 1914. Although many medical and political leaders in the United States believed that much of the problem of drug dependence was due to careless prescribing by physicians, the Harrison Act was not originally intended to interfere with the legitimate practice of medicine or to cause special hardship for those who were already dependent on opiates. For several years after the Harrison Act was passed, a few cities operated clinics that prescribed morphine to persons with established morphine habits. Most of those who were dependent on opiates before the Harrison Act became abstinent within a few years after it was passed, although generally not as a result of treatment at the clinics.

FLUCTUATING ATTITUDES By the 1920s several major changes had taken place in American attitudes and practices. The 18th Amendment to the Constitution, prohibiting the sale of alcohol, became law in 1920 and radically changed drinking behavior in the United States. Within a year after alcohol prohibition was enacted, 14 states also had passed cigarette prohibition laws. Those laws were even less popular than alcohol prohibition; by 1927 they had all been repealed, and by the mid-1920s Americans were smoking 80 billion cigarettes a year. However, cocaine use, which had been prevalent at the turn of the century, was no longer widespread.

Disillusioned by the reluctance of morphine addicts at clinics to seek detoxification, and by repeated relapses to morphine use among those who did, doctors began to recommend (not for the first time) compulsory treatment, with confinement until cure. As the new laws curtailed legitimate supplies of opiates, an illicit traffic developed to provide them to those who could not or would not use the clinics. Increasingly, the drug sold was heroin, introduced for medical use in 1898, but quickly found by drug users to be quite similar to morphine in its actions. Many who patronized the illicit traffickers and used the clinics had histories of delinquency and criminal activity, and eventually that subgroup came to predominate. Reformers, moralists, and the popular press found in the opiate habit, and in the reputation of those who continued to use morphine, proof of the evils inherent in those drugs.

Negative publicity, lurid stories, medical disillusionment, and pressure from law enforcement agents acted in concert to label the morphine clinics as medical folly and brought about their closing, the last in 1923. At the same time a series of United States Supreme Court decisions implied that prescribing even small amounts of opiates or cocaine to an addict for treatment of addiction was not proper medical practice and was, therefore, an illegal sale of narcotic drugs. Several physicians were imprisoned, and numerous others were tried, reprimanded, or otherwise harassed. By the early 1920s persons addicted to opiates were not welcome in doctors' offices, and they were often refused treatment at hospitals. The terms "dope addict" and "dope fiend" had become common, and the average layperson, as well as some otherwise well-informed members of the medical profession, appeared to believe that the opiate molecule was inherently evil. In the late 1930s cannabis acquired a similar reputation, and in 1937 the United States Congress passed legislation prescribing criminal penalties for its use, sale, or possession. However, alcohol prohibition had been repealed in 1933.

NEWER DRUGS Barbital, the first barbiturate sedative, was introduced into clinical medicine in 1903, followed over the next 30 years by scores of congeners, differing primarily in their duration of action. Within a few years after the introduction of each new compound, the first case reports of abuse, dependence, and withdrawal appeared in the medical journals, a pattern that was to be repeated with the nonbarbiturate sedatives, such as glutethimide (Doriden), ethchlorvynol (Placidyl), and meprobamate (Miltown) in the 1950s.

Amphetamine, first synthesized in 1887, was put into clinical use in 1932 as a drug to shrink mucous membranes. By 1935 its central stimulant effects had been recognized and found useful for treating narcolepsy. Dozens of other suggested uses soon followed. Reports of its abuse as a euphoriant first appeared in the late 1930s, but the full significance of its abuse potential was not appreciated until the post-World War II epidemic of intravenous methamphetamine addiction in Japan. That epidemic, precipitated by the sale of surplus methamphetamine tablets intended for combat troops, involved millions of people. Other amphetaminelike drugs were introduced during the 1950s and early 1960s.

Mescaline's psychological effects were known and written about at the end of the 19th century, but public concern about that category of drugs did not reach a high level until the 1960s when the use of a newly discovered and exceedingly potent hallucinogenic compound, lysergic acid diethylamide (LSD), evolved from experimentation by a few college students to more widespread use by younger groups. A local anesthetic developed in the 1950s, phencyclidine (PCP) became a drug of abuse in the 1970s.

Despite repeated reports of abuse and dependence associated with barbiturates, barbituratelike sedatives, and amphetamines and related stimulants, and in spite of concerns about experimentation with LSD and related hallucinogens, no federal criminal sanctions related to these drugs were in force until 1964, when authority for their control was assigned to the Food and Drug Administration (FDA). In contrast, concern about heroin addiction had led in the 1950s to ever harsher criminal penalties for its sale or possession. Although law enforcement efforts aimed at controlling heroin use were increased, both the number of new heroin addicts and the crime rates continued to rise throughout the late 1960s. At about that time there was also a sharp increase in the nonmedical use of other substances, such as cannabis and LSD, and a major epidemic of amphetamine abuse and dependence. In addition to amphetamines diverted from medical channels, supplies came from clandestine laboratories. Drug use, especially cannabis, became linked to antiestablishment attitudes, politics, and life-styles.

CHANGES IN TREATMENT TECHNIQUES Treatment for substance-related problems changed dramatically during the 20th century. The large specialized asylums that were advocated in the 19th century never materialized. Toward the end of the 19th century the medical profession was primarily concerned about how best to manage withdrawal syndromes and whether longer compulsory treatment was needed. With the advent of prohibition, the impetus to develop treatment for alcoholism declined sharply. Interest in treating opioid dependence also declined as the tendency for patients to relapse after detoxification discouraged physicians who treated them, and opioid use and dependence came to be seen more as criminal behavior than as a medical disorder. But some treatment for opioid dependence continued in private sanitoriums, and as drug-addicted prisoners began to fill penitentiaries, two federal hospitals were established in 1930—at Lexington, Kentucky, and at Fort Worth, Texas—to provide treatment for that population and to conduct research on the problem. Treatment of dependence on barbiturates and amphetamines took place largely in state hospitals and in the mainstream of medical practice, but there was no consensus on what constituted effective posthospital care.

In the mid-1930s two recovering alcoholics rediscovered the principles of the Washingtonians, added some new principles, and initiated the self-help movement now known as AA, a movement that by the 1950s had begun to inspire analogous self-help efforts among other types of substance abusers.

The situation changed again in the early 1960s as individual states and the federal government attempted to respond to new outbreaks of heroin use among young persons and to concomitant increases in crime. In California a civil commitment program for addicts was initiated under the administrative control of the Department of Corrections, and in New York City Riverside Hospital was reopened to treat juvenile heroin addicts.

The first follow-up studies of patients treated at the federal hospital at Lexington, published in the early 1960s, revealed exceedingly high rates of relapse after treatment. Doctors and the public demanded new ideas, including a reconsideration of providing addicts with legitimate opioids through medical channels.

In the years from 1958 to 1967 several major new approaches to treating opioid dependence were developed. Synanon, the prototype therapeutic community, was started in California in 1958, and was replicated in New York with the establishment of Daytop Village and Phoenix House; Vincent Dole and Marie Nyswander demonstrated the effectiveness of large daily doses of methadone (Dolophine) in reducing crime and heroin use among selected long-term heroin addicts; and several research groups demonstrated that heroin addicts would voluntarily try treatment with narcotic antagonists. In the mid-1960s New York State and the federal government legislated civil commitment programs modeled after the program in California, with an initial period of prolonged institutional care as a key element. Although many treatment programs initiated in the early 1960s continued to focus on the treatment of opioid dependence, others, especially the therapeutic communities, viewed all nonmedical drug use as stemming from similar defects in character structure and offered a generic approach to treating drug dependence.

Alcohol and nicotine In the 1950s clinicians at Wilmar State Hospital in Minnesota had developed a treatment program for alcoholism built on a synthesis of the medical model and the experiences of recovering alcohol abusers using the 12-step principles of AA. That treatment approach was refined and expanded at the Johnson Institute and Hazelden Foundation, also in Minnesota. The modified programs, widely adopted by other treatment programs, are often referred to as 28-day programs, 12-step programs, or the Minnesota model. In the early 1970s the effort to recognize alcoholism as a disease gained momentum, and the decision of medical insurance carriers to provide coverage for detoxification and inpatient treatment fueled an unprecedented growth of private-sector facilities offering treatment for alcoholism. Almost without exception, they were residential programs using the Minnesota model. The decriminalization of public intoxication spurred a parallel increase in public-sector-supported alcohol treatment programs.

The Surgeon General's Report of 1964 had linked cigarette smoking to lung cancer and had concluded that tobacco smoking was a form of dependence, although not an addiction. But by the 1970s tobacco dependence was becoming more widely accepted as a valid entity, and there was a rise of various treatments for it. By the late 1980s as smoking was becoming socially unacceptable, entire buildings were declared smoke-free, smoking was banned on most airplane flights and in many hospitals, and pharmaceutical companies were marketing new ways of delivering nicotine, such as in nicotine chewing gum and transdermal patches, as aids for smoking cessation.

Two-tiered system When the cocaine epidemic of the early 1980s struck the middle class, many units of the large, private-sector system for treating alcoholism evolved into chemical dependency units offering similar treatments to both alcoholic persons and those with other varieties of substance dependence. By 1990 it was estimated that there were more than 8,000 recognized programs dealing with alcoholism and other substance dependence. The treatment methods used varied widely in terms of the settings, costs, philosophical underpinnings, and populations served. New categories of substance abuse professionals had emerged, and psychiatrists who once had considered the problems to be a low-status area successfully lobbied for the creation of a recognized subspecialty in addiction psychiatry. Treatment capacity was described as being a two-tiered system with private and public sectors, in which the private sector served 40 percent of the population but received 60 percent of the total expenditures for treatment. One response to the escalating cost of substance-abuse services among those with private medical insurance was the rise of a managed-care industry created to control costs on behalf of employers who pay for health insurance, generally by severely limiting the length of stay in hospital settings.

GOVERNMENT RESPONSES: LEGISLATION AND NATIONAL STRATEGIES In 1969 Congress recognized the need to give greater attention to the problem of alcoholism and established the National Institute on Alcohol Abuse and Alcoholism (NIAAA) in the National Institute of Mental Health (NIMH). In 1970 new legislation was passed, reorganizing the jumble of drug regulatory statutes that had evolved since the passage of the Harrison Act, increasing the resources for controlling the availability of illicit drugs, and assigning the task of enforcement to a new agency, the Drug Enforcement Agency (DEA), which incorporated elements of the FDA and the

Bureau of Narcotic and Dangerous Drugs (BNDD). All drugs subject to special controls were included in one of several categories of the Controlled Substances Act.

In 1971, when United States troops in Vietnam were reported to be using heroin heavily, a Special Action Office for Drug Abuse Prevention (SAODAP) was established in the Executive Office of the President to develop and publish an overall national strategy and to coordinate government activities and policies relating to drug abuse. The creation of that office and the associated legislation marked a turning point in United States policy. The notion that opioid dependence was an incurable disorder, which justified the harshest of penalties in the name of prevention, was superseded by a policy that recognized that a substantial proportion of opioid addicts (as well as those with other varieties of drug dependence) could eventually reenter the mainstream of society. New commitments were made to basic research, epidemiology, the development of new treatment methods, and the evaluation of existing treatment approaches. The opioid maintenance approach using methadone was moved, by executive fiat, from the legal limbo of experimental status to a category that recognized its legitimacy. In addition, new regulations were developed to prevent the inappropriate prescribing of opioids. Federal support for the expansion of community treatment programs was also greatly increased. By 1973 about 200,000 substance users, most of them opioid users, were in treatment in community programs. Those programs were repeatedly and intensively evaluated over the subsequent decade. The legislation that established SAODAP also provided the legislative framework for the National Institute on Drug Abuse (NIDA) in the Department of Health, Education and Welfare (HEW). When it was established in 1974 NIDA became the lead agency for implementing federal policy on treatment, research, and prevention.

By the early 1980s it was generally accepted that treatment for opioid dependence had demonstrable impact. However, for the majority of patients in treatment programs, the primary drugs of abuse were no longer opioids, but more typically were cannabis, stimulants, or sedatives. During the early and mid-1970s some groups had argued for the decriminalization or legalization of cannabis. The arguments lost much of their force with the finding that, in 1979, almost 10 percent of high school students were using cannabis on a daily basis. In response to what they perceived as tolerance toward cannabis use, a number of parents' organizations were formed that were committed to making all drug use unacceptable. Those groups forced NIDA to review and remove from all its publications any statements that could be interpreted as being tolerant of drug use. That decreased tolerance for drug use grew in parallel with a more general conservative shift in public attitudes. Even though, in the 1970s, the public and the courts had rejected requiring urine tests to detect drug use as a way to interrupt the heroin epidemic, in 1986 federal employees were required by presidential order to undergo such tests. Similar testing for drug use was encouraged in private industry, giving rise to new industries for testing for the presence of drugs and for interpreting test results and placing drug users in treatment.

Tobacco By the 1970s it had become obvious that the major abuse problems in the United States in terms of social and economic impact and health costs were alcoholism and tobacco dependence. Although the Surgeon General's Report of 1964 linking cigarettes to cancer had not produced any dramatic decrease in smoking, the rate of increase in cigarette consumption among men had begun to level out. The publication of the facts about the health hazards of tobacco did not, however, prevent an increase in smoking among women. By the 1970s the medical and research community increasingly accepted tobacco smoking as a form of drug dependence, and new efforts were made to understand how nicotine gains control of behavior and to develop new treatments for tobacco dependence. In 1988 the Report of the Surgeon General officially defined tobacco dependence as analogous to other varieties of drug dependence. In 1994 the FDA held hearings on the appropriateness of regulating the nicotine in tobacco as an addictive drug.

More laws and reorganization For several years during the 1970s, the excessive use and overprescribing of anxiolytic drugs were also areas of major concern in both the medical and political arenas. But the nation's major illicit drug use problems in the late 1970s and early 1980s were the rapid increase in the use of cocaine and the heavy use of cannabis by adolescents. By 1985, among the illicit drugs, only cannabis was more commonly abused than cocaine. By the late 1980s, as cannabis use was declining steadily among the high school population, new ways of using cocaine (smoking freebase forms such as crack, for example) created unprecedented public concern.

Spurred partly by public concern about the spread of the human immunodeficiency virus (HIV) and AIDS among intravenous drug users, the rising demand for the treatment of cocaine dependence, and the sudden cocaine-induced deaths of several prominent athletes, the Anti-Drug Abuse Act of 1986 was passed. The bill authorized the government to spend nearly \$4 billion to intensify efforts against drugs and drug abuse. Although most of that money was allocated to law enforcement activities, federal resources for the treatment of drug dependence and research were also substantially increased. Recognition of the need to do more about preventing drug dependence, and the rise of the politically active parents' groups with drug abuse prevention as a major concern, led to the creation of the Office for Substance Abuse Prevention (now called the Center for Substance Abuse Prevention [CSAP]) in the Department of Health and Human Services (HHS) in 1986. Rising violence associated with local cocaine distribution networks led to the passage of the 1988 Anti-Drug Abuse Act and the 1989 Emergency Supplemental Appropriation. The 1988 act created the Office of National Drug Control Policy (ONDCP) in the White House, and required the annual publication of a National Drug Control Strategy document. The 1988 act, while still devoting more than two thirds of federal resources to controlling the drug supply, also increased still further the funding for treatment and prevention, which was augmented again by the 1989 supplement. In connection with the latter legislation, and in response to the substantial increase in resources devoted to the expansion and improvement of treatment for drug dependence, primarily dependence on illicit drugs, the Office for Treatment Improvement (now called the Center for Substance Abuse Treatment [CSAT]) was created in HHS.

Despite those changes, the nexus between drug use and crime and the spread of HIV and AIDS continued to spur the public and the federal government to invest even more in treatment and prevention. In 1992 concern that treatment and prevention were not being given adequate emphasis in a research-oriented organizational structure led to still another reorganization of the federal effort. Under the new structure, the three research institutes, NIMH, NIDA, and NIAAA, were shifted to the National Institutes of Health (NIH), while treatment and prevention services for drugs, alcohol, and mental health were reconstituted as a new agency, the Substance Abuse and Mental Health Services Agency (SAMHSA).

EPIDEMIOLOGY

Over the past two decades a number of methods have been developed to gauge the extent of substance use, abuse, and dependence in the United States. The major recurring methods include the National Household Survey on Drug Abuse (Household Survey), the Drug Abuse Warning Network (DAWN), the Drug Use Forecasting (DUF) Program, and the National High School Senior Survey—Monitoring the Future (High School Survey). In addition, data on the street availability and purity of illicit drugs, drug seizures, and arrests for drug offenses are collected nationally from the DEA and the Federal Bureau of Investigation (FBI) and locally from municipal police departments. Each of those data sources has strengths and weaknesses. For example, the Household Survey interviews a representative sample of persons living in households, oversamples minority populations and certain large urban areas, and focuses in detail on drug-using behaviors; however, it does not interview persons who are homeless or are living in dormitories or institutions (jails or hospitals), nor does it attempt to determine whether respondents need treatment or meet the formal criteria for substance dependence. In addition, some respondents may be reluctant to admit to certain types of substance use.

The DUF program interviews and obtains anonymous urine specimens from a sample of arrestees in 24 of the largest cities in the United States. By design, persons charged with the sale or possession of drugs cannot make up more than 25 percent of the sample. Although it does not depend on self-reports to measure use, the DUF results cannot be easily extrapolated to a national population and the information that can be derived from a single urine test is limited.

The DAWN system began obtaining data on drug-related episodes from medical examiners and hospital emergency rooms in 1972. In 1989 the system was modified so that the reporting emergency rooms (770 in 21 metropolitan areas) constitute a representative sample of such facilities in the continental United States. The DAWN data provide useful information on trends in the morbidity associated with various illicit drugs, but those data need to be interpreted with caution because the DAWN system reports only episodes in which a drug is part of the presenting clinical picture. For example, a rising number of emergency room episodes associated with heroin could mean that more heroin users with AIDS-related problems are seeking primary medical care rather than that more persons are using heroin. Similarly, reports by medical examiners of more violent deaths associated with cocaine may signal an escalation of competition among drug dealers rather than more people using cocaine. The analytic methods do not reveal the nature of the linkage by drug use and the presenting problem; which of several drugs present, if any, played a causal role in the episode; or whether the user was a novice or a long-term user.

The High School Survey, which has obtained information since 1975 from forms returned anonymously by high school seniors, recently extended its efforts to former seniors now in college and to students in the 8th and 10th grades. Whereas the survey depends on self-report, and dropouts prior to grade 12 were not sampled until recently, the trend information it provides is exceedingly useful.

In addition to the recurring data-gathering efforts, important epidemiological information is available from two national studies that systematically interviewed representative samples of the population and used DSM-III or DSM-III-R criteria to develop estimates of current and lifetime prevalence of psychiatric disorders, including substance abuse and substance dependence. Those studies are the NIMH Epidemiologic Catchment Area (ECA) Study, conducted in the early 1980s, and the National Comorbidity Survey (NCS), conducted between 1990 and 1992. The ECA interviews in five areas of the United States included persons in institutions (such as mental hospitals, jails, and nursing homes) and used DSM-III criteria to develop estimates of prevalence. The NCS interviews of a nationally representative sample of noninstitutionalized persons used DSM-III-R criteria. Although the ECA was conducted before the cocaine epidemic crested, and the criteria for diagnosis used were somewhat altered in DSM-III-R, it nevertheless remains a landmark study of the extent of drug abuse and dependence and co-occurring psychiatric disorders.

The ECA study found that 16.7 percent of the United States population ages 18 and older met the DSM-III criteria for a lifetime diagnosis of either abuse or dependence on some substance, with 13.8 percent meeting the criteria for an alcohol-related disorder and 6.2 percent meeting the criteria for abuse or dependence of a substance other than alcohol or tobacco.

The lifetime and 12-month prevalence of substance-use disorders found in the NCS are shown in Table 13.1-10. The NCS finding of 26.6 percent lifetime prevalence of substance abuse and dependence is substantially higher than the 16.7 percent found in the ECA study. Some of that discrepancy is probably due to questions in the NCS about prescription drugs that were posed when a patient reported symptoms of dependence and on differences in criteria (DSM-III versus DSM-III-R). However, there may also have been real increases in prevalence. For illegal drugs and the nonmedical use of prescription drugs, the lifetime rate for dependence in the NCS was 7.9 percent, a figure much closer to the 6.2 percent found for such drugs in the ECA study.

Among the major achievements of the NCS analyses were the findings on the proportions of persons who had used drugs at any time in their lives (lifetime users) who became dependent (overall and for each drug category); the demographic factors that predicted use, dependence, and persistence of dependence; and the prevalence and significance of multiple psychiatric diagnoses. It is obvious that dependence cannot develop if a drug is never used. Thus, presenting data on the prevalence of dependence across the population as a whole, including data on those who never used, can obscure the likelihood of developing dependence among those who do use a particular drug. In the NCS the prevalence of lifetime dependence on the broad range of illicit and nonprescribed medications was 14.7 percent, with male *users* only slightly more likely (16.4 percent) than female *users* (12.6 percent) to develop dependence. In a similar analysis of the 12-month prevalence of dependence on those drugs, the rate for the population as a whole was 1.8 percent. However, the 12-month prevalence was 3.5 percent for those who had used any of the drugs at any time in their lives, 10.3 percent for those who had used them in the past 12 months, and 23.8 percent among those who had a lifetime history of dependence. The likelihood of being drug dependent in the past 12 months, given a lifetime history of dependence, was similar for men (24.9 percent) and women (22.2 percent). Lower educational and lower income levels predicted a lifetime history of dependence (odds ratios greater than 2), but race, ethnicity, or living in an urban environment did not. There were also some interesting differences in the likelihood that users would develop dependence (lifetime) across pharmacological classes. For example, among heroin users the lifetime dependence rate was 23 percent; it was 32 percent for tobacco, 16.7 percent for cocaine, and 15.4 percent for alcohol, but only 4.9 percent for psychedelics.

The ECA findings on lifetime prevalence of DSM-III disorders for various drugs are shown in Table 13.1-11. The ECA study has some of the same limitations that apply to the Household Survey, in that it relies on self-report and so may underestimate the extent of drug abuse and dependence.

Table 13.1-12 shows data from the 1993 Household Survey on the percentage of respondents who reported using various drugs. The data are shown for those ages 18 to 25, the group that reported the highest

TABLE 13.1-10
Lifetime and 12-Month Prevalence of UM-CIDI/DSM-III-R Disorders*

	Male				Female				Total			
	Lifetime		12 mo		Lifetime		12 mo		Lifetime		12 mo	
Disorders	%	SE	%	SE	%	SE	%	SE	%	SE	%	SE
Substance use disorders												
Alcohol abuse without dependence	12.5	0.8	3.4	0.4	6.4	0.6	1.6	0.2	9.4	0.5	2.5	0.2
Alcohol dependence	20.1	1.0	10.7	0.9	8.2	0.7	3.7	0.4	14.1	0.7	7.2	0.5
Drug abuse without dependence	5.4	0.5	1.3	0.2	3.5	0.4	0.3	0.1	4.4	0.3	0.8	0.1
Drug dependence	9.2	0.7	3.8	0.4	5.9	0.5	1.9	0.3	7.5	0.4	2.8	0.3
Any substance abuse-dependence	35.4	1.2	16.1	0.7	17.9	1.1	6.6	0.4	26.6	1.0	11.3	0.5
Other disorders												
Antisocial personality	5.8	0.6	...	...	1.2	0.3	...	...	3.5	0.3	...	...
Nonaffective psychosis†	0.6	0.1	0.5	0.1	0.8	0.2	0.6	0.2	0.7	0.1	0.5	0.1
Any NCS disorder	48.7	0.2	27.7	0.9	47.3	1.5	31.2	1.3	48.0	1.1	29.5	1.0

*UM-CIDI indicates University of Michigan Composite International Diagnostic Interview; NCS, National Comorbidity Survey.

†Nonaffective psychosis includes schizophrenia, schizophreniform disorder, schizoaffective disorder, delusional disorder, and atypical psychosis.

Table adapted from R C Kessler, K A McGonagle, S Zhao, C B Nelson, M Hughes, S Eshleman, H-U Wittchen, K S Kendler: Lifetime and 12-month prevalence of DSM-III-R psychiatric disorders in the United States. Arch Gen Psychiatry *51:* 8, 1994. Used with permission.

level of use of illicit drugs during the 30 days preceding the interview. The group of persons ages 26 to 34 had the next highest rate of use in the preceding 30 days and reported a higher lifetime experience with heroin and cocaine. Illicit drug use during the 30 days preceding the interview is far more prevalent among young adults (ages 18 to 34, and particularly those 18 to 25 years old) than among those above age 35 or below age 18. Also, whereas recent use is more common in large metropolitan areas as compared with rural areas, regional, racial, and ethnic differences vary with the age group considered. With the exception of tobacco dependence, all forms of substance abuse or dependence are more common among men than among women. However, as noted, recent data indicate that when adjustment is made for differences in rates of use and experimentation with illicit drugs, women are about as likely as men to become dependent. Overall, the 1993 Household Survey found that 37 percent of Americans over the age of 12 (77 million) had used an illicit drug at least once in their lifetime, 11.8 percent had used an illicit drug in the past year, and 5.6 percent had used an illicit drug within the preceding 30 days. Current illicit drug use (past 30 days) was more common among male respondents (7.4 percent) than among female respondents (4.1 percent) and among the unemployed (11.6 percent). Among other demographic subgroups, it was more common among blacks (6.8 percent) and in the western United States (7.7 percent).

TABLE 13.1-11
Lifetime Prevalence of DSM-III Substance Abuse-Dependence Disorders in Total Population (1980–1984)

Substance	Percent Prevalence
Any drug	6.2
Cannabis	4.4
Stimulants	1.7
Sedatives	1.2
Opioids	0.7
Hallucinogens*	0.4
Cocaine*	0.2
Alcohol	13.8
Tobacco*†	36.0

*Abuse only as per DSM-III.
†One site only.
Table adapted from D B Kandel: Epidemiological trends and implications for understanding the nature of addiction. In Addictive States, C P O'Brien, J H Jaffe, editors, Research Publications: Association for Research in Nervous and Mental Disease, vol 70, p 23. Raven, New York, 1992.

The High School Senior Survey data on self-reported past-30-day drug use indicated that prevalence rates for both cannabis use and illicit drug use in general declined sharply from the high levels reported in 1977 through 1979 to much lower levels in 1991. The decline in cocaine use began in 1987. However, there were no further reductions in the use of cannabis, cocaine, and other illicit drugs in 1992. Prevalence rates increased in 1993 and increased still further in 1994. Lifetime, past year, past month, and daily use of cannabis increased among 8th, 10th, and 12th graders. Other substance use increased also, but levels were still below the peaks observed a decade earlier. More recent annual High School Surveys have begun to monitor the use of crack (inhalable cocaine), as well as of noninhalable forms of cocaine, anabolic steroids, and crystal methamphetamine. In 1993 the annual prevalence rates among high school seniors for use of any illicit drug was 29.4 percent, and for an illicit drug other than cannabis it was 16.2 percent. Annual use rates reported in 1993 for specific drugs were alcohol, 77.7 percent; cannabis, 23.9 percent; stimulants, 8.2 percent; inhalants, 6.6 percent; hallucinogens, 5.8 percent; sedatives, 3.6 percent; cocaine, 3.5 percent; opiates other than heroin, 3.5 percent; heroin, 0.4 percent; and anabolic steroids, 1.4 percent.

The DUF system obtains data from a population in which illicit drug use is high and thus provides trend data not readily available from other sources. In general, current drug use among arrestees is more than 10 times higher than among those sampled by national surveys, despite the fact that urine tests detect drug use for only a few days, whereas surveys typically ask about drug use over the preceding 30 days. For example, in 1988, at the peak of the cocaine epidemic, more than 60 percent of arrestees tested positive for cocaine (80 percent among male arrestees in Manhattan).

Epidemics It is clear that there have been several major overlapping drug abuse epidemics over the past 30 years affecting somewhat

TABLE 13.1-12
Percentages Reporting Lifetime, Past Year, and Past Month Use of Illicit Drugs, Alcohol, and Tobacco in the United States Population Ages 18 to 25: 1985, 1991, 1992, and 1993

	Time Period											
	Lifetime				Past Year				Past Month			
Drug	1985	1991	1992	1993	1985	1991	1992	1993	1985	1991	1992	1993
Any illicit drug[1]	63.7[b]	54.7[a]	51.7	50.9	41.0[b]	29.1	26.4	26.6	25.1[b]	15.4	13.0	13.5
Marijuana and hashish	59.4[b]	50.5	48.1	47.4	36.3[b]	24.5	22.7	22.9	21.9[b]	13.0	11.0	11.1
Cocaine	24.4[b]	17.9[b]	15.8[b]	12.5	15.6[b]	7.7[b]	6.3	5.0	7.5[b]	2.0	1.8	1.5
Crack	—	3.8	3.2	3.5	—	1.0	1.1	1.0	—	0.4	0.4	0.4
Inhalants	13.0[a]	10.9	9.8	9.9	2.1	3.5	2.3	2.8	0.8	1.5	0.8	1.1
Hallucinogens	11.6	13.1	13.4	12.5	4.0	4.7	4.8	4.9	1.8	1.2	1.3	1.3
PCP	5.6	4.2	4.6	4.4	1.4	0.7	1.0	0.7	0.6	0.1[a]	0.2	0.4
Heroin	1.3	0.8	1.3[a]	0.7	0.6	0.3	0.5	0.3	0.3	0.1	0.2	0.1
Nonmedical use of any psychotherapeutic[2]	26.6[b]	17.9[b]	15.4	14.2	15.2[b]	8.6	7.7	7.2	6.3[b]	2.7	2.3	2.9
Stimulants	17.5[b]	9.4[b]	6.8	6.4	9.8[b]	3.3	2.3	3.0	3.8[b]	0.8	0.7	0.9
Sedatives	11.8[b]	4.3[b]	3.2	2.7	5.1[b]	1.9[a]	1.7	1.1	1.6[a]	0.7	0.6	0.6
Tranquilizers	12.6[b]	7.4[a]	6.8	5.4	6.4[b]	2.6	3.0[a]	2.0	1.6[a]	0.6	0.6	0.6
Analgesics	11.5[a]	10.2	8.7	8.7	6.8[a]	5.3	4.8	4.1	2.0	1.4	1.2	1.4
Any illicit drug other than marijuana[3]	38.7[b]	32.0[b]	28.8	27.2	23.7[b]	16.0[b]	13.7	13.0	12.3[b]	6.1	5.2	5.3
Alcohol	92.0[b]	90.2[b]	86.3	87.1	86.4[b]	82.8[b]	77.7	79.0	70.7[b]	63.6[a]	59.2	59.3
Cigarettes	75.2[b]	71.2[b]	68.7	66.7	43.9[b]	41.2	41.1	38.3	36.6[b]	32.2[a]	31.9	29.0
Smokeless tobacco	—	21.9	21.7	19.7	—	8.6	9.2	8.9	—	5.8	6.0	6.4
Anabolic steroids	—	1.3	0.7[a]	1.5	—	0.4	0.1	0.3	—	0.1	0.0	0.2

—Not available.
[1]Nonmedical use of marijuana or hashish, cocaine (including crack), inhalants, hallucinogens (including PCP), heroin, or psychotherapeutics at least once.
[2]Nonmedical use of any prescription-type stimulant, sedative, tranquilizer, or analgesic; does not include over-the-counter drugs.
[3]Nonmedical use of cocaine (including crack), inhalants, hallucinogens (including PCP), heroin, or psychotherapeutics at least once; includes marijuana users who also have used any of the listed drugs; does not include users of marijuana only.
[a]Difference between estimate in this cell and corresponding estimate for 1993 is statistically significant at the .05 level.
[b]Difference between estimate in this cell and corresponding estimate for 1993 is statistically significant at the .01 level.
Table from SAMHSA, Office of Applied Studies, National Household Survey on Drug Abuse.

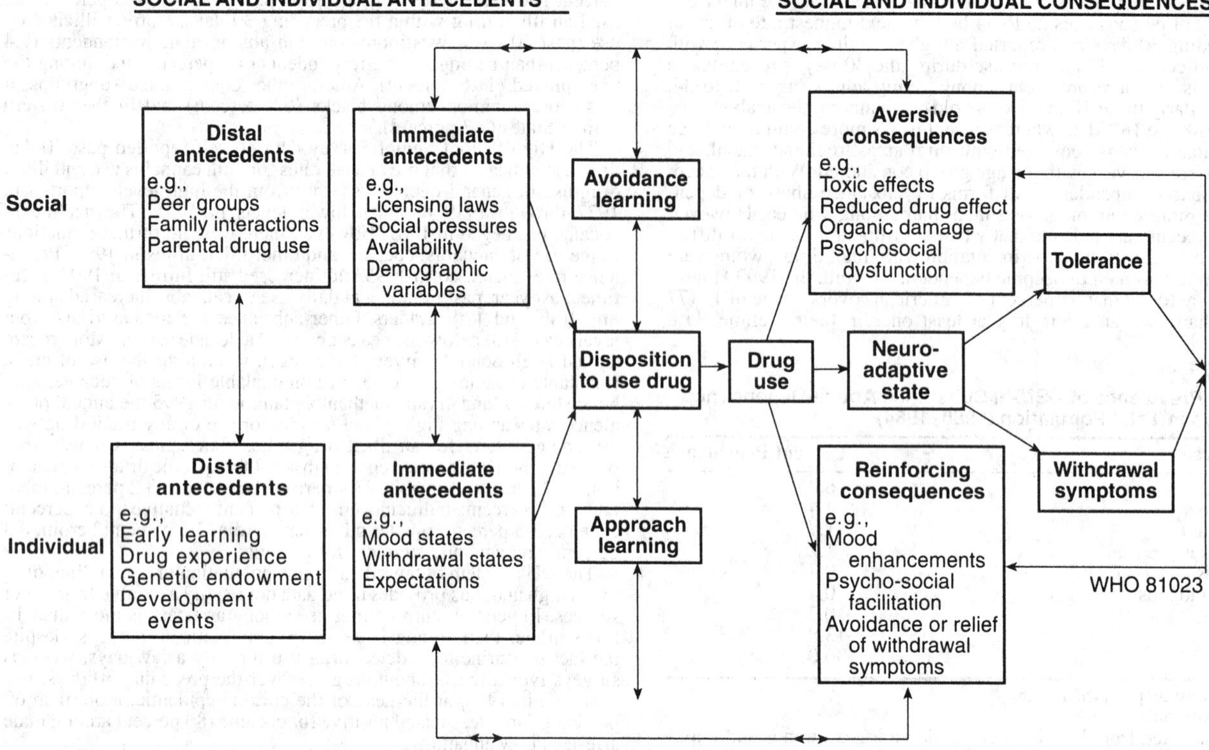

FIGURE 13.1-1 *WHO schematic model of drug use and dependence. (Figure from G Edwards, A Arif, R Hodgson: Nomenclature and classification of drug- and alcohol-related problems. A WHO memorandum. Bull WHO 99: 225, 1981. Used with permission.)*

different populations. Cannabis use, which had been endemic among certain minority groups and some musicians, began to increase in the 1960s, especially among the young, and then spread to other segments of the population. At its peak in 1978-1979, 10 percent of high school seniors were using cannabis on a daily basis, but daily use declined to 5 percent by 1984 and then to 2 percent by 1991. A similar decrease in active users was reflected in the Household Survey. An epidemic of heroin use also began in the early 1960s and peaked from 1969 to 1971. The population of active heroin users reached its highest levels in the early 1970s, but periodic upsurges have occurred as supplies became more available, law enforcement activity waxed and waned, and relapse rates increased among former users. In 1977 the United States government estimated that there were 500,000 opioid abusers and dependent users, and more recently revised the estimate to 700,000. In general, the heroin-using population is an aging one, with a high and still growing prevalence of HIV in some areas. The 1993 Household Survey estimated that about 2.3 million persons had tried heroin at least once and that 245,000 had used it in the past year. However, it is believed that a large percentage of heroin users are outside of the population interviewed by the survey. Since DUF data show that 5 to 15 percent of male arrestees test positive for opioids, the current heroin-using population probably exceeds 700,000.

The cocaine epidemic began in the 1970s and reached its peak around 1985, when it was estimated that 5.8 million persons in the United States (2.9 percent of the population) had used cocaine in the month prior to survey. The epidemic seems to have passed its peak in most segments of society, with current (past-30-days) use rates now at about 0.6 percent. The 1993 Household Survey estimated that about 476,000 persons in the United States had used cocaine weekly or almost weekly at some time in the past year, a figure that, while lower in absolute terms than in 1985, was not viewed as significantly lower. Given the high rate of use among those involved with the criminal justice system, the Household Survey probably underestimates heavy use.

ETIOLOGY

The model of drug dependence from which the DSM-III-R, DSM-IV, and ICD-10 criteria were derived conceptualizes dependence as an aspect of a process in which multiple interacting factors influence drug-using behavior, which may lead to loss of flexibility with respect to decisions about the use of a given drug. Although the actions of a given drug are critical in the process, it is not assumed that all persons who become dependent on the same drug experience its effects in the same way or are motivated by the same set of factors. Furthermore, it is postulated that, at different stages of the process, different factors may be more or less important. Thus, drug availability, social acceptability, and peer pressures may be the major determinants of initial experimentation with a drug, but other factors, such as personality and individual biology, probably are more important in how the effects of a given drug are perceived. Still other factors, including the particular actions of the drug, may be dominant in determining whether drug use will progress to drug dependence, whereas still others may be critical in the likelihood that drug use will lead to adverse effects, or for determining the likelihood of successful recovery from dependence.

Figure 13.1-1 (developed by an ADAMHA-funded WHO collaborative working group) illustrates the way in which various factors might interact in the development of drug dependence. The central element shown is the drug-using behavior itself. The decision to use a drug is influenced by immediate social and psychological situations, as well as by the person's more remote history. The use of the drug initiates a sequence of consequences that can be rewarding or aversive, and which, through a process of learning, can result in a greater or lesser likelihood that the drug-using behavior will be repeated. For some drugs, use also initiates the biological processes associated with tolerance and physical dependence. In turn, tolerance can reduce some of the adverse effects of the drug, permitting or requiring the use of larger doses, which then can accelerate or intensify the development of physical dependence. Above a certain threshold, physical dependence generally acts as a distinct and recurrent motive for further drug use.

For simplicity Figure 13.1-1 shows only drug use as initiating that chain of consequences, but the choices a person makes over and over again are more complex. The decision is whether to use one drug or another or to engage in some behavior that does not involve drug use. Each of those decisions can initiate positive and negative consequences. Changes in the costs and consequences of alternative behaviors can also influence what appears to be compulsive use of a pharmacological agent.

SOCIAL AND ENVIRONMENTAL FACTORS Cultural factors, social attitudes, peer behaviors, laws, and drug cost and availability all influence initial experimentation with substances, including alcohol and tobacco. In the case of initial use of more socially disapproved drugs, such as cocaine and opioids, those factors are still important, but personality factors assume a more important role. Social and environmental factors also influence continued use, although individual vulnerability and psychopathology are important determinants of the development of abuse and dependence. In general, the use of the less socially disapproved substances (alcohol, tobacco, and cannabis) precedes the use of opioids and cocaine, and those antecedent substances are sometimes referred to as gateway drugs.

There is substantial evidence that the consumption of alcohol and tobacco in a population can be altered by changes in their price and availability. When the availability of alcohol is increased by increasing the number of outlets where it can be sold or the hours of sale are lengthened, consumption tends to rise. When the cost of either alcohol or tobacco is increased in relation to disposable income (for example, by increased taxes), consumption falls. Those factors influence the behavior even of dependent persons, although perhaps not to the same degree as for those who are not dependent. Availability can be altered independently of cost, and alterations can be limited to selected populations, as when alcohol sales are prohibited to those under the age of 21.

Social, cultural, and economic factors do not always operate synergistically but may sometimes influence consumption in opposite directions. For example, in the late 1980s increased public awareness of how alcohol use adversely affects health resulted in a decline in its consumption. That decline occurred even though alcohol was more freely available, its cost relative to income remained constant or actually decreased, and social pressures against women drinking (unless pregnant) also decreased.

Illicit drugs Social and cultural factors, including beliefs about the effects of a drug, are frequently more powerful influences on drug-use patterns than are the laws that supposedly reflect such factors. For example, cannabis use increased among high school students from the early 1970s to 1979. It then fell steadily over the next decade, although its use and possession remained illegal throughout the 18-year period and there was no indication that its cost had increased or that it became less available. Some experts believe the decline in use was linked to changing perceptions about the toxic effects of cannabis on health. Similarly, cocaine use increased in the late 1970s, despite the very high costs and risks of criminal penalties. Following several well-publicized deaths from cocaine in the mid-1980s, however, cocaine use fell among high school seniors, as well as in the general population, even as the cost of the drug declined.

Social and cultural factors profoundly influence the availability of illicit drugs, which, in turn, influences which groups in a society are most likely to become users. Currently, illicit opioids and cocaine are more available in the inner cities of large urban areas than in other parts of the country. Such availability not only influences initial and continued use but also influences relapse rates among those who seek treatment but must live in high-availability areas. When a significant number of users of illicit drugs live in one area, a subculture supportive of experimentation and continued use evolves. Many of the areas in which illicit drugs are readily available are also characterized by a high crime rate, high unemployment, and demoralized school systems—all of which serve to reduce the sense of hope and sense of self-esteem that are associated with resistance to use and good prognosis once dependence develops. Those factors, along with family factors, may account for the disproportionately high rates of heroin and cocaine dependence among African-American and Hispanic minorities residing in poor urban areas and the persistence of cocaine use among those groups at a time when such use is decreasing at higher socioeconomic levels. Social and educational factors also affect the likelihood for successful recovery from drug dependence, in that those who can find satisfying alternatives are more likely to be able to abstain from drug use.

Vietnam The experience of United States service personnel who used heroin in Vietnam provided a unique natural experiment in which the influences of availability, vulnerability, and social norms could be observed. During the period 1970 to 1972, high-grade heroin at very low cost was readily available to young persons separated from their families and usual social norms. Among Army enlisted personnel, about half of those who tried heroin became dependent (at least they developed withdrawal symptoms when they attempted to stop using heroin). Of those who used heroin at least five times, 73 percent became dependent. The background factors that were predictors of heroin use in the general civilian population—early deviant behavior, such as fighting, drunkenness, arrest, and school expulsion—also predicted drug use in Vietnam, but those were not the factors that best predicted relapse after the soldiers returned to the United States. Relapse was related to being white, being older, and having parents who had criminal histories or were alcoholic.

Availability and health professionals The important role of availability is also illustrated by the repeated observation that physicians, dentists, and nurses have far higher rates of dependence on controlled substances, such as opioids, stimulants, and sedatives, than have other professionals of comparable educational achievement (for example, accountants or lawyers) who do not have such easy access to the drugs. Compared with controls, physicians appear to be four to five times as likely to take sedatives and minor tranquilizers without supervision by a professional other than themselves. Yet even in that situation other factors play a role. Those physicians who had unhappy childhoods are more likely to self-prescribe than are those who are healthier psychologically.

DRUGS AS REINFORCERS The belief that persons take drugs because of the subjective effects the drugs produce can be traced to antiquity. It is a common experience that different drugs produce distinctive subjective states, and there is extensive laboratory evidence that persons with experience can distinguish one drug class from another and can even rank different classes and doses based on the degree to which they like the effects. Yet the hold that drugs can eventually exert on a user's behavior is not entirely a function of its initial likeable or euphorigenic actions. For example, the effects of cocaine are typically described as powerfully euphorigenic, producing increased self-esteem, alertness, energy, and well-being; the effects of nicotine are more subtle, producing some mixture of alerting and relaxing; and the subjective effects of alcohol are more likely to be described as relaxing, are more variable, and appear to be more dependent on personality. Despite those differences, dependence (or addiction) can occur with each.

Almost all of the drugs that are used for their subjective

effects and are associated with the development of dependence induce some degree of tolerance. In some cases the tolerance to the toxic and aversive effects is more pronounced than is the tolerance to the reinforcing and mood-elevating effects. For example, most opioid users quickly develop tolerance to opioid-induced nausea and vomiting. In some cases that allows users to increase the dose and thus to experience greater euphoric effects. Conversely, those who continue to experience aversive drug effects (such as severe flushing with alcohol) may be less likely to persist in using the drug and are at lower risk for developing dependence. Tolerant opioid users do not continue to self-administer opioids solely to prevent the highly aversive withdrawal phenomena. Interviews with heroin users have indicated that, despite some tolerance to many of the drug's effects, they continue to experience a brief euphoric effect immediately after an injection.

With a few notable exceptions, animals in experimental situations will self-administer most of the drugs that humans tend to use and abuse. Included among the drugs are μ and δ opioid agonists, cocaine, amphetamine and amphetaminelike agents, alcohol, barbiturates, many benzodiazepines, a number of volatile gases and vapors (for example, nitrous oxide and ether), and PCP. Nicotine is self-administered under more specialized conditions; cannabinoid self-administration has been difficult to demonstrate; and LSD-like drugs are not generally found to be reinforcing.

Neural systems For opioids, and probably for other drugs as well, the neural systems involved in drug reinforcement and self-administration are distinct from those responsible for some of the other actions (for example, opioid-induced analgesia), as well as from those that mediate the more visible signs of the withdrawal syndrome characteristic for the drug class. The pathways critical for the reinforcing actions of a number of dependence-producing drugs, such as opioids and cocaine, have their origins in dopaminergic neurons with cell bodies in the ventral tegmental area and processes innervating the nucleus accumbens, which, in turn, projects axons to the ventral pallidum, which then projects to the frontal cortex and other nuclei. The nucleus accumbens is a particularly important site. Dopamine release in the nucleus accumbens may be critical for the reinforcing effects of cocaine, but not for the reinforcing actions of opioids; destruction of dopaminergic terminals in the nucleus accumbens produces extinction of the self-administration of cocaine, but not of heroin. There is some evidence that such drugs as nicotine and cannabinoids also activate dopaminergic pathways linked to the nucleus accumbens. Some workers have proposed that all reinforcement, including that associated with food reward and sex, is critically dependent on the dopaminergic circuit.

Threshold changes In rats cocaine, amphetamines, opioids, and some barbiturates and benzodiazepines lower the threshold for electrical self-stimulation of the brain. The opioid antagonist naloxone (Narcan) not only blocks the threshold-lowering action of opioids, but also attenuates that of cocaine and amphetamine, suggesting that endogenous opioid systems interact with dopaminergic systems in producing reinforcing effects of those stimulants. Furthermore, opioids and amphetamine are synergistic in lowering self-stimulation thresholds in rats and also in producing euphoria in humans. In contrast to the tolerance that develops to some actions of self-administered drugs (for example, analgesic actions of opioids), very little tolerance develops to the threshold-lowering effects of reinforcing drugs.

Drugs can also be reinforcers by terminating aversive states, and some of those actions do not depend on dopaminergic systems. However, several workers argue that compulsive drug use can be explained on the basis of the positive reinforcing effects of drugs without any need to invoke alleviation of withdrawal distress or any obvious source of antecedent pain or dysphoria. Furthermore, those workers argue, craving is primarily associated not with cues that evoke withdrawal but with those that evoke memories of positive reinforcement (euphoria).

Importance of context Reinforcing properties do not reside solely in the drug or in the stimulus. Depending on the previous history of the organism and on the reinforcement schedule, animals will continue to press a lever to self-administer electrical shocks of the same intensity as those they previously had worked hard to avoid. In such an experimental model the high-level shock is a reinforcer in that it maintains the behavior that leads to the shock.

It is not clear whether the neural pathways critical for reinforcement in animals are precisely those that underlie repeated drug use in humans. However, work at several laboratories studying the effects of drugs on brain glucose metabolism and cerebral blood flow in human post-addict volunteers have found that there are striking similarities in the way that different drugs that induce euphoria alter brain function. When such subjects experience euphoria induced by either opioids or cocaine, it is correlated with a decrease in brain glucose metabolism, especially in cortical areas.

LEARNING AND CONDITIONING Drug use, whether occasional or compulsive, can be viewed as behavior maintained by its consequences. Any event that strengthens an antecedent behavior pattern can be considered a reinforcer of that behavior. In that sense certain drugs are positive reinforcers of drug-taking behavior. Drugs can also reinforce antecedent behaviors by terminating some noxious or aversive state, such as pain, anxiety, or depression. In some social situations the use of the drug, quite apart from its pharmacological effects, can be reinforcing if it results in special status or the approval of friends. Social reinforcement can maintain drug use until the effects of primary reinforcement or reinforcement by alleviation of withdrawal symptoms come into play. With each use of the drug, rapid positive reinforcement occurs, either as a result of the rush (the drug-induced euphoria), alleviation of disturbed affects, alleviation of withdrawal symptoms, or any combination of those effects. With short-acting substances, such as heroin, cocaine, nicotine, and alcohol, such reinforcement occurs several times a day, day in and day out, creating powerfully reinforced habit patterns. Eventually, the paraphernalia (needles, bottles, cigarette packs) and behaviors associated with substance use can become secondary reinforcers, as well as cues signaling availability of the substance, and in their presence craving or a desire to experience the effects increases. With socially acceptable substances, such as tobacco, use becomes so woven into the matrix of daily functioning that some users are reminded of the substances when performing ordinary tasks.

Classical conditioning In addition to the operant reinforcement of drug-using and drug-seeking behaviors, other learning mechanisms probably play a role in dependence and relapse. Opioid and alcohol withdrawal phenomena can be conditioned, in the Pavlovian or classic sense, to environmental or interoceptive stimuli. Such conditioning has been demonstrated in both laboratory animals and abstinent and methadone-dependent human volunteers. For a long time following withdrawal (from opioids, alcohol, nicotine, or alcohol), the addict, when exposed to environmental stimuli previously linked with substance use or withdrawal, may experience conditioned withdrawal, conditioned craving, or both. The increased feelings of craving are not necessarily accompanied by symptoms of withdrawal. The conditions that elicit the most intense craving are those conditions associated with the availability or use of the substance, such as watching someone else use heroin, lighting a cigarette, or being offered some drug by a friend, rather than conditions associated with withdrawal. Some workers now believe that the cues that induce memories of drug-induced euphoria are more important for stimulating craving and in predisposing to relapse than either protracted or conditioned withdrawal. Those learning and conditioning phenomena can be superimposed on any preexisting psychopathology, but preexisting difficulties are not required for the development of powerfully reinforced substance-seeking behavior.

WITHDRAWAL SYNDROMES AND NEGATIVE REINFORCEMENT Although positive reinforcement is now viewed as a dominant etiological factor in the genesis of cocaine, amphetamine, and, in some cases, opioid dependence, aversive withdrawal phenomena and negative reinforcement may be equally, if not more, important influences for a number of other drugs. One example of this is seen in most people who become dependent on benzodiazepines taken in the course of treatment for anxiety syndromes. When drug use is interrupted, for some there seems to be a reappearance of the original symptoms; for others there are new distressing symptoms indicative of withdrawal. The use of benzodiazepines alleviates both kinds of aversive states. In either case the drug is acting as a negative reinforcer in perpetuating drug use. Benzodiazepines can induce euphoria in alcoholic patients or in persons with histories of sedative abuse, but they are not reliable euphorigenic agents in normal, nonalcoholic persons. There are instances when benzodiazepine anxiolytics induce euphoria in nondependent, nonanxious persons, but such instances are rare relative to the number of those who experience only relief of anxiety.

One way to determine the contribution of negative reinforcement to the motivation to continue substance use or to relapse after withdrawal is to introduce agents that can modify withdrawal syndromes or aversive states. There is now abundant evidence that, when psychological interventions are held constant, noninhaled nicotine (delivered by transdermal patches or nicotine gum) significantly increases the probability that smokers trying to quit will be successful. Neither nicotine gum nor transdermal patches produce positive reinforcing effects, but they do alleviate aspects of the nicotine withdrawal syndrome. Thus, it is reasonable to infer that, although the symptoms may not be life threatening, nicotine withdrawal plays a significant role in continued smoking and relapse. However, there is evidence that, for some, nicotine acts to control negative affect other than that usually associated with withdrawal. Persons with histories of major mood disorder may experience symptoms of depression when they try to stop smoking, and those symptoms are suppressed by returning to smoking. Heroin addicts treated with oral methadone or buprenorphine (Buprenex) experience a reduction in opioid withdrawal symptoms but little or no euphoric effects from those agents. Yet, such treatment dramatically reduces self-administration of heroin. Such findings support the view that acute and protracted opioid withdrawal (or opioid suppression of aversive affects) is an important factor in the perpetuation of heroin use and relapse after withdrawal.

Conditioned withdrawal In addition to the direct contribution of withdrawal phenomena to the perpetuation of drug use are the indirect effects exerted through learning mechanisms. The regular recurrence of withdrawal-induced aversive states provides ample opportunity for those states to become linked through learning to environmental cues and other mood states, and the rapid relief of withdrawal by drug use results in repeated reinforcement of drug-taking behavior. Long after there are measurable manifestations of acute withdrawal, certain moods or environmental cues can evoke components of the original withdrawal state, along with urges to use the drug again.

It is not clear how long withdrawal phenomena continue to contribute to risk of relapse. There is substantial evidence that for alcohol, opioids, and certain sedatives, a protracted withdrawal syndrome period with subtle disturbances of mood, sleep, and cognition persists for many weeks or months after the acute syndrome subsides.

No easy distinction In most clinical situations, even among users of highly euphoric illicit drugs, the distinction between positive and negative reinforcing effects does not exist. The intravenous heroin user may experience, simultaneously or sequentially, relief of withdrawal, a sense of ease, and alleviation of anger and depression, as well as a sudden rush of intense pleasure. The heavy smoker who inhales deeply on the first morning cigarette probably experiences more than relief of nicotine withdrawal.

BIOLOGICAL FACTORS-VULNERABILITY The children of alcoholic parents are at higher risk for developing alcoholism and drug dependence than are children of nonalcoholic parents. The increased risk is probably due partly to environmental factors (parental modeling, neglect, early child abuse), but there is also evidence that genetic factors are important. The evidence for genetic factors in the vulnerability to alcoholism is derived most convincingly from twin and adoption studies. Several studies of twins have found a higher concordance rate for alcoholism among identical twins than among fraternal twins. Although it is generally believed that identical twins may have more social contact than do fraternal twins, when the effects of environmental factors are adjusted statistically, genetic factors are still found to influence significantly drinking patterns (although not drinking to unconsciousness). Among female twins, concordance of drinking was not influenced by social contact but was powerfully modified by marital status. Genetic factors accounted for far more of the similarities in drinking patterns in unmarried twins than in married twins.

Adoption studies have shown higher rates of alcoholism among sons of alcoholic fathers who were adopted soon after birth as compared with the adopted offspring of fathers who were not alcoholic. Those studies also point toward subtypes of alcoholism among men, one of which results in a later onset of the disorder that is far more sensitive to environmental factors, and another that is associated with criminality in the biological fathers, in which genetic factors seem to account for more of the increased vulnerability. While not contesting the notion that genetics contributes to vulnerability to alcoholism, the hypothesis that there are two genetically distinct types of alcoholism (Type I and Type II) has been criticized on the grounds that it is essentially a relabeling of the older primary-secondary categorization. In the latter alcohol-dependent persons who do not have antisocial personality disorder are designated as having primary alcoholism; those who first exhibit antisocial personality disorder and later develop alcoholism are designated antisocial personality disorder with secondary alcoholism.

Alcoholism can also develop in the absence of detectable family history, and as many as one third of alcohol-dependent persons have no family history of the disorder. Men are more likely to develop alcoholism than are women (fourfold to fivefold in the United States). That is true across every culture studied, probably reflecting, in part, social sanctions on drug use and deviant behavior by women. But it is also postulated that women are less likely to drink heavily because they are less tolerant to alcohol. Women who do drink heavily run the same risk of developing alcoholism as do men who drink heavily, and women who use illicit drugs are as likely to develop dependence as are men who use such drugs.

Since alcohol-dependent persons are at far higher risk for developing other varieties of drug dependence, and drug-dependent persons also are at high risk for alcoholism and often have a family history of alcoholism, it seems reasonable to infer that the genetic factors that increase vulnerability to the disorder may not be specific for alcohol but may represent a more general vulnerability.

While specific genes have not been firmly identified, some studies have reported that a particular allele (A_1) of the gene that codes for the dopamine type 2 (D_2) receptor is more common among persons with histories of severe alcoholism than among controls. A similar higher prevalence of the A_1 allele has been reported among persons with cocaine dependence. Not all studies have confirmed those findings on specific genetic differences, and one meta-analysis has concluded that the initial studies that did find differences overlooked the wide ethnic variability in the occurrence of A_1 allele and did not control for ethnic differences among alcoholic persons and cocaine addicts and normal controls. Most researchers believe that no single gene will be found to account for the complexities of inherited risk for drug and alcohol dependence.

Some genetic factors may act not to increase vulnerability to alcoholism but to decrease it. A genetically determined variation in the activity of enzymes that metabolize alcohol, alcohol dehydrogenase (ADH), and aldehyde dehydrogenase (ALDH), common among some Asian groups, results in high levels of acetaldehyde in response to alcohol ingestion. The effect is to cause alcohol flush reaction and to exert some deterrent effect on alcohol ingestion. Alcoholism is lower among many Asian groups than among whites. Further, Asians with alcoholism are much less likely to have the inactive form of the ALDH enzyme. There is little direct evidence of any specific biological vulnerability to opioid dependence. It has been postulated that some antecedent metabolic deficiency, such as endogenous opioid dysregulation, may increase vulnerability to becoming opioid dependent, but no evidence for such defects has yet emerged.

Biological and behavioral differences Studies exploring how persons with and without family histories of alcoholism might differ have involved measures of personality, drug-use and alcohol-use patterns, psychomotor and cognitive performance, electrical activity of the brain, endocrine responses to challenges with alcohol and other substances, as well as measures of receptor numbers and affinities and enzyme activities (for example, monoamine oxidase) in peripheral tissues (for example, blood platelets and lymphocytes). One finding that has been replicated is that, under some conditions, the electrical response of the brain that occurs about 300 milliseconds after a sensory stimulus (the P_3 wave) is smaller in amplitude in nondrinking sons of alcoholic fathers than in control subjects without family histories of alcoholism. The decrease in amplitude of that wave is believed to reflect a decreased capacity to recognize and interpret complex environmental stimuli. Most studies have not found differences in intelligence among subjects with and without family histories of alcoholism. However, the results are conflicting with respect to personality studies, with some finding no differences and others finding greater impulsivity, adventurousness, and sensation seeking among those with a positive family history. Studies of the drinking patterns of adolescent and young adult sons of alcoholic persons also have not yielded consistent results, with some, but not all, studies showing that sons of alcoholic parents are heavier drinkers. Other studies have compared the subjective, motoric, and endocrine responses of young men with and without family histories of alcoholism following challenge exposures to alcohol and other potentially euphoriant drugs (such as benzodiazepines). Sons of alcoholic fathers seem to be more tolerant to the intoxicating effects of modest doses of alcohol, and in some, but not all, studies, higher doses of alcohol produced smaller changes in prolactin and cortisol levels. Furthermore, in one study sons of alcoholic parents who had the smaller responses to test doses of alcohol at the age of 20 (more tolerant) were fourfold more likely to have developed alcoholism when interviewed 10 years later.

The results of studies using benzodiazepine challenges are also not consistent, one showing a greater euphoric response to alprazolam (Xanax) in sons of alcoholic parents, and another showing no difference between positive family history and negative family history groups after a dose of diazepam. One factor that may account for the inconsistency in the findings is that there appear to be at least two subtypes of alcoholism vulnerability, one characterized by early onset, a high degree of heritability, and alcoholism and criminality in the biological fathers, and the other by later onset, less severity, and alcoholism that manifests itself only when the rearing environment is conducive to heavy drinking. As noted earlier, subjects exhibiting the former pattern seem more likely to exhibit characteristics of antisocial personality disorder as well as alcoholism.

A number of studies have shown that conduct disorder and early childhood aggression are associated with a substantial increase in the likelihood of early involvement with illicit drug use and development of dependence on alcohol and illicit drugs. Recent work suggests that, in addition to having a family history of addictive disorder, antisocial personality disorder represents an independent additional risk factor for addictive disorders. The effects of those risk factors appear to be additive rather than synergistic. It seems possible that in some of the studies of children and young people at high risk for later drug dependence, findings of electrophysiological differences, cognitive deficits, and personality differences may be mediated or associated with the presence of conduct disorder-antisocial personality disorder rather than of family history of alcoholism per se. Thus it may not be enough in such studies to characterize subjects as having family histories positive or negative for alcoholism; it may also be important to characterize the subjects in terms of conduct disorder and antisocial personality disorder.

Animal studies The likelihood that genetics is a factor in drug dependence and its adverse consequences is also supported by research with animals. Strains of laboratory rats have been identified or bred that differ substantially in their preference for alcohol; preferring strains consume to intoxicating levels and develop tolerance more rapidly. The evidence indicates that it is the effect rather than the taste that is preferred. Alcohol causes increased physical activity in preferring rats rather than the sedation that is seen in nonpreferring rats. The alcohol-preferring rats have lower brain levels of serotonin, and their consumption of alcohol is reduced by serotonin-specific reuptake inhibitors, an effect that has also been seen when serotonin reuptake inhibitor antagonists are administered to alcoholic persons. But as is the case with humans with no family history of alcoholism, when environmental factors are changed, even the initially nonpreferring rats will consume as much as the alcohol-preferring strain. Rat and mouse strains also have been identified or selectively bred that exhibit wide differences in their preference for opiates, amphetamines, and cocaine. In one set of experiments comparing two strains of rats, the strain that preferred alcohol also exhibited a greater preference for opioids. In rodent models genetic factors also mediate sensitivity to the toxic and reinforcing effects of cocaine.

PSYCHODYNAMIC FACTORS AND PSYCHOPATHOLOGY Early psychoanalytic formulations postulated that drug users, in general, suffered from either a special form of affective dysregulation—tense depression—that was alleviated by drug use or from a disorder of impulse control in which the search for pleasure was dominant. More recent formulations postulate ego defects, which are manifest in the addict's inability to manage painful affects (guilt, anger, anxiety) and to avoid preventable medical, legal, and financial problems. The newer formulations postulating ego defects are, to some degree, the older formulations with a modest change in terminology that gives greater weight to the inability to cope with painful affects than to the intensity or abnormality of the affects per se. It is postulated that, pharmacologically and symbolically, some substances aid the ego in controlling those affects and that their use can be viewed as a form of self-medication. For example, it has been suggested that opioids help users control painful anger and that nicotine may help some cigarette smokers control symptoms of depression. Although it is conceded that some of those observations may reflect problems produced by long-term use, the psychodynamic perspective is that the psychopathology is the underlying motivation for initial use, dependent use, and relapse after a period of abstinence. However, traditions of passivity and uncovering techniques derived from the psychoanalysis of neurosis are poorly suited to the treatment of most drug addicts. Further, some addicts appear to have great difficulty differentiating and describing what they feel, a difficulty that has been called alexithymia (that is, no words for feelings).

COMORBIDITY (DUAL DIAGNOSIS) Comorbidity (also known as dual diagnosis) is the diagnosis of two or more psychiatric disorders in a single patient. A high prevalence of additional psychiatric disorders among persons seeking treatment for alcohol, cocaine, or opioid dependence has been repeatedly confirmed. Although opioid, cocaine, and alcohol abusers who have current psychiatric problems are more likely to seek treatment, it should not be assumed that those who do not seek treatment are free of comorbid psychiatric problems; such persons may still be able to deny the impact that drug use is having on their lives.

The ECA study, in which more than 20,000 persons in five communities in the United States were interviewed, showed that, even among representative samples of the population, those who meet the criteria for alcohol or drug abuse and dependence (excluding tobacco dependence) are far more likely to meet the criteria for other psychiatric disorders also. In that sample 76 percent of the men and 65 percent of the women who met the criteria for drug abuse or dependence received at least one additional diagnosis. Table 13.1-13 shows that about 60 percent of the men and 30 percent of the women with drug dependence also met the DSM-III criteria for alcohol abuse-dependence, the most common additional diagnosis. Among men the next most common diagnoses were antisocial personality disorder, phobic disorders, and major depression; among women the most common diagnoses after alcohol abuse-dependence were phobic disorders, major depression, and dysthymia. Table 13.1-13 also shows prevalence ratios: the prevalence of a psychiatric disorder among persons with drug abuse-dependence as compared with those without that diagnosis. While every listed psychiatric diagnosis is more common among those who met the criteria for drug dependence, notable increases in odds ratios were seen for alcoholism, antisocial personality disorder, and mania among women, and for mania, antisocial personality disorder, and dysthymia among men. A substantially higher risk for schizophrenia in those with drug abuse-dependence has been found for both men and women.

In general, the probability of comorbidity is higher for those with a lifetime diagnosis of an opioid or cocaine disorder than for those with a diagnosis of cannabis abuse. The ECA findings on comorbidity, which have been confirmed by other studies in smaller community samples and by the NCS, describe rather than explain comorbidity. They do not shed much light on the question of whether (or in which cases) drug use is, at least initially, an adaptive effort at self-medication or whether those with a variety of psychiatric disorders are less able to cope with the effects of substance use and so are more likely to become dependent. It is not clear whether psychiatric disorders increase the vulnerability to drug abuse-dependence, whether drug abuse-dependence contributes to the risk of developing other psychiatric disorders, or whether some common factor contributes to both. In some cases, however, such as the link between cocaine use and panic disorder, the cocaine use does seem to play a causal role.

One way to think about the relation between drug use and other disorders is to examine the odds ratio for developing a drug or alcohol problem given another psychiatric diagnosis. Based on ECA data, 84 percent of persons with antisocial personality disorder also met the criteria for a lifetime diagnosis of some variety of substance abuse-dependence, including alcohol (odds ratio, 29.6); 42 percent also received a diagnosis of drug abuse-dependence other than alcohol (odds ratio, 13.4). For those with any bipolar disorder, 56 percent received a lifetime diagnosis of some form of substance abuse-dependence, including alcohol (odds ratio, 6.6), whereas 33.6 percent received a diagnosis of drug abuse-dependence, excluding alcohol (odds ratio, 8.3). Noteworthy in the ECA study is the very high prevalence (47 percent) of substance abuse-dependence among those meeting the criteria for schizophrenia (odds ratio, 4.6), with about 27.5 percent meeting the criteria for drug abuse-dependence other than alcohol (odds ratio, 6.2).

Among prisoners the comorbidity rates were even higher than in the general population, with addictive disorders found in 92 percent of prisoners with schizophrenia, 90 percent in those with antisocial personality disorder, and 89 percent in those with bipolar disorders. Among persons with mental disorders seeking treatment in specialty settings, 20 percent have a current substance-abuse-disorder diagnosis.

TABLE 13.1-13
Prevalence of Other Psychiatric Disorders Among Men and Women in Total Population Diagnosed as Having Drug Abuse-Dependence Disorders

Specific Additional Diagnoses Among Cases of Drug Abuse-Dependence	Prevalence of Other Disorders		Prevalence Ratios*	
	Men %	Women %	Men %	Women %
Alcohol abuse-dependence	59.8	29.7	2.9	9.0
Antisocial personality disorder	22.2	9.8	7.3	26.6
Phobic disorders	19.2	28.5	2.4	1.9
Major depression	14.0	28.0	4.9	3.6
Dysthymia	8.8	11.8	5.1	3.1
Obsessive-compulsive disorder	6.1	9.4	3.6	3.5
Mania	4.6	6.7	11.3	11.1
Schizophrenia	4.6	8.0	6.2	6.4
Panic disorder	3.2	5.6	4.1	6.4
Any diagnosis	75.6	64.7	2.5	2.5

*Prevalence ratios are derived by dividing diagnosis among drug abuse-dependence cases by prevalence among those with no drug diagnosis.

Table adapted from D B Kandel: Epidemiological trends and implications for understanding the nature of addiction. In *Addictive Studies*, P O'Brien, J H Jaffe, editors, Research Publications: Association for Research in Nervous and Mental Disease, vol 70, p 23. Raven, New York, 1992.

The causal relations among those disorders are complex. There is evidence that, depending on the particular agent, substance abuse can cause or increase the risk for depressive disorder, panic disorder, and schizophrenia, and because some psychiatric disorders, such as mood disorder and antisocial personality disorder, often antedate the development of substance use, those disorders can be viewed as causal or risk factors for substance abuse-dependence. In addition to serving as risk factors for the development of drug-alcohol problems, psychopathology may also serve to modify the course and presentation of the disorder, access to treatment, and the response to treatment. The findings from the NCS largely confirm the observations of the ECA study that those with substance use disorders are substantially more likely to experience other mental disorders and that those with other mental disorders are far more likely to develop substance use disorders. The NCS also underscored the finding that while 52 percent of respondents never experienced any DSM-III-R disorder and 21 percent had one such disorder, 13 percent had two disorders and 14 percent had three or more disorders. In short, 79 percent of those with any disorder had more than one. Furthermore, the 12-month prevalence of a disorder was more likely among those with more than one disorder: 59 percent of all of 12-month disorders occurred in the 14 percent with a lifetime history of three or more disorders, and 89 percent of severe 12-month disorders occurred in the same group.

FAMILY DYNAMICS One family member's substance abuse is often influenced by substance-using behaviors of others in the family and those complex interrelationships can profoundly affect their lives. An understanding of the relationships among substance-using patients and their families is relevant for understanding the etiology of substance dependence and its treatment and for helping other family members to cope with problems associated with the substance-using behavior.

More has been written about the families of alcohol-dependent persons and heroin users than about families affected by users of other drugs. Similarities between the family dynamics in those two prototypical dependencies have led researchers and clinicians to assume that certain general principles apply to all varieties of substance dependence. The observation that alcoholism is commonly found in the families of those seeking treatment for other types of dependence, that alcohol-dependent persons are often dependent on other substances as well, and that those addicted to illicit drugs are often alcoholic suggests that there are common features among families with an addicted member. However, there are not much data to suggest that the families of those dependent on tobacco or benzodiazepines are as dysfunctional as those affected by alcohol, opioids, or cocaine.

It is not always clear to what degree one family member's behavior is the cause of the substance-using behavior of another or is primarily a response to that behavior. Some writers emphasize that the addiction is a symptom that provides a displaced focus for conflict among other family members and that the user (the designated patient) may be playing a role in maintaining the homeostasis of a dysfunctional family. At the same time, it is important to recognize that addiction often arises in families in which one or both parents (and sometimes grandparents) have drug or alcohol problems and other psychopathology. Some characteristics commonly observed both in families of persons who are alcohol-dependent and of those addicted to illicit drugs are: multigenerational drug dependence; a high incidence of parental loss through divorce, death, abandonment, or incarceration; overprotection or overcontrol by one parent (usually the mother), whose life is inordinately dependent on the behavior of the addicted offspring (symbiotic relationships); distant, cold, disengaged, or absent father (when the father is alive); defiant drug-using child, who appears to be engaged with peers but remains unusually dependent on families well into adult life (pseudo-independence). The actual family dynamics are difficult to characterize because the family members' self-reports about their relationships do not reliably correspond to what outsiders observe. Such families typically do not describe themselves in the way that family therapists see them. Some workers have proposed that unresolved family grief plays a role in the genesis of drug addiction in a family member and that such families cannot deal effectively with separation because of previous losses. Despite the pathological interdependence between the addict and other family members, the addict is often described as passive, dependent, withdrawn, and unable to form close relationships.

Despite all the apparent pathology found in families, in many instances the family brings the substance user into treatment, and the patient often believes that it is the family that is most likely to be helpful in recovery. Furthermore, clinicians now generally believe that involving families in treatment is an important, if not essential, element in effective intervention. One aspect of treating the family is dealing with the tendency of some members to shield the patient from the consequences of his or her substance use, a behavior usually labeled by clinicians as enabling, but usually experienced by the family member as loving, supporting, accepting, and protecting.

Codependence The terms "coaddiction," "coalcoholism," or, more commonly, "codependency" or "codependence" have recently come into vogue to designate the behavioral patterns of family members who have been significantly affected by another family member's substance use or addiction. The terms have been used in various ways, and there are no established criteria for codependence. Nevertheless, some professionals (and not just those treating addictive behaviors) have developed specialized programs designed to treat coaddiction or codependence, a concept that some writers have expanded far beyond its origins to encompass any personality disorder that involves difficulty in expressing emotions. However, many have criticized the expanded concept of codependence as a largely invalid notion based solely on anecdote. The following summary of some characteristics frequently described as aspects of codependence is not meant to imply the validity of a unitary syndrome.

ENABLING Enabling was one of the first and more agreed upon characteristics of codependence or coaddiction. Sometimes family members feel that they have little or no control over the enabling acts. Either because of the social support for protecting and supporting family members, or because of pathological interdependencies, or both, enabling behavior is often resistant to modification. Other characteristics of codependence include an unwillingness to accept the notion of addiction as a disease. The family members continue to behave as if the substance-using behavior were voluntary and willful, if not actually spiteful, and that the user cares more for alcohol and drugs than for the members of the family. That results in feelings of anger, rejection, and failure. In addition to those feelings, the family members may feel guilty and depressed because the addict, in an effort to deny loss of control over drugs and to shift the focus of concern away from their use, often tries to place the responsibility for such use on the other family members, who often seem willing to accept some or all of it.

DENIAL Family members, like the substance users themselves, often behave as if the substance use that is causing obvious problems were not really a problem; that is, they engage in denial. The reasons for the unwillingness to accept the obvious vary. Sometimes denial is self-protecting, in that the family members believe that, if there is a drug or alcohol problem, then they are responsible.

Like the addicts themselves, codependent family members seem unwilling to accept the notion that outside intervention is needed and, despite repeated failures, continue to believe that greater will power and greater efforts at control can restore tranquility. When additional efforts at control fail, they often attribute the failure to themselves rather than to the addict or the disease process; and along with failure come feelings of anger, lowered self-esteem, and depression.

OTHER PROBLEMS Some clinicians have reported high levels of somatic disorders, such as ulcers, colitis, and migraine, among family members of alcoholic persons and addicts and have attributed those illnesses to stress or a somatic expression of the feelings engendered by trying to cope with the family member's addiction. However, in light of the findings that there may be a genetic basis for somatization disorders among the daughters of certain subtypes of alcoholic persons, it is not clear that all of the illnesses seen among the family members of substance users are responses to the stresses of living with an addict.

OTHER INFLUENCES In addition to all the factors outlined, and depicted in Figure 13.1-1, there are others that influence the pattern of use and cessation of any given substance. For example, the decision not to use a substance also has consequences that can be aversive or reinforcing, and there is evidence that when the rewards of not using the substance are high, the likelihood of use is reduced. In addition, many of the substances associated with dependence act directly on systems that subserve both motivation and decision making, raising questions about whether use is always influenced solely by its consequences (learning processes). There is evidence that the cognitive processes and skills that would ordinarily subserve decision making are impaired by alcohol, barbiturates, cannabis, and several other categories of self-administered agents. Thus, whereas substance use is influenced by learning, the substances also alter the brain itself. Recognizing that suggests additional problems and possibilities for intervention. Evidence is accumulating that limited cognitive skills reduce the likelihood of successful recovery from substance use and that coping skills can help a person avoid or deal with aversive affective states, environmental stresses, and situations that are associated with a high risk for substance use.

Other factors that influence the course of substance use and dependence are difficult to operationalize or teach or prescribe, but they deserve mention. Studies of the natural history of substance use indicate that recovery is powerfully influenced by the support of family and friends. Many persons report that hope, faith, formal religious affiliation, or the sustaining love of some significant person was more important in their recovery than any specific treatment.

MULTIPLE FACTORS The biopsychosocial general model of substance dependence presented here does not attempt to assign a weight or special significance to any one factor or interaction. The implication is that, for different categories of drugs, different factors may play more or less powerful causal roles in perpetuating substance use or in relapse. For example, positive reinforcing effects may be a more important factor for the development of cocaine dependence, whereas acute and protracted withdrawal phenomena may be more important in the return to opioid use following withdrawal. Even with the same substance, different factors may be more or less important for different persons. Thus, for some cigarette smokers, particularly those with a history of major depressive disorder, the emergence of depressive symptoms may make quitting difficult, and those persons may be helped by antidepressants. Such a multifactorial model implies that different treatments or interventions may be more effective for one substance category than another and that even among persons using the same substances, different treatments may be indicated.

Figure 13.1-1 also implies that the notion of dependence is not a property of any one element, but is an abstraction inferred from the relations among the elements of the system. While it is convenient for clinicians and lay persons to see dependence as something located within a person (and is required by DSM-III-R and DSM-IV), any interpretation that overemphasizes one part of the system, whether the biology of the person, social influences, or behavior, is missing part of the nature of dependence.

TREATMENT

Although the focus here is on the procedures most likely to be used or encountered by mental health professionals, there are many other procedures and interventions that deserve mention. Some of those used in other countries are based on concepts about what causes and perpetuates drug use and dependence that are quite different from those in the United States.

With regard to treatment, it is useful to distinguish among specific procedures or techniques (for example, family therapy, group therapy, relapse prevention, and pharmacotherapy) and treatment programs. Most programs use a number of specific procedures and involve several professional disciplines, as well as nonprofessionals who have special skills or personal experiences with the substance problem being treated. The best treatment programs combine specific procedures and disciplines to meet the needs of the individual patient after a careful assessment. However, there is no generally accepted taxonomy either for the specific procedures used in treatment or for programs making use of various combinations of procedures. That lack of standardized terminology for categorizing programs presents a problem, even when the field of interest is narrowed from substance problems in general to treatment for a single substance, such as alcohol, tobacco, or cocaine. Even the definitions of specific procedures (for example, counseling, group therapy, and methadone maintenance) tend to be so imprecise that it is usually not possible to derive from the terms used just what transactions are supposed to occur. Nevertheless, for descriptive purposes, programs have often been gathered into broad groupings based on one or more of their salient characteristics, such as the environment in which services are provided; whether the program is aimed at merely controlling acute withdrawal and consequences of recent drug use (detoxification) or is focused on longer-term behavioral change; whether the program makes extensive use of pharmacological interventions; and the degree to which the program is based on individual psychotherapy, AA or other 12-step principles, or therapeutic community principles. For example, a framework once commonly used by government agencies to categorize publicly funded treatment programs for heroin dependence divided them into methadone maintenance (mostly outpatient), outpatient drug-free programs, and therapeutic communities. However, those broad descriptions mask as much as they reveal, tend to confuse the setting with the procedures, and obscure differences in the etiological models underlying the treatments used in different programs.

NEED FOR MATCHING Not all interventions are applicable to all varieties of substance use or dependence. For example, some of the interventions used with illicit drugs are not applicable to substances that are legally available, such as alcohol and tobacco, and for some drugs, specific pharmacological agents may be an important component of some interventions (for example, disulfiram for alcoholism, methadone for heroin addiction, nicotine for tobacco dependence). Not all interventions are likely to be useful to health care professionals. For example, many youthful offenders with histories of drug use or dependence are now remanded to shock incarceration facilities (boot camps); other programs for offenders (and sometimes for employees) rely almost exclusively on the deterrent effect of frequent urine testing; still other programs are built around religious conversion or rededication in a specific religious sect or denomination.

In general, for those using illicit drugs, brief interventions (such as a few weeks of detoxification, whether in or out of a hospital) have minimal effects on outcome when measured a few months later. Substantial reductions in illicit drug use, antisocial behaviors, and psychiatric distress are much more likely to be found following treatment lasting at least three months. Such a time-in-treatment effect is seen across very different modalities, from residential therapeutic communities to ambulatory methadone maintenance programs. Unfortunately, a substantial percentage of users of illicit drugs drop out (or are extruded) from treatment before they have achieved significant benefits. Not all of the variance in outcome of treatment can be attributed to differences in the characteristics of patients entering treatment. Outcome is also influenced by events and conditions following treatment. However, it is now clear that there is great variability in the effectiveness of programs based on similar philosophical principles and using what seem to be similar therapeutic procedures. Some of the differences among programs that seem to be similar reflect the range and intensity of services offered. Programs with professionally trained staffs that provide more comprehensive services to patients with more severe psychiatric difficulties are more likely to be able to retain those patients in treatment and to help them to make positive changes. Differences that can powerfully affect outcomes also have been found in the skills of individual counselors and professionals. Such generalizations concerning programs serving illicit drug users may not hold for programs dealing with those seeking treatment for alcohol or tobacco problems uncomplicated by heavy use of illicit drugs.

INFLUENCE OF PHILOSOPHICAL ORIENTATION The kinds of therapeutic procedures deemed valuable or essential by treatment professionals are profoundly affected by their philosophical orientation. For example, one study found that many professionals who adhere to a disease model of substance dependence view reduction of denial, acceptance of disease, need for lifelong abstinence, commitment to recovery, and affiliation with AA as the most important elements of intervention. In contrast, dealing with responsibility, instilling confidence, teaching relapse prevention, and avoiding high-risk situations were rated highest by psychologists espousing a behavioral model of dependence. Although physicians were included among those with a disease perspective, very few of them saw pharmacological therapies (to reduce craving) as having any significant value, and most considered the use of such agents as methadone or medications for cocaine use as detrimental to recovery. At best, there seems to be only a modest correlation between the evidence showing that a given intervention or procedure is effective and the likelihood that it will be widely used.

Currently, whether the patient is a user of illicit drugs or of alcohol or tobacco, entry into a treatment program rarely reflects a truly informed choice in which the characteristics and needs of a given patient are matched to the capacities and skills of a specific program. The notion that a better match between patients and programs would produce better outcomes is being tested in research-supported clinical trials, but until there are systematic changes in the way the treatment is made available, it is likely that the marketplace, chance, and other factors will be the dominant determinants of which user gets what, if any, treatment. For example, although most communities and many health insurers support programs that provide brief, but expensive, hospital-based detoxification for opioid dependence, which rarely leads to lasting behavioral change or abstinence from opioids, there is tremendous resistance to the use of methadone, which has been shown repeatedly to suppress heroin use. And, while a number of studies showed that with appropriate levels of support, outpatient detoxification for alcohol and cocaine are almost as effective as inpatient treatment, the shift from inpatient to outpatient services proceeded at a glacial pace until the advent of managed care.

Despite the persistent problems with developing cost-effective programs and matching patients to the programs, there is some recognition that treatment is often a worthwhile social expenditure. For example, treatment of antisocial illicit drug users in prison settings can produce a decrease in postrelease costs associated with drug use and of rearrests that more than offsets the cost of treatment. Also, treatment of illicit drug users at high risk for acquiring or transmitting HIV has been shown to decrease the rate of seroconversion enough to offset the costs of treatment.

CURRENT STATUS OF RESEARCH It is estimated that more than $858 million is spent annually in the United States on drug, alcohol, and mental health research—and, given the overlap among those areas, the support for research focusing primarily on alcohol and drugs is at least 30 percent of the total. Such an effort generates a wealth of new information on a myriad of questions, ranging from fundamental questions on the molecular mechanisms of action of specific drugs to the efficacy of various approaches to treatment and prevention.

SUGGESTED CROSS-REFERENCES

Individual sections discuss relevant substances in detail, including alcohol-related disorders in Section 13.2, caffeine-related disorders in Section 13.4, cannabis-related disorders in Section 13.5, cocaine-related disorders in Section 13.6, and opioid-related disorders in Section 13.9. Brief psychotherapy is covered in Section 31.9 and methadone in Section 32.17. Drug and alcohol abuse among the elderly is the subject of Section 49.6g.

REFERENCES

Anthenelli R M, Smith T L, Irwin M R, Schuckit M A: A comparative study of criteria for subgrouping alcoholics: The primary/secondary diagnostic scheme versus variations of the Type 1/Type 2 criteria. Am J Psychiatry *151:* 1468, 1994.

Bauer L O, Yehuda R, Meyer R E, Giller E Jr: Effects of a family history of alcoholism on autonomic, neuroendocrine, and subjective reactions to alcohol. Am J Addict *1*: 168, 1992.

Baumohl J: Inebriate institutions in North America, 1840–1920. Br J Addict *85:* 1187, 1990.

Blum K, Noble E P, Sheridan P J, Montgomery A, Ritchie T, Jagadeeswaran P, Nogami H, Briggs A H, Cohn J B: Allelic association of human dopamine D_2 receptor gene in alcoholism. JAMA *263:* 2055, 1990.

Carroll K M, Rounsaville B J: Contrast of treatment-seeking and untreated cocaine abusers. Arch Gen Psychiatry *49:* 464, 1992.

Edwards G, Arif A, Hodgson R: Nomenclature and classification of drug- and alcohol-related problems. A WHO Memorandum. Bull WHO *99:* 225, 1981.

Gelertner J, Goldman D, Risch N: The A_1 allele and the D_2 dopamine receptor gene and alcoholism. JAMA *269:* 1673, 1993.

*Gerstein D R, Harwood H J, editors: *Treating Drug Problems,* vol 1. Committee for the Substance Abuse Coverage Study, Division of Health Care Services, Institute of Medicine. National Academy Press, Washington, 1990.

Goodwin D: Biological factors in alcohol use and abuse: Implications for recognizing and preventing alcohol problems in adolescence. Int Rev Psychiatry *1*: 41, 1989.

Helzer J E: Epidemiology of alcohol addiction: International. In *Comprehensive Handbook of Drug and Alcohol Addiction,* N S Miller, editor, p 39. Marcel Dekker, New York, 1991.

Hesselbrock V, Meyer R E, Hesselbrock M: Psychopathology and addictive disorders: The specific case of antisocial personality disorder. In *Addictive States,* C P O'Brien, J H Jaffe, editors, Research Publications: Association for Research in Nervous and Mental Disease, vol 70, p 179. Raven, New York, 1992.

Holder H, Longabaugh R, Miller W R, Rubonis A V: The cost effectiveness of treatment for alcoholism: A first approximation. J Stud Alcohol *52:* 517, 1991.

*Institute of Medicine: *Broadening the Base of Treatment for Alcohol Problems.* Report of a study by a committee of the Institute of Medicine, Division of Mental Health and Behavioral Medicine, Committee for the Study of Treatment and Rehabilitation Services for Alcoholism and Alcohol Abuse, National Academy of Sciences. National Academy Press, Washington, 1990.

Jaffe J H: Addictions: What does biology have to tell? Int Rev Psychiatry *1*: 51, 1989.

Jaffe J H: Current concepts of addiction. In *Addictive States,* C P O'Brien, J H Jaffe, editors, Research Publications: Association for Research in Nervous and Mental Disease, vol 70, p 1. Raven, New York, 1992.

Johnston L D, O'Malley P M, Bachman J G: National Survey Results on Drug Use from The Monotoring the Future Study, 1975–1993. Volume II. College Students and Young Adults. NIH Publ. No. 94–3810. National Institute on Drug Abuse, Rockville, MD, 1994.

*Kandel D B: Epidemiological trends and implications for understanding the nature of addiction. In *Addictive States,* C P O'Brien, J H Jaffe, editors, Research Publications: Association for Research in Nervous and Mental Disease, vol 70, p 23. Raven, New York, 1992.

Kaufman E: The family in drug and alcohol addiction. In *Comprehensive Handbook of Drug and Alcohol Addiction,* N S Miller, editor, p 851. Marcel Dekker, New York, 1991.

Kessler R C: The epidemiology of psychiatric comorbidity. In *Textbook of Psychiatric Epidemiology,* M Tsuang, M Tohen, G Zahner, editors. J Wiley, New York, 1995.

Kessler R C, McGonagle K A, Zhao S, Nelson C B, Hughes M, Eshleman S, Wittchen H-U, Kendler K S: Lifetime and 12-month prevalence of DSM-III-R psychiatric disorders in the United States. Arch Gen Psychiatry *51:* 8, 1994.

Koob G F: Neurobiological mechanisms in cocaine and opiate dependence. In *Addictive States,* C P O'Brien, J H Jaffe, editors, Research Publications: Association for Research in Nervous and Mental Disease, vol 70, p 79. Raven, New York, 1992.

Morganstern J, Langenbucher J, Labouvie E W: The generalizability of the dependence syndrome across substances: An examination of some properties of the proposed DSM-IV dependence criteria. Addiction *89:* 1115, 1994.

Musto D F: *The American Disease. Origins of Narcotic Control.* Oxford University Press, New York, 1987.

National Institute on Alcohol Abuse and Alcoholism: *Seventh Special Report to the U.S. Congress on Alcohol and Health from the Secretary of Health and Human Services. January 1990.* DHHS Publ No (ADM) 90-1656, Rockville, MD, 1990.

*Nestler E: Molecular neurobiology of drug addiction. Neuropsychopharmacology *11:* 77, 1994.

Nyman D J, Cocores J: Coaddiction: Treatment of the family member. In *Comprehensive Handbook of Drug and Alcohol Addiction,* N S Miller, editor, p 877. Marcel Dekker, New York, 1991.

*Regier D A, Farmer M E, Rae D S, Locke B Z, Keith S J, Judd L L, Goodwin F K: Comorbidity of mental disorders with alcohol and other drug abuse. JAMA *264:* 2511, 1990.

Robins L N: Vietnam veterans' rapid recovery from heroin addiction: A fluke or normal expectation? Addiction *88:* 1041, 1993.

Rounsaville B J, Bryant K, Babor R, Kranzler H, Kadden R: Cross system agreement for substance use disorders: DSM-III-R, DSM-IV and ICD-10. Addiction *88:* 337, 1993.

Schuckit M A: Advances in understanding the vulnerability to alcoholism. In *Addictive States,* C P O'Brien, J H Jaffe, editors, Research Publications: Association for Research in Nervous and Mental Disease, vol 70, p 93. Raven, New York, 1992.

Schuckit M A: Low level of response to alcohol as a predictor of future alcoholism. Am J Psychiatry *151:* 184, 1994.

Substance Abuse and Mental Health Services Administration Office of

Applied Studies. National Household Survey on Drug Abuse: Population Estimates 1993. DHHS Publ. No. (SMA) 94-3017. SAMHSA, Office of Applied Studies, Rockville, MD, 1994.
Weiss R D, Collins D A: Substance abuse and psychiatric illness: The dually diagnosed patient. Am J Addict *1*: 93, 1992.

13.2 ALCOHOL-RELATED DISORDERS

MARC A. SCHUCKIT, M.D.

INTRODUCTION

This section offers clinically relevant information on the drug alcohol, alcoholism (alcohol abuse or dependence), and other alcohol-related disorders. Probably no other topic in this textbook has broader general importance.

Ninety percent of the people in Western societies drink alcoholic beverages at some time during their lives, with the result that the intake of alcohol can affect the course of most psychiatric disorders and alter the absorption and metabolism of most medications. At least 40 percent of men and women have some temporary alcohol-related life impairment, such as (1) absences from school or work caused by drinking and (2) driving when at least moderately intoxicated. Thus, alcohol intake can contribute greatly to work-related and interpersonal problems, even in persons who do not fulfill the criteria for alcohol abuse or dependence. Fully 10 percent or more of men and 5 to 10 percent of women do meet the diagnostic criteria for abuse or dependence on alcohol at some time during their lives. Because people with repetitive alcohol problems are more likely than the general population to seek psychiatric and psychological counseling, probably 25 percent or more of the patients appearing for evaluation in even affluent areas meet the diagnostic criteria for alcohol-related disorders. Perhaps two thirds of alcoholic persons have temporary but potentially severe psychiatric symptoms during intoxication or withdrawal; their clinical pictures resemble major depressive disorder, panic disorder, social phobia, and even psychotic disorders.

The economic costs of alcohol-related difficulties are alarming. For example, *Seventh Special Report to the U.S. Congress on Alcohol and Health* estimated that by 1995 the problem will cost the United States $150 billion. Approximately 60 percent of that sum is likely to be due to lost productivity in the workplace, 15 percent to health costs and treatment, and the remainder to a variety of alcohol-related damages.

DEFINITION

The definition of alcoholism (indicating alcohol abuse or dependence) differs from the formal diagnostic criteria for the syndromes. Each approach indicates evidence of repeated life impairments from alcohol, despite which the person returns to drinking. The distinction between a definition and the diagnostic criteria has been emphasized in the series of definitions that have evolved over the years from the National Council on Alcoholism. The 1992 definition of alcoholism is a chronic and progressive disease characterized by a loss of control over the use of alcohol, with subsequent social, legal, psychological, and physical consequences. A key element of the disorder is the ability to recognize and admit to oneself the life problems caused by alcohol and the relation of those problems to alcohol intake.

A history of the diagnostic criteria appears below, in ''Comparative Nosology.''

COMPARATIVE NOSOLOGY

Most clinicians think that, to be optimally useful, diagnostic criteria must be stated in relatively objective terms (so that they can be used in a similar manner in different settings) and must outline a syndrome that is distinct from other disorders. The goal is to produce diagnostic criteria that indicate whether an intervention is required and to offer information about the pros and cons of various treatment approaches.

DSM-III The emphasis on the use of diagnosis to indicate prognosis and treatment first appeared in the third edition of the American Psychiatric Association's (APA) *Diagnostic and Statistical Manual of Mental Disorders* (DSM-III) in 1980. In that edition, all the substance-use disorders were moved from a heterogeneous section dealing with sexual disorders and personality problems into a separate section, and a list of specific diagnostic criteria was offered. Persons with alcoholism were divided into those with repetitive interference with social, legal, interpersonal, and physical functioning (labeled alcohol abuse) and those with similar levels of life problems who also showed tolerance or physical dependence (labeled alcohol dependence).

DSM-III-R Since DSM-III appeared in 1980, the decision to publish the revised third edition of *Diagnostic and Statistical Manual of Mental Disorders* (DSM-III-R) in 1987 did not give adequate time for extensive testing of any new criteria. Despite the time constraints, the revised edition was used as an opportunity for fairly major changes in the diagnostic approach to substance-use disorders. In DSM-III-R alcohol dependence is a concept based on the expanded dependence syndrome developed by Griffith Edwards and Milton M. Gross in the 1960s. The diagnostic criteria incorporate nine items that emphasize the central and overriding role that alcohol occupies in life, an inability to control its use despite repeated attempts to do so, and several items that measure evidence of tolerance or physical withdrawal. Any combination of three of the nine criteria, even in the absence of tolerance and withdrawal, qualified a person for the diagnosis.

The committee formulating the criteria first envisioned the return to a single alcoholism-type label called ''dependence,'' proposing that the concept of abuse of alcohol be deleted from the manual. That proposal was thought to be justified by the broad nature of dependence, which incorporated many of the elements required for either abuse or dependence in DSM-III. However, under intense pressure from the treatment communities, the concept of abuse was reinserted into the manual. Because most of what could be considered alcoholism was already incorporated in the single broad definition of dependence, abuse was handled as a residual diagnosis to give clinicians a label to use when alcohol interfered with life functioning in someone who did not otherwise fulfill the criteria for dependence. A person could meet the criteria for abuse by the continued use of alcohol despite some level of impairment or by the recurrent use of alcohol in situations that are considered hazardous, including driving while intoxicated (whether arrested or not).

DSM-IV

Dependence and abuse The framers of the alcohol-related disorders section in the fourth edition of *Diagnostic and Statistical Manual of Mental Disorders* (DSM-IV), published in 1994, faced a dilemma. On the one hand, they preferred to avoid offering yet a third unique diagnostic set since 1980. On the other hand, the fairly large change in DSM-III-R for the concepts of both abuse and dependence and the de-emphasis of tolerance and withdrawal raised questions about the validity, the reliability, and the clinical coverage of the DSM-III-R approach. The compromise was to focus on the same basic nine items offered in DSM-III-R and to improve their operational definitions in order to enhance clinical usefulness. The nine DSM-III-R items were decreased to eight by combining into one the two relating to the development of withdrawal symptoms and the use of a substance to avoid or relieve withdrawal. A field trial of over 1,000 persons demonstrated that for most substances those two items performed virtually identically. The original DSM-III-R substance dependence criterion items were further decreased to seven by moving an item that dealt more with social consequences under substance abuse. Thus, as a result of information received from advisors and consultants, extensive literature reviews, and a large field trial, dependence in DSM-IV is defined as any three of seven items.

However, neither data searches nor the field trial established definitively the level of importance that should be placed on the items relating to tolerance or withdrawal. Indeed, those two criteria had high levels of reliability and provided important clinical information about immediate treatment needs. In the field trial, cluster analyses revealed that information relating to tolerance and withdrawal did not clearly stand apart from the five other items listed for dependence. The compromise taken by the DSM-IV committee was to retain the emphasis on any three of the seven items to establish a diagnosis of substance dependence, but to encourage clinicians and researchers to subtype persons with substance dependence into those exhibiting evidence of tolerance or withdrawal (with physiological dependence) and those lacking evidence of these two items (without physiological dependence). It was hoped that this step would encourage both clinicians and researchers to gather data on the potential importance of tolerance with withdrawal in preparation for DSM-V.

For the sake of continuity and to facilitate translation into the 10th revision of the *International Classification of Diseases and Related Health Problems* (ICD-10), DSM-IV maintains separate labels for substance abuse and dependence. However, literature reviews and the field trial demonstrated very low levels of reliability for substance abuse as defined in DSM-III-R, or for harmful use (the rough equivalent of abuse) in ICD-10. Cluster analyses from the field trial suggested that four items dealing with social, occupational, interpersonal, and legal problems might perform together in identifying a less severe substance use disorder. Thus, in DSM-IV substance abuse is defined as any one or more of the four criterion items occurring in an individual who does not meet criteria for substance dependence for that substance or group of related substances. Once again, it was hoped that the time before the publication of DSM-V would allow for more appropriate testing of the criteria set.

Severity and remission The DSM-IV substance-use committee also attempted to better define the concepts of severity and remission. The definition of severity in previous diagnostic manuals was relatively imprecise. The concept was divided into three levels, namely mild (with few symptoms), moderate (with levels of functional impairment intermediate between mild and severe), and severe (with many symptoms). Data reanalyses and field trials were used to test various potential definitions of severity for DSM-IV. Any approach had to be applicable to all substances of abuse (not just alcohol), and the criteria had to be user-friendly in clinical situations. The simplest approach was to take advantage of the more careful definition of the seven items offered in the revised dependence criteria set and to use the data from the literature and the field trial to establish the manner in which the number of diagnostic items correlates with additional and more sophisticated (and difficult to use) severity measures. Unfortunately, none of the approaches tested performed adequately in the analyses. Thus, DSM-IV offers no specific severity criteria.

Remission is a more complex phenomenon. DSM-III-R indicated full remission when, during the previous six months, the person either used no psychoactive substance or used one without symptoms of dependence. Partial remission was indicated by some use of psychoactive substance with one or two symptoms of dependence during the prior six months. The DSM-IV diagnostic criteria for remission were developed by using the data reanalyses and information gathered from the field trial and attempting to create a balance between ease of use and clinical relevance. As shown in Table 13.1-5, the diagnostic criteria distinguish between the high-risk period in the first 12 months of recovery and later time points and ask the clinician to specify whether the patient is totally free of substance-related problems. The criteria also consider agonist treatment and controlled environment.

Comorbid conditions The alcohol-related disorders are highly prevalent conditions, and psychiatric symptoms are common during intoxication and withdrawal. Therefore, if diagnoses are to be used to indicate prognosis and the optimal treatment, a scheme had to be developed to help the clinician disentangle temporary substance-related psychopathology from independent psychiatric syndromes.

Alcohol is an organic agent, and most diagnostic algorithms from Emil Kraepelin through DSM-IV have recognized the potential dangers of labeling psychiatric disorders when the symptoms develop during a condition strongly influenced by an organic cause. That hierarchical approach has many parallels in medicine. For example, pneumonias that develop *de novo* are recognized as having a cause and a long-term prognosis different from those of similar clinical conditions superimposed on congestive heart failure, a bronchus blocked by a carcinoma, or during the course of a severe immune deficiency. Of course, the symptoms of pneumonia must be recognized, but the treatment and the prognostic implications of the label are quite different in the diverse situations. Similarly, in psychiatry, depressive episodes that are observed during hypothyroid states, tremor and symptoms of anxiety seen in hyperthyroidism, and psychotic symptoms observed in connection with a brain tumor must be recognized and are likely to require intervention, but they have prognostic and treatment implications quite different from major depressive episodes, panic disorder, and schizophrenia that developed in the absence of those major preexisting disorders.

That philosophy can also be applied to the alcohol-related disorders. All the diagnostic manuals since DSM-III have warned the clinician that psychiatric disorders developing only during intoxication or withdrawal from substances do not necessarily indicate an independent psychiatric disorder. Recognizing that those caveats are easy to overlook in clinical practice, DSM-IV has added an overall statement about the inadvisability of labeling independent psychiatric disorders based on symptoms observed only during alcohol intoxication or within four weeks of abstinence from alcohol abuse or dependence. Depressions, panic attacks, and psychotic thought processes occurring in the context of alcohol problems do not usually carry the same prognostic implications as actual major depressive episodes, panic disorders, and schizophrenia. Similarly, DSM-IV reminds clinicians that such symptoms of mood disorders or psychoses that are documented before severe life problems from alcohol or that remain beyond four weeks of total abstinence should be carefully evaluated as possible indicators of true comorbidity with the occurrence of two or more independent psychiatric syndromes.

Finally, three psychiatric syndromes—bipolar I disorder, schizophrenia, and antisocial personality disorder—carry heightened risks for subsequent substance-related disorders.

ICD-10 Both ICD-10 and DSM-IV require that diagnoses be based on multiple items from a relatively long list of potential problems, each makes a distinction between a severe pervasive syndrome labeled "dependence" and a less intense level of alcohol-related life problems labeled "abuse" or "harmful use," and each incorporates aspects of the expanded definition of dependence. Data indicate that the same person is highly likely to receive a dependence diagnosis in both systems, especially when five or more of the criterion items are met. However, unlike ICD-10, DSM-IV encourages the clinician to note the potential importance of physiological symptoms by subtyping dependence.

In the past the international system and the United States system differed markedly in their respective definitions of harmful use and abuse. In ICD-10 harmful use involves clear evidence that the use of a substance caused psychological or physical (*not* social or legal) harm to the user. Except for the restriction regarding social and legal problems, ICD-10 appears to be closer to the definition of abuse in DSM-IV than was true of ICD-9 and DSM-III-R. However, it is too soon to know whether the implied high level of concordance will be true in clinical situations.

PHARMACOLOGY

The inclusion of a discussion of pharmacology in a section on alcohol-related disorders is not meant to imply that a disorder can be defined through the use of a substance. After all, most drinkers do not have serious problems related to alcohol, and only a minority of drinkers have difficulties severe and pervasive enough to be labeled abuse or dependence. However, all alcoholic persons have a problem with that potent substance. As a result, clinicians cannot understand the disease or its syndromes without knowing something about alcohol itself.

Ethanol (beverage alcohol) is a simple molecule that is well absorbed through the mucosal lining of the digestive tract in the mouth, the esophagus, and the stomach. The most prominent area of absorption, however, is in the proximal small intestine, which is also the site of absorption of many of the B vitamins. As a result of its high level of solubility in water, ethanol rapidly enters the bloodstream, where it is distributed to almost every body system. As a consequence of its modest fat solubility, alcohol is likely to have effects on body membranes rich in fat, including neurons.

Wine, beer, and such distilled spirits as whiskey, gin, and vodka differ in their content of congeners. *Congeners* are responsible for much of the characteristic taste of the beverage and consist of combinations of methanol, butanol, aldehydes, phenols, tannins, lead, cobalt, iron, and other substances. Under certain circumstances congeners can have physiological effects, but their potency pales in comparison with alcohol.

A drink of an alcoholic beverage is usually defined as between 10 and 12 grams of ethanol. In round figures that is the amount of alcohol contained in approximately 12 ounces of beer (which in the United States has approximately 3.6 percent ethanol), 4 ounces of table wine (containing about 12 percent ethanol), and between 1.0 and 1.5 ounces of 80-proof spirits (containing 40 percent ethanol). For the average 70 kg (155-pound) person who has an average amount of body fat, one drink is likely to raise the blood alcohol level by approximately 15 to 20 mg/dL. The body subsequently metabolizes and excretes approximately one drink an hour. The rate of absorption of alcohol from the digestive tract is likely to be faster on an empty stomach than after a full meal, especially one rich in fats and carbohydrates.

After absorption into the bloodstream from the small intestine, between 2 and 10 percent of the alcohol is then excreted unchanged from the lungs or the kidneys or through sweat; the majority is metabolized in the liver. Liver metabolization occurs mostly through four pathways, with each resulting in the production of acetaldehyde. Most of the process occurs through the actions of alcohol dehydrogenase (ADH) in the cytosol of hepatic cells. Especially at high blood alcohol levels, some of the alcohol is also broken down in the microsomes of the smooth endoplasmic reticulum (the MEOS system). The ADH process is the usual rate-limiting metabolic step, occurring relatively slowly because of the need of the liver to handle the produced hydrogen ions through use of a cofactor that is in relatively short supply, nicotinamide adenine dinucleotide (NAD).

The acetaldehyde produced is then destroyed by the enzyme aldehyde dehydrogenase (ALDH) in both the liver cell cytosol and mitochondria. That step occurs rapidly, with the result that the average person does not have substantial levels of the substance. That is fortunate because, at high levels, acetaldehyde can produce histamine release and, through a variety of mechanisms, contributes to falling blood pressure, nausea, and vomiting. The relative destruction of ALDH by disulfiram (Antabuse) is largely responsible for the alcohol intolerance seen in alcoholic persons treated with disulfiram.

TOLERANCE With repeated administration of alcohol, larger and larger doses of the drug are required to produce the desired effect. That phenomenon, called *tolerance,* is described as the ability to tolerate higher and higher doses of the substance and is the result of at least three processes.

Behavioral tolerance reflects the ability of a person to learn how to perform tasks effectively despite the effects of alcohol. It is a learned behavior and the result of repeated practice. *Pharmacokinetic tolerance* is an adaptation of the metabolizing system to rid the body of alcohol rapidly. After several weeks of daily drinking, the liver produces more ADH than usual and expands the MEOS system, with a resulting increase (up to 30 percent) in the rate of breakdown of ethanol. Finally, *pharmacodynamic or cellular tolerance* is an adaptation of the nervous system so that it can function despite high blood alcohol levels by resisting the actions of alcohol on the cell. Thus, persons have been observed to be awake, relatively alert, and relatively coordinated despite blood alcohol levels of 250 mg/dL, and some persons were awake at blood alcohol levels above 600 mg/dL.

Once a person has tolerance for one of the brain depressants, he or she often shows a similar reaction to a second drug of that class *(cross-tolerance).* Therefore, a person who has been drinking heavily, has tolerance for alcohol, and then stops drinking can be expected to require higher than usual levels of benzodiazepines for sleep induction. Of course, if the person took two depressant drugs at the same time, tolerance is not likely to be observed, and the mixing of the two substances can have lethal effects. Just as tolerance requires a period of days or weeks to develop, the phenomenon is likely to disappear within a similar period of time after ceasing the intake of any depressant drug.

Some clinicians have described a phenomenon of *reverse tolerance*. Clinically, as persons, whether alcoholic or not, grow older, they have increasing levels of sensitivity to most brain depressants, including alcohol. That effect probably reflects a decrease in the rate at which alcohol is metabolized in the liver with increasing age, a decrease in body water as a consequence of an increasing percentage of fat, so that higher blood alcohol levels develop, and neurons have an enhanced sensitivity to the effects of alcohol. Even more dramatic examples of increased sensitivity to alcohol are seen after severe brain damage (the consequence, for example, of an auto accident or alcohol-related brain deterioration) and after impairment in any of the major alcohol-metabolizing systems, as occurs with cirrhosis.

The adaptation of the body to prolonged exposure to high doses of alcohol is likely to produce physical dependence, which is the basis of the alcohol withdrawal syndrome.

EFFECTS ON THE BRAIN All substances of abuse share the ability to produce changes in feeling states and subsequently increase the likelihood that a person will have a psychological drive to continue to take the substance despite potentially severe adverse consequences (psychological addiction or dependence). That effect is distinct from the physical dependence or addiction that produces the withdrawal or abstinence syndrome that characterizes drugs like alcohol. However, the 300 or so diverse psychoactive drugs differ in many important ways. For example, only a few produce physiological tolerance and clinically relevant levels of withdrawal symptoms when someone stops using the substance. Some drugs markedly increase the chances that a person will have temporary psychoses or depressions; other drugs do not. Some are likely to be lethal in overdose; others appear to be relatively safe at high levels. Clinicians, therefore, are presented with a daunting challenge if they attempt to memorize all the attributes for each of the hundreds of psychoactive substances.

A useful shortcut is to place drugs of abuse into categories on the basis of their most prominent effects at the usual doses at which they are taken. In that scheme, substances that have as their most prominent usual effects the production of somnolence and decreased neuronal activity but that are not powerful in attenuating pain are labeled as depressants. They include alcohol, all the benzodiazepines, all the barbiturates, and the carbamate antianxiety drugs, such as meprobamate (Miltown). Those substances produce a similar profile of symptoms during intoxication, are potentially lethal in overdose (especially when multiple drugs in the depressant category are taken at the same time), are cross-tolerant, are physically addicting, and produce similar withdrawal syndromes. The optimal treatment of withdrawal from one drug of that class involves administering a depressant, and regular use of any of those agents is likely to produce severe mood swings during repeated intoxication and severe symptoms of anxiety during withdrawal.

The behavioral and physiological changes observed with any substance differ with the dose, the patient's prior history of exposure to the drug, and clinical conditions, including physiological disorders and the patient's state of fatigue. With a drug like alcohol, the effects also change over time after intake, with more pronounced symptoms observed while the blood alcohol levels are rising than when the blood alcohol levels are falling, a phenomenon called the Mallenby effect.

Despite all the data outlined above, debate continues about the most important mechanisms of action of alcohol on the brain. One of the problems occurs because the drug has a major effect on most neurochemical systems, demonstrating different effects at different doses and sometimes opposite effects during intoxication and withdrawal. One series of theories on the mechanisms underlying intoxication relates to the effects that alcohol has on the cell membrane; alcohol tends to fluidize or decrease the levels of rigidity of the membrane, with subsequent impairments in the ability of the cell to control the influx and the efflux of electrolytes. Other research focuses on changes in dopamine, attempting to tie in the effects of alcohol to the pleasure centers of the limbic system. Still other investigators point to the potential importance of the neurochemical compounds that may, at least theoretically, be formed between acetaldehyde and the neurotransmitters serotonin and dopamine, producing alkaloids that have properties resembling opiates. Another set of investigations point out the indirect effects that alcohol can have on the benzodiazepine-receptor complexes in the brain. With such a diverse range of effects and the absence of an obvious receptor system reacting specifically to alcohol, many leads are promising, but few answers are definitive regarding the most clinically relevant effects of alcohol on the nervous system or the way in which the alterations may relate to abuse or dependence on alcohol.

EFFECTS ON THE BODY Some data indicate that alcohol use is not always harmful and may under some circumstances even have some beneficial effects. However, alcohol is harmful to pregnant persons, to recovering alcoholic persons, and to persons taking medications that may be adversely affected by alcohol or if persons have a relevant medical disorder or have some psychiatric syndrome (such as major depressive disorder or schizophrenia) that may be intensified by alcohol. For other persons a maximum of one or two drinks a day appears to be associated with a decreased risk of cardiovascular disease. That association may be due to an increase in at least one portion of high-density lipoprotein cholesterol (HDLC), although the fraction affected does not appear to be the one most potent in protecting against heart disease. Unfortunately, the intake of more than two drinks a day is likely to increase low-density lipoprotein cholesterol (LDLC) and triglycerides and to raise blood pressure, with the overall result of increasing the risk of cardiac disorders. And even low levels of alcohol intake may increase the risk for breast cancer.

Central nervous system (CNS)

BLACKOUT *Blackout* indicates a memory impairment (anterograde amnesia) for the period of time when the person was drinking heavily but remained awake. This common difficulty is related to the ability of any brain depressant to interfere with the acquisition of memory if the dose is high enough. Perhaps 40 percent of men in their teens and 20s have blackouts, and memory loss does not by itself indicate a high likelihood of alcohol abuse or dependence. The blackout, which is temporary and limited to memory problems involving a short period of time, is not a DSM-IV diagnosis and is distinct from alcohol-induced persisting amnestic disorder.

SLEEP IMPAIRMENT Alcohol intoxication can help a person fall asleep quickly but tends to depress rapid eye movement sleep and inhibit stage 4 sleep. It is likely to be associated with frequent alternations between sleep stages, a process sometimes referred to as sleep fragmentation.

PERIPHERAL NEUROPATHY A more serious and potentially permanent problem is seen in perhaps 10 percent of alcoholic persons after years of heavy drinking. The deterioration of nerve functioning to the hands and feet, called *peripheral neuropathy*, arises through an apparent combination of vitamin deficiencies and the direct effects of alcohol or its metabolites. The symptoms include numbness of the hands and feet, often bilateral, and are frequently accompanied by tingling and paresthesias. Although the condition is usually relatively mild and often improves with abstinence, the pain and the numbness can result in a permanent impairment.

CEREBELLAR DEGENERATION Characterized by unsteadiness of gait, problems with standing, and mild nystagmus, cerebellar degeneration is probably caused by a combination of the effects of ethanol and acetaldehyde, along with vitamin deficiencies. Treatment usually consists of total abstinence and vitamin supplementation, although complete recovery is not common.

OTHER CNS EFFECTS A series of temporary but intense psychiatric syndromes are likely to be observed during alcohol intoxication and withdrawal, including depressed mood, severe anxiety, and psychoses. They often mimic psychiatric disorders but are likely to disappear within weeks of abstinence. Severe amnestic disorders and dementias may also occur.

Gastrointestinal (GI) problems Second only to the nervous system, the GI system is most severely affected by heavy drinking. Probably the most common GI problem associated with alcohol intake is an acute and, at times, severe inflammation of the esophagus or the stomach, with stomach inflammation often accompanied by vomiting and bleeding. If gastritis occurs in the presence of dilated esophageal veins seen with cirrhosis, it can induce potentially lethal bleeding.

The liver and the pancreas are especially vulnerable to alcohol. In the liver, increasing alcohol doses result in the accumulation of fats and proteins in the cells, producing a reversible swelling often described as a fatty liver. Inflammation of the liver cells accompanied by a subsequent intense rise in some liver function tests and other signs of alcoholic hepatitis can lead to the deposition of excessive amounts of hyalin and collagen near blood vessels, an early stage of cirrhosis. As damage progresses, the normal flow of blood through the liver is impaired, dilated veins or varices develop from the increased abdominal venous pressure, and fluid seeps from the liver capsule, accumulating in the abdomen as ascites. As liver failure progresses, secondary cognitive impairment can develop as various levels of hepatic encephalopathy.

Perhaps 15 percent of alcoholic persons respond to acute large doses of alcohol with an inflammation of the pancreas that can present as the abdominal emergency of acute pancreatitis. A chronic irreversible condition of pancreatic destruction, with associated signs of insufficiency in sugar metabolism (a form of diabetes) and digestive enzymes, can then develop.

Cerebrovascular and cardiovascular problems Heavy intake of alcohol increases the blood pressure and elevates both LDLC and triglycerides, thus enhancing the risk for myocardial infarction and thrombosis. At high doses, alcohol is also a striated-muscle toxin with a resulting production of what is usually but not always a reversible deterioration in the heart muscle that manifests itself as beating irregularities and signs of heart failure (*alcoholic cardiomyopathy*). Similar levels of swelling of muscle cells and subsequent muscle pain can be observed in the skeletal muscles.

Blood-producing systems High levels of alcohol intake, often in the range of four to eight drinks a day, decreases the production of white blood cells, impairs the ability of those cells to migrate to sites of infection, and affects the stem cells that produce the red blood components, significantly increasing the average size of the red cell (the mean corpuscular volume or MCV) and can impair the production and the efficiency of blood platelets.

Cancer High rates of many types of cancer are seen in alcoholic persons, especially cancers in the head, neck, esophagus, and stomach. Additional areas of risk include the liver, the colon, and the lungs. The risks probably reflect alcohol-related immune system suppression but may also be a result of the direct effects of ethanol on mucosal membranes. The heightened rates of malignant tumors in alcoholic persons remain significant even when the possible effects of smoking and bad nutrition are considered.

Fetal alcohol effect Alcohol and acetaldehyde can have deleterious effects on the developing fetus. Both substances cross the placenta with ease and in high enough doses can produce fetal death and spontaneous abortion. Surviving infants of heavy-drinking mothers can evidence any mixture of the components of a syndrome that in its full-blown form can include severe mental retardation, a small head, a diminished physical size, facial abnormalities (including a flat bridge of the nose, an absent philtrum, and an epicanthal eye fold), an atrial septal heart defect, and syndactyly. None of those problems is reversible; once present, the cognitive defect and the behavioral problems remain throughout life. Because the exact amount of alcohol required and the most vulnerable periods of pregnancy have not been definitively established, all pregnant women are advised to abstain from any use of alcohol.

EPIDEMIOLOGY

Psychiatrists need to be concerned about the drinking patterns of their patients because alcohol can interact with medications and intensify major psychiatric disorders. Clinicians also need to recognize that a high proportion of their patients have temporary but potentially important alcohol-related problems.

PREVALENCE OF DRINKING At some time during their lives, 90 percent of the population in the United States drinks, with most persons beginning their alcohol intake in the early to mid teens (Table 13.2-1). At any time two out of three men are current drinkers, with a ratio of persisting alcohol intake of approximately 1.3 men to 1 woman. A current drinker is defined most commonly as anyone who has used alcohol during the preceding one to three months and is differentiated from persons with alcohol problems (see below). The age of highest prevalence of drinking and of greatest alcohol intake is from the mid or late teens to the mid 20s.

Different groups in the United States have different propor-

TABLE 13.2-1
Alcohol Epidemiology

Condition	Population (%)
Ever had a drink	90
Current drinker	60–70
Temporary problems	40+
Abuse	Male: 20 Female: 10
Dependence*	Male: 10 Female: 3–5

*20–30 percent of psychiatric patients.

tions of drinkers. Social and cultural factors need to be taken into account when evaluating who is a current drinker. Generally, persons who have high education and high socioeconomic status make up the highest proportion of current drinkers. Among religious groups, Jews have the highest proportion of current drinkers but the lowest number of persons with alcohol problems. Convervative Protestant and Catholic persons use alcohol less frequently than liberal Protestants and Catholics.

Other groups, such as the Irish, have higher rates of severe alcohol problems, but they also have significantly higher rates of abstainers. High rates of alcohol problems are also found among Native Americans and Eskimos.

In the United States the average person over the age of 14 years consumes 2.3 to 2.5 gallons of absolute alcohol a year. That figure translates to 70 gallons of beer, almost 23 gallons of wine, or eight gallons of 80-proof (40-percent) bourbon. Those amounts sound substantial, but they are considerably less than the five-plus gallons of absolute ethanol consumed each year at the time of the American Revolution, and the current figures represent a significant decrease from the amounts consumed during the mid 1970s.

ALCOHOL PROBLEMS Since a high proportion of persons are drinkers, especially in their mid teens to mid 20s, and since the per-capita consumption is high, it is not surprising that a large proportion of persons have alcohol-related problems sometime in their lives. A recent 10-year follow-up study of almost 500 men evaluated at age 33 found that during the preceding decade between one quarter and one third had alcohol-related blackouts, approximately one third admitted to driving after consuming enough alcohol to be impaired, and 20 percent reported missing school or work because of either a hangover or a desire to party with alcohol, rather than work.

As common as those problems are and as much as they contribute to lost work time and to physical morbidity and mortality, most people appear to mature out of alcohol problems with the passage of time. Thus, the proportion of persons with current alcohol-related difficulties is probably lower during their 30s than during their 20s and even lower during their 40s and 50s. Both per-capita consumption and the proportion of persons with problems related to alcohol appear to decrease with increasing age beyond middle adulthood.

Alcohol abuse or dependence The lifetime risk for alcohol dependence is approximately 10 percent for men and 3 to 5 percent for women. The rate of alcohol abuse may be as high as 20 percent for men and 10 percent for women. Those figures tranlate to perhaps a total of 200,000 deaths a year in the United States from accidents (perhaps 25,000 persons a year alone), suicide, cancer, and heart disease—the leading causes of death among alcoholic men and women. Cirrhosis is also found at increased rates; 15 percent of alcoholic persons meet the criteria for cirrhosis. Because alcoholism is associated with numerous medical and psychiatric problems, alcoholic persons are over-represented in psychiatric settings, where they make up one quarter to one third of the usual patient load.

The age of peak onset of alcohol problems severe enough to lead to a diagnosis of alcohol dependence is probably in the mid 20s to approximately 40. Despite multiple difficulties in social relationships, families, and jobs, high functioning in some areas is likely to remain. Thus, the stereotypical alcoholic person living on skid row is likely to be the exception, rather than the rule, representing only 5 percent of all persons with severe, repetitive alcohol-related difficulties.

Age-related differences are found in the pattern of alcohol-related problems. As is true with almost all psychiatric and many medical disorders, the earlier the onset of alcoholism, the greater the chance that the disorder is severe and that another psychiatric disorder preexisted. Therefore, when alcohol dependence is noted in the teens, the person probably has another problem, usually antisocial personality disorder. In that instance the alcohol-related problems are likely to be associated with severe drug difficulties and antisocial problems in school and with family or peers that occurred before the onset of alcohol dependence. At the other extreme, although most alcoholic persons have their problems early in life, perhaps 10 percent or so have an onset of repetitive difficulties after the age of 55. The late onset of the disorder tends to be associated with less severe social difficulties and more subtle signs and symptoms but a greater likelihood of associated medical problems than among younger alcoholic persons.

ETIOLOGY

Many factors probably affect the decision to drink, the development of temporary alcohol-related difficulties in the teens and 20s, and the development of alcohol dependence. The initiation of alcohol intake probably rests with social, religious, and psychological factors, although the high rate of persons who have tried alcohol at some time during their lives indicates that drinking is an almost ubiquitous phenomenon. However, it is important to remember that the factors that influence the decision to drink or those that contribute to temporary problems might be different from those that contribute to the severe repetitive problems of alcohol dependence.

PSYCHOLOGICAL THEORIES A variety of factors relate to the use of alcohol to reduce tension, increase feelings of power, and decrease the effects of psychological pain. Perhaps the greatest interest has been paid to the observation that persons with alcohol-related problems often report that alcohol decreases their feelings of nervousness and helps them cope with day-to-day life stresses. The psychological theories are built, in part, on the observation among nonalcoholic persons that the intake of alcohol in a tense social setting or after a difficult day can, especially in low doses, be associated with an enhanced feeling of well-being and an improved ease of interactions. However, data indicate that in high doses, especially at falling blood alcohol levels, most measures of muscle tension and psychological feelings indicate that heavy drinking is likely to be associated with *increased* nervousness and feelings of tenseness. The theories that focus on the potential of alcohol to enhance feelings of being powerful and sexually attractive and to decrease the effects of psychological pain are difficult to evaluate definitively.

PSYCHODYNAMIC THEORIES Perhaps related to the disinhibiting or anxiety-lowering effects of alcohol, at least at rising blood alcohol levels, is the hypothesis of some theorists that some persons may use alcohol to help them deal with self-punitive harsh superegos as a way of decreasing unconscious stress levels. Also, classical psychoanalytical theory hypothesizes that at least some alcoholic persons have become fixated at the oral stage of development and use alcohol to relieve their frustrations by taking the substance by mouth. Alcoholic persons may also use the drug as part of a need for enhanced feelings of achievement of power. However, hypotheses regarding arrested phases of psychosexual development, as heuristically important as they may be, have had little effect on the usual treatment approaches and are not the focus of extensive ongoing research. Similarly, several hypotheses have questioned the potential importance of addictive personality attributes as they may reflect levels of impulsiveness and sensation seeking. However, careful studies have failed to identify a unique personality profile prone to addictions, with the exception of antisocial personality disorder.

BEHAVIORAL THEORIES Expectations about the rewarding effects of drinking and subsequent actual reinforcement after alcohol intake contribute to the decision to drink again after the first alcohol experience. Those issues are important in efforts to modify drinking behaviors in the general population, and they do contribute to some important aspects of alcoholic rehabilitation, as described below, under "Treatment."

SOCIOCULTURAL THEORIES Sociocultural theories are often based on observations of social groups that have high and low rates of alcoholism. Theorists hypothesize that cultures, such as Jews, that introduce children to modest levels of drinking in a family atmosphere and that eschew drunkenness have low rates of alcoholism. Cultures, such as Irish men, with high rates of abstention but a tradition of drinking to the point of drunkenness among drinkers, are thought to have high rates of alcoholism. One problem is that those theories often depend on stereotypes that are frequently erroneous; another problem is the large number of exceptions to the general rules. For example, some of the theories that are based on observations of the Irish and the French would have predicted high rates of alcoholism among the Italians, although alcohol problems are not generally observed at a high level among Italians.

In the final analysis, social and psychological theories probably have more than heuristic value. They probably outline factors that contribute to the onset of drinking, the development of temporary alcohol-related life difficulties, and even alcoholism. The problem is how to find a way to gather relatively definitive data to support or refute the theories.

BIOLOGICAL THEORIES

Genetic theories The best supported of the biological theories of alcoholism centers on genetics (Table 13.2-2). One finding supporting the genetic conclusion is the threefold to fourfold increased risk for severe alcohol problems in *close relatives of alcoholic persons.* The rate of alcohol problems increases with the number of alcoholic relatives, the severity of their illness, and the closeness of their genetic relationship to the person under study. The family investigations do little to separate the importance of genetics and environment, but *twin studies* take the data a step further. The rate of similarity (or concordance) for severe alcohol-related problems is significantly higher in identical twins of alcoholic parents than in fraternal twins in most studies. The *adoption-type studies,* using both the half-sibling approach and actual adoption records, have all revealed a significantly enhanced risk for alcoholism in the offspring of alcoholic parents, even when the children had been separated from their biological parents close to birth and raised without any knowledge of the problems within the biological family. The risk for severe alcohol-related difficulties is not further enhanced by being raised by an alcoholic adoptive family.

Those data not only support the importance of genetic factors in alcoholism but also highlight the complexity of the phenomenon. The absence of evidence of a single major locus indicates the possibility that a limited number of genes operate with incomplete penetrance or that a combination of genes is required before the disorder expresses itself (a polygenic mode of inheritance). Making matters even more complex is the likelihood that in some phenocopies the disorder is solely an expression of environmental events in some families and the probability that different genetic factors operate in different families to produce a picture of genetic heterogeneity.

TABLE 13.2-2
Data Supporting Genetic Influences in Alcoholism

Close family members have a fourfold increased risk.
The identical twin of an alcoholic person is at higher risk than is a fraternal twin.
Adopted-away children of alcoholic persons have a fourfold increased risk.

Despite those problems, research undertaken during the 1980s has enhanced the understanding of how genetic influences may operate in alcoholism. Most studies have identified men and women at high future risk of alcoholism, usually defined as having an alcoholic parent. Persons at high and low future risk are then compared on psychological and biological parameters. Some protocols then expose young adults to an alcohol challenge, and several investigations have subsequently followed them over time.

Related biological theories Different approaches have highlighted several potential leads to biological factors that may affect the alcoholism risk. Investigations of early-teenage children of alcoholic parents, usually including central-city families or children of persons with the antisocial personality disorder, have shown the potential importance of several neurocognitive test results as possible predictors of an alcoholism risk. Additional leads have come from electrophysiological evaluations of children of alcoholic persons, including the finding that perhaps one third of the sons of severely alcoholic men may have a decreased amplitude of the positive wave observed 300 milliseconds after a rare but unexpected sensory stimulus, the P_3 wave of event-related potential (ERP). Other studies have shown a potential decrease in the amount of power in the slow alpha range on the background cortical electroencephalogram (EEG) or relative deficiencies in beta waves.

An additional potential phenotypic marker involves the intensity of a person's reaction to an alcohol challenge. One study revealed that at age 20 approximately 40 percent of the sons of alcoholic persons showed less intense responses to alcohol than did a matched group of lower-risk controls as measured by EEG, hormone levels, and subjective feelings after consuming three to five drinks. That study includes a 10-year follow-up of both the high risk and the low risk persons, with data generated from 450 persons indicating that a low level of alcohol response at age 20 is a potent predictor of high alcoholism risk by age 30.

Theorists have hypothesized that biological influences, such as the decreased reaction to alcohol and the diminished size of the P_3 wave of the ERP, are factors that interact with environmental events, including the level of exposure to alcohol. In addition, attitudes toward drinking, levels of general life stress, and the ease and the cost with which alcohol was available all interact with the biological factors to produce the final level of risk.

DIAGNOSIS AND CLINICAL FEATURES

Alcoholism is probably the most common of the serious diagnosable behavioral or psychiatric disorders, and the diagnosis of alcoholism requires a high index of suspicion for the disorder in any patient. The usual stereotype of the alcoholic person (the skid-row bum) is inaccurate and misleading. The average man or woman presenting with severe and repetitive alcohol problems is likely to be neatly dressed, to show no signs of severe alcoholic withdrawal, to have a job and a family, and to complain of a variety of physical conditions or temporary but potentially severe psychiatric complaints. Thus, the psychiatrist must gather a history of alcohol-related life problems from both the patient and, whenever possible, a resource person and must try to determine whether alcohol has caused or contributed to the psychiatric or physiological syndrome. Table 13.2-3 lists the alcohol-related disorders.

The first step when the clinical picture is complicated is to obtain a careful history from both the patient and a resource person who knows the patient well. Second, in taking the information, the psychiatrist must emphasize syndromes that meet diagnostic criteria, not just symptoms. Third, the psychiatrist must establish a time line from birth to the patient's current age, noting the approximate age of onset of alcohol problems severe and repetitive enough to justify a diagnosis of alcohol dependence, periods of abstinence of several months or more, and the ages at which the patient met the criteria for any major psychiatric disorders, taking care to emphasize full-blown psychiatric clinical conditions, not isolated symptoms. If a review of the time line reveals no evidence that the additional psychiatric syndromes either antedated the severe alcohol problems or persisted for four or more weeks during a period of abstinence, alcoholism is the major disorder. Under those conditions the other psychiatric syndromes were important but temporary conditions that occurred during alcohol intoxication or withdrawal.

Depressive, anxiety, and psychotic disorders can become part of the differential diagnosis for alcohol-related disorders. However, even if the psychiatric symptoms are intense, they do not indicate a separate psychiatric syndrome when seen only during intoxication or withdrawal. In past editions of DSM, they were referred to as organic mood, anxiety, and delusional disorders. The organic sections of DSM-IV have been thoroughly revised. At least in part as a philosophical statement, the distinction between organic and nonorganic psychiatric syndromes has now been dropped. Then, in an effort to encourage clinicians and researchers to consider the entire span of clinical conditions that might be relevant to any syndrome being observed, all important diagnostic entities related to a specific phenomenon (for example, depressive disorders, anxiety disorders, psychotic disorders) are now listed within the clinically relevant sections of DSM-IV. For the sake of clarity, those disorders associated with substances are now labeled as substance-induced disorders.

As a result, for example, a condition labeled as an organic mood disorder in DSM-III-R is now listed as a substance-induced mood disorder. Although reference to the disorder is offered within the section concerning substance-related disorders, the full criteria and explanation are now offered within the mood disorders section of DSM-IV. As is true of most substance-induced disorders, the syndrome involved must be clinically meaningful and must resemble the type of disorder described within that section (for example, a mood disorder). There must be evidence indicating a likelihood that the clinical condition developed during, or within a month of, substance intoxication or withdrawal from a specific substance, such as alcohol, which would be capable of producing a relevant temporary clinical condition, such as a severe mood disturbance. The clinician and researcher are warned that the substance-induced condition should only be diagnosed when the psychiatric symptoms (for example, depression) are in excess of those usually associated with intoxication or withdrawal. The diagnostic criteria further list the specific substances involved and ask that a distinction be made (whenever possible) indicating whether the condition had an onset during intoxication or withdrawal. Those latter modifiers are important to indicate to the clinician when additional medical and psychiatric treatment might be required. For alcohol-induced mood disorders, diagnoses can also be subtyped regarding the presence or absence of depressive, manic, or mixed features.

DSM-IV offers similar information regarding a substance-induced anxiety disorder, which is listed in the section on anxiety disorders. Again, the condition must be clinically relevant, there must be evidence that a substance, such as alcohol, capable of producing a severe temporary anxiety condition, was involved, and a distinction regarding an onset during intoxication or withdrawal is encouraged. The anxiety conditions can be further subdivided regarding the relevance of generalized anxiety symptoms, repetitive panic attacks, obsessive-compulsive symptoms, or phobic symptoms.

The documentation of hallucinations and delusions associated with intoxication or withdrawal from relevant substances is listed in the section of DSM-IV concerning psychotic disorders. When the condition is clinically relevant and when evidence exists that a substance, such as alcohol, capable of causing the psychotic symptoms, was involved, a label of a substance-induced psychotic disorder—in this instance alcohol-induced psychotic disorder—can be made. Although detailed criteria are not offered here, additional criteria have been developed for substance-induced sexual dysfunction (see Section 21.1a) and sleep disorders (see Chapter 23), both of which syndromes are relevant to alcohol.

TABLE 13.2-3
Alcohol-Related disorders

Alcohol use disorders

Alcohol dependence
Alcohol abuse

Alcohol-induced disorders

Alcohol intoxication
Alcohol withdrawal
Specify if: with perceptual disturbances
Alcohol intoxication delirium
Alcohol withdrawal delirium
Alcohol-induced persisting dementia
Alcohol-induced persisting amnestic disorder
Alcohol-induced psychotic disorder, with delusions
Specify if: with onset during intoxication/with onset during withdrawal
Alcohol-induced psychotic disorder, with hallucinations
Specify if: with onset during intoxication/with onset during withdrawal
Alcohol-induced mood disorder
Specify if: with onset during intoxication/with onset during withdrawal
Alcohol-induced anxiety dirorder
Specify if: with onset during intoxication/with onset during withdrawal
Alcohol-induced sexual dysfunction
Specify if: with onset during intoxication
Alcohol-induced sleep disorder
Specify if: with onset during intoxication/with onset during withdrawal

Alcohol-related disorder not otherwise specified

Table from DSM-IV, *Diagnostic and Statistical Manual of Mental Disorders,* ed 4. Copyright American Psychiatric Association, Washington, 1993. Used with permission.

ALCOHOL DEPENDENCE In DSM-IV all substance-related disorders use the same criteria for dependence and abuse (see

Tables 13.1-2, 13.1-5, and 13.1-6). Dependence concerns a history of a broad array of problems, including compulsive intake of alcohol, an increasingly important place in life occupied by the substance, and evidence of physical withdrawal symptoms. Dependence criteria also concern life impairment related to the substance.

Physical dependence or addiction is a phenomenon that appears to be related to tolerance. As the body changes to resist the effects of alcohol, it is likely to reach a condition in which it cannot function optimally unless the brain depressant is present. That condition takes days or weeks to develop.

The DSM-IV diagnostic criteria presented in Table 13.1-2 are based on the nine basic items from DSM-III-R. As noted briefly above, the field trial for DSM-IV indicated that DSM-III-R items 8 and 9 dealing with two aspects of withdrawal could effectively be combined into one item (item 1) in DSM-IV. Part of item four in DSM-III-R, use in hazardous situations, was moved under abuse with other social, legal, interpersonal, and occupational difficulties, as was evidence of failure in role obligations. Thus, DSM-IV substance dependence criteria include seven items which are subsets of the nine originally listed in DSM-III-R. Those seven items are similar to ICD-10 dependence syndrome criteria, although ICD-10 deals more directly with evidence of a compulsion to use. In addition, while maintaining the broad concept of dependence that appeared in DSM-III-R, DSM-IV asks the clinician to use the two items that deal with tolerance or withdrawal to subdivide dependent persons into those with and those without evidence of physiological symptoms. That division allows clinicians and researchers to determine the treatment and the prognostic implications of tolerance and withdrawal. The framers of DSM-V in the 21st century will then have data to help them decide whether to move back toward the emphasis on physiological symptoms that characterized earlier manuals.

A 39-year-old male junior high school teacher came for evaluation because of deteriorating performance at work. A careful history was taken independently from the patient and from his wife. The history focused on levels of life functioning, problem areas, and the ways in which alcohol may have contributed to the patient's life problems. After establishing a series of life difficulties, the evaluators focused in on the alcohol-use history, looking for evidence of tolerance and symptoms that developed when the patient abstained from alcohol. His history indicated repeated successful efforts to cut down or control the use of alcohol, excessive amounts of time spent using alcohol, and recurrent interference with his ability to fulfill major role obligations. His was a typical case of alcohol dependence.

ALCOHOL ABUSE As shown in Table 13.1-6, the diagnostic criteria for abuse focus on the impairment of social, legal, interpersonal, and occupational functioning. The criteria were developed through careful comparisons of DSM-III and DSM-III-R concepts and were refined through a series of reanalyses of existing data sets and a large field trial of the criteria for abuse and dependence. The field trial involved comparisons of clinical coverage and demographic correlates of DSM-III-R and possible DSM-IV criteria, as applied to more than 1,000 men and women from diverse groups and representing both persons from the general population and those with diverse substance problems in six centers in the United States and four locations in other countries.

ALCOHOL INTOXICATION The description of alcohol intoxication outlined in Table 13.2-4 is straightforward. The diagnostic criteria are based on evidence of recent ingestion of ethanol, maladoptive behavior, and at least one of six possible physiological correlates of intoxication. As a conservative approach to identifying blood levels that are likely to have major effects on driving abilities in the majority of people, the legal definition of intoxication in most states in the United States requires a blood concentration of 80 or 100 milligrams of ethanol per 100 milliliters or deciliter of blood (mg/dL). That is the same as 0.08 to 0.10 grams per deciliter (g/dL). For most people, a rough estimate of the levels of impairment likely to be seen at various blood alcohol concentrations can be outlined. Evidence of behavioral changes, a slowing in motor performance, and a decrease in the ability to think clearly occurs at doses as low as 20 to 30 mg/dL, as shown in Table 13.2-5. Blood levels between 100 and 200 mg/dL are likely to produce a progression of the impairment in coordination and judgment to severe problems with coordination (ataxia), increasing lability of mood, and progressively greater levels of cognitive deterioration. Anyone who does not show significant levels of impairment in motor and mental performance at about 150 mg/dL probably has significant pharmacodynamic tolerance. In that range most persons without significant tolerance also experiences relatively severe nausea and vomiting. With blood alcohol levels in the 200 to 300 mg/dL range, the slurring of speech is likely to become more intense, and memory impairment (anterograde amnesia or alcoholic *blackouts*) becomes pronounced. Further increases in blood alcohol levels result in the first level of anesthesia, and the nontolerant person who reaches 400 mg/dL or higher risks respiratory failure, coma, and death.

Prior editions of DSM also described *alcohol idiosyncratic intoxication*. It was characterized by extreme aggressive behavior occurring within minutes of ingesting relatively small amounts of alcohol, such as two drinks. The person was usually amnestic for the episode, and the aggressiveness was atypical of the person's usual sober comportment. However, a literature review before the publication of DSM-IV revealed little convincing evidence that such a disorder really exists, and it was deleted from the manual.

TABLE 13.2-4
Diagnostic Criteria for Alcohol Intoxication

A. Recent ingestion of alcohol.
B. Clinically significant maladaptive behavior or psychological changes (e.g., inappropriate sexual or aggressive behavior, mood lability, impaired judgment, impaired social or occupational functioning) that developed during, or shortly after, alcohol ingestion.
C. One (or more) of the following signs, developing during, or shortly after, alcohol use:
(1) slurred speech
(2) incoordination
(3) unsteady gait
(4) nystagmus
(5) impairment in attention or memory
(6) stupor or coma
D. The symptoms are not due to a general medical condition and are not better accounted for by another mental disorder.

Table from DSM-IV, *Diagnostic and Statistical Manual of Mental Disorders*, ed 4. Copyright American Psychiatric Association, Washington, 1994. Used with permission.

TABLE 13.2-5
Impairment Likely to Be Seen at Different Blood Alcohol Levels

Level	Likely Impairment
20–30 mg/dL	Slowed motor performance and decreased thinking ability
30–80 mg/dL	Increases in motor and cognitive problems
80–200 mg/dL	Increases in incoordination and judgment errors Mood lability Deterioration in cognition
200–300 mg/dL	Nystagmus, marked slurring of speech, and alcoholic blackouts
>300 mg/dL	Impaired vital signs and possible death

ALCOHOL WITHDRAWAL In persons who have been drinking heavily over a prolonged period of time, any rapid decrease in the amount of alcohol in the body is likely to produce a variety of physical symptoms. That withdrawal or abstinence syndrome is characterized by a group of symptoms that are the opposite of what was initially experienced with intoxication. Therefore, after a person is physically dependent on alcohol, the rapid onset of abstinence is likely to be accompanied by a coarse tremor of the hands, insomnia, anxiety, and increased blood pressure, heart rate, body temperature, and respiratory rate—a condition labeled *alcohol withdrawal* and described in Table 13.2-6. The symptoms rarely include convulsions or delirium. The symptoms are likely to begin within eight hours of relative abstinence, reach a peak intensity on the second or third day, and markedly diminish by the fourth or fifth day. The symptoms can persist in a mild form for three to six months or more as part of a protracted withdrawal syndrome.

A 41-year-old man decided to stop drinking one Saturday night after his wife told him that she would leave him unless he abstained. The next morning he awoke with a tremor of the hands; he felt nauseated and thought he had the flu or a bad hangover. A physical examination confirmed the mild tremor and revealed a pulse rate of 100, a respiratory rate of 21, and a blood pressure reading of 135/90. The patient continued to experience those signs and symptoms at the same level of intensity for two days, after which they rapidly disappeared. His was a typical case of alcohol withdrawal.

ALCOHOL INTOXICATION AND WITHDRAWAL DELIRIUM DSM-IV also contains the diagnoses of alcohol intoxication delirium and alcohol withdrawal delirium (see Chapter 12).

When the symptoms of withdrawal are accompanied by a state of severe agitated confusion or delirium, sometimes associated with tactile or visual hallucinations, the diagnosis of *alcohol withdrawal delirium* (in the past called delirium tremens or DTs) can be made. During withdrawal, some alcoholic persons show one or sometimes several grand mal convulsions, which have sometimes been called rum fits.

A 41-year-old male school principal entered a hospital for gallbladder surgery. His surgeon was not aware of the patient's daily intake of 8 to 12 beers. Thus, the treatment personnel were surprised when, approximately 18 hours postoperatively, the patient had a pulse rate of 120, a respiratory rate of 25, an oral temperature of 101°F, and evidence of extreme agitated confusion. His relatively rare case of delirium, visual hallucinations, and severe autonomic hyperactivity—delirium tremens or DTs—remained intense for approximately 48 hours; after that the signs and symptoms decreased, disappearing by the fourth day. His condition is labeled as alcohol withdrawal delirium in DSM-IV.

TABLE 13.2-6
Diagnostic Criteria for Alcohol Withdrawal

A. Cessation of (or reduction in) alcohol use that has been heavy and prolonged.
B. Two (or more) of the following, developing within several hours to a few days after criterion A:
   (1) autonomic hyperactivity (e.g., sweating or pulse rate greater than 100)
   (2) increased hand tremor
   (3) insomnia
   (4) nausea or vomiting
   (5) transient visual, tactile, or auditory hallucinations or illusions
   (6) psychomotor agitation
   (7) anxiety
   (8) grand mal seizures
C. The symptoms in criterion B cause clinically significant distress or impairment in social, occupational, or other important areas of functioning.
D. The symptoms are not due to a general medical condition and not better accounted for by another mental disorder.

Specify if:
With perceptual disturbances

Table from DSM-IV, *Diagnostic and Statistical Manual of Mental Disorders,* ed 4. Copyright American Psychiatric Association, Washington, 1993. Used with permission.

ALCOHOL-INDUCED PERSISTING AMNESTIC DISORDER One of the most intensely studied alcohol-related CNS syndromes is the relatively rare DSM-IV diagnosis of alcohol-induced persisting amnestic disorder (see Chapter 12), which is the result of a relatively severe deficiency in the B vitamin thiamine. Some persons are at higher risk for this syndrome than are others because of a genetically influenced transketolase deficiency. The condition has been historically subdivided into (1) *Wernicke's syndrome,* with prominent ataxia and palsy of the sixth cranial nerve, a condition that tends to reverse fairly rapidly with vitamin supplementation, and (2) *Korsakoff's syndrome,* which is permanent in at least a partial form in perhaps 50 to 70 percent of the persons affected. Korsakoff's syndrome is characterized by a pronounced anterograde and retrograde amnesia and potential impairment in visuospatial, abstract, and other types of learning. In most cases, the level of recent memory is out of proportion to the global level of cognitive impairment. The 25 percent or so of Korsakoff's syndrome patients who are likely to recover fully and the 50 percent or so who recover partially appear to respond to 50 to 100 mg of oral thiamine a day, usually administered for many months.

ALCOHOL-INDUCED PERSISTING DEMENTIA An alcohol-related CNS diagnosis very relevant to psychiatry is a long-term cognitive problem that can develop in the course of alcoholism, namely alcohol-induced persisting dementia (see Chapter 12). Global decreases in intellectual functioning, cognitive abilities, and memory are observed. At the same time, recent memory difficulties are consistent with global cognitive impairment, an observation that helps to distinguish the syndrome from alcohol-induced persisting amnestic disorder. The decreased brain functioning, including problems with psychomotor performance, tends to improve with abstinence, but perhaps half of all affected patients have long-term and even permanent memory and thinking disabilities. Perhaps 50 to 70 percent of those patients evidence increased size of the brain ventricles and shrinkage of the cerebral sulci, although those changes appear to be partially or, at times, completely reversible during the first year of complete abstinence. In the final analysis, it is unlikely that there is a single alcoholic dementia syndrome. Rather, the problem seems to represent the combined effects of trauma, vitamin deficiencies, and the direct actions of alcohol and acetaldehyde.

ALCOHOL-INDUCED MOOD DISORDER In the context of heavy and repetitive intake of any brain depressant, such as alcohol, symptoms of severe depression are common and may be labeled as an *alcohol-induced mood disorder.* The diagnosis focuses on sadness or mania severe enough to impair functioning that occurred only in the context of repeated heavy drinking and continued for several days to four weeks after abstinence. Experiments in three research laboratories have found that heavy intake of alcohol over several days results in many of the symptoms observed in major depressive disorder, but the intense sadness reverses within days to weeks of abstinence. Consistent with the contention that intoxication with brain depressants can cause severe symptoms of depression is the documentation that 80 percent of alcoholic persons report histories of intense depression; 30 to 40 percent were depressed for two or more weeks, during which they had symptoms that resembled a major depressive episode. However, when information from patients and resource persons was carefully evaluated, only 5 percent of alcoholic men and 10 percent of alcoholic women ever had depressions meeting the criteria for major depressive disorder when they had not been drinking heavily. (The diagnostic criteria for alcohol-induced mood disorder are given in Section 16.6.)

Clinical data reveal that, when even severe depression develops in alcoholic persons, they are likely to improve fairly rapidly without medications or intensive psychotherapy aimed at the depressive symptoms. A recent study of almost 200 alcoholic men found that 40 percent had severe levels of depression after one week of abstinence. However, the percentage with pervasive depressive symptoms decreased to about 5 percent after three additional weeks of abstention from alcohol, even though no treatment was given for the mood symptoms. Thus, intense depressions that mimic major depressive episodes appear to be common in the context of heavy drinking but are likely to improve markedly over a matter of days or weeks.

At the end of several weeks, most alcoholic patients are no longer depressed all day every day. However, they are left with mood swings or intermittent symptoms of sadness that can resemble cyclothymic disorder or dysthymic disorder. Even those mild and intermittent depressive symptoms are likely to diminish and disappear with time. The presence of the dysthymic symptoms usually indicates the normal course of a withdrawal syndrome and not an independent mood disorder.

A 27-year-old male dockworker was brought to an emergency room after telling his family that he was going to kill himself. His history revealed more than two weeks of depressive symptoms, including crying spells, feelings of hopelessness, difficulties in concentrating, insomnia, and loss of appetite. The review of his life problems taken from both the patient and his wife and a series of blood tests all pointed to the regular intake of at least two six-packs of beer on most days for the preceding three months. Because he showed no evidence of daily severe depression interfering with his functioning except in the context of his heavy drinking, the hospital personnel assumed that the hospitalization for severe suicidal thoughts would be relatively short and that the depressive symptoms would begin to lift fairly rapidly without antidepressant medication or cognitive therapy. Indeed, the man turned out to have an alcohol-induced mood disorder and was discharged to an alcohol treatment program four days after his psychiatric admission to the hospital.

ALCOHOL-INDUCED ANXIETY DISORDER Anxiety symptoms fulfilling the diagnostic criteria for *alcohol-induced anxiety disorder* are also common in the context of acute and protracted alcoholic withdrawal. Almost 80 percent of alcoholic persons report panic attacks during acute withdrawal; their complaints can be intense enough for the clinician to consider diagnosing a panic disorder. Similarly, during the first four to six weeks of abstinence, persons with severe alcohol problems are likely to avoid some social situations for fear of being overwhelmed by anxiety (that is, they have symptoms resembling social phobia); their problems can at times be severe enough to resemble agoraphobia. The symptoms of nervousness during acute and protracted withdrawal can also include many of the problems seen in generalized anxiety disorder. However, when psychological or physiological symptoms of anxiety are observed in alcoholic persons only in the several weeks or months after withdrawal, the symptoms are likely to diminish and subsequently disappear with time. (The diagnostic criteria for alcohol-induced anxiety disorder are given in Section 17.5.) Alcoholic persons are no more likely than are people in the general population to have independent major anxiety disorders. They are, however, much more likely to have temporary but intense symptoms of anxiety.

A 52-year-old businessman was referred to a psychiatrist because of repetitive panic attacks. His history revealed a pattern of approximately five typical panic attacks a week during the preceding six weeks. However, no such problems appeared before then, and a physical workup revealed no evidence of physical pathology that might explain the panic episodes. The history gathered from the patient and his spouse revealed a steady increase in alcohol intake over the preceding year. Typically, the man consumed a half bottle of Scotch each Friday night, each Saturday night, and each Sunday, and he drank at much lower levels during the week. The panic attacks were most likely to occur early in the week, and they were observed in the context of a global picture of sweating, a tremor of the hands, and a flulike feeling. The diagnosis was alcohol dependence and an alcohol-induced anxiety disorder with onset during withdrawal. Treatment for the alcohol dependence was instituted, and the panic attacks disappeared within a month of the patient's achieving and maintaining abstinence.

ALCOHOL-INDUCED PSYCHOTIC DISORDER About 3 percent of alcoholic persons have psychotic symptoms in the context of heavy drinking and withdrawal. In DSM-III-R those problems were labeled organic hallucinosis or delusional disorders. Many of the symptoms resemble those seen in schizophrenia, but, when the psychotic features develop only in the context of alcohol problems, they are likely to clear spontaneously. The syndromes are likely to recur only if heavy alcohol intake resumes. (The diagnostic criteria for an alcohol-induced psychotic disorder are given in Section 15.3.)

A 39-year-old male letter carrier was brought to an emergency room by the police after he behaved in an unusual fashion at home and complained that his neighbors were trying to kill him. The history obtained from the patient and his wife revealed that his psychotic thinking developed slowly over the preceding three weeks; he began with feelings that people were looking at him at work, progressed to vague feelings that people were against him, and went on to frank auditory hallucinations that people at work and in the neighboring houses were talking about their plans to kill him. He had no insight into those paranoid delusions and auditory hallucinations. The relatively abrupt onset of the syndrome in his late 30s pointed to a potential organic cause, and further probing documented his daily drinking of between 6 and 18 beers for at least the preceding 10 weeks. A diagnosis of alcohol-induced psychotic disorder with onset during intoxication was made, and both clinical conditions disappeared after three weeks of abstinence. After alcohol treatment, the man stayed sober for the next eight months. Unfortunately, he later resumed heavy drinking and had a reoccurrence of both his hallucinations and his delusions.

LABORATORY AND PHYSICAL EXAMINATION Establishing the diagnosis for a condition centers on obtaining from the patient and a resource person a history of the patient's life problems and the possible role played by alcohol. Up to one third of all psychiatric patients are likely to have an alcohol problem that either caused or exacerbated the presenting clinical condition.

The process of identification can also be facilitated by a series of blood tests, outlined in Table 13.2-7. Those state markers of heavy drinking reflect physiological alterations likely to be observed if the patient regularly ingests four or more drinks a day over many days or weeks. The most sensitive and specific of the markers (perhaps 80 percent sensitivity and specificity)

TABLE 13.2-7
State Markers of Heavy Drinking Useful in Screening for Alcoholism

Test	Relevant Range of Results
Gamma glutamyl transferase (GGT)	>30 U/L
Mean corpuscular volume (MCV)	>91 μm^3
Uric acid	>6.4 mg/dL for men >5.0 mg/dL for women
Serum glutamic-oxaloacetic transaminase (aspartate aminotransferase) [SGOT (AST)]	>45 IU/L
Serum glutamic-pyruvic transaminase (alanine aminotransferase) [SGPT (ALT)]	>45 IU/L
Triglycerides	>160 mg/dL

is a level of 30 or more units of gamma glutamyl transferase (GGT), an enzyme that aids in the transport of amino acids and that is found in most areas of the body. Because that enzyme is likely to return to normal levels after two to four weeks of abstinence, even 20 percent increases in enzyme levels above those observed after four weeks of abstinence can be useful in identifying patients who have returned to drinking after treatment. A second blood test, mean corpuscular volume (MCV), with perhaps 70 percent sensitivity and specificity, is a state marker when the size of the red blood cell is 91 or more cubic mircometers. The 120-day life span of the red cell does not allow the test to be used as an indicator of a return to drinking after a month or so of abstinence. Other tests that can be helpful in identifying patients who are regularly consuming heavy doses of alcohol include those for high normal levels of uric acid (greater than 6.4 mg/dL, with a range that depends on the sex of the person); mild elevations in the usual liver function tests, including aspartate aminotransferase and alanine aminotransferase; and elevated levels of triglycerides or LDLC.

A number of physical findings can also be useful in identifying the otherwise hidden alcoholic patient. Those findings include modest elevations in blood pressure, frequent bruising, cancer of the head and neck and upper digestive tract, an enlarged liver, evidence of cirrhosis, and symptoms consistent with pancreatitis.

A 44-year-old married woman worked part-time as a clerk at a convenience store. She went to a psychiatrist, referred by her family physician, because of irritability, difficulty in getting along with her husband, and complaints of trouble in falling asleep and staying asleep. The evaluation did not reveal evidence of a major depressive episode or an anxiety disorder, but the history focusing on life problems revealed two driving-while-intoxicated arrests, repeated time missed at work because of severe hangovers, evidence of tolerance to alcohol, and difficulties in relationships at home related to her behavior while drinking heavily. Blood tests revealed a GGT level of 45 U/L, a uric acid level of 6.9 mg/dL, and an SGOT level of 55 IU/L. The laboratory results not only confirmed the suspicion of alcohol problems and allowed the psychiatrist to probe further into the patient's alcohol-use history but were also an important tool in trying to help the patient realize that alcohol was a major factor in her life and had begun to produce adverse physical effects.

DIFFERENTIAL DIAGNOSIS

Once the pattern of alcohol-related life problems has been established, the diagnosis of alcohol abuse or dependence is fairly obvious. However, a major difficulty involved in the differential diagnosis of alcoholism is the fact that severe and heavy intake of alcohol and associated withdrawal syndromes can mimic other psychiatric disorders. Another problem is the heightened risk for subsequent alcohol-related disorders seen with the antisocial personality disorder, schizophrenia, and bipolar I disorder.

Family, twin, and adoption studies are consistent with the conclusion that temporary depressive and anxiety syndromes seen in the context of alcoholic intoxication and withdrawal do not usually indicate independent psychiatric disorders. Family investigations controlled for the effects of assortative mating between alcoholic persons and those with other psychiatric disorders have failed to find a heightened risk for severe anxiety and depressive syndromes in relatives of persons with alcohol-related disorders. Similarly, identical twins of primary alcoholic persons are not at high risk for other psychiatric syndromes except when they drink heavily. The adoption studies of the children of alcoholic persons underscore the lack of an enhanced rate of independent psychiatric disorders among relatives of persons with alcohol-related disorders. The half sibling and adoption investigations have failed to find higher than usual rates of depressive, anxiety, or psychotic disorders among alcoholic persons' offspring who were adopted out and raised separately from their alcoholic biological parents.

When the time line reveals a patient who had severe antisocial behaviors in many life areas before the onset of severe alcohol problems, he or she is likely to have antisocial personality disorder, not alcoholism. Similarly, someone with a schizophrenic, manic-depressive, or anxiety syndrome either before the onset of alcoholism or lasting for more than four weeks of abstinence may have an independent psychiatric disorder. In that case, after addressing the patient's medical problems, taking care of any symptoms of withdrawal, and considering the possibility of the eventual need for alcohol rehabilitation, the clinician must pay careful attention to the treatment of the independent psychiatric disorder. However, when psychiatric symptoms are seen only in the course of alcohol abuse or dependence, careful attention to protecting the patients from hurting themselves during the temporary depression or psychotic symptoms and emphasis on alcoholic rehabilitation are probably sufficient to deal with the temporary psychiatric problems.

ALCOHOL-RELATED DISORDER NOT OTHERWISE SPECIFIED DSN-IV allows for the diagnosis of alcohol-related disorder not otherwise specified (NOS) for alcohol-related disorders that do not meet the diagnostic criteria for any of the other disgnoses (Table 13.2-8).

ANTISOCIAL PERSONALITY DISORDER When the emphasis on the chronological development of symptoms is used, at least three diagnoses—antisocial personality disorder, schizophrenia, and bipolar I disorder—are likely to predate alcohol abuse or dependence and to be true comorbid conditions. Antisocial personality disorder, listed on Axis II, begins early in life and has major effects on many aspects of life functioning. The diagnosis is based on evidence of severe antisocial behaviors in many areas beginning before the age of 15 years and continuing into adulthood. Persons with antisocial personality disorder are described as impulsive, frequently violent, highly likely to take risks, and unable to learn from their mistakes or to benefit from punishment. Someone carrying those characteristics into adolescence, the usual time of the initiation of experimentation with alcohol and drugs, can be expected to have difficulty in controlling substance use. Thus, perhaps 80 percent or more of persons with antisocial personality disorder are likely to have severe secondary alcohol problems in the course of their lives. The notation of preexisting antisocial personality disorder with subsequent alcohol dependence indicates someone who is more likely than the average alcoholic person to have severe coexisting drug problems, to be violent during

Table 13.2-8
Diagnostic Criteria for Alcohol-Related Disorder Not Otherwise Specified

The alcohol-related disorder not otherwise specified category is for disorders associated with the use of alcohol that are not classifiable as alcohol dependence, alcohol abuse, alcohol intoxication, alcohol withdrawal, alcohol intoxication delirium, alcohol withdrawal delirium, alcohol-induced persisting demential, alcohol-induced persisting amnestic disorder, alcohol-induced psychotic disorder, alcohol-induced mood disorder, alcohol-induced anxiety disorder, alcohol-induced sexual dysfunction, or alcohol-induced sleep disorder.

treatment, to sign out early from treatment, and to have a much less than optimistic prognosis. Debate continues on the optimal manner of viewing the co-occurrence of antisocial personality disorder and alcoholism, but most researchers agree that the personality disorder is a separate entity worthy of diagnosis, with the probability that the genetic factors that increase the risk for antisocial personality disorder are separate from those that affect the development of alcoholism. In most treatment programs perhaps 5 percent of alcoholic women and between 10 and 20 percent of alcoholic men have preexisting antisocial personality disorder. Other Axis II-type symptoms are often observed during intoxication and as part of the acute and protracted abstinence syndromes, but they have not been documented to predate the alcohol-related disorders.

SCHIZOPHRENIA A second disorder in which secondary alcohol problems are more common than in the general population is schizophrenia. Characterized by what is usually a slow onset of paranoid delusions and auditory hallucinations in a clear sensorium typically beginning in the mid teens to the 20s, schizophrenia is likely to be severe and debilitating. Perhaps related to the lack of long-term treatment facilities is the observation that schizophrenic persons are likely to live in inner-city areas and to spend a great deal of time on the streets. In an effort to decrease feelings of isolation or perhaps in an effort to self-medicate their symptoms, persons with the disorder are more likely than the general population to go on to have severe alcohol-related life problems. Their alcohol intake is likely to undercut the effectiveness of appropriate antipsychotic medications, to increase mood swings and signs of psychoses, and to contribute to a downward course of schizophrenia that entails repeatedly revolving into and out of inpatient care. Because most alcohol treatment programs exclude actively psychotic patients, schizophrenic persons rarely appear in inpatient alcohol treatment programs, although severe alcohol-related disorders are observed in 30 percent or so of schizophrenic persons being treated in public mental health facilities.

A 23-year-old woman was brought in for her sixth hospitalization because of her delusions that her parents were plotting to kill her. Her psychotic disorder developed insidiously at approximately age 17 with a gradual loss of contact with friends, a loss of interest in school work, and decreased attention to her personal hygiene. She was experiencing both auditory hallucinations and paranoid delusions, and a diagnosis of schizophrenia was made. After discharge from a psychiatric hospital, she was sent to a mental health halfway house in a central-city area, where, despite the prescription of antipsychotic drugs, she began to increase her alcohol intake and experimented with other drugs of abuse. The two years before the most recent hospitalization were characterized by repeated episodes of acute psychiatric emergency treatment, stabilization of her situation with antipsychotic medication, discharge from a hospital in a stable condition, and a return to her inner-city living situation. Soon after, she escalated her alcohol intake to a pint of vodka and a six-pack of beer every day. Her drinking was associated with an increase in her paranoid delusions. She would stop taking her medications, have a marked increase in her psychotic behavior, and be brought in for yet another emergency psychiatric hospitalization.

BIPOLAR DISORDER The third disorder in which severe alcohol problems are overrepresented is bipolar I disorder. In a manic episode, the patient is hyperexcited and impulsive, carries out most activities to excess, has poor judgment, and, it is thought, is likely to develop temporary alcohol problems. The severity of the manic symptoms usually precludes inpatient alcohol rehabilitation. However, alcohol-related difficulties must be evaluated in histories taken from persons with manic features entering mental health facilities.

OTHER DISORDERS Debate in the literature continues about whether major depressive episode, panic disorder, social phobia, and other major psychiatric diagnoses are overrepresented in the histories of alcoholic persons. Several studies indicate that, when the time-line method is used and a history is obtained from many informants, little evidence is found of high rates of independent psychiatric disorders among alcoholic persons, other than the three disorders noted above. Similarly, when the alcoholic person does not have multiple independent disorders, the rates of anxiety disorders, psychoses, and major depressive episodes are not found to be elevated in family members. Therefore, although the majority of alcoholic persons have temporary psychiatric symptoms, they are not more likely than are persons in the general population to carry an independent psychiatric syndrome with the three exceptions discussed above.

COURSE AND PROGNOSIS

Details of a clinical course that fit the great majority of persons with any disorder are difficult to describe. However, sufficient data regarding alcohol-related disorders are available to offer a general outline of the typical pattern of problems.

EARLY COURSE Patients with antisocial personality disorder who later go on to alcoholism have an early onset of drinking, intoxication, and alcohol-related problems, but that scenario is not applicable to the other 85 to 90 percent of alcoholic men and 95 percent of alcoholic women. Usually, alcoholic persons have their first drink (other than taking a sip from a parent's glass) between the ages of 13 and 15 years, the first intoxication is likely to occur at 15 or 16 years, and the first evidence of a minor alcohol-related problem is usually observed in the late teens. Those milestones do not differ significantly from what is expected for people in the general population who do not later have alcohol abuse or dependence problems.

For the average person the pattern of severe difficulties becomes apparent in the mid 20s to mid 30s. That is when a constellation of symptoms of relatively great severity is likely to be observed: an alcohol-related breakup of a significant relationship, a second alcohol-related driving or public intoxication arrest, evidence of alcoholic withdrawal, being told by a physician that alcohol has harmed the person's health, or significant interference with functioning at school or work. That pattern probably does not vary much with the type of beverage used, whether beer, wine, or spirits.

The landmarks in Table 13.2-9 are only rough estimates and can differ greatly between people and among various groups. Women, for example, are likely to begin drinking later than men, but their subsequent escalation of symptoms is likely to be more rapid than that seen in men.

LATER COURSE Once alcohol's interference with life functioning has become apparent, the future is likely to include peri-

TABLE 13.2-9
Clinical Course of Alcohol Dependence

Age at first drink*	13–15 years
Age at first intoxication*	15–17 years
Age at first problem*	16–22 years
Age at onset of dependence	25–40 years
Age at death	60 years
Fluctuating course of abstention, temporary control, alcohol problems	
Spontaneous remission in 20 percent	

*Same as general population.

ods of drinking problems that repeatedly alternate with periods of abstinence and evidence of temporary periods of alcohol intake unassociated with problems *(temporary controlled drinking)*. Abstinence often develops in response to some interpersonal, social, or legal crisis and is likely to produce only mild withdrawal symptoms. Average alcoholic persons are then likely to use the temporary cessation of drinking problems to convince themselves that alcohol is not really a cause for concern after all. Those periods of abstinence, lasting days to months, are common in the course of most persons with alcoholism and are usually followed by periods during which drinking rules are established and are temporarily followed. The person is likely to consume only beer or wine (forgetting that a glass of beer, a glass of wine, and a shot of whiskey have similar amounts of alcohol) and tries to drink only at certain times of the day and under certain conditions. That period of temporary control soon leads to an escalation of alcohol intake, the accumulation of a new set of problems, and a subsequent crisis. Those events, in turn, are likely to precipitate a new period of abstinence, and the cycle begins again. Thus, controlled drinking is a common but temporary condition for most alcoholic persons. Those who have less intense alcohol problems, such as those who may fulfill the diagnostic criteria for alcohol abuse in DSM-IV, are probably more likely to have long-term and even permanent periods of control. However, several research projects have indicated that long-term continued control is not likely to be seen once a person meets the diagnostic criteria for alcohol dependence.

An additional attribute important in the course of alcohol dependence is the phenomenon of spontaneous remission. Perhaps in response to nonspecific events or to a crisis, the alcoholic person promises to abstain and keeps the promise forever. Whatever the cause of the abstinence, about 20 percent or more of alcoholic persons, if followed over a long enough period of time, probably do achieve permanent abstinence, even without formal treatment or participation in such self-help groups as Alcoholics Anonymous (AA).

PROGNOSIS Between 10 and 40 percent of alcoholic persons enter some kind of formal treatment program during the course of their alcohol problems. A number of prognostic signs are favorable. First is the absence of preexisting antisocial personality disorder or a diagnosis of drug dependence. Second, evidence of general life stability with a job, continuing close family contacts, and the absence of severe legal problems also bodes well for the patient. Third, if the patient stays for the full course of the initial rehabilitation (perhaps two to four weeks), the chances of maintaining abstinence are good. In fact, the combination of those three attributes predicts a 60 percent chance for one or more years of abstinence. Few studies have documented the long-term course, but researchers agree that one year of abstinence is associated with a good chance for continued abstinence over an extended period of time. However, alcoholic persons with severe drug problems (especially intravenous drug use or cocaine or amphetamine dependence) and those residing on skid row may have only a 10 percent or so chance of achieving one year of abstinence.

Accurately predicting whether any specific person will achieve or maintain abstinence is impossible, but the prognostic factors listed above are associated with a high likelihood of abstinence. However, the factors reflecting life stability probably explain only 20 percent or less of the course of alcohol-use disorders. Many forces that are difficult to measure have significant effects on the clinical course. They are likely to include such intangibles as levels of motivation and the quality of the patient's social support system.

In general, alcoholic persons with preexisting independent major psychiatric disorders—such as antisocial personality disorder, schizophrenia, and bipolar I disorder—are likely to run the course of their independent psychiatric illness. Therefore, clinicians must treat the bipolar I disorder patient who has secondary alcoholism with appropriate psychotherapy and lithium, use relevant psychological and behavioral techniques for the patient with antisocial personality disorder, and offer appropriate antipsychotic medications on a long-term basis to the patient with schizophrenia. The goal is to keep the symptoms of the independent psychiatric disorder as minimal as possible in the hope that a greater level of life stability will be associated with a better prognosis for the patient's alcohol problems.

TREATMENT

The elements of treatment appropriate for patients with severe alcohol problems are fairly straightforward. Much of the clinical challenge comes in recognizing how prevalent alcohol-related disorders are and how often those conditions present with symptoms of other psychiatric syndromes and in learning to use clinical clues, physical findings, and laboratory tests to identify alcoholism.

Three general steps are involved in treating the alcoholic person once the disorder has been diagnosed—confrontation, detoxification, and rehabilitation. Those approaches assume that all possible efforts have been made to optimize medical functioning and to address psychiatric emergencies. Thus, the alcoholic person with symptoms of depression severe enough to be suicidal requires inpatient hospitalization for at least several days until the suicidal ideation disappears; the person presenting with cardiomyopathy, liver difficulties, or gastrointestinal bleeding first needs adequate attention paid to the medical emergency. The patient with alcohol dependence must then be confronted with the disorder, be detoxified if needed, and begin rehabilitation. The essentials of those three steps for an alcoholic person with independent psychiatric syndromes are quite similar to the approaches used for the primary alcoholic person without independent psychiatric syndromes but are applied after the psychiatric disorder has been stabilized to the maximum degree possible.

CONFRONTATION The goal is to break through feelings of denial and to help the patient recognize the adverse consequences likely to occur if the disorder is not treated. Another way of describing confrontation is as a process aimed at increasing the levels of motivation for treatment and for continued abstinence to as high a level as possible.

Confrontation often involves convincing patients that they are responsible for their own actions while reminding them how alcohol has created significant life impairments. The psychiatrist often finds it useful to take advantage of the person's chief complaint, whether it is insomnia, difficulties with sexual performance, an inability to cope with life stresses, depression, anxiety, or psychotic symptoms. Then the psychiatrist can teach the patient how alcohol has either created or contributed to those problems and can reassure the patient that abstinence can be achieved with a minimum of discomfort.

A 38-year-old male college professor had alcohol-related difficulties severe enough to qualify for a diagnosis of alcohol dependence that dated back at least eight years. The pattern of pathological drinking usually involved three or so months of difficulties, followed by several months of abstinence, and then more alcohol-related difficulties. His high level of interpersonal skills allowed him to have close relationships (despite two failed marriages), and his intelligence and personal competence allowed him to function relatively well on the job. However, he had repeated problems, including complaints by each of his ex-wives about the way alcohol interfered with his relationships with them, difficulty in focusing at work as an English teacher, occasional complaints by students regarding his inattentiveness or inability to keep regular office hours, and complaints by his chairperson that he was not publishing enough papers to guarantee continued promotions. The confrontations regarding alcohol dependence were carried out by a close colleague, who often spoke to the patient several days after he had observed inappropriate levels of intoxication at department parties, who called the patient whenever students complained of his lack of availability, and who consulted him when he was passed over for promotion. The confrontations showed the patient that someone could be trusted and understood the problems. When the patient was arrested for the second time on a charge of driving while intoxicated, he called the friend, who arranged for an immediate referral to a knowledgeable physician for evaluation and subsequent treatment.

A physician confronting a patient can use the same nonjudgmental but persistent approach each time an alcohol-related impairment is identified. It is the level of persistence, rather than exceptional confrontation skills, that ususally gets results. A single confrontation is rarely enough. Most alcoholic persons need a series of reminders of how alcohol contributed to each developing crisis before they seriously consider abstinence as a long-term option.

Family The family can be of great help in confrontation. Family members must learn to refrain from protecting the patient from the problems caused by alcohol. Otherwise, the patient may not be able to gather the energy and the concentration necessary to stop drinking.

During the confrontation stage, the family can also suggest that the patient meet with persons who are themselves recovering from alcoholism, perhaps through AA, and they can meet with groups that reach out to family members, such as Alanon. Those support groups for families meet many times a week. They help family members and friends see that they are not alone in their fears, worry, and feelings of guilt. Members share coping strategies and help each other find community resources. The groups can be most important in helping family members rebuild their lives, even if the alcoholic person refuses to seek help.

DETOXIFICATION Most persons with alcohol abuse or dependence have relatively mild symptoms when they stop drinking. If the patient is in relatively good health and adequately nourished and has a good social support system, the depressant withdrawal syndrome usually resembles a mild case of the flu. Even intense withdrawal syndromes rarely approach the severity of symptoms described in some early textbooks in the field.

The essential first step in detoxification is a thorough physical examination. In the absence of a severe medical disorder or combined drug abuse, severe alcohol withdrawal is unlikely. The second step is to offer rest, adequate nutrition, and multiple vitamins, especially those containing thiamine.

Mild withdrawal Withdrawal develops because the brain has physically adapted to the presence of a brain depressant and cannot function adequately in the absence of the drug. Giving enough of a brain depressant on the first day to diminish symptoms and then weaning the patient off the drug over the subsequent five days offers most patients optimal relief and minimizes the possibility that a severe withdrawal will develop. Any depressant—including alcohol, barbiturates, or any of the benzodiazepines—can work, but most clinicians chose a benzodiazepine for its relative safety. Adequate treatment can be given with either short-acting drugs, such as lorazepam (Ativan), or long-acting substances, such as chlordiazepoxide (Librium) and diazepam (Valium).

An example of treatment is the administration of 25 mg of chlordiazepoxide by mouth three or four times a day on the first day, with a notation to skip a dose if the patient is asleep or feeling sleepy. An additional one or two 25-mg doses during that first 24 hours can be used if the patient is jittery or shows signs of increasing tremor or autonomic dysfunction. Whatever the dosage required on the first day, the benzodiazepine can be decreased by 20 percent of the original day's dosage each subsequent day, with a resulting need for no further medication after four or five days. When using a long-acting agent, such as chlordiazepoxide, the clinician must avoid producing excessive sleepiness through overmedication. If the patient is sleepy, the next scheduled dose should be omitted. When taking a short-acting drug, such as lorazepam, the patient must not miss any dose, since rapid changes in blood benzodiazepine levels may precipitate a severe withdrawal.

A social model program of detoxification saves money by avoiding medications while using social supports. That less expensive regimen can be helpful for mild or moderate withdrawal syndromes. Some clinicians have also recommended β-blocker drugs like propranolol (Inderal) or α-agonists like clonidine (Catapres), although those medications do not appear to be superior to the benzodiazepines. In contrast to the brain depressants, those other agents do little to decrease the risk of seizures or delirium.

Severe withdrawal For the 3 percent or so of alcoholic patients with extreme autonomic dysfunction, agitation, and confusion—that is, those with alcoholic withdrawal delirium, also called DTs—no optimal treatment has yet been developed. The key first step is to ask why such a severe and relatively uncommon withdrawal syndrome has occurred; the answer often relates to a severe concomitant medical problem that needs immediate treatment. The withdrawal symptoms can then be minimized either through the use of benzodiazepines (in which case high doses are at times required) or through antipsychotic agents, such as haloperidol (Haldol) and thioridazine (Mellaril). Once again, doses are used on the first or second day to control behavior, and the patient can be weaned off the medication by the fifth day.

Another 3 percent of patients may have a single grand mal convulsion; the rare person has multiple fits. The peak incidence is on the second day of withdrawal. Such patients require a neurological evaluation, but, in the absence of evidence of a seizure disorder, they do not benefit from anticonvulsant drugs.

REHABILITATION For most patients, rehabilitation includes two major components: (1) continued efforts to increase and maintain high levels of motivation for abstinence and (2) work to help the patient readjust to a life-style free of alcohol. Because those steps are carried out in the context of acute and protracted withdrawal syndromes and life crises, treatment requires repeated presentations of similar materials that remind the patient how important abstinence is and that help the patient develop new day-to-day support systems and coping styles.

No single major life event, traumatic life period, or identifiable psychiatric disorder is a unique cause of alcoholism. In addition, the effects of any causes of alcoholism are likely to have been diluted by the effects of alcohol on the brain and the years of an altered life-style, so that the alcoholism has developed a life of its own. Those statements are true even though many alcoholic persons believe that the cause was depression, anxiety, life stress, pain syndromes, and so on. Research, data from records, and resource persons usually reveal that the alcohol contributed to the mood disorder, accident, or life stress, not vice versa.

The same general treatment approach is used for both inpatient and outpatient settings. The selection of the more expensive and intensive inpatient mode often depends on evidence of additional severe medical or psychiatric syndromes, the absence of appropriate nearby outpatient groups and facilities, and the patient's history of having tried but failed in outpatient care. The treatment process in either setting involves confrontation, optimizing physical and psychological functioning, enhancing motivation, reaching out to family, and using the first two to four weeks of care as an intensive period of help. Those efforts must be followed by at least three to six months of less frequent outpatient care. Outpatient care uses a combination of individual and group counseling, the judicious avoidance of psychotropic medications, and involvement in such self-help groups as AA.

Counseling Counseling efforts in the first several months should focus on day-to-day life issues to help patients enhance their levels of functioning. Psychotherapy techniques that provoke anxiety or that require deep insights have not been shown to be of benefit during the early months of recovery and, at least theoretically, may actually impair efforts at maintaining abstinence. Therefore, this discussion focuses on the efforts likely to characterize the first three to six months of care.

Counseling or therapy can be carried out in an individual or group setting; few data indicate that either approach is superior to the other. The technique used is not likely to matter and usually boils down to simple day-to-day counseling or almost any behavioral or psychotherapeutic approach focusing on the here and now. Treatment sessions should explore the consequences of drinking, the likely future course of alcohol-related life problems, and the marked improvement that can be expected with abstinence. Whether in an inpatient or an outpatient setting, individual or group counseling is usually offered for a minimum of three times a week for the first two to four weeks, followed by less intense efforts, perhaps once a week, for the subsequent three to six months.

Much time in counseling deals with how to build a life-style free of alcohol. Discussions cover the need for a sober peer group, a plan for social and recreational events without drinking, approaches for reestablishing communication with family members and friends, and identifying situations in which the risk for relapse is high. The counselor must help the patient develop modes of coping to be used when the craving for alcohol increases or when any event or emotional state makes a return to drinking likely.

An important part of therapy is reminding the patient about the appropriate attitude toward slips. Those short-term experiences with alcohol can never be used as an excuse for returning to regular drinking. The efforts to achieve and maintain a sober life-style are not a game in which all benefits are lost with that first sip. Rather, recovery is a process of trial and error; the patient uses slips when they occur to identify high-risk situations and to develop more appropriate coping techniques.

Most treatment efforts recognize the effects that alcoholism has had on the significant people in the patient's life. Therefore, an important aspect of recovery involves helping family members and close friends understand alcoholism and how rehabilitation is an ongoing process over 6 to 12 months and beyond. Couples and family counseling and support groups for relatives and friends help the persons involved rebuild relationships, avoid protecting the patient from the consequences of any drinking in the future, and be as supportive as possible of the alcoholic patient's recovery program.

Medication If detoxification has been completed and the patient is not one of the 10 to 15 percent of alcoholic persons who have an independent mood disorder, schizophrenia, or anxiety disorder, little evidence supports giving psychotropic medications for the treatment of alcoholism. Lingering levels of anxiety and insomnia as part of a reaction to life stresses and protracted abstinence should be treated with behavior modification approaches and reassurance. Medications for those symptoms, including benzodiazepines, are likely to lose their effectiveness much faster than the insomnia disappears; as a result, the patient may increase the dose and have subsequent problems. Similarly, sadness and mood swings can linger at low levels for several months' time. However, controlled clinical trials indicate no benefit in giving antidepressant medications or lithium to treat the average alcoholic person with no independent psychiatric disorder. The mood disorder will clear before the medications can take effect, and the patients who resume drinking while on the medications face significant potential dangers. With little or no evidence that the medications are effective, the dangers significantly outweigh any potential benefits from their routine use.

One possible exception to the proscription against the use of medications is the alcohol-sensitizing agent disulfiram (Antabuse). Disulfiram is given in dosages of 250 mg a day before the patient's discharge either from the intensive first phase of outpatient rehabilitation or from inpatient care. The goal is to place the patient in a condition in which drinking alcohol precipitates an uncomfortable reaction, including nausea, vomiting, and a burning sensation in the face and stomach. Unfortunately, few data convincingly prove that disulfiram is more effective than a placebo, probably because most people stop taking the disulfiram when they go back to drinking. Many clinicians have stopped routinely prescribing the agent, partly in recognition of the dangers associated with the drug itself: mood swings, rare instances of psychosis, the possibility of an increase in peripheral neuropathies, the relatively rare occurrence of other significant neuropathies, and a potentially fatal cerebral hepatitis. Moreover, patients with preexisting heart disease, cerebral thrombosis, diabetes, and a number of other conditions cannot be given disulfiram, for an alcohol reaction to the disulfiram could be fatal.

Several medications have recently been shown to have potential promise for future treatment of alcohol rehabilitation. These include naltrexone (Trexan), buspirone (BuSpar), and acanysrosate. However, the effects are modest, and long-term trials are required before routine clinical use should be considered.

Self-help groups Clinicians must recognize the potential importance of self-help groups like Alcoholics Anonymous. AA members have help available 24 hours a day, associate with a sober peer group, learn that it is possible to participate in social functions without drinking, and are given a model of recovery by observing the accomplishments of sober members of the group.

Learning about AA usually begins during inpatient or outpatient rehabilitation. The clinician can play a major role in helping patients understand the differences between specific groups. Some groups are composed only of men or women, and others are mixed; some meetings are composed mostly of blue-collar men and women, and others are mostly for professionals;

some groups place great emphasis on religion, and others are eclectic. Patients with coexisting psychiatric disorders may need some additional education about AA. The clinician should remind them that some members of AA may not understand their special need for medications and should arm the patients with ways of coping when group members inappropriately suggest that the required medications be stopped.

SUGGESTED CROSS-REFERENCES

Classification of mental disorders is discussed in Chapter 11, epidemiology in Section 5.1, and the sociocultural sciences in Chapter 4. Delirium and amnestic disorders are discussed in Chapter 12. Other substance-related disorders are discussed in Chapter 13. Mood disorders are discussed in Chapter 16, anxiety disorders in Chapter 17, personality disorders in Chapter 25, and schizophrenia in Chapter 14. Psychotherapies are discussed in Chapter 31.

REFERENCES

Anthenelli R M, Klein J, Tsuang J, Smith T, Schuckit M: The prognostic importance of blackouts in young men. J Stud Alcohol *55:* 290, 1994.

Blane H T, Leonard K E, editors: *Psychological Theories of Drinking and Alcoholism.* Guilford, New York, 1987.

*Brown S A, Irwin M, Schuckit M A: Changes in anxiety among abstinent male alcoholics. J Stud Alcohol *52:* 55, 1991.

Dorus W, Ostrow D G, Anton R, Cushman P, Collins J: Lithium treatment of depressed and nondepressed alcoholics. JAMA *262:* 1646, 1989.

Friedenreich C M, Howe G R, Miller A B, Jain M G: A cohort study of alcohol consumption and risk of breast cancer. Am J Epidemiol *137:* 512, 1993.

Gillin J C, Smith T L, Irwin M, Butters N, Demodena A: Increased pressure for rapid eye movement sleep at time of hospital admission predicts relapse in nondepressed patients with primary alcoholism at 3-month follow-up. Arch Gen Psychiatry *51:* 189, 1994.

Glass I B, editor: *The International Handbook of Addiction Behavior.* Routledge, New York, 1991.

Goedde H W, Agarwal D P, editors: *Alcoholism: Biomedical and Genetic Aspects.* Pergamon, New York, 1989.

Group for the Advancement of Psychiatry: Substance abuse disorders: A psychiatric priority. Am J Psychiatry *148:* 1291, 1991.

Halvorson M R, Campbell J L, Sprague G, Slater K, Noffsinger J K, Peterson C M: Comparative evaluation of the clinical utility of three markers of ethanol intake: The effect of gender. Alcohol Clin Exp Res *17:* 225, 1993.

*Helzer J E, Burnam A, McEvoy L T: Alcohol abuse and dependence. In *Psychiatric Disorders in America,* L N Robins, D A Regier, editors, p 81. Free Press, New York, 1991.

Ishak K G, Zimmerman H J, Ray M B: Alcoholic liver disease: Pathologic, pathogenetic, and clinical aspects. Alcoholism *15:* 45, 1991.

Israel Y, Orrego H, Schmidt W, Popham R E, Escartin P: Trauma in cirrhosis: An indicator of the pattern of alcohol abuse in different societies. Alcoholism *15:* 433, 1991.

Kendler K S, Neale M C, Heath A C, Kessler R C, Eaves L J: A twin-family study of alcoholism in women. Am J Psychiatry *151:* 5, 1994.

Kranzler H R, Burleson J A, Del Boca F K, Babor T F, Korner P, Brown J, Bohn M J: Buspirone treatment of anxious alcoholics: A placebo-controlled trial. Arch Gen Psychiatry *51:* 720, 1994.

Lieber C S: Hepatic, metabolic, and toxic effects of ethanol: 1991 update. Alcoholism *15:* 573, 1991.

Litten R Z, Allen J P: Pharmacotherapies for alcoholism: Promising agents and clinical issues. Alcoholism *15:* 620, 1991.

Martin P R, McCool B A, Singleton C K: Genetic sensitivity to thiamine deficiency and development of alcoholic organic brain disease. Alcohol Clin Exp Res *17:* 31, 1993.

Mello N K, Mendelson J H, Teoh S K: Alcohol and neuroendocrine function. In *Medical Diagnosis and Treatment of Alcoholism,* J H Mendelson and N K Mello, editors. McGraw-Hill, New York, 1992.

Nathan P E: Psychoactive substance dependence. In *The DSM IV Source Book,* T Widiger, A Frances, editors, p 33. American Psychiatric Press, Washington, 1994.

Pohorecky, L A: Stress and alcohol interaction: An update of human research. Alcoholism *15:* 438, 1991.

Roehrs T, Beare D, Zorick F, Roth T: Sleepiness and ethanol effects on simulated driving. Alcohol Clin Exp Res *18:* 154, 1994.

Schuckit M A: *Drug and Alcohol Abuse,* ed 4. Plenum, New York, 1995.

Schuckit M A: Low level of response to alcohol as a predictor of future alcoholism. Am J Psychiatry *151:* 184, 1994.

Schuckit M A: Treatment of anxiety in patients who abuse alcohol and drugs. In *Handbook of Anxiety,* R Noyes, M Roth, G D Burrows, editors, vol 4, p 461. Elsevier, New York, 1990.

Schuckit M A, Hesselbrock V: Alcohol dependence and anxiety disorders: What is the relationship? Am J Psychiatry *151:* 1723, 1994.

Schuckit M A, Irwin M: Diagnosis of alcoholism. Med Clin North Am *72:* 1133, 1988.

Schuckit M A, Irwin M, Smith T L: One-year incidence rate of major depression and other psychiatric disorders in 239 alcoholic men. Addiction *89:* 441, 1994.

Schuckit M A, Slaby A E, editors: *Series in Psychosocial Epidemiology: Alcohol Patterns and Problems,* vol 5. Rutgers University Press, New Brunswick, NJ, 1985.

*Schuckit M A, Smith T L, Anthenelli R, Irwin M: Clinical course of alcoholism in 636 male inpatients. Am J Psychiatry *150:* 786, 1993.

Secretary of Health and Human Services: Eighth Special Report to the US Congress on Alcohol and Health, p 8-1. US Government Printing Office, Washington, 1993.

Shear P K, Jernigan T L, Butters N: Volumetric magnetic resonance imaging qualification of longitudinal brain changes in abstinent alcoholics. Alcohol Clin Exp Res *18:* 172, 1994.

Snow M G, Prochaska J O, Rossi J S: Processes of change in alcoholics anonymous: Maintenance factors in long-term sobriety. J Stud Alcohol *55:* 362, 1994.

*Streissguth A P, Sampson P D, Carmichael Olson H, Bookstein F L, Barr H M, Scott M, Feldman J, Mirsky A F: Maternal drinking during pregnancy: Attention and short-term memory in 14-year-old offspring—A longitudinal prospective study. Alcohol Clin Exp Res *18:* 202, 1994.

Uehsima H. Mikawa K, Baba S, Sasaki S, Ozawa, Tsushima M. Kawaguchi A, Omae T, Katayama Y, Kayamori Y, Ito K: Effect of reduced alcohol consumption on blood pressure in untreated hypertensive men. Hypertension *21:* 248, 1993.

*Vaillant G E: *The Natural History of Alcoholism: Causes, Patterns, and Path to Recovery.* Harvard University Press, Cambridge, 1983.

van Gijn J, Stampfer M J, Wolfe C, Algra A: The association between alcohol and stroke. In *Health Issues Related to Alcohol Consumption,* P M Verschuren, editor, p 43. ILSI Press, Washington, 1993.

Volpocelli J R, Alterman A I, Hayashida M, O'Brien C P: Naltrexone in the treatment of alcohol dependence. Arch Gen Psychiatry *49:* 876, 1992.

Williams G D, Clem D A, Dufour M C: Apparent per capita alcohol consumption: National, state, and regional trends, 1977-91. NIAAA Surveillance Report No 27, November 1993.

Woody G, Schuckit M A, Weinrieb R, Yu E: A review of substance use disorders section of the DSM-IV. In *Psychiatric Clinics of North America,* vol 16, N Miller, editor, p 21. Saunders, Philadelphia, 1993.

13.3
AMPHETAMINE (OR AMPHETAMINELIKE)-RELATED DISORDERS

JEROME H. JAFFE, M.D.

INTRODUCTION

Despite some pharmacological differences between amphetamine (and amphetaminelike drugs) and cocaine their patterns of use, dependence, and toxicity are quite similar and their treatment is currently the same in most instances. The diagnostic criteria for all of the substance use disorders are virtually identical. Among the drugs that produce subjective effects quite similar to those of amphetamine and methamphetamine, and also have some abuse potential, are methylphenidate (Ritalin) and phendimetrazine (Preludin), which are included in Schedule II of the Controlled Substance Act (CSA), and diethylpropion (Tenuate), benzphetamine (Didrex), and phentermine (Ionamin), which are included in Schedules III or IV of the CSA. Those agents will not be considered separately because dependence on them is relatively uncommon and the clinical course of dependence is similar to that seen with the amphetamines.

DEFINITION

Amphetamine use may be associated with a number of distinct disorders, of which dependence and abuse are but two. In the case of amphetamine and amphetaminelike agents, at least 10 other drug-related disorders have been described (Table 13.3-1).

Amphetamine dependence (see Tables 13.1-2 and 13.1-5) is a cluster of physiological, behavioral, and cognitive symptoms that, taken together, indicate that the person continues to use cocaine or amphetaminelike drugs despite significant problems related to such use. Drug dependence in general has also been defined by the World Health Organization (WHO) as a syndrome in which the use of the drugs or class of drugs takes on a much higher priority for a given person than other behaviors that once had a higher value. Both of those brief definitions have as their central features the emphasis on the drug-using behavior itself, its maladaptive nature, and how the choice to engage in that behavior has shifted and become constrained as a result of interaction with the drug over time.

Amphetamine abuse (see Table 13.1-6) is a term used to categorize a pattern of maladaptive use of amphetamine or an amphetaminelike drug leading to clinically significant impairment or distress and occurring within a 12-month period, but one in which the symptoms have never met the criteria for amphetamine dependence (see Table 13.1-2).

The amphetamine-induced disorders include amphetamine intoxication (Table 13.3-2), amphetamine withdrawal (Table 13.3-3), amphetamine-induced psychotic disorder with delusions and amphetamine-induced psychotic disorder with hallucinations (see Section 15.3), amphetamine intoxication delirium (see Chapter 12), amphetamine-induced mood disorder (see Section 16.6), amphetamine-induced anxiety disorder, (see Section 17.5), amphetamine-induced sleep disorder (see Chapter 23), amphetamine-induced sexual dysfunction (see Section 21.1a), and amphetamine-related disorder not otherwise specified (Table 13.3-4).

The coding scheme of the fourth edition of *Diagnostic and Statistical Manual of Mental Disorders* (DSM-IV) provides distinct numbers for amphetamine dependence and amphetamine abuse, but the codes for the other amphetamine-induced disorders are common to several other substance-related disorders. For example, the codes for amphetamine withdrawal and opioid withdrawal are the same.

TABLE 13.3-1
Amphetamine (or Amphetaminelike)-Related Disorders

Amphetamine use disorders

Amphetamine dependence
Amphetamine abuse

Amphetamine-induced disorders

Amphetamine intoxication
Specify if: with perceptual disturbances
Amphetamine withdrawal
Amphetamine intoxication delirium
Amphetamine-induced psychotic disorder, with delusions
Specify if: with onset during intoxication
Amphetamine-induced psychotic disorder, with hallucinations
Specify if: with onset during intoxication
Amphetamine-induced mood disorder
Specify if: with onset during intoxication/with onset during withdrawal
Amphetamine-induced anxiety disorder
Specify if: with onset during intoxication
Amphetamine-induced sexual dysfunction
Specify if: with onset during intoxication
Amphetamine-induced sleep disorder
Specify if: with onset during intoxication/with onset during withdrawal
Amphetamine-related disorder not otherwise specified

Table based on DSM-IV, *Diagnostic and Statistical Manual of Mental Disorders,* ed 4. Copyright American Psychiatric Association, Washington, 1994. Used with permission.

TABLE 13.3-2
Diagnostic Criteria for Amphetamine Intoxication

A. Recent use of amphetamine or a related substance (e.g., methylphenidate).
B. Clinically significant maladaptive behavioral or psychological changes (e.g., euphoria or affective blunting; changes in sociability; hypervigilance; interpersonal sensitivity; anxiety, tension, or anger; stereotyped behaviors; impaired judgment; or impaired social or occupational functioning) that developed during, or shortly after, use of amphetamine or a related substance.
C. Two (or more) of the following, developing during, or shortly after, use of amphetamine or a related substance:
(1) tachycardia or bradycardia
(2) pupillary dilation
(3) elevated or lowered blood pressure
(4) perspiration or chills
(5) nausea or vomiting
(6) evidence of weight loss
(7) psychomotor agitation or retardation
(8) muscular weakness, respiratory depression, chest pain, or cardiac arrhythmias
(9) confusion, seizures, dyskinesias, dystonias, or coma
D. The symptoms are not due to a general medical condition and are not better accounted for by another mental disorder.

Specify if:
With Perceptual Disturbances

Table from DSM-IV, *Diagnostic and Statistical Manual of Mental Disorders,* ed 4. Copyright American Psychiatric Association, Washington, 1994. Used with permission.

TABLE 13.3-3
Diagnostic Criteria for Amphetamine Withdrawal

A. Cessation of (or reduction in) amphetamine (or a related substance) use that has been heavy and prolonged.
B. Dysphoric mood and two (or more) of the following physiological changes, developing within a few hours to several days after criterion A:
(1) fatigue
(2) vivid, unpleasant dreams
(3) insomnia or hypersomnia
(4) increased appetite
(5) psychomotor retardation or agitation
C. The symptoms in criterion B cause clinically significant distress or impairment in social, occupational, or other important areas of functioning.
D. The symptoms are not due to a general medical condition and are not better accounting for by another mental disorder.

Table from DSM-IV, *Diagnostic and Statistical Manual of Mental Disorders,* ed 4. Copyright American Psychiatric Association, Washington, 1994. Used with permission.

TABLE 13.3-4
Diagnostic Criteria for Amphetamine-Related Disorder Not Otherwise Specified

The amphetamine-related disorder not otherwise specified category is for disorders associated with the use of amphetamine (or a related substance) that are not classifiable as amphetamine dependence, amphetamine abuse, amphetamine intoxication, amphetamine withdrawal, amphetamine intoxication delirium, amphetamine-induced psychotic disorder, amphetamine-induced mood disorder, amphetamine-induced anxiety disorder, amphetamine-induced sexual dysfunction, or amphetamine-induced sleep disorder.

Table from DSM-IV, *Diagnostic and Statistical Manual of Mental Disorders,* ed 4. Copyright American Psychiatric Association, Washington, 1994. Used with permission.

HISTORY

Amphetamine agents were not available for clinical use until the 1930s; concern about dependence was first expressed late in that decade. The first cases of amphetamine psychosis were reported in 1938. Between 1932 and 1946 almost three dozen clinical uses of amphetamine were proposed and tried by the medical profession. Some amphetamines were available over the counter in nasal inhalers until 1971.

Although Japan had experienced a large number of cases of intravenous methamphetamine abuse and dependence immediately following World War II, until the end of the 1960s there was reluctance in the United States to view amphetamines and related drugs as capable of causing addiction. However, because the misuse and overuse of these drugs had been a matter of growing concern, they were placed under regulatory control by the Food and Drug Administration (FDA) in the mid-1960s. Despite such controls drugs smuggled into the country or produced illegally in clandestine laboratories increased. The illicit drug supplies on the street (which up to that time had come primarily from the diversion of legitimately produced drugs) were sufficient to fuel a major epidemic of amphetamine and methamphetamine abuse in the late 1960s. The epidemic made clear the potential toxicity of the amphetamines, especially when used intravenously, and such terms as "speed freaks" and "speed kills" left an enduring legacy in the popular vocabulary. Over the next decade regulatory controls on legitimately produced amphetamines were progressively tightened. There is still considerable misuse of amphetamines and amphetaminelike drugs in the United States, with much of the supply coming from illicit laboratories. In the late 1980s there were reports that smoking of crystalline methamphetamine (ice) was on the rise. Although there was concern that methamphetamine abuse might reemerge as a major problem, through the mid-1990s use of amphetaminelike stimulants continued to be overshadowed by cocaine abuse.

Amphetamine is used legitimately almost exclusively for the treatment of narcolepsy and attention-deficit/hyperactivity disorder. Some amphetaminelike agents are still prescribed as appetite suppressants, but the use of amphetamine itself for that purpose has been discouraged and is outlawed in some states. Amphetamines may have use in treating certain atypical depressions, but concern about abuse potential has discouraged the controlled clinical studies that would be necessary to define just which patients, if any, might benefit more from amphetaminelike agents than from tricyclic antidepressants or serotonin-specific reuptake inhibitors.

At the present time amphetamine and methamphetamine, as well as methylphenidate and cocaine, are included in Schedule II of the CSA; phendimetrazine is in Schedule III.

COMPARATIVE NOSOLOGY

The DSM-IV diagnostic criteria for amphetamine dependence are the same generic criteria as applied to other substances (for example, cocaine). The notion of a generic concept of dependence is shared with the revised third edition of DSM (DSM-III-R) and the 10th revision of the *International Classification of Diseases and Related Health Problems* (ICD-10). In making the diagnosis of dependence there is a generally high level of agreement between DSM-IV and ICD-10: they employ similar concepts (the dependence syndrome varying in degree of severity), although the wording of the criteria for determining the presence and severity of the syndrome differ. Both require that three elements of the syndrome occur within a 12-month period. The degree of agreement between DSM-IV and DSM-III-R is even higher, since despite some changes in the wording, the syndromes and criteria in the two editions are quite similar. Although DSM-IV appears to lay greater stress on tolerance and physiological dependence, in practice even if those criteria had been required, that would not have substantially reduced the number of cases meeting the criteria for amphetamine dependence.

The major changes between DSM-III-R and DSM-IV affected the diagnosis of substance abuse. DSM-III-R required the presence of only one of two general criteria whereas DSM-IV requires one of four. Nevertheless, for both amphetamine dependence and amphetamine abuse the agreement between DSM-III-R and DSM-IV is exceedingly high.

There is a major difference between ICD-10 and DSM-IV in the classification of what is called substance abuse in DSM-IV. ICD-10 does not use the term "abuse." Instead, it includes a category of harmful use, which is substantially different from the concept of abuse as used in DSM-IV. The concept of harm is limited to physical and mental health (for example, hepatitis, cardiac damage, episodes of depression, or toxic psychosis). It specifically excludes social impairments as follows: "Harmful patterns of use are often criticized by others and frequently associated with adverse social consequences of various kinds. The fact that a pattern of use of a particular substance is disapproved of by another person or by the culture, or may have led to socially negative consequences such as arrest or marital arguments, is not in itself evidence of harmful use."

Another distinction between ICD-10 and DSM-IV are the coding systems, which limit the number of distinct codes that can be recorded. ICD-10 separates, for record-keeping purposes, cocaine-related disorders from those caused by other stimulants. Because of the limits of the system the code for stimulants includes caffeine with the amphetamines and amphetaminelike stimulants.

EPIDEMIOLOGY

The use of amphetamines has fluctuated dramatically over the past two decades in the United States. Amphetamines and similar drugs are considered together as stimulants in the High School Senior Survey. Self-reported stimulant use has always been higher than for cocaine (and crack), but it also has fallen from the high rates seen in 1982 (lifetime use levels of 28 percent and past-30-days rate of 11 percent) to a lifetime rate of 14 percent and past-30-days rate of 2.3 percent in 1992. The National Household Survey on Drug Abuse (NHSDA), however, found no significant declines in the use of stimulants between 1991 and 1993.

Two relatively recent population surveys that used accepted criteria to measure the extent of drug abuse and dependence were the Epidemiologic Catchment Area (ECA) Study, carried out in the early 1980s, using third edition of DSM (DSM-III) criteria and the National Comorbidity Survey (NCS), carried out from 1990 to 1992, using DSM-III-R criteria. Only the ECA and NCS offer estimates of the prevalence of abuse and dependence as defined by DSM-III and III-R respectively. The ECA report combined categories of dependence and abuse for amphetamine and amphetaminelike drugs. The one-month, six-month, and lifetime prevalences of amphetamine abuse or dependence were 0.1, 0.2, and 1.7 percent, respectively.

ETIOLOGY

Drug dependence, including amphetamine and amphetaminelike substance dependence, is viewed as the result of a process in which multiple interacting factors (social, psychological, cultural, and biological) influence drug-using behavior. That process in some cases leads to the loss of flexibility with respect to use that is the hallmark of dependence. According to that biopsychosocial perspective, the actions of the drug are seen as critical, but not all persons who become dependent experience the effects of a given drug in the same way or are influenced by the same set of factors; even with the same class of pharmacological agents, different factors may be more or less important at different stages of the process.

With amphetamines, as with most substances, it is largely social and cultural factors that influence availability and initial use. In the case of amphetamines and amphetaminelike drugs, however, pharmacological factors are believed to play very important roles in the perpetuation of use and of progression to dependence. Amphetamines have potent mood-elevating and euphorigenic actions in humans and are powerful reinforcers in animal models, particularly when the drug effects are rapid in onset, such as when they are injected or inhaled. Although some degree of physical dependence develops, in contrast to the opioids and sedatives, an aversive withdrawal syndrome probably plays a less prominent role in perpetuating the use of amphetamines and amphetaminelike drugs.

COMORBIDITY Additional psychiatric diagnoses are quite common among those dependent on amphetamines and amphetaminelike drugs. It is not always clear how this comorbidity is linked etiologically to amphetamine dependence, but the epidemiological evidence is clear that the presence of psychiatric disorders not related to substance abuse (for example, mood disorders, schizophrenia, and antisocial personality disorder) substantially increases the odds of developing substance abuse or dependence. For some persons amphetamines and amphetaminelike drugs may alleviate various psychiatric disorders or dysfunctional states. For example, there may be some users (a relative few) who find relief from adult attention-deficit disorders. For others the drugs may alleviate a persistent dysthymic disorder, and for such users the anhedonic state following amphetamine cessation may be experienced as more intense. Still others may have found that the drug facilitated sexual activity that was previously unsatisfactory. Although such factors may explain drug use on more than one occasion, they do not account for progression to dependence or abuse.

It is also postulated that amphetamine use may induce psychiatric syndromes (for example, panic disorders) that may persist, and that persons with certain psychiatric disorders may be prone to experiment with drugs.

Research on the temporal appearance of the syndromes indicates that, in some instances and for some syndromes, drug use antedates the psychiatric disorders. In one component of the ECA study interviewed subjects were reinterviewed one year later. Those who reported use of amphetamines, amphetaminelike drugs, or cocaine in the interval were almost eight times more likely than nonusers to develop a depressive disorder and 14 times more likely to have experienced a panic attack.

GENETIC FACTORS What role genetic factors play in increasing specific vulnerability to amphetamine dependence is unclear. However, the odds of amphetamine dependence are increased among persons with alcohol dependence, schizophrenia, bipolar disorder, or antisocial personality disorder. Since each of those disorders has a genetic predisposition to some degree, it suggests that genetic vulnerability to dependence is a factor that should be considered.

OTHER FACTORS Social, cultural, and economic factors are powerful determinants of initial use, continuing use, and relapse. Excessive use is far more likely in places where amphetamines are readily available.

Since in both human and animal studies alternative positive reinforcers compete with drugs as reinforcers, the absence of such nondrug alternatives can be seen as a causal factor in their use, especially in communities where drugs are available and the social pressures against using them are not strong. Alternative positive reinforcers are not limited to material rewards, but include the kinds of psychological rewards that are associated with satisfying interpersonal relationships and the self-esteem that derives from achievements in socially acceptable roles.

LEARNING AND CONDITIONING Learning and conditioning are also believed to be important factors in the perpetuation of amphetamine use. With each ingestion, inhalation, or injection of the drug the euphoric experience acts to reinforce prior drug-taking behavior. In addition, the environmental cues associated with amphetamine use become associated with the euphoric state so that long after a period of cessation such cues (for example, paraphernalia, friends who use drugs) can elicit memories that reawaken a craving for the drug.

PHARMACOLOGICAL FACTORS The reinforcing and toxic effects of amphetamines and amphetaminelike drugs play an important role in the genesis of amphetamine dependence and other amphetamine-related disorders. As stimulants of the central nervous system (CNS) amphetamines and cocaine produce very similar, if not identical, subjective effects in humans, and similar, although not identical, patterns of toxicity. Both categories of CNS stimulants can produce a sense of alertness, euphoria, and well-being. There may be decreased hunger and need for sleep. Performance impaired by fatigue is usually improved. Both categories of drugs can induce paranoia, suspiciousness, and overt psychosis, which can be difficult to distinguish from the paranoid type of schizophrenia. Both categories can produce major cardiovascular toxicities. However, there are distinct differences in their mechanisms of action at the cellular level, their duration of action, and their metabolic pathways.

Mechanisms of action A critical element in the reinforcing effects of amphetamine and amphetaminelike drugs is the activation of mesolimbic and mesocortical dopaminergic systems. Amphetamines and amphetaminelike drugs inhibit dopamine reuptake, as well as release dopamine from nerve endings.

Common routes of administration Amphetamines and amphetaminelike drugs can be taken orally, by injection, by absorption through nasal and buccal membranes, or by inhalation and absorption through the pulmonary alveoli. As with nicotine, opioids, and phencyclidine (PCP), the inhalation of amphetamine or freebase cocaine produces almost immediate absorption and a rapid onset of effects. Amphetamine and methamphetamine salts can be vaporized without much destruction of the molecule, thus obviating the need for preparing a freebase form for smoking.

As with the opioids the rapid onset of amphetamine effects

from intravenous injection or freebase inhalation produces an intensely pleasurable sensation referred to as a rush. The duration of the amphetamine rush has not been studied in the laboratory, but it is presumed to be shorter than the duration of elevated mood.

Metabolism The pharmacokinetics of amphetamines and amphetaminelike drugs are different from those of cocaine. They are all extensively metabolized in the liver. Unchanged amphetamine, a weak base, is excreted in the urine, and the half-life of amphetamine is considerably shortened when the urine is acidic. The half-life of amphetamine after therapeutic doses ranges from 7 to 19 hours and that of methamphetamine appears to be at least as long. Thus, after toxic dosage, resolution of symptoms may take far longer with amphetamines than with cocaine.

Tolerance and sensitization Most patients seeking treatment report needing progressively more amphetamine to get the same effect. With chronic use some degree of tolerance develops to amphetamine's cardiovascular effects.

Chronic use of either amphetamine or amphetaminelike drugs also produces a form of sensitization in which the response to a given dose is actually enhanced. One theory holds that the sensitization to drug effects is attributable to a variety of kindling in the CNS. In the classic studies of kindling, electrical stimulation of the limbic system, which initially has very little effect, is applied repeatedly; after a matter of days the threshold for effects decreases and major long-lasting seizures appear. In animals similar effects are seen with CNS stimulants, so that repeated doses of amphetamine eventually elicit seizures or stereotyped behaviors not seen with initial doses. The sensitization can be long-lasting.

The paranoid states and toxic psychoses that commonly develop among chronic amphetamine users are believed to be among the phenomena to which sensitization develops. Those who have developed amphetamine psychosis may develop it more rapidly with subsequent exposure.

Withdrawal states Whereas the amphetamine withdrawal syndrome has aversive qualities (for example, dysphoria and anhedonia), it is generally not deemed as aversive as opioid withdrawal and, in most cases, is probably not as critical in perpetuating amphetamine-using behavior. Although withdrawal anhedonia and fatigue usually do not contribute to relapse after brief withdrawal, that does not mean that the problems are not important for some persons. Some users who have come to depend on the drugs for high energy or for helping to project a confident persona may be temporarily unable to function without them. For others withdrawal dysphoria may exaggerate the intensity of an antecedent mood disorder. There does not appear to be a protracted amphetamine withdrawal syndrome.

Other actions Neither the actions of amphetamine nor those of amphetaminelike drugs are selective for dopamine. Amphetaminelike drugs release norepinephrine and serotonin. Some of those actions are relevant to the toxic actions of amphetamine, especially its cardiovascular toxicity.

DIAGNOSIS AND CLINICAL FEATURES

PATTERNS OF USE AND ABUSE

Likelihood of progression Patients with narcolepsy and children with attention-deficit/hyperactivity disorder can take amphetamines and amphetaminelike drugs daily for many years without developing significant tolerance to their therapeutic effects and with little escalation of dose or toxicity. When amphetamine and amphetaminelike drugs were more widely used in the treatment of obesity, relatively few who took them daily developed patterns of drug abuse and dependence. Even when amphetaminelike drugs are taken initially for nonmedical reasons (for example, to reduce fatigue or for euphorigenic effects), not all users progress to abuse and dependence. The absolute risk of such progression is not precisely known, but all estimates suggest that it is high enough to justify a policy that discourages experimentation. One estimate of risk comes from a classic study, carried out in 1974 and published in 1976, of drug use among a representative sample of young men. Seventy-three percent reported having had no experience with amphetamines, but of the 27 percent who had had some experience, almost 10 percent (3 percent of the total) reported daily use.

Varied patterns There are several patterns of abuse of amphetamines and similar agents. Some persons may use the drugs intermittently in relatively low doses; for example, truck drivers or students may use them to overcome fatigue or the need for sleep or to derive some positive mood effects. Some intermittent users become dependent and find it difficult to stop; some may eventually escalate the dosage. Since the drugs are no longer available legitimately for those purposes, persons with that pattern of use are likely to obtain them from illicit sources.

Some persons use amphetamines primarily to induce euphoria. Such users often progress to high dosages, especially if they use the drugs intravenously or by inhalation. Those are obviously the most dangerous patterns of use and commonly lead to compulsive use or toxic effects. Although intravenous use initially may be intermittent with days or weeks elapsing between episodes, such high-dose use often progresses to sprees or speed runs, during which several grams of amphetamine might be injected. The runs can last for days or weeks and are commonly punctuated by episodes of toxicity (amphetamine-induced psychotic disorder with delusions or amphetamine intoxication delirium) or by brief periods of abstinence (crashing), generally precipitated by an interruption in the supply of the drug or exhaustion. High-dose amphetamine users often combine amphetamine with sedatives or opioids to modulate the stimulant effects. Alcohol use and alcohol abuse are common concomitants of high-dose amphetamine abuse and dependence.

Amphetamine-induced disorders All of the disorders listed in DSM-IV for cocaine (intoxication, psychotic disorder, intoxication delirium, mood disorder, anxiety disorder, sleep disorder, and sexual dysfunction) may occur in association with the use of amphetamine or amphetaminelike drugs. The clinical pictures are similar, if not identical; the DSM-IV diagnostic criteria and codes are identical except for the substitution of the words "amphetamine" for the word "cocaine."

Although amphetamine-induced psychotic or delirium syndromes are usually seen only when high doses are used for prolonged periods, such syndromes have been reported in apparently vulnerable persons even after therapeutic doses given for short periods. Haloperidol (Haldol) and phenothiazines have been used to treat the psychotic syndrome. Although with cocaine the delusional syndrome is typically of short duration, with the amphetaminelike drugs it may not resolve for many days after drug cessation. On recovery from either psychotic or delirium syndrome there may be amnesia for the entire episode or for some part of it.

Japanese psychiatrists have presented data showing that amphetamine-induced psychosis may persist for several years, and that, in the acute stage, there may be disturbance of consciousness (confusion, disorientation) in addition to the more typical mood and delusional symptoms. Following recovery such persons seem to be sensitized and will experience acute paranoid psychosis on reexposure to small doses of amphetamines, and some have exacerbations in response to stress.

AMPHETAMINE WITHDRAWAL There are few clear differences between the clinical descriptions of postchronic amphetamine use syndrome and postchronic cocaine use syndrome. In both situations the severity of the syndrome is presumably related to the intensity and duration of the antecedent drug use. Some elements of the syndrome (dysphoria and fatigue) can be seen in amphetamine abusers after relatively brief binges or runs of only a few days. Some aspects of the crashing, albeit less severe, are reported to occur even after 24 hours of use. During phases of the amphetamine withdrawal syndrome users may experience severe depression, which tends to resolve without special treatment when sleep normalizes. Amphetamine users stabilized on amphetamine prior to withdrawal have been studied. Among the findings noted as early as 1963 were a marked shortening of time to first rapid eye movement (REM) sleep and a marked rebound in total REM sleep. A return to normal levels in some cases required several weeks.

The DSM-IV criteria for amphetamine withdrawal and those for cocaine withdrawal are identical. Less is known about the later stages of amphetamine withdrawal, but it is likely that there are periods of increased vulnerability when stimuli previously associated with use elicit memories of drug effects and craving.

COMORBIDITY The frequent co-occurence of other psychiatric disorders and amphetamine dependence was noted among amphetamine abusers starting at about the middle of the 20th century, and that general pattern has not changed. The presence of other psychiatric disorders sharply increases the odds of drug dependence, and drug-dependent persons are more likely than the general population to meet the criteria for additional psychiatric disorders.

Patients with schizophrenia commonly use amphetamine or cocaine and develop both dependence and toxic syndromes. It has been suggested that schizophrenic persons use stimulants to alleviate negative symptoms or side effects of antipsychotics. Special programs involving peer-based support groups seem to be effective in linking drug-using schizophrenic patients with outpatient treatment programs.

TOXICITY AND COMPLICATIONS The amphetamines and cocaine produce a number of similar subjective effects, such as euphoria, mood elevation, and a sense of increased energy (possibly by increasing the actions of dopamine in mesolimbic pathways), but they differ in their mechanisms of action at the cellular level, their metabolic pathways, and the toxic effects they produce. There may even be differences in toxicity between amphetamine and methamphetamine. Like cocaine, amphetamines produce their most dramatic toxic effects on the CNS and the cardiovascular system.

In animals chronically administered high doses of amphetamines produce long-lasting depletion of brain norepinephrine, and more selective but even longer-lasting depletion of dopamine, alterations in dopamine uptake sites, and reduction in serotonergic activity. Methamphetamine in particular seems capable of inducing damage to serotonergic fibers. The long-lasting dopaminergic changes probably account for the altered elevated threshold for self-stimulation in animals and the anhedonia reported by chronic amphetamine users for prolonged periods following cessation. In monkeys the toxic effects of chronic amphetamine use include damage to cerebral blood vessels, neuronal loss, and microhemorrhages. In humans high-dosage amphetamine has also been associated with lethal hyperpyrexia and with destructive deterioration of arterioles. High doses can also produce convulsions, and ultimately coma and death.

Amphetaminelike drugs can cause catastrophes of the cardiovascular system (for example, intracranial hemorrhage, arrhythmias, and acute cardiac failure) as a result of their capacity to release norepinephrine, dopamine, and serotonin, and to raise blood pressure. With amphetamines, considerable tolerance develops to the last effect.

Because amphetamine use can be associated with increased sexual activity, often accompanied by poor judgment, amphetamine users are at elevated risk for venereal diseases, including infection with the human immunodeficiency virus (HIV).

PATHOLOGY AND LABORATORY EXAMINATIONS

Amphetamine and amphetaminelike drugs can be detected for varying lengths of time in urine. Metabolites can also be detected in blood, saliva, and hair. Blood and saliva furnish a better index of current levels, whereas urine provides a longer window of opportunity for detecting use over the previous few days. Hair analysis can reveal drug use over a period of weeks to months but has little applicability in clinical situations.

Such procedures as positron emission tomography (PET) and single photon emission computed tomography (SPECT) have not yet been used during the immediate postamphetamine cessation period, but given the findings seen at autopsy and the pharmacology of amphetaminelike agents, it would not be surprising if there were arteriolar pathology and alterations in dopamine systems.

DIFFERENTIAL DIAGNOSIS

The disorders associated with the use of amphetamine and amphetaminelike drugs need to be distinguished from both primary mental disorders and disorders induced by other classes of drugs. A history of the drug ingestion is important in making those distinctions. However, given the unreliability of self-reports about drug use and the likelihood that many users will deny any drug use at all, laboratory testing for drugs in body fluids and histories from collaterals are very important. Disorders associated with amphetamine use cannot be distinguished from those associated with cocaine except by a reliable history or laboratory tests. Users of amphetamine or cocaine and related drugs may exhibit inappropriate optimism, euphoria, and expansiveness; excessive talkativeness; and a decreased need for sleep sometimes associated with irritability in the context of a clear sensorium, a pattern that is also observed in manic and hypomanic episodes of bipolar I disorder and bipolar II disorder, respectively. Those symptoms, however, may not be obvious enough to suggest their relation to drug use and the first indication of drug dependence may be financial difficulties, an arrest for selling drugs or possessing them, or some drug-induced toxicity.

INTOXICATION Amphetamine intoxication is diagnosed when the effects of the drug exceed the mood-elevating effects that users typically seek when they use amphetamines. The diagnosis of intoxication would be appropriate when the drug effects are problematic enough to require differentiation from hypomanic or manic behavior.

Amphetamine and amphetaminelike drug intoxication can also be confused with PCP intoxication, although the latter is usually associated with nystagmus, motor incoordination, and some cognitive impairment. Endocrine disorders (such as Cushing's disease) and the excessive use of steroids should also be considered.

TOXIC PSYCHOSIS Amphetamine-induced toxic psychosis can be exceedingly difficult to differentiate from schizophrenia and other psychotic disorders characterized by hallucinations or delusions. The presence of vivid visual or tactile hallucinations should raise a suspicion of a drug-induced disorder. In areas and populations where amphetamine use is common it may be necessary to provide only a provisional diagnosis until the patient can be observed and drug test results are obtained. Even then, there may be difficulties because in some urban areas a high percentage of persons with established diagnoses of schizophrenia are also users of amphetamines or cocaine.

AMPHETAMINE-INDUCED ANXIETY DISORDER Amphetamine-induced anxiety disorder must also be distinguished from panic disorder and generalized anxiety disorder.

OTHER SYMPTOMS The symptoms that may emerge during withdrawal—depression, dysphoria, anhedonia, disturbed sleep—need to be distinguished from those of primary mood disorders and primary sleep disorders. Unless the severity of the symptoms is more intense or more prolonged than is typical of amphetamine withdrawal and require independent treatment, the diagnosis should be limited to withdrawal rather than amphetamine-induced mood disorder. When a diagnosis of amphetamine-induced mood disorder is made, it is important to specify whether its onset was during intoxication or in withdrawal. It is also possible to specify the subtype of mood disorder (with depressive, manic, or mixed features). In differentiating amphetamine-induced mood disorder from the primary mood disorder the critical factor is the clinician's judgment that the mood disorder was caused by the drug. In general, an amphetamine-induced mood disorder or mood disorder with onset during intoxication or withdrawal remits within a week or two. It is appropriate, therefore, to withhold judgment about the diagnosis during the early phase of withdrawal. If depressed mood and related symptoms persist beyond a few weeks, the possibility of alternative causes should be entertained. In considering diagnostic possibilities the clinician should consider the age of the patient at the onset of symptoms and a history of episodes of mood disorder that developed before the onset of drug use or during any long intervals when there was no significant drug abuse.

COURSE AND PROGNOSIS

The natural history of amphetamine dependence in the United States is less well documented than that of opioids or cocaine. Some researchers believe that some users of intravenous amphetamines in the 1960s moved on to heroin use in the 1970s. However, it seems likely that many whose use was less severe simply stopped or recovered, whereas others intensified their use of alcohol. Japanese clinicians believe that some amphetamine users may develop persistent psychosis and that those who recover remain at high risk (sensitization) of reexperiencing psychosis if they use amphetamines again.

A three-year to eight-year follow-up study of 110 methamphetamine users hospitalized for drug-related problems in Japan in the 1980s found that 12 former patients had died, a mortality rate 11 times higher than age-matched and sex-matched general population controls. However, 56 percent of those still alive had not used amphetaminelike drugs in the year before interview, and most of them also showed improvements in work and family relationships. Twenty-five percent were thought to have highly or moderately unfavorable outcomes in terms of drug use, work, and family relationships.

The prognosis for Japanese convicted and imprisoned for crimes related to stimulant drug use seems as bleak as in the United States, with 58 percent having again committed crimes within one year after release and 98 percent having again committed crimes within five years.

TREATMENT

There are no specific, well-established treatments for dependence on amphetamine or amphetaminelike drugs.

In contrast to the growing body of controlled studies on the treatment of cocaine dependence, virtually no controlled studies on the treatment of amphetamine dependence have been carried out. It is reasonable to expect that treatments that prove useful with cocaine dependence will be effective in amphetamine dependence as well, and the same general principles described for treating opioid or cocaine dependence are presumed to be appropriate. Differences in approach, if any, will probably be based on differences in the mechanisms of action and toxicity of amphetamine and related substances. For example, in animals drugs that increase the synthesis of 5-hydroxytryptamine (5-HT) (such as L-tryptophan) or block its reuptake (such as fluoxetine [Prozac]) decrease the self-administration of amphetamines but not of cocaine. Thus, although the benefits of fluoxetine remain unclear (in one study it was not found to alter cocaine use or retention in treatment among cocaine users seeking treatment, but in another study it did both), it might still prove useful for amphetamine users. Such agents might also be useful in countering exaggerated mood lability or impulsivity associated with postulated decreases of 5-HT levels that might be caused by high-dose amphetamine abuse. Also, even though tricyclic antidepressants do not have robust and replicable effects on cocaine use, they might be more useful for treating amphetamine dependence. Clinical case reports suggest that such agents can be used during the early weeks following amphetamine withdrawal. In human volunteers pimozide (Orap) has been found to attenuate some of the euphoric effects of oral amphetamine.

SELECTION OF TREATMENT SETTING The general principles of treatment for amphetamine dependence are not very different from those for cocaine and opioid dependence, but there are fewer replicated studies on the efficacy of any particular treatment approach. As is the case with cocaine and opioid dependence, amphetamine dependence that is severe enough to require formal treatment is often associated with other psychiatric diagnoses.

Patient heterogeneity requires thoughtful selection among available alternatives. Not all amphetamine users require extensive treatment; some users who are not dependent respond to external pressures, as when employers insist on careful monitoring of drug use. The executive with little history of psychopathology, a supportive social network, economic assets, and personal skills has a different prognosis and a wider range of options than does a patient who is unemployed and alienated from the family, and who may also be using opioids. Severe depression, psychotic manifestations beyond the initial withdrawal period, and drug use that is completely out of control (that is, repeated failure to respond to outpatient efforts) seem to be the major accepted criteria for hospitalization.

OTHER AGENTS

SUBSTITUTED AMPHETAMINES 3,4-Methylenedioxymethamphetamine (MDMA, also called ecstasy or Adam) is one of a series of substituted amphetamines that includes 3,4-methylenedioxyethylamphetamine (MDEA or MDE also called Eve), 3,4-methylenedioxyamphetamine (MDA), 2,5-dimethoxy-4-bromo-amphetamine (DOB), paramethoxyamphetamine (PMA), and others. The drugs produce subjective effects resembling those of amphetamine and lysergic acid diethylamide (LSD) and in that sense MDMA and similar analogs may represent a distinct category of drugs.

A methamphetamine derivative that came into use in the 1980s, MDMA was not technically subject to legal regulation at the time. Although it has been labeled a designer drug in the belief that it was deliberately synthesized to evade legal regulation, it was actually synthesized and patented in 1914. Several psychiatrists have utilized it as an adjunct to psychotherapy and concluded that it was of value. At one time it was advertised as legal and was used in psychotherapy for its subjective effects. However, it was never approved by the FDA. Its use raised questions of both safety and legality, since the related amphetamine derivatives MDA, DOB, and PMA had caused a number of overdose deaths, and MDA was known to cause extensive destruction of serotonergic nerve terminals in the CNS. Using emergency scheduling authority, the Drug Enforcement Agency made MDMA a Schedule I drug under the CSA, along with LSD, heroin, and marijuana. Despite its illegal status MDMA continues to be manufactured, distributed, and used in the United States, Europe, and Australia.

Mechanisms of action The unusual properties of the drugs may be a consequence of the different actions of the optical isomers, with the R(−) isomers producing LSD-like effects and the amphetaminelike properties linked to S(+) isomers. The LSD-like actions, in turn, may be linked to the capacity to release serotonin. There may be significant differences in subjective effects and toxicity among the various derivatives. Animals in laboratory experiments will self-administer the drugs, suggesting that there are prominent amphetaminelike effects.

Subjective effects After usual doses (100 to 150 mg) users of MDMA experience an elevation of mood and, according to various reports, increased self-confidence and sensory sensitivity; peaceful feelings, coupled with insight, empathy, and closeness to people; and decreased appetite. Difficulty in concentrating and an increased capacity to focus have both been reported. Dysphoric reactions, psychotomimetic effects, and psychosis have also been reported. Higher doses seem more likely to produce psychotomimetic effects. Sympathomimetic effects of tachycardia, palpitation, increased blood pressure, sweating, and bruxism are common. The subjective effects are reported to be prominent for about four to eight hours, but may not last as long or may last longer, depending on the dose and route of administration. The drug is usually taken orally, but it has been snorted and injected. Both tachyphylaxis and some tolerance are reported by users.

The acute untoward effects reported include precipitation of episodes of panic and anxiety. More severe brief psychiatric disturbances can also occur, and preexisting pathology does not appear to be a requisite for severe reactions. A healthy drug-free subject known to be without personal and family psychiatric illness was given a 140 mg dose of the drug and developed a psychosis lasting two and a half hours that included vivid auditory and visual hallucinations and a belief that people were making noise to annoy him intentionally.

Following the acute effects of MDMA there may be a combination of some diminishing residual effects gradually superseded by feelings of drowsiness, fatigue, depression, and difficulty concentrating, somewhat comparable to the crash after the cessation of amphetamines. More persistent neuropsychiatric adverse effects include anxiety, depression, flashbacks, irritability, panic disorder, psychosis, and memory disturbance.

Toxicity Although it is not as toxic as MDA, various somatic toxicities attributable to MDMA have been reported, as well as fatal overdoses. It does not appear to be neurotoxic when injected into the brain of animals, but is metabolized to MDA in both animals and humans. In animals MDMA produces selective, long-lasting damage to serotonergic nerve terminals. It is not certain if the levels of the MDA metabolite reached in humans after the usual doses of MDMA are sufficient to produce lasting damage. Nonhuman primates are more sensitive than are rodents to MDMA's toxic effects, show neurotoxicity at doses not much higher than those used by humans, and the neurotoxicity is either more prolonged or is permanent. Users of MDMA show differences in neuroendocrine responses to serotonergic probes, and although psychological assessment of a small sample of users did not reveal evidence of current anxiety or a mood disorder, eight of nine subjects has at least some impairment on at least one test of neuropsychological function.

Other reported toxicities include arrhythmias, cardiovascular collapse, rhabdomyolysis, acute renal failure, and hepatotoxicity. The role that contaminants in illicit MDMA played in the toxic reactions is uncertain.

Although the abuse of MDMA has continued, dependence does not appear to be a significant problem. Among a sample of Australian MDMA users, 28 percent reported that problems related to the use of the drug were mostly acute reactions, such as panic, paranoia, loss of reality, and hallucinations. Only 2 percent reported feeling dependent (needing to use it every day to cope), but 22 percent claimed that they knew someone who had been dependent and 47 percent believed it was possible to become addicted. MDA, MDMA, PMA, and MDEA have all been linked to psychosis and overdose deaths. The toxic manifestations of overdose include restlessness, agitation, sweating, rigidity, high blood pressure, tachycardia, and hyperpyrexia and convulsions. Chlorpromazine (Thorazine) prevented lethality in dogs but there are no clinical reports of its use for this purpose in humans.

There are currently no established clinical uses for MDMA although before its regulation there were several reports of its beneficial effects as an adjunct to psychotherapy.

KHAT The fresh leaves of *Catha edulis,* a bush native to East Africa, have been used as a stimulant in the Middle East, Africa, and the Arabian peninsula for at least 1,000 years. Khat is still widely used in Ethiopia, Kenya, Somalia, and Yemen. The amphetaminelike effects of khat have long been recognized, and although efforts to isolate the active ingredient were first undertaken in the 19th century, it has only been in the past decade that cathinone [S(−)α-aminopropriophenone or S-2-amino-1-phenyl-1-propanone] was shown to be the substance responsible. Cathinone is a precursor moiety that is normally enzymatically converted in the plant to the less active entities norephedrine and cathine (norpseudoephedrine), which explains why only the fresh leaves of the plant are valued for their stimulant effects. Cathinone has most of the CNS and peripheral actions of amphetamine and appears to have the same mechanism of action. In humans it elevates mood, decreases hunger, and alleviates fatigue. Like amphetamine, it is self-administered by laboratory animals, and produces increased locomotor activity and stereotypy. At high doses it can induce an amphetaminelike psychosis in humans. Because it is typically absorbed buccally after chewing the leaf, and because the alkaloid is metabolized relatively rapidly, high toxic blood levels are not frequently reached. Concern about khat use is linked to its dependence-producing properties rather than to its acute toxicity. It is estimated that five million doses are consumed each day, despite prohibition of its use in a number of African and Arab countries.

In the 1990s several clandestine laboratories began synthesizing methcathinone, a drug with actions quite similar to those of cathinone. Known by a number of street names (for example, CAT, goob, and crank), its popularity is due primarily to its ease of synthesis from ephedrine or pseudoephedrine, which were readily available until placed under special controls. Methcathinone has been moved to Schedule I of the CSA. The patterns of use, side effects, and complications are quite similar to those reported for amphetamine.

SUGGESTED CROSS-REFERENCES

The neural sciences are presented in Chapter 1 and neuropsychiatry and behavioral neurology in Chapter 2. A classification of mental disorders appears in Chapter 11. An introduction to and overview of substance-related disorders is presented in Section 13.1, cocaine-related disorders in Section 13.6, and various drugs in Chapter 32 on biological therapies, particularly sympathomimetics in Section 32.20. Schizophrenia is discussed in

Chapter 14, other psychotic disorders in Chapter 15, and attention-deficit disorders in Chapter 38.

REFERENCES

Frawley P J, Smith J W: One year follow-up after multimodal inpatient treatment for cocaine and methamphetamine dependencies. J Substance Abuse Treatment *9:* 271, 1992.

*Gawin F H, Ellinwood E H: Cocaine and other stimulants. N Engl J Med *318:* 1173, 1988.

Giannini A J, Miller N S, Turner, C: Treatment of khat addiction. J Substance Abuse Treatment *9:* 379, 1992.

Hall W, Hando J: Route of administration and adverse effects of amphetamine use among young adults in Sydney, Australia. Drug Alc Rev *13:* 277, 1994.

*Jaffe J H: Drug addiction and drug abuse. In *Goodman and Gilman's The Pharmacological Basis of Therapeutics,* ed 8, A G Gilman, T W Rall, A S Nies, P Taylor, editors, p 522. Pergamon, New York, 1990.

*Kalant O J: *The Amphetamines.* Charles C Thomas, Springfield, IL, 1973.

Kalix P: Pharmacological properties of the stimulant khat. Pharmacol Ther *48:* 397, 1990.

Kessler R C, McGonagle K A, Zhao S, Nelson C B, Hughes M, Eshelman S, Wittchen H-U, Kendler K S: Lifetime and 12-month prevalence of DSM-III-R psychiatric disorders in the United States. Arch Gen Psychiatry *51:* 8, 1994.

Konuma K, Hirai S, Sasahara M: Treatment of methamphetamine-related mental disorders and follow-up study on its outcome. In *Cocaine and Methamphetamine. Behavioral Toxicology, Clinical Psychiatry and Epidemiology,* S Fukui, K Wada, M Iyo, editors, p 346. Drug Abuse Prevention Center, Tokyo, 1991.

*Seiden L S, Sabol K E, Ricaurte G A: Amphetamine: Effects on catecholamine systems and behavior. In *Annual Review of Pharmacology and Toxicology,* vol 33, A K Cho, T F Blaschke, H H Loh, J L Way, editors, p 639. Annual Reviews, Palo Alto, CA, 1993.

Solowij N, Hall W, Lee N: Recreational MDMA use in Sydney: A profile of "Ecstasy" users and their experiences with the drug. Br J Addict *87:* 1161, 1992.

*Steele T D, McCann, U D, Ricaurte G A: 3,4-Methylenedioxymethamphetamine (MDMA, "Ecstasy"): Pharmacology and toxicology in animals and humans. Addiction *89:* 539, 1994.

13.4 CAFFEINE-RELATED DISORDERS AND NICOTINE-RELATED DISORDERS

JOHN F. GREDEN, M.D.
OVIDE POMERLEAU, Ph.D.

INTRODUCTION

Caffeine and nicotine are two of the three most widely consumed psychoactive agents in the world (the third is ethyl alcohol). Clinical consequences stemming from their use are widespread and real. Diagnosis is not difficult, but discontinuation of use often is, especially for nicotine. Effective intervention strategies are available, but because both agents have been so widely domesticated and accepted, clinical inquiries are often neglected, available interventions are underemployed, and long-term psychological and health consequences ensue.

Caffeine consumers often use nicotine and vice versa, and both agents are metabolized in the cytochrome P_{450} 1A2 system, but they differ in their neurobiological substrates, clinical features, and treatments.

CAFFEINE-RELATED DISORDERS

Caffeine intoxication is caused by caffeine, a xanthine derivative (1-, 3-, 7-trimethlyxanthine) belonging to the chemical class of alkaloids. The drug is found naturally in coffee, tea, cocoa, and maté, and it is a component of soft drinks, chocolate, a number of prescription drugs, and hundreds of over-the-counter drug products, including analgesics, stimulants, diet preparations, and common cold remedies. Despite the introduction and marketing of decaffeinated products, the drug is difficult to avoid, even for those who try. Table 13.4-1 illustrates common sources. Figure 13.4-1 illustrates the "rule of 25s," the simplest approach for calculating caffeine intake in clinical settings. It entails determining concentrations of various caffeine-containing vehicles, rounding off to multiples of 25, and adding intake from all sources.

HISTORY People first began ingesting caffeine-containing berries in Arabic lands approximately 1,000 years ago. The stimulant properties of caffeine were noted, praised, and sought by some, and vigorously criticized by others. Religious leaders generally condemned such use. Government leaders sought to interdict commerce and prohibit the use of caffeine by law or discourage it by high taxes. Some physicians joined the fray, conveying rather frightening descriptions of caffeinism. The chronic consumer was described by an anonymous 18th-century physician as someone who is "tremulous and loses his self-command; he is subject to fits of agitation and depression; he loses his color and has a haggard appearance. The appetite falls off . . . the heart also suffers; it palpitates, or it intermits."

As history documents, such prohibition efforts failed. Rather than disappearing, its use spread throughout every society in the world, encouraged by the introduction of more palatable vehicles for ingestion, such as hot drink preparations of caffeine-containing coffee berries (the first coffee) or tea leaves (the first tea). In the late 1800s, the drug began appearing in soft drinks (Dr. Pepper, Coca-Cola, and Pepsi-Cola), further enhancing its distribution and exposure among younger populations. After 1914 legal statutes required that cocaine be banished from cola drinks and that caffeine be included, one of history's many attempts to deal with one substance of abuse by substituting another deemed less harmful.

The debate about whether caffeine should be considered a drug of abuse persists. The Food and Drug Administration (FDA) has traditionally considered caffeine as one of many substances that are generally recognized as safe (GRAS). In 1978 the FDA decided to reassess the issue, commissioning a committee to investigate GRAS substances and subsequently publishing a report on caffeine. The results, although equivocal, indicated that the scientific debate should continue.

COMPARATIVE NOSOLOGY Caffeine overuse was not considered an official diagnosis by the American Psychiatric Association until 1980 when the third edition of *Diagnostic and Statistical Manual of Mental Disorders* (DSM-III) listed specific criteria for caffeine intoxication. Caffeine intoxication remains the only specific caffeine-related disorder in the fourth edition of DSM (DSM-IV). Caffeine-induced anxiety disorder and caffeine-induced sleep disorder are diagnosed instead of caffeine intoxication only if the symptoms exceed those for caffeine intoxication and warrant independent clinical treatment. Caffeine abuse and dependence have been excluded presumably because of the lack of published clinical evidence that it is difficult to stop caffeine, or a judgment that the withdrawal syndrome following discontinuation is generally not severe enough to warrant clinical attention. Most recent reports disagree with that exclusion. New data emphasize the prevalence of the withdrawal syndrome, its frequent misdiagnosis, the fact that withdrawal can occur even among those whose daily intake is low

TABLE 13.4-1
Sources of Caffeine

Sources	Beverage Sources mg/unit	Rule of 25s
Fresh drip coffee	100-140	(150)
Brewed coffee	90-110	(100)
Decaffeinated coffee	2-4	(0)
Instant coffee	66-100	(75)
Tea (leaf)	30-75	(50)
Tea (bag)	42-100	(50)
Cocoa	5-50	(25)
Caffeinated soft drinks	25-50	(50)

Soft Drink Sources

Sources	Approx amt of caffeine per unit (glass) (in mg)
Traditional cola drink (Pepsi, Coca-cola, Tab, Royal Crown, Dr. Pepper)	25-50
Mountain Dew	25-50
Canada Dry Ginger Ale	0
Caffeine-Free Coca-Cola	0
Caffeine-Free Pepsi	0
7-Up	0
Sprite	0
Squirt	0

Analgesics

Sources	Approx amt of caffeine/unit (tablet) (in mg)
APC (aspirin, phenacetin, and caffeine)	32
Cafergot	100
Darvon Compound	32
Fiorinal	40
Migral	50

Over-the-Counter Medications

Source	Approx amt of caffeine/unit (in mg)
Aspirin compound	32
BC tablet	16
Bromo-seltzer	32.5
Capron	32
Comeback	100
Cope	32
Dolor	30
Easy-Mens	32
Excedrin	60
Goody's Headache Powder	32.5
Medache	32
Moranox	15
Midol	32
Nilain	32
PAC	32
Pre-mens	66
Stanback Tablets	16
Stanback Powder	32
Trigesic	30
Vanquish	32
Many over-the-counter cold preparations	30

Stimulants, Appetite Suppressants, and Cold Tablets (Over-the-Counter)

Source	Approx amts of caffeine/unit (in mg)
Amostat Tablets	100
Anorexin Capsules	100
Appedrine Tablets	100
Caffedrine Capsules	250
Dexatrim Capsules	200
Double-E Alertness	180
Nodoz Tablets	100
Odrinex Tablets	50
Prolamine Capsules	140
Quick-Pep Tablets	150
Spantrol Capsules	150
Tirend Tablets	100

TABLE 13.4.1 (*continued*)

Source	Approx amts of caffeine/unit (in mg)
Verb TD Capsules	200
Vivarin Tablets	200
Wakoz	200
Many over-the-counter cold preparations	30

Over-the-Counter Analgesics Without Caffeine

Source	Approx amt of caffeine/unit (in mg)
Anacin	0
Aspirin	0
Empirin	0
Pamprin	0
Tylenol	0

Chocolate

Source	Approx amt of caffeine/unit (in mg)
Chocolate bar or ounce of baking chocolate	25-35

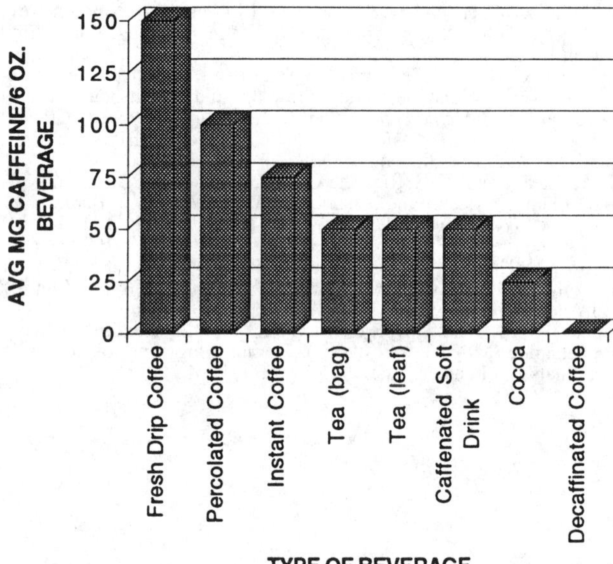

FIGURE 13.4-1 *Illustration of the average caffeine content of beverages in increments of 25. (Figure adapted from J J Barone, H Roberts: Human consumption of caffeine. In* Caffeine, *P B Dews, editor, p 59. Springer-Verlag, New York, 1984.)*

(for example, 100 to 200 mg a day), and the fact that although symptoms are relatively mild, misguided interventions are usually ineffective and can have incremental, deleterious pharmacological consequences. DSM-IV includes suggested research criteria for caffeine withdrawal.

EPIDEMIOLOGY

PATTERNS OF CAFFEINE CONSUMPTION Epidemiological estimates of caffeine-related disorders require assessments of total average daily intake of caffeine from all sources, but consumption data are sketchy for most sources other than coffee. International caffeine consumption appears to exceed several billion kilograms annually. Although similarities outweigh differences, regional and cultural variations are seen. (For example, per capita intake for the entire world's population approximates 70 mg a day, but in the United States that figure exceeds 200 mg.) Approximately 80 percent of adult Americans report regular intake (there are only slight differences in use patterns across various regions of the country). Significant consumption tends to start in the late teens or 20s, to peak in the 30s, and to stabilize thereafter, with use being somewhat greater among men than among women. Ingestion takes place predominantly in the morning hours. As reflected in Figure 13.4-2 the percentage of coffee drinkers dropped significantly just prior to 1985 and remains stable, whereas decaffeinated coffee use simultaneously increased and then also stabilized. Before concluding that caffeine use is on the decline, however, it should be noted that the use of caffeinated tea and soft drinks has increased considerably and that caffeine-containing medications remain popular. Caffeine retains its dubious distinction of being the most consumed psychoactive agent among Americans.

LINKAGES BETWEEN CAFFEINE CONSUMPTION AND CAFFEINE-RELATED DISORDERS It remains difficult to link consumption patterns with actual diagnoses of caffeine intoxication, for several reasons.

First, and most important, there is no clear-cut threshold at which all people can be expected to develop clinically disturbing features. Instead, there is marked individual variation. Most people show characteristic dose-response patterns, but caffeine-related disorders are noted among a few very low users, and yet ostensibly fail to occur among some extremely high consumers.

Second, caffeine-related disorders do not equate with coffee consumption. Although caffeinated coffee is the major source of caffeine for the American population, for many persons other sources represent most, or even all, of their intake; all sources should be considered by clinicians and investigators, but often they are not.

Third, caffeine intoxication is normally associated with recent intake, and the importance of tolerance and chronic use is down played. Most cases of caffeine-related disorders result from chronic ingestion by persons who are tolerant and who have been consuming caffeine for years without apparent difficulty, and then inexplicably start having symptoms. It may be that they have reached a level of intake that is associated with dysphoric symptoms (caffeine has biphasic effects, with pleasurable responses at low doses and dysphoric ones at high doses), or that they have undergone changes in neurobiological substrates (for example, kindling, modifications in receptor sensitivity associated with aging, or up-regulation of adenosine receptors because of chronic consumption).

Fourth, comorbid diagnoses associated with caffeine use often confound an accurate diagnosis. In addition to other psychiatric or medical conditions, concomitant use of other psychoactive agents, such as nicotine, alcohol, or benzodiazepines, is common in caffeine users.

Finally, differing ambient states at the time of ingestion (for example, fatigue, sleep deprivation, and stress), or even consumption at different times of day may obfuscate the question whether a person is caffeine dependent.

ESTIMATED PREVALENCE OF CAFFEINE INTOXICATION Intake exceeding 500 mg a day represents the best marker of high risk for caffeine-related disorders. Twenty to 30 percent of North Americans meet this criterion. An estimated 10 percent are believed to qualify for the diagnosis of caffeine intoxication, a higher rate than for most other substances of abuse. The prevalence rate for psychiatric patients is considerably higher than for the population at large, perhaps as much as double; persons with panic disorders, most of whom report minimal or no use of caffeine, are a notable exception.

ETIOLOGY

NEUROPHARMACOLOGY AND REWARD REINFORCEMENT

Initial exposure For a caffeine-related disorder to occur, one must ingest caffeine. The pattern usually begins during childhood. For most American children, exposure is difficult to avoid because of their consumption of soft drinks, candy, or chocolate products; coffee and tea are infrequent sources. Consumption in children is surprisingly and disturbingly high. When all sources are considered, children between 1 and 5 years of age average 1.20 mg per kg of body weight a day, in contrast to 2.60 mg per kg for persons aged 18 and over. That relatively high dosage is attributable to the small size of children, resulting in a relatively large concentration on a milligram-per-kilogram basis. Parents may ignore this pattern and assume—erroneously—that a 12-ounce cola drink is as innocuous for a 4-year-old as for a 40-year-old. Such is not the case. There is a glaring need for more information on the consequences of caffeine consumption in children.

Escalation Once started, caffeine use generally increases gradually over the years. Such a pattern is consistent with the development of tolerance to certain effects and the involvement of reward-reinforcement mechanisms in the central nervous system (CNS). Consumption often surges during college years, in part for social reasons, but also because of caffeine's well-deserved reputation for enhancing alertness and opposing sleep.

Brain caffeine levels Caffeine is absorbed from the gastrointestinal tract rapidly and completely. Peak plasma levels tend

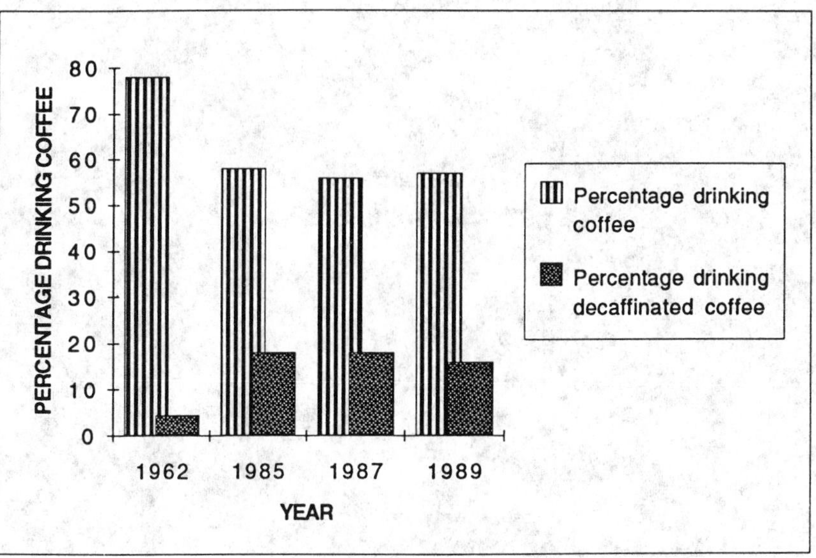

FIGURE 13.4-2 *Consumption trends for coffee and decaffeinated coffee. (Figure based on data from the International Coffee Organization: United States of America coffee drinkers study-winter, London, 1989.)*

to occur within 30 to 45 minutes. Following absorption, the drug promptly crosses the blood-brain barrier; ingested dosages are closely correlated with brain concentrations. Such prompt distribution to the brain is important, since clinical and animal studies indicate that CNS stimulation is what most consumers of caffeine actively seek. Moreover, pharmacological agents that reach the brain's reward pathways promptly (that is, within minutes) are reinforcing and have potential liability for abuse. Paraxanthine is an active metabolite of caffeine. It has many equivalent pharmacological effects and reaches levels about two thirds of those for caffeine.

Neuropharmacological and neuroendocrine effects Caffeine enhances CNS norepinephrine secretion, inhibits phosphodiesterase breakdown of cyclic 3′,5′-adenosine monophosphate (cAMP) at high concentrations, sensitizes central catecholamine postsynaptic receptors (including those for dopamine), enhances cyclic guanosine 3′,5′-monophosphate (cGMP), and modulates acetylcholine and serotonin activity. Caffeine induces significant increases in cortisol, but no meaningful change in prolactin.

Role of dopamine in reinforcement Reinforcement paradigms for most drugs of abuse (for example, cocaine and amphetamines) have been linked to dopaminergic effects on the brain's reward-reinforcement system, located in the median forebrain bundle and hypothalamus. Caffeine seems to be no exception. If tolerance is a factor in the development of caffeinism, then heavy users should find the drug more reinforcing after abstinence; that has been well documented. Tolerance has been shown to develop within days.

Role of adenosine in clinical profile Relatively recent data suggest that caffeine's ability to antagonize adenosine receptors in the brain probably accounts for the most important of the drug's behavioral effects. Adenosine is an important CNS neuromodulator, possessing sedative, anxiolytic, and anticonvulsant properties. Adenosine also dilates blood vessels in cerebral and coronary circulatory networks. Caffeine competes with adenosine for binding at its high-affinity receptor sites, preventing adenosine's normal tranquilizing or sedating effects. Thus, caffeine's stimulant or anxiety-inducing actions appear to be secondary effects of adenosine antagonism. Chronic caffeine exposure has also been shown to induce heterologous upregulation of adenosine receptors in humans. Caffeine's antagonism to vasodilation by adenosine may account for caffeine withdrawal headaches, as well as for its efficacy in treating migraine headaches.

Positron emission tomography (PET) imaging studies confirm that a caffeine dose of 200 mg produces a diffuse decrease in cerebral blood flow of approximately 30 percent within 45 minutes (Figure 13.4-3). Visual portrayals of the phenomenon can be shown to patients and families to illustrate and promote greater acceptance of caffeine's potency.

Genetic predispositions Recent data suggest that some persons may have a genetically inherited susceptibility to the reinforcing aspects of some drugs of abuse, including caffeine, nicotine, and alcohol. There also are suggestions of genetically transmitted variations in sleep after caffeine use.

DIAGNOSIS AND CLINICAL FEATURES Most persons with caffeine-related disorders fail to link symptoms with longstanding ingestion, but instead present with a litany of complaints, most of which they attribute to other causes. Even when a linkage with caffeine is suggested, many vigorously deny any possible connection ("I've always been a big coffee drinker. It

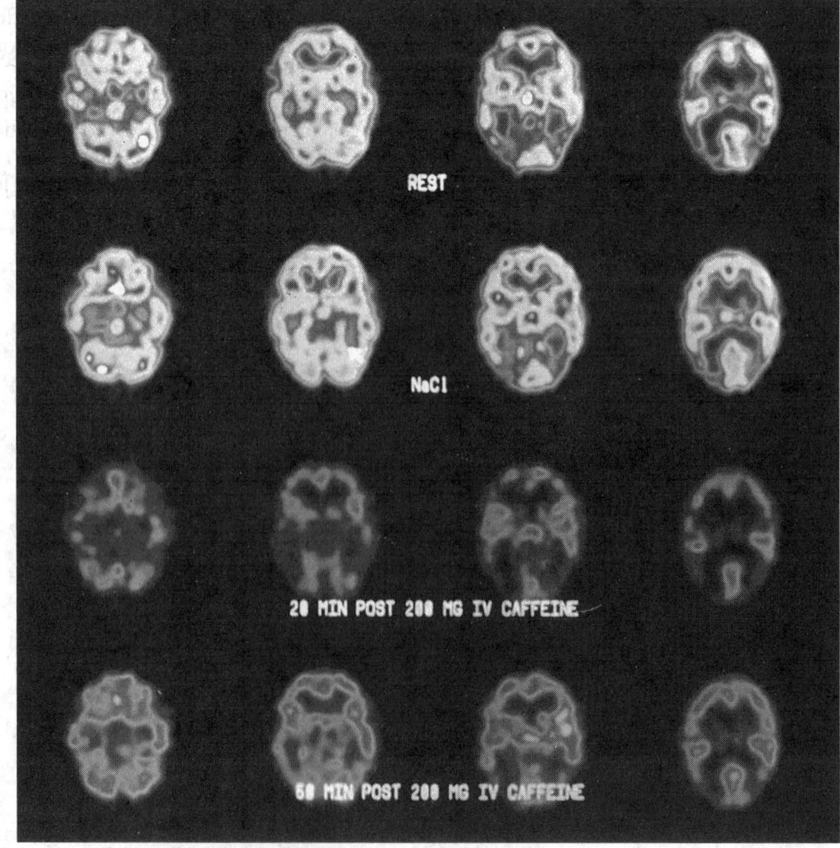

FIGURE 13.4-3 *Positron-emission tomographic measurements of regional cerebral blood flow in a normal adult human subject, using the oxygen-15 water method. Horizontal slices at four brain levels (highest to lowest levels, right to left) were made under four different conditions: (1) resting (top row of four scans); (2) after a saline-NaCl-placebo infusion (second row of scans); (3) 20 minutes after an intravenous infusion of 200 mg of caffeine (third row of scans); and (4) 50 minutes after caffeine infusion. The color scale, highest to lowest blood flow: white, red, orange, green, blue, violet. These results represent a decrease in whole brain blood flow of approximately 30 percent.* (*Courtesy of Oliver G Cameron, MD, PhD. Figure from O G Cameron, J G Modell, M Hariharan: Caffeine and human cerebral blood flow: A positron emission tomography study. Life Sci 47:* 1141, 1990.)

never bothered me before, so it can't be the cause of my problem now''). The diagnosis of caffeine intoxication generally must be ferreted out by the clinician.

DSM-IV lists the caffeine-related disorders (Table 13.4-2) and provides diagnostic criteria for caffeine intoxication (Table 13.4-3), but does not formally recognize a diagnosis of caffeine withdrawal, which is classified as a caffeine-related disorder not otherwise specified (NOS). The diagnostic criteria for other caffeine-related disorders are contained in those sections specific for the principal symptom.

Caffeine intoxication Known conventionally as caffeinism, caffeine intoxication is a multifaceted syndrome produced by acute or chronic overuse of caffeine, usually in the form of coffee, tea, cola, chocolate, cocoa, analgesic medications, or various over-the-counter products. Central nervous system manifestations usually predominate in patients with caffeinism, especially anxiety, sleep disturbances, mood changes, and psychophysiological complaints. Features are largely dose-dependent and are directly related to the drug's established pharmacological actions.

Essential features of caffeine intoxication in DSM-IV include a temporal association between caffeine ingestion, usually in excess of 250 mg (and more commonly in excess of 500 mg) a day, and the development of at least five of the symptoms illustrated in Table 13.4-3.

Caffeine withdrawal Caffeine withdrawal is a physiological state produced by a sudden cessation of the use of caffeine by a regular, dependent consumer. The most common feature is a withdrawal headache. Other symptoms include excessive drowsiness and fatigue. Impaired psychomotor performance, psychophysiological complaints (nausea, excessive yawning), and craving are occasionally described. Although not an official diagnosis in DSM-IV, the withdrawal syndrome is common and is probably responsible for substantial self-medication. The research criteria are presented in Table 13.4-4.

If regular consumption of caffeine is discontinued suddenly, a characteristic withdrawal syndrome develops in 30 to 50 percent of users, usually within 18 to 24 hours. The occurrence of the syndrome is disproportionately high on weekends and during vacations. It was once believed that high daily doses were required for the induction of tolerance and withdrawal, but recent studies illustrate that some persons develop withdrawal manifestations despite very low daily intake (for example, 100 to 200 mg daily). The withdrawal syndrome is further documented by double-blind tests, confirming that a subset of coffee and soda drinkers reliably self-administer caffeinated beverages in preference to uncaffeinated beverages. The caffeine withdrawal syndrome, with its concomitant vascular headache, may account for the fact that so many over-the-counter pain reliever products contain caffeine. Postoperative headache following general anesthesia has been shown to be linked, at least in part, to the caffeine withdrawal syndrome, as have weekend headache attacks in migraine patients, especially those with excessively delayed wakening on Saturdays and Sundays. Those data suggest that caffeine withdrawal justifiably warrants inclusion as an official diagnosis in the nosology.

Mr. E. was a 41-year-old attorney whose internist had referred him for a psychiatric consultation. He had been complaining of fatigue, loss of motivation, sleepiness, headaches, and nausea, and of feeling unsociable and having difficulty concentrating. His symptoms occurred mostly on weekends, and as a result he often begged off from weekend social activities, which caused his wife to become very annoyed with him. She complained that he was fine during the week, but never felt like going out with friends or playing with the children on weekends. He was in good health, with no recent history of medical disorders.

Mr. E. worked a 60-hour week in a busy law practice and barely saw his family during the week. At work he was often anxious, restless, and constantly busy. He frequently had trouble sleeping on weeknights because he worried about his job. He denied marital or family problems, other than those caused by his not wanting to do anything on the weekends.

He had a history of alcohol problems, but had not had a drink for five years. He used to smoke 20 cigarettes a day, but had stopped two months earlier, hoping this would improve his condition. (It did not.) At work he drank four cups of coffee a day. He had stopped using coffee on weekends because he suspected that it might be contributing to his anxiety and sleeplessness.

Discussion Many people recognize that they need a cup of coffee to get going in the morning. What they do not recognize is that often

TABLE 13.4-2
Caffeine-Related Disorders

Caffeine-induced disorders
Caffeine intoxication
Caffeine-induced anxiety disorder
Specify if: with onset during intoxication
Caffeine-induced sleep disorder
Specify if: with onset during intoxication

Caffeine-related disorder not otherwise specified

Table based on DSM-IV, *Diagnostic and Statistical Manual of Mental Disorders,* ed 4. Copyright American Psychiatric Association, Washington, 1994. Used with permission.

TABLE 13.4-3
Diagnostic Criteria for Caffeine Intoxication

A. Recent consumption of caffeine, usually in excess of 250 mg (e.g., more than 2–3 cups of brewed coffee).
B. Five (or more) of the following signs, developing during, or shortly after, caffeine use:
 (1) restlessness
 (2) nervousness
 (3) excitement
 (4) insomnia
 (5) flushed face
 (6) diuresis
 (7) gastrointestinal disturbance
 (8) muscle twitching
 (9) rambling flow of thought and speech
 (10) tachycardia or cardiac arrhythmia
 (11) periods of inexhaustibility
 (12) psychomotor agitation
C. The symptoms in criterion B cause clinically significant distress or impairment in social, occupational, or other important areas of functioning.
D. The symptoms are not due to a general medical condition and are not better accounted for by another mental disorder (e.g., an anxiety disorder).

Table from DSM-IV, *Diagnostic and Statistical Manual of Mental Disorders,* ed 4. Copyright American Psychiatric Association, Washington, 1993. Used with permission.

TABLE 13.4-4
Research Criteria for Caffeine Withdrawal

A. Prolonged daily use of caffeine.
B. Abrupt cessation of caffeine use, or reduction in the amount of caffeine used, closely followed by headache and one (or more) of the following symptoms:
 (1) marked fatigue or drowsiness
 (2) marked anxiety or depression
 (3) nausea or vomiting
C. The symptoms in criterion B cause clinically significant distress or impairment in social, occupational, or other important areas of functioning.
D. The symptoms are not due to the direct physiological effects of a general medical condition (e.g., migraine, viral illness) and are not better accounted for by another mental disorder.

Table from DSM-IV, *Diagnostic and Statistical Manual of Mental Disorders,* ed 4. Copyright American Psychiatric Association, Washington, 1994. Used with permission.

what they are doing by taking one or more cups of coffee is avoiding the development of caffeine withdrawal symptoms. Typically, withdrawal symptoms begin approximately 12 hours after the last cup of coffee. What often happens is that the heavy coffee drinker who has coffee with dinner starts to develop withdrawal symptoms the next morning if he or she, for some reason, does not have coffee at breakfast.

Although caffeine withdrawal is rarely severe enough to cause a person to seek clinical attention, surveys of the general population indicate that 25 percent of people who regularly drink coffee report developing headaches, fatigue, or drowsiness if they miss their usual dose. Interestingly, when actually tested in the laboratory, approximately 50 percent of regular coffee drinkers develop headaches. Even some who regularly drink as little as one cup of coffee a day (100 mg of caffeine) can develop withdrawal symptoms.

It is clear that Mr. E. on weekends, had the characteristic symptoms of caffeine withdrawal, a nonofficial diagnosis that is included in an appendix to DSM-IV.

Follow-up The psychiatrist was impressed with the relationship between the onset of the symptoms of headache, fatigue, difficulty concentrating, sleepiness, and loss of motivation and Mr. E.'s cessation of coffee drinking on weekends. Mr. E. was advised to decrease his consumption of coffee during the week, but he found that he could not function well without his usual dose of coffee. Instead, he decided to resume drinking coffee on the weekends as there was no medical contraindication to his regular use of caffeine. He decided to live with the anxiety and difficulty sleeping that had originally prompted his giving up his weekend coffee. (From *DSM-IV Casebook*. Used with permission.)

Caffeine-induced anxiety disorder Caffeine-induced anxiety disorder, which can occur during caffeine intoxication, is a DSM-IV diagnosis (see Section 17.5). Most items on the list of caffeine intoxication in Table 13.4-3 are anxiety-related. Whenever a patient presents to a psychiatrist with anxietylike features, perhaps one of the most important initial questions to be addressed is whether they might be attributable to concomitant caffeine use. That prioritization is justified for three reasons: (1) both anxiety disorders and caffeine use have high incidence and prevalence and there is considerable overlap between the two (that is, many persons with anxiety features are consuming caffeine); (2) the anxietylike clinical profile associated with caffeinism is indistinguishable from that of general anxiety disorder; and (3) caffeine intoxication is effectively treated by elimination of the causal agent.

Persons with caffeine intoxication often describe themselves as stressed out, uptight, wired, and high-strung. Friends and family members often note that when consuming high doses, the person will talk faster and louder, appear to have excessive energy, complain of not sleeping well, and exhibit greater intolerance, frustration, and irritability. High consumers score significantly higher on levels of both state and trait anxiety. The worst time to increase caffeine intake appears to be during times of stress, since the effects are interactive. Yet, perhaps 30 to 40 percent of persons report increasing intake in the context of stressful situations.

The link between caffeine use and panic attacks is intriguing. Caffeine is not believed to cause panic attacks in normal persons, but 200 mg or more induces onset of panic symptoms in almost three quarters of persons with known panic disorder and intensifies the severity of symptoms when attacks do occur. Considering those aberrations, it is not hard to understand why people with panic disorder report consuming less caffeine than normal controls or patients with other types of psychiatric disorders, or often none at all.

Caffeine-induced sleep disorder Caffeine-induced sleep disorder, which can occur during caffeine intoxication, is a DSM-IV diagnosis (see Chapter 23). Caffeine is associated with a delay in falling asleep, an inability to remain asleep, and early morning awakening. Caffeine interferes with sleep in most persons. Polysomnographic changes are found. The magnitude of interference is greatest among those who have not developed tolerance. Chronic users often fail to associate their sleep impairment with caffeine use earlier in the day, because the pattern develops insidiously, but it is notable that the heaviest caffeine users report significantly greater use of sedative-hypnotic prescription drugs.

Caffeine-related disorder not otherwise specified DSM-IV contains a residual category for caffeine-related disorders, caffeine-related disorder not otherwise specified (Table 13.4-5). The category is for caffeine-related diagnoses that do not meet the criteria for caffeine intoxication, caffeine-induced anxiety disorder, or caffeine-induced sleep disorder.

Comorbid disorders

OTHER SUBSTANCE-RELATED DISORDERS The highest caffeine consumers report greater use of sedative-hypnotics and antianxiety agents than those with moderate, low, or no use. Approximately two thirds of the highest users reported having used an antianxiety agent within the past month. Obviously, patients who have developed anxiety because of caffeine use should discontinue the offending drug rather than add another psychoactive agent to counteract its effects. Despite prevailing myths that caffeine can be used to counteract the effects of alcohol, animal studies reveal that it does not effectively ameliorate, and may worsen, ethanol intoxication.

MOOD DISORDERS High caffeine consumption among psychiatric patients has paradoxically been associated with depressive symptoms. Specifically, depression rating scores were highest among high caffeine users. Causality cannot be generalized to the population at large because no studies have been conducted, but a dose of 450 mg of caffeine has been demonstrated to increase depression scores in patients with panic disorder. Caffeine intake clearly should be considered in every patient with a mood disorder, especially comorbid anxiety and depression.

ATTENTION-DEFICIT/HYPERACTIVITY DISORDER Paradoxically, a small number of people of all ages describe being calmed down by caffeine. The drug has been reported to produce clinical improvement in those with diagnosed attention-deficit/hyperactivity disorder, but it is not considered a first-line treatment.

EATING DISORDERS Caffeine ingestion has been observed to increase during states of starvation. Approximately 15 percent of patients with eating disorders report high caffeine intake (more than 750 mg a day), as well as higher anxiety, a trend toward greater severity of depression (on the Beck Depression Inventory), more frequent binge-eating, and greater use of diet pills, alcohol, and tobacco. Those observations raise the question as to whether some symptoms previously attributed to eating disorders might be linked to concomitant caffeine use. Caf-

TABLE 13.4-5
Caffeine-Related Disorder Not Otherwise Specified

The caffeine-related disorder not otherwise specified category is for disorders associated with the use of caffeine that are not classifiable as caffeine intoxication, caffeine-induced anxiety disorder, or caffeine-induced sleep disorder. An example is caffeine withdrawal.

Table from DSM-IV, *Diagnostic and Statistical Manual of Mental Disorders,* ed 4. Copyright American Psychiatric Association, Washington, 1994. Used with permission.

feine is a primary ingredient in most commercially available diet products.

SCHIZOPHRENIA Some patients with schizophrenia reportedly ingest large amounts of caffeine. Such consumption may worsen positive symptoms of the disorder, perhaps because the drug antagonizes adenosine, a neuromodulator that decreases dopamine release.

Adverse effects Caffeine can induce clinically important actions in most major physiological systems, especially the cardiovascular system (tachycardia and arrhythmias), the gastrointestinal system (epigastric distress, diarrhea, or even peptic ulcer), and the genitourinary system (diuresis, and occasional bladder irritation, leading to frequent and urgent urination). Less common symptoms include excessive perspiration, tingling of fingers and toes, and tinnitus (possibly confounded with concomitant aspirin use through analgesics).

Occasional reports have linked reported coffee or caffeine intake with fibrocystic breast disease, cardiovascular disease, and certain cancers (for example, bladder and pancreatic, although evidence for causality of neoplasms is weak at present). There is emerging evidence that caffeine may accentuate osteoporosis.

PATHOLOGY AND LABORATORY EXAMINATION Caffeine can be measured with liquid chromatography in most body fluids. Since both plasma and brain concentrations are well correlated with oral intake—which can be easily determined—there has been little demand for laboratory assessment of caffeine levels.

DIFFERENTIAL DIAGNOSIS Among primary diagnoses to consider before assigning a diagnosis of caffeine intoxication are general anxiety disorder and related conditions, including panic disorder; medical conditions, such as hyperthyroidism and pheochromocytoma; use of over-the-counter or prescribed stimulant drugs or substances of abuse (especially amphetamines, methylphenidate [Ritalin], cocaine, and phenylpropranolamine [PPA]); other psychiatric diagnoses, such as hypomania, attention-deficit/hyperactivity disorder, coexisting sleep disorders; intake of other pharmacological agents that may occasionally be stimulating, especially yohimbine [Yocon] and anabolic steroids; and sudden withdrawal of antidepressants (especially tricyclics with potent anticholinergic effects).

The clinical history is the key step in diagnosing caffeine intoxication. The "rule of 25s" is helpful in saving time (Table 13.4-1). Caffeine consumption questionnaires—simple, brief, and easily completed and scored—are also extremely effective in screening patients. Persons who report more than 500 mg a day should automatically undergo a more thorough clinical assessment. Urine drug screens may be necessary to rule out other substances of abuse or concomitant use of medications.

Once high intake is documented, the only way to prove a causal relationship is to conduct an A-B-A paradigm, first quantifying symptoms, then totally discontinuing caffeine, a reassessment of symptoms, a two- to three-week wait, and a sudden resumption of caffeine intake. If past symptoms were the result of caffeine intoxication, they generally recur within several days of restarting caffeine.

COURSE AND PROGNOSIS Outcome is favorable, with no known long-term consequences if intake is stopped or dramatically lowered. Relapses are common, however. Caffeine is ubiquitous. It is difficult to avoid consumption entirely, and exposure to even small amounts may prime a relapse in susceptible persons.

TREATMENT Treatment involves discontinuation or marked reduction of intake. Educating patients about sources is essential. Most patients find a list of caffeine-containing agents (Table 13.4-1) helpful as a guide for controlling intake. To enhance effectiveness, availability of decaffeinated alternatives should be encouraged in all major living venues, such as home and work; use of caffeine-containing medications should be reviewed and discontinued where appropriate; and other family members who are caffeine consumers should be encouraged to reduce or preferably to stop intake. If meaningful withdrawal symptoms interfere with the treatment program, a more gradual discontinuation program should be designed. No pharmacological substitutes for withdrawal have been identified, and anxiolytics are not recommended as a long-term solution to treating the syndrome.

Prevention Newborn humans have a limited capacity for caffeine degradation. Fetuses, neonates, infants, and young children have notably less tolerance for caffeine than do adults. The long-term effects of fetal exposure are unknown, but because pregnant women also have decreased ability to metabolize methylxanthines, and early exposure may predispose to subsequent habituation, it is evident that caffeine use should be discouraged throughout pregnancy.

NICOTINE-RELATED DISORDERS

Until quite recently, nicotine dependence resulting from tobacco use was not classified as drug abuse, in part because nicotine agonist effects were not associated with obvious intoxication and because the habit was not considered socially undesirable or disruptive of productive activity. That viewpoint has changed. The cumulative findings of more than 2,500 scientific papers have been summarized in the 1988 *Surgeon General's Report on the Health Consequences of Smoking: Nicotine Addiction.* The unequivocal conclusions were that cigarettes and other forms of tobacco are addicting, that nicotine is the drug in tobacco that causes addiction, and that the pharmacological and behavioral processes that determine tobacco addiction are similar to those that determine addiction to such drugs as heroin and cocaine. The issue of addiction came to the fore dramatically in the 1994 testimony to the United States Congress by the Commissioner of the FDA, who alleged that cigarette manufacturers manipulate the nicotine content of cigarettes for the purpose of making their products addictive.

HISTORY AND COMPARATIVE NOSOLOGY Tobacco products have been consumed since before recorded history, and the similarities in societal responses to both caffeine and nicotine are noteworthy. The earliest known reference to the tobacco plant, native to the New World, is in Mayan stone carvings from about 600 AD. Reports of tobacco smoking are found in Christopher Columbus' diary of 1492, dating the introduction of tobacco to Europe. After that time, despite dismay by some over the rapid spread of tobacco use, no culture to which it was introduced was able to eradicate it. In his famous *Counterblaste to Tobacco* in 1604, King James I of England described the tobacco habit as "a custome lothsome to the eye, hatefull to the Nose, harmefull to the braine, dangerous to the Lungs, and in the blacke stinking fume thereof, neerest resembling the horrible Stigian smoke of the pit that is bottomelesse." To discourage its use in his country, he levied prohibitive taxes. When the exchequer suffered as a result a few years later, he was forced to relent, and he set taxation as high as he could without discouraging use. As one historical commentator observed, governments have been hooked ever since.

EPIDEMIOLOGY Tobacco typically is smoked or is used as snuff, which is either taken into the nasorium or held between the cheek and the gum. Cigarette smokers inhale fairly deeply to bring the nicotine-containing smoke into contact with the small alveoli of the lungs; about 25 percent of the nicotine crosses the alveolar-capillary membrane, reaching the brain in about 15 seconds. Pulmonary absorption factors include inhalation amount, depth, and duration; pH of the smoke; and characteristics of smoke constituents.

Tobacco smoke contains over 3,000 pyrolysis products. In addition to harmful volatile constituents, such as carbon monoxide, the particulate phase contains nicotine, water, and tars (which include radioactive compounds and a number of aromatic hydrocarbons known to be carcinogens, such as nitrosamines, aromatic amines, and benzopyrene).

Cigarette smoking is associated with over 450,000 premature deaths in the United States each year—25 percent of all deaths. Chronic bronchitis and emphysema account for 70,000 deaths per year, 57,000 of which can be attributed to cigarette smoking. Smoking has been proved to be the cause not only of most cases of chronic obstructive pulmonary disease, but also of about 90 percent of bronchogenic carcinoma (106,000 deaths per year) and nearly 35 percent of fatal myocardial infarctions (115,000 deaths a year). Lung cancer is now the leading form of cancer in women, having recently surpassed breast cancer. Although less than 30 percent of Americans currently smoke, the pathophysiological consequences of the habit account for nearly 60 percent of all direct health care costs, with expenditures estimated to exceed one billion dollars a day.

In response to the growing evidence of adverse health effects, the prevalence of smoking has shown a steady decline in the United States. From a peak of 44 percent of adults smoking in 1964, the number had declined to less than 27 percent by the late 1980s. Figure 13.4-4 shows the per capita consumption of cigarettes over the past 70 years. Proportionately fewer women smoke than men, but a linear projection of prevalence trends indicates that more women than men will smoke after 1995. According to recent surveys, 20 percent of adolescent girls smoke, compared with 15 percent of adolescent boys.

ETIOLOGY Initiation into tobacco use was once sufficiently common that it constituted a growing-up ritual, at least among young men. In many parts of the world it is still the case. The smoking status of friends is a good predictor of initiation of smoking, underscoring the importance of social factors in initiation. Smoking by parents and older siblings is also predictive, suggesting the possibility of genetic factors.

With respect to social factors, it should be noted that over the years manufacturers have effectively manipulated the acceptability of tobacco products. For example, smokeless tobacco is marketed in special starter products that have lower concentrations of nicotine, are easier to use (for example, snuff in pouches), and contain nontobacco flavorings, such as mint or cinnamon. Advertising and marketing strategies have involved depicting the use of tobacco by peers in exciting or adventurous settings to imply that the products are social desiderata. The approach was successful, as reflected by the marked rise in the use of smokeless tobacco products by young men in the 1970s.

Nicotine dependence can occur at any age, although use typically begins in adolescence and dependence follows within a few months to a few years. There is evidence that certain users find nicotine's effects to be much more reinforcing (that is, more favorable or adaptive) than do others. Some persons may also be more vulnerable than others to peer pressure and to tobacco advertisements.

Among the reasons people give for smoking are stimulation (increased energy), sensorimotor manipulation (handling and lighting the cigarette), pleasurable relaxation, habit (smoking automatically), reduction of negative affect (smoking to alleviate tension, anxiety, anger, or frustration), and addiction (smoking to avoid or to terminate aversive withdrawal sensations). The subjective effects and observable behavioral consequences of smoking have remarkable concordance with known neuroregulatory actions and effects (Table 13.4-6). The evidence suggests that, by altering the bioavailability of neuroregulators, nicotine serves as a pharmacological coping response to the demands of daily living, providing immediate (although temporary) improvement in affect or performance, as well as relief from the disruptive effects of nicotine withdrawal.

Behavioral genetics A recent review of 18 twin studies found that the concordance rates for smokers were consistently higher in monozygotic than in dizygotic twins (even when the twins were brought up separately), supporting the hypothesis of a genetic component for the smoking habit. In another study, involving 4,960 adult

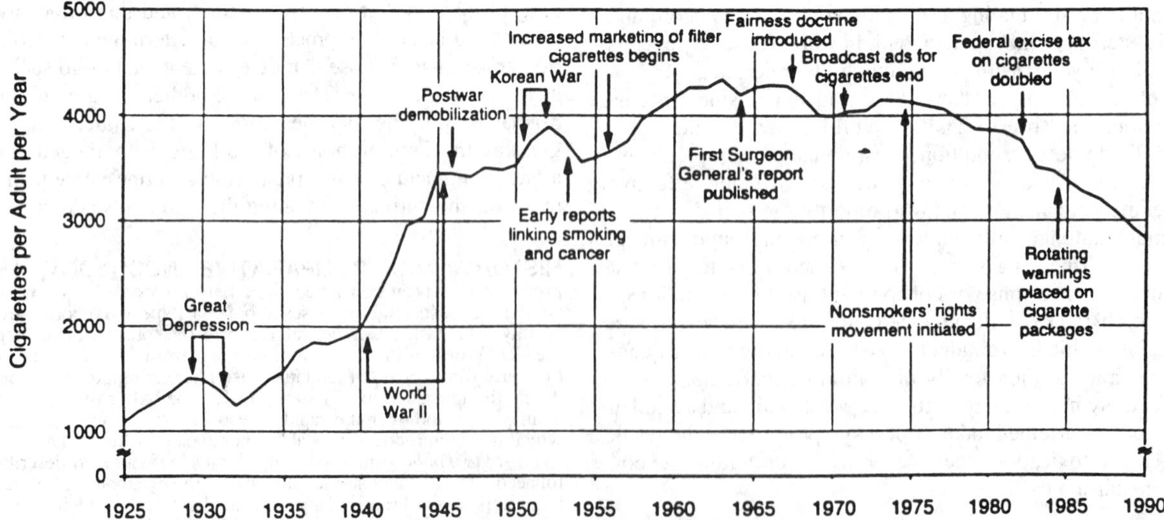

FIGURE 13.4-4 *Per capita consumption of cigarettes among adults in the United States from 1925 to 1990, in relation to certain historical events. (Figure based on data obtained from the United States Department of Health and Human Services: Reducing the Health Consequences of Smoking—25 Years of Progress (A Report of the Surgeon General). Rockville, MD, 1989, and T D MacKenzie, C E Bartecchi, R W Schrier: The human costs of tobacco use. N Engl J Med 330:* 975, 1994.

TABLE 13.4-6
Reinforcement Consequences of Smoking and Putative Neuroregulatory Mechanisms

Positive reinforcement	Negative reinforcement
Pleasure/enhancement of pleasure ↑ dopamine ↑ norepinephrine ↑ β-endorphin	Reduction of anxiety and tension ↑ β-endorphin
Facilitation of task performance ↑ acetylcholine ↑ norepinephrine	Antinociception ↑ acetylcholine ↑ β-endorphin
Improvement of memory ↑ acetylcholine ↑ norepinephrine ↑ arginine vasopressin	Avoidance of weight gain (reduction of hunger) ↑ dopamine ↑ norepinephrine ↑ serotonin
	Relief from nicotine withdrawal ↑ acetylcholine ↑ corticosteroid activity

Table updated from O F Pomerleau, C S Pomerleau: Neuroregulators and the reinforcement of smoking: Towards a biobehavioral explanation. Neurosci Biobehav Rev *8*: 503, 1984.

male twin pairs, heritability was found to be 53 percent for smoking, 45 percent for coffee use, and 36 percent for alcohol use. Using a shared covariance technique to take into account association among drug-taking behaviors, the investigators reported adjusted heritability of 35 percent for smoking, 36 percent for caffeine use, and 29 percent for alcohol use. In a different twin-registry study evidence was found that smoking status and magnitude of dependence have independent heredity factors. Finally, recent animal experimentation involving genetically pure lines of mice has unequivocally demonstrated stable, strain-specific patterns in sensitivity and development of tolerance to nicotine; moreover, those patterns have been linked not only to differences in neuroregulatory activity (that is, the magnitude of the corticosteroid response to nicotine) but also to nicotine receptor variation in different brain regions.

Neuropharmacology With appropriate scheduling of contingencies, nicotine will maintain intravenous self-administration in animals and smokers. Although classified as a sympathomimetic (in keeping with its dominant effect at lower dose levels), nicotine is readily discriminated from other psychomotor stimulants. Drug discrimination involves specific receptors for nicotine and can be blocked by the central nicotinic cholinergic antagonist mecamylamine, although not by muscarinic or adrenergic blocking agents. Although nicotine administration exhibits considerable resistance to extinction once the habit is entrained, nicotine is less potent as a reinforcer than some other substances of abuse, such as amphetamine and cocaine.

After the smoking of one cigarette, circulatory levels of the catecholamines, norepinephrine, and epinephrine rise sharply and then decay; nicotine also alters the bioavailability of dopamine and 5-hydroxytryptamine (5-HT) (serotonin). Nicotine administration in doses produced by smoking a cigarette (5 to 25 ng/mL rise in plasma nicotine) causes a sharp increase in heart rate and blood pressure, an increase in the alerting pattern of the electroencephalogram (EEG), increased tone in some muscle groups (for example, the trapezius), and inhibition of other systems (for example, the patellar reflex).

Nicotine levels in the plasma of regular users are typically maintained at between 10 and 60 ng/mL; plasma values approaching the lower limit typically trigger a compensatory increase in intake, and those approaching the upper limit, a decrease.

As summarized in Table 13.4-6, several of the neuroregulators that exhibit altered bioavailability in response to nicotine have potent behavioral and physiological manifestations. Acetylcholine, for example, has been shown to serve as a neuromodulator of memory and task performance. Norepinephrine may facilitate nicotine's ability to tune out irrelevant stimuli and to focus attention. Nicotine stimulation of cortisol by adrenocorticotropic hormone (ACTH) implicates nicotine in steroid inhibitory feedback mechanisms and the response to stress. Endogenous opioids, such as β-endorphin, not only potentiate vagal reflexes and decrease respiration and blood pressure by opposing the effects of catecholamines, but also may mediate antinociception and anxiety reduction. Finally, nicotine acts on brain reward mechanisms, indirectly through endogenous opioid activity and directly through dopamine pathways.

Neuroendocrinology Nicotine has a pronounced effect on the major stress hormones, and the dose-related effects of nicotine on neuroendocrine responses appear to constitute a critical component of its pharmacological action—effects that may be significantly responsible for both the reinforcement of nicotine use and nicotine dependence. Hypothalamic corticotropin-releasing factor (CRF) is stimulated by nicotine, and levels of hypophyseal hormones—β-endorphin, ACTH, and arginine vasopressin—are increased in a dose-related manner; at higher doses, growth hormone and prolactin are entrained. Corticosteroids are also released in proportion to plasma nicotine concentration.

Pharmacokinetics Given the recent development of several new nicotine-replacement vehicles for the treatment of smoking, knowledge of the pharmacokinetics of administration vehicle assumes great importance for clinicians. When nicotine is inhaled from tobacco smoke, tolerance is readily overcome and the neuroregulatory changes are engaged almost immediately, thereby maximizing the reinforcing effects of the drug. Furthermore, nicotine dosing can be adjusted precisely to obtain desired effects. Small, quick doses are associated with arousal and alertness, whereas large, slow doses are associated with sedation and calming. The metabolism of nicotine is sufficiently rapid (half-life of about two hours) that the effects of a dose do not greatly outlast the situation that prompted use. The kinetic profile of such vehicles as nicotine polacrilex (nicotine gum) or transdermal nicotine delivery systems (nicotine patch) is much more inertial, however, resulting in enhanced tolerance along with diminished reinforcement value.

DIAGNOSIS DSM-IV lists three nicotine-related disorders (Table 13.4-7) but contains specific diagnostic criteria only for nicotine withdrawal (Table 13.4-8). in the nicotine-related-disorders section. The other nicotine-related disorders recognized by DSM-IV are nicotine dependence and nicotine-related disorder not otherwise specified.

Dependence Nicotine dependence is incorporated in DSM-IV as a nicotine use disorder. Criteria (see Tables 13.1-2 and 13.1-5) include the presence of at least three of the following in the same 12-month period: (1) tolerance, made manifest by decreased effect of a given dose or increased dosing to produce the same effect; (2) withdrawal after a period of abstinence; (3)

TABLE 13.4-7
Nicotine-Related Disorders

Nicotine use disorder
Nicotine dependence

Nicotine-induced disorder
Nicotine withdrawal

Nicotine-related disorder not otherwise specified

Table based on DSM-IV, *Diagnostic and Statistical Manual of Mental Disorders,* ed 4. Copyright American Psychiatric Association, Washington, 1994. Used with permission.

TABLE 13.4-8
Diagnostic Criteria for Nicotine Withdrawal

A. Daily use of nicotine for at least several weeks.
B. Abrupt cessation of nicotine use, or reduction in the amount of nicotine used, followed within 24 hours by four (or more) of the following signs:
(1) dysphoric or depressed mood
(2) insomnia
(3) irritability, frustration, or anger
(4) anxiety
(5) difficulty concentrating
(6) restlessness
(7) decreased heart rate
(8) increased appetite or weight gain
C. The symptoms in criterion B cause clinically significant distress or impairment in social, occupational, or other important areas of functioning.
D. The symptoms are not due to a general medical condition and are not better accounted for by another mental disorder.

Table from DSM-IV, *Diagnostic and Statistical Manual of Mental Disorders,* ed 4. Copyright American Psychiatric Association, Washington, 1994. Used with permission.

smoking a greater amount or over a more extended period than intended; (4) a persistent desire to smoke and unsuccessful efforts to cut down; (5) spending considerable time obtaining or using tobacco; (6) giving up or curtailing important social, occupational, or recreational activities because of smoking; (7) continued smoking despite knowledge of risks to health.

Mr. H., a 54-year-old administrator in a midwestern university, was asked to tell the story of his struggle to give up cigarettes. He had not smoked at all for two years, following a six-week treatment with a nicotine patch that was prescribed by a colleague who runs a smoking cessation research program.

Mr. H. began smoking when he was 18, usually smoking one or two packs a day. Beginning in his late 30s, he vowed to stop every morning, but said that by 9:30 AM, "It was over and I was lighting my first cigarette of the day." When he was 45, under a lot of pressure from family, friends, and his cardiologist, he asked his colleague to prescribe an antidepressant that has been used to help smokers break the habit. Over four days the dosage was gradually increased, and he did not smoke. On the fourth day he began to feel like he "was on an LSD trip." His surroundings seemed unreal, and "people opened and closed their mouths, but no words came out." Frightened about what was happening to him, he stopped the drug abruptly. For the next few weeks he still felt drugged, but did not smoke. Back to normal, he began smoking again and was soon up to a pack or two a day.

Over the next five years there was more social pressure for him to stop smoking. Smoking was outlawed in his office building, and his wife and doctor were relentless in their badgering. He also began to notice that he was short of breath when he walked up a few flights of steps. Again he asked his colleague for help, and this time was given a nicotine patch. "I had always thought that I smoked because it was a part of my life, but then I got the patch and didn't need to smoke, and in that moment I realized I was a junkie."

For the six weeks that he wore the patch, life was "beautiful." He was happy, productive, and focused and did not crave cigarettes. He gave up the patch after six weeks, as prescribed, and for months thereafter felt "cranky" and without his usual *joie de vivre*. "One day I was reading an ad for an antidepressant, and I had all the symptoms!" In addition, he began to have frequent, mild viral infections, which he had never experienced before.

Two years later he was still not smoking, and no longer had symptoms of depression, yet felt that something was missing: "The period, the comma, and the exclamation point are missing from my life."

Discussion Because the acute effects of nicotine do not include the maladaptive behavior that is characteristic of intoxication from other commonly abused drugs, such as alcohol or cocaine, it is only recently that the similarity between dependence on nicotine and on other abused drugs has been recognized. Mr. H. referred to himself as a junkie because he recognized that he was as dependent on nicotine as any heroin user might be on heroin. He was repeatedly unable to cut down or control his smoking, he smoked all day, and he smoked despite the knowledge that it was causing him physical problems. Therefore, for many years, Mr. H. had nicotine dependence.

Periodically, as Mr. H. sought to cut down on his smoking, he tried to avoid withdrawal symptoms by using an antidepressant or by using a nicotine patch that slowly administers a low dose of nicotine into the bloodstream.

Although Mr. H. was glad that he was able to kick his nicotine habit, like many other successful former addicts, he missed the pleasure that the drug once gave him. Mr. H. had apparently never had a major depressive disorder. Research has indicated that tobacco users with such a history find it much harder to give up the drug. (From *DSM-IV Casebook.* Used with permission.)

Nicotine withdrawal Nicotine withdrawal is classified as a nicotine-induced disorder. The setting condition is the daily use of nicotine for at least several weeks. Abrupt cessation of nicotine use or reduction in the amount of nicotine taken is followed within 24 hours by a number of characteristic signs, which are typically more intense among persons who smoke cigarettes than among those who use other nicotine-containing products. Table 13.4-8 lists the DSM-IV criteria for nicotine withdrawal.

Nicotine-related disorder not otherwise specified Nicotine-related disorder not otherwise specified (NOS) is a diagnostic category for nicotine-related disorders that do not fit into one of the categories discussed (Table 13.4-9). Such diagnoses may include nicotine intoxication, nicotine abuse, and mood disorders and anxiety disorders associated with nicotine use.

CLINICAL FEATURES

SUBJECTIVE AND BEHAVIORAL EFFECTS The degree of psychiatric impairment from nicotine dependence is minimal, and nicotine withdrawal effects are largely self-limiting, with most symptoms dissipating within a few weeks or months following abstinence.

Nicotine toxicity Clinicians occasionally encounter cases of acute nicotine poisoning (for example, green tobacco sickness in harvesters). Symptoms include nausea, salivation, pallor, weakness, abdominal pain, vomiting or diarrhea, dizziness, headache, and cold sweat. At higher doses (or in persons who are highly sensitive), there may be an inability to concentrate, mental confusion, various sensory disturbances, severe elevations in blood pressure, and a weak, rapid pulse. At lethal doses death usually is caused by respiratory paralysis. Medical treatment is largely supportive, consisting of mechanical assistance for respiration, supplemental oxygen, and short-acting barbiturates to counteract clonic movements. Prenatal exposure to nicotine through smoking is associated with reduced fetal birth weight and complex effects on brain development.

Other clinical considerations There are several reasons for clinicians to determine the nicotine-using status of their patients.

First, smoking is more prevalent among psychiatric patients as compared with the national population, and the percentage is especially high among patients with schizophrenia (88 percent) and mania (70 percent). Although not all findings have been positive, several recent

TABLE 13.4-9
Nicotine-Related Disorder Not Otherwise Specified

The nicotine-related disorder not otherwise specified category is for disorders associated with the use of nicotine that are not classifiable as nicotine dependence or nicotine withdrawal.

Table from DSM-IV, *Diagnostic and Statistical Manual of Mental Disorders,* ed 4. Copyright American Psychiatric Association, Washington, 1994. Used with permission studies indicate a link between depression and smoking, with a history of major depressive disorder associated with greater difficulty giving up smoking.

Second, mood, anxiety, and cognition improve when regular smokers smoke and worsen when they do not.

Third, smoking may decrease the therapeutic effectiveness and exacerbate some of the side effects of psychoactive drugs. For instance, it is pertinent to the treatment of schizophrenia that smoking is associated with decreases in extrapyramidal side effects and with reduction in parkinsonian tremor induced by the long-term use of antipsychotics. However, some investigators have reported an increased prevalence of tardive dyskinesia in smokers treated with antipsychotics.

Finally, because nicotine induces drug-metabolizing enzymes, insufficient plasma levels of antipsychotics or of tricyclic antidepressants may occur in smokers. Accordingly, unless plasma drug levels are monitored, the clinician may find it difficult to distinguish between lack of therapeutic efficacy for a medication and inadequate dosing as a result of enhanced metabolism by nicotine.

Smokers are much more likely than nonsmokers to use or abuse other psychoactive substances. Over 90 percent of alcoholic persons were found to be smokers in one large clinical study. Furthermore, in laboratory studies smoking has been shown to increase as a function of alcohol consumed, an effect that is more pronounced in heavy drinkers and alcoholic persons. Cigarette smokers also generally drink more coffee than do nonsmokers, although laboratory studies have failed to demonstrate the obverse (that is, reliable short-term induction of smoking following caffeine intake). While smoking, smokers may need to consume up to 150 percent more caffeine to obtain the same levels as nonsmokers because of enzyme induction by nicotine, but when they quit, smokers' caffeine levels may be elevated by as much as 250 percent for a while.

COURSE AND PROGNOSIS Within the past decade well-coordinated preventive efforts in the United States, combined with innovative behavioral and pharmacological interventions based on extensive biobehavioral research, have made considerable progress against the tobacco habit. Nevertheless, the public health consequences of chronic nicotine use continue to be devastating.

TREATMENT In only two decades smoking has gone from a habit that was considered nearly unmodifiable (treatment outcome statistics were around 12 percent, the same as the spontaneous quit rate) to one for which there is the most successful of all substance-abuse interventions. Psychological and pharmacological studies conducted on smoking during the past 20 years have shown how behavioral factors and pharmacological effects are thoroughly intertwined in the fabric of daily living. Accordingly, behavioral treatment has focused on learning to carry out ordinary activities, such as eating, driving, or socializing, without smoking, as well as on coping with dysphoric moods, weight gain, or the desire for a cigarette.

Nicotine replacement The objective of nicotine-replacement treatment (agonist therapy) is to transfer nicotine dependence from cigarettes to a vehicle with lower abuse liability, followed by a process of gradual weaning from all sources of nicotine over several months. Although the most extensive experience has been in the use of nicotine polacrilex (chewing gum) for the relief of withdrawal symptoms, new nicotine-replacement products, such as transdermal delivery systems, show promise for equal or better efficacy because of the ease of administration and enhanced compliance. The claims of efficacy are supported by numerous outcome studies. The approach has been shown to be particularly effective when carried out in a habit-change (behavior modification) context: in several reports, nicotine polacrilex in isolation was found to be about as effective as behavior change alone, but when the two were combined, there was a doubling of sustained abstinence rates.

In the hands of skillful practitioners, initial quit rates for nicotine-replacement programs have exceeded 60 percent, and sustained abstinence rates (validated by the use of cotinine, a major metabolite of nicotine) have exceeded 40 percent at six months. A useful feature of nicotine-replacement approaches is that the dosage can be adjusted to provide the desired level of symptom relief. For example, recent studies have shown that some withdrawal symptoms—anxiety, irritability, frustration, anger, difficulty concentrating, and restlessness—in newly quitting smokers were relieved by 2 mg nicotine polacrilex; craving for cigarettes and increased appetite, however, only responded when the 4-mg dose was administered. It is now possible to match treatment to patient characteristics; thus, although smokers who are more nicotine dependent generally have a poorer prognosis than do less dependent smokers, outcomes for more dependent smokers treated 4 mg nicotine polacrilex were equal to or better than outcomes for less dependent smokers treated with 2 mg.

Brief interventions High-technology approaches to treatment show obvious promise, but even simple, brief interventions can have an important effect. For example, unambiguous quit-smoking advice by physicians in an outpatient setting can result in sustained one-year abstinence rates in the 5 percent range. Although the effect of brief advice might seem trivial, it is 17 times more effective than saying nothing. A quit rate of 5 percent, out of 55 million smokers represents 2.75 million persons given a chance to enjoy significantly decreased morbidity and an enhanced quality of life.

Other interventions Various pharmacological adjuncts for smoking cessation are in different stages of development and testing. In addition to new nicotine-replacement vehicles that mimic the fast rise time of plasma nicotine from smoking (for example, nicotine nasal solution and nicotine aerosol), other interventions focusing on the relief of specific symptoms have been tested. For example, corticotropin (for example, depot ACTH) and α-adrenergic agonists (for example, clonidine [Catapres]) have been administered to relieve withdrawal. Serotonin-specific reuptake inhibitors (for example, fluoxetine [Prozac]) have been shown to prevent post–smoking-cessation weight gain. Buspirone (BuSpar) and tricyclic antidepressants have also been tested in clinical trials and may be relevant for the management of symptoms of anxiety or depression that can be unmasked by the termination of nicotine administration. Research on neurohormones has increased the understanding of nicotine's CNS effects, and integration of recent behavioral and biological findings shows great potential for the development of more efficacious interventions based on nicotine neuroregulatory mechanisms.

SUGGESTED CROSS-REFERENCES

Section 13.1 provides an overview of substance use and substance-related disorders. Section 13.2 is devoted to alcohol-related disorders; of related interest to those concerned with symptoms of caffeine-related disorders and nicotine-related disorders are Chapter 22 on eating disorders, Chapter 23 on sleep disorders, and Chapter 38 on attention-deficit disorders. Anxiety disorders are the subject of Chapter 17, and mood disorders are the subject of Chapter 16.

REFERENCES

Balfour D J K: The pharmacology of nicotine in the CNS and its bearing on nicotine replacement therapies. Int J Smoking Cessation *2:* 3, 1993.

Barone J J, Roberts H: Human consumption of caffeine. In *Caffeine,* P B Dews, editor, p 59. Springer-Verlag, New York, 1984.

Benowitz N L: Clinical pharmacology of caffeine. Ann Rev Med *41:* 277, 1990.

*Cameron O G, Modell J G, Hariharan M: Caffeine and human cerebral blood flow: A positron emission study. Life Sci *47:* 1141, 1990.

Charney D S, Heninger G R, Jatlow P I: Increased anxiogenic effects of caffeine in panic disorder. Arch Gen Psychiatry *42:* 233, 1985.

Couturier E G, Hering R, Steiner T J: Weekend attacks in migraine patients: Caused by caffeine withdrawal? Cephalalgia *12:* 99, 1992.

Fennelly M, Galletly D C, Purdie G I: Is caffeine withdrawal the mechanism of postoperative headache? Anesth Analg *72:* 449, 1991.

Goldstein A, Kaizer S, Whitby O: Psychotropic effects of caffeine in man. IV. Quantitative and qualitative differences associated with habituation to caffeine. Clin Pharmacol Ther *10:* 489, 1969.

*Greden J F: Anxiety or caffeinism: A diagnostic dilemma. Am J Psychiatry *131:* 1089, 1974.

Greden J F: Anxiety and depression associated with caffeinism among psychiatric inpatients. Am J Psychiatry *135:* 963, 1978.

Griffiths R R, Bigelow G E, Liebson I A: Human coffee drinking: Reinforcing and physical dependence producing effects of caffeine. J Pharmacol Exp Ther *239:* 416, 1986.

Griffiths R R, Evans S M, Heishman S J, Preston K L, Sannerud C A, Wolf B, Woodson P P: Low-dose caffeine physical dependence in humans. J Pharmacol Exp Ther *255:* 1123, 1990.

Hughes J R: Genetics of smoking: A brief review. Behav Ther *17:* 335, 1986.

Hughes J R, Hatsukami D K, Mitchell J E, Dahlgren L A: Prevalence of smoking among psychiatric outpatients. Am J Psychiatry *143:* 993, 1986.

Hughes J R, Higgins S T, Bickel W K: Caffeine self-administration, withdrawal, and adverse effects among coffee drinkers. Arch Gen Psychiatry *48:* 611, 1991.

Hughes J R, Oliveto A H, Helzer J E, Higgins S T, Bickel W K: Should caffeine abuse, dependence, or withdrawal be added to DSM-IV and ICD-10? Am J Psychiatry *149:* 33, 1992.

Jaffe J: Drug addiction and drug abuse (nicotine and tobacco). In Goodman and Gilman's *The Pharmacological Basis of Therapeutics,* ed 8, A G Goodman, T W Rall, A S Nies, P Taylor, editors, p 545. Pergamon, New York, 1990.

Kessler D A: Testimony by the Commissioner of Food and Drugs to the United States Congress on the Control and Manipulation of Nicotine in Cigarettes. Congressional Record, June 21, 1994.

Kessler D A: Testimony by the Commissioner of Food and Drugs to the United States Congress on Nicotine-Containing Cigarettes. Congressional Record, March 25, 1994.

Kuribara H, Tadokoro S: Caffeine does not effectively ameliorate, but rather may worsen the ethanol intoxication when assessed by discrete avoidance in mice. Jpn J Pharmacol *59:* 393, 1992.

Levinson H C, Bick E C: Psychopharmacology of caffeine. In *Psychopharmacology in the Practice of Medicine,* M D Jarvik, editor, p 451. Appelton-Century-Crofts, New York, 1977.

MacKenzie T D, Bartecchi C E, Schrier R W: The human costs of tobacco use. N Engl J Med *330:* 975, 1994.

Paul S, Kurunwune B, Biaggioni I; Caffeine withdrawal: Apparent heterologous sensitization to adenosine and prostacyclin actions in human platelets. J Pharmacol Exp Ther *267:* 838, 1993.

*Pomerleau C S, Berman B A, Gritz E R, Marks J L, Goeters S: Why women smoke. In *Drug and Alcohol Abuse Reviews,* vol 5: *Addictive Behaviors in Women,* R R Watson, editor, p 39. Humana Press, Totowa, NJ, 1994.

Pomerleau O F, Collins A C, Shiffman S, Pomerleau, C S: Why some people smoke and others do not: New perspectives. J Consult Clin Psychol *61:* 723, 1993

Pomerleau O F, Pomerleau C S: Neuroregulators and the reinforcement of smoking: Towards a biobehavioral explanation. Neurosci Biobehav Rev *8:* 503, 1984.

*Pomerleau O F, Pomerleau C S, editors: *Nicotine Replacement: A Critical Evaluation.* Haworth Press, Binghamton, NY, 1992.

Pomerleau O F, Rosecrans J: Neuroregulatory effects of nicotine. Psychoneuroendocrinology *14:* 407, 1989.

Rand M J, Thurau K, editors: *The Pharmacology of Nicotine* (ICSU Symposium Series, volume 9). IRL Press, Washington, 1988.

Sachs D P L: Smoking cessation strategies: What works, what doesn't. JADA (Suppl): 13S, 1990.

Sachs D P L: Advances in smoking cessation treatment. Cur Pulmonology *12:* 139, 1991.

Siegrist H E: Literary controversy over tea in 18th-century England. Bull Hist Med *13:* 185, 1943.

Silverman K, Evans S M, Strain E C, Griffiths R R: Withdrawal syndrome after the double-blind cessation of caffeine consumption. N Engl J Med *327:* 1109, 1992.

Synder S H, Katims J J, Annau Z, Bruns R F, Daly J W: Adenosine receptors and behavioral actions of methylxanthines. Proc Natl Acad Sci USA *78:* 3260, 1981.

Taylor P T: *The Smoke Ring: Tobacco, Money & Multinational Politics.* Mentor Books (New American Library), New York, 1985.

*United States Department of Health and Human Services. *The Health Consequences of Smoking: Nicotine Addiction (A Report of the Surgeon General).* Office on Smoking and Health, Rockville, MD, 1988.

United States Department of Health and Human Services. *Reducing the Health Consequences of Smoking—25 Years of Progress (A Report of the Surgeon General).* US Government Printing Office, Rockville, MD, 1989.

Winstead D K: Coffee consumption among psychiatric inpatients. Am J Psychiatry, *133:* 1447, 1976.

Wonnacott S, Russell M A H, Stolerman I P: *Nicotine Psychopharmacology: Molecular, Cellular, and Behavioural Aspects.* Oxford

13.5 CANNABIS-RELATED DISORDERS

GEORGE E. WOODY, M.D.
WAYNE MACFADDEN, M.D.

INTRODUCTION

Known in central Asia and China for at least 5,000 years, the Indian hemp plant *Cannabis sativa* is a hardy, aromatic annual herb. The bioactive substances derived from it are collectively referred to as cannabis. By most estimates, cannabis remains the world's most commonly used illicit drug, with approximately 200 to 300 million regular users. Cannabis is indigenous to Asia, and the earliest written reference to its use is in a 15th century BC Chinese medical text, where it is mentioned as a medicinal herb that is to be used for a variety of physical and psychological ailments.

Cannabis sativa is widely cultivated for its fiber, which is used to make rope and cloth; for its seeds, which is used to make oil; and for its psychoactive resin. This resin contains over 60 substances, called cannabinoids, of which Δ-9-tetrahydrocannabinol (THC) is thought to be responsible for most of its psychoactive effects. The term ''marijuana'' most commonly refers to the upper leaves, flowering tops, and stems of the plant, which are cut, dried and chopped, and usually formed into cigarettes. Hashish, named after the Persian founder of the 11th century Assassins, is the dried black-brown resinous exudate from the tops and undersides of the leaves of the female plant. Other names for cannabis or its products include bhang, charas, dagga, and ganja; common slang terms are grass, pot, and weed.

HISTORY

Cannabis was introduced to western Europe for pleasure-seeking purposes in the early 19th century by Napolean's soldiers returning from Egypt. Although some previous knowledge of its use existed, it may have been more widely introduced into the United States by Mexican immigrants in the 1920s. Soon afterward western states pressured the federal government to control cannabis use, because it was linked to violence from foreign, often unwelcome laborers, who were allegedly growing the plant. The Marijuana Tax Act of 1937 established government control over the sale and transfer of the drug, and no stamps or licenses were available for its public use. During that time its use was associated with minority groups, who were not well assimilated into the overall culture, or jazz musicians

Marijuana's image shifted during the 1960s when the youthful counterculture rediscovered cannabis. It became associated with social protest, and its use spread rapidly throughout the general society. Occasional use, even by adolescents, became common. The use of cannabis became normalized throughout United States culture, a fact contributing to the initial difficulty many investigators encountered in associating cannabis with health problems. The favorable attitude toward cannabis reached a peak in about 1978. Since that time its use declined yearly in the overall population until 1993. In attempts to suppress its use, penalties have risen against users and dealers. Although some states decriminalized the use and sale of cannabis during the 1970s it has been recriminalized in many areas, most notably in Alaska after a popular vote in 1990.

The World Health Organization (WHO) and other governmental advisory and regulatory agencies have consistently maintained that cannabis is a drug requiring close monitoring and stringent control. In 1965 WHO declared that "the harm to society derived from abuse of cannabis rests in the economic consequences of the impairment of the individual's social functions and his enhanced proneness to asocial and antisocial behavior." In 1969 WHO regarded cannabis as not physically habit-forming but as a drug of dependence and recommended keeping it under legal control. The classification of cannabis as a highly controlled (Class I) substance by the Drug Enforcement Administration is consistent with that view.

The THC content and concentration of different parts of the plant or between different plant species varies greatly. The effects of THC depend on dosage and on frequency and route of administration, setting, and the experience and expectations of subjects. Most marijuana purchased illicitly varies from about 1 to 5 percent THC content; sinsemilla, a more potent variety may contain 7 to 14 percent THC. Hashish contains up to 10 percent THC, and hashish oil, a concentrated distillate of hashish, has been assayed at up to 15 to 30 percent THC. In addition to genetic variability, the percentage of active THC produced by the plant is related to the amount of sunlight received, humidity, soil condition, and other environmental conditions. Other factors that affect the delivered THC content are smoking technique, the amount destroyed by pyrolysis (about 75 percent), and how quickly the marijuana is used, because the THC deteriorates by about 5 percent per month when stored at room temperature. Assertions that the marijuana available today is much more potent than it was 15 to 20 years ago are difficult to validate. THC content analyzed in some specimens confiscated in the mid-1970s has been reported at 5 percent or higher, which most investigators would consider relatively potent.

Cannabis is most commonly smoked in marijuana cigarettes, or joints. The experienced user inhales deeply and holds his or her breath for as long as possible to extract almost all the THC. Amounts ranging from 2 to 50 percent of the THC may be absorbed by the pulmonary circulation in this manner. Its intoxicating effects may be increased by mixing other drugs or chemicals into the cigarette, such as opium, cocaine paste, or phencyclidine (PCP). It may also be eaten and is often baked in lipid-rich foods, such as brownies.

EPIDEMIOLOGY

It is estimated that the overall use in young Americans has been gradually declining from a high in 1979 to a low in 1992, on the basis of self-reports by high school seniors. In 1978 10.7 percent of seniors reported daily use, and 37.1 percent reported use in the past month. In 1992 comparable figures were 1.9 percent and 11.9 percent, respectively. Lifetime prevalence of use fell from 60.4 percent to 50.2 percent to 42.2 percent during those years. The reasons for that general decline in use may be attributable to a variety of factors, including broad cultural trends away from drugs, adverse effects people may note in their peers who use drugs, and the antidrug parents' movement that is publicized in national and local media campaigns. However, results from a 1993 high school survey demonstrate a reversal of that trend, indicating a rise in marijuana use. Some investigators believe that softening attitudes about the hazards associated with cannabis may be responsible.

Occasional use of cannabis does not imply abuse or dependence. The percentage of users who fulfill criteria for either of these diagnoses is unclear at this time, though it is likely to be relatively low, somewhat analagous to the case with alcohol.

As noted in the high school senior survey, epidemiological data change from year to year. The following epidemiological data for 1991 come from the National Institute on Drug Abuse (NIDA).

PREVALENCE About one third (33.2 percent) of the population reported that they had used marijuana one or more times in their lifetimes, 9.5 percent had used it in the past year, and 4.8 percent had used it in the past month.

Those percentages translate to 67.4 million members of the population who had used marijuana in their lifetimes, 19.2 million in the past year, and 9.7 million in the past month.

Adults aged 26 to 34 were the most likely age group to have ever used marijuana, but those aged 18 to 25 were the most likely to have used marijuana in the past year or the past month. About 60 percent of adults aged 26 to 34 had ever used marijuana, compared with about 51 percent of adults 18 to 25, 24 percent of adults over 34, and 13 percent of youths. An estimated 13 percent of the adults 18 to 25 had used marijuana in the past month, compared with 7 percent of those aged 26 to 34 and smaller percentages of those in other age groups.

Youths aged 12 to 17 were the least likely of the age groups to have used marijuana in their lifetimes, and adults aged 35 and older were the least likely to have used marijuana in the past year and the past month.

DEMOGRAPHIC CORRELATES

Sex The rate of past-month marijuana use by males was almost twice the rate for females. A total of 6.1 million males in the population had used marijuana in the past month, as had 3.6 million females.

Race and ethnicity Blacks were about 1.6 times more likely than whites or Hispanics to have used marijuana in the past month. Even though blacks were proportionately more likely to have used marijuana in the past month, almost three fourths (73.4 percent) of the current users were white. A total of 7.1 million whites had used marijuana in the past month, compared with 1.7 million blacks, 0.7 million Hispanics, and 0.2 million others.

Population density Residents of large and small metropolitan areas were significantly more likely than were residents of nonmetropolitan areas to have used marijuana in the past month. Although 42.9 percent of the United States population live in large metropolitan areas, 48.2 percent of those who had used marijuana in the past month were from large metropolitan areas. A total of 4.7 million residents of large metropolitan areas, 3.3 million from small metropolitan areas, and 1.7 million from nonmetropolitan areas had used marijuana in the past month.

Region Residents of the west were significantly more likely than were residents of the south or north central regions to have used marijuana in the past month. The other regions did not differ significantly. More than 2 million residents of each region had used marijuana in the past month.

PHARMACOLOGY

THC is lipid soluble and rapidly absorbed after inhalation. It is highly protein bound and quickly redistributed from blood into other tissues. That which reaches the liver is almost completely metabolized, primarily into the active 11-hydroxy THC and the inactive 9-carboxy THC. Blood levels of THC peak in about 30 minutes and then decline precipitously as it redistributes through the body to lipid-rich tissues, reaching nearly undetectable levels within three to four hours.

After some equilibrium between concentrations in the blood and other tissues is established, the THC slowly and unevenly reenters the blood stream from its tissue stores. Its concentration declines very slowly in this second phase, with a half-life of three days. That small concentration of THC or its active 11-hydroxy THC metabolite is believed to be below the threshold to produce an effect and is thus clinically insignificant. However, the half-life of those metabolites is at least 50 hours.

Cardiovascular and central nervous system (CNS) effects, such as mood altering properties, begin less than one minute after inhalation. Peak clinical effects may be delayed for 20 to

30 minutes and persist for at least two to three hours. The pharmacological effects of orally ingested cannabis begin after 30 minutes, peak in two to three hours and last three to six hours. Residual effects, such as subtle changes in mood and fine motor control, are measurable for a longer period but only if very sensitive testing procedures are used. An oral dose of approximately 20 mg of marijuana, or the smoking of a cigarette of about 0.5 to 2 percent THC content, will usually produce intoxication. Orally ingested marijuana requires about three times as much THC as smoked marijuana to produce equivalent effects because only 3 to 6 percent of ingested THC is absorbed.

THC interacts with a variety of neurotransmitter systems and neuropeptides. It also demonstrates weak barbiturate-like actions, such as anticonvulsant activity and opioidlike effects, including analgesia, increased catecholamine synthesis, hypothermia, and antidiarrheal activity. Increased limbic system activity has been noted with cannabis use, suggesting that THC may stimulate pleasure-reward mechanisms in the brain.

Cannabis is often used in combination with other drugs. It may alter the effects of amphetamines, atropine, barbiturates, clomipramine (Anafranil), cocaine, ethanol, nicotine, opiates, and phencyclidine. Because of shared hepatic metabolic systems, ethanol and phenobarbital can inhibit metabolism of THC. Similarly, THC can slow the metabolism of a variety of drugs, including theophylline (Theo-Dur), ethanol, and pentobarbital (Nembutal). Cross-tolerance exists between THC and CNS depressant drugs. However, there is no evidence that THC is useful for detoxification from sedative drugs, although they both can enhance or prolong the other's behavioral and psychological effects.

About two thirds of the drug is excreted via the enterohepatic circulation into the feces, and the remaining one third is removed through the kidney. Most of the metabolites of THC are produced by the liver. Among these compounds, one called 11-nor-Δ–9 tetra-hydrocannabinol carboxylic acid has the highest concentration in the urine and is the metabolite usually screened for in routine toxicological analyses. That and other cannabinoid metabolites can be detected in the urine for two to three days after casual use; for daily, heavy users, levels can persist for up to four weeks.

MECHANISM OF ACTION Cannabinoids have been shown to inhibit adenylate cyclase activity centrally in a rapid, reversible, potent, and stereospecific manner. That activity appears to be related to the ability of those compounds to produce CNS effects, especially analgesia, strongly suggesting the presence of unique cannabinoid receptors. Recently such a receptor has been identified in the rat brain, with a protein structure for the binding site. Through a second messenger through a G protein, increased membrane fluidity is ultimately produced.

DIAGNOSIS AND CLINICAL FEATURES

Patterns of use vary widely, the most common being intermittent use of marijuana cigarettes, such as smoking one or two marijuana cigarettes (known as joints) on a weekly or monthly basis, often on social occasions. As with alcohol, a smaller proportion of cannabis users develop the pattern of daily use of high doses that is typically associated with abuse or dependence. The proportion of users who progress to dependence is unknown, but is probably relatively low, as with alcohol.

Marijuana has mild to moderate reinforcing effects, and benign experiences with it may impel users to try other more reinforcing drugs under the belief that drug effects are pleasurable and not to be feared. In fact, initial marijuana usage is a common behavioral pattern in patients who eventually progress to so-called harder drugs, such as opiates, stimulants, and stronger psychedelics. It is unlikely that the relationship is causal, however. The purchase or use of marijuana may imply a willingness to use other illicit substances and may also put the user in contact with people who distribute them.

The fourth edition of *Diagnostic and Statistical Manual of Mental Disorders* (DSM-IV) lists the cannabis-related disorders (Table 13.5-1) but has specific criteria within the cannabis-related disorders section only for cannabis intoxication (Table 13.5-2). The diagnostic criteria for the other cannabis-related disorders are contained in those DSM-IV sections that focus on the major phenomenological symptom—for example, cannabis-induced psychotic disorder, with delusions, in the DSM-IV section on substance-induced psychotic disorder (Section 15.3).

CANNABIS DEPENDENCE AND CANNABIS ABUSE DMS-IV includes the diagnoses of cannabis dependence and cannabis abuse (see Tables 13.1-2, 13.1-5, and 13.1-6). The experimental data clearly show tolerance to many of the effects of cannabis with sustained use of high doses. Tolerance develops to most of the physical effects of cannabis, including tachycardia, decreased skin temperature, increased body temperature, decrease in intraocular pressure, sleep disturbance (decreased rapid eye movement [REM] sleep), electroencephalogram

TABLE 13.5-1
Cannabis-Related Disorders

Cannabis use disorders
Cannabis dependence
Cannabis abuse

Cannabis-induced disorders
Cannabis intoxication
Specify if: with perceptual disturbances
Cannabis intoxication delirium
Cannabis-induced psychotic disorder, with delusions
Specify if: with onset during intoxication
Cannabis-induced psychotic disorder, with hallucinations
Specify if: with onset during intoxication
Cannabis-induced anxiety disorder
Specify if: with onset during intoxication

Cannabis-related disorder not otherwise specified

Table based on DSM-IV, *Diagnostic and Statistical Manual of Mental Disorders,* ed 4. Copyright American Psychiatric Association, Washington, 1994. Used with permission.

TABLE 13.5-2
Diagnostic Criteria for Cannabis Intoxication

A. Recent use of cannabis.
B. Clinically significant maladaptive behavioral or psychological changes (e.g., impaired motor coordination, euphoria, anxiety, sensation of slowed time, impaired judgment, social withdrawal) that develop during, or shortly after, cannabis use.
C. Two (or more) of the following signs, developing within two hours of cannabis use:
 (1) conjunctival injection
 (2) increased appetite
 (3) dry mouth
 (4) tachycardia
D. The symptoms are not due to a general medical condition and are not better accounted for by another mental disorder.

Specify if:
With perceptual disturbances

Table from DSM-IV, *Diagnostic and Statistical Manual of Mental Disorders,* ed 4. Copyright American Psychiatric Association, Washington, 1994. Used with permission.

(EEG) changes (increased alpha waves), and impairment of performance on psychomotor tests. There is less agreement about tolerance to the common mood and behavioral changes, but progressive loss of the so-called high has been reported. Most of the tolerance is due to adaptations of the CNS rather than to more rapid metabolic disposition.

CANNABIS INTOXICATION DSM-IV formalizes the diagnostic criteria for cannabis intoxication (Table 13.5-2). The diagnostic criteria specify that the diagnosis can be augmented with the phrase "with perceptual disturbances." If intact reality testing is not present, the diagnosis is cannabis-induced psychotic disorder.

Cannabis intoxication commonly heightens the user's sensitivity to external stimuli, reveals new details, makes colors seem brighter and richer than in the past, and subjectively slows down the appreciation of time. In high doses, the user may also experience depersonalization and derealization.

THC has well-known deleterious effects on cognition. It impairs short-term memory, attention span, recall, the ability to store knowledge, and the ability to perform tasks requiring multiple mental steps. In addition, the ability to verbalize is often diminished. The term "temporal disintegration" has been coined to characterize THC's effects on the CNS. Intoxicated persons may have difficulty integrating earlier experiences, expectations, and current perceptions to goal-directed action (for example, learning new material is usually impaired). Acute neurophysiological changes include suppression of REM sleep and diffuse slowing of background activity on the EEG. Those acute effects last for a period of minutes up to a few hours, depending on dose and individual sensitivity to the drug. However, they can measurably impair performance if higher levels of cognitive or psychomotor skills are required.

Chronic effects have been more elusive to investigation. Cannabis does not produce chronic cerebral impairment as measurable by current neuropsychological methods, though subtle and chronic impairment cannot be ruled out. Studies of cerebral atrophy have been conflicting and inconclusive. There is no evidence to suggest that cannabis impairs intellectual functioning after the acute effects wear off.

A variety of motor skills are affected, including decreases in muscle strength and hand steadiness, and the performance of simple motor tasks and reflex responses. At higher doses coordination and balance may be impaired. Those effects may last several hours after the subjective effects of the drug have subsided and are additive to those produced by alcohol.

Simple reaction time has not been shown to be adversely affected, but response to complex and unforeseen situations is impaired. Some data suggest that marijuana produces a significant decrease in fast driving (that is, speeding) and other risk-taking behavior, effects opposite to those that often result from alcohol consumption. In a related area, few studies are available on marijuana's effect in causing vehicular accidents. In one report 94 percent of subjects were noted to be intoxicated by trained observers during roadside sobriety tests 90 minutes after smoking moderate amounts of marijuana, and 60 percent after 2½ hours. Despite numbers like these, several studies indicate that marijuana use by itself appears to be a relatively minor risk factor in fatal traffic accidents. Although some observations suggest that there is an increased accident risk in THC-positive drivers, clear interpretation of the data is typically confounded by concurrent alcohol use. Some authors speculate that serious drug and alcohol users gravitate towards marijuana; thus, marijuana testing may be of value as a monitor for hazardous drug use, particularly heavy drinking.

Several controlled studies indicate that the ability to fly airplanes is more impaired than driving by cannabis intoxication. That can be explained by the increased complexity of the tasks involved in flying. For both flying and driving, no correlation has been established between the degree of impairment and blood or urine levels of THC, rendering it very difficult to establish reliable legal levels of intoxication as has been done for alcohol.

In the middle of a rainy October night in 1970, a family doctor in a Chicago suburb was awakened by an old friend who begged him to get out of bed and come quickly to a neighbor's house, where he and his wife had been visiting. The caller, Lou Wolff, was very upset because his wife, Sybil, had smoked some marijuana and was "freaking out."

The doctor, extremely annoyed, arrived at the neighbor's house to find Sybil lying on the couch looking quite frantic, unable to get up. She said she was too weak to stand, that she was dizzy, having palpitations, and could feel her blood "rushing through [her] veins." She kept asking for water because her mouth was so dry she could not swallow. She was sure there was some poison in the marijuana. Sybil was relieved to see the doctor, because she had believed the neighbors would not let her husband call him for fear of being arrested for possession of marijuana, and she was sure that without medical help, she would die.

Sybil, age 42, was the mother of three teenage boys. She worked as a librarian at a university. She was a very controlled, well-organized woman who prided herself on her rationality. She had smoked marijuana, a small amount, only once before, and the only reaction she had detected was that it made her feel "slightly mellow." It was she who had asked the neighbors to share some of their high-quality homegrown marijuana with her, because marijuana was a big thing with the students and she "wanted to see what all the fuss was about."

Her husband said that she took four or five puffs of a joint and then wailed, "There's something wrong with me. I can't stand up." Lou and the neighbors tried to calm her, telling her she should just lie down and she would soon feel better; but the more they reassured her, the more convinced she became that something was really wrong with her, and that her husband and neighbors were just trying to cover it up.

The doctor examined her. The only positive findings were that her heart rate was increased and her pupils dilated. Adopting his best bedside manner, he said to her, "For Christ's sake, Sybil, you're just a little stoned. Go home to bed and stop making such a fuss." Sybil seemed reassured. He then walked into another room and told Lou, "If that doesn't work, we'll have to take her to the emergency room."

Discussion Sybil's bad experience with marijuana (cannabis) includes characteristic physical symptoms, such as dry mouth and increased heart rate. It is the mental symptoms, however, that caused her husband to seek help. Sybil became extremely anxious and had paranoid ideation (thinking that the marijuana was poisoned and that her neighbors would not let her husband call the doctor). That maladaptive reaction to the recent use of cannabis indicates cannabis intoxication.

In diagnosing this case, the doctor considered whether Sybil's paranoid ideation could justify a diagnosis of cannabis-induced psychotic disorder; he decided the answer was no. First of all, the neighbors might well have been reluctant to call the doctor because they would have had to admit that they were smoking an illegal substance. Secondly, Sybil was reassured by the doctor that the marijuana did not contain poison, whereas, by definition, a delusion is a false belief that is firmly held, despite evidence to the contrary.

Follow-up Sybil was helped into her car by Lou (she still couldn't stand up) and went home to bed. She stayed in bed for two days, feeling "spacey" and weak, but no longer terribly anxious. She realized that, because the marijuana was homegrown, there was no reason to think that it contained any poison. However, she still believed her neighbors did not want to call the doctor because they were afraid of the police. She vowed never to smoke marijuana again. (From *DSM-IV Casebook.* Used with permission.)

CANNABIS INTOXICATION DELIRIUM Cannabis intoxication delirium is a DSM-IV diagnosis (see Chapter 12). The delirium associated with cannabis intoxication is characterized by marked impairment on congition and performance tasks. Even modest doses of cannabis result in impairment in memory, reaction time, perception, motor coordination, and attention. High doses that also impair the user's level of consciousness have marked effects on those cognitive measures.

However, there are reports that cannabis may also induce a longer lasting toxic-organic delirium characterized by confusion with disorganization of thought processes, affective lability, delusions, and hallucinations. That reaction is similar to the delirium produced by other psychomimetics, hallucinogens, or toxins and may last up to 10 days. The attribution of cannabis as the primary etiological agent in those cases has been questioned by some investigators, and the final answer continues to be debated.

CANNABIS-INDUCED PSYCHOTIC DISORDER High doses of cannabis are more likely to induce brief psychotic symptoms such as persecutory delusions, or auditory and visual hallucinations, especially in those persons with underlying psychiatric disorders. Those may fulfill the DSM-IV criteria for cannabis-induced psychotic disorder. It is uncertain whether persons with unstable character structures are more susceptible to those brief psychotic episodes.

Cannabis-induced psychotic disorder (see Section 15.3) is diagnosed in the presence of a cannabis-induced psychosis. Cannabis-induced psychotic disorder is rare, but transient paranoid ideation is more common. Florid psychosis is somewhat common in countries in which some persons have long-term access to cannabis of a particularly high potency. The psychotic episodes are sometimes referred to as hemp insanity. Cannabis use is rarely associated with a bad-trip experience, which is often associated with hallucinogen intoxication. When cannabis-induced psychotic disorder does occur, it may be associated with a preexisting personality disorder in the affected person. Efforts to characterize a specific psychotic syndrome unique to cannabis have not been convincing.

It appears likely that cannabis can exacerbate schizophrenia, as is the case with other drugs that have hallucinogenic properties. Cannabis has even been reported as an independent risk factor for the development of schizophrenia and other types of mental illness, but those reports are speculative as a causal association remains unproven. Thus, despite worldwide reports associating cannabis with mental illness, chronic pyschosis has not as yet been reliably and consistently demonstrated to occur more often among cannabis users. Chronic psychotic disorders that may be precipitated by cannabis appear to relate to premorbid vulnerability or psychopathology.

CANNABIS-INDUCED ANXIETY DISORDER Cannabis-induced anxiety disorder (see Section 17.5) is a common diagnosis for acute cannabis intoxication, which in many persons induces short-lived anxiety states that are often provoked by paranoid thoughts. In such circumstances, panic attacks may be induced, based on ill-defined and disorganized fears. The appearance of anxiety symptoms is correlated with the dose and is the most frequent adverse reaction to the moderate use of smoked cannabis. Some cannabis users report occasional unpleasant adverse experiences, most often described as anxiety reactions of mild to moderate intensity. Inexperienced users are much more likely to experience anxiety symptoms than are experienced users.

CANNABIS-RELATED DISORDER NOT OTHERWISE SPECIFIED DSM-IV does not formally recognize cannabis-induced mood disorders; therefore, such disorders are classified as cannabis-related disorders not otherwise specified (Table 13.5-3). Cannabis intoxication can be associated with depressive symptoms, although such symptoms may suggest long-term cannabis use. Hypomania, however, is a common symptom in cannabis intoxication.

TABLE 13.5-3
Cannabis-Related Disorder Not Otherwise Specified

The cannabis-related disorder not otherwise specified category is for disorders associated with the use of cannabis that are not classifiable as cannabis dependence, cannabis abuse, cannabis intoxication, cannabis intoxication delirium, cannabis-induced psychotic disorder, or cannabis-induced anxiety disorder.

Table from DSM-IV, *Diagnostic and Statistical Manual of Mental Disorders,* ed 4. Copyright American Psychiatric Association, Washington, 1994. Used with permission.

DSM-IV also does not formally recognize cannabis-induced sleep disorders or cannabis-induced sexual dysfunction; therefore, both are classified as cannabis-related disorders not otherwise specified (NOS). When either sleep disorder symptoms or sexual dysfunction symptoms are present and related to cannabis use, they almost always resolve within days or a week after the cessation of cannabis use.

Flashbacks Flashbacks, in which feelings and perceptions experienced in the intoxicated state are suddenly thrust into consciousness in the nondrugged condition, have also been reported with cannabis use, although not as often as with lysergic acid diethylamide (LSD) use. It has been suggested that flashbacks result from intermittent release of psychoactive components from the CNS, where they are stored during periods of active use, but that explanation remains highly speculative. A few clinical reports suggest that marijuana use may precipitate flashbacks in persons who have previously used LSD.

Amotivational syndrome An amotivational syndrome associated with chronic cannabis use has been described in some of the older clinical literature from the Middle East, the Orient, and the United States. The syndrome is marked by apathy, poor concentration, social withdrawal, and loss of interest in achievement. Those features may correlate with the reversible decrement in cerebral blood flow that has been documented as an effect of marijuana. However, most of the reports are not rigorously scientific and lack controls so as to distinguish between the effects of cannabis and preexisting psychological and social conditions. Subsequent reports using different populations and better scientific methods have failed to demonstrate the existence of the syndrome. Several authors have noted that it is difficult to determine which came first, the drug or the amotivation. Most plausible perhaps is the suggestion that in certain persons the pharmacological effects of the drug interact with psychological and social factors to retard motivation and productivity.

Thus, the direct causal role of marijuana in the amotivational syndrome has been seriously questioned. Symptoms may be more indicative of ongoing intoxication or represent normal psychosocial variants that predispose to the use of cannabis and other substances. However, because persistent functional and structural changes in hippocampal neurons in animals subjected to long-term THC administration have been observed, the concept that a developing personality can be altered as a consequence of chronic intoxication should not be entirely dismissed. In any event, cessation may lead to gradual improvement. Despite those potential adverse effects, many regard cannabis as a relatively safe drug because lethal doses are unknown in humans.

Withdrawal Withdrawal symptoms have been reported in association with chronic use of high doses. They reach their peak in about eight hours after last use and persist for two to three days. Marijuana withdrawal effects include irritability, anxiety, sleep disturbances, anorexia, weight loss, perspiration, tremors, diarrhea, nausea, vomiting, muscle pains, and increased body temperature. Withdrawal symptoms are usually mild, and no specific treatment is generally required.

ADVERSE EFFECTS THC exerts prominent effects on the CNS. They are highly variable and depend on the user, the dose, and the environment. There is an initial stimulant effect, commonly producing an increased sense of well-being and euphoria and associated with spontaneous laughter, disinhibition, or quiet reverie. Heightened imagination and creative thinking are noted by some. Mood changes vary, and anxiety and depression may also be induced. Those initial effects are often followed by relaxation or lethargy and drowsiness, especially at higher doses. Many users report perceptual and sensory changes, such as a sense that time is passing slowly, an accentuation of auditory and visual perceptions, or actual sensory distortions occasionally involving hallucinations. Because of those perceptual changes, usually only at very high doses, some consider marijuana to be a hallucinogen of very low potency. Dry mouth and throat and increased hunger are also common symptoms.

Most adverse marijuana-induced effects disappear when the acute intoxication has ended, depending on individual vulnerability, environmental factors (whether the user is in a nonthreatening area), and dose. Less common adverse effects are changed sensations of bodily perceptions, depersonalization, derealization, acute panic, and frank paranoia.

Cardiovascular effects Cannabis increases heart rate in a predictable dose-dependent fashion, probably due to an inhibition of vagal tone. That is often one of the first effects of the drug. Along with conjunctival reddening, heart rate correlates with the appearance and duration of psychic effects as well as the plasma concentrations of the drug. Myocardial oxygen demand is increased and exercise tolerance decreased. Those effects can lead to myocardial ischemia if a person with coronary artery disease exercises when intoxicated. Orthostatic hypotension can also occur, especially at high doses. Tolerance to all those cardiovascular effects appears to develop.

Pulmonary effects Smoking is by far the most popular route of cannabis administration. Although not yet subject to the same large-scale, long-term epidemiological analyses which identified tobacco as a carcinogen, cannabis is known to induce pulmonary pathology. Chronic smokers have long demonstrated bronchitis, pharyngolaryngitis, and asthma, most likely from marijuana smoke's highly irritating effect on the bronchial epithelium. Marijuana cigarettes contain far more tar (particulates) and respiratory irritants than tobacco. Tar produced by the burning of marijuana is more carcinogenic to animals than that derived from tobacco, and marijuana smoking is predicted by some to result in human carcinogenesis, as has been seen with tobacco. Adding to the long-term toxic potential is the fact that marijuana smoke is usually inhaled longer and more deeply than cigarette smoke, delivering up to four times more tar to the lungs.

Heavy marijuana smoking has been shown to cause mild but significant large airway obstruction, probably through chronic irritation or inflammation of the bronchial lining, because THC causes bronchodilation to which little tolerance develops.

Immunological and carcinogenic effects Marijuana smoke inhibits pulmonary antibacterial defense systems, primarily alveolar macrophages as well as neutrophils and lymphocytes. Cannabinoids may also suppress cellular and humoral immune responses in animals. The clinical significance of those effects has not been demonstrated.

In vitro and in vivo animal studies using relatively high doses of cannabinoids have shown them to have mutagenic and carcinogenic effects and to impair the synthesis of nucleic acids and proteins. While it is impossible to dismiss the potential clinical significance of those reports, no cytogenic abnormalities have yet been consistently documented in human marijuana smokers.

Hormonal and reproductive effects In animals, cannabis has been shown to disrupt all phases of reproductive functioning by direct action on both the hypothalamic-pituitary axis and the gonads. In humans, all aspects of these effects have been suspected but are difficult to confirm.

Cannabis has been reported to cause reversible inhibition of spermatogenesis with a reduction in the quantity of sperm cells and an increased prevalence of abnormal cells. Decreased levels of testosterone and decreased size of the testes and prostate after heavy use are also seen but are believed to be reversible.

A single marijuana cigarette can suppress plasma leutinizing hormone during the luteal phase of the menstrual cycle. That may account for the higher frequency of anovulatory cycles often associated with marijuana smoking. Those phenonema may be due to THC's central effect of interfering with the release of gonadotropin-releasing hormone at a suprapituitary site and thereby disrupting the release of circulating luteinizing and follicle stimulating hormones.

Cannabinoids cross the placental barrier and appear in maternal milk. Experimentally, cannabis is teratogenic at high doses in some species of animals. However, cannabis' deleterious effects on the human fetus have been difficult to assess because of the frequent concurrent use of other drugs, cigarettes, and alcohol. Studies that have attempted to account for those variables have frequently associated marijuana with low birth weight. Its effects on other types of human fetal abnormalities have been reported, but the correlation is not well documented.

LABORATORY EXAMINATION

Urine testing for marijuana and other drugs has become common in many settings, including drug treatment programs and places of employment. Most laboratories employ the enzyme-multiplied immunoassay (EMIT), although a radioimmunoassay is also commonly used. Both tests, while relatively sensitive and inexpensive, provide an unacceptable level of false positives. Thus confirmation by gas chromatography-mass spectrometry is routinely used. Cannabis and its metabolites may be detected in urine at the usual cutoff level of 100 ng per mL for 42 to 72 hours after the psychological effects subside. Passive inhalation that occurs under unusually crowded conditions may also reveal cannabis metabolites in the urine if the sensitivity of the urine test is increased to 20 ng per mL.

No clear linear relationship between psychoactive effects and urine levels has been determined. Urines containing cannabis metabolites imply nothing more than that cannabis exposure has occurred at an indeterminable time prior to testing. Similarly, there is no clear correlation between THC blood levels and impairment. To avoid problems that may be associated with identifying very low levels of metabolites in the urine, such as can occur with passive inhalation, most labs use a cutoff point of 100 ng per mL or higher.

TREATMENT

Persons who use marijuana are often referred for treatment. Referrals are made for persons with widely varying use patterns and treatment needs. At one extreme is the person who uses cannabis intermittently and at low doses who is identified on a random drug screening test. At the other extreme is the person who uses high doses on a daily basis and meets criteria for dependence. In the former case, periodic urine testing with infrequent supportive counseling may be the only intervention needed. In the later case, referral to a specialized and intensive drug rehabilitation program is probably necessary. Thus, as in other clinical situations involving substance use, treatment should begin only after a complete history is taken and a diagnosis is established. A psychiatric examination is helpful to determine underlying psychopathology and the relationship of drug use to mood states and psychiatric symptoms.

Cannabis dependence and abuse are usually treated by the psychosocial methods that are typically used in drug-free rehabilitation programs. They include attempts to promote realistic and rewarding alternatives to the drug and the associated lifestyles along with a commitment to abstinence from self-administered or unprescribed psychotropic drugs. Treatment usually involves a combination of interventions, including urine testing, participation in 12-step programs, education about drug effects, drug counseling, psychotherapy, and family therapy. Drug-focused group therapy is perhaps the most common treatment technique for all substance-related disorders, including cannabis-related disorders. Common strategies used by the group are social pressure to reinforce abstinence, teaching socialization and problem-solving skills, reducing stress and the sense of isolation often associated with drug use, relapse prevention exercises, and varying degrees of confrontation.

Few people seek treatment for cannabis abuse and dependence alone; other drug abuse usually precipitates treatment. Denial of a drug problem appears common in many persons with cannabis abuse or dependence, as in persons with other substance use disorders.

Treatment of unpleasant adverse reactions, usually anxiety reactions, consists of calm and gentle reassurance in a warm and supportive atmosphere. Short-term use of anxiolytics, such as benzodiazepines, is necessary in some instances where anxiety symptoms are prominent or severe. Short-term use of low doses of antipsychotic medication may be justified if the patient has more persistent and troubling symptoms, such as delusional ideas or frightening flashbacks. Treatment of toxic-delirious states is similarly supportive, symptomatic, and short-term because of their self-limited nature.

THERAPEUTIC USES

Cannabis has been tried as a therapeutic agent for a variety of ailments. In the 20th century, those have included hysteria, anorexia nervosa, epilepsy, rheumatism, bronchial asthma, pain, glaucoma, and nausea. THC has antiemetic effects that are thought to be central in origin. There are anecdotal reports that attempts to use this action to alleviate the nausea and vomiting commonly produced by many cancer chemotherapeutic agents, or to reduce the nausea and diarrhea associated with acquired immune deficiency syndrome (AIDS) or with chemotherapy used to treat human immunodeficiency virus (HIV) infection have met with some success. However, with repeated doses patients experience the typical symptoms of intoxication, such as mood changes and decreases in concentration, coordination, and the ability to estimate time. More controlled studies than currently exist could provide better information than what has been reported in this important and controversial area.

Synthetic cannabinols, such as nabilone and levonantradol, have been reported by most researchers to be of benefit during those treatments because of their antiemetic properties but few euphorogenic attributes. However, the incidence of sedation is high, superiority to older agents, such as the phenothiazines, has not been proved, and the safety of those medications in long-term use has not been established.

Marijuana's ability to lower intraocular pressure has also stimulated interest. Thus far, that effect is mostly short-lived, and there is no evidence as yet that cannabis is more effective than a host of other agents in treating patients suffering from glaucoma. Mild hypothermia, prolongation of barbiturate anesthesia, seizure attenuation, and hyperglycemia are other findings that have not as yet demonstrated clinical utility.

SUGGESTED CROSS REFERENCES

An overview of the substance-related disorders, including substance abuse and substance dependence, appears in Section 13.1. Substance intoxication delirium is discussed in Chapter 12 on cognitive disorders and mental disorders due to a general medical condition. Substance-induced psychotic disorder is discussed in Section 15.3 on acute and transient psychotic disorders and culture-bound syndromes. Substance-induced anxiety disorder appears in Section 17.5 on general anxiety disorder and other anxiety disorders.

REFERENCES

Andreasson S, Allebeck P, Engstrom A, Rydberg U: Cannabis and schizophrenia: A longitudinal study. Lancet *2:* 1483, 1987.

Ashton C H: Cannabis: Dangers and possible uses. Br Med J *294:*141, 1987.

Center for Disease Control: 1990 youth risk behavior survey. MMWR *40:* 776, 1991.

Compton D R, Dewey W L, Martin B R: Cannabis dependence and tolerance production. Adv Alcohol Subst Abuse *9:* 129, 1990.

Council on Scientific Affairs: Marijuana, its health hazards and therapeutic potentials. JAMA *246:* 1823, 1981.

Devane W A, Dysarz F A III, Johnson M R, Melvin L S, Howlett A C: Determination and characterization of a cannabinoid receptor in rat brain. Mol Pharmacol *34:* 605, 1988.

Gieringer D H: Marijuana, driving and accident safety. J Psychoactive Drugs *20:* 93, 1988.

Gruber A J, Pope H G: Cannabis psychotic disorder: Does it exist. Am J Addict *3:* 72, 1994.

Hollister L E: Cannabis-1988. Acta Psychiatr Scand *345:* 108, 1988.

Hollister L E: Health aspects of cannabis. Pharmacol Rev *38:* 2, 1986.

Imade A G T, Ebie J C: A retrospective study of symptom patterns of cannabis induced psychosis. Acta Psychiatr Scand *83:* 134, 1991.

Jaffee J: Drug addiction and drug abuse. In *The Pharmacological Basis of Therapeutics,* ed 8, A G Gilman, T W Rall, A S Nies, P Taylor, editors, p 549. Pergamon, New York, 1990.

*Johnson B A: Psychopharmacological effects of cannabis. Br J Hosp Med *43:* 114, 1990.

Johnston L D, O'Malley P M, Bachman J G: *National Survey Results on Drug Use from Monitoring the Future Study.* US Government Printing Office, Washington, DC, 1993.

*Jones R T: Cannabis and health. Annu Rev Med *34:* 247, 1983.

Melges F T: Temporal disorganization and delusional-like ideation. Arch Gen Psychiatry *30:* 855, 1974.

Mikuriya T H, Aldrich M R: Cannabis 1988- the potency question. J Psychoactive Drugs *20:* 47, 1988.

Miller N S, Gold M S: The diagnosis of marijuana dependence. J Subst Abuse Treat *6:* 183, 1989.
Millman R B: Cannabis abuse and dependence. In *Treatments of Psychiatric Disorders,* B T Karasu editor, p 1241. American Psychiatric Association, Washington, 1989.
*Millman R B, Sbriglio R: Patterns of use and psychopathology in chronic marijuana users. Psychiatr Clin North Am *9:* 533, 1986.
Musto D F: Opium, cocaine and marijuana in American history. Sci Am *265:* 20, 1991.
Nahas G G: Cannabis: Toxicological properties and epidemiological aspects. Med J Aust *145:* 82, 1986.
Negrete J C: Symptoms of cannabis intoxication in a group of users. Toxicomanies 7:7, 1974.
Negrete J C: What's happened to the cannabis debate? Br J Addict *83:* 359, 1988.
*Schwartz R H: Marijuana: An overview. Pediatr Clin North Am *34:* 305, 1987.
Seldon B S, Clark R F, Curry S C: Marijuana. Emerg Med Clin North Am *8:* 527, 1990.
Seth R, Sinha S: Chemistry and pharmacology of cannabis. Prog Drug Res *36:* 71, 1991.
Smiley A: Marijuana: On-road and driving simulator studies. Alcohol, Drugs, Driving: Abstracts and Reviews *2:* 121, 1986.
Thomas H: Psychiatric symptoms in cannabis users. Br J Psychiatry *163:* 141, 1993
Thornicroft G: Cannabis and psychosis. Br J Psychiatry *157:*25, 1990.
Tunving K: Psychiatric aspects of cannabis use in adolescents and young adults. Pediatrician *14:* 83, 1987.
*Tunving K: Psychiatric effects of cannabis use. Acta Psychiatr Scand *72:* 209, 1985.
Weinrieb R M, O'Brien C P: Persistent cognitive deficits attributed to substance abuse. Neurol Clin *11:* 663, 1993.
Weller M P I, Ang P C, Latimer-Sayer D T, Zachary A: Drug abuse and mental illness. Lancet *1:* 997, 1988.
Wert R C, Raulin M L: The chronic cerebral effects of cannabis use. Int J Addict *21:* 605, 1986.

13.6 COCAINE-RELATED DISORDERS

JEROME H. JAFFE, M.D.

INTRODUCTION

Despite some pharmacological differences between cocaine and amphetamines, the patterns of use, dependence, and toxicity are quite similar and the treatment is currently the same in most instances. Furthermore, the diagnostic criteria for all of the substance-related disorders are virtually identical.

DEFINITION

Substance use may be associated with a number of distinct disorders, of which dependence and abuse are but two. In the case of cocaine 10 other substance-related disorders have been described in the fourth edition of *Diagnostic and Statistical Manual of Mental Disorders* (DSM-IV) (Table 13.6-1).

Cocaine dependence is a cluster of physiological, behavioral, and cognitive symptoms that, taken together, indicate that the person continues to use cocaine despite significant problems related to such use. As a generic concept drug dependence has also been defined by the World Health Organization (WHO) as a syndrome in which the use of the drugs or class of drugs takes on a much higher priority for a given person than do other behaviors that once had a higher value. Both of those brief definitions have as their central features the emphasis on the drug-using behavior itself, on its maladaptive nature, and on how the choice to engage in that behavior has shifted and become constrained as a result of interaction with the drug over time.

Cocaine abuse is a term used to categorize a pattern of maladaptive use of cocaine leading to clinically significant impairment or distress and occurring within a 12-month period, but one in which the symptoms have never met the criteria for cocaine dependence.

The disorders induced by cocaine include cocaine intoxication, cocaine withdrawal, cocaine-induced psychotic disorder with delusions or with hallucinations, cocaine intoxication delirium, cocaine-induced mood disorder, cocaine-induced anxiety disorder, cocaine-induced sleep disorder, cocaine-induced sexual dysfunction, and cocaine-related disorder not otherwise specified.

The DSM-IV coding scheme provides distinct code numbers for cocaine dependence and cocaine abuse, but the codes for the other substance-related disorders do not differentiate cocaine-induced disorders from the other substance-induced disorders, with the exception of the alcohol-induced disorders (see Section 11.1). In some cases the same codes must be used for disorders induced by a wide variety of substances.

HISTORY

Purified cocaine became commercially available in 1884; reports in the European literature of compulsive cocaine use and cocaine psychosis appeared as early as the 1880s. Cocaine use and dependence were not uncommon in the United States at the turn of the 20th century. Cocaine was an ingredient of Coca-Cola until 1900, and nonprescription properietary nostrums containing cocaine were widely promoted until passage of the Harrison Act in 1914. With greater public awareness of the physical and legal risks of drug use, both cocaine use and dependence declined. However, it was still common enough in Europe. Hans Maier's classic *Der Kokainismus,* first published in 1926, included descriptions of relatively recent clinical cases. In the United States cocaine use declined gradually, but in the 1920s illicit cocaine was still available for 25 cents for about 100 mg. From the late 1930s through the early 1970s, cocaine use and dependence became quite uncommon. Virtually no cocaine-dependent patients entered the U.S. Public Health

TABLE 13.6-1
Cocaine Use Disorders

Cocaine use disorders

Cocaine dependence
Cocaine abuse

Cocaine-induced disorders

Cocaine intoxication
Specify if: with perceptual disturbances
Cocaine withdrawal
Cocaine intoxication delirium
Cocaine-induced psychotic disorder, with delusions
Specify if: with onset during intoxication
Cocaine-induced psychotic disorder, with hallucinations
Specify if: with onset during intoxication
Cocaine-induced mood disorder
Specify if: with onset during intoxication
with onset during withdrawal
Cocaine-induced anxiety disorder
Specify if: with onset during intoxication/with onset during withdrawal
Cocaine-induced sexual dysfunction
Specify if: with onset during intoxication
Cocaine-induced sleep disorder
Specify if: with onset during intoxication/with onset during withdrawal

Cocaine-related disorder not otherwise specified

Table based on DSM-IV, *Diagnostic and Statistical Manual of Mental Disorders,* ed 4. Copyright American Psychiatric Association, Washington, 1994. Used with permission.

Service Hospital at Lexington, Kentucky, in the 1960s, although there were some heroin users who had used cocaine.

Starting in the 1970s and continuing throughout the 1980s, cocaine availability increased noticeably. During the first few years of its renewed popularity, there were few reports of toxicity or of persons seeking treatment. Some observers, apparently unaware of previous epidemics in which the compulsive nature of cocaine use and its serious toxicity had been repeatedly documented, declared cocaine use to be relatively benign. Cocaine use spread from affluent young adults (who tended to use it intranasally) through all economic and age levels of society. More hazardous routes of administration, including injection and inhalation of freebase forms, such as crack, became common.

By 1985, owing to its increasing availability and declining price, 20 million people had tried cocaine. Its toxicity became quite apparent as the number of emergency room visits rose sharply for cardiovascular, neurological, and psychiatric complications, and its capacity to induce dependence was apparent from the escalating requests for treatment. Increasing numbers of users, overdose deaths, crime, and the images of crack babies damaged in utero by cocaine-using pregnant women gave the drug problem, particularly cocaine use, national visibility. Federal expenditures for law enforcement escalated. Penalties for drug selling and possession were increased and national prevention campaigns were initiated. Drug (urine) testing in the workplace became more common. Toward the end of the decade, there was a decline in casual use and in the number of cocaine-related medical emergency cases seen at hospital emergency rooms. The number of heavy users did not decline as sharply. Urine tests of arrestees showed that a substantial number of criminals were still using cocaine. Cocaine remained relatively available and less costly than in the 1970s. In the early 1990s emergency room visits began to increase again.

COMPARATIVE NOSOLOGY

The DSM-IV criteria for cocaine dependence are the same generic criteria as applied to other psychoactive drugs; the notion of a generic concept of dependence is shared with the revised third edition of DSM (DSM-III-R) and the 10th revision of the *International Classification of Diseases and Related Health Problems* (ICD-10). In making the diagnosis of dependence there is a generally high level of agreement between DSM-IV and ICD-10: they employ similar concepts (the dependence syndrome varying in degree of severity), although the wording of the criteria for determining the presence and severity of the syndrome differs. Both require that three elements of the syndrome be noted within a 12-month period. The degree of agreement between DSM-IV and DSM-III-R is even higher, since, despite some changes in the wording, the syndromes and criteria in the two editions are quite similar. Although DSM-IV appears to lay greater stress on tolerance and physiological dependence, in practice, even if those criteria had been required, that would not have substantially reduced the number of cases meeting the criteria for dependence on cocaine or stimulants. In a study of 399 cocaine abusers a very high proportion (about 83 percent) reported tolerance. Fewer cocaine users reported withdrawal (about half) or using the drug to avoid withdrawal (36 percent).

The major changes between DSM-III-R and DSM-IV affected the diagnosis of substance abuse. DSM-III-R required the presence of only one of two general criteria, whereas DSM-IV requires one of four. Nevertheless, the agreement between DSM-III-R and DSM-IV is exceedingly high.

There is a major difference between ICD-10 and DSM-IV in the classification of what is called substance abuse in DSM-IV. ICD-10 does not use the term "abuse" but instead includes the category of harmful use, which is substantially different from the concept of abuse as used in DSM-IV. However, the concept of harm is limited to physical and mental health (for example, hepatitis, cardiac damage, episodes of depression, or toxic psychosis). It specifically excludes social impairments as follows: "Harmful patterns of use are often criticized by others and frequently associated with adverse social consequences of various kinds. The fact that a pattern of use or a particular substance is disapproved of by another person or by the culture, or may have led to socially negative consequences such as arrest or marital arguments is not in itself evidence of harmful use."

EPIDEMIOLOGY

Cocaine use has fluctuated dramatically over the past two decades, not just in the United States, but also in South America and in western Europe. In the United States among the various activities aimed at estimating the extent and consequences of psychoactive drug use are the annual High School Senior Survey, the National Household Survey on Drug Abuse (NHSDA), reports from a selected group of hospital emergency rooms and medical examiners' offices on drug-related adverse effects and deaths (Drug Abuse Warning Network [DAWN]), and analysis of urine tests of arrestees conducted at selected jails (Drug Use Forecasting [DUF] program) and of applicants for positions at corporations. All of those estimating techniques have sampling limitations, and none apply standardized diagnostic criteria to substance-use patterns or adverse effects. Consequently, although they provide a picture of use over time, these methods do not reveal changes in the incidence and prevalence of specific substance-related disorders, such as dependence and abuse.

The annual High School Senior Survey shows the changes in self-reported cocaine use over time. All indicators of use (lifetime, past year, past month) declined substantially from the high levels seen from 1985 through 1992 to levels lower than or as low as any seen since the survey began in 1975. Use in 1993 was not significantly different from that in 1992.

The NHSDA study found steady declines in the casual use of cocaine from peak levels in 1985 to much lower levels in 1992, and little additional change in 1993. Heavy cocaine users (weekly users) showed relatively little decline over that period. In 1993 there were 1.3 million current users (down from an estimated 5.3 million in 1985) and three million occasional users (less than monthly). Weekly cocaine users remained at about a half million; current crack users were estimated at about a half million, with no decline since 1991.

Two relatively recent population surveys that did use accepted criteria to measure the extent of substance abuse and dependence were the Epidemiologic Catchment Area (ECA) Study, carried out in the early 1980s using third edition of DSM (DSM-III) criteria, and the National Comorbidity Survey (NCS), carried out from 1990 to 1992 using DSM-III-R criteria. Only the ECA and NCS offer estimates of the prevalence of abuse and dependence, as defined by DSM-III and DSM-III-R, respectively. The ECA report combined categories of dependence and abuse for cocaine. The one-month and six-month prevalence rates for cocaine abuse-dependence were too low to be measurable; the lifetime rate was 0.2 percent.

The NCS survey was carried out just after the peak of the cocaine epidemic; it also used DSM-III-R, which did not require tolerance and withdrawal for a diagnosis of dependence. The NCS data for specific drugs have not yet been published.

ETIOLOGY

Substance dependence is currently viewed as the result of a process in which social, psychological, cultural, and biological factors influence substance-using behavior. In that biopsychosocial perspective the actions of the substance are seen as critical. However, not all persons who become dependent experience the effects of a given substance in the same way or are influenced by the same set of factors, and even with the same class of pharmacological agents, different factors may be more or less important at different stages of the process.

Social and cultural factors largely influence the availability and initial use of cocaine and other substances. In the case of cocaine, however, pharmacological factors are believed to play very important roles in the perpetuation of use and of progression to dependence. Cocaine has potent mood-elevating and euphorigenic actions, especially when its effects are rapid in onset, such as when the cocaine is injected or inhaled. Although some degree of physical dependence develops, in contrast to the opioids and sedatives, an aversive withdrawal syndrome probably plays a less prominent role in perpetuating the use of cocaine.

COMORBIDITY Additional psychiatric diagnoses are quite common among those dependent on cocaine. It is not always evident how this comorbidity is linked etiologically to cocaine, but the epidemiological evidence is clear that the presence of psychiatric disorders not related to substance abuse (for example, mood disorders, schizophrenia, and antisocial personality disorder) substantially increases the odds of developing substance abuse-dependence. For some persons cocaine may serve to alleviate various psychiatric disorders or dysfunctional states. Some users, for example, may find relief from dysthymic disorder. Others may find that cocaine facilitates sexual activity that was previously unsatisfactory. However, while such factors may explain substance use on more than one occasion, they do not account for progression to dependence or abuse.

It is also postulated that cocaine use may induce psychiatric syndromes (for example, paranoid psychotic states) that may persist; persons with certain psychiatric disorders may be prone to experiment with cocaine or other substances; or the factors that predispose to psychiatric disorders may also predispose cocaine users to progress to dependence.

Research on the temporal appearance of the syndromes indicates that, in some instances and for some syndromes, substance use antedates the psychiatric disorder. In one component of the ECA study interviewed subjects were reinterviewed one year later. Those who reported cocaine or stimulant use in the interval were almost eight times more likely than were nonusers to experience depression and 14 times more likely to have had a panic attack. Cocaine users were almost 12 times more likely to experience a manic episode.

The ECA data also show a relation between the extent of cocaine use and other psychiatric disorders. Among men 18 to 44 years of age, those who had never used cocaine, or had used it fewer than five times, the lifetime prevalence of major depression was 7.6 percent; it was 11 percent for users who were never daily users and almost 26 percent for those who met the DSM-III criteria for cocaine abuse. Similarly, the lifetime prevalence of panic disorder was related to the extent of cocaine use.

GENETIC FACTORS What role genetic factors play in increasing the specific vulnerability to cocaine dependence is unclear. However, the odds of cocaine dependence are increased among persons with alcohol dependence, schizophrenia, bipolar disorder, or antisocial personality disorder. The fact that each of those disorders has a genetic predisposition suggests that genetic vulnerability to dependence is a factor that should be considered.

OTHER FACTORS Social, cultural, and economic factors are powerful determinants of initial use, continuing use, and relapse. Excessive use is far more likely in countries where cocaine is readily available. Different economic opportunities may influence certain groups more than others to engage in selling illicit drugs, and selling is more likely to be carried out in familiar communities than in those where the seller runs a high risk of arrest.

Since in both human and animal studies alternative positive reinforcers compete with drugs as reinforcers, the absence of such nondrug alternatives can be seen as a causal factor for use, especially where drugs are available and the social pressures against using them are not strong. Alternative positive reinforcers are not limited to material rewards but include the kinds of psychological rewards that are associated with satisfying interpersonal relationships and the self-esteem that derives from achievements in socially acceptable roles.

LEARNING AND CONDITIONING Learning and conditioning are also believed to be important factors in the perpetuation of cocaine use. With each inhalation or injection of cocaine the rush and the euphoric experience act to reinforce the antecedent drug-taking behavior. In addition, the environmental cues associated with substance use become associated with the euphoric state so that long after a period of cessation, such cues (for example, white powder and paraphernalia) can elicit memories of the euphoric state and reawaken craving for cocaine.

PHARMACOLOGICAL FACTORS As a result of actions in the central nervous system (CNS), cocaine can produce a sense of alertness, euphoria, and well-being. There may be decreased hunger and less need for sleep. Performance impaired by fatigue is usually improved. Cocaine can induce paranoia, suspiciousness, and overt psychosis, which can be difficult to distinguish from acute paranoid schizophrenia. It can also produce major cardiovascular toxicities.

Mechanisms of action Cocaine's reinforcing effects and central stimulant actions in the CNS emerge at doses far lower than those needed for local anesthetic action. A critical element in its reinforcing effects is the activation of mesolimbic and mesocortical dopaminergic systems. Cocaine produces such activation primarily by occupying the dopamine transporter mechanism, thereby inhibiting the reuptake of released dopamine.

In animals cocaine is a powerful reinforcer of drug-taking behavior. It is viewed as the most powerful pharmacological reinforcer known; given free access, animals will choose to self-administer cocaine rather than have food, water, or access to other animals. Death from starvation or drug toxicity is the typical consequence of unlimited cocaine access. With limited access (two to six hours a day) cocaine does not gain such control over behavior and animals may select food in preference to cocaine, depending on the dose, the amount of work they must do to get the dose, and the type and amount of food offered as alternative reinforcers.

Common routes of administration Cocaine can be taken orally, by injection, by absorption via nasal and buccal membranes, or by inhalation and absorption through the pulmonary alveoli. Inhalation of freebase cocaine produces almost immediate absorption and a rapid onset of effects. Cocaine hydrochloride, the water-soluble form typically used for snorting or injection, is largely destroyed by the heat of burning and so is not well suited for smoking. Cocaine as freebase sublimates before it is destroyed by the heat. The hydrochloride salt can be converted to the freebase form by treatment with alkali and extraction with organic solvents. In the 1980s users learned to avoid the fire hazard of extracting organic solvents and still produce a crude form of freebase cocaine by heating the cocaine with sodium bicarbonate to yield crack, a hard, white mass that is freebase plus impurities. When smoked, this material gives off a crackling sound. In cocaine-producing countries some users may smoke a crude intermediate product, cocaine sulfate (coca paste, pasta basica, basuca), which is usually contaminated with solvents.

As with the opioids, the rapid onset of cocaine's effects after intravenous injection or freebase inhalation produces an intensely pleasurable sensation referred to as a rush. The cocaine rush lasts only a few minutes, whereas other psychological and physiological effects tend to decline more slowly, in parallel with declining plasma levels.

Metabolism The half-life of a single dose of cocaine in the blood is only about 30 to 90 minutes. It is typically hydrolyzed by plasma pseudocholinesterase and liver esterase into inactive metabolites, the most significant being benzoylecgonine and ecgonine methylester. The metabolite is generally detectable in urine for 24 to 72 hours after brief periods of use. With repeated high doses (for example, 1 to 12 g a day) cocaine or its metabolites may accumulate in body compartments (for example, fat and the CNS), from which it is then slowly released. Consequently, using sensitive measures, cocaine may be detectable in the urine of heavy users for two weeks. In a study of cocaine-dependent patients admitted to an inpatient treatment unit, the average time from last reported cocaine use to first negative urine test (using a cutoff of 300 ng/mL) was 105 hours, and 20 percent had positive tests for 120 hours or longer.

The concurrent use of cocaine and alcohol may result in the accumulation of a distinct metabolite, cocaethylene. The metabolite is active and longer lasting than cocaine itself, and may account for the enhancement of subjective effects and toxicity when the two are used simultaneously.

Tolerance and sensitization Patients seeking treatment often report needing progressively more cocaine to get the same effect. In the laboratory some degree of acute cardiovascular tolerance to cocaine may appear during a series of doses, but it is not clear whether clinically significant tolerance develops to its cardiovascular effects. Even experienced users may sustain significant cardiovascular toxicity.

Chronic use of cocaine also produces a form of sensitization in which the response to a given dose is actually enhanced. One theory holds that the sensitization is attributable to a variety of kindling in the CNS. In the classic studies of kindling, electrical stimulation of the limbic system, which initially has very little effect, is applied repeatedly; after a matter of days the threshold for effects decreases and major long-lasting seizures appear. In animals similar effects are seen with CNS stimulants, so that repeated doses of cocaine eventually elicit seizures or stereotyped behaviors not seen with initial doses. The sensitization can be long lasting.

The paranoid states and toxic psychoses that commonly develop among chronic cocaine users are believed to be among the phenomena to which sensitization develops. Cocaine psychosis develops more rapidly for those who have been chronic users or had developed psychoses previously.

Withdrawal states The cocaine withdrawal syndrome has aversive qualities (for example, dysphoria, anhedonia), but in most cases withdrawal is probably not as critical in perpetuating cocaine using behavior as opioids are in perpetuating opioid-using behavior. Although, in most instances, withdrawal anhedonia and fatigue do not contribute to relapse after brief withdrawal, that does not mean that the problems are not important for some persons. Some users, for example, who have come to depend on cocaine for high energy or for helping to project a confident persona may be temporarily unable to function without it. For others, withdrawal dysphoria may exaggerate the intensity of an antecedent mood disorder. There does not appear to be a protracted cocaine withdrawal syndrome.

Other actions The actions of cocaine are not selective for dopamine. It is almost as potent in blocking the reuptake of norepinephrine, serotonin, and, to some degree, acetylcholine. Some of those actions are relevant to the toxic actions of cocaine, especially its cardiovascular toxicity.

In rats chronic cocaine administration upregulates both μ and κ opioid receptors in selected brain areas without altering the number of δ receptors; chronic, but not acute, cocaine results in the production of novel foslike proteins with relatively long half-lives. Chronic cocaine also produces long-lasting reductions in neuropeptide Y. The clinical significance of those findings is not clear, but the reduction of neuropeptide Y has been postulated to be one mechanism that could account for withdrawal anxiety and depression.

DIAGNOSIS AND CLINICAL FEATURES

PATTERNS OF USE AND ABUSE There are several patterns of cocaine use and abuse. For example, Indians in the Andes chew coca leaves daily, but apparently very few progress to excessive use or toxicity. Although some cocaine users can use it intermittently without becoming dependent, it is not clear how long such intermittent, nondependent use can continue and for what proportion of users. Use of cocaine that does not cause problems for the user does not meet the DSM-IV criteria for either dependence or abuse.

Most cocaine users seeking treatment report that their use was initially intermittent. However, at some stage the use escalated, with episodes of using high doses becoming more frequent. Unlike opioid dependence, the daily use of cocaine is not the most common pattern of use among persons seeking treatment for cocaine dependence. A small percentage of such patients report using high doses, but for only a few days a month over a long period; such persons may still meet the criteria for dependence. That pattern is atypical, but an intermittent pattern of use is not. Intermittent use consists of episodes or binges of use, often starting on weekends and pay days and lasting until the drug supply has been exhausted or toxicity develops. The runs or binges, during which the drug may be used every 15 to 30 minutes, can last seven or more consecutive days, but typically are shorter. Although there appears to be little tolerance between binges, there are changes in the response to the drug during the course of a binge. Euphoric effects seem less prominent, and anxiety, fatigue, irritability, and depression increase. Any pause in the drug use causes blood levels to drop; typically, there is dysphoria rather than a return to normal mood. If cocaine is still available, it is used to dispel the dysphoria. When the binge is interrupted or supplies have been depleted, a cocaine crash quickly follows. The sense of needing more cocaine to get the same effect is reported more commonly by patients than is the experience of pronounced withdrawal. Some users make a distinction between a brief crash and withdrawal. A substantial proportion of cocaine users seeking treatment report daily or almost daily use, which is often associated with daily heroin use.

During the early stages of cocaine use there may be little interference with normal activities. Some persons may even find that the sense of energy and heightened sense of self-confidence facilitate productive activity. Others may find that the cocaine facilitates social interaction, particularly enhancing sexual arousal and enjoyment, at least initially. The development of sexual dysfunction later in the course of use is better documented than is the enhancement.

In addition to feelings of euphoria, cocaine use may also

induce concurrent feelings of anxiety, irritability, and suspiciousness. Users may commit crimes to obtain money to buy cocaine, and such crimes may involve violence. In addition, cocaine can induce paranoid ideation, and there are numerous reports of homicide and attempted homicide during such cocaine-induced toxic states.

Cocaine is especially powerful as a reinforcer when it is taken in ways that produce a rapid onset of effects. Not only do intravenous and intrapulmonary routes of administration produce a rapid rise in blood and brain drug levels and an intense rush but, especially with the smoking of freebase cocaine, there is an almost equally rapid decline in blood and brain drug levels as the cocaine is redistributed and metabolized. Clinicians report that some persons who inhale freebase cocaine appear to move immediately from experimentation to a pattern of regular and compulsive use, limited only by the availability of the drug or of the money to buy it. Even in the laboratory setting it can be shown that craving for cocaine is briefly intensified a few minutes after intravenous use when brain and blood levels are falling. It is important to emphasize, however, that while intravenous and pulmonary cocaine use are far more likely to result in compulsive use and dependence, the intranasal route can also lead to dependence and to the full range of cocaine toxicity (including fatalities).

Cocaine abusers frequently use sedatives or opioids to modulate the stimulant and toxic effects of the cocaine, a practice that can lead to concurrent dependence on sedatives or opioids. Sometimes an opiate, such as heroin, and cocaine are injected intravenously simultaneously; the mixture (speedball) is reported to be especially euphorigenic. As alcohol is probably the substance most commonly used in conjunction with cocaine, it may become associated with cocaine use and can trigger cocaine craving in former users trying to abstain from cocaine. More than 50 percent of cocaine users seeking treatment meet the lifetime Research Diagnostic Criteria (RDC) for alcoholism, and about 29 percent meet the criteria for current alcoholism.

COCAINE DEPENDENCE As use progresses, some persons may place greater priority on obtaining and using cocaine than on meeting other social obligations or on avoiding toxicity or arrest. They may engage in illegal activities to raise money for cocaine or trade sex for it. At that stage the use of cocaine would be viewed as maladaptive and would probably meet the DSM-IV criteria for cocaine abuse or dependence. The DSM-IV criteria for cocaine dependence are the same generic criteria applied to other substances (see Tables 13.1-2 and 13.1-5). For a diagnosis of dependence the drug-use pattern must be maladaptive and must lead to clinically significant impairment or distress as indicated by at least three of seven criteria presented in the table. DSM-IV instructs the clinician to specify whether physiological dependence is present (that is, there is evidence of either tolerance or withdrawal as defined in the diagnostic criteria).

Using the drug to prevent withdrawal is not as dominant a feature of cocaine dependence as it is of opioid dependence. However, the other criteria for dependence are common among heavy users of cocaine. Tolerance to some drug actions (for example, euphorigenic effects) appears to coexist with increased sensitization to other actions (for example, anxiogenic and psychotogenic effects).

COCAINE ABUSE Some cocaine users develop problems or adverse effects related to their drug use (that is, their use is maladaptive), even though such use does not meet the three-criteria requirement for the diagnosis of dependence. Examples of such recurrent maladaptive patterns include use that leads to multiple legal problems; failure to meet major social, school, or work-related obligations; and continued use despite social or vocational difficulties caused by or aggravated by cocaine use. When one or more such substance-related problems occur in a 12-month period, but the pattern has never met the criteria for dependence, the diagnosis of cocaine abuse (see Table 13.1-6) should be made.

COCAINE INTOXICATION Among those who meet the criteria for cocaine abuse or dependence, certain psychiatric toxicities are common. Just as alcohol-dependent persons are frequently intoxicated, during the course of a single binge cocaine users commonly develop the symptoms of cocaine intoxication. Along with the euphoria may come increasing suspiciousness, hypervigilance, anxiety, hyperactivity, talkativeness, and grandiosity. The users may engage in stereotyped and repetitive behaviors (for example, disassembling and reassembling the same object). There are typically other signs and symptoms of central stimulation, such as tachycardia, cardiac arrhythmias, elevated or lowered blood pressure, pupillary dilation, perspiration, or chills. There may also be hallucinations, including tactile hallucinations. Judgment is impaired and there may be confusion, but insight into the drug-induced nature of the hallucinations is retained.

Any of those symptoms following the recent use of cocaine should lead to a consideration of cocaine intoxication, provided they are not better accounted for by some other medical or mental disorder and there are at least two of a number of physiological signs commonly seen with the use of cocaine (such as tachycardia and elevated blood pressure). The DSM-IV diagnostic criteria for cocaine intoxication are shown in Table 13.6-2. The DSM-IV diagnostic criteria for cocaine intoxication are identical to the criteria for amphetamine intoxication except for the substitution of the word "cocaine" for the words "amphetamine or a related substance." Any perceptual disturbances should be specified.

In one study of cocaine abusers in the community just over half reported experiencing paranoia or hallucinations at some

TABLE 13.6-2
Diagnostic Criteria for Cocaine Intoxication

A. Recent use of cocaine.
B. Clinically significant maladaptive behavioral or psychological changes (e.g., euphoria or affective blunting; changes in sociability; hypervigilance; interpersonal sensitivity; anxiety, tension, or anger; stereotyped behaviors; impaired judgment; or impaired social or occupational functioning) that developed during, or shortly after, use of cocaine.
C. Two (or more) of the following, developing during, or shortly after, cocaine use:
  (1) tachycardia or bradycardia
  (2) pupillary dilation
  (3) elevated or lowered blood pressure
  (4) perspiration or chills
  (5) nausea or vomiting
  (6) evidence of weight loss
  (7) psychomotor agitation or retardation
  (8) muscular weakness, respiratory depression, chest pain, or cardiac arrhythmias
  (9) confusion, seizures, dyskinesias, dystonias, or coma
D. The symptoms are not due to a general medical condition and are not better accounted for by another mental disorder.

Specify if:
With perceptual disturbances

Table from DSM-IV, *Diagnostic and Statistical Manual of Mental Disorders,* ed 4.

time, whereas among those who sought treatment 63 percent reported those symptoms. Cocaine intoxication may occur in occasional users who do not meet the criteria for abuse or dependence.

COCAINE DELIRIUM AND COCAINE-INDUCED PSYCHOTIC DISORDER Whereas some degree of paranoia or hypervigilance is typical of cocaine intoxication and tactile and other hallucinations may also occur, the use of cocaine can also induce a toxic delirium and a more persistent toxic psychotic disorder characterized by suspiciousness, paranoia, visual and tactile hallucinations, and loss of insight. The hallucination of bugs (cocaine bugs) or vermin crawling under the skin (formication) is sometimes reported and is often associated with excoriation of the skin. A paranoid syndrome can develop within 24 hours after the beginning of a cocaine binge. When the syndrome develops in the presence of a clear sensorium and the person retains insight into the drug-induced nature of the symptoms, it is designated *cocaine intoxication,* even when there are hallucinations. When insight is lost but the sensorium is clear, the syndrome is designated *cocaine-induced psychotic disorder with delusions* or *with hallucinations* (see Section 15.3).

If consciousness is disturbed (the ability to focus, sustain, or shift attention is reduced) and there are deficits in memory and orientation, the diagnosis would be *cocaine intoxication delirium* (see Chapter 12).

There does not seem to be a predictable relation between the dose of cocaine used and the development of paranoia. Some persons appear to develop the syndrome at far lower doses than used by others who do not develop the syndrome. Furthermore, once it develops, the person seems more likely to develop it again with subsequent cocaine use, a sensitization phenomenon that may be related to kindling in the CNS.

Cocaine use has also been linked to the development of a panic disorder that outlasts the cocaine use; here, too, kindling has been postulated.

COCAINE WITHDRAWAL Cocaine withdrawal phenomena have not been as thoroughly studied as those associated with opioids or alcohol. No experimental studies have been conducted in which patients with known baseline characteristics have been stabilized solely on large doses of cocaine and then abruptly withdrawn. Consequently, most data have been derived from interviews and patients' recollections, or from observations of hospitalized patients whose level of drug ingestion and prior baseline characteristics can only be estimated.

Emil Erlenmeyer reported in 1886 that depression was likely to be seen when cocaine was stopped, and Maier, in *Der Kokainismus,* noted depression and apathy upon cessation. During the cocaine epidemic of the 1980s about 50 percent of cocaine users reported experiencing some type of withdrawal when drug use was interrupted.

Based on interviews with outpatients, researchers at Yale University described a three-phase syndrome in which the first phase, the crash, lasted from nine hours to four days and could itself be divided into several stages. Early in the crash agitation, depression, anorexia, and high cocaine craving were reported, followed by a decrease in cocaine craving, fatigue, depression, and a desire for sleep. That stage was succeeded by symptoms of exhaustion and hypersomnia from which there was intermittent awakening associated with hyperphagia and an absence of cocaine craving. The second phase was reported to be heralded by normalized sleep, improved mood, and low levels of craving, but that relatively benign phase was succeeded by a return of anergia, anhedonia, anxiety, and increased cocaine craving, especially in response to stimuli previously associated with cocaine use. A third phase—extinction (which appears to represent a period of extended vulnerability to relapse rather than a phase of an extended withdrawal syndrome)—was also described.

Such a complex phasic withdrawal has not been reported by others who observed cocaine-dependent patients admitted to clinical and research units. Instead, there was a steady decline in symptoms of depression and craving for cocaine over several weeks. When sleep, weight, and appetite were compared with those of normal controls on the same unit, most symptoms were comparable to those of controls at three weeks. Hypersomnia, disturbed sleep, hyperphagia, and excessive weight gain were not seen, nor was a severe crash observed. It is conceivable that the phases and fluctuations in craving previously reported were related to the effects of environmental stimuli.

Some of the inconsistencies in the findings and symptoms associated with cocaine cessation are probably attributable to differences in the dose and duration of use and to vulnerability factors. In interviews with almost 400 cocaine abusers, including about 100 who were not seeking treatment, some 83 percent reported tolerance to cocaine effects (needing more to get same effect) and 52 percent reported having undergone some type of withdrawal. Those seeking treatment were more likely to report experiencing withdrawal. Based on available data, there seems to be no convincing evidence that a protracted cocaine withdrawal syndrome follows the resolution of the signs and symptoms associated with abrupt cessation. However, abnormalities of brain function are reported to persist for at least 12 weeks.

Drug craving is often part of cocaine withdrawal but is not included among DSM-IV diagnostic criteria. While not commonly observed during recent clinical studies, severe depression, sometimes associated with suicidal ideation, has been reported in the older literature on cocaine withdrawal, and in occasional contemporary clinical reports. To what degree the more severe depressive features are a part of withdrawal or represent the emergence of primary mood disorder is unclear.

The DSM-IV diagnostic criteria for cocaine withdrawal are shown in Table 13.6-3. The criteria specify that the syndrome is one that follows the cessation (or reduction) of cocaine use that has been heavy and prolonged. It is also specified that the dysphoric mood and other symptoms (for example, fatigue and sleep disturbances) be of an intensity that causes significant distress or impairment. Thus, the criteria are structured so that the brief dysphoria and fatigue (crash) that follow a single short

TABLE 13.6-3
Diagnostic Criteria for Cocaine Withdrawal

A. Cessation of (or reduction in) cocaine use that has been heavy and prolonged.
B. Dysphoric mood and two (or more) of the following physiological changes, developing within a few hours to several days after criterion A:
 (1) fatigue
 (2) vivid, unpleasant dreams
 (3) insomnia or hypersomnia
 (4) increased appetite
 (5) psychomotor retardation or agitation
C. The symptoms in criterion B cause clinically significant distress or impairment in social, occupational, or other important areas of functioning.
D. The symptoms are not due to a general medical condition and are not better accounted for by another mental disorder.

binge by an occasional user do not lead to a diagnosis of withdrawal.

Animal models of withdrawal Although there is no easily observable animal model of cocaine withdrawal comparable to that of the syndromes seen with alcohol or opioid withdrawal, animal analogs of the postuse dysphoria and anhedonia often seen in humans have been proposed. In rats cocaine typically lowers the threshold for intracranial electrical self-stimulation. After 24 hours of cocaine self-administration, the thresholds for such self-stimulation are elevated above baseline for several days, which suggests a relative dopaminergic deficiency or insensitivity. The elevated threshold is reversed by bromocriptine (Parlodel), a drug with direct dopaminergic actions.

OTHER COCAINE-INDUCED DISORDERS Other psychiatric syndromes that may develop in the course of cocaine use include cocaine-induced mood disorder (see Section 16.6), cocaine-induced anxiety disorder (see Section 17.5), and cocaine-induced sleep disorder (see Chapter 23). With each of those disorders the clinician should specify whether the onset was during intoxication or during withdrawal. DSM-IV also describes cocaine-induced sexual dysfunction (see Section 21.1a) and a category of cocaine-related disorder not otherwise specified (Table 13.6-4).

Cocaine-induced mood disorder can occur during use or intoxication or during withdrawal. During use and intoxication the disorder is more likely to simulate a manic, hypomanic, or mixed episode; during withdrawal, it is more likely to involve a depressed mood. It is quite difficult to make such diagnoses during periods of active drug use or during the first week or two of withdrawal. Because sexual dysfunction, anxiety, and disturbed sleep are seen so commonly during the course of cocaine use and withdrawal, the diagnoses should be made only when the disturbances or dysfunctions are judged to be in excess of that usually associated with intoxication and withdrawal, and only when they are of sufficient severity to require independent treatment or attention. Panic episodes that develop during cocaine use may persist for many months following its cessation. It has been proposed that lasting vulnerability to panic attacks may be linked to sensitization phenomena.

COMORBIDITY The frequent co-occurrence of other psychiatric disorders and cocaine dependence was noted during the cocaine epidemic in the early part of the 20th century. The presence of other psychiatric disorders sharply increases the odds of substance dependence, and substance-dependent persons are more likely than the general population to meet the diagnostic criteria for additional psychiatric disorders.

Among cocaine users seeking treatment, the rates of additional current and lifetime diagnoses are regularly found to be elevated. In one study about 300 patients in New Haven, Connecticut, were interviewed using the Schedule for Affective Disorders and Schizophrenia (SADS); symptoms occurring within 10 days after the last drug use were not used in making any diagnoses. (Subjects were mostly of lower socioeconomic class, 69 percent were men, and the average age was 28.) The additional psychiatric diagnoses are shown in Table 13.6-5. Note that besides the often-reported high levels of mood disorder, the most common additional diagnosis was alcoholism. An equally striking finding was that depression preceded the onset of drug abuse in only about one third of patients, whereas alcoholism preceded the onset of drug abuse in only 21 percent. The prevalence of antisocial personality disorder was markedly influenced by the diagnostic criteria. (Using DSM-III-R the rate was about 33 percent.)

TABLE 13.6-4
Diagnostic Criteria for Cocaine-Related Disorder Not Otherwise Specified

The cocaine-related disorder not otherwise specified category is for disorders associated with the use of cocaine that are not classifiable as cocaine dependence, cocaine abuse, cocaine intoxication, cocaine withdrawal, cocaine intoxication delirium, cocaine-induced psychotic disorder, cocaine-induced mood disorder, cocaine-induced anxiety disorder, cocaine-induced sexual dysfunction, or cocaine-induced sleep disorder.

Table from DSM-IV, *Diagnostic and Statistical Manual of Mental Disorders*, ed 4. Copyright American Psychiatric Association, Washington, 1994. Used with permission.

TABLE 13.6-5
Additional Psychiatric Diagnoses Among Cocaine Users Seeking Treatment (New Haven Cocaine Diagnostic Study Results, Percent)

Psychiatric Diagnosis	Current Disorder	Lifetime Disorder
Major depression	4.7	30.5
Cyclothymia/hyperthymia	19.9	19.9
Mania	0.0	3.7
Hypomania	2.0	7.4
Panic disorder	0.3	1.7
Generalized anxiety disorder	3.7	7.0
Phobia	11.7	13.4
Schizophrenia	0.0	0.3
Schizoaffective disorder	0.3	1.0
Alcoholism	28.9	61.7
Antisocial personality disorder-RDC	7.7	7.7
Antisocial personality disorder-DSM-III	32.9	32.9
Attention-deficit disorder	—	34.9

Table adapted from B J Rounsaville, S F Anton, K Carroll, D Budde, B A Prusoff, F Gawin: Psychiatric diagnoses of treatment-seeking cocaine abusers. Arch Gen Psychiatry *48:* 43, 1991.

Some studies have found higher rates of depression and adverse consequences of drug use among cocaine users who seek treatment than among those who do not. Another study found that cocaine users not seeking treatment had a comparable severity of cocaine use, comparable rates of lifetime and current psychiatric disorders, and higher rates of polysubstance use and involvement with the legal system, but tended to minimize the adverse consequence of substance use and lacked pressure to seek treatment.

The prevalence of schizophrenia has generally been reported to be low among patients admitted to cocaine treatment programs, but that appears to be due largely to the exclusion of schizophrenics from such programs. In fact, patients with schizophrenia quite commonly use cocaine or amphetamine and develop both dependence and toxic syndromes. Although the diagnosis is not routinely made, estimates of cocaine abuse among schizophrenic persons range from 12 to 30 percent depending on the geographical area. It has been suggested that schizophrenic persons use cocaine and stimulants to alleviate negative symptoms, postpsychotic depressive disorder of schizophrenia, and the side effects of antipsychotics. A substantial proportion of schizophrenic patients admit to having used cocaine during the months before hospital admission, but many are less candid about recent drug use and urine tests frequently reveal recent cocaine use unsuspected by clinicians. Patients who are schizophrenic and using cocaine tend to be younger and more likely to be homeless and unemployed than are psychotic patients who are not abusing drugs. Special programs involving peer-based support groups seem effective in linking substance-using schizophrenic patients to outpatient treatment programs.

TOXICITY AND COMPLICATIONS High doses of cocaine can cause a wide variety of toxic effects, including cardiac arrhythmias, coronary artery spasms, myocardial infarction, and myocarditis. Other reported cardiovascular toxicities include headache, cerebrovascular disorder, and subarachnoid hemorrhage. Toxic effects on the CNS may include seizures, hyperpyrexia, respiratory depression, and death. There also may be fatal arrhythmias and myocardial damage. Rhabdomyolisis is not uncommon after large doses of cocaine and may contribute to renal complications, although vasoconstriction alone may be sufficient to account for renal damage. Sniffing cocaine can cause ulcers of the mucosa in the nose and perforation of the nasal septum as a result of persistent vasoconstriction. Inhaled cocaine freebase is thought to induce lung damage. Gastrointestinal necrosis, caused by vasoconstriction, has been associated with the rupture of swallowed condoms containing large amounts of cocaine. The peripheral actions of high doses of cocaine, especially when injected or smoked, can produce severe hypertension that can lead to cerebral hemorrhages. By producing placental vasoconstriction, cocaine may contribute to fetal anoxia. Table 13.6-6 lists further problems that have been linked to cocaine use.

Seizures and respiratory depression may be related to cocaine's actions as a local anesthetic, and although the cardiovascular complications are due primarily to its effects on the reuptake of catecholamines in the peripheral nervous system, local anesthetic effects may contribute to myocardial depression. Animal studies reveal significant genetically based vulnerability to various kinds of cocaine toxicities, suggesting that some of the observed toxicity in humans may not be predominantly dose dependent and predictable. Furthermore, at high doses cocaine elimination is nonlinear.

Cocaine use is frequently associated with increased sexual activity, and sometimes the exchange of sex for cocaine. Such behaviors put cocaine users at elevated risk for venereal diseases, including infection with the human immunodeficiency virus (HIV).

TABLE 13.6-6
Medical Complications of Cocaine Intoxication and Abuse

Cardiovascular
Hypertension
- Intracranial hemorrhage
- Aortic dissection, rupture

Arrhythmias
- Sinus tachycardia
- Supraventricular tachycardia
- Ventricular tachyarrhythmias

Organ ischemia
- Myocardial ischemia and infarction
- Renal infarction
- Intestinal infarction
- Limb ischemia

Myocarditis
Shock
Sudden death

Central nervous system
Headache
Seizures
Transient focal neurological deficits
Cerebrovascular disorder
- Subarachnoid hemorrhage
- Intracranial hemorrhage
- Cerebral infarction
- Embolic (endocarditis)

Toxic encephalopathy, coma
Neurological complications

Respiratory
Pneumomediastinum
Pneumothorax
Pulmonary edema
Respiratory arrest

Metabolic and other
Hyperthermia
Rhabdomyolysis (muscle breakdown)

Reproductive
Obstetrical
- Spontaneous abortion
- Placental abruption
- Placenta previa

Premature rupture of the membranes
Fetal
- Intrauterine growth retardation
- Congenital malformations

Neonatal
- Crack baby syndrome
- Cerebral infarction
- Delayed neurobehavioral development

*Infectious**
Acquired immune deficiency syndrome (AIDS)
Infectious endocarditis
Hepatitis B
Wound botulism
Tetanus

*Transmitted by contaminated needles or syringes.
Table adapted from N L Benowitz: How toxic is cocaine? In *Cocaine: Scientific and Social Dimensions,* Ciba Foundation Symposium 166, G R Bock, J Whelan, editors, p 125. Wiley, New York, 1992. Used with permission.

Treatment of toxicity The treatment of acute cardiac emergencies is aimed at blocking the sympathomimetic effects of the drug and correcting arrhythmias. Some clinicians have recommended using combined α-β-adrenergic receptor antagonist, or selective β_1-adrenergic receptor antagonists, such as labetalol (Normodyne, Normozide, Trandate). Some studies indicate that labetalol may not alleviate coronary vasoconstriction, although it does control hypertension. Also suggested for myocardial ischemia are calcium channel blockers and nitroglycerine. Grand mal seizures generally respond to diazepam (Valium). In animals μ-agonist opioids reduce cocaine lethality. The fatal hyperpyrexia seen with cocaine has some features in common with neuroleptic malignant syndrome and might respond to similar therapy (for example, dantrolene [Dantrium]).

PATHOLOGY AND LABORATORY EXAMINATIONS

Cocaine metabolites can be detected for varying lengths of time in urine. They can also be detected in blood, saliva, and hair. Blood and saliva provide a better index of current levels, whereas urine provides a longer window of opportunity for detecting use over the previous few days. Hair analysis can reveal drug use over weeks to months but has little applicability in clinical situations.

Most chronic cocaine abusers who are not also alcohol abusers show no evidence of structural damage when examined by computed tomography (CT) scans or magnetic resonance imaging (MRI). However, studies employing positron emission tomography (PET) or single photon emission computed tomography (SPECT) have revealed a variety of functional abnormalities in the brains of recently abstinent cocaine users. As compared with controls, heavy cocaine users showed perfusion defects in the cortex. Considerable improvement in cortical perfusion occurs after several weeks of abstinence, although blood flow in many instances still does not match that of normal controls. Decreased dopamine receptor availability in the basal ganglia appears to persist longer than cortical perfusion deficits. These latter deficits may be related to the vasoconstrictive effects of cocaine but are not necessarily correlated with decreased function, although cognitive deficits have been reported. Dopaminergic activation by cocaine results in a global decrease in cerebral glucose utilization. Cocaine users studied within one week of abrupt cocaine withdrawal had higher levels of cerebral glucose utilization as compared with controls, suggesting decreased dopaminergic activity. In a small sample of patients elevated glucose utilization was no longer significant at two to four weeks. Three to four months after detoxification dopamine type 2 (D_2) receptor availability in basal ganglia and glucose metabolism in areas of the frontal cortex appear to be lower than in controls, but the relationship of these findings to antecedent cocaine use is uncertain.

As compared with normal controls and with patients withdrawn from alcohol, patients withdrawn from cocaine exhibited persistent resting tremor and slower reaction times lasting at least 12 weeks. Compared with age-matched and education-matched controls, chronic cocaine users are more likely to score in the impaired range on a neuropsychological screening battery. Impairment seems most obvious in concentration and memory, with the degree of impairment less in those users who had been abstinent longer. To what extent the abnormalities in brain function are causally related to the signs and symptoms associated with cocaine cessation is uncertain.

A few early studies of cocaine addicts reported that almost all patients exhibited hyperprolactinemia lasting several weeks, a finding that seemed consistent with dopaminergic deficiency. However, several subsequent studies found either no evidence of hyperprolactinemia or a much lower incidence of that effect, and no apparent correlation between hyperprolactinemia and either cocaine craving or the extent of cocaine use.

DIFFERENTIAL DIAGNOSIS

The disorders associated with the use of cocaine need to be distinguished from both primary mental disorders and disorders induced by other classes of substances. A history of substance ingestion is important in making those distinctions. However, given the unreliability of self-reports about substance use and the likelihood that many users will deny any substance use at all, laboratory testing for drugs in body fluids and histories from collaterals are important. Disorders associated with cocaine use cannot be distinguished from those associated with amphetamines and related substances except by reliable history or laboratory tests. Users of cocaine (and amphetamine and related substances) may exhibit inappropriate optimism, euphoria, expansiveness, excessive talkativeness, and a decreased need for sleep sometimes associated with irritability in the context of a clear sensorium, a pattern that is also observed in manic and hypomanic episodes of bipolar disorder. However, those symptoms may not be obvious enough to suggest their relation to substance use and the first indication of substance dependence may be financial difficulties, an arrest for drug sale or possession, or substance-induced toxicity.

INTOXICATION Cocaine intoxication is diagnosed when the effects of cocaine exceed the mood-elevating effects its users typically seek. The diagnosis of intoxication would be appropriate when the effects are problematic enough to require differentiation from hypomanic or manic behavior.

Cocaine intoxication can also be confused with amphetamine intoxication and phencyclidine intoxication, although the last is usually associated with nystagmus, motor incoordination, and some cognitive impairment. Endocrine disorders (such as Cushing's disease) and excessive use of steroids should also be considered.

TOXIC PSYCHOSIS Cocaine-induced toxic psychosis can be exceedingly difficult to differentiate from schizophrenia or other psychotic disorders characterized by hallucinations or delusions. The presence of vivid visual or tactile hallucinations should raise suspicion of substance-induced disorder. In areas and populations where cocaine use is common it may be necessary to provide only a provisional diagnosis until the patient can be observed and substance test results are obtained. Even then there may be difficulties because in some urban areas a high percentage of persons with established diagnoses of schizophrenia are also users of cocaine.

COCAINE-INDUCED ANXIETY DISORDER Cocaine-induced anxiety disorder must also be distinguished from generalized anxiety disorder and panic disorder. Panic disorder that has its onset associated with the use of cocaine may persist well beyond the period of cocaine use.

OTHER SYMPTOMS The symptoms that may emerge during withdrawal—depression, dysphoria, anhedonia, disturbed sleep—need to be distinguished from those of primary mood disorders and primary sleep disorders. Unless the severity of the symptoms is more intense or they are more prolonged than is typical of cocaine withdrawal and so require independent treatment, the diagnosis should be limited to withdrawal, rather than cocaine-induced mood disorder. When a diagnosis of cocaine-induced mood disorder is made, it is important to specify whether the onset was during intoxication or withdrawal. It is also possible to specify the subtype of mood disorder (that is, with depressive, manic, or mixed features). In differentiating cocaine-induced mood disorder from the primary mood disorders the critical factor is the clinician's judgment that the mood disorder was caused by the cocaine. Generally, a cocaine-induced mood disorder, with onset during intoxication or withdrawal, remits in a week or two. It is appropriate, therefore, to withhold judgment about the diagnosis during the early phase of withdrawal. If depressed mood and related symptoms persist beyond a few weeks, alternative causes should be entertained. In reviewing diagnostic possibilities the clinician should consider the age at which symptoms began and a history of mood episodes that developed before the onset of cocaine use or during any long intervals when there was no significant drug abuse.

COURSE AND PROGNOSIS

Not all cocaine users develop cocaine-related disorders. However, cocaine toxicity can occur even among casual users. Among those who do develop some degree of dependence, the time from first use to problematic use ranges from a few months to six or more years. For many the course of cocaine use is marked by shifts from intranasal to intravenous use and inhalation of freebase forms. Some users claim that the reinforcing effects of freebase cocaine are such that they began daily use with the first dose. There are no long-term follow-up studies of cocaine dependence comparable to those for opioid dependence. Since most of those in the United States who tried cocaine did not become dependent, the decrease in cocaine use in the general population in the early 1990s, following the peak rates of self-reported use reached in the 1980s, does not shed much light on the natural history of cocaine dependence.

Chronic, heavy cocaine use does not appear to have decreased substantially over the same period. However, a number of short-term (six-month to two-year) follow-up studies seem to indicate that the course of dependence is more favorable for persons using cocaine who seek treatment than it is for heroin addicts who seek treatment. For example, 26 percent of a sample of 300 male cocaine addicts initially admitted to a Veterans Affairs hospital in California when interviewed a year later reported abstinence from cocaine for the entire year, although 70 percent had had at least one subsequent episode of use. At a two-year interview of a sample of the same group of patients, 77 percent claimed to have been abstinent during the month before the interview. Among veterans on the East Coast randomly assigned to either an inpatient program or a day-hospital program lasting 28 days, 60 percent reported abstinence at four months, which was largely maintained at seven months. About 56 percent of urine specimens were negative for each group at seven months. In a one-year follow-up of almost 300 cocaine users, half treated as outpatients and half treated initially as inpatients, both groups showed reductions in self-reported cocaine use during the 30 days before the interview: from an average 17 days per month at admission to 1.1 days for inpatients; from 10 days per month to 5 days for outpatients. Although the data do not give the percentage of those who were entirely abstinent, the improvement levels were substantial and were different from those typically found among heroin-dependent patients seeking treatment. The prognosis appears to be even better for persons with social support.

In a 12-month to 20-month (average 15.2 months) follow-up of 214 predominantly white, male, employed cocaine-dependent patients treated in several proprietary hospitals with chemical or faradic aversion therapy, 156 were subsequently interviewed or their relapse records at the hospitals were reviewed. Total abstinence was reported to be 53 percent at one year; self-reported current abstinence for the past six-months was 69 percent. The percent abstinence rates for those who used only cocaine were slightly lower, whereas the abstinence rates for patients treated for both alcohol and cocaine dependence were slightly higher. Those who used cocaine intravenously or used freebase did less well than did those who snorted the cocaine. Those findings are similar to follow-up reports on predominantly white, employed men treated by psychological means in a private program.

In a six-month follow-up study by independent evaluators, alcohol and cocaine users (employed, mostly men, and predominantly African-American) referred by employee assistance programs (EAPs) to two outpatient treatment programs showed substantial improvement: 59 percent were completely abstinent and 82 percent were working. However, the prognosis has not always been so benign. A 6-month to 12-month follow-up study of a group of patients (predominantly urban, African-American, male, blue-collar workers) randomly assigned to three types of outpatient psychotherapy found that only 19 percent were not using cocaine at follow-up. There were no differences across therapies, and the investigators said they believed that 19 percent probably reflected the spontaneous recovery rate.

Treatment of cocaine dependence may have various outcomes, including, at the extremes, complete relapse to cocaine dependence or total abstinence from cocaine and related drugs for a prolonged period—more than 12 months (sustained full remission). However, there may also be sustained partial remissions in which, after at least one month when no criteria of dependence have been present, one or more criteria of abuse or dependence are again met, but over the course of 12 months fewer cocaine-dependence criteria have been met than the three required for full relapse. There are also situations in which those patterns are observed but the period of observation is not a full year (early full remission and early partial remission). Any of the patterns of remission may be observed while the person is in a controlled environment, and that fact should be specified.

DSM-IV criteria for both abuse and dependence describe maladaptive use associated with distress or impairment. Technically, it is possible for a person to be in sustained full remission from cocaine dependence despite occasional use, provided the drug use causes no problems or distress and does not escalate. How often such a return to occasional nonproblematic use takes place is unknown.

COCAINE AND CRIME Although the typical interactive relationship between opiate and opioid use and crime generally holds true for cocaine users, there also seem to be some significant differences. As with opioids, there is considerable heterogeneity among cocaine users. Not all who use or become dependent on cocaine engage in crime, although for some meeting the costs of their drug use may create financial distress. As it is for opioids, a history of delinquency or antisocial behavior is often an antecedent to cocaine use. In some cases, however, persons with no previous criminal behavior generate illegal income to buy cocaine by engaging in a variety of activities, ranging from fraud and white-collar crime to drug selling, prostitution, and predatory crime. In a nationwide sample of adolescents 40 percent of serious crimes committed by the entire sample were committed by the 1.3 percent who reported using cocaine. Among persons seeking treatment for substance abuse, cocaine use is correlated with income-generating crime. In the late 1980s, when cocaine use declined in the general population in the United States, among those arrested for a variety of serious offenses it rose or merely stabilized.

Cocaine can induce states of paranoia and aggressive behavior, which is a common reason why cocaine users are brought to emergency rooms. However, pharmacologically induced aggression is not the major reason why cocaine and crime and, more specifically, cocaine and violence are linked. Among those arrested for violent crime, the primary predictors of such crime are past arrests for violent crime, poor education, and poor intellectual ability. Past arrest for violence is also associated with antisocial personality disorder. Studies of violent predatory offenders indicate that most had histories of heavy involvement with multiple substance use and with serious crime as juveniles. Among predatory offenders high-frequency substance users were likely to use many substances, particularly heroin and cocaine, and to engage in a variety of crimes, including violent crimes, at high rates. Cocaine also has a nonpharmacologically based link to violent crime, in that in many urban areas drug dealers who may not themselves use cocaine routinely resort to violence to protect or expand their customer base.

One conceptual framework for thinking about the links between substance use and violence involves three major causal categories: psychopharmacological effects (effects of the substances), economic compulsion (violent crimes committed to obtain money for drugs), and systemic violence (associated with the business methods and life-style of drug dealers).

TREATMENT

SELECTION OF TREATMENT SETTING The general principles of treatment for cocaine dependence are not very different from those for opioid dependence, but there are fewer replicated studies on the efficacy of any particular treatment approach. As is the case with opioid dependence, cocaine dependence that is severe enough to require formal treatment is often associated with other psychiatric diagnoses.

Patient heterogeneity requires thoughtful selection among available alternatives. Not all cocaine users require extensive treatment; some users who are not dependent respond to external pressures, as when employers insist on carefully monitoring substance use. The executive with little history of psychopathology, a supportive social network, economic assets, and personal skills has a better prognosis and a wider range of options than does a patient who is unemployed, alienated from his or her family, and also may be using opioids. Whereas some clinicians favor routine hospitalization for initial detoxification in order to break the cycle of use, some equally experienced clinicians find that many patients do well with entirely outpatient treatment. In a study of working-class veterans seeking treatment for alcohol and cocaine dependence, patients were randomly assigned to either a 28-day inpatient program or a day-hospital program. A somewhat higher proportion of inpatients completed the 28-day program, but at a four-month follow-up there was little difference between the groups in terms of cocaine use or other indexes of social function.

Severe depression, psychotic manifestations beyond the initial withdrawal period, and substance use that is completely out of control (that is, repeated failure to respond to outpatient efforts) seem to be the major accepted criteria for hospitalization. A retrospective study of about 300 patients admitted to inpatient and outpatient treatment programs found that those admitted initially to inpatient treatment had more severe cocaine problems than those admitted to outpatient treatment, suggesting that clinicians were using severity as an important consideration in the decision to hospitalize a patient. The range, intensity, and specificity of treatments offered are not closely correlated with the treatment setting. Some day-hospital and outpatient settings may provide more of certain kinds of services than do many inpatient settings. That is an important point because the intensity and specificity of services for particular problems (that is, medical, psychiatric, and vocational) are now believed to be an important determinant of outcome in the specific areas.

A substantial percentage of cocaine dependent patients are referred by the criminal justice system, many to therapeutic communities (TCs), which seem to be able to alter long-term behavioral patterns, even in persons with histories of antisocial personality disorder and persistent antisocial behavior. Some work indicates that primary cocaine users and crack users (even those not under legal pressure) are as likely to stay in treatment as are those who are primary users of other drugs.

DETOXIFICATION The cocaine withdrawal syndrome is distinct from that of opioid, alcohol or sedative, hypnotic, or anxiolytic dependence. Fatigue, dysphoria, disturbed sleep, and some craving typically are present, but there are no physiological disturbances that would necessitate inpatient or residential withdrawal. Some patients may experience depression; others may simply be unable to stop without help in limiting access to the substance. Thus it is generally possible to engage in a therapeutic trial of outpatient withdrawal before deciding whether a more intensive or controlled setting is required. There are no agents that reliably reduce the intensity of withdrawal, but recovery over a week or two is generally uneventful. It may take longer, however, for sleep, mood, and cognitive function to recover fully.

TREATMENT METHODS Both psychological and pharmacological approaches to the treatment of cocaine dependence have been used in reducing cocaine use and postdetoxification relapse. A generally held consensus is that no use at all of cocaine (total and permanent abstinence) must be the goal of treatment for those who have developed symptoms of dependence; any use is viewed as a prodrome to relapsing into dependence. However, such a perspective may underestimate the benefits that accrue from treatment that results in a substantial and prolonged reduction in drug use but falls short of total abstinence.

Psychotherapy and behavior modification Psychological treatment approaches have used cognitive-behavioral, psychodynamic, and general supportive techniques. One cognitive-behavioral method uses contingency contracting in which there is agreement in advance that, for some finite period (for example, three months), if the patient relapses to cocaine use (as measured by supervised urine testing), the therapist will initiate actions that will have serious adverse consequences for the patient, such as informing an employer or a professional credentials board. In one such study 48 percent of potential patients accepted such a contractual arrangement and 80 percent of those patients successfully abstained from cocaine during the period covered by the contract; many of the successful patients relapsed when the contract expired. Although the technique is not widely used by individual therapists, the general principle of linking drug use and aversive contingencies is central to many employment-based programs or criminal justice programs that use drug (urine) testing. There are no adequate studies comparing such adverse contingency contracts with alternatives. In contrast, there have been studies comparing relapse prevention and contingency contracting using positive rewards with the 12-step type of program for ambulatory cocaine users. For example, a group of predominantly white-collar, mostly caucasian, cocaine abusers were randomly assigned to experienced therapists utilizing 12-step principles or to therapists using behavioral approaches emphasizing contingency management, community reinforcement, and positive reinforcement (for example, vouchers that could be used to purchase goods) for urines negative for cocaine. Retention rates were higher and cocaine use was significantly lower with contingency management and positive rewards. The same researchers found that positive reinforcement was more effective in terms of retention and abstinence than were otherwise identical behavioral treatment methods without positive reinforcement.

Another research group randomly assigned cocaine users (typically white men with more than 12 years of education) to relapse prevention or to 12-step treatment using group techniques. Relapse prevention involved identification of high-risk situations and ways of dealing with negative emotions but did not offer positive material reinforcement of negative urines (such as vouchers or lottery tickets). Also, the 12-step treatment group was not Alcoholics Anonymous (AA) or Narcotics Anonymous (NA), but was led by a man and woman cotherapy team using three of the first 12 steps. There were no differences between groups at six-month follow-up or at end of treatment regarding retention in treatment or reduction in cocaine use. Although initially more in the 12-step group were abstinent from alcohol, that effect did not persist to the six-month follow-up point. In one study relapse prevention was substantially more effective than interpersonal therapy in helping more severely cocaine-dependent ambulatory patients achieve several weeks of complete abstinence.

In another study relapse prevention using cognitive-behavioral coping skills training was compared with clinical management in the context of a pharmacotherapy trial of desipramine (Norpramin) versus placebo. In that case clinical management was intended to foster a supportive doctor-patient relationship, retention in the protocol, and compliance with medication. In contrast to the other two studies, there were more women (27 percent), more minorities (54 percent), fewer high school graduates (24 percent), and fewer patients who were gainfully employed (53 percent). About 40 percent of patients completed the proposed 12-week protocol (mean of 7.2 weekly sessions). Overall, about 70 percent of patients improved, but it did not appear that cognitive-behavioral treatment was better than clinical management. Although there was a trend for more patients receiving relapse prevention or desipramine to complete treatment, the differences were not significant. Relapse prevention appeared to be more helpful with those with more severe cocaine dependence. Desipramine seemed useful primarily for those with less severe dependence and only early in the course of treatment. There were no differences between drug and placebo at 12 weeks.

Supportive therapy In its specific methods supportive therapy overlaps the techniques used by behaviorists. Patients are helped to separate themselves from friends and situations where cocaine is available and which increase drug craving. They are urged to abstain from other substances, such as alcohol and cannabis, because those substances have been reported to increase cocaine craving and the probability of relapse. Patients are also helped in repairing those areas of their lives that once provided satisfaction and may have been damaged by the behaviors associated with cocaine use. In addition, patients may be encouraged to participate in Cocaine Anonymous (CA), AA, or NA as a means of gaining control over other substance use.

Psychodynamic, interpersonal, and combined approaches Psychodynamically oriented clinicians emphasize the patient's unconscious motives for using cocaine (for example, to relieve an inner sense of emptiness or depression). However, experienced clinicians with a wide range of skills believe that a combination of psychological approaches, with the emphasis tailored to the circumstances of the individual patient, is more effective than treatments that emphasize the principles of only one approach.

In treating opioid dependence, combining psychological techniques with newer psychopharmacological treatments seems to be more effective than using only psychological approaches, and it is reasonable to assume that that will also eventually be true for treating dependence on cocaine. For the present, pharmacological treatments cannot be shown to produce robust decreases in cocaine use.

Group psychotherapy techniques At least two distinct approaches to group psychotherapy with cocaine users have been described. Interpersonal group therapy focuses on relationships and uses the group interactions to illustrate the interpersonal causes of individual distress and to offer alternative behaviors. Modified dynamic group therapy is described as emphasizing character, as it manifests itself individually and intrapsychically, and in the context of interpersonal relationships with a focus on affect, self-esteem, and self-care. Both approaches share the view that the group should serve as an interpersonal anchor that leads first to more stable emotional status and enables members to face unresolved life issues. Both approaches recognize the vulnerability of the patients to narcissistic injury and the need for a supportive, empathetic environment. Some psychotherapists emphasize that the focus in the early months of treatment must be exclusively on the disease and on achieving sobriety and recovery, but modified dynamic group therapy asserts that, even early in the process, those goals are not incompatible with attention to characterological problems. An underlying assumption of dynamic group psychotherapy is that substances are used as self-medication, and that the persons most likely to use cocaine include those whose depression, anergia, or boredom is alleviated by it. However, those who place an exaggerated value on assertiveness and self-sufficiency may also find cocaine alluring. Since patients are often required to be abstinent for at least two weeks before participating in group therapy, the technique may be more accurately described as relapse prevention than as a treatment able to induce initial cessation.

Intensive and eclectic treatment The most effective approaches used by private practitioners are best described as intensive and eclectic. The goals of treatment and the techniques shift over time. According to Arnold Washington and Nanette Stone-Washton, the focus of the initial work should be to forge an alliance with the patient and to increase the motivation to achieve abstinence. That may involve several group and individual sessions per week, with the content focused on interrupting the substance-use cycle and on developing detailed plans for avoiding exposure to the substances and high-risk situations. Urine samples should be taken twice weekly so that patients know that they are accountable for their actions. Sometimes patients need a helper to accompany them to meetings and to avoid temptation and to find and dispose of hidden caches of cocaine and drug paraphernalia.

It is not necessary to argue over whether the patient is or is not an addict. Accepting that identity is not a requirement for achieving abstinence from cocaine, and arguing over the issue may drive a patient from treatment. What is critical at both early and later stages is the therapeutic alliance around shared goals and instilling hope, trust, and confidence. Doing so may foster the engagement of even resistant patients. Clinicians who are cognizant of the stages of change will recognize that patients are not always ready to accept program goals. Some may not be ready to give up cocaine entirely. Clinicians need to be able to work with such patients despite their own doubts that they may be enabling substance-using behavior. Change can occur only if the patient stays engaged; hence, the importance of the alliance. The objective is to keep the patient moving in the right direction. Urine testing, which should be supervised to prevent falsification, is designed to be an objective measure of progress, not a device to catch the patient in lies.

Once abstinence has been achieved, the goals of treatment shift to relapse prevention. Slips (occasional use of cocaine), especially during the first 60 days of treatment, are not uncommon and should be used as learning experiences with the focus on how to prevent reoccurrence. In the later stages of treatment a balance must be struck between enabling (tolerating continued use) and being so rigid about use that the patient is extruded from treatment. Sometimes a temporary suspension from the group with continued individual sessions is a useful therapeutic maneuver. Generally, the longer the retention in treatment, the better will be the long-term outcome.

Cocaine use is often linked to compulsive sexual activity. Patients may be ashamed of that linkage, and some practitioners believe that it is important to ask what kinds of sexual behaviors and fantasies are associated with being high on cocaine, since sexual feelings can trigger a craving for cocaine. It is usually not possible to deal with compulsive sexual behavior until cocaine abstinence has been accomplished. It may be appropriate to ask some patients to refrain from sex for the first weeks of treatment. The gap in the patient's life once occupied by cocaine, and subsequently by treatment, should be filled to minimize the likelihood of relapse. Self-help groups can fill the void, but there are other drug-free alternatives.

Pharmacological adjuncts There are currently no pharmacological treatments that produce decreases in cocaine use comparable to those observed when heroin users are treated with methadone (Dolophine, Methadose), levo-α-acetlymethadol (LAAM) [Orlaam]), or buprenorphine (Buprenex). However, a variety of pharmacological agents approved for other uses are being tested clinically for the treatment of cocaine dependence and relapse. Those clinical trials are based on several premises about the etiology of the disorder. Despite the absence of solid evidence of efficacy, some of the agents are being used routinely by clinicians, even though their use for such purposes has not been approved by the Food and Drug Administration (FDA). The most common premises on which pharmacological interventions are based are as follows: (1) chronic cocaine use alters dopaminergic systems, so that discontinuation is associated with a hypodopaminergic state characterized by dysphoria or anhedonia; (2) some cocaine users are using it to ameliorate a preexisting psychiatric disorder, such as major depressive disorder, dysthymic disorder, an attention-deficit disorder, or cyclothymic disorder; and (3) cocaine produces a sensitization or kindling effect that somehow predisposes to continued use.

Cocaine users presumed to have preexisting attention-deficit or mood disorders have been treated with methylphenidate (Ritalin) and lithium (Eskalith), respectively. Those agents are of little or no benefit in patients without the disorders and clinicians are urged to adhere strictly to maximal diagnostic criteria before using either of them in the treatment of cocaine dependence.

Many agents have been explored on the premise that chronic cocaine use alters the function of multiple neurotransmitter systems, especially the dopaminergic and serotonergic transmitters regulating hedonic tone, and that cocaine induces a state of relative dopaminergic deficiency. Although the evidence for such alterations in dopaminergic function has been growing, it has been difficult to demonstrate that agents theoretically capable of modifying dopamine function can alter the course of treatment.

In the early 1980s single-blind trials or nonblind trials of neurotransmitter precursors (for example, tyrosine); dopaminergic agonists (bromocriptine); various antidepressants (desipramine, imipramine [Tofranil], trazodone [Desyrel]); and antiparkinson drugs that may also affect the dopaminergic system (for example, amantadine [Symmetrel]) stimulated more controlled clinical studies, as well as laboratory studies aimed at understanding potential therapeutic and toxic interactions. Those more carefully, controlled clinical trials have forced a more restrained assessment of what can be achieved with adjunctive pharmacological treatment. In general, there is little consistent evidence that any available agent produces practical improvement in the course of inpatient or residential withdrawal. The following material derives primarily from outpatient studies where the goals were to facilitate and help sustain cessation of cocaine use.

DESIPRAMINE Desipramine has been studied in several uncontrolled and several random assignment single-blind and double-blind studies. Despite positive results in one double-blind study, there is no consensus that any difference in outcome produced by desipramine is either robust or reliable enough to justify using it routinely. In a recent double-blind study desipramine seemed to be transiently useful, based on self-report of amount of cocaine used, for patients with less severe levels of dependence. Relapse rates for patients discharged from a four-week, inpatient cocaine-treatment program were not improved by desipramine. In volunteers pretreatment with desipramine (150 mg a day) did not alter the high produced by intravenous cocaine; however, the duration of cocaine craving induced by the intravenous infusion was shortened.

BROMOCRIPTINE Bromocriptine has been used in both ambulatory and hospitalized cocaine users. There are reports that this agent, a direct dopamine receptor agonist, alleviates symptoms of withdrawal and craving. Bromocriptine attenuates decreased brain activity of mesolimbic structures (as measured by glucose utilization) in rats acutely withdrawn after repeated doses of cocaine, and the elevated threshold for intracranial self-stimulation can be normalized. However, as judged by clinical measures of efficacy, such as prevention of relapse after initial abstinence or the proportion of outpatients who reduce cocaine use or remain abstinent for more than a brief period, the evidence is not persuasive. Pretreatment with bromocriptine neither antagonizes nor increases the physiological or subjective effects of cocaine, although in one study it appeared to attenuate the increased craving that briefly follows an intravenous cocaine challenge.

AMANTADINE Amantadine has been tested in cocaine-dependent patients in both open and double-blind outpatient trials. It was expected that it would alleviate cocaine withdrawal by increasing release of dopamine, thereby facilitating cessation of cocaine use. In a double-blind trial reductions in the percentage of urines found positive for cocaine have been greater with amantadine (100 mg twice a day) over the first few weeks than with placebo. Those positive findings have not always been replicated in larger controlled studies.

MAZINDOL In theory mazindol (Mazanor, Sanorex), which binds to a dopamine uptake site, ought to increase synaptic dopamine. Although studies show that animals will self-administer mazindol, humans do not necessarily experience euphoria from high doses. Mazindol did not appear to alter cocaine-induced craving, the subjective effects of cocaine, or cocaine use in a double-blind trial with ambulatory cocaine abusers. The combination of mazindol and cocaine produces larger and more sustained increases in heart rate and blood pressure than does cocaine alone.

FLUPENTHIXOL DECANOATE A long-acting depot preparation of flupenthixol, flupenthixol decanoate was given in an open trial to crack users, who reported a sharp decrease in craving that lasted for several weeks at low doses. The study used no controls.

SEROTONIN-SPECIFIC REUPTAKE INHIBITORS AND AGONISTS Serotonin-specific reuptake inhibitors and agonists have been tried as adjuncts to smoking cessation and cocaine treatment programs. One double-blind study of fluoxetine (Prozac) in ambulatory cocaine users found no differences in cocaine use or retention in treatment between drug and placebo groups. Another controlled trial using similar doses found decreases in cocaine use. However, fluoxetine does attenuate some pleasurable subjective effects of cocaine.

DOPAMINE RECEPTOR ANTAGONISTS Clinical trials are still needed to determine whether the dopamine receptor antagonists will affect the self-administration of cocaine, and if (as appears to be the case with naltrexone [Trexan]) their subtle dysphoric effects will reduce treatment compliance. The agents appear to reduce cocaine's reinforcing effects in animal studies.

CALCIUM CHANNEL INHIBITORS The calcium channel inhibitors appear to diminish some of the subjective and reinforcing effects of cocaine, including the sensation of a rush. In rats trained to self-administer cocaine, pretreatment with nefedipine (Procardia) or nimodipine (Nimotop) consistently increased self-administration, which suggests that the drugs block the reinforcing effects of cocaine to some degree. In human volunteers nimodipine, by increasing α activity and decreasing β activity, normalizes the abnormal EEG patterns seen during cocaine withdrawal. The implications of the findings need further exploration in outpatient studies.

CARBAMAZEPINE Carbamazepine (Tegretol) has been tested in users of cocaine and crack cocaine on the theory that cocaine craving is linked to cocaine-induced kindling. In an open trial patients who were most compliant experienced a significant decrease in cocaine use and craving. However, other studies have shown that compliance itself is usually a powerful predictor of positive outcome for substance-dependent patients, and carbamazepine was not shown to produce significant benefits in a double-blind trial.

BUPRENORPHINE In monkeys trained to self-administer cocaine buprenorphine has been shown to reduce their lever-pressing activity to get cocaine but not to get food. The clinical implications of the study are not clear, since two double-blind outpatient comparisons of buprenorphine and methadone failed to confirm that buprenorphine reduces cocaine use among heroin users who also abuse cocaine.

Acupuncture Auricular acupuncture as a treatment for cocaine and other varieties of dependence behavior has become popular among some groups, including recently organized drug courts and prison-based programs, and has received some support from members of the United States Congress. It has been used as part of the procedure for ambulatory crack withdrawal, and it has also been used in jails during the 30 days before release. Controlled studies of its efficacy for treating cocaine dependence (using sham acupuncture) have been conducted, but are subject to varying interpretations; large differences in cocaine use, as measured by urine tests, have not been shown. In one program treatment is offered in a drop-in outpatient setting; clients are instructed to stay as clean and sober as they can and to come in daily for treatment. Clinic rules are minimal; clients may even prepare their own ears for treatment and remove the needles at the completion of the 45-minute treatment, which usually takes place in groups with patients sitting in comfortable chairs. Dropout rates are generally high. Herbal teas are often consumed as part of the treatment. In a prison setting an acupuncturist can treat about 35 inmates an hour. In one controlled study of acupuncture in the treatment of alcoholic persons, relapse rates were higher among those who were given sham acupuncture (needled at nontherapeutic points), but in another study those results could not be replicated.

Also used for treatment of cocaine dependence are several forms of transcranial electrical stimulation (neuroelectric therapy [NET]). A comparison of NET with sham NET revealed no differences in successful detoxification over a 12-day period of hospitalization. One rationale for both acupuncture and transcranial stimulation is that such stimuli cause the release of endogenous opioids. However, researchers have pointed out that only acupuncture that also employs electrical stimulation has been shown to release endogenous opioids.

SPECIAL POPULATIONS

Patients maintained on methadone Both behavioral techniques and pharmacological agents have been used to reduce cocaine use by patients maintained on methadone. Some methadone programs respond to a patient's cocaine use (measured by urine tests) with progressive sanctions, such as decreased take-home privileges, a decreased methadone dose, and finally, in some cases, discharge from the program. However, in one comparison study, decreasing the methadone dose proved to be far less effective than giving small (5 mg) increases, up to 120 mg a day in some cases, for each cocaine-positive urine. However, at another clinic an analysis of the relation between cocaine use and methadone dose did not find less cocaine use among patients maintained on higher doses of methadone.

Other pharmacological agents that have been tried on methadone patients include bromocriptine, amantadine, desipramine, buproprion (Wellbutrin), carbamazepine, and buprenorphine. In a controlled comparison of amantadine, desipramine, and placebo, self-reports of cocaine abuse were lower for both medication groups at four weeks, but there were no significant differences in cocaine-positive urines; there were no significant group differences at 8 weeks or at 12 weeks. Such findings seem consistent with negative findings of a placebo-controlled study of desipramine in methadone-maintained veterans who were also abusing cocaine, and of studies of cocaine-dependent outpatients not maintained on methadone and treated with desipramine or amantadine.

Buprenorphine has also been studied in cocaine abusers who were dependent on opioids as well. In two double-blind controlled studies comparing buprenorphine and methadone (one of which was not specifically designed to test effects on cocaine use), there were no differences in cocaine use, although buprenorphine and methadone both produced significant decreases in heroin use. In animals buprenorphine appears to antagonize some lethal effects of cocaine and to increase cocaine's reinforcing effects. In humans the combination augments the euphoric effects of cocaine and the effects are reported to be somewhat analogous to the speedball effect seen when heroin and cocaine are combined.

There have been no controlled studies that have shown any specific effect of carbamazepine on cocaine use. Carbamazepine stimulates the metabolism of methadone.

Although buproprion reduced cocaine use among methadone-maintained outpatients in an open pilot trial, in a double-blind inpatient study there was no difference between buproprion and placebo with regard to cocaine craving or depression scores.

In summary, no pharmacological agent has been shown to have reliably robust effects on cocaine use among patients maintained on methadone.

Women, pregnant women, and their children Women who are dependent on cocaine have a number of special needs, especially with respect to their physical health. There are some data suggesting that although women who seek treatment have more severe dependence, they respond as well to treatment as do men. Cocaine use by pregnant women represents a hazard to the fetus. In some urban hospitals 10 to 45 percent of women provided with obstetrical care report cocaine use at some time during the pregnancy. There is some controversy about the frequency and permanence of any damage sustained by the fetus, but there is little question that maternal cocaine use can be associated with some perinatal morbidity and mortality. It is exceedingly difficult to separate cocaine effects from the effects of other substances and of maternal behavior, but it may be that some of the toxicity is due to cocaine-induced hypertension, tachycardia, and vasoconstriction, which lead to impaired placental blood flow and decreased transfer of nutrients and oxygen to the fetus. Some toxicity also results from cocaine's effects on the fetus.

Depending on the severity of the placental and fetal effects and when they occur during gestation, the result may be teratogenic, with destruction of developing tissues or overall retardation of fetal growth. Commonly reported abnormalities in fetuses exposed to cocaine are microcephaly and structural abnormalities in brain and urinary tract development. Ischemic and hemorrhagic lesions in the newborn brain have also been reported. Premature birth, placenta previa, and abruptio placenta are complications of pregnancy that are more common among women who use cocaine than among nonusers; low-birth-weight babies also are common.

Despite the risks, only a minority of infants born to such women exhibit what might be called a neonatal cocaine exposure syndrome, which consists of poor feeding, irritability, tremor, and abnormal sleep patterns. Those abnormalities are most evident on the second day after birth and last for less than a week or two. There are reports that sudden infant death syndrome (SIDS) is more common among infants exposed to cocaine, but controls needed for a clear conclusion are lacking. The long-term neurological, cognitive, and developmental consequences of intrauterine cocaine exposure are still not clear, but after the first few months, most such children appear to be developmentally within normal limits. Unlike opioids, there appears to be no contraindication to abrupt discontinuation of cocaine during pregnancy and prompt abstinence from cocaine should be the goal of treatment.

Patients with other severe psychiatric disorders Cocaine-dependent persons with mood disorders and anxiety disorders are generally managed in programs that focus on the substance-use problem. However, several clinical reports indicate that cocaine users with bipolar disorders generally are not compliant with prescribed lithium.

Patients with a history of an attention-deficit disorder are also likely to have antisocial personality disorder and tend to do poorly in treatment. Clinical trials using methylphenidate (Ritalin), on the assumption that the cocaine use was an attempt to self-medicate an attention-deficit disorder, have led to the caution that in most cases the demand for methylphenidate escalates and it stimulates a craving for cocaine.

Persons with schizophrenia and other psychotic disorders who use cocaine have been managed within either primary drug or psychiatric facilities. In all settings the concurrent use of alcohol further complicates treatment. Although the use of cocaine, amphetamines, and cannabis exacerbates schizophreniform disorder, such use is not an uncommon problem. It has been postulated that some cocaine (or stimulant) use represents an attempt to alleviate negative symptoms, depression, or the side effects of antipsychotic agents. The last problem might be dealt with by using newer antipsychotic agents that have fewer extrapyramidal side effects.

In an open trial cocaine-abusing schizophrenic patients were treated with desipramine (100 to 150 mg a day) in addition to antipsychotic drugs. Compared with patients given only antipsychotic agents, those given desipramine had fewer symptoms, were more likely to stay in treatment, and were less likely to have cocaine-positive urines.

Some clinicians report that with intensive case management that provide the patient with access to social services, schizophrenic patients who abuse cocaine can be treated with non-substance-abusing patients in a day-hospital setting. However, abstinence as a qualification for admission or retention may be unrealistic for such patients, and some of the traditional rules concerning substance abuse and poor attendance may need to be relaxed.

SUGGESTED CROSS-REFERENCES

The neural sciences are presented in Chapter 1 and neuropsychiatry and behavioral neurology in Chapter 2. A classification of mental disorders appears in Chapter 11. The introduction and overview of substance-related disorders are presented in Section 13.1, amphetamine-related disorders in Section 13.3, and various drugs in Chapter 32 on biological therapies, particularly sympathomimetics in Section 32.20. Schizophrenia is discussed in Chapter 14 and other psychotic disorders in Chapter 15. Animal research and its relevance to psychiatry is discussed in Section 5.2. Cognitive-behavioral therapy is discussed in Section 31.6.

REFERENCES

Alterman A I, McLellan A T: Inpatient and day hospital treatment services for cocaine and alcohol dependence. J Substance Abuse Treatment *10:* 269, 1993.

Arndt I O, Dorozynsky L, Woody G E, McLellan A T, O'Brien C P: Desipramine treatment of cocaine dependence in methadone-maintained patients. Arch Gen Psychiatry *49:* 888, 1992.

Benowitz N L: How toxic is cocaine? In *Cocaine: Scientific and Social Dimensions,* Ciba Foundation Symposium 166, G R Bock, J Whelan, editors, p 125. Wiley, New York, 1992.

Berry J, van Gorp W G, Herzberg D C, Hinkin C, Boone K, Steinman L, Wilkins J H: Neuropsychological deficits in abstinent cocaine abusers: Preliminary findings after two weeks of abstinence. Drug Alcohol Depend *32:* 231, 1993.

Budde D, Rounsaville B, Bryant K: Inpatient and outpatient cocaine abusers: Clinical comparisons at intake and one-year follow-up. J Substance Abuse Treatment 9: 337, 1992.

Carroll K M, Rounsaville B J: Contrast of treatment-seeking and untreated cocaine abusers. Arch Gen Psychiatry *49:* 464, 1992.
*Carroll K M, Rounsaville B J, Gordon L T, Nich C, Jatlow P, Bisighini R M, Gawin F H: Psychotherapy and pharmacotherapy for ambulatory cocaine abusers. Arch Gen Psychiatry *51:* 177, 1994.
Frawley P J, Smith J W: One year follow-up after multimodal inpatient treatment for cocaine and methamphetamine dependencies. J Substance Abuse Treatment *9:* 271, 1992.
Gastfriend D R, Mendelson J H, Mello N K, Teoh S K, Reif S: Buprenorphine pharmacotherapy for concurrent heroin and cocaine dependence. Am J Addictions *2:* 269, 1993.
*Gawin F H, Ellinwood E H: Cocaine and other stimulants. N Engl J Med *318:* 1173, 1988.
Gawin F H, Kleber H D: Abstinence symptomatology and psychiatric diagnosis in cocaine abusers: Clinical observations. Arch Gen Psychiatry *43:* 107, 1986.
Higgins S T, Budney A J, Bickel W K, Foerg F, Donham R, Badger G J: Incentives improve outcome in outpatient behavioral treatment of cocaine dependence. Arch Gen Psychiatry *51:* 568, 1994.
Higgins S T, Budney A J, Bickel W K, Hughes J R, Foerg F, Badger G: Achieving cocaine abstinence with a behavioral approach. Am J Psychiatry *150:* 763, 1993.
Holman B L, Mendelson J, Garada B, Teoh S K, Hallgring E, Johnson K A, Mello N K: Regional cerebral blood flow improves with treatment in chronic cocaine polydrug users. J Nucl Med *34:* 723, 1993.
*Jaffe J H: Drug addiction and drug abuse. In *Goodman and Gilman's The Pharmacological Basis of Therapeutics,* ed 8, A G Gilman, T W Rall, A S Nies, P Taylor, editors, p 522. Pergamon, New York, 1990.
Jaffe J H, Cascella N G, Kumor K M, Sherer M A: Cocaine-induced cocaine craving. Psychopharmacology *97:* 59, 1989.
Johnson R E, Jaffe J H, Fudala P J: A controlled trial of buprenorphine treatment for opioid dependence. JAMA *267:* 2750, 1992.
Kang S-Y, Kleinman P H, Woody G E, Millman R B, Todd T C, Kemp J, Lipton D S: Outcomes for cocaine abusers after once-a-week psychosocial therapy. Am J Psychiatry *148:* 630, 1991.
Kessler R C, McGonagle K A, Zhao S, Nelson C B, Hughes M, Eshelman S, Wittchen H-U, Kendler K S: Lifetime and 12-month prevalence of DSM-III-R psychiatric disorders in the United States. Arch Gen Psychiatry *51:* 8, 1994.
Khalsa M E, Paredes A, Anglin M D: Cocaine dependence: Behavioral dimensions and patterns of progression. Am J Addictions *2:* 330, 1993.
*Koob G F: Neurobiological mechanisms in cocaine and opiate dependence. In *Addictive States,* C P O'Brien, J H Jaffe, editors, p 79. Raven P, New York, 1992.
Kosten T R, Morgan C, Falcione J, Schottenfeld R S: Pharmacotherapy for cocaine-abusing methadone-maintained patients using amantadine or desipramine. Arch Gen Psychiatry *49:* 894, 1992.
Kranzler H R, Wallington D F: Serum prolactin level, craving, and early discharge from treatment in cocaine dependent patients. Am J Drug Alcohol Abuse *18:* 187, 1992.
Levin F R, Hess J M, Gorelick D A, Kreiter N A, Fudala P J: Patterns of cocaine use among cocaine-dependent outpatients. Am J Addictions *2:* 109, 1993.
Lipton D S, Brewington V, Smith M: Acupuncture for crack-cocaine detoxification: Experimental evaluation of efficacy. J Substance Abuse Treatment *11:* 205, 1994.
London E D, Cascella N G, Wong D F, Phillips R L, Dannals R F, Links J M, Herning R, Grayson R, Jaffe J H, Wagner H N Jr: Cocaine-induced reduction of glucose utilization in human brain. A study using positron emission tomography and [flourine 18] fluorodeoxyglucose. Arch Gen Psychiatry *47:* 567, 1990.
Maier H W: *Der Kokainismus.* Georg Thieme Verlag, Leipzig, 1926. (Translated and edited by O J Kalant, Addiction Research Foundation, Toronto, 1987.)
Markou A, Koob G F: Bromocriptine reverses the elevation in intracranial self-stimulation thresholds observed in a rat model of cocaine withdrawal. Neuropsychopharmacology *7:* 213, 1992.
McElroy S L, Weiss R D, Mendelson J H, Teoh S K, McAfee B, Mello N K: Desipramine treatment for relapse prevention in cocaine dependence. NIDA Res Monogr *95:* 57, 1990.
McLellan A T, Grissom G R, Brill P, Durell J, Metzger D S, O'Brien C P: Private substance abuse treatments: Are some programs more effective than others? J Substance Abuse Treatment *10:* 243, 1993.
McLellan A T, Grossman D S, Blaine J D, Haverkos H W: Acupuncture treatment for drug abuse: A technical review. J Substance Abuse Treatment *10:* 569, 1993.
Mello N K, Mendelson J H, Bree M P: Buprenorphine suppresses cocaine self-administration by rhesus monkeys. Science *245:* 859, 1989.
Meyer R E: New pharmacotherapies for cocaine dependence . . . revisited. Arch Gen Psychiatry *49:* 900, 1992.
Musto D: Opium, cocaine and marijuana in American history. Sci Am *265:* 40, 1991.
Najavits L M, Weiss R D: The role of psychotherapy in the treatment of substance-use disorders. Harvard Rev Psychiatry *2:* 84, 1992.
Nestler E J: Molecule neurobiology of drug addiction. Neuropsychopharmacology *11:* 77, 1994.
Preston K L, Sullivan J T, Berger P, Bigelow G E: Effects of cocaine alone and in combination with mazindol in human cocaine abusers. J Pharmacol Exp Ther *267:* 296, 1993.
*Regier D A, Farmer M E, Rae D S, Locke B Z, Keith S J, Judd L J, Goodwin F K: Comorbidity of mental disorders with alcohol and other drug abuse. JAMA *264:* 2511, 1990.
Roehrich H, Gold M S: Cocaine. In *Clinical Manual of Chemical Dependence,* D A Ciraulo, R I Shader, editors, p 195. American Psychiatric Press, Washington, 1991.
Rosen M I, Kosten T: Cocaine-associated panic attacks in methadone-maintained patients. Am J Drug Alcohol Abuse *18:* 57, 1992.
Rounsaville B J, Anton S F, Carroll K, Budde D, Prusoff B A, Gawin F: Psychiatric diagnoses of treatment-seeking cocaine abusers. Arch Gen Psychiatry *48:* 43, 1991.
Rounsaville B J, Bryant K: Tolerance and withdrawal in the DSM-III-R diagnosis of substance dependence. Am J Addictions *1:* 50, 1992.
Rounsaville B J, Bryant K, Babor T, Kranzler H, Kadden R: Cross system agreement for substance use disorders: DSM-III-R, DSM-IV, and ICD-10. Addiction *88:* 337, 1993.
Satel S L, Southwick S M, Gawin F H: Clinical features of cocaine-induced paranoia. Am J Psychiatry *148:* 495, 1991.
Shaner A, Khalsa E, Roberts L, Wilkins J, Anglin D, Hsieh S-C: Unrecognized cocaine use among schizophrenic patients. Am J Psychiatry *150:* 758, 1993.
Stine S M, Freeman M, Burns B, Charney D S, Kosten T R: Effect of methadone dose on cocaine abuse in a methadone program. Am J Addictions *1:* 294, 1992.
Strain E, Stitzer M L, Liebson I A, Bigelow G E: Comparison of buprenorphine and methadone in the treatment of opioid dependence. Am J Psychiatry *151:* 1025, 1994.
Unterwald E M, Rubenfeld J M, Kreek M J: Repeated cocaine administration upregulates κ and μ, but not δ receptors. Neuroreport *5:* 1613, 1994.
Volkow N D, Fowler J S, Wang G J, Hitzemann R: Decreased dopamine D2 receptor availability is associated with reduced frontal metabolism in cocaine abusers. Synapse *14:* 169, 1993.
Volkow N D, Fowler J S, Wolf A P, Hitzemann R, Dewey S, Bendriem B, Alpert R, Hoff A: Changes in brain glucose metabolism in cocaine dependence and withdrawal. Am J Psychiatry *148:* 621, 1991.
Volpe J J: Mechanisms of disease: Effect of cocaine use on the fetus. N Engl J Med *327:* 399, 1992.
Wahlestedt C, Reis D J: Neuropeptide Y-related peptides and their receptors—are the receptors potential therapeutic drug targets? In *Annual Review of Pharmacology and Toxicology,* vol 33, A K Cho, T F Blaschke, H H Loh, J L Way, editors, p 309. Annual Reviews, Palo Alto, CA, 1993.
Washton A M, Stone-Washton N: Outpatient treatment of cocaine and crack addiction: A clinical perspective. NIDA Res Monogr *135:* 15, 1993.
Weddington W W, Brown B S, Haertzen C A, Cone E J, Dax E M, Herning R I, Michaelson M A: Changes in mood, craving and sleep during short-term abstinence reported by male cocaine addicts. Arch Gen Psychiatry *47:* 861, 1990.
Weddington W W Jr, Brown B S, Haertzen C A, Hess J M, Mahaffey J R, Kolar A F, Jaffe J H: Comparison of amantadine and desipramine combined with psychotherapy for treatment of cocaine dependence. Am J Drug Alcohol Abuse *17:* 137, 1991.
Wells E A, Peterson P L, Gainey R R, Hawkins J D, Catalano R F: Outpatient treatment for cocaine abuse: A controlled comparison of relapse prevention and Twelve-Step approaches. Am J Drug Alcohol Abuse *20:* 1, 1994.

13.7 HALLUCINOGEN-RELATED DISORDERS

THOMAS J. CROWLEY, M.D.

INTRODUCTION

Hallucinogens include lysergic acid diethylamide (LSD) and related ergot derivatives, phenylalkylamines related to mescaline, indolealkylamines related to N,N-dimethyltryptamine (DMT, a hallucinogenic compound occurring naturally in the human brain), and miscellaneous other indoles or piperidyl benzilate esters. Excluded here are the cannabis principal (tetrahydrocannabinol [THC]), and phencyclidine (PCP); although hallucinogenic, their pharmacology, patterns of use, and clinical presentation set them apart. Also excluded are plants (for example, jimson weed *[Datura stramonium]* and angel's trumpet *[Datura sauveolens]*) and derivative drugs (hyoscyamine, atropine, and scopolamine), which produce hallucinations and delirium in the central anticholinergic syndrome.

DEFINITION

Hallucinogen abuse and hallucinogen dependence are defined by the same criteria used for other drugs. Abuse involves repeated use resulting in physical hazard or adverse social consequences, and dependence adds medically adverse consequences, driven or compulsive use of the drug, and tolerance. Hallucinogen intoxication is a behavioral disorder arising with current or quite recent use of a hallucinogen and abating within hours or a few days. Hallucinogen withdrawal apparently does not occur and is not recognized in the fourth edition of *Diagnostic and Statistical Manual of Mental Disorders* (DSM-IV). Hallucinogen persisting perception disorder (flashbacks) persists long after drug can be detected in the body.

HISTORY

A plant extract called soma, which gave its users visions and a sense of brilliance and strength, is described in a 3,500-year-old Sanskrit text, the Rigveda. Modern ethnobotanists believe soma was prepared from a poisonous mushroom, *Amanita muscaria,* which contains muscimol. Many preliterate societies, especially in the New World, employed hallucinogenic drugs. Guatemalan "mushroom stones," also about 3,500 years old, point to a mushroom cult there. Nutmeg was probably used as a hallucinogen in Southeast Asia, as were its *Virola* relatives in South America. The Aztecs used *Psilocbe* mushrooms, ololiuqui (a morning glory), and the peyote cactus. Early self-experimenters with peyote included the American neuropsychiatrist Weir Mitchell and the English physician Havelock Ellis.

Ergot, a poisonous fungus of grain, took thousands of medieval lives through epidemics of Saint Anthony's fire, with hallucinations, delirium, and severe muscular contractions. In 1938 Albert Hoffman synthesized the ergot alkaloid lysergic acid diethylamide (LSD). In 1943, after taking only 250 μg orally, Hoffman first felt urges to laugh, but then experienced distortions of vision and kinesthesia, the appearance of faces as grotesque masks, and a feeling of possession or of going insane.

Four years later LSD (Delysid) was marketed with suggestions that self-administration would help psychiatrists better to understand psychosis, and that the drug's release of repressed thoughts and feelings could help anxious patients. Psycholytic therapy employed repeated small doses to facilitate expression, and psychedelic therapy used a few doses of over 200 μg to alter experience profoundly. Some favorable reports were published but lacked modern controls.

Aldous Huxley's book on hallucinogens, *The Doors of Perception,* excited artists and intellectuals seeking pharmacologically enhanced creativity. Soon Harvard psychologists Timothy Leary and Richard Alpert, influenced by the poet Allen Ginsberg, encouraged wide use of hallucinogenic drugs, and many responded. The United States government outlawed their sale and use in 1965. The drugs' Schedule 1 classification (indicating no medical use and high abuse potential) has essentially halted human-subject research on them.

COMPARATIVE NOSOLOGY

DSM-IV lists a number of hallucinogen-related disorders (Table 13.7-1) but contains specific diagnostic criteria only for hallucinogen intoxication and hallucinogen persisting perception disorder (flashbacks). The diagnostic criteria for the other hallucinogen-related disorders are contained in the DSM-IV sections that are specific to each symptom—for example, hallucinogen-induced mood disorder is discussed with other mood disorders (see Section 16.6).

TABLE 13.7-1
Hallucinogen-Related Disorders

Hallucinogen use disorders

Hallucinogen dependence
Hallucinogen abuse

Hallucinogen-induced disorders

Hallucinogen intoxication
Hallucinogen persisting perception disorder (flashbacks)
Hallucinogen intoxication delirium
Hallucinogen-induced psychotic disorder, with delusions
Specify if: with onset during intoxication
Hallucinogen-induced psychotic disorder, with hallucinations
Specify if: with onset during intoxication
Hallucinogen-induced mood disorder
Specify if: with onset during intoxication
Hallucinogen-induced anxiety disorder
Specify if: with onset during intoxication

Hallucinogen-related disorder not otherwise specified

Table from DSM-IV, *Diagnostic and Statistical Manual of Mental Disorders,* ed 4. Copyright American Psychiatric Association, Washington, 1994. Used with permission.

Table 13.7-2 compares several diagnostic systems. Differences between the revised third edition of DSM (DSM-III-R) (1987) and DSM-IV are as follows: (1) psychoactive substance abuse was a residual category in DSM-III-R; DSM-IV provides specific diagnostic criteria for substance abuse. (2) The DSM-IV criteria for substance dependence are also modified from those of DSM-III-R. (3) DSM-IV generally permits subtyping of dependence with (or without) physiological dependence, but because hallucinogens produce no withdrawal, that option does not apply here. DSM-IV expands the list of hallucinogen intoxication mental disorders to include (4) hallucinogen intoxication delirium and (5) hallucinogen-induced anxiety disorder. Lower hallucinogen doses may change only feelings and thoughts without perceptual changes. In mid-dose intoxications the person still may recognize that the misperceptions, illusions, or hallucinations are drug induced. Higher doses may cause (6) hallucinogen-induced psychotic disorder, with beliefs that the altered perceptions are real. Hallucinogen-induced psychotic disorder is differentiated from hallucinogen persisting perception disorder in DSM-IV; the latter applies to intermittent flashbacks, recurring long after intoxications end. As discussed below, DSM-IV provides no diagnosis for persisting hallucinogen-induced psychosis.

The ninth revision of the *International Classification of Diseases and Related Health Problems* (ICD-9) provided fewer hallucinogen-induced diagnoses and called intoxication abuse. The ninth revision of the *International Classification of Diseases, Clinical Modifications* (ICD-9-CM), a United States government classification for Medicare and Medicaid billing, also calls intoxication abuse and provides no separate diagnosis of hallucinogen-induced anxiety disorder. The 1992 tenth revision of ICD (ICD-10), names abuse harmful use, and has neither hallucinogen-induced mood disorder nor hallucinogen-induced anxiety disorder diagnoses.

EPIDEMIOLOGY

In the 1991 United States Household Survey 8.2 percent of respondents reported having used hallucinogens (including phencyclidine) at least once; 1.4 percent had used them within

TABLE 13.7-2
Hallucinogen Diagnoses, DSM and ICD

DSM-IV	DSM-III-R	ICD-9	ICD-9-CM	ICD-10
Hallucinogen abuse	Hallucinogen abuse	Nondependent abuse of hallucinogens	Hallucinogen abuse	Hallucinogen harmful use
Hallucinogen dependence	Hallucinogen dependence	Hallucinogen dependence	Hallucinogen dependence	Hallucinogen dependence syndrome
Hallucinogen intoxication	Hallucinogen hallucinosis	Nondependent abuse of hallucinogens	Hallucinogen abuse	Hallucinogen acute intoxication
Hallucinogen intoxication delirium		Acute confusional state	Drug-induced delirium	Hallucinogen acute intoxication
Hallucinogen-induced mood disorder	Hallucinogen mood disorder	Nondependent abuse of hallucinogens	Drug-induced organic affective syndrome	
Hallucinogen-induced anxiety disorder		Nondependent abuse of hallucinogens	Hallucinogen abuse	
Hallucinogen-induced psychotic disorder	Hallucinogen delusional disorder	Hallucinogen paranoid and/or hallucinatory states	Drug-induced organic delusional syndrome	Hallucinogen psychotic disorder
Hallucinogen persisting perceptual disorder	Posthallucinogen perception disorder			Hallucinogen residual psychotic disorder (flashbacks)
Hallucinogen-related disorder NOS	Hallucinogen organic mental disorder NOS		Unspecified drug-induced mental disorder	Other or unspecified mental or behavioral disorder induced by hallucinogen

the preceding year and 0.3 percent within the preceding month. By comparison, cocaine's figures were 11.7, 3.1, and 0.9 percent, respectively. Men accounted for 62 percent of those who had used hallucinogens, but 75 percent of those using within the preceding month (presumably those were more frequent users). Of persons aged 26 to 34, 26 percent had used hallucinogens at least once, the highest of any age group. But recent use was most common among those aged 18 to 25 years; 2 percent of them had used within the preceding month. The percentage of whites reporting use was double that of blacks, with Hispanics between those extremes. Similarly, the proportion of users in the West was double that in the South.

In a 1990 United States survey of high school seniors, 8.7 percent reported having used LSD at least once, and 1.9 percent within the last month.

Hallucinogen problems accounted for only 1 percent of drug-related visits to federally monitored emergency rooms in 1989 (by comparison, 40 percent involved cocaine). Of hallucinogen patients, over three fourths were men. Of all drug-related visits, the proportion of hallucinogen-related visits was highest among whites. Over half of LSD-related visits were by youths 10 to 19 years old, and many were 17 or under. The preponderance of those emergency patients used their drug by the oral route.

Hallucinogens were mentioned as contributing to only one of 5,830 drug deaths (excluding alcohol and tobacco) in a 1990 federal survey of medical examiner reports.

The prevalence in the general population of hallucinogen abuse or hallucinogen dependence (by DSM-III-R or DSM-IV criteria) is unknown, but probably it is much lower than abuse of or dependence on tobacco, alcohol, marijuana, or cocaine.

PHARMACOLOGY

BASIC PHARMACOLOGY Table 13.7-3 lists the more commonly used hallucinogens; many others are known. The table is only a rough guide to overdoses, since purported doses of illegal drugs are unreliable and plants vary greatly in hallucinogenic content. Those drugs are usually taken orally, with good gastrointestinal absorption. Sometimes they are snorted, smoked (especially DMT), or injected intravenously. LSD, the prototype, is metabolized in the liver through hydroxylation and conjugation and mainly excreted through bile into feces.

The drugs' effects vary in onset and duration. The effects of 5-methoxy-3,4-methylenedioxymethamphetamine (MDMA, also known as ecstasy), for example, peak at 30 minutes and last four to six hours. Users first feel LSD's effects within minutes; the effects peak after two to four hours and last 12 to 14 hours. LSD's plasma half-life is about three hours, and plasma concentrations correlate well with scores on simple arithmetic tests. The effects of nutmeg, which must be metabolized to active compounds, begin about five hours after ingestion and may last two to three days.

MECHANISM OF ACTION Cross-tolerance among hallucinogens suggests a common mechanism of action. Although those drugs influence dopamine and other neurotransmitters, their main effect is probably on postsynaptic serotonin (5-hydroxytryptamine) type 2 ($5\text{-}HT_2$) receptors, where most authorities believe they are agonists. Indeed, the drugs' binding affinity to human $5\text{-}HT_2$ receptors correlates very strongly with their human hallucinogenic potency. Repeated LSD administration in rats reduces the number of brain $5\text{-}HT_2$ binding sites, perhaps explaining tolerance. Serotonin blockers prevent animals from identifying LSD in drug discrimination tests, suggesting that such drugs may eventually be useful in hallucinogen intoxications. Autoradiography shows $5\text{-}HT_2$ binding sites throughout the brain, but especially in the olfactory bulb, anterior cortex, nucleus accumbens, caudate, globus pallidus, ventral pallidum, islands of Calleja, mammillary nuclei, inferior olive, and choroid plexus. How $5\text{-}HT_2$ stimulation in those areas produces the hallucinogenic experience is as yet unknown.

PHYSIOLOGICAL AND BEHAVIORAL EFFECTS Stimulant effects (pupillary dilation, tachycardia, and some hypertension or hyperthermia) often begin the hallucinogenic experience, followed by nausea, restlessness, and dizzy, excited, or detached feelings. Low doses then elicit anticipation with feelings of well-being, euphoria, and self-confidence, often without perceptual effects. At slightly higher doses one color may seem particularly bright; edges or cracks in surfaces may seem deeply etched; time seems drawn out. Somewhat higher doses induce

TABLE 13.7-3
Abused Hallucinogens

Class	Common Names	Chemical Name	Source	Usual Dose
1. Ergot derivatives and related compounds	LSD, acid	D-lysergic acid diethylamide	synthesis	50–200 mcg
	morning glory seeds	ergine, isoergine	*Ipomoea tricolor*	200 seeds
	Hawaiian baby woodrose	ergine, isoergine	*Argyreia nervosa*	4–8 seeds
2. Phenylalkylamines	mescaline	3,4,5-trimethoxyphenylethylamine	peyote cactus, *Lophophora williamsii*	6–12 cactus "buttons" or 200–500 mg mescaline
	nutmeg or mace (spices)	myristicin and elemicin, metabolized to 3-methoxy-4,5-methylene-dioxyamphetamine (MMDA) and 3,4,5-trimethoxyamphetamine (TMA)	*Myristica fragrans* (a tree)	1–3 nutmeg seeds
	MDA, love drug, Eve	3,4-methylenedioxyamphetamine	synthesis	75–200 mg
	STP, DOM	2,5-dimethoxy-4-methylamphetamine	synthesis	5 mg
	MDMA, ecstasy, XTC	5-methoxy-3,4-methylenedioxyamphetamine	synthesis	75–200 mg
3. Indole alkaloids	magic mushrooms	psilocybin, psilocin	*Psilocybe sp.*	10–200 mushrooms
	DMT, cohaba snuff	N,N-dimethyltryptamine	synthesis or from *Piptadenia peregrina*	50–100 mg
	bufotenine	5-OH-N,N-dimethyltryptamine	skin of certain toads	uncertain
4. Others	fly agaric mushroom	muscimole, ibotenic acid, others	*Amanita muscaria* or *A. pantheria*	1–4 mushrooms or 30–60 mg ibotenic acid

illusions and visual distortions: flashes of light, moving or zig-zag lines, and moving objects perceived stroboscopically with suspended serial images. With still higher doses faces and familiar objects assume fantastic or grotesque shapes. With synesthesias (the blending of senses) loud noises may be experienced as bright flashes. Perhaps because of the intense experience, performance on cognitive or memory tests is impaired during intoxication.

Euphoria, anxiety, or depression may alternate rapidly, as may feelings of deep fulfillment or union with the universe versus fears of losing control or going insane. True hallucinations, which the person believes to be real, are uncommon; recognition that events are drug induced is usually preserved. Rare attempts to fly or to hold back traffic may be fatal. Many intoxications with intense experience and unclouded consciousness are perceived by users as expanding mind, creativity, and wisdom, but bad trips fraught with the terror of madness, disintegration, and death occasionally drive users to emergency treatment. Such bad trips may occur without explanation in persons with many previous good trips.

Tolerance to hallucinogens develops rapidly with daily use, and it regresses rapidly when administration ceases. Withdrawal (physical dependence) does not occur. Patients seldom complain of hallucinogen use being out of control, or that they continue using despite firm decisions to stop. Such complaints are common among patients dependent on other drugs; hallucinogen use seems less driven or compelled. Hallucinogens (with a few exceptions) are unique among commonly abused drugs in not reinforcing self-administration by animals.

DRUG DIFFERENCES Although the drugs share cross-tolerance and act at the same receptor, they also have differences. The phenylalkylamines are both amphetaminelike and hallucinogenic, but drugs of that group differ in the strength of those two properties. For example, 3,4-methylenedioxyamphetamine (MDA, also known as Eve) and MDMA are closely related chemically, but MDMA is less frequently hallucinogenic in humans, and is sufficiently amphetaminelike to reinforce self-administration by animals. However, one optical isomer of MDA is primarily amphetaminelike, and another is mainly hallucinogenic; their racemic mixture has both properties.

NEURAL DAMAGE, FATAL OUTCOMES Both MDMA and MDA cause long-lasting brain serotonin depletion in rats, apparently as a result of terminal degeneration of serotonin neurons. Brain binding of tritiated LSD is changed for at least a month after chronic LSD administration.

Coma, profound hyperpyrexia, disseminated intravascular coagulopathy, rhabdomyolysis, and acute renal failure have occurred in a number of young adults who used MDMA or MDA during sustained, frenetic dances. The condition resembles both the neuroleptic malignant syndrome and the recently described serotonin syndrome. It is thought to result from derangements of central serotonin homeostasis. Without vigorous treatment the condition is often fatal.

ETIOLOGY

Hallucinogens are widely available (for example, nutmeg can be purchased in most food stores) a fact that contributes to prevalence of use. Demographic factors associated with hallucinogen problems (in emergency rooms) are male sex, age 15 to 40 years, and white race. The greater prevalence of hallucinogen problems in the western versus southern United States suggests that social factors contribute to the risk. Comorbid disorders also increase the chance of hallucinogen problems. Schizophrenic persons may be more likely than others to use hallucinogens, and in a Denver sample of substance-using adolescent boys with conduct disorder, over 40 percent had DSM-III-R diagnoses of hallucinogen dependence.

Curiosity about dramatic effects or a hope for spiritual or philosophical fulfillment probably motivates most initial uses of hallucinogens. Although many Americans have used the drugs, most treatment contacts are for bad-trip intoxications. Few patients seek treatment for hallucinogen abuse or hallucinogen dependence. The reason probably relates to the inability of most hallucinogens to reinforce self-administration by animals, a property that predicts well a drug's tendency to drive compulsive use in humans. Apparently one can use hallucinogens occasionally with little risk of the drug's taking control and compelling escalation of use. Most users who decide to stop apparently can do so without treatment.

Recent years have seen little research on hallucinogen users, and other etiological factors are not well understood.

HALLUCINOGEN ABUSE AND DEPENDENCE

DIAGNOSIS AND CLINICAL FEATURES The cardinal feature of hallucinogen abuse is a maladaptive pattern of repeated hallucinogen use that results in physical risk or adverse social consequences (see Table 13.1-6). If repeated use also causes loss of control over the drug use and tolerance to the drugs' effects (hallucinogens do not produce the withdrawal symptoms of physical dependence), the diagnosis is hallucinogen dependence (see Tables 13.1-2 and 13.1-5). Patients rarely complain of, or seek treatment for, those disorders, which often distress others more than they distress the users. However, the disorders are common among patients (especially adolescents) in treatment for other substance use disorders and among juvenile offenders.

DIFFERENTIAL DIAGNOSIS Since black-market hallucinogens often contain phencyclidine, hallucinogen abuse and hallucinogen dependence must be differentiated from phencyclidine abuse or phencyclidine dependence. The latter often are characterized by more severe intoxications with prominent nystagmus; urinary phencyclidine during intoxication supports those diagnoses. Hallucinogen abuse or hallucinogen dependence may mimic or coexist with schizophrenia. Brief psychotic episodes with a prominence of visual over auditory hallucinations and good interepisode functioning suggest repeated intoxications. Drug identification in urine aids in that differential diagnosis, but only LSD testing is widely available.

COURSE, PROGNOSIS, AND TREATMENT Despite many studies of hallucinogen intoxication and related psychoses, the literature is silent on course, prognosis, and treatment of hallucinogen abuse and hallucinogen dependence. Since few persons seek treatment for the latter disorders, psychiatrists should identify the disorders through history (and urine screening where appropriate) in at-risk patient groups, such as juvenile offenders, youths with conduct disorder, members of socially disaffected groups, and intermittently psychotic or schizophrenic patients. In the absence of research information, general treatment guidelines for patients with phencyclidine abuse or phencyclidine dependence appear applicable to those with hallucinogen abuse or hallucinogen dependence.

HALLUCINOGEN INTOXICATION

DIAGNOSIS AND CLINICAL FEATURES The cardinal feature of hallucinogen intoxication is the development of a reversible, maladaptive behavioral syndrome resulting from recent ingestion of (or exposure to) a hallucinogenic drug. Such syndromes usually develop within minutes to hours after ingestion of the drug and persist for a few hours to a very few days. The most common reason for hallucinogen users to seek treatment is a bad-trip intoxication, and most recover within 24 hours. Table 13.7-4 gives the DSM-IV diagnostic criteria for the condition.

TABLE 13.7-4
Diagnostic Criteria for Hallucinogen Intoxication

A. Recent use of a hallucinogen.
B. Clinically significant maladaptive behavioral or psychological changes (e.g., marked anxiety or depression, ideas of reference, fear of losing one's mind, paranoid ideation, impaired judgment, or impaired social or occupational functioning) that developed during, or shortly after, hallucinogen use.
C. Perceptual changes occurring in a state of full wakefulness and alertness (e.g., subjective intensification of perceptions, depersonalization, derealization, illusions, hallucinations, synesthesias) that developed during, or shortly after, hallucinogen use.
D. Two (or more) of the following signs, developing during, or shortly after, hallucinogen use:
  (1) pupillary dilation
  (2) tachycardia
  (3) sweating
  (4) palpitations
  (5) blurring of vision
  (6) tremors
  (7) incoordination
E. The symptoms are not due to a general medical condition and are not better accounted for by another mental disorder.

Table from DSM-IV, *Diagnostic and Statistical Manual of Mental Disorders,* ed 4. Copyright American Psychiatric Association, Washington, 1994. Used with permission.

DIFFERENTIAL DIAGNOSIS Hallucinogen intoxication is differentiated from other intoxications by the history of what was ingested, characteristic sympathomimetic physical findings (pupillary dilation, tachycardia, hyperthermia, and so on), perceptual changes without clouded sensorium, and laboratory confirmation of LSD (the only widely available test) in bodily fluids. Hallucinogen intoxication should be distinguished from other drug conditions with hallucinations as follows: (1) Patients with anticholinergic intoxications are often described as "hot as a hare, red as a beet, dry as a bone, mad as a hatter, and blind as a bat"; their treatment may require physostigmine (Antilirium). (2) Those intoxicated with amphetamines will also have sympathomimetic signs, but they more commonly have frank delusions and auditory hallucinations. (3) Alcohol withdrawal with perceptual disturbances (alcohol-induced psychotic disorder, with hallucinations) develops soon after cessation (or sharp reduction) of heavy drinking.

Rapid onset after an ingestion, characteristic resolution, and absence of localizing signs help in differentiating hallucinogen intoxications from other neurological disorders but cannot rule them out. Hallucinogen intoxication is differentiated from hallucinogen intoxication delirium, hallucinogen-induced psychotic disorder, hallucinogen-induced mood disorder, and hallucinogen-induced anxiety disorder. Those diagnoses are made instead of hallucinogen intoxication when the additional named symptoms are in excess of those usually associated with hallucinogen intoxication, and when the additional symptoms are sufficiently severe to warrant independent clinical attention.

Schizophrenic patients are more likely than those with hallucinogen intoxication to have poor preepisode functioning and auditory (as opposed to visual) hallucinations, and their episodes resolve more slowly than does hallucinogen intoxication. But schizophrenic persons apparently use hallucinogens more than others do, and so schizophrenia sometimes is comorbid with, and complicates, hallucinogen intoxication.

COURSE AND PROGNOSIS Most hallucinogen intoxications end after a few hours without complications, especially if a trusted guide assists the person, continually orienting to reality and reassuring that the experience is drug induced and temporary. Impaired judgment and motor skills, combined with transcendent self-confidence, occasionally lead intoxicated persons to fatal mistakes when driving automobiles or in high places.

TREATMENT Authorities agree that hallucinogen intoxication is usually best handled by talking down the patient in a quiet room with continuous simple orientation, external focus, and reassurance that the person is neither going insane nor dying. Patients should not be left alone.

Antipsychotics potently block 5-HT_2 receptors, and in more severe cases 5 to 10 mg of haloperidol (Haldol) administered intramuscularly, intravenously, or orally, or 50 mg of chlorpromazine (Thorazine) administered intramuscularly, will probably hasten recovery. Some authorities suggest that antipsychotics complicate recovery from the phenylalkylamine 2,5-dimethoxy-4-methylamphetamine (DOM, also known as STP), but supporting data are very limited. Many physicians recommend 5 to 20 mg of diazepam (Valium) administered orally or intravenously. There are no controlled studies of those treatments.

Cases of coma with severe hyperthermia require rapid cooling, and some experts advocate the use of dantrolene (Dantrium) in a dose of 1 mg per kg of body weight. Although absorption of most hallucinogens is rapid, some experts recommend gavage of an activated charcoal slurry (30 to 40 grams) to decontaminate the gut and block enterohepatic recirculation, or in case more slowly digested plants, such as nutmeg or mushrooms, have been eaten.

HALLUCINOGEN PERSISTING PERCEPTION DISORDER

DIAGNOSIS AND CLINICAL FEATURES The cardinal feature (the flashback) is the intermittent recurrence, long after one or more earlier hallucinogen intoxications, of perceptual experiences like those of the intoxications. In different samples 15 to 77 percent of users reported flashbacks. Some appreciate them as free trips; others are troubled by intrusive misperceptions, illusions, or formed hallucinations. Only those distressed persons meet the criteria in Table 13.7-5.

DIFFERENTIAL DIAGNOSIS Flashbacks are differentiated from psychotic disorders by the absence of other signs of psychosis; also, patients do not believe that flashbacks represent reality. The differential diagnosis includes migraine, seizures, or visual-system disease.

TABLE 13.7-5
Diagnostic Criteria for Hallucinogen Persisting Perception Disorder (Flashbacks)

A. The reexperiencing, following cessation of use of a hallucinogen, of one or more of the perceptual symptoms that were experienced while intoxicated with the hallucinogen (e.g., geometric hallucinations, false perceptions of movement in the peripheral visual fields, flashes of color, intensified colors, trails of images of moving objects, positive afterimages, halos around objects, macropsia, and micropsia).
B. The symptoms in criterion A cause clinically significant distress or impairment in social, occupational, or other important areas of functioning.
C. The symptoms are not due to a general medical condition (e.g., anatomical lesions and infections of the brain, visual epilepsies) and are not better accounted for by another mental disorder (e.g., delirium, dementia, schizophrenia) or hypnopompic hallucinations.

Table from DSM-IV, *Diagnostic and Statistical Manual of Mental Disorders,* ed 4. Copyright American Psychiatric Association, Washington, 1994. Used with permission.

ETIOLOGY, COURSE, AND PROGNOSIS In one study flashbacks were more common among more suggestible users prone to "loose" or illogical thinking. The number of hallucinogen exposures reportedly is not related to flashback occurrence. Episodes may be triggered by entering a dark room, staring at a blank wall, marijuana use, driving, associating with LSD-intoxicated persons, or by flashing lights. Some experts assert that with time flashbacks fade in frequency and intensity, but others present some evidence of persistence.

TREATMENT Case reports suggest that flashbacks may be helped by psychotherapy, antipsychotics, or carbamazepine (Tegretol). A non-blind study of nine benzodiazepine-treated patients and 12 antipsychotic-treated patients suggests a better response in the former.

OTHER HALLUCINOGEN-RELATED DISORDERS

DIAGNOSIS AND CLINICAL FEATURES These diagnoses are made instead of hallucinogen intoxication when the named symptoms are in excess of those usually associated with hallucinogen intoxication, and when the symptoms are sufficiently severe to warrant independent clinical attention.

Hallucinogen intoxication delirium DSM-IV allows for the diagnosis of hallucinogen intoxication delirium (see Chapter 12). The disorder is thought to be relatively rare. It begins during hallucinogen intoxication. However, hallucinogens are often mixed with other substances, and hallucinogen intoxication delirium should be distinguished from delirium induced by such contaminants.

Hallucinogen-induced psychotic disorders If psychotic symptoms are present and the person lacks insight that they are substance-induced, a diagnosis of hallucinogen-induced psychotic disorder may be warranted (see Section 15.3). DSM-IV also allows the clinician to specify whether hallucinations or delusions are the prominent symptoms. The most common adverse effect of LSD and related substances is a bad trip, which resembles the acute panic reaction to cannabis but can be more severe; a bad trip occasionally produces true psychotic symptoms. The bad trip generally ends when the immediate effects of the hallucinogen wear off. However, the course of a bad trip is variable, and occasionally a protracted psychotic episode is difficult to distinguish from a nonorganic psychotic disorder.

Hallucinogen-induced mood disorder DSM-IV provides a diagnostic category for hallucinogen-induced mood disorder (see Section 16.6). Unlike cocaine-induced mood disorder and amphetamine-induced mood disorder, in which the symptoms are somewhat predictable, mood disorder symptoms accompanying hallucinogen abuse can be variable. Abusers may experience maniclike symptoms involving grandiose delusions or depressionlike feelings and ideas or mixed symptoms. As with the hallucinogen-induced psychotic disorder symptoms, the symptoms of hallucinogen-induced mood disorder almost invariably resolve once the drug has been eliminated from the patient's body.

Hallucinogen-induced anxiety disorder Hallucinogen-induced anxiety disorder (see Section 17.5) is also variable in its symptom pattern, and few data regarding symptom patterns are available. Anecdotally, physicians who treat patients who come into emergency rooms with hallucinogen-related disorders have frequently reported panic disorder with agoraphobia.

Hallucinogen use disorder not otherwise specified The residual category in DSM-IV permits coding of unusual additional diagnoses (Table 13.7-6).

WITHDRAWAL DSM-IV does not have a diagnostic category of hallucinogen withdrawal, but some clinicians anecdotally report a syndrome with depression and anxiety that follows the cessation of frequent hallucinogen use. It is not established that such symptoms are linked pharmacologically to cessation of the drug. Such a syndrome may best fit the diagnosis of hallucinogen-related disorder not otherwise specified (NOS).

PERSISTING PSYCHOSES The hallucinogen-induced disorders last a few hours to a very few days. But some authors suggest that hallucinogenic drugs also cause persisting psychoses. Some possibilities are that (1) the drugs by themselves cause persisting psychoses, (2) psychosis or its prodromata cause hallucinogen use, (3) hallucinogen use hastens psychotic decompensation among persons already at risk, or (4) the drug use and the psychosis merely are coincidental in some persons. Schizophrenic patients without drug histories and patients with so-called LSD psychoses reportedly are similar in family loading for schizophrenia and in the phenomenology and course of the illness; that observation reduces the viability of the first explanation. But the connection remains enigmatic, and DSM-IV provides no diagnosis of persisting LSD psychosis. Hallucinogen-induced psychotic disorder describes only brief intoxication-related psychoses.

DIFFERENTIAL DIAGNOSIS, COURSE, AND PROGNOSIS

The differentials for hallucinogen intoxication apply to the other hallucinogen-induced disorders. Also included in the differential diagnosis are mental disorders due to a general medical condition. For example, if mood symptoms are caused by a medication being used to treat a medical condition, mood disorder due to a general medical condition should be diagnosed. Also included are the primary mental disorders. For example, if anxiety symptoms are not causally related to the hallucinogen use, then an anxiety disorder should be diagnosed. Course and outcome are like those of hallucinogen intoxication, but the greater intensity of confusion, panic, delusional thinking, or affect disturbance increases the risk of trauma.

TREATMENT Care for bad trips is similar to that for uncomplicated hallucinogen intoxication, but must be more intense. Careful, continuous watching is essential to prevent injury. Continuous concrete orienting is required, and medication will probably be needed.

SUGGESTED CROSS-REFERENCES

A general discussion of substance use disorders (intoxication, withdrawal, abuse, dependence, and persisting disorders) is found in Section 13.1. Section 11.1 addresses the classification of those disorders in different diagnostic systems. Section 14.7 on schizophrenia highlights differences in the clinical presentation and course between schizophrenia and hallucinogen abuse and hallucinogen dependence, and Section 13.10 on phencyclidine (and related substances) clarifies differences from disorders involving those compounds.

TABLE 13.7-6
Hallucinogen-Related Disorder Not Otherwise Specified

The hallucinogen-related disorder not otherwise specified category is for disorders associated with the use of hallucinogens that are not classifiable as hallucinogen dependence, hallucinogen abuse, hallucinogen intoxication, hallucinogen persisting perception disorder, hallucinogen intoxication delirium, hallucinogen-induced psychotic disorder, hallucinogen-induced mood disorder, or hallucinogen-induced anxiety disorder.

Table from DSM-IV, *Diagnostic and Statistical Manual of Mental Disorders,* ed 4. Copyright American Psychiatric Association, Washington, 1994. Used with permission.

REFERENCES

Abraham H D: Visual phenomenology of the LSD flashback. Arch Gen Psychiatry *40:* 884, 1983.

Abraham H D, Aldridge A M: Adverse consequences of lysergic acid diethylamide. Addiction *88:* 1327, 1993.

Aghajanian G K, Bing O H L: Persistence of lysergic acid diethylamide in the plasma of human subjects. Clin Pharmacol Ther *5:* 611, 1964.

Bowers M B: Psychoses precipitated by psychotomimetic drugs: A follow-up study. Arch Gen Psychiatry *34:* 832, 1977.

Brown R T, Braden N J: Hallucinogens. Pediatr Clin North Am *34:* 341, 1987.

Campkin N J, Davies U M: Treatment of "ecstasy" overdose with dantrolene (letter). Anaesthesia *48:* 82, 1993.

Henry J A: Ecstasy and the dance of death. Br Med J *305:* 5, 1992.

International Statistical Classification of Diseases and Related Health Problems, rev 10, vol 1. World Health Organization, Geneva, 1991.

*Jacobs B L: How hallucinogenic drugs work. Am Scientist *75:* 386, 1987.

Johnston L D, O'Malley P M, Bachman J G: *Drug Abuse Among American High School Seniors, College Students and Young Adults, 1975–1990.* US Department of Health and Human Services, Washington, 1991.

Krystal J H, Price L H, Opsahl C, Ricaurte G A, Heninger G R: Chronic 3,4-methylenedioxymethamphetamine (MDMA) use: Effects on mood and neuropsychological function? Am J Drug Alcohol Abuse *18:* 331, 1992.

*Kulig K: LSD. Emerg Med Clin North Am *8:* 551, 1990.

National Institute on Drug Abuse: Annual data 1989, data from the drug abuse warning network (DAWN). DHHS Publication No. (ADM) 90-1717. US Department of Health and Human Services, Washington, 1990.

National Institute on Drug Abuse: Annual medical examiner data 1990, data from the drug abuse warning network (DAWN). DHHS Publication No. (ADM) 91-1840. US Department of Health and Human Services, Washington, 1991.

National Institute on Drug Abuse: National household survey on drug abuse: Population estimates 1991. DHHS Publication No. (ADM) 92-1887. US Department of Health and Human Services, Washington, 1991.

*Nimmo S M, Kennedy B W, Tullett W M, Blyth A S, Dougall J R: Drug-induced hyperthermia. Anaesthesia *48:* 892, 1993.

Payne R B: Nutmeg intoxication. N Engl J Med *269:* 36, 1963.

Pierce P A, Peroutka S J: Hallucinogenic drug interactions with neurotransmitter receptor binding sites in human cortex. Psychopharmacology *97:* 118, 1989.

Randall T: Ecstasy-fueled "rave" parties become dances of death for English youths. JAMA *268:* 1505, 1992.

Ricaurte G, Bryan G, Strauss L, Seiden L, Schuster C: Hallucinogenic amphetamine selectively destroys brain serotonin nerve terminals. Science *229:* 986, 1985.

*Scanzello C R, Hatzidimitriou G, Martello A L, Katz J L, Ricaurte G A: Serotonergic recovery after (±)3, 4-(methylenedioxy) methamphetamine injury: Observations in rats. J Pharmacol Exp Ther *264:* 1484, 1993.

*Schuckit M A: MDMA (ecstasy): An old drug with new tricks. Drug Abuse & Alcoholism Newsletter *23:* 1, 1994.

Schultes R E: Hallucinogens of plant origin. Science *163:* 245, 1969.

Seymour R B, Wesson D R, Smith D E: MDMA: Proceedings of the conference. J Psychoactive Drugs *18:* 287, 1986.

Simpson D L, Rumack B H: Methylenedioxyamphetamine: Clinical description of overdose, death, and review of pharmacology. Arch Intern Med *141:* 1507, 1981.

Spoerke D G, Hall A H: Plants and mushrooms of abuse. Emerg Med Clin North Am *8:* 579, 1990.

Strassman R J: Adverse reactions to psychedelic drugs: A review of the literature. J Nerv Ment Dis *172:* 577, 1984.

Vardy M M, Kay S R: LDS psychosis or LSD-induced schizophrenia? A multimethod inquiry. Arch Gen Psychiatry *40:* 877, 1983.
Webb C, Williams V: Ecstasy intoxication: Appreciation of complications and the role of dantrolene (letter). Anaesthesia *48:* 542, 1993.

13.8
INHALANT-RELATED DISORDERS

THOMAS J. CROWLEY, M.D.

INTRODUCTION

The recreational inhalation of gases was not uncommon in the 19th century and case reports of vapor inhalation appeared in the 1950s. Larger series were published in the 1960s. Such gases are volatile hydrocarbons and include toluene, n-hexane, methyl butyl ketone, trichloroethylene, trichloroethane, dichloromethane, gasoline, and butane. They make up four commercial classes: (1) solvents for glues and adhesives; (2) propellants for aerosol paint sprays, hair sprays, frying pan sprays, and shaving cream; (3) thinners (for example, for paint products and typing correction fluids); and (4) fuels. Because of their epidemiological and pharmacological differences, the fourth edition of *Diagnostic and Statistical Manual of Mental Disorders* (DSM-IV) excludes anesthetic gases and amyl and butyl nitrites from that group; DSM-IV classifies those as other (or unknown) substance-related disorders.

COMPARATIVE NOSOLOGY

The 1977 ninth revision of the *International Classification of Diseases and Related Health Problems* (ICD-9) mentioned glue sniffing under drug dependence, other, as did ICD-9-CM in its category other specified drug dependence. The 10th revision of ICD (ICD-10) uses the term "harmful use" instead of "abuse," as in DSM-IV. DSM-IV provides no diagnosis of inhalant withdrawal (which is clinically described but probably is rare), whereas that diagnosis apparently can be rendered in ICD-10. Inhalant-related disorders appear in Table 13.8-1. The section on inhalant-related disorders in DSM-IV lists three major categories: inhalant abuse, inhalant dependence, and inhalant intoxication. Table 13.8-2 provides the diagnostic criteria for inhalant intoxication. The other inhalant-related disorders have their diagnostic criteria specified in the DSM-IV sections that specifically address the major symptoms—for example, inhalant-induced psychotic disorders (see Section 15.3).

TABLE 13.8-1
Inhalant-Related Disorders

Inhalant use disorders

Inhalant dependence
Inhalant abuse

Inhalant-induced disorders

Inhalant intoxication
Inhalant intoxication delirium
Inhalant-induced persisting dementia
Inhalant-induced psychotic disorder, with delusions
Specify if: with onset during intoxication
Inhalant-induced psychotic disorder, with hallucinations
Specify if: with onset during intoxication
Inhalant-induced mood disorder
Specify if: with onset during intoxication
Inhalant-induced anxiety disorder
Specify if: with onset during intoxication

Inhalant-related disorder not otherwise specified

Table based on DSM-IV, *Diagnostic and Statistical Manual of Mental Disorders,* ed 4. Copyright American Psychiatric Association, Washington, 1994. Used with permission.

TABLE 13.8-2
Diagnostic Criteria for Inhalant Intoxication

A. Recent intentional use or short-term, high-dose exposure to volatile inhalants (excluding anesthetic gases and short-acting vasodilators).
B. Clinically significant maladaptive behavioral or psychological changes (e.g., belligerence, assaultiveness, apathy, impaired judgment, impaired social or occupational functioning) that developed during, or shortly after, use of or exposure to volatile inhalants.
C. Two (or more) of the following signs, developing during, or shortly after, inhalant use or exposure:
  (1) dizziness
  (2) nystagmus
  (3) incoordination
  (4) slurred speech
  (5) unsteady gait
  (6) lethargy
  (7) depressed reflexes
  (8) psychomotor retardation
  (9) tremor
  (10) generalized muscle weakness
  (11) blurred vision or diplopia
  (12) stupor or coma
  (13) euphoria
D. The symptoms are not due to a general medical condition and are not better accounted for by another mental disorder.

Table from DSM-IV, *Diagnostic and Statistical Manual of Mental Disorders,* ed 4. Copyright American Psychiatric Association, Washington, 1994. Used with permission.

EPIDEMIOLOGY

Inhalants infrequently cause drug-related emergencies, accounting for only 0.3 percent of 1989 drug episodes in federally monitored emergency rooms. Three age groups (10 to 19, 20 to 29, and 30 to 39 years) each accounted for about 30 percent of those visits, and over 20 percent of patients were 10 to 17 years of age. Male patients outnumbered female patients three to one.

Inhalants contributed to 1.0 percent of 1990 drug deaths in federally reviewed medical-examiner reports in the United States. In Great Britain, where toluene-containing compounds are the most popular of the inhalants, toluene deaths are less common than are those from other inhalants, suggesting that they are less toxic. First-time users there are the most likely to die, perhaps because they are inexperienced at that dangerous pastime.

The 1991 United States National Household Survey estimated that 5.6 percent of Americans had used an inhalant at some time in their lives; the estimate was 12 percent for men 18 to 34 years of age. About 0.6 percent had used in the month of the survey. Although reports of inhalant problems often focus on minority groups, in that survey proportionately more whites reported inhalant use than did blacks or Hispanics; however, school surveys in the 1970s and 1980s found prevalence rates in Native Americans to be consistently higher than for other groups. A different survey procedure found that of high school seniors in 1990 about 18 percent had used inhalants, 2.7 percent using within the survey month. Those percentages had risen steadily in successive senior classes since 1975 despite downturns for most other drugs.

Widespread experimentation with inhalants, relatively few current users, and still fewer inhalant emergencies or deaths suggest that most users try the drugs a few times and stop without mishap. But studies indicate a different course for adolescents with conduct disorder or adults with antisocial personality disorder. Their inhalant problems herald serious alcohol and polysubstance use in adulthood, and a few become deteriorated, chronic inhalant-dependent adults. Inhalant use also predicts later injections of drugs, an important consideration for the risk of acquiring the human immunodeficiency virus (HIV). In a general population survey persons reporting any use of inhalants were 45 times more likely than others to have injected drugs and those who had used both inhalants and cannabis were 89 times more likely to have injected drugs.

PHARMACOLOGY

Data on inhalant choice in the United States are limited, but of some 20 abused compounds, toluene and gasoline may be the most popular. Recommended industrial exposure limits for toluene are 100 parts per million (ppm) but inhaled concentrations from a glue-containing bag may reach 10,000 ppm, and several tubes may be consumed daily. About 15 to 20 breaths of 1 percent gasoline vapor produce several hours of intoxication. Sniffing vapor through the nose or huffing (taking deep breaths) through the mouth leads to transpulmonary absorption with very rapid drug access to the brain. Breathing through a solvent-soaked cloth, inhaling fumes from a glue-containing bag, or breathing vapor from a gasoline can are common; putting one's head and a soaked rag into a large plastic bag may cause suffocation.

Toluene blood levels in hospitalized intoxicated persons reportedly range from 0.8 to 8 μg/g. Brain and fat achieve higher levels because the lipophilic compounds preferentially distribute there. The coadministration of alcohol dramatically raises toluene blood levels, increasing toxicity, probably through competition for hepatic metabolizing enzymes. About 20 percent of a toluene dose is excreted unchanged in the breath but most is metabolized in the liver to hippuric acid before urinary excretion. Although toluene may fall to undetectable levels in blood four to 10 hours after exposure, urinary hippuric acid remains measurable somewhat longer; a creatinine-hippurate ratio greater than 1 g/g suggests toluene use but benzoic acid food preservatives may generate false-positive results.

The cellular mechanisms of inhalant action are unclear. Hypotheses include cell membrane fluidization or interactions at γ-aminobutyric acid (GABA)-gated chloride channels but data are very sparse. Behavioral actions in animals suggest that those drugs act like alcohol, barbiturates, and other depressants of the central nervous system (CNS). Like depressants they produce motor stimulation at lower doses and motor suppression at higher doses, as well as ataxia and loss of righting reflex. Inhalants also have anticonvulsant actions and show depressant-like effects in certain behavioral paradigms. Animals will work to self-administer inhalants. And animals trained to press one lever when injected with alcohol or pentobarbital and another when injected with saline will press the depressant-appropriate lever after exposure to toluene vapor, suggesting that the subjective experience after either toluene or a depressant is similar. Moreover, alcohol and benzodiazepines potentiate inhalant effects.

Rodents develop withdrawal seizures after having been exposed for several days to trichloroethane, a frequently abused inhalant. The seizures are blocked by toluene, ethanol, pentobarbital, and midazolam, a benzodiazepine. Thus, inhalants can produce physical dependence, and they show cross-dependence with familiar CNS depressants.

In human subjects low-dose (0, 75, or 150 ppm) toluene exposures for several hours produce dose-related decrements in tests of perception, memory, and manual dexterity, with increases in headaches, mucosal irritation, thirst, and sleepiness.

ADVERSE EFFECTS The inhalants are associated with many potentially serious adverse effects. The most serious adverse effect is death, which can result from respiratory depression, cardiac arrhythmias, asphyxiation, the aspiration of vomitus, or accident or injury (for example, by driving while intoxicated with inhalants). Other serious adverse effects associated with long-term inhalant use include irreversible hepatic or renal damage and permanent muscle damage associated with rhabdomyolysis. The combination of organic solvents and high concentrations of copper, zinc, and heavy metals has been associated with the development of brain atrophy, temporal lobe epilepsy, decreased intelligence quotient (I.Q.), and a variety of electroencephalographic (EEG) changes. Several studies of house painters and factory workers who have been exposed to solvents for long periods have found evidence of brain atrophy on computed tomography (CT) scans and decreases in cerebral blood flow. Additional adverse effects include cardiovascular and pulmonary symptoms (for example, chest pain and bronchospasm), gastrointestinal symptoms (for example, pain, nausea, vomiting, and hematemesis), and other neurological signs and symptoms (for example, peripheral neuritis, headache, paresthesia, cerebellar signs, and lead encephalopathy). There are reports of brain atrophy, renal tubular acidosis, and long-term motor impairment in toluene users. A number of reports concern serious adverse effects on fetal development when the pregnant mother uses or is exposed to inhalant substances.

ETIOLOGY

Inhalants are cheap, available in several forms in most households, easily concealed, legal to possess, and simple to take. They produce a quick high that passes within a few hours, facilitating their use and allowing the users to evade detection or punishment. In animals inhalants pharmacologically reinforce repeated self-administration. Adolescents usually gather in small groups to use inhalants and being a user gains entry to the group, socially reinforcing the use. Finally, living in an impoverished isolated community with few other available reinforcers may increase the attractiveness of inhalants as an exciting, rebellious, and novel experience, which may help to explain the high prevalence of inhalant use at some Indian reservations.

In addition to those extrinsic factors at least one intrinsic factor contributes to inhalant use. A risk-taking propensity that leads some persons to bungee jumping or motorcycle racing may lead others to the at-the-brink excitement and danger of inhalant intoxication. Persons with adolescent conduct disorder or adult antisocial personality disorder are prone to taking extreme risks, and many inhalant users have those disorders. Among youths in grades 7 through 12, in comparison with others who used no drugs or who used only cannabis or alcohol, inhalant users had many characteristics suggesting conduct disorder. They accepted cheating more readily, admitted more stealing, perceived less objection to drug use on the part of their families, liked school less, and reported more sadness, tension, and anger, and a feeling of being blamed by others. In addition, school surveys showed that solvent users were likely to be involved with other drugs. Similarly, among youths referred to court-mandated education for minor alcohol offenses, those who also used inhalants reported fewer school honors and more expulsions, truancy, academic failures, criminal offenses, running away, and associations with troubled peers, as well as many more drug and alcohol problems. More of them also had mothers or siblings with alcohol-related or drug-related problems.

INHALANT DEPENDENCE AND INHALANT ABUSE

DIAGNOSIS AND CLINICAL FEATURES The cardinal feature of inhalant abuse is repeated use of inhalants in ways that produce a physical hazard or adverse social consequences for the user (see Table 13.1-6). Inhalant dependence is characterized by repeated use resulting in some combination of adverse consequences, loss of control of the drug use, and tolerance or withdrawal (see Tables 13.1-2 and 13.1-5). Although DSM-IV provides no diagnosis for inhalant withdrawal, some withdrawal symptoms apparently do occur and complaints of withdrawal probably should contribute to the diagnosis of inhalant dependence.

DIFFERENTIAL DIAGNOSIS Polysubstance use is common in inhalant users, and abuse of or dependence on additional drugs always should be ruled out with a history, physical findings, and toxicological screens. Uncontrolled and impulsive behavior during repeated intoxications may mimic aspects of, or be comorbid with, conduct disorder or antisocial personality disorder. Antisocial behavior before the onset of inhalant abuse or dependence, or in periods of abstinence, suggests the presence of these disorders.

COURSE AND PROGNOSIS Recent studies indicate that inhalant use strongly predicts future diagnoses of antisocial personality disorder and other substance use disorders. However, the high prevalence of inhalant use indicated in high school surveys also suggests that many youthful inhalant users do not progress to other disorders. Such information led one expert to state that inhalant use "should be regarded as a passing phase or fad." It may be so for many youths, but as a comorbid condition with conduct disorder, inhalant abuse and inhalant dependence may herald serious future problems with personality disorders and other substance use disorders. Most of the latter persons will shift from inhalants to other drugs but some continue inhalant use. Such chronic patients may use the drugs for extended periods each day for many years; they demonstrate moderate criminal activity, weight loss, medical disease, slow and slurred speech, and impaired attention and memory, and often are dirty and louse-ridden.

Tolerance occurs and, less commonly, mild withdrawal involving sleep disturbance, irritability, shakiness, sweating, fleeting illusions, and nausea. One observer reported tachycardia, delusions, and hallucinations during withdrawal.

Medical problems in chronic users include (1) muscle weakness, sometimes with myoglobinuria and rhabdomyolysis; (2) gastrointestinal problems, such as pain, nausea, vomiting, or hematemesis; (3) renal dysfunction, often with severe electrolyte imbalance; (4) cardiomyopathy; (5) hepatotoxicity; (6) pulmonary disorders (pulmonary hypertension, increased airway resistance, and acute respiratory distress); and (7) hematopoietic disorders (including elevated carboxyhemoglobin levels, methemoglobinemia, hemolytic anemia, aplastic anemia, and even acute myelocytic leukemia). Neurological problems include (1) headache, (2) paresthesias with peripheral neuropathy, (3) reversible cerebellar signs or cerebellar degeneration, (4) radiological abnormalities of widened sulci and basal cisterns, and (5) dementia (for example, lead encephalopathy from leaded gasoline or white matter dementia from toluene).

Researchers have examined individual cases or small series of cases of mothers who regularly used toluene during pregnancy. The studies, although they need large-scale replication, strongly suggest that such inhalant use, often with accompanying distal renal tubular acidosis in the mother, has devastating effects. Mothers may experience nausea, vomiting, abdominal pain, elevated blood pressure, and early contractions. Preterm delivery is common, and even after correction for gestational age, the infants show intrauterine growth retardation. Growth retardation continues postnatally. Dysmorphic facies, similar to those of the fetal alcohol syndrome, may occur. Perinatal infant deaths are not infrequent. The management of pregnancy in inhalant-using women should aim at cessation of the drug use with attention to the early detection of renal tubular acidosis, preterm labor, and fetal growth retardation.

TREATMENT No controlled studies of inhalant abuse or inhalant dependence guide treatment. Appropriate medical care is required for the disorders' medical sequelae. Very low-key street outreach and extensive social service support have been offered to severely deteriorated inhalant-dependent homeless people. For less seriously disturbed patients numerous psychosocial treatments have been recommended, including family therapy, individual psychotherapy, and group treatment, but outcomes are unclear. The apparent spontaneous resolution of many cases suggests that any treatment will have many favorable outcomes, and recommendations for minimalist, nonalarmist interventions with parental participation seem warranted. But vigorous treatment is needed for patients with comorbid conduct disorder or antisocial personality disorder. Urine monitoring of hippuric acid two or three times a week should reveal relapses to toluene-containing inhalants.

INHALANT INTOXICATION

DIAGNOSIS AND CLINICAL FEATURES Inhalant intoxication is a maladaptive behavioral disorder that develops immediately after inhalant use and (assuming survival) clears a few hours later. Persons intoxicated with inhalants may smell of, or be stained with, the compounds. Perioral eczema from vapor-induced irritation is common. Intoxication signs initially may include vomiting and motor stimulation, followed by slowing, ataxia, depressed reflexes, slurred speech, disorientation, impaired judgment, lethargy, or coma. Bronchospasm, chest pain, cardiac arrhythmias or arrest, trauma, accidental burns, seizures, aspiration of vomitus, or suffocation in a plastic bag may result. Users commonly report such symptoms as slower speech, elated mood, fearfulness, illusions, auditory and visual hallucinations, delusions, and perceptions of altered body size. The DSM-IV diagnostic criteria are listed in Table 13.8-2.

DIFFERENTIAL DIAGNOSIS Its differentiation from other intoxications is aided by a history of inhalant use, the presence of inhalant odor and residues on the skin or clothing or a characteristic perioral rash from contact with organic solvents, and toxicological examination of body fluids. Polysubstance use is common among solvent users and concurrent intoxications with other drugs may be assessed by history and toxicological examinations. Despite evidence of inhalant intoxication other explanations for coma, such as closed head injury, must be considered. Dextrose 50 percent for injection (50 grams) and naloxone

(Narcan) 2 mg intravenously help rule out coma of diabetic or narcotic origin. If delirium develops in the course of an intoxication with inhalants, the diagnosis is inhalant intoxication delirium, rather than inhalant intoxication. If a mood disturbance, anxiety, or psychosis appears very prominently during an intoxication, and if the symptom is severe enough to warrant independent clinical attention, the diagnosis should be inhalant-induced mood disorder, inhalant-induced psychotic disorder, or inhalant-induced anxiety disorder, respectively.

COURSE AND PROGNOSIS The onset of intoxication is almost instantaneous after the inhalation of volatile hydrocarbons, given the rapid absorption of those inhalants across pulmonary membranes and their quick distribution into the brain and other lipids. Inhalant drugs are rapidly metabolized and excreted and inhalant intoxication usually lasts only a few hours. Unless trauma, hypoxia, cardiac arrest, burns, or other serious problems ensue, there probably are no lasting effects from one or a few intoxications, except that each use of a reinforcing drug increases the probability of further use. Prolonged, repeated use causes persisting effects.

TREATMENT Inhalant intoxication, like alcohol intoxication, usually receives no medical attention and resolves spontaneously. However, effects of the intoxication, such as coma, bronchospasm, laryngospasm, cardiac arrhythmias, trauma, or burns, will need treatment. Otherwise, care primarily involves reassurance, quiet support, and attention to vital signs and level of consciousness. Sedative drugs, including benzodiazepines, may potentiate inhalant effects. Following resolution of the intoxication a careful evaluation is needed with appropriate intervention or referral for inhalant abuse or dependence, other substance use disorders, conduct disorder, or antisocial personality disorder.

INHALANT INTOXICATION DELIRIUM

DSM-IV provides a diagnostic category for inhalant intoxication delirium (see Chapter 12). Inhalant intoxication delirium is a disturbance of consciousness and a change in cognition that result from intoxication with inhalants and that are not better explained by dementia. The course and treatment are like those of inhalant intoxication but the additional confusion requires special attention to patient safety. If the delirium results in severe behavioral disturbances, short-term treatment with a dopamine receptor antagonist—for example, haloperidol (Haldol)—may be necessary. Benzodiazepines should be avoided because of the possibility of adding to the patient's respiratory depression.

INHALANT-INDUCED PERSISTING DEMENTIA

DIAGNOSIS AND CLINICAL FEATURES Studies of inhalant-caused cognitive impairment have been equivocal and have been beset by numerous methodological problems, including a focus on adolescent users with briefer lifetime exposures. But clinical and some research evidence suggests that in some adults, repeated use of inhalants causes inhalant-induced persisting dementia (see Chapter 12). For example, among toluene users (average age, 29 years) studied with magnetic resonance imaging a strong correlation existed between the severity of the neuropsychological deficit and the severity of cerebral white matter abnormality.

The cardinal feature of the disorder is dementia resulting from the use of inhalants. Nearly all of those persons meet the criteria for inhalant dependence or inhalant abuse. Patients with inhalant-induced persisting dementia have memory impairment and at least one of the following: aphasia (language disturbance), apraxia (impaired ability to carry out motor activities despite intact motor function), agnosia (failure to recognize or identify objects despite intact sensory function), and disturbed executive functioning (planning, organizing, sequencing, abstracting). The symptoms must significantly impair social or occupational functioning, represent a decrement from earlier functioning, not occur exclusively in the course of a delirium, and persist beyond the usual duration of inhalant intoxication.

DIFFERENTIAL DIAGNOSIS Nearly all of the patients have inhalant dependence and many will be dependent on alcohol, which also produces dementia. Moreover, histories of head injury are very common among such patients. Thus, despite clear evidence of prolonged inhalant use the disorder requires a full evaluation for the multiple causes of dementia.

COURSE AND PROGNOSIS Few of such patients have been studied prospectively. Despite some reports of improvement when patients became abstinent from inhalants, it seems likely that most neuropsychological deficits that have persisted long after an intoxication will continue or worsen. Moreover, as dementia progresses patients become more difficult to treat and each relapse adds to their cerebral toxicity.

TREATMENT There is no established treatment for the cognitive and memory problems of inhalant-induced persisting dementia. Patients may require extensive support within their families or in foster or domiciliary care.

INHALANT-INDUCED PSYCHOTIC DISORDER

The diagnosis applies to patients who qualify for inhalant intoxication but also have additional psychotic symptoms to a greater degree than commonly occurs in inhalant intoxication. The additional symptoms must be sufficiently severe to warrant independent clinical attention. The clinician can specify whether the essential features of substance-induced psychotic disorders (see Section 15.3) are prominent hallucinations or delusions.

The course and treatment of those disorders are like those of inhalant intoxication. The disorders are brief in duration, lasting a few hours to a very few weeks beyond the intoxication. Confusion, panic, or psychosis mandate special attention to patient safety. Vigorous treatment of such life-threatening complications as respiratory or cardiac arrest, together with conservative management of the intoxication itself, is appropriate. Severe agitation may require cautious control with haloperidol (Haldol) 5 mg/70 kg intramuscularly, repeated once in 20 minutes if needed. Sedative drugs, including benzodiazepines, may potentiate inhalant intoxications.

INHALANT-INDUCED MOOD DISORDER AND INHALANT-INDUCED ANXIETY DISORDER

The essential feature of substance-induced mood disorder (see Section 16.6) is a persistent mood disturbance that is predominant in the clinical picture. The essential feature of substance-induced anxiety disorder (see Section 17.5) is prominent anxi-

TABLE 13.8-3
Inhalant-Related Disorder Not Otherwise Specified

The inhalant-related disorder not otherwise specified category is for disorders associated with the use of inhalants that are not classifiable as inhalant dependence, inhalant abuse, inhalant intoxication, inhalant intoxication delirium, inhalant-induced persisting dementia, inhalant-induced psychotic disorder, inhalant-induced mood disorder, or inhalant-induced anxiety disorder.

Table from DSM-IV, *Diagnostic and Statistical Manual of Mental Disorders,* ed 4. Copyright American Psychiatric Association, Washington, 1994. Used with permission.

ety symptoms. The clinician also must judge, in each disorder, that the additional symptoms result from the direct physiological effects of the substance. Depressive disorders probably are the most common mood disorders associated with inhalant use, and panic disorders and generalized anxiety disorder probably are the most common anxiety disorders. Antidepressant or antimanic drugs are seldom needed for substance-induced mood disorder.

INHALANT-RELATED DISORDER NOT OTHERWISE SPECIFIED

The diagnosis of inhalant-related disorder not otherwise specified (NOS) is the DSM-IV diagnosis for inhalant-related disorders that do not fit into one of the above diagnostic categories (Table 13.8-3).

SUGGESTED CROSS-REFERENCES

An overview of substance-related disorders is given in Section 13.1, hallucinogen-related disorders are discussed in Section 13.7, and phencyclidine-related disorders are discussed in Section 13.10. Mood disorders are discussed in Chapter 16.

REFERENCES

Crider R A, Rouse B A: Epidemiology of inhalant abuse: An update. NIDA Res Monogr *85:* 1, 1988.
Crites J, Schuckit M A: Solvent misuse in adolescents at a community alcohol center. J Clin Psychiatry *40:* 39, 1979.
Dinwiddie S H, Reich T, Cloninger C R: Solvent use and psychiatric comorbidity. Br J Addict *85:* 1647, 1990.
*Dinwiddie S H, Reich T, Cloninger C R: The relationship of solvent use to other substance use. Am J Drug Alcohol Abuse *17:* 173, 1991.
*Dinwiddie S H, Reich T, Cloninger C R: Solvent use as a precursor to intravenous drug abuse. Compr Psychiatry *32:* 133, 1991.
Echeverria D, Fine L, Langolf G, Schork A, Sampaio C: Acute neurobehavioral effects of toluene. Br J Ind Med *46:* 483, 1989.
*Evans E B, Balster R L: CNS depressant effects of volatile organic solvents. Neurosci Biobehav Rev *15:* 233, 1991.
Evans E B, Balster R L: Inhaled 1,1,1-trichloroethane-produced physical dependence in mice: Effects of drugs and vapors on withdrawal. J Pharmacol Exp Ther *264:* 726, 1993.
Filley C M, Heaton R K, Rosenberg N L: White matter dementia in chronic toluene abuse. Neurology *40:* 532, 1990.
Jacobs A M, Ghodse A H: Delinquency and regular solvent abuse: An unfavourable combination? Br J Addict *83:* 965, 1988.
Johns A: Volatile substance abuse and 963 deaths. Br J Addict *86:* 1053, 1991.
Johnston L D, O'Malley P M, Bachman J G: Drug abuse among American high school seniors, college students and young adults, 1975-1990. U.S. Department of Health and Human Services, Washington, 1991.
*McHugh M J: The abuse of volatile substances. Pediatr Clin North Am *34:* 333, 1987.
*Morton H G: Occurrence and treatment of solvent abuse in children and adolescents. Pharmacol Ther *33:* 449, 1987.
National Institute on Drug Abuse: National household survey on drug abuse: population estimates 1991. DHHS Publication No. (ADM) 92-1887, 1991.
National Institute on Drug Abuse: Annual medical examiner data 1990, data from the drug abuse warning network (DAWN). DHHS Publication No. (ADM) 91-1840, 1991.
National Institute on Drug Abuse: Annual data 1989, data from the drug abuse warning network (DAWN). DHHS Inhalant. Publication No. (ADM) 90-1717, 1990.
Pearson M A, Hoyme E, Seaver L H, Rimsza M E: Toluene embryopathy: Delineation of the phenotype and comparison with fetal alcohol syndrome. Pediatrics *93:* 211, 1994
Ramsey J, Anderson H R, Bloor K, Flanagan R J: An introduction to the practice, prevalence and chemical toxicology of volatile substance abuse. Hum Toxicol *8:* 261, 1989.
Ron M A: Volatile substance abuse: A review of possible long-term neurological, intellectual and psychiatric sequelae. Br J Psychiatry *148:* 235, 1986.
Rosenberg N L, Kleinschmidt-DeMasters, Davis K A, Dreisbach J N, Hormes J T, Filley C M: Toluene abuse causes diffuse central nervous system white matter changes. Ann Neurol *23:* 611, 1988.
Schutz C G, Chilcoat H D, Anthony J C: The association between sniffing inhalants and injecting drugs. Compr Psychiatry *35:* 99, 1994.
Sharp C W, Rosenberg N L: Volatile substances. In *Substance Abuse: A Comprehensive Textbook,* ed 2. J H Lowinson, P Ruiz, R B Millman, J G Langrod, editors, p 303. Williams & Wilkins, Baltimore, 1992.
Streicher H Z, Gabow P A, Moss A H, Kono D, Kaehny W D: Syndromes of toluene sniffing in adults. Ann Intern Med *94:* 758, 1981.
Westermeyer J: The psychiatrist and solvent-inhalant abuse: Recognition, assessment, and treatment. Am J Psychiatry *144:* 903, 1987.
Wilkins-Haug L, Gabow P A: Toluene abuse during pregnancy: Obstetric complications and perinatal outcomes. Obstet Gynecol *77:* 504, 1991.
World Health Organization: *International Statistical Classification of Diseases and Related Health Problems, Tenth Revision, Volume 1.* World Health Organization, Geneva, 1992.

13.9 OPIOID-RELATED DISORDERS

JEROME H. JAFFE, M.D.

INTRODUCTION

Although there are more than 20 chemically distinct opioid drugs in clinical use, the most prevalent problems are associated with heroin, a drug that is not used for therapeutic purposes in the United States. Dependence on other opioids is limited largely to persons who have developed dependence in the course of medical treatment or to health care professionals who have access to opioids. Virtually all of the dependence and abuse encountered clinically is associated with prototypical μ-agonist opioids. Those agents are included in Schedule I or II of the Controlled Substances Act, although some mixtures (for example, codeine and aspirin) are included in Schedules III or IV of the Controlled Substances Act. Abuse or dependence is occasionally seen with opioids that are not prototypical μ-agonists but have actions at other opioid receptors. Those mixed agonist-antagonists (for example, pentazocine [Talwin], nalbuphine [Nubain]) are either not included in the Controlled Substances Act or are included in Schedule III, IV, or V. Those agents will not be considered separately because dependence on them is relatively uncommon and the clinical course of dependence is not well established. All of the μ-agonists produce similar subjective effects. However, the patterns of opioid use and some aspects of toxicity are powerfully influenced by the route of administration and the metabolism of the specific opioid, as well as by the social conditions that determine its costs and purity and the sanctions attached to its use for nonmedical purposes.

DEFINITIONS

Substance use may be associated with a number of distinct disorders, of which substance dependence and abuse are but two. In the case of the opioid drugs, nine other opioid-related disorders have been described (Table 13.9-1).

Opioid dependence (see Tables 13.1-2 and 13.1-5) is a cluster of physiological, behavioral, and cognitive symptoms that taken together indicate that the person continues to use an opioid drug despite significant problems related to such use. Drug dependence in general has also been defined by the World Health Organization (WHO) as a syndrome in which the use of the drugs or of a class of drugs takes on a much higher priority for a given person than do other behaviors that once had a higher value. Both of those brief definitions have as their central features the emphasis on the drug-using behavior itself, its maladaptive nature, and on how the choice to engage in that behavior has shifted and become constrained as a result of interaction with the drug over time.

TABLE 13.9-1
Opioid-Related Disorders

Opioid use disorders

Opioid dependence
Opioid abuse

Opioid-induced disorders

Opioid intoxication
Specify if: With perceptual disturbances
Opioid withdrawal
Opioid intoxication delirium
Opioid-induced psychotic disorder, with delusions
Specify if: With onset during intoxication
Opioid-induced psychotic disorder, with hallucinations
Specify if: With onset during intoxication
Opioid-induced mood disorder
Specify if: With onset during intoxication
Opioid-induced sexual dysfunction
Specify if: With onset during intoxication
Opioid-induced sleep disorder
Specify if: With onset during intoxication/with onset during withdrawal

Opioid-related disorder not otherwise specified

Table based on DSM-IV, *Diagnostic and Statistical Manual of Mental Disorders,* ed 4. Copyright American Psychiatric Association, Washington, 1994. Used with permission.

TABLE 13.9-2
Diagnostic Criteria for Opioid Intoxication

A. Recent use of an opioid.
B. Clinically significant maladaptive behavioral or psychological changes (e.g., initial euphoria followed by apathy, dysphoria, psychomotor agitation or retardation, impaired judgment, or impaired social or occupational functioning) that developed during, or shortly after, opioid use.
C. Pupillary constriction (or pupillary dilation due to anoxia from severe overdose) and one (or more) of the following signs, developing during, or shortly after, opioid use:
   (1) drowsiness or coma
   (2) slurred speech
   (3) impairment in attention or memory
D. The symptoms are not due to a general medical condition and are not better accounted for by another mental disorder.

Specify if:
With perceptual disturbances

Table from DSM-IV, *Diagnostic and Statistical Manual of Mental Disorders,* ed 4. Copyright American Psychiatric Association, Washington, 1994. Used with permission.

TABLE 13.9-3
Diagnostic Criteria for Opioid Withdrawal

A. Either of the following:
   (1) cessation of (or reduction in) opioid use that has been heavy and prolonged (several weeks or longer)
   (2) administration of an opioid antagonist after a period of opioid use
B. Three (or more) of the following, developing within minutes to several days after criterion A:
   (1) dysphoric mood
   (2) nausea or vomiting
   (3) muscle aches
   (4) lacrimation or rhinorrhea
   (5) pupillary dilation, piloerection, or sweating
   (6) diarrhea
   (7) yawning
   (8) fever
   (9) insomnia
C. The symptoms in criterion B cause clinically significant distress or impairment in social, occupational, or other important areas of functioning.
D. The symptoms are not due to a general medical condition and are not better accounted for by another mental disorder.

Table from DSM-IV, *Diagnostic and Statistical Manual of Mental Disorders,* ed 4. Copyright American Psychiatric Association, Washington, 1994. Used with permission.

TABLE 13.9-4
Opioid-Related Disorder Not Otherwise Specified

The opioid-related disorder not otherwise specified category is for disorders associated with the use of opioids that are not classifiable as opioid dependence, opioid abuse, opioid intoxication, opioid withdrawal, opioid intoxication delirium, opioid-induced psychotic disorder, opioid-induced mood disorder, opioid-induced sexual dysfunction, or opioid-induced sleep disorder.

Opioid abuse (see Table 13.1-6) is a term used to categorize a pattern of maladaptive use of an opioid drug leading to clinically significant impairment or distress and occurring within a 12-month period, but one in which the symptoms have never met the criteria for opioid dependence.

According to the fourth edition of *Diagnostic and Statistical Manual of Mental Disorders* (DSM-IV), the opioid-induced disorders include opioid intoxication (Table 13.9-2), opioid withdrawal (Table 13.9-3), opioid-induced sleep disorder (see Chapter 23), and sexual dysfunction (see Section 21.1a). Those disorders are commonly seen. DSM-IV also includes opioid-induced intoxication delirium (see Chapter 12), which is occasionally seen in hospitalized medical patients. However, opioid-induced psychotic disorder with delusions or with hallucinations (see Section 15.3), opioid-induced mood disorder (see Section 16.6), and opioid-induced anxiety disorder (see Section 17.5) are exceedingly uncommon with μ-agonist opioids, but have been seen with certain mixed agonist-antagonist opioids acting at other receptors. DSM-IV also includes opioid-related disorder not otherwise specified (NOS) for situations that do not meet the criteria for any of the other opioid-related disorders (Table 13.9-4).

The DSM-IV coding scheme provides distinct code numbers for opioid dependence and opioid abuse, but as noted, the codes for the other substance-induced mental disorders do not differentiate among several distinct opioid-induced disorders or from disorders induced by other substances. In some cases the same codes must be used for disorders induced by a wide variety of substances.

HISTORY

Opioids have been used for at least 3,500 years. For most of that time, they were used in the form of crude opium or in alcoholic solutions of opium (containing morphine and codeine). Morphine was first isolated in 1806, and codeine was isolated in 1832. Over the next century, the pure drugs morphine and codeine gradually replaced crude opium for medicinal purposes, although nonmedical use of opium (as for smoking) still persists in some parts of the world. The first semisynthetic derivative—diacetylmorphine, or heroin—was introduced into medicine in 1898. The first purely synthetic opioids, meperidine (Demerol) and methadone (Dolophine), were introduced into medical practice in the 1940s.

Opioid dependence, or at least opioid withdrawal, was first recognized in 1700. Although opioid dependence was common by the middle of the 19th century, it was not until later in the century that it came to be seen as an important medical problem. Public concern about opium smoking among Chinese immigrants, the emergence of more severe forms of dependence associated with the newly introduced hypodermic needle and syringe, and a growing awareness of the problem of allowing opioids to be sold in over-the-counter patent medicines and to be casually dispensed by practitioners with minimal training generated media attention and public debate. The debate, combined with international considerations, led to legislation at the state and federal levels that restricted opioid use to medically recognized purposes and required a legitimate prescription for most use. In the United States the Harrison Act of 1914 had a profound influence on those who were already addicted. The new law was interpreted as excluding the provision of opioids to addicts as a legitimate medical use. Clinics that had been established to provide morphine to addicts were closed, the last in 1923. Doctors were encouraged to avoid opioid addicts entirely. Treatment efforts were a disappointment to both physicians and patients: relapse after detoxification was typical. An illicit traffic arose that provided access to opioids (mostly morphine and heroin) to persons who no longer could use medical channels to get their drugs. Addicts were arrested both for possession and sale. In the early 1930s two federal hospitals were established—at Lexington, Kentucky, and Fort Worth, Texas—to deal with the growing number of federal prisoners who were addicted by providing the long-term residential treatment then believed to be needed, but follow-up studies found that relapse rates were very high despite long periods of treatment.

Although increasingly harsh penalties for the sale or possession of opioids were enacted, heroin addiction persisted and its prevalence rose following World War II. By the early 1960s some thoughtful observers recommended remedicalizing heroin distribution as a way to reduce crime associated with heroin addiction.

However, several new developments in treatment techniques sharply altered the general perception of opioid dependence as an essentially untreatable disorder. They included the development of therapeutic communities based on Synanon (an organization that began in California in 1958), the creation of large-scale civil commitment programs in California (1961) and New York (1965), demonstration by Vincent Dole and Marie Nyswander of the effectiveness of maintenance on oral methadone in decreasing crime and heroin use (1965), and the availability of long-acting opioid antagonists, along with the finding that some addicts were willing to take them.

Starting in the late 1960s, federal and state sources increased support for both research and treatment. In response to the outbreak of heroin addiction among United States military personnel in Vietnam, federal support for treatment was greatly expanded and accelerated. That support was not merely monetary, but included legislation providing for the legitimate use of methadone and protection of the confidentiality of patient records.

In the mid-1970s the four dominant treatment modalities were brief detoxification, methadone maintenance, therapeutic communities, and a heterogeneous category generally designated as drug-free outpatient care. Civil commitment declined in influence and support. In the early 1980s, with the expansion of private insurance to cover treatment for alcohol abuse and drug dependence, in-hospital treatment programs based on the 12-step model pioneered in Minnesota proliferated. While these programs were initially developed as treatments for alcohol abuse, they were gradually broadened to deal with a wider range of dependence, including opioid dependence. For a brief period, chemical dependence programs became an additional significant option in the array of treatments available to persons who were dependent on opioids. By the late 1980s, however, the rising cost of treatment and growing government deficits stimulated the emergence of managed care. The impact of managed-care-mandated changes on the support for the treatment of opioid dependence has not yet been fully felt.

COMPARATIVE NOSOLOGY

The DSM-IV criteria for opioid dependence are the same generic criteria that are applied to other psychoactive drugs; the notion of a generic concept of dependence is shared with the revised third edition of DSM (DSM-III-R) and the 10th revision of the *International Classification of Diseases and Related Health Problems* (ICD-10). In making the diagnosis of dependence, there generally is a high level of agreement between DSM-IV and ICD-10: they employ similar concepts (the dependence syndrome varying in degree of severity), although the wording of the criteria for determining the presence and severity of the syndrome differs. Both require that three elements of the syndrome occur within a 12-month period. The degree of agreement between DSM-IV and DSM-III-R is even higher, since, despite some changes in the wording, the syndromes and criteria in the two editions are quite similar. Although DSM-IV appears to lay greater stress on tolerance and physiological dependence, in practice, even if those criteria had been required, that would not have substantially reduced the number of cases meeting the criteria for dependence on opioids. Virtually all heavy opioid abusers report tolerance and withdrawal at some point in the course of drug use, and continued use to avoid withdrawal symptoms is a hallmark of opioid dependence.

The major changes between DSM-III-R and DSM-IV affected the diagnosis of drug abuse. DSM-III-R required the presence of only one of two general criteria, whereas DSM-IV requires one of four. Nevertheless, for both opioid dependence and abuse, the agreement between DSM-III-R and DSM-IV is exceedingly high.

There is a major difference between DSM-IV and ICD-10 in the definition of what is called substance abuse in DSM-IV. ICD-10 does not use the term "abuse." Instead, it includes a category of harmful use that is substantially different from the concept of abuse in DSM-IV. But the concept of harmful use is limited to physical and mental health (for example, hepatitis, overdose, skin abscess). It specifically excludes social impairments. ICD-10 states: "Harmful patterns of use are often criticized by others and frequently associated with adverse social consequences of various kinds. The fact that a pattern of use or a particular substance is disapproved of by another person or by the culture, or may have led to socially negative consequences such as arrest or marital arguments is not in itself evidence of harmful use."

Another distinction between ICD-10 and DSM-IV is the coding system, which limits the number of distinct drug-induced syndromes that can be recorded (except under the categories "other" and "unspecified") as disorders induced by opioids. In contrast, the ICD-10, which uses a different coding system, separates, for record-keeping purposes, mental and behavioral disorders due to use of opioids from those caused by other categories of drugs.

EPIDEMIOLOGY

In the United States opioid use has not fluctuated as dramatically over the past two decades as has the use of cocaine, but it did rise substantially in Eastern and Western Europe. There are a number of activities aimed at estimating the extent and consequences of psychoactive drug use in the United States. All the regularly recurring estimating techniques have sampling limitations, and none apply standardized diagnostic criteria to substance-use patterns or adverse effects. Consequently, while they provide a picture of substance use over time, the methods do not reveal changes in the incidence and prevalence of specific substance-related disorders, such as substance dependence and substance abuse.

In the annual High School Senior Survey ("Monitoring the Future") heroin use within the past 30 days of answering the survey has been at a very low level (less than 1 percent) over the past 18 years, in contrast to the rise and fall of such drugs as cannabis and cocaine. Self-reported use of opioids other than heroin among high school seniors has always been higher than for heroin. Lifetime use rates for heroin peaked at 2.8 percent in 1975 and fell to 0.9 percent in 1991. The lifetime use rate for other opiates fell from a peak of 10.3 percent in 1977 to 6.6 percent in 1991. For the population as a whole ages 12 and older, the 1993 National Household Survey on Drug Abuse (NHSDA) found the use of heroin within the past year to be 0.2 to 0.3 percent, and use within the past 30 days was less than 0.1 percent. Recent (past 30 days) nonmedical use of analgesics was 0.7 percent.

Two population surveys have used accepted criteria to measure the extent of drug abuse and dependence: the Epidemiologic Catchment Area (ECA) Study, carried out in the early 1980s using criteria from the third edition of DSM (DSM-III), and the National Comorbidity Survey (NCS), carried out from 1990 to 1992 using DSM-III-R criteria. The NCS found the lifetime prevalence of heroin use to be 1.5 percent overall, but with a prevalence of 2.7 percent among 35-year-olds to 44-year-olds, probably reflecting the peak of the heroin epidemic among adolescents and young adults in the late 1960s and early 1970s. Heroin dependence (lifetime) was 0.4 percent overall, but 0.8 percent among 35-year-olds to 44-year-olds. Those findings indicate that about 32 percent of those who used heroin at the peak of the epidemic became dependent at some time in their lives.

Lifetime history of extramedical use of opioid analgesics (other than heroin) was 9.7 percent, with the highest prevalence among 15-year-olds to 34-year-olds, suggesting a different pattern from that of heroin. Overall, only 7.5 percent of those who used opioid analgesics outside of a medical context developed dependence as defined by DSM-III-R. Obviously, the six-month and current prevalence rates of dependence would be lower than these lifetime rates.

The use and dependence rates derived from national surveys do not accurately reflect fluctuations in drug use among opioid-dependent and previously opioid-dependent populations. When the supply of illicit heroin increases in purity or decreases in price, as seemed to be the case in 1994, use among that very vulnerable population tends to increase, with subsequent increases in adverse consequences (emergency room visits) and requests for treatment.

ETIOLOGY

Substance dependence is currently viewed as the result of a process in which multiple interacting factors (social, psychological, cultural, and biological) influence substance-using behavior. The process, in some cases, leads to the loss of flexibility with respect to use that is the hallmark of dependence. In this biopsychosocial perspective the actions of the substance are seen as critical, but not all persons who become dependent experience the effects of a given substance in the same way or are influenced by the same set of factors, and even with the same class or pharmacological agents, different factors may be more or less important at different stages of the process.

With opioids, as with most substances, it is largely social and cultural factors that influence availability and initial use. In the case of opioid drugs, however, pharmacological factors, the initial effects and their consequences, are believed to play very important roles in the perpetuation of use and of progression to dependence. Opioids have potent mood-elevating and euphorigenic actions in humans and are powerful reinforcers in animal models. That is particularly true when the effects are rapid in onset, such as when the opioids are injected or inhaled. The opioids, perhaps more than any other category of drugs, can induce a variety of physical dependence that results in an aversive withdrawal syndrome when brain opioid levels decline. That aversive syndrome appears to play a key role in perpetuating opioid use and in relapse after brief periods of withdrawal.

PHARMACOLOGICAL FACTORS Because the reinforcing and physical dependence-inducing effects of opioid drugs play such an important role in the genesis of dependence (as well as in opioid-induced disorders), the pharmacology of the opioids is briefly summarized here.

Opioids and opioid receptors The discovery of multiple, stereospecific opioid receptors and endogenous ligands for those receptors made it easier to understand the multiple actions of morphinelike drugs and of some of the drugs that only partially resembled morphine. Those discoveries, however, also made it necessary to redefine the term "opioid." Opioid now refers to any exogenous substance that binds specifically to any of several subspecies of opioid receptors and produces some agonistic action. Such opioids may have a pharmacological profile dissimilar to that of morphine (a prototypical μ-agonist), may bind to various receptor subtypes in a pattern distinct from that of morphine, and may not suppress the morphine abstinence syndrome. Drugs that bind to any of the subtypes of receptors, but initiate no actions, are termed opioid antagonists.

During the first few years of research in the area, several opioid receptor subtypes were described, including: (1) μ, where classic opioids such as morphine bind preferentially and produce actions; (2) κ, where drugs such as butorphanol (Stadol) and nalbuphine are believed to exert some of their effects; and (3) δ, which appears to be the preferential binding site for the endogenous pentapeptide met-enkephalin, as well as for several synthetic peptides. With the development of more specific ligands, subtypes of the μ-, δ-, and κ-receptors have also been identified. Several of those distinct receptor subtypes have been cloned in the laboratory.

The σ-receptor was named for the benzomorphan derivative SKF-10,047, which, in dogs, induced excitation and hallucinatory effects but little or no analgesia. Because binding to the σ-receptor is not antagonized by naloxone (Narcan), it is no longer considered an opioid receptor. As is the case with the opioid receptors, several subtypes of σ-receptor have been identified. Since phencyclidine (PCP) may exert some of its actions through that family of receptors, they are discussed at greater length in connection with that drug.

The actions of μ-agonist opioids are exerted primarily at receptors on neural tissues in the central nervous system (CNS), the autonomic nervous system, and, to some uncertain degree, on opioid receptors on white blood cells. The actions of opioids include analgesia, respiratory depression, changes in mood (often euphoria in some persons), indifference to anticipated distress, drowsiness, decreased ability to concentrate, changes in endocrine and other functions regulated by the hypothalamus, and increased tone of smooth muscle in the gastrointestinal tract. μ-Agonists also induce tolerance and neuroadaptive changes in the CNS that result in distressing withdrawal phenomena when the agonist is stopped.

Most of the opioids that are associated with opioid abuse and dependence are typical μ-agonists, having pharmacological profiles that are quite similar to that of morphine and differing primarily in terms of metabolism and pharmacokinetics. Thus heroin is more potent and more lipid soluble than morphine, thereby crossing the blood-brain barrier more rapidly and producing a more rapid onset of subjective effects. However, heroin is hydrolyzed quite rapidly to 6-monoacetylmorphine and morphine. Its actions are probably exerted primarily through those metabolites binding to μ-receptors, although 6-monoacetylmorphine may bind to δ-receptors as well. In contrast, drugs that act at κ-receptors, such as U-50,4884 or ethyl ketocyclazocine, produce some dysphoria and no significant pupillary change, but still induce analgesia.

Codeine (3-methoxymorphine) occurs naturally (0.5 percent) in opium. Codeine is probably a prodrug; after absorption, it is transformed to some degree into morphine, which accounts for its opioid effects. Codeine itself does not bind with great affinity to μ-receptors, but it does cause some toxicity, and that probably accounts for its relatively low abuse potential. Hydrocodone and oxycodone are also prodrugs that require metabolic conversion for full activity. Methadone appears to be a typical μ-receptor agonist, but with an extended duration of action after repeated administration. Meperidine has numerous μ-receptor actions, but probably has some actions at other receptors as well. One of its metabolites, normeperidine, has convulsant properties, and addicts who use excessive amounts may achieve high enough levels of the metabolite to experience delirium and frank seizures. Similar toxicity may be seen in patients receiving meperidine for pain when the excretion of normeperidine is reduced by impaired renal function.

Tolerance and physical dependence appear to be specific for each major receptor type. Thus when tolerance to a given action develops to a μ-agonist, such as morphine, some cross-tolerance will be seen with other μ-agonists. However, when tolerance develops to a selective κ-agonist, such as the investigational drug U-50,488, there is no cross-tolerance to μ-agonists. Furthermore, physical dependence induced by κ-agonists has distinct characteristics and a different pattern of withdrawal signs and symptoms. In animals when physical dependence is induced by δ-agonists, withdrawal is similar to that seen with the μ-agonists.

All of the opioid receptor types are linked by G proteins either to second messenger systems or directly to ion channels. μ-Receptors and δ-receptors are coupled through G_1 proteins to adenylate cyclase or to potassium (K^+) ion channels. Activation of μ-receptors and δ-receptors opens potassium ion channels, thereby decreasing calcium conductance. Activation of κ-receptors results in the closing of calcium ion channels. Decreased calcium conductance is believed to be responsible for decreased transmitter release.

Several analgesics now available have actions at more than one receptor type. Some have antagonist actions at one type and agonist actions at another. For example, pentazocine has reinforcing properties and is self-administered by animals and some addicted persons, but it does not appear to exhibit a significant degree of cross-tolerance with μ-agonists and does not suppress μ-agonist withdrawal to any significant degree. It may be a μ-antagonist or very weak μ-agonist and κ-agonist. Some drug users in the United States inject pentazocine along with tripelennamine (PBZ), an antihistamine that has some euphorigenic effects in its own right. That drug combination is referred to as T's and B's (Talwin and the blue color of tripelennamine).

Buprenorphine (Buprenex) is a partial agonist at the μ-receptor. It supports μ-receptor physical dependence when the degree of physical dependence is low to moderate but precipitates withdrawal when the degree of dependence is high. Since most opioid-dependent persons have a low to moderate level of dependence, buprenorphine typically suppresses withdrawal and maintains dependence. It generally produces neither typical μ-agonist effects nor precipitated withdrawal in patients maintained on doses of methadone below 30 mg. With methadone doses above 60 mg, some withdrawal may occur.

Endogenous opioid substances Three distinct neurobiological opioid peptide systems, or families, have now been described. Each of the systems has a distinct genetic basis, separate biosynthetic pathways, and distinct precursor molecules. The anatomical distributions of the cells that produce and release the respective endogenous peptides are also distinct, but there is sometimes considerable overlap. These three systems are usually referred to as (1) the pro-opiomelanocortin (POMC) system, (2) the proenkephalin system, and (3) the prodynorphin system. Each precursor protein produces more than one active peptide that can be detected in body tissues.

The POMC precursor molecule is a 265-amino-acid protein that contains the 91 amino acid peptide β-lipotropin (β-LPH), as well as adrenocorticotropin hormone (ACTH) and melanocyte-stimulating hormone (MSH). Peptides 61 to 91 in β-lipotropin make up β-endorphin, one of the active opioid fragments produced by the POMC family. The enkephalin system consists primarily of the pentapeptides met-enkephalin (tyr-gly-gly-phe-met) and leu-enkephalin (tyr-gly-gly-phe-leu). In proenkephalin, a 263-amino-acid protein, met-enkephalin or met-enkephalin extended peptides are six times as prevalent as leu-enkephalin. Several additional opioid peptides are also derived from proenkephalin. From the parent pro-dynorphin, the dynorphin system produces the 17-amino-acid peptide dynorphin and several other active dynorphin peptides, all of which are c-terminal extensions of leu-enkephalin. They include dynorphin A (1–17), dynorphin A (1–8), dynorphin B (1–13), α-neoendorphin, and β-neoendorphin, and others.

The processing of the precursor molecules to smaller peptides is tissue specific. For example, in the rat the POMC precursor is processed to different peptides by the anterior and intermediate lobes of the pituitary.

The various endogenous peptides tend to bind preferentially to one or more of the opioid receptor subtypes. For example, met-enkephalin appears to prefer δ-receptors, and the dynorphin family of peptides display their highest affinity for κ-receptors. However, β-endorphin binds to both μ-receptors and δ-receptors and does not appear to be as selective as are other endogenous ligands. Preferential binding is not the same as exclusive binding. Peptides that bind preferentially to one set of receptors can, in high enough concentrations, exert actions at receptors for which they have lower affinities. Researchers have suggested that rather than attempting to categorize an endogenous substance with respect to the receptor at which it acts, it would be preferable to present its binding selectivity profile. Thus far, no endogenous peptide has been found that binds as preferentially to the μ-receptor as do such drugs as morphine. Several laboratories have confirmed the presence of morphine and codeine in mammalian brain and adrenal gland and in human cerebrospinal fluid (CSF). Highest concentrations are found in adrenal glands and spinal cord. Since no exogenous sources could be identified, the morphine and codeine so identified are thought to be of endogenous origin, although the synthetic pathways and possible biological function of those nonpeptide substances are still uncertain. Other findings not yet fully explored are the isolation from brain of natural cleavage products of β-endorphin, which are more potent than naloxone as opioid antagonists; the capacity of certain dynorphin fragments to modify opioid withdrawal; and the likelihood that some of those fragments act at nonopioid receptors.

Also of considerable interest is a family of neuropeptides that is not derived from any of the three precursor molecules described, but appear to act as endogenous opioid antagonists or weak agonists. Those peptides, variously referred to as FMRF-amide peptides, FMRF-related peptides, and neuropeptide FF (NPFF), are the subject of active research. NPFF appears to act at distinct receptors, since it binds poorly to opioid receptors.

TOLERANCE Tolerance does not develop uniformly to all of the actions of opioid drugs. There can be high levels of tolerance to some actions of opioids (such that it requires a 100-fold increase in dose to produce the original effect) when responses to other drug actions show only modest tolerance. With opioids, there can be remarkable tolerance to their analgesic, respiratory depressant, and sedative actions, but markedly less to their miotic effects and their constipating actions on the bowel. Intermediate degrees of tolerance to endocrine actions develop, and there appears to be less tolerance to the capacity of opioids to lower the threshold for electrical self-stimulation of the brain. Opioids occupying the same receptor types exhibit a considerable degree of cross-tolerance.

PHYSICAL DEPENDENCE (OPIOID NEUROADAPTATION) Physical (physiological) dependence is a substance-induced change in a biological system that becomes manifest by a characteristic response pattern, the withdrawal syndrome, when the drug is removed from the body or displaced from its receptor. In general, these responses are opposite in direction to the acute agonistic effects of the drugs, that is, they are rebound hyperexcitabilities. The neuroadaptive changes induced by the repeated administration of opioids occur in cells bearing opioid receptors and in neural systems widespread throughout the organism. In humans the changes begin with the first few doses. For example, if single intramuscular doses of 15 to 18 mg of morphine are given to opiate-naive subjects or abstinent former opiate users, large doses of naloxone (10 to 30 mg) given within 24 hours will precipitate a mild μ-agonist withdrawal syndrome. However, some period of continuous receptor occupation is required before the syndrome reaches a high enough level of intensity that withdrawal responses are obvious to the clinical observer. Withdrawal phenomena are more intense and more readily detectable when the opioid is rapidly removed from its receptor, as happens with opioid antagonist administration.

Opioid withdrawal phenomena can be suppressed by any opioid that occupies the same receptor, as in the phenomenon of cross-dependence. Recent findings suggest that opioid tolerance and neuroadaptive changes are relatively specific to receptor subtypes: κ-agonists do not suppress withdrawal from μ-agonist-induced physical dependence.

Mechanisms of tolerance and physical dependence A variety of mechanisms have been put forth to account for the general observation that opioid tolerance and physical dependence tend to develop in parallel and that withdrawal phenomena tend to be opposite in direction to the acute effects produced by the drugs. Among the mechanisms that have been proposed are changes in gene expression of endogenous opioids, alterations in intracellular Ca^{++} concentration, variations in receptor number or receptor ligand affinities, changes in mechanisms linking receptors to ion channels or second messengers, alterations in neural pathways, and increased concentrations of endogenous peptide antagonists. Those mechanisms are not mutually exclusive. Indeed, they appear to be complementary, and supportive data exist for several of the mechanisms. Opioid drugs can alter the expression of the genes encoding the opioid neurotransmitters. For example, the chronic administration of morphine results in down-regulation of proenkephalin expression in striatal neurons, while administration of opioid antagonists up-regulates pro-enkephalin expression. It has also been found that chronic administration of antagonists produces up-regulation of opioid receptors, following which the response to an opioid agonist becomes greatly increased. (However, the evidence for receptor down-regulation following the administration of opioid agonists is inconsistent.) Other research has focused on guanine-nucleotide-binding proteins (G proteins) that serve as the transducers between receptor activation and ion channels or second messengers. Acute administration of μ or δ opioids (or, in some cells, α_2-adrenergic agonists) results in inhibition of adenylyl cyclase and a decrease in cAMP levels. Opioid-induced changes in the concentrations or activity of G proteins may be the mechanism by which chronic opioid use modifies the rate of synthesis of cAMP. When the opioid is removed, the altered (increased) synthesis rate results in transiently higher cAMP levels. It is postulated that some aspects of withdrawal are attributable to those higher cAMP levels. Drug-induced supersensitivity and alterations in intracellular Ca++ concentrations may also involve alterations in G proteins. Others have hypothesized that chronic opioid administration triggers the activation of endogenous antiopioid peptides.

Chronic treatment with opioids also induces supersensitivity in several distinct transmitter circuits, including the dopaminergic, noradrenergic, cholinergic, and serotonergic systems. Opioids also inhibit the activity of adrenergic neurons in the locus ceruleus, and naloxone causes increased activity in locus ceruleus neurons in opioid-dependent animals. Those and other findings suggested that noradrenergic neurons in the CNS develop changes in sensitivity during chronic morphine treatment and that increased noradrenergic activity plays a role in some aspects of opioid withdrawal. The observation that certain α_2-adrenergic agonists, such as clonidine (Catapres), also inhibit the activity of neurons in the locus ceruleus formed the background for the clinical trials of clonidine in opioid withdrawal. Supersensitivity to neurotransmitters can also be induced by chronic treatment with drugs that are not subject to abuse, such as dopaminergic blockers.

Tolerance and neuroadaptive change can be induced locally, as well as in the whole organism. Thus infusions of opioid limited to the spinal cord induce tolerance and withdrawal limited to spinal structures. Learning and conditioning also play roles in opioid tolerance and, perhaps, in dependence as well. Animals that exhibit marked tolerance to the effects of opioids given repeatedly in one situation may exhibit toxicity when the same dose is administered in a novel environment. Thus adaptations at both the cellular and functional system levels are widespread in animals that are tolerant and physically dependent on opioids.

Chronic administration of cocaine also induces an up-regulation of μ-opioid and κ-opioid receptors, and those changes may underlie some aspects of the dysphoria observed when cocaine is discontinued.

OPIOIDS AS REINFORCERS In laboratory experiments animals will self-administer μ-opioid and δ-opioid agonists, but not κ-agonists, by various routes of administration. In that way opioids have been shown in laboratory situations to be positive reinforcers. Former heroin addicts given opioids report reduced anxiety, increased self-esteem, a better ability to cope with everyday problems, and a decreased sense of boredom. Given intravenously, opioids produce a rush or flash, a sudden, brief sensation that is reported to be exceedingly pleasurable. Although the rush was customarily described as being much like an orgastic sensation felt in the abdomen, in more recent interviews addicts have described it in much more varied terms, although still as a much desired experience. A rush, a far shorter phenomenon than a general sense of euphoria, lasts only a minute or two, and is experienced only with rapid drug intake, as with intravenous or intrapulmonary routes. Heroin addicts who self-administered heroin in a research setting seemed to develop tolerance to the anxiety-relieving and mood-elevating effects of opioids and, over a period of several weeks, developed various somatic complaints and reported feeling increasingly anxious and dysphoric. Nevertheless, they were able to experience brief periods of mood elevation for 30 to 60 minutes each time they received single injections. The loss of mood-elevating effects and the appearance of hypophoria and hypochondriasis have also been observed with the chronic administration of methadone in a research setting.

Tolerant opioid users do not continue to self-administer opioids solely to prevent the highly aversive withdrawal phenomena. Interviews with heroin users indicated that they continue to experience a brief euphoric effect immediately following an injection, despite some tolerance to many of the drug effects.

Opioids are synergistic with either amphetamine or cocaine in lowering self-stimulation thresholds, as they are in inducing euphoria in humans. Some drug users combine opioids with amphetamine or cocaine, a combination often referred to as a speedball. Little tolerance develops to the threshold-lowering effects of euphorigenic drugs.

It is not clear whether the neural pathways critical for reinforcement in animals are the same as those that underlie repeated drug use in humans. However, studies of the effects of drugs on brain glucose metabolism and cerebral blood flow in volunteers have found striking similarities in the way that different drugs that induce euphoria alter brain function. When subjects experienced euphoria induced by either opioids or cocaine, euphoria was correlated with decreased brain glucose metabolism, especially in cortical areas.

OPIOID ACTIONS IN THE ETIOLOGY OF DEPENDENCE Opioid dependence is currently seen as a biopsychosocial disorder in which multiple factors interact to influence initiation of use, continued use, and relapse after periods of abstinence. Those factors—pharmacological, social, environmental, personality, psychopathology, genetic, and familial—are the same that must be considered when looking at abuse and dependence on other categories of drugs. What changes in the case of the opioids is the importance of the various factors. For example, as reinforcers of drug-taking behavior, benzodiazepine anxiolytics are not as powerful as either opioids or cocaine. Consequently, medical attitudes, prescribing patterns, and preexisting psychopathology are more dominant as etiological factors in the dependence on benzodiazepines, whereas pharmacological factors (that is, acute euphorigenic and reinforcing effects, the avoidance of aversive withdrawal states, and perhaps the persistence of some low-level protracted abstinence) play a larger role in dependence on opioids. Some other factors that play important roles in the etiology of opioid dependence are presented here briefly to illustrate their interplay.

SOCIAL AND ENVIRONMENTAL FACTORS Social attitudes, peer pressure, and drug availability are the major determinants of experimentation with the less socially disapproved drugs. Generally, the use of tobacco, alcohol, and cannabis precedes the use of cocaine and opioids. Since in most cases this earlier drug use continues, most opioid or cocaine users are really multiple drug users. Those persons who go on to experiment with the most socially disapproved drugs, such as heroin, generally come from disrupted families or have disturbed relationships with parents, and they often have low self-esteem. A significant proportion of opioid users meet the criteria for antisocial personality disorder, even when those items that are related to illicit drug use are not applied. The importance of availability was seen in the Vietnam experience and in the temporal shifts observed in drug use within families. For example, among a sample of Mexican-American heroin users living in Texas, alcohol abuse was disproportionately high in parents, but opioid use was uncommon. Among the siblings of the heroin users, opioid use was far more common, a finding best understood in the context of the development of heroin trafficking from Mexico through Texas and its increased local availability.

The presence of a significant number of opioid users creates a subculture supportive of experimentation, and continuing use of the drug usually follows. Areas where availability of illicit opioids is high also have high crime rates, high unemployment rates, and demoralized school systems. Those factors all contribute the sense of hopelessness and the low self-esteem that reduce resistance to drug use and militate against a good prognosis once dependence develops. Along with family factors, those factors may contribute to disproportionately high rates of heroin addiction currently seen among African-American and Hispanic minorities.

The experience with United States service personnel who used heroin in Vietnam provided a unique natural experiment where the influences of availability, vulnerability, and social norms could be observed.

PSYCHODYNAMIC FACTORS AND PSYCHOPATHOLOGY The psychodynamic perspective is that psychopathology is the underlying motivation for initial drug use, drug dependence, and relapse after a period of abstinence. Recent psychoanalytic formulations postulate ego defects, which are manifest in the addict's inability to manage painful affects (guilt, anger, anxiety), and to avoid preventable medical, legal, and financial problems. Some addicts also appear to have great difficulty in differentiating and describing what they feel, a difficulty that has been aptly called alexithymia (that is, no words for feelings). It is postulated that, both pharmacologically and symbolically, opioid use helps the ego control those affects and that drug use can be viewed as a form of self-medication.

Epidemiological studies find that persons who use illicit drugs, especially those who use opioids, tend to place more value on independence and less on academic achievement. They are also more tolerant of deviance, and a very substantial number showed significant signs of delinquency before their first experimentation with opioids. The ECA Study and the National Comorbidity Study (NCS) both found that persons with a diagnosis of either drug dependence or alcohol abuse were much more likely than were those without such a diagnosis to also have at least one other mental disorder that was present in the absence of drugs or alcohol. The rates of coexistent psychiatric disorders and substance abuse and findings of high rates of coexistent psychiatric disorders among opioid users seeking treatment do not prove causality; drug use could and does increase the risk of psychopathology. However, those data strongly support the argument that many persons will be left at higher risk for initial treatment failure or relapse if treatment efforts are aimed solely at the drug-using behavior itself and do not address comorbidity.

FAMILY FACTORS More than 50 percent of urban heroin addicts come from single-parent families. Typically, even in two-parent families, there are disturbed family relationships, with one parent, usually of the opposite sex, intensely involved with the addict, and the other parent distant, absent, or punitive. Cross-generational alliances between the drug user and one parent against another parental figure are common. The disability of the drug-using member of the family often serves as a focus for communication among other members, and sometimes, it has been postulated, as the main motive for their remaining together. Thus, it is asserted, the family equilibrium may be threatened by the addict's recovery.

Despite their seeming rebelliousness and precocious efforts to be independent, opioid users often remain dependent on and in close communication with families of origin well into adulthood. Interestingly, both male and female heroin addicts believe that members of their families of origin or their in-laws would be the most helpful to them in their efforts to give up drugs. Rates of alcohol and drug abuse, mental illness, and antisocial personality are higher in the families of heroin users. Relatives of depressed opioid addicts tend to have higher rates of depression and anxiety, but not of other disorders.

OTHER BIOLOGICAL FACTORS At present there is little direct evidence of any specific biological vulnerability to opioid dependence. It has been postulated that some antecedent metabolic deficiency, such as endogenous opioid dysregulation or one induced by chronic opioid use, may increase vulnerability to becoming opioid dependent, but no evidence for such defects has yet emerged. There is some evidence for a genetically transmitted vulnerability to developing alcoholism, and many opioid addicts are alcoholic in addition to being opioid dependent. Many also have biological parents who are alcoholic or drug dependent, or both. In Vietnam, where heroin was readily available, the use of heroin by American service personnel was powerfully predicted by the same factors that predicted use in the United States: the frequency and severity of preservice fighting, truancy, drunkenness, arrest, and school expulsion.

An important distinction between opioids and other classes of pharmacological agents is that physical dependence not only develops rapidly, but there appears to be a protracted period of physiological abnormality that follows the acute opioid withdrawal syndrome. This long-lasting syndrome, characterized by hypophoria, irritability, mood instability, and recurrent urges to use opioids, is postulated to be due to opioid-induced alterations in endogenous opioid peptide systems, opioid receptors, or other intracellular proteins that are produced by neurons exposed to opioids over long periods. It is also postulated that the syndrome is responsible for the high rate of relapse observed when well-motivated patients treated with high-dose methadone are withdrawn from methadone. The relationship of the postulated long-lasting opioid-induced disturbances to antecedent biological vulnerability is, at present, uncertain.

LEARNING AND CONDITIONING Opioids are positive reinforcers of drug self-administration. They can also reinforce antecedent behaviors by terminating noxious or aversive states, such as pain, anxiety, or depression (negative reinforcement).

In some social situations the use of the drug can also be reinforcing if it results in gaining special status among friends. That social reinforcement can serve to maintain drug use until the effects of primary reinforcement or reinforcement by alleviation of withdrawal symptoms come into play. Typically, each time the drug is used, reinforcement occurs. It may be the rush, drug-induced euphoria, alleviation of disturbed affect or of withdrawal symptoms, or any combination of those effects. Use of a short-acting opioid, such as heroin, causes such reinforcement to occur several times a day, day after day, creating a powerfully reinforced habit pattern. Eventually, the paraphernalia and hustling associated with drug use can become secondary reinforcers, as well as cues that signal drug availability, and in their presence craving or desire to experience drug effects increases.

In addition to this operant reinforcement of drug-using and drug-seeking behaviors, classical or Pavlovian conditioning probably plays a role in relapse. In both laboratory animals and human volunteers, opioid withdrawal phenomena can be conditioned to environmental or interoceptive stimuli. For long periods following withdrawal, former opioid addicts may experience conditioned withdrawal or conditioned craving when exposed to environmental stimuli previously linked to drug use or withdrawal. Such conditions as watching someone else use heroin or being offered some drug by a friend, rather than conditions associated with withdrawal, elicit the most intense craving.

DIAGNOSIS AND CLINICAL FEATURES

OPIOID ABUSE AND OPIOID DEPENDENCE Opioid abuse (see Table 13.1-6) is a pattern of maladaptive use of an opioid drug leading to clinically significant impairment or distress and occurring within a 12-month period, but one in which the symptoms have never met the criteria for opioid dependence.

Under DSM-IV, opioid dependence (see Tables 13.1-2 and 13.1-5) is inferred from behaviors that indicate some decrease in volitional control over the use of an opioid drug. A number of criteria have been developed to allow the clinician to decide whether the patient exhibits such a decrease in volitional control. Those criteria are not specific for opioids, but are believed to apply across all psychoactive agents. DSM-IV does not require that any single criterion be met, and none is given special weight. Thus, the presence of tolerance and physical dependence (withdrawal) is not required. However, according to DSM-IV, if tolerance and physical dependence are present, that should be noted specifically.

Because tolerance develops to many of the actions of opioid drugs after chronic use, opioid effects are not readily detected by even the careful observer. Patients maintained on large oral doses of methadone function quite normally. Physicians, nurses, and other medical personnel who use opioids, even by injection, may go undetected by their colleagues for months or years. Thus a candid history obtained from the patient or a reliable informant is needed to made a diagnosis.

Comorbidity The high prevalence of additional psychiatric disorders among treated opioid-dependent patients has now been repeatedly confirmed. Currently no specific subtypology of opioid-dependent patients based on psychopathology has been proposed. However, the type and severity of those additional diagnoses can powerfully influence the course of the disorder and the kind of treatment most likely to be effective.

Among opioid addicts seeking treatment at a Yale University-affiliated program in the 1980s, 87 percent met the Research Diagnostic Criteria (RDC) for a psychiatric disorder, in addition to opioid dependence, at some point in their lives.

TABLE 13.9-5
Lifetime Rates for Psychiatric Disorders Among Opioid-Dependent Patients Using Research Diagnostic Criteria

Type of Disorder	Male (n = 403) (%)	Female (n = 130) (%)
Affective [mood] disorders		
Major depressive disorders	48.9	69.2
Minor depressive disorders	9.4	5.4
Intermittent depression	18.1	20.8
Cyclothymic personality	2.5	6.9
Labile personality	17.1	14.6
Manic disorders	0.5	0.8
Hypomanic disorder	5.5	10.0
Bipolar I or II	3.7	10.8
Any affective [mood] disorder	70.7	85.4
Schizophrenic disorders		
Schizophrenia	0.7	0.8
Schizoaffective, depressed	2.2	0.0
Schizoaffective, manic	0.5	0.0
Anxiety disorders		
Panic	0.5	3.9
Obsessive-compulsive	1.7	2.3
Generalized anxiety	4.7	7.7
Phobic	8.2	13.9
Any anxiety disorder	13.2	25.4
Alcoholism	37.0	26.9
Personality disorders		
Antisocial personality	29.5	16.9
Briquet's syndrome	0.0	0.7
Schizotypal features	8.7	7.7
Other psychiatric disorders	5.7	10.0

Table modified from B J Rounsaville, M M Weissman, H Kleber, C Wilber: Heterogeneity of psychiatric diagnosis in treated opiate addicts. Arch Gen Psychiat *39:* 162, 1982.

The most common diagnoses were mood disorders, alcoholism, antisocial personality, and anxiety disorders (Table 13.9-5). The frequency and distribution of additional psychiatric disorders among opioid users seeking treatment have not changed substantially since that early study and are also observed among such patients in Europe and Australia.

Among women, mood and anxiety disorders were more common, and alcoholism and antisocial personality were less common. If DSM-III criteria, which do not require that the diagnosis of antisocial personality be independent of the need for drugs, had been used, 54 percent of the sample would have received the diagnosis of antisocial personality. The proportion of opioid users meeting the criteria for a current episode of a psychiatric disorder was 70 percent, with mood disorder, antisocial personality, alcohol abuse, and phobia the most common diagnoses. More than half of the patients met the criteria for two or more additional diagnoses, such as alcohol abuse, antisocial personality, and depression. Similar patterns of additional psychiatric disorders have been found by workers at other public clinics and by clinicians in private practice. Among patients in therapeutic communities, 60 percent reported depressive symptoms during the year before entry, 28 percent had contemplated suicide, and 13 percent had made at least one suicide attempt.

The rate of current psychiatric illnesses, such as mood disorders, anxiety disorders, and schizophrenia, will be lower than the lifetime rates shown in Table 13.9-5 and vary with the treatment setting. Rates of current major depressive disorder in the range of 17 to 20 percent are not unusual, as are concurrent rates of alcoholism (alcohol abuse or dependence) of 20 to 30 percent. Although opioid abusers who have current psychiatric problems are more likely to seek treatment, it should not be assumed that those who do not seek treatment are free of comorbid psychiatric problems.

Among the respondents in the ECA, about half of those with a substance (other than alcohol) use disorder had one or more additional psychiatric disorders (odds ratio, 4.5): anxiety disorder, 28.3 percent (odds ratio, 2.5); mood disorder, 26.4 (odds ratio, 4.7); antisocial personality, 17.8 percent (odds ratio, 13.4); schizophrenia, 6.8 percent (odds ratio, 6.2). The probability of comorbidity is higher for those with a lifetime diagnosis of an opioid or cocaine disorder than for those who abuse cannabis. That widespread comorbidity was again found in the NCS; 59 percent of those with a lifetime history of illicit drug abuse or dependence also met DSM-IV criteria for another mental disorder, and 71 percent met the criteria for a lifetime alcohol use disorder.

OPIOID INTOXICATION DSM-IV criteria for opioid intoxication are shown in Table 13.9-2. Intoxication can vary in severity. In severe cases of opioid overdose there is usually coma, severely depressed respiration, and pinpoint pupils. There may be gross pulmonary edema with frothing at the mouth (Figure 13.9-1), but X-ray evidence of pulmonary changes is seen even in less severe cases. Pulmonary edema is an opioid effect and is sometimes seen with overdoses of medically prescribed oral opioids. Depending on when the patient is found, there may also be cyanosis, cold clammy skin, and decreased body temperature. Blood pressure is decreased, but only falls dramatically with severe anoxia, at which point pupils may dilate. Cardiac arrhythmias have been reported and may be related either to anoxia or to the presence of quinine as an adulterant in the opioid.

OPIOID WITHDRAWAL The opioid withdrawal syndrome can vary greatly in intensity, depending primarily on the dose of the opioid used, the degree to which the opioid effects on the CNS were continuously exerted, the duration of the chronic use, and the rate at which the opioid is removed from the receptors. Those generalizations appear to apply as well to other categories of drugs, such as barbiturates and benzodiazepines.

The clinical syndrome observed consists of purposive behavior, which is dependent on the observer and environment (for example, complaints, pleas, and manipulations directed at getting more drug), and nonpurposive behavior, which is not goal oriented and is relatively independent of the observer and environment.

In the case of short-acting drugs, such as morphine or heroin, the first symptoms may be seen within 8 to 12 hours after the last dose of drug. In mild syndromes the symptoms may be limited to craving, anxiety, dysphoria, yawning, perspiration, lacrimation, rhinorrhea, and restless and broken sleep. In the least severe cases, or very early in withdrawal, symptoms may consist only of dysphoria, irritability, restlessness, and general achiness, with few objective signs. In more severe cases, as the syndrome progresses, other signs and symptoms that may be seen include increasing irritability; dilated pupils; aching of bones, back, and muscles; piloerection (waves of gooseflesh, from which comes the term "cold turkey" to describe withdrawal); and hot and cold flashes. In severe syndromes, which, with heroin and morphine, generally reach peak severity at about 48 after the last dose, additional symptoms include nausea, vomiting, diarrhea, weight loss, fever (usually low grade), and increased blood pressure and pulse and respiratory rate. Also often observed are twitching of muscles and kicking movements of the lower extremities, whence comes the phrase "kicking the habit." The DSM-IV diagnostic criteria for opioid withdrawal are shown in Table 13.9-3.

With short-acting drugs, the acute phase of the syndrome, if untreated, runs its course in 7 to 10 days. In research subjects the acute phase was followed by a more subtle but longer-lasting phase, the protracted abstinence syndrome, that persisted for many weeks. During that phase many physiological variables reached subnormal values, such as hyposensitivity to the respiratory stimulant effects of carbon dioxide. There was also

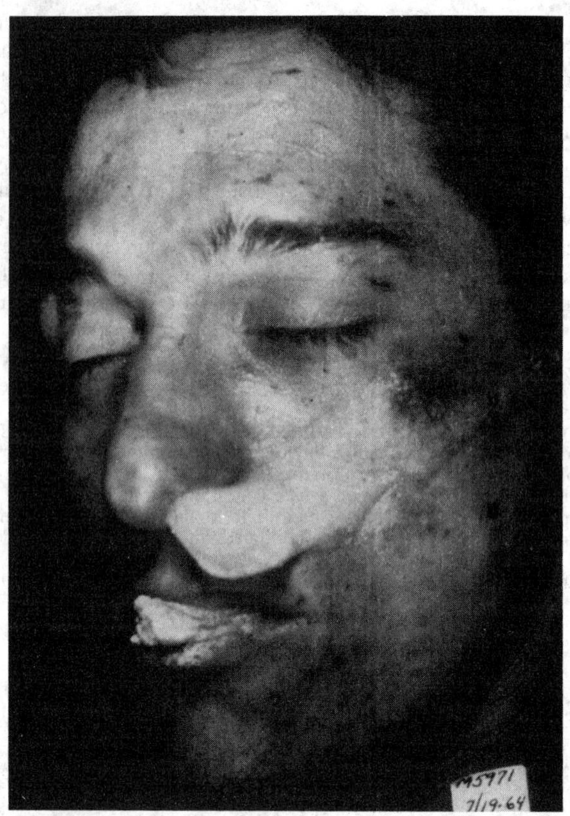

FIGURE 13.9-1 *Pulmonary edema is often associated with heroin overdose. (Figure courtesy of Michael Baden, MD)*

disturbed sleep, overconcern about bodily discomfort, poor self-image, and a decreased capacity to tolerate stress. It is frequently assumed that the protracted abstinence syndrome plays a role in relapse to opioid use.

With longer-acting drugs, such as methadone or L-α-acetylmethadol (LAAM), the onset of withdrawal may be delayed for one to three days following the last dose. Although the syndrome is qualitatively similar, peak symptoms may not occur until the third to eighth day, and the symptoms may persist for several weeks.

Acute withdrawal from methadone, and presumably from LAAM, is also followed by a protracted abstinence syndrome that may last for more than six months. If naloxone is given to a patient dependent on methadone, thereby displacing the drug abruptly from the receptors, the withdrawal is immediate in onset, can be quite severe, and persists until the naloxone is metabolized and the residual methadone reoccupies the receptors.

Withdrawal from analgesics that are presumed to act, in part, as κ-receptor agonists (for example, pentazocine, nalbuphine) is generally rapid in onset, mild, and lasts a few days. The syndrome bears some similarities to the μ-receptor withdrawal syndrome, but there are also some distinct elements. Withdrawal from pure κ agonists is not associated with drug-seeking behavior. Since drug-seeking behavior is sometimes seen with pentazocine, it is likely that it has some low-level agonist actions at receptors other than μ-receptors.

Withdrawal symptoms after chronic administration of buprenorphine, a partial μ-agonist, at doses of 8 mg a day parenterally or sublingually, are generally not severe in intensity, but some patients are uncomfortable enough to request drugs for relief of discomfort and for insomnia. After sublingual administration (8 mg a day), withdrawal symptoms are experienced within a few days after drug use is stopped, and symptoms of the acute phase reach baseline levels by 7 to 10 days. It is usually mild and consists primarily of subjective effects, such as muscle aches, dysphoria, and insomnia, rather than the more dramatic autonomic signs that are measured by the Himmelsbach withdrawal scale.

PATHOLOGY AND LABORATORY EXAMINATION

In opioid abuse and opioid dependence there may be no abnormal laboratory findings at all. Urine tests can usually detect short-acting opioids, such as heroin, for 12 to 36 hours after use. Very potent opioids used, such as fentanyl, may not be detected by standard opioid screens. Standard tests for heroin actually test for its main metabolite, morphine. A positive urine test for morphine can also be caused by therapeutic doses of codeine or by the ingestion of large amounts of poppy seeds.

Persons who have shared injection implements often test positive for hepatitis and for the human immunodeficiency virus (HIV). Other liver enzymes may be elevated if there is active hepatitis. There may be both positive and false-positive tests for syphilis. Chest X-rays may show evidence of pulmonary fibrosis if the person has been using injection materials contaminated with microcrystalline talc or cotton particulates. During withdrawal white cell counts and cortisol levels may be elevated.

Physical findings may be unremarkable if opioids are ingested orally; snorting (insufflation) of heroin may irritate nasal membranes. Drug injectors, however, may show widespread evidence of having used unsterile injection equipment. There may be needle tracks over veins on the arms, legs, and, in some cases, the backs of the hands and the femoral and jugular veins. Infections and venous scleroses and lymph obstruction may lead to severe edema of the hands and feet. There may be skin abscesses or scars on accessible skin surfaces as a result of unsterile subcutaneous injections. There may be rocklike hardening of subcutaneous and muscle tissue as a result of repeated intramuscular injections of meperidine (often seen among health professionals). Endocarditis may produce fever and heart murmurs. In addition, a variety of neurological sequelae of intravenous heroin use may be detected.

DIFFERENTIAL DIAGNOSIS

The diagnosis of opioid dependence can be relatively straightforward when the patient is willing to be candid. It can be quite taxing when the patient is motivated to conceal past patterns of opioid use, as is frequently the case among health-care professionals or persons who obtain opioids from medical sources by simulating disease or greatly exaggerating the painful nature of disease actually present.

The diagnosis of opioid withdrawal is easier when the opioid is short acting and the symptoms are accompanied by obvious physiological signs. That is not the typical case, and the clinician is often confronted by a patient complaining of various aches, pains, anxiety, and insomnia in the absence of obvious signs of withdrawal. It is important to remember that substantial subjective distress can develop before the more obvious physical signs and that, when so motivated, opioid-dependent patients in early withdrawal may exaggerate the severity of distress in the hope that it will elicit higher doses of drugs for relief. Persons who are dependent on opioids may withhold information on the use of other classes of drugs. Since opioid withdrawal does not generally cause tremulousness, confusion, delirium, or seizures, the presence of those signs or the failure of insomnia and anxiety to respond to reasonable doses of an opioid should raise the possibility of dependence on alcohol, barbituratelike agents, or benzodiazepines.

Opioid intoxication must be differentiated from mixed intoxications in which opioids play only a minor role. In general, a failure to respond to modest doses of naloxone suggests that intoxication is due to a nonopioid. Some patients, more typically the elderly, may respond to therapeutic doses of a μ-agonist with dysphoria and confusion. Such reactions are generally short-lived reactions. They are seen more commonly with mixed agonist-antagonists. They should be considered atypical opioid intoxications, rather than opioid-induced intoxication delirium or opioid-induced psychotic disorders, which, although listed in DSM-IV, are quite rare. One possible exception is the toxic state associated with the accumulation of toxic meperidine metabolites. However, even in that case, the syndrome does not usually outlast the metabolites and should probably be considered an intoxication.

COURSE AND PROGNOSIS

Although it was commonly believed that experimentation with illicit opioids invariably led to dependence, it is now apparent that only a fraction of those persons who briefly experimented with illicit opioids developed serious problems. It is still the case that those persons who use opioid drugs heavily—at least once a week—usually go on to use daily, at least for a brief period. It is likely, however, that many of those persons who go on to develop some degree of dependence recover without ever seeking formal treatment. In the St. Louis ECA, only 20 percent of those with a lifetime history of opioid abuse had any symptom during the year prior to interview. Also, the number of opioid users and experimenters in the United States over the past decade is far larger than the total number of persons who have ever entered treatment programs.

Some persons apparently can use opioids occasionally (for example, several times a month) over periods of months or years without becoming dependent. For such users, careful rules about the time and place of use may help in preventing progression to addiction, but the users are still at risk for death from overdose, as well as for infections and other medical complications that affect opioid addicts who inject. When addiction develops, the subsequent course of the syndrome depends on environmental factors, the characteristics of the user, the route of administration, and the specific opioid being used.

HETEROGENEITY OF LIFE-STYLE Opioid addicts seeking or entering treatment in the United States (and in England) exhibit a surprising heterogeneity of life-styles, attitudes toward conventional values, and criminality. Some addicts, except for their drug use, are quite conventional, avoid criminality, work at legitimate occupations, and do not identify with the addict subculture (conformists). At the other extreme, some addicts live exclusively by illicit activities and are highly involved with other addicts (hustlers or junkies). A third group appears to identify with both cultures, engaging in some criminal activities and interacting with other addicts, but living primarily on legitimate earnings (two-worlders). A fourth group of addicts seems not to be involved in either the conventional culture or the addict subculture. They tend to be unemployed, and to live on welfare, rather than on criminal earnings. Those addicts, the uninvolved or loners, often have high levels of psychopathology. Health professionals and those who become addicted to opioids in the course of medical treatment probably constitute additional distinct subgroups.

WHO COMES TO TREATMENT For those users who become dependent in the context of medical treatment, the subsequent course depends largely on the medical problems that generated the opioid use, the willingness of doctors to continue to prescribe drugs for them, and whether the drug is used orally or by injection. Patients who use opioids orally and whose pain is controlled by adequate dosages of legitimately prescribed medication may experience little interference with normal function for many years. If pain is uncontrolled, demands for increased or altered medication schedules will probably lead to repeated diagnostic workups, surgery, and other procedures, punctuated by attempts at withdrawal—voluntary and coerced—and treatment for depression. Health professionals often come to treatment when their drug use is uncovered by colleagues or by drug enforcement agencies. Under supervision, most recover and are able to return to practice. However, return to specialties with easy access to opioids poses a serious hazard. For example, only 34 percent of anesthesiology residents who were abusing opioids were able to return to their specialty. For a significant percentage, the first sign of relapse was a fatal overdose.

In the United States anyone who becomes dependent on illicit opioids, usually heroin, whose use persists for any substantial period, is very likely to come to the attention of the police or to seek medical treatment. Since the development of community-based treatment programs in the early 1970s, the average time from addiction to illicit opioids to first episode of treatment has decreased from six years to about two to three years. For drug users who are arrested, the time from addiction to first arrest may range from six months to five years. Before the advent of community-based treatment programs, a significant proportion of addicts who eventually came to police attention were never voluntarily abstinent, stopping drug use only when incarcerated. Comparisons of heroin addicts who seek treatment with those who do not suggest that the former are more likely to exhibit symptoms of depression, although opioid users in the community are not entirely free of additional psychopathology. It may be that depression (in addition to the pressure from family and law-enforcement agencies) is an important determinant of which drug users enter treatment.

RELAPSE In the early stages of opioid use the most typical course for the user of illicit opioids is one of periods of abstinence, either voluntary or forced (by imprisonment or hospitalization) and lasting from a few weeks to many months, followed by relapse to opioid use and readdiction. Among the addicts who enter treatment, relapse occurs most often in the first three months; a number of studies show that at least two out of three patients relapse within six months. The theme running through the many specific reasons given for periods of voluntary abstinence is a desire to change life patterns and a weariness with the constant difficulty of trying to obtain illicit opioids. At the time of reentry into treatment, addicts are often less seriously impaired than when first treated, suggesting some residual benefit from intermittent treatment. With successful treatment episodes, and with age, the duration of each opioid episode tends to shorten.

Repeated relapse is not an inevitable consequence of opioid dependence. Eighty-eight percent of United States Army enlisted personnel who became addicted during a tour of duty in Vietnam did not become readdicted at any time during the three years following their return to the United States; 56 percent did not use opioids at all. Of the soldiers who did become readdicted in the first year, 70 percent were no longer addicted in the following two years. Only 2 percent of the soldiers who used opioids in Vietnam (6 percent of those who tested positive for opioids at time of departure) entered treatment following return to the United States. However, the relapse rates for those who did enter treatment were as high as for civilians, with two thirds relapsing within less than a year. It is possible that among those who become dependent on opioids, the ones who cannot stop without formal help have a more severe form of the disorder.

In considering the natural history of opioid addiction, a distinction must be made between the course of all those who report a period of dependence (for example, among respondents to a household survey) and the course of those who enter treatment. Those who enter treatment may have additional problems or a greater severity of addiction. Further, opioids are rarely the sole drug class used. During the 1980s a high proportion of opioid-dependent patients also abused or became dependent on cocaine. Abstinence from opioids or recovery from opioid dependence does not mean that the person has no drug problems. Alcohol abuse and abuse of nonopioids is common among those who are no longer using opioids.

LONG-TERM PROGNOSIS Studies from both the United States and Great Britain support the view that opioid addiction is a disorder that eventually ends for many of those addicts who survive. That seems to be so even for those who seek treatment, a group that may have a more severe variety of the disorder. For a substantial number of these persons, it is prolonged incarceration that ends opioid use; others quit opioid use but continue to abuse other drugs. Although there are old opioid addicts in the United States, their numbers are few. Opinion remains divided as to just how many former opioid addicts eventually achieve abstinence outside of an institution. One review of long-term follow-up studies found abstinence rates between 10 and 19 percent for drug-free treatment and 9 and 21 percent following treatment with methadone. A 24-year follow-up of narcotic addicts remanded to the California Civil Commitment Program in the early 1960s classified the 354 survivors into four groups: winners, strivers, those who endure, and the incarcerated. The winners (17 percent) had not used narcotics and had no other serious drug problems over the preceding 36 months; the strivers (13 percent) had been abstinent from narcotics but not from other drugs and they had not been incarcerated. Enduring addicts (41 percent) had avoided incarceration but used narcotics and other drugs. Of the incarcerated (29 percent), many had used drugs during the 12 months prior to interview. Thus 30 percent of the total were free of opioids, although some used other classes of drugs.

The usual measures of treatment outcome—legitimate work, crime, drug use, family relationships, psychological adjustment—are best predicted by different pretreatment variables. Thus pretreatment history of high levels of criminal activity most accurately predicts posttreatment criminal activity, and previous stable work history is more predictive of posttreatment gainful employment. Severity of psychological problems at the beginning of treatment, however, is an important predictor of outcome on all dimensions. Those opioid addicts with the least severe psychological problems appear to respond better to all treatments on all outcome measures. Depression and life crises (especially arguments and interpersonal losses) are associated with relapse to illicit drug use; those factors are additive. The impact of those risk factors is reduced by treatment in drug-abuse programs. Depression is also a risk factor for continued cocaine use among patients in opioid treatment programs, whereas cocaine use itself predicts earlier discontinuation of methadone treatment. Standard methadone maintenance treatment programs do not appear to have any major effect in preventing the emergence of cocaine use among opioid users in treatment.

Follow-up studies of opioid addicts initially treated at public clinics provide some general estimate of the intermediate-term prognosis for opioid dependence. A random sample of addicts receiving heroin at several London clinics in 1969 was studied seven years later: 12 percent were dead; 5 percent were in prison; 5 percent were using illicit opioids regularly; 43 percent were still receiving opioids from clinics, of whom 90 percent were still injecting; 7 percent were entirely abstinent from opioids, but were using alcohol or sedatives daily; 24 percent were entirely abstinent and using no other drugs; and the status of 4 percent was uncertain.

In the United States a sample of men who had been daily heroin users before entering a number of different treatment programs during 1972 and 1973 were followed up six years after initial entry. On average, patients had been out of initial treatment for four years at the time of follow-up. Five percent were known to be dead; 29 percent were not located or could not be interviewed; 3 percent were in jail; 13 percent were using illicit opioids regularly; 8 percent were receiving methadone from clinics; 2 percent had been abstinent, but had relapsed; 5 percent were abstinent from opioids, but were using alcohol or nonopioids heavily; and 32 percent were entirely abstinent from opioids and were not abusing other drugs. By the sixth year, many patients had reentered other treatment programs or had been institutionalized for other reasons. There were no longer any important differences in outcome among patients treated initially in different programs, although over shorter follow-up periods, methadone maintenance, therapeutic communities, and drug-free programs were significantly superior to detoxification programs. More recent studies in the United States and in Australia suggest that addicts electing detoxification or therapeutic communities are younger and have less psychopathology than do those entering more lengthy forms of treatment. While a period of prolonged abstinence is a good predictor of long-term outcome, a study of opioid users in Texas found that 33 percent of those who reported three years of abstinence eventually relapsed. The long-term outcome for opioid dependence among persons with additional major psychiatric disorders, such as schizophrenia or bipolar disorder, is not known. The emergence of HIV and tuberculosis among opioid users will have a major impact on longer-term prognosis regardless of the short-term efficacy of treatment aimed at drug-using behavior.

OPIOIDS AND CRIME The statistical relation between the use of illicit opioids and crime in the United States is unquestionable. Persons who use illicit opioids commit crimes more frequently than do nonusers. There are, however, questions about the degree to which one behavior causes the other. The direct tranquilizing actions of opioids ought to reduce criminal activity, rather than increase it. Indeed, throughout much of history in countries where crude opioids (for example, opium, tincture of opium) were inexpensive and socially acceptable, and were either smoked or taken by mouth, there was little relation between opioid use and criminal behavior. The association between opioid use and crime emerges primarily in countries, such as the United States, that have tried to restrict the use of opioids to legitimate medical indications, but have been unable to eliminate illicit opioid traffic.

In the United States, and Great Britain as well, more than 50 percent of heroin addicts interviewed in prisons and jails or treatment programs had been arrested prior to their first opioid use. In one East Coast city in the United States adolescent boys (ages 11 to 14) who later became opioid addicts exhibited substantially more criminal behavior than did peers or age-matched nonpeers from the same community. Although it might be argued that the criminal behavior seen after the onset of addiction is merely a continuation of a criminal life-style, addicts' self-reports, as well as more objective data, indicate that criminal activity increases sharply after the onset of opioid addiction. Arrest rates for nondrug offenses increase from 1.5-fold to threefold after the onset of addiction, and self-reported property crimes increase to a comparable degree. Other evidence pointing to a causal relationship between opioid use and crime is the sharp reduction in both self-reported criminal activity and arrests during periods of less than daily opioid use. The decrease in crime is seen whether the decrease in opioid use is a result of effective treatment, probation, parole, or spontaneous cessation.

Although most addicts' crimes are directed at generating income for drugs by shoplifting, petty theft, and selling drugs, recently more addicts seem to be engaging in crimes, such as robbery, that involve the potential for violence. However, it has also been suggested that crime is a better predictor of opioid use than opioid use is of crime, and that rather than heavy use causing crime, day-to-day success in crime enables the escalation to heavier opioid use. Among Southeast Asian (Hmong) immigrants who began opium smoking in the United States, crime did not antedate opioid use. Except for a few arrests for the possession of opioids, and despite family displeasure about expenditures for drugs, crime has not yet become a problem for the group. When criminal behavior antedates opioid use, it is unrealistic to expect the successful treatment of opioid dependence to eliminate criminal behavior entirely. Addicts who were criminally active prior to opioid dependence are more likely to persist in criminal acts when abstinent. It is postulated that only more comprehensive treatment directed at social, psychological, and vocational factors, rather than just at illicit drug use, is likely to alter antisocial life-styles.

TOXICITY, MORBIDITY, MEDICAL COMPLICATIONS, AND LIFE EXPECTANCY Oral opioids are relatively nontoxic. Whereas chronic use, as in methadone maintenance, is associated with minor endocrine abnormalities, constipation, and some sleep disturbance, no major organ damage has been noted, and no significant impact on longevity would be expected. The cognitive impairment seen with chronic alcohol and sedative use is not generally found with chronic oral opioid use. Nevertheless, the life expectancy of opioid addicts, especially heroin addicts, is markedly reduced. Before the emergence of HIV infection among opioid injectors, estimates ranged from a twofold to a threefold increase in the expected mortality rate for older addicts to a 20-fold increase in the expected rate among young addicts. Follow-ups of treated opioid addicts in the United States indicate an overall death rate of 1 to 1.5 percent a year. A substantial proportion of those deaths were due to drug overdose, drug-related infections, and suicide. Homicide is also a common cause of death among urban opioid addicts in the United States. In a study of black male heroin addicts in St. Louis, 62 percent of the men had been hospitalized because of narcotics use (12 percent, three or more times); 35 percent reported gunshot or knife wounds; 52 percent reported at least one drug overdose; and 19 percent reported three or more overdoses.

In a British study 128 heroin addicts (93 men, 35 women, average age 25) receiving daily prescriptions for heroin at London drug clinics in 1969 were followed over a 10-year period. Twelve percent had died by the seventh year, and 15 percent (14 men and 4 women) were dead by the 10th year of the study. Eight died because of a drug overdose, four died of renal failure, one died of bronchopneumonia, one committed suicide, two were killed in accidents, and for three, the coroner's verdict was simply addiction to drugs. The death rate at the British clinics providing injectable drugs to young addicts was estimated at 2 to 3 percent a year, at least 20-fold higher than the death rate of comparably aged contemporaries. Mortality rates far higher than for age-adjusted controls were also observed in Italy during a period when heroin use was not a criminal offense.

Although many of the infectious complications are directly related to the use of injectable opioids, death resulting from combining opioids with alcohol or sedatives or from self-destructive behavior is not uncommon among those who are subsequently treated with oral opioids, such as methadone.

The suicide rate among opioid addicts is estimated to be three times higher than that of the general population, but that is probably an underestimate, because it is difficult to determine how many overdose deaths are, to some degree, intentional. However, in the St. Louis population cited only one subject reported that a drug overdose was a suicide attempt.

Medical complications Medical complications associated with the injection of illicit drugs include a variety of pathological changes in the central nervous system (CNS). Degenerative changes in globus pallidus and necrosis of spinal gray matter are usually found at autopsy, but sometimes there are clinical manifestations in those users surviving overdose experiences. Examples are transverse myelitis, amblyopia, plexitis, peripheral neuropathy, parkinsonismlike syndromes, intellectual impairment, and personality changes. Pathological changes in muscles and degeneration of peripheral nerves have also been seen. Illicit laboratories sometimes produce opioidlike agents that are extremely toxic or are so potent that even small doses are lethal. For example, MPTP (1-methyl, 4 phenyl, 1,2,3,6-tetrahydropyridine), a contaminant of illegally produced meperidine, produces a severe form of parkinsonism by selective destruction of dopaminergic neurons. The illicit fentanyl analog, 3-methyl fentanyl (China White), is 1,000 times more potent than morphine and may have been responsible for several hundred overdose deaths.

Because opioid addicts—even physicians who have access to drugs and sterile materials—tend to neglect the hygienic aspects of injecting, infections of skin and systemic organs are quite common. Filtering illicit opioids through cigarette filters or wads of cotton and injection of materials intended for oral use result in the entrance into the bloodstream of starch, talc, and other particulate contaminants; those particulates can cause pulmonary emboli that can eventually result in angiothrombotic pulmonary hypertension and right ventricular failure. Staphylococcal pneumonitis may also be related to septic emboli. Endocarditis and septicemia involving lesions either of the tricuspid or of the aortic and mitral valves is a frequent complication. Less frequent but equally serious complications are meningitis and brain abscess. Other frequently seen infections that can be related to injecting the substance or the sharing of needles include viral hepatitis, malaria, tetanus, osteomyelitis, syphilis, HIV, and the acquired immune deficiency syndrome (AIDS). However, most cases of syphilis are probably acquired in the usual fashion. Many opioid addicts who inject have a low-level chronic hepatitis without jaundice and may have abnormal liver function tests and false-positive tests for syphilis. Seroprevalence surveys conducted by the Centers for Disease Control (CDC) found some marker of hepatitis B infection in sera from 60 to 80 percent of drug injectors. Abnormal liver function tests, which are found in about two out of three heroin addicts, may persist for long periods after the cessation of injection. Excessive use of alcohol may, in some cases, contribute to the liver disease.

HUMAN IMMUNODEFICIENCY VIRUS AND TUBERCULOSIS In 1989 it was estimated that from 5 to 33 percent of intravenous drug users in the United States were infected with HIV. However, despite comparable rates of sharing of injection equipment, there is wide regional variation. Seroprevalence rates were highest in the northeastern United States and Puerto Rico (10 to 65 percent), and lowest (less than 5 percent) in the West, Midwest, and South. Risk of infection appeared to be higher among Hispanics and African Americans. Infection was far lower among former heroin users who had been continuously in methadone treatment.

The finding that not all who shared needles were infected with HIV stimulated vigorous prevention efforts aimed at recruiting patients into treatment and teaching them how to avoid infection by proper cleaning of injection equipment and avoiding both sharing equipment and participating in high-risk sex. Outreach by community workers, coupled with specific instruction, reduces self-reported equipment sharing but has far less effect on high-risk sexual behavior. The question of whether providing injecting drug users with sterile equipment at little or no cost would substantially slow the spread of HIV infection is still controversial, but the available evidence indicates that those who inject drugs will use sterile equipment in order to avoid disease, if the equipment is available at reasonable cost. In England many heroin users now smoke heroin instead of injecting it.

Even before the HIV epidemic, the incidence of tuberculosis was higher among heroin addicts than in the general population. Now a reemergence of tuberculosis poses a major problem for many treatment programs. Patients with compromised immune systems are far more vulnerable to developing active tuberculosis once infected, and poor compliance with antitubercular medication has led to the emergence of drug-resistant strains of the tubercle bacillus. Studies indicate that 4 to 21 percent of AIDS patients are infected with tuberculosis.

μ-Opioid actions at CNS receptors can produce immunosuppressive effects (for example, decreased natural killer cell activity). Opioid receptors are also found on lymphocytes and naloxone-reversible opioid effects can be demonstrated on white cells in vitro. However, the concentrations required are quite high; it seems unlikely that direct actions on white cells mediate effects on the immune system. In heroin addicts there are changes in the ratio of helper-to-suppressor T-cells, and a suppression of cell-mediated immunity. The relation to opioid use is still unclear; the effects are probably more related to unhygienic injection practices. Natural killer activity and immunoglobulin G and M are within normal limits in former heroin users maintained for several years on methadone, although abnormalities are typically observed among heroin addicts.

Even before the HIV-AIDS epidemic lymphadenopathy was seen in 75 percent of addicts and was thought to be related to particulate contaminants; chronic edema of extremities (for example, puffy hands) may be due to lymphatic obstruction caused by contaminants or sclerosis of veins caused by the drugs or their dilutants. Lymphadenopathy in a drug addict who is positive for HIV antibodies now has much more ominous implications. Skin popping may cause widespread ulceration and disfigurement as a result of chemical necrosis or infection (Figure 13.9-2). Some drug users seem determined to experience the effects of the drug used intravenously and switch to the use of femoral and jugular veins when the surface veins of the arms and legs have become sclerosed (Figure 13.9-3).

TREATMENT

INTOXICATION The first task is to ensure an adequate airway; tracheopharyngeal secretions should be aspirated. An airway may be inserted. The patient should be ventilated mechanically until naloxone, a specific opioid antagonist, can be given. Naloxone is administered intravenously at a slow rate—initially, about 0.8 mg/70 kg. Signs of improvement—increase in respiratory rate and pupillary dilation—should occur promptly. In physically dependent addicts too much naloxone may produce signs of withdrawal, as well as reversal of overdosage. If there is no response to the initial dosage, naloxone may be repeated after intervals of a few minutes. In past years it was thought that if no response was observed after 4 to 5 mg, the CNS depression was probably not due solely to opioids. However, buprenorphine, which is now available, is difficult to antagonize with naloxone, and higher doses may be required. The duration of action of naloxone is short compared with that of many opioids, such as methadone and LAAM, and repeated administration may be required to prevent recurrence of opioid toxicity.

WITHDRAWAL

Standard techniques As a general rule, patients who have not been dependent on opioids for more than a year or who

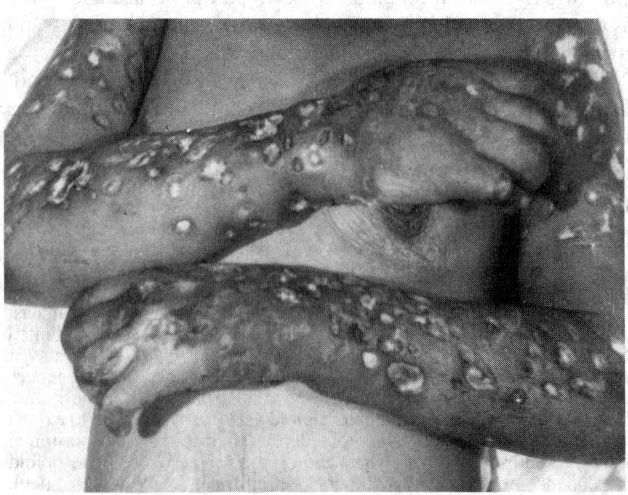

FIGURE 13.9-2 *Skin popper. Circular depressed scars often, with underlying chronic abscesses, can result from skin popping. (Figure courtesy of Michael Baden, MD)*

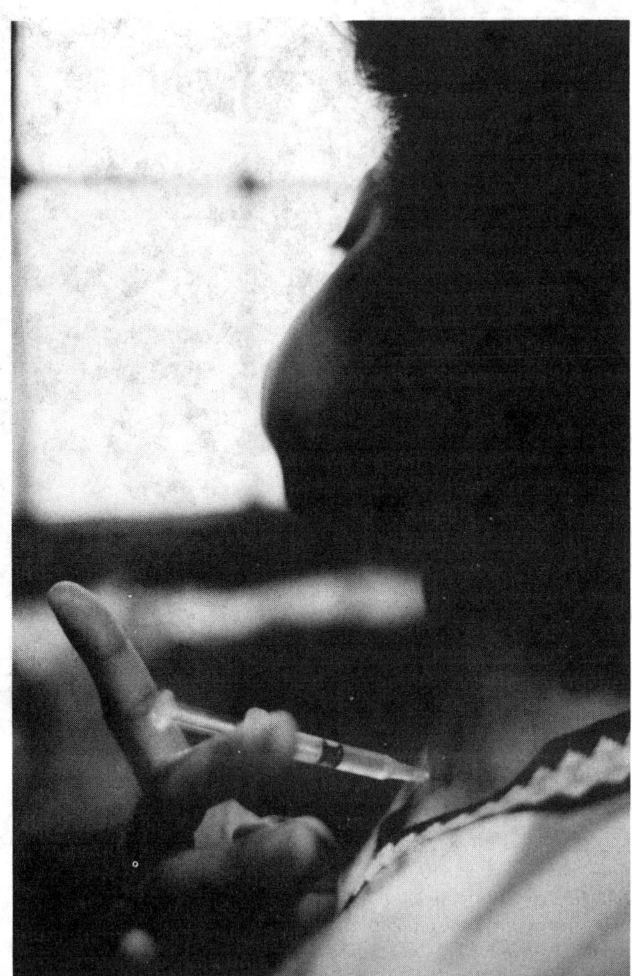

FIGURE 13.9-3 *A heroin user puffs her cheeks to force blood into the jugular vein. (Figure from P T White, S Raymer: The poppy—for good and evil. Nat Geograph* 167: *187, 1985. Used with permission.)*

have not previously made any attempts at withdrawal are not appropriate candidates for prolonged opioid maintenance; therefore, treatment often begins with measures to deal with physical dependence. Detoxification programs may be either outpatient or inpatient. For more than a decade, federal regulations limited the period for prescribing opioid drugs in outpatient detoxification programs to 21 days, although many programs provided for additional psychological support after the three-week period. Those regulations now permit a more gradual detoxification using methadone over a period of 180 days, but some states may have more restrictive regulations.

Currently, the opioid drug most often used to ameliorate the severity of withdrawal is oral methadone. Until the recent introduction of LAAM, it was the only available opioid approved for this purpose by federal regulations. However, theoretically, any opioid can be administered and then gradually reduced. Buprenorphine, a partial μ-agonist opioid, is likely to be approved for use in the treatment of opioid dependence in the near future. In general, the objective in treating hospitalized patients is to make the withdrawal experience tolerable, rather than to suppress all symptoms of withdrawal. Patients should be told to expect some discomfort. For patients using street drugs, the initial dosage of methadone is usually 10 to 20 mg orally. If signs of withdrawal persist, the dose can be repeated after about two hours.

As a general rule, initial stabilization does not require more than 40 mg of methadone during the first 24 hours. Physicians and others who had access to pure drugs are exceptions to that general rule and may require higher doses. If the daily dose of opioid (for example, heroin, meperidine, hydromorphone) is known, the equivalent withdrawal-suppressing dose of methadone can be found in standard pharmacology textbooks or textbooks devoted to addictive disorders. Because the objective of treatment is to prevent severe withdrawal, the current tendency is to base dosage on history, rather than to wait for obvious withdrawal or to precipitate withdrawal with naloxone. Caution should be used when giving doses above 40 mg of methadone a day because the accumulation of methadone can lead to serious toxicity. Once the patient is stabilized, the dose of methadone can be gradually reduced. If patients are hospitalized, the reduction in dose can usually be accomplished within 10 days using dose reductions of 10 to 20 percent per day. In some cases of low-level to moderate dependence, the withdrawal process can be accomplished within one or two days by giving repeated doses of naloxone to precipitate symptoms and ameliorating discomfort with diazepam (Valium) or clonidine. That technique permits rapid transfer to naltrexone. If the detoxification process is to be successful with outpatients, the time required may have to be extended considerably. Some clinicians recommend 10 percent a week as the maximum rate of reduction from high dosage, and reductions of 3 percent a week when the daily dosage is below 20 mg. Patients may be unwilling to accept such a long period of treatment.

Despite the best efforts of clinicians and the use of slow detoxification, all studies to date indicate that many drop out before completing outpatient detoxification and that relapse rates following successful outpatient or inpatient detoxification are high. The relapse rates are particularly high for users of street heroin who attempt to detoxify on an outpatient basis. For such patients, extending the period of withdrawal from three weeks to six weeks or using a longer-acting drug, such as LAAM, does not appear to alter a pattern of almost universal, rapid return to illicit opioid use. In an early study in which drug users were detoxified over a 90-day period with either methadone or low doses (2 mg) of sublingual buprenorphine, both groups did equally poorly in terms of dropping out of treatment and reverting to use of illicit opioids.

Subsequent studies using higher doses of buprenorphine for detoxification found high patient acceptance, good 30-day retention comparable to that with methadone, reduction in illicit opioid use, and withdrawal symptoms that were generally quite mild. The use of buprenorphine may facilitate the transfer to naltrexone. Federal regulations now permit the clinical use of LAAM for detoxification. Despite the problems of initial stabilization, the less frequent need for clinic visits may make LAAM useful for very slow detoxification schedules. Buprenorphine has not yet been approved for the treatment of opioid dependence.

Patients who have formed a relationship with a therapist or who have been maintained for some time on methadone have a far better prognosis for completing detoxification.

Other agents for detoxification Clonidine, an α_2-agonist originally marketed as an antihypertensive, has been shown to suppress some elements of the opioid withdrawal syndrome. With patients stabilized on relatively low doses of opioids—for example, 30 to 40 mg of oral methadone a day—the opioids can be abruptly discontinued and clonidine used to attenuate withdrawal. Clonidine is given orally, starting at doses of 0.1 to 0.3 mg three to four times a day. In outpatient settings a total dosage above 1.0 mg a day is not recommended, although higher doses, 1.5 to 2.5 mg, have been used with hospitalized patients. The major side effects are hypotension, which can be quite extreme, and sedation, and the dosage must be carefully individualized. Patients in outpatient clinics who have been stabilized on methadone and have developed a relationship with the therapists are more successful in achieving abstinence when treated with clonidine than are patients who were taking illicit heroin when clonidine treatment was begun. Some studies have found that outpatient detoxification with clonidine is almost as successful as detoxification using decreasing doses of methadone. In hospitalized patients clonidine permits more rapid detoxification from opioids than does the gradual withdrawal of methadone and patients are more likely to complete the detoxification process.

Clonidine appears to be least effective in suppressing postwithdrawal muscle aches, lethargy, insomnia, restlessness, and craving. There is no evidence that clonidine is useful in preventing relapse after the completion of detoxification. It does appear to facilitate the detoxification of methadone-maintained patients and their stabilization on naltrexone. Properly used, the combination can shorten the period of hospitalization required for detoxification to less than five days. That technique has also been used in a day-hospital outpatient setting. Heroin abusers were given oral clonidine three times a day with dosage (range 0.1 to 0.3 mg) adjusted on the basis of severity of dependence and blood pressure response on the first day, and naltrexone was started on the second day. The naltrexone dose was gradually increased from the initial dose of 1 mg (orally), so that by days 3 to 5 the patients were receiving 40, 50, and 150 mg, respectively. Twelve of 14 subjects so treated were successfully discharged on maintenance naltrexone, but only about one third were still taking naltrexone 30 days later.

α_2-Agonists can also be used with intravenous naloxone to produce accelerated or precipitated detoxification of heroin-using or methadone-maintained patients after first briefly stabilizing them on buprenorphine. In those cases the doses of naloxone and naltrexone are increased to adjust for the greater affinity of buprenorphine for opioid receptors. Initiation of oral naltrexone soon after naloxone-precipitated withdrawal symptoms subside does not appear to result in any additional withdrawal symptoms.

Acetorphan, an enkephalinase inhibitor, is about as effective as clonidine in ameliorating opioid withdrawal.

Other techniques Because opioid withdrawal is rarely life-threatening in healthy adults, a variety of nonpharmacological approaches to drug abstinence have been and continue to be utilized. Abrupt withdrawal (cold turkey) is used in some countries (such as Singapore) as a matter of policy where it is believed that experiencing severe withdrawal is a deterrent to relapse. Abrupt withdrawal, coupled with considerable emotional support, is still used in some therapeutic communities. Since withdrawal stress fatalities can occur in debilitated persons (for example, those with advanced AIDS, tuberculosis, or heart disease), some caution is indicated in selecting accelerated withdrawal or nontreatment for them.

Acupuncture has also been utilized to alleviate opioid withdrawal. The acupuncture-stimulated release of endogenous opioids provides some rational basis for that approach. Whether opioid withdrawal is substantially alleviated by various electrical devices that purport to stimulate the CNS is still not certain despite efforts at controlled studies.

Herbal medicines aimed at ridding the body of toxic substances are sometimes used in a religious or semireligious context (Figure 13.9-4). There is no evidence to indicate that when those traditional approaches are used in their own cultural settings, the outcome is any better or worse than with more medically sophisticated approaches typically used in the United States.

DEPENDENCE Treatment of opioid dependence may involve outpatient, inpatient, residential, or day-care settings. The activities may be centered in hospitals, clinics, prisons, or free-standing, unaffiliated organizations. The staff may consist solely of ex-addicts with considerable personal experience but minimal formal training, correctional officers, formally trained health-care professionals, or some combination of those personnel. The program may emphasize group, individual, or family interactions; all drugs may be proscribed in some programs, whereas other programs may be centered on the use of a drug, such as methadone, or may be designed specifically to target special populations selected by age, gender, culture, race, or special status (for example, pregnant women). Some of the treatment alternatives to be described, such as opioid maintenance, are not currently available in many other countries, and not all options are equally accessible in all parts of the United States. Theoretically, programs with scores of different combinations of environment, staffing, philosophy, target populations, and pharmacological agents are possible, but in practice there are only a handful of major program varieties, each of which may have a few subvarieties.

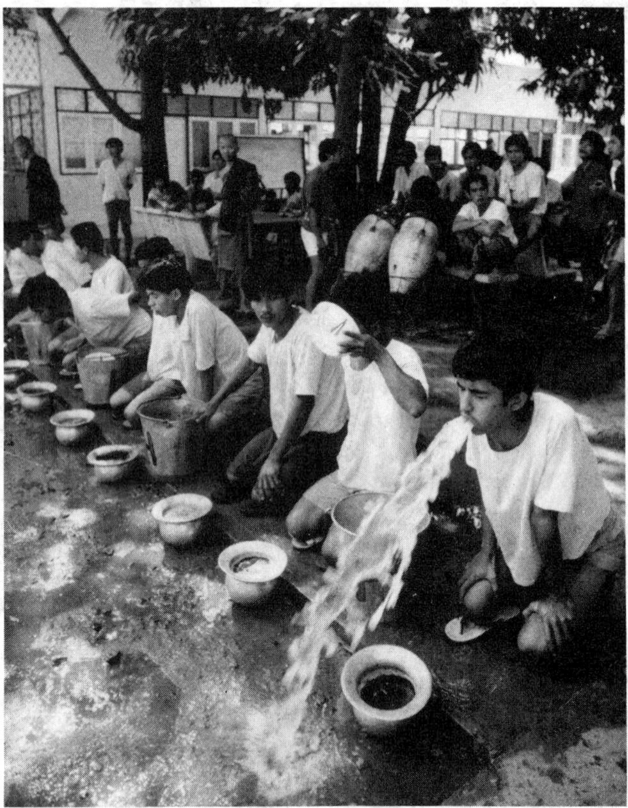

FIGURE 13.9-4 *Treatment of addicts at Tham Krabok Monastery in Thailand results in a 70 percent success rate, according to its records. The 10-day free treatment begins with a vow to Buddha never to use narcotics again. Then patients are given an herbal medicine that makes them vomit immediately. (Figure from P T White, S Raymer: The poppy—for good and evil. Nat Geograph* 167: *187, 1985. Used with permission.)*

Despite a tendency toward a greater diversity of programs for the treatment of addiction in general, most of the opioid users treated annually in the United States are treated in one of four types of programs: detoxification (ambulatory or residential), usually followed by outpatient counseling; methadone maintenance; residential or therapeutic communities; outpatient drug-free programs. Opioid dependence is also treated in chemical-dependency programs based largely on 12-step principles. The outcome for physicians treated in 12-step programs is generally good, but the long-term outcome for persons with backgrounds comparable to those treated in methadone programs or therapeutic communities is not known. Many opioid users benefit from participation in such self-help groups as Alcoholics Anonymous (AA) or Narcotics Anonymous (NA), coupled with participation in a formal program or individual psychotherapy. In some cases such participation is the sole means to begin to maintain control of drug use.

General principles Patients' willingness to accept treatment may change over time as life circumstances, family relationships, and the severity and complications of the dependence change. Consideration should be given not only to the characteristics, wishes, and previous experiences of patients but also to how the patients are likely to react to the particular treatments that are economically and geographically feasible.

The clinician should make it clear that treatment requires a commitment to a long-term change in life-style, attitude, family dynamics, and, sometimes, even geographical location, and that the responsibility for making the changes belongs to the patient. If resources permit, the clinician should not rest content with making a diagnosis of opioid dependence, but should make a complete psychiatric assessment and take a thorough drug-use history. Most opioid users have additional psychiatric disorders (Table 13.9-5). The severity of psychological difficulties (for example, depression, anxiety, paranoid ideation) and patterns of using drugs other than opioids are major predictors of outcome in treatment. Patients, however, should also understand that although antecedent stress, environmental conditions, and underlying psychological difficulties may have played important roles in the genesis of drug dependence, opioid dependence, once established, will not resolve spontaneously even if those conditions are improved. Clinicians must communicate the necessity for treating the pathological drug use as a disorder in its own right. Opioid addicts who enter therapeutic communities under pressure from the criminal justice system are almost as likely to benefit from treatment as are those who enter for other reasons. Court pressure enhances retention in treatment, and retention for more than 90 days is a predictor of positive outcome.

Detoxification as treatment Because brief detoxification alone is generally followed by relapse, some authorities believe that detoxification should be provided only as part of a more comprehensive treatment effort. Other experts feel that brief detoxification should be available for those addicts who want only a limited service. At present it is not clear whether extended ambulatory detoxification (that is, 180 days) should be viewed as detoxification or a distinct treatment approach.

Counseling Counseling and family and individual psychotherapy following opioid withdrawal are usually used but have not been evaluated satisfactorily. Each of those therapeutic techniques has been evaluated in the context of methadone maintenance treatment programs. In such programs scheduled counseling has been shown to reduce illicit drug use substantially and to increase prosocial behaviors. The efficacy of counseling is further supported by studies showing that the quality of counseling and rapport between patient and counselor have a significant impact on outcome measures. When the dosage of methadone was held constant (for example, 60 mg), the addition of drug counseling on a regular basis was distinctly more effective than was emergency counseling in reducing opioid and cocaine use. When patients were provided with on-site medical, psychiatric, employment, and family counseling, the outcome was improved still further. It is reasonable to assume that the quality of counseling, psychiatric, and social services can have an impact on response to treatment among opioid users not maintained on methadone.

Detoxified opioid users assigned to a group-support approach based on the principle that drug users can learn to avoid or cope with situations that provoke drug cravings or feelings of withdrawal (relapse prevention) had lower rates of relapse than did addicts assigned to control groups.

Self-help Narcotics Anonymous is a self-help group of abstinent drug addicts modeled on the principles of AA. Such groups now exist in most large cities and can provide useful group support.

Opioid antagonists The use of opioid antagonists to treat opioid dependence was originally based on the assumption that classically conditioned withdrawal symptoms and operantly reinforced drug-seeking behavior contribute to the high relapse rate typically seen after withdrawal from opioids. Theoretically, by blocking the euphoric effects of opioids, treatment with antagonists would lead to the extinction of operantly reinforced drug seeking; by preventing the reestablishment of physical dependence, treatment with antagonists also leads to the eventual extinction of conditioned withdrawal phenomena. Those drugs do produce the expected blockade of opioid effects, and their toxicity is low. Recently, treatment with antagonists has been based on empirical and laboratory observations that patients taking naltrexone experience less craving in the presence of opioid-related cues, presumably because, on a cognitive basis, they are aware that they are unable to experience the opioid effects.

Naltrexone (Trexan) has been used in a number of clinical trials, but in each, the dropout rate has been high. Curiously, low compliance rates have not been characteristic of alcohol abusers treated with naltrexone.

Naltrexone would appear to be an ideal drug for use in therapy. It is orally effective; when given three times a week (100 mg on weekdays and 150 mg on weekends), it completely blocks the effects of substantial doses of heroin. When naltrexone was tested in a multiclinic, double-blind study, however, very few of those subjects who initially expressed interest in the drug actually took a single dose. In that study about half of the patients already detoxified began treatment with naltrexone, but the dropout rate was quite high: 25 percent of subjects who started treatment dropped out within two weeks; 94 percent stopped by nine months. At the six-month follow-up, few differences were noted between the naltrexone group and the placebo control group, although the naltrexone group had fewer urine specimens positive for opioids while they were in treatment. In other clinical trials subjects continued to take naltrexone for an average of six to eight weeks. A double-blind study in Spain found no differences in drug use or retention in treatment between naltrexone and placebo groups. Former opioid users sometimes report dysphoria, a side effect not reported when the drug is given to alcohol abusers. The only consistent side effect reported is a somewhat higher incidence of nausea.

Experienced clinicians do not think that double-blind placebo trials are the most appropriate way to assess the utility of long-acting antagonists. They believe that to reduce the probability of relapse to opioid use, a period of 30 to 60 days of treatment with naltrexone immediately after detoxification is helpful. In open studies of opioid users on probation who volunteered to take naltrexone, those on active drug were far less likely to violate probation and be reincarcerated than those randomly assigned to placebo. New techniques using clonidine or buprenorphine and clonidine to facilitate the transfer from heroin or methadone to naltrexone may increase the ease of initiating naltrexone treatment, but low compliance and high dropout rates remain unsolved problems. Depot preparations of naltrexone and a somewhat longer-acting antagonist, nalmefine, are under study.

OPIOID MAINTENANCE In the United States about 750 outpatient methadone maintenance programs operating in 40 states and territories are now providing treatment to more than 100,000 patients at any given time. Methadone maintenance is also used in Australia, Hong Kong, and several European countries. Thus methadone maintenance is a major modality for treating opioid dependence.

Initiated by Dole and Nyswander in 1964, the maintenance approach postulated that high doses of methadone would alleviate drug hunger and simultaneously block, by means of cross-tolerance, any euphoria produced by self-administered heroin. Thus opioid users would be freed from the preoccupation with drug-seeking behavior and, with help and rehabilitation, could channel their energies into more productive avenues. The first several hundred chronic heroin addicts treated with that approach showed dramatic decreases in the use of illicit opioids, decreased criminal activity, and increased legitimate, productive work. Furthermore, patients showed little tendency to discontinue treatment, as was the case with other treatment approaches. On the basis of those results, Dole and Nyswander further postulated that opioid dependence is unrelated to antecedent psychological difficulties and that most of the traits of instability and unreliability seen in addicts are the consequence, rather than the cause, of their opioid addiction.

Within the span of a few years, other programs utilizing methadone were established. The results were often less dramatic than those seen by Dole and Nyswander, especially as program criteria for entry were broadened, and more disturbed and less motivated patients were admitted, and also because of changes in program parameters.

General pharmacology Given acutely, methadone is a typical μ-receptor agonist producing euphoria, analgesia, and other typical morphinelike effects. Given chronically by the oral route, however, methadone has several interesting properties that make it unusually useful in maintenance programs. Those qualities include its reliable absorption and bioavailability after oral administration, the delay of peak plasma levels until two to six hours after ingestion, and the apparent nonspecific binding to tissues that creates a large reservoir of methadone in the body. The large reservoir, combined with slow time to peak effects, buffers the patients against sharp peaks in subjective effects after ingestion, which, in any event, are highly attenuated as a result of tolerance. The reservoir of methadone also tends to minimize any sharp declines that would induce withdrawal. Thus not only is the administration of methadone on a once-a-day schedule possible, but minor variations in dosage over short periods do not induce major changes in biological effects. Although the mean plasma half-life in naive subjects is about 15 hours, it ranges from approximately 22 to 56 hours, depending on the measurement technique used, in methadone-maintained subjects. A number of commonly used therapeutic agents can induce liver enzymes and thereby result in more rapid metabolism of methadone and in half-lives significantly less than 22 hours. Some agents can inhibit metabolism.

Standard procedures and government regulations Beginning in 1972, opioid maintenance programs were required to operate according to detailed federal, state, and, sometimes, local regulations. Under recently revised federal regulations, opioid-dependent persons who have been dependent (physiologically addicted) for less than one year can be detoxified using opioids, but cannot be maintained beyond the detoxification period without an opioid-free interval. Persons less than 18 years old must have had two prior treatment failures and verified opioid dependence (physiological dependence) at admission, and have parental consent. Regulations also govern maximum take-home dosage (100 mg without a special exemption from the Food and Drug Administration) and duration of daily clinic treatment before take-home dosage can be provided. Those regulations, and the entire rationale for special regulations, are the subject of a study by the Institute of Medicine of the National Academy of Sciences.

Methadone dose and philosophical differences among programs Methadone maintenance programs vary with respect to dosage, attitudes toward continued antisocial behavior, medical and social services provided, and long-term goals. The original programs emphasized methadone dosage sufficient to suppress opioid drug hunger and to induce a cross-tolerance blockade of the effects of illicit opioids, usually 80 to 120 mg a day. Patients were encouraged to remain on methadone indefinitely on the assumption that the return of opioid drug hunger following detoxification would lead to relapse and the loss of any gains achieved during treatment.

Other programs use lower doses of methadone (20 to 60 mg) that are often adequate for partially suppressing drug seeking, but not for producing adequate cross-tolerance to large doses of heroin. Such programs generally view maintenance as a transitional stage to eventual detoxification. Although patients may remain in treatment in those programs indefinitely, the ambience is often more supportive of efforts at gradual withdrawal. Empirically, patients maintained on lower doses of methadone are far more likely to discontinue treatment. Successful sustained abstinence from opioids is an uncommon result of leaving a methadone maintenance program. Figure 13.9-5, based on data from six different programs, shows that a high proportion of persons are using intravenous heroin again within 12 months after leaving treatment. Since only a small percentage of those persons were actually discharged as having completed treatment, the figure is perhaps a better illustration of what happens to those who drop out.

The influence of methadone dose on outcome has been well studied, and all findings point to the importance of adequate doses. Since there can be wide variations among persons in rates of methadone metabolism, some experts believe that more attention should be given to using laboratory measures of plasma levels to adjust daily dosage. Data suggest that an average level of 400 ng/mL seems adequate and that trough levels below 150 ng/mL are likely to be associated with some degree of withdrawal or drug hunger. Clinicians should be aware that a variety of therapeutic agents can cause a decrease in plasma levels of methadone by inducing hepatic enzymes that metabolize methadone. Among those are rifampin, phenytoin, barbi-

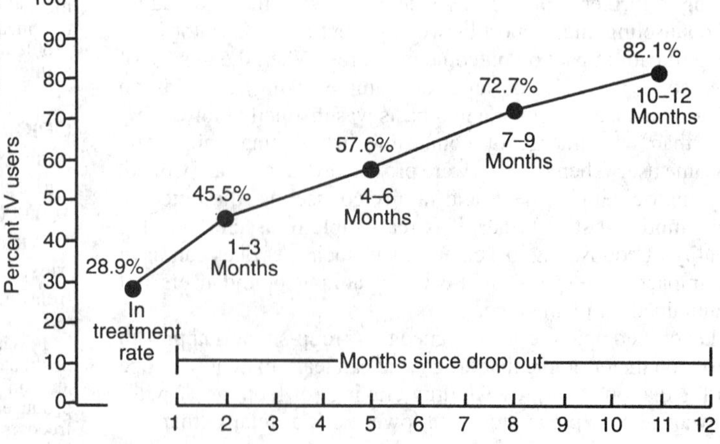

FIGURE 13.9-5 *Relapse to intravenous drug use by 105 men after leaving methadone maintenance treatment. (Figure from J Ball, A Ross:* The Effectiveness of Methadone Maintenance Treatment. *Springer-Verlag, New York, 1991. Used with permission.)*

turates, carbamazepine, and ethyl alcohol. Valproic acid does not accelerate metabolism. Agents that can inhibit methadone metabolism include erythromycin, cimetidine, and ketoconazole. Zidovudine does not alter methadone metabolism, but patients on methadone tend to have higher zidovudine levels than do controls. More methadone is excreted when urinary pH is low than when it is high. Stress and other factors that lower urinary pH can result in lower plasma levels of methadone.

In both high-dose and low-dose methadone programs, there is often a continuing struggle with patients over take-home medication. Patients who do not respond to treatment generally continue to use illicit drugs, both opioid and nonopioid; use alcohol to excess; attend the programs very irregularly; or engage in combative behavior at the clinic. Such patients pose a dilemma to both types of methadone maintenance programs because they would probably fare worse if discharged. However, permitting them to remain demoralizes the staff and other patients and often increases drug use among the latter.

Long-term effects The relative safety of methadone maintenance in terms of organ toxicity has been firmly established. Tolerance to many of the opioid agonist actions of methadone is incomplete, however, and continuing pharmacological effects are observed. Many of those effects, such as euphoria, drowsiness, and somnolence, are more prominent in the first weeks of treatment; if the dosage level is increased too rapidly, the effects even become manifested at later points in treatment. Some effects, however, persist even after many months of treatment. Among the most common long-lasting effects are constipation, which can sometimes result in fecal impaction and intestinal obstruction; excessive sweating; complaints of decreased libido; and sexual dysfunction, for example, an inability to sustain an erection. Opioids reduce plasma levels of testosterone and follicle-stimulating hormone for which tolerance is often incomplete, but the correlation between abnormally low plasma levels of hormones and sexual dysfunction is not high. In general, however, indexes of hypothalamic-pituitary-adrenal axis function are normal in patients maintained on long-term methadone, in contrast with the deranged function typical of active and recently detoxified heroin users. Both sleep abnormalities (insomnia and nightmares) and altered electroencephalogram (EEG) sleep patterns frequently are found during the first months of methadone treatment; the EEG sleep patterns appear to return to baseline, but complaints of sleep abnormalities may persist.

Tolerance does not develop in all patients to the mood-elevating effects of methadone. In double-blind studies some patients regularly report a greater sense of well-being a few hours after ingesting their daily dose. For some patients, that effect may be an important factor in retention in treatment.

In-treatment outcome The majority of patients treated in methadone programs show significantly decreased opioid and nonopioid drug use, criminal behavior, and symptoms of depression and increased gainful employment. Significant differences in effectiveness across programs are due, in some measure, to the characteristics of patients treated, but certain programmatic features tend to make some programs more effective than others. In 1980 the average retention rate for a group of methadone clinics participating in a national prospective study was 81 percent at one month, 67 percent at three months, and 52 percent at six months. Higher retention rates are associated with provision of high-quality social services, especially within the first months; the use of higher doses of methadone (60 mg or more) and allowing patients to know their dosage; the ease of accessibility; no required fees or very low fees; and the use of supportive rather than confrontational techniques.

It has been confirmed repeatedly that positive behavioral change, including decreases in illicit drug use and other criminal behavior, does not typically occur immediately upon entry into treatment, but takes place over a period of many months. Treatments lasting less than 90 days usually have little or no impact; consequently, retention in treatment is critical. Several studies have shown a direct relation between methadone dose and the probability of treatment retention. A study in Australia found that patients on doses of 80 mg or higher were twice as likely to remain in treatment as those at 60 to 79 mg, who were twice as likely to remain as those below 60 mg. Dose has also been shown to have a profound effect on whether or not patients will continue to use illicit heroin. Figure 13.9-6 shows the relation between daily methadone dose and reported heroin use from a study of six different methadone programs. It is somewhat paradoxical that some programs persist in using doses that have been repeatedly shown to be correlated with both high dropout rates and continued illicit drug use.

Other program factors that influence outcome and retention are the perceived range and quality of the social services provided to the patient early in the course of treatment, whether the program is flexible

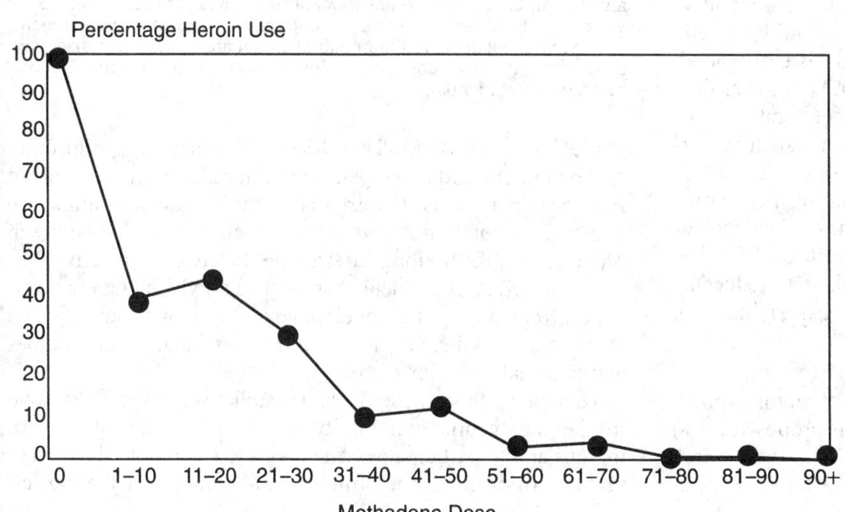

FIGURE 13.9-6 *Heroin use in past 30 days for 407 methadone maintenance patients by current methadone dose. (Figure adapted from J Ball, A Ross:* The Effectiveness of Methadone Maintenance Treatment, *p 248. Springer-Verlag, New York, 1991.*

or confrontational and punitive about occasional illicit drug use, and the competence and quality of the program leadership and the counselors. Outcome correlates with services actually delivered. Some of the better funded programs with better staff-patient ratios did not deliver as many services as did less well-endowed programs. The retention of drug users in programs and the successful reduction of injecting drug use are particularly important in an era when such drug use often results in transmitting or acquiring HIV infection. Older, black, married, and employed patients tend to be retained in methadone programs longer. Those patients with extensive criminal backgrounds tend to drop out sooner and to perform more poorly while in treatment. The severity or duration of opioid use does not correlate with retention or performance in treatment, and patients who enter treatment under what they perceive as legal coercion show improvement comparable to that of patients who report no such external pressure.

Detoxification and long-term outcome Among those patients who successfully detoxify after a period of maintenance, the percentage remaining abstinent at periods of 12 to 36 months ranges from 12 to 28 percent for unselected samples of patients, some of whom were discharged for violation of clinic rules, to 83 percent remaining abstinent from opioids, when analysis is restricted to those patients who elect to be withdrawn with staff and patient consensus that treatment is complete. Predictors of retention and positive outcome in treatment do not necessarily predict success in achieving abstinence or long-term positive outcome once withdrawal has been completed.

In general, patients with shorter drug histories who have been maintained in the program for longer periods but at lower dosages seem more successful than do other patients in detoxifying. In one national, multiclinic follow-up study, 40 percent of former methadone patients interviewed were not using any illicit opioids and did not have any other significant drug problems six years after the completion of initial treatment. Other follow-up studies have found a smaller proportion of former maintenance patients who were opioid abstinent.

Other opioid maintenance drugs L-α-acetylmethadol (LAAM) is a μ-receptor agonist that has been approved for use in the treatment of opioid dependence. It is similar to methadone in its pharmacological actions, and it is converted into active metabolites, nor-acetylmethadol and di-nor-acetylmethadol, that have very long biological half-lives. Consequently, LAAM can be given as infrequently as three times a week, thereby reducing the inconvenience of daily clinic attendance to ingest the drug and simultaneously reducing concerns about illicit diversion. When LAAM is abruptly discontinued, the withdrawal syndrome is slow in onset and relatively mild in intensity, but it is at least as protracted as that of methadone. Over the past 15 years, in both double-blind and large-scale, multicenter, open studies, LAAM has been shown to be equivalent to methadone in terms of suppressing illicit opioid use and encouraging productive activity. It has been consistently found, however, that retention in treatment with LAAM is lower than with methadone. A small percentage of patients complain of side effects not commonly seen with methadone, such as nervousness, stimulation, and amphetaminelike effects. The pharmacology of LAAM is more complex than that of methadone, and its use demands a more skilled clinician than does methadone. Currently, the conditions attached to the use of LAAM prohibit take-home doses. That restriction is likely to reduce its utility, except in situations, such as long-term detoxification, where no take-home methadone is permitted.

BUPRENORPHINE Buprenorphine, a partial μ-receptor agonist, is now available as an analgesic and has been proposed as an alternative to methadone in the treatment of heroin addiction, both for detoxification and for maintenance. It has also been explored in the treatment of concurrent cocaine and opioid dependence. Buprenorphine produces morphinelike effects at low doses, but even when the dose is increased, the intensity of its actions does not seem to exceed that achieved with 30 to 60 mg of morphine. Given sublingually, buprenorphine's opioid-like subjective effects appear to reach a ceiling at about 8 mg, with only modest increases in effects at 16 and 32 mg. Over that dose range, significant respiratory depression was not observed. Because of that apparent ceiling, the risk of overdose may be limited. After chronic administration, buprenorphine attenuates or blocks the subjective effects of parenterally administered morphine or heroin. When buprenorphine given sublingually 8 mg a day for several weeks is abruptly discontinued, a generally mild opioid withdrawal syndrome develops.

Buprenorphine has been compared with methadone as a maintenance agent in several double-blind outpatient studies. Although optimal dose ranges have not been established, one study found 8 mg of buprenorphine sublingually to be comparable to 60 mg of methadone orally on measures of retaining patients in treatment and suppressing heroin use. Buprenorphine and 60 mg of methadone were both superior to 20 mg of methadone on both of these outcome measures. Withdrawal symptoms when buprenorphine was discontinued were mild. In similar studies 8 mg of buprenorphine was significantly less effective than was 80 mg of methadone and was about comparable to 30 mg; in another study 8.9 mg of buprenorphine was comparable to 54 mg of methadone. In none of those double-blind studies did buprenorphine show superiority in reducing cocaine use. Some patients express a clear preference for buprenorphine over methadone. When higher doses of buprenorphine are used, some patients experience no withdrawal for 48 to 72 hours and can reduce clinic visits to less than a daily schedule.

HEROIN VERSUS METHADONE Oral methadone was compared with intravenous heroin at a London clinic in a random assignment study. Most subjects assigned to heroin continued to inject opioids and stayed involved with the drug culture. Some of the heroin subjects sold part of their prescriptions; other subjects supplemented clinic supplies with opioids from illicit sources. Some of the subjects assigned to oral methadone maintenance refused to participate and left treatment immediately; many other subjects left subsequently. At 12 months only 29 percent of oral methadone patients were still at the clinic; of those who left the clinic, 40 percent (28 of those initially assigned to oral methadone) were no longer using opioids regularly at the one year follow-up. Over the 12-month period, more heroin patients than oral methadone patients died or were admitted to hospitals for drug-related problems. A strong relation was found between criminal activity and continued illicit opioid use, although differences in baseline rates of criminality make it difficult to evaluate the net impact of the two types of treatment on crime. As in United States clinics, about one third of the London patients were mildly depressed at admission, 58 percent had a history of depressive episodes, and 38 percent had attempted suicide.

Although the percentage of heroin addicts maintained on methadone who eventually achieve long-term stable abstinence is not high, there is no convincing evidence that the likelihood of abstinence is higher among those treated in other modalities once adjustment is made for various pretreatment predictors of outcome. In one study where methadone treatment appeared to impair eventual abstinence, that disadvantage was offset by substantially lower rates of incarceration among methadone-treated patients.

THERAPEUTIC COMMUNITIES The underlying philosophy of the more than 300 therapeutic communities that have evolved from Synanon is that the drug addict is emotionally immature and requires total immersion in a specialized social structure in order to modify lifelong, destructive behavioral patterns. The goal is to effect a complete change of life-style, including abstinence from drugs, the development of personal honesty and useful social skills, and the elimination of antisocial attitudes and criminal behavior.

To achieve those objectives, the addict was expected to live in the therapeutic community for approximately 12 to 18 months and to participate in frequent group sessions devoted to mutual criticisms of the attitudes and behavior of the participants. The community also acts in many respects as a substitute family. Assumption of responsibility within the community is rewarded with increased personal freedom, material comfort, and the respect of peers. Deviation from community expectations, in terms of behavior or attitude, frequently results in harsh criticisms by staff or, sometimes, by the entire community. Violence and any form of drug use are totally prohibited and may result in expulsion from the community—the ultimate punishment. Although most therapeutic communities avoid the use of drugs even to ease initial withdrawal, some are more flexible regarding treatment with drugs for heavily dependent new entrants. More recently, some therapeutic communities have recognized that a high percentage of addicts have psychopathology in addition to drug dependence. In some cases residents may be prescribed antipsychotic or antidepressant drugs.

Present-day therapeutic communities vary considerably in their attitudes toward professionals and in actual staffing patterns. In every community, however, at least a few ex-addicts are employed as key personnel on the staff; the ex-addicts serve as role models and visible signs that recovery and acceptance are possible and expected. Some therapeutic communities, such as Phoenix House, Odyssey, and Second Genesis, are or were directed by psychiatrists and employ a number of health professionals in key positions. Quite recently, a number of federally supported programs have begun to develop individualized treatment plans and to use health-care professionals, such as physicians, psychologists, or master's-level counselors or social workers, to make initial assessments.

While many therapeutic communities still expect residents to return to the general community after 12 to 18 months, some are experimenting with shorter periods of residence. Because they require so long a period of residence, therapeutic communities obviously have little appeal to those opioid addicts who have stable and gainful employment and satisfactory marital relationships.

Currently, a substantial proportion of entrants into therapeutic communities are referred by the criminal justice system. Criteria for entry have thus been modified, and external pressure to remain in treatment has been increased. Despite the external pressure, dropout rates are still high: 30 to 40 percent in the first 90 days and 50 percent within 6 months. Furthermore, the percentage of new entrants with severe psychopathology has been gradually increasing.

Residence in the therapeutic community results in major reductions in drug-use problems; indicators of depression also decrease significantly. Follow-up studies of graduates and dropouts indicate that patients remaining 90 days or longer exhibit significant decreases in self-reported antisocial behavior, illicit drug use, and recorded arrests, as well as substantial increases in legitimate employment. In general, for those without severe psychopathology, there is a consistent time-in-program effect up to about 12 months; those patients who stay longer exhibit better outcomes along all dimensions at 12-month and 5-year follow-up intervals. In some cases patients found to be doing well have had additional treatment in other programs since leaving the therapeutic community.

OUTPATIENT DRUG-FREE PROGRAMS Such treatment programs often subscribe to the same goals as the residential or therapeutic communities, but they attempt to achieve those goals in a less than 24-hour-a-day setting. The programs vary widely in staffing patterns, philosophy, and program content; they range from highly organized daytime therapeutic communities to drop-in centers offering conversational (rap) sessions and recreational activities. Outpatient drug-free programs tend to deal more with multiple drug abusers than with heavily addicted users of opioids, although heroin addicts are treated by some programs. Long-term follow-up suggests that those programs have an impact beyond that seen with detoxification alone, but differences in patient characteristics make valid comparisons difficult.

Supplements and alternatives to outpatient drug-free therapies must always be mentioned. They include self-help groups, such as AA and NA, as well as non-AA-oriented group therapies focusing on cognitive help in coping with crises and avoiding situations that engender craving (relapse prevention).

PSYCHOTHERAPIES As measured by the use of illicit drugs, need for ancillary psychotropic medicines, scores on scales of psychological distress, and amount of legitimate money earned, patients entering methadone maintenance programs appear to benefit more when individual, analytically oriented, supportive-expressive, or cognitive-behavioral psychotherapy is added to drug counseling than from standard drug counseling alone. With such therapy the very bleak prognosis for patients with the most severe psychopathology can be improved. To best engage patients in individual therapy, the therapy should be started early and be an integral part of the program. In general, patients with antisocial personality without depression do not derive additional benefit, but even among that group, those who seem capable of developing an alliance with the therapist appear to do better than those who do not.

Among methadone-maintained patients, one controlled study suggests that, if urinalysis results are available to monitor drug use, skillful family therapy is superior to standard drug counseling in fostering decreased illicit drug use over a six-month follow-up period.

In contrast to studies on group-based relapse prevention, there are no controlled studies on the efficacy of individual psychotherapy in treating opioid-using patients not stabilized on methadone. Experienced clinicians believe that psychotherapy can influence outcome in opioid users. Some assert that therapists should not be passive, but rather should be willing and able actively and empathetically to help patients look at their vulnerabilities. They also need to be flexible, and be able to communicate respect, empathy, and even admiration. At the same time, therapists must be alert to complex countertransferences that drug-using patients typically provoke. Therapists who see drug-dependent patients in office practice are increasingly recognizing the need to involve the family and to develop a supportive network to aid in their treatment. The therapeutic interventions in such cases are based less on individual psychoanalytic concepts than on cognitive-behavioral techniques that recognize the role of emotional and environmental cues in triggering craving and predisposing to slips and relapses. Although those techniques have been shown to be of value in controlled studies, their efficacy when transferred to office practice is still unclear.

TREATMENT OF SPECIAL POPULATIONS

Criminal justice clients The criminal justice system has complex interactions with drug-dependence treatment systems. Many patients now enter or remain in treatment because of direct coercion by the courts or correctional system. Conversely, some patients on probation or parole may enter treatment against the wishes of their probation officers or in violation of some condition of parole. It was estimated that, in the late 1970s, 15 to 25 percent of opioid-dependent patients treated had some current criminal justice status. The figure for patients entering a methadone program or therapeutic community was above 50 percent. The impact of such coercion on retention in treatment or on outcome has been difficult to estimate because of baseline differences between criminal justice and noncriminal justice patients.

In addition to their relation to the major modalities of treatment, probation or parole, or both, can be viewed as in its own right as a technique that modifies drug-using behavior. Close supervision and drug testing of parolees result in a substantial reduction in daily drug use. The efficacy of such testing and supervision depends in part on the way in which sanctions against use are arranged and the consistency with which such sanctions are exercised. Probation programs that involved use of naltrexone seemed to reduce relapse to opioid use.

Civil commitment programs for opioid users that involved long periods of institutional care, although remaining on the law books, have lost popularity. They were exceedingly expensive as compared with all other treatment modalities, and there was no evidence of their long-term efficacy. In contrast, there is a renewed interest in treatment of incarcerated felons with histories of drug dependence. Those who participated, while incarcerated, in programs based on therapeutic community principles tend to have lower rates of recidivism than do matched controls.

Pregnant women In general, opioid use during pregnancy is associated with decreased fetal growth, but not with any teratological effects. What is clear, however, is that most pregnant women who continue to use heroin do not get prenatal care and deliver low-weight babies with an elevated risk for morbidity and mortality. Babies who survive may be infected with HIV and other diseases as a result of maternal high-risk behavior. Most of those risks can be substantially reduced if the mother can be retained in treatment and provided with prenatal care. Sometimes that can be accomplished in drug-free outpatient or residential programs. Utilizing such programs usually requires initial detoxification, which must be undertaken with considerable caution since severe opioid withdrawal early in pregnancy (before 14 weeks) can induce abortion and late in pregnancy (after week 32) can induce fetal distress. If a woman is already maintained on methadone, it is not necessary to undertake withdrawal, but if withdrawal is elected, it should be done slowly (5 mg every other week) and, if possible, in collaboration with clinicians experienced in perinatal addiction. Dose adjustments (increases) may be needed for pregnant women maintained on methadone because of changes in blood volume and metabolism. Babies born to mothers who have been maintained on methadone usually require treatment for neonatal opioid withdrawal. However, if the use of illicit drugs can be eliminated and adequate prenatal care provided, infant mortality and morbidity are reduced, and in the long run the development and cognitive functioning of the baby are not likely to be impaired.

Other special populations Certain groups of drug users are more likely to enter treatments that seem designed to deal with particular problems, as well as with drug use. For example, some women may feel that only a women's treatment program will deal adequately with issues of childhood sexual abuse, spousal physical abuse, or fears of losing custody of children. Native Americans, Hispanic Americans, or Americans of African or Asian descent may feel more comfortable in programs designed to be sensitive to their cultural values. To what degree such programs are more effective than are less-specialized programs in retaining patients in treatment or producing long-term behavioral change remains undetermined.

OPIOID DEPENDENCE WITH ADDITIONAL PSYCHOPATHOLOGY The severity of psychological disturbances—depression, anxiety, paranoid ideation—are major predictors of the overall outcome of treatment for opioid dependence. Other major predictors of outcome include alcohol abuse and the use of nonopioid drugs.

Mood disorders Some form of affective dysregulation is the most common psychiatric disorder found among opioid addicts in treatment (Table 13.9-5). Clinicians agree that those addicts with manic, hypomanic, or bipolar disorders (the lifetime prevalence among clinic patients is 5 to 10 percent) can benefit from treatment with lithium. Lithium has been used in combination with methadone without adverse interactions.

Although clinicians in private practice often prescribe such antidepressants as amitriptyline (Elavil) or doxepin (Sinequan) for opioid-dependent patients with major depressive disorder and minor depression, publicly supported programs often do not. The reasons for not prescribing those drugs vary. In the past therapeutic communities had a general bias against the use of psychoactive agents; that bias now seems to be decreasing, and some therapeutic communities utilize psychiatric consultants and allow psychoactive medication when indicated. Methadone programs do not have a bias against pharmacotherapy, but most do not commonly assess depressive symptoms, responding only when symptoms become clinically obvious. The efficacy of antidepressants in the treatment of depressed opioid-dependent patients has yet to be clarified. Doxepin, 100 mg daily, mixed with methadone, produced more rapid improvement in depressive symptoms over a four-week period than did a placebo, but the magnitude of the difference was not great. In contrast, imipramine (Tofranil)—an average dose of 140 mg a day—was no better than placebo in methadone-maintained patients; both groups showed significant improvements. Because the pharmacokinetics of imipramine and desipramine (Norpramin) are affected by smoking tobacco and using methadone, adequate plasma levels may not have been achieved. A recent double-blind study of imipramine in methadone-maintained patients with depression that antedated substance use or persisted for more than a month after admission to treatment found significant improvements in mood, as well as decreases in continued illicit drug use.

Depressive symptoms among opioid addicts tend to decrease after entry into treatment, regardless of whether the treatment is an opioid maintenance program or a therapeutic community. Not every patient, however, shows spontaneous improvement. Since the severity of psychological impairment is such a major predictor of overall treatment success, the conscientious clinician will pay particular attention to persistent depression.

Anxiety disorders Anxiety disorders rarely receive specific treatment in programs devoted to opioid dependence. A very high percentage of those addicts with anxiety also have dysphoria. When treatment seems indicated, tricyclic antidepressants, such as doxepin, would appear to be the drugs of choice, because they have antianxiety, antipanic, and antidepressant effects. Also, patients with anxiety disorders may abuse benzodiazepines. Cocaine use can cause cocaine-induced anxiety disorder with panic attacks that persist beyond the period of use. It is not yet clear how cocaine use by opioid users will affect the prevalence of anxiety disorders among that population.

Alcohol abuse Among opioid addicts in treatment, alcoholism (alcohol abuse or dependence) is common, with a lifetime diagnosis rate of 25 to 40 percent. Most addicts who are diagnosed with alcohol abuse or dependence are also diagnosed as having some form of mood disorder. Several studies suggest that there is an inverse relation between alcohol use and heroin use, with alcohol use increasing as heroin use decreases as a result of treatment—a situation that reverses with relapse. Among patients in a methadone program, neither sessions with special AA counselors twice a week nor behavioral modification sessions provided by psychologists were better than a control condition of standard maintenance. However, most alcohol abusers showed decrease in alcohol consumption after entering treatment (despite a decrease in heroin use), and patients and counselors who participated in treatment were enthusiastic about group sessions and expressed the belief that they were beneficial. Disulfiram (Antabuse) can be combined with methadone without adverse effects, and, in small experimental studies, program privileges, such as take-home doses of methadone, have been made contingent on the ingestion of disulfiram. In controlled studies, however, disulfiram was not superior to placebo in modifying alcohol abuse or dependence among methadone-maintained patients. Thus, although alcohol abuse or dependence while in treatment is reported to be a major predictor of reversion to opioid abuse following detoxification from maintenance methadone, it appears that there is no demonstrably effective specific intervention. In programs that do not use methadone continued participation in a residential program sharply reduces alcohol use, but data on long-term outcome are lacking. Both outpatient drug-free and residential programs may employ AA and 12-step approaches to controlling alcohol abuse or dependence along with procedures aimed at opioid use and behavioral change.

Schizophrenia and other psychotic disorders A high percentage of patients (up to 48 percent in some reports) treated in urban hospitals for psychotic disorders, including schizophrenia, also meet the criteria for a substance-use disorder. In most instances, patients are abusing or are dependent on alcohol, cocaine, cannabis, or some combination of those drugs. Even in East Coast urban areas where opioid abuse is common, opioid dependence is relatively uncommon among patients hospitalized for schizophrenia. Two hypotheses have been offered to account for that relatively low level. Either people with schizophrenia are not organized enough to be able to deal with the demands and stresses of obtaining and using heroin, or—in contrast to alcohol, cocaine, and cannabis, which tend to exacerbate schizophrenia—opioids have some ameliorative effects and help persons with schizophrenia avoid hospitalization. There are case reports but, as yet, no controlled studies of opioid users whose psychotic or paranoid states responded to opioids, but responded only poorly to more traditional antipsychotic agents. The endogenous opioids interact with dopaminergic systems, and it has been postulated that methadone has antimanic and antipsychotic actions. Methadone added to antipsychotic medication produces improvement in antipsychotic-resistant patients with paranoid schizophrenia. Heroin addicts treated with methadone may develop tolerance to these postulated antipsychotic effects of opioids so that, after a period on methadone, psychosis may break through again. Although lifetime rates for schizotypal features are 6 to 8 percent among drug-abuse-clinic patients, schizophrenia is uncommon; it is less than 1 percent. For those patients with schizophrenia, dopamine receptor antagonists are probably useful and can be combined with methadone. Some clinicians believe that underlying rage and hostility may play causal roles in opioid dependence and that some addicts use the opioids to control those affects. Clinicians have also observed that, although psychotic patients are reassured by the structure of the usual methadone clinic, borderline patients make the structure and the rules the objects of an all-out war, leading to their rapid and premature discharge from the clinic program.

Opioid dependence with other substance abuse A substantial proportion of opioid users regularly self-administer some other category of drug (for example, amphetamines, cocaine, alcohol, barbiturates, benzodiazepines, or cannabinoids) in amounts sufficient to cause problems. In general, such persons have a greater range and severity of psychiatric problems than do those persons dependent on opioids only. In therapeutic communities such polysubstance abusers create more behavior problems, drop out of treatment sooner, and have poorer posttreatment outcomes than do those who use opioids primarily. Although some polysubstance abusers do not use opioids heavily enough to qualify for treatment in methadone programs, many such persons are eligible. In an attempt to compare outcomes as a function of the category of drugs abused and the treatment received, one study retrospectively matched polysubstance-using male veterans with greater than average psychopathology who entered a therapeutic community with those who entered a methadone maintenance program. The patients were further categorized into opioid-stimulant, opioid-depressant, and opioid-only users. At a six-month follow-up interview, there were clear-cut differences in outcome. Opioid-only patients had better outcomes on all measures than did either of the other groups, and for opioid-only patients, there was no clear superiority of either treatment approach. Opioid-stimulant patients did significantly better in methadone maintenance programs, whereas opioid-depressant patients did significantly better after treatment in a therapeutic community. It was speculated that the hypersensitivity and paranoia of the opioid-stimulant group are alleviated by the effects of methadone and aggravated by the confrontational techniques used in the therapeutic community. It was also inferred that the prolonged abstinence afforded by the therapeutic community was helpful in facilitating recovery from the depression and cognitive impairment that typically accompanies use of sedatives.

SUGGESTED CROSS-REFERENCES

An overview of substance-related disorders is given in Section 13.1. Alcohol-related disorders are discussed in Section 13.2, amphetamine-related disorders in Section 13.3, and cocaine-related disorders in Section 13.6. Methadone is the subject of Section 32.17, and drug and alcohol abuse among the elderly is discussed in Section 49.6g. Posttraumatic stress disorder is discussed in Section 17.4 and sexual dysfunction in Section 21.1a.

REFERENCES

Arndt I O, Dorozynsky L, Woody G E, McLellan A T, O'Brien C P: Desipramine treatment of cocaine dependence in methadone-maintained patients. Arch Gen Psychiatry *49:* 888, 1992.

Bailey R C, Hser Y-I, Hsieh S-C, Anglin M D: Influences affecting maintenance and cessation of narcotics addiction. J Drug Issues *24:* 249, 1994.

Ball J, Ross A: *The Effectiveness of Methadone Maintenance Treatment.* Springer-Verlag, New York, 1991.

Bell J, Hall W, Byth K: Changes in criminal activity after entering methadone maintenance. Br J Addict *87:* 251, 1992.

Caplehorn J R M, Dalton M S Y N, Cluff M C, Petrenas A-M: Retention in methadone maintenance and heroin addicts' risk of death. Addiction *89:* 203, 1994.

Castenada R, Galanter M, Lifshutz H, Franco H: Effects of drugs of abuse on psychiatric symptoms among hospitalized schizophrenics. Am J Drug Alcohol Abuse *17:* 313, 1991.

Cooper J R: Methadone treatment and acquired immunodeficiency syndrome. JAMA *262:* 1664, 1989.

D'Aunno T, Vaughn T E: Variation in methadone treatment practices. Results from a national study. JAMA *267:* 253, 1992.

De Leon G: Treatment of substance abusers in therapeutic communities. In *The Treatment of Substance Abuse,* Galanter M, Kleber H, editors. American Psychiatric Press, Washington, 1994.

Dole V P: Implications of methadone maintenance for theories of narcotic addiction. JAMA *260:* 3025, 1988.

Finnegan L P, Hagan T A, Kaltenbach K: Opioid dependence: Scientific foundations of clinical practice. Proc NY Acad Med *67:* 223, 1991.

Fudala P J, Jaffe J H, Dax E M, Johnson R E: Use of buprenorphine in the treatment of opioid addiction. II. Effects of daily and alternate-day administration and abrupt withdrawal. Clin Pharmacol Ther *47:* 525, 1990.
Galanter M: Network therapy for addiction: A model for office practice. Am J Psychiatry *150:* 28, 1993.
*Gerstein D R, Harwood H J, editors: *Treating Drug Problems.* National Academy Press, Washington, 1990.
Gerstley L, McLellan T, Alterman A, Woody G, Luborsky L, Prout M: Ability to form an alliance with the therapist: A possible marker of prognosis for patients with antisocial personality disorder. Am J Psychiatry *146:* 508, 1989.
Hammersley R, Forsyth A, Morrison V, Davies J: The relationship between crime and opioid use. Br J Addict *84:* 1029, 1989.
Hanlon T E, Nurco D N, Kinlock T W, Duszynski K R: Trends in criminal activity and drug use over an addiction career. Am J Drug Alcohol Abuse *16:* 223, 1990.
Haverkos H W: Infectious diseases and drug abuse. Prevention and treatment in the drug abuse treatment system. J Substance Abuse Treatment *8:* 269, 1991.
Hubbard R L, Marsden M E, Rachal J V, Harwood H J, Cavanaugh E R, Ginzburg H M: *Drug Abuse Treatment: A National Study of Effectiveness.* University of North Carolina Press, Chapel Hill, 1989.
Jaffe J H: Drug addiction and drug abuse. In *Goodman and Gilman's The Pharmacological Basis of Therapeutics,* ed 8, A G Gilman, T W Rall, A S Nies, P Taylor, editors, p 522. Pergamon, New York, 1990.
*Jaffe J H, Epstein S, Ciraulo D A: Opioids. In *Clinical Manual of Chemical Dependence* D A Ciraulo, R I Shader, editors, 95. American Psychiatric Press, Washington, 1991.
Jaffe J H, Martin W R: Opioid analgesics and antagonists. In *Goodman and Gilman's The Pharmacological Basis of Therapeutics,* ed 8, A G Gilman, T W Rall, A S Nies, P Taylor, editors, p 485. Pergamon, New York, 1990.
Johnson R E, Jaffe J H, Fudala P J: A controlled trial of buprenorphine treatment for opioid dependence. JAMA *267:* 2750, 1992.
Kaltenbach K, Silverman H, Wapner R: Methadone maintenance during pregnancy. In *State Methadone Maintenance Treatment Guidelines,* p 173. Center for Substance Abuse Treatment, Substance Abuse and Mental Health Services Administration, U.S. Department of Health and Human Services, Rockville, MD, 1993.
Katims J J, Ng L K Y, Lowinson J H: Acupuncture and transcutaneous electrical nerve stimulation: Afferent nerve stimulation (ANS) in the treatment of addiction. In *Substance Abuse: A Comprehensive Textbook,* ed 2, J H Lowinson, P Ruiz, R B Millman, editors, p 574. Williams & Wilkins, Baltimore, 1992.
Kaufman E R: Countertransference and other mutually interactive aspects of psychotherapy with substance abusers. Am J Addictions *1:* 185, 1992.
Khantzian E, Halliday K S, McAuliffe W I: *Addiction and the Vulnerable Self.* Guilford, New York, 1990.
Kleber H D, Topazian M, Gaspari J, Riordan C E, Kosten T: Clonidine and naltrexone in the outpatient treatment of heroin withdrawal. Am J Drug Alcohol Abuse *13:* 1, 1987.
Koob G F: Neurobiological mechanisms in cocaine and opiate dependence. In *Addictive States,* Research Publications: Association for Research in Nervous and Mental Disease, vol 70. C P O'Brien, J H Jaffe, editors, p 79. Raven, New York, 1992.
Kosten T R, Krystal J H, Charney D S, et al: Rapid detoxification from opioid dependence (letter). Am J Psychiatry *146:* 1349, 1989.
Kreek M J: Rationale for maintenance pharmacotherapy of opiate dependence. In *Addictive States,* Research Publications: Association for Research in Nervous and Mental Disease, vol 70, C P O'Brien, J H Jaffe, editors, p 205. Raven, New York, 1992.
Loimer N, Linzmayer L, Schmid R, Grünberger J: Similar efficacy of abrupt and gradual opiate detoxification. Am J Drug Alcohol Abuse *17:* 307, 1991.
Maddox J F, Desmond D P: Ten year follow-up after admission to methadone maintenance. Am J Drug Alcohol Abuse *18:* 289, 1992.
Maddox J F, Desmond D P: Family and environment in the choice of opioid dependence or alcoholism. Am J Drug Alcohol Abuse *15:* 117, 1989.
Malin D L: The role of non-opioid peptides in opiate dependence. Neuropsychopharmacology *10* (3S/Pt 1): 561S, 1994.
Martin W R, Jasinski D R, Haertzen C A, Kay D C, Jones B E, Mansky P A, Carpenter R W: Methadone—a reevaluation. Arch Gen Psychiatry *28:* 286, 1973.
*McLellan A T, Arndt I O, Metzger D S, Woody G E, O'Brien C P: The effects of psychosocial services in substance abuse treatment. JAMA *269:* 1953, 1993.
McLellan A T, Luborsky L, Woody G E, O'Brien C P, Druley K A: Predicting response to alcohol and drug abuse treatments. Arch Gen Psychiatry *40:* 620, 1983.
*McLellan A T, O'Brien C P, Metzger D, Alterman A I, Cornish J, Urschel H: How effective is substance abuse treatment—compared to what? In *Addictive States.* Research Publications: Association for Research in Nervous and Mental Disease, vol 70. C P O'Brien, J H Jaffe, editors, p 231. Raven, New York, 1992.
Metzger D S, Cornish J, Woody G E, McLellan A T, Druley P, O'Brien C P: Naltrexone in federal probationers. NIDA Res Monogr *95:* 465, 1990.
Najavits L M, Weiss R D: The role of psychotherapy in the treatment of substance-use disorders. Harvard Rev Psychiatry *2:* 84, 1994.
Nestler E J: Molecular neurobiology of drug addiction. Neuropsychopharmacology, *11:* 77, 1994.
Novick D M, Richman B L, Friedman J M, Friedman J E, Fried C, Wilson J P, Townley A, Kreek M J: The medical status of methadone maintenance patients in treatment for 11–18 years. Drug Alcohol Dependence *33:* 235, 1993.
Nurco D N, Kinlock T, Balter M B: The severity of pre-addiction criminal behavior among urban, male narcotic addicts and two non-addicted control groups. J Res Crime Delinquency *30:* 293, 1993.
Payte J T, Khuri E T: Principles of methadone dose determination. In *State Methadone Maintenance Treatment Guidelines,* p 101. Center for Substance Abuse Treatment, Substance Abuse and Mental Health Services Administration, United States Department of Health and Human Services, Rockville, MD, 1993.
Robins L N: Vietnam veterans' rapid recovery from heroin addiction: A fluke or normal expectation? Addiction *88:* 1041, 1993.
*Rounsaville B J, Kosten T R, Weissman M M, Prusoff B, Pauls D, Anton S F, Merikangas K: Psychiatric disorders in relatives of probands with opiate addiction. Arch Gen Psychiatry *48:* 33, 1991.
Rounsaville B J, Weissman M M, Kleber H D, Wilber C: The heterogeneity of psychiatric diagnosis in treated opiate addicts. Arch Gen Psychiatry *39:* 161, 1982.
Salloum I M, Moss H B, Daley D C: Substance abuse and schizophrenia: Impediments to optimal care. Am J Drug Alcohol Abuse *17:* 321, 1991.
Simon E J: Opiates: Neurobiology. In *Substance Abuse: A Comprehensive Textbook,* ed 2, J H Lowinson, P Ruiz, R B Millman, J G Langrod, editors, p 195. Williams & Wilkins, Baltimore, 1992.
Strain E C, Stitzer M L, Liebson I A, Bigelow G E: Comparison of buprenorphine and methadone in the treatment of opioid dependence. Am J Psychiatry *151:* 1025, 1994.
Terenius L T, O'Brien C P: Receptors and endogenous ligands: Implications for addiction. In *Addictive States,* C P O'Brien, J H Jaffe, editors, Research Publications: Association for Research in Nervous and Mental Disease, vol 70, p 123. Raven, New York, 1992.
White P T, Raymer A: The poppy—for good and evil. Nat Geograph *167:* 187, 1985.
Woody G E, O'Brien C P, McLellan A T, Marcovici M, Evans B D: The use of antidepressants with methadone in depressed maintenance patients. Ann NY Acad Sci *398:* 120, 1982.

13.10 PHENCYCLIDINE (or PHENCYCLIDINELIKE)-RELATED DISORDERS

THOMAS J. CROWLEY, M.D.

INTRODUCTION

Phencyclidine (1(1-phenylcyclohexyl)-piperidine), usually referred to as PCP, was first synthesized at Parke-Davis Company as a dissociative anesthetic (Sernyl), that rendered patients comatose, analgesic, and amnesic for surgery. But severe psychiatric effects occasionally marred postsurgical emergence, and the substance never was marketed for use in human anesthesia. It has been used as a veterinary anesthetic (Sernylan) but is no longer marketed in the United States. A less toxic anesthetic analogue, ketamine (Ketalar) is still widely used for human anesthesia. PCP synthesis, which is relatively simple, was described in the lay press, and in 1967 the substance was marketed illegally in San Francisco. It is widely available under such street names as *peace pill*, angel dust, or hog. Adverse

TABLE 13.10-1
Nosology of Phencyclidine-Related Disorders

DSM-IV	DSM-III-R	ICD-9	ICD-9-CM	ICD-10
Phencyclidine abuse	POSAA* abuse	Nondependent abuse of drugs	Nondependent abuse of drugs	Phencyclidine harmful use
Phencyclidine dependence	POSAA dependence	Drug dependence NOS†	Drug dependence	Phencyclidine dependence syndrome
Phencyclidine intoxication (specify if: with perceptual disturbance)	POSAA intoxication	Nondependent abuse of drugs	Nondependent abuse of drugs	Phencyclidine acute intoxication
Phencyclidine intoxication delirium	POSAA delirium	Acute confusional state	Drug-induced delirium	Phencyclidine acute intoxication
Phencyclidine-induced psychotic disorder, with delusions, or with hallucinations (specify if: with onset during intoxication)	POSAA delusional disorder	Drug psychosis	Drug psychosis or drug-induced hallucinosis	Phencyclidine psychotic disorder
Phencyclidine-induced mood disorder (specify if: with onset during intoxication)	POSAA mood disorder		Drug-induced organic affective syndrome	
Phencyclidine-induced anxiety disorder (specify if: with onset during intoxication)				
			Pathological drug intoxication	
Phencyclidine-related disorder NOS	POSAA organic mental disorder NOS		Unspecified drug-induced mental disorder	Other mental or behavioral disorder induced by phencyclidine Unspecified mental or behavioral disorder induced by phencyclidine

*POSAA, phencyclidine or similarly acting arylcyclohexylamine.
†NOS, not otherwise specified.

reactions gave it a bad reputation, and illegal drug dealers often now misrepresent it as tetrahydrocannabinol (THC) or lysergic acid diethylamide LSD.

COMPARATIVE NOSOLOGY

Table 13.10-1 compares several historic diagnostic systems. The fourth edition of *Diagnostic and Statistical Manual of Mental Disorders* (DSM-IV) differs from the revised third edition (DSM-III-R) in several ways. Abuse was viewed as a residual category in DSM-III-R, while DSM-IV provides specific diagnostic criteria for substance abuse. The DSM-IV criteria for substance dependence also are somewhat more specific, and there is an option of subtyping ''with (or without) physiological dependence.'' DSM-IV expands the list of mental disorders arising from PCP intoxication to include phencyclidine-induced anxiety disorder. The DSM-IV phencyclidine (or phencyclidinelike)-related disorders appear in Table 13.10-2.

The ninth revision of the *International Classification of Diseases, and Related Health Problems* (ICD-9) provided many fewer specific diagnostic categories of PCP intoxication and used the term ''abuse'' to include intoxication. ICD-9-CM, an official U.S. government disease classification that modified ICD-9 for purposes of Medicare and Medicaid billing also used the term ''abuse'' interchangeably with intoxication and provided no diagnosis corresponding to phencyclidine-induced anxiety disorder. ICD-10, a revision of ICD-9, replaces the term ''abuse'' with ''harmful use'' and recognizes neither phencyclidine intoxication mood nor anxiety disorders.

Although PCP-treated monkeys show definite withdrawal following drug termination, withdrawal rarely occurs clinically in humans. It is presumed that few people use the frequent high doses required to produce withdrawal. Thus, neither DSM-IV nor DSM-III-R provide for withdrawal diagnoses. The rare instance of PCP withdrawal could be coded in DSM-IV as phencyclidine-related disorder not otherwise specified. The other diagnostic systems mention substance withdrawal states generally, and these presumably could apply to PCP.

TABLE 13.10-2
Phencyclidine (or Phencyclidinelike)-Related Disorders

Phencyclidine use disorders

Phencyclidine dependence
Phencyclidine abuse

Phencyclidine-induced disorders

Phencyclidine intoxication
Specify if: with perceptual disturbances
Phencyclidine intoxication delirium
Phencyclidine-induced psychotic disorder, with delusions
Specify if: with onset during intoxication
Phencyclidine-induced psychotic disorder, with hallucinations
Specify if: with onset during intoxication
Phencyclidine-induced mood disorder
Specify if: with onset during intoxication
Phencyclidine-induced anxiety disorder
Specify if: with onset during intoxication

Phencyclidine-related disorder not otherwise specified

Table from DSM-IV, *Diagnostic and Statistical Manual of Mental Disorders,* ed 4. Copyright American Psychiatric Association, Washington, 1994. Used with permission.

EPIDEMIOLOGY

The extent of use or preference for PCP (alone or in combination with other drugs) among substance abusers varies dramatically in different cities (Figure 13.10-1). Nationally, PCP accounted for about 3.2 percent of 1989 drug-related presentations in federally monitored emergency rooms, totaling only

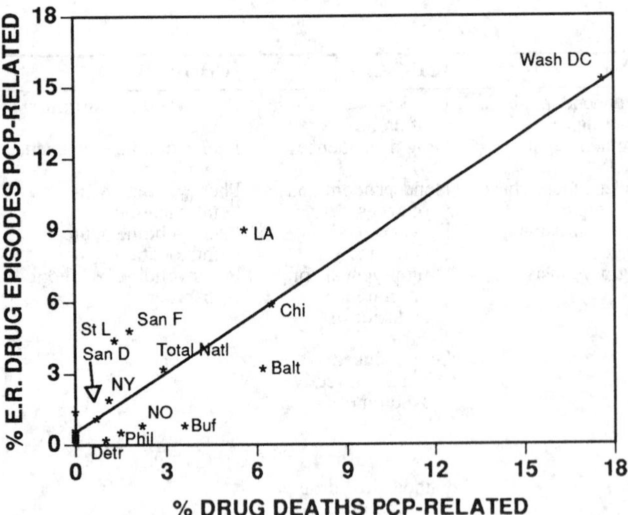

FIGURE 13.10-1 *Plot of PCP-related emergency room visits as a percentage of all drug-related visits versus the proportion of PCP-related drug deaths among all drug deaths. Atlanta, Boston, Dallas, Denver, Miami, Minneapolis, Newark, Phoenix, and Seattle are clumped at 0 drug deaths. Other cities represented are Baltimore, Buffalo, Chicago, Detroit, Los Angeles, New Orleans, New York City, Philadelphia, San Diego, San Francisco, St. Louis, and Washington, DC. Also shown are percentages for the total national sample. Pearson's r = 0.91.* (Data from 1989 Drug Abuse Warning Network, National Institute on Drug Abuse, Washington. Used with permission.)

4.4 percent of drug-related presentations by blacks and Hispanics and only 1.9 percent by whites. Over 80 percent of the patients were aged 20 to 39 years, with few younger or older users. PCP accounted for about 4 percent of drug-related emergency room episodes among men and only about 2 percent among women. Thus, casualties from other drugs are much more common than PCP casualties, and PCP use is concentrated in certain cities, among younger to middle-aged adults, in some minority groups, and in men. Over 90 percent of emergency room episodes (when the route of administration was known) resulted from smoking PCP-laced cigarettes, and cocaine or alcohol was frequently used with the PCP. Selected medical examiners across the country mentioned PCP in about 3 of drug-related deaths (compared, for example, with cocaine in over 50 percent of such deaths). It must be emphasized, however, that PCP estimates in surveys may be particularly unreliable, because PCP, which is easily manufactured but often rejected by users, is especially likely to be sold under false names.

PHARMACOLOGY

PCP, a glistening white solid, is soluble in water and ethanol. Over 30 PCP analogues have been synthesized illicitly, including 1-piperidinocyclohexanecarbonitrile (PCC), 1-(1-2-thienylcyclohexyl) piperidine (TCP), N-ethyl-1-phenylcyclohexyalamine (PCE), 1-(1-phencyclohexyl) pyrrolidine (PHP), and ketamine (which legally is used in anesthesia). Such analogues account for the phrase ''or phencyclidinelike'' in the DSM-IV nomenclature for the PCP group of disorders. However, illicit use of PCP far exceeds that of its analogues. The compounds may be distributed as crystals, paste, liquid, or as a dried blot of liquid on paper. Illicit samples occasionally reach 100 percent purity but are extremely variable.

ROUTE OF ADMINISTRATION, ABSORPTION, AND DISTRIBUTION PCP usually is smoked in tobacco or marijuana cigarettes; with rapid transpulmonary absorption of small incremental doses, users can better titrate the drug effects. PCP is also taken orally, intravenously, or transcutaneously. Bioavailability in those forms is high; at least 70 to 75 percent of an oral or intravenous dose survives initial metabolism and enters the system, whereas about one third of a smoked dose may be absorbed.

Plasma levels of PCP plateau two to four hours after single oral or intravenous test doses and then decline, with a half-life averaging 20 hours but varying considerably among individuals. Only some 15 to 20 percent of a test dose is recovered from urine or feces as intact PCP; the substance is cleared primarily through hydroxylation by the liver.

Because PCP is lipophilic, concentrations in the brain are six to nine times higher than in plasma in animal studies, and adipose-to-plasma ratios are even higher. PCP may be detected in animal brains three weeks after a single injection, and accumulation occurs there with repeated dosing. It has been suggested that accumulated PCP could be mobilized from fat stores by weight loss or stress, and detectable urinary PCP concentrations have recurred after surgery among users who had been abstinent for days or weeks.

BEHAVIORAL AND PHYSIOLOGICAL EFFECTS PCP produces an extraordinary range of effects. First, it reinforces drug self-administration by animals. Monkeys repeatedly press levers to obtain PCP injections until they become too ataxic or lethargic to continue; they later resume self-injecting as soon as possible. They develop physical dependence, and when PCP access ends they undergo withdrawal with vocalizations, bruxism, ocular motor hyperactivity, diarrhea, piloerection, lethargy, tremors, and occasionally with convulsions. Monkeys also develop moderate tolerance to PCP. Human users often report tolerance, but withdrawal is uncommon with the dosing frequency of most human PCP users. Both memory and learning are impaired during intoxication. PCP-treated surgical patients often could not recall their recovery room experiences. Repeated intoxications (poisonings resulting from use of the drug) of chronic users may produce severe deficits of immediate and short-term memory, but some improvement occurs if doses are reduced or eliminated.

Discriminative stimulus studies suggest that the subjective state of an animal during PCP intoxication is unlike that resulting from other drugs. In those studies an animal is reinforced for pressing one lever after receiving PCP injections and a different lever after saline injections. The animal learns to press the correct lever based on its own postinjection feelings. If the animal then is injected with a different drug (such as an amphetamine, pentobarbital, or morphine), the animal does not respond on the PCP lever, pointing to a unique subjective state resulting from PCP use.

In humans PCP produces a reversible psychosis that many observers have likened to acute schizophrenia. Because haloperidol (Haldol) binds at some PCP binding sites in the central nervous system with an affinity about equivalent to its binding at dopamine sites, many speculate that these PCP binding sites may play a role in schizophrenia.

PCP produces amphetaminelike effects (enhanced motility, diminished eating, and reduced prolactin concentrations) and barbiturate-like effects (clumsiness, enhancement of sedation from barbiturates and ethanol, and an anticonvulsant action). Whereas PCP raises seizure thresholds in many model systems, overdoses elicit seizures in humans. Clinical reports emphasize unpredictable aggressiveness during PCP intoxication. On the other hand the drug commonly is termed an animal tranquilizer because it reduces aggressiveness in animals. The basis of this difference is unclear. PCP also protects against cell death after episodes of ischemia or prolonged seizures. Clinical tests of PCP derivatives for acute post-stroke patients are on the horizon.

PCP and ketamine are thought to have less effect on reproductive function than many other anesthetic agents. But in rats serum concentrations of both testosterone and luteinizing hormone are elevated for many days following nine daily PCP treatments. The elevations persist longer among rats treated as they are becoming sexually mature compared to rats treated in adulthood. PCP does cross the placenta, and fetal PCP levels may exceed maternal levels by a wide margin. Babies of PCP-abusing mothers reportedly show neonatal withdrawal with irritability, hypertonic reflexes, diarrhea, poor feeding, inability to track visually, high-pitched cry, and jitteriness. Current evidence does not suggest that maternal PCP use causes congenital anomalies in offspring, but long-term outcome after prenatal exposure or neonatal withdrawal remains unknown.

PCP produces little organ damage. Studies using a general physical examination and a chemistry panel found no differences between control monkeys and monkeys that had self-administered PCP daily for up to eight years. Recent studies in animals, however, revealed neuronal vacuoles in brain tissue for several hours after PCP doses.

A placebo-controlled study of intravenous ketamine (0.1 and 0.5 mg/kg of body weight) documented important behavioral changes induced by this PCP analogue. In a dose-related fashion it produced illusions, ideas of reference, paranoid thoughts, and formal thought disorder. It induced detachment and emotional blunting, despite behavioral activation, and it altered perceptions. Global measures of cognition were not affected, but specific memory tests indicated impairment. Subjects felt a high comparable to that of alcohol intoxication. Most actions ended within one to two hours. Thus, ketamine clearly induces many of the effects of PCP.

MECHANISMS OF ACTION

Dopaminergic Because of its psychosis-producing effects and its amphetaminelike effects on dopamine, PCP has been proposed as a model for the study of schizophrenia. PCP inhibits dopamine uptake into synaptosomes and augments haloperidol-enhanced utilization of dopamine. It inhibits tyrosine hydroxylase activity in vivo and probably causes presynaptic release of dopamine. Its augmentation of locomotor activity in rats is reduced by antidopamine lesioning in the nucleus accumbens. Thus, PCP facilitates the presynaptic release of dopamine and inhibits its reuptake, resulting in amphetaminelike behavioral stimulation. PCP receptors (discussed in the following paragraph) probably are not involved in these dopaminergic effects. Instead, PCP binds with rather high affinity to a "cocaine receptor" that inhibits the dopamine transporter responsible for presynaptic dopamine reuptake. Interestingly ketamine, a PCP derivative that rarely causes psychosis, binds with much less affinity to that receptor.

PCP receptors In the brain PCP binds to receptors now known to be separate from sigma-opioid receptors. At these recognition sites PCP modulates the action of nearby receptors responsive to *N*-methyl-D-aspartate (NMDA) and glutamate. NMDA and glutamate are excitatory, proconvulsant, and neurotoxic amino acids that are released in excess and kill cells during ischemia; PCP and its analogues reduce this toxicity and inhibit the convulsive effects of those amino acids in animals.

The mere existence of phylogenetically old PCP receptors in brain suggests that some endogenous ligands activate them. Several candidate ligands have been isolated from mammalian brains, one of which reportedly produces electrophysiologic and behavioral effects similar to those of PCP. There could be profound implications for the study of mental illness if an endogenous brain compound proves to bind to PCP receptors while mimicking the psychosis-inducing effects of the drug. Postmortem brains from schizophrenic patients reportedly do have more PCP receptor sites than brains from healthy subjects. However, postmortem brains from long-term PCP abusers do not show such changes.

Serotonin and acetylcholine PCP inhibits uptake of serotonin (5-hydroxytryptamine [5-HT]) into synaptosomes, while reducing 5-HT turnover. It also reduces firing rate in some 5-HT neurons. It has mixed cholinomimetic and anticholinergic properties in animals.

ETIOLOGY

Except for reinforcement tests in animals, few studies address the cause of PCP abuse and dependence. However, many factors increase the chances of drug use generally and probably contribute to PCP problems.

EXTRINSIC FACTORS Factors outside of the individual include, first, availability of PCP (presence of local manufacturers, distributors, or dealers; low local cost; PCP-using friends) because drug availability is essential for drug use. Second, PCP use is accepted and relatively prevalent in certain areas and among certain groups, meaning that others are there to initiate a person into PCP use. In addition, the vigorous self-administration of PCP by monkeys demonstrates that PCP use is pharmacologically reinforcing and therefore likely to be repeated after drug use begins. The environment of any given user provides some balance of social punishers and social reinforcers for PCP use or PCP abstinence; if the net influence of others encourages further use, a person is more likely to become involved with the drug. Finally, an absence of competing reinforcers appears generally to increase human propensity to use drugs. A wealth of nondrug-reinforcing activities in the environment reduces the probability of substance abuse. Persons without access to alternative activities may be more likely to abuse substances generally, including PCP.

INTRINSIC FACTORS Factors intrinsic to the person also affect the probability of drug use, and those presumably apply also to PCP use. A general risk-taking propensity, reaching its extreme in conduct disorder and antisocial personality disorder, increases the probability of drug use. PCP is known to be toxic, and those who are willing to take significant risks are probably more likely to use it regularly. In general previous drug experience increases the probability of current and future drug use. Among drug-using adolescents PCP use usually begins after several years of alcohol, marijuana, and tobacco consumption. Genetic factors contribute significantly to the risk of alcohol use, and a recent study of twins suggests that a close genetic relationship to an alcoholic person increases a person's risk for problems with nonalcohol drugs (such as PCP). Age, sex, and ethnicity also are risk factors, with PCP use apparently more common among substance abusers who are male, 20 to 40 years of age, and members of some minority groups.

PHENCYCLIDINE INTOXICATION

DIAGNOSIS AND CLINICAL FEATURES Phencyclidine intoxication is a clinically significant maladaptive behavioral syndrome developing during or shortly after use of PCP or a PCP-related drug and due directly to use of that drug. U.S. Army volunteers and surgical patients have provided information on dose-controlled PCP intoxications from which a profile has been compiled. Doses less than 1 mg were without subjective effect; doses from 5 to 10 mg orally, intravenously, or by inhalation caused difficulty in thinking; changes in body image and sensory perception; disorganized thought; and feelings of unreality, estrangement, depersonalization, euphoria or affective dullness, loquacity, and a lack of concern. Nystagmus was common, together with mild increases in blood pressure and heart rate. Doses to 15 mg produced alcohollike intoxication with vertigo, ataxia, nausea and vomiting, weakness, slowed reaction times, mental depression, and analgesia. Effects lasted up to 14 hours. Doses above 15 mg intravenously produced amnesia, analgesia, and anesthesia. Seizures followed doses of 30 to 60 mg.

In a large series of patients 57 percent had horizontal, vertical, or rotatory nystagmus, and 57 percent had mild to moderate hypertension. These two symptoms, together with behavioral abnormalities, have been considered cardinal manifestations of PCP intoxication, but clearly, many patients lack these symptoms. Diagnostic criteria appear in Table 13.10-3.

DIFFERENTIAL DIAGNOSIS Phencyclidine intoxication is differentiated from other intoxications by patient history and drug identification in bodily fluids. History or laboratory evidence of drug use, sudden onset, relatively rapid resolution, and usually an absence of localizing neurologic signs differentiate this disorder from traumatic, vascular, neoplastic, and degenerative neurological problems. This disorder is differentiated from phencyclidine intoxication delirium. If delirium is present in any intoxication, that diagnosis always takes precedence, even though the presumed causative agent is named first.

TABLE 13.10-3
Diagnostic Criteria for Phencyclidine Intoxication

A. Recent use of phencyclidine (or a related substance).
B. Clinically significant maladaptive behavioral changes (e.g., belligerence, assaultiveness, impulsiveness, unpredictability, psychomotor agitation, impaired judgment, or impaired social or occupational functioning) that developed during, or shortly after, phencyclidine use.
C. Within an hour (less when smoked, "snorted," or used intravenously), two (or more) of the following signs:
   (1) vertical or horizontal nystagmus
   (2) hypertension or tachycardia
   (3) numbness or diminished responsiveness to pain
   (4) ataxia
   (5) dysarthria
   (6) muscle rigidity
   (7) seizures or coma
   (8) hyperacusis
D. The symptoms are not due to a general medical condition and are not better accounted for by another mental disorder.

Specify if:
With perceptual disturbances

Table from DSM-IV, *Diagnostic and Statistical Manual of Mental Disorders,* ed 4. Copyright American Psychiatric Association, Washington, 1994. Used with permission.

Phencyclidine intoxication also is differentiated from phencyclidine-induced mood or anxiety disorders. Symptoms of those disorders do arise during intoxications, but those diagnoses are made when the additional named symptoms are in excess of those usually associated with phencyclidine intoxication and when the additional symptoms are sufficiently severe to warrant independent clinical attention. If the patient experiences hallucinations or altered perceptions but believes that they are unreal, the diagnosis is phencyclidine intoxication with the specifier, with perceptual disturbances. If the patient believes the hallucinations or delusions to be real, the diagnosis is phencyclidine-induced psychotic disorder.

COURSE AND PROGNOSIS Phencyclidine intoxication begins soon after dosing. The effects peak within minutes after intravenous or transpulmonary use or within a few hours after oral use. Intoxication usually abates over four to 15 hours, but may persist for some days. Resolution usually is complete, but because use of the substance is reinforcing, each intoxication increases the probability of further self-dosing episodes. Severe phencyclidine intoxication lasting more than two to three days may result from continued absorption of the drug; smugglers sometimes swallow drug-laden condoms, which then may leak slowly for days. Intoxication may result in injury or death secondary to diminished judgment or motor skills, belligerence, drowning, or other impairment.

TREATMENT Treatment mainly is supportive and expectant.

Agitation In a large series of patients about one third were considered violent and one third agitated. Such patients are maintained and protected in quiet, dimly lit rooms with little stimulation. Most experts discourage with PCP the talking down or reassurance that frequently is recommended for hallucinogen intoxication. Frequent monitoring of vital signs permits rapid response to worsening effects. If the time of peak effect has passed, no other treatment may be needed. But in severe cases a large, well-trained staff may need to overpower and secure a patient in full restraints. Marked agitation is reduced with haloperidol (Haldol), 5 mg intramuscularly, repeated after 20 minutes if needed. Diazepam (Valium) 5 mg intravenously, repeated as needed up to 30 mg, may be used instead, but resulting respiratory depression may require artificial ventilation.

Stupor or coma Stupor or coma occurred in about 15 percent of a large group of PCP-intoxicated patients. Most comas lasted two to 24 hours, but some persisted up to a week. Respiratory support may be required. Positioning the patient on the side may avoid aspiration of vomitus. Intensive life-support may be needed for prolonged coma. Other causes of coma, such as narcotic overdose or closed head injury, must be ruled out even if phencyclidine intoxication is proved.

Hypertension Although common, hypertension accompanying PCP use usually is modest. Dangerous hypertension requires appropriate antihypertensive intervention.

Hypothermia or hyperthermia Body temperature fell below 36.67°C in 6.4 percent and rose above 38.89°C in 2.6 percent of a large series of PCP-intoxicated patients. Some temperatures exceeded 41°C. External heating or cooling may be required to control those conditions.

Seizures Seizure occurred in about 3 percent of patients in a large series of cases. PCP seizures usually are controlled with diazepam 5 to 10 mg intravenously, repeated as needed (usual maximum, 30 mg); the resulting respiratory depression may require supported ventilation. Because continued seizures may cause hypoxia, metabolic acidosis, or hypothermia, and may worsen rhabdomyolysis, neuromuscular blockade may be required for status epilepticus.

Rhabdomyolysis Some 70 percent of a large series of PCP-intoxicated patients had at least mild elevations of creatinine phosphokinase (CPK), indicating muscle damage of uncertain origin. About 2 percent experienced rhabdomyolysis and severe kidney impairment. Urine should be screened for myoglobin by heme dipstick testing; serum CPK should be measured in heme-positive patients. Urinary alkalization may be required to protect the kidneys (even though it may slow urinary excretion of PCP), and some authors recommend the use of mannitol, furosemide (Lasix), and sodium bicarbonate in these patients.

Abnormal involuntary movements, posturing A variety of dystonias and dyskinesias, including athetosis, occurred in about 7 percent of a group of hospitalized PCP-intoxicated patients. Dystonias responded well to diphenhydramine (Benadryl) 50 mg intravenously. Catalepsy with mutism and staring, as well as stereotyped repetitious movements, also occurred.

Enhanced detoxification Because PCP is concentrated in acidic media it may be excreted into acidic stomach contents and subsequently reabsorbed from the basic medium of the small intestine. Similarly, it is more rapidly excreted in acidic urine than in neutral urine. Thus, some experts recommend continuous nasogastric suction (especially for comatose patients) to withdraw PCP contained in acidic gastric contents. Others recommend placing 30 to 40 g of activated charcoal slurry into the stomach every six to eight hours to bind the PCP being excreted there. Some experts administer ammonium chloride, about 2.75 mEq/kg in 2 to 3 oz of saline or water through a gastric tube, repeated every six hours until urinary pH falls below 5. (Awake, cooperative patients can take ammonium chloride capsules). Those experts also advise the acute use of ascorbic acid, 2 grams in 500 mL of intravenous fluid every six hours (or orally in awake patients), as well as continued urinary acidification with three to four glasses of cranberry juice daily for several weeks to speed PCP excretion. Other clinicians eschew urinary acidification. Only a small proportion of PCP is excreted in urine; most is metabolized in the liver. Thus, large increases in urinary excretion reflect relatively small changes in total PCP disposition. Metabolic acidosis may have its own complications, and acidic urine increases the risk of myoglobinuric renal failure in rhabdomyolysis. No controlled studies have examined patient outcome after acidification, but in animals ammonium chloride and charcoal reduce manifestations of PCP intoxication (the combination is more effective than either alone).

Other signs and symptoms Conditions occurring in 10 percent or fewer of PCP-intoxicated patients include mutism, staring, nudism, no apparent behavioral effects, muscular rigidity, dystonias, grimacing or athetosis, diaphoresis, bronchospasm, bronchorrhea, hypersalivation, pupillary constriction or enlargement, urinary retention, and (very rarely) cardiac arrest.

PHENCYCLIDINE INTOXICATION DELIRIUM

DIAGNOSIS AND CLINICAL FEATURES The diagnosis of PCP intoxication delirium (see Chapter 12) applies to patients who simultaneously meet the specifications for both phencyclidine intoxication and substance-induced delirium. The disorder supersedes other phencyclidine intoxication diagnoses; therefore, a patient qualifying for both this diagnosis and, for example, phencyclidine-induced psychotic disorder, would receive only the diagnosis of phencyclidine intoxication delirium.

DIFFERENTIAL DIAGNOSIS The differential diagnoses for both phencyclidine intoxication and delirium apply to this disorder. Helpful indicators of phencyclidine intoxication delirium versus other deliria include the patient's history or laboratory findings indicating use of PCP (or a related substance), nystagmus or hypertension, and an absence of other drug use or central nervous system disease.

COURSE AND PROGNOSIS About 25 percent of patients in a large series of PCP intoxications manifested delirium. Concomitant problems were labile and inappropriate affect; agitated, violent, or bizarre behavior; and anxiety or fearfulness. Delirium usually lasted a few hours to a few days, but sometimes persisted for several weeks. Injuries occurred in about one fifth of patients. Some observers also note that cognitive dullness persisting for several weeks complicates recovery in many PCP users.

TREATMENT Delirium requires special attention to the patient's physical safety, but treatment otherwise is similar to that for phencyclidine intoxication.

PHENCYCLIDINE-INDUCED PSYCHOTIC DISORDER

DIAGNOSIS AND CLINICAL FEATURES Patients who appear to experience phencyclidine intoxication but have psychotic symptoms in excess of those usually associated with that condition are diagnosed as having phencyclidine-induced psychotic disorder (see Section 15.3). The psychotic symptoms must be sufficiently severe to warrant independent clinical attention. Such patients show prominent intoxication-related hallucinations or delusions and impaired reality testing, without delirium. DSM-IV encourages the use, when appropriate, of the diagnostic specifier, with onset during intoxication; the specifier applies to essentially all cases.

DIFFERENTIAL DIAGNOSIS The differential diagnosis for phencyclidine intoxication applies here. This condition is differentiated from phencyclidine intoxication by the presence of prominent delusions or hallucinations that the patient accepts as real. It is differentiated from phencyclidine intoxication delirium by the absence of impaired consciousness and cognition, which are prominent in delirium. The delirium diagnosis takes precedence. Criterion D for the diagnosis of substance-induced psychotic disorder requires that the condition not occur exclusively during the course of a delirium. Therefore, patients qualifying for phencyclidine intoxication delirium receive that diagnosis rather than PCP-induced psychotic disorder even if delusions or hallucinations are present. The condition is differentiated from schizophrenia or other psychotic disorders by the patient history or by laboratory evidence of recent intoxication with PCP or a related substance, by the absence of a premorbid history suggesting schizophrenia, and by relatively rapid resolution of symptoms. However, schizophrenic persons using PCP do experience intoxication, and the drug worsens schizophrenic symptoms; these two conditions may coexist.

COURSE AND PROGNOSIS About 6 percent of a large sample of PCP-intoxicated patients had delusions or hallucinations without delirium. Bizarre behavior, agitation, religiosity, and paranoid ideas were common. Hallucinations were both auditory and visual. Of these patients, about 40 percent had either hypertension or nystagmus. Some 10 percent had been injured, but other medical complications were rare. Symptoms persisted from one to 30 days, averaging 4.3 days.

Long-term prognosis is unclear. A few patients have persisting psychoses for many weeks. Repeated drug use and rehospitalizations were common in a group of 10 such patients followed for eight years after intoxication; six had schizophrenic diagnoses at follow-up study. It is unknown whether such patients have true schizophrenia unmasked during PCP intoxication, or whether PCP induces prolonged schizophreniclike psychoses.

TREATMENT Patients in several controlled studies of this disorder some improvement in less than one hour after 5-mg doses of haloperidol were given intramuscularly twice, 20 minutes apart. Most authorities recommend use of haloperidol in frequently repeated intramuscular doses (up to about 30 mg total in one hour or less, depending on symptom intensity). There are no reports of outcome after several days of antipsychotic treatment, and there are no controlled studies of long-term outcome with neuroleptic medications in prolonged or recurring cases. One case report suggests benefit from 10 electroconvulsive treatments in a patient whose PCP-related psychosis had continued for one month despite antipsychotic treatment.

PHENCYCLIDINE ABUSE AND PHENCYCLIDINE DEPENDENCE

DIAGNOSIS AND CLINICAL FEATURES Phencyclidine abuse (see Table 13.1-6) is characterized by repeated use of PCP or a related drug in ways that produce physical risk or adverse social effects for the user. Phencyclidine dependence (See Tables 13.1-2 and 13.1-5) is characterized by repeated use of PCP or a related substance in a pattern reflecting some combination of adverse consequences from the drug use, loss of control of drug use, and tolerance (a withdrawal syndrome from these drugs is seldom if ever observed in human beings).

DIFFERENTIAL DIAGNOSIS Abuse and dependence disorders of PCP use may be comorbid with, or mistaken for, abuse or dependence on other drugs; because PCP often is misrepresented as another substance by drug dealers, users may be unaware of what they are taking. The characteristic severity of intoxications should suggest PCP, and urine testing may confirm its use. The repeated PCP intoxications of phencyclidine abuse or dependence also may mimic some aspects of, or be comorbid with, antisocial personality disorder; the differential diagnosis is aided by a childhood history of conduct disorder and an absence of PCP-positive urine tests in antisocial personality disorder. Phencyclidine abuse or dependence is differentiated from schizophrenia by the patient's history or by laboratory evidence of drug taking, relatively rapid symptom resolution after intoxications, and lack of signs or symptoms of schizophrenia between intoxications.

COURSE AND PROGNOSIS There are no reports on course, prognosis, or treatment of patient groups with phencyclidine abuse or dependence, as defined by DSM-III-R or DSM-IV criteria. However, studies of patients with phencyclidine intoxication undoubtedly include many who would meet those criteria. Course in treatment probably is similar to that of demographically comparable users of other nonopioid drugs.

TREATMENT There are no well-controlled studies, or even uncontrolled prospective descriptions, of treatment outcome in phencyclidine abuse or dependence. In the absence of such information, approaches developed for other substance use disorders are followed. Seriously disturbed, suicidal, confused, or psychotic patients should be hospitalized in a supportive and quietly nonstimulating milieu. Patients without community supports (including lack of abstinence-supporting associates) or with previous failures in outpatient treatment receive community residential care or intensive (several hours per day, several days per week) outpatient care. Phencyclidine-induced psychotic disorder should be treated with neuroleptic drugs; the response of phencyclidine-induced mood disorder to antidepressant drugs is unclear. In the absence of other comorbid psychiatric disorders, medications are avoided and treatment emphasizes total abstinence from PCP.

Individual and group supportive therapy is oriented initially toward problems of daily living such as working, reintegrating into the family, avoiding associates who use or sell drugs, finding drug-free associates and leisure activities, and resuming financial and other responsibilities. Vigorous confrontations or intellectually complex verbal therapies are inappropriate to the emotional lability and mild cognitive dullness of recently detoxified patients. Family therapy should educate family members about the chronic relapsing nature of substance dependence, specifying a goal of preventing or aborting future relapse before adverse outcomes develop. The patient and family must plan in advance their responses to the frequent problem of treatment drop-out. Therapists should support family allies favoring abstinence, while counteracting those directly or indirectly encouraging continued drug use. Participation in Narcotics Anonymous meetings is recommended strongly. Specialized evaluations and rehabilitation may help with specific work or school problems. Urine samples are obtained frequently under direct observation and are analyzed for PCP and other abused substances, although samples may remain weakly and intermittently positive for several weeks after chronic or high-dose use. Patients who relapse frequently may benefit from contingency contracts.

PHENCYCLIDINE-INDUCED MOOD DISORDER

CLINICAL FEATURES AND DIFFERENTIAL DIAGNOSIS Patients with phencyclidine-induced mood disorder (see Section 16.6) meet the criteria for phencyclidine intoxication but have mood disturbance in excess of that usually associated with phencyclidine intoxication; the mood problem must be sufficiently severe to warrant independent clinical attention. DSM-IV encourages the use of the specifier with onset during intoxication when appropriate. This specifier applies to essentially all cases. If the patient also qualifies for a diagnosis of phencyclidine intoxication delirium, that diagnosis is made instead, since DSM-IV forbids making the diagnosis of phencyclidine mood disorder if the mood disturbance occurs exclusively during the course of a delirium.

COURSE AND PROGNOSIS About 3 percent of a group of hospitalized patients with PCP intoxications had elated, euphoric moods; most could be released within hours, after observation and minimal treatment. Others, despite being alert and oriented, became violent and combative. Of the latter patients 41 percent suffered injury, and most remained hospitalized for more than one day. Some reports suggest that depression of several weeks' duration may follow phencyclidine psychotic disorder.

TREATMENT Treatments for agitation are the same as for phencyclidine intoxication. No studies document the efficacy of antidepressant medications for PCP-related depression, and clinicians should not expect that mood disorders arising during intoxications will necessarily respond to treatment in the same way that major depressive disorder does. In the absence of clear data conservative management for several weeks seems warranted, since depressions related to other substances usually are self-limited. Suicidal ideation may require inpatient treatment.

PHENCYCLIDINE-INDUCED ANXIETY DISORDER

CLINICAL FEATURES AND DIFFERENTIAL DIAGNOSIS

Patients with phencyclidine-induced anxiety disorder (see Section 17.5) meet the criteria for phencyclidine intoxication but have anxiety in excess of that usually associated with phencyclidine intoxication; the anxiety must be sufficiently severe to warrant independent clinical attention. DSM-IV encourages the use of the specifier, with onset during intoxication when appropriate. This specifier applies to essentially all cases. If the patient also qualifies for a diagnosis of phencyclidine intoxication delirium, that diagnosis is made instead, since DSM-IV forbids making the diagnosis of phencyclidine induced anxiety disorder in the anxiety disturbance occurs exclusively during the course of a delirium.

COURSE AND PROGNOSIS Among a series of patients hospitalized with PCP intoxications fewer than 5 percent had restless agitation and anxiety without delirium. They frequently showed tachycardia and increased respiratory rate. The condition usually ended within six hours. Medical complications were rare, except for injury in a few patients.

TREATMENT General treatments for phencyclidine intoxication apply. Diazepam 5 mg orally or intravenously, repeated as needed, may reduce anxiety and agitation. Intravenous diazepam occasionally induces apnea, requiring ventilatory assistance.

PHENCYCLIDINE-RELATED DISORDER NOT OTHERWISE SPECIFIED

The residual category permits coding of phencyclidine diagnoses not covered by the other phencyclidine-related disorders (Table 13.10-4).

TABLE 13.10-4
Phencyclidine-Related Disorder Not Otherwise Specified

The phencyclidine-related disorder not otherwise specified category is for disorders associated with the use of phencyclidine that are not classifiable as phencyclidine dependence, phencyclidine abuse, phencyclidine intoxication, phencyclidine intoxication delirium, phencyclidine-induced psychotic disorder, phencyclidine-induced mood disorder, or phencyclidine-induced anxiety disorder.

Table from DSM-IV, *Diagnostic and Statistical Manual of Mental Disorders,* ed 4. Copyright American Psychiatric Association, Washington, 1994. Used with permission.

SUGGESTED CROSS-REFERENCES

A general introduction to substance-related disorders is provided in Section 13.1. PCP disorders may mimic or be comorbid with schizophrenia, which is discussed in Chapter 14. Chapter 12 reviews delirium and its differential diagnosis. Section 13.7 covers hallucinogenic drugs, which share some properties with PCP. Receptors and neurotransmitters are reviewed in detail in Chapter 1, on neuroscience. There is a discussion of conduct disorder in Chapter 39 and a discussion of antisocial personality disorder in Section 28.3.

REFERENCES

*Baldridge E B, Bessen H A: Phencyclidine. Emerg Med Clin North Am *8:* 541, 1990.

Balster R L: The behavioral pharmacology of phencyclidine. In *Psychopharmacology: The Third Generation of Progress,* H Y Meltzer, editor, p 1573. Raven Press, New York, 1987.

Carroll M E: PCP and hallucinogens. Adv Alcohol Subst Abuse *9:* 167, 1990.

Cook C E, Brine D R, Jeffcoat A R, Hill J M, Wall M E, Perez-Reyes M, Di Guiseppi S R: Phencyclidine disposition after intravenous and oral doses. Clin Pharmacol Ther *31:* 625, 1982.

Cosgrove J, Newell T G: Recovery of neuropsychological functions during reduction in use of phencyclidine. J Clin Psychol *47:* 159, 1991.

Done A K, Aronow R, Miceli J N: Pharmacokinetic bases for the diagnosis and treatment of acute PCP intoxication. J Psychedelic Drugs *12:* 253, 1980.

*Fram D H, Stone N: Clinical observations in the treatment of adolescent and young adult PCP abusers. NIDA Res Monogr *64:* 252, 1986.

Giannini A J, Nageotte C, Loiselle R H, Malone D A, Price W A: Comparison of chlorpromazine, haloperidol and pimozide in the treatment of phencyclidine psychosis: da-2 receptor specificity. Clin Toxicol *22:* 573, 1984-85.

Glantz J C, Woods J R: Cocaine, heroin, and phencyclidine: Obstetric perspectives. Clin Obst Gynecol *36:* 279, 1993.

*Gorelick D A, Wilkins J N: Inpatient treatment of PCP abusers and users. Am J Drug Alcohol Abuse *15:* 1, 1989.

International Statistical Classification of Diseases and Related Health Problems, 10th revision, vol 1. World Health Organization, Geneva, 1992.

Javitt D C, Zukin S R: Recent advances in the phencyclidine model of schizophrenia. Am J Psychiatry *148:* 1301, 1991.

Johnson K M, Jones S M: Neuropharmacology of phencyclidine: Basic mechanisms and therapeutic potential. Annu Rev Pharmacol Toxicol *30:* 707, 1990.

Johnston L D, O'Malley P M, Bachman J G: Drug abuse among American high school seniors, college students and young adults, 1975-1990. U.S. Department of Health and Human Services, Rockville, MD, 1991.

Junien J L, Leonard B E: Drugs acting on sigma and phencyclidine receptors: A review of their nature, function, and possible therapeutic influence. In *Clinical Neuropharmacology,* 12, p 353. Raven, New York, 1989.

Kornhuber J, Mack-Burkhardt F, Riederer P, Hebenstreit G F, Reynolds G P, Andrews H B, Beckmann H: [^{3}H]MK-801 binding sites in postmortem brain regions of schizophrenic patients. J Neural Transm *77:* 231, 1989.

Krystal J H, Karper L P, Seibyl J P, Freeman G K, Delaney R, Bremner J D, Heninger G R, Bowers M B, Charney D S: Subanesthetic effects

of the noncompetitive NMDA antagonist, ketamine, in humans. Arch Gen Psychiatry *51:* 199, 1994.
Lyddane J E, Thomas B F, Compton D R, Martin B R: Modification of phencyclidine intoxication and biodisposition by charcoal and other treatments. Pharmacol Biochem Behav *30:* 371, 1988.
*McCarron M M, Schulze BW, Thompson G A, Conder M C, Goetz W A: Acute phencyclidine intoxication: Clinical patterns, complications, and treatment. Ann Emerg Med *10:* 290, 1981.
McCarron M M, Schulze B W, Thompson G A, Conder M C, Goetz W A: Acute phencyclidine intoxication: Incidence of clinical findings in 1,000 cases. Ann Emerg Med *10:* 237, 1981.
National Institute on Drug Abuse: Annual data 1989, data from the drug abuse warning network (DAWN). Department of Health and Human Services publication (ADM) 90-1717, 1990.
National Institute on Drug Abuse: Annual medical examiner data 1990, data from the drug abuse warning network (DAWN). Department of Health and Human Services publication (ADM) 91-1840, 1991.
National Institute on Drug Abuse: National household survey on drug abuse: population estimates 1991. Department of Health and Human Services publication (ADM) 92-1887, 1991.
Pradhan S N: Phencyclidine (PCP): Some human studies. Neurosci Biobehav Rev *8:* 493, 1984.
*Smith D E, Wesson D R: PCP abuse: Diagnostic and psychopharmacological treatment approaches. J Psychedelic Drugs *12:* 293, 1980.
Wright H H, Cole E A, Batey S R, Hanna K: Phencyclidine-induced psychosis: Eight-year follow-up of ten cases. South Med J *81:* 565, 1988.
Young J D, Crapo L M: Protracted phencyclidine coma from an intestinal deposit. Arch Intern Med *152:* 859, 1992.

13.11 SEDATIVE-, HYPNOTIC-, OR ANXIOLYTIC-RELATED DISORDERS

DOMENIC A. CIRAULO, M.D.
DAVID J. GREENBLATT, M.D.

INTRODUCTION

The problem of sedative, hypnotic, or anxiolytic dependence is best understood not only in terms of the pharmacology of the drugs, but also in the context of the beliefs and values of physicians, patients, and society at large, which in turn are influenced by the moral, economic, and political views of the time.

Several cultural attitudes have shifted since the 1960s when benzodiazepines were first marketed. A sense of trust in the medical profession and the pharmaceutical industry has eroded, accompanied by the devaluing of medical technology in favor of alternative forms of healing. Concerns about illicit drugs have led to irrational fears of all psychoactive agents and have resulted in the promulgation of regulations and restrictions that limit even the appropriate use of psychotropic drugs, particularly hypnotics and anxiolytics. An example is the triplicate prescription program recently enacted by New York that has resulted in a decrease in prescriptions for benzodiazepines, but an increase in prescriptions for the older, less effective, and more hazardous sedatives.

Some have observed that as the politics of the United States has become more conservative, a puritanical moral tone has developed that emphasizes self-reliance and minimizes the significance of emotional suffering. In that view anxiety becomes a sign of moral weakness rather than an illness. Medication treatment is seen as the easy way out. Some have referred to it as pharmacological Calvinism or, "If it feels good, it's wrong."

Politics enters into the physician's prescribing decisions in even a more basic way. As the government controls expenditures for pharmaceuticals in its entitlement programs (for example, Medicare, Medicaid, and state mental and federal veterans' hospitals in the United States and the National Health Service in Canada and the United Kingdom), the availability of certain drugs has been limited. For example, before generic alprazolam became available, the higher cost of Xanax made it the focus of special restrictions in the Medicaid program in Massachusetts and at several Department of Veterans Affairs medical centers.

The prescription of anxiolytic medication forces clinicians to take society's values into account in a way that differs from the prescription of other medications. In the treatment of hypertension, for example, it would be ludicrous to suggest that if dietary and life-style changes failed to lower blood pressure, a patient with hypertension would be better off without medication. Nevertheless, an antimedication bias is often expressed in discussions of the therapy of anxiety disorders.

Several factors contribute to the opinion that it is better to overcome anxiety without the aid of drugs. Some hold the mistaken belief that since anxiety is part of the common experience, pathological anxiety is no different from the apprehension that everyone experiences in certain situations. An example of such thinking is expressed in an article about the dangers of alprazolam that appeared in the January 1993 *Consumer Reports:* "If anxiety is an inevitable part of the human condition, then the wish for a magic potion to banish anxiety is probably a timeless human desire." Experienced clinicians recognize that pathological anxiety is not an inevitable part of the human condition.

Some conceptualize anxiety as a defense and not as an illness that requires a search for, and treatment of, underlying intrapsychic etiological factors. With this model anxiety should not be treated with medication because the exploration of anxiety is grist for the psychotherapeutic mill. The problem with that approach is that it promotes needless suffering. Various forms of psychotherapy help some but not all types of anxiety, and for most serious forms of anxiety, a combination of medication and psychotherapy is usually required.

Clinical experience with patients who abuse those drugs may also influence the clinician's attitude toward prescribing benzodiazepines. The psychiatrist who serves as an attending physician on a chemical-dependence treatment unit sees about one in four patients who use or abuse benzodiazepines as part of a mixed-drug dependence syndrome. The opinions concerning benzodiazepine abuse that emerge from that experience differ substantially from those of the anxiety clinic physician whose patients typically use the drugs according to their doctors' instructions.

Prescribing may be influenced by a physician's inadequate fund of knowledge, poor judgment, or unethical behavior. Even the most competent physicians sometimes feel the demand to do something and may offer a prescription when more specific treatments are unavailable. At other times more subtle influences may be at play—physicians from a working class background and those practicing in relative isolation are the highest prescribers of anxiolytics.

The negative publicity in the lay media, in which isolated incidents of adverse effects or idiosyncratic reactions (which often are coincidental rather than causally related to the medication) receive attention far out of proportion to their clinical significance, may influence both physician prescribing habits and patient acceptance. Moreover, some physicians misinterpret the extant literature on the benzodiazepines as demonstrating a high risk for adverse effects or dependence.

Patients have beliefs about the medication that may influence their usage patterns. Those who view the drug as critical to their coping in life take it on a chronic basis and are unlikely to try to stop it on their own or to request tapering. Another group of patients uses the anxiolytic in crisis situations; those patients will use it for brief periods and discontinue it when the crisis passes. As one patient put it, "It's like having a good relief pitcher in the bullpen. Just because he's warming up doesn't mean you've got to use him, but it's good to know he's available."

DEFINITION

DETERMINING ABUSE LIABILITY Any study of sedative, hypnotic, or anxiolytic dependence is limited by the operational definitions of abuse and dependence. Drug abuse is a behavioral and social phenomenon, albeit with significant pharmacological origins and medical consequences.

Any set of criteria established to determine abuse of necessity will be subjective, based on society's values. Even when there is agreement on what makes a drug abusable, society's attitude toward the drugs that meet the criteria for abuse will vary. For example, most persons would probably agree that a drug that is frequently associated with overdose or emergency room treatment is dangerous. The top two drugs in the last National Institute on Drug Abuse (NIDA) Drug Abuse Warning Network (DAWN) report that account for over 70 percent of emergency room mentions are one illicit drug, cocaine, and one legal drug, ethanol. Diazepam (Valium) accounts for about 3 percent of mentions, less than aspirin or acetaminophen (Tylenol), drugs considered to have little abuse potential (Tables 13.11-1 and 13.11-2). The DAWN report is frequently cited in assessments of abuse liability; however, it more accurately reflects how commonly a drug is used in overdose attempts.

Abuse liability is established by asking a series of questions about a drug or class of drugs. Those questions that have their origins in society's values lead to studies of illicit trafficking; population surveys of nonprescription use; audits of prescribing practices; monitoring of diversion from physicians' offices, pharmacies, or manufacturing sites; emergency room treatment; and overdose deaths.

Questions regarding pharmacological characteristics also predict abuse liability: drug-induced euphoria and the development of tolerance, an abstinence syndrome, or cross-tolerance with known abusable substances may all predict risk of abuse. Finally, a number of ingenious methods for determining drug preferences in humans and animal models have been developed to determine abuse liability.

The terms "abuse" and "misuse" are used synonymously; they refer to the use of a drug in a manner that is not consistent with generally accepted medical practice or social and legal custom (for example, use without a valid prescription or delib-

TABLE 13.11-1
Drugs Mentioned Most Frequently by Medical Examiners in 1989 (Drugs with Less Than 10 Mentions Excluded)

Rank	Drug Name	Number of Mentions	Percent of Total Episodes
1	Cocaine	3,618	50.52
2	Alcohol-in-combination	2,778	38.79
3	Heroin, morphine	2,743	38.30
4	Codeine	840	11.73
5	Methadone	450	6.28
6	Diazepam	428	5.98
7	Amitriptyline	382	5.33
8	Nortriptyline	304	4.24
9	D-Propoxyphene	282	3.94
10	Marijuana/hashish	246	3.43
11	Diphenhydramine	238	3.32
12	Acetaminophen	217	3.03
13	Lidocaine	212	2.96
14	PCP, PCP combinations	211	2.95
15	Desipramine	192	2.68
16	Doxepin	191	2.67
17	Methamphetamine, speed	191	2.67
18	Unspec. benzodiazepine	177	2.47
19	Phenobarbital	173	2.42
20	Aspirin	127	1.77
20	Imipramine	127	1.77
24	Secobarbital	89	1.24
26	Chlordiazepoxide	72	1.01
27	Alprazolam	61	0.85
29	Butalbital	55	0.77
31	Glutethimide	50	0.70
33	Amobarbital	41	0.57
33	Flurazepam	40	0.57
37	Temazepam	35	0.49
41	Triazolam	33	0.46
46	Pentobarbital	22	0.31
52	Oxazepam	18	0.25
57	Lorazepam	15	0.21

Table from Drug Abuse Warning Network (DAWN) Annual Data 1989, National Institute on Drug Abuse.

TABLE 13.11-2
Drugs Mentioned Most Frequently by Emergency Rooms in 1989 (Drugs with Less Than 10 Mentions Are Excluded)

Rank	Drug Name	Number of Mentions	Percent of Total Episodes
1	Cocaine	61,665	40.13
2	Alcohol-in-combination	46,735	30.42
3	Heroin, morphine	20,566	13.38
4	Marijuana, hashish	9,867	6.42
5	Acetaminophen	6,456	4.20
6	Aspirin	5,048	3.29
7	PCP, PCP combinations	4,899	3.19
8	Diazepam	4,874	3.17
9	Ibuprofen	3,944	2.57
10	Alprazolam	3,567	2.32
11	Methamphetamine, speed	2,715	1.77
12	Acetaminophen with codeine	2,245	1.46
13	OTC sleep aids	1,766	1.15
14	Amitriptyline	1,754	1.14
15	Diphenhydramine	1,661	1.08
16	Methadone	1,609	1.05
17	Lorazepam	1,518	0.99
18	D-Propoxyphene	1,404	0.91
19	LSD	1,351	0.88
20	Hydantoin	1,208	0.79
21	Triazolam	1,194	0.78
22	Phenobarbital	1,067	0.69
23	Lithium carbonate	1,066	0.69
24	Oxycodone	1,054	0.69
25	Haloperidol	1,016	0.66
28	Theophylline	905	0.59
30	Fluoxetine	819	0.53
34	Flurazepam	724	0.47
35	Butalbital combinations	703	0.46
44	Clonazepam	584	0.38
54	OTC diet aids	390	0.25
59	Meperidine HCl	317	0.21
67	Butabarbital combination	245	0.16
73	Glutethimide	197	0.13
76	Methaqualone	178	0.12
79	Ethchlorvynol	160	0.10
85	Meprobamate	152	0.10
91	Oxazepam	132	0.09
97	Secobarbital	115	0.07
110	Chloral hydrate	98	0.06
112	Prazepam	98	0.06
119	Butalbital	86	0.06
133	Secobarbital, amobarbital	59	0.04
148	Primidone	44	0.03
156	Theo/ephed/phenobarbital	41	0.03
160	Pentobarbital	39	0.03

Table from Drug Abuse Warning Network (DAWN) Annual Data 1989, National Institute on Drug Abuse.

erately to produce intoxication, pleasure, or a high). The fourth edition of *Diagnostic and Statistical Manual of Mental Disorders* (DSM-IV) defines abuse as a ''maladaptive pattern of substance use manifested by recurrent and significant adverse consequences related to repeated use.'' Some authorities limit misuse to situations in which a drug is taken for a legitimate medical or psychiatric disorder, but is used in a way that is not consistent with medical practice. The distinction between abuse and misuse is not widely accepted and the terms are used interchangeably here. Recreational use refers to the use of drugs solely for their hedonic value. According to DSM-IV substance dependence is ''a cluster of cognitive, behavioral, and physiological symptoms indicating that the individual continues use of the substance despite significant substance-related problems. There is a pattern of repeated self-administration that usually results in tolerance, withdrawal, and compulsive drug-taking behavior.'' The term ''physiological dependence'' is used according to the definition of the World Health Organization (WHO): a pathological state brought about by repeated administration of a drug and that leads to the appearance of a characteristic and specific group of symptoms, termed an ''abstinence syndrome'' (or ''discontinuance syndrome'') when the drug is discontinued or, in the case of certain drugs, significantly reduced. The abstinence syndrome has specific characteristics referable to the autonomic nervous system (such as tremor, sweating, tachycardia, and startle response) and must be clearly distinguished from recurrence of the features of the underlying disease for which the drug was originally given. It can be reversed or attenuated by readministration of the discontinued drug or by administration of a drug with cross-tolerance. Some authorities reserve the term ''discontinuance syndrome'' for withdrawal syndromes that develop with therapeutic agents, to distinguish physiological dependence that develops in the course of treatment from dependence that develops as part of drug abuse. The terms are used interchangeably here.

SUBSTANCES The drugs discussed in this section are referred to as anxiolytics or sedative-hypnotics. The terminology for that group of drugs has not been clearly established. Their sedative or calming effects are on a continuum with their hypnotic or sleep-inducing effects. Anxiolytic drugs cover a wide spectrum of pharmacological agents, and the terminology implies more specificity than actually exists. For most of the drugs the differentiation of their sedative, hypnotic, and anxiolytic activities has more to do with marketing than with pharmacology. In the broad group of drugs that historically has been included in that class there is considerable variation in clinical utility, toxicity, risk for abuse, and potential for diversion or recreational use. In this section the abuse liability of those agents will be considered using the following classification: (1) benzodiazepines (and nonbenzodiazepine agonists that act at the benzodiazepine receptor), (2) barbiturates, and (3) miscellaneous sedative-hypnotics with limited clinical use (meprobamate [Miltown], chloral hydrate [Noctec], ethchlorvynol [Placidyl], glutethimide [Doriden], and methaqualone [Quaalude]). In the practice of both psychiatry and addiction medicine the drugs that are most important clinically are the benzodiazepines.

ETIOLOGY AND NEUROPHARMACOLOGY

The benzodiazepines, barbiturates, and barbituratelike substances all have their primary effects on the γ-aminobutyric acid (GABA) type A ($GABA_A$) receptor complex, which contains a chloride ion channel, a binding site for GABA, and a well-defined binding site for benzodiazepines. The barbiturates and barbituratelike substances are also believed to bind somewhere on the $GABA_A$ receptor complex. When a benzodiazepine, barbiturate, or barbituratelike substance does bind to the complex, the effect is to increase the affinity of the receptor for its endogenous neurotransmitter, GABA, and to increase the flow of chloride ions through the channel into the neuron. The effect of the influx of negatively charged chloride ions into the neuron is inhibitory, since it hyperpolarizes the neuron relative to the extracellular space.

Although all the substances in the class induce tolerance and physical dependence the mechanisms behind those effects are best understood for the benzodiazepines. After long-term benzodiazepine use there is an attenuation of the receptor effects caused by the agonist. Specifically, after the long-term use of benzodiazepines GABA stimulation of the $GABA_A$ receptors results in less influx of chloride than was caused by GABA stimulation before the benzodiazepine administration. That down-regulation of receptor response is not caused by a decrease in receptor number or a decrease in the affinity of the receptor for GABA, but its basis seems to be in the coupling between the GABA binding site and the activation of the chloride ion channel. That decreased efficiency in coupling may be regulated in the $GABA_A$ receptor complex itself or by other neuronal mechanisms.

ABUSE LIABILITY

Surveys of prescribing practices, patient-initiated dosage changes, and recreational or nonmedical benzodiazepine use, along with reports from emergency rooms, medical examiners, and law enforcement agencies, all suggest that benzodiazepine abuse is not a major public health problem. They are rarely used for recreational purposes and most studies suggest that they are not commonly the sole drug of abuse. The vast majority of medical and psychiatric patients use benzodiazepines appropriately, although they may be abused by patients who are dependent on alcohol or other drugs.

Abuse liability is evaluated, in part, by measuring the reinforcing properties of the drug. If its pharmacological effects increase a behavior, such as the self-administration of a dose or the work required to permit self-administration, then the drug is a positive reinforcer and has abuse liability. Both animal and human studies have assessed the reinforcing properties of the benzodiazepines.

ANIMAL STUDIES Animal studies have demonstrated that benzodiazepines have minimal reinforcing effects. Although a few studies show that animals will self-administer benzodiazepines more frequently than other drugs, they are consistently less potent in that regard than are drugs of abuse, such as cocaine or even many other sedative-hypnotics, including most barbiturates.

Animal studies employing schedule-induced polydipsia (the use of intermittent food administration to the experimental animal, which promotes ingestion of fluids, including drug solutions) indicate that midazolam (Versed) is ingested more often than water, but self-administration of chlordiazepoxide (Librium) and flurazepam (Dalmane) is not significantly different from that of water. Prior exposure to ethanol or sedative-hypnotics may increase the reinforcing effects of benzodiazepines, but some studies do not support that finding. Baboons have a clear preference for ethanol but not for diazepam or

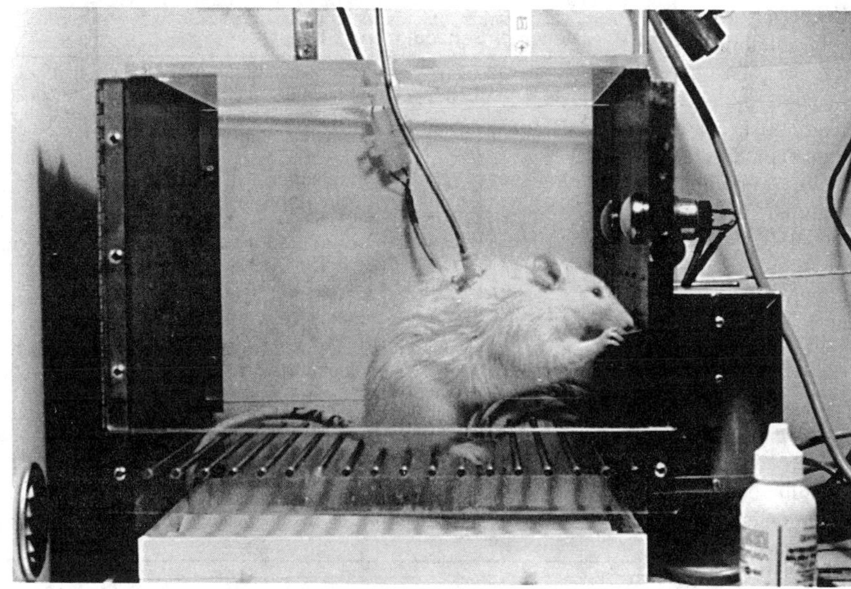

FIGURE 13.11-1 *Animal in an operant chamber self-administers a drug by pressing a bar to receive an infusion of a predetermined dose that is delivered from a syringe pump via a cannula implanted in its jugular vein. (Figure courtesy of Dr. Conan Kornetsky, Boston University School of Medicine.)*

triazolam (Halcion), using the schedule-induced polydipsia model.

Another animal model predictive of abuse liability consists of drug infusion in response to activity by the animal, such as lever pressing (Figure 13.11-1). Drug infusion may allow either continuous or intermittent drug availability, and rates of administration of the drug are compared with those of vehicle, other sedative-hypnotics, and standard drugs of abuse, such as cocaine. Studies with continuous drug access suggest that triazolam, diazepam, midazolam, clobazam, and chlordiazepoxide have reinforcing effects, whereas those with intermittent drug availability show that diazepam, midazolam, triazolam, alprazolam (Xanax), lorazepam (Ativan), chlordiazepoxide, and bromazepam maintain responses at a level higher than vehicle, which indicates abuse liability. With the possible exception of triazolam and midazolam, in studies using that model, the benzodiazepines consistently demonstrate lower abuse liability than do barbiturates other than phenobarbital, which also has relatively low abuse liability. Partial benzodiazepine receptor agonists such as abecarnil and bretazenil have low abuse liability in those models.

Animal studies support the lower abuse liability of the benzodiazepines as compared with that of most barbiturates. Among the benzodiazepines there is some indication that triazolam and midazolam may have the greatest potential for abuse, but more studies are required to define differences within the class.

HUMAN STUDIES The assessment of abuse liability in humans relies on two predictive models: self-administration of benzodiazepines by experimental subjects who have a history of drug abuse and subjective responses that correlate with high abuse potential.

In the first paradigm one type of study allows subjects with a history of sedative-hypnotic dependence to self-administer orally (that is, sample) different color-coded drugs and placebo under double-blind conditions in a simulated social environment. During subsequent sessions they are permitted to self-administer the drug they like the best. Some studies require that the subjects perform a task, such as riding a stationary bicycle, to earn doses. The abuse liability of different drugs is assessed by how often they are chosen for self-administration or by how much work a subject does to earn a dose. Scales measuring drug effect are also administered. The paradigm has the advantage of directly observing the behavior involved with ingesting the drug, albeit under somewhat artificial circumstances. It works best for subjects who are former sedative-hypnotic abusers without psychiatric illness. In those subjects it is probably safe to infer that they are administering the drug to get high. For other subjects the reason for self-administration may not be clear. Do patients with anxiety disorder self-administer the drugs because they are effective anxiolytics or because they induce euphoria? Similarly, if subjects are in withdrawal from sedative-hypnotics or ethanol, do they choose the most effective agent for alleviating their withdrawal symptoms or do they select the drug that produces the greatest euphoria? An additional problem with this design is that it exposes subjects to multiple doses of potentially addictive drugs.

An alternative strategy is to administer only a single dose of the test drugs and then compare subjective responses associated with abuse liability. A set of scales, which differs slightly among laboratories, usually consists of the Morphine Benzedrine Group subscale of the Addiction Research Center Inventory (ARCI-MBG); self-reports of sedation, liking, and intensity of drug effect; monetary street value of the drug; and similarity to reference drugs of abuse. Studies demonstrate that estimates of abuse liability using that paradigm are consistent with assessments based on the self-administration model. One disadvantage of the single-dose paradigm is that it measures only subjective effects, not behavior. It also has some of the same limitations as the self-administration paradigm. Does the subject like the drug because it has a therapeutic effect or because it is intoxicating? Both designs attempt to circumvent the problem by including an adequate battery of scales that measure several different dimensions of drug effect. Dosage equivalency and homogeneity of the subjects (especially with respect to a personal or family history of psychoactive substance abuse and psychiatric illness) are critical factors in the study design and in the interpretation of data from both models.

The predictive models in humans clearly establish that benzodiazepines occupy an intermediate position on the spectrum of abuse liability of sedative-hypnotics. Methaqualone and barbiturates generally produce higher ARCI-MBG and drug-liking scores than do benzodiazepines. Buspirone (BuSpar) a nonbenzodiazepine anxiolytic (that is, it is essentially devoid of benzodiazepine agonist activities), has little or no abuse liability in those models. With respect to differences among the benzodiazepines, the weight of the evidence suggests that diazepam has greater abuse liability than halazepam (Paxipam), oxazepam (Serax), chlordiazepoxide, or clorazepate (Tranxene). Diazepam, lorazepam, alprazolam, and triazolam produce very similar profiles of abuse potential using those paradigms. The clinical relevance of the findings has not been adequately studied. Also requiring further study is the relative role of pharmacokinetic and pharmacodynamic factors in determining the abuse liability of various benzodiazepines. Some drugs, such as diazepam, may appear to have high abuse liability because of a rapid rate of absorption from the gastrointestinal tract after oral doses. Little is known about differences in abuse liability between full and partial agonists or among drugs that have preferential effects on specific subtypes of the benzodiazepine receptor. Zolpidem (Ambien), for example, is an imidazopyridine hypnotic that has a rapid onset of action and a short elimination half-life. Although some evidence suggests that it is selective for the Type 1 central benzodiazepine receptor, other studies suggest that zolpidem and triazolam depress energy metabolism in the same areas of the brain. With respect to subjective, psychomotor, and memory effects, there are no significant differences between a single 10-mg dose of zolpidem and a single 0.25-mg dose of triazolam. High doses of triazolam (0.75 mg) are identified more often as similar in effect to barbiturates, benzodiazepine, or alcohol as compared with high doses of zolpidem (45 mg). Zolpidem also produces nausea and vomiting but whether those characteristics lead to lower abuse liability is not known.

Recent work investigating patient characteristics that influence abuse liability shows that alcoholic persons and their sons when given a single dose of alprazolam or diazepam have greater increases on abuse potential scales than do nonalcoholic controls without a family history of alcoholism. Supporting the validity of those findings are data from a survey of 5,000 male college students that showed that 23 percent of those with a positive family history of alcohol abuse reported using benzodiazepines as compared with 0.9 percent of those without such a family history. Findings from another study indicate that moderate drinkers self-administer higher doses of diazepam than do light drinkers. It is not known whether those results are drug specific or apply to the class of benzodiazepines as a whole.

When using a self-administration model subjects with anxiety do not choose diazepam more frequently than they do placebo, but when anxious subjects seeking treatment are tested they show a high rate of diazepam selection. As there is no evidence from survey data or clinical experience to suggest that patients with uncomplicated anxiety disorders have high rates of benzodiazepine abuse, those seemingly contradictory findings point out the limits of the self-administration model in differentiating the various motives for self-administration in nondependent subjects (that is, whether subjects with psychic distress take the drug for its therapeutic or euphoric effects).

TABLE 13.11-3
Prevalence of Benzodiazepine Use

- Retail sales of benzodiazepines reached their highest level in 1973–1975 at 87 million a year but have declined gradually since then.
- The United States has the greatest volume of sales in the world, but per capita sales are at the median of the nine countries with the largest sales.
- Sales of drugs with short elimination half-lives (e.g., alprazolam) have increased compared with drugs with long half-lives (e.g., diazepam).
- The National Institute on Drug Abuse Household Survey reported that nonmedical use of tranquilizers was 1.5 percent in 12- to 17-year-olds, 2.4 percent in 18- to 25-year-olds, and 1.3 percent in persons 26 years old or older.
- A survey of the United States population showed that self-reported medical use of a tranquilizer declined from 10.9 percent to 8.3 percent from 1970 to 1990. Hypnotic use declined from 3.5 to 2.6 percent during the same period.
- In 1990 over half of the patients surveyed in the United States who were taking tranquilizers took them for a month or less and 25 percent took them for a year or longer. Seventy percent of users of hypnotics took them for less than a month and 14 percent for a year or longer.
- Persons who abuse alcohol and drugs use and abuse benzodiazepines at higher rates than do anxiety disorder patients without substance abuse histories.

EPIDEMIOLOGY

Several surveys have been conducted to determine the extent of benzodiazepine use by prescription and by illicit means. Drug sales to retail pharmacies provide one measure of benzodiazepine use. Between 1980 and 1983 sales of benzodiazepines to retail pharmacies in the United States declined from 17.5 to 15.8 DDD per 1,000 persons a day (the average maintenance dose for the major indication per 1,000 persons a day), but by 1985 was back up to 17.1 DDD per 1,000 persons a day. Sales of drugs with long half-lives such as diazepam and flurazepam decreased, whereas sales of drugs with shorter half-lives, such as alprazolam, triazolam, and temazepam (Restoril) increased. The prevalence of benzodiazepine use is presented in Table 13.11-3.

In 1989 the United States accounted for the greatest volume of retail sales of benzodiazepines, but per capita exposure was at the median of the nine countries with the largest number of sales (United States, France, Japan, Italy, United Kingdom, Germany, Spain, Brazil, and Canada). The United States had a per capita exposure of 16.9 dosage units a year for benzodiazepines used as tranquilizers as compared with France, which had the highest, 55 dosage units a year, and with Brazil, which had the lowest of the nine countries at 7.3 dosage units a year. Despite having the lowest total sales volume Canada had a per capita exposure of 30.9 dosage units a year. Rates of per capita exposure to benzodiazepine tranquilizers were three to five times higher than were rates of exposure to benzodiazepine hypnotics, except in the United Kingdom, where hypnotic use was greater than tranquilizer use (12.4 versus 8.9 per capita exposure). In 31 countries surveyed benzodiazepine tranquilizer sales increased by 13 percent and benzodiazepine hypnotic sales by 47 percent from 1981 through 1989. Notable exceptions were the United Kingdom, where sales of both tranquilizers and hypnotics declined, and Germany, where a decline in tranquilizer sales was almost offset by an increase in hypnotic sales. In 1989 lorazepam had 20.7 percent of the world market share, diazepam had 17.1 percent, and alprazolam had 10.5 percent.

In the United States sales of benzodiazepines are monitored by IMS America Ltd., and its data indicate that benzodiazepine tranquilizer sales peaked in the period 1973 to 1975, when annual sales were approximately 87 million. After 1986 there was a gradual decline in benzodiazepine tranquilizer sales to about 56 million prescriptions in 1989. Alprazolam accounted for 33 percent of the United States market share in 1989, diazepam for 25 percent, and lorazepam for 19 percent. Of the benzodiazepine hypnotics triazolam had a 49 percent market share in 1989, temazepam had 30 percent, and flurazepam had 21 percent.

Interview data are important supplements to prescription monitoring. Despite the problems with validity and reliability, self-report data offer insight into the appropriateness of benzodiazepine use. In surveys of the United States population self-reported tranquilizer use declined slightly from a 1970-1971 survey in which 10.9 percent of the adult population reported using anxiolytics during the previous year as compared with 8.3 percent in a 1990 survey. Hypnotic use declined from 3.5 percent to 2.6 percent during the same period, with little change since 1979. Long-term users were more likely to be older and to be women, and they had high levels of emotional distress and chronic health problems.

Over half of the patients surveyed in 1990 took benzodiazepines for a month or less and 25 percent took them for longer than 12 months, which represents an increase from the 15 percent of the population who were long-term users in 1979. The reasons for the increase are not clear, but may represent chronic benzodiazepine treatment for panic disorder, an aging population that is more likely to take benzodiazepines, or a decrease in the number of short-term users.

Seventy percent of hypnotic users took the drugs for less than a month in 1990 and 14 percent used them for 12 months or longer. That shows a slight increase from the 1979 survey, which reported 11 percent of users taking the drug for 12 months or longer.

A survey of unsupervised changes in dosage indicated that 12 percent of patients had decreased their anxiolytic dosage and 6 percent had increased it; 9 percent of patients taking hypnotics decreased their dosage and 8 percent increased it. To put those unauthorized increases in perspective, the same survey indicated that 13 percent of patients had unauthorized increases in antidepressant dosages and those drugs have low abuse liability. A prospective study found that patients were more likely to use antidepressants than benzodiazepines on a long-term basis, suggesting that long-term use should not, in itself, be a measure of abuse liability.

The NIDA National Household Survey indicated that nonmedical use of tranquilizers was not a major public health problem. In 1990 1.5 percent of 12- to 17-year-olds, 2.4 percent of 18- to 25-year-olds, and 1.3 percent of those over 26 years of age reported nonmedical use of tranquilizers in the previous year. Surveys of psychiatric patients have demonstrated high rates of benzodiazepine prescription, but almost uniformly low abuse. In one study of 2,719 outpatients none of the 178 patients who had received benzodiazepines were diagnosed with abuse or dependence based on the revised third edition of DSM (DSM-III-R) criteria. Studies of inpatient psychiatric patients suggest that the rate of benzodiazepine abuse or dependence ranges from 0.4 percent to 13 percent of admissions. A study from the University of Munich found that 6.7 percent of 9,408 admissions had a diagnosis of benzodiazepine abuse or dependence, approximately half of whom were dependent on benzodiazepines alone. Lorazepam was the most commonly abused benzodiazepine and oxazepam was the least, even though the latter drug was the most commonly prescribed benzodiazepine in the country.

There is substantial evidence that benzodiazepines are frequently used by patients who abuse other drugs. A survey of drug abuse treatment centers across the United States in 1979 through 1981 found that 22.6 percent of patients used minor tranquilizers (primarily benzodiazepines) on a weekly or more frequent basis. In a survey of opioid abusers in Sheffield, England, 90 percent reported benzodiazepine use on a daily or mostly daily basis. Use began with a prescription in one third of the sample. The most commonly used benzodiazepine was diazepam and the primary goal was relief from such symptoms as insomnia, withdrawal, and anxiety rather than to get high. Lower rates of benzodiazepine use were reported in French (50 percent) and German (30 percent) studies. An interesting observation in the last two studies was that heroin addicts underreported benzodiazepine use, with toxicological studies required to detect such use.

Since the mid-1980s reports from Scotland have indicated that intravenous drug abusers were using temazepam, often in combination with buprenorphine (Buprenex). One study reported that 92 percent of intravenous drug abusers had used temazepam in the year preceding the survey and most of them had injected the drug intravenously. Marketed as a liquid-filled capsule, the fluid was extracted by a syringe and injected. That formulation was changed to a gel-filled capsule, which drug abusers now boil with water or heat in a microwave oven to liquify it before injecting it. Several cases of ischemia secondary to vasculitis and venous thrombosis have been reported as a consequence of intravenous or intraarterial injection of the new formulation.

Several studies have examined rates of benzodiazepine use among patients at methadone clinics. Three different United States clinics reported that 22 percent, 40 percent, 44.7 percent of their patients had urines positive for benzodiazepines. European clinics report comparable rates. Flunitrazepam, in countries where it is marketed, appears to be the preferred benzodiazepine. In other countries diazepam, alprazolam, and lorazepam are the most commonly abused. In a recent study from Austria patients in a methadone clinic rated their preference for the effects of a variety of drugs. Benzodiazepines were rated behind heroin, cocaine, all opiates, cannabis, barbiturates, and stimulants. Flunitrazepam and diazepam were the highest rated benzodiazepines but at the time the survey began alprazolam was not available in Austria. In a study of three United States cities patients on methadone (Dolophine) maintenance rated diazepam as producing the best high, with lorazepam and alprazolam also valued for their effects, and all three as significantly different from clorazepate, oxazepam, and chlordiazepoxide. Concerns have been raised about alprazolam abuse in methadone clinics and at least one clinic reported that its use has surpassed that of diazepam. Patients taking methadone presumably use benzodiazepine to boost the effects of the methadone, but some studies have suggested that self-medication may also be an important motivation.

Cocaine abusers appear less likely to use benzodiazepines than are patients in methadone clinics, with alcohol and opioids the preferred secondary drugs of abuse. Benzodiazepines are used to attenuate the cocaine crash or to alleviate anxiety during cocaine use. Such patients generally employ therapeutic doses of benzodiazepines on an intermittent basis.

Surveys of alcoholic persons indicate that many of them have taken or are currently taking benzodiazepines. They receive the benzodiazepines for the treatment of the alcohol withdrawal syndrome or coexisting anxiety or sleep disorders, and often present for such treatment without revealing the extent of alcohol use to the prescribing physician. Physicians must be cautious because evidence suggests that there is an increased risk of benzodiazepine abuse in alcoholic persons; however, there are also case reports documenting the efficacy of benzodiazepines in selected alcoholic persons with anxiety disorders.

Experimental studies have shown that moderate drinkers self-administer diazepam and that alcoholic persons have greater euphoric responses to a single dose of alprazolam than do control subjects. Both diazepam and alprazolam increase euphoria and liking scores in alcoholic persons and increase the desire for ethanol as measured by self-reports on visual analog scales. The changes in euphoria and liking are minimal with halazepam (Paxipam) as compared with diazepam, suggesting that its abuse liability may be lower than that of diazepam in such patients.

Most survey data indicate that the concurrent use of benzodiazepines by alcoholic persons who enter treatment is between 12 percent and 33 percent. Alcoholic women may have higher rates of concurrent use than alcoholic men. It is not entirely clear how many alcoholic patients misuse the benzodiazepines, but one study found that of alcoholic outpatients who also used sedatives (mostly benzodiazepines), only 15 percent were judged to have used them as prescribed, 24 percent to have both used them appropriately and abused them, and 61 percent to have abused them. Another study reported that a little more than half of the alcoholic outpatients with positive urine drug screens for benzodiazepines were abusing them. Those data should be regarded with caution because the treatment population surveys are biased to select only those patients for whom previous therapy has failed.

If it is that the higher estimates of 33 percent use of benzodiazepines by alcoholic patients are accurate and that between 50 and 60 percent of those patients are abusing them, then approximately 15 to 20 percent of all alcoholic persons presenting for treatment may be abusing benzodiazepines. Benzodiazepines are used to self-medicate withdrawal symptoms or anxiety disorders, to produce euphoria, and to enhance the effects of ethanol.

TABLE 13.11-4
Sedative-, Hypnotic-, or Anxiolytic-Related Disorders

Sedative, hypnotic, or anxiolytic use disorders
Sedative, hypnotic, or anxiolytic dependence
Sedative, hypnotic, or anxiolytic abuse

Sedative-, hypnotic-, or anxiolytic-induced disorders
Sedative, hypnotic, or anxiolytic intoxication
Sedative, hypnotic, or anxiolytic withdrawal
Specify if: with perceptual disturbances
Sedative, hypnotic, or anxiolytic intoxication delirium
Sedative, hypnotic, or anxiolytic withdrawal delirium
Sedative-, hypnotic-, or anxiolytic-induced persisting dementia
Sedative-, hypnotic-, or anxiolytic-induced psychotic disorder, with delusions
Specify if: with onset during intoxication/with onset during withdrawal
Sedative-, hypnotic-, or anxiolytic-induced psychotic disorder, with hallucinations
Specify if: with onset during intoxication/with onset during withdrawal
Sedative-, hypnotic-, or anxiolytic-induced mood disorder
Specify if: with onset during intoxication/with onset during withdrawal
Sedative-, hypnotic-, or anxiolytic-induced anxiety disorder
Specify if: with onset during withdrawal
Sedative-, hypnotic-, or anxiolytic-induced sexual dysfunction
Specify if: with onset during intoxication
Sedative-, hypnotic-, or anxiolytic-induced sleep disorder
Specify if: with onset during intoxication/with onset during withdrawal

Sedative-, hypnotic-, or anxiolytic-related disorder not otherwise specified

Table based on DSM-IV, *Diagnostic and Statistical Manual of Mental Disorders,* ed 4. Copyright American Psychiatric Association, Washington, 1994. Used with permission.

DIAGNOSIS AND CLINICAL FEATURES

DIAGNOSIS DSM-IV lists a number of sedative-, hypnotic-, or anxiolytic-related disorders (Table 13.11-4) but contains specific diagnostic criteria only for sedative, hypnotic, or anxiolytic intoxication (Table 13.11-5) and sedative, hypnotic, or anxiolytic withdrawal (Table 13.11-6). Other sedative-, hypnotic-, or anxiolytic-related disorders have their diagnostic criteria outlined in those DSM-IV sections that are specific for the major symptom—for example, sedative-, hypnotic-, or anxiolytic-induced psychotic disorder (see Section 15.3).

Dependence and abuse Sedative, hypnotic, or anxiolytic dependence and sedative, hypnotic, or anxiolytic abuse are diagnosed according to the general criteria in DSM-IV for substance dependence and substance abuse (see Tables 13.1-2, 13.1-5, and 13.1-6 in Section 13.1).

Intoxication DSM-IV contains a single set of diagnostic criteria for intoxication by any sedative, hypnotic, or anxiolytic substance (Table 13.11-4). Although the intoxication syndromes induced by all those drugs are similar, subtle clinical differences are observable, especially with intoxications that involve low doses. The diagnosis of intoxication by one of that class of substances is best confirmed by obtaining a blood sample for substance screening.

Withdrawal DSM-IV contains a single set of diagnostic criteria for withdrawal from any sedative, hypnotic, or anxiolytic substance (Table 13.11-5). The clinician can specify ''with perceptual disturbances'' if illusions, altered perceptions, or hallucinations are present but are accompanied by intact reality testing. Two important issues to remember about withdrawal are that benzodiazepines are associated with a withdrawal syndrome and that withdrawal from barbiturates can be life threatening. Withdrawal from benzodiazepines can also result in serious medical complications, such as seizures.

TABLE 13.11-5
Diagnostic Criteria for Sedative, Hypnotic, or Anxiolytic Intoxication

A. Recent use of a sedative, hypnotic, or anxiolytic.
B. Clinically significant maladaptive behavioral or psychological changes (e.g., inappropriate sexual or aggressive behavior, mood lability, impaired judgment, impaired social or occupational functioning) that developed during, or shortly after, sedative, hypnotic, or anxiolytic use.
C. One (or more) of the following signs, developing during, or shortly after, sedative, hypnotic, or anxiolytic use:
  (1) slurred speech
  (2) incoordination
  (3) unsteady gait
  (4) nystagmus
  (5) impairment in attention or memory
  (6) stupor or coma
D. The symptoms are not due to a general medical condition and are not better accounted for by another mental disorder.

Table from DSM-IV, *Diagnostic and Statistical Manual of Mental Disorders,* ed 4. Copyright American Psychiatric Association, Washington, 1994. Used with permission.

Delirium DSM-IV allows for the diagnosis of sedative, hypnotic, or anxiolytic intoxication delirium and sedative, hypnotic, or anxiolytic withdrawal delirium (see Chapter 12). Delirium that is indistinguishable from delirium tremens associated with alcohol withdrawal is more commonly seen with barbiturate withdrawal than with benzodiazepine withdrawal. Delirium

TABLE 13.11-6
Diagnostic Criteria for Sedative, Hypnotic, or Anxiolytic Withdrawal

A. Cessation of (or reduction in) sedative, hypnotic, or anxiolytic use that has been heavy and prolonged.
B. Two (or more) of the following, developing within several hours to a few days after criterion A:
  (1) autonomic hyperactivity (e.g., sweating or pulse rate greater than 100)
  (2) increased hand tremor
  (3) insomnia
  (4) nausea or vomiting
  (5) transient visual, tactile, or auditory hallucinations or illusions
  (6) psychomotor agitation
  (7) anxiety
  (8) grand mal seizures
C. The symptoms in criterion B cause clinically significant distress or impairment in social, occupational, or other important areas of functioning.
D. The symptoms are not due to a general medical condition and are not better accounted for by another mental disorder.

Specify if:
With perceptual disturbances

Table from DSM-IV, *Diagnostic and Statistical Manual of Mental Disorders,* ed 4. Copyright American Psychiatric Association, Washington, 1994. Used with permission.

TABLE 13.11-7
Diagnostic Criteria for Sedative-, Hypnotic-, or Anxiolytic-Related Disorder Not Otherwise Specified

The sedative-, hypnotic-, or anxiolytic-related disorder not otherwise specified category is for disorders associated with the use of sedatives, hypnotics, or anxiolytics that are not classifiable as sedative, hypnotic, or anxiolytic dependence; sedative, hypnotic, or anxiolytic abuse; sedative, hypnotic, or anxiolytic intoxication; sedative, hypnotic, or anxiolytic withdrawal; sedative, hypnotic, or anxiolytic intoxication delirium; sedative, hypnotic, or anxiolytic withdrawal delirium; sedative-, hypnotic-, or anxiolytic-induced persisting dementia; sedative-, hypnotic-, or anxiolytic-induced persisting amnestic disorder; sedative-, hypnotic-, or anxiolytic-induced psychotic disorder; sedative-, hypnotic-, or anxiolytic-induced mood disorder; sedative-, hypnotic-, or anxiolytic-induced anxiety disorder; sedative-, hypnotic-, or anxiolytic-induced sexual dysfunction; or sedative-, hypnotic-, or anxiolytic-induced sleep disorder.

Table from DSM-IV, *Diagnostic and Statistical Manual of Mental Disorders,* ed 4. Copyright American Psychiatric Association, Washington, 1994. Used with permission.

associated with intoxication can be seen with either barbiturates or benzodiazepines if the dosages are high enough.

Persisting dementia DSM-IV allows for the diagnosis of sedative-, hypnotic-, or anxiolytic- induced persisting dementia (see Chapter 12). The existence of the disorder is controversial inasmuch as there is uncertainty as to whether a persisting dementia is due to the substance use itself or to associated features of the substance use. It will be necessary to evaluate the diagnosis further, using DSM-IV criteria to ascertain its validity.

Persisting amnestic disorder DSM-IV allows for the diagnosis of sedative-, hypnotic-, or anxiolytic-induced persisting amnestic disorder (see Chapter 12). Amnestic disorders associated with sedatives, hypnotics, and anxiolytics may have been underdiagnosed. One exception has been the increased number of reports associated with amnestic episodes associated with the short-term use of benzodiazepines with short half-lives (such as triazolam).

Psychotic disorders The psychotic symptoms of barbiturate withdrawal can be indistinguishable from those of alcohol-associated delirium tremens. Agitation, delusions, and hallucinations are usually visual, but sometimes tactile or auditory features develop after about one week of abstinence. Psychotic symptoms associated with intoxication or withdrawal are much more common with barbiturates than with benzodiazepines and are diagnosed as sedative-, hypnotic-, or anxiolytic-induced psychotic disorders (see Section 15.3). The clinician can further specify whether delusions or hallucinations are the predominant symptoms.

Other disorders Sedative, hypnotic, and anxiolytic use has also been associated with mood disorders (see Section 16.6), anxiety disorders (Section 17.5), sleep disorders (see Chapter 23), and sexual dysfunctions (Section 21.1a). When none of those diagnostic categories are appropriate for a person with a sedative, hypnotic, or anxiolytic use disorder, the appropriate diagnosis is sedative-, hypnotic-, or anxiolytic-related disorder not otherwise specified (NOS) (Table 13.11-7).

CLINICAL FEATURES

PATTERNS OF ABUSE

Oral use The sedatives, hypnotics, and anxiolytics can all be taken orally, either occasionally to achieve a time-limited specific effect or regularly to obtain a constant, usually mild, intoxication state. The occasional-use pattern is associated with young persons who take the substance to achieve specific effects—relaxation for an evening, intensification of sexual activities, and a short-lived period of mild euphoria. The user's personality and expectations about the substance's effects and the setting in which the substance is taken also affect the substance-induced experience. The regular-use pattern is associated with middle-aged, middle-class people who usually obtain the substance from the family physician as a prescription for insomnia or anxiety. Abusers of that type may have prescriptions from several physicians, and the pattern of abuse may go undetected until obvious signs of abuse or dependence are noticed by the person's family, coworkers, or physicians.

Intravenous use A severe form of abuse involves the intravenous use of this class of substances. The users are mainly young adults intimately involved with illegal substances. Intravenous barbiturate use is associated with a pleasant, warm, drowsy feeling, and users may be inclined to use barbiturates more than opiates or opioids because of the low cost of barbiturates. The physical dangers of injection include the transmission of the human immunodeficiency virus (HIV), cellulitis, vascular complications from accidental injection into an artery, infections, and allergic reactions to contaminants. Intravenous use is associated with a rapid and profound degree of tolerance and dependence and with a severe withdrawal syndrome.

BENZODIAZEPINES Since the introduction of chlordiazepoxide in 1960 benzodiazepines have become the primary class of drugs used in the treatment of anxiety and insomnia, largely replacing barbiturates and other sedative-hypnotics. Zolpidem is an imidazopyridine hypnotic that is chemically distinct from the benzodiazepines but has similar clinical effects and acts at the $GABA_A$-benzodiazepine receptor complex. The benzodiazepines have lower abuse liability than most barbiturates, pose a much lower risk when taken in overdose, and have fewer interactions with other drugs. The advantages of the benzodiazepines must be weighed against the risk for abuse and physiological dependence.

Intoxication Benzodiazepine intoxication can be associated with behavioral disinhibition, potentially resulting in hostile or aggressive behavior in some persons. The effect is perhaps most common when benzodiazepines are taken in combination with alcohol. Benzodiazepine intoxication is associated with less

Discontinuance syndrome

SIGNS AND SYMPTOMS Studies in the early 1960s by Leo Hollister established that the abrupt discontinuation of high doses of chlordiazepoxide or diazepam could lead to a discontinuance syndrome. More recent studies have shown that therapeutic doses given for periods of weeks to months may also be associated with a discontinuance syndrome.

The signs and symptoms of the benzodiazepine discontinuance syndrome (which are presented in Table 13.11-8) have been classified as major or minor, along the lines of the alcohol withdrawal syndrome. According to that classification minor symptoms include anxiety, insomnia, and nightmares, and major symptoms, which are extremely rare, include grand mal seizures, psychosis, hyperpyrexia, and death.

The discontinuance syndrome may also be divided into the separate symptom categories of rebound, recurrence, and withdrawal. Rebound symptoms are defined as those symptoms for which the benzodiazepine was originally prescribed that return in a more severe form than they were in before treatment. They have a rapid onset following termination of therapy and are of brief duration. Recurrence refers to the return of the original symptoms at or below their original intensity. The pattern and course of those symptoms will reflect the anxiety disorder for which treatment was originally instituted. The Task Force Report on Benzodiazepine Dependence, Toxicity, and Abuse of the American Psychiatric Association defined withdrawal as a true abstinence syndrome consisting of "new signs and symptoms and worsening of preexisting symptoms following drug discontinuance that were not part of the disorder for which the drugs were originally prescribed." Many authorities have taken issue with that definition of withdrawal and prefer to distinguish withdrawal only from recurrence, not from rebound symptoms, conceptualizing the true abstinence syndrome as consisting of rebound symptoms plus new signs and symptoms.

TABLE 13.11-8
Signs and Symptoms of the Benzodiazepine Discontinuation Syndrome

The following signs and symptoms may be seen when benzodiazepine therapy is discontinued. They reflect the return of the original anxiety symptoms (recurrence), worsening of the original anxiety symptoms (rebound), or emergence of new symptoms (true withdrawal).

Disturbances of mood and cognition:
Anxiety, apprehension, dysphoria, pessimism, irritability, obsessive rumination, paranoid ideation

Disturbances of sleep:
Insomnia, altered sleep-wake cycle, daytime drowsiness

Physical signs and symptoms:
Tachycardia, elevated blood pressure, hyperreflexia, muscle tension, agitation—motor restlessness, tremor, myoclonus, muscle and joint pain, nausea, coryza, diaphoresis, ataxia, tinnitus, grand mal seizures

Perceptual disturbances:
Hyperacusis, depersonalization, blurred vision, illusions, hallucinations

Withdrawal symptoms are loosely categorized into four types: (1) disturbances of mood and cognition, (2) disturbances of sleep, (3) physical signs and symptoms, and (4) perceptual disturbances. Mood and cognitive symptoms are anxiety, apprehension, dysphoria, irritability, obsessive ruminations, and paranoia. Sleep disturbances include insomnia, altered sleep-wake cycle, and daytime drowsiness. Somatic symptoms are agitation, tachycardia, palpitations, motor restlessness, muscle tension, tremor, myoclonus, nausea, coryza, diaphoresis, lethargy, muscle and joint pain, hyperreflexia, ataxia, tinnitus, and seizures. Among perceptual disturbances are hyperacusis, depersonalization, blurred vision, illusions, and hallucinations.

The temporal sequence of symptom development is not well established, but upon the abrupt cessation of benzodiazepines with short elimination half-lives, symptoms may appear within 24 hours and peak at 48 hours. Symptoms arising from abrupt discontinuance of benzodiazepines with long half-lives may not peak until two weeks later. Although some investigators suggest that there is a subgroup of patients with withdrawal syndromes that last for many months, there is no medical or scientific evidence to validate the existence of such a syndrome. Prolonged symptoms are almost certainly attributable to recurrence of the original anxiety or to the progression of the anxiety disorder itself.

RISK FACTORS Factors influencing the development of the discontinuance syndrome are listed in Table 13.11-9. Studies on both humans and animals have attempted to identify risk factors for the development of physiological dependence. Animal studies demonstrate that the severity of withdrawal is greater with higher doses and longer periods of drug administration, but that has not been as consistently demonstrated in clinical populations. When patients are stratified into high- and low-dose groups, the withdrawal syndrome is seen to be more severe in the high-dose group. However, two recent studies, one using a daily 21-mg dose of diazepam equivalent as the cutoff separating high- and low-dose groups and the other using three groups based on diazepam dose (less than 6 mg, between 6 and 10 mg, and greater than 10 mg), indicate no significant differences in withdrawal symptoms between groups. One possible explanation for the failure consistently to demonstrate a relation between dose and withdrawal symptoms is that subjects in clinical studies are being treated for an anxiety disorder, and when the benzodiazepine is discontinued the reemergence of the original anxiety symptoms may be confused with withdrawal symptoms. Furthermore, the dose of the drug is probably higher in those patients with the most severe disease, complicating any relation between dose and the intensity of the discontinuance syndrome.

According to one study there is a relation between withdrawal symptoms and the duration of treatment when the length of the treatment is less than eight months but not when it is a year or longer. The findings of another group indicate that patients taking benzodiazepines for more than five years have more withdrawal symptoms than those taking them for less than five years.

TABLE 13.11-9
Factors Influencing the Development of the Benzodiazepine Discontinuation Syndrome

- Dose of benzodiazepine
- Duration of benzodiazepine treatment
- Rate of drug taper
- Psychopathology

Mild withdrawal symptoms may occur with abrupt discontinuation of therapeutic doses after four weeks of benzodiazepine treatment. There is a risk of rebound insomnia after a few days to one week of treatment with benzodiazepine hypnotics with short elimination half-lives. Those benzodiazepine hypnotics with longer elimination half-lives are less likely to induce rebound insomnia upon abrupt discontinuation. The likelihood of a serious withdrawal syndrome increases as treatment continues and many authorities see four months of treatment at therapeutic doses as a critical point in the development of clinically significant physiological dependence. That does not imply, however, that four months constitutes an upper limit for the duration of treatment.

Also influencing the risk of a discontinuance syndrome is the rate at which the drugs are discontinued. Gradual tapering of the benzodiazepines with short elimination half-lives is associated with fewer withdrawal symptoms than is their abrupt discontinuation. Clinical research shows less distinct differences between gradual and abrupt discontinuation of benzodiazepines with long half-lives, either because those drugs have a self-tapering action or because the period of tapering and observation in many studies is insufficient.

If benzodiazepines are abruptly discontinued, the discontinuance syndrome related to short half-life agents appears earlier and may be more intense than with long half-life drugs. Differences in intensity have not been proved because most studies do not monitor withdrawal symptoms for two weeks, which may be the time of peak symptoms with some drugs with long half-lives. Furthermore, any difference in withdrawal severity between short and long half-life agents is not entirely supported by animal studies. There is no difference in symptom severity of the withdrawal syndrome after animals are treated with either midazolam or chlordiazepoxide, for example, because essentially all benzodiazepines, regardless of their pharmacokinetic properties in humans, are eliminated very rapidly in small-animal species.

There are also differences in the development of physiological dependence resulting from benzodiazepine partial agonists as compared with that of full agonists. In animal models the partial agonists bretazenil and abecarnil are associated with fewer withdrawal symptoms than are classic agonists such as diazepam or clorazepate (the prodrug for desmethyldiazepam). Clinical studies in anxious patients, however, indicate that the abrupt termination of abecarnil is associated with withdrawal symptoms in some patients.

Some studies in animals indicate that periodic administration of the benzodiazepine antagonist flumazenil (Mazicon) during the chronic administration of lorazepam, diazepam, triazolam, or clobazam may attenuate the withdrawal syndrome.

Personality traits may be a risk factor for the development of the benzodiazepine withdrawal syndrome. Withdrawal severity is greater in patients with higher scores on the dependence scale of the Minnesota Multiphasic Personality Inventory (MMPI), high prewithdrawal levels of anxiety and depression, lower educational level, and passive-dependent personality disorder.

Overdose The benzodiazepines, in contrast to the barbiturates and the barbituratelike substances, have a large margin of safety when taken in overdoses, a feature that contributed significantly to their rapid acceptance. The ratio of lethal-to-effective dose is about 200 to 1 or higher because of the minimal degree of respiratory depression associated with the benzodiazepines. Even when grossly excessive amounts (more than 2 grams) are taken in suicide attempts, the symptoms include only drowsiness, lethargy, ataxia, some confusion, and mild depression of the user's vital signs. A much more serious condition prevails when benzodiazepines are taken in overdose in combination with other sedative-hypnotic substances, such as alcohol. In such cases small doses of benzodiazepines can cause death. The availability of flumazenil, a specific benzodiazepine antagonist, has reduced the lethality of the benzodiazepines, since flumazenil can be used in emergency rooms to reverse the effects of the benzodiazepines.

BARBITURATES Since the advent of the benzodiazepines the barbiturates have had a limited role in modern medicine. Phenobarbital is still prescribed as an anticonvulsant and as a sedative, especially for children. It is also a common component of many combination products and reduces the stimulating effects of sympathomimetic agents. Butalbital (for example, Fiornal) is an intermediate-acting barbiturate that is found in a widely used combination product that also contains acetaminophen and caffeine and is approved for the treatment of muscle contraction headaches. Given the limited availability of barbiturates it is uncommon, at least in the United States, for addiction units to treat patients dependent on barbiturates other than butalbital and phenobarbital. The barbiturates marketed currently in the United States are listed in Table 13.11-10.

A major disadvantage of the use of the barbiturates is the development of pharmacokinetic and pharmacodynamic tolerance. Tolerance is defined as reduced drug response as a result of either decreased drug concentration at the site of action, usually the result of increased drug metabolism (pharmacokinetic), or of cellular adaptive changes with unchanged or higher drug concentrations at the site of action (pharmacodynamic). Pharmacodynamic tolerance begins after acute doses and continues to develop over weeks to months. Tolerance to the mood-altering and sedative effects develops to a greater extent than does tolerance to the lethal effects, increasing the risk of accidental overdose.

Intoxication When barbiturates and barbituratelike substances are taken in relatively low doses, the clinical syndrome of intoxication is indistinguishable from that associated with alcohol intoxication. The symptoms include sluggishness, incoordination, difficulty in thinking, poor memory, slowness of speech and comprehension, faulty judgment, disinhibition of sexual and aggressive impulses, a narrowed range of attention, emotional lability, and an exaggeration of basic personality traits. The sluggishness usually resolves after a few hours, but

TABLE 13.11-10
Barbiturates and Other Sedative-Hypnotics

The substitution technique for sedative-hypnotic withdrawal requires calculation of equivalent doses of phenobarbital to replace the sedative-hypnotic that the patient is taking. The following are doses of various sedative-hypnotics for which a 30-mg dose of phenobarbital should provide adequate coverage of a withdrawal syndrome. Daily doses of phenobarbital should rarely exceed 600 mg using this protocol.

Generic Name	Trade Name	Dose (mg)
Amobarbital	Amytal	100
Aprobarbital	Alurate	40
Butabarbital	Butisol	100
Butalbital	Many combination products (e.g., Fiorinal)	100
Pentobarbital	Nembutal	100
Secobarbital	Seconal	100
Chloral hydrate	Generic	500
Ethchlorvynol	Placidyl	500
Glutethimide	Generic	250
Meprobamate	Miltown	400

the impaired judgment, distorted mood, and impaired motor skills may remain for 12 to 24 hours, depending primarily on the half-life of the abused substance. Other potential symptoms are hostility, argumentativeness, moroseness, and, occasionally, paranoid and suicidal ideation. The neurological effects include nystagmus, diplopia, strabismus, ataxic gait, positive Romberg's sign, hypotonia, and decreased superficial reflexes.

Dependence and withdrawal Physiological dependence may develop after a daily dose of 400 mg of pentobarbital for three months; abrupt discontinuation results in paroxysmal abnormalities on the electroencephalogram (EEG) in about 30 percent of patients. At a daily dose of 600 mg of pentobarbital for one to two months, a withdrawal syndrome characterized by anxiety, insomnia, anorexia, tremor, and EEG changes occurs in about half of the patients and 10 percent may have a single seizure. At higher doses of 800 to 2,200 mg a day for several weeks to months, abrupt discontinuation leads to minor symptoms within 24 hours of the last dose, which include apprehension and uneasiness, insomnia, muscular weakness, twitches, coarse tremors, myoclonic jerks, postural faintness and orthostatic hypotension, anorexia, vomiting, and EEG changes. Minor symptoms may persist for up to two weeks. At high doses major symptoms develop. As many as 75 percent of patients may have grand mal seizures on the second or third day after withdrawal and two thirds will have more than one seizure. The interictal EEG shows 4-per-second spike-wave discharges. Two thirds of those patients develop delirium between the third and eighth day of withdrawal, and it is sometimes accompanied by hyperthermia, which may be fatal. Disorientation, visual hallucinations, and frightening dreams may precede the onset of full delirium. Once delirium has developed it may be exceedingly difficult to reverse, even with large doses of a barbiturate, and thus clinicians should never wait for the appearance of withdrawal symptoms before instituting therapy. The duration of the withdrawal syndrome is between 3 and 14 days, with most ending by the eighth day.

Overdose Barbiturates are lethal when taken in overdose because of their induction of respiratory depression. In addition to intentional suicide attempts, accidental or unintentional overdoses are common. Barbiturates in home medicine cabinets are a common cause of fatal drug overdoses in children. As with benzodiazepines the lethal effects of the barbiturates are additive to those of other sedative-hypnotics, including alcohol and benzodiazepines. Barbiturate overdose is characterized by the induction of coma, respiratory arrest, cardiovascular failure, and death.

The lethal dose varies with the route of administration and the degree of tolerance for the substance after a history of long-term abuse. For the most commonly abused barbiturates the ratio of lethal-to-effective dose ranges between 3 to 1 and 30 to 1. Dependent users often take an average daily dose of 1.5 grams of a short-acting barbiturate, and some have been reported to take as much as 2.5 grams a day for months. The lethal dose is not much greater for the long-term abuser than it is for the neophyte. Tolerance develops quickly to the point at which withdrawal in a hospital becomes necessary to prevent accidental death from overdose.

MISCELLANEOUS SEDATIVE-HYPNOTICS The drugs discussed here have little or no role in modern therapeutics. Unfortunately, prescriptions for some have been increasing, especially in New York, where a 1989 triplicate prescription program has led to a decline in benzodiazepine prescribing by 44 percent in retail pharmacies, 60 percent in the Medicaid program, and 30 percent in Blue Cross-Blue Shield programs. Corresponding prescription increases of 125 percent for meprobamate, 84 percent for methyprylon (Noludar), 29 percent for ethchlorvynol, and 136 percent for chloral hydrate have been reported.

The older sedative-hypnotics are similar in effect to the barbiturates, and they lead to tolerance and physiological dependence. The withdrawal syndrome is similar to the barbiturate withdrawal syndrome and the protocols described for barbiturates should be used to safely withdraw patients dependent on those drugs.

Meprobamate Meprobamate is a carbamate derivative that has weak efficacy as an antianxiety agent. At clinical doses in humans it has minimal muscle-relaxant effects, but it may have a mild analgesic effect in musculoskeletal pain and may potentiate analgesics. Typical daily doses are between 1,200 mg and 1,600 mg, with a maximum of 2,400 mg, in three or four divided daily doses. A discontinuance syndrome will occur after several weeks of treatment with a daily dose of 2,400 mg and mild symptoms may be seen with long-term therapy at doses of 1,600 mg daily. Onset of the discontinuance syndrome takes place within 12 to 48 hours after abrupt discontinuation and lasts for an additional 12 to 48 hours. Seizures may be common in withdrawal from meprobamate and reports published in the 1970s suggest that serious withdrawal symptoms are more common with meprobamate than with barbiturates. Fatalities from overdose have been reported after doses as low as 12 grams. The manufacturer offers the following guidelines for blood levels: levels of 0.5 to 2.0 mg percent (5 to 20 μg per mL) are the normal range with recommended doses; levels of 3.0 to 10 mg percent are associated with mild to moderate overdosage with patients in stupor or light coma; levels of 10 to 20 mg percent are associated with serious overdose, deeper coma, and fatalities; levels over 20 mg percent are associated with more fatalities than survivals. Meprobamate induces microsomal enzymes and may exacerbate intermittent porphyria.

Chloral hydrate Chloral hydrate is used as a hypnotic, in doses of 0.5 to 2.0 g. After oral administration it is rapidly transformed to trichloroethanol, the metabolite that is responsible for its pharmacological activity. It is also effective in blocking experimentally induced seizures; however, anticonvulsive and hypnotic doses are similar in humans, making the benzodiazepines and barbiturates better choices for anticonvulsive medications.

At high doses chloral hydrate may produce respiratory depression, hypotension, gastric necrosis, depressed cardiac contractility, and shortened refractory period. Even at therapeutic doses it is associated with gastric distress and flatulence. In some instances somnambulism, disorientation, and paranoid ideation occur. Tolerance and physiological dependence develop with long-term use, and the withdrawal syndrome is similar to the barbiturate abstinence syndrome. Several drug interactions occur with chloral hydrate, including displacement of oral anticoagulants and acidic drugs from protein binding sites by the metabolite trichloroacetic acid. When combined with furosemide, flushing, tachycardia, hypotension or hypertension, and diaphoresis have been reported. It potentiates the effects of ethanol, and it should not be used in patients with intermittent porphyria. Fatalities from overdose may occur with as little as 4 g, although patients have survived after taking 30 g.

Ethchlorvynol Ethchlorvynol is a rapidly acting sedative-hypnotic with anticonvulsant and muscle-relaxant properties. Recommended doses are 500 to 1,000 mg. Initial effects, which may include euphoria, occur 15 to 30 minutes after an oral dose and plasma levels peak at 1 to 1.5 hours. The elimination half-life of the parent compound is 10 to 20 hours. The duration of the hypnotic effect is about five hours. Long-term use of ethchlorvynol has been associated with toxic amblyopia, scotoma, nystagmus, and peripheral neuropathy, which are usually reversible upon drug discontinuation. Intravenous self-administration may cause pulmonary edema.

Idiosyncratic reactions of excitement and stimulation have been described. Hypersensitivity reactions with urticaria and rare fatal thrombocytopenia may also arise. It should not be used in patients with intermittent porphyria. Tolerance, physiological dependence, and a withdrawal syndrome are seen with long-term administration. Lethal doses are typically between 10 and 25 g; one person was reported to have died after taking 2.5 g with ethanol and one patient survived but was in a coma for seven days after taking 50 g.

Glutethimide and methyprylon Glutethimide and methyprylon (no longer marketed in the United States) are piperidinedione sedative-hypnotics that have high liability for abuse. Glutethimide is similar to the barbiturates in most respects, but differs from them in having significant anticholinergic activity. An overdose can cause ileus, bladder atony, mydriasis, hyperpyrexia, myoclonic jerks, and convulsions. A lethal dose is between 10 and 20 g; intoxication may be seen at a dose of 5 g. An unusual characteristic of glutethimide is that a withdrawal syndrome can occur in patients taking therapeutic doses (0.5 to 3.0 g daily) even when they have not stopped taking the drug. The abstinence syndrome includes tremulousness, nausea, tachycardia, fever, tonic muscle spasms, and grand mal seizures. Withdrawal from a combination of glutethimide and antihistamine has caused catatonia and dyskinesia. When glutethimide is taken with codeine (the street name is a load) a euphoria similar to that with heroin results. In those cases detoxification may require opioid withdrawal in addition to sedative withdrawal.

Methaqualone Methaqualone is no longer available in the United States and much of what is sold on the street as methaqualone is actually diazepam. Methaqualone is a quinazoline with sedative, anticonvulsive, local anesthetic, and antispasmodic activity. It has antitussive effects comparable to those of codeine and weak antihistaminic activity. During the 1960s and 1970s it was considered by the drug culture to be the ultimate high of all sedative-hypnotics, producing euphoria comparable to that from heroin. Chronic users may take daily doses of between 75 mg and 2 g, with an average daily dose of 775 mg. Adverse effects include peripheral neuropathy, nightmares, somnambulism, gastric discomfort, and urticaria. Death has been reported after 8 g, but one report suggested that most deaths that took place under the influence of methaqualone were caused by accidents due to impairment produced by the drug. Tolerance and physiological dependence are seen with chronic dosing.

An overdose of methaqualone may result in restlessness, delirium, hypertonia, muscle spasms, convulsions, and, in very high doses, death. Unlike barbiturates methaqualone rarely causes severe cardiovascular or respiratory depression, and most fatalities result from combining methaqualone with alcohol.

TREATMENT

WITHDRAWAL

Benzodiazepines Guidelines for the treatment of benzodiazepine discontinuance syndrome and the clinical management of withdrawal are presented in Table 13.11-11. The most common clinical situations that require medically supervised withdrawal from the benzodiazepines involve patients with anxiety disorders or chronic insomnia who have been maintained on therapeutic doses of benzodiazepines for several months or years, patients taking supratherapeutic doses of benzodiazepines for treatment-resistant types of anxiety or because of inappropriate dosage escalation, and patients who abuse benzodiazepines as part of a mixed abuse pattern (for example, those who use benzodiazepines to self-medicate alcohol withdrawal or to end a cocaine run).

To plan a rational withdrawal clinicians should keep in mind the factors that influence the development of physiological dependence. The risk of withdrawal is greatest in patients taking high doses over long periods. The onset of withdrawal and its peak severity are earlier with agents with short half-lives, and if they are not tapered, the withdrawal from them may be more severe than from agents with long elimination half-lives, although the last point has not been definitively established. The concurrent use of other sedative-hypnotics, such as barbiturates or ethanol, may alter both the time course and severity of the benzodiazepine withdrawal syndrome.

TAPERING The basic principle underlying safe withdrawal is gradual tapering of the benzodiazepine. In cases of detoxification from therapeutic doses, the daily dosage will be known and the tapering protocol is easily calculated. Anyone taking a ben-

TABLE 13.11-11
Guidelines for Treatment of Benzodiazepine Discontinuance Syndrome

1. Evaluate and treat concomitant medical and psychiatric conditions.
2. Obtain drug history and urine and blood sample for drug and ethanol assay.
3. Determine required dose of benzodiazepine or barbiturate for stabilization, as guided by history, clinical presentation, drug-ethanol assay, and, in some cases, challenge dose.
4. Detoxification from supratherapeutic doses:
   a. Hospitalize if there are medical or psychiatric indications, poor social supports, or polysubstance dependence, or the patient is unreliable.
   b. Some clinicians recommend switching to longer-acting benzodiazepine for withdrawal (e.g., diazepam, clonazepam), while others recommend stabilizing on the drug that patient was taking or on phenobarbital.
   c. After stabilization make an initial dosage reduction of 30 percent on the second or third day and evaluate the response, keeping in mind that symptoms that occur after decreases in benzodiazepines with short elimination half-lives (e.g., lorazepam) will appear sooner than with those with longer elimination half-lives (e.g., diazepam).
   d. Reduce dosage further by 10 to 25 percent every few days if tolerated.
   e. Use adjunctive medications if necessary (e.g., carbamazepine, β-adrenergic receptor antogonists, valproate, clonidine, and sedative antidepressants have been used but their efficacy in the treatment of the benzodiazepine abstinence syndrome has not been established).
5. Detoxification from therapeutic doses:
   a. Initiate 10 to 25 percent dose reduction and evaluate response.
   b. Dose, duration of therapy, and severity of anxiety will influence the rate of taper and need for adjunctive medications.
   c. Most patients taking therapeutic doses will have uncomplicated discontinuation.
6. Psychological interventions may assist patients in detoxification from benzodiazepines and in the long-term management of anxiety.

zodiazepine for two weeks or longer should be tapered from the drug. Initially, the dosage is reduced by approximately 10 to 25 percent, and the patient is observed for any signs and symptoms of withdrawal. It should be emphasized that the appearance of withdrawal signs will be earlier for drugs with short half-lives as compared with drugs with long half-lives. Subsequent reductions will depend on how the patient responds to initial changes and will require individualization based on careful observation of the patient's condition following each dosage change.

In some cases patients taking high therapeutic doses of a benzodiazepine for a year or more may require several months or longer to stop the medication completely, not primarily because of pharmacological factors, but rather to teach patients alternative strategies for coping with anxiety. The majority of patients taking midrange therapeutic doses for a shorter time will tolerate weekly reductions ranging from 10 to 25 percent. Most authorities agree that the last phases of drug discontinuation are the most difficult for the patient, and it may be necessary to slow the taper rate or to stop the taper entirely. The adjunctive use of nonbenzodiazepine medications may also be useful in those circumstances.

Detoxification from supratherapeutic doses of benzodiazepines may require a slightly different approach. Most clinicians hospitalize such patients owing to the greater medical risks associated with supratherapeutic dose withdrawal. Patients may be tapered using the benzodiazepine they have been taking or switched to a drug with a long elimination half-life, such as diazepam or clonazepam (Klonopin), using the dose equivalencies listed in Table 13.11-12 to determine the initial daily dose. The estimated equivalent dose is then administered in divided doses on day 1 to be certain that an accurate history and appropriate equivalency are established. Some clinicians stabilize patients on that dose for two to three days, others prefer to reduce the dose by 30 percent on the second day, followed by 5 to 10 percent daily reductions. The use of carbamazepine (Tegretol) in high-dose withdrawal often permits even larger daily reductions in the benzodiazepine dose. Most high-dose detoxification can be completed in two weeks or less using that protocol. For some patients the dose cannot be reduced that rapidly, however, and slower, longer tapers are sometimes necessary. The efficacy of carbamazepine for the treatment of the benzodiazepine discontinuance syndrome has not been established, although clinical experience to date has been encouraging.

When the physician knows the patient has been taking supratherapeutic doses but is unable to determine the exact dose, 20 mg of diazepam may be given to estimate tolerance. The dose should be repeated every two hours until mild sedation occurs. The total dose required to induce mild sedation is considered the initial dose and the detoxification proceeds as described above.

Some concerns have been raised regarding a lack of cross-tolerance between triazolobenzodiazepines and other benzodiazepines. Those concerns are based entirely on anecdotal reports and are not supported by controlled trials or experimental data. Case reports suggest that diazepam does not adequately treat the withdrawal syndrome from alprazolam, and the combination of chlordiazepoxide and diazepam fails to attenuate withdrawal symptoms from triazolam, although questions have been raised concerning the adequacy of the diazepam doses in those cases. Others report that lorazepam can successfully treat triazolam withdrawal and clonazepam can be substituted for alprazolam in patients with panic disorder. If the primary drug that the patient is taking is not going to be used in the withdrawal protocol, clonazepam or lorazepam may be the best drugs to use when detoxifying patients who have been taking supratherapeutic doses of triazolobenzodiazepines. It is not clear whether higher doses of diazepam would have alleviated the alprazolam withdrawal syndrome in the published case reports. Some authorities recommend the use of phenobarbital in such cases.

DETOXIFICATION FROM MULTIPLE DRUGS OF ABUSE Polysubstance abuse may present special problems for safe withdrawal. The most common polysubstance abuse pattern that influences the medical management of detoxification from benzodiazepines is the concurrent use of alcohol, opioids, and cocaine. Combination with alcohol alters the time course and increases the severity of the sedative withdrawal syndrome. Adequate doses of a benzodiazepine are usually sufficient for safe withdrawal; however, in rare instances even large doses of diazepam can be ineffective and switching to a barbiturate becomes necessary.

When supratherapeutic doses of benzodiazepines are abused with large amounts of opioids it is best to discontinue the former drug first and then stabilize the patient on methadone or some other oral opioid. When the period of risk for major symptoms of sedative-hypnotic withdrawal passes opioid withdrawal may begin. Addiction to low or moderate doses of benzodiazepines or opioids often permits simultaneous withdrawal from both classes of drugs.

Benzodiazepines are often used to terminate a cocaine or other psychostimulant run or to decrease anxiety induced by cocaine. Benzodiazepines used intermittently in that manner usually do not require detoxification. The chronic use of high doses of benzodiazepines with cocaine is less common, but does require medically supervised benzodiazepine taper. The cocaine abstinence syndrome is characterized by depression, irritability, lethargy, amotivation, hypersomnolence, confusion, and drug craving. The clinical presentation of the sedative-hypnotic withdrawal syndrome may be altered in the presence of recent cocaine use and is best monitored by the careful measurement of vital signs (for example, increases in pulse, temperature, and blood pressure).

Some clinicians prefer to use phenobarbital for detoxification in cases of mixed-drug abuse. A dose of phenobarbital equivalent to the benzodiazepine and other sedatives the patient is taking is calculated (Tables 13.11-10 and 13.11-12) or, preferably, the dose is determined from a challenge test and the patient is stabilized on that amount in divided daily doses for

TABLE 13.11-12
Approximate Therapeutic Equivalent Doses of Benzodiazepines

Generic Name	Trade Name	Dose (mg)
Alprazolam	Xanax	1
Chlordiazepoxide	Librium	25
Clonazepam	Klonopin	0.5–1
Clorazepate	Tranxene	15
Diazepam	Valium	10
Estazolam	ProSom	1
Flurazepam	Dalmane	30
Lorazepam	Ativan	2
Oxazepam	Serax	30
Prazepam	Paxipam	80
Temazepam	Restoril	20
Triazolam	Halcion	0.25
Quazepam	Doral	15
Zolpidem*	Ambien	10

*An imidazopyridine benzodiazepine agonist.

the period of peak risk of withdrawal. The maximum daily dose of phenobarbital is 600 mg. After stabilization phenobarbital is reduced by 30 to 60 mg every two to three days.

ADJUNCTIVE MEDICATIONS Several adjunctive medications are used to treat the benzodiazepine withdrawal syndrome, but in no case has their efficacy consistently been supported in controlled trials nor is there evidence that any specific adjunctive medication is superior to another.

Carbamazepine, given in doses that achieve the therapeutic levels for treatment of seizures, may partially attenuate the withdrawal syndrome from benzodiazepines. Initial doses are 200 mg twice a day, although some clinicians recommend a single dose of 400 mg at bedtime to take advantage of the sedative effect. If initial doses are well tolerated, carbamazepine is increased to 600 mg on the second or third day. Typical total daily doses range between 400 and 800 mg. After several days of treatment benzodiazepines are tapered. In spite of reports that such tapering can be completed within a week, even from supratherapeutic doses, some patients will still require a slow taper that lasts several weeks. Carbamazepine can be quickly tapered two to four weeks after the last benzodiazepine dose. It has been suggested that carbamazepine may not be successful in withdrawing patients with panic disorder because it is ineffective in blocking panic attacks, but its use has seen some success even in those patients, as long as a slow benzodiazepine taper is used. The efficacy of other anticonvulsants is undetermined, but one report suggests that sodium valproate (Depakote) may reduce withdrawal symptoms as well.

The β-adrenergic receptor antagonists may also attenuate withdrawal symptoms. Propranolol (Inderal) in doses of 60 to 120 mg may reduce the symptoms of benzodiazepine withdrawal, although tachycardia and elevated blood pressure are the primary symptoms affected, while the subjective sense of discomfort and dysphoria persists. The β-adrenergic receptor antagonists do not have prophylactic effects against seizures and should not be used as the sole drug treatment of withdrawal. Nevertheless, in some cases propranolol or atenolol (Tenormin) (50 to 100 mg) may be helpful adjuncts to withdrawal treatment.

Clonidine (Catapres), 0.1 mg administered twice a day to 0.2 mg three times a day or as a patch, has been used in the treatment of low-dose benzodiazepine withdrawal with variable results. Clonidine does not provide protection against withdrawal seizures. It may be effective only when used before withdrawal symptoms develop.

Although antidepressants have not been rigorously studied in the treatment of benzodiazepine withdrawal, many experienced clinicians prescribe them. Agents with well-established antipanic and sedative effects may be very useful as adjunctive medications in patients in whom anxiety recurs during taper or after drug discontinuation. Imipramine (Tofranil), amitriptyline (Elavil), doxepin (Adapin, Sinequan), trazodone (Desyrel), serotonin-specific reuptake inhibitors, and monoamine oxidase inhibitors may all be useful in that role.

PSYCHOLOGICAL TREATMENTS Specific psychological treatments for withdrawal have not been widely studied. Cognitive behavioral strategies for anxiety management have been applied to patients withdrawing from benzodiazepines with mixed results. Patients who meet the criteria for generalized anxiety disorder are poor candidates for relaxation training.

Many practitioners believe that a critical factor in successful withdrawal is transmitting to the patient a sense of control over the withdrawal symptoms. Supporting that belief is the finding that placebo substitution is associated with fewer withdrawal symptoms after drug discontinuation than is withdrawal without placebo. Apparently the belief that one is taking an effective medication is enough to reduce symptoms.

One way to foster a sense of control over withdrawal symptoms is to link the symptoms of anxiety to environmental or intrapsychic stressors. Cognitive restructuring educates the patient about the withdrawal syndrome and helps the patient to identify and relabel withdrawal symptoms as anxiety, thus permitting the implementation of adaptive coping strategies, which include systematic desensitization, in vivo graded exposure, and group problem solving. The use of a diary to record mood states and their precipitants sometimes helps to develop the process of cognitive restructuring. A diary may also help to alert the clinician to maladaptive responses to benzodiazepine withdrawal, such as increased alcohol consumption.

The concept of cognitive coping should be introduced to patients and examples of self-statements ("talking to yourself") that are applicable to withdrawal and anxiety management should be discussed and provided as flash cards. They include such statements as, "I feel nervous now but it won't last" or "I feel bad but it's no worse than when I had the flu" or "I feel uncomfortable, but nothing bad is going to happen to me." Self-statements should be short, simple, and relevant to the patient.

Patients are encouraged to be active participants in the development of their withdrawal schedule. Clinicians should be flexible as to the rate of taper and should encourage the patient to be a partner in the withdrawal process, especially those who are withdrawing from therapeutic doses. It is often useful to request that the patient choose which doses should be decreased or eliminated according to his or her perceived need. For some patients it may be necessary to set a maximum permissible daily dose.

LONG-TERM OUTCOME Only a few adequately designed follow-up studies have been carried out on patients who terminated benzodiazepine treatment. Many of the studies suffer from sample selection bias, diagnostic heterogeneity of the sample, and failure to assess environmental factors or to control for concurrent psychotherapy or psychoactive medication. But despite those shortcomings several interesting findings have emerged.

In one study of patients who had discontinued benzodiazepines from 10 months to 3.5 years earlier, 70 percent were no longer taking benzodiazepines and had few or no symptoms, 22 percent were not taking benzodiazepines but required other psychotropic medications, and 8 percent had returned to benzodiazepine use. Another study assessed patients who were evaluated for a discontinuation program three to six years earlier and found that 45 percent were not using benzodiazepines, although some were using other psychoactive medication. Of those who successfully completed the tapering program, 73 percent were benzodiazepine-free at follow-up, compared with 39 percent of patients who entered but did not complete the program and 14 percent of patients who did not participate in the program. Yet another study of patients who had been treated for benzodiazepine dependence found that 56 percent of benzodiazepine-free (no use during the preceding month) patients had moderate to severe anxiety and 38 percent had moderate to severe depression at one to five years follow-up. A different study found that even though 66 percent of patients were not taking benzodiazepines at follow-up, 75 percent had taken them at some time during the five years after entering a discontinuation program.

The follow-up studies suggest that most patients can successfully discontinue benzodiazepines. They also indicate that some patients will experience a recurrence of anxiety that will require alternative psychoactive medication or reinstitution of the benzodiazepine. However, a subgroup of patients who discontinue benzodiazepines will actually show improvement in anxiety over pretapering levels, which suggests that those who continue to have significant symptoms of anxiety or depression while taking a benzodiazepine should probably undergo a drug-free trial period. The value of a structured program for discontinuation and the substitution of medications with low abuse liability are supported in several studies. There does not appear to be a relation between long-term outcome (that is, not using benzodiazepines at follow-up) and the dose or duration of treatment or the specific benzodiazepine that was discontinued.

Barbiturates There are three common methods of establishing the dose of a barbiturate required for safe withdrawal: (1) administration of a test dose of pentobarbital (Nembutal) to determine tolerance, (2) calculation of required doses based on estimated equivalencies, and (3) administration of phenobarbital loading doses.

In the first method the initial step is to determine tolerance. Once intoxication has subsided but before withdrawal symptoms have developed, an oral dose of 200 mg of pentobarbital is administered on an empty stomach and the effects are observed after one hour to determine the stabilization dose (Table 13.11-13). If no changes are observed, the test dose is repeated three hours later using 300 mg. If there is still no response, the total requirement may be more than 1,600 mg a day. The calculated daily dose is divided and given every four to six hours for a two- to three-day stabilization period. Daily dose reductions are usually 10 percent of the stabilization dose, but withdrawal regimens must be individualized. Phenobarbital may be substituted for pentobarbital for stabilization and withdrawal at one third the dose.

The second method of barbiturate detoxification requires the calculation of the equivalent hypnotic dose of phenobarbital based on the dose of barbiturate or other sedatives the patient reports taking, also taking into consideration any alcohol consumed. A dose of 30 mg of phenobarbital is substituted for an equivalent hynotic dose of the sedative. The patient is stabilized for the period of peak vulnerability to withdrawal, which is two to three days for sedative-hypnotics with short half-lives, and reductions of 30 to 60 mg of phenobarbital are made every two or three days. Clinicians using that method report that only rarely are daily doses of phenobarbital greater than 600 mg required. The procedure is not recommended, however, because published equivalencies are only approximations and patients will vary greatly in their metabolism and pharmacodynamic responses to the same dose of the sedative. Furthermore, animal studies indicate that cross-tolerance among the various anxiolytics and sedative-hypnotics is not complete. An additional weakness of the method is that it relies on the patient's history of drug use, which is often unreliable. Plasma levels can establish which sedatives have been ingested and may indicate the degree of tolerance when clinical correlations are made. Estimation of tolerance, and thus determination of dosage requirements, is best made after either a test dose or a loading dose is administered. Tables 13.11-10 and 13.11-12 list approximate equivalencies of selected barbiturates, benzodiazepines, and sedatives.

The final method for medical withdrawal from barbiturates involves using loading doses of phenobarbital. According to the original protocol, doses of 120 mg are administered every one to two hours until three of five signs are present—nystagmus, drowsiness, ataxia, dysarthria, emotional lability—or if patients are in withdrawal, until abstinence symptoms abate. No additional drug is administered, and because of its long half-life, the drug self-tapers. Patients are assessed before each dose. Some clinicians have modified the protocol to use doses of 60 mg every one to two hours and to use a gradual taper rather than abrupt discontinuation. The originators of the protocol reported a mean loading dose of 1,440 mg, with hourly doses sometimes required for 15 to 20 hours. They have also administered phenobarbital intravenously at 0.3 mg per kga minute, with close medical supervision, for medically ill patients.

TABLE 13.11-13
Pentobarbital Test Dose Procedure for Barbiturate Withdrawal

Symptoms After Test Dose of 200 Mg Oral Pentobarbital	Estimated 24-Hour Oral Pentobarbital Dose (mg)	Estimated 24-hour Oral Phenobarbital Dose (mg)
Level I: Asleep but arousable; withdrawal symptoms not likely	0	0
Level II: Mild sedation; patient may have slurred speech, ataxia, nystagmus	500–600	150–200
Level III: Patient is comfortable; no evidence of sedation; may have nystagmus	800	250
Level IV: No drug effect	1,000–1,200	300–600

Table modified from D A, Ciraulo, R I Shader, editors: *Clinical Manual of Chemical Dependence,* p 164. American Psychiatric Press, Washington, 1991. From data in Ewing J A, Bakewell W E: Diagnosis and management of depressant drug dependence. Am J Psychiatry *123:* 909, 1967.

OVERDOSE The treatment of overdose of the general class of substances involves gastric lavage, activated charcoal, and careful monitoring of vital signs and central nervous system activity. Overdose patients who come to medical attention while awake should be kept from slipping into unconsciousness. Vomiting should be induced, and activated charcoal should be administered to delay gastric absorption. If the patient is comatose, the clinician must establish an intravenous fluid line, monitor the patient's vital signs, insert an endotracheal tube to maintain a patent airway, and provide mechanical ventilation, if necessary. Hospitalization of a comatose patient in an intensive care unit is usually required during the early stages of recovery from such overdoses.

SUGGESTED CROSS-REFERENCES

Substance-related disorders are discussed throughout Chapter 13, with an introduction and overview and relevant general tables in Section 13.1. Biological therapies are the focus of Chapter 32; benzodiazepines in Section 31.6, monoamine oxidase inhibitors in Section 32.18, and serotonin-specific reuptake inhibitors in Section 32.19.

REFERENCES

Berlin I, Warot D, Hergueta T, Molinier P, Bagot C, Puech A J: Comparison of the effects of zolpidem and triazolam on memory functions. J Clin Psychopharmacol *13:* 100, 1993.

Busto U, Sellers E M, Naranjo C A, Cappeli H, Sanchez-Craig M, Sykora K: Withdrawal reaction after long-term therapeutic use of benzodiazepines. N Engl J Med *315:* 854, 1986.

Ciraulo D A, Barnhill J G, Ciraulo A M, Greenblatt D J, Shader R I: Parental alcoholism as a risk factor in benzodiazepine abuse: A pilot study. Am J Psychiatry *146:* 1333, 1989.
Ciraulo D A, Barnhill J G, Greenblatt D J, Shader R I, Ciraulo A M, Tarmey M F, Molloy M A, Foti M E: Abuse liability and clinical pharmacokinetics of alprazolam in alcoholic men. J Clin Psychiatry *49:* 333, 1988.
Ciraulo D A, Sands B F, Shader R I: Critical review of liability for benzodiazepine abuse among alcoholics. Am J Psychiatry *145:* 1501, 1988.
*De Wit H, Griffiths R R: Testing the abuse liability of anxiolytic and hypnotic drugs in humans. Drug Alcohol Depend *28:* 83, 1991.
De Wit H, Pierri J, Johanson C E: Reinforcing and subjective effects of diazepam in nondrug-abusing volunteers. Pharmacol Biochem Behav *33:* 205, 1989.
DuPont R L: Abuse of benzodiazepines: The problems and the solutions. Am J Drug Alcohol Abuse *14:* 1, 1988.
Evans S M, Critchfield T S, Griffiths R R: Abuse liability assessment of anxiolytics/hypnotics: Rationale and laboratory lore. Br J Addict *86:* 1625, 1991.
Evans S M, Funderburk F R, Griffiths R R: Zolpidem and triazolam in humans: Behavioral and subjective effects and abuse liability. J Pharmacol Exp Ther *255:* 1246, 1990.
*Gabe J: Towards a sociology of tranquilizer prescribing. Br J Addict *85:* 41, 1990.
Gillin J C, Spinweber C L, Johnson L C: Rebound insomnia: A critical review. J Clin Psychopharmacol *9:* 161, 1989.
Greenblatt D J, Allen M D, Noel B J, Shader R I: Acute overdosage with benzodiazepine derivatives. Clin Pharmacol Ther *21:* 497, 1977.
Greenblatt D J, Harmatz J S, Engelhardt N, Shader R I: Pharmacokinetic determinants of dynamic differences among three benzodiazepine hypnotics. Arch Gen Psychiatry *46:* 326, 1989.
Greenblatt D J, Harmatz J S, Shapiro L, Engelhardt N, Gouthro T A, Shader R I: Sensitivity to triazolam in the elderly. N Engl J Med *324:* 1691, 1991.
Greenblatt D J, Harmatz J S, Zinny M A, Shader R I: Effect of gradual withdrawal on the rebound sleep disorder after discontinuation of triazolam. N Engl J Med *317:* 722, 1987.
Griffiths A N, Jones D M, Richens A: Zopiclone produces effects on human performance similar to flurazepam, lormetazepam and triazolam. Br J Clin Pharmacol *21:* 647, 1986.
Griffiths R R, Bigelow G, Liebson I: Human drug self-administration. Double-blind comparison of pentobarbital, diazepam, chlorpromazine, and placebo. J Pharmacol Exp Ther *210:* 301, 1979.
Griffiths R R, Lamb R J, Ator N A, Roache J D, Brady J V: Relative abuse liability of triazolam: Experimental assessment in animals and humans. Neurosci Biobehav Rev *9:* 133, 1985.
Griffiths R R, Lamb R J, Sannerud C A, Ator N A, Brady J V: Self-injection of barbiturates, benzodiazepines and other sedative-anxiolytics in baboons. Psychopharmacology *103:* 154, 1991.
Kales A, Bixler E O, Soldatos C R, Vela-Bueno A, Jacoby J A, Kales J D: Quazepam and temazepam: Effects of short-term and intermediate-term use and withdrawal. Clin Pharmacol Ther *39:* 345, 1986.
Kales A, Manfredi R L, Vgontzas A M, Bixler E O, Vela B A, Fee E C: Rebound insomnia after only brief and intermittent use of rapidly eliminated benzodiazepines. Clin Pharmacol Ther *49:* 468, 1991.
Kales A, Soldatos C R, Bixler E O, Goff P J, Vela B A: Midazolam: Dose-response studies of effectiveness and rebound insomnia. Pharmacology *26:* 138, 1983.
Lader M: History of benzodiazepine dependence. J Subst Abuse Treat *8:* 53, 1991.
Lader M, Lawson C: Sleep studies and rebound insomnia: Methodological problems, laboratory findings, and clinical implications. Clin Neuropharmacol *10:* 291, 1987.
Malcolm R, Brady K T, Johnston A L, Cunningham M: Types of benzodiazepines abused by chemically dependent inpatients. J Psychoactive Drugs *25:* 315, 1993.
Miller L G, Greenblatt D J, Barnhill J G, Shader R I: Chronic benzodiazepine administration. I. Tolerance is associated with benzodiazepine receptor downregulation and decreased gamma-aminobutyric acid A receptor function. J Pharmacol Exp Ther *246:* 170, 1988.
Miller L G, Greenblatt D J, Lopez F, Schatzki A, Heller J, Lumpkin M, Shader R I: Chronic benzodiazepine administration: Effects *in vivo* and *in vitro*. Adv Biochem Psychopharmacol *46:* 167, 1990.
Miller L G, Greenblatt D J, Roy R B, Summer W R, Shader R I: Chronic benzodiazepine administration. II. Discontinuation syndrome is associated with upregulation of gamma-aminobutyric acid A receptor complex binding and function. J Pharmacol Exp Ther *246:* 177, 1988.
Miller L G, Woolverton S, Greenblatt D J, Lopez F, Roy R B, Shader R I: Chronic benzodiazepine administration. IV. Rapid development of tolerance and receptor downregulation associated with alprazolam administration. Biochem Pharmacol *38:* 3773, 1989.
Nutt D J, Costello M J: Rapid induction of lorazepam dependence and reversal with flumazenil. Life Sci *43:* 1045, 1988.
Pecknold J C, Swinson R P, Kuch K, Lewis C P: Alprazolam in panic disorder and agoraphobia: Results from a multicenter trial. III. Discontinuation effects. Arch Gen Psychiatry *45:* 429, 1988.
Piercey M F, Hoffman W E, Cooper M: The hypnotics triazolam and zolpidem have identical metabolic effects throughout the brain: Implications for benzodiazepine receptor subtypes. Brain Res *554:* 244, 1991.
Rall T W: Hypnotics and sedatives; ethanol. In *Goodman and Gilman's the Pharmacological Basis of Therapeutics,* A G Gilman, T W Rall, editors, p 345. Pergamon, New York, 1990.
Rickels K, Case W G, Schweizer E, Garcia-Espana F, Fridman R: Benzodiazepine dependence: Management of discontinuation. Psychopharmacol Bull *26:* 63, 1990.
Rickels K, Case W, Schweizer E, Garcia-Espana F, Fridman R: Long-term benzodiazepine users 3 years after participation in a discontinuation program. Am J Psychiatry *148:* 757, 1991.
Rickels K, Case W G, Schweizer E E, Swenson C, Fridman R B: Low-dose dependence in chronic benzodiazepine users: A preliminary report of 119 patients. Psychopharmacol Bull *22:* 407, 1986.
Rickels K, Fox I L, Greenblatt D J, Sandler K R, Schless A: Clorazepate and lorazepam: Clinical improvement and rebound anxiety. Am J Psychiatry *145:* 312, 1988.
Rickels K, Schweizer E, Case W G, Greenblatt D J: Long-term therapeutic use of benzodiazepines. I. Effects of abrupt discontinuation. Arch Gen Psychiatry *47:* 899, 1990.
Roy-Byrne P P, Dager S R, Cowley D S, Vitaliano P, Dunner D L: Relapse and rebound following discontinuation of benzodiazepine treatment of panic attacks: Alprazolam versus diazepam. Am J Psychiatry *146:* 860, 1989.
*Sellers E M, Ciraulo D A, Dupont R L, Griffiths R L, Kosten T R, Romach M K, Woody G E: Alprazolam and benzodiazepine dependence. J Clin Psychiatry *54:* 64, 1994.
*Shader R I, Greenblatt D J, Ciraulo D A: Treatment of physical dependence on barbiturates, benzodiazepines, and other sedative-hypnotics. In *Manual of Psychiatric Therapeutics,* R I Shader, editor, p 87. Little, Brown, Boston, 1994.
Tyrer P, Rutherford D, Huggett T: Benzodiazepine withdrawal symptoms and propranolol. Lancet *1:* 520, 1981.
Uhlenhuth E H, De Wit H, Balter M B, Johanson C E, Mellinger G D: Risks and benefits of long-term benzodiazepine use. J Clin Psychopharmacol *8:* 161, 1988.
*Woods J H, Katz J L, Winger G: Benzodiazepines: Use, abuse, and consequences. Pharmacol Rev *44:* 151, 1992.

CHAPTER 14 SCHIZOPHRENIA

14.1 SCHIZOPHRENIA: INTRODUCTION AND OVERVIEW

WILLIAM T. CARPENTER, JR., M.D.
ROBERT W. BUCHANAN, M.D.

INTRODUCTION

Schizophrenia is a clinical syndrome that exacts enormous personal and economic costs worldwide. An editorial in *Science* described it as the worst disease affecting mankind, not excepting even acquired immune deficiency syndrome (AIDS). Schizophrenia is a disease of the brain that manifests with multiple signs and symptoms involving thought, perception, emotion, movement, and behavior. Those manifestations combine in various ways, creating considerable diversity among patients, but the cumulative effect of the illness is always severe and usually long-lasting.

HISTORY

Insanity has afflicted mankind throughout history. Written descriptions of schizophrenic symptoms date back to the 15th century BC. In the first and second centuries AD, Greek physicians described the deterioration in cognitive functions and personality commonly observed in schizophrenic patients today, as well as delusions of grandeur and paranoia. The observation and treatment of the schizophrenic patient receded during the Dark Ages. Schizophrenia did not reemerge as a medical condition worthy of study and treatment until the 18th century. By the 19th century, the various psychotic disorders were generally viewed as either insanity or madness, with principal conceptual issues relating to the polemic over regrettable affliction versus reprehensible behavior. Mid- to late 19th-century clinical descriptions of insanity contained many descriptive categories, but no general approach was capable of integrating the widely diverse manifestations of the various forms of mental aberration into discernible illness groups.

A major impediment to distinguishing between the illness patterns of bipolar disorder and schizophrenia was the existence of another common form of insanity. The symptom manifestations of general paresis were quite diverse and overlapped extensively with the symptoms of schizophrenia. The cause of syphilitic insanity was subsequently traced to a spirochetal infection, and antibiotics were eventually found to be effective in treatment and prevention. The identification of syphilitic insanity enabled Emil Kraepelin to delineate two other major patterns of insanity, manic-depressive psychosis and dementia precox (or dementia of the young), and to group together under one diagnostic category the previously disparate categories of insanity such as hebephrenia, paranoia, and catatonia. Kraepelin, in differentiating dementia precox from manic-depressive illness, emphasized what he believed to be the characteristic poor long-term prognosis of dementia precox, as compared to the relatively nondeteriorating course of manic-depressive illness. In *Dementia Praecox and Paraphrenia,* published in 1919, Kraepelin described the two principal pathophysiological or disease processes occurring in dementia precox:

> On the one hand we observe a weakening of those emotional activities which permanently form the mainsprings of volition. In connection with this, mental activity and instinct for occupation become mute. The result of this part of the process is emotional dullness, failure of mental activities, loss of mastery over volition, of endeavor, and of ability for independent action. The essence of personality is thereby destroyed, the best and most precious part of its being, as Griesinger once expressed it, torn from her. . . . The second group of disorders, which gives dementia praecox its peculiar stamp, . . . consists in the loss of the inner unity of the activities of intellect, emotion, and volition in themselves and among one another. Stransky speaks of an annihilation of the "intrapsychic coordination." . . . This annihilation presents itself to us in the disorders of association described by Bleuler, in incoherence of the train of thought, in the sharp change of moods as well as in desultoriness and derailments in practical work. But further, the near connections between thinking and feeling, between deliberation and emotional activity on the one hand, and practical work on the other is more or less lost. Emotions do not correspond to ideas.

The description of those processes provided the conceptual framework for what are now termed the negative and positive symptoms of schizophrenia, respectively.

In 1911 Eugen Bleuler, recognizing that dementia was not a usual characteristic of dementia precox, suggested the term "schizophrenia" (splitting of the mind) for the disorder. Bleuler introduced the concept of primary and secondary schizophrenic symptoms; his four primary symptoms (the four A's) were abnormal associations, autistic behavior and thinking, abnormal affect, and ambivalence. Of those four symptoms Bleuler viewed as central to the illness the loss of association between thought processes and among thought, emotion, and behavior. Typical examples of the loss of association are silly giggling on receiving news of the death of a loved one, the introduction of magical thinking and peculiar concepts into an ordinary discussion, the sudden display of angry behavior without experiencing anger (or an understandable provocation), and the like.

Bleuler's view that a dissociative process is fundamental to schizophrenia and that it underlies a wide variety of the symptom manifestations of schizophrenia has supported a major paradigm for conceptualizing the illness, namely, that despite its various manifestations, schizophrenia is a single disease entity in which extensive similarity in etiology and pathophysiology is seen across all patients with the disorder. According to that view, a neurophysiological disturbance of indeterminate origin and nature occurs that manifests as a dissociative process adversely influencing the development of mental capacities in the areas of thought, emotion, and behavior. Depending on the individual's adaptive capacity and environmental circumstances, the fundamental dissociative process could lead to secondary disease manifestations such as delusions, hallucinations, social withdrawal, and diminished drive.

There are many parallels in medicine for the single disease model. Diabetic patients have in common an impairment in glucose metabolism, but the secondary manifestations vary considerably, depending on which organ systems are involved. Similarly, seizure disorders may share a common pathophysiological mechanism, but the location of the lesion leads to different signs and symptoms. One patient may experience a momentary lapse in consciousness, a second may have full-body convulsions, and a third may experience strange sexual sensations and excessive religiosity. The diverse manifestations of syphilitic insanity illustrate the potential utility of the single disease model in schizophrenia.

The major alternative paradigm conceptualizes schizophrenia as a clinical syndrome rather than a single disease entity. In that view, although a commonality of signs and symptoms groups patients with schizophrenia in a category that is distinct from other categories of psychosis (for example, mood disorders and toxic psychoses), more than one disease entity will eventually be found within the syndrome of schizophrenia. The demonstration that mental retardation is a clinical syndrome rather than a single disease entity illustrates that construct. Specific etiologies and pathophysiologies of the multiple disease entities leading to mental retardation have been well-defined. With regard to schizophrenia, it is necessary to accept the clinical syndrome designation because proof of a single disease entity is lacking. Almost all schizophrenia experts consider it prudent to designate schizophrenia as a clinical syndrome, and most expect that more than one disease entity will eventually be defined.

There are other competing models for conceptualizing schizophrenia which, although seriously debated in the past, are currently dismissed as demonstrably invalid or so seriously reductionistic as not to account for major observations associated with the illness. The facts that schizophrenia meets all definitions of an illness or disease, and that society subscribes to both scientific and humane imperatives to identify and treat persons who are ill, militate against the use of nondisease models. Earlier formulations, such as the societal reaction theory (which held that schizophrenia was a sane reaction to an insane world), cannot account for central facts of the illness, nor do they lead to effective intervention. For example, Thomas Szasz's theory that schizophrenia is a myth enabling society to manage deviant behavior is vacuous in that it cannot account for facts central to schizophrenia, such as its distribution among biological relatives, the myriad of associated brain abnormalities, and the restorative effects of drug treatment. Narrow-framework disease models that attempt to account for the illness solely at the level of psychological mechanisms are also inadequate in accommodating the known facts of the illness. Genetic or immunovirological causal factors cannot be addressed by reductionistic theories operating at the psychological or social levels. The many biological, psychological, and social factors relevant to the understanding and treatment of schizophrenia require a broad medical model and rule against reduction to any single level of the functioning organism.

Thus, schizophrenia is appropriately conceptualized as a disease process. Although a unifying etiology and pathophysiology may eventually be uncovered that would account for all (or almost all) cases, it is more likely that more than one disease entity exists within the clinical syndrome of schizophrenia, with each entity having its own distinguishable etiology and pathophysiology. A broad medical model that integrates factors ranging from the molecular to the psychosocial is necessary to describe schizophrenia, account for the range of pathogenic influences, and create a framework for treatment and rehabilitation.

EPIDEMIOLOGY

The essential facts about the prevalence and impact of schizophrenia are important. Schizophrenia affects just under 1 percent of the world's population (approximately 0.85 percent). The number of affected persons markedly increases if schizophrenia spectrum disorders are included in prevalence estimates. The concept of schizophrenia spectrum disorders is derived from observations of illness manifestations in the biological relatives of patients with schizophrenia. Although the full picture of schizophrenia is manifest at an increased rate in relatives, more frequently only a partial manifestation is observed. Diagnoses and approximate lifetime prevalence rates by percent of population are as follows: schizoid personality disorder, fractional percentage; schizotypal personality disorder, 1 to 4 percent; schizoaffective disorder, 0.7 percent; and the atypical psychoses and delusional disorder, 0.7 percent.

The manifestations of schizophrenia are observed in individuals in all societies and geographical areas evaluated to date. Although comparable data are difficult to obtain, incidence and lifetime prevalence are roughly the same anywhere in the world. The psychosis usually manifests during late adolescence and early adulthood, although there is a difference associated with sex. The incidence in men peaks during ages 15 to 25 years, whereas the peak incidence in women occurs between 25 and 35 years. The incidence figures are probably similar in rural and urban populations, but the prevalence of schizophrenia is higher among urban and lower socioeconomic populations. The increased prevalence is generally attributed to the social drift phenomenon, in which afflicted or vulnerable persons tend to lose their job and social niche and drift toward pockets of poverty and inner city areas. Occasional geographical areas exhibiting an increased prevalence of schizophrenia are interesting in terms of illness etiology. For example, an isolated population in northern Scandinavia appears to have a gene pool enriched for schizophrenia vulnerability, probably brought to the region generations ago by two immigrating families.

Because schizophrenia begins early in life, causes significant and long-lasting impairments, makes heavy demands for hospital care, and requires ongoing clinical care, rehabilitation, and support services, the financial cost of the illness in the United States is estimated to exceed that of all cancers combined. The financial cost for all mental illnesses for 1988 was an estimated $129.3 billion, of which almost $40 billion was spent on schizophrenia. In 1955 about 500,000 hospital beds in the United States were occupied by the mentally ill—the majority with a diagnosis of schizophrenia. That figure is now approximately 268,000. Schizophrenic patients also had a total of 369,402 psychiatric admissions to hospitals in the 12 months preceding April 1, 1986. The locus of care has shifted dramatically to acute hospital care and community-based services. Many patients in need of services lose touch with care services, but as of April 1, 1986, 298,808 outpatients were under care in the United States.

Deinstitutionalization has been a dramatic success in terms of reducing the number of beds in custodial facilities, but overall its consequences are disheartening. Many patients have simply been transferred to alternative forms of custodial care (in contrast to treatment or rehabilitative services), including nursing home care and poorly supervised shelter arrangements. Others have been released to communities unable or unwilling to provide minimal clinical care or humane support. For the more fortunate patient, the burden of care has shifted to the family, creating a difficult burden for large numbers of families in the United States. The overall cost to those families in 1985 was estimated at $2.5 billion. The less fortunate patient may have no place to live or may be forced to live in circumstances of extreme isolation and hopelessness. Patients with a diagnosis of schizophrenia are reported to account for 33 to 50 percent of homeless Americans.

ETIOLOGY

Detailed knowledge of the cause or causes of schizophrenia is lacking. Genetic factors are important in some (perhaps all) cases, but it is not yet clear which genes are deviant, how they contribute to pathophysiology, or whether the same or different genes are involved in all cases that have a genetic etiology.

Other early influences, variously marked by gestational and birth complications and winter birth excess, must be involved in the causal pathways for schizophrenia, but the pathophysiological mechanisms underlying the involvement of those factors are not yet known. Various versions of viral and immune theories of causation are plausible, but no virus or immune mechanism has yet been established as an etiological factor in schizophrenia.

For about a decade a central question underlying the investigation of the etiology of schizophrenia has been whether schizophrenia is a neurodevelopmental or neuropathological disorder. Is the cause of schizophrenia to be found in failure of the brain to develop normally, or is it to be found in a disease process that alters a normally developed brain? Both causes, of course, may be true, for the schizophrenia syndrome probably represents more than one etiological and disease process, and a developmental abnormality may increase the risk for subsequent disease pathogeneity. However, although there are sporadic reports of gliosis in schizophrenic brains that may indicate the presence of a disease process and subsequent neuropathological response, the preponderance of evidence is consistent with the hypothesis that schizophrenia is a neurodevelopmental disorder. The consistency with which the known data point to early deviations in the development of the central nervous system (CNS) has been useful in focusing theory and investigative work.

Increasing information on the neurobiology of brain development has led to considerable new knowledge of the mechanisms of pathogenic influences. It is now clear that subtle deviations in brain development could create dysfunctions associated with specific behaviors. Postmortem findings of abnormalities in pyramidal cell density and alignment, although not always replicated, support the proposition that the developmental process of cell migration underlying the establishment of normal brain cytoarchitecture may go awry in schizophrenia. Alternatively, it is known that the brain has extensive redundancy during the developing years, and that the fine-tuning necessary for efficient functioning involves eliminating certain nerve cells and many of the synapses connecting cells. Inadequate pruning of nerve cells and synapses or errors in selection for pruning could, in theory, underlie dysfunctions that later lead to schizophrenia symptoms.

Principal hypotheses regarding causation include the altered expression of genes, neuroimmunovirology factors, and hypoxic damage during gestation and birth.

GENETIC HYPOTHESES Schizophrenia and schizophrenialike manifestations occur at an increased rate among the biological relatives of patients with schizophrenia. The increased rate is most evident in the case of monozygotic twins, who have an identical genetic endowment and a concordance rate for schizophrenia between 40 and 50 percent. That rate is four to five times the concordance rate in dizygotic twins or the rate of occurrence in other first-degree relatives (siblings, parents, or offspring). The finding of a higher rate of schizophrenia among the biological relatives of an adopted-away person who develops schizophrenia than among adoptive, nonbiological relatives who rear the patient has added further support to pedigree and twin study evidence suggesting a significant genetic contribution to the etiology of schizophrenia. However, the modes of genetic transmission in schizophrenia are unknown. No current model (for example, single gene dominant or recessive, the polygenetic model, or the multifactorial model) satisfactorily accounts for the data. Further, the monozygotic twin data demonstrate that persons who are genetically vulnerable to schizophrenia do not inevitably become schizophrenic; environmental factors must be involved in determining a schizophrenia outcome. If the vulnerability model of schizophrenia is correct in its postulation of an environmental influence, then other factors may prevent or cause schizophrenia in the genetically vulnerable individual. Environmental causal factors include gestational and birth complications, and probably substance abuse. Other aspects of the biological and psychosocial environment will probably be found to alter risk in the vulnerable person.

Determining the mode of transmission in a putative genetic disorder requires a known phenotype and genetic homogeneity across pedigrees. Neither of those conditions is met in schizophrenia. Nonetheless, to understand the role of genes in the etiology of schizophrenia, it will eventually be necessary to identify the actual genes and their products, and how they are expressed in the brain. The delineation of the different phenotypic manifestations of the schizophrenic gene or genes is important for case ascertainment. Physiological markers of the phenotypes would move genetic inquiry closer to the neuronal effects of schizophrenia-related genes. Measures of smooth pursuit eye movements (SPEMs), information processing, and sensory gating are the most prominent candidate markers. SPEM and information-processing tasks (such as the continuous performance task and forced span of apprehension test) have been found to distinguish schizophrenic probands and their biological relatives from control groups. Similarly, patients and their biological relatives are more likely than comparison groups to fail to inhibit neuronal response to a repeated stimulus (measured by a peak amplitude in electrical signal at about 50 milliseconds—the P50 sensory gating phenomenon). That phenomenon is of particular interest because it captures a basic neuronal property whose dysfunction could explain schizophrenic pathophysiology.

It has proved difficult to progress from evidence confirming a genetic contribution to the etiology of schizophrenia to evidence implicating specific genes in the disease. Nonetheless, genetic investigation is highly promising, for there is unequivocal evidence of a genetic contribution to some, perhaps all, forms of the illness, and knowledge and techniques relevant to discovering the genetic basis for human disease are advancing rapidly. Linkage analysis has moved from a few marker probes to banks of hundreds, and the entire genome will soon be examined with probes spaced along all chromosomes. Analytical techniques have been developed to evaluate polygenetic disorders, and gene substructure techniques now enable investigators to focus on candidate genes found to distinguish schizophrenic brains.

NEUROIMMUNOVIROLOGY HYPOTHESES Immune and viral hypotheses of schizophrenia are as old as scientific knowledge in those areas. That a virus could cause neuropsychiatric disease was confirmed when Louis Pasteur isolated the rabies virus in 1881. But schizophrenia is not an acute encephalitis or a fulminating infection. More subtle pathophysiological mechanisms are involved, which makes it more difficult to establish etiology. Moreover, the epidemiological data supporting an infectious etiology, although interesting, are weak. Schizophrenia may have a north to south prevalence gradient in the Northern hemisphere (south to north in the Southern hemisphere), may be endemic to a few areas (for example, northern Sweden), is associated with a winter birth excess, and, like multiple sclerosis, exhibits monozygotic twin discordance. However, it has been difficult to conduct definitive studies of immunovirological hypotheses because any potential marker of an immune or viral process associated with schizophrenia is relevant only to some cases of schizophrenia and could be construed as secondary to conditions associated with the disease (for example, crowding of chronically hospitalized patients, exposure of chronically ill patients living in low socioeconomic circumstances, poor health habits).

Viral theories remain popular despite the difficulty of validating any particular version. Their popularity stems from the fact that several specific viral theories have the power to explain the particular localization of pathology necessary to account for a range of manifestations in schizophrenia without requiring extensive infection. The six general pathogenic models of viral and immune pathophysiology relevant to schizophrenia are described below.

Retroviral infection A retrovirus can insert itself into, and thereby alter, the genome—a process that could initiate a genetic contribution to schizophrenia. It is postulated that the retrovirus inserts itself into the genome and alters the expression of the host's own genes and the genes of the host's offspring toward the development of schizophrenia (the virogene hypothesis). Presently, no evidence supports the retrovirus theory of schizophrenia.

Current or active viral infection Many investigators have postulated that viruses with an affinity for the CNS are involved in the etiology of schizophrenia. It is envisioned that either a neurotropic virus infects nerve cells in discrete parts of the brain and causes sustained alterations in the functioning of the involved neural systems, or that by-products of a viral infection have direct toxic effects on nerve cell functioning. Abnormal immune indices have been reported in schizophrenia and could be indicative of an active infectious process; however, most investigators have considered the viral factor an early event resulting in brain damage that has a long-lasting effect.

An alternative formulation of the current viral infection hypothesis is based on the observation that so-called slow viruses can infect the brain, with substantive disease manifestations appearing only years later. In theory, that could account for the subtle early manifestations frequently observed in schizophrenic patients, which are followed by more intense symptom manifestations 10 to 30 years later.

A substantial challenge to either formulation of the current or active viral infection hypothesis is the absence of direct evidence substantiating a viral etiology, including the lack of physical signs of active viral infection in postmortem tissue.

Inactive viral infection According to the inactive viral infection hypothesis, a virus may either infect certain brain tissues early in life, to create vulnerability to schizophrenia, or act as a causal mechanism for the initial illness processes that later lead to the classic picture of schizophrenia. The resulting tissue damage produces long-lasting alterations in neural systems, leading to schizophrenia manifestations without concurrent viral infection. Gliosis, sometimes observed in postmortem tissue, would support the proposition of an earlier, now dormant viral infection; a dormant infection would help account for the fact that signs of active viral infection are not ordinarily observed in postmortem brain tissue. A limited number of experiments have not been successful in using material from brains of schizophrenic patients as a source for transmitting CNS viral infection into the brain tissue of other species, further supporting the proposition that, if a virus is relevant to the etiology of schizophrenia, it is not causing active infection at the time of death.

Virally activated immunopathology Two general mechanisms have been proposed for a virally activated immunopathology. The first is based on the observation that viruses are normally endogenous to the human brain and develop specific foci in the brain. Periodic viral reactivation of those foci of colonization normally does not result in psychotic symptoms. However, in an individual with a genetically or environmentally determined abnormal immune response to viruses, it is hypothesized that viral reactivation could result in an induction of schizophrenic psychopathology. The theory regards the products of immunoreactivity, such as interferon-α (INF-α), as mediators of the pathogenic influence. That recently proposed theory has little direct evidence to support it but receives indirect support from findings of abnormalities in INF-α responsiveness in schizophrenic patients as compared with normal controls.

The second mechanism proposed is that the virus may induce the host to fail to recognize its own tissues as self and subsequently to mount a destructive immune response. The virus may knock out the normal recognition pattern by altering some cellular component, such as normally cryptic neural cell surface proteins, causing the component to stimulate a host response. An antibody response would directly interfere with nerve cell function either by destroying the cells or, in the case of receptor proteins, by altering neurotransmission.

Autoimmune pathology Viral inducement of autoimmune pathology, discussed above, is an example of the autoimmune pathogenic model. Another example would be a model similar to that operative in several known autoimmune diseases, where, for reasons not entirely clear but probably involving genetics, some tissues are not recognized as self and become the target of the immune response.

Secondary influence of maternal viral infections on fetal brain development Reports of an increased risk of schizophrenia associated with fetal exposure to maternal influenza during the second trimester of pregnancy raise the possibility that some attribute of maternal infection (for example, fever and cytokine production) perturbates normal brain development during a period of active neural cell migration.

BIRTH AND PREGNANCY COMPLICATION HYPOTHESES Infants born with a history of pregnancy or birth complications are at increased risk for developing schizophrenia as adults. The reason for the increase in risk is not known. The following plausible explanations, which are not mutually exclusive, guide present-day research.

1. The genes that create vulnerability for schizophrenia may also alter early embryonic development in a manner that increases the likelihood of gestational and birth complications.

2. Adverse influences on the developing brain early in gestation create a risk for birth complications and later for schizophrenia. Possible instances of the latter proposition are the findings that (a) fetuses in the second trimester of gestation during influenza epidemics are at substantially increased risk of developing schizophrenia as adults, and (b) female fetuses exposed to severe food deprivation during the first trimester are at increased risk for developing schizophrenia.

3. The proposed mechanism whereby gestational or birth complications may alter brain development is diminished oxygen supply (hypoxia). The oxygen-deprivation theory is attractive for two reasons: First, many of the reported pregnancy and birth complications can be associated with temporary hypoxia, and second, the hippocampus, a component of the limbic sys-

tem, the cerebral cortex, and the basal ganglia—brain regions most frequently implicated as deviant in schizophrenia—are among the areas in the developing brain most sensitive to the adverse effects of hypoxia.

PATHOPHYSIOLOGY

The pathophysiological question of how the brain is involved in schizophrenia is different from the etiological question of why deviations in brain function occur. Because the illness represents disturbances in some, but not all, brain functions, it is reasonable to suppose that specific areas or neural circuits of the brain are involved. The manifestations of schizophrenia must then involve altered physiological processing, which, in turn, reflects altered cytoarchitectural, biochemical, and electrophysiological properties of the neural systems.

It is easier to assert that schizophrenia must involve deviations in brain physiology than to clearly document the pathophysiology. Throughout most of the 20th century, examination of postmortem brain tissue has been the principal source of data on the neuroanatomy of schizophrenia. Early in the century, schizophrenia was referred to as the graveyard of neuropathology—not because of a lack of neuropathological findings, for abnormalities were observed with considerable frequency, but because of the lack of a discernible pattern to the pathological findings and the possibility that deviations were either artifactual or were a consequence, rather than a cause, of the disease. For example, head trauma and viral infections affecting the brain would be more common in crowded custodial hospitals than in typical comparison groups. Moreover, the widespread use of antipsychotic drugs in the treatment of schizophrenia introduced another potential artifact into studies of brain pathophysiology. Finally, brain-behavior relations were not sufficiently detailed to guide neuropathological inquiry during much of the 20th century.

Scientists have long been aware of the need for noninvasive techniques to study the functioning brain of living patients. Such techniques are particularly important in the absence of valid animal models. During the middle third of the 20th century, pneumoencephalography (PEG) provided substantial evidence of enlarged brain ventricles, suggesting diminished tissue in schizophrenic patients compared to controls. Electroencephalography (EEG) provided information on cortical surface activity, but neither PEG nor EEG allowed a comprehensive evaluation of the functioning human brain.

A more detailed view of brain structure and metabolism has become possible only with the recent development of in vivo structural imaging techniques, such as computed tomography (CT) and magnetic resonance imaging (MRI), and functional studies, such as positron emission tomography (PET) and single photon emission computed tomography (SPECT). The availability of those techniques coincided with the recognition that a better understanding was needed of the interconnections between subcortical structures and cortical areas and their implications for brain-behavior relations. CT studies have recorded the enlarged ventricles observed with PEG and have further shown that a substantial proportion of schizophrenic patients, in comparison with healthy control subjects, exhibit cortical atrophy. Those results suggest that schizophrenic patients have relatively less brain tissue, a condition that could represent either a failure in development or the subsequent loss of tissue. MRI, with its enhanced gray and white matter resolution, allows a more detailed assessment of specific brain structures. Studies employing MRI have found evidence in schizophrenic patients for decreased cortical gray matter, especially in the temporal cortex; a decreased volume of limbic system structures, such as the amygdala, hippocampus, and parahippocampus; and an increased volume of basal ganglia nuclei. Those findings are consistent with findings on neuropathological (including ultrastructural) examinations of postmortem tissue that in some cases indicate cell loss, misalignment of cells, altered structure in specific brain regions, or gliosis suggestive of trauma.

Structural findings can also help clarify the interpretation of altered metabolic patterns observed with dynamic imaging procedures such as xenon-133 regional cerebral blood flow (rCBF) studies and PET studies with glucose and oxygen metabolism. The latter studies have suggested diminished metabolism in frontal cortical structures, with preliminary evidence suggesting a differential association of metabolic indices with the positive psychotic symptoms and primary, enduring negative symptoms.

Present-day knowledge is acquired from structural imaging, dynamic imaging, and anatomically relevant neuropsychological techniques in living subjects, supplemented by postmortem biochemical and structural evaluation. An understanding of the findings in aggregate may be enhanced by viewing their integration into the several major neuroanatomical theories of schizophrenia. Those theories, while different in important aspects, are not mutually exclusive.

MAJOR NEUROANATOMICAL THEORIES The past 20 years have seen a gradual evolution from the concept of schizophrenia as a disorder involving discrete areas of the brain to a disorder of brain neural circuits. A major stimulus for the change in perspective was the development of neuroanatomical theories based on knowledge of dopamine pathways in the brain and of brain-behavior relations (Figure 14.1-1). Delineation of the mesolimbic and mesocortical dopaminergic pathways in the brain led to hypotheses postulating the involvement of the limbic system, the frontal cortex, or both in the pathophysiology of schizophrenia. Those and other more recent neuroanatomical models share the same essential premise, namely, that the brain is organized in neural circuits, and either a structural or functional lesion somewhere in the circuit disrupts the functional integrity of the entire circuit.

The limbic system is integral to perception, motivation, gratification, memory, thought, and many other behaviors whose disturbance is often associated with schizophrenia. Dopaminergic neurons from the ventral tegmental area (VTA) project to both the nucleus accumbens and the amygdala. Lesions in primate amygdaloid nuclei can cause impairments in drive, social function, and emotional arousal that are reminiscent of the negative symptoms of schizophrenia. The prefrontal cortex also receives dopaminergic input from the VTA and plays a primary role in many of the higher executive functions. Lesions of the prefrontal cortex in animals and humans result in apathy, decreased emotional expressiveness, and a loss of initiative and spontaneity, behaviors also reminiscent of the negative symptoms of schizophrenia. Studies reporting diminished metabolism in the frontal cortices and impaired performance on neuropsychological tasks that place demands on frontal lobe function have encouraged the view that prefrontal cortex dysfunction is involved in schizophrenia.

Limbic and prefrontal neuroanatomical models of schizophrenia have been integrated into a single unifying neurodevelopmental theory of schizophrenia. The integration of those models is based on data derived from animal studies, in which lesions of the mesocortical dopaminergic tracts result in increased dopaminergic activity in limbic system structures,

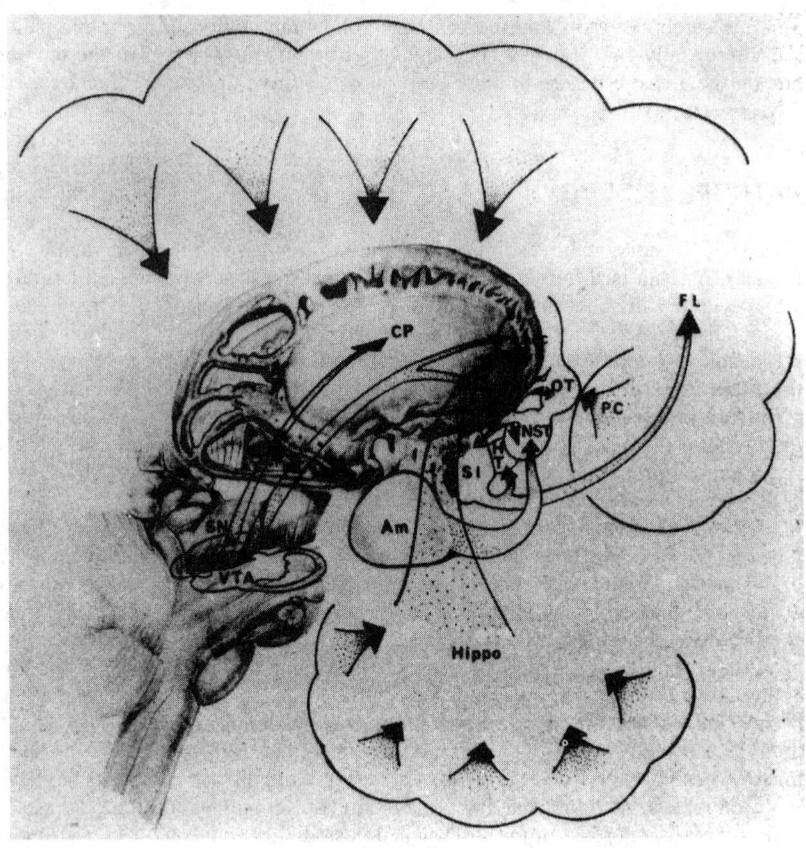

FIGURE 14.1-1 *Diagrammatic representation of fan-like confluence of neocortical structures on caudate putamen* (CP), *which receives dopamine axons form substantia nigra* (SN). *A similar confluence toward limbic striatum includes projection of amygdala* (Am) *to bed nucleus of stria terminals* (NST), *hippocampus to nucleus accumbens* (Acc), *piriform cortex* (PC) *to olfactory tubercle* (OT), *and a separate dopamine projection ascending from the ventral tegmental area.* (VTA). *Output from neostriatum via globus pallidus to thalamus (not shown) parallels limbic striatal efferents that exit via substantia innominata* (SI) *to frontal lobe* (FL) *and hypothalamus* (HT). *(Figure from J R Stevens: An anatomy of schizophrenia? Arch Gen Psychiatry* 29: *177, 1973.) Used with permission. Orginally adapted from J Klingler, P Gloor: The connections of the amygdala and the anterior temporal cortex. J Comp Neurol* 115: *333, 1960 and drawing by Walle J Nauta, Massachusetts Institute of Technology, Cambridge.)*

suggesting that the prefrontal cortex provides inhibitory feedback to limbic system structures. An early developmental lesion of the dopaminergic tracts to the prefrontal cortex would hypothetically result in the appearance of the negative symptoms of schizophrenia, and the reduction in inhibitory feedback to limbic structures and subsequent increased activation would result in psychotic symptoms (Figure 14.1-2).

Parallel basal ganglia-thalamocortical neural circuits Recent investigations of the basal ganglia have revealed that those nuclei are integral components of a series of segregated parallel neural circuits connecting the cerebral cortex with the thalamus by way of the basal ganglia (Figure 14.1-3). Projections from the thalamus to the frontal cortex complete the circuit. Each of the circuits is hypothesized to subserve a discrete range of functions. A number of investigators have used those circuits as a starting point for developing hypotheses of schizophrenic pathophysiology. The various hypotheses differ from each other primarily in their point of emphasis.

Integrating data from animal studies and neurobehavioral and functional and structural imaging studies in humans, investigators have hypothesized that dysfunction of the anterior cingulate basal ganglia-thalamocortical circuit underlies the production of psychotic symptoms and dysfunction of the dorsolateral prefrontal circuit underlies the production of primary and enduring negative, or deficit, symptoms. Dysfunction in one of the circuits may be independent of dysfunction in the other.

The basal ganglia-thalamocortical neural circuits have also served as a starting point for the articulation of a hypothesis proposing disruption of the interaction between the glutamate neurons projecting from the cerebral cortex and the dopamine projections to the basal ganglia. The cerebral cortex, through glutamate projections from the cortex to the basal ganglia, facilitates the performance of selected behaviors while inhibiting others. The excitatory glutamatergic neurons terminate on γ-aminobutyric acid (GABA) ergic and cholinergic neurons, which, in turn, suppress or excite dopaminergic and other neurons. The regulatory activity of the neural circuits enables the cortex to protect itself from overstimulation from thalamocortical neurons (Figure 14.1-4). A dysfunction in the system could account for failure to protect the brain from endogenous neurotoxicity and from phencyclidine (PCP)like effects mediated by the *N*-methyl-D-aspartate (NMDA) receptor complex. Data from clinical and preclinical studies, including observations of PCP-induced effects, support such a construal of the anatomy of schizophrenia.

Another model involving basal ganglia-thalamocortical neural circuits is derived from studies of attention dysfunction and blood flow in schizophrenic patients. The hypothesis is based on three observations. First, PET imaging with $H_2{}^{15}O$ has shown increased blood flow in the left globus pallidus in schizophrenic patients who have never been medicated. Because increased blood flow is thought to reflect changes in the function of the nerve fibers projecting to the globus pallidus rather than changes in the pallidal nerve cells themselves, the result suggested that there was decreased input to the left globus pallidus from either the caudate and putamen, subthalamic nucleus, and nucleus accumbens (potentially more than one of those areas). Second, schizophrenic patients are less able to shift visual attention, an impairment that may be indicative of left cerebral hemisphere involvement. Third, animals with unilateral lesions of midbrain dopaminergic neurons have behavioral impairments analogous to those seen in schizophrenic patients. Those dopaminergic neurons project to the caudate, putamen, and nucleus accumbens, the brain areas implicated in the PET study. Those three lines of evidence have led to the hypothesis

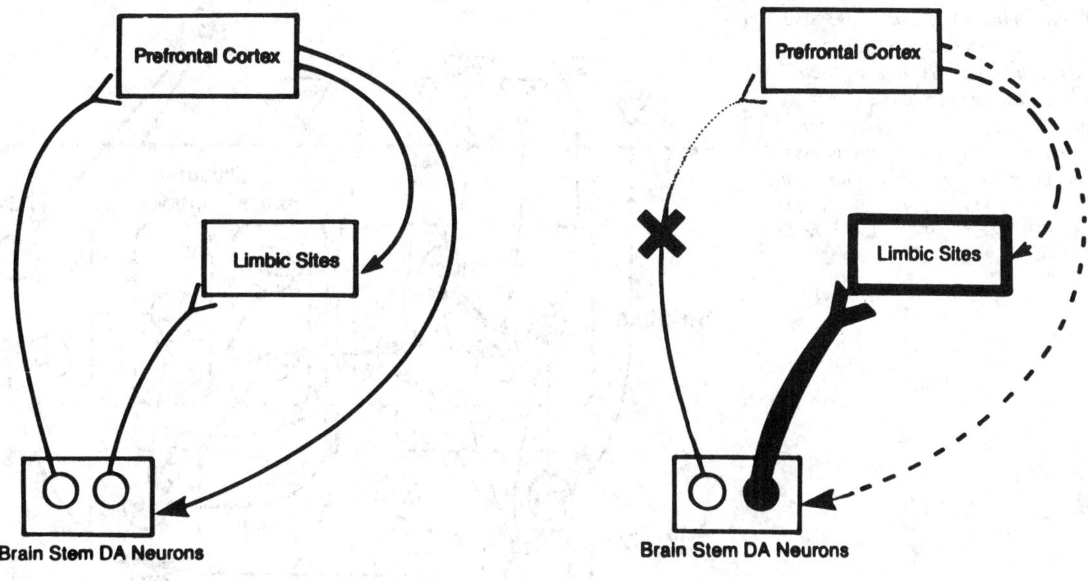

FIGURE 14.1-2 *Schematized interactions between mesolimbic and mesocortial dopamine system in normal state* (left) *and after selective lesioning of dopamine input to prefrontal cortex* (right), *based on the work of Pycock et al. Broken line indicates that specific effect of lesion corticolimbic feedback (for example, decreased inhibition or increased excitation) is known.* DA, *dopamine. (Figure from D R Weinberger: Implications of normal brain development for the pathogenesis of schizophrenia. Arch Gen Psychiatry 44: 660, 1987. Used with permission.)*

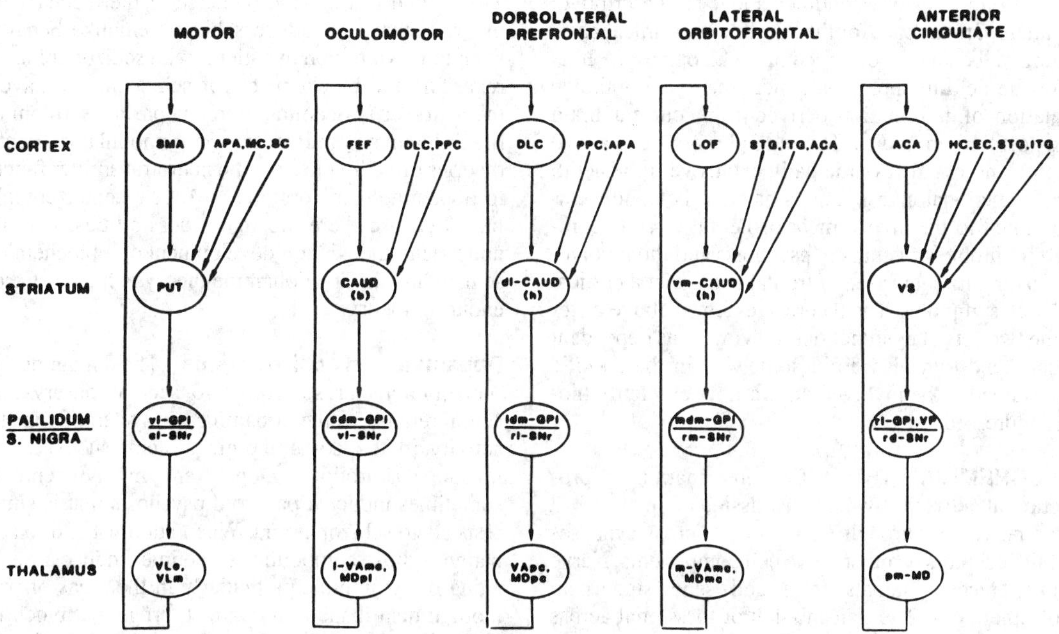

FIGURE 14.1-3 *Parallel organization of the five proposed basal ganglia-thalamocortical circuits. Each circuit engages specific regions of the cerebral cortex, striatum, pallidum, substantia nigra, and thalamus.* ACA, *anterior cingulate area;* APA, *arcuate premotor area;* CAUD, *caudate:* (b), *body;* (h), *head;* DLC, *dorsolateral prefrontal cortex;* EC, *entrohinal cortex;* FEF, *frontal eye fields;* GPi, *internal segment of globus pallidus;* HC, *hippocampal cortex;* ITG, *inferior temporal gyrus;* LOF, *lateral orbitofrontal cortex;* MC, *motor cortex;* MDpl, *medialis dorsails pars paralamellaris;* MDmc, *medialis dorsalis pars magnocellularis;* MDpc, *medialis dorsalis pars parvocellularis;* PPC, *posterior parietal cortex;* PUT, *putamen;* SC, *somatosensory cortex;* SMA, *supplementary motor area;* SNr, *substantia nigra pars reticulata;* STG, *superior temporal gyrus;* VAmc, *ventralis anterior pars magnocellularis;* Vapc, *ventralis anterior pars parvocellularis;* VLm, *ventralis lateralis pars medialis;* VLo, *ventralis lateralis pars oralis;* VP, *ventral pallidum;* VS, *ventral striatum;* cl-, *caudolateral;* cdm-, *caudal dorsomedial;* dl-, *dorsolateral;* l-, *lateral;* ldm-, *lateral dorsomedial;* m-, *medial;* mdm-, *medial dorsomedial;* pm, *postermedial;* rd-, *rostrodorsal;* rl-, *rostrolateral;* rm-, *rostromedial;* vm-, *ventromedial;* vl-, *ventrolateral. (Figure from G E Alexander, M R DeLong, P L Strick: Parallel organization of functionally segregated circuits linking basal ganglia and cortex. Ann Rev Neurosci 9: 357, 1986. Used with permission.)*

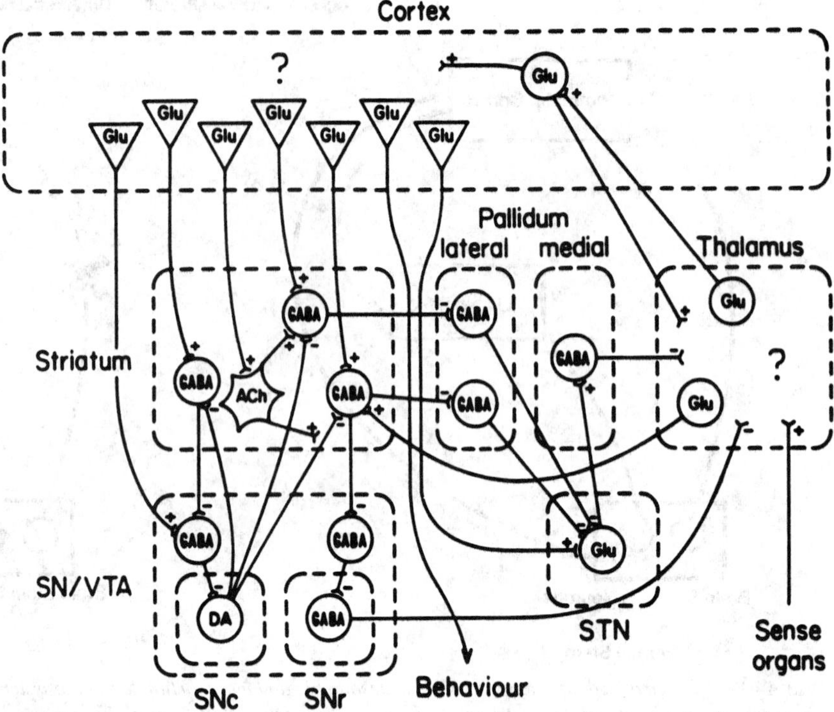

FIGURE 14.1-4 *A tentative scheme of interactions between glutamate and DA in the basal ganglia.* DA, *dopamine;* Glu, *glutamate;* SNc, *substantia nigra pars compacta;* SNr, *substantia nigra pars reticulata;* STN, *subthalamic nucleus;* VTA, *ventral tegmental area. (Figure from M Carlsson, A Carlsson: Interactions between glutamatergic and monoaminergic systems within the basal ganglia: Implications for schizophrenia and Parkinson's disease. Trends Neurosci* 13 *(7): 272, 1990. Used with permission.)*

that schizophrenia is related to impaired basal ganglia-thalamocortical circuit function secondary to decreased dopaminergic innervation of basal ganglia.

The neuroanatomical theories outlined above are descriptive; that is, they attempt to account for the possible anatomical basis for the disturbed behaviors observed in schizophrenia. It is important for the field to apply anatomical theory to optimize the interpretation of information derived from current brain imaging and postmortem studies. The examples provided above are overlapping and not always mutually exclusive. In general, structural and functional investigations of brain-behavior relations have pointed to the involvement of neural circuits comprised of certain limbic structures in psychosis and the involvement of neural circuits comprised of frontal and parietal cortical regions in deficit symptoms. The theories reviewed above differ in whether the two sets of dysfunctions are viewed as dependent or independent, and they also differ somewhat in the specific structures presumed to be involved and in how explicitly biochemistry is addressed.

MAJOR BIOCHEMICAL THEORIES Information is processed in neuronal networks by the transmission of an electrical signal from a nerve cell through its axon and across synapses to postsynaptic receptors on other nerve cell components. Nerve cells generally receive signals from and send signals to thousands of other cells. The transmission of the signal across the synapse requires a complex series of biochemical events. (The entire operation in the cell involves a number of steps requiring large amounts of energy and the synthesis and degradation of protein.) The physiological function in any brain system involves the chemistry of that system, and dysfunction can emanate from any of the biochemical processes. Thus, the biochemistry of the brain would be expected to play a fundamental role in the disruptions of brain function involved in schizophrenia.

The move from a general concept of the biochemistry of schizophrenia to specific theories is based on two principal sources of knowledge. The first is an ever-increasing understanding of the neurotransmitter systems involved in various brain circuits and of how those circuits are related to behavior. The second source is knowledge of the mechanisms of action of drugs that can induce schizophrenialike behaviors or alter symptom expression in patients with schizophrenia. Hypotheses regarding the biochemistry of schizophrenia have considered the actions of dopamine, norepinephrine, serotonin, acetylcholine, glutamate, and several neuromodulatory peptides. Those theories often invoke specific neurotransmitter functions related to dopamine receptors, the NMDA receptor complex, and the like. Because there are many possibilities, it is important to understand the general development of a biochemical theory of schizophrenia. The dopamine theory is the most prominent and enduring theory.

Dopamine and schizophrenia The dopamine hypothesis of schizophrenia arose from two sets of observations of drug action relating to the dopaminergic system. Drugs that increase activity in the dopaminergic system, such as amphetamine, levodopa (Larodopa, Dopar) and methylphenidate (Ritalin), sometimes induce a paranoid psychosis that is similar in some respects to schizophrenia. When administered to schizophrenic patients, those compounds sometimes induce a transitory worsening of symptoms, particularly in the areas of psychosis and thought disturbance. In contrast, drugs that block postsynaptic dopamine receptors reduce the symptoms of schizophrenia. There is an impressive correlation between a drug's potency in blocking those receptors and its degree of antipsychotic effect. Substantial evidence supports the role of postsynaptic dopamine blockade as an initiating factor in a cascade of events responsible for the mode of action of antipsychotic drugs. Other mechanisms, such as depolarization blockade, have been implicated as plausible explanations for long-term antipsychotic effects. That those actions are actually corrective for the pathophysiological disturbances in schizophrenia is suggested by the capacity of dopamine-stimulating drugs to worsen schizophrenic symptoms or to induce psychosis. In aggregate, the evidence for the role of dopamine, especially dopamine excess, in at least the cognitive and psychotic aspects of schizophrenia is compelling. However, clinical studies testing the dopamine hypothesis have proved problematic, as they have been characterized by marked variability in results, regardless of the indices of dopamine metabolism used.

The most decisive clinical testing of the dopamine hypothesis has been at the level of observed drug action and symptom manipulation. Studies aimed at measuring abnormal concentrations of dopamine or its metabolites in blood, urine, and cerebrospinal fluid (CSF) face problems that are almost insurmountable. Regardless of which substance is sampled, any alteration associated with schizophrenia will have only a minor effect on the dopamine measured. CSF necessarily provides a summation of total brain activity, most of which is not considered germane to schizophrenia, and blood and urine provide even more diluted measures. Nevertheless, positive correlations have been found between plasma homovanillic acid (HVA) measurements (a principal breakdown product of dopamine) and treatment response in patients with schizophrenia. HVA is elevated in plasma during acute psychotic exacerbations and decreases as symptoms improve during antipsychotic therapy.

Indirect evidence of dopamine involvement is potentially available from examining altered metabolic rates in dynamic imaging studies in systems where dopamine is an important neurotransmitter. Some of the data confirming metabolic alterations in limbic anatomy may be supportive, but it is not possible to determine the extent to which that reflects an alteration of dopamine biochemistry rather than an alteration of any one of a number of interacting neurotransmitter and neuromodulatory systems. PET demonstration of an increased quantity of dopamine receptors in the caudate nucleus in drug-free schizophrenic patients is also interesting support for the dopamine theory, but the finding has yet to be replicated.

Finally, relatively precise biochemical studies can be carried out on postmortem tissue, but sources of artifact and imprecision have been difficult to manage in those studies as well. The concentration of a neurotransmitter in any tissue is altered as cellular components break down after death and as small differences in dissection arise from brain to brain. The administration of antipsychotic drugs during life almost always confounds the biochemistry of postmortem tissue, and the investigator can rarely be sure of the extent to which any biochemical finding is secondary, rather than primary, to the schizophrenic disease process. In addition, there are a large number of candidate areas for brain dysfunction, so that the investigator may easily examine the wrong location. It is also possible that areas of biochemical dysfunction earlier in life are no longer abnormal in their functioning at the time of death, or that the biochemistry of death may obscure the biochemistry of life.

Although postmortem studies have not been definitive, some studies have reported differences between the brains of schizophrenic patients and control subjects. For example, an increased concentration of dopamine has been found in the left amygdala (a limbic system structure) in autopsied brains of schizophrenic patients. The finding has been replicated, and, because it is lateralized and specific to the amygdala, it is not likely to be an artifact. There has also been a report of an increase in dopamine postsynaptic receptors in postmortem tissue from schizophrenic patients whose medical records provided a diagnosis of schizophrenia but did not reveal antipsychotic drug use. Thus, several routes of investigation suggest that the increase in binding (receptor) number is not secondary to antipsychotic drug use.

The dopamine excess hypothesis remains a viable explanation for the psychosis, or positive symptoms, of schizophrenia. It is particularly robust for explaining the antipsychotic effect of antipsychotic drugs. However, recent studies have suggested that a dopamine deficiency may also occur in schizophrenic patients. For example, an inverse correlation between CSF HVA concentration and negative symptoms has been reported. Also, patients with influenza encephalitis who were mistaken for being schizophrenic tended to have emotional dullness and low drive. Similarities in those cases with aspects of Parkinson's disease (which is known to involve loss of dopamine neurons) and the fact that some of the postencephalitic patients developed Parkinson's disease lend support to a dopamine deficiency hypothesis for aspects of schizophrenia. In addition, antipsychotic drugs, which are dopamine-blocking agents, produce behaviors suggestive of the deficit symptoms of schizophrenia in animals and humans free of mental illness. A modification of the dopamine hypothesis that incorporates the possibility of concomitant dopamine excess and deficiency would restrict dopamine excess to the dopaminergic pathways projecting to the basal ganglia and the limbic system and dopamine deficiency to the mesocortical pathways. Hypofunction of the mesocortical neurons would account for the negative symptoms of schizophrenia.

Other neurotransmitter and neuromodulatory hypotheses Any neurotransmitter involved in neural systems subserving behaviors whose disruption could result in symptoms of schizophrenia are of interest in schizophrenia theory and research. Serotonergic deficiency in schizophrenia was proposed in the early 1950s. Lysergic acid diethylamide (LSD), which is chemically similar to serotonin and occupies serotonin receptor sites, was proposed as a model for psychosis and furthered the hyposerotonin hypothesis. However, drugs that diminish serotonin activity (for example, reserpine [Serpasil], ritanserin, and clozapine [Clozaril]), tend to reduce schizophrenic symptoms. Of greater current interest are hypotheses positing a serotonin excess as causative of schizophrenic psychopathology.

The rich innervation of the frontal cortex with serotonergic neurons, the modulatory effect of these neurons on dopaminergic neurons (serotonin 5-HT_{2a} receptor-mediated effects generally inhibit dopamine systems), and the hypothesized role of the frontal cortex in the production of negative (or deficit) symptoms make the serotonin excess theory attractive with regard to understanding the pathophysiology of deficit symptoms. The robust action of clozapine as a serotonin antagonist, coupled with its demonstrated effectiveness in chronically ill, treatment-resistant patients and its putative but not yet demonstrated effectiveness in reducing primary negative symptoms, has contributed to the current interest in the serotonin excess theory. As with the dopamine hypothesis, support for the hyperserotonin hypothesis is derived from reasoning from knowledge of brain-behavior relations, the anatomy of neural transmitter systems, and drug mechanisms of action. Support from clinical and postmortem studies is weak.

In general, pharmacological modification of serotonin systems has not produced impressive clinical benefits in schizophrenia. Drawing inferences from peripheral biochemistry is even more problematic with serotonin than with dopamine, and postmortem tissue studies are inconclusive.

Hypotheses implicating norepinephrine in the psychopathology of schizophrenia have been of interest in schizophrenia for some time. Anhedonia, or the impaired capacity for emotional gratification and the decreased ability to experience pleasure, has long been noted to be a prominent feature of schizophrenia.

A selective neuronal degeneration within the norepinephrine reward neural system could account for much of schizophrenic symptomatology. However, biochemical and pharmacological data bearing on that proposal are inconclusive. As with dopamine and serotonin, both noradrenergic excess and deficiency pathophysiological hypotheses have been proposed.

Neuromodulatory hypotheses focus on the fact that neuropeptides, such as substance P and neurotensin, are colocalized with the catecholamine and indolamine neurotransmitters and influence the action of those neurotransmitters. Alterations in neuromodulatory mechanisms could facilitate, inhibit, or otherwise alter the pattern of firing in those neuronal systems. Explorations of neuromodulator hypotheses are preliminary and inconclusive.

An interesting recent emphasis has been placed on the possible role of excitatory amino acids in schizophrenia because of their potential for neurotransmission and neurotoxicity. The general neuroinhibitory role, throughout the brain, of GABA and the intrinsic relation between that system and the catecholamine systems make plausible a role for excitatory amino acids in schizophrenia.

An emerging hypothesis of considerable heuristic value combines neuromodulation, dopaminergic interaction, and excitatory amino acid elements relating to the NMDA receptor complex. PCP is active in that complex, occupying receptors within open calcium ion (Ca^{2+}) channels to block ion flow. PCP can cause toxic effects that mimic both positive and negative symptoms of schizophrenia and can exacerbate symptoms in schizophrenic patients. In the NMDA receptor complex, PCP and PCP analogues interfere with glutamatergic transmission, while glycine is facilitory. Activation of dopamine receptors inhibiting glutamatergic neurons or decreased NMDA-mediated inhibition of dopamine neurons could be associated with a dopamine excess psychosis, a psychosis potentially reversed by glycine site activation in the NMDA receptor complex. It could also be the case that glutamate acts independently of dopamine in the GABA-mediated inhibition of thalamocortical pathways. Although there are some supportive data, the theory basically reflects the opening of a door in schizophrenia research made possible by advances in basic neuroscience and the implementation of new drug-animal models.

In fact, a major transition has occurred recently in the biochemistry of schizophrenia. Previously, observations of drug actions in schizophrenia first led to clinical treatment and then to the pathophysiological theory of schizophrenia. With increasing knowledge of the neural organization of the brain and of the various properties and receptor sites of neurotransmitter, it is now possible to postulate pathophysiological theory first and then attempt to derive new clinical treatment from theory. New treatment approaches may be developed more rapidly in the future, based on a broader range of pathophysiological theory and the availability of more precise animal models. Dopamine-blocking drugs will be joined by compounds with other modes of therapeutic action in the treatment of schizophrenia.

DIAGNOSIS

The history of the diagnosis of schizophrenia is often misunderstood, a circumstance that has led to erroneous conclusions about the validity of the diagnostic process. Throughout most of the 20th century, there has been substantial agreement among diagnosticians throughout the world and between seemingly divergent diagnostic approaches in the recognition of typical cases of schizophrenia. There has also been no difficulty in distinguishing schizophrenia from normality. Diagnostic systems in place when effective drug treatment was introduced in 1952 were capable of identifying suitable subjects for therapy, although useful refinements have evolved.

Areas of disagreement between diagnostic approaches were principally concerned with how broad the definition of schizophrenia should be, whether psychosis was required, and whether psychosis in the absence of known organic cause always signified schizophrenia. In general, the broader the definition, the greater the likelihood that more subtle cases would be included and the greater the likelihood that disagreement would arise regarding the diagnosis of such cases. Even here, there was little disagreement regarding the presence of psychopathology. Rather, disagreement, when present, focused on whether the psychopathology observed was part of schizophrenia. That difference in viewpoint did create problems, which became important as different classes of drugs were found to be effective for different classes of illness.

The success of the scientific search for more effective drugs for specific disease classes made it urgent to establish an agreed-on diagnostic approach to schizophrenia and the mood disorders in order to maximize appropriateness of treatment. The need for such agreement was also highlighted by the results of an influential study comparing diagnostic approaches in the United Kingdom with those in New York City, which demonstrated that United States diagnosticians employed a much broader and less defined construct of schizophrenia than their British counterparts.

For a time in North America, particularly in the northeastern United States, a broad definition of schizophrenia tended to include two categories of patients ill-suited for the pharmacological treatment that had become standard for schizophrenia. In the first category were patients with bipolar or unipolar disorders with psychotic features who, if erroneously considered to have schizophrenia, were administered antipsychotic medication rather than the more specific and effective treatments for patients with mood disorders (antidepressant drugs, lithium [Eskalith], and electroconvulsive therapy [ECT]). In the second category were patients with personality disorders, particularly the schizoid, schizotypal, and borderline types. Those patients were sometimes misdiagnosed as having schizophrenia and, as a consequence, were likely to be administered drug treatments designed for schizophrenia psychosis that provided little benefit and subjected them to substantial risk.

A considerable body of research during the 1960s and 1970s clarified many diagnostic issues and set the stage for the development of a diagnostic system implemented in the third edition of *Diagnostic and Statistical Manual of the Mental Disorders* (DSM-III). This approach, with specified diagnostic criteria and demonstrated reliability, is the accepted diagnostic system in North America and throughout the international research community. Adherence to that system has led to a reliable and consistent approach to the differential diagnosis of schizophrenia that has enhanced scientific and clinical communication and has substantially increased the likelihood of the effective use of diagnosis-specific treatments. DSM-III and the revised third edition of DSM-III (DSM-III-R) have had a major impact on scientific research and clinical thinking throughout the world, and an extensive integration between the American system and that employed in the *International Classification of Diseases and Related Health Problems* (ICD) has been achieved with publication of the fourth edition of DSM (DSM-IV) and the 10th revision of ICD (ICD-10).

BEYOND DIAGNOSIS A valid diagnostic system for schizophrenia has considerable utility for clinical and epidemiological purposes. It is now possible to accurately estimate the occurrence of the syndrome in populations, to identify persons suffering from the illness process, to guide treatment and rehabilitation considerations, and to differentiate other forms of illness similar in some manifestations but differing importantly in treatment requirements. However, diagnosis at the syndrome level has not been an adequate guide to the scientific study of the causes of and mechanisms underlying schizophrenia or to the development of treatments for all key features of the illness.

The traditional approach to reducing the heterogeneity of the schizophrenia syndrome has been to delineate subtypes and attempt to confirm or disprove their validity. The classic subtypes—hebephrenia, paranoid, catatonic, and simple schizophrenia—represent the most frequently used approach to reducing heterogeneity. Although important differences, such as age at onset and the pattern of symptom development, validate those subtypes, the classic subtypes have not provided a strong heuristic framework for the study of differential etiology, neuroanatomy, and pathophysiology. In light of the limitations of those subtypes, alternative approaches have been sought to reduce syndromal heterogeneity. One approach that has received considerable attention is the proposition that specific symptom complexes define pathological entities that differ from one another in neuroanatomical pathophysiology, in course and onset, in treatment requirements, and, possibly, in etiology and pathophysiology. Interest in the proposition that symptom complexes, or domains of psychopathology, represent semi-independent underlying disease processes emerged from the extensive study of the longitudinal patterns of symptom manifestation and impairment in patients with schizophrenia. For example, a number of studies have demonstrated that the extent of psychosis is only modestly associated with the extent of negative symptoms and that both negative and positive symptoms are only moderately related to cognitive impairments. It follows that the etiology and pathophysiology of specific symptom complexes, such as positive or psychotic symptoms (hallucinations, delusions, and the like), cognitive and attentional impairments, and negative or deficit symptoms, can be examined separately from other symptom complexes and that the presence or absence of those complexes can be used to define valid subcomponents of schizophrenia. Extensive study over the past 10 years, particularly with regard to negative symptoms, has supported that proposition. There is now preliminary evidence that the major symptom complexes differ from one another in their heritability, alterations in brain structure, treatment response characteristics, age at onset, course, and eventual outcome. Recognition of those differences will greatly strengthen research designs in the future. Study questions can now be aimed at hypotheses relating to specific domains of psychopathology rather than at the schizophrenia syndrome itself, thus avoiding false-negative findings or failures of replication that are caused by including patients in the study sample who do not actually have the disorder under investigation. Because the clinical syndrome of schizophrenia probably represents more than one pathological process, specifically addressing the etiology, pathophysiology, and treatment of specific symptom domains offers important new power to research designs.

COURSE, PROGNOSIS, AND OUTCOME

Extensive data on the long-term course of schizophrenia have been accrued following the introduction of antipsychotic drug treatment to supplement observations on the natural course of the disease made prior to the availability of effective therapy. Despite evidence to the contrary, there has been a long-standing tendency to presume the inevitability of a deteriorating course, with the outcome being exceptionally poor in most cases. In their pioneering descriptions, Kraepelin and Bleuler emphasized poor prognosis with devastating outcomes, but neither realized the extent to which his observations were skewed toward chronic, hospitalized populations. Although schizophrenia is always severe in its manifestations, the long-term course varies among patients, and is sometimes relatively benign. Although the disease does not always progress to a deteriorated end state, there are substantial and enduring adverse consequences for most patients.

The course of the illness of schizophrenia can be divided into three general epochs. The first epoch is onset. Onset is insidious in about half of patients, with the earliest signs of involvement occurring many years before the more blatant manifestations of psychosis appear. In other cases onset is relatively sudden or acute, with the onset of psychotic symptoms marking a sharp deviation in development. The insidious onset of schizophrenia tends to be characterized by increasing emotional withdrawal, diminishing social engagement and social drive, and idiosyncratic responses to ordinary events or circumstances. School performance, social interaction, and emotional responsivity gradually erode, well in advance of the onset of hallucinations, delusions, and disorganized thought processes. Patients with an insidious onset of illness are likely to have both a poor intermediate and a poor long-term course. In contrast, patients with normal development and ordinary personality attributes who experience the relatively sudden appearance of hallucinations, delusions, and disorganized thought vary widely in terms of intermediate and long-term outcome, some having good and others poor long-term outcomes.

The second epoch in the course of the illness includes those years immediately following the onset of psychotic symptoms. There are two typical patterns to that epoch. One is the continuous presence of the psychotic process, with a certain ebb and flow in the severity of signs and symptoms, but with the patient never achieving full recovery. The other is an episodic pattern of psychotic manifestations followed by complete or relatively complete recovery.

Recent studies have shown that the underlying deterioration associated with schizophrenia occurs principally during the first and second epochs of illness rather than over the remaining course. However, complications caused by the illness lead to ever-increasing impediments to normal existence, so that secondary effects may be progressive even though the primary pathology has reached a plateau. For example, patients hospitalized or sheltered in relative isolation for many years will lose social skills and work capabilities even if their symptom level improves. Effective treatment late in the course of a chronic disease will diminish illness, but it will not restore lost experience and opportunity—nor will it overcome stigma. A history of disabling schizophrenia is a serious social and occupational burden regardless of the degree of recovery.

The third epoch refers to the long-term course and outcome. Some surprising findings have emerged relevant to the third epoch. The intensity of psychosis tends to diminish with age, and many patients with long-term impairments regain some degree of social and occupational competence. Although the illness becomes less disruptive and easier to manage, the effects of years of dysfunction are rarely overcome. It would be highly unusual for a person with a chronic form of schizophrenia to gain the niche in society and the quality of personal life that would have been possible had the illness not been present. More typically, patients continue to manifest direct signs of the illness process throughout their life. Several 20- to 40-year follow-up studies of patients with schizophrenia provide a basis for estimates of about 55 percent with moderately good outcomes on global measures of symptoms and functioning, and 45 percent with severe outcomes on those measures. Those figures are more optimistic than earlier views, for at least two reasons. First, sample selection was broader and more representative, and second, effective treatments, which make a considerable difference in the short-term course and outcome of the illness, have also had a modest impact on the long-term course.

Although no present treatment approach can prevent or cure schizophrenia, some have had remarkable remedial effects on the course of illness. Although not subject to scientific verification, there is considerable evidence from a large body of clinical experience that a form of schizophrenia referred to as devastating schizophrenia, which represented about 15 percent of cases before the introduction of antipsychotic medication, now represents only about 5 percent of cases. That form of the illness begins suddenly and without prior insidious impairments, but, paradoxically, leads to an unrelenting deteriorating course. There is another line of evidence, also difficult to substantiate experimentally, which suggests that the earlier antipsychotic medication is administered in the initial course of illness, the more benign the course. Other, more verifiable evidence suggests that in patients who have an episodic course (one that is characterized by periodic relapses), the prophylactic use of antipsychotic medication reduces the relapse rate by one half. Finally, because treatment reduces symptoms in the majority of patients, it has been possible to substantially reduce inpatient care in favor of community-based treatment. The level of success associated with that major shift in the setting in which schizophrenia is treated and the serious shortcomings associated with shifting care to unprepared communities are noted in the discussion on treatment and rehabilitation.

There are interesting results from the World Health Organization studies on the social determinants of outcome in different cultures. Those studies have documented that the course of schizophrenia tends to be more benign in developing countries than in developed countries. That difference in course is generally understood as representing a psychosocial influence on course rather than cultural differences in the causes of schizophrenia. The incidence and lifetime prevalence of the disease appear to be relatively comparable across cultures and societies. One compelling construct is that the sociocentric structures of developing countries place less demand on individual performance and provide a more broadly supportive interpersonal environment than do the egocentric cultures of the more developed nations. The more developed nations, with their marked emphasis on individual accomplishment and productivity, are more demanding and stressful for those with impaired drive or impaired mental functioning. Rather than finding an appropriate, usually reduced level of functioning in society, the schizophrenic patient in Western industrialized societies tends to be isolated, with greatly reduced opportunities for work and meaningful social contacts. Indicative of the lack of involvement, unemployment rates for patients with schizophrenia are above 70 percent in the United States.

TREATMENT AND REHABILITATION

There is a large body of literature and scientific data on the treatment of schizophrenia and significant literature on rehabilitative efforts and the evaluation of their effects. For the present discussion, *treatment* refers to specific interventions aimed at reducing direct manifestations of illness. *Rehabilitation* refers to specific interventions and general support intended to minimize impairments that are secondary to the illness process. Drug therapy and psychotherapy are examples of treatment; social skills training, vocational training, and supervised living are examples of rehabilitation.

The history of the care and treatment of patients with schizophrenia is replete with instances of both humane and inhumane approaches. From a practical and moral standpoint, the value of humane care is intrinsic and does not rest on scientific evaluation of specific efficacy. Before 1952 there was no generally applicable treatment of demonstrated effectiveness. Reserpine had been used with some limited success, and ECT was important in reducing symptoms in the most acutely disturbed cases. It was not until the introduction of chlorpromazine (Thorazine) in France in 1952 and in North America in 1954 that the modern era of effective medical therapy for schizophrenia began.

The antipsychotic drugs used to treat schizophrenia have a wide variety of mechanisms of action, but all share the capacity to occupy postsynaptic dopamine receptors in the brain. The clinical effect of those compounds is to diminish symptom expression and reduce relapse rates. They are particularly effective with the psychotic aspects of the illness and are also effective in treating psychosis associated with illnesses other than schizophrenia. Pharmacologically, the drugs are related to each other and are sometimes referred to as neuroleptics, because of their neuronal effect, or more usually, as antipsychotics, because of their principal clinical effect. Although sedation may be a side effect and diminished anxiety a clinical effect, the value of antipsychotics lies not in their sedating or tranquilizing properties but in their remedial effect on the psychosis itself. The fact that such medications are effective in psychosis regardless of etiology means that they are best considered antipsychotic rather than antischizophrenic. Also, some aspects of schizophrenia, such as long-standing negative (deficit) symptoms, have not proved responsive to antipsychotic treatment.

Antipsychotic drugs are used throughout the world for four primary clinical purposes: (1) to manage acute symptomatic disturbances, (2) to induce remission from psychotic exacerbation, (3) to maintain the achieved clinical effect over prolonged periods of time (maintenance therapy), and (4) to prevent relapses or new episodes of symptom expression (prophylactic therapy). Recently, attempts have been made to reduce the dosage of antipsychotic drugs administered, in the hope of diminishing adverse side effects without losing clinical benefit. The intent is also to administer the drugs in a manner that increases patient compliance and avoids illness exacerbations due to patients discontinuing their medication. It is now recognized that optimal treatment involves the integration of antipsychotic drug treatment with psychosocial treatment approaches and rehabilitation techniques.

Clozapine, referred to as an atypical antipsychotic because of its unique mechanism of action, was shown during the 1970s to have a differential effect in patients resistant to the therapeutic effects of standard antipsychotic drugs. However, there is an approximately 1 to 2 percent risk of agranulocytosis associated with the use of clozapine. The potentially lethal cessation in the production of white blood cell elements was associated with a series of deaths in Finland during the mid-1970s and led to the decreased use of clozapine in Europe and failure to market the drug in the United States. Interest in clozapine in the United States was rekindled by the results of a recent large-scale multicenter study that yielded convincing evidence of clozapine's effectiveness in ameliorating psychotic symptoms in approximately one third of schizophrenic patients who had previously been nonresponsive to antipsychotics. Consistent with the worldwide experience in the 1980s, the study also showed that clozapine could be used with relative safety within the context of careful monitoring for agranulocytosis. The development of clozapine represents the first incremental gain in the effectiveness of the pharmacological agents used to treat schizophrenia since the original introduction of chlorpromazine.

The demonstration that clozapine can be effective in some patients in whom typical antipsychotics are not generated interest in the development of new treatments for schizophrenia. Clozapine is only the first of a new generation of novel antipsychotic agents whose development is based on increasing knowledge of the brain's neurotransmitter systems and biochemical functioning. New agents, such as risperidone (Risperdal), provide hope for antipsychotic efficacy in combination with reduced adverse effects. Simultaneously, the recognition that schizophrenia is comprised of discrete psychopathological processes has increased the interest of basic scientists in developing models that may prove useful for screening potential treatments for psychopathological processes other than psychoses. Developing new animal models useful for screening drugs for various antischizophrenic effects will combine with rapidly advancing knowledge of brain biochemistry to generate new drug treatments.

A number of pharmacological approaches other than antipsychotics have been used in the treatment of schizophrenia, but they have only been modestly successful. Aspects of clinical management are improved with the use of lithium, antiseizure and antianxiety drugs, and a series of medications that counteract the side effects of antipsychotics. However, none of these compounds has proved to be an effective alternative to antipsychotic therapy, nor are substantially enhanced benefits observed when they are used in combination with antipsychotics. Some small subgroup of patients may be differentially responsive to a class of drugs other than antipsychotics, but in the absence of the capacity to identify in advance which patients will respond favorably, it is difficult to prove or disprove this proposition.

ECT was frequently used in the treatment of patients with schizophrenia prior to the 1952 introduction of antipsychotic drugs. ECT is particularly effective in the treatment of catatonic stupor and excitement, but generally produces results similar to those obtained with antipsychotics, namely, a reduction in psychosis rather than a reversal of long-term functional impairments. Although ECT is now safe and painless, its use is restricted, in part by litigation and societal attitudes but also because any therapeutic advantage gained in an initial series of treatments is not easily maintained. Also, there is no indication that ECT is effective in antipsychotic-resistant patients. For a number of reasons, then, drug treatment approaches are generally preferred.

During the middle third of the 20th century, intensive psychotherapy was often advocated for the treatment of schizophrenia, but it was used only in a relatively small number of cases. Recent controlled clinical trials have demonstrated that intensive psychotherapy is less effective than drug treatment, however, and it is no longer considered as an alternative to the use of antipsychotic drugs. The major question now is whether psychotherapy is effective in patients receiving antipsychotic medication. The answer from studies published to date is in the affirmative, at least with regard to certain types of psychosocial approaches. From a scientific point of view, the question is one of determining the optimal integration of drug and psychosocial treatments rather than regarding their use as mutually exclusive.

Intensive exploratory psychotherapy, derived from psychoanalysis, has not proved to be superior to less expensive, less ambitious psychosocial forms of psychotherapy. Supportive psychotherapy and family therapy and education, which help patients and their families understand the illness, reduce stress, and enhance coping capabilities, have proved more successful for the treatment of schizophrenic patients. Empirical data from well-designed clinical studies have established that supportive forms of psychosocial treatment are entirely compatible with drug treatment and can increase the effectiveness of overall treatment, reduce the amount of medication necessary, and enhance patient participation in the full range of treatment.

Rehabilitation usually addresses long-term impairments in an effort to minimize the consequences of illness rather than to directly treat the illness itself. There is a wide range of models for which there is evidence of enhanced social and occupational outcome for patients with schizophrenia. Rehabilitation programs in schizophrenia are essential. However, it has proved difficult to establish the comprehensive continuity of care systems necessary to effectively integrate pharmacotherapy, psychosocial therapies, and rehabilitation.

OPPORTUNITIES FOR NEW KNOWLEDGE

It has been difficult to accumulate new knowledge on schizophrenia. A few years ago the number of investigators was too small, research funding was inadequate, the basic science foundation was too incomplete, animal and drug models were not compelling, and the technology for studying living human brain systems was inadequate for decisive progress. The situation has rapidly changed. Gene mapping, linkage, and other new genetic strategies provide an opportunity to move from the general pedigree, twin, and adoptive studies that affirm a genetic component to the actual identification of involved genes. Brain imaging techniques, including computerized electrical mapping, CT, and MRI; dynamic imaging with PET, magnetic resonance spectroscopy, and SPECT; and potential developments with magnetoencephalography permit direct study of the living human brain and the testing of theories previously untestable. Recent emphasis on postmortem work with enhanced methods for studying gene expression and for investigating the ultrastructure of neuronal components creates opportunities to gain new knowledge and to verify antemortem clinical studies with postmortem examination. The recognition of discrete symptom clusters in schizophrenia that represent distinguishable pathophysiological processes creates a new opportunity for decisive clinical studies and for developing animal models for heuristic purposes. Finally, newly differentiating clinical phenomena can be described at the level of information processing, providing more detailed knowledge of what is wrong in schizophrenia.

The study of schizophrenia is taking place within the context of an explosion of information from the basic neurosciences and behavioral sciences. The potential for gaining new knowledge of complex brain diseases is substantially greater now than it was a generation ago. Problems of the validity and reliability of case identification have been largely resolved and no longer pose an important barrier to research. Finally, recent attention to infrastructure considerations, particularly National Institute of Mental Health's *National Plan for Schizophrenia Research* and *The Decade of the Brain*, has rapidly increased the momentum of research activity devoted to the study of schizophrenia.

SUGGESTED CROSS-REFERENCES

More detailed discussions of etiology, brain structure and function, clinical features, and somatic and psychosocial treatments are presented in other sections of Chapter 14. A detailed introduction to areas of neuroscience and cognitive science relevant to schizophrenia is provided in Section 1.2 on functional neuroanatomy, Section 1.10 on principles of neuroimaging, Section 1.14 on basic molecular neurobiology, and Section 3.1 on perception and cognition.

REFERENCES

*Alexander G E, DeLong M R, Strick P L: Parallel organization of functionally segregated circuits linking basal ganglia and cortex. Annu Rev Neurosci *9:* 357, 1986.

Andreasen N C, Arndt S, Swayze V, Cizadio T, Flaum M, O'Leary D, Ehrhardt J C, Yuh W T C: Thalamic abnormalities in schizophrenia visualized through magnetic resonance image averaging. *Science: 266:* 294, 1994.

Barr C E, Mednick S A, Munk-Jorgensen P: Exposure to influenza epidemics during gestation and adult schizophrenia: A 40-year study. Arch Gen Psychiatry *47:* 869, 1990.

Bellack A S, Mueser K T: Psychosocial treatment for schizophrenia. Schizophr Bull *19:* 317, 1993.

Bleuler E: *Dementia Praecox or the Group of Schizophrenias.* J Zinken, translator. International Universities Press, New York, 1950.

Bogerts B: Recent advances in the neuropathology of schizophrenia. Schizophr Bull *19:* 431, 1993.

Braff D L, Saccuzzo D P, Geyer M A: Information processing dysfunctions in schizophrenia: Studies of visual backward masking, sensorimotor gating, and habituation. In *Handbook of Schizophrenia,* vol 5, S R Steinhauer, J H Gruzelier, J Zubin, editors, p 303. Elsevier, Amsterdam, 1991.

Buchanan R W, Carpenter W T: Domains of psychopathology: An approach to the reduction of heterogeneity in schizophrenia. J Nerv Ment Dis *182:* 193, 1994.

Carlsson M, Carlsson A: Interactions between glutamatergic and monoaminergic systems within the basal ganglia: Implications for schizophrenia and Parkinson's disease. Trends Neurosci *13:* 272, 1990.

*Carpenter W T, Buchanan R W: Domains of psychopathology relevant to the study of etiology and treatment of schizophrenia. In *Schizophrenia: Scientific Progress,* S C Schulz, C A Tamminga, editors, p 13. Oxford University Press, New York, 1989.

Carpenter W T, Buchanan R W: *Schizophrenia.* N Engl J Med *330:* 681, 1994.

Cornblatt B, Winters L, Erlenmeyer-Kimling L: Attentional markers of schizophrenia: Evidence from the New York high-risk study. In *Schizophrenia: Scientific Progress,* S C Schulz, C A Tamminga, editors, p 83. Oxford University Press, New York, 1989.

*Creese J, Burt D R, Snyder S N: Dopamine receptor binding predicts clinical and pharmacological potencies of antischizophrenic drugs. Science *192:* 481, 1976.

Dohrenwend B P, Dohrenwend B S, Gould M S, Link B, Neugebauer R, Wunsch-Hitzig R: *Mental Illness in the United States: Epidemiological Estimates.* Praeger, New York, 1980.

Greden J F, Tandon R, editors: *Negative Symptoms: Pathophysiology and Clinical Implications.* American Psychiatric Press, Washington, 1991.

Holzman P S, Kringlen E, Matthysse S: A single dominant gene can account for eye tracking dysfunctions and schizophrenia in offspring of discordant twins. Arch Gen Psychiatry *45:* 641, 1988.

Jaskiw G, Kleinman J E: Postmortem neurochemistry studies in schizophrenia. In *Schizophrenia: Scientific Progress,* S C Schulz, C A Tamminga, editors, p 264. Oxford University Press, New York, 1989.

Javitt D C, Zukin S R: Recent advances in the phencyclidine model of schizophrenia. Am J Psychiatry *148:* 1301, 1991.

Kane J, Honigfeld G, Singer J, Meltzer H: Clozapine for the treatment-resistant schizophrenic: A double-blind comparison with chlorpromazine. Arch Gen Psychiatry *45:* 789, 1988.

Kane J M, Marder S R: Psychopharmacologic treatment of schizophrenia. Schizophr Bull *19:* 287, 1993.

Kaufman C A, Ziegler R J: The viral hypothesis of schizophrenia. In *Receptors and Ligands in Psychiatry,* A K Sen, T Lee, editors, p 187. Cambridge University Press, Cambridge, MA, 1987.

Kendler K S, Diehl S R: The genetics of schizophrenia: A current, genetic-epidemiologic perspective. Schizophr Bull *19:* 261, 1993.

Kovelman J A, Scheibel A B: A neurohistological correlate of schizophrenia. Biol Psychiatry *19:* 1601, 1984.

*Kraepelin E: *Dementia Praecox and Paraphrenia.* R M Barclay, translator. Robert R. Krieger, Huntington, NY, 1971.

Liddle P F, Friston K J, Frith C D, Hirsch S R, Jones T, Frackowiak R S: Patterns of cerebral blood flow in schizophrenia. Br J Psychiatry *160:* 179, 1992.

Marder S R, Meibach R C: Risperidone in the treatment of schizophrenia. Am J Psychiatry *151:* 825, 1994.

McGlashan T H: A selective review of recent North American long-term followup studies of schizophrenia. Schizophr Bull *14:* 515, 1988.

McHugh P R, Slavney P R: *The Perspectives of Psychiatry.* Johns Hopkins University Press, Baltimore, 1983.

McNeal T F: Perinatal influences in the development of schizophrenia. In *Biological Perspectives of Schizophrenia,* H Helmchen, T A Henn, editors, p 125. Wiley, New York, 1987.

Nemeroff C B: Neuropeptides and schizophrenia: A clinical review. In *Advances in Neuropsychiatry and Psychopharmacology,* vol 1, C A Tamminga, S C Schulz, editors, p 77. Raven, New York, 1991.

Pickar D, Breier A, Hsiao J K, Doran A R, Doran M D, Wolkowitz O M: Cerebrospinal fluid and plasma monoamine metabolites and their relation to psychosis. Arch Gen Psychiatry *47:* 641, 1990.

Regier D A, Boyd J H, Burke J D, Rae D S, Myers J K, Kramer M, Robins L N, George L K, Karno M, Locke B Z: One month prevalence of mental disorders in the United States. Arch Gen Psychiatry *45:* 977, 1988.

Shapiro R M: Regional neuropathology in schizophrenia: Where are we? Where are we going? Schizophr Res *10:* 187, 1993.

Stevens J R: An anatomy of schizophrenia. Arch Gen Psychiatry *29:* 177, 1973.

Szasz T S: *The Myth of Mental Illnesses: Foundations of a Theory of Personal Conduct.* Hoeber-Harper, New York, 1961.

Tamminga C A, Thaker G K, Buchanan R W, Kirkpatrick B, Alphs L D, Chase T N, Carpenter W T: Limbic system abnormalities identified in schizophrenia using positron emission tomography with fluorodeoxyglucose and neocortical alterations with deficit syndrome. Arch Gen Psychiatry *49:* 522, 1992.

Torrey E F, Bowler A E, Taylor E H, Gottesman I I: *Schizophrenia and Manic Depressive Disorder: The Biological Roots of Mental Illness as Revealed by the Landmark Study of Identical Twins.* Basic Books, New York, 1994.

*Weinberger D R: Implications of normal brain development for the pathogenesis of schizophrenia. Arch Gen Psychiatry *44:* 660, 1987.

Wong D F, Wagner H N, Tune L E, Dannals R F, Pearlson G D, Links J M, Tamminga C A, Broussole E P, Ravert H T, Wilson A A: Positron emission tomography reveals elevated D_2 dopamine receptors in drug-naive schizophrenics. Science *234:* 1558, 1986.

Wyatt R J: Neuroleptics and the natural course of schizophrenia. Schizophr Bull *17:* 325, 1991.

Zigun J, Weinberger D R: In vivo studies of brain morphology in patients with schizophrenia. In *New Biological Vistas on Schizophrenia,* J P Lindenmayer, S R Kay, editors. Brunner/Mazel, New York, 1991.

14.2
SCHIZOPHRENIA: EPIDEMIOLOGY

MARVIN KARNO, M.D.
GRAYSON S. NORQUIST, M.D.

INTRODUCTION

In a discussion of the frequency and causes of dementia precox in his classic textbook of psychiatry, Emil Kraepelin noted, "Dementia praecox is without doubt one of the most frequent of all forms of insanity." He added the important observation that "As the patients neither quickly die off like the paralytics, nor become in considerable number again fit for discharge like the manic-depressive cases, they accumulate more and more in the institutions and thus impress on the whole life of the institution its peculiar stamp." He also bleakly noted that "The causes of dementia praecox are at the present time still wrapped in impenetrable darkness." Although science has begun to illuminate the complex etiology of the mental disorder known today as schizophrenia, its epidemiology was for decades the subject of greater study than that of any other mental disorder.

The epidemiological study of a mental disorder is critically dependent on the definition of "caseness" (that is, who among a population under study does or does not represent a case of that disorder). Epidemiological definitions of "caseness" rely closely on the rules or practices of clinical diagnosis, even though the procedures for such definition differ from those employed in clinical diagnosis. The clinical diagnosis of schizophrenia has been a veritable battleground of competing personalities and concepts throughout most of this century in Western medicine.

Kraepelin's formulation of the disease dementia precox was based on extensive and meticulous longitudinal clinical observations, with descriptions of many hundreds of patients. He emphasized the "loss of the inner unity of the activities of intellect, emotion and volition in themselves and among one another" produced by the disease. He also remarked on the customary onset of the disease in the second and third decades of life and its generally deteriorating course to apparent dementia. Although Kraepelin did acknowledge that cases might commence in early childhood or in middle and late years and that a small proportion of cases did not show a progressive course, Eugen Bleuler's term schizophrenia came into permanent use because it did not imply an invariantly early onset and deteriorating course and it did compactly describe the schism or fragmentation of mental functioning characteristic of the disease.

Bleuler conceived of schizophrenia as characterized by fundamental symptoms that directly expressed the destructive process of the disorder and accessory symptoms which, though common, are not invariably present and might be transient or never present. He considered the four "A's"—disturbances of association and affect and symptoms of autism and ambivalence—to be invariable and fundamental symptoms. Unless present to a marked degree, any one or combination might not, however, be expressed in behavior which today would be considered "psychotic." The definition of the term psychotic given in Appendix C (Glossary of Technical Terms) in the fourth edition of *Diagnostic and Statistical Manual of Mental Disorders* (DSM-IV) refers to narrow and broader definitions of the term. The narrowest definition "is restricted to delusions or prominent hallucinations, with the hallucinations occurring in the absence of insight into their pathological nature." Hallucinations and delusions were considered by Bleuler to be accessory symptoms. Thus, for Bleuler, a person suffering from schizophrenia need never be psychotic in the strictest sense. Bleuler postulated a category of "simple" schizophrenia, lacking accessory (psychotic) symptoms, which he considered to be far more common in the community than other types of the disorder, and rarely found in hospitals.

Although Kraepelin agreed that disturbances of association and affect were invariable and fundamental symptoms of dementia precox, he did not consider autism and ambivalence to be involved. Most importantly, although he recognized what Bleuler termed simple schizophrenia, Kraepelin was cautious about that category and expressed concern that it be delimited ". . . as a special clinical form." Not only did Bleuler not delimit simple schizophrenia, but in the words of Wyrsh, a student of Bleuler,

> Around 1920 and even during the subsequent decade, we in Switzerland had a rather wide concept of schizophrenia, much wider than Kraepelin in Germany, where I understand people mocked that Bleuler just shakes schizophrenia out of his sleeve.

That appears not to be an exaggeration. Bleuler expressed the unfortunately class-conscious and mysogynistic opinion that

> "On the lower levels of society, the simple schizophrenics vegetate as day laborers, peddlers, even as servants. They are also vagabonds and hoboes as are other types of schizophrenics of mild grade. On the higher levels of society, the most common type is the wife (in a very unhappy role we can say), who is unbearable, constantly scolding, nagging, always making demands but never recognizing duties."

This historical competition of a broad versus narrow concept of schizophrenia had important sequellae for epidemiological investigations until the 1980s. The diagnoses of pseudoneurotic, latent, mild, and incipient schizophrenia came to characterize the broad perspective, which profoundly influenced American psychiatric thought and practice. It found expression in the first edition of DSM (DSM-I, 1952) in the definition of "schizophrenic reactions," which were problematically ambiguous and heavily derivative from Bleuler's emphasis on fundamental symptoms. The second edition of DSM (DSM-II, 1968) included mention of those symptoms differentiating schizophrenia from paranoid and affective disorders, but otherwise provided little clarification.

In 1980 the American Psychiatric Association (APA) published the third edition of DSM (DSM-III) as an "official" diagnostic system, with rules for specifiable inclusions and exclusions of symptoms, their severity, and the temporal boundaries for diagnoses. Prior to 1980 the APA diagnosis of schizophrenia was strongly condemned in several quarters for its requirement of the presence of psychotic symptoms and its heavy reliance on the first-rank symptoms considered by Kurt Schneider to be pathognomonic of schizophrenia in the absence of primary organic disease. With the publication of DSM-III, the revised third edition (DSM-III-R), and now the fourth edition (DSM-IV), the official diagnosis of schizophrenia must include the occurrence of active psychotic symptoms at some time during the course of the illness. However, research does continue actively on extended genetic studies and on a broad array of information processing and psychophysiological assessments of persons who are believed to share in some degree of schizophrenic vulnerability (that is, they lie somewhere on a schizophrenic spectrum) but who are neither clinically nor epidemiologically diagnosable as suffering from schizophrenia.

In the following presentation of prevalence and incidence data are two important and delimiting decisions: (1) community rather than clinical populations are the focus, and (2) epidemiological data based on standardized instruments incorporating DSM-III, DSM-III-R, or DSM-IV criteria are used primarily. The former decision is based on the well-known fact that patients in clinical settings are rarely representative in frequency or characteristics of the total population at risk for a specific disease or disorder. The latter decision is based on the authors' wish to exclude from discussion the ongoing controversies concerning the true nature of schizophrenia. In psychiatry, diagnosis—and hence epidemiological caseness—must ultimately depend on consensus definitions grounded in empirical observations, in the same way in which medical science deals with complex disorders such as collagen diseases. Disagreements and alternative viewpoints may still remain forces that motivate further valid and important research, which may continue to refine prevailing concepts and diagnosis.

The World Health Organization (WHO)-sponsored Determinants of Outcome of Severe Mental Disorders (DOSMD) study (1978–1984) provides the most careful and comprehensive international multisite effort to date regarding the incidence (and natural history) of schizophrenia in geographically and culturally diverse community populations. The National Institute of Mental Health (NIMH)-sponsored Epidemiologic Catchment Area (ECA) study, which was carried out during the same time period, has resulted in the publication of detailed data concerning the prevalence of schizophrenia and other mental disorders in a large population of community household residents in the United States. The two studies employed different diagnostic instruments and diagnostic systems, and although each is acknowledged to have important limitations, they provide the best data to date concerning the prevalence and incidence of schizophrenia in the United States and worldwide.

The recently completed National Comorbidity Survey (NCS) of selected DSM-III-R defined disorders among a household population has not reported on prevalence rates for schizophrenia to date. Data are given for a summary category termed "nonaffective psychosis" (NAP), which includes delusional disorder, atypical psychosis, schizoaffective disorder, and schizophreniform disorder as well as schizophrenia. The preliminary results and the methodology of this study bear importantly on interpreting the earlier-obtained ECA prevalence data.

DIAGNOSIS AND CASE ASSESSMENT

Various diagnostic criteria for schizophrenia are in use throughout the world. All entail observing and interviewing patients or subjects and obtaining clinical histories from persons significant in their lives. No laboratory tests or biological markers are available to date for the diagnosis of schizophrenia, despite earlier promising theories such as levels of platelet monoamine oxidase, or recent research findings concerning smooth pursuit eye tracking, performances on attentional or information processing tasks, and neuroimaging indicators.

The WHO, in a series of three international epidemiological studies of schizophrenia commencing in the early 1970s, has relied on a diagnostic instrument of British origin, the Present State Examination (PSE). The PSE is a semistructured inventory of a wide range of psychiatric symptoms common in schizophrenia and other mental disorders. The PSE includes detailed questions on the positive symptoms of schizophrenia, particularly those symptoms emphasized by Schneider, and is recommended for use by doctoral level clinicians who have been carefully trained in its administration. The exact wording of probes to clarify the severity, presence, or absence of symptoms is left to the discretion of the interviewer. The responses to the PSE may be used to establish a clinical diagnosis according to the *International Statistical Classification of Diseases, and Related Health Problems,* or may be subjected to the CATEGO computer program analysis, which identifies cases with the clinical characteristics of schizophrenia. The PSE uses a time frame only for the month prior to the interview in its inventory of symptoms.

The ECA study utilized the Diagnostic Interview Schedule (DIS), which had been designed specifically for community use by carefully trained lay interviewers. The DIS is a totally structured, detailed inventory of symptoms that incorporates within computer algorithms specific DSM-III criteria in order to produce DSM-III equivalent diagnoses. The ECA results presented in this section are based on DSM-III criteria. The principal changes in schizophrenia criteria from DSM-III to DSM-III-R were the specification of one week for psychotic symptoms (less if successfully treated) and the omission of a maximum age of onset. The former modification would perhaps have decreased the ECA prevalence estimates by eliminating cases of very brief, reactive symptoms, and the latter change may have increased ECA prevalence figures by including a small number of very late onset cases.

The changes introduced in DSM-IV regarding the diagnosis of schizophrenia include (1) an active-phase required duration of one month instead of one week; (2) a simplified criterion A list, with the inclusion of the negative symptoms of alogia and avolition in addition to the prior specified affective flattening; (3) simplification of prodromal and residual phase criteria; and (4) changed course of illness descriptors to match those from the 10th revision of the *International Classification of Diseases and Related Health Problems* (ICD-10).

The one-month duration requirement for the active phase of the illness will undoubtedly eliminate an unknown number of false-positive cases from future prevalence and incidence studies. The other changes are unlikely to affect future estimates significantly. However, the inclusion of cultural considerations in the diagnostic discussions of schizophrenia and other mental disorders for the first time in DSM-IV may also tend to reduce culturally misinterpreted other false-positive cases, again tending to lower future prevalence and incidence estimates. Greater diagnostic rigor and stricter definitions may quite significantly lower community prevalence rate estimates.

DEFINITIONS

The term "prevalence" refers to the number of cases of a disorder present either at a particular point in time (point prevalence) or during a particular period of time (the week, month, or year prior to evaluation: period prevalence). Lifetime prevalence generally is determined only by retrospective recall of whether the disorder had ever occurred during the person's life. *Incidence* refers to the number of new cases of a disorder or illness that appear in a population during a specified period. The most frequently utilized incidence period is one year (annual incidence). *Crude incidence* refers to crude estimates of the occurrence of new cases of a disorder, based on admission rates to hospitals, clinics, or other clinical facilities. The crudeness derives from the potential sources of discrepancy between the number of cases that actually occur and the number that come to clinical attention during a given period.

CASE FINDING

COMMUNITY SURVEYS *Community surveys* entail face-to-face interviews of every accessible member of a community or of a selected sample of respondents from that community. The former approach has been feasible with small, insulated, clearly defined populations such as residents of an island, members of a cohesive religious sect, or inhabitants of a village or town. The results of such studies are of limited use in establishing generalizations. Studies of large populations require some form of stratified or random sampling in order to limit cost of data collection and volume of collected data. A total survey of a small, well-defined population presumably cannot be discredited for not being as representative of the group as might a sample from a large population. Total or large-sample surveys of large populations are rendered more economically feasible by a two-stage approach, in which the entire population or sample is first given a brief screening interview, after which only potential cases are pursued with a detailed interview. The relatively low lifetime prevalence of schizophrenia—traditionally estimated at less than one in 100 persons—demands that large populations be studied in order to find enough cases to generate statistically significant information about the many factors associated with the disorder.

CASE REGISTERS Case registers are the product of regular reporting of all cases of a disorder and all clinical contacts with those patients in a defined geographical area or community. The degree to which all cases of schizophrenia come to clinical attention and are faithfully reported to the central case register is unknowable; thus, the authority of a case register as a source of epidemiological data is limited.

KEY INFORMANTS The *key informant* approach, historically a staple of ethnographic investigations in cultural anthropology, identifies persons whose characteristics are of interest to the investigator. A key informant is a person who is known in the community for having intimate knowledge of that culture and wide social contacts. The key informant has been essential for locating persons with mental disorders in nonliterate societies or those in which mental disorders are not routinely defined according to Western medical parameters.

CLINICAL FACILITY REPORTS OR SEARCHES Clinical records provide a wealth of epidemiological data, but the cases reported or identified by search may (1) represent a significant undercount of the cases in the community served by the facility and (2) report cases that have uniquely skewed clinical or sociodemographic characteristics not representative of all persons who have the disorder in question. Psychiatric clinical samples typically are not representative of the age, sex, ethnicity, socioeconomic, religious, and demographic characteristics of the population at risk, and may overreport relatively severe cases. Given the large homeless population in the United States (estimates range from 300,000 to 3 million) and recent evidence for high rates among them of severe mental disorders and infrequent contacts with health care resources, case register or clinical facility reports would miss many cases of schizophrenia.

PREVALENCE OF SCHIZOPHRENIA

Prior to the ECA program, over 50 studies of the prevalence of schizophrenia worldwide conducted between 1931 and 1983 revealed point prevalences of 0.6 to 7.1 cases per 1,000 population and lifetime prevalence from 0.9 to 11.0 cases per 1,000 population. Lifetime prevalence data include some rates adjusted for what has been considered the period of susceptible risk (approximately ages 15 to 45). These studies used diverse methodologies and case criteria, and all but a few predated the introduction of structured diagnostic criteria. The extreme variation in these rates is more likely the result of methodological differences than of true differences in prevalence.

EPIDEMIOLOGIC CATCHMENT AREA PROGRAM The largest and most carefully controlled psychiatric epidemiological study yet undertaken in the United States is the NIMH-sponsored ECA Program, in which face-to-face interviews were conducted in households with 17,803 persons residing in New Haven, Connecticut; Baltimore, Maryland; St. Louis, Missouri; the North Carolina piedmont; and greater Los Angeles, California, from 1980 through 1984. All respondents were randomly selected from the designated catchment areas. Additionally, 1,379 persons residing in nursing homes, prisons and psychiatric hospitals were interviewed, an important innovation. Earlier community surveys that omitted institutionalized residents are likely to have missed substantial numbers of mentally ill persons. Although neither the catchment areas nor the five communities are representative of the entire population of the United States, the inclusion of large numbers of elderly, black, Hispanic, and rural respondents in this study, the geographical distribution of the sample, and the inclusion of institutional residents strongly suggest that the data obtained provide the best estimates available of rates of DSM-III-defined mental disorders in the United States.

The DIS was developed for the ECA study. The DIS inquires about the presence or absence of specific psychiatric symptoms, and responses are scored by computer algorithm to produce diagnoses for about 40 disorders defined in DSM-III, including subcategories. The interview was administered by trained lay interviewers and included specific probes to ascertain the severity of symptoms and whether the reported symptoms were not likely to result from mental disorder. Approximately 76 percent of those contacted and selected agreed to be interviewed.

The questions intended to assess the presence or absence of schizophrenia included a requirement for the verbatim recording of any positive symptom reported by the respondent. Information about the duration of symptoms allowed for the diagnosis of either schizophreniform disorder (if present less than six months) or schizophrenia.

As noted in Table 14.2-1 the one-year and lifetime prevalence rates for schizophrenic disorders among the combined five-site household population were 1.0 percent and 1.4 percent, respectively. The sharply higher rates for the institutional population indicate the importance of their inclusion in community studies.

DEMOGRAPHIC CORRELATES OF PREVALENCE RATES Although women were initially found to have higher rates of schizophrenia than men, their lower socioeconomic status (SES) and greater frequency of separation and divorce, factors independently correlated with higher prevalence for schizophrenia, were found to account for this differential. Similarly, the apparently higher rates for blacks indicated in Table 14.2-2, disappear when SES and marital status are controlled. The low rates for Hispanics, the great majority of whom were Mexican Americans residing in Los Angeles, cannot be so explained. An at least partial explanation may be the factor of selective immigration. The majority of Mexican-American respondents were first-generation immigrants, who had gener-

TABLE 14.2-1
Prevalence of Schizophrenic Disorders by Place of Residence

	% Prevalence (Standard Error)	
Resident Status (% of study)	**One-Year**	**Lifetime**
Household population(98.7)	1.0 (0.1)	1.4 (0.1)
Institutional population(1.3)	4.5 (0.6)	5.6 (0.1)
Mental hospitals(0.1)	16.7 (4.9)	20.4 (5.8)
Nursing homes(0.9)	3.0 (0.5)	3.8 (0.7)
Prisons(0.3)	5.4 (1.6)	6.7 (1.9)

Table from S J Keith, D A Regier, D S Rae: Schizophrenic disorders. In *Psychiatric Disorders in America,* L N Robins, D A Regier, editors, p 37. Free Press, New York, 1991. Used with permission.

TABLE 14.2-2
Prevalence of Schizophrenic Disorders by Ethnic Group

	% Prevalence (Standard Error)		
Ethnic Group	**One-Year**	**Lifetime**	**% Remission**
White and other	0.9 (0.1)	1.4 (0.1)	34
Black	1.6 (0.2)	2.1 (0.2)	25
Hispanic	0.4 (0.2)	0.8 (0.3)	46

Table from S J Keith, D A Regier, D S Rae: Schizophrenic disorders. In *Psychiatric Disorders in America,* L N Robins, D A Regier, editors, p 41. Free Press, New York, 1991. Used with permission.

ally lower rates of mental disorder at the Los Angeles ECA site than did Mexican Americans born in the United States or non-Hispanic whites. The stresses and coping demands of immigration may tend selectively to prevent those with mental disorder, particularly a disorder as disabling as schizophrenia, from successfully immigrating and residing in this country.

Marital status was found to be significantly related to the likelihood of schizophrenia. As indicated in Table 14.2-3, separated or divorced persons were three to four times more likely to be so diagnosed in the ECA study compared to those who were married at the time of interview. Prevalence rates were intermediate in persons who had never married. The cross-sectional nature of the ECA data prevents determination of the extent to which schizophrenic disorders tend to prevent marriage or to result from the severe stresses attendant on marital dissolution.

A similar cause-effect paradox that cannot be resolved in the ECA data is the strikingly marked inverse correlation between SES and prevalence rates for schizophrenia disorders. Those with DSM-III DIS diagnoses of schizophrenia were 10 times more likely to be in the lowest SES quintile than in the highest. That confirms a long-observed association that has fueled the continuing controversy of social selection (''downward drift'') versus causation by social stress to account for the association.

NATIONAL COMORBIDITY SURVEY A household survey interview study of over 8,000 respondents, aged 15 to 54 years, was carried out in 1990 to 1992 on a stratified, multistage area probability sample designed to represent major demographic variations in the United States. The NCS was congressionally mandated to assess the comorbidity of substance use and non-substance use mental disorders, and its design advances over the decade-earlier ECA study included the use of DSM-III-R criteria; the use of the Composite International Diagnostic Interview; which was derived from the earlier DIS; and (important in regard to schizophrenia and other nonaffective psychotic disorders) reinterviews by experienced clinicians using a version of the Structured Clinical Interview for DSM-III-R (SCID) of respondents who reported any psychotic symptoms. The SCID had earlier demonstrated its reliability in the diagnosis of schizophrenia.

The NCS reported a lifetime prevalence of 0.7 percent for the summary diagnostic category of NAP. Although the specific prevalence for schizophrenia, partialed out from the additional four other NAP psychotic diagnoses, is not yet available, it is reasonable to assume that it is no more than 0.6 percent. That would particularly be likely if the more restrictive DSM-IV criteria had been employed.

The discrepancy between the NCS and ECA prevalence estimates will be clarified by future research reports. At this time it is reasonable to conclude that the ECA study results did likely include a significant number of schizophrenia cases that would today be considered false-positive results. Those cases would have been eliminated by the use of careful clinician reinterviews and the more precise and restrictive criteria of DSM-III-R. There is still, however, no way of knowing how much of the discrepancy is due to such potential cases. For the present a range in the lifetime United States household prevalence rate of schizophrenia of 0.6 percent to 1.4 percent must be considered and weighed in the light of future findings.

TABLE 14.2-3
Prevalence of Schizophrenic Disorders by Marital Status

	Prevalence in % (Standard Error)		
Marital Status	**One-Year**	**Lifetime**	**Remission**
Married	0.6 (0.1)	1.0 (0.2)	45%
Single	1.5 (0.3)	2.1 (0.3)	27%
Widowed	0.6 (0.2)	0.7 (0.2)	22%
Separated or divorced	2.4 (0.4)	2.9 (0.5)	19%

Table from S J Keith, D A Regier, D S Rae: Schizophrenic disorders. In *Psychiatric Disorders in America,* L N Robins, D A Regier, editors, p 44. Free Press, New York, 1991. Used with permission.

INCIDENCE OF SCHIZOPHRENIA

Crude incidence estimates have usually been based on rates of initial psychiatric clinic or hospital contacts, and have suffered from major methodological limitations. A review of 13 such studies carried out before 1980 revealed crude annual incidence rates ranging from 0.11 to 0.70 per 1,000 population.

DETERMINANTS OF OUTCOME OF SEVERE MENTAL DISORDERS STUDY This WHO-sponsored study undertook the ambitious goal of identifying every new case of schizophrenia in 12 sites in 10 nations: Aarhus (Denmark), Agra and Chandigarh (India), Cali (Colombia), Dublin (Irelend), Honolulu and Rochester (United States), Ibadan (Nigeria), Moscow (the former Union of Soviet Socialist Republics), Nagasaki (Japan), Nottingham (United Kingdom), and Prague (Czech Republic). Those catchment areas, ranging in population from a little over 100,000 to almost 3 million, were subjected to a case-finding and screening process to identify every person from age 15 through 54 who presented to a helping agency with signs or symptoms suggestive of a psychotic illness, during a two-year period. Over 1,500 individuals passed screening criteria that led to a second-stage comprehensive evaluation, including a PSE administered by a trained research psychiatrist. All instruments in the non-English-speaking sites were translated into the local language and back-translated to provide culturally appropriate and equivalent meanings. The final study population in whom the onset of illness could be dated was 1,218. Extensive family, life event, medical, and social data were obtained concerning each subject.

Annual incidence rates for those cases with a restrictive core or nuclear schizophrenic symptom profile (characterized by Schneiderian, first-rank positive symptoms) were remarkably similar at about 10 cases per 10,000 population, across the eight sites considered to have carried out the most satisfactory case findings. The broader diagnostic categories, inclusive of a greater range of positive and negative symptoms, provided an annual incidence range of 1.5 per 10,000 in Aarhus to 4.2 in rural Chandigarh.

The DOSMD investigators have been impressed by the support their data provide to the belief that the more restricted syndrome of schizophrenia, characterized by the positive symptoms emphasized by Schneider and the DSM-III, DSM-III-R and DSM-IV, may occur at a similar rate in diverse cultures and nations around the world.

Given the complex and probably multiple etiological factors underlying even a core schizophrenia syndrome, this possibility of a similar worldwide incidence is certainly counter-intuitive. However, two other common syndromes of a neurobehavioral nature have also been noted to have a surprisingly similar worldwide incidence, namely, mental retardation and epilepsy—which are both known to have multiple causes.

Further research is needed to arrive with confidence at what are the basic incidence and prevalence rates for schizophrenia. For the present however, the data from the DOSMD and ECA studies (the latter carefully tempered by consideration of initial NCS results) appear to give the most reliable data.

RISK FACTORS

The term ''risk'' refers to the likelihood that a person who does not currently have schizophrenia will develop the disorder after exposure to certain factors (risk factors). Thus, a *risk factor* is an inherent or acquired characteristic or an external condition associated with an increased probability of developing schizophrenia. Epidemiological studies in schizophrenia seek to determine the most important risk factors for this disorder.

The concept of risk can be expressed in several ways. The most common is a report of the absolute number of new schizophrenia cases detected in a population exposed to a postulated risk factor. Relative risk (risk ratio) and risk difference (attributable risk)—expressions of the relationship of the incidence in those exposed to the risk factor to that of those not exposed—are also often used.

Significant risk factors are identified through the use of several different study designs. One type, cross-sectional studies, report descriptive data at a defined point in time, such as the increased presence of a particular risk factor in a population with a higher prevalence of schizophrenia. Case control studies compare schizophrenia patients with matched controls and determine whether those who express the disease were exposed to a given risk factor. The most informative (and expensive) study design is the prospective cohort study, which follows a group over time to determine whether those exposed to certain risk factors have a higher incidence of schizophrenia.

Risk factors are categorized in several different ways: demographic and concomitant factors (such as age, sex, race, social class), precipitating factors that operate immediately before the onset of schizophrenia (such as life events, migration), and predisposing factors that act for long periods of time or during an earlier part of life (such as genes, perinatal complications, infections). Another schema describes risk factors as either familial influences or sociodemographic factors. The latter can be further subdivided into mutable factors (such as social class, marital status, immigration) and immutable ones (such as ethnic group, sex, birthplace); mutable sociodemographic factors could be a result and not a cause of the disease.

Several cautions are necessary before one considers reports from studies of schizophrenic risk factors. First, a high prevalence of schizophrenia in a particular area may be the result of protracted illness rather than an increased incidence of schizophrenia (that is, prevalence is roughly equal to incidence × duration). Second, studies that report only the prevalence of schizophrenia may have failed to control other confounding factors that might increase prevalence. Third, designating something as a risk factor does not imply that everyone exposed to it is at personal risk to develop schizophrenia. It means that a group of people exposed to the risk factor at some time are likely to show a higher incidence of schizophrenia than a similar group who were not exposed. Risk does not imply causation but rather an association between that risk factor and the development of schizophrenia. Fourth, schizophrenia may be an etiologically heterogeneous disorder involving many risk factors and many protective factors.

Earlier studies of risk factors had many methodological problems, the most important being the failure to standardize diagnostic criteria for selection of schizophrenia cases. However, those studies have helped in the continued search to understand the complicated disorder.

GENETIC FACTORS Identification of a genetic influence is a major challenge in the understanding of schizophrenia. The search for a genetic risk factor has been examined through studies of twins, of families, and of children of schizophrenic parents who were adopted by others. Twins studies have shown a concordance of 33 to 78 percent among monozygotic twins, but of only 8 to 28 percent in dizygotic twins. Those results may be affected by selection bias if monozygotic twins are more likely to come to the attention of researchers than are dizygotic twins. Also, monozygotic twins may have greater environmental similarity. Family studies reveal that first-degree relatives of a schizophrenic person have approximately a fivefold to 10-fold greater chance of developing schizophrenia than nonrelatives. Children have about a 35 percent chance of schizophrenia if both parents have schizophrenia compared with about a one percent lifetime risk if neither parent has schizophrenia. Although the results from family studies are thought to indicate genetic influences, similar environmental factors among relatives cannot be discounted. Adoption studies are conducted in an effort to control environmental influences. Those studies show that the adopted-away offspring of persons with schizophrenia are at increased risk for schizophrenia and schizophrenia-spectrum disorders.

Although there are methodological problems with all three study approaches, the findings suggest some type of genetic influence in schizophrenia, the significance of which has yet to be delineated. Likewise, the mode of transmission has not been found. Recent efforts have focused on linkage analyses and attempts to locate specific genes. Genetic and environmental factors play a role in the development of schizophrenia, and further refinement in methodology should help to identify the environmental and genetic components of schizophrenia.

ETHNICITY AND RACIAL FACTORS Several studies have discovered differences in the prevalence and number of new cases of schizophrenia among various ethnic and racial groups. The findings are not consistent and may result from failure to control for confounding factors such as social class, age, sex, and immigration status. Data from the NIMH-ECA study confirm that if potential confounding factors such as education are controlled, the difference in prevalence across races disappears.

Previous studies of different geographic areas have found a higher prevalence and a larger number of new cases in different countries (for example, Ireland) and within countries (for example, the Istrian Peninsula of Yugoslavia). Most studies comparing geographical areas are usually flawed because they fail to validate diagnostic methods in different ethnic groups and localities. The recent WHO Outcome study reported that the incidence of schizophrenia is similar in various cultures, especially when a restricted definition is used. If true differences in incidence can be shown, perhaps differences in environmental characteristics, genetic characteristics, or both, can be found in these areas.

AGE Early studies showed mean ages of onset for schizophrenia well below 45 in men and women. However, recent data indicate that onset after age 45 is not as rare as was previously assumed. Data from the NIMH-ECA study reveal that failure to diagnose schizophrenia in the elderly may result because the disease has a different presentation in this age group. When compared with younger persons, most elderly people with delusions or hallucinations may not have the typical pattern of chronic progressive schizophrenia and are less likely to be significantly impaired or to be under the care of a mental health specialist.

SEX Studies that do not separate groups by age of onset show a male to female ratio of close to one, but this changes when various age cohorts are examined. Men are most likely to have the onset of symptoms between ages 15 and 25; women are at highest risk at ages 25 to 35. The reasons for this difference are not clear. The disease may manifest differently in the two sexes, or sociocultural factors may predispose men to earlier case findings.

As data from the recent WHO Outcome study show, when different cultures are examined, the findings (earlier date for first treatment and first hospitalizations for men) are the same. More asocial premorbid characteristics, birth complications, and cerebral structural changes (especially in the left or dominant hemisphere) have been reported in men than in women, and schizophrenia in men may have a more chronic and disabling course. The findings are not conclusive and are limited by methodological problems such as failure to control for sociocultural factors.

SEASON AND BIRTH ORDER Studies have shown that a disproportionate number of schizophrenic persons are born during winter months (seasonal excess of approximately 10 percent); that, together with a birth pattern in their nonschizophrenic siblings that is similar to that seen in the general population, suggest the presence of a seasonal factor. Proposed explanations for this seasonal effect include deleterious environmental factors in the winter (such as temperature, nutritional deficiencies, infectious agents); a genetic factor in those with a propensity for schizophrenia that protects against infection and other insults and thus increases the likelihood of survival; and more frequent conception in the spring and summer by the parents of schizophrenic persons.

Although no experimental testing has been conducted, studies appear to favor the harmful-effects hypothesis that schizophrenia involves infectious agents, but the other hypotheses have not been ruled out conclusively. Although some studies in the Southern Hemisphere confirm a higher birth rate for schizophrenic persons in winter than in other seasons, further study of that hypothesis is needed. There are a number of methodological problems with previous studies. If there are statistically significant increases of schizophrenic births during the Southern Hemisphere winter, environmental factors should be favored over sociocultural ones. Whether winter- and summer-born schizophrenic persons differ is not clear, but that would not necessarily be expected if the causative agent is active all year but more active in the colder months.

Early studies also reported a characteristic birth order pattern for schizophrenic persons, but the results have not been consistent and family size can affect the findings. For example, some have found schizophrenia to be unusually common in the youngest children of large families and in first-born sons of small families. Again, methodological problems limit the value of the studies.

BIRTH AND FETAL COMPLICATIONS When compared with controls, schizophrenic persons as a group experience a greater number of birth complications, especially male infants. Some studies have also reported a relationship between perinatal complications and early onset of disease, negative symptoms, and poorer prognosis. The crucial factor appears to be transient perinatal hypoxia, although not all infants so affected later develop a psychiatric disorder. There is, however, a general trend toward psychopathology in persons who have suffered obstetrical complications; such events appear to increase the vulnerability to development of schizophrenia and probably are not a specific cause. Some have proposed that complications at birth may be the result of preexisting fetal neurodevelopmental abnormalities or a vulnerability to such abnormalities. No prospective studies have been done, and retrospective case-control studies may be biased if informants interviewed about a schizophrenic relative try harder to remember birth complications than do informants reporting on healthy controls. Obstetrical records often refer only to severe complications.

SOCIAL CLASS Social class can be specified in various ways using some combination of income, occupation, education, and place of residence. In previous studies the prevalence and number of newly identified cases of schizophrenia have been reported to be higher among members of lower social classes than upper social classes. Two different explanations have been proposed. One explanation is that socioenvironmental factors found at lower socioeconomic levels are a cause of schizophrenia (social causation theory). Those factors include more life event stressors, increased exposure to environmental and occupational hazards and infectious agents, poorer prenatal care, and fewer support resources if stress does occur.

The other explanation is that lower socioeconomic status is a consequence of the disorder (social selection or drift theory). The insidious onset of inherited schizophrenia is believed to preclude elevating one's status or to cause a downward drift in status. Prospective studies have shown that persons with schizophrenia have less upward mobility from generation to generation than do the general population and that there is downward drift after the onset of symptoms. Many continue to argue this unsettled question, but a recent study strongly suggests that social drift processes are more important than social causation.

MARITAL STATUS Reports based on first hospital admissions have shown higher rates of schizophrenia for unmarried than for married patients, and some have inferred that single status contributes to the development of schizophrenia. However, the phenomenon may be similar to that described under social class; that is, the disease lessens the chance of marriage and increases the chance of divorce. Studies have not shown marriage to have a protective effect against schizophrenia and have not shown an excess of schizophrenia in widowed persons. Previous research using subjects hospitalized for the first time may have been flawed because unmarried and married men appear to have different hospital utilization patterns.

IMMIGRATION A higher risk for schizophrenia among recent immigrants than in native populations has been reported, but no study to date has confirmed that immigration stress leads to schizophrenia. Indeed, as indicated earlier, the ECA study found a low prevalence of schizophrenia among Mexican Americans studied in Los Angeles, most of whom were immigrants. The generally reported increased prevalence of schizophrenia among immigrants could result from selection (that is, schizophrenic persons may be more likely to leave their families); from the failure to control for such other factors as social class, age, and sex; or from the failure to compare immigrant patients to nonimmigrant controls from the same homeland. These methodological issues limit any conclusions that can be drawn from current reports.

URBANIZATION AND INDUSTRIALIZATION The prevalence of schizophrenia has been reported to be higher in urban environments than in rural areas. That is consistent with widely held beliefs that cities are places of rapid change and social disorganization, whereas rural areas are more socially stable and the inhabitants more integrated. However, data from the NIMH-ECA study show no difference in the prevalence of schizophrenia between urban and rural areas when such factors as race, sex, and age are controlled.

The assertion that the prevalence and incidence of schizophrenia have increased in the 20th century has been tested by comparing less developed cultures with those in industrialized nations, but such studies are fraught with methodological problems. For example, because infant mortality is lower in industrialized countries, those likely to develop schizophrenia may survive more frequently. Families are smaller and more insular, and ill members may be more obvious. The question of whether schizophrenia is more prevalent in modern times has also been studied by analyzing the reported number of new cases over time. However, it is difficult to control for probable diagnostic or recognition bias across centuries, especially for a disease that was first defined only in the late 1800s.

LIFE STRESSORS The association between stressful life events (such as loss of job, divorce) and the etiology and course of schizophrenia has been much studied. Schizophrenia or relapse of preexisting disorder often follows extraordinary stress, so it has been suggested that such stress might provoke acute schizophrenia in a healthy person. Others argue that stress plays only a marginal role in the pathogenesis of the disorder or simply triggers schizophrenia in vulnerable persons. The few studies that have considered the issue have suffered the usual methodological problems of retrospective case-control studies and have had difficulty in outlining predispositional factors in schizophrenia. The stressor might have triggered the onset of a disorder that would have occurred without the stressor. The issue is not settled and will require further studies, especially prospective reviews in which the role and severity of stressors in individual cases can be considered.

INFECTIONS Anatomical changes suggestive of viral infection of the central nervous system have been reported in some schizophrenia patients. A viral hypothesis is consistent with seasonal excesses and geographical differences. Viruses could also interact with a genetic predisposition, familial transmission, or both, in complex ways in the development of the disease. Recent studies have reported that exposure to viral infections during the second trimester may increase the risk for development of schizophrenia. As yet no study has conclusively shown an association between viral infection and the onset of schizophrenia. Further studies, especially those that can show evidence of viral transmission, are needed.

SUICIDE RISK Suicide is a leading cause of mortality in people suffering from schizophrenia. Estimates very, but as many as 10 percent of people with schizophrenia may die because of a suicide attempt. Although the risk for suicide is greater in people with schizophrenia than in the general population, some risk factors—such as being male, white, and socially isolated—are similar in both groups. Factors such as depressive illness, a history of suicide attempts, unemployment, and recent rejection also increase the risk for suicide in both populations. Previous studies have revealed other risk factors that are unique to this disorder. Among these are being young and male and having a chronic illness with numerous exacerbations. A history of postdischarge course involving high levels of psychopathology and functional impairment increases the risk for suicide. In addition, people who have a realistic awareness of the deteriorative effects of the illness and a nondelusional assessment of their future are at increased risk for suicide. Other factors such as fear of further mental deterioration, hopelessness, excessive treatment dependence, or loss of faith in treatment increase the risk of suicide in people with schizophrenia. The risk of mortality is especially high in the young, during the early postdischarge period, and early in the course of illness, although the risk persists across the patient's life span. Risk factors identified in previous studies may be helpful in assessing acute suicidal risk in a specific individual. Further research is needed to understand better what risk factors are most predictive of future suicide in the general schizophrenic population and various schizophrenic subpopulations, and what interventions are most helpful in preventing suicide.

CHILDHOOD SCHIZOPHRENIA As with adult-onset schizophrenia, different diagnostic criteria can affect the interpretation of results from studies of childhood-onset schizophrenia. Early definitions of childhood-onset schizophrenia tended to be broad and often included patients with autistic disorder. Recent diagnostic systems have departed from the earlier broad definitions by using the more restrictive criteria applied to adults that emphasize hallucinations and formal thought disorder. This restrictive definition, however, fails to consider developmental issues, such as the nature of delusions in childhood, and how a formal thought disorder can be diagnosed in a child under 8 years of age whose formal cognitive processes are not fully developed. Others have considered developmental stages in diagnosing childhood-onset schizophrenia, but no consensus has been reached. The accuracy of any reported epidemiological data on childhood-onset schizophrenia is compromised by differences in diagnostic criteria.

No large-scale population study has used rigorous, standardized criteria for diagnosis. Therefore, the prevalence of childhood-onset schizophrenia is not clear, but it is probably less than that of early infantile autism and is estimated to be less than that of adult-onset schizophrenia. There does not appear to be a greater incidence in boys than girls, as there is in infantile autism.

The risk factors in childhood-onset schizophrenia are not well known, and many investigators have simply extrapolated from adult findings. However, environmental stressors, perinatal complications, and central nervous system dysfunction have all been reported to occur more frequently in children who are diagnosed as schizophrenic.

FUTURE DIRECTIONS

Future epidemiological work in schizophrenia should use multisite, collaborative, long-term, and international study. The WHO studies provide some of the foundations for such proposed efforts. We recommend, however, that longitudinal prospective studies of persons at risk be carried out, from before or near birth, and extending through the ages of major risk (early adult years). Such studies, with appropriate controls, should incorporate opportunities for genetic mapping of families at risk; chromosomal studies; and current laboratory measures of potential psychophysiologic vulnerability such as continuous performance and sensory discrimination testing, eye tracking, neuroimaging, and other measures evolving with methodological advances. The expense of such studies would not be greater than that of comparable multisite, long-term studies of risk factors for cardiovascular and other diseases and would be small compared to the extraordinary direct and indirect costs of this most devastating of mental disorders.

SUGGESTED CROSS-REFERENCES

Some of the methods and concepts relevant to the content of this chapter are discussed in Section 5.1 on epidemiology and Section 5.3 on statistics and experimental design. The genetics of schizophrenia is discussed in detail in Section 14.5. More detailed discussions of other aspects of schizophrenia, including clinical diagnosis and treatment and basic research findings, are presented throughout the other sections of Chapter 14. Other nonmood psychotic disorders are reviewed in Sections 15.1 through 15.4. Postpsychotic depressive disorder of schizophrenia is discussed in Section 16.6. Clinically similar conditions resulting from substance use are discussed in Section 13.3 on amphetamine-related disorders, Section 13.7 on hallucinogen-related disorders, and 13.10, phencyclidine-related disorders. Childhood-onset schizophrenia is discussed in Chapter 45.

REFERENCES

Beiser M, Iacono W G: An update on the epidemiology of schizophrenia. Can J Psychiatry *35:* 657, 1990.

Bleuler E: *Dementia Praecox or the Group of Schizophrenias.* International Universities Press, New York, 1950.

Bojholm S, Stromgren E: Prevalence of schizophrenia on the island of Bornholm in 1935 and in 1983. Acta Psychiat Scand *79* (Suppl 348): 157, 1989.

Caldwell C B, Gottesman I I: Schizophrenics kill themselves too: A review of risk factors for suicide. Schizoph Bull *16:* 571, 1990.

Cannon T, Mednick S, Parnas J, Schulsinger S, Praestholm J, Vestergaard A: Developmental brain abnormalities in the offspring of schizophrenic mothers. Arch Gen Psychiatry *50:* 551, 1993.

Castle D J, Murray M: The epidemiology of late-onset schizophrenia. Schizophr Bull *19:* 691, 1993.

Cohen A: Prognosis for schizophrenia in the third world: A reevaluation of cross-cultural research. Cult Med Psychiatry *16:* 53, 1992.

Day R, Nielsen J A, Korten A, Ernberg G, Dube K C, Gebhart J, Jablensky A, Leon C, Marsella A, Olatawura M, Sartorius N, Stromgren E, Takahashi R, Wig N, Wynne L C: Stressful life events preceding the acute onset of schizophrenia: A cross-national study from the World Health Organization. Cult Med Psychiatry *11:* 123, 1987.

*Dohrenwend B P, Levov I, Shrout P E, Schwartz S, Noveh G, Link B G, Skodol A E, Stueve A: Socioeconomic status and psychiatric disorders: The causation—selection issue. Science *255:* 946, 1992.

Eaton W W: The epidemiology of schizophrenia. In *Handbook of Studies on Schizophrenia,* G D Burrows, T R Norman, G Rubinstein, editors, p 11. Elsevier, New York, 1986.

Edgerton R B, Cohen A: Culture and schizophrenia: The DOSMD challenge. Br J Psychiatry 164: *222,* 1994.

Haffner H: What is schizophrenia? Changing perspectives in epidemiology. Eur Arch Psychiatry Neurol Sci *238:* 63, 1988.

Harrison G, Mason P: Schizophrenia—falling incidence and better outcome? Br J Psychiatry 163: *535,* 1993.

*Jablensky A, Sartorius N, Ernberg G, Anker M, Korten A, Cooper J E, Day R, Bertelsen A: Schizophrenia: Manifestations incidence and course in different cultures. Psychol Med *20:* 38, 1992.

*Keith S J, Regier D A, Rae D S: Schizophrenic disorders. In *Psychiatric Disorders in America,* L N Robins, D A Regier, editors, p 33. Free Press, New York, 1991.

*Kendell R E, Adams W: Unexplained fluctuations in the risk for schizophrenia by month and year of birth. Br J Psychiatry *158:* 758, 1991.

Kendell R E, Kemp I W: Maternal influenza in the etiology of schizophrenia. Arch Gen Psychiatry *46:* 878, 1989.

Kendler K S, Diehl S R: The genetics of schizophrenia: A current, genetic-epidemiologic perspective. Schizophr Bull *19:* 261, 1993.

Kessler R C, McGonagle K A, Zhao S, Nelson C B, Hughes M, Eshleman S, Wittchen H U, Kendler K: Lifetime and 12-month prevalence of DSM-III-R psychiatric disorders in the United States. Results from the National Comorbidity Survey. Arch Gen Psychiatry *51:* 8, 1994.

Kraepelin E: *Dementia Praecox and Paraphrenia.* Livingstone, Edinburgh, 1919.

Kringlen E, Cramer G: Offspring of monozygotic twins discordant for schizophrenia. Arch Gen Psychiatry *46:* 873, 1989.

Leon C A: Clinical course and outcome of schizophrenia in Cali, Colombia: A 10-year follow-up study. J Nerv Ment Dis *177:* 593, 1989.

Lewis M S: Age incidence and schizophrenia: Part I. Beyond age incidence. Schizophr Bull *15:* 59, 1989.

Lewis M S: Age incidence and schizophrenia: Part II. The season of birth controversy. Schizophr Bull *15:* 75, 1989.

*McGue M, Gottesman I I: The genetic epidemiology of schizophrenia and the design of linkage studies. Eur Arch Psychiatry Neurol Sci *240:* 174, 1991.

Mednick S A, Mochon R A, Huttunen MO, Bonett D: Adult schizophrenia following prenatal exposure to an influenza epidemic. Arch Gen Psychiatry *45:* 189, 1989.

Muller H G, Kleider W: A hypothesis on the abnormal seasonality of schizophrenic births. Eur Arch Psychiatry Neurol Sci *239:* 331, 1990.

Murphy J M, Helzer J E: Epidemiology of schizophrenia in adulthood. In *Psychiatry, vol 5, Social, Epidemiologic and Legal Psychiatry,* G L Klerman, M M Weissman, P S Appelbaum, L H Roth, editors, p 181. Basic Books, New York, 1986.

Norman R M, Malla A K. Stressful life events and schizophrenia. Br J Psychiatry *162:* 161, 1993.

O'Callaghan E, Gibson T, Colohon H A, Walshe D, Backley P, Lorkin C, Waddington J L: Season of birth in schizophrenia. Br J Psychiatry *158:* 764, 1991.

O'Callaghan E, Sham P, Glover G, Murray R M: Schizophrenia after prenatal exposure to 1957 A2 influenza epidemic. Lancet *337:* 1248, 1991.

Regier D A, Myers J K, Kramer M, Robins L N, Blazer D G, Hough R L, Eaton W W, Locke B Z: The NIMH Epidemiologic Catchment Area Program. Arch Gen Psychiatry *41:* 934, 1984.

Sartorius N, Jablensky A, Korten A, Ernberg G, Anker M, Cooper J E, Day R: Early manifestations and first-contact incidence of schizophrenia in different cultures. Psychol Med *16:* 909, 1986.

Stevens J R, Wyatt R J: Similar incidence worldwide of schizophrenia: Case not proven (letter). Br J Psychiat *151:* 131, 1987.

Torrey E F, Bowler A E: Geographical distribution of insanity in America: Evidence for an urban factor. Schizophr Bull *16:* 591, 1990.

Torrey E F, Bowler A E, Rawlings R, Terrazas A: Seasonality of schizophrenia and stillbirths. Schizophr Bull *19:* 557, 1993.

Walker E F, Lewine R R J: Sampling biases in studies of gender and schizophrenia. Schizophr Bull *19:* 1, 1993.

Wing J K, Cooper J E, Sartorius N: *Measurement and Classification of Psychiatric Symptoms: An Instruction Manual for the Present State Examination and CATEGO Program.* Cambridge University Press, Cambridge, 1974.

World Health Organization: *Report on the International Pilot Study of Schizophrenia.* World Health Organization, Geneva, 1973.

14.3
SCHIZOPHRENIA: BRAIN STRUCTURE AND FUNCTION

KAREN FAITH BERMAN, M.D.
DAVID G. DANIEL, M.D.
DANIEL R. WEINBERGER, M.D.

INTRODUCTION

Whether schizophrenia is an organic disease with underlying physical brain pathology has been an important question for researchers and clinicians for as long as the illness has been studied. The search for a central nervous system (CNS) lesion has been greeted with varying enthusiasm over the past century. Attempts during the first half of the present century to find a site of pathological structure or function resulted in a large body of literature in which virtually every brain structure was implicated. However, many methodological problems attended those early studies and no consistent area of pathology was found.

During the 1950s and 1960s it became increasingly popular to emphasize psychological and social factors in conceptualizations of schizophrenia. The fact that, despite many years of postmortem examinations, no single underlying neuropathological or neurophysiological factor common to most patients with schizophrenia had yet been identified compounded the prevailing skepticism with which the concept of biological contributions to mental illness was viewed during that period. Schizophrenia was held to be functional rather than organic, and rigorous attempts to link the illness to the brain languished.

Over the past two decades several factors have resulted in a resurgence of interest in a neuropathological basis of schizophrenia and a renewed research effort to find it. One force behind the resurgence has been the emergence of medical treatments, especially pharmacological ones, that incontrovertibly ameliorate major psychotic symptoms. Another factor is the increasing availability of neuroimaging tools that have made it possible to study brain structure and function in great detail during life with little or no risk, discomfort, or inconvenience to the patient. No longer is the search for a neurobiological substrate of schizophrenia limited to indirect or peripheral measurements of trace substances in cerebrospinal fluid (CSF), urine, or serum—measurements that may or may not relate to brain physiology.

Concurrent with the advent of new tools for the direct examination of the brain have been advances in the understanding of human functional neuroanatomy, which, in turn, have resulted in a more enlightened and refined approach to postmortem investigations. At the same time the development and acceptance of reliable, explicit diagnostic criteria that allow greater consensual definition of psychiatric populations helped overcome a major methodological problem that plagued earlier research efforts.

Schizophrenia is increasingly believed to be based in organic conditions primarily affecting the CNS. Such features as peculiarities of gait and posture, disordered smooth-pursuit eye movements, minor (or soft) neurological signs, and subtle electroencephalographic (EEG) abnormalities all suggest a link between schizophrenia and CNS pathology. More compelling evidence is offered by neuropsychological, neuroradiological, and neurophysiological studies. Although no single pathognomonic neurostructural or neurophysiological abnormality has yet been delineated in schizophrenia, certain cerebral concomitants of the illness have been demonstrated in a consistent fashion. Increasingly, it appears that cerebral dysfunction of a system of interconnected cortical and subcortical brain regions may be present to a lesser or greater degree and may produce more or less psychopathology in individual patients.

POSTMORTEM STUDIES OF BRAIN STRUCTURE IN SCHIZOPHRENIA

NEUROPATHOLOGICAL ATTEMPTS TO LINK SCHIZOPHRENIA TO THE BRAIN Over the past century hundreds of studies have been devoted to a search in autopsy material from patients with schizophrenia for gross and microscopic CNS structural abnormalities. In several 19th-century neuropathological reports of anatomical pathology in the brains of hebephrenic and catatonic persons actually predate the conceptualization by Emil Kraepelin of dementia precox as a clinical entity. Although abnormalities of virtually every area of the CNS have been reported over the years, no consensus as to a pathognomonic brain lesion has been reached. The heterogeneity of findings has been interpreted in various ways: (1) that schizophrenia is a heterogeneous disorder with differing pathologies; (2) that methodological refinements are required before conclusions can be reached on the basis of postmortem studies; and (3) that there is no association between schizophrenia and brain pathology. With regard to the last interpretation an equally tenable stance is that, in the face of so many positive findings, the notion of brain structural abnormalities in schizophrenia cannot be ruled out.

THEORETICAL ISSUES

Diagnostic and clinical heterogeneity The classic approach to neuropathology has yielded a great deal of information about neurological disorders and about the normal function of various brain structures. Searching for the brain pathology underlying an illness relies on the assumption that the illness is a single entity with regard to the underlying pathology. Such a search in schizophrenia is complicated by the possibility that etiological heterogeneity underlies the ostensible clinical homogeneity seen in the disorder. Eugen Bleuler's concept of schizophrenia as a syndrome of etiologically distinct disorders has gained wide acceptance and has been interpreted by some to imply that schizophrenia cannot be traced to a single, finely circumscribed locus of brain abnormality. In the light of new data, however, including in vivo brain imaging studies of monozygotic twins discordant for schizophrenia (vide infra), the pendulum has begun to swing toward the case for neuropathological homogeneity in schizophrenia.

Changing notions of clinical and diagnostic subtypes of schizophrenia, inconsistent nomenclature, and lack of standardized or useful diagnostic criteria have complicated the search for such neuropathology. Those factors have rendered comparison of findings across the years and across studies difficult and have added to the variability of the results. The nosological confusion of the early part of the 20th century may in part explain the inconsistent findings and may have contributed to premature closure on the question of structural brain pathology in schizophrenia.

Relevance of understanding functional neuroanatomy The clinical relevance of structural neuropathological findings lies in their effect on brain function and behavior. At the turn of the century the brain areas targeted for neuropathological examination in schizophrenia were in the neocortex, a reasonable first choice based on Emil Kraepelin's notion of a profound deterioration of personality (be it called dementia precox or schizophrenia) and the fact that the neocortex was the primary site of pathology in the other dementias to which schizophrenia was likened at the time. However, targeting brain areas on the basis of clinical correlates depends on a knowledge of the precise function of the areas being studied. Until relatively recently little was known about the anatomical sites of higher cognitive and psychological functions. For example, the functions of and interrelationships between the largest and most complex areas of the neocortex, the frontal and temporal lobes, are only beginning to be elucidated. Also, knowledge of the limbic areas and diencephalon had been limited. New tools for examining the human brain directly during life have helped to refine current concepts of the roles of some of those brain regions in human behavior and have offered new impetus for their study in postmortem specimens of patients with schizophrenia.

METHODOLOGICAL ISSUES IN POSTMORTEM STUDIES

As compared with in vivo methods studies of postmortem tissue have the advantage of microscopic and even subcellular resolution, but methodological problems and artifacts may obscure subtle neuropathology and contribute to the inconsistency of the results. Consistent diagnosis, always a pivotal point in psychiatric research, assumes a role of particular importance in postmortem studies of the brain in schizophrenia. Diagnostic criteria and the rigor with which the criteria are applied have varied extensively since the concept of dementia precox was first put forth. Moreover, even with the relatively rigorous and standardized diagnostic criteria in use today, making diagnoses on the basis of chart review after death may be unreliable.

Because the pathology in schizophrenia is likely to be subtle, there are other critical methodological issues. Control specimens must be matched not only on the basis of age, sex, and other demographic variables, but also for methods of tissue processing, the interval between death and autopsy (postmortem interval), concurrent illnesses, and agonal events. The latter factors can produce brain structural changes that are not directly related to the illness itself; that is, postmortem interval and the processes of fixation, staining, and sectioning of brain tissues may produce tissue distortion and other artifacts. Agonal events, particularly hypoxia, infection, and trauma, may also cause structural alterations. The possible effects of pharmacological or other somatic treatments, such as electroconvulsive therapy (ECT) or, in early cases, insulin coma and leukotomy, must also be controlled for. Once appropriately matched patient and control samples have been collected, assessments must be done by a blind investigator (one who does not know which specimens come from which group of patients).

EARLY HISTOPATHOLOGICAL EXAMINATIONS OF THE BRAIN IN SCHIZOPHRENIA The first half of the century saw a period of vigorous research in which a plethora of abnormalities occurring in the brains of patients with schizophrenia (or dementia precox) were described, but from which few conclusions can be drawn. The important features of study design discussed in the foregoing were not appreciated by most early investigators in this field. The early studies, whose results were often confounded by small patient populations without proper controls, were rarely consistent with respect to diagnostic criteria, selection of patients and controls, choice of brain area to be studied, or methods of tissue preparation and processing. In view of those problems it is perhaps not surprising that virtually no histopathological findings from the period were rigorously replicated.

A number of studies focused on the cortex, then presumed to be the site of higher cognitive function and thus a likely candidate for pathology in schizophrenia. Although the studies were largely anecdotal in many instances they implicated frontal cortex and cortical layers II and III (that is, those projecting primarily intracortically). Also, a variety of histopathological changes were described in many other cortical regions and also in the thalamus, basal forebrain, globus pallidus, corpus striatum, and many other areas. They included alterations and loss of neurons; changes in oligodendroglia, astrocytes, and microglia; and vascular and perivascular changes. However, none of the abnormalities were noted consistently.

One explanation for both the diversity of the findings and their inconsistency was offered by investigators who presented topographical analyses of specific types of symptoms. Some believed that loss of cortical neurons and accompanying gliosis was the primary histopathology of dementia precox and that specific psychotic symptoms might be generated in specific cortical areas. For example, delusions, catatonia, and auditory hallucinations were postulated to be associated with frontal, parietal, and temporal lobe lesions respectively. The researchers noted that, given the clinical heterogeneity of the patient population, different patterns of histopathology would be expected, an idea that is again in vogue but does not wholly account for the confusing and inconsistent range of findings.

The efforts of the era culminated in the First International Congress of Neuropathology in 1952 in Rome, which was attended by many leading neuropathologists. The meeting was fraught with bitter disagreements and controversy regarding the lack of consensus about CNS pathology in schizophrenia. However, it did serve to highlight many of the methodological pitfalls that had been encountered; and it paved the way for a more cohesive approach to neuropathological studies of postmortem tissue.

RECENT POSTMORTEM STUDIES OF THE BRAIN IN SCHIZOPHRENIA Unlike the earlier investigations, which tended to search for a qualitatively pathognomonic lesion, more recent studies have aspired to more conservative goals, such as ascertaining whether any neuropathological process has occurred. Central to that goal has been a shift toward quantitative analysis, such as cell counting and neuronal morphometry. Special stains and advanced technology, including electron microscopy and computer-assisted image analysis, have been developed. New approaches to the analysis of postmortem tissue that are based on the rapidly advancing field of molecular biology are also emerging. In addition, there has been more consistency of focus on several brain areas suggested by various hypotheses and by the findings of in vivo brain imaging studies.

Basal ganglia The basal ganglia are a group of functionally and structurally interrelated subcortical gray-matter structures lying in the forebrain and midbrain. Typically, the caudate, claustrum, globus pallidus, putamen, subthalamic nucleus, and substantia nigra are included in the group. Their function is to integrate input from sensorimotor and association cortices. They are of interest in schizophrenia research because of (1) their dense aminergic innervation, especially dopaminergic; (2) the peculiarities of motor function in schizophrenic patients (that is, stereotypies, mannerisms, and bizarre movements); and (3) their role in modulating frontal lobe activity, which neuropsychological testing indicates is often disordered in schizophrenia.

STRUCTURAL STUDIES Results of traditional neuropathological searches for cell loss or reduction in volume of the basal ganglia have been inconsistent. The Cecile and Oskar Vogt collection of postmortem tissue is useful because it was collected before antipsychotic drug therapy became available. Studies utilizing the material have shown evidence of a reduced volume of segments of the globus pallidus and substantia nigra, but additional studies are required before firm conclusions can be drawn.

NEUROCHEMICAL STUDIES Dopaminergic activity has been of interest in postmortem schizophrenia research since the relative potencies of antipsychotics were demonstrated to correlate directly with their in vitro dopamine type 2 (D_2) receptor blocking activity. On that basis it was proposed that an increase in density (B_{max}) or increased affinity of D_2 receptors played a primary role in schizophrenic symptomatology. The increased density of D_2 receptors in the basal ganglia (caudate and putamen) and nucleus acumbens has become the most replicable postmortem neurochemical finding in schizophrenia research. However, interpretation of those findings is clouded by the antemortem use of antipsychotics because animal and human postmortem studies have demonstrated that long-term D_2 receptor blockade causes dopaminergic supersensitivity and proliferation of D_2 receptors. That raises the question of whether the increase in D_2 receptor density in schizophrenia is a primary characteristic of the disorder or is secondary to antipsychotic treatment. Examples of evidence supporting the notion that increased D_2 receptor activity in schizophrenia occurs independently of antipsychotic exposure include three studies of drug-naive patients with schizophrenia that found an increase in D_2 receptor density and evidence that the severity of positive symptoms correlates with the quantity of D_2 receptors. However, at least two studies involving drug-free periods did not find evidence of increased D_2 density. The differences in results may be secondary to variations in research methodology, but the question remains unresolved. In schizophrenia research dopamine type 1 (D_1) receptors have been much less thoroughly studied in the basal ganglia than have D_2 receptors. Two studies found normal density of D_1 receptors in the caudate and putamen, while a third found decreased densities. All three found a relative increase in the ratio of D_2 to D_1 receptors. As with the D_2 receptors the potential effects of antipsychotic medication are unresolved. Recent evidence suggests that a selective increase in density of the D_2-like dopamine type 4(D_4) receptor may occur in schizophrenia and may be associated with abnormal coupling of dopamine receptors. Further work in the area is necessary but data regarding the dopamine family of receptors now being cloned underscore the importance of molecular biological approaches to the research.

Postmortem investigations of neurochemical measures of dopamine activity (that is, concentrations of dopamine, its metabolites, and degradatory enzymes) in the basal ganglia have not produced consistent findings. Studies of serotonin activity in the basal ganglia have consistently reported increases in serotonin levels in the globus pallidus, but not in the caudate or putamen. The implications of the findings in the globus pallidus are unclear but could be related to serotonin's regulatory role in dopaminergic activity. There are no consistent reports of alterations in basal ganglia norepinephrine, γ-aminobutyric acid (GABA), glutamate, glycine, opiates, substance P, or cholecystokinin.

Limbic system The limbic system includes several anatomically and functionally interconnected structures, including the hippocampus, amygdala, nucleus acumbens, septum, hypothalamus, cingulate, anterior thalamus, and olfactory cortices and bulbs. The limbic system is of interest in schizophrenia research because of its role in the modulation of the emotional aspects of behavior.

STRUCTURAL STUDIES At least six independent groups of investigators have reported structural abnormalities, including reduced volume and cytoarchitectural abnormalities, in the hippocampal region in schizophrenic patients, making that the most consistently replicated postmortem finding in schizophrenia research. When viewed with existing confirmatory evidence from in vivo magnetic resonance imaging (MRI) studies (vide infra), pathology of the hippocampal region appears to be a robust research finding in schizophrenia. Investigations of the microscopic pathology underlying those macroscopic changes suggest cytoarchitectural disarray in the parahippocampal gyrus, which is consistent with a developmental abnormality. A report of disarray of the dendritic arborizations of hippocampal pyramidal cells has not been independently replicated.

The hypothalamus is of interest in part because it surrounds the anterior third ventricle, which in vivo imaging studies have consistently shown to be enlarged in schizophrenia. Although the possibility has been raised that the enlargement could be secondary to a loss of volume of the hypothalamus, there is no consistent evidence to support it. Unconfirmed findings include thinning of the periventricular hypothalamic gray matter and extensive gliosis in the periventricular hypothalamus, but those are likely to be epiphenomena that are not found in most patients. The nucleus acumbens is difficult to measure because of its relatively indistinct boundaries. There are no replicated findings despite a single report of volume reduction and decreased neuronal size.

NEUROCHEMICAL STUDIES There are no replicated findings of neurochemical abnormalities in the limbic system. The areas of the limbic system that have received the most scrutiny are the hypothalamus, amygdala, hippocampus, and nucleus acumbens. The most consistent (but still disputed) finding in the hypothalamus is of increased norepinephrine levels.

In the amygdala increases in dopamine and its principal dopamine metabolite, homovanillic acid (HVA), have been reported. An unreplicated report suggesting that cholecystokinin concentrations are reduced in the amygdala and hippocampus of patients with a preponderance of negative symptoms is of interest because cholecystokinin appears to be localized in dopaminergic neurons. There are also preliminary suggestions of dysfunction of the glutamate system and increased levels of *N*-methyl-D-aspartate (NMDA) in the amygdalohippocampal region.

The nucleus acumbens is of interest because of its putative role in interconnecting the limbic system with the basal ganglia and thalamus and because of its dense dopaminergic innervation. In the nucleus acumbens increased numbers of D_2 receptors have been a consistent finding. Three of four groups that investigated norepinephrine levels also found increases. There is a suggestion of a link between norepinephrine elevations and the chronic paranoid subtype. Again, the relation of those findings, if any, to antemortem antipsychotic exposure is unresolved. Studies of serotonin and other neurotransmitters, metabolites, and enzyme levels in the acumbens have not produced replicable positive findings.

The interconnectedness of the limbic system and cortex has received increased scrutiny. For example, recent data suggest that a neonatal lesion of the ventral hippocampus in rodents can produce differential changes in cortical and limbic dopaminergic activity. That model may prove useful in exploring theories about schizophrenia.

Cerebral cortex

STRUCTURAL STUDIES The executive functions of the cerebral cortex are usually impaired in schizophrenia. The search for structural abnormalities in the cortex of schizophrenic patients, however, has produced scattered and inconsistent findings, including the possibility of cortical gray matter thinning, reduced cell counts, and reductions in neuronal number and density in the prefrontal cortex. A series of findings in the frontal and cingulate cortex, including a reduction in pyramidal and interneuronal cell populations and increases in neuropil, have been reported, but they require independent confirmation. Also, a single study reported abnormal gyral patterns in the frontal lobe and axonal thickening in the cerebral cortex and adjacent subcortical white matter and thalamus. The MRI findings of reduced temporal lobe volume have yet to be confirmed in postmortem investigations.

Some have interpreted anatomical findings as suggesting that abnormalities in the pattern of neuronal migration during development in schizophrenia disrupt cortical connectivity and associative function. Support for that notion is offered by recent immunocytochemistry studies of postmortem specimens of schizophrenic patients in whom the distribution of nicotinamide-adenine dinucleotide phosphate-diaphorase staining cells in frontal and temporal cortex was found to be shifted from superficial to deep white matter. Those findings were thought to be consistent with a disturbance of the subplate, an early formed but transitory structure that plays a key role in cortical development and connection formation.

NEUROCHEMICAL STUDIES No clear patterns of receptor or neurotransmitter abnormalities have been delineated in the cortex of schizophrenic patients. Among the formidable methodological problems that have complicated interpretation of the existing studies are variance in the precise location of the anatomical areas sampled by different investigators and in the subtypes of receptors assayed. One of the most consistent neurochemical findings has been an increase in glutamate receptors in the frontal cortex. Glutamate, an excitatory transmitter, may have neurotoxic effects and has been implicated in other psychotic states related to Huntington's disease and phencyclide (PCP)-induced psychotic disorder.

Brainstem The brainstem is the primary source of catecholamine and indolamine input for the remainder of the brain, and the thalamus and cerebellum have critical information-processing functions in a number of cognitive and motor domains. Nevertheless, postmortem investigations of the brainstem in schizophrenia are relatively lacking.

There are single reports of increased D_2 receptors in the substantia nigra, increased ratios of dopamine to norepinephrine in the thalamus, increased norepinephrine in the pons, and decreased serotonin in the medulla and mesencephalon. The ventral tegmental area of the midbrain, which is of interest because it contains dopaminergic cell bodies that project to the cerebral cortex and limbic structures, has been reported to contain smaller cell bodies in schizophrenic patients. All of the reports are unreplicated and their significance is uncertain.

There are no independently replicated structural findings, although the ventral tegmental area of the midbrain, the source of dopamine afferents to the midbrain, has been reported to contain smaller cells in patients with schizophrenia than in controls. Gliosis has been reported in the pons and periaqueductal gray.

Several in vivo imaging studies suggest that atrophy of the vermis of the cerebellum is more common in patients with schizophrenia than in controls, which is consistent with the results of a postmortem morphometric study. Those findings must be viewed with caution considering the effects of numerous toxic factors on the cerebellum, including certain medications. Decreased numbers of small neurons and diminished volume have been reported in various parts of the thalamus. Reduced volume in the dorsomedial thalamus is of potential relevance to schizophrenia because of its functions in relaying information between the hypothalamus and nucleus acumbens and prefrontal cortex. All of the findings must be considered tentative.

IN VIVO STRUCTURAL BRAIN IMAGING STUDIES IN SCHIZOPHRENIA

In the decades since the initial demonstration of the anatomical contours of the living brain by pneumoencephalography (PEG), increasingly incisive structural imaging techniques have revolutionized clinical research and practice in psychiatry by providing noninvasive methods of directly observing the anatomy of the living brain. The value of in vivo brain imaging techniques lies in the potential for comparison of findings with concurrent clinical evaluations and correlation with other diagnostic tests, such as neurological examinations and neuropsychological testing. Longitudinal studies and examinations of persons at high risk for schizophrenia are also possible. Convincing evidence has emerged suggesting that the techniques are capable of associating disorders of behavior and cognition with quantifiable neurostructural pathology in schizophrenia.

Although the techniques remain primarily in the research domain, they may play a role in the psychiatric clinical workup. One investigator has suggested that among the indications for a psychiatrist to order an X-ray, computed tomography (CT) scan or (MRI) study are a first episode of a psychosis of unknown etiology, confusion or dementia of unknown cause, movement disorder of unknown etiology, prolonged catatonia, and a first episode of personality change or mood disorder after the age of 50.

METHODS The first radiological modality for imaging the living brain, PEG, involved the injection into the subarachnoid space of a volume of air, which migrated into the cerebral ventricular system, displacing CSF. That resulted in sufficient differences in X-ray attenuation to provide a rudimentary two-dimensional image on photographic film of the boundaries of the CSF-filled spaces by simple geometrical projection of X-rays onto roentgenographic film. As early as 1927 PEG reports suggested that patients with schizophrenia had enlarged CSF spaces. Numerous replications appeared over the next 40 years, but the finding tended to be overlooked or disregarded, largely because of uncertainties concerning potential methodological artifacts. Newer methods are noninvasive and produce vastly superior, virtually artifact-free image quality. In CT and MRI, respectively, a detector device is used to measure the energy passed through (CT) or given off (MRI) by the tissue and a mathematical model is used to reconstruct a three-dimensional representation of the tissue in the form of slices.

Computed tomography Scanning by CT became widely available for clinical use early in the 1970s. To image a slice of brain a collimated (thin-beamed) X-ray source rotates around the head and detectors are arrayed to measure nonabsorbed X-rays as they emerge on the other side. Creation of a graphic representation of the tissue depends on the fact that tissues of different densities differentially attenuate the X-rays. A computer determines the amount of X-ray attenuation from many directions simultaneously, and from that information reconstructs the density of the structures encountered by the X-rays as they pass through the head. A two-dimensional map of tissue density is created by the computer for each slice of tissue. The most common slice orientation used, transaxial, is located perpendicular to the rostral-caudal axis. Ionizing radiation exposure to the patient is typically 3 to 5 rads. Electron-dense iodinated contrast materials that do not cross the intact blood-brain barrier may be used for image enhancement, particularly when disruption of the blood-brain barrier or abnormal vascular structures are suspected.

Magnetic resonance imaging MRI became widely available as a clinical tool in the mid-1980s. It has a number of advantages over CT. It does not employ ionizing radiation and so is more suitable for studies of children and for longitudinal studies requiring multiple repeat scans. The only known contraindication to MRI is the presence in the patient's body of metal objects, such as cardiac pacemakers and aneurysm clips. Its spatial resolution and the clarity with which anatomical details are visualized are far superior to CT, and gray and white matter can be clearly differentiated. In addition to the transaxial planes to which CT is usually limited, MRI can be used to reconstruct sagittal or coronal sections, and it permits complete three-dimensional reconstruction. Relatively small structures of interest in schizophrenia, such as the hippocampus and thalamus, can be visualized in detail.

Based on the principles of nuclear magnetic resonance (NMR) long utilized in analytical chemistry, MRI exploits the fact that atoms with odd numbers of nucleons (protons and neutrons) exhibit net magnetization and act as small dipoles. In the natural state those dipoles are randomly distributed and produce no net magnetic direction. However, when placed in a strong magnetic field, the dipoles will tend to align with the lines of force of the field. Images are produced by exposing tissue to a strong magnetic field, which causes the atoms with unpaired nucleons (most commonly hydrogen 1, but to a lesser extent carbon 13, sodium 23, fluorine 17, and others) temporarily to become artificially aligned, pointing in the same direction. Typically magnets used for that purpose have a field strength of 0.1 to 2.0 teslas. Next, brief shortwave frequency electromagnetic energy in the form of radio waves is broadcast through the tissue, increasing the atoms' energy state and tilting them out of alignment. For each type of atom in a given magnetic field there is a specific radio frequency, called the Larmour frequency, at which that occurs. When the nuclei are allowed to return to their original relaxed state in the magnetic field, the previously absorbed excitation energy is emitted in the form of element-specific radio-wave signals that can be measured by a radio frequency receiver and computer processed into a spatial image. In MRI the word "resonance" refers to the excitation effect of the atom-specific Larmour frequency.

By producing anatomical detail approaching that achieved with postmortem tissue specimens MRI has gained recognition as the foremost tool for the investigation of soft-tissue anatomy in vivo. It can image physiological information as well as structural detail, an approach that holds great promise for the future.

STRUCTURAL FINDINGS IN SCHIZOPHRENIA In the pioneering studies in which PEG was used to search for neuropathology in schizophrenia, enlargement of the third and lateral cerebral ventricles and widening of the cortical sulci were observed and correlated with clinical phenomenology. Since then independently replicated observations about the brains of schizophrenic patients as compared to controls include enlargement of the cortical sulci and lateral and third ventricles, overall reduction in gray matter and whole brain volume, diminution in size of temporal lobe structures, thinning of the cerebellar folia, alterations in corpus callosum size and shape, changes in cerebral asymmetry, and altered brain density. It is important to emphasize that none of those structural markers can confirm a diagnosis of schizophrenia in an individual patient; none have been found exclusively in patients with schizophrenia or in every patient with the illness. The diagnosis of schizophrenia remains a clinical one to be rendered by the clinician on the basis of the current examination and past history.

Enlargement of the cerebral ventricles Enlargement of the lateral ventricles has become one of the most frequently replicated findings in the field of schizophrenia research, with approximately 75 percent of such studies demonstrating significant enlargement as compared to a control group. The percentage may actually rise to 90 percent when only studies that utilize relatively sensitive measures of ventricular size, rigorously diagnosed diagnostic groups, and normal controls are considered. The cerebral ventricles have received such extensive study because they are easily measured and their size is a sensitive indicator of cerebral pathology that may be either diffuse or localized to the adjacent structures (that is, limbic and diencephalic nuclei). Many of those structures have been implicated, at least in theory, in the pathophysiology of schizophrenia. Figures 14.3-1 and 14.3-2 contrast lateral ventricular size in the MRI scans of normal controls and of patients with schizophrenia. Enlargement of the ventricular system in schizophrenia is usually much more subtle than in noncommunicating hydrocephalus or dementia of the Alzheimer's type.

Studies utilizing the superior anatomical detail of MRI have confirmed earlier CT findings of lateral ventriculomegaly and provided the first in vivo volumetric analyses of relatively small anatomical structures, such as the hippocampus and corpus callosum, which were never before accessible in the living brain. In a recent study of the MRI scans of 15 sets of monozygotic twins who were discordant for schizophrenia, the twin with schizophrenia could be identified by visual inspection of the CSF spaces in 12 of 15 discordant pairs. Quantitative measurements using a computerized image-analysis system indicated that in the twins with schizophrenia as compared with their normal cotwins, the lateral ventricles were larger on the left in 14 and on the right in 13 of the 15 discordant pairs. Figure 14.3-2 illustrates that even when the size of the affected twin's ventricle appears normal, it may be enlarged relative to its genetic baseline.

As with the lateral ventricles, studies utilizing MRI to measure the third ventricle have confirmed earlier CT studies indicating increased size in schizophrenic patients. Like the lateral ventricles the third ventricles are of interest because enlargement may reflect damage to the structures surrounding them (hypothalamus, thalamus, and midline limbic nuclei and tracts). Enlargement of the third ventricles appears to be as consistent a finding in schizophrenia as is enlargement of the lateral ventricles, suggesting that the structural changes underlying enlarged ventricles may involve a variety of brain regions. The recent discordant monozygotic twin study noted that the third ventricle was larger in the schizophrenic twin in 13 of the 15 twin pairs. That study provided the most definitive evidence to date that subtle increases in both lateral and third ventricular size are a relatively ubiquitous finding in schizophrenia and are, at least in part, not genetic.

The clinical relevance of structural brain imaging findings has been tested in a number of studies that explored their impact on selected measures of brain function. In schizophrenia enlargement of the lateral ventricles has been correlated with (1) clinical observations, including increased frequency of deficit or negative symptoms, decreased frequency of positive symptoms, cognitive impairment, poor premorbid social adjustment, and poor prognosis; and (2) parameters related to cerebral dopamine activity, including diminished response to antipsychotics, increased extrapyramidal side effects of antipsychotic medication, and reduced CSF levels of HVA and dopamine β-hydroxylase. While such correlations have not been found in every study, they have been independently replicated in every case, indicating that the correlations, albeit subtle, are probably not spurious. Relations between third ventricular size and age, length of illness, and other clinical and neuropsychological variables have not been reproduced with consistency.

It was apparent from the earliest quantitative CT study that only a minority of schizophrenic patients have enlarged ventricular size as defined by the normal limits of variability; the

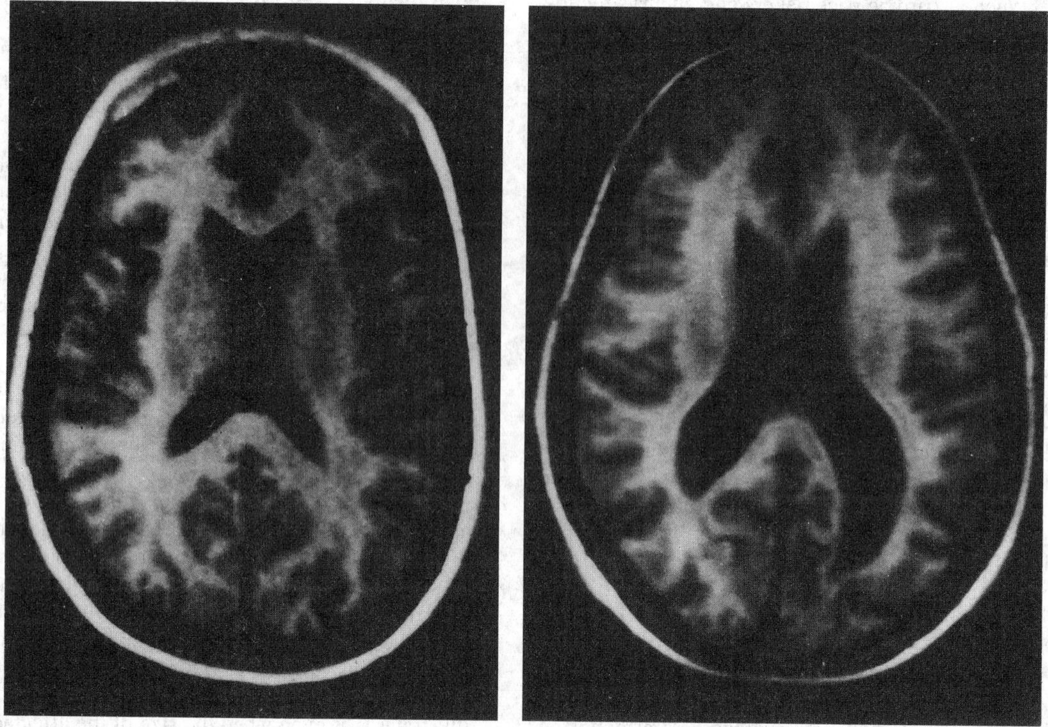

FIGURE 14.3-1 *Axial MRIs contrasting ventricular size in the MRI scan of a normal control (left) with that of a patient with schizophrenia (right). The scan on the right shows an unusual degree of lateral ventricular enlargement. The left hemisphere is pictured on the right side of the scan.*

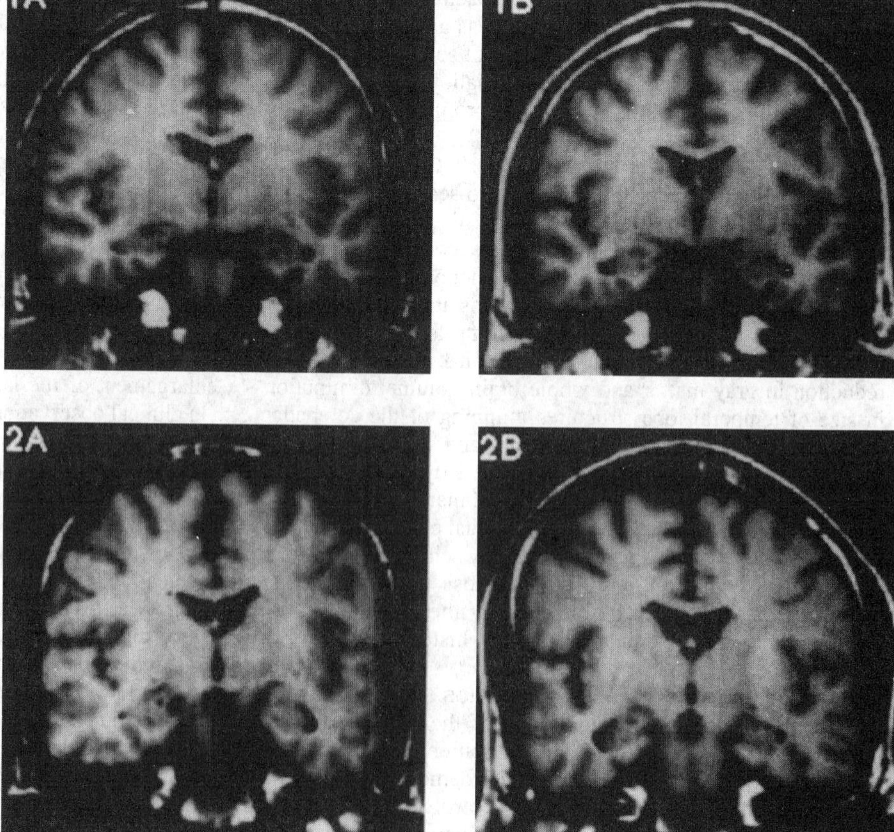

FIGURE 14.3-2 *Subtle differences in lateral ventricular size in the coronal MRI scan of the unaffected (1B and 2B at right) and affected (1A and 2A at left) members of two monozygotic twin pairs discordant for schizophrenia. Note that the ventricular size of the schizophrenic twin may appear normal or even small, but is larger than that of the unaffected twin.*

scans of most patients would not be read as qualitatively abnormal by most neuroradiologists. Depending on which quantitative cutoff point is used the prevalence of ventriculomegaly in a given schizophrenic population has varied from 6 to 62 percent. The interpretation of those findings is controversial and has been taken by some to imply that a pathological process affects the ventricles of only a minority of patients with schizophrenia and that ventriculomegaly defines a specific subtype of schizophrenia. Another view is that ventricular size exists on a continuum in which enlarged ventricles are associated with a more severe but qualitatively indistinct form of the disorder. Recent evidence suggests that with the use of adequately matched controls almost all patients with schizophrenia are seen to have at least a slight increase in ventricular size. That is best illustrated by the studies of monozygotic twin pairs discordant for schizophrenia in which even when the schizophrenic twin had normal or small ventricles, they were larger than those of the well twin. Statistical analyses of very large aggregated samples of schizophrenic patients do not support the notion of distinct populations based on ventricular size.

An important caveat that must be considered in interpreting the findings is that cerebral ventricular enlargement is a nonspecific phenomenon that has also been reported in several other neuropsychiatric disorders and so cannot be considered as diagnostic of schizophrenia. It is also a nonspecific finding that can reflect diminution of tissue anywhere in the brain.

The origin of ventricular enlargement in schizophrenia is unclear. It has been suggested that ventriculomegaly is a by-product of antipsychotic medication or the psychosocial stresses of repeated psychological decompensations and hospitalizations. That seems unlikely in view of (1) the PEG literature that found ventriculomegaly in schizophrenia prior to the introduction of antipsychotics, (2) the lack of a relation between ventricular size and either length of illness or amount of treatment, and (3) studies of first-break schizophrenic patients that found the changes to be present at the onset of the illness. Occasional reports have suggested that the imaging findings may exist even before the diagnosis is made. For example, enlargement of the lateral, third, and fourth ventricles was reported in a 10-year-old with recent onset of schizophrenia. Another case report described ventricular enlargement serendipitously observed in a CT scan of a patient 18 months before the emergence of a schizophreniform episode.

The preponderance of evidence appears to support the following conclusions about lateral ventricular enlargement in schizophrenia: (1) ventricular enlargement is present at the onset of schizophrenia and is a static, nonprogressing lesion; (2) its presence is weakly predictive of cognitive and psychosocial impairment; and (3) it is probably present to some degree in most patients with the illness.

Cerebrospinal fluid spaces on the cortical surface Expansion of the cortical fissures and sulci is of interest in schizophrenia because it may reflect diminution of volume of the cortical gyri. Numerous writers have observed widened, deepened, and more prominent sulci and fissures in schizophrenic patients relative to control subjects, especially the sylvian and interhemispheric fissures. Figure 14.3-3 illustrates sulcal dilation in a patient with schizophrenia. The results of several investigations addressing whether cortical sulcal dilation as viewed with CT can be localized have been mixed, some suggesting relatively prominent frontotemporal involvement and others suggesting more widespread changes. Despite the fact that surface markings have been shown to increase in prominence with aging in normal controls, in patients with schizophrenia no relation between cortical markings and age or length of illness has been documented. That is consistent with studies indicating that lateral ventricular enlargement is not progressive. However, it is puzzling that in contrast to findings of lateral ventricular enlargement in first-break schizophrenic patients, cortical sulcal dilation has not been generally observed in such studies. Interpretation of those studies is complicated by measurement-related methodological problems.

Reports of associations between schizophrenia and cortical changes in the CT literature have been supported by MRI volumetric measurements of the temporal lobes, but not as consistently of the frontal lobes. Although one study found no reduction in temporal lobe volume in schizophrenia, a subsequent

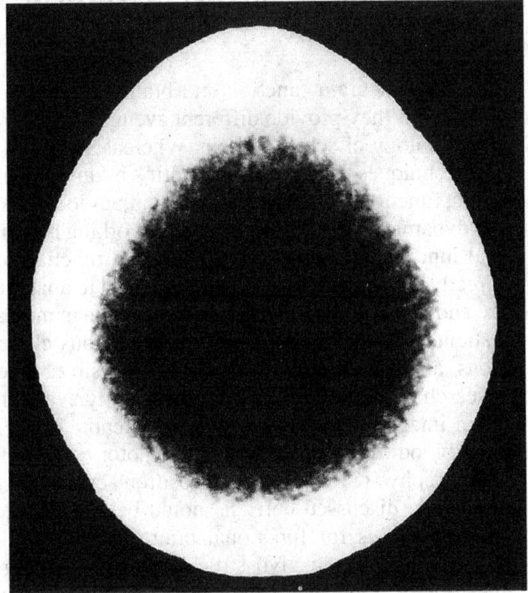

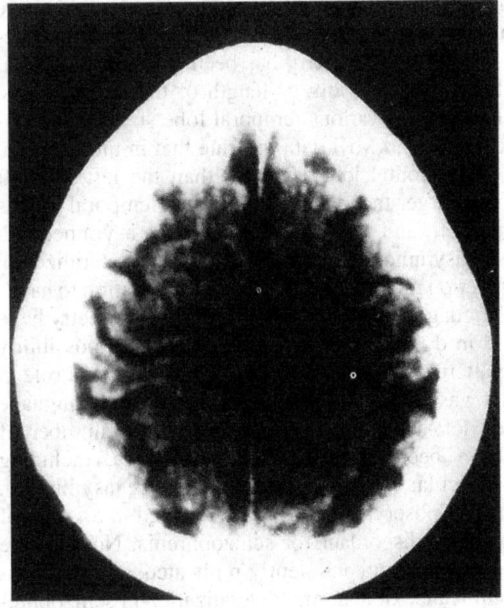

FIGURE 14.3-3 *CT scan illustrating increased sulcal size and decreased width of the gyri in the cortex of a patient with schizophrenia (right) compared with a normal control.*

study using a more sophisticated computerized image-analysis system found reduced temporal lobe gray matter bilaterally and reduced overall temporal lobe volume in the right hemisphere. Moreover, the finding in that study of a negative correlation between the amount of temporal lobe gray matter and the magnitude of lateral ventricular enlargement suggests that the ventriculomegaly is an ex-vacuo phenomenom secondary to temporal lobe volume loss. Two independent investigators recently found enlargement in the temporal horns of the lateral ventricles, further supporting the notion of temporal lobe volumetric reductions in schizophrenia. The superior spatial resolution of MRI in conjunction with sophisticated computerized measurement techniques permits analysis of small temporal lobe structures in order to further localize the pathology. In the *aforementioned* twin studies quantitative analysis of sections through the level of the pes hippocampus showed the hippocampus to be smaller on the left in 14 of 15 and smaller on the right in 13 of 15 affected twins as compared with the well twins. That is consistent with earlier in vivo and postmortem reports of limbic system pathology in patients with schizophrenia. A recent study of the posterior hippocampus in first-episode schizophrenics suggested that the changes are not secondary to medication, chronic hospitalization, or other secondary aspects of the illness.

In contrast to the relatively consistent temporal lobe findings, MRI studies have less clearly implicated changes in the frontal lobe, and notions about focal changes have been challenged. A recent CSF volume study and a gray matter volumetric study have again suggested that the volume increases and decreases, respectively, are widespread. Recent postmortem, CT, and MRI evidence suggests that the volumetric deficits found in the cortex of schizophrenic patients are primarily of gray rather than white matter. Neurodevelopmental models of schizophrenia propose that subtle abnormalities during fetal maldevelopment result in abnormal development of limbic-prefrontal cortex pathways that become manifest clinically as dysfunctional cognitive processing.

Variations in patterns of anatomical asymmetry Dating perhaps to the discovery that human language has a distinct, consistent anatomical substrate with primacy in the left hemisphere, studies of lateralization of brain function and structure have been an important focal point in the field of human functional neuroanatomy. Asymmetry has been quantified by measuring the differences in width or length of the frontal lobes, the occipital lobes, and various temporal lobe structures. Neuropathological, CT, and MRI data indicate that in most normal persons the right frontal lobe is larger than the left, the left occipital lobe is larger than the right, the right temporal lobe is larger than the left, and the sylvian fissures are asymmetrical. Morphological asymmetry has been linked to the lateralization of cerebral function most intensively studied in relation to handedness and language, and reversed patterns of asymmetry have been reported in dyslexia and autisic disorder. The possibility that altered patterns of cerebral asymmetry might play a role in schizophrenia was raised by observations of impaired language and increased left-handedness in the disorder. A number of alterations have been reported in schizophrenia, including abnormal ventricular, lobar, and sylvian fissure asymmetry. However, the last observation was not replicated in a group of monozygotic twins discordant for schizophrenia. None of the other findings have been consistently replicated, and the existence and significance of abnormal lateralization in schizophrenia remain to be established.

Cerebellar pathology The cerebellum is of interest in schizophrenia research because of its anatomical connections to limbic-diencephalic areas thought to be involved in emotion and psychosis and because of occasional reports of psychotic states developing in patients with cerebellar pathology. Measurement techniques vary from subjective visual comparison to computerized methods of measuring the area of the fourth ventricle, cisterna magna, and cerebellar vermis.

A number of studies using CT and more recently MRI have reported evidence of cerebellar atrophy in schizophrenia. The reported prevalence of such cerebellar atrophic changes has ranged from 0 to 50 percent, with most studies clustering in the range of 5 to 17 percent. In contrast, the prevalence of cerebellar atrophic changes in normal controls with no neurological history is reported to be from 1 to 2.5 percent. Like ventriculomegaly, cerebellar atrophy is not specific to schizophrenia and has been reported in a number of disorders that affect brain function, including alcohol-use disorders, mood disorders, degenerative dementias, autistic disorder, hypothyroidism, and use of phenytoin. Thus the choice of control group (that is, medical controls) may heavily influence whether a comparison with schizophrenic patients has a positive outcome. The finding of cerebellar atrophy in schizophrenia has been confirmed by at least one postmortem study. However, in the only study to examine the cerebellum at the onset of schizophrenic illness, no abnormalities were detected. It could be speculated, therefore, that considering the known sensitivity of the cerebellum to toxic influences, the changes seen in more chronic patients are caused by medication or other secondary factors. Further work is necessary in the area.

Alterations in tissue density Measurement of tissue density has been purported to be an indirect way of assessing the health of both white and gray matter structures in the brain. The method depends on pixel-by-pixel quantification of CT attenuation values, which reflect the extent of tissue absorption of X-rays. Studies of patients with schizophrenia have produced such disparate results that the only conclusion that can be drawn is that the method requires additional refinement to be credible.

PHYSIOLOGICAL BRAIN FUNCTION IN SCHIZOPHRENIA

The roles of brain function and brain structure are intimately linked, but they provide different avenues to understanding the neurobiology of schizophrenia. Whereas structural brain imaging techniques localize and quantify brain anatomy, which is static, functional brain imaging techniques localize and quantify the dynamic properties of the living, working human brain. Several innovative approaches allow brain function to be studied directly during life and offer the potential to anatomically localize and physiologically to characterize human mental processes. Patients also can be assessed during various clinical interventions and longitudinal studies are possible. The results of research carried out with several currently available functional brain imaging techniques, including xenon 133 regional cerebral blood flow (rCBF), single photon emission computed tomography (SPECT), and positron emission tomography (PET) are discussed here. It should be emphasized that all of the procedures for functional brain imaging remain research tools; unlike the in vivo structural brain imaging procedures they do not, at present, have a place in a routine clinical workup in psychiatry. The results of all functional brain imaging studies must be interpreted in light of the conditions under which they were carried out, the mental and cognitive state of the subjects, limitations of the instrumentation, and sampling biases in the experimental population.

TECHNICAL ISSUES IN FUNCTIONAL BRAIN IMAGING

Measurable parameters of brain function There is no single parameter that completely or even best describes the functional status of the brain. Any measurement of brain activity subsumes a complex set of physiological and biochemical phenomena subserving diverse neuronal activities, such as cellular homeostasis, neuronal excitation and inhibition, maintenance of membrane potentials, and even plastic change at the cellular or subcellular level. The choice of which parameter to measure in a given study of schizophrenia must be largely guided by the particular research question to be asked. The most common parameters of general neuronal function are rCBF and the local cerebral metabolic rate of glucose. An exciting and relatively newer approach is to measure the functional activity of components of various specific neurochemical systems, such as neuroreceptors and enzymes.

REGIONAL CEREBRAL BLOOD FLOW The measurement of rCBF, as a marker of neuronal activity and metabolism, is perhaps the oldest approach to neurofunctional quantitation. It is well grounded on a firm theoretical base, beginning with observations in the late 1800s that an augmented level of a tissue's function is sustained by increasing its rate of oxygen consumption and, therefore, the flow of oxygenated blood to the tissue. An extensive body of basic research and clinical studies has demonstrated that the concept is applicable to the brain: in the grossly intact brain brain work, neuronal metabolism, and blood flow are tightly coupled. An important implication of those observations is that cerebral blood flow (CBF) not only can be studied just to elucidate cerebral hemodynamics per se, but can serve as a marker for brain activity.

Current methods for measuring rCBF include the nontomographic xenon 133 inhalation method; xenon 133 and xenon 127 inhalation SPECT; SPECT with a variety of less quantifiable intravenously administered radiopharmaceuticals, such as technetium 99m hexamethylpropyleneamineoxime (HMPAO) and technetium 99m ethyl cysteinate dimer (ECD); and PET using an intravenous bolus of oxygen 15 water or inhaled $^{15}O_2$ or $C^{15}O$. Each has advantages and disadvantages.

Recent work with MRI suggests that high spatial and temporal resolution studies of regional cerebral perfusion may be possible with rapid sequence MRI scans and special contrast agents, noninvasively, with no radiation exposure to the subject and thus no limit to the number of studies that could be done on a single person. If shown to be feasible, the approach may prove to be closest to the ideal blood flow imaging technique for studying schizophrenia.

LOCAL CEREBRAL METABOLIC RATE OF GLUCOSE UTILIZATION The brain's energy requirements are among the highest of any organ system in the body. In the normal state blood glucose provides the main substrate for that high level of cerebral energy metabolism. Cerebral glucose metabolism (lCMRGlu) is currently best measured with the fluorodeoxyglucose 18 (FDG^{18}) technique and PET. The FDG technique is based on several important properties of deoxyglucose. Deoxyglucose and glucose are transported across the blood-brain barrier by the same carrier, but in the cerebral tissues they are phosphorylated to deoxyglucose-6-phosphate and glucose-6-phosphate, respectively, which have differing fates. The latter is metabolized to carbon dioxide (CO_2) and water whereas the former is trapped (that is, not further metabolized) in the cerebral tissues, at least long enough to be imaged if it is tagged with a radiolabel such as fluorine 18 or carbon 11. The FDG PET method typically involves the intravenous injection of FDG^{18}, periodic sampling of arterial blood levels, and a single 20- to 30-minute scan performed approximately 40 minutes postinjection (at which time the glucose metabolic rate of the brain is assumed to have reached a steady state).

Because of certain features of the fluorine 18 positron and the relatively prolonged scanning time that is possible with it, the FDG^{18} method affords perhaps the best spatial resolution and the most anatomical detail of any currently available functional brain imaging technology. Its drawbacks include (1) the relatively high radiation exposure, which limits each subject to two to four studies per year; and (2) the long measurement period, which limits its temporal resolution and sensitivity to cognitive and acute pharmacological activations.

MEASUREMENT OF NEUROCHEMICAL SYSTEMS Imaging and quantitation of neuroreceptors with PET and SPECT has many features in common with autoradiography and with in vitro receptor binding techniques. A specific receptor ligand (or binding agent) with desirable pharmacological characteristics is labeled with a single photon or positron emitter and injected into the subject. The anatomical distribution of the radioligand in the brain is determined with tomographic scanning techniques (PET or SPECT). A quantitative estimate of specific receptor binding can be achieved by compartmental modeling to take into account the kinetic behavior of the ligand between extracerebral and intracerebral plasma and tissue, as well as the nonspecific binding and extraneuronal concentration. Alternatively and more simply, the radioligand concentration in a brain area that is known to have little or no specific binding (such as the cerebellum for dopamine receptors) can be used to estimate the nonspecific binding. At present SPECT and PET ligands are available for imaging the dopamine, opioid, serotonin, benzodiazepine, and other systems.

Cerebral concentration and distribution of neurotransmitter turnover and of enzymes of interest in schizophrenia can also be measured with PET and SPECT, such as [^{11}C]clorgyline and L-[^{11}C]deprenyl (irreversible inhibitors of monoamine oxidase [MAO]) for mapping MAOA and MAOB, respectively, and [^{18}F]dopa, a radiolabeled analog of the dopamine precursor, for studying the rate of presynaptic dopamine turnover. The PET technique has also been used to investigate brain distribution and kinetics of pharmacological agents, such as [^{11}C]chlorpromazine, [^{11}C]benztropine, and [^{11}C]cocaine. Those studies emphasize the power of PET and SPECT to study directly the neurochemistry of the living human brain and their potential to monitor and guide pharmacological treatments.

Methods for functional brain imaging The ideal functional brain imaging technique for studying schizophrenia would have a number of special features. It would be noninvasive to avoid creating extraneous cognitive sets (that is, those not of primary interest, such as anxiety or discomfort) that might be reflected in the physiological data and thus contaminate the cerebral physiological landscape being investigated. It should be procedurally easy for patients who might not be able to cooperate with long, invasive procedures and with motor restraint or other discomforts. It would have short enough temporal resolution to allow transient mental phenomena to be studied. Finally, its spatial resolution would be sufficient to allow small structures, such as the hippocampus and the basal ganglia, to be investigated. At the present time none of the readily available techniques for functional brain imaging completely fulfill those criteria, and each involves a trade-off. Xenon 133 rCBF exposes the subject to less radioactivity and is less expensive and more convenient than PET. However, PET has considerably superior spatial resolution, and it can measure a number of indicators of neuronal activity in addition to rCBF, including regional glucose metabolism, oxygen utilization, and specific neurochemical metabolism. A new approach that is as yet restricted to only a few major research centers, using MRI to measure rCBF, may come closest to the ideal. Electroencephalography is another method of assessing brain function.

TWO-DIMENSIONAL XENON 133 STUDIES The concept of utilizing rCBF measurements to indicate brain activity is based on the fact that brain work, neuronal activity, and local blood flow are coupled in the grossly intact brain; therefore, measurements of blood flow, for the most part, reflect brain metabolism. The theory underlying that homeostatic relation was first applied to investigating the physiology of the human brain by studying the exchange between capillary and brain tissue of nonmetabolized (inert), diffusible molecules, such as nitrous oxide, between capillary and brain tissue. The rate of the exchange would be a function of blood flow, and in 1945 researchers first demonstrated that average blood flow could be measured for the human brain as a whole by ascertaining the difference between arterial and venous concentrations of the inert tracer arriving and leaving the brain. Regional blood flow measurements by extracranial monitoring of the delivery and washout of radioisotopes of inert substances soon followed.

In the 1960s a method for measuring the blood flow of many cortical regions in one hemisphere was developed. It involved the injection into the carotid artery of a saline solution of the inert radioisotope xenon 133 gas. Extracranial detectors were used to monitor the rates of arrival and disappearance of gamma rays from various cortical areas, which allowed the calculation of regional blood flow to each area. It was quickly noted that rCBF measurements carried out in that fashion, albeit invasive, were sensitive to functional activation of specific cortical areas.

Schizophrenia research during the 1980s saw the introduction of a completely noninvasive, atraumatic, and quick technique, in which xenon 133 gas was administered to the subject by inhalation and which was particularly well suited to studying psychotic persons. The major disadvantages include poor spatial resolution (approximately 2 centimeters [cm]) and the fact that it is a nontomographic technique and so cannot differentiate between radiation counts originating in superficial brain structures as compared with deep brain structures. In recent years the following tomographic techniques have come into more widespread use and have largely supplanted nontomographic xenon measurements.

SINGLE PHOTON EMISSION COMPUTED TOMOGRAPHY In the early 1960s a method was proposed for using the data from numerous planar (two-dimensional) images taken at different angles to reconstruct a three-dimensional picture of the distribution of a radioisotope in the brain. Major technological advances in that area culminated in the development of SPECT and PET as used today. The term "single photon emitting radioisotope" refers to any radionuclide that produces only one photon per disintegration. They include technetium 99m, iodine 123, and the radioxenons (xenon 133 and xenon 127), which are commercially available and widely used for imaging. Although most commonly available SPECT scanners have spatial resolution of the order of 1 cm, some dedicated head scanners can resolve objects as small as 6 millimeters (mm).

SPECT has several advantages over other available methods. Compared with the two-dimensional rCBF technique, it has the obvious advantages of a tomographic approach and better spatial resolution. Since single photon emitting isotopes have longer half-lives than do positron emitters, an on-site cyclotron or other radionuclide production is not necessary. For the same reason scans with the iodine 123 and technetium 99m radiopharmaceuticals can be performed many hours after the radiotracer, giving SPECT greater procedural flexibility than PET. The cost of SPECT falls between that of PET and the two-dimensional technique. In general, SPECT is less invasive than PET.

There are also several disadvantages, including difficulties in the absolute quantitation of data obtained with any sort of tomographic imaging. Attenuation of radiation counts refers to the fact that since the energy of a photon is diminished as it travels through matter, which slows or even stops it, fewer photons originating in deep structures reach the extracranial detectors than do photons originating in superficial structures. That may produce artificially lower values for deep brain regions (such as the basal ganglia), which may be important in schizophrenia, and relatively higher values at the surface. The problem is greatest for photons of low energy, such as xenon 133. No completely satisfactory method for dealing with the issue has been found for SPECT scanning.

Another problem that is common to both SPECT and PET concerns the so-called partial-volume effect. It results from the fact that when a structure that is smaller than the spatial resolution of the scanner is imaged, that structure only partially occupies the volume that the detectors see. That may result in an underestimation of the structure's activity level, and is a particularly serious confound for imaging the brain, in which there are numerous small structures with heterogeneous functions. The better the spatial resolution of the imaging system, the smaller will be the partial-volume effect. The nontomographic (two-dimensional) technique does not have that problem.

POSITRON EMISSION TOMOGRAPHY The use of PET involves the administration of certain cyclotron-produced radioisotopes. Unlike those used for SPECT the radioisotopes for PET emit very short-lived positrons that are rapidly annihilated, producing two characteristic photons of equal energy that can be simultaneously detected outside the head. Those twin photons confer upon PET its superior spatial resolution. Several PET radioisotopes are in use. Fluorine 18 fluorodeoxyglucose is used to measure cerebral glucose metabolism, whereas oxygen 15 incorporated into water or oxygen-containing gases is employed to measure cerebral oxygen utilization and CBF. Carbon 11 compounds, positron emitter labeled neuroreceptor ligands (such as 11C-methylspiperone for dopamine receptors), and neurotransmitter precursors (such as fluorine-18-fluorodopa) have also been developed.

The main advantage of PET is its excellent spatial resolution (about 6 mm in most new scanners and 3 mm in some experimental machines). Also, PET is more quantitative than SPECT because it is possible to measure directly the amount of attenuation of radiation counts by each person's brain. Another advantage is that PET scanners are sensitive enough that sequential scans of very short duration (for example, 5 to 20 seconds) can be acquired, providing detailed information about the kinetic behavior of the radiotracer. That characteristic has been particularly important in studying neuroreceptors, and it allows very rapid measurement of the very short-lived oxygen 15 blood flow agents (for example, total scanning time of 40 seconds for oxygen 15 water). Preliminary results suggest that some high-sensitivity SPECT scanners may also be capable of rapid, sequential scanning.

The major disadvantage of PET lies in its invasiveness and expense, and in the limitations of short-lived radiotracers. For fully quantitative studies radial arterial lines are necessary to monitor continuously the amount of radioisotope being delivered to the brain by the arterial blood supply. However, for paired studies in which the main interest is in the difference between the two data sets or their relative values, adequate information can be obtained by simply comparing the regional count rates, obviating the need for the arterial catheter. The problem with relatively short-lived tracers is that studies must be performed quickly. In practice that is a concern only in pharmacological studies in which the radiotracers do not have a chance to reach equilibrium, necessitating the application of complex and controversial theoretical kinetic models. Short studies are desirable for investigating mental phenomena, such as cognition; for performing multiple measurements in the same person; and for studying uncooperative patient populations.

FUNCTIONAL MAGNETIC RESONANCE IMAGING The traditional use of MRI methodology for anatomical imaging is being expanded to include MRI measurement of many aspects of biological function. Advances in two areas, spectroscopy and ultrafast imaging, will allow researchers to probe brain biochemistry and blood flow at close to a microscopic level. The application of those techniques to research in psychiatric disorders is now in its infancy and a body of research data has yet to emerge, but the approach promises to offer nonivasive, high spatial and temporal resolution information without exposure to radiation.

Traditional MRI measures the unpaired protons of water and of fat (both extremely proton rich), yielding valuable anatomical information, but little information about the biochemistry of the brain. Magnetic resonance spectroscopy (MRS) masks the huge signal from the unpaired protons of water and fat to look at the much smaller signal from such elements as phosphorus and sodium. Many of the various compounds containing phosphorus (such as adenosine triphosphate (ATP) and phosphocreatine) can be measured, giving detailed data about the energy state for small areas of brain.

With the advent of ultrafast scanning, blood flow images can be acquired in under one second using readily available techniques and under 50 milliseconds (ms) using more sophisticated echo-planar imaging. In conjunction with the development of paramagnetic tracers (such as gadolinium-diethylenetriamine pentaacetic acid [DTPA]) those techniques can be used to measure the minute changes in cerebral blood volume related to neuronal activity. In contrast to rCBF imaging and measurement with other techniques, the MRI approach has the potential for spatial resolution of 1 ms in all three planes, temporal resolution of the order of seconds, and unlimited repeated scans on a single person since there is no radiation exposure. At present only qualitative blood flow information can be obtained using MRI methods, but accurate quantification will almost certainly be achieved in the near future. In addition, new advances may also make it possible to take advantage of the different magnetic properties of oxyhemoglobin and deoxyhemoglobin to measure brain function in real time with excellent resolution.

Research design: pitfalls, challenges, solutions The facet of the techniques that renders them so potentially powerful, their ability to measure physiological changes underlying transient mental phenomena, also makes their application to psychiatric research complex. Since a subject's sensory input, cognitive and motor outputs, mental state, and the ambient conditions in the testing environment all have potential neurophysiological repercussions, they must be rigorously controlled. It is now quite clear that testing conditions cannot be considered too carefully in research design and in the interpretation of the resulting data. Studies carried out at rest, when there is no prescribed sensory, motor, or cognitive activity, produce extremely variable results. That variability may obscure subtle physiological changes that might be related to psychopathology in schizophrenia.

A less variable and more meaningful approach is to measure brain function during conditions that predictably activate specific brain areas in normal subjects and that may have clinical relevance, such as during cognitive activities. Measuring brain function for each person under several different conditions, as is possible with rCBF measurements, allows each subject to be used as his or her own control. That approach minimizes the large interperson variability in cerebral function that exists, and in paired task designs serves to highlight the metabolic concomitants of complex behaviors and cognitive activities.

Additional potential methodological problems in some functional brain imaging studies include poorly matched patient and control groups and failure to study patients who are not being treated with medication. While pharmacological treatments have not definitively been shown to affect brain structure as measured by in vivo imaging techniques, there are definite neurophysiological effects.

BRAIN FUNCTIONAL ALTERATIONS IN SCHIZOPHRENIA The extensive body of literature attempting to localize and characterize physiological brain dysfunction in schizophrenia does not always present a cohesive picture, perhaps in part because of differences in instrumentation and the application of techniques. In some cases poor research design has also contributed to the variability in the literature. However, several consistent themes have emerged.

Alterations in global metabolism or cerebral blood flow Reductions in blood flow and metabolism to the entire brain have been consistently demonstrated in primary degenerative dementias (in which there are also more severe localized functional decrements in temporoparietal and sometimes frontal regions) and, to a lesser extent, in normal aging. Although the question of whether schizophrenia presents a similar pathophysiological picture of globally reduced function is an important one, the data are less clear. Early studies using intracarotid techniques rarely found reduced flow, but the results of inhalation rCBF and PET studies have been mixed. A review of some 27 studies across all methodological modalities found that although 70 percent were negative, 30 percent did find global reductions. Some of the positive findings in the area may be accounted for by differences in patient populations or important methodological problems. A potential problem for some blood flow studies is the failure to take into account the subjects' arterial CO_2 levels, which can alter blood flow. Many PET studies avoid the use of arterial lines and, therefore, report only relative values (for example, regional data expressed as a percentage of some global measure rather than absolute values). In those PET studies that do report absolute values an additional problem is the possibility that, since patients with schizophrenia may have relatively less brain tissue and enlarged CSF spaces as compared with normal controls, more values for CSF may be averaged in with values for tissue in those patients (the so-called partial-volume artifact), producing lower apparent tissue values.

Whether those factors can explain all of the positive findings is unclear, but the bulk of the available evidence indicates that, if there is reduced global brain function in schizophrenia, the changes are not of the magnitude present in typical dementias, such as dementia of the Alzheimer's type. That is perhaps not surprising given that most neurological illnesses in which marked decreases in global brain function have been unequivocally demonstrated are characterized by either gross structural or physiological pathology and more gross neurological signs than have been demonstrated in schizophrenia.

Alterations in patterns of functional asymmetry The notion that schizophrenia may involve disordered lateralization of brain activity has been explored for many years using a variety of methods. However, even among those studies that support the notion there is little agreement as to which hemisphere is implicated or whether the putative aberration may involve both hemispheres. Similarly, if there is an abnormality, it is unclear whether it consists of increased or decreased activity on the affected side or an increase in one side and a decrease on the other side. The existing functional brain imaging data concerning the question are relatively sparse and do little to resolve it. A number of xenon 133 resting rCBF studies do not support the notion of altered laterality in schizophrenia. However, two studies performed during cognitive activation specifically designed to explore laterality in schizophrenia suggested that there is left hemisphere overactivity. Very few PET reports of altered lateralization have been published, but left hemisphere overactivation and increased left temporal metabolism, with particular focus on the hippocampus and parahippocampal areas, have been reported.

A report of over 400 xenon 133 rCBF studies comparing laterality indexes in medication-free patients with schizophrenia and controls during 11 different cognitive conditions (Figure 14.3-4) reflects the inconsistent findings in the literature and illustrates several problems encountered in that line of research. No consistent differences between patients and controls were found in the study, but several isolated differences could be demonstrated if a very liberal statistical approach (multiple univariate comparisons) were employed. There was one instance of greater left mean hemispheric rCBF in schizophrenia in the context of a right hemisphere preponderance in the normal subjects (during an attentional task), one instance of a greater degree of left prefrontal lateralization in the patients in the context of a lesser lateralization in the same direction in the normals (during a resting condition), and one instance of greater right temporal lobe activation in the patients in the context of normal left temporal lateralization (during an abstract reasoning task). The diversity of the findings highlights the state dependency of functional laterality and the need for careful control of state variables. Whether normal lateralization is to the left or to the right, and whether patients and controls differ, depends on what the subjects are doing during the scans and what region is examined. Although it cannot be ruled out that some patients with schizophrenia may have disordered lateralization in some brain areas during some conditions, there are few consistent findings, and further research is necessary to ascertain the role of functional laterality in schizophrenia.

Metabolic hypofrontality Several lines of converging evidence suggest that impaired frontal cortical function may play a role in schizophrenia. For example, clinical signs and symptoms of patients with gross frontal lobe lesions (including minor or soft neurological signs, disordered smooth-pursuit eye movements, impaired problem solving and abstract thinking, and such clinical features as bizarre behavior, poor social functioning, and inadequate hygiene) are also seen in schizophrenia. Studies of subhuman primates indicate a role for the prefrontal cortex (especially the dorsolateral aspect) in higher-order cognitive processes analogous to those impaired in schizophrenia.

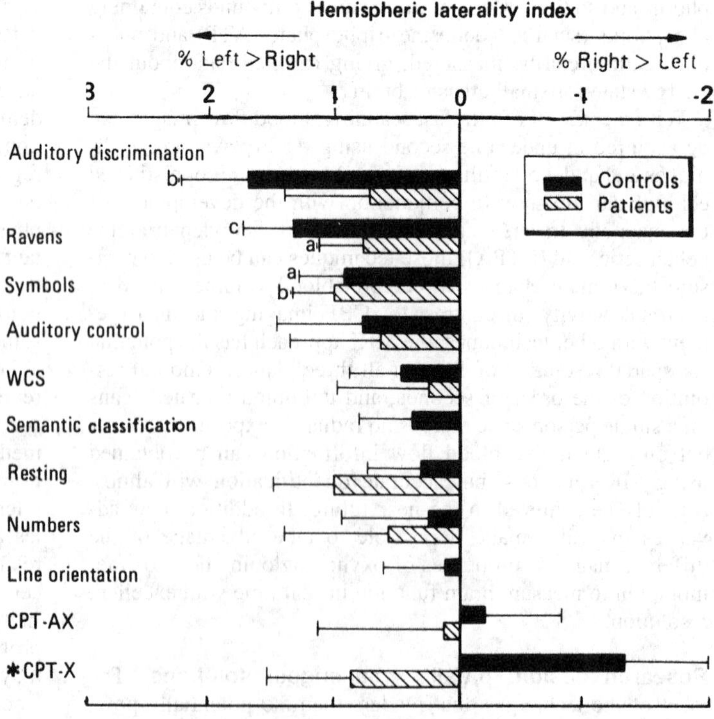

FIGURE 14.3-4 *Relative right versus left hemisphere gray cortical blood flow values for normal subjects and patients with schizophrenia during 11 different cognitive conditions. Note that laterality values vary widely with different behavioral states. Hemispheric laterality index values were calculated as follows: (Left hemisphere − Right hemisphere) × 100/Whole brain mean CBF. (Figure from K F Berman, D R Weinberger: Lateralisation of cortical function during cognitive tasks: Regional cerebral blood flow studies of normal individuals and patients with schizophrenia. J Neurol Neurosurg Psychiatry 53: 150, 1990. Used with permission.)*

Although those lines of reasoning are inferential more direct evidence for frontal cortical involvement in schizophrenia emerged from intracarotid rCBF studies in the 1970s. The early studies noted that patients with schizophrenia had relatively lower blood flow to frontal regions and relatively greater flow to postcentral regions. The patients who were most indifferent, most inactive, and showed the greatest degree of autistic disorder were the most hypofrontal, whereas the most cognitively disturbed patients showed the highest postcentral rCBF. In addition to those observations it was noted that rCBF measurements could be made during cognitive activation. During a simple picture test normal subjects showed changes in rCBF whereas the more deteriorated patients did not.

Those pioneering research findings heralded the beginning of the modern era of functional brain imaging in psychiatry and refocused interest on the frontal lobes in schizophrenia. However, the intracarotid technique of xenon 133 administration was not well suited to clinical research. More recent attempts to confirm hypofrontality in schizophrenia using the noninvasive inhalation technique have met with inconsistent results. Possible explanations for the lack of consensus in the literature may include differences in instrumentation and methodology, differences in patient populations, and, most important, failure to control testing conditions adequately. Studies carried out during the resting state have proved variable.

IS HYPOFRONTALITY IN SCHIZOPHRENIA BEHAVIORALLY SPECIFIC? A series of xenon 133 inhalation experiments in which rCBF was measured during a number of different cognitive activation conditions, some linked to prefrontal cortex and others that were not, indicated that patients do have prefrontal cortical dysfunction, but that it may not become apparent unless the brain is called on to increase the level of physiological activity in the region. In those studies normal subjects increased prefrontal rCBF while performing a neuropsychological test linked to prefrontal cortex and requiring abstract reasoning (the Wisconsin Card Sorting Test), but neither medication-free nor antipsychotic treated patients showed the change. During tasks not specifically linked to prefrontal cortex, including simple matching tasks and paradigms involving attention and vigilance, hypofrontality was not as consistently and robustly observed. Attempts were made in the experiments to control nonspecific and state-dependent epiphenomenological factors that often confound interpretation of such studies. They included the use of a baseline activation measurement in addition to regionally specific cortical activation and the monitoring of peripheral indicators of autonomic arousal, such as pulse, blood pressure, and respiratory rate. The studies highlight the importance of controlling state factors in functional brain imaging studies.

As with xenon studies the most consistent finding in schizophrenia to emerge from PET technology is decreased frontal lobe function. A recent review of more than 35 functional brain imaging studies of schizophrenia found that over 60 percent were positive. However, of those studies that attempted to control behavior during the scans by having subjects perform a task that was in some way linked to the frontal lobe, 100 percent demonstrated hypofrontality.

The results suggest that the degree to which patients appear hypofrontal as compared with controls during a functional brain imaging study depends on whether they are engaged in an activity that in normal persons is associated with the activation of the prefrontal cortex. If true, that conjecture would have important implications for understanding the pathophysiological mechanism, and ultimately the neural specificity, of prefrontal failure in schizophrenia, and the observation may explain a number of the inconsistencies in the PET and rCBF literature. The fact that prefrontal cortical dysfunction in schizophrenia may be condition dependent is not inconsistent with the clinical picture of psychopathology that waxes and wanes under various circumstances.

IS HYPOFRONTALITY IN SCHIZOPHRENIA AN EFFECT OF MEDICATION? The majority of rCBF and PET studies have been carried out in patients who were either receiving antipsychotic drugs at the time of the study or who had been previously treated and then withdrawn from antipsychotics for some time before the study. That, along with the fact that hypofrontality could not be demonstrated in several resting state PET studies of small numbers of patients who had never received medications, suggested to some investigators that antipsychotic treatment is responsible for hypofrontality in schizophrenia. However, a growing body of evidence refutes this notion.

First, two xenon 133 rCBF studies of young patients who had never received antipsychotics did find hypofrontality. That finding has been confirmed by two SPECT studies and a number of PET studies of antipsychotic-naive patients, most during a behavioral-cognitive task. Hypofrontality has also been observed in patients regardless of whether they are receiving or have been withdrawn from haloperidol (Haldol) but those results do not rule out the possibility of long-term effects of antipsychotic treatment on prefrontal physiology. However, a study of patients with Huntington's disease, some of whom had been chronically maintained on antipsychotic drugs, found no differences in prefrontal blood flow between such patients and those who were naive to antipsychotics. A study of eight pairs of monozygotic twins who were concordant for schizophrenia, but whose lifetime histories of antipsychotic drug intake differed greatly, found that in most pairs the twin who had been exposed to more antipsychotics was the more hyperfrontal of the pair during a prefrontally linked task.

Finally, a number of studies have examined the metabolic or rCBF changes that occur when patients go from the unmedicated state to the medicated state. Those studies have reported either no change in values or an increase in parameters of relative or absolute prefrontal activity. Such a result might be predicted on the basis of animal research showing that lCMRGlu correlates mainly with activity in presynaptic terminals, since dopaminergic projections to prefrontal cortex appear to become overactive and to remain overactive following antipsychotic treatment. There are little convincing data to support antipsychotic treatment as a major factor in hypofrontality. However, further work, including longitudinal studies and examinations of more patients early in their course, will be necessary to resolve the question definitively.

HOW PREVALENT IS HYPOFRONTALITY IN SCHIZOPHRENIA? Is hypofrontality a consistent characteristic of schizophrenia, or does it just affect a subgroup of patients who may have different pathophysiologies and etiologies underlying their illnesses? The approach of most studies has been to compare the mean value for a group of patients with schizophrenia with the mean value for an unrelated group of normal subjects. The results of such a comparison often confirm that, on the whole, patients have decreased parameters of frontal lobe function. However, there may be a great deal of overlap between the two groups, with only a minority of patient values actually falling beyond the lower limit of the normal values. One interpretation could be that hypofrontality is restricted to only a small subgroup of outliers. But since there is great variability in normal physiological values, and since what a given patient's potential value would have been if he or she did not have schizophrenia is not known, the true prevalence of hypofrontality in the schizophrenic population cannot be estimated.

Recent rCBF studies of monozygotic twins (Figure 14.3-5) discordant for schizophrenia shed light on the question. Assuming that the rCBF measurements for the well cotwin of a monozygotic pair may reflect the values that would have characterized the ill twin if he or she did not have schizophrenia, the former can be used as a genetically (as well as socioeconomically and environmentally) perfect control to determine the pathophysiological changes that have occurred in each patient. During a task linked to the frontal lobe the twin with schizophrenia was more hypofrontal than his or her well cotwin in every case. That would seem to suggest that if the experimental conditions are properly controlled, hypofrontality can be demonstrated in most, if not all, patients.

Hypofrontality was the first functional abnormality to be shown in schizophrenia, and it remains the most frequently observed. However, data regarding the pathophysiologic mechanism of hypofrontality are just beginning to emerge.

Other regional changes In addition to the results of studies addressing major hypotheses several other findings have been reported. For the most part they represent the results of single reports that have not been replicated. For example, one study found increased left globus pallidus rCBF relative to whole brain mean values in two groups of five drug-naive patients each as compared to 10 normal controls. Another study found decreased left lentiform nucleus glucose metabolism in medication-free patients, whereas yet another found decreased rCBF in the basal ganglia of patients. Other investigators have suggested that striatal glucose metabolism is increased in schizophrenia, and one study reported that the ratio of cortical to subcortical (primarily basal ganglia) glucose metabolism was reduced in schizophrenia. However, the weight of the evidence suggests that the phenomenon is related to antipsychotic treatment.

Structural abnormalities of the temporal-limbic system have been confirmed by postmortem and MRI studies, but it is difficult to predict what the functional implications of the structural changes reported in schizophrenia would be. While temporal lobe abnormalities have been infrequently found, both increased metabolism and decreased metabolism have been reported. One PET study found slightly reduced glucose metabolism in the right amygdala in medication-free patients, but many regional comparisons were performed. Another reported a direct correlation between degree of psychopathology and rCBF in the left parahippocampal gyrus. Further study of that area is necessary.

Several investigators have suggested that schizophrenia is characterized by increased posterior cortical activity. The first rCBF study of schizophrenia in the mid-1970s suggested that the hypofrontal pattern represented a redistribution of flow with relatively lower flow to frontal areas and relatively higher flow to posterior cortex. In that study the patients who were the most indifferent, the most inactive, and the most autistic had the lowest frontal flows, whereas the most cognitively disturbed patients showed the highest postcentral rCBF. That finding suggested that schizophrenia includes a hypointentional component related to hypofrontality as well as a hypergnostic component related to increased postcentral blood flow.

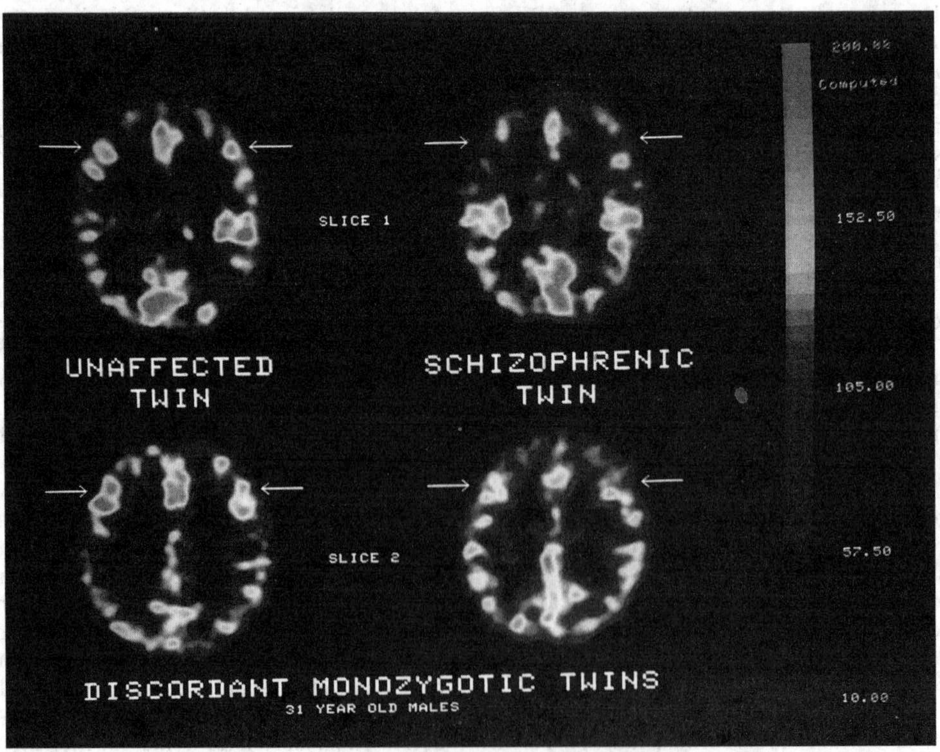

FIGURE 14.3-5 *Oxygen 15 water PET scans of a pair of monozygotic twins discordant for schizophrenia during performance of a prefrontal task. Two slices through the dorsolateral prefrontal cortex are shown for each twin; the more inferior slice is shown at the top. The affected twin is hypofrontal (that is, has less activity in dorsolateral prefrontal cortex [arrows]) compared with his well cotwin.* * = P ≤ *.05 for between-group comparison of laterality index. a,b,c,d* = P ≤ *.05, .01, .005, .001, respectively, for within-group comparison of left versus right hemisphere relative CBF. (See Color Plate 9.)*

An early FDG[18] study performed while patients received mild forearm shock suggested that the decreased ratio of anterior to posterior metabolism found in schizophrenia was caused by increased posterior flow rather than by lower frontal flow. However, later studies by the same investigators also demonstrated decreased frontal activity, and no other investigators have shown similar findings; in contrast an isolated report found a reversal of the pattern with relatively increased frontal and decreased posterior glucose metabolism in unmedicated patients during resting. Another study performed during a task that activates posterior cortical areas in normal subjects, a situation that might be expected to evoke posterior abnormalities in patients if present, failed to demonstrate any such changes. All those miscellaneous abnormalities remain, for the most part, sporadic findings and await further confirmation.

Alterations in neuroreceptors The ability to examine neuroreceptors and other parameters of specific neurochemical function in vivo with PET and SPECT represents one of the most exciting applications of functional brain imaging. Alterations in neuroreceptors in schizophrenia are suggested by the facts that (1) such alterations, particularly elevations of dopamine receptors in the striatum, have been found in postmortem studies; and (2) neurochemical therapeutic interventions, such as dopamine antagonists, remain the mainstay of treatment. The postmortem observations, however, have been complicated by potential artifacts having to do with receptor alterations after death, the effects of agonal events leading to death, and, to an even greater extent, the fact that most patients will have received extensive treatment with antipsychotic medication by the time of death. The last is a problem because it has been shown that the antipsychotics themselves produce an elevation of dopamine receptors in the striatum, making it difficult to conclude whether the observed increases in dopamine receptors are associated with the disease or are the effects of the antipsychotic medication. Since SPECT and PET studies have the potential to investigate patients while they are young and early in their course of illness, perhaps even before antipsychotic treatment, many of the problems can be circumvented, and a more meaningful assessment of receptor status may be obtained. Several studies have measured striatal D_2 receptors in vivo in schizophrenia, with mixed results. The first was carried out using SPECT and bromine 77 bromospiperone with semiquantitative methods. The patients had been medication-free for at least six months (which some studies suggest is not long enough to negate the antipsychotic effect) and four had never received antipsychotics. A small but statistically significant increase (11 percent) in radioactivity counts was seen in the patients. However, another SPECT study found no consistent alteration in the patients on the whole.

Two PET studies have also been reported, one using [^{11}C]N-methylspiperone, a ligand with high affinity for both D_2 and 5-hydroxytryptamine type 2(5-HT_2) receptors, and the other using the selective D_2 receptor antagonist carbon 11 raclopride. Both studies were of patients reported to have never received antipsychotic treatment. In the former study the patients' values were elevated two to three times over those of the controls; the findings were the same for antipsychotic-treated patients. In contrast the latter study found no difference from normal controls. Differences in patient selection, radioligands, and modeling methods may have played a role in the discrepancy. With regard to the role of radioligands in the discrepant findings, differences in the degree to which the ligands are displaced by endogenous dopamine in the synapse and differences in their binding to D_4 receptors have both been cited. Thus no definitive conclusion can be drawn at present and further studies will be necessary to resolve the question. There have been few demonstrations of clinical correlates of metabolic alterations as assessed by PET; those that have been reported do not form a cohesive story, and the area requires further study.

UNDERSTANDING FUNCTIONAL ABNORMALITIES IN SCHIZOPHRENIA There is a wealth of diverse functional abnormalities in schizophrenia, but there is also a lack of consensus about the findings. There may be a number of reasons for that dichotomy but chief among them are the difficulty of controlling the behavior of the subjects during the procedures and the complexity of interpreting functional abnormalities.

Functional effects of distant lesions Functional abnormalities of a specific brain area can result from a variety of pathological situations, including structural abnormalities in the area itself (intrinsic abnormalities) or in its afferent or efferent pathways, as well as neurochemical aberrations in any of those locations. Any single structural or neurochemical lesion can result in a variety of spatially disparate functional abnormalities, which, in turn, may lead to other functional problems downstream and which may become manifest under some conditions (for example, afferent input or physiological load), but not under others. Therefore, a given functional problem may actually be a reflection of distant pathology and may appear to be an inconsistent finding.

Several examples of distant effects of lesions are well documented in the neurology literature. Perhaps the most commonly seen is the phenomenom of crossed-cerebellar diaschisis in which supratentorial lesions, such as infarction or tumor, can produce rCBF and lCMRGlu reductions in the contralateral cerebellar hemisphere. Those linked structural-functional abnormalities reflect anatomical connections between the affected areas. Cases in which the symptoms of patients with cerebrovascular disorders were related to functional changes distant from the structural infarct have also been reported. The reports clearly show that structural lesions can lead to deafferentation or disconnection syndromes with distant physiological repercussions and associated clinical sequelae.

In schizophrenia, where no overt structural aberrations such as infarcts or tumors are apparent, the functional repercussions may be expected to be even more subtle and more difficult to measure, but the same principles apply.

What is the pathophysiological mechanism of hypofrontality? A highly simplified scheme might consider three possible pathophysiological mechanisms for hypofrontality in schizophrenia—deefferentation of prefrontal cortex, deafferentation, and intrinsic prefrontal abnormality—operating either alone or in combination. Although it remains unproved as to which, if any, of the mechanisms may play a role in the behaviorally related pathophysiology of the prefrontal cortex in the illness, some clues are offered by the collective results of the functional and structural imaging literature.

Animal and human studies suggest a role for dopamine in the activation of prefrontal cortex and in prefrontally linked behaviors. One study demonstrated a direct correlation between CSF levels of the dopaminergic metabolite HVA and prefrontal rCBF during a prefrontal task in schizophrenia, and several groups have reported the reversal of hypofrontality with the administration of dopaminergic agonists.

There is also evidence for a link between prefrontal physiological hypoactivity and anatomical pathology in schizophrenia. One study observed a correlation between prefrontal rCBF during a prefrontal task and ventricular size on CT. The relationship was not observed during nonprefrontally specific tasks. Consistent with that finding is a recent monozygotic twin study that found that in the affected twins the volume of the hippocampus (the structural variable that best differentiated the well from the ill twins) strongly predicted the degree of dorsolateral prefrontal activation during prefrontal cognition (the physiological variable that best differentiated the cotwins). The smaller the hippocampus, the less is the prefrontal activity, suggesting that there may be dysfunction of neocortical-limbic connectivity in schizophrenia. It is tempting to think that the anatomical, functional, and neurochemical alterations highlighted by those studies might be linked, but further work will be necessary to delineate the specifics of such a hypothesis.

Interpretation of physiological abnormalities can be complex. However, the wealth of information offered by brain imaging studies, particularly considered in conjunction with correlative data, provide important and heretofore unavailable clues. Future technological developments and new applications of the techniques will undoubtedly provide new insights.

SUGGESTED CROSS-REFERENCES

The Neural basis of schizophrenic psychopathology is further discussed in Section 1.1 an introduction and overview of neural sciences, in Section 1.2 on functional neuroanatomy, in Section 1.3 on monoamine neurotransmitters, in Section 1.14 on basic molecular neurobiology, and in Section 3.6 on brain models of mind. Neuroimaging is presented in Section 1.10 on the principles of neuroimaging. Schizophrenia is also discussed in Section 14.1 on introduction and overview of schizophrenia; in Section 14.2 on epidemiology of schizophrenia; in Section 14.4 on neurochemical, viral, and immunological studies of schizophrenia; in Section 14.5 on genetics of schizophrenia; and in Section 14.7 on clinical features of schizophrenia. Antipsychotics are presented in Section 32.15 on dopamine receptor antagonists.

REFERENCES

Akbarian S, Bunney W E, Potkin S G, Wigal S B, Hagman J O, Sandman C A, Jones E G: Altered distribution of nicotinamide-adenine dinucleotide phosphatase-diaphorase cells in frontal lobe of schizophrenics implies disturbances of cortical development. Arch Gen Psychiatry *50:* 169, 1993.

Akbarian S, Vinuela A, Kim J J, Potkin S G, Bunney W E, Jones E G: Distorted distribution of nicotinamide-adenine dinucleotide phosphatase-diaphorase neurons in temporal lobe of schizophrenics implies disturbances of cortical development. Arch Gen Psychiatry *50:* 178, 1993.

Andreasen N C: Brain imaging: Applications in psychiatry. Science *239:* 1381, 1988.

Bartley A J, Jones D W, Torrey E F, Zigun J R, Weinberger D R: Sylvian fissure asymmetries in monozygotic twins: A test of laterality in schizophrenia. Biol Psychiatry *34:* 853, 1993.

Benes F M, Davidson J, Bird M D: Quantitative cytoarchitectural studies of the cerebral cortex in schizophrenia. Arch Gen Psychiatry *43:* 31, 1986.

*Berman K F, Torrey E F, Daniel D G, Weinberger D R: Regional cortical blood flow in monozygotic twins discordant and concordant for schizophrenia. Arch Gen Psychiatry *49:* 927, 1992.

Berman K F, Weinberger D R: Lateralisation of cortical function during cognitive tasks: Regional cerebral blood flow studies of normal individuals and patients with schizophrenia. J Neurol Neurosurg Psychiatry *53:* 150, 1990.

Berman K F, Weinberger D R: The prefrontal cortex in schizophrenia and other neuropsychiatric disorders: In vivo physiological correlates of cognitive deficits. Prog Brain Res *85:* 511, 1990.

*Berman K F, Weinberger D R: Functional localization in the brain in schizophrenia. In *American Psychiatric Press Review of Psychiatry,* vol 10, A Tasman, S M Goldfinger, editors, p 24. American Psychiatric Press, Washington, 1991.

Berman K F, Zec R F, Weinberger D R: Physiological dysfunction of dorsolateral prefrontal cortex in schizophrenia: II. Role of neuroleptic treatment, attention, and mental effort. Arch Gen Psychiatry *43:* 126, 1986.

Bogerts B, Meetz E, Schonfeldt-Bausch R: Basal ganglia and limbic system pathology in schizophrenia. Arch Gen Psychiatry *42:* 784, 1985.

Buchsbaum M S, Haier R J: Functional and anatomical brain imaging: Impact on schizophrenia research. Schizophr Bull *13:* 115, 1987.

Christison G W, Casanova M F, Weinberger D R, Rawlings R, Kleinman J E: A quantitative investigation of hippocampal pyramidal cell size, shape variability or orientation in schizophrenia. Arch Gen Psychiatry *46:* 1027, 1989.

Corsellis J A N: Psychoses of obscure pathology. In *Greenfield's Neuropathology,* ed 3, W Blackwood, J A N Corsellis, editors. Edward Arnold, London, 1976.

Daniel D G, Kim E, Kostianovsky D, Goldberg T E, Casanova M F, Kleinman J E, Weinberger D R: Computed tomography measurements of brain density in schizophrenia. Biol Psychiatry *29:* 745, 1991.

*Daniel D G, Zigun J, Weinberger D R: Brain imaging in neuropsychiatry. In *Textbook of Neuropsychiatry,* S C Yodofsky, R C Hales, editors, p 165. American Psychiatric Press, Washington, 1992.

Davidson K, Bagley C R: Schizophrenia-like psychoses associated with organic disorders of the central nervous system. Br J Psychiatry, *4* (Suppl): 113, 1969.

Friston K J, Liddle P F, Frith C D, Hirsch S R, Frackowiak R S J: The left medial temporal region and schizophrenia: A PET study. Brain *116:* 367, 1992.

Gur R E, Mozley D, Resnick S M, Shtasel D, Kohn M, Zimmerman R, Herman G, Atlas S, Grossman R, Erwin R, Gur R C: Magnetic resonance imaging in schizophrenia I: Volumetric analysis of brain and cerebrospinal fluid. Arch Gen Psychiatry *48:* 407, 1991.

*Hyde T M, Cassanova M F, Kleinman J E, Weinberger D R: Neuroanatomical and neurochemical pathology and schizophrenia. In *The American Psychiatric Press Review of Psychiatry,* vol 10, A Tasman, editor, p 7. American Psychiatric Press, Washington, 1991.

Ingvar D H, Franzen G: Abnormalities of cerebral blood flow distribution in patients with chronic schizophrenia. Acta Psychiatr Scand *50:* 425, 1974.

Jaskiw G E, Andreasen N C, Weinberger D R: X-ray computed tomography and magnetic resonance imaging in psychiatry. In *American Psychiatric Association Annual Review,* vol 6, A J Frances, R E Hales, editors. American Psychiatric Press, Washington, 1987.

Kety S S, Woodford R B, Harmel M H, Freyham K E, Appel E E, Schmidt C E: Cerebral blood flow and metabolism in schizophrenia. Am J Psychiatry *104:* 765, 1948.

Kovelman J A, Scheibel A B: Biological substrates of schizophrenia. Acta Neurol Scand *73:* 1, 1986.

Liddle P F, Friston K J, Frith C D, Hirsch S R, Jones T, Frackowiak R S W: Patterns of cerebral blood flow in schizophrenia. Br J Psychiatry *160:* 179, 1992.

Lipska B K, Jaskiw G E, Chrapusta S, Karoum F, Weinberger D R: Ibotenic acid lesion of the ventral hippocampus differentially affected dopamine and its metabolites in the nucleus accumbens and prefrontal cortex in the rat. Brain Res *585:* 1, 1992.

Nasrallah H A, Weinberger D R, editors: *Handbook of Schizophrenia* vol 1: *The Neurology of Schizophrenia.* Elsevier, Amsterdam, 1986.

Nieto D, Escobar A: Major psychoses. In *Pathology of the Nervous System,* vol 3, J Minckler, editor. McGraw-Hill, New York, 1972.

Seeman P, Hong-Chang G, Van Tol H H M: Dopamine D_4 receptors elevated in schizophrenia. Nature *365:* 441, 1993.

Seidman L F: Schizophrenia and brain dysfunction. Psychol Bull *94:* 195, 1983.

Shapiro R M: Regional neuropathology in schizophrenia: Where are we? Where are we going? Schizophr Res *10:* 187, 1993.

Stevens J R: Schizophrenia: Neuropathological changes in the brain. In *Receptors and Ligands in Psychiatry and Neurology,* A K Sen, T Lee, editors. Cambridge University Press, Cambridge, 1988.

Suddath R L, Cassanova M F, Goldberg T E, Daniel D G, Kelsoe J R, Weinberger D R: Temporal lobe pathology in schizophrenia: A quantitative magnetic resonance imaging study. Am J Psychiatry *46:* 464, 1989.

Suddath R L, Christisen G W, Torrey E F, Cassanova M F, Weinberger D R: Anatomical abnormalities in the brains of monozygotic twins discordant for schizophrenia. N Engl J Med *322:* 789, 1990.

Weinberger D R: Brain disease and psychiatric illness: When should a psychiatrist order a CAT scan? Am J Psychiatry *141:* 1521, 1984.

*Weinberger D R, Berman K F, Suddath R, Torrey E F: Evidence for dysfunction of a prefrontal-limbic network in schizophrenia: An MRI and rCBF study of discordant monozygotic twins. Am J Psychiatry *149:* 890, 1992.

Weinberger D R, Berman K F, Zec R F: Physiological dysfunction of dorsolateral prefrontal cortex in schizophrenia: I. Regional cerebral blood flow (rCBF) evidence. Arch Gen Psychiatry *43:* 114, 1986.

Zigun J R, Weinberger D R: In-vivo studies of brain morphology in schizophrenia. In *New Biological Vistas on Schizophrenia,* J P Lindenmayer, R K Stanley, editors, p 57. Brunner/Mazel, New York, 1992.

Zipursky R B, Lim K O, Sullivan E V, Brown B W, Pfefferbaum A: Widespread cerebral gray matter volume deficits in schizophrenia. Arch Gen Psychiatry *49:* 195, 1992.

14.4 SCHIZOPHRENIA: NEUROCHEMICAL, VIRAL, AND IMMUNOLOGICAL STUDIES

RICHARD JED WYATT, M.D.
DARRELL G. KIRCH, M.D.
MICHAEL F. EGAN, M.D.

INTRODUCTION

Despite numerous studies suggesting an association with genetic, toxic-metabolic, endocrine, viral-immunological, and other biological factors, the etiology of schizophrenia is not known. Whatever its primary cause, the pathophysiology of schizophrenia is probably mediated by neurochemical alterations. Although the characteristic psychopathology of schizophrenia at first glance may appear far removed from neurotransmitters, mental phenomena take place in the brain and may therefore be driven by abnormalities in neurochemical systems. This section reviews the evidence for underlying neurochemical abnormalities associated with schizophrenia and discusses the more prominent theories regarding a primary viral or immunological etiology of schizophrenia.

HISTORY The examination of schizophrenic patients from a biochemical perspective dates back at least to the 19th century, when psychiatry and biochemistry were in their infancy. In the 1890s at the Maryland Hospital for the Insane and at the turn of the century at McLean Hospital near Boston, investigators reported measurements of 24-hour urine constituents. Substances such as urea, uric acid, ammonia, creatinine, total chlorides, total sulfates, neutral sulfur, ethereal sulfates, indican, and total nitrogen, as well as specific gravity, volume, and acidity, were found to be normal in schizophrenic patients. At the same time Italian scientists noted that in chronically ill patients, many of whom had schizophrenia, the leukocyte count was increased, while the erythrocyte count was decreased during excitation. Another experimenter added *Bacillus anthracis* to three culture plates and found that the plate that contained the blood of schizophrenic patients had an increased number of colonies, which led him to believe that the blood of schizophrenics added to the growth of the bacteria.

In 1922 John C. Whitehorn, who later became head of the psychiatry department at Johns Hopkins University, injected a number of substances intradermally and found that schizophrenic patients had smaller wheal responses to histamine than other patients or healthy subjects, a finding that was replicated in the 1940s and 1950s. Whitehorn speculated that the reason for the decreased histamine response in schizophrenic patients was an excess of an adrenalinelike (catecholamine) substance. Today, after decades of intensive investigation, the major hypothesis concerning the neurochemical basis of schizophrenia postulates an excess of the catecholamine dopamine; the issue of abnormal histamine metabolism remains unresolved. Unfortunately, the reliability of early findings (through the 1940s) is complicated by the historical presence in psychiatric hospitals of patients with various infectious and metabolic disorders that either mimicked schizophrenia or occurred concurrently. Furthermore, until a few years ago the bioassays that were used to detect the presence of chemical substances were often nonspecific and unreliable.

Nevertheless, the value of a hypothesis such as that of dopaminergic excess in schizophrenia largely depends on the interest it generates and the possibility of designing experiments to refute or support it. In most areas of human biology, particularly neuropsychiatry, understanding of the relevant systems is too poor to permit substantiation or refutation of hypotheses that can be refuted by only one or even a series of experiments. Therefore, hypotheses—including those related to the pathophysiology and the etiology of schizophrenia—tend to linger. Some are revised in light of new knowledge; others are merely pushed aside by the aggressiveness of new techniques and their proponents. Nevertheless, any comprehensive hypothesis of schizophrenia must take into consideration what is known about the disorder. The strongly supported observations detailed below are ones that should be explained by a comprehensive hypothesis of schizophrenia.

FACTS ABOUT SCHIZOPHRENIA

GENDER DIFFERENCES Although the lifetime risk of developing schizophrenia is approximately equal for males and females, males are younger at onset and have a poorer outcome than females. Female patients also respond better to antipsychotic medications. Monozygotic twin studies indicate a higher concordance rate for schizophrenia among females than among males.

AGE AT ONSET Identifiable symptoms of schizophrenia are rare before puberty. The peak age at onset for males is between 18 and 25 years, and for females between 26 and 45. Although schizophrenia can begin after age 45, late onset is uncommon.

GENETICS There is strong evidence that schizophrenia is, at least in part, a genetic disorder. It is not clear, however, if a genetic diathesis is necessary for developing schizophrenia or if there is a pure genetic form. A simple autosomal dominant model of inheritance is unlikely. Several genes may be involved that could have variable penetrance and phenotypic expression. That could involve, for example, genes that are determined by mitochondrial deoxyribonucleic acid (DNA), which have been found to be altered in a number of neurological disorders.

Other possible genetic contributions might come from the effect of in utero events produced by genetically controlled interactions between the mother and fetus, such as Rh incompatibility.

ENVIRONMENT Because schizophrenia cannot be entirely accounted for by a genetic contribution, an environmental—social, psychological, or physical—factor must play a significant role. Schizophrenic exacerbations are often related to stress. In addition, schizophrenia is more prevalent in large urban environments and in persons of low socioeconomic status, although geographical or socioeconomic drift may be factors.

SEASON OF BIRTH Birth dates of schizophrenic patients show a modest peak during the late winter and early spring months, above that found in the general population. Some studies associate the winter-spring excess with viral epidemics, particularly if they occur during the second trimester of pregnancy. There are other plausible explanations for seasonality. For example, it is possible that the parents of future schizophrenic persons conceive more often in the late spring and early summer because of increased sexual activity.

COURSE OF ILLNESS The course of schizophrenia is extremely variable. Some patients have one or several episodes and return to normal functioning; others have a gradually deteriorating course. Rarely, even patients who have been ill for many years have complete, spontaneous recoveries. Many more of the chronically ill gradually improve during middle age.

STRUCTURAL AND FUNCTIONAL BRAIN ABNORMALITIES The high prevalence of abnormal electroencephalograms (EEGs), abnormal computed tomography (CT), magnetic resonance imaging (MRI), and positron emission tomography (PET) scans, and subtle neurological abnormalities associated with the disorder is a strong indication that schizophrenia involves central nervous system (CNS) structural defects, CNS functional abnormalities, or both.

PHARMACOLOGICAL TREATMENT Medications that block dopamine type 2 (D_2) receptors are effective in treating the positive symptoms of schizophrenia (such as delusions, hallucinations, and thought disorder). They may also have some effect on the deficit, negative, or core symptoms (such as restricted affect, loss of drive, and poverty of speech). Clozapine (Clozaril), a unique, atypical antipsychotic agent, is sometimes effective when other antipsychotic medications are not, which suggests that something other than D_2 receptor blockade is at work. Cognitive deficits in memory and conceptual thinking respond poorly, if at all, to current treatments.

The success of any theory of schizophrenia depends in part on how well it explains the essential clinical facts outlined above. Current theories have their foundations in a large experimental data base that includes studies of neurochemical, viral, and immunological abnormalities in patients with schizophrenia. The most important neurotransmitter systems are the dopamine, norepinephrine, serotonin, and glutamate systems. The basic neurobiology of those systems and the abnormalities they exhibit in association with schizophrenia are described below. Also described are a number of other neurochemical abnormalities that at one time or another have been studied in connection with schizophrenia. Because many of those neurochemical systems probably operate within interconnected neural networks, a broader view of the implications of neurochemical abnormalities on information processing is presented. Finally, studies suggesting that the dysfunctional neural networks arise from viral or immunological abnormalities (or both) are described.

DOPAMINE

A relation between a functional excess of dopaminergic activity and the development of schizophrenia has been the most promising and widely accepted hypothesis of schizophrenia. It is also one of the most generative yet perplexing hypotheses in the schizophrenia literature.

The dopamine hypothesis of schizophrenia in its most basic form states that an excess of dopamine neurotransmission in the brains of persons with schizophrenia leads to psychotic symptoms. Evidence supporting the dopamine hypothesis comes from a variety of sources. Some of the most compelling studies supporting the dopamine hypothesis showed that the relative clinical potency of antipsychotic medications is closely correlated with their ability to block D_2 receptors. That observation suggests that the mechanism of action of antipsychotic medications is attributable to a reduction in dopamine neurotransmission.

Many investigators have proposed variations of the basic dopamine hypothesis. One is that dopaminergic activity is reduced in the prefrontal and other cortical regions and increased in subcortical and limbic regions. Reduced cortical dopamine may explain impaired cognition and other negative symptoms (such as anhedonia and lack of motivation). Increased subcortical and limbic dopamine levels, on the other hand, could be related to positive symptoms (such as hallucinations and delusions). The prefrontal cortex appears to regulate subcortical and limbic dopaminergic neurotransmission, leading to speculation that a primary cortical deficit produces a secondary increase in subcortical and limbic dopamine. A variant hypothesis is that initial increases in prefrontal cortical dopamine levels lead to progressive down-regulation or depletion in the prefrontal cortex. Several studies have shown that prefrontal dopamine levels are increased with stress. That observation suggests that stress-induced increases in prefrontal dopamine could lead to chronic depletions in the prefrontal regions and secondary increases in the subcortical and limbic regions. Numerous studies have sought evidence of those changes in the dopamine system. To appreciate the results of those studies, it is helpful to understand the basic biology of the dopamine systems.

NEUROBIOLOGY OF DOPAMINE Dopamine is synthesized from tyrosine through levodopa (Larodopa, Dopar) (the rate-limiting step for dopamine formation is the synthesis of levodopa from tyrosine by tyrosine hydroxylase) (Figure 14.4-1). Dopamine is metabolized to inactive products that can be removed from the CNS. Those inactive products include 3-methoxytyramine (3-MT), dihydroxyphenylacetic acid (DOPAC), and homovanillic acid (HVA). Levels of those metabolites have been examined in the brain, cerebrospinal fluid (CSF), plasma, and urine of patients with schizophrenia in search of evidence of increased or decreased dopamine neurotransmission.

The cell bodies of the dopamine-containing neurons are primarily located in two small mesencephalic nuclei. The dopamine cell bodies that form the nigrostriatal tract are primarily in the substantia nigra (pars compacta). Slightly more anterior and medial, in the decussation of the superior cerebellar peduncle, are the nonpigmented dopamine neurons of the ventral tegmental area (VTA). Those neurons project to the nucleus accumbens and the prefrontal cortex and make up the mesolimbic and mesocortical systems, respectively. A fourth dopamine tract is found entirely within the hypothalamus. That tract includes two parts, the incertohypothalamic system and the tuberoinfundibular tract. The latter gives dopaminergic innervation to the median eminence and pituitary gland. The arcuate system may be useful for studies of schizophrenia because it can be studied by relatively noninvasive techniques. For example, serum concentrations of prolactin and growth hormone, which reflect hypothalamic dopaminergic activity, have often been studied in schizophrenia.

There are at least five types of CNS dopamine receptors, D_1 through D_5, identified on the basis of their DNA sequence. Most pharmacological functions of dopamine receptors characterized so far are attributed to D_1 and D_2 receptors. Little is known about the actions of the D_3, D_4, and D_5 receptors. D_1 receptors can be differentiated from D_2 receptors using pharmacological probes. Binding studies indicate that the D_1 and D_2 receptors may themselves exist in two forms, one with high affinity (the degree to which the agonist or antagonist binds), the other with low affinity. One important difference is that D_1 receptors stimulate whereas D_2 receptors inhibit the activity of the enzyme adenylate cyclase through interactions with the receptor-linked G proteins. Adenylate cyclase in turn synthesizes the second messenger, cyclic adenosine monophosphate (cAMP). Activation of dopamine receptors may also activate third messengers and immediate early genes, such as c-fos and c-jun. Those early genes may regulate a variety of changes in gene expression.

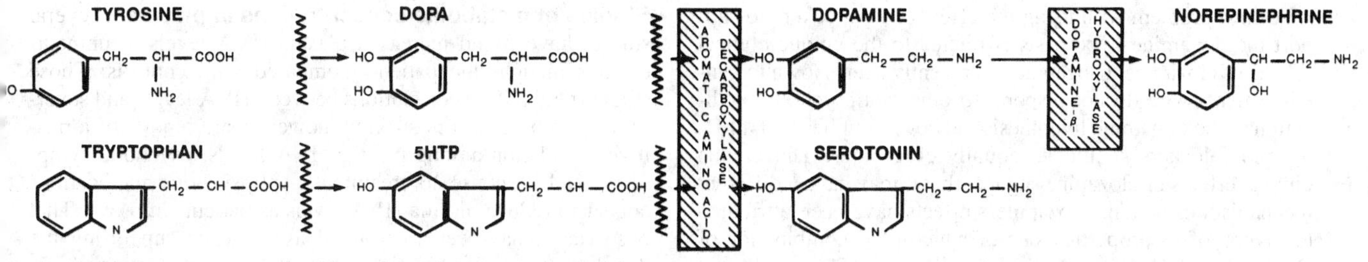

FIGURE 14.4-1 *Structures and metabolic pathways of serotonin and of the catecholamines dopamine and norepinephrine.*

D_1 and D_2 receptors are found predominantly in areas that receive innervation from dopaminergic neurons. The highest concentrations occur on the primary efferent neurons of the prefrontal cortex, striatum, and limbic system (in particular the nucleus accumbens). D_2 receptors are also located on the presynaptic dopamine terminal, where they appear to affect dopamine synthesis and release. The function of dopamine receptors on postsynaptic neurons (γ-aminobutyric acid [GABA]-ergic medium spiny neurons) is unclear. In the striatum the primary efferent (outflow) neurons have D_1 or D_2 receptors, or both. The effect of dopamine receptor activation in those neurons appears to be inhibitory under some conditions, although excitation has also been reported. Inhibition versus excitation may depend on whether D_1 or D_2 receptors predominate. The medium spiny neurons are heterogeneous, containing a variety of neuropeptide transmitters, or neuromodulators, in addition to GABA. The function of those peptides appears to be regulated in part by dopamine. Alterations in peptide neurotransmission could play a role in schizophrenia. Less is known about the effects of dopamine in limbic and prefrontal cortical regions. The prefrontal cortex is relatively rich in D_1 receptors, compared with the D_2 receptor-rich areas of the striatum. That observation has led to attempts to improve cortical function with D_1 stimulators while blocking subcortical D_2 receptors.

EVIDENCE FOR ALTERED DOPAMINE NEUROTRANSMISSION IN SCHIZOPHRENIA Evidence for the dopamine hypothesis of schizophrenia comes from a variety of sources. One approach has been to examine the effects of different medications on schizophrenic symptoms. As mentioned previously, sustained treatment with antipsychotic medications that block D_2 receptors relieves psychotic symptoms. Dopamine agonists, on the other hand, may worsen symptoms. A second approach has been to look at various indices of dopaminergic activity in patients with schizophrenia. Those indices include measures of presynaptic activity, such as the major dopamine metabolites DOPAC and HVA, as well as postsynaptic markers, primarily dopamine receptors. Metabolite studies have examined HVA in the CSF, plasma, urine, and autopsied brain. Receptor studies have been performed on postmortem brain tissue and, more recently, in living patients using PET and a related technology, single photon emission computed tomography (SPECT). Newer methods are being developed that can also assess presynaptic dopamine levels and dopamine release using those two neuroimaging techniques. Dopamine neurotransmission could be altered by changes in any one of a number of neuronal functions, including synthesis, degradation, release, uptake, receptor binding or activity, or even presynaptic-postsynaptic receptor mismatch. Although several decades of research have not definitively affirmed the dopamine hypothesis, investigators are beginning to appreciate the complexity of the dopamine systems and are finding new ways to study and modulate dopaminergic activity.

Clinical effects of dopaminergic agents The hypothesis of a dopamine excess in schizophrenia is best supported by clinical observations on the effects of drugs that modulate dopaminergic transmission. First, medications that reduce psychotic symptoms appear to do so by decreasing dopamine neurotransmission. Second, those that increase dopamine, such as amphetamine, when given in high doses or for prolonged periods of time are capable of producing a paranoid psychosis similar to paranoid schizophrenia. Although both observations are compelling and strongly implicate dopamine, neither ultimately supports the view that schizophrenia is due simply to increased dopamine neurotransmission.

In 1963 Arvid Carlsson and M. Lindquist reported that antipsychotic medications such as chlorpromazine (Thorazine) and haloperidol (Haldol) increased brain 3-MT, a major metabolite of dopamine. Medications that did not alter the symptoms of schizophrenia did not increase 3-MT. Carlsson and Lindquist proposed that antipsychotic medications block dopamine receptors, thereby increasing the production of dopamine metabolites. That hypothesis was supported by the observation that antipsychotic agents produced parkinsonian side effects, symptoms that had recently been linked to deficits in striatal dopamine. Finally, 14 years later two groups reported a striking correlation between the relative clinical potencies of antipsychotics and their ability to bind to D_2 receptors in in vitro preparations of striatum. Those landmark studies demonstrated that at least some antipsychotic effects were mediated by D_2 receptor blockade.

Although the correlation between clinical potency and D_2 receptor blockade for antipsychotic medications was compelling evidence for the dopamine hypothesis, several problems remained. D_2 receptor blockade occurs within hours of administration of antipsychotic medications, but the antipsychotic effects of the medications often take days or weeks to fully develop. The delay suggests that a secondary process is required. One possibility is depolarization inactivation. After several weeks of treatment, dopamine neurons become depolarized and no longer fire. That phenomenon was thought to produce a marked reduction in dopamine release and suggests that reduced dopamine neurotransmission mediates antipsychotic efficacy. A number of studies, however, have not found reduced dopamine release after chronic treatment with antipsychotic medication, suggesting that some process other than reduced dopamine release must underlie the therapeutic effects of those medications.

Another problem with invoking the mechanism of action of antipsychotic medications to support the dopamine hypothesis is that at times those medications work minimally or not at all. Not only are some patients refractory to treatment, but many patients continue to have cognitive deficits and negative symptoms despite having had a marked response to treatment. That finding suggests that schizophrenia involves more than a simple increase or alteration in dopamine neurotransmission.

A third problem with using the effect of D_2 blockers to support the dopamine hypothesis is related to the unique clinical effects of clozapine. Clozapine has recently been shown to benefit patients who do not respond to other antipsychotic medications. The dopamine hypothesis, however, implies that all D_2 receptor blockers should be equally efficacious. The unique clinical effects of clozapine suggest that it may have a different mechanism of action. Clozapine's effects have been attributed to several of its properties, one of which is its combination of D_1 and D_2 blockade. A second possibility involves serotonin (discussed later under serotonin). The pharmaceutical industry has developed a number of relatively selective D_1 and D_2 antagonists, some of which are in preclinical or clinical trials.

A second line of evidence supporting the dopamine hypothesis comes from observations on the effects of dopamine agonists. Chronic amphetamine ingestion, for example, can lead to a paranoid psychosis similar to paranoid schizophrenia. The process is thought to be mediated by amphetamine-induced release of dopamine. Amphetamine-induced psychoses, however, lack a number of features commonly associated with schizophrenia, such as the presence of negative symptoms, the specific kinds of auditory hallucinations that occur in schizophrenia, and a chronic course. Furthermore, psychotic symptoms develop only after prolonged use (or with very high doses), whereas dopamine neurotransmission is increased shortly after amphetamine administration. Those differences suggest that repeated increases in dopamine release may induce other changes that are more directly responsible for producing a paranoid psychosis.

Occasionally, patients with Parkinson's disease develop a psychosis that is attributed to treatment with levodopa, although it is unclear if the psychosis is related to the release of dopamine or norepinephrine. Perhaps more important are case reports of dopamine agonists such as bromocriptine (Parlodel) producing psychosis. Although those drug-induced psychotic conditions again implicate dopamine, they are seen in only a minority of patients, usually following chronic treatment.

Studies of metabolite concentrations in cerebrospinal fluid A large number of studies have looked for changes in CSF dopamine, HVA, and DOPAC levels. Although most studies have failed to find elevated levels, several have reported positive correlations between HVA concentration and the severity of positive symptoms. That finding suggests that increased dopamine transmission may be related to the production of active symptoms. On the other hand, studies of medication-free patients have found that concentrations of dopamine metabolites are decreased. Negative correlations have been found between HVA concentrations and ventricular enlargement or the severity of negative symptoms (for example, poor-prognosis anhedonia, flat affect, cognitive impairment).

Several methodological issues make the interpretation of those studies problematic. First, dopamine and metabolite concentrations in the CSF are affected by a number of variables that have not always been controlled, among them diet, time of day, height, and motor activity. Second, increased ventricular volume itself could affect the concentration of HVA. Third, CSF monoamine levels may have little relation to actual neurotransmission in a specific brain region. Certainly, if dopamine transmission in the prefrontal cortex is reduced and subcortical transmission is increased, it is difficult to predict what would happen to CSF levels. Nevertheless, CSF data are often interpreted as supporting the supposition that too much dopamine is related to positive symptoms and too little underlies negative symptoms.

Studies of metabolite concentrations in plasma Several studies have found increased plasma HVA levels in unmedicated schizophrenic patients compared with controls. Those studies tend to find correlations between HVA levels and severity of psychosis. More striking, however, are reports of a positive correlation among plasma HVA levels, psychotic symptoms, and response to treatment. Antipsychotic medications appear to reduce plasma HVA levels as patients improve. That observation has been interpreted as evidence supporting the depolarization inactivation hypothesis of antipsychotic medication.

As with CSF studies, methodological problems cloud the interpretation of plasma HVA levels. It is unclear whether plasma HVA levels correlate with HVA levels in limbic brain regions—the area most likely to underlie the production of psychotic symptoms. More problematic, however, are reports that HVA concentration, whether measured in the plasma, CSF, or brain, is not correlated with actual dopamine neurotransmission or release. It is more likely an index of dopamine metabolism that may or may not be related to alterations in release.

Studies of metabolite concentrations in urine There are surprisingly few studies of urinary dopamine and its metabolites in patients with schizophrenia. One study found that when the molar sum of dopamine and its metabolites was expressed as a ratio over the sum of norepinephrine and its metabolites, medication-free schizophrenic patients had a lower mean ratio than a group of normal controls. The ratio normalized after treatment with antipsychotic medications. That finding suggests an overall reduction in body and perhaps brain dopamine metabolism. Again, the significance of that change for alterations in dopamine neurotransmission in different brain regions is not known.

Studies of metabolite concentrations in brain A number of postmortem studies of patients with schizophrenia and control subjects have found increased dopamine or HVA concentrations in a variety of brain regions, although the reports are often inconsistent. One investigation found increased dopamine concentrations in the left amygdala in schizophrenic patients, whereas a second reported increases in the nucleus accumbens. Often, changes in patients as compared with control subjects are attributed to the effects of antipsychotic medications.

Studies of brain dopamine receptors A number of studies using postmortem brain tissue show increased numbers of D_2 receptor binding sites in the brains of schizophrenic patients. A major issue is whether the increase is a primary alteration in schizophrenia or represents a reaction to the antipsychotic medication. Studies in nonmedicated and medication-naive patients are conflicting. A number of studies of patients off medication for at least one month have found increased numbers of D_2 receptors, although several have not. Philip Seeman and coworkers have suggested that treatment with antipsychotic medications cannot account for the marked increase in and bimodal distribution of D_2 receptors seen in patients who had been treated. Imbalances between D_1 and D_2 receptors have also been reported. Recently, Seeman and others found that D_4 receptors, which are blocked by clozapine, may also be elevated in patients with schizophrenia.

PET has been used in living human patients to measure striatal D_2 receptors. Here, too, results have been conflicting. One study of medication-naive patients found increased numbers of receptors, while two others did not. Of the latter, one found higher D_2 densities on the left than on the right in schizophrenic patients. The asymmetry was not seen in the control group. Methodological refinements may produce more consistent studies in the future. PET and SPECT are relatively new technologies that hold promise for addressing the issue in the future.

Brain and peripheral enzymes involved in dopamine metabolism Increased levels or activity of enzymes in the synthetic pathway of dopamine might indicate that the brain is capable of making excess dopamine. On the other hand, a reduction in enzymes involved in dopamine degradation could also lead to a dopamine excess. Tyrosine hydroxylase, the enzyme responsible for converting tyrosine to levodopa, has been found to be normal in several postmortem studies of different areas of the brain in schizophrenics. Decreased monoamine oxidase in autopsied brains of patients with schizophrenia was first described in 1941. Although all but one of the subsequent studies failed to confirm that finding, decreased monoamine oxidase activity has been found in the majority of studies of platelet, lymphocyte, and muscle samples from schizophrenic patients. However, the size of the decrease (usually less than 40 percent, compared with 99 percent in most genetic enzymatic defect diseases) makes it unlikely that the alteration is of direct physiological importance. Furthermore, a number of studies have indicated that, at least in platelets, monoamine oxidase activity can be significantly decreased by antipsychotic medication.

Animal models Animal studies have been invaluable in efforts to understand normal and abnormal function of the dopamine system. Those studies have shown that striatal dopamine regulates motor activity and a variety of other functions. Mesolimbic dopamine neurotransmission is important for modulating motivation and reward. Prefrontal dopamine activity has been linked with higher cognitive function, such as working memory, planning, and problem solving. Of particular relevance for schizophrenia research are studies of environmental factors or insults that can produce long-term alterations in dopamine function.

Initial attempts to model schizophrenia employed chronic treatment with stimulants (such as amphetamine or cocaine). Administration of those stimulants may mimic, to some extent, the repeated stressors that can trigger psychotic relapses (and perhaps initial psychotic breaks) in patients with schizophrenia. The model has shown that dopaminergic agonists increase the sensitivity of the mesolimbic dopamine system (sensitization), which suggests that stress-induced dopamine release could play a role in psychotic decompensation. At higher doses stimulants may also reduce presynaptic indices of dopamine activity. Amphetamine and methamphetamine (Desoxyn) in particular have been shown to produce degeneration of dopamine axons. That finding led to speculations that chronic increases in dopaminergic transmission might eventually lead to long-term reductions or alterations in dopaminergic function. Stimulant-induced alterations could therefore have some aspects of increased as well as decreased dopaminergic activity. The representation could vary depending on brain region and environmental conditions.

Another promising line of animal research suggests an imbalance between dopamine activity in different brain regions. Dysfunction in one region may alter dopamine levels in another. Frontal lobe damage, for example, may lead to increased subcortical dopamine levels. Within the limbic system itself, hippocampal lesions, amygdala kindling, and lesions appear to increase dopamine indices in the nucleus accumbens. Prefrontal cortical dopamine levels, on the other hand, may be reduced. Of note, hippocampal pathology has been found in a number of neuroimaging and neuropathological studies of schizophrenia, which suggests that the hippocampus could mediate dopamine abnormalities in schizophrenia.

Animals have also been used to model psychophysiological and cognitive abnormalities in patients, such as backward masking, waveforms of the auditory evoked potential (such as P50), prepulse inhibition, and poor performance on delayed alternation tasks. In general, dopamine was found to modulate those phenomena in animal models. That finding suggests that information-processing abnormalities in schizophrenia are due in part to abnormal dopaminergic neurotransmission.

Animal research has implicated stress, stimulants, and limbic or prefrontal cortical abnormalities as factors that can alter dopamine function. Clinical research with patients tends to support the proposition that those factors may play some role in psychotic decompensation or in the initiation of illness. Animal homologues of the psychophysiological and cognitive abnormalities found in patients are also mediated by dopamine. Those models offer indirect support for the dopamine hypothesis and provide valuable tools to explore how such alterations in dopamine (and other neurotransmitter systems) could be corrected with new therapeutic agents.

Location of changes Numerous studies with pneumoencephalography, CT, and MRI and postmortem measurements have shown that localized alterations in brain structure are present in some patients with schizophrenia. Those alterations include enlargement of the lateral and third ventricles, widened cortical sulci, and decreased hippocampal and amygdala size. In some patients there may be reductions in prefrontal cortical size even when there is little evidence of alterations in other cortical areas. The structural abnormalities are consistent with studies demonstrating relatively decreased regional cerebral blood flow and metabolism in the prefrontal cortex (hypofrontality), particularly when the prefrontal cortex has been specifically activated. The structural abnormalities are also consistent with poor performance on neuropsychological tests of prefrontal function.

Structural abnormalities could be related to altered dopamine neurotransmission. As mentioned earlier, animal studies have shown that subcortical dopamine is regulated by limbic and frontal cortical areas. The subtle pathology demonstrated in those areas could induce alterations in subcortical dopamine in patients with schizophrenia. Furthermore, frontal cortical pathology and hypofrontality raise the possibility of an underlying deficit in cortical dopamine. Unfortunately, preliminary attempts to increase cortical dopamine with D_1 agonists have not been encouraging.

INTEGRATIVE DOPAMINE HYPOTHESES The dopamine hypothesis has been of great heuristic value, generating thousands of basic science and clinical experiments. A number of hypotheses have been generated to synthesize what is known about dopamine with other important clinical facts about schizophrenia. Two kinds of hypotheses that have recently been proposed are described below.

Neurodegeneration hypotheses Neurodegeneration hypotheses suggest that a neurodegenerative process produces the structural alterations and cognitive deficits common in patients with schizophrenia. MRI and CT have shown a variety of structural abnormalities, such as enlarged ventricles and reduced volume of such temporal lobe structures as the hippocampus and amygdala. Most patients exhibit a marked cognitive decline early in the illness, when positive psychotic symptoms are most prominent. Progressive dysfunction or degeneration in key areas, such as the prefrontal cortex or hippocampus, could lead to alterations in mesolimbic and mesocortical dopamine systems. Prospective neuroimaging studies should help identify the course of structural brain changes. Several initial studies suggest that ventricular abnormalities may predate the onset of psychotic symptoms and that temporal lobe and limbic changes may develop later.

Alternatively, a primary dopamine abnormality could induce neurodegenerative changes. Schizophrenic patients could have a vulnerable dopaminergic system (perhaps genetic) that, under repeated stress, could lead to overactivity and a subsequent loss of dopaminergic terminals, similar to the situation produced by high doses of amphetamine. The theory of a primary dopamine abnormality suggests that a vulnerable stress-response system is initially responsible for increased dopamine turnover and the positive psychotic symptoms of schizophrenia. The progressive loss of dopamine terminals is ultimately responsible for negative symptoms and the burned-out state. Structural abnormalities and cognitive deficits could result from secondary alterations in the glutamatergic system. Excessive glutamate has been shown to produce neurodegeneration.

Neurodegenerative hypotheses take into consideration structural and dopaminergic abnormalities, account for the role of stress, and are consistent with the observation that patients whose illness begins with predominantly positive symptoms often subsequently develop predominantly negative symptoms. It does not readily explain season of birth or age at onset. The lack of solid evidence for neuronal degeneration (that is, gliosis) argues against those hypotheses.

Neurodevelopmental hypothesis The neurodevelopmental hypothesis suggests that an insult early in development, perhaps in utero, is responsible for the cortical abnormalities described in patients with schizophrenia, including a variety of cognitive deficits and structural abnormalities. Psychotic symptoms are not expressed until late adolescence, owing to maturational changes in the brain. Cognitive functions such as those subserved by the prefrontal cortex may not fully develop until late adolescence. Late development may be related to the delayed myelination of the prefrontal cortex. As the prefrontal cortex comes on line in late adolescence, abnormal function becomes manifest. Dopamine systems may become involved at that point. With reduced prefrontal function, mesolimbic dopamine systems may also become dysfunctional, as described in animal models. Increased or altered mesolimbic dopamine may account for positive symptoms.

The neurodevelopment hypothesis accounts for age at onset of schizophrenia and for structural and dopaminergic abnormalities. It may also accommodate observations on the effects of stress and season of birth. It less easily accounts for the course of illness, particularly the reduction in I.Q. and marked neuropsychological impairment that develop within the first few years of the illness. Furthermore, the existence of childhood schizophrenia is difficult to explain.

NOREPINEPHRINE

NOREPINEPHRINE IN THE BRAIN Like dopamine, norepinephrine, the neurotransmitter of the sympathetic autonomic nervous system, is widely distributed in the brain. It is most highly concentrated in the hypothalamus, thalamus, limbic system, and cerebellum. Cell bodies of noradrenergic neurons are located primarily in the locus ceruleus, located beneath the floor of the fourth ventricle. The first proposed subdivision of noradrenergic receptors was into two types—α-receptors, found in cortical and limbic structures, and β-receptors, found in cortical projections and in the cerebellum. Responses attributed to α-adrenergic receptor activation are primarily excitatory; responses attributed to β-adrenergic receptor activation are inhibitory, with the exception of myocardial stimulant effects. α-Noradrenergic receptors have been further subdivided into α_1- and α_2-receptors. Presynaptic receptors are α_2; postsynaptic neurons contain α_1-receptors. All three receptors are linked to the activation of the second messenger cAMP. The presynaptic α_2-adrenergic receptor, known as an autoreceptor, mediates feedback through its sensitivity to the product (norepinephrine) released by the neuron, and decreases both the firing of norepinephrine neurons and norepinephrine release.

Hypotheses concerning the normal functioning of CNS norepinephrine neurons include a role in learning and memory, mood and affect, reinforcement, sleep-wake cycle regulation, anxiety, and nociperception, as well as a more general role in the regulation of CNS blood flow and metabolism. Animal behavior studies support the idea that norepinephrine, along with dopamine, may play a role in the reward system. Activation of the locus ceruleus with electrodes produces such behaviors as reward-directed, self-stimulating lever pressing.

NOREPINEPHRINE AND SCHIZOPHRENIA David Wise, Larry Stein, and Michael Baden proposed that schizophrenia may be related either to a defect in the noradrenergic reward system or to selective norepinephrine neuron degeneration, producing the anhedonia (or lack of self-initiated goal-directed behavior) characteristic of many chronic schizophrenic patients. Wise and Stein's original hypothesis of reduced dopamine-β-hydroxylase has not been confirmed. Exploration of other aspects of noradrenergic dysfunction in schizophrenia continues, motivated in part by frequent clinical observations of increased autonomic arousal during both the prodromal phase and the psychotic phases of some schizophrenic patients' courses. Those observations are consistent with initial reports of the successful treatment of schizophrenia with propranolol (Inderal), a medication that blocks β-adrenergic receptors. Unfortunately, propranolol has not proved to be consistently efficacious in subsequent studies.

There have been many studies of both peripheral and central noradrenergic metabolism in schizophrenia. Early studies on periodic catatonia, a questionable form of schizophrenia, generally did not find the norepinephrine metabolite 3-methoxy-4-hydroxyphenylglycol (MHPG) to be elevated in the CSF. In the early 1970s studies showed that patients with periodic catatonia excreted more norepinephrine in their urine when they were in a stuporous phase than when they were in remission, and excreted more norepinephrine than healthy subjects. In a study that examined the genetic contribution to urinary catecholamine excretion, other investigators found that although MHPG was not elevated in schizophrenic patients, dopamine, norepinephrine, and epinephrine were elevated in the urine of both the schizophrenic and nonschizophrenic cotwins of monozygotic twin pairs when compared with normal subjects. Further, the values for the discordant twins were highly correlated with each other. One recent report of urinary norepinephrine and MHPG in medication-free schizophrenic patients reported unaltered levels; in contrast, studies of urinary norepinephrine in patients with mood disorders have reported low levels. Plasma norepinephrine and MHPG levels in medication-free patients with acute and chronic schizophrenia have been reported to be increased. It is possible, however, that those measurements can be affected by the position of the patient's body and perhaps by antipsychotic medication. Several studies have shown an association between the clinical state and such peripheral measures.

At least five studies have reported higher concentrations of norepinephrine in the CSF of some patients with chronic schizophrenia (particularly those with paranoid schizophrenia) than in control subjects. Of particular interest is the finding of Daniel van Kammen and Mary Kelley that patients who decompensated following withdrawal of haloperidol had higher CSF norepinephrine levels, both before and after medication withdrawal, than patients who did not relapse. Other studies have found an increase in norepinephrine levels with the activation of psychosis. It appears, however, that antipsychotic medications may increase norepinephrine concentrations by inhibiting metabolism. It is possible, therefore, that studies that reported norepinephrine data on patients two or three weeks after the withdrawal of antipsychotics were still seeing some of the long-term effects of medication. Nevertheless, a recent study from Japan suggests that plasma MHPG is elevated in acute schizophrenia prior to treatment with antipsychotic medications.

In postmortem brain studies of patients with paranoid schizophrenia, one group reported increased norepinephrine concentrations in the limbic region, and a second found increases in the mesencephalon. A third study, which did not include paranoid schizophrenic patients, found high levels of both norepinephrine and MHPG in the nucleus accumbens. Although the studies together suggest an alteration in norepinephrine metabolism in at least a subgroup of schizophrenic patients, the issue of the effect of medication, particularly in the postmortem studies, has not been resolved.

Investigations of noradrenergic receptors have also been conducted. In some areas their juxtaposition of dopaminergic neurons has led to interesting hypotheses of feedback loops and inhibitory-excitatory mechanisms. There is little information about β-adrenergic receptors in schizophrenics, but van Kammen recently found a negative correlation between β-adrenergic receptor activity on lymphocytes and the antipsychotic effects of propranolol. α_2-Adrenergic receptor function on platelets has been studied in medication-free schizophrenic patients as a model for α_2-adrenergic receptor function in the brain. Elevated numbers of α_2-adrenergic receptors have been found to be associated with a deficiency in prostaglandin E_1-stimulated cAMP production, a function known to be inhibited by α_2-adrenergic receptor stimulation. Although it is not known whether those peripheral findings parallel brain metabolism, one study found increased α_2-adrenergic receptor numbers in the autopsied brains of schizophrenic patients. It is also of interest that α_1-adrenergic receptors in rat brain are uniformly elevated after long-term treatment with a variety of antipsychotic medications, including clozapine. Another indication of an abnormality in norepinephrine function in schizophrenic patients is that clonidine (Catapres) (a presynaptic α_2-receptor agonist that, in low doses, reduces norepinephrine release) suppresses plasma MHPG in healthy persons but not in schizophrenic patients. A series of studies found that patients who are likely to relapse when taken off antipsychotic medications have a larger response to challenges with stimulants such as methylphenidate (Ritalin). Such stimulants are usually thought to affect the dopamine system but may also stimulate the norepinephrine system. Finally, antipsychotic medications have been found to consistently increase the number of α_1-adrenergic receptors in animals treated with those medications for prolonged periods, although there is no correlation between α_1-adrenergic receptor binding and the relative clinical potencies of the antipsychotic medications.

In clinical medication trials norepinephrine agents have had mixed success. In one study clonidine produced a transient reduction in symptoms in some schizophrenic patients while concurrently reducing plasma norepinephrine and MHPG concentrations. A second study reported clonidine to be as effective as a typical antipsychotic medication for the reduction of schizophrenic symptoms; however, several additional reports found no therapeutic benefit. Although relatively few studies have been performed with clonidine, it appears to have a more noticeable effect when given without antipsychotic medications. One group recently added the α_2-adrenergic receptor antagonist idazoxane to fluphenazine (Prolixin) in chronic schizophrenic patients and found some improvement, compared with treatment with fluphenazine alone. On the other hand, one study reported that yohimbine (Yocon), also an α_2-adrenoceptor antagonist, made acutely ill schizophrenic patients worse. In another study of yohimbine, more stable patients were not affected. Phenoxybenzamine (Dibenzyline), a mixed α-adrenergic receptor antagonist, has not been of benefit in schizophrenia. The results of the three studies are clearly inconsistent.

The studies reviewed here do not contain sufficient evidence to suggest that a defect in the norepinephrine system is primary to the development of schizophrenia. Although elevations in plasma, CSF, and brain norepinephrine levels, particularly in patients with paranoid schizophrenia have been reported by a number of investigators, the reasons for the elevations are unclear. In aggregate, however, the studies implicate an alteration in norepinephrine metabolism or response to stress in at least some schizophrenic patients. The noradrenergic system not only is integral to the body's response to stress but is also involved in modulating the dopaminergic system.

SEROTONIN

Although the link between serotonin and depression is well accepted, a possible role for serotonin in schizophrenia is more speculative. Such a role was first hypothesized when the hallucinogen lysergic acid dethylamide (LSD) was found to block serotonin receptors. Subsequent studies looking for evidence of altered serotonin neurochemistry had mixed results. Clinical medication trials are more intriguing. Some data suggest that altering serotonergic function could improve patients with schizophrenia, or at least reduce antipsychotic-induced motoric side effects. Even if no clear role is identified for serotonin in the neurochemistry of schizophrenia, serotonergic agents may eventually play a significant role in the treatment of psychosis.

BASIC NEUROBIOLOGY Serotonin (5-hydroxytryptamine [5-HT]) is synthesized from tryptophan and broken down into 5-hydroxyindoleacetic acid (5-HIAA) (Figure 14.4-1). Synthesis of 5-HT depends on tryptophan concentrations. Indeed, some studies have shown that plasma tryptophan concentration is the rate-limiting factor for central serotonin synthesis. Tryptophan is an essential amino acid that is found in the diet and is transported into the brain. Although low dietary tryptophan intake markedly reduces central 5-HT neurotransmission, an increase in dietary intake does not appear to significantly increase 5-HT neurotransmission. The synthesis of 5-HT is also modulated by autoreceptor inhibition from 5-HT itself.

The serotonergic system is part of the brainstem reticular formation. 5-HT neuronal cell bodies are located primarily in nine separate nuclei of the raphe and reticular region. Most ascending 5-HT pathways originate in the medial and dorsal raphe. Axons from those nuclei course through the median forebrain bundle to project to forebrain structures such as the cortex, striatum, cingulate, and a variety of limbic structures. In the rat, cortical projections are distributed in a uniform pattern, whereas in humans there is marked variability from one cortical area to another.

Serotonin cells fire in a regular, slow, rhythmic pattern that is autoregulated by inhibitory feedback axon collaterals and dendritic autoreceptors. Cell firing is also controlled by feedback from a variety of target regions such as the prefrontal cortex, the substantia nigra, and limbic regions. Substantial cross-innervation exists between 5-HT, norepinephrine, and dopamine systems, and the activities of those systems may be coordinated. 5-HT cell firing rates correlate with levels of arousal, can be altered by extreme external stimuli, and are inhibited during rapid eye movement sleep.

The effect of 5-HT on target neurons is excitatory or inhibitory, depending on which receptors are expressed by the postsynaptic neuron. Currently, four classes of 5-HT receptors have been characterized, 5-HT_1 through 5-HT_4. As many as five subtypes of 5-HT_1 receptors, 1a through 1e, have been described. There may be two 5-HT_2 receptors, 5-HT_{2a} and 5-HT_{2b}. Some authors have suggested that the 5-HT_{1c} receptor, with its structural similarity with 5-HT_2 receptors, also belongs in the 5-HT_2 group. 5-HT_2 receptors are found in the prefrontal cortex, nucleus accumbens, striatum, and, peripherally, in platelets. Platelet concentrations have been used to assess 5-HT levels, receptor number, and uptake because they are more accessible than brain regions and have been hypothesized to reflect central synaptic activity. 5-HT_3 receptors are also found in a variety of cortical and subcortical areas, including the amygdala, hippocampus, and nucleus accumbens. 5-HT receptor activation can produce alterations in second messenger systems, including cAMP and phosphoinositide, and can suppress potassium conductance.

The serotonergic system modulates a wide variety of physiological processes and behaviors. One of the best-studied effects is its regulation of dopaminergic neurotransmission. 5-HT_2 antagonists, for example, increase dopaminergic neuronal firing. 5-HT receptors on striatal dopaminergic terminals inhibit dopamine release. Behaviorally, 5-HT appears to be important in modulating movement, emesis, sexual behavior, and pain perception. 5-HT agonists induce resting tremors, head weaving, and other postural and movement abnormalities. In humans, 5-HT uptake blockers are effective antidepressants and offer one of the few treatments for severe obsessions and compulsions. Further, a so-called hyperserotonergic syndrome has been described that includes fever, delirium, seizures, and death. Lesions of 5-HT raphe neurons produce hyperactivity and hyperresponsivity.

Specific receptor agonists and antagonists are increasing clinicians' understanding of serotonergic function and its role in psychiatric disorders. In rats, 5-HT_1 agonists have anxiolytic and antiaggressive properties. In humans, the partial 5-HT_{1a} agonist buspirone (BuSpar) is marketed as an anxiolytic. On the other hand, the 5-HT_2 antagonist ritanserin reduces depression and anxiety and improves sleep in humans. Blockade of 5-HT_3 receptors with odansetron appears to have antiemetic properties. 5-HT_{1a} agonists and 5-HT_2 and 5-HT_3 antagonists either have been used or are being used in treatment studies for patients with schizophrenia.

EVIDENCE FOR ALTERED SEROTONERGIC NEUROTRANSMISSION IN SCHIZOPHRENIA Speculation that reduced 5-HT neurotransmission could underlie psychotic symptoms in patients with schizophrenia began with the discovery that the hallucinogen LSD binds to 5-HT receptors. Schizophrenic symptoms could be due, for example, to the formation of endogenous methylated biogenic amines that could, like LSD, have hallucinogenic properties. Since initial attempts to find such compounds were not fruitful, subsequent studies looked for differences in the parameters of 5-HT neurotransmission between patients with schizophrenia and normal subjects. Relevant parameters have included levels of 5-HT or its metabolite 5-HIAA in platelets, blood, CSF, and brain. Recently, postmortem brain studies have begun to quantify receptor subtypes in various brain regions. Specific 5-HT receptor antagonists have also been tried clinically in psychotic patients.

Studies measuring 5-HT levels in peripheral fluids have not clearly demonstrated differences between patients with schizophrenia and controls. At least eight groups have found increased 5-HT levels in platelets or blood, although several other studies have not. The reasons for a possible increase are unknown. Platelet uptake of 5-HT, on the other hand, has occasionally been reported to be reduced. The reduced uptake could be an effect of medication. CSF levels may be more relevant to serotonergic neurotransmission in the brain, although most studies have not found differences between patients and controls. Three groups, however, have reported reduced CSF 5-HIAA levels in drug-free patients with enlarged ventricles. Other studies have reported elevated levels of CSF-HIAA in schizophrenic patients with family histories of schizophrenia. Interpretation of the conflicting data is both problematic and complicated by the fact that the relation of blood, platelet, and CSF 5-HT levels to regional 5-HT neurotransmission in the CNS is unknown.

Studies of 5-HT in the brain have been mixed. The only two findings that have consistently been replicated are increased levels of 5-HT in the putamen and in the globus pallidus. Inconsistencies with other findings as a result of a variety of methodological problems, such as cause of death, time from death to autopsy, medication status, and reliability of postmortem diagnoses, underscore the difficulties of human postmortem studies. Brain receptor studies have so far produced one finding that has been replicated, a reduction in prefrontal cortical 5-HT_2 receptors. Several studies that failed to replicate that finding have been criticized for methodological problems. Reductions in uptake sites have also been reported in the dorsolateral prefrontal cortex, putamen, and caudate, but it is unclear if the reductions were due to the effects of treatment with antipsychotic medications.

Serotonergic function in patients with schizophrenia has been studied in vivo by studying neuroendocrine response to acute challenges with serotonergic agents. The secretion of cortisol, prolactin, renin, oxytocin, vasopressin, and growth hormone are all regulated by central serotonin input. Higher prolactin peaks and blunted growth hormone response have been reported in patients with schizophrenia following intravenous L-tryptophan. However, the inconsistent results and the unclear effects of antipsychotic medications make further studies necessary before conclusions can be drawn.

Some of the most intriguing data suggesting that serotonin may play a role in schizophrenia come from studies that looked at the mechanism of action of atypical antipsychotics, such as clozapine. Clozapine markedly improves symptoms in some patients who do not respond to other treatments. The atypical therapeutic effects suggest that it has a unique mechanism of action. Clozapine has several properties that could account for its atypicality, including weak D_2 affinity, relatively potent D_1 affinity, or D_4 binding. Another candidate is clozapine's 5-HT binding. Clozapine blocks 5-HT_{1c}, 5-HT_2, and 5-HT_3 receptors acutely. Like many antidepressants, it also produces a subsequent down-regulation of 5-HT_2 receptors.

Clozapine is similar to a number of other antipsychotic agents that are considered atypical because they produce few if any motoric side effects (such as dystonia and parkinsonism). Herbert Meltzer and colleagues have shown that such motorically atypical agents, when compared with typical antipsychotic medications, have greater 5-HT_2 affinity relative to D_2 affinity. That finding has led to speculation that clozapine's unique antipsychotic effects could also be due to 5-HT_2 blockade.

Efforts at producing medications similar to clozapine are ongoing. Risperidone (Risperdal) and setoperone, both of which block 5-HT_2 and D_2 receptors, appear to be fairly effective antipsychotics that produce fewer extrapyramidal side effects than typical antipsychotic medications. It is unclear whether or not they, like clozapine, have atypical antipsychotic effects as well. Typical antipsychotic medications have been combined with the 5-HT_2 antagonist ritanserin in attempts to produce atypical results. Some studies have shown significant improvement with ritanserin, particularly improvement in negative symptoms and motoric side effects, but others have not. Typical antipsychotic medications have also been combined with the 5-HT_3 antagonist odansetron. The results similarly suggested some antipsychotic efficacy and a reduced liability for motoric side effects.

A variety of other strategies have been used to alter 5-HT neurotransmission in schizophrenia. 5-HT precursors such as L-tryptophan and 5-HT have generally been ineffective antipsychotics, although they may reduce aggressiveness. Drugs that deplete 5-HT, including fenfluramine (Pondimin) and parachlorophenylalanine, have also been ineffective, as has methysergide (Sansert), a 5-HT_1 antagonist. 5-HT_{1a} agonists such as buspirone and eltoprazine appear to be anxiolytics. Some have suggested that those agents could also have antipsychotic or antiaggressive properties in patients with schizophrenia, although no clinical trials have yet been published to support that possibility.

Studies of patients with schizophrenia have failed to convincingly demonstrate that abnormalities in 5-HT neurotransmission mediate the expression of symptoms. Nevertheless, some data are suggestive. Postmortem receptor studies in particular have implicated frontal cortical 5-HT_2 abnormalities. Increased 5-HT levels in the nuclei of the basal ganglia suggest that that region could be involved as well. Finally, preliminary data from medication trials support the notion that specific 5-HT receptor blockers, particularly 5-HT_2 and 5-HT_3 antagonists, could play a future role in the pharmacotherapy of schizophrenia.

GLUTAMATE

Interest in glutamate's role in the pathophysiology of schizophrenia has developed only recently. That interest was spurred primarily by two observations. First, phencyclidine (PCP, angel dust) produces a clinical syndrome similar to schizophrenia, probably by blocking glutamate neurotransmission. Second, glutamate is an essential neurotransmitter in those neural networks that are thought to be involved in schizophrenia (discussed later under neural circuits). Thus, some alterations in glutamate neurotransmission are likely to underlie abnormalities in information processing in those brain circuits.

BASIC NEUROBIOLOGY Glutamate is one of the most prevalent neurotransmitters in the brain. Virtually all neurons in the brain are affected when glutamate is applied. A nonessential amino acid that does not cross the blood-brain barrier, glutamate can be synthesized in the brain from glutamine or, in the Krebs cycle, from α-ketoglutarate. The relative contributions of those pathways to the pool of glutamate that is relevant to neurotransmission are unclear. The dominant mode of inactivation of synaptic glutamate is via reuptake by a specific, high-affinity uptake site. Several agents block those uptake sites, but none have become pharmacological tools.

The three main classes of ionotropic glutamate receptors are named after their affinity for the following compounds: *N*-methyl-D-aspartate (NMDA), quinolinic acid, and kainic acid. Those receptors have been implicated in neurotoxicity through ischemia. The NMDA receptor is functionally different from the others and has been implicated in long-term potentiation (a process related to memory) in the hippocampus.

The NMDA receptor is a complex protein of particular relevance for schizophrenia research. Blockade of the NMDA receptor with phencyclidine, a noncompetitive antagonist, produces symptoms similar to those seen in schizophrenia. Of note, NMDA receptor density is highest in the hippocampus and prefrontal cortex, two areas that are implicated in schizophrenia. NMDA receptor activation opens an ion channel, permitting cationic flux. Cationic flux reduces the membrane potential, thus exciting postsynaptic neurons. The NMDA receptor has at least two modulatory sites that bind either to opioids at the σ opioid site or to glycine. Phencyclidine binds to a third site within the open ion channel, resulting in the blockade of ionic flux. Drugs that bind to the σ site also reduce NMDA activation and can produce psychotic symptoms. The mechanism by which NMDA antagonism produces psychotic symptoms is unclear but could be related to NMDA receptor effects on striatal and limbic dopaminergic neurotransmission.

Glutamate may be relevant to the neurochemistry of schizophrenia because of its role in key neural networks (discussed later under neural circuits). Descending projections from cortical and hippocampal pyramidal neurons use glutamate as their primary neurotransmitter. They include projections to subcortical structures, such as the striatum, nucleus accumbens, and VTA, whose outputs are strongly modulated by glutamate. Arvid Carlsson and Maria Carlsson have put forth an elegant proposal regarding the possible role of glutamate in schizophrenia. Based on their work and the work of others, it has become apparent that information flow through corticostriatothalamocortical loops may be altered in schizophrenia. Information flow through those loops depends heavily on glutamatergic neurotransmission and on numerous other transmitters such as dopamine, serotonin, and norepinephrine. Thus, by its position in key neural networks glutamate is probably involved in altered information processing in schizophrenia.

GLUTAMATE IN SCHIZOPHRENIA The observation that the NMDA antagonist phencyclidine produces a schizophrenialike syndrome has implicated glutamatergic circuits in schizophrenia. Phencyclidine abuse can lead to hallucinations, thought disorder, negative symptoms, and cognitive deficits. Acute phencyclidine intoxication reduces frontal cortical metabolism in control subjects, a finding similar to the hypofrontality seen in schizophrenia. In comparison, dopamine agonists such as amphetamine produce paranoid delusions. The differences in those drug-induced psychoses imply that reductions in glutamate neurotransmission may underlie some schizophrenic symptoms that are not produced by dopamine agonists and could thus be dopamine independent. Those symptoms, which include negative symptoms and cognitive deficits, are usually unresponsive to treatment with D_2 antagonists.

Studies of glutamate levels in the CSF and brain tissue of patients with schizophrenia have not been encouraging. One study found low levels of glutamate in the CSF of patients compared with controls. Possible methodological problems make the data difficult to interpret, and two subsequent studies were unable to replicate the finding. One study that used postmortem brain tissue found no differences in glutamate content between patients and controls in several regions, including the frontal cortex, nucleus accumbens, and caudate nucleus.

Postmortem receptor studies have been more promising. One study reported increased kainate binding in the medial frontal cortex but not in other cortical areas, such as the putamen. A second study reported increased kainate binding in both the medial and orbitofrontal cortex and increased glutamate uptake sites in the cortex. Other studies have reported an increased number of NMDA receptors (MK-801 binding) in the putamen and reduced kainate binding in the left hippocampus. The latter, however, was not seen on the right side. A quantitative autoradiography examination of kainate, NMDA, and quisqualate binding in the hippocampus also found a loss of kainate binding sites, with significant reductions in the CA4-CA3 mossy fiber termination zone of the cornu ammonis and bilateral reduction in the dentate and parahippocampal gyri. No alterations were seen in NMDA binding. In aggregate, the data suggest a loss of glutamatergic neurons in temporal areas. Increased receptors in the cortex and putamen could be due to reduced glutamatergic inputs or neurotransmission.

The clinical similarity between phencyclidine intoxication and schizophrenia, combined with data from postmortem studies, has stimulated clinical trials of glutamatergic agents in patients with schizophrenia. One problem with such clinical trials is the neurotoxic and epileptogenic potential of glutamate or NMDA agonists. To avoid those effects, agents that affect the regulatory subunits of the NMDA receptor have been used. Two preliminary, open-label studies using glycine were not strongly supportive. Milacemide, a glycine prodrug, has also been used, with similarly discouraging results. Antagonists of the σ opioid binding site have likewise not proved promising. Other compounds that have been considered for clinical use include cycloserine (a glycinelike agent) and polyamines, such as spermidine and spermine. Despite early negative reports, research in glutamate continues to hold promise for illuminating the neurochemical abnormalities that underlie schizophrenia.

NEURAL CIRCUITS

Abnormalities in the neurotransmitter systems described above implicate disordered information processing in several interconnected neural networks in individuals with schizophrenia (Figure 14.4-2). A brief overview describes how neurochemical abnormalities could result in the altered functioning of those neural circuits.

Dopamine abnormalities suggest that nigrostriatal (path 2 to 3), mesolimbic (path 2 to 1), or mesocortical (path 2 to 4) dopamine neurons and the pathways that regulate their activity may be dysfunctional. A simplified view of those circuits, some of the most widely studied circuits in the brain, is shown in Figure 14.4-2A. Dopamine cell bodies in the substantia nigra and VTA, both of which are in the midbrain, send axons to forebrain regions. The substantia nigra primarily projects to the striatum (caudate and putamen) (path 2 to 3). Those areas in turn send GABAergic projections back to the substantia nigra (path 3 to 2). VTA projections are regulated by projections from such limbic areas as the nucleus accumbens, ventral pallidum, and, most likely, from cortical regions (not shown). Further, cortical regions that receive dopaminergic innervation, such as the prefrontal cortex, amygdala, and hippocampus, also appear to regulate dopamine release in the nucleus accumbens and striatum (path 4 to 1), possibly through a presynaptic mechanism. That suggestion has led to speculation that dysfunction in those regions may increase limbic (for example, nucleus accumbens) dopamine levels (Figure 14.4-2B).

Dopamine projections to striatal, limbic, and cortical areas may play a role in modulating information flow through a larger group of circuits, shown in Figure 14.4-2C. A group of circuits sends information from the cortex through subcortical regions. The subcortical regions in turn project to the thalamus (path 5 to 6), which then projects the information back to the cortex (path 6 to 4). The nature of the information processing that occurs in those circuits is not clear. Garrett Alexander, Mahlon DeLong, and Peter Strick hypothesized that at least five functionally segregated parallel loops compose the corticostriatothalamic circuit, subserving functions related to movement, oculomotor activity, higher cognitive processing (such as spatial memory and behavioral sets), and limbic (emotional) processing. Impairments in many of those operations have consistently been demonstrated in patients with schizophrenia. The impairments are reflected in abnormal voluntary and involuntary movements, abnormal eye tracking, poor performance on prefrontal cognitive tasks, and reduced emotional responsivity (flat or blunted affect and poor motivation). Functional neuroimaging studies, such as SPECT and PET, have also shown reduced metabolism in parts of the circuit, such as the prefrontal cortex and thalamus.

A variety of neurotransmitter systems are involved in regulating information flow through the corticostriatothalamocortical loops, and some of those systems could be altered in schizophrenia. The primary input to the corticostriatothalamocortical loops comes from glutamatergic cortical neurons (4). Those neurons project first to the striatum and nucleus accumbens, where they synapse primarily on the main striatal output neurons, the GABAergic medium spiny neurons (1). The latter also receive dopaminergic innervation (path 2 to 1), most likely on the same dendritic spines. That allows dopamine and the glutamatergic input to mutually regulate each other and the outflow from the striatum.

The medium spiny striatal neurons project in two major outflow pathways. The two pathways may be antagonistic, each counterbalancing the output of the other. Both eventually project to the substantia nigra, and from there to the thalamus. The thalamic neurons complete the circuit by projecting back to the cortex (path 6 to 4). The balance between the two opposing output pathways from the striatum are important in determining how the thalamus regulates cortical activity. Imbalances in the motor loops, for example, produce parkinsonian symptoms or hyperkinetic movements such as choreathetosis. A number of neuropeptides, including enkephalin, substance P, somatostatin, and dynorphin, are colocalized in the GABAergic medium spiny neurons and may regulate their activity. Thus, output from the system is modulated by those peptides in addition to dopamine, norepinephrine, serotonin, cholecystokinin, glutamate, and GABA.

Dysfunction of the interconnected neural networks could arise from a variety of insults and could be reflected in the alteration of many neurotransmitter systems. Figure 14.4-2B, for example, describes the potential impact of dysfunction of the prefrontal cortex. Glutamatergic projections from the prefrontal cortex may alter dopamine neurotransmission in limbic regions—in Figure 14.4-2 through the nucleus accumbens (path 4 to 1). Figure 14.4–2D includes representation of the hippocampus and amygdala. Damage (presumably prenatal) to the hippocampus and amygdala could result in increased glutamatergic activity in neurons projecting from those structures (path

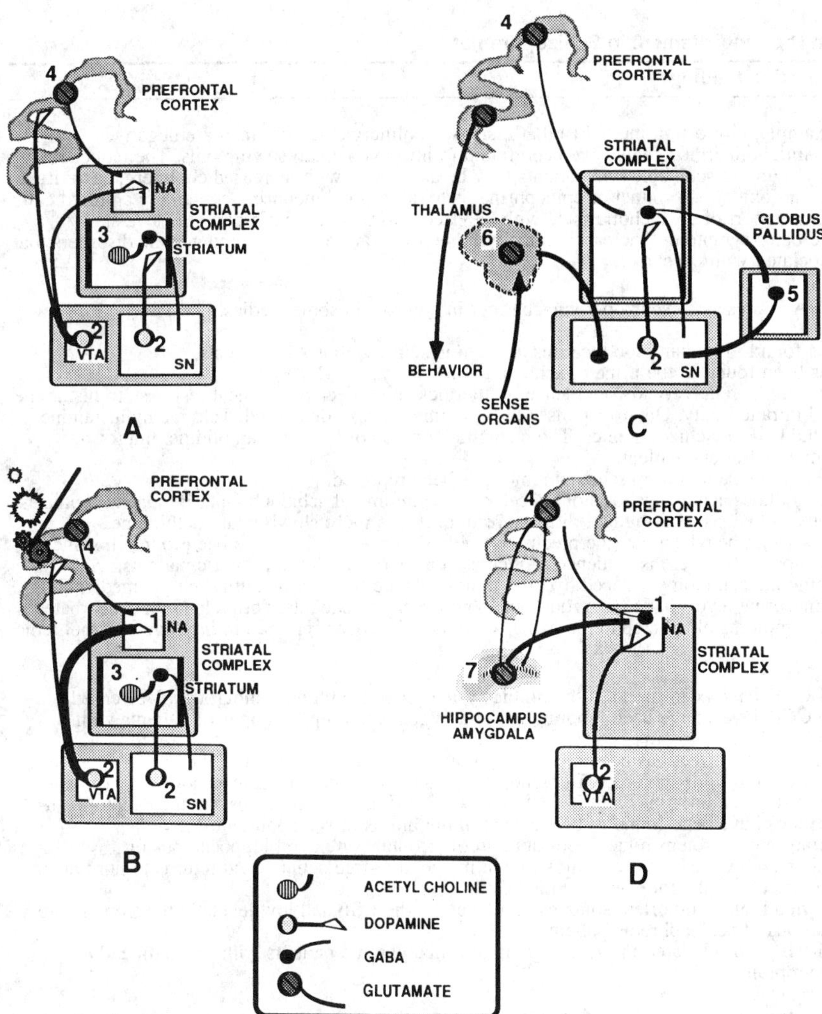

FIGURE 14.4-2 *Diagram of some of the brain circuitry that has been implicated in the pathophysiology of schizophrenia (see text). NA = nucleus accumbens, VTA = ventral tegmental area, SN = substantia nigra.*

7 to 1) to the nucleus accumbens. Consequently, dopaminergic transmission in the nucleus accumbens is altered. As a result of dopaminergic activity, dopamine D_2 receptors are increased. When the person becomes stressed, dopamine turnover increases in response to the stress; the result is an acute psychotic state from the excess dopamine transmission. Additional changes from prefrontal or hippocampal damage could also produce changes in serotonin, norepinephrine, glutamate, and other transmitters, such as peptides.

OTHER NEUROCHEMICAL ABNORMALITIES AND POTENTIAL CLUES

Table 14.4-1 lists some of the other neurochemical systems that have been associated with schizophrenia. Presenting all the affirmative and negative data for each system is beyond the scope of the present discussion. Nevertheless, some understanding of both the range of concepts that have been investigated and the evidence that at one time supported those concepts can be gained from Table 14.4-1. The more active hypotheses were reviewed above.

Table 14.4-2 lists some diseases and disorders that imitate schizophrenia. Because many can mimic one or more aspects of schizophrenia, they have sometimes been confused with schizophrenia. Because they may affect brain structures or neurochemical systems in a similar manner as schizophrenia, some of them may be of considerable theoretical and diagnostic interest.

VIRUSES AND AUTOIMMUNITY IN SCHIZOPHRENIA

THE VIRAL-AUTOIMMUNE HYPOTHESIS This section has focused on the numerous neurochemical systems that might be involved in schizophrenia. Several environmental insults and simple genetic abnormalities that could play a role in the development of those neurochemical alterations were mentioned briefly. The question of etiology, however, remains. Although it is generally assumed that there is a significant genetic contribution to the development of schizophrenia, genetic models have heretofore not adequately explained the observed distribution of the illness in families and throughout the population. Investigators are now focusing on complex models that emphasize a possible interaction between genes predisposing for schizophrenia and other environmental factors. In regard to the latter, it has been proposed that infection or an autoimmune reaction against CNS tissue may be etiologically involved in at least some cases of schizophrenia.

The hypothesis that schizophrenia may be the result of a brain infection is not new. Nearly a century ago investigators con-

TABLE 14.4-1
Agents and Some of the Supporting Evidence for Their Involvement in Schizophrenia*

Agent	Claimed Supporting Findings
Biogenic Amines	
Acetylcholine (ACh)	Agents (for example, physostigmine, DFP) that increase cholinergic activity increase negative symptoms. Anticholinergic agents have been found to improve negative symptoms. The reduced REM latency found in schizophrenic patients may be associated with increased cholinergic activity.
Adrenochrome	Adrenochrome, an oxidation product of epinephrine, is toxic to norepinephrine-containing cultured cells.
Asparagine	There is one case report of a psychotic male with elevated plasma and CSF asparagine levels.
Cysteine, homocysteine	Cysteine exacerbates symptoms. Increased homocysteine levels are found in some genetic disorders that are also associated with psychosis.
Endogenous psychotogenes	
Dimethoxyphenylethylamine (DMPEA; pink spot)	Urinary DMPEA is present in schizophrenics but not in controls in some studies.
Dimethyltryptamine (DMT)	DMT, which is found in human blood, causes acute, transient psychosis in normals.
Bufotenine	Bufotenine has been found in the urine of schizophrenics.
Histamine	Schizophrenics have a relatively low incidence of allergies and a decreased wheal response to histamine administered intradermally. Other responses to histamine are also decreased. Tele-methylhistamine is elevated in the CSF of schizophrenics. The histamine-2 receptor blocker, famotidine, improved negative symptoms in one patient.
Kynurenine	Excessive kynurenine excretion by schizophrenics has been reported.
Methionine, betaine	Methionine precipitates acute psychosis or exacerbates symptoms of schizophrenia. Betaine accentuates hallucinations, delusions, and thought disorganization. It acts more slowly than methionine.
Phenylethylamine (PEA)	Higher fasting serum phenylalanine (the precursor to PEA) concentrations have been found in some schizophrenic patients. There is evidence of increased urinary PEA in psychiatric patients. Hallucinogeniclike symptoms induced by PEA in animals are blocked by antipsychotic medications.
Serine, glycine	Elevated plasma serine levels have been found in some psychotic patients. Serine loading exacerbates some of the symptoms of schizophrenic patients. Glycine has been reported to improve schizophrenic symptoms.
Neuropeptides	
Cholecystokinin (CCK)	High levels of CCK have been found in the limbic system of schizophrenic subgroups. Decreased postmortem CCK levels have been reported in the amygdala and hippocampus of patients with predominantly deficit symptoms.
Endogenous opioids, endorphins	A delayed antipsychotic effect has been observed following the administration of the opioid antagonist naloxone (Narcan) to schizophrenics. Buprenorphine (Buprenex) has an antipsychotic effect in some patients. The γ-type endorphins and FK 33-824 have been found to reduce psychotic symptoms. α- and γ-endorphins have been found to be elevated in the brains of schizophrenics.
Neurotensin	Increased postmortem neurotensin has been found in the frontal cortex and hippocampus of schizophrenic patients. CSF neurotensin is low in medication-free patients and returns to normal when they are treated with antipsychotic medications.
Somatostatin	One study reported high postmortem somatostatin levels in the CSF and low levels in the frontal cortex and hippocampus of schizophrenic patients.
Vasoactive intestinal peptide (VIP)	A study found VIP to be elevated in the amygdala of schizophrenic patients with predominantly productive symptoms.
Miscellaneous	
α_2-Haptoglobin	Haptoglobin has been found to be elevated in the CSF of schizophrenic patients. There has also been a report of a possible alteration in gene frequency in some schizophrenic subtypes.
Creatinine phosphokinase (CK, CPK)	High levels of CK have been found in the serum of schizophrenic patients, especially those with acute schizophrenia, periodic catatonia, and depressive psychoses. Some family members who have not been psychotic also have elevated levels. Schizophrenia has been associated with some muscle abnormalities.
Folic acid (vitamin B_{12})	Folic acid administration has been shown in a few studies to improve schizophrenic symptoms. A genetic defect in folic acid metabolism produces a schizophrenialike illness.
Free radicals	Free radicals are thought to be produced by an overactive dopaminergic system. The enzyme glutathione peroxidase, which is involved in the degradation of the toxic by-products of oxidative metabolism, is decreased in the platelets of schizophrenics. Decreased amounts of the norepinephrine-synthesizing enzyme dopamine-β-hydroxylase have been found in the brains and CSF of schizophrenic patients. Vitamin E (a free radical scavenger) is useful in treating tardive dyskinesia.
GABA	Some benzodiazepines (for example, diazepam [Valium], clonazepam [Klonopin], alprazolam [Xanax]) that potentiate GABA activity have antipsychotic effects.
Gluten	There were a decreased number of psychiatric admissions during World War II when the diet was gluten deficient. There is a high prevalence of schizophrenia in individuals with coelic disease. Improvement can be seen in patients on a gluten-free diet.
Human leukocyte-associated antigen (HLA)	Various HLA types have been claimed to be associated with schizophrenia.
2,4-Dimethyl-3-ethylpyrrole (mauve factor)	This substance appeared as a mauve-colored spot on chromatographs of urine from schizophrenic patients and was later identified as a pyrrole. Elevated urinary excretion is considered to identify patients with pyridoxine and zinc deficiency.
Neural cell adhesion molecule (N-CAM)	N-CAM has been found to be elevated in the serum of schizophrenic patients. N-CAM is possibly related to increased synaptic turnover.
Nicotinic acid and nicotinamide	In early studies nicotinic acid was found to decrease the amount of methyl donor substances available for transmethylation. Nicotinic acid and nicotinamide have been used to treat schizophrenia.
Pineal gland extract	Since the early 1920's there have been sporadic reports of crude extracts of beef pineal gland producing an improvement when injected into schizophrenic patients.
Porphyria	The condensation product of catecholamines is thought to be toxic. There is some indication of increased herozygosity for porphyria among schizophrenic patients.
Prostaglandin E_2	PGE_2 has been reported to be decreased in the plasma of schizophrenics.
Pyruvate-dehydrogenase complex	Decreased brain carbon dioxide production from glucose and increased lactate has been reported. There has been one report of acetazolamide plus thiamine (which should correct metabolic abnormality) decreasing symptoms in schizophrenic patients.
Taraxein	Taraxein produces catatonia and abnormal symptoms when injected into monkeys and humans.

*Negative findings are not presented, but some of the suggested neurochemical findings are no longer tenable. Some agents are discussed in greater detail in the text.

TABLE 14.4-2
Diseases and Disorders That Imitate Schizophrenia

Brain Injury or Disease
Embolism
Aqueductal stenosis
Ischemia
Trauma
Tumor
Epilepsy
Encephalitis
Narcolepsy
Obstructive hydrocephalus
Cerebrovascular infarction
Neoplasms
Metabolic or Systemic Disorders
Vitamin B_{12} deficiency
Acquired immune deficiency system
Syphilis
Tuberculous meningitis
Pellagra
Hypoglycemia
Hepatic encephalopathy
Hyperthyroidism
Lead poisoning
Lupus erythematosus
Multiple sclerosis
Uremia
Cotard's syndrome
Herpetic encephalitis
Cysticercosis
Cushing's disease
Genetic or chromosomal disorders
XXY karyotype (Klinefelter's syndrome)
XO karyotype (Turner's or Noonan's syndrome)
$18q^-$ deletion (missing piece of long arm of chromosome 18)
5,q11-q13 triplication
Huntington's disease
Acute intermittent porphyria
Metachromatic leukodystrophy
Familial basal ganglia calcification
Homocystinuria
Phenylketonuria
Wilson's disease
Albinism
Congenital adrenal hyperplasia
Glucose-6-phosphate dehydrogenase deficiency (favism)
Kartagener's syndrome

ducted studies that showed increased white blood cell counts in schizophrenic patients. Early in the 20th century a link was described between a schizophrenialike psychosis and infection with the influenza virus. Over 50 years ago investigators found increased CSF protein concentrations, a possible indicator of CNS infection or immune activation (or both), in schizophrenic patients as a group. Recent developments have stimulated further exploration of the infectious-autoimmune hypothesis of schizophrenia. One is the rapid evolution of new immunological laboratory techniques. Another is the realization that schizophrenia may be a heterogeneous group of disorders involving multiple etiological factors that may interact to cause the illness. In fact, there are several variations of the infectious-autoimmune hypothesis. They include not only the possibility that a virus may directly infect the brain and actively cause schizophrenic symptoms, but also the possibility that viruses, or autoantibodies stimulated after a viral infection, may interfere in more subtle ways with CNS development and function.

VIRUSES, AUTOANTIBODIES, AND THE BRAIN A number of schizophrenia researchers have focused on the affinity of certain viruses for CNS tissue. Among those neurotropic viruses are cytomegalovirus (CMV), herpes simplex virus type 1 (HSV-1), other DNA viruses in the herpes family, and the newly discovered human retroviruses. In addition to their neurotropism, the ability of those viruses to be reactivated from latency has raised the possibility that they are involved in schizophrenia.

It has long been known that some psychotic disorders that clinically resemble schizophrenia may be caused by CNS infection or autoimmunity. Patients with tertiary neurosyphilis, a disorder that can present as a schizophrenialike psychosis, filled psychiatric hospitals prior to the development of effective antibiotic treatment. Cases are also seen in which herpes encephalitis or infection with the human immunodeficiency virus causes a psychosis resembling schizophrenia. Systemic lupus erythematosus is an autoimmune disorder that may profoundly affect the CNS, causing a schizophrenialike illness.

Those clinical prototypes, paired with growing knowledge regarding virus-brain interactions, suggest that some cases now labeled schizophrenia may result from an interaction between a virus (or autoantibodies generated subsequent to a viral infection) and CNS tissue.

EVIDENCE SUPPORTING A ROLE FOR INFECTION OR AUTOIMMUNITY

Epidemiology A number of different approaches have been used to look at the distribution of schizophrenia around the world and over time in search of evidence supporting infection as a factor in the disorder. Although the prevalence of schizophrenia is relatively constant around the world, pockets of unusually high or low prevalence exist. In addition, there are reports of greater prevalence in urban areas, which may be independent of socioeconomic factors. The greater prevalence could be due to the greater likelihood of viral infections in the more crowded urban regions relative to rural areas. Alternatively, other variables might also explain those differences.

As mentioned earlier, the season-of-birth effect that has repeatedly been observed in schizophrenia may reflect exposure in utero to infections that are more common in the late fall and early winter months.

A compelling finding, replicated in some but not all studies, is an association between in utero exposure to influenza epidemics and the later development of schizophrenia. Persons exposed during the second trimester of fetal development, a crucial period of cortical neuronal migration, are at significantly increased risk for subsequent schizophrenia. The association with schizophrenia may not be specific to exposure to viral effects. For example, another recent study noted that first-trimester exposure to famine was associated with an increased risk for the later development of schizophrenia.

Clinical findings A number of clinical facts regarding schizophrenia may be consistent with infection or autoimmunity, although they do not specifically confirm that viruses or autoantibodies are etiologically involved in schizophrenia. Although the structural and functional deficits in schizophrenic patients could be due to brain damage or to a failure in brain development related to early exposure to an infection or autoantibodies, other perinatal insults could also play a role. Similarly, reported increases in minor physical anomalies in patients with schizophrenia could reflect in utero exposure to infection. That possibility could also explain the observation of an increased frequency of dermatoglyphic changes in schizophrenic patients.

IMMUNOLOGICAL ABNORMALITIES

Cellular immune function Numerous disturbances in cellular immunity have been reported in schizophrenia, including morphologically atypical lymphocytes, deficient natural killer cell production, and abnormalities in helper-suppressor cell ratios. Unfortunately, those cellular disturbances have not been consistently replicated and may have been influenced by treatment with antipsychotic medications. The assessment of cellular immune function has advanced with the recent introduction of monoclonal antibodies to label specific lymphocyte subsets. Using such techniques, investigators have recently reported that schizophrenic patients may have an increase in one subset, CD5 + B-lymphocytes, which might be consistent with a state of autoimmune activation. Those findings are preliminary, and questions remain regarding their diagnostic specificity as well as the possible effects of antipsychotic or nonprescribed medications on lymphocyte parameters.

Antibody production Studies have been conducted regarding immunoglobulin levels in the serum and CSF of schizophrenic patients. Using quantitative indices that correct for abnormalities in blood-CSF permeability, investigators have reported increases in endogenous CNS immunoglobulin production in a subset of schizophrenic patients. That finding, which demonstrates overall increased immunoglobulin production in CSF, has not been replicated by all groups, and studies have been inconsistent regarding immunoglobulin levels in the serum. Another approach has been to search for antibodies to particular infectious agents, especially the herpesviruses and other neurotropic agents, in schizophrenic patients. Those studies have also produced equivocal results, in part probably attributable to the ubiquitous exposure to many of the viruses among adults. Although a number of investigators have reported indications of autoantibodies against constituents of CNS tissue in schizophrenic patients, no consistent pathogenic autoantibody has been demonstrated. The possibility also exists that autoantibodies might be generated secondarily to some process of CNS tissue pathology in schizophrenia, rather than being primary etiological factors.

Immune mediators Assays are now available to determine concentrations of the cytokines, including the interferons and interleukins, in blood and CSF. The cytokines are key immune system mediators. A number of groups have reported abnormalities in interleukin production in schizophrenia, including decreased soluble interleukin-2 receptors. Although one group reported increased interferon in the blood of schizophrenic patients, that finding has not been consistently replicated. Nevertheless, abnormalities in cytokine production or receptor levels may reflect abnormal immunological function in some schizophrenic patients.

SEARCHING FOR A VIRUS

Antigens One way to look directly for the presence of a virus in brain tissue is to search for antigenic viral proteins. A number of studies of postmortem tissue samples from schizophrenic patients have used antibodies developed to label such antigens in the brain. One problem in those studies has been the possibility of false-positive results due to nonspecific binding, and studies searching for antigenic components of both CMV and HSV-1 have not produced definitive positive results.

Viral nucleic acids A specific way to search for the presence of viral material is to use nucleic acid probes complementary to viral genomic sequences. The labeled probes may then bind to viral DNA or ribonucleic acid (RNA), if it is present. Again, the results of those studies have been equivocal because of the methodological problem of nonspecific binding. The recent development of the polymerase chain reaction technique makes it possible to search specifically for very low numbers of viral nucleic acid sequences. That technique has been used to search for CMV and other herpesviruses in brain tissue from schizophrenic patients, but no unequivocally positive cases have been identified.

Transmission Even if one is not targeting a specific virus, it is still possible to conduct transmission experiments in which brain tissue or CSF from schizophrenic patients is inoculated into the CNS of laboratory animals or applied to cell cultures in an attempt to transmit an infectious agent. Transmission studies have been successful in the study of other degenerative disorders, specifically the spongiform encephalopathies of kuru and Creutzfeldt-Jakob disease caused by unconventional viruses. Using both in vivo and in vitro approaches, no investigators have conclusively proved the existence of a transmissible, infectious particle in schizophrenia.

IMPLICATIONS FOR THE PATHOGENESIS OF SCHIZOPHRENIA Although no convincing proof of the involvement of either an infectious agent or an autoantibody response in schizophrenia has come forth, the search continues. It is increasingly apparent that multiple etiological factors may be involved in schizophrenia, perhaps in some cases acting independently and in other cases interacting with genes that contribute to vulnerability. It may also be that viruses, autoantibody responses, or both are important etiological factors only in relation to the timing of the insult. The studies on second trimester exposure to influenza epidemics are particularly interesting in that regard. A development of great importance in schizophrenia research is the emphasis on abnormalities in brain development. Neurodevelopmental models stress that there are key windows during which phases of CNS maturation must occur in a highly structured way. As the more subtle details of viral pathogenesis are elucidated, it may become apparent that it is only a relatively covert interaction between viral particles or an autoantibody and the brain during those crucial phases of CNS development that can, in some individuals, result in schizophrenia. The probable clinical heterogeneity of schizophrenia makes it important that viruses and autoantibodies continue to be considered as potential etiological factors.

INTEGRATIVE FRAMEWORK

The facts of schizophrenia, presented at the beginning of the section, may now be adumbrated with the clinical findings and research hypotheses detailed subsequently.

Schizophrenia is a clinical syndrome without known cause. Although there appears to be a genetic predisposition, the mode of transmission is not known. Interactions of environmental forces on genetically vulnerable individuals may precipitate the disorder, yet it is not certain whether either alone is sufficient to do so. The season-of-birth phenomenon suggests a possible role for seasonal environmental factors and is one of the strongest pieces of evidence in favor of the involvement of a prenatal viruslike agent in schizophrenia.

A viral hypothesis of schizophrenia is not incompatible with the existence of some type of biochemical dysfunction. For example, monoamine metabolism in mouse brain has been shown to be altered by herpes simplex infection, although it can only be speculated as to which class (or classes) of viruses is likely to be involved in schizophrenia. One hypothesis integrates genetic and viral etiologies by proposing a prominent role for retroviruses. Retroviruses are a special class of RNA viruses that carry the enzyme reverse transcriptase. Reverse transcriptase allows the viral RNA to be transcribed intracellularly into DNA, which then enters the host cell genome, transmitting the viral information. Retroviruses, by virtue of their infectious nature, may also produce characteristics of a typical viral infection. The possibility that a viral infection is a pathogenic factor in schizophrenia, either by direct neuronal injury or by stimulation of autoantibodies, merits further exploration. The peak onset in early adulthood, the illness's course of exacerbations and recoveries, and the evidence of structural cerebral damage are reminiscent of the infections produced by known neurotropic viruses that persist within neurons, periodically altering their function and causing cellular damage. Alternatively, the fluctuations in course could be explained by periodic production of autoantibodies, like that which occurs in the accepted autoimmune diseases. The genetic disorder intermittent porphyria could also be a model for a nonviral illness with similar exacerbations and remissions.

Sex differences and the peak age at onset should be further clues to the biochemical pathophysiology of schizophrenia. The estrogen-testosterone differences between males and females may explain some of the differences in age at onset, outcome, and the clinical features of schizophrenia between the sexes. Studies of normal development show sex differences in the rate of brain growth and differentiation, as well as structural differences in specific parts of the adult brain, that may be produced in part by sex hormone regulation of brain growth. Brain development on a cellular and biochemical level may reach its peak in males in their early 20s and somewhat later in females. In animal studies, some estrogens appear to have antipsychotic effects, and estrogens are known antagonists of D_2 receptors. Conversely, dopamine regulates the biological effects of estrogen by decreasing the binding of that hormone to its receptors. Some studies have also shown greater serotonergic activity in females. Surges in serotonin levels may actually initiate the onset of puberty by exerting a regulatory effect on steroid hormone production. Little is known of the possible effects of androgens on catecholamines and indoleamines. Testosterone may increase aggressiveness and could thus aggravate symptoms of psychosis. Perhaps those effects are enough to modify the expression of the primary pathogenic agent. The crucial factor initiating the schizophrenic process, however, remains unknown, although it is likely that the interactions of steroid hormones with catecholamines and indoleamines play a role. In addition to the biochemical changes that take place during adolescence and young adulthood, there are numerous social demands that could interact with an already altered substrate to increase the risk of developing schizophrenia.

The peak age at onset of schizophrenia, in the early to mid-20s, may relate to peak changes in monoamines and receptor responsivity or other parallel neurochemical events that are modified by gonadal hormones. Onset may be related to subtle alterations in neuroendocrine regulation at a time when hormone levels are peaking. Although there is some evidence for neuroendocrine dysfunction in schizophrenia, based on measurements of hypothalamic releasing hormones and postmortem studies of peptides, more investigation in pursuit of a neuroendocrine hypothesis is needed. Alternatively, since age at onset has been found in several studies to be correlated among siblings with schizophrenia, age at onset may be genetically programmed or at least related to an incubation period subsequent to the occurrence of an earlier environmental event. An insult to the brain during crucial periods of embryonic and perinatal growth and differentiation may affect certain cells of the brain whose functions are not expressed until early adulthood.

The overwhelming beneficial effect of antipsychotic medications in schizophrenia cannot be overlooked. Regardless of the original cause of the illness, the neurochemical outcome appears to be a perturbation of the dopamine neurotransmitter system. Although other neurochemical systems, including the norepinephrine, serotonin, and glutamate systems, may also be altered, they appear to be less important. From a review of the neural systems in which those transmitters function, it is apparent that none of them operates in isolation. Thus, schizophrenia is no longer regarded as a defect in one neurotransmitter.

The brain is a complex biochemical organ, with multiple anatomical as well as biochemical networks playing a final role in behavior. Many researchers, studying the neurochemistry of schizophrenia, have tried to place their work into a structural and functional context. The more that can be learned about the role of each substance in normal neurophysiological function and behavior, the more that will be understood of the mechanism of neurobehavioral disorders.

SUGGESTED CROSS-REFERENCES

Section 1.4 on amino acid neurotransmitters and Section 1.3 on monoamine neurotransmitters discuss some of the receptors relevant to etiological theories of schizophrenia. Section 1.2 on functional neuroanatomy and Chapter 2 on neuropsychiatry and behavioral neurology provide additional information on those subjects. Section 1.7 on basic electrophysiology discusses dopamine neurons and the effects of antipsychotic medications. Section 14.1, which provides an overview of schizophrenia, and Section 14.2, which discusses epidemiology, contribute to understanding those areas.

REFERENCES

Alexander G E, DeLong M R, Strick P L: Parallel organization of functionally segregated circuits linking basal ganglia and cortex. Annu Rev Neurosci *9:* 357, 1986.

Alexander R C, Spector S A, Casanova M, Kleinman J, Wyatt R J, Kirch D G: Search for cytomegalovirus in the postmortem brains of schizophrenic patients using the polymerase chain reaction. Arch Gen Psychiatry *49:* 47, 1992.

Bell D: Comparison of amphetamine psychosis and schizophrenia. Am J Psychiatry *111:* 701, 1965.

Benes F M, Vincent S L, Alsterberg G, Bird E D, SanGiovanni J P: Increased GABAA binding in superficial layers of cingulate cortex in schizophrenics. J Neurosci *12:* 924, 1992.

*Carlsson M, Carlsson A: Interactions between glutamatergic and monoaminergic systems within the basal ganglia: Implications for schizophrenia and Parkinson's disease. Trends Neurosci *13:* 272, 1990.

Carlsson A, Lindquist M: Effect of chlorpromazine and haloperidol on formation of 3-methoxytyramine and norepinephrine in mouse brain. Acta Pharmacol Toxicol *20:* 140, 1963.

Chiodo L A, Bunney B S: Typical and atypical neuroleptics: Differential effects of chronic administration on the activity of A-9 and A-10 midbrain dopaminergic neurons. J Neurosci *3:* 1607, 1983.

Creese I, Burt D R, Snyder S H: Dopamine receptor binding predicts clinical and pharmacological potencies of antischizophrenic drugs. Science *192:* 481, 1975.

*Crow T J: Positive and negative schizophrenic symptoms and the role of dopamine. Br J Psychiatry *137:* 383, 1980.

Csernansky J G, Murphy G M, Faustman W O: Limbic/mesolimbic connections and the pathogenesis of schizophrenia. Biol Psychiatry *30:* 383, 1991.

Davis K L, Kahn R S, Ko G, Davidson M: Dopamine in schizophrenia: A review and reconceptualization. Am J Psychiatry *148:* 1474, 1991.

Friedhoff A J: A dopamine-dependent restitutive system for the maintenance of mental normalcy. Ann NY Acad Sci *463:* 47, 1986.

Ganguli R, Brar J S, Chengappa K N R, Yang Z W, Nimgaonkar V L, Rabin B S: Autoimmunity in schizophrenia: A review of recent findings. Ann Med *25:* 489, 1993.

Ganguli R, Rabin B S: Increased serum interleukin 2 receptor concentration in schizophrenic and brain-damaged subjects. Arch Gen Psychiatry *46:* 292, 1989.

Glowinski J, Tassin J P, Thierry A M: The mesocorticoprefrontal dopaminergic neurons. Trends Neurosci 7: 415, 1984.
Grace A A, Bunney B S: Induction of depolarization block in midbrain dopaminergic neurons by repeated administration of haloperidol: Analysis using in vivo intracellular recording. J Pharmacol Exp Ther *238:* 1092, 1986.
Hyde T M, Casanova M F, Kleinman J E, Weinberger D R: Neuroanatomical and neurochemical pathology in schizophrenia. *American Psychiatric Press Review of Psychiatry,* vol 10, A Tasman, editor, p 7. American Psychiatric Press, Washington, 1991.
*Kirch D G: Infection and autoimmunity as etiologic factors in schizophrenia: A review and reappraisal. Schizophr Bull *19:* 355, 1993.
Kirch D G, Alexander R C, Suddath R L, Papadopoulos N M, Kaufmann C A, Daniel D G, Wyatt R J: Blood-CSF barrier permeability and central nervous system immunoglobulin G in schizophrenia. J Neural Transm *89:* 219, 1992.
McAllister C G, Rapaport M H, Pickar D, Podruchny T A, Christison G, Alphs L D, Paul S M: Increased numbers of CD5+ B lymphocytes in schizophrenic patients. Arch Gen Psychiatry *46:* 890, 1989.
Mednick S A, Machon R A, Huttunen M O, Bonett D: Adult schizophrenia following prenatal exposure to an influenza epidemic. Arch Gen Psychiatry *45:* 189, 1988.
Meltzer H Y, Matsubara S, Lee J C: Classification of typical and atypical antipsychotic drugs on the basis of dopamine D_1, D_2 and serotonin$_2$ pK_i values. J Pharmacol Exp Ther *251:* 238, 1989.
Murray A M, Waddington J L: The interaction of clozapine with dopamine D_1 versus D_2 receptor-mediated function: Behavioural indices. Eur J Pharmacol *186:* 79, 1990.
Pycock C J, Kerwin R W, Carter C J: Effect of lesion of cortical dopamine terminals on subcortical dopamine in rats. Nature (London) *286:* 74, 1980.
Rapaport M H, McAllister C G: Neuroimmunological factors in schizophrenia. In *Psychoimmunology Update,* J M Gorman, R M Kertzner, editors. American Psychiatric Press, Washington, 1991.
Reynolds G P: Beyond the dopamine hypothesis: The neurochemical pathology of schizophrenia. Br J Psychiatry *155:* 305, 1989.
Seeman P: Dopamine receptor sequences: Therapeutic levels of neuroleptics occupy D2 receptors, clozapine occupies D4. Neuropsychopharmacology *7:* 261, 1992.
Seeman P, Lee T, Chau-Wong M, Wong K: Antipsychotic drug doses and neuroleptic/dopamine receptors. Nature *261:* 717, 1977.
Stevens J R: An anatomy of schizophrenia? Arch Gen Psychiatry *29:* 177, 1973.
Stevens J R, Hallick L M: Viruses and schizophrenia. In *Neuropathogenic Viruses and Immunity,* S Specter, M Bendinelli, H Friedman, editors. Plenum, New York, 1992.
Suddath R L, Christison G W, Torrey E F, Casanova M F, Weinberger D R: Anatomical abnormalities in the brains of monozygotic twins discordant for schizophrenia. N Engl J Med *322:* 789, 1990.
van Kammen D P, Kelley M: Dopamine and norepinephrine activity in schizophrenia: An integrative perspective. Schizophr Res *4:* 173, 1991.
*Weinberger D R: Implications of normal brain development for the pathogenesis of schizophrenia. Arch Gen Psychiatry *44:* 660, 1987.
White F J, Wang R X: Differential effects of classical and atypical antipsychotic drugs on A9 and A10 dopamine neurons. Science *221:* 1054, 1983.
Whitehorn J C: Aporrhegma reactions in psychoses. Am J Psychiatry 2: 421, 1923.
Wise C D, Baden M M, Stein L: Postmortem measurement of enzymes in human brain: Evidence of a central noradrenergic deficit in schizophrenia. J Psychiatr Res *11:* 185, 1974.
Wyatt R J: The dopamine hypothesis: Variations on a theme. In *Research in the Schizophrenic Disorders: The Stanley R. Dean Award Lectures,* R Cancro, S R Dean, editors. Spectrum, Jamaica, NY, 1985.
Wyatt R J: Neuroleptics and the natural course of schizophrenia. Schizophr Bull *17:* 235, 1991.
*Wyatt R J, Alexander R C, Egan M F, Kirch, D G: Schizophrenia, just the facts: What do we know, how well do we know it? Schizophr Res *1:* 3, 1988.

14.5 SCHIZOPHRENIA: GENETICS

KENNETH S. KENDLER, M.D.
SCOTT R. DIEHL, Ph.D.

INTRODUCTION

The goal of this section is to provide an overview of the current state of knowledge regarding the genetics of schizophrenia. The discussion will focus on the following key questions: Is schizophrenia a familial disorder? To what extent is any familial aggregation of schizophrenia due to genetic versus environmental factors? How narrow or broad are the psychiatric disorders that are transmitted within families? Because genetic factors play an important role in the familial transmission of schizophrenia, the following additional questions are also pertinent: What kinds of genetic transmission mechanisms appear most likely? What is the current status of and the future prospects for identifying specific genes that predispose a person to schizophrenia?

IS SCHIZOPHRENIA FAMILIAL?

The most basic question in the genetics of schizophrenia is whether the disorder aggregates (or runs) in families. Technically, familial aggregation means that a close relative of a person with a disorder is at increased risk for that disorder compared with a matched person chosen at random from the general population. Family studies of schizophrenia have examined primarily first-degree relatives (parents, full siblings, and offspring), and little systematic information on more distant relationship has been gathered in recent years.

In a 1967 review paper Edith Zerbin-Rüdin listed 17 major family studies of schizophrenia involving first-degree relatives. By 1980 at least nine other major family studies had been reported. Parental relationships are exceptional and are not considered here because it is well established that persons affected by schizophrenia exhibit reduced fertility. Since, by definition, a parent must have successfully reproduced at least once, parents of schizophrenic offspring are less likely to have expressed the symptoms of the disorder, despite carrying predisposing risk factors that may have been transmitted to their offspring. Aside from parental relationships the studies consistently showed a much greater risk for schizophrenia in the close relatives of schizophrenic persons than would be expected in the general population.

However, nearly all studies suffered from three important methodological limitations. First, no control groups were used, so the rates of schizophrenia in the general population required for comparison had to be derived from the literature. Second, diagnoses were made nonblind, with the investigator or coworkers always knowing that the person evaluated was a relative of a schizophrenic person. Third, neither structured personal interviews nor operationalized diagnostic criteria were used. In fact in many of the early studies it is unclear how many persons were personally examined and how many were evaluated from indirect information such as reports of relatives or doctors, or from hospital notes.

RECENT FAMILY STUDIES In the early 1980s several research groups questioned the validity of earlier family studies of schizophrenia. They suggested that the evidence for the familial aggregation of schizophrenia may have resulted from consistent biases in the previous studies. In addition, they were concerned that the diagnostic approach to schizophrenia in earlier studies might have been overly broad. They argued that the familial aggregation of schizophrenia might be weak or absent when narrowly diagnosed. Since 1980, 11 major family studies of schizophrenia have been reported that used blind diagnoses, control groups, personal interviews, and operationalized diagnostic criteria. Those studies have permitted a more rigorous evaluation than has hitherto been possible of the degree to which schizophrenia aggregates in families.

The key results from those studies are summarized in Table 14.5-1. The table lists the diagnostic criteria used in the study, the nature of the control proband group, and the *p* value (that is, the probability of observing such a difference in the rates of schizophrenia in the two groups by chance, if the true rates were identical). The term "proband" refers to the person through whom the family was identified for study. A typical family study of schizophrenia would then begin with two types of probands: those with schizophrenia, and a matched group of control probands. Relatives of those probands are then systematically assessed. Table 14.5-1 also presents data on lifetimes at risk in the assessed relatives of schizophrenia probands and control probands, and the morbid risk for schizophrenia in the two groups. *Lifetimes at risk* is the sum for all assessed relatives of the proportion of their lifetime risk for schizophrenia that they have thus far completed. *Morbid risk* (MR) is a statistic commonly used in genetics and equals the total proportion of persons who would be expected to be affected with a disorder in a given population if all members of that population have completed their age at risk. Finally, the table includes the correlation of liability. If schizophrenia is due to several genetic and environmental factors that act approximately additively in influencing a person's liability or predisposition to schizophrenia, then this figure represents the degree of correlation between first-degree relatives in overall risk of the disease. The correlation of liability is a useful figure because it combines into a single easily understood statistical number the risk figures for schizophrenia in relatives of schizophrenic and control probands. The higher the correlation of liability, the stronger is the degree of familial aggregation of schizophrenia.

Three comments aid to an understanding of the major results summarized in Table 14.5-1 data. First, three of the studies reported in the table used nonschizophrenic psychiatric patients as control probands, while the remaining studies used various normal or screened nonpsychiatric controls. The use of psychiatric controls represents a potentially significant methodological limitation, because the risk of schizophrenia in relatives of other psychiatric patients may differ from that expected in the general population. Second, the sample size of relatives studied varies widely in the different investigations. For example, the lifetimes

TABLE 14.5-1
Summary Results of Major Recent Family Studies of Schizophrenia That Included a Control Group, Personal Interviews With Relatives, and Blind Diagnosis of Relatives*

			First-Degree Relatives of Schizophrenic Probands			First-Degree Relatives of Control Probands				
Senior Author and Year	Diagnostic Criteria	Controls	BZ	N	Schizophrenia MR (%)	BZ	N	Schizophrenia MR (%)	*p*	Correlation in Liability (r) ± SE
Scharfetter 1980	ICD-9	Affective illness	550	49	8.9	451	15	3.3	.0003	0.23 ± 0.03
Tsuang† 1980	Consensus Senior Iowa Clinicians	Screened surgical controls	362	20	5.5	475	3	0.6	.00002	0.36 ± 0.04
Guze‡ 1983	Modified Washington University	Nonschiz psychiatric patients	111	9	8.1	1076	18	1.7	.00001	0.32 ± 0.07
Baron 1985	RDC DSM-III	Normal persons	329	19	5.8	337	2	0.6	.0001	0.37 ± 0.04
Kendler† 1985	DSM-III	Screened surgical patients	703	26	3.7	931	2	0.2	8×10^{-8}	0.38 ± 0.03
Frangos 1985	DSM-III	Normal persons	478	26	5.4	536	6	1.1	.0001	0.28 ± 0.04
Coryell 1988	RDC	Never-ill volunteers	72	1	1.4	160	0	0	NS	0.23 ± 0.12
Gershon 1988	RDC chronic schiz	Volunteer controls	97	3	3.1	349	2	0.6	.038	0.25 ± 0.09
Maier 1990	RDC	Never-ill matched controls	463	23	5.0	294	1	0.4	.0004	0.38 ± 0.03
Onstad 1991	DSM-III-R	Affective illness	136	10	7.4	45	0	0	.06	0.35 ± 0.06
Kendler 1992	DSM-III-R	Unscreened matched controls	276	18	6.5	428	2	0.5	.000004	0.41 ± 0.04

*BZ indicates *bezugsziffer* (total lifetime equivalents of risk); MR, morbid risk; SE, standard error; ICD-9, ninth revision of *International Classification of Diseases;* DSM-III, third edition of *Diagnostic and Statistical Manual of Mental Disorders;* RDC, Research Diagnostic Criteria; schiz, schizophrenia; nonschiz, nonschizophrenic; NS, nonsignificant.

†Studies on partially overlapping data sets; results include relatives with only hospital records.

‡Prevalence rather than MR reported.

at risk in relatives of schizophrenics range nearly 10-fold, from over 700 to 72. On average, larger studies provide more stable statistical estimates for the true risk of schizophrenia in relatives of schizophrenic and control probands. Third, various diagnostic criteria were utilized in the studies. However, seven studies used criteria from either the third edition of *Diagnostic and Statistical Manual of Mental Disorders* (DSM-III), Washington University, Research Diagnostic Criteria (RDC) (for chronic schizophrenia) or revised third edition of DSM (DSM-III-R) criteria, all of which require, in addition to specified psychotic symptoms, at least six months of illness, usually with functional impairment.

Five major conclusions can be drawn from the large body of work summarized in Table 14.5-1. First, the risk for schizophrenia in first-degree relatives of schizophrenic probands varies widely across studies, from a low of 1.4 percent to a high of 8.9 percent. Much of the fluctuation can probably be explained by differences in diagnostic criteria or statistical fluctuations in small samples (the lowest risk is found in the smallest study). However, it remains possible that there are true population differences in the risk for schizophrenia in relatives of schizophrenic probands.

Second, the risk for schizophrenia in the relatives of nonpsychiatric control probands is relatively similar across studies, ranging from only 0.2 to 1.1 percent, which corresponds closely to the range of risks for schizophrenia found in general population studies. However, higher rates are found in two studies that employed psychiatric control groups.

Third, in every study the risk for schizophrenia was higher in the relatives of schizophrenic probands than in relatives of control probands. On average the first-degree relatives of schizophrenic probands had a risk for schizophrenia 5-fold to 10-fold higher than that found in the relatives of the control probands. Fourth, in all but two studies, the difference in risk for schizophrenia in the relatives of schizophrenic and control probands was quite unlikely to occur by chance (*p* less than .05). The two studies that had higher *p* values were the two with the smallest sample sizes. In a number of studies, the *p* values were very low (for example, less than .001), indicating that such differences in risk would be extremely unlikely to occur by chance.

Finally, although there was some variation, the correlation in liability for all studies fell in a relatively narrow range from +0.23 to +0.41. Furthermore, most of the largest studies that used relatively narrow diagnostic criteria for schizophrenia obtained correlations of liability in the narrow range of +0.32 to +0.41. Those results suggest that many of the studies can be seen as replications of one another because they provide similar results in regard to the observed degree of familial aggregation of schizophrenia. Although beyond the scope of this discussion, the correlation of liability between first-degree relatives in the range of +0.30 to +0.40 indicates a relatively strong degree of familial aggregation.

The data allow one to address questions raised in the early 1980s about the degree of familial aggregation of schizophrenia. The results of a large number of recent, carefully performed family studies support the conclusions of earlier and less methodologically rigorous investigations in finding that schizophrenia strongly aggregates in families. The familial aggregation of schizophrenia appears to be substantial when schizophrenia is defined using relatively narrow diagnostic criteria such as those found in DSM-III and DSM-III-R. On average, the risk for schizophrenia in the relatives of controls is between 0.5 and 1.0 percent, compared with between 3 and 7 percent in relatives of schizophrenic probands. The best estimate of the correlation in liability to schizophrenia in first-degree relatives is probably between +0.3 and +0.4.

TO WHAT EXTENT IS THE FAMILIAL AGGREGATION DUE TO GENETIC VERSUS ENVIRONMENTAL FACTORS?

TWIN STUDIES Resemblance among relatives can generally be ascribed to two principal mechanisms: shared environment and shared genes. A major goal in psychiatric genetics is to determine the degree to which familial aggregation for a disorder like schizophrenia results from environmental versus genetic mechanisms. While sophisticated analysis of family data can begin to make this discrimination, nearly all current knowledge regarding that distinction in schizophrenia comes from twin and adoption studies.

Twin studies are based on the assumption that monozygotic (MZ) and dizygotic (DZ) twins share a common environment to approximately the same degree. However, monozygotic twins are genetically identical, whereas dizygotic twins (like full siblings) share on average only half of their genes in common. While the validity of the second assumption is beyond question, the first (the equal environment) assumption has been a focus of controversy.

Several studies have shown that measures of the social environment (such as sharing friends, attitudes of parents and teachers) are more highly correlated among young monozygotic twins than among young same-sex dizygotic twins. The results at first appear to suggest that the equal environment assumption is false. However, another interpretation is possible. While similarity in environment might make monozygotic twins more similar, it is also plausible that, by behaving alike, monozygotic twins seek out or create similar environments for themselves. Those two alternative hypotheses have been subjected to empirical evaluation in a number of studies, nearly all of which suggest that the environmental similarity of monozygotic twins is the result and not the cause of their behavioral similarity. Current evidence supports the general validity of the equal environment assumption of twin studies.

Results are available from 12 major twin studies of schizophrenia (Table 14.5-2). None, however, meets all of the methodological criteria outlined earlier for family studies and an additional criterion that zygosity assignment be made blind with respect to psychiatric diagnosis. Some studies come closer than others. For example, a variety of different clinicians made diagnoses from blind case abstracts in the original report from the Maudsley twin series of Irving Gottesman and James Shields. Those same case records have more recently been examined using modern operationalized criteria, with similar overall results. In the study by Kenneth Kendler and Dennis Robinette from the National Academy of Sciences-National Research Council (NAS-NRC) Registry, psychiatric diagnoses were collected from a variety of clinical settings in which clinicians could not possibly have been aware of any research hypotheses. Furthermore, it could be shown that zygosity assignment was not biased with respect to psychiatric diagnosis. The recent study from Norway used structured psychiatric interviews which, however, were performed nonblind.

While all these studies agree that probandwise concordance for schizophrenia (the risk for schizophrenia in the cotwin of a schizophrenic proband twin) is much higher in monozygotic twins than in dizygotic twins, the absolute rates of concordance vary widely. Two factors are probably responsible for most of the variation. First, some studies employed a broader definition

TABLE 14.5-2
Concordance With Respect to Probands and the Heritability of Liability in the Major Twin Studies Reported to Date

			Probandwise Concordance*				
			MZ		Same-Sex DZ		Heritability of Liability
Author	Country	Year	N	%	N	%	(± SE)
Luxenburger	Germany	1928	14/22	64	0/13	0	†
Rosanoff et al	United States	1934	25/41 to 50/66	61	7/53 to 14/60	13	0.84 ± 0.26 to
				76		23	0.63 ± 0.26
Essen-Moller	Sweden	1941	7/11	64	4/27	15	0.87 ± 0.36
Kallmann	United States	1946	191/245	78	59/318	19	0.90 ± 0.13
Slater	England	1953	28/41	68	11/61	18	0.73 ± 0.21
Inouye	Japan	1963	33/55	60	2/11	18	0.66 ± 0.35
Kringlen	Norway	1967	31/69	45	14/96	15	0.61 ± 0.20
Fischer	Denmark	1973	14/23	61	12/43	28	0.41 ± 0.29
Gottesman and Shields	England	1972	15/26	58	4/34	12	0.86 ± 0.32
Tienari	Finland	1975	7/21	33	6/42	14	0.53 ± 0.33
Kendler and Robinette	United States	1983	60/194	31	18/277	6	0.71 ± 0.04‡
Onstad et al	Norway	1991	15/31	48	1/28	4	0.87 ± 0.08‡

*Concordance rates are not age-corrected. Estimates of the heritability of liability are based on population risks for schizophrenia either provided in the study or estimated by the reviewer. For further details regarding figures in this table see the Kendler et al (1983) studies with multiple reports; the latest or most complete report was chosen for analysis.
†Cannot be calculated because none of the DZ twin pairs were concordant.
‡Correlation in liability in MZ twins are reported rather than the standard heritability of liability.

of schizophrenia than others. Second, some studies obtained most of the proband twins from chronically hospitalized populations whereas others used population-based registries where milder cases would commonly occur. Twin studies have often, but not always, found a positive relationship between concordance and severity of illness.

Heritability of liability Both the diagnostic approach to schizophrenia and the method of ascertaining probands should equally affect concordance rates in monozygotic and dizygotic twins. Therefore, a better method of comparing results across studies would be a summary statistic based on concordance in both monozygotic and dizygotic twins. One of the best of those is the heritability of liability as calculated from the correlations in liability in monozygotic and dizygotic twins. That statistic ranges from 0.0 if genetic factors play no role in susceptibility to a disorder to a maximum of 1.0 if genes entirely determine disease risk. Because the statistic is based on the polygenic multifactorial threshold model, which may or may not be appropriate for schizophrenia, the results should be regarded as only one plausible way of approximating reality. Nonetheless, the major twin studies of schizophrenia agree in estimating the heritability of liability of schizophrenia at between 0.6 and 0.9 (Table 14.5-2). The results suggest that genetic factors play a major role in the familial transmission of schizophrenia.

Genetic theory predicts that if all the familial aggregation of schizophrenia were attributable to genetic factors, then the heritability of liability should be approximately double the correlation in liability found in first-degree relatives (because, on average, first-degree relatives share half of their genes in common). Comparison of the results shown in Tables 14.5-1 and 14.5-2 indicates that, at least as a rough approximation, the hypothesis is supported. The range of the heritability of liability to schizophrenia calculated from twin studies is approximately twice the range of the correlation in liability to schizophrenia found in first-degree relatives in most family studies.

Nongenetic familial transmission Twin studies also provide two powerful tests for the role of nongenetic familial transmission in the liability to schizophrenia. First, one can ask whether the correlation in liability in dizygotic twins is more than half that which would be predicted in monozygotic twins if only additive genetic factors were operating. A review of all major twin studies to date suggests that nongenetic factors may play a modest role in the transmission of schizophrenia. The estimates of the proportion of liability to schizophrenia attributable to familial nongenetic factors range, in all but one study, between 0 and +0.30, with a weighted mean of about 0.18. Second, the risk for schizophrenia in dizygotic cotwins can be compared with that in siblings of schizophrenic probands. Although having the same degree of genetic relationship to the affected proband, dizygotic cotwins share more of the familial environment than do ordinary siblings. Several twin studies have suggested than a difference in risk does exist between the two groups. However, such a difference has not been consistently found across all studies and was not found in the recent Norwegian small-sample twin family study of schizophrenia.

ADOPTION STUDIES Adoption studies can clarify the role of genetic and environmental factors in the transmission of schizophrenia by studying two kinds of rare but particularly informative relationships: (1) persons who are genetically related but do not share familial-environmental factors, and (2) persons who share familial-environmental factors but are not genetically related. Table 14.5-3 summarizes, in the order discussed, the major adoption studies of schizophrenia, reporting raw data and statistical tests. The summary here is organized by the kind of adoption design utilized.

Affected biological parent design Three studies have compared the adopted-away offspring of schizophrenic parents with the adopted-away offspring of matched controls. In the first of these Leonard Heston found a significant excess of schizophrenia in adopted-away offspring of schizophrenic mothers than in those of control mothers. The second such study, performed in Denmark under the direction of David Rosenthal, found similar results which, however, fell short of statistical significance, particularly when only parents with a consensus diagnosis of schizophrenia or schizophrenia spectrum were included. That study has been the subject of a blinded reanalysis using DSM-III criteria, which, when including only biological parents with a consensus diagnosis of schizophrenia from the original investigators, found a significant excess of schizophrenia spectrum in adopted-away offspring of schizophrenic parents versus those of control parents. The third and by far the largest study is still under way in Finland under the direction of Pekka Tien-

TABLE 14.5-3
Summary Results of Major Adoption Studies of Schizophrenia*

Study and Year	Location	Diagnosis in Relatives	Relationship of Index Group to Schizophrenic Proband	Affected N	Affected %	Control Group	Affected N	Affected %	p	Comments
Heston 1966	Oregon	Schiz	AAO	5/47	10.6	AAO of normals	0/50	0	0.01†	
Rosenthal et al 1971	Denmark	Schiz spect	AAO controls	14/52	26.9	AAO of controls	12/67	17.9	0.12†	Including only parents where judges agreed on a schiz spect dx
Lowing et al 1983	Denmark	Schiz spect	AAO	11/39	28.2	AAO	4/39	10.3	0.02‡	Independent analysis of the study by Rosenthal et al; biological parents restricted to DSM-II schiz; spectrum in offspring defined by DSM-III as schizophrenia and as schizotypal and schizoid personality disorders
Tienari 1992	Finland	Schiz	AAO	6/125	4.8	AAO of normals	2/178	1.1	0.02†	Preliminary report from ongoing study using matched index and control adoptees
Kety et al 1975	Denmark	Schiz spect	BRAS	24/173	13.9	BRAC	6/174	3.4	0.0003†	Greater Copenhagen sample, utilizing both hospital abstracts and personal interviews; biological rels of schiz adoptees include both first- and second-degree rels; results reported excluding schizoid personality from spectrum
			ARAS	2/74	2.7	ARAC	5/91	5.5	NS§	
Kety 1994	Denmark	Schiz spect	BRAS	22/171	12.9	BRAC	3/121	2.5	<0.005	The Provincial Danish Adoption Study, based on personal interviews
			ARAS	0/71	0	ARAC	0/55	0	NS§	
Kendler and Gruenberg 1994	Denmark	Schiz spect	BRAS	9/38	23.7	BRAC	5/107	4.7	0.001‡	Independent analysis of personal interviews from Kety's Copenhagen and Provincial studies, using DSM-III criteria; results from index adoptees with DSM-III schiz; only first-degree biological rels considered. In rels, schiz spect is defined as schizophrenia, schizoaffective disorder, mainly schizophrenic, and schizotypal and paranoid personality disorders
			ARAS	0/30	0	ARAC	1/102	1.0	NS§	

*Schiz indicates schizophrenia or schizophrenics; spect, spectrum; dx, diagnosis; AAO, adopted-away offspring; BRAS, biological relatives of adopted schizophrenics; BRAC, biological relatives of adopted controls; ARAS, adoptive relatives of adopted schizophrenics; ARC, adoptive relatives of adopted controls; rels, relatives.

†Represents statistical test for genetic transmission of liability to schizophrenia. Values of *p* are one-tailed.

‡Represents independent analyses of previous studies, not new investigations.

§Represents statistical test for cultural transmission of liability to schizophrenia. Values of *p* are two-tailed.

For references, see Kendler K S: The genetics of schizophrenia: An overview. In *Handbook of Schizophrenia,* vol 3, *Nosology, Epidemiology, and Genetics,* M T Tsuang, J C Simpson, editors. Elsevier, The Netherlands, 1988.

ari. Preliminary results indicate a statistically significant excess of schizophrenia in 125 adopted-away offspring of schizophrenic mothers compared with the 178 adopted-away offspring of matched control mothers.

Affected adoptee design Another major adoption strategy used for studying schizophrenia begins with ill adoptees rather than with ill parents. The full implementation of that design permits two separate experiments: (1) a test for the etiological role of shared environmental factors by comparing the nonbiological adoptive relatives of the schizophrenic and the control adoptees, and (2) a test for the etiological role of genetic factors by comparing the biological relatives of the schizophrenic and control adoptees who were raised in households away from their ill relatives. That strategy has been used by Seymour Kety and colleagues in a series of adoption studies carried out in Denmark. The first, or Copenhagen, sample began with 34 adoptees located in Copenhagen who received a consensus diagnosis of chronic, borderline, or acute schizophrenia. Those adoptees and their matched controls had been separated from their biological parents at an early age and raised by persons with whom they had no biological relationship. The first report on that series was based on hospital abstracts of all relatives located by the population and psychiatric registries available in Denmark. Schizophrenia and related disorders were significantly concentrated only in the biological relatives of the schizophrenic adoptees. The next phase of that project involved personal interviews of all available and cooperative relatives. After the interviews had been dictated into English and blinded a diagnostic review of those records also indicated a substantial concentration of schizophrenia spectrum disorders only in the biological relatives of the schizophrenic adoptees.

The final results of the sample, which were recently published, replicate all the major findings of the Copenhagen sample. Both chronic schizophrenia and schizophrenia spectrum disorders were significantly more common in the biological relatives of schizophrenic probands than in the biological relatives of control adoptees. No concentration of schizophrenia spectrum illness was seen in the adoptive relatives of schizophrenic adoptees. Interviews from the Copenhagen sample have been subject to several reanalyses. However, only one (by Kendler and Alan Gruenberg) reviewed all available interviews with adoptees and relatives. Using DSM-III criteria, those investigators replicated all the key findings of Kety and coworkers. Kendler and Gruenberg also blindly reviewed all interviews from the Provincial sample and recently reported on those results as well as findings from the two combined studies—termed the ''National Sample.'' Using diagnostic concepts closely related to the fourth edition of DSM (DSM-IV) they found strong evidence for the genetic transmission of schizophrenia and a clear genetic relationship between schizophrenia and schizoaffective disorder and schizotypal personality disorder.

Vertical cultural transmission Because studies of twins contain no parent-offspring pairs, they are not helpful in clarifying whether parents influence their children's risk for schizophrenia in ways other than passing on genes. However, several adoption strategies have been used to clarify the role of parent-offspring environmental transmission (termed vertical cultural transmission [VCT]) in schizophrenia. First, if offspring of schizophrenic persons in part learn schizophrenia from their parents, then decreasing the amount of contact between schizophrenic parents and their children should decrease their risk for illness. Two studies have produced results inconsistent with this hypothesis. Jerry Higgins and coworkers compared the adopted-away offspring of schizophrenic parents with naturally reared offspring of other schizophrenic parents. Although the sample size was small (23 offspring in each group), follow-up personal interviews indicated a nonsignificant excess of schizophrenia in the adopted-away offspring compared with those children reared by a schizophrenic parent. In a variation of a full adoption study, a similar design was utilized in Israel to compare (1) 25 offspring of schizophrenic persons reared in a kibbutz (where children are raised together in children's houses, although still having considerable contact with their parents) with (2) 25 offspring of schizophrenic parents raised in conventional nuclear family settings in towns elsewhere in Israel. A follow-up interview in adulthood with all offspring revealed that the risk for DSM-III schizophrenia was actually higher (nonsignificantly) in the kibbutz-reared offspring (13.0 percent) than in the town-reared offspring (8.7 percent). When schizophrenia spectrum disorders were included, that difference was even greater (26.1 percent versus 13.0 percent), although still short of statistical significance. Both sets of results are inconsistent with the vertical cultural transmission hypothesis.

A second way to address the vertical cultural transmission hypothesis is to look at the risk for schizophrenia in the adopted-away offspring of normal individuals reared by schizophrenic parents. Although limited by a small sample size and a small number of parents with typical schizophrenia, Paul Wender and coworkers found no evidence for increased rates of illness in such adoptees.

Third, vertical cultural transmission of schizophrenia would predict that among adopted individuals who become schizophrenic, schizophrenia should be overrepresented in their adoptive parents, who would culturally ''transmit'' schizophrenia. In Kety's Copenhagen and Provincial samples, no excess cases of schizophrenia or related spectrum conditions were seen in the adoptive parents of the schizophrenic adoptees. In separate samples, Wender and associates twice studied psychopathology in the adoptive parents of schizophrenic adaptees. The first of those studies found evidence for an excess of severe psychopathology in the adoptive parents of schizophrenics. In the second study, which the authors believed to be better controlled, no such increase was found.

Fourth, because the step-siblings of schizophrenics would be exposed to the same schizophrenogenic rearing environment as the schizophrenic person but would lack a biological relationship to the parents, vertical cultural transmission would also predict an excess of schizophrenia in step-siblings of schizophrenic persons. Two studies have been unable to find an excess risk for schizophrenia in the relatively small samples of step-siblings of schizophrenic probands.

In summary, twin and adoption studies provide strong, consistent evidence that genetic factors have a major role in the familial aggregation of schizophrenia. Evidence for a role for nongenetic familial factors is less clear. Some studies suggest that nongenetic factors may contribute modestly to the familial aggregation of schizophrenia, but the majority of studies find no evidence for significant nongenetic familial factors for schizophrenia.

HOW NARROW OR BROAD ARE THE PSYCHIATRIC DISORDERS THAT ARE TRANSMITTED WITHIN FAMILIES?

The first systematic family study of schizophrenia, performed by Ernst Rüdin in Emil Kraepelin's Psychiatric Institute in Munich in 1916, found that siblings of schizophrenic patients had increased rates not only of schizophrenia but also of other potentially related psychotic disorders. Since that time, a major focus of family, twin, and adoption studies of schizophrenia has been to clarify more precisely the nature of the psychiatric syndromes that occur in excess frequency in relatives of schizophrenic patients. That effort has been greatly aided by the emergence of operationalized diagnostic criteria in psychiatry, which permit more precise and reliable diagnoses.

HYPOTHESES On the level of psychopathological syndromes, four heuristic hypotheses can be articulated about the nature of the liability to schizophrenia that is transmitted in families: (1) a general liability to all psychiatric illnesses; (2) a liability to poor psychosocial functioning, oddness, and suspiciousness; (3) a liability to many forms of psychosis; and (4) a specific liability to typical schizophrenia. Those hypotheses are useful because each generates a different prediction about the kinds of psychiatric disorders that should be seen in excess in families of schizophrenic persons.

Nonspecific liability toward all psychiatric illness The first hypothesis predicts that the risk for all major forms of psychiatric illness should be increased in relatives of schizophrenic probands. The hypothesis is consistent with the unitary hypothesis of mental disorders, which postulates that all psychiatric illness is on a single continuum, with schizophrenia at the most deviant end. That hypothesis can be best evaluated in modern family studies and in reanalyses of major adoption studies that have used similar diagnostic criteria and normal control groups.

In the six modern family studies of schizophrenia that meet those criteria five examined anxiety disorders, and none found that anxiety disorders occurred in significant excess in relatives of schizophrenic versus matched control probands. All six studies examined the risk for mood disorder illness, and four studies found no significant excess risk for affective illness in relatives of schizophrenic probands. However, two studies found that major depressive disorder was significantly more common in relatives of schizophrenic probands. Five studies examined the risk for alcoholism, four of which found no significant difference in risk for that disorder in relatives of schizophrenic and control probands, while one study found a significant deficiency of cases of alcoholism in relatives of schizophrenic probands. Similar results on a smaller sample size were found in the reanalysis of the Copenhagen sample of the Danish adoption study where no excess risk for either anxiety disorders or depression was found in the biological relatives of the schizophrenic adoptees versus the control adoptees. The familial liability to schizophrenia appears to possess some specificity and does not increase the risk for anxiety disorders or alcoholism and probably does not increase the risk for mood disorder.

Schizophrenia-related personality disorders Both of the two chief architects of the concept of schizophrenia, Kraepelin and Eugen Bleuler, noted that some close relatives of patients with schizophrenia, though never psychotic, had odd or eccentric personalities that were clinically reminiscent of schizophrenia. Since that time similar observations have been made by a number of clinicians and researchers. The first and probably most influential rigorous study of what may be termed "schizophrenia-related personality disorders" was made by Kety and colleagues in the Danish adoption studies. Based on a blind diagnostic review with their own diagnostic criteria, Kety and colleagues found a statistically significant excess rate of borderline and uncertain schizophrenia in the biological relatives of schizophrenic adoptees versus control adoptees.

More recent applications of operationalized criteria have replicated and extended those earlier findings in support of the second hypothesis. Since 1983 eight family studies have examined the risk for schizophrenia spectrum, defined as schizotypal or paranoid personality disorder by DSM-III or DSM-III-R criteria, in relatives of schizophrenic probands and matched normal control probands (Table 14.5-4). Those studies included two reanalyses of different Danish adoption samples, three family studies conducted in the United States, one family study conducted in Greece, one in Denmark, and one in Ireland. The absolute rates of schizotypal and paranoid personality disorders in both relatives of schizophrenic persons and control probands differed widely across the studies. That might be expected because different approaches are used for assessment of these personality disorders. However, every study found that schizotypal or paranoid personality was more common in relatives of schizophrenic persons than in control probands, and that difference was statistically significant in six of the eight studies. In aggregate those results provide strong support for the second hypothesis articulated earlier: that the familial liability to schizophrenia is in part reflected by a set of personality traits related to social isolation, oddness, and suspiciousness.

General liability to psychosis Recent family and adoption studies of schizophrenia have also provided substantial data with which to evaluate the third hypothesis. If the familial liability to schizophrenia increases the risk of a variety of nonaffective psychoses, then the risks for nonschizophrenic psychotic disorders should be increased in relatives of schizophrenic probands and also the risk for schizophrenia should be increased in relatives of probands with the other nonschizophrenic psychotic disorders.

The literature on family studies of schizoaffective disorder is complex and confusing. However, if schizoaffective disorder is defined, as in DSM-III-R, to include patients who, in addition to episodes of concurrent prominent affective symptoms and psychosis, also have periods of psychotic symptoms without prominent affective symptoms, the results are relatively consistent. Three family studies have found a significant excess of such cases of schizoaffective illness in relatives of schizophrenic probands versus relatives of control probands. Four family studies have reported an excess risk for schizophrenia in the relatives of probands with schizoaffective disorder versus control probands. In their reanalysis of the Copenhagen sample of the Danish adoption study Kendler and associates found an excess risk for schizophrenia spectrum psychopathology in the biological relatives of adoptees with a diagnosis of schizoaffective disorder.

Evidence regarding a familial relationship between schizophrenia and delusional disorder and schizophrenia and the remitting or atypical psychoses is somewhat less clear. Several studies beginning with delusional disorder probands have found

TABLE 14.5-4
Summary Results of Major Family and Adoption Studies Using Personal Interviews to Examine Risk for DSM-III and DSM-III-R Schizotypal or Paranoid Personality Disorder in First-Degree Relatives of Schizophrenic and Normal Control Probands

		Relatives of Schizophrenic Probands			Relatives of Control Probands			
			SPD or PPD			SPD or PPD		
Author and Year	Study Group	BZ*	N	MR ± SE	BZ*	N	MR ± SE	*p*
Lowing 1983	Adopted-away offspring	39	6	15.4 ± 5.8	39	3	7.7 ± 4.3	.29
Kendler 1994†	Biological relatives of adoptees	35	6	17.1 ± 6.4	106	4	3.8 ± 1.9	.01
Baron 1985	Nuclear family study	329	72	21.9 ± 2.3	337	16	4.7 ± 1.2	$<10 \times 10^{-9}$
Frangos 1985	Nuclear family study	478	13	2.7 ± 0.7	536	3	0.6 ± 0.3	.006
Coryell 1988	Nuclear family study	72	3	4.2 ± 2.3	160	4	2.5 ± 1.2	.49
Gershon 1988	Nuclear family study	108	3	2.8 ± 1.6	380	0	0	.01
Kendler 1993	Nuclear family study	319	26	8.2 ± 1.5	580	10	1.7 ± 0.5	.000003
Parnas 1993	Nuclear family offspring only	192	41	21.3 ± 3.0	101	5	5.0 ± 2.2	<.0001

*BZ indicates *bezugsziffer* (lifetimes at risk); SPD, schizotypal personality disorder; PPD, paranoid personality disorder; MR, morbid risk; SE, standard error.

†Reanalyses of adoption studies, reporting prevalence rather than MR.

no significant excess risk for schizophrenia in their relatives. However, at least two large sample family studies of schizophrenia have found a significantly increased risk for delusional and atypical psychoses in the relatives of schizophrenic probands versus control probands. The asymmetry of results may be the result of differing levels of diagnostic accuracy in probands versus secondary cases (cases found in relatives).

Another specific test of the third hypothesis is to examine the frequency of psychotic mood disorders in relatives of schizophrenic probands. In large-scale family studies both in Iowa and in Ireland, Kendler and colleagues found that while relatives of schizophrenic persons were not at increased risk for mood disorders, if affectively ill, they were more than twice as likely to become psychotic as the mood-disordered relatives of controls. Furthermore, in both studies, relatives of probands with psychotic mood disorders were at increased risk for schizophrenia compared with relatives of controls.

Results to date provide strong evidence against the validity of hypotheses one and four. The familial predisposition to schizophrenia is neither completely nonspecific nor highly specific. Results are available to support the second hypothesis strongly and also to provide some evidence in favor of the third hypothesis. Current evidence suggests that the familial liability to schizophrenia increases not only the risk for narrowly defined schizophrenia but also for schizotypal and paranoid personality disorder and probably for several nonschizophrenic psychotic illnesses. Those findings provide an increasingly complex but informative picture of the nature of the transmitted liability to schizophrenia.

GENETIC TRANSMISSION MECHANISMS

The conclusion that genes account for the majority of risk for schizophrenia and related psychiatric disorders naturally leads to an interest in understanding the detailed mechanisms underlying genetic transmission. What is the genetic architecture of schizophrenia? Do very many genes of very small individual effect exert a cumulative effect in the transmission of genetic risk or, do single genes act alone to transmit a major risk of developing schizophrenia? If such major genes exist, do they function in a dominant or recessive manner?

In addition to those relatively simple questions, other important issues ultimately need to be addressed. Among those are the possible complex ways that specific genes may interact with each other and with specific factors in the cultural and biological environment. For many years genetic epidemiological studies have been carried out with the goal of answering such questions; unfortunately, most have not yet been definitively solved.

STATISTICAL TECHNIQUES In brief, statistical genetic techniques used to investigate the genetic architecture of schizophrenia, such as segregation analysis, involve comparing the observed patterns of co-occurrence of schizophrenia among family members of close genetic relationship versus more distant genetic relationship with the degree of sharing expected under the assumptions of alternative genetic model. For example, a single-locus-dominant model of genetic transmission would predict that schizophrenia will occur in half of the children of families where one parent is schizophrenic and the other parent is not affected by schizophrenia or any genetically related disorder. From the familial aggregation data reviewed above it is immediately clear that that simple model can be rejected as implausible as a complete explanation of the genetic architecture of schizophrenia. However, more realistic models become complex, and that complexity leads to much greater difficulty in either accepting or rejecting their validity with any degree of confidence.

Some studies that have been carried out with the aim of discriminating the genetic mechanisms underlying familial transmission of schizophrenia are detailed in Table 14.5-5. The methods used to address that important question have grown increasingly sophisticated since the time when Rüdin first focused his attention on the problem shortly after the laws of simple mendelian transmission were rediscovered at the beginning of the 20th century. Since the late 1960s a controversy has persisted between those who have favored the polygenic or multifactorial threshold hypothesis in which genetic liability is transmitted by many genetic loci (presumably hundreds), each of very small effect, versus the proponents of the single major locus hypothesis, which in the extreme proposes that all differences in genetic risk among persons are the result of allelic variation at a single locus of necessarily major effect. Compounding this dichotomy are arguments regarding how and to what extent biological and cultural environments interact with the genetic factor or factors. Inspection of Table 14.5-5 shows that to date the segregation analysis approach has yielded only inconclusive and inconsistent results. At best, only some extreme genetic models (such as exclusively simple mendelian transmission) can be ruled out, and even that modest conclusion requires an assumption of the unlikely hypothesis of homogeneity in the genetic factors responsible for schizophrenia in all of the families studied.

COMPLICATING FACTORS The answer to why the segregation analysis approach has failed to shed much light on the genetic architecture of schizophrenia might best be illustrated by considering what sorts of parameters a biologically realistic segregation analysis of the disorder might need to incorporate. A list of those parameters probably should include the following:

1. Allowance for incomplete penetrance for any major loci considered (that is, some persons who are carriers of high-risk genotypes may not express clinically recognizable symptoms of the disorder, especially as a function of age)
2. Allowance for phenocopies (that is, some persons recognized to have classic clinical symptoms may not carry any significant predisposing genes, but may simply be affected as a consequence of environmental insult)
3. Comparison of models having only one major susceptibility gene, or several major genes that interact either additively or more complexly, with allowances made for a multitude of alleles at the major genes that potentially have different patterns of dominance and interaction with other loci
4. Inclusion of polygenic components that may interact with one or more of the major genes if the latter are present (that is, the mixed model)
5. Different kinds of environmental effects, including some that are transmitted familially and some that may interact with any or all of the genes present in the model
6. Account of the known occurrence of positive assortative mating (Persons affected by schizophrenia are more likely to choose mates who are also schizophrenic than would be expected to occur by chance.)
7. Allowance for reduced fitness of schizophrenic persons (especially men), to reflect the observed reduction in reproduction that occurs after the onset of the disorder
8. Consideration of a range of possible diagnostic criteria (multiple disease thresholds) as a definition of the illness—

TABLE 14.5-5
Studies of the Mode of Transmission of Schizophrenia

Study and year	Method of Analysis*	Conclusion
Rüdin et al 1916	Simple inspection of family histories	Reject simple fully penetrant dominant or recessive transmission; propose causation by two fully penetrant recessive genes
Gottesman and Shields 1967	MFT	Data found to be compatible with polygenic model
Kidd and Cavalli-Sforza 1973	SML	Favor partially recessive SML with environmental influence and existence of some nongenetic cases
Matthysse and Kidd 1976	SML versus MFT	Neither simple model adequate; both models predict genetic heterogeneity
Elston et al 1978	SML with AOO	Reject both simple SML and purely environmental modes of transmission
Carter and Chung 1980	MM	Inconclusive; preference for polygenic model
Tsuang et al 1982	SML with AOO	Reject simple SML model and purely environmental modes of transmission; suggest genetic heterogeneity
O'Rourke et al 1982	SML with AOO	Reject simple SML model
Risch and Baron 1984	MM	Data compatible with either polygenic or (largely) SML transmission
Risch 1990	Risk in relatives	Data indicate risk due to interaction among multiple loci
Vogler et al 1990	MM	Inconclusive

*MFT indicates multifactorial threshold (polygenic) model; SML, single major locus model; AOO, variable age of onset of schizophrenia; MM, mixed model, which combines SML and MT parameters with allowance for common sibling environment.

ranging from very narrowly defined schizophrenia to a much broader range of related psychiatric disorders

9. Adjustment for potential biases in how the sample of families being examined was originally identified and further studied (that is, ascertainment bias), which may be straightforward in theory but impossible in practice under the conditions encountered in field studies.

10. The high likelihood of the existence of heterogeneity among different families included in any study (that is, different families have different underlying disease etiologies that have led to indistinguishable clinical phenotype lumped together as schizophrenia.).

None of the complicating factors alone—nor their effect together—invalidates the segregation analysis approach to elucidation of the genetic etiology of schizophrenia in theory. A major problem exists, however, which becomes apparent when considering the very limited sample sizes that even the most ambitious family study of schizophrenia could ever produce. Incorporation of more than one or two of the 10 biological factors listed above into a statistical genetic model requires the model to become extremely complicated, requiring that a large number of parameters be estimated from the study data itself. In addition, parameter estimates become confounded as there are not enough degrees of freedom to resolve so many interacting factors. The attempt to ask so many questions of any limited data set quickly complicates the analysis such that its statistical power becomes quite small. Another way of stating that is to say that the only questions that can be answered with adequate confidence are too simple to be of much interest because such a large body of other evidence argues too strongly against any simple explanations for the genetic etiology of schizophrenia. On the other hand, the really interesting questions are probably beyond the ability to address by a statistical approach alone.

But, fortunately, review of the genetics of schizophrenia need not end on such a pessimistic note. New developments in molecular genetic technologies, combined with advances in statistical methods and refined diagnostic procedures offer hope for resolving the dilemma. All studies summarized thus far are based on observations about the occurrence of schizophrenia in various familial relationships. The studies have attempted to draw conclusions about the mode of action of genes using knowledge about the proportions of genes that are expected by statistical principles to be identical among close relatives versus distant relatives versus unrelated individuals. That approach has been called the unmeasured genotype approach. Note that in those studies actual genes are never tracked through the families to see whether or to what extent sharing of a specific gene product correlates with the chance of sharing the schizophrenia clinical phenotype. Rather, it is becoming increasingly feasible technically to follow the transmission of specific genes and chromosomes through families to apply a measured genotype approach to the study of complex disorders such as schizophrenia, using measurements of genes made at the deoxyribonucleic acid (DNA) level. That approach offers substantial promise for bridging the current gap between a conclusion that genes appear to be important in transmitting the risk for schizophrenia, and the ultimate goal of research, which is to understand the cause of the disorder at the cellular, physiological, and biochemical levels.

CURRENT STATUS AND FUTURE PROSPECTS FOR IDENTIFYING SPECIFIC GENES THAT PREDISPOSE TO SCHIZOPHRENIA

Two fundamentally distinct strategies have been employed in attempts to find specific genes that confer susceptibility to schizophrenia: tests of association and linkage. The former has traditionally been carried out using unrelated schizophrenic probands as subjects, while the latter is inherently a family based study. To date, no widely replicated reports that identify specific susceptability genes for schizophrenia have yet appeared despite considerable efforts expended.

ASSOCIATION STUDIES The association studies approach tests whether persons affected by a disease more frequently have a particular allele at some candidate genetic locus than persons not affected by the disease. The classic genetic system used for many association tests is the immune system histocompatibility genes, known as the human lymphocyte antigen (HLA) region. If one suspects that defects in immune regulation might underlie the pathology of a disorder it is reasonable to ask whether any allele at an HLA locus (or combinations of adjacent alleles, known as a haplotype) occurs more frequently among persons affected by the disease than persons not affected. For example, it has been clearly demonstrated that insulin-dependent diabetes is associated with alleles in the HLA region. The DNA sequence differences that actually distinguish alleles at a candidate gene being tested in an association study (for example, restriction fragment recognition site differences) need not necessarily directly confer altered biological function of the candidate gene, although that could occur in some cases. If the DNA differences that distinguish the marker alleles do not directly alter the function of the candidate gene, they must themselves be associated (technically, in disequilibrium) with neighboring DNA sequences in the candidate gene that actually influence susceptibility to the disease. That requirement places a major limitation on the power of association tests.

Application of the association strategy to schizophrenia has included only a limited number of candidate gene loci thus far. Only one relatively consistent association has been found: that between the HLA A9 allele and the paranoid subtype of schizophrenia. Even that finding is not entirely consistent across repeated studies of ethnic and racial groups, and risk associated with this marker is only elevated by 60 percent. In addition to loci in the HLA region possible associations have been sought according to blood group and serum proteins. The development of DNA-based polymorphisms now offers the potential to substantially expand the scope of association studies of schizophrenia to include a large number of neurotransmitter and neuroreceptor genes, as well as other genes associated with the development and regulation of the central nervous system. Several investigators have recently examined the association between schizophrenia and alleles at dopamine receptors. Preliminary evidence of a positive association between schizophrenia and certain dopamine type 3 (D_3) receptor alleles has not been widely replicated. There is limited interest in pursuing the association strategy in recent studies, because of some inherent drawbacks in that approach.

Limitations of association studies An association between a disease and allelic variation at a candidate gene is insufficient evidence for concluding that the candidate gene causes the disease. If a study finds a statistically significant association between a disease and alleles at a candidate gene the result must be interpreted with great caution because there are several population genetic mechanisms and statistical artifacts that might bring about an association even if the candidate gene has nothing to do with the disease. For example there is the possibility of association due to ethnic differences between the patient and control groups. If a particular marker allele at a candidate gene is more common in some ethnic group (perhaps as a result of random genetic drift as the group was genetically isolated from other groups) and if that ethnic group happens to be more frequently represented in the patient group than in the control group, an association with the candidate gene and schizophrenia would be observed. The allele associated in that case, however, has nothing to do with causing the disease but simply reflects the biased sampling in the construction of the patient and control groups. Therefore, it is necessary to be careful in matching subjects between the two groups, which makes the assembly of very large groups for such comparisons more difficult to achieve. Other ways that noncausal associations can arise include failure to correct adequately for multiple comparisons and the possibility of recent population admixture. While multiple comparisons can be corrected relatively easily, such correction comes at an increasingly higher cost in terms of reduced statistical power to detect real associations, especially if one contemplates carrying out association tests using hundreds of DNA-based polymorphisms. Population admixture can lead to a noncausal association. Consider a scenario in which two human populations that differ both in the frequency of some gene that has a major influence on susceptibility to schizophrenia and in the frequency of alleles at a candidate locus have been combined in recent historical time by migration. That admixture creates an association between the schizophrenia gene and the candidate gene even if the candidate gene has nothing to do with causing the disorder. Even if the candidate gene is located on a different chromosome than the schizophrenia susceptibility gene and if there is random mating, the association created by admixture is only reduced by 50 percent in each generation. Given the dramatic movements and mixing of human populations during the past century, the possibility of admixture-induced associations will have to be considered.

Alternatively, if a study fails to find any evidence of an association it is by no means safe to conclude that the candidate gene in question can be eliminated as a potential cause of the disease. The DNA sequence variation that is responsible for distinguishing the alleles of the candidate gene must directly cause differences in the function of the candidate gene's product (for example, cause amino acid substitutions or differences in the level of expression of the gene), or the allelic differences themselves must be in association with other DNA sequence differences that bring about these biologically significant changes. Thus, it is entirely possible that some of the DNA sequences that distinguish alleles used for association studies may reside within or very near a gene that actually does predispose to the development of schizophrenia, but may simply not be in association with the neighboring DNA sequences that result in the important biochemical variation in the gene's product. That would be especially likely to occur if the allelic variation occurred within portions of a gene that do not code for amino acids within the protein product but rather within portions of genes called "introns" that are simply spliced out of the gene sequence prior to the start of protein synthesis. The vast majority of DNA-based polymorphisms identified thus far reside within noncoding regions.

Genetic recombination during meiosis acts continually to reduce the degree of association (disequilibrium) that may initially exist between any DNA polymorphisms that flank the actual functional DNA sequence variation within a disease candidate gene. For that reason only polymorphisms that are very close to the candidate gene and therefore experience only very infrequent recombination are expected to be found in association with the disease. The phenomenon requires either that the investigator has already identified candidate loci that are very likely *a priori* to be involved etiologically with the disease or that he or she contemplates genotyping an unrealistically large number of marker polymorphisms in order to search the entire human genome adequately. In contrast, for linkage analysis polymorphic DNA markers can be distributed up to tens of millions of DNA bases apart from each other and still provide considerable power to detect genetic effects of specific loci that reside between those distantly spaced markers. For that reason, and also because of the difficulty of obtaining any solid conclusions from either positive or negative association study results, most efforts to identify specific loci that underlie the etiology of schizophrenia have focused on the linkage analysis approach.

LINKAGE ANALYSIS Linkage studies differ from association studies in that, for the former, persons from different families that are affected by the disease are not expected to share similar alleles at the polymorphic marker locus being studied. If a marker locus is linked to a particular disease gene, however, affected persons within a family will generally share the same marker alleles. The term linkage simply means that the disease gene and the marker locus occur together in relatively close proximity on the same chromosome. Because adjacent pieces of human chromosomes are usually passed as a unit from parent to offspring (in the absence of recombination), inheritance of the disease susceptibility gene will be correlated with inheritance of particular marker alleles within a family. However, in unrelated families the disease gene may happen to reside on a chromosome that contains a different marker allele, and so within that family, inheritance of the disease will be correlated with inheritance of the alternative marker allele.

Linkage analysis has been well developed and applied with great benefit for improving an understanding of both animal and plant genetic systems since the turn of the century. Until recently, however, its use in human genetic studies was limited because of the availability of only a few polymorphic marker loci. To search a particular chromosomal region for a schizophrenia gene, it is necessary to have marker loci that ideally are highly variable among different persons and that can be easily and reliably distinguished. The recent developments in molecular genetic technology have now provided researchers with such markers, enabling searches to be undertaken throughout the entire human genome. Previously, the only variable marker loci available were for the HLA region, the blood group antigens, and a few serum enzymes and other proteins. With so few marker polymorphisms, only a very small fraction of the human genome could be examined using the linkage analysis approach.

Linkage studies A selection of linkage studies of schizophrenia are summarized in Table 14.5-6. The table is not exhaustive. Prior to the development of DNA-based polymorphisms only limited efforts to map genes responsible for schizophrenia were undertaken (with inconclusive results).

In 1988 that situation changed dramatically. First, a cytogenetically visible chromosomal abnormality (an unbalanced partial trisomy) in the proximal region of the long arm of chromosome 5 was observed in a child and his maternal uncle, both of whom had schizophrenia and physical anomalies. That finding led other investigators to carry out linkage analyses using polymorphic DNA markers that reside in the abnormal trisomic region of chromosome 5. A study reported by Sherrington and colleagues in 1988 used five pedigrees from Iceland and two pedigrees from England that contained a high density of schizophrenic patients. Statistical analyses indicated strong support for linkage to that region on chromosome 5 in most or all of the families studied, far beyond results that might be expected to arise by chance alone in the absence of any true linkage.

One unexpected aspect of the report was the fact that support for linkage increased substantially as the definition of the affected phenotype was widened to include not only broadly defined schizophrenia but also many other psychiatric disorders such as alcoholism or eating disorders. That indication of a broad susceptibility to many psychiatric disorders is inconsistent with many family and adoption studies and was judged by some as evidence against the validity of the conclusion that a major gene for schizophrenia actually could be located in that chromosomal region. It is entirely possible that the type of illness present in these particular studies studied may not be typical of most cases of schizophrenia, but even the identification of such an atypical, broadly acting gene might still be immensely valuable. Consider, for example, the beneficial insights that have come from studies of families affected by severe hypercholesterolemia and coronary artery disease. The severe and atypical form of coronary artery disease found in those families is clearly not representative of the manifestation of this disease in the general population. Nevertheless, the genetic variation at the lipoprotein receptors that was identified as causing the severe cases is also highly relevant to the risk of coronary artery disease in the general population. That strategy is partly responsible for the ongoing attempt to identify and study many high-density schizophrenia families. Although those families may not accurately represent the genetic etiology of schizophrenia in the general population, they may substantially increase the ability to detect the effects of genes that have a major influence on susceptibility to the disorder.

Unfortunately, many attempts to replicate the original positive report of linkage on chromosome 5q11-q13 have all provided evidence against linkage. However, many reasons can be suggested to explain the lack of inconsistency. For example, most of the follow-up studies used only one or a very limited number of genetic models to test for linkage (such as dominant transmission only or failure to adjust penetrance values for delayed age of onset). It is theoretically possible, but extremely unlikely, that those analytical differences could account for such a major discrepancy. Another study demonstrated that any multiple comparisons bias in the original study—because logarithm of the odds (LOD) scores were maximized by sequentially testing 18 somewhat different genetic models (different disease definitions and penetrance levels)—was unlikely to generate such strong evidence of linkage falsely.

It is possible that the defective gene responsible for schizophrenia in the Icelandic families does not exist in other populations. Alternatively, the 5q11-q13 gene may be present in some of those populations, but may occur in only a relatively small subset of families. Given the small numbers of families studied in most of the follow-up reports, it is conceivable that this could be the case. With one exception no study has had sufficient statistical power to detect linkage that is present in a minority proportion of families (that is, locus heterogeneity). Most studies included only a few families and at most 200 marker genotypes. The exception is the study reported by Ying Su et al., which included 112 Irish families and over 2,000 marker genotypes. The greater sample size of that study provided statistical power to go beyond addressing the unrealistic hypothesis (to which all of the other studies are limited) that a schizophrenia gene is present in the candidate chromosomal region in all or most families in the population under study. Instead, the more realistic hypothesis that a major gene in the candidate region could be present in as few as 25 percent of the Irish families was excluded by the results of the study.

In fact, recent studies using additional DNA markers in the originally reported families, as well as other Icelandic families, indicate that the 5q11-q13 linkage finding was most likely a false positive. Given the strength of statistical support for the original data, an adequate explanation for its subsequent dramatic decline has not yet been provided. The unfolding of this situation is certainly an apparent setback to the goal of finding genes that have a major influence on susceptibility to schizophrenia. On the other hand, the outcome can also be viewed as

TABLE 14.5-6
Linkage Studies of Schizophrenia

Study and Year	Locus/Region*	Exclusion or Support of Linkage
McGuffin and Sturt 1986†	HLA/6p21.3	Exclusion assuming homogeneity
McGuffin and Sturt 1986†	20 protein loci	Either exclusion assuming homogeneity or inconclusive
Sherrington et al 1988	ADM/5q11-13	Strong support assuming either homogeneity or heterogeneity
Kennedy et al 1988	ADM/5q11-13	Exclusion assuming homogeneity
St. Clair et al 1989	ADM/5q11-13	Exclusion assuming homogeneity
Detera-Wadleigh et al 1989	ADM/5q11-13	Exclusion assuming homogeneity
Aschauer et al 1990	ADM/5q11-13	Exclusion assuming homogeneity
McGuffin et al 1990	ADM/5q11-13	Exclusion assuming homogeneity
Crowe et al 1991	ADM/5q11-13	Exclusion assuming homogeneity
Byerley et al 1991	ADM/5q11-13	Exclusion assuming homogeneity
Su et al 1991	ADM/5q11-13	Exclusion assuming 25 to 50 percent proportion linked
Aschauer et al 1991	ADM/2q	Weak support assuming homogeneity or heterogeneity
Byerley et al 1991	DRD1/5q34-35	Exclusion assuming homogeneity
Kennedy et al 1991	DRD1/5q34-35	Exclusion assuming homogeneity
Moises et al 1991	DRD2/11q23	Exclusion assuming homogeneity
Byerley et al 1991	DRD2/11q23	Exclusion assuming homogeneity
Su et al 1991	DRD2/11q23	Exclusion assuming 25 to 50 percent proportion linked
Kennedy et al 1991	DRD4/11p15.5	Exclusion assuming homogeneity
Byerley et al 1991	ADM/150 loci	Exclusion assuming homogeneity or inconclusive
Polymeropoulos et al 1991	ADM/30 loci	Exclusion assuming homogeneity or inconclusive
Collinge et al 1991	ADM/XYpter	Suggestion of linkage
Delisi et al 1991	ADM/Xq27-28	Exclusion assuming homogeneity
St. Clair et al 1990	CR/1q43-11q21	Suggestion of linkage (for broadly defined psychiatric illness)
Hallmayer et al 1992	5-HT_2/13	Exclusion in one pedigree
Byerley et al 1993	TH/11p15.5	Exclusion assuming homogeneity
Coon et al 1993	DRD1-5	Exclusion assuming homogeneity
Wang et al 1993	ADM/XYpter	Exclusion assuming homogeneity
Wang et al 1993	ADM/11q	Exclusion assuming homogeneity
Gill et al 1993	ADM/11q	Exclusion assuming homogeneity
Polymeropoulos et al 1994	ADM/22q	Weak evidence for linkage
Pulver et al 1994	22q12-13.1	Initial positive finding not replicated by other groups

*Locus indicates name of locus for markers that are genes or proteins of known function: ADM if anonymous DNA marker, and CR if chromosome rearrangement; Region, chromosomal location of marker loci.
†Review of several independent studies.

a demonstration of the robustness of the linkage analysis approach, in that false-positive findings can and will be refuted. Any positive reports of linkage will continue to be viewed with caution, and researchers in this field have shown that they are capable of quickly following up on positive reports to determine their validity.

The other studies listed in Table 14.5-6 include the following: (1) a suggestion of linkage on the long arm of chromosome 2, a region that was again initially of interest due to a chromosomal rearrangement correlated with schizophrenia; (2) studies of several dopamine receptor genes that have recently been cloned and for which there are now DNA-based polymorphisms; (3) two genome-wide searches using polymorphic markers located on many different chromosomes without any *a priori* hypothesis regarding the region; (4) a suggestion of linkage to the pseudoautosomal region of the X and Y chromosomes (a region of interest because of a reported sex concordance among schizophrenic siblings), and an exclusion of the distal portion of the X chromosome (abnormalities of the sex chromosome are sometimes associated with various forms of psychosis); (5) suggestion of linkage to the long arm of chromosome 11 using the segregation of a chromosome rearrangement within a large extended family with illness defined broadly; and (6) suggestion of possible linkage between schizophrenia and a region on the long arm of chromosome 22. Those suggestive positive results are now being followed by many laboratories. It should again be emphasized that because of the small number of families studied, the many results that have excluded various candidate genes or chromosomal regions (with the exception of the studies by Su et al.) have thus far only excluded the unrealistic hypothesis of linkage in most or all families in each report. It will require studies on a larger scale to address the crucial questions of whether those genes and regions may be important for significant but minority subsets of families.

It is appropriate to ask why the linkage analysis approach is robust to the long list of complexities presented as impediments to segregation analysis. The answer lies in the goal of linkage analysis, which in some sense is more limited than that of segregation analysis. A linkage test simply addresses the question of whether a given polymorphic marker locus cosegregates with schizophrenia among close or distant relatives. The test can be performed either by using multiple analyses assuming different possible modes of transmission (with straightforward ways to adjust *p* values) or by using nonparametric methods that do not even require those assumptions. Furthermore, some factors that can drastically confound results of segregation analyses (such as ascertainment bias and fitness effects) have either little or no effect on the outcome of linkage tests.

Heterogeneity One aspect of schizophrenia that affects both linkage and segregation analyses is the likely existence of heterogeneity, especially locus heterogeneity, which means that a gene of major effect only segregates in a subset of all families. Most linkage analyses of schizophrenia have not taken that important factor into proper account. That is especially true for reports of exclusion of linkage to particular loci or chromosomal regions. Most of the studies listed in Table 14.5-6 have addressed exclusion only in terms of the homogeneity hypothesis: the evidence in support of linkage in all of the families under study is compared to a null hypothesis of linkage in none of the families. Because few if any researchers of the genetics of schizophrenia expect that the disorder could be caused by a single malfunctioning gene in all families, rejection of the simple homogeneity hypothesis is not very interesting.

The influence of heterogeneity on both positive findings of linkage as well as exclusion of linkage is illustrated in the following set of figures. The data were generated using computer simulation techniques in which it is possible to control the underlying genetic parameters and the extent of genetic heterogeneity exactly. For the analysis, 25 medium-sized families were generated, each having three schizophrenic children, three unaffected children, one schizophrenic parent, and one unaffected parent. One computer simulation run consisted of generating the expected distribution of two alleles at two marker loci that were located on either side of a schizophrenia-predisposing gene at a distance of 0.05 recombination fraction. That resulted in 25 simulated families, 100 percent of which contained a gene for schizophrenia located between the two marker loci. The linkage analysis of that data set is shown in Figure 14.5-1, with four separate analyses showing the expected results under the homogeneity hypothesis of a proportion of 1.0 of the families linked (actually true for this example), as well as reduced proportions at 0.75, 0.50, and 0.25. The LOD score is plotted for tests of alternative hypotheses, and it can be seen that strong evidence of linkage is found for all hypotheses with the true hypothesis of 100 percent of the families linked receiving the strongest support.

For a second example, another 25 families were simulated using the same pedigree structure used above but with the schizophrenia gene unlinked to either of the two marker loci. Twelve of the unlinked families were combined with 13 of the linked group of families from above into a total data set of 25 families. That data set, in which about 50 percent of the families are actually linked, was then analyzed under the four alternative heterogeneity hypotheses, as shown in Figure 14.5-2. The results differ dramatically from those obtained when 100 percent of the families are linked. In fact, the highest LOD score is obtained under the true situation of a 0.50 proportion of families linked, but the statistical support in favor of the linkage hypothesis has been greatly weakened (a maximum LOD score of 2.6 versus 11.8). The important conclusion to be drawn from the result is that it is much harder to identify linkage if the disease gene is responsible for causing the disease in only a subset of all families in the study. In addition, note that the LOD score curve is actually negative in the close vicinity of the truly linked gene if an incorrect analysis assuming homogeneity (1.0 proportion linked) is applied to the heterogeneous data.

Last, a model was developed that considered the situation that exists if no disease-causing genes actually are linked to the region being tested. The analysis used all 25 families that were simulated as having no linkage between the disease gene and the marker loci. The data were again analyzed under the four alternative hypotheses regarding the proportion of families actually linked to the marker loci region. The results are plotted in Figure 14.5-3. The data strongly exclude the hypothesis that 100 percent of the families are linked to the region (LOD score < -2 required for exclusion). The curve generated represents the type of analyses described in Table 14.5-6 as "exclusion assuming homogeneity." However, that hypothesis is not realistic for a complex disorder such as schizophrenia (perhaps more appropriately referred to as "the schizophrenias"). When addressing the more realistic hypotheses of linkage of only a subset of families, the results very quickly lose statistical power. In fact, the results cannot rule out the possibility that as many as half of the families studied could be linked to the candidate region, although there is no positive evidence in support of that conclusion as was obtained for the example shown in Figure 14.5-2. It would require a study of many more families to begin to address some of the tenable hypotheses regarding the genetics of schizophrenia, such as the possibility that major genes may be segregating in 25 percent or even in only 10 percent of families. The conclusion to be drawn from both Figures 14.5-2 and 14.5-3 is that large-scale studies will be required in order to achieve reasonable power to map complex and heterogeneous disorders, such as schizophrenia. Such studies will require both very many families (as large as possible and ideally spanning three generations or more, with many affected persons). In addition, because there is at present no strong *a priori* candidate genes or regions for the disorder, researchers will have to genotype hundreds of highly informative DNA marker loci dispersed throughout the entire human genome.

Future prospects The prospects during the next decade for finding genes that confer susceptibility to schizophrenia are very substantial. The three principal tools that are necessary to provide a good chance (though not a guarantee) of success in this endeavor are becoming increasingly more refined and pow-

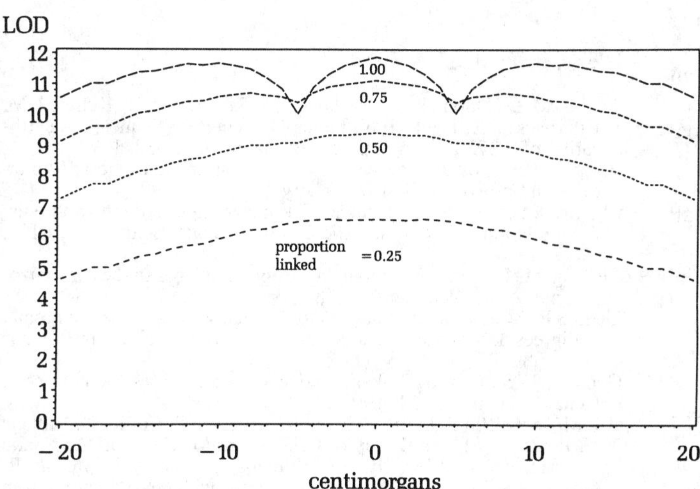

FIGURE 14.5-1 *Linkage with homogeneity. LOD scores were obtained from computer analysis of 25 simulated nuclear families (described in the text) in which a disease gene is located at the 0.0 centimorgan map position in all families (genetic homogeneity) and flanked on both sides by genetic marker loci located about 5 centimorgans on either side. Support for four alternative tests of linkage are shown. The hypotheses differ in the hypothesized proportion of families in the collection of families that might contain a major gene conferring susceptibility to schizophrenia. Those hypotheses of linkage with varying levels of genetic heterogeneity are contrasted with the null hypothesis that none of the families contains such a gene (proportion linked = 0.0). When all families are actually linked to the candidate region, as in this example, all four hypotheses show strong support for linkage. However, because LOD scores are based on a $\log_{10}$ scale, the LOD score of 12.0 in support of the true hypothesis (proportion linked = 1.00) provides over one million times (10^6) greater odds of linkage than the hypothesis that receives the lowest support (proportion linked = 0.25), which has a LOD score of 6.0.*

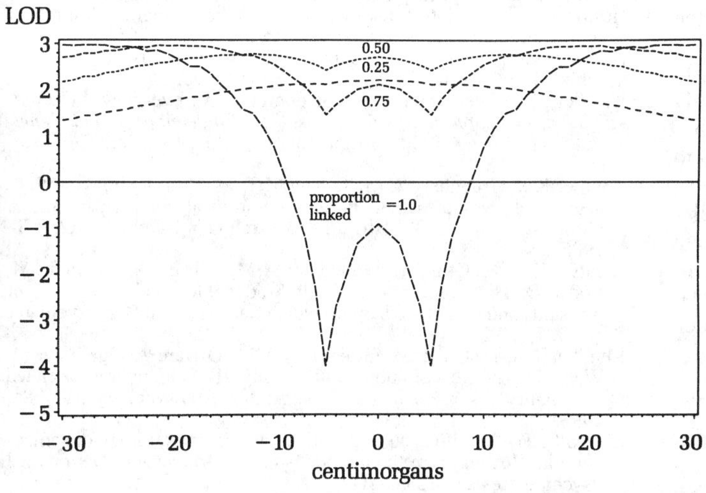

FIGURE 14.5-2 *Linkage with heterogeneity. For the example, only half of the 25 families in the sample actually contain a major disease susceptibility gene at the 0.0 centimorgan map position. The correct hypothesis of genetic heterogeneity (proportion linked = 0.50) receives the highest support among the four hypotheses tested. However, the strength of support (LOD score of 2.6) is greatly reduced from that obtained when all families are linked as in Figure 14.5-1, and would not meet even the standard criterion (LOD score > 3.0) that has come to be considered a minimum necessary for demonstration of linkage. Analyses performed under the incorrect hypothesis of linkage homogeneity (proportion linked = 1.00) would actually provide evidence against the conclusion that there might be a gene in the location where it actually resides in half of the families (negative LOD scores).*

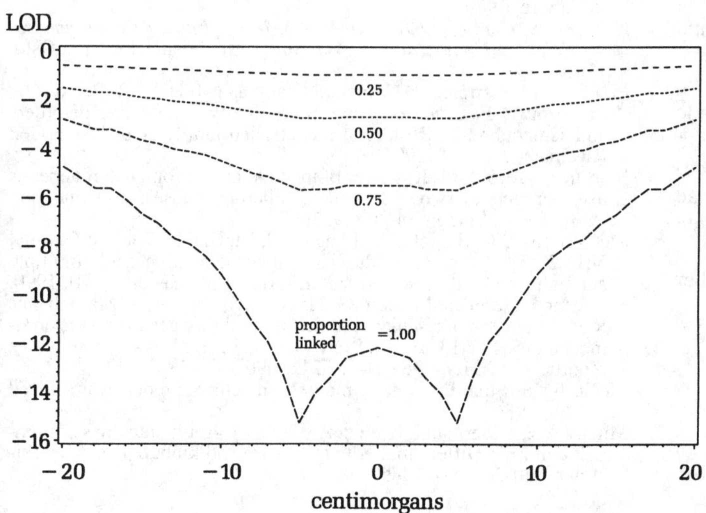

FIGURE 14.5-3 *Exclusion of linkage under heterogeneity. In this example, none of the 25 families actually has a gene located in the chromosomal region shown. The four linkage tests demonstrate the difficulty of ruling out the possibility that a sizable minority of such families could actually contain such a gene. The hypothesis of homogeneous linkage (proportion linked = 1.00) is strongly excluded applying the traditional criterion for exclusion: LOD < −2. However, the possibility that even 40 percent of the sample of families could be linked to that region cannot be ruled out with confidence.*

erful. First, several large-scale field studies that are necessary to identify, sample, and carefully diagnose the many families required to provide adequate statistical power are now under way. For example, DNA samples from over 1,400 persons have already been obtained in a collaborative study being carried out by the authors in Ireland focused on high-density schizophrenia families. Second, molecular genetic methods that make it possible to genotype many highly informative marker loci throughout the human genome are constantly improving at a rapid pace. Especially promising is the trend towards automation in all aspects of sample handling, genotype assays, and data management and analyses that have been pursued as part of the Human Genome Initiative. Third, continued progress has been made in the design of improved methods of statistical analysis, which increase the power to detect linkage for complex and heterogeneous disorders.

Complementing those advances in the methods of linkage analysis, basic studies being carried out through the Human Genome Initiative should also eventually improve the ability to find schizophrenia susceptibility genes. One example is the recent report of the partial DNA sequence characterization of over 2,500 genes expressed in the human brain. That project, carried out in one laboratory within a short period of time, doubled the number of human genes characterized by DNA sequence analysis, and may have included as many as 5 percent of all human genes. One especially noteworthy feature of the results is that 83 percent of those genes were totally new in the sense that their sequence did not match any previously described DNA sequences. The finding suggests that it is likely that the presently undiscovered genes that underlie susceptibility to schizophrenia (which are presently undiscovered) fall into that previously unknown category. Ultimately, there is reason to expect that improved knowledge of the basic genetic architecture for the development and functioning of the human brain will converge with increasingly more powerful measured genotype genetic epidemiological approaches to provide the fundamental insights into the etiology of schizophrenia that have been sought for so long.

The evidence is strong that schizophrenia is a familial disorder and that the familial aggregation of schizophrenia is due largely, although probably not entirely, to genetic factors. Whatever the familial predisposition that operates for schizophrenia, it not only codes for the classic, psychotic disorder but also increases liability to ''schizophrenialike'' personality disorders and probably for some other nonschizophrenic nonaffective psychoses. Two decades of research using the unmeasured genotype approach (segregation analysis and related methods) have failed to delineate clearly the fundamental genetic architecture of schizophrenia, a result that is understandable given the complexity of the task. Large scale gene mapping studies now under way using tools recently made available from basic molecular genetic research, together with improved statistical analysis strategies and diagnostic procedures, offer substantial promise for finding at least some of the specific genes that underlie susceptibility to the disorder. Even limited success in that pursuit has potential for ultimately revolutionizing future approaches to the treatment and further study of schizophrenia.

SUGGESTED CROSS-REFERENCES

A general review of molecular genetic mechanisms is in Section 1.14. Population genetics in psychiatry is discussed in Section 1.15, and genetic linkage analysis of the psychiatric disorders is discussed in Section 1.16.

REFERENCES

Adams M D, Dubnick M, Kerlavage A R, Moreno R, Kelley J M, Utterback T R, Nagle J W, Fields C, Venter C: Sequence identification of 2,375 human brain genes. Nature *355:* 632, 1992.

Baron M, Endicott J, Ott J: Genetic linkage in mental illness: Limitations and prospects. Br J Psychiatry *157:* 645, 1990.

Chen W J, Faraone S V, Tsuang M T: Linkage studies of schizophrenia: A simulation study of statistical power. Genet Epidemiol *9:* 123, 1992.

Cloninger C R: Turning point in the design of linkage studies of schizophrenia. Am J Med Genet *54:* 83, 1994.

*Diehl S R, Kendler K S: Strategies for linkage studies of schizophrenia: Pedigrees, DNA markers, and statistical analyses. Schizophr Bull *15:* 403, 1989.

Gershon E S: Genetic linkage and complex diseases: A comment. Genet Epidemiol *7:* 21, 1990.

Gill M, McGuffin P, Parfitt E, Mant R, Asherson P, Collier D, Vallada H, Powell J, Shaikh S, Taylor C, Sargeant M, Clements A, Nanko S, Takazawa N, Llewellyn D, Williams J, Whatley S, Murray R, Owen M: A linkage study of schizophrenia with DNA markers from the long arm of chromosome 11. Psychol Med *23:* 27, 1993.

Gottesman I I: *Schizophrenia Genesis: The Origins of Madness.* Freeman, New York, 1991.

*Gottesman I I, Shields J: *Schizophrenia: The Epigenetic Puzzle.* Cambridge University Press, New York, 1982.

Guze S B, Cloninger C R, Martin R L, Clayton P J: A follow-up and family study of schizophrenia. Arch Gen Psychiatry *40:* 1273, 1983.

Heston L L: Psychiatric disorders in foster home reared children of schizophrenic mothers. Br J Psychiatry *112:* 819, 1966.

Kendler K S: Overview: A current perspective on twin studies of schizophrenia. Am J Psychiatry *140:* 1413, 1983.

*Kendler K S: The genetics of schizophrenia: An overview. In *Handbook of Schizophrenia,* vol. 3, *Nosology, Epidemiology, and Genetics,* M T Tsuang, J C Simpson, editors, p 437. Elsevier, The Netherlands, 1988.

Kendler K S, Gruenberg A M, Tsuang M T: Psychiatric illness in first-degree relatives of schizophrenic and surgical control patients: A family study using DSM-III criteria. Arch Gen Psychiatry *42:* 770, 1985.

Kendler K S, McGuire M, Gruenberg A M, O'Hare A, Spellman M, Walsh D: The Roscommon Family Study: I. Methods, diagnosis of probands and risk of schizophrenia in relatives. Arch Gen Psychiatry *50:* 527, 1993.

Kendler K S, McGuire M, Gruenberg A M, O'Hare A, Spellman M, Walsh D: The Roscommon Family Study: III. Schizophrenia-related personality disorders in relatives. Arch Gen Psychiatry *50:* 781, 1993.

Kety S S: The significance of genetic factors in the etiology of schizophrenia: Results from the national study of adoptees in Denmark. J Psychiatr Res *21:* 423, 1987.

Kety S S, Rosenthal D, Wender P H, Schulsinger F, Jacobsen B: Mental illness in the biological and adoptive families of adopted individuals who have become schizophrenic: A preliminary report based on psychiatric interviews. In *Genetic Research in Psychiatry,* R Fieve, D Rosenthal, H Brill, editors, p 147. Johns Hopkins University Press, Baltimore, 1975.

Kringlen E: *Heredity and Environment in the Functional Psychoses: An Epidemiolgical-Clinical Twin Study.* Universitetsforlaget, Oslo, 1967.

Maier W, Lichtermann D, Minges J, Hallmayer J, Heun R, Benkert O, Levinson D F: Continuity and discontinuity of affective disorders and schizophrenia: Results of a controlled family study. Arch Gen Psychiatry *50:* 871, 1993.

Martinez M, Goldin L R: Power of the linkage test for a heterogeneous disorder due to two independent inherited causes: A simulation study. Genet Epidemiol *7:* 219, 1990.

McGillivray B C, Bassett A S, Langlois S, Pantzar T, Wood S: Familial 5q11.2-q13.3 segmental duplication cosegregating with multiple anomalies, including schizophrenia. Am J Med Genet *35:* 10, 1990.

*McGuffin P, Sargeant M, Hetti G, Tidmarsh S, Whatley S, Marchbanks R M: Exclusion of a schizophrenia susceptibility gene from the chromosome 5q11-q13 region: New data and a reanalysis of previous reports. Am J Hum Genet *47:* 524, 1990.

McGuffin P, Sturt E: Genetic markers in schizophrenia. Hum Hered *36:* 65, 1986.

Mirsky A F, Silberman E K, Latz A, Nagler S: Adult outcomes of high-risk children: Differential effects of town and kibbutz rearing. Schizophr Bull *11:* 150, 1985.

Onstad S, Skre I, Edvardsen J, Torgersen S, Kringlen E: Mental disorders in first-degree relatives of schizophrenics. Acta Psychiatr Scand *83:* 463, 1991.
Onstad S, Skre I, Torgersen S, Kringlen E: Twin concordance for DSM-III-R schizophrenia. Acta Psychiatr Scand *83:* 395, 1991.
Owen M J: Will schizophrenia become a graveyard for molecular genetics? Psychol Med *22:* 289, 1992.
Parnas J, Cannon T D, Jacobsen B, Schulsinger H, Schulsinger F, Mednick S A: Lifetime DSM-III-R diagnostic outcomes in the offspring of schizophrenic mothers: Results from the Copenhagen high-risk study. Arch Gen Psychiatry *50:* 707, 1993.
Pulver A E, Karayiorgou M, Lasseter V K, Wolyniec P, Kasch L, Antonarakis S, Housman D, Kazazian H H, Meyers D, Nestadt G, Ott J, Liang K-Y, Lamacz M, Thomas M, Childs B: Follow-up of a report of a potential linkage for schizophrenia on chromosome 22q12-113.1: Part 2. Am J Med Genet *54:* 44, 1994.
*Risch N: Genetic linkage and complex diseases, with special reference to psychiatric disorders. Genet Epidemiol *7:* 3, 1990.
Sherrington R, Brynjolfsson J, Petursson H, Potter M, Dudleston K, Barraclough B, Wasmuth J, Dobbs M, Gurling H: Localization of a susceptibility locus for schizophrenia on chromosome 5. Nature *336:* 164, 1988.
Smith C: Concordance in twins: Methods and interpretation. Am J Hum Genet *26:* 454, 1974.
Su Y, Burke J, O'Neil A, Murphy B, Nie L, Kipps B, Bray J, Shinkwin R, Ni Nuallain M, MacLean C J, Walsh D, Diehl S R, Kendler K S: Exclusion of linkage between schizophrenia and the D_2 dopamine receptor gene region of chromosome 11q in 112 Irish multiplex families. Arch Gen Psychiatry *50:* 205, 1993.
Watson J D: The human genome project: Past, present, and future. Science *248:* 44, 1990.
Weeks D E, Brzustowicz L, Squires-Wheeler E, Cornblatt B, Lehner T, Stefanovich M, Bassett A, Gilliam T C, Ott J, Erlenmeyer-Kimling L: Report of a workshop on genetic linkage studies of schizophrenia. Schizophr Bull *16:* 673, 1990.
Weeks D E, Lehner T, Squires-Wheeler E, Kaufmann C, Ott J: Measuring the inflation of the lod score due to maximization over model parameter values in human linkage analysis. Genet Epidemiol *7:* 237, 1990.
White R, Lalouel J-M: Chromosome mapping with DNA markers. Sci Am *258:* 40, 188.
Zerbin-Rüdin E: Endogene Psychosen. In *Humangenetik: ein kurzes Handbuch in fünf Bande, vol 2,* P E Becker, editor, p 446. Thieme, Stuttgart, 1967.

14.6 SCHIZOPHRENIA: PSYCHODYNAMIC TO NEURODYNAMIC THEORIES

THOMAS H. McGLASHAN, M.D.
RALPH E. HOFFMAN, M.D.

INTRODUCTION

By its mind-twisting pathophysiologies, schizophrenia destroys the lives of those it afflicts, often in the springtime of their adult seasons. By holding fast to the secrets of its causes, schizophrenia also taunts those who would study and understand how it wreaks its devastation. Thus, the most aberrant and obvious of human mental illnesses remains the most mysterious, challenging theorists to postulate more and more creative hypotheses and eluding definition as each hypothesis fails to stand the test of time and replication.

To patients, schizophrenia threatens the loss of what almost everyone takes completely for granted—self hood, the ontological sense of being someone and something. Only when that sense is missing is its importance, its survival value, and its function of endorsing people as sentient creatures appreciated. Because schizophrenia often invades that core of human narcissism, people have always regarded it with intense ambivalence. On the one side lies fascination because of the secrets it holds for the understanding of the brain, the uniquely human organ of understanding. On the other side lies horror because it threatens the ultimate paralysis—living meaninglessness. To clinicians and scientists, schizophrenia generates a sense of confusion and helpless ignorance time and again, thus assaulting another fortress of human narcissism—pride in knowing.

HISTORY

Perhaps because it creates such double jeopardy for the capacity to understand, schizophrenic madness has had more explanations thrown at it and has been the object of more attempts to render it meaningful than has any other mental illness. Before Galileo Galilei most of those explanations were found in religious texts. From Galileo to Emil Kraepelin the explanations were found in medical texts alongside neurological disorders and idiocy. By the early 20th century and under the influence of psychoanalytic thinking, the nature and the cause of schizophrenia turned functional. No longer supernatural or organic in cause, schizophrenia became a clash of ideas, of wishes, of learned habits—that is, psychological in its genesis and manifestations. From that milieu came the various *psychodynamic* theories of schizophrenia. By the late 20th century, the organic structures underlying psychological processes received greater attention, leading to models focusing on the mind-body interface, here labeled the *neurodynamic* theories of schizophrenia.

Neurodynamic theories assert that, in addition to psychodynamics, one must look at the neurobiological structures that generate psychology to comprehend symptom formation in schizophrenia. In the computer metaphor, symptoms arise in schizophrenia because of shifts or defects in the hardware of mentation and because of conflicts and warps in the software of psychology. That hardware consists of biologically programmed neuronal networks in dynamic communication through chemical and electrical connections, hence the term neurodynamic.

Although purely psychological theories have advanced the understanding of schizophrenia to some degree, that body of thought has not progressed much in the past 20 years. Modern thinking about the psychodynamic contributions to psychopathology has increasingly recognized the central influence of both nature and experience. Schizophrenia, more than any other psychiatric disorder, challenges the boundaries of what is meant by psychodynamic. A broad definition, one that includes both organic and psychological contributions to mental phenomena, is the one most valid definition, certainly for schizophrenia and possibly for many other mental disorders as well.

Historically, the 1911 publication of Sigmund Freud's analysis of Daniel Paul Schreber probably marks the formal beginning of the systematic psychodynamic theories of schizophrenia. For the next 50 years, virtually all thinking in that realm emerged from within the various psychoanalytic schools, here labeled the classical, interpersonal, and developmental schools. The next major body of theory grew out of psychoanalysis around the middle of the century as family transaction models. Shortly thereafter, after the biological revolution in psychiatry and the genetic studies of schizophrenia, the neurodynamic theories emerged, introduced by the stress-diathesis or vulnerability-stress hypothesis. The advent of artificial intelligence and computer simulations of brain functioning gave rise to the parallel distributed processing model of schizophrenic symptom formation.

DEFINITION

A rigorous and operationally oriented definition of *theory* envisions it as a set of assumptions and definitions that can generate testable and refutable hypotheses or predictions about a phenomenon. That form of theory constitutes the backbone of modern scientific empiricism. According to Joseph Lichtenberg, a broader, esthetically oriented definition of theory regards it as a set of assertions explaining something in a manner that is "balanced, logical, and comprehensive while at the same time parsimonious in its assumptions." That form of theory characterizes most psychodynamic theories of schizophrenia.

Either type of theory can serve as a useful cognitive framework. As Robert Cancro noted, "Theory imposes boundaries and a filter on the potential data set of observation and decreases and sharpens it to manageable size." Furthermore, theories and hypotheses predict relations that are not immediately or intuitively obvious. Theory informs the task of observation and makes it finite. No serious clinician approaches the schizophrenic patient in a theoretical vacuum; organizing principles are required to avoid being overwhelmed. Theory may foster selective inattention and exclude important alternate meanings or observations. On balance, however, such risks are minor compared with the chaos that greets any therapist without an explicit or implicit model.

PSYCHODYNAMIC THEORIES

The disorders gathered under the term "schizophrenia" arise (etiology), develop over time (pathogenesis), emerge in certain forms (manifest illness), and undergo vicissitudes over the patient's life span (course). Relevant theories may address any of those facets. Generally, they cluster into two paradigms: descriptive-homeostatic theories and etiological-facilitative theories.

Descriptive-homeostatic theories are focused on the here and now and stay closest to manifest phenomenology. The theories label, order, and integrate the data on the basis of observed or hypothesized relations (for example, Eugen Bleuler's division of schizophrenic symptoms into those that are primary and those that are secondary). Those theories also introduce causation and attempt to explain or understand how the disease works as a homeostatic system. An example is Sigmund Freud's postulate that paranoia represents reversed and projected latent homosexual wishes.

Etiological-facilitative theories are concerned with the broader view of schizophrenia over the course of a lifetime. How is it generated? What forces shape its expression? Such theories are more comprehensive in scope and usually more hypothetical than are descriptive-homeostatic theories. An example is Melanie Klein's postulate that schizophrenia arises from fixations engendered at the paranoid-schizoid phase of development in early infancy. Such theories are often labeled psychogenic because they try to explain the genesis of schizophrenia.

Most psychodynamic theories of schizophrenia are of the broad, esthetically oriented variety. Few of those considered here can be operationalized and tested. They are too abstract or are based on data collected empathically, rather than objectively. Their validity does not rest on empirical validation. Although the theories must, in general, conform to the rules of evidence, their truthfulness basically derives from their capacity to help one understand schizophrenia. The verity of the theories is proportional to the degree to which they generate meanings about schizophrenia that make communicable sense and that are useful in one's empathic encounters with afflicted patients. Validity here stems from a theory's vividness, connectedness, and depth, as well as from its parsimonious integration of complexity. Validity also derives from the theory's usefulness in alerting doctor and patient as listeners and hunters for what is missing from the patient's experience.

PSYCHOANALYTIC MODELS: CLASSICAL SCHOOL

Sigmund Freud The classical psychoanalytic model postulates that manifest psychopathology is generated by active and sustained psychological conflict between drive-created wishful impulses and antithetical wishes, reality, or conscience. The conflict generates defenses against the wishful impulses, and those defenses can often be seen in the form of symptoms. All or any part of the drama may be carried on outside of awareness—that is, unconsciously.

The model finds its most complete elaboration in the *structural theory,* which postulates the existence of three functional entities in the mind. The *id* is the wellspring of peremptory sexual and aggressive drives and wishes. It is largely unconscious and primitive in its structure. The *superego* or conscience and ego-ideal is the repository of rules and values learned (internalized) from parents and society during development. It is also largely unconscious but makes its presence known through the affects of guilt and shame. The *ego* is a group of psychological functions that mediate adaptation between the person and the environment (for example, reality testing) and among conflicting psychological forces within the person (for example, the repression of forbidden impulses). The ego is complex and develops slowly over the course of life. Many of its functions, such as defense, are activated by *anxiety,* the danger signal generated by conflict among psychological forces or with reality. Ego functions, too, operate mostly out of awareness.

Freud postulated that the structures develop during infancy and childhood and are in place by the end of the oedipal period (ages 3 to 5). The person at that point has a stable, integrated ego, which is seen as a sense of self that is enduring and cohesive. Conflict within and among the structures produces the symptomatic and character neuroses. Freud regarded schizophrenia as deriving from psychological development that is arrested before the oedipal stage, before the development of an integrated ego. Such an arrest, Freud believed, severely compromises the schizophrenic patient's capacity to relate and renders treatment by psychoanalysis difficult, if not impossible.

Although he had virtually no clinical experience with schizophrenic patients, Freud was the first analyst to elaborate a systematic psychodynamic model for the syndrome. He may be said to have formulated two models, one emphasizing conflict and defense and the other emphasizing deficiency as the cause of schizophrenic symptoms.

The conflict-defense model basically explains schizophrenic symptoms by using the structural model. In that model, schizophrenia, like all psychopathologies, is the result of conflict and defense. The difference between schizophrenia and the neuroses is purely quantitative, not qualitative. Schizophrenic conflict is more intense than neurotic conflict and requires the frequent use of primitive (that is, developmentally early) defenses, such as denial and projection, which frequently involve a break with reality. The ego functioning of the schizophrenic patient regresses to developmentally early stages or levels of organization, the exact level being determined (or fixated) by one or more past psychological traumas. The difference between schizophrenia and neurosis lies in the depth of the regression and the point of fixation, which Freud placed in the preoedipal phase of development.

Freud used a deficiency or deficit model to explain schizophrenic symptom formation in the analysis of Schreber. Freud worked from Schreber's published autobiographical account of his paranoid psychosis. Clinically, Schreber's illness began with hypochondriacal preoccupations. That phase was followed by an apocalyptic panic, leading to catatonia, a personality change, and symptoms of psychosis, particularly grandiose and paranoid delusions.

Freud, who was elaborating his libido theory at the time, explained Schreber's psychosis as follows: Conflict initiates the sequence, as it does in all psychopathologies. In schizophrenia, however, another process supersedes defense. That process is the patient's withdrawal of libidinal or energic investments *(cathexes)* from the real outside world, especially from people (*objects,* in psychoanalytic parlance). The patient concomitantly withdraws libidinal investments from the inner, fantasied, mental representations or images of that world and those people. In the developing schizophrenic process the withdrawn libidinal energy increasingly becomes invested in the patient's self-image, seen clinically as self-aggrandizement or megalomania, or invested in the patient's body image, seen clinically as hypochondriasis. In neurosis a similar process of withdrawal from real, external relations occurs in response to conflict, but the withdrawn libido remains invested in the fantasied objects.

That withdrawal reaches a state so profound as to constitute a break with external reality and relationships and with internal object representations and relationships in fantasy. At that stage, one can see the apocalyptic panic clinically. It represents a projection outward of the internal catastrophe or collapse of psychological investments. The collapse and the profound withdrawal constitute the deficit of schizophrenia. It renders the patient incapable of relationships, including transference, and thus precludes treatment by psychoanalysis. After the catastrophe the patient tries to recover and to reinvest libido. Since there has been a break with reality, however, the efforts produce the well-known symptoms of schizophrenia, especially hallucinations, delusions, and disordered thinking. The patient has reinvested interest and attention but in objects that are not part of the real world.

In Freud's defense theory the sequence of conflict, anxiety, and defense is regarded as sufficient to account for schizophrenic psychopathology. In the deficit theory, conflict and anxiety initiate pathogenesis but trigger a withdrawal process that is qualitatively different from defense. Freud never resolved the difference between his two theories. He seemed to say that schizophrenic people are very much like normal and neurotic people in some ways but profoundly different in others. His two theories formed the nidus for much subsequent controversy.

Freud's other theoretical contributions to schizophrenia concern the psychodynamics of delusion formation. Early in his career he postulated the mechanism of projection, whereby a person's wish is disavowed and projected onto or attributed to another person (the object). Later he suggested that delusions of persecution arise from latent homosexual impulses that undergo reversal and projection. Thus, the situation, "I (a man) love him (a man)" is reversed to, "I do not love him; I hate him" and projected into, "He hates (and persecutes) me." Later in his career Freud maintained that the hostility inherent in any form of intense ambivalence toward an object can be projected into feelings of being persecuted by that object.

Paul Federn If Freud was the first major psychodynamic theoretician of schizophrenia, Paul Federn was the first major psychodynamic clinician of schizophrenia. A contemporary of Freud's, Federn disagreed with his Viennese colleague's pessimism about the schizophrenic patient's capacity for transference and for treatment by psychoanalytically informed therapy. Federn treated many schizophrenic patients and developed techniques that were virtually half a century ahead of his time.

Federn greatly expanded the idea of ego set down by Freud in the structural theory. He was perhaps the first psychoanalytic theoretician to introduce the notion of self. To Federn the ego was not just a collection of psychological functions but also had its own existential being or ego feeling. The various ego functions aggregate into a sum or a self that has a feeling of permanence and continuity vis-à-vis time, space, and causality. That is ego feeling, the totality of feeling that a person has of his or her own living being. Ego feeling as subject is *I*. Ego feeling as object is *self*.

Federn also elaborated the concept of ego boundary originally introduced by Viktor Tausk. To Federn, each person possesses an inner ego boundary and an outer ego boundary. The outer boundary consists of the ego versus the external world; it divides and distinguishes mental phenomena from real phenomena. The inner boundary consists of the repression barrier or the line between conscious experience and unconscious experience. According to his scheme, which uses Freud's libido theory, schizophrenia is a disease of the ego. The psychopathological process involves a loss of energic investments in ego boundaries. Attenuation at the inner boundary means derepression or a reemergence of developmentally early (archaic) ego states. Attenuation at the outer boundary means a loss of the distinction between mental and real, as seen in the typical schizophrenic symptoms. Mature and archaic ego states, however, can coexist, making it possible for the patient to adjust to the real world while symptomatic and to engage in psychodynamically oriented therapeutic discourse despite illness.

Federn's basically descriptive model follows the theme of defect. Nevertheless, his concepts prefigure the later distinction between psychotic and nonpsychotic aspects of the patient's personality. For him the schizophrenic process is never total. Furthermore, by highlighting the self phenomenology in the ego of Freud's structural model, Federn anticipated the development of self psychology.

Heinz Hartmann Working within Freud's classical structural theory, Heinz Hartmann was impressed with the ego's complexity and versatility, its strength in opposition to the drives, and its primary aim of serving reality adaptation and survival. Defenses like intellectualization and sublimation, for example, can also be coping devices. He regarded humans as biological organisms phylogenetically equipped at birth for adaptation to an average expectable environment. That equipment includes primary ego functions like perception, memory, and motility that are not derived from conflict. Also, ego functions developing later out of conflicts can become autonomous of id and superego or free of conflict to function independently and to serve adaptation. Such functions include language, intellect, thinking, will, judgment, attention, affectivity, reality testing, intention, and object relations, in addition to the defenses and the primary functions already mentioned. The existence of psychopathology indicates that the ego functions can become reinstinctualized or involved in conflict situations.

The ego, according to Hartmann, also possesses a synthetic function, its aim being to promote homeostasis, a harmonious equilibrium between the drives of sex and aggression, among the intrapsychic tripartite systems of id, ego, and superego and between the person and the environment. That supraordinate integrative function carries echoes of Federn's ego feeling. Hartmann, however, regarded the self as an idea (representation), rather than as an entity or functioning mental system.

In comparison with his extensive contributions to general psychodynamic theory, Hartmann's specific postulates regarding schizophrenia are abbreviated, perhaps because such patients did not constitute a large part of his practice. His theory was a mixture of defense and defect. Like Freud, Hartmann thought that schizophrenic symptoms can result from conflicts secondary to intolerable realities or amplified drive pressures. In addition, he postulated an inborn primary defect in the ego of the preschizophrenic patient that renders the ego incapable of neutralizing certain drive pressures, especially aggression. Aggression generated later in life by conflict or narcissistic injury floods the ego (especially its synthetic functioning) and draws it easily into conflict. The ensuing regression is substantial and mobilizes primitive defenses, such as denial and projection, which are viewed as the symptoms of schizophrenia. However, not all ego functions regress to the same extent, thus accounting for the heterogeneity of the clinical picture.

Hartmann's theory added the importance of aggression to the pathogenesis of schizophrenia. It also placed the source of the syndrome in the preschizophrenic patient's constitution, thus marking such people as qualitatively different from those who are normal or become neurotic. Hartmann conceptualized the ego as multidimensional. Schizophrenia affects ego functioning selectively and can, therefore, be graded in severity. In Hartmann's scheme it is possible to have degrees of schizophrenia. Overall, he emphasized the biological underpinnings of many psychological functions and presaged later neurodynamic theories of schizophrenia.

PSYCHOANALYTIC MODELS: INTERPERSONAL SCHOOL

Harry Stack Sullivan The interpersonal model of Harry Stack Sullivan, although psychodynamic in its structure, is fundamentally different from psychoanalytic drive theory in its content. Drive theory works from the perspective of the person as an individual encountering and shaping the world according to inner drives and satisfactions. Interpersonal theory elaborates the perspective of the person as a social creature who, from the beginning, is object-related and relationship seeking. Sullivan's model still postulates motivational drives and needs—namely, the needs for satisfaction (mostly biological, in the form of hunger and lust) and the needs for security (mostly psychosocial, in the form of power). However, all those needs require interaction with at least one other human being and serve to mediate the interpersonal exchange.

The developmental aspect of Sullivan's theory regards the human infant as being without a psychology separate from the initial mother-infant dyad. Psychological awareness consists of successive discoveries of one's self in relationship with significant others (objects). The first self consists of a we, not an I. Development proceeds according to an increasingly complex hierarchy of needs, all interactional in nature—the needs for maternal contact in infancy, parental mirroring in childhood, peer play in latency, chum closeness in early adolescence, and sexual intimacy in late adolescence and beyond.

Sullivan viewed anxiety, the affect that drives psychopathology, as external to the infant but imparted to the infant by an anxious parent, usually the mother. Anxiety in the interpersonal situation develops three self-states: a good me (low anxiety), a bad me (high anxiety), and a not me (intolerable anxiety). Not-me anxiety is extreme awe, dread, loathing, or panic that is so dysphoric that it is experienced rarely, as in nightmares or during severe schizophrenic end-of-the-world panic experiences.

Anxiety leads to the organization of defensive structures, which Sullivan described as self dynamisms or *self systems.* The systems function to maximize satisfactions and to maintain security or to minimize anxiety through the use of such security operations as selective inattention (dissociation), sublimation, and projection. The self system in its content is what one takes oneself to be. It is largely secondary to what others take one to be—that is, it consists mostly of reflected appraisals. The self system security operations operate to establish and protect the content of the self system. In the face of anxiety, the security operations lead to the creation of fantasied defensive self-other constellations, such as the self as helpless but deserving and the other as magical and merciful, the self as victimized and hurt and the other as powerful and persecutory, and the self as special and the other as idealizing. Such illusory configurations are superimposed on a person's here-and-now relationships, distorting them, a process akin to transference that Sullivan labeled *parataxic distortion.*

Sullivan's psychodynamic theory of schizophrenia was informed by extensive clinical experience with acutely and subacutely affected inpatients. He regarded the disorders in the Meyerian tradition as purely functional reactions to encounters between the person and the environment. Central to the psychopathological process is a disturbance in the capacity to relate to others that is not biological in origin but reflects the history of the patient's interactions with significant others, especially with the mother in the formative years. The syndrome itself represents a massive dissociation secondary to the intense anxiety generated by low self-esteem during interpersonal experiences. Sullivan acknowledged the probable existence of hereditary or organic determinants in some disorders, such as chronic process schizophrenia. However, he did not consider them to be schizophrenia per se or, at least, the type of schizophrenia to which he thought his theory applied.

The pathogenesis of schizophrenia, according to Sullivan's scheme, begins with a mother who is more anxious than normal and who imparts tension to her child as excessive not-me experiences. The child's self system, developing around the time of speech acquisition, overcompensates with excessive dissociation and warps its own further development. The adolescent surge of new sexual needs (lust dynamisms) assault that compromised self system. The defensive wall of selective inattention fractures; not-me disorganizing anxiety returns, and panic ensues. That state of terror is characterized not only by the uncanny eruption into awareness of developmentally primitive states of mind but also by a collapse of the integrated self system into what Sullivan described as "an exceedingly unpleasant form of nothingness." The afflicted person's primary urgencies at that point are to avoid the not-me menace and to reorganize the self in order to reestablish meaning and become human again. The reorganization, known as schizophrenia, is effected at the price of reality.

According to Sullivan, schizophrenia is more than a disorder. It is also an adaptive strategy for avoiding fragmentation and chaos (panic and terror) and for reconstructing a self with human identity, meaning, and purpose, no matter how fantastic that defensive self-other constellation is. It is better, for example, to be the hapless victim of tyrannical persecutors than to be nothing at all. One must have character, even if it manifests as caricature. With schizophrenia the needs for satisfaction and reality are secondary to the needs for security and self-meaning.

The descriptive-homeostatic aspects of Sullivan's theory highlight the self, both as a content (idea) and as a functional system. Although Federn may have been the first to describe the self as part of a psychodynamic system (as ego feeling), Sullivan was the first to postulate its functional centrality to human psychology. To him, creating and maintaining the integrity and functional alacrity of a self is one of the human's primary motivating forces. With schizophrenia, in fact, the drive for meaning exerts hegemony over all other needs. Sullivan viewed schizophrenia as the result of cumulative experiential traumas during development. His own bias was to regard the preschizophrenic infant as a tabula rasa on which the mother's anxieties were etched. The source of pathogenic anxiety is clearly external to the infant, and schizophrenia is seen as an adaptive attempt to cope with that dysphoric milieu.

British object relations theorists The British object relations school operated independently of Sullivan but pursued many of the same ideas, regarding humans as inherently social or object-related. Their major spokespersons are Melanie Klein, W. R. D. Fairbairn, and D. W. Winnicott.

MELANIE KLEIN For Melanie Klein psychodynamic conflict involved love versus hate in relationships (rather than the tension between wish and reality of more classical psychoanalysis). Her descriptive-homeostatic theories were key contributions to classical psychoanalytic dynamics. She emphasized the importance of fantasy, both conscious and unconscious, in determining behavior. Fantasy usually takes the form of a drama involving the self relating with another—constellations that have come to be known as internal object relationships. She added two important coping or defense mechanisms to the ego's repertoire: splitting and projective identification. During infancy those mechanisms promote development and adaptation. During adulthood they signal trouble. Klein related psychopathology to an overabundance of aggression and hate in relationships. Envy (mostly innate) is especially pathogenic, because it is directed at good objects and their capacity to give, thus destroying hope by devaluing healthy relationships.

Klein conceived of human development as a hierarchy of relational patterns—that is, positions, rather than phases. Two positions, both within the first year of life, are central to normal development or to later psychopathology: the *paranoid position,* in which aggressive, dysphoric interpersonal experiences are split off and projected onto significant others, who are then regarded anxiously as persecutory, and the *depressive position,* the infant's guilty recognition of personal responsibility for being the aggressive persecutor at times. The accuracy of that scheme may be questionable vis-à-vis contemporary infant observation, but it is compelling in its description of two mental constellations frequently encountered in patients with severe psychopathology.

Klein's theory of schizophrenia closely followed her developmental scheme. She regarded the potential schizophrenic patient as endowed with strong sadistic and envious impulses that render the infant prone to intense paranoid anxieties and, therefore, to the overuse of withdrawal, splitting, and projective identification. Such infants never negotiate the depressive position and remain fixated at the paranoid position, to which they regress in the face of later stress after further development through adolescence.

W. R. D. FAIRBAIRN To W. R. D. Fairbairn the primary aim of human behavior is contact with another, even if it is unpleasant. He viewed psychopathology entirely from a developmental perspective as the product of failure to establish good object relationships in infancy. Maternal absence or withdrawal during the paranoid-schizoid position leads the infant to regard love as noxious or bad. The resultant schizoid conflict—to love or not to love—sets off a withdrawal from relatedness in reality with compensatory investments in defensive internal object relations. Those internal object relations, like Sullivan's fantasied self-other constellations, provide a sense of security and continuity that is missing in real relationships, especially the earliest ones with the parents. Fairbairn conceived of schizophrenia on a continuum with schizoid psychopathology, the difference being one of degree. The schizophrenic patient withdraws loving investments to such an extent that emotional contact with others and with external reality is renounced.

Both Klein and Fairbairn saw the mind as a consequence of development over time. Psychological structures and functions are built almost entirely out of internalized (learned) experiences with significant others, especially the mother. Accordingly, severe psychopathology derives from problems in the early nurturing relationship between the mother and the infant. Klein emphasized heightened constitutional aggression in the infant, whereas Fairbairn emphasized maternal withdrawal and deprivation. Both, however, conceived of the human infant as an undifferentiated mound of clay, passively and helplessly waiting to be shaped by the forces of inner drives and external reality. The third major figure of the British object relations school, Winnicott, saw the infant as possessing power and influence from the start.

D. W. WINNICOTT To D. W. Winnicott the infant is an equal partner with the mother in the early drama of the dyadic relationship. The mother, through primary maternal empathy, provides a proper holding environment for her infant. She responds appropriately to her infant's needs at the moment of excitation when the infant signals them to her. That is, she receives and promotes her infant's initiative. Equally important, she does not impinge on her infant's quiescent states to fulfill her own needs. The environment (as the mother) finds the child and promotes a fitting together that is true to the child's innate potential and uniqueness. For the infant those are experiences of omnipotence, power, or control over the mother or the environment. The experiences form the basis of a healthy, competent sense of self. The infant learns about reality little by little over time through the mother's natural failures to shape the world perfectly according to the infant's demands. The soothing illusion of omnipotence and magic, however, remains alive and healthy within the realm of transitional objects and experiences.

Winnicott never articulated a theory of schizophrenia per se. However, according to his scheme as interpreted by others, schizophrenia can be viewed as a failure in the development of the spontaneous and competent or true self out of its relational matrix. Because of an improper fit, the infant is exposed to realities that are out of phase with its needs and states of activation and, therefore, is exposed to the premature destruction of the illusion of power. That destruction leads to the development of a false self that compliantly reacts to external realities and the needs of others. Increasingly, needed omnipotence derives from defensive, internal, or autistic fantasy, rather than from transitional interaction with the environment. In schizophrenia the fantasy finally replaces reality.

The importance of Winnicott's ideas derives not so much from their contribution to a theory of schizophrenia as from their elaboration of a theory of self. Like Sullivan, Winnicott regarded the self as a central psychodynamic force and entity. Winnicott went beyond Sullivan, however, in postulating the importance of illusion to normal growth and development. To Winnicott the omnipotent self, as played out in fantasy or in transitional space, is a sign of health and only later a signal of possible trouble. To Sullivan such fantasies or self systems are always defensive, a sign of pathological adaptation. Winnicott's perspective also introduced an entirely new dimension to psychodynamic treatment theory. To the classical search for truth and insight (that is, reality), Winnicott advocated the need for the treatment dyad to create and internalize a protective sense of illusion. He provided the theoretical underpinning for adding the facilitating environment to the analytic situation. Supportive psychotherapeutic techniques, commonly used clinically with schizophrenia and severely character-disordered patients by dynamic clinicians since Federn, now had a proper theoretical rationale.

PSYCHOANALYTIC MODELS: DEVELOPMENTAL SCHOOL Latter-day American theorists contributing to the psychodynamic understanding of schizophrenia include Margaret Mahler, Edith Jacobson, and Ping-Nie Pao. As a group, they have drawn heavily on observations of and theories about human development.

Margaret Mahler Margaret Mahler clearly related early developmental experiences to later mental function. Her developmental phases of autism, symbiosis, and separation-individuation captured the attention and the imagination of many theorists who saw different forms of psychopathology corresponding to different levels in her developmental progression. Schizophrenia, for example, is regarded as corresponding to Mahler's autistic phase of development. It is assumed or postulated that the preschizophrenic infant fails to form an adequate and stable symbiosis with the mothering object; that developmental failure renders the child's image of the mother inconstant and leaves the person vulnerable to regression when facing the second and final phase of individuation in late adolescence. The regression itself goes back to the preverbal, presymbiotic stage of autism, with loss of ego boundaries, merger experiences, and replacement of reality by autistic fantasy.

Edith Jacobson Edith Jacobson saw schizophrenia as a disturbance of the sense of self or identity, defined as the observable capacity of the person to remain the same in the midst of change. Although schizophrenic patients have difficulties with object relationships, their primary problems lie with maintaining a stable sense of self-sameness and self-cohesion. The breakdown of that sense is one of the most painful and traumatic experiences known to humans, provoking preservation efforts that often abandon allegiance to reality.

Ping-Nie Pao Ping-Nie Pao wove together theoretical threads of many forebears. On the basis of extensive clinical experience, he typed schizophrenic patients into acute cases, for whom conflict plays a pivotal role, and chronic cases, with high genetic-biological loading. Pao, like Freud, was impressed with the catastrophic panic experience that signaled the onset of the schizophrenic process and symptom formation. That process is precipitated by psychodynamic conflicts no different in content from those experienced by all other people. In the schizophrenia-vulnerable person, however, the conflicts no longer generate neurotic levels of anxiety but at some point catalyze a crisis known as *organismic panic,* the term being modeled after Mahler's developmental observations of states of extreme infantile distress. That panic brings with it paralysis of the ego's integrative capacity and fragmentation of the sense of continuity of self, which constitutes an unbearable loss of a basic sense of safety. The ego mobilizes primitive or regressive defenses to reestablish and protect a sense of self, albeit pathologically. The result of that attempt at adaptation or recovery is the postpanic emergence of a different personality, either pieced together with or distorted by psychotic symptoms. Typical delusions, for example, help construct a new sense of meaningful self and, although often unpleasant, are clung to tenaciously because their loss leads to a threatened return of disorganization and panic.

Pao's etiological-developmental theory attempts to explain the origin of the schizophrenic vulnerability to organismic panic and regression. Like other relationalists, he placed the cause in the experiences of early development. An aberrant constitution and inappropriate mothering combine to generate a series of failed emotional cuings within the dyad, leading to frequent episodes of infantile organismic distress or "pain in being held and pain in being laid down." Cumulative exposures to such distress bend further development in maladaptive directions, including a tendency to use primitive defenses, impaired capacity for instinctual neutralization, inability to maintain a sense of reality constancy, heightened aggressive responses to frustration, and heightened wishes for closeness with others coupled with a dread of self-dissolution in symbiosis (the need-fear dilemma). Those vulnerabilities lie dormant and do not produce symptoms until the advent of adolescent drive demands and stress.

PSYCHOANALYTIC THEORIES: CRITIQUE Psychoanalytic theories of schizophrenia have in recent years fallen into obscurity, mainly because the traumatic-developmental perspective on causes appears to lack credibility. Virtually all psychoanalytic theorists postulate an experiential disharmony between the mother and her preschizophrenic infant. Whether that disharmony derives from genetic or constitutional factors in the infant or from psychological factors in the parent is secondary, as the purported central pathogenic elements are dysphoric experiences that become internalized as aberrant psychological structures. Explicitly or implicitly, the psychogenic models of schizophrenia regard those experiences as sufficient to explain most, if not all, cases of the syndrome.

Several considerations cast doubt on that postulate. First, recent findings from infant research challenge many of the assumptions put forth by psychoanalytic developmentalists. For example, normal development is not like pathological stages projected backward. Infants are active, stimulus-seeking, and socially oriented from day one. Stages such as the narcissistic, autistic, symbiotic, and schizoid-paranoid are not observed, so it is doubtful that schizophrenia represents regression to one of them. Also, infants are far more powerfully and intricately preprogrammed for adaptation and survival than the psychoanalytic theorists assumed; almost without exception the theorists saw infants as helpless, utterly dependent, and mindless creatures of infinite malleability. The fact that many infants survive despite unusually bleak or traumatic rearing suggests that factors orthogonal to nurture may be operative.

Second, some people who have schizophrenia as adults come from basically healthy families and undergo normal growth and development—a direct challenge to the traumatic hypotheses. Furthermore, the childhood suffering in the histories of schizophrenic patients is often no more severe or profound than that of patients with other forms of mental illness, suggesting the necessary presence of nonexperiential pathogenic factors. Why, for example, do similar adverse life circumstances result in anxiety or depression in one person and hallucinations and thought disorder in another?

Third, the psychogenic theories have difficulty in explaining why, in most cases of schizophrenia, some two decades pass between the purported pathogenic infantile traumatic experiences and the onset of overt symptoms. If the experiences postulated by the theories do occur, one might expect to see symptom formation at the time, followed by predictable and nonrepressible (that is, observable) deformities in subsequent development, at least in some cases. An infantile catastrophe severe enough to produce an illness of the magnitude of schizophrenia is not likely to go unnoticed, yet such catastrophes and their immediate behavioral consequences have not been documented.

Generally, psychoanalytic theories of schizophrenia, especially those with a descriptive-homeostatic perspective, continue to inform the clinical eye and help clinicians understand the patients they encounter. In that context they are vital and worthy of study. Furthermore, while exploring the past with schizophrenic patients may no longer be expected to yield causative or historical truth, it does provide meaningful metaphors that can be useful in the empathic dialogue between the doctor and the patient.

FAMILY TRANSACTION MODELS The family transaction models of schizophrenia represent attempts to understand and explain the syndrome as the transmission of aberrant interactions from the family to the patient. The models are compatible with object-relation-oriented psychoanalytic psychogenic theories in assuming psychopathology to be determined largely by experience and learning within the family during growth and development. The models are different, however, in their respective hypothesis-generating and hypothesis-validating data bases. For psychoanalytic theories the data are the associations of individual patients; for family transaction theories the data are observed interactions in families with one or more schizophrenic members.

Family transaction models emerged after World War II from the context of clinical work with the families of schizophrenic patients; it was noted with increasing frequency that irrationality was not limited to the identified patient. Unusual and unpredictable interactions were observed between persons within the family or among family members as an entire unit. Motivated by the idea that those interactions may be schizophrenogenic, several clinical investigators began to describe the families and their transaction patterns in some detail.

Gregory Bateson and Donald Jackson Gregory Bateson and Donald Jackson outlined a form of family interaction that they labeled the *double bind.* The interaction usually occurs between a parent and the schizophrenic offspring; it consists of the parent giving the child incompatible (if not antithetical) messages (for example, stiffly avoiding a physical embrace while saying, "Why don't you show me more affection?"). That sets up an inescapable damned-if-you-do-and-damned-if-you-don't situation, a double bind, in which the offspring feels paralyzed. Bateson and Jackson hypothesized that repeated exposure to such a dilemma generates or aggravates the schizophrenic state.

Ruth and Theodore Lidz Ruth and Theodore Lidz systematically studied the characteristics of families with a schizophrenic offspring. Using a psychoanalytically oriented psychodynamic perspective, they looked for and observed disorders in the role and affective relationships among family members, especially the triad of the mother, the father, and the schizophrenic child. They described several irrational patterns, such as marital schism between parents who remain married because of pathological interdependence, despite considerable overt conflict; marital skew between parents who hide chronic disagreement behind a facade of harmony; permeable generational boundaries, in which one parent requires the schizophrenic child to assume a parental role; eroticized parent-child relatedness, in which one parent treats the schizophrenic child as a peer or a contemporary; and emotional divorce, in which family members fail to acknowledge and confirm one another's psychological integrity. The Lidzes asserted that such irrational family functioning is sufficient to account for schizophrenia in certain offspring exposed to it during their formative years.

Lyman Wynne and Margaret Singer Lyman Wynne, Margaret Singer, and their colleagues explored the nature of communication and cooperation among families with a schizophrenic offspring. From their observational work came the concept of communication deviance, which includes parental communications that lack commitment to ideas and percepts; parental communications that are unclear, as they are filled with idiosyncratic themes and ideas, language anomalies, discursive speech, and problems with closure; and parental communications that reflect an inability to establish or maintain a shared focus of attention during transactions with another family member. They identified an amorphous style, in which communications are vague, indefinite, and loose, and a fragmented style, in which communications are easily disrupted, are poorly integrated, and lack closure. They also described familial displays of mutuality or hostility or both that serve as facades hiding antithetical themes and conflicts.

Unlike most other family transactional theorists, Wynne and Singer were able to operationalize their concepts into reliable measures, thus allowing their hypotheses to be tested systematically. They found communication deviance to be more specific to the families of schizophrenic patients than to the families of offspring with depressive disorders, personality disorders, neuroses, or no pathology. Furthermore, amorphous patterns of communication deviance correlated frequently with process schizophrenia, and fragmented patterns correlated frequently with reactive schizophrenia. They also found significant quantitative correlations between the amount of communication deviance in the parents and the severity of psychopathology in their offspring. For example, schizophrenic offspring came from families in which both parents had high levels of communication deviance, normal and neurotic offspring came from families in which both parents had low levels of communication deviance, and borderline offspring came from families in which one parent's communication deviance level was high and the other parent's level was low.

Expressed emotion and the family milieu Recently, family investigators have described several family factors that interact powerfully with schizophrenia either to precipitate its emergence or to aggravate its course. One factor, called *expressed emotion,* consists of critical or emotionally overinvolved (or both) attitudes and behaviors displayed by parents toward their ill offspring. Another family transactional factor of interest and current study is *negative affective style.* It includes four kinds of parental behavior: criticism, guilt induction, intrusiveness, and inadequate support. It has been shown and replicated that schizophrenic patients living with high expressed emotion or negative affective style families relapse with a significantly higher frequency than do schizophrenic patients living in families with low expressed emotion or normal affective style.

Critique Like the psychoanalytic theories of schizophrenia, the family transaction theories have come under considerable criticism as causative models. With the exception of communication deviance, few of the family transactions described above are demonstrably specific to schizophrenia. Furthermore, the observed irrational transactions among families may derive from the necessity of dealing with an overtly deviant child, thus reversing the direction of the hypothesized causal vector. In the absence of hard causative data, the assumption that families transmit and concentrate their irrationalities on a designated family member-victim becomes a nonproductive assignment of blame that does little to advance understanding but much to undermine the working alliances of professionals and afflicted families.

Like the psychoanalytic theories of schizophrenia, the family transaction theories remain viable and useful as descriptive-homeostatic models. Although irrational behaviors in the families of schizophrenic patients may not cause the illness, those behaviors are nevertheless present and real in their evocative effects. As demonstrated by the expressed emotion and affective style studies, the family's emotional milieu can profoundly influence the onset or the course of schizophrenia. Family transactional stress may not be causative; however, it can be powerfully facilitative in both pathological and therapeutic directions. The family theories also fit well into the earliest neurodynamic theory of schizophrenia: the vulnerability-stress hypothesis.

NEURODYNAMIC THEORIES

VULNERABILITY-STRESS MODEL The first neurodynamic model, the vulnerability-stress hypothesis (also known as the stress-diathesis model), views schizophrenia dynamically as a product of interacting forces, some genetic or biological and some psychological, some innate or constitutional and some learned through experience. Unlike the purely psychodynamic theories, the vulnerability-stress model regards nature as important, as suggested by genetic studies and the efficacy of biological treatments. Both nature and experience, however, are considered necessary to describe and to understand schizophrenia.

A Finnish adoption study illustrates the model. Comparing adopted-away children of schizophrenic mothers (high-genetic-risk probands) with adopted-away children of nonschizophrenic mothers (low-genetic-risk controls), the researchers found that schizophrenia developed only in the probands with genetic vulnerability who were raised in adoptive families in which the emotional environment was demonstrably unhealthy. None of the high-genetic-risk probands raised in healthy adoptive families had psychosis. Likewise, none of the low-genetic-risk probands raised in unhealthy adoptive families had psychosis, although many had other forms of psychopathology. Those results strongly suggest that both a disturbed rearing environment and an innate vulnerability to schizophrenia are necessary to generate the syndrome.

The concept of such an interaction began with Freud. Describing the origin of neurosis in "On the History of the Psycho-Analytic Movement," he wrote:

> Disposition and experience are here linked up in an indissoluble aetiological unit. For *disposition* exaggerates impressions which otherwise have been completely commonplace and have no effect, so that they become traumas giving rise to stimulations and fixations; while *experiences* awaken factors in the disposition which, without them, might have long remained dormant and perhaps never have developed.

Freud could well have been writing about the origins of psychosis. Certainly, subsequent psychoanalytic theorists took the model seriously in explaining schizophrenia, especially those who emphasized deficit. The true conceptual fathers of today's vulnerability-stress model of schizophrenia, however, are Sandor Rado and Paul Meehl.

Rado hypothesized that schizophrenia begins with an inherited disposition or genotype. The interaction of the genotype with the environment produces the schizophrenic phenotype, a personality type or trait called the *schizotype.* Central to that trait is an inherent incapacity to experience pleasure. As Rado wrote:

> In the schizotype the machinery of psychodynamic integration is strikingly inadequate, because one of its essential components, the organizing action of pleasure—its motivational strength—is innately defective.

That defect impairs the development of initiative and leads to schizo-adaptations, such as compensatory overdependence on others (especially parents) and the elaboration of intricate cognitive processes devoid of affect. Anhedonia results in weak emotional bonds and leads to attenuated relationships. The well-compensated schizotype remains a stable schizoid personality. The poorly compensated schizotype develops exaggerated, bizarre behaviors. Schizophrenia proper represents a decompensated schizotype with adaptive incompetence. The nature and the severity of the schizo-adaptation depends on the genotypic loading and on the degree of familial and environmental stress.

To Meehl the inherited schizophrenic genotype (which he labeled *schizotaxia*) consists of a defect in neural integration. That defect, plus social learning (environment), leads to an abnormally organized personality (the schizotype) characterized by cognitive slippage (thought disorder), anhedonia, ambivalence, and aversion to human relationships. Further progression from schizotypy to schizophrenia depends on the nature and the severity of the environmental stress versus the availability of help and support.

That hypothetically pathogenic interaction between nature and experience came to be known as the stress-diathesis or the vulnerability-stress model. As currently conceived, the model accepts the idea that the relative roles of nature and nurture in the cause of schizophrenia will remain obscure until markers are available for the genetic predisposition or the constitutional vulnerability. The model shifts the emphasis from the role of psychodynamic factors in causing schizophrenia to their role in facilitating and preventing the expression of the disease process.

The vulnerability to schizophrenia is seen as a relatively enduring proclivity toward developing clinical symptoms. It is a stable trait independent of nonenduring psychopathological states, meaning that its features are present premorbidly, at onset, during symptomatic efflorescence, and in remission. However, the trait should not be regarded as developmentally static or fixed. Rather, it is shaped epigenetically by transactions with the environment at each developmental phase. Aspects of vulnerability are undoubtedly genetic. Some aspects may be acquired biologically through intrauterine, birth, and postnatal complications. The season of birth may also contribute, for reasons yet to be ascertained. The evidence for psychosocially acquired vulnerability is meager at present, but it cannot be ruled out.

The stress side of the model postulates that a variety of stressors—that is, internal and external events requiring adaptation—can convert vulnerability into symptoms. Therefore, coping strengths and supports that diminish stress should minimize or prevent the clinical expression of vulnerability.

In the model the vicissitudes of schizophrenia are determined by the nature of the vulnerability and the stress and by the person's strengths and environmental supports. The interaction of sufficient stress with sufficient vulnerability can lead to transient, intermediate (prodromal) states of dysfunction that amplify existing cognitive, affective-autonomic, and social-coping deficits. Those transient states interact negatively with stressors, magnifying their effects in a downward-spiraling deterioration that culminates in a full-blown clinical syndrome.

Vulnerabilities to schizophrenia The list of specific vulnerabilities to schizophrenia is extensive. A few have been demonstrated, and many are postulated. First are deficits in the processing of complex information, in maintaining a steady focus of attention, in distinguishing between relevant and irrelevant stimuli, and in forming consistent abstractions. Second are dysfunctions in psychophysiology, suggesting deficits in sensory inhibition and poor control over autonomic responsivity, especially to aversive stimuli. Third are impairments in social competence, such as in processing interpersonal stimuli, eye contact, assertiveness, and conversational capacity. Those deficits probably reflect both a core disturbance of schizophrenia (vulnerability) and the social outcomes of severe psychopathology. In the past the sources of those difficulties were often attributed to such external elements as antipsychotic drugs and institutions, a perspective that unduly diverted attention from their primacy in the disorder. Fourth are general coping deficits, such as overevaluating threat, underestimating internal resources, and the extensive use of denial.

Finding, mapping, and integrating those vulnerabilities have become central efforts in current schizophrenia research. Virtually all investigation has focused on demonstrable phenotype manifestations of hypothetical genotypic vulnerabilities in children and adolescents at risk for schizophrenia. An additional possibility is a genotypic vulnerability with variable onset of its expression. Huntington's disease, for example, is an adult-onset neurological deterioration leading to psychosis and dementia; in a similar fashion, many cases of schizophrenia may result from a genotype whose phenotypic expression is not triggered until late adolescence or early adulthood. The phenotype may be a deficit in the neurophysiological maturation of self systems during adolescence or a still later-onset neural deterioration or inhibition of those same systems in adulthood. Early-onset genotypes may help account for cases with easily identifiable phenotypic deviations that begin in childhood as schizotypal aberrations and progress to chronic process cases of schizophrenia later on. Late-onset genotypes may help explain the acute occurrence of schizophrenia later in life in persons with normal growth and development and healthy premorbid personalities.

Stressors in schizophrenia Systematic studies of the stresses that affect the course of schizophrenia, aside from the family environment, have focused on social class and culture, social networks, and life events.

Socioeconomic and cultural factors have a long history of empirical association with schizophrenia. One of the most replicated findings in the schizophrenia literature is the clustering of schizophrenic patients in the lowest social classes, especially in urban communities. Few now hold that a poor socioeconomic environment causes schizophrenia, but few doubt that it has a major effect on its course. Poverty, ignorance, unemployment, social isolation, poor nutrition, and marginal health care are powerful chronic stressors that lead to frequent breakdowns in vulnerable persons.

Schizophrenia and the social network are highly interactive, cross-sectionally and longitudinally. Compared with other people, schizophrenic patients usually have social networks that are smaller, less interconnected, simpler, and more dependent, casual, nonintimate, and peopled with family, as opposed to peers. The interplay between schizophrenia and social networks appears to be circular, rather than linear. Initially, the major influence is schizophrenia on the social network. After the appearance of clinical symptoms, however, the social network is likely to exert a powerful influence on the subsequent vicissitudes of schizophrenia.

Stressful life events have a demonstrated association with schizophrenia, but the association may not always be necessary or direct. Questions often arise concerning whether stress differs in its effects on disease onset versus recurrence and whether a stressful event precedes illness or represents a product of symptom exacerbation. Convention dichotomizes stressful events into those that are ambient, nonindependent, or chronic and those that are independent or acute. The chronic stresses are associated with everyday living, such as family, work, poverty, physical disability, and mental deficit; the acute stresses are associated with largely external or unusual changes, such as loss, death, acute illness, and moves, especially if those changes are unanticipated, undesired, and uncontrolled. Research suggests a high frequency of such events shortly before schizophrenia onset or symptom exacerbation. Furthermore, there appears to be an important interaction between maintenance antipsychotic medication and life-event stress. Patients in the community without medication are vulnerable to both acute and chronic stress. Patients taking medication, however, appear to be protected against either type of stress alone but are likely to suffer relapse if the two types occur concurrently.

PARALLEL-DISTRIBUTED PROCESSING MODEL The latest neurodynamic model of schizophrenia hypothesizes with specificity the neuroanatomical nature of the vulnerability to schizophrenia and its biophysical contribution to symptom formation. The model is built on postulates that most human mentation arises from neuronal networks organized in parallel-distributed processing systems. Furthermore, the systems can, under certain physiological conditions, generate thoughts or feelings in ways orthogonal to the normal processes by which psychology is generated. The aberrant development, called *memory parasitism,* can produce mentations that are literally products or short circuits in the wiring apparatus of the brain and that are experienced and interpreted psychodynamically as unintended and alien by the bearer of the brain. The physical conditions conducive to such developments are unknown but are hypothesized to involve a loss of neural circuit density because of perinatal insults or a genetically or developmentally programmed excessive pruning of the connections between cortical nerve cells.

Mental events are basically neuronally constructed representations of experience as memory. Memories, in general, are accessible to consciousness in a manner that is content-addressable—that is, the brain is able to use part of a memory to access the memory in its entirety. Artificial intelligence researchers, such as John Hopfield, James McClelland, and David Rumelhart, have discovered that certain types of computer-assisted computations achieve content-addressable information retrieval in a fashion that partially simulates nature. Those systems are composed of many simple computing units, generally referred to as "neurons," which are densely interconnected by synapses. There is no single command unit; the effectiveness of the network as a whole reflects the cooperative interactions of its parts. Each neuron simultaneously receives information from many other neurons and computes its response to those inputs in parallel with the computations of the system's other neurons. There is no one-to-one correspondence between a memory and the activation of a particular neuron. Instead, a memory corresponds to a pattern of activation involving many neurons; memories are stored by modifying functional connections between neurons. Networks that store and retrieve information on the basis of distributed patterns of activation are referred to as parallel-distributed processing systems.

An increasing body of neurobiological research suggests that the functional architecture of the mammalian cerebral cortex can be broken down into a number of linked neuronal assemblies. Of special interest is the long-term memory system, which probably involves the brain's hippocampal and cortical areas. The hippocampus is active during a critical gestational period (ranging from minutes to hours), during which input information is distributed to interconnected circuits linking frontal, parietal, and sensory-association cortical areas. If the functioning of the hippocampus is temporarily impaired, memories in gestation are permanently lost. However, once information is functionally linked within the cortex, its retrieval does not seem to require an intact functioning hippocampus. Activating a posterior sensory area with an image representation or a frontal area with an abstract concept, such as a goal or a generalization, can immediately seed widely distributed cortical circuits to yield complex memories.

Parallel-distributed processing systems with content-addressable mnemonic representations probably constitute the working neuronal hardware generating normal mental activity and psychology. The psychoanalytic method of free association, for example, relies on the content-addressability of mental representations. Freud first observed that human mentation follows patterns that are seldom logical or governed by the rational rules of secondary process. More often than not, mental representations are connected by condensations, displacements, and symbolizations of mnemonic content, whether that content be concrete imagery, stories, or abstract theories. Those are the *primary processes* of mentation postulated by Freud to underlie the formation of dreams and neurotic-level symptoms. Content-addressability is a new term for an old psychoanalytic postulate that every mental event (thinking, feeling, acting) is overdetermined and can be arrived at by multiple pathways. In Robert Waelder's principle of multiple function, a vast array of related factors (for example id, ego, superego) must be considered in trying to understand any behavior. The functional dynamics of parallel-distributed processing systems also suggests that an enormous amount of neuronal and mental activity accompanies any single mental event or idea, thus assuming or accounting for the dynamic unconscious of psychoanalysis.

Memory parasitism Most psychiatric syndromes include some form of repetitively reproduced mental content, ranging from obsessional thoughts to the idée fixe of psychotic delusions. Such repetitive memories can be produced in computer-simulated parallel-distributed processing systems on the basis of attractor dynamics. The systems tend to be attracted to particular activation patterns that are low-energy states of the system. Energy here is defined on the basis of a branch of physics known as statistical mechanics. Statistical *energy* corresponds to the degree of disorder in the system. Neurons that freely interact in a neuronal network tend to be attracted to those activation patterns that minimize its statistical energy. The patterns correspond to the memories of the system that tend to be reproduced because of the energy minima. Particularly strong memories correspond to deep energy minima that tend to pull the system into its own activation pattern to the exclusion of other activation patterns. That is, a memory with a particularly deep energy minimum relentlessly strives to express itself. As such, it is parasitic in nature because it coercively transforms a wide range of input information into a single memory-activation pattern.

Computer-simulated models can provide an account of how such pathological memories are induced. Under varying circumstances, a memory can be created that does not reflect any specific prior experience. Those spurious memories are not linked to naturally occurring and stored input-activation patterns but are created de novo by the brain itself and can be triggered by the most irrelevant internal or external cues. The memories link or condense disparate contents and may appear at times to be the products of primary process. However, they cannot be grasped by the empathic primary processes of others—that is, they remain strange and beyond understanding in Karl Jaspers's sense of being self-evident or common to human experience. The memories tie together representations or fragments of representations that are ordinarily not linked, even by the weakest and most remote of primary process pathways, hence the term "loose association." They are, in a sense, violations of content-addressability; associations are no longer free but are constrained by disturbed attractor dynamics.

Parasitic memories are the product of biophysical energic processes, not primary and secondary psychological processes. At the same time, they arise in the midst of other neural networks that are not compromised and that generate normal and abnormal psychology in the usual way—that is, by primary and secondary processes. Persons experiencing such parasitic memories may feel as though parts of the brain or mind are functioning out of their control. They may experience the unintended mental events as though someone else were putting thoughts into their minds. Such post hoc reasoning that an outside force is inserting thoughts into one's mind may reflect the difficult task of describing and making sense of the experience of one's mind being repeatedly captured by a perseverative attractor seemingly acting according to its own will. In that fashion parasitic memories in a parallel-distributed processing system can account for many of the seemingly bizarre symptoms of schizophrenia.

Pathophysiology How do such memories come about? In computer-based parallel-distributed processing systems, parasitic memories derive from two types of pathology. First, parasitic memories can be produced when the system attempts to store memories whose number exceeds its capacity. Second, parasitic memories can be produced when an insufficient number of synaptic connections link the neurons of the system. Those two types of pathology may be located in the system of long-term memory storage and recall involving the hippocampus and diffuse cortical circuits of the brain.

Considerable interest involves the hippocampus in schizophrenia. Neuroradiological and postmortem studies have suggested a reduced volume of the hippocampus and a disarray of its pyramidal cells in some schizophrenic patients. Reductions in the pyramidal cell number, functional efficiency, or information transfer capacity—perhaps occurring secondary to prenatal complications, such as viral infection—may downsize memory storage capability in the hippocampus, thereby rendering it vulnerable to the induction of memory parasitism.

A second form of schizophrenia may reflect abnormalities in postnatal brain development. Considerable evidence in humans and other primates indicates that after birth an overproduction of corticocortical connections occurs over time; those connections are then selectively pruned and shaped during later developmental periods. In humans, pruning of cortical synapses seems to extend well into adolescence for connections involving the frontal areas. Moreover, the continued elaboration and pruning away of cortical synapses probably continues, albeit at a much reduced rate, throughout adulthood.

Developmental studies, when considered in light of parallel-distributed processing simulations, suggest a second mechanism leading to parasitic and spurious memories—reductions in corticocortical connections that are induced as an extension of the developmental processes. If excessive developmentally induced pruning of the connections leads to a form of schizophrenia, a ready explanation for its age of onset and the involvement in the frontal areas is provided: the pruning of synapses is most prolonged in the frontal areas, and the end of adolescence is when the effects of that pruning process are first fully felt.

Implications The parallel-distributed processing paradigm is neurodynamic in scope because it postulates the creation of symptoms, at least in part, on the basis of defects in the hardware of the brain. Purely psychodynamic paradigms account for pathology solely as a reflection of aberrant software or conflicting functional programs in the mind. The parallel-distributed processing model regards psychodynamics as necessary but often not sufficient to explain most schizophrenic symptoms. It is a model at the mind-body interface, and it views psychotic psychopathology as the product of a complex interraction of skewed mentation arising organically, with normal or abnormal psychology arising psychodynamically.

The model remains speculative but offers an advantage of being falsifiable. Many of the functional and neuroanatomical predictions of the model may be subject to hypothesis testing and validation, thus bringing theorizing about schizophrenia closer to the realm of scientific empiricism.

OVERVIEW

In the 20th century psychiatry has seen the elaboration of four major psychodynamic models of schizophrenia: psychoanalytic, family transaction, vulnerability-stress, and parallel-distributed processing. All have provided useful descriptions of this mysterious disease and have elaborated the psychopathological and homeostatic functions of schizophrenia in ways that are meaningful and clinically useful.

In terms of sheer volume, the bulk of psychodynamic theories belong to psychoanalysis. In terms of content, the major issues have not changed much since Freud posited two theories—the structural-conflict theory and the withdrawal-deficit theory. By never integrating those two theories, Freud seemed to be saying that schizophrenia may be both, explained in part by intrapsychic conflict and in part by something else. Psychodynamic theories became more elaborate and sophisticated over the ensuing years, yet one can still follow the thematic threads of Freud's original explanations. Conflict theory has seen a line of development polarized toward object relations, experiential learning within the family, the stressors that interact with vulnerability, and the psychological sequelae of organically disturbed neural circuitry. Deficit theory has seen a line of development polarized toward individual drives, complex constitutional inborn factors, the physical vulnerabilities of the vulnerability-stress model, and the hard-wiring defects of parallel-distributed processing neural networks. Today, those two threads are each regarded as valid facets of the overall phenomenon. Both threads are necessary for a comprehensible and potentially workable theory of schizophrenia.

None of the psychodynamic models of schizophrenia has solved the mystery of its cause, but each model has offered cogent hypotheses or educated guesses. The neurodynamic models see nature as primary or, at least, as initiating a process of negative interaction with environmental experience that becomes pathogenic sooner or later in life, depending on the onset trigger of the genotype. The family transactional model, at least as originally conceived, sees nurture or experience as primary and, frequently, as sufficient for generating schizophrenia. Psychoanalytic models have posited one or the other or both. Since Sullivan and Mahler, however, the emphasis has shifted toward traumatic nurturing experiences during early development, a shift that has come under increasing criticism.

Overall, the impressive evidence for the existence of genetic and constitutional factors in schizophrenia has raised questions about the causative hegemony of experience and learning in early development. Hypothetically, some (if not many) cases of schizophrenia arise from an adolescent-onset neurological dysfunction or deterioration in people who are, up to that point, developmentally normal. Such a process, along the model of overpruned parallel-distributed processing neural networks, selectively inhibits or destroys later developmental levels of personality, especially those neuronal networks involved with the structures, the functions, and the representations of the self. In response, the person falls back on primitively organized levels of personality and development. Such regression is compensatory and adaptive, rather than primary and motivating. The regression occurs not because of developmental fixation but because simpler developmental levels and patterns may be the only ones left.

THERAPEUTIC IMPLICATIONS

Psychodynamic theories of schizophrenia carry with them distinct implications for treatment. Early proponents of the psychoanalytic conflict model advocated the classic techniques of clarification, confrontation, and interpretation. Early proponents of the psychoanalytic deficit model introduced additional strategies. Federn, for example, thought that the usual psychoanalytic techniques aim at *de*repression, whereas, with schizophrenia, the goal is to foster *re*repression. He encouraged positive transference, avoided negative transference, protected patients from undue anxiety and insomnia, taught them to improve their capacities for attention and thinking, exhorted them to give up unrealistic life goals, provided support beyond analytic hours in the form of a skilled nurse-assistant available to the patients at home, and offered consultation to the patient's family (recognizing the importance of the home environment to the outcome).

Proponents of the family transactional theories uniformly advocate family therapy in some form. Those who view the family milieu as causing schizophrenia usually regard the entire family as the patient or as the problem and focus their interventions accordingly. Those who regard the family as facilitative, rather than causative, emphasize the positive and negative effects that domestic tensions can have on the course of the identified patient. Technical strategies in the first instance are interpretive; in the second instance they are psychoeducational.

Proponents of the vulnerability-stress and parallel-distributed processing models advocate any intervention that enhances strength and support and that minimizes stress and vulnerability. Interventions include both psychobiological and psychodynamic treatments. The neurodynamic models are the only ones that formally (that is, theoretically) incorporate biology and endorse it therapeutically. The models also define psychodynamic treatment liberally. Any and all forms of psychosocial intervention, from individual psychotherapy to social skills training, are potentially useful, depending on the modality's track record of efficacy with the specific clinical situation or condition.

Conflict psychodynamic models, in keeping with their bias toward object relations and development in the family, emphasize the therapeutic centrality of the doctor-patient relationship. That relationship is facilitating, parental, soothing, mirroring, and protective, and the patient grows by internalizing the interactions that transpire within the dyad. The patient's actual interpersonal experience of the therapist is crucial; the therapist's reality and benignity serve to reality-test the patient's transferentially distorted images.

Deficit psychodynamic models, in keeping with their bias toward the patient as an individual with phenotypic abnormalities, emphasize the therapeutic centrality of insight. The goal of treatment is to enhance the power of the ego by expanding its knowledge and control over the inner drives and the psychopathological idiosyncrasies. Enlightenment replaces unconscious defense with conscious choice. Therapy from that perspective focuses primarily on developing the patient's cognitive systems through interpretation, psychoeducation, training, and rehabilitation. The patient realizes that something is wrong, what that something is, and how it can be dealt with.

The conflict psychodynamicists once eschewed deficit theories as therapeutically nihilistic, insisting that there was no way to make up for a biological defect by psychological means. Such an assertion may be literally correct but operationally erroneous. For example, psychological manipulation cannot make paraplegics walk under their own power, but it can train them in prosthetic ambulation, and it can enhance their adaptation and their quality of life. Whatever the origin of schizophrenia, its successful psychological treatment involves both the resolution of intrapsychic conflict through insight and the acquisition of a psychic structure through affective relationships. If the core of schizophrenia is psychological, treatment addresses the sick self; if the core is defect, treatment addresses the healthy self. In the psychological view, treatment minimizes weakness; in the defect view, treatment maximizes strength. In most cases it does both.

INTEGRATIVE MEDICAL MODEL

One theory encompasses all the foregoing 20th-century trends—the biopsychosocial medical model. According to that model, each patient consists of and participates in multiple systems that are related but also distinct from each other. Common systems are subatomic particles, atoms, molecules, organelles, cells, tissues, organs, organ systems, the central nervous system, the individual, the dyad, the family, the community, the culture-subculture, the society-nation, and the biosphere. In health and disease, all systems are relevant. Each system of the biopsychosocial medical model has a functional structure, one of its purposes being the reduction of complexity and randomness to protect the system's integrity. The functional structure of the psychological systems in the model consist of meanings that order experience through understanding and explanation.

Schizophrenia presents most dramatically at the psychological level as a loss or a distortion of the self as a meaningful entity. Despite that, schizophrenia is not entirely or even essentially psychological in its nature. Accordingly, proper medical attention to the disorder should be aimed at any and all relevant systems in the biopsychosocial hierarchy. Whatever schizophrenia may be, it is profoundly disabling and usually chronic. Anything therapeutic that works with sufficient safety is relevant, whether it be biological, psychological, or sociological. Psychodynamic approaches to treatment should not ignore biology because biology exists outside the realm of empathy and meaning. Biological approaches to treatment should not justify psychological retreat from patients because conflicts cannot be teased apart by electrophoresis. Finally, treatment advocates of both approaches should be aware of patients' social, cultural, and political needs for a place of dignity and safety within society. That is, they also require adequate attention at the social level of the biopsychosocial system.

SUGGESTED CROSS-REFERENCES

The relevance of brain structure and function in schizophrenia is discussed in Section 14.3; neurochemical, viral, and immunological studies are discussed in Section 14.4; and genetics in schizophrenia is discussed in Section 14.5. Somatic treatment is discussed in Section 14.8, psychosocial treatment in Section 14.9, and individual psychotherapy in Section 14.10. Theories of personality and psychopathology are discussed in Chapters 6, 7, and 8. Schizophrenia in childhood is discussed in Chapter 45, and schizophrenia in late life is discussed in Section 49.6c.

REFERENCES

Burnham D L, Gladstone A I, Gibson R W: *Schizophrenia and the Need-Fear Dilemma.* International Universities Press, New York, 1969.

Cancro R: General considerations relating to theory in the schizophrenic disorders. In *Towards a Comprehensive Model for Schizophrenic Disorders,* D B Feinsilver, editor, p 97. Analytic Press, Hillsdale, NJ, 1986.

Cohen J D, Servan-Schreiber D: Context, cortex, and dopamine: A connectionist approach to behavior and biology in schizophrenia. Psychol Rev *99:* 45, 1992.

Engel G A: The need for a new medical model: A challenge for biomedicine. Science *196:* 129, 1977.

Federn P: *Ego Psychology and the Psychoses.* Basic Books, New York, 1952.

Feinberg I: Schizophrenia: Caused by a fault in programmed synaptic elimination during adolescence? J Psychiatr Res *4:* 319, 1982.

Freud S: The interpretation of dreams. In *Standard Edition of the Complete Psychological Works of Sigmund Freud,* vol 5, p 94. Hogarth Press, London, 1953.

Freud S: On the history of the psycho-analytic movement. In *Standard Edition of the Complete Psychological Works of Sigmund Freud,* vol 14, p 3. Hogarth Press, London, 1957.

*Freud S: Psychoanalytic notes on an autobiographical account of a case of paranoia (dementia paranoides). In *Standard Edition of the Complete Psychological Works of Sigmund Freud,* vol 12, p 9. Hogarth Press, London, 1958.

Greenberg J R, Mitchell S A: *Object Relations in Psychoanalytic Theory.* Harvard University Press, Cambridge, MA, 1983.

Hoffman R E: Computer simulations of neural information processing and the schizophrenia/mania dichotomy. Arch Gen Psychiatry *44:* 178, 1987.

Hoffman R E: The mechanism of positive symptoms in schizophrenia. Behav Br Sci *14:* 33, 1991.

Hoffman R E, Dobscha S B: Cortical pruning and the development of schizophrenia: A computer model. Schizophr Bull *15:* 477, 1989.

Hoffman R E, McGlashan T H: Corticocortical connectivity, autonomous networks, and schizophrenia. Schizophr Bull *20:* 257, 1994.

*Hoffman R E, McGlashan T H: Parallel distributed processing and the emergence of schizophrenic symptoms. Schizophr Bull *19:* 119, 1993.

Hopfield J J: Neural networks and physical systems with emergent collective computational abilities. Proc Natl Acad Sci USA *79:* 2554, 1982.

Jaspers K: *General Psychopathology.* Grune & Stratton, New York, 1959.

Lichtenberg J D: Pao's theory: Origins and future directions. In *Towards a Comprehensive Model for Schizophrenic Disorders,* D B Feinsilver, editor, p 75. Analytic Press, Hillsdale, NJ, 1986.

Lidz T: *Schizophrenia and the Family.* International Universities Press, New York, 1965.

McGlashan T H: Psychosocial treatments of schizophrenia: The potential of relationships. In *Schizophrenia: From Mind to Molecule,* N C Andreasen, editor, p 189. American Psychiatric Press, Washington, 1994.

McGlashan T H, Fenton W S: Subtype progression and pathophysiologic deterioration in the course of early manifest schizophrenia. Schizophr Bull *:* 71, 1993.

*Meehl P E: Toward an integrated theory of schizotaxia, schizotypy, and schizophrenia. J Pers Disord *4:* 1, 1990.

Mesulam M M: Large-scale neurocognitive networks and distributed processing for attention, language, and memory. Ann Neurol *28:* 567, 1990.

Pao P-N: *Schizophrenic Disorders.* International Universities Press, New York, 1979.

Pettegrew J W, Keshavan M S, Minshew N J: ^{31}P nuclear magnetic resonance spectroscopy: Neurodevelopment and schizophrenia. Schizophr Bull *19:* 35, 1993.

Rado S: *Psychoanalysis of Behavior.* Grune & Stratton, New York, 1956.

Rumelhart D E: McClelland J L: *Parallel Distributed Processing: Explorations in the Microstructure of Cognition,* vol 1. MIT Press, Cambridge, MA, 1986.

Scheibel A B, Conrad A S: Hippocampal dysgenesis in mutant mouse and schizophrenic man: Is there a relationship? Schizophr Bull *19:* 21, 1993.

Segal H: *Introduction to the Work of Melanie Klein.* Basic Books, New York, 1973.

*Spring B, Zubin J: Vulnerability to schizophrenic episodes and their prevention in adults. In *Primary Prevention in Psychopathology: The Issues,* G W Albee, J M Joffee, editors, vol 1, p 254. University Press of New England, Hanover, N H, 1977.

Stern D: *The Interpersonal World of the Infant.* Basic Books, New York, 1985.

*Sullivan H S: *Clinical Studies in Psychiatry.* Norton, New York, 1956.

Tienari P, Sorry A, Lahti I, Narala M, Wahlberg K-E, Ronkko T, Pohjola J, Moring J: The Finnish adoptive family study of schizophrenia. Yale J Biol Med *58:* 227, 1985.

Waelder R: The principle of multiple function. Psychoanal Q *5:* 45, 1936.

Wynne L C, Singer M: Thought disorder and family relations of schizophrenics: II. Classification of forms of thinking. Arch Gen Psychiatry *9:* 199, 1963.

14.7 SCHIZOPHRENIA: CLINICAL FEATURES

ALAN A. LIPTON, M.D., M.P.H.
ROBERT CANCRO, M.D., Med.D.Sc.

INTRODUCTION

The group of disorders that constitute schizophrenia are the major public health problem faced by psychiatry, for they affect approximately 1 percent of the population. The disorders usually have their onset in early adult life and usually leave varying degrees of residual impairment. Persons with schizophrenia frequently do not attain their full psychosocial potential. They are usually unable to perform complex work and sometimes are not able to work at all. Their interpersonal relationships are altered negatively to varying degrees. Their sense of personal worth is almost invariably diminished.

All known societies identify the adult role in terms of work and procreation. Persons who are not able to perform the work responsibilities expected by their society and who are also impaired in the interpersonal skills that are required as part of the procreative process do not achieve full adult recognition in their societies. The combination of early onset, long duration, and significant psychosocial impairment defines the public health problem.

The financial cost of schizophrenia is monumental. The cost is not primarily a function of the medical and social care rendered, although such care costs billions of dollars a year in the United States alone. The major economic cost is the inability of persons with schizophrenia to make their full contribution to society. There are no measures to express the cost of the human suffering of the patient, family, and friends. Schizophrenia and other psychotic disorders are associated with a high rate of attempted and completed patient suicide because of the unbearability of the symptoms.

CONCEPTUALIZATION

Until the middle of the 19th century observers of the mentally ill generally restricted their classificatory efforts to an individual or group phenomenologically based nosology. In the second half of the 19th century the drive to create scientific classifications had become more powerful. That thrust was influenced in part by the contributions of microbiologists to the study of infectious diseases. As specific causes of infectious diseases were discovered, clinicians were able to identify cases that had been falsely included or falsely excluded in the previous diagnostic efforts.

The revolutionary change from a descriptive nosology to an etiopathogenic classification of infectious diseases inspired workers in psychiatry as well. Although the initial search for microorganisms and pathognomonic postmortem changes in psychiatric patients failed, the concepts inherent in Robert Koch's postulates carried the day. It was assumed that mental disease entities existed and that their existence could eventually be demonstrated. Emil Kraepelin (1856–1926) created a hypothetical disease entity called dementia precox. He argued that although it went through many phases and stages, it was a single disease with a natural course and a predictable, poor outcome. The disease entity approach to mental disorders has remained a powerful and popular one.

Eugen Bleuler rejected the unitary disease entity approach and substituted a syndrome or multiple entity concept. In addition, he changed the name from dementia precox to the group of the schizophrenias, believing that dementia precox subsumed multiple disorders that differed in etiology and pathogenesis but had certain clinical features in common.

In a third and fundamentally different approach, illnesses were seen as reactive disorders to life events. That approach was typified by the work of Adolf Meyer, who saw the schizophrenic disorders as reactions to occurrences in the patient's life. Meyer, however, recognized the importance of biological predisposition. The reaction pattern approach was carried to an extreme by some workers who believed that if enough of the right stresses were applied, anyone would develop a schizophrenic disorder. Those workers de-emphasized the importance of the preexisting diathesis.

The first edition of *Diagnostic and Statistical Manual of Mental Disorders* (DSM-I) was heavily influenced by Meyer's thought and referred to schizophrenic reactions. The second edition of DSM (DSM-II) moved toward a disease entity model, whereas the third (DSM-III) and fourth (DSM-IV) editions attempted to be atheoretical. Nevertheless, the unspoken assumptions implicit in any nosology influence it in real ways. One of the most important nosological assumptions is that the traditional disease model is the one that should be followed. More recent understanding of the nervous system reveals a dynamic system that is continuously influenced by internal and external inputs and that is self-organizing and self-conscious. A dynamic, self-organizing system can malfunction for a variety of reasons, some of which differ from traditional conceptualizations of pathogenesis. Presently, the traditional stress-diathesis disease model for schizophrenia reigns supreme, but as developmental neurobiology evolves, other, more sophisticated models may prove useful.

OTHER THEORISTS

Ernst Kretschmer Ernst Kretschmer's data supported the idea that schizophrenia is more common in patients with asthenic, athletic, and dysplastic body types than in patients with pyknic body types, who are more likely to have bipolar disorders. Although that observation seems unusual, it is not inconsistent with a superficial impression regarding the body types of many homeless persons.

Gabriel Langfeldt Langfeldt divided the patients with major psychotic symptoms into two groups, those with true schizophrenia and those with schizophreniform psychosis. Langfeldt emphasized the importance of depersonalization, autism, emotional blunting, an insidious onset, and feelings of derealization in his description of true schizophrenia. True schizophrenia also came to be known as nuclear schizophrenia, process schizophrenia, and nonremitting schizophrenia in the literature that followed Langfeldt's papers.

Karl Jaspers Karl Jaspers was a psychiatrist and a philosopher, and he was a major contributor to existential psychoanalysis. Jaspers approached psychopathology with the idea that there are no firm conceptual frameworks or fundamental principles. In his theories regarding schizophrenia, therefore, Jaspers attempted to remain unencumbered by traditional concepts, such as subject and object, cause and effect, and reality and fantasy. One specific development of that philosophy was his interest in the content of psychiatric patients' delusions.

DIAGNOSTIC CRITERIA

The early efforts at diagnosing schizophrenia relied on general behavioral descriptions and clinical experience rather than on highly specified criteria. Kraepelin's lengthy descriptions were intended to produce mental templates of the variety of clinical presentations that could be called schizophrenia. The clinician could then compare an actual patient with the mental templates and arrive at a diagnosis.

Bleuler listed specific criteria that he identified as the *fundamental symptoms* of schizophrenia. Those fundamental symptoms—Bleuler's four A's—included disturbances of association, disturbances of affect, ambivalence, and autism. Bleuler also described *accessory symptoms,* which included hallucinations and delusions, symptoms that had been a prominent part of Kraepelin's conceptualization of the disorder. The Bleulerian symptoms, however, are not exclusive to schizophrenia. For example, autism and ambivalence are present in all humans in varying degrees. A quantitative clinical judgment had to be made as to whether the degree of autism and ambivalence present in a given patient was sufficient to warrant the diagnosis of schizophrenia. Bleuler also argued that the associational and affective disturbances seen in schizophrenia occurred on a spectrum of severity that ranged from perfectly normal to normal aberrations, such as those seen in sleep-deprived persons, to very subtle pathological signs that did not warrant hospitalization (latent schizophrenia), to florid presentations that necessitated hospital care. Bleuler's criteria were relatively simple to understand, but applying them clinically tended to lead to arbitrary decisions. The effort to develop diagnostic criteria continued to deteriorate through the 1940s as different nosological systems appeared and competed with each other, each having its own adherents. By the time DSM-I was published in 1952, there were three competing nosological systems officially in use in the United States.

DSM-I stated that the schizophrenic reactions were,

> a group of psychotic reactions characterized by fundamental disturbances in reality relationships and concept formations, with affective, behavioral, and intellectual disturbances in varying degrees and mixtures. The disorders are marked by a strong tendency to retreat from reality, by emotional disharmony, unpredictable disturbances in stream of thought, regressive behavior, and in some, by a tendency to "deterioration."

Although DSM-I emphasized that the schizophrenic disorders were reactive illnesses, DSM-II, published in 1968, construed them as a group of disorders whose theoretical origin was not implicit in the label. DSM-II emphasized the disturbances of thinking and behavior, with the mood changes seen as a corollary of the thinking disturbance.

UNITED STATES-UNITED KINGDOM CROSS-NATIONAL PROJECT The application of DSM-II led to diagnostic practices that were highly idiosyncratic. That variability was highlighted by the United States-United Kingdom Cross-National Project, completed in 1970. Standardized interviews were used to establish project diagnoses in New York and London, and the diagnoses were compared with those made by local hospital psychiatrists. The study revealed that the criteria used in the United States for the diagnosis of schizophrenia were significantly more inclusive than those used in London and that, if standardized criteria were used, the prevalence rates in New York and London would be essentially identical.

INTERNATIONAL PILOT STUDY OF SCHIZOPHRENIA Concomitantly, the International Pilot Study of Schizophrenia, conducted by the World Health Organization, utilized the Present State Examination (PSE) and its computerized classification system in nine international field centers to evaluate over 1,000 patients. The PSE, developed in Great Britain, emphasized an empirical approach to the clinical phenomenology of schizophrenia and, in the service of operational reliability, included many first-rank symptoms developed by Kurt Schneider. Although those first-rank symptoms were no longer assigned pathognomonic status, they were more easily objectified and more reliably rated than the softer, more subjective appraisals of affective state and thought processes used in DSM-II.

OTHER DIAGNOSTIC SYSTEMS A number of other diagnostic systems for schizophrenia have been developed (Table 14.7-1). Among them was the Flexible System, derived from the International Pilot Study of Schizophrenia, which used discriminant function analysis to develop 12 discriminators—restricted affect, poor insight, hearing thoughts aloud, absence

TABLE 14.7-1
Essential Features of Various Diagnostic Criteria for Schizophrenia

KURT SCHNEIDER CRITERIA

1. First-rank symptoms
   a. Audible thoughts
   b. Voices arguing or discussing or both
   c. Voices commenting
   d. Somatic passivity experiences
   e. Thought withdrawal and other experiences of influenced thought
   f. Thought broadcasting
   g. Delusional perceptions
   h. All other experiences involving volition, made affects, and made impulses
2. Second-rank symptoms
   a. Other disorders of perception
   b. Sudden delusional ideas
   c. Perplexity
   d. Depressive and euphoric mood changes
   e. Feelings of emotional impoverishment
   f. "... and several others as well"

GABRIEL LANGFELDT CRITERIA

1. Symptom criteria
   Significant clues to a diagnosis of schizophrenia are (if no sign of cognitive impairment, infection, or intoxication can be demonstrated):
   a. Changes in personality, which manifest themselves as a special type of emotional blunting followed by lack of initiative, and altered, frequently peculiar behavior. (In hebephrenia, especially, the changes are characteristic and are a principal clue to the diagnosis.)
   b. In catatonic types, the history and the typical signs in periods of restlessness and stupor (with negativism, oily facies, catalepsy, special vegetative symptoms, etc.)
   c. In paranoid psychoses, essential symptoms of split personality (or depersonalization symptoms) and a loss of reality feeling (derealization symptoms) or primary delusions
   d. Chronic hallucinations
2. Course criterion
   A final decision about diagnosis cannot be made before a follow-up period of at least five years has shown a long-term course of disease

NEW HAVEN SCHIZOPHRENIA INDEX

1. a. Delusions: not specified or other-than-depressive	2 points
b. Auditory hallucinations c. Visual hallucinations d. Other hallucinations	any one: 2 points
2. a. Bizarre thoughts b. Autism or grossly unrealistic private thoughts c. Looseness of associations, illogical thinking, overinclusion	any one: 2 points
d. Blocking e. Concreteness	either: 2 points
f. Derealization g. Depersonalization	each: 1 point
3. Inappropriate affect	1 point
4. Confusion	1 point
5. Paranoid ideation (self-referential thinking, suspiciousness)	1 point
6. Catatonic behavior a. Excitement b. Stupor c. Waxy flexibility d. Negativism e. Mutism f. Echolalia g. Stereotyped motor activity	any one: 1 point

Scoring: To be considered part of the schizophrenic group, the patient must score on Item 1 or Item 2a, 2b, or 2c and must receive a total score of at least 4 points.

FLEXIBLE SYSTEM

Minimum number of symptoms required can be four to eight, depending on investigator's choice:
1. Restricted affect
2. Poor insight
3. Thoughts aloud
4. Poor rapport
5. Widespread delusions
6. Incoherent speech
7. Unreliable information
8. Bizarre delusions
9. Nihilistic delusions
10. Absence of early awakening (one to three hours)
11. Absence of depressed facies
12. Absence of elation

RESEARCH DIAGNOSTIC CRITERIA

Criteria 1 through 3 required for diagnosis:
1. At least two of the following for definite illness and one for probable (not counting those occurring during period of drug or alcohol abuse or withdrawal):
   a. Thought broadcasting, insertion, or withdrawal
   b. Delusions of being controlled or influenced, other bizarre delusions, or multiple delusions
   c. Delusions other than persecution or jealousy lasting at least one month
   d. Delusions of any type if accompanied by hallucinations of any type for at least one week
   e. Auditory hallucinations in which either a voice keeps up a running commentary on subject's behaviors or thoughts as they occur or two or more voices converse with each other
   f. Nonaffective verbal hallucinations spoken to subject

TABLE 14.7-1 (*continued*)

RESEARCH DIAGNOSTIC CRITERIA (*continued*)

g. Hallucinations of any type throughout day for several days or intermittently for at least one month
h. Definite instances of marked formal thought disorders accompanied by blunted or inappropriate affect, delusions, or hallucinations of any type or grossly disorganized behavior

2. One of the following:
   a. Current period of illness lasted at least two weeks from onset of noticeable change in subject's usual condition
   b. Subject has had previous period of illness lasting at least two weeks, during which he or she met criteria, and residual signs of illness have remained (e.g., extreme social withdrawal, blunted or inappropriate affect, formal thought disorder, or unusual thoughts or perceptual experiences)
3. At no time during active period of illness being considered did subject meet criteria for probable or definite manic or depressive syndrome to the degree that it was a prominent part of illness

ST. LOUIS CRITERIA

1. Both necessary:
   a. Chronic illness with at least six months of symptoms before index evaluation without return to premorbid level of psychosocial adjustment
   b. Absence of period of depressive or manic symptoms sufficient to qualify for mood disorder or probable mood disorder
2. At least one of the following:
   a. Delusions or hallucinations without significant perplexity or disorientation
   b. Verbal production that makes communication difficult owing to lack of logical or understandable organization (in presence of muteness, diagnostic decision must be deferred)
3. At least three for definite, two for probable, illness:
   a. Never married
   b. Poor premorbid social adjustment or work history
   c. Family history of schizophrenia
   d. Absence of alcohol or other substance abuse within one year of onset
   e. Onset before age 40

TAYLOR AND ABRAMS CRITERIA

All criteria must be met for diagnosis:

1. Duration of episode greater than six months
2. Clear consciousness
3. Presence of delusions, hallucinations, or formal thought disorder (verbigeration, non sequiturs, word approximations, neologisms, blocking, and derailment)
4. Absence of broad affect
5. Absence of signs and symptoms sufficient to make diagnosis of mood disorder
6. No alcohol or other substance abuse within one year of index episode
7. Absence of focal signs and symptoms of coarse brain disease or major medical illness known to produce significant behavioral changes

PRESENT STATE EXAMINATION

The following 12 items from the Present State Examination correspond to a 12-point diagnostic system for schizophrenia, with varying levels of certainty of diagnosis based on the cut-off score determined by the examiner. Nine of the symptoms are scored 1 point each when present (+), and three are scored 1 point each when absent (−).

1. Restricted affect (+)
2. Poor insight (+)
3. Thoughts aloud (+)
4. Awaking early (−)
5. Poor rapport (+)
6. Depressed facies (−)
7. Elation (−)
8. Widespread delusions (+)
9. Incoherent speech (+)
10. Unreliable information (+)
11. Bizarre delusions (+)
12. Nihilistic delusions (+)

TSUANG AND WINOKUR CRITERIA

I. Hebephrenic (A through D must be present):
   A. Age of onset and sociofamilial data (one of the following):
      1. Age of onset before 25 years
      2. Unmarried or unemployed
      3. Family history of schizophrenia
   B. Disorganized thought
   C. Affect changes (either 1 or 2):
      1. Inappropriate affect
      2. Flat affect
   D. Behavioral symptoms (either 1 or 2):
      1. Bizarre behavior
      2. Motor symptoms (either a or b):
         a. Hebephrenic traits
         b. Catatonic traits (if present, subtype may be modified to hebephrenia with catatonic traits)

II. Paranoid (A through C must be present):
   A. Age of onset and sociofamilial data (one of the following):
      1. Age of onset after 25 years
      2. Married or employed
      3. Absence of family history of schizophrenia
   B. Exclusion criteria:
      1. Disorganized thoughts must be absent or of mild degree, such that speech is intelligible
      2. Affective and behavioral symptoms, as described in hebephrenia, must be absent or of mild degree
   C. Preoccupation with extensive, well-organized delusions or hallucinations

The criteria of Schneider and Langfeldt from World Psychiatric Association: *Diagnostic Criteria for Schizophrenic and Affective Psychoses.* American Psychiatric Press, Washington, 1983. Used with permission. The criteria of St. Louis, RDC, NHSI, Flexible, and Taylor and Abrams from J Endicott, J Nee, L Fleiss, J Cohen, J B W Williams, R Simon: Diagnostic criteria for schizophrenia. Arch Gen Psychiatry *39:* 884, 1982. Used with permission. The criteria for Tsuang and Winokur from M T Tsuang, G Winokur: Criteria for hebephrenic and paranoid schizophrenia. Arch Gen Psychiatry *31:* 43, 1974. Used with permission.

of early awakening, poor rapport, absence of depressed facies, absence of elation, widespread delusions (fixed, false beliefs), incoherent speech, unreliable information, bizarre delusions, and nihilistic delusions. The minimum number of discriminators (symptoms) required for a diagnosis of schizophrenia could be four to eight, depending on the investigator's choice and need for comprehensiveness and specificity.

The New Haven Schizophrenia Index, another diagnostic approach, used a symptom checklist heavily weighted in the areas of disturbed thought and cognition, delusions, and hallucinations. The Feighner (St. Louis) Criteria included longitudinal features, notably the requirement of a six-month period of continuous symptoms. The Research Diagnostic Criteria (RDC), continuing in the attempt to minimize the probability of false-positive diagnoses, established diagnoses with varying degrees of certainty, that is, definite, probable, or not present. An interview schedule, the Schedule for Affective Disorders and Schizophrenia (SADS), was developed to assist in the RDC diagnosis. Subsequently, other interview schedules were published, among them the Diagnostic Interview Schedule (DIS), the Structured Clinical Interview for DSM-III (SCID), and the Comprehensive Assessment of Symptoms and History (CASH).

DSM-III and the revised third edition of DSM (DSM-III-R) represented major efforts to increase reliability over prior nosological efforts. As investigators recognized that validity was not yet attainable, the goal of reliability became even more important. That consideration was reflected in the development of DSM-IV. DSM-IV requires the presence of at least two characteristic symptoms for a significant portion of time during a one-month period, or less if the patient was successfully treated. The list of characteristic symptoms includes delusions, hallucinations (sensory perceptions in the absence of corresponding stimuli), disorganized speech, grossly disorganized or catatonic behavior, and negative symptoms. One symptom is sufficient for diagnosis if that one symptom consists of bizarre delusions, or hallucinations of a voice sustaining a running commentary on the person's behavior or thoughts, or hallucinations of two or more voices conversing with each other.

DSM-IV also requires the presence of social and occupational dysfunction. From the beginning of the onset of illness, there must be a diminishment in the functional level present before the onset of illness. There should be continuous signs of functional disturbance for at least six months. That six-month period must include the one month of symptoms necessary to fulfill the requirement of characteristic symptoms, plus either prodromal or residual symptoms. Additionally, DSM-IV requires the exclusion of schizoaffective disorder and mood disorder with psychotic features. Finally, it requires that the schizophrenic illness not be a consequence of substance abuse or of a general medical condition. The DSM-IV diagnostic criteria for schizophrenia appear in Tables 14.7-2 and 14.7-3.

TABLE 14.7-2
Diagnostic Criteria for Schizophrenia

A. *Characteristic symptoms:* Two (or more) of the following, each present for a significant portion of time during a one-month period (or less if successfully treated):
(1) delusions
(2) hallucinations
(3) disorganized speech (e.g., frequent derailment or incoherence)
(4) grossly disorganized or catatonic behavior
(5) negative symptoms, i.e., affective flattening, alogia, or avolition

Note: Only one criterion A symptom is required if delusions are bizarre or hallucinations consist of a voice keeping up a running commentary on the person's behavior or thoughts, or two or more voices conversing with each other.

B. *Social/occupational dysfunction:* For a significant portion of the time since the onset of the disturbance, one or more major areas of functioning such as work, interpersonal relations, or self-care are markedly below the level achieved prior to the onset (or when the onset is in childhood or adolescence, failure to achieve expected level of interpersonal, academic, or occupational achievement).

C. *Duration:* Continuous signs of the disturbance persist for at least six months. This six-month period must include at least one month of symptoms (or less if successfully treated) that meet criterion A (i.e., active-phase symptoms) and may include periods of prodromal or residual symptoms. During these prodromal or residual periods, the signs of the disturbance may be manifested by only negative symptoms or two or more symptoms listed in criterion A present in an attenuated form (e.g., odd beliefs, unusual perceptual experiences).

D. *Schizoaffective and mood disorder exclusion:* Schizoaffective disorder and mood disorder with psychotic features have been ruled out because either (1) no major depressive, manic, or mixed episodes have occurred concurrently with the active-phase symptoms; or (2) if mood episodes have occurred during active-phase symptoms, their total duration has been brief relative to the duration of the active and residual periods.

E. *Substance/general medical condition exclusion:* The disturbance is not due to the direct physiological effects of a substance (e.g., a drug of abuse, a medication) or a general medical condition.

F. *Relationship to a pervasive developmental disorder:* If there is a history of autistic disorder or another pervasive developmental disorder, the additional diagnosis of schizophrenia is made only if prominent delusions or hallucinations are also present for at least a month (or less if successfully treated).

Classification of longitudinal course (can be applied only after at least one year has elapsed since the initial onset of active-phase symptoms):

Episodic with interepisode residual symptoms (episodes are defined by the reemergence of prominent psychotic symptoms); *also specify if:* **with prominent negative symptoms**
Episodic with no interepisode residual symptoms
Continuous (prominent psychotic symptoms are present throughout the period of observation); *also specify if:* **with prominent negative symptoms**
Single episode in partial remission; *also specify if:* **with prominent negative symptoms**
Single episode in full remission
Other or unspecified pattern

Table from DSM-IV, *Diagnostic and Statistical Manual of Mental Disorders,* ed 4. Copyright American Psychiatric Association, Washington, 1994. Used with permission.

NATURAL HISTORY

It is difficult to speak of the natural history of a heterogeneous group of disorders that differ in etiology, onset, pathogenesis, course, and outcome. Nevertheless, it is possible to speak of the more common clinical patterns, even though they do not attain the frequency necessary to become pathognomonic patterns.

MODE OF ONSET Schizophrenia usually first becomes manifest during adolescence or early adulthood. Most often a psychotic episode is preceded by a period of subtle but progressive behavioral symptoms, although a florid psychotic state can appear suddenly in a person who has shown no discernible prior alteration in personal and social adjustment. The behavioral symptoms, when examined retrospectively, usually reveal diminutions in effective adaptations in almost all functional areas—personal, social, and school or work functioning. In other cases retrospective evaluation often reveals a person who was seemingly different from birth—physically awkward, emotionally restricted, and not in tune with the mother, with those differences setting in motion a parent-child interaction fraught with the possibility of unhappiness and eventually illness. Although such descriptions lack precision, they appear often enough in clinical experience to warrant inclusion. Further, they emphasize the need for rigorous phenomenological descriptions.

The person with schizophrenia often evinces steady patterns of withdrawal, moodiness, and a disinclination to relate emo-

TABLE 14.7-3
Diagnostic Criteria for Course Specifiers for Schizophrenia

The following specifiers may be used to indicate the characteristic course of symptoms of schizophrenia over time. These specifiers can be applied only after at least one year has elapsed since the initial onset of active-phase symptoms. During this initial one-year period, no course specifiers can be given.

Episodic with interepisode residual symptoms. This specifier applies when the course is characterized by episodes in which criterion A for schizophrenia is met and there are clinically significant residual symptoms between the episodes. **With prominent negative symptoms** can be added if prominent negative symptoms are present during these residual periods.

Episodic with no interepisode residual symptoms. This specifier applies when the course is characterized by episodes in which criterion A for schizophrenia is met and there are no clinically significant residual symptoms between the episodes.

Continuous. This specifier applies when characteristic symptoms of criterion A are met throughout all (or most) of the course. **With prominent negative symptoms** can be added if prominent negative symptoms are also present.

Single episode in partial remission. This specifier applies when there has been a single episode in which criterion A for schizophrenia is met and some clinically significant residual symptoms remain. **With prominent negative symptoms** can be added if these residual symptoms include prominent negative symptoms.

Single episode in full remission. This specifier applies when there has been a single episode in which criterion A for schizophrenia has been met and no clinically significant residual symptoms remain.

Other or unspecified pattern. This specifier is used if another or an unspecified course pattern has been present.

Table from DSM-IV, *Diagnostic and Statistical Manual of Mental Disorders,* ed 4. Copyright American Psychiatric Association, Washington, 1994. Used with permission.

tionally to family members during adolescence and early adulthood. Personal grooming may deteriorate or, conversely, may become an overriding preoccupation. Health concerns are often expressed that range from unusual dietary restrictions to the conviction that a disease exists despite the absence of any medical findings. Friends may be ignored or rejected, and school and work performance flags. Parents, friends, and teachers frequently view those changes as part of normal adolescence and expect them to dissipate as the young person matures.

The person undergoing such behavioral changes often feels perplexed, unfocused, and increasingly strange. Feelings, values, and perceptions previously taken for granted now appear dissociated from each other, requiring verification and confirmation of their validity. Bodily sensations may assume unfamiliar and frightening qualities, and the entire body itself, its boundaries and position in space, may seem distorted and unstable. Such phenomena are generally subsumed under the concepts of self, ego boundaries, and identity. They include proprioceptive organization as well as the complex demarcations and recognition of the relation between the body and the world.

The person responds to those disrupting experiences with nascent or established patterns of psychological adaptation ranging from attempts at denial, compartmentalized control, and symbolic altered expression to an almost unlimited range of desperate rational explanations that ultimately become blatantly implausible or frankly bizarre. Those responses, however, do not provide the restitutive balance necessary to integrate the person's emotional and ideational behavior. Concomitant with those ideational constructs are emotional responses that combine, in various degrees, fearfulness, perplexity, and progressive demoralization.

The prodromal period may continue for weeks to years before the psychotic symptoms sufficient for diagnosis appear. Recent studies have more clearly exposed the long duration of behavioral manifestations, which may precede by years the onset of psychosis. In contrast, the premorbid period of behavioral symptoms may be very short and may precede a psychotic state by only a short interval.

Those affected persons who appear different early in childhood characteristically are excessively shy, introverted, difficult to relate to, emotionally restricted, and bland. They may exhibit motor awkwardness and an uneven developmental progression that sometimes combines cognitive precocity in some areas with inexplicable deficiencies in other, seemingly less complex areas. They seldom develop close friendships, become more intensely isolated with time, and, although unusually vulnerable to stress, are generally described as good children, obedient and nonconfrontational. The progression from that pattern to obvious psychosis occurs almost imperceptibly. Although seldom attributable to an obvious precipitating event, the first episode of psychosis often occurs in association with situational or environmental changes (for example, leaving home for school).

CHARACTERISTIC SYMPTOMS Bleuler's definition, "the disease is characterized by a specific alteration of thinking, feeling and relation to the external world which appears nowhere else in this particular fashion," established a precedent for the diagnosis of schizophrenia based on his designated altered fundamental symptoms. Bleuler required that those symptoms occur in the absence of primary disturbances of perception, orientation, or memory. He described delusions and hallucinations as accessory symptoms, insufficient and unnecessary for establishing the diagnosis. Bleuler's subdivisions—simple, hebephrenic, catatonic, and paranoid—reflected a gradation of the preponderance of the fundamental symptoms, from their exclusive presence in simple schizophrenia to their lesser presence in paranoid schizophrenia, where delusions and hallucinations dominated the clinical picture.

The designation of altered fundamental symptoms established for the first time apparently precise criteria for the diagnosis of schizophrenia, criteria that were interpreted by clinicians as pathognomonic. Thus, the clinical findings of restricted, blunted, or inappropriate affect; or of impoverished, illogical, tangential, or blocked thought processes; or of ambivalence; or of the pathological predominance of fantasy over reality (autism) were sufficient to make the diagnosis.

In the current era of ongoing modifications and combinations of criteria for the diagnosis of schizophrenia, and because of the unlikelihood of identifying pathognomonic symptoms, the altered fundamental symptoms retain considerable clinical significance in both the diagnosis and prognosis of schizophrenia. Those symptoms are now generally subsumed under the group of negative or deficit symptoms—apathy, avolition, alogia, and affective flattening.

Certain delusions and hallucinations, in contrast to their secondary designation by Kraepelin, Bleuler, and Sigmund Freud, were assigned pathognomonic significance by Schneider. He assigned first-rank significance to such positive symptoms as audible thoughts, voices arguing or discussing, commenting voices, experiences of somatic passivity, thought withdrawal, thought insertion, and thought broadcasting. Other diagnostic systems use combinations of those criteria in their respective classifications. The question of pathognomonic symptoms remains uncertain, although DSM-IV permits the diagnosis when only one characteristic symptom is sufficiently typical.

A psychotic episode is often heralded by an increasing dissonance between the person and the social environment. Usually precipitated by a succession of behaviors seen as intolerable by the family or social environment, the ensuing conflict frequently evokes responses from the affected person that are interpreted as dangerous either to the person or to others. It is common for some form of coercion, ranging from intense persuasion to involuntary legal action, to be exerted to bring the person to medical attention.

The presenting clinical picture is significantly influenced by concomitant substance abuse, identified in about 50 percent of patients with schizophrenia admitted to urban hospitals. Stimulants, in particular, tend to amplify the quality of delusions and hallucinations and intensity of the underlying emotional state. Patients may have to be observed for days to weeks in a controlled setting before symptoms can be attributed to substance abuse or to an underlying schizophrenic process.

Clinicians' awareness of confounding issues and their sensitivity to the uniquely estranged state of the patient experiencing a psychotic episode will usually determine the quality of the information obtained during a clinical examination. The task of evoking trust from an individual who sees the world in a distorted fashion and whose emotional responsivity is asynchronous with that of the examiner is daunting. Time is necessary to achieve trust. Sensitive clinicians avoid intrusiveness and remain aware of their personal reactions to communicating with a person with schizophrenia.

MENTAL STATUS

GENERAL APPEARANCE AND BEHAVIOR Persons with schizophrenia often seem uniquely odd. Their general appearance and behavior reflect varying aspects of an apparent defective integration of those qualities that make a person whole. They are characteristically not well put together. Clothing combinations, for example, while not necessarily disheveled, may be incongruous and untasteful. Attitude may vary from general perplexity to oppositional hostility or a seemingly naive sense of confusion. An intense and strongly pointed statement may be unexpectedly followed by a different emotional tone. Frequently, an emptiness is sensed in patients, who demonstrate an emotional moat that seems impossible to cross. Dealing with such patients may cause the examiner to feel unconnected to the patient, the so-called precox feeling. Although such descriptions are anathema to nosologists, who emphasize low-inference data, those qualities have nonetheless been described by clinicians for almost a century and deserve consideration.

Deteriorated appearance and manners The personal appearance of a patient with chronic schizophrenia tends to deteriorate. Efforts at grooming and self-care may become minimal, and patients may have to be reminded to wash, bathe, shave, and change their clothes; in general, they show poor regard for the social amenities. They may fail to return a greeting or a smile or carry on their part in a conversation and may exhibit idiosyncratic table manners or offensive behavior.

Social withdrawal and relationship to examiner Social withdrawal is a common symptom in schizophrenia. The examiner feels unable to establish rapport with the patient, as do others in the patient's life. This symptom often prevents others from feeling empathy or sympathy toward the patient, thereby further isolating the patient. Health care providers, family, and friends should be educated about the symptom and encouraged consciously to try to overcome the tendency not to feel warmth toward schizophrenic persons. Conversely, some patients with schizophrenia are bizarrely intrusive, demonstrating no appreciation for the usual social and interpersonal boundaries and conventions.

Lack of motivation Lack of motivation may first be evident to a clinician when the patient seems not to care about talking to the doctor or about his or her illness or situation. Further questioning of patient, friends, and family may disclose a pervasive lack of planning and volition. The patient may have stopped working at a job, completing schoolwork, or doing household chores. The patient may show complete disinterest in planning what to do during the coming day, let alone the next week or year.

DISORDERS OF THOUGHT AND SPEECH Formal disorders of speech and the inferred underlying disorders of thought processes are manifested by a variety of pathological features. Most important, the integrity of the thought process becomes distorted and continuity is disrupted. The associations are logically unrelated to antecedents (loosening of associations). Separate ideas can be incomprehensibly combined, apparently based on sound rather than on meaning (clang association). New words may be formed (neologisms). Words or statements may be stereotypically repeated (verbigeration), or the examiner's words may be repeated (echolalia). The patient may experience sudden and inexplicable blocking of thoughts and may be unable to pursue the original train of thought. Other clinical examples of disordered speech associated with schizophrenia are perseveration, tangential thinking, circumstantiality, and stilted language.

Loosening of associations Loosening of associations, a classic Bleulerian concept, was derived from late 19th-century association theory. The patient's associations appear to lose their continuity, suggesting that thought itself has become illogical, even bizarre. Loosening of associations extends symptomatically from mild slippage or derailment of thought sequence to utter incoherence and word salad. In Bleuler's work the most important determination of associations is purpose; schizophrenic speech reveals an absence of the concept of purpose. A sentence completion test illustrates the point. The sentence to be completed was, "The man fell on the street. . . ." The patient's response was "because of World War I." Although the thought of falling might be associated with falling in combat, it was an inappropriate association for the stimulus.

It can be helpful to look at disorders of association as disorders of the word and disorders of the sentence. Disorders of the word range from loss of symbolic meaning of a word (as in clang associations), to inability to maintain the correct semantic context for a word, to approximate use of words, to the creation of new words. Disorders of the sentence include associative failures and failures of system placement. Most language has multiple meanings. Even a simple question such as "Where is your husband?" must be answered in terms of the frame of reference. In one context the question might ask for the physical location of the husband, and in another context it might ask for his identification in his graduating class picture. An example of system shifting was reported by Silvano Arieti in 1955. Commenting on the Japanese attack on Pearl Harbor, a patient said, "The next time they may attack at Diamond Harbor or Emerald Harbor." The patient had lost the contextual system of Pearl Harbor as a geographical place and had substituted the contextual system in which pearls are precious stones.

Incomprehensibility Schizophrenic patients do not seem to be aware that their verbal communication is abnormal even when it reaches the point of incomprehensibility.

The following proclamation was written by a schizophrenic woman. The phrases are repetitive, and the syntax is distorted, which, together with numerous non sequiturs, renders the text sometimes incoherent.

> The French Force orders from now on to the German Force to respect the Queen Sacre in Christianity as well as the Queens in France & in other countries, ill treated and destroyed in all countries since the beginning of this century in Europe and allied countries. The Queens are the co-partners in masonry of the order of Grand Masters and by doing so the prosperity and balance of the world have been destroyed, they have been destroyed for homosexuality which is the emblem of grand mystery really instead of being distinguished from the criminals who kill the soul and commit the crime of homosexuality of destroying

the emblem of grand mastery. The attack on the Queen Sacre in Masonry comes from an inversion in data in the German spying service in 1903 in the class of sorcerers of this organization, deciding that the Chateau de Chambord en France was going to be the Castle not of the saint to be, but of the sorceress and killing in soul that child many times without the effect desired obtained.

The following is a patient's short apologetic note to a psychiatrist whom she had bluntly propositioned on frequent occasions. It expresses her sexually laden message briefly and, in her way, to the point. She had previously inserted a screwdriver into her vagina and later expressed continuing guilt feelings for having done so.

Dear . . .
I wasn't thinking too well when I was speaking to you but I do believe you were the postman whom I spent the night with. It is still Dr. David . . . in my heart. Am sick because of the screw driver. Please no hard feelings. Kiss your penis did. I would not harm you. . . .
Sincere regards,

The following brief transcript from a videotaped interview with a young man with schizophrenia illustrates his autistic preoccupation with sex and death; there seems to be some clang association between "feet" and "foetus." The patient was puzzled that his interviewer had difficulties following him.

the fleur de Lys is a castrated ace—you see, the design is the feet—the same as a woman's foetus—now you take five French safes and you put them together between four coffins—that's what it represents. . . .

Thought blocking When a patient's thoughts seem to stop suddenly and without warning, the phenomenon is referred to as *thought blocking*. The patient may cease speaking in the middle of a sentence and may remain silent for seconds or minutes. When questioned about the experience, patients sometimes report the physical sensation of having had their thoughts taken out of their heads.

Poverty of content The examiner may feel that he or she has received no information from the patient, despite having listened intently to the patient for several minutes. That is referred to as *poverty of content*. Conversely, some clinicians claim to be able to understand virtually every verbal production of their patients with schizophrenia.

Ability to utilize abstract concepts An impairment in the ability of patients with schizophrenia to utilize abstract concepts has often been emphasized. The interpretation of proverbs is traditionally used to test that ability. A patient with schizophrenia may interpret "A stitch in time saves nine" as meaning, "I should sew nine buttons on my coat," both personalizing the proverb and missing the abstract concept about procrastination. The clinician should be cautioned that proverb interpretation is not a particularly reliable test in uncontrolled clinical settings and that many other factors (for example, motivation, intelligence, culture) can affect the patient's responses. Moreover, an inability to conceptualize abstract concepts is not pathognomonic for schizophrenia.

Prosody In addition to disorders of form and process, the accessory behaviors and intonations of speech may be abnormal. The patient may lack the usual expressive gestures, such as hand waving and head movements. Even more obvious, the patient may demonstrate both productive and receptive aprosodia, that is, an inability to understand or to create the usual emotional inflections of speech. The patient's speech may have an abnormal modulation of emphasis and volume, producing speech that is too loud, too soft, or unusually accented.

Mutism Mutism, an inhibition of speech and vocalization, may last for hours or days, but before the days of modern treatment methods, it often lasted for years in patients with chronic schizophrenia of the catatonic type. Many patients with schizophrenia tend to be monosyllabic and to answer questions as briefly as possible. They may attempt to restrict contact with the interviewer as much as possible without being altogether uncooperative.

Neologisms A woman with schizophrenia who had been hospitalized for several years kept repeating, in an otherwise quite rational conversation, the word "polamolalittersjittersstittersleelitla." She explained that "polamolalitters" was intended to recall the disease poliomyelitis, because the patient wanted to indicate that she felt she was suffering from a serious disease affecting her nervous system; the component "litters" stood for untidiness or messiness, the way she felt inside; "jitterstitters" reflected her inner nervousness and uneasiness; "leelitla" was a reference to the French *le lit là* (that bed there), meaning that she was both dependent on and feeling handicapped by her illness.

Stilted language The following excerpt from a letter written by a physician with schizophrenia who had been hospitalized for more than 15 years but is now living alone in an apartment is an example of stilted language.

My dear friend and Professor: A hearty and cheerful. (Please turn page over) and a real magnanimous good-morning to you on this first Wednesday of our glorious New Year: And I do hope that our great and our good Lord, and our dearly beloved and kind Shepherd. (Kindly read page three, now). Will be gracious unto both me and thee. I am sure that He will be gracious unto both of us; if He has some sound common sense in His Being, this morning . . . I have not yet heard (Kindly turn over to p4 now) from any one of my own colleagues when I am leaving this noble institution of the healing arts; Nor with whom: Nor through which of the portals. Though I am sure that you—as much as any (Kindly turn to page five, now) one else—must be able to enlighten me; very soon, my good old friend. . . .

Echolalia A patient demonstrates echolalia when he or she repeats exactly the words of another person. Examiner: "I heard that you played well in the softball game." Patient: "I heard that you played well in the softball game."

Loss of ego boundaries This phrase describes a patient's lack of a clear sense of where his or her own body, mind, and influence end and where those aspects of other animate and inanimate objects begin. For example, the patient may have *ideas of reference*—that other people, the television, or the newspapers are talking about him or her. Other symptoms include the sense of having fused with outside objects (for example, a tree, another person) or of having disintegrated completely. Depersonalization and derealization can be conceptualized as stemming from a loss of clear ego boundaries. Given that state of mind, it is not surprising that patients with schizophrenia may have doubts as to which sex they are or what their sexual orientation is. Those symptoms should not be confused with transvestism, transsexuality, or homosexuality.

DISORDERS OF AFFECT The difficulties in evaluating the characteristic disturbances of affect in schizophrenia are often compounded by cultural differences. Ethnic diversities, even within one nationality, are often accompanied by different styles and standards of emotional expression. Sensitivity to those variations is required of the clinician, just as awareness of culturally sanctioned unusual beliefs and perceptions is vital in distinguishing such experiences from delusions.

Schizophrenic disorders of emotional state are often difficult to evaluate precisely because of overlapping characteristics with the affective displays in mood disorders. Classically, however, a flat or blunted affect in the absence of major depressive disorder is common. Affect that is inappropriate to or incongruent with the associated content of speech can often be identified clinically even when mild in extent. Disparities between emotion and ideational content range from subtle incongruities to blatant inappropriateness. The cadence and modulation of communication is similarly distorted, resulting in varieties of aprosodia.

The more dramatic emotional displays, such as exaltation, expansiveness, and oceanic feelings, may be more common in mania but are seen in schizophrenia as well.

Reduced emotional responses Many patients with schizophrenia seem to be indifferent (or, at times, totally apathetic). Others with less marked emotional restriction, or *blunting,* show emotional shallowness. Inexperienced observers, however, should be extremely careful in assessing emotional depth. For example, what is normal emotional expression in Anglo-Saxon culture may suggest a flattened emotional response in a person from a Mediterranean culture. Evaluating the degree of normal emotional responses can be difficult in urban emergency rooms that serve a large variety of cultural groups. *Anhedonia* is an extreme form of reduced emotions in which the patient is incapable of experiencing, or even imagining, any pleasure; the result is a sense of profound emotional barrenness. Patients themselves often offer valuable and valid information about their own gradually increasing inability to experience emotions.

Inappropriate responses Many times the emotional reaction of a person with schizophrenia is incongruous or inappropriate to the ideational content or situation. A patient may talk about a morbid subject with a smile or answer a straightforward question with anger. In some patients with schizophrenia, disorganized type, a profound silliness can color all interpersonal interactions. Again, it should be remembered that the patient's outward affect may not represent his or her internal emotional tone.

Bizarre emotions Schizophrenia not only alters emotional reactions; it may induce strange emotions that are rarely experienced by normal persons. A patient may feel, for example, states of exaltation, feelings of omnipotence, oneness with the universe, religious ecstasies, terrifying apprehensions about the disintegration of personality or body, or anxiety about impending destruction of the universe.

Emotional sensitivity Many clinicians have described a particular sensitivity to emotional trauma in patients with schizophrenia. It has been clinically noted that schizophrenic patients are very easily hurt by even slightly aggressive or rejecting behavior by others, behavior that in most cases would not be noticed by a person of normal emotional sensitivity. That observation is particularly germane to less experienced clinicians, who, feeling frustrated in their therapeutic efforts to treat a patient with schizophrenia, may say or do something that is unconsciously aggressive. Such behavior on the part of a therapist can provoke an exacerbation of psychotic symptoms. Emotional sensitivity also needs to be considered when the person with schizophrenia is at home with his or her family or in the workplace.

DISORDERS OF AMBIVALENCE Bleuler's definition, ". . . the tendency of the schizophrenic psyche to endow the most diverse psychisms with both a positive and a negative indicator at one and the same time . . . ," included three types of ambivalence: ambivalence of affect, ambivalence of will, and ambivalence of intellect. Experienced clinicians emphasize the significance of ambivalence in schizophrenia while acknowledging the imprecision of its definition. The yes-no and seemingly simultaneous contradictions of feelings, thoughts, and actions are possibly qualitatively, but usually quantitatively, distinct from the mixed feelings and broodings of the obsessive. Translated into behavior, schizophrenic ambivalence is the hallmark of the catatonic subtype.

DISORDERS OF BEHAVIOR Bizarre behavior associated with schizophrenia includes mannerisms, echopraxia (repeating or mirroring another's actions), stereotyped behavior (repeating the same actions for short or extended periods of time), negativism, automatic obedience, waxy or rigid catalepsy, and posturing. Most of those symptoms can be grouped under catatonic excitement or stupor.

Stereotyped behavior Stereotyped behavior is more often seen in chronic patients with schizophrenia than in acutely ill ones. It may present as repetitive patterns of moving or walking (for example, walking the same circle every day), repetitive performance of strange gestures, or endless repetitions of the same phrase or question. For more than five years, a 36-year-old man with schizophrenia greeted his doctor, whenever they met, with the question, "Is it going to rain?" (in the summer) or "Is it going to snow?" (in the winter). It may be difficult to distinguish stereotyped behavior from obsessive-compulsive symptoms that also occur in schizophrenia. Both types of symptoms are thought to carry a poor prognosis.

Stuporous states Until the mid-1930s, mental hospitals were filled with stuporous catatonic patients, many of whom would lie motionless for weeks or months, unresponsive to almost every stimulus. They had to be fed by gavage twice a day and catheterized regularly. For some unknown reason, stuporous states are quite rare now. Such stuporous patients were also known to erupt with episodes of excited catatonia. Also rare today is *waxy flexibility* (catalepsy), which was present in many patients 50 years ago. It consisted of waxlike yielding of the limbs and trunk, such that a patient put into even an awkward and apparently uncomfortable position would remain so for very long periods of time.

Eating disorders Eating disorders (which meet some, but usually not all, of the criteria for anorexia nervosa, bulimia nervosa, or pica) are not rare in schizophrenia. Obesity, a common clinical problem, especially in female patients, is exacerbated by many psychotropic medications. Approximately one half of schizophrenia-related eating disorders are in response to psychotic experiences—for example, the belief that the food is poisoned.

Self-induced water intoxication It is sometimes noted on routine laboratory tests that a patient has a low urine specific gravity and a low serum sodium concentration. It may retrospectively be noted that the patient seems always to be at the water fountain. The syndrome of self-induced water intoxication should be considered in the differential diagnosis of seizures in schizophrenic patients, and the workup for increased water intake should include tests for inappropriate secretion of antidiuretic hormone, which is sometimes caused by treatment with antipsychotics, carbamazepine (Tegretol), lithium (Eskalith), or other drugs.

Echopraxia Echopraxia, the motor analog of echolalia, consists of the imitation of the movements and gestures of the person the patient with schizophrenia is observing.

Negativism A patient's refusal to cooperate with even the most simple and reasonable requests constitutes negativism. Sometimes the patient may even do the opposite of what is asked.

Somatic symptoms Plausible and relatively mild somatic complaints are quite common during the prodromal phase of schizophrenia, and more extreme and even bizarre somatic concerns occur during later phases of the illness. However, the profoundly uncommunicative nature of some patients may cause them not to complain about potentially serious medical symptoms. For example, severely regressed patients with schizophrenia may suffer silently form abdominal pain that, without adequate medical care, can result in a ruptured appendix; a woman with schizophrenia may not report symptoms of pregnancy.

DISORDERS OF PERCEPTION Delusions, hallucinations, and illusions (false interpretations of actual sensory stimuli), despite their accessory significance to Bleuler, have assumed increasing importance in contemporary diagnostic schemata. Auditory hallucinations, the most common clinically observed hallucinations in schizophrenia, are subdivided according to duration, intensity, and content. Delusions are characterized according to standards of content and bizarreness.

Hallucinations Hallucinations may occur in any sensory modality—auditory, visual, tactile, olfactory, and gustatory. Cenesthesic hallucinations—sensations of altered body states—are not uncommon and are often difficult to differentiate from somatic delusions. Diagnostically significant auditory hallucinations include a voice keeping up a running commentary on the patient's behavior or thoughts, or two or more voices conversing with each other. Although every form of hallucination has been reported in schizophrenia, clinical experience emphasizes the need for an intense differential diagnosis, especially the exclusion of brain toxicity or pathology, when hallucinations other than auditory dominate the clinical picture.

Patients may be reluctant to discuss their hallucinations; therefore, clinicians need to take a particularly nonthreatening and nonjudgmental approach in order to elicit the information. Sometimes the voices are those of God or the devil; sometimes they are voices of deceased relatives, neighbors, or unrecognized individuals. Two or more voices may discuss the patient in the third person; voices may make threatening or obscene comments about the patient. Patients can often be observed talking aloud to their hallucinated voices, as if in conversation. The hallucinations may also be merely of identifiable or unidentifiable sounds.

Illusions may also occur in schizophrenia, but the clinical differentiation between hallucinations and illusions may be quite difficult when discussing a particular sensory experience of an individual patient.

Unusual perceptual sensations Patients with schizophrenia may experience a haunting unfamiliarity with their normal environment, sometimes causing them to feel a sensory jolt, or a remoteness and lack of contact with the world through the usual five senses.

Delusions Delusions are generally of the referential, persecutory, or grandiose type. Especially characteristic are delusions dominated by themes of outside control—outside forces controlling the patient's thoughts, feelings, or behavior, either influencing the content of these experiences or withdrawing or broadcasting one's thoughts. Common paranoid delusions of patients are that they are being spied upon, talked about, or at risk of being harmed. The experiences of thought broadcasting, thought insertion, thought withdrawal, and thought control (for example, "by X-rays") are common in schizophrenia and can be variously conceptualized as delusions, disorders of perception, or the result of a loss of ego boundaries. Frequently, in patients with schizophrenia delusions of imminent doom take the form of a delusional scientific or political insight that the patient believes can prevent or counteract the threat. The patient may be driven by an urgent need to get that important message to scientific or government authorities, who should then be able to put it into action for the protection of humankind. Such patients often use excessive scientific jargon, and the schemes may seem almost rational at first glance.

A common characteristic of schizophrenic delusions is the direct, immediate, and total certainty with which the patient holds these beliefs. If asked why he or she believes such an unlikely idea, a schizophrenic patient will often simply say, "I know it." Although delusions can occur in any psychotic illness, the clinical impression is that schizophrenic delusions are consistently more bizarre.

Increasing evidence points to more subtle distortions of perception in schizophrenia—unusual responses to stimuli, for example, short of illusions or hallucinations. It may be that the content of some delusions is initiated by unusual perceptions rather than by purely inner conflicts.

SENSORIUM Schizophrenia is characterized by a clear consciousness on traditional clinical examination. Although ordinary clinical appraisals of orientation for time, place, and person, in the absence of delusional contamination, usually do not reveal abnormalities, increasing evidence of cognitive brain dysfunction requires a more complete clinical examination than has heretofore been customary. The examination should include an assessment of attention, language, memory, constructions, and executive functions. That assessment and the variations in findings over time can contribute significantly to the clinician's appraisal of the patient's adaptive capacities in addition to the status of the psychotic symptoms.

NEUROLOGICAL AND PSYCHOLOGICAL TESTING

Although normal findings on neurological examination and the absence of sensorial and cognitive abnormalities were, until recently, part of the clinical description of schizophrenia, consistent findings now point to both neurological and psychological abnormalities in a significant portion of patients with schizophrenia.

NEUROLOGICAL TESTING Neurological dysfunction is identified in over 50 percent of patients with schizophrenia when the examination includes extensive testing of brain function. Although uncertainty persists over the precision of the diagnosis in a number of cases, and although neurological findings are observed in other psychiatric disorders, the findings in schizophrenia appear presumptively strong. Attempts to localize the neurological dysfunction to frontal, parietal, or cerebel-

TABLE 14.7-4
Soft Signs and Frontal Items

Dominance: L = 1, R = 2	Comb ______ Write ______ Throw ______ Brush ______ Hole ______ Telescope ______ Step on roach ______
R-L discrimination: 0 = Correct 1 = Incorrect	Right hand ______ Left hand ______ Right hand to right ear ______ Left hand to left ear ______ Right hand to left ear ______ Left hand to right ear ______ Identify right and left on examiner ______
Hopping: 0 = Normal 1 = Abnormal	Right ______ Left ______
Standing balance: ______ 0 = Normal 1 = Abnormal	Walking: ______ 0 = Normal 1 = Abnormal Romberg's: ______ 0 = Normal 1 = Abnormal
Tandem gait: ______ 0 = Normal 1 = Abnormal	
Finger-thumb opposition: 0 = Normal 1 = Suggestive 2 = Yes	One hand right ______ One hand left ______ Overflow right ______ Overflow left ______ Two hands right ______ Two hands left ______
Extinction: 0 = Correct 1 = Extinguishes left 2 = Extinguishes right 3 = Irrelevant answer	RF–LH ______ LF–RH ______ F–F ______ H–H ______
Graphesthesia: 0 = Correct 1 = Incorrect	3 Right ______ 8 Left ______ 1 Right ______ 7 Left ______ 8 Right ______ 1 Left ______ 7 Right ______ 3 Left ______
Astereognosis: 0 = Correct 1 = Incorrect	Key right ______ Quarter left ______ Penny right ______ Comb left ______ Key left ______ Quarter right ______ Penny left ______ Comb right ______
Face-hand test:	Right face-right hand ______ Left face-left hand ______
Fist-ring: 0 = Normal 1 = Suggestive 2 = Abnormal	Left arm imitate ______ Left continue ______ Right arm imitate ______ Right arm continue ______
Fist-edge-palm: 0 = Normal 1 = Suggestive 2 = Abnormal	Left arm imitate ______ Left continue ______ Right arm imitate ______ Right arm continue ______
Fist stretch: 0 = Normal 1 = Suggestive 2 = Abnormal	Left arm imitate ______ Left continue ______ Right arm imitate ______ Right arm continue ______

lar areas are inconclusive, and the precise clinical relevance of those soft signs is unclear. The suggestive relation between frontal lobe abnormalities and negative symptoms is receiving much attention from the field, as are the different responses of patients with such deficits to antipsychotic treatment. Table 14.7-4 presents a scale used to evaluate neurological abnormalities.

Neurological history A critical part of a neurological examination is a complete history. Questions should be asked regarding perinatal events, including prematurity, complicated labor, infections, seizures, and Apgar scores. The patient's childhood developmental milestones should be ascertained, and school and work performance should be evaluated. Any history of head trauma, central nervous system (CNS) infections, and drug abuse should be carefully noted. Information should be obtained regarding family history of epilepsy, dementia, other neurological diseases and of psychiatric, immune, and endocrine disorders.

Motor system One of the earliest signs of incipient schizophrenia can be a loss of the natural gracefulness of body movements. Choreoathetoid movements of the extremities and involuntary movements of the orobuccal area can be symptoms of tardive dyskinesia, but similar abnormal movements were reported in patients with schizophrenia before the advent of antipsychotic drugs. An estimated 10 to 25 percent of patients with schizophrenia have abnormal movements that are not related to antipsychotic drug treatment. Somewhat less obvious motor abnormalities seen in schizophrenia include abnormal gait, stereotypies, mannerisms, grimacing, abnormal motor tone (increased or decreased), impaired fine motor skills, and abnormal reflexes (glabellar, grasp, palmomental, pollicomental, decreased gag reflex, and abnormal vestibular reflexes). Patients may also exhibit an apraxia, that is, difficulty in carrying out a purposeful, organized, somewhat complex task, such as drawing a picture, dressing, or following a command to strike and blow out a match.

Abnormal eye signs There are two major ocular abnormalities in schizophrenia: unusually frequent blinking and abnormal rapid eye movements. The rate of blinking, thought to reflect dopaminergic CNS activity, decreases with antipsychotic medication and the remission of psychotic symptoms. Abnormal rapid eye movements (saccades) during attempts to follow a moving object smoothly are seen in approximately 50 to 80 percent of patients. Saccades are seen on smooth pursuit in only 8 percent of normals but in approximately 40 percent of first-degree relatives of schizophrenic patients, including children of parents with schizophrenia. Abnormal smooth pursuit may be a neurophysiological marker for some aspect of the pathophysiology of schizophrenia. Abnormal saccades are also seen in some patients with mood disorders, in patients with cerebellar lesions, and in some drug-induced states. It has been hypothesized that the site of pathology may be the frontal lobe input to the basal ganglia and superior colliculus.

Nonlocalizing neurological signs Nonlocalizing neurological signs, sometimes referred to as soft neurological signs, are seen in patients with schizophrenia more frequently than in normals and about equally commonly in patients with schizophrenia and organic mental syndrome. Those signs include dysdiadochokinesia, astereognosis, poor right-left discrimination, and extinction on the face-hand test. Although those signs are nonlocalizing, they are consistent with brain injury to the frontal or parietal lobes.

Speech disorders Some investigators who approach schizophrenia as a neurological disorder consider a disorder of thought to be a forme fruste of aphasia, perhaps implicating the dominant parietal lobe. Schizophrenic patients' inability to perceive the prosody of speech or to inflect their own speech (for example, aprosodia) can be conceptualized as a neurological symptom of the nondominant parietal lobe. Other symptoms in schizophrenia that implicate the parietal lobes include the apraxias, right-left disorientation, and lack of concern about the illness (anosognosia).

Autonomic abnormalities During an acute schizophrenic episode, a patient often presents with dilated pupils, moist palms, moderate tachycardia, and a systolic blood pressure 10 to 20 mm Hg above the norm. Those signs of sympathetic excitation may be present even if the patient shows no outward signs of emotional excitation, and initially they may point toward an erroneous diagnosis of sympathomimetic drug ingestion.

PSYCHOLOGICAL TESTING Traditional psychological testing of the projective type, such as the Thematic Apperception Test (TAT) and the Rorschach test, remains useful in explicating psychodynamic aspects of a person's life but are of little value in diagnosing schizophrenia in the absence of clinical findings. The same is true of other questionnaire tests, such as the Minnesota Multiphasic Personality Inventory (MMPI), where categorical standards were established based on criteria that have since been critically modified.

Neuropsychological testing, on the other hand, which may identify process rather than content abnormalities, reveals deficit patterns in chronic schizophrenia similar to those found in brain-damaged patients. In general, such findings are grouped under the headings of attention, memory, executive functions, language, and motor functions.

Attentional deficits, especially those of selective attention, have been found especially in the nonparanoid group. Those deficits are consistent with frontal lobe dysfunction and are not related to chronicity.

Consistent deficits have been reported in working memory unrelated to attention, motivation, or cooperativeness. Recent studies indicate comparable impairment of working memory in first-episode and chronic schizophrenia.

The planning, sequencing, concept formation, cognitive set shifting, and maintenance of responses to environmental cues have been found to be impaired in groups of patients with schizophrenia. Although such findings again suggest frontal lobe dysfunction, further investigations are needed to confirm the results.

Although no compelling evidence exists of basic language deficits in schizophrenia, several studies have revealed thought process disturbances, which currently are interpreted as a secondary symptom.

The clinical experience of abnormal motor functioning in schizophrenia is confirmed by a series of studies, particularly of simple reaction time slowing. Increased volitional saccadic latency, an eye-tracking measure, is a frequent finding.

The following representative neuropsychological tests are used in clinical protocols:

> (1) intelligence (Wechsler Adult Intelligence Scale-Revised [WAIS-R]) vocabulary, information, picture completion, and digit symbol; (2) memory (Wechsler Verbal Paired Associates I and II, Wechsler Visual Reproduction I and II); (3) attention (Visual Search and Attention Test, Symbol Digit Modalities Test, Trail Making Test A and B, Stroop Test); (4) language (sentence repetition, nonsense sentences, test of reading comprehension, and controlled word association); (5) visual perceptual functioning (facial recognition); (6) motor functioning (finger tapping); and (7) tactile perception (stereognosis, graphesthesia).

It seems likely that with refined data, neuropsychological testing may become a standardized element of clinical diagnosis, useful for subtyping and investigational correlations.

SUBTYPES

In the absence of etiological and phenomenological clarity, Kraepelinian subtyping has been maintained in both the 10th revision of the *International Classification of Diseases and Related Health Problems* (ICD-10) and DSM-IV classifications. Paranoid type (Table 14.7-5), disorganized type (previously called hebephrenic type) (Table 14.7-6), catatonic type (Table 14.7-7), undifferentiated type (Table 14.7-8), and residual type (Table 14.7-9) are the DSM-IV subtypes of schizophrenia. Simple schizophrenia, included as a subtype in ICD-10, is designated simple deteriorative disorder (Table 14.7-10) in an appendix of DSM-IV.

Recent longitudinal studies suggest that many acute cases are not clearly differentiated until after several years of illness, following which, as negative symptoms increase, differences again diminish.

Several investigators have noted a decrease in the number of catatonic and disorganized cases in industrialized societies.

TABLE 14.7-5
Diagnostic Criteria for Schizophrenia, Paranoid Type

A type of schizophrenia in which the following criteria are met:
A. Preoccupation with one or more delusions or frequent auditory hallucinations.
B. None of the following is prominent: disorganized speech, disorganized or catatonic behavior, or flat or inappropriate affect.

Table from DSM-IV, *Diagnostic and Statistical Manual of Mental Disorders,* ed 4. Copyright American Psychiatric Association, Washington, 1994. Used with permission.

TABLE 14.7-6
Diagnostic Criteria for Schizophrenia, Disorganized Type

A type of schizophrenia in which the following criteria are met:
A. All of the following are prominent:
  (1) disorganized speech
  (2) disorganized behavior
  (3) flat or inappropriate affect
B. The criteria are not met for catatonic type.

Table from DSM-IV, *Diagnostic and Statistical Manual of Mental Disorders,* ed 4. Copyright American Psychiatric Association, Washington, 1994. Used with permission.

TABLE 14.7-7
Diagnostic Criteria for Schizophrenia, Catatonic Type

A type of schizophrenia in which the clinical picture is dominated by at least two of the following:
(1) motoric immobility as evidenced by catalepsy (including waxy flexibility) or stupor
(2) excessive motor activity (that is apparently purposeless and not influenced by external stimuli)
(3) extreme negativism (an apparently motiveless resistance to all instructions or maintenance of a rigid posture against attempts to be moved) or mutism
(4) peculiarities of voluntary movement as evidenced by posturing (voluntary assumption of inappropriate or bizarre postures), stereotyped movements, prominent mannerisms, or prominent grimacing
(5) echolalia or echopraxia

TABLE 14.7-8
Diagnostic Criteria for Schizophrenia, Undifferentiated Type

A type of schizophrenia in which symptoms that meet criterion A are present, but the criteria are not met for the paranoid, disorganized, or catatonic type.

Whether that decrease represents, as in the case of hysteria, the influence of culture on symptoms, changes of diagnostic criteria, or effects of antipsychotic medications remains unclear. It does appear, however, that the disorganized and undifferentiated types tend to show onsets that are insidious, continuous, and less obviously reactive to life events.

PARANOID TYPE The utility of subtypes is most evident in the paranoid type, which is commonly characterized by a later and more acute onset, a higher premorbid occupational and social achievement, and a more clearly reactive component to the illness than the other subtypes of schizophrenia. The prognosis of the paranoid subtype is demonstrably better, in both the short and the long term.

A highly educated white man in his early 30s became convinced over a one-year period that he was the Messiah. The conviction was associated with experiences of thought insertion from people and message reception from the television set. In addition, he began to interpret a number of routine occurrences as signs from God instructing him as to what he should do. He informed his family of those beliefs, and they brought him to a local hospital for evaluation.

The patient was diagnosed as having an acute episode of schizophrenia, paranoid type, and a regimen of antipsychotic medication was begun. Within a month he had improved considerably and was discharged. He was continued on antipsychotic medication for several years with a marked resolution of the symptoms. The patient's only residual impairment was that he was slightly more withdrawn and not as productive at work. It became necessary to work in the family business. He spent less time with his friends than he had prior to the illness but otherwise was functioning normally.

Medication was withdrawn, and the patient had one recurrence approximately six months after the medication was stopped. Subsequently, he remained asymptomatic, functioning at slightly below premorbid psychosocial levels and free of medication for over five years.

The following case vignette illustrates a second paranoid individual with schizophrenia, paranoid type whose outcome was not as good but who also showed minimal deterioration from premorbid psychosocial functioning.

A 32-year-old white, unmarried male engineer had been having an affair with a married woman whose husband was on active war duty. The engineer was an Orthodox Jew and felt remorse and shame over his behavior. He decided to terminate the affair. Several weeks later he experienced 12 hours of continuous auditory and visual hallucinations in which God revealed to him not only the secrets of the world but that he, the patient, was the long awaited Messiah. Thereupon the patient undertook a more intensive study of religious texts and began to write letters to his government giving both unsolicited advice and warnings as to the negative consequences that would result should they not heed his advice. Those warnings were perceived as threats and resulted in his arrest and examination by government authorities. He was found to be suffering from an acute schizophrenic reaction, and his family arranged for him to immigrate to the United States in return for the dismissal of charges.

The patient came to the United States, lived with relatives, abandoned his work, and continued his religious studies. He began to write advice and warnings to the President of the United States. Once again he came to the attention of the authorities, was examined, and was found mentally ill. The authorities found he did not represent an imminent threat, and he was released after a period of inpatient examination.

His American relatives sought further private psychiatric evaluation. Despite the passage of almost 10 years, the patient remained convinced that he was not mentally ill, was in fact the Messiah, and had special powers that could be used for good or evil. He refused both medication and to stop haranguing the government. When confronted with the reality that he would continue to be harassed (as he saw it) by the United States Secret Service, the patient decided to go to South America and start his own church. He was successful in establishing a church with a number of followers and had no further difficulty with the authorities. He apparently lost interest in the politics of this world and emphasized the importance of an orthodox religious revival. He died in his mid-60s of natural causes, still convinced that he was the Messiah but in no legal difficulty.

Spontaneous remissions with and without psychotherapy do occur, particularly in later life. The following vignette illustrates spontaneous remission in a female patient.

A 28-year-old married woman, after the birth of her second child, began to have the idea that she had been selected to perform a mission involving world education. As the initial thought became a conviction, she also became convinced that people were staring at her, talking about her, and making jealous and critical comments. Gradually, she began to hear voices of people commenting on her behavior and criticizing her for not doing more than she was doing.

She consulted a psychiatrist who was well known for a deep explorative psychodynamic approach to the psychotic disorders and who was

TABLE 14.7-9
Diagnostic Criteria for Schizophrenia, Residual Type

A type of schizophrenia in which the following criteria are met:
A. Absence of prominent delusions, hallucinations, disorganized speech, and grossly disorganized or catatonic behavior.
B. There is continuing evidence of the disturbance, as indicated by the presence of negative symptoms or two or more symptoms listed in criterion A for schizophrenia, present in an attenuated form (e.g., odd beliefs, unusual perceptual experiences).

TABLE 14.7-10
Research Criteria for Simple Deteriorative Disorder (Simple Schizophrenia)

A. Progressive development over a period of at least a year of all of the following:
   (1) marked decline in occupational or academic functioning
   (2) gradual appearance and deepening of negative symptoms such as affective flattening, alogia, and avolition
   (3) poor interpersonal rapport, social isolation, or social withdrawal
B. Criterion A for schizophrenia has never been met.
C. The symptoms are not better accounted for by schizotypal or schizoid personality disorder, a psychotic disorder, a mood disorder, an anxiety disorder, a dementia, or mental retardation and are not due to the direct physiological effects of a substance or a general medical condition.

opposed to the use of medication. She worked with him for a period of over 12 years, until his death. By the time of his death, her hallucinations had long ceased but her delusional preoccupations remained active. Furthermore, she was involved in very elaborate rituals that were necessary to ward off her anxiety. The rituals essentially took all of her waking hours and left little time for her to meet her day-to-day obligations.

She consulted a new psychiatrist who recommended medication, which she refused. He gave her supportive and reality-oriented psychotherapy for an additional 10 years. During treatment, she undertook, with his encouragement, regular volunteer work. She made new friends and strengthened previous friendships that had been neglected. By the time she terminated treatment in her early 50s, she was essentially free of all major symptoms, although residual effects included adhedonia, rituals, and diminished psychosocial functioning compared with her premorbid state. The patient continued in good remission despite the normal stresses and strains of living.

CATATONIC TYPE Catatonic schizophrenia occurs as inhibited (or stuporous) catatonia and as excited catatonia.

Stuporous catatonia Stuporous catatonic patients with schizophrenia may be in a state of complete stupor or may show a pronounced decrease in spontaneous movements and activity. They may be mute or nearly so and may show distinct negativism, stereotypies, echopraxia, or automatic obedience. After standing or sitting motionless for long periods of time, they may suddenly and without provocation have a brief outburst of violence. Occasionally, catatonic patients with schizophrenia exhibit catalepsy or waxy flexibility.

An 18-year-old student was admitted for the first time to the psychiatry service because for three days she had not spoken and would not eat. According to her parents, she had been a normal teenager, with good grades and friends, until about one year earlier when she began to stay at home more, alone in her room, and seemed preoccupied and less animated. Six months before admission she began to refuse to go to school, and her grades became barely passing. About a month later she started to talk gibberish about spirits, magic, the devil—things that were totally foreign to her background. For the week preceding admission to the hospital she had stared into space, immobile, only allowing herself to be moved from her bed to a chair or from one room to another. (Adapted from *DSM-III Case Book.* Used with permission.)

Excited catatonia Excited catatonic patients are in a state of extreme psychomotor agitation and talk and shout almost continuously. Verbal productions are often incoherent, and behavior seems to be influenced more by inner stimuli than by responses to the environment. Patients in catatonic excitement urgently require physical and medical control because they are often destructive and violent toward others, and their excitement can cause them to injure themselves or to collapse from complete exhaustion. In the past, excited catatonic states that could not be controlled by sedation were called pernicious or fatal catatonia. It is likely, however, that many of the patients previously thought to have excited catatonia were actually in a manic phase of bipolar disorder.

An unmarried man of 27, a teacher, was admitted to a psychiatric hospital after having become increasingly agitated and irrational after several nights of wakefulness. He was extremely talkative and ran about aimlessly. His behavior at home was bizarre: He tried to clean everything in the house, wore his wristwatch up on his shoulder, stripped his clothes off, chewed large wads of paper in the belief that it was good for him, talked about killing himself, then said he might already be dead.

He heard voices constantly ordering him about, and he frequently laughed for no apparent reason. After chewing the paper, he would spit in it and then drink his saliva. He rolled into odd postures on the bed, sticking out his tongue. He started to jump and dance when taken to the bathroom for a shower, and destroyed the bathroom furnishings. His gait was manneristic. His speech was utterly incomprehensible. He refused to take any medication and had to be sedated parenterally.

Periodic catatonia A rare but intriguing form of catatonia has been called periodic catatonia (a subtype not specified in DSM-IV). Patients with the syndrome have periodic episodes of stuporous or excited catatonia that have been correlated with shifts in thyroid hormone levels and nitrogen balance. Such patients respond to administration of thyroxine in combination with antipsychotics. The vast majority of patients who present with catatonia do not have periodic catatonia.

DISORGANIZED TYPE The disorganized or hebephrenic type is characterized by primitive, disinhibited, and unorganized behavior. The hebephrenic patient is usually active but aimlessly and nonconstructively so. Thought disorder is pronounced; contact with reality is extremely poor. Personal appearance is slipshod, and social behavior is primitive. Emotional responses are inappropriate, and there is explosive laughter without apparent reason. Incongruous grinning and grimacing are common in this type of patient.

Emilio was 40 but looked 10 years younger. He was brought to the hospital (his 12th hospitalization) by his mother, because she was afraid of him. He was dressed in a ragged overcoat, bedroom slippers, and a baseball cap and wore several medals around his neck. His affect ranged from anger at his mother—"She feeds me shit . . . what comes out of other people's rectums"—to a giggling, obsequious seductiveness toward the interviewer. His speech and manner had a childlike quality, and he walked with a mincing step and exaggerated hip movements. His mother reported that he had stopped taking his medication about a month ago and had since begun to hear voices and to look and act more bizarrely. When asked what he had been doing, he said, "eating wires and lighting fires." His spontaneous speech was often incoherent and marked by frequent rhyming and clang associations.

Emilio's first hospitalization occurred after he dropped out of school at 16; since that time he had never been able to attend school or hold a job. He was living with his elderly mother, but sometimes disappeared for several months at a time, eventually to be picked up by the police as he wandered in the street. He had no known history of drug or alcohol abuse. (Adapted from *DSM-III Case Book.* Used with permission.)

UNDIFFERENTIATED TYPE Frequently, patients who clearly have schizophrenia cannot be easily fitted into one of the other types. DSM-IV classifies those patients as the undifferentiated type.

RESIDUAL TYPE According to DSM-IV, the residual type is characterized by the presence of continuing evidence of the schizophrenic disturbance, in the absence of a complete set of active symptoms or sufficient symptoms to meet another type of schizophrenia. Emotional blunting, social withdrawal, eccentric behavior, illogical thinking, and mild loosening of associations are common in the residual type. If delusions or hallucinations are present, they are not prominent and are not accompanied by strong affect.

POSITIVE-NEGATIVE DISTINCTION

The distinction between manifestations of schizophrenia that appear to represent a loss of function (for example, emotional blunting, poverty of speech, and such symptoms as delusions and hallucinations) has been part of the diagnostic process at least since Kraepelin, whose concept of an avolitional syndrome was the predecessor of the concept. Bleuler's division of symptoms into fundamental and accessory may be seen as supporting that separation, with certain of the negative symptoms assigned diagnostic primacy. It should be remembered, however, that Kraepelin agreed in principle with Bleuler on the distinction between fundamental and accessory symptoms. In 1913 Kraepelin stated,

the former [fundamental symptoms] constitute the real characteristics of the clinical state and can be demonstrated in each individual case more or less distinctly; the latter [accessory symptoms] may be present but may also be absent; they are not caused by the character of the morbid process but by circumstances which are in loose connection with it. . . . [F]rom this point of view the weakening of judgment, of mental activity and of creative ability, the dulling of emotional interest and the loss of energy, lastly, the loosening of the inner unity of the psychic life would have to be reckoned among the fundamental disorders of dementia praecox, while all the remaining morbid symptoms, especially hallucinations and delusions . . . would be regarded more as secondary accompanying phenomena. . . .

As psychiatric nosology has been modified over the past decades, largely in the service of greater reliability, the positive symptoms (accessory symptoms as designated by Bleuler) have assumed principal importance in the diagnostic criteria used internationally and in the United States from DSM-III onward.

Two distinct psychopathological processes were postulated in 1980. Type I schizophrenia was characterized by predominantly positive symptoms, good premorbid functioning, acute onset, normal brain structures on computed tomography (CT), good response to treatment, and a better long-term course. Type II schizophrenia was characterized by mainly negative symptoms, an insidious onset, poor premorbid functioning, abnormalities on CT scans, a tendency to drug resistance, and a poorer long-term course and outcome, often resulting in behavioral deterioration (Table 14.7-11). Other similar groupings include negative and positive schizophrenia and deficit and nondeficit forms of schizophrenia. The past decade saw a large number of investigations into possible relations between those syndromes and a variety of issues, including course and outcome, neurotransmitter hypotheses, brain imaging findings, family studies, and so forth.

Scales have been developed to measure negative symptoms that have acceptable interrater reliability. Those scales invariably designate flat affect and poverty of speech among the negative symptoms and generally also include anhedonia, apathy, and avolition. Thought disorder, bizarre behavior, and inappropriate affect are more variable in such classifications.

A recent review summarized and compared findings in patients with negative and positive symptoms. Those with negative symptoms experienced an earlier onset of schizophrenia, tend to be male and unmarried, had a worse premorbid level of functioning, had more motor abnormalities, and were more likely to be concordant for illness if an identical twin. In view of those findings, negative symptoms have been reintroduced into the diagnostic classifications as one of the characteristic symptom complexes necessary for the diagnosis of schizophrenia.

Certain manifestations simulate negative symptoms but are a consequence of medication, depression, institutionalization, or other life circumstances. Those manifestations must be distinguished from the core negative symptoms of schizophrenia. Moreover, most patients present with a mixture of positive and negative symptoms, the degrees of which vary over time.

TABLE 14.7-11
Percentage of Patients with Negative and Positive Symptoms (111 Consecutively Admitted Schizophrenic Patients)

Symptoms	Mild or Moderate	Severe or Extreme
Negative symptoms		
Affective flattening		
Unchanging facial expression	54	33
Decreased spontaneous movements	37	14
Paucity of expressive gestures	34	24
Poor eye contact	39	16
Affective nonresponsivity	18	18
Inappropriate affect	29	22
Lack of vocal inflections	40	9
Alogia		
Poverty of speech	20	20
Poverty of content of speech	33	6
Blocking	12	3
Increased response latency	17	6
Avolition-apathy		
Grooming and hygiene	33	41
Impersistence at work or school	13	74
Physical anergia	36	31
Anhedonia-asociality		
Recreational interests, activities	38	41
Sexual interest, activity	11	23
Intimacy, closeness	24	35
Relationship with friends, peers	25	63
Attention		
Social inattentiveness	25	32
Inattentiveness during testing	33	19
Positive symptoms		
Hallucinations		
Auditory	19	51
Voices commenting	22	12
Voices conversing	27	12
Somatic-tactile	10	6
Olfactory	5	1
Visual	16	15
Delusions		
Persecutory	19	47
Jealousy	2	1
Guilt, sin	16	2
Grandiose	15	15
Religious	12	11
Somatic	11	11
Delusions of reference	13	21
Delusions of being controlled	25	12
Delusions of mind reading	19	14
Thought broadcasting	11	2
Thought insertion	15	4
Thought withdrawal	11	6
Bizarre behavior		
Clothing, appearance	8	4
Social, sexual behavior	17	7
Aggressive-agitated behavior	14	6
Repetitive-stereotyped behavior	7	4
Positive formal thought disorder		
Derailment	30	4
Tangentiality	28	4
Incoherence	9	1
Illogicality	10	1
Circumstantiality	14	0
Pressure of speech	14	0
Distractible speech	12	1
Clanging	1	0

Table adapted from N C Andreasen: The diagnosis of schizophrenia. Schizophr Bull *13:* 9, 1987. Used with permission.

OTHER SUBTYPES

The subtyping of schizophrenia has had a long history, and other subtyping schemes can be found in the literature, especially from countries other than the United States.

The names of some of those subtypes are self-explanatory—for example, childhood and process. Schizophrenia with a *childhood onset* is simply called schizophrenia in DSM-IV, although even the literature in the United States tends to refer to childhood schizophrenia. *Process schizophrenia* means schizophrenia with a particularly debilitating and deteriorating course.

***BOUFFÉE DÉLIRANTE* (ACUTE DELUSIONAL PSYCHOSIS)** This French diagnostic concept is differentiated from schizophrenia primarily on the basis of a symptom duration of less than three months. The diagnosis is similar to the DSM-IV diagnosis of schizophreniform disorder. French clinicians report that about 40 percent of patients with a diagnosis of *bouffée délirante* progress in their illness and are eventually classified as having schizophrenia.

LATENT The concept of latent schizophrenia developed during a time when there was a broad diagnostic conceptualization of schizophrenia. Currently, patients must be very mentally ill to warrant a diagnosis of schizophrenia; however, with a broad diagnostic conceptualization of schizophrenia, patients who would not today be seen as severely ill can receive a diagnosis of schizophrenia. Latent schizophrenia, for example, was often the diagnosis used for patients with what now may be called schizoid and schizotypal personality disorders. Those patients may occasionally present peculiar behaviors or thought disorders but do not consistently manifest psychotic symptoms. The syndrome was also termed borderline schizophrenia in the past.

ONEIROID The oneiroid state is a dreamlike state in which the patient may be deeply perplexed and not fully oriented in time and place. The term "oneiroid schizophrenic" has been used for patients with schizophrenia who are particularly engaged in their hallucinatory experiences to the exclusion of involvement in the real world. When an oneiroid state is present, the clinician should be particularly careful to examine the patient for a medical or neurological cause of the symptoms.

PARAPHRENIA This term is sometimes used as a synonym for "paranoid schizophrenia." In other usages the term is used for either a progressively deteriorating course of illness or the presence of a well-systemized delusional system. The multiple meanings of the term render it not very useful in communicating information.

PSEUDONEUROTIC Occasionally, patients who initially present such symptoms as anxiety, phobias, obsessions, and compulsions later reveal symptoms of thought disorder and psychosis. Those patients are characterized by symptoms of pananxiety, panphobia, panambivalence, and sometimes a chaotic sexuality. Unlike patients suffering from anxiety disorders, they have anxiety that is free-floating and that hardly ever subsides. In clinical descriptions of the patients, they rarely become overtly and severely psychotic.

SIMPLE SCHIZOPHRENIA As with "latent schizophrenia," the term "simple schizophrenia" was used during a period when schizophrenia had a broad diagnostic conceptualization. Simple schizophrenia was characterized by a gradual, insidious loss of drive and ambition. Patients with the disorder were usually not overtly psychotic and did not experience persistent hallucinations or delusions. The primary symptom is the withdrawal of the patient from social and work-related situations. The syndrome may reflect depression, a phobia, a dementia, or an exacerbation of personality traits. The clinician should be sure that the patient truly meets the diagnostic criteria for schizophrenia before making that diagnosis. In spite of those reservations, simple deteriorative disorder (simple schizophrenia) appears as a diagnostic category in an appendix of DSM-IV.

LATE-ONSET SCHIZOPHRENIA Late-onset schizophrenia is usually defined as schizophrenia that has an onset after age 45. However, the DSM-III criteria for schizophrenia required onset before age 45, DSM-III-R and DSM-IV, in consonance with clinical experience and international standard, removed that age requirement. Although less common than an earlier onset, the active symptoms of schizophrenia can first appear late in life. In general, late onset schizophrenia occurs more frequently in women than in men, is often characterized by paranoid symptoms, and tends to respond to antipsychotic therapy. Clinical considerations emphasize the importance of differential diagnosis in the elderly and the explicit need to exclude other possible causes of brain disorder.

ALTERNATIVE DIMENSIONAL DESCRIPTORS FOR SCHIZOPHRENIA

DSM-IV states:

> Because of limitations in the classical subtyping of schizophrenia, a three-factor dimensional model (psychotic, disorganized, and negative) has been suggested to describe current and lifetime symptomatology. The psychotic factor includes delusions and hallucinations. The disorganized factor includes disorganized speech, disorganized behavior, and inappropriate affect. The negative factor includes the various negative symptoms. Studies suggest that the severity of symptoms within each of these three factors tends to vary together, both cross-sectionally and over time, whereas this is less true for symptoms across factors.

The research criteria for alternative dimensional descriptors for schizophrenia appear in Table 14.7-12.

SCHIZOAFFECTIVE DISORDER Schizoaffective disorder appears to lie between schizophrenia and the mood disorders. The category is surrounded by uncertainty. Family and outcome studies suggest a relation between schizophrenia and the mood disorders, further confounding the Kraepelinean disease dichotomy. Following the absence in DSM-III of criteria for schizoaffective disorder, DSM-III-R stressed the relative duration and degree of temporal overlap between psychotic and mood disorder symptoms in the diagnostic distinction. DSM-IV requires concurrent symptoms that meet criterion A for schizophrenia and a major depressive episode, manic episode, or mixed episode. During the same period of illness there must be at least two weeks of characteristic delusions or hallucinations in the absence of prominent mood symptoms.

SCHIZOPHRENIA SPECTRUM DISORDERS The schizophrenia spectrum disorders are a cluster of personality disorders, including schizotypal, schizoid, and paranoid personality disorders, that are characterized by odd or eccentric behavior. Working with relatives of patients with schizophrenia, investigators have accumulated evidence of higher rates of schizophrenia spectrum disorders in the families of patients with schizophrenia than in the families of normal subjects. In addition, rates for schizophrenia are higher in siblings of patients

TABLE 14.7-12
Research Criteria for Alternative Dimensional Descriptors for Schizophrenia

Specify: absent, mild, moderate, severe for each dimension. The prominence of these dimensions may be specified for either (or both) the current episode (i.e., previous six months) or the lifetime course of the disorder.

psychotic (hallucinations/delusions) dimension: describes the degree to which hallucinations or delusions have been present

disorganized dimension: describes the degree to which disorganized speech, disorganized behavior, or inappropriate affect have been present

negative (deficit) dimension: describes the degree to which negative symptoms (i.e., affective flattening, alogia, avolition) have been present.
Note: Do not include symptoms that appear to be secondary to depression, medication side effects, or hallucinations or delusions.

Table from DSM-IV, *Diagnostic and Statistical Manual of Mental Disorders,* ed 4. Copyright American Psychiatric Association, Washington, 1994. Used with permission.

with schizophrenia if the parents have schizotypal personality disorder and various neurophysiological abnormalities, such as eye-tracking, information-processing, and attention deficits resembling those found in schizophrenia.

NOSOLOGICAL LIMITATIONS Psychiatry's newer scientific nosology has not come about without certain losses and the probability of further losses. The emphasis on easily observable manifestations has excluded many traditional clinical considerations, especially those derived from inferential and introspective data. It has also tended to organize diagnostic criteria at their simplest and most easily communicated level, potentially omitting complex criteria when the latter might be more true to the fund of knowledge.

The nosology also serves administrative and political functions that add little to the search for scientific truth. How they may contaminate that process remains to be more clearly evaluated. Ironically, the very phenomenology, the precise description of psychopathology, that serves as the benchmark of the new system is in danger of progressive constriction and limitation as the diagnostic criteria become traditions of their own. Openness to new observations requires disciplined avoidance of theoretical constructs. The psychiatric clinician should remember that contemporary nosology is an elaborate series of compromises, even if informed. The clinician should remain open to new and fresh observations.

SUICIDE

Suicide is a frequent event in the schizophrenic population. Estimates of suicide attempts vary by up to 40 percent; however, at least 10 percent of schizophrenic persons commit suicide, mostly during the first 10 years of illness. Their suicide rate is 20 times higher than that of the general population.

The risk of suicide appears greater in men with the paranoid type. The clinical picture, often of later onset and with more florid symptoms, may afford the patient both a demoralizing awareness of the illness and the volitional capacity to act on a self-destructive impulse.

VIOLENCE

The literature on violence and schizophrenia is subject both to the methodological difficulties associated with unreliable diagnostic appraisals, patient selection and setting, concomitant mental disorders (especially substance abuse), and cultural variations, as well as to a lack of precision in the definition of violence itself.

Recent investigators, however, highlight certain observations. Well-planned and directed violence, often dangerous, generally follows the delusions of paranoid schizophrenia. Violence that is the product of more disorganized psychotic states tends to be poorly focused and less dangerous. Command hallucinations seem to play less of a role in psychotic violence than was previously believed. On the other hand, delusional misidentification of an object has been associated with violence.

Violence during hospitalization is a function of the stage and type of illness and the interaction of the patient and the environment. Generally, the violence associated with acute illness subsides as the symptoms are treated and remit. Of those who remain persistently assaultive, some 50 percent respond when treated in specially staffed units providing a more structured program and environmental space. Interestingly, the 50 percent nonresponders differ most in demonstrating higher neurological impairment, show less response to antipsychotic medications, and may actually experience worsening of symptoms as medications are increased.

The National Institute of Mental Health's Epidemiologic Catchment Area (ECA) survey that pooled data on over 10,000 respondents who had reported violent behavior during the previous year revealed that 12.7 percent of all those with schizophrenia reported violence (Table 14.7-13). In contrast, 25 percent of those with alcoholism (alcohol abuse or dependence) reported violence.

TABLE 14.7-13
Percentage of Psychiatric Patients Violent in Previous Year in Epidemiologic Catchment Area Sample, by Diagnosis

Diagnosis	% Violent
No disorder	2.1
Schizophrenia	12.7
Major depression	11.7
Mania or bipolar disorder	11.0
Alcohol abuse/ dependence	24.6
Drug abuse/dependence	34.7

COURSE AND OUTCOME

Until the past two decades, clinical pessimism dominated the discussion of prognosis in schizophrenia. Kraepelin revised his original recovery rate of 13 percent downward to no more than 4 percent, ultimately suggesting that a full recovery brought the original diagnosis into question. Bleuler, while acknowledging the fact of recovery, described the patient as never achieving full *restitutio ad integrum.* That belief was sustained in DSM-III, which described a complete return to premorbid functioning as unusual. DSM-III-R continued that view by stating, "A return to full premorbid function in this disorder is not common. . . . Residual impairment often increases between episodes. . . . There is some evidence, however, that in many people with the disorder, the residual symptoms become attenuated in the later phases of the illness." More recent data, however, have considerably modified that view. It is convenient to organize those data under a discussion of short-term and long-term outcome.

SHORT-TERM OUTCOME Early work comparing various therapeutic efforts in newly admitted patients with schizophrenia demonstrated convincingly that drug treatment, singly or in combination, produced significantly better responses than patients not treated with medication as measured by clinical, social, and psychological test standards. The group not initially treated with medication generally had a poorer response over a three-year follow-up period even if they had later been treated with medication. Recent analysis has shown that patients who did not receive antipsychotics yet who recovered sufficiently to be discharged within six months had more rehospitalizations than patients who received antipsychotics initially. That finding supported earlier work indicating that relapse rates after hospital discharge were higher in patients who had been ill for more than a year before treatment. In that group, only 18 percent remained free of relapse after two years. Overall, pooled data from 13 international studies indicated that approximately one third of first-admission patients with schizophrenia were relapse free during the first two years after admission. The relapse rate after two years of illness was around 60 percent.

Contemporary outcome investigations are focusing on longitudinal studies of first-episode psychosis in an attempt to overcome the diverse methodological problems associated with most previously reported studies. The new patient cohorts are being subjected to careful diagnostic, clinical, psychological, and neurological evaluations and are screened for potentially confounding comorbid conditions, particularly substance abuse. Preliminary data indicate that between one third and two thirds of those patients never regain their premorbid level of functioning after the first episode and that approximately one fifth ultimately require continued hospitalization.

In studies describing the symptoms that appeared or worsened before hospitalization, the following symptoms occurred in over two thirds of patients: appeared tense and nervous, ate less than usual, had trouble concentrating, had trouble sleeping, and enjoyed things less. Approximately 50 percent of patients reported a similar pattern of symptoms before repeated episodes of relapse.

In general, symptom progression appears limited by time, often reaching a plateau by about five years of illness. That finding seems consistent over a variety of studies.

The World Health Organization's International Pilot Study of Schizophrenia, begun in 1968 and carried out in nine countries, demonstrated the feasibility of carrying out an elaborately designed study cross-culturally. Follow-up assessments were performed at two and five years in all centers. For the study as a whole, 26 percent of patients belonged to the best outcome group and 18 percent to the worst outcome group. Of interest was the reporting of a significantly higher proportion of best outcomes in the developing countries of India and Nigeria, 48 percent and 57 percent, respectively, whereas the industrialized Western countries reported a low percentage of best outcome patients (6 to 26 percent). The disparity in outcomes between developing and developed countries appears to be holding up over time.

Clinical factors predicting a favorable outcome in the short term include the following:

- A good premorbid adjustment. The usual areas of adjustment—personal, social, and employment (or school)—are the guidelines employed in this determination.
- Marital status. Being married carries an independently more favorable prognosis in men. Women have a better prognosis than men but are also more likely to be married. The implications of marital status are complex and have not been clearly separated, but marital status is not prognostically useful in females.
- Symptomatic presentation. A long-standing clinical observation, confirmed in a number of studies, is that a florid symptomatic presentation bodes better for favorable outcome.
- Number and duration of psychotic episodes. Fewer and briefer psychotic episodes are correlated with better outcomes. It is instructive to recall the American Worcester State Hospital report on the outcome of patients admitted to that hospital from 1833 to 1852 who had been ill for less than one year before admission. Of that group, some 71 percent were discharged as recovered or improved, in contrast to 45 percent of those whose illness had exceeded one year before admission. Antedating the era of antipsychotic medications by over a century, those results occurred under the general philosophy of moral treatment in America and the removal of patients from the stresses of their prehospital life situations.
- Expressed emotion. High levels of exposure to hostile, critical, or emotionally overinvolved relatives are correlated with higher relapse rates. Although the issue remains somewhat controversial in longer-term follow-up, it deserves recognition and further evaluation, especially in rehabilitation research, where psychoeducational programs are used to lower the expressed emotion in families. Expressed emotion may be an important variable in outcome differences reported between developing and developed countries.
- Continued medication. Continued use of antipsychotic medication is correlated with better outcomes over at least a two-year period. Relapse rates are higher during this time interval when medications are discontinued.
- Female sex. Female patients have later ages of onset and better short-term outcomes than male patients.
- Timing of symptoms. The time interval between the onset of behavioral symptoms and the onset of psychotic symptoms, called the mode of onset by some writers, may be related to outcome. The shorter that time interval, the better the prognosis that may be expected.

LONG-TERM OUTCOME All of the major long-term follow-up studies of schizophrenia, including the European and North American studies, describe a heterogeneous course characterized by remissions and relapses. Nonetheless, the relentlessly pessimistic view of the past has turned more optimistic with the demonstration of significant possibilities for remission and an illness course often characterized as undulating. Studies suggesting cautious optimism emphasize the heterogeneity of outcome measures in such areas as occupational functioning and social competence.

The benefits of antipsychotic medications early in the illness are less clear once the acute episodes have been controlled. The risk-benefit considerations of long-term antipsychotic treatment must include not only the drug-induced movement disorders and drug-induced deficitlike symptoms but, increasingly, the question of progressive cognitive impairment.

Taken together, the long-term studies support the following conclusions:

- Although not inevitably leading to deterioration, schizophrenia is usually a chronic and disabling disease.
- On average, the outcome of schizophrenia is worse than the outcome of other so-called functional mental disorders. In that sense the Kraepelinian dichotomy appears to be valid.
- Schizophrenia is associated with an increased risk for suicide, physical illness, and mortality. The average life span of affected patients is shortened by about 10 years.
- The disease does not inevitably worsen over the long term but appears to plateau after about five years.
- The effect of any treatment on the long-term course of the illness is not yet established.
- Outcome seems influenced by sociocultural factors, with the urban-rural contrast perhaps playing a greater role than simple economic considerations.

Only about a dozen longitudinal studies following patients across decades have appeared in the literature. Many of those studies are hampered by a number of methodological problems, including inconsistent diagnostic standards and the unresolved questions of clinical and adaptive artifacts produced by insti-

TABLE 14.7-14
Long-Term Studies of Schizophrenia

Burgholzli Hospital Study
(M. Bleuler, 1972—Switzerland)
208 patients, 23-year study
Results: 66% recovered or significantly improved

Lausanne Study
(Ciompi and Müller, 1976—Switzerland)
289 patients, average 37 years of study
Results: 27% recovered
22% mildly dysfunctional
Total: 49% favorable outcome

Vermont Longitudinal Project
(Harding and colleagues, 1987)
269 patients, 22–59 years of study
Results: 34% considerably recovered
34% fully recovered
Total: 68% favorable outcome

tutionalization. An extensive review of such North American studies is available. With the exception of the Vermont study, however, outcomes were poor; in general, less than 25 percent of patients achieved a satisfactory adjustment in the community. During the past two decades, however, three long-term studies have been completed, each following patients for at least 20 years (Table 14.7-14). Extending back for 20 to 40 years, those studies report rates of recovery or significant improvement ranging from 49 to 68 percent, with the highest percentage reported by the Vermont study.

DIFFERENTIAL DIAGNOSIS

The syndromic nature of schizophrenia is such that schizophrenic signs and symptoms may occur in the course of any process or disease affecting the brain, ranging from environmental to the most intrinsically anatomical process. Therefore, the DSM-IV requirement to exclude any disturbance that is due to the direct effects of a substance (for example, drugs of abuse and medication) or to a general medical condition requires a deep knowledge of medicine.

The causal link between substances of abuse or general medical conditions and an episode of psychosis phenomenologically similar to schizophrenia can vary from an apparently explicit relation to an uncertain one. When the clinical picture of psychosis occurs synchronously with conditions known to generate the syndrome, the clinical assumption is that the substance or medical condition is primary and that the mental disorder is a secondary manifestation. That assumption is substantiated when the psychotic symptoms remit in conjunction with effective treatment for the primary conditions. Some examples are the classical psychotic syndrome occurring in tertiary syphilis, hypoparathyroidism, and certain brain tumors.

The specificity of that assumption, however, varies through a hierarchy of medical conditions wherein disorders of mental status reflect unique combinations of the particular condition and the person's vulnerability to a schizophrenic syndrome. The relation between many conditions—infectious, toxic, metabolic, traumatic, neurological, convulsive—and a schizophrenialike syndrome is often problematical. Medically, however, any such possibility must be excluded before schizophrenia is diagnosed. That medical requirement remains consistent for a first episode or a recurrence. The clinician must also be sensitive to the possibility of such a condition occurring during an already established course of schizophrenia. It follows, therefore, that the medical evaluation includes a complete medical and family history (especially regarding psychiatric and neurological disease) and systematic laboratory and chemistry evaluations. To the extent appropriate, the evaluation may include brain imaging.

The striking comorbidity of substance abuse and psychosis poses many vexing problems of differential diagnosis. Although anecdotal reports vary, clinical experience indicates that the psychotic episodes associated with the hallucinogens (lysergic acid diethylamide [LSD] and phencyclidine [PCP]), usually vivid in expression, generally subside after approximately 48 hours. The use of stimulant drugs, including amphetamine and cocaine, often produces a paranoid psychosis that similarly resolves within a few days. Persistence of the psychosis, when it occurs, probably reflects a greater personal vulnerability to that form of mental decompensation. The relation between cannabis use and schizophrenia has not been clearly demonstrated. Although reports often document high levels of comorbidity, a causal relation has not been firmly established.

Table 14.7-15 lists the differential diagnosis of schizophrenia and schizophrenialike symptoms.

SELECTED CROSS-REFERENCES

Substance-related disorders (including alcohol-, cocaine-, and hallucinogen-related disorders) are discussed in Chapter 13.

TABLE 14.7-15
Differential Diagnosis of Schizophrenialike Symptoms

Medical or neurological
- Substance-induced psychotic disorder, especially amphetamines, alcohol hallucinosis, anticholinergic, barbiturate withdrawal, belladonna alkaloids, cimetidine, cocaine, digitalis, disulfiram, hallucinogens, L-dopa, phencyclidine (PCP)
- Epilepsy, especially of temporal lobe origin
- Tumors, especially frontal or limbic
- CNS infections, especially herpes encephalitis, Creutzfeldt-Jakob disease, neurosyphilis, AIDS
- Acute intermittent porphyria
- Dementia of the Alzheimer's type
- B_{12} deficiency
- Carbon monoxide poisoning
- Endocrinopathies, especially adrenal and thyroid
- Fabry's disease
- Fahr's syndrome
- Hallervorden-Spatz disease
- Heavy metal poisoning (arsenic, manganese, mercury, thallium)
- Homocystinuria
- Huntington's disease
- Metachromatic leukodystrophy
- Normal-pressure hydrocephalus
- Pellagra
- Pick's disease
- Systemic lupus erythematosus
- Wernicke-Korsakoff syndrome
- Wilson's disease

Psychiatric
- Malingering
- Factitious disorder with predominantly psychological symptoms
- Autistic disorder
- Schizophrenia
- Schizophreniform disorder
- Brief psychotic disorder
- Mood disorder
- Schizoaffective disorder
- Psychotic disorder NOS (atypical psychosis)
- Delusional disorder
- Personality disorder, especially schizotypal, schizoid, borderline, paranoid
- Obsessive-compulsive disorder

Schizoaffective disorder, schizophreniform disorder, and brief psychotic disorder are discussed in Section 15.1. The clinical features of mood disorders are discussed in Section 16.6. Dissociative disorders are discussed in Chapter 20. Adult antisocial behavior and criminality are discussed in Section 28.3

REFERENCES

Andreasen N C, Olsen S: Negative versus positive schizophrenia: Definition and validation. Arch Gen Psychiatry *39:* 789, 1982.

Arieti S: *Interpretation of Schizophrenia.* Brunner, New York, 1955.

*Bleuler E: *Dementia Praecox, or, the Group of Schizophrenias,* H Zinkin, translator. International Universities Press, New York, 1950.

Bleuler M N: *The Schizophrenic Disorders: Long-Term Patient and Family Studies.* Yale University Press, New Haven, 1978.

Carpenter W T Jr, Strauss J S, Mulek S: Are there pathognomonic symptoms in schizophrenia? An empiric investigation of Kurt Schneider's first-rank symptoms. Arch Gen Psychiatry *28:* 847, 1973.

Crow T J: Molecular pathology of schizophrenia: More than one disease process? Br Med J *280:* 66, 1980.

Fenton W S, McGlashan T H: Natural history of schizophrenia subtypes. Arch Gen Psychiatry *48:* 969, 1991.

Freud S: *Standard Edition of the Complete Psychological Works of Sigmund Freud.* Hogarth Press, London, 1953–1966.

*Grinker R R: Diagnosis and schizophrenia. In *The Schizophrenic Reactions,* R Cancro, editor. Brunner/Mazel, New York, 1970.

Harding C M, Brooks, G W, Ashikaga T, Strauss J S, Breier A: The Vermont Longitudinal Study: II. Long term outcome for subjects who retrospectively met DSM-III criteria for schizophrenia. Am J Psychiatry *144:* 718, 1987.

Jaspers K: The phenomenological approach in psychopathology. Br J Psychiatry *114:* 1313, 1968.

Kay S R, Fiszbein A, Opler L A: The positive and negative syndrome scale (PANSS) for schizophrenia. Schizophr Bull *13:* 261, 1987.

*Kraepelin E: Dementia praecox and paraphrenia. In *The 8th German Edition of the Textbook of Psychiatry,* vol III, part 2: *Endogenous Dementias,* R M Barclay, translator. Livingstone, Edinburgh, 1919.

Langfeldt G: *The Schizophreniform States.* Munksgaard, Copenhagen, 1939.

Lieberman J A, Koreen A R: Neurochemistry and neuroendocrinology of schizophrenia: A selective review. Schizophr Bull *19:* 371, 1993.

May P R A, Tuma A H, Dixon W J: Schizophrenia: A followup study of the results of five forms of treatment. Arch Gen Psychiatry *38:* 776, 1981.

McGlashan T H, Fenton W S: The positive-negative distinction in schizophrenia: A review of natural history validations. Arch Gen Psychiatry *49:* 63, 1992.

Monahan J: Mental disorder and violent behavior. Am Psychol *47:* 511, 1992.

*Pope H, Lipinski J: Diagnosis of schizophrenia and manic-depressive illness: A reassessment of the specificity of schizophrenic symptoms in the light of current research. Arch Gen Psychiatry *35:* 811, 1978.

Rado S: Understanding the adaptive struggles of schizophrenic patients. In *Psychopathology of Schizophrenia,* P H Hoch, J Zubin, editors. Grune & Stratton, New York, 1966.

Sartorius N, Jablensky A, Shapiro R: Cross-cultural differences in the short-term prognosis of schizophrenic psychoses. Schizophr Bull *4:* 102, 1978.

Schneider K: *Clinical Psychopathology,* M W Hamilton, translator. Grune & Stratton, New York, 1959.

Seeman P, Guan H-C, Van Tol H H M: Dopamine D4 receptors elevated in schizophrenia. Science *365:* 441, 1993.

Siegel B V, Buchsbaum M S, Bunney W E, Gottschalk L A, Haier R J, Lohr J B, Lottenberg S, Najafi A, Nuechterlein K H, Potkin S G, Wu J C: Cortical-striatal-thalamic circuits and brain glucose metabolic activity in 70 unmedicated male schizophrenic patients. Am J Psychiatry *150:* 1325, 1993.

Stoll A L, Tohen M, Baldessarini R J, Goodwin D C, Stein S, Katz S, Geenens D, Swinson R P, Goethe J W, McGlashan T: Shifts in diagnostic frequencies of schizophrenia and major affective disorders at six North American psychiatric hospitals, 1972–1988. Am J Psychiatry *150:* 1668, 1993.

Volavka J: Schizophrenia and violence. Psychol Med *19:* 559, 1989.

Wing J K, Cooper J E, Sartorius N: *The Measurement and Classification of Psychiatric Symptoms.* Cambridge University Press, Cambridge, England, 1974.

*World Health Organization: *The International Pilot Study of Schizophrenia,* vol 1. World Health Organization, Geneva, 1973.

14.8 SCHIZOPHRENIA: SOMATIC TREATMENT

S. CHARLES SCHULZ, M.D.

INTRODUCTION

Schizophrenia is considered to be one of the most devastating of the psychiatric disorders because of its marked impact on a person's ability to function, and because persons with schizophrenia suffer from frightening perceptions and delusions as well as anxiety and depression. In addition, the families of schizophrenic patients are dramatically affected as parents and siblings try to deal with the troublesome symptoms of the disorder and what they generally describe as the loss of their relative to an illness that robs a person of interpersonal ability. Therefore, comprehensive and appropriate treatments need to be instituted to reduce a patient's suffering from symptoms, to offer the best chance at rehabilitation, and to help those who are close to the patient.

The clinical use of somatic treatments for schizophrenia has been demonstrated through empirical research to decrease symptoms of schizophrenia. In addition, the past decade has brought increased knowledge about the variability of response of schizophrenic patients to somatic treatments, the treatment of refractory and comorbid conditions, and the integration of somatic and psychosocial treatments.

HISTORY

The history of somatic treatments of schizophrenia parallels the history of the various theories regarding the causes of mental illnesses and the frustration of scientists at not being able to discover the causes of mental disorders. During the Middle Ages, when theories of abnormal behavior were grounded in religious dogma, there were no appropriate social or somatic treatments as the insane were frequently the targets of inquisition and execution. Whether for religious or practical reasons, many psychotic persons were locked in prisonlike institutions where therapy was not a consideration.

The movement of moral therapy, which many date to Philippe Pinel's historic unchaining of the insane in Paris in 1792, led to pastoral sites of treatment. Documents of the day indicate pride of the staff of such institutions in the discharge of patients and a hopefulness that mental illness was not an invariably progressive disorder. Of interest are the indications that somatic treatments, such as a relaxation chair, were seen as adding to the therapeutic armamentarium. Another somatic treatment was the technique of dropping patients into cold water as a type of shock technique. It appears that for nearly two centuries the field of psychiatry has been attempting interventions aimed at jarring patients out of their symptoms.

Pharmacology of the 19th century brought amazing advances to the field of medicine with the introduction of morphine as a painkiller and ether as an anesthetic. The mood-altering abilities of the exogenous opiates were soon appreciated, and the hypothesized relationship of the opiate system to schizophrenia remains to this day. In the 1970s there was excitement about the potential of endorphin infusions or opiate antagonists for the treatment of schizophrenia.

Other 19th century advances were the introduction of the bromides as sleeping pills and sedatives and the discovery of barbiturates for the same indication. Sedative pharmacological agents were useful to a field that had no clues as to the cause of schizophrenia and had no treatments specific to the symptoms. However, sedatives dulled the senses and motivations of patients and were thus seen as interfering with other forms of treatment.

In desperation investigators in the first half of the 20th century turned to numerous somatic interventions in hopes of reversing or curing schizophrenia. Removal of the colon was attempted in the early part of this century, based on the theory that impurities had passed into the patient's body. Based on observations that stress increased schizophrenic symptoms, one team of investigators tried removal of the adrenals. That latter dramatic intervention was not successful in helping patients but caught the attention of the legal world and led to significant advances in the cause of informed consent for research.

Since the 1920s some scientists have returned to the idea that symptoms of psychosis may be secondary to an endogenous substance. The first exchange transfusion experiments were conducted during that decade, and although reports of mild success were noted, enthusiasm for the procedure was low. Hemodialysis as a treatment for schizophrenia captured the attention of the field for a few years in the 1970s. Sparked by the report of success of hemodialysis in an open trial, a number of centers tried the treatment while others tested it in controlled trials. Final results of the placebo-controlled studies did not confirm the initial observations, and that somatic treatment is no longer pursued.

Based on a theory that schizophrenia and epilepsy are mutually exclusive, the induction of convulsions to reduce symptoms of schizophrenia was introduced in the 1930s. The theory was not borne out by observation, but by treatment. Electroconvulsive therapy (ECT) is still an effective and safe treatment for mood disorders. Its use in the treatment of schizophrenia has waned since the introduction of the antipsychotic medications, but it may still hold some promise for patients who are not fully responsive to medications.

The induction of coma to treat schizophrenia was a common somatic treatment from the late 1930s to the time of the introduction of the antipsychotic medications and in some parts of the world lingered as a treatment until the 1980s. Although a common treatment for two decades, it was never tested with the scientific rigor that ECT and pharmacological treatments have undergone.

Also prior to the introduction of the antipsychotic agents, psychosurgery (including prefrontal lobotomy) was used frequently on patients with schizophrenia. Although it was observed to calm patients and to make their management easier, there was and remains a repugnance for an irreversible symptomatic treatment. That attitude toward psychosurgery has grown all the more strong since the empirical evidence for the usefulness of antipsychotic agents, both in the specific reduction of psychotic symptoms and the nonspecific decrease in agitation.

Perhaps one of the most significant historic trends of the 20th century has been the schism that still exists between proponents of psychodynamic psychotherapy and those who espouse somatic interventions. During the current century much has been learned that has helped patients with schizophrenia, and there is a noticeably more humane approach to patients than in previous centuries.

With the introduction of antipsychotic medications in the latter half of the 20th century there has been an unprecedented ability to reduce the most serious symptoms of schizophrenia. However, those who propound psychodynamic theories have at times done so to the exclusion of the evidence for the somatic treatments, while those with extreme views on the usefulness of medications have downgraded other forms of treatments as soft. That schism has led to a decrease in the ability of schizophrenic patients to receive the full benefit of attention from the field that is the proponent of their care. Although the schism has diminished in recent years, it is not yet historical. It is hoped that the contributions of both areas of endeavor will be melded in to comprehensive treatment in the future.

The history of the development of antipsychotic medications has been interwoven with the history of somatic treatments for schizophrenia since the discovery of chlorpromazine (Thorazine) in 1949. This first antipsychotic medication was administered to patients with schizophrenia after the medicine had been demonstrated to be a useful sedative in France by Henri Laborit. Over the next few years, it was recognized that the new medicine was not only a sedative but also reduced the symptoms of psychosis. Chlorpromazine was introduced to North America by Heinz Lehman in the early 1950s and was quickly taken into the United States. The late Nathan Kline was awarded the Lasker prize for his work with the antipsychotic medications during that decade. Wide usage of the antipsychotic medications has been credited with the beginning of the dramatic decrease in utilization of psychiatric hospitals in this country.

Demonstration of the usefulness of chlorpromazine led to another phenomenon that has been a hallmark of the past three decades of psychiatric research: the investigation of the mechanism of action of an efficacious drug. With the landmark work in 1963 of Arvid Carlsson and M. Lindqvist, who noted the impact of antipsychotic medication on dopamine metabolism, the field of psychiatry has utilized the strategy of investigating how medications work as they try to discover the etiology of schizophrenia. Now with agents such as clozapine (Clozaril), investigators are using similar strategies to discover clues to its cause.

At the beginning of the era of discovery of pharmacological agents (tricyclic antidepressants and benzodiazepines, soon followed the discovery of antipsychotic medications) there was the important emphasis on the use of the controlled clinical trial to investigate the efficacy of the new agents. The initial trials, sponsored by the National Institute of Mental Health, demonstrated the efficacy over placebo, and subsequent studies by Philip May showed the newly introduced antipsychotic medications to be better than insight-oriented psychotherapy, milieu therapy, and electroconvulsive therapy. The controlled clinical trial has been the backbone for the continued development of somatic treatments from the demonstration of clozapine as an efficacious treatment of refractory patients to trials demonstrating the usefulness of combined medication and psychosocial interventions.

CLINICAL USE OF ANTIPSYCHOTIC MEDICATIONS

Currently, the antipsychotic medications are the mainstay of somatic treatments for schizophrenia. Treatments used before the discovery of antipsychotic drugs are no longer used in the acute stages of treatment.

DIAGNOSIS It is clearly recognized that the antipsychotic medications are useful in treating many forms of psychosis ranging from psychotic features of a mood disorder to anesthesia-induced psychotic disorder. However, the extended use of antipsychotic medications is generally limited to schizophrenia. Because of that and because there are other very useful and safe medications (such as lithium [Eskalith]) for bipolar I disorder, it is important to be accurate in the diagnostic formulation of the psychotic patient suspected of having schizophrenia. There must be careful and thoughtful discussion with the patient and the family to elicit symptoms and course of illness. Utilization of the fourth edition of *Diagnostic and Statistical Manual of Mental Disorders* (DSM-IV) is important to avoid idiosyncratic diagnostic practices and needless assignment of a patient to antipsychotic medication. In patients with psychotic disorders the initial diagnosis does not always pertain throughout the illness, so that each clinician should remain vigilant for changes in symptom patterns or the emergence of new symptoms that would change the diagnostic impression. Also, it appears that psychiatry is changing in its philosophy of nosology from a pattern of parsimonious diagnosis to a pattern of multiple or comorbid diagnoses. That change may hold special relevance for somatic treatments, as recent trials have shown combined medication treatments to be of superior efficacy for comorbid schizophrenia and depression.

Evaluation for somatic causes of a schizophrenialike disorders (for example, schizophreniform disorder and psychotic disorders due to temporal lobe epilepsy, vitamin B12 deficiency, and tumors) remains critical. The use of structural imaging can be an invaluable aid in the assessment of psychosis. Furthermore, testing on admission to inpatient service for the presence of psychotomimetic agents, such as cocaine, cannot be ignored.

The increased impact of controlled clinical trials and the various editions of DSM have made the field more aware of structured diagnostic instruments used for research. Such instruments provide scientists with the documentation and routine essential for research and can even be useful in practice for training and documentation. They do not serve as a substitute for the establishment of a relationship with the patient and the family and assessment of other information that may assist in evaluation.

ASSESSMENTS The assessment of change after the initiation of medication treatment can appear complicated because of the diversity of the patient's feelings and behavior. Because there are many ways that a person can be diagnosed as having schizophrenia; listing the target symptoms and assessing them at regular intervals has been a recommended strategy. Target symptoms, such as multiple voices commenting on the patient's behavior, should be clearly described and able to be elicited by other examiners. Target symptoms that call on the inference of the clinician or are complex tend to be less reliable.

During the past 10 years, there has been an increase in attention to negative symptoms of schizophrenia: those symptoms that represent an absence of a function. Such symptoms as the loss of usual affect, anhedonia, and amotivation had been felt to be not amenable to change. Recent investigations have shown that such symptoms may change during the course of antipsychotic treatment by either improving or worsening. However, inclusion of negative symptoms in the target list may prove helpful to the clinician following schizophrenic patients over the long term.

Rating scales of behavior and emotions have been used for a number of decades in the conduct of medication trials of all types of medications, including the antipsychotic drugs. In clinical trials such scales provide objective measures of change over time and are generally constructed to address the major symptoms of the disorder in question. As medication studies have become a larger part of the psychiatric literature, psychiatrists are more aware of their usage and have incorporated them into practice. Some scales of symptoms, such as the Hopkins Symptom Checklist-90, are instruments completed by the patient, whereas other scales call for the clinician to address the symptoms and decide on the rated value. The Brief Psychiatric Rating Scale (BPRS) is an example of the latter and has been used as the major repeated assessment tool of most studies of antipsychotic medication. The use of a rating scale such as the BPRS may be useful to the clinician, but there are two caveats to be considered: (1) that the clinician receive training in the use of the instrument; and (2) that both the patient and clinician recognize that the scale is not a substitute for a relationship.

The emphasis on symptom reduction in the use of somatic treatments had diminished interest in the quality of life of patients with schizophrenia. During the past decade, however, first with investigation of quality of life associated with dose-lowering strategies, and then with atypical antipsychotic treatments, there has been renewed interest in that parameter of treatment. Assessment of quality of life has been addressed by rating scales for reasons of objectively and quantitatively examining the effects of treatments. Such scales as the Quality of Life Scale developed at the Maryland Psychiatric Research Center address satisfaction with life role, function in employment, and with the family. Whether a rating scale is employed or those issues are part of assessment and therapy, they clearly belong as part of the comprehensive treatment of the patient with schizophrenia.

The assessment of comorbid symptoms, such as depression and panic, are of equal importance, especially as there is evidence for their reduction with augmenting medications. In addition awareness of the potential for suicide is a crucial part of the clinician's responsibility. Estimates of the prevalence of completed suicides in the United States range from 10 to 17 percent of schizophrenic patients. The group at highest risk appears to be patients in the first five years of their illness who are experiencing hopelessness about their disorder. Recognition of depression and an assessment of suicidality are part of the assessment process.

Substance abuse in all psychiatric patients, including those with schizophrenia, cannot be ignored, as several reports have indicated that there is a high prevalence on admission and at clinic visits. Obviously, many drugs of abuse can mimic psychiatric symptoms, including psychosis, panic, and mania. Awareness of the possibility and discussion with the patient and his or her family is a start in the evaluation and ongoing assessment of patients with schizophrenia. Laboratory screening of urine or blood may aid in the detection of illegal drug use, with the testing conducted in a helpful rather than policing manner. Somatic treatments for substance abuse are not in common use at this time in a field that may be in its formative stages. Some patients may be using illegal drugs to self-medicate. For example, schizophrenic patients may use marijuana to calm anxiety or panic, while others with feelings of depression may use cocaine. Use of prescribed drugs to treat depression may be helpful in this situation.

ANTIPSYCHOTIC MEDICATIONS When first introduced, the antipsychotic medications were termed major tranquilizers in comparison to the antianxiety medications of the day, such as meprobamate (Miltown). Shortly thereafter, especially after the relationship of antipsychotic medications to dopamine neurotransmission was established, the medications were frequently termed neuroleptics. That term was also used because of the then-observed invariable association of neurological side effects and antipsychotic medication treatment. Currently, the medications are called antipsychotic medications, although a change in terms could occur. With the demonstration of the efficacy of clozapine an antipsychotic medication without movement disorder side effects, the term atypical antipsychotic medication was first used, and the older medications were then referred to as ''atypical antipsychotics.'' As new strategies for antipsychotic medication development have been employed by pharmaceutical companies, other agents with actions different from both the typical medications and from the archetypal atypical agent, clozapine, will appear. Continued drug development will lead to further refinement of nomenclature.

The early trials of antipsychotic medications were frequently designed to test whether antipsychotics were equivalent to psychotherapy. Following landmark studies by Philip May and then Lester Grinspoon it became clear that the antipsychotic medications are the mainstay of the treatment of schizophrenia. Currently, there is not another somatic treatment that is indicated before beginning a trial of antipsychotic medications. Also, there is no empirical support for the use of a psychosocial intervention before or without antipsychotic medication treatment. Recently there has been investigation into the possibility that the length of time before antipsychotic medication treatment may have a negative influence on long-term outcome. Although not conclusive, such a theory would indicate that it is not appropriate to have a long period between diagnosis of schizophrenia and initiation of antipsychotic medication treatment. Therefore, in the early stages of treatment, the decisions about antipsychotic medication treatment is not whether to use, but which agent, at which dose. Strategies for long-term care can follow later.

Selection of specific medication During the period of the development of antipsychotic medications, a number of claims were made for the efficacy of specific antipsychotic medications. The medications that were sedating were thought to be best for agitated patients, whereas withdrawn patients were thought to do best with nonsedating or activating agents. Neither empirical research nor investigations of mechanism of action of the antipsychotic medications have supported such a view. It is now believed that the antipsychotic medications are of equal efficacy when used at equipotent doses. As there is no reason to pick one antipsychotic medication over another based on efficacy, the initial decision is based on side-effect profiles of the medications.

During the acute stage of treatment or during acute exacerbations of schizophrenia there are various philosophies for the choice of antipsychotic medications. Many psychiatrists now lean toward the initiation of the nonsedating antipsychotic medications because patients complain about sedation and because it is easier to measure a patient's progress when they are not sedated. Also, because the nonsedating drugs are less likely to cause hypotension, they are frequently preferred in the older population. Concerning initial selection of an antipsychotic medication for the very agitated and out-of-control patient, studies have shown that nonsedating agents are as efficacious and may be preferred to high doses of sedating medications.

Despite the statements about nonsedating agents, there are situations in which an antipsychotic medication of medium potency (for example, trifluoperazine [Stelazine] or perphenazine [Etrafon]) may be employed. It has been repeatedly observed that young male schizophrenic patients have difficulty with the dystonic and parkinsonian side effects of the high-potency agents and that midpotency agents can be started for them.

Early in the treatment of patients with schizophrenia, some patients may exhibit neuroleptic intolerance to the initial medication chosen—an event that occurs more frequently with high-potency medications. Neuroleptic intolerance is a term used to describe side effects such as akathisia and parkinsonism that are so troubling that the dose of antipsychotic medication cannot be raised to the point that a fair trial of the drug can be made. Changing to a medium-potency medication can be useful in some, but not all, of such cases.

Dosing strategies The past decade has seen intense research interest in the dosing strategies for the treatment of schizophrenia with a focus on utilization of the lowest effective dose of antipsychotic medication. Perhaps because of the large margin of safety of the antipsychotic medications, doses in the United States for the treatment of schizophrenia were very much higher than those used in other countries around the world. In addition, during the 1970s a dosing strategy termed "rapid neuroleptization" was described that posited that by frequent doses of antipsychotic medications resulting in high initial doses, patients would benefit faster than by usual strategies. Based on similar strategies using digitalis or phenytoin, the strategy was attractive, but empirical research did not support its use. Interestingly, as research of the rapid neuroleptization strategy was conducted, the equal efficacy of usual doses (500 chlorpromazine equivalents per day or haloperidol [Haldol] 10 milligrams [mg] per day) was demonstrated. Such studies also underscored an important point about time to response to antipsychotic medication: that a four- to five-week period of treatment was needed for significant reduction in symptoms no matter what the dose. That research has led to two tenets about the use of antipsychotic medication: (1) that high doses of medication are not needed and may confer extra side effects; and (2) response to treatment is time-dependent, and changing doses upward quickly is not necessary.

Currently, a beginning dose of medication is selected that gives the patient a fair trial of the drug (not so low that symptoms are not treated and not so high as to lead to unnecessary side effects). An analysis of studies of antipsychotic medications indicates that below 300 chlorpromazine equivalents, the medications are no more successful than placebo. Beginning doses in the range of 300 to 500 chlorpromazine equivalents is considered by many as a usual procedure. Dosing may then be increased or decreased depending on side effects or less than full response to treatment.

In many areas of medicine as well as in psychiatry blood levels of medication are used to guide dosing. Most familiar to psychiatrists is the use of lithium levels to assist in dosing decisions and monitoring of medication for safety. Many studies have investigated the possibility that measuring concentrations of antipsychotic medications could aid in dosing strategies. Such studies have centered attention on a concept of the therapeutic window hypothesis. That hypothesis states that low doses and high doses are less effective than an optimal dose. Therefore, even though there is not a perfectly predictable relationship between dose and blood level, the blood level could be measured to achieve optimal dosing. To date such studies have been equivocal, although there is suggestive evidence that a therapeutic window exists.

Other research groups have pointed out that perhaps the therapeutic window pattern of response in patients occurs because of increased side effects of the higher doses. Such investigators would posit that poor symptomatic improvement at higher doses (or blood levels) is secondary to the stress and discomfort of neuroleptic-induced acute akathisia and neuroleptic-induced parkinsonism.

In practice, measurement of blood levels is used infrequently. Some feel that blood testing might be used more often, especially in the assessment of the poorly responsive patient. When used to evaluate treatment response, a range of medication concentration of 5 to 15 nanograms per milliliter of haloperidol may be considered. Case reports and some studies have indicated that poor response may occur with medication blood levels far below the therapeutic range or far above it. The clinician embarking on using medication levels in practice would need to be familiar with the metabolism of the medication he or she is using and aware of the accuracy of laboratory measurement of the drug.

Transition to maintenance treatment After symptoms have been reduced during the acute stage of treatment the transition to maintenance medication is started. The early evidence of the efficacy of antipsychotic medication focused on the acute phase of the illness, and it was not until later that the importance of continued somatic treatment was appreciated. It has been demonstrated in controlled clinical trials that nearly 80 percent of patients assigned to placebo in a study of maintenance treatment will relapse in the first year. Therefore, continued medication treatment is the rule rather than the exception.

Lower doses of medication can be used to help keep symptoms at the level of that achieved with acute treatment—on the order of 150 to 200 chlorpromazine equivalents. Also, following a few weeks of divided dose regimens, oral medication during the maintenance phase of treatment can be taken once a day, usually in the evening, because of the long half-life of the antipsychotic medications. Such a strategy can help diminish missed doses and may also decrease some side effects.

Many patients continue to use oral medication during the maintenance phase of the illness; however, long-lasting injectable medication is frequently used during the maintenance phase of treatment. The first injectable medication—fluphenazine decanoate (Prolixin Decanoate)—is a preparation of an antipsychotic medication dissolved in an oil that allows for slow release of the active medication. Initially, injectable medication was used for patients who were noncompliant with their oral regimen. That has changed in recent years as the convenience of injectable medications has become more apparent. Now there is a second injectable medication—haloperidol decanoate—which gives the clinician more options in designing treatment, as once-a-month dosing is recommended.

Numerous recent studies have indicated that, as with acute treatment of psychosis in the United States, many patients may have been receiving more medication than was needed to keep their symptoms under control. Whereas many patients were started on fluphenazine decanoate at 25 mg intramuscularly every two weeks, research has demonstrated that 12.5 mg every two weeks is as effective for some patients. In addition the strategies of lower doses have led to decreased side effects for patients who can be managed in that way.

In the management of schizophrenic patients with injectable medications adjustment of dosage should be done slowly, as the time from dose change to change of blood level of the medication is long—on the order of 3 months. Rapid changes in the injectable medications does not make sense. Some recent work in the field has indicated that the addition of oral medication during a crisis may be more useful.

In attempts to use the least amount of medication some research sites have investigated the use of intermittent strategies during the maintenance phase of treatment. Such an approach would utilize the appearance of prodromal symptoms to reinitiate antipsychotic medications. To date controlled trials have not supported the usefulness of that strategy to reduce medication exposure and forestall relapse.

Persistently psychotic patients Despite the statistical evidence that the antipsychotic medications are more effective than placebo in the acute treatment of schizophrenia and that they prevent relapse during maintenance treatment, nearly one third of the schizophrenic patients given an adequate trial of medication remain persistently psychotic. Poor response to medication is a significant problem in psychiatry because such patients require increased hospitalization, are probably more frequently homeless, and still suffer from disabling symptoms. Recently, there has been significant interest in attempting to understand the nature of the problem of poor response and to identify treatments.

Although research into the problem of chronic illness is by no means new, the research utilizing brain imaging has led to renewed interest in this area. Research a decade ago indicated that patients with enlarged ventricles on computed tomographic scans had a poorer response to medication. Other correlates of poor response were also identified such as neurological soft signs: poor performance on neuropsychological testing, family history of schizophrenia, abnormal electroencephalogram (EEG), changes in blood levels of homovanillic acid during the early stage of antipsychotic treatment, and altered response to stimulant challenge (both behavioral and neuroendocrinological). No characteristic has been shown to be pathognomonic of poor response, but research indicates that one or perhaps multiple characteristics that may indicate increased brain dysfunction are associated with persistent illness. As such research progresses, it is hoped that the prediction of medication response can become more accurate.

The initial approach to the patient who is persistently ill is to ensure that he or she has had a complete evaluation of the illness and does not suffer from an underlying disease causing a schizophrenialike psychosis. The next step is to ensure that the person has had an adequate trial of antipsychotic medication. Considerable progress has been made since the trials of clozapine were begun in the United States in the early 1980s. Now most treatment centers consider that an adequate trial of antipsychotic medication includes trials of two or three different medications given at dosages of least 1,000 chlorpromazine equivalents, for at four to six weeks each. Further, poor response is considered to be characterized by BPRS scores of greater than 35 and a Clinical Global Impression score of 4 (a score indicating moderate illness). Such characteristics are part of the research of the past decade and have not yet been completely translated into clinical practice. For example, there is no empirical evidence that changing to another class of antipsychotic medication will change response, which is not surprising as the typical antipsychotic medications exert their therapeutic action through dopamine blockade. Also, the BPRS score is not directly related to the debility of a patient, so that the clinician needs to make a complicated decision about proceeding to further somatic treatments of the persistently ill patient.

The approach to the poorly responsive patient is currently in a stage of flux because of the explosion in research of the atypical antipsychotic medications. Because of the risk of agranulocytosis (1 to 1.5 percent) with the use of clozapine, the choice of whether to move forward with clozapine or to begin with augmenting medications is not settled. Also, there has been no empirical trial of clozapine versus an augmenting strategy to inform the decision.

AUGMENTING AGENTS TO ANTIPSYCHOTIC TREATMENT

Psychiatry has had an interesting history in its view of combining medications to achieve optimal response. In the early era of psychopharmacology combined medication strategies were common. However, as the understanding of how the medications worked improved, it became clear that medicines with the same action were being given at the same time, thus conferring only increased susceptibility to side effects. Also, medications with opposite effects were being given together. An interesting example of the latter was the preparation of chlorpromazine and amphetamine. For some time the use of multiple agents was frowned on and given the name polypharmacy. Clinicians were trained to avoid the situation. Starting in the 1970s, however, a number of investigators began to explore whether adding non-neuroleptic agents to the regular medication could improve response. Most trials indicated an advantage of the augmenting agent over control conditions. The tested medication augmentation strategies are summarized in (Table 14.8-1). In the treatment of schizophrenia the use of augmenting strategies is viewed as a conservative first approach to poor response of the patient to antipsychotic medications.

LITHIUM Shortly after the introduction of lithium in the United States, Joyce Small and colleagues demonstrated that a significant proportion of schizophrenic patients in a state hospital benefitted when lithium was added to their antipsychotic regimen. Her group also noted that the combination was safe and that psychosis, not just agitation, was reduced with the augmenting treatment. All of the other controlled trials have confirmed that initial observation to a greater or lesser degree.

When lithium is used usual doses and serum levels are aimed for. Some clinicians find that when lithium is administered, the dose of antipsychotic medication can be reduced. Also, there may be increased sedation. Because there have been no longitudinal studies for the administration of lithium as part of such an augmentation strategy, a conservative approach would indicate that finding the lowest dose of the antipsychotic drug and perhaps occasional trials off lithium could be indicated for long-term treatment. One of the clinical trials of the augmentation strategy examined the effects of discontinuing the antipsychotic medication after improvement was seen with the combination of drugs. Return of symptoms was seen in three of the four patients, leading to the conclusion that the medications were synergistic. Not all recent controlled studies of lithium aug-

TABLE 14.8-1
Augmenting Agents Added to Antipsychotic Medication in Persistently Psychotic Patients

Medication	Dose (Blood Level)	Indications	Side Effects	Comments
Lithium	900–1,800 mg/day (0.8–10 mEq/L)	Persistent psychosis, schizoaffective disorder	Neuropathological effects may be more likely with high neuroleptic dose	Can reduce both excitement and psychosis
Carbamazepine	200–500 mg/8 hours (4–10 mg/mL)	Persistent psychosis with aggression, abnormal electroencephalogram	Carbamazepine lowers haloperidol concentrations in blood	Monitoring of carbamazepine and antipsychotic blood concentrations useful
Benzodiazepines	Alprazolam 2.5 mg/day (average dose)	Persistent psychosis, behavioral management after adequate neuroleptic dose, comorbid panic	Possible disinhibition, difficulty discontinuing	Useful agent in early management
Reserpine	1.5–3.5 mg/day	Persistent psychosis	Hypotension, depression	Little controlled trial evidence
Electroconvulsive therapy	Same as for mood disorder; maintenance may be indicated	Persistent psychosis, schizoaffective disorder	Anesthesia effects	Still few controlled trials, outpatient maintenance may hold promise

mentation have confirmed the earlier reports; that may be the result of improved diagnostic practices or other factors.

Although a number of reports have noted the safety of combining lithium with antipsychotic medications, patients administered the combination should be closely observed for tremor and stiffness. High doses of antipsychotic drugs while using lithium should probably be avoided.

CARBAMAZEPINE As the psychoactive properties of carbamazepine were increasingly appreciated following reports of its usefulness in bipolar I disorder, investigators interested in schizophrenia began to examine its use. By itself carbamazepine does not seem to relieve symptoms of schizophrenia. In the early 1980s some groups noted that by using carbamazepine as an augmenting agent, symptoms of schizophrenia could be reduced. Further analysis of the characteristics of patients most successfully treated indicated that those who exhibited violent behavior or who had an abnormal EEG appeared to benefit the most. Studies of persistently psychotic patients who did not have those characteristics did not show consistent advantage over placebo.

In using carbamazepine as an augmenting agent the clinician must remember that blood levels of the medication need to be monitored. Doses of carbamazepine that produce blood levels that are appropriate for anticonvulsant treatment are used. Carbamazepine is a medication that induces an acceleration in its own metabolism, so that levels need to be serially monitored. In addition to known pharmacokinetic factors some reports have indicated that carbamazepine can lead to reduced levels of the antipsychotic medication haloperidol. Those findings indicate that monitoring of the antipsychotic medication would also be important.

BENZODIAZEPINES Benzodiazepines are known to increase γ-aminobutyric acid (GABA) activity in the brain and thus theoretically could reduce dopaminergic overactivity. There have been reports over the years that benzodiazepines are helpful when used in the acute phases of schizophrenia; therefore, they were tried in combination with antipsychotic drugs for those who were persistently ill. Reports of the strategy to date indicate that the addition of benzodiazepines can be useful and in addition there are thoughts that negative symptoms of schizophrenia may also decrease.

High doses of benzodiazepines are not needed to utilize the strategy, and in one of the larger trials in which alprazolam was tested, efficacious doses were in the range of 2.5 mg. One of the concerns of those who have worked with the augmenting strategy is that there may be a rebound in psychotic symptoms when benzodiazepines are withdrawn. That may not be a problem for the successfully treated patient, but tapering benzodiazepines in the patient who does not benefit can take weeks. When using benzodiazepines with a short half-life, sudden withdrawal should be avoided.

RESERPINE By itself reserpine (Serpasil) is known to have antipsychotic properties, but it is also well known for its ability to lead to symptoms of depression. Therefore, it has not been used as an antipsychotic by itself. Occasional reports of its usefulness as an augmenting agent have been seen in recent years, but the old problem of depression with reserpine use remains. In addition as reserpine is an effective antihypertensive, some patients are unable to tolerate its hypotensive effects.

ECT ECT has been used to treat schizophrenia since the 1930s. Prior to the introduction of the antipsychotic medications, it was used successfully by itself for the reduction of symptoms of schizophrenia. Even after antipsychotic medications were in wide use, it was extensively used, and perhaps the most rigorous trial of ECT versus antipsychotics and psychotherapy found it useful, but not as effective as antipsychotic medications, for acutely ill patients. The treatment effect for schizophrenia was found to be transient after the first weeks of treatment in acute cases, so that as the need for maintenance treatment became more clear, ECT was used less. It should also be noted that during the 1960s and 1970s there was less emphasis on somatic treatments, so that even though ECT was effective for some patients with schizophrenia and new techniques increased its safety, it was rarely performed in some areas of the United States.

With the increased recognition of the suffering of persistently psychotic patients attention has again turned to ECT. A few small and uncontrolled trials of have indicated that for persistently ill patients it can reduce psychotic symptoms in the short term. When used with antipsychotics, there may be some more sustained improvement in some cases. Further research is needed for that special class of schizophrenic patients.

AUGMENTING STRATEGIES FOR PATIENTS WITH COMORBID DISORDERS

Conflicting views about the use of medications from more than one class have been prominent over the past three decades. During the period of introduction of the antipsychotic and antidepressant medications, combinations were marketed to treat a number of complex symptom patterns. Later, the field turned to specific medications for specific disorders—rightly so, as it appears that antipsychotic medications were overused in non-schizophrenic disorders. However, combinations of medications for such entities as major depression with psychotic features have shown that antipsychotic and antidepressant medications together are superior to the use of either alone.

Since the introduction of the third edition of DSM (DSM-III) and continuing with DSM-IV and the ensuing structured interviews, there has been a recognition of the phenomenon of comorbidity. Empirical trials of medication combinations have been performed in the past decade that indicate that the strategy is useful and bears further expansion.

The most extensively studied comorbid condition is that of schizophrenia and depression. Results of controlled trials indicate that the addition of a classic tricyclic antidepressant to antipsychotic medication can reduce symptoms of depression without increasing the symptoms of psychosis. As the morbidity of depression with schizophrenia is severe and there may even be increased mortality in this comorbid condition, the strategy should be carefully considered in such patients. Preliminary, but not controlled, trials of newer antidepressants (such as fluoxetine [Prozac]) indicate their usefulness, and those may become the treatment of choice as there is less cholinergic effect and significantly less lethal effect if used in an overdose attempt.

Benzodiazepine antianxiety medications have been shown over three decades to be useful as an adjunctive treatment for persistent psychosis. With attention to the concept of comorbidity, some groups have noted that some schizophrenic patients fulfill criteria for panic disorder and that the use of added benzodiazepines help reduce the symptoms of panic. That area is far from fully established but warrants consideration with such patients.

Comorbidity with substance abuse has been widely recognized and perhaps just as widely ignored by pharmacologic investigators. As different substances of abuse have different actions (for example, alcohol has a sedative effect and cocaine has a stimulating effect), patients with schizophrenia and substance abuse probably are composed of many subtypes. Recognition that patients abusing illicit drugs may be trying to relieve untreated symptoms may help guide future studies. Currently, there is no recognized somatic approach to such patients.

ATYPICAL ANTIPSYCHOTIC MEDICATION

In 1990 a new antipsychotic medication, clozapine, was introduced in the United States after extensive testing as a treatment of last resort for persistently psychotic patients with schizophrenia. In addition to the excitement and controversy regarding whether the new medication could be helpful to treatment-resistant patients, there was significant interest in the new drug because it could reduce symptoms of psychosis without causing movement disorder side effects. Therefore, it was labeled an atypical antipsychotic medication, because it had antipsychotic activity without neuroleptic effects. When testing of clozapine demonstrated that antipsychotic activity was not inexorably linked to the process of neurological side effects, a number of pharmaceutical companies began to investigate novel compounds that acted in new ways. Some of those medications, which are in development, are also termed atypical antipsychotic medications even if they do have some movement side effects. Some experimental compounds have clozapinelike activities, while others seem to act with fewer side effects by being more specific for dopamine type 2 receptor blocking than the traditional antipsychotic medications. A clear consensus of a nosology of the new medications has not been reached, but will complicate our understanding of the antipsychotic agents for some time to come.

The second atypical antipsychotic medication to be released in the United States was risperidone (Risperdal). Trials in Europe were encouraging as they showed the new medication to be efficacious in decreasing symptoms of schizophrenia while being less likely to cause extrapyramidal side effects. A recent multicenter trial in the United States has confirmed and extended those findings. Controlled trials addressing risperidone as a treatment of last resort have as yet to be completed.

CLOZAPINE First tested in the 1970s, clozapine was found at that time to be an efficacious if not superior antipsychotic medication as compared with the traditional drugs. Although a number of cases of fatal agranulocytosis in Finland led some countries, including the United States, to withdraw the medication and to stop testing, interest in the drug continued around the world and led to a treatment of last resort trial in the 1980s that showed that carefully characterized treatment nonresponders did well on clozapine. The large multicenter trial reported by John Kane and colleagues demonstrated that 33 percent of patients who had previously been unresponsive met criteria for response after six weeks of clozapine treatment. Other trials from around the world have indicated that schizophrenic patients who are poorly responsive to traditional antipsychotic medications who receive the medication sooner or have a trial longer than six weeks show higher rates of response. It is now clear that psychiatrists treating patients with schizophrenia should be familiar with the use of clozapine and its indications.

Clozapine treatment In the United States clozapine treatment is indicated for those patients who are poorly responsive to traditional antipsychotic medication treatment. Many investigators and clinicians use the guidelines of the multicenter study that defined that three antipsychotics from different classes be given in adequate doses. Some clinicians would further state that neuroleptic intolerance—the phenomenon of the patient having intolerable side effects at doses below those that would provide an adequate trial—and severe persistent neuroleptic-induced tardive dyskinesia constitute a rationale for clozapine treatment. It should be noted that outside the United States many countries use clozapine much earlier in the process of poor response. Also, there is currently no empirical study of the role of augmentation strategies prior to a clozapine trial.

When clozapine is indicated, careful physical and laboratory evaluation should be performed, focusing on the assessment of hematological status and history, neurological history (especially history of seizures), and cardiac evaluation including electrocardiography and blood pressure. During the period of time that clozapine was used in the United States in compassionate use protocols, washout periods were indicated. Now, after significant clinical use, simultaneous transition from typical agents is frequently performed. Some caveats of the beginning stage of clozapine are that nonsedating traditional agents be used at the lowest dose that helps in symptom reduction. Other medications that may have been used should be discontinued.

Because of the sedation and hypotension caused by clozapine, the initial dosing strategy is different from the usual strategy for traditional drugs. Beginning with 12.5 mg to 25 mg on the first day of treatment, dosing is increased by 25 mg per day as tolerated by the patient. The side effects to be monitored during the period of dose increase are mostly sedation and blood pressure, as those effects limit increases to usual therapeutic doses. For most patients, 250 to 300 mg per day of clozapine significantly reduces symptoms. Some patients have been found to require less, while others may have their best response when a dose of 900 mg per day is achieved. Empirical titration is currently the best method to find the lowest effective dose. To date the levels of clozapine have not provided further guidance in dosing, but it could be expected that blood level measurements could determine patients who do not have amounts of medication in their bloodstream that are effective.

Because of the side effect of agranulocytosis, most clinical users of clozapine felt that a short trial of clozapine was indicated so that if a person was not a responder, he or she would not be unnecessarily exposed to the potential of a serious side effect. Further studies have indicated that such a response may not occur until 12 or 24 weeks from starting the drug, so that an adequate trial may be longer than originally thought.

Almost all patients who have been tried on clozapine and had the medication discontinued because of agranulocytosis or other side effects have not done well on traditional antipsychotic medications, indicating that once clozapine response has been achieved, the medication needs to be continued indefinitely.

Recent reports have indicated that patients who are diagnosed as having schizoaffective disorder and have been refractory to treatment do well with clozapine. At this time such reports are considered preliminary, but hopeful, for patients with that difficulty.

An important point in the treatment of persistently ill patients is the psychosocial support needed for the re-entry period. Families and patients require understanding as they deal with issues related to long hospitalizations and persistent disability.

Clozapine mechanism of action Because clozapine is clinically effective without the side effect of movement disorder, there has been intense interest in exploring the mechanism of action of clozapine. Investigators think that by understanding how the atypical drugs (such as clozapine) work, they may find clues to the pathophysiology of schizophrenia. Currently, investigators are examining hypotheses focused on regional specificity of atypical antipsychotic medications. That hypothesis states that the atypical medications preferentially act on limbic areas of the brain, which may be the relevant dopamine tracks involved in schizophrenia. Other investigators have noted that the atypical medications interact with the dopamine and serotonin systems in ways that are different from the typical drugs. That observation has led to hypothesis about the balance of dopamine and serotonin in the pathophysiology of schizophrenia.

RISPERIDONE TREATMENT Risperidone is the first atypical antipsychotic medication to be released for the first line treatment of schizophrenia. As with the other medications previously described careful assessment needs to be performed prior to treatment. Although controlled trials of risperidone indicate that a dose of 6 mg per day is optimal, clinicians using the new medication still begin at a lower dose to assess for efficacy and raise the dose to the range of 6 to 8 mg per day if needed.

Side effects to be noted include orthostatic hypotension during the early stage of treatment. Tachycardia can be seen as well. Extrapyramidal symptoms are observed in some cases, including tremor, akathisia, and rigidity. Agranulocytosis has not been associated with risperidone.

SIDE EFFECTS OF ANTIPSYCHOTIC MEDICATIONS

The use of antipsychotic medications has constituted a revolution in the treatment of patients with schizophrenia, but the side effects of the medications are significant, ranging from mild to moderate discomfort to permanent movement disorders. The side effects of antipsychotic medications can be subdivided into neurological and nonneurological groups (Table 14.8-2).

NEUROLOGICAL SIDE EFFECTS AND THEIR MANAGEMENT Neurological side effects that are the most common involve the blockade of basal ganglia dopamine receptors. Those side effects are relatively time dependant, and anticipation of their appearance can lead to timely early intervention or to prevention.

Neuroleptic-induced acute dystonia appears in the very early stages of neuroleptic treatment, especially in the neuroleptically naive patient. Dystonic reactions to antipsychotic medication are characterized by muscle spasms in discrete groups, such as the neck or eye muscles: torticollis or oculogyric crisis, respectively. Because the side effect occurs at the initiation of treatment in psychotic patients, it can lead to noncompliance with medications and with other treatment. Therefore, some clinicians start treatment of never-medicated schizophrenic patients by also administering anticholinergic agents to minimize the reaction. Others think that the most appropriate strategy is to be observant and to treat dystonia quickly after its emergence and then to begin anticholinergic medications only in those who have a dystonic reaction or develop parkinsonian side effects. Either approach is acceptable and is superior to being unaware and allowing a dystonic reaction to go untreated. It must also be noted that a case report exists implicating haloperidol at a very high dose (200 mg per day) in laryngeal dystonia and resulting sudden death.

TABLE 14.8-2
Side Effects of Antipsychotic Medications (Typical Agents)

Symptom or Syndrome	Intervention
Neurological	
Dystonia	Benadryl (diphenhydramine) intramuscular or intravenous; begin anti-Parkinson treatment
Parkinsonism	Anticholinergic or dopamine-stimulating medication; use lowest effective dose of antipsychotic drug
Tardive dyskinesia	Lowest effective dose, clozapine in selected cases
Akathisia	β-blocker treatment, consider lower potency agent
Seizure	Evaluation for cause, anticonvulsant treatment
Neuroleptic malignant syndrome	Immediate discontinuation of antipsychotic drug, close observation and supportive care, consider dopamine agonist, may restart antipsychotic under close observation
Nonneurological	
Sedation	Change to nonsedating agent or to lower dose
Hypotension (severe hypotension)	Change to nonsedating agent, use norepinephrine or phenylephrine
Jaundice	Evaluate for other causes of liver illness, change to another agent
Retinitis pigmentosa	Avoid high doses of thioridazine (Mellaril)
Galactorrhea	Consider bromocriptine

When dystonic symptoms occur, they can be relieved by the use of diphenhydramine (Benadryl) intramuscularly or intravenously. Following acute treatment, the use of an anticholinergic medication should be instituted to prevent return of symptoms. Some clinicians have also indicated that the use of mid-potency antipsychotic medications may be useful in prevention of dystonic reactions in schizophrenic patients, especially teenagers, even though there are no clinical trials to support this practice.

Neuroleptic-induced parkinsonism is frequently observed after the initial weeks of treatment with antipsychotic medication and symptomatically resemble Parkinson's disease: shuffling gait, masked facies, muscle stiffness, and drooling. In many patients the presentation may be subtle; thus, careful observation of the patient is important, as he or she may be somewhat unaware of the syndrome.

Treatment of early drug-induced movement disorders can be approached by using the lowest effective dose of medication that abates psychosis. That strategy may not work in all cases, so that antiparkinsonian medications, such as the anticholinergic drugs, are used (Table 14.8-2). Because of concerns that the anticholinergic medications may mask the ability of the clinician to detect symptoms of tardive dyskinesia and because of concerns about cognitive effects of anticholinergic medications, the need for such medications should be monitored closely. That may involve collaborating with the patient in stopping antiparkinsonian drugs. In the past decade there has been significant work on the use of dopamine receptor-stimulating medications to treat parkinsonian side effects. Medications such as amantadine (Symmetrel) have been the most frequently used and offer advantages of not causing cholinergic side effects. Interestingly, use of those dopamine stimulating agents does not appear to exacerbate psychosis.

Neuroleptic-induced tardive dyskinesia is a late-appearing side effect of antipsychotic medications, although there are reports of its emergence in the first year of treatment. Tardive dyskinesia is characterized by abnormal involuntary movements that are slowly rhythmic or choreatic. In some instances tardive dystonia characterized by a stiff posturing of a muscle group may be observed, such as an unusual carrying angle of the arm or hand. Perhaps the most common onset of tardive dyskinesia is abnormal mouth movements: lip-smacking or tongue-protrusion. Tardive dyskinesia is the most carefully studied of the antipsychotic medication side effects, and occurs in 4 percent of the patients per year. After a seven-year period there may be a plateau of incidence, and epidemiological studies indicate that approximately one quarter of treated patients will develop tardive dyskinesia. Although even low doses of antipsychotic medication have been associated with tardive dyskinesia, use of the lowest effective dose is recommended as a preventative measure. Also, as patients with an affective disorder are more susceptible to tardive dyskinesia, careful diagnostic assessment and reassessment is another important prevention strategy.

When tardive dyskinesia appears, the most conservative approach is to adjust the dose of medication to the lowest effective dose, if that has not already been done. A number of studies have indicated that such a strategy leads to nonprogression of symptoms in most of the patients. The strategy of abruptly stopping medications carries the risk of relapse of psychotic symptoms and possibly of rehospitalization. Attempting to determine whether a patient still requires antipsychotic medication can be done by tapering the dose. To date there are no medications that when added to antipsychotic medications have been demonstrated to reverse tardive dyskinesia. Because clozapine has not or is very rarely associated with tardive dyskinesia, some research groups have shown that when their medication is changed to clozapine, many patients have a reduction or cessation of tardive dyskinesia symptoms. Because symptoms have returned after clozapine discontinuation in some of those patients, the role of clozapine in curing tardive dyskinesia is not clear at this time. The increased interest in the development of atypical antipsychotic medications holds the promise of antipsychotic treatment without tardive dyskinesia.

Neuroleptic malignant syndrome is a serious and frequently lethal condition seen in association with antipsychotic medication treatment. Characterized by muscle rigidity, high temperature, increase in levels of muscle enzymes, and leukocytosis, the side effect is observed in approximately 0.1 to 1 percent of patients treated with neuroleptics, although there are occasional reports that it may be more prevalent. It appears that no antipsychotic medication is exempt from leading to neuroleptic malignant syndrome and that it can occur during any portion of treatment. The condition may resemble catatonia in some factors, especially muscle stiffness, but a number of clinicians indicate that the muscle stiffness is more like rigor than catatonia.

If symptoms of neuroleptic malignant syndrome appear antipsychotic medication should be stopped, and if symptoms are severe, supportive treatment should begin immediately. There is significant importance in establishing a clear diagnosis, investigating for infection, for example. Many patients with the syndrome are observed in intensive care units. Recent reports indicate that use of dopamine agonists are useful in the treatment of neuroleptic malignant syndrome and should be strongly considered.

Once the crisis of the acute episode is resolved, treatment of the psychosis remains an issue. Some patients appear to be able to tolerate antipsychotic treatment again, whereas others have another episode. At this time it is worthwhile to treat the symptomatic schizophrenic patient again under careful observation.

Neuroleptic-induced acute akathisia is a common side effect of antipsychotic medications. It is characterized by restlessness in the legs, but motor restlessness may be experienced in other parts of the body. Pacing and jiggling of the legs are frequently observed as patients attempt to relieve the troublesome symptom. Akathisia is often associated with the higher potency antipsychotic medications in higher doses, and some investigators feel that it is a major factor in noncompliance and perhaps even aggressive in episodes on inpatient services.

Akathisia has not been responsive to anticholinergic medications used to treat parkinsonian side effects. Benzodiazepines and benadryl have also been tested with some limited success. During the past few years, β-blocking medications have been found to be useful for treating akathisia. Low doses are required for treatment; for example, 80 grams per day of propranolol in divided doses is usually sufficient. Usual care in the use of propranolol should be observed, such as assessment of blood pressure and electrocardiographic testing.

Seizures may occur with the use of the typical antipsychotic medications in some cases. The incidence of seizures is low so that risk factors are difficult to assess, but seizures may be associated with high doses of antipsychotic medications. For a patient with a seizure disorder who has schizophrenia (or psychotic disorder due to temporal lobe epilepsy) an anticonvulsant should be continued.

OTHER SIDE EFFECTS Nonneurological side effects appear to be less common, perhaps because there has been an increase in use of higher potency antipsychotic medications. In the early years of use of antipsychotic medication frequent cases of liver dysfunction characterized by jaundice were observed. Also, sedation was common in treated schizophrenic patients, as the initial medications are more frequently associated with this side effect. For some time, the sedating quality of the lower potency antipsychotic medications was thought to be helpful, even though patients find that side effect troublesome.

Hypotension, liver abnormalities, blood dyscrasia, and hormonal effects such as hyperprolactinemia are the most common nonneurological side effects (Table 14.8-2). Hypotension occurs most commonly with the lower potency medications. That effect can still be problematic, although it was perhaps more prevalent when low-potency medications were used in high doses to manage emergency situations. In the emergency situation of severe hypotension resulting from the use of antipsychotic medication supportive measures should be instituted and norepinephrine or phenylephrine considered. Epinephrine is not to be used as a pressor agent, as it may cause an exacerbation of hypotension. Cholestatic jaundice can occur with the use of antipsychotic medications and should be watched for. With the current focus on the incidence of agranulocytosis associated with clozapine administration there has been a reexamination of the incidence of blood dyscrasia in the use of traditional agents. The reexamination has revealed that although traditional medications are less commonly associated with leukocytosis and with agranulocytosis, those side effects still occur. Patients taking the medications and their families need to participate in discussions about the need to contact the physician in the event of an unusual or protracted infection. A complete blood count examination before starting an antipsychotic medication is indicated.

Because antipsychotic medications block dopamine receptors, they also interrupt the dopamine regulation of prolactin. All patients treated with a traditional antipsychotic medication have prolactin increase, and some of those patients have physical effects such as gynecomastia (in men) or disturbance in menses (in women) and galactorrhea. Thus, a lowest effective dose strategy is indicated and helps most patients. Bromocriptine has been used for galactorrhea.

SIDE EFFECTS OF CLOZAPINE The side effects of clozapine are discussed separately because of the significant difference of this medication from the traditional agents and to underscore the importance of monitoring for agranulocytosis (Table 14.8-3). As medication development continues, clinicians will find that side effect profiles will become more complex.

TABLE 14.8-3
Side Effects of Antipsychotic Medications (Atypical Agents; Clozapine)

Symptom or Syndrome	Intervention
Agranulocytosis	Weekly monitoring; with white blood cell count (WBC) < 3,000, monitor daily (assess neutrophils), and with WBC < 2,000, discontinue clozapine immediately
Increased temperature	Observe, rule out infection
Salivation	Consider benztropine
Sedation	Lowest effect dose, most patients will develop tolerance
Tachycardia	Electrocardiography before initiating treatment, monitor dose and pulse
Hypotension	Careful screening prior to initiating treatment, monitor dose and blood pressure
Neuroleptic malignant syndrome	Same management as with typical agents
Seizures	Doses above 400 mg per day only when necessary, anticonvulsant with clozapine after seizure

Agranulocytosis associated with clozapine use was first noted in the mid-1970s following a series of cases in which that condition led to eight deaths. When clozapine was determined to have superior efficacy compared to traditional medications for nonresponsive patients, a monitoring program was required for use of the medication. Current estimates for the prevalence of agranulocytosis are 1.5 to 2.0 percent of patients, with most cases occurring in treatment (first 12 to 24 weeks). Some research has indicated that there may be a risk factor associated with a human leukocyte antigen (HLA) subtype, but that has not reached application in the clinical arena. Others have explored the possibility of a toxic clozapine metabolite leading to agranulocytosis, which, if confirmed, would perhaps allow clinicians to measure the offending chemical. Currently, the policy in the United States for the use of clozapine is that evaluation of hematological status be performed by history and complete blood count prior to the initiation of clozapine. Thereafter, weekly monitoring the white blood cell count needs to be performed or the patient is not to receive continued medication. Guidelines for monitoring are that increased frequency of white blood cell counts need to be performed when the count is below 3,000 white blood cells per cubic meter. When such low counts occur, it is important to obtain a differential count so the amount of neutrophils can be assessed. Medication should be stopped immediately when absolute counts reach 2,000 white blood cells per cubic meter or when neutrophil counts reach 1,000 per cubic meter.

In the United States the monitoring mechanism has been effective in dramatically reducing a fatal outcome. When agranulocytosis occurs, hospitalization is indicated and the patient needs to be observed for signs of infection while receiving daily complete and differential blood cell counts.

Seizures are more commonly associated with clozapine treatment than with traditional antipsychotic medications, but that side effect is dose related. When doses of clozapine are over 400 mg per day, there can be as high as 4 to 5 percent incidence of a seizure. That incidence lessens with doses below 400 mg per day but does not disappear. That is another reason for collaborating with the patient to find the lowest effective dose of medication. Patients with seizures may take clozapine, but clinicians need to consider the hematological side effects of the anticonvulsant being used.

Sedation as an early side effect is one of the important factors in the initial dosing strategy of clozapine. Many patients sleep as much as 14 hours per day during the initial dose-finding period; however, most patients soon adapt to that effect. There are occasional patients who have considerable sedation even after months of clozapine treatment, so that collaboration in dosing is required.

Hypotension and tachycardia are also side effects to be monitored early during treatment with clozapine. Obviously, when a medication such as clozapine is used, careful evaluation of hypotension and electrocardiographic studies are required before beginning treatment. Antihypertensive medication should also be carefully evaluated. Some patients do not need antihypertensive medications while on clozapine. When clozapine treatment is initiated, hypotension may limit the rate of increase of dosing; however, most patients are able to reach a therapeutic dose with slower increases. The geriatric population is perhaps the most at risk for hypotension, but there has been little empirical research on the use of clozapine in that group.

Other side effects of clozapine include increased temperature without infection and dramatically increased salivation. Increased temperature must be observed, and signs of infection sought. Increased temperature by itself is not a cause for discontinuation of the medication. Salivation with clozapine can be a bothersome problem to which some accommodation by the patient's body does occur. One group has empirically investigated the use of benztropine for the treatment of hypersalivation with positive results.

The definition of atypical antipsychotic medication includes the caveat that there are no movement effects. Tardive dyskinesia is not associated with clozapine treatment. As there is some weak binding of clozapine to basal ganglia dopamine receptors, there is the possibility of early movement disorder effects. Most clinical experience is that movement disorders are rare and mild with clozapine use.

INFORMED CONSENT WITH SOMATIC TREATMENTS

The issue of consent in medicine and psychiatry has changed dramatically in the past few decades, from little discussion of treatment with the patient to elaborate informed consent procedures for research and clinical care. Psychiatry has been a forum for extended discussions of the merits of disclosing diagnosis and discussing treatment options in objective language. A number of different forces have combined to make objective informed consent to diagnosis and treatment a crucial part of the use of somatic treatments for schizophrenia, including demands by patients and their families, the legal climate related to medical malpractice, legislation for treatment planning signed by patients, and the reports by clinicians of improved medication outcome and compliance by collaboration around informed consent.

Despite the movement toward a psychoeducational approach to the somatic treatment of schizophrenia, the implementation of imparting information to a patient with psychosis requires an integrated and sensitive clinical approach. In the initial stages of interaction with a patient with schizophrenia who is receiving medication for the first time, the psychiatrist and the treatment team are dealing with a number of issues in the consent process, such as the meaning of taking a medication for a mental illness, the role of the psychosis in the patient's understanding of the consent process, and the time-dependent relevance of the information about side effects. Clear discussions about the role of medications in the reduction of symptoms—and not as a punishment or intervention for personal inadequacy—are important initial discussions. Discussion of side effects that are relevant to the initial stages of treatment can be presented without unduly frightening the patient and can allow for the initial collaboration between the treatment team and the patient. In the early stages of medication administration, assessment for side effects by questions and examination provides a venue for further matter-of-fact discussion.

The concept of ongoing consent was introduced in psychiatry by William Carpenter as he described the issue of consent on a research ward. The practice of ongoing consent in the somatic treatment of schizophrenia has become an integral part of many schizophrenia programs. Usually in groups, sometimes with family members present, the issues of somatic treatments and side effects are discussed and experiences of other patients are shared. Such an approach reinforces the collaborative relationship between the psychiatrist, and patient, and the patient's family.

The issue of informed consent about tardive dyskinesia is complex, as that side effect is not a result of acute treatment, and many feel that discussion about a possibly permanent side effect at the initiation of treatment could deter initiation of a needed intervention. However, as treatment progresses, the diagnosis is confirmed, and longer term treatment is indicated, clear discussion of tardive dyskinesia is indicated. It should be noted that some hospitals have policies about documentation of a patient's status as it relates to tardive dyskinesia through such scales as the Abnormal Involuntary Movement Scale. Some groups have noted that because of the repeated examination for it as a side effect, an awareness of the potential of tardive dyskinesia is increased in both the clinician and the patient. One group has found that explicit examination of patients in long-term treatment did not deter them from treatment with antipsychotic medications.

INTEGRATION WITH PSYCHOSOCIAL TREATMENT

A number of tensions have emerged since the introduction of psychotropic medications, not the least of which has been the interplay between medication treatment and psychological and social interventions. Early studies focused on the question of whether medications interfered with talking therapy, which they did not. The publication by May of one of the most comprehensive controlled studies of medication treatments indicated that medication treatment was a successful intervention and that it was not statistically less effective than medication treatment and psychotherapy combined. That finding was misinterpreted by many in the mental health field as indicating that psychosocial interventions were not additive to somatic treatments.

Fortunately, a large number of well-designed studies, characterized by objective definition of psychosocial intervention and outcome measures, have clearly demonstrated that comprehensive treatment programs for the treatment of schizophrenia are superior to medication treatment alone. Following the work of an English research group a number of centers in England and the United States have studied the impact of family interventions as they relate to relapse rates in patients with schizophrenia. Table 14.8-4 is a list of the studies performed to date, which demonstrate the advantage for groups in which family therapy was included. Approaches include use of psychoeducational workshops for patients and families, multiple family

TABLE 14.8-4
Outcome of Family Treatment Trials for Schizophrenia

	Relapse Ratio Over 6-12 Months (%)	
Study	**Control**	**Experimental**
Goldstein et al (1978)	48	0
Falloon et al (1982)	44	6
Leff et al (1982)	50	8
Hogarty et al (1986)	41	0
Tarrier et al (1987)	53	12
Leff et al (1989)	—	8*
	—	17†

*Family therapy.
†Relatives group attenders.
The Table lists the relapse rates of schizophrenic patients treated with antipsychotic medication who received family therapy versus other psychosocial interventions. The reduced relapse rates for patients whose families were in treatment is apparent and underscores the importance of combining pharmacological and psychosocial treatments. Table from J Leff: Family Factors in Schizophrenia. Psychiatr Ann *19:* 542, 1989. Used with permission.

groups, social skills training, and vocational rehabilitation. Utilization of such approaches can significantly reduce the relapse rate of patients with schizophrenia.

SUGGESTED CROSS-REFERENCES

For further information related to assessment of the schizophrenic patient see Section 9.3 on typical signs and symptoms of psychiatric illness and Section 9.8 on psychiatric rating scales. Chapter 14 on schizophrenia is important for a full understanding of the syndrome. To appreciate the antipsychotic medications see Section 32.15 on antipsychotic drugs. As other medicines are used to augment antipsychotic medications, see the other sections of Chapter 32 on biological therapies.

REFERENCES

*Andreasen N C, Olsen S: Negative vs positive schizophrenia: Definition and validation. Arch General Psychiatry *39:* 789, 1982.

*Angrist B, Schulz S C: *The Neuroleptic-Nonresponsive Patient: Characterization and Treatment.* American Psychiatric Press, Washington, 1990.

Baldessarini R J, Cohen B M, Teichner M H: Significance of neuroleptic dose and plasma level in the pharmacological treatment of psychosis. Arch Gen Psychiatry *45:* 79, 1988.

Breier A, Wolkowitz O M, Pickar D: Stress and schizophrenia. In *Schizophrenia Research: Advances in Neuropsychiatry and Psychopharmacology,* C A Tamminga, S C Schulz, editors, vol 1, p 141. Raven, New York, 1991.

Carlsson A., Lindqvist M: Effect of chlorpromazine or haloperidol on formation of 3-methoxytyramine and normetanephrine in mouse brain. Acta Pharmacol Toxicol *20:* 140, 1963.

Carpenter W T Jr: Approaches to knowledge and understanding of schizophrenia. Schizophr Bull *13:* 17, 1987.

Carpenter W T Jr, Heinrichs D W, Wagman A M: Deficit and nondeficit forms of schizophrenia: The concept. Am J Psychiatry *145:* 578, 1988.

Cole J O, Goldberg S C, Klerman G L: Phenothiazine treatment in acute schizophrenia. Arch Gen Psychiatry *10:* 246, 1964.

Davis J M, Schaffer C B, Killian G A, Kinard C, Chan C: Important issues in the drug treatment of schizophrenia. Schizophr Bull *6:* 70, 1980.

*Falloon I R, Boyd J L, McGill C W, Razani J, Moss H B, Gilderman A M: Family management in the prevention of exacerbations of schizophrenia. A controlled study. N Engl J Med *306:* 1347, 1982.

Goldstein M J: Psychosocial issues. Schizophr Bull *13:* 171, 1987.

Hirsch S R, Emami J, Bowen J T, Cramer P: The contribution of life events to schizophrenic relapse: An event history analysis. Schizophr Res *6:* 172, 1992.

*Kane J, Honigfeld G, Singer J, Meltzer H Y, and the Clozaril Collaborative Study Group: Clozapine for the treatment-resistant schizophrenic: A double-blind comparison versus chlorpromazine/benztropine. Arch Gen Psychiatry *45:* 789, 1988.

Kane J M, Lieberman J A: Maintenance pharmacotherapy in schizophrenia. In *Psychopharmacology: The Third Generation of Progress,* H Y Meltzer, editor, p 1103. Raven, New York, 1987.

Kane J M: Treatment of schizophrenia. Schizoph Bull *13:* 147, 1987.

Land W, Salzman C: Risperidone: A novel antipsychotic medication. Hosp Community Psychiatry *45:* 434, 1994.

Lieberman J A, Kane J M, Johns C A: Clozapine: Guidelines for clinical management. J Clin Psychiatry *50:* 329, 1989.

Marder S R, Mebane A, Chien C P: A comparison of patients who refuse and consent to neuroleptic treatment. Am J Psychiatry *140:* 470, 1983.

Marder S R, Meibach R C: Risperidone in the treatment of schizophrenia. Am J Psychiatry *151:* 825, 1994.

*Marder S R, Van Putten T, Mintz J, Lebelle M, McKenzie J, May P R: Low and conventional-dose maintenance therapy with fluphenazine decanoate: Two year outcome. Arch Gen Psychiatry *44:* 518, 1987.

May P R: *Treatment of Schizophrenia.* Science House, New York, 1968.

McGlashan T H: The schizophrenia spectrum concept: The Chestnut Lodge follow-up study. In *Schizophrenia Research: Advances in Neuropsychiatry and Psychopharmacology,* C A Tamminga, S C Schulz editors, p 193. Raven, New York, 1991.

Mueser K T, Douglas M S, Bellack A S, Morrison R L: Assessment of enduring deficit and negative symptom subtypes in schizophrenia. Schizophr Bull *17:* 565, 1991.

Munetz M R, Roth L H: Informing patients about tardive dyskinesia. Arch Gen Psychiatry *42:* 866, 1985.

Rifkin A, Seshagiri D, Basawaruj K, Borenstein M, Wachspress M: Dosage of haloperidol for schizophrenia. Arch Gen Psychiatry *48:* 166, 1991.

Roback A A, Kiernan T: *Pictorial History of Psychology and Psychiatry.* Philosophical Library, New York, 1969.

Schulz S C, Conley R R, Kann E M, Alexander J: Non-responders to neuroleptics: A distinct subtype. In *Schizophrenia: Scientific Progress,* S C Schulz, C A Tamminga, editors, p 341. Oxford University Press, New York, 1989.

Tamminga C A, Gerlach J: New neuroleptics and experimental antipsychotics in schizophrenia. In *Psychopharmacology: The Third Generation of Progress,* H Meltzer, editor, p 1129. Raven, New York, 1987.

Volavka J, Cooper T B: Review of haloperidol blood level and clinical response: Looking through the window. J Clin Psychopharmacol *7:* 25, 1987.

Weinberger D R, Bigelow L B, Kleinman J E, Klein D F, Rosenblatt J E, Wyatt R J: Cerebral ventricular enlargement in chronic schizophrenia: An association with poor response to treatment. Arch Gen Psychiatry *37:* 11, 1980.

Wyatt R J: Early intervention with neuroloptics may decrease the long-term morbidity of schizophrenia. Schizophr Res *5:* 201, 1991.

Zwelling S S: *Quest for a Cure: The Public Hospital in Williamsburg, 1773–1885.* The Colonial Williamsburg Foundation, Williamsburg, VA, 1985.

14.9 SCHIZOPHRENIA: PSYCHOSOCIAL TREATMENT

ANTHONY F. LEHMAN, M.D.

INTRODUCTION

Schizophrenia exerts a broad range of effects on the lives of persons it afflicts. Schizophrenia and its treatment have baffled and challenged clinicians for generations. Much scientific research and controversy about the nature of the disorder have dominated the past several decades. One conceptual dichotomy that has preoccupied the field has been the debate about biological versus psychosocial factors in both the cause and the treatment of schizophrenia. Theories about schizophrenia during the past 50 years have focused on such diverse causal mechanisms as poverty, parenting style, family communication style, viruses, autoimmune disorders, genetics, and various specific neurotransmitters. On the basis of those presumed causal theories, a wide variety of therapies have been developed and applied to treat schizophrenia. Polemic schisms within the field have often diverted researchers and clinicians from a comprehensive view of schizophrenia and the treatment of persons with it.

Fortunately, from that turmoil have emerged integrative theories about the cause, course, and treatment of schizophrenia that allow the clinician to use a combination of therapeutic interventions in treating patients with schizophrenia. The process has been accelerated by recent scientific advances in biological and psychosocial treatments. Although the causes of the schizophrenia syndrome remain unclear, considerable consensus views schizophrenia from a vulnerability-stress (also called stress-diathesis) or biopsychosocial perspective. Those views emphasize the underlying biological vulnerabilities that predispose a person to schizophrenia and the importance of psychological and social factors in the onset and the course of the disorder. The integrative models form the basis for comprehensive treatment of schizophrenia and have set the stage for many therapeutic advances in the treatment of patients.

THEORETICAL ISSUES AND DEFINITIONS

The many different types and levels of complexity of psychosocial treatments for schizophrenia and the wide range of outcomes that they must address pose impediments to clinicians who wish to understand and use them. Therefore, this discussion warrants a road map to provide a clear perspective on their purpose and practice.

First, ''psychosocial'' implies the use of psychological and social procedures to intervene on behalf of the patient; specifically, it excludes somatic interventions. ''Psychosocial'' refers neither to the cause of the problem nor to the mechanisms by which the treatment exerts its effects. The mechanisms by which the treatments exert their influences may be at psychosocial or at biological levels. For example, a psychosocial treatment may improve patients' understanding of their illness, which in turn enhances compliance with medications, thus exerting a cascade of mediating effects on the underlying physiology of the disorder. ''Psychosocial'' defines the treatment modality, not its mechanism of action or the nature of its targeted outcome.

The term ''treatment'' may be more difficult to define in this context than the term ''psychosocial.'' Because the broad range of psychosocial treatments used for persons with schizophrenia are delivered by an equally diverse range of professionals and agencies, philosophical disagreements exist about what does and does not constitute treatment. Who can deliver treatment? Do treatment and rehabilitation differ? Such questions are important to interdisciplinary debates and philosophical arguments about the nature of what is being treated (disease or disability) but in practice bear little relevance to the needs of the persons suffering from a schizophrenic disorder. Therefore, in this discussion, treatment is viewed broadly to include clinical and rehabilitation interventions conducted with the patient or the patient's social environment for the purpose of sustaining or improving the person's condition. The psychosocial treatments reviewed include individual and group psychotherapies, family treatments, vocational rehabilitation, residential treatment, psychosocial rehabilitation, and case management.

Second, the outcomes targeted by various psychosocial treatments must be defined. The several dimensions of outcome include symptoms, cognitive impairments, functional disabilities, social handicaps, patient responses to illness, and societal responses to illness. The *symptoms* of schizophrenia are the common manifestations defined in the fourth edition of *Diagnostic and Statistical Manual of Mental Disorders* (DSM-IV), including delusions, hallucinations, bizarre behaviors, disorganized speech, inappropriate affects, avolition, and alogia. *Cognitive impairments* are the underlying disruptions in brain functions, such as disturbances in attention span, memory, and information processing. *Functional disability* is the loss of or the failure to develop the capacity for certain role functions, such as self-care, work, parenting, and spouse roles. *Social handicaps* are the diminished opportunities to participate in social roles and activities; the term refers to the interactive effects of individual and social factors. It reflects both the patient's disabilities and the reduced access to resources and opportunities afforded by society to disabled persons. *Patient and societal responses to illness* are the psychological reactions and attitudes of the patient and key persons in the patient's social environment to the symptoms, impairments, disabilities, and handicaps that occur because of schizophrenia. Those responses can profoundly affect the patient's course of illness and quality of life and include such negative reactions as stigma, shame, and demoralization, as well as positive reactions characterized by resiliency, courage, and realistic adaptation to disabilities and strengths.

Psychosocial treatments may address any variety of outcomes, and ideally the choice of treatments reflects the specific outcome problems faced by the patient. Table 14.9-1 provides a guide to the relations between psychosocial treatments and the outcomes that they target.

PSYCHOLOGICAL TREATMENTS

Psychological treatments for schizophrenia include both individual and group therapies. Traditional individual and group therapies target the symptoms of schizophrenia and the patient's responses to the disorder. Recently developed group approaches also aim at the amelioration of underlying cognitive impairments and functional disabilities. In general, interest in psychological treatments for schizophrenia has undergone consider-

TABLE 14.9-1
Psychosocial Treatments and Their Primary Target Outcomes*

Treatment	Symptoms	Cognitive Impairment	Functional Disability	Social Handicap	Patient Responses to Illness	Social Responses to Illness
Individual and group therapies						
Supportive	x				x	
Cognitive	x	x			x	
Social skills	x		x		x	
Family treatments	x					x
Vocational rehabilitation			x	x		
Residential care				x		
Psychosocial rehabilitation			x	x	x	
Case management						
Basic model				x		
Intensive clinical	x		x	x	x	x
Rehabilitation			x	x	x	x

*The primary target outcomes are those that are theoretically most proximal to the focus of the intervention and are marked by ''x'' in the table. In some cases the efficacy of the treatment for alleviating the target problem has been demonstrated. In others the relation remains unproved. Excluded are potential secondary effects of the treatments; for example, residential treatment may reduce symptoms, but that is not the primary focus of housing.

able decline in recent years because of disappointing research results, the rise of knowledge about the biological vulnerabilities underlying the disorder, and the efficacy of pharmacotherapy in alleviating symptoms. However, as the heat of the biological versus psychosocial debate has cooled and as the importance of comprehensive treatment approaches has gained wide acceptance, interest in psychological treatments in combination with pharmacotherapies has grown.

INDIVIDUAL THERAPIES Most discussions of individual therapy for schizophrenia have focused on comparisons of psychodynamically oriented and supportive psychotherapies.

Psychodynamic therapies Used mainly before the 1960s, psychodynamic therapies emphasized an understanding of the developmental experiences and the psychological conflicts and defense mechanisms that were thought to underlie the symptoms and the inner experiences associated with schizophrenia. Regressive techniques, interpretation, and transference-countertransference issues were emphasized. During the 1960s a series of studies failed to show any advantage of that type of psychotherapy for schizophrenia compared with supportive, less intensive, reality-oriented approaches. For example, the 1984 Boston Psychotherapy Study compared an exploratory, insight-oriented psychotherapy, provided two to three times weekly, with reality-adaptive, supportive therapy offered in weekly or biweekly sessions. All the patients met the research diagnostic criteria for schizophrenia, received the usual pharmacotherapy and aftercare services in addition to psychotherapy, and were randomized to the two psychotherapy conditions. The results revealed minimal outcome differences between the two treatments and did not support the hypothesized advantage of exploratory, insight-oriented therapy over reality-adaptive, supportive therapy.

Such studies led to the common misunderstanding that psychotherapy in general is not helpful in the treatment of schizophrenia. Unfortunately, that conclusion overlooks the fact that some patients in the studies did experience improvement with psychotherapy, despite the fact that no major differential outcome effects were found among alternative psychotherapies. Furthermore, the studies in no way demonstrated that a strong therapeutic relationship with a patient with schizophrenia does not enhance the treatment process. Nonetheless, research and development of psychological therapies for schizophrenia became largely dormant for the next several years. Interest in psychotherapy for schizophrenia has increased again with the acceptance of the vulnerability-stress model of the disorder and the recognition that currently available medications do not alleviate many of the adverse effects of the illness on patients' lives. However, current research on individual psychotherapy for schizophrenia remains essentially nonexistent.

Supportive therapy The most widely accepted and practiced form of individual therapy for patients with schizophrenia today is supportive. Supportive therapy emphasizes empathic listening; active problem solving around issues of everyday life; education about the illness, treatment, and individual risk factors for relapse; and a generally supportive relationship with the therapist. The theory underlying that approach is that schizophrenia impairs the patient's capacity to relate to others and to recognize and cope with stresses that may result in relapse or other problems. The purpose of the therapeutic relationship is to offset those deficits with emotional support, practical advice and training about everyday life, and enduring contact with someone who is objective yet knows and cares about the patient.

The major problem with the practice of supportive therapy for schizophrenia is that it remains largely undefined and unstudied in the literature. No supportive therapy manuals have been published, and no data give its specific indications. Who needs it when, under what conditions, and for which problems? The paucity of information has left the practice of supportive therapy for schizophrenia in a nether realm, often devalued or claimed as a nonspecific activity by everyone or no one. Much needed is knowledge about what elements of a supportive therapeutic relationship are essential to improve or sustain specific outcomes among the various groups of patients with schizophrenia.

Despite the absence of research, certain potential benefits of supportive therapy can be identified. First, such a relationship may be essential to the practice of good pharmacotherapy by permitting a sensitive and individualized approach to the patient. The supportive therapeutic relationship provides a context to educate the patient about schizophrenia, the role of prescribed medications, and the importance of recognizing early signs of relapse. The relationship allows the patient to ask questions and to raise concerns about the medications and gives the clinician the opportunity to respond to those issues to make needed adjustments in the medication and to correct patient misunderstandings. The net effect may be improved medication compliance and symptom control.

Second, support and practical advice can help reduce the distress experienced by the patients in the course of everyday life problems. Failure to deal effectively with such stresses can lead to symptom relapse. Thoughtful listening and suggestions from the therapist can enhance the patient's sense of hope and competence in the face of those problems. Patient education about the association of symptoms with stress and the importance of managing distress can improve the patient's sense of control and ability to cope.

Third, perhaps the least articulated reason for supportive therapy is the importance of understanding patients' psychological and social development and their illness experiences within the broad context of their lives. The motive for that understanding is not to explain the cause of schizophrenia but to clarify and share the patients' experiences with their illness and to reinforce their sense of themselves and their connections to the world around them. Such a relationship fosters recognition that the therapist cares about the patient, not just about symptoms and medication effects. That recognition can be critical for patients who often feel alienated and devalued because of their illness.

A 33-year-old man from a middle-class family experienced the onset of paranoid delusions and auditory hallucinations at age 17, shortly after graduating from high school. Before that he was an introverted but good student. The first six years of his illness were marked by four hospitalizations totaling nearly three years, recurrent aggressive acts toward others, and frequent noncompliance with medications. Despite those problems he completed one year of community college during that time but was unable to hold a job for more than four months or to live on his own.

Six years ago, after his last hospitalization, which spanned six months and during which he was highly assaultive, a more intensive effort at supportive psychotherapy was implemented. The initial sessions focused on educating him about his diagnosis and the reasons for continuing the antipsychotic medication—at the time, 1 cc of fluphenazine decanoate (Prolixin) every two weeks. He was reluctant to continue the medication because he felt too sleepy and did not entirely believe that he had a mental illness. Instead, he believed that his problems arose from the social abuse that he had experienced from other students in high school several years earlier. However, he agreed to work with the psychiatrist to gradually decrease the dosage, rather than stop the medication abruptly.

After the establishment of that medication contract, the patient spent several therapy sessions talking about his feelings of paranoia and of being out of control of his life, his rage at perceived past harassment by others, and his extreme frustration about feeling like a "wimp and a loser.'' He stated that his frequent aggressive outbursts and fights in the hospital had been conscious efforts to prove his manhood. To increase the patient's sense of control, the therapist switched the medication from depot to tablet form and gradually reduced the dosage until mild paranoia reemerged. Thereafter, the patient was compliant with the medication at a dosage of 5 mg oral fluphenazine a day.

Over the past three years the patient has continued to discuss his feelings of rage as an adolescent, his poor self-esteem, and his feelings of shame. He has remained nonpsychotic, and, although frustrated frequently about his general level of disability relative to his much more successful brothers, he completed a vocational rehabilitation training program, works full-time at a manual labor job, and lives in his own apartment. Supportive therapy sessions have decreased gradually from weekly to monthly, with the option of scheduling extra sessions when needed. In those sessions he continues to seek advice about practical problems—such as dating, dealing with a boss he does not like, and techniques for feeling relaxed with others—and about such psychological issues as his shame about his illness, his ambivalence about his parents' attempts to continue to support him, and his confusion about how to integrate his intense emotional experiences of alienation in high school with the concept of having a brain disorder, schizophrenia.

GROUP THERAPIES A variety of group therapies exist for schizophrenia. They have the same outcome goals as individual therapies—namely, symptom reduction and improvement in patients' responses to their illness. Some new types of group therapies address other outcomes as well, specifically targeting cognitive deficits and functional disabilities.

Patient education and support groups for schizophrenia are common in many clinical settings. The purpose of the groups is much the same as for supportive individual therapy. They use a group context to provide patients with opportunities for mutual support, the sharing of common experiences, feedback about their social behaviors, a setting to practice new social skills, and an efficient educational forum to learn about schizophrenia and its treatment. The therapist acts as a facilitator of the group process and uses natural group dynamics to encourage support, learning, and change. In view of the ubiquity of the groups in clinical settings, it is disappointing that a supporting body of controlled research does not exist. An exception is one randomized study in Sweden assessing the value of adding communication-oriented group therapy to a regimen of antipsychotic medication and social skills training. The results revealed little additional effect of the group therapy on symptoms but favorable effects of the group on social functioning.

A specific and structured type of group therapy that has developed in recent years is *social skills training*. Largely designed by investigators at the University of California at Los Angeles (UCLA) Center for Schizophrenia and Psychiatric Rehabilitation, the social skills training groups target the social disabilities that accompany schizophrenia. The group uses structured behavioral techniques, including role playing, modeling, feedback, rehearsal, behavioral coaching, and rewards to enhance the patients' skill levels. The types of skills taught vary widely and include communication skills (listening, processing, and sending), assertiveness skills, problem-solving skills, and skills related to specific activities of daily living (medication management, shopping, the use of transportation, money management, leisure-time activities, and the use of community resources). Research indicates that patients with schizophrenia can learn to improve the behaviors that are targeted in those groups but that generalization to real-life settings has been disappointing. For that generalization to occur, training in the actual settings in which the patients will use the skills may be needed—that is, the store, the bus, the bank, the home. Figure 14.9-1 charts the steps in the UCLA social skills training model.

Recently, attention has been turned to therapeutic group techniques that address *cognitive impairments*. Such groups are still experimental but aim, through the use of structured educational techniques, to improve patients' underlying cognitive functions, including perception, attention span, memory, concept formation, and the recognition and modulation of affects. The groups are similar to social skills training groups in their level of structure but focus on basic cognitive processes, rather than functional skills. One European technique outlines dysfunctions that patients with schizophrenia show in various stages of information processing and prescribes group techniques to help patients master the steps of information processing. A cognitive group therapy technique currently under study at the University of Nebraska derives from the hierarchy-collapse model of schizophrenia, which postulates that, under stress, the vulnerable person's hierarchy of appropriate cognitive responses collapses because of inherent neurological deficits or reduced tolerance for heightened arousal. Interventions are aimed at the remediation of those deficits. Those strategies are quite new and have not yet been put to any rigorous empirical tests.

FAMILY TREATMENT

During the past decade a variety of similar family interventions have been described that are based on the premise that what families of persons with schizophrenia need are support, information, practical advice, and training in how to cope with the challenges posed by the illness. The family interventions focus on two major outcome areas: symptom reduction and societal (family) reactions to the illness.

Early studies in Great Britain found that patients with schizophrenia who returned to families with a highly charged negative emotional climate, so-called high expressed emotion, relapsed at a much higher rate than did patients who returned to families with positive emotional climates. That association between relapse and family environment has been replicated in the United States and appears to be robust. That finding has stimulated considerable controversy as to why high expressed emotion correlates with illness relapse, in particular whether the negative family environment precipitates the relapse or whether patient characteristics and behaviors that predict relapse also elicit negative family responses. That debate misses the basic points that schizophrenia is a stressful illness for both patients and their families and that the emotional turmoil that sometimes arises from the illness is detrimental to all involved. Both families and patients suffer considerably under such circumstances; therefore, there is good reason to try to help families and patients in such situations.

Several types of family interventions have been developed in response to the original observation about expressed emotion and have been evaluated in well-controlled studies with consistent findings. The programs differ in terms of various characteristics but share a common focus on educating the family about schizophrenia and its treatment and on assisting the family in the resolution of everyday problems that arise because of the illness.

British investigators developed a program for families of persons with schizophrenia consisting of educational sessions, multifamily groups, and meetings with individual families and patients. The educational materials covered diagnosis, symptoms, causes, course of illness, and prognosis. In-home assessments were conducted with each family and the patient to identify areas of conflict and to discuss ways for resolution. An ongoing relatives group, which excluded patients, provided the families with opportunities for mutual support and problem sharing. A randomized evaluation of that approach versus routine clinical care found a clear reduction in relapse for the experimental group compared with controls during the ensuing nine

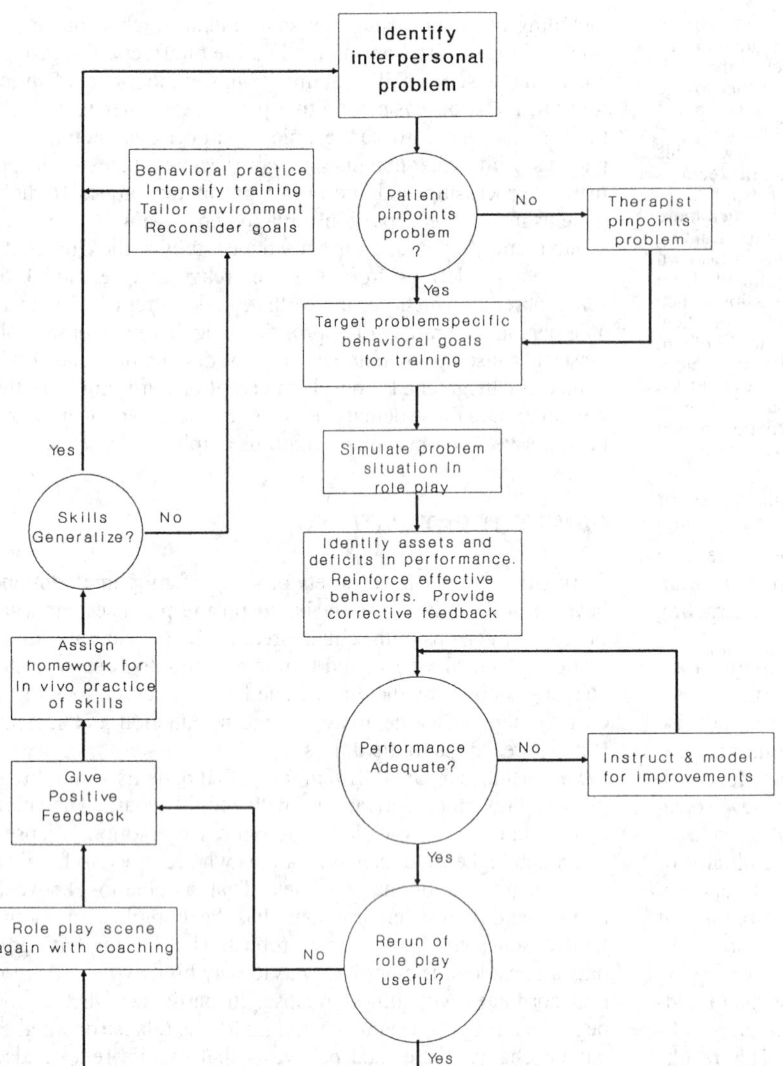

FIGURE 14.9-1 *Flow chart for conducting social skills training. (From R L Liberman, editor: Psychiatric Rehabilitation of Chronic Mental Patients,* p 167. American Psychiatric Press, Washington, 1988. Used with permission.)

months (9 percent versus 50 percent symptom relapse, respectively).

Investigators at UCLA developed and evaluated a short-term crisis-oriented family therapy program in the aftercare of acute schizophrenia. It consisted of six weekly sessions conducted with individual patients and their families and focused on conflict resolution and stress reduction through the development of specific coping strategies. They found that patients receiving the family intervention, plus a standard dosage of fluphenazine decanoate, had fewer relapses during the next six months than did patients who did not receive the family intervention or who received a low-dosage antipsychotic. A second group of Los Angeles investigators implemented a behavioral family program for outpatients with schizophrenia and their families. That home-based intervention also reduced relapse rates compared with a standard treatment regimen.

Researchers in Pittsburgh have developed an extensive family intervention program consisting of family sessions without the patient, a survival skills workshop, family sessions with the patient, and a maintenance phase over an extended period (6 to 12 months). Individual patients and their families participate in regular family sessions that stress increasing the structure in the home, strengthening interpersonal and intergenerational boundaries, and a close relationship between the family and community supports. Beyond that, families who continue to have significant difficulties move on to intensive individual family therapy; those who are improving gradually reduce the frequency of the sessions. Evaluations of the family interventions, combined with antipsychotic medication, have shown an effect of the family program on reductions in symptomatic relapses. Combinations of medication, family program, and social skills training for the patient yielded the best results; medication and either family intervention or patient skills training yielded the next best result, and medication alone yielded the poorest result.

The research findings in randomized experimental studies comparing those innovative family programs with various control treatment conditions for the reduction of symptom relapse have been remarkably consistent. The results are summarized in Figure 14.9-2.

Despite the consistency across diverse interventions, the components critical to the success of such family psychoeducational programs have not been identified. Little is known about the relative efficacy of alternative family interventions. The programs vary, for example, in their duration, whether they focus on individual families or on multifamily groups, whether the patient is included in the sessions, and whether they occur

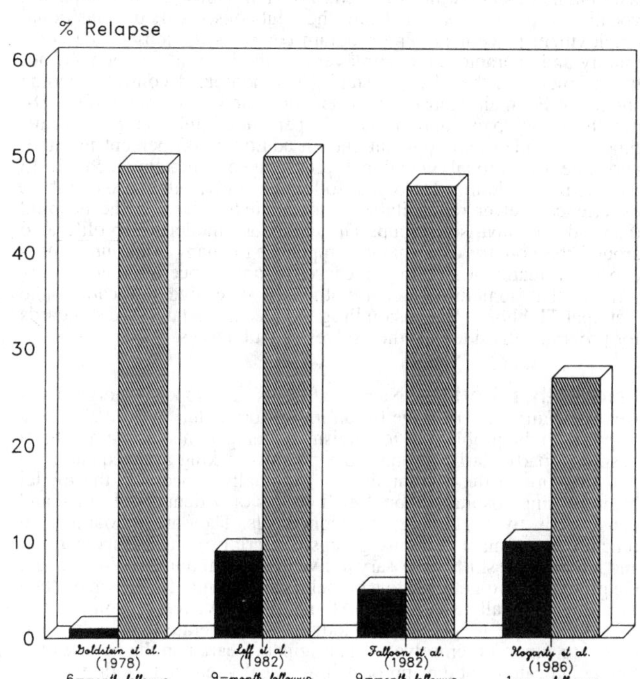

FIGURE 14.9-2 *Relapse rates from four studies of family therapy for schizophrenia. (From M J Goldstein: Psychosocial treatment of schizophrenia. In* Schizophrenia: Scientific Progress, *S C Schulz, C A Tamminga, editors, p 320. Oxford University Press, New York, 1989. Used with permission.)*

in the clinic or in the family's home. Research is needed to clarify the relative cost-effectiveness of different models of family treatment for various patient groups and types of problems.

REHABILITATION

With the mass relocation over the past four decades of the care for persons with schizophrenia from the hospital to the community, community-based psychosocial rehabilitation programs for the patients have expanded. Rehabilitation has the dual primary objectives of reducing functional disabilities through patient training and education and reducing social handicaps through support for the patients' social environment and advocacy for adequate resources and opportunities for them. Rehabilitation programs and services include vocational rehabilitation services, residential treatment and housing, and psychosocial rehabilitation centers.

VOCATIONAL REHABILITATION Surveys of patients with schizophrenia have consistently identified unemployment as a major factor in their reduced quality of life. Programs to improve their work functioning have existed for a long time, dating back to the rural public asylums of the last century, which often included a functional farm on which patients worked. In modern times the concern about work has translated into vocational rehabilitation programs. The types of programs include hospital-based workshop programs, lodge programs with a focus on work, sheltered workshops, vocational counseling programs, job clubs, psychosocial clubhouse programs, and supportive employment. Those programs can be subsumed under two general types: train-and-place programs and place-and-train programs. The target outcomes of the programs are improvement in patient functional disabilities (specifically work disability) and, through the actions of the placement or job-finding services of vocational rehabilitation programs, reduction in the barriers to employment for the patients, a type of social handicap.

The traditional *train-and-place model,* which includes all transitional and sheltered vocational rehabilitation programs, first assesses and trains patients with regard to general work habits and particular job skills. The patients are assessed for their work aptitudes, preferences, and skills. Then they are assisted in improving their work habits (keeping regular work hours, staying on the job, completing the job according to specifications) and trained to do a certain kind of work, such as a clerical, computer, or maintenance job. Once they have achieved a certain level of competence and consistent performance, they are placed at a regular job site. The advantages of that model are that it provides the opportunity to assess and work with the patients before they are exposed to the rigors of a real job setting, permits patients to make midcourse changes in their job-training preferences before committing to real jobs, and takes advantage of the efficiency of serving large numbers of patients in a rehabilitation center. The major problems with the model are that it may not adequately prepare patients for the transition from the shelter of the rehabilitation center to the regular work world, and patient choices about the types of work are limited to the specific types of jobs for which the rehabilitation center offers training. At times, patients complain about the delays before they are able to work for pay and about having to work in menial sheltered jobs for extended periods of time.

In response to those problems, rehabilitation specialists have developed a new model of vocational rehabilitation in recent years, the *place-and-train model.* Under that approach, patients work with a vocational counselor to identify their vocational goals and the type of jobs they would like to have that fit with their abilities. Patients then identify, with the help of a counselor, the specific mainstream job settings where they would like to work and where the employer is interested in on-the-job rehabilitation. Patients are then placed at those job sites and are trained to do that specific job in that specific setting. The intent is for the patient to remain permanently on that job. In that model, often referred to as supported employment, the patient works with a job coach, who assists the patient in whatever way is necessary to learn and keep that job. The advantages of that approach are that it is highly individualized and avoids the stressful transition from sheltered to unsheltered work settings. Patients also begin earning a wage more quickly than in the train-and-place model and may be less likely to perceive the job as menial or demeaning. The disadvantages are its costs and the dependence on employers who are willing to support that type of on-the-job training for disabled persons.

Well-controlled research on vocational rehabilitation for persons with schizophrenia is relatively sparse, given the long time that the programs have been in existence and the potential importance of work for improved outcome. Employment rates for persons with schizophrenia are generally reported to be in the range of 25 percent and consist primarily of part-time minimal-wage work. A review of the controlled evaluations of vocational rehabilitation programs for persons with psychiatric disabilities, predominantly schizophrenia, found disappointing results. Although patients involved in vocational rehabilitation programs consistently had higher forms of any paid employment than did patients without the programs (51 percent versus 29 percent), only one of 13 studies found that vocational rehabilitation programs had a significant effect on competitive employment. Those studies focused primarily on the traditional train-and-place approach.

RESIDENTIAL TREATMENT AND HOUSING PROGRAMS

Housing services are perhaps one of the most important yet least studied aspects of psychosocial treatment for schizophrenia. Residential care generally aims to improve patient functional disabilities and, by providing affordable and supportive housing, to reduce the social handicap of limited access to appropriate residential settings arising from patients' disabilities and social stigma.

Two major paradigm shifts in providing housing for persons with schizophrenia during the past 40 years have been defined by housing specialists in Boston. The first shift involved the discharge of large numbers of persons from mental hospitals to live in the community; that shift began in the early 1950s and peaked in the 1970s. That first wave of community-based residential care has been referred to as the paradigm of the linear continuum. Central to that paradigm was the development of a graduated continuum of residential treatment programs in the community through which a person progresses toward higher functioning and less restrictive settings.

Considerable variety characterizes that linear continuum of community residential-care settings for persons with schizophrenia, and the literature is replete with terminologies for referring to those settings. Eight basic types have been identified: transitional halfway houses, long-term group residences, cooperative apartments, intensive-care community residences, nursing homes, foster care, board-and-care homes, and total rural environments. Those types of residential care differ according to the length of time a person is allowed to stay, the intensity of on-site staff supervision, the degree to which they emphasize clinical or rehabilitation services versus simply housing, and the level of aggregation of patients in the living space.

Transitional halfway houses provide 24-hour daily supervision, a planned program, and the expectation that the patient will move on to

TABLE 14.9-2
Paradigms of Residential Services for Persons with Schizophrenia

Supported Housing	Linear Continuum
A home	Residential treatment settings
Choice	Placement
Normal roles	Client role
Client control	Staff control
Social integration	Grouping by disability
In vivo learning in permanent settings	Transitional preparatory settings
Individualized flexible services and supports	Standardized levels of service
Most facilitative environment, long-term supports	Least restrictive environment, independence

Table adapted from P Ridgway, A M Zipple: The paradigm shift in residential services: From the linear continuum to supported housing approaches. Psychosoc Rehab J *13:* 11, 1990. Used with permission.

permanent housing in the community. The houses are conceived as a bridge between the hospital and the community. In contrast, *long-term group residences* are designed to offer 24-hour daily supervision on a long-term basis and may be the sequel setting for a transitional halfway house resident who is unable to move on to independent living. *Cooperative apartments* typically have no on-site supervision but provide regular staff oversight and supervision for a small number of residents living together in an apartment. *Intensive-care or crisis residences* offer a short-term alternative to hospitalization and are staffed by clinicians. *Nursing homes* offer a long-term version of clinically supervised residential care for those persons needing ongoing intensive nursing care and supervision. Under the *foster care* model, private families or citizens in the community take mentally disabled persons into their homes. *Board-and-care homes* are proprietary homes that provide room, board, and some minimal but ongoing supervision. Typically, they are converted apartment buildings, hotels, or motels. *Total rural environments,* a rare version of residential care, are residential farms that are supervised by staff members and that emphasize rehabilitation through working and living together.

The research on those alternative residential settings in the linear continuum is limited and leaves many unanswered questions—in particular, their relative efficacy for various patient groups. However, in general, the research indicates that many of the settings offer viable and preferable alternatives to long-term hospitalization for those patients able to leave the hospital.

Because of a variety of problems with that linear continuum paradigm, a second major shift in housing for persons with schizophrenia is now underway. It is referred to as the paradigm of supported housing. The paradigm emphasizes mainstream housing settings fully integrated into the community with support services provided as needed but not on site. The housing is conceived as a normal living environment, not a treatment or service setting. Because the paradigm emphasizes individual choice and normalization of the patient's living environment, it has attracted considerable attention and advocacy throughout the country. However, research needs to clarify when and for whom it is a viable alternative to the traditional and restrictive linear continuum settings and how support services need to be linked for its success. The philosophical differences between the two paradigms are summarized in Table 14.9-2.

PSYCHOSOCIAL REHABILITATION MODELS At least four organized models of psychosocial rehabilitation can be identified: the Fountain House clubhouse model, the Fairweather Lodge model, the Boston University model, and the UCLA social skills training model. The target outcomes of psychosocial rehabilitation are reductions in functional disabilities and handicaps.

Fountain House Founded in 1948 in New York City, Fountain House is one of oldest and best known psychosocial rehabilitation programs in the United States. It grew out of a consumer self-help group and emphasizes consumer involvement in its operation. Although essentially atheoretical, the model seeks to enhance patients' sense of hope and competence through self-help assisted by staff and other supports as needed. The clubhouse program offers a variety of activities, including problem-solving groups, assistance with basic needs (clothing, food), and vocational services. Activity in the clubhouse itself revolves around three work areas—clerical, maintenance, and kitchen—in which patients, referred to as members, work to sustain the operation of the clubhouse as a part of their recovery. Staff work with the members but not for them. Fountain House also developed a vocational program apart from the clubhouse, called transitional employment placement. The program contracts for jobs in the community and guarantees the employer that the job will be done—if not by the member, then by the staff. No randomized control outcome studies of Fountain House have been conducted. One uncontrolled 18-month follow-up evaluation found 16 percent of club members in full-time independent employment and an additional 45 percent in either part-time transitional vocational programs or attending school. In another nonrandomized two-year follow-up study, clubhouse members experienced fewer rehospitalizations and fewer days in the hospital than did a comparison group. The clubhouse model has proliferated around the country as a major component of many community psychosocial treatment systems. Because of some concern about the distortions that sometimes occur with such extensive replication, the National Clubhouse Expansion Program recently established standards for programs that identify themselves as clubhouses.

Fairweather Lodge Named after its developer, George Fairweather, Fairweather Lodge began in California during the 1960s as a response to the problem of recidivism among patients discharged from hospitals, particularly among those patients lacking an adequate support network in the community. As originally conceived, the model begins during hospitalization. Small groups of patients are formed and taught daily living, coping, and work skills. They are encouraged to function as semiautonomous groups, fostering mutual responsibility and learning the skills necessary to live in the community. When ready, the group move together into a homelike community lodge, where they function essentially as a family. All members have responsibilities and roles within the lodge, and the lodges often operate their own businesses to support themselves. The original research on the Fairweather Lodge indicated that the approach dramatically reduced recidivism and increased the rates of full-time employment. Subsequent evaluations have tended to support those initial results. Some data indicate that mature patients may do better than young patients in the programs.

Unfortunately, the Fairweather Lodge model has not been extensively replicated, other than in Texas and Michigan, probably because of the additional implementation barriers posed by having to coordinate the preparation and the discharge of a group of patients, rather than individual patients, as is typically done.

Boston University and UCLA models Two major centers for the development of psychosocial rehabilitation models for schizophrenia and other disabling mental disorders are the Boston University Center for Psychiatric Rehabilitation and the UCLA Center for Schizophrenia and Psychiatric Rehabilitation. Those programs emphasize behavioral and social learning theories to develop specific packages and programs to teach patients social skills and techniques for developing resources in the community. The UCLA model relies heavily on the techniques of social skills training. The Boston University model emphasizes a similarly structured process of rehabilitation and identifies three phases of the process: rehabilitation diagnosis, rehabilitation planning, and rehabilitation interventions. The rehabilitation diagnosis flows from rehabilitation goals identified by the patient. Examples of those goals include obtaining a specific place to live and getting a specific paid job. With a well-defined goal in mind, the patient and a rehabilitation counselor proceed through a detailed and explicit review of the patient's functioning and resource status relevant to achieving the goal. That assessment of skills and resources leads to a rehabilitation plan that assigns specific interventions and objectives and that monitors progress toward those objectives. Interventions include direct skills teaching and resource coordination and modification.

Comparisons Although all those psychosocial rehabilitation models emphasize learning and support, the Fountain House and the Fairweather Lodge models do so through broadly organized support networks (clubhouses and lodges) designed to foster growth. The UCLA and Boston University models assume a much more structured approach and produce rehabilitation technologies that can be packaged, transported, and implemented in various settings. Much needed are studies that evaluate the efficacy of those rehabilitation models relative to no organized rehabilitation effort and that evaluate their efficacy relative to each other.

CASE MANAGEMENT

Case management now commands wide conceptual acceptance as a bulwark for organizing effective services for persons with schizophrenia, but systematic research on it has been impeded by great diversity in its definition and implementation.

A wide variety of potential activities have been subsumed under the term "case management." Those activities include outreach, patient assessment, case planning, referral to service providers, advocacy for the patient, direct casework, developing natural support systems, reassessment, advocacy for resource development, monitoring quality, public education, and crisis intervention. Various models of case management have been proposed: minimal, coordination, comprehensive, clinical, and rehabilitation-oriented. Those models can be provided by individuals, teams, or systems. The great variability in the definition of the dimensions of case management contributes to much of the ambiguity and confusion in the field. The generic target outcome of all case-management models is reduction in social handicaps through improved access to services, resources, and opportunities. As shown in Table 14.9-1. the various models of case management may target additional problems, including symptoms, functional disability, and patient and societal responses to the illness.

The empirical literature on the effectiveness of case management has grown in recent years. The best-known experimental study is the evaluation of assertive community treatment (also referred to as intensive clinical case management) by researchers in Madison, Wisconsin. In a 14-month randomized comparison of hospital treatment and standard aftercare versus an innovative assertive outreach and community-based treatment program, the patients in the experimental program, compared with the control cases, had lower rates of hospitalization, higher levels of functioning, greater life satisfaction, and no differences in levels of family burden. Costs for the two programs were essentially equivalent. Those results have been replicated elsewhere.

Other studies have also produced promising results regarding case management. An Indiana study compared assertive case management (again essentially an intensive clinical case-management model) with standard aftercare for severely mentally ill patients at risk for hospitalization (predominantly patients with schizophrenia) in a randomized experiment in three community mental health centers in Indiana. In the six-month follow-up period the assertive-case-management patients had fewer hospital days and fewer rehospitalizations compared with controls. However, no group differences were found in the quality of life, medication compliance, involvement in community mental health center programs, or contacts with the legal system. Direct and indirect treatment costs for the case-management group varied by a factor of 2.5 across the three community mental health centers. Another study compared a rehabilitation-oriented case-management program with a standard aftercare program after an episode of inpatient treatment in Canada. Case-management patients were compared with matched controls who received standard aftercare before the initiation of the new case-management program. At two-year follow-up, the case-management group had better occupational functioning and more independent living settings and were less socially isolated. No differences were found in hospitalizations.

Other studies of case management have yielded less favorable results. In a randomized comparison of case management (type not clearly specified) and standard community-based care without formal case management, Texas researchers found that the case-managed patients at 12-month follow-up had received more services, incurred higher service costs, and had more hospitalizations but had no better quality of life outcomes compared with the standard-treatment group. In another study a cohort of young severely mentally ill patients, mainly with schizophrenia, were followed over a seven-year period covering two years before intensive case management and five years with case management. The researchers found that, with case management, patient hospital days were reduced by 75 percent but that the resultant reduction in inpatient costs were offset by a 183 percent increase in structured residential care days. No significant changes in the level of functioning or in the total cost of services were noted.

Together, those studies indicate that, under the right circumstances with appropriately targeted patients, intensive case management can be highly effective in sustaining patients with schizophrenia in the community and in enhancing outcomes. However, case management is not a panacea. The major unanswered questions pertain to which patients require that type of service at what intensity and at what time points in their illness.

INTEGRATING SOMATIC AND PSYCHOSOCIAL TREATMENTS

The vulnerability-stress model of schizophrenia and the need to remediate the broad range of deleterious effects that schizophrenia has on patients' lives lead to the importance of understanding how to integrate somatic and psychosocial treatment to yield optimum results. Research on such treatment integration remains limited.

One study exemplifies what may be accomplished with such linkage. Researchers at the University of Pittsburgh randomized patients with schizophrenia to four treatment groups with various combinations of fluphenazine decanoate and two psychosocial treatments: family psychoeducation and social skills training. The four treatment groups received (1) fluphenazine only, (2) fluphenazine and family psychoeducation, (3) fluphenazine and social skills training, and (4) fluphenazine and both family psychoeducation and social skills training. During the first 12 months of follow-up, the relapse rates were 46 percent, 23 percent, 30 percent, and 9 percent, respectively. Two-year follow-up relapse rates were 66 percent, 32 percent, 57 percent, and 35 percent, respectively, showing particular promise for the combination of medication and family psychoeducation. A secondary finding was that, among unrelapsed patients, those who received the family treatment were more likely to be competitively employed or in school than were those who did not receive family treatment (77 percent versus 41 percent, respectively). Although the study focused primarily on symptom outcomes, it lends optimism to the possibility that combining somatic and psychosocial treatments will also enhance outcomes in other domains.

LOCUS OF PSYCHOSOCIAL TREATMENT

In this era of brief hospitalization, psychosocial treatments occur primarily in community-based settings, including clinics, private offices, day treatment programs, psychosocial rehabilitation centers, vocational rehabilitation centers, and residential-care settings. Indeed, research on alternatives to long-term hospitalization for persons with schizophrenia has shown no advantages for extended hospital care when community-based care is a feasible alternative.

Although the psychosocial treatments for schizophrenia appropriately emphasize life outside the hospital, some of those treatments can and must be adapted to the needs of patients so disabled as to require long-term institutional care. Individual and group therapies, family intervention programs, and various rehabilitation approaches can all be applied to address the needs of long-stay patients, with the goal of either eventual discharge to the community or enhancement of functioning and well-being in the hospital.

Milieu treatment is the use of the hospital environment itself as a therapeutic intervention. Early hospital milieu treatment concepts were embodied in the mental asylums of the 19th century. Recently, hospital-based milieu treatment approaches have included *therapeutic communities,* which emphasize peer support and help and democratic decision making, and behavioral milieus, such as token economies. *Token economies* rely heavily on techniques that reinforce desired behaviors and extinguish undesirable behaviors through the use of tokens that can be earned by patients and spent for rewards. In one classic study, published in 1977, of milieu treatment for treatment-refractory, long-stay patients with schizophrenia, researchers showed the efficacy of a social-learning token-economy approach compared with a therapeutic community approach and with a traditional psychiatric ward approach. Efficacy measures included improved functional status and successful discharge to the community. That study was the culmination of many years of research on improving hospital-based care for patients with schizophrenia. That line of research essentially halted with the dramatic advance of deinstitutionalization in the 1970s. Interest in what to do for patients who require extended hospitalization despite deinstitutionalization must be revived.

Even in the community, new pressures are arising to shift the locus of care from centers of treatment to mainstream community contexts. Several examples of that trend are evident: the move from clinic-based treatment to mobile clinical services (exemplified by the assertive community treatment programs based on the Madison, Wisconsin, model), the move from family treatment in the clinic to home-based family training programs, the move from residential treatment programs to mainstream supported housing, and the move from train-and-place vocational rehabilitation centers to place-and-train models of supported employment. Such trends are inevitably influenced by economics, political philosophy, and the vested interests of competing service providers. Much needed is research to guide the further development of a continuum of approaches that foster the comprehensive integration of individualized treatments for persons with schizophrenia.

SUGGESTED CROSS-REFERENCES

Somatic treatment of schizophrenia is discussed in Section 14.8, individual psychotherapy for schizophrenia in Section 14.10, group psychotherapy in Section 31.4, family therapy in Section 31.5, cognitive therapy in Section 31.6, and hospital and community psychiatry in Chapter 50, including psychiatric rehabilitation in Section 50.4.

REFERENCES

*Anderson C M, Reiss D J, Hogarty G E: *Schizophrenia and the Family.* Guilford, New York, 1986.

Anthony W A, Blanch A: Research on community support services: What have we learned? Psychosoc Rehab J *12:* 55, 1988.

*Anthony W A, Liberman R P: The practice of psychiatric rehabilitation: Historical, conceptual, and research base. Schizophr Bull *12:* 542, 1986.

*Bellack A S, editor: *A Clinical Guide for the Treatment of Schizophrenia.* Plenum, New York, 1989.

Bellack A S, editor: *Schizophrenia: Treatment, Management, and Rehabilitation.* Grune & Stratton, Orlando, FL, 1984.

Bellack A S, Mueser K T: Psychosocial treatment for schizophrenia. Schizophr Bull *19:* 143, 1993.

Bernheim K F, Lehman A F: *Working with Families of the Mentally Ill.* Norton, New York, 1985.

Braun P, Kochansky G, Shapiro R, Greenberg S, Gudeman J E, Johnson S, Shore M F: Overview: Deinstitutionalization of psychiatric patients: A critical review of outcome studies. Am J Psychiatry *138:* 736, 1981.

Brenner H D, Boker W, Hodel B, Wyss H: Cognitive treatment of basic pervasive dysfunctions in schizophrenia. In *Schizophrenia: Scientific Progress,* S C Schulz, C A Tamminga, editors, p 358. Oxford University Press, New York, 1989.

Chiardello J A, Bell M D, editors: *Vocational Rehabilitation of Persons with Prolonged Psychiatric Disorders.* Johns Hopkins University Press, Baltimore, 1988.

Corrigan P W, Storzbach D M: Behavioral interventions for alleviating psychotic symptoms. Hosp Community Psychiatry *44:* 341, 1993.

Dincin J, Wasmer D, Witheridge T F, Sobeck L, Cook J, Razzano L: Impact of assertive community treatment on the use of state hospital inpatient bed-days. Hosp Community Psychiatry *44:* 833, 1993.

Dion G L, Anthony W A: Research in psychiatric rehabilitation: A review of experimental and quasi-experimental studies. Rehab Counsel Bull *30:* 177, 1987.

Fairweather G W, editor: *The Fairweather Lodge: A Twenty-Five Year Retrospective.* Jossey-Bass, San Francisco, 1980.

Falloon I R H, Boyd J L, McGill C W, Razani J, Moss H B, Gildeman M A: Family management in the prevention of exacerbations of schizophrenia. N Engl J Med *306:* 1437, 1982.

Goldstein M J, Rodnick E H, Evans J R, Phillip R A M, Steinberg M: Drug and family therapy in the aftercare of acute schizophrenia. Arch Gen Psychiatry *35:* 1169, 1978.

Group for the Advancement of Psychiatry: *Beyond Symptom Suppression: Improving Long-Term Outcomes of Schizophrenia.* American Psychiatric Press, Washington, 1992.

Gunderson J G, Frank A F, Katz H M, Vannicelli M L, Frosch J P, Knapp P H: Effects of psychotherapy in schizophrenia: II. Comparative outcome of two forms of treatment. Schizophr Bull *10:* 564, 1984.

Hatfield A B, Lefley H P, editors: *Families of the Mentally Ill: Coping and Adaptation.* Guilford, New York, 1987.

Hatfield A B, Lefley H P: *Surviving Mental Illness: Stress, Coping, and Adaptation.* Guilford, New York, 1993.

*Herz M I, Keith S J, Docherty J P, editors: *Psychosocial Treatment of Schizophrenia: Handbook of Schizophrenia,* vol 4. Elsevier, New York, 1990.

Hogarty G E, Anderson C M, Reiss D J, Kornblith S J, Greenwald D P, Javna C D, Madonia M J, EPICS Schizophrenia Research Group: Family psychoeducation, social skills training, and maintenance chemotherapy in the aftercare treatment of schizophrenia: I. One-year effects of a controlled study on relapse and expressed emotion. Arch Gen Psychiatry *43:* 633, 1986.

Hogarty G E, Anderson C M, Reiss D J, Kornblith S J, Greenwald D P, Ulrich R F, Carter M: Family psychoeducation, social skills training, and maintenance chemotherapy in the aftercare treatment of schizophrenia: II. Two-year effects of a controlled study on relapse and adjustment. Arch Gen Psychiatry *48:* 340, 1991.

Hornstra R K, Bruce-Wolfe V, Sagduyu K, Riffle D W: The effect of intensive case management on hospitalization of patients with schizophrenia. Hosp Community Psychiatry, *44:* 844, 1993.

Intagliata J: Improving the quality of community care for the chronically mentally disabled: The role of case management. Schizophr Bull *8:* 655, 1982.

Leff J P, Kuipers L, Berkowitz R, Eberlein-Vreis R, Sturgeon D: A controlled trial of social interventions in the families of schizophrenic patients. Br J Psychiatry *141:* 121, 1982.

Liberman R P, editor: *Psychiatric Rehabilitation of Chronic Mental Patients.* American Psychiatric Press, Washington, 1988.

McEvoy J P, Schooler N R, Friedman E, Steingard S, Allen M: Use of psychopathology vignettes by patients with schizophrenia or schizoaffective disorder and by mental health professionals to judge patients' insight. Am J Psychiatry *150:* 1649, 1993.

McFarlane W R, editor: *Family Therapy in Schizophrenia.* Guilford, New York, 1983.

McGurrin M C: An overview of the effectiveness of traditional vocational rehabilitation services in the treatment of long term mental illness. Psychosoc Rehab J *17:* 37, 1994.

*Meyerson A T, Fine T, editors: *Psychiatric Disability: Clinical, Legal, and Administrative Dimensions.* American Psychiatric Press, Washington, 1987.

Newman S J: The housing and neighborhood conditions of persons with severe mental illness. Hosp Community Psychiatry *45:* 338, 1994.

Olfson M: Assertive community treatment: An evaluation of the experimental evidence. Hosp Community Psychiatry *41:* 634, 1990.
Paul G L, Lentz R J: *Psychosocial Treatment of Chronic Mental Patients: Milieu versus Social Learning Programs.* Harvard University Press, Cambridge, MA, 1977.
Spaulding W D, Storms L, Goodrich V, Sullivan M: Applications of experimental psychopathology in psychiatric rehabilitation. Schizophr Bull *12:* 560, 1986.
Stein L, Test M A: An alternative to mental hospital treatment: I. Conceptual model, treatment program, and clinical evaluation. Arch Gen Psychiatry *37:* 392, 1980.
Stuve P, Erickson R C, Spaulding W: Cognitive rehabilitation: The next step in psychiatric rehabilitation. Psychosoc Rehab J *15:* 9, 1991.
Tarrier N, Beckett R, Harwood S, Baker A, Yusupoff L, Ugarteburu I: A trial of two cognitive-behavioral methods of treating drug-resistant residual psychotic symptoms in schizophrenic patients: Outcomes. Br J Psychiatry *162:* 524, 1993.
Wasylenki D A: Psychotherapy of schizophrenia revisited. Hosp Community Psychiatry *43:* 123, 1992.
Weiden P, Havens L: Psychotherapeutic management techniques in the treatment of outpatients with schizophrenia. Hosp Community Psychiatry *45:* 549, 1994.
Zubin J, Spring B: Vulnerability: A new view of schizophrenia. J Abnorm Psychol *86:* 103, 1977.

14.10 SCHIZOPHRENIA: INDIVIDUAL PSYCHOTHERAPY

WAYNE S. FENTON, M.D.
THOMAS H. McGLASHAN, M.D.

INTRODUCTION

Despite significant advances in the knowledge of schizophrenia's neurobiology and the development of new pharmacological treatments and treatment strategies, schizophrenia remains a catastrophic illness with a substantial risk of lifelong disability. Even with optimal pharmacological intervention, relapse and rehospitalization rates are substantial; the reported incidence of noncompliance with prescribed pharmacological regimens ranges from 11 to 80 percent of patients treated. If a professional consensus exists about anything concerning schizophrenia, it is that no treatment alone is capable of ameliorating the disorder. Therapeutic efforts need to be comprehensive, multimodal, and individualized, including attention to the provision of basic human services, the pharmacological reduction of specific target symptoms, the rehabilitation of social and vocational skills, the provision of structure (someplace to be, something productive to do), and the provision of education and support to the patient's family and other caretakers.

Individual psychotherapy is defined broadly as a professional relationship in which the technical expertise of the physician is brought to bear in an effort to promote a patient's recovery or to relieve suffering. Individual psychotherapy is often the cornerstone of treatment efforts in schizophrenia. Minimally, the physician-patient relationship provides the context in which symptoms and disabilities are assessed, consent and collaboration for treatment are obtained, and the effects of interventions are evaluated. More ambitious goals, appropriate for selected patients in settings where time and resources allow, include the exploration of maladaptive patterns of living through a careful scrutiny of relationships with others and the therapeutic relationship itself. As practiced, most psychotherapy falls somewhere in between, requiring from the therapist a broad base of medical and psychological skills. A psychiatrist providing psychotherapy for schizophrenic patients should probably be prepared to give an intramuscular injection one day, interpret transference the next day, and give a patient a ride to work on the third day. With few exceptions relatively little has been written recently addressing the work from a broad perspective.

HISTORY

Prevailing psychiatric and psychoanalytic thinking in the early decades of the 20th century viewed schizophrenia as a fundamentally irreversible and untreatable process. Organic psychiatry, as represented by Emil Kraepelin, saw schizophrenic personality disintegration as an inevitable product of neurological deterioration. Sigmund Freud, representing the mainstream of psychoanalysis, considered dementia precox an effort at adjustment on the part of the patient, but he came to view the disorder as a narcissistic neurosis in which libido is directed inward, away from others. As a result, transference and analytic treatment were considered impossible. The diagnosis of dementia precox most often led to therapeutic nihilism and to the recommendation of lifelong institutional care.

Despite the misgivings of classical adherents to Freud, individual psychotherapy for schizophrenia in the United States originated as a modification of psychoanalysis. Early psychoanalysts, such as A. A. Brill, observed that, in treating schizophrenia with psychoanalysis, the therapist cannot be a passive listener. Instead, the therapist needs to make an active effort to promote rapport and to arouse the patient's interest in the malady. Brill described, for example, providing didactic reading material, visiting a patient at home, at times frankly labeling false beliefs as delusions, and providing direct advice about work and relationships. In time, Brill observed, confidence in and a passive attachment to the physician can develop; the physician may become a bridge between the patient and reality.

SULLIVAN Between 1922 and 1930 Harry Stack Sullivan set up and ran a small treatment unit for male schizophrenic patients at Sheppard and Enoch Pratt Hospital in Towson, Maryland. He was influenced by the early psychobiological perspectives of Adolf Meyer and William Allison White, who emphasized that personality is influenced by life events not only in childhood but also over the entire course of development. On the basis of his intuition that like cures like, Sullivan staffed the unit with sensitive, shy, introverted male attendants who possessed a natural proclivity and ease of rapport with isolated and withdrawn patients. Stressing that the patients' difficulties were not qualitatively different from those of so-called normal people, Sullivan promoted the development of closeness or benevolent intimacy in the milieu. He observed that providing an experience of reciprocal trust—which, he hypothesized, many patients had missed during important periods of development—can be beneficial by allowing a "validation of all components of personal worth."

In that setting careful observation of the difficulties his patients had in maintaining relationships with others led Sullivan to formulate a new paradigm of interpersonal psychiatry. He de-emphasized the prevailing psychoanalytic view that personality is formed and behavior motivated by drives pressing for expression from within. He recast psychopathology as difficulties in living, which he saw arising largely from personal and social relations, and as personality warps, which he regarded as the lasting residue of early unsatisfactory interpersonal experiences.

Over a period of years, Sullivan elaborated his ideas further in a series of seminars at Chestnut Lodge Hospital in Rockville, Maryland, where, under the leadership of Dexter Bullard, a group of psychoanalysts and social scientists interested in the intensive study of schizophrenia assembled during the 1940s. There the influence of interpersonal patterns among patients and between patients and staff members were observed to have a powerful effect on the patients' psychopathology. Covert tension and disagreements among staff members, for example, often appeared to be associated with the worsening of the patients' psychotic symptoms; improvement followed when those tensions were resolved. Such observations drew attention to the influence of psychosocial factors on schizophrenia and raised the idea that the disorder may be caused and potentially cured by psychosocial means.

FROMM-REICHMANN Drawing on her European psychoanalytic background, her guidance by Sullivan, and her clinical work with psychotic patients at Chestnut Lodge, Frieda Fromm-Reichmann integrated the available knowledge concerning the intensive psychotherapy of schizophrenia into a relatively comprehensive body of theory and technique. In *Principles of Intensive Psychotherapy* she articulated a modified form of psychoanalysis that is applicable to patients with severe mental illness, including schizophrenia. The ideas embodied in her writings and clinical work represent the first elaboration of what has come to be known as intensive psychodynamic psychotherapy.

RECENT DEVELOPMENTS The predecessors of ego psychology and self psychology, interpersonal psychiatry and psychodynamic psychotherapy became dominant paradigms in American psychiatry in the 1940s and the 1950s and beyond. Their hopeful and humanistic perspectives were adopted by many influential psychiatric treatment centers. Intensive individual psychotherapy came to be viewed as the treatment of choice and, at times, the only effective treatment of schizophrenia. Its practitioners kept the field's interest focused on severely ill patients during the decades before the widespread availability of effective pharmacological treatments. Exposure to a second generation of charismatic teachers and clinicians (Otto Will, Ted and Ruth Lidz, Steve Fleck, Elvin Semrad, and Harold Searles, to name a few) kindled interest in treating and studying schizophrenia among psychiatric residents and trainees throughout the country.

INVESTIGATIVE PSYCHOTHERAPY

Although issues of efficacy (reviewed later) have replaced debates about theory and technique over the past two decades, intensive individual psychotherapy for schizophrenia continues to be widely practiced. A review of the voluminous clinical literature in the area suggests that, differences in language and terminology notwithstanding, a consistent orientation and approach have been articulated. The approach can be outlined in terms of the nature of investigative psychotherapy and the nature of schizophrenia from the psychotherapist's point of view, elements of the psychotherapeutic situation, general technical interventions, and general technical attitudes.

NATURE OF INVESTIGATIVE PSYCHOTHERAPY Sullivan defined the psychiatric interview as a two-person transaction that is more or less voluntarily initiated on a progressively unfolding expert-client basis. Its purpose is to elucidate the patient's characteristic patterns of living, the revealing of which is assumed to be useful. The psychotherapeutic encounter is an actual interpersonal experience in which the doctor and the patient are both participant observers. According to Fromm-Reichmann, the goals of intensive psychotherapy are the alleviation of the patient's emotional difficulties and the elimination of symptoms. Those goals are met by undertaking a thorough scrutiny of the patient's life history (especially the history of interpersonal relationships), reviewing in close detail the realities of the patient's current relationships and life situation, and understanding the genetic (historical) roots and the current ramifications of maladaptive interpersonal patterns, as reflected in the doctor-patient relationship and in daily life. Important emotional experiences from which the patient's difficulties spring are assumed to have been forgotten, and their recovery during the therapeutic process is expected. That process is expected to result in a durable remodeling of maladaptive interpersonal patterns—personality change.

Specific assumptions concerning the intelligent nature of humans underlie the intensive psychotherapy of schizophrenia, including the following assumptions: (1) Behaviors, including symptoms, are multidetermined and goal-directed; seemingly inexplicable symptoms have an original context in which they make sense. (2) Past experience is a major factor in determining current behavior. (3) People are never fully aware of the reasons for their feelings and actions and often resist such awareness. (4) The therapist becomes a transference target, and the patient's memory of and emotions associated with important past interpersonal experiences can be reached by examining their repetition in the doctor-patient relationship. (5) Behavior can be modified through learning and by expanding the patient's awareness of unconscious motivation. (6) The patient is responsible, in part, for producing predicaments and is more than a victim. (7) The benefits of treatment are proportional to the degree of the patient's active participation in the process. (8) Treatment involves patient initiative, the exercise of will, and willingness to suffer.

NATURE OF SCHIZOPHRENIA The literature on intensive psychotherapy emphasizes the influence of the environment and learning in the causes and pathogenesis of schizophrenia. Characteristic difficulties in interpersonal relationships among schizophrenic patients are said to include a basic mistrust and expectation of harm from others; marked ambivalence in relationships, with endless oscillations between longing for merger, based on an intolerance of loneliness, and withdrawal and isolation, based on a terror of closeness; weak or absent ego boundaries, with resulting difficulty in differentiating one's own thoughts and impulses from those of others; the absence of a sense of self, often compensated for by an effort to ferret out the expectations of others and to mold oneself accordingly (false self) or, alternatively, to organize in fixed opposition to the wishes of others; a pervasive posture of passivity (things happen to one, and others are the cause of all difficulties); fear that strong emotional arousal of any sort (anger, pleasure, wants, desires) will escalate uncontrollably and lead to panic or catastrophe, with compensating constriction and repression of drives or affects and a resultant inability to express affects or desires to others; fragmented or idiosyncratic thinking; frequent misinterpretation of the motives of others; and an antipathy toward reality, with intolerance of frustration and withdrawal into fantasy.

Extrapolating backward from those key aspects of schizophrenic psychopathology, many early proponents of intensive psychotherapy postulated real or fantasized negative first experiences between the infant patient and its primary caregivers. Those experiences are regarded as causative of schizophrenia and are thought to involve a rejecting or ambivalent mother, a defective infant rendered incapable of using adequate mothering because of excessive inborn aggression or a defective stimulus barrier, or a temperamental mismatch between the infant and its caregiver. Whatever the source, the result is a central unconscious conflict that Lewis Hill described as "that of a small child dependent on a person by whom he feels persecuted and who is, in his opinion, unstable and uncertain." That position represents the patient's conviction concerning the nature of human relationships, and it dominates all the patient's thoughts, feelings, and behaviors.

Subsequent research has failed to substantiate the role of bad parenting in the cause of schizophrenia, and such causative theories are now rightfully rejected as stigmatizing and blaming families. Nonetheless, the clinical descriptions of schizophrenic patients' basic mistrust of others and difficulty in forming relationships remain in many instances valid.

Phases of emotional development A developmental perspective and hierarchical model of the mind is implicit in the clinical theory underlying intensive psychotherapy. A variety of specific developmental schemes have been offered, but most suggest some version of the following phases in emotional development:

1. In the *autistic phase,* during the first weeks of life, the presence of others is not recognized, satisfaction of biological needs is hallucinated, and only undifferentiated states of anxiety, activation, and satiation are present.

2. In the *symbiotic phase* a boundaryless state of bliss is present, with an empathic caregiver who can anticipate and fulfill all needs. The successful completion of the phase is thought to form the substrate of basic trust.

3. The *separation-individuation phase* begins with the ability to ambulate, when the image of the good-enough caregiver becomes progressively internalized, allowing a feeling of security during physical separations. Early in the phase experiences of frustration with the caregiver are emotionally separate from experiences of satisfaction, and the good object and the bad object seem to be different people. Aggression and anger deriving from frustrations are projected onto and attributed to the bad object. The good-enough caregiver accepts those projections without responding with excessive retaliatory anger or anxiety and, thus, contains and soothes the frustrated child. Those experiences of containment or holding form the basis for the child's later capacity to soothe himself or herself, modulate affect, and develop comfort with emotional arousal. By the end of the phase, cognitive and emotional development allow for the recognition that the frustrating caregiver and the satisfying caregiver are the same person (libidinal object constancy), a recognition that forms the basis for seeing others as separate and complex persons.

4. The *oedipal phase* is the major focus of psychoanalysis with neurotic patients. It involves the mastering of triadic relationships, competitive urges, and identifications with the same-gender parent.

Although no writers about intensive psychotherapy consider the schizophrenic patient's mental functioning to be equivalent to that of an infant, primitive adaptive levels of functioning derived from early phases of development are thought to be ever present, hierarchically underlying sophisticated adaptive levels acquired later in development. During states of psychotic regression, developmentally primitive states of mind are thought to gain ascendancy, and higher capacities are thought to be temporarily lost. Nonetheless, the retention of some nonpsychotic functioning is assumed, no matter how sick the patient.

PSYCHOTHERAPEUTIC SITUATION

Participants Although the characteristic difficulties of schizophrenic patients are elaborated at length in the literature, attributes of the optimal psychotherapist are less well defined. Among the therapist attributes cited as important are an interest in and a capacity to tolerate intense affect, dependency, confusion, and ambiguous communication. Basic respect for the patient is a prerequisite, especially respect that stems from a conviction that the patient's problems are not much different from one's own. Aloofness, rigidity, and critical pomposity are especially discouraged. Psychotherapists should be flexible, creative, and willing to admit when they are wrong.

The match between patient and therapist is thought to be central, but it defies easy categorization. When present, a good match is characterized by a developing sense of specialness, a poor match by negativism and oppositionality. Many authors emphasize that physicians working with schizophrenic patients must possess sufficient self-esteem and sources of satisfaction in their nonprofessional lives to avoid using patients to meet personal needs for admiration or prestige. Personal psychotherapy or psychoanalysis is often recommended.

Setting Intensive psychotherapy must be conducted in a setting of mutual safety. Within an organized care setting, the milieu must be ideologically supportive. The frequency of visits can range from one to five a week. Use of the couch and free association, as in psychoanalysis, are generally discouraged as aggravating disorganization and thought disorder.

The use of a two-person team approach—the therapist-administrator split—is sometimes advocated, particularly in inpatient settings. The administrative therapist (often the inpatient unit chief) assumes responsibility for all pragmatic decisions—such as passes, consequences of behavioral difficulties, and medications—allowing the patient to speak freely with the individual psychotherapist without the urgency of meeting some immediate need.

As part of creating the setting for individual psychotherapy, the therapist endeavors to achieve consensus with the patient early on regarding the nature of the patient's problems, the treatment required, and the rules governing therapy, including attendance, fees, contact between hours, proscribed behaviors, and confidentiality.

Process The process elements in psychotherapy for schizophrenia are the expectable developments in the doctor-patient relationship as it evolves, including transference and countertransference. The management of those elements is central to the therapeutic endeavor.

TRANSFERENCE In transference the perception of persons in the present is shaded or distorted by important past relationships. It is thought to be ever present, a natural but often unconscious aspect of all human relationships. Examining transference as it develops and unfolds in the doctor-patient relationship is a major task in exploratory (as opposed to supportive) psychodynamic therapy. The examination is expected to be useful in allowing patients to understand their current difficulties and to respond realistically and productively to people in their current lives. Examining transference should also facilitate the recovery of lost memories, some of which may be accessible only through their re-creation or repetition in the transference relationship.

In nonpsychotic transferences the patient perceives or responds to the therapist *as if* the therapist resembled some important figure from the patient's past. The patient retains, however, the capacity to recognize the transferences as misperceptions, to separate the real aspects of the therapist from the distorted aspects, and to trace the distortions back to their origin in the patient's past experiences.

Sally, a 19-year-old young woman with schizophrenia who, as a child, had been sexually abused by her stepfather, sought intensive psychotherapy as an outpatient after discharge from a hospital. After several weeks of treatment, she expressed her fear that her male psychotherapist would soon demand sexual relations with her. She could readily accept the therapist's interpretation that the fear was unwarranted in the present but reflected the patient's traumatic experiences as a child. The therapist noted that Sally nearly always held her arms and hands in an awkward posture, an observation he attributed to schizophrenic mannerisms. After many months of therapy, Sally told the therapist that she feared the wrong kind of hand movements would be taken by him as an invitation to a sexual liaison. Exploration of that fear allowed her to remember her conviction many years earlier that her hand and body gestures across the dinner table signaled to her stepfather her willingness to engage in sexual activity. Shortly after the recovery of that memory, Sally's self-consciousness about her hands improved, and her mannerisms became more fluid.

The capacity to recognize early experiences as the source of current distortions is often absent or lost in schizophrenia, leading to *transference psychosis,* in which the patient believes or behaves as if the therapist actually were or were like some figure from the past.

Marcy, a woman in her 20s with paranoid schizophrenia, had been raised by a mother who had had many hospitalizations for an intermittent psychotic disorder and who blamed all her difficulties on Marcy. Marcy felt persecuted and wrongfully accused of being mentally ill. She recalled that, when she was upset and in need of comforting from her mother, her mother would often lock herself in her own bedroom until Marcy's upset ran its course and gave way to exhaustion. During the course of psychotherapy as an inpatient, Marcy held the conviction that her female psychotherapist was at the center of a plot to drive her crazy. During one session Marcy assaulted the therapist in a rage; when Marcy stepped out of the office briefly, the therapist was able to lock herself in her office to gain protection from further attack.

Transference, even transference psychosis, is an inevitable and unavoidable development in intensive psychotherapy. Nonpsychotic transference can usually be resolved with time, support, and interpretation. Psychotic transference is more difficult to remove, and a therapeutic relationship must often accommodate that distortion yet remain useful to the patient.

COUNTERTRANSFERENCE Countertransference involves the therapist's thoughts and feelings about the patient; some are distortions arising from the therapist's personal past, and many derive from the interaction with the patient. Feelings that arise in work with schizophrenic patients can be particularly intense and uncomfortable and may include discouragement, fear, worthlessness, hatred, contempt, guilt, rage, envy, and lust. Awareness of countertransference and the ability through introspection to understand its sources are crucial functions for the psychotherapist.

Countertransference is often an important source of information about the patient's state of mind, particularly in patients unable to talk.

John, a recently hospitalized mute young male schizophrenic patient, had not responded to psychotropic medications and was referred for long-term residential treatment. Moments after seating him for an initial psychotherapeutic interview, the therapist found himself feeling trapped and terrified by the sudden recognition that John, with a paranoid glare, was on the verge of assault. After ruling out a run for the door as too risky, the therapist looked at John and asked, "Are you afraid of me?" "Yes," said a perceptibly relieved patient; "I think something bad is going to happen, and you're part of it." "Well, you're scaring the hell out of me," said the therapist. Now appreciably calmer, John said, "I'm sorry," and a conversation ensued. Some time later, John explained that on the day of his arrival he felt that he had been brought to the hospital to be executed and expected at any moment to be shot in the head. The therapist learned to conduct his initial assessments of hospitalized patients in a place where help could be readily obtained if needed.

The therapist's reaction may also be a good barometer for understanding how others typically react and respond to the patient.

By the end of the first week of therapy with Grace, a schizophrenic woman in her 50s, her therapist felt hopelessly overwhelmed by Grace's endless demands for reassurance regarding imagined physical illnesses. Telephone interviews with Grace's two daughters, who had broken off all contact with their mother five and three years before, revealed that they had found their mother's physical complaints and demands so discouraging that both felt no contact whatsoever was the only alternative to constant harassment.

Successful management of countertransference allows the therapist to create a holding or containing relationship with the patient that is postulated to be central to the mutative action of psychotherapy.

Frank, a schizophrenic man in his early 30s who lived in the community, had ambivalent feelings about his 20-hours-a-week job as a dishwasher at a hotel. Frank often found his interaction with coworkers stressful and, hence, was prone to avoid work; he was also plagued by unrelenting guilt about his inability to move up to full-time work on any sustained basis. Frank's father often reinforced that view by telling him that his illness amounted to little more than laziness and that with willpower and strong character Frank should certainly be able to handle a full-time job. Over a period of years, a clear pattern in Frank's illness was detectable: Frank would work part-time and be stable for a period. Driven by his guilt, he would increase his work hours. The stress and overstimulation of the heavier work schedule would lead to an exacerbation of his symptoms and, finally, a full-blown relapse. He would have to quit work altogether for a period and then seek another new part-time job; and the cycle would begin anew. During Frank's relapses, his primary symptom was the delusional fear that he would be damned and persecuted for his moral weaknesses.

Over years of outpatient psychotherapy, Frank's interactions with his therapist about work were of great interest. (The therapist himself was a workaholic.) Whenever Frank contemplated missing a day's work (and there were many such times), he would call the therapist at home the evening before for permission, often presenting the flimsiest of excuses and rationales about why he should not work the next day. Receiving those calls late in the evening, when he himself was still working, the therapist often felt the intense urge to tell Frank to shape up, be a man, show some character, and quit acting as though a little work would kill him. Recognizing that urge as countertransference (derived in part from Frank's seemingly unconscious effort to re-create his relationship with his father with the therapist), the therapist was able to refrain from such moralistic admonishments, discuss matters calmly, and allow Frank to decide on his own about work the next day.

After some years Frank came to realize that his illness was real, rather than a moral weakness. With that realization he was able to accept the fact that, for him, full-time work was probably not going to be possible. The frequent relapses ceased, and Frank was able to sustain long periods of stability. The therapist thought that his recognition of the countertransference allowed him to hold Frank's self-loathing about his work disability and to reflect that acceptance back to Frank in a benign manner, without being overly accusatory or moralistic. To the therapist, that attitude seemed to be an important factor leading to Frank's benign and accepting view of his own disabilities.

TRANSFERENCE-COUNTERTRANSFERENCE CONFIGURATIONS Transference and countertransference tend to mirror each other at any given time, and over the course of treatment a range of transference-countertransference configurations are traversed. The configurations may re-create early development epochs. Typical configurations can include (1) an *autistic* relationship in which the patient does not express the slightest interest or even recognize the existence of the therapist; the therapist, in turn, feels devalued as a nonhuman object; (2) an *idealizing,* symbiotic interaction in which the therapist is perceived by the patient as an omnipotent, protective, and loving figure and in which negative feelings are projected onto others outside the dyad; here the therapist is likely to feel that he or she alone can truly understand the patient, whose problems clearly stem from the insensitivities of others; (3) a *hostile,* paranoid relationship in which the therapist is perceived as a bad object—untrustworthy, engulfing, and intent on harming the patient; here the therapist often feels hatred and rage at the patient's accusations and is tempted to become defensive or retaliatory, thus fulfilling the patient's expectation of others as untrustworthy. Searles has written about the range of transference and countertransference experiences arising in intensive psychotherapy with schizophrenic patients with unusual candor.

TECHNICAL INTERVENTIONS The literature on intensive psychotherapy lists categories of interventions that roughly correspond to the phases of therapy. Although the tasks and strategies may be relevant at any point in treatment, they are often ordered sequentially: (1) establishing a relationship with the patient, (2) elucidating the patient's experience in the here and now, (3) tolerating the mobilized transference and countertransference, (4) integrating the patient's experiences into an expanded perspective of the self, and (5) working through. If therapy progresses, the accomplishment of early tasks allows attention to be paid to subsequent tasks.

Establishing a relationship with the patient Therapy must begin where the patient is. Because of suspiciousness, disorganization, indifference, or ambivalence about human attachments, establishing a relationship with a schizophrenic patient is often a major challenge. Therapists should be aware that, irrespective of conversation or behavior, patients are checking them out and attempting to answer for themselves such questions as, "Who is this person?" and "What is therapy?"

The patient and the therapist must find some way to be comfortable enough with each other to allow therapy to progress. Analytic strategies of passive neutrality and anonymity can easily be misinterpreted as disinterest or dislike and are generally discouraged. Consistency, straightforwardness, and an active effort to establish rapport are advocated. Within bounds, a reasonable degree of self-disclosure by the therapist can help counter distortions by allowing the patient to get a fix on the therapist as a person. If the patient initially wants the therapist only to meet some immediate need (for example, to secure the patient's discharge from a hospital or to intervene for the patient with the family), that is taken as the starting point and is viewed positively as a sign that the therapist is seen as potentially useful. At times, engaging in activity (walking or playing a game), finding a neutral topic of common interest (sports, music), or placidly accepting periods of silence can further the establishment of a relationship. Flexibility, creativity, and patience are the only rules.

If the initial encounters are traversed successfully, a background feeling of security and predictability increasingly characterizes the therapy.

By the end of his first interview with John (see above), a young schizophrenic man who had not responded to antipsychotic medication, it was clear to the therapist that sitting in an office talking with him was too anxiety-provoking for both of them to be of much value. Because John was confined to an inpatient unit, he was interested in taking walks and getting fresh air, so the therapist initiated a regular schedule of walks. In a large, nonconfined space both the patient and the therapist were more comfortable than in the office. They negotiated a regular route through the local neighborhood and, to an extent bounded by John's frequent incoherence, traded small talk. The therapist learned that John was interested in martial arts and rock music and, before becoming ill, had driven a motorcycle. After a short time the therapist noticed that the stride and the rhythm of his and John's gaits almost automatically became synchronized, so that the two walked together with comfort.

On a visit to the hospital recreation hall, John asked the therapist if he could play pool and recounted that his grandfather, whom he remembered with great fondness, had had a pool table in his basement and had taught him how to play many years before. That revelation allowed the therapist to inquire further about John's family members, hometown, and interests.

After many weeks the therapist suggested that they visit his office, acknowledging that a visit to the scene of their early tense encounter would likely feel awkward for each of them. The therapy shifted gradually to the office, although walks were still relied on from time to time during particularly upsetting periods.

ACTIVE PARTICIPATION At times, an engaging style can promote the establishment of a relationship. Some have advocated active participation or playing with a patient's communications or symptoms as a means of capturing their attention.

Tony, a male patient in his early 20s, was hospitalized because, despite a variety of interventions, his thought and conduct remained entirely dominated by the fixed delusion that he was married to and had children by a famous female rock star. During walks with his male therapist, Tony would often remark about pretty women the two passed. The therapist lightheartedly admonished Tony for having such thoughts, reminding him that, as a married man with children, more fitting and important considerations ought to concern him. Tony reacted with a smile; over time it became an inside joke between the patient and the doctor.

INTELLECTUAL CONVERSATION Intellectual conversation often obscures important emotional reactions, but it may be promoted to further the goal of establishing a relationship.

Daniel, a 25-year-old man with a schizoaffective disorder, had not left his family's home for three months. His family finally persuaded him to visit a psychiatrist. During the interview Daniel explained his conviction that store clerks, people on the street, and nearly everyone he met could read his thoughts, which were shameful and humiliating. Over the past several months Daniel spent much of his time studying psychology books, attempting to find out what was wrong with him. During the first two interviews he appeared most comfortable when discussing abstract psychological theories gleaned from his reading and solipsistic reveries. The psychiatrist readily engaged in those discussions, which took on the quality of a discussion between a student and a professor. Daniel clearly prided himself on being able to read and understand psychology texts.

Daniel did not appear for his third appointment; 15 minutes after the hour was to begin, the psychiatrist called the patient's home and reached him by phone. Daniel explained that, since it was clear the psychiatrist did not really like him, there was no sense in returning for therapy. The psychiatrist said that, although it was certainly Daniel's choice whether to continue in therapy or not, one more session to discuss the important decision could not hurt. The patient agreed to a final visit, scheduled for the next day.

During that meeting, Daniel said that he had been quite certain that the psychiatrist had been laughing at him at several junctures and attempting to hide his laughter. The psychiatrist suggested that they review their last meeting, so that the specific moments Daniel felt that he had been laughed at could be identified. Daniel's recall of the session was excellent, and it appeared that he felt the psychiatrist was laughing when he had been describing the breakup of a relationship with his girlfriend that resulted, months before, in his return to his parents' home. The psychiatrist told Daniel with sincerity and honesty that he had not been laughing at those moments and, to the contrary, had found Daniel's description of the breakup to be moving and sad. The psychiatrist wondered aloud whether it was possible that in other situations Daniel had misinterpreted people's reactions to him. Referring back to their discussions of psychological theory, the psychiatrist pointed out that Daniel knew that distorted perceptions were often a topic for doctors and patients in psychotherapy and suggested the following psychological experiment: Every time, in the course of their dealings with each other, that Daniel felt the psychiatrist was laughing or otherwise thinking poorly of him, Daniel would agree to stop at that moment and let the psychiatrist know. For his part the psychiatrist would agree to report to Daniel with candor what, in fact, he was thinking at those moments. In that way Daniel might discover the role of distortions in his dealings with the psychiatrist. Daniel found the experiment intriguing and decided, for the moment, to continue in treatment.

Elucidating the patient's experience in the here and now Semrad viewed the three core tasks of psychotherapy as helping patients to acknowledge, to bear, and to put into perspective their feelings and painful life experiences. Acknowledging the patient's feelings and painful experiences in the present becomes particularly pertinent once a relationship has been established. Acknowledging first requires elucidating affects. Strategies for elucidating include listening, narrowing the focus, seeking concrete details, acknowledging feelings (especially loss, anger, and sadness), and naming or labeling affects. The therapist may act as a comforter, an inquisitor, or a teacher, conveying to the patient that experiencing feelings will neither overwhelm the patient nor hurt others. Psychotic symptoms, when expressed, are thought to signal an affective reaction to some actual event that the patient and the doctor do not yet understand. Examining the patient's day-to-day life in detail allows the therapist to develop a vivid picture of the patient's difficulties, frustrations, and characteristic reactions to others. The aim is to help the patient organize and communicate, to guide the patient into sharpened conceptualizations, and to promote a tolerance of life experience as it is.

If those efforts are successful, the therapist and the patient then share a common language with which to talk about the patient's difficulties. Increasingly, the patient independently reports important life events and emotional reactions to them.

During a therapy hour in his therapist's office, John (see above) reported that a nuclear attack under his control had just been launched in Europe and that, as he and the therapist sat, millions of people were being killed. With single-minded persistence, despite John's evasive disorganization, the therapist attempted to find out what John had been doing that morning before his therapy appointment. The therapist was able to piece together that, immediately preceding the "nuclear attack," John had been listening to the radio, and another patient on his unit had, without asking, changed the station. The therapist suggested and John acknowledged that that had irritated him. The therapist suggested that perhaps there was a connection between John's anger at the other patient and his current concern with millions being killed. The therapist wondered whether, the next time something like that happened, it would be possible for John to temperately register his protest to the other patient. John said that was out of the question; he did not want to be tried for murder. The therapist said that, in his view, a mild protest was quite different from murder.

Suspecting the importance of Daniel's (above) breakup with his girlfriend, his psychiatrist endeavored to collect a detailed descriptive history of the relationship during a series of therapy hours. While living in an apartment with his girlfriend in a different city, Daniel had become increasingly unable to leave the apartment, fearful that anyone who saw him would readily see he was too immature to be having a relationship and would submit him to ridicule. He stopped going to work and, jealous of his girlfriend's ability to go out and meet people, began to interrogate her suspiciously about her activities. Eventually, physical altercations ensued, and the girlfriend, Francine, ended the relationship. Daniel told his psychiatrist that he now spent the bulk of his time in guilty despair and remorse about having ruined what was his only relationship and that he spent many hours a day attempting to communicate telepathically with his girlfriend so that she would reestablish contact with him. The psychiatrist acknowledged the immense sadness of what had happened. Citing Freud's "Mourning and Melancholia," which Daniel had read, the psychiatrist suggested that it would help to talk in detail about Daniel's relationship with his girlfriend, so that he would in time let go of her and perhaps learn from his mistakes.

Tolerating mobilized transferences and countertransferences Tolerating affects, transference, and countertransference corresponds to Semrad's concept of bearing painful feelings that have been acknowledged. As illustrated above in the case illustration of Frank, tolerance is achieved first by the therapist and then, through example, by the patient. The concept of holding or containment is relevant and is thought to be central in the mutative effect of psychotherapy. The patient is thought of as putting negatively valenced affects and self-representations into the therapist, who, by processing those feelings in a mature way, contains, holds, or metabolizes them and makes them available in a benign form for reinternalization by the patient.

Holding and containment operate through projective identification, an intrapsychic and interpersonal process with three component phases. The first phase involves the projection by the patient into the therapist of some unwanted aspect of the self. (Patient: ''I'm not the angry or aggressive one here, Doc; you are!'') The second phase involves the acceptance of the projection; it is often accompanied by interpersonal pressure by the patient on the therapist to accept and think of the content of the projection as his or her own. The third phase involves modulating and processing the projection through the therapist's personality to detoxify it so that it can be reintrojected by the patient in a less disruptive form at the appropriate time. (Therapist: ''Sure, I get angry from time to time. So does everyone. It's also true that I find your unwillingness to take medication at times irritating because I think it would help you more than hurt you. I also think you sometimes don't take the medicine *in order* to get me irritated, just as you did with your parents.'') Simply stated, patients experience themselves as being accepted, negative emotions and all, and learn from the therapist's example to accept unwanted aspects of themselves. Thus, the patient's identification with the therapist and his or her functioning is a major factor in the therapeutic action of psychotherapy.

After Marcy's (see above) attack on her, the therapist seriously wondered whether to continue treating the disagreeable patient, who, after months of therapy, did not seem one iota closer to establishing a trusting relationship than she had before the therapy began. On reflection, the therapist became vividly aware of the manner in which Marcy's view of herself as hated and persecuted by nearly everyone had become a self-fulfilling prophecy. Marcy's suspiciousness, hostility, and accusations were so irritating that the accusations, if not true today, would be tomorrow. The therapist or anyone else who had to deal with Marcy would soon find her despicable and impossible to deal with. Sensing that Marcy's attack and accusations were driven by guilt and self-hatred that had been projected onto her, the therapist found her contempt for Marcy tempered by an understanding of her suffering. The therapist hoped that, if that understanding could be conveyed to Marcy, the vicious cycle of turning nearly everyone against her might be interrupted. When she next saw Marcy in a more secure setting, the therapist did not deny her anger at Marcy for the attack but indicated that the episode, although serious, could be talked about and learned from.

Daniel's discussion of the way in which his jealousy and suspiciousness had ruined his relationship with his girlfriend led to further elaboration of the many ways in which, nearly as long as he could remember, he had been disabled by a fear of others, by ideas of reference, and by the terrifying belief that his thoughts were readily readable by anyone who saw him. As a result of those disabilities, he had not had a single friend throughout elementary school, and months would pass without his uttering a single word in class. At the same time, he reported that at home he would entertain his family with stories (all made up) of his friendships and brilliant academic performances at school.

In recounting that history, the patient alternated between sadness and self-pity, blaming himself for his dismal social failures, and righteous indignation, blaming his parents for not having seen through his act and found some effective way to help him. In listening to the material, the psychiatrist often felt tempted to admonish Daniel to stop unproductively blaming his problems on his parents and stop wallowing in self-pity. Sensing those urges as a response to Daniel's provocation, the psychiatrist saw his task was to empathize with Daniel's plight, to acknowledge both the sadness of his history and his current resentments while conveying a moderate degree of hopefulness, and to blame neither Daniel nor his parents for his sad condition. The psychiatrist hoped that in time both Daniel's self-blame and the provocative resentment toward his parents would be diminished and replaced by an interest in what Daniel himself could do to improve his lot.

Integrating the patient's experience into an expanded perspective of self Broadening patients' understanding of themselves and their situations corresponds to the third part of Semrad's triad: helping patients put into perspective their painful affects, life experiences, and maladaptive solutions. Sullivan said, ''No one has grave difficulties in living if he has a very good grasp of what is happening to him.'' Providing insight is another way in which psychotherapy is thought to be useful, complementing identification with the therapist. Integrating the patient's experience entails a change in the therapeutic relationship and enlists interpretation as its major technical tool. Patients able to traverse this phase of therapy may resolve many of their difficulties and resume emotional growth; those who cannot may remain chronically handicapped.

At that phase in therapy, the nature and the tenor of the therapeutic relationship changes; the therapist becomes more demanding, frustrating, and insistent on adaptation, reality testing, and health. Although remaining supportive, the therapist increasingly confronts or analyzes defenses, frustrates wishes, and interprets transference. The therapist's major task is to accept the patient but reject the psychosis and maladaptive interpersonal maneuvers. Insight can occur at several depths: (1) as simple recognition of the fact of illness, (2) as knowledge about the nature of the illness (for example, hallucinations come from one's own mind), (3) as recognition of the dynamics of the illness (symptoms occur in relation to personal difficulties), and (4) as recognition that symptoms and illness solve problems and conflicts. Emotional insight, gained by direct experience in the doctor-patient relationship, is emphasized.

INTERPRETATION Interpretations point out the transferential nature of the patient's feelings about the doctor, including their origin in the patient's past experience and their inappropriate application in the patient's current everyday life. The what, how, and when of interpretation stem from an empathic attunement to the patient's tolerance, although certain recommendations recur repeatedly. Most psychotherapists are reluctant to interpret content (particularly sexual), since patients are often flooded with unwanted thoughts and impulses. Rather, interpretations focus on defensive operations, resistances to therapy, and the link between symptoms and everyday stresses. Especially targeted for interpretation are negative transference, aggressive impulses, depressive concerns, and dependency issues, since those are the issues often warded away from consciousness out of the patient's fear that their emergence would be overwhelming. Interpretations are presented in a way to help patients learn to formulate interpretations on their own. They are presented as tentative observations in the spirit of mutual inquiry. Short, simple, and nontechnical language is used, and the patient is considered the final judge of the interpretations' validity and usefulness.

PATIENT REACTIONS If traversed successfully, this phase of therapy leaves patients with an accepting and complex view of themselves as persons capable of experiencing the full range of human emotions. Patients no longer view all their difficulties as the product of mistreatment at the hands of others; they assume responsibility for their own treatment and health. Passivity and indecision are seen as active choices, and patients recognize that continued progress depends on their willingness to attempt new solutions, both inside and outside treatment. Gaining perspective involves a gradual renunciation of the therapist as an object of gratification as the patient renews meaningful relationships outside treatment. Losses are faced with a recognition that growth carries pain, as well as pleasure; that life's early losses cannot be undone; and that a magical cure is an illusion.

Over the course of four years of psychotherapy, Daniel's (see above) functioning had in many ways improved; he had moved out of his parents' home, found and kept part-time work, and shared an apartment with a roommate. Although comfortable with his therapist, Daniel still found himself suspecting that others thought ill of him and was fearful lest his inner feelings show. He often found himself caught between intense loneliness and isolation on the one hand and the anxiety of letting himself get close to anyone on the other hand. That conflict was painfully obvious to him, particularly as he compared himself with his roommate, who with seeming effortlessness entertained a long series of female friends and acquaintances. Lying in bed, listening to his roommate visit with a guest, the patient would often hear or imagine he heard them speaking disparagingly of him. The envy Daniel sometimes felt toward his roommate was a great source of shame for him, as was his own adult interest in the opposite sex.

His psychiatrist encouraged the discussion of Daniel's envy and sexual interests in countless psychotherapy sessions, reasoning that, if Daniel could accept the fact that he, like all other human beings, felt envy and lust, he would be less plagued by ideas of reference and the fear that his sexual interest would show.

Working through With improvement in the psychosis and with maturation of the patient's nonpsychotic personality, the phase of integrating evolves into the phase of working through. The patient becomes able to help the therapist perform functions and eventually becomes capable of performing those functions alone. Psychotic transferences are mastered as the patient sees the therapist as real, different, and imperfect. Technical interventions at that time are similar to those used with neurotic patients. Each step toward independence and autonomy generates separation anxiety, and a two steps forward and one step back trajectory can be anticipated. Regressions and symptomatic exacerbations recur but should be shorter, less intense, and more readily influenced by interpretation than they were in the past. The end of treatment may be negotiated, but many authors have noted that patients often remain attached to their therapists and may contact them during crucial junctures many years after therapy has ended.

SUPPORTIVE PSYCHOTHERAPY

AIMS Although perspectives from intensive investigative psychotherapy have dominated the literature for most of the past 50 years, supportive forms of psychotherapy have also been practiced and described. Supportive psychotherapy, historically favored by biologically and pharmacologically oriented clinicians, is firmly grounded in the medical model, in which the patient is seen as suffering from an organically based illness that requires treatment from a physician who will actively prescribe and do something for the patient.

In contrast with the ambitious aim of personality change that is associated with intensive investigative therapy, the short-term and long-term goals of supportive psychotherapy are comparatively modest. Those goals include (1) relief from the immediate crisis or direct reduction of the acute disequilibrium, (2) the reduction of the symptoms to premorbid levels, (3) the reestablishment of psychic homeostasis through a strengthening of defenses, (4) the sealing over of psychotic experiences and conflicts, (5) the circumscribed fostering of adaptation, (6) the mobilization and the preservation of healthy aspects of the patient to enable optimal functioning with any continuing deficit. Functional or social recovery, rather than personality change, is the primary aim of treatment.

TECHNIQUES The overall technical approach of supportive psychotherapy is one of pragmatism and management; the physician, using medical and psychiatric expertise, helps the patient interpret and adapt to reality. The therapist uses techniques that include defining reality, offering direct reassurance, giving advice on current problems of living, urging modification of expectations, and actively organizing the environment for patients who cannot do so themselves. To help stabilize the patient's environment, the therapist often maintains close contact with the patient's family or other treaters and may intervene on the patient's behalf with family, employers, and social agencies.

A major task in the supportive psychotherapeutic session is the eliciting and the tracking of symptoms and the targeting of symptoms for psychopharmacological intervention. Psychopathology is interpreted in a medical context as the unwanted emergence of signs of illness. The basic content of psychotherapy focuses on teaching and relearning; patients are educated regarding the nature of their illness, taught to monitor symptoms and to act promptly to suppress exacerbation. The therapist fosters positive transference as a benign authority; positive feelings are treated as real. Negative transference is avoided. The therapist may become active in helping the patient learn new ways of adapting and may use or prescribe cognitive, behavioral, and social skills training techniques.

RESEARCH STUDIES

EFFICACY OF INDIVIDUAL PSYCHOTHERAPY In the decades after the introduction of phenothiazines, psychiatry became increasingly divided into adherents of the psychodynamic paradigm and adherents of the biological paradigm. Disagreements about the value of intensive psychotherapy became a focal point of often acrimonious ideological and scientific debates. Randomized clinical-trial methods unambiguously showed the value of pharmacological interventions in schizophrenia and came to be seen as the optimal standard for evaluating all treatments. Five studies conducted during the 1960s and the 1970s attempted to empirically evaluate the efficacy of various forms of individual psychotherapy compared with treatment programs not specifically featuring psychotherapy. Although criticized by proponents of intensive psychotherapy on a number of methodological grounds, together the results of those randomized clinical trials provided little or no evidence for the efficacy of psychotherapy as the sole treatment for schizophrenia. Supporting that conclusion were the results of recent long-term follow-up studies at Chestnut Lodge, where many of the techniques of intensive individual psychotherapy were developed, and at Columbia University's Psychiatric Institute, where a group of schizophrenic patients received intensive psychotherapy three times a week. Exceptions notwithstanding, the long-term follow-up of schizophrenic patients in those settings found that the majority of patients treated remained seriously and chronically ill.

The Boston Psychotherapy Study, begun in the late 1970s, was designed to address the methodological weaknesses of earlier clinical trials. Reflecting the then extant ideological rivalry between psychodynamically and biologically oriented clinicians, the study aimed to evaluate the comparative effectiveness of psychodynamic expressive, insight-oriented individual psychotherapy and reality-adaptive, supportive psychotherapy against a backdrop of high-quality inpatient milieu and pharmacological treatment provided to both patient groups. The objectives and the methods of the respective therapies are sum-

TABLE 14.10-1
Boston Psychotherapy Study Description of Reality-Adaptive, Supportive and Expressive, Insight-Oriented Psychotherapy

	Reality-Adaptive, Supportive Psychotherapy	Expressive, Insight-Oriented Psychotherapy
Objectives	Symptom relief by drug management and strengthening of existing defenses	Self-understanding: how one feels and thinks and how those factors influence the course of one's life
Interview focus	Management, complaints, interpersonal problems, current situational problems	Relationship to therapist and significant others, exploration of feelings and conflicts
Psychic arena	Focus on current awareness, no hidden agendas	Look for current meaning, hidden motivation, unconscious factors
Temporal focus	Present and future	Present and past
Techniques	Support, reassurance, limits, clarification, direction, suggestions for environmental manipulation, use of community resources	Support, reassurance, limits, clarification, interpretation, catharsis
Transference	Encourage positive transference to further alliance; actively discourage negative transference	Accept positive transference and work through negative transference
Countertransference	Positive feelings important and expressible; control negative feelings	Mixed feelings expected and generally not disclosed

From A H Stanton, J G Gunderson, P H Knapp, A F Frank, M L Vannicelli, R Schnitzer, R Rosenthal: Effects of psychotherapy in schizophrenia: 1. Design and implementation of a controlled study. Schizophr Bull *10:* 535, 1984.

marized in Table 14.10-1. Contrary to the investigators' expectations, neither therapy emerged as clearly superior, although differential effects across outcome domains were noted: reality-adaptive, supportive psychotherapy was preferentially effective in the areas of recidivism and role performance; expressive, insight-oriented psychotherapy exerted a modest preferential effect on ego functions and cognition.

The disappointing results of randomized clinical trials and follow-up studies contributed substantially to a decline in the prestige and the influence of the psychodynamic paradigm generally and of intensive individual psychotherapy for schizophrenia in particular. An additional challenge came from infant observational research, which indicated that infants are far more active, stimulus seeking, and socially oriented from birth than was suggested by early psychodynamic theory. Likewise, such stages as the autistic and the symbiotic were not observed, and the infants' plasticity, resilience, and capacity for adaptation appeared to be far greater than was thought. Those findings challenged the validity of psychosocial theories of cause, at least as articulated by psychodynamic thinkers. Because of those and other factors, individual psychotherapy research and psychological theorizing about schizophrenia slowed to a near halt. The biological paradigm decisively gained ascendancy as the most influential in the field.

REAPPRAISAL OF INDIVIDUAL PSYCHOTHERAPY

Rancorous debates about the relative value of drugs and psychotherapy have largely given way to the recognition that no single approach can claim to be the definitive treatment of schizophrenia and that optimal patient care is comprehensive and individualized. Significant among the findings from the Boston Psychotherapy Study was the degree to which, despite theoretical differences, the techniques used by the therapists tended to converge. Both types of therapy, for example, were found to use substantial supportive elements. Sobering but also significant was the substantial difficulty that patients assigned to both types of therapy had remaining in treatment. Although those who remained in therapy continued to accrue benefits, after 12 months more than half (56 percent) and after two years more than two thirds (69 percent) of all patients had unilaterally dropped out of treatment.

Having found few differences in overall outcome between patients treated with expressive, insight-oriented therapy and those treated with reality-adaptive supportive therapy, investigators from the Boston Psychotherapy Study searched for common factors in the treatments associated with positive therapeutic change and good outcome. The results indicated that patients able to form a good alliance with the therapist in the first six months of treatment are more likely to remain in therapy, comply with medication, and achieve better outcomes after two years with less medication than are those who do not form a good alliance. Looking at therapist activity, the investigators found in both therapies a strong positive correlation between, on the one hand, reductions in patient denial of illness and retardation-apathy and, on the other hand, the therapist's demonstration of a sound dynamic understanding and accurate attunement to the patient's underlying concerns. Directive activity was associated with reductions in anxiety and depression.

FLEXIBLE PSYCHOTHERAPY

The results of empirical research clearly call for a reformulation of psychotherapeutic techniques. Findings from the Boston Psychotherapy Study suggest that the historical distinction between supportive therapy and exploratory therapy may no longer be salient. A broad and pragmatic approach to psychotherapy that relies on a variety of strategies applied flexibly, depending on the individual patient's type of schizophrenia and phase of illness, likely represents the best that can be recommended. Such an approach may at various times include supportive, directive, educational, investigative, and insight-oriented activity that is provided in the context of an ongoing and stable doctor-patient relationship. The relationship should be characterized by empathy and a sound dynamic understanding of schizophrenia on the part of the physician. Dogmatic or rigid adherence to a single approach applied to all patients is probably the method least likely to be of value.

ASSUMPTIONS A comprehensive approach to the psychotherapy for schizophrenia specific to illness phase and subtype has yet to be articulated, operationalized, or tested. Therefore, largely on the basis of clinical experience and scant data, the authors can present only general principles and strategies that must be considered tentative.

A flexible approach to psychotherapy is based on a revised set of assumptions about the nature of schizophrenia that recognizes the joint contributions of biological, psychological, social, and environmental factors.

Vulnerabilities The stress-diathesis or vulnerability-stress model represents one of the best available integrations of data pertinent to the cause, course, and outcome of schizophrenia. The model postulates that schizophrenia results from a dynamic interaction between environmental stress and experiential stress in a person who is vulnerable to react to those stresses with schizophrenic symptom formation.

The vulnerabilities to schizophrenia are likely to be multiple and heterogeneous. Aspects of vulnerability are undoubtedly genetic, but some may be acquired biologically through intrauterine, birth, and postnatal complications. Although a variety of specific vulnerabilities have been postulated, few have been demonstrated, and none have been shown to be ubiquitous. Some of the relatively enduring difficulties observed among subgroups of patients are (1) deficits in information processing and maintaining a steady focus of attention; (2) dysfunctions in psychophysiology, suggesting deficits in sensory inhibition and autonomic responsivity; (3) impairments in social competence; and (4) general coping deficits, such as overvaluing threat, underappraising abilities, and the extensive use of denial.

Vulnerability to schizophrenia is seen as a relatively enduring proclivity to overt clinical symptoms; vulnerability is likely to be manifest as a set of stable traits that are present premorbidly, at onset, during acute episodes, and during remissions. At the same time, vulnerability is not static; it is shaped epigenetically over time by environmental influences; a stress sufficient to precipitate a relapse at one time, for example, may be less likely to do so at a later time, when new coping strategies or better supports have been acquired.

Stressors The stress side of the vulnerability-stress model postulates that a variety of stressors (internal and external events requiring adaptation) can precipitate the emergence of symptoms in a vulnerable person. With biologically based vulnerability, the onset, the course, and the outcome of a person's disorder may be shaped largely by interactions between the person and the environment. Among psychosocial factors, stressful life events, cultural milieu (egocentric versus sociocentric), social class, social network size and density, and emotional quality of the living environment are associated with the onset and the course of schizophrenia.

The vicissitudes of illness are best understood as a dynamic product of the affected person's adaptive assets and vulnerabilities interacting over time with various stresses. In a highly vulnerable person, sufficient stress can precipitate intermediate (prodromal) states of dysfunction that amplify preexisting cognitive, affective-autonomic, and social coping deficits. In the absence of adaptive strategies or environmental supports, those deficits interact negatively with the existing stressors to magnify their effect in a downwardly spiraling process that ends in a full-blown clinical syndrome.

Clinical experience indicates that the stresses associated with illness onset or exacerbation are highy individualized, rendering generalization about the typical nature of such stresses difficult. Stresses may be primarily biochemical (as in substance abuse), environmental (as in leaving for college, joining the armed services, breaking up with a girlfriend), or social (as in poverty, unemployment).

Heterogeneity Schizophrenia is heterogeneous, as are the persons afflicted with it. The clinical diversity of schizophrenia—considered in relation to vulnerabilities, risk factors, age, type of onset, manifest signs and symptoms, longitudinal course, and long-term outcome—suggests that the disorder is heterogeneous in regard to underlying causes. That heterogeneity may be partially captured by currently available subtyping systems. Paranoid schizophrenia, for example, is associated with good premorbid functioning, late age of onset, many positive symptoms (delusions, hallucinations), intermittent illness over the first several years, and a comparatively high likelihood of good outcome, despite a high risk of suicide; the deficit form of schizophrenia is characterized by poor premorbid functioning, early onset, severe and enduring negative symptoms (flat affect, anhedonia, poverty of speech), a low risk of suicide, and often persistent lifelong disability. A method of subtyping based on cause that allows for precise longitudinal prediction for individual patients is not, however, available. At a minimum, schizophrenic illnesses of greater and lower severity and virulence can be identified, and the biological vulnerability of patients may differ.

Like the illness itself, persons afflicted with schizophrenia differ substantially in adaptive capacities, intelligence, and instrumental and verbal competence. Furthermore, the degree of social support available to them varies greatly. In general, the greater the level of instrumental skills acquired before the onset of illness (work or educational experience, experience with relationships, experience living independently), the better positioned the person is to recover or to maintain functioning once the illness has become established. For some patients the failure to acquire much in the way of adaptive skills may represent the product of the lifelong vulnerability underlying the tendency to the illness. For other patients a particularly virulent form of schizophrenia may catastrophically erode adequate premorbid skills, resulting in substantial permanent disability. Other patients with good premorbid abilities may be left after an episode with their skills and competence largely intact.

Phases Schizophrenia is often phasic in course. Systematic investigations of the longitudinal course have only recently begun, and understanding of the illness phases is preliminary. The phases may include (1) prodromal periods, during which a highly individualized constellation of symptoms that represent early manifestations of clinical decompensation emerge; (2) acute or active phases, often associated with the full-blown emergence of positive symptoms superimposed on preexisting deficits; (3) convalescent phases, characterized by the gradual restoration of some functioning, perhaps associated with postpsychotic depression; (4) moratoriums or adaptive plateaus, characterized by a gradual reconstitution of identity, a gathering of support, and a strengthening of skills; (5) change points, shifts in functioning over a relatively brief period, initiated by the patient's own desires or by pressure from others and associated with the potential for either significant improvement or decompensation; and (6) end state or stable plateaus, relatively enduring periods of stability characterized by fixed deficits or chronic levels of positive symptoms.

CLINICAL TASKS AND TECHNICAL STRATEGIES To treat schizophrenia, the therapist must use a variety of interventions and strategies. The crucial question becomes which interventions are of potential value for a particular patient at a particular phase of the illness. All interventions aim to minimize the effect of vulnerabilities, to bolster adaptive capacities, and to reduce the extent and the effects of stress. The range of therapeutic tasks and techniques can be ordered hierarchically. As outlined in Table 14.10-2, the therapeutic tasks can be roughly linked to illness phases. In addition, some tasks are clearly rel-

TABLE 14.10-2
Flexible Individual Psychotherapy for Schizophrenia: Therapeutic Levels and Tasks

Therapeutic Levels and Tasks	Salient Issues	Interventions	Goals	Phase
Medical assessment and stabilization	Medical, diagnostic, safety, acute symptom management	Clinical, medical, neurological evaluation; hospitalization or community alternative; legal commitment; short-term pharmacological treatment; directive, structured, and supportive interventions; limit setting	Rule out medical and neurological disorders; rapid symptom reduction; maintain safety, and minimize destructive effects of psychotic behavior on life situation	Prodromal-acute phase
Psychosocial assessment and case management	Adaptive capacities, social supports, stresses, and vulnerabilities; daily activities, living situation	Skilled psychological and psychosocial assessment, leading to accurate understanding of patient's human service needs; environmental manipulation	Mobilization of social support, structured activities, entitlements; tentative plan for postepisode return to living, including necessity of other modalities (day treatment, supportive housing)	Subacute and convalescence
Establishing supportive ongoing treatment	Damage to self-esteem, mistrust, denial, disorganization	Continued medication; attention to complaints, situational problems, support, reassurance, bolstering defenses, positive regard; encourage benign positive transference; promote comfort with and in treatment	Sufficient acceptance of illness to comply with treatment, establishing treatment routine, supporting strengths, and promoting highest functioning possible; monitoring for relapse	Moratorium or adaptive plateau
Psychoeducation	Acceptance of and adaptation to chronic disorder; human concerns associated with disability, self-management of illness, adaptation to residual deficits	Supportive didactic instruction, understanding of particularly potent individual stresses, patterns of prodromal symptoms, maintenance of medication	Better self-monitoring and management of illness; early recognition of prodome; avoidance of relapse; determination of lowest effective prophylactic medication	Moratorium change points
Habilitative and rehabilitative tasks	Learning or relearning social, vocational, living skills; establishing realistic expectations; adaptation to defects	Practicing, modeling; attention to details of daily social and occupational functioning, direct support, intervention with family and employers; specialized cognitive and social skills enhancement; maintenance medication	Promoting and maintaining highest adaptive functioning possible within limits of deficits; enhancement of self-esteem; maximize quality of life	End state stable plateau
Investigative psychotherapeutic tasks	Transference, countertransference, unconscious motivation, conflicts	Exploration of relationship to therapist; exploration of feelings and conflicts; focus on unconscious, hidden meanings; interpretation	Integrating psychosis into expanded conception of self; construction of narrative history; working through conflicts; improved capacity for intimacy and productivity	Selected patients during clinically stable periods

evant for all patients receiving individual treatment; other tasks, particularly those relating to the goals of intensive psychotherapy, are pertinent for only a small group of patients. The strategic Rosetta stone here is the therapist's capacity to shift gears flexibly and to change roles with all patients on the basis of changing circumstances, always holding in mind the goal of helping the patient accept, learn about, and self-manage what may often be a chronic and devastating illness.

Consideration of schizophrenia subtype, the patient's current and premorbid functioning, and the individual patient's self-defined treatment goals are all relevant to the determination of appropriate treatment tasks. For patients with severe disorganized (hebephrenic) schizophrenia and deficit types of schizophrenia, for example, the most humane and practical goal may be to establish a supportive ongoing treatment within a sheltered setting that minimizes stress and provides for basic human needs for an indefinite period. For the majority of patients who reside in the community amid varying supportive structures, some degree of psychoeducation and rehabilitative tasks should be planned with the aim of minimizing relapses and promoting maximal functioning and quality of life. A primary focus on investigative tasks should probably be reserved for patients who (1) have developed or are maintaining a reasonably secure sense of self, (2) use a minimum of denial, (3) have established a good working relationship with their therapist, and (4) exhibit an interest in the tasks and an ability to make constructive use of the techniques. Those patients are likely to have good premorbid functioning, intermittent and less severe forms of schizophrenia, minimal residual deficits, and retention of some capacity for self-observation, curiosity, frustration tolerance, and humor.

Many treatment modalities are required, and they need someone to orchestrate and coordinate them. In many instances a psychiatrist is best at providing individual therapy and continuity of care over a prolonged period. As is true in medicine generally, the quality of the individual doctor-patient relationship is a major factor in the success of the therapeutic endeavor. A focus on the skillful use of that relationship usefully informs all tasks at all levels. Removed from outmoded causative assumptions and overly ambitious aims, the substantial clinical knowledge derived from the tradition of intensive psychotherapy can be applied pragmatically in a contemporary context.

Many of the tasks overlap with the concerns and the expertise of other service providers; however, all the tasks should be the concern of the individual psychotherapist and a focus for individual psychotherapy. A common mistake made by trainees is to focus on high-level psychological tasks and to ignore overwhelming difficulties at the level of basic human services. Thus, the necessary first goal of psychotherapy with a homeless person is usually direct assistance in finding suitable housing.

The following general treatment strategies are common to all therapeutic tasks.

Evaluation A thorough evaluation of the patient initiates the treatment process. At the level of medical assessment and stabilization, the evaluation includes ruling out the role of identifiable physical conditions, assessing the patient's competence to consent to treatment, and determining the responsivity of the patient's symptoms to short-term pharmacological intervention. Psychosocial assessment inventories the patient's available supports and aims to measure the degree to which the patient's adaptive capacities measure up against the stresses and the demands of his or her living environment. Efforts to establish a supportive ongoing treatment test the patient's capacity to trust and rely on another human being for support and guidance. When applicable, psychoeducational, rehabilitative, and investigative interventions are preceded by an assessment of the patient's cognitive strengths and deficits, allowing interventions to be formulated that match the patient's talents.

Continuous reevaluation The fluid nature of schizophrenia and of patients' adaptation to it over time demands periodic reassessment of the course, the prognosis, the illness phase, and the target problems. As those change, so do treatment goals. Providing concrete support in the form of a ride to work may be helpful early in the effort to promote vocational rehabilitation, but later in therapy the ride may promote unwarranted dependency and prolong disability.

Timing The phasic natural history of schizophrenia requires attention to when particular therapeutic tasks are attempted. To minimize stress and forestall relapse in many patients, the therapist should attempt relatively little beyond assessment, stabilization with medication, and the establishment of a supportive ongoing treatment during the first 6 to 12 months after an episode. Once the patient is asymptomatic and shows signs of revitalization, the therapist may gradually introduce rehabilitation and complex psychoeducational elements.

Titration The therapist should apply treatment interventions with graded increases of intensity and complexity. High-level therapeutic tasks should be attempted and high levels of work or social functioning expected only after the patient has completed and consolidated earlier gains. Substantial rehabilitation, for example, is rarely possible until progress has been made in attaining a stable, supportive treatment relationship. Likewise, early, active, and ambitious psychologically oriented treatment may be disorganizing or toxic for certain patients. In general, the therapist should pursue treatment changes cautiously, modifying only one element at a time.

Integration with psychopharmacology Each of the tasks outlined above takes as a given short-term and prophylactic antipsychotic drugs for most patients. The control and prevention of psychotic symptoms, using the lowest effective dosage of medication, is the overall treatment goal. Decisions regarding pharmacological management are often linked to the relative success or failure of accomplishing various psychotherapeutic tasks. Considerable psychoeducation, for example, should be accomplished before attempting maintenance-medication dosage reduction or the initiation of a targeted (intermittent) medication strategy. Long-acting injectable antipsychotics may be useful for patients unable to tolerate the daily reminder of illness associated with oral medication and for patients unable to maintain a reliable treatment relationship.

MEDICATION NONCOMPLIANCE Noncompliance with effective psychopharmacological treatment during both short-term and maintenance therapy is a major cause of morbidity among patients with schizophrenia. When prolonged or repeated, noncompliance contributes to a downwardly spiraling cycle of relapse, recidivism, and deterioration of social and instrumental functioning. Patient characteristics typically identified as associated with medication noncompliance include severe anxiety, paranoia, grandiosity, depression, hostility, global psychopathology, coexisting personality disorders, and substance abuse. Available research underscores the multiplicity of explanations for reduced compliance and highlights the necessity of an individualized assessment that includes careful attention to practical barriers to compliance (complex drug schedules, uninviting treatment settings, transportation problems), conceptual disorganization or forgetfulness, and aversive side effects. Of unique relevance to psychotherapy, however, are the psychological meanings attached by patients to their illness and its treatment.

Psychological meanings Among the psychological meanings associated with medication noncompliance are the following: (1) pervasive denial about having an illness and needing treatment; (2) reactive efforts to regain control of one's life and to maintain a sense of self-cohesion by organizing in opposition to the will of others; (3) the concrete equation of taking medication with being ill ("If I need drugs, I must be sick. The higher the dose, the sicker I am. I'll stop being ill if I stop taking drugs"); (4) lack of knowledge or incorrect beliefs about medications ("Taking drugs is a sign of weakness"); (5) paranoid views of medication as being poison, controlling, or damaging; (6) secondary gains from psychosis—grandiose delusional gratification, escape from normal expectations and responsibilities; (7) pain and anguish accompanying symptom reduction with its attendant recognition that one has been ill and that the illness is severe; (8) displacement from transference (for example, discontinuing medication as an expression of anger toward the therapist or the patient's family); (9) an expression of unconscious ambivalence or fear of autonomy, as in discontinuing medication immediately before beginning a new job or a rehabilitation program.

The variety of possible meanings underscores the need for a broad and flexible approach that applies a range of interventions based on current knowledge of psychopharmacology and sound dynamic understanding of the individual patient. General recommendations for improving compliance in the context of psychotherapy include (1) conveying interest and concern about medication by asking specific questions about how much medication is being taken, its effects, and its side effects; (2) assuming that many patients will at times take more or less medication and creating a therapeutic environment where such experiments are legitimized and can be talked about; (3) involving patients to the greatest extent possible in their own medication treatment (for example, allowing the self-regulation of dosage within bounds); (4) arranging for the taking of medication under the supervision of family, friends, or others and enlisting their support for medication compliance; (5) direct praise and support for medication compliance; (6) education in the areas of medication side effects, relapse prevention, and the biological basis of major mental disorders; (7) promoting self-monitoring through record keeping and other behavioral interventions; (8) attending to the therapeutic relationship and building it as a lever for change; and (9) helping the patient engage in activities that promote self-esteem and compete with psychosis as sources of gratification. When lack of knowledge and cognitive deficit are major factors in noncompliance, specific cognitive and behavioral procedures can enhance cognitive mastery and skills attainment. When noncompliance represents an unconscious wish to regress or to act out transference, dynamic exploration and interpretation are required.

Countertransference Some patients who appear to be clear candidates for medication continue to refuse it, despite all efforts. Those circumstances typically arouse countertransference reactions, such as telling patients out of anger to seek treatment elsewhere, wishing to hurt patients through abandonment, and withholding advice or support that may be of use to patients in order to see them ''learn their lesson'' by experiencing a full-blown relapse.

Circumstances requiring the therapist to initiate commitment proceedings or the involuntary administration of medication also typically evoke powerful countertransference. After such coercive interventions, the humanistically oriented psychotherapist may experience considerable guilt or fear of the patient. At such a time the therapist is tempted to discontinue all contact and to turn the patient over to another clinician, rationalizing that a therapeutic alliance will never again be possible after such heavy-handed acts. Such an assessment is usually a distortion that more often serves the needs of the therapist than the needs of the patient. After the resolution of such an episode, many patients express gratitude for the therapist's action. If such a painful episode can be accepted, endured, and borne by both participants, the event can become an important part of the shared history of experiences that is psychotherapy.

SUGGESTED CROSS-REFERENCES

General discussions of the psychotherapies appear in Chapter 31. Various aspects of schizophrenia and its treatment are discussed in the other sections of Chapter 14.

REFERENCES

Amandor X F, Strauss D H, Yale S A: Awareness of insight in schizophrenia. Schizophr Bull *17:* 113, 1991.

Berman A L: Case consultation: The suicide of Marigold Perry. Suicide Life Threat Behav *22:* 396, 1992.

Book H E: Some psychodynamics of non-compliance. Can J Psychiatry *32:* 115, 1987.

Brill A A: Schizophrenia and psychotherapy. Am J Psychiatry *9:* 519, 1929.

Burnham D L, Gladstone A I, Gibson R W: *Schizophrenia and the Need-Fear Dilemma.* International Universities Press, New York, 1969.

Caldwell C B, Gottesman I I: Schizophrenics kill themselves too: A review of risk factors for suicide. Schizophr Bull *16:* 571, 1990.

Corrigan P W, Liberman R P, Engel J D: From noncompliance to collaboration in the treatment of schizophrenia. Hosp Community Psychiatry *41:* 1203, 1990.

Coursey R D: Psychotherapy with persons suffering from schizophrenia: The need for a new agenda. Schizophr Bull *15:* 349, 1989.

Diamond R J: Enhancing medication use in schizophrenic patients. J Clin Psychiatry *44:* 8, 1983.

*Dingman C W, McGlashan T H: Psychotherapy. In *A Clinical Guide for the Treatment of Schizophrenia,* A S Bellack, editor, p 263. Plenum, New York, 1989.

Eckman T A, Liberman R P, Phipps C C, Blair K E: Teaching medication management skills to schizophrenic patients. J Clin Psychopharmacol *10:* 33, 1990.

Falloon I R H: Early intervention for first episodes of schizophrenia: A preliminary exploration. Psychiatry *55:* 4, 1992.

Fenton W S, McGlashan T H: Natural history of schizophrenia subtypes: I. Longitudinal study of paranoid, hebephrenic, and undifferentiated schizophrenia. Arch Gen Psychiatry *48:* 969, 1991.

Fenton W S, McGlashan T H: Natural history of schizophrenia subtypes: II. Positive and negative symptoms and long-term course. Arch Gen Psychiatry *48:* 978, 1991.

Frank A F, Gunderson J G: The role of the theraputic alliance in the treatment of schizophrenia: Relationship to course and outcome. Arch Gen Psychiatry *47:* 228, 1990.

*Fromm-Reichmann F: *Principles of Intensive Psychotherapy.* University of Chicago Press, Chicago, 1950.

Glass L L, Katz H M, Schnitzer R D, Knapp P H, Frank A F, Gunderson J G: Psychotherapy of schizophrenia: An empirical investigation of the relationship of process to outcome. Am J Psychiatry *146:* 603, 1989.

Goering P N, Strauss J S: Intensive studies of patients and the experiences of investigators and clinicians. Psychiatry *57:* 166, 1994.

*Greenfeld D: *The Psychotic Patient: Medication and Psychotherapy.* Free Press, New York, 1985.

Gunderson J G, Frank A F, Katz H M, Vannicelli M L, Frosch J P, Knapp P H: Effects of psychotherapy in schizophrenia: II. Comparative outcome of two forms of treatment. Schizophr Bull *10:* 564, 1984.

Hill L B: *Psychotherapeutic Intervention in Schizophrenia.* University of Chicago Press, Chicago, 1955.

Levine I L, Wilson A: Dynamic interpersonal processes and the inpatient holding environment. Psychiatry *48:* 341, 1985.

McGlashan T H: Intensive individual psychotherapy of schizophrenia: A review of techniques. Arch Gen Psychiatry *40:* 909, 1983.

McGlashan T H: Schizophrenia: Psychosocial treatments and the role of psychosocial factors in its etiology and pathogenesis. In *Annual Review of Psychiatry,* vol 5, A Frances, R Hales, editors, p 96. American Psychiatric Press, Washington, 1986.

McGlashan T H, Keats C J: *Schizophrenia: Treatment Process and Outcome.* American Psychiatric Press, Washington, 1989.

McGlashan T H, Nayfack B: Psychotherapeutic models and the treatment of schizophrenia: The records of three successive psychotherapists with one patient at Chestnut Lodge for 18 years. Psychiatry *51*: 340, 1988.

*Meehl P E: Schizotaxia, schizotypy, schizophrenia. Am Psychol *17:* 827, 1962.

Nuechterlein K H, Dawson M E: Vulnerability and stress factors in the developmental course of schizophrenic disorders. Schizophr Bull *10:* 158, 1984.

Perry H S: *Psychiatrist of America: The Life of Harry Stack Sullivan.* Belknap, Cambridge, MA, 1982.

Rako S, Mazer H, editors: *Semrad: The Heart of a Therapist.* Aronson, New York, 1980.

Searles H F: *Collected Papers on Schizophrenia and Related Topics.* International Universities Press, New York, 1965.

Searles H F: *Countertransference.* International Universities Press, New York, 1979.

Stanton A H, Gunderson J G, Knapp P H, Frank A F, Vannicelli M L, Schnitzer R, Rosenthal R: Effects of psychotherapy in schizophrenia: I. Design and implementation of a controlled study. Schizophr Bull *10:* 520, 1984.

Strauss J S, Goering P N: Introduction. Psychiatry *57:* 165, 1994.

Strauss J S, Hafez H, Lieberman P, Harding C M: The course of psychiatric disorder: III. Longitudinal principles. Am J Psychiatry *142:* 289, 1985.

*Sullivan H S: *The Psychiatric Interview.* Norton, New York, 1970.

Weiden P, Havens L: Psychotherapeutic management techniques in the treatment of outpatients with schizophrenia. Hosp Community Psychiatry *45:* 549, 1994.

CHAPTER 15 OTHER PSYCHOTIC DISORDERS

15.1 SCHIZOAFFECTIVE DISORDER, SCHIZOPHRENIFORM DISORDER, AND BRIEF PSYCHOTIC DISORDER

SAMUEL G. SIRIS, M.D.
MICHAEL R. LAVIN, M.D.

INTRODUCTION

Throughout the 20th century, psychiatry has traditionally categorized the functional psychoses as belonging to one of two basic groups of disorders, either to the group of disorders now known as schizophrenia or to the group of disorders now known as mood disorders. That diagnostic distinction has been based on two arenas of observation: symptoms and longitudinal course. Patients with predominantly perceptual and cognitive problems (hallucinations, impaired reality testing, and thought disorders) and with a deteriorating social or vocational course have come to be classified as having schizophrenia. Patients whose symptoms are predominantly in the realm of a disorder of mood regulation (either in the direction of depression or in the direction of euphoria or irritability) and who tend to have a more fully remitting course have come to be classified as having mood disorders.

That characterization, however, does not work well for all patients encountered in clinical practice. Some patients present with mixtures of those characteristics. That is, some patients have symptoms that have prominent and persistent aspects of both perceptual-cognitive disturbances and mood disturbances. Other patients seem to have predominantly perceptual-cognitive symptoms but have a favorable psychosocial course, with full remission after an episode of relatively short duration. Still other patients present with symptoms that are predominantly in the realm of mood, but the disorders fail to remit or the patients experience deteriorating psychosocial courses. Those observations have led to the hypothesis that a so-called third psychosis exists, and to the alternative formulation that all psychoses are on a spectrum reaching from pure schizophrenia at one extreme to pure mood disorders at the other. Adhering to a nontheoretical approach, the editors of *Diagnostic and Statistical Manual of Mental Disorders* (DSM) have grouped patients with mixed characteristics into the larger and potentially heterogeneous category of psychotic disorders not otherwise specified.

Over time, many patients with prominent or persistent symptoms in both the perceptual-cognitive and affective realms have come to be spoken of as having schizoaffective disorder, a term that itself implies the two notions. However, many definitions of schizoaffective disorder have been used over the years, greatly complicating its conceptualization and the accumulation of an empirical data base concerning patients with the disorder. Indeed, at times the existence of schizoaffective disorder as a proper diagnostic category has been challenged. Nevertheless, the presenting symptoms and histories of a sizable number of patients seem to force the use of the diagnostic category, which the first part of this section considers.

The later parts of the section, concerning schizophreniform disorder and brief psychotic disorder, address those patients whose presenting psychotic symptoms are consistent with schizophrenia but whose remitting courses and favorable psychosocial outcomes do not conform to the typical longitudinal patterns of schizophrenia.

SCHIZOAFFECTIVE DISORDER

DEFINITION Schizoaffective disorder is defined by the fourth edition of DSM (DSM-IV) as a psychiatric illness that includes significant and enduring mood symptoms, thus satisfying criteria that, in the absence of psychotic symptoms, would qualify for a diagnosis of a major mood disorder. In schizoaffective disorder, however, the mood symptoms overlap with prominent psychotic symptoms that are also persistent and that continue to be present during a substantial interval of illness when the patient lacks prominent mood symptoms. However, the symptoms that meet criteria for a mood episode must also be present for a substantial portion of the total duration of active and residual periods of that episode of illness. In addition, if the mood episode is a major depressive episode, pervasive depressed mood must be present. The specific DSM-IV diagnostic criteria are listed in Table 15.1-1.

DSM-IV also specifies the diagnosis of schizoaffective disorder in two ways. It distinguishes between a bipolar type and

TABLE 15.1-1
Diagnostic Criteria for Schizoaffective Disorder

A. An uninterrupted period of illness during which, at some time, there is either a major depressive episode, a manic episode, or a mixed episode concurrent with symptoms that meet criterion A for schizophrenia.
 Note: The major depressive episode must include criterion A1: depressed mood.
B. During the same period of illness, there have been delusions or hallucinations for at least two weeks in the absence of prominent mood symptoms.
C. Symptoms that meet criteria for a mood episode are present for a substantial portion of the total duration of the active and residual periods of the illness.
D. The disturbance is not due to the direct physiological effects of a substance (e.g., a drug of abuse, a medication) or a general medical condition.

Specify type:
 Bipolar type: if the disturbance includes a manic or a mixed episode (or a manic or a mixed episode and major depressive episodes)
 Depressive type: if the disturbance only includes major depressive episodes

a depressive type on the basis of whether the interval of illness includes a manic or mixed episode (bipolar type) or only a depressive episode or episodes (depressive type).

HISTORY At the end of the 19th century, Emil Kraepelin proposed a two-entity model for functional psychiatric disorders. The elegant simplicity of that model and the massive scholarship underlying it have dominated psychiatric nosology ever since. According to that model, a deteriorating course and an otherwise poor prognosis were intimately linked with dementia precox (later defined as schizophrenia by Eugen Bleuler); a favorable or remitting course of illness was associated with a manic-depressive (that is, mood disorder) diagnosis.

The practical clinical world, however, was not to be divided up that easily; a substantial number of patients did not fit cleanly into one category or the other. The term "schizoaffective" was first used by Jacob Kasanin in 1933 to describe a group of patients with acute psychoses that contained both schizophrenic and affective features. The patients' premorbid functioning tended to be good, their psychotic episodes brief, and their prognoses relatively favorable. Four years later Gabriel Langfeldt, exploring apparently schizophrenic patients who atypically experienced recovery or otherwise good outcomes, coined the term "schizophreniform." That grouping of patients, otherwise thought to have important features of schizophrenia, who experience relatively favorable outcomes persists to this day.

COMPARATIVE NOSOLOGY

DSM-I, DSM-II, and DSM-III The first edition of DSM (DSM-I), published in 1952, continued the tradition of classifying schizoaffective disorder as a subtype of schizophrenia, which was consistent with the tendency to overdiagnose schizophrenia in the United States during the mid-20th century, in comparison with European practices. During the next decade and a half the antipsychotic drugs that were discovered and that began to revolutionize many aspects of psychiatry were often thought of as being antischizophrenic; consequently, the second edition of DSM (DSM-II), published in 1968, made few changes in the diagnostic position of schizoaffective disorder. However, the progressive development of lithium (Eskalith) in the 1960s and the early 1970s as a treatment for mania helped stir a reassessment of the nosological position of schizoaffective disorder. Citing the usefulness of lithium in at least some cases of schizoaffective disorder and the early studies of outcome and family history, several authors began to propose that schizoaffective disorder be classified with affective illnesses. Other authors, challenging the simplistic two-entity model, suggested the existence of a third entity or, alternatively, a spectrum model of psychosis with no point of rarity between the purely affective and the purely schizophrenic types. That position was supported when several symptom cluster analyses failed to reveal clear bimodal or trimodal aggregates of characteristics. Other authors persisted with the argument that schizoaffective disorder was really a misnomer and that patients so classified had been misdiagnosed. Throughout the 1970s opinion was divided on the issue, and the modest amount of empirical data was sufficiently contradictory that, when the third edition of DSM (DSM-III) was published in 1980, a category was inserted for schizoaffective disorder, but it was the only specific disorder for which no operationalized diagnostic criteria were included.

Research diagnostic criteria, DSM-III-R, and DSM-IV Reflecting additional research, the revised third edition of DSM (DSM-III-R), published in 1987, resolved DSM-III's ambiguity by adopting operationalized diagnostic criteria for schizoaffective disorder. Those criteria were descriptively similar to the Research Diagnostic Criteria (RDC), which had been in existence since the mid-1970s. In contrast to the RDC, though, DSM-III-R recognized the difficulty of making a purely cross-sectional diagnosis of schizoaffective disorder and incorporated certain longitudinal characteristics in the definition (for example, a requirement for at least two weeks of psychotic symptoms in the absence of major mood symptoms).

The bulk of the meaningful research currently available concerning schizoaffective disorder has used either the RDC or the DSM-III-R system of classification. The RDC further subdivides schizoaffective disorder into mostly affective and mostly schizophrenic on the basis of (1) core schizophrenic symptoms being present for at least one week in the absence of manic or depressive features and (2) features of deterioration—such as social withdrawal, impaired occupational functioning, eccentric behavior, and unusual thoughts or perceptual experiences—having occurred before the onset of the affective features. If either or both of those two characteristics are present, the patient is classified as mostly schizophrenic. The DSM-III-R criteria for schizoaffective disorder basically resemble the RDC criteria for the mostly schizophrenic subtype of schizoaffective disorder. Most patients meeting the RDC for the mostly affective type of schizoaffective disorder have been classified by DSM-III (or later by DSM-III-R) as having affective (or mood) disorders with mood-incongruent psychotic features.

DSM-IV retains the fundamental structure of the DSM-III-R diagnostic criteria for schizoaffective disorder but resolves some of the temporal ambiguities concerning the relationship of psychotic and mood symptoms. DSM-IV retains the DSM-III-R subdivision of schizoaffective disorder into a bipolar type and a depressive type on the basis of whether the patient has ever had a manic or mixed episode. That subdivision in DSM-III-R was originally based on the informative nature of the bipolar-unipolar distinction among patients with mood disorders. It has been continued in DSM-IV because empirical data have emerged that the distinction may correlate with certain family history, outcome, and treatment response data.

EPIDEMIOLOGY Changes in diagnostic standards over time have left studies of the epidemiology of schizoaffective disorder difficult to interpret. Depending on which of the various diagnostic criteria have been used, patients with schizoaffective disorder have been reported to constitute between 10 and 30 percent of psychiatric hospital admissions for functional psychosis. Studies have estimated the annual incidence of schizoaffective disorder to be 0.3 to 5.7 per 100,000 population and the lifetime prevalence of the disorder to be 0.5 to 0.8 percent. Those figures may be underestimates, however, inasmuch as one study (based on RDC criteria) that prospectively followed patients with an operationalized admission diagnosis of schizophrenia and rediagnosed them on a weekly basis found that in 20 percent of such patients the diagnosis was changed to schizoaffective disorder before discharge. Nevertheless, schizoaffective disorder is generally thought to be less common than schizophrenia.

The age at onset of schizoaffective disorder, as for schizophrenia, is typically late adolescence or early adulthood. No specific associations have been reported with sex, race, geographic area, or social class.

ETIOLOGY Psychological, psychodynamic, environmental, and interpersonal factors may play precipitating or triggering roles when they coincide with the biomedical diathesis that creates the vulnerability for decompensations of a schizoaffective nature. Little has been written concerning which psychological or interpersonal stresses are the most noxious to specifically schizoaffective persons, so hypotheses remain speculative in that regard. Issues considered to be important for patients with schizophrenia in particular and psychoses in general may well be applicable. Those issues include concerns regarding boundaries and difficulties in processing information overload because of a faulty stimulus barrier for external and internal stimuli. Similarly, themes known to be important in depression and mania, such as loss, loss of love, and internal standards, may also be important in schizoaffective disorder.

Proposed models of the diathesis Several hypotheses have been advanced concerning the nature of the underlying biological diathesis of schizoaffective disorder: (1) Schizoaffective disorder is a variant of schizophrenia. (2) It is a variant of a mood disorder. (3) It is a third psychosis, distinct from both schizophrenia and affective disorder. (4) Schizoaffective disorder is heterogeneous and consists of a subtype related to schizophrenia, a subtype related to a mood disorder, and perhaps a subtype that represents a third psychosis. (5) A unitary spectrum of functional psychosis extends from schizophrenia at one extreme to mood disorders at the other extreme, and schizoaffective disorder occupies an intermediate position on that spectrum. (6) Schizoaffective disorder is an interaction of schizophrenic and major mood disorder diatheses (a shared-diathesis model). Because no tissue diagnosis exists for either schizophrenia or mood disorders, those six hypotheses remain speculative, and the data relevant to them must be regarded inferentially. The evidence has also tended to vary, not unexpectedly, with the definition of schizoaffective disorder used.

The family study and outcome data associated with the DSM-III-R definition of schizoaffective disorder, especially the depressive subtype, have often tended to suggest a relation to schizophrenia. That has also been the case for the RDC definition of the mostly schizophrenic schizoaffective disorder. For example, studies using each of those definitions have found that the relatives of schizoaffective patients have a rate of schizophrenia similar to the rate occurring in relatives of schizophrenic patients. Similarly, a twin-pair study found schizoaffective disorder to assort with schizophrenia, not with mood disorders. Studies using the cross-sectional RDC definition of schizoaffective disorder in general or the RDC mostly affective type in particular have tended to find a closer familial association of schizoaffective disorder with mood disorders than did studies that used DSM-III-R criteria. Earlier studies involving schizoaffective disorder patients with good outcomes had led to similar results, as did a more recent study involving schizomanic patients. Still other studies have provided evidence that atypical psychoses breed true—that is, although schizophrenic patients tend to have schizophrenic relatives and mood disorder patients tend to have relatives with mood disorder, schizoaffective patients were found to have relatives with schizoaffective disorder and *not* either schizophrenia or mood disorder. Those results support the third-psychosis hypothesis; however, the findings have not always been replicated. Several studies have found schizoaffective patients to have more relatives with mood disorder than do schizophrenic patients or controls, but fewer relatives with mood disorder than do patients with primary mood disorder. Analogous intermediate results were also found regarding schizophrenic relatives for those patients. Those results support the spectrum hypothesis, the heterogeneity hypothesis, or the diathesis interaction hypothesis.

The heterogeneity hypothesis has been supported by an argument that, although at least some data support each of the other hypotheses, other data argue against each of the other hypotheses, and no data clearly contradict the heterogeneity hypothesis. That argument, however, is weakened by the fact that it is hard to contradict a heterogeneity hypothesis—that is, many different findings can be considered to be part of the heterogeneity. Furthermore, almost all the genetic and family data can also be interpreted as consistent with a shared diathesis hypothesis.

Shared diathesis model The shared diathesis hypothesis is based on the assumption, supported by neuropsychiatric data, that the diathesis for schizophrenia is itself a continuum or a spectrum. A small number of patients have a high loading for the biological diathesis of schizophrenia, and presumably they will go on to develop schizophrenia, no matter what else occurs. A much larger number of persons have progressively smaller loadings with the schizophrenia diathesis. That relation is depicted by the curve in Figure 15.1-1. Toward the extreme left on the figure are those few persons who have such a massive biological loading for the perceptual and cognitive dysfunctions of schizophrenia that they are destined to develop that disorder virtually independently of any other circumstances they encounter. Toward the right side of the figure are the many persons with such a small loading for schizophrenia that they will probably never manifest any symptoms resembling the disorder. However, in the intermediate region are a substantial number of persons with some loading but not enough to make the occurrence of the disorder inevitable. For those people, psychotic symptoms reflecting their schizophrenic diathesis become manifest in the presence of additional biopsychosocial insults of sufficient magnitude. For patients who come to manifest schizophrenia (or, in milder cases, schizophreniform disorder), those insults may result from early brain injury (obstetrical complications); early viral infection (consistent with season of birth findings); early poor nutrition, psychological traumas, and social deprivations (all associated with poverty); substance abuse; or major psychological or social stresses at the time of the onset of the episode (the stress-diathesis model). Similarly, according to the shared diathesis model, an episode of a major mood disorder may constitute a sufficient stressor to activate (or, in combination with other insults, help activate) the underlying psychotic diathesis.

Such a model explains the close proximity of most psychotic symptoms to episodes of mood dysregulation in schizoaffective patients yet does not require the full diathesis of schizophrenia to be present in schizoaffective patients. Lack of requirement for a full diathesis in this situation is consistent with schizoaffective patients' more favorable premorbid course and outcome than schizophrenic patients. It is also congruent with the larger number of schizoaffective patients identified clinically than would be predicted on the basis of a requirement for a full schizophrenia diathesis coinciding with a full mood disorder diathesis. Therefore, the shared-diathesis model, although speculative, appears to be consistent with available family and genetic findings.

DIAGNOSIS AND CLINICAL FEATURES Considerable variability is possible in the presenting symptoms of schizoaffective disorder. All or any of the psychotic symptoms commonly associated with schizophrenia may be present during an acute episode. Those symptoms include delusions of various sorts, hallucinations, and evidence of thinking disturbances. The delusions are often paranoid in nature, although any kind of delusion is possible, including delusions of thought insertion or

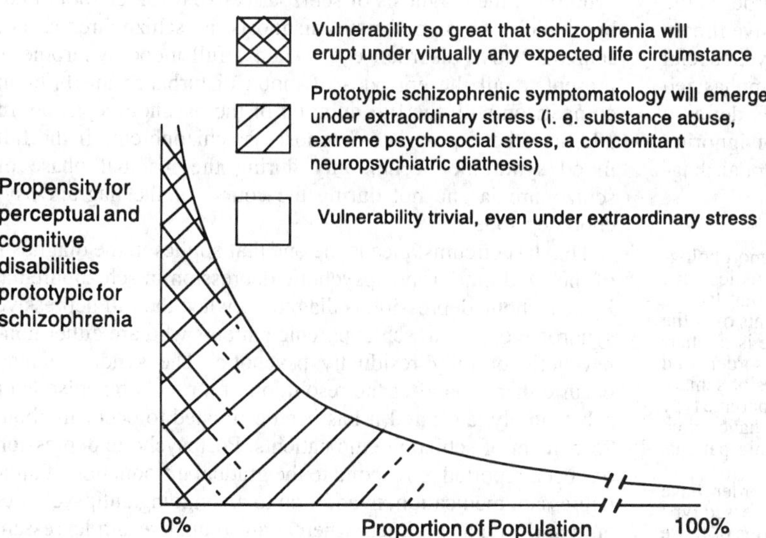

FIGURE 15.1-1 *Vulnerability to schizophrenic psychosis and its interaction with other stress factors.*

withdrawal, delusions of control, and fantastic or bizarre delusions. In addition, the delusions may be either congruent or incongruent with the patient's prevailing mood state. In the realm of perceptual aberrations, auditory hallucinations are the most common, followed in order by visual, tactile, olfactory, and gustatory hallucinations. Illusions or other perceptual distortions are also possible. Many of the disturbances of thinking in patients with schizoaffective disorder are also similar to those of schizophrenic patients. Although schizoaffective manic patients, like manic patients, have been noted to produce a substantial number of responses, the productions of schizoaffective patients often lack the humor or playfulness of those of manic patients. Schizoaffective patients also tend to generate a high percentage of idiosyncratic verbalizations, autistic thinking, and confusion. Schizoaffective depressed patients have also been noted to produce idiosyncratic and absurd responses on occasion.

Prominent mood disorder symptoms are also present in schizoaffective disorder. The symptoms may be of either the manic or the depressive variety (or both) and reach full and sustained syndromal proportions. Manic episodes include a distinct period of consistently elevated or irritable mood, with such associated features as grandiosity, a decreased need for sleep, overtalkativeness, racing thoughts, distractibility, increased activity or agitation, and a tendency toward excess without proper regard for the consequences. Patients in that manic state generally have a driven or excited quality. When they are in the throes of a manic episode, their behavioral aberrations are often fully ego-syntonic, doubt is absent, and they may exhibit an impenetrable sense of self-righteousness. Depressive episodes, however, are dominated by a blue mood, with such accompanying features as sleep or appetite disturbances; diminished level of interest or pleasure in usual activities; psychomotor retardation or agitation; subjective sense of energy loss; excessive or inappropriate guilt; feelings of worthlessness; diminished ability to think, concentrate, or make decisions; and recurrent thoughts of death or suicide. Depressive patients often feel hopeless and helpless, and their minds tend to be filled with the most negative images of themselves and upsetting, pessimistic, or otherwise gloomy thoughts. Although not all the characteristics of mania or depression are present in all patients, the clear gestalt is present and overlaps significantly with the time during which the patient is flagrantly psychotic. The psychotic and mood disorder symptoms are also of sufficient magnitude to impair social, occupational, and self-care functioning.

Also central to the concept of schizoaffective disorder is the episodic nature of the disturbance. Intervals of intensive illness tend to punctuate quiescent periods during which psychosocial functioning is adequate. Several researchers have emphasized the importance of that course-related characteristic in defining schizoaffective disorder, despite the convenience of ignoring that issue and making a symptom-based cross-sectional diagnosis at the time of a specific episode.

Pathology and laboratory examination Specific morphological, physiological, neuropsychological, and biochemical studies have usually not been undertaken in schizoaffective disorder. That lack is probably due to diagnostic inconsistencies and disagreements over the years and to the general assumption that the wisest course is to characterize such issues first in the well-defined pure mood disorders and schizophrenia. Nevertheless, a number of biological studies of schizophrenia have included patients with the RDC mostly schizophrenic type of schizoaffective disorder, because internal data analyses have failed to distinguish them from the larger group of schizophrenic patients studied.

Several neuroendocrine studies of schizoaffective disorder have been undertaken, and they have tended to show that the depressed type of schizoaffective disorder assorts with schizophrenia in terms of those parameters. Specifically, the rate of nonsuppression on the dexamethasone suppression test (DST) has been reported to be as low in patients with schizoaffective depression as it is in patients with schizophrenia or in normal control subjects and distinguishable from the higher rate noted in major depressive disorder. Similarly, the response of thyroid-stimulating hormone (TSH) and prolactin to an infusion of thyrotropin-releasing hormone (TRH) in schizoaffective patients has been observed to be similar to the response in schizophrenic patients and normal controls and not blunted, as is the case in many patients with major depressive episodes. Nevertheless, those schizoaffective patients who do have neuroendocrine responses paralleling endogenous depression are more likely to fully recover than are other schizoaffective patients. That observation appears to be independent of any family loading for mood disorders. Few studies have been undertaken in schizoaffective manic patients, though, and at least one of those studies presented results suggesting that the results of DST and TRH tests more closely approximate the results seen in patients with mood disorders than in nonmanic schizoaffective disorder patients. One study also found schizoaffective patients to resemble patients with bipolar disorder, rather than schizophrenic patients, in their rate of urinary 3-methoxy-4-hydroxyphenylglycol (MHPG) excretion.

DIFFERENTIAL DIAGNOSIS Schizoaffective disorder must be differentiated from mood disorders, schizophrenia, and other psychotic states with which it could be confused diagnostically.

Mood disorders Mood disorders that need to be differentiated include mania and psychotic depression. Manic patients can be flagrantly psychotic on occasion, manifesting hallucinations, delusions, and thought disorders, along with their full manic syndromes; thus, they resemble schizoaffective manic patients. The difference is that patients with pure mania do not have extended intervals (two weeks or more) during which hallucinations or delusions persist in the absence of prominent mood disorder symptoms. Similarly, although psychoticly depressed patients may manifest either mood-congruent or mood-incongruent delusions and hallucinations, those features do not continue for as much as two weeks at a stretch in the absence of prominent mood disorder symptoms, as they do in schizoaffective disorder. In the midst of an episode, therefore, the diagnosis may not be clear, so the definitive assessment should be reserved for a time when the episode has concluded.

Schizophrenia One key to the differential diagnosis of schizoaffective disorder from schizophrenia is that a full affective syndrome—mania or depression—must be present in schizoaffective disorder. Mood symptoms of various types may be present or even prominent in the course of an episode of schizophrenia, but, in the absence of a full and sustained mood syndrome, the diagnosis of schizoaffective disorder should not be made. The appropriate diagnosis is schizophrenia, not schizoaffective disorder, even when a full mood syndrome is present, if all the episodes of mood disturbance are brief in comparison with the full duration of the psychotic episode. In addition, the appropriate diagnosis is schizophrenia if the full mood syndrome occurs only during the residual phase of schizophrenia and not during the course of the flagrant psychotic episode.

That last circumstance is the one that applies in the diagnosis of the syndrome of postpsychotic depression in schizophrenia. Postpsychotic depression is diagnosed when the full depressive syndrome occurs in schizophrenic patients who are either nonpsychotic or only residually psychotic. The syndrome may occur either soon after the resolution of a psychotic episode or substantially later; and it has been estimated to occur in about 25 percent of schizophrenic patients. Postpsychotic depression has been reported to respond to the gradual introduction of antidepressant medication, in addition to an ongoing antipsychotic-antiparkinsonian regimen, whereas an adjunctive antidepressant may not be indicated in acute episodes of schizoaffective depression.

Akinesia Schizoaffective depression (or postpsychotic depression, depending on the temporal sequence involved) must also be differentiated from the neuroleptic-induced extrapyramidal side effects of akinesia. The akinesia syndrome may manifest with a lack of spontaneity (impairment in the initiation or the sustaining of behaviors), even in the absence of other obvious motor side effects, such as stiffness, cogwheeling, or reductions in accessory motor movements. The presentation of akinesia can easily be confused with the lack of energy or the anhedonia of depression. Furthermore, patients with neuroleptic-induced akinesia sometimes manifest a sad mood and experience guilt or self-blame for their condition—features that can accentuate the degree to which their state resembles a form of depression. Fortunately, neuroleptic-induced akinesia is often quickly responsive (that is, within several days) to full dosages of anticholinergic antiparkinsonian medications, and a trial of those compounds is often the most effective way to make the diagnosis.

The negative symptoms of schizophrenia can easily be confused with depression or akinesia. Anhedonia and anergia are often prominent and central components of the negative symptom syndrome, and they can be clear phenocopies of the anhedonic and anergic states that are common in depression. Blue mood, however, is not a component feature of the negative symptom syndrome. In fact, some have described flat affect as the central aspect of negative symptoms.

Akathisia Akathisia is another neuroleptic-induced side effect that can mimic mood disorder symptoms. The motor restlessness of severe akathisia can resemble mania in the way the patient stays in almost constant motion. In akathisia, however, the patient experiences the state of constant activity as uncomfortable or unpleasant. The patient wishes to stop or rest but feels unable to do so. In mania, by contrast, the patient feels that the motor activity, however excessive, is something originating in the patient's own initiative and is behavior the patient wishes to engage in. Neuroleptic-induced akathisia may also resemble the agitation that is sometimes a component of the depressive syndrome. Because akathisia is unpleasant, often markedly so, the associated dysphoria can be mistaken for depression. Suicidal impulses have been described in states of akathisia and can mimic depression. Obviously, increasing the dosage of neuroleptics only makes akathisia worse. Decreasing the neuroleptic dosage, if possible, is the best treatment, and a positive response to that intervention helps make the diagnosis. Benzodiazepines and propranolol (Inderal) are the adjunctive medications most often effective in controlling neuroleptic-induced akathisia.

Substance abuse Substance abuse, both acute intoxication and chronic states, can result in clinical presentations indistinguishable in cross section from schizoaffective disorder. Psychostimulants can initially generate excited psychotic states resembling schizoaffective mania, but the crash that may follow can also resemble the depressed form of schizoaffective disorder if psychotic features persist into that interval. The amotivational syndrome associated with chronic cannabis use can easily be mistaken for depression. Use of psychotomimetics, other street substances, and even alcohol can cause mixed psychotic and mood states in various stages of intoxication or withdrawal. That is true for patients in whom substance abuse occurs alone and for patients with either pure schizophrenia or a pure mood disorder who may appear schizoaffective under the influence of various substances. A screen for substances of abuse is indicated with any patient in whom the diagnosis of schizoaffective disorder is being considered.

Medical illnesses A variety of medical illnesses can lead to mixed states of mood and psychotic symptoms. A proper medical workup therefore needs to be performed to rule out the possibility of a medical illness.

COURSE AND PROGNOSIS The course and the outcome of schizoaffective disorder, on the whole, tend to be more favorable than the course and the outcome of schizophrenia but less favorable than those of a pure mood disorder. Bipolar schizoaffective patients who also have histories of pure mood disorder episodes have been reported to have outcomes no less favorable than patients with major mood disorders, although other patients with schizoaffective mania have been noted to manifest more psychotic symptoms, more subsequent maniclike episodes, and poorer social outcomes than do pure manic patients.

Patients with a number of schizoaffective depressive episodes and those who have histories of both schizoaffective depressed and schizophrenic episodes tend to have significantly poorer outcomes than patients who do not. Studies have also found that, when a full schizophrenic syndrome is present in schizoaffective disorder patients, along with the mood syndrome (only a full affective syndrome is required for the diagnosis of schizoaffective disorder, not a full schizophrenic syndrome), poorer outcomes occur than in schizoaffective disorder patients without a full schizophrenic syndrome. Overall, a substantial degree of outcome heterogeneity is found in general, and notable inconsistencies are seen within and between patients in terms of social, vocational, and symptomatic domains of outcome.

TREATMENT

Schizoaffective mania

ACUTE TREATMENT Antipsychotics and lithium are the psychopharmacological agents most often used in the treatment of schizoaffective mania, and both have value in controlling the acute symptoms. In the studies that have made the comparison, associations have usually not been found between the most prominent symptoms and the specific degree of usefulness of one or the other of those two agents within the diagnostic category. An important distinction was found in one large collaborative study, however, when patients were subdivided on the basis of level of activation. In that study, highly active patients were found to benefit more from treatment with the antipsychotic agent—in that case, chlorpromazine (Thorazine)—than from lithium, and the two drugs were found to have equivalent efficacy among moderately active patients. Low-potency antipsychotic compounds have the side effect of sedation, which can be clinically useful in controlling excited patients. Other side effects, such as constipation, dry mouth, blurred vision, and orthostatic hypotension, also accompany the use of low-potency antipsychotic agents. As always, clinical judgment is required to balance the medication effects and side effects that best match the patient's psychiatric and medical status.

Certain studies have suggested that the combination of lithium and an antipsychotic may be more effective than the use of either agent alone. Although the side effects are increased by combined treatment, the best evidence is that the effects are merely additive. Reports indicate that the benefit of adding lithium to antipsychotics in the treatment of schizoaffective manic patients extends throughout the entire range of the patients' symptoms and is not restricted to the mood component. In all cases of the use of antipsychotics or lithium or their combination, the standard dosages recommended for their use in schizophrenia and mania are recommended, and monitoring of blood lithium levels is required. An episode of schizoaffective mania, however, can be expected to resolve more slowly than an episode of mania, and the resolution may be less complete in schizoaffective mania than in mania.

Electroconvulsive therapy (ECT) can also be an effective acute treatment of schizoaffective mania, and its use should be considered when the most rapid possible response is important (for example, in dangerous situations) and when the patient appears to be refractory to other interventions. Carbamazepine (Tegretol) and valproic acid (Depakene) are alternative adjunctive medications that may be effective when added to the antipsychotic or to lithium (or both) in difficult cases.

CONTINUATION AND MAINTENANCE TREATMENT Lithium is effective in the prophylactic management of schizoaffective mania or the bipolar type of schizoaffective disorder when it is used at plasma levels of 0.60 mEq/L or above. It is most useful in patients with the most severe affective symptoms. As is the case with other patients receiving long-term lithium treatment, consistency of fluid and sodium intake and routine surveillance of lithium levels and kidney and thyroid function are indicated. Patients, their families, and other caretakers should be informed about the early signs of lithium toxicity and what to do should the signs occur.

Because tardive dyskinesia is a risk with long-term antipsychotic treatment, perhaps especially in patients with mood disorder features, it is reasonable to discontinue antipsychotic medications and attempt a long-term treatment trial of lithium alone for schizoaffective mania. However, lithium by itself may not prove adequate. In that case, antipsychotics should be titrated down to the lowest dosages that provide suitable protection. Indeed, small antipsychotic dosages may allow for the optimal level of psychosocial functioning while slowing the progression of new episodes, even if the antipsychotics do not abort the episodes entirely. A strategy of intermittent antipsychotic dosing may be appropriate for patients who themselves or in conjunction with their support systems are able to detect impending episodes and instigate treatment.

Schizoaffective depression

ACUTE TREATMENT Although the combination of an antipsychotic and an antidepressant may be a good choice of treatment in psychotic depressions, support for such a strategy is much more meager in schizoaffective depression. One controlled study did show an advantage for that combination over either component given alone, but the most recent, carefully controlled, prospective study indicated that the addition of an antidepressant to the antipsychotic actually slowed the improvements of acutely psychotic schizoaffective depressed patients. Lithium also does not have a high likelihood of being helpful for schizoaffective depressions, especially in patients who do not have a history of bipolar disorder-type mood changes. Therefore, the best initial approach to a psychotic patient with the diagnosis of schizoaffective depression is likely to be treatment with a simple antipsychotic-antiparkinsonian combination, with a dosage strategy similar to that used for schizophrenia. In many cases the symptoms of depression disappear coincident with the fading of the psychotic symptoms. If the psychotic symptoms resolve but the depressive symptoms remain, the first course of action should be to rule out the possibility of neuroleptic-induced akinesia with antipsychotic dosage reduction (if feasible). Alternatively or in conjunction, a vigorous trial of antiparkinsonian medication may be undertaken. If a syndrome of depression persists in a consistent fashion, a trial of an antidepressant medication, gradually increasing to the full dosage used in primary depression, added to the antipsychotic-antiparkinsonian combination is appropriate. The patients, therefore, are treated much the same as patients meeting the DSM-IV criteria for postpsychotic depression.

ECT is also worth considering in schizoaffective depression. Although empirical studies with modern diagnostic criteria are lacking, a trial of ECT is appropriate in refractory cases.

CONTINUATION AND MAINTENANCE TREATMENT The best course of treatment is probably to continue whatever treatment was useful in leading to the remission of an acute episode. As noted earlier, lithium is less likely to be effective in schizoaffective depression than in schizoaffective mania. The same cautions referred to earlier regarding the use of antipsychotics and other agents for the long-term treatment of schizoaffective mania also apply to schizoaffective depression.

Adjunctive medications Antiparkinsonian medications are indicated when antipsychotic medications are used for the treatment of acute schizoaffective episodes. That precaution helps avert acute dystonias and other acute and unpleasant extrapyramidal side effects that may be associated with antipsychotics. That action is also helpful in avoiding lack of compliance with antipsychotic regimens (or with treatment altogether) because of how unpleasant the side effects can be. Even in continuation and maintenance phases, adjunctive antiparkinsonian agents may be essential for the same reasons. And in the later stages of treatment, adjunctive antiparkinsonian drugs may be crucial to prevent neuroleptic-induced akinesia, which can at times closely resemble negative symptoms or depression.

Benzodiazepines may be valuable adjuncts for the treatment of anxiety or insomnia during acute schizoaffective episodes. In that role they may also contribute to the antipsychotic effects or allow for a lower dosage of antipsychotic medication than might otherwise be possible. Benzodiazepines can also be useful in the treatment of neuroleptic-induced akathisia, should that occur, although other medications, such as propranolol, may also be useful in that situation. During maintenance treatment, an adjunctive benzodiazepine or propranolol may be indicated for similar reasons.

During the maintenance phase, adjunctive antidepressants may be useful in the treatment of secondary depressive episodes that emerge in patients with schizoaffective disorder during intervals in which they are not flagrantly psychotic. After the confounding syndrome of neuroleptic-induced akinesia is ruled out, the treatment of such a depressive episode is similar to the treatment of postpsychotic depression in schizophrenia, with the gradual addition of full dosages of antidepressant medications to an ongoing antipsychotic-antiparkinsonian regimen.

Psychosocial interventions Although somatic treatments directly address the biological diatheses that are involved in schizoaffective disorder, prominent morbidities occur in the course of the illness that are fundamentally psychological or social. Those morbidities need to be addressed with appropriate interpersonal modalities to help patients and their familial, social, and vocational support networks cope with the onslaught of acute episodes and the recuperative and reconstructive tasks involved during the postacute phases of treatment. Psychodynamic issues deserve careful attention, inasmuch as intrapsychic conflicts can be important triggers or perpetuators of psychotic symptoms in accordance with the stress-diathesis concept. Supportive interventions are indicated, but uncovering or exploratory techniques are generally to be avoided, especially during the acute stages of illness. Psychotic patients often have trouble organizing the turmoil generated by the uncovering of powerful primitive instinctual drives that are ordinarily held outside the domain of conscious awareness. Instead, structured, integrated, and problem-solving psychotherapeutic interventions should be used, although the therapist should remain alert to and respectful of important psychodynamic issues.

Psychiatric hospitalization is often required at the time of acute psychotic episodes since the patients' loss of reality testing, judgment, and thinking ability and the overwhelming press of their affectivity may have outstripped their (and their support networks') ability to attend to their immediate needs. A hospital provides 24-hour structure and guidance designed to protect patients from their own impulses and lack of judgment, which otherwise may result in harm to themselves or others, whether that harm is physical (suicide, assaultiveness), financial, legal, vocational, or social. A hospital also provides protection or, quite literally, asylum from outside stressors that may be triggering or exacerbating the patients' conditions.

During hospitalization, coincident with somatic treatments, an evaluation of the patient's life situation and coping capacities takes place, and interventions are instituted to reinforce the most constructive aspects of those capacities to allow the reinstitution of appropriate autonomies. Simultaneously, the patient's psychosocial support network is examined, both to enhance the treatment team's understanding of the tasks with which the patient has to cope and to interact with that network, when possible, to allow the network to provide a good fit with the patient's adaptive needs through such interventions as psychoeducation, the reduction of expressed emotion, and the provision of concrete social services.

Hospitalization should not be continued longer than required so as not to foster unnecessary regression and dependence. Step-down levels of care, such as partial hospitalization, continued day treatment, or halfway houses, can be valuable psychosocial supports and can provide patients with a more normative environment than a hospital and the opportunity to resume responsibilities for which they have regained capability. In those environments and in the clinic environments to which patients may then progress, suitable programs of rehabilitation should be provided for building and practicing social and vocational skills that they either previously lacked or did not fully regain after the resolution of the acute episode. In those programs, respect for and attention to the patients' natural skills, interests, and aspirations become as important as the recognition of their problems and deficits.

A 25-year-old male teacher directing a high school play involving a murder became convinced that the murder in the play reflected a real one. He also believed that he was in danger from the unknown perpetrator and several cast members. That state persisted for three weeks, during which time he gradually stopped talking to his associates. His need for sleep diminished, and he started wandering the streets at night, searching for clues. He became increasingly excited as he concluded that an international intrigue underlay the murder he was solving. At that point he felt the "pressure of world history," and his behavior became frenzied. His speech was accelerated, he had the subjective sense that his thoughts were racing with great clarity, and he got into heated and irrational arguments with other teachers who offered to help with the play. When he finally confided to his girlfriend that his directing the play to a surprise ending would result in the release of Middle Eastern hostages, she arranged for his hospitalization.

On admission to the hospital, his physical examination and laboratory results were normal, and a substance abuse screen was negative. After three weeks of chlorpromazine treatment, the patient's sleep pattern normalized. He appeared to be relaxed, and he began conversing with staff members. He continued to suspect that the play had a hidden meaning but acknowledged that it did not have international implications. Lithium was added to his regimen, and after two more weeks he was discharged. As an outpatient, he continued to do well as the chlorpromazine was gradually tapered, and he successfully returned to his teaching.

Three years later, after stopping the lithium medication on his own, the patient suffered a similar psychotic decompensation. Hospitalized, he again responded to an antipsychotic plus lithium. Subsequently, he has continued to take lithium for six years without further episodes. He has continued to teach and has several good friends. However, he has lost interest in theater activities and remains unmarried.

SCHIZOPHRENIFORM DISORDER

Schizophreniform disorder was first described in relatively broad terms in patients with abrupt onsets of psychotic illness and favorable prognoses, but it has since been redefined to include a more restricted group of patients. The impetus for the diagnostic term stemmed from the observation that some patients diagnosed as having schizophrenia did not progress to a chronic disorder or display deterioration in functioning. The term allows the clinician to guard against the premature diagnosis of schizophrenia and may help the patient avoid unnecessary treatment and stigma. Studies assessing the validity of the contemporary definition of schizophreniform disorder have yielded conflicting results, and additional studies and experience are needed to establish the disorder's existence, boundaries, and characteristics.

DEFINITION DSM-IV defines schizophreniform disorder as identical to schizophrenia with the prime exceptions of duration of illness and the requirement for a deterioration in social or occupational functioning (Table 15.1-2). During the acute episode, psychotic symptoms—including delusions, hallucinations, disorganized thinking, and catatonic behavior—may all be present, as in schizophrenia, but the total episode of disturbance—including prodromal, active, and residual phases—is defined as between one and six months' duration. When the diagnosis of schizophreniform disorder must be made without waiting for recovery, it should be qualified as provisional. If symptoms then persist for longer than six months, subchronic schizophrenia becomes the accurate diagnosis. Although many patients experience dysfunction in various areas of daily living, impairment in social or occupational functioning is not required to diagnose schizophreniform disorder. Schizophreniform disorder is not to be diagnosed if the disturbance is substance-induced or due to a general medical condition or if the disorder, including the prodromal and residual phases, lasts less than one month. Patients may be further classified as having good prognostic features or not.

HISTORY Gabriel Langfeldt first coined the term "schizophreniform disorder" in 1939 to classify a group of psychotic patients with

TABLE 15.1-2
Diagnostic Criteria for Schizophreniform Disorder

A. Criteria A, D, and E of schizophrenia are met.
B. An episode of the disorder (including prodromal, active, and residual phases) lasts at least one month but less than six months. (When the diagnosis must be made without waiting for recovery, it should be qualified as "provisional.")

Specify if:

Without good prognostic features
With good prognostic features: as evidenced by two (or more) of the following:
(1) onset of prominent psychotic symptoms within four weeks of the first noticeable change in usual behavior or functioning
(2) confusion or perplexity at the height of the psychotic episode
(3) good premorbid social and occupational functioning
(4) absence of blunted or flat affect

Table from DSM-IV, *Diagnostic and Statistical Manual of Mental Disorders,* ed 4. Copyright American Psychiatric Association, Washington, 1994. Used with permission.

good prognoses. It represented an attempt to classify patients who had been described as schizophrenic but who did not display deterioration in overall functioning. They had, for example, acute reactions that were often precipitated by stress. Many of the patients exhibited good premorbid functioning, depressive or hysterical features, and clouding of consciousness during the acute psychosis. The original concept of schizophreniform disorder included several other conditions, and Langfeldt wrote that both schizoaffective disorder and brief reactive psychosis should be included under the term. His intention was to differentiate patients with "genuine schizophrenia" from others who did not experience a poor outcome and a declining course.

Subsequent investigators continued to use the term "schizophreniform disorder" for a number of conditions, including schizoaffective disorder. With the introduction of DSM-III, however, the original concept of schizophreniform disorder was altered. Since then, the term has been used for a condition considered identical to schizophrenia except for its duration.

COMPARATIVE NOSOLOGY Schizophreniform disorder was not included in DSM-I or DSM-II. DSM-II defined a heterogeneous condition, acute schizophrenic episode, that included acute schizophrenic symptoms accompanied by confusion, emotional turmoil, excitement, and depression in some cases. Some patients were noted to recover within weeks, but others progressed much more slowly. The eighth and ninth revisions of the *International Classification of Diseases and Related Health Problems* (ICD-8 and ICD-9) did not use the term "schizophreniform disorder." "Schizophreniform" appeared in the glossary of ICD-9 but was not defined.

In 1980 DSM-III defined schizophreniform disorder in much the same terms as schizophrenia except that the total duration of symptoms was limited to six months. It also excluded patients with mood disorder and brief reactive psychosis. In 1987 DSM-III-R sought to define schizophreniform disorder more carefully than in the past by including the term "provisional" so that the clinician could make the diagnosis before waiting for the six-month period to elapse. It also allowed for the specification of with and without good prognostic features, with at least two of four features required to define good prognosis. Those features, however, had been the subject of few studies and appeared to be relatively nonspecific in terms of outcome. Differentiating schizophreniform disorder of less than one month's duration from brief reactive psychosis in DSM-III and DSM-III-R also proved to be difficult. DSM-IV has set a one-month requirement for active symptoms to appear after the first noticeable change in behavior or functioning.

EPIDEMIOLOGY Few studies have examined the incidence or the distribution of schizophreniform disorder as defined by DSM-III, DSM-III-R, or DSM-IV. True schizophreniform disorder seems to be a rare condition, and in many studies more than half of the patients are reclassified at follow-up as suffering from schizophrenia. One large review suggested that a small subgroup of patients (0 to 29 percent) exhibit a remitting nonaffective psychosis. Community studies have reported a lifetime prevalence of schizophreniform disorder of approximately 0.2 percent and a one-year prevalence of 0.1 percent. The age at onset of schizophreniform disorder is believed to be similar to that found in schizophrenia—primarily adolescence and early adulthood. Little information is available concerning sex, race, or social class distribution. Family studies have used small numbers of patients, differing definitions of schizophreniform disorder, and mostly retrospective reviews. Their conflicting data have left it unclear whether the relatives of patients with schizophreniform disorder have an increased risk of schizophrenia, although some evidence supports an increased risk of psychotic mood disorders among the relatives. Although the rate of schizophreniform disorder has been observed to be less than 5 percent of all patients with a first episode of psychosis, the rate may be higher in developing countries, where recovery from psychotic episodes may be more rapid than in developed countries.

ETIOLOGY The cause of schizophreniform disorder is unknown. A number of hypotheses have been generated for schizophrenia and mood disorders, but it is unclear whether similar theories of cause or pathophysiology should be applied to schizophreniform disorder. Of the existing hypotheses concerning the pathophysiological mechanism of schizophreniform disorder, dopamine receptor supersensitivity is probably the leading candidate.

Because existing family studies are limited by methodological flaws, it is also unknown whether there is a genetic predisposition for the development of schizophreniform disorder. In general, the relatives of patients with schizophreniform disorder do not seem to share an identical pattern of psychiatric illness when compared with the relatives of patients with schizophrenia. Much of the early literature suggested a familial link with mood disorders, and, since the publication of DSM-III, the majority of family studies of patients with schizophreniform disorder favor the idea that their relatives are at increased risk for mood disorders. A couple of those studies also concluded that relatives of probands with schizophreniform disorder have an intermediate risk for schizophrenia when compared with the relatives of patients with schizophrenia (who had the greatest risk) and mood disorders.

Biological and laboratory markers validating the presence of schizophreniform disorder and distinguishing it from other forms of psychiatric illness have not appeared. In several studies, computed tomography (CT) scans failed to detect significant differences between patients with schizophreniform disorder and those with schizophrenia, although both types of patients displayed increased ventricular brain ratios when compared with controls or patients with other types of psychiatric illness, including mood disorders. However, in a study of neuroendocrine markers, patients with schizophreniform disorder exhibited abnormal dexamethasone suppression at a rate intermediate between the rate of those with schizophrenia and those with mood disorders and a frequency of blunted TSH response to TRH that was similar to that of patients with mood disorders and greater than that of schizophrenic patients. In another study involving growth hormone (GH) response to apomorphine, patients with schizophreniform disorder had larger GH responses than did schizophrenic patients, again suggesting biological dissimilarities. A study of abnormalities of smooth-pursuit eye movements found that schizophreniform patients and their relatives had similarly low rates of abnormalities as compared with normal control subjects and a schizophrenic control group. In another study, a battery of neuropsychological tests revealed that schizophreniform patients performed significantly worse than normal subjects but had similar cognitive deficits as patients with chronic schizophrenia.

Although many patients with schizophreniform disorder experience significant psychological or social stressors before the onset of their disorders, the role of specific psychosocial stressors has not been carefully evaluated in controlled studies of those patients. Psychodynamic and other psychological or social factors presumably can function as triggers of psychotic episodes in accordance with the stress-diathesis model.

DIAGNOSTIC AND CLINICAL FEATURES Patients with schizophreniform disorder often appear in a floridly psychotic state, with a relatively abrupt onset of auditory or visual hallucinations, delusional thinking, and bizarre behavior. That state may manifest in an agitated or threatening manner or as a withdrawn or catatonic condition. In the short term, patients with schizophreniform disorder do not differ from schizophrenic patients in their manifest psychopathology or severity of symptoms. Acute affective symptoms may be present, but a full affective syndrome is not sustained. By definition, the active phase of the illness persists for at least one month. At present, no specific imaging techniques or laboratory studies are able to distinguish schizophreniform disorder from other psychiatric illnesses.

The total duration of an episode of schizophreniform disorder—including prodromal, active, and residual phases—is at least one month but less than six months. Although the patients may have multiple episodes or hospitalizations, their social and occupational functioning is generally intact at other times, as the patients tend to recompensate well after the episode.

Several prognostic features have been proposed, although they have been the subject of few controlled studies. At least two of the following criteria allow for the specification of the good prognosis subtype in DSM-IV: (1) the onset of prominent psychotic symptoms within four weeks of the first noticeable change in the patient's usual behavior or functioning; (2) confusion, disorientation, or perplexity at the height of the psychiatric episode; (3) good premorbid social and occupational functioning; and (4) the absence of blunted or flat affect. Many patients present with one or more of those features.

DIFFERENTIAL DIAGNOSIS Distinguishing schizophreniform disorder from other medical and psychiatric conditions that may present in a floridly psychotic state can be challenging. A detailed history should focus on the time of symptom onset, the course, the patient's premorbid functioning, the precipitants, the patient's physical health, the use of medications, the patient's use of alcohol and other substances, the family history, and the presence of any previous episodes. Such a detailed history may require the assistance of family members or others familiar with the patient. The often abrupt onset of symptoms, coupled with the lack of previous episodes in many cases, underscores the need for a toxicological and medical evaluation.

Substance abuse is one of the most common causes of the abrupt onset of psychotic symptoms, and a toxicology screen is indicated in any such case to aid in the diagnosis. A number of medical and neurological disorders may also manifest with symptoms characteristic of schizophreniform disorder. Those conditions include various metabolic and endocrine disorders, cerebral tumors, meningitis, and temporal lobe epilepsy. If the mental status examination reveals an absence of a clear sensorium or difficulty in maintaining attention, a general medical condition and delirium should be considered.

Dating the exact onset of such an illness can be difficult, and prodromal symptoms may be subtle. When symptoms clearly persist for more than six months, though, the diagnosis of another psychiatric disorder must be made. The possibilities include schizophrenia, schizoaffective disorder, a mood disorder with psychotic features, delusional disorder, substance-induced psychotic disorder, and psychotic disorder due to a general medical condition. An especially difficult distinction to make occurs in patients with affective symptoms in the setting of an acute psychosis. Insomnia, fatigue, irritability, and decreased concentration may be secondary events, for example, in a patient struggling with persistent auditory hallucinations. Although patients with schizophreniform disorder sometimes meet the criteria for mood disorders, the psychotic symptoms are the most prominent. When symptoms have been present for less than one month and there is a stressful precipitant, the diagnosis of brief psychotic disorder should preempt the diagnosis of schizophreniform disorder.

COURSE AND PROGNOSIS By definition, schizophreniform disorder is marked by a short course, with symptoms present from one to six months. Patients usually display good premorbid functioning, and at least a fourth recover fully, returning to their baseline social and vocational states on resolution of the psychotic episode. In general, although most outcome studies indicate that patients with schizophreniform disorder do significantly better than schizophrenic patients, they do not do as well longitudinally as patients with mood disorders. A significant number of patients relapse, and long-term follow-up studies suggest that more than half of patients with schizophreniform disorder are reclassified at a later time as having schizophrenia, schizoaffective disorder, or a mood disorder with psychotic features. As a group, patients with schizophreniform disorder have higher mortality and suicide rates than the general population.

DSM-III-R and DSM-IV specify several prognostic signs and symptoms in an effort to predict the course of the illness. The abrupt onset of symptoms, confusion or perplexity at the height of the psychotic episodes, a brief duration of illness at index admission, good premorbid social and occupational functioning, and the absence of blunted or flat affect are all thought to be favorable prognostic signs.

Few available biological indicators suggest whether an acute first-episode psychosis will become chronic, although neuroendocrine dysfunction may provide some prognostic information. One study found that a high percentage of patients with schizophreniform disorder in whom symptoms remitted had an abnormal DST or TRH-stimulating test. However, that finding may have been confounded by underlying mood disorders in some of the patients studied.

The patient's response to antipsychotic medication may also prove useful in determining the course of the disorder. A recent limited study showed that patients with schizophreniform disorder responded faster than schizophrenic patients to antipsychotic medication. Further, those with a delayed response seemed to have a longer illness course than did rapid responders.

TREATMENT No controlled studies of the treatment of schizophreniform disorder are available to help guide clinicians. As a result, the prevailing approach to treatment for the acute psychotic condition comes from what is known about the short-term responses of schizophrenic patients. In general, the aims are to protect and stabilize the patient, minimize the psychosocial consequences, and resolve the target symptoms with minimal side effects. Another study suggested that left ventricular enlargement in patients with schizophreniform disorder correlated with progression to schizophrenia or schizoaffective disorder at a one-year follow-up.

The patient often needs hospitalization, which not only allows for complete diagnostic evaluation but helps ensure the safety of the patient, who may be at risk of harming himself or herself or others. A supportive environment with minimal stimulation is most helpful. As improvement progresses, help with coping skills, problem-solving techniques, and psychoeducational approaches may be added for patients and their families.

When patients are actively hallucinating and delusional, antipsychotic medications are the psychopharmacological agents of choice. If patients are extremely agitated, the intramuscular route of administration is preferred for prompt relief of symptoms. Prophylactic antiparkinsonism medication should also be offered to help reduce the likelihood of acute extrapyramidal symptoms. That medication not only helps improve compliance but may also help preserve the therapeutic alliance at that early stage of treatment. The adjunctive use of small dosages of benzodiazepines may also be beneficial at times of increased anxiety or agitation. If the patient or a family member has a history of response to treatment, that may prove to be a valuable guide. Other medications, such as lithium and antidepressants, may be indicated after further observation and the gathering of additional history.

At present, it is unclear how long patients should be maintained on medication after the resolution of their florid symptoms. The regimen needs to be based on characteristics of the individual case and consideration of medication side effects, such as tardive dyskinesia. By definition, schizophreniform disorder is limited in duration and should not require prophylactic antipsychotic medication. However, gradual tapering of medications is more likely to be a successful strategy than abrupt discontinuation. Further, patients need to be monitored during and after medication termination because a substantial proportion experience a recurrence of symptoms.

After the acute psychotic episode has resolved, psychosocial interventions, including individual, group, and family therapy, may be useful. Supportive psychotherapy can be targeted to improve patients' self-esteem and restore their sense of autonomy. In general, clinicians should focus on problem-solving strategies, improving communication skills, and reducing stress. Doing so enables patients to cope in the world outside the hospital. Patients may benefit from a structured intermediate environment, such as a day hospital, during the initial phases of returning to the community. Involvement of the patients' external support systems in the treatment plan is also beneficial. Efforts should be made to educate both the patients and their families about the early signs of relapse and the need for continuing treatment. Those approaches advance the overall aim of helping patients regain productive roles in society while reducing the risk of relapse.

A 21-year-old single male college sophomore who had previously worked steadily and had a pilot's license was referred for psychiatric hospitalization after the onset of auditory hallucinations and paranoid thinking one month previously. He complained to his parents about neighbors calling him names for unknown reasons and about their children wanting to harm him. In addition, he claimed to hear criticizing voices in his head. He often stayed awake at night, pacing, and was unable to continue his studies, withdrawing into his room. He was aware of no clear precipitants other than feeling stressed by the recent sickness of his father. He had no previous psychiatric or medical history, and he denied any drug or alcohol use.

On admission to the hospital, the results of a laboratory workup, including CT of the brain and an electroencephalogram (EEG), were unremarkable. The results of the toxicology screen for substances of abuse were negative. The patient responded markedly within three weeks after starting to take an antipsychotic medication. He no longer noted any hallucinations and denied any paranoid ideation. He also seemed to benefit from a combination of individual, group, and family therapies. He continued taking the medication for six months after discharge from the hospital and was able to return to school and obtain his degree. At follow-up three years later, he remained symptom-free.

BRIEF PSYCHOTIC DISORDER

Brief psychotic disorder, a new diagnostic category in DSM-IV, incorporates brief reactive psychosis, the designation for a disorder that is clearly a response to markedly stressful events.

Brief psychotic disorder is one of the least understood and least investigated forms of functional psychosis. Although the diagnosis of brief psychotic disorder started to gain increased consideration by American psychiatrists, it has traditionally been the subject of study by Scandinavian researchers. As defined by DSM-IV, brief psychotic disorder includes active psychotic symptoms that persist for periods ranging from at least one day to one month. By definition, that period is followed by a full return to premorbid levels of functioning. The onset is often abrupt and, according to some, serves as a defense reaction to avoid the pain associated with a traumatic event. The illness has been called by various names over time and in different countries, and it remains a concept plagued by much confusion, with most studies hampered by unclear diagnostic criteria and other methodological flaws.

DEFINITION DSM-IV defines brief psychotic disorder as an illness lasting from one day to one month, with eventual return to premorbid levels of functioning. At least one of the following symptoms indicative of impaired reality testing is required: delusions, hallucinations, disorganized speech, catatonia, or grossly disorganized behavior. When symptoms occur after and in response to one or more events that, singularly or together, would be markedly stressful to almost anyone in similar circumstances in that person's culture, then the further designation of brief reactive psychosis is appropriate (called brief psychotic disorder with marked stressors in DSM-IV). The exclusion criteria include the presence of a full mood syndrome (mood disorder with psychotic features), schizoaffective disorder, and any substance-induced psychotic disorder or psychotic disorder due to a general medical condition. If the diagnosis must be made without waiting for the expected recovery, it should be qualified as provisional. The DSM-IV diagnostic criteria are listed in Table 15.1-3.

That definition modifies the DSM-III and DSM-III-R diagnostic criteria to make them less restrictive. Emotional turmoil or confusion is no longer necessary during the reaction. Cases in which a precipitating stressor is absent are included under the rubric brief psychotic disorder, but the specifier, without marked stressor, should be noted. An additional specifier, with postpartum onset, notes the onset of psychotic symptoms within four weeks postpartum.

HISTORY For well over a century, investigators have used various terms to define psychotic states that seem to occur in response to a stressful life event. Such terms have included hysterical psychosis, *bouffée délirante*, psychogenic psychosis, reactive schizophrenia, good-prognosis schizophrenia, cycloid psychosis, transient psychosis, and atypical psychosis. In nonindustrialized countries such terms as yak, latah, koro, amok, and whitigo psychosis have been used to describe psychotic states precipitated by stressful events.

In 1913 Karl Jaspers offered specific criteria for reactive psychosis. First, a precipitating factor should have occurred shortly before the onset of the reactive state. Second, it should be an adequate factor and should have a meaningful connection with the abnormal reaction. Third, the psychosis should remit when that factor is removed. Over time, the "understandability" of the symptoms in regard to the stress has been emphasized. Although Scandinavian psychiatrists were instrumental in further defining the disorder, an international acceptance has grown, although, in certain cases, culture-specific conditions may limit generalizability.

COMPARATIVE NOSOLOGY Brief psychotic disorder is a new diagnosis in DSM-IV. The diagnosis of brief reactive psychosis was first incorporated into the world psychiatric nomenclature in ICD-8 in 1967 and first appeared in DSM-II in 1968, although neither of those classifications provided distinct diagnostic criteria. In ICD-8 a special class was created, under the title "other psychoses," in which psychotic conditions attributable to a recent life experience were noted. In DSM-II several subtypes were designated: psychotic depressive reaction, reactive excitation, reactive confusion, acute paranoid reaction, and reactive psychosis unspecified. ICD-9 also did not provide criteria.

TABLE 15.1-3
Diagnostic Criteria for Brief Psychotic Disorder

A. Presence of one (or more) of the following symptoms:
   (1) delusions
   (2) hallucinations
   (3) disorganized speech (e.g., frequent derailment or incoherence)
   (4) grossly disorganized or catatonic behavior
   Note: Do not include a symptom if it is a culturally sanctioned response pattern.
B. Duration of an episode of the disturbance is at least one day but less than one month, with eventual full return to premorbid level of functioning.
C. The disturbance is not better accounted for by a mood disorder with psychotic features, schizoaffective disorder, or schizophrenia, and is not due to the direct physiological effects of a substance (e.g., a drug of abuse, a medication) or a general medical condition.

Specify if:
- **With marked stressor(s)** (brief reactive psychosis): if symptoms occur shortly after and apparently in response to events that, singly or together, would be markedly stressful to almost anyone in similar circumstances in the person's culture
- **Without marked stressor(s):** if psychotic symptoms do *not* occur shortly after, or are not apparently in response to events that, singly or together, would be markedly stressful to almost anyone in similar circumstances in the person's culture
- **With postpartum onset:** if onset within four weeks postpartum

Table from DSM-IV, *Diagnostic and Statistical Manual of Mental Disorders*, ed 4. Copyright American Psychiatric Association, Washington, 1994. Used with permission.

It listed brief reactive psychosis as a subtype of other and unspecified reactive psychoses. The disorder was listed in the glossary as a florid psychosis of at least a few hours' duration but not longer than two weeks, having a sudden onset soon after a severe stressor, and involving full recovery to the previous baseline state.

DSM-III described a disorder of sudden onset with a total duration limited to two weeks. It required at least one psychotic symptom, a recognizable precipitating stressor, and a full return to premorbid functioning. DSM-III-R lengthened the duration criterion to include cases lasting up to one month. In addition, the psychotic symptoms needed to occur apparently in response to the stressful life event. That criterion not only emphasized the chronological relationship but also required that a clinical judgment be made about the causal relation. DSM-III-R also adjusted the stressor criteria to allow the precipitant to be a series of events, no one of which was highly stressful but that in aggregate yielded an overwhelming state. DSM-III-R excluded mood disorders, schizotypal personality disorder, and the prodromal symptoms of schizophrenia.

The DSM-III and DSM-III-R diagnostic criteria drew criticism from some investigators, who felt that the concept delineated by Scandinavian psychiatrists had been altered and the criteria made too restrictive. They argued that doing so limited the clinician's ability to study an appropriate cohort of patients. For example, it was unclear what fraction of patients historically met the criteria for emotional turmoil or overwhelming perplexity during the reactive episode. Also, if prodromal symptoms were taken out of the context of schizophrenia, they could be broad and ill-defined, even representing certain elements of personality that made the patient vulnerable to a reactive psychosis. DSM-III-R also contained an apparent contradiction: Schizotypal personality disorder was cited as making patients particularly vulnerable to brief reactive psychosis, yet the diagnostic criteria specifically excluded patients with that personality disorder.

DSM-IV now allows for a broadly defined disorder under the rubric brief psychotic disorder. Cases may be specified to occur in response to marked stressors or not. The exclusion criteria for the prodromal symptoms of schizophrenia and the presence of schizotypal personality disorder have been eliminated. With the duration requirement increased to one month for schizophreniform disorder, those criteria are no longer thought to be necessary to clarify the boundary between the disorders. The criteria for emotional turmoil or overwhelming perplexity and confusion also are no longer required. DSM-IV's criteria allow for increased flexibility of diagnosis and should help reduce the number of cases diagnosed in the residual category of psychotic disorders not otherwise specified. The criteria are also compatible with ICD-10, which uses the general term "acute and transient psychotic disorders," with further subtyping based on the presence of stress, to define reactive psychosis.

EPIDEMIOLOGY Brief psychotic disorder appears to be an uncommon condition. Because of variations in diagnostic criteria and other methodological differences, wide discrepancies exist across studies that have attempted to define the incidence and the prevalence of brief reactive psychosis. It has not been diagnosed often by American psychiatrists, and it was found to be relatively uncommon in DSM field trials. Its onset is most frequently reported in young adults, with the average age at onset being in the late 20s or early 30s, although cases have also been recognized later in life. No reliable data are available on sex, race, or social class associations.

ETIOLOGY Little is known about the etiology of brief psychotic disorder. Historically, the presence of a markedly stressful event was thought to precipitate brief reactive psychosis. Along with posttraumatic stress disorder and adjustment disorders, brief reactive psychosis is one of the few diagnoses in DSM-IV in which a specific causative agent is identified (that is, a psychosocial stressor). However, no well-controlled studies have assessed the causal role of various forms of stress or other factors in causing brief reactive psychosis. Conflict may arise from domestic strife, employment problems, accidents, illness, or the death of a family member. Immigrants may be vulnerable to the condition and may appear in a state of culture shock. The magnitude of a stressor has classically been emphasized, but the cumulative effect of several events may prove to be more important than one event. In addition, the meaning that a specific event has for a person in a given psychosocial setting should be clinically appreciated. Severe intrapsychic conflicts have also been posited as potential triggers for brief psychotic disorder.

Stressors are generally considered to be nonspecific and seem to influence most directly the timing of the onset of the disorder. Many investigators think that preexisting psychopathology helps predispose a patient to its development, and people with paranoid, histrionic, narcissistic, schizotypal, or borderline personality disorders are thought to be particularly vulnerable. Various explanations have been offered, including psychodynamic formulations. For example, some cases of "hysterical psychosis" have been described as an extreme presentation of a hysterical personality disorder in which the ego's ability to function has been overwhelmed by unconscious material that erupts into consciousness. In borderline personality disorder patients, psychotic reactions have been noted at times of threatened abandonment and are seen by some clinicians as an attempt to provide temporary distance in the relationship. Other explanations may involve immature ego development, the use of primitive defenses, and the lack of external supports. A causative role of stress is not assumed, however, in the DSM-IV category of brief psychotic disorder.

A number of family studies have supported a genetic vulnerability to brief reactive psychosis. Although the studies are often limited by methodological flaws, the evidence shows that reactive psychosis tends to run true in families. Although brief psychotic disorder may have a relation to mood disorders, no evidence supports a genetic relation to schizophrenia.

DIAGNOSIS AND CLINICAL FEATURES Patients with brief psychotic disorder have an abrupt onset of impaired reality testing and may present with a variety of associated symptoms, including delusions, hallucinations, bizarre behavior and postures, disorganized speech, and catatonic behavior. Such patients may also appear highly confused and their affect may shift rapidly, although those features are no longer required for diagnostic purposes. In cases of brief reactive psychosis, symptoms can often be understood in the context of the patient's psychosocial surroundings, although the clinician may require some knowledge of different cultures. Culturally sanctioned response patterns are important to recognize and to consider prior to making a diagnosis of brief psychotic disorder. The precipitating event may be a major stress, such as the loss of a loved one or the psychological trauma of combat. Alternatively, a series of life stresses may have the cumulative effect of causing patients to exceed a stress threshold, a point at which they begin to exhibit psychotic symptoms. On cross-sectional viewing, the diagnosis is difficult to differentiate from other types of acute psychosis.

Scandinavian investigators have defined several subtypes of reactions based on the predominant symptoms. The subtypes include acute paranoid reactions, reactive confusions with disturbances in attention and orientation, reactive excitations or manias, and reactive depressive psychosis; the majority of cases in the literature are of the depressive subtype. By definition, the symptoms persist from one day to one month, and the patient usually has a prompt recovery, with a full return to the premorbid level of functioning and personality, which may include a personality type, such as histrionic or borderline, that can predispose to further episodes of brief psychotic disorder.

DIFFERENTIAL DIAGNOSIS Given the often abrupt onset of symptoms, clinicians must consider the possibility of a psychotic disorder due to a general medical condition, a substance-induced psychotic disorder, or delirium. The initial history, physical examination, and laboratory studies, including a toxicology screen, should help rule out a number of those conditions. When the patient appears confused and unable to sustain attention, the diagnosis of delirium needs to be considered. Further testing with modalities such as CT, magnetic resonance imaging (MRI), or EEG should also be considered.

If the psychiatric disorder persists for more than one month, the diagnosis has to be changed to schizophreniform disorder, schizophrenia, schizoaffective disorder, mood disorder with psychotic features, delusional disorder, or psychotic disorder not otherwise specified. The differential diagnosis between brief psychotic disorder and schizophreniform disorder may be especially difficult to make when the psychotic symptoms have remitted before one month in response to pharmacological treatment. In that case, longitudinal observations to rule out the possibility of a recurrent psychotic disorder should be considered. When symptoms are present for less than one month, the presence of a clear stressor and an abrupt onset suggest brief reactive psychosis (called brief psychotic disorder, with marked stressor, in DSM-IV), but factitious disorder, with predominantly psychological signs and symptoms, may be present (if the symptoms are intentionally produced), and malingering should also be considered. Some personality disorders, such as borderline personality disorders, have transient psychotic symptoms. However, if psychotic symptoms persist for at least one day, an additional diagnosis of brief psychotic disorder may be appropriate. In a few cases a dissociative disorder is a valid diagnosis when the patient is unable to recall personal information as a result of a severe stressor. However, the presence of florid psychotic symptoms makes the diagnosis of dissociative disorder unlikely.

COURSE AND PROGNOSIS By definition, brief psychotic disorder is of short duration (less than one month), and the patient makes a full return to baseline functioning. Follow-up studies have been done mainly in Scandinavia and are limited by methodological flaws, such as retrospective designs. About 50 percent of patients who have received the diagnosis of brief reactive psychosis seem to retain that diagnosis at long-term follow-up. A substantial number of other cases, however, go on to a long-term course and are rediagnosed as schizophrenia or mood disorder. At present, there is no initial way to distinguish brief psychotic disorder from acute-onset schizophrenia or mood disorders with psychotic features. Certain features prognostic of a good outcome have been identified in the literature, although those features have been inconsistent. The good prognostic features include an acute onset of symptoms, good premorbid functioning, the presence of affective symptoms, a short duration of symptoms, and confusion during the episode of psychosis.

A recent study shows a higher mortality risk for patients with brief reactive psychosis than for the population in general. That risk seems to be highest for young patients in the first years after the resolution of the psychotic reaction. Other studies show that some patients experience significant psychosocial disability and suggest the need for continued follow-up after the treatment of the brief psychotic disorder. Few data are available on the recurrence of reactive episodes.

TREATMENT Acute psychotic disorder requires both immediate and long-term treatment. In the short term, patients with the disorder may be a danger to themselves or others, and hospitalization should be considered. Hospitalization facilitates both close observation and a full examination for possible medical conditions. A quiet, well-structured environment with reduced stimulation is usually helpful. At times, behavioral disturbances may necessitate physical or chemical restraints.

No controlled studies are available to guide the clinician in the treatment of the disorder. If medication is necessary, a low dosage of a high-potency antipsychotic, preferably with a prophylactic antiparkinsonism agent, is one option. That regimen reduces the likelihood of acute extrapyramidal side effects, such as akathisia, which has been linked to episodes of agitation and violent behavior. Benzodiazepines are another alternative. They may be used alone or in combination with an antipsychotic. In general, benzodiazepines are safe and may have antipsychotic efficacy in the acute situation. Their use helps minimize patient exposure to antipsychotic medication side effects and may be less likely than the antipsychotics to obscure the clinical situation. However, benzodiazepines can lead to behavioral disinhibition and may create the risk of withdrawal seizures, although the seizures seem to be of greatest concern with prolonged use at high dosages. The role of lithium, antidepressants, and other medications is unclear at this time, although scattered reports favor their use.

Once the acute episode has subsided, the clinician must work with patients to clarify their vulnerability to stress and to enhance their coping mechanisms. The therapist may need to understand a wide array of sociocultural and interpersonal issues, and a tailored treatment plan is needed for each case. Emphasis on problem-solving skills is valuable, and psychotherapy may help strengthen personality weaknesses. Supportive psychotherapy can also help restore the patient's morale and self-esteem. Longer-term therapy is suggested after the acute psychosis has resolved.

In general, maintenance antipsychotic treatment has no role in brief psychotic disorder. If the patient continues to require antipsychotics for many months, an alternative diagnosis should be considered.

A 52-year-old registered nurse was brought to an emergency room by a friend because of visual hallucinations (seeing colors and numbers), referential thinking concerning colors, and persecutory delusions. The patient had been well until one week before, when her family noticed that she started to throw things away, including food, for no apparent reason. One evening she stood in a doorway, staring for several minutes. She had been talking a lot about family problems, including being the sole support for several children, but she was most upset by her brother's recent prison release, fearing that he was going to harm her.

She had no history of drug or alcohol use and no medical problems, and she was using no medications. On two previous occasions she had requested help for anxiety related to different sets of stressors. In each case she remained in treatment for a short period and did not receive medication.

On admission to the hospital, she kept questioning staff member identification cards, and she felt that she was about to be harmed. She displayed a strange gait at times and histrionically demanded to know what the cause was. Her physical examination and laboratory results were unremarkable, as were the findings of brain MRI, EEG, and urine toxicology tests. After receiving lorazepam (Ativan) for several days, her thought disorder improved, and she no longer experienced hallucinations. She was responsive to the ward milieu, benefiting from individual and group therapies. In a family meeting she was able to discuss her concerns and develop effective coping strategies. After her discharge from the hospital, she did well at work and continued in supportive psychotherapy without the need of medication.

SUGGESTED CROSS-REFERENCES

Material relevant to this section is presented in Chapter 14 on schizophrenia and Chapter 16 on mood disorders. Relevant information concerning treatment can be found in Chapter 32 on biological therapies and Chapter 31 on psychotherapies. Psychiatric rehabilitation is discussed in Section 50.4. Psychosocial treatment of schizophrenia is discussed in Section 14.9, and individual psychotherapy of schizophrenia is discussed in Section 14.10. Psychosocial treatments of mood disorders are discussed in Section 16.8. Psychodynamic concepts relevant to the causes of schizophrenia and mood disorders are found in Section 14.6 and Section 16.5, respectively. Medical illnesses that can lead to mixed states of affective and psychotic symptoms are discussed in Section 26.12 on consultation-liaison psychiatry.

REFERENCES

Bartels S J, Drake R E: Depressive symptoms in schizophrenia: Comprehensive differential diagnosis. Compr Psychiatry *29:* 467, 1988.

Beiser M, Fleming J A E, Iacono W G, Lin T: Refining the diagnosis of schizophreniform disorder. Am J Psychiatry *145:* 695, 1988.

Bergen A L M, Dahl A A, Guldberg C, Hansen H: Langfeldt's schizophreniform psychoses fifty years later. Br J Psychiatry *157:* 351, 1990.

*Coryell W, Keller M, Lavori P, Endicott J: Affective syndromes, psychotic features, and prognosis: I. Depression. II. Mania. Arch Gen Psychiatry *47:* 651, 1990.

Coryell W, Tsuang M T: Outcome after 40 years in DSM-III schizophreniform disorder. Arch Gen Psychiatry *43:* 324, 1986.

Goldstein J M, Faraone S V, Chen W J, Tsuang M T: The role of gender in understanding the familial transmission of schizoaffective disorder. Br J Psychiatry *163:* 763, 1993.

Hoff A L, Riordan H, O'Donnell D W, Morris L, DeLisi L E: Neuropsychological functioning of first-episode schizophreniform patients. Am J Psychiatry *149:* 898, 1992.

*Jauch D A, Carpenter W T: Reactive psychosis: I. Does the pre-DSM-III concept define a third psychosis? J Nerv Ment Dis *176:* 72, 1988.

Jauch D A, Carpenter W T: Reactive psychosis: II. Does DSM-III-R define a third psychosis? J Nerv Ment Dis *176:* 82, 1988.

Jorgensen P, Jensen J: An attempt to operationalize reactive delusional psychosis. Acta Psychiatr Scand *78:* 627, 1988.

Kasanin J: The acute schizoaffective psychoses. Am J Psychiatry *90:* 97, 1933.

Kendler K S, Spitzer R L, Williams J B W: Psychotic disorders in DSM-III-R. Am J Psychiatry *146:* 953, 1989.

Langfeldt G: *The Schizophreniform States.* Munksgaard, Copenhagen, 1939.

Lapensée M A: A review of schizoaffective disorder: I. Current concepts. II. Somatic treatment. Can J Psychiatry *37:* 335, 1992.

Lavin M R, Rifkin A: Prophylactic antiparkinsonian drug use: I. Initial prophylaxis and prevention of extrapyramidal side effects. II. Withdrawal after long-term maintenance therapy. J Clin Pharmacol *31:* 763, 1991.

Levinson D F, Levitt M E M: Schizoaffective mania reconsidered. Am J Psychiatry *144:* 415, 1987.

*Levitt J J, Tsuang M T: The heterogeneity of schizoaffective disorder: Implications for treatment. Am J Psychiatry *145:* 926, 1988.

Maier W, Lichtermann D, Minges J, Hallmayer J, Heun R, Benkert O, Levinson D F: Continuity and discontinuity of affective disorders and schizophrenia: Results of a controlled family study. Arch Gen Psychiatry *50:* 871, 1993.

Maj M, Starace F, Pirozzi R: A family study of DSM-III-R schizoaffective disorder, depressive type, compared with schizophrenia and psychotic and nonpsychotic major depression. Am J Psychiatry *148:* 612, 1991.

Marneros A, Rohde A, Deister A: Factors influencing the long-term outcome of schizoaffective disorders. Psychopathology *26:* 215, 1993.

Marneros A, Tsuang M T: *Affective and Schizoaffective Disorders: Similarities and Differences.* Springer, New York, 1990.

McDermott B E, Sautter F J, Garver D L: Heterogeneity of schizophrenia: Relationship to latency of neuroleptic response. Psychiatry Res *37:* 97, 1991.

Modestin J, Bachmann K M: Is the diagnosis of hysterical psychosis justified? Clinical study of hysterical psychosis, reactive/psychogenic psychosis, and schizophrenia. Compr Psychiatry *33:* 17, 1992.

Nuechterlein K H, Dawson M D: A heuristic vulnerability/stress model of schizophrenic episodes. Schizophr Bull *10:* 300, 1984.

Okasha A, Seif El Dawla A, Khalil A H, Saad A: Presentation of acute psychosis in an Egyptian sample: A transcultural comparison. Compr Psychiatry *34:* 4, 1993.

Procci W R: Schizoaffective psychosis: Fact or fiction? A survey of the literature. Arch Gen Psychiatry *33:* 1167, 1976.

Pulver A E, Brown C H, Wolyniec P S, McGrath J A, Tam D: Psychiatric morbidity in the relatives of patients with DSM-III schizophreniform disorder: Comparisons with the relatives of schizophrenic and bipolar disorder patients. J Psychiatr Res *25:* 19, 1991.

Rubin P, Møller-Madsen S, Hertel C, Juvl-Povlsen U, Norang U, Hemmingsen R: Computerized tomography in newly diagnosed schizophrenia and schizophreniform disorder: A controlled blind study. Br J Psychiatry *163:* 604, 1993.

Samson J A, Simpson J C, Tsuang M T: Outcome studies of schizoaffective disorders. Schizophr Bull *14:* 543, 1988.

Sautter F, McDermott B, Garuer D: The course of DSM-III-R schizophreniform disorder. J Clin Psychol *49:* 331, 1993.

Shenton M E, Solovay M R, Holzman P: Comparative studies of thought disorders: II. Schizoaffective disorders. Arch Gen Psychiatry *44:* 21, 1987.

Siris S G: Adjunctive medication in the maintenance treatment of schizophrenia and its conceptual implications. Br J Psychiatry *163* (Suppl): 66, 1993.

*Siris S G: Diagnosis of secondary depression in schizophrenia: Implications for DSM-IV. Schizophr Bull *17:* 75, 1991.

Siris S G: The treatment of schizoaffective disorder. In *Current Psychiatric Therapy,* D L Dunner, editor, p 160. Saunders, Philadelphia, 1993.

Stephens J H, Shaffer J W, Carpenter W T: Reactive psychosis. J Nerv Ment Dis *170:* 657, 1982.

Strakowski S M: Diagnostic validity of schizophreniform disorder. Am J Psychiatry *151:* 815, 1994.

Strauss J S: Schizoaffective disorders: 'Just another illness' or key to understanding the psychoses? Psychiatria Clin *16:* 286, 1983.

*Taylor M A: Are schizophrenia and affective disorder related? A selective literature review. Am J Psychiatry *149:* 22, 1992.

Tsuang D, Coryell W: An 8-year follow-up of patients with DSM-III-R psychotic depression, schizoaffective disorder, and schizophrenia. Am J Psychiatry *150:* 1182, 1993.

Weinberger D R: The pathogenesis of schizophrenia: A neurodevelopmental theory. In *Handbook of Schizophrenia,* H A Nasrallah, D R Weinberger, editors, vol 1, p 397. Elsevier, New York, 1986.

15.2 DELUSIONAL DISORDER AND SHARED PSYCHOTIC DISORDER

THEO C. MANSCHRECK, M.D.

INTRODUCTION

Delusional disorder is the current classification for a group of disorders of unknown cause, the chief feature of which is the delusion (Table 15.2-1). Although the specific content of the delusion may vary from one case to the next, it is the occurrence of the delusion, its persistence, its impact on behavior, and its prognosis that unify these seemingly different disorders. In considerable agreement with Emil Kraepelin's concept of paranoia, the revised third edition of *Diagnostic and Statistical Manual of Mental Disorders* (DSM-III-R) provided reliable criteria for identifying cases and collecting systematic information about these conditions. That development in classification reestablished the clinical importance of this group of disorders and may have reversed a trend of diagnosing them infrequently. The criteria use the term "delusional" to avoid the ambiguity of the term "paranoid" used earlier in the third edition of DSM (DSM-III) classification, "paranoid disorders," and to emphasize that the category includes disorders in which delusions other than those of the persecutory or jealous type are present. The fourth edition of DSM (DSM-IV) attempts to refine the definitions and the boundaries with other disorders, including substance-induced disorders, mental disorders due to general medical conditions, mood disorders, and schizophrenia. The DSM-IV definition, like its predecessors, hinges on the presence of a nonbizarre delusion. DSM-IV acknowledges the difficulty of judging whether a delusion is bizarre, meaning clearly

TABLE 15.2-1
DSM-IV Definition of Delusion and Certain Common Types Associated with Delusional Disorders

delusion A false belief based on incorrect inference about external reality that is firmly sustained despite what almost everyone else believes and despite what constitutes incontrovertible and obvious proof or evidence to the contrary. The belief is not one ordinarily accepted by other members of the person's culture or subculture (e.g., it is not an article of religious faith). When a false belief involves a value judgment, it is regarded as a delusion only when the judgment is so extreme as to defy credibility. Delusional conviction occurs on a continuum and can sometimes be inferred from an individual's behavior. It is often difficult to distinguish between a delusion and an overvalued idea (in which case the individual has an unreasonable belief or idea but does not hold it as firmly as is the case with a delusion).

Delusions are subdivided according to their content. Some of the more common types are listed below:

bizarre—A delusion that involves a phenomenon that the person's culture would regard as totally implausible.
delusional jealousy—The delusion that one's sexual partner is unfaithful.
erotomanic—A delusion that another person, usually of higher status, is in love with the individual.
grandiose—A delusion of inflated worth, power, knowledge, identity, or special relationship to a deity or famous person.
mood-congruent *See* mood-congruent psychotic features.
mood-incongruent *See* mood-incongruent psychotic features.
of being controlled—A delusion in which feelings, impulses, thoughts, or actions are experienced as being under the control of some external force rather than being under one's own control.
of reference—A delusion whose theme is that events, objects, or other persons in one's immediate environment have a particular and unusual significance. These delusions are usually of a negative or pejorative nature, but also may be grandiose in content. This differs from an *idea of reference,* in which the false belief is not as firmly held nor as fully organized into a true belief.
persecutory—A delusion in which the central theme is that one (or someone to whom one is close) is being attacked, harassed, cheated, persecuted, or conspired against.
somatic—A delusion whose main content pertains to the appearance or functioning of one's body.
thought broadcasting—The delusion that one's thoughts are being broadcast out loud so that they can be perceived by others.
thought insertion—The delusion that certain of one's thoughts are not one's own, but rather are inserted into one's mind.
mood-congruent psychotic features—Delusions or hallucinations whose content is entirely consistent with the typical themes of a depressed or manic mood. If the mood is depressed, the content of the delusions or hallucinations would involve themes of personal inadequacy, guilt, disease, death, nihilism, or deserved punishment. The content of the delusion may include themes of persecution if these are based on self-derogatory concepts such as deserved punishment. If the mood is manic, the content of the delusions or hallucinations would involve themes of inflated worth, power, knowledge, or identity, or a special relationship to a deity or a famous person. The content of the delusion may include themes of persecution if these are based on concepts such as inflated worth or deserved punishment.
mood-incongruent psychotic features—Delusions or hallucinations whose content is not consistent with the typical themes of a depressed or manic mood. In the case of depression, the delusions or hallucinations would not involve themes of personal inadequacy, guilt, disease, death, nihilism, or deserved punishment. In the case of mania, the delusions or hallucinations would not involve themes of inflated worth, power, knowledge, or identity, or a special relationship to a deity or a famous person. Examples of mood-incongruent psychotic features include persecutory delusions (without self-derogatory or grandiose content), thought insertion, thought broadcasting, and delusions of being controlled whose content has no apparent relationship to any of the themes listed above.

implausible, not understandable, and not derived from ordinary life experiences. In contrast, the nonbizarre delusion involves situations or circumstances that can occur in real life (for example, being followed, infected, or deceived by a lover). DSM-IV also emphasizes the differential diagnosis of schizophrenia, mood disorders, substance-induced disorders, and mental disorders due to a general medical condition before the diagnosis of delusional disorders can be made. Those conceptual refinements and demarcations from other conditions have increased the usefulness of the delusional disorder criteria.

Despite those advances, clinicians are relatively unaware of delusional disorders. There are several possible reasons. Persons with the conditions do not regard themselves as mentally ill and actively oppose psychiatric referral. Because they may experience little impairment, they generally remain outside hospital settings, appearing reclusive, eccentric, or odd, rather than ill. If they do have contact with professionals, it is more likely to be with lawyers regarding litigious concerns; with medical specialists regarding health concerns; or with the police regarding complaints of trespass, persecution, or threat, rather than psychiatric clinicians regarding complaints of emotional disorder. It is a hallmark of those disorders that the patient does not believe that he or she is deluded or in need of psychiatric assistance. In the infrequent psychiatric encounter the tendency among clinicians is to diagnose them as other conditions, often schizophrenia or mood disorders.

Delusional disorders are uncommon, but probably not as rare as previously thought. While many individuals with such disorders seek assistance from medical specialists, judges, or the police, they are increasingly being recognized as psychiatrically ill. The relationship of these disorders to other psychoses remains unclear, and much about them is a puzzle. The DSM-IV requirement of excluding other conditions is prudent given the special importance of differential diagnosis. Though the DSM-IV criteria are not definitive, they have provided a sound basis for clinical and research investigation. Systematic studies based on larger samples of these disorders are needed to anchor classification with sound information, although such studies may be difficult to achieve. A biological basis for these disorders is proposed on many grounds, but its definition has been elusive and remains distant.

DEFINITION

DELUSIONAL DISORDER According to DSM-IV, the diagnosis of delusional disorder can be made when a person exhibits nonbizarre delusions of at least one month's duration that cannot be attributed to other psychiatric disorders. Definitions of the term ''delusion'' and types relevant to delusional disorders are presented in Table 15.2-1. Diagnostic criteria for delusional disorder are presented in Table 15.2-2. Nonbizarre means that the delusions must be about situations that can occur in real life, such as being followed, infected, loved at a distance, and so on. There are several types of delusions, and the predominant type is specified when making the diagnosis.

In general, the patient's delusions are well systematized and have been logically developed. The person may experience auditory or visual hallucinations, but those are not prominent features. Tactile or olfactory hallucinations may be both present and prominent if they are related to the delusional content or theme. The sensation of being infested by bugs, associated with delusions of infestation, and the belief that one's body odor is foul, associated with somatic delusions, are examples. The per-

TABLE 15.2-2
Diagnostic Criteria for Delusional Disorder

A. Nonbizarre delusions (i.e., involving situations that occur in real life, such as being followed, poisoned, infected, loved at a distance, or deceived by spouse or lover, or having a disease) of at least 1 month's duration.
B. Criterion A for schizophrenia has never been met. Note: Tactile and olfactory hallucinations may be present in delusional disorder if they are related to the delusional theme.
C. Apart from the impact of the delusion(s) or its ramifications, functioning is not markedly impaired and behavior is not obviously odd or bizarre.
D. If mood episodes have occurred concurrently with delusions, their total duration has been brief relative to the duration of the delusional periods.
E. The disturbance is not due to the direct physiological effects of a substance (e.g., a drug of abuse, a medication) or a general medical condition.

Specify type (the following types are assigned based on the predominant delusional theme):
Erotomanic type: delusions that another person, usually of higher status, is in love with the individual
Grandiose type: delusions of inflated worth, power, knowledge, identity, or special relationship to a deity or famous person
Jealous type: delusions that the individual's sexual partner is unfaithful
Persecutory type: delusions that the person (or someone to whom the person is close) is being malevolently treated in some way
Somatic type: delusions that the person has some physical defect or general medical condition
Mixed type: delusions characteristic of more than one of the above types but no one theme predominates
Unspecified type

TABLE 15.2-3
Diagnostic Criteria for Shared Psychotic Disorder

A. A delusion develops in an individual in the context of a close relationship with another person(s), who has an already-established delusion.
B. The delusion is similar in content to that of the person who already has the established delusion.
C. The disturbance is not better accounted for by another psychotic disorder (e.g., schizophrenia) or a mood disorder with psychotic features and is not due to the direct physiological effects of a substance (e.g., a drug of abuse, a medication) or a general medical condition.

son's behavioral and emotional responses to the delusion appear to be appropriate. Impairment of functioning or personality deterioration is minimal, if it occurs at all. General behavior is neither obviously odd nor bizarre.

SHARED PSYCHOTIC DISORDER Shared psychotic disorder is defined in Table 15.2-3. This unusual condition has also been called *folie à deux* and induced psychotic disorder. It develops in an individual in the context of a close relationship with another person who has an established delusion, and requires an absence of psychotic disorder prior to the onset of the induced delusion. It has usually been classified with paranoid disorders.

HISTORY OF THE PARANOID CONCEPT

Nineteenth century psychiatry devoted much attention to the description of paranoid disorders, in which delusions are a cardinal feature. Karl Ludwig Kahlbaum's description of paranoia in 1863 was the first in a series of contributions that culminated in the classification of paraphrenia, *folie à deux,* morbid jealousy, the better known schizophrenias, and mania. His work also led to a recognition that paranoid features are nonspecific characteristics of many diseases. Subsequent work has led to refined criteria for paranoid and related disorders and has reestablished awareness of less common paranoid presentations such as delusional disorder.

Many clinicians remember being taught that paranoia is so rare that most would not examine a single patient during an entire career. That widespread belief has compromised interest in paranoid disorders. The fact that most persons with delusional disorder live in the community and do not generally seek psychiatric care have made it difficult to carry out systematic case studies. Indeed, knowledge of these conditions has been scanty and frequently anecdotal. However, case series such as those of Alistair Munro (for delusional disorder, somatic type, or for hypochondriacal delusional disorder) or those of Nils Retterstol have been influential in shaping understanding and awareness. What they tell us is that there are persons with these disorders, that the disorders are complex forms of psychiatric illness, and that much remains to be learned.

A major change in the classification of delusional disorders in DSM-III-R and DSM-IV has been to emphasize the central role of delusions in those disorders and to steer away from the vague label of paranoid, which has become synonymous with suspicious. Indeed, suspiciousness may be less common than expected in those disorders. The history of the concept of paranoia indicates that lack of clarity in its use is not new. The word "paranoia" was coined by the ancient Greeks from roots meaning beside and self. Hippocrates applied this term to delirium associated with high fever, but other writers used it to describe demented conditions and madness. It sometimes meant thinking amiss, folly, and the like. Hence, its meaning was unclear. For centuries the term fell into disuse until a revival of interest in the 19th century.

Kahlbaum in 1863 classified paranoia as a separate mental illness: "a form of partial insanity, which, throughout the course of the disease, principally affected the sphere of the intellect." Influenced by the new scientific methods of empirical medicine, Kahlbaum emphasized the importance of natural history in mental illness and restricted the term paranoia to a persistent delusional illness that remained largely unchanged throughout its course. Delusions, he noted, could occur in other medical and psychiatric conditions.

Kraepelin found the paranoid concept troublesome and altered his thinking on it with each edition of his textbook. His final view advocated three types of paranoid disorder. Like Kahlbaum, Kraepelin based his conclusions on analysis of the natural history of mental disorders, particularly on outcome. He restricted the definition of paranoia to an uncommon, insidious, chronic illness (he saw 19 cases during his career) characterized by a fixed delusional system, an absence of hallucinations, and a lack of deterioration of the personality. The types of delusions noted included persecutory, grandiose, somatic, jealous, and possibly hypochondriacal. He considered this illness to derive from defects in the capacity of judgment, a disorder of personality caused by constitutional factors and environmental stress. Paraphrenia was a second paranoid disorder that developed later than dementia precox and was milder. There were hallucinations (auditory in particular) but no mental deterioration (dementia). Finally, there was dementia paranoides, an illness that initially resembled paranoia but had an earlier onset and showed a deteriorating course. Because of this latter feature Kraepelin considered dementia paranoides a form of dementia precox that arose from disorders of thought, cognition, and emotion. Kurt Mayer's follow-up of Kraepelin's 78 paraphrenia cases challenged the validity of this category because the vast majority in fact showed an outcome indistinguishable from that of dementia precox, casting doubt on the separability of this group. Karl Kolle's follow-up of Kraepelin's paranoia cases indicated some overlap with dementia precox. Kraepelin also emphasized that isolated paranoid symptoms occurred in a variety of psychiatric and medical illnesses.

Eugen Bleuler also recognized paranoia (though he broadened its definition to include cases with hallucinations); a paranoid form of dementia precox, which he called schizophrenia; and an intermediate group, but thought that the paranoia described by Kraepelin was so rare that it did not warrant a separate classification. Further, he argued that schizophrenic symptoms must be suspected and carefully sought after even in those cases. Paraphrenia and intermediate conditions, he held, were forms of schizophrenia linked by "much that was identical," and in particular a common disturbance in associative processes. He also emphasized that paranoid symptoms occurred in other conditions and that to label them schizophrenic required at least one of the fundamental symptoms: loosened associations, ambivalence, inappropriate affect, and autism.

Sigmund Freud used the autobiographical writings of Judge Daniel Schreber to illustrate the role of psychological defense mechanisms in the development of paranoid symptoms. He proposed that Schreber's illness involved a process of denial or contradiction of repressed homosexual impulses toward his father. Persecutory and other delusions result from projecting these denied yearnings into the environment. He did not differentiate subtypes of paranoid disorder, and he added to the confusion by proposing that the term "paraphrenia" be substituted for dementia precox or schizophrenia. The major impact of Freud's work was to suggest hypotheses that indicated the relationship between certain delusions and personality.

Ernst Kretschmer's work on the theory of paranoia emphasized that certain sensitive personalities, characterized by depressive, pessimistic, and narcissistic traits, developed paranoid features acutely when key or precipitating experiences occurred at critical moments in their lives. He observed that those individuals did not develop schizophrenia and had a favorable prognosis. A number of other observers, predominantly but not exclusively European (for example, the American concept of hysterical psychosis) proposed connections between personality and delusion development. Those efforts, based on various theories of course of paranoid disturbance, have persisted despite modest empirical support. Out of such work have come terms, such as reactive and psychogenic psychosis, which have figured in various classification schemes, adding further confusion to the effort to bring about international consistency in definition.

Current views are based on those historical antecedents. DSM-III introduced greater rigor in the assessment by requiring clearer criteria boundaries among the varied disorders with delusions. And the awareness that delusions result from numerous conditions has had a positive influence on the diagnostic process. Yet much of current clinical and research writing on paranoid conditions has characteristically avoided defining the term "paranoid," apparently because it has assumed that everyone knows what paranoid means. In popular and literary usage the term "paranoid" has come to mean insane, angrily suspicious, distrustful, or irrationally irritable. The paranoid concept, however clumsy it may be, continues to be used in clinical work. Because it is necessary to differentiate conditions with paranoid features, a useful concept of the term is fundamental.

SHARED PSYCHOTIC DISORDER Jules Baillarger first described the syndrome, calling it *folie à communiquée,* in 1860, although the first description is commonly attributed to Ernest Charles Lasègue and Jules Falret, who described the condition in 1877 and gave it the name of *folie à deux.* The syndrome has also been called communicated insanity, contagious insanity, infectious insanity, psychosis of association, and double insanity. Marandon de Montyel divided *folie à deux* into three groups (*folie imposée, folie simultanée,* and *folie communiquée*), and Heinz Lehmann added a fourth group, *folie induite.*

CLARIFICATION OF THE PARANOID CONCEPT

Paranoid features (signs and symptoms) are among the most dramatic and serious disturbances in psychiatry and medicine. Nevertheless, the term "paranoid" refers to a variety of behaviors that are often not psychopathological and are not necessarily related to schizophrenia. Hence, the meaning of the term "paranoid" has become obscure. Some clinicians label ordinary suspiciousness paranoid. Others restrict use of the term to persecutory delusions. Still others apply the term only to grandiose, litigious, hostile, and jealous behavior, despite the fact that those behaviors may be within the normal behavioral spectrum. To make the paranoid concept useful and less vague requires the consideration of several points.

1. The term "paranoid" is a clinical construct used to interpret observations, and in order to apply this construct effectively, the clinician must know its meaning and be able to make accurate observations of potentially paranoid behavior.
2. Use of the term "paranoid" means the clinician has judged that the person's behavior is psychopathological. This judgment is usually based on the discovery that the person who displays such features is either disturbed or disturbing to others.
3. Although many contributions to understanding paranoid phenomena have focused on conditions in which paranoid features are central (for example, schizophrenia for Bleuler, paranoia for Kraepelin, and dementia paranoides), those features are not necessarily associated with schizophrenia and can appear in other psychiatric and medical disorders. Hence, paranoid features indicate psychopathology, but no specific cause (Table 15.2-4), chronicity, or curability.
4. The observations that form the basis for judging behavior to be paranoid are of two kinds: subjective (part of the private mental experience of the patient, for example, a delusion) and objective (observable as a manifest form of behavior, such as litigiousness, guardedness, grandiosity). Table 15.2-5 is a list of the subjective and objective features that have traditionally been labeled paranoid and that are frequently found in association. Some can be manifestations of normal behavior. The judgment that such features are paranoid may rest on their extremeness or inappropriateness, their presence in combination or association with other behaviors on the list, and the presence of delusions.
5. The term paranoid delusions has traditionally referred to a wide variety of delusions, not simply those of grandeur, persecution, or jealousy. Because of recent confusion that term probably should not be used. The term "paranoid" and associated terms are defined in Table 15.2-6.

TABLE 15.2-4
Conditions and Agents Associated with Delusions and Other Paranoid Features

Neurological disorders	Infections
Arteriosclerotic psychoses	Acquired immune deficiency syndrome
Blunt head trauma	Encephalitis lethargica
Brain tumors	Creutzfeldt-Jakob disease
Cerebrovascular disease	Malaria
Delirium	Syphilis
Dementia	Toxic shock syndrome
Fat embolism	Trypanosomiasis
Hearing loss	Typhus
Huntington's chorea	Viral encephalitides
Hydrocephalus	Psychiatric disorders
Hypertensive encephalopathy	Brief psychotic disorder
Idiopathic basal ganglia calcification	Delusional disorder (including classic paranoia)
Idiopathic Parkinson's disease	Shared psychotic disorder
Intracranial hemorrhage	Mood disorders
Marchiafava-Bignami disease	Schizoaffective disorder
Menzel-type ataxia	Schizophrenia (all subtypes)
Metachromatic leukodystrophy	Schizophreniform disorder
Migraine	Alcohol and drugs
Motor-neuron disease	Alcohol withdrawal
Multiple sclerosis	Amphetamine
Muscular dystrophy	Anesthetic nitrous oxide
Narcolepsy	Atropine toxicity
Postencephalitic parkinsonism	Barbiturate
Presenile psychoses (Alzheimer's and Pick's diseases)	Chronic alcohol hallucinosis
Roussy-Levy syndrome	Chronic bromide intoxication
Senile psychoses	Cocaine
Spinocerebellar degeneration	Ephedrine
Subarachnoid hemorrhage	Marijuana
Subdural hematoma	Mescaline and other hallucinogens
Temporal lobe epilepsy	Perbitine
Metabolic and endocrine disorders	Withdrawal from minor tranquilizers and hypnotic medications
Acute intermittent porphyria	Toxic agents
Addison's disease	Arsenic
Complication of surgical portacaval anastomosis for cirrhosis	Carbon monoxide
Cushing's syndrome	Manganese
Folate deficiency	Mercury
Hemodialysis	Thallium
Hypercalcemia	Pharmacological agents
Hypoglycemia	Adrenocorticotropic hormone
Hyponatremia	Amphetamine and related compounds
Hypopituitarism	Anticholinergic drugs
Liver failure	Antimalarials
Malnutrition	Antitubercular drugs
Niacin deficiency	Bromocriptine
Pancreatic encephalopathy	Bupropion
Parathyroid disorders	Cimetidine
Pellagra	Cortisone
Pernicious anemia	Diphenylhydantoin
Phenylketonuria	Disulfiram
Systemic lupus erythematosus	L-Dopa
Thiamine deficiency	Imipramine and other tricyclic antidepressants
Thyroid disorders	Mephentermine
Uremia	Methyldopa and imipramine (combination)
Vitamin B_{12} deficiency	Methyltestosterone
Wilson's disease	Pentazocine
Sex chromosome disorders	Phenylpropanolamine
47 XXY	Propylhexedrine
Klinefelter's syndrome	
Turner's syndrome	

COMPARATIVE NOSOLOGY

Certain advances have been made in the nosology of delusional disorders, but the variety of current definitions illustrates that consensus has not yet been achieved. The reasons for such differences are multiple. The principal reason is simply a lack of relevant data; delusional disorders occur infrequently or are easily misdiagnosed and have minimal overt identifying characteristics. Because only limited knowledge, largely from case reports, has accumulated; systematic, larger scale studies are uncommon. Those studies that exist have generally been European and have employed varied classifications. Also, the fundamental concept that the disorders are distinct from schizophrenia and mood disorders has until recently been unacceptable to many psychiatrists.

Kahlbaum was the first to use the term paranoia to designate a diagnostically separate group of disorders. Kraepelin developed this diagnostic concept further by emphasizing the chronic and unremitting nature of paranoia and the lack of other features such as hallucinations that distinguished it from schizophrenia. The first diagnostic manual of the American Psychiatric Association (DSM-I) incorporated those ideas in 1952 and defined paranoid reactions as conditions in which there are persecutory or grandiose delusions, with emotional responses and behavior consistent with the delusions, but generally lacking hallucinations. The subtypes were paranoia (a chronic disorder with sys-

TABLE 15.2-5
Paranoid Features

Objective features
- Anger
- Critical, accusatory behavior
- Defensiveness
- Grandiosity or excessive self-importance
- Guardedness, evasiveness
- Hate
- Hostility
- Humorlessness
- Hypersensitivity
- Inordinate attention to small details
- Irritability, quick annoyance
- Litigiousness (letter writing, complaints, legal action)
- Obstinacy
- Resentment
- Seclusiveness
- Self-righteousness
- Sullenness
- Suspiciousness
- Violence, aggressiveness

Subjective features*
- Delusions of self-reference, persecution, grandeur, infidelity, love, jealousy, imposture, infestation, disfigurement
- Overvalued ideas

*Part of private mental experience. The patient often discloses those features during the clinical interview, but may not do so, even with specific questioning.

tematized delusions) and paranoid state (a more acute, less persistent condition with less systematized delusions). The second edition of DSM (DSM-II) in 1968 largely preserved these concepts.

DSM-III Although new definitions were established in DSM-III in 1980, earlier concepts are still evident. The essential features of paranoid disorders in DSM-III are persistent persecutory delusions or delusional jealousy not due to any other mental disorder. Included in the group of paranoid disorders were paranoia; shared paranoid disorder; acute paranoid disorder; and a residual category, atypical paranoid disorder. The boundaries between these conditions and other disorders, such as paranoid personality disorder or paranoid schizophrenia, were noted to be vague. Different types of paranoid disorders were classified on the basis of chronicity. The criteria narrowed the bounds of previous classifications by not including cases with marked hallucinations or certain delusions (for example, hypochondriacal, erotomania, and others).

DSM III-R In 1987, DSM-III-R simplified the DSM-III definition, attempted to minimize the confusion associated with the term paranoid, and highlighted the view that the formation of delusions in the absence of schizophrenia, mood disorder, or organic disorder is the essential feature of these conditions. In contrast to DSM-III, diagnosis in DSM-III-R and DSM-IV requires a one-month's duration of symptoms. Subtyping is based on the predominant type of delusion, which is specified (such as jealous, erotomanic, somatic). This latter feature broadens the category to include a variety of unusual delusions as well as the more common persecutory type. In many respects these criteria are virtually identical to Kraepelin's formulation of paranoia. The two exceptions were Kraepelin's reluctance to endorse a subtype of somatic or hypochondriacal paranoia or to permit cases with hallucinations to be given this diagnosis. He believed cases with hypochondriacal delusions rarely occurred alone.

Shared paranoid disorder was renamed induced psychotic disorder in DSM-III-R and was placed in the category psychotic disorders not elsewhere classified, along with schizophreniform and schizoaffective disorders and brief reactive psychosis. This represents a fundamental departure from DSM-III, which placed this disorder in the paranoid disorders. In patients with this disorder, the delusional content may concern not only persecution or jealousy but virtually any form of delusion, hence, the change in terminology. The term "induced" may more accurately describe the nature of the condition, but hardly resolves the puzzle of causation.

DSM-IV

DELUSIONAL DISORDER DSM-IV makes modest changes in the DSM-III-R criteria in attempting to refine the definition

TABLE 15.2-6
Terminology Connected with Paranoia

Term	Description
Delusional disorders	DSM-III-R category emphasized that the cardinal feature of these conditions is delusions; DSM-IV criteria is one or more nonbizarre delusion lasting for more than one month
Paranoia	Old term for an insidiously developed disorder in which persons suffer from an unshakable delusional system but have no disturbance in the clarity or form of their thinking; also known as paranoia vera, simple delusional disorder, delusional monomania
Paranoic or paranoiac	Old adjectives used to describe persons with paranoia
Paranoid	Broad term meaning suspicious to most people. In psychiatry it is a clinical construct used to describe various objective and subjective features of behavior deemed to be psychopathological (Table 15.2-5); refers to no specific condition (e.g., to be paranoid does not mean that schizophrenia is present)
Paranoid delusion	Older term used to refer to persecutory and grandiose delusions because of their occurrence in the paranoid subtype of schizophrenia; this term has suffered from the confusion associated with the paranoid concept; DSM-III-R recommended that it no longer be used
Paranoid disorders	DSM-III term for an idiopathic group of conditions including paranoia, acute paranoid disorder, shared paranoid disorder, and atypical paranoid disorder; no longer used
Paranoid personality	Enduring traits of paranoid behavior not due to schizophrenia or other mental disorder; generally, there is no evidence of delusions or other features of psychosis
Paranoid syndrome	Term applied to constellations of paranoid features that occur together and can arise from multiple sources, including depression, general medical condition, substance-induced disorders, and schizophrenia
Paraphrenia	Old term for conditions lying theoretically between schizophrenia and paranoia and sharing features of both (hallucinations but no deterioration). It, too, remains controversial and probably should not be used until research validates its meaning

of delusional disorders. In DSM-III-R, the distinction between schizophrenia and delusional disorders had been unclear and controversial. In DSM-III-R, this boundary was defined by the nonbizarre qualities of delusions in delusional disorder and the absence of other active phase symptoms of schizophrenia. Also important was the required absence of other odd or bizarre behavior apart from the delusion. Because the distinction between bizarre and nonbizarre is difficult to define and therefore to apply reliably, other terms such as systematized and prominent were suggested. In practice, however, those terms also have limitations. The quandary has helped promote the case for modifying the criteria in another way: specifically, to use the level of impaired functioning as a means of characterizing the distinction between schizophrenia and delusional disorders. However, given the variability of outcomes in both disorders, this strategy also has limitations. In DSM-IV the suggestion is made that when poor functioning occurs in delusion disorder, it is the result of the delusional beliefs themselves. For example, a person quits a job because he or she believes that the fumes in the workplace are causing a cancerous growth. That person's financial situation worsens with repeated medical consultations. In contrast, poor functioning in schizophrenia is the result of positive and negative symptoms, especially avolition. The resolution of how to make modifications, however, must rest on the effectiveness of the criteria in defining homogeneous and valid subsets of psychotic disordered patients. For this purpose field trials and data analyses have been used to inform the decision scientifically. While the DSM-IV criteria reflect some progress, their validity remains only partly established.

SHARED PSYCHOTIC DISORDER DSM-IV renamed the DSM-III-R category induced psychotic disorder (shared paranoid disorder), calling it shared psychotic disorder. That change reflects the attempt to avoid the term "paranoid" and to identify the condition without reference to any presumed cause or mechanism. The criteria incorporate efforts to define the boundaries between this condition and more common ones, such as other psychotic disorders, mood disorders with psychotic features, substance-induced psychotic disorder, and psychotic disorder due to a general medical condition.

ICD The ninth revision of *International Classification of Diseases and Related Health Problems* contained a larger number of categories for paranoid disorder than the American schemes. Most paranoid disorders fall under the rubric paranoid state, including simple paranoid state, paranoia, paraphrenia, and induced psychosis. Additional subcategories include other and unspecified paranoid states. Acute paranoid reactions and psychogenic paranoid psychosis are classified separately. DSM-III, DSM-III-R, and DSM-IV generally reflect an atheoretical position with respect to the causes of these disorders, whereas ICD-9 was less neutral. For example, psychogenic paranoid psychosis implies a kind of causal mechanism. The categories of paranoid disorder according to these classifications are summarized in Table 15.2-7.

In the tenth revision of ICD (ICD-10), more attention has been paid to creating classifications similar to DSM-III-R and DSM-IV (Table 15.2-8). Paraphrenia, for example, is subsumed under delusional disorder. On the other hand, delusions must be present for about three months to diagnose delusional disorder. For those conditions of less duration, acute and transient psychotic disorder is diagnosed.

EPIDEMIOLOGY

Delusional disorder has been considered an uncommon, if not rare, condition from its earliest descriptions. Epidemiological information is meager. Recent demographic evidence covering a period from 1912 to the 1970s provides an estimate of incidence, prevalence, and related statistics (Table 15.2-9). However, this evidence was assembled using definitions that are not the same as those of DSM-III, DSM-III-R, or DSM-IV. Subsequent data will in all likelihood be somewhat different using the newer criteria. Clearly, the estimates are merely indications, but can be useful guidelines to future appraisals.

Certain features of the data are, nevertheless, remarkable. For example, the stability of estimated incidence has been striking over extended periods of time in this century. The prevalence of these disorders substantiates the widely held clinical impression that they are uncommon conditions (compared with mood disorders and schizophrenia) but are not rare. Most studies indicate that the disorder accounts for 1 to 2 percent of inpatient psychiatric admission. Patients with delusional disorders are somewhat more likely to be women, (but this is an inconsistent feature) and to be relatively more disadvantaged socially and educationally compared to patients with mood disorders. There

TABLE 15.2-7
Comparative Nosology of Delusional Disorder

ICD-9 (1979)	DSM-III (1980)	DSM-III-R (1987)	ICD-10 (1992)	DSM-IV (1994)
Paranoid state, simple	—	—	Delusional disorder	—
Paranoia	Paranoia	Delusional (paranoid) disorder	Delusional disorder	Delusional disorder
Paraphrenia (involuntional paranoid state, late paraphrenia)	—	—	Delusional disorder	—
Induced psychosis (folie à deux, induced paranoid disorder)	Shared paranoid disorder	Induced psychotic disorder	Induced delusional disorder	Shared psychotic disorder
Other specified states (paranoia querulans, Sensitiver Beziehungswahn)	—	—	Delusional disorder	—
Unspecified paranoid states	Atypical paranoid disorder	—	Persistent delusional disorder, unspecified	—
Acute paranoid reaction (bouffée délirante)	Acute paranoid disorder	—	Paranoid reaction	—
Psychogenic paranoid psychosis (protracted reactive paranoid psychosis)	—	—	—	—

is suggestive evidence that immigrant status is associated with delusional disorder. Yet all such observations remain subject to the need for unambiguous replication.

ETIOLOGY

The cause of delusional disorders is unknown. Paranoid features, including the types of delusions encountered in these disorders, occur in a large (and growing) number of conditions (Table 15.2-4). Differences in approach to classifying idiopathic delusional disorder add to the problems of understanding causation. Theories and explanations of delusions abound in the literature; empirical evidence to support those theories is limited. With so many uncertainties, conclusions concerning the cause of delusional disorder must be modest.

The problem can be stated in this fashion. We are dealing with an uncommon, probably heterogeneous, group of illnesses, the validity of which has been questioned since Kahlbaum published his views. The major phenomenologic feature of these conditions is the formation and persistence of delusions. It is well known that delusions occur in a variety of psychiatric and medical conditions, the pathogenesis of which is not fully understood. Hence, discussion of etiology in the delusional disorders can proceed on two lines: (1) the distinctiveness of the category itself, and (2) the theories proposed to account for delusion formation per se.

DISTINCTIVENESS OF DELUSIONAL DISORDER An issue that is central to attributing causation is whether delusional disorder represents a separate group of conditions or, instead, atypical forms of schizophrenic and mood disorders. The relevant data come from a limited number of studies. Despite this, certain consistencies are apparent. Epidemiological data suggest that delusional disorder is a separate condition: delusional disorder is far less prevalent than schizophrenic or mood disorders; age of onset is later than in schizophrenia; and the sex ratio is different from that of mood disorder, which occurs primarily in women. Findings from family or genetic studies also support the concept of separateness. If delusional disorder is simply an unusual form of schizophrenic or mood disorder, the incidence of these latter conditions in family studies of delusional disorder patients should be higher than that of the general population. However, this has not been a consistent finding. Moreover, a recent study concluded that patients with delusional disorder are more likely to have family members who show suspiciousness, jealousy, secretiveness, even paranoid illness, than families of controls. Other investigative efforts have found paranoid personality disorder and avoidant personality disorder to be more common in relatives of delusional disorder patients than in relatives of controls or of schizophrenic patients.

Natural history investigations also lend support to the separateness of the delusional disorder category. Though fraught with methodological shortcomings, premorbid personality data indicate that schizophrenic patients and patients with delusional disorder differ early in life. The former are more likely to be introverted, schizoid, and submissive; the latter, more extroverted, dominant, and hypersensitive. Delusional disorder patients may have below average intelligence. Precipitating factors, especially related to social insolation, conflicts of conscience, and immigration, are more closely associated to delusional disorder than schizophrenia. These characteristics support Kraepelin's view that environmental factors may have an important etiological role. Recent observations of successful treatment with pimozide (Orap) in several subtypes of delusional disorders suggest the possibility of a common pathogenetic mechanism in these disorders. Follow-up studies indicate that the diagnosis of delusional disorder remains stable: only a small proportion of cases (3 to 22 percent) are diagnosed later as schizophrenia, and even fewer (6 percent) are diagnosed later as a mood disorder. Outcome in terms of hospitalization and occupational adjustment are markedly more favorable for delu-

TABLE 15.2-8
ICD-10 Diagnostic Criteria for Persistent Delusional Disorders

Persistent Delusional Disorders
This group includes a variety of disorders in which long-standing delusions constitute the only, or the most conspicuous, clinical characteristic and which cannot be classified as organic, schizophrenic, or affective. They are probably heterogeneous, and have uncertain relationships to schizophrenia. The relative importance of genetic factors, personality characteristics, and life circumstances in their genesis is uncertain and probably variable.

Delusional Disorder
This group of disorders is characterized by the development either of a single delusion or of a set of related delusions which are usually persistent and sometimes lifelong. The delusions are highly variable in content. Often they are persecutory, hypochondriacal, or grandiose, but they may be concerned with litigation or jealousy, or express a conviction that the individual's body is misshapen, or that others think that he or she smells or is homosexual. Other psychopathology is characteristically absent, but depressive symptoms may be present intermittently, and olfactory and tactile hallucinations may develop in some cases. Clear and persistent auditory hallucinations (voices), schizophrenic symptoms such as delusions of control and marked blunting of affect, and definite evidence of brain disease are all incompatible with this diagnosis. However, occasional or transitory auditory hallucinations, particularly in elderly patients, do not rule out this diagnosis, provided that they are not typically schizophrenic and form only a small part of the overall clinical picture. Onset is commonly in middle age but sometimes, particularly in the case of beliefs about having a misshapen body, in early adult life. The content of the delusion, and the timing of its emergence, can often be related to the individual's life situation, e.g. persecutory delusions in members of minorities. Apart from actions and attitudes directly related to the delusion or delusional system, affect, speech, and behavior are normal.

Diagnostic Guidelines
Delusions constitute the most conspicuous or the only clinical characteristic. They must be present for at least three months and be clearly personal rather than subcultural. Depressive symptoms or even a full-blown depressive episode may be present intermittently, provided that the delusion persists at times when there is no disturbance of mood. There must be no evidence of brain disease, no or only occasional auditory hallucinations, and no history of schizophrenic symptoms (delusions of control, thought broadcasting, etc.).

Includes: paranoia
paranoid psychosis
paranoid state
paraphrenia (late)
sensitiver Beziehungswahn

Excludes: paranoid personality disorder
psychogenic paranoid psychosis
paranoid reaction
paranoid schizophrenia

Other Persistent Delusional Disorders
This is a residual category for persistent delusional disorders that do not meet the criteria for delusional disorder. Disorders in which delusions are accompanied by persistent hallucinatory voices or by schizophrenic symptoms that are insufficient to meet criteria for schizophrenia should be coded here. Delusional disorders that have lasted for less than three months should, however, be coded, at least temporarily, under acute and transient psychotic disorders.

Includes: delusional dysmorphophobia
involutional paranoid state
paranoia querulans

Persistent Delusional Disorder, Unspecified

Table from World Health Organization: *The ICD-10 Classification of Mental and Behavioural Disorders: Clinical Descriptions and Diagnostic Guidelines.* World Health Organization, Geneva, 1992. Used with permission.

TABLE 15.2-9
Epidemiological Features of Delusional Disorder

Incidence*	0.7–3.0
Prevalence*	24–30
Age at onset (range)	35–45 (18–80)
Sex ratio M:F	0.85

Table adapted from K S Kendler: Demography of paranoid psychosis (delusional disorder). Arch Gen Psychiatry *39:* 890, 1982.
*Incidence and prevalence figures represent cases per 100,000 population.

sional disorder than for schizophrenic disorder. As previously noted, when social or occupational functioning is poor in delusional disorder, it occurs as the result of the delusional beliefs themselves, not because of negative symptoms.

The evidence argues for distinctiveness of delusional disorder, but it is likely that at least some patients diagnosed as having delusional disorder will develop schizophrenia or mood disorders. Hence, current clinical criteria have limitations and need improvement, possibly with the use of laboratory techniques or more specified clinical definitions. Furthermore, the data suggest that delusional disorder is relatively chronic and is probably biologically distinct from other psychotic disorders.

THEORIES OF DELUSION FORMATION While a clear understanding of the pathogenesis of delusions remains an unfulfilled hope, several major theories have been advanced. Any adequate hypothesis for delusion formation must deal with certain facts: (1) delusions occur in a variety of medical and psychiatric diseases; (2) not all persons with such conditions develop delusions; (3) the content of delusions constitutes a relatively short list of types and is strikingly repetitious despite the variety of diseases; (4) delusions can clear rapidly with treatment of the underlying condition or its termination; (5) delusions can persist, and even become systematized; (6) delusions often accompany perceptual changes such as hallucinations or impaired sensory input; (7) delusions may be highly encapsulated features in persons such that their functioning may not be compromised socially, intellectually, or emotionally. Further, any adequate hypothesis must respond to two questions. First, why does the patient have a delusion? This is a question concerning the form of the psychopathology. Second, why does the patient have this particular delusion? This is a question concerning the content of the psychopathology.

There are three categories of theory in delusion formation.

1. Delusions arise in an otherwise intact cognitive system because a deviant pattern of motivational interest is present (psychodynamic mechanism, social attribution theory).
2. Delusions arise as the result of a fundamental cognitive defect that impairs the patient's capacity to draw valid conclusions from evidence (disorder of reasoning).
3. Delusions arise from normal cognitive processes directed at explaining abnormal perceptual experiences (psychobiological mechanism, anomalous experience hypothesis).

These theories need not be mutually exclusive. It is probable that delusional beliefs are the result of different processes involving one or more of the proposed mechanisms.

Psychodynamic mechanism In 1911 Freud published "Psychoanalytic Notes Upon an Autobiographical Account of a Case of Paranoia (Dementia Paranoides)." His interpretation of this case, which became the foundation of the psychodynamic theory of paranoia, was based on his reading of the memoirs of the presiding judge of a Dresden appeals court, Daniel Paul Schreber, who had suffered episodes of psychiatric illness in 1884, in 1885, and in 1893. The second episode led to two prolonged hospitalizations from which the patient obtained discharge in 1902 following legal action, although he was still delusional. Freud asserted that Schreber's 1903 account, *Memoirs of My Nervous Illness,* offered a legitimate basis for theory, as "paranoiacs cannot be compelled to overcome their internal resistances, and . . . in any case they only say what they choose to say. . . ." Freud argued that the written case report can take the place of personal acquaintance; and in the case of Schreber, Freud never saw the patient. Freud asserted that Schreber's case illustrated a general mechanism of delusion formation involving denial or contradiction and projection of repressed homosexual impulses that break out from the unconscious. The forms of delusion in paranoia can be represented as contradictions of the proposition "I (a man) love him (a man)." The following examples illustrate the forms of illogic.

1. Delusion of persecution. In the contradiction "I do not love him, I hate him," a hatred that persons deem unacceptable at the conscious level is transformed and becomes, instead, "He hates (elaborated to persecutes) me." Patients can then rationalize their anger by consciously hating those persons whom they perceive to hate them.
2. Delusion of erotomania. The proposition "I do not love him—I love her" is transformed through projection to "She loves me—and so I love her."
3. Delusional jealousy. To protect against unwarranted, threatening impulses, the patient transforms the proposition in this manner: "I do not love him—she (a wife, lover) loves him." Hence, jealous delusions represent the transformed attractions of the deluded for the lover.
4. Delusion of grandiosity (megalomania). Here the contradiction made is, "I do not love him—I love myself."

The essence of the theory is that delusions represent attempts to manage the stirrings of unconscious homosexuality. The dynamics of unconscious homosexuality are similar for female as well as male patients in the classic theory.

COMMENT Many theorists have added to the psychodynamical lore on delusion formation from the standpoint of understanding personality factors. For example, some of the vulnerability to delusion formation may be related to deficiently developed trust, to narcissistic dynamics, or to exaggerated traits such as hypersensitivity.

CRITIQUE Freud's mechanism of delusions sidesteps the distinction between form and content in psychopathology. He proposes an inferential process to account for the particular delusion but does not clearly address the issue of why a delusion is formed rather than another symptom, such as hallucination. Verification of the hypothesized mechanism clearly rests on finding evidence that delusions are associated with indications of homosexual tendencies. The theory has been perpetuated in part because an absence of homosexuality can never be proved, and such tendencies can be used as a pillar, even if not a scientifically or empirically demonstrable pillar, in the psychodynamic argument. The few experimental attempts made to test the hypothesis have been inconclusive or equivocal. Moreover, though homosexual concerns have been found among some delusional patients, the variety of conditions with such delusions argues against a common mechanism of unconscious homosexuality in all. Indeed those persons who delusional patients say are persecuting them are not always known by them. Neither is the persistence of such delusions adequately accounted for in that formulation. Nevertheless, the classic approach has had immense influence and has provided important psychoanalytical concepts, such as projection, and an awareness that developmental experiences may operate to influence the content of delusional thinking. Systematic empirical study would be valuable.

Disordered reasoning Related to the psychodynamic formulation is the proposal that delusions arise on the basis of defects in formal logical reasoning. Popular in the 1950s and 1960s, this view, promulgated by Eilhard Von Domarus among others, suggested that errors in logic such as the principle of identity (two subjects are identical on the grounds of identical predicates) have an etiological role. For example, "Charles Manson used drugs; I use drugs; therefore, I am Charles Manson." The empirical assessment of that proposal has failed to establish that deluded patients exhibit more defects in reasoning; rather it appears that normal and deluded persons both make similar and frequent errors of reasoning.

Two other proposals involving disturbance in reasoning have been studied recently. The first portrays the difficulty underlying delusion formation as a failure in the application of Bayesian reasoning. According to this model of developing beliefs, making choices, and drawing conclusions, deluded patients accept conclusions at levels of probability too low for acceptance by nondelusional persons. However, attempts to demonstrate that failure have had equivocal results. The second proposal suggests that the reasoning processes of deluded patients are influenced by the person's tendency to assign meaning in a biased manner. The bias arises in making judgments about a person's behavior that assigns causes of the behavior to characteristics of the person concerned regardless of the social situation or circumstances involved. That model, based on social attribution theory, has been tested, but the results do not provide strong support for this formulation.

Other psychological mechanisms In *Manic Depressive Insanity and Paranoia,* Kraepelin considered the delusions of paranoia to be the "morbidly transformed expression of the natural emotions of the human heart" and, more specifically, "a kind of psychological compensation for the disappointments of life." He dismissed the Freudian psychodynamic mechanism on the grounds that it did not refer to a clear concept of paranoia and that it was not supported by evidence. He also emphasized constitutional factors in his formulation, including, especially, disturbances of judgment. Other authors have made similar suggestions about the role of need fulfillment in the development of paranoia. For example, delusions of persecution might serve to maintain the self-esteem of the deluded person, according to a social attribution view about delusion formation in which a normal bias—that of assigning blame for negative outcomes to other persons or circumstances—is exaggerated.

CRITIQUE Those contributions also fail to address the issue of pathogenesis rigorously. They help one to reach an understanding of the delusion, especially its content, but fail to provide an explanation of its form. The commonness of the risk factors or antecedent features cited repeatedly as central to delusion formation contrasts dramatically with the uncommonness of delusional disorder.

Psychobiological mechanism The French psychiatrist Gaëtan G. de Clerambault proposed in 1942 that chronic delusions resulted from abnormal neurological events. Infections, lesions, intoxication, and other forms of damage produce automatisms that puzzle or distress the patient initially, and eventually demand explanation. The explanations take the form of delusions. Automatisms include hallucinations, a constant parade of memories, feelings of familiarity, false recognition, arresting of thought, disturbances in attention, bizarre tactile sensations, and even kinesthetic sensation.

The view that delusions offer an explanation for hallucinations is an old concept in psychiatry that has not been well formulated. The fact that hallucinations have been introduced into and retracted from the definition of paranoia over the years also reflects a lack of clarity regarding a possible connection between the two forms of psychopathology.

Brendan Maher has proposed a similar hypothesis that conceptualizes delusions as explanations of anomalous experiences that arise in the environment, the peripheral sensory system, or the central nervous system. A central tenet of his view is that the processes whereby delusional beliefs are formed are similar in their essential nature to those that operate in the formation of normal beliefs and scientific hypotheses. Integral to the hypothesis is the assumption that components of this normal operational sequence have a neural substrate. The neural substrate may be activated either by sensory input (as in hallucinatory effects of drugs) or by the effects of brain damage (as in alcoholism). The activation of any part of the sequence demands explanation and may thus give rise to delusions. The sequence, activated by disturbances in sensory experience, emotional incongruity, or central nervous system abnormalities, has the following stages: (1) anomalous experience, (2) feelings of significance, (3) testing for reality of experience, (4) developing tentative hypothoses, (5) additional observation, (6) exploring insights, and (7) confirmation of the insight by selective observation.

In Maher's explanation, the patient is delusional because he or she actually experiences anomalies that demand explanation. The particular content of the delusion is drawn from the past or current circumstances, experience, and personal and cultural background of the patient. The explanation answers questions such as the following: What is happening? Why? Why do other people deny it is happening? Why is it only happening to me? Who is responsible for it? The delusional explanation offers relief from puzzlement, and that relief works against abandonment of the explanation.

CRITIQUE Although the psychobiological formulation has gone largely unstudied, there is supporting evidence. Studies of altered perception among patients and healthy controls experiencing sensory impairment or sensory deprivation, and among persons taking various drugs of abuse have demonstrated a high incidence of delusion formation. The failure to detect a fundamental defect in the cognitive process of delusional patients or to identify basic differences in belief formation between persons with delusions and normal controls provides indirect support as well. Clearly, this hypothesis warrants further examination, and it remains to be seen how applicable it is to conditions, such as delusional disorder, where the occurrence of hallucinations is debated. Sensory impairment and central nervous dysfunction, though apparently likely, have not been established for the disorder.

While the anomalous experience hypothesis focuses on the psychological mechanisms underlying delusion formation, a complementary proposal concerns the anatomic loci associated with delusional thinking. Jeffrey Cummings and others have used the growing data on psychopathological consequences of neurological disease to suggest that delusions occur in diseases involving the limbic system—in particular, temporal lobe structures and caudate nuclei. Diseases characterized by excessive dopaminergic activity or reduced cholinergic activity also carry a heightened risk of delusion formation. Cummings further hypothesizes that the common locus of delusion formation is limbic dysfunction that leads to misinterpretation of the environment accompanied by inappropriate perception of threat. Both disease- and patient-related factors influence the content, complexity, and timing of the delusion.

Other relevant factors Delusions have been linked to a variety of additional factors such as social and sensory isolation, socioeconomic deprivation, and personality disturbance. The deaf, the visually impaired, and possibly immigrant groups with limited ability in a new language may be more vulnerable to delusion formation than the normal population. Vulnerability is heightened with advanced age. Delusional disturbance and other paranoid features are common in the elderly. In short, multiple factors are associated with the formation of delusions, and the source and pathogenesis of delusional disorders has yet to be specified.

DIAGNOSIS AND CLINICAL FEATURES

DELUSIONAL DISORDER

CLINICAL PRESENTATION DSM-IV defines the core psychopathological feature of delusional disorder as persistent, nonbizarre delusions not explained by other psychotic disorders (Table 15.2-2). Onset can be acute, following a precipitating event, or the disorder may emerge gradually and may become chronic. Behavioral and emotional responses are generally appropriate; neither a mood disorder nor the volitional, thinking, and emotional disturbances of schizophrenia are present. In general, patients with delusional disorder show little disorganization or impairment in their behavior or in the clarity of their thinking.

The delusions are unusual yet they refer to aspects of life that might occur, such as being conspired against, cheated on, physically ill, in love, jealous, and the like. They are, as Winokur has suggested, "possible," rather than totally incredible and bizarre as are many of the delusions of schizophrenia. The types of delusions are specified according to their content; the most common concern persecution and jealousy. The delusions are fixed (persistent) and unarguable. Patients interpret facts to fit the delusion rather than modifying the delusion to fit the facts. There is systematization in the delusional thinking, meaning that a single theme or series of connected themes is present with links to the predominant delusion.

Many have proposed that there is a descriptive continuum between paranoid personality disorder, delusional disorder, and the paranoid subtype of schizophrenia in terms of degrees of disorganization and impairment. However, there is little evidence to support the concept that these disorders share more than overlapping psychopathology.

The presence of hallucinations in delusional disorder has been debated, some arguing that schizophrenia is a more likely diagnosis in such cases, others are not so concerned as long as the hallucinations are not marked and persistent. The resolution of this issue remains distant, but it is reasonable to consider infrequent hallucinations that are not a prominent part of the psychopathology to be a feature of delusional disorder. The hallucinations are usually auditory but may be visual and tend to be more common in acute cases. Other types of hallucinations are possible; however, tactile or olfactory hallucinations may be present and even prominent if they are related to the delusional theme.

The person's emotional contact and behavior are generally intact. The emotional response is usually consistent with the delusional concern, and the mood is often appropriately depressed. Restlessness and agitation may be present. Loquaciousness and circumstantiality, usually accompanying descriptions of the delusions, are found in some patients, but formal thought disorder as sometimes found in schizophrenia is absent. Persons with delusional disorder may behave in a remarkably normal way much of the time; they become strikingly different when the delusion is focused on, at which time thinking, attitude, and mood may change direction abruptly. Social and marital functioning are more likely to be compromised than intellectual and occupational functioning.

Associated features in delusional disorder include those of the paranoid syndrome (Table 15.2-5). The degree of hostility and suspiciousness may be such that violent or aggressive behavior results. Litigious behavior is common among such patients. However, some patients, notably those with somatic delusions, may not display hostility, anger, or even suspiciousness to any considerable degree.

DIAGNOSIS Making the diagnosis of delusional disorders requires that the clinician match the features of the case to the appropriate criteria. When the clinician has successfully ruled out other disorders, certain features of the case can help substantiate the diagnosis of delusional disorder.

MENTAL STATUS EXAMINATION The patient's complaints are brought to the attention of the clinician by the patient or a third party, such as police, family, neighbors, or a consulted physician or attorney. The patient may have acted to draw attention by asking for protection, quarreling with neighbors, visiting too many clinics, or similar behavior. The complaint focuses on the distressing behavior and possibly on incidental symptoms. The patient will not complain of a psychiatric condition; in fact, he or she will deny that or the presence of any psychiatric symptoms. Examination of the patient leads to the discovery (often to the surprise of those expecting to observe a range of mental deviances) that thinking, orientation, affect, attention, memory, perception, and personality are intact. The patient's thinking is so clear and the delusional features are so central to his or her concerns that the clinician begins to anticipate precisely the responses of the patient to the point that accurate predictions of specific actions and reactions are possible. Such predictability may distinguish the behavior of the delusional disorder patient from that associated with other psychotic conditions. The patient's behavior and responses to the interview are consistent with the range of features in other paranoid conditions. There may be hostility, anger, lack of cooperation, and a sarcastic or challenging quality to most of what the patient says.

The capacity to act in response to delusions is an important dimension of the evaluation. Level of impulsiveness should be assessed and related to any potential for violence or suicidal behavior. The patient's self-righteousness, the intensity of the delusional experience, and its emotional impact on the patient may be clues to possible violent behavior; and any plans for harming others, including homicide, should be inquired about. Jealousy and erotomania are perhaps especially important concerns in the assessment of possible aggression and violence. If such thoughts exist, the patient should be asked how they were handled in the past. Careful judgment and diplomatic interviewing are especially important in such presentations.

ASSESSMENT OF DELUSIONS The detection of delusions solidifies the judgment that a paranoid condition is present. Delusions are usually easy to detect. Features of behavior (Table 15.2-5) may suggest their presence. Associated psychopathological symptoms such as hallucinations, disturbed form of thought, and mood disorder may also provide clues that delusions are part of the clinical picture.

The clinical challenge is clear in subtle cases. Fundamentally, the clinician must make a judgment based on available observations and the reported private mental experience of the patient. Attempts to dissuade the patient with counterevidence and counterarguments may be useful in determining whether the patient's beliefs can be influenced with evidence usually sufficient to alter the belief of a nondelusional person. Spending time in discussion with the patient to grasp the nature of delusional thinking in terms of its themes, impact on the patient's life, complexity, systematization, and related features may be crucial in making the judgment. The most sensible guideline for all cases of suspected delusional thinking is to establish as comprehensive a picture as possible concerning the condition of the patient, including the patient's subjective private experience and evidence of psychopathological symptoms. Such information should reduce much of the uncertainty in the evaluative process.

Persecutory type The delusion of persecution is a classic symptom of delusional disorder. Persecutory type and jealousy type delusions are probably the forms seen most frequently by psychiatrists. In contrast to persecutory delusions in schizophrenia, the clarity, logic, and systematic elaboration of the persecutory theme in delusional disorder leave a remarkable stamp on this condition. The absence of other psychopathology, of deterioration in personality, or of deterioration in most areas of functioning also contrast with manifestations of schizophrenia.

A 29-year-old single, white man with a college background had been drifting from one clerical position to another. For years he had been convinced that a close relative was trying to get rid of him to take over the family business. He based his conviction on various remarks, coincidences, and ''putting two plus two together.'' He appeared at a friend's apartment in an acutely agitated, fearful, and demoralized state. After trying to reassure him, the friend brought the patient to the psychiatric emergency room. The patient had made an anonymous phone call one week before to the police informing them that he had once mailed a postcard that contained a vague threat to the relative intending to scare him. Worry that advanced technologies would enable the police to trace the phone call to him had so distressed the patient that he had become preoccupied and constantly apprehensive. For several days he had been unable to sleep. However, there was no evidence of hallucinations, thought disorder, or other emotional change. The patient was reluctant to return for a follow-up visit to discuss his adjustment; he refused all medication, nor did he appear reassured by discussion of his guilt and the likelihood that the matter was not of interest to the police. He left the emergency room less agitated, however. Five years later, the patient requested consultation to discuss his preoccupation that the police were likely to determine the source of the phone call and were about to discover him. His level of functioning had not changed dramatically. He continued to have the same concerns and said he was troubled only from time to time by the worry that his cousin would contact the police. But when such thoughts did occur, he was made miserable. During those episodes of intense concern about the delusion, he was able to work but would find himself constantly distracted from his duties. It was under those circumstances that he sought out further professional attention.

Jealous type Delusional disorder with delusions of infidelity has been called conjugal paranoia when it is limited to the delusion that a spouse has been unfaithful. The eponym ''Othello syndrome'' has been used for the condition. The delusion usually afflicts men, often those with no prior psychiatric illness. It may appear suddenly and serve to explain a host of present and past events involving the spouse's behavior. The condition is difficult to treat and may diminish only on separation, divorce, or death of the spouse.

Richard Krafft-Ebing described the symptom of delusional jealousy in alcoholics in 1891 and believed that extreme jealousy was pathognomonic for alcoholism. Other disorders with this symptom were later described. A recent retrospective analysis of 8,134 psychiatric inpatients disclosed a prevalence of delusional jealousy of 1.1 percent among the major diagnostic groups. Among paranoid disorders (ICD-9 classification) a 6.7 percent prevalence was determined. Delusional disorder with alcohol dependence frequently shows the single delusion of jealousy, a persistent feature that sometimes remits if alcohol abuse is brought under control. In personality disorders the symptom may be confused with extreme jealousy, but other psychotic features should be absent. The prevalence of delusional jealousy among hospitalized mood disorder patients was a surprisingly low 0.1 percent. A study of 26,000 psychiatric inpatients using DSM-III-R criteria yielded a 0.17 percent rate of delusional disorder, jealous type. Jealous delusions occur much more frequently in other disorders than in delusional disorder, which is a very uncommon condition.

Marked jealousy is thus a symptom (usually termed pathological or morbid jealousy) of many disorders—including schizophrenia (where female patients more commonly display this feature), epilepsy, mood disorders, drug abuse, and alcoholism—for which treatment is directed at the primary disorder. Jealousy is a powerful emotion; when it occurs in delusional disorder or as part of another condition it can be a potentially dangerous feature and has been associated with violence, notably both suicide and homicide. The forensic aspects of the symptom have been noted repeatedly, especially its role as a motive for murder. However, physical and verbal abuse appear more frequently than extreme actions among individuals with this symptom. Caution and care in deciding how to deal with such presentations are essential not only for diagnosis but also for safety concerns.

A 39-year-old truck driver was admitted to the hospital through efforts of the police and courts following complaints by his neighbors that he was verbally abusing his wife and physically beating her. The patient vehemently denied psychiatric illness and reported that there was no reason for him to see a psychiatrist. He claimed that he was responding to his wife's long-term secret affair with another man. He asked to speak to his lawyer and refused to cooperate in the psychiatric examination except to defend his actions. He related that he had spent a great deal of time trying to assess the nature of his wife's affair. He had hired a detective and had set up a variety of electronic video and eavesdropping devices to monitor his wife's activity over the preceding weeks in an effort to document her transgressions. The patient claimed that episodes of infidelity had begun years ago both before and after his marriage. The patient was at the hospital briefly and received a trial of antipsychotic medications. The emotional turmoil he was experiencing began to diminish. The patient became more calm, but the delusional thinking persisted. The patient was able eventually to leave the hospital, free of medication. Meanwhile, his wife had decided to divorce him. At follow-up some months later he remained convinced about her infidelity, but he admitted that it did not bother him or not quite so much.

Erotomanic type Patients with erotomania have delusions of secret lovers. Most frequently the patient is a woman, but men are also susceptible to the delusion. The patient believes that a suitor, usually more socially prominent than herself, is in love with her. The delusion becomes the central focus of the patient's existence. Onset can be acute.

Erotomania, the *psychose passionelle,* is also referred to as de Clerambault's syndrome to emphasize its occurrence in different disorders. Besides being the key symptom in some cases of delusional disorder, it is known to occur in schizophrenia, mood disorder, and other organic disorders. There was no mention of erotomania in DSM-III; the diagnosis was atypical psychosis. DSM-III-R reinstated the condition, and it remains in DSM-IV.

Patients with erotomania frequently show certain characteristics; they are generally but not exclusively women, unattractive in appearance, with low-level employment positions, who lead withdrawn, lonely lives, with single status and limited sexual contacts. They select secret lovers with substantially contrasting features. They exhibit what has been called paradoxical conduct, the delusional phenomenon of interpreting all denials of love, no matter how clear, as secret affirmations of love. The course may be chronic, recurrent, or brief. Separation from the love object may be the only satisfactory means of intervention. Although men are less commonly afflicted by this condition than women, they may be more aggressive and possibly violent in their pursuit of love. The object of aggression may not be the loved individual but a companion or protector of the love object. The tendency toward violence among male erotomanic cases may lead initially to police rather than psychiatric contact.

A 25-year-old woman was brought to the hospital by the police at the request of the court following a complaint of harassment made against her by a local priest. The patient had seen the priest during services. Several months later she had developed a passionate love for him which she was convinced he had for her as well. The priest had noticed that he was being followed by the patient when he left the rectory on errands. Eventually, he decided to confront her. In response she protested that she would do anything for him, and as the priest finally walked away in exasperation she concluded that his behavior was in reality an endorsement of his enduring love. She began to stand outside the rectory for long periods daily and to phone the priest at all hours. Eventually, the priest felt there was no other alternative but to turn the matter over to the police. She was arrested, and when interrogated about the purpose of her harassing behavior, disclosed her feelings. The hospital psychiatrist examined the patient and could find no evidence of perceptual disturbance, confusion, thought or emotional incongruity or other abnormalities in the patient's mental state besides intensity of emotional responses. The psychiatrist recommended further evaluation, and she was treated with antipsychotic medications. The treatment provided limited benefit, although the patient's general level of demoralization improved. On the other hand, the patient continued to contact the priest from the inpatient unit of the hospital by calling on the public telephone in the corridor until she was finally restricted from telephone use. There ensued a period when the patient was writing letters secretly to the priest. The patient's harassing behavior finally abated so that she could be released. She was warned that she should not approach the priest in the future. She seemed to have some understanding of the nature of the situation and said that she would abide by this recommendation. Several months later the patient was arrested again for trespassing at the priest's rectory.

Somatic type Delusional disorder with hypochondriacal delusions has been called monosymptomatic hypochondriacal psychosis. The condition differs from others with hypochondriacal symptoms in degree of reality impairment. In delusional disorder, the delusion is fixed, unarguable, and presented intensely, because the patient is totally convinced of the physical nature of the disorder. In contrast, hypochondriacs are often aware that their fear of illness is groundless. The content of the delusion may vary widely from case to case. Munro has described the largest series of cases and has used the content of delusions to define three main groups of patients: (1) those with delusions of infestation (including parasitosis); (2) those with delusions of dysmorphophobia, such as of misshapenness, personal ugliness, or exaggerated size of body parts; and (3) those with delusions of foul body odors and/or halitotis.

The frequency of these conditions is low, but they may be underdiagnosed, as patients present to dermatologists, plastic surgeons, and infectious disease specialists more often than to psychiatrists in the unremitting search for curative treatment. That feature may partially account for Kraepelin's skepticism about the occurrence of this form of paranoia. Several recent reports indicate that pimozide (a diphenylbutyliperidine and highly specific dopamine blocker) and certain serotonin-specific reuptake inhibitors may be effective in treatment of such disorders, even in cases with a variety of delusional themes. There may be a heightened association of shared psychotic disorder involving primary cases of hypochondriacal delusion. One series reported a quarter of cases with such an association.

This condition has a poor prognosis without treatment. It affects both sexes roughly equally. A previous history or family history of psychotic disorder is uncommon. In younger patients, a history of substance abuse or head injury is frequent. Although anger and hostility are commonplace, shame, depression, and avoidant behavior are even more characteristic. Suicide, apparently motivated by anguish, is not uncommon.

A 43-year-old married woman with no children was admitted with a presenting complaint of acute agitation associated with blindness. Her vision and eyes had been examined repeatedly at the local emergency room. Because she refused to accept the clinical judgment that there was no evidence of pathology, she was finally referred to the psychiatric clinic. The patient appeared to have no difficulty seeing but regarded herself to be blind and in need of various aids to manage this disability. At the hospital the patient's behavior was remarkably litigious: she demanded her own room in the hospital; she requested further eye examinations; and she indicated that she would follow only certain rules in her hospitalization. While she did complain about the blindness, it often appeared that the main concern was being able to complain and to complain to the appropriate authorities. The patient wrote a series of letters to the police, judges, and federal and state authorities urging all to become involved in her case to help in her release from an unjustified hospitalization. The patient was treated with a variety of antipsychotic and antidepressant agents with no success. She said she preferred to be without medication (claiming that she was not mentally ill). After supportive counseling and several months of hospitalization she was discharged from the hospital in fair condition, still acting as if she were blind. Months later, the patient, still apparently unable to see, was involved in a political campaign on behalf of a major presidential candidate. She had created enough difficulty in the campaign headquarters to arouse the concern of the campaign manager for the election committee. She sought no further psychiatric intervention.

Grandiose type Delusions of grandeur (megalomania) have been noted for years. They were described in Kraepelin's paranoia and have been associated with conditions fitting the description of delusional disorder.

A 51-year-old man was arrested for disturbing the peace. Police had been called to a local park to stop him from carving his initials and those of a recently formed religious cult into various stately trees surrounding a pond in the park. Confronted, he had scornfully argued that, having been chosen to begin a new townwide religious revival, it was necessary for him to publicize his intent in a permanent fashion. The police were unsuccessful at preventing the man from cutting another tree and made the arrest. Psychiatric examination was ordered at the state hospital, and the patient was observed there for several weeks. He denied any emotional difficulty and had never received psychiatric treatment. There was no history of euphoria or mood swings. The patient was angry about being hospitalized and only gradually permitted the doctor to interview him. In a few days, however, he was busy preaching to his fellow patients and letting them know that he had been given a special mandate from God to bring in new converts through his ability to heal. Eventually, the preoccupation with special powers diminished. No other evidence of psychopathology was observed. The patient was discharged, having received no medication at all. Two months later he was arrested at a local theater, this time for disrupting the showing of a film that depicted subjects he believed to be satanic.

Mixed type The category of mixed type applies to patients with two or more delusional themes. However, the diagnosis of mixed type should be reserved for cases in which no single delusional type predominates.

Unspecified type The category of unspecified type is reserved for cases in which the predominant delusion cannot be subtyped in the previous categories. An example is certain delusions of misidentification—for example, Capgras's syndrome, named after the French psychiatrist who described the *illusion des sosies* or the illusion of doubles. The delusion in Capgras's syndrome is the belief that imposters have replaced a familiar person or persons. Others have described variants of the Capgras's syndrome, namely the delusion that persecutors or familiar persons could assume the guise of strangers (Fregoli's delusion) and the very rare delusion that familiar persons could change themselves into other persons at will (intermetamorphosis) have also been described. Each disorder is not only rare but is highly associated with schizophrenia, dementia, epilepsy, and other organic disorders. Reported cases have been predominantly in women, have had associated paranoid features, and have included feelings of depersonalization or derealization. The delusion may be short-lived, recurrent, or persistent. It is unclear whether delusional disorder can appear with such a delusion. Certainly, the Fregoli and intermetamorphosis delusions have bizarre content and are unlikely; but the delusion in Capgras's syndrome is a possible candidate. The role of hallucination or perceptual disturbance in this condition needs to be explicated.

SHARED PSYCHOTIC DISORDER Shared psychotic disorder (also referred to as shared paranoid disorder, induced psychotic disorder, *folie à deux,* and double insanity) was first described by Lasegue and Falret in 1877. It is probably rare, but incidence and prevalence figures are lacking, as the literature consists almost entirely of single case reports. The disorder is characterized by the transfer of delusions from one person to another; both persons have been closely associated for a long time and typically live together in relative social isolation. In its most common form, *folie imposée* (which is covered by the DSM-IV criteria), the individual who first has the delusion (the primary case) is often chronically ill and typically is the influential member of a close relationship with a more suggestible person (the secondary case) who also develops the delusion. The secondary case is frequently less intelligent, more gullible, more passive, or more lacking in self-esteem than the primary case. If the pair separates, the secondary case may abandon the delusion, but that outcome is not uniformly seen. The occurrence of the delusion is attributed to the strong influence of the more dominant member. Old age, low intelligence, sensory impairment, cerebrovascular disease, and alcohol abuse are among the factors associated with this peculiar form of psychotic disorder. A genetic predisposition to idiopathic psychoses has also been suggested as a possible risk factor.

Other special forms have been reported, such as *folie simultanée,* where two people become psychotic simultaneously and share the same delusion. Occasionally, more than two individuals are involved (for example, *folie à trois, quatre, cinq;* also *folie à famille*), but those cases are especially rare. The most common relationships in *folie à deux* are sister-sister, husband-wife, and mother-child, but other combinations have also been described. Almost all cases involve members of a single family.

There is some question whether patients with such conditions are truly delusional rather than highly impressionable, as frequently there is merely passive acceptance of the delusional beliefs of the more dominant person (primary case) in the relationship until they are separated, at which point the unusual belief may remit spontaneously. In the DSM-IV criteria the requirement that the secondary case not have a psychotic disorder prior to onset of the induced delusion illustrates the relevance of this question. The psychopathology of secondary cases in fact varies. In DSM-III such patients were required to meet the criteria for paranoid disorder (that is, show evidence of disturbed personality and perhaps evidence of other psychiatric disorder, mental subnormality, or dementia). Probably, some cases will fit the definition of delusional disorder.

A 40-year-old woman consulted physicians to help cure her problem of disagreeable body odor. The physicians failed to satisfy the woman's hopes of diagnosis and treatment, because they found nothing wrong with her. They did occasionally recommend psychiatric consultation, which she refused. Her husband, a quiet, retiring man of 35, accompanied his wife to all medical specialist consultations. When questioned, he shared his wife's concerns about body odor and provided many examples of how distressing this problem had become. When he was told that there really was nothing wrong with his wife, he objected repeatedly and proclaimed that the doctors were incompetent. A psychiatrist was called to the clinic to see the couple and found consistent stories from both. The woman accepted a recommendation for hospitalization on the psychiatry-medical unit, and the husband returned home. After weeks of evaluation and treatment, the woman was discharged. The husband had stopped visiting, however, and when informed that his wife would be coming home, commented that he thought she had been cured of her problem. Three months later, however, the couple was again making rounds to different specialists.

A 52-year-old man was referred by the court for inpatient psychiatric examination, charged with disturbing the peace. He had been arrested for disrupting a trial, complaining of harassment by various judges. He had walked into a courtroom, marched to the bench, and begun to berate the probate judge. While in the hospital, he related a detailed account of conspiratorial goings-on in the local judiciary. A target of certain judges, he claimed he had been singled out for a variety of reasons for many years: he knew what was going on; he had kept records of wrongdoings; and he understood the significance of the whole matter. He refused to elaborate on the specific nature of the conspiracy. He had responded to it with frequent letters to newspapers, the local bar association, and even to a Congressional subcommittee. His mental state, apart from his story and a mildly depressed mood, was entirely normal. A family interview revealed that his wife and several grown children shared the belief in a judicial conspiracy directed against the patient. There was no change in delusional thinking in the patient or the family after 10 days of observation. The patient refused follow-up treatment.

The intensity of conviction is governed by the presence of the primary case in the life of the secondary case. Protection is provided by others who share the delusion and believe in the reasonableness of the response. Munro has found that shared psychotic disorder is frequently associated with delusional disorder, somatic type.

PATHOLOGY AND LABORATORY EXAMINATION

PATHOLOGY As in most psychiatric conditions, there is no evidence of localized brain pathology to correlate with clinical psychopathology. Patients with delusional disorder seldom die early and show no consistent abnormalities on neurological examination. Delusions can complicate many disorders and virtually all brain disorders. Certain disorders produce delusions at rates greater then the expected in the general population; for example, in patients with epilepsy (especially involving temporal lobe), degenerative dementias (Alzheimer's and vascular dementias), cerebrovascular disease, extrapyramidal disorders, and traumatic brain injury.

While many types of delusions have been reported in patients with brain disorders, there appear to be particular connections between delusion phenomenology and certain kinds of brain dysfunction. For example, patients with more severe cortical impairment tend to experience more simple, transient, persecutory delusions. This type of delusional experience is characteristic of conditions such as Alzheimer's multiinfarct dementia, and metabolic encephalopathy. Those disorders are also associated with significant cognitive disturbance. More complex (that is, elaborate and systematic) delusional experiences tend to be more chronic, intensely held, resistant to treatment, and associated with neurological conditions producing less intellectual impairment and strong affective components. Those features occur in patients with neurological lesions involving the limbic system or subcortical nuclei rather than cortical areas. That, coupled with the observation of response of some patients to drug treatment, such as pimozide and other medications, provides a rational basis on which to hypothesize the presence of subcortical pathology, possibly involving systems subserving temporolimbic areas.

Although investigators are far from a neuropathology of delusional disorders, the available evidence suggests that if there is such a finding it will be subtle. Nevertheless, future empirical studies, guided by etiological hypotheses, could lead to breakthroughs. Given the uncommoness of delusional disorder, intensive studies of specific cases and of conditions with delusions from known causes (and with identifiable neuropathologies) offer useful beginning points.

LABORATORY EXAMINATION A range of assessments is often necessary, but several have a high likelihood of detecting key factors in the case. The use of drug screening measures is particularly valuable given the marked delusional responses induced by a number of substances, especially alcohol, amphetamine, cocaine, and other central nervous system stimulants.

Neuropsychological assessment may help disclose evidence of impaired intellectual functioning that suggests brain abnormalities. The assessment of intelligence may show discrepancies between verbal and performance scores as well as scatter in overall performance. Limited data on delusional disorder (especially the more chronic forms) suggest that average or marginally low intelligence is characteristic. Projective testing such as the Rorschach has limited value in making the diagnosis but may confirm features consistent with it. The Minnesota Multiphasic Personality Inventory (MMPI) has among its clinical scales the paranoia (Pa) scale, developed to identify paranoid symptoms. Deviation on this scale has strong correlations to paranoid features and may help substantiate the diagnosis or raise it as a possibility.

DIFFERENTIAL DIAGNOSIS

DELUSIONAL DISORDER Because delusional disorders are uncommon, idiopathic, and possess features characteristic of the full range of paranoid illnesses, differential diagnosis has a clear-cut logic: namely, delusional disorder is a diagnosis of exclusion. There are many conditions to consider (Table 15.2-10). To avoid premature diagnosis, a comprehensive strategy of careful evaluation is required.

This clinical assessment of paranoid features requires three steps. Initially, the clinician must recognize, characterize, and judge as pathologic the presence of paranoid features. Next, the clinician should determine whether they form a part of a syndrome or are isolated. Finally, the clinician should develop a differential diagnosis.

The first of the three steps must be pursued systematically. The clinician must be aware that a range of objective traits or behaviors (Table 15.2-5) is often found in paranoid illness and may constitute the only clue that a paranoid illness is present. Paranoid patients are frequently unwilling to reveal their subjective experiences to examiners or to cooperate in the clinical investigation. Careful interviewing of the patient and other informants may disclose further evidence that the behavior is clearly psychopathologic; in other cases, however, that conclusion must await further observations. Sometimes the plausibility of the delusion requires investigating to determine whether the belief is indeed delusional or not. Premature acceptance that the patient is deluded has at times been an embarrassment to some clinicians who learn that the patient was not deluded. If the judgment that the patient is delusional seems unassailable, then careful elaboration of the nature of the delusion is called for. The delusional thinking should be examined for its fixity, logic, encapsulation, degree of systematization and elaboration, and its effect on action and planning.

Having determined that a paranoid condition is present, the clinician should attend to the premorbid characteristics, the course, and associated symptoms to detect patterns of psychopathology. The discovery of clouded consciousness, perceptual disturbance, other psychopathology, physical signs, or confusing symptoms may suggest different causes for paranoid features. Isolated acute paranoid symptoms, on the other hand, often appear early in medical illness.

Finally, the clinician should avoid the temptation to make the diagnosis of schizophrenia and delusional disorder prematurely in cases where paranoid features are present, as those features occur regularly in a variety of psychiatric and medical illnesses. Consequently, awareness of the multiple causes of paranoid features (step one) is essential to completing the differential diagnosis (step three).

Certain principles should guide effective assessment. First, it

TABLE 15.2-10
Differential Diagnosis of Delusional Disorder

Disorder	Delusions	Hallucinations	Awareness	Other Features
Delusional disorder	+	Occasionally	Alert	Free of psychopathology generally
Psychotic disorder due to a general medical condition, with delusions	+	+	May be impaired	Cognitive changes; substance abuse history; impairment frequent
Schizophrenia	+ (bizarre)	+	Alert	Emotional changes, pervasive thought disorder; impairment
Major depressive episode	+ (mood congruent)	+/−	Alert	Concerted changes in mood and neurovegetative features
Manic episode	+ (mood congruent)	+/−	Alert	Concerted changes in mood, need for sleep, activity, energy, lack of inhibition
Personality disorders	−	−	Alert	Not psychotic
Obsessive-compulsive disorder	−	−	Alert	Not psychotic; impairment present often
Somatoform disorders	−	−	Alert	Not psychotic
Shared psychotic disorder	+	−	Alert	Close associate has some delusions

is important to have knowledge of the paranoid features and patterns of the clinical conditions in which they occur. For example, a small percentage (10 to 20 percent) of schizophrenia cases begin after age 40, and most idiopathic psychiatric problems do not begin after age 50. Second, the premorbid status of the patient should be determined. Generally, a normal premorbid state suggests that acute paranoid features are the consequence of medical disease. Third, an abrupt change in personality, mood, ability to function, and mental state should be noted as this may indicate complications resulting from medical disease. Fourth, in those cases in which there is evidence that the patient has been refractory to psychotropic medication or psychotherapy, the continuing presence of paranoid features should alert the clinician to consider alternative diagnoses.

The final diagnosis in cases where paranoid features are prominent should be made only following: (1) a complete medical and psychiatric history with special attention to alcohol and drug history (including drugs of abuse, prescribed drugs, and over-the-counter medication history); (2) a thorough physical examination, including neurological and mental status examinations; (3) appropriate laboratory studies, particularly serological, toxicological, endocrine, microbiological, radiological, and electroencephalographic studies.

There are certain delusional conditions that, because of their frequency and seriousness, should be routinely considered in the differential diagnosis, as among the most likely sources of delusions. Delirium, dementia, psychotic disorder due to a general medical condition, and substance-induced psychotic disorder should receive special attention.

Psychotic disorder due to a general medical condition, with delusions Delusions arise in a number of organic diseases and syndromes. Many are listed in Table 15.2-4. What they frequently have in common is a disturbance of perception particularly of visual and auditory functioning. Physical, neurological, and mental status study, and laboratory examinations, will usually enable detection of organic causes of delusions. A special focus in each evaluation should be on perceptual disturbance. Medical conditions associated with delusions should be searched for, according to the guidelines outlined concerning differential diagnosis.

Substance-induced psychotic disorder, with delusions Drug intoxications are particularly relevant. Abused drugs, such as amphetamines and cocaine; over-the-counter drugs, such as sympathomimetics; and prescribed drugs, such as steroids and L-dopa, can cause substance-induced psychotic disorder, with delusions, often without cognitive impairment. A careful drug history and screen may establish the diagnosis. A history of alcohol abuse or dependence is so common that it should always be considered. Alcoholism is often associated with jealousy, presecutory ideas, and poor impulse control.

Cognitive disorders Dementia should be considered when paranoid features occur, particularly in older persons. Mental status examination should uncover characteristic cognitive changes absent in delusional disorder. Delirium, with its fluctuating course, confusion, memory impairment, and transient delusions, contrasts with the clarity of mental functioning and the persistence of delusions in delusional disorder, and should be considered in acute cases with paranoid features.

Schizophrenia Delusions may be the presenting feature of schizophrenia. That diagnosis should be considered when the delusions are implausible or bizarre, affect is blunted or incongruous with thinking, auditory or visual hallucinations are prominent, thought disorder is pervasive, and role functioning is impaired. Paranoid schizophrenic persons may have somewhat less bizarre delusions, but role functioning is impaired, and prominent auditory hallucinations are often present, in contrast with delusional disorder.

Shared psychotic disorder The delusions and symptoms of shared psychotic disorder may resemble those of delusional disorder; but the delusions arise in the context of a close relationship with a delusional person, are identical in content to the delusions of that person, and diminish or disappear when secondary and primary case are separated.

Mood disorders with psychotic features The persistent and profound dysphoric mood of depressed patients often points to the proper diagnosis; in delusional disorder, affect may be intense, but is not itself an overwhelming or preoccupying experience to the patient. Delusions in depression, if present, are frequently related to mood (mood congruent delusions). For example, the patient with feelings of worthlessness or guilt may consider that persecution against him or her is justified as a punishment for evil ways. Somatic delusions may be puzzling to differentiate if the clinician fails to consider associated psychopathological features. If delusions occur exclusively during mood episodes, the diagnosis is mood disorder with psychotic features. Depression refers to a host of signs and symptoms, and usually has a constellation of neurovegetative features (affecting appetite, sleep, libido, energy, and so forth) that are not part of delusional disorder. Moreover, depression is frequently cyclical and is often associated with a positive family history of mood disorder. Delusional disorder, in contrast, is remarkably free of symptoms other than the delusion. Occasionally, mood symptoms that meet the criteria for a mood episode are present in a delusional condition. Delusional disorder is diagnosed only if the total duration of all mood episodes remains brief relative to the total duration of the delusional disturbance.

Manic episode Manic delusions, often grandiose and therefore mood congruent, occur in the severest stages of this illness. This could mislead the diagnostician, but the cyclical nature, the marked change in mood (often euphoric or irritable at a very intense level), the reduced need for sleep, increased energy, easy distractibility and lack of focused concentration ability, lack of social inhibition, and increased activity level of manic episodes should be decisive in distinguishing that condition from delusional disorder.

Obsessive-compulsive disorder Severe forms of this disorder should be considered in the differential diagnosis, especially obsessive-compulsive disorder with poor insight. Preoccupation with fear, unusual rituals, and obsessional beliefs may be puzzling, yet the pervasive effects of the condition on functioning differ from the experience of delusional disorder. Moreover, delusions and hallucinations should be absent. In practice, that differential may be difficult without a long period of observation.

Somatoform disorders Severe forms of body dysmorphic disorder may be difficult to distinguish from delusional disorder. The degree of conviction about imagined physical disfigurement may be the only guideline for the differential diagnosis.

Lack of other features of psychopathology, often present in such cases, may also help make the distinction.

Hypochondriasis may also be distinguished on the basis of absence of delusions, although many of the behaviors associated with delusional disorders, somatic type, may occur. Usually such patients reveal some doubt or uncertainty about the validity of their health preoccupations. Their overvalued beliefs about disease or affliction may clearly resemble delusional disorder, somatic type; severe cases may require considerable diagnostic effort.

Paranoid personality disorder Individuals with paranoid personality disorder by definition have abundant paranoid features. They are persistently oversensitive, ready to take offense, suspicious, resentful, rigid, and frequently self-centered. Rather than delusions, such persons tend to have strongly held ideas (overvalued ideas). Generally, however, they are believed to be free of delusions. This is the most useful differential feature. There is some evidence that this personality pattern occurs often enough in families of probands with delusional disorder to suggest a possible genetic connection between the two. This relationship remains unclear at present.

Schizoid personality disorder and schizotypal personality disorder Paranoid features may occur in these personality disorders as well. The pervasive disturbance in personality functioning and the absence of delusions and other psychotic features are usually definitive distinguishing characteristics.

Disorders of aging Any discussion of differential diagnosis of paranoid features is incomplete unless consideration is given to the occurrence of paranoid features in the elderly. Paranoid features develop frequently in the elderly, and assessment in such cases should be particularly thorough. Our understanding of paranoid features among the aged is limited. There are several facts worth knowing: (1) the association of depressive illness with paranoid features is high enough to warrant suspicion of mood disorder in all cases with paranoid features; (2) there appears to be a late-occurring form of schizophrenia sometimes labeled late paraphrenia or late-onset schizophrenia in which paranoid characteristics frequently occur (this controversial diagnosis, however, would be warranted only when no other disorders could be diagnosed); (3) the sudden onset of acute paranoid features in the elderly can be a sign of cerebrovascular injury or other medical illness; (4) many of the medical conditions associated with delusions have increased incidence in the elderly population; (5) perhaps most important for the general clinician is to recognize sources of increased risk of paranoid disorder among older individuals. It is now known that many factors contribute to the incidence of paranoid features in the aged, including lack of stimulating company, isolation, physical illness, the aging process itself, loss of hearing, and loss of visual acuity, each of which should be carefully assessed. Delusional disorder may be present in the elderly, may even have its onset in the elderly, but the frequency of other causes of paranoid features calls for a prudent, systematic search.

SHARED PSYCHOTIC DISORDER Malingering, factitious disorder with predominantly psychological signs and symptoms, psychotic disorder due to a general medical condition, and substance-induced psychotic disorder need to be considered in the differential diagnosis of shared psychotic disorder. The boundary between shared psychotic disorder and generic group madness, such as the Jonestown massacre in Guyana, is unclear.

COURSE AND PROGNOSIS

DELUSIONAL DISORDER Onset can begin in adolescence but generally occurs from middle to late adulthood on with variable patterns of course, including lifelong disorder in some cases. Studies generally indicate that delusional disorder does not lead to severe impairment or change in personality, but rather to a gradual, progressive involvement with the delusional concern. Suicide has been associated with such disorders, although most patients live the normal life span. The base rate of spontaneous recovery may not be as low as previously thought. Retterstol's personal follow-up investigation of a large series of cases has provided much of the viewpoint on the natural history of the disorder, but other studies have added information.

The more chronic forms of the illness (patients presenting with features for more than six months) have their onset early in the fifth decade. Onset is acute in nearly two thirds of the cases, and gradual in the remainder. In 53 percent the delusion has disappeared at follow-up study, is improved in 10 percent, and is unchanged in 31 percent. In more acute forms of the illness the age of onset is in the fourth decade, a lasting remission occurs in over half of patients, and a pattern of chronicity develops in only 10 percent. A relapsing course occurred in 37 percent.

Thus the more acute and earlier the onset, the more favorable the prognosis. The presence of precipitating factors signifies a positive outcome, as does being a woman and married. In terms of prognosis, the persistence of delusional thinking is most favorable for cases with persecutory delusions, and somewhat less favorable for delusions of grandeur and jealousy. Outcome in terms of overall functioning appears, however, somewhat more favorable for the jealousy subtype. Such patients may experience fewer hospitalizations and are less likely to be complicated by more severe psychotic or schizophrenic deteriorations. Work status at follow-up has indicated that the vast majority of patients are employed. These observations, though limited to few cases, provide some basis for optimism: perhaps half of cases with delusional disorders may remit, but relapse and chronicity are common.

SHARED PSYCHOTIC DISORDER The nature of the disorder suggests that separation of the submissive person who has shared psychotic disorder (the secondary case) from the dominant person (the primary case) should result in the resolution and the disappearance of the psychotic symptoms in the submissive person. Often, the submissive person requires treatment with antipsychotic drugs, just as the dominant person needs antipsychotic drugs for his or her psychotic disorder. Because the persons are almost always from the same family, they usually move back together after release from a hospital. If separated, the patient will experience a possible remission. If not separated, the patient may have a similar prognosis as the primary case.

TREATMENT

DELUSIONAL DISORDER The goals of treatment are to establish the diagnosis, to decide on appropriate interventions, and to manage complications. Fundamental to the success of those goals is an effective and therapeutic doctor-patient relationship. Establishing that is far from simple. The patients do not complain about psychiatric symptoms and often enter treatment against their will. Even the psychiatrist may be brought into their delusional nets.

Psychosocial treatments There is not enough evidence to substantiate the claims for any particular school or approach in talking with the patient. Insight-oriented therapy is usually contraindicated, but a combination of supportive psychotherapeutic approaches and possibly cognitive-behavioral interventions is sensible. It is unlikely that there is any psychiatric condition that requires greater diplomacy, openness, and reliability from the therapist. Considerable skill is required in dealing with the profound and intense feelings that accompany these disorders.

Awareness of the fragile self-esteem and unusual sensitivity of these patients is essential for general management and somatic treatment. Direct questioning about the veracity of the delusion, apart from carefully establishing its nature and the evidence to support it during clinical evaluation, is seldom helpful. Although forging an alliance may be especially difficult, responding to the patient's concerns rather than the delusion itself may be effective. Understanding that fear and anxiety serve to stimulate hostility may be the key to adopting a flexible approach that promotes empathy but maintains physical and emotional distance. Patients with the disorder suffer. They often feel demoralized, miserable, isolated, and abandoned. They may face rejection at home or on the job. However, they can be approached, and their treatment focused on such experiences.

The goals of supportive therapy are to allay anxiety, initiate discussion of troubling experiences and consequences of the delusion, and thereby gradually to develop a collaboration with the patient. In some patients this strategy allows the psychiatrist to suggest means of coping more successfully with the delusional thinking. For example, the psychiatrist might encourage the patient to keep those ideas to oneself as they might lead to surprise, dismay, or amazement in others at considerable cost to the patient. For others, if the patient is amenable, it may be possible to provide educational intervention to help the patient understand how factors such as sensory impairment, social and physical isolation, and stress contribute to making matters worse. In all such approaches, the overriding aim is to assist in a more satisfying general adjustment.

Cognitive approaches have attempted to reduce delusional thinking through modification of the belief itself, focusing on the reasoning or the reality testing of the deluded patient. Unlike noncognitive behavioral approaches that center attention on reduction of verbal behavior (talking about the delusion), this strategy seeks a more lasting and clinically meaningful intervention through multiple techniques that keep the relationship with the patient collaborative. Those techniques include distancing, homework, and exploration of emotions associated with various delusion. The effectiveness of cognitive and behavioral therapies has not been studied enough to justify recommendation. It is important to determine the long-term as well as the short-term impact of these treatments. Nevertheless, they are promising enough to continue assessment.

Somatic treatment Delusional disorder is a psychotic disorder by definition, and the natural presumption has been that the condition would respond to antipsychotic medication. Because controlled studies are lacking and the disorder is uncommon, the results required to support this practice have not yet been obtained. Munro and others have reported beneficial responses with pimozide, in monosymptomatic hypochondriacal psychosis especially and in certain other delusional disorder subtypes. The impression remains that antipsychotic drugs are effective, and a trial especially with pimozide may be warranted. Certainly, trials of antipsychotic medication make sense when the agitation, apprehension, and anxiety that accompany delusions are prominent.

Delusional disorders respond less well generally to electroconvulsive treatment than do major mood disorders with psychotic features. According to case reports, some cases may respond to serotonin-specific reuptake inhibitors. In cases where differential diagnosis is unclear between delusional disorder and psychotic depression, a trial of combined antipsychotic and antidepressant therapy may be worthwhile. In cases where standard strategies are unsuccessful, trials of lithium or of anticonvulsant medication (for example, carbamazepine [Tegretol]) probably should be considered. However, we have no systematic information to support such approaches.

Use of somatic treatment is difficult on two levels. The patients' insistence on lack of psychiatric problems may be an insurmountable barrier to initiating treatment, and their sensitivity to all side effects may constitute an additional frustrating factor in their care. An open and clear approach to warn patients about and to assist them through possible unpleasant experiences is essential.

In general, some patients, especially younger delusional patients, respond to supportive management and somatic treatment. Unfortunately, others, especially the elderly, are refractory to attempts to reduce their delusional thinking. In all cases goals that are realistic and modest are the most sensible. As most of the difficulty in this disorder results from the effects of the patient's actions concerning the delusions, any preventive approach has considerable potential value.

Hospitalization Most delusional disorder patients can be treated effectively in outpatient settings. Hospitalization may be necessary when there is potentially dangerous behavior or unmanageable aggressiveness. The patient may show signs of poor impulse control, excessive motor and psychic tension, unremitting anger, brooding, and even threats. Suicidal ideation and planning are also potential grounds for hospitalization. Patients with erotomania, jealousy, and persecutory delusions are particularly at risk. Once the psychiatrist decides on hospitalization, it is preferable to inform the patient tactfully that voluntary hospitalization is necessary. If this strategy fails, legal means to commit the patient to a hospital must be undertaken.

SHARED PSYCHOTIC DISORDER The initial step in treatment is the separation of the affected person from the source of the delusions, the dominant partner. The patient may need significant support to compensate for the loss of that person. The patient with shared psychotic disorder should be observed for the remission of the delusional symptoms. Antipsychotic drugs can be used if the delusional symptoms have not abated in one or two weeks.

Psychotherapy with nondelusional members of the patient's family should be undertaken, and psychotherapy with both the patient with shared psychotic disorder and the dominant partner may be indicated later in the course of treatment. In addition, the mental disorder of the dominant partner should be treated.

To prevent the recurrence of the syndrome, the clinician must use family therapy and social support to modify the family dynamics and to prevent the redevelopment of the syndrome. It is often useful to make sure that the family unit is exposed to input from outside sources to decrease the family's isolation. In short, a comprehensive approach emphasizing support and, when necessary, medication is useful.

SUGGESTED CROSS-REFERENCES

Conditions to be differentiated for delusional disorders are discussed in Chapter 14 on schizophrenia, in Chapter 16 or mood disorders, in Chapter 18 on somatoform disorders, in Chapter 25 on paranoid personality disorder, in Section 17.3 on obsessive-compulsive disorder; and in Chapter 12 on mental disorders due to a general medical condition. Aging is discussed in Section 49.4, and psychiatric disorders in the elderly in Section 49.6i.

REFERENCES

Alford B A, Beck A T: Cognitive therapy of delusional beliefs. Behav Res Ther *32:* 369, 1994.

Bentall R P, Kaney S, Dewey M E: Paranoia and social reasoning: An attribution theory analysis. Br J Clin Psychiatry *30:* 13, 1991.

Chadwick P D, Lowe C F: A cognitive approach to measuring and modifying delusion. Behav Res Ther *32:* 355, 1994.

Crowe B R, Clarkson C, Tsai M, et al: Delusional disorder: Jealous and non-jealous types. Eur Arch Psychiatry Neurol Sci *237:* 179, 1988.

*Cummings J L: Psychosis in neurologic disease: Neurobiology and pathogenesis. Neuropsychiatr Neuropsychol Behav Neurol *5:* 144, 1992.

Cummings J: Organic delusions: Phenomenology, anatomical correlation, and review. Br J Psychiatry *146:* 184, 1985.

de Clérambault G G: *Les Psychoses Passionelles. Oeuvre Psychiatrique.* Presses Universitaires de France, Paris, 1942.

DeLeon J, Antelo R E, Simpson G: Delusion of parasitosis or chronic tactile hallucinosis: Hypothesis about their brain physiopathology. Compr Psychiatry *33:* 25, 1992.

Driscoll M S, Tothe M J, Grant-Kels J M, Hale M S: Delusional parasitosis: A dermatologic, psychiatric, and pharmacologic approach. J Am Acad Dermatol *29:* 1023, 1992.

Enoch M D, Trethowan W H: *Uncommon Psychiatric Syndromes,* ed 2. John Wright, Bristol, 1979.

*Freud S: Psychoanalytic notes upon an autobiographical account of a case of paranoia (dementia paranoides). In *Collected Papers,* vol 3. Hogarth, London, 1950. Originally published, 1911.

Huq S F, Garety P A, Hemsley D R: Probabilistic judgments in deluded and non-deluded subjects. Q J Exp Psychol *40:* 801, 1988.

Kolle K: *Die Primare Verrucktheit: psychopathologische, klinische und geneologische Untersuchungen.* Thieme, Leipzig, 1931.

Kolle K: *Der Wahnkranke in Lichte alter und neuer Psychopathologie.* Thieme, Stuttgart, 1957.

Kendler K S: Demography of paranoid psychosis (delusional disorder). Arch Gen Psychiatry *39:* 890, 1982.

Kendler K S: The nosologic validity of paranoia (simple delusional disorder). Arch Gen Psychiatry *37:* 699, 1980.

Kraepelin E: *Manic Depressive, Insanity and Paranoia.* Livingstone, Edinburgh, 1921.

Krafft-Ebing R V: Über Eifersuchtswahn beim Manne. Jahrb Psychiatrie *10:* 212, 1891.

Lewis A: Paranoia and paranoid: A historical perspective. Psychol Med *1:* 2, 1970.

Maher B A: Delusional thinking and perceptual disorder. J Individ Psychol *30:* 98, 1974.

Maher B A: Delusions: contemporary etiological hypotheses. Psychiatr Ann *22:* 260, 1992.

Maher B A: Ross J: Delusions. In *Comprehensive Handbook of Psychopathology,* H E Adams, P B Sutker, editors, p 383. Plenum, New York, 1983.

*Maher B A, Spitzer M: Delusions. In *Comprehensive Handbook of Psychopathology,* ed 2. H E Adams, P B Sutker, editors, p 263. Plenum, New York, 1993.

*Manschreck T C: Delusional disorders: Clinical concepts and diagnostic strategies. Psychiatr Ann *22:* 241, 1992.

Manschreck T C: Pathogenesis of delusions. Psychiatr Clin N Amer, 1995.

Manschreck T C: The assessment of paranoid features. Compr Psychiatry *20:* 370, 1979.

Manschreck T C, Petri M: The paranoid syndrome. Lancet *2:* 251, 1978.

McAllister T W: Neuropsychiatric aspects of delusions. Psychiatr Ann *22:* 269, 1992.

Mowat R R: *Morbid Jealousy and Murder.* Tavistock, London, 1966.

*Munro A: Psychiatric disorders characterized by delusions: Treatment in relation to specific types. Psychiatr Ann *22:* 232, 1992.

Munro A: Monosymptomatic hypochondriacal psychosis. Br J Psychiatry *153:* 37, 1988.

Opler L A, Feinberg S S: The role of pimozide in clinical psychiatry: A review. J Clin Psychiatry *52:* 221, 1991.

Retterstol N: *Paranoid and Paranoiac Psychoses.* Charles C Thomas, Springfield, IL, 1966.

Segal J H: Erotomania revisited: From Kraepelin to DSM-III-R. Am J Psychiatry *146:* 1261, 1989.

Schreber D: *Memoirs of My Nervous Illness.* Bentley R, Cambridge, MA, 1955. Originally published, 1903.

Shepherd M: Morbid jealousy: Some clinical and social aspects of a psychiatric syndrome. J Ment Sci *107:* 687, 1961.

Soyka M, Haber G, Völcker A: Prevalence of delusional jealousy in different psychiatric disorders. Br J Psychiatry *158:* 549, 1991.

Spier S A: Capgras syndrome and the delusion of misidentification. Psychiatr Ann *22:* 279, 1992.

Winokur G: Delusional disorder (paranoia). Compr Psychiatry *18:* 511, 1977.

Winokur G: Familial psychopathology in delusional disorder. Compr Psychiatry *26:* 241, 1985.

15.3
ACUTE AND TRANSIENT PSYCHOTIC DISORDERS AND CULTURE-BOUND SYNDROMES

JUAN E. MEZZICH, M.D., Ph.D.
KEH-MING LIN, M.D., M.P.H.

INTRODUCTION

Psychotic disorders not only are severe forms of psychopathology with major implications for both clinical care and public health, but are also quite intricate and complex in their range of symptomatology, course, and context. Although schizophrenia and bipolar disorders are the major psychotic categories in the 10th revision of the World Health Organization's (WHO's) *International Classification of Diseases and Related Health Problems* (ICD-10) and the fourth edition of the American Psychiatric Association's *Diagnostic and Statistical Manual of Mental Disorders* (DSM-IV), a number of other psychotic conditions are recognized and delineated within those classifications.

Schizoaffective disorder has been regarded for decades as the intermediate psychosis *par excellence.* More recently, several additional categories have emerged, based on acuteness and response to stress (for example, schizophreniform disorder and brief psychotic disorder). Even more recently, ICD-10 has incorporated under the umbrella of acute and transient psychotic disorders a number of multiform and relatively short-lived conditions originally described in northern European countries and in traditional societies in Asia, Africa, and Latin America. The internationally informed and conceptually flexible framework of the acute and transient psychotic disorders also render them highly relevant for the discussion of culture-bound syndromes with psychoticlike features. Those variously delineated conditions characteristically emerge or adopt distinctive forms in certain societies or cultures, indicating the need always to consider cultural factors when assessing psychiatric patients.

HISTORY

As depicted in ancient times, madness often took the form of short-lived insanity. In ancient Greek mythology, for example, Ajax experienced a brief madness when he was refused the armor of Achilles, and Agave tore her son Pentheus to pieces and then recovered. Before the 19th century clinicians tended to attribute madness either to psychosocial stressors or to somatic illnesses (particularly fevers) and mental hospitalizations were much briefer than at the end of that century.

There are two major antecedents for the current ICD-10 concept of acute and transient psychotic disorders. One encompasses a group of special psychoses identified in northern European countries. The other is the acute psychoses observed in traditional or developing countries.

ACUTE PSYCHOSES IN NORTHERN EUROPE Particularly conspicuous are the French category of *bouffée délirante,* the Scandinavian concept of psychogenic psychosis, and the cycloid psychoses described in Germany by Karl Leonhard. Those psychotic conditions have sometimes been regarded as intermediate, in the sense that they are not schizophrenic or bipolar disorders.

Bouffée délirante was only one of more than 20 terms used in 19th-century France to describe transient psychoses, reflecting protean and alternating manifestations. Frequently, the disorder starts abruptly, presenting polymorphic phenomenology (multiple and disorganized delusions, with or without hallucinations; depersonalization or derealization, with or without confusion; depression; or elation), with symptoms changing from day to day or even from hour to hour. Some cases seem to represent a response to a psychosocial stressor, whereas others do not. *Bouffée délirante* is typically transitory (with manifestations disappearing completely in a few weeks or months), but it may recur.

The concept of psychogenic psychosis was described by the Danish psychiatrist August Wimmer in 1916, building on Karl Jaspers' psychopathology background. It is a reactive psychosis that arises in immediate response to psychosocial trauma (the nature of which determines the content of the psychosis) in persons with particularly vulnerable personalities. It tends to have a benign course of a few weeks, followed by complete recovery. Studies suggest that it was diagnosed in 10 to 25 percent of all psychotic cases in Scandinavian countries. In the eighth and ninth revisions of ICD (ICD-8 and ICD-9) the use of the diagnosis was minimal.

Cycloid psychoses were one of the various types of endogenous psychoses described by Leonhard. He indicated that cycloid psychoses had a benign long-term prognosis and presented a periodic course oscillating between particular extremes, which characterized their three subtypes: anxiety-happiness, motility (hyperkinesia-hypokinesia), and excited-inhibited confusion. That complex diagnosis influenced research and clinical care in various countries, as shown by the work of Carlo Perris in Sweden, for whom its main feature was polymorphic symptomatology, and that of Kimura and Yamashita in Japan.

ACUTE PSYCHOSES IN ASIA, AFRICA, AND LATIN AMERICA There is a high prevalence of acute and transient psychoses in traditional societies and nonindustrialized countries. For example, a major multicentric study conducted by the Indian Council of Medical Research, involving over 300 persons presenting a psychotic picture that had started during the previous two weeks, found that more than 75 percent of the patients had fully recovered, with no relapse, during the course of a one-year follow-up.

Studies in sub-Saharan Africa produced acute psychotic pictures similar to those described in Asia and Latin America, with acute onset, amorphous phenomenology (excitement, disorganized behavior, confusion, affective changes, thought disturbances), and frequent precipitation by life events. Those psychoses were more common in underprivileged persons with a background of poor physical health and living in a social setting where such behavior under stress is culturally acceptable. The duration of psychosis was usually brief with or without antipsychotic medication.

A major collaborative study was recently organized by the WHO using the Schedule for Clinical Assessment of Acute Psychotic States. It entered over 1,000 cases of acute first-episode psychosis in India (where about half of all cases were seen at several centers), Denmark, Indonesia, Nigeria, the Philippines, the United Kingdom, and the United States (Hawaii). A large proportion of patients with acute psychoses had typically schizophrenic symptoms, about half showed evidence of an immediate precipitating stress, and subjects tended to be young adults of both genders from below-average socioeconomic groups. On follow-up it was observed that recovery was rapid, often within weeks, and that during the first year about two thirds of the patients had remained well, with no relapse. Those patients with schizophrenialike symptoms were as likely to have a favorable outcome as those with only affective symptoms.

Very recent analyses from the WHO Determinants of Outcome Study revealed that the incidence of nonaffective acute remitting psychotic disorders in developing countries was 10 times greater than in industrialized countries. To put that in perspective, one must remember that over 80 percent of the world population reside in developing countries.

DEFINITION AND COMPARATIVE NOSOLOGY

ICD-10 The acute psychoses described in northern European and in developing countries have been, for the first time, accommodated and organized in ICD-10, under the category of acute and transient psychotic disorders.

The conditions are formulated and arranged according to the following principles, in order of priority:

1. An acute onset (less than two weeks) as the key criterion for the whole group. Acute onset denotes a change within two weeks or less from a state without psychotic features to a clearly abnormal psychotic state (not necessarily at its peak severity).
2. The presence of typical syndromes. Those include, first, a rapidly changing and variable state, called polymorphic, prominent in acute psychoses described in several countries, and, second, the presence of typical schizophrenic symptoms.
3. The presence or absence of associated acute stress (within two weeks of the first psychotic symptoms).

Complete recovery usually occurs within one to three months (depending on the specific disorder), often within a few weeks or days. Only a small proportion of patients with those conditions develop persistently disabling states.

More details on the clinical use of acute and transient psychotic disorders can be obtained from WHO's *ICD-10 Classification of Mental and Behavioral Disorders: Clinical Descriptions and Diagnostic Guidelines.* Table 15.3-1exhibits the corresponding, more rigorous Diagnostic Criteria for Research for acute and transient psychotic disorders.

DSM-IV The evaluation of a psychotic patient requires the consideration of the possibility that the psychotic symptoms are the result of a general medical condition (for example, a brain tumor) or the ingestion of a substance (for example, phencyclidine).

Those two situations are classified in DSM-IV as *psychotic disorder due to a general medical condition* and *substance-induced psychotic disorder,* respectively. DSM-IV also includes a diagnosis of *catatonic disorder due to a general medical condition* to emphasize the special considerations regarding the differential diagnosis of catatonic symptoms (Chapter 12).

DSM-IV also includes psychotic disorder not otherwise specified (NOS) for psychotic disorders that do not meet the criteria for any other specific psychotic disorder. In previous editions of DSM, those were called atypical psychoses.

CULTURE-BOUND SYNDROMES A variety of culture-bound syndromes have been described in the literature. The culture-bound syndromes can often be fitted into one or another DSM-IV diagnosis, including psychotic disorder not otherwise specified. Other syndromes in addition to those discussed below are listed in Table 15.3-2.

EPIDEMIOLOGY

Relevant epidemiological data about acute and transient psychotic disorders, psychotic disorder due to a general medical condition, and substance-induced psychotic disorder are lacking.

TABLE 15.3-1
ICD-10 Diagnostic Criteria for Research for Acute and Transient Psychotic Disorders

F23 **Acute and transient psychotic disorders**

G1 There is acute onset of delusions, hallucinations, incomprehensible or incoherent speech, or any combination of these. The time interval between the first appearance of any psychotic symptoms and the presentation of the fully developed disorder should not exceed two weeks.

G2 If transient states of perplexity, misidentification, or impairment of attention and concentration are present, they do not fulfil the criteria for organically caused clouding of consciousness as specified for F05.-, criterion A.

G3 The disorder does not meet the symptomatic criteria for manic episode (F30.-), depressive episode (F32.-), or recurrent depressive disorder (F33.-).

G4 There is insufficient evidence of recent psychoactive substance use to fulfil the criteria for intoxication (F1x.0), harmful use (F1x.1), dependence (F1x.2), or withdrawal states (F1x.3 and F1x.4). The continued moderate and largely unchanged use of alcohol or drugs in amounts or with the frequency to which the individual is accustomed does not necessarily rule out the use of F23; that must be decided by clinical judgment and the requirements of the research project in question.

G5 *Most commonly used exclusion clause.* There must be no organic mental disorder (F00–F09) or serious metabolic disturbances affecting the central nervous system (not including childbirth).

A fifth character should be used to specify whether the acute onset of the disorder is associated with acute stress (occurring two weeks or less before evidence of first psychotic symptoms):

F23.x0 Without associated acute stress
F23.x1 With associated acute stress

For research purposes it is recommended that change of the disorder from a nonpsychotic to a clearly psychotic state is further specified as either abrupt (onset within 48 hours) or acute (onset in more than 48 hours but less than two weeks).

F23.0 **Acute polymorphic psychotic disorder without symptoms of schizophrenia**

A. The general criteria for acute and transient psychotic disorders (F23) must be met.
B. Symptoms change rapidly in both type and intensity from day to day or within the same day.
C. Any type of either hallucinations or delusions occurs, for at least several hours, at any time from the onset of the disorder.
D. Symptoms from at least two of the following categories occur at the same time:
(1) emotional turmoil, characterized by intense feelings of happiness or ecstasy, or overwhelming anxiety or marked irritability;
(2) perplexity, or misidentification of people or places;
(3) increased or decreased motility, to a marked degree.
E. If any of the symptoms listed for schizophrenia (F20.0–F20.3), criteria G(1) and (2), are present, they are present only for a minority of the time from the onset (i.e., criterion B of F23.1 is not fulfilled).
F. The total duration of the disorder does not exceed three months.

F23.1 **Acute polymorphic psychotic disorder with symptoms of schizophrenia**

A. Criteria A, B, C, and D of acute polymorphic psychotic disorder (F23.0) must be met.
B. Some of the symptoms for schizophrenia (F20.0–F20.3) must have been present for the majority of the time since the onset of the disorder, although the full criteria need not be met (i.e., at least one of the symptoms in criteria G1 (1) a to G1 (2) c).
C. The symptoms of schizophrenia in criterion B above do not persist for more than one month.

F23.2 **Acute schizophrenialike psychotic disorder**

A. The general criteria for acute and transient psychotic disorders (F23) must be met.
B. The criteria for schizophrenia (F20.0–F20.3) are met, with the exception of the criterion for duration.
C. The disorder does not meet criteria B, C, and D for acute polymorphic psychotic disorder (F23.0).
D. The total duration of the disorder does not exceed one month.

F23.3 **Other acute predominantly delusional psychotic disorders**

A. The general criteria for acute and transient psychotic disorders (F23) must be met.
B. Relatively stable delusions or hallucinations are present but do not fulfil the symptomatic criteria for schizophrenia (F20.0–F20.3).
C. The disorder does not meet the criteria for acute polymorphic psychotic disorder (F23.0).
D. The total duration of the disorder does not exceed three months.

F23.8 **Other acute and transient psychotic disorders**

Any other acute psychotic disorders that are not classifiable under any other category in F23 (such as acute psychotic states in which definite delusions or hallucinations occur but persist for only small proportions of the time) should be coded here. States of undifferentiated excitement should also be coded here if more detailed information about the patient's mental state is not available, provided that there is no evidence of an organic cause.

F23.9 **Acute and transient psychotic disorder, unspecified**

Table from World Health Organization: *The ICD-10 Classification of Mental and Behavioural Disorders: Diagnostic Criteria for Research.* World Health Organization, Geneva, 1992. Used with permission.

ETIOLOGY

CULTURAL FACTORS The diagnosis of psychotic disorders depends primarily on the accurate and thoughtful assessment of delusions, hallucinations, and bizarre psychomotor behaviors. Culture profoundly influences the meaning and nature of symptoms in all those areas, frequently leading to misdiagnosis and diagnostic ambiguity in cross-cultural clinical situations. Lacking adequate information on what constitutes normal behavior patterns or culturally sanctioned idioms of distress, clinicians evaluating patients with different cultural, ethnic, or religious backgrounds are likely to misidentify less severe complaints or behaviors as delusional, hallucinatory, or bizarre. Similarly, they are likely to suspect the existence of major psychopathology in patients with fleeting psychotic manifestations.

Spiritual and religious beliefs can present major sources of diagnostic dilemma for clinicians. Beliefs in witchcraft and sorcery are common in many societies and may or may not be delusional. Spiritism, Santeria, and various other religious movements, and different forms of shamanism practiced in many parts of the world, encourage and sanction personal communication and active involvement with the dead, with spirits, and with various deities. Such supernatural and mystical practices and experiences are not necessarily indicative of psychopathology. However, such culturally congruent beliefs often also exert substantial pathoplastic influences on symptom formation in psychotic patients. Similarly, possession and trance phenomena are frequently seen in most non-Western societies, and it is often difficult to determine whether those experiences, in a particular case, are part of an ongoing psychotic process or are culturally and contextually appropriate.

SOCIOPOLITICAL FACTORS Sociopolitical factors can also significantly influence symptom formation in psychiatric patients, thereby complicating the diagnosis of psychotic conditions. Sustained exposure to racist and discriminatory behaviors tends to increase levels of vigilance and suspiciousness among members of ethnic minorities, and it may contribute to a higher propensity for paranoid symptoms in such persons. Paranoid symptoms also are more prevalent among those, such as refugees, who are forced to live in an unfamiliar cultural milieu. Fear of political persecution is a reality of life for persons living under oppressive regimes, and it may contribute to a higher prevalence of paranoid ideation in such societies.

TABLE 15.3-2
Culture-Bound Syndromes

amok A dissociative episode characterized by a period of brooding followed by an outburst of violent, aggressive, or homicidal behavior directed at persons and objects. The episode tends to be precipitated by a perceived slight or insult and seems to be prevalent only among men. The episode is often accompanied by persecutory ideas, automatism, amnesia, exhaustion, and a return to premorbid state following the episode. Some instances of amok may occur during a brief psychotic episode or constitute the onset or an exacerbation of a chronic psychotic process. The original reports that used this term were from Malaysia. A similar behavior pattern is found in Laos, Philippines, Polynesia (*cafard* or *cathard*), Papua New Guinea, and Puerto Rico (*mal de pelea*), and among the Navajo (*iich'aa*).

ataque de nervios An idiom of distress principally reported among Latinos from the Caribbean, but recognized among many Latin American and Latin Mediterranean groups. Commonly reported symptoms include uncontrollable shouting, attacks of crying, trembling, heat in the chest rising into the head, and verbal or physical aggression. Dissociative experiences, seizurelike or fainting episodes, and suicidal gestures are prominent in some attacks but absent in others. A general feature of an ataque de nervios is a sense of being out of control. Ataques de nervios frequently occur as a direct result of a stressful event relating to the family (e.g., news of the death of a close relative, a separation or divorce from a spouse, conflicts with a spouse or children, or witnessing an accident involving a family member). Persons may experience amnesia for what occurred during the ataque de nervios, but they otherwise return rapidly to their usual level of functioning. Although descriptions of some ataques de nervios most closely fit the DSM-IV description of panic attacks, the association of most ataques with a precipitating event and the frequent absence of the hallmark symptoms of acute fear or apprehension distinguish them from panic disorder. Ataques span the range from normal expressions of distress not associated with having a mental disorder to symptom presentations associated with the diagnoses of anxiety, mood, dissociative, or somatoform disorders.

bilis and **colera** (also referred to as *muina*) The underlying cause is thought to be strongly experienced anger or rage. Anger is viewed among many Latino groups as a particularly powerful emotion that can have direct effects on the body and can exacerbate existing symptoms. The major effect of anger is to disturb core body balances (which are understood as a balance between hot and cold valences in the body and between the material and spiritual aspects of the body). Symptoms can include acute nervous tension, headache, trembling, screaming, stomach disturbances, and, in more severe cases, loss of consciousness. Chronic fatigue may result from the acute episode.

bouffée délirante A syndrome observed in West Africa and Haiti. The French term refers to a sudden outburst of agitated and aggressive behavior, marked confusion, and psychomotor excitement. It may sometimes be accompanied by visual and auditory hallucinations or paranoid ideation. The episodes may resemble an episode of brief psychotic disorder.

brain fag A term initially used in West Africa to refer to a condition experienced by high school or university students in response to the challenges of schooling. Symptoms include difficulties in concentrating, remembering, and thinking. Students often state that their brains are "fatigued." Additional somatic symptoms are usually centered around the head and neck and include pain, pressure or tightness, blurring of vision, heat, or burning. "Brain tiredness" or fatigue from "too much thinking" is an idiom of distress in many cultures, and resulting syndromes can resemble certain anxiety, depressive, and somatoform disorders.

dhat A folk diagnostic term used in India to refer to severe anxiety and hypochondriacal concerns associated with the discharge of semen, whitish discoloration of the urine, and feelings of weakness and exhaustion. Similar to *jiryan* (India), *sukra prameha* (Sri Lanka), and *shen-k'uei* (China).

falling-out or **blacking out** Episodes that occur primarily in southern United States and Caribbean groups. They are characterized by a sudden collapse, which sometimes occurs without warning but is sometimes preceded by feelings of dizziness or "swimming" in the head. The person's eyes are usually open but the person claims an inability to see. The person usually hears and understands what is occurring around him or her but feels powerless to move. This may correspond to a diagnosis of conversion disorder or a dissociative disorder.

ghost sickness A preoccupation with death and the deceased (sometimes associated with witchcraft) frequently observed among members of many American Indian tribes. Various symptoms can be attributed to ghost sickness, including bad dreams, weakness, feelings of danger, loss of appetite, fainting, dizziness, fear, anxiety, hallucinations, loss of consciousness, confusion, feelings of futility, and a sense of suffocation.

hwa-byung (also known as **wool-hwa-byung**) A Korean folk syndrome literally translated into English as "anger syndrome" and attributed to the suppression of anger. The symptoms include insomnia, fatigue, panic, fear of impending death, dysphoric affect, indigestion, anorexia, dyspnea, palpitations, generalized aches and pains, and a feeling of a mass in the epigastrium.

koro A term, probably of Malaysian origin, that refers to an episode of sudden and intense anxiety that the penis (or, in women, the vulva and nipples) will recede into the body and possibly cause death. The syndrome is reported in south and east Asia, where it is known by a variety of local terms, such as *shuk yang, shook yong,* and *suo yang* (Chinese); *jinjinia bemar* (Assam); or *rok-joo* (Thailand). It is occasionally found in the West. Koro at times occurs in localized epidemic form in east Asian areas. The diagnosis is included in the second edition of *Chinese Classification of Mental Disorders* (CCMD-2).

latah Hypersensitivity to sudden fright, often with echopraxia, echolalia, command obedience, and dissociative or trancelike behavior. The term *latah* is of Malaysian or Indonesian origin, but the syndrome has been found in many parts of the world. Other terms for the condition are *amurakh, irkunii, ikota, olan, myriachit,* and *menkeiti* (Siberian groups); *bah tschi, bah-tsi, baah-ji* (Thailand); *imu* (Ainu, Sakhalin, Japan); and *mali-mali* and *silok* (Philippines). In Malaysia it is more frequent in middle-aged women.

locura A term used by Latinos in the United States and Latin America to refer to a severe form of chronic psychosis. The condition is attributed to an inherited vulnerability, to the effect of multiple life difficulties, or to a combination of both factors. Symptoms exhibited by persons with locura include incoherence, agitation, auditory and visual hallucinations, inability to follow rules of social interaction, unpredictability, and possible violence.

mal de ojo A concept widely found in Mediterranean cultures and elsewhere in the world. *Mal de ojo* is a Spanish phrase translated into English as "evil eye." Children are especially at risk. Symptoms include fitful sleep, crying without apparent cause, diarrhea, vomiting, and fever in a child or infant. Sometimes adults (especially women) have the condition.

nervios A common idiom of distress among Latinos in the United States and Latin America. A number of other ethnic groups have related, though often somewhat distinctive, ideas of nerves (such as *nevra* among Greeks in North America). Nervios refers both to a general state of vulnerability to stressful life experiences and to a syndrome brought on by difficult life circumstances. The term *nervios* includes a wide range of symptoms of emotional distress, somatic disturbance, and inability to function. Common symptoms include headaches and brain aches, irritability, stomach disturbances, sleep difficulties, nervousness, easy tearfulness, inability to concentrate, trembling, tingling sensations, and *mareos* (dizziness with occasional vertigo-like exacerbations). Nervios tends to be an ongoing problem, although variable in the degree of disability that is manifest. Nervios is a very broad syndrome that spans the range from cases free of a mental disorder to presentations resembling adjustment, anxiety, depressive, dissociative, somatoform, or psychotic disorders. Differential diagnosis will depend on the constellation of symptoms experienced, the kind of social events that are associated with the onset and progress of nervios, and the level of disability experienced.

piblokto An abrupt dissociative episode accompanied by extreme excitement of up to 30 minutes' duration and frequently followed by convulsive seizures and coma lasting up to 12 hours. It is observed primarily in arctic and subarctic Eskimo communities, although regional variations in name exist. The person may be withdrawn or mildly irritable for a period of hours or days before the attack and will typically report complete amnesia for the attack. During the attack the person may tear off his or her clothing, break furniture, shout obscenities, eat feces, flee from protective shelters, or perform other irrational or dangerous acts.

qi-gong psychotic reaction A term describing an acute, time-limited episode characterized by dissociative, paranoid, or other psychotic or nonpsychotic symptoms that may occur after participation in the Chinese folk health-enhancing practice of qi-gong (exercise of vital energy). Especially vulnerable are persons who become overly involved in the practice. This diagnosis is included in the second edition of *Chinese Classification of Mental Disorders* (CCMD-2).

TABLE 15.3-2 (*continued*)

rootwork A set of cultural interpretations that ascribe illness to hexing, witchcraft, sorcery, or the evil influence of another person. Symptoms may include generalized anxiety and gastrointestinal complaints (e.g., nausea, vomiting, diarrhea), weakness, dizziness, the fear of being poisoned, and sometimes fear of being killed (voodoo death). Roots, spells, or hexes can be put or placed on other persons, causing a variety of emotional and psychological problems. The hexed person may even fear death until the root has been taken off (eliminated), usually through the work of a root doctor (a healer in this tradition), who can also be called on to bewitch an enemy. Rootwork is found in the southern United States among both African American and European American populations and in Caribbean societies. It is also known as *mal puesto* or *brujeria* in Latino societies.

sangue dormido (''sleeping blood'') A syndrome found among Portuguese Cape Verde Islanders (and immigrants from there to the United States). It includes pain, numbness, tremor, paralysis, convulsions, stroke, blindness, heart attack, infection, and miscarriage.

shenjing shuairuo (''neurasthenia'') In China a condition characterized by physical and mental fatigue, dizziness, headaches, other pains, concentration difficulties, sleep disturbance, and memory loss. Other symptoms include gastrointestinal problems, sexual dysfunction, irritability, excitability, and various signs suggesting disturbance of the autonomic nervous system. In many cases the symptoms would meet the criteria for a DSM-IV mood or anxiety disorder. The diagnosis is included in the second edition of *Chinese Classification of Mental Disorders* (CCMD-2).

shen-k'uei (Taiwan); **shenkui** (China) A Chinese folk label describing marked anxiety or panic symptoms with accompanying somatic complaints for which no physical cause can be demonstrated. Symptoms include dizziness, backache, fatigability, general weakness, insomnia, frequent dreams, and complaints of sexual dysfunction, such as premature ejaculation and impotence. Symptoms are attributed to excessive semen loss from frequent intercourse, masturbation, nocturnal emission, or passing of white turbid urine believed to contain semen. Excessive semen loss is feared because of the belief that it represents the loss of one's vital essence and can thereby be life threatening.

shin-byung A Korean folk label for a syndrome in which initial phases are characterized by anxiety and somatic complaints (general weakness, dizziness, fear, anorexia, insomnia, gastrointestinal problems), with subsequent dissociation and possession by ancestral spirits.

spell A trance state in which persons ''communicate'' with deceased relatives or with spirits. At times the state is associated with brief periods of personality change. The culture-specific syndrome is seen among African Americans and European Americans from the southern United States. Spells are not considered to be medical events in the folk tradition, but may be misconstrued as psychotic episodes in clinical settings.

susto (''fright,'' or ''soul loss'') A folk illness prevalent among some Latinos in the United States and among people in Mexico, Central America, and South America. Susto is also referred to as *espanto, pasmo, tripa ida, perdida del alma,* or *chibih.* Susto is an illness attributed to a frightening event that causes the soul to leave the body and results in unhappiness and sickness. Persons with susto also experience significant strains in key social roles. Symptoms may appear any time from days to years after the fright is experienced. It is believed that in extreme cases, susto may result in death. Typical symptoms include appetite disturbances, inadequate or excessive sleep, troubled sleep or dreams, feelings of sadness, lack of motivation to do anything, and feelings of low self-worth or dirtiness. Somatic symptoms accompanying susto include muscle aches and pains, headache, stomachache, and diarrhea. Ritual healings are focused on calling the soul back to the body and cleansing the person to restore bodily and spiritual balance. Different experiences of susto may be related to major depressive disorder, posttraumatic stress disorder, and somatoform disorders. Similar etiological beliefs and symptom configurations are found in many parts of the world.

taijin kyofu sho A culturally distinctive phobia in Japan, in some ways resembling social phobia in DSM-IV. The syndrome refers to a person's intense fear that his or her body, its parts or its functions, displease, embarrass, or are offensive to other people in appearance, odor, facial expressions, or movements. The syndrome is included in the official Japanese diagnostic system for mental disorders.

zar A general term applied in Ethiopia, Somalia, Egypt, Sudan, Iran, and other North African and Middle Eastern societies to the experience of spirits possessing a person. Persons possessed by a spirit may experience dissociative episodes that may include shouting, laughing, hitting the head against a wall, singing, or weeping. They may show apathy and withdrawal, refusing to eat or carry out daily tasks, or may develop a long-term relationship with the possessing spirit. Such behavior is not considered pathological locally.

Table adapted from DSM-IV, *Diagnostic and Statistical Manual of Mental Disorders,* ed 4. Copyright American Psychiatric Association, Washington, 1994. Used with permission.

Because of those complications, it is often difficult to determine whether paranoid experiences among recent immigrants and sojourners are reactive in nature or indicate a more serious psychotic process.

PHYSIOLOGICAL FACTORS Physical conditions—such as cerebral neoplasms, particularly of the occipital or temporal areas—can induce hallucinations. Sensory deprivation, as occurs in blind and deaf persons, can also result in hallucinatory or delusional experiences. Lesions involving the temporal lobe and other cerebral regions, especially the right hemisphere and the parietal lobe, are often associated with delusions.

Psychoactive substances are common causes of psychotic syndromes. The most commonly involved substances are alcohol, indole hallucinogens—for example, lysergic acid diethylamide (LSD), amphetamine, cocaine, mescaline, phencyclidine (PCP), and ketamine. Many other substances, including steroids and thyroxine, can be associated with substance-induced hallucinations.

DIAGNOSIS AND CLINICAL FEATURES

ICD-10

Acute polymorphic psychotic disorder without symptoms of schizophrenia Acute polymorphic psychotic disorder without symptoms of schizophrenia is characterized by obvious but variable and rapidly changing hallucinations, delusions, and perceptual disturbances, often accompanied by emotional turmoil (happiness and ecstasy or anxiety and irritability). The criteria for manic episode, depressive episode, or schizophrenia are not met. The disorder tends to have an abrupt onset (less than 48 hours) and then a rapid resolution of symptoms. If those persist for more than three months, the diagnosis should be changed (for example, to persistent delusional disorder or some other nonorganic psychotic disorder). It accommodates the concepts of *bouffée délirante* and cycloid psychosis, both either unspecified or without symptoms of schizophrenia.

Acute polymorphic psychotic disorder with symptoms of schizophrenia Acute polymorphic psychotic disorder with symptoms of schizophrenia is as polymorphic as the preceding disorder, but is additionally characterized by the consistent presence of typical schizophrenic symptoms. If the schizophrenic symptoms last more than one month, the diagnosis should be changed to schizophrenia. The disorder accommodates the concepts of *bouffée délirante* and cycloid psychosis, both with symptoms of schizophrenia.

Acute schizophrenialike psychotic disorder Acute schizophrenia-like psychotic disorder is characterized by the consistent and stable presence of typical schizophrenic symptoms, without the polymorphic character of the foregoing disorders. If the schizophrenic symptoms last more than one month, the diagnosis should be changed to schizophrenia.

Other acute predominantly delusional psychotic disorders The other disorders are characterized by relatively stable delusions or hallucinations, without fulfilling the criteria for either schizophrenia or the acute polymorphic psychotic disorders. If the delusions persist for more than three months, the diagnosis should be changed to persistent delusional disorder, and if only the hallucinations persist, to other nonorganic psychotic disorder. The disorder accommodates the concepts of psychogenic paranoid psychosis and paranoid reaction.

Other acute and transient psychotic disorders The category includes other acute psychotic disorders not classifiable under the preceding categories, provided there is no evidence of an organic cause. Examples include acute psychoses with definite but fleeting delusions or hallucinations, and states of undifferentiated excitement.

Acute and transient psychotic disorder, unspecified The residual category accommodates such concepts as brief reactive psychosis not otherwise specified.

DSM-IV

Psychotic disorder due to a general medical condition The DSM-IV diagnosis of psychotic disorder due to a general medical condition (Table 15.3-3) combines into one diagnosis the two similar diagnostic categories in the revised third edition of DSM (DSM-III-R), organic delusional disorder and organic hallucinosis. The phenomena of the psychotic disorder are defined in DSM-IV by further specifying the predominant symptoms. When the diagnosis is used, the medical condition, along with the predominant symptom pattern, should be included in the diagnosis—for example, psychotic disorder due to a brain tumor, with delusions. The DSM-IV criteria further specify that the disorder does not occur exclusively while the patient is delirious or demented and that the symptoms are not better accounted for by another mental disorder.

Substance-induced psychotic disorder DSM-IV has combined the various DSM-III-R diagnostic categories that relate to psychoactive substance-induced psychotic disorders into a single diagnostic category, substance-induced psychotic disorder (Table 15.3-4). The diagnosis is reserved for persons who have substance-induced psychotic symptoms in the absence of reality testing. Persons who have substance-induced psychotic symptoms (for example, hallucinations) but who have retained reality testing should be classified as having a substance-related disorder—for example, phencyclidine intoxication with perceptual disturbances. The intent of including the diagnosis of substance-induced psychotic disorder with the other psychotic disorder diagnoses is to prompt the clinician to consider the possibility that a substance is causally involved in the production of the psychotic symptoms. The full diagnosis of substance-induced psychotic disorder should include the type of substance involved, the stage of substance use when the disorder began (for example, during intoxication or withdrawal), and the clinical phenomena (for example, hallucinations or delusions).

Psychotic disorder not otherwise specified The psychotic disorder not otherwise specified (NOS) category is used for patients who have psychotic symptoms (for example, delusions, hallucinations, and disorganized speech and behavior)

TABLE 15.3-3
Diagnostic Criteria for Psychotic Disorder Due to a General Medical Condition

A. Prominent hallucinations or delusions.
B. There is evidence from the history, physical examination, or laboratory findings that the disturbance is the direct physiological consequence of a general medical condition.
C. The disturbance is not better accounted for by another mental disorder.
D. The disturbance does not occur exclusively during the course of a delirium.

Code based on predominant symptom:
- **With delusions:** if delusions are the predominant symptom
- **With hallucinations:** if hallucinations are the predominant symptom

Coding note: Include the name of the general medical condition on Axis I, e.g., psychotic disorder due to malignant lung neoplasm, with delusions; also code the general medical condition on Axis III.

Coding note: If delusions are part of a preexisting dementia, indicate the delusions by coding the appropriate subtype of the dementia if one is available, e.g., dementia of the Alzheimer's type, with late onset, with delusions.

Table from DSM-IV, *Diagnostic and Statistical Manual of Mental Disorders,* ed 4. Copyright American Psychiatric Association, Washington, 1994. Used with permission.

TABLE 15.3-4
Diagnostic Criteria for Substance-Induced Psychotic Disorder

A. Prominent hallucinations or delusions. **Note:** Do not include hallucinations if the person has insight that they are substance-induced.
B. There is evidence from the history, physical examination, or laboratory findings of either (1) or (2):
   (1) the symptoms in criteria A developed during, or within a month of, substance intoxication or withdrawal
   (2) medication use is etiologically related to the disturbance
C. The disturbance is not better accounted for by a psychotic disorder that is not substance induced. Evidence that the symptoms are better accounted for by a psychotic disorder that is not substance induced might include the following: the symptoms precede the onset of the substance use (or medication use); the symptoms persist for a substantial period of time (e.g., about a month) after the cessation of acute withdrawal or severe intoxication, or are substantially in excess of what would be expected given the type or amount of the substance used or the duration of use; or there is other evidence that suggests the existence of an independent non-substance-induced psychotic disorder (e.g., a history of recurrent non-substance-related episodes).
D. The disturbance does not occur exclusively during the course of a delirium.

Note: This diagnosis should be made instead of a diagnosis of substance intoxication or substance withdrawal only when the symptoms are in excess of those usually associated with the intoxication or withdrawal syndrome and when the symptoms are sufficiently severe to warrant independent clinical attention.

Code: [Specific substance]-induced psychotic disorder (Alcohol, with delusions; alcohol, with hallucinations; amphetamine [or amphetaminelike substance], with delusions; amphetamine [or amphetaminelike substance], with hallucinations; cannabis, with delusions; cannabis, with hallucinations; cocaine, with delusions; cocaine, with hallucinations; hallucinogen, with delusions; hallucinogen, with hallucinations; inhalant, with delusions; inhalant, with hallucinations; opioid, with delusions; opioid, with hallucinations; phencyclidine [or phencyclidinelike substance], with delusions; phencyclidine [or phencyclidinelike substance], with hallucinations; sedative, hypnotic or anxiolytic, with delusions; sedative, hypnotic or anxiolytic, with hallucinations; other [or unknown] substance, with delusions; other [or unknown] substance, with hallucinations)

Specify if:
- **With onset during intoxication:** if criteria are met for intoxication with the substance and the symptoms develop during the intoxication syndrome
- **With onset during withdrawal:** if criteria are met for withdrawal from the substance and the symptoms develop during, or shortly after, a withdrawal syndrome

Table from DSM-IV, *Diagnostic and Statistical Manual of Mental Disorders,* ed 4. Copyright American Psychiatric Association, Washington, 1994. Used with permission.

TABLE 15.3-5
Diagnostic Criteria for Psychotic Disorder Not Otherwise Specified

This category includes psychotic symptomatology (i.e., delusions, hallucinations, disorganized speech, grossly disorganized or catatonic behavior) about which there is inadequate information to make a specific diagnosis or about which there is contradictory information, or disorders with psychotic symptoms that do not meet the criteria for any specific psychotic disorder.
Examples include:
1. Postpartum psychosis that does not meet criteria for mood disorder with psychotic features, brief psychotic disorder, psychotic disorder due to a general medical condition, or substance-induced psychotic disorder
2. Psychotic symptoms that have lasted for less than one month but that have not yet remitted, so that the criteria for brief psychotic disorder are not met
3. Persistent auditory hallucinations in the absence of any other features
4. Persistent nonbizarre delusions with periods of overlapping mood episodes that have been present for a substantial portion of the delusional disturbance
5. Situations in which the clinician has concluded that a psychotic disorder is present, but is unable to determine whether it is primary, due to a general medical condition, or substance induced

Table from DSM-IV, *Diagnostic and Statistical Manual of Mental Disorders,* ed 4. Copyright American Psychiatric Association, Washington, 1994. Used with permission.

but who do not meet the diagnostic criteria for other specifically defined psychotic disorders. In some cases the diagnosis of psychotic disorder not otherwise specified may be used when not enough information is available to make a specific diagnosis. DSM-IV has listed some examples of the diagnosis to help guide clinicians (Table 15.3-5).

CULTURE INFLUENCES ON THE MANIFESTATION OF PSYCHOSES In addition to those enumerated above, there are many factors that make the cross-cultural assessment of psychotic patients particularly challenging. Cross-ethnic differences in emotional expressiveness have been well documented in the literature and may hinder the assessment of affect and behavior in such a way that a culturally appropriate range of expression may be mistaken as evidence of flat affect or emotional withdrawal. Relative to the clinician's standard for the normal range of affect, the patient's reports may be either overestimated or underestimated in their significance.

The clinician's interpretation of the patient's complaints tends to be framed by the official nosological system. That raises the question of the validity of the diagnostic system used. Although greater efforts have been made to base the construction of the new standard manuals on sounder epidemiological data and to reflect greater attention to cultural factors, major limitations remain in both the balance of conceptualization and the adequacy of field trials.

Ms. A., a 27-year-old, single woman, was brought to the emergency room of a community hospital in California because of acute onset of agitation, shouting, refusal of food and drink, and fear of impending death. Brought up in Ethiopia as a Coptic Christian, she had lived a sheltered life until approximately five years before evaluation, when the family (parents and 11 siblings) became victims of civil war. Along with some relatives, she escaped to Kenya and eventually resettled in the Los Angeles area, joining a brother who had migrated there many years earlier. They had apparently lost contact with the rest of the family.

Her life in the United States in the past three years had not been easy. Her attendance at classes in English as a Second Language was erratic, with limited progress. She was, in general, quite isolated, not only from mainstream society, but also from the local Ethiopian community. Several months earlier, she had started working as a housekeeper, but quit abruptly just prior to the current episode, apparently because of persecutory fears. She had no prior history of contact with psychiatric services. However, in Kenya she was once taken to see a "medicine man," who told her that there were people around her who were trying to "poison" her. Since arriving in the United States, she had mentioned several times that someone might try to poison and kill her, without describing those suspicions in detail.

In the hospital she at first appeared extremely agitated and delusional, and she reported that her mother, who she thought had died in Ethiopia, had talked to her and warned her of impending dangers. She also admitted to Schneiderian-like thought insertion and to hearing voices commenting on her behavior. However, language difficulties made questionable the validity of those symptoms. Two days after treatment with small doses of antipsychotics most of the symptoms had disappeared. She became calm and cooperative, with some restriction in affect. She was promptly discharged and followed up at a local outpatient clinic where the medication was discontinued because of her complaints of side effects. Three months later she dropped out of the clinic. At her last visit she was asymptomatic and was working again as a housekeeper.

Diagnostic assessment presented a challenge to the clinicians involved. Although a schizophrenic process was suspected, there were many quandaries. Paranoid symptoms were partially explainable by the woman's life experiences and her culturally sanctioned beliefs about sorcery, reinforced by the medicine man she had seen in Kenya. Hearing her deceased mother's voice could be culturally congruent. Although her social isolation and low level of functioning before the episode could be construed as prodromal signs of schizophrenia, they could equally be the result of her difficulty in adjusting to an alien, technologically complex culture. Last, the clinical course was also not congruent with a diagnosis of schizophrenia. With an abrupt onset, rapid response to treatment, and almost complete recovery, the case more closely resembled the archetype of *bouffée délirante* often observed in West Africa and Haiti. It could perhaps be accommodated within ICD-10 as an acute polymorphic psychotic disorder with symptoms of schizophrenia.

CULTURE-BOUND SYNDROMES Perhaps the most dramatic example of the difficulties in applying Western-based nosological concepts and criteria cross-culturally can be found in the ongoing controversy surrounding the culture-bound syndromes.

As pointed out recently by the United States National Institute of Mental Health Culture and Diagnosis Group, the term "culture-bound syndrome" denotes recurrent, locality-specific patterns of aberrant behavior and troubling experiences that appear to fall outside conventional Western psychiatric categories. Those include categories in folk nosological systems (often organized in relation to perceived cause and symptom clusters) as well as idioms of distress or culturally salient expressions for securing social support and communicating symptoms. Terms formerly used to refer to such phenomena include "cultural and ethnic psychoses and neuroses" and "atypical and exotic psychotic syndromes." Because the experience and expression of psychiatric illness are always influenced by cultural factors, those terms are evidently problematic.

Amok Although "running amok" has become a common English expression, most people are not aware of its origin as a Malayan term referring to a violent or furious fit with homicidal intent. The syndrome of amok may be defined by four major characteristics: prodromal brooding, homicidal outburst, persistence in reckless killing without apparent motive, and a claim of amnesia. The attack, which often results in multiple casualties, is usually terminated only when the afflicted person becomes totally exhausted or is captured or killed.

Amok and its related terms, *mengamok* (the act of running amok), *pengamok* (the amoker), *gila mengamok* (amok psychosis), and *mata gelap* (darkened eye), are familiar concepts to the Malays. The amokers are believed almost always to be young men whose self-esteem has been severely injured. Although they traditionally are not held responsible for their acts, they nevertheless are either confined or ostracized for fear of recurrences. It has been suggested that amok constitutes a behavioral alternative in reaction to the heavy emphasis in Malay culture on hierarchy, appropriateness, and nonaggression. The belief that someone may actually become an amoker (if pushed to the extreme) may also serve to curb the excessive use of power by those in positions of authority.

Attacks of sudden mass assault with amoklike behavior and consequences are not limited to the Malay cultural sphere, having been reported throughout Southeast Asia, as well as in North America and the Caribbean area. Similar syndromes are *mal de pelea* in Puerto Rico and *iich'aa* among the Navajos. The available literature suggests that those cases share with Malay amokers some important demographic (age and gender), psychosocial (perceived humiliation as precipitant), and perhaps psychodynamic (difficulties with independence and aggression) characteristics.

Koro Koro is usually manifest as an episode of sudden and desperate fear that the penis (or less commonly, the vulva and breasts in women) is shrinking and may recede into the abdomen, possibly causing death. During the attack patients typically experience intense fear and panic associated with cold sweat, paresthesias, palpitations, weakness, skin pallor, visual blurring, and faintness. In their attempt to prevent the complete retraction of the penis, and hence death, they hold on to the penis either manually or with the aid of strings or clamps. Family members, relatives, and friends often take turns holding the penis to prevent its shrinking.

Koro is a Malay term of uncertain origin. First reported by Dutch physicians working in western Sulawesi (formerly known as Celebes, an island of Indonesia), in recent years the condition has been observed predominantly among Chinese residing in Southeast Asia and southern China, where it has been known as *suoyang* (*suo:* retract; *yang:* penis). More recently, korolike conditions have also been observed in Mindanao (an island in the southern part of the Philippines, neighboring Indonesia), northern Thailand, and northeast India. Among the Chinese, the syndrome is deeply imbedded in traditional medical theories, including the yin-yang humoral balance, the importance of the conservation of vital energy, the value of semen as the purest (and thus most precious) form of vital energy, and the belief that the complete retraction of the penis results in death. Practically all Chinese koro (suo yang) cases report preexisting worries about what the sufferers consider sexual excesses, such as nocturnal emission, masturbation, or sexual overindulgence. Many cases are precipitated by unhealthy coitus (for example, with prostitutes), sudden exposure of the penis to cold water or cold air, or hearing about people dying from koro. Reflecting its widely held importance, the condition is included in the second edition of the *Chinese Classification of Mental Disorders* (CCMD-2).

In addition to individual cases, koro has also been observed in epidemic forms, typically in communities experiencing heightened social or political tension. For example, in 1967, at the height of the Malay-Chinese conflict in Malaysia, more than 400 Chinese developed koro within five days after hearing the rumor that the pork that they had eaten had been deliberately infected with swine fever. More recent epidemics in Thailand and India were similarly precipitated by political rumors (for example, that Vietnamese soldiers had poisoned the water to make Thai men impotent).

Sporadic cases involving intense fear of penile retraction have been reported in Western countries and in Africa. However, those cases lack the cultural elaboration of true koro cases. Sufferers do not associate their experiences with the belief of impending death, and episodes are more likely to appear in the context of major psychiatric conditions, such as organic brain syndromes, schizophrenia, drug-induced psychosis, and mood disorders.

Latah *Latah* is a Malay term for the hypersensitivity to sudden fright or startle. In those afflicted a sudden stimulus typically provokes the suspension of all normal activities and triggers involuntary motor and verbal reactions that are stereotypical and socially inappropriate (for example, coprolalia). In more severe cases the hypersensitivity to startle is also accompanied by mimetic or echo symptoms, including echolalia, echopraxia, and automatic obedience.

Latah affects both men and women although most are middle-aged women of relatively low or marginal social status. The syndrome is often precipitated by major stressful life events. Social conditioning may also contribute to the onset of the condition, because in a Malayan setting those with a tendency to startle are repeatedly poked or teased. Most latah sufferers are embarrassed and ashamed of their problems, and many tend to shy away from social interactions to avoid the teasing and the provocation of latah behavior. Others appear to enjoy the attention they receive with their latah performances. For them latah may provide an important social role that satisfies their intrapsychic needs.

Conditions similar to latah have been reported in other cultures, including *imu* among the Ainu in northern Japan; *myriachit, ikota,* and *amurakh* in Siberia; *bah tschi* in Thailand, and *mali-mali* in the Philippines.

Taijin kyofu sho The Japanese term means "fear of facing or interacting with other people," not necessarily fear of people. Patients suffering from the condition experience a profound fear—often reaching seemingly psychotic proportions—of hurting the feelings of others, with certain shortcomings within themselves. Those shortcomings include a real or imagined propensity to blush, to gaze inappropriately at others, to emit (most often imaginary) body odors, or to shake or to tense up involuntarily in front of others. Most taijin kyofu sho (TKS) patients are adolescent boys and young adult men. Despite the intensity of their symptoms and the near-delusional quality of their obsessions, they are typically engaging and eager to cooperate during clinical interviews, and they show a strong desire to be with other people rather than to avoid them. Clinicians have great difficulty placing TKS patients in any standard diagnostic category because their symptoms are simultaneously suggestive of obsessive-compulsive disorder, somatoform disorder, and even psychotic disorder. Although the core symptom of the condition, the fear of social situations, is similar to what is seen in standard social phobia, the conditions are distinctively different. Differences include not only the prevalence and severity of symptoms, the degree of disability associated with the condition, and demographic characteristics (predominantly younger men), but the subjective meaning of the symptoms. TKS patients' primary concern not to embarrass or inconvenience others reflects the group orientation of Japanese culture, and it is harder to understand within the Western individualistic context, where most patients with social phobia are primarily worried about being embarrassed or ridiculed. The syndrome is included in the *Japanese Clinical Modification* of ICD-10.

Piblokto Occurring among Eskimos and sometimes referred to as Arctic hysteria, *piblokto* is characterized by attacks lasting from one to two hours, during which patients (usually women) begin to scream and to tear off and destroy their clothing. While imitating the cry of some animal or bird, the patients may throw themselves on the snow or run wildly about on the ice, although the temperature may be well below zero. After the attack the person appears to be normal and usually has no memory of the episode. The Eskimos are reluctant to touch afflicted persons during the attacks because they believe that the attacks involve evil spirits. Piblokto appears to be a hysterical state of a dissociative disorder. It has become much less frequent than it used to be among Eskimos.

Qi-gong psychotic reaction Qi-gong (exercise of vital energy) is an age-old Chinese self-healing practice with features of meditation and kung-fu that in recent years has gained a great deal of popularity in practically all Chinese communities, including mainland China, Hong Kong, Taiwan, and those in North America. In mainland China an estimated 10 percent of the more than one billion citizens practice qi-gong on a regular basis. Based on the traditional Chinese belief in the importance of *qi* (or *chi,* which means vital energy) circulation, both within the body and between the body and its natural environment, such exercises are supposed to improve one's physical, mental, and spiritual health by reducing the stagnation of the qi circulation. While performing the exercises, practitioners often experience a special sensation of qi's following the meridian routes through the body. Since the belief also involves the exchange of qi between the exerciser and the environs and, through the environs, with other people, some qi-gong practitioners also believe that it is not only a self-healing practice but can also be used to heal others.

Regular practice of qi-gong is believed to result in a sense of well-being and to be effective in reducing stress and various psychological and psychophysiological symptoms. However, qi-gong is clearly not an innocuous practice because if done inappropriately (according to its enthusiasts), it can induce adverse side effects, ranging from transient, minor symptoms (for example, an increase in anxiety) to persistent psychotic symptoms, including hallucinations and delusions. With the growing popularity of the practice in China, the prevalence of the qi-gong psychotic reaction has apparently greatly increased, to the extent that it has become necessary for Chinese psychiatrists to include it in CCMD-2.

Voodoo, rootwork, and related states Behavioral disturbances associated with possession phenomena are observed in many cultural settings and are given different names (for example, *zar, mal puesto, shin-byung*). Voodoo hexing is the most widely known and discussed, not only by anthropologists and psychiatrists, but also by popular writers and others. Originating in West Africa, voodoo cult practices can be found in many parts of Africa, the Caribbean region, and Latin America, and they are particularly widespread in Haiti. Victims of voodoo curses are believed to succumb to voodoo death, and then to be brought to life again by voodoo doctors or those who possess the voodoo power. The living dead are believed totally to lack self-awareness and self-initiation and to be controlled completely by those with the voodoo power. The phenomenon of voodoo death has been the subject of intense research and speculation, and various explanatory theories have been postulated, including poisoning, dehydration, stress-induced cardiac arrhythmia, the overstimulation of the sympathetic and parasympathetic nervous systems, and the giving up–given up complex.

Voodoo death is a relatively rare event even in voodoo-endemic areas, such as Haiti. However, the belief in voodoo power is widespread and deeply rooted among persons of African descent in the Caribbean area. The same appears to be true in the case of rootwork, a similar belief prevalent in certain parts of the South in the United States.

Wihtigo *Wihtigo,* or windigo psychosis, is a psychiatric disorder confined to the Cree, Ojibwa, and Salteaux Indians of North America. Affected persons believe that they may be transformed into a wihtigo, a giant monster that eats human flesh, and during times of starvation, may feel and express a craving for human flesh. Because of the patient's belief in witchcraft and in the possibility of such a transformation, symptoms affecting the alimentary tract, such as loss of appetite and nausea from trivial causes, may cause the patient to become greatly excited for fear of being transformed into a wihtigo.

PATHOLOGY AND LABORATORY EXAMINATION

A large number of general medical problems may cause or exacerbate patients' psychotic conditions, often involving confusing and puzzling presentations. They include such conditions as infections (including human immunodeficiency virus [HIV] infection), head trauma, endocrine disorders (Cushing's and Addison's diseases and disorders of the thyroid and parathyroid glands), autoimmune diseases (systemic lupus erythematosus), vitamin deficiencies, seizure disorders, genetic diseases (Wilson's disease, acute intermittent porphyria), drug and toxin exposures, and the effects of psychoactive drugs. Those conditions are usually included in the differential diagnosis of any psychotic disorder, but they should be given more careful consideration when the patient's symptom profile is polymorphic or inchoate. For such patients laboratory tests should include not only the routine chemistry panels (electrolytes, glucose, complete blood counts, renal and liver functions) and urinalysis, but also thyroid function tests, syphilis tests, and determination of serum cortisol levels, vitamin B_{12} and foliate levels, and calcium and phosphate levels. In addition to a chest X-ray and an electrocardiogram (ECG), an electroencephalogram (EEG) should also be considered. An EEG with sleep deprivation and nasopharyngeal leads also has been recommended. Computerized EEG (brain mapping), magnetic resonance imaging (MRI), single photon emission computered tomography (SPECT), and neuropsychological testing may yield useful information.

Psychosocial assessment should include a careful review of the patient's life history, with special attention to the patient's personality traits and recent stresses. A detailed assessment of family history and dynamics should also be included. Contextual factors, such as psychosocial stressors and supports, should be carefully appraised, along with the ability of the person to perform basic roles (for example, occupationally, with family, and socially).

COURSE AND PROGNOSIS

In patients with an acute and transient psychotic disorder, complete recovery usually occurs within one to three months (depending on the specific disorder), often within a few weeks or days, and only a small proportion of patients develop persistently disabling states.

Limited data on the longitudinal course of patients with culture-bound syndromes have suggested that some of them eventually develop clinical features compatible with a diagnosis of schizophrenia, bipolar disorder, cognitive disorder, or other psychotic disorders. It is thus crucial to gather information from all possible sources. Since clinical pictures evolve over time, thorough reevaluations should be conducted periodically to enable an accurate diagnosis and effective clinical care.

TREATMENT

Careful evaluation, clinical observation, and comprehensive information gathering are the cornerstones of treatment planning for any psychiatric or general medical disorder. Comprehensive and longitudinal assessments are of particular importance in the management of patients who are experiencing acute and transient psychotic disorders and culture-bound disorders.

A multiaxial assessment using such schemas as those in ICD-10 and DSM-IV can be very helpful in effective treatment planning. A complementary cultural formulation, such as the one recommended in DSM-IV, can substantially enhance diagnosis and clinical care. Such a formulation involves appraising the cultural identity of the patient, the cultural framework of illness and its context and implications, and intercultural elements in the clinician-patient relationship.

The treatment plan for any patient must be individualized, but that principle is particularly important when dealing with cases of acute and transient psychotic disorders and culture-bound psychotic disorders. Because of the intricate and heterogeneous nature of those conditions, there is no standard treatment strategy that can be applied to the majority of the cases.

Because a common denominator of all the disorders discussed in this section is the presence of psychosis, pharmacotherapy frequently involves the use of antipsychotic drugs. There is some evidence that the dosage of antipsychotics necessary for acute transient psychotic disorders is significantly lower than that required for other psychotic conditions, especially schizophrenia. It is thus prudent to use the lowest dose that can control the patient's symptoms. Since acute and transient psychotic disorders are often episodic, the intermittent use of antipsychotics, guided by the emergence of psychotic symptoms, is worth considering.

Depending on the clinical features of particular cases, many other psychiatric medicines have also been recommended. They include benzodiazepines for controlling agitation, lithium (Eskalith) for modulating mood swings, and antidepressants for ameliorating depressive symptoms, and are often used in conjunction with antipsychotics. Anticonvulsants, such as carbamazepine (Tegretol), have been reported to have been effective in treating a number of psychotic patients with atypical features.

Limited research has been conducted to date on the efficacy of various psychosocial interventions for managing acute and transient psychotic disorders and culture-bound disorders. It appears reasonable to consider findings from studies involving other psychotic conditions. Those include approaches based on expressed emotion concepts, psychoeducational and skill-competence training, and Thomas McGlashan's phase-specific theory on the need for stimulation in schizophrenic patients (the avoidance of excessive stimuli in the acute phase and the uses of structured activities and stimuli in later phases). It is important to consider involving the family in therapy and to establish a supportive and trusting therapeutic relationship.

The importance of cultural issues in the evaluation and treatment of atypical psychoses can hardly be exaggerated, especially when dealing with patients from non-Western and ethnic minority populations. Cultural information not only is crucial for accurate diagnosis, but also is indispensable in the formulation of treatment plans. Treatment approaches that do not take the patient's sociocultural background into account are likely to fail no matter how well intentioned the therapists may be. For example, in cultures in which family and group harmony and unity are valued over individual independence, the rigid application of Western-based psychotherapeutic techniques may exacerbate, rather than ameliorate, the patient's psychopathological condition. Consideration of the intercultural elements in the clinician-patient relationship is also fundamental for the establishment of rapport and the effective engagement of the patient and the family in the treatment process.

One promising avenue is collaboration with indigenous healers. Several researchers have reported on their success in the use of indigenous and traditional healers in the treatment of psychiatric patients, especially those whose psychotic conditions are substantially connected to culture-specific beliefs (for example, fear of voodoo death). Others have mentioned the potential pitfalls and problems in such collaboration. Decisions about involving indigenous healers should be individualized and thoughtfully planned, taking into consideration the setting, the sophistication and flexibility of the available healers, the type of psychopathology, and the patient's characteristics. The WHO has long advocated the implementation at the local level of a policy of close collaboration between the health system and traditional medicine, and, in particular, between individual health professionals and traditional practitioners.

SUGGESTED CROSS-REFERENCES

The influences of culture on the nature of and responses to psychiatric disorders are discussed in Section 4.2 on sociology and psychiatry. Section 4.3, on sociobiology and psychiatry, is also relevant. Section 11.2 concerns international perspectives on psychiatric diagnosis. Section 15.1 is devoted to other psychotic disorders, including brief psychotic disorder. Sociocultural aspects of geriatric psychiatry are the subject of Section 49.4b.

REFERENCES

Adebimpe V R: Overview: White norms and psychiatric diagnosis of black patients. Am J Psychiatry *138:* 279, 1981.

Akerele O: The best of both worlds: Bringing traditional medicine up to date. Soc Sci Med *24:* 177, 1987.

Bustamante J A: *Psiquiatría Ciencia y Técnica.* Instituto Cubano del Libro, La Habana, 1972.

Cohen L S, Rosenbaum J F: Clonazepam. New uses and potential problems. J Clin Psychiatry *48*(Suppl): 50, 1987.

*Cooper J E, Jablensky A, Sartorius N: WHO collaborative studies on acute psychoses using the SCAAPS schedule. In *Psychiatry: A World Perspective,* C N Stefanis, A D Rabavilas, C R Soldatos, editors. Elsevier, Amsterdam, 1990.

Fabrega H: An ethnomedical perspective on Anglo-American psychiatry. Am J Psychiatry *146:* 588, 1989.

Farmer A E, Falkowski W F: Maggot in the set, the snake factor, and the treatment of atypical psychosis in West African women. Br J Psychiatry *146:* 446, 1985.

Fisher W, Piazza C C, Page T J: Assessing independent and interactive effects of behavioral and pharmacological interventions for a client with dual diagnosis. J Behav Ther Exp Psychiatry *20:* 241, 1989.

German G A: Aspects of clinical psychiatry in sub-Saharan Africa. Br J Psychiatry *121:* 461, 1972.

Guinness E A: Patterns of mental illness in the early stages of urbanization. Br J Psychiatry *160* (16, Suppl): 4, 1992.

Indian Council of Medical Research: *Collaborative Study on the Phenomenology and Natural History of Acute Psychosis.* Author, New Delhi, 1989.

Jablensky A, Sartorius N, Ernberg G, Anker M, Korten A, Cooper J E, Day R, Bertelsen A: *Schizophrenia: Manifestations, Incidence and Course in Different Cultures; A World Health Organization Ten-Country Study.* Psychol Med [Monogr Suppl] *20,* 1992.

Johnson F A: African perspectives on mental disorder. In *Psychiatric Diagnosis: A World Perspective,* J E Mezzich, Y Honda, M C Kastrup, editors. Springer-Verlag, Berlin and New York, 1994.

Jorge M R, Mezzich J E: Latin American contributions to psychiatric nosology and classification. In *Psychiatric Diagnosis: A World Perspective,* J E Mezzich, Y Honda, M C Kastrup, editors. Springer-Verlag, Berlin and New York, 1994.
Karno M, Jenkins J H: Cultural considerations in the diagnosis of schizophrenia and related disorders and psychotic disorders not otherwise classified. In *DSM-IV Source Book,* T A Widiger, A Frances, H A Pincus, M B First, R Ross, W Davis, editors. American Psychiatric Press, Washington, 1994.
Kimura B: Longitudinal study of the relationship between EEG changes and clinical picture of atypical psychosis. Psychiatr Neurol Japonica *83:* 823, 1981.
*Kleinman A: *Rethinking Psychiatry.* Free Press, New York, 1988.
Leonhard K: *Aufteilung der Endogenen Psychosen.* Akademic Verlag, Berlin, 1957.
Lin K-M: Cultural influences on the diagnosis of psychotic and organic disorders. In *Culture and Psychiatric Diagnosis,* J E Mezzich, A Kleinman, H Fabrega, D L Parron, editors. American Psychiatric Press, Washington, 1995.
Lin K-M, Kleinman A M: Psychopathology and clinical course of schizophrenia: A cross-cultural perspective. Schizophr Bull *14:* 555, 1988.
Manschreck T C, Petri M: The atypical psychoses. Cult Med Psychiatry *2:* 233, 1978.
Mezzich J E, Jorge M R: Psychiatric nosology: Achievements and challenges. In *International Review of Psychiatry,* J A Costa e Silva, C C Nadelson, editors. American Psychiatric Press, Washington, 1993.
*Mezzich J E Kleinman A, Fabrega H, Parron D L: *Culture and Psychiatric Diagnosis.* American Psychiatric Press, Washington, 1995.
Mezzich J E, Kleinman A, Fabrega H, Parron D L, Good B J, Lin K-M, Manson S, editors: Cultural issues section. In *DSM-IV Source Book,* T A Widiger, A Frances, H A Pincus, M B First, R Ross, W Davis, editors. American Psychiatric Press, Washington, 1995.
Murphy H B M: *Comparative Psychiatry: The International and Intercultural Distribution of Mental Illness.* Springer-Verlag, Berlin and New York, 1982.
Perris C: *A Study of Cycloid Psychoses.* Munksgaard, Copenhagen, 1974.
Pull C B, Chaillet G: The nosological views of French-speaking psychiatry. In *Psychiatric Diagnosis: A World Perspective,* J E Mezzich, Y Honda, M C Kastrup, editors. Springer-Verlag, Berlin and New York, 1994.
Sartorius N, DeGirolamo G, Andrews G, German G A, Eisenberg L: *Treatment of Mental Disorders: A Review of Effectiveness.* World Health Organization and American Psychiatric Press, Washington, 1993.
Seguín C A: Psiquiatría Folklórica. Ediciones Errmar, Lima, Peru, 1979.
Shen Y C: On the second edition of the Chinese Classification of Mental Disorders. In *Psychiatric Diagnosis: A World Perspective,* J E Mezzich, Y Honda, M C Kastrup, editors. Springer-Verlag, Berlin and New York, 1994.
*Simons R C, Hughes C C: *The Culture-Bound Syndromes: Folk Illnesses of Psychiatric and Anthropological Interest.* D. Reidel, Dordrecht, Holland, 1985.
Strömgren E: Scandinavian contributions to psychiatric nosology. In *Psychiatric Diagnosis: A World Perspective,* J E Mezzich, Y Honda, M C Kastrup, editors. Springer-Verlag, Berlin and New York, 1994.
Susser E, Wanderling E: Epidemiology of non-affective acute remitting psychosis vs schizophrenia. Arch Gen Psychiatry *51:* 294, 1994.
Takahashi S: Diagnostic classification of psychotic disorders in Japan. In *Psychiatric Diagnosis: A World Perspective,* J E Mezzich, Y Honda, M C Kastrup, editors. Springer-Verlag, Berlin and New York, 1994.
Westermeyer J: *Mental Health for Refugees and Other Migrants.* Charles C Thomas, Springfield, IL, 1989.
*Wig N N, Parhee R: Acute and transient psychoses: A view from the developing countries. In *International Classification in Psychiatry: Unity and Diversity,* J E Mezzich, M von Cranach, editors. Cambridge University Press, Cambridge, 1988.
World Health Organization: *The ICD-10 Classification of Mental and Behavioral Disorders. Clinical Descriptions and Diagnostic Guidelines.* World Health Organization, Geneva, 1992.
World Health Organization: *The ICD-10 Classification of Mental and Behavioral Disorders. Diagnostic Criteria for Research.* World Health Organization, Geneva, 1993.
Yamashita I: *Periodic Psychosis of Adolescence.* Hokkaido University Press, Hokkaido, Japan, 1993.
Yamashita I: *Taijin Kyofu or Delusional Social Phobia.* Hokkaido University Press, Hokkaido, Japan, 1993.
Yap P M: *Comparative Psychiatry.* University of Toronto Press, Toronto, Canada, 1974.

15.4 POSTPARTUM PSYCHIATRIC SYNDROMES

BARBARA L. PARRY, M.D.

INTRODUCTION

Postpartum psychiatric illnesses are an underrecognized, undertreated, and underresearched area. One reason for the lack of attention to the disorders may be that postpartum psychiatric illnesses were not recognized as specific disorders before the fourth edition of the American Psychiatric Association's *Diagnostic and Statistical Manual of Mental Disorders* (DSM-IV), reportedly because the disorders were not considered to have distinguishing features.

Postpartum psychiatric syndromes are listed as onset specifiers under mood disorders. The specifier with postpartum onset can also be applied to brief psychotic disorder. Unfortunately, going against the recommendation of the advisory members, the work group specified that the onset of the episode must be within four weeks postpartum. Although most psychotic episodes do have their onset within four weeks postpartum, many depressive episodes occurring postpartum have an insidious onset beginning three to four months postpartum.

DEFINITION

Postpartum psychiatric syndromes are mental illnesses that occur primarily as psychotic and nonpsychotic mood disorders. By the definition of the Marcé Society (an international society for the understanding, prevention, and treatment of mental illness related to childbearing), the illnesses have their onset within the first year after childbirth (in contrast to DSM-IV's cutoff point of four weeks). Most postpartum psychiatric syndromes, once organic factors are ruled out, are mood disorders. In DSM-IV, both psychotic and nonpsychotic major depressions and manias that occur postpartum are categorized as specifiers under the mood disorders section. In the revised third edition (DSM-III-R) postpartum psychiatric illness was not listed as a separate category but was listed under psychotic disorder not otherwise specified (atypical psychosis). Little attention was paid to postpartum psychiatric illness in the ninth and tenth revisions of the International Classification of Diseases (ICD-9 and ICD-10). Table 15.4-1 presents the DSM-IV criteria for postpartum onset specifier.

TABLE 15.4-1
Criteria for Postpartum Onset Specifier

Specify if:
With postpartum onset (can be applied to the current or most recent major depressive, manic, or mixed episode in major depressive disorder, bipolar I disorder, or bipolar II disorder; or to brief psychotic disorder)
Onset of episode within four weeks postpartum

Table from DSM-IV, *Diagnostic and Statistical Manual of Mental Disorders,* ed 4. Copyright American Psychiatric Association, Washington, 1994. Used with permission.

HISTORY

Psychiatric illnesses after childbearing have many unique qualities that distinguish them from other kinds of psychiatric illnesses. The phenomenon was noticed and documented by the French physician Louis Victor Marcé, whose 1858 treatise on peripartum mental illness dominated world thinking on those matters for a half-century. Marcé noted that postpartum illness displays a wide variety of symptoms, many of which appear in illnesses unrelated to childbearing. He noted, however, that the combinations of symptoms and signs, the syndromes of postpartum illness, are unique, as are the ways in which syndromes change, go into remission, only to be followed by an exacerbation or a different syndrome. He also noted that the manifestations of postpartum illness move in tandem with the then-known changes in female anatomy and physiology as women move from the pregnant to the nonpregnant state. Assessing those associations and the pervasive occurrence of confusion and delirium, Marcé was convinced that he was dealing with conditions with organic causes, conditions in which known physical and chemical factors interfere with cerebral functioning: fevers, toxins, and psychological states associated with known medical disorders. He saw the rapid changes in the generative system as a cause, but he was unable to find the mechanism that bridges the gap between the physical phenomena and the mind. He was so certain of the connection that he gave it a name, *sympathie morbide*. He wrote and died a quarter of a century before the outlines of the endocrine system began to become apparent. For the rest of the 19th century and a decade into the 20th century, many astute observers and investigators supplied many details regarding the unique and wide-ranging presentations of psychiatric illness after childbearing.

Some time after the turn of the century, a substantial part of the psychiatric profession shifted its interest from the care of severely and acutely ill patients to intensive psychotherapy for neurotic patients. Patients who required hospitalization were cared for in state and private facilities, where patients and staff members were at some distance from the mainstream of modern medicine. Classification became a dominant concern in the psychiatric facilities, and psychiatrists found little basis to follow the medical practice of naming and classifying patients according to cause. They fell back on a second choice, classification according to constellations of symptoms. Postpartum patients exhibited a wide and widely changing array of symptoms and syndromes. The complex and changing presentation of symptoms was regarded as threatening to the new classification system. The simple solution advocated by some leaders of psychiatry and affirmed officially in 1952 by the American Psychiatric Association in DSM-I was to strike out the term "postpartum" and all its synonyms from the nomenclature and to recommend that psychiatric disorders after childbearing be classified and named according to the symptoms or syndrome that was predominant at the time of the examination.

The consequences were a setback for patient care and for the advancement of knowledge in postpartum psychiatric illnesses. The vast majority of physicians, especially those in the fields of psychiatry and obstetrics, decided that responsible committees of knowledgeable physicians had come to the conclusion that postpartum illnesses did not exist and that childbirth had simply exposed latent functional illnesses, such as schizophrenia and bipolar disorder. That conclusion led to precepts that dominated most of medical thinking until the early 1980s: (1) It is folly to look for unique qualities in postpartum cases; at most, the cases are epiphenomena and only questionably relevant to etiology or treatment. (2) The developing armamentarium of psychotropic drugs is appropriate and sufficient for psychiatric illness after childbearing.

Research on postpartum psychiatric illness was almost nonexistent for most of the 20th century. Some suggestive leads from the late 19th century were disregarded. The vast majority of patients were treated with the same drugs and methods as their sisters with functional disorders. That situation continued until 1980, when Ian Brockington called a conference on postpartum mental illness in Manchester, England. Worldwide interest and concern were disclosed. Two hundred clinicians and investigators with interest in the matters formed the Marcé Society, an international scientific organization devoted to the psychiatric illnesses of new mothers. As a result, research throve, and ideas germinated.

Fifteen years is insufficient for a final doctrine of diagnosis, etiology, and treatment. Some competent investigators opine that there are many possible morbid mechanisms and that it is too early to select those most likely to be responsible for postpartum illness. They believe that many years of extensive experimentation must precede the decision to introduce specific medications directed toward presumed disease mechanisms.

Nevertheless, a historical perspective lends itself to the following observations: When clinical cases are studied and when data from related areas in clinical medicine, endocrinology, and clinical chemistry are reviewed, a remarkably simple pattern of pathophysiology emerges. The pattern has had a number of clinical trials and standard experimental tests. There is support from many directions for the hypothesis that a causal relation exists between transitory hormonal deficits and two principal syndromes of postpartum mental illness, postpartum psychoses and postpartum major depression.

EPIDEMIOLOGY

POSTPARTUM PSYCHOSIS The frequency of postpartum psychosis in primiparous women (women who have given birth for the first time) is about 1 in 500. After a subsequent delivery, the risk for previously affected women is about 1 in 3.

POSTPARTUM NONPSYCHOTIC DEPRESSION The risk of nonpsychotic depression in primiparous women is 10 to 15 percent. The risk of recurrence is 50 percent in women without a prior history of a mood disorder and may approach 100 percent in those women with both a history of a mood disorder and a history of a previous postpartum major depressive disorder.

Maternity blues is not considered a disorder, since it generally occurs in 50 to 80 percent of women postpartum and because of the absence of major symptoms.

As several large-scale epidemiological studies have shown, the risk for major, hospitalizable mental illness during pregnancy is low—much lower than the expected rate in women not in the pregnant or postpartum state. However, the incidence of mental illness rises dramatically in the month after childbirth. That increased risk continues for six months to a year and in one study for up to two years postpartum. It is as though a protective factor against the onset of mental illness during pregnancy is released after childbirth.

ETIOLOGY

HORMONAL

Estradiol Since there is a marked elevation in estradiol during pregnancy, followed by an abrupt decline after parturition, a reasonable place to begin examining hormonal hypotheses of postpartum disorders is with this endocrine system. However, studies do not consistently show correlations between estradiol concentrations and postpartum blues, depression, or psychoses.

Progesterone One investigator claimed progesterone withdrawal as a cause of postpartum dysphoria on the basis of reports of the efficacy of progesterone treatment for the disorder and for premenstrual syndrome. However, that claim has not been substantiated by controlled clinical trials. Further substantive evidence for a progesterone deficiency as a basis for treating postpartum psychiatric syndromes is lacking. However, there are anecdotal reports of the efficacy of progesterone as a prophylactic treatment, although recent studies and progesterone's potential depressogenic side effects make it much less a viable prophylactic treatment than is lithium (Eskalith, Lithobid). Perhaps the therapeutic success achieved in those cases can be attributed to a change in progesterone-receptor sensitivity. The question needs rigorous clinical and biochemical evaluation.

Androgens In women both the ovaries and the adrenal cortex secrete the androgens testosterone and androstenedione. During pregnancy and lactation the cyclic variation of the ovarian secretion of those androgens is absent. Some studies report changes in levels of androgens associated with mood changes during the menstrual cycle and menopause. However, androgen therapy, given its masculinizing and depressive side effects, is warranted in postpartum depressive illness only for severe disorders and in those women who choose to refrain from breast feeding.

Cortisol Some of the hypotheses proposed to account for postpartum psychiatric disorders and possibly for other less severe syndromes include the following: The loss of the placenta at delivery is followed by a precipitous fall in both serum estrogen and progesterone. Those changes are not directly responsible for extensive psychological symptoms, but they initiate processes that lead eventually to symptoms. The circulation, the mass, and the secretory activity of the pituitary gland are decreased markedly during the days immediately after delivery. Serum cortisol is elevated during the last trimester. The sluggish postpartum pituitary decreases its adrenocorticotropic hormone (ACTH) stimulation of the adrenal cortex, and that diminution acts to decrease the serum cortisol, with the free and physiologically active cortisol decreasing more rapidly than the cortisol bound to transcortin. The symptoms of the early, florid postpartum psychosis may be a response to a deficit below the threshold of cortical neuron tolerance. Extreme anxiety symptoms, often prominent in the early cases, is the result of stimulation of the autonomic centers in the hypothalamus by the extensive and repeated discharge of adjacent neurons that are sensors of low serum cortisol. The insomnia that is characteristic of the disorder follows the stimulation of the sleep centers adjacent to the cortisol sensors. The rapid but usually temporary remissions may be attributable to irregular discharges of ACTH that temporarily remedy the cortisol deficit.

Another chain of evidence indicates that temporary cortisol deficit plays a role in many cases of postpartum psychiatric illness. In 1858 Marcé noted that postpartum patients who failed to recover tended to have weakness, anemia, and peripheral edema. Other observers noted headache, sleep disturbances, decrease in blood pressure, hair and skin changes, amenorrhea, and marked weight changes, either gains or losses. Those physical signs are similar to the signs seen in chronic disorders of the pituitary and adjacent brain areas. In the mid-1950s an investigator noted a similarity between patients with early postpartum illness and patients who became psychotic after withdrawal from cortisone treatment. The investigator administered 10 to 15 mg of prednisolone daily for two to three weeks and reported successful treatment of 16 patients, as compared with a fairly comparable group of 16 control patients. In 1984 the investigator reported on 10 additional cases of early postpartum illness treated successfully with prednisolone.

SHEEHAN'S SYNDROME In 1967 the endocrine pathologist Howard Sheehan began reporting on postpartum necrosis of the anterior pituitary, a condition in which blood loss at delivery is followed by circulatory collapse of the pituitary. That collapse produces a wide array of multiglandular disorders as pituitary tropic hormones are lost. Worldwide research in the field was summarized in a 1982 monograph. Among the sequelae described are a wide variety of psychiatric syndromes, including agitation, delirium, hallucinations, delusions, and depression. The similarities to the range and the quality of postpartum illness are notable. The symptoms and the syndromes tend to group themselves into two major patterns, an early agitated condition and a dull depressive condition. The physical stigmata of postpartum necrosis of the pituitary, Sheehan's syndrome, are like those described as characteristic of cases of postpartum psychiatric illness that become chronic.

The foregoing findings and observations lead directly to the hypothesis that postpartum psychiatric illness may be related to Sheehan's syndrome, with the postpartum psychiatric illness caused by a temporary deficit in pituitary-controlled hormones from a sluggish postpartum pituitary and Sheehan's syndrome following extensive destruction of pituitary secretory cells. After decades of experimentation, it was determined that fairly effective treatment of Sheehan's syndrome was a daily dose of 35 mg of cortisone acetate and 0.3 mg of thyroxine. With that medication the psychiatric symptoms of Sheehan's syndrome were said to disappear within a few days. Those are virtually the same hormones as those reported to be effective for the late depression, the desiccated thyroid, and the early agitated state. The combination of thyroxine and a steroid has never been reported with psychiatric patients. For definitely established Sheehan's syndrome, neither thyroid alone nor cortisone alone yields satisfactory results.

The concept of Sheehan's syndrome and postpartum psychiatric illness now can be extended. They could be opposite poles of a continuum, with Sheehan's syndrome following extensive infarction and cellular destruction of the pituitary and with the psychiatric disorders reflecting a sluggish postpartum pituitary with temporary deficits in the production of hormones from glands responsive to deficits in pituitary tropic hormones. Both in Sheehan's syndrome and in the psychiatric disorders, the most important hormones in deficit appear to be cortisol and thyroxine.

OTHER PITUITARY DEFICITS If the psychiatric disorders and Sheehan's syndrome are on a continuum, intermediate cases can be expected. When they are looked for, they seem to appear. Two investigators described a case of postpartum depression that was later found to have a half-empty sella turcica. In retrospect, some of the cases of chronic psychiatric illness described probably had pituitary damage. Marcé cited extensive loss of blood at delivery as one of the causes of postpartum *folie*.

Excessive bleeding is not necessary for a marked diminution of pituitary function to occur. Exquisite drawings of pituitary changes during pregnancy and the normal puerperium were published early in this century. Between delivery and a few days postpartum, the pituitary exhibits a markedly diminished size and blood supply and a marked decrease in the number of secretory cells. Secretory granules all but disappear.

The sequence of psychiatric symptoms relates to the possible influence of hormonal deficit. After three days but during the first fortnight after delivery, florid psychotic symptoms tend to make their appearance. After three weeks, depressive syndromes develop. Some cases have both types of psychiatric disorder, with an early florid psychosis moving gradually into a depression.

The hormonal sequence in the puerperium is this: Both serum cortisol and thyroxine are high at delivery and then begin to fall. Both hormones are still well above the prepregnancy level at the third day. Nevertheless, psychiatric symptoms of the early agitated syndrome or psychosis may emerge rapidly at or soon after the third day. However, physiologically significant deficits may occur in free cortisol. After delivery, free cortisol tends to fall off more rapidly than does bound cortisol. Cerebral impairment from free cortisol deficit could be the critical factor in the production of the mercurial early postpartum psychosis.

Recent studies do not consistently show differences in measurable cortisol between symptomatic and asymptomatic patients, although most of the symptomatic patients sampled were suffering from maternity blues, not postpartum psychoses. The studies, however, are limited by the lack of circadian sampling, which may indicate changes in the diurnal profile of cortisol secretion. Furthermore, patients with maternity blues, although more accessible to study, are not suffering from a major mood disorder, in which altered neuroendocrine profiles may be readily apparent.

Since baseline studies often do not indicate abnormalities that reveal themselves only when the system in question is challenged by experimental perturbations, it is worth examining the results of the dexamethasone-suppression test (DST), which challenges the glucocorticoid system, in patients with postpartum mood disturbances. However, since normal control women show a high incidence of altered DST responses in the immediate postpartum period, the DST cannot be considered a valid descriminator of postpartum depression, psychoses, and normal mood states during the postpartum period.

Thyroid hormones Postpartum depression of late onset has been attributed to thyroid disturbances. Thyroxine, which is high during the third trimester, decreases gradually as thyroid-stimulating hormone (TSH) from the pituitary diminishes after childbearing. After two or three weeks the declining thyroxine reaches a serum level near that of prepregnancy. The drop in thyroxine continues past the prepregnancy level and through a symptom threshold level in some cases. Depressive symptoms are frequent in hypothyroidism and myxedema. Somatic symptoms and signs characteristic of postpartum depression—including diminution of energy, peripheral edema, loss of hair, amenorrhea, and loss of sexual responsiveness—may also occur.

HISTORY The clues that support the foregoing thyroid hypothesis began to accumulate during the 19th century. Marcé reported a host of physical signs and symptoms in cases of depression of late onset, especially those that failed to recover quickly. He made the astute observation that the physical symptoms tended to precede the psychological symptoms. The medical condition of myxedema had not been explored in Marcé's time.

As early as the 16th century, a variety of mentally retarded, edematous dwarfs were reported to live in some of the valleys of the Swiss Alps. Some said that the creatures were the result of the mating of animals with maidens. Others insisted that the dwarfs were the progeny of human fathers and mothers; the dwarfs were human. In the local dialect "Christian" was synonymous with "human," so the dwarfs were called *crestin*. French physicians translated the designation of the dwarfs to "cretin," but not until the second half of the 19th century was it known that the dwarf owed a bizarre body and mental deficiency to a deficit of iodine in the Swiss valleys.

The occurrence of thyroid deficit as a sequel to pregnancy was first noted by the British physician William Withey Gull in 1874. The condition was briefly known as Gull's disease, but the surgeon William Miller Ord insisted that a descriptive term, myxedema, be used. (In *myxedema* a sticky, clear mucuslike fluid exudes when the edematous skin is punctured.) Ord prevailed, since he was chairman of a committee of the Clinical Society of London assigned to study the condition. The committee's report, published in 1883, described 109 dwarfs, 94 of whom were females. Half of the dwarfs had severe psychiatric disorders, described as melancholia, mania, and dementia. Insomnia and occipital headaches were frequent. Of the women, nearly all dated their illness to childbirth.

By the late 1890s biologically active desiccated thyroid became available, and a host of papers reported on trials of the new medication for many disorders. In 1901 an investigator summarized 42 reports on the administration of thyroid to a total of 638 patients who had myxedema and psychiatric symptoms for many years. Overall 50 percent were reported as recovered, with the investigator noting that patients resistant to treatment were those who had been ill for a long time. A wide range of psychiatric symptoms were reported to be benefited or cured. The most common symptoms were chronic depression and a stuporous condition the investigator described as that of a hibernating animal. Other frequent syndromes were delirium, hallucinations, flight of ideas, delusions, and dementia.

Thus, at the turn of the century, associations between childbearing, thyroid deficit, and psychiatric illness had been discovered. Nevertheless, dominant psychiatric thinking resisted and continues to resist the notion that postpartum diminution of serum thyroxine may be an important factor in postpartum psychiatric illness. A few physicians accidentally discovered the thyroid connection. In 1910 an investigator reported on a case with dramatic relief of postpartum depression after childbirth, and another clinician used thyroid extensively for depression of mood with loss of energy, diminished sexual responsiveness, and insufficient lactation. James Alexander Hamilton in the 1960s reported on the apparently successful use of thyroid in 29 cases of postpartum depression, later extended to more than 200 cases. When triiodothyronine was made available in 1957, it was seen as an opportunity to achieve a thyroid effect quickly and thereby facilitate controlled experimentation with postpartum depression. However, when that approach was attempted in a double-blind study, the rapid changes in mood between drug administration and placebo administration resulted in unacceptable suicidal hazards.

THYROID HORMONE DEFICITS Serum thyroxine, markedly elevated at the end of the third trimester, falls after delivery. On average it reaches and crosses the prepregnancy level three weeks postpartum, but there are individual differences. Recently, work suggests that some women with autoimmune thyroiditis may exhibit a postpartum peak, but that peak is followed by a drop in serum thyroxine. Ten percent of women have postpartum hypothyroidism peaking at four to five months postpartum; the extent of the hypothyroidism can be predicted by the measurement of thyroid antibodies early in pregnancy. The postpartum fall in thyroxine may pass through a threshold of symptom vulnerability to produce the physical and depressive symptoms noted more than 100 years ago.

Thyroid disturbances, particularly hypothyroidism and blunted TSH responses to thyrotropin-releasing hormone (TRH), tend to occur late, rather than early, in the course of postpartum mood disturbances. Large-scale studies examining sensitive thyroid tests in patients most likely to show disorders—that is, patients with late-onset major postpartum depression—are indicated. The limits of being able to do such studies, however, are apparent.

Other biological hypotheses Other hormonal systems that have been implicated in the pathophysiology of postpartum mood disorders but that are too premature to serve as the basis of treatment strategies include prolactin, tryptophan, beta-endorphin, oxytocin, and such neurotransmitters as norepinephrine, dopamine, and serotonin. In view of the disruption of normal daily and biological rhythms with the birth of an infant, consideration of chronobiological hypotheses and treatment strategies are in order and are currently under experimental investigation.

PSYCHOSOCIAL FACTORS Like other medical and psychiatric illnesses, postpartum psychiatric disorders can exacerbate under stress. The disruption of the mother's previous lifestyle and the strain the child can place on the marital relationship constitute significant stressors. However, the clinician should not regard stress alone as a precipitant to the major postpartum psychiatric disorders. Unfortunately, cases of postpartum psychoses have occurred after well-meaning physicians told their patients to reduce the stress in their lives to prevent the onset or the exacerbation of postpartum mood problems. As large-scale epidemiological studies have suggested, women who have significant stressors, such as those who are unmarried or who are from poor socioeconomic backgrounds, do not have higher than usual rates of postpartum psychiatric disorders. A history of infertility may be a risk factor. Particularly in the United States, the lack of an extended family in the home or nearby may precipitate a sense of isolation in the new mother, exacerbate her symptoms, and keep her from getting the help and the support she needs to care for a new infant. Such isolation can also inhibit the early recognition and treatment of postpartum mood disorders by a mental health professional. Psychological precipitants that can aggravate symptoms can be averted by sending a health care worker into the home, a custom endorsed in the United Kingdom. Psychodynamic theories—although they may be helpful, for example, in understanding the need for perfectionism in the mother and the resulting anxiety when perfection is inevitably thwarted by the child—do not provide encompassing explanations for the range, the domain, and the course of symptoms that are currently thought to have a predominantly hormonal cause.

Psychoanalytic explanations for postpartum depressions include a narcissistic loss of the independent self, which must now provide nurturance, rather than be the sole recipient of it. The loss of pregnancy is seen as a loss of closeness with the fetus and may be reminiscent of the loss of some other family member or loved one. In those cases the mother sees the baby as a version of herself. The shift of attention from the mother as a child to her being the source of comfort and gratification contributes to a sense of loss, deprivation, and fatigue. In delusional states the baby is seen as someone else, perhaps a sibling or a lost person with whom the mother shared an ambivalent relationship. Ambivalence in the relationship of the mother to her own mother may also be stimulated during the postpartum period, irrespective of the sex of the child. The infant may engender fantasies, meanings, dependency, and loss issues not unique to the particular mother-infant dyad. In psychoanalytic thinking, obsessional thoughts to hurt the child may derive from previously unacknowledged hostility feelings within the self that were not able to be tolerated by the self concept. Such psychoanalytic concepts have more bearing on the nonpsychotic depressions in the postpartum period than on the spectrum of psychotic postpartum psychiatric disorders, which warrant biological understanding and treatment.

PREDISPOSING FACTORS Primiparous women, women with personal or family histories of mood disorders, and women with previous episodes of depression or psychosis after childbirth are at higher than usual risk for the disorder. Large-scale epidemiological studies do not show that breast-feeding women versus nonbreast-feeding women show different incidences of postpartum psychiatric illness, although there are anectodal reports of women having more than usual mood disturbances after the cessation of breast feeding. Generally, studies show that obstetric variables (length of gestation or delivery, whether vaginal or cesarean, birth weight, dystocia) do not correlate with postpartum psychiatric problems. Obviously, perinatal death is a major loss and, thereby, a cause of depression in the mother, but that depression has a different cause and a different course than hormonally mediated postpartum psychiatric syndromes.

DIAGNOSIS AND CLINICAL FEATURES

Postpartum mood syndromes are listed, along with their clinical features and courses, in Table 15.4-2.

POSTPARTUM PSYCHOSIS The most severe postpartum disorder is an agitated, highly changeable psychosis that develops usually between the 3rd and the 14th day postpartum. The disorder may begin with confusion, depersonalization, and insomnia and then move rapidly to delirium, with prominent hallucinations and transitory delusions. The changeability is marked, so that the term "mercurial" has been applied to the

TABLE 15.4-2
Postpartum Mood Syndromes

	Frequency (all deliveries)	Clinical Features	Course
Maternity blues	50–80%	Crying Irritability Euphoria	3–10 days postpartum
Postpartum depression	10–15%	Melancholia Neurasthenia Insomnia (↓ stage 4 sleep)	80% have onset within six weeks postpartum (not before third postpartum day) Duration: 6–9 months
Postpartum psychosis	0.1%	90% mood disorders 40% mania Core schizophrenic symptoms absent Delirium, confusion	Acute onset within two weeks postpartum Good prognosis Duration: 2–3 months

psychosis. Syndromes may change rapidly. A manic state may appear to clear, only to be followed by a deep depression, which may continue for several days or weeks, followed by recovery or gradual evolution into a moderate depression. The course may be punctuated by occasional outbursts of florid psychosis. Eventually, after weeks or months, the disorder may clear.

Mrs. A was the 32-year-old wife of a physician. She had no personal or family history of psychiatric illness. She had been in good health, and there had been no complications during her pregnancy or delivery. She and her husband had planned for and been looking forward to the birth of their first child. There were no reported major life stressors. The four-year marital relationship was described as stable, and Mrs. A's husband appeared to be supportive.

One week postpartum Mrs. A began to be agitated and confused at certain times of the day. She said to her husband at one point that she had given birth to twin baby girls, rather than a baby boy. Those symptoms disappeared at other times of the day, and Mrs. A appeared to be perfectly normal. The patient was given haloperidol (Haldol), 2 mg at bedtime. Within one week her agitation and delusional symptoms resolved. The patient was followed at weekly intervals for six weeks before the medication was withdrawn. The patient continued to do well but was followed closely throughout the remainder of the postpartum period. Had her symptoms not been treated in their early stages, more severe consequences might have followed.

Informally, the terms "postpartum psychosis" and "puerperal psychosis" are applied to the disorder. The author has suggested that it be called "postpartum psychotic depression" to identify the depressive component. The initial risk for a postpartum psychosis is 1 in 500. However, once a woman has had an episode of postpartum psychosis, her risk for another psychotic episode after a subsequent delivery is about 1 in 3. It appears that women do not develop a tolerance for the disorder; rather, the course of the illnesses appears to obey the model of kindling and behavioral sensitization in that untreated episodes may become more severe and occur spontaneously with increasing frequency over time. One of the most unfortunate consequences of the disorder is that about 4 percent of women with a postpartum psychosis (not depression alone without psychosis) may commit infanticide. Thus, postpartum psychosis is the most severe of the postpartum psychiatric syndromes not only because of the nature of its symptoms but also because, if not recognized early and treated appropriately, it is likely to recur in the future and have potentially devasting consequences for the infant, the mother, her family, and society.

POSTPARTUM DEPRESSION The second postpartum disorder is a moderate to severe depression that begins insidiously after the second or third week postpartum, develops slowly for weeks or months, and then reaches a plateau or improves. The disorder is unofficially called "postpartum depression." The author has suggested "major postpartum depression." A common characteristic of the disorder is the frequency of somatic complaints, especially excessive fatigue. Studies generally indicate that the incidence of postpartum depression is approximately 10 to 15 percent. The disorder may not become apparent until the fourth or fifth month postpartum (the peak incidence of postpartum hypothyroidism) and thus may be missed or at least not attributed to the postpartum state. The risk of developing a postpartum psychosis or depression may continue for a year or, according to some investigators, up to two years postpartum.

Mrs. B was a 36-year-old previously employed primipara with no personal or family history of mood disorders, but she had a father with alcoholism. No problems were reported during the planned pregnancy, and the delivery was uncomplicated. On the fifth day postpartum the patient reported feeling anxious, shaky, and jittery. Over the next week to 10 days, the symptoms progressed until she felt she could not sit still. She had trouble sleeping, and she lost her appetite. She had never had symptoms like those before. She complained of episodes, lasting 1½ to 2 hours, characterized by tightness in her chest, palpitations, and shortness of breath—all associated with a sense of doom.

Her family physician prescribed lorazepam (Ativan) 1 mg as needed. After she had used it for a week, it was deemed not appropriate to continue the medication. Since she was also describing symptoms of depersonalization, she was given perphenazine (Trilafon) 4 mg for sedation and nortriptyline (Aventyl, Pamelor) 50 mg at bedtime for what was seen as an anxious, agitated depression. Her agitated symptoms resolved over the next two weeks. The periphenazine was subsequently withdrawn. The patient appeared to stabilize, but about the third month postpartum the symptoms of a retarded depression began to appear. The nortriptyline dosage was increased to 75 mg to obtain values in the upper range of therapeutic levels. Her depressive symptoms improved. She still noted her increased vulnerability to daily stressors. Therapeutic strategies were discussed and developed to help her get help in the home and to decrease her sense of isolation. She joined a support group and started addressing her own issues of perfectionism and control, derived from her alcoholic family background, that were being frustrated by the inevitable chaos resulting from having an infant in the home. At almost a year postpartum she was dealing with the issues of returning to work, her mood was stabilized, and she felt that she had a good support structure behind her to deal with the added stressors and vicissitudes of returning to the work force. She felt that she could not have addressed the work issues, as well as the home issues, before that time.

That case illustrates how postpartum psychiatric syndromes can initially present with anxious, agitated features resembling a panic disorder and then progress to a retarded depression later in the postpartum course. It also points to the need for longitudinal follow-up in patients. Often, the dynamic issues present themselves and the patients are ready to deal with those issues only after the acute symptoms are treated with pharmacological measures.

MATERNITY BLUES Postpartum major depressive disorder and psychosis need to be distinguished from a condition known as the maternity blues or baby blues, which is not considered to be a disorder; it does not impair functioning, and it occurs in a majority of women. The maternity blues may occur in 50 to 80 percent of women. The condition is characterized by crying, irritability, rapid mood shifts, and even euphoria; it generally appears after the third day postpartum and usually resolves spontaneously within a week. Education and reassurance are indicated, rather than pharmacological treatment, which is generally not needed unless the condition develops subsequently (but rarely) into a severe disorder.

Mrs. C returned home after the delivery of her first child. Her husband was concerned because she would burst into tears at the drop of a pin. He had previously known her to be sound, stable, and not prone to outbursts. He knew how much she had looked forward to the birth of their child, so he could not understand why she would suddenly get upset. She would say that nothing was bothering her and that she did not know why she was tearful. At times, she appeared to be perfectly happy—in fact, unusually boisterous and euphoric. At other times, she would get irritable over the least little things.

The patient and her husband were given reassurance and education that hers was a normal reaction and that it would most likely resolve on its own over the course of the next week to 10 days, which it did.

DIFFERENTIAL DIAGNOSIS

Although postpartum psychiatric disorders are predominantly mood disorders, they may manifest in a variety of clinical syndromes. They may appear as anxiety disorders, obsessive-compulsive disorders, rapid-cycling mood disorders or cyclothymia, schizophreniform disorders, and such organic disorders as Cushing's syndrome and hypothyroidism, which may present as a delirium. The key to making the diagnosis is recognition of the onset and the course of symptoms having their onset within the first 12 months postpartum.

COURSE AND PROGNOSIS

Postpartum psychosis usually has its onset within the first two weeks postpartum. If treated early and aggressively, it generally has a good prognosis. It may develop into a depression later in its course during the postpartum period. Like psychosis, postpartum depression has a good prognosis with early recognition and treatment, although its onset may be more insidious than postpartum psychosis and not appear until the third or fourth month postpartum. If left untreated, both postpartum depression and postpartum psychosis may become chronic and refractory to treatment, extend into the second and third year postpartum, and cause significant impairment, morbidity, and even mortality.

TREATMENT

A rational treatment plan for postpartum depression and postpartum psychosis cannot be developed from double-blind, placebo-controlled crossover trials of pharmacological or psychotherapeutic interventions. Because the illnesses can be devastating to the mother and her family, clinicians have used whatever interventions have been immediately useful and available. In the literature the majority of the scientifically rigorous treatment studies are confined to studies of patients with maternity blues—that is, women without severe disorders. By necessity, suggested treatment approaches discussed here reflect clinical experience more than information derived from research investigations.

The first principle of treating postpartum depression and postpartum psychosis is that organic illnesses must be ruled out. An initial presentation of postpartum psychiatric illness may be due to an underlying Sheehan's syndrome, thyrotoxicosis (if presenting as an acute psychosis in the first month after delivery), or hypothyroidism (if presenting as a major depression in the fourth or fifth month postpartum). All too often those medical emergencies are overlooked, with disastrous consequences. One of the first crucial steps in the initial evaluation and treatment of postpartum disorders, as in other medical and psychiatric disorders, is a thorough history, physical examination, and laboratory tests.

The other important principle guiding treatment is that the earlier the symptoms are recognized and treated, the better. For example, postpartum psychosis may initially present with symptoms of depersonalization: the patient may feel distant from her child and from the situation at hand. She may feel that she is just an onlooker (portrayed in the film "Rosemary's Baby"). The phenomenon may be interpreted as a failure to bond, but it more likely represents the initial presentation of an emerging psychosis. Patients may then have strange and bizarre sensations or may think that the child's head is separate from the baby's body. If treatment is instituted with small doses of an antipsychotic medication, the symptoms may resolve without a few days or a week. However, if not recognized and treated in its initial stages, the symptoms may rapidly progress to paranoid delusions and a frank agitated psychosis, which may become severe, refractory to treatment, and likely to recur over the next six months to a year. Without aggressive management and early detection, the symptoms may extend into the second and third years postpartum.

Because of the changing nature of postpartum psychiatric illness, different treatments at different stages of the illness are indicated. For example, an early presentation of psychosis is best treated with antipsychotic medication. However, the psychosis may resolve, and the patient may then have symptoms of major depression that require antidepressant medication. Furthermore, the initial presentation of the depression may appear in an agitated form, with many anxious features and insomnia. Then treatment with a sedative antidepressant, such as imipramine (Tofranil), is indicated, whereas later the patient may present with symptoms of a retarded, anergic depression, sometimes with obsessive-compulsive features, in which an activating or serotonergic compound, such as fluoxetine (Prozac), may be indicated. Different treatment modalities may have differential effects and efficacies, depending on when in the course of the illness those treatments are administered.

POSTPARTUM PSYCHOSIS One of the most important aspects of the management of postpartum psychosis is that the earlier it is recognized and treated, the more likely it is to respond to treatment and to have a positive outcome and prognosis. Since most postpartum psychoses have an onset within the first two weeks postpartum (generally not until after the third postpartum day) and 80 percent of them occur within one month postpartum, clinicians should be on the alert for early signs of depersonalization, delusional thinking, mania, or bizarre behavior, especially if the woman has a previous history of postpartum psychiatric illness or a mood disorder. The clinician should hospitalize any patient with symptoms of an impending postpartum psychosis. Early hospitalization can prevent infanticide and suicide, which may occur when mothers at risk are left alone at home to care for their infants.

Often, small (2 to 5 mg) doses of antipsychotics—such as haloperidol or, if that is too potent, perphenazine or loxapine (Loxitane)—may decrease the symptoms and prevent the development of a severe psychosis.

If the symptoms of an emerging postpartum psychosis are recognized and treated early, they may resolve within a week. Cases in which the symptoms are not recognized and treated in their initial stages may become refractory to treatment and take a long time to resolve. In general, however, the postpartum psychoses have a good prognosis, resolve in two to three weeks, and are amenable to treatment. Postpartum psychosis is the condition under which women are most likely to commit infanticide; an estimated 4 percent of women with postpartum psychoses commit infanticide. That consequence generally does not occur unless the woman is psychotic. The tragedy is made all the more poignant by the recognition that the disorder is otherwise amenable to treatment, and the tragedy is, thereby, preventable.

Although dosages of antipsychotics can be reduced after the initial episode of psychosis is resolved, the reduction should be done gradually and cautiously. Women remain at risk for recurrences, particularly those women with a previous history of psychiatric illness, for at least 6 months and sometimes up to 12 months postpartum. Data from a large-scale epidemiological study in Edinburgh, Scotland, suggest an increased risk for psychiatric admissions for up to two years postpartum. Although the clinician need not maintain a patient on antipsychotic medication for that length of time, the clinician should be on the alert for early signs of recurrence and should remember that a patient who initially presents with symptoms of a postpartum psychosis within the first few weeks after delivery may have symptoms of a postpartum depression later in the course of her illness—for example, four or five months postpartum. In an early onset of psychoses, patients should probably continue to take antipsychotics for at least six weeks postpartum. Antipsychotics are not contraindicated with breast feeding.

As in other psychiatric illnesses, postpartum psychosis responds best to psychopharmacological measures when they are combined with psychotherapeutic interventions. Pharmacological intervention is urgently needed to keep the mother from becoming increasingly psychotic and committing infanticide. At that point the patient is not cognitively and emotionally available to participate in a psychotherapeutic interaction until the medications reduce the hallucinations, delusions, and agitated behavior. However, as most clinicians and even psychotic patients appreciate, medications are most likely to be received and taken willingly when the patient and her family perceive some sense of rapport, trust, and support from the physician.

POSTPARTUM DEPRESSION In contrast to postpartum psychosis, which has an onset early in the postpartum period, postpartum depression generally has an insidious onset that may occur later, such as four to five months postpartum, and may range from mild to moderate dysthymia and anxiety disorders to major melancholia. As with the postpartum psychoses, organic abnormalities—particularly hypothyroidism, which occurs in 10 percent of women postpartum, with a peak incidence at four to five months—need to be ruled out. Transient hyperthyroidism may appear early in the postpartum course. Indications for the use of antidepressant medication are similar to those for other mood disorders and include the presence of neurovegetative signs. Untreated episodes tend to become severe, frequent, and often refractory to treatment. The depressive episodes should be treated aggressively with both pharmacological and psychotherapeutic strategies early in the course to prevent untoward biological and psychological consequences. Since many of the depressions may appear with obsessive-compulsive features, implicating serotonergic mechanisms, recent clinical experience suggests the efficacy of the serotonergic antidepressants, such as fluoxetine. However, side effects, particularly agitation, need to be monitored closely, and fluoxetine should not be the first line of treatment in the anxious depressions often seen early in the postpartum state.

For patients who present with symptoms of agitated and anxious depressions, such sedative antidepressants as imipramine are appropriate. If agitated depressive symptoms occur early in the postpartum state, small doses of antipsychotics can be beneficial. Anxiolytics are best avoided because of their risk for the development of physiological dependence, withdrawal, and exacerbation of agitation and because of their inadvisability for use in breast-feeding women. When using an antidepressant, the clinician should advise the woman to stop breast feeding, as some studies indicate that small amounts of the drug may be excreted into the breast milk. If administering antidepressant drugs to a postpartum patient, the clinician should rule out hypothyroidism, closely follow the course and the timing of the patient's mood changes, and discontinue the antidepressant if the woman shows evidence of drug-induced rapid cycling. In the potentially hypothyroid postpartum state, antidepressants may induce rapid cycling and are not recommended in breast-feeding women. Being female, being in the postpartum state, and being hypothyroid are all risk factors for tricyclic-induced rapid cycling.

Recently, estrogen skin patches have been reported to be beneficial in severe postpartum depression. For postpartum dysphoria one investigator has recommended progesterone treatment (100 mg intramuscularly [IM] for the first postpartum week and then 400 mg twice a day by suppository for two or more months postpartum). However, some clinicians and investigators find that progesterone may exacerbate depression.

For severe or psychotic postpartum depression or mania refractory to pharmacotherapy, electroconvulsive therapy (ECT) remains the treatment of choice. Sleep deprivation has therapeutic efficacy in a majority of patients with major depressive disorders. The efficacy of sleep deprivation in postpartum mood disorders is currently under experimental investigation. The relapse that may occur after sleep deprivation may be averted with lithium.

Since the experience of a postpartum depression can be cognitively and emotionally disruptive for the woman and her family, the disorder, like other psychiatric disorders, is best treated with a combination of pharmacological and psychotherapeutic management. The clinician should provide education, support, and cognitive structuring so that the patients and their families can find some method out of the madness that stems from the confusing, disorienting, and emotionally traumatic cataclysm in their lives.

Anthropological studies indicate that other cultures have rituals allowing for 40-day rest periods for the mother after the birth of a baby in which to mother the mother. During that time period, the focus is on allowing the mother time to rest, recuperate, eat, and sleep. Female relatives come to the home to prepare meals, do housework, and care for the infant. Thus, social support, education, child care services, and social recognition of the new motherhood status is ensured. In this country in the past a one-week hospital stay for the mother was required after delivery. Now, the mother usually goes home a day after delivery and often without an extended family or neighbors to help with infant care. In that isolated environment, the woman does not receive the supportive therapeutic factors that would help mitigate the development or the exacerbation of a spectrum of nonpsychotic depressions.

MATERNITY BLUES As mentioned earlier, the maternity blues is not considered a disorder, since it occurs in 50 to 80 percent of women and because of the absence of major symptoms. The blues is best treated with reassurance that the symptoms occur in a majority of women and that they generally improve spontaneously in a week to 10 days. In rare instances the symptoms may progress to a severe postpartum disorder, a fact that stresses the necessity of making frequent follow-up visits. However, that progression is the exception, rather than the general rule.

In contrast to postpartum psychosis, pharmacological intervention is generally not warranted for the maternity blues. Instead, psychotherapeutic intervention in the form of education, support, and reassurance is needed.

PROPHYLAXIS Since there is a high recurrence rate for both postpartum psychosis (initial risk, 1 in 500; recurrent risk, 1 in 3) and postpartum depression (initial risk, 1 in 10; recurrent risk, 1 in 2), prophylactic treatment for women, particularly for those who have a previous history of mood disorders, is an integral part of the management of the disorders.

Patients with a previous history of nonpuerperal mood disorders are three times more likly to have postpartum mood disorders, particularly mania, than are women who had no history of mood disorders. One of the most effective prophylactic interventions is lithium. Although lithium dosage should be halved about one week before delivery because of marked fluid and electrolyte changes occurring in the woman then, it can be restarted shortly after delivery. However, lithium, in contrast to antipsychotic medication, is contraindicated in breast-feeding women. Clinicians should be particularly alert for lithium-induced hypothyroidism in postpartum women, since 90 percent of lithium patients with hypothyroidism are women and since the postpartum period presents a particular risk factor for the development of hypothyroidism. Furthermore, postpartum hypothyroidism may induce rapid mood cycling.

Patients with a previous history of mood disorders may have an exacerbation of their illness during pregnancy. Although lithium is contraindicated during the first trimester because of the infant's risk for Ebstein's anomaly of the heart, in severe cases lithium may be administered cautiously, checking particularly for fluid and electrolyte changes in the woman, during the third trimester. For mania occurring during pregnancy, antipsychotics or ECT can be given without undue risk to the fetus.

Another prophylactic treatment that has received attention, although it is controversial, is progesterone (100 mg IM after labor, daily for seven days, then progesterone suppositories for two months or until the return of menstruation). Since progesterone is essentially an anesthetic in animals, its use in humans is probably more effective for the agitated than for the depressive symptoms of postpartum psychiatric syndromes. It may exacerbate depressive symptoms.

One additional body of information supports the hypothesis that postpartum illnesses are unique and organic in cause: reports of the successful use of three different substances for prophylaxis in high-risk patients—that is, patients who have had previous postpartum psychoses or depressions. The three substances are long-acting parenteral estrogen, long-acting progesterone, and pyridoxine, although lithium prophylaxis is at present the mainstay of treatment for recurrent mood disorders.

SUGGESTED CROSS-REFERENCES

Further information on the reproductive endocrinology of pregnancy and the postpartum period and guidelines for the use of psychotropics during pregnancy and lactation can be found in Section 29.4 on psychiatry and reproductive medicine. Mood disorders are discussed at length in Chapter 16, and brief psychotic disorder is discussed in Section 15.1.

REFERENCES

Boyd D A: Mental disorders associated with childbearing. Am J Obstet Gynecol *43:* 148, 1942.

*Brockington I F, Kumar R, editors: *Motherhood and Mental Illness.* Academic Press, London, 1982.

Cox J L, Murray D, Chapman C: A controlled study of the onset, duration and prevalence of postnatal depression. Br J Psychiatry *163:* 27, 1993.

Dalton K: *Depression after Childbirth.* Oxford University Press, Oxford, 1980.

Glover V, Liddle P, Taylor A, Adams D, Sandler M: Mild hypomania (the highs) can be a feature of the first postpartum week—association with later depression. Br J Psychiatry *164:* 517, 1994.

Gull W W: On a cretinoid state supervening in adult life in women. Trans Clin Soc London *7:* 180, 1874.

*Hamilton J A: *Postpartum Psychiatric Problems.* Mosby, St. Louis, 1962.

*Hamilton J A, Harberger P N: *Postpartum Psychiatric Illness: A Picture Puzzle.* University of Pennsylvania Press, Philadelphia, 1992.

Harris B: A hormonal component to postnatal depression. Br J Psychiatry *163:* 403, 1993.

Henderson A F, Gregoire A J P, Kumar R C, Studd, J W W: Treatment of severe postnatal depression with oestradiol skin patches. Lancet *338:* 816, 1991.

*Kendall R E, Chalmers J C, Platz C: Epidemiology of puerperal psychoses. Br J Psychiatry, *150:* 662, 1987.

Kitamura T, Shima S, Sugawara M, Toda M A: Psychological and social correlates of the onset of affective disorders among pregnant women. Psychol Med *23:* 967, 1993.

*Kumar R, Brockington I F: *Motherhood and Mental Illness,* ed 2: *Causes and Consequences.* Butterworth, London, 1988.

Lovestone S, Kumar R: Postnatal psychiatric illness: The impact on partners. Br J Psychiatry *163:* 210, 1993.

Marcé L V: *Traite de la folie des femmes encientes, des nouvelles accouchees et des nourrices.* Bailliere, Paris, 1858.

Parry B L, editor: *Women's Disorders.* Saunders, Philadelphia, 1989.

Pedersen C A, Stern R A, Pate J, Senger M A, Bowes W A, Mason G A: Thyroid and adrenal measures during late pregnancy and the puerperium in women who have been major depressed or who become dysphoric postpartum. J Affect Disord *29:* 201, 1993.

Railton I: The use of corticoids in postpartum depression. J Am Med Wom Assoc *16:* 450, 1961.

Sheehan H L, Davis J C: *Postpartum Hypopituitarism.* Thomas, Springfield, IL, 1982.

Strecker E A, Ebaugh F G: Psychoses occurring during the puerperium. Arch Neurol Psychiatry *15:* 239, 1926.

Whiffen V E, Gotlib I H: Comparison of postpartum and nonpostpartum depression—clinical presentation, psychiatric history, and psychosocial functioning. J Consult Clin Psychol *61:* 485, 1993.

Wisner K L, Peindl K, Hanusa B H: Relationship of psychiatric illness to childbearing status—a hospital-based epidemiologic study. J Affect Disord *28:* 39, 1993.

Wisner K L, Peindl K, Hanusa B H: Symptomatology of affective and psychotic illnesses related to childbearing. J Affect Disord *30:* 77, 1994.

Wisner K L, Perel J M, Wheeler S B: Tricyclic dose requirements across pregnancy. Am J Psychiatry *150:* 1541, 1993.

CHAPTER 16 MOOD DISORDERS

16.1 MOOD DISORDERS: INTRODUCTION AND OVERVIEW

HAGOP S. AKISKAL, M.D.

PRESENT SCOPE OF MOOD DISORDERS

PUBLIC HEALTH SIGNIFICANCE Known for nearly 2,500 years, mood disorders continue to command major public health interest. Especially in their depressive forms, they are among the most common maladies, affecting at least 12 percent of women and 8 percent of men at some time during life. Those figures are extrapolated from the National Institute of Mental Health (NIMH) Epidemiologic Catchment Area studies performed in five sites in the United States. Despite the availability of effective treatment, many persons with mood disorders are disabled, and rates of suicide, a complication occurring in about 15 percent of depressive disorders, are high in young and, especially, elderly men. Thus, although depressive disorders are more common in women, more men than women die of suicide.

The epidemiological trends cannot be ascribed to underdiagnosis and undertreatment alone. The arguments are several. First, Gerald Klerman and colleagues suggest that the incidence of mood disorders may be increasing in younger age groups, especially in cohorts born in the 1960s, and may be associated with rising rates of alcohol and substance abuse. Second, mood disorders, once believed to be essentially adult disorders, are increasingly diagnosed in children and adolescents. Third, clinical studies suggest higher rates of chronicity, recurrence, and refractoriness than previously believed. For instance, chronicity, reported by Emil Kraepelin to be no more than 5 percent at the turn of the century in Germany, is now seen in about 15 percent of cases of mood disorders in Western countries.

BROADENING THE BOUNDARIES OF MOOD DISORDERS Current conceptualization of mood disorders in the United States embraces a wide spectrum of disorders, including many conditions previously diagnosed as schizophrenia, personality disorder, or neurosis. The diagnostic shift occurred in part as a result of the United States-United Kingdom Diagnostic Project, which demonstrated that schizophrenia was being diagnosed at the expense of mood disorders (Figure 16.1-1). The broadening of the conceptual boundaries was further stimulated by the availability of new and effective treatments, both somatic and psychotherapeutic, and by the high risk for tardive dyskinesia and suicide in persons with mood disorders incorrectly given other diagnoses. Present research interest in mood disorders emanated from a landmark NIMH conference on the psychobiology of affective illnesses, published in 1972. The NIMH Collaborative Depression Study—a long-term prospective project deriving directly from recommendations made at the conference—has legitimatized the broader perspective. Nevertheless, current data (summarized by Martin Keller and collaborators) suggest widespread undertreatment of mood disorders.

In Europe, where the concept of mood disorders has historically embraced a broad spectrum of disorders, the work of two British schools of thought has been influential. The Maudsley school—Aubrey Lewis and his followers—has promoted a continuum model from anxiety disorders to mild neurotic depressions to severe endogenous and psychotic depressions, whereas the Newcastle school, led by Martin Roth, has sharply demarcated those conditions from one another. Although vestiges of both approaches are still influential in clinical and basic research, their significance seems overshadowed by continental European studies that subdivide mood disorders on the basis of polarity: unipolar (depressive episodes only) and bipolar (depressive episodes plus manic or hypomanic episodes). That subdivision, supported by studies in the United States, has served as the basis for much recent research into and classification of mood disorders, as reflected in the fourth edition of *Diagnostic and Statistical Manual of Mental Disorders* (DSM-IV) and the 10th revision of the *International Classification of Diseases and Related Health Problems* (ICD-10).

CONCEPTS AND DEFINITIONS

Mood disorders encompass a large group of psychiatric disorders in which pathological moods and related vegetative and psychomotor disturbances dominate the clinical picture. Known in previous editions of DSM as affective disorders, the term "mood disorders" is preferred today because it refers to sustained emotional states and not merely to the external (affective) expression of the present emotional state. Mood disorders are best considered as syndromes (rather than discrete diseases) that consist of a cluster of signs and symptoms that are sustained over a period of weeks to months, represent a marked departure from a person's habitual functioning, and tend to recur, often in periodic or cyclical fashion.

MAJOR DEPRESSIVE DISORDER AND BIPOLAR DISORDERS Major depressive disorder, sometimes called unipolar depression (not a DSM-IV term), is the most common mood disorder. It may manifest as a single episode or as recurrent episodes. The course may be somewhat protracted—up to two years or longer—in those with the single episode form. Whereas the prognosis for recovery from an acute episode is good for most patients with major depressive disorder, two out of three patients experience recurrences throughout life, with varying degrees of residual symptoms between episodes.

Bipolar disorder, previously called manic-depressive disorder (not a DSM-IV diagnosis), consists of at least one excited (manic or hypomanic) episode; although some patients experience only manic episodes, most end up having one or more depressive episodes. During the numerous recurrences of the

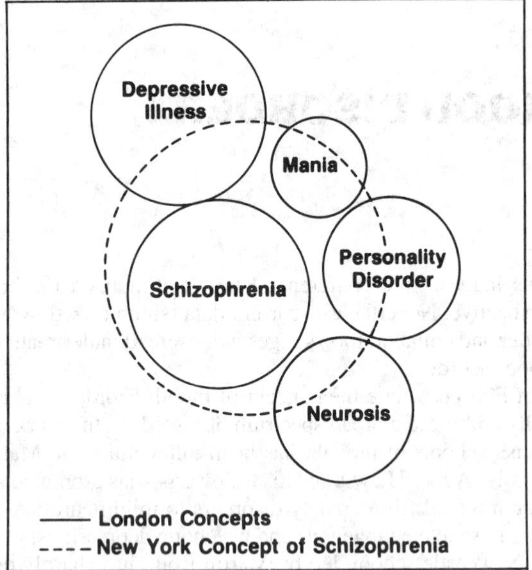

FIGURE 16.1-1 *Comparison of British (London) and United States (New York) concepts of schizophrenia. (Figure from J E Cooper, R E Kendell, B J Garland, L Sharpe, J R M Copeland, R Simon:* Psychiatric Diagnosis in New York and London. *Oxford University Press, London, 1972. Used with permission).*

alternating or cyclical phases, about one third of patients also develop mixed states, comprising simultaneous depressive and manic symptoms. The bipolar disorders were classically described as psychotic mood disorders with both manic and major depressive episodes (now termed bipolar I disorder), but recent clinical studies have shown the existence of a spectrum of ambulatory depressive states that alternate with milder and short-lived periods of hypomania rather than full-blown mania (bipolar II disorder). Those subdivisions within the larger group of bipolar disorders have focused attention on the entire range of bipolar disorders. Bipolar II disorder, which is not always easily discriminable from recurrent major depressive disorder, illustrates the need for more research to elucidate the relationship between bipolar disorders and major depressive disorder.

CYCLOTHYMIC DISORDER AND DYSTHYMIC DISORDER Clinically, it is observed that major depressive episodes often arise from low-grade intermittent or chronic depression known as dysthymic disorder. Likewise, many instances of bipolar disorders, especially ambulatory forms, represent episodes of mood disorder superimposed on a cyclothymic background, that is, numerous brief periods of hypomania alternating with numerous brief periods of depression. Dysthymia and cyclothymia were two of the basic temperaments described by Kraepelin and Ernst Kretschmer as predisposing persons to affective illness. Cyclothymic disorder and dysthmic disorder frequently coexist with borderline personality disorder.

It is not always easy to demarcate full-blown syndromal episodes of depression and mania from their subsyndromal temperamental counterparts commonly observed during the interepisodic periods. The subsyndromal episodes appear to be fertile ground for interpersonal conflicts and postaffective pathological character developments that may ravage the lives of patients and their families. In North America many such patients end up being labeled with borderline personality disorder.

Cyclothymic disorder and dysthymic disorder also exist in the community as subaffective disorders without progression to full-blown mood disorder episodes. However, at least one out of three persons with those disorders does make the transition to a major mood disorder. Understanding the factors that mediate the transition is important for preventing manic and depressive episodes.

COMORBID DISORDERS Mood disorders, especially depressive disorders, overlap considerably with anxiety disorders. As summarized in an NIMH monograph edited by Jack Maser and Robert Cloninger, anxiety disorders can occur during an episode of depression, may be a precursor to the depressive episode, and, less commonly, may occur during the future course of a mood disorder. Those findings suggest that at least some depressive disorders share a common diathesis with certain anxiety disorders. Other NIMH epidemiological research indicates that comorbidity of mood (especially bipolar) disorder and substance and alcohol abuse is common. In some cases the alcohol or substance abuse may represent an attempt at self-treatment of the mood disorder. Finally, physical illness—both systemic and cerebral—occurs in association with mood disorders with a frequency greater than would be expected by chance alone.

NEED FOR CLINCAL INTEGRATION Research on comorbid conditions is in early stages and is not further elaborated in this section. Instead, the discussion focuses on the major conceptual developments that have shaped current views of mood disorders and have contributed to an integrative pathogenetic framework that takes into account the interactions of social, psychological, and biological factors as originally formulated by the author and William McKinney in 1973. An integrated framework of pathogenesis is necessary for understanding psychopharmacological, somatic, and psychotherapeutic approaches in the clinical management of patients with mood disorders.

CLASSICAL DESCRIPTIONS OF MELANCHOLIA AND MANIA

Much of what is known today about mood disorders was described by the ancient Greeks and Romans. The terms "melancholia" and "mania" were coined and their relation was noted. The ancients also hypothesized a temperamental origin for those disorders. Much of modern thinking about mood disorders, as exemplified by the work of the French and German schools in the middle and latter part of the 19th century—which influenced current British and American concepts—can be traced back to these ancient concepts.

MELANCHOLIA Hippocrates (460–357 BC) described melancholia ("black bile") as a state of "aversion to food, despondency, sleeplessness, irritability, [and] restlessness." Thus, in choosing the name of the condition, Greek physicians, who may have borrowed the concept from ancient Egyptians, postulated the earliest biochemical formulation of any mental disorder. They further believed the illness often arose from the substrate of the somber melancholic temperament, which, under the influence of the planet Saturn, made the spleen secrete black bile, which ultimately darkened the mood through its influence on the brain. Greek descriptions of the clinical manifestations of depression and of the temperament prone to melancholia are reflected in the DSM-IV and in the subdepressive lethargy, self-denigration, and habitual gloom of the person with dysthymic disorder.

One of the Hippocratic aphorisms recognized the close link between anxiety and depressive states: "Patients with fear . . . of long-standing are subject to melancholia." According to Galen (AD 131–201), melancholia manifested in "fear and depression, discontent with life, [and] hatred of all people." A few hundred years later another Roman, Aurelianus, citing the now lost works of Soranus of Ephesus, amplified the role of aggression in melancholia (and its link to suicide) and described how the illness assumed delusional coloring: "Animosity toward members of the household, sometimes a desire to live and at other times a longing for death, suspicion on the part of the patient that a plot is being hatched against him."

In addition to natural melancholia, which arose from an innate predisposition to overproduce the dark humor and led to a more severe form of the malady, Greco-Roman medicine recognized such nonnatural (environmental) contributions to melancholia as immoderate consumption of wine, perturbations of the soul due to the passions (for example, love), and disturbed sleep cycles. Autumn was considered to be the season most disposing to melancholy.

MANIA A state of raving madness with exalted mood was noted by the ancient Greeks, although it referred to a somewhat broader group of excited psychoses than in modern nosology. Its relation to melancholia was probably noted as early as the first century BC, but according to Aurelianus, Soranus discounted it. Nonetheless, Soranus had observed the coexistence of manic and melancholic features during the same episode, consisting of continual wakefulness and fluctuating states of anger and merriment, sometimes of sadness and futility. Soranus thus seemed to have described what today are called mixed episodes in DSM-IV. Although natural melancholy was generally considered a chronic disorder, Soranus noted the tendency for attacks to alternate with periods of remission.

Although others prior to him hinted at it, Aretaeus of Cappadocia (circa AD 150) is generally credited with making the connection between the two major mood states: "It appears to me that melancholy is the commencement and a part of mania." He described the cardinal manifestations of mania as it is known today:

> There are infinite forms of mania but the disease is one. . . . If mania is associated with joy, the patient may laugh, play, dance night and day, and go the market crowned as if victor in some contest of skill. . . . The ideas the patients have are infinite. . . . [They] believe they are experts in astronomy, philosophy, or poetry. . . .

Aretaeus described the extreme psychotic excitement that could complicate the foregoing clinical picture of mania:

> The patient may become excitable, suspicious, and irritable. . . . [H]is hearing may become sharp. . . . [S]ome get noises and buzzing in the ears . . . or may have visual hallucinations . . . bad dreams and his sexual desires may get uncontrollable. . . . [I]f aroused to anger, he may become wholly mad and run unrestrainedly, roar aloud . . . kill his keepers, and lay violent hands upon himself.

Noting the fluctuating nature of symptoms in the affectively ill, Aretaeus commented:

> They are prone to change their mind readily; to become base, mean-spirited, illiberal, and in a little time . . . extravagant, munificent, not from any virtue of the soul, but from the changeableness of the disease.

Aretaeus was thus keenly aware of the characterological distortions so commonly manifested during the different phases of cyclical mood disorders.

Finally, consolidating the knowledge of several centuries, Aretaeus described mania as a disease of adolescent and young men given intermittently to "active habits . . . drunkenness, lechery" and an immoderate life-style (what today might be called cyclothymic disorder). Exacerbations were most likely to occur in the spring.

AFFECTIVE TEMPERAMENTS The concept of health and disease in Greco-Roman medicine was based on harmony and balance of the four humors, of which the sanguine humor was deemed the healthiest. But even a desirable humor like blood, which made people habitually active, amiable, and prone to jest, could in excess lead to the pathological state of mania. The melancholic temperament, dominated by black bile and predisposed to pathological melancholia, was described as lethargic, sullen, and given to brooding or contemplation; its modern counterparts are depressive personality disorder and dysthymic disorder. A long tradition dating back to Aristotle (384–322 BC) attributed creative qualities to the otherwise tortured melancholic temperament in such fields as philosophy, the arts, poetry, and politics. The remaining two temperaments, choleric and phlegmatic, were less desirable, as yellow bile made people choleric (irritable, hostile, and given to rage) and phlegm made them phlegmatic (indolent, irresolute, and timid). The choleric and phlegmatic temperaments would probably be recognized today as borderline and avoidant personality disorders, respectively.

Many of the original Greek texts on melancholia were transmitted to posterity through medieval Arabic texts such as those of Ishaq Ibn Imran and Avicenna (and their Latin rendition by Constantinus Africanus). In describing different affective states, Avicenna developed the theory of the temperaments to its fullest. He speculated that a special form of melancholia supervened "if black bile . . . be mixed with phlegm" when the illness was "coupled with inertia, lack of movement, and quiet." Further, mania was not necessarily linked to the sanguine (hypomanic) temperament, as many forms of excited madness were believed to represent a mixture of black and yellow bile. Avicenna further observed that the appearance of anger, restlessness, and violence heralded the transition of melancholia to mania. Those elaborations on Galen's tempermental types might be considered the forerunners of current personality dimensions, deriving mood states from various mixtures of neuroticism and introversion-extroversion. Finally, the speculation on how diverse depressive phenomena could be understood as a mix of humors anticipated modern multiple-transmitter hypotheses of depression.

Ishaq Ibn Imran summarized the existing knowledge of melancholia by considering the interaction of genetic factors ("injured prenatally as the result of the father's sperm having been damaged") with a special temperament given to "mental overexertion"—though not necessarily physical overactivity—and that in turn was associated with "disruption of the correct rhythms . . . of sleeping and waking." Those views, too, have a very modern ring to them.

BEGINNINGS OF MULTIFACTORIAL CONCEPTUALIZATION The first English text (Figure 16.1-2) entirely devoted to affective illness was Robert Burton's *Anatomy of Melancholy,* published in 1621. A scholarly review of two millennia of medical and philosophical wisdom, the text also gives a sufferer's perspective. The concept of affective disorder endorsed by Burton was rather broad—as it always has been in the United Kingdom—embracing mood disorders and many of the disorders today considered somatoform disorders, including hypochondriasis. Although he described "causeless" melancholias, Burton also categorized the various forms of love melancholy and grief. Particularly impressive was his catalog of causes, culminating in a grand conceptualization:

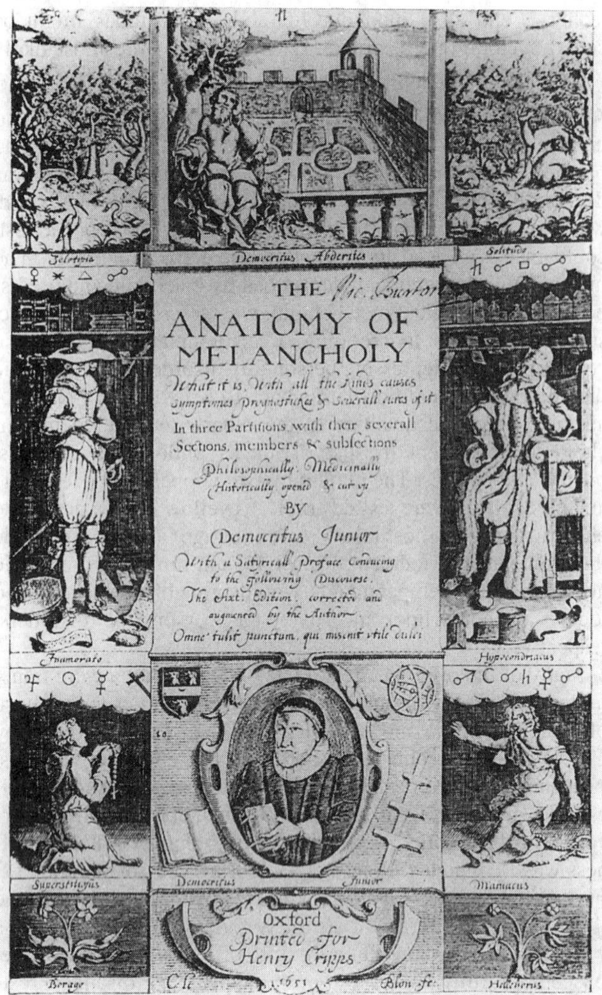

FIGURE 16.1-2 *Frontispiece of Robert Burton's* Anatomy of Melancholy *(1621).*

> Such as have . . . Saturn . . . misaffected in their genitures . . . such as are born of melancholy parents . . . as offend in those six non-natural things, are of a high sanguine complexion . . . are solitary by nature, great students, given to much contemplation, lead a life out of action, are most subject to melancholy. Of sexes both, but men more often. . . . Of seasons of the year, autumn is most melancholy. Jobertus excepts neither young nor old. . . .

Burton's six nonnatural things referred to such environmental factors as diet, alcohol, biological rhythms, and perturbations of the passions such as intense love. Burton himself did not definitively indicate age prevalences. Like nearly all of his predecessors, he favored male (rather than the currently reported female) preponderance. Finally, Burton considered both the melancholic (contemplative) and the sanguine (hot-blooded) temperaments to be substrates of melancholia. Burton's work clearly links certain forms of depression with the softer expressions of the manic disposition, or bipolar II disorder.

EARLY MODERN ERA

CONCEPT OF AFFECTIVE DISORDER Although Celsus (circa AD 30) had described forms of madness that go no further than sadness, the French alienist Jean-Philippe Esquirol (1772–1840) may have been the first psychiatrist in modern times to suggest that a primary disturbance of mood might underlie many forms of depression and related paranoid psychoses. Until Esquinol's work melancholia had been categorized as a form of insanity—that is, ascribed to deranged reasoning or thought disturbance. Esquirol's observations on melancholic patients led him to postulate that their insanity was partial—dominated by one delusion, a monomania—and that "the symptoms were the expression of the disorder of the affections. . . . [T]he source of the evil is in the passions." He coined the term "lypemania" (from the Greek, "sorrowful insanity") to give nosological status to a subgroup of melancholic disorders that were affectively based. Esquirol cited Benjamin Rush (1745–1813), the father of American psychiatry, who had earlier described tristimania, a form of melancholia in which sadness predominated.

Esquirol's influence led other European psychiatrists to propose milder states of melancholia without delusions, which were eventually categorized as simple melancholias and, ultimately, as primary depressions. Such descriptions culminated in the Anglo-Saxon psychiatric term "affective disorder." The term was coined by Henry Maudsley (1835–1918), the renowned British psychiatrist after whom the London hospital is named:

> The affective disorder is the fundamental fact. . . . [I]n the great majority of cases it precedes intellectual [delusional] disorder. . . . [I]t frequently persists for a time after this has disappeared.

MANIC-DEPRESSIVE ILLNESS AND THE QUESTION OF PSYCHOGENIC DEPRESSIONS Although the connection between mania and depression had been sporadically rediscovered since it was first described 2,000 years ago, the clinical work that finally established "circular insanity" (Jean-Pierre Falret's term) as *folie à double forme* (Jules Baillarger's term) was undertaken by those two Esquirol disciples in the 1850s. That accomplishment built on Philippe Pinel's reforms, which championed the humane treatment of the mentally ill in Paris around the turn of the 18th century and emphasized systematic clinical observations of patients, detailed in case records. French alienists made longitudinal observations on the same patient from one psychotic attack into another. Further, Esquirol had introduced the chronicling of events in statistical tables. Thus, the Hippocratic approach to defining a particular case by its onset, circumstances, course, and outcome was applied by French alienists in studying the affectively ill. The humanitarian reforms introduced in the 19th century ensured that standards of general health and nutrition would improve the outlook for the mentally ill—especially those with potentially reversible disorders like affective disorders—who could now be discharged from the asylums. The French school, then, by segregating the nondeteriorating mood disorders from the dementing types of insanity, paved the way for the Kraepelinian system.

Kraepelin's (1856–1926) unique contribution was not so much his grouping together of all the forms of melancholia and mania, but his methodology and painstaking longitudinal observations, which established manic-depressive illness as a nosological and, he hoped, a disease entity. His rationale was as follows: (1) The various forms had a common heredity measured as a function of familial aggregation of homotypic and heterotypic cases. (2) Frequent transitions from one form to the other occurred during longitudinal follow-up. (3) A recurrent course with illness-free intervals characterized most cases. (4) The superimposed episodes were commonly opposite to the patient's habitual temperament; that is, mania was superimposed on a depressive temperament and depression was superimposed on a hypomanic temperament. (5) Both depressive and manic features could occur during the same episode (mixed states). Kraepelin's synthesis was developed as early as the sixth (1899) edition of his *Lehrbuch der Psychiatrie* and most explicitly stated in the opening passages of the section on manic-depressive psychosis in the eighth edition (published in four volumes, 1909–1915):

> Manic-depressive insanity . . . includes on the one hand the whole domain of so-called periodic and circular insanity, on the other hand simple mania, the greater part of the morbid states termed melancholia and also a not inconsiderable number of cases of [confusional insanity]. Lastly, we include here certain slight and slightest colorings of mood, some of them periodic, some of them continuously morbid, which on the one hand are to be regarded as the rudiment of more severe disorders, on the other hand, pass over without . . . boundary into the domain of personal predisposition.

For Kraepelin, the core pathology of clinical depression consisted of lowering of mood and slowed (retarded) physical and mental processes. In mania, by contrast, the mood was elated and both physical and mental activity accelerated. Although his earlier observations on what he termed "involutional melancholia" (referring to 40- to 65-year-old patients with extreme anxiety, irritability, agitation, and delusions) had led him to separate that entity from the broader manic-depressive rubric, in the eighth edition of *Lehrbuch der Psychiatrie* he united it with the manic-depressive group with the justification that it was a special form of mixed state.

The classification of depressive disorders is still evolving. Karl Leonhard in 1957, Jules Angst in 1966, Carlo Perris in 1966, and George Winokur, Paula Clayton, and Theodore Reich in 1969, working independently in four different countries, proposed that depressive disorders without manic or hypomanic episodes (major depressive disorder) that appear in middle age and later are distinct from depressive episodes that begin at earlier ages and alternate with manic or hypomanic episodes (bipolar disorder). The main difference between the two disorders is the greater familial loading for mood disorder, especially for bipolar disorder.

Kraepelin had conceded the occurrence of psychogenic states of depression occasioned by situational misfortune. Manic-depressive illness, on the other hand, he believed to be hereditary. Yet he could not document postmortem anatomopathological findings in the brains of manic-depressive patients. Therefore, manic-depression had to be conceptualized as a functional mental disorder in which brain disturbances were presumed to lie in altered physiological functions. Such biological factors were deemed absent in the psychogenic depressions. Thus, Kraepelin's classification of mood disorders is both dualistic and unitary. It is dualistic to the extent that he divided them as either psychologically occasioned or somatically caused. It is unitary with respect to disorders in the latter group, which have been termed endogenous affective disorders (that is, due to internal biological causes). In other words, Kraepelin restricted the concept of clinical depression to what DSM-IV terms "major depressive disorder with melancholic features." Moreover, he postulated a continum between that condition and what DSM-IV terms "bipolar disorder."

As summarized in Table 16.1-1, in the past century endogenous depressions have been contrasted with those of exogenous cause (that is, external and, presumably, psychogenic causes). Transitions between the two groups are so frequent, however, that the two-type thesis of depression has been largely abandoned in official classifications in North American psychiatry. The endogenous-exogenous dichotomous grouping still has many adherents in the United States, Europe, and elsewhere in the world who continue to research actively its potential for clinical predictions. Those research endeavors generally attempt to validate the various subtypes based on their clinical characteristics rather than presumed etiology. Indeed, most clinical researchers today would probably agree that most forms of depression have endogenous and exogenous etiological components. Consensus would be less likely on how to delimit clinical depressive disorder from potentially comorbid disorders such as the various anxiety disorders, substance use disorders, and personality disorders. Clarifying the boundaries between those disorders has emerged as a principal challenge in the classification of mood disorders.

TABLE 16.1-1
Overlapping Dichotomies of Affective Disorders That Are Not Necessarily Synonymous

Manic-depressive	Psychogenic
S (somatic) type	J (justified) type
Autonomous	Reactive
Endogenous	Exogenous
Psychotic	Neurotic
Acute	Chronic
Major	Minor
Melancholic	Neurasthemic
Typical	Atypical
Primary	Secondary
Biological	Characterological

Cartesian thinking in 17th-century France conceptually separated mind from body, thereby providing physicians autonomy over the somatic sphere, freed from interference by the Church. The dichotomous paradigm ensured that study of the two aspects of the human organism would be unconfounded by the complexities of mind-body interactions. That is one reason why Kraepelin's descriptive observations have proved valuable to subsequent generations of clinicians. Further, his approach exemplifies the best tradition of scientific humanism in medicine: Description and diagnostic categorization of an individual patient are necessary if the physician is to offer the patient the fruits of knowledge gained from past observations made on similarly described and diagnosed patients. One limitation to the Kraepelinian approach is its biological reductionism, as a result of which it is not sufficiently articulate to account for mind-body interactions in the genesis of mental disorders.

DEPRESSIONS AS PSYCHOBIOLOGICAL AFFECTIVE REACTION TYPES Bridging the divide between psyche and soma was the ambition of the Swiss-born Adolf Meyer (1866–1950), who dominated psychiatry from his chair at Johns Hopkins University during the first half of the 20th century. Meyer coined the term "psychobiology" to emphasize that both psychological and biological factors could enter into the causation of depressive disorders and other mental disorders. Because of the nascent state of brain science during Meyer's time, he was more adept at biography than biology and therefore paid greater attention to psychosocial causation. He preferred the term "depression" ("pressed down") to "melancholia" because of its lack of biological connotation. He conceived of depressive states in terms of unspecified constitutional or biological factors interacting with a series of life situations beginning at birth or even at conception. From that viewpoint arose the unique importance accorded to personal history in depressive reactions to life events.

Meyer's terminological revision left a somewhat confusing legacy in that the term "depression" is now applied to a broad range of affective phenomena ranging from sadness and adjustment disorders to clinical depressive disorders and bipolar disorders. Repercussions can be seen in the low threshold for diagnosing major depressive disorder in DSM-IV, which renders difficult the differentiation of major depressive disorder from transient life stresses that produce adjustment disorder with depressed mood. Nosological nuances to which Meyerians paid little attention, such as the difference between melancholic depression and more mundane depressions, are not just a matter of semantics. To the extent that those two forms of depression are seen in different clinical settings, hypotheses based on one population may not apply to the other. For instance, study subjects may have learned, as a consequence of uncontrollable traumatic events in their biography, to feel helpless or to view the world in a negative light, but that does not equate with clinical illness. Failure to make such nosological distinctions further clouds interpretations of the results of trials of psychotherapy versus pharmacotherapy for depressive disorders.

The Meyerian emphasis on biographical factors and their meaning for the patient represented a more practical approach to depth psychology. Recent sociological interpretations of depression can also be traced to Meyer's work. But in the final analysis the Meyerian concern for the uniqueness of the individual has proved heuristically sterile. It de-emphasizes what is diagnostically common to different individuals, thereby obscuring the relevance of accrued clinical wisdom for the index patient. For that reason the Meyerian approach, after enjoying clinical popularity for several decades in North America, has given way to neo-Kraepelinian rigor. However, the psychobiological vision of bridging biology and psychology, one of the major preoccupations of psychiatric thought and research today, represents a Meyerian legacy.

CONTEMPORARY ETIOLOGICAL MODELS OF DEPRESSION

From classical times through the early part of the 20th century, advances in understanding mood disorders broadly involved conceptual shifts from supernatural to naturalistic explanations, from reductionistic, unitarian theories of causation to pluralistic theories, and from dualism to psychobiology. Knowledge of those conceptual developments provides a useful base from which to scrutinize more recent models and concepts of mood disorder, developed later in the 20th century. The new approaches, derived from competing theoretical positions, have generated models for understanding various aspects of mood disorders, particularly depressive disorders (Table 16.1-2).

The formative influence of early experience as it is dynamically shaped by emerging mental structures during development is the common denominator for the psychoanalytic concepts of psychopathological phenomena. By contrast, behavioral approaches in their more traditional formulations focus on the pathogenetic impact of proximate contexts. The cognitive approaches, which are akin to the behavioral-pathogenetic tradition, nonetheless concede that negative styles of thinking might mediate between proximate stressors and more remote experiences. All three schools—psychoanalytic, behavioral, and cognitive—emphasize psychological constructs in explaining the origin of mood disorders. The biological models, on the other hand, are concerned with defining the somatic mechanisms that underlie or predispose to morbid affective experiences. The schism between psychological and biological conceptualizations is an instance of the mind-body dichotomy that has characterized the Western intellectual tradition since Descartes. It must not be forgotten that psychological and somatic approaches represent merely convenient investigational strategies that attempt to bypass the methodological gulf between neural and mental structures. The ultimate aim is to understand how mood disorders develop within the psychoneural framework of a given person.

AGGRESSION - TURNED - INWARD MODEL Sigmund Freud was initially interested in a psychoneural project for all mental phenomena. Limitations of the brain sciences of the day led him to adopt instead a model that relied on a concept of mental function borrowed from physics. The notion that depressed affect is derived from retroflexion of aggressive impulses directed against an ambivalently loved internalized object was actually formulated by his Berlin disciple, Karl Abraham, and later elaborated by Freud. Abraham and Freud hypothesized that turned-in anger was intended as punishment for the love object that had thwarted the depressed patient's need for dependency and love. Because, in an attempt to prevent the traumatic loss, the object had already been internalized, the patient now became the target of his or her own thanatotic impulses. A central element in those psychic operations was the depressed patient's ambivalence toward the object, which was perceived as a frustrating parent. Aggression directed at a loved object (parent) was therefore attended by considerable guilt. In the extreme such ambivalence, guilt, and retroflexed anger could lead to suicidal behavior.

According to that model, depression was an epiphenomenon of the transduction of thanatotic energy, a reaction that took place in the closed hydraulic space of the mind. In Freud's earlier writings anxiety had similarly been viewed as derived from the transformation of dammed-up sexual libido. Although Freud envisioned that neuroanatomical localization of psychoanalytic constructs would one day be realized, the hydraulic mind is a metaphor that does not refer to actual physiochemical space in the brain.

The conceptualization of emotional behavior as an arena of incompatible forces confined to a psyche that is relatively impervious to current influences outside the organism is the major liability of the aggression-turned-inward model and perhaps of orthodox psychoanalysis itself. Although the sexual energy transduction hypothesis of anxiety has been discarded in modern psychoanalytic thought, in modified version the aggression-turned-inward model continues to be used in clinical conceptualization today. The lingering popularity of the model may be due in part to its compatibility with the clinical observation that many depressed patients suffer from lack of assertion and outwardly directed aggressiveness. Yet a substantial number of hostile depressed patients are also encountered in clinical practice, and clinical improvement typically leads to a decrease rather than increase in hostility. Those observations shed doubt on the aggression-turned-inward mechanism as a universal explanation for depressive behavior. Finally, there is little evidence to support the contention that the outward expression of anger is of therapeutic value in clinical depression.

Outwardly directed hostility in depression is not a new clinical observation—the Greco-Roman physicians cited earlier noted as much—and can be considered a common manifestation rather than cause of depressive disorder, especially when the disorder is attended by mixed bipolar features. The hostility of the depressed patient can also be understood as an exaggerated reaction to frustrating love objects, as secondary to self-referential attributions, or simply as nonspecific irritability of an ego in affective turmoil. Such commonsense explanations that do not invoke unobservable hydraulic transmutations have greater appeal from heuristic and clinical perspectives.

OBJECT LOSS AND DEPRESSION Object loss refers to traumatic separation from significant objects of attachment. Ego-psychological reformulations of the Abraham-Freud conceptualization of depression have paid greater attention to the impact of such losses on the ego, de-emphasizing the id-libid-

TABLE 16.1-2
Contemporary Major Models of Depression

Proponents (Year)	Model	Mechanism	Scientific and Clinical Implications
Karl Abraham (1911)	Aggression-turned-inward	Transduction of aggressive instinct into depressive affect	Hydraulic mind closed to external influences Nontestable
Sigmund Freud (1917) John Bowlby (1960)	Object loss	Disruption of an attachment bond	Ego-psychological Open system Testable
Edward Bibring (1953)	Self-esteem	Helplessness in attaining goals of ego ideal	Ego-psychological Open system Social and cultural ramifications
Aaron Beck (1967)	Cognitive	Negative cognitive schemata as intermediary between remote and proximate causes	Ego-psychological Open system Testable Predicts phenomenology Suggests treatment
Martin Seligman (1975)	Learned helplessness	The belief that one's responses will not bring relief from undesirable events	Testable Predicts phenomenology Predicts treatment
Peter Lewinsohn (1974)	Reinforcement	Low rate of reinforcement, or reinforcement presented noncontingently; social deficits might preclude responding to potentially rewarding events	Testable Predicts phenomenology Predicts treatment
Joseph Schildkraut (1965) William Bunney and John Davis (1965) Alec Coppen (1968) I. P. Lapin and G. F. Oxenkrug (1969) David Janowsky et al (1972) Arthur Prange et al (1974) Larry Siever and Kenneth Davis (1985)	Biogenic amine (neurochemical)	Impairment or dysregulation of aminergic transmission	Testable Reductionistic Explains phenomenology and opposite episodes Suggests treatment
Alec Coppen and D. M. Shaw (1963) Peter Whybrow and Joseph Mendels (1968) Robert Post (1990)	Neurophysiological	Electrophysiological disturbances leading to neuronal hyperexcitability and kindling	Testable Reductionistic Explains phenomenology and recurrence Suggests treatment
Hagop Akiskal and William McKinney (1973) Peter Whybrow and Anselm Parlatore (1973) Frederick Goodwin and Kay Jamison (1990)	Final common pathway	Stress-diathesis interaction converging on midbrain mechanisms of reward and biological rhythms	Testable Integrative, psychobiological Pluralistic Explains phenomenology Suggests treatment

The dates provided for the models refer to the original paper or work in which they first appeared. In some instances, the bibliography at the end of the section provides references reflecting more updated thinking by those authors.

Table adapted from H Akiskal, W McKinney: Overview of recent research in depression: Integration of 10 conceptual models into a comprehensive clinical frame. Arch Gen Psychiatry *32:* 285, 1975.

inal and related hydraulic aspects. It is often noted that the depressant impact of separation events resides in their symbolic meaning for a person rather than in any arbitrary objective weight that the event may have for clinical raters. However, love loss, bereavement, and other exits from the social scene, as defined by the London psychiatrist Eugene Paykel, are presently the concepts most commonly used in practice and research.

Although love melancholy had been described since antiquity, it was in Freud's 1917 paper on mourning and melancholia that grief and melancholia were systematically compared for the first time. According to current data, the transition from grief to pathological depression occurs in no more than 2 to 5 percent of adults and 10 to 15 percent of children. Those figures suggest that such transition occurs largely in persons predisposed to mood disorders.

The work of John Bowlby of the Tavistock Clinic, London, is a comprehensive clinical investigation of the attachment that the child establishes with the mother or mother substitutes during development; that bond is considered the prototype for all subsequent bonds with other objects. Like many psychoanalytic explanations of adult symptom-formation, the object loss model is formulated as a two-step hypothesis, consisting of early breaks in affectional bonds, which provide the behavioral predisposition to depression, and adult losses, which are said to revive the traumatic childhood loss, thereby precipitating depressive episodes. However, the role of proximate separations in provoking depressive reactions rests on more solid clinical evidence than the hypothesized sensitization resulting from developmental object loss. That realization has led Bowlby to regard childhood sensitization resulting from early deprivation as a generic characterological vulnerability to a host of adult psychopathological conditions.

Compared with aggression turned inward, object loss is more directly relevant to clinical depression; yet it is still pertinent to question whether it is an etiological factor. Studies at the Wisconsin Primate Center have indicated that optimal homeostasis with the environment is most readily achieved when the individual is securely attached to significant others, and the dissolution of such ties appears relevant to the emergence of a broad range of psychopathological disturbances rather than depression per se. A related methodological question is whether object loss operates independently of other etiological factors. For instance, a history of early breaks in attachment may reflect the fact that one or both of the patient's parents had mood disorder, with resultant separation, divorce, suicide, and so forth.

On balance, the ego-psychological object loss model is conceptually superior to its id-psychological counterpart. In postulating an open system of exchange between a person and the environment, the model permits consideration of etiological factors other than separation—such as heredity, character structure, and adequacy of social support—all of which might modulate the depressant impact of adult separation events. Conceptualizing the origin of depression along those lines is in the mainstream of current ideas of adaptation, homeostasis, and disease. An important treatment implication is the value of social support in preventing relapse and mitigating chronicity of depression. That is indeed an ingredient in the interpersonal psychotherapy of depression, which can be conceptualized as a form of brief, focused, and practical psychodynamic therapy.

DEPRESSION AS LOSS OF SELF-ESTEEM Reformulation of the dynamics of depression in terms of the ego suffering a collapse of self-esteem represents a further conceptual break with the original id-psychological formulation: Depression is said to originate from the ego's inability to give up unattainable goals and ideals. The model further posits that the narcissistic injury that crushes the depressed patient's self-esteem is imposed by the internalized values of the ego rather than the hydraulic pressure of retroflected thanatotic energy deriving from the id. Because the construct of the ego is rooted in social and cultural reality, loss of self-esteem may result from symbolic losses involving power, status, roles, identity, values, and purpose for existence. Thus, the existential and sociocultural implications of depression conceived as a derivative ego state provide the clinician with a far more flexible and pragmatic tool for understanding depressed persons than the archaic hydraulic metaphors related to libidinal vicissitudes. That model represents one of the first attempts to formulate depression in terms that subsequent psychological theory and research could operationalize in more testable form.

Self-esteem is part of the habitual core of the individual and as such is integral to the personality structure. Indeed, low self-esteem conceived as a trait is a major defining attribute of the depressive (melancholic) personality. While it is understandable how such individuals can easily sink into melancholia in the face of environmental adversity, it is not obvious why persons with apparently high self-esteem, such as those with hypomanic and narcissistic personalities, also succumb to melancholy with relative ease. To explain such cases, one must invoke an underlying instability in the system of self-esteem that renders it vulnerable to depression. The opposite is also known to occur; that is, manic episodes may develop from a baseline of low self-esteem, as sometimes occurs in patients with dysthymic disorder.

The foregoing considerations suggest that the vicissitudes of self-esteem deemed central to the model of depression as loss of self-esteem are manifestations of a more fundamental mood dysregulation. In classical psychoanalysis it is conceded that such dysregulation is of constitutional origin. In general, attempts by psychoanalytic writers to account for bipolar oscillations have not progressed beyond metapsychological jargon, with the possible exception of denial of painful affects as a mechanism in the phenomenology of mania.

COGNITIVE MODEL The cognitive model, developed by Aaron Beck at the University of Pennsylvania, hypothesizes that thinking along negative lines (for example, thinking that one is helpless, unworthy, or useless) is the hallmark of clinical depression. In effect, depression is redefined in terms of a cognitive triad, according to which the patient thinks of him- or herself as helpless, interprets most events in an unfavorable light vis-à-vis the self, and believes the future to be hopeless. In more recent formulations in academic psychology, those cognitions are said to be characterized by a negative attributional style that is global, internal, and stable and to exist in the form of latent mental schemata that generate biased interpretations of life events.

Because the cognitive model is based on retrospective observations of already depressed persons, it is virtually impossible to prove that causal attributions such as negative mental schemata precede and hence predispose to clinical depression; they can just as readily be regarded as clinical manifestations of depression. The importance of the cognitive model lies in the conceptual bridge it provides between ego-psychological and behavioral models of depression. It has also led to a new system of psychotherapy that attempts to alter the negative attributional style, to alleviate the depressive state, and, ultimately, to fortify the patient against future lapses into negative thinking, despair, and depression.

The cognitive model therefore has the cardinal virtue of focusing on key reversible clinical dimensions of depressive illness, such as helplessness, hopelessness, and suicidal ideation, while providing a testable and practical psychotherapeutic approach. That approach, however, is less likely to succeed in patients with the full-blown melancholic manifestations of a depressive disorder. It is doubtful that negative cognitions alone could account for the profound disturbances in sleep, appetite, and autonomic and psychomotor functions encountered in melancholic depressions. Further, to conceptualize a multifaceted malady such as depression largely or solely as a function of distorted cognitive processes is reminiscent of pre-Esquirolian notions that emphasized impaired reasoning in the development of depression.

LEARNED HELPLESSNESS The learned helplessness model is in some ways an experimental analog of the cognitive model. The model proposes that the depressive posture is learned from past situations in which the person was unsuccessful in initiating action to terminate undesirable contingencies. The model is based on experiments in dogs that were prevented from taking adaptive action to avoid unpleasant electrical shock and subsequently showed no motivation to escape such aversive stimuli, even when escape avenues were readily available. Armed with evidence from many such experiments, the University of Pennsylvania psychologist Martin Seligman postulated a trait of learned helplessness—a belief that it is futile to initiate personal action to reverse aversive circumstances—that is formed from the cumulation of past episodes of uncontrollable helplessness.

The learned helplessness paradigm is a general one and refers to a broader mental disposition than depression. Thus, it is potentially useful in understanding such diverse conditions as social powerlessness, defeat in sporting events, and posttraumatic stress disorder. In addition, past events might shape a characterological cluster, consisting of passivity, lack of hostility, and self-blame, relevant to certain depressive phenomena. The low hostility observed in some patients during clinical depression could, for instance, be ascribed to the operation of such factors. Learned helplessness could thereby provide plausible links between aspects of personal biography and clinical phenomenology in depressive disorders. Therapeutic predictions for alleviating depression and related psychopathological states capitalize on new cognitive strategies geared to modifying expectations of uncontrollability and the negative attributional style. That is an illustration on how insights gained from experimental paradigms can be fruitfully combined to address clinical disorders.

Nonetheless, the clinician should be wary of unwarranted clinical extrapolations. For instance, some clinicians have argued that the depressed patient's passivity is manipulative, serving to obtain interpersonal rewards. It has also been claimed that such factors have a formative influence on the development of the depressive character. That interpretation appears more relevant to selected aspects of depression than to the totality of the disorder. Depressive behavior and verbalizations clearly have a powerful interpersonal impact, but to speculate that depression represents merely a masochistic life-style developed for the purpose of securing interpersonal advantages represents a circular argument that is mechanistic and could be viewed as disrespectful of the clinical agony of patients with mood disorders. Finally, although most formulations focusing on helplessness have emphasized acquisition through learning, recent experimental research in animals tends to implicate genetic factors in the vulnerability to learning to behave helplessly.

REINFORCEMENT AND DEPRESSION Other behavioral investigators, notably Peter Lewinsohn, have developed clinical formulations of depression that hinge on certain deficits in reinforcement mechanisms. According to the reinforcement model, depressive behavior is associated with lack of appropriate rewards and, more specifically, with the receipt of noncontingent rewards. The model identifies several contributory mechanisms. Some environments may consistently deprive persons of rewarding opportunities, thereby placing them in a chronic state of boredom, pleasurelessness, and, ultimately, despair. That reasoning, however, may offer more insight into social misery than clinical depression. A more plausible postulated mechanism is the provision of rewards that are not in response to the recipient's actions; in other words, the gratis provision of what a person considers undeserved rewards may lead to lowering of self-esteem. Predisposition to depression is formulated in terms of deficient social skills, which are hypothesized to decrease a person's chances of responding to potentially rewarding contingencies in any environment. Indeed, recent research on the relation between personality and mood disorder suggests that such deficits might contribute to certain nonbipolar depressions. Therefore, psychotherapeutic approaches designed to enlarge a patient's repertoire of social skills may prove valuable in preventing depressive episodes.

The concepts of depression that have been derived from behavioral methodology and developed in the past three decades are scientifically articulate and therefore testable approaches to the clinical phenomena of depression. Yet in the behavioral literature the distinction between depression on self-report inventories and clinical depression is sometimes overlooked. Further, the behavioral model does not address the distinct possibility that reinforcement deficits may simply represent the psychomotor inertia of depressive illness. Nevertheless, by focusing on reward mechanisms, the behavioral model provides a conceptual bridge between purely psychological and emerging biological conceptualizations of depression.

BIOGENIC AMINE IMBALANCE

Chemistry of the emotional brain The formulation of sophisticated biological explanations of mood disorders had to await the development of neurobiological techniques that could probe parts of the brain involved in emotions. Although the complex physiology of the limbic-diencephalic centers of emotional behavior is generally inaccessible to direct observation in humans, much has been learned from animal work. The limbic cortex is linked with both the neocortex, which subserves higher symbolic functions, and the midbrain and lower brain centers, which are involved in autonomic control, hormonal production, and sleep and wakefulness. Norepinephrine-containing neurons are involved in many of the functions that are profoundly disturbed in melancholia, including mood, arousal, appetite, reward, and drives. Other biogenic amine neurotransmitters that mediate such functions are the catecholamine dopamine, especially important for psychomotor activity, and the indoleamine serotonin, involved in mood and sleep and inhibitory control. Cholinergic neurons, secreting acetylcholine at their dendritic terminals, are generally antagonistic in function to catecholaminergic neurons. Although the opioid system might, on experimental and theoretical grounds, also serve as one of the neurochemical substrates for mood regulation, in the author's opinion no cogent model of mood disorders involving that system has appeared to date.

Biogenic amine hypotheses Joseph Schildkraut at Harvard University and William Bunney and John Davis at NIMH published the first reports formally hypothesizing a connection between depletion or imbalance of biogenic amines, specifically norepinephrine, and clinical depression. The serotonin counterpart of the model was emphasized in the models proposed by Alec Coppen in England and I.P. Lapin and G.F. Oxenkrug in Russia. Both catecholamine and indoleamine hypotheses were essentially based on two sets of pharmacological observations. First, reserpine, a medication that decreases blood pressure by depleting biogenic amine stores, was known to precipitate clinical depression in some patients. Second, antidepressant medications, which alleviate clinical depression, were found to raise the functional capacity of the biogenic amines in the brain. That style of thinking is known as the pharmacological bridge, extrapolating from evidence on mechanism of drug action to the neurotransmitter pathologies presumed to underlie a given psychiatric disorder. Such pharmacological strategies have been of heuristic value in developing research methods for the investigation of mood disorders and schizophrenia. Indeed, the research methodology developed by the relatively few investigators working in the area in the past three decades is among the most elegant in the history of psychiatry.

Different variations of the biogenic amine model give somewhat different importance to the relative weight of the biogenic amines norepinephrine and serotonin in the development of pathological mood states. Arthur Prange and colleagues at the University of North Carolina formulated a permissive biogenic amine hypothesis according to which serotonin deficits permit the expression of catecholamine-mediated depressive or manic states. That hypothesis was supported by subsequent animal research showing that an intact serotonin system is necessary for the optimal functioning of noradrenergic neurons. In a recent study, the omission of tryptophan from the diet of antidepressant-responsive depressed patients annulled the efficacy of the antidepressant. Although that finding is intriguing, the precursor-loading strategy to increase the brain stores of serotonin (for example, with L-tryptophan) has not been unequivocally successful in addressing clinical depression. Dietary loading with catecholamine precursors has fared even worse than serotonin precursor loading in the treatment of depression.

The cholinergic-noradrenergic imbalance hypothesis as proposed by David Janowsky and colleagues represents yet another attempt to elucidate the roles of biogenic amines. More recent formulations by Larry Siever and Kenneth Davis at the Mount Sinai Hospital in New York have hypothesized noradrenergic dysregulation as an alternative neurochemical mechanism for depressive disorders. The model envisions oscillation from one output mode to the other at different phases of depressive illness. In a provocative extrapolation from that model, bipolar depression would emerge as being of low noradrenergic output, but many instances of major depressive disorder, like some anxiety disorders, could be biochemically conceptualized as high-output conditions.

Despite three decades of extensive research and indirect evidence, however, it has not been proved that a deficiency or excess of biogenic amines in specific brain structures is necessary or sufficient for the occurrence of mood disorders. The role of dopamine, though less extensively studied than that of norepinephrine, deserves greater recognition: It might have relevance to atypical and bipolar depression as well as mania. The putative permissive role of serotonin appears more relevant to aggressive suicide attempts than to depression per se. It is also of theoretical and clinical interest that serotonergic dysfunction might subserve other conditions characterized by lack of inhibitory control, among them obsessive-compulsive and panic phenomena, bulimia nervosa, certain forms of insomnia, alcoholism, and a host of impulse-ridden personality disorders. Such considerations have led the Dutch psychiatrist Herman van Praag and his colleagues to postulate a dimensional neurochemical disturbance generic to a large group of disorders within the traditional nosology. That hypothesis might be variously regarded as a challenge to psychiatric nosology or as a statement of the need to supplement clinical classification with biochemical parameters.

The biogenic amine models provide meaningful links with the clinical phenomena of, and the pharmacological treatments currently employed in, mood disorders. Although the predisposition to mood disorder is not specified in those models, it is implied that the biochemical faults are genetically determined.

Neuroendocrine links Inadequate or excessive mobilization of neurotransmitters such as noradrenaline in the face of continued or repeated stress, as reflected in pathological modification of noradrenergic receptor function, could represent a neurochemical final common pathway of homeostatic failure. Such mechanisms could also provide links with psychoendocrine dysfunction; the hypothesized neurotransmitter deficits may underlie the disinhibition of the hypothalamic-pituitary-adrenal axis, characterized by steroidal overproduction, the most widely studied endocrine disturbance in depressive illness. When challenged with dexamethasone, the altered axis has been found resistant to suppression, thereby offering Bernard Carroll and colleagues at the University of Michigan the possibility of developing the dexamethasone suppression test (DST) for melancholia (the test is currently of uncertain specificity for melancholia). That line of research has culminated in the demonstration by Charles Nemeroff and other investigators of increased concentrations of corticotropin-releasing factor (CRF) in the cerebrospinal fluid of patients with major depressive disorder. CRF also appears relevant to the pathophysiology of anxiety disorders, such as panic disorder.

Another neuroendocrine index of noradrenergic dysregulation—blunted growth hormone response to the α_2-adrenergic receptor agonist clonidine—likewise points to limbic-diencephalic disturbance. However, studies performed in the United States suggest that it is positive in both endogenous depression and severe anxiety disorder (panic disorder). Thyroid-stimulating hormone (TSH) blunting upon thyrotropin (TRH) stimulation, another common neuroendocrine disturbance in depression, is also of limited specificity (it is often positive in alcoholism).

What is remarkable, however, is that the DST, clonidine, and TRH challenge data in aggregate identify the majority of persons with clinical depression. The more relevant point is that such evidence of midbrain disturbance argues for considering clinical depression a legitimate illness. Finally, the data tend to argue for shared mechanisms between certain mood and anxiety disorders.

Stress, biogenic amines, and depression The concept of a pharmacological bridge implies two-way traffic. The hypothesized chemical aberrations may be primary or biologically induced. Provision should also be made, however, for the likelihood that psychological events, which serve as precipitants of clinical depression, might induce or initiate neurochemical imbalance in vulnerable subjects. That suggestion is supported by studies in animals, where separation and inescapable frustration are known to effect profound alterations in the turnover of biogenic amines and in postsynaptic receptor sensitivity. It is conceivable that, in genetically predisposed persons, environmental stressors might more easily lead to perturbations of limbic-diencephalic neurotransmitter balance. Finally, it is plausible that in vulnerable individuals, especially during the formative years of childhood, the psychological mechanisms discussed earlier might more easily perturb midbrain neurochemistry.

NEUROPHYSIOLOGICAL APPROACHES

Electrolyte metabolism and neuronal hyperexcitability

Abnormalities in neuronal electrolyte balance (an excess of residual sodium, defined by radioisotope techniques) and hypothesized secondary neurophysiological disturbances were the focus of investigations by Coppen and colleagues in the early 1960s. The existing data appear compatible with the hypothesized movement of excess sodium into the neuron during an episode of mood disorder and redistribution toward the preillness electrolyte balance across the neuronal membrane during recovery; intraneuronal leakage of sodium is postulated in both depressive and manic disorders but deemed more extreme in the latter. Because the harmonious activity of the neuronal cell—and, by implication, that of a group of neurons—depends on the electrical gradient maintained across its membrane by the differential distribution of sodium, abnormalities in sodium concentrations and transport are hypothetically relevant to the production of an unstable state of neurophysiological hyperexcitability.

The view that mania represents a more extreme electrophysiological dysfunction in the same direction as depression violates the commonsense notion of symptomatological opposition between the two kinds of disorder, yet it may in part account for the existence of mixed states in which symptoms of depression and mania coexist. That many depressed patients with a bipolar substrate respond to lithium salts—a provocative finding first documented by the NIMH team led by Frederick Goodwin—further supports the concept of a neurophysiological common denominator to mania and depression.

Rhythmopathy and depression Recent neurophysiological formulations by Thomas Wehr and Norman Rosenthal, working at NIMH, have focused on abnormalities in the circadian regulation of temperature, activity, and sleep cycles, thereby paving the way for new theoretical constructs and therapeutic possibilities. It has been found that depressed patients are phase-advanced in many of their biological rhythms, including the latency to first rapid eye movement (REM) in sleep. Shortening of REM latency, which has been extensively studied by David Kupfer and colleagues at the University of Pittsburgh, has been proposed as another biological test for depressive disorder. Finally, it has been hypothesized that sleep deprivation (originally developed by European investigators) and exposure to bright white light (demonstrated by NIMH research) might correct phase disturbances and thereby terminate depressive episodes, especially in patients with periodic and seasonal illness. Although the specificity and efficacy of those neurophysiological indices and manipulations for mood disorders require more extensive research, cumulatively they point to midbrain dysregulation as the likely common neurophysiological substrate of depressive disorders.

The foregoing considerations further suggest that the ancient Greeks, who ascribed melancholia to malignant geophysical influences, did not indulge in mere poetic metaphor. It is also striking that the ancients had observed the disturbed circadian patterns and advocated their readjustment to restore euthymia.

Affective dysregulation as the fundamental pathology
The ultimate challenge for research in mood disorders is to characterize the basic molecular mechanisms that underlie the neurophysiological rhythmopathies, which in turn might account for the recurrent nature of the affective pathology as envisioned by Kraepelin. This means that in the most typical recurrent forms of the disorders, the constitutional foundations—manifested as cyclothymic and dysthymic temperaments—are so unstable that the illness may run its entire course more or less autonomously, with the environment largely serving the role of turning on and off the more florid phases (episodes). The Parisian psychiatrist Jean Delay also emphasized affective dysregulation as the fundamental pathology in the spectrum of mood disorders. Robert Post, at NIMH, has hypothesized that the electrophysiological substrates could be kindled, such that an oligoepisodic disorder, initially triggered by environmental stressors, could assume an autonomous and polyepisodic course. The monograph on manic-depressive illness by Goodwin and Kay Jamison presents eloquent arguments for a fundamental cyclical thymopathy, based on current psychobiological understanding.

CONCEPTUAL INTEGRATION

TOWARD PATHOPHYSIOLOGICAL UNDERSTANDING

Modern psychobiology attempts to link experience and behavior to the central nervous system. To build sturdy conceptual bridges between the psychological and biological approaches to mood disorders, sophisticated strategies are needed that go beyond the Cartesian notion of limited mind-body interactions through the pineal gland and the more pedestrian generalizations of the Meyerian school.

In collaboration with Peter Whybrow at the University of Pennsylvania, William McKinney and the author have further developed the conceptual framework that considers the syndromes of melancholia and mania as the final common pathway of various psychological and biological processes. The overarching hypothesis is that psychological and biological etiological factors converge in reversible deficits in the diencephalic substrates of pleasure and reward. Those areas of the brain subserve the functions that are disturbed in melancholia and mania. The integrative model links the central chemistry and physiology of reward mechanisms with the object loss and behavioral models of depression, both of which give singular importance to the depressant role of loss of rewarding interpersonal bonds; an essential element of the model is the circadian disturbances observed since ancient times in both depressive and manic syndromes. Both syndromes then are conceptualized as the clinical manifestations of a disordered limbic system with its subcortical and prefrontal extensions. Multiple factors converge in producing dysregulation in the system and are described below.

Predisposing heredity Current evidence indicates that genetic factors play a significant role in the causation of bipolar and recurrent major depressive disorders. Genetic heterogeneity is likely, and may involve single-gene-dominant inheritance with variable penetrance or polygenic inheritance. Although it is not known exactly what is inherited, recent research by Kenneth Kendler and associates suggests that heritability involves a broad spectrum of disorders, including milder depressive episodes.

Developmental predisposition As parents with mood disorders are often in conflict, which may lead to separation, divorce, and suicide, it can be said that heredity often determines the type of environment into which the child predisposed to mood disorder is born. Developmental object loss, although not causing mood disorder, might modify the expression of the illness, possibly by leading to earlier onset, more severe episodes, and an increased likelihood of personality disorder and suicide attempts.

Temperament Since ancient times, persons prone to mania and melancholia have been described as possessing certain temperamental attributes, representing variations on the theme of what today is subsumed under cyclothymia and dysthymia. The fact that many monozygotic twins discordant for mood disorders studied by Aksel Bertelsen's Danish research team exhibited affective instability along such temperamental lines strongly suggests that such attributes represent genetically determined traits. That research and research conducted by Kendler and associates suggest that many of the temperamental attributes might be transmitted as part of the overall genetic liability to mood disorders. The author's research has identified those temperaments in the prepubertal offspring of parents with bipolar (manic-depressive) disorders, suggesting that they precede by years to decades the onset of major mood disorder episodes. Those temperaments in turn generate much interpersonal friction, emotional arousal, and sleep loss, and thereby might give rise to many of the life stressors that precipitate episodes of mood disorders. The use of stimulant drugs—either to self-treat lethargy or enhance hypomanic episodes—can also precipitate such episodes.

Life events Most individuals do not develop clinical depression when exposed to environmental adversity. Such adversity seems to play a pathogenic role in those with an affective diathesis. Thus, current data suggest that social stressors in the onset of depression are more relevant to the early course of the illness. The evidence linking such events to mania is less robust. At any rate, socially stressful events often appear to be triggered by the temperamental instability that precedes clinical episodes. Interpersonal losses are common events in the lives of individuals with intense temperaments. Indeed, a recent study by Peter McGuffin and associates at the Institute of Psychiatry, London, raised the possibility that one mechanism by which heredity produces depression is by creating environmental adversities in the lives of individuals predisposed to this illness. Whatever the origin of environmental adversity, it is common clinical experience that loss represents an important—perhaps even central—theme in clinical depression. Variables that seem to modulate the impact of adult losses include concurrent life events, resultant changes in life-style, lack of interpersonal support, deficient social skills, and the symbolic meaning of the loss.

Biological stressors Many physical diseases and pharmacological agents are known to precede the onset of both depressive and manic episodes. Like psychosocial stressors, however, they do not generally seem to cause de novo episodes but mobilize them in those persons with a personal and family history of mood disorders.

Sex Clinical and epidemiological studies concur in suggesting that women are at higher risk for mood disorders, with the risk highest for the milder depressive states. Although it is customary to ascribe the increased risk to social and interpersonal variables, biological factors appear equally relevant. Women have higher levels of brain monamine oxidase (the enzyme that breaks down monamine transmitters), have more precarious thyroid status (often associated with chronic and rapid-cycling mood episodes), experience postpartum precipitation, experience premenstrual accentuation of dysphoric mood, and are vulnerable to the depressant effect of steroidal contraceptives. Recent data reported by Giulio Perugi and associates at the University of Pisa, Italy, have raised the hypothesis that female sex might also favor the greater expression of dysthymic attributes, whereas hypomanic traits appear favored by male sex. Those considerations tend to parallel, respectively, the ruminative and active cognitive response styles reported by Stanford's Susan Nolen-Hoeksema to distinguish the sexes. What specific sex-related biographical factors might interact with sex-related biological factors to produce such trait differences is presently unknown.

The model presented here (Figure 16.1-3) goes beyond the general provisions of the unified approach developed two decades earlier. It is submitted that, at least in the highly recurrent forms of the malady, affective temperaments represent the intermediary stage between remote (for example, hereditary) and proximate (for example, stressful) factors, and that limbic-diencephalic dysfunction is best characterized as the biological concomitant of the clinical manifestations of the affective syndromes. Like the temperamental dysregulations, those biological disturbances represent a stage in the pathogenetic chain: They emerge as temperamental instabilities that react to, provoke, or invite life events, substance use, and rhythmopathies, which in turn usher in the behavioral and subjective manifestations of the illness.

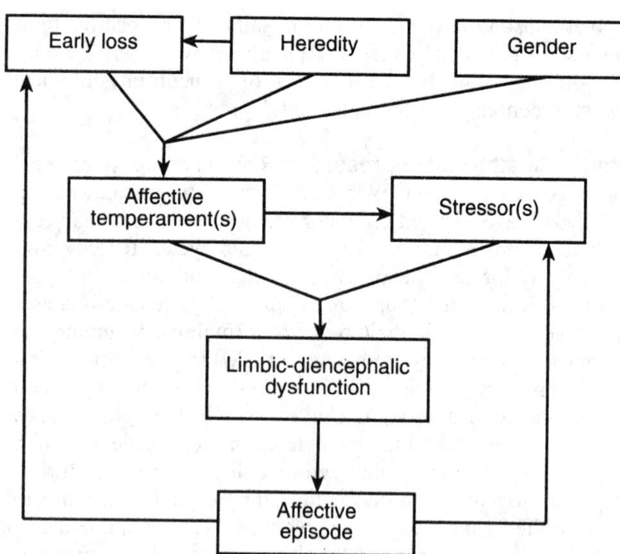

FIGURE 16.1-3 *An integrative pathogenetic model of mood disorders.*

IMPLICATIONS FOR TREATMENT AND PREVENTION

The foregoing integrative model envisions the joint use of somatic-pharmacological and psychosocial interventions. Although the milder forms of mood disorders can be managed with psychotherapy, somatic treatments are usually required for reversing the biological disturbances in melancholia before the patient can respond to interpersonal feedback. Depressive disorders with psychotic features often necessitate more definitive somatic interventions such as electroconvulsive therapy. Continued psychopharmacological treatment is also effective in decreasing rates of relapse and future recurrence.

Psychosocial therapy by skilled therapists can provide support, combat demoralization, change maladaptive self-attributions, and improve conjugal and vocational functioning. Whether such therapy can also modify personality traits to fortify the patient against new episodes is a future research challenge. In the author's view, it may prove more profitable to attempt to help patients explore professional and object choices that match their temperamental proclivities and assets and that in turn might provide them greater harmony and adaptation in life. Although much needs to be learned about the indications for medication and psychotherapy in different subtypes of mood disorders, research to date not only does not indicate a negative interaction between the two forms of treatment but in some instances suggests additive and even synergistic interaction.

The challenge for psychiatric research in the decade ahead is to elucidate the basic mechanisms whereby the predisposing, precipitating, and mediating variables reviewed here, and others yet to be identified, interact to produce the final common path of decompensation in melancholia. Because of the heterogeneity of depressive conditions presenting as a psychobiological final common syndrome, and because antidepressant agents, irrespective of specificity to one or another biogenic amine, are about equally effective in two thirds of those with depressive disorder with melancholic features, the antidepressant agents, effective as they are, may be acting not on the primary lesions of the depressive disorders but on a neurochemical substrate distal to the underlying biological faults. The choice of antidepressants is still very much guided by the side effect profile least objectionable to a given patient's constitution, physical condition, and life-style.

Current evidence suggests that in depressed patients with bipolar disorder antidepressants might provoke mixed episodes, hypomanic episodes, or both and, possibly, increased cycling in the subsequent course of the disorder. The value of lithium in such cases does suggest some biochemical specificity. The kindling-sensitization model further suggests the utility of anticonvulsant medication on escalation of the disorder and represents another example of pathophysiology-based intervention. Interventions geared to disturbed rhythms of the disorder represent yet another example. Thus, mood clinics should educate patients and their significant others on how to dampen stimulation so that it is kept at an optimal level for depressed patients with cyclothymic disorder. All offending drugs (for example, cocaine, caffeine) should be eliminated and circadian disruptions and sleep loss minimized. The greater challenge is how to curb the tempestuous romantic liaisons or ill-fated financial ventures that periodically jolt the lives of patients with cyclothymic disorder. Psychoeducation and psychotherapy have the task of ameliorating the resulting social problems. Assuring compliance to a lithium regimen—which in many would have attenuated episodes and prevented such sequelae—is not easily achieved. Research on both compliance-enhancing techniques and the physiochemical mechanisms of lithium is needed before the drug can be used efficiently in the large number of patients who might benefit from it.

It is tempting to suggest that biogenic amines, the humors of modern psychobiology, play the same heuristic role as the ancient humors did for many centuries. The black humor, appropriately evoked in the construct of melancholia in DSM-IV, may not have the same claim for etiological relevance to depressive disorders as biogenic amines but at least has a classical heritage. In any discipline, scientific truth is a function of its technology, but understanding the phenomena under consideration is a matter of philosophical temperament that seeks integration and the hope for a unified vision. Research into the causes and treatment of mood disorders has generated an abundance of recent data suitable for integration into theory and practice, and conceptualizing the origin and treatment of mood disorders can no longer be justified on the ground of ideological preference alone.

SUGGESTED CROSS-REFERENCES

The other sections of Chapter 16 cover the various aspects of mood disorders in detail. Epidemiology is the subject of Section 16.2; biochemical aspects are the focus of 16.3; Section 16.4 is a discussion of genetic aspects; psychodynamic etiology is the subject of Section 16.5. Clinical features are covered in Section 16.6, somatic treatment in Section 16.7, and a discussion of psychosocial treatments concludes the chapter in Section 16.8.

REFERENCES

Abraham K: Notes on the psychoanalytical investigation and treatment of manic-depressive insanity and allied conditions. In *Selected Papers of Karl Abraham,* p 137. Hogarth Press, London, 1948.

Akiskal H S: Temperament, personality, and depression. In *Research in Mood Disorders: An Update,* H Hippius, C Stefanis, editors, p 45. Hogrefe & Hubes, Gottingen, 1994.

*Akiskal H S, McKinney W T: Depressive disorders: Toward a unified hypothesis. Science *182:* 20, 1973.

Angst J: The etiology and nosology of endogenous depressive psychoses. Foreign Psychiatry 2: 1, 1973.

Aretaeus of Cappadocia: *The Extant Works of Aretaeus, the Cappadocian,* F Adams, editor-translator. Sydenham Society, London, 1856.

*Beck A T: *Depression: Causes and Treatment.* University of Pennsylvania Press, Philadelphia, 1967.

Bertelsen A, Harvald B, Hauge M: A Danish twin study of manic-depressive disorders. Br J Psychiatry *130:* 330, 1977.

Bowlby J: Process of mourning. Int J Psychoanal *45:* 317, 1961.

Bunney W E Jr, Davis J M: Norepinephrine in depressive reactions: A review. Arch Gen Psychiatry *13:* 483, 1965.

Carroll B J, Feinberg M, Greden J F, Tarika J, Albala A A, Haskett R F, James N M, Kronfol Z, Lohr N, Steiner M, de Vigne J P, Young E: A specific laboratory test for the diagnosis of melancholia: Standardization, validation, and clinical utility. Arch Gen Psychiatry *38:* 15, 1981.

Coppen A: The biochemistry of affective disorders. Br J Psychiatry *113:* 1237, 1967.

Delay J: *Les Dérèglements de L'humeur.* Presses Universitaires de France, Paris, 1946.

Freud S: Mourning and melancholia. In *Standard Edition of the Complete Psychological Works of Sigmund Freud,* vol 4, J Strachey, editor, p 152. Hogarth Press, London, 1975.

*Goodwin F K, Jamison K R: *Manic-Depressive Illness.* Oxford University Press, New York, 1990.

Jackson S W: *Melancholia and Depression: From Hippocratic Times to Modern Times.* Yale University Press, New Haven, 1986.

Janowsky D S, El-Yousef M K, Davis J M, Sekerke H J: A cholinergic-adrenergic hypothesis of mania and depression. Lancet 2: 632, 1972.

Keller M B, Klerman G L, Lavori P W, Fawcett J A, Coryell W, Endicott J: Treatment received by depressed patients. JAMA *248:* 1848, 1982.

Kendler K S, Neale M C, Kessler R C, Heath A C, Eaves L J: A longitudinal twin study of personality and major depression in women. Arch Gen Psychiatry *50:* 853, 1993.

Klerman G L, Lavori P W, Rice J, Reich T, Endicott J, Andreasen N C, Keller M B, Hirschfield R M: Birth-cohort trends in rates of major depressive disorder among relatives of patients with affective disorder. Arch Gen Psychiatry *42:* 689, 1985.

*Klibansky R, Panofsky E, Saxl F: *Saturn and Melancholy.* Nendeln, Kraus Reprint, Liechtenstein, 1979.

*Kraepelin E: *Manic-Depressive Insanity and Paranoia,* R M Barclay, translator, G M Robertson, editor. Livingstone, Edinburgh, 1921.

Kupfer D J: REM latency: A psychobiologic marker for primary depressive disease. Biol Psychiatry *11:* 159, 1976.

Lapin I P, Oxenkrug G F: Intensification of the central serotoninergic processes as a possible determinant of the thymoleptic effect. Lancet *1*: 132, 1969.

Leonhard K: *The Classification of Endogenous Psychoses,* R Berman, translator. Irvington, New York, 1979.

Lewinsohn P M, Youngren M A, Grosscup S J: Reinforcement and depression. In *The Psychobiology of Depressive Disorders; Implications for the Effects of Stress,* R A Depre, editor. Academic Press, New York, 1979.

Lewis A: States of depression: Their clinical and aetiological differentiation. Br Med J 2: 875, 1938.

Maser J D, Cloninger C R, editors: *Comorbidity of Mood and Anxiety Disorders.* American Psychiatric Press, Washington, 1990.

McGuffin P, Katz R, Bebbington P: The Camberwell Collaborative Depressive Study: III. Depression and adversity in the relatives of depressed probands. Br J Psychiatry *152:* 775, 1988.

Nemeroff C B, Widerlov E, Bissette G: Elevated concentrations of CSF corticotropin-releasing factor-like immunoreactivity in depressed patients. Science *226:* 1342, 1984.

Nolen-Hoeksema S, Morrow J, Fredrickson B L: Response styles and the duration of episodes of depressed mood. J Abnorm Psychol *102:* 20, 1993

Perris C: A study of bipolar (manic-depressive) and unipolar recurrent depressive psychoses. Acta Psychiatr Scand Suppl *45,* 1966.

Perugi G, Musetti L, Simorini E, Piagentini F, Cassano G B, Akiskal H S: Gender mediated clinical features of depressive illness: The importance of temperamental differences. Br J Psychiatry *157:* 835, 1990.

Post R M: Transduction of psychosocial stress into the neurobiology of recurrent affective disorder. Am J Psychiatry *149:* 999, 1992.

Prange A J Jr, Wilson I C, Lynn C W, Alltop L B, Stikeleather R A: L-tryptophan in mania: Contribution to a permissive hypothesis of affective disorders. Arch Gen Psychiatry *30:* 56, 1974.

Robins L N, Regier D A, editors: *Psychiatric Disorders in America.* Free Press, New York, 1991.

Roth R M, Barnes T R: The classification of affective disorders: A synthesis of old and new concepts. Compr Psychiatry *22:* 54, 1981.

Schildkraut J J: The catecholamine hypothesis of affective disorders: A review of supporting evidence. Am J Psychiatry *122:* 509, 1965.

Seligman M D: *Helplessness: On Depression, Development and Death.* Freeman, San Francisco, 1975.

Siever L J, Davis K L: Overview: Toward a dysregulation hypothesis of depression. Am J Psychiatry *142:* 1017, 1985.

van Praag H M, Kahn R S, Asnis G M, Wetzler S, Brown S L, Bleich A, Korn M L: Denosologization of biological psychiatry or the specificity of 5-HT disturbances in psychiatric disorders. J Affective Disord *13:* 1, 1987.

Wehr T A, Rosenthal N E: Seasonality and affective illness. Am J Psychiatry *146:* 829, 1989.

Whybrow P C, Akiskal H S, McKinney W T Jr: *Mood Disorders: Toward a New Psychobiology.* Plenum Press, New York, 1984.

Williams T A, Katz M M, Shields J S, editors: *Recent Advances in the Psychobiology of Depressive Illness.* US Government Printing Office, Washington, 1972.

Winokur G, Clayton P J, Reich T: *Manic-Depressive Illness.* Mosby, St Louis, 1969.

16.2
MOOD DISORDERS: EPIDEMIOLOGY

DAN BLAZER II, M.D., Ph.D.

INTRODUCTION

The epidemiological study of mood disorders complements clinical investigation of those disorders by completing the clinical picture in breadth and through time. The clinician's experience with a chronic syndrome, such as depression, is limited to the hospital and the outpatient setting. The epidemiologist broadens the study to community populations and studies the natural history of those syndromes through time. The tasks of epidemiology have been applied to the mood disorders by many investigators in recent years. Those tasks include: identification of cases (for example, What is a case of major depressive disorder?), distribution of cases (for example, Do blacks experience more depressive disorders than nonblacks?), historical trends (for example, Is major depressive disorder becoming more prevalent in the population as one nears the end of the 20 century?), identification of causes (for example, Does low socioeconomic status predispose to the onset of major depressive disorder?), prognosis (for example, What is the likelihood of disability from a major depressive episode within the first year after a case is diagnosed?), and need demand, supply, and use of psychiatric services (for example, What percentage of persons with mood disorders in the community receive care from a mental health specialist?).

Most of the data presented here derive from studies of depressive symptoms and the diagnosis of major depressive disorder. Bipolar disorders will receive less attention than they do in clinical studies because the community-based epidemiological data are sparse. The lifetime prevalence of some mood disorders, including dysthymic disorder and cyclothymic disorder, appears in Table 16.2-1.

CASE IDENTIFICATION

Clinicians who treat patients experiencing mood disorders must distinguish normal variations in mood from the mood disorders. The diagnostic criteria for the specific mood disorders in the fourth edition of *Diagnostic and Statistical Manual of Mental Disorders* (DSM-IV) and its predecessors are not always easily applied in epidemiological studies. Some of the diagnostic categories, such as adjustment disorder with depressed mood, cannot be operationalized in standardized interviews because the criteria require a subjective clinical judgment (for example, the mood disturbance must be related to a specific stressor). Other diagnoses are too inclusive when applied to community samples, such as major depressive disorder. Cases identified using current diagnostic criteria are therefore a heterogeneous mix that has little clinical relevance beyond symptom severity. In other words, the borderline between clinical depression and normal fluctuation in mood is fuzzy. Even the presence or absence of a symptom may be disputed.

TABLE 16.2-1
Lifetime Prevalence of Some DSM-IV Mood Disorders

Mood Disorder	Lifetime Prevalence
Depressive disorders	
Major depressive disorder (MDD)	10-25% for women; 5-12% for men
Recurrent, with full interepisode recovery, superimposed on dysthymic disorder	Approximately 3% of persons with MDD
Recurrent, without full interepisode recovery, superimposed on dysthymic disorder (double depression)	Approximately 25% of persons with MDD
Dysthymic disorder	Approximately 6%
Bipolar disorders	
Bipolar I disorder	0.4-1.6%
Bipolar II disorder	Approximately 0.5%
Bipolar I disorder or bipolar II disorder, with rapid cycling	5-15% of persons with bipolar disorder
Cyclothymic disorder	0.4-1.0%

Data from DSM-IV, *Diagnostic and Statistical Manual of Mental Disorders,* ed 4. Copyright American Psychiatric Association, Washington, 1994.

Some persons in community samples may present with depressive syndromes that do not fit the DSM diagnostic system (for example, for major depressive disorder or dysthymic disorder) but they nevertheless suffer disabling depressive symptoms. Much attention has been focused in recent years on so-called minor depressive disorder, a syndrome defined by symptoms that are less severe than major depressive disorder and of shorter duration than dysthymic disorder. Persons identified in community surveys as experiencing minor depressive disorder have been shown in prospective studies to be at greater risk for time lost at work and increased use of general health services than persons without depressive symptoms.

The process of case identification in community studies also may contribute to bias. Recall of past symptoms is only modestly accurate when compared with clinical records of previous depressive episodes. The threshold for reporting a symptom of depression may be higher in a community setting than in a clinical one because clinicians often probe for evidence of a symptom that the patient initially denies. Most of the interview instruments that are used in epidemiological surveys to identify DSM diagnoses, such as the Diagnostic Interview Survey (DIS) and the Schedule for Affective Disorders and Schizophrenia (SADS), were developed in clinical settings and were standardized using classic cases that present to psychiatric treatment settings. Depressive symptoms that are disabling to persons in the community may not always be identified by diagnostic techniques that are effective in clinical settings.

Comorbidity presents another problem to psychiatric epidemiologists who study mood disorders in community settings. More often than not, symptoms of anxiety and depression overlap. Many subjects receive concurrent diagnoses of major depressive disorder, dysthymic disorder, and generalized anxiety disorder. Most community survey subjects cannot accurately remember whether the depression or the anxiety was the first syndrome experienced. Do major depressive disorder and generalized anxiety disorder coexist, or is anxiety an epiphenomenon of major depressive disorder? That question remains unanswered.

Those problems in case identification in community surveys for psychiatric morbidity have stimulated clinical and community-based investigators to seek better case finding and case identification methods. Standardized diagnostic interviews have greatly improved the reliability of symptom identification. (For example, clinical investigators may not agree upon the utility of the diagnosis of mood disorder with seasonal pattern, also known as seasonal affective disorder, but they can test their disagreement using the same criteria for case identification and findings are therefore comparable across studies.) Explicit diagnostic criteria, such as the Research Diagnostic Criteria and its successors, provide hypotheses for testing. (For example, is bipolar I disorder, as defined by DSM-IV, more heritable than major depressive disorder? If so, then those criteria differentiate, to some extent, two different psychobiological entities.)

DISTRIBUTION OF CASES

The prevalence of the most common mood disorders by age and sex is presented in Figure 16.2-1. Those data are derived from the largest community-based epidemiological case finding

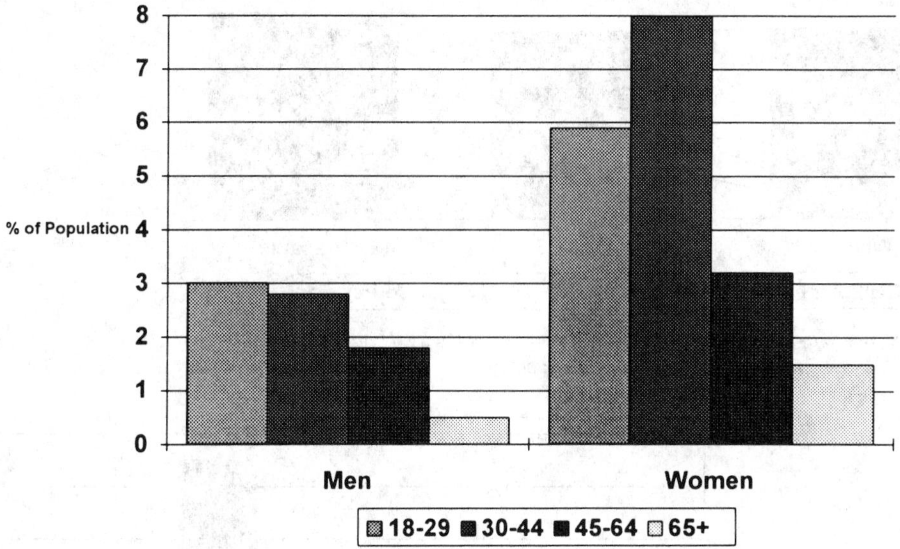

FIGURE 16.2-1 *Prevalence of the most common mood disorders by age and sex. Data derived from the Epidemiologic Catchment Area study.*

study fielded in western society—the Epidemiologic Catchment Area (ECA) Study. The Diagnostic Interview Schedule was administered to over 18,000 community and institutionalized subjects at five sites throughout the United States—New Haven, East Baltimore, St. Louis, the Piedmont of North Carolina, and Los Angeles. By virtue of the large numbers of subjects and the oversampling of subjects not accurately represented in previous studies, such as blacks, Hispanics, and the elderly, much better estimates of the actual distribution of cases were possible.

AGE AND SEX The most striking finding from the ECA study was the much higher prevalence of all the mood disorders among persons under the age of 45 compared with persons over 45 years of age. Manic episodes are about equally prevalent in men and women, whereas major depressive disorder and dysthymic disorder are more prevalent in women than in men. Rates were comparable across ECA sites, except for a lower prevalence in North Carolina. The North Carolina sample was composed of both urban and rural residents. Persons in urban areas were as likely to be diagnosed with a mood disorder in North Carolina as in urban areas at other ECA sites. In contrast, rural subjects in North Carolina had much lower rates of major depressive disorder than rural subjects at other ECA sites.

The most consistent finding across epidemiological studies of the mood disorders, confirmed by the ECA study, is the relatively higher prevalence of major depressive disorder in women than in men. The sex differences are consistent across the life cycle, but are much more prominent in young adult and middle-aged persons than in the elderly and children. Many factors have been suggested to account for this sex difference, such as endocrine physiology and genetics. Although the endocrine system of women differs significantly from that of men, there is no consistent endocrinological theory to account for the sex differences in depressive disorders. Because alcohol abuse and mood disorders are often inherited in the same family, and alcohol abuse and dependence are more prevalent in men than in women, perhaps depressive disorder and alcohol abuse and dependence are phenotypic variants of the same genotype. Little evidence, however, supports that hypothesis. Consistent findings across community-based epidemiological studies have nullified the hypothesis that depressive disorder appears to be more prevalent in women because they are more likely to seek services for depression than men. Psychosocial explanations for the higher prevalence of depressive disorders among women are currently considered the most promising. For example, the greater stress for women of maintaining multiple roles, such as homemaker, professional, wife, and mother is one possible explanation.

RACE As illustrated in Figure 16.2-2, the prevalence of the mood disorders does not vary significantly by race. In most epidemiological studies of psychiatric disorders, racial differences in the rates can be explained by socioeconomic and educational differences. The ECA was the first study in western society that permitted direct comparison of whites with blacks and Hispanics. Previous comparisons, which could not control for geographical differences, were subject to significant bias, because prevalence estimates clearly vary by place of residence.

LIFETIME PREVALENCE The overall lifetime prevalence of mood disorders from the ECA study is 6 percent. Distribution by age and gender is presented in Figure 16.2-3. Lifetime prevalence (which include current cases) follows a similar distribution as current rates. The lower lifetime prevalence of major depressive disorder in the elderly strongly suggests methodological problems and a significant cohort effect. One would expect that the longer a person lives (that is, the more years at risk for a psychiatric disorder), the more likely the person would experience that disorder.

A recent study of a national sample of over 8,000 persons from 15 to 54 years of age, the National Comorbidy Study estimates the prevalence rate of mood disorders to be higher than what was found in the ECA study. The current 30-day prevalence of major depressive disorder was estimated at 4.9 percent overall, and the lifetime prevalence was estimated at 17.1 percent. A different method of case ascertainment, however, rather than any change in actual prevalence since the ECA study, probably accounts for the higher estimates. The distribution of cases by sex and ethnic groups was similar to that found in the ECA study.

The findings of the ECA study and the National Comorbidity Study have tended to parallel earlier epidemiological studies in the United States, such as the Stirling County Study (current prevalence of major depression was 4.7 percent in men and 6.0 percent in women) and the New Haven Study (3.2 percent in men and 5.2 percent in women). Most studies in developed

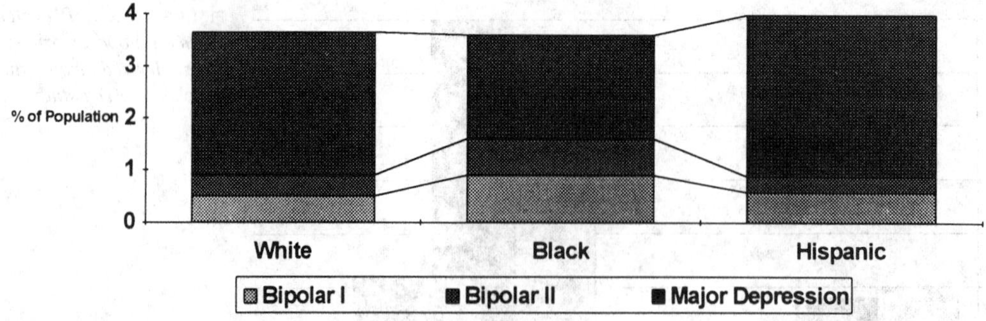

FIGURE 16.2-2 *Current (one year) prevalence of mood disorders by ethnicity. Data derived from the Epidemiologic Catchment Area study.*

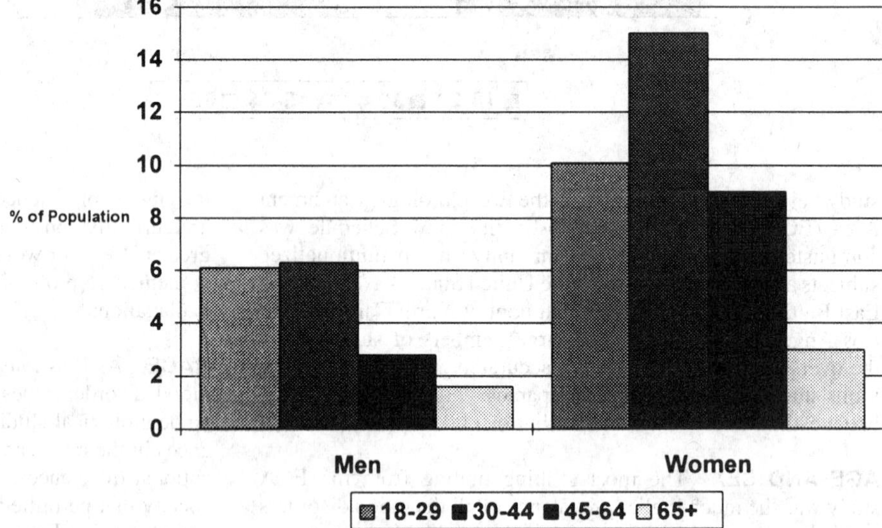

FIGURE 16.2-3 *Lifetime prevalence of mood disorders by age and sex. Data derived from the Epidemiologic Catchment Area study.*

countries estimate the distribution of major depressive disorder to be greater in women than in men, in young adulthood than in midlife and old age, in urban residents than in rural residents, and among single or divorced persons than among married persons. Few studies document a racial difference when social class and education are controlled.

DEPRESSIVE SYMPTOMS The prevalence and distribution of clinically significant depressive symptoms parallels that of major depressive disorder, although the age differences are not nearly so great. In most studies, between 8 and 20 percent of community samples report depressive symptoms at a level above the cutoff used to screen for major depressive disorder, such as 16+ on the Center for Epidemiologic Studies Depression Scale (CES-D). Many of those persons do not meet criteria for specific DSM-IV mood disorders. Those depressive symptoms, however, have been associated with higher mortality rates, higher disability rates, and poor social functioning.

INCIDENCE The incidence of the mood disorders is the percentage of new cases of the disorder which emerge in a population at risk for the disorder (that is, persons not experiencing the disorder at the beginning of the study) over a specified period of time (usually one year). Because major depressive disorder is common and tends to remit and recur, the incidence is relatively high. The annual incidence of major depressive disorder in the ECA study was 1.59 percent overall. The distribution by age and sex is presented in Figure 16.2-4. A survey in Lundby, Sweden, revealed an annual first incidence of depression (cases of depression in persons who never experienced depression before) of 0.43 percent in men and 0.76 percent in women. Up to the age of 70, the cumulative probability of a first episode of depression was 27 percent in men and 45 percent in women, making depression one of the most important public health problems.

SETTING The prevalence of major depressive disorder is much higher in treatment settings than in the community at large. Most investigators find that 10 to 15 percent of persons in acute hospital settings and in long-term care facilities meet the criteria for the diagnosis of major depressive disorder. An additional 20 to 30 percent of persons in treatment settings report clinically significant, subsyndromal depression (minor depression). The similarities between those cases of major depressive disorder to cases found in psychiatric treatment settings has yet to be documented. Although some of the depressed and medically ill patients respond to antidepressant therapy and brief psychotherapy, many of them have comorbid conditions which render traditional therapies ineffective.

Depression is also more prevalent in primary care settings than in the general population. Using methods of case identification similar to the ECA study, the current prevalence of depression is about double that found in the general population. In most surveys of primary care clinics, over 20 percent of the patients report clinically significant depressive symptoms. Major depressive disorder is diagnosed in one third to one half of those outpatients—a prevalence of 5 to 10 percent. Young women are at greatest risk for depression in primary care, and

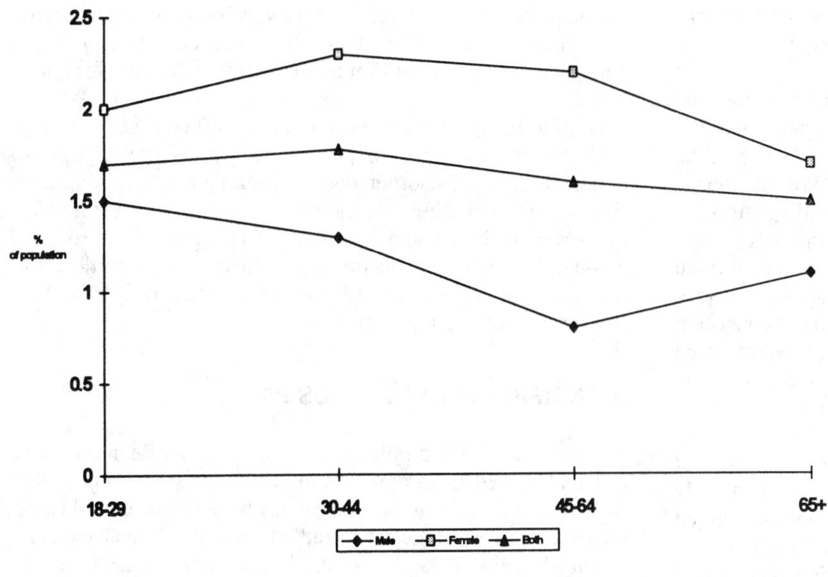

FIGURE 16.2-4 *Annual incidence of major depressive disorder by age and sex. Data derived from the Epidemiologic Catchment Area study.*

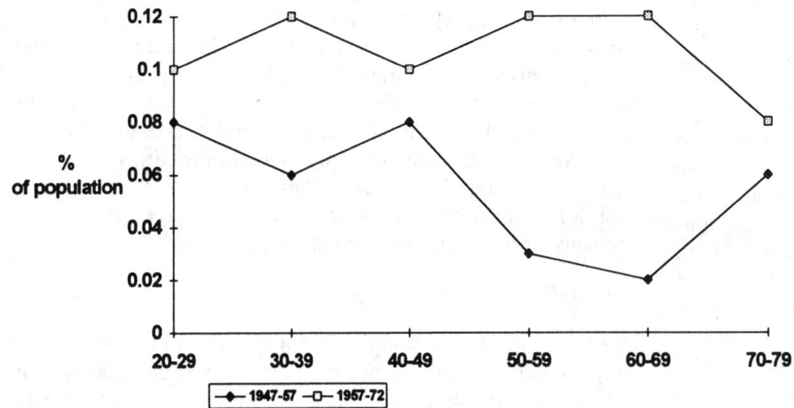

FIGURE 16.2-5 *Risk of contracting a first-onset depressive disorder for younger birth cohorts compared with older birth cohorts in Sweden. Data derived from O Hagnell, J Lanke, B Rorsman, L Ojesjo: Are we entering an age of melancholy? Depressive illnesses in a prospective epidemiological study over 25 years: The Lundby Study, Sweden. Psychol Med 12: 279, 1982.*

most persons who report depressive symptoms to a health care professional report them to a primary care physician. Unlike the depressive syndromes that present in hospital and long-term care settings, the depressive syndromes that present in outpatient medical settings may be prime targets for psychotherapeutic and pharmacotherapeutic treatment.

HISTORICAL TRENDS

The higher prevalence of depression in younger than in older age groups has led to the hypothesis that birth cohorts born after World War II are at appreciably greater risk for major depressive disorder than older birth cohorts in advanced Western society. The trend has been observed not only in the United States, but also in Sweden, Germany, Canada, and New Zealand. (Higher prevalence among older persons has not been observed in comparable community surveys in Korea, Puerto Rico, and Mexican Americans living in the United States.) When the findings were originally reported, many researchers attributed them to bias in case identification, such as problems of recall, selective mortality, and diagnostic criteria more applicable to a younger age. Thorough evaluation of the case finding methods, however, coupled with adjustments for selective mortality, do not substantiate bias as the sole explanation for the differences in prevalence across age groups.

A number of observations made prior to the ECA study suggested that rates of depressive disorders were changing. Relevant factors included a progressively lower age of onset of depressive disorders reported in community studies; an increase in childhood mood disorders seen by pediatricians and mental health workers; a decrease in deaths from suicide among the elderly; and a fall in the average age of onset for depressive disorders in clinical samples since World War II. For example, the risk of first-onset depression was higher for younger birth cohorts than for older birth cohorts in Sweden (Figure 16.2-5). The trends in suicide data parallel the trends in mood disorders (that is, suicide rates are much higher in younger persons today than they were 30 years ago, whereas suicide rates for older persons are lower today than they were 30 years ago (although suicide rates in older adults have increased by 25 percent since 1980).

FACTORS THAT INFLUENCE HISTORICAL TRENDS

Three factors influence the historical trends in the relative prevalence of mood disorders by age—period effects, age effects, and cohort effects.

Period effects *Period effects* are changes in the prevalence of an illness secondary to environmental stressors on the population, or particular age groups within the population, at a specific period in history. (For example, the uncertainty of employment among college graduates and the trend among younger persons to delay marriage during the 1990s may place young adults at greater risk for depression and suicide because of economic impairment and lack of affiliative relations.)

Age effects *Age effects* are the biological and psychosocial factors that predispose an individual to develop a particular disorder during a specific part of the life cycle. (For example, the genetic predisposition to develop major depressive disorder is probably greatest during the 30s, whereas the predisposition to develop a bipolar disorder is greatest during the 20s.) Age-related changes in the brain, such as the increase in subcortical hyperintensities on brain magnetic resonance imaging, may also be associated with mood disorders. Perhaps the most consistent age effect relevant to the mood disorders that has been observed during the 20th century is the positive association between age and suicide among white males in the United States.

Cohort *Cohort effects* are the relative differences in rates of illness across different generations. The cohort is usually defined by the year or decade of birth. A person born in a given year may be at greater risk for an illness, such as major depressive disorder, throughout his or her life. Suicide data reveal marked cohort trends throughout the 20th century. (For example, persons currently 70 to 80 years of age [approximately the birth cohorts of 1915 to 1925] have exhibited lower suicide rates at all ages than the 1900 and 1940 birth cohorts.)

Interaction of effects There are considerable statistical and methodological problems in sorting out the relative contribution of period, age, and cohort effects upon the prevalence and incidence of mood disorders by age. First, those effects undoubtedly interact. Stressors during a particular period interact with age-related vulnerability. (For example, the current high rate of substance abuse among adolescents may be secondary, in part, both to the vulnerability of adolescents to substance abuse and to the greater availability of drugs to adolescents.) Second, older persons may not recognize major depressive episodes as such and so do not report them. Yet age does not appear to affect the rate of hospitalization for mood disorders. The more severe cases of major depressive disorder are hospitalized, regardless of age. The relative cohort differences persist in hospitalization rates.

Although most investigators have explained the current data as reflecting a cohort effect, some have suggested that they reflect a period effect. They argue that the risk for depressive disorders increased dramatically for all ages from about 1965 to 1975, but has since stabilized. Young persons are more vulnerable to that period effect, however, and therefore carry the greatest burden of depressive disorders. A young person who experiences a major depressive episode is likely to exhibit ongoing and severe depressive episodes for many years. Therefore, clinicians can expect to see the current cohort of younger persons bear the burden of major depressive disorder for a long time.

Despite being the healthiest and most affluent generation of the 20th century, younger persons may be at greater risk for major depressive disorder due to a number of environmental risk factors, including: (1) increased urbanization; (2) increasing social isolation and anomie; (3) changes in the roles of women; (4) changes in occupational roles and career trajectories for both men and women; (5) increased secularization; and (6) greater geographic mobility.

IDENTIFICATION OF CAUSES

The risk factors for bipolar disorders and major depressive disorder identified from epidemiological studies are summarized in Table 16.2-2. Some of the findings have not been replicated, but others have emerged repeatedly from both clinical and community-based studies. (For example, an increased risk for major depressive disorder was discovered in an isolated community of the Hutterites who live near the border between the United States and Canada, suggesting that the rigid moral control they exert predisposes community members to depression.) Most community studies, however, fail to find that identification with or participation in particular religious groups is associated with an increased risk for major depressive disorder. In contrast, virtually every community survey has demonstrated an increased risk for major depressive disorder and depressive symptoms in persons who report negative life events.

DEMOGRAPHIC FACTORS

Sex Almost all community-based epidemiological surveys of mood disorders find that women are twice as likely as men to be experiencing an episode of major depressive disorder. Few investigators discount the finding as an artifact of prejudice in the diagnostic criteria for major depressive disorder or of increased help-seeking behavior among women. Yet female sex has not been demonstrated to be a risk factor per se. The social environment of women and a higher threshold for reporting depressive symptoms in men may account for the increased association.

Age The average age of onset for both major depressive disorder and bipolar disorders falls between the ages of 20 and 40 years. Recent studies confirm that major depressive disorder can occur in childhood. Bipolar I disorder typically has an earlier age of onset than major depressive disorder, with an average of

TABLE 16.2-2
Risk Factors for Bipolar I Disorder and Major Depressive Disorder

Risk Factor	Bipolar I Disorder	Major Depressive Disorder
Sex	No difference	Women at greater risk than men
Race	No difference	Blacks at somewhat less risk than whites
Age	Young at greater risk	Young at greater risk
Socioeconomic status (SES)	Higher SES at somewhat greater risk	Lower SES at greater risk for depressive symptoms and for major depressive disorder
Marital status	Separated and divorced have highest rates	Separated and divorced have highest rates
Family history	Persons with family history have higher rates	Persons with family history have higher rates
Childhood experiences	Bipolar patients may come from families with low perceived prestige in their community	Evidence that early parental death and disruptive childhood environment leads to major depression
Stressful life events	No known difference	Negative stressful events associated with increased risk
Absence of a confidant	No known difference	Absence of confidant leads to increased risk, especially in women
Residence	Greater risk in suburbs than in inner city	Greater risk in urban areas than in rural areas

30 years. Yet both major depressive disorder and bipolar disorders can first occur at any time during adulthood. Nothing suggests that young age, in itself, places a person at greater risk for the mood disorders (though genetic factors may have their greatest influence at a younger age). Social factors appear to place younger persons at greater risk than the elderly. Biological predisposition to major depressive disorder may actually increase with age.

Race Race has not proved to be a significant risk factor for either bipolar I disorder or major depressive disorder. In many community surveys, blacks experience a higher prevalence of depressive symptoms. The racial difference usually disappears, however, when other factors, such as socioeconomic status, age, and residence, are controlled. Because treatment for mood disorders is less common for blacks than for whites, prevalence studies based on treatment samples usually contain proportionally more whites. Recent findings from the ECA study suggest that major depressive disorder may be less common among blacks than among whites and Hispanics. Investigators must not overgeneralize from these results, because the case finding methods used in the ECA study may be biased against finding cases among blacks. (For example, blacks may be more likely to somatize the experience of depression, although there was no evidence that blacks somatize overall more than whites.)

SOCIOECONOMIC STATUS The findings from community-based studies relating to socioeconomic status (SES) as a risk factor for depression are mixed. In the overall ECA studies, there was only a weak correlation between major depressive disorder or bipolar disorders and lower SES. In the North Carolina ECA study, however, there was a consistent relation between SES and major depressive disorder, even when multiple potential confounders, such as race and residence, were controlled. Studies prior to the ECA found a consistent positive relation between lower SES and depression. In one classic study reported by August Hollingshead and Fredrick Redlich, depressive symptoms were strongly associated with the lower social classes. In a more recent study, working-class women from an eastern suburb of London were much more likely to suffer depressive symptoms than women from higher social classes.

MARITAL STATUS Marital status appears to be one of the most consistent risk factors for both depressive symptoms and major depressive disorder. Rates for major depressive disorder are highest among separated and divorced persons, and lowest among single and married persons. Recent widowhood is associated with higher rates of major depressive disorder across the life cycle.

The risk appears to vary with sex. Single women have been found to have lower rates of depression than married women, whereas married men have lower rates than single men. However, the investigator must not confound marital status with the loss of a spouse through death or divorce (a stressful life event). If a subject was widowed during the six months prior to the study, then the event, not the status, is the causative factor. In addition, cause and effect may be reversed (for example, depressive illness may place a person at greater risk for divorce). In most studies, however, the separated or divorced status places the person at greater risk for depression, even if the marital breakup occurred long before the assessment.

The ECA studies, unlike previous studies, also documented a much higher prevalence of bipolar disorders among the separated and divorced than among single persons. The highest rates, however, were found among those who were cohabiting, even when adjusting for age, sex, and race or ethnicity. The association of the mood disorders and marital status is also reflected in the association of mood disorders with household size. Major depressive disorder is twice as common among persons living alone than among those who live with others. In persons not living alone household size is not associated with depression.

Marital status may not be the proximal causative factor. The perception of social support and lack of conflict within the social network are critical factors in protecting against mood disorders. Longitudinal studies of the social network and neuroses have shown that the most important predictors of depression are not the objective characteristics of the network, but rather the perception of how adequately the network assisted the person. Large-scale community-based investigations of the risk factors for major depressive disorder and bipolar I disorder cannot disentangle the subtleties of the complex interactions between persons and their social network. (For example, the dissolution of a difficult marriage may relieve long-standing depressive symptoms.)

FAMILY HISTORY Most epidemiological studies of treatment samples have shown a consistent increase in family history of mood disorders among subjects, especially in first-degree relatives. A family history of suicide and alcoholism has also been repeatedly demonstrated to be more common among the depressed subjects than among controls. Most experts attribute the increased risk for depression when family history is positive to a genetic predisposition. Yet the shared family environment may also contribute to the increased risk. Genetic transmission is much more firmly established for bipolar I disorder than for major depressive disorder. In family members of bipolar subjects, both bipolar I disorder and major depressive disorder are more prevalent.

EARLY CHILDHOOD EXPERIENCE Much attention has been directed to the association of early childhood experience with the onset of mood disorders later in life. Although the complexities of a psychodynamic investigation of childhood traumas cannot be applied in community-based epidemiological studies, even cursory investigation of childhood experiences has revealed correlates. Parental loss before adolescence has been well documented as a risk factor for adult-onset depression. A deprived and disrupted home environment also constitutes a risk. Methodological problems make objective study of childhood trauma and deprivation difficult. Some events, such as divorce or separation of parents, can be documented reliably, but others, such as parental neglect, are very subjective. The report of parental neglect by the depressed adult may vary depending on the respondent's emotional state at the time of the interview.

PERSONALITY ATTRIBUTES Personality attributes are closely related to early childhood experience as a risk for mood disorders in later life. Personality emerges early in life and is formed by biological tendencies coupled with the child's social environment. Persons predisposed to develop a depressive disorder have been shown to lack energy, to be more introverted, to worry, to be more dependent, and to be hypersensitive. Major depressive disorder has also been found to be frequently comorbid with the Axis II disorders. Yet the study of the relation of depression and personality is confounded by the time at which personality is studied. Epidemiologists rarely have the opportunity to assess personality before the onset of the first episode of depression. If personality is assessed during an episode of depression, then the depressive symptoms mask certain personality traits and exaggerate others. When a person has experienced and recovered from a depressive episode its impact on personality makes an accurate assessment of premorbid personality difficult. (For example, the personality characteristics that are associated with depression are exactly those which might emerge in response to the experience of a difficult mental disorder.)

SOCIAL STRESS Social stress has received more attention than most of the other risk factors for major depressive disorder across the life cycle. Three kinds of social stress can be distinguished: life events, chronic stress, and daily hassles. *Life events* are the kind most often used in epidemiological studies. They are identifiable, discrete changes in life patterns that disrupt the usual behavior and threaten the person's well-being. Bereavement, the stress reaction to the loss of a loved one, is the prototype stressful life event. *Chronic stress* includes long-term conditions that challenge the person, including financial deprivation, ongoing interpersonal difficulties (such as conflict in the workplace), and persistent threat to security (such as living in a dangerous neighborhood). *Daily hassles* are ordinary but stressful occurrences that are ubiquitous in modern life, such as managing household finances and unpleasant interactions with neighbors.

Life events Most epidemiological studies reveal a relation between stressful life events, especially negative events, and the onset and outcome of major depressive disorder. Nevertheless, the use of stressful life event scales, such as the Schedule of Recent Events, introduces many potential biases into the study of stressors and depression. Such scales usually tally the number of events and weight them according to a predetermined algorithm. Most schedules weight events based on normative data from the population. Because the data usually derive from weightings provided by young adults, they do not apply across the life cycle. (For example, retirement in late life may be a very positive event, whereas premature retirement in midlife may present major problems that can precipitate a depressive disorder.)

The perception of the event is probably more important than the event itself. More sensitive measures of stressful events document not only the event itself but the subject's response to it. Was the event perceived to be positive or negative? Even the death of a spouse may be viewed as a positive event if it occurred after a protracted and disabling illness during which the subject was the caretaker. Was the event perceived to be important or unimportant? For some older persons a move may be extremely traumatic, especially if it is the first move in half a century. For others, a move may be a usual and relatively unimportant event, especially in a society where mobility is becoming more the norm. Was the event expected or unexpected? If income decreases at retirement at a rate expected by the retiree, then the loss of income is much less stressful than if a person is forced to take an unexpected cut in salary while still in the workforce.

The accumulation of stressful negative life events does appear to predispose a person to episodes of major depressive disorder. In a study from New Haven, depressed patients had an average increased frequency of eight life events during the six months before the onset of depressive symptoms. Those events included marital arguments, marital separation, starting a new type of work, change in work conditions, serious personal illness, death of an immediate family member, serious illness of family members, and a family member leaving home. Stressful events are also associated with the persistence of depressive disorders. In a study from England, adverse events during the year following the initial episode of depression were associated with a poorer outcome of the episode. The adverse effects of life events may be offset by neutralizing events. (For example, if a woman loses her job but soon after finds another job with equal pay and benefits, then the adverse event is neutralized.) However, persons experiencing a recurrent major depressive disorder are less likely to report a stressful event associated with the onset of episodes after the first two episodes of depression.

Chronic stress Chronic stress can place a subject at greater risk for major depressive disorder than specific stressful life events. The stress of a chronic illness, for example, frequently manifests itself in the symptoms of a major depressive episode. As long as the stressor of the illness persists, the individual has difficulty recovering from the major depressive episode. Persons usually have more difficulty coping with ongoing stressors than with specific events, to which they can adapt.

Daily hassles Few studies document the association of daily hassles with the onset of major depressive disorder. Impulsive acts, such as a suicide attempt, may be closely associated with daily hassles to which the subject cannot adapt within the context of a stressful life event or chronic stress. That is, daily hassles may be the straw that breaks the camel's back.

SOCIAL SUPPORT Factors in the social environment that may modify the effects of social stress have received increased attention in the epidemiological investigation of both physical and psychiatric disorders. One factor is social support, the provision of meaningful, appropriate, and protective feedback from the social environment that enables a person to negotiate environmental stressors. In theory, social support is an attractive concept, for it is potentially more amenable to interventions than environmental stressors. The roots of the construct social support go back at least to the early 20th century, when Émile Durkheim proposed that persons who are not integrated into society (the condition called "anomie") are at greater risk for suicide.

Social support has four components: the social network, social interaction, perceived social support, and instrumental support. The *social network* consists of those individuals or groups of individuals, such as a spouse and children, who are available to the subject. The absence of a spouse is a risk factor for major depressive disorder. *Social interactions* may be assessed by documenting the frequency of interactions between the subject and other network members. A number of studies confirm that social isolation (that is, a deficit of social interaction) places a subject at greater risk for depression. Yet the quality of the interaction appears to be more important than the frequency of the interaction. *Perceived social support* is the subjective evaluation by the individual of the dependability of the social network, the ease of interaction with the network, the sense of belonging to the network, and the sense of intimacy with network members. The association of major depressive disorder and lack of a confidant is an example of the relation between perceived inadequate support and depression.

Instrumental support consists of concrete and observable services that are provided to the subject by the social network (for example, cooking meals, financial assistance, and nursing services for the physically ill). Although such support is essential to the well-being of the young and the elderly in society few studies document the association of depression with a deprivation of instrumental support. The physical health of the person is a confounding factor. Instrumental support is usually not obvious unless the person exhibits an actual need for such services. In addition, the perception of the availability of those services in a time of crisis may not reflect the actual availability.

Social integration The construct of social support is strongly influenced by the construct of social integration. An integrated society is a social system which insures the patterns of interpersonal behavior that are essential to the survival and welfare of the society. Those patterns enable the group to obtain what is needed for subsistence, protection against weather and disease, control of hostility and other forms of social disruption, creation of new members and their education, disposal of the dead, communication, storage of information, and ways for arriving at decisions and taking united action. Alexander Leighton and his colleagues undertook the most ambitious epidemiological studies of social integration and mental health in a study of communities in Nova Scotia. Social scientists and anthropologists studied each community to determine its relative integration versus disintegration. At all ages, the rates of depressive disorders (and other psychiatric disorders) were higher in disintegrated communities. Studies of social integration are not as proximal to the individual as studies of social stressors and social support, because measures of social integration are not specific to the individual. Those studies are ecological, for they document that the overall level of social disintegration in a community is associated with the overall level of psychopathology.

Residence Most studies of social integration have been limited to comparisons of communities by traditional parameters, the most common of which is urban versus rural residence. The hypothesis is that rural communities are more integrated and less stressful than urban communities. In the ECA study of North Carolina, major depressive disorder was two times more common in the urban community, with the largest differences among the young (under 45 years of age) and among women. Those urban-rural differences in prevalence persisted even when the comparison was controlled for race, socioeconomic status, marital status, and age. The prevalence of major depressive disorder was also lower in North Carolina than in the other ECA sites, suggesting that geographical location may contribute to differences in the prevalence of major depressive disorder.

Unemployment Another risk factor for depression is unemployment. At present, most men and women under the age of 65 are in the labor force. Men and women who were unemployed for at least six months during the five years prior to the ECA survey were more than three times as likely as others to report the symptoms of an episode of major depressive disorder during the year prior to the survey.

The multiple risk factors for mood disorders form a web of causation. Each factor can not only affect the subject directly but can interact with other factors. Mathematical models of causative factors are therefore useful for determining the relative importance and the complex interaction of those factors. Models include linear and logistic regression analyses.

An example is presented in Table 16.2-3. Three variables in the multivariate model are significant—urban residence, younger age, and female sex. The coefficients in the logistic-regression model are equivalent to an odds ratio (that is, the odds of a risk factor being associated with major depressive disorder when the comparison factor has a risk of 1). For example, when the comparison factor for age is the over 65 age group, then the middle-aged (25 to 44) are over three times as likely to be depressed. Each of the risk factors is presented while accounting for the other factors (that is, all other factors are controlled).

TABLE 16.2-3
Logistic-Regression Effects (Odds Ratios) of Urban/Rural Residence and Control Variables on Major Depressive Disorder

Variable	Coefficient (Odds Ratio)	Significance
Urban residence	1.983	<.05
Age (25-44)	3.143	<.05
Separated or divorced	1.434	NS*
Widowed	0.738	NS
Never married	1.576	NS
Female	2.695	<.05
Nonwhite	1.130	NS
Education	1.033	NS
Moved in last 5 years	1.109	NS

*NS = Not significant

Table adapted from D G Blazer, L K George, R Landerman, M Pennybacker, M L Melville, M Woodbury, K G Manton, K Jordan, B Locke: Psychiatric disorders: A rural/urban comparison. Arch Gen Psychiatry *42:* 651, 1985. Used with permission.

Therefore the risk for depression is increased in younger ages, even when education, marital status, and sex are taken into account.

PROGNOSIS

Two recent studies have concentrated on the public health impact of depressive disorders because of their chronic and disabling nature.

In the first, over 11,000 outpatients in a variety of primary care settings were screened for depression. Patients with either depressive disorders or depressive symptoms (without a diagnosis of a specific mood disorder) tended to have worse physical, social, and role functioning. When their objective health status was controlled, they perceived their current health to be worse than patients who were not depressed, and they reported greater physical pain. The poor functioning associated with depressive symptoms, with or without a diagnosis of a mood disorder or not, was comparable with or worse than in eight major chronic medical conditions. The number of days in bed with depressive symptoms was significantly greater than with hypertension, diabetes, or arthritis.

In a second study, from the ECA sample in North Carolina, persons with the diagnosis of major depressive disorder or dysthymic disorder and with symptoms of minor depressive disorder were followed for one year. Compared with asymptomatic individuals, persons with major depressive disorder had a five-times greater risk of disability and persons with minor depressive disorder had a one-and-one-half-times greater risk. Persons with minor depressive disorder were at greater risk of developing an anxiety syndrome and major depressive disorder at one-year follow-up.

Both studies demonstrate the need not to limit the cases in epidemiological investigations of depressive morbidity to existing nosological categories. They also demonstrate two key factors relating to the outcome of mood disorders in the community. First, depressive symptoms and major depressive disorder are important public health concerns. When distributing funds for research and clinical care, policymakers should recognize the costs of medical care, time lost from work, and the decreased life satisfaction associated with depressive disorders. The mood disorders are treatable despite their chronicity, and treatments have improved dramatically over the past 25 years. Yet the stigma of mental illness continues to affect coverage for the treatment of psychiatric disorders, and much less money is allotted for research on mood disorders than for many chronic and disabling illnesses that carry less stigma.

Second, the studies emphasize the risk among persons with less severe symptoms of developing more severe or additional psychiatric disorders, as well as to experience a poorer outcome from physical disorders. Mortality rates among the depressed are greater than among age-matched controls, even greater than are accounted for by suicide.

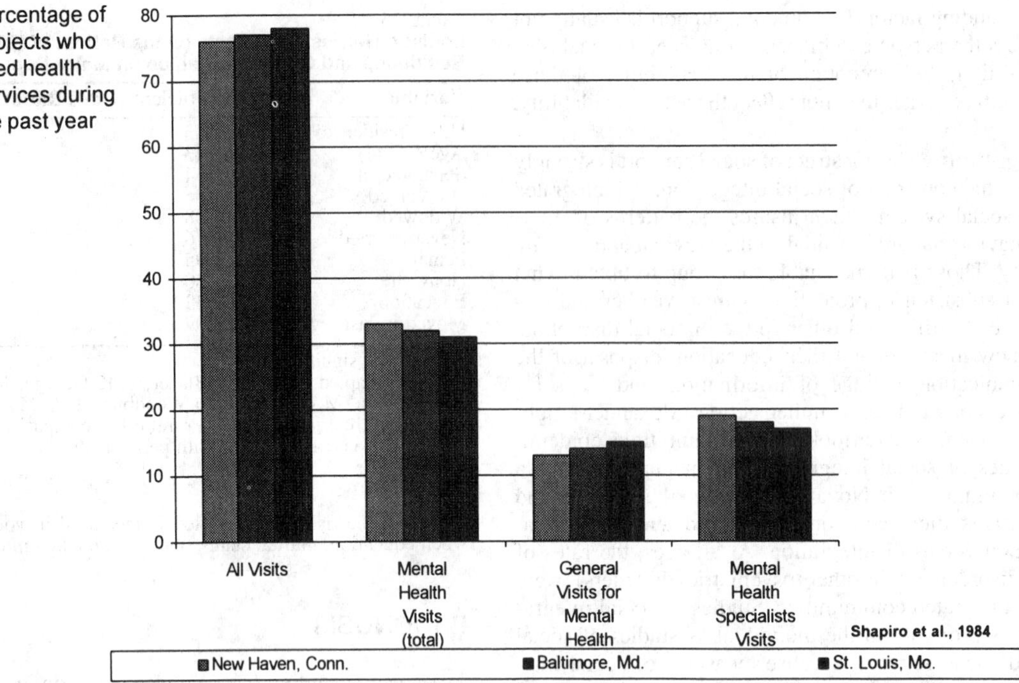

FIGURE 16.2-6 *Utilization of outpatients visits by persons with mood disorders (percentage use by category from three ECA sites).*

A number of natural history studies of mood disorders have been performed on clinical samples. The most extensively studied cohort derives from the Psychobiology of Depression Study of over 500 young adult and middle-aged subjects diagnosed with either bipolar I disorder or major depressive disorder. During the years following diagnosis, about 50 percent of patients recovered during the first year, but less than 30 percent of the others recovered during subsequent years. Comorbid dysthymic disorder with a slow onset, accompanying psychotic symptoms, and severe symptoms were associated with less likelihood for recovery. Relapse rates are high for major depressive disorder immediately following recovery. Superimposed dythymic disorder and a history of three or more major depressive episodes were associated with relapse. Bipolar I disorder patients with only manic episodes had a better outcome than those with major depressive disorder. However, bipolar I patients with a mixed episode (depression and manic) or with rapid cycling had a worse outcome than those with major depressive disorder.

USE OF HEALTH SERVICES

Use of health services for mood disorders occurs in general health care settings and in specialty settings. Most mental health visits reported by subjects in the ECA study, regardless of disorder, occur in primary care settings for older persons and in specialty settings for younger persons. Women use mental health services in both settings about twice as often as men. The pattern of mental health visits and general health visits at three ECA sites among subjects diagnosed with dysthymic disorder and major depressive disorder are presented in Figure 16.2-6. Visits are about equally distributed between general medical providers and mental health specialists in all three settings. All visits and all mental health visits are more frequent in persons who are depressed than for persons with no disorder identified in the ECA surveys.

SUGGESTED CROSS-REFERENCES

An overview of epidemiology is given in Section 5.1. Social origins of mood disorders are discussed in Section 4.2. Classification of mental disorders is presented in Chapter 11. Specific review of the genetics of mood disorders can be found in Section 16.4. The role of stress in the etiology of psychiatric disorders is discussed in Section 26.9. Suicide is discussed in detail in Section 30.1. The epidemiology of psychiatric disorders in late life is reviewed in Section 49.2.

REFERENCES

Blacker C V R, Clare A W: Depressive disorder in primary care. Br J Psychiatry *150:* 737, 1987.

Blazer D G, Bachar J R, Manton K G: Suicide in late life: Review and commentary. J Am Geriatr Soc *34:* 519, 1986.

Blazer D G, George L K, Landerman R, Pennybacker M, Melville M L, Woodbury M, Manton K G, Jordan K, Locke B: Psychiatric disorders: A rural/urban comparison. Arch Gen Psychiatry *42:* 651, 1985.

*Blazer D G, Kessler R C, McGonagle K A, Swartz M S: The prevalence and distribution of major depression in a natural community sample: The National Comorbidity Survey. Am J Psychiatry *151:* 979, 1994.

*Broadhead W E, Blazer D G, George L K, Tse C K: Depression, disability days, and days lost from work in a prospective epidemiologic survey. JAMA *264:* 2524, 1990.

Coryell W, Aksikal H S, Leon A C, Winokur G, Maser J D, Mueller T L, Keller M B: The time course of nonchronic major depressive disorder. Arch Gen Psychiatry *51:* 405, 1994.

Durkheim É: *Suicide: A Study in Sociology.* Free Press, New York, 1951.

Eaton W W, Kramer M, Anthony J C, Dryman A, Shapiro S, Locke B Z: The incidence of specific DIS/DSM-III mental disorders: Data from the NIMH Epidemiologic Catchment Area Program. Acta Psychiatr Scand *79:* 163, 1989.

Eaton J W, Weil R J: *Culture and Mental Disorders.* Free Press, New York, 1955.

Endicott J, Spitzer R L: A diagnostic interview: The Schedule for Affective Disorders and Schizophrenia. Arch Gen Psychiatry *35:* 837, 1978.

*Hagnell O, Lanke J, Rorsman B, Ojesjo L: Are we entering an age of melancholy? Depressive illnesses in a prospective epidemiological

study over 25 years: The Lundby Study, Sweden. Psychol Med *12:* 279, 1982.
Hirschfeld R M A, Klerman G L: Personality attributes and affective disorders. Am J Psychiatry *136:* 67, 1979.
Hollingshead A B, Redlich F C: *Social Class and Mental Illness.* Wiley, New York, 1958.
Jorm A F: Sex and age differences in depression: A quantitative synthesis of published research. Aust N Z J Psychiatry *21:* 46, 1987.
Keller M B, Shapiro R W, Lavori P W, Wolfe H: Recovery in major depressive disorder. Arch Gen Psychiatry *39:* 905, 1982.
Kessler R C, McGonagle K A, Zhao S, Nelson C B, Hughes M, Eshleman S, Wittchen H, Dendler K S: Lifetime and 12-month prevalence of DSM-III-R psychiatric disorders in the United States: Results from the National Comorbidity Survey. Arch Gen Psychiatry *51:* 8, 1994.
Klerman G L, Weissman M M: Increasing rates of depression. JAMA *261:* 2229, 1989.
Koenig H G, Meador K, Cohen H J, Blazer D: Depression in elderly hospitalized patients with medical illness. Arch Intern Med *148:* 1929, 1988.
*Leighton A H: *My Name Is Legion.* Basic Books, New York, 1959.
Leighton D C, Harding J S, Macklin D B, MacMillan A M, Leighton A H: *The Character of Danger: Psychiatric Symptoms in Selected Communities.* Basic Books, New York, 1963.
Morris J N: *Uses of Epidemiology, ed 3.* Churchill Livingstone, London, 1975.
Paykel E S: Life stress and psychiatric disorder. In *Stressful Life Events: Their Nature and Effects,* B S Dohrenwend, B P Dohrenwend, editors, p 135. Wiley, New York, 1974.
Robins L N, Helzer J E, Croughan J, Ratcliff K: National Institute of Mental Health Diagnostic Interview Schedule: Its history, characteristics, and validity. Arch Gen Psychiatry *38:* 381, 1981.
Rorsman B, Grasbeck A, Hagnell O, Lanke J, Ohman R, Ojesjo L, Otterbeck L: A prospective study of first-incidence depression: The Lundby Study, 1957-1972. Br J Psychiatry *156:* 336, 1990.
Shapiro A, Skinner E A, Kessler L G, Von Korff M, German P S, Tischler G L, Leaf P J, Benham L, Cottler L, Regier D A: Utilization of health and mental health services: Three Epidemiologic Catchment Area sites. Arch Gen Psychiatry *41:* 971, 1984.
Somervell P D, Leaf P J, Weissman M M, Blazer D G, Bruce M L: The prevalence of major depression in black and white adults in five United States communities. Am J Epidemiol *130:* 725, 1989.
Tennant C: Female vulnerability to depression. Psychol Med *15:* 733, 1985.
Weissman M M, Livingston B, Leaf P J, Florio L P, Holzer C: Affective disorders. In *Psychiatric Disorders in America: The Epidemiologic Catchment Area Study,* L N Robins, D A Regier, editors, p. 53. Free Press, New York, 1991.
*Weissman M M, Merikangas K R, Boyd J H: Epidemiology of affective disorders. In *Psychiatry,* R Michels, A M Cooper, S B Guze, L L Judd, G L Klerman, A J Solnit, A J Stunkard, P J Wilner, vol 1, section 60, p 1. New York, Lippincott, 1991.
Wells K B, Stewart A, Hays R D, Burnam A, Rogers W, et al: The functioning and well-being of depressed patients: Results from the Medical Outcomes Study. JAMA *262:* 914, 1989.

16.3 MOOD DISORDERS: BIOCHEMICAL ASPECTS

ALAN I. GREEN, M.D.
JOHN J. MOONEY, M.D.
JOEL A. POSENER, M.D.
JOSEPH J. SCHILDKRAUT, M.D.

INTRODUCTION

The biochemistry of affective disorders, called mood disorders in the fourth edition of *Diagnostic and Statistical Manual of Mental Disorders* (DSM-IV), has been an active area of scientific investigation since the introduction of the first clinically effective antidepressant drugs—imipramine (Tofranil) and the monoamine oxidase inhibitors (MAOIs)—in the late 1950s. In the decades since then, those first antidepressant drugs, as well as the newer ones as they have come along, have themselves become major research tools. Research into their mechanisms of action has provided the basis for various working hypotheses about the biochemistry of depressions and has led to more fundamental discoveries about the neurobiology of the central nervous system (CNS) itself. This section delineates the several lines of current research on the biochemistry of depressive disorders and provides a guide for understanding existing theoretical frameworks.

The brain contains billions of neurons, each one interacting with others by electrochemical means. When a neuron is stimulated, the resulting impulse, or electrical action potential, causes a release of a chemical substance (a neurotransmitter) from a specialized region in close proximity to a neighboring neuron. The neurotransmitter is released into a space between the two neurons, called the synaptic cleft. The neuron leading to the synaptic cleft is called the presynaptic neuron, and the neuron leading away from the synaptic cleft is called the postsynaptic neuron. The neurotransmitter released into the synaptic cleft from the presynaptic neuron briefly interacts with a receptor on the postsynaptic neuron. This interaction may produce electrical stimulation (increasing the likelihood of an action potential) or electrical inhibition (decreasing the likelihood of an action potential) of the postsynaptic neuron, as well as intracellular biochemical and physiological changes within the postsynaptic neuron.

Many different substances apparently can act as neurotransmitters in the brain, and many other brain chemicals can be regulators or modulators of the process. Pharmacological agents, such as the antidepressants or environmental stimuli of many kinds, ultimately exert their effects by altering neurotransmitter-mediated or neuromodulator-mediated interactions between neurons.

Genetic factors may have biochemical expressions at the synapse, and environmental or psychological factors may act in that way as well. Neurochemical and neurophysiological changes secondary to such factors can alter a person's vulnerability to depressive episodes or even precipitate a depressive episode; therefore, sharp distinctions cannot be drawn between genetically and environmentally induced depressions or between biological and psychological depressions. Similar neurochemical and neurophysiological changes are probably involved to a greater or lesser degree in virtually every type.

Most biological research involving the mood disorders aims ultimately at learning more about the workings of the CNS in these disorders. As an offshoot of that research, however, investigators are utilizing various biochemical measures in an attempt to subtype the mood disorders. Biological subtyping, if successful, may allow the differentiation of groups of patients who appear similar clinically but differ biochemically. The existence of such subtypes may have important clinical implications.

HISTORY

The two major classes of antidepressant drugs, the MAOIs and the tricyclic antidepressants, were first used in psychiatry nearly 40 years ago. Within a few years after their introduction, several lines of evidence began to suggest that these medications worked at least in part through effects on catecholamines (norepinephrine, epinephrine, and dopamine) or indoleamines (such as serotonin), two of the many groups of chemical substances that function as neurotransmitters within the CNS. One of the catecholamines, norepinephrine, seemed to have particular importance in that regard. The first clue was that the MAOIs increased concentrations of norepinephrine in the brain by blocking one of its metabolic pathways. Shortly thereafter the drug imipramine, a tricyclic antidepressant, was found to enhance the effects of norepinephrine by blocking a major inactivation mechanism—the reuptake of norepinephrine into presynaptic neurons after release into the synaptic cleft. At about the same time reserpine (Serpasil), a drug then used for hypertension, was noted to deplete catecholamines in the brain and to cause clinical depressions in some patients.

On the basis of these and other data, the catecholamine hypothesis of affective disorders was formulated and introduced into the literature by Joseph Schildkraut in the mid-1960s. In its simplest form, the hypothesis proposed that some depressive disorders may be associated with an absolute or relative deficiency of catecholamines, particularly norepinephrine, at functionally important synapses in the brain, whereas manias may be associated with an excess of such catecholamines. The focus on levels of catecholamines in the simplest statement of the hypothesis was based on the research techniques of the day, which only allowed for the measurement of the output and metabolism of norepinephrine released by presynaptic neurons. Nevertheless, the possibility of abnormalities in receptor function was also considered in the general formulation of the hypothesis, because it was known that in the event of receptor subsensitivity a relative functional deficiency of norepinephrine could occur even with normal or elevated presynaptic output.

Because the broad clinical and biological heterogeneity of depressive disorders was recognized, it was apparent from the outset that a focus on catecholamine metabolism was, at best, an oversimplification of complex biological mechanisms. Alterations in many other neurotransmitter or neuromodulator systems were envisioned, as were ionic changes, endocrine changes, and other biochemical abnormalities. Nonetheless, the possibility that different subgroups of depressed patients might ultimately be characterized by differences in the metabolism of norepinephrine or in the physiology of noradrenergic (norepinephrine-containing) neuronal systems was raised in the initial formulation of the catecholamine hypothesis of affective disorders. Subsequent studies by many research groups provided considerable data to support this possibility. Other research has looked at the role of other neurotransmitters, neuromodulators, and neurohormones in patients with mood disorders. For example, there have been numerous studies on the relationship of serotonin, dopamine, acetylcholine, and corticotropin-releasing hormone (CRH) to the mood disorders.

In the past, many investigations attempted to separate the depressive disorders into noradrenergic or serotonergic depressions, according to certain biochemical data and particular responses to various tricyclic antidepressant drugs. This approach, based in part on presumed differences between various tricyclic antidepressant drugs in the inhibition of norepinephrine and serotonin reuptake, no longer seems tenable. Recent findings from studies of depressed patients, and data on the physiological interactions between noradrenergic and serotonergic neurons and the complex neuropharmacological effects of antidepressant drugs, make it obvious that such separations are overly simplistic and artificial.

Acetylcholine, another classic neurotransmitter, also may play a role in the pathophysiology of certain depressive disorders. Drugs that stimulate acetylcholinergic activity have been found to induce depressions in control subjects, to exacerbate depressions in depressed patients, and to decrease manias in manic patients. Recent studies have also suggested that some depressed patients may have supersensitive acetylcholinergic receptors. Thus, the anticholinergic effects of the commonly prescribed antidepressant drugs may be responsible for more than side effects; they may be of some importance in the drug's actual antidepressant effects as well.

Neurotransmitters interact with specific receptors to exert their effects. Recent studies have shown that alterations in the biochemical and physiological properties of these receptors may be involved both in the mechanisms of action of antidepressant drugs and in the pathophysiology of depressive disorders. These possibilities have been investigated in many laboratories throughout the world.

It is becoming increasingly clear that the pathophysiology of depressive disorders is not restricted to abnormalities in brain function. Rather, the depressive disorders must be conceptualized as complex neuroendocrinometabolic disorders that involve many different organ systems throughout the body. In particular, the close connection to the endocrine system has become increasingly clear over the past 25 years. Many specialized laboratory tests are now being used in psychiatry, and it is expected that such clinical laboratory tests will play an increasingly important role in the diagnostic evaluation and treatment of patients with depressive disorders.

BIOGENIC AMINES

The term "biogenic amine" generally refers to four compounds—the catecholamines norepinephrine, epinephrine, and dopamine and the indoleamine serotonin. All four compounds have a single amine group on the side chain and consequently are also called monoamines. The neuronal systems utilizing the monoamines originate as relatively small collections of cell groups located mainly in the brainstem. From there the cell groups project widely into other brain regions, where they regulate neuronal processing of information and the tone and coloring of behavior. The widespread projections of these neuronal systems make them logical targets for psychiatric research, since small changes in them can have diverse behavioral effects.

At the synapse, the biogenic amines are released into the synaptic space and act at presynaptic and postsynaptic receptor sites. Most of the neurotransmitter is inactivated by reuptake into the presynaptic neuron; however, a portion may be metabolized outside the neuron after release into the synaptic space. The mitochondrial enzyme monoamine oxidase (MAO) is involved in the metabolism of neurotransmitters within the presynaptic neuron; such intraneuronal metabolism of neurotransmitter can occur independent of neurotransmitter release into the synaptic cleft.

NOREPINEPHRINE METABOLISM AND PHYSIOLOGY

The noradrenergic cell bodies containing norepinephrine are found in the locus ceruleus, medulla oblongata, and pons. They distribute projections by two major pathways to the entire neocortex, limbic structures, thalamus, hypothalamus, reticular formation, dorsal raphe nucleus, cerebellum, sensory and motor brainstem nuclei, and spinal cord. Individual locus ceruleus neurons can simultaneously send collateral branches to the neocortex, hippocampus, cerebellum, and spinal cord. The norepinephrine projections from the locus ceruleus also regulate brain blood flow and capillary permeability.

Many lines of evidence suggest that some patients with depressive disorders have abnormalities in catecholamine physiology or metabolism. Studies in animals have shown that many clinically effective antidepressants alter the reuptake, metabolism, and turnover of norepinephrine in the brain. Recent longitudinal clinical studies measuring norepinephrine and its metabolites in the urine of depressed patients during six weeks of treatment with the antidepressant desipramine (Norpramin) showed that desipramine produces time-dependent changes in the metabolism and turnover of norepinephrine, which may help to explain the well-known two- to six-week lag time in clinical response to antidepressant drugs. Total norepinephrine synthesis and turnover were decreased during the entire course of treatment with desipramine, as reflected in sustained decreases in urinary levels of the major deaminated O-methylated metabolites of norepinephrine, 3-methoxy-4-hydroxymandelic acid (VMA), and 3-methoxy-4-hydroxyphenylglycol (MHPG), that in part reflect intraneuronal metabolism by MAO (see above). By contrast, urinary norepinephrine and its O-methylated metabolite normetanephrine, which are derived from physiologically active norepinephrine released extraneuronally into the synaptic space, were decreased during the first week of treatment with desipramine but increased in subsequent weeks. These data suggest that the clinical response to desipramine may be related in part to an increased release of norepinephrine extraneuronally (that is, into the synapse) that occurs after the first week of treatment.

Tyrosine hydroxylase is the rate-limiting enzyme in the biosynthesis of norepinephrine, and recent evidence suggests that this enzyme may be involved in the pathophysiology of depression. For example, one recent study reported decreased levels of tyrosine hydroxylase protein in the brains of suicide victims. Another study noted that administration of α-methylparatyrosine, an inhibitor of tyrosine hydroxylase, produced an exacerbation of symptoms in patients whose depression had been improved by antidepressant treatment with the norepinephrine reuptake inhibitors desipramine and mazindol (Mazanor, Sanorex).

One method of studying the activity of noradrenergic neurons in the brain of living patients is to measure the level of MHPG in the urine. Known to be a major metabolite of norepinephrine originating in the brain, MHPG also derives in part from the peripheral sympathetic nervous system. MHPG from either source may undergo conversion to VMA. Thus, the fraction of urinary MHPG that is derived from brain norepinephrine is uncertain. Despite that uncertainty, measurement of urinary MHPG has been used in attempts to elucidate the pathophysiology of depressions and to discriminate among biologically distinct subgroups of depressive disorders.

Urinary MHPG levels In longitudinal studies of patients with naturally occurring classic bipolar (manic-depressive) disorder or amphetamine-induced manic-depressive episodes, many investigators have found that under antidepressant drug-free conditions, levels of urinary MHPG are low during periods of depression and high during periods of mania or hypomania. Comparably low MHPG values, however, do not occur in all types of depressions. This observation has raised the possibility that MHPG or other catecholamine metabolites may provide a biochemical basis for differentiating among subgroups of depressive disorders.

In early studies urinary MHPG levels were found to be significantly lower in patients with classic bipolar manic-depressive depressions than in patients with unipolar nonendogenous chronic characterological depressions. Subsequent studies confirmed the presence of reduced urinary MHPG levels (and plasma norepinephrine levels) in patients with classic bipolar depressions—that is, bipolar I (but not bipolar II) depressive disorders—when compared with mean values in patients with various subtypes of unipolar depression, including major depressive disorder, or in nondepressed control subjects. One study suggested that the differences in urinary MHPG levels between patients with bipolar depression and control subjects became more pronounced when the peripheral contribution to urinary MHPG was reduced with carbidopa (Sinemet), a decarboxylase inhibitor that does not cross the blood-brain barrier.

In contrast to the reduction in urinary MHPG levels in depressed patients with bipolar disorder as compared with unipolar depressive disorder, a number of studies reported no differences in urinary VMA levels. This finding is important, because studies reporting that circulating MHPG may be converted to VMA have raised questions concerning the specific value of urinary MHPG (for example, in contrast to VMA) as an index of norepinephrine metabolism in the brain or as a biochemical marker in studies of depressed patients.

A wide range of plasma norepinephrine, plasma MHPG, and urinary MHPG levels have been reported in patients with unipolar depressions, including major depressive disorder. Low, intermediate, and high levels of urinary MHPG have been found in various studies. The range of findings may be due to diagnostic heterogeneity among patients with major depressive disorder and other unipolar depressions: In some patients levels of urinary MHPG are as low as those seen in patients with bipolar disorder; in others values are sometimes above the normal range. Because urinary MHPG values in normal control subjects also tend to exhibit a broad range, they cannot be used to diagnose depression per se but may help in the differentiation of depressive subgroups.

Recent studies have described a subgroup of patients with severe unipolar depressive disorder in whom urinary MHPG and urinary free cortisol (UFC) levels were both very high. In this subgroup of severely depressed patients with high catecholamine and cortisol output, increased acetylcholinergic activity could conceivably be a primary factor in the depression, with elevated urinary MHPG and UFC levels as a secondary response. This suggestion is particularly intriguing when certain other data are considered: (1) physostigmine (Antilirium, Eserine), an anticholinesterase, and other pharmacological agents that increase brain cholinergic activity exacerbate depressive symptoms in normal control subjects; (2) physostigmine produces an increase in plasma cortisol levels in normal controls; (3) physostigmine can overcome suppression of the hypothalamic-pituitary-adrenocortical (HPA) axis by dexamethasone in normal subjects, thereby mimicking the abnormal escape from dexamethasone suppression seen in some depressed patients with cortisol hypersecretion; and (4) physostigmine produces an increase in cerebrospinal fluid (CSF) levels of MHPG in healthy subjects. These observations have led to speculation about a possible adrenergic-cholinergic imbalance in some depressed patients and raise the possibility that the anticholinergic effects of some antidepressant drugs, commonly regarded as side effects, may actually contribute to their antidepressant action in patients with this depressive subtype.

There may be at least three distinct subtypes of what appear to be unipolar depressive disorder that can be distinguished by urinary MHPG levels. Subtype I, characterized by low pretreatment urinary MHPG levels, may have low norepinephrine output as the result of a decrease in norepinephrine synthesis or its release from noradrenergic neurons. (Many patients included in subtype I may be patients with underlying bipolar I [manic-depressive] disorders who have not yet experienced a first episode of mania or hypomania.) In contrast, subtype II, characterized by intermediate urinary MHPG levels, may have normal norepinephrine output but abnormalities in other biochemical systems. Subtype III, characterized by high urinary MHPG levels, may have high norepinephrine output in response to alterations in noradrenergic receptors, an increase in cholinergic activity, or an increase in CRH activity (described below). Further research is required to confirm these findings and to explore physiological abnormalities that may be associated with the different subtypes of unipolar depressive disorder.

D-type equation Although MHPG levels alone help differentiate subtypes of depression, multivariate discriminant function analysis has been used to explore the possibility that the inclusion of levels of norepinephrine (NE), epinephrine (E), normetanephrine (NMN), metanephrine (MN), and VMA might provide an even better differentiation. This analysis led to the development of an empirically derived equation, termed the depression-type (D-type) equation, that distinguishes even more precisely between depressed patients with classic bipolar (manic-depressive) disorder and unipolar nonendogenous chronic characterological depression than urinary MHPG alone. The discrimination equation is of the form:

$$\text{D-type score} = C_1\,(\text{MHPG}) - C_2\,(\text{VMA}) + C_3\,(\text{NE}) - C_4\,\frac{(\text{NMN} + \text{MN})}{\text{VMA}} + C_0.$$

The metric for the equation was established so that patients with bipolar depressions would tend toward a score of 0 and patients with unipolar nonendogenous depressions would tend toward a score of 1.

In a subsequently studied validation sample of 114 depressed patients whose data had not been used to derive the equation, the D-type score (using a criterion of D-type score ≤ 0.5) had a sensitivity of 0.85 and a specificity of 0.83 in identifying depressed patients with clinically diagnosed bipolar (manic-depressive) disorder and bipolar-related schizoaffective depressions. A wide range of D-type scores was seen in patients with clinically diagnosed (putative) unipolar endogenous depressions (that is, depressed patients with no prior history of mania). Preliminary findings using the equation suggest that low D-type scores in patients with such putative unipolar depressions may identify patients with latent bipolar disorders who have not yet had a clinical episode of mania.

D-type scores may be an even better predictor than urinary MHPG levels alone of responses to imipramine or alprazolam (Xanax) in patients with unipolar depressions. When a model or equation that was derived to describe or account for observations in one domain is found to have more general applicability in predicting observations in another domain, confidence in the explanatory power of that model is enhanced. The D-type equation was initially derived to separate depressed patients with bipolar (manic-depressive) depressions from depressed patients with other subtypes of depressive disorders. The finding that D-type scores also appear to predict differential clinical responses to certain antidepressant drugs in patients with unipolar depressions thus extends the potential clinical utility of the D-type equation, and also enhances its heuristic value.

Urinary MHPG levels as predictors of differential responses to antidepressant drugs Studies from a number of laboratories have indicated that pretreatment levels of urinary MHPG may help predict responses to certain tricyclic and tetracyclic antidepressant drugs. In many, though not all, studies depressed patients with low pretreatment urinary MHPG levels have been found to respond more favorably to treatment with imipramine, desipramine, nortriptyline (Pamelor), or maprotiline (Ludiomil) than patients with high MHPG levels. In contrast, some but not all studies have found that depressed patients with high pretreatment levels of urinary MHPG respond more favorably to treatment with amitriptyline or alprazolam than do patients with lower MHPG levels. As noted above, D-type scores may be a better predictor of response to some antidepressant drugs than urinary MHPG levels alone. Further research is required.

Urinary MHPG values trichotomized into the three subtypes described above may be useful in predicting treatment responses. Preliminary data have shown that although depressed patients with elevated MHPG levels may be more responsive to treatment with imipramine or maprotiline than patients with intermediate levels, neither group was as responsive as patients with low MHPG levels. Moreover, patients with low pretreatment urinary MHPG levels responded rapidly to relatively low doses of maprotiline, whereas those with elevated MHPG levels required significantly higher doses and longer periods of drug administration, if they responded to maprotiline at all. This finding suggests a differential response, or that the antidepressant drug maprotiline may exert different pharmacological properties in high doses than in low doses. The concept of relative sensitivity of different subtypes of depressions to antidepressant drugs may be analogous to the concept of relative sensitivity of different infectious diseases to antibiotic drugs.

At present, it is not possible to draw valid inferences about biochemical predictors of differential antidepressant drug responses on the basis of hypothesized pharmacological mechanisms of action, as it is known that antidepressant drugs have multiple, complex effects on many neurotransmitter systems. Consequently, empirical clinical trials are needed to assess the value of particular biochemical measures, such as urinary MHPG levels, as clinically useful predictors of responses to each specific antidepressant drug. But because the patients referred for study in academic centers today may be more refractory to the commonly used antidepressant drugs than the patients studied some years ago, when antidepressant drugs were less widely used in medicine and psychiatry, caution must be exercised when comparing new data with earlier findings.

DOPAMINE METABOLISM AND PHYSIOLOGY A role for dopamine in the pathophysiology of depression is suggested by the fact that certain antidepressant drugs produce effects on dopaminergic systems. More direct evidence that dopamine is involved in depressive pathophysiology comes from studies of homovanillic acid (HVA), the major metabolite of dopamine, in patients with mood disorders. Studies have found that levels of HVA in the CSF are reduced in many depressed patients (especially those with psychomotor retardation and suicidality) compared to controls. However, depressed patients with delusions of a history of psychosis may have higher CSF HVA levels than patients with nonpsychotic depressions. An increase in dopamine turnover in response to increased corticosteroid output has been proposed as a mechanism that could account for the increased CSF HVA levels in patients with delusional depressions.

SEROTONIN METABOLISM AND PHYSIOLOGY The cell bodies of serotonergic neurons are located in the raphe nuclei and superior central nucleus, and their axons project widely throughout the CNS—to the entire neocortex, rhinal cortex, thalamus, hypothalamus, limbic structures, reticular formation, locus ceruleus, cerebellum, and spinal cord. As for noradrenergic neurons, the widespread projection of serotonergic neurons makes them logical candidates for psychiatric research. In many regions the serotonergic and noradrenergic projections overlap with each other, and there is at least one major interface between the raphe nuclei of the serotonergic system and the locus ceruleus of the noradrenergic system.

Certain lines of evidence suggest that some patients with depressive disorders have abnormalities in serotonin physiology or metabolism. Studies in animals have shown that treatment with many clinically useful antidepressants alters the reuptake, metabolism, and turnover of serotonin in the brain. And in depressed patients, successful treatment with serotonin-specific reuptake inhibitor (SSRI) antidepressants may be reversed by consumption of a diet augmented with neutral amino acids, which block transport of tryptophan, the amino acid precursor of serotonin, into the brain.

A number of studies have found that some depressed patients have reduced levels of 5-hydroxyindoleacetic acid (5-HIAA), the principal metabolite of brain serotonin, in the CSF. Other studies have noted an association between low CSF 5-HIAA levels and an increased incidence of completed suicide, attempted suicide, or impulsive acts of aggression. Among unipolar depressed patients, those who attempt or complete suicide often have lower CSF 5-HIAA levels than those who are not suicidal.

Reduced concentrations of serotonin or 5-HIAA have been found in postmortem brain tissue taken from depressed and suicidal patients. Some, but not all, studies looking at the brains of suicide victims have found that the binding of tritiated (H^3)-imipramine, which binds to reuptake sites on presynaptic serotonergic nerve terminals, is decreased. Moreover, some but not all studies have found increased postsynaptic 5-hydroxytryptamine (5-HT_2) serotonin receptor densities in the brains of suicide victims. Taken together, these findings have led a number of investigators to suggest that there may be a serotonin deficiency in suicide victims or in depressed patients who attempt suicide.

Decreased serotonin uptake into platelets has been observed in patients with depressive disorders. H^3-imipramine binds to serotonin uptake sites in platelets as well as brain, and a highly significant decrease in the number of H^3-imipramine-binding sites with no significant change in the apparent affinity constant has been observed in platelets from depressed patients compared with those from control subjects. While it has been proposed that the decreased platelet H^3-imipramine binding observed in depressed patients may reflect a deficiency in the platelet serotonin transport mechanism in those patients, recent studies employing H^3-paroxetine cast some doubt on this proposal. Paroxetine is a more specific ligand than imipramine for labelling the serotonin transporter protein. And in several recent studies, there was no difference in the binding of H^3-paroxetine in platelets when values in depressed patients and control subjects were compared.

Another research strategy for evaluating serotonin physiology in depressed patients involves the use of challenge tests in which the endocrine responses to serotonin-releasing agents, such as fenfluramine (Pondimin), or to serotonin receptor agonists are evaluated. These studies have suggested that the primary abnormality of serotonin neurotransmission in depression may be decreased serotonin release rather than altered sensitivity of postsynaptic serotonin receptors.

Last, the introduction in recent years of new antidepressant drugs (fluoxetine [Prozac], sertraline [Zoloft], and paroxetine [Paxil]) that are relatively specific blockers of serotonin reuptake into presynaptic nerve terminals has highlighted the importance of serotonin systems in the pathophysiology and treatment of depression. Further studies are required to elucidate whether the specific serotonin reuptake blocking drugs have a mechanism of action that is truly distinct from that of older agents or whether the drugs all share one or more common pathways of action.

STUDIES OF RECEPTORS Many investigators have suggested that alterations in receptor sensitivity may play a role in both the mechanism of action of antidepressant drugs and the pathophysiology of the depressive disorders. The time course of the clinical effects of antidepressants has been linked to changes in receptor functioning. Moreover, it is possible that various subtypes of depressive disorders may be distinguished by particular receptor characteristics.

Receptors are studied by in vivo or in vitro techniques. In vivo study involves the use of pharmacological challenges to affect physiological processes thought to reflect the action of particular receptors. For example, the α_2-adrenergic receptor agonist clonidine (Catapres) stimulates growth hormone (GH) release, which is thought to occur via the postsynaptic α_2-adrenergic receptor. In many depressed patients the GH response is blunted, suggesting decreased sensitivity of these receptors.

Direct studies of brain receptors have been performed on postmortem tissue. The finding of increased serotonin 5-HT_2 receptor density in the brains of suicide victims was discussed earlier. There have also been studies of noradrenergic β- and α-receptors in various regions of the cortex and in subcortical regions of the brain. Although the findings are of interest, to date they are not consistent and thus do not allow definitive interpretation. Clearly, additional research in this area is required.

The study of adrenergic receptors on human blood cells allows in vitro measurement of adrenergic receptors from psychiatric patients. These receptors may not reflect similar changes in the CNS; however, they do provide a valuable research tool. For example, the number of β-adrenergic receptor binding sites on lymphocytes has been found to be decreased in some depressed and manic patients compared to control subjects or euthymic patients. Some studies also suggest that β-adrenergic receptor-mediated stimulation of cyclic adenosine monophosphate (cAMP) production by isoproterenol (Isuprel) is reduced in leukocytes and lymphocytes from depressed patients. One investigator noted a lack of responsiveness in depressed patients with psychomotor agitation but not in those with psychomotor retardation. More research is needed to clarify the significance of findings suggesting decreased β-adrenergic receptor function in lymphocytes from some depressed patients.

There also have been studies of platelet α_2-adrenergic receptors, which suppress the activity of prostaglandin-stimulated adenylate cyclase, in depressed patients. Some studies of depressed unipolar patients with depressive disorder have reported that both prostaglandin-stimulated and α_2-adrenergic suppression of prostaglandin-stimulated adenylate cyclase were decreased, while other studies have reported platelet adenylate cyclase (whether basal, prostaglandin-stimulated, or α_2-adrenergic suppression of prostaglandin-stimulated) to be unchanged. The discrepancies between these sets of observations may reflect differences in platelet adenylate cyclase activity in subgroups of depressed patients.

Several studies have reported that the total numbers of platelet α_2-adrenergic receptors were either unchanged or increased (but not decreased) in depressed patients. In light of the findings of decreased platelet α_2-adrenergic suppression of adenylate cyclase, the failure to find a decrease in the number of platelet

α_2-adrenergic receptors suggests a defect in the coupling between platelet α_2-adrenergic receptors and platelet adenylate cyclase in some patients with unipolar depressive disorder. This deficiency may involve the guanine nucleotide regulatory proteins that link neurotransmitter or hormone receptors to the catalytic unit of adenylate cyclase.

Thus, the evidence suggests that depressive disorders may be associated with a decrease in the absolute number or function of a diverse range of adrenergic receptors. Also, several laboratories have found increased catecholamine output in some depressed patients. In the presence of increased catecholamine levels, catecholamine-receptor interactions tend to become desensitized over time. One group of investigators has suggested that the changes in receptor coupling and functioning seen in some depressed patients may be the result of heterologous desensitization. The term ''heterologous desensitization'' (or agonist-nonspecific desensitization) refers to the process whereby long-term exposure to one particular agonist (such as a neurotransmitter, neuromodulator, or hormone) produces diminished responsiveness to multiple agonists in many different receptor systems because of a reversible alteration in the guanine nucleotide regulatory proteins that link or couple all of those receptors to the catalytic unit of adenylate cyclase. This concept raises the possibility that many of the physiological and neuroendocrine-metabolic alterations observed in patients with depressive disorders (including some of the psychoneuroendocrine abnormalities described below) may be the result of catecholamine-induced heterologous desensitization.

PLATELET MAO ACTIVITY To explore further the pathophysiology of the depressive disorders, investigators have studied the enzyme MAO, which deaminates biogenic amines in many body tissues, including the nervous system and the blood platelet. A growing body of literature suggests that levels of platelet MAO activity may help discriminate among subtypes of depressive disorders.

In the early 1970s platelet MAO activity was reported to be increased in a heterogeneous group of depressed patients (most of whom had unipolar depressive disorder) and to be decreased in a group of bipolar depressed patients. Subsequent results have not been as clear. For example, some investigators have reported increased platelet MAO activity in patients with unipolar endogenous depressions; others have reported increased platelet MAO activity in patients with unipolar nonendogenous depressions. Because each study used different criteria for the diagnosis of endogenous or nonendogenous depressions and different methods to determine platelet MAO activity, it is not possible to reconcile the conflicting data at the present time.

One study, however, suggested that bipolar disorder and unipolar depressive disorder may show differences in the relation between platelet MAO activity and the severity of clinical symptoms. In bipolar depression greater severity was associated with low platelet MAO activity, and in unipolar depression greater severity was associated with high platelet MAO activity. (That study systematically excluded patients with schizotypal features, such as unusual perceptions, ideas of reference, impairment in communication, and a history of social isolation. This was done because the presence of such schizotypal features would raise the question of schizophrenia-related disorders, with associated changes in platelet MAO activity, which might otherwise confound the data.)

Several studies have reported an unexpected association between increased platelet MAO activity and increased activity of the HPA axis in depressed patients. Elucidation of the clinical and pathophysiological significance of this intriguing association may help clarify aspects of the confusing and seemingly contradictory literature on platelet MAO activity in relation to subtypes of depressive disorders.

In some studies of patients with unipolar depressive disorder platelet MAO activity correlated both with the severity of the depression and with anxiety symptoms and somatic complaints. The clinical items that correlated with platelet MAO activity in these studies corresponded to symptoms reported by other investigators to be associated with favorable responses to treatment with MAOIs. Other studies have found an association of high platelet MAO activity with social introversion or asociality and of low platelet MAO activity with social extraversion or sensation-seeking.

Despite the interesting data about platelet MAO activity, further research needs to be done. For example, additional studies are needed to determine whether such clinical (psychometric) variables may help to account for the differences in platelet MAO activity that have been observed in various subgroups of depressions. Research is also needed to compare kinetic parameters (and other properties) of platelet mitochondrial MAO with other biological indices in patients with various subtypes of depressive disorders and in control subjects. Recently developed molecular genetic strategies for studying the MAO enzymes should be used to help elucidate the possible linkage of MAO genes to various subtypes of mood disorders and to explore the mechanisms by which those genes are regulated by neurotransmitters, hormones, and other neuroregulators.

PSYCHONEUROENDOCRINOLOGY

Because many endocrinopathies present with psychiatric symptoms, particularly affective symptoms, clinicians and investigators have long considered the possible connection between the endocrine system and mood disorders. The discovery that peptides from the hypothalamus, under the control of various neurotransmitters linked with the pathophysiology of these disorders, regulate the release of pituitary hormones prompted further speculation about this relationship. Recent advances, including the development of sensitive hormonal assays and the isolation of many hypothalamic peptides, have enabled psychoneuroendocrinology to emerge as an important research discipline.

The possibility that hormones might be related to affective states was raised with the earliest clinical descriptions of Cushing's disease and hypothyroidism, both of which are associated with changes in mood. The exact relationship between the endocrine system and the brain as a mediator of behavior, however, was unclear for years. It was not until the late 1940s that the neurovascular model linking the hypothalamus and the pituitary was first proposed, and not until the mid-1950s that the existence of a substance in pituitary extract that stimulated the release of adrenocorticotropic hormone (ACTH) was demonstrated. This substance was called corticotropin-releasing factor (CRF)—and later corticotropin-releasing hormone (CRH)—but its structure eluded investigators until 1981. In the past 20 years a number of hypothalamic peptides controlling the anterior pituitary have been isolated and synthesized, among them thyrotropin-releasing hormone (TRH), gonadotropin-releasing hormone (GnRH), growth hormone-releasing factor (GHRF), growth hormone release-inhibiting factor (GHRIF or somatostatin), and CRH itself.

The activity of the limbic system—long suggested to be the CNS site of affective states—is regulated by many of the neurotransmitters thought to be involved in the pathophysiology and, possibly, the etiology of affective states. The limbic system in turn regulates the hypothalamus, a key element in the endocrine network. Thus, many investigators have examined endocrine changes in affective illness in an attempt to obtain information concerning possible functional alterations of certain CNS neuronal systems that use one or another neurotransmitter or neuromodulator. This strategy has been likened to looking at the brain through a neuroendocrine window. Another strategy in recent psychiatric studies has been more practical: the search for one or more laboratory tests of endocrine function that might distinguish certain affective subtypes from other subtypes of mood disorders, or mood disorders from other psychiatric illnesses.

The neuroendocrine network is a highly complex, well-integrated system. It involves the release of anterior pituitary hormones by various hypothalamic factors, a feedback control of that release by circulating target organ hormones, and an overriding control on the entire system by internal biological rhythms or external events affecting the hypothalamus.

The methods used for studying the endocrine network as it relates to mood disorders are multifaceted. First, because each bodily hormone is released according to a circadian rhythm, the study of possible changes in rhythm in an affective disease state is of interest. Second, the response of the anterior pituitary to the introduction of a hypothalamic factor can also be measured in affected patients and compared with normal subjects. Third, direct challenges to the hypothalamus itself, such as insulin-induced hypoglycemia, provide further information about the functioning of the endocrine axes. Fourth, provocative neuropharmacological challenges with such drugs as the amphetamines, clonidine, or physostigmine can also be used to test for changes in neurotransmitter systems in affective disease states.

Hundreds of studies using one or another of these strategies have resulted in an enormous volume of information. The studies are often conflicting, yet one conclusion seems sure: Various endocrine changes are associated with affective disorders. The best-documented changes involve the hypothalamic-pituitary-adrenal (HPA), the hypothalamic-pituitary-thyroid (HPT), and the hypothalamic-pituitary-growth hormone (HPGH) axes.

The material below details particular disturbances. Most of the work has involved patients with unipolar (including major) depressive disorder, but studies on patients with bipolar disorder are noted where applicable. Because the field is changing rapidly, the material is best read as a guide to the status of the field in mid-1994.

HYPOTHALAMIC-PITUITARY-ADRENAL AXIS CRH, the hypothalamic neuropeptide identified in 1981, is the principal regulator of ACTH release from the anterior pituitary and exerts a stimulatory effect on ACTH release. ACTH in turn stimulates the synthesis and release of cortisol from the adrenal cortex. Cortisol feeds back to inhibit the release of both CRH from the hypothalamus and ACTH from the pituitary. An additional, important point of regulation involves feedback of cortisol to the hippocampus, which exerts a tonic inhibitory effect on CRH release. The entire HPA axis has a circadian rhythm; most of the cortisol released from the adrenal glands comes in periodic bursts in the early morning hours.

CRH has been a focus of intense research interest over the past decade. Primarily, this interest stems from the discovery that CRH is widely distributed in the brain outside of the hypothalamus and has neurotransmitter function independent of its role in the HPA axis. High concentrations of CRH are found in the neocortex, limbic system, and regions involved in regulation of the autonomic nervous system; CRH receptors are also found in high concentration near the locus ceruleus. CRH activates the peripheral sympathetic and adrenomedullary systems, increases both norepinephrine and dopamine turnover throughout the brain, and produces behavioral changes in experimental animals similar to those seen following stress; these changes are generally independent of the effects of CRH on the HPA axis. These latter observations have led some investigators to propose that CRH is a central integrative mediator of the stress response. CRH release from the hypothalamus is itself stimulated by noradrenergic, serotonergic, and cholinergic inputs and is inhibited by γ-aminobutyric acid (GABA). The reciprocal interactions between CRH and catecholaminergic systems and the complex central functions of this neuropeptide make it a natural candidate for consideration as a factor in psychiatric pathophysiology.

Corticoid levels in depression Hypersecretion of cortisol, documented by 24-hour urinary corticoid output or serum cortisol levels, has been consistently reported in depressed patients over the past two decades; such abnormalities are found in approximately half of the depressed patients studied. The cortisol hypersecreters show a characteristic flattening of the circadian cycle, such that they secrete cortisol during the time of day when such secretion is normally at a minimum. The cortisol abnormality seems related to the depression and not merely due to stress or hyperactivity. In most studies the hypercortisolic state has been reported to revert to normal with clinical remission, although one study suggested that in some depressed patients elevated urinary cortisol levels may persist after resolution of the depression. Interestingly, plasma cortisol levels in depressed patients at one-year follow-up have been found to predict poor social and occupational functioning, independent of the degree of residual depression.

Dexamethasone suppression test The dexamethasone suppression test (DST) has been used extensively to study the HPA axis in patients with affective disorder. First introduced in 1960 for the study of Cushing's disease, the procedure determines whether administration of dexamethasone results in normal suppression of the HPA axis as determined by lowered concentrations of cortisol in blood at various times after the administration of dexamethasone. Two groups of investigators, working independently, began applying the DST to depressed patients in the late 1960s; both groups found abnormal DST results (failure of dexamethasone to suppress cortisol secretion) in some of the patients with endogenous depressions. A number of seminal reports in the early 1980s led to widespread interest in the use of the DST in psychiatric research and practice. Those reports specified (1) an optimal method (1 mg of oral dexamethasone, with 4 PM and 11 PM plasma cortisol measurements); (2) sensitivity (67 percent); (3) specificity (96 percent, if strict exclusion criteria are followed); and (4) a cutoff for normal postdexamethasone plasma cortisol levels (5 μg/dL). Some recent studies have reported data utilizing other dexamethasone dosages; a few investigations have suggested that a 2-mg dose may provide a more valid measure of the cortisol hyperactivity.

The more recent literature contains many reports both confirming and questioning various aspects of the early DST findings. The reported sensitivity level for the 1-mg dose has been confirmed by many other investigators for patients variously described as having major depressive disorder, primary depression, or endogenous depression. The percentage of positive (abnormal) tests in patients with unipolar psychotic depressions or in older depressed patients has been found to be higher than in nonpsychotic melancholic patients or in younger depressed patients; the actual cortisol concentration in 4 PM postdexamethasone blood samples may be significantly higher in psychotic and elderly depressed patients as well. The percentage of abnormal results on the DST is often reported to be lower than 50 percent in outpatients, perhaps because outpatients may be more heterogeneous and, as a group, have less severe depressions. The association of abnormal DST results with a family history of depression has been reported by some investigators but not by others. Some investigators, moreover, have suggested that the DST abnormality cuts across many different diagnostic categories and may define a diagnostically broader, but biologically more homogeneous, group of disorders than melancholia per se.

The DST abnormality appears to be stable over the course of a depressive episode and often remits with clinical recovery. Subsequent depressions in a particular patient seem to run true; suppressors in one depression tend to be suppressors in the next. The change in DST results with treatment precedes the clinical recovery; some have suggested that an incomplete normalization of the DST, irrespective of clinical symptoms, indicates incomplete resolution of the depressive process. Others have advocated serial use of the DST to determine the safe period for withdrawing antidepressant medication because a number of studies report that incomplete normalization of the DST predicts a higher likelihood of poor outcome. After electroconvulsive therapy (ECT), however, the picture does not appear to be clear; the possibility has been raised that ECT itself may interfere, at least temporarily, with the DST. A recent meta-analysis of the literature on the DST as a predictor of clinical course in depression concluded that baseline DST status does not predict response to treatment, with the exception that baseline nonsuppression predicts a poor placebo response; however, persistent nonsuppression after treatment was found to be a strong predictor of poor outcome.

The issue of the specificity of the DST for depression is an important one; in large measure it determines the test's clinical utility. The rate of false-positive results on the DST in normal subjects has varied from 4 percent to over 10 percent in different reports. One study suggested that the variability in those reports may have been due to an unrecognized history of mood disorders in the subjects or their relatives. In patients and normal subjects, variations in plasma dexamethasone levels after a fixed oral dexamethasone dose may contribute to some inconsistency in the DST data. Depressed patients may have lower dexamethasone levels than controls, but that difference alone does not appear able to explain the DST abnormality in depression. Differences in laboratory assay techniques and accuracy may also account for some of the reported variability in the DST data. Compliance with taking the dexamethasone is an obvious but sometimes overlooked potential confound. In addition, a number of medical disorders and pharmacological agents can produce false-positive or false-negative results. Weight loss per se, often an accompaniment of major depressive disorder, may also cause an abnormal DST result.

The literature on psychiatric conditions other than depressions that may be associated with an abnormal DST is considerable. The DST may be abnormal in some patients with panic disorder and obsessive-compulsive disorder, especially in severe cases in which secondary depression is suspected. Patients with anorexia nervosa and bulimia may also have abnormal DST results, even in the absence of major weight change. An abnormal DST is observed in many patients with depressionlike states after strokes, and also in persons withdrawing from alcohol. Although a number of investigators have found normal results on the DST in schizophrenic patients, the literature contains a few reports of a significant percentage of abnormalities on the DST in that group. High rates of DST nonsuppression have also been observed in manic patients.

As may be expected from the conflicting published reports, the possible clinical utility of the DST has attracted considerable controversy. Known factors that can produce a false-positive DST are expanding. Some investigators have suggested that postdexamethasone plasma cortisol levels may be of greater value than the mere qualitative assessment of the test as normal or abnormal. There is a reasonable consensus of opinion that the DST has little value as a diagnostic screening test for depression. But many investigators suggest that it may be helpful in difficult clinical situations (for example, in differentiating psychotic depression from schizophrenia). The ability of the DST to predict treatment response is limited. However, some investigators have taken the finding that an abnormal DST predicts a poor placebo response to suggest that a truly abnormal DST in a depressed patient may indicate the need for pharmacological treatment.

Other HPA axis abnormalities Over the past 10 years, abnormalities at a number of levels of the HPA axis have been identified in depressed patients. A number of studies have found that depressed patients have a greater output of cortisol in response to administration of synthetic ACTH than do controls. Moreover, the volume of the adrenal gland is increased in depressed patients compared with controls, suggesting that hyperplasia of the adrenal cortex may be responsible for the exaggerated response to ACTH. Another challenge strategy involved stimulation of the HPA axis by CRH. Studies have shown quite consistently that compared to healthy control subjects, depressed patients have a blunted output of ACTH in response to exogenous CRH (despite an apparent increased volume of the pituitary in these patients). An important finding, and one that has been replicated in independent samples, is that patients with major depressive disorder have increased levels of CRH in the CSF. This finding suggests that the blunted response to administered CRH may be due to down-regulation of pituitary CRH receptors. It has been proposed that the fundamental HPA axis abnormality in depression is hypersecretion of CRH; this putative defect is able to explain the abnormalities observed at lower levels of the axis. Hypersecretion of CRH itself could be due to a number of other abnormalities, including a defect in response to cortisol feedback at the level of the limbic system; abnormal feedback responses to administered cortisol have in fact been observed recently in depressed patients. CRH hypersecretion could also be caused by and could influence abnormalities in monoaminergic and other neuromodulatory systems that regulate CRH.

The relationship of HPA axis abnormalities to other biological variables is an important area for current and future research. Some reports have described a subgroup of patients with severe unipolar depressions who have increased catecholamine output (as reflected in very high levels of urinary MHPG) and evidence of high HPA axis activity (documented by elevated UFC levels or an abnormal DST). As noted earlier, the subgroup of depressed patients with high levels of urinary MHPG (subtype III) may have high norepinephrine output because of increased CRH activity in some cases. Investigators have also observed an association of increased platelet MAO activity with HPA axis hyperactivity, as detected by the DST, in some depressed patients. As with much of the data on the

HPA axis, further study is needed to clarify the meaning of this association.

HYPOTHALAMIC-PITUITARY-THYROID AXIS Interest in the thyroid and its function in emotion dates back centuries. Modern investigation can be traced to a 1938 report that suggested that some patients with periodic catatonia improved when they received thyroid extract. Approximately 40 years later it was suggested that small doses of triiodothyronine (T_3) (Cytomel) potentiated the antidepressant effects of tricyclics, a finding that has recently been confirmed in a well-controlled study. In recent years, a number of subtle changes in the thyroid axis have been detected in patients with mood disorders.

The HPT axis, like the HPA axis, is a complex and highly integrated network. The hypothalamic peptide TRH is carried to the anterior pituitary by the pituitary portal circulation. TRH stimulates the release of the pituitary hormone thyrotropin (TSH), which regulates the production of the thyroid hormones L-thyroxine (T_4) and L-triiodothyronine (T_3). The thyroid hormones exert a feedback control over the axis.

Symptoms of depression have long been known to occur in patients with frank hyperthyroidism or hypothyroidism; the psychiatric symptoms generally revert with normalization of the thyroid status. Many psychiatric patients may exhibit transient changes in thyroid function test results at the time of hospitalization. These abnormalities, which generally revert to normal within a matter of weeks, may simply reflect the stress of acute illness. Some (but not all) recent studies have found that as a group, depressed patients have significantly lower TSH and higher free T_4 values than controls; some studies also suggest that response to antidepressant medication may be associated with a decrease in free T_4 level.

Some individual depressed patients, especially those with bipolar disorder, may exhibit persistent mild, or subclinical, hypothyroidism, detected by an elevated TSH value, an elevated TSH response to injected TRH, or the presence of antimicrosomal thyroid or antithyroglobulin antibodies. The relationship of these subclinical thyroid abnormalities to the effects of thyroid hormone augmentation of antidepressant medication is not clear, although a recent report suggests that depressed patients with subclinical hypothyroidism do benefit from the addition of thyroid hormone to their antidepressant regimen. Frank or subclinical hypothyroidism has been well documented in patients with rapid-cycling bipolar disorders. Interestingly, most patients with rapid-cycling disorders appear to benefit from hypermetabolic doses of thyroid hormone, regardless of whether the patient actually has subclinical hypothyroidism. The adjunctive benefit gained from the use of thyroid hormone in patients with affective disorder may derive, in part, from the thyroid modulation of adrenergic receptors.

TRH stimulation test The TRH stimulation test, a standard endocrine procedure, has been used to probe the HPT axis in patients with mood disorders but apparently normal thyroid functioning. In medicine, the test is used mainly for the evaluation of subtle dysfunction in the HPT axis. Often helpful in pinpointing the source of the dysfunction, it is considered to be a safe clinical procedure. The TRH test has become a useful research tool in psychiatry, one that may have clinical applications as well. Using the test, many investigators have consistently reported a decreased or blunted TSH response to TRH in depressed patients.

The test has been standardized and is generally performed as follows. After an overnight fast, the patient is placed in a recumbent position. An intravenous (IV) line is started in the morning and a baseline blood sample for TSH is drawn. TRH is then injected IV, and multiple blood samples are taken at intervals over the next 90 minutes for TSH measurements. The test result is usually expressed as ΔTSH, or the highest TSH value after the TRH infusion minus the TSH value before TRH infusion. Because in depression the TSH values are likely to be low, the laboratory assay (generally a radioimmunoassay) must be sensitive to low levels.

The data on the TSH response have been reported either as group means or as a percentage of blunting for individual patients. Studies using group means have clearly indicated that, as a cohort, depressed patients have a lower TSH response to TRH than normal persons. Reports on percentage of blunting vary from about 25 to 70 percent, depending on the definition of blunting and the diagnostic groups studied. One group of investigators performed TRH stimulation tests at 8 AM and 11 PM the same day in patients with major depression and in healthy control subjects. The difference between ΔTSH values at the two time points (11 PM minus 8 AM) defined as ΔΔTSH, was significantly lower in the patients. Setting the criterion for ΔΔTSH blunting at less than 3 mU/L, the test had a diagnostic sensitivity of 89 percent and specificity of 95 percent. Some groups have found that those patients with a blunted TSH response to TRH also have a blunted prolactin response or an abnormal GH response, but other groups have not had the same results. The possibility of differences in the blunting of the TSH response to TRH in bipolar versus unipolar depressions has been raised but not resolved in the literature.

Several factors are known to cause blunting in normal persons. Most important for the use of the test in psychiatry are increasing age and male sex. Many of the studies reported in depressed patients are hard to interpret because of lack of adequate controls. Other factors that may be related to blunting include acute starvation, chronic renal failure, Klinefelter's syndrome, repeated TRH tests, and administration of somatostatin, neurotensin, dopamine, thyroid hormone, or glucocorticoids. Because of the effect of glucocorticoids on the TRH test, it was suggested that the blunted TRH test in patients with depressive disorders might be an epiphenomenon related to an elevated plasma cortisol level. A number of recent studies, however, have separated these two factors. At times, TRH blunting and an abnormal DST occur in the same depressed patient. However, some patients exhibit only one abnormality, while others may have neither.

The possible diagnostic significance of TSH blunting has been a subject of some debate. Some 25 to 70 percent of patients variously described as having endogenous depression, primary depression, or major depression have a blunted TSH response to TRH. In two separate studies patients with TSH blunting were found not to be within particular familial subtypes of depression. Only a few studies have reported specifically on the TSH response to TRH in neurotic or minor depressions; in these studies the TSH response was normal, although one recent study found a 50 percent rate of TSH blunting in patients with subaffective dysthymic disorder. The TRH stimulation test has been normal in groups of patients with secondary depressions, schizophrenia, and acute paranoid reactions. Normal TSH responses, but with delayed time course, have been reported in patients with anorexia nervosa. Alcoholics, both during and after withdrawal, have been reported to have TSH blunting in the range of 25 to 60 percent. Some patients with borderline personality disorder may have blunting as well.

Thus, a blunted TSH response to TRH is not specific for

endogenous depression. Some have suggested, however, that with the proper exclusion criteria, it may be useful in the differential diagnosis of dysphoric states. Others do not agree. The recent findings of abnormalities in the diurnal variation of the TSH response to TRH suggest that this procedure may be more specific, but replication of these results will be important.

The TRH test has great potential utility for research. An important research question is that of normalization of the TSH blunting with clinical improvement. In some depressed patients the TSH response seems to change with symptoms. A number of studies, however, have found that not all of the blunted responses in depressed patients return to normal with clinical improvement. Similarly, TSH responses have been reported to be blunted in some alcoholics both during and long after withdrawal. It has been suggested, therefore, that the TSH response to TRH may have trait as well as state characteristics. The possibility that TSH blunting may be a partial trait marker has stimulated studies of nondepressed relatives of TSH-blunted, depressed patients.

Some investigators have studied the prognostic value of the TRH test. One group reported that a blunted TSH response may predict a more favorable response to antidepressant drugs. Another group followed a cohort of clinically recovered depressed patients to determine relapse rates based on a ΔΔTSH index, defined as ΔTSH on a TRH stimulation test subsequent to a favorable treatment response minus ΔTSH on a TRH stimulation test performed before treatment began. In their studies, a ΔΔTSH above 2 mU/L was associated with no relapse within six months in 93 percent of cases, whereas a value of 2 mU/L or lower predicted a relapse within six months in 83 percent of cases. In all cases no maintenance treatment was continued after the clinical response. These investigators suggested that the ΔΔTSH index might be helpful in determining when to stop treatment. Other studies have confirmed the value of ΔΔTSH as a predictor of relapse, but it has not been clear that antidepressant therapy would prevent it.

A number of investigators have reported on the relationship of TRH test blunting to other biological measurements in depressed patients, but clear-cut, replicated findings have not yet emerged. Studies such as these, combining multiple biological tests, are likely to become increasingly common.

It is not known what relationship the TRH test blunting has to the augmented TSH response to TRH that may be seen in depressed patients with subclinical hypothyroidism. Moreover, the pathophysiological significance of the TSH blunting in mood disorders is not clear. Hypersecretion of TRH could lead to down-regulation of pituitary TRH receptors and produce TSH blunting. This possibility is supported by one report in the literature of elevated TRH in the CSF of depressed patients; however, a more recent study failed to replicate this finding.

HYPOTHALAMIC-PITUITARY-GROWTH HORMONE AXIS

The third endocrine system studied in patients with mood disorders is the HPGH axis. Investigators have looked at levels of GH and somatostatin (GHRIF), as well as the GH response to various stimuli, such as insulin hypoglycemia, L-dopa, 5-hydroxytryptophan, apomorphine, *d*-amphetamine, clonidine, growth hormone-releasing hormone (GHRH), and TRH. The findings in patients with mood disorders have been, in general, confusing; the HPGH axis is very complex.

GH is elevated during stress and in relation to the first nightly cycle of slow-wave sleep, but GH also seems to be released in 6-hour intervals throughout each 24-hour day. Adrenergic, serotonergic, cholinergic, and opioidergic inputs modify the production of hypothalamic GHRH and GHRIF, but the relationship of these factors to the pulsatile secretion is unclear.

Basal GH levels in depressed patients are generally reported to be grossly normal, despite the apparent stress of the illness. However, a reduction in mean GH levels (when measured every 15 minutes over 24 hours) has been observed. This overall reduction appears due to a decrease in GH secretion during sleep. An intermittent increase in daytime release of GH in depressed patients has also been noted.

Although a number of lines of evidence suggest that GH regulation may be abnormal in patients with depression, the picture is far from clear. Sleep-associated GH release may be low, and daytime GH secretion in depressed patients may be intermittently elevated. A number of studies have found that CSF levels of somatostatin (GHRIF) are decreased in depressed patients, but one study has not confirmed this finding. In addition, although some challenge tests of the GH system have substantiated the suspicion of abnormalities in depressed patients, others have not.

One challenge test, involving stimulation of the GH system with clonidine, has been reported fairly consistently to be abnormal in depression, although there have been recent negative findings. In this test, which measures the responsiveness of postsynaptic α_2-adrenergic receptors, depressed patients have a decreased GH response compared to controls. There have been suggestions that the abnormality persists after treatment and thus may represent a trait marker of depression or perhaps a severe form of depression. Another recently studied challenge test (measuring the GH response to desipramine, which also measures α_2-receptor sensitivity) has also been reported to show a decreased GH response among depressed patients.

Results from most other challenge tests of the GH system have been conflicting. As noted above, stimulation by L-dopa (Larodopa, Dopar) has been used as a measure of GH response. An early report suggested that depressed patients had a lower GH response to L-dopa; however, in a subsequent study that controlled for age, sex, and menopausal status, the diminished GH response to L-dopa disappeared.

Similarly, the use of amphetamine as a probe in patients with mood disorders has produced data the interpretation of which has changed in recent years. An early study reported that GH release after IV amphetamine administration was lower in patients with endogenous depression and higher in those with reactive depression as compared with normal controls. A subsequent report, however, suggested that age or estrogen status greatly influenced the amphetamine effect on GH. A restudy of GH release after amphetamine employing adequate control groups did not confirm the original findings.

There has been an interesting series of reports about abnormal positive GH responses to TRH in depressed patients. TRH normally causes the release of TSH and prolactin only. According to three separate groups, GH increases can be detected in approximately 50 percent of patients with either unipolar or bipolar depressions but in no patients with minor depression. The abnormality remits with clinical recovery. However, at least three other groups have not found an abnormal GH response to TRH in depressed patients. It is unclear why the findings are inconsistent. Further studies are required.

The availability of GHRH in recent years has allowed this peptide to be used in a challenge test with depressed patients. Again, the data are discordant. Some studies noted a blunted GH response to GHRH, others did not. Differences in methodology and in the form of synthetic GHRH used may explain the differing results. Further investigations with the procedure are needed.

A number of investigators have noted a reduced GH response to insulin administration in some depressed patients. It may be more dramatic in psychotic depression and, in some cases may persist after clinical recovery. One report noted the GH reduction to be more pronounced in bipolar than in unipolar depressions; another report found just the opposite. One recent study, which controlled for adequacy of the hypoglycemic response to insulin, reported no evidence of an abnormal GH response, but a second investigation, which also assured an adequate hypoglycemic response, did note blunted GH secretion. Correcting for the hypoglycemic response to insulin is essential since some investigators have noted that unipolar depressed patients have a blunted hypoglycemic response to insulin. This latter effect, too, may be associated with more severe depressions.

The HPGH axis may provide intriguing clues to the pathophysiology of depressions but requires more intensive study. It must also be recognized that putative abnormalities in the HPGH system may be exceedingly difficult to interpret because of the complexity of the HPGH axis and its relationship with other neuroendocrine and neurotransmitter systems.

MELATONIN Melatonin, a hormone derived from the pineal gland, is synthesized from serotonin under the regulatory control of norepinephrine. Although the function of melatonin in humans is poorly understood, investigators have utilized it in the study of psychiatric disorders. For example, many, but not all, recent studies have suggested a relationship between light-induced changes in melatonin secretion and depressive symptoms. There has also been interest in nocturnal melatonin levels based in part on the fact that nocturnal synthesis and secretion of melatonin are controlled primarily by noradrenergic input to the pineal gland. A number of investigators have reported decreased nocturnal melatonin levels in depression. However, the only two studies that matched depressed patients and control subjects for age, sex, and menstrual status, variables known to affect melatonin secretion, failed to find significant differences in nocturnal melatonin concentrations between patients and controls; in fact, both studies showed trends toward significant increases in melatonin among the patients. There is a need for additional, well-controlled research on melatonin in depression; longitudinal studies of patients in different clinical states are particularly important.

OTHER BIOCHEMICAL ASPECTS OF MOOD DISORDERS

NEUROPEPTIDES In the past 20 years dozens of neuropeptides have been isolated and sequenced. The study of their multiple and complex actions throughout the nervous system has become a major thrust of neuroscience research. Possible relations between neuropeptides and psychiatric disorders have also been examined. Studies with the peptides CRH and TRH have added important information to the understanding of neuroendocrine axes in patients with mood disorders. Many other neuropeptides, including β-endorphin, β-lipotropin, somatostatin, arginine vasopressin, cholecystokinin, substance P, bombesin, vasoactive intestinal peptide, δ-sleep-inducing peptide, calcitonin, neuropeptide Y, and diazepam-binding inhibitor, have also been studied in patients with mood disorders. Unfortunately, the information reported for these neuropeptides is conflicting and, for some, quite sparse. Those that have been studied the most are β-endorphin, somatostatin, and arginine vasopressin.

The well-known effects of administered opioids and the discovery of endogenous opioid peptides led to questions about the role of the opioid peptides in mood disorders. Some have suggested that administered opioids might have antidepressant effects, or that opioid antagonists might worsen depression and lessen mania. A number of studies have failed to provide evidence supporting these ideas; there is, however, one study suggesting that a high dose of the opioid antagonist naloxone (Narcan) may exacerbate depression.

ACTH and β-endorphin are cleavage products of a common precursor, pro-opiomelanocortin (POMC), and this posttranslational processing occurs under the regulation of CRH. For that reason, changes in β-endorphin have been studied to provide further information about the integrity of the HPA axis in depressed patients. Some investigators have reported elevated plasma levels of β-endorphin in depressed patients, although negative findings have also been reported. There may be a negative correlation between β-endorphin levels and symptom severity. Plasma levels of β-endorphin have also been used as an index of pituitary response to dexamethasone. High rates of failure to suppress β-endorphin (after dexamethasone) have been found in depressed patients, and some depressed patients who suppress cortisol fail to suppress β-endorphin. Studies of CSF β-endorphin or total opioid binding in depressed patients have not shown the same changes seen with plasma measures.

As noted above, somatostatin (GHRIF) has been studied in patients with mood disorders as an indicator of GH axis regulation. Somatostatin, however, is a neuromodulator with complex actions impinging on many other neurotransmitter systems. Because of its widespread actions, somatostatin has been thought to play a role in the behavioral, physiological, and endocrine changes in patients with mood disorders. At least four separate studies have shown decreases in CSF somatostatin levels in patients with depression, but one study has reported no decrease. Any relationship, however, will be complex, as somatostatin levels are also related to sleep, which is frequently disturbed in depressed patients.

Arginine vasopressin (AVP) is known to be widely distributed throughout the CNS, where it functions as a neuromodulator and produces complex behavioral effects. Preclinical studies have suggested that the actions of AVP may be related to memory, rapid-eye-movement sleep, biological rhythms, and neuroendocrine function, all thought to be altered in patients with mood disorders. In clinical research, one study found CSF AVP levels to be significantly lower in depressed patients than in controls and to be significantly higher in manic than in depressed patients. In another study, when the vasopressin analogue 1-desamino-8-D-arginine vasopressin (desmopressin, DDAVP [Adiuretin]) was given to four depressed patients, their cognitive function improved without a change in mood. Because ACTH release by the pituitary is regulated in part by AVP, the ACTH response to AVP administration has been examined in depressed patients. In contrast to the blunted ACTH response to administration of CRH found in depressed patients, AVP administration does not appear to produce a decreased ACTH response in depressed patients compared with controls; there is even a suggestion that depressed patients may have an exaggerated ACTH response to a low dose of AVP.

PSYCHOIMMUNOLOGY Although some studies suggest that bereavement and depression can interfere with immunological competence, the findings in this area of research have been diverse and often inconsistent. Studies of bereaved men and women have reported reduced in vitro lymphocyte response to mitogen stimulation, with normal levels of circulating immunoglobulins and normal responses on delayed hypersensitivity skin tests; the reduced lymphocyte response is most dramatic in bereaved patients with depressive symptoms. A recent meta-analysis of methodologically sound studies addressing cellular immunity in depression found that the immune abnormalities reliably associated with depression were (1) decreased proliferative response of lymphocytes to mitogen stimulation, (2) decreased natural killer cell activity, and (3) abnormalities of different white blood cell lines. The magnitude of these immune system abnormalities correlated with the intensity of depressed mood. However, one review cautioned that methodological concerns limit the interpretation and generalizability of much of the available data on the immune system in depression, and another review, noting the high incidence of failure to replicate findings, concluded that specific or reproducible abnormalities of the immune system in depression have not been demonstrated.

A potential explanation for some of the diverse findings may involve high catecholamine output and the increased production of prostaglandins, each of which has been observed separately in studies of depressed patients. Catecholamines, acting through β-adrenergic receptors, are known to suppress the activity of human natural killer cells. Prostaglandins, functioning through a complex interaction between second messenger systems, may inhibit in vitro mitogen-induced lymphocyte proliferation. Because recent animal work suggests that prostaglandin production is increased by catecholamines through a nonreceptor-mediated mechanism, the diminished immunological competence reported in depressed patients may be a result of the dysregulation of the catecholaminergic system.

GABA METABOLISM AND PHYSIOLOGY Recent studies have found that plasma levels of GABA, which reflect brain GABA activity, may be decreased in certain patients with unipolar or bipolar depressions or during manic episodes. In the patients with unipolar depression and low GABA levels, the GABA level did not appear to correlate with severity or duration of illness, and the low plasma levels persisted after remission of the depressive illness. This finding raises the possibility that, in some patients, plasma GABA may be a trait marker of depression.

INTRACELLULAR CALCIUM Several recent studies have suggested that abnormalities of intracellular calcium are associated with mood disorders. Basal concentrations of intracellular free calcium ion appear to be elevated in platelets and lymphocytes obtained from patients with bipolar disorders during either manic or depressed episodes; in contrast, patients with unipolar depression appear to have normal basal levels of calcium in these cells.

BEYOND THE CATECHOLAMINE HYPOTHESIS: TOWARD A BIOCHEMICAL CLASSIFICATION OF DEPRESSIVE DISORDERS

The mood disorders include a heterogeneous group of conditions. Clinical subtyping of these disorders has been only partially successful in identifying homogeneous categories; even within categories (such as major depressive disorder) the natural history of the disorder may vary, as may the response to treatment. It is also generally recognized that the clinical categories do not necessarily represent distinct biologically homogeneous entities. For these reasons, studies have examined various biochemical characteristics that might serve as independent variables for classifying subtypes of mood disorders.

Studies of the biogenic amines have revealed important clues about the pathophysiology underlying the heterogeneity of mood disorders. For almost 30 years the catecholamine hypothesis proved to have heuristic value. It gave both investigators and clinicians a frame of reference for understanding much of the available data on mood disorders, and it stimulated new research on their biochemistry.

The field continues to evolve, and much new information is being accumulated, not all of which can be fitted into any one theoretical framework. Intriguing clues across the biological variables have begun to appear. The process of norepinephrine-induced heterologous desensitization, if confirmed, may provide a useful link among some of those variables. But that work, like much of the new research, is still preliminary. Perhaps the best synthesis that can be currently offered should emphasize two facts: The mood disorders are most likely a group of interrelated neuroendocrinometabolic disorders, and biochemical procedures will be required to subdivide and classify them.

The development of a biochemical classification of depressive disorders will require, in part, empirically derived clinical laboratory tests that reflect one or another aspect of the pathophysiology of these disorders. It seems highly unlikely, however, that there will be a truly comprehensive understanding of the etiology and pathophysiology of the depressive disorders until a parallel description of the functional neurochemistry and neurophysiology of the normal human brain becomes available. Eric Kandel's pathfinding studies using animal models to explore specific forms of behavior at the cellular and molecular levels demonstrated the feasibility of such an undertaking but also underscored how far away is the attainment of that goal. Thus, in the foreseeable future, psychiatric practice may be guided by the use of specialized clinical tests that may not be meaningfully integrated into the theory of psychiatry for many years. In this regard, however, psychiatrists are in a position quite similar to that of their colleagues in other medical specialties.

It may be useful to compare the pneumonias and the depressions. Both disorders are diagnosed on the basis of clinical data, and both are treated more effectively using information gleaned from clinical tests. In the case of pneumonias, the physician makes a diagnosis on the basis of the history and physical examination (including a chest X-ray). After the diagnosis is made, sputum cultures are obtained to aid in determining the specific type of pneumonia that the patient may have and the specific antibiotic or other forms of treatment that may be most effective, irrespective of why the pneumonia developed. Similarly, in the case of depressions, the physician diagnoses depression on the basis of the clinical history and findings on physical and mental status examinations. Having made a diagnosis of depression, a physician can then use specialized clinical laboratory tests to obtain further information to assist in determining the type of depression the patient may have and the forms of treatment most likely to be effective in the care of that patient.

Although the biochemical tests available today do not necessarily enable physicians to select a clinically effective treatment on the first trial, the use of clinical laboratory tests can increase the probability of their doing so. Considering the time it takes for antidepressant drugs to exert their clinical effects, even a small increase in the percentage of patients who receive an effective drug on the first clinical trial of treatment would represent a major advance in the treatment of patients with depressive disorders.

SUGGESTED CROSS-REFERENCES

Monoamine neurotransmitters are discussed in Section 1.3, and the contributions of the neural sciences in general are the focus of the other sections of Chapter 1. Biological therapies are covered in Chapter 32.

REFERENCES

American Psychiatric Association Task Force on Laboratory Tests in Psychiatry, A H Glassman, chairman: The dexamethasone suppression test: An overview of its current status in psychiatry. Am J Psychiatry *144:* 1253, 1987.

Arana G W, Baldessarini R J: Clinical use of the dexamethasone suppression test in psychiatry. In *Psychopharmacology: The Third Generation of Progress,* H Y Meltzer, editor, p 609. Raven, New York, 1987.

Avissar S, Schreiber G: The involvement of guanine nucleotide binding proteins in the pathogenesis and treatment of affective disorders. Biol Psychiatry *31:* 435, 1992.

Bauer M S, Whybrow P C: Rapid-cycling bipolar affective disorder: II. Treatment of refractory rapid cycling with high dose levothyroxine. A preliminary study. Arch Gen Psychiatry *47:* 435, 1990.

Bauer M S, Whybrow P C, Winokur A: Rapid-cycling bipolar affective disorder: I. Association with grade I hypothyroidism. Arch Gen Psychiatry *47:* 427, 1990.

Calabrese J R, Kling M A, Gold P W: Alterations in immunocompetence during stress, bereavement, and depression: Focus on neuroendocrine regulation. Am J Psychiatry *144:* 1123, 1987.

Carroll B J: Dexamethasone suppression test: A review of contemporary confusion. J. Clin Psychol *46:* 13, 1985.

Cowen P J: Serotonin receptor subtypes in depression: Evidence from studies in neuroendocrine regulation. Clin Neuropharmacol *16* (Suppl 3): S6, 1993.

Delgado P L, Miller H L, Salomon R M, Licinio J, Heninger G R, Gelenberg A J, Charney D S: Monoamines and the mechanism of antidepressant action: Effects of catecholamine depletion on mood of patients treated with antidepressants. Psychopharmacol Bull *29* (3):389, 1993.

Duval F, Macher J P, Mokrani M-C: Difference between evening and morning thyrotropin responses to protirelin in major depressive episode. Arch Gen Psychiatry *47:* 443, 1990.

Duval F, Mokrani M-C, Crocq M-A, Bailey P, Macher J-P: Influence of thyroid hormones on morning and evening TSH response to TRH in major depression. Biol Psychiatry *35:* 926, 1994.

Gold P W, Rubinow D R: Neuropeptide function in affective illness: Corticotropin-releasing hormone and somatostatin as model systems. In *Psychopharmacology: The Third Generation of Progress,* H Y Meltzer, editor, p 617. Raven Press, New York, 1987.

Golden R N, Markey S P, Risby E D, Rudorfer M V, Cowdry R W, Potter W Z: Antidepressants reduce whole-body norepinephrine turnover while enhancing 6-hydroxymelatonin output. Arch Gen Psychiatry *45:* 150, 1988.

Goodwin F K, Jamison K R: *Manic-Depressive Illness.* Oxford University Press, New York, 1990.

Green A I: Thyroid function and affective disorders. Hosp Community Psychiatry *35:* 1188, 1984.

*Holsboer F: Neuroendocrinology of Mood Disorders. In *Psychopharmacology: The Fourth Generation of Progress,* F E Bloom, D J Kupfer, editors, p 957. Raven Press, New York, 1994.

Hudson C J, Young L T, Li P P, Warsh J J: CNS signal transduction in the pathophysiology and pharmacotherapy of affective disorders and schizophrenia. Synapse *13:* 278, 1993.

Irwin M: Psychoneuroimmunology of Depression. In *Psychopharmacology: The Fourth Generation of Progress,* F E Bloom, D J Kupfer, editors, p 983. Raven Press, New York, 1994.

Janowsky D S, Khaled El-Yousef M, DAvis J M, Sekerke H J: A cholinergic-adrenergic hypothesis of mania and depression. Lancet *2:* 632, 1972.

Janowsky D S, Overstreet D H: The Role of Acetylcholine Mechanisms in Mood Disorders. In *Psychopharmacology: The Fourth Generation of Progress,* F E Bloom, D J Kupfer, editors, p 945, Raven Press, New York, 1994.

Joffe R T, Levitt A L: The thyroid and depression. In *The Thyroid Axis and Psychiatric Illness,* R T Joffe, A J Levitt, editors, p 195. American Psychiatric Press, Washington, 1993.

Kafka M S, Paul S M: Platelet alpha$_2$-adrenergic receptors in depression. Arch Gen Psychiatry *43:* 91, 1986.

Kandel E R: From metapsychology to molecular biology: Explorations into the nature of anxiety. Am J Psychiatry *140:* 1277, 1983.

Kirkegaard C: The thyrotropin response to thyrotropin-releasing hormone in endogenous depression. Psychoneuroendocrinology *6:* 189, 1981.

Krog-Meyer I, Kirkegaard C, Kijne B L: Prediction of relapse with the TRH test and prophylactic amitriptyline in 39 patients with endogenous depression. Am J Psychiatry *141* (8):945, 1984.

Langer G, Koinig G, Hatzinger R, Schonbeck G, Resch F, Aschauer H, Keshavan M S, Sieghart W: Response of thyrotropin to thyrotropin-releasing hormone as predictor of treatment outcome. Arch Gen Psychiatry *43:* 861, 1986.

Lesch K P, Manji H K: Signal-transducing G proteins and antidepressant drugs: Evidence for modulation of α subunit gene expression in rat brain. Biol Psychiatry *32:* 549, 1992.

Maes M, Meltzer H Y: The serotonin hypothesis of major depression. In *Psychopharmacology: The Fourth Generation of Progress,* F E Bloom, D J Kupfer, editors, p 933, Raven Press, New York, 1994.

Miles A, Philbrick D R S: Melatonin and psychiatry. Biol Psychiatry *23:* 405, 1988.

Mooney J J, Schatzberg A F, Cole J O, Kizuka P P, Salomon M, Lerbinger J, Pappalardo K M, Gerson B, Schildkraut J J: Rapid antidepressant response to alprazolam in depressed patients with high catecholamine output and heterologous desensitization of platelet adenylate cyclase. Biol Psychiatry *23:* 543, 1988.

Mooney J J, Schatzberg A F, Cole J O, Samson J A, Gerson B, Pappalardo K M, Schildkraut J J: Urinary MHPG and the depression-type score as predictors of differential responses to antidepressants. J Clin Psychopharmacol *11:* 339, 1991.

*Nemeroff C B, Krishnan K R R: Neuroendocrine alterations in psychiatric disorders. In *Neuroendocrinology,* C B Nemeroff, editor. CRC, Ann Arbor, MI, 1992.

Owens M J, Nemeroff C B: Physiology and pharmacology of corticotropin-releasing factor. Pharmacol Rev *43:* 425, 1991.

*Owens M J, Nemeroff C B: Role of serotonin in the pathophysiology of depression: Focus on the serotonin transporter. Clin Chem *40:* (2): 288, 1994.

Petty F, Kramer G L, Hendrickse W: GABA and depression. In *Biology of Depressive Disorders,* Part A: *A Systems Perspective,* J J Mann, D J Kupfer, editors, p 79. Plenum, New York, 1993.

Plotsky P M, Owens M J, Nemeroff C B: Neuropeptide alterations in mood disorders. In *Psychopharmacology: The Fourth Generation of Progress,* F E Bloom, D J Kupfer, editors, p 971, Raven Press, New York, 1994.

Post R M, Ballenger J C: *Neurobiology of Mood Disorders.* Williams & Wilkins, Baltimore, 1984.

Potter W Z, Manji H K: Catecholamines in depression: An update. Clin Chem *40* (2): 279, 1994.

Prange A J Jr, Garbutt J C, Loosen P T: The hypothalamic-pituitary-thyroid axis in affective disorders. In *Psychopharmacology: The Third Generation of Progress,* H Y Meltzer, editor, p 629. Raven, New York, 1987.

Ribeiro S C M, Tandon J, Greenhaus L, Greden J F: The DST as a predictor of outcome in depression: A meta-analysis. Am J Psychiatry *150:* 1618, 1993.

Roy A, Linnoila M: Monoamines and suicidal behavior. In *Violence and Suicidality: Perspectives in Clinical and Psychobiological Research,* H M van Pragg, R Plutchik, A Apter, editors, p 141. Brunner/Mazel, New York, 1990.

Samson J A, Gudeman J E, Schatzberg A F, Kizuka P P, Orsulak P J, Cole J O, Schildkraut J J: Toward a biochemical classification of depressive disorders: VIII. Platelet MAO activity and subtypes of depressions. J Psychiatr Res *19:* 547, 1985.

Schatzberg A F, Orsulak P J, Rosenbaum A H, Maruta T, Kruger E R, Cole J O, Schildkraut J J: Toward a biochemical classification of depressive disorders: V. Heterogeneity of unipolar depressions. Am J Psychiatry *139:* 471, 1982.

Schatzberg A F, Rothschild A J, Gerson B, Lerbinger J E, Schildkraut J J: Toward a biochemical classification of depressive disorders: IX. DST results and platelet MAO activity in depressed patients. Br J Psychiatry *146:* 633, 1985.

Schatzberg A F, Rothschild A J, Langlais P J, Bird E D, Cole J O: A corticosteroid/dopamine hypothesis of psychotic depression and related states. J Psychiatr Res *19:* 57, 1985.

*Schatzberg A F, Schildkraut J J: Recent studies on norepinephrine systems in mood disorders. In *Psychopharmacology: The Fourth Generation of Progress,* F E Bloom, D J Kupfer, editors, p 911, Raven Press, New York, 1994.

*Schildkraut J J: The catecholamine hypothesis of affective disorders: A review of supporting evidence. Am J Psychiatry *122:* 509, 1965.

Schildkraut J J, Keeler B A, Grab E L, Kantrowich J, Hartmann E: MHPG excretion and clinical classification in depressive disorders. Lancet *1*: 1251, 1973.

Schildkraut J J, Orsulak P J, LaBrie R A, Schatzberg A F, Gudeman J E, Cole J O, Rohde W A: Toward a biochemical classification of depressive disorders: II. Application of multivariate discriminant function analysis to data on urinary catecholamines and metabolites. Arch Gen. Psychiatry *35:* 1436, 1978.
Schildkraut J J, Orsulak P J, Schatzberg A F, Gudeman J E: Cole J O, Rohde W A, LaBrie R A: Toward a biochemical classification of depressive disorders: I. Differences in urinary MHPG and other catecholamine metabolites in clinically defined subtypes of depressions. Arch Gen Psychiatry *35:* 1427, 1978.
Schildkraut J J, Schatzberg A F, Mooney J J, Orsulak P J: Depressive disorders and the emerging field of psychiatric chemistry. In *Psychiatry Update: The American Psychiatric Association Annual Review*, vol 2, L Grinspoon, editor, p 457. American Psychiatric Press, Washington, 1983.
Siever L J: Role of noradrenergic mechanisms in the etiology of the affective disorders. In *Psychopharmacology: The Third Generation of Progress*, H Y Meltzer, editor, p 493. Raven, New York, 1987.
Stein M, Miller A H, Trestman R L: Depression, the immune system, and health and illness: Findings in search of meaning. Arch Gen Psychiatry *48:* 171, 1991.
Weisse C S: Depression and immunocompetence: A review of the literature. Psychol Bull *111:* 475, 1992.
Willner P: Dopaminergic mechanisms in depression and mania. In *Psychopharmacology: The Fourth Generation of Progress*, F E Bloom, D J Kupfer, editors, p 921. Raven Press, New York, 1994.

16.4 MOOD DISORDERS: GENETIC ASPECTS

KATHLEEN RIES MERIKANGAS, Ph.D.
DAVID J. KUPFER, M.D.

INTRODUCTION

Rapid developments in molecular biology have introduced a new era in human genetics. Although only a decade ago linkage depended on inferences about the underlying genetic alleles from phenotypic expression of known markers, advances in the identification of polymorphic deoxyribonucleic acid (DNA) markers and the methods for processing and sequencing the DNA have enhanced dramatically the ability to detect linkage between those markers and diseases for which no aberrant gene product has been identified. Family pedigrees may be examined to determine whether a particular disease or trait is associated with a specific DNA marker (linkage). Since the exciting discovery of a linked marker for Huntington's disease, studies of numerous other diseases have followed, and the primary gene defect has now been discovered for Duchenne's muscular dystrophy and cystic fibrosis. Those dramatic discoveries have led to a new focus on the role of genes in the etiology of major psychiatric illness.

In a field plagued by complexity of expression and lack of valid definitions of discrete disorders, coupled with the little progress in uncovering the cause of psychiatric disorders, the application of molecular biological approaches has provided a renewed opportunity for researchers to identify markers for psychiatric disorders. Such markers may serve as vulnerability or disease indicators with which to circumvent the exclusive reliance on clinical signs and symptoms to diagnose psychiatric illness. However, the initial enthusiasm engendered by the potential yield of these methods has diminished after five years of inconsistent and disappointing results involving labor-intensive and costly research.

The major psychiatric disorders consist of disorders for which the validity of definitions has yet to be established, the cause is unknown, and the pathway from genotype to the phenotype is complex and probably heterogeneous. The new field of genetic epidemiology, with an integration of knowledge from clinical psychiatry, neurobiology, molecular biology, immunology, and endocrinology, provides hope of unraveling some of the complexity that continues to obscure the etiology and pathogenesis of the psychiatric conditions. The disorders are among the most prevalent and distressing of all chronic human diseases. Specification of the role of genetic factors for a disease may also lead to the identification of critical environments for its expression. In fact, knowledge of the role of genetic factors may lead to prevention and amelioration of the diseases by purely environmental methods. Even without accomplishing the ultimate aim of specification of causation, a considerable degree of optimism is warranted that the current generation of genetic epidemiology studies may yield information that will enable prevention and intervention efforts to minimize the effects of the disorders.

Although caution is warranted in the investigation of the cause of complex disorders, that does not imply that discovery of the role of genes is a phenomenon in the distant future. Recent developments in the understanding of human cancers, including retinoblastoma and an early-onset form of breast cancer, demonstrate the importance of inheritance of genetic factors which, in the presence of particular environmental factors, lead to the development of disease.

BACKGROUND

HUMAN GENETICS Human genetics, the scientific study of heredity, began in the early 1900s with the integration of mendelian theory and the basic principles of population genetics. The major subdivisions of human genetics that have evolved include biochemical genetics, population genetics, cytogenetics, molecular genetics, and immunogenetics. Genetic epidemiology is primarily derived from the division of population genetics.

Each normal human being has 23 pairs of chromosomes, the cellular components that are bearers of heredity, which are found exclusively in the nucleus of all living cells. Humans have 22 pairs of autosomes and one pair of sex chromosomes, with one member of each pair deriving, respectively, from maternal and paternal lines. Chromosomes have two components: DNA, and a class of small, positively charged proteins called histones. DNA is comprised of two complementary strands of nucleotides. There are four nucleotides—adenine and thymine, guanine and cytosine—each of which pairs exclusively with only one of the other three. Various combinations of three of the nucleotides code for amino acids, which are then joined sequentially to form specific proteins. The two intermediate steps in the process involve (1) in the nucleus, transcription of one of the DNA strands to its complement or messenger ribonucleic acid (mRNA) (which is identical to DNA except that the nucleotide uracil replaces thymine, and the sugar is ribose rather than deoxyribose), and (2) translation of the mRNA into a sequence of amino acids with the assistance of transfer-RNA (t-RNA) on the ribosomes in the cytoplasm of the cell.

All sequences of DNA are not active coding regions. Within genes, active coding sequences, or exons, are interspersed among introns, the noncoding sequences and intervening sequences. Enhancers, promoters, and control sequences are located at one end of a gene. Control of gene activity (protein synthesis) is a complex process that can occur at several different levels. The signals that turn genes on and off are mediated by or generated within the cytoplasm of the cell by the presence of activating or inhibiting molecules, such as hormones.

However, even after a protein has been manufactured, there still remains a complex pathway to its final expression in the phenotype, which may depend on the presence or absence of a variety of other genetic and environmental factors. For example, the disease phenylketonuria (a homozygous recessive condition resulting from a mutation in the gene coding for the enzyme phenylalanine hydroxylase, which converts the amino acid phenylalamine to tyrosine) results in permanent brain damage only if the vulnerable individual is exposed to typical levels of phenylalanine in the diet.

One-to-one correspondence between genotype and disease is often absent, even for traits that are produced by known genetic loci. Examples of this phenomenon include the following: epistasis, the interaction between distinct genes; variable expressivity, variation in the effects of a particular gene; genotype-environment interaction, genotypes that produce different phenotypes depending on the environment in which they are expressed; and reduced penetrance, the situation in which persons with a relevant genotype express a phenotype mildly *(formes fruste)* or not at all. Conversely, a single gene can have multiple effects (pleitropy). Because the complexity of the genotype is expected to exceed that of the phenotype, which only has a limited repertoire of expression, some investigators recommend that studies should begin at a phenotypic level and proceed backward toward the level of the genotype. Alternatively, other scientists argue that genetic heterogeneity, together with the other factors that are related to a lack of one-to-one correspondence between the genotype and the phenotype, strongly limit the ability of phenotypic studies to identify the underlying gene mechanisms. Instead, they suggest that molecular genetics studies of single large pedigrees are more likely to yield information on the genetic factors involved in a complex disorder.

GENETIC EPIDEMIOLOGY Although there have been major advances in the fields of epidemiology and human genetics, particularly in biostatistical methods (spurred by the integration of molecular biology and population genetics), there has been little communication between researchers in the fields of genetics and epidemiology. Although the goal of epidemiology is to study the interaction between host, agent, and environment, epidemiologists have tended to neglect "host" characteristics other than demographics. Similarly, geneticists have often neglected to consider the environment as a potential etiological agent, either randomizing or controlling for it in their analyses. Geneticists consider the environment as "noise" and heredity as "signal," whereas epidemiologists do the opposite.

Despite their history of independence, the two fields share much common ground. Both are interested in determining the causes of complex human disorders and predicting familial recurrence risks for such disorders. The advent of the new field of genetic epidemiology, defined as a science that deals with the cause, distribution, and control of disease in groups of relatives, and with inherited (biological or cultural) causes of disease in populations, has served to bridge the gap between the two fields. Newton Morton notes that the "synthesis of genetics and epidemiology is necessary before diseases of complex etiology can be understood and ultimately controlled." Hogben in 1933, quoted by Harris in 1977, has noted that in metaphoric terms, stating: ". . . our genes cannot make bricks without straw. The individual differences which men and women display are partly due to the fact that they receive different genes from their parents and partly due to the fact that the same genes live in different houses. . . ."

Genetic epidemiology is a relatively new discipline that has emerged from an integration of methods from the fields of population and clinical genetics, and chronic disease epidemiology. Until relatively recently, studies currently within the domain of genetic epidemiology were conducted within the realm of clinical genetics or behavior genetics. However, with the increasing awareness of the importance of simultaneous consideration of the relationship between the background population characteristics and the role of environmental factors in gaining understanding of the pathophysiology of disease, the discipline of epidemiology has become a critical component of genetic studies. During the past 10 years, the discipline of genetic epidemiology has grown rapidly, as exemplified by the introduction of the journal *Genetic Epidemiology* and the publication of several new textbooks describing a wide variety of applications and methods in the field. The application of the techniques of the new field of genetic epidemiology, which is without either environmentalist or hereditarian bias, should result in substantial contributions to the understanding of psychiatric disorders.

The most common misconception regarding the role of genetic factors in the manifestation of a particular trait or disease is that the term "genetic" implies determinism by innate factors with a subsequently unalterable course. Nothing has impeded progress in knowledge of the development of human traits and disorders more than the nature versus nurture controversy. The concept was originally introduced by Francis Galton in 1894 as nature and nurture. The majority of known genetic traits are not totally independent from the environment in which they are expressed. An illustrative example of gene-environment interaction is glucose-6-phosphate dehydrogenase (G6PD) deficiency, an X-linked disorder caused by a mutation on the long arm of the X chromosome. The expression of the disorder manifests as hemolytic anemia only when the susceptible individual is exposed to certain drugs or to fava beans. Genes may also be involved in the response or resistance to purely environmental agents such as diet, stress, exercise, drugs, and nutritional deficiencies, through the activity of immunogenetic factors of the major histocompatibility complex.

Not only is the expression of genes modified by the environment, but there is now substantial evidence that numerous environmental factors may actually alter the genotype. For example, environmental agents may induce chromosomal mutations that lead to carcinoma, such as the role of Epstein-Barr virus in Burkitt's lymphoma, or tobacco smoking in small cell carcinoma of the lung.

Design and analysis of genetic epidemiological studies

Descriptive epidemiological studies are important in specifying the rates and distribution of disorders in the general population. The data can be applied to identify biases that may exist in treated populations and case registries from which persons who serve as probands in family, twin, and adoption studies are selected. Such persons often constitute the tip of the iceberg of the disease and are not representative of the general population of similarly affected persons with respect to demographic, social, or clinical characteristics.

The traditional case-control study, an epidemiological study design, has been employed to study familial aggregation of disease in two ways: one in which the frequency of a positive family history among the cases is compared with that among the controls, and one in which the retrospectively assessed course of relatives of the cases is compared with that of the controls (retrospective cohort study).

After familial transmission of a trait has been established, the immediate goal of genetic epidemiological studies is to identify the relative degree of phenotypic variance that can be attributed to genetic factors and to transmissible and nontransmissible environmental factors. The ultimate purpose of such studies is to identify the specific agents that play an etiological or contributing role to the development of the trait.

The two chief study paradigms for studying gene-environment interactions involve holding either the genetic background or the environment constant and evaluating systematic changes in the other. Examples of studies that hold the genetic background constant while observing differential environmental exposures include studies of discordant twins; migrant population studies; relatives exposed to a particular agent, such as a virus; twins reared separately; or the family set design, in which comparisons are made among families of similar structure living in distinct environments. Examples of paradigms in which the environment is held constant and genetic factors are allowed to vary include monozygotic twins of affected individuals compared with dizygotic twins and nontwin siblings; offspring of consanguineous matings compared with offspring of nonconsanguineous matings; half-siblings compared with full siblings living in the same home; and first-degree relatives of affected persons. In both types of studies, observations can be made regarding time-space clustering of disease, which can provide information regarding environmental agents, or a characteristic age of onset and course, which may provide information on genetic factors.

Application of the genetic-epidemiological approach has also yielded information on risk and etiological factors for a number of disorders such as diabetes, hyperlipidemia, and coronary heart disease. An exemplary study of monozygotic twins who were concordant for heart disease but discordant for cigarette smoking demonstrated that smoking was not a risk factor for coronary heart disease. However, the twin pairs were found to be discordant for lung disease, which was found to be strongly related to cigarette exposure.

The importance of the integration of epidemiological methods in genetic studies is underscored by the results of family, twin, and adoption studies of numerous complex human disorders which suggest the importance of both genetic and nongenetic contributions to their causation. Such an approach is illustrated by the identification of the causes of specific types of cancer, such as retinoblastoma, which results from an interaction between an inherited gene defect and an environmentally induced mutation of the second allele at that locus.

It is often difficult to distinguish between transmitted and genetic factors, because environmental factors are often confounded with genetic susceptibility to those factors. The effects of putative exogenous factors such as drugs, dietary factors, and physical factors such as stress, fever, and exercise, may be modified by immunogenetic factors or by genetic variation in enzymes, hormones, fatty acids, or neurochemicals. In addition, factors that may appear to be purely environmental may actually be a result of transmissible factors.

GENETICS OF MOOD DISORDERS: REVIEW OF EMPIRICAL EVIDENCE

EPIDEMIOLOGY OF MOOD DISORDERS The lifetime prevalence of bipolar disorder ranges from 0.6 to 0.9. The incidence rates of bipolar disorder range from 9 to 15.2 new cases per 100,000 population per year for men and 7.4 to 32 new cases per 100,000 per year for women. For major depressive disorder the lifetime prevalence is 2.0 to 12.0 for men and 5.0 to 26.0 for women. The aggregate incidence rates of major depressive disorder are 247 to 598 per 100,000 per year for women and 82 to 201 for men. The results derived from the Epidemiologic Catchment Area Study, a large epidemiological survey of psychiatric disorders in the United States, yielded rates within the above-cited ranges for both bipolar disorder and major depressive disorder.

The demographic distribution of bipolar disorder and depressive disorders exhibits several differences: The sex ratio favors women for depressive disorders, whereas there is a nearly equal distribution of men and women for bipolar disorder. A family history of depression is the most important risk factor for both mood disorders, and both generally begin in early adulthood, with bipolar disorder having an earlier age of onset than major depressive disorder.

METHODS AND STUDY DESIGNS IN GENETIC EPIDEMIOLOGY There are four types of evidence that genetic factors contribute to a disease of unknown cause: (1) significant aggregation of the illness within families; (2) a higher concordance among monozygotic twins than among dizygotic twins; (3) a higher incidence of the trait, irrespective of home environment, among biological offspring of affected persons than among biological offspring of unaffected persons (that is, positive adoption study); and (4) linkage of the illness with an identifiable allele at a marker locus.

The types of studies that have been conducted to assess the role of genetic factors in the etiology of illnesses include the following: (1) family studies, which assess the degree of aggregation of a trait among relatives of affected probands compared with expected rates from the general population; (2) twin studies, which compare concordance rates for monozygotic twins, who have identical genotypes, with those among dizygotic twins, who share an average of half of their genes in common; (3) adoption studies, which compare the degree of similarity between an adoptee and his or her biological parents, from whom he or she was separated, and between the adoptee and the adoptive parents. Those comparisons yield relative risks of the genetic and environmental factors and their interaction in producing a disease; and (4) association and linkage studies of genetic markers, which examine the relationships between a known genetic trait and disease status either across families or within pedigrees.

Specific analytical techniques that are applicable to each type of study include comparison of morbid risk or correlations among relatives of a proband with risk in the population-at-large; path analysis, which partitions the total variance of the pairwise correlations between different types of relatives into genetic, cultural, and random environmental components; computation of pair or proband concordance for monozygotic versus dizygotic twins; comparison of correlations of adoptees with their biological siblings or parents and with their adoptive siblings or parents; and the sibling pair and LOD (logarithm of the odds) score methods of linkage analysis (described later). After the involvement of a genetic component in a disease has been established, there are numerous analytical methods for the detection and identification of the role of major genes, such as segregation analysis, disease-marker association studies, and linkage analysis.

FAMILY STUDIES

Designs and methods Familial aggregation of a disease is generally the initial source of evidence suggesting the involvement of genetic factors in its causation. However, common environmental factors such as diet, infection, shared behavioral patterns, or stress may also lead to familial clustering of a disease. The major goal of family studies is to understand the magnitude and patterns of familial aggregation of a particular disease.

Although family studies cannot yield direct evidence for the involvement of genes in the causation of a disease, they are a rich source of evidence for examining the correspondence between the observed patterns of expression of a disease and the patterns predicted by specific modes of transmission. A second application of family studies is the investigation of the validity of diagnostic categories and their subtypes through inspection of the degree to which particular symptoms or symptom constellations breed true in families. Whereas the homogeneity of expression of disorders is the goal of the latter studies, information on heterogeneity of expression within families may also be employed to identify variable expressivity of transmitted disorders.

A major advantage of studying diseases within families is that the assumption of homotypy of the underlying factors eliminates the effects of heterogeneity that are present in comparisons made between families. However, all individuals within a particular sibship are not expected to share equal genetic risk because of independent segregation of genes. Nevertheless, if two members are affected, similar etiological factors can be assumed, and variable forms of expression can be identified.

The three major designs of family studies are as follows: (1) increased prevalence of a disease among relatives of an affected proband compared with disease occurrence in the population from which they were selected; (2) increased prevalence of a disease among the relatives of an affected proband compared with a comparable group of relatives of controls; and (3) patterns of disease expression that do not differ from the predictions of specific genetic models of disease transmission.

Family studies may be analyzed as either traditional case-control studies in which the family history is classified dichotomously according to the presence or absence of a disorder in at least one of the first-degree relatives of persons with the disease compared with those without the disease, or through the calculation of rates of the disorder among the first-degree relatives of probands compared with rates among controls. The advantage of the latter approach is that information on the full pedigree may be employed, whereas the former approach eliminates possible bias associated with the lack of independence of observations obtained within families.

Modes of familial transmission Table 16.4-1 summarizes the major models of disease transmission and the expected patterns of illness within pedigrees according to each model. Adequate fit of the models to the observed data does not provide positive evidence regarding the mode of transmission of a disorder. Rather, those models that do not provide an adequate fit to the data can be excluded as explanations of the mode of transmission of a particular disorder if the assumptions of the model are not violated.

The traditional single major locus mendelian models have rarely fit family data for the major psychiatric disorders (with the exception of some bipolar disorder pedigrees, described later). However, the models may still provide a good fit to subtypes of the psychiatric disorders. Despite the recent progress in the development of standardized diagnostic nomenclature, definitions of psychiatric disorders still suffer from a lack of established reliability and validity, thereby casting doubt on assignment of disease status in probands and their families. The lack of adequate models of disease transmission is one of the major obstacles to progress in linkage studies of those conditions. Furthermore, the probable genetic heterogeneity or different genetic factors resulting in similar phenotypic expression of the major psychiatric disorders also compromises current attempts to identify the role of genes in these conditions.

The multifactorial model of disease transmission, first proposed by Douglas Falconer, specifies that there are numerous genes and transmissible and nontransmissible cultural factors that are additively and independently (without epistasis) involved in producing a phenotype. There is assumed to be a continuous underlying distribution, or liability, which is defined as the propensity for expressing a disease. The total liability includes a genetic (transmitted) component and a nontransmitted component of the variance. The liability is assumed to be normally distributed, with mean = 0 and a variance = 1. The disorder becomes apparent after the accumulation of vulnerability factors surpass the threshold, or the point on the distribution beyond which the disorder becomes manifest.

The analytical technique that has been frequently applied to resolve the polygenic and cultural components under multifactorial transmission is path analysis. The basic parameters are paths, copaths, and correlations between pairs of relatives throughout an extended pedigree. Allowance is made for assortative mating, correlated environments between pairs of individuals, and unique environments of individuals. The observed and expected values of the correlations are compared and tested for statistical significance. Resolution of cultural and biological inheritance requires either extended familial relationships (monozygotic twins, half siblings), or the identification of a relevant index of inherited environment.

TABLE 16.4-1
Observed Patterns of Transmission for the Major Genetic Models

Model	Observed Patterns
Autosomal dominant	Every generation, no skipping Unilineal transmission Half of the relatives affected
Autosomal recessive	Horizontal transmission One fourth of siblings affected Equally affects men and women Consanguinity increased in parents
X-linked recessive	Men are affected to a greater extent than women Absence of male-to-male transmission Half the sons of female carriers are affected All daughters of affected men are carriers
X-linked dominant	Women are affected more than men Affected women transmit trait to half of their sons and half of their daughters Affected men transmit to all daughters, but not to sons
Multifactorial	One Gene (polygenic) and more than one nongenetic factor Risk among relatives increased according to severity of the proband disorder Bilineal transmission common Mean for offspring midway between parents and population values (continuous traits) Recurrence risk (dichotomous traits) or correlation (continuous traits) among relatives proportional to the degree of the genetic relationship
Mixed model: single major locus (SML) and multifactorial	Three distributions within a single skewed distribution

Methodological standards for family studies of psychiatric disorders Several large-scale family studies during the past decades have developed standard methods for conducting family studies of the major psychiatric disorders. The following design features are included: recruitment of a well-characterized homogeneous group of probands with a particular disorder; selection of a control group of persons who are comparable with the affected probands on all possible confounding factors except the disorder itself; systematic enumeration of all living and deceased relatives according to the degree of relationship to the probands and controls; use of structured diagnostic interviews with relatives using predetermined diagnostic criteria and reliable and valid diagnostic instruments; maintenance of blindness with respect to the diagnostic status of the proband in collecting diagnostic information from the relatives and formulating the final diagnostic estimates; collection of information regarding relatives unavailable for interview in a standardized format from as many informants as possible; inclusion of ancillary information to supplement interview and family history data; development of reliable procedures to integrate material from direct interviews, family history reports, and ancillary medical or psychiatric information in deriving the diagnostic assignment of the probands and relatives; and application of sophisticated statistical techniques to control for confounding variables and simultaneously adjust for length of observation of the relatives.

Empirical evidence: family studies For centuries, depression has been known to occur often in closely related family members. The tendency for melancholia to pass from parent to offspring was noted by Hippocrates in ancient Greece. Numerous family studies of manic depression conducted in Europe during the first half of the 20th century have shown that manic depression was familial. The first systematic family studies which separated bipolar and unipolar depression revealed that bipolar depression was familial, but that unipolar depression was not increased among the relatives of bipolar probands and the converse.

Although numerous family studies of both bipolar disorder and major depressive disorder have been conducted during the past 30 years it is remarkable that only four family studies of bipolar disorder and five studies of major depressive disorder meet the previously cited standards of family study methodology—including inclusion of control probands and relatives, application of standardized diagnostic criteria with structured diagnostic instruments, and blindness with respect to the diagnosis of the probands.

Table 16.4-2 summarizes the series of controlled family studies of probands with bipolar disorder. The results of the studies consistently reveal a significantly greater risk (range, 3.7 to 17.5 percent) of bipolar disorder among the relatives of bipolar probands compared with risk among the relatives of controls. The absolute rates of bipolar disorder among the relatives of bipolar probands are quite similar, ranging from 3.8 to 6.8 percent. The rates of major depressive disorder among the relatives of bipolar probands are also consistently elevated but of a much lower magnitude than those of bipolar disorder. In accordance with expectations derived from epidemiological studies, the rates of major depressive disorder are greater than those of bipolar disorder, with a range from 6.8 to 16.7 percent. There is an average twofold increase in the relative risk of major depressive disorder among the relatives of bipolar probands compared with risk in relatives of controls.

Investigations of the familial aggregation of mood disorders among the relatives of probands with major depressive disorder compared to controls are shown in Table 16.4-3. The magnitude of rates of bipolar disorder among the relatives of major depressive disorder probands is about half that of relatives of bipolar probands. Similarly, the relatives' risks, although significantly elevated in two of the studies, appear to be attributable to extremely low rates of bipolar disorder in the relatives of controls (0.2 percent, which is significantly less than expectation of bipolar disorder in the general population). Thus, the evidence for transmission of bipolar disorder among probands with major depressive disorder is weak and may be an artifact of differences in control samples.

In contrast, rates of major depressive disorder are significantly greater among the relatives of patients with the disorder compared with relatives of controls. There is an average twofold increase in the risk of major depressive disorder among the relatives of patients with that condition, thereby suggesting some degree of specificity of transmission of both bipolar disorder and major depressive disorder in families.

Factors associated with familial transmission of affective disorders The transmission of mood disorders may vary according to polarity, degree of relationship to the proband, age of onset of disorder in the proband, and the sex of the proband and of the relative. Many of the family studies cited have explored the relationship between the proband characteristics and those in their relatives.

RELATIONSHIP TO THE PROBAND Numerous studies have presented the rates of mood disorders among both the first- and second-degree relatives of mood disorder probands. According

TABLE 16.4-2
Controlled Family Studies of Bipolar Probands

Author and Year	Status	Number of Relatives	% Bipolar Disorder in Relatives	Relative Risk	% Major Depressive Disorder in Relatives	Relative Risk
Gershon et al 1975	Cases	341	3.8	17.5	6.8	9.7
	Controls	518	0.2		0.7	
Tsuang et al 1980	Cases	100	5.3	17.7	12.4	1.7
	Controls	160	0.3		7.5	
Winokur and Crowe 1983	Cases	196	1.5	5.0	12.8	1.8
	Controls	344	0.3		7.3	
Gershon et al 1982	Cases	401	4.6	—	14.0	2.4
	Controls	217	0		5.8	
Maier et al 1991	Cases	389	4.4	3.7	11.1	1.6
	Controls	419	1.2		6.9	

Data compiled from Taylor M A, Berenbaum S A, Jampala V C, Cloninger C R: Are schizophrenia and affective disorder related? Preliminary data from a family study. Am J Psychiatry *150:* 278, 1993; Maier W, Lichtermann D, Minges J, Hallmeyer J, Heun R, Benkert O, Levinson D F: Continuity and discontinuity of affective disorders and Schizophrenia. Results of a controlled family study. Arch Gen Psychiatry *150:* 871, 1993.

TABLE 16.4-3
Controlled Family Studies of Probands with Major Depressive Disorder

Author and Year	Status	Number of Relatives	% Bipolar Disorder in Relatives	Relative Risk	% Major Depressive Disorder	Relative Risk
Gershon et al	Cases	96	2.1	10.5	11.5	18.9
1975	Controls	518	0.2		0.7	
Tsuang et al	Cases	225	2.2	11.0	11.0	2.0
1980	Controls	160	0.2		4.8	
Gershon et al	Cases	112	1.5	—	12.8	2.9
1982	Controls	217	—		5.8	
Weissman et al	Cases	133	2.3	1.4	14.9	3.1
1982	Controls	82	1.6		5.6	
Winokur and Crowe	Cases	305	1.0	3.3	11.2	1.5
1983	Controls	344	0.3		7.3	
Maier et al	Cases	221	1.4	1.2	11.3	1.6
1991	Controls	419	1.2		6.9	

Data compiled from Taylor M A, Berenbaum S A, Jampala V C, Cloninger C R: Are schizophrenia and affective disorder related? Preliminary data from a family study. Am J Psychiatry *150:* 278, 1993; Maier W, Lichtermann D, Minges J, Hallmeyer J, Heun R, Benkert O, Levinson D F: Continuity and discontinuity of affective disorders and schizophrenia. Results of a controlled family study. Arch Gen Psychiatry *150:* 871, 1993.

to expectations of traditional genetic models, risks to all classes of first-degree relatives should be equal for dominant traits, whereas siblings should have increased rates of disorders for recessive traits. The aggregate data for bipolar disorder reveal that the risk of bipolar disorder among parents and siblings are approximately equal for both bipolar and major depressive disorder. However, the offspring tend to have elevated rates of bipolar disorder and equal rates of major depressive disorder when compared with parents and siblings. In the absence of control data, it is difficult to interpret the latter finding. However, the elevation in the risk among offspring could result from comorbidity, recall bias, a cohort effect, or assortative mating in the parental generation.

Most genetic models predict a decrement in risk of disease according to the degree of relationship to the affected proband. Although a large number of studies have reported rates of mood disorder among both the first- and second-degree relatives, there is only a single controlled study in which the rates of mood disorders were compared between the first- and second-degree relatives and with controls. The results of that study revealed that the rates of bipolar disorder among first-degree relatives of bipolar probands were approximately twice those of second-degree relatives, which in turn were greater than those of controls. In contrast there was no elevation in the rates of either major depressive or bipolar disorder among the second-degree relatives of major depressive disorder probands, nor was there an increased rate of major depressive disorder among the second-degree relatives of bipolar probands.

AGE OF ONSET The effect of age of onset on the familial aggregation of mood disorders was first described by Stenstedt and was subsequently confirmed in several studies. However, numerous possible confounding factors have not been adequately addressed in those studies including: recurrence, comorbidity, biased recall, and personality factors. Moreover, the conclusions of the studies have been based on a dichotomous classification of the age of onset of probands, rather than on significant correlations between the age of onset of probands and relatives.

SEX OF PROBAND The effect of the sex of the proband and relative has been systematically investigated for both bipolar and major depressive disorder. In general there is little deviation in family study data from the sex ratio for bipolar disorder and major depressive disorder reported in epidemiological studies. The rates of occurrence of bipolar disorder are nearly equal in male and female relatives, whereas there is a female preponderance of mood disorders among the relatives with major depressive disorder. However, the transmission of both bipolar disorder and major depressive disorder has been shown to be unrelated to the sex of the proband, with equal rates of mood disorders among the relatives of male and female bipolar disorder and major depressive disorder probands.

In summary the family studies of bipolar disorder and major depressive disorder demonstrate a strong degree of familial aggregation of both mood disorders. However, the evidence is inconclusive regarding the role of shared underlying factors in the expression of the disorders. The transmission of mood disorders appears to be associated with an early age of onset of mood disorder in probands, bipolar disorder, and major depressive disorder with recurrent episodes, but not with the sex of the proband.

MODES OF TRANSMISSION OF MOOD DISORDERS No single mode of transmission of either bipolar disorder or major depressive disorder has been consistently reported. Of the more than 25 segregation and pedigree analyses of patterns of familial transmission of the mood disorders, few studies have reported an adequate fit of the observed familial transmission data to the predictions of most of the traditional genetic models. The threshold models have been found to provide the best fit to the data, with two threshold models for polarity, or two for sex, being the most consistently nonrejected hypotheses. Bipolar disorder is the only mood disorder for which there is an approximately 50 percent decrement in the risk of depression by the degree of relationship to the proband. However, the average recurrence risk of bipolar disorder in first-degree relatives (five percent to 10 percent) is far lower than the 50 percent risk predicted by single major genes with high penetrance as a causative factor. In a 1982 review of the aggregate data on the transmission of bipolar disorder Risch and Baron concluded that the data did not deviate from the expectations of X-linked transmission recessive inheritance because of the low frequency of father-to-son transmission and because the sex ratio seems equal. However, a recent review of the X-linkage studies of bipolar disorder revealed that few of the pedigrees exhibited the hallmarks of X-linked transmission for segregation: that is, a lack of occurrence in offspring of affected males. Moreover, several of the pedigrees used to analyze X-linkage include instances of possible male-to-male transmission.

TWIN STUDIES OF MOOD DISORDERS Numerous studies have compared the rates of mood disorders among monozygotic and dizygotic twins. The majority of the earlier studies selected probands from inpatient settings or treatment registries. Table 16.4-4 reviews data on the twin studies of probands with bipolar and major depressive disorder in which there were at least 15 twin pairs. The average concordance for mood disorders among monozygotic twins was 60 percent and that for dizygotic twins was 12 percent. There is a fivefold greater rate of concordance for mood disorders among monozygotic than dizygotic twins, thereby indicating the importance of the role of genetic factors in the familial aggregation of bipolar disorder.

There are two recent twin studies of major depressive disorder defined according to criteria of the third edition of *Diagnostic and Statistical Manual of Mental Disorders* (DSM-III) or the revised third edition of DSM (DSM-III-R). The evidence for the role of genes in the cause of major depressive disorder is much weaker than for a genetic role in bipolar disorder. The relative risks, comparing monozygotic and dizygotic twins in the two studies, were 1.9 and 1.2, respectively. Nevertheless, the application of quantitative models that estimate the relative components of the variance attributable to shared genes, common environment, or unique nonshared environment yielded significant degrees of heritability in both studies (.39 in the former and .84 in the latter). Differences in the results of the two studies could be attributable to difference in sampling (hospitalized patients were included in the study by McGuffin and colleagues; only women from the general population were included in the study by Kendler and colleagues) or to other methodological differences.

Early studies of the specificity of transmission of polarity in twin studies were reviewed by Edith Zerbin-Rüdin in 1969. The largest twin study that systematically investigated differences in concordance among bipolar and unipolar twins was presented by A. Bertelsen and colleagues in 1977. Table 16.4-5 presents a summary of the studies that examined the concordance rates among twins by polarity. The data provide support for a strong degree of specificity of transmission of the two mood disorders, with little cross-transmission between bipolar disorder index twins with major depressive disorder cotwins, and the converse. The average relative risk for cross-transmission for probands with either depressive or bipolar disorder was 1.5. In contrast, bipolar disorder was found to exhibit a strong degree of specificity, with an eightfold greater risk of bipolar disorder occurring among the cotwins of bipolar monozygotic probands compared with occurrence in their dizygotic counterparts.

The major conclusion that can be drawn from the current evidence from twin studies is that mood disorders are strongly heritable, with bipolar disorder exhibiting a much greater degree of involvement of genetic factors in its etiology than major depressive disorders. Moreover, there is little evidence for the cross-transmission of the two mood disorders. One study calculated the aggregate variance components from the twin studies of major depressive disorder then available and found a significant degree of heritability (.51), a significant contribution of the common environment of the twins (variance, .42), and nearly no effect of the unique environment in the development of mood disorders. Twin studies of milder mood disorders are difficult to interpret because of differences in diagnostic definitions and inconsistent application of the criterion of hospitalization for mood status.

ADOPTION STUDIES OF MOOD DISORDERS Adoption studies are the most powerful design to test the relative contributions of genetic and environmental factors to the causation of the mood disorders. The small number of adoption studies regarding mood disorders is surprising if one considers the rich adoption data on schizophrenia. Of the four adoption studies of mood disorders, three examined the rates of disorders in the biological and adoptive parents of affected and nonaffected adoptees, and only one had bipolar disorder subjects. Two of the three studies yielded strong evidence for transmission of mood disorder after adoption irrespective of the degree of exposure to the biological affected parent (Table 16.4-6). The study by Julien Mendlewicz and John Rainer in 1977 examined both bipolar disorder adoptees and bipolar disorder nonadoptees to control for the factors associated with adoption that may bias

TABLE 16.4-4
Studies of Mood Disorders in Twins*

Author and Year	Monozygotic No.	Monozygotic % Concordance	Dizygotic No.	Dizygotic % Concordance	Relative risk
Bipolar Disorder					
Rosanoff et al (1935)	23	70	67	16	4.4
Kallman (1953)	27	93	55	24	3.9
Harvald and Hauge (1965)	15	67	40	5	13.4
Allen et al (1974)	15	33	34	0	—
Bertelsen et al (1977)	55	51	11	14	3.6
Major Depression					
McGuffin et al (1991)†	62	53	79	28	1.9
Kendler et al (1992)†‡	590	48	440	42	1.2

*Studies with ≥ 15 twin pairs.
†Women only.
‡DSM-III-R criteria.

TABLE 16.4-5
Specificity of Twin Concordance Rates by Polarity

Index Twin	Co-Twin	Monozygotic No.	Monozygotic % Concordance	Dizygotic No.	Dizygotic % Concordance	Relative Risk
Bipolar	Bipolar	42	39	4	5	7.8
	Unipolar	13	12	7	9	1.3
Unipolar	Bipolar	4	11	1	6	1.8
	Unipolar	15	43	3	18	2.4

Data compiled from Zerbin-Rüdin E: Zur genetik der depressiven erkrankurnen. In *Das depressive Syndrom,* H Hippius, H Selbach, editors, p 37. Urban and Schwarzenberg, Berlin, 1969; Bertelsen A, Harvald B, Hauge M: A Danish twin study of manic-depressive disorder. Br J Psychiatry *130:* 330, 1977.

TABLE 16.4-6
Adoption Studies of Mood Disorder

Author and Year	Study Population	% Mood Disorder in Parents: Biologic	% Mood Disorder in Parents: Adoptive
Mendlewicz and Rainer 1977	29 bipolar disorder adoptees	31	12
	31 bipolar disorder nonadoptees	26	—
	22 normal adoptees	2	10
Von Knorring et al 1983	56 adoptees	5	3
	115 controls	5	—
Wender et al 1986	71 adoptees	29	6
	75 controls	5	4

the results. The study reported nearly identical rates of mood disorders among the biological parents of the bipolar adoptees and nonadoptees: 31 percent and 26 percent, respectively. That indicates that the adoptees do not comprise a biased sample with respect to the development of mood disorders. The rate of depression among the biological parents of the control adoptees was only 2 percent, nearly 15 times less than the rates reported among the parents of bipolar disorder subjects.

Paul Wender and associates in 1986 reported the results of a similar adoption study of bipolar adoptees compared with control adoptees. In accordance with the results of Mendlewicz and Rainer, Wender found that whereas 29 percent of the adoptees of biological parents with mood disorder developed mood disorders themselves, only 5 percent of the parents of control adoptees reported mood disorders. Rates of mood disorders in the adoptive parents were also low: 6 percent and 4 percent, respectively. Therefore both studies provide strong evidence of the role of genetic factors in the pathogenesis of mood disorders. The only exception to the positive adoption studies was the 1983 study of Anne-Liis Von Knorring and colleagues, which revealed no evidence of transmission of mood disorders among parents with the condition and their adopted offspring.

Only a single study (Table 16.4-7) employed the adoption study paradigm in which the rates of disorders among the adopted offspring of biological parents with and without mood disorders were investigated. The number of cases was small. The study showed that major depressive disorder among adoptees was positively, but not significantly, associated with a biological background of major depressive disorder. Instead, several environmental factors in the adoptive home, such as death of an adoptive parent before the child reached age 19, or the presence of a behavioral disturbance in a member of the adoptive family, seemed to be related to a predisposition to depression in the adoptee. Nevertheless, the data provide preliminary support for a moderate role of genetic factors in the cause of mood disorders.

The aggregate data from adoption studies of mood disorders clearly indicate that genetic factors are involved in the causation of mood disorders, but that the moderate degree of concordance between biological parents and their adopted-out offspring suggest that common environmental factors also contribute to the expression of mood disorders.

STUDIES OF GENETIC MARKERS

ASSOCIATION STUDIES OF MOOD DISORDERS

Methods The search for markers for the mood disorders has been under way for nearly 40 years. A trait must meet the following criteria in order to be constituted a biologic marker: (1) it should be associated with an increased risk of illness; (2) it should be observable during phases of illness or recovery; and (3) it should be shown to be independent of treatment. Genetic markers are a specific class of biological markers that exhibit clear mendelian modes of inheritance, may be assigned or are assignable to a specific chromosomal location, and are polymorphic, with at least two alleles with a gene frequency of at least 1 percent.

TABLE 16.4-7
Percentage of Mood Disorders in Adopted Offspring by Parental Diagnostic Status

Adoptive Parent	Number	% Mood Disorder in Adoptees
Mood disorders	8	38
Other psychiatric disorders	75	5
Controls	43	9

Data compiled from Cadoret R J, O'Gorman T W, Heywood E, Troughton E: Genetic and environmental factors in major depression. J Affective Disord 9: 155, 1985.

Association studies investigate the relationship between disease status and a particular marker or allele across families and individuals. Most association studies employ the traditional case-control design in which the prevalence of a putative disease marker is compared among persons with a disorder and persons without the disorder. The most common methodological error in association studies is the lack of equivalence between the cases and controls on factors that may confound the association between the purported marker and disease.

After exclusion of spurious associations resulting from methodological factors or population stratification, associations between a disease and a marker could be attributed to either linkage disequilibrium between genes for the disease and for the marker, or the effect of a single gene that encodes both the marker and the disease.

The loci for several biochemical parameters that are suspected to be involved in either the cause or outcome of psychiatric disorders have been identified. However, many of those assignments are based on a single study, and replication is clearly necessary. Identification of new loci is occurring at such a rapid rate that it is necessary to update the human map monthly. It is estimated that more than 10,000 gene loci will have been assigned to particular sites on chromosomes by the year 2000. Application of the methodology to investigations of psychiatric disorders may be particularly fruitful in identifying major genes that are segregating in informative families.

Review of evidence: association studies There have been numerous studies of associations between biological markers and mood disorders. In the past the general approach was to study the relationship between the expression of a known genetic factor at a particular locus and disease status among probands, their relatives, and the general population. The most commonly studied genetic traits have been the human erythrocyte blood groups (ABO), the human leukocyte antigens (HLA), and the enzyme monoamine oxidase (MAO). The results of association studies regarding mood disorders have been inconsistent. There are no markers for which significant associations have been found in more than a handful of studies.

The association between MAO and all of the major psychiatric disorders has been widely studied. Two major forms of MAO have been studied in human populations: MAO_A, in plasma, and MAO_B, in platelets, with varying proportions in most tissues. Low levels of plasma MAO have been reported for major depressive disorder and bipolar disorder. The lack of specificity for a particular disorder suggests that the enzyme cannot be used to identify susceptibility to a specific disorder. Rather, it may be a nonspecific response to dysregulation of another neurochemical system. Furthermore, there may be little or no relationship between the activity of MAO in brain and the periphery of humans, because of the possibility of the involvement of different genes, or differential regulation in the central nervous system than in the periphery. This principle may also apply to other neurotransmitters, neuromodulators, hormones, and enzymes as well. That underscores the importance of including subjects with other psychiatric illnesses as controls, in addition to mood disorder controls, when studying associations between markers and a particular psychiatric disorder. A recent review of biological markers for depression concluded that the most promising candidate biological markers are rapid-eye-movement sleep, cation transport, and blunted growth hormone response to clonidine.

In contrast to earlier studies, which relied on the expression of inferred underlying genetic mechanisms, it is now possible to apply the techniques of molecular biology to study biological markers in psychiatry. Several recent studies have investigated the association between bipolar disorder and specific DNA markers including tyramine hydroxylase gene on chromosome 11p4 and the dopamine receptor genes on chromosome 5q as shown in Table 16.4-8. Lionel C. C. Lim and associates recently reported confirmation of earlier associations between MAO_A activity and bipolar disorder using DNA polymorphisms. A study of the association between bipolar disorder and the dopamine type 1 (D_1) receptor gene on chromosome 5q and the dopamine type 2 (D_2) receptor gene on chromosome 11q revealed no significant difference in the proportion of cases and controls with specific alleles of the D_1 and D_2 receptor genes. Although one study reported an association between bipolar disorder and the tyramine hydroxylase gene and on chromosome 11p, numerous other studies have failed to replicate the finding. Likewise, studies of other markers yielded no significant association with bipolar mood disorder.

Despite the inconsistent findings of the association studies conducted thus far, the study paradigm comprises an important strategy for identifying genes that may be involved in the cause of the mood disorders. A 1991 study noted that the application of molecular genetic techniques to association studies of depression could actually yield more information than linkage studies regarding the specific functions of genetic abnormalities that contribute to the cause of depression. Moreover, studies of the molecular mechanisms of state markers could yield valid information on the cause of particular symptoms.

LINKAGE STUDIES OF MOOD DISORDERS

Methods Linkage is based on the principle that two genes that lie in close proximity on a chromosome are transmitted to their progeny together. However, if the loci are far apart, crossing-over between the maternal and paternal chromosomes may take place during meiosis, thereby producing new combinations of alleles. The farther apart the loci, the greater the probability that crossing-over will occur and that the offspring may inherit a recombinant of the two parental chromosomes. Crossovers can be detected by inspection of the maternal and paternal genome; when a particular chromosome is not identical to the parental chromosome, a crossover or recombination between the maternal and paternal chromosomes has occurred.

Linkage studies differ from association studies in that linkage is based on an association between genetic markers and putative disease genes within families, whereas association is the co-occurrence of a marker and disease at the level of the general population. Linkage does not imply that the adjacent gene is etiologically related to the disease, only that it can be used to track possible genes in families. Therefore, one allele at a particular locus may be linked to a disease in some families, whereas the other allele may cosegregate with the same disease in other families. In contrast, associations are detected in case-control studies that compare the prevalence of a marker in patients with a particular illness with the proportion of control subjects who possess the marker. Thus, an association found in patient samples may not extend to their families. For example, a strong association between HLA-DR2 and HLA-DQw1 antigens and narcolepsy has been found in 90 percent of patients with narcolepsy compared with 20 to 35 percent of the general population; however, those markers may not cosegregate with narcolepsy in their families.

TABLE 16.4-8
Association Studies of Bipolar Disorder and DNA Markers

Author and Year	Marker	Association
Todd and O'Malley (1989)	Tyramine hydroxylase	No
Korner et al (1990)	Tyramine hydroxylase	No
Leboyer et al (1990)	Tyramine hydroxylase	Yes
Nöthen et al (1990)	Tyramine hydroxylase	No
Nöthen et al (1992)	Dopamine (D_1) 5q	No
	Dopamine (D_2) 11q	No
Inayama et al (1993)	Tyramine hydroxylase	No
Lim et al (1994)	Monoamine oxidase-A	Yes

Two major methods of genetic linkage analysis are the LOD score method and the sib-pair method, derived from Penrose. The LOD score is defined as the ratio of the logarithmic odds of the likelihood of a linkage between two loci within a pedigree to that of the likelihood of independent segregation of the two loci, or a recombination frequency of 0.5. A LOD score $> +3$ represents a probability of .001 of falsely concluding that linkage exists when it is absent, and a LOD score < -2 indicates significant evidence for a lack of linkage between the putative marker and disease. Scientific evidence for acceptance of linkage between a disease and genetic marker was described by Neil Risch, who stated that in addition to a LOD score $> +3$, a linkage finding should be replicated in a different sample in a different laboratory.

The mood disorder sib-pair method examines the sharing of marker alleles at a locus among affected sibling pairs. The null hypothesis of no linkage specifies probabilities of one quarter, one half, and one quarter for sharing 2, 1, and 0 marker alleles among mood disorder sibling. Excess sharing of two haplotypes (or conversely, diminished sharing of haplotypes) provides evidence for linkage. The sib-pair method is a powerful design if the gene is rare and requires no assumption regarding the mode of inheritance of the disorder.

Although previous linkage studies were hampered by the limited number of known polymorphic markers, recent advances in molecular genetics have resulted in the identification of markers across the human genome. Those markers, restriction fragment length polymorphisms (RFLPs), have enabled geneticists to identify disease loci for several major diseases, with Huntington's disease and cystic fibrosis being dramatic examples.

Designs of linkage studies Linkage studies of psychiatric disorders involve interdisciplinary collaboration and are labor intensive. The studies are comprised of three major components, as illustrated in Figure 16.4-1. Clinical psychiatry is involved in defining the phenotype, in diagnoses in probands and relatives, and in the collection of information on families of affected and unaffected probands. The genetic epidemiology component is engaged in study design, determining the optimal sampling procedures both within and between families, defining the population parameters, and conducting statistical analyses of the data. The role of the molecular geneticist is the definition of the genotypes through application of the methods of molecular biology.

In 1988 a workshop on "Linkage and Clinical Features in Affective Disorders" was organized and supported by the MacArthur Foundation, Mental Health Research Network I on the Psychobiology of Depression, in order to review the status and methodology of the linkage studies of mood disorders available at that time. The group examined the comparability of studies in the published literature, identified the major features of mood disorders that were hampering linkage studies, and identified

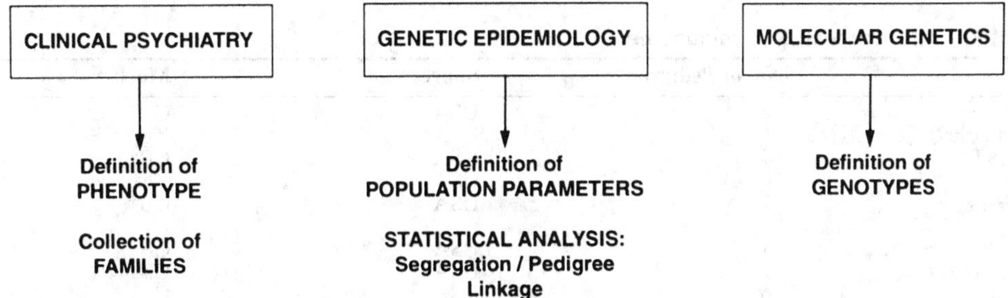

FIGURE 16.4-1 *Major components of linkage studies.*

several key analytical questions regarding mood disorders that needed to be studied thoroughly. The recommendations regarding standards for linkage studies of psychiatric disorders are summarized in Table 16.4-9. Another Task Force was subsequently convened to investigate the specific analytical issues through simulation and theoretical studies. A summary report of the results and recommendations of that group has recently been published.

ETHICAL ISSUES As in any family study of psychiatric disorders, ethical issues apply to genetic linkage studies as well. However, the complexity of the goals and findings of linkage studies require more thoughtful explanations than those of family studies. The results of linkage studies could be easily misinterpreted by the lay audience as implying that the gene that causes bipolar disorder will be identified in specific families. Whereas the sample in family studies usually consists of a large number of nuclear families, linkage studies are often limited to a few large families. Confidentiality is critical and must be maintained, particularly in linkage studies of extended pedigrees that may possess identifying characteristics.

A recent review of the ethical issues in linkage studies enumerates and discusses the following issues in genetic linkage studies: protecting the privacy of the proband in the ascertainment process; opposition by one relative to contact another; specific problems associated with informed consent; and therapeutic intervention. Those are best avoided by the use of experienced clinical interviewers who can explain the specific implications of the study and the importance of the cooperation of as many relatives as possible. Rather than completing a diagnostic evaluation, drawing blood, and thanking the subjects, the investigator should include resources necessary to assist the family members in need of treatment or facilitate contact with mental health professionals, provide results of the individual diagnostic evaluations to treatment professions (on request of the subjects), and supply a personally written letter to convey the results of the study findings to the subjects at their request. Such interaction enhances the relationship between subjects and research staff.

TABLE 16.4-9
Recommended Standards for Linkage Studies*

Advance specification of specific phenotypic definitions
Clear description of ascertainment strategies of probands and relatives
Systematic assessment of both paternal and maternal lines of the pedigree
Collection of extensive clinical information on all members of pedigree
Application of consistent diagnostic criteria, instrumentation, and procedures across studies
Maintenance of blindness to marker and diagnostic status of probands and relatives
Inclusion of sufficient information on methods in publication to allow replicability
Use of longitudinal study designs to validate diagnoses

*Modification of Recommendations of Task Force on Linkage Studies of Affective Disorders Sponsored by MacArthur Foundation Network I on the Psychobiology of Depression and Other Affective Disorders. Arch Gen Psychiatry *46:* 1137, 1989.

TABLE 16.4-10
Sibling Pair Linkage Studies of Mood Disorders: HLA

Author and Year	No. of Pairs	Source	LOD Score
Smeraldi et al (1978)	26	Italy	*
Targum et al (1979)	9	USA	NS†
Smeraldi and Bellodi (1981)	26	Italy	NS
Suarez and Croughan (1982)	26	USA	NS
Kruger et al (1982)	2	USA	‡
Goldin et al (1982)	18	USA	§
Weitkamp et al (1981)	21	USA	NS
Kidd et al (1984)	59	USA	§
Suarez and Reich (1984)	15	USA	§

*> +2
†NS indicates not significant.
‡> +3
§< −2

Review of evidence

The sib-pair method has been applied extensively to investigate the association between HLA haplotypes and mood disorders (Table 16.4-10). The majority of studies do not provide support for linkage between HLA markers and mood disorder. Only two studies yielded significant findings for a positive association, whereas eight other studies concluded that there was either no association or a negative association between mood disorder and HLA. Despite the negative findings to date, the use of DNA markers as candidate genes in association studies may yield information of the involvement of specific genes in mood disorders. In general, however, the power of association studies is lower than that of linkage studies.

Linkage studies of pedigrees of probands with mood disorder have focused on X-chromosome markers and those on the short arm of chromosome 11 (Tables 16.4-11 and 16.4-12). Linkage studies of mood disorders and X-chromosome markers were first reported 20 years ago by Theodore Reich and colleagues, who found significant LOD scores between color blindness and affective disorders in two large pedigrees. Subsequent attempts to replicate that finding yielded contradictory evidence; of a total of 10 additional studies of color blindness, Mendlewicz and colleagues and Baron and colleagues confirmed the finding of linkage between color blindness and mood disorders in a total of 28 families. However, subsequent studies of a subset of the same families using DNA markers failed to confirm it. Other X-chromosome markers for which linkage with affective disorders was investigated were the Xg blood group, factor IX,

TABLE 16.4-11
Linkage Studies of Bipolar Disorders: X Chromosome

Author and Year	No. of Pedigrees	Source	Marker	LOD Score*
Reich et al (1969)	2	USA	CB†	‖
Winokur and Tanna (1969)	6	USA	Xg‡	NS
Mendlewicz et al (1972)	7	USA	CB†	‖
Fieve et al (1973)	4	USA	Xg‡	NS
Mendlewicz and Fleiss (1974)	7	USA	CB†	¶
Baron (1977)	1	USA	CB†	‖
Johnson and Leeman (1977)	2	USA	CB†	NS
Gershon et al (1979)	6	USA	CB†	#
Mendlewicz et al (1979)	8	Belgium	CB†	‖
Gershon et al (1980)	16	Europe, USA	CB†	NS
Mendlewicz et al (1980)	1	Belgium (Iranian)	G6PD	¶
Del Zompo et al (1984)	2	Sardinia	G6PD	NS
Kidd et al (1984)	4	USA	CB†	NS
			Xg‡	NS
Mendlewicz et al (1987)	10	Belgium	Factor IX	¶
Baron et al (1987)	5	Israel	G6PD	¶
			CB†	#
Berrettini et al (1990)	9	USA	Xg28	#
Neiswanger et al (1990)§	3	USA	Dxδ52	#
Gejman et al (1990)	1	USA	—	#
Nanko et al (1991)	2	Japan	Xq	NS
Gill et al (1992)	1	United Kingdom	F9	NS
Lucotte et al (1992)	1	France	F9	¶
Curtis et al (1993)	5	Iceland	DBH	#
Bredbacka et al (1993)	1	Finland	F9	#
			DXS548	
Baron et al (1993)	3	Israel	Xq28	#

*Significance of LOD score at $\theta = .05$. NS indicates not significant.
†Color blindness.
‡Xg blood group.
§Major depressive disorder.
¶> +3.
‖> +2.
#< −2.

G6PD, dopamine β hydroxylase (DBH) and an RFLP marker Xq28. As shown in Table 16.4-11, most of the studies yielded negative results.

The dramatic announcement of linkage between bipolar disorder and the Harvey-*ras* oncogene on the short arm of chromosome 11 in the Amish spurred the current generation of linkage studies of schizophrenia and mood disorders. As shown in Table 16.4-12, all subsequent attempts have failed to replicate the original finding, including reanalyses of the original pedigree with follow-up data and additional extensions of the pedigree. Another recent study of the D_2 receptor gene on chromosome 11 in five Icelandic pedigrees also failed to yield evidence for linkage.

In summary, linkage studies of mood disorder based on inferred expression of an underlying gene through investigation of the phenotype do not consistently support linkage between mood disorders and any genetic marker. A possible exception is the observation of linkage between bipolar illness and loci on the long arm of the X chromosome. Although that too has been controversial, Neil Risch and Miron Baron in 1982 reanalyzed the published studies on X-linkage in bipolar disorder and confirmed that there was a subset of pedigrees in which there was cosegregation for the color-blindness and G6PD loci on the X chromosome and bipolar disorder. Those studies have nearly exclusively focused on probands with bipolar disorder because of the strength of evidence regarding the genetic etiology of the condition. Subsequent attempts to investigate major depressive disorder have also failed to yield evidence for linkage.

CHROMOSOMAL ABERRATIONS The focus on linkage and association studies of psychiatric disorders has led to a relative neglect of studies of possible chromosomal abnormalities that may play a role in their causation (Table 16.4-13). Cytogenetic abnormalities may be of critical importance for identifying regions in which to begin genome searches for linkage and association studies. Stimulated by Ann Bassett's work on chromosomal aberrations in schizophrenia, several investigations have conducted cytogenic studies of bipolar disorder patients. A recent review of that work identified four genomic regions of potential interest including chromosome 11q 21-25, 15q 11-13, 21q, and Xq 28 based on the results of 28 published chromosomal studies of bipolar disorder.

COMPLEXITY OF MOOD DISORDERS

FACTORS INVOLVED IN COMPLEXITY With the aggregate evidence overwhelmingly indicating the involvement of genetic factors in the causation of the mood disorders, why is so little known about their specific role, the magnitude of their contribution, and the mechanisms through which they exert their influence? Moreover, why are the results of the linkage and association so inconclusive?

There are several critical differences between mood disorders and the disorders to which the molecular biologists' tools have been successfully applied. Linkage has been reported for diseases that are extremely rare (<.01 percent population prevalence); exhibit mendelian patterns of inheritance, and are clearly diagnosed with extremely high specificity and sensitivity.

In contrast, the mood disorders are complex disorders, defined as conditions characterized by high population prevalence, a lack of clear distinction between affected and unaf-

TABLE 16.4-12
Linkage Studies of Bipolar Disorders: Chromosome 11

Author and Year	No. of Pedigrees	Source	Marker*	LOD Score†
Egeland et al (1987)	1	USA (Amish)	HRAS INS	§
Hodgkinson et al (1987)	3	Iceland	HRAS	‖
Detera-Wadleigh et al (1987)	3	USA	HRAS	‖
Gill et al (1988)	1	Ireland	HRAS	NS
Kelsoe et al (1989)	1	USA (Amish)	HRAS INS	NS
Neiswanger et al (1990)†	3	USA	HRAS INS	‖
Mitchell et al (1991)	2	Australia	TH HRAS INS	NS
Mendlewicz et al (1991)	1	Belgium	TH HRAS INS	NS
Holmes et al (1991)	5	Iceland	DRD2 TH	‖
Nanko et al (1991)	2	Japan	INS HRAS	NS NS
Mendlewicz et al (1991)	1	Belgium	INS HRAS	‖
Law et al (1992)	1	Amish	INS HRAS	‖ ‖
Byerley et al (1992)	8	USA	TH	‖
Mitchell et al (1992)	2	Australia	DRD2	‖
Curtis et al (1993)	5	Iceland	TH DRD2	‖ ‖
Kelsoe et al (1993)	3 1	Iceland (Amish)	D2 D11S21	‖ NS
Gurling et al (1993)	6	UK	TH DRD4	NS
Lim et al (1993)	6	Iceland	TH DRD4	NS ‖
Debruyn et al (1994)	14	Belgium	DRD4 TH TYR DRD2 HRAS INS	‖ ‖ ‖ ‖ ‖ ‖

*HRAS indicates Harvey-*ras* oncogene; INS, insulin gene; TH, tyrosine hydroxylase; DRD2 (4), dopamine receptor gene; TYR, tyrosinase; +, nonbipolar major depression.
†Significance of LOD score at $\theta = .05$. NS indicates not significant.
§> +3
‖< −2

TABLE 16.4-13
Linkage Studies of Mood Disorders: Other Loci

Author and Year	No. of Pedigrees	Source	Chromosome	LOD* Score
Detera-Wadleigh et al (1992)	14	USA	5q	†
Mitchell et al (1993)	9	Australia	3q13	†
(1992)	2	Australia	5q (DRD1)	†
Eiberg et al (1993)	2	Denmark	16p13	‡
Curtis et al (1993)	5	Iceland	8q 5q 9q	† † †
Coon et al (1993)	8	USA	5q	†

*Significance of LOD score at $\theta = .05$.
†< −2.
‡> +2.

fected (with the threshold for case definition being somewhat arbitrary), and failure to adhere to mendelian patterns of transmission. The high frequency of the mood disorders in the general population complicate analyses of familial aggregation and patterns of transmission. Even bipolar disorder, which is believed to be a rare condition, is considered to be common by geneticists, who generally deal with conditions with prevalence rates that are 10 to 100 times less frequent than 1 percent. The high prevalence of the conditions in a population increases the probability that family members of both patients and controls will exhibit mood disorders by chance, thereby making it more difficult to discriminate between true cases and phenocopies (that is, persons who express the disease but do not possess the underlying genetic factors).

Despite the inclusion of bipolar disorder as an X-linked disorder (#30920) in the catalogue of *Mendelian Inheritance in Man,* the aggregate evidence from segregation analyses does not consistently reveal evidence favoring any specific mendelian pattern of transmission over another. Nevertheless, convergent evidence suggests that the mood disorders, and bipolar disorder in particular, are familial, with genetic factors playing at least some role in the familial aggregation of the condition.

Other major features of mood disorders that complicate genetic analyses are (1) lack of valid definition(s) of the phenotype and subtypes; (2) heterogeneity of expression of symptoms, (that is, variable underlying syndromes); (3) nonrandom mating patterns among persons with mood disorders, in which probands with affective disorders are more likely to have a spouse with a mood disorder than predicted by population expectations; (4) co-occurrence of other major psychiatric disorders, including primary anxiety disorders, and substance abuse; and (5) lack of evidence for a specific mode of transmission.

METHODS FOR INVESTIGATING COMPLEX DISORDERS

Such methods are critical not only to the identification of genes, but also to all of the research domains that purport to examine the pathways between the genotype and phenotype, such as neurobiologic, imaging, psychophysiology, or challenge strategies, which may be examining as many disease subtypes as patients. The basic approach of genetic epidemiology is the use of the within-family design to minimize the probability of heterogeneity, assuming that the cause of a disease is likely to be homotypic within families. This design reduces or eliminates the danger of genetic heterogeneity that is likely to characterize the mood disorders.

A recent study, in which the results of complex segregation analyses were consistent with a single recessive gene for attending medical school, serves as a reminder of the dangers of overeager acceptance of simple explanations of the transmission of complex phenotypes. The study concluded that the application of segregation or linkage analysis are not a panacea for the problems of complex phenotypes and that the formulation of genetic studies must be developed in the context of information gleaned from the application of classical methods of genetic epidemiology including family, twin, and adoption studies.

IMPLICATIONS OF GENETIC EPIDEMIOLOGIC STUDIES IN PSYCHIATRY

A summary of the clinical and research applications of linkage studies in psychiatry is presented in Table 16.4-14.

TABLE 16.4-14
Application of Linkage Studies in Psychiatry

Identification of aberrant expression or regulation of a gene
Genetic counseling
Identification of subtypes of disorders
Understanding effects of neuropsychopharmacology
Identification of the role of environmental factors

CLINICAL IMPLICATIONS Inquiry regarding the family history is an important component of a thorough clinical evaluation of a patient. Because of the high proportion of false-negative rates in family history studies, information from knowledgeable informants is the best way to enhance the quality of family history data. Several studies have shown that proper collection of family history requires inquiry about each of the first-degree relatives individually, and specific patterns of symptoms and longitudinal course should also be elicited, rather than a global history of the presence or absence of mood disorder.

Because mood disorders are not genetically lethal or associated with a strong increase in mortality, genetic counseling is rarely appropriate for the condition. However, patients may sometimes seek advice regarding the risk of depression in their offspring. In the absence of any genetic or trait markers for depression, such advice should be based on the aggregate data on the familial transmission of depression. Risk estimates should be based on a combination of the age, sex, family history, and risk factors for mood disorders in the individual. Because the mode of transmission of the mood disorders is not known, genetic counseling of couples-at-risk now involves specification of the empirical recurrence risks that have been derived from previous studies of the familial transmission of the disorder. The empirical recurrence risk should be refined according to the family's or individual's sociodemographic characteristics such as age, sex, socioeconomic status, and ethnicity, and the consultant's clinical characteristics including age-at-onset, comorbidity, severity of illness, illness in the coparent, and other factors that may be related to transmission of the disorder. It is also important to consider patterns of transmission in previous generations of the pedigree in estimating recurrence risks.

Approximate empirical recurrence risks for mood disorders among the offspring of probands with bipolar disorder is 12 percent, and among those of probands with major depressive disorder, seven percent. Those estimates have been derived from reviews of controlled family studies that specify the risk of recurrence in offspring of one psychiatrically ill parent. When both parents have mood disorders the estimates may double or triple.

The presence of some disorders can be detected in utero by biochemical means if the defect is known, or through linked markers (with a certain confidence level) if the precise defect is not yet known by assessment of markers in the fetal chromosomes. If the ongoing molecular genetics studies of the psychiatric disorders succeed in identifying disease markers, such markers could ultimately be used to detect a disease-predisposing genotype.

Although the mood disorders have been consistently found to be related to major disruption in familial functioning, it has been difficult to identify whether the disruption in social functioning is causal, contributory, or residual to the illness. Nevertheless, such detrimental environments tend to be transmitted through families, and such combinations of vulnerable genotypes and negative environments are likely to interact in increasing the likelihood that offspring will have mood disorders. The results of recent studies of populations at high risk for the disorders may yield information on premorbid indicators that may permit prediction of persons who are likely to develop a particular disorder. To date, there are no consistent premorbid biological trait markers that allow clinicians to identify vulnerable individuals for any of the major psychiatric disorders.

Finally, clinicians are often called on by family members or prospective spouses to provide data on the course of a particular psychiatric illness. Again, a summary of empirical data relevant to that person's combination of demographic, social, and clinical characteristics should be carefully prepared. Unfortunately, the course of psychiatric disorders and their subtypes have been too often neglected in recent systems of diagnostic nomenclature. That is in direct contrast to the diagnostic approach prescribed by Emil Kraepelin, in which the course of illness was considered to be an essential element of diagnostic definitions.

Because treatment response may also be similar in families, knowledge regarding the treatment history may provide important information in decisions regarding choice of treatment modalities. For example, C.M.B. Pare and J.W. Mack found that relatives of probands with mood disorders shared the pattern of drug response or nonresponse with the proband. In eliciting a family history of a psychiatric disorder, clinicians should also examine the efficacy of specific pharmacological agents among other family members with similar psychiatric syndromes to the patient under evaluation. The application of such information may conserve considerable time and effort in treatment decisions.

RESEARCH IMPLICATIONS In terms of research, application of the within-family design can minimize the heterogeneity that is likely to characterize samples of unrelated patients. That approach, which controls for both shared genetic and environmental factors within families, comprises an extremely powerful method with which to identify the underlying neurobiological mechanisms involved in the pathogenesis of the mood disorders. Moreover, application of other genetic epidemiological study paradigms—such as those of discordant monozygotic twins, monozygotic twins concordant for patterns of expression of depression and associated neurobiological abnormalities, half-sibling studies, and migrant studies—may yield important information for classification, course, risk factors, treatment, and ultimately for the cause of the mood disorders.

Another critical complication of family studies in elucidating the role of genetic factors in mood disorders is the focus on the specific symptoms and symptoms clusters, particularly those that can be assessed quantitatively. The use of family study paradigms to examine the specificity of transmission of the components of mood disorders or putative markers is a necessary step before attempting to employ linkage analyses of the pedigrees. Moreover, the data may also be required for the development of definitions of mood illness and its subtypes, for which the lack of validity appears to be the rate-limiting step in applying the powerful tools of molecular biology and statistical genetics.

Perhaps the most important long-term implication of linkage studies is the potential for identifying individuals with vulnerability to a particular disorder. That would permit identification of the role of environmental factors in either protecting or enhancing the expression of a mood disorder in vulnerable persons. At the same time, there is great danger in the future ability of such studies to identify DNA markers for psychiatric illness. Although such markers comprise valuable indicators of vulnerability, they also could be potentially used as negative labels resulting in social and occupational discrimination.

RECOMMENDATIONS FOR FUTURE RESEARCH

VALIDATION OF DIAGNOSTIC CATEGORIES OF MOOD DISORDERS There is an urgent need for evidence regarding the validity of the mood disorders, particularly the milder forms and those which can be measured on a continuum. Genetic-epidemiological studies designed specifically to test the validity of diagnostic categories and the overlap between comorbid disorders are necessary to define homogenous subgroups to which the tools of molecular biology may be applied.

INTERDISCIPLINARY APPROACH During the coming decade, as the pathways involved in the expression of genes involved in the central nervous system structure and function become elucidated and genetic markers for the mood disorders and categories thereof become available, researchers can routinely investigate the role of such markers in the transmission of the mood disorders and the mechanisms by which those markers exert their influence; furthermore, as the modification of gene expression through the immune and endocrine systems becomes more clearly elucidated, an interdisciplinary approach in the design of genetic studies will be imperative. That approach will permit simultaneous consideration of the roles of genetic vulnerability factors, nontransmissible factors including the biological environment of the individual, and nontransmissible environmental factors in the expression of underlying vulnerability for depression.

STUDY DESIGNS Application of hybrid and novel designs are forthcoming, such as twin and offspring studies, combinations of family and high-risk paradigms, and half-sibling and extended pedigree studies, all of which are not limited to estimating the heritability of particular disorders but also include identification of specific environmental factors that may be involved in the pathogenesis of these diseases. Substantial work in statistical genetics will be involved, together with the development of creative study designs to investigate gene-environment interactions.

GENETIC LINKAGE STUDIES Genetic linkage studies of psychiatric disorders need to be conducted to resolve the discrepant results obtained thus far, particularly for traits with known loci. The linkage studies that employ RFLPs or polymorphic markers with no known function should also be conducted on selected large pedigrees with clear segregation patterns. Collaborative studies will be the most efficient way to unravel the role or roles of genes in the mood disorders through the sharing of resources, laboratory facilities, and methodological standards in order to prevent the repetition of inconsistent findings that have emerged from the past two decades of linkage studies directed by single investigators. The Gene Bank Initiative of the National Institute of Mental Health in the United States and the Network on the Molecular Biology of Mental Illness of the European Science Foundation are examples of the types of collaborative effort that will be necessary to maximize the application of molecular biology to the study of the mood disorders.

SUGGESTED CROSS-REFERENCES

A general review of molecular genetic mechanisms is provided in Section 1.14. Population genetics in psychiatry is discussed in Section 1.15, and genetic linkage analysis of the psychiatric disorders is discussed in Section 1.16. Genetic epidemiological approaches are also discussed in Section 14.5, with reference to schizophrenia.

REFERENCES

Alexander J R, Lerer B, Baron M: Ethical issues in genetic linkage studies of psychiatric disorders. Br J Psychiatry *160:* 98, 1992.

Angst J: On the etiology of the endogenous depressive psychoses. In *Monograph on Neurology and Psychiatry.* Springer-Verlag: Berlin, 1966.

Baron M, Risch N, Hamburger R, Mandel B, Kushner S, Newman M, Drumer D, Belmaker R H: Genetic linkage between X-chromosome markers and bipolar affective illness. Nature *326:* 289, 1987.

Bertelsen A, Harvald B, Hauge M: A Danish twin study of manic-depressive disorders. Br J Psychiatry *130:* 330, 1977.

Cadoret R J, O'Gorman T W, Heywood E, Troughton E: Genetic and environmental factors in major depression. J Affective Disord *9:* 155, 1985.

Cowen P J, Wood A J: Biological markers of depression (editorial). Psychol Med *21:* 831, 1991.

Craddock N, Owen M: Chromosomal aberrations and bipolar affective disorder. Br J Psychiatry *164:* 507, 1994.

Egeland J A, Gerhard D S, Pauls D L, Sussex J N, Kidd K K, Allen C R, Hostetter A M, Housman D: Bipolar affective disorders linked to DNA markers on chromosome II. Nature *325:* 783, 1987.

Falconer D S: The inheritance of liability to certain diseases, estimated from the incidence among relatives. Ann Hum Genet *29:* 51, 1965.

Galton F: *Natural Inheritance.* Macmillan, New York, 1894.

Gershon E S: The genetics of affective disorders. In *Psychiatric Update,* vol 2, p 434. American Psychiatric Press, Washington, DC, 1983.

Gershon E S, Hamovit J, Guroff J J, Dibble E, Leckman J F, Sceery W, Targum S D, Nurnberger J I Jr, Goldin L R, Bunney W E Jr: A family study of schizoaffective bipolar I, bipolar II, unipolar and normal control probands. Arch Gen Psychiatry *39:* 1157, 1982.

Gershon E S, Mark A, Cohen N, Belizon N, Baron M, Knobe K E: Transmitted factors in the morbid risk of affective disorders: A controlled study. J Psychiatr Res *12:* 283, 1975.

Goldin L R, Gershon E S: Association and linkage studies of genetic marker loci in major psychiatric disorders. In *Psychiatric Developments: Advances and Prospects in Research and Clinical Practice,* S B Guze, M Roth, editors, p 387. Oxford University Press, Oxford, 1983.

Gurling H: Application of molecular biology to mental illness: Analysis of genomic DNA and brain RNA. Psychiatr Dev *3:* 257, 1985.

Harris H: Nature and nurture. N Engl J Med *297:* 1399, 1977.

Harvald B, Hauge M: Hereditary factors elucidated by twin studies. In *Genetics and the Epidemiology of Chronic Diseases,* US Public Health Service publication 1163, J V Neel, editor, p 61. US Government Printing Office, Washington, DC, 1965.

Hebebrand J: A critical appraisal of X-linked bipolar illness: Evidence for the assumed mode of inheritance is lacking. Br J Psychiatry *160:* 7, 1992.

Hogben LT: *Nature and Nurture.* Allen and Unwin, London, 1933.

Kallmann F J: *Heredity in Health and Mental Disorder.* Norton, New York, 1953.

Kelsoe J R, Ginns E E, Egeland J A, Gerhard D S, Goldstein A M, Bale S J, Pauls D L, Long R T, Kidd K K, Conte G, Housman D E, Paul S: Re-evaluation of the linkage relationship between chromosome 11p loci and the gene for bipolar affective disorder in the Old Order Amish. Nature *16:* 238, 1989.

Kendler K S, Neale M C, Kessler R C, Heath A C, Eaves L J: A population-based twin study of major depression in women: The impact of varying definitions of illness. Arch Gen Psychiatry *49:* 257, 1992.

King M C, Lee G M, Spinner N B, Thomson G, Wiensch M R: Genetic epidemiology. Annu Rev Public Health *5:* 1, 1984.

Kraepelin E: *Manic-depressive Insanity and Paranoia,* G Roberson, editor. E and S Livingston, Edinburgh, 1921.

Leboyer M, McGuffin P: Collaborative strategies in the molecular genetics of major psychoses. Br J Psychiatry *158:* 605, 1990.

Lyness J M, Conwell Y, Nelson J C: Suicide attempts in elderly psychiatric inpatients. J Am Geriatr Soc *40:* 320, 1992.

Maier W, Hallmayer J, Lichtermann D, Philipp M, Klingler T: The impact of the endogenous subtype on the familial aggregation of unipolar depression. Eur Arch Psychiatry Clin Neurosci *240:* 355, 1991.

Maier W, Lichtermann D, Minges J, Hallmeyer J, Heun R, Benkert O, Levinson D F: Continuity and discontinuity of affective disorders and schizophrenia. Results of a controlled family study. Arch Gen Psychiatry *50:* 871, 1993.

McGuffin P, Huckle P: Simulation of mendelism revisited: The recessive gene for attending medical school. Am J Hum Genet *46:* 994, 1990.

McGuffin P, Katz R: The genetics of depression and manic-depressive disorder. Br J Psychiatry *155:* 294, 1989.

McGuffin P, Katz R, Rutherford J: Nature, nurture and depression: A twin study. Psychol Med *21:* 329, 1991.

McKusick V: Mendelian inheritance in man. Johns Hopkins University Press, Baltimore, 1988.

*Mellon CD: Genetic linkage studies in bipolar disorder: A review. Psychiatr Dev *2:* 143, 1989.

Mendlewicz J, Rainer J D: Adoption study supporting genetic transmission in manic-depressive illness. Nature *268:* 327, 1977.
Mendlewicz J, Sevy S, Mendelbaum K: Minireview: Molecular genetics in affective illness. Life Sci *52:* 231, 1993.
Mendlewicz J, Simon P, Sevy S, Charon F, Brocas H, Legros S, Vassart G: Polymorphic DNA marker on X chromosome and manic depression. Lancet 1230, 1987.
*Merikangas K R: Genetic epidemiology of psychiatric disorders. In *Psychiatric Update,* vol 6, R E Hales, A J Frances, editors, pp 625-646. American Psychiatric Press, Washington, DC, 1987.
Merikangas K R, Spence A, Kupfer D J: Linkage studies of bipolar disorders: Methodologic and analytic issues. Arch Gen Psychiatry *46:* 1137, 1989.
Merikangas K R, Spiker D G: Assortative mating among inpatients with primary affective disorder. Psychol Med *12:* 753, 1982.
Merikangas K R, Weissman M M, Pauls D L: Genetic factors in the sex ratio of major depression. Psychol Med *15:* 63, 1985.
Morton N E: *Outline of Genetic Epidemiology.* S Karger, Basel, 1982.
Pare C M B, Mack J W: Differentiation of two genetically specific types of depression by the response to antidepressant drugs. J Med Genet *8:* 306, 1971.
Penrose L S: The detection of autosomal linkage in data which consists of pairs of brothers and sisters of unspecified parentage. Ann Eugen *6:* 133, 1935.
Perris C: A study of bipolar (manic-depressive) and unipolar recurrent depressive psychoses. Acta Psychiatr Scand [Suppl] *42* (94 Suppl): 1, 1966.
Rao D C, Morton N E, Gottesman II, Lew R: Path analysis of qualitative data on pairs of relatives: Application to schizophrenia. Hum Hered *31:* 325, 1981.
Reich T, Clayton P J, Winokur G: Family history studies: V. The genetics of mania. Am J Psychiatry *125:* 64, 1969.
*Rice J, McGuffin P: Genetics of schizophrenia and affective disorders. In *Psychiatry,* vol 1, J O Cavenar, editor. Lippincott, Philadelphia, 1985.
Rieder R O, Gershon E S: Genetic strategies in biological psychiatry. Arch Gen Psychiatry *35:* 866, 1978.
*Risch N: Genetic linkage and complex disease, with special reference to psychiatric disorders. Genet Epidemiol *7:* 3, 1990.
Risch N, Baron M: X-linkage and genetic heterogeneity in bipolar-related major affective illness: re-analysis of linkage data. Am J Hum Genet *46:* 153, 1982.
Roy A: Genetic and biologic risk factors for suicide in depressive disorders. Psychiatr Q *64:* 345, 1993.
Shapiro R W: A twin study of non-endogenous depression. Acta Jutlandica *42:* 1, 1970.
Simpson S G, Folstein S E, Meyers D A, McMahon F J, Brusco D M, DePaulo J R: Bipolar II: the most common bipolar subtype? Am J Psychiatry *150:* 901, 1993.
Smeraldi E, Bellodi L: Possible linkage between primary affective disorder susceptibility locus and HLA haplotypes. Am J Psychiatry *139:* 1232, 1981.
Spence M A, Bishop D T, Boehnke M, Elston R C, Falk C, Hodge S E, Ott J, Rice J, Risch N, Merikangas K, Kupfer DJ: Methodological issues in linkage analyses for psychiatric disorders: Secular trends, assortative mating, bilineal pedigrees. Report of the MacArthur Foundation Network I Task Force on Methodological Issues. Hum Hered *43:* 166, 1993.
Stenstedt A: Genetics of neurotic depression. Acta Psychiatr Scand *42:* 392, 1966.
Suarez B K, Cox N J: Linkage analysis for psychiatric disorders: I. Basic concepts. Psychiatr Dev *3:* 219, 1985.
Susser M: Separating heredity and environment. Am J Prev Med *1:* 5, 1985.
*Tsuang M, Faraone S V: *The Genetics of Mood Disorders.* Johns Hopkins University Press, Baltimore, 1990.
Tsuang M T, Winokur G, Crowe R R: Morbidity risks of schizophrenia and affective disorders among first-degree relatives of patients with schizophrenia, mania, depression, and surgical conditions. Br J Psychiatry *137:* 497, 1980.
Von Knorring A L, Cloninger C R, Bohman M, Sigvardsson S: An adoption study of depressive disorders and substance abuse. Arch Gen Psychiatry *40:* 943, 1983.
Weissman M M, Bruce M L, Leaf P J, Florio L P, Holzer C III: Affective disorders. In *Psychiatric Disorders in America: The Epidemiologic Catchment Area Study,* L N Robins, D A Regier, editors, p 53. Free Press, New York, 1991.
Weissman M M, Merikangas K R, John K, Wickramaratne P, Prusoff B A, Kidd K K: Family-genetic studies of psychiatric disorders. Arch Gen Psychiatry *43:* 1104, 1986.
Weitkamp L R, Stancer H C, Persad E, Flood C, Guttormsen S: Depressive disorders and HLA: A gene on chromosome 6 that can affect behavior. N Engl J Med *305:* 1301, 1981.
Wender P H, Kety S S, Rosenthal D, Schulsinger F, Ortmann J, Lundel I: Psychiatric disorders in the biological and adoptive families and adopted individuals with affective disorders. Arch Gen Psychiatry *43:* 923, 1986.
Wesner R B, Tanna V L, Palmer P J, Goedken R J, Crowe R R, Winokur G: Linkage of c-Harvey-*ras*-1 and INS DNA markers to unipolar depression and alcoholism is ruled out in 18 families. Eur Arch Psychiatry Neurol Sci *239:* 356, 1990.
Winokur G, Crowe R R: Bipolar illness: The sex-polarity effect in affectively ill family members. Arch Gen Psychiatry *40:* 57, 1983.
Winokur G, Tanna V L: Possible role of X-linked dominant factor in manic depressive disease. Dis Nerv Syst *30:* 89, 1969.
Wolpert L: DNA and its message. Lancet *2:* 853, 1984.
Zerbin-Rüdin E: Zur genetik der depressiven erkrankugen. In *Das Depressive Syndrom,* H Hippius, H Selbach, editors, p 37. Urban and Schwarzenberg, Berlin, 1969.

16.5 MOOD DISORDERS: PSYCHODYNAMIC ETIOLOGY

GLEN O. GABBARD, M.D.

INTRODUCTION

The terms "affective disorder" and "mood disorder" are often used interchangeably. However, in psychodynamic parlance "mood" and "affect" have somewhat different meanings. "Affect" is a more specific term than "mood," in that affect is a subjective emotion or feeling attached to a specific idea or an internal representation of the self or of an object. By contrast, a mood is a complex internal feeling state that is pervasive, stable, and sustained by the continuing influence of unconscious fantasy.

In any discussion of the psychodynamic causes of depression or mania, one must avoid consideration of the psychodynamic factors in isolation from the biological and neurophysiological factors. Psychological concerns—such as real or imagined loss, failure to live up to one's expectations, and problematic relationships—may trigger neurochemical and neurophysiological changes in the brain that result in significant alterations in the balance of neurotransmitters. Empirical research suggests that, even in severely depressed patients with melancholia, as many as three fourths have experienced a stressful life event in the months preceding the onset of the illness that is deemed causatively relevant by both the patient and a family member or significant other in the patient's life. Hence, one can conclude that in many cases of depression the cause of the illness may be identified in interpersonal, environmental, and psychological stressors and that the pathogenesis involves actual brain dysfunction in response to the causative influences.

Psychosocial stressors and interpersonal events must also be taken into account in treatment. Attention to relationships in a psychotherapeutic treatment appears to have a specific prophylactic effect in preventing relapse. Compliance with prescribed medication may also be influenced by psychosocial factors. The official Depression Practice Guidelines note that psychotherapeutic management should be part of every treatment for depression.

DEPRESSION

Substantial empirical data support the idea that life events and environmental stressors are relevant to the development of clinically significant depression. The loss of a spouse, for example, is the environmental stressor most often associated with the onset of an episode of depression. The most impressive piece of evidence linking loss to subsequent depression is the finding that loss of a parent before age 11 places adults at a higher than usual risk of depression. Some investigators have postulated that early childhood losses or separations actually sensitize neuronal receptor sites in the brain, thereby producing a vulnerability to mood disorders in adulthood. Persons who grow up with that enhanced vulnerability may be highly sensitive to images or ideas linked to depressive states, so that an episode of depression may be precipitated without requiring a catastrophic external loss. Chronic stress or deprivation of environmental origin may produce alterations in the catecholaminergic system in response to stimulation from the corticotropin-releasing hormone-adrenocorticotropic hormone (ACTH) axis. The end result of the changes may be the clinical picture of depression.

The effects of psychosocial influences on neurophysiological factors have been amply demonstrated in primate research. Infant squirrel monkeys who are separated from their mothers experience long-lasting and, in some cases, permanent neurobiological changes. The changes include lasting alterations in the sensitivity of noradrenergic receptors, changes in hypothalamic serotonin secretion, and persistently elevated plasma cortisol levels. The sensitivity and the number of brain opiate receptors are also significantly affected by repeated separations. Some of the changes are reversible if the infant monkeys are reunited with their mothers or siblings; other changes are not. Moreover, the separations appear to be more or less damaging during certain developmental periods, possibly because of the correlation with myelinization in the nervous system.

In the ensuing discussion of psychodynamic factors in the etiology of depression, the reader must keep in mind that psychological influences work in concert with genetic vulnerability and neurophysiological alterations to produce the characteristic clinical picture of depression. Those characteristics include psychomotor retardation, sleep changes, loss of appetite, diminished sex drive, anhedonia, loss of energy, inappropriate guilt feelings, and suicidal ideation. Similarly, comprehensive treatment planning must take into account both the psychodynamic factors and the alterations of neurotransmitters.

One of the most sophisticated efforts to define the relative contributions of psychological vulnerability, genetics, and environmental stressors in major depressive disorder was a prediction study involving female twins. Multiple assessments of 680 female-female twin pairs of known zygosity were made over time, and the findings allowed the investigators to develop an etiological model to predict major depressive episodes. One of the most influential predictors was the presence of recent stressful events. Genetic factors were also important in prediction of depression. Two other factors, neuroticism and interpersonal relations, also played a substantial etiological role. Neuroticism seemed to contribute in part by reducing the level of social support for an individual. Interpersonal dimensions of social support, recent difficulties, and parental warmth all were involved in predicting a major depressive episode.

PSYCHODYNAMIC THEORIES OF DEPRESSION

Anger turned inward A common finding in depressed patients is profound self-depreciation. Sigmund Freud, in his classic 1917 paper "Mourning and Melancholia," attributed that self-reproach to anger turned inward, which he related to object loss. The object loss may or may not be real. A fantasied loss may be sufficient to trigger a severe depression. Moreover, the patient may actually be unaware of any specific feelings of loss in light of the fact that the fantasied loss may be entirely unconscious.

Freud drew an analogy between serious melancholic states and normal grief. Both may be time-limited, but Freud cited two principal differences. In cases of *grief,* there is an *actual* object loss in external reality; in *depression* the lost object is more likely to be *emotional* than real. The second difference is that persons with depression experience profound loss of self-esteem, but the self-regard of persons engaged in a mourning process is not diminished.

The observational differences between grief and depression were pivotal in Freud's theory. He reasoned that one way of dealing with the loss of a beloved person is to become like the person. Freud defined that process as *introjection,* a defense mechanism central to the psychodynamics of depression, in which the patient internalizes the lost object so that it becomes an internal presence. Freud later noted that introjection is the only way that the ego can give up a valued and loved object.

Because depressed persons perceive the departed love object as having abandoned them, feelings of hatred and anger are intermingled with feelings of love. Freud suggested that ambivalence of that nature, involving the coexistence of love and hate, is instrumental in the psychodynamics of depression. As a result of introjecting the lost object, the negative part of the depressed patient's ambivalence—the hatred and anger—is directed inward and results in the pathognomonic picture of self-reproach. In that manner a suicidal act may have the unconscious meaning of murder.

Karl Abraham, one of Freud's early colleagues, shared Freud's view of depression but also extended and elaborated it further. Abraham viewed the process of introjection as a defense mechanism that takes two forms. First, he thought that the introjection of the original love object is the basis for building one's ego-ideal, so that the role of the conscience is eventually taken over by the introjected object. In that conceptualization much of pathological self-criticism is seen as emanating from the introjected love object. In the second form of introjection, more in keeping with Freud's idea, the content of self-reproach is merciless criticism directed at the object. In other words, Abraham viewed the two processes of introjection as instrumental in the creation of the superego. Abraham also linked depression to early fixations at the anal and the oral levels of psychosexual development. He viewed oral sadistic tendencies as the primary source of self-punishment in depressed patients, and he inferred that inadequate mothering during the oral stage of development was involved.

The psychodynamic understanding of depression defined by Freud and expanded by Abraham is known as the classical view of depression. That theory involves four key points: (1) Disturbances in the infant-mother relationship during the oral phase (the first 12 to 18 months of life) predispose to subsequent vulnerability to depression. (2) Depression can be linked to real or imagined object loss. (3) Introjection of the departed object is a defense mechanism invoked to deal with the distress connected with the object loss. (4) Because the lost object is regarded with a mixture of love and hate, feelings of anger are directed inward at the self.

Depressive position Although Melanie Klein understood depression as involving the expression of aggression toward loved ones, much as Freud did, the developmental theory on which her view was based is quite different from Freudian theory. During the first year of life, Klein believed, the infant progresses from the paranoid-schizoid position to the depressive position. In the first few months of life, according to Klein, the infant projects highly destructive fantasies into its mother and then becomes terrified of the mother as a sadistic persecutor. That terrifying "bad" mother is kept separate from the loving, nurturing "good" mother through the defense mechanism of splitting. In that manner the infant's blissful feeding experience remains uncontaminated and undisturbed by persecutory fears of attack by the "bad" mother. In the course of normal development, according to Klein, the positive and the negative images of the mother are integrated into a more ambivalent view. In other words, the infant recognizes that the "bad" mother it fears and hates is the same mother as the "good" mother it loves and adores. The recognition that one can hurt loved ones is the essence of the depressive position.

Klein connected clinical depression with an inability to successfully negotiate the depressive position of childhood. She regarded depressed persons as fixated or stuck at a developmental level in which they are extraordinarily concerned that loved good objects have been destroyed by the greed and destructiveness they have directed at them. In the absence of those good objects, depressed persons feel persecuted by the hated bad objects. In short, Klein's view was that depressed patients are longing or pining for the lost love objects while being persecuted by bad objects. In that theoretical framework the feelings of self-depreciation are linked to the fear that one's good parents have been transformed into violent persecutors as a result of one's own destructive tendencies. Also, the bad internal objects are internalized into the superego, which then makes sadistic demands on the patient. Hence, in the Kleinian view, the self-reproaches experienced by depressed patients are directed against the self and internal impulses, rather than toward an introjected object, as in Freud's view.

Tension between ideals and reality Whereas most psychodynamic theories of depression incorporate the superego as a significant part of the conceptual understanding, Edward Bibring viewed depression as tension arising from within the ego itself, rather than between the ego and the superego. According to Bibring, the ego has three highly invested narcissistic aspirations—to be good and loving, to be superior or strong, and to be loved and worthy. Those ideals are held up as standards of conduct. Depression sets in when a person becomes aware of the discrepancy between those ideals and reality. Helplessness and powerlessness result from the feeling that one cannot measure up to such high standards. Any blow to the self-esteem or any frustration of the strivings toward those aspirations precipitates depression. Bibring's theory, unlike Freud's and Klein's, does not regard aggression as playing a primary role in depression. The depressed person may ultimately experience anger turned inward, resulting from the awareness of helplessness; however, such expressions of aggression are secondary, rather than primary. The essence of depression, in Bibring's view, is a primary affective state arising within the ego and is based on the tension between what one would like to be and what one is.

Ego as victim of superego Edith Jacobson compared the state of depression to a situation in which the ego is a powerless, helpless child, victimized by the superego, which becomes the equivalent of a sadistic and powerful mother who takes delight in torturing the child. Like Freud, Jacobson assumed that depressed persons have identified with ambivalently regarded lost love objects. The self is experienced as identified with the negative aspects of the object, and ultimately the sadistic qualities of the lost love object are transformed into the cruel superego. Hence, depressed persons feel that they are at the mercy of a sadistic internal tormentor that is unrelenting in its victimization. Jacobson also noted that the boundary between self and object may disappear, resulting in a fusion of the bad self with the bad object.

Dominant other Silvano Arieti studied the psychodynamic underpinnings of depression in severely ill patients who were unresponsive to most somatic treatments. He observed a common psychological theme in those patients that involved living for someone else, rather than for themselves. He referred to the person for whom depressed patients live as the dominant other. In most cases the dominant other is the spouse or a parent, but Arieti also noted that sometimes a principle, an ideal, or an organization serves a similar psychodynamic function. In such cases he referred to the entity as the dominant ideology or the dominant goal.

Depression often sets in when patients realize that the person for whom they have been living is never going to respond in a manner that will meet their expectations. The goal of their lives is regarded as unattainable, and a profound feeling of helplessness sets in. In Arieti's conceptualization of depression, he stressed a marked rigidity in the thinking of depressed persons, so that any alternative to living for the dominant other or the dominant ideology is viewed as unacceptable and even unthinkable. Depressed patients feel locked into an inflexible perspective on how they should live their lives and how gratification or fulfillment can be obtained. Even though they are depressed because living for someone or something other than themselves has been a failure, they nevertheless feel paralyzed and unable to shift their approach to life. If the dominant other will not respond to them in the way they have longed for, they feel that life is worthless, and that rigidity is often involved in a decision that suicide is the only alternative.

CASE EXAMPLE A 19-year-old college student consulted a psychiatrist after one semester in school. He told the psychiatrist that he was depressed and discouraged with college and with himself. College was not what he had expected, and he had not performed up to his expectations. He was seriously questioning whether he should return for the second semester, and he had a sense of hopelessness about changing his feelings. Suicidal thoughts had occasionally crossed his mind, although he was not planning to act on them. His sleep was disturbed by awakening in the middle of the night and ruminating about what he should do. He felt a significant diminution in his energy level, and he commented that things he used to find enjoyable no longer gave him pleasure.

The patient attended a prestigious college on the West Coast, but he indicated that he had actually wanted to get into Harvard. His application to Harvard had resulted in his being placed on the waiting list, but he had not been accepted. The psychiatrist he consulted commented that the college he had chosen to attend was certainly a highly regarded one. The patient responded, "It's not Harvard." When the psychiatrist asked the patient how he had done academically during the first semester, the patient appeared embarrassed and replied, "I only got a 3.25 grade-point average—one A and three Bs." The psychiatrist asked him why he seemed embarrassed to reveal such a solid academic record. The patient explained that he had wanted to make the dean's list but that he had fallen short of it, since the list required a 3.5 grade-point average.

The psychiatrist asked the patient if he hoped to be in a different situation after one semester of college. The patient's answer revealed that he had an extraordinarily high internal expectation of himself. He had wanted to be "a star," a straight-A student at Harvard. He explained that his father had gone to Harvard, and he hoped that, by being a standout there, he would finally achieve the praise and recognition from his father that he had always longed for but had never received. His father seemed disappointed that his son had not been accepted to Harvard, and the patient was convinced that his father was ashamed of his son for not making the dean's list.

EXPLANATION The above case example illustrates the psychodynamic theories of both Arieti and Bibring. The patient was living his life for a dominant other—his father. He tried to perform beyond his abilities to extract an approving and loving response from his father that was never forthcoming. That longed-for response was rigidly construed as the only thing that mattered in life; even though he was succeeding at a highly competitive college, his success did not result in his feeling good about himself. Moreover, the patient's depression can also be linked to his awareness of the disparity between his idealized expectations of himself and the reality of his situation, as described by Bibring. Being a straight-A student at Harvard was his own aspiration; the reality was that he was a B+ student at a college that did not measure up to Harvard.

The vignette also reflects two other key elements in the psychodynamic etiology of depression. First, in accord with the psychoanalytic notion of multiple causation, more than one psychodynamic theory may be pertinent in understanding an individual patient's depression. Clearly, both the dominant other and the tension between ideals and realities were significant determinants in causing the patient's depression. Second, the precipitating factors that produce depression do not have to be catastrophic events involving obvious external disasters. To a casual observer the college student had no apparent reason to be depressed, since he was performing successfully at a highly regarded college. Nonetheless, the *intrapsychic meaning* of his academic performance was such that the patient felt hopeless and despairing as a result. In assessing the psychodynamic factors in depression, clinicians must always attend to idiosyncratic personal meanings of events to fully understand the effects they have on the patient. Otherwise, clinicians run the risk of responding in the same unempathic manner that often characterizes the responses of family members. In the absence of objective evidence of any disastrous events in the depressed person's life, loved ones often react by saying: "You have no reason to be depressed. Everything is going so well in your life."

Selfobject failure The ego and the superego do not figure in Heinz Kohut's conceptualization of depression. Kohut's theory, known as self psychology, rests on the assumption that the developing self has specific needs that must be met by parents to give the child a positive sense of self-esteem and self-cohesion and that similar responses are required from others throughout the course of the life cycle. He referred to those needs as mirroring, twinship, and idealization. The *mirroring* responses required by the self are equated with the gleam in the mother's eye when the child exhibitionistically shows off for the mother. Admiration, validation, and affirmation are responses that are included under the category of mirroring. *Twinship* responses refer to the child's need to be like others. A small boy who is outside playing with his toy lawn mower while his father is mowing the lawn is meeting important psychological needs in asserting his commonality with his father. Finally, the need for *idealization* is an important aspect of the development of the self. Children who grow up with parents they can respect and idealize develop healthy standards of conduct and morality.

Kohut referred to those three needs collectively as selfobject needs. In other words, the responses demanded from others are required by the self, and the needs of the object as a separate person are not taken into account. The other person serves as an object who meets the needs of the self. Selfobject needs essentially refer to certain functions that persons in the environment provide, rather than to those persons themselves. Kohut felt that selfobject responses continue to be needed throughout life and are as necessary for emotional health as oxygen is for physical health. Within that conceptual framework, depression involves the failure of selfobjects in the environment to provide the self of the depressed person with mirroring, twinship, or idealizing responses necessary for the self to feel whole and sustained. The massive loss of self-esteem seen in depression is regarded by Kohut and the self psychologists as a serious disruption of the self-selfobject connection or bond.

Depression as affect and compromise formation Among contemporary ego psychologists a widely held view is that depression is not truly a psychiatric disorder or illness. Instead, depression is regarded as an affect reflecting conflict and compromise formation. Charles Brenner, the principal architect of that view, suggested that concern about such childhood calamities as object loss, loss of love, castration, and punishment are associated with two kinds of unpleasure. One form of unpleasure is anxiety, which involves an *anticipated* calamity or danger. The other form of unpleasure, depressive affect, involves a calamity that has *already happened.* That theory of depressive affect differs sharply from the classical views of Freud and Abraham. Brenner pointed out that depression is not always related to object loss or to oral wishes. He also asserted that identification with a lost object is found in some depressed persons but not in all and that anger turned inward is a *result* of depression, rather than a cause. Depressive affect, in Brenner's view, can be linked to any of the childhood calamities, rather than uniquely to object loss. People can experience depressive affect because they feel unloved, because they feel castrated, or because they feel punished in a variety of ways. Depressive affect is a normal and universal part of the human condition.

A critical feature in Brenner's formulation is the idea of compromise formation, in which a symptom is viewed as simultaneously expressing an unconscious wish or drive and a defense against that wish or drive. A particular compromise formation may be more or less successful in eradicating depressive affect in the same manner as it may succeed to varying degrees in dealing with anxiety. A dog phobia, for example, is a symptomatic compromise formation that succeeds in eliminating anxiety as long as dogs are avoided. Similarly, certain forms of compromise formation may eradicate depressive affect while others do not.

The central point of Brenner's psychodynamic theory is that depressive affect is a universal feature in every pathological conflict, whether it is apparent on the surface or buried in the depths of the compromise formation. Depressive affect is a universal factor in all cases of psychiatric illness. From that standpoint, Brenner believed that classifying certain forms of mental illness as depression simply because depressive affect is part of the conscious symptoms does not make sense. The conscious experience of depression provides information about the efficacy and the nature of a patient's defensive maneuvers and compromise formations, in Brenner's view, but it does not reveal much about the underlying causes of the patient's illness.

Early deprivation Several investigators have noted that consistent, loving, nurturant parental involvement appears to have some value in preventing the development of depression. Conversely, separation from parents early in life or the actual loss of a parent may predispose one to depression. Edith Zetzel observed that adverse experiences in the formative years of childhood, particularly those involving separation and loss, make it difficult for children to tolerate depressive affects without resorting to primitive defensive operations. If caretakers fail to assist children in identifying and tolerating painful feelings that result from an adverse life experience, the child will grow up with inadequate coping mechanisms. That impaired adaptation may contribute to the subsequent development of depression.

Empirical research has provided some corroboration for the view that early deprivation is relevant to the cause of depression. René Spitz demonstrated that infants separated from their mothers during the second six months of life have overt signs of depression. In some cases the infants in Spitz's studies wasted away and died in response to the separations. Margaret Mahler and her colleagues, who studied the interactions between normal and abnormal mother-infant pairs, found that children's emotional dependence on their parents is instrumental in the development of their capacity to grieve and mourn. That capacity, in turn, influences children's feelings of self-esteem and helplessness. Although the development of depression may involve genetic and constitutional factors, as well as environmental stressors, most theorists agree that the early relationship between child and parent plays a significant role in causing depression.

Premorbid personality factors A comprehensive psychodynamic understanding of depression must include premorbid personality factors in the equation. All persons may become depressed, given sufficient environmental stress, but certain personality types or traits appear to dispose one to depression. For example, the harsh, perfectionistic superego characteristic of persons with obsessive-compulsive personality disorder may lead them to feel that they are always falling short of their own excessive expectations of themselves. As noted earlier, that intrapsychic constellation may be critical in the development of a major depressive episode. Similarly, Axis II personality disorders involving dependent yearnings for care—such as dependent, histrionic, and borderline personality disorders—may also be more vulnerable to depression. Those personality disorders that use projection and other externalizing defense mechanisms, such as antisocial and paranoid personality disorders, are less likely to decompensate into depression. No particular premorbid personality type has been associated with the development of bipolar disorder.

Evidence is accumulating that an Axis II diagnosis of a personality disorder may complicate the course and treatment of depression. Depressed patients with personality disorders generally have poorer outcomes in the area of social functioning than those without personality disorders. Furthermore, residual depressive symptoms are more likely to present in recovering depressed patients who have an Axis II diagnosis. Psychoanalytic clinicians have observed that personality factors frequently serve to maintain a depressed state once it has occurred. In clinical practice the complicating factors of a comorbid personality disorder diagnosis are quite common. One study found that 42 percent of persons with major depressive disorder and 51 percent of patients with dysthymic disorder have an accompanying Axis II diagnosis.

CHARACTEROLOGICAL DEPRESSION Many patients encountered in clinical practice report feelings of depression even though they lack symptoms of a well-defined Axis I disorder, such as major depressive episode. Many of those patients have a primary diagnosis of a personality disorder on Axis II and experience characterological depression, a feeling of pervasive loneliness or emptiness associated with the perception that others are not meeting one's emotional needs. They can be distinguished from patients with an Axis I diagnosis of major depressive episode by the absence of vegetative symptoms (such as psychomotor retardation, loss of libido, diminished appetite, lack of energy, and sleep disturbance) and by the presence of certain qualitative features of their complaint of depression. Loneliness, emptiness, and boredom are often chronic complaints in characterological depression but are much less common in Axis I illnesses. In addition, a conscious sense of rage at not having their needs met may be present. The patients often describe childhood experiences in which they felt deprived of appropriate emotional nurturance from their parents. As a result, they continue to seek parental substitutes in adult life.

Characterological depression is differentiated from Axis II personality disorders by the fact that it is an affective state occurring within the context of certain personality disorders, rather than a constellation of traits forming an overarching personality type.

A 29-year-old woman came to psychotherapy complaining that she was "empty" inside and "needed to be filled up" by a positive experience with a psychotherapist. She said that, while she was growing up, her mother never had time for her and that her mother loved her two sisters more than her. The patient had had a series of romantic relationships with men, but she never felt that she was getting the kind of attention and love that she needed from any of them. The men often ended the relationship because they felt that she was too demanding and that they could not possibly meet all her needs. Her last therapist had "given up" on her because he, too, felt that he was unable to be of help to her. The patient also indicated that she had called her previous therapist almost every night because she would begin to feel lonely and need his reassurance that he still cared. She feared that she had turned off her therapist by being too demanding. She also described several angry outbursts directed at him when he would not talk with her for lengthy periods of time on the phone during the evening. She wondered if her outbursts made him hate her.

The patient had taken four different antidepressive medications with no improvement. She did not meet the diagnostic criteria for an Axis I dysthymic disorder or major depressive episode. However, she did have characteristics in keeping with two different Axis II diagnoses—dependent personality disorder and borderline personality disorder.

OTHER CLINICAL ENTITIES In addition to the existence of characterological depression in the presence of other Axis II personality disorders, another clinical entity is described by psychoanalysts as depressive personality or depressive character. That disorder may be a form of chronic depression closely related to the Axis I diagnosis of dysthymic disorder. Persons suffering from the disorder exhibit the following symptoms: helplessness; chronic feelings of guilt; relationships characterized by dependency; persistent low self-esteem; an inclination to be self-punitive, self-denying, and hypercritical; and a conviction that things are hopeless and will never change. Patients with that character structure do not allow themselves to have any form of gratification in life because of disturbed relationships in childhood with parents or parental substitutes.

A related form of characterological depression has been labeled depressive-masochistic personality disorder by Otto Kernberg. Patients with the disorder are characterized by an extremely demanding superego that results in humorless, overly conscientious, self-critical tendencies. The patients have excessive needs for approval, love, and acceptance from others, and they unconsciously cause others to feel guilty because of their inability to meet the patient's demands. The consequences of that pattern of interaction are further feelings of rejection because others do not want to be part of a relationship in which they never meet the expectations of the patient. People with depressive-masochistic personalities are also characterologically prone to turn anger inward to avoid any expression of aggression and anger toward others.

Clinicians must remember that depression spans the entire spectrum of pathology and health. In addition to being a discrete psychiatric disorder, depression refers to an emotional state that can be present in normal persons at certain times, as well as in persons with characterological or psychotic conditions. Moreover, simply because the patient does not have sufficient symptoms to be given an Axis I diagnosis of a mood disorder does not mean that the depression is benign. In one study, employees with minor forms of depression that did not meet Axis I criteria had 51 percent more disability days than did persons with a diagnosis of major depressive episode.

MANIA

Even though the standard treatment of bipolar disorder is pharmacological, a psychodynamic understanding of patients with mania is of value in the overall treatment and management of bipolar disorder. Genetic vulnerability and biochemical abnormalities are clearly involved in the illness, but psychological factors have repeatedly been observed to play roles in the precipitation of manic episodes. One 10-year follow-up study identified two different groups of treatment failures in a cohort of patients with bipolar disorder. One group of patients were shown to relapse because the treating psychiatrist had failed to increase the lithium (Eskalith) dose in response to increased physiological activation before the onset of a manic episode. In the other group of treatment failures, psychological issues that were clearly involved in precipitating manic episodes had not been given appropriate attention by the responsible psychiatrists, and manic episodes had resulted from the stress of those psychological factors.

Patients with bipolar disorder have been studied from the perspective of ongoing psychoanalysis and psychoanalytic psychotherapy, and those clinical investigations have revealed specific psychodynamic factors at work in the onset of manic episodes. In one series of patients, unconscious sexual urges and fantasies seemed to overpower ego defense mechanisms, leading to a clinical picture of hypersexuality and other symptoms of mania. Increasing the lithium dosage resulted in a decline of the sexual behavior and a reinstitution of the ego defense mechanisms that were present before the manic episode. In the course of continued psychotherapeutic or psychoanalytic treatment, those patients became consciously aware of their unconscious sexual desires and of the defenses brought to bear to deal with those desires. That conscious awareness enabled the patients to identify early warning signals of increased sexual impulses, so that future manic episodes could be avoided by increasing the lithium dose.

Those studies reflect how a psychodynamic understanding of patients with bipolar disorder may be crucial to the effective treatment of the disorder. Most manic patients cannot make use of psychotherapy interventions in the midst of a full-blown manic episode because the essence of mania is a denial of psychological problems. However, after the patient has become euthymic as a result of pharmacological stabilization, psychotherapeutic interventions may have value both in preventing subsequent episodes and in dealing with the feelings of shame and guilt associated with embarrassing behavior that took place during the manic episode.

PSYCHODYNAMIC THEORIES OF MANIA The psychodynamic understanding of mania is usefully applied to clinical instances of hypomania because the differences between the two entities are quantitative, rather than qualitative. Just as mania and depression have been linked from a neurophysiological standpoint, they are similarly connected from a psychodynamic perspective.

Karl Abraham Most theories of mania view manic episodes as defensive against underlying depression. Karl Abraham, for example, believed that manic episodes may reflect an inability to tolerate childhood depression in reaction to a developmental tragedy, such as the loss of a parent. The manic state, in Abraham's view, is understood as a way of removing the shackles of a tyrannical superego through the merger of the ego and the superego. Self-criticism is then replaced by euphoric self-satisfaction.

Bertram Lewin Bertram Lewin regarded the hypomanic patient's ego as a purified pleasure ego. The defense mechanism of denial is appropriated by the ego to disregard unpleasant perceptions and affects, as well as distressing psychic realities that may result in self-punishment or self-criticism.

Melanie Klein Melanie Klein also viewed mania and hypomania as defensive reactions to depression, but she linked the mechanism to the depressive position, rather than to an overriding of the superego. The essence of the depressive position is intense anxiety that one's own aggression has resulted in the destruction of important love objects, such as parents. In Klein's own words, "Persecution (by 'bad' objects) and the characteristic defenses against it, on the one hand, and pining for the loved ('good') object, on the other, constitute the depressive position." She thought that manic defenses are necessary both to control and master the dangerous bad objects and to restore and save the loved good objects.

Those manic defenses include omnipotence, denial, idealization, and contempt. *Omnipotence* serves to deny the need for good objects, to delude oneself into feelings of self-containment and grandiosity, and to help one feel insulated and protected from assault by internal persecutors. *Idealization and denial* work together in such a way that idealization of self and others serves to deny any destructiveness or aggression in relationships. The euphoric disposition of the manic or hypomanic patient reflects the tendency to gloss over any unpleasant aspects of reality and to treat everything with a sense of humor and a striking disregard for the tragic dimensions of reality, even if the situation is tragic. Idealization, however, may rapidly give way to *contempt,* which is also linked to denial because it is a way of disregarding the importance of love objects and, therefore, denying the concern that damage has been done to them and reparation is needed. Moreover, the manic patient can then minimize any distressing feelings of sorrow or regret that may arise in connection with concerns about having destroyed love objects.

Klein also observed that a wish to triumph over parents is often an integral part of the manic defensive posture. She noted that a frequent childhood fantasy is to reverse the child-parent relationship and that the fantasy produces feelings of guilt and anxieties of a depressive nature related to the wish to destroy and replace the parents. Feelings of depression may develop after a job promotion or other professional success because the person's unconscious wish to triumph over and to surpass one's parents has been fulfilled.

The Kleinian conceptualization of mania as defensive against feelings of depression is useful in understanding the phenomenon of dysphoria in manic patients when depression breaks through a manic episode, requiring a resurgence of manic denial. That formulation is also useful in understanding the commonly observed phenomenon of elation after the death of a loved one.

A patient received a phone call that informed him of his mother's death. Rather than feeling grief-stricken or shocked, he noted a sense of expansiveness and power. As he discussed the odd reaction with his psychotherapist, he was able to recognize that the high feeling he experienced was related to a sense that he was finally liberated from feelings of slavish dependence on a tyrannical mother.

TREATMENT The psychodynamic theory of Klein also informs psychotherapeutic approaches to bipolar-disorder patients. Because manic defenses are evoked by difficulties in working through the depressive position, the psychotherapist must assist the patient in integrating the loving and aggressive sides of both object representation and self-representation within. The process of integration facilitates the work of mourning. An auspicious moment for that form of therapeutic work may be after a manic episode, when patients feel remorseful about the damage they have done to others and to their own reputations by ill-advised behavior. Klein observed that, through a positive relationship with a therapeutic figure, patients may be able to restore the lost love objects by the internalization of the therapist and thereby lessen the fear of persecution from the bad objects. Manic defenses are less important then because the need for them has profoundly changed.

Other Theories Other views of mania include Bibring's conceptualization that manic elation is essentially a compensatory reaction secondary to severe depression or an unconscious fulfillment of a person's narcissistic aspirations to be loved, worthy, superior, and virtually flawless. Jacobson understood mania as a transformation of the sadistic superego figure from a punitive tormentor into a loving and forgiving object who is thoroughly idealized. This dramatically altered superego is then projected into persons in the outside world with whom the manic patient establishes idealized relationships that are free from any negative characteristics, such as hatred and anger.

CLINICAL IMPLICATIONS The overthrow of the superego characteristic of manic states manifests itself clinically as lack of conscientiousness, disregard for laws or rules of conduct, and hypersexuality.

A 45-year-old dentist in the throes of a manic episode was admitted to a psychiatric hospital. The psychiatry resident who was on duty attempted to take a history of the patient, who refused to cooperate in any way with the examination. Instead, he told jokes, most of which contained sexual innuendoes, and tried to engage the female resident in seductive banter. When a male nurse arrived at the scene to assist with the admission, the patient suggested that the resident could have sex with him while the nurse watched. He denied having any problems that required hospitalization and said that his wife had forced him to come to the hospital because she was a prude and did not like any of his sexual demands. He said he had the largest penis in the city and that he had to fight off women who were dying to sleep with him.

Some manic patients induce a sense of giddiness in clinicians, so that serious and even tragic dimensions of the clinical situation are minimized or glossed over. Also, the grandiose and expansive sense of self is often an obvious compensatory reaction to feelings of profoundly low self-esteem. As in the case of the manic dentist, patients may attempt to convince others that they have extraordinary sexual prowess or that they are besieged by admirers; such attempts are ways of dealing with feelings of sexual inadequacy or loneliness. Some manic patients write novels or "scientific" treatises that are hundreds of pages long and characterize their creative products as brilliant works of genius. When others read them and do not understand them, the patients suggest that other people lack the intelligence to comprehend their sophisticated thinking.

OTHER PSYCHOLOGICAL THEORIES

ADOLF MEYER Meyer viewed depression as a person's reaction to a distressing life experience, such as a financial setback, the loss of a job, the death of a loved one, or a serious physical illness. He believed that depression must always be understood in the context of the patient's life history, as an event that has psychic causality.

KAREN HORNEY Horney believed that children raised by parents who are rejecting and unloving are prone to feelings of insecurity and loneliness. In her view, children need to be loved but fear criticism and rejection, which makes them susceptible to feelings of depression and helplessness.

SANDOR RADO Rado linked depression to a profound feeling of helplessness. He believed that anhedonia, the inability to experience pleasure, is a central phenomenon in depression that develops when persons are not aware of their capacities or are unable to provide feelings of emotional self-gratification. Rado connected severe depression with a punitive superego that punishes the patient for unconscious hostility toward a deceased loved one.

JOHN BOWLBY Bowlby saw depression from an ethological perspective that emphasized disturbances of the mother-infant attachment bond. He believed that separations of infants from mothers (or other caretakers) early in life lead to feelings of depression and hopelessness that may in some cases continue throughout the life cycle.

HARRY STACK SULLIVAN Although Sullivan concentrated his efforts on schizophrenia more than on mood disorders, his interpersonal perspective applies to both. He thought that adverse interactions between persons and their psychosocial environments were critical to the development of depression.

COGNITIVE-BEHAVIORAL THEORY According to the theory developed by Aaron Beck, depression results from specific cognitive distortions that are present in persons prone to depression. Those distortions are referred to as *depressogenic schemata,* which are cognitive templates that perceive both internal and external data in ways that are altered by early experiences. Those schemata are associated with four systematic errors in logic: overgeneralization, magnification of negative events with a simultaneous minimization of positive events, arbitrary inference, and selective abstraction.

LEARNED HELPLESSNESS The learned helplessness theory of depression connects depressive phenomena to the experience of uncontrollable events. For example, when dogs in a laboratory were exposed to electrical shocks from which they could not escape, they showed certain behaviors that differentiated them from dogs who had not been exposed to such uncontrollable events. After exposure to the shocks, they would not cross a barrier to stop the flow of electric shock when put in a new learning situation. According to the learned helplessness theory, the dogs learned that outcomes were independent of responses, so they had both cognitive motivational deficit (meaning they would not make attempts to escape the shock) and emotional deficit (indicating a decreased reactivity to the shock). In the reformulated view of learned helplessness as applied to human depression, internal causal explanations are thought to produce a loss of self-esteem after adverse external events. Behaviorists who subscribe to the theory stress that improvement of depression is contingent on the patient's learning a sense of control and mastery of the environment.

SUGGESTED CROSS-REFERENCES

Further discussion of psychoanalytic theory can be found in Section 6.1. For additional material on characterological depression, see the discussion of borderline personality disorder in Chapter 25.

REFERENCES

Abraham K: Notes on the psycho-analytical investigation and treatment of manic-depressive insanity and allied conditions. In *Selected Papers of Karl Abraham, M.D.*, p 137. Basic Books, New York, 1953.

American Psychiatric Association: Practice guidelines for major depressive disorder in adults. Am J Psychiatry (Suppl) *150:* 126, 1993.

*Arieti S: Psychotherapy of severe depression. Am J Psychiatry *134:* 864, 1977.

*Bibring E: The mechanism of depression. In *Affective Disorders: Psychoanalytic Contributions to Their Study*, P. Greenacre, editor, p 13. International Universities Press, New York, 1953.

*Brenner C: A psychoanalytic perspective on depression. J Am Psychoanal Assoc *39:* 25, 1991.

Broadhead W E, Blazer D G, George L K, Tse C K: Depression, disability days, and days off from work in a prospective epidemiologic survey. JAMA *264:* 2524, 1990.

Coe C L, Glass J C, Wiener S G, Levine S: Behavioral but not physiological adaptation to repeated separation in mother and infant primates. Psychoneuroendocrinology *8:* 401, 1983.

Coe C L, Mendoza S P, Smotherman W P, Levine S: Mother-infant attachment in the squirrel monkey: Adrenal responses to separation. Behav Biol *22:* 256, 1978.

Coe C L, Wiener S G, Rosenberg L T, Levine S: Endocrine and immune responses to separation and maternal loss in nonhuman primates. In *The Psychobiology of Attachment and Separation,* M Reite, T Field, editors, p 163. Academic Press, Orlando, 1985.

Depression Guideline Panel: *Depression in Primary Care*, vol 2, *Treatment of Major Depression.* US Department of Health and Human Services, Rockville, MD, 1993.

Feinstein S C, Wolpert E A: Juvenile manic-depressive illness: Clinical and therapeutic considerations. J Am Acad Child Psychiatry *12:* 123, 1973.

Freud S: The ego and the id. In *Standard Edition of the Complete Psychological Works of Sigmund Freud,* vol 19, p 3. Hogarth Press, London, 1961.

*Freud S: Mourning and melancholia. In *Standard Edition of the Complete Psychological Works of Sigmund Freud,* vol 14, p 237. Hogarth Press, London, 1963.

Gabbard G O: *Psychodynamic Psychiatry in Clinical Practice: The DSM-IV Edition.* American Psychiatric Press, Washington, 1994.

Gabbard G O: Psychodynamic psychiatry in the decade of the brain. Am J. Psychiatry *149:* 991, 1992.

Gold P W, Goodwin F K, Chrousos G P: Clinical and biochemical manifestations of depression: Relation to the neurobiology of stress, part I. N Engl J Med *319:* 348, 1988.

Gold PW, Goodwin F K, Chrousos G P: Clinical and biochemical manifestations of depression: Relation to the neurobiology of stress, part II. N Engl J Med *319:* 413, 1988.

Jacobson E: Psychotic identifications. In *Depression: Comparative Studies of Normal, Neurotic, and Psychotic Conditions,* p 242. International Universities Press, New York, 1971.

Jacobson E: Transference problems in depressives. In *Depression: Comparative Studies of Normal, Neurotic, and Psychotic Conditions,* p 284. International Universities Press, New York, 1971.

Kendler K S, Kessler R C, Neale M C, Heath A C, Eaves L J: The prediction of major depression in women: Toward an integrated etiological model. Am J Psychiatry *150:* 1139, 1993.

*Klein M: Mourning and its relation to manic-depressive states. In *Love, Guilt, and Reparation and Other Works 1921–1945,* p 344. Free Press, New York, 1975.

Klerman G L, Weissman M M, editors: *New Applications of Interpersonal Therapy.* American Psychiatric Press, Washington, 1993.

Kohut H: *The Analysis of the Self: A Systematic Approach to the Psychoanalytic Approach of Narcissistic Personality Disorders.* International Universities Press, New York, 1971.

Kohut H: *How Does Analysis Cure?* A Goldberg, editor. University of Chicago Press, Chicago, 1984.

Marin D B, Kocsis J H, Frances A J: Personality disorders in dysthymia. J Per Dis *7:* 223, 1993.

Miller M D, Frank E, Cornes C: Applying interpersonal psychotherapy to bereavement-related depression following loss of a spouse in late life. J Psychother Prac Res *3:* 149, 1994.

Lewin B D: *The Psychoanalysis of Elation.* Norton, New York, 1950.

Loeb F F, Loeb L R: Psychoanalytic observations on the effect of lithium on manic attacks. J Am Psychoanal Assoc *35:* 877, 1987.

Phillips K A, Gunderson J G, Hirschfeld R M A, Smith L E: A review of the depressive personality. Am J Psychiatry *147:* 830, 1990.

Slavney P R: The mind-brain problem, epistemology, and psychiatric education. Acad Psychiatry *17:* 59, 1993.

Suomi S J: The development of affect in rhesus monkeys. In *The Psychobiology of Affective Development,* N Fox, R Davidson, editors, p 119. Erlbaum, Hillsdale, NJ, 1984.

Suomi S J: Early stress and adult emotional reactivity in Rhesus monkeys. In *Childhood Environment and Adult Disease: Symposium No. 156,* Ciba Foundation Symposium Staff, editors, p 171. Wiley, Chichester, England, 1991.

16.6
MOOD DISORDERS: CLINICAL FEATURES

HAGOP S. AKISKAL, M.D.

HETEROGENEITY OF MOOD DISORDERS

NOSOLOGY Mood disorders are characterized by pervasive dysregulation of mood and psychomotor activity as well as by related biorhythmic disturbances. The rubric of affective disorder—which in some European classifications also subsumes morbid anxiety states—increasingly is being replaced by the nosologically more delimited concept of mood disorder. Thus the term "mood disorder" is now the preferred term in both the World Health Organization's 10th revision of the *International Classification of Diseases and Related Problems* (ICD-10, 1992) and the American Psychiatric Association's (APA) fourth edition of *Diagnostic and Statistical Manual of Mental Disorders* (DSM-IV, 1994) for bipolar disorder (with manic or hypomanic and depressive episodes) and major depressive disorders and their respective attenuated variants known as cyclothymic and dysthymic disorders.

Conditions that in earlier editions of those manuals were categorized as endogenous depression, involutional melancholia, and psychotic depressive reaction have been incorporated into major depressive disorder, whereas depressive neurosis has been largely absorbed by dysthymic disorders. Although the neurotic-endogenous distinction has been officially deleted, the term "melancholic features" is now used as a qualifying phrase for those major depressive disorders where biological concomitants predominate. While both the American and international classifications recognize the common occurrence of mixed anxiety-depressions, it is unresolved as to whether they should be classified with mood disorders or with anxiety disorders. It is equally uncertain how to classify the classic neurasthenic conditions, which have reemerged under the name "chronic fatigue syndrome."

DESTIGMATIZATION The reshuffling and reclassification of various affective conditions into the mood disorders section of the third edition of DSM (DSM-III) and DSM-IV has, on balance, led to considerable broadening of their boundaries. That reflects, in part, new developments in pharmacotherapy that have resulted in considerable alleviation of suffering for persons with classic mood disorders. As a result many persons with recurrent mood disorders who would have been otherwise disabled are now able to lead productive lives. Those gratifying results have, in turn, helped to destigmatize that group of disorders. Destigmatization has been further facilitated by published self-revelations of famous persons with depressive disorder and bipolar disorder.

SPECTRUM OF MOOD DISORDERS As often happens when new therapeutic interventions prove successful, the past decade has witnessed an increased readiness to diagnose mood disorders—and their variants—even where clinical features are atypical. Those developments should not be dismissed as mere therapeutic fad, however. External validating strategies, such as familial-genetic studies and prospective follow-up, can now be used to buttress the broadened concept of mood disorders. New research comparing monozygotic and dizygotic twins has demonstrated that the genetic potential to mood disorders embraces entities that extend beyond the narrow concept of endogenous depression (melancholia in DSM-IV) to subsume a larger variety of depressions, including many affected persons in the community who have never received psychiatric treatment. Although such data might seem counterintuitive to those who would restrict depression to a core primary biological disease, they suggest that the constitutional predisposition for mood dysregulation occurs in as many as one of every three persons. That ratio is similar to the proportion of those who develop a full depressive disorder following bereavement or to that of rhesus monkeys developing depressivelike behavior following a separation paradigm. Those figures, in turn, suggest that many subjects possess protective factors against major depressive breakdowns; alternatively, such data suggest that other factors mediate which person with emotional distress will progress to a clinical case. A great deal thus might be learned about the nature of pathological affective processes by studying self-limiting affective conditions on the border of mood disorders.

The suffering and dysfunction resulting from mood disorders are among the most common reasons advanced for consulting psychiatrists and other physicians. All great physicians of the past, beginning with Hippocrates, have devoted considerable space in their general medical texts to the clinical characterization of such disorders. Those classic texts provided detailed clinical portrayals of both melancholia and mania, as well as their cyclic alterations in the same patient. Greek physicians recognized a broad spectrum of affective disturbances, ranging from the relatively mild temperamental forms (which in the official nosology is represented by dysthymic disorder and cyclothymic disorder) to the more severe illnesses (including what today is considered mood disorder with mood-congruent and mood-incongruent psychotic features). The ancients were also aware of the intimate relation of morbid states of fear to melancholia. Finally, they noted that melancholia and certain physical diseases shared seasonal incidence, and described the common occurrence of alcohol indulgence, especially in those prone to mania.

BOUNDARIES The boundaries between temperament (personality) and mood disorder, grief and melancholia, anxiety and depressive states, depressive and bipolar disorders, mood-congruent and mood-incongruent psychotic features, and other (schizophrenic) psychotic conditions are still unresolved. Since the earliest descriptions in ancient medical treatise, mood disorders have been known to be highly comorbid with alcohol use and somatic disease. These trends continue to be true today, with the addition of substance use disorders.

AFFECTS, MOODS, TEMPERAMENTS, AND MORBID MOOD STATES

ETHOLOGICAL CONSIDERATIONS Affects and moods refer to different aspects of emotion. Affect is communicated through facial expression, vocal inflection, gestures, and posture, and, according to current ethological research, is intended to move people to appraise whether a person is satisfied, distressed, disgusted, or in danger. Thus joy, sadness, anger, and fear are basic affects that serve a communicative function in humans and other primates, as well as many mammalian species.

Affects tend to be short-lived expressions, reflecting momentary emotional contingencies. Moods convey sustained emotions; their more enduring nature means that they are experienced long enough to be felt inwardly. Moods are made manifest in subtle ways, and their accurate assessment often requires empathic understanding by the interviewer. The words that subjects use to describe their inner emotions may or may not coincide with the technical terms used by researchers or clinicians. Furthermore, the inward emotion and the prevailing affective tone may conflict. That conflict could be due to deliberate simulation (that is, the subject does not wish to reveal his or her inner emotion), or it could be the result of a pathological lesion or process that is affecting the emotions and their neural substrates. Thus evaluating moods and affective expression requires considerable experience.

SADNESS AND JOY The normal emotions of sadness and joy are part of everyday life and should be differentiated from major depressive disorder and mania. Sadness, or normal depression, is a universal human response to defeat, disappointment, or other adversities. The response may be adaptive, in an evolutionary sense, by permitting withdrawal to conserve inner resources, or it might signal the need for support from significant others.

Transient depressive periods also occur as reactions to certain holidays or anniversaries, as well as during the premenstrual phase and the first week postpartum. Termed, respectively, holiday blues, anniversary reactions, premenstrual dysphoric disorder (see Section 15.4) and maternity blues, the conditions are not in themselves psychopathological, but those predisposed to mood disorder may develop clinical depression during such times.

In view of the higher prevalence of depression in women, premenstrual affective changes—tension, irritability, hostility, and labile mood—have received much attention. The attempt to establish a late-luteal-phase dysphoric disorder has neglected the not uncommon occurrence of premenstrual eutonia, increased energy, and sexual drive. Those mixed affective manifestations tend to point toward a biphasic phenomenon. Available data do not support the existence of a distinct premenstrual mood disorder. Rather, women with severe premenstrual complaints appear to have higher rates of lifetime major mood disorders. Furthermore, such events as epileptic attacks, panic states, and the perpetration of violent crimes might, in some instances, be associated with the premenstrual phase. Those considerations suggest the hypothesis that psychobiological changes occurring premenstrually exacerbate, in a nonspecific way, a large spectrum of neuropsychiatric disorders to which the women are otherwise predisposed. In other words, the exaggerated premenstrual variability in emotional equilibrium is unlikely to be the primary factor or cause of those neuropsychiatric manifestations.

GRIEF Also known as normal bereavement, grief is considered to be the prototype of reactive depression, and occurs in response to significant separations and losses, such as death, divorce, romantic disappointment, leaving familiar environments, forced emigration, or civilian catastrophes. (Unfortunately, DSM-IV tends to limit the concept of normal grief to loss due to death.) In addition to depressed affect appropriate to the loss, bereavement reactions are characterized by the prominence of sympathetic arousal and restlessness, believed to represent, from an evolutionary perspective, physiological and behavioral mechanisms to facilitate the search for the lost object. Like other adversities, bereavement and loss do not generally seem to cause depressive disorder, except in those predisposed to mood disorder.

ELATION The positive emotion of elation is popularly linked to success and achievement. However, paradoxical depressions may also follow such positive events, possibly because of the increased responsibilities that often have to be faced alone. Elation is conceptualized psychodynamically as a defense against depression or as a denial of the pain of loss, as exemplified by the so-called maniacal grief, a rare form of bereavement reaction in which elated hyperactivity may replace the expected grief.

Other pseudomanic states include the brief energetic and unusually lucid periods encountered in dying patients or in those who need to take superhuman action in the face of unusual duress, both of which have been conceptualized as flights into health. It is also conceivable that in predisposed persons those reactions might be the prelude to a genuine manic episode. Given such predisposition, sleep deprivation (which commonly accompanies major stressors) might represent one of the intermediary mechanisms between stressor and adverse clinical outcome.

AFFECTIVE TEMPERAMENTS Another mediating factor between normal and pathological moods is temperament. Most persons have a characteristic pattern of basal affective oscillations that defines their temperament. For instance, some are easily moved to tears by sad or happy circumstances, whereas others tend to remain placid. Normally, oscillations in affective tone are relatively minor, tend to resonate with day-to-day events, and do not interfere with functioning. Some exhibit greater variability of emotional responses whereby, with no obvious provocation, the person alternates between normal mood and sadness or elation, or both. They tend to cluster into basic temperamental types: the depressive temperament (where the person easily swings into the sad direction), the hyperthymic temperament (where the person is naturally inclined toward cheerful moods), and the cyclothymic temperament (where the person swings between cheerful and sad moods). All three temperaments typically have an early onset and tend to persist throughout life.

An examination of the traits associated with those temperaments can provide the rationale for Ernst Kretschmer's hypothesis about the social functions they served. Thus, the person with a depressive temperament (Table 16.6-1) is hard-working, dependable, and suitable for jobs that require long periods of devotion to meticulous detail. Some such persons shoulder the burdens of existence without experiencing its pleasures. The hyperthymic temperament (Table 16.6-1), endowed with high levels of energy, extraversion, and humor, will assume leadership positions in society or excel in the performing arts or entertainment. In talented persons the cycloid temperament, which alternates between sadness and elation, could provide the inspiration and the intensity needed for composing music, painting, or writing poetry. The danger with such temperaments is that they could swing too far in one or the other direction, or in both directions. Such substances as alcohol, caffeine, and other stimulants when used by those persons might further destabilize their affect regulation.

Temperaments then are best regarded as variations of normal emotional expressiveness, which might continue throughout life without significant impairment, or they might be accentuated in the teenage and early adult years, and become manifest as a dysthymic disorder or a cyclothymic disorder with its attendant interpersonal, academic, and vocational problems. Finally, they might be the point of departure for major mood disorders.

MORBID MOOD STATES Mood disorders are morbid mood states characterized by the following features.

Pathological mood change Pathological moods are distinguished from their normal counterparts by being out of proportion to any concurrent stressor or situation; being unresponsive to reassurance; being sustained for weeks, months, and sometimes years; and having a pervasive effect on the person, such that judgment is seriously influenced by the mood.

Endoreactive moods Major depression and mania are diagnosed respectively, when, sadness or elation is overly intense and continues beyond the expected impact of a stressful life event; indeed, the morbid mood might arise without apparent or significant life stress. Thus the pathological process in mood disorders is in part defined by the ease with which an intense emotional state is released, and especially by its tendency to

TABLE 16.6-1
Attributes of Depressive and Hyperthymic Temperaments

Depressive	Hyperthymic
1. Gloomy, incapable of fun, complaining	1. Cheerful and exuberant
2. Humorless	2. Articulate and jocular
3. Skeptical, pessimistic, and given to brooding	3. Overoptimistic and carefree
4. Guilt-prone, low self-esteem, and preoccupied with inadequacy or failure	4. Overconfident, self-assured, boastful, and grandiose
5. Introverted with restricted social life	5. Extroverted and people seeking
6. Sluggish, living a life out of action	6. High energy level, full of plans and improvident activities
7. Few interests, but which, nonetheless, can be pursued with relative constancy	7. Versatile, with broad interests
8. Passive	8. Overinvolved and meddlesome
9. Reliable, dependable, and devoted	9. Uninhibited and stimulus seeking
10. Habitual long sleeper (more than 10 hours a night)	10. Habitual short sleeper (less than six hours a night)

persist autonomously even when the offending stressor is no longer operative. Rather than being endogenous (that is, occurring in the absence of precipitants), mood disorders are best conceptualized as endoreactive (that is, once released, they tend to persist autonomously). The homeostatic dyscontrol of mood, which is part of a more pervasive mood dysregulation, resists reversal to the habitual or baseline affective tone. DSM-IV, which tends to disparage theory and adhere to a descriptive level of operationalization, gives insufficient weight to this fundamental characteristic of mood disorders.

Syndromal illness In a more descriptive vein what sets mood disorders apart from their normal emotional counterparts is the clustering of signs and symptoms into discrete syndromes that typically recur on an episodic basis or pursue a course of intermittent chronicity. Such cyclicity—and in some cases regular recurrence known as periodicity—represents other signs of mood dysregulation particularly relevant to bipolar disorder.

Impairment Normative reactions to adversity and stress, including biological stress, typically consist of transient admixtures of anxiety and dysphoria that are best captured under the DSM-IV rubric of adjustment disorder with mixed emotional features. That is, the self-limiting reactions are best qualified broadly as normal affective states that produce little, if any, impairment in the main areas of functioning.

Although anxiety, irritability, and anger do occur in various types of mood disorders, it is pathologically sustained mood states of depression and elation that characterize those disorders. Morbid mood states (mood disorders) then consist of protracted emotional reactions that deepen or escalate, respectively, into clinical depression or mania, with a tendency to recur or to evolve, in as many as a third of cases, into chronicity. The contribution of temperamental peculiarities to such outcomes should be apparent. The impaired functioning characteristic of mood disorders is thus based on a combination of factors, which include severity, autonomy, recurrence, and chronicity of the clinical features.

To recapitulate, dysregulation in mood disorders can take different forms. It could become manifest as a single severe episode that persists autonomously for months and sometimes for years, or it might recur with episodes of varying severity, years apart or in rapid succession, and with or without interepisodic remission. In general, the earlier the age at onset, the more likely it is that there will be recurrences, especially those that are bipolar in nature. Thus, depending on the course of the illness, impairment could be state dependent, occurring during an episode, or it could extend into the interepisodic period. National Institute of Mental Health (NIMH) estimates suggest that, on the average, a woman with bipolar disorder spends 12 years in florid episodes (often hospitalized), loses 14 years from a productive career and motherhood, and has her life curtailed by 9 years.

Recent observations have also revealed another pattern of impairment. In dysthymic disorder and cyclothymic disorder, which represent an intensification of temperamental instability, impairment is not due to the severity of the mood disturbance per se, but to the cumulative impact of the dysregulation beginning in the juvenile or early adult years and continuing unabated or intermittently over long periods; hence the frequent confusion with character pathology. Here the impairment is more subtle but nonetheless pervasive. Persons with cyclothymic disorder tend to be perpetual dilettantes whereas those with dysthymic disorder often lead morose and colorless lives.

PSYCHOPATHOLOGY AND CLINICAL PRESENTATION

DEPRESSIVE SYNDROME Like other illnesses, depressive disorder clusters into signs and symptoms that constitute what DSM-IV and ICD-10 term major depressive episode (Table 16.6-2). Those criteria attempt to set an operational threshold for depressive disorder based on a specified number of items and their temporal patterns. It is only after taking an in-depth phenomenological approach that a clinician can ascertain the presence of a depressive disorder. The DSM-IV diagnostic criteria for major depressive disorder (Tables 16.6-3 and 16.6-4) provide only a general guide. Disturbances in all four spheres—mood, psychomotor activity, cognitive, and vegetative—should be ordinarily present for a definitive diagnosis of major depressive disorder, although that is not specified in DSM-IV.

Mood disturbances Mood change, usually considered the sine qua non of morbid depression, becomes manifest in a variety of disturbances, including (1) painful arousal, (2) hypersensitivity to unpleasant events, (3) insensitivity to pleasant events, (4) insensitivity to unpleasant events, (5) reduced anticipatory pleasure, (6) anhedonia or reduced consummatory pleasure, (7) affective blunting, and (8) apathy. The phenomenology and psychometric properties of that broad range of mood distur-

TABLE 16.6-2
Criteria for Major Depressive Episode

A. Five (or more) of the following symptoms have been present during the same two-week period and represent a change from previous functioning; at least one of the symptoms is either (1) depressed mood or (2) loss of interest or pleasure.
Note: Do not include symptoms that are clearly due to a general medical condition, or mood-incongruent delusions or hallucinations.
(1) depressed mood most of the day, nearly every day, as indicated by either subjective report (e.g., feels sad or empty) or observation made by others (e.g., appears tearful). **Note:** In children and adolescents, can be irritable mood.
(2) markedly diminished interest or pleasure in all, or almost all, activities most of the day, nearly every day (as indicated by either subjective account or observation made by others)
(3) significant weight loss when not dieting or weight gain (e.g., a change of more than 5% of body weight in a month), or decrease or increase in appetite nearly every day. **Note:** In children, consider failure to make expected weight gains.
(4) insomnia or hypersomnia nearly every day
(5) psychomotor agitation or retardation nearly every day (observable by others, not merely subjective feelings of restlessness or being slowed down)
(6) fatigue or loss of energy nearly every day
(7) feelings of worthlessness or excessive or inappropriate guilt (which may be delusional) nearly every day (not merely self-reproach or guilt about being sick)
(8) diminished ability to think or concentrate, or indecisiveness, nearly every day (either by subjective account or as observed by others)
(9) recurrent thoughts of death (not just fear of dying), recurrent suicidal ideation without a specific plan, or a suicide attempt or a specific plan for committing suicide

B. The symptoms do not meet criteria for a mixed episode.
C. The symptoms cause clinically significant distress or impairment in social, occupational, or other important areas of functioning.
D. The symptoms are not due to the direct physiological effects of a substance (e.g., a drug of abuse, a medication) or a general medical condition (e.g., hypothyroidism).
E. The symptoms are not better accounted for by bereavement, i.e., after the loss of a loved one, the symptoms persist for longer than two months or are characterized by marked functional impairment, morbid preoccupation with worthlessness, suicidal ideation, psychotic symptoms, or psychomotor retardation.

Table from DSM-IV, *Diagnostic and Statistical Manual of Mental Disorders,* ed 4. Copyright American Psychiatric Association, Washington, 1994. Used with permission.

TABLE 16.6-3
Diagnostic Criteria for Major Depressive Disorder, Single Episode

A. Presence of a single major depressive episode.
B. The major depressive episode is not better accounted for by schizoaffective disorder and is not superimposed on schizophrenia, schizophreniform disorder, delusional disorder, or psychotic disorder not otherwise specified.
C. There has never been a manic episode, a mixed episode, or a hypomanic episode. **Note:** This exclusion does not apply if all of the manic-like, mixed-like, or hypomaniclike episodes are substance or treatment induced or are due to the direct physiological effects of a general medical condition.

Specify (for current or most recent episode):
Severity/psychotic/remission specifiers
Chronic
With catatonic features
With melancholic features
With atypical features
With postpartum onset

Table from DSM-IV, *Diagnostic and Statistical Manual of Mental Disorders,* ed 4. Copyright American Psychiatric Association, Washington, 1994. Used with permission.

TABLE 16.6-4
Diagnostic Criteria for Major Depressive Disorder, Recurrent

A. Presence of two or more major depressive episodes.
Note: To be considered separate episodes, there must be an interval of at least two consecutive months in which criteria are not met for a major depressive episode.
B. The major depressive episodes are not better accounted for by schizoaffective disorder and are not superimposed on schizophrenia, schizophreniform disorder, delusional disorder, or psychotic disorder not otherwise specified.
C. There has never been a manic episode, a mixed episode, or a hypomanic episode. **Note:** This exclusion does not apply if all of the maniclike, mixed-like, or hypomaniclike episodes are substance or treatment induced or are due to the direct physiological effects of a general medical condition.

Specify (for current or most recent episode):
Severity/psychotic/remission specifiers
Chronic
With catatonic features
With melancholic features
With atypical features
With postpartum onset

Specify:
Longitudinal course specifiers (with and without interepisode recovery)
With seasonal pattern

Table from DSM-IV, *Diagnostic and Statistical Manual of Mental Disorders,* ed 4. Copyright American Psychiatric Association, Washington, 1994. Used with permission.

bances are under investigation at the Salpêtrière Hospital in Paris. The focus here will be primarily on painfully aroused mood (depression) and diminished capacity for pleasure (anhedonia), two mood disturbances given selective weight in DSM-IV and ICD-IO.

DEPRESSED MOOD The term "depressed mood" refers to negative affective arousal, variously described as depressed, anguished, mournful, irritable, or anxious. Those terms tend to banalize a morbidly painful emotion that is typically experienced as worse than any physical pain. There is thus a physical quality to depressed mood, which in the extreme is indescribably painful. Even when not so severe, depressive suffering is qualitatively distinct from its neurotic counterparts, taking the form of groundless apprehensions with severe inner turmoil and torment. That description is particularly apt for middle-aged and elderly persons, who were once considered to be suffering from involutional melancholia. The sustained nature of the mood permits no respite, although it tends to be less intense in the evening. Suicide may represent an attempt to find deliverance from such unrelenting psychic torment: death can be experienced as comforting.

Patients with a milder form of the malady typically seen in primary care settings might deny experiencing mournful moods and instead complain of physical agony in the form of headache, epigastric pain, precordial distress, and so on, in the absence of any evidence of physical illness. Such conditions have been described as *depressio sine depressione,* or masked depression. In such cases, commonly observed in older patients, the physician should corroborate the presence of mood disturbance by the depressed affect in the patient's facial expression, voice, and overall appearance.

ANHEDONIA AND LOSS OF INTEREST Paradoxically, the heightened perception of pain in many persons with depressive disorder is accompanied by an inability to experience normal emotions. Patients exhibiting the disturbance may lose the capacity to cry, a deficit that is reversed as the depression is lifting.

In evaluating anhedonia it is not enough to inquire whether the patient has lost the sense of pleasure; the clinician must document that the patient has actually given up previously enjoyed pastimes. When mild, anhedonia evidences with decreased interest in life. Later, patients complain that they have lost all interest in things that gave them pleasure. In the extreme they lose their feelings for their children or spouses, who once were a source of joy. Thus the hedonic deficit in clinical depression might represent a special instance of a more pervasive inability to experience emotions.

Some patients emotionally cut off from others, experience depersonalization, and the world seems strange to them (derealization). The impact of the loss of emotional resonance can be so pervasive that patients may surrender values and beliefs that had previously given meaning to their lives. For instance, a member of the clergy might present with the complaint that he or she no longer believes in the work, that he or she has lost God. The inability of the person with depressive disorder to experience normal emotions—commonly observed among young depressed patients—is different from the schizophrenic patient's flat affect in that the loss of emotions is itself experienced as painful, that is, the patient suffers immensely from the inability to experience emotions.

Psychomotor disturbances In depression refer to psychomotor changes consisting of abnormalities in the motor expression of mental activity.

AGITATION Although agitation (pressured speech, restlessness, wringing of hands, and pulling of hair) is the more readily observed abnormality, it appears less specific to the illness than does retardation (slowing of psychomotor activity). Psychophysiological studies have documented that such slowing often coexists with agitation.

PSYCHOMOTOR RETARDATION Underlying many of the deficits seen in clinical depression, some authorities believe psychomotor retardation to be the core or primary pathology in mood disorders. Morbid depression—what patients describe as being "down"—can be understood in terms of extreme psychomotor slowing. The patient experiences inertia, being unable to act physically and mentally. Recent brain imaging research that has revealed subcortical (extrapyramidal system) disturbances in mood disorders tends to support the centrality of psychomotor dysfunction in these disorders.

Long neglected in psychopathological research, psychomotor retardation has now been measured with precision. In the Salpêtrière Retardation Scale special emphasis is placed on the following disturbances: (1) paucity of spontaneous movements; (2) slumped posture with downcast gaze; (3) overwhelming fatigue—patients complain that "everything is an effort"; (4) reduced flow and amplitude of speech and increased latency of responses, often giving rise to monosyllabic speech; (5) a subjective feeling that time is passing slowly or has stopped; (6) poor concentration and forgetfulness; (7) painful rumination—thinking that dwells on a few (usually unpleasant) topics; and (8) indecisiveness, which refers to an inability to make simple decisions.

DSM-IV places greater emphasis on the more easily observable objective or physical aspects of retardation. For the patient, however, the subjective sense of slowing is often its more pervasive and disabling aspect. That psychological dimension of retardation is most reliably elicited from depressed persons with good verbal skills.

Ms. A., a 34-year-old literature professor, presented to a mood clinic with the following complaint: "I am in a daze, confused, disoriented, staring. My thoughts do not flow, my mind is arrested . . . I seem to lack any sense of direction, purpose . . . I have such an inertia, I cannot assert myself. I cannot fight, I have no will."

A patient with lesser linguistic sophistication would simply complain of an inability to perform household chores or a difficulty in concentrating on his or her studies. Such psychomotor deficits in turn underlie depressed patients' diminished efficiency or their inability to work.

PSEUDODEMENTIA AND STUPOR In elderly persons the slowing of mental functions can be so pronounced that the patient may experience memory difficulties, disorientation, and confusion. In young persons psychomotor slowing is sometimes so extreme that the patient might slide into a stupor, unable to participate even in such basic biological functions as feeding himself or herself; such an episode often represents the precursor of bipolar disorder, which later declares itself by mania. (In the author's view, it is terminologically and historically misleading to label those phenomena as catatonic features, as stipulated by DSM-IV.) Today depressive disorder is diagnosed in its earlier stages, and subtle degrees of stupor are much more likely to be encountered clinically, as illustrated by the following vignette:

A 20-year-old male college student seen in the emergency room spoke of "being stuck—as if I have fallen into a black hole and can't get out." Further evaluation revealed that the patient was speaking metaphorically of his total loss of initiative and drive, and as having been engulfed by the disease process. To a clinician without the requisite phenomenological training, such a patient might be considered bizarre, and perhaps even psychotic. Yet the patient responded dramatically to fluoxetine (Prozac) and in two weeks was back in school.

Cognitive disturbances According to the cognitive view of depression, negative evaluations of the self, the world, and the future are central to understanding depressed mood and behavior. It is equally likely, however, that the depressed mood colors perceptions of the self and others or that disturbed psychomotor activity leads to negative self-evaluations. Therefore, it is best to approach cognitive changes in depression empirically as key clinical manifestations of depression. Clinically those faulty thinking patterns become manifest as follows: (1) ideas of deprivation and loss; (2) low self-esteem and self-confidence; (3) self-reproach and pathological guilt; (4) helplessness, hopelessness, and pessimism; and (5) recurrent thoughts of death and suicide.

The essential characteristic of depressive thinking is that the sufferer views everything in an extremely negative light. The self-accusations are typically unjustified or are blown out of proportion, as in the case of a middle-aged woman who was tormented by guilt because as a child she had not repaid 5 cents she had borrowed from a classmate. Some of the thoughts may verge on the delusional. For instance, an internationally renowned scientist complained that he was "nothing." Such self-evaluations, which indicate an extremely low image of self, might nonetheless reflect an accurate perception of the impairment due to psychomotor retardation.

MOOD-CONGRUENT PSYCHOTIC FEATURES In depressive disorder with psychotic features negative thinking acquires grossly delusional proportions, being maintained with such conviction that the thoughts are not amenable to change by evidence to the contrary. Classically, delusional thinking in depression derives from humankind's four basic insecurities, those regarding health, financial status, moral worth, and relationship to others. Thus severely depressed patients may have delusions of worthlessness and sinfulness, reference, and persecution. They believe they are being singled out for their past mistakes and that everyone is aware of their errors. Persecutory ideation in depression is often *prosecutory* in nature in that it derives from the belief that the person deserves punishment for such transgressions. A severely depressed man may feel so incompetent in all areas of functioning, including the sexual sphere, that he may suspect his wife of having an affair (delusion of infidelity).

Other depressed persons believe that they have lost all their money and that their children will starve (delusions of poverty); or that they harbor an occult illness, such as cancer or the acquired immune deficiency syndrome (AIDS) (delusions of ill health); or that parts of their bodies are missing (nihilistic delusions). In more severe illness the patient might feel that the world has changed, that calamity and destruction await everyone. In rare instances a parent with such delusions might kill his or her young children, to save them from moral or physical decay, and then commit suicide. Finally, a minority of depressed persons may have fleeting auditory or visual hallucinations with extremely unpleasant content along the lines of their delusions (for example, hearing accusatory voices or seeing themselves in coffins or graveyards). All of those psychotic experiences are genuine affective delusions or hallucinations. They are mood congruent in the sense that they are phenomenologically understandable in light of the prevailing pathological mood.

The DSM-IV criteria for severity-psychotic-remission specifiers for current (or most recent) major depressive episode, including mood-congruent and mood-incongruent psychotic features, appear in Table 16.6-5.

MOOD-INCONGRUENT PSYCHOTIC FEATURES It is possible that so-called first-rank or Schneiderian-type symptoms could arise in the setting of a major depressive episode.

A 42-year-old civil servant said she was so paralyzed by depression that she felt that she had no personal initiative and volition left; she believed some malignant force had taken over her actions, and that it would comment on every action that she would undertake. The patient fully recovered with thymoleptic medication. There is no reason to believe that the feelings of somatic passivity and running commentary were indicative of a schizophrenic process.

Thus with proper phenomenological probing, certain classes of apparently mood-incongruent psychotic experiences listed in DSM-IV, can be understood as arising from the pathological mood and the profound changes in psychomotor activity that

TABLE 16.6-5
Criteria for Severity/Psychotic/Remission Specifiers for Current (or Most Recent) Major Depressive Episode

Note: Code in fifth digit. Can be applied to the most recent major depressive episode in major depressive disorder and to a major depressive episode in bipolar I or II disorder only if it is the most recent type of mood episode.

Mild: Few, if any, symptoms in excess of those required to make the diagnosis and symptoms result in only minor impairment in occupational functioning or in usual social activities or relationships with others.
Moderate: Symptoms or functional impairment between "mild" and "severe."
Severe without psychotic features: Several symptoms in excess of those required to make the diagnosis, **and** symptoms markedly interfere with occupational functioning or with usual social activities or relationships with others.
Severe with psychotic features: Delusions or hallucinations. If possible, specify whether the psychotic features are mood-congruent or mood-incongruent:
  Mood-congruent psychotic features: Delusions or hallucinations whose content is entirely consistent with the typical depressive themes of personal inadequacy, guilt, disease, death, nihilism, or deserved punishment.
  Mood-incongruent psychotic features: Delusions or hallucinations whose content does not involve typical depressive themes of personal inadequacy, guilt, disease, death, nihilism, or deserved punishment. Included are such symptoms as persecutory delusions (not directly related to depressive themes), thought insertion, thought broadcasting, and delusions of control.
In partial remission: Symptoms of a major depressive episode are present but full criteria are not met, or there is a period without any significant symptoms of a major depressive episode lasting less than two months following the end of the major depressive episode. (If the major depressive episode was superimposed on dysthymic disorder, the diagnosis of dysthymic disorder alone is given once the full criteria for a major depressive episode are no longer met.)
In full remission: During the past two months, no significant signs or symptoms of the disturbance were present.
Unspecified.

Table from DSM-IV, *Diagnostic and Statistical Manual of Mental Disorders,* ed 4.

accompany them. (In other instances, the clinician must search history of alcohol and/or substance use disorder or withdrawal as putative explanation for mood-incongruence in psychotic depression.)

HOPELESSNESS AND SUICIDE Given that most, if not all, clinically depressed patients find themselves locked in the private hell of their negative thoughts, it is not surprising that up to 15 percent of untreated or inadequately treated patients give up hope that they will ever recover and so kill themselves. The suicide attempt is not, however, undertaken in the depth of melancholia. One severely depressed patient, when asked if she had any suicide plans, replied, "Doctor, I don't exist—I am already dead."

Thus the risk of suicide is less pronounced during acute severe depression. Emil Kraepelin has observed that it is when psychomotor activity is improving, and yet mood and thinking are still dark, that the patient is most likely to muster the requisite energy to commit the suicidal act. Profound hopelessness on mental status evaluation should alert the clinician to the possibility of such an outcome.

There is no basis for the common belief that inquiring about suicide would provoke such behavior. On the contrary, the patient is often relieved that the physician is aware of the magnitude of his or her suffering. Suicidal ideation is commonly expressed indirectly, such as in a wish not to wake up. Some depressed persons are tormented with suicidal obsessions in the sense that they are constantly resisting unwanted urges or impulses to destroy themselves. Others might yield to such urges passively, as by careless driving or by walking among high-speed traffic. A third group will harbor elaborate plans, carefully preparing their will and taking out insurance. Such deliberate planning indicates a very high suicidal risk. The examples are not exhaustive, however, but are meant to remind clinicians in charge of depressed patients to be always alert to the possibility of suicide.

Vegetative disturbances The Greeks believed that depression was a somatic illness and ascribed it to black bile, and hence the term "melancholia." The mood change in depressive disorder is accompanied by measurable alterations of biorhythms that implicate limbic-diencephalic dysfunction. Once the changes occur, they tend to become autonomous of the environment throughout much of the episode, which means that they do not respond to interpersonal feedback of a pleasant and upbeat nature. The biological concomitants of melancholia include profound reductions in appetite, sleep, and sexual functioning, as well as alterations of other circadian rhythms, especially morning worsening of mood and psychomotor performances. Those disturbances are central to the DSM-IV concept of melancholia (Table 16.6-6), a form of depression in which such biological concomitants predominate. In a smaller subgroup of depressed persons, there is a reversal of the vegetative and circadian functions whereby there are increases in appetite and sleep—and sometimes in sexual functioning—along with an evening worsening of mood; in that atypical pattern (Table 16.6-7), now recognized in DSM-IV, patients often exhibit mood reactivity and sensitivity to rejection.

ANOREXIA AND WEIGHT LOSS Among the most reliable somatic indicators of depressive disorder are anorexia and weight loss. In addition to the presumed hypothalamic disturbance of depression, anorexia might be secondary to blunted olfactory or taste sensations or a decreased enjoyment of food, or, rarely, it might be due to a delusional belief that the food has been poisoned.

If weight loss is severe, especially after the age of 40, the psychiatrist should first rule out, through appropriate medical consultation, the likelihood of an occult malignancy. Inanition, especially in elderly persons, can lead to malnutrition and electrolyte disturbances, which represent medical emergencies.

TABLE 16.6-6
Criteria for Melancholic Features Specifier

Specify if:
With melancholic features (can be applied to the current or most recent major depressive episode in major depressive disorder and to a major depressive episode in bipolar I or bipolar II disorder only if it is the most recent type of mood episode)

A. Either of the following, occurring during the most severe period of the current episode:
   (1) loss of pleasure in all, or almost all, activities
   (2) lack of reactivity to usually pleasurable stimuli (does not feel much better, even temporarily, when something good happens)
B. Three (or more) of the following:
   (1) distinct quality of depressed mood (i.e., the depressed mood is experienced as distinctly different from the kind of feeling experienced after the death of a loved one)
   (2) depression regularly worse in the morning
   (3) early morning awakening (at least two hours before usual time of awakening)
   (4) marked psychomotor retardation or agitation
   (5) significant anorexia or weight loss
   (6) excessive or inappropriate guilt

Table from DSM-IV, *Diagnostic and Statistical Manual of Mental Disorders,* ed 4.

TABLE 16.6-7
Criteria for Atypical Features Specifier

Specify if:
With atypical features (can be applied when these features predominate during the most recent two weeks of a major depressive episode in major depressive disorder or in bipolar I or bipolar II disorder when the major depressive episode is the most recent type of mood episode, or when these features predominate during the most recent two years of dysthymic disorder)

A. Mood reactivity (i.e., mood brightens in response to actual or potential positive events)
B. Two (or more) of the following features:
 (1) significant weight gain or increase in appetite
 (2) hypersomnia
 (3) leaden paralysis (i.e., heavy, leaden feelings in arms or legs)
 (4) long-standing pattern of interpersonal rejection sensitivity (not limited to episodes of mood disturbance) that results in significant social or occupational impairment
C. Criteria are not met for with melancholic features or with catatonic features during the same episode.

Table from DSM-IV, *Diagnostic and Statistical Manual of Mental Disorders,* ed 4. Copyright American Psychiatric Association, Washington, 1994. Used with permission.

WEIGHT GAIN Overeating, decreased activity, or both may result in weight gain. In middle-aged patients it may aggravate preexisting diabetes, hypertension, or coronary artery disease. In younger patients, especially women, weight problems may conform to a bulimic pattern. That is sometimes the expression of the depressive phase of a bipolar disorder with infrequent hypomanic periods (bipolar II disorder). It does not mean, however, that all bulimia nervosa is the result of a mood disorder.

INSOMNIA Sleep disturbance, a cardinal sign of depression, often becomes manifest in insomnia that is characterized by multiple awakenings, especially in the early hours of the morning, rather than by difficulty falling asleep. The light sleep of a depressed person, in part a reflection of the painful arousal of the disorder in general, tends to prolong the depressive agony over 24 hours. Thus deep stages of sleep (3 and 4) are either decreased or deficient. The attempt to overcome the problem by drinking alcohol may initially meet with success, but ultimately will lead to an aggravation of the insomnia. That also is true for sedative-hypnotic agents, which are often prescribed by the busy general practitioner who has not spent enough time in diagnosing the depressive condition. Sedatives, including alcohol, while effective in reducing the number of awakenings in the short term, are not effective in the long run because of a further diminution of stage 3 and stage 4 sleep. They are not antidepressants and tend to prolong the depression.

HYPERSOMNIA Young depressed persons, especially those with bipolar tendencies, often complain of hypersomnia, and will have difficulty getting up in the morning.

Kevin, a 15-year-old boy, was referred to a sleep center to rule out narcolepsy. His main complaints were fatigue, boredom, and a need to sleep all the time. Although he had always been somewhat slow to get going in the morning, he now could not get out of bed to go to school. That alarmed his mother, prompting the sleep consultation. Formerly a B student, he had been failing most of his courses in the six months before referral. Psychological counseling, predicated on the premise that his family's recent move from another city had led to Kevin's isolation, had not been beneficial. He had also received an extensive neurological and general medical workup, with negative results. He slept 12 to 15 hours a day, but denied cataplexy, sleep paralysis, and hypnagogic hallucinations. During the interview he denied being depressed, but admitted that he had lost interest in everything except his pet. He had no drive, participated in no activities, and had gained 30 pounds in six months. He believed he was brain damaged and wondered whether it was worth living like that. The question of committing suicide disturbed him as it was contrary to his religious beliefs. In view of the findings he was prescribed desipramine (Norpramin) in a dosage that was gradually increased to 200 mg a day over three weeks. Not only did the desipramine reverse the presenting complaints, but it pushed him to the brink of a manic episode.

The affective nature of the disorder in such patients often goes unrecognized, and their slothful behavior and tendency to slumber may be ascribed to laziness.

CIRCADIAN DYSREGULATION Many circadian functions, such as temperature regulation and cortisol rhythms, are disrupted in major depressive disorder. Disturbances of sleep rhythms, however, have received the greatest research focus. Whether suffering from insomnia or hypersomnia, nearly two thirds of patients with depressive disorder exhibit a shortening of rapid-eye-movement (REM) latency, the period from the onset of sleep to the first REM period. That abnormality is observed throughout the depressive episode and, in persons with recurrent depression, may be seen in relatively euthymic periods as well. Their occurrence in the well relatives of the affectively ill suggests that circadian abnormalities might precede the psychological manifestations of the disorder. Other REM abnormalities include longer REM periods and increased density of eye movements in the first third of the night.

There are little data on the consistency of sleep electroencephalogram (EEG) abnormalities in patients examined from episode to episode. However, clinical experience suggests that the same patient observed over time (even during the same episode) may exhibit insomnia and morning worsening of mood and activity at one period of the disorder and hypersomnia extending to late morning hours at another period. In either case persons with depressive disorder are characteristically tired in the morning, which means that even prolonged sleep is not refreshing for them. The propensity to exhibit such divergent patterns of sleep disturbance is more likely in bipolar illness. Patients with major depressive disorder tend to exhibit insomnia in a more stereotypical fashion, episode after episode; despite extreme fatigue, even with thymoleptic medication, they rarely oversleep. Such fatigue coexisting with negative affective arousal is exhausting.

SEASONALITY Another biorhythmic disturbance in mood disorders is seasonal (especially autumn-winter) accentuation or precipitation of depression; many, if not most, of those patients experience hypomania in the spring and thus should be classified as having bipolar II disorder. In the fall and winter the patients complain of fatigue, tend to crave sugars, and overeat and oversleep. The hypersomnia in some of those patients is associated with delayed (rather than short) REM latencies. Such data suggest that circadian abnormalities in depressive disorders are characterized by dysregulation rather than by mere phase advance. The DSM-IV criteria for seasonal pattern specifier are listed in Table 16.6-8.

SEXUAL DYSFUNCTION Decreased sexual desire is seen in both depressed men and women. In addition, some women experience a temporary interruption of their menses. Depressed women are typically unresponsive to lovemaking or are disinclined to participate in it, a situation that could lead to marital conflict; psychotherapists may mistakenly ascribe the depression to the marital conflict, resulting in unnecessarily zealous psychotherapeutic attention to conjugal issues. A decrease in or loss of libido in men often results in erectile failure, which may prompt endocrinological or urological consultation. Again, depression may be ascribed to the sexual dysfunction rather than the reverse, and definitive treatment may be delayed due to the physician's focus on the sexual complaint. Some men with depressive disorder have even been subjected to permanent penile implants before having received a more definitive treatment for their depression.

Among a small subgroup of persons with depressive disorder, there may be increased sexual drive of a compulsive nature. Such patients tend to have other atypical features as well, and hence the symptom of increased sexual drive can be considered the fifth reverse vegetative sign in those patients (after evening or morning worsening of mood, initial insomnia, hypersomnia, and weight gain). In other depressed persons, increased sexual drive may indicate a mixed episode in bipolar disorder.

MANIC SYNDROME As with clinical depression, the psychopathology of mania can be conveniently discussed under mood, psychomotor, circadian, and cognitive disturbances. The clinical features of mania are generally the opposite of those of depression. Thus instead of lowered mood, thinking, activity, and self-esteem, there is elevated mood, a rush of ideas, psychomotor acceleration, and grandiosity. Despite those contrasts the two disorders also share such symptoms as irritability, anger, insomnia, and agitation; an excess of such symptoms suggests a mixed phase or mixed state of mania and depression occurring simultaneously. Manic and mixed manic episodes represent the hallmark of what was once termed manic-depressive psychosis and currently are recognized as bipolar I disorder.

Although milder degrees of mania (hypomania) can contribute to success in business, leadership roles, and the arts, recurrences of even mild manic symptomatology could be disruptive. The elated mood tends to produce overoptimism concerning abilities, and coupled with the impulsivity characteristic of mania, could lead to disaster. Thus accurate and early diagnosis is paramount.

Classic mania—as formulated in the DSM-IV operationalization of manic episode (Table 16.6-9)—is relatively easy to recognize. However, misdiagnosis is still common in North American practice, with clinicians' confusing severe mania with schizophrenia and its milder variants with normality or with narcissistic or sociopathic disorders. As with the misdiagnosis of depressive disorder, such errors in clinical judgment are often attributable to a lack of familiarity with the phenomenology of the classic illness. Again, DSM-IV criteria provide only a guideline. The actual diagnosis requires empathic understanding. The manic patient lifts the observer's mood, makes the person smile and even laugh, and can be irritating as well. The patient's speech is fast, and may even appear loose, but it also can be witty. Finally, the behavior is often dramatic, expansive, and jesting. The overall gestalt experienced in the presence of such patients is emotionally and qualitatively distinct from that of persons with schizophrenia. Those considerations become clearer when clinicians familiarize themselves with the psychopathology of mania in the area of mood, behavior, and thinking.

TABLE 16.6-8
Criteria for Seasonal Pattern Specifier

Specify if:
With seasonal pattern (can be applied to the pattern of major depressive episodes in bipolar I disorder, bipolar II disorder, or major depressive disorder, recurrent)

A. There has been a regular temporal relationship between the onset of major depressive episodes in bipolar I or bipolar II disorder or major depressive disorder, recurrent, and a particular time of the year (e.g., regular appearance of the major depressive episode in the fall or winter).
Note: Do not include cases in which there is an obvious effect of seasonal-related psychosocial stressors (e.g., regularly being unemployed every winter).
B. Full remissions (or a change from depression to mania or hypomania) also occur at a characteristic time of the year (e.g., depression disappears in the spring).
C. In the last two years, two major depressive episodes have occurred that demonstrate the temporal seasonal relationships defined in criteria A and B, and no nonseasonal major depressive episodes have occurred during that same period.
D. Seasonal major depressive episodes (as described above) substantially outnumber the nonseasonal major depressive episodes that may have occurred over the person's lifetime.

TABLE 16.6-9
Criteria for Manic Episode

A. A distinct period of abnormally and persistently elevated, expansive, or irritable mood, lasting at least one week (or any duration if hospitalization is necessary).
B. During the period of mood disturbance, three (or more) of the following symptoms have persisted (four if the mood is only irritable) and have been present to a significant degree:
   (1) inflated self-esteem or grandiosity
   (2) decreased need for sleep (e.g., feels rested after only three hours of sleep)
   (3) more talkative than usual or pressure to keep talking
   (4) flight of ideas or subjective experience that thoughts are racing
   (5) distractibility (i.e., attention too easily drawn to unimportant or irrelevant external stimuli)
   (6) increase in goal-directed activity (either socially, at work or school, or sexually) or psychomotor agitation
   (7) excessive involvement in pleasurable activities that have a high potential for painful consequences (e.g., engaging in unrestrained buying sprees, sexual indiscretions, or foolish business investments)
C. The symptoms do not meet criteria for a mixed episode.
D. The mood disturbance is sufficiently severe to cause marked impairment in occupational functioning or in usual social activities or relationships with others, or to necessitate hospitalization to prevent harm to self or others, or there are psychotic features.
E. The symptoms are not due to the direct physiological effects of a substance (e.g., a drug of abuse, a medication, or other treatment) or a general medical condition (e.g., hyperthyroidism).

Note: Maniclike episodes that are clearly caused by somatic antidepressant treatment (e.g., medication, electroconvulsive therapy, light therapy) should not count toward a diagnosis of bipolar I disorder.

Mood elevation The mood in mania is classically one of elation, euphoria, and jubilation, typically associated with laughing, punning, and gesturing.

Mood lability and irritability The prevailing positive mood in mania is not stable, and momentary tearfulness is common. Also, for many patients the high is so excessive that it is actually dysphoric. When opposed, the patient can become extremely irritable and hostile. Thus lability and irritable hostility are as much features of the manic mood as are the elated mood.

Psychomotor acceleration Accelerated psychomotor activity, the hallmark of mania, is characterized by an overabundance of energy and activity and by rapid and pressured speech. Subjectively, the patient experiences an unusual sense of physical well-being (eutonia).

FLIGHT OF IDEAS Thinking processes are accelerated, experienced as flight of ideas, and thinking and perception are unusually sharp. The patient may speak with such pressure that it is difficult to follow the associations; such clang associations are often based on rhyming or chance perceptions, and could flow with lightning rapidity. The pressure to speak may continue despite the development of hoarseness.

IMPULSIVE BEHAVIOR Manic patients are typically impulsive, disinhibited, and meddlesome. They are intrusive in their increased involvement with other persons, leading to friction with family members, friends, and colleagues. They are distractible and move quickly, not only from one thought to another, but from one person to another, showing heightened interest in every new activity that strikes their fancy. They are indefatigable and engage in various activities in which they usually display poor social judgment. Examples include preaching or dancing in the street; abuse of long distance calling; buying new cars, hundreds of records, expensive jewelry, or other unnecessary items; impulsive marriages; engaging in risky business ventures; gambling; and sudden aimless trips. Such pursuits can lead to personal and financial ruin.

DELIRIOUS MANIA An extremely severe expression of mania (also known as Bell's mania), delirious mania involves frenzied physical activity that continues unabated, leading to a medical emergency that is life threatening; that complication, the manic counterpart of stupor, is rare, however. (There is no need to invoke here the concept of catatonic features [Table 16.6-10], as advocated by DSM-IV. The DSM-IV position is terminologically confusing and phenomenologically imprecise.)

Vegetative disturbances

Such disturbances are more difficult to evaluate in mania as compared with depression.

HYPOSOMNIA The cardinal sign is decreased need for sleep—the patient sleeps for only few hours but feels energetic on awakening. Some patients may actually go sleepless for several days. That practice could lead to a dangerous escalation of manic activity, which might continue despite signs of physical exhaustion.

INATTENTION TO NUTRITION There does not seem to be a clinically significant level of appetite disturbance as such, but weight loss may occur because of increased activity and neglect of nutritional needs.

SEXUAL EXCESSES The sexual appetite is typically increased and may lead to sexual indiscretion. Married women with previously unblemished sexual lives may associate with men below their social status. Men typically overindulge in alcohol, frequenting bars and visiting prostitutes on whom they squander their savings. The sexual misadventures of manic patients result in marital disasters, and hence the multiple separations or divorces that are almost pathognomonic of the disorder. Such sexual impulsivity is even more problematic now, in view of the AIDS epidemic.

TABLE 16.6-10
Criteria for Catatonic Features Specifier

Specify if:
With catatonic features (can be applied to the current or most recent major depressive episode, manic episode, or mixed episode in major depressive disorder, bipolar I disorder, or bipolar II disorder)
The clinical picture is dominated by at least two of the following:
(1) motoric immobility as evidenced by catalepsy (including waxy flexibility) or stupor
(2) excessive motor activity (that is apparently purposeless and not influenced by external stimuli)
(3) extreme negativism (an apparently motiveless resistance to all instructions or maintenance of a rigid posture against attempts to be moved) or mutism
(4) peculiarities of voluntary movement as evidenced by posturing (voluntary assumption of inappropriate or bizarre postures), stereotyped movements, prominent mannerisms, or prominent grimacing
(5) echolalia or echopraxia

Table from DSM-IV, *Diagnostic and Statistical Manual of Mental Disorders,* ed 4. Copyright American Psychiatric Association, Washington, 1994. Used with permission.

Cognitive distortions

Manic thinking is overly positive, optimistic, and expansive.

GRANDIOSITY, LACK OF INSIGHT, AND DELUSION FORMATION The patient presents an inflated self-esteem and a grandiose sense of confidence and achievements. Behind that façade, however, there may be a vague and painful recognition that the positive self-concepts do not represent reality. However, such insight, if present at all, is transient, and manic patients are notoriously refractory to self-examination and insight. Denial and lack of insight, cardinal psychological derangements of mania, are not listed in the DSM-IV criteria for manic episode or bipolar disorders. It is because of their lack of insight that manic patients engage in activities that harm them and their loved ones. It also explains, in part, their noncompliance with medication regimens during the manic phase. Finally, because of their lack of insight, manic experiences can easily acquire delusional proportions. Those include delusions of exceptional mental and physical fitness and exceptional talent; delusions of wealth, aristocratic ancestry, or other grandiose identity; delusions of assistance (that is, well-placed persons or supernatural powers are assisting in their endeavors); or delusions of reference and persecution, based on the belief that enemies are observing or following them out of jealousy at their special abilities. At the height of mania patients may even see visions or hear voices congruent with their euphoric mood and grandiose self-image; for instance, they might see images of heaven or hear cherubs chanting songs to praise them. (The denial characteristic of mania—and the frequently psychotic nature of episodes—means that clinicians must routinely obtain diagnostic information about past episodes from significant others.)

MOOD-INCONGRUENT MANIC PSYCHOSIS Psychosis in the setting of mania is typically mood congruent. The sense of physical well-being and mental alacrity is so extraordinary that it is understandable why manic persons believe that they possess superior powers or perhaps are great scientists or famous reformers. Moreover, their senses are so vivid that reality appears richer and more exotic, and can be easily transformed into a vision; likewise, their thoughts are so rapid and vibrant that they feel they can hear them. Thus certain first-rank Schneiderian-type symptoms, which have been traditionally considered mood incongruent, can be understood phenomenologically to arise from the powerful mental experiences of mania.

Mr. Z., a 37-year-old engineer, had experienced three manic episodes for which he had been hospitalized; all three episodes were preceded by several weeks of moderate psychomotor retardation. Although each time he had responded to lithium (Eskalith, Lithobid), once outside the hospital, he had been reluctant to take it and eventually refused to do so. Now that he was euthymic, following his third and most disruptive episode during which he had badly beaten his wife, he said that he could better explain how he felt when manic. Mania, he felt, was "like God implanted in him," so he could serve as "testimony to man's communication with God." He elaborated as follows: "Ordinary mortals will never, never understand the supreme manic state which I'm privileged to experience every few years. It is so vivid, so intense, so compelling. When I feel that way, there can be no other explanation: To be manic is, ultimately, to be God. God himself must be supermanic: I can feel it, when mania enters through my left brain like laser beams, transforming my sluggish thoughts, recharging them, galvanizing them. My thoughts acquire such momentum, they rush out of my head, to explain the true nature of mania to psychiatrists and all others concerned. That's why I will never accept lithium—to do so is to obstruct the divinity in me." Although he was on the brink of divorce, he would not yield to his wife's plea to go back on lithium.

The vignette illustrates the possibility that even some of the most psychotic experiences in mania represent explanatory delusions, the patient's attempt to make sense of the mania. The DSM-IV criteria for severity-psychotic-remission specifiers for manic episode (Table 16.6-11) are more concerned with operational rigor than phenomenological sophistication needed to understand such core manic experiences. (Some manic patients abuse alcohol and stimulants in order to enhance their mental state and, therefore, mood-incongruence can sometimes be explained on that basis.)

Mania versus hypomania Nonpsychotic and nondisruptive variants of mania are much more common and are recognized by DSM-IV as hypomanic episodes (Table 16.6-12). Diagnostically, it is important to obtain information from others who have observed the patient: the experience is often pleasant and the subject may either be unaware of it or tend to deny it. Although DSM-IV states that treatment-emergent hypomania does not count towards a diagnosis of bipolarity, prospective observations have shown that all such episodes are followed eventually by spontanious hypomania.

DIAGNOSIS AND CLINICAL SUBTYPES

The classification of mood disorders in DSM-IV subsumes a large variety of patients seen in private and public, ambulatory, and inpatient settings. The main demarcation in that large clinical terrain is that between bipolar and depressive (unipolar) disorders. Thus bipolar disorder ranges from the classic manic and depressive episodes of psychotic intensity (bipolar I) through recurrent major depressive episodes, hypomanic episodes (bipolar II disorder), and cyclothymic mood swings. Likewise, depressive disorders include those with psychotic severity, melancholia, atypical features, and dysthymic variants.

The distinction between major and specific attenuated subtypes depends on the disorder's depth and duration. In dysthymic disorder and cyclothymic disorder a partial mood syndrome—consisting of subdepressive features in the former and subdepressive and hypomanic features in the latter—is maintained, either intermittently or continuously, for at least two years. The onset is typically in adolescence or childhood, and most persons with those attenuated diagnoses seen in young adulthood have had low-grade mood symptoms for 5 to 10 years. Major mood disorders, which on the average begin much later in life, require the presence of either a full manic episode or a full depressive episode—sustained for at least one or two weeks, respectively—and an episodic course, typically permitting recovery or remission from episodes. DSM-IV recognizes that nearly 20 percent of persons with major depressive disorders fail to achieve full symptomatic recovery and, therefore, should be qualified as chronic (Table 16.6-13) or in partial remission (Table 16.6-15). They will no longer be considered dysthymic, as was the misleading convention in the DSM-III.

DICHOTOMY OR CONTINUUM? Although, in the extreme, bipolar and depressive (unipolar) disorders are discriminable clinically and therapeutically (Table 16.6-14), clinical observations testify to a vast area of overlap between those extremes.

TABLE 16.6-11
Criteria for Severity/Psychotic/Remission Specifiers for Current (or Most Recent) Manic Episode

Note: Code in fifth digit. Can be applied to a manic episode in bipolar I disorder only if it is the most recent type of mood episode.
Mild: Minimum symptom criteria are met for a manic episode.
Moderate: Extreme increase in activity or impairment in judgment.
Severe without psychotic features: Almost continual supervision required to prevent physical harm to self or others.
Severe with psychotic features: Delusions or hallucinations. If possible, specify whether the psychotic features are mood-congruent or mood-incongruent:
 Mood-congruent psychotic features: Delusions or hallucinations whose content is entirely consistent with the typical manic themes of inflated worth, power, knowledge, identity, or special relationship to a deity or famous person.
 Mood-incongruent psychotic features: Delusions or hallucinations whose content does not involve typical manic themes of inflated worth, power, knowledge, identity, or special relationship to a deity or famous person. Included are such symptoms as persecutory delusions (not directly related to grandiose ideas or themes), thought insertion, and delusions of being controlled.
In partial remission: Symptoms of a manic episode are present but full criteria are not met, or there is a period without any significant symptoms of a manic episode lasting less than two months following the end of the manic episode.
In full remission: During the past two months no significant signs or symptoms of the disturbance were present.
Unspecified.

Table from DSM-IV, *Diagnostic and Statistical Manual of Mental Disorders,* ed 4. Copyright American Psychiatric Association, Washington, 1994. Used with permission.

TABLE 16.6-12
Criteria for Hypomanic Episode

A. A distinct period of persistently elevated, expansive, or irritable mood, lasting throughout at least four days, that is clearly different from the usual nondepressed mood.
B. During the period of mood disturbance, three (or more) of the following symptoms have persisted (four if the mood is only irritable) and have been present to a significant degree:
 (1) inflated self-esteem or grandiosity
 (2) decreased need for sleep (e.g., feels rested after only three hours of sleep)
 (3) more talkative than usual or pressure to keep talking
 (4) flight of ideas or subjective experience that thoughts are racing
 (5) distractibility (i.e., attention too easily drawn to unimportant or irrelevant external stimuli)
 (6) increase in goal-directed activity (either socially, at work or school, or sexually) or psychomotor agitation
 (7) excessive involvement in pleasurable activities that have a high potential for painful consequences (e.g., the person engages in unrestrained buying sprees, sexual indiscretions, or foolish business investments)
C. The episode is associated with an unequivocal change in functioning that is uncharacteristic of the person when not symptomatic.
D. The disturbance in mood and the change in functioning are observable by others.
E. The episode is not severe enough to cause marked impairment in social or occupational functioning, or to necessitate hospitalization, and there are no psychotic features.
F. The symptoms are not due to the direct physiological effects of a substance (e.g., a drug of abuse, a medication, or other treatment) or a general medical condition (e.g., hyperthyroidism).

Note: Hypomaniclike episodes that are clearly caused by somatic antidepressant treatment (e.g., medication, electroconvulsive therapy, light therapy) should not count toward a diagnosis of bipolar II disorder.

Table from DSM-IV, *Diagnostic and Statistical Manual of Mental Disorders,* ed 4. Copyright American Psychiatric Association, Washington, 1994. Used with permission.

TABLE 16.6-13
Criteria for Chronic Specifier

Specify if:
 Chronic (can be applied to the current or most recent major depressive episode in major depressive disorder and to a major depressive episode in bipolar I or II disorder only if it is the most recent type of mood episode)
 Full criteria for a major depressive episode have been met continuously for at least the past two years.

Table from DSM-IV, *Diagnostic and Statistical Manual of Mental Disorders,* ed 4. Copyright American Psychiatric Association, Washington, 1994. Used with permission.

TABLE 16.6-14
Differentiating Characteristics of Bipolar and Unipolar Depressions

	Bipolar	Unipolar
History of mania or hypomania (definitional)	Yes	No
Temperament—personality	Cyclothymic—extroverted	Dysthymic—introverted
Sex ratio	Equal	More women than men
Age of onset	Teens, 20s, and 30s	30s, 40s, 50s
Postpartum episodes	More common	Less common
Onset of episode	Often abrupt	More insidious
Number of episodes	Numerous	Fewer
Duration of episode	Three to six months	Three to twelve months
Psychomotor activity	Retardation > agitation	Agitation > retardation
Sleep	Hypersomnia > insomnia	Insomnia > hypersomnia
Family history		
Bipolar	Yes	±
Unipolar	Yes	Yes
Alcoholism	±	Yes
Pharmacological response		
Cyclic antidepressants	Induce hypomania-mania	±
Lithium carbonate	Acute antidepressant effects	Ineffective

TABLE 16.6-15
Course Specifiers That Apply to Mood Disorders

	With/Without Interepisode Recovery	Seasonal Pattern	Rapid Cycling
Major depressive disorder, single episode			
Major depressive disorder, recurrent	X	X	
Dysthymic disorder			
Bipolar I disorder, single manic episode			
Bipolar I disorder, most recent episode hypomanic	X	X	X
Bipolar I disorder, most recent episode manic	X	X	X
Bipolar I disorder, most recent episode mixed	X	X	X
Bipolar I disorder, most recent episode depressed	X	X	X
Bipolar I disorder, most recent episode unspecified	X	X	X
Bipolar II disorder, hypomanic	X	X	X
Bipolar II disorder, depressed	X	X	X
Cyclothymic disorder			

Table from DSM-IV, *Diagnostic and Statistical Manual of Mental Disorders,* ed 4. Copyright American Psychiatric Association, Washington, 1994. Used with permission.

TABLE 16.6-16
Criteria for Longitudinal Course Specifiers

Specify if (can be applied to recurrent major depressive disorder or bipolar I or II disorder):

With full interepisode recovery: if full remission is attained between the two most recent mood episodes

Without full interepisode recovery: if full remission is not attained between the two most recent mood episodes

Table from DSM-IV, *Diagnostic and Statistical Manual of Mental Disorders,* ed 4. Copyright American Psychiatric Association, Washington, 1994. Used with permission.

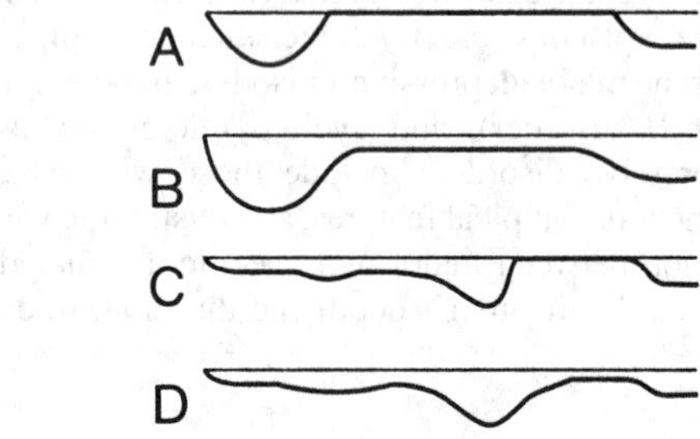

FIGURE 16.6-1 *The four graphs depict prototypical courses.* (A) *The course of major depressive disorder, recurrent, in which there is no antecedent dysthymic disorder and there is a period of full remission between the episodes. That pattern predicts the best future prognosis.* (B) *The course of major depressive disorder, recurrent, in which there is no antecedent dysthymic disorder but in which prominent symptoms persist between the two most recent episodes—that is, no more than partial remission is attained.* (C) *shows the rare pattern (present in fewer than 3 percent of persons with major depressive disorder) of major depressive disorder, recurrent, with antecedent dysthymic disorder but with full interepisode recovery between the two most recent episodes.* (D) *The course of major depressive disorder, recurrent, in which there is antecedent dysthymic disorder and in which there is no period of full remission between the two most recent episodes. This pattern, commonly referred to as double depression, is seen in about 20–25 percent of persons with major depressive disorder. (Figure from DSM-IV,* Diagnostic and Statistical Manual of Mental Disorders, *ed 4. Copyright American Psychiatric Association, Washington, 1994. Used with permission.)*

Thus the distinctions between the various affective subtypes are not as hard and fast as DSM-IV attempts to portray. For instance, full-blown bipolar disorder can be superimposed on cyclothymic disorder which tends to persist after the resolution of manic or major depressive episodes. Even more common is major depressive disorder complicating cyclothymic disorder. Likewise, recent evidence indicates that dysthymic disorder may precede major depressive disorder in as many as a third of cases. Moreover, one of four persons with major depressive disorder subsequently develop hypomanic or manic episodes and so should be reclassified as having bipolar disorder. Finally, unexpected crossing from dysthymic disorder to manic episodes has also been described, suggesting that some forms of dysthymic disorder are subaffective precursors of bipolar disorder. Such observations are in line with Kraepelin's historic attempt to bring all mood disorders under one rubric.

Undoubtedly, heterogeneity exists in the realm of mood disorders. What the foregoing observations suggest, however, is that a large chunk of the unipolar terrain might be pseudo-unipolar—to wit, soft bipolar. The clinical significance of those considerations lies in the fact that many of the DSM-IV subtypes of mood disorders are not pure entities, and that considerable overlap and switches in polarity take place. They also provide some rationale, for instance, as to why lithium (or lithium augmentation) may be effective in some apparently unipolar depressions; such patients do not experience spontaneous hypomanic episodes, but instead often exhibit a high baseline level of hyperthymia. Finally, there seems to be an emerging consensus that persons with bipolar disorders whose premorbid adjustment and interepisodic adjustment are cyclothymic are at risk for antidepressant-induced rapid cycling, defined as a rapid succession of major episodes with few or no intervals of freedom. Those considerations further testify to the wisdom of supplementing major mood diagnoses with temperamental attributes. DSM-IV makes subtle or oblique hints concerning that.

The course specifiers that apply to DSM-IV mood disorders are listed in Table 16.6-15. The DSM-IV criteria for longitudinal course specifiers are presented in Table 16.6-16. Four prototypical courses of depressive disorders are shown in Figure 16.6-1. Those course specifiers and patterns do not represent an exhaustive list.

DEPRESSIVE DISORDERS

The broad category of depressive disorders includes major depressive disorder, dysthymic disorder, and depressive disorder not otherwise specified (NOS) (Table 16.6-17).

MAJOR DEPRESSIVE DISORDER Episodes usually begin over a prodromal period of weeks to months. The DSM-IV diagnosis of major depressive disorder requires (1) dysphoric mood or decreased interest in usual activities and (2) at least four additional classic depressive signs and symptoms, (3) which must be sustained for at least two weeks, and (4) cannot be explained by a process known to cause depressive symptoms, such as normal bereavement or certain physical conditions commonly associated with depression.

Nature of comorbid physical disease Those considerations raise the question of whether major depressive disorder should be limited to depressions of unknown etiology (for example, those without documented physical causes). The DSM-IV approach has basically taken the position that whenever the etiology is known, the condition should be diagnosed as mood disorder due to a general medical condition, which must be specified (Table 16.6-18) or substance-induced mood disorder (Table 16.6-19). The problem with that approach lies in the fact that many common medical factors associated with depression—for example, use of reserpine—do not seem to be causative in the etiological sense but rather are triggering agents in otherwise predisposed persons. That is analogous to the situation with life events, which no longer are used in making distinctions between subtypes of depression. A more troubling implication is that major depressive disorders without demonstrable physical disease are not medical or otherwise biological. There appears to be no reliable or valid way in which a clinician can decide that a depressive condition is due to a specified medical condition. For that reason it is generally more practical to diagnose the depressive disorder on Axis I and to specify the contributing physical condition on Axis III. In brief, the designation "due to a general medical condition" is both cumbersome and redundant. It is the author's position that major depressive disorder represents a syndrome which is the final common pathway of multifactorial interacting factors, and should be diagnosed irrespective of presumed etiology.

Diagnostic threshold Another question concerning the DSM-IV definition of major depressive disorders relates to the threshold at which a constellation of depressive features can be said to constitute a condition distinct from the ordinary blues. According to the current definition it is sufficient for a person to experience, in response to a setback, a lowering of the spirits, self-doubt, difficulty in sleeping and concentration, and

TABLE 16.6-17
Diagnostic Criteria for Depressive Disorder Not Otherwise Specified

The depressive disorder not otherwise specified category includes disorders with depressive features that do not meet the criteria for major depressive disorder, dysthymic disorder, adjustment disorder with depressed mood, or adjustment disorder with mixed anxiety and depressed mood. Sometimes depressive symptoms can present as part of an anxiety disorder not otherwise specified. Examples of depressive disorder not otherwise specified include

1. Premenstrual dysphoric disorder: in most menstrual cycles during the past year, symptoms (e.g., markedly depressed mood, marked anxiety, marked affective lability, decreased interest in activities) regularly occurred during the last week of the luteal phase (and remitted within a few days of the onset of menses). These symptoms must be severe enough to markedly interfere with work, school, or usual activities and be entirely absent for at least one week postmenses.
2. Minor depressive disorder: episodes of at least two weeks of depressive symptoms but with fewer than the five items required for major depressive disorder.
3. Recurrent brief depressive disorder: depressive episodes lasting from two days up to two weeks, occurring at least once a month for 12 months (not associated with the menstrual cycle).
4. Postpsychotic depressive disorder of schizophrenia: a major depressive episode that occurs during the residual phase of schizophrenia.
5. A major depressive episode superimposed on delusional disorder, psychotic disorder not otherwise specified, or the active phase of schizophrenia.
6. Situations in which the clinician has concluded that a depressive disorder is present but is unable to determine whether it is primary, due to a general medical condition, or substance induced.

TABLE 16.6-18
Diagnostic Criteria for Mood Disorder Due to a General Medical Condition

A. A prominent and persistent disturbance in mood predominates in the clinical picture and is characterized by either (or both) of the following:
   (1) depressed mood or markedly diminished interest or pleasure in all, or almost all, activities
   (2) elevated, expansive, or irritable mood
B. There is evidence from the history, physical examination, or laboratory findings that the disturbance is the direct physiological consequence of a general medical condition.
C. The disturbance is not better accounted for by another mental disorder (e.g., adjustment disorder with depressed mood in response to the stress of having a general medical condition).
D. The disturbance does not occur exclusively during the course of a delirium.
E. The symptoms cause clinically significant distress or impairment in social, occupational, or other important areas of functioning.

Specify type:
With depressive features: if the predominant mood is depressed but the full criteria are not met for a major depressive episode
With major depressivelike episode: if the full criteria are met (except criterion D) for a major depressive episode
With manic features: if the predominant mood is elevated, euphoric, or irritable
With mixed features: if the symptoms of both mania and depression are present but neither predominates

Coding note: Include the name of the general medical condition on axis I, e.g., mood disorder due to hypothyroidism, with depressive features; also code the general medical condition on axis III.

Coding note: If depressive symptoms occur as part of a preexisting dementia, indicate the depressive symptoms by coding the appropriate subtype of the dementia if one is available, e.g., dementia of the Alzheimer's type, with late onset, with depressed mood.

TABLE 16.6-19
Diagnostic Criteria for Substance-Induced Mood Disorder

A. A prominent and persistent disturbance in mood predominates in the clinical picture and is characterized by either (or both) of the following:
   (1) depressed mood or markedly diminished interest or pleasure in all, or almost all, activities
   (2) elevated, expansive, or irritable mood
B. There is evidence from the history, physical examination, or laboratory findings of either (1) or (2):
   (1) the symptoms in criterion A developed during, or within a month of, substance intoxication or withdrawal
   (2) medication use is etiologically related to the disturbance
C. The disturbance is not better accounted for by a mood disorder that is not substance induced. Evidence that the symptoms are better accounted for by a mood disorder that is not substance induced might include the following: the symptoms precede the onset of the substance use (or medication use); the symptoms persist for a substantial period of time (e.g., about a month) after the cessation of acute withdrawal or severe intoxication or are substantially in excess of what would be expected given the type or amount of the substance used or the duration of use; or there is other evidence that suggests the existence of an independent non-substance-induced mood disorder (e.g., a history of recurrent major depressive episodes).
D. The disturbance does not occur exclusively during the course of a delirium.
E. The symptoms cause clinically significant distress or impairment in social, occupational, or other important areas of functioning.

Note: This diagnosis should be made instead of a diagnosis of substance intoxication or substance withdrawal only when the mood symptoms are in excess of those usually associated with the intoxication or withdrawal syndrome and when the symptoms are sufficiently severe to warrant independent clinical attention.

Code [Specific Substance]-Induced Mood Disorder:
(alcohol; amphetamine [or amphetaminelike substance]; cocaine; hallucinogen; inhalant; opioid; phencyclidine [or phencyclidinelike substance]; sedative, hypnotic, or anxiolytic; other [or unknown] substance)

Specify type:
With depressive features: if the predominant mood is depressed
With manic features: if the predominant mood is elevated, euphoric, or irritable
With mixed features: if symptoms of both mania and depression are present and neither predominates

Specify if:
With onset during intoxication: if the criteria are met for intoxication with the substance and the symptoms develop during the intoxication syndrome
With onset during withdrawal: if criteria are met for withdrawal from the substance and the symptoms develop during, or shortly after, a withdrawal syndrome

Table from DSM-IV, *Diagnostic and Statistical Manual of Mental Disorders,* ed 4. Copyright American Psychiatric Association, Washington, 1994. Used with permission.

decreased sexual interest for 14 days to qualify for a diagnosis of a major depressive disorder of mild intensity. Some authorities would consider such a condition to represent instead a minor depression, probably no more than an adjustment disorder. It would appear that criteria other than signs and symptoms and duration would be necessary to differentiate a depressive disorder from adjustment reactions to life situations. The presence of the following characteristics might assist in such a differentiation.

1. By definition a major depressive disorder should be incapacitating. Previously, much attention had been paid to the interpersonal consequences of depression. Recent evidence indicates that measurable deficits in work performance are often early manifestations. Afflicted persons are also unable to benefit from taking leisure time, and hence the futility of prescribing vacations.

2. Depressive disorder is usually perceived as a break from a person's usual or premorbid self, which can be so striking that the sufferer may feel as though he or she is losing his or her mind. The important point is that both the patient and significant others can usually relate the onset of the illness to a given month or quarter of a year, which is not true, for instance, for dysthymic disorder.

3. Depressive disorder is often experienced by the sufferer as qualitatively distinct from grief or other understandable reactions to loss or adversity. William James described it as follows:

> There is a pitch of unhappiness so great that the goods of nature may be entirely forgotten, and all sentiment of their existence vanish from the mental field. For this extremity of passion to be reached, something more is needed than [adversity] . . . the individual must in his own person become the prey of pathological melancholy . . . such sensitiveness and susceptibility of mental pain is a rare occurrence where the nervous constitution is entirely normal: one seldom finds it in a healthy subject even where he is the victim of the most atrocious cruelties of outward fortune . . . it is an . . . active anguish, a sort of psychical neuroglia wholly unknown to healthy life.

Two additional features, when present, would further validate the diagnosis of major depressive disorder.

4. Recurrence—especially periodicity or regular seasonal occurrence.

5. Consecutive-generation family history of mood disorder—especially when a large number of family members are afflicted with depression or mood disorder—is characteristic of clinical depression. For instance, in one study in which minor or neurotic depressive persons were prospectively followed, it was found that such pedigrees predicted the development of major episodes. DSM-IV makes no provision for considering such familial factors in diagnostic decisions. In clinical practice those factors often do influence diagnostic decisions.

Single episode and recurrent subtypes About a third of all major depressive episodes do not recur. Such patients tend to be older, they are less likely to have a positive family history for mood disorders, and the course of the disorder is more protracted (one to two years). Patients with major depressive disorder, single episode (Table 16.6-3), should be distinguished from those experiencing their first episodes of major depressive disorder, recurrent (Table 16.6-4). The latter group tends to be younger, and the disorder is more likely to have been preceded by a depressive temperament or dysthymic disorder.

Research has also established that recurrent major depressive disorders are more familial than are their single-episode counterparts. The average length of episodes is six months, whereas the mean interval between episodes tends to vary (typically years). The mean number of major episodes over a lifetime, according to retrospective and prospective studies, is five to six, as contrasted with an average number of eight to nine major episodes in bipolar disorder.

Melancholic features In DSM-III the neurotic-endogenous distinction was deleted. Neurotic depression was absorbed by dysthymic disorder and the major depressive disorders that complicate it; endogenous depression became melancholic features, a qualifying phrase for those major depressive disorders in which anhedonia, guilt, and psychomotor-vegetative disturbances dominate the clinical picture (Table 16.6-6). DSM-IV has retained those conventions.

Although the foregoing conventions have received much criticism, they are based on solid data from independent studies in the United States and Germany. Thus neurotic depression, defined as a reactive (that is, precipitated) nonpsychotic depression of mild to moderate intensity with predominant anxiety and characterologic pathology, does not seem to constitute a distinct nosological entity. Although such a presentation is com-

TABLE 16.6-20
Three- to Four-Year Prospective Follow-up in Neurotic Depressions (N = 100)

Diagnosis and Outcome	N*
Manic episode	4
Hypomanic episode	14
Psychotic depression	21
Endogenous depression	36
Episodic course	42
Unstable characterological features	24
Social invalidism	35
Suicide	3

*The total exceeds 100 because more than one outcome was possible in each patient.

Table from H Akiskal, A Bitar, V Puzantian, T Rosenthal, P Walker. The nosological status of neurotic depression: A prospective 3-to-4 year examination in light of the primary-secondary and unipolar-bipolar dichotomies. Arch Gen Psychiatry *35:* 756, 1978. Used with permission.

mon in clinical practice, the prospective follow-up course of those patients is heterogeneous (Table 16.6-20). The progression of a precipitated, relatively mild depression (reactive illness) to severe psychotic depression—or one with a melancholic autonomy—during prospective observation suggested that so-called endogenous depressions may have their onset in milder depressions, that neurotic and psychotic depressions do not necessarily refer to distinct disorders but to disorders that differ in severity, and that the presence of precipitating stress carries little diagnostic weight in differentiating subtypes of depression (although the absence of such stress might be used to support a melancholic level of major depressive disorder).

At the heart of the concept of morbid depression is its autonomy from stresses that may have precipitated it and its general unresponsiveness to other environmental input. That is embodied in Donald Klein's concept of endogenomorphic depression, which could be precipitated and mild (endoreactive, as discussed earlier) while exhibiting disturbances of hedonic mechanisms refractory to current interpersonal contexts. Many authorities believe that autonomy dictates the need to use somatic approaches to reverse the maladaptive autonomy and restore response to interpersonal feedback; that is, psychotherapeutic approaches are deemed largely ineffective until the autonomy is somatically lysed.

Given the somatic connotation of the ancient concept of melancholia, the (APA) classification has officially adopted it as the preferred nosological term for the revised concept of endogeneity, and hence the prominence of the vegetative and biorhythmic features accorded to it in both DSM-III and DSM-IV. However, the APA diagnostic schema risks confusing endogeneity with another classic concept of mood disorder, that of involutional melancholia.

Psychotic features About 15 percent of major depressive disorders, usually those with melancholic features, develop into delusional depressions. In young persons they tend to be retarded, even stuporous, and are best considered as initial episodes of bipolar disorder. When psychotic depression develops for the first time after the age of 50, it often presents with severe agitation, delusional guilt, hypochondriacal preoccupations, early-morning awakening, and weight loss. The premorbid adjustment of those patients has classically been characterized as obsessoid. Their mournful-anxious mood and agitation are autonomous, being refractory to psychological interventions, and they endure great suffering. Except for the fact that the frequency of episodes is generally in the range of one to two in late-onset (so-called involutional) depressions, they represent the closest approximation to the DSM-IV melancholia. In view of Kraepelin's postulation of a cerebral basis for such cases, it is of interest that ventricular enlargement and white matter opacities have been reported in psychotic depressions. Their etiological specificity for persons with late-onset psychotic depression has been controversial, however, given similar findings in younger (more bipolar) persons with psychotic depression. Brain imaging findings tend to be correlated with the neurocognitive deficits observed in psychotic depressions. Those features do not seem to define a distinct depressive subtype, but one of greater severity. Finally, despite attempts to suggest a neurochemical uniqueness, based largely on the need for antipsychotic treatment in the acute phase of many of those patients, familial and other external validators have failed to support psychotic depression as a separate entity, and hence the decision in DSM-IV to use psychotic features merely as a specifier for major depressive episode (Table 16.6-5). Emerging data, nonetheless, might eventually force a change in this convention. For instance, William Coryell and collaborators in the National Institute of Mental Health (NIMH) collaborative study of depression have shown psychotic depression to be the most consistent unipolar subtype across episodes.

Chronic depression The symptom profile in chronic depressions is usually one of low-grade intensity rather than one of severe syndromal chronicity. Severe depressive disorder in its psychotic forms is so agonizing that the sufferer is at risk of committing suicide before the disorder has a chance to become chronic. More commonly, the psychotic symptoms respond to medication or to electroconvulsive therapy (ECT), but residual depressive symptoms may linger for a long time. In other persons with chronic depressions the chronicity arises from more mundane (nonpsychotic) major depressive episodes, depressive residua following one or several clinical episodes that fail to remit fully. Thus instead of the customary remission within a year, the patients are ill for years. The level of depression varies, fluctuating between syndromal illness and milder symptoms. The patients often show a sense of resignation, a generalized fear of an inability to cope, adherence to rigid routines, and inhibited communication.

Rather than exhibiting a frankly depressive mood, many persons with chronic depression suffer from deficits in their ability to enjoy leisure and display an attitude of irritable moroseness. Those leisure deficits and the irritable humor tend to affect their conjugal lives: their marriages are typically in a state of chronic deadlock, leading neither to divorce nor to reconciliation. In other patients the residual phase is dominated by somatic features, such as sleep and other vegetative or autonomic irregularities. Thus self-treatment with ethanol or iatrogenic benzodiazepine dependence is commonly observed. That those interpersonal, conjugal, and autonomic manifestations represent unresolved depression is shown by persistent sleep EEG—especially REM and delta phase—abnormalities that are indistinguishable from their acute counterparts.

Failure to recover from major depressive disorder is associated with increased familial loading for depression, disabled spouses, deaths of immediate family members, concurrent disabling medical disease, use of depressant antihypertensive agents, and excessive use of alcohol and sedative-hypnotic agents. Social support is often eroded in persons with residual depression, through either the death or the illness of significant others. Therefore, a thorough medical evaluation and socially supportive interventions should be essential ingredients of the overall approach to those patients.

Interpersonal disturbances in such patients are usually secondary to the distortions produced by long-standing depression.

Therefore, observed pathological characterological changes—clinging or hostile dependence, demandingness, touchiness, pessimism, and low self-esteem—are best considered as constituting postdepressive personality changes. There exists a dangerous stereotypical thinking that because a patient has not responded adequately to standard treatments (the illness has become chronic), there must be a characterological substrate to the disorder. The long duration of the disorder often leads to the patient's identification with the failing functions of depression, producing the self-image of being a depressed person. Such a self-image itself represents a malignant cognitive manifestation of the depressive disorder and dictates vigorous treatment targeted at the mood disorder.

The DSM-IV criteria for chronic specifier appear in Table 16.6-14.

DYSTHYMIC DISORDER Dysthymic disorder (Table 16.6-21) is distinguished from depressive disorder by the fact that it is not a sequel to well-defined major depressive episodes. Instead, in the most typical cases, patients complain that they have always been depressed. Thus most cases are of early onset, beginning in childhood or adolescence, and certainly by the time the persons reach their 20s. A late-onset subtype is much less prevalent and has not been well characterized clinically, but has been identified largely through epidemiological studies in the community among middle-aged and geriatric populations.

TABLE 16.6-21
Diagnostic Criteria for Dysthymic Disorder

A. Depressed mood for most of the day, for more days than not, as indicated either by subjective account or observation by others, for at least two years. **Note:** In children and adolescents, mood can be irritable and duration must be at least one year.

B. Presence, while depressed, of two (or more) of the following:
(1) poor appetite or overeating
(2) insomnia or hypersomnia
(3) low energy or fatigue
(4) low self-esteem
(5) poor concentration or difficulty making decisions
(6) feelings of hopelessness

C. During the two-year period (one year for children or adolescents) of the disturbance, the person has never been without the symptoms in criteria A and B for more than two months at a time.

D. No major depressive episode has been present during the first two years of the disturbance (one year for children and adolescents); i.e., the disturbance is not better accounted for by chronic major depressive disorder, or major depressive disorder, in partial remission.
Note: There may have been a previous major depressive episode provided there was a full remission (no significant signs or symptoms for two months) before development of the dysthymic disorder. In addition, after the initial two years (one year in children or adolescents) of dysthymic disorder, there may be superimposed episodes of major depressive disorder, in which case both diagnoses may be given when the criteria are met for a major depressive episode.

E. There has never been a manic episode, a mixed episode, or a hypomanic episode, and criteria have never been met for cyclothymic disorder.

F. The disturbance does not occur exclusively during the course of a chronic psychotic disorder, such as schizophrenia or delusional disorder.

G. The symptoms are not due to the direct physiological effects of a substance (e.g., a drug of abuse, a medication) or a general medical condition (e.g., hypothyroidism).

H. The symptoms cause clinically significant distress or impairment in social, occupational, or other important areas of functioning.

Specify if:
Early onset: if onset is before age 21 years
Late onset: if onset is age 21 years or older
Specify (for most recent two years of Dysthymic Disorder):
With atypical features

Although the dysthymic disorder category in DSM-IV can occur as a secondary complication of other psychiatric disorders, the core concept of dysthymic disorder refers to a subaffective disorder with the following characteristics: (1) low-grade chronicity for at least two years, (2) insidious onset with origin often in childhood or adolescence, and (3) persistent or intermittent course. Although not part of the formal definition of dysthymic disorder, the family history is typically replete with both depressive and bipolar disorders, which is one of the more robust findings supporting its link to primary mood disorder.

Social adjustment Dysthymic disorder is typically an ambulatory disorder compatible with relatively stable social functioning. However, the stability is precarious; recent data have documented that many of the patients invest whatever energy they have in work, leaving none for leisure and family or social activities, which results in the characteristic marital friction. Those empirical findings on the work orientation of persons with dysthymic disorder echo earlier formulations in the German and Japanese literature. For instance, Kraepelin described such persons as follows: "Life with its activity is a burden which they habitually bear with dutiful self-denial without being compensated by the pleasure(s) of existence."

It has been suggested that the dedication to work on the part of persons with dysthymic disorder represents an overcompensation in that it is a defense against their battle with disorganization and inertia. Nevertheless, Kretschmer suggested that such persons are the backbone of society, dedicating their lives to jobs that require dependability and great attention to detail. Epidemiological studies have demonstrated that some persons with protracted dysthymic complaints, extending over many years, have never experienced clear-cut depressive episodes. Some of them may seek outpatient counseling and psychotherapy for existential depressions, with feelings of being empty and of lacking any joy in life outside their work. Such persons have been described as leading monocategorical existences. Others present clinically because of an intensification of their low-grade dysphoria into major depressive disorder.

Course An insidious onset of depression dating back to late childhood or the teens, preceding any superimposed major depressive episodes by years, or even decades, represents the most typical developmental background of dysthymic disorder. A return to the low-grade depressive pattern is the rule following recovery from superimposed major depressive episodes, if any, and hence the designation "double depression" as a prominent DSM-IV course pattern for depressive illness. That pattern is commonly seen in clinical practice and consists of the baseline dysthymic disorder fluctuating in and out of depressive episodes.

Patients with dysthymic disorder often complain of having been depressed since birth or of feeling depressed all the time. They seem to view themselves as belonging to an aristocracy of suffering. Those descriptions of chronic gloominess in the absence of more objective signs of depression earn such patients the label of characterological depression. The description is further reinforced by the fluctuating depressive picture that merges imperceptibly with the patient's habitual self, and thus the uncertainty as to whether dysthymic disorder belongs in Axis I or in Axis II.

Clinical picture The profile of dysthymic disorder overlaps with that of major depressive disorder, but differs from it in that symptoms tend to outnumber signs (more subjective than objective depression). Thus marked disturbances in appetite and libido are uncharacteristic, and psychomotor agitation or retardation is not observed. All of that translates into a depression that is attenuated in symptomatology. However, subtle endogenous features not uncommonly are observed: psychomotor inertia, lethargy, and anhedonia that are characteristically worse in the morning. Because patients presenting clinically often fluctuate in and out of a major depressive episode, the core DSM-IV criteria for dysthymic disorder tend to emphasize vegetative dysfunction, whereas the alternative criterion B for dysthymic disorder (Table 16.6-22) in a DSM-IV appendix lists cognitive symptoms.

Although dysthymic disorder as defined here represents a more restricted concept than does its parent, neurotic depression, it is still quite heterogeneous. Anxiety is not a necessary part of its clinical picture, yet dysthymic disorder is often diagnosed in patients with anxiety and neurotic disorders. That clinical situation is perhaps to be regarded as a secondary or anxious dysthymic disorder or even as a general neurotic syndrome. For greater operational clarity it is best to restrict dysthymic disorder to a primary disorder, one that cannot be explained by another psychiatric disorder. The essential features of such primary dysthymic disorder include habitual gloom, brooding, lack of joy in life, and preoccupation with inadequacy. Dysthymic disorder then is best characterized as long-standing fluctuating low-grade depression, experienced as part of the habitual self and representing an accentuation of traits observed in the depressive temperament (Table 16.6-1). Thus dysthymic disorder can be viewed as a more symptomatic form of that temperament (introduced in a DSM-IV appendix as a depressive personality disorder [see Chapter 25]). Sleep EEG data indicate that many persons with dysthymic disorder at baseline exhibit the sleep patterns of those with acute major depressive disorder, providing further support to the constitutional nature of the disorder. Yet further evidence for that position comes from studies demonstrating high rates of familial affective disorder in dysthymic disorder and depressive temperament or depressive personality.

The clinical picture of dysthymic disorder thus is varied, with some patients proceeding to major depressive disorder, whereas in others the pathology becomes manifest largely at the personality level. In contrast with these continuously morbid dysthymic conditions, community studies have revealed intermittent forms of dysthymiclike manifestations. Some have been considered recurrent brief depressive disorder (Table 16.6-23), in a DSM-IV appendix, because they do not meet the duration criterion for major depressive disorder, while pursuing a protracted intermittent course like that of dysthymic disorder; the group includes persons who make frequent suicide attempts. In so-called minor depressive disorder (Table 16.6-24), observed in primary care settings, the depression is subthreshold in that it is milder than major depression and yet is not protracted enough to be considered dysthymic. Those varied manifestations of depression argue for a continuum model (Figure 16.6-2) as originally envisaged by Kraepelin. Judd and collaborators have recently suggested that subthreshold depressive symptoms—without necessarily meeting the criterion for mood change, might actually represent the most common expressions of depressive disorders. From such a base, individuals predisposed to depressive illness, would fluctuate in and out of the various DSM-IV subtypes of depressive disorders.

Prospective studies on children with dysthymic disorder have demonstrated that they frequently experience major depressive episodes, some of which progress to hypomanic episodes, manic episodes, or mixed episodes (Tables 16.6-25 and 16.6-26) during puberty or adolescence. Persons with dysthymic disorder presenting clinically as adults more often pursue a unipolar course, which can be disabling without treatment.

TABLE 16.6-22
Alternative Research Criterion B for Dysthymic Disorder

B. Presence, while depressed, of three (or more) of the following:
  (1) low self-esteem or self-confidence, or feelings of inadequacy
  (2) feelings of pessimism, despair, or hopelessness
  (3) generalized loss of interest or pleasure
  (4) social withdrawal
  (5) chronic fatigue or tiredness
  (6) feelings of guilt, brooding about the past
  (7) subjective feelings of irritability or excessive anger
  (8) decreased activity, effectiveness, or productivity
  (9) difficulty in thinking, reflected by poor concentration, poor memory, or indecisiveness

TABLE 16.6-23
Research Criteria for Recurrent Brief Depressive Disorder

A. Criteria, except for duration, are met for a major depressive episode.
B. The depressive periods in criterion A last at least two days but less than two weeks.
C. The depressive periods occur at least once a month for 12 consecutive months and are not associated with the menstrual cycle.
D. The periods of depressed mood cause clinically significant distress or impairment in social, occupational, or other important areas of functioning.
E. The symptoms are not due to the direct physiological effects of a substance (e.g., a drug of abuse, a medication) or a general medical condition (e.g., hypothyroidism).
F. There has never been a major depressive episode, and criteria are not met for dysthymic disorder.
G. There has never been a manic episode, a mixed episode, or a hypomanic episode, and criteria are not met for cyclothymic disorder. **Note:** This exclusion does not apply if all of the manic-, mixed-, or hypomaniclike episodes are substance or treatment induced.
H. The mood disturbance does not occur exclusively during schizophrenia, schizophreniform disorder, schizoaffective disorder, delusional disorder, or psychotic disorder not otherwise specified.

TABLE 16.6-24
Research Criteria for Minor Depressive Disorder

A. A mood disturbance, defined as follows:
  (1) at least two (but less than five) of the following symptoms have been present during the same two-week period and represent a change from previous functioning; at least one of the symptoms is either (a) or (b):
    (a) depressed mood most of the day, nearly every day, as indicated by either subjective report (e.g., feels sad or empty) or observation made by others (e.g., appears tearful). **Note:** In children and adolescents, can be irritable mood.
    (b) markedly diminished interest or pleasure in all, or almost all, activities most of the day, nearly every day (as indicated by either subjective account or observation made by others)
    (c) significant weight loss when not dieting or weight gain (e.g., a change of more than 5% of body weight in a month), or decrease or increase in appetite nearly every day. **Note:** In children, consider failure to make expected weight gains.
    (d) insomnia or hypersomnia nearly every day
    (e) psychomotor agitation or retardation nearly every day (observable by others, not merely subjective feelings of restlessness or being slowed down)
    (f) fatigue or loss of energy nearly every day
    (g) feelings of worthlessness or excessive or inappropriate guilt (which may be delusional) nearly every day (not merely self-reproach or guilt about being sick)
    (h) diminished ability to think or concentrate, or indecisiveness, nearly every day (either by subjective account or as observed by others)

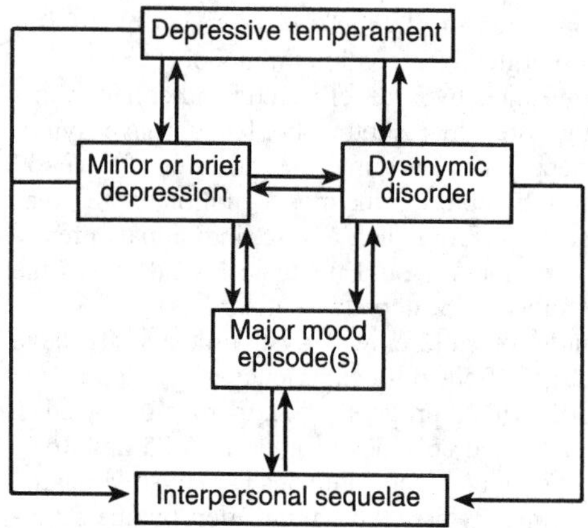

FIGURE 16.6-2 *Relation of various depressive conditions supporting a spectrum concept. (Figure from H S Akiskal: Dysthymia; Clinical and external validity. Acta Psychiatr Scand 89 (Suppl): 19, 1994. Used with permission.)*

TABLE 16.6-25
Criteria for Mixed Episode

A. The criteria are met both for a manic episode and for a major depressive episode (except for duration) nearly every day during at least a one-week period.
B. The mood disturbance is sufficiently severe to cause marked impairment in occupational functioning or in usual social activities or relationships with others, or to necessitate hospitalization to prevent harm to self or others, or there are psychotic features.
C. The symptoms are not due to the direct physiological effects of a substance (e.g., a drug of abuse, a medication, or other treatment) or a general medical condition (e.g., hyperthyroidism).

Note: Mixedlike episodes that are clearly caused by somatic antidepressant treatment (e.g., medication, electroconvulsive therapy, light therapy) should not count toward a diagnosis of bipolar I disorder.

Table from DSM-IV, *Diagnostic and Statistical Manual of Mental Disorders,* ed 4. Copyright American Psychiatric Association, Washington, 1994. Used with permission.

TABLE 16.6-26
Criteria for Severity/Psychotic/Remission Specifiers for Current (or Most Recent) Mixed Episode

Note: Code in fifth digit. Can be applied to a mixed episode in bipolar I disorder only if it is the most recent type of mood episode.

Mild: No more than minimum symptom criteria are met for both a manic episode and a major depressive episode.
Moderate: Symptoms or functional impairment between "mild" and "severe."
Severe without psychotic features: Almost continual supervision required to prevent physical harm to self or others.
Severe with psychotic features: Delusions or hallucinations. If possible, specify whether the psychotic features are mood-congruent or mood-incongruent:

Mood-congruent psychotic features: Delusions or hallucinations whose content is entirely consistent with the typical manic or depressive themes.

Mood-incongruent psychotic features: Delusions or hallucinations whose content does not involve typical manic or depressive themes. Included are such symptoms as persecutory delusions (not directly related to grandiose or depressive themes), thought insertion, and delusions of being controlled.

In partial remission: Symptoms of a mixed episode are present but full criteria are not met, or there is a period without any significant symptoms of a Mixed Episode lasting less than two months following the end of the mixed episode.
In full remission: During the past two months, no significant signs or symptoms of the disturbance were present.
Unspecified.

Table from DSM-IV, *Diagnostic and Statistical Manual of Mental Disorders,* ed 4. Copyright American Psychiatric Association, Washington, 1994. Used with permission.

A 27-year-old, male grade-school teacher presented with the chief complaint that life was a painful duty and that it had always lacked luster for him. He said he felt enveloped by a sense of gloom that was nearly always with him. Although he was respected by his peers, he felt, he said, "like a grotesque failure, a self-concept I have had since childhood." He stated that he merely performed his responsibilities as a teacher, and that he had never derived any pleasure from anything he had done in life. He said he had never had any romantic feeling: sexual activity, in which he had engaged with two different women, had been one of pleasureless orgasm. He said he felt empty, going though life without any sense of direction, ambition, or passion, a realization that itself was tormenting. He had bought a pistol, to put an end to what he called his useless existence, but did not carry his suicide out, believing that it would hurt his students and the small community in which he lived.

Patients with dysthymic disorder who present clinically as adults rarely develop mania. However, when treated with antidepressants some of them may develop brief hypomanic switches that typically disappear when the antidepressant dose is decreased. DSM-IV would not allow the occurrence of such switches in dysthymia; yet systematic clinical observation have verified their occurrence in as many as a third of dysthymic patients. In that special subgroup of persons with dysthymic disorder the family histories are often positive for bipolar disorder. Such patients represent a clinical bridge between depressive disorder and bipolar II disorders.

BIPOLAR DISORDERS

Four bipolar disorders are included in DSM-IV: bipolar I (manic-depressive) disorder, bipolar II disorder, cyclothymic disorder, and bipolar disorder NOS (Table 16.6-27).

BIPOLAR I DISORDER Typically beginning in the teenage years, the 20s, or the 30s, the first episode could be manic, depressive, or mixed. One common mode of onset is mild retarded depression, or hypersomnia, for a few weeks or months, which then switches into a manic episode. Others begin with a severely psychotic manic episode that presents schizophreniform features; it is only when a more classic manic episode occurs that the affective nature of the disorder is clarified. In a third group several depressive episodes take place before the first manic episode. A careful history taken from significant others will often reveal dysthymic or cyclothymic traits that antedated the frank onset of major episodes by several years. In DSM-IV there are six ways to subcategorize bipolar I patients: single manic episode (Table 16.6-28), most recent episode hypomanic (Table 16.6-29), most recent episode manic (Table 16.6-30), most recent episode mixed (Table 16.6-31) most recent episode depressed (Table 16.6-32) and most recent

TABLE 16.6-27
Diagnostic Criteria for Bipolar Disorder Not Otherwise Specified

The bipolar disorder not otherwise specified category includes disorders with bipolar features that do not meet criteria for any specific bipolar disorder. Examples include

1. Very rapid alternation (over days) between manic symptoms and depressive symptoms that do not meet minimal duration criteria for a manic episode or a major depressive episode
2. Recurrent hypomanic episodes without intercurrent depressive symptoms
3. A manic or mixed episode superimposed on delusional disorder, residual schizophrenia, or psychotic disorder not otherwise specified
4. Situations in which the clinician has concluded that a bipolar disorder is present but is unable to determine whether it is primary, due to a general medical condition, or substance induced

Table from DSM-IV, *Diagnostic and Statistical Manual of Mental Disorders,* ed 4. Copyright American Psychiatric Association, Washington, 1994. Used with permission.

TABLE 16.6-28
Diagnostic Criteria for Bipolar I Disorder, Single Manic Episode

A. Presence of only one manic episode and no past major depressive episodes.
Note: Recurrence is defined as either a change in polarity from depression or an interval of at least two months without manic symptoms.
B. The manic episode is not better accounted for by schizoaffective disorder and is not superimposed on schizophrenia, schizophreniform disorder, delusional disorder, or psychotic disorder not otherwise specified.

Specify if:
Mixed: if symptoms meet criteria for a mixed episode
Specify (for current or most recent episode):
Severity/psychotic/remission specifiers
With catatonic features
With postpartum onset

Table from DSM-IV, *Diagnostic and Statistical Manual of Mental Disorders,* ed 4. Copyright American Psychiatric Association, Washington, 1994. Used with permission.

TABLE 16.6-29
Diagnostic Criteria for Bipolar I Disorder, Most Recent Episode Hypomanic

A. Currently (or most recently) in a hypomanic episode.
B. There has previously been at least one manic episode or mixed episode.
C. The mood symptoms cause clinically significant distress or impairment in social, occupational, or other important areas of functioning.
D. The mood episodes in criteria A and B are not better accounted for by schizoaffective disorder and are not superimposed on schizophrenia, schizophreniform disorder, delusional disorder, or psychotic disorder not otherwise specified.

Specify:
Longitudinal course specifiers (with and without interepisode recovery)
With seasonal pattern (applies only to the pattern of major depressive episodes)
With rapid cycling

Table from DSM-IV, *Diagnostic and Statistical Manual of Mental Disorders,* ed 4. Copyright American Psychiatric Association, Washington, 1994. Used with permission.

episode unspecified (Table 16.6-33). According to DSM-IV, bipolar I disorder, Single manic episode, is used to describe patients who are having a first episode of mania (most such patients eventually develop depressive episodes). The remaining subcategorization is used to specify the nature of the current or most recent episode in patients who have had recurrent mood episodes. For clinicians and researchers alike it is more meaningful to chart a patient's course in color over time—for example, red rectangles for manic, blue for depressive, and violet for mixed episodes; hypomanic, dysthymic and cyclothymic periods can be drawn in the appropriate colors on a smaller scale between the major episodes. Life events, biologic stressors, and treatment can be indicated by arrows on the time axis. This approach, championed by Kraepelin, is routinely used in mood clinics.

On the average, manic episodes predominate in youth and depressive episodes in the later years. Although the overall sex ratio is about one to one, men on the average undergo more manic episodes and women experience more mixed and depressive episodes. Bipolar I disorder in children is not as rare as previously thought; however, most reported cases are boys, and mixed-manic (dysphoric-explosive) presentations are the most common mode.

Manic phase Mania, typically begins acutely over a period of one to two weeks; more sudden onsets have also been described. The DSM-IV criteria (Table 16.6-9) stipulate (1) a

TABLE 16.6-30
Diagnostic Criteria for Bipolar I Disorder, Most Recent Episode Manic

A. Currently (or most recently) in a manic episode.
B. There has previously been at least one major depressive episode, manic episode, or mixed episode.
C. The mood episodes in criteria A and B are not better accounted for by schizoaffective disorder and are not superimposed on schizophrenia, schizophreniform disorder, delusional disorder, or psychotic disorder not otherwise specified.

Specify (for current or most recent episode):
Severity/psychotic/remission specifiers
With catatonic features
With postpartum onset
Specify:
Longitudinal course specifiers (with and without interepisode recovery)
With seasonal pattern (applies only to the pattern of major depressive episodes)
With rapid cycling

Table from DSM-IV, *Diagnostic and Statistical Manual of Mental Disorders,* ed 4. Copyright American Psychiatric Association, Washington, 1994. Used with permission.

TABLE 16.6-31
Diagnostic Criteria for Bipolar I Disorder, Most Recent Episode Mixed

A. Currently (or most recently) in a Mixed Episode.
B. There has previously been at least one Major Depressive Episode, Manic Episode, or Mixed Episode.
C. The mood episodes in criteria A and B are not better accounted for by schizoaffective disorder and are not superimposed on schizophrenia, schizophreniform disorder, delusional disorder, or psychotic disorder not otherwise specified.

Specify (for current or most recent episode):
Severity/psychotic/remission specifiers
With catatonic features
With postpartum onset
Specify:
Longitudinal course specifiers (with and without interepisode recovery)
With seasonal pattern (applies only to the pattern of Major Depressive Episodes)
With rapid cycling

Table from DSM-IV, *Diagnostic and Statistical Manual of Mental Disorders,* ed 4. Copyright American Psychiatric Association, Washington, 1994. Used with permission.

TABLE 16.6-32
Diagnostic Criteria for Bipolar I Disorder, Most Recent Episode Depressed

A. Currently (or most recently) in a major depressive episode.
B. There has previously been at least one manic episode or mixed episode.
C. The mood episodes in criteria A and B are not better accounted for by schizoaffective disorder and are not superimposed on schizophrenia, schizophreniform disorder, delusional disorder, or psychotic disorder not otherwise specified.

Specify (for current or most recent episode):
Severity/psychotic/remission specifiers
Chronic
With catatonic features
With melancholic features
With atypical features
With postpartum onset
Specify:
Longitudinal course specifiers (with and without interepisode recovery)
With seasonal pattern (applies only to the pattern of major depressive episodes)
With rapid cycling

Table from DSM-IV, *Diagnostic and Statistical Manual of Mental Disorders,* ed 4. Copyright American Psychiatric Association, Washington, 1994. Used with permission.

TABLE 16.6-33
Diagnostic Criteria for Bipolar I Disorder, Most Recent Episode Unspecified

A. Criteria, except for duration, are currently (or most recently) met for a manic, a hypomanic, a mixed, or a major depressive episode.
B. There has previously been at least one manic episode or mixed episode.
C. The mood symptoms cause clinically significant distress or impairment in social, occupational, or other important areas of functioning.
D. The mood symptoms in criteria A and B are not better accounted for by schizoaffective disorder and are not superimposed on schizophrenia, schizophreniform disorder, delusional disorder, or psychotic disorder not otherwise specified.
E. The mood symptoms in criteria A and B are not due to the direct physiological effects of a substance (e.g., a drug of abuse, a medication, or other treatment) or a general medical condition (e.g., hyperthyroidism).

Specify:
Longitudinal course specifiers (with and without interepisode recovery)
With seasonal pattern (applies only to the pattern of major depressive episodes)
With rapid cycling

Table from DSM-IV, *Diagnostic and Statistical Manual of Mental Disorders,* ed 4. Copyright American Psychiatric Association, Washington, 1994. Used with permission.

distinct period that represents a break from premorbid functioning, (2) a duration of at least one week, (3) an elevated or irritable mood, (4) at least three to four classic manic signs and symptoms, and (5) the absence of any physical factors that could account for the clinical picture. The irritable mood in mania can deteriorate to cantankerous behavior, especially when the person is rebuffed. Such patients are among the most aggressive seen in the emergency room. Extreme psychotic disorganization, a common presentation of mania, further contributes to the aggression. Alcohol use, which is observed in at least 50 percent of bipolar I patients (typically in the manic phase), further disinhibits the patient and might lead to a dangerous frenzy. Such patients may attack loved ones and hurt them physically. So-called crimes of passion have been committed by patients harboring delusions of infidelity on the part of spouses or lovers, usually when under the influence of alcohol.

The genesis of delusional and hallucinatory, even first-rank, psychotic experiences in mania have already been described. Recent research has also documented that most types of formal thought disorders are common to both schizophrenic and mood psychoses: only poverty of speech content (vagueness) emerges as significantly more common in schizophrenia. Finally, posturing and negativism have been shown to occur in mania (and, in the author's view, do not warrant the designation of catatonic features as advocated by DSM-IV). Although not specifically mentioned in the DSM-IV definition, confusion, even pseudodemented presentations, can occur in mania.

Mania is most commonly expressed as a phase of bipolar I disorder, which has strong genetic determinants. Available evidence does not permit separating recurrent mania without depressive episodes as a distinct nosological entity from that form.

Secondary mania Although there is some suggestion that postpartum mania without depression is distinct from familial bipolar I disorder, in which both depressive and manic episodes can sometimes occur in the postpartum period, the evidence for a distinct puerperal mania is not compelling at this time (hence the decision in DSM-IV to use postpartum-onset as a specifier, rather than a separate mood disorder subtype [see Section 15.4]). It has also been known for some time that mania without prior bipolarity can arise in the setting of such somatic illnesses as influenza, thyrotoxicosis, systemic lupus erythematosus or its treatment with steroids, rheumatic chorea, multiple sclerosis, Huntington's disease, cerebrovascular disorder, diencephalic and third ventricular tumors, head trauma, complex partial seizures, and most recently, AIDS. The family history is reportedly low in such cases, suggesting a relatively low genetic predisposition and thus a lower risk of recurrence. The patients do not easily fit into the DSM-IV category of mood disorder due to a general medical condition (Table 16.6-18) because most of the conditions appear to be cerebral.

Less well-defined forms of mania are the so-called reactive manias. Personal loss and bereavement are hypothesized to be triggering factors, and the reaction is conceptualized in psychodynamic terms as a denial of loss. Although such explanations may be plausible in individual cases, no systematic data are available to suggest that the patients differ in family history from persons with other manias. The same is generally true for depressed patients who switch to hypomania or mania after the abuse of stimulant drugs, treatment with antidepressants, or sleep deprivation; in all of those situations a bipolar diathesis is usually manifest, either in a family history of mania or in spontaneous excited episodes during prospective observation. First-onset manic episodes have also been seen in persons who abstained from alcohol after one or two decades of abuse and who evolved into having classic bipolar I disorder.

Chronic mania DSM-IV does not specifically address the diagnostic questions posed by the 5 percent of bipolar I patients characterized by a chronic manic course. That course most commonly represents deterioration of course dominated by recurrent manic episodes. Noncompliance with pharmacological treatment is the rule. Recurrent excitement is personally reinforcing, subjective distress is minimal, and insight is seriously impaired; therefore, the patient sees no reason to adhere to treatment. Episodic or chronic alcohol abuse, which is prevalent in such patients, has been suggested as a contributory cause of the chronicity. Some authorities consider comorbid cerebral pathology to be responsible for nonrecovery from manic excitements occurring in late life.

Grandiose delusions, such as delusions of inventive genius or aristocratic birth, are not uncommon in chronic mania, and may lead to the mistaken diagnosis of paranoid schizophrenia. Because of their social deterioration, Kraepelin had subsumed such patients under the category "manic dementia." Nonschizoid premorbid adjustment and a family history of bipolar I disorder, as well as the absence of flagrant formal thought disorder, can be marshaled in establishing the affective basis of those poor-prognosis manic states.

Mixed phase Momentary tearfulness, depressed mood, and even suicidal ideation are commonly observed at the height of mania or during the transition from mania to retarded depression. Another common mixed feature is racing thoughts in the context of a retarded depression. Those transient labile periods, which occur in most bipolar I patients, must be contrasted with the mixed episodes experienced by 30 to 40 percent of patients in the long-term course of bipolar I disorder.

The mixed episodes proper (Table 16.6-25)—variously referred to as mixed mania or dysphoric mania—are characterized by dysphorically excited moods, anger, panic attacks, pressured speech, agitation, suicidal ideation, severe insomnia, grandiosity, and hypersexuality, as well as by persecutory delusions and confusion. Mixed states, when of mild to moderate intensity, could be misdiagnosed as major depressive disorder, or as atypical or neurotic depression, whereas severely psychotic forms that involve hallucinations and Schneiderian symptoms, can be misdiagnosed as schizoaffective disorder, or even schizophrenia. A correct diagnosis is mandatory for proper management because most classes of antidepressants may further aggravate the mixed pathology of those patients, whereas antipsychotics could exacerbate the depressive component. Thus misdiagnosis and inappropriate treatment can prolong the patient's suffering, leading to a protracted course over many months. That is especially likely to happen when the patient is nondelusional and the clinical picture is confused with agitated depressive disorder, and the patient is subjected to aggressive antidepressant therapy.

Depressive phase Psychomotor retardation, with or without hypersomnia, is the hallmark of the depressive phase of bipolar I disorder. Symptoms typically begin over a period of several weeks, although sudden onsets over one or two days are also seen. Although bipolar depressive episodes do not always acquire full-blown melancholic features, the autonomy of the episodes is a fundamental characteristic. Delusional and hallucinatory experiences are less common in the depressive phase of bipolar I disorder as compared with the manic and mixed phases. Stupor is the more common mode of psychotic presentation of bipolar depression, particularly in adolescents and young adults, where the mistaken diagnosis of catatonic stupor is often made. Pseudodemented organic presentations appear to be the counterpart of stupor in the elderly.

CYCLOTHYMIC DISORDER An attenuated bipolar disorder that typically begins insidiously before the age of 21, it is characterized by alternating short cycles of subsyndromal depression and hypomania (Table 16.6-34). That list, which reflects findings from the author's research, is more explicit than are the DSM-IV criteria (Table 16.6-35). The course of cyclothymia is continuous or intermittent, with infrequent periods of euthymia. Shifts in mood are typically endoreactive, such as suddenly falling in love or feeling profoundly dejected without adequate cause. Circadian cycles seem to play a role in the sudden mood changes, such as the person's going to sleep in good spirits and waking up early with suicidal urges.

In these ambulatory patients mood swings are overshadowed by the chaos that such swings produce in their personal lives. Repeated marital failures or romantic breakups are common, due to interpersonal friction and episodic promiscuous behavior. Uneven performance at school and work is another common characteristic. Thus persons with cyclothymic disorder are dilettantes: they show great promise in many areas, but rarely are able to bring any of their efforts to fruition. Their lives are often a string of improvident activities. Geographical instability is a characteristic feature: easily attracted to a new location, a new job, or a new love partner, they soon lose interest and leave in dissatisfaction. Polysubstance abuse, a complication occurring in 50 percent of such persons, is often an attempt at self-treatment.

TABLE 16.6-34
Clinical Features of Cyclothymic Disorder

Biphasic dysregulation characterized by abrupt endoreactive shifts from one phase to the other, each phase lasting for few days at a time, with infrequent euthymia.

Behavioral manifestations:
- Hypersomnia versus decreased need for sleep
- Introverted self-absorption versus uninhibited people seeking
- Taciturn versus talkative
- Unexplained tearfulness versus buoyant jocularity
- Psychomotor inertia versus restless pursuit of activities

Subjective manifestations:
- Lethargy and somatic discomfort versus eutonia
- Dulling of senses versus keen perceptions
- Slow-witted versus sharpened thinking
- Shaky self-esteem alternating between low self-confidence and overconfidence
- Pessimistic brooding versus optimism and carefree attitudes

Summarized from H S Akiskal, M Khani, A Scott-Strauss: Cyclothymic temperamental disorders. Psychiatr Clin North Am 2: 527, 1979.

TABLE 16.6-35
Diagnostic Criteria for Cyclothymic Disorder

A. For at least two years, the presence of numerous periods with hypomanic symptoms and numerous periods with depressive symptoms that do not meet criteria for a major depressive episode. **Note:** In children and adolescents, the duration must be at least one year.
B. During the above two-year period (one year in children and adolescents), the person has not been without the symptoms in criterion A for more than two months at a time.
C. No major depressive episode, manic episode, or mixed episode has been present during the first two years of the disturbance.
Note: After the initial two years (one year in children and adolescents) of cyclothymic disorder, there may be superimposed manic or mixed episodes (in which case both bipolar I disorder and cyclothymic disorder may be diagnosed) or major depressive episodes (in which case both bipolar II disorder and cyclothymic disorder may be diagnosed).
D. The symptoms in criterion A are not better accounted for by schizoaffective disorder and are not superimposed on schizophrenia, schizophreniform disorder, delusional disorder, or psychotic disorder not otherwise specified.
E. The symptoms are not due to the direct physiological effects of a substance (e.g., a drug of abuse, a medication) or a general medical condition (e.g., hyperthyroidism).
F. The symptoms cause clinically significant distress or impairment in social, occupational, or other important areas of functioning.

Table from DSM-IV, *Diagnostic and Statistical Manual of Mental Disorders,* ed 4. Copyright American Psychiatric Association, Washington, 1994. Used with permission.

BIPOLAR II DISORDER (AND THE SOFT BIPOLAR SPECTRUM) Research conducted during the past 15 years has shown that between the extremes of classic manic-depressive illness defined by at least one acute manic episode (bipolar I disorder) and strictly defined major depressive disorder without any personal or family history of mania, there exists a large group of intermediary forms characterized by recurrent major depressive episodes and hypomanic episodes (variously termed as atypical, bipolar II, or unipolar II). Table 16.6-36 summarizes those nosological concepts. The most accepted of the subtypes is bipolar II disorder, elevated to the status of a nosological entity in DSM-IV (Table 16.6-37). Bipolar II disorder may actually be more common than bipolar I disorder. That certainly appears to be the case in the outpatient setting, where as many as 30 percent of persons with major depressive disorder might conform to the bipolar II pattern.

The self-description provided by a 34-year-old poet illustrates the pattern: "I have known melancholy periods, lasting months at a time, when I would be literally paralyzed: All mental activity comes to a screeching halt, and I cannot even utter one word. I become so dysfunctional that I was once hospitalized. Although the paralysis creeps into me insidiously—often lasting months—it typically reverses within hours. I am suddenly alive and vibrant, I cannot turn off my brain neither during the day nor at night; I usually go on celebrating like this for many weeks, needing no more than few hours of slumber each day."

The hypomania at the end of depressive episodes in most bipolar II disorders does not persist that long; it is usually measured in days. Another common form of bipolar II disorder is major depressive disorder superimposed on cyclothymic disorder, where hypomania precedes and follows major depres-

TABLE 16.6-36
Spectrum of Bipolar Disorders Compared with Unipolar Depression

	Bipolar I:	At leat one manic episode
Soft bipolar	Bipolar II:	Recurrent depressions with hypomania and cyclothymic disorder
Soft bipolar	Bipolar III: (pseudo-unipolar)	Recurrent depressions without spontaneous hypomania but often with hyperthymic temperament and bipolar family history
	Unipolar depressions:	No evidence for hypomania, cyclothymic disorder, hyperthymic disorder, or bipolar family history

TABLE 16.6-37
Diagnostic Criteria for Bipolar II Disorder

A. Presence (or history) of one or more major depressive episodes.
B. Presence (or history) of at least one hypomanic episode.
C. There has never been a manic episode or a mixed episode.
D. The mood symptoms in criteria A and B are not better accounted for by schizoaffective disorder and are not superimposed on schizophrenia, schizophreniform disorder, delusional disorder, or psychotic disorder not otherwise specified.
E. The symptoms cause clinically significant distress or impairment in social, occupational, or other important areas of functioning.

Specify current or most recent episode:
- **Hypomanic:** if currently (or most recently) in a hypomanic episode
- **Depressed:** if currently (or most recently) in a major depressive episode

Specify (for current or most recent major depressive episode only if it is the most recent type of mood episode):
- **Severity/psychotic/remission specifiers** **Note:** Fifth-digit codes cannot be used here because the code for bipolar II disorder already uses the fifth digit.
- **Chronic**
- **With catatonic features**
- **With melancholic features**
- **With atypical features**
- **With postpartum onset**

Specify:
- **Longitudinal course specifiers (with and without interepisode recovery)**
- **With seasonal pattern** (applies only to the pattern of major depressive episodes)
- **With rapid cycling**

sion, the entire interepisodic period being characterized by cyclothymic mood swings.

Hypomania in bipolar II disorder can be defined as minimanic episodes occurring spontaneously. Thus bipolar II disorder can be characterized as cyclical depression. In bipolar III disorder (which is not an official nosological term) evidence of bipolarity is softer, such as a single brief episode of antidepressant-mobilized switch. In a related subgroup of cryptic bipolar disorders, strong evidence for familial bipolarity raises the hypothesis that some phenotypically unipolar depressions might actually be genotypically bipolar. In such cases, also referred to as pseudounipolar, hypomania as such is not observed; instead the patient's habitual temperamental baseline is sunny, overenergetic, and overoptimistic (hyperthymic). Depending on the threshold of traits used in determining the presence of hyperthymia, those patients may constitute 10 to 20 percent of those with major depressive disorder. Recurrent hypomanic episodes without intermittent depressions (example 2 in the DSM-IV criteria for bipolar disorder NOS [Table 16.6-27]) are almost never observed clinically.

The depressive episodes of bipolar II or III patients often have mixed admixtures—for example, flight of ideas, increased drives and impulsivity. These are depressive mixed states completely ignored by DSM-IV. Their existence explains why antidepressants often fail in these patients.

Hypomania The common denominator of the soft spectrum of bipolar disorders is the occurrence of hypomania. Hypomania refers to a distinct period of at least few days of mild elevation of mood, sharpened and positive thinking, and increased energy and activity levels, typically without the impairment characteristic of manic episodes. It is not merely a milder form of mania. Hypomania occurring as part of bipolar II disorder rarely progresses to manic psychosis. Thus distractibility is uncommon in hypomania, and there is relative preservation of insight. Hypomania is distinguished from mere happiness by the fact that it tends to recur (happiness does not!), and can sometimes be mobilized by antidepressants. In cyclothymic disorder it alternates with minidepressions, whereas in hyperthymic disorder it constitutes the person's habitual baseline. Those definitions then recognize three patterns of hypomania: brief episodes heralding the termination of a retarded depressive episode (bipolar II disorder), cyclic alternation with minidepressions (cyclothymic disorder), and an elevated baseline of high mood, activity, and cognition (hyperthymic disorder or chronic hypomania).

Because hypomania is experienced either as a rebound relief from depression or as pleasant, short-lived, ego-syntonic moods, persons with bipolar II disorder rarely report them spontaneously. Skillful questioning thus is required in making the diagnosis of soft bipolar conditions; as in mania, collateral information from family members is crucial. In interviewing the patient the following probes have been found useful to elicit hypomania: "Have you had a distinct sustained high period (1) when your thinking and perceptions were unusually vivid or rapid, (2) your mood was so intense that you felt nervous, and (3) you were endowed with such energy that others could not keep up with you?" The clinician must ascertain that, when endorsed by the patient, those experiences were not due to stimulant abuse.

When in doubt, direct clinical observation of hypomania—sometimes elicited by antidepressant pharmacotherapy—will provide definitive evidence for the bipolar nature of the disorder. However, in some cases depressive and hypomanic periods are not easily discerned because chronic caffeinism or stimulant abuse complicates the depression. In such instances, diagnosis should be based on clinical observation at least one month beyond detoxification.

Seasonal patterns Another characteristic observed in many cyclic depressions is seasonality, which often becomes manifest with autumn or winter anergic depression and energetic or frankly hypomanic periods in the spring. Thus seasonal depressions conform, in large measure, to the bipolar II or III pattern. Preliminary evidence suggests that when treated with classic antidepressants, such persons exhibit a disruption of their baseline seasonality, with the depressive phase appearing in the spring and summer. The changes induced by antidepressants in seasonal depressions probably represent a special variant of the phenomenon of rapid cycling.

Temperament and polarity of episodes New research from collaboration between the University of Tennessee and the University of Pisa has shown that bipolar II disorder (characterized predominantly by depressive attacks) appears to arise more often from a hyperthymic or cyclothymic baseline, whereas bipolar I disorder (defined by manic attacks) not uncommonly arises from the substrate of a depressive temperament. Bipolarity is conventionally defined by the alternation of manic (or hypomanic) and depressive episodes. Those data on temperaments suggest that a more fundamental characteristic of bipolarity is the reversal of temperament into its opposite episode (that is, from the depressive temperament to mania and from the hyperthymic temperament to depression).

Those considerations have implications for preventing recurrence. For instance, in a prospective study of the onset of bipolar disorder in the offspring or sibs of adults with the disorder, it was found that children with onsets of depression (treated with antidepressants) had significantly higher rates of recurrence than did those with manic or mixed onsets (treated with lithium) during a three-year prospective observation. Such data suggest the hypothesis that temperamental instability in the depressive group might have predisposed them to the cycling effect of antidepressants.

Alcohol, substance abuse, and suicide New evidence supports the high prevalence of alcohol and substance abuse in mood disorder subtypes, especially those with cyclothymic and hyperthymic temperaments. The relation appears particularly strong in the teenage and early adult years, at which time the use of such substances often represents self-medication. It is not to be viewed just as self-treatment for selected symptoms associated with the down or up phases (for example, alcohol to alleviate the insomnia and nervousness characteristic of both phases), but also as augmenting certain desired ends (for example, stimulants to enhance high-energy performance and sexual behavior associated with hypomania). The exact proportion of those with alcohol and substance abuse secondary to an underlying bipolar diathesis is a question for future research, and is of public health significance in view of findings suggesting a link between adolescent polysubstance abuse and suicide in those with bipolar familial backgrounds. Although alcohol and substance use often continues into adult years in a considerable number of bipolar patients, such use does not appear related to familial alcoholism and, in many instances, tends to dwindle during long-term follow-up. Those data provide support for the self-medication hypothesis. To complicate matters, in a substantial minority of cases, bipolar mood swings appear for the first time following abrupt cessation of long-term alcohol use.

Rapid-cycling bipolar disorder Rapid cycling is defined as the occurrence of at least four episodes—both retarded depression and hypomania (or mania)—a year. That means that rapid cyclers are rarely free of affective symptoms, resulting in serious vocational and interpersonal incapacitation. Lithium is often only modestly helpful to those patients, as are antipsychotics; tricyclic antidepressants readily induce excited episodes and thereby aggravate the rapid cycling pattern. A balance among lithium, antipsychotics, and antidepressants may be difficult to achieve. The patients require frequent hospitalization because they develop explosive excitement and precipitously descend into severe psychomotor inhibition. The disorder is a roller-coaster nightmare for the patient, significant others, and the treating physician.

As expected, rapid cycling commonly arises from a cyclothymic substrate, which means that most rapid cyclers have bipolar II disorder. Factors favoring its occurrence include (1) female gender; (2) hypothyroidism; (3) menopause; (4) temporal lobe dysrhythmias; (5) alcohol, minor tranquilizer, stimulant, or caffeine abuse; and (6) long-term use of antidepressant medications. The DSM-IV criteria for rapid-cycling specifier are presented in Table 16.6-38.

Rapid-cycling uncommonly arises from a bipolar I baseline. These patients might resemble examples 1 and 3 listed under bipolar disorder NOS (Table 16.6-27).

TABLE 16.6-38
Criteria for Rapid-Cycling Specifier

Specify if:
With rapid cycling (can be applied to bipolar I disorder or bipolar II disorder)
At least four episodes of a mood disturbance in the previous 12 months that meet criteria for a major depressive, manic, mixed, or hypomanic episode.
Note: Episodes are demarcated either by partial or full remission for at least two months or a switch to an episode of opposite polarity (e.g., major depressive episode to manic episode).

Table from DSM-IV, *Diagnostic and Statistical Manual of Mental Disorders,* ed 4. Copyright American Psychiatric Association, Washington, 1994. Used with permission.

Leadership and creativity Persons with hyperthymic temperament, and soft bipolar conditions in general, possess assets that permit them to assume leadership roles in business, the professions, civic life, and politics. Increased energy, sharp thinking, and self-confidence represent the virtues of an otherwise stormy life.

Creative achievement is relatively uncommon among those with the manic forms of the disorder, which is too severe and disorganizing to permit the necessary concentration and dedication. It is among those with the soft bipolar disorders, especially cyclothymic disorders, that notable artistic achievements are found. Psychosis, including severe bipolar swings, is generally incompatible with creativity. That conclusion, based on recent systematic studies, tends to refute the romantic tendency to idolize insanity as being central to the creative process. As talent is the necessary ingredient of creativity, how might soft bipolarity contribute? The simplest hypothesis is that depression could provide insights into the human condition, which, however, requires the activation associated with hypomania to produce the artistic work. A more profound interpretation would suggest that the repeated self-doubt that comes with recurrent depression might be an important ingredient of creativity, because original artistic or scientific expression is often initially rejected, and the self-confidence that accompanies repeated bouts of hypomania can help in rehearsing such ideas or expressions until they are perfected. Finally, the tempestuous object relations associated with bipolarity often create the unique life situations that might be immortalized in an artistic medium.

MOOD DISORDER NOT OTHERWISE SPECIFIED After all diagnostic information has been obtained, some depressed and bipolar or otherwise affective patients do not meet the criteria for the mood disorders described thus far. The author prefers to consider them as undiagnosed mood disorders rather than using the DSM-IV rubrics of depression disorder NOS, bipolar disorder NOS, or mood disorder NOS. The DSM-IV criteria for mood disorder NOS appear in Table 16.6-39.

TABLE 16.6-39
Diagnostic Criteria for Mood Disorder Not Otherwise Specified

This category includes disorders with mood symptoms that do not meet the criteria for any specific mood disorder and in which it is difficult to choose between depressive disorder not otherwise specified and bipolar disorder not otherwise specified (e.g., acute agitation).

Table from DSM-IV, *Diagnostic and Statistical Manual of Mental Disorders,* ed 4. Copyright American Psychiatric Association, Washington, 1994. Used with permission.

What follows are descriptions of conditions that are commonly used in the epidemiological, clinical, or pharmacological literature, but do not easily fit into the classic nosology of mood disorders. They probably subsume many, but not all, of the situations implied in the DSM-IV NOS concepts.

Recurrent brief depressive disorder The disorder (now in a DSM-IV appendix) derives largely from epidemiological studies conducted in young adult cohorts in Zurich. The description is that of short-lived depressions that recur on a monthly basis but are not menstrually related. They could coexist with major depressive disorder and dysthymic disorder. It is believed that such patients are more prevalent in primary care than in psychiatric settings. The minority seen in psychiatric settings present with repeated suicide attempts, and are likely to be given Axis II diagnoses, such as borderline personality disorder. The research criteria for recurrent brief depressive disorder appear in Table 16.6-23.

The current nosological status of those patients is uncertain, but they testify to Kraepelin's observation that many transitional forms link the depressive temperament to affective episodes:

> A permanent gloomy stress in all the experiences of life . . . usually perceptible already in youth, and may persist without essential change throughout the whole of life . . . (or) there is actually an uninterrupted series of transitions to periodic melancholia . . . in which the course is quite indefinite with irregular fluctuations and remissions.

Given the high rate of brief depressive recurrences among the patients observed in the Zurich cohort, it is likely that brief hypomanic episodes have been missed during evaluations performed by nonclinicians. Some, if not most patients meeting the Zurich description might actually belong to the soft bipolar spectrum.

Reactive depression Classically such a depression is defined as resulting from a specific life event. In an ideal case the depression would not have occurred without the event (for example, love loss) to which it is a reaction, it would continue for as long as the event were present, and it would terminate with the reversal of the event (for example, the return of the lover). Depressions exhibiting all of those features are almost never seen in clinical practice. With interpersonal support most people are able to face life's reverses, which explains why reactive depression tends to be self-limiting. Hence, adjustment disorder would be the more appropriate diagnosis in most cases of reactive depression.

Conceptually, however, it is possible to envision chronically unsatisfactory life situations that might lead to chronic demoralization. However, such a condition, which could warrant the designation of chronic reactive depression, is a contradiction in terms. The question often raised is why a person would continue to stay in the situation. Sometimes the concept of masochism is invoked by psychodynamic authors to explain why certain persons are unable to rid themselves of painful life situations, the implication being that they somehow contribute to their maintenance. Current thinking is that many of those presumed self-defeating traits, believed to be indicative of masochism, are more situation specific than previously believed, and might resolve with the elimination of the situation. So-called self-defeating features then are best conceptualized as psychodynamic mechanisms, rather than as being indicative of a specific personality. At the present stage of knowledge, they do not deserve to be raised to the level of a nosological entity. Chronic adjustment disorder, seemingly a contradiction in terms, might describe the chronic demoralization observed among some individuals stuck in chronically unsatisfactory life situations. Others might fullfill the criteria for dysthymia.

Mixed anxiety-depressive disorder The inclusion of anxious depressive states in a DSM-IV appendix acknowledges the simultaneous occurrence of anxious (for example, the threat loss represents) and depressive (for example, the despair of loss) cognition when confronted with a major aversive life situation. The admixture implies that the progress of psychopathology is from anxiety to depression, that the patient's mental state is still in flux, and that the ongoing dynamics in part explains the subacute or chronic nature of the disorder. Anxious depression serves to point to the common presence of anxiety in depressive states, and especially its greater visibility when the depression is less prominent. Patients with the latter presentation are reportedly most prevalent in general medical settings. According to DSM-IV, persons whose presentation meets those research criteria would be diagnosed as having anxiety disorder not otherwise specified (see Section 17.5).

Some authorities argue that neurotic depressions arise in that fashion (that is, as maladaptive response to anxiety) and, on that etiological ground, suggest retaining the neurotic depressive rubric. Recent preliminary genetic data tend indirectly to support the contention that certain (unipolar) depressive and (generalized) anxiety states are related. However, more research needs to be conducted in the area before such an entity can be unequivocally accepted as an official nosological category. The difficulty lies in the fact that, as currently defined, anxious depressions are heterogeneous.

Neurasthenia Neurasthenia, a century-old term developed by the American neuropsychiatrist George Beard, refers to a more chronic stage of anxious-depressive symptomatology. The anxiety generated by overstimulation is so excessive that it is replaced by a chronic disposition to irritability, fatigue (especially mental fatigue), lethargy, and exhaustion. It is as if the sufferer's mind refuses to take on new stresses. The clinical picture described by Beard suggests that anxious manifestations were preeminent in his time. They included headache, scalp tenderness, backache, heavy limbs, vague neuralgias, yawning, dyspepsia, palpitations, sweating hands and feet, chills, flushing, sensitivity to weather changes, insomnia, nightmares, pantaphobia, asthenopia, and tinnitus.

Although the diagnosis of neurasthenia itself is now used more in China than it is in the United States, the recent worldwide upsurge in the popularity of the concept of chronic fatigue states attests to the clinical acumen of classic physicians. Despite much energy invested in a viral or immunological etiology, current descriptions tend to suggest an anxiety or mood disorder basis for many, if not most, of those with the syndrome. However, under what circumstances anxiety or depression would become manifest primarily in fatigue is as elusive as it was 100 years ago.

Like other patients presenting to primary care settings with somatic complaints, those with chronic fatigue tend to denounce psychiatric diagnoses as inadequate explanations for their ills. Empathic listening, perhaps in a group therapy format, might be a reasonable approach to that difficult group of patients, who can be quite disabled.

Atypical depression Although a delimited version of the construct has been incorporated into DSM-IV as atypical features (Table 16.6-7) to qualify the cross-sectional picture of depressive disorders, the construct is much broader in the clinical research literature and warrants further discussion. The rubric, originally developed in England and currently under investigation at Columbia University in New York, refers to fatigue superimposed on a history of somatic anxiety and phobias, together with reverse vegetative signs (mood worse in the evening, insomnia, tendency to oversleep and overeat). Given that nighttime sleep is disturbed in the first half of the night in many persons with atypical depressive disorder, irritability, hypersomnolence, and daytime fatigue would seem to represent expected daytime stigmata of sleep deprivation due to intermittent initial insomnia. The temperaments of those patients are characterized by inhibited-sensitive traits. There seems to be some specificity of the MAOIs (and possibly serotonergic antidepressants) for such patients, which is the main reason that atypical depression is taken seriously.

Other research suggests that reverse vegetative signs can be classified as either (1) the anxious type just described, or (2) a subtle bipolar subtype with protracted hyperphagic-hypersomnic-retarded dysthymic disorder with occasional brief extroverted hypomanic-type behavior, often elicited by antidepressants. There is some affinity between atypical depression and bipolar II and III disorders. Many patients with dysthymic disorder at various times exhibit atypical features.

Hysteroid dysphoria The category combines reverse vegetative signs with the following characteristics: (1) giddy responses to romantic opportunities, and an avalanche of dysphoria (angry-depressive, even suicidal responses) upon romantic disappointment; (2) impaired anticipatory pleasure, yet the capability to respond with pleasure when such is provided by others (that is, preservation of consummatory reward); (3) craving for chocolate and sweets, which contain phenylethylamine compounds and sugars believed to facilitate cellular and neuronal intake of the amino-acid L-tryptophan, hypothetically leading to the brain's synthesis of endogenous antidepressants. The use of the epithet "hysteroid" was meant to convey that what appeared to be a character pathology was secondary to a biological disturbance in the substrates governing affect, drives, and reward. The hysteroid dysphorics' intense, giddy, and unstable life suggests links to cyclothymic disorder or bipolar II disorder. That suggestion is further supported by the Columbia group's tendency to subsume those patients under atypical depressions (some of which, as indicated, have bipolar affinities). Finally, like bipolar depressives, they show preferential response to MAOIs.

Postpsychotic depressive disorder of schizophrenia In DSM-IV the description of postpsychotic depressive disorder of schizophrenia appears as follows:

> The essential feature is a Major Depressive Episode that is superimposed on, and occurs only during, the residual phase of Schizophrenia. The residual phase of Schizophrenia follows the active phase (i.e., symptoms meeting Criterion A) of Schizophrenia. It is characterized by the persistence of negative symptoms or of active-phase symptoms that are in an attenuated form (e.g., odd beliefs, unusual perceptual experiences). The superimposed Major Depressive Episode must include depressed mood (i.e., loss of interest or pleasure cannot serve as an alternate for sad or depressed mood). Most typically, the Major Depressive Episode follows immediately after remission of the active-phase symptoms of the psychotic episode. Sometimes it may follow after a short or extended interval during which there are no psychotic symptoms. Mood symptoms due to the direct physiological effects of a drug of abuse, a medication, or a general medical condition are not counted toward postpsychotic depressive disorder of Schizophrenia.

TABLE 16.6-40
Research Criteria for Postpsychotic Depressive Disorder of Schizophrenia

A. Criteria are met for a major depressive episode.
   Note: The major depressive episode must include criterion A1: depressed mood. Do not include symptoms that are better accounted for as medication side effects or negative symptoms of schizophrenia.
B. The major depressive episode is superimposed on and occurs only during the residual phase of schizophrenia.
C. The major depressive episode is not due to the direct physiological effects of a substance or a general medical condition.

Table from DSM-IV, *Diagnostic and Statistical Manual of Mental Disorders,* ed 4. Copyright American Psychiatric Association, Washington, 1994. Used with permission.

According to DSM-IV, persons whose presentation meets those research criteria (Table 16.6-40) would be diagnosed as having depressive disorder NOS. In the author's opinion, mood or depressive disorder NOS represent such a hodgepodge of clinical situation that the designation of NOS is at best meaningless and at worst confusing.

DIFFERENTIAL DIAGNOSIS

Missing a mood disorder diagnosis, with the result that the disorder does not receive specific treatment, can have serious consequences. Many persons drop out of school or college, lose their jobs, are divorced, or commit suicide. Those with unexplained somatic symptoms are frequent utilizers of the general health system. Still others are unwell despite interminable psychotherapy. Some develop tardive dyskinesia unnecessarily. As with other medical disorders for which specific treatments are available, accurate diagnosis and early treatment are within the purview of all physicians. All psychiatrists, clinical psychologists, and psychiatric social workers should be competent in the detection of mood disorders. Despite massive educational efforts, underdiagnosis of mood disorders and their undertreatment are still serious problems worldwide.

Although much enthusiasm was generated a decade earlier about the potential utility of certain biological markers (such as REM latency, dexamethasone suppression test, and the thyrotropin-releasing-hormone test) as corroborating evidence in the differentiation of mood disorder from adjacent disorders, no definitive progress has been made along those lines that would justify their routine use in clinical practice. Faced with unusual or confusing presentations, a systematic clinical approach is still the only method in differential diagnosis (1) to characterize in great detail all the clinical features of the current episode, (2) to elicit a history of more typical major mood episodes in the past, (3) to assess whether the presenting complaints recur in a periodic or cyclical fashion, (4) to substantiate the adequacy of social functioning between periods of illness, (5) to obtain a positive family history for classic mood disorder and to construct a family pedigree, and (6) to document a history of unequivocal therapeutic response to thymoleptic medication or ECT in either the patient or in the family.

Using the foregoing validating approach, it is possible to examine the affective links of many DSM-IV disorders currently listed under conditions other than mood disorders. They include (1) conduct disorders; (2) borderline personality disorder; (3) impulse-control disorder; (4) polysubstance abuse; (5) psychotic disorder not otherwise specified; (6) pain disorder; (7) hypochondriasis; (8) hypoactive sexual desire disorder; (9) circadian rhythm sleep disorder, delayed sleep phase type; (10) bulimia nervosa; and (11) adjustment disorder (with work inhibition). It is apparent that those conditions place special emphasis on selected affective features, such as disinhibited behavior, temperamentality, lability, vegetative disturbances, and psychomotor retardation. What follows is a systematic examination of the differential diagnosis of mood disorders with their more classic boundaries.

ALCOHOL AND SUBSTANCE USE DISORDERS The high comorbidity of those disorders with mood disorders cannot be explained merely as the chance occurrence of two prevalent disorders. Self-medication for mood symptoms is insufficiently appreciated by both psychiatrists and addictionologists. Given the clinical dangers of missing an otherwise treatable disorder, mood disorder should be given serious consideration as the primary diagnosis if marked affective manifestations continue beyond the period of detoxification (for example, two months). That consideration also pertains to cyclothymic disorder and dysthymic disorder, which are common substrates for self-medication. The clinical validating strategies listed can further buttress a mood disorder diagnosis.

The DSM-IV category of substance-induced mood disorder (Table 16.6-20) is difficult to validate clinically because, in the absence of an affective diathesis, detoxification will usually clear affective disturbances occurring in persons who abuse substances. In the author's view, a dual diagnosis of both a mood disorder and a substance use disorder is a better alternative than is the DSM-IV construct.

PERSONALITY DISORDERS The state dependency of most personality measures is well documented. Accordingly, as exhorted by DSM-IV, clinicians should refrain from using personality disorder labels in describing patients with active affective illness, but should focus instead on treating the disorder. As discussed earlier, even in those with chronic or intermittent subsyndromal mood disorders, personality maladjustment is postaffective, arising from the distortions and conflicts that mood disturbances produce in the life of the sufferer. The most problematic of the personality labels used in those with mood disorders is borderline personality disorder, usually applied to teenage and young adult patients. The DSM-IV diagnostic criteria for the disorder indicate a liberal assemblage of low-grade affective symptoms. As shown in Table 16.6-41, the overlap between borderline personality disorder and mood disorders is extensive, so that giving a borderline personality disorder diagnosis to a person with mood disorder is redundant. When personality disorder diagnoses are used, they lead to neglect of the mood disorder. Although much more research needs to be done on the complex interface of personality disorders and mood disorders, clinically they may be inseparable. As with alcohol and substance use disorders, it appears preferable to diagnose mood disorders at the expense of personality disorders, which should not be difficult to justify in most cases where the validating strategies outlined are satisfied. Although not all personality disturbances recede with the competent treatment of mood disorders, so many experienced clinicians have seen such disturbances disappear with the successful resolution of the mood disorder that erring in favor of mood disorders is justified.

TABLE 16.6-41
Overlap of Borderline Personality Disorder and Mood Disorders

Familial:	High rates of mood disorder
Phenomenology:	Dysthymic disorder
	Cyclothymic disorder
	Bipolar II disorder
	Mixed state
Pharmacological response:	Worsening on tricyclic antidepressants
	Stabilization on anticonvulsants
Prospective course:	Major mood episodes
	Suicide

Summarized from H Akiskal, S Chen, G Davis, V Puzantian, M Kashgarian, M Bolinger: Borderline: An adjective in search for a noun. J Clin Psychiatry *46:* 41, 1985.

TABLE 16.6-42
Misdiagnosis in the Affectively Ill Juvenile Kin of Adults with Bipolar Disorder

Total (N = 44)	Percent
Adjustment disorder	35
Conduct disorder	15
Attention-deficit/hyperactivity disorder	9
Mental retardation	6
Separation anxiety disorder	9
Overanxious disorder	11
Schizophrenia	15

Table adapted from H S, Akiskal, J Downs, S Watson, D Daugherty, D B Pruitt: Affective disorders in referred children and younger siblings of manic-depressives. Arch Gen Psychiatry *43:* 996, 1985.

The interface of mood disorders and behavioral disorders in children is even more problematic than in adult psychiatry. Some progress has occurred in recognizing certain behavioral manifestations as possible signs of depression in juvenile patients, including (1) decline in school performance; (2) restlessness and pulling or rubbing hair, skin, or clothing; (3) outbursts of complaining, shouting, or crying; and (4) aggressive or antisocial acts. Examined carefully, many of the children will meet the specific criteria for the diagnosis of major depressive disorder or dysthymic disorder. It is important, however, to note that many children do not complain of subjective dysphoria; instead, the clinician can observe the depressed affect in the child's facial expressions or overall demeanor. In brief, after much resistance, many child clinicians have come to accept the existence of childhood depression. Bipolar disorder in children, even among adolescents, is still grossly underdiagnosed at the expense of so-called externalizing disorders. Table 16.6-42 lists those and related conditions often confused with bipolar disorders in juvenile patients. In many of the children bipolar disorder is expressed in explosive outbursts of irritable mood and behavior (that is, as a mixed or dysphoric manic state). Another common pattern is intermittent hypomania and cyclothymia. The correct diagnosis depends on the index of suspicion by a clinician who is convinced that bipolarity exists in childhood.

NORMAL BEREAVEMENT As bereaved persons exhibit many depressive symptoms during the first one or two years after their loss, how can the 5 percent of bereaved persons who have progressed to a depressive disorder be identified? Here are some points on which they differ:

1. Whereas grieving persons, and their relatives, perceive bereavement as a normal reaction, those with depressive disorder often view themselves as sick, and may actually believe they are losing their minds.
2. Unlike the melancholic person, the grieving person is reactive to the environment, and tends to show a range of positive affects.
3. Marked psychomotor retardation is not observed in normal grief.
4. Although bereaved persons sometimes feel guilty about not having done certain things that might have saved the life of the deceased loved one, they typically do not experience guilt of commission.
5. Delusions of worthlessness or sin, and psychotic experiences in general, point toward mood disorder.
6. Active suicidal ideation is rare in grief but common in major depressive disorder.

7. Mummification, which refers to keeping the belongings of the deceased person exactly as they were before his or her death, is indicative of psychopathology.

8. Severe anniversary reactions should alert observers to the possibility of psychopathology.

In another form of bereavement depression, the sufferer simply pines away, unable to live without the departed person, usually a spouse. Although not necessarily pathological by the foregoing criteria, such persons do have a serious medical condition. Their immune function is often depressed and their cardiovascular status is precarious. Death within a few months of that of a spouse can ensue, especially among elderly men. Such considerations suggest that it would be clinically unwise to withhold antidepressants from certain persons experiencing an intensely mournful form of grief.

ANXIETY DISORDERS Anxiety symptoms—including panic attacks, morbid fears, and obsessions—are common during depressive disorders, and depression is a common complication of anxiety states. Systematic British studies have shown that early-morning awakening, psychomotor retardation, self-reproach, hopelessness, and suicidal ideation are the strongest clinical markers of depression in that differential diagnosis. On follow-up of depressed patients, the manifestations tend to remit, whereas those with anxiety states continue to exhibit marked tension, phobias, panic attacks, vasomotor instability, feelings of unreality, and perceptual distortions, as well as hypochondriacal ideas. A predominance of such anxiety features antedating the present disorder suggests the diagnosis of an anxiety disorder. Given that anxiety disorders rarely make their first appearance after the age of 40, such late appearance of marked anxiety features strongly favors the diagnosis of melancholia. The clinical picture is often one of morbid groundless anxiety with somatization, hypochondriasis, and agitation. The patient's depressive nature is further supported by the superior response to ECT.

Periodic monosymptomatic phobic and obsessional states also exist that can be regarded as affective equivalents, based on a family history of mood disorders and the response to thymoleptic agents, including lithium. There are also social phobias that usher in an adolescent depression, even a bipolar disorder.

The psychopathological differentiation of anxiety and depressive states has not been entirely resolved. Cognitive factors may best differentiate them (Table 16.6-43). Although recurrent (especially retarded) major depressive disorder is a distinct disorder from anxiety states, at least some forms of depression may share a common diathesis with anxiety disorders. Before assigning patients to such a putative mixed anxiety-depressive group (not yet an official nosological entity), the clinician must note that anxiety that arises primarily during depressive episodes is best considered as exiphenomenal to depressive disorder. The same is generally true for anxiety symptoms that occur in a person with depressive disorder who is using alcohol or sedative-hypnotic or stimulant drugs. Finally, anxiety symptoms could be prominent features of mixed bipolar states as well as of complex partial seizures.

TABLE 16.6-43
Unique Cross-Sectional Profiles of Clinical Anxiety and Depression

Anxiety	Depression
Hypervigilance	Psychomotor retardation
Severe tension and panic	Severe sadness
Perceived danger	Perceived loss
Phobic avoidance	Loss of interest—anhedonia
Doubt and uncertainty	Hopelessness—suicidal
Insecurity	Self-deprecation
Performance anxiety	Loss of libido
	Early-morning awakening
	Weight loss

Table from H S Akiskal: Toward a clinical understanding of the relationship of anxiety and depressive disorders. In *Comorbidity of Mood and Anxiety Disorders,* J P Maser, C R Cloninger, editors, p 597. American Psychiatric Press, Washington, 1990. Used with permission.

PHYSICAL DISEASE Somatic complaints are common in depressive disorders. Some, such as vegetative disturbances, represent the hypothalamic pathology that presumably underlies a depressive disorder. Autonomic arousal, commonly associated with depression, could explain such symptoms as palpitations, sweating, and headache. In some instances the physical symptoms might reflect delusional experiences.

Depression in the setting of physical disease The clinician must be alert, however, to the fact that somatic complaints in depression could also reflect an underlying physical illness. Table 16.6-44 lists the most common medical conditions that have been associated with depression. When depressive symptoms occur in the setting of physical illness, it is not always easy to determine whether they constitute a genuine depressive disorder. Before diagnosing depression, psychiatrists must make sure that they are not dealing with pseudodepression: (1) functional loss due to physical illness; (2) vegetative signs, such as anorexia nervosa, as manifestations of such an illness; (3) stress and demoralization secondary to the hospitalization; (4) pain and discomfort associated with the illness; and (5) medi-

TABLE 16.6-44
Pharmacological Factors and Physical Diseases Associated with Onset of Depression

Pharmacological	Steroidal contraceptives
	Reserpine; α-methyldopa
	Anticholine-esterase insecticides
	Amphetamine or cocaine withdrawal
	Alcohol or sedative-hypnotic withdrawal
	Cimetidine; indomethacin
	Phenothiazine antipsychotics
	Thallium; mercury
	Cycloserine
	Vincristine; vinblastine
Endocrine	Hypothyroidism and hyperthyroidism
	Hyperparathyroidism
	Hypopituitarism
	Addison's disease
	Cushing's disease
	Diabetes mellitus
Infectious	General paresis (tertiary syphilis)
	Toxoplasmosis
	Influenza; viral pneumonia
	Viral hepatitis
	Infectious mononucleosis
	AIDS
Collagen	Rheumatoid arthritis
	Lupus erythematosus
Nutritional	Pellagra
	Pernicious anemia
Neurological	Multiple sclerosis
	Parkinson's disease
	Head trauma
	Complex partial seizures
	Sleep apnea
	Cerebral tumors
	Cerebrovascular disorder
Neoplastic	Abdominal malignancies
	Disseminated carcinomatosis

cation side effects. The presence of the following might be useful in supporting a mood disorder diagnosis in the presence of physical illness: (1) persistent anhedonia; (2) social withdrawal; (3) observed depressed mood with frequent crying; (4) observed psychomotor retardation or agitation; (5) indecisiveness; (6) convictions of failure, worthlessness, or guilt; (7) suicidal ideation; (8) nonparticipation in the process of medical care.

One of the most difficult problems making the interface of mood disorder and physical disease is the rare development of malignancy in patients with an established mood disorder. The patient who had responded well to a given antidepressant during previous episodes will now evince an unsatisfactory response to the same medication. Even a small dose (for example, imipramine [Tofranil], 25 mg) may cause such alarming symptoms as agitation, dizziness, depersonalization, and illusions, which might be indicative of an occult malignancy, perhaps in the abdomen or the brain. Thus the psychiatrist should always be vigilant about the appearance of life-threatening physical diseases in patients with preestablished depressive disorder.

Stupor Although less common today, stupor still raises a diagnostic problem in differentiating between a mood disorder and somatic disease, as well as other psychiatric disorders. It is relatively easy to distinguish depressive stupor from so-called hysterical mutism or nonresponsiveness; in the latter, behavior is meaningfully directed to significant others in the patient's environment. The rubric of catatonic stupor is best reserved for a phase of schizophrenia; in such patients the schizophrenic origin of the catatonia might be apparent from the patient's history. Otherwise, most acute-onset stupors are probably affective in origin. The main differential diagnosis here is from organic stupor (due to drugs or acute intracranial events); the physical and neurological examination is not always decisive in such cases, and diagnosis depends on a high index of suspicion concerning possible somatic factors.

Depressive pseudodementia The geriatric equivalent of semistupor in younger persons with depressive disorder, it is distinguished from primary degenerative dementia by (1) its acute onset; (2) a history of past affective episodes; (3) self-reproach; (4) diurnality of the cognitive dysfunction (worse in the morning); (5) the circumscribed nature of those deficits, which, with proper coaching, can be reversed; and (6) a tendency to improve with sleep deprivation.

Chronic fatigue syndrome The syndrome represents a complex differential diagnostic problem in view of the subtle nature of the immunological disturbances presumably associated with it. The following self-report by such a patient illustrates many of the uncertainties marking the present knowledge of the interface between the syndrome and mood disorders.

> I am a 39-year-old, never-married woman, trained as a social worker, but currently on disability. I have experienced extreme lethargy and fatigue for many years. I have always felt foggy headed and had trouble thinking and concentrating. My complaint is of fatigue, not of depression. My body feels like lead and aches all over. My brain feels achy and sore. I feel much worse in the morning and I can't get out of bed; I feel better at night. I feel bad every day. I ache all over, as though someone had beaten me up. Exercise has been prescribed to me, but it makes me worse. Also, I am very sensitive to hot and cold. My sexual drive is low. I have a general feeling of anhedonia. As far back as I remember—in junior high school—I was always exhausted. I always complained about fatigue, *not* depression, because that has been the overwhelming problem. I feel the depression is secondary to the fatigue. In high school I was a compulsive overeater and I was bulimic for a few years, but it was never severe and I was only about 10 pounds overweight. In those days I would sleep 10 or 12 hours a night on the weekend and still feel exhausted; I could not get up for school on Monday. As an adolescent, I felt inferior. I couldn't make decisions, I didn't want to go to camp or leave home for long periods of time—I felt so insecure. Recently I had a sleep study done, which showed a short latency to stage REM sleep (49 minutes). I was diagnosed as having dysthymic disorder, and began taking antidepressants. When I took tranylcypromine (Parnate), it was the first time in my life that I felt like a normal person. I could play sports, I had a sex drive, I had energy, and I was able to think clearly. But the benefits lasted for barely two months. My response was equally short-lived to phenelzine (Nardil), imipramine (Tofranil), seligeline (Eldepryl), and bupropion (Wellbutrin). I have not responded to serotonin-specific reuptake inhibitors (SSRI) at all. I also wish to point out that I had never experienced high periods before I took antidepressants. My main problem has always been one of exhaustion. When I responded to medications, they worked very quickly (within a few days) and I felt great, but they all stopped working after a short time. The dose would be raised, and again I would feel better. Eventually, when I got to high doses, I either could not tolerate the high dose or the drug would no longer help. I have taken different combinations of drugs for 10 years and I haven't been able to feel well for more than six weeks at a time. Recently, I went to an immunologist. He said I have an abnormality in regulating antibody production and recommended gammaglobulin shots. They did not help. When I first started working, I always felt tired and foggy headed, so it was difficult to be sharp while at work. At times I would close the door to my office and put my head down. Working has become increasingly difficult for me. I had two great jobs, which I blew. As of last year I had to go on disability. I am desperate for relief, as my condition has drastically affected my life. Disability has been hard for me. I am single and have no other financial resources. I am very despondent, as I feel that my life is passing by without the hope of my ever really improving.

Many mood disorder experts will consider that the foregoing clinical picture is compatible with pseudounipolar (bipolar III) disorder with an endogenous dysthymic disorder base. Some virologists and immunologists, and some psychiatrists, believe that abnormal humors circulate in the bloodstream that bathes the brains of such patients. Pending the positive identification of those humors, a mixture of phlegm and black bile is as adequate an explanation as any other! While awaiting more definitive research on the etiology of chronic fatigue, the psychiatrist can cautiously consider certain patients for thymoleptic trials. That decision can be bolstered by the following considerations: (1) fatigue is not alleviated by sleep or rest; and (2) the patient wakes up with it; (3) fatigue is part of a more generalized psychomotor inertia or lack of initiative; (4) fatigue is associated with anhedonia, including sexual anhedonia; and (5) fatigue coexists with anxious and pessimistic ruminations. Although none of the foregoing alone is pathognomonic for depression, in aggregate they point in that direction. The occurrence of hypomaniclike periods (as in the above vignette) further supports the link between chronic fatigue and mood disorder. Lithium and valproate, though not yet formally tested in such patients, represent rational choices.

SCHIZOPHRENIA Cross-sectionally, young bipolar patients might seem psychotic and disorganized and thus appear schizophrenic. Their thought processes are so rapid that they may seem loose, but, unlike in schizophrenia, it will be in the setting of expansive and elated affect. By contrast, the severely retarded bipolar depressive person, whose affect may superficially seem flat will almost never exhibit major fragmentation of thought. The clinician, therefore, should place greater emphasis on the pattern of symptoms, rather than on individual symptoms, in the differential diagnosis of mood and schizophrenic psychoses. There actually are no pathognomonic differentiating signs and symptoms. Differential diagnosis should be based on the overall clinical picture, phenomenology, family history, course, and associated features. Because the two groups of disorders entail radically different pharmacological treatments on a long-term basis, the differential diagnosis is of major clinical importance. Table 16.6-45, summarizing the author's research in the area, lists the most common pitfalls in the task of diagnosis.

TABLE 16.6-45
Misdiagnosis of Mood Disorder as Schizophrenia

Common pitfalls:
- Reliance on cross-sectional rather than longitudinal picture
- Incomplete interepisodic recovery equated with schizophrenic defect
- Equation of bizarreness with schizophrenic thought disorder
- Ascribing of irritable and cantankerous mood to paranoid delusions
- Mistaking of depressive anhedonia and depersonalization for schizophrenic emotional blunting
- Flight of ideas perceived as loose associations
- Lack of familiarity with the phenomenological approach in assessing affective delusions and hallucinations
- Heavy weight given to incidental Schneiderian symptoms

In the past many bipolar patients, especially those with prominent manic features at onset, were labeled as having acute schizophrenia or schizoaffective schizophrenia. Such misdiagnosis, which typically led to long-term treatment with antipsychotics, has proved very costly in view of the likelihood of tardive dyskinesia, vocational and social decline, and even suicide. Thus some patients with postpsychotic depressive disorder of schizophrenia in the DSM-IV scheme (Table 16.6-40) represent postmanic depressions that have been treated with antipsychotics.

Modern treatments, which tend to keep many persons with schizophrenia out of the hospital, do not seem to prevent an overall downhill course; by contrast, the intermorbid periods in bipolar illness are relatively normal or even supernormal, yet over time some social impairment may result from the accumulation of divorces, financial catastrophes, and ruined careers. (Although rapid-cycling disorders, which seem to be on the rise during the past decade, cause considerable social impairment, mood symptoms are of such prominence that differentiation from schizophrenia is generally not difficult; also, in such cases there is usually a more classic bipolar phase before the rapid cycling).

The postpsychotic depressions among persons with established schizophrenia are sometimes due to inadequate control of schizophrenic symptomological or pharmacological features. In other patients, especially more intelligent young schizophrenic patients, they reflect the experience of losing one's ego and sanity. It would be more meaningful to diagnose such patients with both schizophrenia and a depressive disorder. The concept of postpsychotic depression is too vague.

SCHIZOAFFECTIVE DISORDER The diagnosis should not be made for depressions in the setting of well-established schizophrenia as discussed above, but the concept of schizoaffective (or cycloid) psychosis should be restricted to recurrent psychoses with full affective and schizophrenic symptoms occurring nearly simultaneously during each episode. Such a diagnosis should not be considered in a mood psychosis where mood-incongruent psychotic features (for example, Schneiderian and Bleulerian symptoms) can be explained on the basis of one of the following: (1) affective psychosis superimposed on mental retardation, giving rise to extremely hyperactive and bizarre manic behavior; (2) affective psychosis complicated by concurrent brain disease, substance abuse, or substance withdrawal, known to give rise to numerous Schneiderian symptoms; (3) mixed episodes of bipolar disorder, which are notorious for signs and symptoms of psychotic disorganization.

In official diagnostic systems such as that of DSM-IV, the category of schizoaffective disorder is used broadly. Thus patients with clear-cut manic episodes will receive a schizoaffective diagnosis if delusions or hallucinations occur in the interepisodic period, in the absence of prominent affective symptoms. As discussed earlier, many psychotic symptoms in mood disorders often are of an explanatory nature, albeit delusional, whereby the patient tries to make sense of the core experiences of the illness. In patients with recurrent episodes, delusional thinking can be carried over into the interepisodic period. Such patients would thus be delusional in the absence of prominent mood symptoms and, technically (that is, by research diagnostic or DSM-IV criteria), might be considered schizoaffective. The author does not concur with that convention. Affective illness is typically a lifelong process, and it is artificial to limit its features to discrete episodes. Although antipsychotics might be prescribed on an as needed basis to reduce the strong affective charge of those interepisodic delusions, they are not effective in eliminating the affect-laden experiences. Continued thymoleptic treatment (resorting to ECT, if necessary) in the context of an empathic psychotherapeutic approach is more rewarding in the long run.

A 29-year-old female college graduate, mother of two children and married to a bank president, had experienced several manic and retarded depressive episodes that had responded to lithium carbonate. She was referred to the present writer, because she had developed the delusion that she had been involved in an international plot. Careful probing revealed that the delusion represented further elaboration, in a rather fantastic form, of a grandiose delusion she had experienced during her last postpartum manic episode; she believed she had played an important role in uncovering the plot, thereby becoming a national hero. Nobody knew about it, she contended, as the affair was top secret. She further believed that she had saved her country from the international scheme, and suspected that she was singled out for persecution by the perpetrators of the plot. At one point she had even entertained the idea that the plotters sent special radio communications to intercept and interrupt her thoughts. As is typical in such cases, she was on a heavy dosage of a lithium-antipsychotic combination. The consultation was requested because the primary mood symptoms were under control, and yet she had not given up her grandiose delusion. She flippantly remarked that one should be "crazy" to believe in her involvement in an international plot, but she could not help but believe in it. Over a period of several months, seen typically in 60 minute to 90-minute sessions weekly, the patient had developed sufficient trust that the author could gently challenge her beliefs.

She was, in effect, told that her self-professed role in the international scheme was highly implausible, and that someone with her superior education and high social standing could not entertain a belief, to use her own words, "as crazy as that." She eventually broke into tears, saying that everyone in her family was so accomplished and famous that, to keep up with them, she had to be involved in something grand; in effect, the international scheme, she said, was her only claim to fame: "Nobody ever gives me credit for raising two kids, and throwing parties for my husband's business colleagues. My mother is a dean, my older brother holds high political office, my sister is a medical researcher with five discoveries to her credit [all true], and who am I? Nothing. Now, do you understand why I need to be a national hero?" As she alternated, over subsequent months, between such momentary flashes of insight and delusional denial, antipsychotic medication was gradually discontinued. Maintained on lithium, she now only makes passing reference to the grand scheme. She was encouraged to pursue her career goal toward a master's degree in library science.

The vignette illustrates how phenomenological understanding, rational pharmacotherapy, and practical sociotherapeutic or vocational guidance can be fruitfully combined in the approach to patients with psychotic mood disorders. At a more fundamental level it suggests that clinical diagnoses in psychiatry cannot be entirely based on operational criteria, as what one thinks of patient's illnesses not infrequently changes based on how they respond to treatment. In the author's opinion, DSM-IV represents something good (operationalization of diagnostic criteria) carried to a ridiculous extreme (arbitrary precision often divorced from clinical reality).

SUGGESTED CROSS-REFERENCES

Diagnosis and psychiatry are discussed in Chapter 9, the clinical manifestations of psychiatric disorders are covered in Chapter

10, and the classification of mental disorders is presented in Chapter 11. Schizophrenia is the subject of Chapter 14. The somatic treatment of mood disorders is discussed in Section 16.7 and their psychosocial treatment in Section 16.8. Mood disorders and suicide in children are the topic of Chapter 44, anxiety disorders are presented in Chapter 17, and mood disorders in geriatric psychiatry are discussed in Section 49.6b.

REFERENCES

Akiskal H S: Dysthymic and cyclothymic depressions; therapeutic considerations. J Clin Psychiatry *55:* 46, 1994.
Akiskal H S, Akiskal K: Re-assessing the prevalence of bipolar disorders: Clinical significance and artistic creativity. Psychiatr Psychobiol *3:* 29s, 1988.
*Akiskal H S, Maser J D, Zeller P, Endicott J, Coryell W, Keller M, Warshaw M, Clayton P, Goodwin F K: Switching from "unipolar" to bipolar II: An 11-year prospective study of clinical and temperamental predictors in 559 patients. Arch Gen Psychiatry *52:* 114, 1995.
Andreasen N C, Akiskal H S: The specificity of Bleulerian and Schneiderian symptoms: A critical reevaluation. Psychiatr Clin North Am *6:* 41, 1983.
Beard G M: *A Practical Treatise on Nervous Exhaustion (Neurasthenia): Its Nature, Sequences, and Treatment.* Wood, New York, 1881.
Cassano G B, Akiskal H S, Savino M, Musetti L, Perugi G, Soriani A: Proposed subtypes of bipolar II disorder: With hypomanic episodes and/or with hyperthymic temperament. J Affect Disord *26:* 127, 1992.
Clayton P J: The sequelae and nonsequelae of conjugal bereavement. Am J Psychiatry *136:* 1530, 1979.
Coryell W, Winokur G, Shea T, Maser J, Endicott J, Akiskal H S: The long-term stability of depressive subtypes. Am J Psychiatry *151:* 701, 1994.
Davidson J R, Miller R D, Turnbull C D, Sullivan J L: Atypical depression. Arch Gen Psychiatry *39:* 527, 1982.
Himmelhoch J M, Mulla D, Neil J F, Detre T P, Kupfer D J: Incidence and significance of mixed affective states in a bipolar population. Arch Gen Psychiatry *33:* 1062, 1976.
James W: *The Varieties of Religious Experience.* Random House, New York, 1902.
Jouvent R, Hardy P, Bouvard M, Braconnier A, Roumengous V, Grasset F, Widlocher D: Heterogeneity of the depressive mood. Construction of a polydimensional scale. Encephale *13:* 233, 1987.
Judd L L, Rapaport M H, Paulus M P and Brown J L: Subsyndromal Symptomatic Depression: A New Mood Disorder? J Clin Psychiatry *55:* 18, 1994.
Kendler K S, Neale M C, Kessler R C, Heath A C, Eaves L J: A population-based twin study of major depression in women. The impact of varying definitions of illness. Arch Gen Psychiatry *49:* 257, 1992.
Klein D F: Endogenomorphic depression. A conceptual and terminological revision. Arch Gen Psychiatry *31:* 447, 1974.
*Kraepelin E (translated by R M Barclay): *Manic-Depressive Insanity and Paranoia,* G M Robertson, editor. Livingstone, Edinburgh, 1921.
*Kretschmer E (translated by E Miller): *Physique and Character.* Kegan, Paul, Trench, Trubner, London, 1936.
Nelson J C and Charney D S: The symptoms of major depressive illness. Am J Psychiatry *138:* 1, 1981.
*Nesse R M: What good is feeling bad? Sciences Nov/Dec: 30, 1991.
Rosenthal N E: *Winter Blues,* New York, Guilford Press, 1993.
Taylor M A and Abrams R: The phenomenology of mania: a new look at some old patients. Arch Gen Psychiatry *29:* 520, 1973.
*Widlocher D J: Psychomotor retardation: Clinical, theoretical, and psychometric aspects. Psychiatr Clin North Am *6:* 27, 1993.
Zisook S, Shuchter S R, Sledge P A, Paulus M and Judd L L: The spectrum of depressive phenomena after spousal bereavement. J Clin Psychiatry *55:* 29, 1994.

16.7 MOOD DISORDERS: SOMATIC TREATMENT

ROBERT M. POST, M.D.

INTRODUCTION

Treatment of the mood disorders has entered into a new era of therapeutics based on a variety of factors. There is increasing recognition that mood disorders have a prominent genetic component with well-documented neurobiological alterations that have been elucidated on biochemical, neuroendocrinological, and functional brain imaging measures. The descriptive and diagnostic aspects of the illness have been explicated, and it is recognized that in most cases the mood disorders are recurrent and have the potential for severe morbidity and even mortality. Thus, treatment requires the utmost in clinical management skills.

As knowledge of the classification, course, and mechanisms underlying acute episodes and their recurrences has increased, so also has the array of effective psychopharmacotherapeutic modalities and related somatic treatments. Although single drugs in one or two classes were available for the treatment of depression several decades ago, multiple therapeutic modalities now exist, often with many agents within each class. Thus, the treating physician should be aware of the nuances in the management of patients with acute and recurrent mood disorders so that treatment can be optimized from the outset and the impact of the illness on patients, their lives, and their families can be minimized.

There is also increasing consensus on several new treatment principles. Early recognition and intervention in an acute episode not only may save the patient months of pain and suffering but also may be lifesaving. More careful assessment of the efficacy of an agent at early and regular intervals, with early revision of the treatment modality if it is not optimal, is an important new guideline that applies not only to somatic treatments, but also to psychotherapeutic approaches and combination psychotherapy-pharmacotherapy when treatment is not proceeding optimally.

A large body of evidence supports the efficacy of long-term prophylactic management of recurrent mood disorders. Early institution of long-term prophylaxis is now recognized as a critical approach for the patient with recurrent mood disorders. Such an approach holds promise for reducing the morbidity of the illness and for altering favorably its subsequent course and treatment responsiveness. There is increasing consensus that a patient with a first episode of bipolar disorder is a candidate not only for continuation therapy following the resolution of that episode, but also for long-term prophylaxis, particularly if the patient has a family history of bipolar illness. Correspondingly, in major depressive disorder there is a new appreciation for the recommendation of prophylaxis after the third episode or two closely occurring episodes.

Thus, a variety of factors and guidelines shape the physician's approach to the patient with an acute episode of mood disorder. The illness should be treated with the same respect as is given to the early diagnosis and treatment of a malignancy, with the same skills brought to bear in choosing targeted and, at times, multimodal therapeutics. In a parallel fashion, early and effective intervention may be lifesaving, whereas delayed or inadequate treatment may be associated with considerable acute and long-term morbidity from both the illness and its secondary consequences. The recurrent mood disorders should be conceptualized not as trivial, mental, or illusory phenomena that can easily be modified by patients' acts of will, but as serious and potentially life-threatening medical illnesses that have clearly defined mood, cognitive, motor, somatic, and neurobiological concomitants.

Major depressive disorder is a common illness, occurring in 7 to 12 percent of male patients and 20 to 25 percent of female patients during their lifetimes. Although bipolar disorder occurs in approximately 1 percent of the population, that percentage translates into 2.5 million people in the United States alone. The bipolar disorders are disabling in the short and long term. For example, it is estimated that the average woman with onset of a bipolar disorder at age 25 will lose 14 years of effective lifetime functioning as a result of the illness. In addition, up to 15 to 20 percent of patients with inadequately treated mood disorders commit suicide. Thus, diagnosis and treatment should be approached with the knowledge that the patient is experiencing a potentially recurrent, disabling medical illness.

HISTORY

Until the middle of the 20th century the available treatments for mood disorders were largely supportive and palliative. Electroconvulsive therapy (ECT) then emerged as efficacious treatment for major depressive disorder. In the following decades, the monoamine oxidase inhibitors (MAOIs) and tricyclic antidepressants were introduced. Today, second- and third-generation treatment modalities are available. The latter preparations include drugs with novel structures, different mechanisms of action, and more benign side-effect profiles than the original agents. Those agents include the serotonin-specific reuptake inhibitors (SSRIs) (fluoxetine [Prozac], sertraline [Zoloft], paroxetine [Paxil], fluvoxamine [Luvox]), the mixed serotonergic-noradrenergic drug venlafaxine (Effexor), and the dopaminergic-noradrenergic agent bupropion (Wellbutrin). The emergence of a new range of acute antidepressant psychopharmacological agents raises important treatment issues for the clinician, particularly when those agents must be chosen on the basis of an inadequate literature on potential clinical and biological markers of responsiveness to a given drug in a given person. There is general consensus in the field that, with the possible exception of ECT, no antidepressant modality is more effective or more rapid in onset than another. Thus, agents may be chosen based on their side-effect profile, acceptability in long-term prophylaxis, and clinical lore regarding possible syndromal selectivity of response.

A similar revolution has occurred in the treatment of bipolar disorder. In the first half of the 20th century no adequate treatment for bipolar disorder was available, whereas in the second half lithium (Eskalith) emerged as a wonder drug for the acute and prophylactic management of the disorder. It is noteworthy, however, that there were marked oscillations in the assessment of the efficacy and utility of lithium, and it was initially abandoned as unsafe (until adequate monitoring of blood levels was devised so as to eliminate cardiovascular and central nervous system [CNS] toxic effects). After many decades of use, the limitations of lithium are better recognized. As many as 50 percent of patients do not show adequate response to lithium even when conservative criteria for clinical response, such as one episode of illness during a two-year follow-up, are employed. Fortunately, as the limitations of lithium were increasingly recognized, a variety of other treatment modalities became available, particularly the anticonvulsants carbamazepine (Tegretol) and valproate (Depakene, Depakote). However, as is the case of matching treatment to patient in the depressive disorders, there is even less evidence in the bipolar disorders for clinical and biological predictors of acute and long-term responsiveness to the mood-stabilizing agents.

In treating patients with bipolar disorders the clinician often has to resort to educated guesses and to systematic, sequential clinical trials to delineate optimal responsivity. Even with the availability of new treatment modalities, episodes of illness can emerge through otherwise partially successful pharmacoprophylaxis, necessitating adjunctive measures. The role of combination therapies is well recognized in many branches of medicine; for example, it is central to the treatment of congestive heart failure, tuberculosis, and most malignancies. By comparison, research on combination therapies in the mood disorders has lagged behind clinical practice, and clinicians are often left to their own devices without the aid of controlled studies as a guide for determining the optimal algorithm in cases refractory to standard treatments.

This section reviews the knowledge base gleaned from both systematic controlled clinical trials and anecdotal observations, and delineates novel treatment interventions that may be employed when patients fail to respond to first-, second-, and third-line treatment options. Although many of the specific recommendations may change in the years to come as the results of new, more systematic research are reported, the principles enunciated here should provide useful guidelines for physicians formulating optimal treatment options for acute and long-term prophylaxis for patients with mood disorders.

INITIAL DIAGNOSTIC AND THERAPEUTIC APPROACHES

IMPEDIMENTS TO ACUTE AND LONG-TERM TREATMENT Although the mood disorders are treatable, several illness-related variables complicate access to treatment and the ability of the patient to follow through. It is estimated that as many as 25 percent of patients with major depressive disorder do not receive treatment. Depressed patients often do not recognize their constellation of symptoms as a medical illness, and the symptoms of depression, such as motor retardation, apathy, inertia, and hopelessness, may preclude the patient's becoming involved in treatment. Thus, the patient's family, acquaintances, and medical physician may have to play active roles in encouraging the patient to initiate treatment.

Treatment must be conducted against the backdrop of the patient's distorted depressive cognitions, sense of hopelessness, and view of the untreatability of the illness. Patients should be informed that such beliefs and feelings are symptoms of the illness and that a positive response to treatment is likely, based on the literature and the physician's own experience with the illness. However, the physician's empirically based hope for recovery should be conveyed to the patient without the promise of immediate results. The physician should also explain that lags in onset of treatment efficacy are expected so that the patient does not misinterpret such delays as confirmation that the illness is untreatable. Finally, the risk for suicide during each phase of a depressive illness must be continually reassessed.

Similar impediments to the effective treatment of manic patients exist. For example, in the early stages of hypomania the sense of well-being and increased productivity may lead the patient to ignore more severe consequences of the illness, including irritability, intrusiveness, insomnia, poor judgment, engagement in high-risk behaviors without appropriate appreciation of the consequences, and other activities and behaviors that may be detrimental to the patient's social structure, marriage, and employment. Early recognition of those symptoms as part of the illness may be crucial to instituting appropriate treatment and to preventing full-blown manic episodes in patients with bipolar I disorder.

There are important roles for the family in both the diagnostic evaluation and the ongoing treatment of a patient with a bipolar disorder. Family participation may be needed to assist the patient in confronting the denial of illness and the thought disorder that are associated with hypomania and mania and that can be just as great impediments to adequate treatment as are the apathy and hopelessness of depression. Therefore, therapeutic activism, engagement of the family, and early and aggressive treatment of mood disorders are important. The patient and family should receive immediate and regular information about the medical aspects of the illness, its course, and its response to treatment. The long-term goals of education are to increase compliance and destigmatize the illness. Compliance and destigmatization may become focal issues later in therapy when the physician considers recommendations for long-term prophylaxis; at that time society's negative attitudes toward taking psychotropic medications may have to be addressed. The conceptualization of mood disorders as medical illnesses that deserve the same attention and respect as other medical disorders may be important to the patient and family in choosing and committing to a long-term treatment option.

Thus, a variety of societal, attitudinal, and illness-related variables may interfere with appropriate help-seeking and maintenance behavior in the various phases of treatment of mood disorders. During each of the successive phases—acute care, continuation treatment, and long-term prophylaxis—the patient and family should be assisted in their evaluation of the medical data and the potential impact of the disorder on the patient. The variables affecting treatment should be addressed sequentially as they arise in each phase of the illness rather than in aggregate at the start of treatment. For example, the importance of continuation therapy, which should have a duration of four to nine months following the resolution of acute symptoms, should be discussed once the patient has begun to respond to treatment, rather than being raised with the acutely depressed patient, who may feel hopeless about ever achieving a therapeutic outcome.

Similarly, education on the importance of long-term treatment, with appropriate provision of data to the patient and family, may be critical for achieving an optimal outcome. Patients taking medications long term for any reason may decide to test the need for therapy by discontinuing the medication. As an example, even with an illness such as juvenile diabetes, in which it is unequivocally demonstrated that the patient cannot survive without adequate insulin treatment, many adolescents nevertheless feel compelled to test the long-term need for insulin and consequently experience periods of marked hyperglycemia that often lead to hospitalization. In parallel fashion, it should be anticipated that patients with bipolar mood disorders are likely to be tempted to discontinue their recommended treatment, all the more so because data on the potential lethality of the regimen or its morbid consequences may be less well delineated. Consequently, the treating clinician has the educational responsibility of providing patients and families with information on the high likelihood of a recurrence in a relatively short time in patients with several prior episodes and with information on the ability of a variety of antidepressant agents and bimodal mood-stabilizing agents to prevent recurrences of major depressive disorder and bipolar disorder, respectively.

After several prior episodes of major depressive disorder, the likelihood of a new episode after successful, acute antidepressant treatment and placebo substitution is approximately 50 percent in the first year and increases with time. Maintenance treatment can reduce that rate by more than half. Although often a helpful adjunct, long-term psychotherapy cannot substitute for pharmacotherapy in the prophylaxis of either major depressive disorder or bipolar disorder.

In bipolar disorder the high likelihood of relapse (80 to 90 percent) following lithium discontinuation is widely recognized. In addition, although it had previously been assumed that if a well-treated patient experienced a relapse following drug discontinuation, the patient would readily respond again once treatment was reinstituted, several reports of lithium discontinuation-induced refractoriness have been noted. After long periods of successful lithium treatment, the patients discontinued the drug, experienced a relapse, and did not re-respond once treatment was restarted at similar or higher doses. Other patients may not respond as rapidly as they did to the first treatment sequence. Several studies suggest that lithium may be less effective in patients who experienced more than three or four episodes prior to lithium initiation than in those in whom lithium is initiated earlier in the illness sequence. Thus, in recommending long-term preventive therapy, the physician should consider not only the potential morbidity and mortality of an episode recurrence, but also the possibility that new episodes could affect the subsequent course of the illness and its pharmacological responsivity.

PSYCHIATRIC HISTORY A thorough history and medical examination is paramount. Because several medical conditions may mimic both manic and depressive syndromes, the diagnosis should be approached from the perspective that a medical cause may exist for the illness until proved otherwise. Throughout the history taking and physical examination, attention should be paid to obvious and subtle hallmarks of associated pathology. The physician should be alert to the signs and symptoms indicative of CNS neuropathology, underlying endocrinopathy, and associated medical illness. Although aggressive in exploring those themes with the patient and family, the physician should directly state that the patient's somatic and vegetative symptoms are most likely indicative of a typical depressive process.

Thus, even the earliest parts of the history taking can be used not only for diagnostic purposes but also to begin educating the patient about the types of symptoms that are characteristic of mood disorders, the likely course of remission of episodes, and the likely response to somatic and pharmacological interventions. Simultaneously, the physician should be isolating the target symptoms for future assessment of the efficacy of psychological and pharmacological interventions and constructing a framework for longitudinal monitoring of the patient. The same symptoms are likely to appear in future recurrences and thus may provide an early warning system to aid in early detection and the aggressive institution of treatment. The medical history and examination should also look for evidence of glaucoma (a relative contraindication to anticholinergic antidepressants) and cardiac, renal, and thyroid abnormalities that may preclude certain treatments.

A detailed family history of medical and psychiatric illness is crucial to the initial diagnostic assessment of the patient. It is recommended that a formal family tree be graphically constructed and information recorded on the potential diagnosis, course of illness, and response to therapy of each first-degree relative, as that information may provide a guide to current treatment of the patient. Patients with a positive family history of bipolar disorder should be more strongly considered for prophylaxis after the first manic episode than those without such a family history. Similarly, patients with a family history of major depressive disorder should be strongly considered for prophylaxis after two depressive episodes. Some data suggest that clinical response to a given agent may generalize across family members or generations; in the absence of other clinical predictors, that may provide a reasonable initial treatment guideline.

Graphing the course of illness The author suggests developing a graphical representation of the patient's prior depressive and manic episodes (Figures 16.7-1 through 16.7-4). A formal graphical representation of the patient's longitudinal course of illness is useful for several reasons: (1) It provides a clear-cut picture of the earlier course of illness (which appears to be the best predictor of the future pattern of episodes). (2) It clarifies medication responsiveness (by indicating the efficacy of previous treatments, if any) and helps in the medicalization of the history taking and management process (with regard to current and future prescriptions). (3) It encourages the patient to collaborate and thus may enhance the doctor-patient relationship by bringing the patient into the process as an active rather than passive participant. (4) If a number of past recurrences are uncovered in the history, that information may help in determining the subsequent long-term approach to the illness and in identifying the patient's willingness to comply with prescribed regimens. (5) Graphing the course of illness often uncovers important psychosocial events and possible precipitants of the illness; unique characteristics of the illness, such as seasonal variation and relation to anniversaries; and other patterns that cannot be discovered easily without systematic and graphical representation of the prior course. Elucidation of periods of increased vulnerability to illness provides a template for future intensification of observation and augmentation of therapeutic modalities as appropriate.

With a little practice the course of an illness can be graphed easily. It is suggested that graphing be done as part of the initial intake session and be the primary mode of history taking, rather than a verbal account that is later converted to graphical form. A graphical rather than verbal representation immediately and systematically focuses the patient and physician on the longitudinal course of the illness and its variation over time. The graphical approach and its associated temporal landmarks can also facilitate recall of important events, dates, and episodes that would otherwise be obscured or forgotten.

Levels of severity Physicians can devise their own ways of plotting the longitudinal course of illness or can adopt a system like the one the author and his colleagues have used successfully over the past decade. That consists of graphing three levels—mild, moderate, and severe—of mania or depression, based on the degrees of associated functional incapacity, and can easily be assessed retrospectively (Figures 16.7-1 and 16.7-2).

MILD LEVEL The mild level is one in which the patient or family notes a distinct change from the patient's usual behavior without a notable impairment in the patient's functional status. This state is readily discerned by depressed patients and may represent the baseline of double depression from which more severe episodes erupt. Hypomanic patients, however, may deny a mild state, and the physician may have to obtain additional information from family members and relatives. (That observation underscores the utility of an initial nonanalytic approach

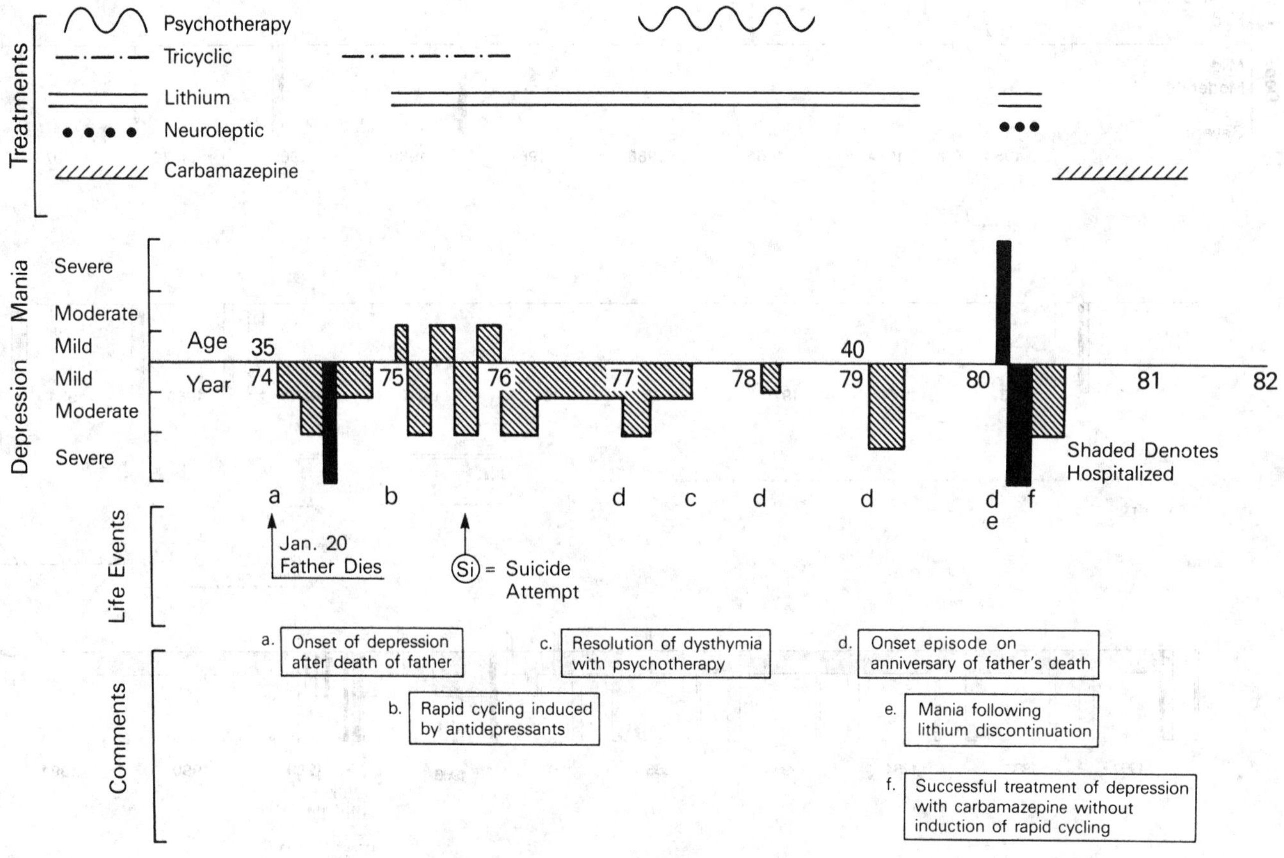

FIGURE 16.7-1 *Graphing the course of affective illness: Prototype of a life chart.*

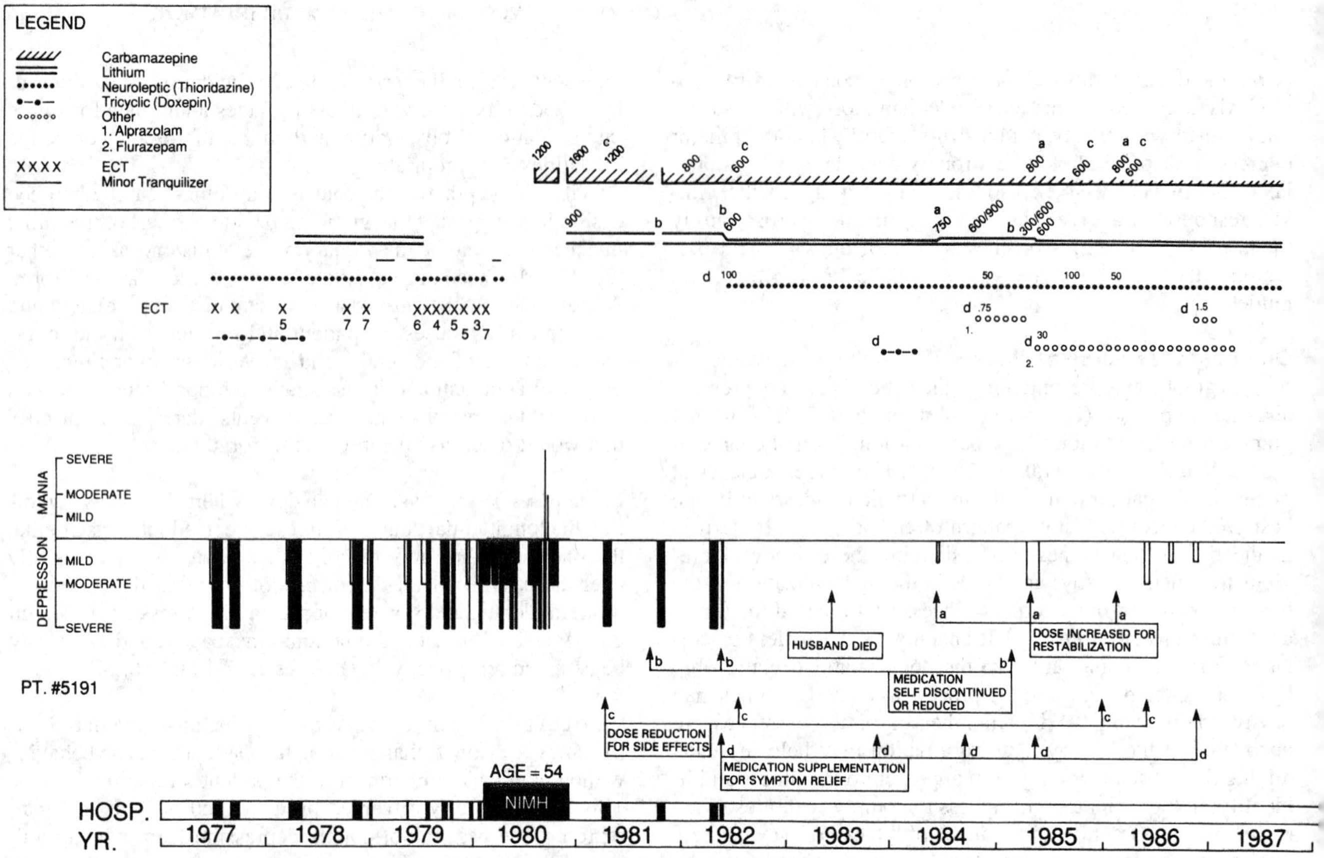
LEGEND
Carbamazepine
Lithium
Neuroleptic (Thioridazine)
Tricyclic (Doxepin)
Other
1. Alprazolam
2. Flurazepam
XXXX
ECT
Minor Tranquilizer
ECT
MANIA
DEPRESSION
SEVERE
MODERATE
MILD
PT. #5191
HUSBAND DIED
DOSE INCREASED FOR RESTABILIZATION
MEDICATION SELF DISCONTINUED OR REDUCED
DOSE REDUCTION FOR SIDE EFFECTS
MEDICATION SUPPLEMENTATION FOR SYMPTOM RELIEF
AGE = 54
NIMH
HOSP.
YR.
1977
1978
1979
1980
1981
1982
1983
1984
1985
1986
1987

FIGURE 16.7-2 *Carbamazepine prophylaxis maintained with optimal management of dose titration against side effects.*

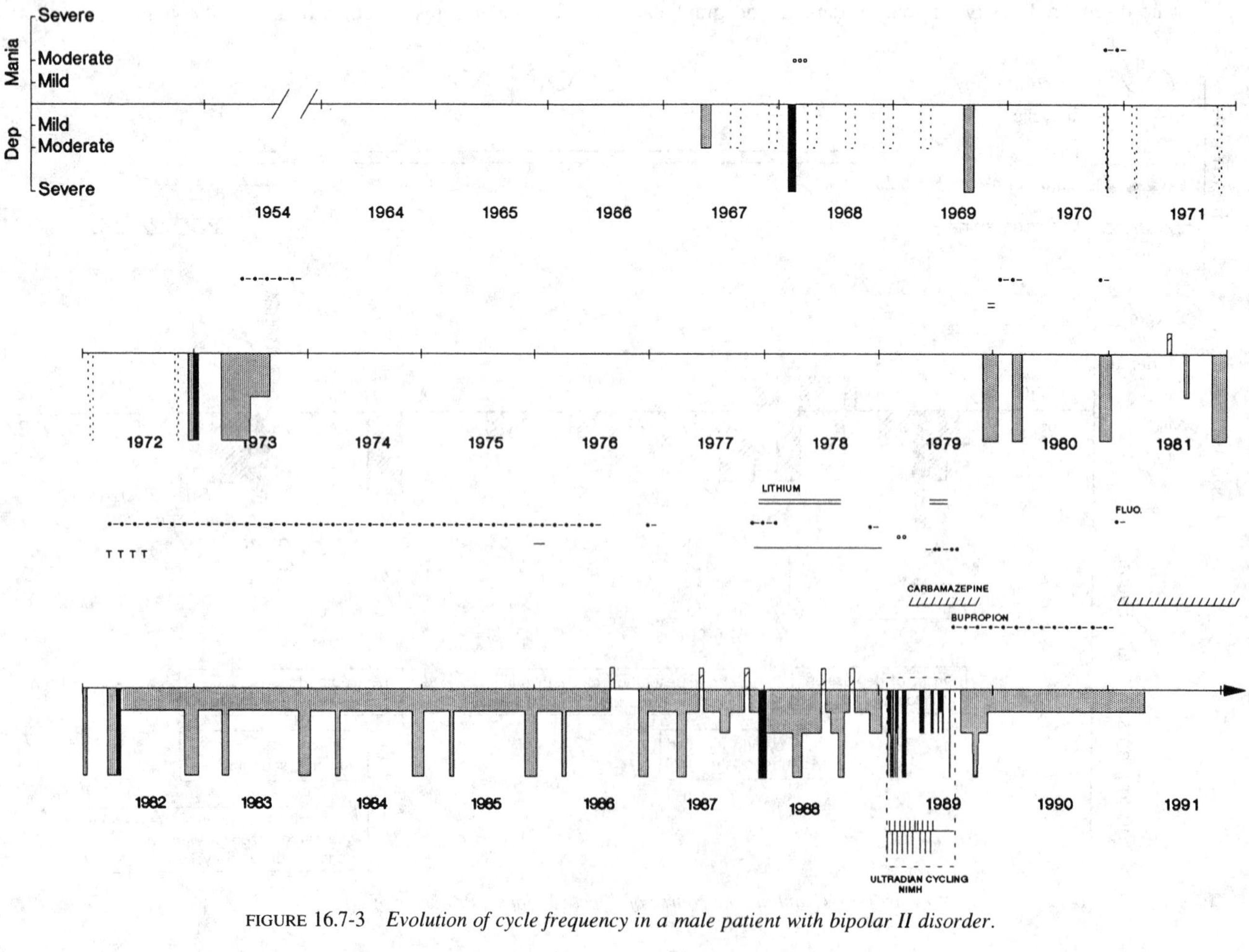
Mania
Dep
Severe
Moderate
Mild
1954
1964
1965
1966
1967
1968
1969
1970
1971
1972
1973
1974
1975
1976
1977
1978
1979
1980
1981
LITHIUM
FLUO.
TTTT
CARBAMAZEPINE
BUPROPION
1982
1983
1984
1985
1986
1987
1988
1989
1990
1991
ULTRADIAN CYCLING
NIMH

FIGURE 16.7-3 *Evolution of cycle frequency in a male patient with bipolar II disorder.*

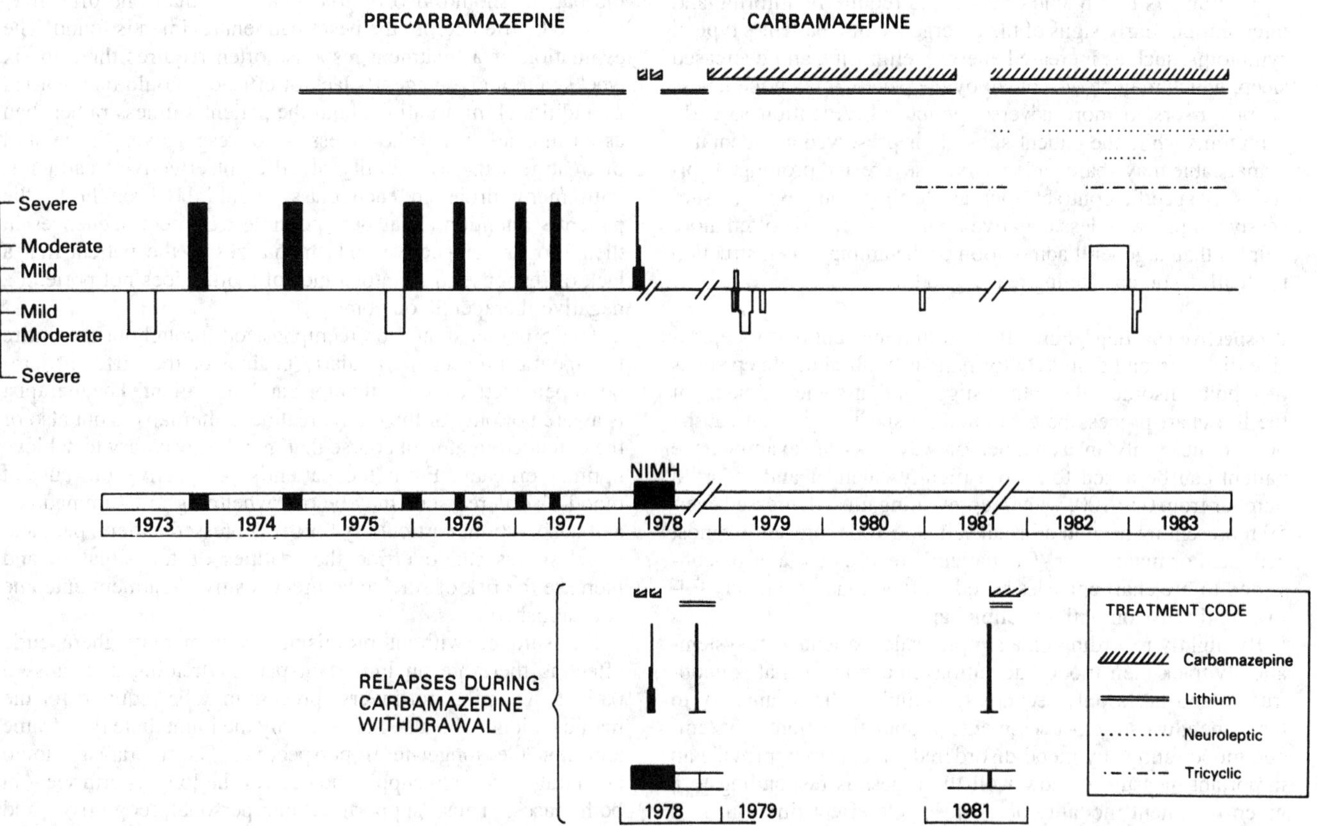

FIGURE 16.7-4 *Response to acute and prophylactic treatment with carbamazepine in a lithium nonresponder.*

to the patient's illness and its diagnosis and the value of family participation and support from the outset.) Information from the family may be of value in both gaining historical information and in managing the potential suicidality of depression and the denial of the adverse consequences of hypomania and mania. Hypomanic signs and symptoms such as distinct periods of increased energy, productivity, creativity, and decreased need for sleep should be asked about in a nonpejorative fashion. Those milder periods may also be easier to explore once the more severe phases of a patient's illness have been detected and the characteristic components of the early presentation agreed on.

MODERATE LEVEL Moderate levels of depression and mania can be graphed at the next level to represent illness with distinct functional impairment. Patients have difficulties continuing their social or employment responsibilities, showing absences from work or performance deficits on routine social tasks.

SEVERE LEVEL The third or severe level of impairment is graphed when patients are functionally incapacitated and are unable to perform consistently in their usual roles (that is, they are no longer able to go to work or to perform socially). Hospitalization can be indicated by shading in the severe manic or depressive episode. When an episode has occurred in the past but its precise timing is not available, it can be indicated on the life chart with dotted lines.

Earlier psychopharmacological interventions Superimposed on this template of mood fluctuations can be the history of prior psychopharmacological interventions, which is plotted above the mood disorder episodes, as illustrated in Figure 16.7-1 (life chart schema) and in Figures 16.7-2 and 16.7-3 (case examples). When plotted in this fashion, the efficacy of earlier treatments is often reclassified. A treatment previously deemed ineffective may, on careful reexamination, be shown to be partially effective (that is, a decreased frequency or severity of prior episodes compared with the pretreatment baseline may emerge). If that is the case, the reassessment may suggest supplementing this partially effective treatment rather than abandoning it. Previous psychotherapeutic interventions should also be included so that their impact on the illness and patient satisfaction can be assessed. Important psychosocial events (for example, anniversaries, suicide attempts) and other notes about drug side effects, dosages, reasons for discontinuation of medications, and the like can be noted below the mood graph (Figure 16.7-1).

Descriptive symptoms The anamnestic account of symptomatology provides a basis for following clinical improvement during an acute episode and possible subsequent episodes. The clinician should develop a sense for the major symptoms that are the best descriptors of a patient's episodes. In some patients impaired sleep with early morning awakening may be the major symptom; in others it may be inability to concentrate, decreased energy or increased agitation, isolation, anxiety, a change in appetite, or weight gain. The sequential ebbing of symptoms during a treated episode may be a clue to the duration of maintenance treatment required and to the earliest symptoms that may recur during a subsequent episode. Should the more difficult or residual symptoms emerge during prophylaxis, or should they recur or become more profound as medication is tapered, they can be used as indicators for renewed, more aggressive management of a potential episode.

Similarly, clinicians should decide on and make a contract with their patients in advance about specific symptoms that may be forerunners to a manic episode and require monitoring and intervention. Early signs of the emergence of a patient's typical symptoms, such as increased energy, religiosity, and decreased sleep, which may be welcomed by the patient, may nonetheless be precursors to more adverse symptoms. Attention to early symptoms while the patient's insight is preserved and denial is manageable may spare patients more severe and prolonged episodes. A specific contract, such as "Call if you have two successive nights with less than five hours of sleep," is often more helpful than a general admonition or the ambiguous instruction to "call if you are feeling really good."

Prospective charting For patients with recurrent major depressive disorder, and definitely for patients with multiple episodes of bipolar disorder, the author suggests that some elements of the life chart process be continued prospectively. That can be done quite easily in a number of ways. As an example, the patient can be asked to keep a nightly calendar and record a number from 0 to 100, with 0 representing most depressed ever, 50 representing normal or usual self, and 100 representing most activated or manic ever. The patient's record can later be converted to life chart episodes based on functional incapacity following discussion with the clinician.

By nightly recording on a simple scale, patients can systematically track their mood fluctuations in a manner that is unobtrusive and takes only seconds to complete. In an analogy to the urine glucose self-assessments of diabetic patients, systematic mood ratings by mood-disordered patients may provide an important measure of how well the illness is responding to a given treatment modality or of dose-side effect titration. It is worth reemphasizing that the morbidity and mortality of the mood disorders can be no less severe than those of many medical illnesses in which a great deal more attention is paid to the longitudinal and systematic monitoring of fluctuations in symptoms, biochemistry, and underlying pathology. Patients should be encouraged to help in the life chart process, if they are amenable to it, and should receive copies of the ongoing or completed chart, as it may be helpful in any future transfer of medical care, orientation of hospital staff, or consultation should they move or experience future episodes requiring review of treatment.

Subjective and objective differences Asking patients to make a calendar and rate their moods with a specific number from 0 to 100 has an additional, secondary benefit: It addresses the possibility of becoming attuned to the major subjective or objective differences in the assessment of a patient's illness. Many patients with major depressive disorder can detect mood changes and side effects before the therapist observes them. Conversely, many patients with bipolar disorder show remarkable objective improvement in major symptom areas, including sleep, appetite, energy, spontaneity, and sociability, without any subjective sense of clinical improvement attending those changes. If patients do not recognize that their depression is improving, it may lead to further therapeutic pessimism and may increase the possibility of suicide as the patient may have more energy to carry out such a plan while still convinced that improvement is not imminent. Moreover, return to previous levels of social and occupational functioning may lag even further behind the patient's objective and subjective appreciation of symptomatic improvement, and the patient should be adequately supported and encouraged during that time.

Time frame of education Although a hopeful perspective on the treatability of a patient's episode should be maintained, the patient should also be told that more than one drug may have to be tried before the best treatment regimen is found. The evaluation of a treatment response often requires three to six weeks, and a given agent's lack of efficacy should be regarded as additional information about the patient's illness rather than as an indication that the illness is not responsive. At the start of treatment the availability of different effective treatments, with many drugs in each class, should be brought to the patient's attention. That puts possible treatment sequences in their proper perspective and emphasizes to the patient that a lack of response to or intolerance of a drug does not portend a negative therapeutic outcome.

Those points should be reemphasized throughout the entire therapeutic process, particularly in light of the different temporal perspectives of the therapist and the patient. The therapist is aware not only of the many treatment alternatives but also of the extended treatment course that may be necessary to achieve optimal efficacy. From the patient's perspective the current mood-disordered state may be overwhelming in its immediacy and desperation. Particularly for the depressed patient, pain and hopelessness can override the realities of the situation and increase the risk of suicide before a positive treatment outcome is established.

Reassurance without promising an immediate therapeutic effect is therefore an important part of treating a depressed patient. A similar but inverse process may be required for the manic patient, who also may see only the immediate time frame and not the longer-term perspective. The therapist should encourage and help supply the ego for the longer-term view in both cases. Thus, supportive, interpersonal, cognitive, and behavioral approaches to the psychopharmacotherapy of the mood disorder may be essential. The patient should be counseled not to make important long-term decisions on the basis of a distorted view of himself or herself during an acute manic or depressive episode.

Stressing the time frame of possible improvement and the need to evaluate a given treatment over a matter of weeks to months may not only aid in maintaining patients' and families' morale but may also be helpful in obtaining adequate informed consent and avoiding malpractice litigation. In regard to the latter, it is important to indicate the possible side effects of each drug treatment so that they are seen as expected and not worrisome or, conversely, can be recognized as out of the ordinary and something that merits a call to the physician.

Hospitalization The decision to hospitalize severely depressed or manic patients depends on a variety of clinical and pharmacological issues. Hospitalization is often indicated for the acutely suicidal patient, but it may also be considered for a patient with associated medical problems or one who needs close management and monitoring of complicated or novel psychopharmacological regimens. For the knowledgeable patient with a supportive family, it may be possible to institute psychopharmacological approaches on an outpatient basis, particularly if there is close coordination between patient and physician regarding dosage, titration, side effects, and the like. Despite societal criticisms of ECT, that modality should be given higher than usual priority when the physician is faced with an extremely suicidal patient, one with associated medical illnesses, one whose profile of side effects from routine psychopharmacological agents precludes use of those agents, or one in whom other medical and psychological situations pose a therapeutic emergency necessitating the most rapid treatment response available.

For the patient with recurrent, severe episodes of mania, who may refuse voluntary hospitalization at the height of an episode, obtaining informed consent in advance during a well interval for a future hospitalization may avoid many practical and medicolegal difficulties should another manic episode occur that requires hospitalization.

PSYCHOTHERAPY AND PHARMACOTHERAPY

Depression is a serious, potentially life-threatening medical illness, and patients and their families deserve much support. The author emphasizes the importance of combining psychosocial and pharmacological approaches in a majority of patients, not only because of evidence of the efficacy of both treatment modalities, but also because of the potential for mutual interaction and support of the patients and their social system in the context of ongoing pharmacotherapy.

Although psychotherapy may not be considered an appropriate primary treatment modality for severe depression, it may behoove the clinician to use combined treatment, for several reasons. Not only does initial evidence suggest that the two types of therapy may target different symptoms, but the therapeutic process may provide support for the patient before the psychopharmacological interventions are effective, especially if several agents must be tried before a successful one is found. Psychosocial issues and stresses not only may play important etiological roles in the onset and amelioration of some types of depression, they may also indicate the need for more aggressive pharmacological management during a period of high vulnerability.

Frequent meetings with the patient may also help in assessing the progress of pharmacotherapy, titrating the dose against blood levels and side effects, and facilitating compliance in the face of pessimism. Finally, if a depressed patient experiences severe pain and suffering, frequent meetings may encourage the physician to apply maximum clinical and therapeutic leverage and to revise regimens as appropriate within the shortest time frame (generally two to four weeks) if improvement is not forthcoming in optimal fashion. Combined treatment may also be helpful in instances of only partial response to extensive pharmacotherapy, if an episode is very protracted, or if there is poor interepisode recovery of function, associated personality disorder, or the presence of acute psychosocial stressors.

THEORETICAL ASSUMPTIONS AND RATIONALE: NEUROTRANSMITTER THEORIES Because most of the effective treatments for mood disorders were discovered by serendipity or empiricism, the effectiveness of somatic treatments has propelled theoretical formulations rather than vice versa. Neurotransmitter theories of the basis of depression and the transmitters involved have included serotonergic (5-hydroxytryptamine [5-HT]), noradrenergic (NE), cholinergic (ACh), dopaminergic (DA), and γ-aminobutyric acid (GABA)-ergic theories, each based on presumed mechanisms of effective pharmacotherapeutic interventions. For example, the findings that several drugs (which acutely potentiated catecholamines and indoleamines) were antidepressants and that reserpine (Serpasil) (which depleted these neurotransmitters) could exacerbate depression and treat mania led to the amine hypotheses of deficiencies in depression and excesses in mania.

Insofar as relatively selective manipulations of each of several different neurotransmitter systems (5-HT, NE, DA) appear to be associated with antidepressant effects (Table 16.7-1), a critical psychopharmacological question is raised as to whether a patient may respond to one type of treatment targeting one neurotransmitter system but not to another that targets an alternative system. Because definitive studies that would answer that question are lacking, the sequential use of drugs that act differently within or among classes of agents may be appropriate (for example, changing from a relatively more serotonergic drug to a relatively more noradrenergic tricyclic reuptake blocker or from a tricyclic to an MAOI to lithium). Because relatively few validated clinical or biological markers of responsivity to given treatment agents exist, the clinician must move through various treatments or adjuncts for a patient with a refractory condition until an effective one is found, with the process largely being trial and error. In mania, a similar strategy of using agents with different mechanisms of action may also be warranted.

TREATMENT OF DEPRESSIVE DISORDERS

ACUTE AND CONTINUATION THERAPY FOR MAJOR DEPRESSIVE DISORDER The drugs of choice may vary for an agitated, retarded, or psychotic depression. Because clinical trials of many weeks' duration are needed to evaluate the clinical efficacy of any individual drug, before switching treatment modalities the physician might attempt to potentiate a specific drug treatment once adequate blood levels have been reached. Thus, thyroid or lithium potentiation warrants earlier emphasis in the treatment sequence than do multiple trials with single alternative agents (Figure 16.7-5).

Once a detailed history from the patient and, perhaps, a friend or relative has revealed no prior personal or family history of mania, the acute and prophylactic treatment of a patient with major depressive disorder proceeds very differently from that for a patient with bipolar disorder. The acute approaches form a backdrop to continuation treatment and longer-term prophylaxis of either recurrent major depressive disorder or bipolar disorder. When an antidepressant treatment modality is found to help alleviate an acute episode of major depressive disorder, treatment should be continued for six to nine months—a period during which vulnerability to relapse is high. The presence of residual symptoms (such as minor sleep disturbance, anergy, lack of concentration, or minor early morning awakening) suggests continued and more aggressive treatment with higher doses or potentiation. Minor increases in depression after a gradual reduction in dosage may also suggest the need for continuing the therapy. (Tapering of cyclic and MAOI antidepressants may also help in avoiding minor drug withdrawal symptoms, which include sleeplessness, nausea, vomiting, and irritability, as well as rapid eye movement [REM] rebound with the MAOIs.)

Although more research is needed on biological predictors of treatment response, initial data suggest that the failure to normalize on the dexamethasone suppression test may be associated with a higher risk of relapse. Thus, a positive test may point to continuing antidepressant treatment even though the patient is clinically asymptomatic. Some evidence indicates that the sleep electroencephalogram (EEG) may remain abnormal for a long time after remission, although that test does not appear to be a practical marker for continuation therapy. The course of an episode may best be predicted from scrutiny of past episodes. Therefore, if the history reveals earlier, protracted episodes with some evidence of relapse before medication was stopped, the treatment of the current episode should be extended.

Serotonin-specific reuptake inhibitors Fluoxetine, sertraline, and paroxetine are available in the United States for the treatment of acute and recurrent depressions, and fluvoxamine is likely to be approved soon. Fluoxetine is one of the leading

TABLE 16.7-1
Side-Effect Profiles of Some Commonly Prescribed Antidepressants

Drug (Dose Range, mg/day)	Sedation/ Weight Gain	Hypo-tensive	Antichol-inergic	Lethality from Overdose	Inhibits Reuptake of Ne/ 5-HT	Dosage	Elimination Half-life (hr)	Blood Levels, nmol/L (ng/mL)	Other
Serotonin-Specific Reuptake Inhibitors (SSRIs)									
Fluoxetine (Prozac) (5–80)	±/0	–	0	Low	0/+++	AM	24–96	660–2,300 (15–55)	Following discontinuation, wait 6 wk before starting MAOI; enzyme inhibition (increased drug interactions) Long-acting metabolite (elimination half-life = norfluoxetine 4–16 days)
Sertraline (Zoloft) (50–200)	±/0	–	0	Low	0/+++	AM or PM	24	(50–200)	Some enzyme induction rather than inhibition; no active metabolite
Paroxetine (Paxil) (20–50)	±/0	–		Low	0/+++	AM or PM	21	(1–150)	Most potent of SSRIs for binding at 5-HT uptake site (6× more potent than fluoxetine) moderate enzyme inhibition
Serotonin-Nonselective Reuptake Inhibitors									
Venlafaxine (Effexor) (75–375)	±/0	–	±	Low	++/+++	3× a day	5 Metabolite: 11 hr		Some anticholinergic side effects despite low binding potency at this receptor; moderate effects on dopamine; mild increases in blood pressure
Dopamine Active									
Bupropion (Wellbutrin) (225–480)	0/– –	++	++	Low	+/0	3×–4× a day	10–14	100–400 (25–75)	Divided dose required; increased risk of seizures at doses above 450 mg/day Consider for depressive episodes in bipolar disorder
Norepinephrine Active									
Desipramine (Norpramin) (75–300)	+/+	+++	+	High	+++/0	Bedtime	12–76	470–1,125 (125–300)	(?) Less weight gain than with other TCAs
Maprotiline (Ludiomil) (100–225)	++/++	++	++	High	+++/0	Bedtime	27–58	720–2,160 (50–350)	Increased risk of seizures
Secondary Amines									
Nortriptyline (Pamelor, Aventyl) (40–200)	++/+	+	++	High	+++/++	Bedtime	13–88	190–570 (50–150)	Inverted U shape of blood levels-response curve; increased levels in blacks; persons of Japanese ancestry require one-half the dose
Protriptyline (Vivactyl) (15–60)	±/?	++	+++	High	+++/+	AM	54–124	260–990	
Trimipramine (Surmontil) (75–300)	+++/++	++	+	High			7–30	(70–260)	Blocks D_2–D_4 receptors

Other									
Trazodone (Desyrel) (150–600)	++/+	+++	0	Low	0/++	3× a day,	4–9	2,150–4,300 (800–1,600)	Priapism; no prolongation of cardiac conduction, but possibly arrhythmogenic
Amoxapine (Asendin) (100–600)	++/±	+	++	Low	+++/++		8		Extrapyramidal side effects and tardive dyskinesia
Buspirone (BuSpar) (5–35) (?)	+/	0		?		3×–4× a day	2–3	(200–600)	5-HT_{1A} selective; generalized anxiety disorder
Alprazolam (Xanax) (2–6)	+++/0	0	0	Low		3×–4× a day	6–27	(20–55)	Generalized anxiety disorder; panic; (?) dependence and withdrawal
Lithium (Eskalith) (900–2,400)	±/+++	0	0	Low to high		Bedtime	10–40	0.5–1.5	Low therapeutic index; careful blood monitoring required; excellent adjunct to other antidepressants
Clonazepam (Klonopin) (1–4)	+++/0	+	+	None		3× a day	18–50		
ECT (6–10 Rxs)	NA/0	0	0	—		AM		NA	Rapid onset, especially for delusional depression; transient confusion and memory loss common
Tertiary Amines									
Clomipramine (Anafranil) (75–300)	+++/++	+++	+++	High	+/+++	Bedtime	17–28	650–2,300	Only approved agent for obsessive-compulsive disorder; relatively 5-HT selective
Amitriptyline (Elavil) (75–300)	+++/+++	+++	+++	High	+/+++	Bedtime	14–46	300–925 (75–250)	Typical TCA side effects common (dry mouth, drowsiness, dizziness, constipation, fatigue, and blurred vision)
Imipramine (Tofranil) (75–300)	++/++	+++	+++	High	++/+++	Bedtime	14–34	630–1,050 (150–300)	Same as above
Doxepin (Adapin, Sinequan) (75–300)	+++/++	++	++	High	++/+	Bedtime	8–36	550–920 (30–250)	Useful block of H_2 receptors; does not reverse guanethidine
MAOIs									
Tranylcypromine (Parnate) (20–60)	+/++	+++	0	?	NA	AM/3× a day	1–3		Dietary restrictions necessary, especially for refractory depressive and retarded bipolar depression Wait 6 wk after discontinuing fluoxetine before starting MAOI
Deprenyl (Eldepryl) (10)		++		High		AM/lunch	2–20		

Abbreviations: NE, norepinephrine; 5-HT, 5-hydroxytryptamine; MAOIs, monoamine oxidase inhibitors; —, unknown; NA, not applicable; TCA, tricyclic antidepressants.

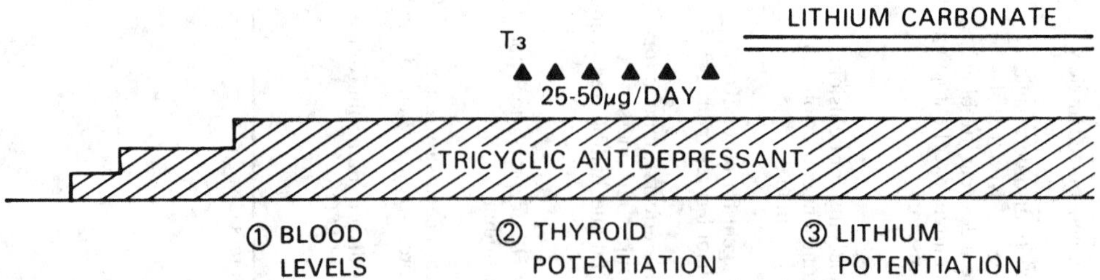

FIGURE 16.7-5 *Maximizing and potentiating antidepressant treatment.*

antidepressants sold in the United States, not so much because of its unique profile of therapeutic efficacy, but because of its relatively benign side-effect profile (Table 16.7-1). In contrast to many of the first-generation tricyclic antidepressants, which affect multiple receptor systems (α_1, α_2, ACh, histamine, and the like), fluoxetine use is not associated with weight gain, orthostatic hypotension, anticholinergic side effects, and high lethality when taken in an overdose. Its side effects are more likely to include increased agitation with insomnia, an internal sense of being driven, headache, tremor, gastrointestinal (GI) upset, and sexual dysfunction. To avoid a potentially lethal serotonergic syndrome, it is mandatory to wait six weeks after fluoxetine discontinuation before initiating MAOI treatment. The wait is necessary because of the long-acting metabolite of fluoxetine, norfluoxetine, which has an elimination half-life of five to seven days.

Sertraline has a shorter half-life than fluoxetine and does not have a long-lasting metabolite. Despite those differences, sertraline shares most of the side effects seen with fluoxetine, including GI distress and sexual dysfunction. In contrast to fluoxetine, sertraline exhibits first-order kinetics (that is, it does not inhibit its own metabolism). Further, some patients intolerant of fluoxetine may respond to and tolerate sertraline. It does not increase the blood levels of other drugs. The most prominent side effects are GI effects (nausea, diarrhea, dyspepsia) and sexual effects (anorgasmia).

Serotonin nonselective reuptake inhibitors Venlafaxine is a mixed serotonin, norepinephrine, and, to a lesser extent, dopamine reuptake inhibitor with a novel phenylethylamine structure. Unlike the specific SSRIs fluoxetine, sertraline, and paroxetine, venlafaxine provides substantial inhibition of norepinephrine reuptake. Like other antidepressants, venlafaxine decreases locus coeruleus firing. A single dose in rats produces down-regulation of β-adrenergic receptors, suggesting the possibility of more rapid onset of action than with existing agents, although clinical data are inconclusive. Unlike many older antidepressants, venlafaxine lacks significant binding to adrenergic, serotonergic, dopaminergic, histaminergic, and cholinergic receptors. That may explain why venlafaxine therapy is less likely to yield the orthostasis, sedation, weight gain, tachycardia, dry mouth, and constipation seen during therapy with older-generation antidepressants.

The mixed serotonergic, noradrenergic, and dopaminergic action of venlafaxine makes it a potentially useful agent in the treatment of patients with depression who are refractory to agents that affect only one of those monoamine systems. A 40 percent response rate to venlafaxine has been reported in patients who have failed adequate trials of other treatments, including MAOIs and ECT. MAOIs (which also affect all three monoamine systems) have been found effective in treating refractory depression, but side effects, dietary restrictions, and drug interactions have limited their utility.

Venlafaxine has a plasma elimination half-life of about five hours, requiring administration two or three times a day. Its principal metabolite, O-desmethylvenlafaxine, is active and has a half-life of about 11 hours. Venlafaxine is metabolized by and is a weak inhibitor of the cytochrome P-450 2D6 isoenzyme, so that pharmacokinetic interactions with other drugs (including some antidepressants) metabolized by that system may occur. Knowledge of the pharmacokinetic interactions of venlafaxine with other psychotropic agents is preliminary.

Venlafaxine is generally well tolerated, with a side-effect profile similar to that of the SSRIs. The most frequent side effects include nausea, weight loss, sweating, sedation, dry mouth, and sexual dysfunction. Except for nausea, side effects appear to be dose-related, and most attenuate over time or with a decrease in dosage. Infrequently, they require discontinuation of the medication. Increases in supine diastolic blood pressure have been reported with venlafaxine. Such increases are generally mild, but are more common with higher doses (mean increase of about 7 mm Hg at 375 mg a day). About 3 percent of patients develop a rash that requires discontinuation of the drug. Approximately 0.25 percent of patients develop seizures, an incidence similar to that seen with other antidepressants. In addition, about 1 in 200 patients experience hypomania or mania while taking venlafaxine.

The recommended dosage titration in the clinical treatment of depression includes starting with 25 mg three times a day (75 mg a day) and increasing by 75 mg a day at four-day intervals until the dosage reaches 125 mg three times a day (375 mg a day), if necessary.

Heterocyclics The antidepressant properties of bupropion do not involve potent effects on brain 5-HT. Bupropion does increase levels of dopamine in the nucleus accumbens and striatum. Preliminary reports in patients with bipolar disorders suggest that it may have prophylactic effects without increasing the risk of mania in those patients. A positive effect on motor retardation has been reported. Bupropion has few anticholinergic side effects, and its administration is not associated with weight gain. The risk of seizures is increased at doses above 450 mg; the dose should be divided and generally should not exceed 150 mg at a given time.

Despite sporadic claims to the contrary, there is little convincing evidence that one particular antidepressant works more rapidly than another. That statement remains true for the newer second- and third-generation heterocyclic (tetracyclic and bicyclic) antidepressants. Although further research may uncover some exceptions to the rule, clinicians should be familiar with several different antidepressants in the heterocyclic class and their dose-response and dose-side effects characteristics. The clinical response profiles and side effects of heterocyclic and other antidepressants are summarized in Table 16.7-1. Given the relatively uniform incidence and time of onset of efficacy, the side-effect profile may be the deciding factor in the choice of antidepressants for both acute treatment and long-term prophylaxis. A benign side-effect profile not only may help the patient achieve adequate therapeutic levels in the relative absence of side effects, it may also facilitate optimal compliance during the more difficult phases of continuation therapy and long-term prophylactic therapy.

Thus, for the first antidepressant, a second- or third-generation antidepressant compound with a relatively benign side-effect profile or a secondary amine tricyclic antidepressant might be selected over the better studied but less well-tolerated primary amine compounds. One possible exception to that general recommendation is the use of clomipramine (Anafranil) in the patient with comorbid obsessive-compulsive disorder, as clomipromine, unlike desipramine (Norpramin), is highly effective in the treatment of obsessive-compulsive disorder.

Monoamine oxidase inhibitors MAOIs may be started shortly after the termination of tricyclic antidepressant therapy, but the converse is not recommended, as MAO inhibition can persist for two weeks or more after cessation of treatment. Treatment with an MAOI should not be started until five weeks after termination of fluoxetine therapy because of the possibility of a lethal serotonergic syndrome. The lag in onset of relief with the MAOIs is similar to that of the heterocyclics. Consequently, three to six weeks may be required to assess the treatment's effectiveness. Doses in the higher range (phenelzine [Nardil], 60 to 90 mg; tranylcypromine [Parnate], 30 to 60 mg) should be given to achieve adequate MAO inhibition in the absence of clinical response and side effects at lower doses. Antidepressant effects may be more closely associated with inhibition of MAO type A (MAO_A) (clorgylinelike), primarily affecting NE (and 5-HT). Thus, high doses of MAO type B (MAO_B)-selective agents such as L-deprenyl (30 to 60 mg), may be required to achieve antidepressant effects. Phenelzine and tranylcypromine are A,B nonselective. The potentiation of antidepressant efficacy during MAOI therapy has also been reported for both L-triiodothyronine (T_3, liothyronine) (Cytomel) and lithium carbonate.

Side effects Conventional wisdom suggests using initial minor selection criteria to choose one agent over the next. For example, among the tricyclics the clinician might consider protriptyline (Vivactil) or desipramine for a patient with retarded depression and a more sedating drug, such as amitriptyline (Elavil) or doxepin (Adapin, Sinequan), for a patient with agitated depression. In general, the tertiary amine antidepressants, such as amitriptyline, imipramine, trimipramine (Surmontil), and doxepin, tend to be more sedating than the secondary amines desipramine, nortriptyline (Pamelor), and protriptyline (Vivactil).

The SSRIs fluoxetine, sertraline, and paroxetine, and bupropion, venlafaxine, desipramine, and possibly trazodone (Desyrel) may be considered for the overweight depressed patient or one with a history of weight gain during previous tricyclic administration, as preliminary evidence suggests that those drugs may be less likely to induce weight gain than most tricyclics. Bupropion and the SSRIs may even be associated with weight loss rather than gain. Isocarboxazid (Marplan), which is no longer generally available, was thought to be less likely to cause weight gain than tranylcypromine and phenelzine.

Anticholinergic effects (dry mouth, blurred vision, sweating, constipation, urinary hesitancy and retention, delayed ejaculation) tend to be more prominent with the tertiary amine tricyclics and less so with trazodone, desipramine, amoxapine (Asendin), maprotiline (Ludiomil), and the MAOIs, SSRIs, and lithium.

Orthostatic hypotension, particularly in the elderly, may be associated with the administration of imipramine, amitriptyline, desipramine, trazodone, and the MAOIs but less frequently with the SSRIs, bupropion, nortriptyline, amoxapine, maprotiline, and doxepin (or lithium and carbamazepine). The heterocyclics amoxapine, maprotiline, and trazodone, touted for their less sedating and possibly less anticholinergic and less cardiotoxic profile, are not consistent in that regard.

Orthostatic hypotension may become more prominent in the second and third weeks of MAOI treatment. Salt loading, the use of pressure stockings, and fludrocortisone (Florinef) administration may prove effective in the treatment of MAOI-induced hypotension. MAOIs can be given in a single morning dose or in divided doses. If marked insomnia occurs, nighttime doses of trazodone have been recommended by some authorities. Bouts of daytime drowsiness and sedation may also become problematic. The clinician might attempt to titrate the dose against side effects, as variations in dosage or timing of administration may be helpful.

The necessity of restricting substances that release tyramine or catecholamines and can produce hypertensive crises during MAOI treatment should be emphasized to the patient. Hypertensive crises may be clinically manifested as explosive headaches, flushing, palpitations, perspiration, and nausea. Immediate treatment with a slow infusion of phentolamine (Regitine), 5 mg given intravenously in an emergency room, is the recommended treatment (Tables 16.7-2 through 16.7-4).

TABLE 16.7-2
Instructions for Patients Taking Monoamine Oxidase Inhibitors (MAOIs)

Background Information

Foods rich in tyramine and some related amines have been known to cause serious side effects and hypertensive responses in patients taking MAOIs. Tyramine is an amino acid found in many protein substances and is produced by fermentation, aging, spoiling, or pickling. The enzyme MAO found in the liver normally inactivates tyramine. In the presence of an MAOI, tyramine is not deactivated by MAO and is allowed to circulate and indirectly cause the release of norepinephrine from nerve endings. This may lead to detrimental side effects, especially hypertensive responses.

Summary of Guidelines to Follow While Taking an MAOI

1. The foods in the "high tyramine" category should be completely avoided. If you consume small quantities of foods in this category without symptoms, do not assume that you can repeat this. These foods vary greatly in tyramine content and their ability to cause a severe reaction. You may have a reaction the second time.
2. You are allowed foods with moderate to low tyramine content (categories 2 and 3). These foods should be eaten in moderation. Try to avoid eating combinations of foods in these categories because of the possible additive effects of tyramine.
3. Avoid aged, spoiled, improperly refrigerated, or frozen foods. Do not eat tuna fish that has been in the refrigerator for 2 or 3 days. Eat only fresh food or freshly prepared frozen or canned foods. Beware of many foods that derive their flavor from aging, smoking, or pickling. Also note that cooking of degraded protein does not alter the tyramine content of these foods.
4. Avoid any foods that have previously caused adverse side effects.
5. Cheeses have been responsible for the greatest number of reported hypertensive responses. Observe that many foods contain cheese as an ingredient, such as cheese crackers, pizza, and cheese bread.
6. There are certain prescription and nonprescription medicines that should be avoided. See list of MAOI Drug Incompatibilities [Table 16.7-4]. Be certain to tell your physician, dentist, or pharmacist that you are taking an MAOI.
7. Call your physician immediately or go to your nearest emergency medical facility if you should suffer from the following symptoms: a throbbing, explosive headache of sudden onset associated with flushing, visual disturbances, nausea or vomiting. Major muscle jerks, confusion, or excitement may also occur, and in the case of a reaction with another drug, sometimes without a severe headache.

Table from D L Murphy, T Sunderland, R M Cohen: Monoamine oxidase-inhibiting antidepressants: A clinical update. Psychiatr Clin North Am *7:* 549, 1984. Used with permission.

TABLE 16.7-3
MAOI Dietary Restrictions

High Tyramine Content—Not Permitted	
Aged, matured cheeses (unpasteurized)	Cheddar, Camembert, Stilton, bleu, Swiss
Smoked or pickled meats, fish, or poultry	Herring, sausage, corned beef
Aged putrefying meats, fish, and poultry	Chicken or beef liver, paté, game
Yeast or meat extracts	Bovril, marmite, brewer's yeast (beware of drinks, soups, and stews made with those products)
Red wines	Chianti, burgundy, sherry, vermouth
Italian broad beans	Fava beans
Moderate Tyramine Content—Limited Amounts Allowed	
Meat extracts	Bouillion, consommé
Pasteurized light and pale beers	
Ripe avocado	
Low Tyramine Content—Permissible	
Distilled spirits (in moderation)	Vodka, gin, rye, scotch
Cheese	Cottage cheese, cream cheese
Chocolate- and caffeine-containing beverages	
Fruits	Figs, raisins, grapes, pineapple, oranges
Soy sauce	
Yogurt, sour cream (made by reputable manufacturers)	

Table from D L Murphy, T Sunderland, R M Cohen: Monoamine oxidase-inhibiting antidepressants: A clinical update. Psychiatr Clin North Am *7:* 549, 1984. Used with permission.

TABLE 16.7-4
MAOI Drug Incompatibilities

Generally Contraindicated Hazardous Potentiations*	
Stimulants	Weight-reducing or antiappetite drugs; amphetamines, cocaine
Decongestants	Sinus, hay fever, and cold tablets; nasal sprays or drops; asthma tablets or inhalants, cough preparations (or any products containing ephedrine, phenylephedrine, or phenylpropanolamine)
Antihypertensives	Methyldopa, guanethidine, reserpine
TCAs	Imipramine, desipramine, clomipramine
MAOIs	Tranylcypromine, after other MAOIs
Sympathomimetics	Dopamine, Metaraminol
Amine precursors	L-dopa, L-tryptophan
Narcotics	Meperidine (Demerol)
Some Potentiation Possible	
Narcotics	Morphine, codeine
Sedatives	Alcohol, barbiturates, benzodiazepines
Local anesthetics containing vasoconstrictors	
Sympathomimetics	Ephedrine, norepinephrine, isoproterenol
General anesthetics	

*Under certain circumstances, some of these drugs may be used together with MAOIs in specialized treatment approaches and with additional precautions. For example, TCAs and L-tryptophan have been used with MAOIs in antidepressant regimens. Also of note, other agents from these drug classes are safely used (for example, the antihypertensive agent chlorothiazide) as only mild potentiation occurs.

Table from D L Murphy, T Sunderland, R M Cohen: Monoamine oxidase-inhibiting antidepressants: A clinical update. Psychiatr Clin North Am *7:* 549, 1984. Used with permission.

Blood levels Blood levels of tricyclics above 450 μg/mL may be cardiotoxic, and doses of tricyclics equivalent to 2,500 mg or more of imipramine may be fatal. Electrocardiographic (ECG) monitoring should be considered in patients on high-dose tricyclic therapy (above 300 mg a day). The risk of seizures increases with increasing dosages of many cyclic antidepressants, especially maprotiline (above 225 mg a day). Maprotiline should therefore be avoided in patients with an abnormal EEG or a family history of epilepsy. Many of those guidelines are based on anecdotal evidence and may not stand the test of time and careful clinical research evaluation.

As a general rule, blood levels among patients treated with the same dose of a tricyclic or heterocyclic agent vary widely. Thus, giving all patients doses within the conventional range will leave some with subtherapeutic blood levels and others with very high levels. That may be important for nortriptyline, for which there is evidence of an inverted U-shaped curve (that is, there is a therapeutic window for clinical improvement below and above which patients do not do well). Thus, with the exception of nortriptyline, it appears clinically useful to increase doses slowly, titrating against side effects with blood level monitoring at (maintenance) doses in patients who do not show an adequate therapeutic effect. During nortriptyline treatment with a moderate to a high, but ineffective, dose, one might decrease the dose to bring blood levels back into the therapeutic range, which is highly variable across studies.

It may be useful to assess the blood level of a heterocyclic agent in a patient who fails to show adequate therapeutic response to conventional doses of the drug. Evaluation may be done once steady-state blood levels have been reached and a clinical response can be expected, generally two to three weeks after initiation of the drug. Blood levels may also be helpful in assessing the patient with substantial side effects at the lower dosage ranges. Finally, a single blood level determination in the well-maintained patient may be prudent, as a score of medicolegal cases are pending in which massive blood levels of tricyclic antidepressants were associated with sudden death. Although general blood level guidelines for some agents are given in Table 16.7-1, the clinician should remember that blood level-response relations are obscure for most drugs and that laboratories may differ widely in the accuracy of the determination and in the agreed-upon therapeutic range. Nonetheless, blood levels may be helpful in the general assessment of the nonresponsive patient and may provide an opportunity for discussing issues such as fast metabolism and noncompliance when unexpectedly low levels are ascertained. In contrast, blood level monitoring may be less important for the SSRIs.

Time frame With the traditional tricyclics and other antidepressants, initial improvement in sleep in the first weeks of treatment is not necessarily predictive of subsequent clinical outcome. Nevertheless, the patient may be comforted by the fact that sleep is improving. Antidepressants often require two to four weeks to produce substantial effects and four to eight weeks to produce maximal effect; however, gradual improvement often begins in the first and second weeks of treatment. Thus, there may not be an absolute lag in time to onset of clinical efficacy, only in time to onset of substantial or maximal change.

Potentiation Because antidepressants have to be administered for several days to weeks before the response can be evaluated, the clinician should consider antidepressant potentiation in either the first or second antidepressant trial before switching antidepressants, even if the category of agents seems to lack efficacy in the patient under treatment. Thus, if a patient is

TABLE 16.7-5
Approaches to Refractory Depression

Level of Refractoriness	Therapeutic Strategies
I Failure to respond	Optimize dosage; assess blood levels
II Failure to respond to adequate trial of first agent	Consider potentiation or switch to new antidepressant with different mechanism of action, or to one in a new class
III Failure to respond to second agent	Potentiate with T_3. If no response, discontinue and potentiate with lithium Switch to a third agent Strongly consider an MAOI Add or revise psychotherapy
IV Failure to respond to third agent	Definitely consider an MAOI, with or without potentiation with T_3 and lithium Consider ECT, depending on severity and suicidality Add or revise psychotherapy Consider consultation and reexamination of compliance and diagnosis, especially previously unrecognized physical, psychiatric, or substance abuse comorbidity If comorbidity is present, treatment should be better targeted to that comorbid condition (i.e., medical therapy, revised pharmacotherapy, and adjunctive group work such as Alcoholics Anonymous, a related ''12-step'' program, or a self-help group)
V Failure to respond to numerous clinical trials of agents with different mechanisms of action, MAOIs and ECT	Consider novel therapies, including • extreme doses of MAOIs (80–120 mg tranylcypromine) • carbamazepine or valproate with or without an adjunct antidepressant such as bupropion (especially if recurrent or rapid cycling) • alprazolam (especially if increased anxiety) • bromocriptine (dopamine-acting, especially for retarded depression) • TCA plus MAOI (in this but not reverse order) • MAOI plus stimulant (pemoline, amphetamine, methylphenidate). *Use stimulant or MAOI only with great care and after appropriate informed consent has been obtained* • adjunctive folate

receiving the maximal tolerated dose or has adequate blood levels of the drug and is not responding adequately, the clinician might consider adding thyroid hormone or lithium carbonate (Table 16.7-5 and Figure 16.7-5).

There is a sizable literature on the efficacy of thyroid potentiation in converting antidepressant nonresponders to responders, but only in some 20 to 30 percent of patients. This appears to be independent of an initial clinical thyroid status or any evidence of hypothyroidism. A response to the addition of T_3 (25 to 50 μg a day in the morning) may occur within days and usually occurs within the first week or two of treatment. If no response to antidepressant potentiation occurs during that time frame, the clinical trial of T_3 can be exchanged for other options. Side effects are unusual but may include tachycardia, hypertension, anxiety, and flushing.

A second option is potentiation with lithium carbonate. An extensive literature, including several controlled clinical trials, reveals that the addition of lithium carbonate to a variety of antidepressant modalities, including tricyclic, heterocyclic, and MAOI antidepressants and carbamazepine, is often accompanied by a rapid clinical improvement in 50 to 60 percent of patients. Improvement may begin within 24 to 48 hours but may be slower in onset and stretch over the first week to 10 days. Doses of lithium that are slightly lower than those conventionally used for monotherapy are generally effective (that is, 600 to 900 mg in a single dose taken at bedtime may be sufficient). When lithium is used in that fashion, its side-effect profile appears to be quite benign. Lithium potentiation may be effective in all subtypes of depression. The initial reports of estrogen potentiation of antidepressant response do not appear as promising as those of either thyroid or lithium potentiation.

Drug sequence The clinician might consider exchanging one type of antidepressant for another should unacceptable side effects appear before adequate blood levels or clinical response have been achieved. If an adequate dose and adequate blood levels have been achieved but the clinical response is inadequate, the clinician may switch to a drug with a different biochemical profile within the same class or to a different class altogether, such as an MAOI.

APPROACHES TO DEPRESSIVE SYMPTOMS AND SUBTYPES

Comorbid anxiety disorder and panic disorder DSM-IV notes the existence of a mixed anxiety-depressive disorder among the anxiety disorders. It is not known whether patients with significant symptoms of both anxiety and depression are affected by two different disease processes or by one disease process that produces both kinds of symptoms.

If panic disorder coexists with a depressive disorder, an SSRI, tricyclic antidepressant, or MAOI should be tried initially, as those drugs are among the best for treating primary panic disorder. If symptoms of panic or anxiety remain prominent despite apparently adequate antidepressant treatment, the physician might consider the acute adjunctive use of a benzodiazepine-active agent such as alprazolam (Xanax) or the less well-studied clonazepam (Klonopin), which has also been reported to be useful in treating primary panic disorder. Those benzodiazepine agents may also have a role in the first weeks of tricyclic treatment, when anxiety symptoms occasionally increase. Alprazolam should be used with caution in patients with borderline personality disorder as it may be associated with an increased incidence of dyscontrol acts. Patients with panic or marked anxiety symptoms have often been reported to respond to MAOIs, with or without lithium potentiation. Trazodone and bupropion should be avoided as first-line treatments as they are ineffective in patients whose primary diagnosis is panic disorder or anxiety disorder. Trazodone should be avoided in male patients because of the risk of irreversible priapism that requires surgical intervention.

The new antianxiety drug buspirone (BuSpar) has recently been reported to produce moderate to marked antidepressant effects in 50 percent of patients with depressive disorders without melancholic features, although it had no effect on those with melancholic features, and responses were not associated with baseline anxiety scores. Buspirone has been used to potentiate and to maintain response to fluoxetine, and vice versa.

The early literature suggested a response to MAOIs in atypical depressed patients with rejection sensitivity, leaden paralysis, hypersomnia, and hyperphagia, although a recent study reported characteristics of typical depression as predictive of a positive response to tranylcypromine. Those characteristics included greater initial severity of depressed mood, psychomotor retardation, weight loss, but less middle and late insomnia (early morning awakening). Thus, the MAOIs should be considered for patients in whom multiple agents have failed, regardless of the subtype of clinical presentation. Five to six weeks must elapse following the discontinuation of fluoxetine before an MAOI is initiated.

Psychosis A growing literature suggests that if a patient's depression has reached psychotic proportions and delusions are present, the adjunctive use of low to moderate doses of antipsychotics may help produce an antidepressant response and alleviate delusional symptoms. Preliminary evidence also suggests that lithium carbonate may be useful and that a triple drug regimen consisting of a heterocyclic agent, an antipsychotic, and lithium may be needed in some patients. When using antipsychotic potentiation in delusional depression, the physician should taper and discontinue the antipsychotics as early as possible in the continuation phase in order to lessen the risk of tardive dyskinesia. Amoxapine may also be considered for agitated, delusionally depressed patients as it has some inherent antipsychotic (dopamine receptor-blocking) properties that may be advantageous, although it, too, has been associated with the development of tardive dyskinesia.

ECT is more likely to be successful in treating delusionally depressed patients and has a more rapid onset than most psychopharmacological regimens. Thus, ECT may be considered earlier for depressed patients with delusions rather than as a treatment of last resort after psychopharmacological trials have failed. An absolute contraindication to ECT is the presence of a cerebral aneurysm or increased intracranial pressure, but a recent myocardial infarction is only a relative contraindication. Additional indications for implementing ECT may include severe medical or suicidal risk, cardiac problems (which make tricyclics dangerous), and, possibly, severe mood episodes associated with pregnancy.

Insomnia Persistent insomnia may accompany an inadequate antidepressant response but should begin to resolve as the treatment begins to take effect. Giving more sedating antidepressants in a once-a-day evening dose is usually an effective strategy for the insomniac depressed patient because of the long half-life of most cyclic antidepressants. That regimen makes positive use of the sedation at bedtime and increases the likelihood of compliance with a single nighttime dose. Acute adjunctive treatment with a benzodiazepine may be warranted in rare instances of severe sleep loss, although the physician should be cautious about prescribing benzodiazepines and related sedatives on a long-term basis because of the possibility of habituation and addiction. Benzodiazepines should not be used as the primary antidepressant modality, as is still common in many general practice settings. The physician may also consider adjunctive nighttime medication with such agents as nortriptyline or buspirone in the patient experiencing insomnia while taking SSRIs.

Paradoxically, sleep deprivation may be an adjunctive procedure, whether or not there is severe sleep loss. An acute but transient antidepressant response to one night of sleep deprivation has been consistently reported in studies from different laboratories. Although many patients relapse after one night's recovery of sleep, sleep deprivation may be used in combination with more traditional tricyclic antidepressant or lithium carbonate treatment. Lithium may help sustain the sleep deprivation response. Moreover, preliminary evidence suggests that deprivation of sleep in the last half of the night (from 3 to 7 AM) may be just as effective as total sleep deprivation and thus may be more convenient for clinical use in outpatient treatment. The rapid onset of effects achieved in approximately one half of severely depressed patients is different from the slower but sustained effects following selective deprivation of REM sleep, which is not amenable to easy clinical induction.

Lethargy and retardation Extreme morning lethargy and retardation may be an indication for the use of SSRIs, bupropion, venlafaxine, or secondary amine tricyclic antidepressants. In the face of unsuccessful drug trials, including T_3 and lithium potentiation, the short-term supplementation of cyclic antidepressants (not MAOIs) with psychomotor stimulants has been recommended by some until there is an adequate antidepressant response to the other agents. Small doses of methylphenidate (Ritalin, 5 to 10 mg) or an amphetamine in the morning may help the otherwise incapacitated, severely retarded depressed patient face the day with more energy. Stimulants as a primary antidepressant modality in elderly depressed patients have been recommended by some authorities but remain relatively understudied.

For depressed patients with decreased appetite and associated decreased nutritional intake, the physician may consider potentiating with folic acid supplements, as a folic acid deficiency has been reported to cause refractory depression in patients receiving anticonvulsants and, presumably, could also occur because of decreased dietary intake. Moreover, intracellular deficits can occur in the setting of apparently normal plasma levels.

Obsessive-compulsive symptoms The associated occurrence of marked obsessive-compulsive symptoms may lead to the consideration of clomipramine, which has been reported to be highly effective in adults and children with primary obsessive-compulsive symptoms when more traditional antidepressants are ineffective. Fluoxetine and the other SSRIs may share that positive effect on obsessive-compulsive symptoms.

Double depression It is important to assess the possible occurrence of a double depression, defined by DSM-IV as the condition in which major depressive disorder is superimposed on dysthymic disorder. As the patient's superimposed depressive symptoms are alleviated, a core of chronic, minor depression may be left. In such a case the physician may erroneously conclude that the superimposed episode has not been successfully treated. Psychopharmacological approaches to the baseline level of the double depression have not been adequately delineated, but the physician might consider drugs used for the cyclic mood disorders (for example, lithium) in addition to the more traditional antidepressant agents and the SSRIs. Psychotherapy may also be indicated for some patients.

Atypical depressive features The occurrence of atypical features or reverse or vegetative symptoms, such as hypersomnia, carbohydrate craving, and weight gain, suggests a careful reevaluation for the possible bipolar II disorder and seasonal affective disorder (SAD) (called mood disorder with seasonal pattern in DSM-IV). The atypical features may be effectively targeted with the SSRIs, bupropion, venlafaxine, and the MAOIs.

A clear-cut diagnosis of SAD with increased depression that is selectively associated with decreased daylight hours in the winter months suggests the use of light treatment. The syndrome responds well over a period of several days to high-intensity light given in the morning or evening. Light treatment can be used prophylactically throughout the winter months in a patient with marked SAD. Ordinary light is not effective; rather, light in the intensity of 2,500 lux or greater is required to achieve a therapeutic response. It is unclear whether light treatment could be an effective adjunct for nonseasonal depressions.

APPROACHES TO REFRACTORY DEPRESSION A sequence of treatment reevaluations and options for different levels of refractoriness is outlined in Table 16.7-5. During each sequence the physician should consider optimizing a given regimen by appropriately maximizing the dose and titrating blood levels against the emergence of side effects, and using appropriate augmentation strategies. Switching among different classes of antidepressants or, within the heterocyclic class of agents, among drugs with different mechanisms of action appears most appropriate, although occasionally response to one but not another of the SSRIs may be observed. A trial of an MAOI should definitely be considered in a patient in whom multiple previous trials have failed. Venlafaxine also has a relatively positive response profile in patients who have not responded to multiple previous clinical trials. With increasing levels of refractoriness the physician should reevaluate the diagnosis (with careful assessment of possible physical, psychological, and substance use comorbidity) and should consider consultation, psychotherapy revision, ECT, and combination modalities.

Clinical trials have suggested some antidepressant efficacy of the direct dopamine agonist bromocriptine (Parlodel), which is used to treat parkinsonian patients. One double-blind study indicated that bromocriptine was equally as effective as imipramine. A related dopamine agonist, piribedil (Trivastal), has also been effective for the occasional patient with treatment-refractory depression. Dopamine-active drugs had been reported to be more effective in patients with low cerebrospinal fluid (CSF) levels of the dopamine metabolite homovanillic acid (HVA). Whether that relation holds for bupropion, with its ability to increase dopamine levels in the nucleus accumbens and striatum, remains to be explored. A similar relation between low levels of the serotonin metabolite 5-hydroxyindoleacetic acid (5-HIAA) and a better response to the serotonin-active compounds clomipramine and sertraline has been reported. The results are inconsistent as to whether urinary levels of the norepinephrine metabolite 3-methoxy-4-hydroxyphenylglycol (MHPG) can predict the response to noradrenergically active antidepressants, such as desipramine, maprotiline, and venlafaxine. Consistent endocrine or other biochemical markers of antidepressant response have not yet been found.

Although the acute antidepressive effects of lithium have been repeatedly reported, especially in patients with bipolar disorders, they remain controversial; nonetheless, consideration of lithium for patients with unresponsive major depressive disorder, particularly in augmentation trials, appears reasonable. The lag in onset to full antidepressant response is often two to four weeks or longer when lithium is used as monotherapy. Combination treatment with a tricyclic antidepressant and an MAOI has been advocated by some for patients with treatment-resistant major depressive disorder, although the superiority of that combination regimen to single-agent treatment remains controversial and virtually unstudied in a systematic fashion. If used (under extreme circumstances), both drugs can be started together (at low doses), or the MAOI can be added later. The reverse order should be avoided. The tricyclic nortriptyline may have a better safety record than imipramine or protriptyline.

Carbamazepine has been reported to be effective when used acutely and prophylactically in some patients with major depressive disorder in whom multiple trials with traditional antidepressants have failed, especially those with a history of head trauma or EEG abnormalities. For patients with treatment-refractory bipolar disorder the anticonvulsants carbamazepine and valproate may be used in combination with bupropion. Those and other combination treatments for the patient with refractory depression warrant further systematic research to provide adequate statistical and sequence-ordering guidance for the clinician.

OTHER ANTIDEPRESSANT MODALITIES A host of studied but unproven antidepressant modalities have been reported; many are unavailable in the United States and are not generally accepted treatments. Among them are *S*-adenosylmethionine (SAM), β-noradrenergic agonists, GABA agonists (such as progabide [Gabrene]), the opiate agonist buprenorphine (Temgesic), the α_2 antagonist idazoxan, very high parenteral doses of reserpine, anticholinergics, thyrotropin-releasing hormone (TRH), melanocyte inhibitory factor (MIF-1), vasopressin, and circadian-phase interventions.

Because of the rapid onset of effects of SAM in a high percentage of patients and the relative absence of side effects in a large number of controlled studies, that agent warrants further clinical and theoretical investigation. In double-blind studies SAM in doses of 400 mg a day produced rapid effects.

Compounds active in the dopamine biosynthetic pathway—phenylalanine, tyrosine, and levodopa (Larodopa, Dopar)—have each been reported effective in small groups of depressed patients. Levodopa may be more activating in retarded depressed patients with low CSF HVA levels, but its effectiveness is limited by increases in agitation, psychosis, and the switch into mania in patients with bipolar disorders. The precursors of 5-HT, tryptophan and 5-hydroxytryptophan (5-HTP), also have been reported to have antidepressant effects. Surprisingly favorable results in 12 of 14 studies have been reported with 5-HTP in 53 percent of a total of 547 depressed patients. The status of those agents remains in considerable doubt, however, especially in light of a reported association with malignant eosinophilia.

PHARMACOPROPHYLAXIS Although ongoing interpersonal psychotherapy may delay the onset of subsequent episodes in patients with recurrent major depressive disorder, only maintenance, standard-dose pharmacotherapy appears highly effective in preventing subsequent relapses and the emergence of new episodes. There is a high rate of relapse in depressed patients who have been entered into controlled studies after having had two or more previous episodes (Table 16.7-6). When effective treatment with an antidepressant agent has been followed by placebo substitution, the rate of recurrence of depressive episodes has averaged 55 percent by one year, 74 percent by two years, and 85 percent by three years. Double-blind maintenance of the original effective treatment reduced the rate of relapse by more than half at each of those time points. Statistically significant results have been obtained using a variety of treatment agents, among them the tricyclics imipramine and amitriptyline, the SSRIs fluoxetine, sertraline, and paroxetine; noradrenergic selective agents, such as maprotiline (whose effects were shown to be dose-dependent); and other agents,

TABLE 16.7-6
Impact of Prophylaxis on Relapse Rates in Major Depressive Disorder

	% Relapsed	
	Placebo	Active
1-yr trials (12 studies)	55	21
2-yr trials (6 studies)	74	32
3-yr trials (3 studies)	85	35
All trials (21 studies)	**65**	**26**

including lithium and buspirone. Based on a meta-analysis of 18 studies, John Davis and colleagues calculated that the likelihood that those results are due to chance is the astronomically low value 1×10^{-32}.

Given those data, the physician should strongly recommend pharmacoprophylaxis to patients with recurrent major depressive disorder who have had three or more prior episodes or several closely occurring episodes in the past two years. Prophylaxis should be strongly considered for the patient with two prior depressive episodes in the past five years. The strength of the recommendation should be highly integrated with a variety of other factors, including prior episode severity, refractoriness, degree of incapacitation, and the likelihood of suicidal risk if another depressive episode should occur. The recommendation should be strengthened if there is a family history of mood disorder.

Investigators in the field have observed the phenomenon of lithium-induced discontinuation refractoriness when effective prophylactic treatment was stopped in patients with bipolar disorder (Figure 16.7-6). Though the question of whether a similar phenomenon could occur in the treatment of major depressive disorder has not been systematically examined, it is at least possible that repeated depressive episodes after discontinuation of effective treatment with an antidepressant might lead not only to the reemergence of new episodes (Table 16.7-6) but also, in some percentage of patients, to refractoriness. Repeated episodes, in addition to carrying their own morbidity and potential for mortality (through suicide), may affect the subsequent course of illness. Thus, recurrent episodes could render the patient more vulnerable not only to subsequent relapses, but also to the possibility of decreased responsiveness to medications.

Patients should be specifically educated about the known risks for recurrence on a percentage basis (Table 16.7-6), and their negative attitudes concerning prophylaxis should be addressed and discussed. Negative attitudes include viewing the need for long-term prophylaxis as reflecting weakness, lack of effort, a character defect or flaw, and the like. Those attitudes need to be explored and countered. Societal stigma against open recognition of psychiatric illness and its short- and long-term treatment should also be addressed.

The risks of recurrence should be weighed against the relative lack of evidence of long-term side effects when the agents are used for prophylaxis, acknowledgment of the few potential side effects that can occur (such as the effects of lithium on the kidney and thyroid), and evidence for the lack of habituation

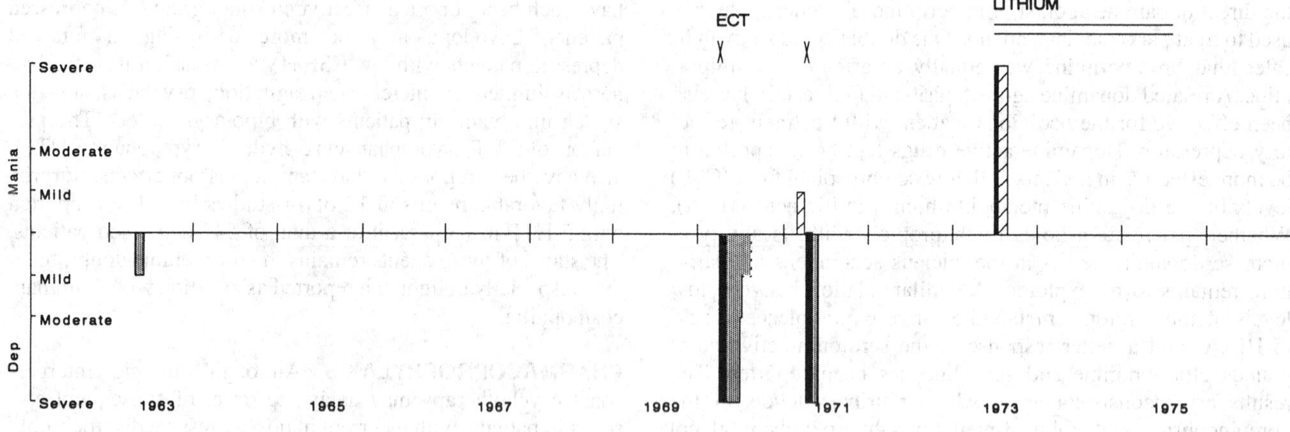

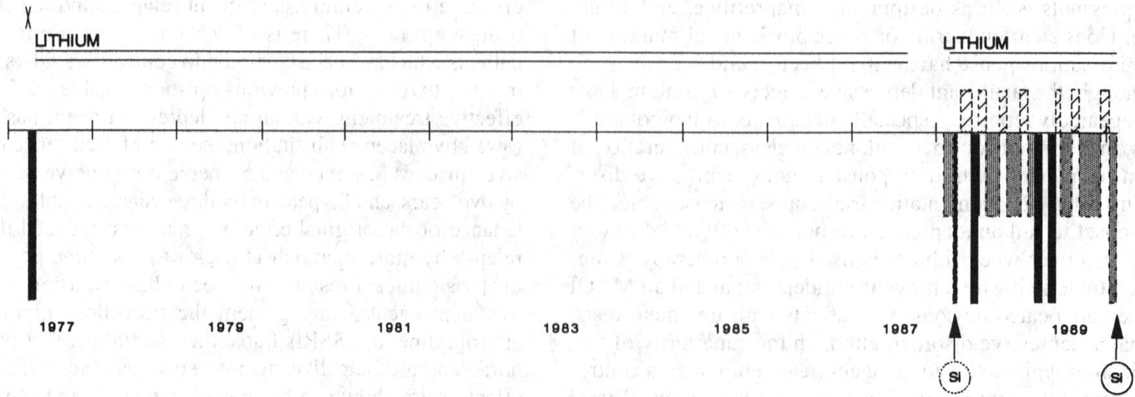

FIGURE 16.7-6 *Loss of drug responsiveness following lithium discontinuation—a fatal outcome.*

or addiction to those medical regimens. Analogies to long-term prophylaxis for other medical diseases may help dissipate negative stereotypes regarding the long-term medical management of psychiatric disorders. For example, most patients do not consider it useful to attempt a clinical trial of digitalis discontinuation in order to give their hearts a renewed experience of congestive failure and the associated potential for the occurrence of severe, even irreversible changes in the size and function of the heart muscle. In parallel fashion, it may be equally unreasonable for a patient to practice having depressive episodes, because of the chance that the neurochemical changes underlying the episodes may similarly be progressively facilitated.

If the patient chooses to discontinue prophylaxis, it is recommended that the drug treatment be very slowly tapered. Slow tapering avoids withdrawal insomnia and may serve other functions as well. If minor episodic symptoms begin to reemerge, treatment can be reinstituted early, before a full-blown episode has occurred and gained a momentum of its own. Thus, a specific contract should be made with the patient to contact a physician should symptoms reemerge. Reminding the patient of the long time frame to clinical response in prior episodes and his or her associated despair and incapacitation may also help the patient arrive at the decision for prophylaxis. In analogy to a fully loaded tanker, it is much easier to deal with a depression before it gains a full head of steam than to try stopping it once it has gained full speed and a momentum of its own.

Regular psychiatric visits during the prophylactic phase are recommended at intervals ranging from one to four months, depending on a variety of ancillary circumstances, including completeness of response, lack of psychosocial crises, excellent history of compliance, lack of ambivalence about the process, absence of side effects, and the financial constraints and wishes of the patient. In addition to periodic assessment of all of those issues, regular treatment visits are recommended to assess separately the potential risks of suicide, independent of the occurrence of discrete episodes. Periodic assessment of suicidal risk is particularly important if there is a family history of suicide or if other risk factors are present, among them male sex, older age, comorbid alcohol abuse, and prior suicide attempts (particularly if they were severe). One study of maprotiline, for example, indicated that although patients showed a substantial and highly significant ($P < 0.0001$) decreased likelihood of recurrence of depressive episodes during treatment with that agent compared to placebo, there was a small but statistically significant increased likelihood of suicide attempts in the patient group that remained on active treatment. Thus, suicidal impulses and acts may not always vary directly with either severity of depression or reemergence of a full-blown episode that requires hospitalization, and the assessment of such risks should be part of the ongoing clinical assessment of each patient in all phases of the illness and treatment. A specific contract for communicating with the clinician on reemergence of suicidal thoughts should be considered for patients with some of the risk factors described above.

TREATMENT OF BIPOLAR DISORDER

ACUTE MANIA

Lithium carbonate Lithium remains the paradigmatic treatment for acute mania. In comparative studies with antipsychotics, it demonstrates better overall improvement in all aspects of manic symptomatology, including psychomotor activity, grandiosity, manic thought disorder, insomnia, and irritability.

The typical clinical profile of the manic patient most responsive to lithium carbonate consists of (1) a classic presentation and euphoric mania rather than severe or dysphoric mania, (2) a pattern of mania followed by depression and then a well interval (MDI) rather than DMI (depression-mania-well interval) or continuous cycling, (3) a history of few prior episodes and no rapid cycling illness (defined as four episodes a year), and (4) a positive family history of primary mood disorder in first-degree relatives. Lithium doses should be administered to achieve blood levels between 0.8 and 1.2 mEq/L. Although a high-dose strategy (to 1.5 mEq/L) is advocated by some investigators, the author has not seen many patients who, after failing to respond at more typical blood levels of lithium, responded well when the dosage was pushed to higher, potentially toxic levels. Dose-limiting side effects may include GI disturbances, particularly diarrhea, and neuropsychiatric syndromes, including tremor, confusion, and myoclonic twitches. For the inadequate responder the author recommends potentiation with other agents rather than increasing lithium to toxic levels. Blood levels of lithium achieved at a given dose may also increase further if the patient switches from mania to depression, thus leading to greater side effects.

Lithium's antimanic action may take several weeks to manifest, even with aggressive dosing, and so, for acutely deteriorating, aggressive, or psychotic manic patients, lithium may need to be supplemented in the early phases of treatment. In a recent collaborative study that used the liberal criterion of 50 percent improvement in manic severity, only 50 percent of patients treated with lithium (or valproate) had improved at the end of the three-week monotherapy trial in an intent-to-treat analysis. That figure speaks to the frequent need for combination strategies, particularly as short stays and rapid discharges from inpatient units are increasingly mandated by managed care. Augmentation has traditionally been accomplished with antipsychotics, including the phenothiazines and butyrophenones, such as haloperidol (Haldol). Because of growing evidence of the acute antimanic efficacy of carbamazepine and valproate, it is suggested that those agents or the high-potency benzodiazepines be used for initial supplementation (rather than an antipsychotic), for reasons discussed below.

Double-blind controlled evaluations reported from different laboratories have indicated that the onset of antimanic efficacy is often as rapid with carbamazepine as it is with traditional antipsychotics, including chlorpromazine (Thorazine), thioridazine (Mellaril), pimozide (Orap), and haloperidol. As of 1994, 19 double-blind studies of carbamazepine in acute mania had indicated clinical efficacy. Fewer controlled studies have been performed with valproate, but those available, including a recent large collaborative study, also indicate acute antimanic efficacy. Because initial acute antimanic response may be a guide to subsequent prophylaxis (the major focus of therapeutics in bipolar disorders), the author encourages the investigation of an individual patient's response to those alternative anticonvulsant agents. Antipsychotics can be employed later in the sequence if there is a lack of clinical response to the mood stabilizers.

Antipsychotics Long-term maintenance treatment with traditional antipsychotics should be avoided, if possible, in patients with bipolar disorder, as they are reported to have an increased risk for tardive dyskinesia. The strategy of rapid tranquilization with suprathreshold doses of antipsychotics should clearly be avoided. Many double-blind evaluations of that high-dose strategy in acutely psychotic and manic patients have shown it to be no more efficacious than traditional dose regimens, and it may be associated with toxic effects. Particularly for extremely manic patients, the use of heroic doses to decrease psychomotor activation may not be justifiable because of the added risk of ordinary toxic effects, the risk for neuroleptic malignant syndrome, and the risk for sporadic syndromes of reversible and irreversible organic impairment when used in conjunction with lithium.

Carbamazepine Several preliminary studies have suggested that some of the variables associated with a poor response to lithium may be associated with a good antimanic response to carbamazepine. Thus, the drug should be considered for lithium-nonresponsive manic patients.

Typical doses of carbamazepine to treat mania have ranged between 600 and 1,600 mg a day and are associated with blood levels ranging from 6 to 12 μg/mL. However, within that dose and blood level range, there does not appear to be a clear relation to the degree of clinical response across patients. For an individual patient, however, clinical response and side effects are typically dose-related. Thus, it is important to individualize dose administration, as there is wide variability in the dose and blood level at which side effects occur. Increasing the dose to achieve a clinical effect while titrating the increases against the emergence of side effects is an appropriate strategy for a drug with such wide dose-response variability.

Valproate Typical dose levels are 750 to 2,000 mg a day, to achieve blood levels between 50 and 120 μg/mL. Oral loading with 20 mg per kg a day from the outset is likely to be well tolerated and rapidly effective. In several case series patients with more typical manic syndromes and fewer schizoaffective symptoms appeared to show a high frequency of response. Dysphoric manic patients and rapid cyclers may also be responsive. Carbamazepine and valproate have been used in combination to treat epilepsy, and preliminary evidence for the efficacy of that combination in the acute and prophylactic management of the patient with refractory bipolar disorder is available. Valproate may act by enhancing GABAergic tone, although it also has actions shared by carbamazepine and lithium. Typical side effects are listed in Table 16.7-7.

TABLE 16.7-7
Comparative and Differential Clinical and Side-Effect Profile of Lithium Carbonate, Carbamazepine, and Valproate

	Lithium Carbonate	Carbamazepine	Valproate
Clinical Profile			
Mania (M)	+ +	+ +	+ +
Dysphoric	±	(+ +)	+ +
Rapid cycling	+	+ +	+ +
Family history negative	±	+	±
Depression (D)	(+)	(+)	(+)
M D prophylaxis	+ +	+ +	+ +
Epilepsy	0	+ +	+ +
Pain syndromes	0	+ +	0 (+ +)
Side Effects			
White blood cell count	↑*	↓	–
Diabetes insipidus	↑*	↓	–
Thyroid hormones (T_3, T_4)	↓	↓	↓
TSH	↑*	–	?
Serum calcium	↑	↓	?
Weight gain	↑	(–)	↑
Tremor	↑	–	↑
Memory disturbances	(↑)	(↑)	(↑)
Diarrhea, GI symptoms	(↑)	(↑)	(↑)
Teratogenic	(?)	(↑)	(↑)
Psoriasis	(↑)	–	–
Pruritic rash	–	↑	–
Alopecia	–	–	(↑)
Agranulocytosis	–	(↑)	–
Aplastic anemia	–	(↑)	–
Thrombocytopenia	–	(↑)	(↑)
Hepatitis	–	(↑)	↑
Hyponatremia, water intoxication	–	↑	–
Dizziness, ataxia, diplopia	–	↑	(+)
Hypercortisolism, escape from dexamethasone suppression	–	↑	–

Key: Clinical efficacy:
0 = None
± = Equivocal
+ = Effective
+ + = Very effective
( ) = Ambiguous or insubstantial data base
* = Effect of lithium predominates in combination with carbamazepine

Side effects:
↑ = Increase
↓ = Decrease
( ) = Inconsistent or rare
– = Absent

Clonazepam and lorazepam Benzodiazepine anticonvulsants that have been studied in acute mania include clonazepam and lorazepam (Ativan). The sedating side effects of clonazepam may be problematic in some outpatients but may be useful in the management of inpatients or for bedtime medication for severely insomnic manic patients. The two anticonvulsants work at the central-type benzodiazepine receptor; in contrast, carbamazepine is not active at that receptor and appears to act at the peripheral-type benzodiazepine receptor. Classic central-type benzodiazepine receptors are associated with GABA receptors and surround the chloride ionophore through which chloride influx mediates neuronal inhibition. In contrast, the peripheral-type benzodiazepine receptor appears to be more closely associated with calcium fluxes and neurosteroid biosynthesis. Those findings may have ramifications for a possible differential clinical response between the two classes of anticonvulsants.

Calcium channel antagonists A series of preliminary reports suggest that the calcium channel antagonist verapamil (Calan), and possibly also nifedipine (Procardia) and nimodipine (Nimotop), have acute antimanic efficacy. The clinical utility of the calcium channel antagonists appears promising but needs to be more systematically documented.

Other anticonvulsants The clinical utility of other anticonvulsants, such as the GABA agonist progabide or the traditional anticonvulsant phenytoin (Dilantin), also requires further evaluation. Acetazolamide (Diamox) has been reported to be effective in patients who were not responsive to lithium or carbamazepine, especially those with atypical psychoses associated with dreamy confusional states occurring premenstrually or in the puerperium. The efficacy of the newly approved anticonvulsants felbamate and gabapentin and those about to be approved, such as lamotrigine, remains to be studied.

Electroconvulsive therapy Older clinical observations and recent controlled clinical trials have demonstrated the efficacy of ECT in acute mania. Bilateral treatments are necessary; unilateral, nondominant treatments have been reported to be ineffective and to exacerbate manic symptoms in some studies. Because of the many effective pharmacological treatments that are available, assessing their usefulness for long-term preventive therapy, based on their acute antimanic efficacy, should be emphasized. ECT may then be reserved for the rare refractory patient or one with medical complications, extreme exhaustion, lethal catatonia, or malignant hyperthermia. Otherwise, after a course of successful ECT the clinician still faces the task of deciding on the most likely effective pharmacological approach to prophylaxis.

Antiadrenergic drugs Several other nonanticonvulsant compounds with some neurotransmitter selectivity have been reported to be effective in the treatment of mania. Clonidine, an α_2-adrenergic receptor agonist, is used to treat hypertension. It acutely inhibits the firing of the noradrenergic locus ceruleus and has been reported to have acute antimanic efficacy in some, but not all, controlled trials. However, response in the first few days of treatment may not be associated with the ultimate outcome. Another agent that inhibits noradrenergic function is the β-adrenergic receptor antagonist propranolol (Inderal). Because very high doses of propranolol in either the *d*- or *l*-isomer form have been effective, it is not known whether the β-antagonist properties or some other membrane-stabilizing effects of the drug account for its acute antimanic efficacy.

Cholinomimetics Intravenous administration of the indirect-acting cholinergic agonist physostigmine (Antilirium, Eserine) has an almost immediate antimanic effect. Physostigmine inhibits acetylcholine esterase function, making more acetylcholine available at the synapse. Although intravenous administration can produce rapid decreases in manic symptoms, physostigmine also has a short half-life and can be associated with marked increases in dysphoria and other side effects such that its long-term utility is doubtful. The success of attempts to increase cholinergic function chronically through other methods, such as lecithin, deanol, or direct acetylcholine agonists, has not been adequately delineated.

Overview of antimanic agents The ability to achieve rapid antimanic effects with intravenous physostigmine suggests that, with appropriate pharmacological intervention and pharmacokinetics, there is no theoretical reason why an acute antimanic response cannot be achieved extremely rapidly, even though most of the other antimanic treatments have a moderate delay in onset. Manipulations of a variety of neurotransmitter systems (inhibition of noradrenergic and dopaminergic systems, but potentiation of cholinergic, benzodiazepinergic, GABAergic, and, perhaps, serotonergic systems) are all capable of inducing antimanic effects. The antipsychotics block dopamine receptors; clonidine and propranolol appear to decrease α- and β-noradrenergic function, respectively; lithium, ECT, and carbamazepine each alter DA, NE, and GABA function, among others. Reserpine, which depletes catecholamines and indoleamines, has also been reported to have antipsychotic and antimanic effects. The literature on tryptophan-induced altered serotonergic function in relation to antimanic efficacy is ambiguous. Awareness of the multiple neurotransmitter approaches to the treatment of mania not only may be clinically useful in changing treatments that target different systems in nonresponsive patients, but it also suggests the current weakness of any hypothetical single neurotransmitter defect in mania.

Alterations in endogenous neuropeptide function also have been postulated in mania. Although manipulations of opiates or cholecystokinin (CCK) have not produced consistent results in psychotic schizophrenic patients, calcitonin has been reported successful in treating excited psychotic states including mania. Preliminary evidence suggests that other calcium-active treatments may also be effective in treating acute mania. The clinical efficacy of calcitonin and other peptide interventions in mania remains to be confirmed but is mentioned because peptides could represent the next generation of antimanic treatments, particularly in light of increasing evidence that peptide neurotransmitters coexist in the same neurons with the more classic neurotransmitter substances that have been indirectly linked to the manic syndromes.

MAINTENANCE TREATMENT OF BIPOLAR DISORDER

Lithium prophylaxis Lithium carbonate originally appeared to be effective in some 70 to 80 percent of bipolar patients, but current estimates suggest that even with adjunctive use of antidepressants and antipsychotics, a figure of 40 to 50 percent efficacy in many lithium clinics is more accurate.

Although early studies indicated the need for blood levels between 0.8 and 1.2 mEq/L, some case studies have suggested that lower levels, in the range of 0.5 to 0.8 mEq/L might also be effective in maintenance treatment. However, a recent controlled study found that the lower levels of side effects are achieved at the cost of a three-times-higher relapse rate when a low lithium level range (0.4 to 0.6 mg/L) is used in comparison to higher levels (0.8 to 1.0 mg/L). Monitoring of trough levels (performed in the early morning, before the morning dose is given) at one- to two-month intervals, or more frequently if the patient's course is unstable, is recommended.

Because of the overwhelming data on long-term efficacy, it is important to consider preventive treatment after a single severe episode of mania particularly if there is a family history of mood disorder. The development of a life chart, outlined above, so that the frequency, severity, and interval between episodes can be accurately assessed, may also assist in arriving at the decision for prophylaxis. If previous episodes were severe—that is, socially incapacitating and requiring hospitalization, or associated with extremely adverse events for the patient and family—the physician should consider prophylaxis earlier rather than later, despite moderately long well intervals between episodes. Those factors should be discussed with the patient during a euthymic interval so that the appropriate risk-benefit ratios can be weighed intelligently and adequate informed consent can be obtained. New data from several studies indicate that a history of more than three or four prior episodes is associated with a poor response to lithium prophylaxis; therefore, a delay in instituting prophylaxis may have consequences not only for morbidity during recurrence but also for ultimate treatment response.

Lithium-induced side effects The profile of lithium-induced side effects has proved to be generally benign even in the long-term maintenance treatment of patients over several decades. Several of lithium's effects deserve comment, however.

THYROID FUNCTION Lithium can impair thyroid function by several different mechanisms, and it has even been used to treat hyperthyroidism. Lithium lowers T_3 and T_4 levels circulating in the plasma and, in some patients, increases the production of thyroid-stimulating hormone (TSH). TSH increases above normal can be indicative of the hypothalamic-pituitary-adrenal axis working overtime to maintain normal levels of thyroid hormones. Thus, thyroid replacement with T_4 might be considered when TSH levels are substantially elevated, even when thyroid hormone indices are still within the lower limits of normal. Thyroid function should be assessed at six-month intervals, and more frequently if there is a breakthrough of depressive symptoms during otherwise adequate lithium maintenance treatment. Treatment of underlying hypothyroidism can, in those instances, help alleviate a depression that is linked to this hormonal deficit. Whereas T_4 is generally used for suppression of TSH and for replacement therapy, anecdotal evidence suggests that the addition of T_3 to T_4 replacement therapy may help some patients with refractory depression or cycling.

RENAL FUNCTION By the 1980s, the scare regarding the possible high incidence of long-term adverse consequences of lithium on the kidneys had largely dissipated. Original reports of severe nephrotoxicity and pathology induced by lithium were in part related to the absence of an age-matched control group of psychiatric patients not treated with lithium. Thus, although lithium impairs vasopressin function at the level of adenylate cyclase and often produces a syndrome of diabetes insipidus, it is less consistently associated with other evidence of renal toxicity. Preliminary data suggest that less renal toxicity may occur with single nighttime dosing, which produces higher peaks but lower nadirs than conventional dosing regimens. Single nighttime dosing may also facilitate compliance.

Current practice suggests that frequent monitoring of renal function is not indicated. It is important, however, to obtain baseline measures of renal function, including the creatinine clearance rate, before beginning lithium treatment, particularly in patients with a history of renal alterations. Because of the induction of diabetes insipidus syndrome related to the blockade of antidiuretic hormone actions, patients must have adequate fluid intake to maintain an appropriate fluid and electrolyte balance. Several cases have been reported in which high levels of lithium during intoxication were associated with irreversible cerebellar toxicity. Thus, lithium levels, fluid and electrolyte status, or both should be monitored closely during periods of febrile illness, decreased fluid intake, or greater than ordinary fluid loss (such as during extreme athletic stress or GI illnesses accompanied by vomiting or diarrhea). Amiloride (Midamor, 5 to 10 mg) has been useful in the treatment of lithium-induced diabetes insipidus. If diuretics (furosemide [Lasix] or thiazide [Diuril]) are used, lower doses of lithium may be indicated.

TREMOR Tremor can be problematic for a small but substantial percentage of patients treated with lithium. Tremor is frequently exacerbated by social stress. When the tremor persists at doses at the lower end of the therapeutic range or at the minimum doses necessary for therapeutic efficacy, attempts can be made to treat it symptomatically. Some investigators find that 10 to 40 mg of the β-blocker propranolol in divided daily doses may reduce lithium tremor. Relief may occur within 30 minutes and may last from four to six hours.

GASTROINTESTINAL EFFECTS GI side effects (diarrhea and indigestion) can be problematic for many patients but may be attenuated by reducing the dose or giving it at meal times (for indigestion). Antidiarrheal agents should be restricted to acute treatment.

MENTAL EFFECTS Patients may express concern about the effects of lithium on their memory, spontaneity, and creativity. Although impairment can be objectively delineated on some, but not all, types of detailed neuropsychological testing, most patients either do not experience that effect or do not find it unduly impairing. In fact, productivity and creativity may, overall, be enhanced during lithium treatment because it prevents unproductive manic and depressive episodes. Though no adequate approach to measuring the subjective cognitive effects of lithium has been reported, it is important to rule out associated causes for cognitive impairment, including possible hypothyroidism or an inadequately treated coexisting depression, and to consider a careful dose reduction. Many so-called drug-related side effects occur during placebo treatment and thus appear to be more closely associated with illness-related variables than with a particular psychopharmacological treatment. That perspective on lithium maintenance treatment needs to be explored with the patient to avoid premature discontinuation of treatment or noncompliance.

WEIGHT GAIN Lithium-induced weight gain is a problem in a small percentage of patients. If there is a reactive hypoglycemic component, carbohydrate restriction may help avoid the problem. Thyroid indices should be rechecked and the patient reminded not to use calorie-containing beverages to maintain the necessary increased fluid intake associated with diabetes insipidus. The role of bupropion for weight loss in the context of antidepressant augmentation remains to be studied systematically.

Dose reduction Dose reduction may be a first maneuver in treating a variety of lithium-induced problems (for example, tremor, weight gain, thirst, urinary frequency, diarrhea, and psychomotor slowing). If lower doses are not adequate for prophylaxis, combination or alternative treatment, especially with carbamazepine (which has a different side-effect profile) or valproate, may be indicated. Other lithium-related effects during combination treatment with carbamazepine are discussed below. Because the renal clearance of lithium appears to decrease with age, a lower dose may be adequate and necessary in the older patient on lithium maintenance therapy. The calcium channel blockers may be effective in lithium responsive patients, yet avoid most lithium-related side effects.

Treatment of depressive breakthrough episodes during lithium prophylaxis The treatment of a depressive episode in an untreated patient with bipolar disorder or of an episode emerging during lithium prophylaxis is very different from the treatment for major depressive disorder. Although SSRIs, cyclic antidepressants, and MAOIs are the mainstays of treatment of major depressive disorder, they should be used cautiously in patients with bipolar disorder. Some studies have reported an increased incidence of switches into hypomania or mania during tricyclic or MAOI therapy, above that expected for the patient's natural course of illness (Figures 16.7-3 and 16.7-7). Although it is unknown whether the increased incidence of switching is sufficient cause to reduce the use of unimodal antidepressants in patients with bipolar disorder, it is clear that treatment with those compounds can speed up the rate of cycling in rapid-cycling patients. Thus, a depressive episode may be shortened at the cost of more rapid onset of the subsequent manic episode. Withdrawal of antidepressants has also attenuated cycle frequency in some patients.

Some uncontrolled observations implicate tricyclics and related compounds in the development of continuous cycling phases (that is, successive episodes without a well-interval) (Figures 16.7-3, 16.7-7, and 16.7-8). Continuous cycling is difficult to treat and tends to be refractory to lithium. There is anecdotal evidence (requiring further investigation) that bupropion may not be associated with the same tendency toward cycle induction as are other antidepressant modalities (Figure 16.7-3). The SSRIs (or venlafaxine) may have the same effect on the switch phenomenon and on cycle induction as the tricyclics, but that conjecture requires further investigation.

Once a switch has been observed while the patient was taking

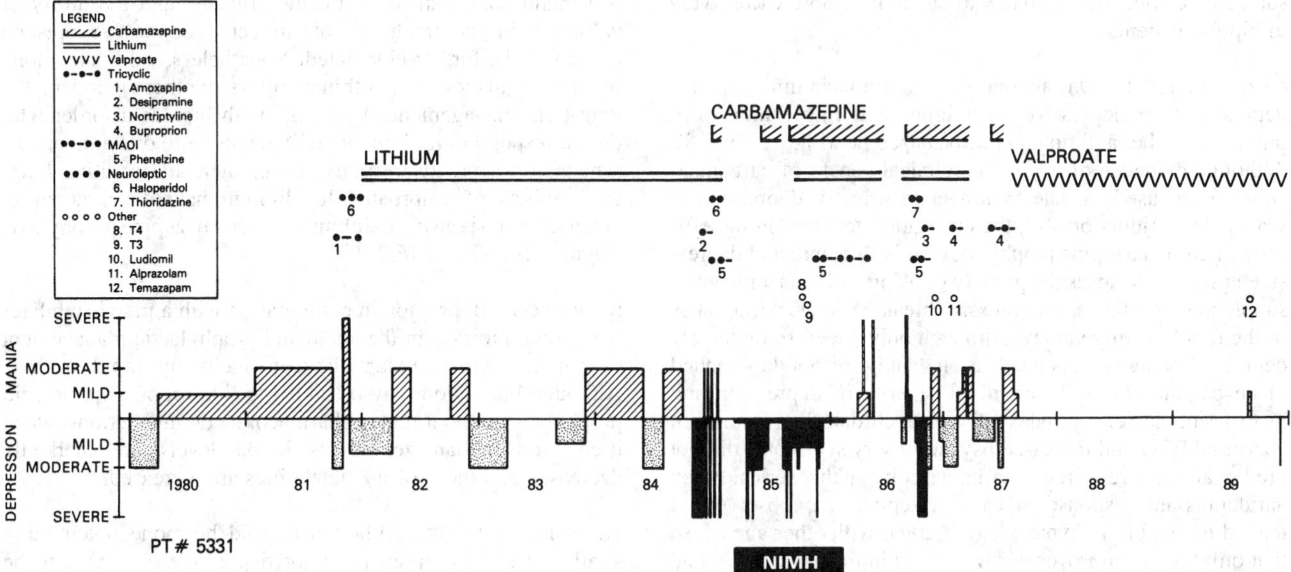

FIGURE 16.7-7 *Prophylactic response to valproate in a nonresponder to lithium and carbamazepine.*

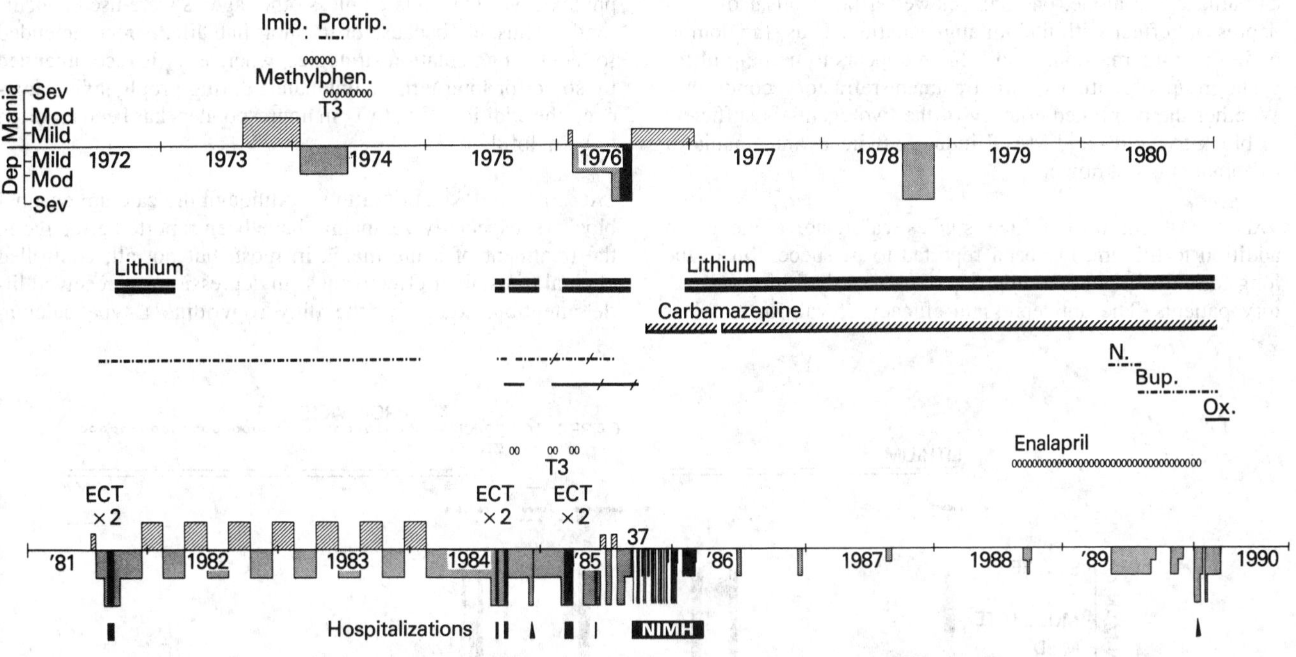

FIGURE 16.7-8 *Loss of prophylactic efficacy in a woman with rapid-cycling bipolar II disorder.*

an MAOI, reexposure, even to a different MAOI, has been reported to lead to earlier onset of a switch, perhaps reflecting the occurrence of sensitization. It is unclear whether a drug-induced switch occurs only in those predestined to have spontaneous switches or whether it predisposes to the development of further spontaneous manic episodes.

Therefore, the unimodal antidepressants should be used with caution in treating the depressive episodes of bipolar disorder, particularly if there is a history of drug-induced switches. In addition, other options should be considered, such as adding another mood stabilizer (for example, lithium, carbamazepine, or valproate). Women appear to be particularly predisposed to heterocyclic- and antidepressant-induced cycling. If unimodal antidepressants are used for a bipolar depressive episode, they should be tapered and discontinued as soon as possible to avoid the potential for drug-induced switches and cycle acceleration. Lithium and other mood stabilizers may not be able to prevent those phenomena entirely. Several case reports suggest that alprazolam may induce switches into hypomania and mania even in nonpredisposed patients.

The MAOIs in general may be less likely to induce switches than the tricyclics (Figure 16.7-7). They should be given relatively greater consideration, especially for anergic, hypersomnic, hyperphagic patients with bipolar disorders. A substantially higher rate of antidepressant response has been reported in one controlled series for tranylcypromine (81 percent) compared with imipramine (48 percent) in patients with bipolar disorder. Clorgyline, a selective MAO type A inhibitor that is not yet clinically available, has been reported to slow the cycling frequency. The efficacy of other type A-selective drugs, such as meclobemide, remains to be studied more extensively in bipolar patients.

CARBAMAZEPINE One alternative to traditional unimodal antidepressants for depressive breakthroughs during lithium prophylaxis is the addition of carbamazepine (Figure 16.7-8). Although evidence of the overall clinical benefit of carbamazepine when used as sole treatment in primary depression is scanty, in conjunction with the emerging literature on the efficacy of carbamazepine prophylaxis for both manic and depressive episodes, it raises the priority of using carbamazepine as a supplement to lithium in depressive breakthroughs, particularly of the rapid-cycling variety. Although only one third of acutely depressed patients responded in one study, responders tended to be patients with greater initial severity of depression and histories of discrete episodes rather than chronic depression. An abnormal EEG and increased psychosensory symptoms did not predict an acute response to carbamazepine in that series. When antidepressant response to carbamazepine was observed, it tended to exhibit the typical lag observed with other agents, so that only minor improvement was noted in the first and second weeks of treatment, whereas considerable improvement was observed after the third and fourth weeks.

In a small series of patients who responded inadequately to carbamazepine alone, one half showed a rapid onset of antidepressant effect with lithium augmentation. Thus, the combination of carbamazepine and lithium appears to be helpful for a subgroup of patients with treatment-refractory conditions. Whether the combined efficacy of the two agents is sufficient to block tricyclic- and MAOI-induced switches into mania or hypomania is unknown.

VALPROATE In uncontrolled studies valproate, alone or in addition to lithium, has been reported to be successful in the long-term treatment of a subgroup of previously lithium-refractory patients. The antidepressant efficacy of valproate is less well delineated than its antimanic efficacy, and the utility of valproate in the treatment of an acute depressive episode remains to be further elucidated. Nonetheless, valproate, alone or in combination with lithium, offers another option in the long-term management of patients with bipolar disorder who do not respond to lithium alone. A response to one anticonvulsant may not predict response to another, and positive long-term effects of valproate plus lithium have been noted in patients not responsive to lithium or carbamazepine prophylaxis (Figures 16.7-7 and 16.7-9).

BUPROPION Bupropion in combination with a mood stabilizer has shown promise in the acute and prophylactic management of patients with bipolar disorder, including rapid cyclers. Although bupropion may be added to lithium or valproic acid prophylaxis without major pharmacokinetic interactions, when used with carbamazepine its blood levels are markedly decreased and those of its metabolites are increased.

THYROID HORMONE Although thyroid hormone potentiation similar to that observed in major depressive disorder can be attempted, treatment with greater than suppressive doses should be approached with caution. Medical toxic effects have been reported with high-dose thyroid treatment, and long-term prophylaxis was inadequate unless other agents were used concurrently. Thus, T_3, because of its short half-life, is recommended for acute augmentation strategies, whereas T_4 is recommended by some for long-term maintenance during prophylaxis. However, the addition of T_3 to T_4 in nonresponders has been reported to be helpful.

CALCIUM CHANNEL BLOCKERS Although the calcium channel blockers, especially verapamil, have been reported effective in the treatment of acute mania in most, but not all, controlled clinical trials, their effectiveness in depression has received little attention. Recently, the dihydropyridine L-type calcium

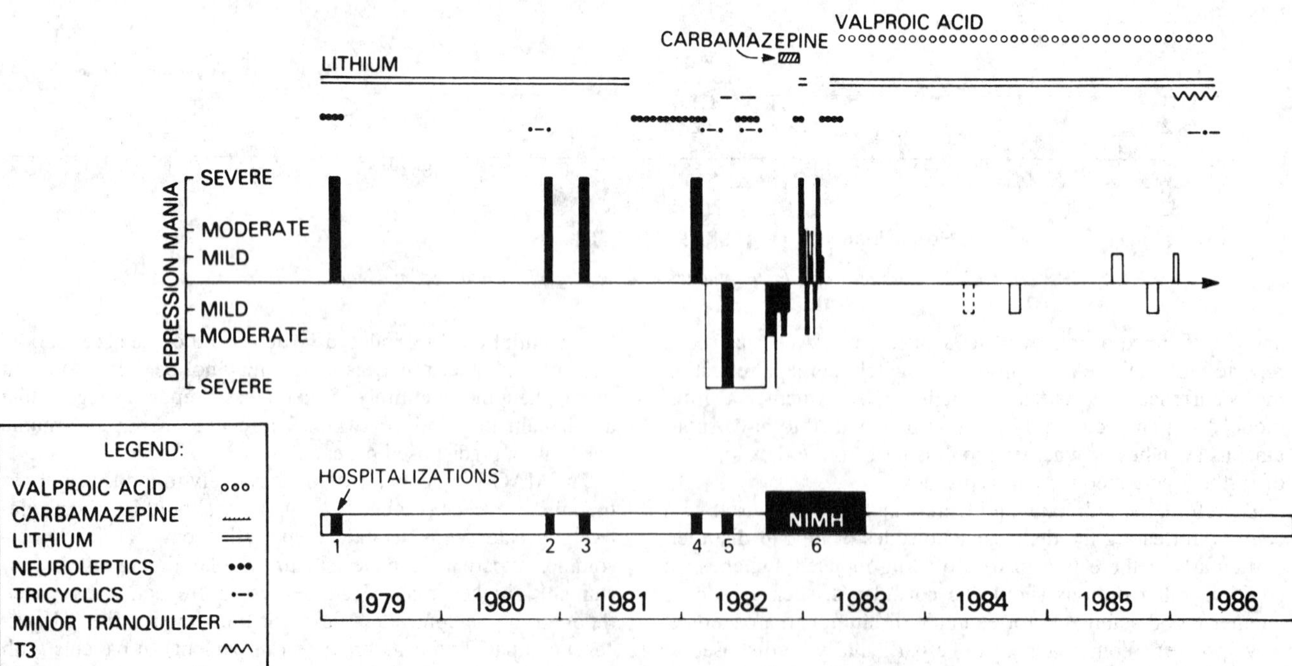

FIGURE 16.7-9 *Prophylactic response to valproate in a carbamazepine nonresponder.*

channel blocker nimodipine was studied in placebo-controlled designs and appeared to be effective in approximately one third of patients with treatment-refractory bipolar disorder.

Among those showing responses, confirmed with the use of blind off-on-off-on (placebo-drug-placebo-drug) designs, were those with bipolar refractory depression, rapid and ultradian cycling, and recurrent, brief episodes of major depressive disorder. All of the patients with bipolar disorder who responded to nimodipine failed to respond to verapamil, but did respond to the dihydropyridine isradipine. Studies on the use of nimodipine in combination with lithium or carbamazepine for inadequate responders to those agents alone are promising.

SPIRONOLACTONE Spironolactone (Aldactone) was reported to be effective in six lithium-intolerant patients. It has received no further systematic study.

FOLIC ACID A single investigation reported that folic acid supplementation in the dose range of 300 to 400 μg a day significantly reduced affective morbidity, compared with results in a placebo group maintained on lithium. The promising result and the benign nature of folic acid treatment suggest that it be considered while awaiting further clinical investigation.

ELECTROCONVULSIVE THERAPY ECT may be useful for bipolar depressed patients who do not respond to lithium and adjunctive agents. Whether ECT would help abbreviate recurrent depressive episodes in rapid-cycling patients and whether it would be useful in long-term prophylaxis are questions that await further investigation.

Treatment of manic breakthroughs during lithium prophylaxis A wide range of drugs is available for breakthrough manic episodes occurring during lithium treatment. They include the entire spectrum of drugs indicated for the treatment of acute mania, and particularly carbamazepine and valproate because of their longer-term prophylactic efficacy. Clonazepam or lorazepam may also be useful acute alternatives to antipsychotic supplementation even though the benzodiazepines (and antipsychotics) appear to have a lesser role in the long-term management of bipolar disorders than does carbamazepine or valproate.

Other approaches to the manic breakthrough include the judicious use of antipsychotics at minimal doses and for the shortest period of time. The use of clozapine for refractory bipolar and schizoaffective patients (that is, those unresponsive to lithium, carbamazepine, and valproate) appears promising in light of preliminary reports of its efficacy and its lack of induction of tardive dyskinesia.

Lithium augmentation with carbamazepine or valproate Supplementing the clinical effects of lithium with anticonvulsants such as carbamazepine and valproate is often more effective than using the anticonvulsant alone. Because lithium treatment is continued, evaluation of the anticonvulsant's efficacy is not confounded by a lithium withdrawal-induced episode, and time may be saved in the assessment of one clinical trial of the combination rather than two sequential trials (the anticonvulsant alone and then the combination). For patients who are unable to tolerate lithium carbonate, carbamazepine or valproate alone may be useful in preventing both manic and depressive episodes when given as long-term maintenance treatment. The literature on open clinical trials with carbamazepine is substantial, and several double-blind studies support the preliminary evidence of its long-term efficacy. Most of the data on valproate are based on clinical case series. The choice of carbamazepine or valproate may depend on the development of better clinical predictors or on the current assessment of their relative side-effect profiles.

Side Effects During Combination Therapy

HEMATOLOGICAL EFFECTS The side-effect profile of carbamazepine tends to be quite different from that of lithium or valproate (Table 16.7-7). As a rule of thumb, whenever lithium and carbamazepine act on a common target system, the effects of lithium tend to override those of carbamazepine. In almost every instance that is a clinical disadvantage except in terms of white blood cell (WBC) count suppression: The ability of lithium to increase the WBC count and override the count-suppressing effects of carbamazepine may be useful. Lithium is effective only against carbamazepine's benign suppression of the WBC count, and its effects are doubtful if there is evidence of more problematic interference by carbamazepine in hematological function in other cell lines, such as platelets or red cells, indicative of a pancytopenic or aplastic process. If levels of those other blood elements are normal, potentiation with lithium to reverse the benign WBC count suppression of carbamazepine may be attempted. Valproate has been associated with thrombocytopenia; the potential impact of lithium on that syndrome has not been reported.

VASOPRESSIN FUNCTION AND ELECTROLYTES Because carbamazepine appears to act as a vasopressin agonist, either directly or by potentiating vasopressin effects at the receptor, it is not sufficient to reverse lithium-induced diabetes insipidus, which occurs by an action of lithium below the receptor level at the adenylate cyclase second-messenger system. Lithium may counter the hyponatremic effects of carbamazepine, however. To the extent that the minor cognitive impairments of lithium are, in part, related to its ability to impair vasopressin function in the brain, those data suggest not only that carbamazepine would be less likely to cause that side effect but that during combination treatment the side effects of lithium would override those of carbamazepine. Carbamazepine tends to induce a benign hypocalcemia that is generally not associated with bone demineralization. In contrast, lithium often produces a transient increase in serum calcium levels.

THYROID FUNCTION Not only does carbamazepine tend to decrease T_4, free T_4, and T_3 levels, as does lithium, but, when the two drugs are given in combination, the decreases are potentiated. However, during carbamazepine treatment there is a negligible incidence of clinical hypothyroidism or above-normal increases in TSH. Consequently, thyroid supplementation of carbamazepine is rarely needed, but when the two drugs are used in combination, lithium's effect on TSH will override that of carbamazepine and the patient may require thyroid supplementation.

ALLERGIC RASH Carbamazepine induces an allergic rash in 5 to 15 percent of patients treated. In most instances the drug should be discontinued. However, if carbamazepine has shown efficacy and other available agents have not, prednisone (40 mg a day) has been reported to be effective in suppressing uncomplicated carbamazepine-induced rashes.

HEPATITIS There are extremely rare cases of carbamazepine-induced hepatitis. Routine monitoring for that side effect does not appear to be indicated.

Valproate has been associated with reports of severe hepatitis in the neurological literature; most of the fatalities have been in children, particularly those under the age of 2 years and on polytherapy. Few serious hepatic side effects have been reported in the adult psychiatric patients so far studied with valproate, but liver function should be monitored periodically when that agent is used, and the patient should be warned to report symptoms that might be referable to hepatitis, such as fever, right upper quadrant pain, malaise, nausea, anorexia, and jaundice. Benign elevation of values on liver function tests (to two or three times normal) can be followed without drug discontinuation, however. Selenium vitamin supplements may be helpful in avoiding valproate-induced hepatitis-pancreatitis.

NEUROTOXICITY There have been occasional reports of neurotoxicity when lithium and carbamazepine were used together. Because both agents can cause neurotoxic effects at or below clinically accepted dose ranges, they may occasionally occur from the combination treatment as well. In most studies the combination appears to be well tolerated, without producing side effects greater than those seen with either agent alone. Many of the side effects reported in the literature appear to have been caused by starting with relatively large doses of carbamazepine (rather than increasing the dosage slowly) in combination with other agents and assuming that the side effects were related to the combination treatment rather than to carbamazepine alone. Lithium and valproate are generally well tolerated in combination, but effects on tremor or GI distress may be additive.

PHARMACOKINETIC INTERACTIONS There do not appear to be major pharmacokinetic interactions between carbamazepine and lithium. However, that is not the case with carbamazepine and haloperidol, as haloperidol blood levels are markedly reduced by carbamazepine. Nevertheless, most studies report improvement with carbamazepine supplementation, which suggests that carbamazepine might potentiate antipsychotic effects because of its action on systems not involving dopamine receptor blockade.

Agents commonly employed in medical practice can markedly increase carbamazepine levels and produce attendant toxicity. The most frequent dose-related toxic manifestations are dizziness, drowsiness, ataxia, diplopia, and confusion. Those effects may occur in a patient who may tolerate carbamazepine well until another agent is added. Erythromycin, troleandomycin, isoniazid (but apparently not other MAOIs), and the calcium channel blockers verapamil and diltiazem (Cardizem) (but not nifedipine or nimodipine) increase blood levels of carbamazepine. Less marked increases occur during cotreatment with propoxyphene (Darvon), fluoxetine and fluvoxamine, and, transiently, cimetidine (Tagamet). Carbamazepine lowers the blood levels of various agents (especially oral contraceptives, so that higher-dose formulations or other contraceptive strategies are indicated) and interfere with some tests that are dependent on protein binding.

In contrast to the multiple pharmacokinetic interactions between carbamazepine and other drugs—in large part owing to carbamazepine's metabolism by and its ability to be an inducer of hepatic P-450 enzymes—valproate is largely without those effects. If carbamazepine and valproate are used together, the clinician should consider reducing the dose of carbamazepine (because valproate displaces carbamazepine from protein-binding sites, increases levels of free drug, and increases levels of the -10,11-epoxide metabolite) and increasing the dose of valproate (because carbamazepine lowers levels of valproate).

TERATOGENIC EFFECTS Cardiac and great vessel (Ebstein's) anomalies have been reported to occur with a higher frequency than expected in patients treated with lithium during pregnancy. However, recent retrospective and prospective studies have indicated that the risk may be only minimally greater than in control patients not exposed to lithium and in the normal population. In light of those data and the substantial risk of episode recurrence and its possible effects on the subsequent course of illness should lithium be stopped, routine discontinuation of lithium in all patients wishing to become pregnant should be reevaluated.

Lithium may be safer than valproate or carbamazepine for the patient with prior frequent, severe, psychotic, or suicidal episodes that might render discontinuation inadvisable. If lithium is to be discontinued for a planned pregnancy, discontinuation should be done so slowly, since a taper is less likely than rapid discontinuation to be associated with episode re-occurrence. Recently, an increased risk of inducing minor congenital malformations and developmental delay has been reported for carbamazepine. A substantial and increased risk of spina bifida has been reported for valproate. The risk is only slightly lower with carbamazepine, and use of those mood-stabilizing agents should be avoided in pregnancy if possible.

Using the lowest effective doses and supplementing with folic acid should be considered in patients who need those agents during pregnancy. Consultation with a specialist for fetal monitoring and assessment of possible defects with ultrasound and other techniques is also recommended. Persisting biochemical alterations have been found in some animal studies of fetal exposure to antipsychotics, but have not been assessed systematically in follow-up studies in humans. ECT may have the lowest risk to the fetus among the somatic treatments, but risks to the fetus from maternal seizures have not been adequately elucidated.

SENSITIZATION EFFECTS ON THE MOOD DISORDERS

Early clinical observations and more recent systematic controlled studies suggest that recurrent major depressive disorder and bipolar disorders may undergo a transition from initial episodes that are often precipitated by psychosocial stressors to later episodes that tend to occur more spontaneously. The transition often occurs in the context of an overall pattern of cycle acceleration with decreasing well intervals between successive episodes. It has been postulated that psychosocial stressors and recurrent episodes of mood disorder themselves not only may cause acute biological perturbations but also may leave behind residual biological memory traces, based on their ability to alter gene expression. It is thought that, following stress- and episode-induced changes in neurotransmission, a cascade of neurobiological effects takes place that includes not only short-term adaptations but also longer-lasting alterations initiated by a variety of transcription factors, including immediate early genes such as c-fos and c-jun. Those transcription factors are then capable of inducing changes in the long-term regulation of transmitters, receptors, nerve growth factors, neuropeptides, and possibly even in the microstructural synaptic organization of the brain, as demonstrated in many models of learning and memory.

If that conceptualization proves to be correct, it suggests the potential twofold importance of preventing episodes of mood disorder. Not only would the associated morbidity and potential mortality be prevented, but the longer-lasting neurobiological vulnerabilities associated with the experience of repeated episodes of mood disorder (sensitization) might be attenuated as well. In light of increasing evidence that greater numbers of episodes of mood disorder are a poor prognostic sign and may be associated with relative resistance to effective treatment with lithium, the clinical and theoretical data speak to the importance of early institution and long-term maintenance of prophylaxis, particularly in patients already identified as being at high risk for episode recurrence. A specific focus on education and other practical ways of avoiding noncompliance is similarly important.

Treatment efficacy may vary as a function of the stage or severity of evolution of illness. For example, pharmacotherapies such as lithium may be more effective in initial and midphases of the illness, but with the emergence of rapid and ultrarapid cycling, alternative and adjunctive treatments with the anticonvulsants may be required. Similar treatment alterations may be necessary in patients with major depressive disorder, for whom psychotherapy may be effective in the early, milder forms of the illness, but, with major recurrent episodes (and particularly melancholic and psychotic syndromes), aggressive acute and maintenance pharmacotherapy may be mandatory. Adjunctive interpersonal, cognitive, and behavioral psychotherapeutic techniques may also play important roles in the late and severe stages of illness as problem-solving, remoralization, and suicide prevention techniques and in facilitating compliance with prescribed pharmacological regimens.

If two or more episodes of major depressive disorder have occurred, the clinician should strongly consider recommending long-term pharmacoprophylaxis, whether or not the patient is in ongoing psychotherapy, as recent data unequivocally support the long-term efficacy of a variety of antidepressant agents. In contrast, psychotherapy appears to be of only minor utility in delaying the onset of the next episode.

The mood disorders involve multiple areas of brain dysfunction and affect a variety of organ systems, producing alterations not only in mood but also in motor, cognitive, sleep, appetite, reward, and other somatic systems. Neurobiological alterations are evident at the level of endocrine dysfunction, as reflected not only in alterations in the regulation of glucocorticoids, corticotropin-releasing hormone, TRH, and somatostatin, but also in the size of the pituitary and the adrenals. Brain imaging has revealed alterations in blood flow and glucose utilization reflecting hypofrontality in primary and secondary depression in many studies in direct proportion to the severity of the depressive syndrome. Thus, patient and clinician should be reminded of the wealth of evidence indicating that the mood disorders are grave, potentially life-threatening, medical illnesses not different from those that afflict other major organ systems of the body and as such should be treated with equal respect.

SUGGESTED CROSS-REFERENCES

Biological therapies are discussed in Chapter 32. Obsessive-compulsive disorder is covered in Section 17.3. The range of psychotherapeutic modalities and techniques useful in treating depressed patients is discussed in Section 16.8. The rest of Chapter 16 can be consulted for other aspects of mood disorders.

REFERENCES

Aronson T A, Shukla S, Hirschowitz J: Clonazepam treatment of five lithium-refractory patients with bipolar disorder. Am J Psychiatry *146:* 77, 1989.

Baldessarini R J: Antidepressant agents. In *Chemotherapy in Psychiatry: Principles and Practices,* R J Baldessarini, editor, Harvard University Press, Cambridge, MA, 1985.

Basco M R, Rush A J: *Cognitive Behavioral Treatment of Manic Depressive Disorder.* Guilford, New York, 1994.

Blumenthal S J: Suicide: A guide to risk factors, assessment, and treatment of suicidal patients. Med Clin North Am *72:* 937, 1988.

Bowden C L, Brugger A M, Swann A C, Calabrese J R, Janicak P G, Petty F, Dilsaver S C, Davis J M, Rush A J, Small J G, Garza-Trevino E S, Risch S C, Goodnick P J, Morris D D: Efficacy of divalproex vs lithium and placebo in the treatment of mania. JAMA *271:* 918, 1994.

Calabrese J R, Markovitz P J, Kimmel S E, Wagner S C: Spectrum of efficacy of valproate in 78 rapid-cycling bipolar patients. J Clin Psychopharmacol *12:* 53S, 1992.

Cohen L S, Friedman J M, Jefferson J W, Johnson E M, Weiner M L: A reevaluation of risk of in utero exposure to lithium. JAMA *271:* 146, 1994.

Cooke R G, Joffe R T, Levitt A J: T_3 augmentation of antidepressant treatment in T_4-replaced thyroid patients. J Clin Psychiatry *53:* 16, 1992.

Davis J M, Wang Z, Janicak P G: A quantitative analysis of clinical drug trials for the treatment of affective disorders. Psychopharmacol Bull *29:* 175, 1993.

Dubovsky S L: Calcium antagonists in manic-depressive illness. Neuropsychobiol *27:* 184, 1993.

Faedda G L, Tondo L, Baldessarini R J, Suppes T, Tohen M: Outcome after rapid vs gradual discontinuation of lithium treatment in bipolar disorders. Arch Gen Psychiatry *50:* 448, 1993.

Fawcett J, Kravitz H M, Zajecka J M, Schaff M R: CNS stimulant potentiation of monoamine oxidase inhibitors in treatment-refractory depression. J Clin Psychopharmacol *11:* 127, 1993.

*Frank E, Kupfer D J, Perel J M, Cornes C, Jarrett D B, Mallinger A G, Thase M E, McEachran A B, Grochocinski V J: Three-year outcomes for maintenance therapies in recurrent depression. Arch Gen Psychiatry *47:* 1093, 1990.

Gelenberg A J, Kane J M, Keller M B, Lavori P, Rosenbaum J F, Cole K, Lavelle J: Comparison of standard and low serum levels of lithium for maintenance treatment of bipolar disorder. N Engl J Med *321:* 1489, 1989.

*Goodwin F K, Jamison K R: *Manic-Depressive Illness.* Oxford University Press, New York, 1990.

Gupta S, Ghaly N, Dewan M: Augmenting fluoxetine with dextroamphetamine to treat refractory depression. Hosp Community Psychiatry *43:* 281, 1992.

Hoschl C: Do calcium antagonists have a place in the treatment of mood disorders? Drugs *42:* 721, 1991.

Joffe R T, Schuller D R: An open study of buspirone augmentation of serotonin reuptake inhibitors in refractory depression. J Clin Psychiatry *54:* 269, 1993.

Joffe R T, Singer W, Levitt A J, MacDonald C: A placebo-controlled comparison of lithium and triiodothyronine augmentation of tricyclic antidepressants in unipolar refractory depression. Arch Gen Psychiatry *50:* 387, 1993.

Keller M B: Diagnostic and course-of-illness variables pertinent to refractory depression. In *Review of Psychiatry,* vol 9, A Tasman, S M Goldfinger, C A Kaufmann, editors, p 10. American Psychiatric Press, Washington, 1990.

Kramlinger K G, Post R M: The addition of lithium carbonate to carbamazepine: Antidepressant efficacy in treatment-resistant depression. Arch Gen Psychiatry *46:* 794, 1989.

*Kupfer D J, Frank E, Perel J M, Cornes C, Mallinger A G, Thase M E, McEachran A B, Grochocinski V J: Five-year outcome for maintenance therapies in recurrent depression. Arch Gen Psychiatry *49:* 769, 1992.

Maj M, Pirozzi R, Kemali D: Long-term outcome of lithium prophylaxis in patients initially classified as complete responders. Psychopharmacology (Berlin) *98:* 535, 1989.

McElroy S L, Keck P E, Pope H G, Hudson J I: Valproate in the treatment of bipolar disorder: Literature review and clinical guidelines. J Clin Psychopharmacol *12:* 42S, 1992.

Montgomery S A, Dufour H, Brion S, Gailledreau J, Laqueille X, Ferrey G, Moron P, Parant-Lucena N, Singer L, Danion J M, Beuzen J N, Pierredon M A: The prophylactic efficacy of fluoxetine in unipolar depression. Br J Psychiatry *153:* 69, 1988.

Montgomery S A, Roberts A, Patel A G: Placebo-controlled efficacy of antidepressants in continuation treatment. Int Clin Psychopharmacol *9:* 49, 1994.

Murphy D L, Sunderland T, Cohen R M. Monoamine oxidase-inhibiting antidepressants: A clinical update. Psychiatr Clin North Am *7:* 549, 1984.

Nolen W A, Van de Putte J J, Dijken W A, Kamp J S, Blansjaar B A, Kramer H J, Haffmans J: Treatment strategy in depression: I. Non-tricyclic and selective reuptake inhibitors in resistant depression. A double-blind partial crossover study on the effects of oxaprotiline and fluvoxamine. Acta Psychiatr Scand *78:* 668, 1988.

O'Connell R A, Mayo J A, Flatow L, Cuthbertson B, O'Brien B E: Outcome in bipolar disorder of long-term treatment with lithium. Br J Psychiatry *159:* 123, 1991.

Okuma T: Effects of carbamazepine and lithium on affective disorders. Neuropsychobiology *27:* 138, 1993.

Okuma T, Yamashita I, Takahashi R, Itoh H, Kurihara M, Otsuki S, Watanabe S, Sarai K, Hazama H, Inanaga K: Clinical efficacy of carbamazepine in affective, schizoaffective, and schizophrenic disorders. Pharmacopsychiatry *22:* 47, 1989.

Peselow E D, Fieve R R, Difiglia C, Sanfilipo M P: Lithium prophylaxis of bipolar illness: The value of combination treatment. Br J Psychiatry *164:* 208, 1994.

*Post R M: Alternatives to lithium for bipolar affective illness. In *Review of Psychiatry,* vol 9, A Tasman, S M Goldfinger, C A Kaufmann, editors, p 170. American Psychiatric Press, Washington, 1990.

Post R M: Prophylaxis of bipolar affective disorders. Int Rev Psychiatry *2:* 277, 1990.

Post R M: Sensitization and kindling perspectives for the course of affective illness: Toward a new treatment with the anticonvulsant carbamazepine. Pharmacopsychiatry *23:* 3, 1990.

Post R M: Transduction of psychosocial stress into the neurobiology of recurrent affective disorder. Am J Psychiatry *149:* 999, 1992.

Post R M, Leverich G S, Altshuler L, Mikalauskas K: Lithium discontinuation-induced refractoriness: Preliminary observations. Am J Psychiatry *149:* 1727, 1992.

Post R M, Weiss S R B: Endogenous biochemical abnormalities in affective illness: Therapeutic vs. pathogenic. Biol Psychiatry *32:* 469, 1992.

Preskorn S H: Pharmacokinetics of antidepressants: Why and how they are relevant to treatment. J Clin Psychiatry *54:* (Suppl): 14, 1993.

Price L H, Charney D S, Heninger G R: Variability of response to lithium augmentation in refractory depression. Am J Psychiatry *143:* 1387, 1986.

Quitkin F M, McGrath P J, Stewart J W, Harrison W, Tricamo E, Wager S G, Ocepek-Welikson K, Nunes E, Rabkin J G, Klein D F: Atypical depression, panic attacks, and response to imipramine and phenelzine. Arch Gen Psychiatry *47:* 935, 1990.

Ribeiro S C, Tandon R, Grunhaus L, Greden J F: The DST as a predictor of outcome in depression: A meta-analysis. Am J Psychiatry *150:* 1618, 1993.

Rouillon F, Phillips R, Serrurier D, Ansart E, Gerard M J: Recurrence of unipolar depression and efficacy of maprotiline. Encephale *15:* 527, 1989.

Rouillon F, Serrurier D, Miller H D, Gerard M J: Prophylactic efficacy of maprotiline on unipolar depression relapse. J Clin Psychiatry *52:* 423, 1991.

Schou M: Relapse prevention in manic depressive illness: Important and unimportant factors. Can J Psychiatry *36:* 502, 1991.

Shea M T, Pilkonis P A, Beckham E, Collins J F, Elkin I, Sotsky S M, Docherty J P: Personality disorders and treatment outcome in the NIMH treatment of depression collaborative research program. Am J Psychiatry *147:* 711, 1990.

*Suppes T, Baldessarini R J, Faedda G L, Tohen M: Risk of recurrence following discontinuation of lithium treatment in bipolar disorder. Arch Gen Psychiatry *48:* 1082, 1991.

Thase M E, Frank E, Mallinger A G, Hamer T, Kupfer D J: Treatment of imipramine-resistant recurrent depression: III. Efficacy of monoamine oxidase inhibitors. J Clin Psychiatry *53:* 5, 1992.

White K, Simpson G: Combined MAOI-tricyclic antidepressant treatment: A reevaluation. J Clin Psychopharmacol *1:* 264, 1981.

16.8 MOOD DISORDERS: PSYCHOSOCIAL TREATMENTS

ROBERT M. A. HIRSCHFELD, M.D.
M. TRACIE SHEA, Ph.D.

INTRODUCTION

Although psychoanalytic approaches were the predominant mode of treatment for depression in the early to middle part of this century, now many types of psychotherapy based on a variety of concepts are in use. Psychotherapeutic approaches have been developed specifically for depression that aim to correct specific manifestations, including cognition, behavior, and affect. In general, those treatments are short-term and seek to alleviate the depressive condition, not to change the character of the patient.

PSYCHOANALYSIS AND PSYCHOANALYTIC APPROACHES

THEORETICAL CONCEPTS The interpersonal nature of depression was noted and emphasized in the earliest psychoanalytic writings on depression, as was the centrality of the regulation of self-esteem. In *Mourning and Melancholia* Sigmund Freud stated that a vulnerability to depression caused by an interpersonal disappointment early in life led to future love relationships marked by ambivalence. Actual or threatened interpersonal losses in adult life trigger a self-destructive struggle in the ego that is manifested as depression. That theory was significantly refined by later psychoanalysts who described the depression-prone personality as one needing constant reassurance, love, and admiration, and as being dependent on others for narcissistic gratification and maintenance of self-esteem. Frustration of those dependency needs leads to a plummet in self-esteem and to subsequent depression. That notion was later expanded to include any person with a fragile self-esteem system. Another dynamic approach focuses on the cognitive aspects of depression, highlighting the recognition of the disparity between one's actual and idealized situation. That realization leads to a sense of helplessness and powerlessness and ultimately to depression.

GOALS All psychoanalytic contributions to studies of depression derive from the theory that a disturbance in interpersonal relations in early childhood, usually involving a loss or disappointment, impairs subsequent interpersonal relations. The affected person is especially vulnerable to interpersonal disappointments and losses later in life, which may result in depressive illness. The goal of traditional psychoanalytic psychotherapy is to elicit changes in personality structure, not simply to alleviate symptoms. It aims to improve the patient's potential for interpersonal trust, intimacy, and generativity; coping mechanisms, the ability to experience a wide range of emotions; and the capacity to grieve. Treatment may often require the patient to experience heightened anxiety and distress during the course of therapy, which usually continues for several years. Early psychoanalytic treatments were of short duration compared with current practice, usually lasting no more than a few months. Freud, for example, cured the composer Gustav Mahler of a sexual problem in one four-hour session. Psychoanalytic treatment lengthened in duration as the development and interpretation of the transference relationships became the core of the therapy and as the therapists became more passive in their behavior. Several clinicians, including Franz Alexander in Chicago, attempted to reverse those trends, but have had relatively little impact on their colleagues. In the past two decades, however, several specific short-term psychoanalytic approaches have evolved that are applicable to the treatment of depression. These approaches seek to reduce symptoms, resolve neuroses, and improve the patient's quality of life. Perhaps the most seminal work was by Michael Balint and his colleagues in the 1950s at the Tavistock Clinic in London. Since the death of Balint, David Malan has continued that work. Other contributors include Habib Davanloo in Montreal, Peter Sifneos in Boston, Hans Strupp in Tennessee, and Lester Luborsky in Philadelphia (Table 16.8-1).

Short-term psychoanalytic therapies for depression are distinguished from other psychotherapeutic approaches by the use of the transference relationship. The therapeutic relationship has two aspects: the real and the transferred. The real relationship refers to thoughts, feelings, and behaviors that are relevant and appropriate to the current interaction between patient and therapist. The transferred aspect is used to identify and reexperience

TABLE 16.8-1
Features of Short-Term Psychoanalytic Approaches

Name	Treatment Duration (No. of Sessions)	Specific Time Limit	Indications	Notes
Brief psychotherapy (Malan)	20-40	Yes	Patients with a focal life problem who respond to trial interpretations	Significant personality changes in suitable patients
Short-term dynamic psychotherapy (Davanloo)	15-30	No	Oedipal problems; neurotic problems where the focus is loss; obsessional and phobic neuroses; long-standing, characterological problems without a single focus	Highly confrontational, recommended for resistant patients; not recommended for patients with significant dependency or separation problems
Short-term anxiety provoking psychotherapy (Sifneos)	12-15	No	Oedipal triangular interpersonal problems	Avoids regression into pregenital characterological issues; change attributed to interpretation of Oedipal issues
Time-limited dynamic psychotherapy (Strupp)	<25	Yes	Avoidant, dependent, compulsive, and passive-aggressive personality disorders associated with depression, anxiety, and resentment	Focus on interpersonal themes, use of transference in a here-and-now way, not genetically
Supportive-expressive treatment (Luborsky)	12-25	Yes	Broad range of problems from mild situational maladjustments to borderline psychotic	Techniques flexible so that a wide range of patients can benefit from treatment

problems and patterns that developed in important relationships early in life and have been re-created in current important relationships. Transference is considered to be the key to all psychoanalytic approaches. The various treatments differ in how they deal with transference, although most relate patterns of therapist-patient interactions to current interpersonal situations. The development of a transference neurosis in which there is a regression into early childhood relationships is usually discouraged in those short-term therapies.

The short-term treatments depart in other ways from classic psychoanalytic practice. All involve active participation by the therapist and discourage free-association techniques. In general, they identify and emphasize a single focal issue. That issue, usually an interpersonal problem, is selected, and both the patient and therapist agree to deal primarily with the one problem. That focus is considered dynamic because it is used as a link with core conflicts arising from early life. The current conflict becomes a microcosm for the patient's earlier, more substantial, and long-lasting conflicts.

Active collaboration between patient and therapist involves the establishment of a working alliance. The therapist seeks to convey interest in the patient's problems, respect, and warmth, and attempts to elucidate explanations from the patient regarding behavior and feelings in addition to using interpretations.

Most short-term psychoanalytic approaches discourage regression, principally because emergence of such material as pregenital characterological issues often leads to a significant therapeutic impass that may not be resolved in a short period of time.

Identification of suitable patients for the short-term psychoanalytic therapies is given preeminence by all proponents. Patient selection criteria are similar, although there are some differences among the therapies. The patients selected should be intelligent; be capable of introspection; be able to see a connection among thoughts, feelings, and behavior; have a strong motivation for change; and be flexible. Motivation can be tested by assessment of the patient's responsiveness to interpretations early in therapy. A capacity for meaningful human relationships must have been demonstrated at some time during life. Finally, the capacity to tolerate anxiety and frustration is required. Obviously, those criteria exclude a significant proportion of psychiatric patients, leaving only the most desirable, verbal therapy candidates. Nonetheless, the proponents of these therapies point out that, for such patients, serious personality problems can be addressed in a relatively short time.

STRATEGIES AND TECHNIQUES Among the specific techniques used in the short-term approaches are the active interpretation of the transference, the identification of and emphasis on the specific dynamic focus, the active collaboration between patient and therapist, and the discouragement of regression.

In the short-term approaches, the transference is actively developed and interpreted, often from the outset of therapy. That approach is illustrated in an excerpt from an initial session with Davanloo in which he immediately challenges a patient's passivity.

Therapist: How do you feel about talking to me about yourself?

Patient: I feel uncomfortable. I have never done this before, so I don't really, you know . . . I feel I don't really know how to answer some of your questions.

Therapist: Um-hum. But have you noticed that in your relationship here with me you are passive, and I am the one who has to question you repeatedly?

Patient: No.

Therapist: Um-hum. What do you think about this? Is this the way it is with other people, or is it only here with me? . . . This passivity, lack of spontaneity.

Another vignette illustrates the interpretation of the transference relationship.

Patient: Since we talked about it last week, I've been noticing how much I try to impress people at work.

Therapist: Can you describe any of those times from last week?

Patient: Well, when I went to lunch with a colleague, I was continually telling him about all my latest accomplishments in an attempt to impress him. It's sort of how I feel in here sometimes.

Therapist: So sometimes when we're talking you find yourself thinking about how I feel about you, and whether I am impressed with you?

Patient: Yes.

Therapist: Why do you suppose that matters to you?

Patient: I guess because I want you to like me.

Therapist: Do you remember when you first had this feeling with another person?

Patient: Yes. I remember I felt this way when I talked to my father. He was always putting me down when I talked. I remember how I was constantly trying to impress him with the things I did like playing sports and bringing home good grades, but nothing I ever did seemed to be good enough for him.

Therapist: It is interesting that you are doing the same things with me to impress me that didn't work with your father.

In his manual, Strupp describes a married woman in her 30s who sought treatment for recurrent depressive episodes. The woman's manner in the interview was aloof and curt, which led the therapist to want to discuss facts rather than elicit feelings. When this inclination was pointed out to her, the patient responded that she could not imagine that anything she said could be of interest to anyone, and acted in this way to protect herself from being hurt. The dynamic focus then became an exploration of her expectation that she was of no interest to anyone. A link was subsequently made with the patient's childhood, during which her parents seemed to prefer her sisters to her.

Sifneos gives an example of a patient who became angry and demanding about making up a canceled session. Instead of encouraging associations to childhood orality and dependency the therapist confronted the patient's maladaptive and self-destructive current behavior and encouraged the patient to request an extra session rather than being angry and withdrawn.

EFFICACY Eleven studies of brief psychodynamic psychotherapy in the treatment of depression have been reported in the past 15 years. Most included the psychodynamic treatments as controls, not as the experimental groups. In one study dynamic therapy was reported to have a better outcome than a waiting list control. In four studies the outcome for dynamic psychotherapy was found to be no different than that for cognitive therapy, behavior therapy, or pharmacotherapy. In one study psychodynamic therapy was less efficacious than combined pharmacotherapy and cognitive therapy; in three studies it was less efficacious than behavior therapy and cognitive therapy. All studies were published prior to 1988 (most were considerably earlier).

INTERPERSONAL THERAPY

THEORETICAL CONCEPTS Interpersonal therapy (IPT) was developed by Gerald Klerman and Myrna Weissman as part of their extensive research on the nature and treatment of depression over the past two decades. The theoretical basis of IPT includes the work of Adolf Meyer and Harry Stack Sullivan. In contrast with the predominantly intrapsychic orientation of classic psychoanalysis and Emil Kraepelin's biomedical model, Meyer's psychobiological approach emphasizes the interaction between the individual and the psychosocial environment over the patient's entire life course. The patient's current interpersonal experiences and attempts to adapt to environmental change and stress are seen as critical factors in psychiatric illness. Sullivan's interpersonal theory, which views interactions between people as the focus for study and treatment in psychiatry, draws heavily from the social sciences, including anthropology and sociology. A second major influence comes from John Bowlby's studies of attachment. These studies demonstrate the importance of attachment and social bonding to human functioning and the connection between disruption of these bonds and vulnerability to depression.

IPT conceptualizes depression from a medical model: depression is something that happens to the person that requires treatment. The depressed person is allowed to assume the "sick role" and is not blamed for the affliction any more than someone would be blamed for having cancer, heart disease, or pneumonia. The issue of attribution of blame is important. Many other approaches view depression as something the patient has brought on and must end by his or her own efforts.

The IPT approach to depression involves three interacting components: symptom formation, social and interpersonal experiences, and enduring personality patterns. Medication may be recommended for symptom reduction; psychotherapy focuses on improving the patient's interpersonal functioning. Although the causes of depression may vary with regard to a person's biological vulnerability, personality predispositions, or psychosocial precipitants, depression always occurs in a psychosocial and interpersonal context. Depression can predispose a patient to interpersonal problems, or interpersonal problems can precipitate depression. An interpersonal focus in the treatment process is thus presumed as essential for recovery.

GOALS IPT sets two therapeutic goals. The first is to reduce the patient's depressive symptoms and improve self-esteem. The second is to help the patient develop more effective strategies for dealing with current social and interpersonal relations. As a short-term psychotherapy, IPT does not attempt to restructure the patient's personality. IPT does, however, recognize the importance of early developmental experiences and assumes that historical conflicts are manifested in current relationships.

GENERAL CONSIDERATIONS IPT, a short-term psychotherapy, normally consisting of 12 to 16 weekly sessions, was developed specifically to treat nonbipolar, nonpsychotic ambulatory patients suffering depressive disorders. It is characterized by an active approach on the part of the therapist and by an emphasis on current issues and social functioning in the life of the patient. Intrapsychic phenomena such as defense mechanisms or internal conflicts are not addressed. Discrete behaviors such as lack of assertiveness, social skills, or distorted thinking may be addressed, but only in the context of their meaning or effect on interpersonal relationships.

STRATEGIES AND TECHNIQUES

General strategies For goal 1, reduction of symptoms, an educational approach is used. The patient is told about the clinical syndrome of depression, including its components and course. The therapist reviews the symptoms with the patient, gives a sense of optimism and hope, and emphasizes that depression is a common disorder with a good prognosis. Pharmacotherapy may be considered for symptom reduction if appropriate.

For goal 2, IPT defines four major problem areas commonly presented by depressed patients: grief, interpersonal role disputes, role transitions, and interpersonal deficits (Table 16.8-2). Associated therapeutic goals and recommended treatment strategies are outlined for each.

The choice of specific IPT strategies and techniques depends on the problem area defined as most salient for the patient. The four areas are not mutually exclusive, and patients may have multiple problems in more than one area; however, only one or two current interpersonal problems are selected for focus in order to set realistic goals and productive treatment strategies.

Cases of abnormal grief may involve delayed or distorted mourning, or both. The following example is cited in the IPT manual. A 68-year-old woman became depressed following the death of her husband, who had suffered a long course of physical and mental deterioration that resulted in considerable constraints and isolation on the part of the patient. Her symptoms included pervasive sadness and preoccupation with feelings of guilt and hopelessness. The first aim of treatment was to help the patient successfully mourn the loss, as the mourning process had been blocked by anger. The second aim was to help her to reestablish interests and relationships to substitute for what she had lost.

Interpersonal issues in a troublesome and conflicted marriage may include role disputes or role transitions. The choice between the two problem areas depends on whether the patient believes that the marriage is salvageable and whether the patient wants to stay in the marriage. If the patient decides to leave the marriage and the problem area is defined as role transition, the therapist will attempt to help the patient make that transition. That goal may include working on identifying

TABLE 16.8-2
Focal Problem Areas of Interpersonal Therapy

Problem Areas	Definition	General Goals and Strategies
Grief	Abnormal grief reactions occur because of failure to go through normal mourning following the death of a person important to the patient	Facilitate the mourning process; help reestablish interests and relationships to substitute for the loss
Interpersonal role disputes	Nonreciprocal expectations are occurring in patient's relationships with others	Help patient identify the dispute, guide in choices as to plans of action, encourage modification of maladaptive communication patterns, encourage reassessment of expectations
Role transitions	Feeling of inability to cope with change in life role (may be experienced as threatening to self-esteem, sense of identity, or both)	Help patient regard role in a more positive and less restrictive manner, restore self-esteem by helping patient develop sense of mastery with regard to demands of new role
Interpersonal deficits	History of inadequate or unsustaining interpersonal relationships	Reduce patient's social isolation by focusing on past relationships and relationship with therapist and by helping patient form new relationships

new sources of emotional support, overcoming irrational fears and regarding the new role more positively, and helping the patient master the demands of the new role. Alternatively, if the problem area is defined as a role dispute, the treatment strategies will include identifying the dispute and working toward its resolution, improving communication patterns, examining appropriateness of expectations, outlining various options, and deciding on a plan of action.

The interpersonal deficit problem area is appropriate for patients who are socially isolated or who have a sufficient number of relationships but feel unable to enjoy them. Interpersonal deficits may exist in patients who are chronically depressed and experience chronically impaired interpersonal functioning. Problems with social isolation may be long-standing or temporary; for each, treatment strategies aim to reduce social isolation. In the absence of current relationships discussion of positive and negative features of past relationships may be used as a model for the development of new relationships. Treatment may also focus on the relationship between therapist and patient.

An example of an interpersonal deficit cited by the IPT manual is as follows:

A 22-year-old unmarried man became severely depressed one month after the breakup of a three-year relationship with his girlfriend. The patient, a part-time student employed as a cook, lived with his mother, who had stopped working after being hospitalized for physical problems, and subsequently, he had become depressed. Discussion of the patient's current relationship revealed that he felt close to no one except to his mother.

The patient's history revealed inadequate social relationships and lack of interpersonal skills. Treatment focused on past significant relationships and on conflicts over his relationship with his mother. The patient-therapist relationship provided a direct source of information about the patient's style of relating to others, and that information was used to modify maladaptive interpersonal patterns and improve his ability to form relationships with others.

Specific techniques The specific techniques used in IPT may be applied to any of the four interpersonal problem areas. In the general order of their use in the course of treatment, they are (1) exploratory techniques, (2) encouragement of affect, (3) clarification, (4) communication analysis, (5) use of therapeutic relationship, and (6) behavior change techniques (Table 16.8-3).

TABLE 16.8-3
Interpersonal Therapy Techniques

Techniques	Definition
Exploratory techniques	Collect (by directive or nondirective methods) information about the patient's symptoms and problems
Encouragement of affect	Help patient recognize and accept painful affects, help patient use and manage affects positively in interpersonal relationships, encourage expression of suppressed affect
Clarification	Restructure and feed back patient's communications
Communication analysis	Identify maladaptive communication patterns, help patient communicate more effectively
Use of therapeutic relationship	Examine patient's feelings and behaviors in therapeutic relationship as model of patient's interactions in other relationships
Behavior change	Use to help patient solve simple life problems, teach patient to consider range of options for solving problems, use role playing to explore and understand patient's relationship with others and train patient in new ways of interacting with others

EFFICACY The efficacy of IPT has been tested in two large controlled studies. The first involved four groups (approximately 25 outpatients) treated by IPT alone, IPT plus amitriptyline (Elavil), amitriptyline alone, and a nonscheduled treatment comparison group. All active treatment groups, including that using IPT alone, were significantly more effective at reducing depressive symptoms than nonscheduled treatment; the combination of IPT and amitriptyline proved most effective. In addition, the IPT conditions had much lower dropout rates than did those without IPT.

In the second study, the National Institute of Mental Health (NIMH) Treatment of Depression Collaborative Research Program, 250 outpatients with major depressive disorder were randomly assigned to one of four 16-week treatment conditions: IPT, cognitive-behavioral therapy, imipramine (Toframil) with clinical management (IMI-CM), and placebo with clinical management (PLA-CM). In this study all four treatment conditions significantly reduced depressive symptoms. For severely depressed patients IPT was significantly more effective than PLA-CM in achieving remission of symptoms at 16 weeks. IMI-CM, however, tended to have the best outcome, particularly for patients with impairment in functioning. Imipramine was more rapid in its effects, with significantly better outcome than all other conditions at 12 weeks.

BEHAVIORAL APPROACHES

THEORETICAL CONCEPTS Although there are a number of behavioral approaches to depression, each with somewhat different theoretical assumptions and specific treatment methods, they have a common source in the work of B. F. Skinner, who incorporated the principles of classical and operant conditioning in an empirical analysis of behavior. Skinner's research provides the basic framework, methodology, and assumptions for the current behavioral theories and their clinical applications. Application of that model to complex human behavior led some theorists to expand the framework. For example, social learning theory includes cognitive phenomena, such as emphasizing the role of subjective expectations and value in reinforcement. Although interested in the role of cognition, behavioral theorists assume that cognitions follow the same laws of learning as do more observable behavioral events and, while related, do not determine behavior in a causal sense. This assumption distinguishes behavioral approaches from the cognitive-behavioral approach described later. Despite some differences in focus, behavior therapies are commonly characterized by an emphasis on (1) the links between an observable or operationally definable behavior and the conditions that control or determine it and (2) the role of rewards or reinforcement as determinants of behavior and behavioral change.

The application of the behavioral approach to depression first occurred in 1965 with an analysis of depression by Charles B. Ferster, who proposed that depression is caused by a person's loss of positive reinforcement (for example, through separation, death, or sudden environmental change), which results in reduction of the entire behavioral repertoire, depressed behavior, and dysphoric feelings. That concept of depression is central to all behavioral approaches. A change in the rate of reinforcement is believed to be a key factor in the origin and maintenance of depression (through lack of available reinforcers or when the available reinforcers are not contingent on the person's behavior) and also in its reversal. Ferster also proposed that a social skills deficit—characterized by difficulty in obtaining social reinforcement—might increase a person's difficultly in coping with the loss of the usual supply of reinforcement.

GOALS The goals of the behavior therapies are to increase the frequency of the patient's positively reinforcing interactions with the environment and to decrease the number of negative interactions. Some behavioral treatments aim also at improving social skills. Alteration of personal behavior is believed to be the most effective way to change the associated depressed thoughts and feelings.

GENERAL CONSIDERATIONS Several behavior therapies devised to treat depression are characterized by overlapping behavioral and cognitive intervention strategies. One extensively studied approach was developed by Peter Lewinsohn on the basis of social learning theory. In addition to the individual-based social learning approach, Lewinsohn developed a "Coping with Depression Course" designed to deliver the specific behavioral strategies in a group format. The focus of Lewinsohn's approach, whether in individual or group format, is on increasing pleasant activities and interactions with the environment. A second prominent behavioral approach, based on a self-control model of behavior, was developed by Lynn Rehm to treat depression. Key components of this approach include techniques designed to correct deficits in the patient's ability to realistically and productively self-monitor, self-evaluate, and self-reinforce. A third approach focuses on the training of social skills in parents to increase positive social interactions and reinforcements (Table 16.8-4). These therapies share certain assumptions and strategies:

1. The treatment program is highly structured and generally short term.
2. The principle of reinforcement is seen as the key element in depression.
3. Changing behavior is considered to be the most effective way to alleviate depression.
4. The focus is on the articulation and attainment of specific goals.

Some behavioral treatments combine a variety of behavioral techniques and tailor the techniques to the individual needs of

TABLE 16.8-4
Behavioral Approaches to Depression

Treatment Approach	Basic Approach and Strategies	Tactics
Self-control therapy (Rehm)	Self-monitoring—gain control over and increase positive activities Self-evaluation—learn to set realistic goals; learn to make more accurate attributions regarding causes of successes and failures Self-reinforcement—learn to increase and maintain level of positive activities	Monitor mood Schedule pleasurable activities Set realistic goals and operational subgoals Schedule activities related to goals and monitor progress Learn to make correct self-attributions Construct individualized self-reinforcement programs to increase and maintain level of positive activities
Social learning therapy (Lewinsohn)	Initial two-week diagnostic phase leading to behavioral diagnosis Treatment designed to increase activity level and enhance social skills	Home observation Daily monitoring of mood and activity Increased participation in pleasant events Environmental interventions (environmental shifts, change consequences of certain behaviors) Assertion training through modeling and rehearsal Set goals for increasing social activities Relaxation training Time management Cognitive techniques (including thought interruption, worrying time, disputing irrational thoughts, noticing accomplishments, and positive self-rewarding thoughts)
Social skills training (Michel Hersen, Alan S. Bellack)	Skills training—patient is taught positive assertion, negative assertion, and conversational skills Social perception training—patient learns to attend to relevant context and cues of interpersonal interactions Practice—newly learned responses are carried out in the natural environment	Didactic instruction Modeling, guided practice of skills Role playing Homework assignments Monitoring and recording of homework performance by patient
	Self-evaluation and self-reinforcement—patient is trained to evaluate responses more positively and to provide self-reinforcement	Patient's evaluation of role-playing responses with letter grade; therapist's correction of inappropriately low responses; therapist's modeling of positive self-statement

each patient. Normally, there are core ingredients in conjunction with a number of optional techniques.

STRATEGIES AND TECHNIQUES Although the major behavioral approaches to depression vary in their focus and emphasis in treatment and in the frequency of use of specific techniques, the following eight strategies are commonly used. Detailed manuals specify treatment regimes for most of these approaches.

Maintain records Recording mood and activities, both positive and negative, is essential to most behavioral therapies. Patients may also monitor the immediate and long-term consequences of specific behavior.

Increase general activity level, particularly pleasant events On the basis of the daily mood and activity recordings, the therapist encourages the patients to increase their participation in those activities rated as most pleasant by demonstrating a relationship between increased pleasant activities and lower levels of depression.

Decrease or manage unpleasant events From the daily ratings, negative interactions or situations that trigger feelings of depression are identified. Patients learn to avoid and decrease unpleasant events when possible. Patients are also taught to manage their reactions to negative events by learning to substitute more positive thoughts, to prepare for unpleasant events, and to prepare for failure.

Develop new self-reinforcement patterns Patients learn to reward themselves or to increase goal-related activities with material rewards or activities.

Enhance social skills Deficits in social skills and interaction patterns may be addressed through assertiveness training, modeling, and role playing with feedback and rehearsal or by providing graduated performance assignments to promote rewarding social interaction and to decrease social avoidance. A combination of approaches can be used. Group therapy sessions may be used to improve communication skills or to resolve specific interpersonal problems.

Relaxation training Relaxation techniques may aid in achievement of other goals, such as increasing social interaction, reducing the aversiveness of unpleasant situations, or producing a mood state incompatible with depression. Patients are taught relaxation of the major muscle groups; they are encouraged to practice relaxation twice a day and are instructed to keep a written log of relaxation activity.

Time management Training patients to plan ahead and make preparations necessary to participate in pleasant events (for example, obtaining a baby-sitter) is part of time management. An effort is made to work out an appropriate balance between activities that the patients want to do and activities they feel they have to do.

Cognitive skills training Cognitive skills training is generally geared toward decreasing negative thinking and increasing positive thinking. Patients are taught to monitor their thinking and to discriminate between positive and negative thoughts, necessary and unnecessary thoughts, and constructive and destructive thoughts. Specific techniques include thought-stopping, disputing irrational thoughts, and correcting errors in attribution regarding causes of successes and failures.

EFFICACY Behavior therapy has been tested in a number of studies of depressed subjects. Eight published studies involve random assignment and either a waiting list or nonspecific treatment group as control. Behavior therapy methods significantly reduced depressive symptoms in three quarters of the studies.

COGNITIVE-BEHAVIORAL THERAPY

THEORETICAL CONCEPTS Cognitive-behavioral therapy stems from four major previous theories: psychoanalytic theory, phenomenological philosophy, cognitive psychology, and behavioral psychology. One salient common feature is the recognition of the importance of the subjectiveness of conscious experience (one's perceptual experience of reality rather than the objective reality); another is the recognition of the emotional consequences of irrational beliefs and thoughts.

Aaron Beck, the originator of cognitive-behavioral therapy, developed a comprehensive, structured theory of depression. According to this theory, depression is associated with negative thought patterns, specific distorted schemas, and cognitive errors or faulty information processing (Table 16.8-5). Such cognitive dysfunctions form the core of depression while affective and physical changes and other associated features of depression are its consequences.

Cognitive theory conceptualizes depression as involving negative cognitions regarding the cognitive triad (ideas of oneself, the world, and one's future). The self is perceived as being defective, inadequate, deprived, worthless, and undesirable. The world appears as a negative, demanding, and defeating place, and one expects failure and punishment, continued hardship, suffering, deprivation, and failure in the future. Underlying the negative conditions are stable cognitive structures, called schemas, that include core beliefs or assumptions through which one interprets experience. Schemas associated with depression are analogous to viewing the world through dark glasses (for example, the core belief that one is unlovable). Cognitive errors, or systematic errors in thinking, allow the persistence of negative schemas despite contradictory evidence. A cognitive error frequently associated with depression is dichotomous thinking, the tendency to view one's experiences as black or white without shades of gray, or to believe that people

TABLE 16.8-5
Elements of Cognitive Theory

Element	Definition
Cognitive triad	Beliefs about oneself, the world, the future
Schemas	Ways of organizing and interpreting experiences
Cognitive distortions	
Arbitrary inference	Drawing a specific conclusion without sufficient evidence
Specific abstraction	Focus on a single detail while ignoring other more important aspects of an experience
Overgeneralization	Forming conclusions based on too little and too narrow experience
Magnification and minimization	Over- or undervaluing the significance of a particular event
Personalization	Tendency to self-reference to external events without a basis
Absolutist, dichotomous thinking	Tendency to place experience into all-or-none categories

are either all bad or all good. Symptoms of depression follow from the cognitive error. For example, apathy and low energy are results of the individual's expectation of failure in all areas. Similarly, a paralysis of will stems from the individual's pessimism and feelings of hopelessness.

GOALS The goal of cognitive-behavioral therapy is to change the way a person thinks and, subsequently, to alleviate the depressive syndrome and prevent its recurrence. This is accomplished by helping the patient (1) identify and test negative cognitions; (2) develop alternative, more flexible schemas; and (3) rehearse both new cognitive and new behavioral responses.

GENERAL CONSIDERATIONS Cognitive-behavioral therapy is a short-term, structured therapy that involves active collaboration between the patient and the therapist toward achieving set goals. It is oriented toward current problems and their resolution. Therapy is usually conducted on an individual basis, although group techniques have been developed and tested. Cognitive-behavioral therapy may be used in conjunction with pharmacotherapy.

STRATEGIES AND TECHNIQUES As with other psychotherapies, the attributes of the therapist are fundamental to successful cognitive-behavioral therapy. Therapists must be empathatic, able to understand the life experience of each patient, and capable of being genuine and honest with themselves and their patients. Therapists also must be able to relate skillfully to patients in their own experiential world in an interactive way. As a highly structured therapeutic approach, cognitive-behavioral therapy involves setting the agenda at the beginning of each session, assigning homework to be performed between sessions, and teaching specific new skills. The active collaboration between the therapist and the patient provides a genuine sense of teamwork.

Cognitive-behavioral therapy has three basic components: didactic aspects, cognitive techniques, and behavioral techniques (Table 16.8-6).

Didactic aspects The didactic aspects include explaining to the patient the nature of the cognitive triad, schemas, and faulty logic. The therapist informs the patient that they will formulate hypotheses together and will test them over the course of treatment. The therapist presents a full explanation of the relationship between depression and thinking, affect, and behavior, as well as the rationale for all aspects of the treatment. This contrasts with the more psychoanalytically oriented therapies in which very little explanation is involved.

TABLE 16.8-6
Components of Cognitive Behavioral Therapy

Didactic issues
Learning rationale and strategy of the therapy
Cognitive techniques
Eliciting automatic thoughts
Testing automatic thoughts
Identifying maladaptive underlying assumptions
Analyzing validity of maladaptive assumptions
Behavioral techniques
Scheduling activities
Mastery and pleasure
Graded task assignment
Cognitive rehearsal
Self-reliance training
Role playing
Diversion techniques

Cognitive techniques The cognitive approach has four strategies: eliciting automatic thoughts, testing automatic thoughts, identifying maladaptive underlying assumptions, and testing the validity of maladaptive assumptions.

ELICITING AUTOMATIC THOUGHTS Automatic thoughts are cognitions that intervene between external events and the individual's emotional reaction to the event. For example, a person invited to go bowling may think, negatively, "everyone is going to laugh at me when they see how badly I bowl," before he actually bowls with this group of people. Another example is when a person thinks "he doesn't like me" if someone passes the person in the hall without saying hello.

TESTING AUTOMATIC THOUGHTS The therapist, acting as a teacher, helps the patient test the validity of the automatic thought. The goal is to encourage the patient to formulate alternative possible interpretations and reject inaccurate or exaggerated automatic thoughts, after carefully examining them. For example, patients often set unrealistic expectations for themselves, then blame themselves when they are unable to live up to these expectations. The case of a 32-year-old depressed computer programmer with self-denigrating thoughts about his ability to complete homework assignments illustrates this point.

Patient: I don't know what's been wrong with me this week. I just don't seem to be as interested in doing my homework assignments. I don't know if I'm ever going to get better.

Therapist: Can you think of a specific time this week that you had problems doing homework because of disinterest?

Patient: Yes, on Thursday I tried to do my relaxation exercises, but I eventually gave up.

Therapist: Can you tell me what you were thinking at the time?

Patient: Well, I started doing my breathing, but I couldn't calm my thoughts and stop thinking about other things, like the instructions in the manual said. Then I started thinking about how long I've been working on this and how I should know how to do it by now.

Therapist: And how long have you been working on the breathing technique?

Patient: Uh, one week.

Therapist: Let's review the evidence that supports your statement that you should be performing this exercise with no problems at this time.

In this example, when the patient and therapist carefully reviewed the situation, it became apparent that the patient's expectation that he should be able to perform this exercise perfectly after one week of practice was unreasonable. On consideration that the ability to breathe and maintain calm thoughts is a skill that normally takes many weeks to perfect, the patient realized that his belief about his inability to learn was distorted and incorrect.

Generating alternative explanations is another technique used to undermine inaccurate and distorted automatic thoughts.

A 29-year-old secretary with a two-year history of depression reported that she frequently experienced feelings of sadness and hurt at work because of the curt and gruff manner in which her boss interacted with her. The automatic thought that she reported following one interaction with her boss—in which he stated "I wish things around here ran smoother"—was "He doesn't like me. He doesn't think I'm doing a good job." The therapist helped the patient generate a list of other interpretations of her employer's statement and behavior including the possibility that he interacted with all people this way, that he was a generally unhappy person, that he did not like his job and was allowing his unhappiness about his work situation to influence how he interacted with the patient, and that he was having personal problems that were preoccupying him and causing him to be unhappy at work and inattentive to the manner in which he interacted with his employees.

IDENTIFYING MALADAPTIVE ASSUMPTIONS As the patient and therapist continue to identify automatic thoughts, patterns usually become apparent, representing underlying rules or maladaptive general assumptions that guide the patient's life. Examples of such rules include, "To be happy, I must be perfect" or "If everyone doesn't like me, I'm not lovable." Such rules inevitably lead to disappointment, to failure, and subsequently to depression.

ANALYZING MALADAPTIVE ASSUMPTIONS Similar to testing the validity of automatic thoughts is testing the accuracy of maladaptive assumptions. One particularly effective technique is for the therapist to ask the patient to defend the validity of an assumption.

Patient: I guess I believe that I should always work up to my potential.
Therapist: Why is that?
Patient: Otherwise I would be wasting time.
Therapist: What is the long-range goal in working up to your potential?
Patient: I've never really thought about that. I've just assumed that I should.
Therapist: Are there any positive things you give up by always having to work up to your potential?
Patient: I suppose it makes it hard to relax or take a vacation.
Therapist: What about living up to your potential to enjoy yourself and relax? Is that important at all?
Patient: I've never really thought of it that way.
Therapist: Maybe we can work on giving yourself permission not to work up to your potential at all times.

In this example, the therapist is helping the patient recognize how maladaptive it is to strive to work up to one's potential at all times.

Behavioral techniques Behavioral techniques are used conjointly with cognitive techniques to test and change maladaptive or inaccurate cognitions in order to help patients understand the inaccuracy of their cognitive assumptions and to learn new strategies and ways of dealing with issues. A repertoire of behavioral techniques are utilized in cognitive-behavioral therapy.

1. Among the first things done is to schedule activities on an hourly basis. The patient keeps a record of these activities and reviews it with the therapist.
2. Patients are asked to rate the amount of mastery of and pleasure derived from those activities; they are often surprised at how much more mastery and pleasure they gain from the activities than they had otherwise believed.
3. To simplify the situation and allow for mini-accomplishments, tasks are often subdivided into subtasks, as in graded task assignments, to demonstrate to patients that they can succeed.
4. Cognitive rehearsal involves having the patient imagine the various steps involved in meeting and mastering a challenge and rehearsing the various aspects of it.
5. Self-reliance training involves encouraging patients to become more self-reliant, by doing such simple things as making their own beds, doing their own shopping, or preparing their own meals, rather than relying on other people.
6. Role playing is a particularly powerful and useful technique used to elicit automatic thoughts and learn new behaviors.
7. Diversion techniques are useful in helping patients get through particularly difficult times by means of physical activity, social contact, work, play, or visual imagery.

The techniques used are highly structured and goal oriented and require active collaboration between the therapist and the patient. Emphasis is on identifying maladaptive, inaccurate cognitions in various forms, seeking alternative explanations, and learning new behaviors to reverse the affective and drive disturbances and other associated features of depression and, it is hoped, help prevent their recurrence.

EFFICACY Cognitive therapy has been studied extensively in the treatment of outpatients with major depressive disorder. Of 34 such reports nine included a pill placebo, waiting list, or nonspecific treatment as a control group. In most studies, cognitive-behavioral therapy was superior to the control group in reducing depressive symptoms. The one notable exception is the NIMH Treatment of Depression Collaborative Research Program (TDCRP), in which cognitive-behavioral therapy did not differ significantly from the placebo clinical management condition (see prior section on IPT). Compared with pharmacotherapy alone, cognitive-behavioral therapy was found to be superior in two studies conducted in the 1970s. In three more recent studies, including the TDCRP, there were no differences in efficacy between antidepressant medication and cognitive-behavioral therapy. In six studies that compared cognitive-behavioral therapy with that therapy plus pharmacotherapy, five found no differences between the two outcomes and one found that the combined treatment was superior to cognitive-behavioral therapy alone.

In summary, cognitive-behavioral therapy has been shown to be an effective treatment for many outpatients with major depressive disorder. It is particularly effective among mild to moderately depressed patients and may be less effective than pharmacotherapy among more severely depressed patients.

DISCUSSION

Several issues influence the choice of treatment for depression, the duration of treatment, and whether or not to use more than one treatment modality at the same time. These issues include the phase of illness, diagnosis and patient characteristics, the presence of chronicity and dysthymia, the presence of bipolar disorder, and use of combined pharmacological-psychotherapeutic treatments.

PHASE OF ILLNESS Nearly all studies of psychosocial treatments for depression have focused on the acute phase of treatment; that is, they have tested the performance of a specific psychotherapeutic approach in resolving depressive symptoms within 12 to 16 weeks. These studies have generated considerable evidence of the efficacy of IPT, cognitive-behavioral therapy, and behavioral therapy in certain groups of patients during this time period. An episode of depression, however, does not necessarily end when the acute symptoms have abated. In fact, a relapse of symptoms may occur if treatment is discontinued too soon after the initial control of symptoms. That happens presumably because the acute treatment (especially pharmacotherapy) has not cured the illness, but rather ameliorated or reduced the symptoms temporarily. This situation is analogous to the effect of insulin on diabetes mellitus. Depression is now recognized as a recurrent, and often chronic, illness. Therefore, withdrawal of the treatment may result in return of illness.

An important consequence of our recognition of the long-term nature of the illness is the need for treatment beyond the acute phase and into the continuation and maintenance phases. Continuation treatment is the ongoing treatment from the point of clinical remission to the point at which spontaneous remission is expected to occur in untreated patients (that is, to the putative true end of an untreated episode). For depression, the continuation phase in pharmacological treatments generally lasts approximately six to nine months following acute treatment. Maintenance treatment is longer-term, and is intended to prevent future depressive episodes or decrease their intensity. The model for psychotherapeutic treatments, in contrast, is that the strategies and techniques change maladaptive patterns that are linked to depression, and thus should result in a reduced risk for future episodes or symptoms of depression.

There are two sets of questions with regard to continuance of short-term psychotherapies over the long term. First, do the therapies confer a prophylactic effect in the future? Second, is it helpful to continue the treatments following a positive response into the continuation and maintenance phases?

Prophylactic effect of short-term therapies Follow-up studies of patients responding positively to acute treatment for depression have attempted to address the question of whether treatment offers long-term prophylactic effects.

For IPT, one study reported no differences in relapse or recurrence at a one-year follow-up between patients in a 16-week clinical trial treated with IPT, amitriptyline, amitriptyline plus IPT, and nonscheduled treatment in terms of relapse or recurrence. However, patients treated with IPT did have better social functioning at the one-year reevaluation point.

The majority of the follow-up studies have examined relapse rates in patients successfully treated with cognitive therapy or antidepressant medication. Those studies have shown a clear pattern of lower relapse rates for patients treated with cognitive-behavioral therapy than for those treated with short-term pharmacotherapy. However, the naturalistic designs of these studies precludes conclusions regarding the reasons for the differences found (that is, whether the results represent some enduring effects of the cognitive therapy, or to differences in risk for relapse among patients who respond to drugs versus psychotherapy).

Despite the positive findings for short-term psychotherapy in terms of decrease in symptoms and the possibly lower relapse rates with use of cognitive-behavioral therapy, the success of these approaches, as a well as of pharmacological treatments, depends on how outcome is defined. When outcome is defined optimally as complete remission of symptoms and maintenance of symptom-free remission for an extended period following treatment, it becomes clear that 12 to 16 weeks of treatment (with psychotherapy or pharmacotherapy) is insufficient for the majority of patients who present with major depression. This is illustrated by findings from the NIMH TDCRP, which reported the proportion of all patients starting treatment who achieved this stringently defined outcome. Complete remission (at least 8 weeks without symptoms) at the end of treatment and maintenance of remission for 18 months following treatment was achieved by 30 percent of patients after cognitive-behavioral therapy, by 26 percent after IPT, by 19 percent after imipramine with clinical management, and by 20 percent after placebo with clinical management. Considering outcome in this optimal way highlights the need for longer periods of treatment for full recovery as well as the need for continuation and maintenance treatments.

Treatment during the continuation phase Does continuing treatment after successive resolution of symptoms help to prevent relapses and recurrences? This clinically important question has received relatively little attention, but has been addressed in one study on cognitive-behavioral therapy. Forty-two subjects who received acute therapy were followed for one year. At three months into the follow-up study, half of those who responded to treatment were given additional treatment (''booster'' sessions) until completion of the study while the other half of the responder group was given no additional treatment. The authors found no difference in relapse rates or depressive symptoms between the two groups at one year, suggesting that continued treatment with cognitive therapy after successful resolution of symptoms does not improve outcome. It must be emphasized that this is a single study and further research is needed. There are no studies on the use of IPT or behavior therapy in the continuation phase.

Treatment during the maintenance phase Does therapy continued a year or more after successive treatment help to prevent the occurrence of new episodes? In a landmark study by Ellen Frank and colleagues, a group of 128 patients with recurrent major depressive disorder who had responded to a combined short-term and continuation treatment of imipramine and IPT were randomly assigned to different maintenance treatment groups. Those treated with IPT alone had a significantly lower relapse rate than those receiving placebos. However, those treated with imipramine, with or without IPT, did significantly better than the IPT without imipramine groups. This study strongly supports continued treatment, especially pharmacotherapy, over a long period in time of patients with a history of recurrent episodes of depression.

There is some evidence that, in patients with recurrent depression, long-term treatment is useful in delaying or preventing recurrences. However, the value of continuation and maintenance treatment with psychotherapy remains unresolved and awaits further research.

DIAGNOSIS AND PATIENT CHARACTERISTICS The psychotherapeutic treatment approaches described above were developed for use with outpatients with nonbipolar, nonpsychotic depression. They should generally not be used as a sole treatment for severely depressed inpatients or for patients with bipolar depression, although their use when combined with pharmacotherapy for such patients has begun to be evaluated.

Whether these treatment approaches should be used without medication for outpatients with major depressive disorder has been controversial. The general clinical belief is that antidepressants should be part of the treatment when patients are more severely depressed, or have endogenous depressions. Findings from the NIMH Treatment of Depression Collaborative Research Program have suggested that IPT may be effective for at least some of the more severely depressed outpatients, and thus may be a feasible treatment for such patients if an alternative to medication is needed or desired. Endogenous depression was not found to differentially predict outcome in this study. Findings from other studies regarding endogenous depression have been mixed, but most do not find that outpatients with endogenous depression (as defined by the Research Diagnostic Criteria) respond better to pharmacotherapy than to psychotherapy. Treatment for patients meeting criteria for melancholia, however, should typically include medication.

Other findings from the NIMH Treatment of Depression Collaborative Research Program regarding patient characteristics and treatment outcome included better outcomes with IPT for patients with less impairment in social functioning, and better outcome with cognitive-behavioral therapy and with imipramine for patients with less distortion in cognitions (dysfunctional attitudes). Other studies have also shown that high scores on measures of dysfunctional attitudes predict a poorer outcome in cognitive-behavioral therapy. Together, these findings suggest that patients may require a minimal level of proficiency in the area of functioning that the treatment targets in order to benefit from the treatment (at least in the short term). That is an important question for future research.

Some patient characteristics have been found to be predictive of response across treatments in general. Longer duration of the current episode, and also the diagnosis of dysthymic disorder prior to the onset of the major depressive disorder (double depression) have been shown to predict a poorer response; higher expectations of improvement have been associated with a better outcome to different forms of treatment.

The beliefs and expectations of the patient regarding depression and treatment should also be considered. Some patients who consider depression to be a psychological disorder that should be amenable to psychotherapeutic approaches are resistant to using medication. Others consider their depression to be a biochemical disturbance that will require medication if it is to be corrected, and not psychotherapy. A good therapist may be able to modify such expectations when necessary, but a positive attitude toward treatment on the part of the patient may be significantly important to a successful outcome.

In general, the therapist should be cautious in making attributions about premorbid personality problems during the depressed phase. Many interpersonal and cognitive styles may appear different to the patient and the therapist after the acute phase of the disorder has been alleviated. Nonetheless, several studies have found that the presence of a personality disorder is associated with a slower or generally worse response to treatment. For depression, such patients are likely to need longer periods of treatment.

DYSTHYMIC DISORDER AND CHRONICITY Most of our knowledge on the treatment of depression comes from the study of patients with acute major depression, and we know far less about the treatment of chronic depression. This is unfortunate, given the prevalence of dysthymic disorder. Over 3 percent of adults in the United States suffer from dysthymic disorder during any six-month period, according to the Epidemiologic Catchment Area (ECA). In addition, approximately one third of psychiatric outpatients suffer from dysthymic disorder. Nearly one in five patients with a major depressive episode fails to recover and becomes chronically depressed.

The importance and potential usefulness of psychosocial treatments for such patients is demonstrated by (1) the notable morbidity and impairment of quality of life associated with dysthymic disorder, which has been shown to exceed that associated with most medical illnesses; (2) the fact that a substantial proportion of patients with dysthymic disorder either fail to respond to medication or cannot tolerate the side effects; and (3) with or without medication, the long-standing patterns of social withdrawal; lack of assertiveness; impairment in family, marital, and occupational functioning; and chronic pessimism and hopelessness associated with dysthymic disorder need to be addressed. When depression is severe, pharmacological treatments are encouraged to alleviate suffering and increase the ability of the person to engage in the therapy. There are no controlled studies of the effectiveness of this treatment approach; however two naturalistic follow-up studies have suggested that long-term analytic therapy can have long-term beneficial effects.

More recent developments in the treatment of dysthymic disorder include the modification of psychotherapeutic approaches specifically for the treatment of dysthymic disorder, as well as preliminary open trial studies investigating the effectiveness of the modified psychotherapies for dysthymic patients. The chronic interpersonal and social deficits associated with dysthymic disorder provide a strong rationale for the use of IPT with dysthymic patients, and a manual has recently been developed. Aspects of dysthymic disorder that distinguish it from acute depression, requiring modification of IPT, include the lack of an acute precipitant, the characterological features often associated with the presence of a chronic mood disorder (such as paucity of interpersonal relationships, lack of self-assertion, poor social skills), and the lack of euthymic memories. Given the typical absence of an acute precipitant in dysthymic disorder the choice of a focus of treatment becomes more difficult. While all of the four IPT problem areas do occur in dysthymic patients, their frequency as a primary focus differs from acute depression. Grief is rarely the primary focus, whereas interpersonal deficits more frequently are. The frequent absence of interpersonal relationships in the patient's life requires an increased focus on the therapeutic relationship, which is used as a model for other interpersonal interactions. Social isolation is addressed by encouraging occupational and social activities involving contact with others. Participation in activities are used to examine social behaviors, expectations, and desires.

When relationships do exist, they are often unsatisfactory, in light of the difficulty these individuals have in asserting themselves, expressing anger, or setting limits. IPT for these patients emphasizes exploration of what the patient desires from the relationships and of what options are available to alter the relationships. The patient is helped to begin to identify personal needs, to begin to assert them, and to set limits. The expression of anger is encouraged and supported. Preliminary support for the use of IPT for dysthymic disorder has been provided by a nonrandomized pilot study of 19 patients treated with IPT, desipramine (Norpramin), or both.

Another psychotherapeutic approach that has recently been developed specifically for the treatment of dysthymic disorder is the Cognitive-Behavioral Analysis System of Psychotherapy (C-BASP). The focus of this treatment approach is on problematic cognitive and behavioral patterns associated with dysthymic disorder. A situational analysis procedure that includes performance feedback is a central part of the approach. Patients are taught to evaluate the adequacy of their behavior in various situations, particularly those involving interactions with others, and to target and modify self-defeating behaviors. Beliefs of helplessness and absence of control are challenged by the experience of mastery in producing desired outcomes. The treatment is conducted in stages, with the requirement that the patient demonstrates mastery at each stage before moving on to the next. The duration of treatment thus differs for different patients, but is typically short-term (less than six months). Ten dysthymic patients treated in a naturalistic study were reported as having a successful outcome, with nine of these remaining in remission for dysthymic disorder at follow-up of two years or more.

Despite these important recent advances, it is clear that controlled studies are needed to more clearly determine the nature, degree, and duration of benefits derived from these psychotherapeutic approaches in the treatment of dysthymic disorder and chronic depression.

PSYCHOSOCIAL TREATMENT OF BIPOLAR DISORDER

The clinical and research literature on major depressive disorder is replete with both psychotherapeutic and psychopharmacologic approaches. In sharp contrast is the literature on treatment of bipolar disorder, which focuses almost exclusively on psychopharmacology and, specifically, on the use of lithium carbonate (Eskalith) as the overwhelming treatment of choice. The introduction of lithium has influenced the diagnostic system, the clinical practice, and the therapeutic outcome of patients with bipolar disorder for 20 years. It is as close to a wonder drug as has been experienced in psychiatry.

However, lithium is not the absolute cure for bipolar disorders. About one third of patients either do not respond or only partially respond to lithium. Even for those who respond fully, many serious social, occupational, familial, and marital problems often remain. Psychological and behavioral problems are frequently associated with bipolar disorder, and alcohol and substance abuse, violence, and suicide can result from inadequate treatment. Psychotherapeutic interventions may be particularly relevant for these problems.

Another major rationale for adjunctive psychotherapy is to improve medication compliance. An estimated 20 to 50 percent of patients with bipolar disorder who are on a prescribed medication regimen either do not fully comply with their doctor's instructions or discontinue treatment altogether. Physical side effects, as well as the psychological unwillingness to take pills, adds to the noncompliance problem. Lithium noncompliance or discontinuation increases relapse. Psychotherapy combined with lithium may result in increased medication compliance and a better clinical outcome.

Adjunctive psychotherapy can also be used to provide important educational benefits. It can help the patient and family members to learn to identify early warnings of an impending mania so that more rapid interventions can occur, and to identify problems that exacerbate or precipitate episodes.

Treatments Little has been written about the psychotherapeutic treatment of bipolar disorders since the report of 12 cases by Mabel Blake Cohen in 1954. In recent years, however, several approaches have been developed for psychosocial and psychotherapeutic treatment of bipolar disorder. Unfortunately there is no empirical research published on the efficacy of these approaches as yet, but they are sufficiently important that a description of each is included here.

These approaches, designed as short-term, outpatient interventions, were inspired by the well-documented success of similar programs used with schizophrenic patients.

Miklowitz and Goldstein The first treatment package, developed by David J. Miklowitz and Michael J. Goldstein, is based on behavioral family management techniques. Based on the premise that the same family attributes thought to be important in predicting the course of schizophrenia are also associated with the course of bipolar disorders, the focus of the program is on educating the family about bipolar disorders and aiding in the development of communication and problem-solving skills. This approach (like all psychosocial approaches for bipolar disorders) is not intended to serve as a substitute for a traditional medication regimen but rather as adjunctive therapy. The program for patients recently discharged after an episode of hypermania includes 21 one-hour sessions conducted in the patient's home over a nine-month period. These sessions are divided into seven sessions dealing with family education, seven on communication skills training, and seven on problem-solving skills training.

In a pilot trial with nine patients, only one patient relapsed over the nine-month posthospitalization period during which treatment was implemented. In comparison, a 61 percent relapse rate was reported from a naturalistic outcome study using traditional medication regimens without family management.

Basco and Rush The second treatment package, developed by Monica R. Basco and A. John Rush, is designed around four goals: (1) to educate the patient regarding bipolar disorder; (2) to teach cognitive-behavioral skills for coping with the psychosocial stressors, as well as the cognitive and behavioral problems associated with manic and depressive symptoms; (3) to facilitate compliance with a prescribed medication regimen; and (4) to monitor the occurrence, severity, and course of manic and depressive symptoms. The protocol is divided into three phases corresponding with these goals. The first phase, consisting of one-hour sessions, once a week for five weeks, educates the patient about the causes, symptoms, and treatment of bipolar disorder. The second phase, which teaches cognitive-behavioral skills, consists of weekly sessions lasting approximately 75 to 90 minutes. The third phase—maintenance—provides an opportunity to monitor the patient's symptoms, reinforce skills, and facilitate medication compliance. This final phase is held in one-hour sessions no less than once a month and no more than four times a month.

The treatment protocol is highly structured. Each session covers one component of the treatment package, and includes (1) a summary of the intention and direction of the session, (2) background information about the intervention technique, (3) goals of the session, (4) a step-by-step description of the intervention procedures, and (5) a homework assignment to reinforce what was learned in the session or to prepare for the next session.

COMBINED PHARMACOLOGIC-PSYCHOTHERAPEUTIC TREATMENT It is common practice for many psychiatrists to provide combined pharmacotherapy and psychotherapy for their patients with nonbipolar depression. The prevailing clinical opinion is that antidepressant medication is most effective for depressive symptoms, especially such vegetative symptoms as sleep disturbance, appetite disturbance, and loss of interest, whereas psychotherapy targets and improves marital and family relationships, social functioning, and occupational performance. However, the empirical evidence supporting this belief is minimal.

Is combined treatment more efficacious than either treatment modality alone? And does combined therapy treat a broader range of outcomes than either modality alone? Research addressing these questions is fraught with methodologic difficulties. Nonetheless, nearly 15 studies on combined therapy have been completed over the past 20 years. In general they have not found substantial increased efficacy of combined treatment over either treatment alone.

Seven studies of combined treatment with cognitive therapy have been conducted. These have all involved tricyclic antidepressants. Several compared the combined treatment with both medication alone and psychotherapy alone. Others compared the combined treatment against only one modality. Overall the results are inconsistent and do not demonstrate the superiority of combined treatment over that using a single modality. Three studies of combined behavior therapy and tricyclic antidepressants versus either medication alone or psychotherapy alone found no differences between the combined and single-modality treatments. Two studies of combined IPT and amitriptyline are also inconsistent, with one showing a trend for better outcome for the combined treatment, and the other showing no differences between outcomes of combined and single-modality treatments. As noted, Frank and colleagues, studying combined imipramine and maintenance IPT in patients with severe recurrent depression, found that imipramine with or without maintenance IPT was clearly superior to all other treatment modalities in the maintenance phase of the illness. However, in addition to studying a different phase of treatment, this study addressed a different sample (patients with highly recurrent disease who were responsive to combined treatment) than the other studies of combined treatment.

SUGGESTED CROSS-REFERENCES

Information regarding related aspects of mood disorders are discussed further in Chapter 16. Chapter 31 on psychotherapies also outlines behavioral and cognitive therapies and other psychosocial treatments. Psychiatric treatments of adolescents are reviewed in Chapter 46 and treatments in the elderly population are included in Section 49.7. Application of psychosocial treatment to schizophrenia may be found in Section 14.9.

REFERENCES

Basco M R, Rush A J: Cognitive-behavioral therapy for bipolar disorder. In *Cognitive Behavioral Treatment of Manic Depressive Disorder*. Guilford, New York, 1995.

Beck A T, Rush A J, Shaw B F, Emery G: *Cognitive Therapy of Depression*. Guilford, New York, 1979.

Bellack A S, Hersen M, Himmelhoch J S: Social skills training for depression: A treatment manual. Cat Sel Doc Psychol *10:* 2156, 1980.

Bemporad J R: Long-term analytic treatment of depression. In *Handbook of Depression*, Beckham E E, Leber W R, editors, p. 82. Dorsey, Homewood, IL: 1985.

Crits-Christoph P: The efficacy of brief dynamic psychotherapy: A meta-analysis. Am J Psychiatry *149:* 151, 1992.

Conte H R, Karasu T B: A review of treatment studies of minor depression: 1980–1991. Am J Psychother *46:* 58, 1992.

Davanloo H: *Short-Term Dynamic Psychotherapy*, vol 1. Aronson, New York, 1980.

Elkin I, Parloff M B, Hadley S W, et al: NIMH treatment of depression collaborative research program: Background and research plan. Arch Gen Psychiatry *42:* 305, 1985.

*Elkin I, Shea M T, Watkins J T, Imber S D, Sotsky S M, Collins J F, Glass D R, Pilkonis P A, Leber W R, Docherty J P, Fiester S J, Parloff M B: National Institute of Mental Health Treatment of Depression Collaborative Research Program: General effectiveness of treatments. Arch Gen Psychiatry *46:* 971, 1989.

Evans, M D, Hollon S D, DeRubeis R J, Plasecki J M, Grove W M, Garvey M J, Tuason V B: Differential relapse following cognitive therapy and pharmacotherapy for depression. Arch Gen Psychiatry *49:* 802, 1992.

Ferster C B: A functional analysis of depression. Am Psychol *10:* 857, 1973.

*Frank E, Kupfer D J, Perel J M, Cornes C, Jarrett D B, Mallinger A G, Thase M E, McEachran A B, Grochocinski V J: Three-year outcomes for maintenance therapies in recurrent depression. Arch Gen Psychiatry *47:* 1093, 1990.

*Frank E, Kupfer D J, Wagner E F, McEachran A B, Cornes C: Efficacy of interpersonal psychotherapy as a maintenance treatment of recurrent depression. Arch Gen Psychiatry *48:* 1053, 1991. [Contributing factors (published erratum) Arch Gen Psychiatry *49:* 401, 1992.]

Gaylin W, editor: *The Meaning of Despair*. Aronson, New York, 1968.

Jarrett R B: Psychosocial aspects of depression and the role of psychotherapy. J Clin Psychiatry *51:* 26, 1990.

Jarrett R B, Rush A J: Cognitive therapy for depression. *Directions Clin Psychol,* 1995.

Kavanagh D J, Wilson P H: Prediction of outcome with group cognitive therapy for depression. Behav Res Ther *27:* 333, 1989.

Kazdin A E: Comparative outcome studies of psychotherapy: Methodological issues and strategies. J Consult Clin Psychol *54:* 95, 1986.

Keitner G I, Miller I W: Combined psychopharmacological and psychosocial treatment of depression. RI Med J *76:* 415, 1993.

Klerman G L: Drugs and psychotherapy. In *Handbook of Psychotherapy and Behavior Change: An Empirical Analysis,* Garfield, A Bergin, editors. Wiley, New York, 1986.

Klerman G L, Dimascio A, Weissman M, Prusoff B, Paykel E S: Treatment of depression by drugs and psychotherapy. Am J Psychiatry *131:* 186, 1974.

Klerman G L, Weissman M W, Rounsaville B J, Chevron E S: *Interpersonal Psychotherapy of Depression.* Basic Books, New York, 1984.

Lewinsohn P M, Antonuccio D, Steinmetz J L, Teri L: *The Coping With Depression Course: A Psychoeducational Intervention for Unipolar Depression.* Castalia, Eugene, OR, 1984.

Lewinsohn P M, Sullivan J M, Grosscup S J: Changing reinforcing events: An approach to the treatment of depression. Psychother Theor, Res Pract *17,* Fall 1980.

Luborsky L: *Principles of Psychoanalytic Psychotherapy—A Manual for Supportive-Expressive Treatment.* Basic Books, New York, 1984.

Malan D H: *Individual Psychotherapy and the Science of Psychodynamics.* Butterworth, London, 1979.

Markowitz J C, Klerman G L: *Manual for Interpersonal Therapy With Dysthymic Patients.* Payne Whitney Clinic, New York, 1991.

McCullough J P: Psychotherapy for dysthymia: A naturalistic study of ten patients. J Nerv Ment Dis *179:* 734, 1991.

Miklowitz D, Goldstein M, Neuchterlein K, Snyder K, Mintz J: Family factors and the course of bipolar affective disorder. Arch Gen Psychiatry *45:* 225, 1988.

Moreau D, Mufson L, Weissman M M, Klerman G L: Interpersonal psychotherapy for adolescent depression: Description of modification and preliminary application. J Am Acad Child Adolesc Psychiatry *30:* 642, 1991.

Rehm L P: Self-management therapy for depression. Adv Behav Res Ther *6:* 83, 1984.

Rush A J, Beck A T, Kovacs M: Comparative efficacy of cognitive therapy and pharmacotherapy in the treatment of depressed outpatients. Cogn Ther Res *I*: 17, 1977.

Rush A J, editor: *Short-Term Psychotherapies for Depression.* Guilford, New York, 1982.

*Rush A J: Short-term psychotherapeutic approaches to depression. *The Medical Psychotherapist,* 1995.

Shea M T, Elkin I, Hirschfeld, R M A: Psychotherapeutic treatment of depression. In *Review of Psychiatry,* R E Frances, A J Hales, editors. American Psychiatric Press, Washington, DC, 1988.

*Shea M T, Elkin I, Imber S D, Sotsky S M, Watkins J T, Collins J F, Pilkonis P A, Beckham E, Glass D R, Dolan R T, Parloff M B: Course of depressive symptoms over follow-up: Findings from the National Institute of Mental Health treatment of depression collaborative research program. Arch Gen Psychiatry *49:* 789, 1992.

Sifneos P E: *Short-Term Dynamic Psychotherapy: Evaluation and Technique,* ed 2. Plenum, New York, 1987.

Simons A D, Murphy G E, Levine F L, et al: Cognitive therapy and pharmacotherapy for depression: Sustained improvement over one year. Arch Gen Psychiatry *43:* 43, 1986.

Sotsky S M, Glass D R, Shea M T, Pilkonis P A, Collins J F, Elkin I, Watkins J T, Imber S D, Leber W R, Moyer J, Oliveri M E: Patient predictors of response to psychotherapy and pharmacology: Findings in the NIMH Treatment of Depression Collaborative Research Program. Am J Psychiatry *148:* 997, 1991.

Strupp H, Binder J L: *Psychotherapy in a New Key: A Guide to Time-Limited Dynamic Psychotherapy.* Basic Books, New York, 1984.

Thase M E: Long-term treatments of recurrent depressive disorders. J Clin Psychiatry: 32, 1992.

Watkins J T, Leber W R, Imber S D, Collins J F, Elkin I, Pilkonis P A, Sotsky S M, Shea M T, Glass D R: Temporal course of change of depression. J Consult Clin Psychol *61:* 858, 1993.

Weissman M M, Jarrett R B, Rush A J: Psychotherapy and its relevance to the pharmacotherapy of major depression: A decade later (1976–1985). In *Psychopharmacology: The Third Generation of Progress,* H Meltzer, editor, p 1059. Raven, New York, 1987.

Weissman M M, Klerman G L, Prusoff B A, Sholomskas D, Padian N: Depressed outpatients: Results one year after treatment with drugs and/or interpersonal therapy. Arch Gen Psychiatry *38:* 1981.

Weissman M M, Prusoff B A, Dimascio A, Neu C, Goklaney M, Klerman G L: The efficacy of drugs and psychotherapy in the treatment of acute depressive episodes. Am J Psychiatry *136:* 555, 1979.

Wells K B, Stewart A, Hays, R D: The functioning and well-being of depressed patients: Results from the Medical Outcomes study. JAMA *262:* 914, 1989.

CHAPTER 17 ANXIETY DISORDERS

17.1
PANIC DISORDERS AND AGORAPHOBIA

ABBY J. FYER, M.D.
SALVATORE MANNUZZA, Ph.D.
JEREMY D. COPLAN, M.D.

INTRODUCTION

Panic disorder is a common, chronic illness associated with considerable morbidity and social cost. Its central features are recurrent unexpected panic attacks (sudden rushes of fear accompanied by several somatic symptoms such as difficulty breathing, palpitations, and dizziness) and associated avoidance and worry related to the possible recurrence, consequences, or health implications of the attacks. Although panic symptoms have been well described for over a century, only in the past decade has panic disorder become widely recognized as a distinct psychiatric illness. Moreover, although several effective treatments are now available, as many as half of panic disorder sufferers are either undiagnosed, misdiagnosed, or untreated.

One reason for the underdiagnosis and undertreatment is that most patients with panic disorder are initially seen by general practitioners, internal medicine subspecialists, or emergency room physicians with complaints of sudden and overwhelming somatic symptoms (for example, palpitations, difficulty breathing, chest pain, dizziness). The somatic symptoms of panic often mimic those of such common catastrophic medical events (for example, myocardial infarction). Making an accurate diagnosis in the face of the patient's evident distress usually requires that the physician be aware of the possibility of a psychiatric etiology and have the time for careful, specific questioning. Unfortunately, in the current medical environment many persons with panic disorder undergo elaborate, expensive, but inconclusive medical workups or receive ineffective treatment for nonspecific anxiety.

DEFINITION

Anxiety may take several forms. It may be experienced as an inexplicable feeling of impending doom, or as unfounded worries about numerous things (the health of one's child, the success of one's business, the fate of one's marriage), or as an irrational fear of a situation (attending a party), activity (driving), or object (animals).

In *panic disorder* anxiety manifests as recurrent panic attacks—sudden rushes of fearfulness accompanied by a number of physical and cognitive signs and symptoms, such as rapid heartbeat, trembling, feelings of unreality, and fears of dying. Different from generalized or free-floating anxiety, panic attacks are experienced as discrete periods that reach peak intensity within seconds or minutes and subside soon afterward. Panic attacks differ from phobic anxiety in that they are not always predictable; at least some attacks are unexpected. The criteria for panic attacks appear in Table 17.1-1.

Panic attacks are ubiquitous in psychiatry. They may occur in anxiety disorders other than panic disorder, in mood disorders, in certain intoxication and withdrawal syndromes—in fact, in any mental disorder. In addition, panic attacks may be observed in certain nonpsychiatric medical conditions. However, if a pattern of recurrent, unexpected panic attacks is experienced and the individual becomes distressed in anticipation of future attacks, their consequences, or implications (for example, underlying heart disease), or if there is a significant change in the individual's behavior that is associated with the attacks, then that individual is said to have panic disorder without agoraphobia (Table 17.1-2).

In some persons, the fear of having a panic attack becomes associated with certain situations. Characteristically, those situations include the use of public transportation, driving across a bridge, being in a crowd, waiting in line, or leaving familiar settings alone. Concerns about those situations revolve around whether the person will be able to flee from them quickly and get help in the event a panic attack should occur. Consequently, the person begins to avoid the situations or must force himself or herself to enter them while experiencing intense anxiety. The person might also insist on being accompanied by a friend or relative when traveling on a bus or driving. A person with that form of panic disorder is said to have panic disorder with agoraphobia. The criteria for agoraphobia are listed in Table 17.1-3. The diagnostic criteria for panic disorder with agoraphobia appear in Table 17.1-4.

There are also cases in which agoraphobia is observed without a history of panic disorder (Table 17.1-5). In those cases the fears and avoidance are associated with the possibility of suddenly developing a paniclike symptom or symptoms in the

TABLE 17.1-1
Criteria for Panic Attack

Note: A panic attack is not a codable disorder. Code the specific diagnosis in which the panic attack occurs (e.g., panic disorder with agoraphobia).
A discrete period of intense fear or discomfort, in which four (or more) of the following symptoms developed abruptly and reached a peak within 10 minutes:
(1) palpitations, pounding heart, or accelerated heart rate
(2) sweating
(3) trembling or shaking
(4) sensations of shortness of breath or smothering
(5) feeling of choking
(6) chest pain or discomfort
(7) nausea or abdominal distress
(8) feeling dizzy, unsteady, light-headed, or faint
(9) derealization (feelings of unreality) or depersonalization (being detached from oneself)
(10) fear of losing control or going crazy
(11) fear of dying
(12) paresthesias (numbness or tingling sensations)
(13) chills or hot flushes

TABLE 17.1-2
Diagnostic Criteria for Panic Disorder without Agoraphobia

A. Both (1) and (2):
   (1) recurrent unexpected panic attacks
   (2) at least one of the attacks has been followed by one month (or more) of one (or more) of the following:
      (a) persistent concern about having additional attacks
      (b) worry about the implications of the attack or its consequences (e.g., losing control, having a heart attack, "going crazy")
      (c) a significant change in behavior related to the attacks
B. Absence of agoraphobia.
C. The panic attacks are not due to the direct physiological effects of a substance (e.g., a drug of abuse, a medication) or a general medical condition (e.g., hyperthyroidism).
D. The panic attacks are not better accounted for by another mental disorder, such as social phobia (e.g., occurring on exposure to feared social situations), specific phobia (e.g., on exposure to a specific phobic situation), obsessive-compulsive disorder (e.g., on exposure to dirt in someone with an obsession about contamination), posttraumatic stress disorder (e.g., in response to stimuli associated with a severe stressor), or separation anxiety disorder (e.g., in response to being away from home or close relatives).

TABLE 17.1-3
Criteria for Agoraphobia

A. Anxiety about being in places or situations from which escape might be difficult (or embarrassing) or in which help may not be available in the event of having an unexpected or situationally predisposed panic attack or paniclike symptoms. Agoraphobic fears typically involve characteristic clusters of situations that include being outside the home alone; being in a crowd or standing in a line; being on a bridge; and traveling in a bus, train, or automobile.
   Note: Consider the diagnosis of specific phobia if the avoidance is limited to one or only a few specific situations, or social phobia if the avoidance is limited to social situations.
B. The situations are avoided (e.g., travel is restricted) or else are endured with marked distress or with anxiety about having a panic attack or paniclike symptoms, or require the presence of a companion.
C. The anxiety or phobic avoidance is not better accounted for by another mental disorder, such as social phobia (e.g., avoidance limited to social situations because of fear of embarrassment), specific phobia (e.g., avoidance limited to a single situation like elevators), obsessive-compulsive disorder (e.g., avoidance of dirt in someone with an obsession about contamination), posttraumatic stress disorder (e.g., avoidance of stimuli associated with a severe stressor), or separation anxiety disorder (e.g., avoidance of leaving home or relatives).

Note: Agoraphobia is not a codable disorder. Code the specific disorder in which the agoraphobia occurs (e.g., panic disorder with agoraphobia or agoraphobia without history of panic disorder).

kinds of situations described above. For example, a person might avoid all public transportation out of fear of losing bladder control. In some cases of agoraphobia without panic disorder there might not be a single, unitary focus of fear. However, the disorder would be apparent from the characteristic cluster of agoraphobic situations described above.

HISTORY

Although the terms used to identify the syndrome have varied considerably, panic disorder has been described in the literature for well over a century. During the American Civil War of the 1860s, Jacob Mendes DaCosta observed "a peculiar form of functional disorder of the heart" among soldiers in military hospitals. The disorder, which he called irritable heart, was characterized by intense, often incapacitating chest pain, violent palpitations, and other cardiac signs in the absence of any identifiable structural lesions of the heart. The diagnosis of irritable

TABLE 17.1-4
Diagnostic Criteria for Panic Disorder with Agoraphobia

A. Both (1) and (2):
   (1) recurrent unexpected panic attacks
   (2) at least one of the attacks has been followed by one month (or more) of one (or more) of the following:
      (a) persistent concern about having additional attacks
      (b) worry about the implications of the attack or its consequences (e.g., losing control, having a heart attack, "going crazy")
      (c) a significant change in behavior related to the attacks
B. The presence of agoraphobia.
C. The panic attacks are not due to the direct physiological effects of a substance (e.g., a drug of abuse, a medication) or a general medical condition (e.g., hyperthyroidism).
D. The panic attacks are not better accounted for by another mental disorder, such as social phobia (e.g., occurring on exposure to feared social situations), specific phobia (e.g., on exposure to a specific phobic situation), obsessive-compulsive disorder (e.g., on exposure to dirt in someone with an obsession about contamination), posttraumatic stress disorder (e.g., in response to stimuli associated with a severe stressor), or separation anxiety disorder (e.g., in response to being away from home or close relatives).

TABLE 17.1-5
Diagnostic Criteria for Agoraphobia without History of Panic Disorder

A. The presence of agoraphobia related to fear of developing paniclike symptoms (e.g., dizziness or diarrhea).
B. Criteria have never been met for panic disorder.
C. The disturbance is not due to the direct physiological effects of a substance (e.g., a drug of abuse, a medication) or a general medical condition.
D. If an associated general medical condition is present, the fear described in criterion A is clearly in excess of that usually associated with the condition.

heart (or DaCosta's syndrome) was made frequently during the Franco-Prussian and Boer Wars of the mid- to late 1800s.

In his 1895 paper, "On the Grounds for Detaching a Particular Syndrome from Neurasthenia Under the Description 'Anxiety Neurosis,' " Sigmund Freud argued that George Miller Beard's use of the term "neurasthenia" was overly inclusive and lacked general validity. Freud coined the term "anxiety neurosis" and described a syndrome characterized by symptoms such as general irritability, anxious expectation, vertigo, paresthesias, heart spasms, sweating, and breathing difficulties. He also indicated that the syndrome could take a chronic form or manifest as discrete attacks ("sudden onslaughts of anxiety").

During World War I, irritable heart returned as "disordered action of the heart," the official British Army term for the disorder. In 1918 Sir Thomas Lewis proposed the term "effort syndrome" to reflect the individual's labored response to mild exertion. B. S. Oppenheimer later suggested "neurocirculatory asthenia" to better represent cardiac symptoms and physical exhaustion as key features.

By World War II, soldiers who complained of symptoms previously considered to have resulted from functional heart disorders were referred to military psychiatrists rather than to internists. Also, diagnoses of anxiety reaction were considered.

The association between panic attacks and agoraphobia similarly has been known for nearly a century. In his 1895 paper, "Obsessions and Phobias," Freud stated: "In the case of agoraphobia . . . we often find the recollection of an anxiety attack; and what the patient actually fears is the occurrence of such an attack under the special conditions in which he believes he cannot escape it." However, despite that early observation, for many years agoraphobia was viewed simply as a phobic disorder.

COMPARATIVE NOSOLOGY

FROM DSM-II TO DSM-III Although detailed descriptions of panic anxiety were published over 100 years ago, panic disorder did not become an officially recognized diagnosis until 1980, with publication of the third edition of *Diagnostic and Statistical Manual of Mental Disorders* (DSM-III). Anxiety neurosis, the diagnosis listed in the second edition of DSM (DSM-II), published in 1968, was split into two diagnoses in DSM-III, panic disorder and generalized anxiety disorder. That decision was based in part on the finding that imipramine (Tofranil) blocks panic attacks but has little or no immediate effect on anticipatory anxiety or avoidance behavior. Several subsequent family, twin, treatment, and biological studies have supported the view that panic disorder is a distinct clinical entity.

DSM-III AND DSM-III-R Panic disorder and agoraphobia underwent a major reconceptualization in the revised third edition of DSM-III (DSM-III-R). DSM-III included the diagnoses agoraphobia with and without panic attacks, and panic disorder. In DSM-III-R those categories were changed to panic disorder with and without agoraphobia, and agoraphobia without a history of panic disorder. The revisions were prompted by the clinical observation that agoraphobia is usually a complication of recurrent panic attacks. Thus, the DSM-III-R categories more accurately reflected the central role of panic attacks in the typical development of agoraphobia.

Since the publication of DSM-III-R in 1987, several studies have shown that (1) in subjects who experience both agoraphobic avoidance and panic attacks, the panic attacks usually but not invariably precede the avoidant behavior in the development of the syndrome; (2) agoraphobia without panic attacks is uncommon in clinical settings; and (3) when agoraphobia occurs without panic attacks, many individuals report limited symptom attacks or other spontaneous, episodic, and incapacitating somatic symptoms. In conclusion, most studies have supported the association of agoraphobia and panic attacks. However, some controversy remains about the central role of panic attacks in causality.

A second change from DSM-III to DSM-III-R concerned the definition of agoraphobia. DSM-III required an "increasing constriction of normal activities until the fears or avoidance behavior dominate[d] the individual's life." That restrictive criterion precluded the diagnosis of a large group of clinically impaired individuals who exhibited only partial avoidance or endurance with intense anxiety. DSM-III-R rectified the problem by providing categories of mild, moderate, severe, in partial remission, and in full remission to specify the current severity of agoraphobic avoidance.

DSM-IV Individuals who experience a clustering of attacks during a circumscribed period would fulfill DSM-III (three panic attacks in a three-week period) or DSM-III-R (four attacks in four weeks) panic disorder criteria. However, many infrequent panickers also exhibit functional impairment and help-seeking. Consequently, DSM-III-R and the fourth edition of DSM (DSM-IV) incorporated provisions for irregular patterns of panic attacks. DSM-III-R required *either* four attacks in four weeks *or* a single attack followed by at least a month of fear of having additional attacks. DSM-IV requires "recurrent unexpected panic attacks" plus a month or more of persistent concern about having other attacks, or about the implications of attacks, or the demonstration of a significant behavioral change. However, no numerically defined cluster, such as three attacks in three weeks, is stipulated. The revisions were prompted by DSM-IV literature reviews, data reanalyses, and field trial findings. The decision made in DSM-III-R to include agoraphobia as a subtype of panic disorder was retained in DSM-IV.

ICD VERSUS DSM The ninth edition of *International Classification of Diseases and Related Health Problems* (ICD-9), published in 1978, included the categories anxiety states and phobic state, with no guidelines for diagnosing individuals with both panic disorder and agoraphobia. Thus, it is not surprising that attempts to equate DSM and ICD anxiety diagnoses were unsuccessful. In one study some patients with DSM-III-R panic disorder with agoraphobia were diagnosed as having ICD-9 anxiety states, whereas others were classified as having a phobic state. In a second study patients with DSM-III panic disorder received a wide range of ICD-9 diagnoses, most often anxiety states, affective psychoses, and depressive neuroses.

Different from DSM-III-R and DSM-IV, the 10th edition of ICD (ICD-10) gives precedence to agoraphobia (which is listed under the group of phobic disorders) over panic disorder when both are present. ICD-10 considers panic attacks in phobic situations as indicators of phobic severity and explicitly restricts the diagnosis of panic disorder to cases in which no phobia is observed. Consistent with DSM-IV categories, ICD-10 includes panic disorder and generalized anxiety disorder as separate categories.

EPIDEMIOLOGY

Several epidemiological studies completed in the past decade at diverse sites throughout Europe and North America consistently report lifetime prevalence rates of DSM-III panic disorder of 1.5 to 2 percent. Six-month prevalence rates are lower, 0.6 to 1.1 percent. An additional 3 to 4 percent of the population report panic attacks but do not meet full DSM-III criteria. Many of those subdisorder panickers report significant panic-related morbidity, and some seek treatment. They fail to meet DSM-III criteria only because they have never had a dense cluster of at least three attacks in three weeks.

In response to that dilemma, DSM-III-R and DSM-IV criteria for panic disorder allow diagnosis of individuals who have less frequent or more irregular patterns of panic attacks than stipulated by DSM-III. Therefore, prevalence rates are expected to be slightly higher. For example, the one published epidemiological study using DSM-III-R panic disorder criteria found a lifetime prevalence of 3.5 percent.

The prevalence of agoraphobia has been a subject of some discussion. Lifetime rates for agoraphobia in epidemiological studies using DSM-III or closely related operationalized criteria vary more widely (2.5 to 6.5 percent) than those for panic disorder or attacks. Moreover, in sharp contrast to observations in clinical populations, only one third to one half of cases of agoraphobia identified in epidemiological samples also have a history of panic attacks or disorder. In clinical populations agoraphobia is almost never seen without an accompanying history of panic attacks or disorder.

Several, in some cases contradictory, interpretations of the data have been proposed. One possibility is methodological variation between clinical and epidemiological settings. Some epidemiological studies have used lower thresholds for agoraphobia than those defined by DSM-III or DSM-III-R. That difference may have led to including individuals with DSM simple phobia who would not be expected to have had unexpected panic attacks. Failure to inquire about the specific cause of avoidance behavior may also have led to overdiagnosis in the epidemiological studies. For example, assessment of fear attribution is necessary to distinguish agoraphobia from both social phobia (in which fear of going out is due to concern over embarrassment at being observed by others) and depression (in which loss of interest, negative self-evaluation, and anhedonia may all lead to avoidance of leaving home).

Alternatively, the discrepancy may be an example of Berkson's fallacy: Individuals who suffer from agoraphobia without panic attacks may not be seen in clinical settings because they do not seek treatment as a result of an intervening unascertained variable, such as cultural beliefs. Definitive resolution of the problem requires further clinical interview and follow-up studies of epidemiological populations.

Women are two to three times more likely than men to be affected with panic disorder, panic attacks, or agoraphobia. Significant socioeconomic or ethnic risk factors have not been identified. However, in several studies divorce or separation were associated with increased rates of both panic disorder and panic attacks. Family history also represents a significant risk factor.

FAMILY AND GENETIC STUDIES A series of direct interview studies using DSM-III or similar operationalized diagnostic criteria found a four- to eightfold increased risk for panic disorder among first-degree relatives of panic disorder patients as compared with first-degree relatives of never mentally ill control subjects. Rates of panic disorder in relatives of panic probands were 2 to 21 percent, compared with 2 to 4 percent in relatives of controls.

Although only a limited amount of twin study data is available, the findings are consistent with a genetic contribution. A small clinical interview study found that the concordance rate for anxiety with panic attacks was significantly higher in monozygotic twins (4 of 13) than in dizygotic twins (0 of 16). The concordance rate for anxiety disorders without panic attacks did not differ between the two groups. A second study, using a population-based twin sample, found a moderate genetic contribution with a heritable liability of 30 to 40 percent.

Adoption studies of panic disorder have not been reported. Several genetic linkage studies using polymorphic deoxyribonucleic acid (DNA) markers are in progress. However, to date, only exclusion data have been reported.

The mode of inheritance of panic disorder is not known. Segregation analyses have been reported, but results are inconsistent. One study suggested a single dominant locus. A second study excluded the possibility but could not distinguish between heterogeneity and polygenic models.

Agoraphobia A number of studies confirm a heritable contribution to agoraphobia. The heritable interrelationships of agoraphobia and panic disorder are not well studied. However, two recent reports suggest that panic disorder with agoraphobia is a more severe form of panic disorder.

ETIOLOGY

The etiology of panic disorder has been addressed by three theoretical schools—psychoanalytic, cognitive-behavioral, and biological.

PSYCHOANALYTIC THEORIES Freud's theories concerning the causes of anxiety evolved over the course of his career. Only in the very early neurophysiological model did he describe an etiologically defined syndrome (anxiety neurosis) that phenomenologically parallels the DSM-IV definition of panic disorder. During that early period Freud divided neuroses into two major types: actual neuroses (including neurasthenia, anxiety neurosis, and hypochondriasis) and psychoneurosis (hysteria and obsessions). Psychoneuroses were regarded as psychological in origin, in which undischarged excitation was generated in connection with an unacceptable sexual idea. In contrast, in actual neuroses anxiety and its somatic manifestations resulted from the transformation of an incomplete discharge of central nervous system (CNS) neuronal excitation. Anxiety neurosis specifically developed from an immediate physiological cause, the interruption of sexual activity. Freud's description of anxiety neuroses, in which anxiety attacks occurred without apparent eliciting factors over a background of free-floating or generalized anxiety and apprehension, is strikingly similar to DSM-IV criteria for panic disorder.

Although in his early work Freud believed that anxiety neurosis and attacks had a somatic etiology, he later abandoned that view in favor of a psychological theory of origin. In the three theoretical constructs of anxiety—evolutionary, learning, psychological—anxiety attacks were largely regarded by Freud as a nondiscrete entity occupying a position at the severe end of the continuum of anxiety states. For example, in his final and most influential psychological model, Freud proposed that anxiety was a signal of danger from the threatened emergence into consciousness of repressed infantile wishes, invariably of an unacceptable, sexual nature. That view was further elaborated by Freud with the inclusion of either internal (for example, the action of the id or superego on the ego) or external (for example, environmental) events as potential danger signals. If the ego's defense mechanisms are incapable of deactivating unconsciously perceived threats of danger, symptomatic anxiety ensues. Modern psychoanalytic theorists have proposed that if the defense mechanisms are totally overwhelmed, the anxiety may progress to a state of panic.

That evolution has been summarized by John Nemiah as follows:

> Anxiety appears clinically in two forms: First, as a state of panic, it is manifested as a massive, global, and intense discharge of autonomic functions that overwhelms and disorganizes ego functions and renders the individual helpless to behave adaptively. Second, as a signal of danger, internal or external, anxiety is a less intense experience that enables the individual to anticipate the threat of danger and to take defensive action against it.
>
> In Freud's initial theory of anxiety as a transformation of libido into somatic, autonomic discharge, he viewed the intensity of the discharge as matching the intensity of the libido from which it was derived. This economic theory of anxiety explained its source and magnitude but could not account for its formal characteristics. Initially, Freud proposed that the somatic manifestations of acute anxiety were in many ways similar to those of orgasmic discharge. This explanation, however, did not account for the significant difference between the ecstatic pleasure of orgasm and the overwhelmingly painful affect of panic. Accordingly, Freud subsequently suggested that anxiety recapitulated the affective and somatic response of the infant to the trauma of the birth process, which acted as a template for the form of all later anxious reactions to severe traumatic situations. Ultimately, Freud generalized his concept of anxiety to include traumatic anxiety, the response to an actually present overwhelming and dangerous traumatic situation, and to signal anxiety, which as an ego affect alerts the individual to anticipate the threat of a traumatic situation. In signal anxiety, anxiety occurs as a response to cognitive processes, such as the perception of indicators of potential danger and the memory of past experiences of psychic trauma. This form of anxiety is derived from those cognitions, not from a transformation of repressed affects, libidinal or otherwise, and its intensity cannot be economically equated with the intensity of the repressed affects. With the development of the concept of anticipatory anxiety, the economic theory of anxiety was replaced by what has come to be called the signal theory of anxiety.

Psychoanalytic views of agoraphobia In Freud's earlier work, agoraphobia was viewed as a pseudophobia, in contrast to real phobias such as fear of animals, people, or contamination (as seen in modern-day simple phobia, social phobia, or obsessive-compulsive disorder, respectively). Freud's distinction between real phobias and pseudophobias arose from his belief that the anxiety attacks that accompanied anxiety neurosis were responsible for agoraphobia. Thus agoraphobia, like anxiety neurosis, was viewed as originating from somatic causes. Real phobias, however, represented symbolic substitutions for suppressed wishes and were addressed in treatment through psychological explanations. In later years Freud did not stringently adhere to his distinction of phobic subtypes. Consequently, agoraphobia was subsumed by Freud and his followers under the general heading of real phobias and, like real phobias, was regarded as arising from a symbolic substitution of a suppressed wish. The latter view of the causation of agoraphobia persists in modern-day psychoanalysis.

COGNITIVE-BEHAVIORAL APPROACHES Psychological theorists have proposed a variety of conditioning, personality, and cognitive hypotheses as alternatives to a purely biological or psychoanalytic theory of panic. In particular, they have argued that biological explanations are insufficient to account for the full clinical picture observed in panic disorder. Like Freudian theory, cognitive-behavioral models have also undergone progressive modification and refinement. Those models include (1) classic conditioning, (2) the "fear of fear" principle and interoceptive conditioning, (3) catastrophic misinterpretation theory, and (4) anxiety sensitivity.

Classical conditioning Systematic exposure of agoraphobic patients to feared situations typically reduces avoidance and may also attenuate panic attacks. To explain that phenomenon, researchers invoke two-way classic conditioning as an etiology for the disorder. The first step is the acquisition of fear by the occurrence of a noxious event (unconditioned stimulus), such as an electric shock, in contiguous association with a previously neutral stimulus (unconditioned stimulus), such as visiting a supermarket or crossing a bridge. The second step is learning to avoid the fear response elicited by the harmless situation (conditioned response) by escape or avoidance. The major limitation to the model is that in a majority of patients, no noxious external event or trauma leading to phobic avoidance can be identified.

The fear of fear principle and interoceptive conditioning A key observation for the further development of cognitive-behavioral theory was the realization that, rather than fearing specific external situations, what panic disorder patients most feared were internal events, namely panic attacks. That recognition led to the fear of fear formulation of panic disorder. Consequently, investigators suggested that panic attacks were the result of pavlovian interoceptive conditioning. In that model usually innocuous somatic events such as a mild dizzy sensation or bowel discomfort may, through learned association, become cues for an impending panic attack. The internal cues are then established as conditioned stimuli for the prediction of a conditioned fear response, a panic attack. As a result, patients subsequently closely monitor their internal sensations for any evidence of possible panic.

Theorists have argued against the model's validity primarily because of an overlap between the conditioned stimuli and conditioned responses. As an example, palpitations may serve as an internal cue for a panic attack (conditioned stimulus), but they may also be a symptom of a panic attack (conditioned response).

Catastrophic misinterpretation Expanding on the fear of fear construct, one group of investigators posited that misinterpretation of certain bodily sensations as catastrophic is essential for the production of panic attacks. According to that model, palpitations, for instance, may be misinterpreted as representing an imminent heart attack and dizziness as impending insanity. The perception of approaching physical disaster helps precipitate panic.

Although the model is appealing on clinical grounds, important limitations include the presence of sleep panic attacks (which occur during non-rapid eye movement [REM], dream-free sleep) and the reported absence of an awareness of catastrophic misinterpretation preceding the panic attacks in many patients.

Anxiety sensitivity Another model suggests that panic patients develop or maintain misattribution of innocuous somatic sensations because of high anxiety sensitivity. That construct purportedly accounts for why certain persons tend to respond specifically to anxiety symptoms with fear. Although high trait anxiety describes a person who may become readily anxious when faced with a range of stressors, anxiety sensitivity is posited to reflect pathological beliefs about anxiety symptoms and is thought both to antedate the panic attacks and to predispose to them. Because high trait anxiety may exist without anxiety sensitivity, the model explains why not all anxious patients panic.

Supporters of the anxiety sensitivity model cite evidence for pathological fear-oriented memory structures leading to a bias for retrieving anxiety-related information. The studies providing that evidence have not been extensively replicated.

BIOLOGICAL HYPOTHESES Biological theories of panic have rested on the observations that pharmacological treatments were capable of blocking panic attacks, and that induction of panic in the laboratory was feasible through administration of various compounds.

Laboratory provocation of panic A major advance in the field of panic research has been the development of a range of pharmacological provocation procedures capable of inducing panic attacks in the laboratory. To be considered accurate models, the challenge procedures should induce panic that is phenomenologically similar to naturally occurring panic, and the panic induced should be specific to patients with a history of panic; it should not occur in healthy or psychiatric controls. Recognition of the panic-provoking properties of a particular compound has usually been followed by hypotheses linking the putative chemical effects of the panic-provoking agent to an underlying neurobiological defect in panic disorder.

Panic-provoking compounds A host of panic-provoking agents (sometimes called panicogens) has been reported. The most widely studied are a group of naturally occurring compounds with physiological effects on acid-base and cardiorespiratory status that induce prominent dyspnea. The group includes racemic sodium lactate, carbon dioxide, sodium bicarbonate, and sodium D-lactate. Because compounds in that group induce dyspnea and hyperventilation, they have been postulated to interact with a so-called false suffocation alarm system that is aberrantly activated in patients with panic disorder.

Another major group of compounds appear to act on specific central neurochemical systems to induce panic-provoking effects. Among that group yohimbine (Yocon), which stimulates noradrenergic activity through its action as a central α_2-receptor antagonist, has supported a noradrenergic hypothesis of panic disorder. Although isoproterenol (Isuprel), a β-receptor agonist, also induces panic attacks in patients with panic disorder but not healthy volunteers, it poorly crosses the blood-brain barrier and is thought to mediate panic by peripheral cardiovascular activation. Stimulation of serotonergic function by means of direct (methchlorophenylpiperazine [mCPP]) or indirect (fenfluramine [Pondimin]) agonists has also been shown to induce paniclike states. The panic-provoking effects of flumazenil (Mazicon), a γ-amino butyric acid (GABA)-benzodiazepine antagonist, has supported the view of GABA-benzodiazepine dysfunction in panic disorder. Neuropeptides also play a role in inducing panic responses, as exhibited by the panic-provoking properties of the gut polypeptide, cholecystokinin. Curiously, compounds that act on specific neurochemical systems are more likely to induce hypothalamus-pituitary-adrenal (HPA) axis activation without dyspnea, whereas compounds with acid-base or cardiorespiratory effects tend to induce dyspnea without HPA axis activation.

Thus, challenge paradigms have stimulated a range of neurotransmitter-based hypotheses for panic, although the mechanism of action of some panic-provoking agents has been argued to be nonspecific. For instance, sodium lactate reliably provokes panic in people with panic disorder, but a plausible explanation for its effects is lacking. In fact, some evidence suggests that sodium lactate, like the β-agonist isoproterenol, may not cross the blood-brain barrier in appreciable amounts during standard laboratory procedures.

MECHANISMS OF ACTION Psychological theorists have argued that the panic-provoking effects of compounds like sodium lactate may be nonspecific and may depend on their ability to produce somatic sensations that are erroneously interpreted to signal impending catastrophe. An alternative biologically based hypothesis posits that peripheral baroreceptors and chemoreceptors are activated by sodium lactate infusion and other peripherally acting agents. Viscerosensory stimuli are carried by the vagus or glossopharyngeal nerves to the nucleus tractus solitarius and the nucleus paragigantocellularis of the medulla. At the medullary level, autonomic stimuli are abnormally integrated, leading to a false detection of serious autonomic dysfunction. In addition to provoking a rapid autonomic outflow, the signal of serious autonomic dysfunction is also transmitted to the pontine locus ceruleus and may then be carried by projections to limbic structures, where fear responses are putatively produced. Cognitive modulation of those processes is feasible by projections from the prefrontal cortex to limbic areas and the medulla.

Despite the plethora of evidence implicating abnormal function in a range of neurochemical systems, it remains unclear which abnormalities are indicative of pathophysiological processes in contrast to etiological determinants. Further, the likely heterogeneity of panic disorder may result in subgroups of patients in which different neurobiological systems are affected.

Brain imaging studies in panic disorder The development of noninvasive imaging techniques has made brain imaging one of the most promising areas of psychiatric research. The introduction of three-dimensional techniques has rendered the whole brain, including subcortical structures, accessible. Brain imaging studies in panic disorder are of two basic types: (1) structural studies, such as computed tomography (CT) and magnetic resonance imaging (MRI), which may provide evidence of potential structural abnormalities in panic disorder, and (2) functional studies, such as positron emission tomography (PET) and single proton emission computed tomography (SPECT), which may suggest functional differences between patients with panic disorder and control subjects.

In general, PET and SPECT studies have indicated that patients with an asymmetrical increase in regional cerebral blood flow (right greater than left) in the parahippocampal areas of the temporal lobe and inferior prefrontal areas appear differentially susceptible to the effects of lactate-induced panic. Anxiety itself, irrespective of the mode of induction, is usually accompanied by a reduction in frontal cerebral blood flow. The specificity of such findings to panic disorder remains questionable. Available MRI studies have also indicated greater rates of temporal lobe abnormalities in patients with panic disorder than in healthy volunteers. However, the results of those studies should be considered preliminary, and the techniques employed are recommended only as research tools.

DIAGNOSIS AND CLINICAL FEATURES

PANIC ATTACK The essential feature of panic disorders is the panic attack. A panic attack is a discrete period of intense fear, discomfort, or apprehension during which at least 4 of the 13 symptoms listed in Table 18.1-1 develop abruptly, reaching a crescendo within 10 minutes after onset.

DSM-IV distinguishes three types of panic attacks on the basis of the context in which the attacks occur:

1. **Unexpected** (uncued, spontaneous): The onset of the panic attacks is not associated with a situational trigger (that is, the attacks occur totally unpredictably, "out of the blue").
2. **Situationally bound** (cued and invariably occurring): The attack invariably (or almost invariably) results immediately on exposure to, or in anticipation of, a situational trigger or cue (these attacks are totally predictable).
3. **Situationally predisposed** (cued but variably occurring): The attack is more likely to occur on exposure to the situational trigger but does not invariably occur and may not occur immediately after the exposure.

In the above definitions, the situational trigger may be any phobic stimulus, such as a dog (in the case of a specific phobia of animals), an activity (for example, speaking before an audience, in an individual with social phobia, or driving, in an individual with agoraphobia), or a place (high places in a person with a specific phobia of heights).

Determining the type of panic attack is critical for formulating an accurate differential diagnosis. In general, situationally bound attacks are most often observed in patients with specific and social phobias, situationally predisposed attacks are most common in patients with panic disorder with agoraphobia, and unexpected attacks are required for the diagnosis of panic disorder (with or without agoraphobia).

AGORAPHOBIA Agoraphobia may occur as a complication of panic disorder or, more rarely, in the absence of a history of panic disorder. In panic disorder with agoraphobia, the person avoids, or endures with intense anxiety, places or situations in which escape might be difficult or embarrassing, or in which help may not be available should a panic attack occur. Less commonly, the person may not avoid such situations but may need the presence of a companion (Table 17.1-3). Impairment is usually moderate to severe, and the disorder may be incapacitating.

PANIC DISORDER Several patterns may be observed in the development of the syndrome. Some patients experience recurrent, spontaneous panic attacks that are infrequent at first (months apart) but whose rate of occurrence soon spirals upward to weekly or daily. Others experience bursts of attacks during certain periods (called "bad days"), with few if any attacks during intermittent intervals (called "good days"). Still others report fairly regular attacks over long periods of time (for example, two to three attacks per month for nine months). There may also be isolated attacks (separated by years) that precede the full development of the syndrome.

Panic disorder may occur with or without agoraphobia. Even in the absence of agoraphobic avoidance, however, the degree of distress and disruption of functioning can be significant.

Panic disorder without agoraphobia A 26-year-old woman came to the clinic complaining of waves of terror and the effect they were having on her life. About one year earlier, while sitting at home watching television, she had experienced an inexplicable rush of anxiety ("like someone injected me with large doses of adrenaline") that was accompanied by a pounding heart, gasping for air, chest pain ("like someone was sitting on top of me"), numbness in her fingers and toes, and violent shaking. Although the attack subsided in minutes, she rushed to the emergency room of a local hospital, believing she had experienced a heart attack. All test results were negative.

About five months after the first attack she experienced another episode while walking to her job as a legal secretary. Again, the attack seemed to come out of nowhere. She took the day off from work and consulted a cardiologist. The results of all examinations were negative. The cardiologist told her that she was suffering from anxiety, and prescribed a mild tranquilizer.

A third attack with the same symptoms occurred three months later while the patient was in a supermarket. She became terrified, dropped her groceries, and ran home.

The attacks quickly escalated in frequency, from one every few weeks to weekly, then daily. There was no escaping them—they occurred at home, in restaurants, at work. Soon, she became so preoccupied with having the attacks that she could not concentrate on her work. When she was seen at the clinic, she had been experiencing multiple attacks daily for nearly two months.

Note that the patient's attacks were described by her as "inexplicable" and "seem[ing] to come out of nowhere" (that is, they were unexpected, uncued, spontaneous). The results of medical examinations were negative; no organic factor could be identified that initiated and maintained the disturbance. The patient's reactions to the attacks (rushing to an emergency room, consulting a cardiologist) are often observed in patients with panic disorder, who (understandably) think they are having a heart attack. Further, the patient became preoccupied with having the attacks. Although functional impairment was minimal (she had difficulty concentrating on her work, but there was no major disruption of occupational, home, or daily routine functioning), the panic attacks were a significant source of distress in her life.

Panic disorder with agoraphobia A 30-year-old college professor came to the clinic escorted by his wife. "I have to get my life back together. I have been out of work for nearly a month and, if it weren't for my wife accompanying me, I wouldn't be here now," he said.

About four months earlier, while attending a family picnic, he had suddenly become "nervous." His heart began to race "a mile a minute" and he began to perspire profusely, felt nauseated, experienced a tightness in his chest, and felt he was suffocating, "as if someone was smothering me with a pillow." The attack came on for no apparent reason and continued for about 15 minutes. It terrified him ("I thought that I was going to die"), so much so that he asked his wife to drive home for fear that he might have another attack while driving. Later that day he experienced a second attack while sitting on the porch with a neighbor.

During the next three weeks he underwent numerous examinations by different specialists (cardiologists, endocrinologists, gastroenterologists, and so forth), but the results of all tests were negative.

The attacks continued at a rate of two or three a week. The patient noticed that the attacks were more likely to occur in trains, although they did not always occur in that situation. He had already stopped driving to work (for fear of having an attack) and needed the train to get to work. He began to take early trains (6:00 AM) to work and late trains (7:00 PM) from work to avoid crowds that might block his escape route. Also, he would limit himself to local trains (versus expresses) "since they make more stops, and therefore the doors open more frequently." The anxiety experienced in anticipation of having an attack was almost as intense as the attacks themselves. Soon, he could no longer bear the extreme discomfort of riding in a train, and consequently took a leave of absence from work. In addition, his fear generalized to all crowded places (stores, banks, offices, streets) to the extent that he needed his wife to accompany him whenever he left the house.

When seen at the clinic, he was experiencing three or four attacks a week, was essentially housebound, and was in constant fear of having a fatal episode.

The second case history exemplifies several of the features that are typically observed in the development of panic disorder with agoraphobia. Although the initial attacks were spontaneous, some of the later attacks were situationally predisposed. That is, the patient noticed that the likelihood of having an attack was increased when he was on a train, although the attacks did not occur invariably in that situation. Also, he altered his daily routine (taking early and late trains) to enable him to escape rapidly in the event of an attack. (Some individuals with panic disorder report sitting in an aisle seat that is close to an exit in a movie theater for the same reason.) In addition to avoidance of driving, trains, and crowds, the patient experienced extreme anticipatory anxiety (worry about what would happen if he had an attack driving or while on the train). His inability to leave home unaccompanied is observed in severe cases of the disorder.

AGORAPHOBIA WITHOUT HISTORY OF PANIC DISORDER Agoraphobia in the absence of panic disorder is similar to panic disorder with agoraphobia. In both disorders the individual fears the sudden development of a symptom (or symptoms) and consequently avoids, endures with dread, or requires a companion in certain situations (Table 17.1-4). However, in the former, there is no history of panic disorder, and the focus of fear does not involve having a full panic attack.

A 60-year-old widowed proprietor of a large manufacturing company came to the clinic escorted by two of her employees. Until two years earlier her life had been rewarding and fulfilling. She and her husband had built a small company into a major enterprise. "I made all the decisions and fielded all the criticism and pessimism expressed by others; he supplied the money," she said. The patient continued to develop the business after her husband's death 15 years earlier. However, at age 58 she began to experience sudden spells of dizziness that came over her suddenly, for no known reason, and that continued for 5 to 10 minutes. Tests conducted by her neurologist and otolaryngologist failed to identify any organic cause for the spells.

Although the patient had not experienced an episode for nearly a year before she came to the clinic, the fear of becoming dizzy (and of falling and being injured) continued to have a profound effect on her life. For example, her housekeeper escorted her to the limousine each morning. When she arrived at her firm, she was met and escorted to her office by an employee. She could not walk down the hallway to the lavatory without being accompanied. All of her dependency needs revolved around the fear of sudden incapacitation and consequent injury resulting from a fall. Although that fear did not impair her keen business sense or her long-standing social relationships, it clearly pervaded her life.

Recently, her manufacturing company had experienced major financial difficulties beyond her control, and she was concerned about what her life would be like without a staff of housekeepers and business employees to rely on. "I cannot travel, shop, or even leave the house alone. The only time I feel safe is when I'm sitting down. I am even afraid to live at home alone, for fear that I may become dizzy and no one will be there to help me. What will become of me?"

If it were not for her relatively unique situation, in all likelihood the patient would have been totally incapacitated. Her entire life was arranged around her fear of sudden dizzy spells and their consequences. She became completely dependent on others, and even the thought of living alone, with no one around to help her in the event of a fall, terrified her.

Other symptoms that may be observed in agoraphobia without a history of panic disorder include fear of vomiting, fear of loss of bowel or bladder control, and any of the associated symptoms of panic attacks, among them depersonalization, choking, and palpitations (Table 17.1-1).

PATHOLOGY AND LABORATORY EXAMINATION

It is important for the clinician to rule out any medical condition that may present as panic disorder. On the other hand, it is not helpful to request exhaustive workups when the clinical presentation is best explained by panic disorder. A determination may be difficult since patients with panic disorder present with a plethora of somatic complaints. A careful history and physical examination may arouse suspicion of any potential medical problems. The general medical screening should include a complete blood cell count; electrolyte, fasting blood sugar, urea, creatinine, and calcium level determinations; liver panel; thyroid screen (for triiodothyronine [T_3], thyroxine [T_4], and thyroid-stimulating hormone [TSH]); urinalysis; and electrocardiography (ECG). Such a screen will rule out thyroid disease, hypoparathyroid disease, hypoglycemia, and certain cardiac conditions. Drug screens are advised if substance abuse is suspected. Further tests are warranted only if the clinical presentation suggests an organic etiology. In patients with chest pain and other risk factors for cardiac or pulmonary disease, a stress test, chest X-ray and cardiac enzyme determinations may be indicated. In patients with palpitations consisting of an irregular or rapid heartbeat, 24-hour ECG monitoring is recommended. Mitral valve prolapse (MVP) is confirmed by echocardiography but is of doubtful clinical significance. If hyperventilation is accompanied by organic features, chest radiography and pulmonary function tests may be required. Suspicious neurological symptoms, such as weakness, loss of consciousness, disorientation, olfactory hallucinations, and other symptoms suggestive of temporal lobe epilepsy, space-occupying lesions, or multiple sclerosis, should be investigated by careful neurological or otoneurological examination and, if indicated, by EEG, CT, or MRI. Less common conditions, such as carcinoid syndrome, pheochromocytoma, and porphyria, can be ruled out by 24-hour urine assay for 5-hydroxyindoleacetic acid (5-HIAA) and catecholamines or urine assay for porphobilinogen, respectively.

No currently available laboratory tests are diagnostic for panic disorder. Although challenge procedures using intravenous sodium lactate or oral yohimbine may produce panic attacks in the majority of individuals with the disorder, those tests should not be employed for diagnostic purposes. Similarly, neuroimaging techniques, such as PET, that indicate abnormal limbic activity in certain patients with panic disorder have significant research implications but are not adequately refined for routine diagnostic purposes.

DIFFERENTIAL DIAGNOSIS

MEDICAL CONDITIONS Several nonpsychiatric medical conditions and organic factors can mimic the symptoms of panic disorder (Table 17.1-6).

The onset of panic disorder after age 45 years is rare. Therefore, if a patient reports that the first spontaneous panic attack (in a series of attacks) occurred after age 45, an organic factor should be considered.

The presence of atypical symptoms during an attack is also a red flag, even if the full criteria for a panic attack (Table 17.1-1) are met. Such atypical symptoms include true vertigo; loss of balance, consciousness, or bladder or bowel control; headaches; slurred speech; amnesia; and hunger pangs.

TABLE 17.1-6
Medical Conditions and Other Organic Factors that Can Present as Panic Disorder

Thyroid dysfunction
Hyperthyroidism
Hypothyroidism
Parathyroid dysfunction
Hyperparathyroidism
Adrenal dysfunction
Pheochromocytoma
Vestibular dysfunction
Seizure disorders
Central nervous system stimulant (e.g., cocaine, amphetamines) intoxication
Central nervous system depressant (e.g., alcohol, barbiturates) withdrawal
Cardiac conditions (e.g., arrhythmias, supraventricular tachycardia, mitral valve prolapse)
Hypoglycemia(?)

Thyroid dysfunction Anxiety is commonly described by patients with hyperthyroidism and hypothyroidism. Thus, patients presenting with panic attacks should undergo routine thyroid function tests, including those that assess TSH levels.

Parathyroid dysfunction Less often, hyperparathyroidism may present as panic disorder. Tests for serum calcium levels are needed to rule out the condition.

Adrenal dysfunction Pheochromocytoma is a rare condition in which a tumor of the adrenal medulla causes hypersecretion of catecholamines. Symptoms include anxiety, headaches, tachycardia, sweating, flushes, trembling, and hypertension. When a pheochromocytoma is suspected, urinary catecholamine metabolite concentrations should be monitored for 24 hours.

Vestibular dysfunction The vestibular system includes the labyrinths, the vestibular nerve, the nuclei within the medulla, and the pathways to the cerebellum and cerebrum. Interruption of the vestibular system can produce vertigo (spinning sensation), often accompanied by nausea, vomiting, ataxia, and anxiety. When vestibular dysfunction is suspected, an otolaryngologist or neurologist should be consulted.

Seizure disorders Seizure disorders, notably temporal lobe epilepsy, may also manifest with symptoms of panic anxiety. Patients who report other symptoms that suggest an organic syndrome (for example, olfactory hallucinations) should undergo EEG, and a neurologist should be consulted.

Intoxication and withdrawal syndromes Panic attacks may result from CNS stimulant intoxication (for example, by amphetamines, caffeine, cocaine), as well as from CNS depressant withdrawal (from alcohol, barbiturates). Although the recent use of those substances is easily detected on urine or serum tests, it must be determined whether the substance initiated and maintained the disturbance before panic disorder can be ruled out. The relation of the substance to the disturbance can be established by obtaining a detailed history and by prospective monitoring. Many persons with panic disorder and other anxiety syndromes may abuse alcohol and other substances to combat their symptoms.

Cardiac conditions Numerous cardiovascular conditions can mimic a panic attack, among them cardiac arrhythmias (irregular heart rhythms or beats) and supraventricular (atrial or nodal) tachycardia. In such cases the patient's chief complaint usually is severe chest pain, skipped beats, or an accelerated heart rate. ECG is warranted.

MVP, a condition characterized by a displacement or bowing of the mitral valve back into the left atrium during systole, is mentioned here because considerable research has focused on the condition's relationship to panic disorder. Those studies reported widely discrepant findings, probably as a result of different methods for diagnosing MVP, poor interrater reliability within the same method, nonblind assessments, sample selection biases, inadequate control groups, and a host of other factors. In general, the studies suggest that (1) a significant minority of patients with panic disorder have MVP; (2) the prevalence of panic disorder in patients with MVP does not differ significantly from that in the general population; and (3) the identification of MVP in patients with panic disorder has little or no clinical or prognostic significance regarding the treatment of spontaneous panic attacks. DSM-IV specifically indicates that the diagnosis of panic disorder is not precluded if MVP is observed.

Hypoglycemia During the 1950s several popular books purported that idiopathic hypoglycemia was implicated in the development of numerous mental disorders. Recent, methodologically refined studies have not supported those claims. A substantial minority of persons in the normal (nonanxious) population have at least one blood sugar value in the abnormal range when administered a standard five-hour glucose tolerance test (GTT). The test-retest reliability of the GTT is often below acceptable standards, and false positives may result from chronic dieting and other factors. Finally, provocative testing with insulin in patients with panic disorder has not supported a relationship. Taken together, the data suggest it is highly unlikely that hypoglycemia plays a role in the pathogenesis of panic disorder.

A number of medical conditions can produce hypoglycemia, among them insulin overdose, unusually strenuous activity in a diabetic patient, liver dysfunction (for example, cirrhosis), and pancreatic cancer. The hypoglycemia that occurs in those conditions may manifest with somatic symptoms that partially overlap the symptoms experienced during a panic attack. However, a full medical history usually clarifies the differential diagnosis by revealing symptoms or other evidence of the coexisting medical condition. In addition, although certain symptoms (such as sweating, trembling, palpitations, and paresthesias) can occur during both panic attacks and hypoglycemic episodes, others (slurred speech, blurred vision, hunger pangs, sedation) are specific to hypoglycemia.

MENTAL DISORDERS Although laboratory examinations can generally be relied on to rule out medical conditions that mimic panic disorder, there are no definitive tests that would rule out other psychiatric disorders. Panic attacks are ubiquitous in psychiatry, and they often occur in patients with anxiety as well as in those with nonanxiety mental disorders. Further, there is substantial comorbidity among patients with panic disorder: Those individuals frequently have concurrent mood, substance abuse, or (other) anxiety syndromes. Therefore, the differential diagnosis of panic disorder requires a skilled, careful, and comprehensive interview evaluation.

Panic attack type DSM-IV distinguishes three types of panic attacks—unexpected, situationally bound, and situationally predisposed. Distinguishing among the three is critical for formulating an accurate differential diagnosis.

Panic disorder is always associated with spontaneous or unexpected panic attacks. Although panic attacks may occur intermittently in any syndrome, spontaneous attacks are required for a diagnosis of panic disorder.

Situationally bound attacks are most often observed in persons with specific phobia and persons with social phobia. For example, persons with a specific phobia of enclosed spaces might become panic-stricken whenever they enter a small room with no windows, and persons with a social phobia of writing in public might experience a full-blown panic attack when required to sign a check in the presence of a bank teller.

Situationally bound panic attacks are also observed in other anxiety and nonanxiety disorders. Patients with obsessive-compulsive disorder might experience panic attacks whenever they attempt to resist obsessions or compulsions; patients with posttraumatic stress disorder, whenever they are exposed to situations that resemble the trauma; and patients with psychotic disorder, whenever they experience distressing hallucinations.

Situationally predisposed panic attacks are most often observed in the later stages of panic disorder with agoraphobia but may also occur in social and specific phobias. By definition, the probability of having those attacks is increased in certain situations. For example, an individual with social phobia might state, "I get nervous, but usually don't panic, when eating in the presence of others. However, my chances of having an anxiety attack are greatest in this situation."

A second aspect of situationally predisposed panic attacks is that the attacks may not occur immediately after exposure to the situational trigger. For example, a person with panic disorder with agoraphobia might state, "I never know when, or if, I will panic when in a crowded room. Sometimes the attack comes on shortly after I enter the room, sometimes 20 minutes later, and sometimes not at all."

In the usual development of panic disorder with agoraphobia, the patient initially experiences recurrent, spontaneous panic attacks that later become associated with certain situations (situationally predisposed attacks). Anticipatory anxiety (anxiety about having future attacks) and avoidance (of agoraphobic situations) follow.

Focus of fear and avoidance Another important aspect of establishing an accurate differential diagnosis of panic disorder with agoraphobia is determining what the patient fears. In general, all phobic disorders (specific phobia, social phobia, and agoraphobia) are characterized by a fear of what will happen in the situation rather than by the phobic stimulus itself. In specific phobia of heights, the individual fears falling, not tall buildings, ladders, or mountains; in specific phobia of driving, the individual fears hitting someone or having an accident, not automobiles; in specific phobia of flying, the individual fears crashing, not planes.

In social phobia, although phobic situations are associated with concerns about scrutiny, humiliation, and embarrassment, actual fears vary across situations. For example, in the social phobia of eating in public, the individual fears dribbling or spilling a drink, not restaurants; in the social phobia of speaking in public, the individual fears becoming tongue-tied or forgetting lines; of attending social affairs, the individual fears saying something stupid or not knowing how to act, not the affair itself.

In panic disorder with agoraphobia, the individual fears the inability to escape, becoming embarrassed, or not being able to get help in the event of having a panic attack. In a sense, the particular agoraphobic situations are inconsequential. For example, fear of crowds by itself is diagnostically uninterpretable unless the focus of fear is known. The fear may represent specific phobia, social phobia, or agoraphobia, depending on what the individual fears will happen when in the situation.

The logic may also be extended to avoidance behavior. A patient with obsessive-compulsive disorder may avoid public lavatories because of concern over not being able to resist hand washing compulsions. A patient with a major depressive disorder may avoid social gatherings as a result of low self-esteem and diminished interests. A patient with paranoid schizophrenia may exhibit pervasive avoidance (become housebound) because of persecutory delusions.

The main point is that symptoms are of limited diagnostic value when viewed out of context, and determining the focus of fear is critical for establishing a diagnosis of panic disorder with agoraphobia.

Comorbid disorders and secondary or associated symptoms With the suspension of most diagnostic hierarchies, which was implemented in DSM-III-R and retained in DSM-IV, diagnoses of comorbid (or dual) disorders are permitted provided that the criteria for both (or all) are fully met. For example, prior to 1987 (DSM-III-R), panic attacks that were limited to a period of major depression were considered associated features of the depressive syndrome, regardless of the type and frequency of the attacks. Presently, if the criteria for panic disorder and major depressive disorder are fulfilled, both disorders are diagnosed.

Dysphoric mood is common in patients with panic disorder, and intermittent panic attacks are not uncommon in patients with major depressive disorder. However, both disorders are diagnosed only if the complete panic and mood syndromes are present.

Several studies of community and clinic samples have shown that panic and mood disorders often coexist. Further, there is considerable comorbidity among the anxiety disorders. However, caution must be exercised when formulating dual diagnoses. Consider the diagnoses of panic disorder and social phobia. As panic disorder develops, the person begins to avoid the usual agoraphobic situations (public transportation, bridges, crowds, and the like); in addition, the person begins to avoid large, formal affairs (such as weddings) for the same reason—fear of not being able to escape rapidly in the event of experiencing a panic attack. When asked, "Are you concerned that you might become humiliated at weddings?" the individual responds, "Sure. Wouldn't you be embarrassed if you had a panic attack in front of a large group of people?" No new syndrome has developed in that case, for the individual's fear of having a panic attack has been the core disturbance throughout. Although large, formal affairs are generally considered social situations (because others are present), the individual's focus of fear clearly discounts an additional diagnosis of social phobia.

Substance intoxication and withdrawal syndromes can present with panic attacks. However, individuals with panic disorder often self-medicate, and comorbid substance abuse (particularly of marijuana, alcohol, or cocaine) is not uncommon. If it can be established that the substance initiated and maintained the panic syndrome, then the diagnosis of panic disorder would be ruled out. However, a panic disorder diagnosis may be appropriate if, although the first panic attack occurred in conjunction with drug use (for example, cocaine), attacks continue in the absence of further use.

In somatization disorder, complaints of palpitations, shortness of breath, chest pain, dizziness, and nausea are common. Those symptoms are described in the context of a chronic disturbance that is characterized by recurrent and multiple somatic complaints involving several organ systems. However, panic disorder may coexist with somatization disorder, in which case both diagnoses are made.

COURSE AND PROGNOSIS

Relatively little information is available on the course and long-term prognosis of panic disorder. Prospective, large-scale, epidemiologically sampled studies that would answer those questions have not been done. The available information is derived from retrospective life history and naturalistic follow-up studies of treated patients.

Panic disorder usually begins in late adolescence or early adulthood. Some studies suggest a bimodal age at onset, with a second, smaller peak occurring between ages 35 and 40 years. Childhood onset has been increasingly reported. Because specific effective treatments for panic disorder are readily available, panic disorder is an important consideration in the differential diagnosis of children and young adolescents presenting with anxiety and phobias.

The lifetime course of panic disorder in clinical settings is often chronic but fluctuating. In some individuals a pattern associating particular types of life events (for example, the loss of a significant interpersonal relationship through death or separation) with relapse is observed. In general, however, risk factors associated with relapse or remission are not well understood.

Despite its chronicity, the long-term prognosis of panic disorder is good. A recent review of naturalistic studies indicated that at one- to eight-year follow-up, 30 to 40 percent of patients were well, 30 to 50 percent were symptomatic but able to lead relatively normal lives, and only 10 to 20 percent were still significantly ill and impaired. However, as the naturalistic follow-up methodology used to collect those data did not control for treatment type or duration, the extent to which outcome reflects inherent characteristics of the illness versus variations in treatment, compliance, or other unknown confounding variables is not known.

COMPLICATIONS AND COMORBIDITY Phobic avoidance and agoraphobia are common complications of recurrent panic attacks. In clinical settings, avoidance is reported by 70 to 90 percent of patients with panic disorder, and agoraphobia is reported by 30 to 40 percent.

A lifetime history of major depressive disorder is reported by 40 to 80 percent of patients with panic disorder. In most cases the depression follows the onset of panic attacks. However, in one fourth to one third of clinical cases, the depressive disorder is reported to have occurred before or simultaneous with the onset of panic attacks.

Alcohol and substance abuse are also frequent sequelae. Individuals with panic disorder often report use of alcohol or unprescribed benzodiazepines or sedative-hypnotics to alleviate anxiety and enable them to carry out their normal routine. In some cases the alleviation is only temporary and tolerance may develop; repeated use may lead to substance abuse and substance dependence.

A series of recent studies indicated an association between a lifetime history of panic disorder and an increased risk for suicide attempts, as compared to the risk in the general population without psychiatric disorders. Whether that finding reflects an association or predictive risk has not been established.

TREATMENT

Three main approaches are currently employed in the treatment of panic disorder: pharmacotherapy, cognitive-behavioral therapy, and a combination of the two modalities. The relative merits of the varied strategies have prompted widespread and unresolved controversy. Unfortunately, neither definitive comparative outcome data nor empirically based guidelines for optimum matching of patients to specific treatments are available. In that context the National Institute of Mental Health Consensus Conference on Treatment of Panic Disorder has recommended that at the time of the diagnostic evaluation, the clinician should provide the patient with information about procedures and the advantages and disadvantages of each of the various treatment approaches. The decision about which treatment to use should be made in conjunction with the patient and his or her specific history and concerns.

Almost all panic disorder patients can achieve marked improvement with appropriate treatment. If the initial treatment approach does not produce clear change in 8 to 10 weeks, then reevaluation is essential.

Dynamically based treatments may be useful as an adjunctive modality but, because of a lack of systematic evidence supporting their efficacy, they should not be considered a primary or exclusive treatment form.

PHARMACOLOGICAL TREATMENT

Treatment strategy The context in which medication is administered is as critical to the successful psychopharmacological treatment of panic disorder as are the correct choice and dosage of medication. At the start of treatment it is important to establish a physician-patient relationship that ensures respectful attention to the patient's many worries, realistic reassurance, and a willingness to be available should any unexpected problems arise. Many panic patients are particularly apprehensive about taking medication. Therefore, it is important to carefully ascertain each individual's fear regarding medication. Reassurance, particularly with regard to the safety of the medication and the physician's availability and responsiveness should problems arise, is emphasized.

During the initial visits the physician provides an explanation of the treatment and what the patient can expect to happen. To establish a common vocabulary between patient and physician, the three components of the disorder—panic attacks, anticipatory anxiety, and avoidance—are defined and the patient's specific experience of each is reviewed. It is explained that the medication is used to block the core psychophysiological component of recurrent unexpected panic attacks. Anticipatory anxiety and avoidance arise from concerns about the implications of the attacks and a desire to avoid situations in which attacks are likely to occur. Once the panic attacks are blocked by medication, the patient will be able to venture into phobic situations without risking a panic attack. In most cases the persistence of the panic blockade over time in the face of increasing range of activity leads to a gradual decrease in both avoidance and worry.

Patients vary in the degree to which they need encouragement to tackle further phobic situations once protected from the risk of panic. In most cases the addition of systematic exposure or instruction in cognitive exercises is helpful.

Antipanic medications Several types of medications (tricyclic antidepressants, monoamine oxidase inhibitors [MAOIs], and high-potency benzodiazepines) have been demonstrated in controlled studies to be effective in the acute treatment of panic. Several serotonergic agents, although less systematically studied, also show promise.

TRICYCLIC DRUGS The antipanic efficacy of imipramine has been demonstrated in over a dozen placebo-controlled double-blind studies. The acute effect of imipramine administration is to block the reuptake of the neurotransmitters norepinephrine and serotonin from the synaptic cleft into the presynaptic neuron. Despite a large body of research, the ultimate mechanism of imipramine's antipanic effect, which occurs three to six weeks later, remains undetermined.

Starting doses for treating panic disorder should be lower than those used for depression. Imipramine is started at 10 mg a day, and the dosage is increased by cautious titration. For example, 10 mg a day may be given for three days, followed by 20 mg a day for three days, with the dosage then increased by 10 mg a day every two to four days, depending on the patient's tolerance. Patients with panic disorder are notoriously sensitive to tricyclics, and if the initial dose is not sufficiently low, the trial may be aborted by the patient. Despite that, many patients require at least 200 mg a day to block panic attacks. Therefore, careful dosage titration up to 300 mg a day is indicated if an adequate response is not achieved at lower doses. Plasma levels of tricyclics can also be obtained; the reader is referred to other sources regarding their indication.

Other tricyclics, such as desipramine (Norpramin), amitriptyline (Elavil), doxepin (Adapin, Sinequan), and nortriptyline (Pamelor), may be effective in panic disorder, although double-blind studies have not been performed on these agents. Clomipramine (Anafranil), a tricyclic recently introduced into the United States, is distinguished from other tricyclics by its highly selective serotonin reuptake blockade. Clomipramine appears at least as effective as imipramine in comparative double-blind, placebo-controlled studies, and there is some evidence that it may be superior to imipramine in blocking panic symptoms. The usual antipanic doses of clomipramine range from 10 to 100 mg a day. As in the case of imipramine, a low starting dose (10 mg) and slow titration (10 to 20 mg a week) are important.

Tricyclic drugs are not well tolerated by all patients. Besides the uncomfortable anticholinergic side effects (dry mouth, constipation), cardiac conduction and hepatic effects, orthostasis, and weight gain may preclude their usage. They are also extremely dangerous in overdose. Paradoxical excitement and nervousness can also be a problem but may usually be diminished or avoided by using low doses and increasing the dosage slowly.

MONOAMINE OXIDASE INHIBITORS The MAOIs (for example, phenelzine [Nardil]) are also effective antipanic agents. The MAOIs, similar to tricyclic drugs, increase synaptic norepinephrine, serotonin, and dopamine by inhibiting the extraneuronal enzyme MAO from metabolizing monoamines. As with the tricyclic antidepressants, the mechanism of antipanic activity remains undetermined. Three to six weeks of drug administration is necessary for the onset of action. The MAOIs are started in low dosages (such as 15 mg a day of Nardil) but may require dosages comparable to those used in depression for effectiveness (for example, 75 to 90 mg a day). The main drawback of the MAOIs is their propensity to produce the tyramine effect. Blockade of gut MAO allows pressor substances, such as tyramine, to enter the systemic circulation and produce a hypertensive crisis. Patients taking MAOIs must therefore adhere to a strict diet in which tyramine-rich foods (such as cheese and red wine) and medications that contain pressor substances (nasal decongestants) are avoided. Other side effects include orthostasis, weight gain, and sexual dysfunction. Although not generally used as first-line agents, MAOIs can be extremely effective in patients with panic and atypical depression (that is, characterized by mood reactivity) or who are otherwise nonresponsive to treatment.

BENZODIAZEPINES The initial view was that benzodiazepines were effective in decreasing anticipatory anxiety but not in blocking panic. That idea has been revised with the advent of high-potency benzodiazepines (for example, alprazolam [Xanax], clonazepam [Klonopin]) that are effective antipanic medications. Those agents are believed to attach to benzodiazepine receptors in the brain, components of the ubiquitous central benzodiazepine-GABA receptor complex. Activation of the benzodiazepine receptor enhances affinity of the GABA receptor for GABA. Activation of GABA receptor sites produces inhibitory effects on the neuron by enhancing chloride conductance through neuronal membrane chloride ionophores. The precise site of action necessary for the antipanic effects of the benzodiazepines is unknown.

The starting dose for alprazolam is 0.25 to 0.5 mg three times a day. If tolerated, the dosage is gradually increased by 0.25 to 0.5 mg every two to three days. Most patients are maintained on a daily dose of 2 to 6 mg divided into a three or four times a day schedule, although dosages up to 8 mg a day may be needed in some cases.

Antipanic doses of clonazepam are slightly lower, and a twice daily dose schedule is generally well tolerated. Clonazepam is usually started at a dosage of 0.25 to 0.5 mg twice a day and increased by 0.25 to 0.5 mg every three to five days. Most patients with panic can be maintained on 1 to 3 mg a day.

Recent studies indicate that conventional benzodiazepines (for example, diazepam [Valium], lorazepam [Ativan]) may, in high doses, also block panic attacks in some patients. However, sufficient supporting data are not yet available to justify recommending those medications as primary treatment for panic disorder.

The main side effect of the benzodiazepines is sedation, but patients usually accommodate over three to four days. Because therapeutic effects are observed within the first week of treatment, benzodiazepines are particularly useful when therapeutic effects are rapidly desired. Because of the possibility for dependence and abuse, the benzodiazepines should be avoided in patients with a history of substance or alcohol abuse. Gradual tapering is necessary when discontinuing those drugs, as abrupt cessation may result in seizures, and even rapid tapering may result in severe discomfort (anxiety, headaches, tremor, muscle aches, insomnia). Clinicians are generally advised to taper the dosage of alprazolam or clonazepam by approximately 0.25 to 0.5 mg a week. Tapering in even smaller decrements may be necessary in the final phases. Cross-tolerance between high-potency and conventional-potency benzodiazepines has been incompletely studied, and switching between those classes of drugs should be done carefully.

SEROTONIN-SPECIFIC REUPTAKE INHIBITORS The SSRIs, a recently developed group of agents characterized by their ability to selectively inhibit the reuptake of serotonin, also have powerful antipanic properties. Published double-blind studies have been performed with only two of those agents, fluvoxamine (Luvox) and zimelidine, although zimelidine has been withdrawn because it produced Guillain-Barré syndrome. Fluvoxamine appears as effective as clomipramine in blind comparative trials, which suggested an efficacy similar to that of the tricyclics. Fluoxetine (Prozac), sertraline (Zoloft), and paroxetine (Paxil) are agents of the SSRI class now available in the United States. Although SSRIs appeared effective in open trials, controlled studies have not been published. Like the tricyclics, SSRIs should be started in very low doses (for example, 2.5 mg a day for fluoxetine) to avoid initial excitement or stimulation, and increased slowly. For fluoxetine, the effective dosage ranges from 5 to 60 mg a day. For sertraline, a starting dosage of 25 mg every other day is recommended, with slow titration up to 50 to 100 mg a day. For paroxetine, a starting dosage of 10 mg every other day is recommended, with slow titration up to 20 to 40 mg a day. Besides anxiety induction, SSRIs may also cause gastrointestinal distress, hypomania, headaches, sexual dysfunction, and insomnia. The major advantages of SSRIs over tricyclic drugs are the absence of anticholinergic side effects, less or no weight gain, less orthostasis, and no cardiac conduction defects. They are also relatively safe in overdose.

DRUGS NOT EFFECTIVE IN PANIC DISORDER Certain drugs are not effective in panic disorder. Buproprion (Wellbutrin), an antidepressant with dopaminergic effects, does not block panic. The tetracyclic antidepressant maprotiline (Ludiomil), a specific noradrenergic reuptake inhibitor, and deprenyl (Eldepryl), a selective MAO_B inhibitor, are also antidepressants without significant antipanic effects. Results with trazadone (Deseryl), an agent with complex serotonergic effects, are conflicting. Buspirone (BuSpar), a serotonin type 1A ($5\text{-}HT_{1A}$) partial receptor antagonist, and ritanserin, a $5\text{-}HT_2$ antagonist, both anxiolytics, are also ineffective. β-Adrenergic receptor antagonists, such as propranolol (Inderal), may block palpitations and other cardiovascular symptoms but do not block actual panic attacks. In general, because of dependency and toxicity factors, other anxiolytics, such as barbiturates and meprobamate (Miltown), should be avoided.

COGNITIVE-BEHAVIORAL TREATMENTS Early behavioral techniques focused primarily on in vivo exposure with the intention of ameliorating agoraphobic avoidance. The field has subsequently evolved to include specific antipanic strategies involving a number of treatment modalities. The best studied cognitive-behavioral approaches have been demonstrated as effective in controlled clinical trials. The relative effectiveness, however, of psychological versus pharmacological therapy or of a combination of both remains controversial. It is also unclear whether severity of illness may determine differential responsivity. Four main forms of treatment have been proposed: (1) cognitive therapy and psychoeducation, (2) applied relaxation, (3) respiratory control techniques, and (4) in vivo exposure.

Cognitive therapy Patients are initially informed that their panic attacks are the result of a misinterpretation of bodily sensations as more dangerous than they actually are and do not represent an immediately impending physical or mental disaster. Cognitive restructuring techniques have therefore been developed to address the beliefs and misattributions that may contribute to the induction and maintenance of panic attacks. The first step is to provide the patient with accurate information concerning the likelihood that their somatic symptoms are innocuous. The second step is to explain to the patient that, even in the event of a panic attack, the symptoms are invariably time-limited and are not as disruptive as the patient predicts. Cognitive techniques are continued in conjunction with other techniques.

Applied relaxation Relaxation training employs exercises to reduce arousal levels and may help instill a sense of control over panic attacks if and when they do occur. Relaxation training includes progressive muscle relaxation and imaginative techniques. Paradoxically, for some patients, relaxation may, at times and through unknown mechanisms, precipitate panic.

Respiratory control techniques Respiratory control techniques are employed to address the hyperventilation that consistently accompanies panic attacks. In fact, a range of symptoms experienced during panic attacks have been attributed to hyperventilation, including dizziness, breathlessness, faintness, and paresthesias. The main objective of breathing retraining is to increase the pressure of carbon dioxide in the blood by reducing the amount (rate or depth) of respiration. That effect is believed to mediate panic reduction.

Exposure therapy Exposure-based techniques have long been employed for avoidance symptoms. The fundamental premise is confrontation with the feared stimulus. Although exposure has traditionally consisted of exposure to external stimuli, as in the case of agoraphobia, the focus has now shifted to additional exposure to feared internal stimuli. Interoceptive exposure may therefore reduce panic attacks by exposing subjects to their feared somatic sensations. For example, if a patient is afraid of dizziness, deliberate encouragement of hyperventilation will show the patient that symptoms can be brought on without threatening survival. Although imaginal techniques have been effectively used in exposure treatments, in vivo techniques appear superior with respect to agoraphobia.

COMBINED PHARMACOLOGICAL AND COGNITIVE-BEHAVIORAL TREATMENT Studies of combination treatments that use medication and various cognitive-behavioral therapies have yielded discrepant results, possibly because of methodological flaws, patient selection, or investigator bias. The available data suggest that in the aggregate, combined pharmacotherapy (imipramine) plus behavioral treatment may be modestly more effective than either approach alone. However, as most patients respond extremely well to a single treatment modality, at present the decision to use combined treatment is probably best made on a case-by-case basis and in response to specific clinical needs. Methodologically rigorous studies are under way that address those issues and compare more specific panic control therapies with imipramine, and their combination.

Selection of patients for cognitive-behavioral treatments Cognitive-behavioral approaches may be particularly useful for patients who fear or are opposed to medications or for medically ill patients in whom side effects from medications may be dangerous. However, certain patients with panic disorder, including those with clinical depression or substance abuse, should not receive cognitive-behavioral therapy as primary treatment. Comorbid psychopathology that is not directly addressed is likely to interfere with antipanic treatment. In such cases initial evaluation for pharmacotherapy may be advisable. Cognitive-behavioral treatment for panic disorder, if appropriate, may be started after comorbid conditions have been removed.

OTHER PSYCHOTHERAPEUTIC APPROACHES Prior to the development of effective specific interventions, supportive psychotherapy was frequently used in the treatment of panic disorder and agoraphobia. Some patients reported reduction in anxiety and improvement in other areas of their life (such as interpersonal relationships). However, there is no evidence that such treatment led to the resolution of specific panic or phobic symptoms. Some studies suggest that supportive psychotherapy is as effective an adjunct to medication as specific cognitive-behavioral techniques. Recent preliminary work suggests that supportive psychotherapy in conjunction with education about panic disorder may be as helpful as some specific cognitive-behavioral treatments. Comparisons with medication alone or with a combination of medication plus cognitive-behavioral treatment have not been reported. However, supportive psychotherapy alone is not recommended as primary treatment for panic disorder or agoraphobia.

SUGGESTED CROSS-REFERENCES

Other anxiety disorders are covered in the other sections in Chapter 17. Learning theory and conditioning are the subject of Section 3.3. Psychoanalysis is treated in Section 31.1, behavior therapy in Section 31.2, and cognitive therapy in Section 31.6. Various biological therapies are reviewed in Chapter 32.

REFERENCES

Angst J, Vollrath M: The natural history of anxiety disorders. Acta Psychiatr Scand *84:* 446, 1991.

Ballenger J C, editor: *Neurobiology of Panic Disorder.* Wiley-Liss, New York, 1990.

*Ballenger J C, Burrows G D, DuPont R L, Lesser I M, Noyes R, Pecknold J C, Rifkin A, Swinson R P: Alprazolam in panic disorder and agoraphobia: Results from a multicenter trial. I. Efficacy in short-term treatment. Arch Gen Psychiatry *45:* 413, 1988.

Ballenger J C, Fyer A J: DSM-IV in progress: Examining criteria for panic disorder. Hosp Community Psychiatry *44* (3): 226, 1993.

Barlow D H: *Anxiety and Its Disorders: The Nature and Treatment of Anxiety and Panic.* Guilford, New York, 1988.

Breier A, Charney D S, Heninger G R: Major depression in patients with agoraphobia and panic disorder. Arch Gen Psychiatry *41:* 1129, 1984.

Carey G, Gottesman I I: Twin and family studies of anxiety, phobic, and obsessive disorders. In *Anxiety: New Research and Changing Concepts,* D F Klein, J G Rabkin, editors, p 117. Raven, New York, 1981.

Coplan J D, Gorman J M, Klein D F: Serotonin-related function in panic disorder: A critical overview. Neuropsychopharmacology *6* (3): 189, 1992.

Crowe R R: The genetics of panic disorder and agoraphobia. Psychiatr Dev *2:* 171, 1985.

*Freud S: Inhibitions, symptoms and anxiety. In *Standard Edition of the Complete Psychological Works of Sigmund Freud,* vol 20, p 77. Hogarth Press, London, 1966.

Freud S: Obsessions and phobias. In *Standard Edition of the Complete Psychological Works of Sigmund Freud,* vol 3, p 71. Hogarth Press, London, 1966.

Freud S: On the grounds for detaching a particular syndrome from neurasthenia under the description "anxiety neurosis." In *Standard Edition of the Complete Psychological Works of Sigmund Freud,* vol 3, p 90. Hogarth Press, London, 1966.

*Fyer A J, Sandberg D, Klein D F: Psychopharmacological treatment of panic disorder and agoraphobia. In *Panic Disorder and Agoraphobia: A Comprehensive Guide for the Practitioner,* G R Norton, C Ross, J R Walker, editors, p 211. Brooks-Cole, Pacific Grove, CA, 1991.

Gorman J M, Liebowitz M R, Fyer A J, Stein J: A neuroanatomical hypothesis for panic disorder. Am J Psychiatry *146:* 148, 1989.

Hirschfeld R M A: The clinical course of panic disorder and agoraphobia. In *Handbook of Anxiety,* vol 5, G D Burrows, editor. Elsevier Science, Amsterdam, 1990.

*Katon W: *Panic Disorder in the Medical Setting.* National Institute of Mental Health, Washington, 1989.

Kendler K S, Neale M C, Kessler R C, Heath A C, Eaves L J: Panic disorder in women: A population based twin study. Psychol Med *23* (2): 397, 1993.

Kessler R C, McGonagle K A, Zhao S, Nelson C B, Hughes M, Esh-

leman S, Wittchen H U, Kendler K S: Lifetime and 12-month prevalance of DSM-III-R psychiatric disorders in the United States: Results from the National Comorbidity Survey. Arch Gen Psychiatry *51:* 8, 1994.
*Klein D F: Delineation of two drug-responsive anxiety syndromes. Psychopharmacology *5:* 397, 1964.
Klein D F: False suffocation alarms, spontaneous panics, and related conditions: An integrative hypothesis. Arch Gen Psychiatry *50:* 306, 1993.
Klein D F, Rabkin J G, editors: *Anxiety: New Research and Changing Concepts.* Raven, New York, 1981.
Klerman G L, Weissman M M, Ouellette R, Johnson J, Greenwald S: Panic attacks in the community: Social morbidity and health care utilization. JAMA *265:* 742, 1991.
Mannuzza S, Fyer A J, Liebowitz M R, Klein D F: Delineating the boundaries of social phobia: Its relationship to panic disorder and agoraphobia. J Anx Disord *4:* 41, 1990.
Markowitz J S, Weissman M M, Ouelette R, Lish J D, Klerman G L: Quality of life in panic disorder. Arch Gen Psychiatry *46:* 984, 1989.
Marks I M: *Fears and Phobias.* Academic Press, New York, 1969.
Maser J D, Cloninger C R, editors: *Comorbidity of Mood and Anxiety Disorders.* American Psychiatric Press, Washington, 1990.
Maser J D, Wolfe B E: Origins and overview of the Consensus Development Conference on the Treatment of Panic Disorder. In *Treatment of Panic Disorder,* J D Maser, B E Wolfe, editors, p 3. American Psychiatric Press, Washington, 1994.
Noyes R, Crowe R R, Harris E L, Hamra B J, McChesney C M, Chaudhry D R: Relationship between panic disorder and agoraphobia: A family study. Arch Gen Psychiatry *43:* 227, 1986.
Papp L A, Coplan J D, Gorman J M: Biological markers in anxiety disorders. In *Review of Psychiatry,* vol 13, J M Oldham, M B Riba, editors. American Psychiatric Press, Washington, 1994.
Pollack M H, Otto M W, Rosenbaum J F, Sachs G S, O'Neil C, Asher R, Meltzer-Brody S: Longitudinal course of panic disorder: Findings from the Massachusetts General Hospital naturalistic study. J Clin Psychiatry *51* (12, Suppl A): 12, 1990.
Roth M: The phobic-anxiety-depersonalization syndrome. Proc R Soc Med *52:* 587, 1959.
Schneier F R, Liebowitz M R, Davies S O, et al: Fluoxetine in panic disorder. J Clin Psychopharmacol *10* (2): 119, 1990.
Torgersen S: Genetic factors in anxiety disorders. Arch Gen Psychiatry *40:* 1085, 1983.
Uhde T W, Boulenger J P, Roy-Byrne P P, Geraci M R, Vittone B J, Post R M: Longitudinal course of panic disorder. Prog Neuropsychopharm Biol Psychiatry *9:* 39, 1985.
Von Korff M R, Eaton W W: Epidemiologic findings on panic. In *Panic Disorder: Theory, Research and Therapy,* R Baker, editor, p 183. Wiley, New York, 1989.
Weissman M M: Family genetic studies of panic disorder. J Psychiatr Res *24* (Suppl, 1): 19, 1990.
Weissman M M, Wickramaratne P, Adams P B, Lish J D, Horwath E, Charney D, Woods S W, Leeman E, Frosch E: The relationship between panic disorder and major depression: A new family study. Arch Gen Psychiatry *50:* 767, 1993.
Zitrin C M, Klein D F, Woerner M G, Ross D C: Treatment of phobias: I. Comparison of imipramine hydrochloride and placebo. Arch Gen Psychiatry *40,* 125, 1983.

17.2 SPECIFIC PHOBIA AND SOCIAL PHOBIA

DAVID H. BARLOW, Ph.D.
MICHAEL R. LIEBOWITZ, M.D.

INTRODUCTION

Most people fear various objects or situations to some degree, but according to epidemiological reports for about 5 to 10 percent of the population those fears are severe enough to be labeled ''phobia,'' making it the most common mental disorder in the United States. The variety of names contrived to describe those often obscure fears or phobias is limited only by the number of Greek and Latin prefixes describing modern-day objects or situations (for example, anemophobia, or the fear of air currents, wind, and drafts).

Despite the fascination with phobias and widespread public knowledge of their nature (as opposed to other psychiatric conditions), until recently, those potentially serious disorders aroused little interest among clinicians and even less among researchers. For example, a 1985 review called social phobia a ''neglected anxiety disorder.'' Its prevalence was unknown, its clinical characteristics were poorly described, and the resulting disability was grossly underestimated. In addition, there were no known psychopharmacological treatments and no controlled trials of medication specifically for patients with social phobia.

HISTORICAL NEGLECT OF PHOBIAS In the case of specific phobias there are several reasons for the lack of attention. First, relatively few persons with phobias seek treatment despite the large number who report phobias in epidemiological studies. When they do come for treatment they seldom complain only of an isolated specific phobia. Such persons usually present with a variety of additional anxiety or mood disorders, making it difficult to decide whether the phobia is the principal problem even if it is relatively severe.

Second, relatively few types of specific phobias present for treatment. Of those that do, the most common are claustrophobia, blood-injection-injury phobia, dental phobia, and some small animal phobias, if very severe.

RECENT INCREASE IN INTEREST IN PHOBIAS The relative lack of interest in phobias has begun to change, however, as new developments in conceptualizations of the nosology, etiology, and treatment of both specific phobia and social phobia have taken place. Social phobia is now understood to be a common disorder with two principal subtypes, performance anxiety or discrete social phobia and a more widespread or generalized form of social phobia. Performance anxiety is perhaps the most widespread phobia in the American population. The generalized form of social phobia can be chronic and disabling, resulting in marked social, vocational, and academic impairment. Social phobia starts early, may give rise to other anxiety and depressive disorders, and frequently leads to substance (particularly alcohol) abuse. Controlled trials suggest that both pharmacological and cognitive-behavioral approaches are useful. In addition, because of its prevalence, disabling qualities, low placebo-response rate, and pharmacological responsivity, various new pharmacological approaches are now being used to study social phobia.

Investigation of social phobia also leads to ethological issues, such as dominance and submission. Childhood temperament, as shown by Jerome Kagan's work with behavioral inhibition, may be a precursor of social anxiety. Social phobia forces the confrontation of often ignored similarities between childhood and adult psychiatric disorders; social anxiety and social phobia present in children, adolescents, young adults, and the elderly, usually with similar features. In addition, the generalized form of social phobia overlaps substantially with avoidant personality disorder, raising the issue of the sometimes nebulous boundary between Axis I and Axis II conditions.

DEFINITION

SPECIFIC PHOBIA In the fourth edition of *Diagnostic and Statistical Manual of Mental Disorders* (DSM-IV) specific phobia refers to fear cued by the presence (or anticipation) of a specific object or situation, such as flying, heights, animals, receiving an injection, or seeing blood. Moreover, the object or situation must be avoided or else endured with marked distress, and the fear of it must be recognized by the person as excessive or unreasonable and result in a significant disruption of the person's life.

SOCIAL PHOBIA DSM-IV defines social phobia as "a marked and persistent fear of one or more social or performance situations in which the person is exposed to unfamiliar people or to possible scrutiny by others. The individual fears that he or she will act in a way (or show anxiety symptoms) that will be humiliating or embarrassing." The key to the definition is that feelings of anxiety or avoidance are experienced in situations in which a person feels that he or she is being evaluated or scrutinized. Such situations can involve performance, such as public speaking, auditioning, looking for a job, or even eating, drinking, or signing one's name in front of others; or social interaction, such as asking someone for a date, going out with friends, attending a party, or talking to a boss or to a colleague. DSM-IV also requires that in social phobia the feared situations be avoided or else be endured with intense anxiety or distress; that the person recognize that his or her fear is excessive or unreasonable (although that might not be true of children); and that the anxiety and avoidance significantly interfere with the person's normal routine, occupational (or academic) functioning, usual social activities or relationships, or that there be marked distress about having the phobic fear.

HISTORY AND COMPARATIVE NOSOLOGY

Despite the general awareness of phobic reactions historically, as late as 1959 only three of nine systems for classifying psychiatric disorders in various countries listed phobic disorder as an independent diagnosis. During the past several decades phobias have become more prominent in systems of classification, but only in a very general sense. For example, the ninth revision of the *International Classification of Diseases and Related Health Problems* (ICD-9) listed phobic states under categories for which anxiety is a major defining feature. Parenthetically, it was noted that phobic state "includes agoraphobia, animal phobias, anxiety-hysteria, claustrophobia, phobia NOS (not otherwise specified)."

ICD-10 In the 10th revision of the ICD (ICD-10) phobias are defined as follows:

> A group of disorders in which anxiety is evoked only, or predominantly, by certain well defined situations or objects (external to the subject) which are not currently dangerous. As a result, these situations or objects are characteristically avoided or endured with dread. Phobic anxiety is indistinguishable subjectively, physiologically and behaviourally from other types of anxiety and may vary in severity from mild unease to terror.

ICD-10 describes specific phobias as follows:

> These are phobias restricted to highly specific situations such as proximity to particular animals, heights, thunder, darkness, flying, closed spaces, urinating or defecating in public toilets, eating certain foods, dentistry, the sight of blood or injury, and the fear of exposure to specific diseases. Although the triggering situation is discrete, contact with it can evoke panic as in agoraphobia or social phobias.

The ICD-10 approach to social phobia is somewhat similar to that of DSM-IV, although it does not include the latter's subtypes. In general ICD-10 emphasizes a fear of scrutiny by other people that leads to the avoidance of social situations. More pervasive social phobias are recognized and thought to be associated with low self-esteem and a fear of criticism. Typical presentations are said to include complaints of blushing, hand tremor, nausea, or urgency to urinate. It is recognized that the symptoms may progress to panic attacks, but subtypes of panic attacks are not distinguished. ICD-10 also notes the frequent co-occurrence of symptoms of depressive disorder and the fact that some patients may become so globally socially avoidant that they are virtually housebound.

DISTINGUISHING SOCIAL PHOBIA AND AGORAPHOBIA A distinction between social phobia and agoraphobia must be made. Patients with social phobia will usually go out alone if they are sure that they will not meet someone with whom they will have to converse whereas patients with panic disorder with agoraphobia would be uncomfortable in such isolation. Patients with panic disorder with agoraphobia find the presence of others to whom they might turn for help reassuring whereas those with social phobia relieve their anxiety by fleeing the presence of others.

> A 29-year-old male office worker applied for treatment of what he described as panic attacks, which often occurred while he was riding on the subway. He was treated with imipramine (Tofranil) for panic disorder, but despite a vigorous trial with good blood levels, he failed to respond. On clinical reexamination he revealed that he only felt panicky if others on the subway were looking at him and that he was very comfortable on the train when alone. He was rediagnosed as having social phobia and did very well on a subsequent trial of phenelzine (Nardil).

DSM DSM has now appeared in its fourth edition but it was the third edition that departed radically from its predecessors in its descriptions of most disorders, including phobias. Table 17.2-1 compares the specifications of anxiety disorders from DSM-II through DSM-IV. In its overarching organization DSM-IV is seen to be largely unchanged from DSM-III-R with the exception that anxiety-related disorders previously classified under organic mental disorders and psychoactive substance use disorders have now been grouped with the anxiety disorders. They are anxiety disorder due to a general medical condition (for example, anxiety disorder due to hyperthyroidism) and substance-induced anxiety disorder (for example, cocaine-induced anxiety disorder with panic attacks). In addition, acute stress disorder was introduced in DSM-IV to capture posttraumatic stress disorderlike features occurring immediately after a severe trauma.

Specific phobia DSM-II mentioned phobic neuroses in its section on neuroses but did not provide a further breakdown of phobic disorders. DSM-III further divided DSM-II phobic neuroses into agoraphobia with panic attacks, agoraphobia without panic attacks, social phobia, and simple phobia. The term "simple" was introduced to differentiate the residual phobias from agoraphobia and social phobia where fear of panic attacks or of humiliation or embarrassment, respectively, were key presenting features in addition to situational fear. In DSM-III-R simple phobia was largely unchanged but underwent a rather radical revision in DSM-IV. First, the term "specific phobia" was adopted to improve definitional clarity and to maintain compatibility with ICD-10. Second, important information emerging in the past several years supported the value of subtyping specific phobias into different categories on the basis of age of onset, sex ratio, family history, and physiological responsiveness to exposure to the phobic stimulus—all of which have treatment implications. Finally, the role of panic attacks in specific phobias, which was ambiguous in previous versions, is

TABLE 17.2-1
Classification of Anxiety Disorders in DSM-II, DSM-III, DSM-III-R, and DSM-IV

DSM-II	DSM-III	DSM-III-R	DSM-IV
Phobic neurosis	Phobic disorders (or phobic neuroses) Agoraphobia with panic attacks Agoraphobia without panic attacks Social phobia Simple phobia	Phobic disorders Social phobia Simple phobia Agoraphobia without history of panic disorder	Phobic disorders Social phobia Specific phobia Agoraphobia without history of panic disorder
Anxiety neurosis	Anxiety states (or anxiety neuroses) Panic disorder Generalized anxiety disorder	Anxiety states Panic disorder with agoraphobia Panic disorder without agoraphobia	Anxiety states Panic disorder with agoraphobia Panic disorder without agoraphobia
Obsessive-compulsive neurosis	Obsessive-compulsive disorder (or obsessive-compulsive neurosis)	Generalized anxiety disorder Obsessive-compulsive disorder	Generalized anxiety disorder Obsessive-compulsive disorder
	Posttraumatic stress disorder Acute Chronic or delayed	Posttraumatic stress disorder Anxiety disorder not otherwise specified	Posttraumatic stress disorder Acute stress disorder
	Atypical anxiety disorder		
Neuroses not classified as anxiety disorders in DSM-III (or DSM-III-R)			Anxiety disorder due to a general medical condition
Hysterical neurosis	Somatoform disorders Dissociative disorders		Substance-induced anxiety disorder
Depressive neurosis	Affective disorders		Anxiety disorder not otherwise specified
Neurasthenic neurosis	[Eliminated]		

Table adapted from D H Barlow: *Anxiety and Its Disorders: The Nature and Treatment of Anxiety and Panic*, Guilford, New York, 1988.

specified in greater detail. That specification also may have treatment implications.

The DSM-IV criteria for specific phobia are presented in Table 17.2-2. In addition to the change in terminology from "simple" to "specific" two other revisions will have far-reaching implications. First, there now exists, for the first time, a typing schema for phobia specifying animal type; natural environment type; blood-injection-injury type; situational type (for example, situations from which escape may be difficult, such as methods of transportation, claustrophobic circumstances, or bridges); and a residual type for specific phobias not categorized, which is referred to as "other type" with specific examples of phobic avoidance of situations that may lead to choking, vomiting, or contracting an illness. Illness phobia is noteworthy in that the condition was previously described in hypochondriasis. It is also placed among the specific phobias in ICD-10 but is termed disease phobia.

Social phobia DSM-III was the first to incorporate social phobia into its official nomenclature. The specification of social phobia as a separate type was based on Isaac Marks's work in the 1960s, which suggested that agoraphobia, specific phobia, and social phobia were distinct disorders. Marks's original definition of social phobia was a broad one and included a range of performance and interpersonal situations. However, DSM-III took a narrower view, suggesting that persons with social phobia had only one or two types of fear. Also, the examples given in DSM-III were, for the most part, performance related. Persons with more widespread social fears were considered to have avoidant personality disorder, which was an exclusion for the diagnosis of social phobia. It is important to note that there was no empirical basis for that decision.

Research in the early and mid-1980s by the second author and others demonstrated that many patients with social phobia had widespread social fears, and suggested that such patients should be considered as having a generalized subtype of social phobia. Liebowitz and colleagues distinguished between patients who experienced performance anxiety in such situa-

TABLE 17.2-2
Diagnostic Criteria for Specific Phobia

A. Marked and persistent fear that is excessive or unreasonable, cued by the presence or anticipation of a specific object or situation (e.g., flying, heights, animals, receiving an injection, seeing blood).
B. Exposure to the phobic stimulus almost invariably provokes an immediate anxiety response, which may take the form of a situationally bound or situationally predisposed panic attack. **Note:** In children, the anxiety may be expressed by crying, tantrums, freezing, or clinging.
C. The person recognizes that the fear is excessive or unreasonable. **Note:** In children, this feature may be absent.
D. The phobic situation(s) is avoided or else is endured with intense anxiety or distress.
E. The avoidance, anxious anticipation, or distress in the feared situation(s) interferes significantly with the person's normal routine, occupational (or academic) functioning, or social activities or relationships, or there is marked distress about having the phobia.
F. In individuals under age 18 years, the duration is at least 6 months.
G. The anxiety, panic attacks, or phobic avoidance associated with the specific object or situation are not better accounted for by another mental disorder, such as obsessive-compulsive disorder (e.g., fear of dirt in someone with an obsession about contamination), posttraumatic stress disorder (e.g., avoidance of stimuli associated with a severe stressor), separation anxiety disorder (e.g., avoidance of school), social phobia (e.g., avoidance of social situations because of fear of embarrassment), panic disorder with agoraphobia, or agoraphobia without history of panic disorder.

Specify type:
- **Animal type**
- **Natural environment type** (e.g., heights, storms, water)
- **Blood-injection-injury type**
- **Situational type** (e.g., airplanes, elevators, enclosed places)
- **Other type** (e.g., phobic avoidance of situations that may lead to choking, vomiting, or contracting an illness; in children, avoidance of loud sounds or costumed characters)

Table from DSM-IV, *Diagnostic and Statistical Manual of Mental Disorders,* ed 4. Copyright American Psychiatric Association, Washington, 1994. Used with permission.

tions as speaking, eating, writing, or drinking in public and patients whose fears were more interactional or interpersonal and who suffered from a more generalized form of social phobia. The latter type was shown to be highly responsive to monoamine oxidase inhibitors (MAOIs). The researchers argued strongly that those persons should be thought of as suffering a form of social phobia rather than avoidant personality disorder, which would direct clinicians away from both cognitive-behavioral and pharmacological treatments.

DSM-III-R accepted the findings and defined social phobia more broadly, establishing a generalized subtype for persons whose fears involved most social situations. In that regard DSM-III-R took a quantitative rather than a qualitative approach to distinguishing among social phobia subtypes.

Western psychiatry did not recognize social phobia until fairly recently, but Japanese investigators have long been interested in interpersonal phobias, going back to at least the 1920s. The Japanese recognize a variety of interpersonal phobic fears and reactions that they call *taijin kyofusho,* which range from the fear of blushing or eye-to-eye confrontation to quasi-delusional states in which a person believes that others avoid him or her because he or she emits a bad body odor or has a piercing gaze.

Although DSM-III-R represented a significant improvement over DSM-III in terms of social phobia criteria, the DSM-IV Anxiety Disorders Work Group discovered a number of uncertainties and problems regarding the DSM-III-R definition of social phobia. The first had to do with the issue of subtypes. DSM-III-R used a quantitative approach to define the generalized subtype, that is, as having excessive fears involving most social or interpersonal situations. An alternative, more qualitative, approach is whether the focus of concern is on performance-related issues or on social interactions. DSM-IV considered both the quantitative and qualitative approaches, as well as a subtyping scheme that would combine both types of distinctions to create three subtypes: a performance subtype, a limited situational or interactional subtype (one or two interpersonal or social situations), and a generalized subtype (most interpersonal or social situations). In the end there were not enough empirical data to merit changing the DSM-III-R subtyping schema. The DSM-IV criteria for social phobia are presented in Table 17.2-3.

In DSM-III-R social anxiety or avoidance secondary to a minor medical condition, such as parkinsonian tremor or stuttering, was excluded from social phobia. Again, there was no empirical basis for doing this. The social phobia subgroup for DSM-IV examined the validity of the exclusion and considered three ways to handle it. The first was its continued exclusion, the second was to abolish the exclusion completely, and the third was to include in social phobia persons whose social anxiety or performance anxiety was due to a minor medical condition, if the anxiety or avoidance clearly exceeded what most persons with a similar medical disability would experience. That is, excessive social anxiety or avoidance in reaction to a medical disability would be social phobia and it would be left to clinical judgment to make the distinction. Available evidence suggested relaxing the exclusion but was too preliminary to be conclusive, so the DSM-III-R format was carried over into DSM-IV.

TABLE 17.2-3
Diagnostic Criteria for Social Phobia

A. A marked and persistent fear of one or more social or performance situations in which the person is exposed to unfamiliar people or to possible scrutiny by others. The individual fears that he or she will act in a way (or show anxiety symptoms) that will be humiliating or embarrassing. **Note:** In children, there must be evidence of the capacity for age-appropriate social relationships with familiar people and the anxiety must occur in peer settings, not just in interactions with adults.
B. Exposure to the feared social situation almost invariably provokes anxiety, which may take the form of a situationally bound or situationally predisposed panic attack. **Note:** In children, the anxiety may be expressed by crying, tantrums, freezing, or shrinking from social situations with unfamiliar people.
C. The person recognizes that the fear is excessive or unreasonable. **Note:** In children, this feature may be absent.
D. The feared social or performance situations are avoided or else are endured with intense anxiety or distress.
E. The avoidance, anxious anticipation, or distress in the feared social or performance situation(s) interferes significantly with the person's normal routine, occupational (academic) functioning, or social activities or relationships, or there is marked distress about having the phobia.
F. In individuals under age 18 years, the duration is at least six months.
G. The fear or avoidance is not due to the direct physiological effects of a substance (e.g., a drug of abuse, a medication) or a general medical condition and is not better accounted for by another mental disorder (e.g., panic disorder with or without agoraphobia, separation anxiety disorder, body dysmorphic disorder, a pervasive developmental disorder, or schizoid personality disorder).
H. If a general medical condition or another mental disorder is present, the fear in criterion A is unrelated to it (e.g., the fear is not of stuttering), trembling in Parkinson's disease, or exhibiting abnormal eating behavior in anorexia nervosa or bulimia nervosa.

Specify if:
Generalized: if the fears include most social situations (also consider the additional diagnosis of avoidant personality disorder)

Table from DSM-IV, *Diagnostic and Statistical Manual of Mental Disorders,* ed 4. Copyright American Psychiatric Association, Washington, 1994. Used with permission.

EPIDEMIOLOGY AND FAMILIAL PATTERNS

SPECIFIC PHOBIA

Prevalence Phobia is the most common mental disorder in the country according to results of the Epidemiologic Catchment Area (ECA) study, with specific phobia heading the list. Six-month prevalence rates for specific phobia range from 4.5 to 11.8 per 100 population. In the aggregate the data show that the female-to-male ratio for specific phobia is about two to one. It is the most common mental disorder in women and also the second most common in men, following only substance abuse. There is also evidence that many persons who suffer from substance abuse began by using medications to alleviate an underlying anxiety disorder, which in many cases might be a phobia.

Age at onset Different specific phobias may begin at somewhat different ages. Figure 17.2-1 presents data from Sweden on the age at onset of persons with four specific phobias and includes agoraphobia and social phobia for the sake of comparison. The sample is interesting as it comprised a large number of persons whose phobias were severe enough to compel them to seek treatment over an eight-year period.

Specific phobias in general had a much earlier age of onset than social phobia. It was earliest in animal phobia (mean of 7 years of age), followed by blood phobia (mean of 9 years of age) and dental phobia (mean of 12 years of age). What is interesting about those data, as well as other data collected on the same topic, is that the mean age of onset in claustrophobia (20 years of age) was much closer to that in agoraphobia, where the age of onset also peaked in the 20s, than to that in other specific phobias.

Heterogeneity Those data, along with recent important reanalyses by George Curtis and his colleagues, have led to a reconsideration of the homogeneity of specific phobia. Some of the

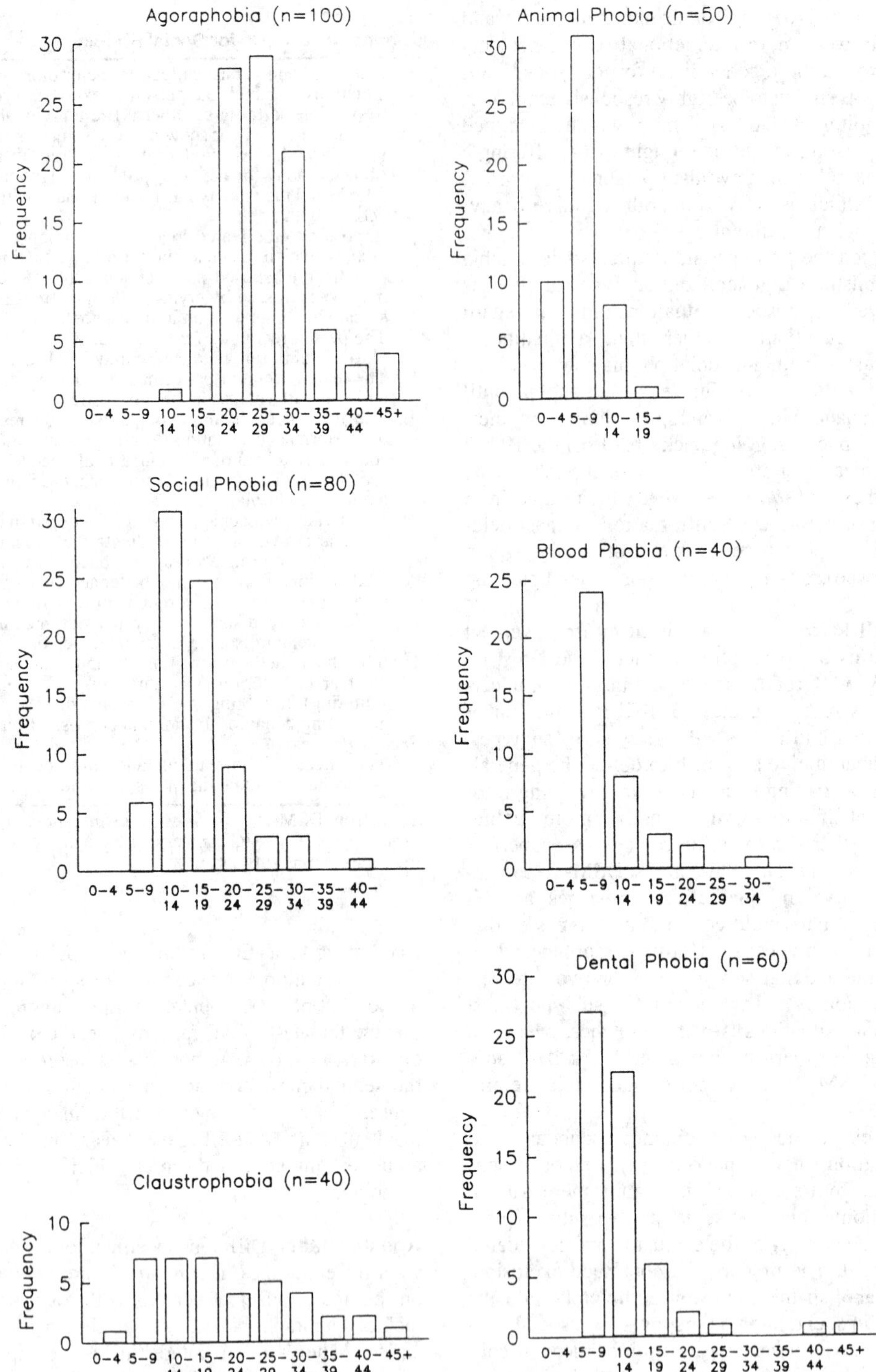

FIGURE 17.2-1 *Ages of onset for four specific phobias, agoraphobia, and social phobia. (Figure adapted from L G Öst: Age at onset in different phobias. J Abnorm Psychol* 96: *223, 1987. Also in D H Barlow:* Anxiety and Its Disorders: The Nature and Treatment of Anxiety and Panic. *Guilford, New York, 1988.)*

reanalyses suggested that marked heterogeneity exists across the specific phobias. On the basis of the suggestions Curtis and his group reanalyzed much of the published data on age of onset and sex ratio as well as the etiology and familial aggregation of the specific phobias.

In the first study prepared for the DSM-IV subgroup on specific phobia the investigators examined all previously published work meeting the standards necessary for inclusion in the analyses. They grouped phobias into animal phobias, height phobias, and specific phobias of situations often associated with agoraphobia, such as fear of driving, flying, being in tunnels and other enclosed places, bridges, and heights. They found that the age of onset for situational phobias was similar to that for agoraphobia (early to mid-20s) and in contrast to the onset in very early childhood of animal phobias. The exception was height phobias, which tend to develop in late childhood or early adolescence.

The researchers noted similarities in sex ratios between situational phobias and agoraphobia in that the percentage of men, although still clearly the minority, was somewhat higher for situational phobias than was the percentage of male subjects who had animal phobias. Curtis and his group also observed that persons with situational phobias were more likely to report an etiology consisting of an initial unexpected panic attack that did not develop into a panic disorder. Animal phobics were less likely to report that etiology and more likely to report a traumatic etiology consisting of an unpleasant encounter with an animal.

Finally, the specific phobias were reported to evidence familial aggregation by type of phobia. Probands with animal phobias thus were likely to have first-degree relatives with animal phobias (although not usually involving the same animal). Similarly, probands with situational phobias tended to have relatives with phobias of other types of situations. However, the data were very limited in that area and further investigation is needed.

In addition, Curtis and his group reanalyzed the ECA data set for phobias further to assess the relation of situational phobias to agoraphobia. Various forms of statistical clustering, followed by stepwise logistic regressions, were conducted on the ECA data. Three main clusters were identified: an agoraphobia cluster consisting of being alone, going out of the house alone, and crowds; a childhood cluster consisting of animals, storms, and being in water; and an inconsistent clustering of items that were somewhat difficult to interpret. However, fear of heights stood out in the last cluster, particularly in terms of the sex of the phobics, in that it is the only phobia that affects men more than it does women. Nevertheless, it appears to be more similar to situational phobias than it does to other phobias.

Types On the basis of the data reanalysis, which largely confirmed and extended previous published reports, specific phobias subsumed under the designation ''natural environment'' were differentiated from situational phobias. Furthermore, DSM-IV further separated animal phobias from other natural environment phobias (for example, water and storms) to form a third type.

To those three types was added a fourth type, blood-injection-injury phobia. That decision was based on a variety of published reports, as well as on a literature review submitted to the DSM-IV subgroup on specific phobia by Lars-Goran Öst. Öst reported that the prevalence of blood phobia is rather high, in the range of 3 to 4.5 percent of the population, although the data are still somewhat tentative. The sex ratio seems to be more nearly 50 to 50 with approximately 9 years of age the mean age at onset. Blood-injection-injury phobia is highly familial. For example, interviews with first-degree relatives of 25 persons with blood phobia in Sweden showed that 64 percent had at least one relative who also had blood phobia. More important, persons with blood-injection-injury phobia present with a distinct physiological response characterized by decreased heart rate and blood pressure rather than the more usual pattern of increased blood pressure. Consequently, approximately 75 percent reported a history of fainting in the phobic situation. The combination of a somewhat different age of onset, a very high and distinct familial aggregation, and the characteristic vasovagal physiological response suggests the importance of according blood-injection-injury phobia its own type.

Evidence for other types, including phobias of choking or space phobia (in which the person is fearful of falling when away from walls or other sources of support), is too preliminary to warrant subtyping.

Family studies More sophisticated analyses of familial aggregation of specific phobia have shown that 73 percent of the families of a proband with specific phobia include at least one relative with specific phobia as compared with 29 percent of the families of a proband without specific phobia. Those important pilot data form the basis for an ongoing larger investigation into the familial and possible genetic contributions to the transmission of specific phobia.

The data suggest that specific phobia is a highly familial disorder whose transmission is distinct from that of other anxiety disorders. However, it is not yet clear whether the increased risk reflects an overriding intergenerational transmission that is independent of phobic stimulus or the combined effect of several transmissionally distinct subtypes (for example, animal, situational). But preliminary data indicate that both persons with animal phobia and those with situational phobia appear to transmit an increased risk for their own subtype to their relatives as compared with the relatives of controls.

SOCIAL PHOBIA

Prevalence A variety of epidemiological studies of social phobia have been carried out, and findings vary considerably. The largest investigation, the ECA study, used lay interviewers. In the study three questions screened for social phobia, which was defined as ''an unreasonable fear or avoidance of a particular situation which interfered a lot with activities.'' Subjects were questioned as to whether they had such difficulty when eating in front of other people, when speaking in public or speaking to strangers, or when meeting new people. Across the sites the rates of positive diagnoses based on the latest analyses varied from 1.9 to 3.2 per 100 population with an overall mean of 2.4 per 100 population. Age of onset tended to be early, with most phobias beginning before the age of 20. The most frequent age at onset was between 11 and 15 years of age. The prevalence was greater for women than for men, which is the reverse of what is seen in clinical samples where men tend to predominate over women. The most likely explanation is that men preferentially seek treatment because having social phobia is a greater impediment to carrying out their expected social roles so that they are overrepresented in clinical samples in comparison with their prevalence in community samples.

A more recent study, the National Comorbidity Survey, used more probes for social phobia and found much higher one-year and lifetime prevalences. In that study social phobia was the third most common mental disorder after substance abuse and major depressive disorder. The findings suggest that the ECA figures are underestimates because of the failure to elicit all affected persons. Data from a telephone survey in a Canadian city support that premise. Social phobia prevalence was a function of the number of assessment questions asked.

In terms of age-specific features it has been noted in clinical samples that adults generally say they have a fear of or avoid social or performance situations whereas children may more readily acknowledge discomfort in the situation but do not realize what it is that makes them uncomfortable until they are specifically asked. Children also have less opportunity to avoid a situation, often being compelled to perform, to go to school, or to interact with peers. Thus younger patients usually evidence a distress rather than an avoidance pattern. However, social phobia is a frequent cause of school avoidance for teenagers.

Family studies In 1993 Abby Fyer and coworkers did a direct family interview study of social phobia, comparing affected probands with not-ill controls. They found a significantly elevated rate of social phobia in the first-degree relatives of the proband group. Relative risk was more than three times that of the normal controls. Relatives of persons with social phobia also had a high risk for major depressive disorder, which persisted even if proband comorbidity was factored out. It should be noted that the sample was clinical rather than epidemiological and that twin and adoption studies will be necessary to separate genetic and environmental influences.

ETIOLOGY

SPECIFIC PHOBIA, BLOOD-INJECTION-INJURY TYPE

As with most disorders few would suppose that a phobia is inherited directly as is hair or eye color. Rather, if the findings are confirmed, what is inherited is a vulnerability or disposition that then must interact with psychosocial events to produce the phobia. In blood-injection-injury phobia, for example, a person might inherit a strong vasovagal response to the sight of blood or a low threshold for such a response. Because the vasovagal response is thought to be a special defensive reaction, a tendency to respond in that manner should be distributed normally among the population. The extreme reactors would be located at the end of the distribution and would be most likely to faint when confronted with minimal blood stimuli. That reaction would constitute a vulnerability. The response has a strong familial component, which probably is the result of underlying genetic contributions.

The vulnerability alone would not be sufficient to cause a phobia. The person must sense that the reaction is out of control and be susceptible to becoming anxious about its recurrence for a severe phobic reaction to develop. Sudden and unexpected fainting is likely to provoke that response in susceptible persons, but there probably are many who have learned to cope with (control) the fainting response and so do not develop a disorder.

EVOLUTIONARILY PREPARED OBJECTS AND SITUATIONS The etiology of most phobic disorders, according to retrospective descriptive evidence, seems to involve the association of an alarm (that is, a marked fear response or panic attack) with an object or situation that has a high probability of acquiring phobic properties. The alarms may be either true alarms, as when a traumatic event is experienced, or false alarms, as when no objective danger exists (that is, an unexpected panic attack). Some of the potential phobic objects or situations may have danger or pain inherently associated with them or otherwise be predisposed in an evolutionary sense to that type of association or learning (for example, snakes, violent storms, or other natural environment phobias). Other objects or situations may have been the focus of mild anxious apprehension because of vicarious experiences or transmission of information prior to the association with an alarm. For example, a child may have been warned repeatedly of the dangers of dogs and have observed a parent's avoidance of all dogs.

MODES OF ACQUISITION Öst ascertained various modes of acquisition by means of a structured questionnaire administered to six groups of persons with phobias. The results are presented in Table 17.2-4. In the table the word "conditioning" would mean either confrontation with a traumatic experience (resulting in a true alarm) or the experience of an initial false alarm (unexpected panic) while in the potentially phobic situation. Another study examined a series of persons with driving phobias and noted that 40 percent reported an initial false alarm while driving; an additional 30 percent reported traumatic experiences that presumably resulted in a true alarm, such as a collision. In one case involving a true alarm a woman's headlights stopped functioning while she was driving at night on a winding mountain road with no guardrail. That leaves 30 percent of persons with driving phobias who could recall no specific adverse experience while driving, but had been warned repeatedly that driving could be dangerous (instruction-information mode) or had witnessed or heard about someone who had undergone difficulties while driving (modeling). Finally, some of the persons with phobias could recall nothing that might have precipitated or even made more probable the phobic response. The large number of subjects questioned and the structured nature of the questionnaire make this the best information to date on the various modes of acquisition. Nevertheless, these data are based on retrospective recall, sometimes of events that happened 20 or 30 years earlier, and so must be considered preliminary.

The distribution of persons with each of the retrospectively recalled modes of acquisition of a phobia is also presented in Table 17.2-4. Different phobias are seen to be associated with different modes of transmission. Blood phobia seems particularly prone to modeling influences, perhaps reflecting the fact that a strong underlying biological predisposition associated with the phobia is easily triggered by observation.

There are also cases in which the transmission of information seems the sole means of acquisition in the absence of alarm responses of any kind. Öst describes a woman with extremely severe snake phobia who had never encountered a snake in her life. Instead, while she was growing up she had been warned repeatedly of the dangers of snakes in high grass and was encouraged to wear rubber boots to guard against the threat.

MODES OF ACQUISITION The etiology of phobia is varied and complex. The various hypothetical methods of acquisition are outlined in Figure 17.2-2. In that etiological model a nonspecific biological vulnerability to experiencing fear and anxiety or a specific biological vulnerability to one or more types of anxiety may interact with either a direct or vicarious experience with the phobic object or situation. The experience may be of a traumatic nature, resulting in a true alarm. In addition, misinformation about the phobic object or situation may precede a traumatic interaction (true alarm) with the phobic object, further increasing the possibility of phobic activation as the person already would have been somewhat anxious about the phobic object or situation. Occasionally, it would seem that someone who is highly stressed as a result of negative life events or receives misinformation that results in anxiety might experience a false alarm spontaneously that becomes associated with or attributed to a specific object or situation. For example, a person might experience an unexpected panic attack while driving or flying although he or she had been driving or flying comfortably for years. More rarely, a person who is repeatedly warned of a rarely occurring situation or seldom-seen object might never experience a discrete alarm but simply develop intense anxious apprehension (anticipatory anxiety) about the possibility of encountering the phobic object or situation, as in the example of the woman who was afraid of snakes although she had never seen one.

Alarms thus can quickly become associated with the phobic object or situation, leading to anxious apprehension (anxiety) about future encounters and phobic behavior.

VULNERABILITY TO SOCIAL PHOBIA Other, more specific vulnerabilities have been hypothesized for social phobia. As a group persons with social phobia perceive their parents as having been less caring, more rejecting, and more overprotective as compared with the perceptions of normal controls; however, no contrasting study has been carried out with persons

TABLE 17.2-4
Ways of Acquisition for the Different Groups of Phobias

Ways of Acquisition	Animal		Social		Claustro-phobia		Agora-phobia		Blood		Dental		Total	
	No.	%	No.	%	No.	%	No.	%	No.	%	No.	%	No.	%
Conditioning	19	48	18	58	24	69	65	81	10	45	35	68	171	66
Modeling	11	27	4	13	3	9	7	9	7	32	6	12	38	15
Instruction-information	6	15	1	3	4	11	0	0	2	9	3	6	16	6
No recall	4	10	8	26	4	11	8	10	3	14	7	14	34	13

Table from L G Öst: Mode of acquisition of phobias. *Acta Universitatis Uppsaliensis (Abstracts of Uppsala Dissertations from the Faculty of Medicine), 529,* 1. Copyright 1985 by the Faculty of Medicine, University of Uppsala, Sweden. Used with permission. Also appears in D H Barlow: *Anxiety and Its Disorders: The Nature and Treatment of Anxiety and Panic.* Guilford, New York, 1988.

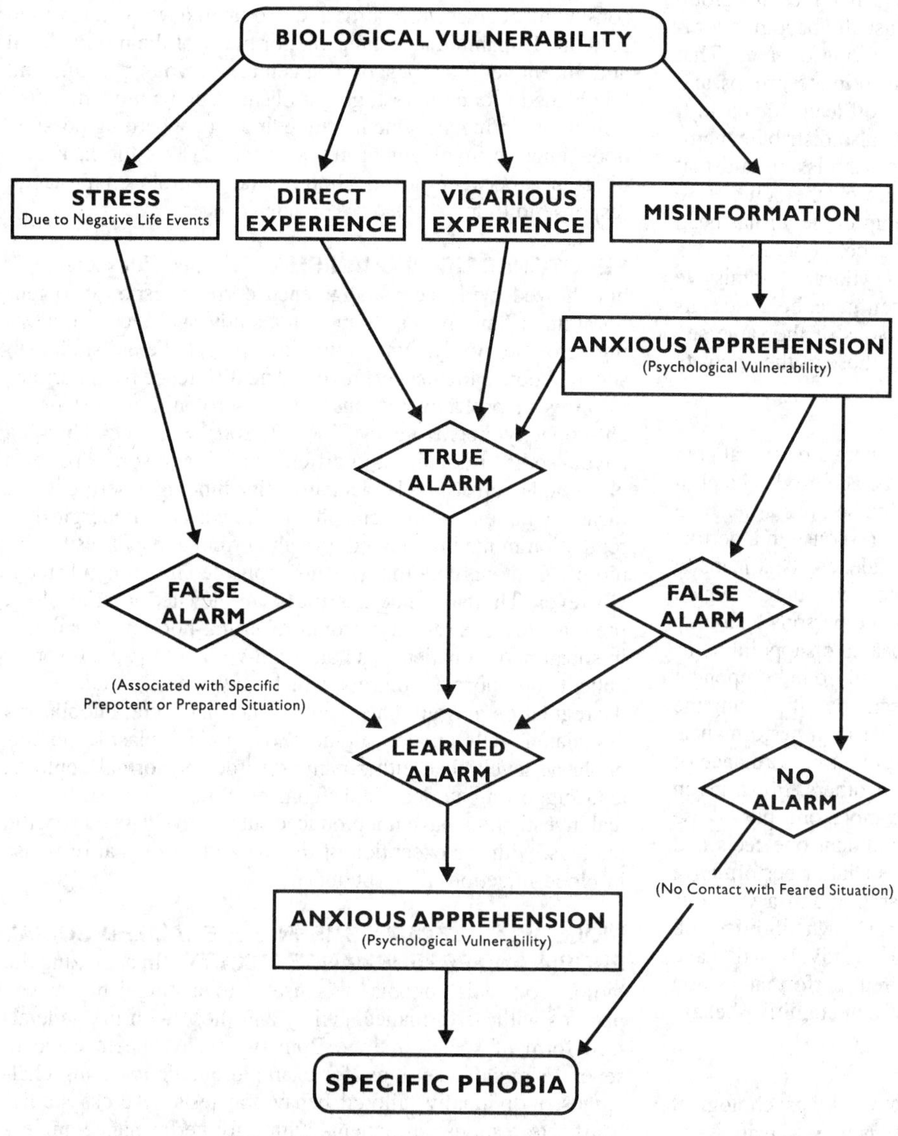

FIGURE 17.2-2 *Model of the etiology of simple phobia. (Figure from D H Barlow:* Anxiety and Its Disorders: The Nature and Treatment of Anxiety and Panic. *Guilford, New York, 1988. Used with permission.)*

with other phobias and so the specificity of the findings for social phobia is uncertain. Also, those assessments were retrospective and do not resolve the issue of cause and effect.

One intriguing line of evidence is Kagan and colleague's work with behavioral inhibition in young children. Upon being examined at the age of 18 months when their mothers bring them into a room in which there are other people, toys, and objects, children react in one of several ways. One group, perhaps 15 percent, will be very exploratory. Most of the rest, or 70 percent, of the children will be somewhat exploratory, and the remaining 15 percent will be very shy and withdrawn. The last group has been labeled as having behavioral inhibition, which appears to be a stable trait that continues through at least the first decade of life. In addition, it is more frequently seen in the offspring of adults with panic disorder. As they age the children also begin to show some of the signs of social phobia, especially if their parents are also overprotective toward them. Severe shyness and perhaps generalized social phobia might be associated with behavioral inhibition, but definitive studies are lacking. If the trait is inherited, as seems likely, it could confer a predisposition, either specifically for social phobia or for anxiety disorders in general. In the latter situation, the prevalence of any specific anxiety disorder would still be influenced by environmental experience.

ETHOLOGICAL MODEL OF SOCIAL PHOBIA There is an ethological model for social phobia that involves dominance and submission. In any mammalian species that lives in a group or herd setting one member of the group usually becomes dominant and the others have to submit to varying degrees. That tendency has been studied extensively in primate groups and also in wolf packs, where an alpha male wolf leads the pack. It is possible to speculate that human beings also distribute themselves along a range from dominance to submission and that persons with generalized social phobia are on the submissive end of the spectrum. Keeping one's chin up in the air has been called a human manifestation of dominance, equivalent to a wolf's keeping its tail up. Most persons who are submissive keep their chins down. They also avert their gaze, because staring is considered a challenge among persons of the same sex and an indication of interest on the part of those of the opposite sex.

ACQUISITION OF SOCIAL PHOBIA There are several possible ways in which social phobia might be acquired. The phobia might be traumatic in origin when a person has a negative experience, and perhaps a resulting alarm response in a performance or social encounter, and loses confidence. That leads to anxiety and poor performance in subsequent encounters, which gradually progresses to social phobia. Some persons also may have social skills deficits that lead to repeated disappointments and failures. Cognitive factors, although only one component of anxiety, can affect self-confidence directly by influencing the way in which a person interprets his or her own performance, predicts the likelihood of being successful in a performance or social situation, or views the reactions of others. For a given degree of competence and practice, the more one puts those factors in a favorable light, the more confident one feels and the better one performs. Whereas a little social or performance anxiety is useful to ensure proper preparation and a vigorous performance, persons who denigrate their own abilities too much or interpret others' reactions too negatively will have much more anxiety, leading to impaired performance and avoidance. Those are the substrates on which cognitive-behavioral therapy tries to work.

HYPERSENSITIVITY TO REJECTION A psychological antecedent and correlate of social anxiety is hypersensitivity to rejection and criticism, whereby affected persons overreact emotionally and are devastated by any perceived negative reactions on the part of others. That feeling is closely related to what has been hypothesized for atypical depression, where criticism or rejection by others provokes a severe depressive reaction. Interestingly, atypical depressive patients respond very well to MAOIs, which have also been found to work well in social phobia. Rejection hypersensitivity appears to be a link between the generalized form of social phobia and atypical depression.

DOPAMINERGIC MECHANISMS Hypersensitivity to rejection has been thought to be dopaminergically mediated. Dopaminergic mechanisms have been postulated for social phobia. First, although further controlled trials are needed, preliminary evidence suggests that tricyclic antidepressants are not as effective for social phobia as are MAOIs. MAOIs differ from tricyclics in that they have more potent effects on the dopaminergic system. Dopaminergic deficits have been found in genetically shy strains of mice and those were the only biological differences that distinguished them from more aggressive strains. In addition, when the dopamine systems of the aggressive mice were muted pharmacologically the animals became more submissive. In another study spinal-fluid dopamine metabolite levels were found to be elevated in extroverted persons with depressive disorders as compared with introverted patients. Dopamine is responsible for many of the motivational and incentive functions of the central nervous system, and heightened social interest, gregariousness, and confidence may reflect that influence. One negative finding concerning possible dopaminergic involvement in social phobia was the lack of a difference between social phobics and controls on prolactin response to L-dopa, noted by Manuel Tancer.

SEROTONERGIC MECHANISMS Patients with social phobia showed evidence of heightened cortisol response to fenfluramine (Pondimin) challenge in a study by Tancer, suggesting serotonergic dysregulation. However, challenge studies in social phobia patients have revealed no difference from normals in terms of prolactin response to the serotonin agonist meth-chlorophenylpiperazine (MCPP). Persons with social phobia have also been found not to differ from panic disorder patients or normal controls in platelet paroxetine binding, a serotonergic measure. Patients with social phobia showed noradrenergic dysregulation in having blunted growth hormone responses to clonidine (Catapres) but that was not replicated in a second study. However, Thomas Uhde has found an elevated arterial blood pressure response to thyrotropin-releasing-hormone challenge in social phobia patients as compared with both panic disorder patients and normal controls, which may reflect noradrenergic dysregulation as well. One study found that social phobia was associated with greater supine and standing plasma norepinephrine levels than either panic disorder or normal controls, also suggesting autonomic differences. Similar lines of biological investigation have not produced substantive data on specific phobias, with the exception of the marked vasovagal response in blood-injection-injury phobia.

BIOLOGICAL MECHANISMS IN GENERALIZED SOCIAL PHOBIA AND PERFORMANCE ANXIETY In analyzing the biology of social phobia it is useful to distinguish between patients with performance anxiety and those with the generalized form of social anxiety. Both types have been tested in several simulated settings (for example, public speaking challenges, individually tailored behavioral tests). Across studies heart rate response in patients with only performance anxiety was higher than that in patients with generalized social phobia. That finding is consistent with the belief that β-adrenergic receptor antagonists help with public speaking anxiety but not with the generalized form of social phobia.

In performance anxiety either an excess of epinephrine is secreted (although that was not demonstrated in a recent study) or affected persons are more sensitive to normal epinephrine surges, responding with characteristic rapid heartbeat, sweating, and tremor. Certain highly negative cognitions may generate such physiological responses as well. In normal persons the high physical arousal attenuates rapidly within or across performances but those with severe performance anxiety do not show either kind of attenuation. Instead, the physical symptoms mount and become distracting. The person becomes afraid that others will notice his or her discomfort, which further heightens anxiety. That generates more physical symptoms, more impaired performance, and more embarrassment in a positive feedback cycle until the person becomes so incapacitated that he or she loses the ability to perform. Such an experience then generates anxiety about and avoidance of the next performance. To clarify these mechanisms further more studies of social phobia, including detailed studies of catecholamines and other chemical systems, are needed.

PSYCHOANALYTIC THEORIES Psychoanalytic theories of phobias are now mainly of historical interest but are included for purposes of completeness. John Nemiah's description of those theories in the fifth edition of the *Comprehensive Textbook of Psychiatry* was the basis for the following material.

Freud viewed the phobic disorder, or anxiety hysteria, as he continued to call it, as resulting from conflicts centered on an unresolved childhood oedipal situation. In the adult, because the sexual drive continued to have a strong incestuous coloring, its arousal tended to cause anxiety that was characteristically a fear of castration. The anxiety then alerted the ego to exert repression to keep the drive away from conscious representation and discharge, but when repression was not entirely successful, it was necessary for the ego to call on auxiliary defenses. In patients with phobias the defenses, arising from an earlier phobic response during the initial childhood period of the oedipal conflict, primarily used displacement; that is, the sexual conflict was transposed or displaced from the person who evoked the conflict to a seemingly unimportant, irrelevant object or situation, which now had the power to arouse the entire constellation of affects, including signal anxiety. A psychoanalytic tenet was that on examination it could be determined that the phobic object or situation thus selected had a direct associative connection with the primary source of the conflict and had come naturally to symbolize it. Furthermore, the situation or object was usually such that the patient was able to keep out of its way and, by this additional mechanism of the defense of avoidance, could escape suffering serious anxiety.

Since Freud's formulation other investigators, without altering its basic structure, extended or made changes in the details of the theory to bring it into agreement with observations that often seemed initially to contradict what Freud proposed. Those revisions fall into three main categories: (1) Writers such as Kurt Lewin developed the theory of the processes by which the phobic facade is created, pointing out the similarity between the manifest content of dreams and the associative links that tie the phobic object or situation to the basic conflict—an observation that Freud himself had recognized. (2) Clinical observation suggested that aggression and pregenital sexual drives, as well as oedipal sexuality, contributed to the formation of phobic symptoms, such as the scoptophilic impulse in its relation to erythrophobia (fear of blushing). (3) It has been demonstrated that, in addition to castration anxiety, other forms of anxiety, notably separation anxiety, were prominent in many phobias.

DIAGNOSIS AND CLINICAL FEATURES

SPECIFIC PHOBIA

Panic attacks The emergence of a variety of new data has indicated that panic attacks may occur in the context of specific phobias, which is also consistent with ICD-10. Criterion B in the DSM-IV criteria for specific phobia makes that explicit by noting "exposure to the phobic stimulus almost invariably provokes an immediate anxiety response, which may take the form of a situationally bound or situationally predisposed panic attack." Furthermore, at the onset of the phobia the attack might be unexpected. For example, a person who had traveled by airplane for 20 years without fear one day experiences an unexpected panic attack while flying. The person may then avoid planes or else endure them with intense dread, but reports that the phobic behavior is limited to the particular situation and that panic attacks never occur outside of that situation. Similarly, a person might be bitten by a dog and then experience panic attacks upon the sight of all dogs encountered after the incident, even those that are known to be harmless and friendly. Phenomenologically, the panic attack seems to be the same in both instances; that is, there is a sudden burst of intense fear or dread with the accompanying autonomic symptoms. For the person with the dog phobia, however, the cue is clear from the beginning, whereas in the person with the flying phobia the panic attack is reported as unexpected but quickly becomes associated with traveling by air. In unexpected panic attacks associated with agoraphobia or panic disorder shortness of breath or a feeling of suffocation often is a prominent symptom but is less prominent in the severe anxiety that accompanies specific phobia anxiety responses. The symptom pattern of isolated, unexpected panic attacks that initiate a specific phobia needs further study in this regard. The role of panic attacks in specific phobia leads to some ambiguities in differential diagnoses with other anxiety disorders.

Apprehension It is clear that specific phobias are anxiety disorders and the experience of anxiety or anxious apprehension is a marked component of the disorder, in addition to the experience of true or false alarms. Criterion E notes that the "avoidance, anxious anticipation, or distress in the feared situation(s) interferes significantly with the person's normal routine, occupational (or academic) functioning, or activities or relationships. . . ." The criterion reflects the fact that a major part of any severe phobic disorder is severe anxiety whenever one is faced with even the possibility of having to encounter the phobic object or situation. For example, if a person with a phobia about flying finds it necessary to fly, the anxiety may begin as soon as the necessity becomes apparent, perhaps months before the actual event. If the flight is canceled at the last minute, the person still will have endured months of intense anxiety and dread without ever actually confronting the phobic situation.

SPACE PHOBIA In addition to the major types of specific phobias, at least two other interesting varieties exist. Isaac Marks and colleagues have described a condition referred to as space phobia. Marks's initial observation concerned a patient who presented with what appeared to be an agoraphobic pattern. On closer examination it was ascertained that the patient's fear revolved around falling when no support was nearby, as would happen when the patient was in the middle of a room or a corridor away from the walls. Occasionally, such persons resort to crawling on their hands and knees across an open space. The phobia seems to be found more often in older people who have experienced a bad fall. One study found some evidence of mild right hemisphere dysfunction in space phobia, supporting the possibility of a disturbance in visual-perceptual spatial functioning that may underlie the disorder. It is such symptoms of unsteadiness that become the focus of fear and anxiety.

ILLNESS PHOBIA Another development in DSM-IV is the designation of illness phobia as a specific phobia classified under other type. Controversy has existed for years on the boundary between hypochondriasis and specific phobia. Paul Salkovskis, Hillary Warwick, and David Clark reviewed the literature in that area for the DSM-IV specific phobia subgroup to determine where the boundary might best be placed and also collected other data on the issue. What they found in the literature, as well as in their own data, was a rather clear difference between the fear of contracting an illness or worry about getting a disease and the belief that one has an illness or is worried about having a disease. The definition of hypochondriasis in DSM-III-R seemed to incorporate two phenomenologically distinct entities of illness phobia and disease conviction. Thus it seemed reasonable that persons with a phobia about developing or being exposed to such illnesses as the acquired immune deficiency syndrome (AIDS) or cancer or who anxiously avoided stimuli associated with such illnesses were more properly placed in the specific phobia category, as long as they did not believe that they were currently suffering from the illness. The diagnostic criteria for hypochondriasis emphasize the disease conviction component in the context of medical reassurance to the contrary. Persons with obsessive-compulsive disorder sometimes report fear of disease in the form of intrusive thoughts regarding contamination, but in the prototypical case, the intrusive thoughts are more ego dystonic and elaborate stereotypical rituals follow the obsessional thoughts. Nevertheless, diagnosis may be difficult at the boundary of obsessive-compulsive disorder and illness phobia.

SOCIAL PHOBIA Social phobia in DSM-IV has the following features:

> Criterion A: "A marked and persistent fear of one or more social or performance situations in which the person is exposed to unfamiliar people or to possible scrutiny by others. The individual fears that he or she will act in a way (or show anxiety symptoms) that will be humiliating or embarrassing."

Criterion A is the key feature of social phobia in that it highlights the situations that generate it (that is, those involving scrutiny or evaluation) and the characteristic fear that someone will show anxiety or otherwise act in a way that will be embarrassing or humiliating.

> Criterion B: "Exposure to the feared social situation almost invariably provokes anxiety, which may take the form of a situationally bound or situationally predisposed panic attack."

What is meant here is that it is a situational fear. Every time the person is in the social or performance situation, he or she experiences severe anxiety symptoms and perhaps a panic attack (this does not mean unexpected panic attacks).

> Criterion C: "The person recognizes that the fear is excessive or unreasonable."

Insight is maintained, since we are not dealing with delusional or paranoid kinds of fears. However, the feature may be absent in children.

> Criterion D: "The feared social or performance situations are avoided or else are endured with intense anxiety or distress."

That is meant to differentiate social phobia from the less intense kinds of anxiety that most persons feel in social or performance situations.

> Criterion E: "The avoidance, anxious anticipation, or distress in the feared social or performance situation(s) interferes significantly with the person's normal routine, occupational (academic) functioning, or social activities or relationship, or there is marked distress about having the phobia."

Criterion E is a distress or impairment criterion, which was included to help distinguish social phobia from ubiquitous but milder social and performance anxiety in the general population.

> Criterion G: "The fear or avoidance is not due to the direct physiological effects of a substance (for example, a drug of abuse, a medication) or a general medical condition and is not better accounted for by another mental disorder (e.g., panic disorder with or without agoraphobia, separation anxiety disorder, body dysmorphic disorder, a pervasive developmental disorder, or schizoid personality disorder)."

The aim of the criterion is to serve as a reminder that several other conditions frequently give rise to clinical syndromes with features of social phobia and that clinical judgment must be relied on to make the differential diagnosis.

SOCIAL PHOBIA AND SOCIAL EMBARRASSMENT DSM-IV considered several options for dealing with the relationship to social phobia of social embarrassment secondary to such medical conditions as stuttering or tremor. DSM-III-R had made it a total exclusion so that such secondary social fears were not part of social phobia. A drawback of that approach was that persons with those secondary social phobic phenomena do not receive the same kinds of treatment as do those with primary social phobias even though preliminary clinical trials have shown that they can benefit from them.

> A 35-year-old unmarried professional man presented with the following history. He was born with retrolental fibroplasia related to premature birth and oxygen therapy, and a visual-angle kappa condition with disconjugate gaze strabismus, and cataracts. At least partly because he anticipated negative comments from others about his physical disabilities, while in high school he developed a fear of public speaking and of meeting people. He developed an intention tremor while in his early 20s, which led to anxiety and marked avoidance of eating or writing in public. When he presented for treatment he was virtually unable to work and was extremely isolated socially.
>
> He was put in a placebo-controlled treatment study of social phobia and received phenelzine (Nardil) on a double-blind basis. Within four to six weeks he was substantially less socially anxious and avoidant. Within several months he was able to return to work and had developed a much fuller social life. Improvement has persisted for two years with continued phenelzine treatment, although efforts to taper medication have led to symptom flare-ups.

An alternative diagnostic approach is to waive the exclusion completely and consider any secondary social anxiety as social phobia. A concern with that approach was that the prevalence of social phobia might increase, potentially trivializing the diagnosis. However, recent epidemiological studies of social phobia did not explicitly exclude secondary cases. In addition, certain medical conditions, such as highly disfiguring burns or scars, would cause almost anyone to become socially avoidant. A third option is to include as social phobia social avoidance secondary to medical problems where there is clearly an emotional overreaction that exceeds what most persons with the same medical problem would exhibit. An example might be severe avoidance secondary to a mild tremor or stutter. Although that approach seems reasonable, more studies of such persons and their responses to treatment are needed. Also, such a solution would depend on clinical judgment as to when a reaction is an overreaction and the interrater reliability would need to be studied. Therefore, this option was not adopted for DSM-IV, which elected instead to maintain the DSM-III-R convention (criterion H).

Social phobia and avoidant disorder of childhood and adolescence DSM-IV eliminates the diagnosis of avoidant disorder of childhood and adolescence. The DSM-IV diagnostic criteria for social phobia now subsumes avoidant disorder of childhood and adolescence.

In DSM-III-R a problem in the diagnosis of social phobia was its relationship to avoidant disorder of childhood or adolescence. The criteria overlapped those in social phobia so that the latter diagnosis could be used more frequently for both children and adolescents. The problem, however, was with the wording. Children could not acknowledge fear of social situations so much as be uncomfortable in them. A situation might cause them discomfort even though they were not fully aware of why it was so. In addition, they could not always avoid such situations because they did not have as much control over their behavior as did adults.

Generalized type With regard to subtypes of social phobia DSM-IV allows the clinician to specify whether the fear is generalized. In the generalized subtype, as defined in DSM-IV, the phobic fears involve most social situations. That contrasts with nongeneralized social phobia, which may involve only performance fears, such as auditioning, performing, writing, eating, and drinking in public, or interactional fears limited to one or two life domains.

DIFFERENTIAL DIAGNOSIS

SPECIFIC PHOBIA The diagnosis of a specific phobia is seldom as straightforward as it would appear because very few persons present for treatment with just a specific phobia. Most have several phobias as well as comorbid diagnoses. Therefore, the first task required of a clinician is to assess whether the phobia is an independent problem or an associated feature of another disorder.

A woman presented with a fear of sharp, pointed objects, particularly kitchen knives. Although she acknowledged only a phobia of knives, further detailed assessment revealed a severe obsessional process that was difficult for her to admit. The woman was repeatedly called by her daughter to care for her grandchildren and found it difficult to refuse. One day while babysitting she was preparing dinner and she felt a fleeting urge to stab one of the children, who was being particularly disruptive. The horrific thought was totally unacceptable and marked the beginning of what developed into an obsessive-compulsive disorder. The sight of knives called up the true source of her concern, her obsessional thoughts about killing her grandchildren.

Panic disorder with agoraphobia Research and data reanalyses for DSM-IV revealed that one of the more ambiguous differential diagnoses concerns the relation between specific phobia and panic disorder with agoraphobia, particularly the situational type of specific phobia. Both types of patients experience panic attacks that have similar symptom profiles. In addition, at least initially, the attacks might be unexpected in both conditions. Furthermore, even patients with a very circumscribed specific phobia might report fearing the possibility of having a panic attack. For example, the person who fears flying might report anxiety focused on the possibility of panicking while flying rather than on the plane's crashing. Despite those findings the issues need further study.

However, several differences seem to form a boundary between specific phobia and panic disorder with agoraphobia. First, persons with specific phobia feel immediate panic or anxiety upon being exposed to the phobic stimulus (or its representation). Second, they do not have panic attacks outside of the context of the specific phobic situation as do patients with panic disorder with agoraphobia. Finally, persons with specific phobia do not experience anxiety or anxious apprehension between panic attacks unless contact with the phobic object or situation once again becomes imminent. Patients with panic disorder with agoraphobia seem to suffer from more chronic anxiety, never knowing when their next panic attack might occur.

Agoraphobia Another issue concerns the differential diagnosis between situational specific phobia and agoraphobia without a history of panic disorder. Agoraphobia is defined in DSM-IV as a fear of being in places or situations from which escape might be difficult or embarrassing or in which help may not be available in the event of the sudden development of paniclike symptoms. The focus of the anxiety is not on the situation but rather on the feared symptoms, even if the symptoms do not meet the criteria for panic attack. In addition, patients with agoraphobia tend to fear and avoid a broader range of situations than do those with specific phobia. In any case the issue is probably moot for most clinicians since agoraphobia without a history of panic disorder is rarely encountered clinically.

Posttraumatic stress disorder and acute stress disorder There is considerable overlap among specific phobia patients whose phobia was precipitated by a clear traumatic event phobia (for example, a car accident) and those with other disorders involving trauma (for example, posttraumatic stress disorder and acute stress disorder). Although additional criteria are specified for a diagnosis of posttraumatic stress disorder (for example, flashbacks) it now seems clear that those disorders must be distinguished on the basis of specific symptom profiles. For example, posttraumatic stress disorder and acute stress disorder are associated with the persistent reexperiencing of the trauma (for example, flashbacks and nightmares) whereas such reexperiencing of the trauma is rarely a feature of specific phobia.

SOCIAL PHOBIA Distinguishing social phobia from normal shyness is a quantitative issue in the sense that social phobia is disabling whereas shyness may not be. Many persons describe themselves as shy; some of them will have social phobia whereas others will exhibit the same features to a lesser degree that does not cause severe distress or impairment. However, as current research is revealing, forms of social phobia that have significant academic and vocational ramifications, in the sense of how far one goes in school and what career one chooses, are much more common than previously thought.

Panic disorder with agoraphobia DSM-IV also attempts to clarify the boundary between social phobia and panic disorder or agoraphobia. DSM-III took a historical approach to the effect that if a disorder began with unexpected panic attacks and social or performance anxiety followed from that, the person was considered to be suffering from panic disorder or agoraphobia. However, much as with patients with specific phobia, there are persons in whom the illness may have begun as unexpected panic but years later the only avoidance they show is of social or performance situations and the only panic attacks they suffer are situationally caused. Such persons may be more appropriately regarded as having social phobia than agoraphobia. DSM-IV allows for clinical judgment in such instances. It excludes from social phobia those cases in which the social avoidance is part of current agoraphobia, but otherwise relies on the phrase "not better accounted for by another mental disorder" to emphasize the need for clinical judgment in deciding whether a historical or a cross-sectional perspective serves best as the guideline for making the diagnosis.

Ultimately, what are needed are external validating criteria to help make such decisions. Those criteria could include treatment response, course, family history, or biological data, but none is yet sufficiently known or precise enough to validate their use as a guide in diagnosing social phobia. Whereas most cases will not be difficult to diagnose clinically, there are a number of persons whose clinical presentations will not meet the prototypical definitions.

Other disorders Social phobia also must be distinguished from schizoid personality disorder, which is characterized by a lack of interest in social interactions rather than by anxiety-generating avoidance. Some persons will also appear socially avoidant during episodes of depression but such avoidance is state rather than trait related and resolves when the depression remits.

Quasi-delusional conditions that appear to be similar to social phobia have been reported to be common in Japan, where they are called *taijin kyofushu.* Affected persons believe that they give off an abnormal smell or that there is something wrong with their gaze that makes other people uncomfortable and they thus become socially avoidant. Whether it is actually a delusion or is a manifestation of Japanese culture that places more emphasis on other people's comfort than one's own is not clear. For example, the Japanese usually will be uncomfortable about blushing, not because it shows their own embarrassment, but because it makes others uncomfortable.

COURSE AND PROGNOSIS

Both specific phobia and social phobia can be disabling conditions. Recent additional analyses of ECA data found that even uncomplicated social phobia can lead to increased financial dependence and heightened utilization of medical treatment. The data also showed that it was associated with more suicidal thoughts, although no excess of suicide attempts characterized such patients unless they had other psychiatric disorders as well. In general, social phobia tends to be chronic, to begin at an early age (often in the teenage years) (Figure 17.2-1), and to result in academic impairment (suboptimal performance in school or avoidance of further schooling). It is a cause of dropout in the high school years and leads to vocational impairment, at least in part, by limiting the person's choice of a career. It also leads to social impairment. Persons with social phobia often have no friends and commonly are unable to marry. Social phobia results in depression and demoralization and substance (particularly alcohol) abuse. Many persons who abuse alcohol report preexisting social phobia. The use of alcohol complicates social phobia more often than it does any other anxiety disorder. Disabilities stemming from social phobia need much further study given its prevalence and the fact that many affected persons have subtle kinds of vocational, academic, and social impairments of which they are not fully cognizant, or are not aware of as having been caused by social or performance anxiety.

Similar conclusions can be drawn for specific phobia. Blood-injection-injury phobia can result in the avoidance of even necessary medical and dental care. Unlike agoraphobia specific phobia and social phobia fluctuate very little in intensity during their chronic course.

TREATMENT

SPECIFIC PHOBIA Despite the complexities of its etiology and the variety of presentations of specific phobia, what is known about its treatment is relatively straightforward. There is near unanimity of opinion among biological and psychological clinicians and investigators on the appropriateness of exposure-based procedures for specific phobias. That was not always the case. Early in the development of psychoanalysis most believed that dynamically oriented psychotherapies were the treatment of choice for phobia. The treatments were recommended on the basis of theoretical conceptions of phobia that considered early oedipal-genital conflicts important in the etiology of those conditions. It was soon recognized, however, that directing therapy at the unconscious conflicts while ignoring the phobic behavior did little to reduce either the anxiety or the behavior. Freud himself, along with his pupils, recognized that no progress would be made without direct, active, exposure-based treatments.

Near unanimity of opinion also exists on the seeming lack of benefit of adding drugs to those procedures. For that reason very little serious investigation of the possible benefits of drugs in the treatment of specific phobias has taken place.

Exposure therapy Exposure-based and similar procedures have been quite successful in treating specific phobias. They are best administered by arranging for a gradual self-paced exposure to a hierarchy of in vivo situations that ultimately results in exposure to the most intensely feared object or situation. For example, the treatment of a person with claustrophobia would begin with the patient's exposure to situations rated rather low on a self-rated scale of fear and anxiety, such as the patient's spending time in a small room in his or her own home. That procedure would then progress slowly (the pace and number of situations depending on the clinician's and the patient's judgment) until the patient faced the most difficult situation, such as riding an elevator to the top of a tall building. During exposure sessions the patient might practice such anxiety-reducing techniques as relaxation, diaphragmatic breathing, and identifying and changing automatic strong fearful thoughts through cognitive therapy processes. It must be made clear to the patient that he or she should not engage in any distracting activities during the exposure procedure.

If the problem is blood phobia, one other procedure should be added. In that technique, referred to as applied tension, patients with blood phobia are instructed to tense their bodies during exposure sessions (and to maintain a seated or reclining position, if at all possible). The additional procedure counteracts the hypotension (and possible fainting) that characterizes the vasovagal response.

Focusing on panic One possibility that is being evaluated is the use of either drugs with antipanic properties or structured psychosocial approaches that attack panic directly to treat panic attacks that occur in the context of specific phobia. Those specific phobias are found predominantly among the situational phobias. Preliminary evidence indicates that, in the case of psychosocial treatments, patients with a primary focus on experiencing a panic attack in the context of their situational phobia may benefit more from treatments focusing on that fear than from more broadly construed exposure treatments, although exposure presumably would also be necessary. Similar evaluations of appropriate drugs for panic are also being undertaken.

SOCIAL PHOBIA

Pharmacotherapy Treatments that have demonstrated efficacy for social phobia can be divided into pharmacological and psychotherapeutic modalities. The most effective medications appear to be the MAOIs, notably phenelzine, which in four double-blind placebo-controlled trials significantly helped an average of two thirds of each patient sample as compared with one third who benefitted from placebo. One study suggests that it is patients with generalized social phobia who do particularly well on MAOIs. The dosage is similar to that used to treat a depressive disorder and positive responses are seen in six weeks, which persist as long as the medication is continued. The discontinuation of phenelzine is associated with some relapse, but the rates vary across studies.

An 18-year-old man was referred for treatment because he had dropped out of high school owing to social and performance anxiety. He was virtually housebound; he went out for walks only at night when he felt he would not meet anyone with whom he would have to converse. He was initially treated with the cardioselective β-adrenergic receptor antagonist atenolol (Tenormin), up to 100 mg a day, with moderately favorable results. He returned to school and began a part-time job but still would not talk to other students or speak in class. With the discontinuation of the atenolol he expressed a strong wish to again drop out of school and he was started on phenelzine. Within six weeks he was much more comfortable in all social interactions. On 75 mg a day he was slightly disinhibited, causing some behavioral disturbance. After the dosage was lowered to 45 mg a day he was able to interact comfortably with peers and teachers and eventually graduated from high school and went on to college.

The reversible MAOIs selective for the A isoenzyme of monoamine oxidase appear to have better safety and side-effects profiles than do standard MAOIs and may be useful for social phobia as well. The initial experience with moclobemide (Aurorix) was promising, but more recent studies have been less positive. Initial studies with brofaramine are also promising, but further controlled trials are needed.

The other class of drugs with demonstrated efficacy in controlled trials of social phobia is the benzodiazepines. Placebo-controlled trials suggest that both clonazepam (Klonopin) and alprazolam (Xanax) are effective for social phobia. In separate trials alprazolam's benefits did not quite measure up to those seen with phenelzine but clonazepam appeared to be as effective as phenelzine. On the basis of limited data tricyclics do not seem to be useful. Serotonin-specific reuptake inhibitors such as fluoxetine (Prozac), sertraline (Zoloft), paroxetine (Paxil), and fluvoxamine (Luvox) have shown efficacy in open or small controlled trials, but further studies are needed. Buspirone (BuSpar) also showed modest efficacy in an open trial.

The β-adrenergic receptor antagonists have received only limited study. In one placebo-controlled comparative trial with phenelzine the cardioselective peripherally acting β-adrenergic receptor antagonist atenolol was not effective but most of the patients had generalized social phobia. β-adrenergic receptor antagonists should be most helpful for performance anxiety but in the study under discussion the performance anxiety subgroup was not large enough to permit the assessment of atenolol's effects. Propranolol (Inderal) seems effective anecdotally when taken on an as-needed basis for performance anxiety. In one small placebo-controlled trial on social phobia propranolol did not seem to be effective, but it was administered on a maintenance rather than as-needed basis and all patients also received behavior therapy. It is not clear whether the sample consisted of persons with generalized or discrete social phobias.

Psychosocial treatment Cognitive-behavioral therapy uses cognitive retraining, as well as desensitization through rehearsal, homework, and relaxation training, and is often carried out in a group setting. It may be more effective for patients with performance anxiety than for those with highly generalized social phobia or avoidant personality disorder but seems helpful for the latter groups as well. With cognitive-behavioral therapy there may be less relapse when treatment is discontinued because active coping and mastery are encouraged. Ultimately, combinations of medication and specific therapies may prove best for severely disturbed patients who are highly impaired.

In controlled comparisons of phenelzine and cognitive-behavioral group therapy carried out by the second author and R. G. Heimberg, the MAOI worked faster and demonstrated greater acute efficacy than the group therapy, but the therapy appeared to be more durable than phenelzine after treatment discontinuation.

SUGGESTED CROSS-REFERENCES

Panic disorders and agoraphobia are discussed in Section 17.1, obsessive-compulsive disorder is discussed in Section 17.3, and generalized anxiety disorder is discussed in Section 17.5. Biological therapies are discussed in Chapter 32, especially β-adrenergic receptor antagonists in Section 32.3 and monoamine oxidase inhibitors in Section 32.18. Anxiety disorders in the geriatric population are discussed in Section 49.6d.

REFERENCES

Agras S, Sylvester D, Oliveau D: The epidemiology of common fears and phobias. Compr Psychiatry *10:* 151, 1969.

*Barlow D H: *Anxiety and Its Disorders: The Nature and Treatment of Anxiety and Panic.* Guilford, New York, 1988.

Barlow D H, Craske M G: *Mastery of Your Anxiety and Panic.* Graywind, New York, 1994.

Davidson J R T, Hughes D L, George L K, Blazer D G: The epidemiology of social phobia: Findings from Epidemiologic Catchment Area Study. Psychol Med *23:* 709, 1993.

Davidson J R T, Potts N, Richichi E, Krishnon L, Ford S M, Smith R, Wilson W R: Treatment of social phobia with clonazepam. J Clin Psychopharmacol *13:* 423, 1993.

Fyer A J, Mannuzza S, Chapman T, Liebowitz M R, Klein D F: A direct interview family study of social phobia. Arch Gen Psychiatry *50:* 286, 1994.

Fyer A J, Mannuzza S, Gallops M S, Martin L Y, Aaronson C, Gorman J M, Liebowitz M R, Klein D F: Familial transmission of simple phobias and fears. Arch Gen Psychiatry *47:* 252, 1990.

Heimberg R G, Barlow D H: New developments in cognitive-behavioral therapy for social phobia. J Clin Psychiatry *52:* 21, 1991.

Himle J A, McPhee K, Cameron O F, Curtis G C: Simple phobia: Evidence for heterogeneity. Psychiatry Res *28:* 25, 1989.

Kagan J, Reznick J S, Snidman N: Behavioral inhibition to the unfamiliar. Child Dev *55:* 2212, 1984.

Kiessler R C, McGonagle K A, Zhao S, Nelson C B, Hughes M, Eshleman S, Wittchen H U, Kendler K S: Lifetime and 12-month prevalence of DSM-III-R psychiatric disorders in the United States. Arch Gen Psychiatry *51:* 8, 1994.

Levin A P, Saoud J, Straumen T, Gormen T, Fyer A J, Crawford R L, Liebowitz M R: Responses of "generalized" and "discrete" social phobics during public speaking. J Anx Disord, *7:* 207, 1993.

*Liebowitz M R, Gorman J M, Fyer A F, Klein D F: Social phobia: Review of a neglected anxiety disorder. Arch Gen Psychiatry *42:* 729, 1985.

Liebowitz M R, Quitkin F M, Stewart J W, McGrath P J, Harrison W M, Markowitz J S, Rabkin J G, Tricamo E, Goetz D M, Klein D F: Antidepressant specificity in atypical depression. Arch Gen Psychiatry *45:* 129, 1988.

*Liebowitz M R, Schneier F, Campeas R, Hollander E, Hatterer J, Fyer A, Gorman J M, Papp L, Davies S, Gully R, Klein D F: Phenelzine vs. atenolol in social phobia: A placebo controlled comparison. Arch Gen Psychiatry, *49:* 290, 1992.

*Marks I M: *Fears and Phobias.* Heinemann, London, 1969.

Marks I M, Bebbington P: Space phobia: Syndrome or agoraphobic variant? Br Med J *2:* 345, 1976.

Marks I M, Gelder M G: Different ages of onset in varieties of phobia. Am J Psychiatry *123:* 218, 1966.

McCaffrey R J, Rapee R M, Gansler D A, Barlow D H: Interaction of neuropsychological and psychological factors in two cases of "space phobia." J Behav Ther Exp Psychiatry *21:* 113. 1990.

Munjack D J: The onset of driving phobia. J Behav Ther Exp Psychiatry *15:* 305, 1984.

Myers J K, Weissman M M, Tischler C E, Holzer C E III, Orvaschel H, Anthony J C, Boyd J H, Burke J D Jr, Kramer M, Stoltzman R:

Six-month prevalence of psychiatric disorders in three communities. Arch Gen Psychiatry *41:* 959, 1984.
Oberlander E, Liebowitz M R, Schneier F R: Physical disability and social phobia. J Clin Psychopharmacol *14:* 136, 1994.
*Öst L G: Age of onset of different phobias. J Abnorm Psychol *96:* 223, 1987.
Öst L G: Ways of acquiring phobias and outcome of behavioral treatment. Behav Res Ther *23:* 683, 1985.
Öst L G, Sterner U: Applied tension: A specific behavioural method for treatment of blood phobia. Behav Res Ther *25:* 25, 1987.
Reiger D A, Myers J K, Kramer M, Robbins D G, Hough R L, Eaton W W, Locke B Z: The NIMH Epidemiologic Catchment Area (ECA) program: Historical context, major objectives, and study population characteristics. Arch Gen Psychiatry *41:* 934, 1984.
Schneier F R, Johnson J, Horning C D, Liebowitz M R, Weissman M M: Social phobics: Comorbidity and morbidity in an epidemiological sample. Arch Gen Psychiatry *49:* 282, 1992.
Seligman M E P: Phobias and preparedness. Behav Ther *2:* 307, 1971.
Stein M B, Tancer M E, Uhde T W: Heart rate and plasma norepinephrine response severity to orthostatic challenge and anxiety disorder. Arch Gen Psychiatry *49:* 311, 1992.
Stein M B, Walker J R, Ford D R: Setting diagnostic threshold for social phobia: Considerations from a community survey of social anxiety. Am J Psychiatry *151:* 408, 1994.
Tancer M E: Neurobiology of social phobia. J Clin Psychiatry *54* (12, Suppl): 26, 1993.
Uhde, T W, Tancer M E, Black B, Brown T M: Phenomenology and neurobiology of social phobia: Comparison with panic disorder. J Clin Psychiatry *52:* 31, 1991.

17.3 OBSESSIVE-COMPULSIVE DISORDER

MICHAEL A. JENIKE, M.D.

INTRODUCTION

Obsessive-compulsive disorder (OCD) was, until recently, considered to be a rare disorder, but new data have revealed that it is in fact a common illness. "I know it's stupid. I feel like a crazy person, but I know that I'm not crazy!" Those are examples of statements from a typical patient with OCD who may spend hours a day washing his hands, although he recognizes that there is no real reason to do so. Some OCD patients check and recheck that a stove is turned off, that a door is locked, or that some disaster has not befallen their children. An internist with OCD may repeatedly call the laboratory to be absolutely certain that he heard the results correctly. Some patients do not have rituals, but they endure endless hours of intrusive obsessive thoughts. The disorder may be so severe that patients are unable to work. If untreated, patients may be disabled for life. Although a complete cure is extremely rare there are now treatments (behavior therapy and psychotropic medication) that result in considerable improvement for the majority of patients. Comorbidity of OCD with depressive disorders and other anxiety disorders is common and often complicates the diagnosis. Before beginning treatment, it is important for the clinician to understand the entire clinical picture.

DEFINITION The fourth edition of *Diagnostic and Statistical Manual of Mental Disorders* (DSM-IV) requires that a patient have either obsessions or compulsions that are a significant source of distress; are time-consuming; or interfere significantly with the person's normal routine, occupational functioning, or usual social activities or relationships. At some point during the course of the illness, the adult patient must recognize that the obsessions or compulsions are excessive or unreasonable. According to DSM-IV, *obsessions* are defined by the following features:

1. Recurrent and persistent thoughts, impulses, or images that are experienced at some time during the disturbance as intrusive and inappropriate and that cause marked anxiety or distress.
2. Thoughts, impulses, or images that are not simply excessive worries about real-life problems.
3. Attempts to ignore or suppress such thoughts or impulses or to neutralize them with some other thought or action.
4. Recognition that the obsessional thoughts, impulses, or images are a product of one's own mind, not imposed from without as in thought insertion.

Clinically, the most common obsessions are repetitive thoughts of violence (for example, killing one's child), contamination (for example, becoming infected by shaking hands), and doubt (for example, repeatedly wondering whether one has performed some act, such as having hurt someone in a traffic accident).

Compulsions are defined as follows:

1. Repetitive behaviors that the person feels driven to perform in response to an obsession or according to rules that must be rigidly applied.
2. Behaviors or mental acts aimed at preventing or reducing distress or preventing some dreaded event or situation. Those behaviors or mental acts are either unconnected realistically with what they are designed to neutralize or prevent, or clearly excessive.

Typical compulsions include handwashing, ordering, and checking. A significant change from DSM-III-R to DSM-IV is reflected in the addition of mental compulsions, such as praying, counting, and repeating words silently. In DSM-III-R, those were called obsessions, but because such repetitive mental actions generally serve to decrease anxiety, it was felt that they would be better characterized as mental compulsions. Obsessions are usually anxiety-provoking, whereas compulsions are usually anxiety-relieving (at least over the short term).

DSM-IV also notes that if another Axis I disorder is present, a diagnosis of OCD is appropriate only if the content of the obsessions or compulsions is not restricted to it (for example, preoccupation with food in the presence of an eating disorder, hair pulling in the presence of trichotillomania, concern with appearance in the presence of body dysmorphic disorder, preoccupation with drugs in the presence of a substance use disorder, preoccupation with having a serious illness in the presence of hypochondriasis, or guilty ruminations in the presence of major depressive disorder). Furthermore, to meet the diagnostic criteria for OCD, the symptoms must not be due to the direct effects of a substance, such as a drug of abuse or a medication, or to a general medical condition.

DSM-IV also allows the specification of poor insight type if, for most of the time during the current episode, the person does not recognize that the obsessions and compulsions are excessive or unreasonable. That uncommon subtype has been referred to in the past psychiatric literature as "OCD psychotic" or "schizo-obsessive" and has generally been considered to have a poor prognosis.

HISTORY

Centuries ago, persons with obsessive blasphemous or sexual thoughts were considered to be possessed. That religious view of obsessions was consistent with the contemporary world view, and the logical treatment was designed to expel evil from the unfortunate soul who was possessed. Exorcism was the treatment of choice, with the person being subjected to torture in an effort to drive out the intruding entity. Surprisingly, those treatments were occasionally successful. Obsessions and hand-washing rituals resulting from guilt were immortalized in the 17th century in Shakespeare's character, Lady Macbeth.

With time, the explanation of obsessions and compulsions moved from a religious view to a medical one. OCD was first described in the psychiatric literature by Jean Étienne Dominique Esquirol in 1838, and by the end of the 19th century, it was generally regarded as a manifestation of melancholy or depression.

By the beginning of the 20th century, theories of obsessive-compulsive neurosis shifted towards psychological explanations. Pierre Janet reported successful treatment of rituals with behavioral techniques; but with Sigmund Freud's writings on psychoanalysis of the Rat Man, OCD came to be conceptualized as resulting from unconscious conflicts and from the isolation of thoughts and behaviors from their emotional antecedents. As a result of those theories, treatment of OCD turned from attempts to modify the obsessional symptoms themselves toward the resolution of the unconscious conflicts presumed to underlie the symptoms. With the rise of behavior therapy in the 1950s, learning theories which had proved useful in dealing with phobias were applied to OCD, and, although they clearly did not account for all OCD phenomenology, they led to the development of the powerful techniques of exposure and response prevention for reducing compulsive rituals.

Over the last few years research on the biology of OCD has accelerated, with ongoing studies of pharmacological agents, neurosurgical treatments, brain imaging, genetics, neuropsychological dysfunction, and the association of OCD symptoms with Tourette's disorder and other possibly related illnesses, such as trichotillomania and body dysmorphic disorder. Theories of basal ganglia and frontal lobe dysfunction have been developed that lead to testable hypotheses about the underlying pathophysiology of OCD.

EPIDEMIOLOGY

PREVALENCE Even within the past decade, OCD was considered to be extremely rare (approximately 0.05 percent of the population). But more recent studies, including the Epidemiologic Catchment Area study, have demonstrated a six-month point prevalence of about 1.5 percent and a lifetime prevalence of 2 to 3 percent. That means that in the United States alone, between five and seven million people suffer from OCD. Recent pharmaceutical data indicate that far fewer than half of those patients are being treated.

AGE OF ONSET The mean age of onset for OCD in one study was in the early 20s, with over half of the patients becoming symptomatic by age 25, and three quarters by age 30. Fewer than 5 percent of the patients had onset past age 40. Another study of 83 patients arrived at similar findings: 65 percent of the sample had onset prior to 25 years of age. Another group found that 27 OCD patients had a mean onset of 25.6 years. A more recent report found a mean age of onset in 44 OCD patients of 19.8 years. From those data, it is quite apparent that OCD usually begins in early adulthood.

In an effort to see if patients with different symptoms of OCD (for example, checking, obsessions only, mixed symptoms) had different ages of onset, the author recently studied 138 consecutively evaluated OCD patients. Those with obsessions only or cleaning rituals only had a mean age of onset of about 27, while patients with checking rituals only or mixed rituals (for example, washing and checking) had an earlier onset of about age 18 or 19. In agreement with previous studies, the author found a significantly earlier mean age of onset for men (20 years) than for women (25 years).

ETIOLOGY

NEUROBIOLOGY In rare cases, one can identify a brain insult, such as encephalitis or head injury, as an antecedent to OCD, but typically there is no identifiable neurological precipitant. With the advent of precise neuroimaging techniques, such as morphometric magnetic resonance imaging (mMRI) and positron emission tomography (PET), new ways to look at the brain are now available. PET scans have indicated abnormalities in the frontal lobes, cingulum, and basal ganglia of OCD patients when compared with depressed persons and normal controls. In addition, volumetric computed tomographic measurements have demonstrated decreased caudate volumes bilaterally in OCD patients compared with normal controls (although that was not confirmed by a later magnetic resonance imaging [MRI] study), and other investigators have reported occasional patients with demonstrable lesions in the striatum. MRI has also found longer mean T_1 values for frontal white matter in OCD patients than in controls. Another study compared mMRI scans of the brains of 10 OCD patients to the scans of 10 normal controls matched for age, sex, and handedness and found that OCD patients have significantly more gray matter and less white matter, suggesting a developmental abnormality. The combination of findings from several high-technology imaging studies supports a neurological hypothesis for OCD.

Clinically, there is much overlap among patients with OCD, chronic motor tics, and Tourette's disorder, and a genetic relation among those disorders seems likely. Researchers find that about 20 percent of OCD patients exhibit tics.

Serotonin There is evidence that serotonin-specific reuptake inhibitors (SSRIs) are partially effective treatments for OCD. In one study comparing clomipramine (Anafranil) to nortriptyline (Aventyl) and placebo, only clomipramine was significantly superior to placebo in reducing OCD symptoms. In addition, response to clomipramine was strongly correlated with lowering of cerebrospinal fluid (CSF) concentrations of 5-hydroxyindoleacetic acid (5-HIAA), a metabolite of serotonin, suggesting that changes in the serotonergic system had something to do with the good clinical outcome. In another OCD study, clomipramine was compared to a monoamine oxidase inhibitor (MAOI) (clorgyline) in a double-blind placebo-controlled crossover manner. Again, clomipramine significantly reduced OCD symptoms in comparison with both clorgyline and placebo, with improvement correlating with plasma concentrations of clomipramine. Other researchers found clomipramine to be clearly superior to desipramine (Norpramin) in the treatment of children and adolescents with OCD. In the majority of drug studies to date, although there has been significant comorbidity with major depressive disorder, the depressed subjects showed no difference in treatment response of OCD symptoms.

Open and double-blind trials of other SSRIs, such as fluvoxamine (Luvox), paroxetine (Paxil), sertraline (Zoloft), and fluoxetine (Prozac), have yielded comparable beneficial results. Because differences in efficacy among these agents are probably quite small, only large-scale trials would be likely to demonstrate that any one drug is superior to another. It can be concluded that several agents that selectively block serotonergic uptake diminish OCD symptoms, while pharmacologically similar agents without serotonergic selectivity are not nearly as effective.

Although research suggests that alteration of brain serotonergic systems may be one mechanism through which SSRIs have their therapeutic effects, there is no evidence of baseline serotonergic dysfunction in OCD patients. No significant difference in imipramine (Tofranil) binding or serotonergic uptake in platelets has been found, but CSF 5-HIAA has inconsistently been found to be elevated in OCD patients compared with normal controls, implying a higher rate of serotonin turnover.

One study found that the Bmax (estimate of receptor density in a tissue sample) determined by 3H-imipramine binding was significantly reduced in an OCD group compared with controls. If confirmed, that would suggest a lower density of 5-hydroxytryptamine (5-HT) receptors in OCD, a conclusion inconsistent with the hypothesis that treatment with SSRIs has its effect via down regulation of 5-HT receptors. Another study of childhood OCD subjects and age-matched normal controls found no differences in platelet 5-HT binding, monoamine oxidase activity, or plasma epinephrine, or plasma norepinephrine concentrations between the two groups.

Some data suggest that serotonergic perturbations can modify symptoms of OCD. M-chlorophenylpiperazine (mCPP), a putative 5-HT agonist, has been shown to decrease brain 5-HIAA in rats when administered intraperitoneally, but the effects of mCPP on human subjects are problematic. A comparison of the effects of *intravenously* administered mCPP was performed on OCD subjects and normal controls. It did not exacerbate OCD symptoms. The effects of *orally* administered mCPP, studied in a double-blind placebo-controlled comparison between OCD subjects and normal controls, exacerbated OCD symptoms in OCD patients, who also became significantly more anxious, depressed, and dysphoric in comparison with controls. It is difficult to explain the disparity between the various findings. Possibilities include the differential route of administration (that is, oral versus intravenous) or some difference in the population of OCD subjects studied. A subsequent experiment studied the effects of oral mCPP versus placebo in nine OCD subjects, challenged in a double-blind crossover paradigm, before and during (after four months) clomipramine treatment. The baseline effects of mCPP replicated the previous findings (that is, worsening of OCD symptoms). However, after four months of clomipramine, mCPP no longer exacerbated OCD symptoms. The investigators regarded their findings as consistent with the hypothesis that clomipramine acts via down-regulation of 5-HT receptors.

Other Neurotransmitters A number of studies support the hypothesis that the serotonergic system is not the only system involved in the pathophysiology of OCD. The clinical ineffectiveness of the potent serotonergic agent, zimelidine, and of the anxiolytic 5-HT_{1A} partial agonist buspirone (BuSpar), for example, are difficult to explain within a strictly serotonergic model. It is possible that a balance of adrenergic and serotonergic action is necessary. A meta-analysis of four studies of potent serotonergic agents (fluvoxamine, sertraline, fluoxetine, and clomipramine) in obsessive-compulsive patients revealed that greater effect size (that is, improvement in OCD symptoms) was actually associated with *less* serotonergic selectivity. The results suggest that a comprehensive model of OCD must be based on a multiple neurotransmitter system.

PSYCHODYNAMIC THEORIES Although psychoanalysis and psychodynamically oriented psychotherapy are not effective in the treatment of obsessions and compulsions, a number of interesting hypotheses are raised by theorists in that area. Many of the psychoanalytic theorists do not clearly distinguish obsessive-compulsive personality disorder from OCD and may see these disorders on a continuum. The psychoanalytic theories, described by John Nemiah and Thomas Uhde in the previous edition of this textbook are summarized below.

Nemiah and Uhde noted that, from a psychoanalytic perspective, three major psychological defensive mechanisms determine the form and quality of obsessive-compulsive symptoms and character traits: isolation, undoing, and reaction formation.

Isolation Isolation is a defense mechanism that protects an individual from anxiety-provoking affects and impulses. Under ordinary circumstances, an individual experiences in consciousness both the affect and the imagery of an emotion-laden idea, whether it be a fantasy or the memory of an event. When isolation occurs, the affect and the impulse from which it derives are separated from the ideational component and pushed out of consciousness. If isolation is completely successful, the impulse and its associated affect are totally repressed, and the patient is consciously aware of only the affectless idea that is related to it. Sometimes, however, the isolation is less effective, and the total quantity of energy accruing to the impulse and its associated affect cannot be completely restrained by the repressing forces from entering the patient's consciousness. Patients experience a partial awareness of the impulse without fully recognizing its meaning or significance. For example, they may have frightening and compelling murderous impulses toward strangers or casual acquaintances; here, the impulse makes itself felt as an urge to violent action, but the direction of the urge is displaced from the true object of the patients' aggression. At the same time, isolation makes patients unaware that they are angry, so that they are puzzled and disturbed by their compulsions. Alternatively, patients may be obsessed with images and thoughts of violence and destruction; here again, the energy from the partially repressed impulse gives the thoughts their compelling quality, and the continuing partial functioning of the mechanism of isolation prevents patients from becoming aware that beneath the surface they harbor intense aggression.

Undoing Nemiah and Uhde noted that, in the face of the impulse's constant threat to escape the primary defense of isolation, further defensive operations are required to combat the impulse and to quiet the anxiety aroused by its imminent eruption into consciousness. The anxiety-allaying function of compulsive acts can readily be noted in the clinical manifestations of OCD. The compulsive act is the manifestation of a defensive operation aimed at reducing anxiety and at controlling the underlying impulse that has not been sufficiently contained by isolation. A particularly important secondary defensive operation of that sort is the mechanism of undoing. As the word suggests, undoing refers to a compulsive act that is performed in an attempt to prevent or undo the consequences that the patient irrationally anticipates from a frightening obsessional thought or impulse.

Reaction formation Both isolation and undoing are defensive maneuvers that are intimately involved in the production of clinical symptoms. Reaction formation, a third mechanism closely associated with OCD, according to Nemiah and Uhde, results in the formation of character traits rather than symptoms. As the term implies, reaction formation involves manifest patterns of behavior and consciously experienced attitudes that are exactly the opposite of the underlying impulses. Often these patterns appear to an observer to be highly exaggerated and sometimes quite inappropriate. Reaction formation is thought to be responsible for many of the personality traits characterized by control that make up some elements of obsessive-compulsive personality disorder.

Psychogenetic factors Nemiah and Uhde noted that one of the striking features of patients with OCD is the degree to which they are preoccupied with aggression or dirt, either overtly in the content of their symptoms or in the associations that lie behind them. That and other observations have led to the psychodynamic proposition that the psychogenesis of OCD lies in disturbances in normal growth and development related to the anal-sadistic phase. According to that conceptualization, the impulses associated with the anal-sadistic phase are normally modified in the oedipal and succeeding stages of development. If that developmental process is disturbed, unmodified anal-sadistic impulses will persist as components of the individual's psychological makeup. Ordinarily, impulses of that type are controlled and disguised by character traits and do not significantly affect the person's day-to-day functioning. However, they remain as fixation points that may give rise to difficulties under certain circumstances.

Regression According to Nemiah and Uhde, the psychoanalytic concepts of disturbances in development and fixation points permit an understanding of the process of regression. In the classic analytic formulation, regression is the central mechanism in the formation of obsessive-compulsive symptoms and determines that a person will develop that disorder rather than a conversion disorder. According to psychoanalytic theory, the person with conversion disorder has repressed oedipal genital libido, and the energy from that undischarged impulse is converted into somatic symptoms. A different process occurs in the obsessive-compulsive reaction. OCD patients may begin with a conflict over the oedipal genital impulse, when, for example, it is aroused by an environmental stimulus. Instead of repressing and converting that impulse, they avoid the associated anxiety by abandoning the genital impulses and regressing to the earlier anal-sadistic phase. Regression is facilitated by the fixation points that remain from the distortions that occurred during childhood development. By giving up genital urges, patients are no longer confronted with the conflicts and problems resulting from these urges.

Ambivalence Nemiah and Uhde noted that ambivalence is the direct result of a change in the characteristics of the impulse life. Ambivalence is an important feature during the normal anal-sadistic developmental phase. Children in that phase feel both love and murderous hate toward the same person. One emotion follows the other in such rapid succession that they appear temporarily to exist side by side. In normal development much of the aggression is neutralized, and what remains is the desire to win out over, rather than to destroy, the other person. As a result, in a mature person, love for the object is dominant, and aggression plays a minor role. When regression occurs, there is a return to the earlier level of functioning, in which ambivalence is a characteristic mode of feeling. OCD patients often consciously experience both love and hate towards others. The conflict of opposing emotions may be seen in the doing-undoing patterns of behavior and in the paralyzing doubt in the face of choices that are so frequently found in persons with OCD.

Magical thinking In the phenomenon of magical thinking, Nemiah and Uhde reported that the regression uncovers earlier modes of thought rather than impulses; that is, ego functions, as well as id functions, are affected by regression. The phenomenon of the omnipotence of thought is inherent in magical thinking. Individuals believe that merely by thinking about an event in the external world they can cause it to occur, without intermediate physical actions. It is that feeling that makes aggressive thoughts so frightening to OCD patients. The phenomenon is related to the incantations and rituals that are central to organized magic in all ages and cultures. The same mode of thinking is present in primitive peoples who fear the evil thoughts of others and ward off the bad consequences of such thoughts by special formulas, or who try to influence natural forces, such as rain and fertility, by magic. The same kind of magical thinking can be seen in children's rituals, games, and fears, which at times reach a degree that is suggestively pathological.

Changes in the superego Nemiah and Uhde described the psychoanalytic view of OCD as a regression to developmentally earlier stages of the infantile superego (sometimes called the archaic superego), the harsh, exacting, punitive characteristics of which now reappear in the mental functioning of neurotic adults. The appearance of symptoms in OCD is attributed to a defensive regression of the psychic apparatus to the preoedipal anal-sadistic phase, with the consequent emergence of earlier modes of functioning of the ego, superego, and id. Those factors, along with the use of specific ego defenses—isolation, undoing, displacement—combine to produce the clinical symptoms of obsessions and compulsions.

DIAGNOSIS AND CLINICAL FEATURES

PSYCHIATRIC EXAMINATION OCD patients usually present with specific complaints, such as pronounced obsessions or compulsive rituals, that allow the clinician to make the diagnosis easily. With nonpsychiatric physicians and even with psychiatrists who do not specialize in anxiety disorders, patients may be reluctant to discuss symptoms that they find embarrassing or disgusting. Some patients in intensive psychodynamic psychotherapy or psychoanalysis do not even mention their OCD symptoms. For that reason, clinicians should question new patients specifically about intrusive repetitive thoughts or rituals. Sometimes paper and pencil questionnaires, such as the Maudsley Obsessive-Compulsive Inventory (Table 17.3-1) and the Yale-Brown Obsessive-Compulsive Scale (Table 17.3-2) allow patients to respond positively to questions that the clinician can later discuss more fully. Sometimes patients cannot resist performing rituals in front of the physician, or they refuse to shake hands for fear of contamination. Most patients, however, can resist their urges when they are in public or in the physician's office. Patients usually appear completely normal to the casual observer.

Patients who divulge the nature of their obsessions may appear bizarre or irrational, but they almost always retain full insight and recognize that their thoughts and impulses are unreasonable and alien to the rest of their personality structure. No generalizations can be made about the personality types of OCD patients, and their demeanor may range from histrionic crying to obsessive fussiness and controlling. The majority meet criteria at least for mild personality disorders when first presenting to the physician, but those features usually subside as OCD symptoms improve. Conclusions cannot be drawn, therefore, about personality disorders or personality type when the patient is actively ill with OCD or with any other severe psychiatric or medical illness.

The DSM-IV diagnostic criteria for obsessive-compulsive disorder are given in Table 17.3-3.

SUBTYPES Symptoms can usually be placed into one of several categories: checking rituals, cleaning rituals, obsessive thoughts, obsessional slowness, or mixed rituals. Checking and cleaning rituals are the most common and multiple symptoms are the rule.

Cleaning compulsions A 20-year-old woman feared contamination from touching various things she considered dirty. She had to wear gloves or use paper towels to touch various "dirty objects." If, however, she did happen to touch her laundry, her bed, the door handles in public restrooms, shoes, the gas cap on her car, or other "dirty" objects, she experienced vague dirty and uncomfortable feelings, and she would engage in prolonged washing of her hands and would wash any clothing that had come into contact with the object. As a result of those symptoms, she was unable to work full-time and her social life was almost nonexistent.

Checking compulsions A 46-year-old woman checked when unsure whether she had performed an action correctly. She plugged and unplugged electric appliances many times to make sure that she actually took the plug out of the socket, and she turned light switches on and off repeatedly until she was convinced that she in fact had turned them off. She would stare at a closed door for up to 20 minutes to ensure that she had actually closed and locked it. She completely avoided financial paperwork because of a compulsion to check numbers over and over again, and she could no longer work in her previous job as a bookkeeper. She was no longer able to read because she continually reread sentences to be sure she had not missed any crucial ideas.

Primary obsessional disorder Perhaps as many as 15 percent of OCD patients have only obsessive thoughts, with few or no rituals.

TABLE 17.3-1
Maudsley Obsessive-compulsive Inventory

INSTRUCTIONS: Please answer each question by putting a circle around the "TRUE" or the "FALSE" following the question. There are no right or wrong answers and no trick questions. Work quickly and do not think about the exact meaning of the question.

1.	I avoid using public telephones because of possible contamination.	TRUE	FALSE
2.	I frequently get nasty thoughts and have difficulty in getting rid of them.	TRUE	FALSE
3.	I am more concerned than most people about honesty.	TRUE	FALSE
4.	I am often late because I can't seem to get through everything on time.	TRUE	FALSE
5.	I don't worry unduly about contamination if I touch an animal.	TRUE	FALSE
6.	I frequently have to check things (e.g., gas or water taps, doors) several times.	TRUE	FALSE
7.	I have a very strict conscience.	TRUE	FALSE
8.	I find that almost every day I am upset by unpleasant thoughts that come into my mind against my will.	TRUE	FALSE
9.	I do not worry unduly if I accidentally bump into somebody.	TRUE	FALSE
10.	I usually have serious doubts about the simple everyday things I do.	TRUE	FALSE
11.	Neither of my parents was very strict during my childhood.	TRUE	FALSE
12.	I tend to get behind in my work because I repeat things over and over again.	TRUE	FALSE
13.	I use only an average amount of soap.	TRUE	FALSE
14.	Some numbers are extremely unlucky.	TRUE	FALSE
15.	I do not check letters over and over again before mailing them.	TRUE	FALSE
16.	I do not take a long time to dress in the morning.	TRUE	FALSE
17.	I am not excessively concerned about cleanliness.	TRUE	FALSE
18.	One of my major problems is that I pay too much attention to detail.	TRUE	FALSE
19.	I can use well-kept toilets without any hesitation.	TRUE	FALSE
20.	My major problem is repeated checking.	TRUE	FALSE
21.	I am not unduly concerned about germs and diseases.	TRUE	FALSE
22.	I do not tend to check things more than once.	TRUE	FALSE
23.	I do not stick to a very strict routine when doing ordinary things.	TRUE	FALSE
24.	My hands do not feel dirty after touching money.	TRUE	FALSE
25.	I do not usually count when doing a routine task.	TRUE	FALSE
26.	I take rather a long time to complete my washing in the morning.	TRUE	FALSE
27.	I do not use a great deal of antiseptics.	TRUE	FALSE
28.	I spend a lot of time every day checking things over and over again.	TRUE	FALSE
29.	Hanging and folding my clothes at night does not take up a lot of time.	TRUE	FALSE
30.	Even when I do something very carefully I often feel that it is not quite right.	TRUE	FALSE

Table from S J Rachman, R J Hodgson: *Obsessions and Compulsions,* p 222. Prentice-Hall, Englewood Cliffs, NJ, 1980.

The thoughts are typically of an aggressive, sexual, or religious nature and are upsetting and repulsive to the patient. For example, an 18-year-old man could no longer go to public places because of obsessive thoughts and impulses to shout obscenities. Similarly, a 32-year-old woman no longer went to church because she would experience intolerable sexual thoughts about people she saw there and felt that she would blurt out obscenities at the priest.

Other less common subtypes Some patients spend inordinate periods of time placing objects in a specific order. Others suffer with primary obsessional slowness and become stuck for hours while performing everyday tasks, such as dressing and eating. Relatively rare subtypes are being identified, such as patients with obsessions and compulsions primarily aimed at controlling an overwhelming fear of having a bowel movement or urinating in public or young women who have face-picking bouts which can last for hours. Other disorders that may be closely related to OCD are monosymptomatic hypochondriasis, body dysmorphic disorder, and obsessive fear of acquired immune deficiency syndrome (AIDS), cancer, or some other illness.

DIFFERENTIAL DIAGNOSIS

OBSESSIVE-COMPULSIVE PERSONALITY DISORDER Obsessive-compulsive disorder is frequently confused with obsessive-compulsive *personality* disorder. OCD is an Axis I disorder in DSM-IV, while obsessive-compulsive personality disorder is an Axis II disorder. Occasionally, patients with OCD also have compulsive personality traits, and some (roughly 6 percent when assessed by a standardized structured interview generating DSM-III criteria) also meet criteria for obsessive-compulsive personality disorder.

PHOBIC DISORDERS The essential feature of specific phobia is persistent fear of a circumscribed object or situation. The essential feature of social phobia is persistent fear of humiliation or embarrassment in certain social situations. Common specific phobias include fear of small animals (for example, dogs, snakes, insects, mice), blood, closed spaces, heights, and air travel. In patients with OCD, phobic avoidance of certain situations that are associated with anxiety about dirt or contamination is frequent, but the concomitant presence of typical obsessions or rituals clarifies the diagnosis of OCD.

DEPRESSIVE DISORDERS Classic compulsive rituals are not generally part of the picture of depression, but depressed patients occasionally ruminate about a particular topic and may appear to have obsessions. Careful history will usually reveal that the depression preceded the obsessions or ruminations. In addition, the ruminations of the depressed person are more likely to have a realistic basis. For example, a depressed patient may constantly think about losing his or her job during hospitalization and may be unable to focus on anything else. In fact, the job may be jeopardized, and the concerns may be exaggerated but well-founded. About a third of the patients with OCD develop clinically significant secondary depression; fortunately, most antiobsessional drugs are also potent antidepressant agents.

SCHIZOPHRENIA Occasionally, the obsessions in OCD become so severe that the patient seems truly uncertain whether his or her concerns are realistic. Such obsessions are called *overvalued ideas;* for example, patients may hold the almost unshakable belief that they are contaminating other people unless they wash their hands for three hours after urinating. However, OCD patients with overvalued ideas can, after considerable discussion, usually acknowledge the possibility that their beliefs are unfounded. In contrast, the person with a true delusion usually has a fixed conviction that cannot be shaken and is also likely to have other psychotic symptoms, such as ideas of reference, paranoia, and hallucinations.

TABLE 17.3-2
Yale-Brown Obsessive-compulsive Scale

1. Time occupied by obsessive thoughts	0 =	None
	1 =	Mild (less than 1 hr/day), or occasional intrusion (occur no more than 8 times a day).
	2 =	Moderate (1 to 3 hrs/day), or frequent intrusion (occur more than 8 times a day, but most hours of the day are free of obsessions).
	3 =	Severe (greater than 3 and up to 8 hrs/day), or very frequent intrusion (occur more than 8 times a day and occur during most hours of the day).
	4 =	Extreme (greater than 8 hrs/day), or near constant intrusion (too numerous to count and an hour rarely passes without several obsessions occurring)
2. Interference due to obsessive thoughts	0 =	None
	1 =	Mild, slight interference with social or occupational activities, but overall performance not impaired.
	2 =	Moderate, definite interference with social or occupational performance, but still manageable.
	3 =	Severe, causes substantial impairment in social or occupational performance.
	4 =	Extreme, incapacitating.
3. Distress associated with obsessive thoughts	0 =	None
	1 =	Mild, infrequent, and not too disturbing.
	2 =	Moderate, frequent, and disturbing, but still manageable.
	3 =	Severe, very frequent, and very disturbing.
	4 =	Extreme, near constant, and disabling distress.
4. Resistance against obsessive thoughts	0 =	Makes an effort to always resist, or symptoms so minimal doesn't need to actively resist.
	1 =	Tries to resist most of the time.
	2 =	Makes some effort to resist.
	3 =	Yields to all obsessions without attempting to control them, but does so with some reluctance.
	4 =	Completely and willingly yields to all obsessions.
5. Control over obsessive thoughts	0 =	Complete control.
	1 =	Much control, usually able to stop or divert obsessions with some effort and concentration.
	2 =	Moderate control, sometimes able to stop or divert obsessions.
	3 =	Little control, rarely successful in stopping obsessions, can only divert attention with difficulty.
	4 =	No control, experienced as completely involuntary, rarely able to even momentarily divert thinking.
6. Time spent performing compulsions	0 =	None
	1 =	Mild (less than 1 hr/day performing compulsions), or occasional performance of compulsive behaviors (no more than 8 times a day).
	2 =	Moderate (1 to 3 hrs/day performing compulsions), or frequent performance of compulsive behaviors (more than 8 times a day, but most hours are free of compulsive behaviors).
	3 =	Severe (spends more than 3 and up to 8 hrs/day performing compulsions), or very frequent performance of compulsive behaviors (occur more than 8 times a day and compulsions performed during most hours of the day).
	4 =	Extreme (more than 8 hrs/day performing compulsions), or near constant compulsive behaviors (too numerous to count and an hour rarely passes without several compulsions being performed).
7. Interference due to compulsive behaviors	0 =	None
	1 =	Mild, slight interference with social or occupational activities, but overall performance not impaired.
	2 =	Moderate, definite interference with social or occupational performance, but still manageable.
	3 =	Severe, causes substantial impairment in social or occupational performance.
	4 =	Extreme, incapacitating.
8. Distress associated with compulsive behaviors	0 =	None
	1 =	Mild, only slightly anxious if compulsions prevented, or only slight anxiety during performance of compulsions.
	2 =	Moderate, reports that anxiety would mount but remain manageable if compulsions prevented, or that anxiety increases but remains manageable during performance of compulsions.
	3 =	Severe, prominent, and very disturbing anxiety if compulsions interrupted, or prominent and very disturbing anxiety when performing compulsions.
	4 =	Extreme, incapacitating anxiety from any intervention aimed at modifying activity, or incapacitating anxiety develops during performance of compulsions.
9. Resistance against compulsions	0 =	Makes an effort to always resist, or symptoms so minimal doesn't need to actively resist.
	1 =	Tries to resist most of the time.
	2 =	Makes some effort to resist.
	3 =	Yields to all compulsions without attempting to control them, but does so with some reluctance.
	4 =	Completely and willingly yields to all compulsions.
10. Degree of control over compulsive behaviors	0 =	Complete control.
	1 =	Much control, experiences pressure to perform the behavior, but usually able to voluntarily control it.
	2 =	Moderate control, strong pressure to perform behavior, must be carried to completion, can only delay with difficulty.
	3 =	Little control, very strong drive to perform behavior, can only delay with difficulty.
	4 =	No control, drive to perform behavior experienced as completely involuntary and overpowering, rarely able to even momentarily delay activity.

TABLE 17.3-3
Diagnostic Criteria for Obsessive-compulsive Disorder

A. Either obsessions or compulsions:
Obsessions as defined by (1), (2), (3), and (4):
(1) recurrent and persistent thoughts, impulses, or images that are experienced, at some time during the disturbance, as intrusive and inappropriate and that cause marked anxiety or distress
(2) the thoughts, impulses, or images are not simply excessive worries about real-life problems
(3) the person attempts to ignore, or suppress such thoughts, impulses, or images, or to neutralize them with some other thought or action
(4) the person recognizes that the obsessional thoughts, impulses, or images are a product of his or her own mind (not imposed from without as in thought insertion)
Compulsions as defined by (1) and (2):
(1) repetitive behaviors (e.g., handwashing, ordering, checking) or mental acts (e.g., praying, counting, repeating words silently) that the person feels driven to perform in response to an obsession, or according to rules that must be applied rigidly
(2) the behaviors or mental acts are aimed at preventing or reducing distress or preventing some dreaded event or situation; however, these behaviors or mental acts either are not connected in a realistic way with what they are designed to neutralize or prevent, or are clearly excessive
B. At some point during the course of the disorder, the person has recognized that the obsessions or compulsions are excessive or unreasonable. Note: this does not apply to children.
C. The obsessions or compulsions cause marked distress; are time-consuming (take more than an hour a day); or significantly interfere with the person's normal routine, occupational (or academic) functioning, or usual social activities or relationships.
D. If another Axis I disorder is present, the content of the obsessions or compulsions is not restricted to it (e.g., preoccupation with food in the presence of an eating disorder; hair pulling in the presence of trichotillomania; concern with appearance in the presence of body dysmorphic disorder; preoccupation with drugs in the presence of a substance use disorder; preoccupation with having a serious illness in the presence of hypochondriasis; preoccupation with sexual urges or fantasies in the presence of a paraphilia; or guilty ruminations in the presence of major depressive disorder).
E. The disorder is not due to the direct effects of a substance (e.g., a drug of abuse, a medication) or a general medical condition.
Specify if:
with poor insight: if, for most of the time during the current episode, the person does not recognize that the obsessions and compulsions are excessive or unreasonable

Table from DSM-IV, *Diagnostic and Statistical Manual of Mental Disorders,* ed 4. Copyright American Psychiatric Association, Washington, 1994. Used with permission.

TOURETTE'S DISORDER Obsessive-compulsive disorder is often found in patients with Tourette's disorder, and in that case both diagnoses are given. There is much confusion in the terminology used by neurologists, who often see Tourette's disorder patients, and that used by psychiatrists, who are more likely to see OCD patients. For example, rituals are sometimes referred to as complex tics in the neurological literature.

COURSE AND PROGNOSIS

The mean age of onset of OCD is between ages 20 and 24; over 80 percent of patients develop symptoms before age 35. Some patients describe the onset of symptoms after a stressful event, such as a pregnancy, a sexual problem, or the death of a relative, and in many cases the onset is sudden. Because many patients manage to keep their symptoms secret, there is often a delay of 5 to 10 years before patients receive psychiatric attention.

The precise course and prognosis of OCD cannot be predicted since details of its natural history are unknown. No carefully conducted studies have evaluated its longitudinal course. In general, OCD is a chronic illness that exhibits a waxing and waning course, even with treatment. Complete cures are unusual. However, approximately 90 percent of patients can expect moderate to marked improvement with optimum treatment. Some evidence indicates that good premorbid functioning is an optimistic prognostic sign, but hard evidence of this is lacking. The actual obsessional content does not seem to be related to prognosis.

FAILURE TO IMPROVE Poor compliance with treatment instructions is the most common reason for failure with behavior therapy. Behavior therapists make specific demands on patients, and compliance with behavioral instructions both during treatment sessions and also during homework assignments is imperative if patients are to improve as much as possible. Family members or friends often act as surrogate therapists in helping OCD patients to carry out homework assignments.

Patients who hold overvalued ideas that their compulsive rituals are necessary to prevent a catastrophe seem to have a poor outcome with behavioral treatments. For example, the patient who believes that her daughter will die if she does not wash all of her daughter's clothes every day is unlikely to give up washing rituals with behavior therapy alone. Antiobsessional medication may produce changes in such fixed beliefs, and behavior therapy may then be helpful.

In severely depressed patients, physiological habituation to a feared stimulus does not usually occur, regardless of the length of exposure, but such patients often respond well to behavior therapy once depression is controlled pharmacologically.

Patients meeting criteria for both OCD and schizotypal personality disorder seem not to respond well to either behavior therapy or pharmacotherapy. Those patients may really believe that their rituals are necessary to prevent some terrible event. In addition, they have difficulty complying with assigned behavioral and record keeping instructions. Such patients may benefit from a structured environment, such as a day treatment center or halfway house. Behavioral treatment may produce modest decreases in their obsessive and compulsive symptoms, along with moderate improvements in overall functioning. Even though the patients themselves may benefit only slightly, treatment often allows the rest of the family to lead a more normal life.

Even when responsive to behavioral techniques, patients with checking rituals appear to respond more slowly than those with cleaning rituals. Patients with checking rituals, especially those who check excessively at home, are often unable to engage in prescribed response prevention. Patients with primary obsessional slowness respond more slowly to behavior therapy than do patients with either cleaning or checking rituals.

TREATMENT

The treatment of patients suffering from OCD is an example of the need to integrate various approaches to maximize patient outcome. They must generally receive medication in combination with other approaches, particularly behavior therapy. That combined approach can be expected to improve the condition of most patients substantially, and occasionally completely, within a few months.

PSYCHOTHERAPY In the absence of any adequate studies of psychotherapy for OCD, it is difficult to make valid generalizations about its effectiveness. Nemiah and Uhde noted that, early in the development of psychoanalysis, psychotherapy was the treatment of choice, because, like conversion hysteria, OCD was regarded as a transference neurosis and should theoretically therefore respond to psychoanalytical techniques. Nemiah and Uhde noted that some analysts have seen striking and lasting improvements in patients with obsessive-compulsive personality disorder traits, especially when the patients were able to come to terms with aggressive impulses behind those traits.

Traditional psychodynamic psychotherapy is not considered an effective treatment for obsessions and rituals occurring in patients who meet the criteria for OCD in DSM-IV; there are no reports of patients who stopped ritualizing when treated with that method alone. Such treatment may be helpful for patients with obsessive-compulsive *personality* disorder. Conversely, there is no evidence that behavior therapy and medications are helpful for patients with the personality disorder. Many traditional psychotherapists find themselves becoming more directive with OCD patients and adopt techniques similar to those used by behavior therapists.

Supportive psychotherapy is often helpful. Regular contact with a kind, warm, and understanding therapist can help the patient to comply with behavior therapy and to cope with medication side effects. Whether or not OCD patients involve family members in their rituals, families may be very troubled by patients' behaviors. Any psychotherapeutic endeavors must include attention to family members through the provision of emotional support, reassurance, explanation, and advice on how to manage and respond to the patient. In addition, family members can be very helpful to the patient by serving as surrogate home behavior therapists.

PHARMACOTHERAPY The typical randomized prospective placebo-controlled trial, which proved so useful in depression research, was until recently almost impossible because of the small numbers of OCD patients available to any one researcher. The number of controlled trials is increasing, however, as OCD clinics are seeing growing numbers of patients. Currently, pharmacotherapy (combined with behavior therapy for patients with rituals) is considered a treatment of choice for OCD.

Cyclic and atypical antidepressants Case reports of successful treatment of OCD have involved almost every antidepressant on the market, including imipramine (Tofranil), clomipramine, amitriptyline (Elavil, Endep), doxepin (Adapin, Sinequan), desipramine, sertraline, zimelidine, fluoxetine, trazodone (Desyrel) and fluvoxamine. Recent double-blind placebo-controlled trials have revealed that clomipramine (up to 250 mg a day), fluvoxamine (up to 300 mg a day), sertraline (up to 200 mg a day), paroxetine (up to 60 mg a day), and fluoxetine (up to 80 mg a day) are effective.

The best studied antiobsessional agent is clomipramine, a tricyclic antidepressant, that has been available in Europe and Canada for many years. It has specific antiobsessional properties in addition to its antidepressant qualities. The optimum dose is unknown, but the majority of researchers believe that dosage should be increased to 250 mg a day if patients can tolerate the side effects. Many carefully controlled studies have confirmed preliminary results that clomipramine is indeed superior to placebo in the treatment of OCD. In one study, almost 60 percent of patients on clomipramine had at least a moderate response, and another 25 percent reported at least some improvement. The main drawback to clomipramine is its substantial anticholinergic side effects. Sexual difficulties are common, and a small incidence of seizures occur at higher doses. Most patients, however, tolerate it well.

Monoamine oxidase inhibitors Anecdotal evidence suggests that MAOIs are particularly helpful for patients who suffer concomitantly from OCD and panic attacks or severe anxiety. Affective illness in patients or their families does not appear to be a good predictor of responsiveness to MAOIs.

Lithium One double-blind crossover trial of six OCD patients carried out in Denmark reported that lithium (Eskalith) was not effective in OCD. On the other hand, there are a few case reports of patients with classic OCD who improved with lithium carbonate.

Obsessive-compulsive behaviors are sometimes found in patients suffering from bipolar disorder. A recent report of two patients who met criteria for both disorders, who were treated with a combination of therapist-aided and self-administered exposure and response prevention, demonstrated that behavior therapy was effective only after their major affective disorder was effectively controlled with lithium and antipsychotics.

A 22-year-old woman did not respond to clomipramine alone, but improved greatly a few days after lithium carbonate was added with a stabilized blood level of 0.9 mEq/L. Whether or not lithium augmentation of other tricyclic antidepressants or MAOIs for obsessive-compulsive symptoms is helpful, has yet to be shown.

Antipsychotic agents Only a few case reports outline success with antipsychotic agents. Most of the patients were atypical, and some fit the clinical picture of schizophrenia rather than classic OCD. The schizophrenic features may have been partly, or even substantially, responsible for the good results. One group of researchers reported that antipsychotics enhanced the effects of fluvoxamine alone or in combination with lithium carbonate in OCD patients with concomitant tics, while it did not help OCD patients without tics. However, in view of the scarcity of data on the efficacy of those agents and the frequency of their toxic side effects, their use can be recommended only for acutely disturbed obsessional patients for the shortest possible period.

Anxiolytic agents Anxiolytic agents are of little use in the treatment of obsessions or compulsions, but they do help with anxiety that many OCD patients report. If antiobsessional agents improve OCD, anxiety usually decreases without the use of anxiolytics. The literature contains a few case reports of success and a couple of controlled trials where outcome criteria were unclear. Buspirone was ineffective in one open trial, while another study reported that both buspirone and clomipramine led to similar and statistically significant improvement in OCD symptoms. The resolution of those conflicting results awaits further data, but most researchers are skeptical about the usefulness of buspirone in treating OCD symptoms.

ELECTROCONVULSIVE THERAPY Historically, many OCD patients received trials of electroconvulsive therapy (ECT). Most did not suffer from a major mood disorder, and the primary reason for administering ECT was for treatment of OCD.

A few studies report that ECT in combination with other treatment modalities was helpful. One atypical patient (obsessions only which developed after his wife's death) had a good response to ECT after not responding to a number of treatments, including a 12-week trial of clomipramine. One group assessed the combined effects of ECT, modified narcosis, and antidepressants on obsessional neurotics (unclear diagnostic criteria) and found that 40 percent of the patients improved; however, the relative effect of each form of treatment separately was obscure. Another author studied 100 patients with obsessional symptoms, which were also poorly defined, and concluded that

ECT had little effect on obsessional states. The general consensus is that ECT is not useful in the OCD patient who is not endogenously depressed, although scant literature exists concerning the effects of ECT alone on OCD.

PSYCHOSURGERY With the advent of restricted and relatively safe psychosurgical operations, such as cingulotomy and capsulotomy, and the recognition that some patients are severely disabled and remain refractory to modern treatments, interest in psychosurgery has reawakened. Since most OCD patients who undergo psychosurgery have had very severe illness that has not responded to multiple therapeutic approaches (including pharmacotherapy and behavior therapy), the results of surgical intervention are impressive.

A recent study confirmed the relative safety and partial efficacy (at least 25 to 30 percent of patients improved) of stereotactic cingulotomy as a treatment for refractory, severely disabled OCD patients. The main complication, seizures, which occurred in 3 (9 percent) patients, was easily controlled by phenytoin (Dilantin). Four patients committed suicide, but each was very ill with complicating disorders, especially severe depressive disorder, in which suicide is a common complication. All four patients were known to be severely depressed with strong suicidal ideation at the time of operation. It is possible that disappointment in the failure of the last-resort treatment contributed to suicide in those patients. There is some evidence that other treatments, including pharmacotherapy and behavior therapy, are more likely to be successful after psychosurgery than before, but more research is needed in that area. Psychosurgical patients often benefit only a few weeks to months after the operation.

A number of operations are used for the treatment of disabling OCD. A review of four neurosurgical procedures (anterior cingulotomy, limbic leucotomy, tractotomy, and anterior capsulotomy) reveals that anterior cingulotomy has a very low complication rate and a moderate success rate. Limbic leucotomy combines bilateral cingulate lesions with lesions in the orbitomedial frontal areas containing fibers of a fronto-caudate-thalamic tract that may be critical in the formation of obsessive-compulsive symptoms. Anterior capsulotomy and tractotomy also produce significant improvement rates.

The identification of patient subgroups with a good prognosis after neurosurgical procedures merits further study. Currently, it is impossible to predict which patients might improve and which procedure is the best for a particular patient. It is still unclear which OCD patients should be referred for surgical procedures, and definite recommendations must await the results of ongoing prospective studies. However, currently, psychosurgery does appear to have a role for the severely disabled and treatment-refractory OCD patient.

BEHAVIOR THERAPY The behavioral techniques most consistently effective in reducing compulsive rituals and obsessive thoughts are *exposure* to the feared situation or object, and *response prevention,* in which the patient resists the urge to perform the compulsion after exposure. Simple relaxation therapy is an ineffective treatment for OCD symptoms. Behavior therapy produces the most significant changes in rituals, such as compulsive cleaning or checking, whereas changes in obsessive thoughts are less predictable. That difference reflects the specific effects of behavioral treatment, in which the behaviors themselves are the targets of treatment. Behavior therapy (in combination with pharmacotherapy) is now regarded as the treatment of choice when behavioral rituals predominate.

Behavioral techniques have been understood for over a century; in fact, Pierre Janet gave a remarkably accurate description of what is now called exposure therapy, including the name itself:

> The guide, the therapist, will specify to the patient the action as precisely as possible. He will analyze it into its elements if it should be necessary to give the patient's mind an immediate and proximate aim. By continually repeating the order to perform the action, that is, exposure, he will help the patient greatly by words of encouragement at every sign of success, however insignificant, for encouragement will make the patient realize these little successes and will stimulate him with the hopes aroused by glimpses of greater successes in the future. Other patients need strictures and even threats and one patient told [Janet], 'Unless I am continually being forced to do things that need a great deal of effort I shall never get better. You must keep a strict hand over me.'

Inexperienced clinicians are sometimes fearful of the effects or unaware of the potential of behavior therapy. A number of common misconceptions have developed. The clinician needs to know that: behavior therapy will not lead to the formation of substitute symptoms; interrupting compulsive rituals is not dangerous in any way to the patient; the patient's thoughts and feelings are not ignored in behavior therapy; modern behavior therapists do not assume that all maladaptive behavior is learned through simple conditioning processes; the use of medication is not incompatible with behavior therapy; and behavior therapists recognize that their therapeutic techniques are not equally effective for all patients. Controlled outcome studies of exposure and response prevention for OCD over the past 15 years with more than 200 patients in various countries have found that 60 to 70 percent of OCD patients were much improved after behavioral treatment. At follow-up of two or more years, reduction in rituals were maintained in almost all patients. Preliminary results of a recent study indicate that behavior therapy may be more effective than pharmacotherapy. Patients with only obsessive thoughts and no rituals have been studied separately, with unpredictable results. Although the technique of thought-stopping is widely used to treat obsessive thoughts, there is no clear empirical support for its usefulness.

A few studies have attempted to tease apart the differential effects of the exposure and the response prevention components of behavior therapy. For example, with washers, exposure therapy was found to help mainly in reducing the anxiety component, while response prevention had its greatest effect in reducing the ritualistic washing. The combined treatment was more effective than either component in isolation.

In patients with checking rituals, combined imaginal exposure (that is, having the patient vividly imagine the most feared consequences of not ritualizing) and response prevention are superior to response prevention alone. That approach is necessary for some patients because the catastrophic consequences that many checkers fear never actually occur, so habituation must be carried out in their imagination.

Because OCD patients engage in obvious cognitive errors in inference and in assessing the probability of danger, the use of cognitive therapy to modify those cognitive processes would seem to be useful. Unfortunately, the treatment outcome with cognitive therapy has been less predictable than the combination of exposure and response prevention. The only controlled study found that cognitive therapy did not add significantly to the effects of in vivo exposure.

SUGGESTED CROSS-REFERENCES

Neurotransmitters are discussed in Sections 1.3 and 1.4 and learning theory in Section 3.3. Personality disorders, including obsessive-compulsive personality disorder, are discussed in Chapter 25. Behavior therapy is discussed in Section 31.2. Biological therapies are discussed in Chapter 32; electroconvulsive therapy is discussed in Section 32.28, and psychosurgery in Section 32.29.

REFERENCES

Baer L, Jenike M A, Ricciardi J, Holland A, Seymour R, Minichiello W E, Buttolph L: Personality disorders in patients with OCD. Arch Gen Psychiatry *47:* 826, 1990.

*Baer L: *Getting Control.* Little Brown, Boston, 1991.

Baer L, Minichiello W E: Behavior therapy for OCD. In *Obsessive Compulsive Disorders: Theory and Management,* ed 2, M A Jenike, L Baer, W E Minichiello, editors, p 203. Year Book Publishing, Chicago, 1990.

*Baxter L R, Schwartz J M, Mazziotta J C, Phelps M E, Pahl J J, Guze B H, Fairbanks L: Cerebral glucose metabolic rates in nondepressed patients with obsessive-compulsive disorder. Am J Psychiatry *145:* 1560, 1988.

The Clomipramine Collaborative Study Group. Efficacy of clomipramine in OCD: Results of a multicenter double-blind trial. Arch Gen Psychiatry *48:* 730, 1991.

Flament M, Rapoport J L: Childhood OCD. In *New Findings in Obsessive-Compulsive Disorder,* T R Insel, editor, p 183. American Psychiatric Press, Washington, 1984.

Foa E B: Failure in treating obsessive-compulsives. Behav Res Ther *17:* 169, 1979.

Foa E B, Steketee G, Milby J R: Differential effects of exposure and response prevention in obsessive-compulsive washers. J Consult Clin Psychol *48:* 71, 1980.

Freud S: *Standard Edition of the Complete Psychological Works of Sigmund Freud.* Hogarth Press, London, 1953–1966.

Jenike M A: OCD: A hidden epidemic. N Engl J Med *321:* 539, 1989.

Jenike M A: OCD: A question of a neurologic lesion. Compr Psychiatry *24:* 298, 1984.

Jenike M A, Baer L, Ballantine H T, Martuza R L, Tynes S, Giriunas I, Buttolph L, Cassem N: Cingulotomy for refractory obsessive-compulsive disorder: A long-term follow-up of 33 patients. Arch Gen Psychiatry *48:* 548, 1991.

*Jenike M A, Baer L, Minichiello W E: *Obsessive-Compulsive Disorders: Theory and Management,* ed 2. Year Book Publishing, Chicago, 1990.

Jenike M A, Baer L, Minichiello W E, Schwartz C E, Carey R J: Concomitant obsessive-compulsive disorder and schizotypal personality disorder: A poor prognostic indicator. Arch Gen Psychiatry *43:* 296, 1986.

Jenike M A, Hyman S E, Baer L, Buttolph L, Summergrad P, Minichiello W E, Holland A, Seymour R, Ricciardi J: A controlled trial of fluvoxamine for obsessive-compulsive disorder: Implications for a serotonergic theory. Am J Psychiatry *147:* 1209, 1990.

*Marks I M: Review of behavioral psychotherapy, I: Obsessive-compulsive disorders. Am J Psychiatry *138:* 584, 1981.

Martuza R L, Chiocca E A, Jenike M A, Giriunas I E, Ballantine H T: Stereotactic radiofrequency thermal cingulotomy for obsessive-compulsive disorder. J Neuropsychiatry Clin Neurosci *2:* 331, 1990.

Minichiello W E, Baer L, Jenike M A, Holland A: Age of onset of major subtypes of obsessive-compulsive disorder. J Anx Disord *4:* 147, 1990.

Moniz E: Prefrontal leucotomy in the treatment of mental disorders. Am J Psychiatry *93:* 1379, 1937.

Murphy D L, Zohar J, Benkelfat C, Pato M T, Pigott T A, Insel T R: OCD as a 5-HT subsystem-related behavioural disorder. Br J Psychiatry *155* (Suppl 8): 15, 1989.

Rachman S J, Hodgson R J: *Obsessions and Compulsions.* Prentice-Hall, Englewood Cliffs, NJ, 1980.

*Rapoport J L: *The Boy Who Couldn't Stop Washing.* Dutton, New York, 1989.

Rauch S L, Jenike M A: Neurobiological models of obsessive compulsive disorder. Psychosomatics *34:* 20, 1993.

Rauch S L, Jenike M A, Alpert N M, Baer L, Breiter H C R, Fischman A J: Regional cerebral blood flow measured during symptom provocation in OCD using 15-O labeled CO_2 and positron emission tomography. Arch Gen Psychiatry *1:* 62, 1994.

17.4 POSTTRAUMATIC STRESS DISORDER AND ACUTE STRESS DISORDER

JONATHAN R. T. DAVIDSON, M.D.

INTRODUCTION

The diagnosis of posttraumatic stress disorder (PTSD) first appeared in 1980 in the third edition of *Diagnostic and Statistical Manual of Mental Disorders* (DSM-III). It underwent some revision in 1987 in the revised third edition (DSM-III-R). The fourth edition (DSM-IV) defines it in six parts: (1) The person must have experienced, witnessed, or been confronted with an event involving death, serious injury, or a threat to the physical integrity of the self or others. (2) The traumatic event must be persistently reexperienced in the form of distressing images, thoughts, perceptions, dreams, or reliving; intense psychological or physiological reactivity may also be present on being reminded of the event. (3) Persistent avoidance of stimuli associated with the trauma and numbing of responsiveness must be present since the trauma. (4) Persistent symptoms of increased arousal should be present since the trauma. (5) Duration should be at least four weeks. (6) The disturbance should cause clinically significant distress in social, occupational, or other important areas of functioning.

The diagnostic criteria for PTSD are given in Table 17.4-1. The diagnostic criteria for acute stress disorder are given in Table 17.4-2.

HISTORY

Shakespeare recognized the features of the traumatic stress response. In *Henry IV* he described what are essentially the same three symptom clusters now represented in the DSM-IV definition—that is, recurrent intrusive features, avoidance, and hyperarousal. Other artistic and literary representations of the disorder abound from the past. The first medical reference can be traced to Silas Weir Mitchell, who observed traumatic stress responses in male Civil War veterans and female civilians, both of whom self-medicated with alcohol and opiates to deal with their symptoms. During the 19th century, debates ensued between those, like Hermann Oppenheim, who believed that traumatic syndromes are of organic structural origin and those, like Jean Charcot, who believed the syndromes to be psychogenically derived. Those debates have not yet been properly resolved.

Theories of the syndrome's psychological cause began to compete with physical causation theories in the early 1900s. Under the influence of psychodynamic theory, traumatic neurosis was viewed as the result of the reactivation of an unresolved conflict in a predisposed person. Childhood traumas and conflicts that might lie dormant out of the person's consciousness were emphasized. The stressor was considered to be not of primary importance but, rather, an event that brought previously unresolved conflicts to awareness. That theory was consistent with the view that objective trauma itself cannot cause a neurosis without significant childhood predisposition.

Military conflict invariably kindles interest in traumatic neurosis, although often after an initial denial by the authorities that such problems have occurred. In World War I the disorder was referred to as "shell shock" and "soldier's heart." Experimental studies revealed that the patients exhibited intolerance of carbon dioxide and exaggerated psychological and physiological responses to epinephrine.

In World War II traumatic responses were referred to as "operational fatigue" and "combat neurosis." Abraham Kardiner, who saw many World War II casualties, recognized a set of symptoms common to all extreme stressors. Accordingly, he established the first set of operational criteria for a condition that he referred to as a physioneurosis: (1) atypical dream life, (2) preoccupation with the trauma, (3) constriction of personality, (4) startle response, and (5) irritability.

Military psychiatry in World War II contributed substantially to the

TABLE 17.4-1
Diagnostic Criteria for Posttraumatic Stress Disorder

A. The person has been exposed to a traumatic event in which both of the following were present:
  (1) the person experienced, witnessed, or was confronted with an event or events that involve actual or threatened death or serious injury, or a threat to the physical integrity of self or others
  (2) the person's response involved intense fear, helplessness, or horror.
  Note: In children, this may be expressed instead by disorganized or agitated behavior
B. The traumatic event is persistently reexperienced in one (or more) of the following ways:
  (1) recurrent and intrusive distressing recollections of the event, including images, thoughts, or perceptions. **Note:** In young children, repetitive play may occur in which themes or aspects of the trauma are expressed.
  (2) recurrent distressing dreams of the event. **Note:** In children, there may be frightening dreams without recognizable content.
  (3) acting or feeling as if the traumatic event were recurring (includes a sense of reliving the experience, illusions, hallucinations, and dissociative flashback episodes, including those that occur on awakening or when intoxicated). **Note:** In young children, trauma-specific reenactment may occur.
  (4) intense psychological distress at exposure to internal or external cues that symbolize or resemble an aspect of the traumatic event
  (5) physiologic reactivity on exposure to internal or external cues that symbolize or resemble an aspect of the traumatic event
C. Persistent avoidance of stimuli associated with the trauma and numbing of general responsiveness (not present before the trauma), as indicated by three (or more) of the following:
  (1) efforts to avoid thoughts, feelings, or conversations associated with the trauma
  (2) efforts to avoid activities, places, or people that arouses recollections of the trauma
  (3) inability to recall an important aspect of the trauma
  (4) markedly diminished interest or participation in significant activities
  (5) feeling of detachment or estrangement from others
  (6) restricted range of affect (e.g., unable to have loving feelings)
  (7) sense of a foreshortened future (e.g., does not expect to have a career, marriage, children, or a normal life span)
D. Persistent symptoms of increased arousal (not present before the trauma), as indicated by two (or more) of the following:
  (1) difficulty falling or staying asleep
  (2) irritability or outbursts of anger
  (3) difficulty concentrating
  (4) hypervigilance
  (5) exaggerated startle response
E. Duration of the disturbance (symptoms in criteria B, C, and D) is more than one month.
F. The disturbance causes clinically significant distress or impairment in social, occupational, or other important areas of functioning.

Specify if:
  Acute: if duration of symptoms is less than three months
  Chronic: if duration of symptoms is three months or more
Specify if:
  With delayed onset: if onset of symptoms is at least six months after the stressor

Table from DSM-IV, *Diagnostic and Statistical Manual of Mental Disorders,* ed 4. Copyright American Psychiatric Association, Washington, 1994. Used with permission.

understanding of treatment methods in acute traumatic stress states. Investigators conducted pioneer work using barbiturates, amphetamines, insulin, ether, and carbon dioxide abreactions. They also observed clinical symptoms associated with chronicity and recognized the importance of general treatment principles, including the need for brevity, centrality (that is, the administration of treatment at one location), and the expectation of a return to military action (that is, the undesirability of avoidance behavior).

Early investigators of the survivors of death camps described symptoms of anxiety, motor restlessness, hyperapprehensiveness, difficulty in sleeping, night terrors, fatigue, phobic reactions, and a constant preoccupation with recollections of persecutory experiences. Those symptoms became known as the concentration camp syndrome. Some investigators regarded as the significant factor an organic brain disease as a result of physical injury. The concentration camp syndrome occurred, however, so regularly without evidence of predisposition among a high proportion of survivors that it became clear the symptoms were almost

TABLE 17.4-2
Diagnostic Criteria for Acute Stress Disorder

A. The person has been exposed to a traumatic event in which both of the following were present:
  (1) the person experienced, witnessed, or was confronted with an event or events that involved actual or threatened death or serious injury, or a threat to the physical integrity of self or others
  (2) the person's response involved intense fear, helplessness, or horror
B. Either while experiencing or after experiencing the distressing event, the individual has three (or more) of the following dissociative symptoms:
  (1) a subjective sense of numbing, detachment, or absence of emotional responsiveness
  (2) a reduction in awareness of his or her surroundings (e.g., "being in a daze")
  (3) derealization
  (4) depersonalization
  (5) dissociative amnesia (i.e., inability to recall an important aspect of the trauma)
C. The traumatic event is persistently reexperienced in at least one of the following ways: recurrent images, thoughts, dreams, illusions, flashback episodes, or a sense of reliving the experience; or distress on exposure to reminders of the traumatic event.
D. Marked avoidance of stimuli that arouse recollections of the trauma (e.g., thoughts, feelings, conversations, activities, places, people).
E. Marked symptoms of anxiety or increased arousal (e.g., difficulty sleeping, irritability, poor concentration, hypervigilance, exaggerated startle response, motor restlessness).
F. The disturbance causes clinically significant distress or impairment in social, occupational, or other important areas of functioning or impairs the individual's ability to pursue some necessary task, such as obtaining necessary assistance or mobilizing personal resources by telling family members about the traumatic experience.
G. The disturbance lasts for a minimum of two days and a maximum of four weeks and occurs within four weeks of the traumatic event.
H. The disturbance is not due to the direct physiological effects of a substance (e.g., a drug of abuse, a medication) or a general medical condition, is not better accounted for by brief psychotic disorder, and is not merely an exacerbation of a preexisting Axis I or Axis II disorder.

Table from DSM–IV, *Diagnostic and Statistic Manual of Mental Disorders,* ed 4. Copyright American Psychiatric Association, Washington, 1994. Used with permission.

entirely the result of the psychological trauma itself. The existential factors involved in surviving the concentration camp were vividly described by Viktor Frankl in his book *From Death Camp to Existentialism.* Robert Lifton emphasized in *The Broken Connection* the death imagery and resultant symptoms among civilians after the bombing of Hiroshima.

Partly because of the effects of World War II and the effects of the disastrous Coconut Grove fire in 1941, psychological trauma was recognized as an important and legitimate mental disorder. It was accordingly included in the first edition of *Diagnostic and Statistical Manual of Mental Disorders* (DSM-I), published in 1952.

COMPARATIVE NOSOLOGY

DSM-I DSM-I assigned traumatic stress responses to a separate category, calling them gross stress reactions and subdividing them into civilian and combat types. The reactions were viewed as self-limiting—that is, no chronic form of the disorder was permitted. When symptoms failed to remit, it was believed that such continuity reflected some preexisting disorder.

DSM-II In the second edition (DSM-II), published in 1968, traumatic stress responses were relegated in importance, being subsumed under the rubric of "adjustment disorder of adult life." As with DSM-I, DSM-II did not permit a chronic form of the illness.

DSM-III The third edition (DSM-III), published in 1980, incorporated many of the advances that had been made in the field of psychological trauma during the 1970s. DSM-III also acknowledged the serious traumatizing effects of the Vietnam War.

In establishing the new category of posttraumatic stress disorder, the framers of DSM-III included five elements. First, the event had to be a recognizable stressor that would evoke distress in most people. Second, it was necessary to have at least one symptom in which the trauma was reexperienced. Third, two or more symptoms of numbing or reduced involvement with the world were required (for example, efforts to avoid activities or thoughts related to the trauma, estrangement from others). Fourth, at least one of a miscellaneous symptom cluster was required; therefore, at least four symptoms were required out of a possible total of 12 symptoms. And fifth, DSM-III did not require a minimum duration for symptoms but stipulated an acute form (that is, less than six months), a chronic form (at least six months), and a delayed form.

DSM-III-R In the revised third edition (DSM-III-R), published in 1987, six additional symptoms were defined, and one (guilt) was removed. The six new symptoms were psychogenic amnesia, avoidance of thoughts associated with the trauma, avoidance of feelings associated with the trauma, sense of foreshortened future, irritability, and anger. In addition, two DSM-III features were subdivided in four criteria: intensification of symptoms by exposure to reminders of the event were separated into physiological and psychological distress on exposure to reminders of the trauma, and hyperalertness or exaggerated startle response became two separate items. Furthermore, the DSM-III criterion of memory impairment or trouble in concentrating became simply difficulty in concentrating in DSM-III-R.

DSM-III-R also took a coherent approach to the symptom groupings, reflecting the work of those who recognized that reactions to trauma often follow a phasic course: intrusive symptoms may alternate with or be followed by avoidance and denial. Furthermore, DSM-III-R required that a traumatic stress be outside usual human experience.

The DSM-III-R definition of a traumatic event has posed problems. Normative—that is, reliability—data do not exist with regard to whether an event is outside normal experience or unusually distressing to almost anyone. And the definition rules out some low-magnitude stresses that may give rise to PTSD in susceptible people. Therefore, in DSM-IV the definition incorporates objective characteristics of the event and the type of response that the event induces in the victim.

Another criticism of DSM-III-R is its heavy emphasis on avoidant symptoms in the C criteria. Some clinicians believe that the required minimum of three symptoms is too high a threshold; it disenfranchises many victims of disasters and other trauma who otherwise have PTSD. In addition, some of the avoidant symptoms are difficult to use (for example, foreshortened future and reduced interest since the traumatic event). Yet another problem with DSM-III-R is its lack of a category for acute nonpsychotic responses to extreme stress.

A final consideration is where PTSD belongs in the nomenclature. DSM-III and DSM-III-R both accepted the strong evicence that PTSD is a form of anxiety and included it in the anxiety disorders category. Growing evidence indicates that, as a causatively defined disorder, it properly belongs in its own category of stress disorders, as it was in DSM-I and in the ninth revision of the *International Classification of Diseases* (ICD-9) and as it is now in the tenth revision of ICD (ICD-10). Such a category can either be broadly based and include any form of stress response, including adjustment disorder, or be narrowly focused on disorders related to extreme psychological trauma.

DSM–IV In DSM–IV, the principal changes have been to alter the definition of the traumatic stressor, basing the new criteria on characteristics of the event itself and the emotional response induced in the victim. The intrusive symptoms remain as they were in DSM-III-R, with the addition of physiological hyperreactivity upon exposure to a reminder of the trauma. Instead of having to meet criteria for either avoidance or numbing, both elements are now required for the diagnosis of PTSD. The hyperarousal symptoms remain unchanged except that physiological hyperreactivity was transferred to the intrusive category. Duration of symptoms remains the same, but the acute and chronic subtypes have been reintroduced, as they had previously been in DSM-III. Delayed PTSD remains unchanged. An additional requirement is that the disturbance causes clinically significant distress or impairment in functioning, as is the case for all other anxiety disorders in DSM-IV.

Other differences in the description of PTSD in DSM-IV include the addition of some stressors which were previously disqualified (for example, life-threatening illness, non-physically threatening, developmentally inappropriate sexual experiences, and parental bereavement for a child).

Associated features elaborate upon the more diffuse symptomatology and behavioral changes which follow exposure to prolonged interpersonal stress, the culture- and age-specific emphasis on somatic symptoms, and, in the case of children, reenactment by play or disorganized behavior.

PTSD is one of the few conditions in DSM-IV where mention is made of the possible diagnostic value of psychophysiological measures of arousal. While those are far from being established as a diagnostic test, they promise to bring psychiatry one step nearer to the laboratory.

Associated physical examination findings are addressed. Although few are specific to PTSD, particular attention should be paid to the effects of head injury and burns.

Prevalence rates are included in the DSM–IV text on PTSD, citing figures ranging from 1 to 14 percent in the community, and 3 to 58 percent in at-risk populations.

The diagnoses of acute stress disorder is introduced into DSM-IV for the following reasons: First, emergence of major psychopathological states in the immediate aftermath of trauma may help with case detection of people more highly at risk for developing subsequent chronic morbidity. Second, in themselves, the disorganized behaviors that may be seen after extreme stress often leave the victims unable to properly look after themselves, and as a result treatment interventions are indicated. Third, ICD-10 and DSM-IV attempt to be as compatible as possible; since ICD-10 already included a disorder similar to acute stress disorder, its inclusion in DSM-IV brings these two documents closer together. A number of studies support the notion that an acute dissociative type of reaction exists after extreme stress and that common symptoms include distortions of time; alterations in cognition, memory, and somatic sensation; and derealization and depersonalization. Moreover, those symptoms are predictive of ongoing morbidity several months later.

Acute stress disorder is described as a disorder following traumatic stress as defined in PTSD. Persons with acute stress disorder show a decrease in emotional responsiveness, may feel detached from their bodies or their surroundings, or have dissociative amnesia. Associated features include hopelessness to a degree compatible with major depressive disorder, survival guilt, and problems arising from the patient's neglect of basic health and safety needs in the aftermath of trauma. Impulsiveness and risk-taking behaviors are often found.

The severity of response and the type of symptoms may be modulated by cultural differences. The prevalence of acute stress disorder is currently undetermined, but it is thought to be a function of severity and persistence of the trauma and degree of exposure to it.

Acute stress disorder is defined as being brief in duration, lasting from at least two days up to a maximum of four weeks. If the symptom picture persists at the end of a month, then the diagnosis of PTSD or other appropriate disorder is commonly given.

Differential diagnosis includes the need to rule out mental disorder due to a general medical condition such as head trauma, substance-induced disorder, brief psychotic disorder, and major depressive episode. It is important to establish that symptoms appearing immediately after trauma are not merely an exacerbation of a preexisting mental disorder. Some subjects may develop symptoms following exposure to extreme stress which does not conform to either acute stress disorder or PTSD: In many cases, a diagnosis of adjustment disorder would be therefore appropriate. Malingering needs to be ruled out both for acute stress disorder and PTSD.

ICD-10 The tenth revision of ICD contains a category of stress-related disorders, including (1) adjustment disorder, (2) acute stress disorder, (3) chronic stress disorder "following exposure to an exceptional mental or physical stressor, either brief or prolonged," and (4) enduring personality change after exposure to a traumatic event.

EPIDEMIOLOGY

A number of studies have examined the prevalence of PTSD; they can be grouped into studies of community populations and studies of high-risk groups exposed to a trauma. The epidemiological studies take into account nontreatment-seeking populations, since treatment-seekers are probably atypical for the disorder. For example, one researcher noted that only 1 out of 20 community-based cases had received psychiatric treatment.

The most widely used instrument, the Diagnostic Interview Schedule (DIS), may have underestimated the prevalence of PTSD, although a recent modification probably yields a sensitive and accurate estimate. Studies using the old version of the DIS suggest a lifetime prevalence in the 1 to 3 percent range; an additional 6 to 14 percent of the population have experienced subclinical forms of the disorder. A study using a revised version of the DIS found a 9 percent lifetime prevalence of the disorder and a lifetime 39 percent prevalence of exposure to a traumatic event.

Among populations who were chosen on the basis of exposure to a stressor, lifetime prevalence rates for PTSD range from 3.6 to 75 percent with various instruments. The National Vietnam Veterans Readjustment Study, in many ways a model epidemiological study, found lifetime rates for PTSD to be 30 percent for male Vietnam theater veterans and 26 percent for female Vietnam theater veterans. An additional 22 percent of veterans had experienced partial or subclinical forms of PTSD.

Early reports showed high rates of psychiatric morbidity after exposure to extreme trauma. Unfortunately, those studies could not apply contemporary diagnostic criteria for PTSD, so it is unclear just what the prevalence of the disorder would have been. However, reports were almost certainly describing states akin to PTSD. Included in the reports were an 85 percent prevalence of concentration camp syndrome in survivors of Nazi death camps and a 100 percent prevalence of some form of psychopathology. Fifty-seven percent (26 out of 46 survivors) had psychiatric complications after the 1941 Coconut Grove nightclub fire. Those early studies were important in highlighting the heavy toll taken after exposure to disaster.

Clearly, PTSD is common, as are traumatic stressors, using the DSM-IV definition; those events as a group are not outside normal human experience.

ETIOLOGY

PTSD is one of only a few disorders in DSM-IV that is defined by its cause. Without a stressor, the disorder cannot exist, but the trauma is not sufficient; many traumatized people do not have the disorder. The relative importance and the predisposing elements of the trauma are not clearly understood; the same is true for other causative factors. An interactive relation may exist between one event and one victim. At all events, no model of the cause of PTSD would be complete unless it took into account pretrauma (that is, personal vulnerability), trauma (stressor characteristics), and posttrauma variables.

STRESSOR A consistent relation emerges between the magnitude of the stress exposure and the risk of PTSD. The relation holds true across several kinds of trauma, including combat, homicidal crime, and sexual trauma. No evidence suggests that a certain threshold of severity must be met, nor does good evidence suggest that low-magnitude stress (for example, divorce, loss of income, chronic illness in the family) gives rise to PTSD to any appreciable extent.

Besides the events involving actual or threatened death or injury or a threat to the physical integrity of the self or others, cognitive appraisal factors are probably important. For example, one study noted that a rape victim's perception of being in a safe place at the time of the assault predicted high levels of symptoms. The experience of being intensely afraid, helpless, or horrified is a likely risk factor. Extreme shame or guilt may also be a risk factor, as in the participants in a brutal atrocity.

BIOLOGICAL FACTORS Numerous psychophysiological and neurochemical systems appear to be implicated in PTSD. Although not proved, the assumption is that changes in those systems were absent before the trauma and that the trauma itself is the inciter of short-term and long-term functional and structural changes. Some indirect evidence supports the contention.

Sympathetic activity Several studies show that enduring autonomic arousal exists in chronic PTSD arising from both civilian and military trauma. Elevated heart rate and elevated 24-hour urinary catecholamines both suggest increased sympathetic tone. Comparable with that interpretation are findings of lowered platelet monoamine oxidase (MAO) activity and of α-adrenoreceptor activity. However, there is some debate as to whether tonic increases of catecholamines are present in PTSD once the duration of baseline is taken into account. Studies which employed longer baseline rest periods did not find an increase in norepinephrine.

Further evidence of abnormal noradrenergic functioning in PTSD comes from studies which show increased psychophysiological reactivity to yohimbine (Yocon), an α_2 antagonist. Symptoms of PTSD are increased when yohimbine is given to patients with PTSD.

Heightened sympathetic arousal in combat veterans with PTSD is seen when they are exposed to reminders of their original trauma, as shown by heart rate, blood pressure, electromyography, and sweat activity. Enduring arousal in response to combat cues occurred in veterans with PTSD but not in combat veterans without PTSD but with other forms of anxiety. That finding confers a specificity to the diagnosis that allows the conclusion that cue-specific arousal in PTSD is more than a nonspecific index of anxiety-proneness. Recent studies have indicated a promising application of that paradigm to the diagnosis of PTSD as part of a multimodal assessment. Enduring arousal is accompanied not only by anxiety but also by anger and depression. The fact that those emotions may be primal can be taken to support the view that PTSD is best classified not as an anxiety disorder but in a separate category.

Neuroendocrine functions Several studies have examined hypothalamo-pituitary-adrenal (HPA) function in PTSD. Both reduced and elevated levels of 24-hour urinary cortisol have been reported, an inconsistency that has not been satisfactorily resolved. Possible explanations include (1) differences in the collection or assay procedure, (2) differences in the type of PTSD, and (3) differences in the symptomatic state (that is, acute exacerbation versus chronic stable symptoms). One study found basal plasma cortisol to correlate with increased PTSD severity; lowered cortisol may bespeak a pattern of denial. Therefore, conceivably some people with the disorder have decreased guilt and relative lack of denial and, perhaps, increased urinary cortisol levels.

One study found a blunted adrenocorticotropic hormone (ACTH) response after a challenge with corticotropin-releasing hormone (CRH). That finding was correlated with PTSD symptom severity but not with depression severity, suggesting a specific relation between PTSD symptoms and HPA axis dysfunction.

Recently, some researchers found a supersensitivity and an increase in glucocorticoid receptors in combat veterans with PTSD. Furthermore, a relation was found between HPA axis dysfunction and the disorder's symptom severity.

Other biological factors Opioid system abnormalities, including a naloxone (Narcan)-reversible analgesia in combat veterans who were exposed to reminders of trauma, have been seen. The degree of analgesia so induced was comparable to the analgesia produced by an 8 mg dose of morphine sulfate. The full relevance of such findings is unclear; perhaps the numbing and dissociative components of PTSD are mediated by changes in the opiate system.

Animal models and the clinical effects of fluoxetine (Prozac) in PTSD both suggest that serotonin is implicated. In further support is evidence that some serotonin agonists can evoke symptoms of PTSD in combat veterans with that diagnosis.

Abnormal event-related potential (ERP) indices of information processing have been found in PTSD, indicative of problems distinguishing target and distractor (that is, relevant and irrelevant) stimuli. Those may form the basis of concentration and memory impairment, and be reflective of an underlying noradrenergic fault.

Sleep studies Studies of prisoners of war from World War II, 30 years after their exposure to trauma, and studies of Vietnam veterans with PTSD have revealed increased rapid eye movement (REM) sleep and decreased stage 2 sleep. Following treatment with doxepin (Adapin), REM sleep measures were reduced, while the restorative stages 3 and 4 sleep increased.

Of importance to the separation of PTSD from major depressive disorder is the fact that the REM alterations of PTSD do not share many of the characteristics found in major depressive disorder, such as shortened latency or increased early sleep REM.

PSYCHOLOGICAL FACTORS Three relevant psychological models—based on psychodynamic, cognitive and information-processing, and behavioral theories—have been advanced.

Psychodynamic theory Sigmund Freud and other early analysts made several attempts to explain the symptoms and the cause of traumatic neurosis. An early formulation contended that trauma revives the original childhood neurosis through regression. Later, an energy model was postulated in which a strong external trauma causes a disturbance in the organism's energy. The stimulus barrier or protective shield is exceeded. Defensive mechanisms, such as repression of the event and undoing (in dreams and compulsive repetition of the trauma), are the ego's attempts to cope with the event and to drain off excess energy. Fixation on the trauma is important to the theory. Severe trauma with a chronic course and a poor response to treatment may lead to two unmodifiable ego changes: ego exhaustion and changes in the ego-superego boundary as a result of overwhelming guilt and shame.

Other analysts revised the concept of a stimulus barrier, changing it from a passive shield to an active attempt by the ego to protect itself against traumatization: The trauma must be understood in terms of the person's psychic reality and how the person interprets and reacts to the experience. Psychic trauma may result in the person's being overwhelmed with emotion and becoming terrified of the emotion's uncontrollable elements. The central role of affect in the theory explains such phenomena as affective blocking, alexithymia, and chronic depression.

Cognitive and information-processing theory After severe stress some persons are unable to process and assimilate the event adequately or to deal effectively with its effects. Because trauma may require its victims to make unaccustomed changes in their plans, satisfactory assimilation of the experience may be difficult, prolonged, and sometimes incomplete. Unfortunately, the experience is kept alive as an active memory and repeatedly intrudes into awareness. Because such experiences are painful, the person attempts to deny or to avoid the experience; by such avoidance, levels of anxiety may be reduced. In PTSD, those intrusive and avoidance phases alternate. The degree of distress, the impact of the event, can be measured by a 15-item self-rating scale (Table 17.4-3).

Information-processing models have been invoked to account for the development of the disorder. Fear may be stored as a memory network that contains information about danger-related stimuli. Because life-threatening trauma evokes a powerful response, that particular fear structure remains intense and easily activated. Distinctions between what is safe and what is dangerous are unclear, and persons who are strongly influenced by such fear structures may feel both lack of control and lack of predictability with respect to their environments.

Behavior theory Behavior theory posits a two-factor learning process in PTSD. In the first phase, persons exposed to a trauma (the unconditioned stimulus) learn by association to be upset by central events, images, thoughts, or situations that occur in proximity to the trauma (the conditioned stimulus).

Instrumental learning leads to the second factor, avoidance of both the unconditioned stimulus and the conditioned stimulus; that process is sustained because it leads to a decrease in anxiety. High-order conditioning occurs; ultimately, a wide range of stimuli elicit arousal (stimulus generalization). Although the two-factor theory has been criticized, it provides a theoretical basis for treating PTSD by means of direct therapeutic exposure to cues of the original trauma, an approach that may be beneficial.

OTHER CAUSATIVE FACTORS Many stressors can give rise to PTSD, although certain features are probably common to all stressors. Those features include objective qualities (for example, exposure to actual or threatened death, physical injury, or threat to physical integrity) and subjective responses (perceived helplessness, fear, or horror). Common examples of traumatic events include violent crime, sexual trauma, chronic physical abuse, military combat, natural disasters, manufactured disasters (acts of either commission or omission), complicated and unexpected bereavements, accidents, and captivity.

Such events can affect individuals or groups; they may leave a person's community and support system either intact or lost; they can occur as one-time, repetitive, or continuous events; they can occur at all ages in the life cycle; they can occur at varying levels of intensity. All those factors can affect the level of morbidity, the response to treatment, and the cause of the illness. Repeated traumatization in childhood may produce

TABLE 17.4-3
Impact of Event Scale

Below is a list of comments made by people after stressful life events. With respect to your own experiences of __________, please indicate how frequently these comments were true for you during the past __________. If they did not occur during that time, please mark the "not at all" column.

	Not at All (0)	Rarely (1)	Sometimes (3)	Often (5)
1. I thought about it when I didn't mean to.	____	____	____	____
2. I avoided letting myself get upset when I thought about it or was reminded of it.	____	____	____	____
3. I tried to remove it from my memory.	____	____	____	____
4. I had trouble falling asleep or staying asleep, because of pictures or thoughts about it that came into my mind.	____	____	____	____
5. I had waves of strong feeling about it.	____	____	____	____
6. I had dreams about it.	____	____	____	____
7. I stayed away from reminders of it.	____	____	____	____
8. I felt as if it hadn't happened or wasn't real.	____	____	____	____
9. I tried not to talk about it.	____	____	____	____
10. Pictures about it popped into my mind.	____	____	____	____
11. Other things kept making me think about it.	____	____	____	____
12. I was aware that I still had a lot of feelings about it, but I didn't deal with them.	____	____	____	____
13. I tried not to think about it.	____	____	____	____
14. Any reminder brought back feelings about it.	____	____	____	____
15. My feelings about it were kind of numb.	____	____	____	____

I* Total = ______ A† Total = ______ Totals I + A = ______

I: 1, 4, 5, 6, 10, 11, 14
A: 2, 3, 7, 8, 9, 12, 13, 15

*I = Intrusive
†A = Avoidance
Table from M Horowitz, N Wilner, W Alvarez: Impact of Event Scale: A study of subjective stress. Psychosom Med *41:* 209, 1979. Used with permission.

long-lasting states and may adversely affect interpersonal relationships and development; exposure to the most extreme kinds of trauma (for example, prisoner-of-war and death camps) may result in particularly severe and persistent states of PTSD.

Group trauma and the loss of the community may complicate the course of PTSD, as may engagement in litigation and extensive media coverage. The media serve as constant and often uncontrolled reminders of the trauma and as evokers of negative affect. The nature of a particular trauma can be both a pathological risk factor for PTSD and a determinant of symptom expression. For example, being in extremely confined spaces, such as underground tunnels in wartime, can give rise to panic symptoms. Participation in abusive violence leads to a predominance of denial and numbing, whereas witnessing such acts as a nonparticipant results in a predominance of reexperiencing symptoms.

Social support consistently relates to the risk of developing PTSD. The presence of social support has a buffering effect; lack of support serves as a vulnerability factor. Lack of support can be a preexisting vulnerability factor, or it can develop when trauma victims become separated from their social support networks (for example, in a natural disaster or mass genocide).

Additional premorbid risk factors from epidemiological and treatment-seeking samples include a family history of psychiatric illness in general and of anxiety disorder in particular, previous psychiatric disorders, personality traits of high neuroticism and poor self-confidence, early separation of parents, parental poverty, behavioral misconduct in childhood, abuse in childhood, limited education, adverse life events before the trauma, being female, and the quantity of alcohol ingested.

Epidemiologic data identify the risk factors for exposure to trauma, as they are somewhat different from the risk factors for posttraumatic stress disorder once the trauma has occurred. One study found the six strongest predictors of exposure to trauma to be male sex, absence of a college education, extroversion, neuroticism, early misconduct, and family psychiatric illness. By contrast, the six strongest predictors for risk of PTSD are female sex, neuroticism, early separation from parents, prior anxiety or depression, familial anxiety, and familial antisocial personality disorder.

Knowledge of the causative and the risk factors of the disorder can guide the efforts at early recognition and prevention of the disorder.

DIAGNOSIS AND CLINICAL FEATURES

In the immediate aftermath of trauma, a polymorphic symptom picture may emerge; the full complex of PTSD may not appear until several weeks later. A marked level of dissociation may be seen within the first few days of exposure to an extreme trauma, giving rise to the clinical diagnosis of acute stress disorder, which was introduced in DSM-IV for the first time. In other instances no clear-cut symptoms may emerge until some later time, when PTSD appears as a delayed response. Yet other manifestations may develop in which only some elements of PTSD appear, such as intrusive and arousal symptoms.

The stressor must meet two criteria: (1) be life-threatening or associated with serious injury or threat in physical integrity; and (2) evoke intense fear, helplessness, or horror in the victim.

Symptoms are grouped into three categories: (1) intrusive, painful, persistent, and recurrent reexperiencing of the trauma (the B criteria); (2) persistent avoidance of stimuli associated with the trauma and numbing of general responsiveness (the C criteria); and (3) persistent increased arousal that was not present before the trauma (the D criteria). Besides being conversant with the symptoms themselves, an assessor of PTSD must pay attention to the qualifying adjectives: ''persistent,'' ''recurrent,'' and ''distressing.'' The assessor must also decide whether or not numbed responsiveness and hyperarousal occurred subsequent to the trauma. In cases of chronic PTSD and in cases of early traumatization, arriving at such judgments is not easy; indeed, the validity of such a construct can be questioned when traumatic events like incest and childhood abuse were the causes of PTSD. Unless proper attention is given to those points, PTSD may be overdiagnosed.

The 17 symptoms of PTSD are listed in Table 17.4-1. At least one of five possible intrusive symptoms is required for B criteria, which represent the essential and distinctive set of symptoms by which PTSD is distinguished from all other forms of anxiety and depression.

A combat veteran had participated in atrocities involving the murder of civilians by a firing squad and had observed many rapes of civilian women. For years afterward he experienced vivid nightmares in which the scenes were reenacted in graphic detail. At other times he engaged in conversation with imaginary people, and during those conversations he relived the episodes. Often, he withdrew even from those to whom he felt close.

At least three of seven possible avoidance (C criteria) symptoms are required. The first three criteria—(1) avoiding thoughts or feelings associated with the trauma; (2) avoiding activities, situations, or play associated with the trauma; and (3) inability to recall an important aspect of the trauma—specifically relate to the trauma. The remaining four criteria are not specific to PTSD and may be found in other disorders, such as depression. Both avoidance and numbing are required for the diagnosis.

A woman in her early 20s had been raped seven years before. For several years after the trauma, the patient was unable to use the word ''rape,'' she avoided any conversation that dealt with sexual trauma, and she stayed away from her hometown to avoid exposure to any persons or any place that reminded her of the event. She went to considerable lengths, even spending her summer vacations in another state.

At least two of five possible hyperarousal symptoms (D criteria) are required. Those symptoms may also be seen in other disorders, such as generalized anxiety disorder.

A woman had been held up at gunpoint during an armed robbery. Although she had no previous history of psychiatric symptoms, for several years after the event she found herself unable to relax; she was on edge, had insomnia, and had to sleep in her mother's room with a gun beside her.

On the basis of literature surveys, no compelling reasons lead one to believe that the symptom picture differs substantially according to the age, sex, or ethnicity of the patient or the type of trauma. However, somatic expressions of PTSD may be seen more commonly in populations from other cultures, as well as in children. A number of associated symptoms can occur and may prove important in the treatment of individual patients. Those symptoms include survival and behavioral guilt, somatic distress, paranoia, interpersonal alienation, and the vegetative changes of depression. Victims of prolonged interpersonal abuse can exhibit impaired modulation of affect, impulsive behavior, and feelings of ineffectiveness and hopelessness.

Psychometric testing may reveal elevated neuroticism scores on the Eysenck Personality Inventory and elevated Sc, D, F, and Ps scores on the Minnesota Multiphasic Personality Inventory (MMPI). Rorschach testing may reveal the presence of aggressive and violent thoughts. For the most part, however, those psychometric studies are based on studies of combat veterans.

DIFFERENTIAL DIAGNOSIS

GENERALIZED ANXIETY DISORDER The hyperarousal symptoms described in the D criteria set are similar to those present in generalized anxiety disorder, but that disorder lacks a traumatic origin and the intrusive symptoms found in criteria B. Nonetheless, if any anxious patient presents with ready startle, remains on guard, and does not respond to the usual measures for generalized anxiety disorder, the clinician should consider a diagnosis of PTSD.

DEPRESSION Depressive features of reduced interest, estrangement, numbing, poor concentration, and insomnia occur in PTSD. Intrusive trauma-bound symptoms are not a feature of depression. However, after exposure to trauma, posttraumatic reactions are seen, and the clinician needs to address the traumatic component. Polysomnographs and neuroendocrine studies may help in the differential diagnosis of PTSD and major depressive disorder.

PANIC DISORDER Panic attacks resemble the autonomic hyperactivity in PTSD (criteria D). To distinguish the two, the interviewer should establish whether the panic attacks are related to the trauma or to reminders of it.

OBSESSIVE-COMPULSIVE DISORDER PTSD and obsessive-compulsive disorder both share the occurrence of repetitive, distressing recollections, images, or thoughts. To distinguish between the two disorders, the clinician must obtain a careful history, asking about the occurrence of the trauma and establishing whether the intrusive phenomena are thematically linked to the event.

DISSOCIATIVE DISORDERS Flashbacks, numbing, and amnesia may suggest dissociative disorders. When those symptoms are prominent or presenting features, the clinician must elicit a clear history of the additional intrusive, avoidant, and hyperarousal features that occur in PTSD but not in dissociative disorders.

BORDERLINE PERSONALITY DISORDER The diagnosis of borderline personality disorder is often made when PTSD is a more appropriate diagnosis or, at least, a necessary concomitant diagnosis. A clinician who makes the diagnosis of borderline personality disorder must inquire further into possible early trauma and ensuing symptoms.

MEDICAL DISORDERS After a patient sustains a head injury, the clinician must evaluate the degree of any brain damage and its possible contribution to some of the symptoms (for example, impaired memory and concentration, hyperarousal, dissociative symptoms). Close collaboration with a neurologist is advisable.

The clinican should also clarify the role of alcohol or psychoactive substance intoxication and withdrawal, since those disorders can aggravate PTSD symptoms.

FACTITIOUS DISORDERS PTSD must sometimes be distinguished from factitious disorders. Helpful clues are corroborative evidence that a trauma did occur and that the patient is usually distressed about the trauma and often reluctant at first to discuss its details. Factitious symptoms often vary in response to the immediate environment.

MALINGERING The clinician should evaluate the parameters of factitious disorders. Moreover, the motivational factors for malingering are usually quite clear.

COURSE AND PROGNOSIS

In the immediate aftermath of a trauma, a high percentage of persons have acute stress disorder or a similar set of symptoms. Those reactions are normally short-lived, but, by one month after the traumatic event, 70 to 90 percent of the victims may show the full symptom picture of PTSD. Such findings have been reported, for example, in rape victims.

About 30 percent of patients recover completely, 40 percent continue to have mild symptoms, 20 percent continue to have moderate symptoms, and 10 percent remain unchanged or become worse. Relative proportions of the intrusive, avoidant, and hyperarousal symptoms vary over time. The intrusive features may be prominent initially, with the avoidant features becoming prominent later. During World War II the observation was made that marked startle and hypervigilance—when persisting beyond the acute reaction, despite treatment—was a sign of a relatively poor prognosis.

Unfortunately, the passage of time does not always bring with it automatic improvement, and symptoms often worsen with age. Particular symptoms that increase with time include startle, nightmares, irritability, and depression.

DELAYED-ONSET POSTTRAUMATIC STRESS DISORDER

Although delayed-onset PTSD is rare, its existence is clearly established in a variety of victim groups. It is particularly well described among veterans of combat and victims of early sexual trauma. For reasons not fully understood, the disorder may arise de novo as long as 30 to 40 years after the trauma. In such cases an inciting trigger may activate unresolved aspects (unintegrated memories) of the original trauma. In other cases coping mechanisms, such as working and physical activity, may have successfully allowed denial; when those mechanisms are no longer available, because of retirement or physical illness, the memories appear. In addition, PTSD usually coexists with other psychiatric disorders; activation of the comorbid state can activate PTSD.

TREATMENT

Acute states of the disorder are best handled by immediate treatment geared to promote the integration of the traumatic experience. Chronic states of the disorder require multimodal individual or group treatments that are often but not invariably trauma-focused and aimed at integration. Medications should be offered to most patients with a diagnosis of chronic PTSD, although some patients may choose not to use drugs. Long-term supportive therapy measures are often indicated.

ACUTE STRESS DISORDER Acute traumatic reactions are traditionally treated in a way that encourages ventilation (or abreaction) of affects and images connected with the trauma. Telling of the tale is often desirable, and may help to minimize dissociation, which could otherwise lead to severe chronic morbidity. By encouraging that, the clinician enables the patient to confront, accept, process, and begin to integrate repressed or overwhelming material. Abreaction can be achieved in a number of ways—including individual therapy, group therapy, and hypnosis—and with intravenous barbiturate or benzodiazepine drugs. In addition, the clinician may need to treat agitated states by means of rest, sedation, and hypnotics.

The principles that are followed in treating acute PTSD include brevity, immediacy, centrality, proximity (close to the event), expectancy of return to full functioning, and superficiality (avoidance of dredging up deep issues).

CHRONIC POSTTRAUMATIC STRESS DISORDER Chronic PTSD can be treated by several techniques; in general, relying exclusively on one approach is likely to prove insufficient.

Initially, explanation and destigmatization are important; such explanations can be provided to the patient and the family members. The explanations include a description of the symptoms and the course of PTSD, the responses that occur after a severe trauma, and the general treatment principles. The clinician can also give information on appropriate reading, local support groups and resources, and the names and addresses of nationally based advocacy organizations. Attention to those initial issues helps promote trust and also affords reassurance that the therapist has a good understanding of the problem.

Pharmacotherapy Chronic PTSD is accompanied by enduring neurochemical and psychophysiological changes; its symptoms are distressing and lead to substantial psychosocial dysfunction. Symptom intensity is sometimes so distressing that it precludes effective trauma-focused psychotherapy. For those reasons the use of medication should not be delayed unnecessarily.

Tricyclic drug therapy with amitriptyline (Elavil) or imipramine (Tofranil) remains the most solidly established form of effective treatment; two double-blind studies of more than 100 patients support the drugs' efficacy. Both studies demonstrated efficacy on core intrusive features and showed that the benefits were not merely due to antianxiety or antidepressant effects. Studies with poor results for pharmacotherapy—using desipramine (Norpramin), phenelzine (Nardil), and alprazolam (Xanax)—either used inadequate dosages or too short a treatment term. At least eight weeks of treatment may be needed to show drug efficacy in chronic PTSD. Maintenance treatment should probably continue at least one year, although controlled studies are lacking. One group found that the maximum benefits of amitriptyline and psychotherapy took seven to nine months.

Open studies and one double-blind study attest to the value of phenelzine in PTSD, although the side effects may be a problem. Other drugs that may help include carbamazepine (Tegretol), fluoxetine (Prozac), bupropion (Wellbutrin), propranolol (Inderal), clonidine (Catapres), lithium (Eskalith), clonazepam (Klonopin), and valproic acid (Depakene). Controlled trials of those agents have yet to be performed. Since they encompass wide-ranging differences in mechanism, it is important to learn more about the unique advantages of each drug in PTSD; doing so may lead to a better recognition of the disorder's types.

Noteworthy is the relative lack of indications for antipsychotics in PTSD. Alprazolam may have only a limited application in PTSD, since one study found its therapeutic effects to be negative, and withdrawal from the drug proved to be stormy in a number of cases. Predictors of response to amitriptyline were examined by one group who noted that higher intensity of exposure to original combat trauma, as well as higher baseline Hamilton depression score, were particularly strong predictors of poor outcome.

At this stage, dogmatic assertions as to the specific effects of pharmacotherapy are premature. However, the data suggest that the intrusive symptoms respond to tricyclic drugs, MAO inhibitors, and β-blocker drugs. The avoidant symptoms appear to be less responsive than the intrusive symptoms, although some evidence suggests that serotonergic antidepressants (amitriptyline, fluoxetine) can help the avoidant symptoms. Hyperarousal may respond to MAO inhibitors, tricyclic drugs, azaspirones and benzodiazepines, although tricyclics may not effectively reduce increased startle responses.

Recommended drugs and doses are given in Table 17.4-4.

TABLE 17.4-4
Drug Treatment of Chronic Posttraumatic Stress Disorder

Drug	Dose Ranges (mg/day)
Antidepressant	
Amitriptyline (Elavil)	50–300
Imipramine (Tofranil)	50–300
Phenelzine (Nardil)	30–90
Fluoxetine (Prozac)	20–60
Sertraline (Zoloft)	50–200
Paroxetine (Paxil)	20–50
Bupropion (Wellbutrin)	225–450
Mood Stabilizer	
Lithium carbonate (Eskalith)	300–1,500
Anxiolytics	
Clonazepam (Klonopin)	0.25–3
Propranolol (Inderal)	40–160
Clonidine (Catapres)	0.2–0.6
Anticonvulsants	
Valproic acid (Depakene)	750–1,750
Carbamazepine (Tegretol)	200–1,200

Individual psychotherapy Crisis intervention is important in the immediate aftermath of a trauma and may reduce the development of chronic PTSD or other complications. Such treatment is geared to (1) establish support, (2) promote an acceptance of what happened, (3) provide education and information, and (4) attend to general health needs.

Individual trauma-focused psychotherapy can be given as a time-limited series of exposure-based cognitive behavioral treatments. Present evidence suggests that the magnitude of therapeutic effect from direct therapeutic exposure (DTE) is somewhat greater than the effect of pharmacotherapy in PTSD. However, that conclusion is confounded by the fact that DTE has been studied in somewhat different populations than has pharmacotherapy. As a result, the role of trauma and patient type still needs to be clarified. Such treatment, given during nine sessions, has been successfully used for rape victims with PTSD. Another approach is to provide a brief, time-limited course of stress-inoculation training, which has also proved effective in a controlled treatment trial of rape-induced chronic PTSD. Those methods have not been so well evaluated in other PTSD groups.

Implosive therapy, a related but initially more intense form of exposure therapy, is used to treat PTSD. The criteria to be met may include (1) the ability to tolerate intense levels of emotional or physiological arousal, (2) reactivity to specific and clearly defined traumatic memories, (3) adequate ability to produce imagery, (4) the absence of comorbid depression or any other major Axis I disorder, and (5) a high level of motivation and good compliance.

Systematic desensitization (graded exposure) can be of benefit in overcoming phobic avoidance related to the trauma (the C cluster of symptoms). The treatment uses repeated exposure to situations of gradually increasing fear levels to achieve habituation at each level. Such treatment, usually time-limited, can be either in vivo or imagined.

A much-used model of treatment is a phase-oriented approach. Overwhelmingly intrusive symptoms are counteracted by means of structuring, and avoidant and numbing tendencies are met with procedures to minimize such behavior. With the model the establishment of a safe therapeutic alliance is essential; medications are used sparingly. The model strives toward an end point in which the trauma is meaningfully integrated into the survivor's life schema and toward the reduction of the distressing intrusive and avoidant phases of PTSD. While the approach awaits controlled testing for efficacy, it aspires to reduce all aspects of the disorder's symptoms.

Although integration of the trauma and working through powerful affects are laudable goals, in many cases the goals are not fully attainable. Limiting factors include the patient's personality type, degree of personality pathology, ability to express and to tolerate affect, available support systems, and compliance with treatment; the nature of the trauma; the level of persisting arousal, which may limit habituation; and the impairment of concentration and memory. The therapist and the patient may choose to settle for modest but no less worthwhile goals. The patient may need supportive long-term treatment that accepts the limitations imposed by the disorder but at the same time maximizes those adaptive behaviors and coping skills unique to that patient. The clinician needs to decide on an ongoing basis whether to hospitalize, whether to medicate, when to involve a family member, whether to refer the patient to a substance or alcohol abuse program, whether some other emergent comorbid disorder needs managing, whether to address employment concerns, and whether to refer the patient to a support group. Hospitalization may be necessary at times of crisis—for example, during suicidal or homicidal risk, acute drug intoxication, and severe depression. When first-line treatments have failed or if a comprehensive evaluation is needed, elective hospitalization may be recommended. Specialty units for the disorder can be helpful, too.

Medications are generally needed at some point in the treatment of chronic PTSD, which in this sense is analogous to other chronic Axis I disorders, such as schizophrenia and obsessive-compulsive disorder. In all those states, treatment is usually multimodal, and residual symptoms often persist even after a useful treatment response. Treatment needs do not remain static; they should be subject to constant review but not hasty change.

Group therapy Several authorities recommend group therapy. The advantages of the modality include (1) the availability of understanding and support that can be provided only by fellow victims of a trauma, (2) the intense affects that can be generated and processed in a group, (3) the presence of an alternative when individual therapy is unavailable or the patient has problems relating to a therapist, (4) the presence of an alternative when individual therapy is not the preferred treatment, and (5) its possibly greater effect on the avoidance and numbing symptoms in comparison with drug treatment and individual therapy.

Relaxation training Applying relaxation training to patients with PTSD can lead to control over the physiological and motor components of the disorder. Progressive muscle relaxation, hypnosis, and biofeedback may be useful techniques, but further controlled studies are needed.

SUGGESTED CROSS-REFERENCES

Some of the syndromes associated with trauma are described in Section 15.1 on brief psychotic disorder, Chapter 23 on sleep disorders, Section 24.2 on adjustment disorders, Chapter 20 on dissociative disorders, and Chapter 25 on personality disorders.

REFERENCES

Archibald H C, Tuddenham H: Persistent stress reaction after combat: A twenty-year follow-up. Arch Gen Psychiatry *12:* 475, 1965.

*Breslau, N, Davis G C, Andreski P, Peterson E: Traumatic events and posttraumatic stress disorder in an urban population of young adults. Arch Gen Psychiatry *48:* 216, 1991.

Cardena E, Spiegel D: Dissociative reaction to the San Francisco Bay Area earthquake of 1989. Am J Psychiatry *150:* 474, 1993.

Davidson J R T, Foa E B: Diagnostic issues in posttraumatic stress disorder: Considerations for the DSM-IV. J Abnorm Psychol *100:* 346, 1991.

Davidson J R T, Hughes D L, Blazer D G, George L K: Posttraumatic stress disorder in the community: An epidemiological study. Psychol Med *21:* 713, 1991.

*Davidson J R T, Kudler H S, Smith R D, Mahorney S L, Lipper S, Hammett E B, Saunders W B, Cavenar J O: Treatment of posttraumatic stress disorder with amitriptyline and placebo. Arch Gen Psychiatry *47:* 25, 1990.

Davidson J R T, Kudler H S, Saunders W B, Erickson L, Smith R D, Stein R M, Lipper S L, Hammett E B, Mahorney S L, Cavenar J O Jr: Predicting response to amitriptyline in posttraumatic stress disorder. Am J Psychiatry *150:* 1024, 1993.

Davidson L M, Baum A: Chronic stress and posttraumatic stress disorders. J Consult Clin Psychol *54:* 303, 1986.

Feinstein A, Dolan R: Prediction of posttraumatic stress disorder following physical trauma: An examination of the stressor criterion. Psychol Med *21:* 85, 1991.

Flannery R: From victim to survivor: A stress management approach in the treatment of learned helplessness. In *Psychological Trauma,* B A van der Kolk, editor, p 216. American Psychiatric Press, Washington, 1987.

Frankl V: *From Death Camp to Existentialism.* Beacon Press, New York, 1959.

Giller E L: *Biological Assessment and Treatment of Posttraumatic Stress Disorder.* American Psychiatric Press, Washington, 1990.

Horowitz M: *Stress Response Syndromes.* Aronson, Northridge, NJ, 1986.

Horowitz M, Wilner N, Alvarez W: Impact of Event Scale: A study of subjective stress. Psychosom Med *41:* 209, 1979.

*Jones J C, Barlow D H: The etiology of posttraumatic stress disorder. Clin Psychol Rev *10:* 299, 1990.

Kilpatrick D G, Saunders B, Amick-McMullen A: Victim and crime factors associated with the development of posttraumatic stress disorder. Behav Res Ther *20:* 199, 1989.

*Krystal J H, Kosten T R, Perry B D, Giller E L Jr: Neurobiological aspects of PTSD: Review of clinical and preclinical studies. Behav Res Ther *20:* 177, 1989.

Kulka R A, Schlenger W E, Fairbank J A, Hough R L, Jordan K, Marmar C, Weiss D: *Contractual Report of Findings from the National Vietnam Veterans Readjustment Study.* Research Triangle Institute, Research Triangle Park, NC, 1988.

Lifton R J: *The Broken Connection.* Simon & Schuster, New York, 1979.

Litz B T, Blake D D, Gerardi R J, Keane T M: Decision making guidelines for the use of direct therapeutic exposure in the treatment of posttraumatic stress disorder. Behav Ther *13:* 91, 1990.

Malloy P F, Fairbank J A, Keane T M: Validation of a multimethod assessment of posttraumatic stress disorder in Vietnam veterans. J Consult Clin Psychol *51:* 488, 1983.

March J S: The nosology of posttraumatic stress disorder. J Anx Disord *4:* 61, 1990.

McFall, M E, Veith R C, Murburg M M: Basal sympathoadrenal function in posttraumatic stress disorder. Biol Psychiatry *31:* 1050, 1992.

McFarlane A C, Weber D L, Clark C R: Abnormal stimulus processing in posttraumatic stress disorder. Biol Psychiatry *34:* 311, 1993.

*McFarlane A C: The etiology of posttraumatic morbidity: Predisposing, precipitating and perpetuating factors. Br J Psychiatry *154:* 221, 1989.

McFarlane A C: The phenomenology of posttraumatic stress disorders following a natural disaster. J Nerv Ment Dis *176:* 22, 1988.

Pitman R K, Orr S P: Psychophysiologic testing for posttraumatic stress disorder: Forensic psychiatric application. Bull Am Acad Psychiatry Law *21:* 37, 1993.

Pitman R K, Orr S P, Forgue D F, de Jong J B, Claiborn J M: Psychophysiologic assessment of posttraumatic stress disorder imagery in Vietnam combat veterans. Arch Gen Psychiatry *44:* 970, 1987.

Pitman R K, van der Kolk B A, Orr S P, Greenberg M: Naloxone-reversible analgesic response to combat-related stimuli in posttraumatic stress disorder: A pilot study. Arch Gen Psychiatry *47:* 541, 1990.

Pynoos R S, Frederick C, Nader K, Arroyo W, Steinberg A, Eth S, Nuñez F, Fairbanks L: Life threat and posttraumatic stress in school-age children. Arch Gen Psychiatry *44:* 1057, 1987.

Ross R J, Ball W A, Dinges D F, Dribbs N B, Morrison A R, Silver S M, Mulvanes F D: Rapid eye movement sleep disturbance in posttraumatic stress disorder. Biol Psychiatry *35:* 195, 1994.

Rothbaum B O, Foa E B: Subtypes of posttraumatic stress disorder and duration of symptoms. In *Posttraumatic Stress Disorder: DSM-IV and Beyond,* J R T Davidson, E B Foa, editors, p 23. American Psychiatric Press, Washington, 1993.

Smith M A, Davidson J R, Ritchie J C, Kudler H S, Lipper S, Chappell P, Nemeroff C B: The corticotropin-releasing hormone test in patients with posttraumatic stress disorder. Biol Psychiatry *26:* 349, 1989.

Solomon S D, Gerrity E T, Muff A M: Efficacy of treatment for posttraumatic stress disorder: An empirical review. JAMA *238:* 633, 1992.

Southwick S M, Krystal J H, Morgan C A, Johnson D, Nagy L M, Nicolaou A, Heninger G R, Charney D S: Abnormal noradrenergic function in posttraumatic stress disorder. Arch Gen Psychiatry *50:* 266, 1993.

Weisaeth L: Posttraumatic stress disorders after an industrial disaster: Point prevalences, etiological and prognostic factors. In *Psychiatry: The State of the Art,* ed 6, P Pichot, R Berner, R Wolf, K Og Thau, editors, p 299. Plenum, New York, 1985.

Yehuda R, Boisoneau D, Mason J W, Giller E L Jr: Glucocorticoid receptor number and cortisol excretion in mood, anxiety and psychotic disorders. Biol Psychiatry *34:* 18, 1993.

17.5
GENERALIZED ANXIETY DISORDER

LASZLO A. PAPP, M.D.
JACK M. GORMAN, M.D.

INTRODUCTION

Until 1980 disagreements about the nature of anxiety produced confusing and idiosyncratic nomenclatures not only within psychiatry but also across other medical specialties. Anxious patients with primarily cardiovascular complaints but no organic abnormalities were given diagnoses of irritable heart, nervous tachycardia, and neurocirculatory asthenia. The anxious patient with prominent gastrointestinal symptoms received the diagnosis of irritable bowel syndrome, but the coexistence of respiratory symptoms and anxiety virtually guaranteed the diagnosis of hyperventilation syndrome.

The diversity of opinions made research and the comparison of data almost impossible. Spearheaded by psychiatry for the past two decades, clinicians are slowly developing a consensus on the optimal approach to patients with anxiety disorders. In close collaboration with cardiologists, gastroenterologists, pulmonary physiologists, endocrinologists, neurologists, and urologists, psychiatric researchers have revealed relevant biological and psychological abnormalities in patients with anxiety disorders. Through education of the lay and professional public, the stigma attached to anxiety disorders has begun to fade, and an increasing proportion of anxious patients takes advantage of improved treatment options.

DEFINITION

Generalized anxiety disorder (GAD) is defined in the fourth edition of *Diagnostic and Statistical Manual of Mental Disorders* (DSM-IV) as excessive anxiety and worry for six months, or longer, accompanied by at least three of six somatic symptoms. The anxiety is difficult to control and causes significant impairment in social or occupational functioning or marked distress in the patient. The diagnosis of GAD is not made if the anxiety is only one feature of another Axis I disorder or is due to a substance or a general medical condition.

DSM-IV eliminates the revised third edition of DSM (DSM-III-R) category of overanxious disorder of childhood and modifies the diagnostic criteria for GAD to include overanxious children and adolescents.

HISTORY

Anxiety as a separate diagnostic entity was not recognized by medicine until the late 1800s. Instead, anxiety was simply considered a common but not causally relevant feature of medical conditions like cardiopulmonary and gastrointestinal abnormalities. Most physicians viewed anxiety as a normal human trait that did not require specific attention.

In 1871 Jacob DaCosta was the first to describe chronic cardiac symptoms with no apparent organic cause. Subsequently, the syndrome irritable heart or DaCosta's syndrome became a frequently observed phenomenon among soldiers in the Boer War. "Neurasthenia" was a related term used at about the same time for patients who complained of a mixture of exhaustion, anxiety, and depression. At the turn of the century, Sigmund Freud recognized the central role of anxiety in these disorders and presented the first case studies of patients with anxiety neuroses. The term "anxiety neurosis," encompassing all types and degrees of anxiety remained in use in American psychiatry until the publication of the third edition of DSM (DSM-III) in 1980. The rest of medicine has been slow to adopt the anxiety disorder concept when anxiety, rather than a physiological abnormality, is primary.

COMPARATIVE NOSOLOGY

The term "generalized anxiety disorder" (GAD) was first introduced in 1980 in DSM-III. It marked the official beginning of an ongoing process of dividing the traditional anxiety neuroses category into clinically meaningful diagnostic groups. The phenomenological approach in DSM-III represented a conscious effort to steer clear of theoretical debates concerning the cause of anxiety.

In DSM-III GAD, along with atypical anxiety disorder, was considered a residual category reserved for disorders not meeting the criteria for any other anxiety category. The diagnosis of GAD was not applicable if the symptoms were due to another physical or mental disorder. At the same time, many patients with subthreshold Axis I symptoms still received the GAD diagnosis. According to DSM-III, patients with GAD suffered from persistent, increased levels of diffuse anxiety of at least one month's duration and manifested symptoms from three of four categories: motor tension, autonomic hyperactivity, apprehensive expectation, and vigilance and scanning.

In an attempt to heighten diagnostic reliability, DSM-III-R changed the duration of symptoms necessary to meet the criteria for GAD from one to six months, emphasized the importance of excessive or unrealistic worry, and required the presence of at least 6 of 18 anxiety symptoms. Recognizing the high level of comorbidity of GAD with other anxiety and mood disorders, DSM-III-R eliminated some of the hierarchical rules and allowed the diagnosis of GAD in the presence of other Axis I disorders. The DSM-IV diagnostic criteria are listed in Table 17.5-1. DSM-IV places the emphasis on the pervasiveness and uncontrollability of the worry rather than on the specific sphere of the worry and simplifies the criteria for somatic symptoms. The distinction between GAD and normal anxiety is emphasized by the use of the words "excessive" and "difficult to control" in the criteria and by the specification that the symptoms cause significant impairment or distress.

The changes in diagnostic thinking through the succession of DSMs were instrumental in the revision of the anxiety categories in the ninth revision of the *International Classification of Diseases* (ICD-9). Although ICD-9 acknowledges only generic anxiety states under the category "Neurotic disorders," ICD-10 is fully compatible with the terminology used in DSM-IV.

TABLE 17.5-1
Diagnostic Criteria for Generalized Anxiety Disorder

A. Excessive anxiety and worry (apprehensive expectation), occurring more days than not for at least six months, about a number of events or activities (such as work or school performance).
B. The person finds it difficult to control the worry.
C. The anxiety and worry are associated with three (or more) of the following six symptoms (with at least some symptoms present for more days than not for the past six months). **Note:** Only one item is required in children.
   (1) restlessness or feeling keyed up or on edge
   (2) being easily fatigued
   (3) difficulty concentrating or mind going blank
   (4) irritability
   (5) muscle tension
   (6) sleep disturbance (difficulty falling or staying asleep, or restless unsatisfying sleep)
D. The focus of the anxiety and worry is not confined to features of an Axis I disorder (e.g., the anxiety or worry is not about having a panic attack [as in panic disorder], being embarrassed in public [as in social phobia], being contaminated [as in obsessive-compulsive disorder], being away from home or close relatives [as in separation anxiety disorder], gaining weight [as in anorexia nervosa], having multiple physical complaints [as in somatization disorder], or having a serious illness [as in hypochondriasis], and the anxiety and worry do not occur exclusively during posttraumatic stress disorder.
E. The anxiety, worry, or physical symptoms cause clinically significant distress or impairment in social, occupational, or other important areas of functioning.
F. The disturbance is not due to the direct physiological effects of a substance (e.g., a drug of abuse, a medication) or a general medical condition (e.g., hyperthyroidism) and does not occur exclusively during a mood disorder, a psychotic disorder, or a pervasive developmental disorder.

Table from DSM-IV, *Diagnostic and Statistical Manual of Mental Disorders,* ed 4. Copyright American Psychiatric Association, Washington, 1994. Used with permission.

DSM-IV is a *categorical* diagnostic system. If the criteria are met, the condition is present; if the criteria are not met, the condition is absent. An alternative approach to psychopathology is the *dimensional* system. According to the dimensional approach, most symptoms—such as anxiety and depression—are present in most psychiatric conditions. The degree and the proportion of the symptom determine the clinical picture. In a dimensional system, generalized or chronic anxiety is a component of most psychiatric illnesses. Characterologic anxiety disorder, based on Thomas Widiger's concept of characterologic affective disorder, is a testable dimensional alternative to the current approach to anxiety. Some argue in favor of adopting the dimensional approach, but others insist it will lead to impressionistic rather than reliable diagnoses.

The diagnostic reliability of lifetime GAD, using DSM-III-R criteria, has been found to be acceptable even in the presence of a comorbid mood or anxiety disorder. However, a number of problems and questions remain unanswered. Is pathological worry, the core feature of GAD, distinguishable from normal and other Axis I disorder worries? If there is a difference, is it quantitative or qualitative? How can one define excessive and unrealistic worry?

Although it is not yet supported by biological data, GAD, on the basis of field trials and clinical experience, seems to be a legitimate and distinct anxiety disorder. The sources of poor reliability for current GAD are inconsistent ratings of the 18 anxiety symptoms, poor and inconsistent recall by patients, overlap of GAD features with comorbid conditions, and disagreements about the nature of GAD worry. The diagnostic reliability of GAD as modified in DSM-IV could improve by the increased emphasis on the pathological nature rather than the specific sphere of the worry.

EPIDEMIOLOGY

In view of the radical diagnostic changes in DSM-III, epidemiological surveys conducted prior to 1980 have limited relevance to generalized anxiety disorder. Nevertheless, the early surveys do support the current conclusion that anxiety disorders are one of the most common psychiatric disorders. The Epidemiologic Catchment Area (ECA) study, based on large community samples, found the one-year prevalence rate for generalized anxiety disorder to range from 2.5 to 8 percent. GAD, probably the most common anxiety disorder, is estimated to be four times more prevalent than panic disorder and three times more prevalent than simple phobia. Women are approximately twice as likely to be affected as are men. Most patients with GAD report that they have been anxious all their lives. Thus, determining the age of onset for GAD is frequently impossible. Interviews conducted to assess childhood and family factors in the development of the illness have been unsuccessful in differentiating patients with GAD from patients with panic disorder. In those surveys an abundance of adverse life events was experienced by both patient groups but no comparisons were made with normal controls.

ETIOLOGY

The anxiety response clearly involves both psychological and physiological processes, but many have attempted to characterize anxiety, along with most other human emotions, as a purely physiological or purely psychological phenomenon. Even though the debate continues between purists and eclectics, advocates of the dichotomous view are confronted with a growing body of evidence that make their position increasingly untenable. The comparable results of psychological and biological research suggest that a valid hypothesis of anxiety has to consider both areas.

PSYCHOANALYTIC THEORY During his early work Freud understood anxiety as a manifestation of a physiologically induced tension state. With the 1909 publication of the case of Little Hans, Freud reversed his earlier opinions and adopted a psychological theory of anxiety. That theory was restated in the context of the structural theory in the 1926 book *Inhibitions, Symptoms, and Anxiety* (published in America as *The Problem of Anxiety*). There, Freud concluded that anxiety is a symptom of an unresolved unconscious conflict between the impulses for libidinal or aggressive gratification and the ego's recognition of the external danger that could result from that gratification. Mobilized by signal anxiety and acting according to the pleasure principle, the ego uses various defenses to avoid the anxiety produced by both intrapsychic conflict and potential external danger. The experience of anxiety is the result of a failure of the ego to use effective defenses. Signal anxiety occurs outside awareness, felt anxiety is consciously experienced and can reach traumatic proportions. Freud's description of traumatic anxiety closely correlates with the current definition of a panic attack.

Freud does not appear to have reconciled his early clinical observations with his later psychological and metapsychological theories, in which distinctions between types of anxiety are quantitative, rather than qualitative.

According to psychoanalytic theory, *anxiety* arises from a conflict between instinctual drive and internal inhibition. Real external dangers evoke *fear,* which is distinct from anxiety. However, in clinical practice, fear and anxiety cannot always be differentiated, and in most cases the two coexist. Analysts as a group disagree about whether various types of anxieties should be viewed on a continuum or understood as distinct and separate phenomena.

COGNITIVE BEHAVIOR THEORY The basic cognitive theory of anxiety, represented by the work of Aaron Beck, suggests that anxiety is a response to perceived danger. Consistent distortions in information processing lead to misperceiving danger and experiencing anxiety. Pathological anxiety is related to selective information processing of a threat. Anxious patients also perceive their resources as inadequate to cope with the threat. Lack of control over the environment is a major factor in the maintenance of anxiety. According to David Barlow, who differentiates anxiety and fear, GAD is characterized by anxiety related to a perception of loss of control, rather than to fear of a threat.

Other psychological mechanisms stipulated as instrumental in the development and maintenance of GAD include selective allocation of attentional resources to threat, particularly to the threat to the self (self-schemas); easy access to and quick retrieval of threat-related information; self-consciousness or excessive worry about how one is perceived by others; exaggerated, excessive fear of bodily sensations associated with anxiety; and a faulty perception of the degree of stress or the difficulty of the task and an inappropriate level of applied effort to cope. The prominent worry in GAD has been explained as a defense against the intrusive and difficult to dismiss thoughts of anticipated trauma.

Although these theories are stimulating, the empirical evidence to confirm or to refute the validity and the relevance of the underlying mechanisms are still largely lacking. However, research based on chronic or trait anxiety, rather than on GAD, suggests that information processing may be different in anxious patients and in controls. Anxious patients seem to allocate more attention to threat stimuli, remember threat-related information more, and perceive themselves as having less control over external and internal stimuli than do nonanxious controls.

BIOLOGICAL THEORIES Since benzodiazepines are a widely accepted and effective pharmacological treatment for GAD, abnormalities of the benzodiazepine receptor system in the brain have been suggested as a possible biological mechanism of anxiety. High-affinity benzodiazepine-binding sites are an integral part of the complex consisting of a γ-aminobutyric acid (GABA) receptor and a chloride ionophore. Benzodiazepines bind to the receptor complex potentiating the effect of GABA, the major inhibitory neurotransmitter in the brain. Benzodiazepine agonists enhance the inhibitory effects of GABA by increasing the frequency of openings of the chloride channel. Benzodiazepine antagonists like flumazenil (Mazicon) and reverse agonists like the β-carbolines are anxiogenic in both animals and humans.

Because the concentration of benzodiazepine receptors is highest in the occipital lobe, that region of the human brain has been suggested as a possible anatomical locus for GAD. A few functional and structural brain-imaging studies have confirmed the presence of abnormalities in the occipital cortex of GAD patients, but the findings are never specific or exclusive enough to draw definite conclusions. Preclinical and clinical brain imaging has also implicated the limbic lobe, the basal ganglia, and the prefrontal cortex in the generation of various types of anxieties and stress responses.

The efficacy of azaspirones, a new class of antianxiety medications unrelated to benzodiazepines, suggests a significant role for the serotonergic system in GAD. Buspirone (BuSpar), the only currently available azaspirone, works primarily on the 5-hydroxytryptamine (5-HT) system as a 5-HT_{1A} agonist.

Although mostly untested in patients with GAD, other neurotransmitter systems have shown promising leads into the understanding of the biology of panic disorder, obsessive-compulsive disorder, and posttraumatic stress-related anxiety. The further investigation of the serotonergic, noradrenergic, L-glutamic acid, and cholecystokinin (CCK) systems in patients with GAD is clearly warranted.

GENETIC THEORIES Most anxiety disorders run in families. Structured diagnostic interviews conducted in family members of patients with GAD have confirmed that about 20 percent of the relatives suffer from GAD. The approximate respective ratios for panic disorder, specific phobia, and social phobia are 50 percent, 31 percent, and 7 percent. The few available twin studies in patients with anxiety disorder also suggest that the genetic basis of GAD, compared with panic disorder, is less important and probably different. In one twin study, changing the duration criteria from one month to six months further reduced the significance of genetic factors in GAD. The concordance rate for clinical anxiety is approximately four times higher in monozygotic twins than in dizygotic twins. The absence of panic attacks in patients with GAD eliminates the differences in concordance rates between monozygotic twins (17 percent) and dizygotic twins (20 percent). Linkage between the GAD gene and genetic markers has not yet been attempted. The few linkage studies conducted in panic disorder patients have not been successful.

DIAGNOSIS AND CLINICAL FEATURES

As evidenced by the long list of diagnostic criteria in Table 175-1, the symptoms of generalized anxiety disorder are numerous and fluctuating. The symptoms are categorized under three general areas: (1) motor tension, (2) autonomic hyperactivity, and (3) hyperarousal. Motor tension manifests itself as shakiness, inability to relax, restlessness, and fatigue, frequently accompanied by back and neck pain. Headaches are common, mostly presenting as pressure or tension headaches. The signs of autonomic hyperactivity include shortness of breath, palpitation, sweating, dizziness, hot and cold flashes, and frequent urination. Gastrointestinal symptoms may include upset stomach, nausea, heartburn, belching, and flatulence with occasional loose bowel movements. The signs of hyperarousal include vigilance and scanning. Patients with GAD are irritable and easily startled. They constantly monitor the environment for danger signs and frequently have difficulty in falling or staying asleep. The number of symptoms required for the diagnosis of GAD was significantly reduced in DSM-IV. Central to the diagnosis is the presence of excessive worry about minor day-to-day problems. Premenstrual worsening of the disorder is commonly reported. Chronic, generalized anxiety can be demoralizing and frequently the cause of significantly disturbed social and vocational functioning.

Most patients with GAD are first seen by general practitioners, family physicians, and internists after the patients have had symptoms for many years. The clinical picture of a patient with florid symptoms involving at least two separate organ systems should raise the suspicion of an anxiety disorder. Restlessness, perspiration, frequent sighing, tachycardia, and brisk reflexes in the context of an otherwise unremarkable physical examination are the norm. Quite appropriately, a number of standard laboratory assessments—such as complete blood count, routine chemistries, thyroid function tests, and an electrocardiograph (ECG)—are performed at the first consultation. Rarely is a clinically significant abnormality found. Unless some compelling and unusual symptom is present, a further workup is not necessary, and the patient should be referred for a psychiatric evaluation. Unfortunately, most patients are only offered tranquilizers, and only a small fraction are ever referred.

If the patient is seen by a psychiatrist first, the same medical workup should be performed. Although the test results rarely explain the patient's dysfunction, anxiety disorder patients can have concomitant physical illnesses. Once the diagnosis of generalized anxiety disorder is established, treatment recommendations can be made.

A 27-year-old married electrician complained of dizziness, sweating palms, heart palpitations, and ringing of the ears of more than 18 months' duration. He also experienced dry mouth and throat, periods of extreme muscle tension, and a constant "edgy" and watchful feeling that often interfered with his ability to concentrate. These feelings had been present most of the time over the previous two years; they had not been limited to discrete periods. Although these symptoms sometimes made him feel "discouraged," he denied feeling depressed and continued to enjoy activities with his family.

Because of these symptoms the patient had seen a family practitioner, a neurologist, a neurosurgeon, a chiropractor, and an ear-nose-throat specialist. He had been placed on a hypoglycemic diet, received physiotherapy for a pinched nerve, and told he might have "an inner ear problem."

He also had many worries. He constantly worried about the health of his parents. His father, in fact, had a myocardial infarction two years previously, but was now feeling well. He also worried about whether he was "a good father," whether his wife would ever leave him (there was no indication that she was dissatisfied with the marriage), and whether he was liked by coworkers on the job. Although he recognized that his worries were often unfounded, he could not stop worrying.

For the past two years the patient had had few social contacts because of his nervous symptoms. Although he sometimes had to leave work when the symptoms became intolerable, he continued to work for the same company he joined for his apprenticeship following high school graduation. He tended to hide his symptoms from his wife and children, to whom he wanted to appear "perfect," and reported few problems with them as a result of his nervousness.

DISCUSSION This man consulted numerous physicians for his symptoms, but the absence of preoccupation with fears of having a specific physical disease precluded a diagnosis of hypochondriasis. He recognized that his worries were often excessive, but they did not have the intrusive and inappropriate quality that characterizes the obsessions of obsessive-compulsive disorder.

His predominant symptom was excessive and uncontrollable anxiety and worry for most of the time over the past two years. This suggests the diagnosis of GAD. He also had the characteristic associated symptoms of feeling on edge, difficulty concentrating, and muscle tension. His worries caused him significant distress and impaired his social functioning. The diagnosis of GAD was made in this case because the worries were not confined to the features of another Axis I disorder (for example, worrying about having a panic attack, as in panic disorder, or being embarrassed in public, as in social phobia), the symptoms did not occur only during the course of a mood or psychotic disorder, they were not the direct effects of a substance (for example, drugs of abuse or medication) or a general medical condition (for example, hyperthyroidism), and the disturbance had persisted for more than six months.

The diagnosis of GAD first appeared in DSM-III when panic disorder was separated out of what previously had been called anxiety neurosis. Since that time there has been controversy as to how best to define the condition. The current definition emphasizes the cognitive component of excessive worry and deemphasizes autonomic symptoms. However, many patients, particularly in medical settings, present with primarily somatic symptoms of anxiety and deny excessive worry. It is not at all clear that these patients, who are not eligible for this diagnosis, have a different disorder. (From *DSM-IV Casebook.* Used with permission.)

BIOLOGICAL FEATURES Compared with the extensive literature on the biological features of panic disorder, biological research of generalized anxiety disorder has been sparse. The relative lack of interest is due to a number of factors. First, GAD represents a heterogeneous diagnostic category with substantial symptomatic overlap with many other Axis I disorders. Second, treatment is far less successful in controlling the symptoms of GAD than in controlling the symptoms of panic disorder. Third, most of the patients with GAD are seen by internists, general practitioners, and cardiologists and are not readily available for psychiatric research. Therefore, most of the knowledge concerning the biological features of GAD is based on studies that used GAD patients as a comparison group, rather than on research with the focus of attention on GAD.

RESPONSE TO NORMAL STRESS Because of substantial symptomatic overlap, the response to normal stress has traditionally been considered the prototype of chronic anxiety.

Therefore, many biological investigations of chronic generalized anxiety have used normal stress reactions as their paradigm. The inconsistency of the results from that type of research is easily explained by the multitude of genetic, emotional, and personality factors that determine the biological response of normal volunteers to stress. Despite those limitations the data suggest that physiological reactions to stress include increased blood pressure, heart rate, and minute volume. Skin conductance, muscle tension, and plasma levels of epinephrine, norepinephrine, growth hormone, cortisol, and prolactin also rise.

Research findings Research with a variety of anxious patients before DSM-III resulted in inconsistent biological findings: elevated, labile, or normal resting heart rate and blood pressure; elevated, not different or decreased, skin conductance; increased or not different electromyographic activity; decreased or not different exercise tolerance; increased or not different respiration, as evidenced by lower or not different carbon dioxide concentrations; decreased, increased, or not different thyroid function; elevated or normal plasma prolactin levels; stronger and weaker catecholamine responses to stress; and higher resting plasma cortisol and 17-adrenocorticotropine levels compared with controls. The findings of elevated resting catecholamine levels in anxious psychiatric patients and exaggerated catecholamine responses during agitation prompted the administration of epinephrine infusions to anxious patients. The infusions reproduced the physiological responses but resulted in a psychological experience ranging from fear to amusement.

The most consistent findings in those studies before DSM-III were high interindividual and intraindividual variability, the inability of anxious patients to habituate to stress, and their delay in reaching baseline again after a challenge.

Perhaps as an indicator of continued problems with diagnostic reliability and specificity, biological studies conducted since 1980 in patients with DSM-III or DSM-III-R diagnoses for GAD have not yielded significant breakthroughs in understanding the pathophysiology of the disorder. The results of the few relevant studies are still inconsistent. Resting catecholamine and 3-methoxy-4-hydroxyphenylglycol (MHPG) levels and platelet monoamine oxidase (MAO) activity in GAD patients were found to be high in some studies, but others failed to find patient-control differences. Both hyperthyroidism and euthyroidism have been reported in GAD patients. So far unreplicated findings in GAD patients include decreased platelet α_2-adrenergic receptor binding, compared with normal controls and patients with depression, and blunted growth hormone response to clonidine (Catapres), compared with controls, suggesting postsynaptic α_2-receptor subsensitivity in GAD patients. However, no GAD-control differences in clonidine-induced blood pressure, heart rate, and MHPG changes were registered, nor were there blood pressure, heart rate, anxiety, cortisol, or MHPG-level differences between GAD patients and controls in response to oral yohimbine (Yocon).

As possible evidence for benzodiazepine subsensitivity, diazepam (Valium) has been recently shown to slow the velocity of saccadic eye movements in patients with panic disorder and with GAD but not in normal controls. Thus, altered central benzodiazepine receptors may be responsible for anxiety and arousal in patients with GAD.

Two studies found higher nonsuppression rates in the dexamethasone-suppression test in GAD patients, compared with controls. The rate of nonsuppression was comparable to that in depressed patients and was unrelated to the presence of depression in the GAD patients.

Similarly inconsistent results have been reported on *psychophysiological* variables. In contrast to prior reports of increased resting autonomic arousal in GAD patients, no patient-control differences were found in resting blood pressure, heart rate, minute volume, and skin conductance.

The two reported sleep EEG studies in GAD patients conflict on the length of stage 2 sleep, one reporting more stage 2 sleep and the other finding less stage 2 sleep. GAD patients seem to have longer rapid eye movement (REM) latency, less REM activity, and less total sleep time than do depressed patients.

Brain imaging This relatively new technique has allowed the direct assessment of the effects of anxiety on the brain. However, most of the results of the few promising studies in patients with GAD are preliminary and in need of replication.

The complex and highly variable association between anxiety and cerebral blood flow (CBF) is influenced by a multitude of factors, such as age, sex, handedness, blood pressure, pulse rate, acid-base status, blood viscosity, blood-brain barrier status, level of circulating catecholamines, and acclimatization to the scanning procedure. Different types of anxiety (stress-induced, anticipatory, free-floating, panic, somatic, and psychic) may manifest in characteristic CBF responses.

In general, mild to moderate arousal produces a significant increase in cerebral blood flow and metabolism, but severe anxiety results in cerebral vasoconstriction. Resting CBF measurements have revealed no global GAD patient-control differences, but state anxiety has shown a significant inverse correlation with CBF in patients. Five percent CO_2 inhalation for 30 minutes has also shown an inverse relation between anxiety and CBF in nine GAD patients, but no patient-control differences in anxiety levels were found. Anxiety-induced hyperventilation, which reduces CBF, may obscure the differential CBF response to CO_2 inhalation. Relative cerebral hypoxia may be the mechanism behind a number of severe anxiety symptoms, such as light-headedness, confusion, and derealization.

Surprisingly, in spite of inducing significant anxiety, epinephrine infusions did not result in detectable changes in regional or hemispheric CBF in 20 GAD patients. Sodium lactate infusion, the gold standard of laboratory induction of panic in panic disorder patients, induced more anxiety in GAD patients than in normal controls but did not result in panic attacks. The effects of sodium lactate infusion on CBF have not been assessed in patients with GAD.

A number of structural and functional brain-imaging studies have addressed the effects of benzodiazepine treatment on the brains of anxious patients. Benzodiazepine-naive controls were not assessed as controls, but increased ventricular-brain ratio has been reported to correlate consistently with the length of benzodiazepine use in one computed tomography (CT) scan study of patients with anxiety disorders. Electroencephalographic (EEG) abnormalities in benzodiazepine-treated GAD patients were limited to the occipital and temporal regions. A positron emission tomography (PET) study of benzodiazepine-treated GAD patients found reduced metabolism in the visual cortex and increased metabolism in the basal ganglia and the thalamus. Benzodiazepine treatment of GAD patients was also associated with decreased right frontal and right occipital glucose metabolism. The clinical implications of those findings are limited. GAD patients may or may not exhibit CBF and cerebral metabolism patterns clearly distinct from those of normal controls and patients with other anxiety disorders.

DIFFERENTIAL DIAGNOSIS

Since the introduction of generalized anxiety disorder as a new diagnostic category, its reliability and validity as a separate entity have been repeatedly challenged. The frequent comorbidity of GAD with other anxiety disorders and a number of mood disorders, its prolonged duration, and the seeming absence of a unique symptom profile and of clear boundaries with other anxiety and mood disorders have prompted suggestions that GAD be abolished and classified as a phase of chronic mood disorders, as a mild form of panic disorder, or as a separate personality disorder.

Since DSM-III assigned a low hierarchical status to residual categories, GAD was rarely diagnosed as a comorbid condition before DSM-III-R. The few available comorbidity studies since 1987 show that about two thirds to nine tenths of the patients with the principal diagnosis of GAD had an additional Axis I disorder, with social phobia and dysthymic disorder leading the list. GAD as a comorbid condition is most common in depression and dysthymic disorder. Up to one fifth of patients with depression have comorbid GAD, but less than one tenth of patients with other anxiety disorders manifest the picture of GAD as a secondary diagnosis. On a dimensional level the symptom of generalized anxiety is part of most anxiety and mood disorders without meeting the categorical criteria for the full syndrome of GAD.

PANIC DISORDERS Most of the studies attempting to distinguish GAD from other Axis I disorders compare GAD with panic disorders. The age of onset seems to be similar, but panic disorder patients seek treatment significantly earlier than do patients with GAD. Panic disorder patients are usually more disabled by their symptoms than are patients with GAD. Unlike the sudden, unexpected panic attack marking the beginning of panic disorder, the onset of generalized anxiety disorder is usually insidious. Patients with GAD are usually unable to recall the beginning of their anxiety and tend to be vague about the usually protracted course of their illness. When searching for precipitants, the clinician frequently finds enduring, nonspecific environmental stressors like financial, social, and work difficulties, but a clear relation between symptoms and stressors is rarely established.

In a comparison of the symptoms of the two disorders, somatic complaints–such as nausea, headache, tension, and insomnia—are more common in GAD patients. Patients with panic disorder report more severe overall, especially cognitive, symptoms and more derealization, depersonalization, hypochondriasis, and fear of death or of losing control.

DEPRESSION Depression, especially dysthymic disorder and GAD share numerous features. Dysthymic disorder and GAD are both chronic conditions, with episodic exacerbations frequently representing the prodromal stage to major depression or panic disorder. Episodic depression is common in GAD, and episodic anxiety frequently complicates depression, especially early-onset dysthymic disorder. About one quarter to one third of the patients with GAD present with comorbid depression, and the same proportion of patients with depression meet the criteria for GAD. Some studies have identified underlying Axis II disorders in both anxiety and mood disorders, but no comparison has been made between personality traits specific to GAD and those specific to dysthymic disorder. Therefore, the explanation that the significant comorbidity is due to personality factors cannot be substantiated.

Some investigators have concluded that depression and GAD may be indistinguishable. Recently, however, a comparison was made between pure (no depressive comorbidity) GAD and pure (no anxiety disorder comorbidity) dysthymic disorder patients. More severe depressive symptoms—such as depressed mood, suicide tendencies, work and activity impairment, and hopelessness—lower ratings of respiratory symptoms, and vigilance and scanning in dysthymic disorders compared with GAD, clearly differentiated the two groups.

HYPOCHONDRIASIS Hypochondriasis presents a differential diagnostic dilemma because of considerable symptomatic overlap, worry as a prominent feature in both conditions, and health as the key area of worry in hypochondriasis and an important sphere of concern in GAD. Unfortunately, no current guidelines regarding hierarchy are available when both conditions are diagnosable. Making disease conviction the key feature of hypochondriasis and disease fear a feature of GAD are potential solutions requiring further research.

PSYCHOLOGICAL FACTORS AFFECTING MEDICAL CONDITION Similar overlaps between GAD and this category can be remedied by allowing the latter diagnosis only in the absence of other Axis I diagnoses.

SUBSTANCE-RELATED DISORDERS Marked comorbidity has been reported between most anxiety disorders and substance abuse. Up to two thirds of patients treated for alcohol-related disorders report clinically significant anxiety, including GAD. In contrast, alcohol problems are not overrepresented in patients with GAD. GAD patients do self-medicate their anxiety with alcohol and other substances, but that practice is much less frequent in GAD patients than in patients with agoraphobia and social phobia. The relatively low rate of self-medication in GAD patients is supported by the finding that, in more than half the comorbid cases of GAD and alcohol problems, GAD started after the alcohol problems. Prolonged drinking-induced anxiety, the consumption of large amounts of alcohol or other substances, and alcohol and other substance withdrawal states represent serious differential diagnostic dilemmas.

Alcoholic persons who drink for days at a time report acute anxiolytic effects but experience increased anxiety and dysphoria as they continue to drink. Alcohol withdrawal manifests in symptoms indistinguishable from the autonomic symptoms of GAD and occurs 12 to 48 hours after heavy, prolonged drinking. When asked to voluntarily hyperventilate, alcoholic patients cannot differentiate between the resulting symptoms and those experienced during acute withdrawal. The toxic effects of prolonged exposure to alcohol include gastrointestinal, acid-base, and sleep disturbances similar to those described by GAD patients. The chronic consumption of caffeine can also mimic the symptoms of GAD. The manifestations of chronic caffeine intoxication include restlessness, a variety of motor tics, diarrhea, and psychomotor agitation. The pattern of alcohol and substance use problems in patients with comorbid GAD seems to be different from the pattern seen in patients with comorbid agoraphobia and social phobia. GAD is usually the consequence, rather than the initiating factor, in substance use problems.

PERSONALITY DISORDERS Although a specific GAD personality disorder has not been identified, personality disorders may be present in up to half of the patients with GAD; in cases of treatment-resistant GAD, the percentage may be as high as 80 percent. The average rate of all personality disorders in the general population is less than 10 percent.

Theories abound to explain the significance of the association. Some believe that a personality disorder represents vulnerability for an attenuated subsyndromal form or a complication of an anxiety disorder. Others suggest that both personality disorder and anxiety disorder originate from a common diathesis. In the absence of data, those theories can only be speculative at present.

A six-year prospective study found no difference in the rate of baseline personality disorder between patients who later had depression and those who had an anxiety disorder. Thus, premorbid personality disorders do not seem to predispose to anxiety disorders. Since personality traits seem to improve with anxiety disorder specific treatments, some personality disorders may be secondary to an anxiety disorder.

COURSE AND PROGNOSIS

Prospective follow-up data regarding the natural course of GAD are not available. The age of onset is thought to be in the late teens or early 20s. Antecedent features include anxiety, apprehension, behavioral inhibition to unfamiliar situations, and a history of overanxious disorder in childhood. GAD patients in their 40s report an average 20-year history of severe anxiety. Without treatment of the anxiety, extended periods of remission are unlikely. Retrospective surveys conclude that GAD tends to run a chronic and fluctuating course, with periodic exacerbations and quiescence. Clinical experience suggests that GAD patients have fewer symptoms and become less disabled as they age.

Since pure GAD alone rarely lands the patient in psychiatric treatment, psychiatrists identify GAD mostly as a comorbid condition. As mentioned above, the most frequent comorbid conditions are depression and dysthymic disorder, followed by social and simple phobias. Additional Axis I and Axis II diagnoses make the prognosis of GAD variable. Clinical lore, rather than controlled studies, suggests that the long-term outcome of GAD depends on environmental stress, including the strength and the nature of the patient's social support, the biology of the disorder, the patient's ego functions, and the duration of the illness.

TREATMENT

As is the case for most anxiety disorders, the available treatments for GAD can be divided into psychological and pharmacological approaches. For many years, researchers and clinicians devoted to one or the other have claimed their method to be superior. Diagnostic differences and methodological and treatment variations have made comparisons of the treatments impossible. The artificial fragmentation of the field and the developing hostility between biological and psychological approaches have slowed scientific progress and confused the patient.

The division of the homogeneous anxiety neuroses into specific anxiety disorders in DSM-III generated renewed interest in anxiety research. Anxiety-disorder-specific medications and psychotherapies were developed, and their success in most cases reinforced the new diagnostic thinking. The process of comparing anxiolytic medications and specific psychotherapies in carefully screened patient populations finally began. While the process continues, preliminary results suggest that the biology-psychology division is unjustified. An increasing number of clinicians and researchers recognize the shortcomings of purity and advocate an eclectic approach.

Diverse and highly effective treatments are now available to manage most anxiety disorders. Unfortunately, two thirds of those diagnosed with an anxiety disorder and judged to be in need of treatment never receive it.

PSYCHOTHERAPY A number of psychotherapies are said to be effective for treating GAD. Although possibly correct, most of the claims are in need of scientific substantiation. The findings of psychotherapy research in GAD are limited by small sample sizes and by a focus on GAD patients with relatively mild symptoms. However, since clinical experience suggests that psychotherapy augments the efficacy and shortens the length of time of pharmacotherapy, psychotherapeutic techniques, ranging from relatively simple stress management and problem-solving assistance to more complex cognitive and psychodynamic treatments, should be applied for almost every patient with GAD.

Dynamic psychotherapy The assumption underlying the dynamic approach to treating GAD is that the nature of the symptoms is relatively unimportant compared with the various factors determining the strength of the patient's ego. Since anxiety is a manifestation of an internal conflict, the treatment should focus on dysfunctional relationships, maladaptive defenses, and the patient's capacity for introspection and insight. Once the conflict is resolved, usually through transference, the anxiety should lift. Unfortunately, data regarding the efficacy of analytic treatment for GAD is not available.

Supportive psychotherapy Regular contact with a sympathetic and concerned clinician, repeated reassurance about the harmless nature of anxiety, the removal or the alleviation of environmental stress, and support when confronting anxiety-inducing situations usually lead to a significant reduction of anxiety. Although not necessarily curative, supportive techniques by themselves or in combination with other treatments do increase the efficacy of most antianxiety approaches.

Cognitive behavior therapy Cognitive behavior theorists and clinicians have developed an impressive variety of techniques in dealing with various anxiety disorders. Cognitive restructuring, psychoeducation, relaxation, breathing retraining, exposure, graded practice, flooding, and self-instructional training are but a few highly efficacious procedures used in both individual and group therapies. Compared with the long-established and highly successful behavior therapy for specific phobias, cognitive behavioral therapy for GAD is recent. A number of treatment studies have been completed in GAD patients, but missing follow-up data, unknown medication status, and relatively small sample sizes limit the possible conclusions.

Relaxation techniques, regardless of whether used as progressive muscle relaxation or with frontal electromyographic (EMG) biofeedback, result in small but significant drops in anxiety. However, one study did not find relaxation techniques to be more effective than transcendental meditation. Success in most relaxation programs seems to depend on the regularity of the practice. A quarter to a third of GAD patients report increased tension, rather than reduced tension, during progressive muscle relaxation. Cognitive theory explains that paradoxical response as a fear of loss of control. Relaxation in that context can work as a form of exposure.

Cognitive restructuring is almost invariably added to relaxation techniques in the treatment of GAD. Two studies found the combination of cognitive and behavior techniques superior to simply being on a waiting list for treatment, and one study found the combination superior to a drug placebo in reducing generalized anxiety. The improvements were maintained after three and six months in the majority of the patients. Although both treatments proved to be effective, only marginal differences were found when cognitive behavior therapy was compared with behavior therapy alone. Nondirective therapy with or without relaxation was also indistinguishable from cognitive behavior therapy on most measures in reducing anxiety in GAD patients. Most of the comparative studies clearly suffer from the lack of control for the nonspecific components of therapy, such as empathy, attention, and monitoring.

Overall, cognitive behavior therapy appears to reduce symptom severity in GAD but does not induce complete remission. The claim that the therapy is superior to medication at long-term follow-up has not been substantiated. It is not known which of the many and varying components of the numerous types of cognitive behavior therapy is therapeutic or essential. The reported efficacy of nonspecific supportive treatments in GAD patients is also puzzling. Studies are currently underway to identify the therapeutic components, using the so-called dismantling research strategy. That strategy consists of the removal of a key element of the treatment and the use of the rest of the treatment package unchanged. The preliminary results suggest that providing the patient with a sense of control and dealing with chronic worry should be central aspects of any psychotherapeutic approach.

PHARMACOTHERAPY Alcohol, the oldest antistress drug, remains the most favored nonspecific tranquilizer. The approximately 100-year history of modern pharmacological anxiolytics began with the introduction of paraldehyde, followed shortly by the first uses of bromides and barbiturates. The obvious shortcomings of barbiturates prompted the development of a series of nonbarbiturate, nonbenzodiazepine anxiolytics, such as glutethimide (Doriden), meprobamate (Miltown), methaqualone (Quaalude), methyprylon (Noludar), and tybamate (Benvil, Solacen). At present, those drugs should be avoided, as they turned out to be highly addicting and fatal in overdose and to possess a low therapeutic index. Paraldehyde and some of the barbiturates retain some specialized usefulness in the treatment of alcohol withdrawal, seizures, and congenital hyperbilirubinemia.

During the first 20 years after their introduction in the 1960s, benzodiazepines replaced most pharmacological agents in the management of anxiety. According to recent surveys, about 1 out of every 10 American adults take benzodiazepines at least once a year. Unfortunately, the safety, efficacy, ease of administration, and mild side effects of benzodiazepines led to occasional indiscriminate use. Benzodiazepines became the quick-fix remedies for all types of mental distress. The recognition of dependence and the discontinuance syndrome, coupled with growing public and professional concern over their misuse, resulted in increased governmental control of benzodiazepine prescriptions. The misguided triplicate law in New York State resulted in a 57 percent drop in benzodiazepine prescriptions and a concomitant 130 percent increase in meprobamate use. Contrary to public perception, scientific data conclusively show that benzodiazepines are safe, not overused, and that tolerance to their therapeutic effects is rare. The number of prescriptions filled by retail pharmacies had leveled off many years before the enactment of limiting legislative actions.

Recent research with azapirones, a new class of anxiolytics completely unrelated neurobiologically to the benzodiazepines, and a number of treatment studies with heterocyclic antidepressants have suggested that safe and efficacious alternatives to benzodiazepines exist to treat patients with generalized anxiety disorder.

Benzodiazepines For the overwhelming majority of patients with GAD, the pharmacological treatments of choice are benzodiazepines and triazolobenzodiazepines. Those medications are unquestionably effective in relieving the symptoms of GAD. Opinions based on clinical experience differ, but the data do not support the advantage of any particular benzodiazepine over another. An adequate trial of benzodiazepines results in significant improvement in about 70 percent of patients. Most patients with GAD respond to a daily dose equivalent of 15 to 25 mg of diazepam (Valium). No correlation has been established between clinical response and dose or plasma level. One study found that GAD patients with severe cardiovascular symptoms required higher doses of benzodiazepine than did GAD patients with low levels of cardiovascular complaints, in spite of comparable levels of psychic anxiety. Most responders experience both somatic and psychic symptom relief within the first week of treatment. Unfortunately, data regarding the length and the dosage of an adequate trial, the predictors of response, and the differential efficacy of the various benzodiazepines are not yet available.

Tolerance to the sedative and psychomotor effects of benzodiazepines develop within a few weeks, but tolerance to their antianxiety effects is rare. The beneficial effects of a given dose appear to be well-maintained over time. The side effects are relatively mild and usually disappear a few days to weeks after drug discontinuation. The drugs are safe when taken in overdose. Prolonged use of benzodiazepines produces physiological dependence, manifested by the discontinuance syndrome on lowering or discontinuing the drug. The symptoms are divided into withdrawal, rebound, and relapse symptoms. Most discontinuance symptoms are relatively mild and similar to the original symptoms, such as anxiety, dysphoria, nausea, and insomnia. Serious discontinuance symptoms—such as psychosis, delirium, and seizure—are of concern if high-potency, high-dose benzodiazepines are abruptly discontinued after prolonged use. Benzodiazepines must be tapered gradually, usually by one eighth to one quarter of the daily dose weekly or even more slowly.

A lack of response to benzodiazepine treatment is frequently due to unrecognized concomitant Axis I pathology. The relapse rate in successfully treated GAD patients is high after drug discontinuation. In one study almost two thirds of the patients relapsed at one-year follow-up after drug discontinuation.

Azapirones Buspirone (BuSpar), the only currently available azapirone, has been shown to be effective in the treatment of GAD. Azapirones exert their effects on the serotonin system; buspirone is thought to achieve its anxiolytic action as a partial 5-HT_{1A} agonist. Like benzodiazepines, buspirone appears to cause little tolerance over time to its antianxiety effects. On discontinuation of buspirone, the original anxiety symptoms return rapidly. Also like benzodiazepines, buspirone produces relatively few side effects and no known irreversible somatic effects with long-term administration. Buspirone is less sedating than benzodiazepines, does not alter cognitive or psychomotor functions, does not interact with alcohol, has no discernible abuse liability, and is not a muscle relaxant or an anticonvulsant.

Buspirone has a two-to-four-week lag in clinical efficacy, whereas the antianxiety effects of benzodiazepines are apparent within the first week of treatment. Clinical efficacy of benzodiazepines and buspirone seem to be indistinguishable during maintenance, but buspirone may be less effective in patients previously exposed to benzodiazepines. A major advantage of buspirone compared with benzodiazepines is the lack of withdrawal symptoms on drug discontinuation.

The usual dosage of buspirone ranges from 30 to 60 mg daily in three divided doses. Response rates between 60 and 80 percent can be expected. That response rate is comparable to the response rates with benzodiazepine treatment, but significantly more patients with GAD drop out of buspirone treatment than out of benzodiazepine treatment.

The clinical success of buspirone has led to studies with a number of related compounds. Gepirone and ipsapirone, not yet available commercially, seem to demonstrate efficacy comparable to that of buspirone in GAD patients.

Antidepressants Several recent studies confirm the beneficial effects of cyclic antidepressants in the treatment of GAD patients. The dosage is comparable to that required in panic disorder and depression, with an onset of effect of several weeks. Paradoxically, the subjective improvement with antidepressants may coincide with increased anxiety-related physiological symptoms, possibly induced by the side effects of the antidepressants. That effect contrasts with the response pattern to benzodiazepines, in which the subjective improvement in anxiety is accompanied by decreased physiological distress.

Some of the studies comparing cyclic antidepressants with benzodiazepines and a placebo in GAD patients failed to control for the presence of significant depression and panic attacks. Therefore, at present, the antianxiety effects of the tested antidepressants in GAD are not known to be independent of their antidepressant and antipanic effects.

β-Blockers Palpitation, tremor, and perspiration may respond to β-blockers alone, but the full symptoms of GAD usually require benzodiazepines, azaperones, or antidepressants. The dosage of β-blockers, most commonly atenolol (Tenormin) or propranolol (Inderal), has to be titrated to a level that reduces the heart rate by 5 to 10 beats a minute. If effective, β-blockers work within the first week of treatment. Their side effects include depression, weakness, light-headedness, nausea, fatigue, and loss of concentration. Patients with bradycardia, heart block, and asthma should not take β-blockers.

Long-term pharmacological treatment Since the pharmacological treatment of GAD is usually long-term, the lowest dosage of medication that controls the patient's symptoms should be prescribed. In view of the natural periods of relative symptom remission in GAD, the clinician should try approximately every six months to discontinue the medication. Benzodiazepines should be tapered slowly; buspirone, antidepressants, and β-blockers can be discontinued more rapidly. Frequently, emerging depression and other mood disorder symptoms require vigorous treatment. The clinician should use a variety of psychotherapeutic techniques, as they may reduce the need for antianxiety medication.

Most patients with GAD are not able to remain symptom-free for long periods without taking medications. GAD is a chronic illness that requires chronic treatment. Fortunately, the medications recommended for GAD are overwhelmingly safe, even when given for long periods of time. Failures to taper antianxiety drugs or apply psychotherapeutic techniques should be explained by the nature of the disease, rather than considered the fault of the doctor or the patient.

COMBINATION TREATMENTS Some claim that medication and psychotherapy may interfere with each other, but clinical wisdom suggests that the combination has advantages compared with a single-treatment approach. According to anecdotal evidence, the combination of benzodiazepines with antidepressants, buspirone, or β-blockers may result in rapid symptom relief. Once the antidepressant or buspirone becomes effective, the benzodiazepine can be tapered off. The confirmation of those possibilities requires controlled studies.

OTHER ANXIETY DISORDERS

DSM-IV lists the following anxiety disorders: panic disorder with and without agoraphobia, agoraphobia without a history of panic disorder, specific and social phobias, obsessive-compulsive disorder, posttraumatic stress disorder, acute stress disorder (all discussed in other sections in this chapter), generalized anxiety disorder, anxiety disorder due to a general medical condition, substance-induced anxiety disorder, and anxiety disorder not otherwise specified, including mixed anxiety-depressive disorder (all discussed in this section).

Virtually everyone who drinks alcohol has on at least a few occasions used alcohol to reduce anxiety, most often social anxiety. In contrast, carefully controlled studies have found that the effects of alcohol on anxiety are variable and can be significantly affected by gender, the amount of alcohol ingested, and cultural attitudes. Nevertheless, alcohol use disorders and other substance-related disorders are commonly associated with anxiety disorders. Alcohol use disorders are about four times more common among patients with panic disorder than among the general population, about 3.5 times more common among patients with obsessive-compulsive disorder, and about 2.5 times more common among patients with phobias. Several studies have reported data indicating that genetic diatheses for both anxiety disorders and alcohol use disorders may cosegregate in some families.

ANXIETY DISORDER DUE TO A GENERAL MEDICAL CONDITION Anxiety disorder due to a general medical condition was listed in DSM-III-R as organic anxiety syndrome, one of the organic mental disorders associated with Axis III physical disorders or conditions. As with other major syndromes (for example, psychosis and mood disorder symptoms), anxiety disorder due to a general medical condition has been included within the relevant section to encourage the formulation and the consideration of a complete differential diagnosis. However, the inclusion of the disorder does not imply that the other anxiety disorders are not also medical conditions.

Epidemiology The occurrence of anxiety symptoms related to general medical conditions is common, although the incidence of the disorder varies for each specific general medical condition.

Etiology A wide range of medical conditions can cause symptoms similar to those seen in anxiety disorders (Table 17.5-2). Hyperthyroidism, hypothyroidism, hypoparathyroidism, and vitamin B_{12} deficiency are frequently associated with anxiety symptoms. In the authors' opinion, however, vitamin B_{12} deficiency has a poor correlation with anxiety. A pheochromocytoma produces epinephrine, which can cause paroxysmal episodes of anxiety symptoms. Certain lesions of the brain and postencephalitic states reportedly produce symptoms identical to those seen in obsessive-compulsive disorder. Some other medical conditions, such as cardiac arrhythmia, can produce physiological symptoms of panic disorder.

Diagnosis The DSM-IV diagnosis of anxiety disorder due to a general medical condition (Table 17.5-3) requires the presence of symptoms of an anxiety disorder. DSM-IV allows clinicians to specify if the disorder is characterized by symptoms of generalized anxiety, panic attacks, or obsessive-compulsive symptoms.

The clinician should have an increased level of suspicion for the diagnosis when chronic or paroxysmal anxiety is associated with a physical disease that is known to cause such symptoms in some patients. Paroxysmal bouts of hypertension in an anxious patient may indicate that a workup for a pheochromocytoma is appropriate. A general medical workup may reveal dia-

TABLE 17.5-2
Disorders Associated with Anxiety

Neurological disorders	Miscellaneous conditions
Cerebral neoplasms	Hypoglycemia
Cerebral trauma and postconcussive syndromes	Carcinoid syndrome
Cerebrovascular disease	Systemic malignancies
Subarachnoid hemorrhage	Premenstrual syndrome
Migraine	Febrile illnesses and chronic infections
Encephalitis	Porphyria
Cerebral syphilis	Infectious mononucleosis
Multiple sclerosis	Posthepatitis syndrome
Wilson's disease	Uremia
Huntington's disease	Toxic conditions
Epilepsy	Alcohol and drug withdrawal
Systemic conditions	Amphetamines
Hypoxia	Sympathomimetic agents
Cardiovascular disease	Vasopressor agents
Cardiac arrhythmias	Caffeine and caffeine withdrawal
Pulmonary insufficiency	Penicillin
Anemia	Sulfonamides
Endocrine disturbances	Cannabis
Pituitary dysfunction	Mercury
Thyroid dysfunction	Arsenic
Parathyroid dysfunction	Phosphorus
Adrenal dysfunction	Organophosphates
Pheochromocytoma	Carbon disulfide
Virilization disorders of females	Benzene
Inflammatory disorders	Aspirin intolerance
Lupus erythematosus	Idiopathic psychiatric disorders
Rheumatoid arthritis	Depression
Polyarteritis nodosa	Mania
Temporal arteritis	Schizophrenia
Deficiency states	Anxiety disorders
Vitamin B_{12} deficiency	Generalized anxiety
Pellagra	Panic attacks
	Phobic disorders
	Posttraumatic stress disorder

Table from J L Cummings: *Clinical Neuropsychiatry,* p 214. Grune & Stratton, Orlando, 1985. Used with permission.

TABLE 17.5-3
Diagnostic Criteria for Anxiety Disorder Due to a General Medical Condition

A. Prominent anxiety, panic attacks, or obsessions or compulsions predominate the clinical picture.
B. There is evidence from the history, physical examination, or laboratory findings that the disturbance is the direct physiological consequence of a general medical condition.
C. The disturbance is not better accounted for by another mental disorder (e.g., adjustment disorder with anxiety, in which the stressor is a serious general medical condition).
D. The disturbance does not occur exclusively during the course of a delirium.
E. The disturbance causes clinically significant distress or impairment in social, occupational, or other important areas of functioning.

Specify if:

With generalized anxiety: if excessive anxiety or worry about a number of events or activities predominates in the clinical presentation

With panic attacks: if panic attacks predominate in the clinical presentation

With obsessive-compulsive symptoms: if obsessions or compulsions predominate in the clinical presentation

Coding note: Include the name of the general medical condition on Axis I, e.g., anxiety disorder due to pheochromocytoma, with generalized anxiety; also code the general medical condition on Axis III.

betes, an adrenal tumor, thyroid disease, or a neurological condition. For example, some patients with complex partial epilepsy have extreme episodes of anxiety or fear as their only manifestation of the epileptic activity.

Clinical features

GENERALIZED ANXIETY A high prevalence of generalized anxiety symptoms in patients with Sjögren's syndrome has been reported, and that may be related to the effects of Sjögren's syndrome on cortical and subcortical functions and on thyroid function. The highest prevalence of generalized anxiety symptoms in a medical disorder seems to be Graves' disease, in which as many as two thirds of all patients meet the criteria for generalized anxiety disorder.

OBSESSIVE-COMPULSIVE SYMPTOMS Reports in the literature have associated the development of obsessive-compulsive symptoms with Sydenham's chorea and multiple sclerosis.

PANIC ATTACKS Patients who have cardiomyopathy may have the highest incidence of panic attacks secondary to a general medical condition. One study reported that 83 percent of cardiomyopathy patients awaiting cardiac transplantation had panic disorder symptoms. In some studies, about 25 percent of patients with Parkinson's disease and chronic obstructive pulmonary disease have symptoms of panic disorder. Other medical conditions associated with panic disorder include irritable bowel syndrome, thyroid abnormalities, chronic pain, primary biliary cirrhosis, and epilepsy, particularly when the focus is in the right parahippocampal gyrus.

A 78-year-old, retired, lumber-company president sought help for the onset of a series of attacks in which he experienced marked apprehension, restlessness, and the need to be outdoors to relieve his sense of discomfort. He described the most recent event as having occurred at 3:00 A.M. a week earlier: he awoke from sleep and felt "the walls were caving in" on him. He denied that this was related to dreaming and said that he was fully awake at the time. He arose, dressed, and went outside in subzero weather; once outside, he noted gradual improvement (but not full resolution) of his symptoms. Complete resolution took a full day.

In response to pointed questioning, the patient denied dyspnea, palpitations, choking sensations, paresthesias, and nausea. He reported trembling and some sweating, together with intermittent dizziness. He imagined that he would die (or lose consciousness) if he could not "escape" from his house. He spoke of a need "to be active."

On questioning, the patient recalled a similar series of attacks almost 30 years earlier following eye surgery for an injury. He described bilateral patching of his eyes and being confined to bed for days, with his head sandbagged to preclude movement. Once ambulatory, he had experienced these attacks for more than a year.

The patient denied recent sleep dysfunction, change in appetite or weight, crying spells, or decreased energy. He had been taking diazepam for approximately two months for feelings of increased nervousness and tension. He had noted mild memory problems of late.

Further inquiry established a problem with balance and intermittent pain in the right arm, and a complaint of indigestion and intermittent diarrhea. The patient had stopped gardening the past summer because of his balance problem. On examination he was found to have a "beefy" red tongue (which he said was painful), difficulty with tandem gait and rapid alternating motion, and a mild intention tremor. He denied urinary incontinence.

Laboratory studies revealed a macrocytic anemia, and vitamin B_{12} deficiency. The patient was given B_{12} replacement, and his attacks did not recur.

Discussion This patient describes fairly typical, unexpected panic attacks, suggesting a diagnosis of panic disorder. However, careful physical examination and laboratory findings indicate the characteristic features of vitamin B_{12} deficiency caused by pernicious anemia, an acquired vitamin B_{12} malabsorption syndrome. Because the panic attacks disappeared with treatment of the vitamin deficiency, it is reasonable to assume that the correct diagnosis is anxiety disorder due to pernicious anemia, with panic attacks.

What is puzzling was the history of similar episodes of panic many years ago. In the absence of any known general medical condition or substance causing the panic attacks, at that time we assume that he had panic disorder. The current anxiety disorder due to pernicious anemia may be a manifestation of an underlying vulnerability to panic attacks.

Differential diagnosis Anxiety as a symptom can be associated with many psychiatric disorders, in addition to the anxiety disorders themselves. A mental status examination is necessary to determine the presence of mood symptoms or psychotic symptoms that may suggest another psychiatric diagnosis. For the clinician to conclude that a patient has an anxiety disorder due to a general medical condition, the patient should clearly have anxiety as the predominant symptom and should have a specific causative nonpsychiatric medical disorder. To ascertain the degree to which a general medical condition is causative for the anxiety, the clinician should know how closely the medical condition and the anxiety symptoms have been related in the literature, the age of onset (primary anxiety disorders usually have their onset before age 35), and the patient's family history of both anxiety disorders and relevant general medical conditions (for example, hyperthyroidism). A diagnosis of adjustment disorder with anxiety must also be considered in the differential diagnosis.

Course and prognosis The unremitting experience of anxiety can be disabling, interfering with every aspect of life, including social, occupational, and psychological functioning. A sudden change in the level of anxiety may prompt the affected person to seek medical or psychiatric help more quickly than when the onset is insidious. The treatment or the removal of the primary medical cause of the anxiety usually initiates a clear course of improvement in the anxiety disorder symptoms. In some cases, however, the anxiety disorder symptoms continue even after the primary medical condition is treated—for example, in continuing anxiety after an episode of encephalitis. Also, some symptoms, particularly obsessive-compulsive disorder symptoms, linger for a longer time than do other anxiety disorder symptoms. When anxiety disorder symptoms are present for a significant period after the medical disorder has been treated, the remaining symptoms should probably be treated as if they were primary—that is, with psychotherapy or pharmacotherapy or both.

Treatment The primary treatment for anxiety disorder due to a general medical condition is the treatment of the underlying medical condition. If the patient also has an alcohol or other substance use disorder, that disorder must also be therapeutically addressed to gain control of the anxiety disorder symptoms. If the removal of the primary medical condition does not reverse the anxiety disorder symptoms, treatment of those symptoms should follow the treatment guidelines for the specific mental disorder. In general, behavioral modification techniques, anxiolytic agents, and serotonergic antidepressants have been the most effective treatment modalities.

SUBSTANCE-INDUCED ANXIETY DISORDER DSM-IV includes the substance-induced mental disorders in the categories for the relevant mental disorder syndromes. Substance-induced anxiety disorder, therefore, is contained in the category of anxiety disorders. In DSM-III-R, patients with the disorder were classified as having a psychoactive substance-induced organic mental disorder.

Epidemiology Substance-induced anxiety disorder is common, both as the result of the ingestion of so-called recreational drugs and as the result of prescription drug use.

Etiology A wide range of substances can cause symptoms of anxiety that can mimic any of the DSM-IV anxiety disorders. Although sympathomimetics (for example, amphetamine, cocaine, and caffeine) have been most associated with the production of anxiety disorder symptoms, many serotonergic drugs (for example, lysergic acid diethylamide [LSD] and 3,4-methylene dioxymethamphetamine [MDMA]) can also cause both acute and chronic anxiety syndromes in users of those drugs. A wide range of prescription medications are also associated with the production of anxiety disorder symptoms in susceptible persons.

Diagnosis The DSM-IV diagnostic criteria for substance-induced anxiety disorder require the presence of prominent anxiety, panic attacks, obsessions, or compulsions (Table 17.5-4). The DSM-IV guidelines state that the symptoms should have developed during the use of the substance or within a month of the cessation of substance use. However, DSM-IV encourages the clinician to use appropriate clinical judgment to assess the relation between substance exposure and anxiety symptoms. The structure of the diagnosis includes specification of the substance (for example, cocaine), specification of the appropriate state during the onset (for example, intoxication), and mention of the specific symptom pattern (for example, panic attacks).

Clinical features The associated clinical features vary with the particular substance involved. Even infrequent use of psychostimulants can result in anxiety disorder symptoms in some persons. Associated with the anxiety disorder symptoms may also be impairments in comprehension, calculation, and memory. Those cognitive deficits are usually reversible if the substance use is stopped.

Differential diagnosis The differential diagnosis includes the primary anxiety disorders, anxiety disorder due to a general medical condition (for which the patient may be receiving an implicated drug), and mood disorders, which are frequently accompanied by symptoms of anxiety disorders. Personality disorders and malingering must be considered in the differential diagnosis, particularly in some urban emergency rooms.

TABLE 17.5-4
Diagnostic Criteria for Substance-Induced Anxiety Disorder

A. Prominent anxiety, panic attacks, or obsessions or compulsions predominate in the clinical picture.
B. There is evidence from the history, physical examination, or laboratory findings of either (1) or (2):
   (1) the symptoms in criterion A developed during, or within one month of, substance intoxication or withdrawal
   (2) medication use is etiologically related to the disturbance
C. The disturbance is not better accounted for by an anxiety disorder that is not substance induced. Evidence that the symptoms are better accounted for by an anxiety disorder that is not substance induced might include the following: the symptoms precede the onset of the substance use (or medication use); the symptoms persist for a substantial period of time (e.g., about a month) after the cessation of acute withdrawal or severe intoxication or are substantially in excess of what would be expected given the type or amount of the substance used or the duration of use; or there is other evidence suggesting the existence of an independent non-substance-induced anxiety disorder (e.g., a history of recurrent non-substance-related episodes).
D. The disturbance does not occur exclusively during the course of a delirium.
E. The disturbance causes clinically significant distress or impairment in social, occupational, or other important areas of functioning.

Note: This diagnosis should be made instead of a diagnosis of substance intoxication or substance withdrawal only when the anxiety symptoms are in excess of those usually associated with the intoxication or withdrawal syndrome and when the anxiety symptoms are sufficiently severe to warrant independent clinical attention.

Code [Specific Substance]-induced anxiety disorder (alcohol; amphetamine (or amphetamine-like substance); caffeine; cannabis; cocaine; hallucinogen; inhalant; phencyclidine (or phencyclidine-like substance); sedative, hypnotic, or anxiolytic; other [or unknown] substance)

Specify if:
- **With generalized anxiety:** if excessive anxiety or worry about a number of events or activities predominates in the clinical presentation
- **With panic attacks:** if panic attacks predominate in the clinical presentation
- **With obsessive-compulsive symptoms:** if obsessions or compulsions predominate in the clinical presentation
- **With phobic symptoms:** if phobic symptoms predominate in the clinical presentation

Specify if:
- **With onset during intoxication:** if the criteria are met for intoxication with the substance and the symptoms develop during the intoxication syndrome
- **With onset during withdrawal:** if criteria are met for withdrawal from the substance and the symptoms develop during, or shortly after, a withdrawal syndrome

Table from DSM-IV, *Diagnostic and Statistical Manual of Mental Disorders,* ed 4. Copyright American Psychiatric Association, Washington, 1994. Used with permission.

Course and prognosis The course and the prognosis generally depend on the removal of the causally involved substance and the long-term ability of the affected patient to limit the use of the substance. The anxiogenic effects of most drugs are reversible. When the anxiety does not reverse with the cessation of the drug, the clinician should reconsider the diagnosis of substance-induced anxiety disorder or consider the possibility that the substance causes irreversible brain damage.

Treatment The primary treatment for substance-induced anxiety disorder is the removal of the causally involved substance. Treatment then must focus on finding an alternative treatment if the substance was a medically indicated drug, on limiting the patient's exposure if the substance was introduced through environmental exposure, or on treating the underlying substance-related disorder. If anxiety disorder symptoms continue even though the substance use has stopped, treatment of the anxiety disorder symptoms with appropriate psychotherapeutic or pharmacotherapeutic modalities may be appropriate.

ANXIETY DISORDER NOT OTHERWISE SPECIFIED

Some patients have symptoms of anxiety disorders that do not meet the criteria for any specific DSM-IV anxiety disorder or adjustment disorder with anxiety or mixed anxiety and depressed mood. Such patients are most appropriately classified as having anxiety disorder not otherwise specified (NOS). DSM-IV includes four examples of conditions that are appropriate for the diagnosis (Table 17.5-5). One of the examples is mixed anxiety-depressive disorder.

Mixed anxiety-depressive disorder DSM-IV follows the lead of ICD-10 by including, in the DSM-IV appendix and as an example of anxiety disorder NOS, mixed anxiety-depressive disorder. That disorder covers patients who have both anxiety and depressive symptoms but who do not meet the diagnostic criteria for either an anxiety disorder or a mood disorder. The combination of depressive and anxiety symptoms results in a significant functional impairment for the affected person. The condition may be particularly prevalent in primary care practices and outpatient mental health clinics. Opponents have argued that the mere availability of the diagnosis discourages clinicians from taking the necessary time to obtain a complete psychiatric history to differentiate true depressive disorders from true anxiety disorders.

EPIDEMIOLOGY The coexistence of major depressive disorder and panic disorder is common. As many as two thirds of all patients with depressive symptoms have prominent anxiety symptoms, and one third may meet the diagnostic criteria for panic disorder. Researchers have reported that from 20 to 90 percent of all patients with panic disorder have episodes of major depressive disorder. Those data suggest that the coexistence of depressive and anxiety symptoms, neither of which meet the diagnostic criteria for other depressive or anxiety disorders, may be common. At this time, however, formal epidemiological data on mixed anxiety-depressive disorder are not available. Nevertheless, some clinicians and researchers have estimated that the prevalence of the disorder in the general population is as high as 10 percent and in primary care clinics as high as 50 percent, although conservative estimates suggest a prevalence of about 1 percent in the general population.

ETIOLOGY There are several hypotheses that suggest anxiety symptoms and depressive symptoms are causally linked in some affected patients. First, a number of investigators have reported similar neuroendocrine findings in depressive disorders and anxiety disorders, particularly panic disorder, including blunted cortisol response to adrenocorticotropic hormone (ACTH), blunted growth hormone response to clonidine, and blunted thyroid-stimulating hormone (TSH) and prolactin responses to thyrotropin-releasing hormone (TRH). Second, several investigators have reported data indicating that hyperactivity of the noradrenergic system is causally relevant to some patients with depressive disorders and to some patients with panic disorder. Specifically, those studies have found elevated concentrations of the norepinephrine metabolite 3-methoxy-4-hydroxyphenylethyleneglycol (MHPG) in the urine, the plasma, or the CSF of depressed patients and panic disorder patients who were actively experiencing a panic attack. As with other anxiety and depressive disorders, serotonin and GABA may also be causally involved in mixed anxiety-depressive disorder. Third, many studies have found that serotonergic drugs, such as fluoxetine (Prozac) and clomipramine (Anafranil), are useful in treating both depressive and anxiety disorders. Fourth, a number of family studies have reported data indicating that anxiety and depressive symptoms are genetically linked in at least some families.

DIAGNOSIS The DSM-IV research criteria (Table 17.5-6) are similar to the ICD-10 criteria for mixed anxiety and depressive disorder, which require the presence of subsyndromal symptoms of both anxiety and depression and the presence of some autonomic symptoms, such as tremor, palpitations, dry mouth, and the sensation of a churning stomach. Some preliminary studies have indicated that the sensitivity of general practitio-

TABLE 17.5-5
Diagnostic Criteria for Anxiety Disorder Not Otherwise Specified

This category includes disorders with prominent anxiety or phobic avoidance that do not meet criteria for any specific anxiety disorder, adjustment disorder with anxiety, or adjustment disorder with mixed anxiety and depressed mood. Examples include

1. Mixed anxiety-depressive disorder: clinically significant symptoms of anxiety and depression but the criteria are not met for either a specific mood disorder or a specific anxiety disorder.
2. Clinically significant social phobic symptoms that are related to the social impact of having a general medical condition or mental disorder (e.g., Parkinson's disease, dermatological conditions, stuttering, anorexia nervosa, body dysmorphic disorder).
3. Situations in which the clinician has concluded that an anxiety disorder is present but is unable to determine whether it is primary, due to a general medical condition, or substance induced.

TABLE 17.5-6
Research Criteria for Mixed Anxiety-Depressive Disorder

A. Persistent or recurrent dysphoric mood lasting at least one month.
B. The dysphoric mood is accompanied by at least one month of four (or more) of the following symptoms:
   (1) difficulty concentrating or mind going blank
   (2) sleep disturbance (difficulty falling or staying asleep, or restless unsatisfying sleep)
   (3) fatigue or low energy
   (4) irritability
   (5) worry
   (6) being easily moved to tears
   (7) hypervigilance
   (8) anticipating the worst
   (9) hopelessness (pervasive pessimism about the future)
   (10) low self-esteem or feelings of worthlessness
C. The symptoms cause clinically significant distress or impairment in social, occupational, or other important areas of functioning.
D. The symptoms are not due to the direct physiological effects of a substance (e.g., a drug of abuse, a medication) or a general medical condition.
E. All of the following:
   (1) criteria have never been met for major depressive disorder, dysthymic disorder, panic disorder, or generalized anxiety disorder
   (2) criteria are not currently met for any other anxiety or mood disorder (including an anxiety or mood disorder, in partial remission)
   (3) the symptoms are not better accounted for by any other mental disorder

ners to a syndrome of mixed anxiety-depressive disorder is low, although that lack of recognition may reflect the lack of an appropriate diagnostic label for the patients.

CLINICAL FEATURES The clinical features of mixed anxiety-depressive disorder are a combination of some of the symptoms of anxiety disorders and some of the symptoms of depressive disorders. In addition, symptoms of autonomic nervous system hyperactivity, such as gastrointestinal complaints, are common and contribute to the high frequency with which the patients are seen in outpatient medical clinics.

DIFFERENTIAL DIAGNOSIS The differential diagnosis includes other anxiety and depressive disorders and personality disorders. Among the anxiety disorders, generalized anxiety disorder is the one most likely to overlap with mixed anxiety-depressive disorder. Among the mood disorders, dysthymic disorder and minor depressive disorder are the ones most likely to overlap with mixed anxiety-depressive disorder. Among the personality disorders, avoidant, dependent, and obsessive-compulsive personality disorders may have symptoms that resemble those seen in mixed anxiety-depressive disorder. A diagnosis of a somatoform disorder should also be considered. Only a psychiatric history, a mental status examination, and a working knowledge of the specific DSM-IV criteria can help the clinician differentiate among those conditions.

COURSE AND PROGNOSIS On the basis of clinical data to date, patients seem to be equally likely to begin with prominent anxiety symptoms, prominent depressive symptoms, or an equal mixture of the two symptoms. During the course of the illness, anxiety or depressive symptoms may alternate in their predominance. The prognosis is not known at this time.

TREATMENT Since adequate studies comparing treatment modalities for mixed anxiety-depressive disorder are not currently available, the clinician is probably most likely to treat the patient on the basis of the symptoms present, their severity, and the clinician's own level of comfort and experience with various treatment modalities. Psychotherapeutic approaches may involve time-limited approaches, such as cognitive therapy or behavior modification, although some clinicians use a less structured psychotherapeutic approach, such as insight-oriented psychotherapy. Pharmacotherapy for mixed anxiety-depressive disorder may include antianxiety drugs or antidepressive drugs or both. Among the anxiolytic drugs, some data indicate that the use of triazolobenzodiazepines (for example, alprazolam) may be indicated because of their effectiveness in treating depression associated with anxiety. However, the authors believe that the antidepressant effect of alprazolam is weak. A drug that affects the serotonin type-1A (5-HT_{1A}) receptor, such as buspirone, may also be indicated. Among the antidepressants, in spite of the noradrenergic theories linking the anxiety disorders and the depressive disorders, the serotonegric antidepressants (for example, fluoxetine) may be most effective in treating mixed anxiety-depressive disorder, although the data to support that assumption are lacking.

SUGGESTED CROSS-REFERENCES

Further nosological issues concerning the diagnosis of GAD are presented in Section 11.1 on classification of mental disorders. Section 6.1 on psychoanalysis provides the background for the description of the analytic theory and treatment of GAD. The description of learning theory in Section 3.3 forms the basis of cognitive behavior theory and therapy for GAD. Chapter 1 on the neural sciences describes the neuroanatomy, the neurobiology of neurotransmission, and the basis of brain imaging underlying the biological theories and treatment of GAD. The sections in Chapter 32 on antianxiety drugs detail the pharmacology of the specific agents recommended in the treatment of GAD.

REFERENCES

*American Psychiatric Association Task Force: *Benzodiazepine Dependence, Toxicity, and Abuse*. American Psychiatric Association Press, Washington, 1990.

Borkovec T D, Inz J: The nature of worry in generalized anxiety disorder: A predominance of thought activity. Behav Res Ther *28:* 153, 1990.

Bradwejn J: Benzodiazepines for the treatment of panic disorder and generalized anxiety disorder: clinical issues and future directions. Can J Psychiatry *38* (Suppl 4): S109, 1993.

Butler G, Fennell M, Robson P, Gelder M: Comparison of cognitive behavior therapy in the treatment of generalized anxiety disorder. J Consult Clin Psychol *59:* 167, 1991.

Charney D S, Woods S W, Heninger G R: Noradrenergic function in generalized anxiety disorder. Psychiatry Res *27:* 173, 1989.

Clark D A, Beck A T, Beck J S: Symptom differences in major depression, dysthymia, panic disorder, and generalized anxiety disorder. Am J Psychiatry *151:* 205, 1994.

Di-Nardo P, Moras K, Barlow D H, Rapee R M, Brown T A: Reliability of DSM-III-R anxiety disorder categories. Using the Anxiety Disorders Interview Schedule-Revised (ADIS-R). Arch Gen Psychiatry *50:* 251, 1993.

*Gorman J M, Papp L A, editors: Anxiety disorders. In *Annual Review of Psychiatry*, vol 11, A Tasman, editor, American Psychiatric Association Press, Washington, 1992.

Gorman J M, Papp L A: Chronic anxiety: Deciding the length of treatment. J Clin Psychiatry *5:* 11, 1990.

Gross P R, Eifert G H: Components of generalized anxiety: The role of intrusive thoughts vs worry. Behav Res Ther *28:* 421, 1990.

Jarrell M P, Ballenger J C: Psychiatric comorbidity in patient with generalized anxiety disorder. Am J Psychiatry *150:* 1216, 1993.

Liebowitz M R, Fyer A J, Gorman J M, Campeas B, Sandberg D P, Hollander E, Papp L A, Klein D F: Tricyclic therapy of the DSM-III anxiety disorders: A review with implications for further research. J Psychiatr Res *22* (1, Suppl): 7, 1988.

Manuzza S, Fyer A J, Martin L Y, Gallops M P, Endicott J, Gorman J, Liebowitz M R, Klein D F: Reliability of anxiety assessment: I. Diagnostic agreement. Arch Gen Psychiatry *46:* 1093, 1989.

Martin M, Williams R M, Clark D M: Does anxiety lead to selective processing of threat-related information? Behav Res Ther *29:* 147, 1991.

Massion A O, Warshaw M G, Keller M B: Quality of life and psychiatry morbidity in panic disorder and generalized anxiety disorder. Am J Psychiatry *150:* 600, 1993.

McLeod D R, Hoehn-Saric R, Foster G V, Hipsley P A: The influence of premenstrual syndrome on ratings of anxiety in women with generalized anxiety disorder. Acta Psychiatr Scand *88:* 248, 1993.

McLeod D R, Hoehn-Saric R, Zimmerli W D, De Souza E B, Oliver L K: Treatment effects of alprazolam and imipramine: Physiological versus subjective changes in patients with generalized anxiety disorder. Biol Psychiatry *28:* 849, 1990.

Nisita C, Petracca A, Akiskal H S, Galli L, Geppent I, Cassano G B: Delimitation of generalized anxiety disorder: Clinical comparisons with panic and major depressive disorders. Compr Psychiatry *31:* 409, 1990.

Papp I A, Zitrin C M, Coplan J, Gorman J M: The role of personality in anxiety disorders. Psychiatr Med *8:* 107, 1990.

*Rapee R M, Barlow D H, editors: *Chronic Anxiety*. Guilford, New York, 1991.

Rickels K, Downing R, Schweizer E, Hassman H: Antidepressants for the treatment of generalized anxiety disorder: A placebo-controlled comparison of imipramine, trazodone, and diazepam. Arch Gen Psychiatry *50:* 884, 1993.

*Rickels K, Schweizer E: The clinical course and long-term management of generalized anxiety disorder. J Clin Psychopharmacol *10:* 101S, 1990.

Roy-Byrne P P, Cowley D S, Hommer D, Ritchie J, Greenblatt D,

Nemeroff C: Neuroendocrine effects of diazepam in panic and generalized anxiety disorders. Biol Psychiatry *30:* 73, 1991.
*Sanderson W C, Barlow D H: A description of patients diagnosed with DSM-III-R generalized anxiety disorder. J Nerv Ment Dis *178:* 588, 1990.
Spitzer R L, Gibbon M, Skodol A E, Williams J B W, First M B: DSM-IV Casebook. American Psychiatric Press, Washington, 1994.
Starcevic V, Fallon S, Uhlenhuth E H: The frequency and severity of generalized anxiety disorder symptoms: Toward a less cumbersome conceptualization. J Nerv Ment Dis 1994 *182:* 80, 1994.
Weissman M M: Panic and generalized anxiety: Are they separate disorders? J Psychiatr Res 24 (2, Suppl): 157, 1990.
Woodman C L: The genetics of panic disorder and generalized anxiety disorder. Ann Clin Psychiatry *5*: 231, 1993.
Wu J C, Buchsbaum M S, Hershey T G: PET in generalized anxiety disorder. Biol Psychiatry *29:* 1181, 1991.

CHAPTER 18 SOMATOFORM DISORDERS

FREDERICK G. GUGGENHEIM, M.D.
G. RICHARD SMITH, M.D.

INTRODUCTION

Somatoform disorders represent a relatively new clustering of time-weathered psychiatric conditions in which bodily sensations or functions are influenced by a disorder of the mind. Gathered together and renamed in 1980 by the third edition of *Diagnostic and Statistical Manual of Mental Disorders* (DSM-III) were five clinical syndromes: (1) somatization disorder; (2) conversion disorder; (3) psychogenic pain disorder; (4) hypochondriasis; and (5) atypical somatoform disorder. In the fourth edition of DSM (DSM-IV), there are now five specific and two residual categories, with some significant changes improving clinical applicability.

As the name ''somatoform'' implies, the disorders are at the mind-body interface: bodily symptoms, with concerns as a psychiatric disorder. Somatoform disorders also exemplify mind-brain interactions: the brain, in ways only recently delineated and still not clearly understood, sending various signals that impinge on the patient's awareness to indicate a serious problem in the body proper.

CORE FEATURES Characteristic of somatoform disorders are two enduring clinical features: (1) somatic complaints that suggest major medical maladies yet have no associated serious, demonstrable, peripheral organ disorder; and (2) psychological factors and conflicts that seem important in initiating, exacerbating, and maintaining the disturbance.

Because of their intense bodily perceptions, restricted level of physical functioning and morbid beliefs, the patients have become convinced they harbor serious physical problems. Moreover, their symptoms are not willfully controlled. Whatever their faults and problems, the patients are not malingerers. Yet their physicians' physical and laboratory examinations persistently fail to evince significant substantiating data about physical infirmity save for the patients' vigorous and sincere complaints.

However true be the demeaning phrase, ''It's all in your head,'' somatoform patients have been persuaded by their symptoms that their suffering comes from some type of presumably undetected and untreated bodily derangement.

DIAGNOSTIC ISSUES When a somatoform disorder occurs without another comorbid psychiatric condition, the primary care physician and the patient usually do not initially consider a psychiatric condition. The patient's morbid preoccupation with bodily concerns is paramount, not emotional feelings or disordered interpersonal relationships. Often that preoccupation is so severe that it interferes with the patient's capacity for living, loving, or working.

Because of the patient's focus on bodily issues, the psychiatrist's questions (should referral ever occur) about stress and family matters might seem wide of the mark to the patient. But the research literature, as well as clinical experience from seasoned psychiatric consultants, has demonstrated the utility of psychiatric input into managing somatoform patients from the perspective of physical health status, mental health status, global outcome, and cost.

PRIMARY PHYSICIAN'S DIAGNOSTIC PROCESS Physicians are trained to record faithfully the patient's medical history, to perform a physical examination and to make use of laboratory tests. Often during the evaluation process an underlying psychiatric condition is spotted by the astute primary care clinician sensing considerable emotional turmoil. The clinician then elicits specific findings on the mental status examination.

In the ordinary practice of medicine, as long as the patient can render a concise chronicle of events and present a straightforward account of bodily perceptions underlying pathophysiological events, the primary care physician has a remarkably good chance of making an appropriate diagnosis and instituting corrective treatment. However, it becomes understandably difficult for the physician to develop an accurate diagnosis when the somatoform patient forgets (represses) or refuses (suppresses) to share with the physician certain medically relevant, critical events, or when the somatoform patient magnifies or diminishes internal stimuli in a fashion that is not usual and customary for a given medical or surgical condition.

Moreover, when the physician's expectations about the patient's disease are not substantiated by results of the physical examination and laboratory findings, then the highly charged issue of the somatoform patient's competency, motivation, or integrity is raised. Is this account of suffering actually purposeful distortion? Is it simple forgetfulness when the patient fails to tell the physician that there was a similar episode of such symptoms 10 years ago (with benign outcome)?

To the probing clinician it might appear at first that somatoform patients are guilty of blatant, intentional manipulation, or at the least of considerable distortion. Most physicians are not primed to consider that the lack of concordance between subjective suffering and objective physical findings can stem from a set of distorted internal perceptions and unusual beliefs.

In an emergency room or office practice setting the application of specific diagnostic criteria for the somatoform disorders can be helpful. Each set of symptoms and signs needs to be investigated in an appropriate fashion to delineate relevant mechanisms. Even patients with somatoform disorders do get ill and eventually die of something. In the past physicians have been far too ready to attribute atypical presentations of certain protean medical diseases to psychiatric causes—coupling such reductionistic thinking with the conclusion that a putative psychiatric disorder does not merit further investigation or even referral.

Over the past decade the inclusion criteria for the diagnosis of somatoform disorders have been considerably narrowed and simplified. Of course, what must be avoided is the use of a psychiatric diagnosis by exclusion just because no other medical diagnosis can yet be ruled in. Table 18-1 lists a few of the disorders commonly confused with somatoform disorders, especially early in their course.

TABLE 18-1
Conditions Commonly Confused With Somatoform Disorder

Multiple sclerosis	Acute intermittent porphyria
Central nervous system syphilis	Lupus erythematosus
Brain tumor	Hyperthyroidism
Hyperparathyroidism	Myasthenia gravis

THEORETICAL BIOMEDICAL FORMULATIONS There has been little dissemination to the field of those few research findings on somatoform disorders that do bear on relevant underlying physiological or structural brain abnormalities. That makes the internist's task of explaining to the patient that he or she has a psychiatric disorder even more complicated.

To comprehend the underlying basis of the somatoform disorders it may be helpful to view the brain both as a transducer of experience and as a practiced, highly trained organizer of perceptions from the milieu interieur and the milieu exterieur. The brain filters, amplifies, or dampens afferent and efferent stimuli from all parts of the body and from the brain itself. It then produces signals that form the matrix of the patient's experiential world. That is, the brain sends out signals about bodily function that it then interprets in light of past incidents. Somatoform disorders presumably can involve a considerable variety of neuronal pathways—from brain-brain signals to pain pathways and perceptual pathways—in addition to efferent signals to motor apparatus, blood vessels, and the like.

CONVERSION DISORDER

INTRODUCTION AND DEFINITION A conversion disorder is a disturbance of bodily functioning that does not conform to current concepts of the anatomy and physiology of the central or the peripheral nervous system. It typically occurs in a setting of stress and produces considerable dysfunction. DSM-IV diagnostic criteria are shown in Table 18-2.

Many conversion disorders simulate acute neurological pathology (for example, strokes and disturbances of speech, hearing, or vision). But conversion disorders are not associated with the usual pathological neurodiagnostic signs. Conversion symptoms (for example, anesthesias and paresthesias produced by a conversion disorder) do not conform to usual dermatome distribution of the underlying peripheral nerves. Rather the signs and symptoms of a conversion disorder conform to the patient's concept of the medical condition.

Conversion disorders seem to come about with alchemy, changing psychic energy from the turmoil of acute conflict into a bodily manifestation. Turbulence of the mind is transformed into a somatic statement, condensing and focusing concepts, role models, and communicative meanings into one or several physical signs or symptoms of dysfunction. Those somatic representations often simulate an acute medical calamity; initiate urgent, often expensive medical investigation; and produce disability. In primitive settings, however, conversion symptoms have been taken as tokens of religious faith and even as expressions of witchcraft.

While most conversion reactions are transient (hours to days), some can linger. Chronic conversion disorders can actually produce permanent conversion complications, such as disuse contractures of a ''paralyzed'' limb, that can remain long after the psychic strife of the conversion has been resolved.

Conversion disorders challenge the diagnostic competence of internists, neurologists, otolaryngologists, and ophthalmologists. In addition to sensorimotor symptoms, marked autonomic

TABLE 18-2
Diagnostic Criteria for Conversion Disorder

A. One or more symptoms or deficits affecting voluntary motor or sensory function that suggest a neurological or other general medical condition.
B. Psychological factors are judged to be associated with the symptom or deficit because the initiation or exacerbation of the symptom or deficit is preceded by conflicts or other stressors.
C. The symptom or deficit is not intentionally produced or feigned (as in factitious disorder or malingering).
D. The symptom or deficit cannot, after appropriate investigation, be fully explained by a general medical condition, or by the direct effects of a substance, or as a culturally sanctioned behavior or experience.
E. The symptom or deficit causes clinically significant distress or impairment in social, occupational, or other important areas of functioning or warrants medical evaluation.
F. The symptom or deficit is not limited to pain or sexual dysfunction, does not occur exclusively during the course of somatization disorder, and is not better accounted for by another mental disorder.

Specify type of symptom or deficit:
With motor symptom or deficit
With sensory symptom or deficit
With seizures or convulsions
With mixed presentation

Table from DSM-IV, *Diagnostic and Statistical Manual of Mental Disorders,* ed 4. Copyright American Psychiatric Association, Washington, 1994. Used with permission.

disturbances such as protracted (psychogenic) vomiting, hyperemesis gravidarum, urinary retention, and pseudocyesis are also seen, but less commonly.

Conversion disorders are not volitional. Rather, ego defense mechanisms of repression and dissociation act outside of the patient's awareness. Most patients experience *la belle indifférence,* an emotional unconcern or even flatness in a setting of catastrophic illness; but some patients do experience considerable anguish with their new symptoms.

A conversion disorder can be considered when a patient manifests a loss or alteration in physical functioning suggesting a medical or neurological disorder and the condition cannot be explained by any other known medical disorder or pathophysiological process. A conversion disorder cannot be diagnosed just because a medical disorder cannot be ruled in. Failure to prove a physical illness is a necessary, but not sufficient, condition for making the diagnosis of conversion disorder.

HISTORY Until the middle of the 19th century, somatization disorder and conversion disorder (which often travel together) were considered to be one condition called hysteria. The term was derived from the Greek word *hystera,* meaning uterus. Descriptions of conversion disorders appeared as far back as 1900 BC when multiple symptoms were attributed by Egyptian physicians to a wandering of the uterus within the body.

Paul Briquet, in the middle of the 19th century, originated the modern concept of conversion disorder. He considered the disorder to result from a dysfunction of the central nervous system. He proposed that conversion symptoms occurred in those with a constitutional predisposition, when a receptive part of the brain was impacted by extreme stress. Later Russel Reynolds described clinical cases in which the loss of function, or the persistence of severe pain, could be attributed to an idea that the patient had about the body.

Jean-Martin Charcot then expanded on the biological concepts of Briquet and psychological constructs of Reynolds, adding heredity to factors that influence predisposition. Moreover, he suggested that a traumatic event planted the idea which then lead to the brain's dynamic dysfunction. Charcot also contributed the notion that the idea could be produced in the brain by hypnosis.

The term "conversion" was first used by Sigmund Freud and his associate Josef Breuer to describe the clinical case of Anna O., when a somatic symptom was converted or substituted for a repressed thought. Freud then worked out his concept of talking therapy as a catharsis through which unconsciously repressed material might become conscious. With catharsis in psychotherapy and with hypnotic suggestion, somatic conversion symptoms were shown to diminish and even disappear.

Pierre Janet in 1929, following from Charcot, observed that conversion disorders were preceded by a lowering of conscious threshold and were associated with dissociation.

COMPARATIVE NOSOLOGY In 1952 the American Psychiatric Association's first edition of the DSM (DSM-I) used the diagnostic term "conversion reaction," stressing the reactive part of the disorder as well as issues of symbolism, symbols or ciphers from the individual's unconscious that relate to significant life experiences, and secondary gain, tangible benefits that accrue to the individual upon assumption of the sick role. In 1967 the second edition of DSM (DSM-II) changed the diagnostic term to "hysterical psychoneurosis, conversion type." Important in this formulation was *la belle indifférence*. Follow-up studies of specific phenomena associated with conversion disorder were constructed by assigning relative weights to certain features associated with conversion studies. Those studies indicated that there is no pathognomonic validity (using outcome as a gold standard) to symbolism of the symptom, secondary gain, hysterical personality and *la belle indifférence*.

In 1980, DSM-III revised the diagnostic term again to conversion disorder. Removed from the cluster of symptoms was psychogenic pain disorder, a symptom-based pain disorder with criteria otherwise comparable to that of conversion disorder. DSM-III and DSM-III-R required that conversion disorder must be judged by the clinician to be etiologically related to the conversion symptom because of a temporal relationship between it and a significant psychosocial stressor or a demonstrated coupling of conflict and psychological need and the initiation or the exacerbation of a preexisting symptom. That is, it was one of the few diagnoses where the judgment of the clinician was explicitly sought in the making of a diagnosis based on psychodynamic mechanisms. A subjective rather than an objective component was written into the diagnostic criterion. Obviously, that raised the issue of inter-rater reliability in the diagnostic process.

One of the major changes from DSM-III and DSM-III-R to DSM-IV is the further removal of the etiological inference of unconscious mechanisms and psychodynamics involved in the productions of symptoms, with the statement now that "psychological factors are judged to be associated with the symptom or deficit because [it was] preceded by conflicts or other stressors."

A second difference in DSM-IV from DSM-III-R is in the category surrounding the concept of "not fully explained by a known physical disorder" that is now broadened to include culturally sanctioned behavior or experience, general medical condition, and the direct use of substance.

A third change is in the distress-disability category, in which the concept has been broadened to also include important areas of functioning to the individual other than just social and occupational; and the phrase "warrants further medical attention" has been added (for example, distress to family or physician because of potential medical implications associated with the symptom or deficit).

A fourth change focuses on wording to eliminate factitious disorder and malingering. The term "not conscious of intentionally producing the symptom" has been removed in favor of the simple concept "not intentionally produced or feigned."

The ninth revision of the *International Classification of Diseases and Related Health Problems* (ICD-9) in 1978 used the term "hysteria" to include both conversion disorder and dissociative phenomena. Both were defined as mental disorders in which a mechanism out of the patient's awareness produced either a restriction of the field of awareness or a disturbance of motor or sensory function. Hysteria was, as such, associated with psychological advantage or symbolic value. Conversion symptoms involved the body's function, whereas dissociative symptoms involved the mind's function.

When the 10th revision of ICD (ICD-10) considered the somatoform disorders, it listed somatization disorder and its subthreshold companion diagnosis, undifferentiated somatoform disorder, plus hypochondriacal disorder, persistent somatoform pain disorder, autonomic (psychogenic aerophagia) and nonautonomic (psychogenic pruritus) somatoform disorders as part of the group of the somatoform disorders. However, ICD-10 has now assigned conversion disorder to another cluster of disorders, the dissociative disorders.

EPIDEMIOLOGY Conversion disorders are the most frequently occurring of the somatoform disorders. The ages of those with the disorder range from early childhood into old age. The annual incidence of conversion disorders seen by psychiatrists in a New York county has been estimated to be 22 cases per 100,000 population. In a general hospital setting 5 percent to 16 percent of all psychiatric consultation patients manifest some conversion symptoms. In a study of a rural Veterans Administration general hospital, 25 to 30 percent of all male patients had a conversion symptom at some time during their admission. In a psychiatric emergency room or psychiatric clinic by contrast, the incidence of conversion disorder is far lower (one percent of all psychiatric admissions), as different selection factors supervene. Lifetime figures for ever having any conversion symptom, even if only on a transient basis, are far higher, with some studies reporting a 33 percent prevalence rate. Conversion disorder occurs mainly in women, with a ratio of 2 to 1 up to 5 to 1. Among children, however, there may not be an overrepresentation of females.

The prevalence of the disorder is highest in rural areas and among the undereducated and the lower socioeconomic classes. It is more prevalent in military populations, especially those exposed to combat. It is also more common in primitive persons, in those of subnormal intelligence, and in industrial settings where compensation neurosis may become an issue. There may be a tendency for familial aggregation and for the patient to be the youngest sibling in the family. The incidence of the disorder may be declining.

ETIOLOGY

Biological factors Recent etiological research on conversion disorder has involved event-related potentials, structural and functional brain imaging, and neuropsychological testing to investigate aspects of corticofugal inhibition of afferent stimuli.

IMAGING Pierre Flor-Henry's important work on the etiopathology of conversion disorder emphasizes (1) hypofunction of the dominant hemisphere systems, (2) a consequent dysfunctional overactivity of the nondominant hemisphere, and (3) abnormal interhemispheric relations. Defects in both processing of endogenous somatic signals and integrating sensorimotor signals appear to be the consequence of altered dominant hemispheric systems. Particularly in women there seems to be a secondary disorganization of the contralateral hemisphere that in turn is capable of producing the characteristic somatic symptoms.

NEUROPSYCHOLOGICAL TESTS Impaired vigilance-attention and short-term memory have been demonstrated. Localizing studies using the Halstead-Reitan battery of neuropsychological tests have manifested dysfunction of both nondominant right and especially dominant left hemispheres. Increased field dependency and heightened suggestibility is also present.

UNILATERAL SYMPTOMS AND LOCALIZATION Taken together, the findings suggest that patients with conversion disorder, under extraordinary circumstances, can experience impaired intercortical communication and blockade of ordinary channels of verbal associations. The preponderance of left-sided, unilateral symptoms seen in conversion disorder, plus the strong association of conversion disorders with depressive disorders, point to nondominant right hemispheric vulnerability. Additionally, the left hemisphere is phylogenetically associated with inhibitory influences. Thus, the motor and sensory symptoms of conversion suggest defects in processing and in analysis of sensorimotor signals, leading to a failure in the integration of endogenous somatic signals. The proposed defect in understanding of the signals in conversion is in some ways analogous to the failure of comprehension in a stroke (that is, with receptive and expressive aphasia when acoustic-motor coordination of auditory signals involving language fails to occur).

GENDER AND BRAIN LOCALIZATION The fact that conversion disorders occur mainly in women becomes still another piece of evidence used to construct a theory of brain localization. Studies from a variety of sources indicate that women have greater instability of right hemispheric organization. Thus it has been proposed that a primary defect in the left hemisphere interferes with the normal transcallosal inhibitory stabilizing functions of the unstable contralateral right hemisphere. Those circumstances then could account for the symptoms of conversion disorders and for its almost exclusive restriction to the female pattern of cerebral organization.

Much more clinical and experimental work remains to be done if these heuristic hypotheses are to have widespread clinical relevance. The phenomena of both conversion disorder and hypnosis have been considered to be due to blockade of corticofugal impulses induced by emotional rapport or intense emotional experience. Both conditions can lead to selective diminution of awareness of a bodily function. Interestingly, hypnosis can bring about temporary remission of conversion symptoms. Hypnosis can also produce a mimicry of conversion symptoms in those not afflicted with the condition.

Those biomedical theories account for the how, but not the what or the why of conversion disorder. Obviously a multifactorial explanation is needed to render an understanding of the patient's plight and to serve as a framework for testing the most effective and efficient methods of treatment. Conversion symptoms represent a common pathway for the expression of a complex biopsychosocial event. A conversion disorder patient, having a specific diathesis, experiences and creates (outside of his or her level of awareness) an illness in a setting of stress that is shaped to some extent on his or her model of disease.

Psychosocial constructs Long before neuropsychological, neurophysiological, and imaging evidence was available to contribute to an understanding of symptoms of conversion, astute 19th century clinicians focused their attention on the psychological aspects of their patients' internal and external worlds. Psychoanalysts carefully studied their neurotic patients' ongoing emotional struggles and relevant life circumstances immediately antecedent to conversion symptom. In such a fashion the context of the acute psychic trauma and other aspects of the patient's life story often could be coupled meaningfully to the development and maintenance of the patient's conversion symptoms. Moreover, psychoanalytic and hypnotic techniques at times produced dramatic and sometimes permanent remission of the patient's symptoms.

PSYCHOANALYTIC THEORY According to psychoanalytic theory, a conversion disorder results when the anxiety of unconscious intrapsychic conflict is converted into somatic symptoms. When aggressive or sexual impulses emerge in a field of strong inhibition of their expression, the resultant conflict overwhelms the person's ordinary ego defense mechanisms. In such a setting unconscious mechanisms facilitate a compromise as conversion symptoms emerge. The settlement allows a partial expression of the primitive impulse but disguises it so that the individual is unaware of the unconscious wish and the unacceptable desire. The symptom formation, however, may impose a considerable price. Suffering and disability then serve as atonement for having had the unacceptable wish or impulse.

The decrease in anxiety and psychological distress after formation of the conversion symptom is the primary gain. Benefits that also accrue to the individual after the sick role is assumed are the secondary gain. Both primary and secondary gain are typically part of the syndrome associated with conversion disorder. Its permanence and severity can be reinforced by the patient's being enmeshed in irresolvable conflict for which he or she feels no responsibility.

In psychodynamic terms conversion symptoms represent a solution to an unconscious conflict between instinctual drives and superego prohibitions to their expression. The formation of the specific conversion symptom may embody a symbolic aspect of the intrapsychic conflict. Sometimes the conversion symptoms derive from identification with a significant individual, often someone whom the patient associates with loss and who has also experienced such a symptom (a conversion model).

SOCIOCULTURAL THEORY Viewed by itself or as complementary to psychoanalytic theory, conversion symptoms can be understood in sociocultural terms as a form of communication concerning an emotionally charged feeling or idea blocked from expression by personal or cultural restraints. Conversion symptoms can express the forbidden, using mimicry or pantomime instead of words. Moreover, the symptoms of a conversion disorder allow the individual to enter into the sick role, avoiding certain responsibilities or noxious situations. As such, the patient can control or otherwise manipulate the behavior of others.

LEARNING THEORY In terms of conditioned learning theory a conversion symptom can be seen as a piece of classically conditioned learned behavior: symptoms of illness, learned in childhood, then are called forth as a means of coping with an otherwise impossible situation.

DIAGNOSIS AND CLINICAL FEATURES A frequent but not invariable common denominator of conversion disorder is the pseudoneurological nature of the symptom. Common types of conversion symptoms are listed in Table 18-3.

Motor symptoms Abnormal gait, weakness, and paralysis may occur. There can be involuntary-type movements, rhythmical tremors, episodic jerks, tics, seizures, and falling. When patients with conversion symptoms fall, they rarely are severely hurt. Blepharospasm, torticollis, and opisthotonos may happen. All such symptoms tend to grow more intense when observed. Of course, many neurological symptoms of patients with a known pathophysiological basis, such as Parkinson's disease, also tend to intensify when the individual experiences increased anxiety.

Astasia-abasia A staggering, ataxic gait with gross jerks and thrashing or wild waving of the upper extremities, often with an inability to stand without support, is called astasia-abasia. Surprisingly, such patients sometimes can dance to music after the clinician suggests that the ability to successfully perform a dance such as the Fox Trot or the Texas Two-Step is not impacted by the patient's inability to stand or walk.

Pseudoseizures Convulsions associated with conversion disorders often take place when the clinician walks into the patient's room or just when the family visits. After the pseudoseizure terminates the patient usually does not have a period of sluggishness, sleepiness, or confusion typically seen following a true convulsion. Although tongue-biting, urinary incontinence, injury during falls, and seeming loss of consciousness do not usually occur with a pseudoseizure, all can occur. However, the preservation of corneal, pupillary, and gag reflexes, plus the absence of extensor plantar responses and the preservation of normal color during the attack all hint at the diagnosis of a pseudoseizure. The eyes of a patient in a pseudoseizure reportedly deviate toward the ground when the patient is placed on his or her side.

The proportion of pseudoseizures in a given study typically reflects the nature of the referral source and their relationship with the evaluation. From a clinician's perspective about one third of patients evaluated for a pseudoseizure do not have a convulsive disorder or pseudoseizures but rather have some other neurological condition. Another third have both true convulsions and pseudoseizures; and another third have just pseudoseizures.

Other common motor symptoms Other symptoms include paralysis or paresis, more frequently on the patient's nondominant side (left side if right-handed). Paralyses can occur in one limb, several, or in all. In contrast to a patient with neuropathy, the reflexes in a conversion disorder patient with anesthesia or paralysis remain normal. There is no fasciculation, no other electromyograph abnormality, and no atrophy. However, in cases of long-standing pseudoparalysis, disuse atrophy and even contractures can occur as a conversion complication.

Sensory symptoms Anesthesias, hypesthesias, and paresthesias are common conversion symptoms, especially in the extremities (Table 18-4). The pattern of distribution of the anesthesia does not conform to the underlying central or peripheral nerve distribution. Typical are glove or stocking and strict midline anesthesias. Despite a claimed loss of total sensation in the legs and feet, for example, conversion patients can walk in the dark without stumbling (unlike those with tabes dorsalis who lack position sense). Conversion patients told to answer "yes" if they can feel anything when pricked with a pin in the anesthetic zone often will respond "no" when pricked, even when they are not looking at the area being tested.

Hysterical blindness Other sensory modalities can also be affected. Patients with hysterical blindness typically do not hurt themselves seriously when they bump into stationary objects. Despite their "lack" of vision, their pupils react to light and their visual evoked potentials on the electroencephalogram (EEG) are consistent with those of normal vision.

Hallucinations Patients with conversion disorder can have positive or negative hallucination. With positive hallucinations the patient perceives an image or hears a sound that is not there. Hallucinations in conversion disorder are usually associated with intact insight, and the hallucinations are often visual, auditory, and tactile. They tend to be described by the person as part of an interesting story. Conversely, with a negative hallucination the patient with an intact nervous system does not see an object that others can see or hear a sound that others are aware of. When generalized to more than a specific object that, for example, is not seen, then the individual seems to be blind while the visual apparatus is still working.

Visceral symptoms Psychogenic vomiting can occur as a conversion disorder (Table 18-5). Typically such a vomiting patient will not suffer significant weight loss while observed for a week on an inpatient medical service; gastrointestinal workup will show no significant disease or disorder. Another visceral conversion disorder is urinary retention. On urological workup, conversion patients show normal intracystometric dynamics. Conversion as pseudocyesis manifests as a cessation of menses, a protuberant abdomen, and an elevation of serum hormones seen in usual phases of early pregnancy. Other visceral con-

TABLE 18-3
Common Motor Symptoms of Conversion Disorder

Involuntary movements
Tics
Blepharospasm
Torticollis
Opisthotonos
Seizures
Abnormal gait
Falling
Astasia-abasia
Paralysis
Weakness
Aphonia

TABLE 18-4
Common Sensory Deficits of Conversion Disorder

Anesthesia, especially of extremities
Midline anesthesia
Blindness
Tunnel vision
Deafness

TABLE 18-5
Common Visceral Symptoms of Conversion Disorder

Psychogenic vomiting
Pseudocyesis
Globus hystericus
Swooning or syncope
Urinary retention
Diarrhea

versions include *globus hystericus,* syncope, urinary retention, and diarrhea.

Comorbidity Medical and especially neurological disorders occur frequently among patients with conversion disorders. Indeed in some series the majority of conversion patients have a well-documented neurological condition. What is typically seen in these comorbid neurological or medical conditions is an elaboration of symptoms stemming from the original organic lesion. Whether this tells the clinician something about the nature of the sick role or about the nature of the brain with compromised functioning and an altered state of consciousness remains an important open question.

Preexisting or emerging psychopathology also seems to predispose an individual to the development of a conversion disorder. Among Axis I psychiatric conditions, especially noted for their association with conversion are depressive disorders, anxiety disorders, schizophrenia, and somatization disorders. Studies of patients admitted to a psychiatric hospital for conversion disorder reveal that, on further study, one quarter to one half have a clinically significant mood disorder or schizophrenia.

Axis II personality disorders also frequently accompany a conversion disorder, especially the histrionic type (in 5 to 21 percent of cases); the passive-dependent type (9 to 40 percent of cases); and the passive-aggressive type of personality disorder. However, conversion disorders can occur in persons with no predisposing medical, neurological, or psychiatric disorder.

Important caveats As with all disorders with a low specificity and no confirmatory laboratory test, substantiation of the diagnosis is facilitated by the passage of time with no other countervening diagnosis evolving. Also helping to confirm the diagnosis of conversion disorder is the development of another bout of conversion symptoms. About 25 percent of conversion patients will develop another episode during the following one to six years.

The diagnosis of a conversion disorder is made more secure if one can elicit details of a prior set of conversion symptoms. Complicating the collecting of the past medical history, however, in many patients with somatoform disorders is their frequent use of repression. Such patients thus may not recall important pieces of historical data. In adding collateral information a review of the patient's old clinical chart can be very helpful.

Another important caveat is that the diagnosis cannot be based solely on inexplicable neurological findings accompanied by relevant psychological factors. Patients with lesion-based neurological disorders also wrestle with the acceptance or the rejection of the sick role. Moreover, although suggestibility is often seen in patients with conversion, some patients with organic disorders can also respond to suggestion, briefly altering their symptoms.

Critical review of the literature finds little or no empirical support for the necessity of a number of previously widely accepted classic accompaniments of conversion disorder including: *la belle indifférence,* hysterical personality, the presence of secondary gain, the symptom as symbolism, sibling position, disturbed sexuality and conversion V pattern on the Minnesota Multiphasic Personality Inventory (MMPI) (elevated hysteria and hypochondriasis scales, even higher than the depression scale). When taken by itself, no one associated finding is pathognomonic for the diagnosis of conversion disorder. However, a number of features taken together help the clinician determine the likelihood (that is, possible, probable, definite) of a conversion disorder.

Setting of the conversion disorder Marked psychological stress is almost always present. Precipitants typically may have been acute rage, truncated grief, sexual abuse, or physical abuse. Somatic symptoms may develop abruptly following a dramatic psychological blow, mechanical trauma, or a life-threatening experience. Yet studies on patients with conversion disorder demonstrate that their life experiences are not more extreme than those with other types of psychiatric disorders.

The conversion patient's initial mental status examination may prove to be quite unremarkable: a calm person who may or may not be troubled by his or her new somatic symptom, with no insight into the symptom's underlying dynamics. At first glance the patient's family may appear to be happy and integrated, with the family predicament (if present) being covert. Family difficulties are common in patients with conversion disorders, but not more so than for families of patients with other psychiatric disorders attending a psychiatric clinic.

Mrs. A was a 22-year-old right-handed fundamentalist farmer's wife, home-maker, and mother of three from a sparsely settled Western state. Her past medical history was benign except for a history of a motor vehicle accident two years previously that produced a sharp blow to the right temporal area, resulting in several hours' loss of consciousness. She had an unremarkable behavioral history without substance abuse, prolonged depressions, or unexplained somatic symptoms. Her demeanor had always been placid and unassuming. There was no family history of antisocial behavior or substance abuse.

On Thanksgiving Day, while taking her usual solitary afternoon walk along the creek behind the kitchen, she came upon the floating, lifeless bodies of two of her children. She shrieked, swooned, and fell to the ground. Relatives in the house rushed out to assist but were unable to revive the children. When she was helped up, she asked that her husband guide her back to her room. Later that afternoon she seemed calm, even detached, as others scurried about making arrangements. She admitted to a visitor that she seemed to have lost the gift of sight.

That same evening the family physician was called to examine the newly sightless woman. He noted that her pupils were round, equal, and constricted briskly with a bright light; she was unable to touch the tips of her index fingers together in front of her; she failed to look at her own hands when instructed to do so; and she had no other neurological abnormalities, asymmetries, or complaints. The physician explained to the gathered family and patient that: she was suffering from nervous shock, needed kindly quiet support, and should refrain from routine household chores for the moment. The physician also suggested that her eyesight would gradually return over the next week or so, perhaps following the funerals of her children. The patient's vision did slowly return over the next days and bit-by-bit she resumed her usual level of care for home, her surviving child, and other members of the family.

PSYCHOPATHOLOGY AND LABORATORY EXAMINATION Diagnostic workup is a multistep process that begins with a very thorough history and physical examination. There are a number of simple but specialized examinations that can be worked into a seemingly routine physical examination. Although some diagnoses can be made from the foot of the bed (or chair or stretcher), with substantiating data collected in just a few minutes, it is not infrequent for an initial workup of a patient with a conversion disorder to take many hours even when conducted by a skilled clinician. Collateral sources need to be included to build a case based on circumstantial evidence of what was going on in the patient's life at the time of the acute shock. Table 18-6 lists examples of important tests on the physical examination relevant to conversion disorder symptoms.

There are also a few specialized laboratory-based procedures that can assist in the diagnostic workup of some patients with conversion disorder. Helpful in specific instances are simultaneous EEG and videotaping of behavior along with lack of elevation of serum prolactin levels in pseudoseizures; optokinetic drum test in conversion blindness; cortical evoked potentials for auditory and visual deficits; and electromyogram for fasciculation in lower motor neuron paralysis.

TABLE 18-6
Distinctive Findings on Physical Examination in Conversion Disorder

Condition	Test	Conversion Findings
Anesthesia	Map dermatomes	Sensory loss does not conform to recognized pattern of distribution
Hemianesthesia	Check midline	Strict half body split
Tunnel vision	Visual fields	Changing pattern on multiple examinations
Astasia-abasia	Walking, dancing	With suggestion, those who can't walk may be able to dance; alteration of sensory or motor findings with suggestion
Paralysis, paresis	Drop paralyzed hand onto face	Hand falls next to face, not on it
	Hoover test	Pressure noted in examiner's hand under paralyzed leg when attempting straight leg raising
	Motor strength	Give-away weakness
Aphonia	Request a cough	Essentially normal coughing sound indicates cords are closing

DIFFERENTIAL DIAGNOSIS Many serious neurological diseases can be mistaken for conversion disorders listed in Table 18-7; and a number of psychiatric conditions need to be considered in the differential diagnosis of conversion disorder, listed in Table 18-8.

Until the diagnosis is clarified, ongoing evaluation by a psychiatrist and a neurologist may be useful. Premature closure obviously aborts further diagnostic consideration.

COURSE AND PROGNOSIS Clinicians may erroneously think the patient has a psychiatric illness such as conversion because of an inexplicable neurological signs and coincidence of emotional conflict, missing an underlying neurological-medical disease.

Diagnostic errors in series of conversion patients followed for 2 to 20 years have not been uncommon because clinicians, using subjective criteria, proved to be too liberal in their use of the diagnosis. Some long-term follow-up studies have shown that 25 percent of patients on psychiatric wards who subsequently died had, in retrospect, inaccurate initial psychiatric diagnoses of conversion disorder. Long-term follow-up studies using selection criteria heavily weighted to psychodynamic issues (symbolism, secondary gain, *la belle indifférence*) from DSM-I, DSM-II, ICD-9, and even DSM-III have shown an appalling lack of diagnostic consistency. A British inpatient study, for example, reported that over half of their patients had an organic disease 7 to 11 years later that accounted for the symptoms of the supposed conversion disorder. Further, many cases from that inpatient study who did not develop neurological disease instead developed some other type of disabling psychiatric disorder.

In an American study investigators found that neurological disease explained the original conversion symptoms in more than one fifth of the cases. The emergence of neurological disease was more frequent in those conversion patients who did not have somatization disorder as a comorbid condition. Another study with a 20-year follow-up noted that fully one third of patients later experienced a psychotic illness, often paranoid schizophrenia. In that sample central nervous system disease, especially epilepsy, was often mistaken for hysteria. A third major study with a 10-year follow-up noted that a quarter of patients developed organic disorders over time that accounted for the presenting conversion symptoms: mainly degenerative diseases of the spinal cord, peripheral nerves, bones, muscle, and connective tissue.

Thus, follow-up studies show a high likelihood of the emergence of other medical, neurological, or disabling psychiatric disorders to account for the original DSM-I, DSM-II, or DSM-III conversion symptoms. That would seem to indicate either that the inclusion criteria used for the initial diagnosis of conversion disorder was far too inclusive, or else that much more humility needs to be used when pronouncing the diagnosis of conversion disorder.

TABLE 18-7
Neurological Conditions in the Differential Diagnosis of Conversion Disorder

Myasthenia gravis	Subdural hematoma
Periodic paralysis	Acquired and hereditary dystonias
Brain tumor	Drug-induced dystonia
Multiple sclerosis	Creutzfeldt-Jacob disease
Optic neuritis	Early manifestations of acquired immune deficiency syndrome (AIDS)
Partial vocal cord paralysis	
Guillain-Barré syndrome	
On-off syndrome of Parkinson's disease	
Degenerative diseases of basal ganglia and peripheral nerves	
Acquired myopathies including polymyositis	

TABLE 18-8
Psychiatric Conditions in the Differential Diagnosis of Conversion Disorder

Major depressive episodes
Catatonic schizophrenia
Pain disorder
Somatization disorder
Histrionic personality disorder
Adjustment disorder
Posttraumatic stress disorder
Malingering

Prognosis For those conversion patients without comorbid neurological or medical disorders 90 of 100 patients recovered by time of psychiatric hospital discharge in one retrospective study. On follow-up five years later, 75 percent remained well. A general hospital study demonstrated that half of patients on a medical surgical unit found to have a conversion disorder during a psychiatric consult experienced remission of their conversion symptoms by medical discharge. In another study of conversion patients with a one-year follow-up, only one fifth had relapsed. Symptom substitution was minimal.

A favorable prognosis of conversion disorder is associated with acute onset; readily identifiable stressful events; good premorbid health with no comorbid psychiatric, medical, or neurological disease; and no ongoing compensation litigation.

TREATMENT Most conversion symptoms remit either spontaneously or after behavioral treatment, suggestion, and a supportive environment. Thus, for symptoms of very recent onset a variety of other therapies have also been utilized successfully. In practice clinicians tend to choose therapies that reflect their training. Irrespective of technique used, most approaches seem to work when symptoms are not reinforced and when the patient and his or her psychosocial plight is the focus of attention.

Common denominators of success What seems least likely to be effective is trying to get the newly afflicted patient to accept the therapist's opinion that the somatic symptom is a direct manifestation of a psychosocial problem (for example, that the physical disability is the representation of a psychiatric problem). Rather, the common denominator of successful treatment (irrespective of the clinician's theoretical framework) is the building of a caring, authoritative relationship. It is important to supply the patient with a safe environment to facilitate the gradual decrease in symptoms. The clinician can then deal indirectly with interpretations of the conversion symptom while trying to minimize or eliminate the symptom. It is not helpful to argue with the patient about the cause of the conversion disorder.

A multiplicity of types of therapies have their adherents (Table 18-9). When successful, some common elements in many of these treatments are the following: (1) nonconfrontational approach; (2) discouraging retention symptoms; and (3) manipulating the environment.

On some occasions, parenteral injections of amobarbital (Amytal) or lorazepam (Ativan) have been seen as helpful. Medications may reduce anxiety and allow the patient to engage in a psychotherapeutic process that might otherwise be too overwhelming to handle. Decreasing the need for secondary gain by opening up other channels of communication seems to help. Eventually the more emotionally healthy patients seem to be able to gain insight into the meaning of their symptoms. Working at resolving the patient's problems as well as eliminating the conversion symptom seems to be the best approach, using a variety of techniques.

Poor outcomes Not all symptoms remit in hours or days. Some linger tenaciously even despite skilled inpatient treatment. In such instances other psychopathology and immutably malignant social pathology are often present. Symptom substitution may occur if the patient still needs the conversion symptom, but most authors assert that substitution is usually not seen if one works patiently and with tact. Symptom removal seems to be least successful if compensation is at issue.

TABLE 18-9
Therapies Used in Conversion Disorder

Faradic stimulation	Hypnosis and other suggestive techniques
Physical therapy	Behavioral approach to symptom elimination
Electrosleep	Family therapy
Inexact interpretations	Long-term insight-oriented psychotherapy

SOMATIZATION DISORDER

INTRODUCTION The essential feature of somatization disorder is recurrent, multiple somatic complaints requiring medical attention but not associated with any physical disorder. The diagnosis requires a history of many physical complaints of several years' duration and a lifetime history, beginning before age 30, which result in medical treatment or alteration in life-style. The symptoms must not be fully explained by a known nonpsychiatric medical condition, or the resulting complaints or impairment must be excessive. The symptoms must meet a specific pattern: four different sites of pain; two different gastrointestinal symptoms; one sexual or reproductive symptom other than pain; and one neurological symptom. The subjective severity of the symptoms must be sufficient such as to lead the patient to consult a physician, take medicine, or make life-style changes.

HISTORY The history of somatization disorder is complex. Essentially, over the centuries two complementary syndromes have been described: one monosymptomatic and the other polysymptomatic. The monosymptomatic syndrome is currently recognized as conversion disorder, while the polysymptomatic syndrome has become known as somatization disorder. Historically, the two disorders have often been interrelated and commingled.

Hysteria Somatization disorder has had many names and many antecedents. One such predecessor has been referred to in older texts as hysteria, first recognized by the ancient Egyptians. As previously mentioned, the Egyptians believed that hysteria was caused by upward dislocation of the uterus and displacement of other organs. Migration of the uterus throughout the body thus provided the basis for the multiple symptoms.

Doubts about the uterine origin of hysteria began in the 17th century. Thomas Syndenham not only dissociated hysteria from the uterus but also associated it with a psychological disturbance known at that time as "antecedent sorrows," therein recognizing the emotional origin of the disorder. Further, Sydenham was also the first to recognize the disorder in men.

In 1859 Briquet emphasized the multisymptomatic aspects of the disease and a protracted course. His report of the 430 cases observed at the Hospital de la Charité in Paris focused on polysymptomatic aspects of the disorder. Briquet also recognized the disorder in men, and attributed the disorder to emotional causes.

Modern era An important series of papers published between 1951 and 1953 presented the first modern conceptualization of the multisymptomatic concept of hysteria. The Washington University, St. Louis, group concluded that hysteria is a definable syndrome with a characteristic clinical picture that begins before the age of 35. Using objectifiable criteria, they defined a prevalence of the multisymptomatic disorder in the general hospital of 2.2 percent of all admissions. While noting the similarities of their work to Briquet's, they initially deviated by suggesting that men did not have the disorder.

A decade later two studies confirmed the original findings of a definable clinical syndrome, demonstrating diagnostic stability of the multisymptomatic concept of hysteria. In 1970 the eponym "Briquet's syndrome" or "Briquet's disease" was proposed to denote multisymptomatic hysteria. The disorder, characterized by at least 25 symptoms from 10 symptom groups, was known as Briquet's syndrome until the publication of the DSM-III. Ironically, after the decision was made to incorporate Briquet's syndrome as part of the new diagnostic nomenclature, an unrelated decision was made to drop all eponyms. Hence a new name had to be created: somatization disorder.

DSM-III streamlined the criteria to 14 lifetime symptoms in women (12 in men) from a list of 37 symptoms; moreover, a requirement that for symptom grouping (by organ systems) was dropped. With the advent of DSM-III-R and further time for detailed follow-up studies, the number of symptoms required for men and women were both changed to 13.

COMPARATIVE NOSOLOGY There have been multiple predecessors to the current diagnosis of somatization disorder. The best validated of these has been Briquet's syndrome. Later studies have demonstrated only a moderate degree of diagnostic concordance between Briquet's syndrome and somatization disorder. In spite of those limitations, in most situations it appears reasonable to apply the findings from the Briquet's literature and somatization disorder patients. Somatization disorder did not appear in DSM-I or DSM-II. It first appears in DSM-III and later in DSM-III-R.

For DSM-IV the diagnostic criteria were simplified to require one or more symptoms from each of four symptom groups.

The ICD-10 criteria require (1) at least two years of multiple and variable physical symptoms with no adequate physical explanation; (2) persistent refusal to accept advice, and (3) some degree of impairment of functioning.

EPIDEMIOLOGY Several studies based on large populations have estimated the prevalence of somatization disorder as 0.13 percent of the general population, or roughly one person per thousand. However scholars feel that this underestimates the true prevalence of somatization disorder. One group found the prevalence in the Piedmont region of North Carolina to be approximately 0.4 percent.

Because patients with somatization disorder believe themselves to be medically ill, one assumes they congregate in physicians' offices. Recent work indicates that as many as 5 percent of patients seen in family practice settings meet criteria for the disorder.

ETIOLOGY Numerous theories have been advanced to explain the psychosocial mechanisms involved in the process of somatization. By contrast few theories have been yet proposed to account for the biological basis of somatization disorder. The act of somatization can be understood as a social communication and emotional communication. It can also be explained as the result of an intrapsychic dynamic with somatization carried to an extreme.

Social communication Somatization as social communication includes the use of bodily symptoms to manipulate or control relationships (for example, an adolescent girl's developing unexplained abdominal pain to prevent her parents from going away for the weekend).

Somatizing also can serve as emotional communication. Patients may be unable to verbally express their emotions; therefore, they use somatic symptoms and somatic complaints to express their emotional state. Symptoms may be used to symbolically communicate emotions, as they are in conversion symptoms. Some patients also use medical complaints as a coping device to deal with stress. Finally, physical symptoms may be used as a solution to an intrapsychic conflict, again as in conversion symptoms.

Studies of psychological tests in somatization disorder have reported that, compared to sex and age-matched controls, the patients have significantly many more scale elevations on the MMPI.

Psychoanalytic theory Classic psychoanalytic theory has held that hysteria represents a substitution of somatic symptoms for repressed instinctual impulses. Freud postulated that the conflict was a phallic Oedipal one. However, more recent articles in the analytic literature now emphasize a pregenital conflict as well.

Biomedical mechanisms Interesting data are now finally available concerning the biomedical underpinnings of somatization disorder. Neuropsychological testing demonstrates equal bifrontal impairment of the cerebral hemispheres and nondominant hemispheric dysfunction in patients with somatization disorder. Preliminary evidence indicates that patients with somatization disorder may have an abnormality in cortical functioning, as evidenced by abnormal auditory-evoked potentials. In contrast to controls somatization patients responded similarly to both relevant and irrelevant stimuli, suggesting an impairment in selective attention. The data require much more extensive follow-through.

Considerable evidence now also points to familial and genetic associations in somatization disorder. Some data support the findings that groups of patients with somatization disorder have a higher than expected prevalence of antisocial personality disorder or, at the very least, manifest a considerable amount of antisocial personality traits. Other data, however, do not support such a strong association. One theory holds that antisocial personality disorder and somatization disorder may have a common genetic background. Some scholars consider that somatization disorder is the female expression of a genetic tendency, with antisocial personality disorder being its male counterpart.

DIAGNOSIS AND CLINICAL FEATURES Table 18-10 presents the diagnostic criteria of somatization disorder according to DSM-IV. It is important to note that specific symptoms do not need to be considered legitimate by the clinician. Rather, patients' reports that they have the symptom is sufficient, as long as the symptom meets the severity criteria. Moreover, a patient can have somatization disorder even if a current or presenting symptom did not begin before the age of 30 years. A careful review for an early onset of any of the unexplained symptoms for which the patient has had problems is necessary to make the diagnosis. At least one of these symptoms must begin before age 30.

Patients with somatization disorder consider themselves to be severely ill. In fact, they report their health is worse than those with chronic, lesion-based medical conditions. In contrast, the mortality rate of somatization patients is similar to that of the general population and is substantially less than patients with major depressive disorder.

Ms. D. is a 52-year-old white woman who was referred to a general internist in the city for evaluation of persistent back pain and multiple other complaints. At hospitalization it was noted that the patient was disabled from her job as a machine operator at a shoe factory. Ms. D. gave a history of 10 operations: removal of a tumor from her right wrist, a dilation and curettage, a hysterectomy, three abdominal gastric operations, three breast biopsies, and leg surgery. She had received care from five different hospitals and seven different physicians in the past two years.

On physical examination, Ms. D. was an obese, chronically ill-appearing woman who came to the hospital wearing her transcutaneous electrical nerve stimulation unit. She was cooperative and showed her various scars with a certain amount of enthusiasm. The remainder of her physical examination was within normal limits except for a

TABLE 18-10
Diagnostic Criteria for Somatization Disorder

A. A history of many physical complaints beginning before age 30 years that occur over a period of several years and result in treatment being sought or significant impairment in social, occupational, or other important areas of functioning.
B. Each of the following criteria must have been met, with individual symptoms occurring at any time during the course of the disturbance:
   (1) *four pain symptoms:* a history of pain related to at least four different sites or functions (e.g., head, abdomen, back, joints, extremities, chest, rectum, during menstruation, during sexual intercourse, or during urination)
   (2) *two gastrointestinal symptoms:* a history of at least two gastrointestinal symptoms other than pain (e.g., nausea, bloating, vomiting other than during pregnancy, diarrhea, or intolerance of several different foods)
   (3) *one sexual symptom:* a history of at least one sexual or reproductive symptom other than pain (e.g., sexual indifference, erectile or ejaculatory dysfunction, irregular menses, excessive menstrual bleeding, vomiting throughout pregnancy)
   (4) *one pseudoneurological symptom:* a history of at least one symptom or deficit suggesting a neurological condition not limited to pain (conversion symptoms such as impaired coordination or balance, paralysis or localized weakness, difficulty swallowing or lump in throat, aphonia, urinary retention, hallucinations, loss of touch or pain sensation, double vision, blindness, deafness, seizures; dissociative symptoms such as amnesia; or loss of consciousness other than fainting)
C. Either (1) or (2):
   (1) after appropriate investigation, each of the symptoms in Criterion B cannot be fully explained by a known general medical condition or the direct effects of a substance (e.g., a drug of abuse, a medication)
   (2) when there is a related general medical condition, the physical complaints or resulting social or occupational impairment are in excess of what would be expected from the history, physical examination, or laboratory findings
D. The symptoms are not intentionally produced or feigned (as in factitious disorder or malingering).

Table from DSM-IV, *Diagnostic and Statistical Manual of Mental Disorders,* ed 4. Copyright American Psychiatric Association, Washington, 1994. Used with permission.

decreased range of motion in the area of her lumbar spine and local muscle guarding with some tenderness in that area as well. Spinal radiographs revealed some degeneration of vertebral bodies L-2 to L-5. On mental status examination she was cooperative and pleasant, and her behavior was somewhat seductive. There was no pressure or eccentricities in her speech. She showed little hesitation in discussing intimate details of her life. Her mood was euthymic; her affect was appropriate to mood but possibly a little shallow. The remainder of her mental status examination was within normal limits.

Disallowing all back-related symptoms, Ms. D. was positive for eight pain symptoms: four gastrointestinal symptoms, two sexual symptoms, and two pseudoneurological symptoms with an age of onset of 26 years. During the previous 12 months, Ms. D. reported that she had been in bed 21 days, had made seven office visits to four physicians, and had been hospitalized for a total of 52 days.

Ms. D.'s case illustrates that the diagnosis of somatization disorder can and should be made in the presence of comorbid medical conditions. Patients with somatization disorder do become ill, and their problems need to be appropriately diagnosed and treated. However, the management of somatization disorder should continue unchanged.

Comorbid psychiatric conditions Frequent concomitants of somatization disorder are major depressive disorder, anxiety disorders, and personality disorders. Over half of somatization patients have a lifetime history of a mood disorder in addition to their somatization disorder. The anxiety disorders prevalent in somatization patients are phobias, panic disorder, and generalized anxiety disorder. A number of different comorbid personality disorders are also found in somatization disorder. Earlier studies had only reported an association with histrionic personality and antisocial personality disorder. Many patients with somatization disorder also have conversion symptoms.

Suicide threats are common in patients with somatization disorder, as are suicide gestures; however, suicide attempts rarely are lethal or near-lethal. Doctor shopping is frequent, with patients moving from one doctor to another. Typically, somatization patients have very chaotic social lives with frequent divorces, separations, and remarriages. Similarly, they have trouble maintaining jobs and often become too disabled to hold gainful employment.

Gender Early reports found somatization disorder exclusively in women. However, it is now recognized that somatization disorder afflicts men, but less commonly than women. Men comprise 5 to 20 percent of those with somatization disorder.

PATHOLOGY AND LABORATORY EXAMINATION There are no known neuropathological or routine laboratory findings specific for somatization disorder.

DIFFERENTIAL DIAGNOSIS An important aspect of the differential diagnosis is distinguishing a somatic symptom secondary to another psychiatric disorder from a symptom of somatization disorder. Table 18-11 explains how somatic complaints in other disorders differ from those found in somatization disorder.

COURSE AND PROGNOSIS By definition, somatization disorder is a chronic relapsing condition. No cure for the disorder has been found. It usually begins in middle to late adolescence, but may start as late as the third decade of life.

Typically, patients develop a new symptom, or symptoms, during times of emotional distress. No research data are yet available as to how long a modal episode of illness lasts. Clinical wisdom indicates that a typical episode lasts 6 to 9 months, with quiescent periods lasting 9 months to a year. It is unlikely that patients with somatization disorder go more than a year without developing a new symptom and seeking some type of health care. Periods of psychosocial distress seem to coincide either with the onset of new symptoms or with increased health care-seeking behavior associated with some preexisting symptom. While no research data exist on whether stress precipitates the relapse, anecdotally there does seem to be an association. That association is especially problematic for the patients because somatization disorder considerably disrupts social aspects of living.

Long-standing poor health Somatization disorder patients typically consider their health to be poor. When standard measures for health status are applied, the patients report that all aspects of their health—physical, social, and mental—as well as their general health perceptions are severely impaired. Somatization disorder patients report worse health than do those with chronic medical conditions. Further, because somatization disorder patients perceive themselves to be sicker than the sick, it

TABLE 18-11
Nonsomatization Somatic Symptoms

Anxiety or depressive disorders	Usually one or two somatic symptoms of acute onset and short duration
Panic disorder	Somatic symptoms experienced only during panic episode
Hypochondriasis	Patient's focus is on fear of disease, not focus on a symptom
Conversion disorder	Only one or two complaints
Pain disorder	One or two unexplained pain complaints, not a lifetime history of multiple complaints

is not at all incongruous that they usually deem themselves disabled from work.

TREATMENT Because the cause of somatization disorder is unknown and no curative or ameliorative treatment has been found, the clinician needs to focus on management rather than treatment.

Management of somatization disorder has only been tested empirically in two studies. Those findings revealed that when certain specific management strategies were undertaken by the primary care physician, patients with somatization disorder improved their physical functioning. Simultaneously, their health care utilization decreased. Table 18-12 suggests helpful management strategies on somatization disorder.

Doctor-patient relationship The cornerstone for successful management of the somatization disorder patient is establishing a trusting relationship between the patient and one community physician. The constant doctor-hopping that frequently occurs in somatization disorder patients is both frustrating and countertherapeutic.

Recently, a form of group treatment was shown to be effective in somatization patients. The intervention tested was a time-limited, behaviorally oriented group with a structured protocol. The overall goals of the group were to be a source of peer support, to share methods of coping, to increase the ability to perceive an expressed emotion, and to allow the patient to enjoy the group experience. The study demonstrated that in the year following treatment the experimental group of somatization patients demonstrated better physical and emotional health and evidenced decreased health care charges than untreated somatization disorder controls.

HYPOCHONDRIASIS

INTRODUCTION Hypochondriasis is a disorder characterized by preoccupation with the fear of developing a serious disease or the belief that one has it. The fear is based on the patient's interpretation of physical signs or sensations as evidence of disease. Yet the physician's physical examination does not support the diagnosis of any physical disorder. The unwarranted fear of, or belief in, a diseased state persists in spite of medical reassurance. Still, the belief does not have the certainty of delusional intensity.

HISTORY The concept of hypochondriasis has been a part of medical lore since ancient times. Prior to the early 19th century the area of the body below the rib cage, the abdomen, was called the hypochondrium. Thus, hypochondriasis referred to somatic complaints occurring in the abdomen. In the late 1920s, R. D. Gillespie provided the first modern description of the disorder.

TABLE 18-12
Helpful Management Strategies for Somatization Disorder

- Establish primary care physician as patient's main and (if possible) only physician
- Set up regularly scheduled visits every four to six weeks
- Keep outpatient visits brief
- Perform at least a partial physical examination during each visit directed at the organ system of complaint
- Understand symptoms as emotional communication rather than the harbinger of new disease
- Look for signs of disease rather than being symptom focused
- Avoid diagnostic tests, laboratory evaluations, and operative procedures unless clearly indicated
- Set a goal of getting at least selected somatization disorder patients referral-ready for mental health care

COMPARATIVE NOSOLOGY Hypochondriacal symptoms can be a part of another disorder such as major depression, dysthymia, generalized anxiety disorder, or adjustment disorder. However, primary hypochondriasis, or hypochondriacal disorder, is a chronic and somewhat disabling disorder with hypochondriacal symptoms, not merely a part of another psychiatric condition.

Hypochondriasis was a diagnostic entity in DSM-I. The diagnostic criteria continued to be revised in DSM-II, DSM-III, and DSM-III-R; however, the changes have been primarily of language, not substance. The only change between DSM-III-R and DSM-IV is the addition of a specifier to note that the patient has poor insight during the current episode. The ICD-10 criteria for hypochondriases are essentially the same as those of DSM-IV.

EPIDEMIOLOGY Recent work indicates that in a six-month period of observation, 4 to 6 percent of the general medical population may have a hypochondriacal disorder. The prevalence in either sex is comparable to that within the general medical population. There are no specific tendencies for overrepresentation based on social position, education, marital status, or other sociodemographic descriptors. There is a wide range of ages at onset. Although the disorder can begin at any age, onset is thought to be most common between 20 and 30 years of age.

ETIOLOGY There are four major etiological theories concerning hypochondriasis: (1) amplification of normal bodily sensations; (2) psychodynamic formulations; (3) social learning concepts; and (4) syndromic variant of some other psychiatric disorder.

Amplification The amplification hypothesis posits that hypochondriasis results from the augmentation of normal bodily sensations. Of the four hypotheses it has the most research support: hypochondriacal patients amplify their normal somatic sensations and misattribute pathological meanings. For instance, a change in a patient's perception of his or her peristalsis might be interpreted as abnormal, hence, representing disease.

Psychodynamics A variety of hypotheses purport that intrapsychological factors are responsible for hypochondriasis. Those factors run the gamut from Freud's early theories about disturbed object relations and intensive preoccupation with the self, through the concept of hypochondriasis as ego defense mechanisms against guilt.

Some advocate that in hypochondriasis aggressive and hostile wishes toward others are transferred into physical complaints through either repression or displacement. Anger that the patients express may be caused by past losses, rejections, or disappointments. At times, the anger is expressed by these patients by first soliciting, then rejecting, the help and concern of others. Alternatively, hypochondriasis may be viewed as a defense against guilt, a result of low self-esteem, or a sign of excessive self-concern. Pain and somatic suffering then symbolically become a means of atonement or can be experienced as deserved punishment for past real or imagined wrongdoing.

Learning theory Learning theory postulates that psychosocial learning has a strong etiological component in hypochondriacal disorder. The concept contends that a patient learns the sick role and that role is sufficiently reinforced through either social contact or some need gratification. The sick role then becomes a ticket of admission to caretaking.

Variants Finally, the variant theory holds that hypochondriasis is a modification of some other psychiatric disorder, such as depressive disorders, anxiety disorders, and certain personality disorders, such as obsessive-compulsive personality disorder. Although some scholars have maintained that hypochondriasis is a variant of a depressive condition, current research has not supported that hypothesis. Research that hypochondriasis is a variant of an anxiety disorder is more compelling.

DIAGNOSIS AND CLINICAL FEATURES Table 18-13 lists DSM-IV criteria for the diagnosis of hypochondriasis. Patients typically present for the first time with the complaint of a symptom, pain, or sensation. With some gentle questioning they quickly move from concern about the symptom to fear of a disease. Almost uniformly the patients are not concerned transiently about a minor disease, but rather are persistently worried about a serious disease. The specific disease may change from time to time. The duration of an episode of a feared disease may run from months to years. Alternatively, the feared disease may not change at all throughout the course of the disorder.

PATHOLOGY AND LABORATORY EXAMINATION At present there are no known pathological features of the disorder, nor are there known routine laboratory tests.

DIFFERENTIAL DIAGNOSES Basic to the process of differential diagnoses is ruling out underlying organic disease. In the vast majority of cases that can be completed by the primary care physician without referral to a specialist. The workup is usually a straightforward process and typically focuses around the disease of the patient's concern.

Somatization disorder is the main somatoform disorder that needs to be differentiated from hypochondriasis. While there are numerous differences between somatization disorder and hypochondriasis, the major distinction is that patients with somatization disorder are concerned about their symptoms and are relatively indifferent to concerns about underlying disease.

TABLE 18-13
Diagnostic Criteria for Hypochondriasis

A. Preoccupation with fears of having, or the idea that one has, a serious disease based on the person's misinterpretation of bodily symptoms.
B. The preoccupation persists despite appropriate medical evaluation and reassurance.
C. The belief in Criterion A is not of delusional intensity (as in delusional disorder, somatic type) and is not restricted to a circumscribed concern about appearance (as in body dysmorphic disorder).
D. The preoccupation causes clinically significant distress or impairment in social, occupational, or other important areas of functioning.
E. The duration of the disturbance is at least six months.
F. The preoccupation is not better accounted for by generalized anxiety disorder, obsessive-compulsive disorder, panic disorder, a major depressive episode, separation anxiety, or another somatoform disorder.

Specify if:
With poor insight: if, for most of the time during the current episode, the person does not recognize that the concern about having a serious illness is excessive or unreasonable

Table from DSM-IV, *Diagnostic and Statistical Manual of Mental Disorders,* ed 4. Copyright American Psychiatric Association, Washington, 1994. Used with permission.

Patients with hypochondriasis have an exactly opposite preoccupation; they are fearful of an underlying disease, and concern about the symptom quickly fades. Typically, hypochondriacal patients do not have the plethora of symptoms present in somatization disorder. Hypochondriasis needs to be distinguished from factitious disorder with predominantly physical signs and symptoms and from malingering. In hypochondriasis patients actually experience the symptoms they report rather than simulating them.

Patients with psychotic disorders, particularly major depressive disorder and schizophrenia, may have somatic delusions or concerns about the presence of a disease. Hypochondriacal concerns secondary to major psychiatric disorders are categorized with the more serious disorders. Candidate conditions include major depressive disorder, dysthymic disorder, generalized anxiety disorder, obsessive-compulsive disorder, and panic disorder.

COURSE AND PROGNOSIS Hypochondriasis is a chronic, relapsing condition with waxing and waning symptoms. The disorder is usually long-standing, frequently over several years. Episodes typically last months and even a few years. There are often quiescent periods between episodes; however, frequently there will be recurrences during times of psychosocial distress.

Symptom severity of the disease is such that some degree of psychosocial impairment occurs. Typically, familial and spousal relationships become strained by living with a patient who persistently fears disease. The ability to work may or may not be affected.

Historically, hypochondriasis has been given a pessimistic prognosis; however, that reputation may be erroneous. Some authors now state that approximately 50 percent of patients show improvement; the remainder show a chronic, fluctuating course. Unfortunately, there are no controlled clinical trials on which to make a judgment.

Generally, the following characteristics, which bode well for a patient's general health status, bode well for patients with hypochondriasis: a high socioeconomic status; the presence of other treatable conditions, such as an anxiety or depressive disorder; an acute onset; an absence of a personality disorder; and the absence of comorbid organic disease.

TREATMENT To date there are no controlled clinical trials on which to base rational treatment. Therefore, inferences have to be made from the treatment of other disorders and from clinical lore used in treating hypochondriasis. The simplest treatment approach is to look for and treat any comorbid psychiatric conditions, such as anxiety disorder and depressive disorder. When those conditions are treated, the hypochondriasis often will improve.

The management of hypochondriasis is typically in the domain of the primary care physician especially, because the patients initially strongly resist psychiatric referral. To date, those management suggestions which have been shown to be effective in somatization disorder (Table 18-12) seem reasonable to be tried in patients with hypochondriasis.

After their medical workup is completed, patients with hypochondriasis may accept referral for psychiatric care when the reason for referral is framed in the context of stress associated with their medical problems or some other euphemism for psychiatric symptoms. Similarly, the patients may accept referral for treatment of a comorbid psychiatric condition, which can then lead to treatment for hypochondriasis as well.

Another approach that seems reasonable is group treatment. A cognitive-educational group treatment has recently been proposed which at face value appears to have validity, especially given the success demonstrated by a similar approach in patients with somatization disorder.

UNDIFFERENTIATED SOMATOFORM DISORDER

INTRODUCTION Undifferentiated somatoform disorder is characterized by one or more unexplained physical complaints of at least six months' duration. Those symptoms impair the patient in some domain and are temporally associated with a stressor. Psychological factors are assumed to be associated with the symptoms or complaints because of a contemporaneous relationship between the initiation or exacerbation of the symptoms and stressors, conflicts, or needs. The complaint must be unattributable to any other known psychiatric condition or pathophysiological mechanism or, when it is related to a nonpsychiatric condition, the physical complaints or resulting social and occupational impairment is grossly in excess of what would ordinarily be expected from the findings.

HISTORY Undifferentiated somatoform disorder was introduced to the psychiatric lexicon in DSM-III-R because somatization disorder was considered to be too restrictive by primary care providers to provide adequate coverage for many patients with significant somatoform complaints. Thus the sub-syndromic grouping was formalized to facilitate learning about the natural course of a large cluster of patients.

COMPARATIVE NOSOLOGY Many who work in the general medical setting find the diagnosis of undifferentiated somatoform disorder helpful. Research indicates the validity distinguishing undifferentiated somatoform disorder from somatization disorder. The disorder was not included in DSM-I, DSM-II, and DSM-III. It was first introduced in DSM-III-R and remains unchanged in DSM-IV. The criteria for undifferentiated somatoform disorder in ICD-10 are similar to the diagnostic criteria in DSM-IV.

Somatizing syndrome The disorder, characterized by a lifetime history of four unexplained somatic complaints for men and six for women, has been called various names. It forms a subset of patients with undifferentiated somatoform disorder. All research data to date have used the term "somatization syndrome" rather than the broader term "undifferentiated somatoform disorder." The remainder of the section therefore refers to data from research on somatizing syndrome.

EPIDEMIOLOGY Undifferentiated somatoform disorder has at least 30 times greater prevalence than somatization disorder. There is an estimated lifetime prevalence of between 4 and 11 percent, and there is an estimated 1 percent six-month prevalence.

The disorder is typically found with women. Undifferentiated somatoform disorder has also been shown in some reports to be associated with lower socioeconomic status, older age, and Hispanic or African-American origin. One study found a slight association with antisocial personality disorder; however, other studies have not confirmed this.

ETIOLOGY There are multiple theories about the process of somatization. Those theories are covered in the discussion on somatization disorder. None of the theories are specific to undifferentiated somatoform disorder.

DIAGNOSIS AND CLINICAL FEATURES The DSM-IV diagnostic criteria are listed in Table 18-14. Patients with undifferentiated somatoform disorder have more comorbid psychiatric diseases than do general medical patients without the disorder. These comorbid conditions are primarily depressive and anxiety disorders. Approximately 50 percent of patients with the disorder have comorbid psychiatric conditions compared with 7 percent in the general population.

PATHOLOGY AND LABORATORY EXAMINATION There are no specific pathological or routine laboratory features for undifferentiated somatoform disorder.

DIFFERENTIAL DIAGNOSIS In the differential diagnosis of undifferentiated somatoform disorder care must be taken to differentiate somatic symptoms that could be a part of many other psychiatric disorders. For example, somatic symptoms frequently occur in major depression. Similarly, the somatic delusion of schizophrenia and major depressive disorder also needs to be differentiated from undifferentiated somatoform disorder.

Several other psychiatric disorders need to be differentiated from undifferentiated somatoform disorder. Somatization disorder is a more severe disorder characterized by a chronic history of multiple unexplained somatic complaints which fit a specific pattern and begin before the age of 30. Adjustment disorder with physical symptoms may also have unexplained somatic complaints; however, the duration of that disorder is by definition less than six months. Finally, the diagnosis of psychological factors affecting medical condition may at first appear similar; however, the disorder effects a known Axis III disorder rather than mimicking an Axis I disorder.

COURSE AND PROGNOSIS In general, the course of undifferentiated somatoform disorder is chronic and relapsing; however, little systematic research on the disorder has been accomplished to date. It is likely that some cases of the disorder can resolve after a single episode. There is substantial disability, work impairment, and excessive health care utilization in undifferentiated somatoform disorder. The dysfunction is not seen to the same extent as in somatization disorder.

TREATMENT Recent studies have indicated that patients with undifferentiated somatoform disorder respond to the same treatment or management approach as patients with somatization disorder (Table 18-12).

TABLE 18-14
Diagnostic Criteria for Undifferentiated Somatoform Disorder

A. One or more physical complaints (e.g., fatigue, loss of appetite, gastrointestinal or urinary complaints).
B. Either (1) or (2):
   (1) after appropriate investigation, the symptoms cannot be fully explained by a known general medical condition or the direct effects of a substance (e.g., a drug of abuse, a medication)
   (2) when there is a related general medical condition, the physical complaints or resulting social or occupational impairment is in excess of what would be expected from the history, physical examination, or laboratory findings
C. The symptoms cause clinically significant distress or impairment in social, occupational, or other important areas of functioning.
D. The duration of the disturbance is at least six months.
E. The disturbance is not better accounted for by another mental disorder (e.g., another somatoform disorder, sexual dysfunction, mood disorder, anxiety disorder, sleep disorder, or psychotic disorder).
F. The symptom is not intentionally produced or feigned (as in factitious disorder or malingering).

Table from DSM-IV, *Diagnostic and Statistical Manual of Mental Disorders,* ed 4. Copyright American Psychiatric Association, Washington, 1994. Used with permission.

NEURASTHENIA

Neurasthenia, literally a lack of nerve energy, is not included in DSM-IV, nor was it included in DSM-III or DSM-III-R. In DSM-I the condition was called psychologic nervous system reaction and in DSM-II it was called neurasthenic neurosis. It is diagnosed with some frequency in countries other than the United States and is included in ICD-10.

PAIN DISORDER

INTRODUCTION With their expertise in the use of psychoactive medication plus their interest in the personal and family dynamics of patients with chronic medical disorders, psychiatrists have long been involved in the treatment of patients with chronic pain. It has long been recognized by astute clinicians that some patients use their pain as a way of seeking human relationships; they then may become reinforced in maintaining that pain. Other clinicians have noted that pain syndromes sometimes dissipate when an accompanying psychiatric disorder is treated, both receding together.

It has always been difficult to specify just how much chronic pain ought to be associated with a given lesion. Assessing the degree to which emotional factors are intensifying the patients' complaints is also complicated. Moreover, patients with chronic pain are not always immediately motivated to give an intricate personal history. Finally, many studies in the pain literature have demonstrated conclusively that different personalities and different cultures experience and express themselves in divergent fashions.

Hence Wilder Penfield's clinical wisdom about patients with chronic pain has now become rather widely accepted in the field: if the patient is not a malingerer, the complaints about the extent of the pain are to be believed. The issues that need to be explored clinically are: (1) how disabled by the pain is the patient and (2) to what extent are there complicating emotional factors and comorbid psychiatric conditions. Still, the physician attendant to the suffering of a patient with chronic pain needs to render a diagnosis that (1) communicates important underlying aspects of the case and (2) leads to a treatment plan encompassing the patient's emotional needs.

COMPARATIVE NOSOLOGY There have been a variety of informal and formal diagnostic terms associated with pain. For example, the euphemistic term "atypical" has been used, as in atypical facial pain, or atypical pelvic pain, to indicate that psychiatric issues needed to be considered in the cause or the maintenance of the severe pain syndrome. ICD-9 used the term "psychalgia," while DSM-III incorporated the term "psychogenic pain."

DSM-III-R employed the term "somatoform pain disorder" as a formal psychiatric diagnosis for those pain disorders in which psychological factors play a pronounced role.

DSM-III-R required preoccupation with pain for at least six months and either no organic pathology or no pathophysiological mechanism found after appropriate evaluation; or if organic pathology is present, then the extent of the complaints about the pain or the degree of social-occupational disability should be greater than could be expected by the examiner based on the physical findings.

Applying the diagnostic terminology of DSM-III and DSM-III-R, however, has proved difficult. Even when diagnostic criteria required only no organic pathology or impairment in excess of what would be expected, precise application of criteria became problematic. Judging whether the amount of a patient's subjective pain is excessive became a daunting task.

DSM-IV provides a more focused approach, not relying on the extent of the pain as a criteria but asking the clinician to make a judgment as to whether psychological factors have a major role in the onset, severity, exacerbation, or maintenance of the pain, and as to whether there are or are not factors from the general medical condition that also make a major contribution to the symptoms.

Pain disorders have newly been split into three subtypes: pain disorder associated with psychological factors, pain disorder associated with both psychological factors and a general medical condition, and pain disorder associated with a general medical condition (which is not considered to be a mental disorder but is included to help in the differential diagnosis).

ICD-10 does not subdivide pain into subtypes in which psychological factors play a major role along with a general medical condition and in which psychological factors are the determinant of pain. As to emotional factors involved in the cause of the pain, ICD-10 is compatible with the DSM-III-R definition of pain disorder, using the phrase "pain occurs in association with emotional conflict or psychosocial problems that are sufficient to allow the conclusion that they are the main causative influences." Moreover, ICD-10 does not indicate that emotional factors can impinge on certain aspects of the pain condition (onset, severity, exacerbation, or maintenance).

EPIDEMIOLOGY Pains of one sort or another are among the most frequent reasons that patients consult their physician. Most pain is remediable, but chronic pain carries with it a high price: more than $10 billion was spent in 1980 in disability payments for chronic pain problems. Low back pain currently affects more than 7 million Americans.

Because diagnostic criteria for the disorder have been changing (from DSM-III to DSM-III-R to DSM-IV), detailed investigations that pull together the data bases are still lacking. Studies seem to indicate that there are twice as many women as men with pain disorder, with peak incidence in the fourth and fifth decades, especially in those with blue collar occupations. There is also some tendency for familial aggregation, along with more depression and more chemical dependency use disorders in those families.

ETIOLOGY Pain comes from many sources, but almost always involved are peripheral afferent nerves, central nervous system processing, and central nervous system interpretation of the localization and the severity of the pain. In some cases of pain disorder of the psychological or the combined type, a purely neurosurgical approach (eliminating a painful lesion and its connectivity) can successively chop away at parts of a person's peripheral and central nervous system until the cortex is no longer in contact with the relevant nerves or the involved spinal cord from an afflicted area. Yet the pain can still continue.

No adult registers an experience on a *tabula rasa.* Rather, persons all encounter life happenings in a context of (1) personal training based on critical developmental incidents; (2) family-centered culture transmitted early in life; and (3) societal values about appropriate behaviors, including the expression of feelings. Those past experiences all interact with a person's constitutional hard wiring, including preprogrammed response modes.

Chronic pain syndromes are among the most frustrating conditions in all of medicine for patient and physician. For clinicians to even have a chance at being successful in dealing with patients in pain they need to be able to appreciate the patient in a biopsychosocial context. Successful academic pain clinics have discovered the necessity of using a multidisciplinary approach. Indeed, physicians caring for such a patient need to do more than just take a detailed history. They also need to understand the patient's life both from the patient's and the family's perspective.

Some persons (for reasons they may or may not be aware of) magnify a given pain. Others pay little attention to it, diminishing their responsiveness to a lesion that might otherwise cause great discomfort. Pain thresholds, which can be clinically measured, vary from person to person. Pain tolerance, likewise, has considerable latitude. Moreover, there is a broad range of ways that individuals express their discomfort or even agony. Some with a broken ankle will be stoic; others with the same fracture will scream out in agony, facies pinched, arms flailing.

Although there are conditions in which persons do not have pain fibers (familial dysautonomia), that is so rare that it does not come into play in everyday practice. It is easier for our understanding of the pain experience to divide the discussion of issues in pain into three categories: intrapersonal factors, interpersonal factors, and biological factors.

Intrapersonal factors Intrapersonal factors can impact how pain is experienced. Psychodynamically formative events in the early years can carry over later into how one processes illness and other types of distress. Having pain and expressing distress attracts others to deliver needed attention. In later years the experience of pain can be associated with obtaining love from an otherwise absent significant caregiver. Or painful experiences, such as repeated severe corporal punishment from an abusive parent, can set the stage many years later for the person's response to a wrongful piece of behavior with self-imposed retribution. Thus a pain disorder may be used to pay for some self-perceived sin or transgression. However, simple interpretation (illuminating the repressed, suppressed, or even grudgingly embellished facts) rarely serves to dramatically remove the pain.

Some patients can be vaguely, or poignantly, aware of the associations between past life events and being pain-prone or even being overresponsive to a painful experience. For other pain patients, the recollection of associated early life experiences of pain are deeply buried, coming out only through a lengthy process of free association, dream work, or psychological testing.

Not every one with severe pain and unusual pain behavior has had dysfunctional early life experiences leading to a psychopathological organization of the character structure. But astute clinicians are always alert to the possibility that there may be important masochistic, dependent, or narcissistic features to the personality that impact how a given patient handles pain.

No one psychological test can accurately delineate the extent of the psychological component in a pain syndrome. Any painful chronic disease highlights, and even changes, certain personality components. Psychological testing, as well as patient interviews, can give clear evidence that some patients with considerable emotional overlay to their pain are (at least initially) resistant to suggestions that pain symptoms are due to anything other than physical causes.

Interpersonal factors Interpersonal factors may also impact on the pain experience. Behaviors can be reinforced or inhibited. For example, reinforcements given by others important to the pain-afflicted person can play a major role in day-to-day and even second-to-second experiences. Lavishing attention on an individual when chronic pain intensifies creates a different inner and outer world than when pain is either ignored or treated with additional painful experiences.

Some persons use their pain manipulatively. Clinicians often observe that when there is a chaotic and otherwise inattentive family or when there is a dysfunctional marriage that becomes reorganized around the continued crisis of chronic pain. Surprisingly, in some persons the persistence of pain is far less important than what it is traded for: a relationship far more to the patient's liking.

The consequences of pain are often gain. Secondary gains, such as monetary rewards or avoidance of distasteful activities, are not an unusual consequence of having prolonged pain. At times it is only when the interpersonal and other rewards are stripped away from the pain experience and its attendant disability that the individual with pain can develop a more normal life.

Just as somatizing can become a way of life that alters the behavior of another, so it can be with pain disorder. The caring physician must always be aware of interpersonal factors. Family, financial, and legal dynamics of a situation can have a dramatic influence on the patient's pain experience and pain behavior.

Biological factors Biological factors also play a large role in the onset and perpetuation of chronic pain. Cortical and subcortical centers process and filter afferent impulses. Sensory and limbic structural abnormalities can determine the severity of a pain experience. The gate control theory purports that a gating mechanism in the dorsal horn of the spinal cord handles afferent pain signals; competing signals as well as neurotransmitters then can open or close the gate on painful perceptions. Endorphin deficiency seems to correlate with the augmentation of afferent stimuli. Serotonin, presumably relatively diminished in some forms of depression, has now been implicated as the main neurotransmitter in descending inhibitory pathways. Indeed a number of neurotransmitter systems, including substance P, are involved in altering the pain threshold.

Thus the underlying psychodynamic and neurobiological framework can impact on the complex ways a given person experiences and reexperiences pain.

DIAGNOSIS AND CLINICAL FEATURES Pain disorder as a psychiatric condition is diagnosed when a patient's preoccupation with pain is consuming and to some extent disabling. That is, pain becomes the predominant focus of the clinical presentation and the pain itself causes clinically significant distress or impairment. Another crucial point without clear guidelines is that psychological factors are judged to play a role. Table 18-15 lists the diagnostic criteria for pain disorder.

Pain patients make repeated visits to physicians, often successively or even concomitantly. There is a risk of excessive use of narcotic or sedative hypnotic agents, as the patients are enveloped by pain and often have associated complaints of anxiety, depression, and insomnia.

The major feature of pain disorder is an all-encompassing focus on the pain. As such, any other concern takes on less than its ordinary significance. It is ascribed by the patient as the source for all the patient's misery. If the patient is depressed or has insomnia, those symptoms are almost always considered by the patient to be secondary to the pain. Other ancillary symptoms include changes in appetite, loss of energy, decreased interest in social activities, decline in sexual interest, diminished physical exercise, and even diminished exertion. Also often noted are a change in normal recreational pursuits, a breakdown

TABLE 18-15
Diagnostic Criteria for Pain Disorder

A. Pain in one or more anatomical sites is the predominant focus of the clinical presentation and is of sufficient severity to warrant clinical attention.
B. The pain causes clinically significant distress or impairment in social, occupational, or other important areas of functioning.
C. Psychological factors are judged to have an important role in the onset, severity, exacerbation, or maintenance of the pain.
D. The symptom or deficit is not intentionally produced or feigned (as in factitious disorder or malingering).
E. The pain is not better accounted for by a mood, anxiety, or psychotic disorder and does not meet criteria for dyspareunia.

Code as follows:

Pain disorder associated with psychological factors: psychological factors are judged to have the major role in the onset, severity, exacerbation, or maintenance of the pain. (If a general medical condition is present, it does not have a major role in the onset, severity, exacerbation, or maintenance of the pain.) This type of pain disorder is not diagnosed if criteria are also met for somatization disorder.

Specify if:
Acute: duration of less than six months
Chronic: duration of six months or longer

Pain disorder associated with both psychological factors and a general medical condition: both psychological factors and a general medical condition are judged to have important roles in the onset, severity, exacerbation, or maintenance of the pain. The associated general medical condition or anatomical site of the pain (see below) is coded on Axis III.

Specify if:
Acute: duration of less than six months
Chronic: duration of six months or longer

Note: The following is not considered to be a mental disorder and is included here to facilitate differential diagnosis.

Pain disorder associated with a general medical condition: a general medical condition has a major role in the onset, severity, exacerbation, or maintenance of the pain. (If psychological factors are present, they are not judged to have a major role in the onset, severity, exacerbation, or maintenance of the pain.) The diagnostic code for the pain is selected based on the associated general medical condition if one has been established or on the anatomical location of the pain if the underlying general medical condition is not yet clearly established—for example, low back, sciatic, pelvic, headache, facial, chest, joint, bone, abdominal, breast, renal, ear, eye, throat, tooth, and urinary.

Table from DSM-IV, *Diagnostic and Statistical Manual of Mental Disorders,* ed 4. Copyright American Psychiatric Association, Washington, 1994. Used with permission.

in family relationships, an increased amount of time spent in bed or lying down, an increased amount of self-absorption (including hypochondriasis), and multiple drug use or abuse. Multiple visits to physicians and requests for relief from medical or even surgical approaches are commonplace.

Sites of pain Typical sites and types of pain involved in pain disorder are headache, atypical facial pain, low back pain, and chronic pelvic pain. But any site is a potential target. Pain can emanate from almost any point source in the body or it can be a conversion symptom involving just pain, using a previous pain pattern from organic disease as a conversion pain model. If the pain is used as a metaphor for psychic turmoil converted into a somatic form, it may bring to the afflicted person primary and secondary gains that reinforce the initiation, maintenance, and even exacerbation of pain symptoms for psychological purposes. When pain is a conversion, then its distribution may not conform to known anatomical patterns.

Mrs. L., 72-year-old married, Ukrainian-born, pious, wealthy retailer and father of a large family from an East Coast city was admitted to the orthopedic service of a general hospital for evaluation of unbearable pain in the arches of his feet. He had fled his native country following a pogrom when he was 9. During the year of flight, he had endured enormous physical hardships, starvation, and beatings until the surviving family members finally were able to emigrate to the United States. With incessant hard work, he had prospered economically; married a patient, supportive wife; and witnessed his six children develop promising careers. He became the major contributor to his temple and gave unstintingly to local charities for the needy and unfortunate. He had little time for personal enjoyment. Indeed, over the years each time he and his wife had time alone and she had been affectionate with him, shortly thereafter he would develop some sort of excruciating bodily pain: blinding headache, severe back spasm, abdominal pain, facial pain, pelvic pain. Those pains usually receded several days after the weekend was over, or the trip completed. Some pains occurred more frequently than others. He sought medical attention rarely except for these pains, which occurred every few months to yearly. His mood varied from glum to gloomy, but he denied that he was depressed. On the contrary, often he claimed that he had been blessed with good fortune. He led a temperate life, drank little, and had relatively good health in between episodes of pain.

Over four decades that his physicians cared for him, they had become frustrated with this unassuming and humble man: his ardent complaints of pain were always so nonspecific and fluctuating in nature that they could not describe adequately for themselves the pathophysiological mechanisms that accounted for his pain; nor were their diagnostic tests revealing; and he usually refused their offers of narcotic or other analgesic relief. Laboratory workup for pains in the arches was noncontributory, and he was discharged when his symptoms cleared in three days. Four months later, he was readmitted to the surgical service of the general hospital with severe, unrelenting, left-side upper abdominal pain. In contrast to his illusive descriptions of his other myriad pains, this time he described this new pain in meticulous detail. A brief workup revealed far-advanced carcinoma of the tail of the pancreas. He took the news from his physician stolidly and asked to be discharged home that day.

DIFFERENTIAL DIAGNOSIS All pain is subjective and only obvious if the patient tells the physician. Acute pain tends to distort the facies in a grimace, causes muscle tightening, and causes elevation of autonomic measures, such as pulse and blood pressure. Chronic pain, however, produces none of these signs. Clinicians trying to explore the extent of psychiatric involvement have used a number of clues, the validity of which still remains to be proved. Those are listed in Table 18-16. Judgment about underlying dynamics and the presence or absence of conflicts and stressors are open to multiple interpretations. Only careful long-term follow-up studies of large series of patients will help increase validity.

Patients deal with their chronic illnesses in ways characteristic of their dynamics and their own psychopathology. Those with a histrionic nature exaggerate. Those who use a history of ill luck to manipulate their environment will no doubt make the most of their pain for their own ends. Those with a need for punishment for real or imagined sins may fulfill their needs for atonement.

Both acute and chronic pain tend to be very field dependent. For example, soldiers who have survived fierce fighting on the battlefield typically need far less morphine for relief than their civilian counterparts with the same degree of tissue injury. Absolute pronouncements about no somatic pathology or no emotional components to the clinical picture must be looked on with a critical eye. Nor will a positive response to a trial of placebo medication indicate anything about the organic nature of the patient's pain or the extent of the underlying psychopathology. The placebo response is positive in about one third of

TABLE 18-16
Clues to Underlying Psychopathology in Pain Disorder

- Antecedent history of poor premorbid adjustment: alcohol or drug abuse, sexual difficulties, multiple marriage, inability to hold a job
- Temporal relationship between an environmental stimulus, relevant intrapsychic conflict, and pain
- Utility of pain in either gaining compensation or avoiding situation deemed noxious by the patient
- Lack of variation in the amount of pain from distraction, suggestion, or fear

whatever population is tested. Pain associated with both melancholia and metastases can respond to placebo.

The patients and their clinical syndromes need to be treated without too much loss of time deliberating about whether the pain caused the depression or the depression caused the pain. Those with personality disorders with chronic pain tend to have a more difficult time coping with any type of difficulty, both in the hospital and at home. They will also challenge their physicians' abilities. Fortunately, intensive inpatient treatment of refractory chronic pain has had some success.

Depression Depression is the most common of the psychiatric diseases that present as a pain disorder. At times the individual will have had previous depressive episodes with an altogether different clinical presentation that has no associated pain. Sometimes the best clue to the presence of an affective disorder is just the family history of severe depression, with or without pain as part of the clinical picture. There is no specific type of pain picture to alert the clinician to the presence of depression. Moreover the sadness accompanying the pain disorder can almost always be ascribed to being a pain victim.

But supporting the diagnosis of a mood disorder are the vegetative signs of depressive disease, especially sleep and libidinal disturbances. Cognitive signs of an accompanying depression include apathy, decreased interest in work, suicidal ideation, and a preoccupation with death. Collaborative sources of information are often needed to get the total concept of the patient's functioning.

Sometimes the best way to make the diagnosis of depressive disorder in a patient presenting with pain is to initiate a treatment trial of an antidepressant in addition to nonspecific modalities. Dramatic clinical relief of both the pain and the vegetative signs of depression provides the answer to the clinical question. Suicide in chronic pain patients must always be kept in mind, especially during the first 10 days of antidepressant treatment, when the patient begins to look better and has more energy; that state often occurs before the feeling of despair has lifted.

Conversion When a conversion mechanism is involved in the pain disorder, the clinician determines that (1) details of the pain picture have symbolic or other specific meaning for the patient; (2) there is a conversion model, often a parent or other close family member; and (3) the pain follows no known anatomical pathway.

Treatment here is similar to the psychotherapy of a patient with a conversion disorder. In addition, the clinician will use the same nonspecific treatment that one might give to many or all pain disorder patients: physiotherapy, water pool massage, infrared heat, nonsteroidal anti-inflammatory agents, and the like.

Psychosis When a psychosis associated with schizophrenia, medical disorder, or a dementing illness presents with pain, the pain itself is delusional and the pain pattern will be atypical in quality and in distribution. Treatment must relieve the underlying psychiatric disorder. Delusional beliefs, however, may prevent the patient from cooperating with the treatment plan.

Malingering When someone is purposely lying about pain, the pain is hard to detect. Those persons are not interested in the same outcome as the physician: relief of pain. Sometimes old records betray that the patient has tried to malinger in other settings and in other ways. Unlike the patient with Munchausen's syndrome, who is interested in staying in the sick role, the malingerer is consciously interested in some other benefit. Some clinicians have found that Munchausen patients will willingly agree to painful procedures, whereas the malingerer will not.

The late Thomas Hackett was long interested in defining the extent of the emotional component associated with chronic pain. Such a determination was helpful, and a care plans could then be effected, along with appropriate expectations and appropriate treatment. His well-known MADISON scale (Table 18-17) has not been rigorously validated but has been of considerable help to those working in the field.

COURSE AND PROGNOSIS Once diagnosis is complete, treatment on an outpatient basis can be carried out by concerned physicians who will see the patient on a regular basis, be interested in the patient's complaints, and assure the patient that treatment will continue without abandonment if there is some improvement. Those pain disorder patients with pending litigation often attain no, or only minimal, relief until after the legal proceedings are finished.

Pain-prone Persons who are pain-prone often have their pain in response to losses or other stresses, presumably as a way of dealing with unresolved guilt. Outcomes from treating the pain-prone are typically described as transient or poor. Techniques that are most promising are supportive therapy, a modicum of insight, and, when indicated, antidepressant medication.

TREATMENT Many patients, especially those with considerable depression, can be helped considerably. The key to dealing with the pain disorder patient is accurate diagnosis and focus on the patient's level of functioning. The patient's pain and predicament are always acknowledged at each visit, but the major focus is in moving on, regaining function. Pain clinics and inpatient pain treatment units both have had their share of successes.

Treatment of the patient with any of the pain disorder subtypes needs to be multidisciplinary and multidimensional. Treatment team planning is important from the onset, coordinated as needed on a periodic basis. Multiple regimens often help in reducing pain intensity. Tailored to the person, options include nonsteroidal anti-inflammatory agents, tricyclics, nerve blocks, localized electrical stimulation, visual imaging, relaxation, physical therapy, hypnosis, counseling, and medical psychotherapy. If narcotics have been used for chronic refractory

TABLE 18-17
Madison Scale for Markers of Considerable Emotional Overlay

M = Multiplicity: Pain is either in more than one place or of more than one variety; when treated, may recur elsewhere.
A = Authenticity: More interested in clinician's acceptance of pain as genuine than in a cure.
D = Denial: Especially exaggerated marital or family harmony; when admitting depression or anxiety, no impact on pain is admitted.
I = Interpersonal relationship: Although the connection to the presence of any particular person's company as worsening the pain may be denied, observation of the patient's nonverbal and interactive behavior indicates otherwise.
S = Singularity: When the pain is described as unlike that of anyone else, ever.
O = "Only you": When the patient immediately idealizes the physician as savior, despite numerous failures by other competent experts.
N = Nothing helps, or no change: When there is no relief whatsoever from any type of intervention, although all are tried (including narcotics) and there is no hour-to-hour or day-to-day fluctuation under a variety of circumstances.

Table adapted from T P Hackett, N H Cassem: *Massachusetts General Handbook of General Hospital Psychiatry,* p 53. Mosby, St. Louis, 1978.

pain, they are tapered and discontinued, because obviously they weren't helping and may have been interfering.

Price of chronic pain The clinician needs to be aware that any type of chronic pain can alter the patient's personality, family dynamics, and the way the patient relates to the environment. At the onset of treatment the clinician needs to set guidelines for continuing and for discontinuing treatment. Grounds for termination of treatment are no improvement in any way over six months. If improvement is shown, the patient will need continued support. Often the patient's objective improvement far exceeds the subjective improvement.

BODY DYSMORPHIC DISORDER

INTRODUCTION Body dysmorphic disorder focuses on the patient's feelings of malaise or even loathing about some aspect of the body. Despite the starkness of the complaint, few empirical data about the condition have been gathered.

DEFINITION Patients with body dysmorphic disorder have a pervasive subjective feeling of ugliness despite a normal appearance (Table 18-18). The core of the disorder is the person's strong belief or fear that he or she is unattractive or even repulsive. That fear is rarely assuaged by reassurance or compliments. Yet the typical patient with the disorder is quite normal in appearance. Although a minority of patients with the disorder do have a minor defect, the patient's concern is disproportionate to the degree of defect. So great is the individual's preoccupation that there is significant impairment in social or occupational functioning, or there is marked personal distress. Finally, the preoccupation is not better accounted for by any other mental disorder.

HISTORY Body dysmorphic disorder has been described in the European, Japanese, and Russian psychiatric literature for almost a century with various names. Emil Kraepelin considered it to be a compulsive neurosis. Pierre Janet called it an obsession of shame of the body, and Freud's famous case of the Wolf-Man was obsessively concerned about the size of his nose. In the United States it has been referred to as an atypical somatoform disorder, labeled first as dysmorphophobia; but until the past decade it has been little used and little studied in this country.

COMPARATIVE NOSOLOGY In the United States body dysmorphic disorder first appeared in DSM-III with the term ''dysmorphophobia'' in the residual category of atypical somatoform disorder. Because dysmorphophobia implied inaccurately the presence of a behavioral pattern of phobic avoidance of the body, the term ''body dysmorphic disorder'' was introduced in DSM III-R, as a nondelusional somatoform disorder of undue preoccupation with imagined defects of appearance. Clinicians have had difficulty wrestling with the concept of whether a patient's strong conviction about a feature of appearance was or was not of delusional intensity (that is, did the patient have a somatoform disorder or a delusional disorder with somatoform features). DSM-IV resolves that issue by not requiring that the conviction be defined in intensity as a criteria for inclusion. It was first incorporated into ICD-9 with the somatoform disorders and is grouped with them in ICD-10.

TABLE 18-18
Diagnostic Criteria for Body Dysmorphic Disorder

A. Preoccupation with an imagined defect in appearance. If a slight physical anomaly is present, the person's concern is markedly excessive.
B. The preoccupation causes clinically significant distress or impairment in social, occupational, or other important areas of functioning.
C. The preoccupation is not better accounted for by another mental disorder (e.g., dissatisfaction with body shape and size in anorexia nervosa).

Table from DSM-IV, *Diagnostic and Statistical Manual of Mental Disorders,* ed 4. Copyright American Psychiatric Association, Washington, 1994. Used with permission.

EPIDEMIOLOGY The average age of patients with body dysmorphic disorder is 30 years. Patients with the disorder first develop symptoms in adolescence or young adulthood. Typically they come from middle class families and constitute a tiny but distinct group of patients in the general population. Only about 2 percent of those attending a university hospital plastic surgery clinic meet criteria for the disorder. Too few patients with the disorder have been studied over time to form a clear picture of prevalence, sociodemographic variables, gender predominance, and long-term outcome.

ETIOLOGY The cause of body dysmorphic disorder is unknown. The high comorbidity with depressive disorders, a higher-than-expected family history of mood disorders and obsessive-compulsive disorder, and the reported responsiveness to serotonin-specific reuptake inhibitors indicates that, in at least some patients, the pathophysiology of the disorder may involve serotonin and may be related to other disorders. There may be significant cultural or social effects on body dysmorphic disorder patients because of the emphasis on stereotyped concepts of beauty that may be emphasized in certain families and within the culture at large. In psychodynamic models, body dysmorphic disorder is seen as reflecting the displacement of a sexual or an emotional conflict onto a nonrelated body part. Such an association occurs through the defense mechanisms of repression, dissociation, distortion, symbolization, and projection.

DIAGNOSIS AND CLINICAL FEATURES There are two likely places to find patients with this uncommon disorder: in a mood disorders clinic and in a plastic surgery clinic. A patient with a body dysmorphic disorder might be requesting rhinoplasty; removal of facial sags, jowls, wrinkles, or puffiness; or breast reduction or augmentation. In a clinic for refractory and recurrent depression a patient with the disorder might request relief from a depression caused by an imagined but burdensome bodily defect. Frequent accompanying symptoms, presumably related to suffering from discomfort about appearance in social situations, are insomnia, depression, and anxiety.

Facial flaws are the most common defect in body dysmorphic disorder. Other body parts that sometimes become a focus include hair, breasts, and genitalia. Commonly associated with the distorted belief about appearance is an unrealistic concept of how much one's image can be improved by surgical intervention. However, magical thinking concerning the degree to which the operation will change the person's life (for example, improving job or marital opportunities) is uncommon.

Family histories of obsessive-compulsive disorder and mood disorder are common in reported cases. Also predisposing to the disorder may be certain types of personality characteristics, especially a mixture of obsessional and schizoid traits, but no single personality pattern predominates. Reportedly the patients are shy, self-absorbed and self-centered, narcissistic, and overly sensitive to their imagined defect as a focus of notice or criticism. As adolescents, typically they had few friends and seldom dated.

Although there may be some ideas of reference, there are no frank delusions of reference or persecution. Nor is there any formal thought disorder. In summary, the major abnormality on mental status examination is the lack of insight into the nature of the problem.

DIFFERENTIAL DIAGNOSIS Body dysmorphic disorder patients have an overvalued idea about their defective appearance. A number of other psychiatric disorders are also accompanied by odd or at least unusual ideas about the body. In general such patients are best accounted for diagnostically by considering other major psychiatric disorders as primary, adding that they also have body dysmorphic symptoms. For example, some patients, especially in the early phases of schizophrenia, may have somatic delusions for which they seek correction by cosmetic surgery. In such cases there is an absolute conviction of ugliness plus other bizarre delusional material and perhaps even hallucinations.

Other disorders with body dysmorphic symptoms include mood disorder, narcissistic personality disorder, and anorexia nervosa. Melancholically depressed patients often have additional delusions about some aspect of their body's inadequacy or defect. The presence of a mood disorder, if suspected, can be further elucidated through the taking of the appropriate medical history. Patients with narcissistic personality disorder have a continual interest in their appearance and a long history of interpersonal difficulties that overshadows body image problem. Constant preoccupation with both feared obesity and inadequacy in an obviously malnourished person may be best classified as anorexia nervosa.

With obsessive-compulsive disorder there can also be recurrent and persistent thoughts and images about one's ugly appearance. However, in obsessive-compulsive disorder the person may realize that the preoccupation is a product of an overworrisome mind and may struggle to suppress such thinking. By contrast, the patient with body dysmorphic disorder conceptualizes the problem as not with the thinking apparatus but with physical appearance—often, for example, seeking a surgical cure for an almost imperceptible anomaly. Even if the patient has obsessions about appearance and associated compulsive behaviors (such as mirror checking), the diagnosis of obsessive-compulsive disorder is not given if the obsessions only concern aspects of appearance.

Isolated somatic delusions unrelated to appearance and accompanied by absolute certainty without other evidence of thought disorder are best classified with the delusional disorders. The belief that one's gender is not rightly assigned (according to the appearance of external genitalia at birth) is better accounted for by a diagnosis of gender identity disorder. Opinions still vary as to whether monosymptomatic hypochondriacal psychosis (a delusion about a disease or disfigurement in a body part) and body dysmorphic disorder are one or two disorders.

COURSE AND PROGNOSIS Onset of the disorder may be gradual, during adolescence or in the 20s. Discontentment may build for several years before the person may consider some type of definitive surgical correction. However, surgical treatment produces no panacea. Several long-term follow-up series of those patients undergoing cosmetic surgery have indicated the frequent later emergence of even more severe psychopathology.

TREATMENT Neither surgical nor psychotherapeutic intervention has had any significant long-term impact on decreasing preoccupation with defective bodily appearance in most patients with body dysmorphic disorder. Psychotherapy can benefit some patients with this disorder: presumably those helped most with that treatment modality are the more emotionally intact.

Case reports have documented the efficiency of tricyclic antidepressants; monoamine oxidase inhibitors; and pimozide (Orap), a dopamine receptor antagonist. Both the family histories of depressive disorder in some patients and favorable responses to a variety of antidepressant agents have raised the issue that body dysmorphic disorder may be a variant of an atypical depressive disorder.

Some patients refractory to the older antidepressive agents have recently been shown in open trials to respond to antidepressant and antiobsessional agents with potent 5-HT receptor blockade, such as fluoxetine (Prozac) and clomipramine (Anafranil). Many of those patients have family histories of obsessive-compulsive disorder. Together, that has suggested that body dysmorphic disorder may be an ego-syntonic variant of obsessive-compulsive disorder (the latter, however, is usually associated with ego-dystonic thoughts).

Potent serotonin-specific reuptake inhibitors have recently been reported to be effective in symptomatic relief of some of the patients. After maximal treatment response, some patients with body dysmorphic disorder may still retain remnants of their bodily preoccupation, but symptom intensity is often diminished enough to allow resumption of full social and personal lives. Relapse when taken off medication, however, is common.

SOMATOFORM DISORDER NOT OTHERWISE SPECIFIED

This is the second of the residual categories for the somatoform disorders. Like the first residual category, undifferentiated somatoform disorder, this category was created in order to classify certain somatoform disorder patients whose symptoms and associated disability do not fit the full criteria for other somatoform disorders. The diagnostic criteria for somatoform disorder not otherwise specified are presented in Table 18-19. Patients with this disorder have clinically significant distress or

TABLE 18-19
Diagnostic Criteria for Somatoform Disorder Not Otherwise Specified

This category includes disorders with somatoform symptoms that do not meet the criteria for any specific somatoform disorder. Examples include

1. Pseudocyesis: a false belief of being pregnant that is associated with objective signs of pregnancy, which may include abdominal enlargement (although the umbilicus does not become everted), reduced menstrual flow, amenorrhea, subjective sensation of fetal movement, nausea, breast engorgement and secretions, and labor pains at the expected date of delivery. Endocrine changes may be present, but the syndrome cannot be explained by a general medical condition that causes endocrine changes (e.g., a hormone-secreting tumor).
2. A disorder involving nonpsychotic hypochondriacal symptoms of less than six months' duration.
3. A disorder involving unexplained physical complaints (e.g., fatigue or body weakness) of less than six months' duration that are not due to another mental disorder.

disabilities in social, occupational or other important areas of functioning.

SUGGESTED CROSS-REFERENCES

Related disorders are discussed in Chapters 19, Factitious Disorders, and Chapter 20, Dissociative Disorders. Section 26.12 on consultation-liaison psychiatry, Section 28.1 on noncompliance with treatment, and Section 28.2 on malingering also have relevant information.

REFERENCES

Adler R H, Zlot S, Hurny C, Minder C: Engel's psychogenic pain and the pain-prone patient: A retrospective, controlled clinical study. Psychosom Med *51:* 87, 1989.

Barsky A J, Wood C: Histories of childhood trauma in adult hypochondriacal patients. Am J Psychiatry *151:* 3, 1994.

*Barsky A J, Wyshak G, Klerman G L: Hypochondriasis. Arch Gen Psychiatry *43:* 493, 1986.

Barsky A J, Klerman G L: Overview: Hypochondriasis, bodily complaints, and somatic styles. Am J Psychiatry *140:* 273, 1983.

Barsky A J, Wool C, Barnett M C, Cleary P D: Histories of childhood trauma in adult hypochondriacal patients. Am J Psychiatry *151:* 3, 1994.

Barsky A J: *Worried Sick: Our Troubled Quest for Wellness.* Little, Brown, Boston, 1988.

Bates M S, Edwards W T: Ethnocultural influences on variation in chronic pain perception. Pain *52:* 101, 1993.

Bendefeldt F, Miller L L, Ludwig A M: Cognitive performance in conversion hysteria. Arch Gen Psychiatry *33:* 1250, 1976.

Corbishley M A, Hendrickson R, Beutler L E, Engle D: Behavior, affect, and cognition among psychogenic pain patients in group expressive psychotherapy. J Pain Symptom Management *5:* 241, 1990.

Drake M E Jr: Conversion hysteria and dominant hemisphere lesions. Psychosomatics *34:* 524, 1993.

Flor-Henry P, Fromm-Auch D, Tapper M, Schopflocher D: A neuropsychological study of the stable syndrome of hysteria. Biol Psychiatry *16:* 601, 1981.

Ford C V: The somatizing disorders. Psychosomatics *27:* 327, 1986.

Ford C V: *The Somatizing Disorders: Illness as a Way of Life.* Elsevier, New York, 1983.

Ford C V, Folks D G: Conversion disorders: An overview. Psychosomatics *26:* 371, 1985.

Hackett T P: The pain patient: Evaluation and treatment. In *The Massachusetts General Hospital Handbook of General Hospital Psychiatry,* T P Hackett, N H Cassem, editors, p 41. Mosby, St. Louis, 1978.

Hendler, N H, Kozikowski J G: Overlooked physical diagnoses in chronic pain patients involved in litigation. Psychosomatics *34:* 494, 1993.

*Hollander E, Neville D, Frenkel M, Josephson S, Liebowitz M R: Body dysmorphis disorder: Diagnostic issues and related disorders. Psychosomatics *33:* 156, 1992.

James L, Gordon E, Kraiuhin C, Howson A, Meares R: Augmentation of auditory evoked potentials in somatization disorder. J Psychiatr Res *24:* 155, 1990.

Jenkins P L G: Psychogenic abdominal pain. Gen Hosp Psychiatry *13:* 27, 1991.

Kellner R: Hypochondriasis and somatization. JAMA *258:* 2718, 1987.

Kellner R: *Somatization and Hypochondriasis.* Praeger, New York, 1986.

Kirmayer L J, Robbins J M, editors: *Current Concepts of Somatization: Research and Clinical Perspectives.* American Psychiatric Press, Washington, DC, 1991.

*Lipowski Z J: Somatization: The concept and its clinical application. Am J Psychiatry *145:* 1358, 1988.

McElroy S L, Phillips K A: Body dysmorphic disorder: Does it have a psychotic subtype? J Clin Psychiatry *54:* 389, 1993.

Noyes R Jr, Kathol R G: The validity of DSM-III-R hypochondriasis. Arch Gen Psychiatry *50:* 961, 1993.

Newman N J: Neuro-ophthalmology and psychiatry. Gen Hosp Psychiatry *15:* 102, 1993.

Phillips K A, McElroy S L: Body dysmorphic disorder: 30 cases of imagined ugliness. Am J Psychiatry *150:* 302, 1993.

*Pilowsky I, Barrow C G: A controlled study of psychotherapy and amitriptyline used individually and in combination in the treatment of chronic intractable, 'psychogenic' pain. Pain *40:* 3, 1990.

Rost K, Kashner T M: Effectiveness of psychiatric intervention with somatization disorder patients: Improved outcomes at reduced costs. Gen Hosp Psychiatry *16:* 381, 1994.

Sackeim H A: Lateral asymmetry in bodily response to hypnotic suggestions. Biol Psychiatry *17:* 437, 1982.

Simon G E, Von Korff M: Somatization and psychiatric disorder in the NIMH epidemiologic catchment area study. Am J Psychiatry 148: 1494, 1991.

*Smith G R: *Somatization Disorder in the Medical Setting.* American Psychiatric Press, Washington, DC, 1991.

Smith G R, Monson R A, Ray D C: Psychiatric consultation in somatization disorder. New Engl J Med *314:* 1407, 1986.

Valdes M, Garcia L, Treserra J, Pablo J, Flores T: Psychogenic pain and depressive disorders: An empirical study. J Affective Disord *16:* 21, 1989.

Von Korff M, Resche L L: First onset of common pain symptoms: A prospective study of depression as a risk factor. Pain *55:* 251, 1993.

Wexler B E: Cerebral laterality and psychiatry: A review of the literature. Am J Psychiatry *137:* 279, 1980.

CHAPTER 19 FACTITIOUS DISORDERS

REBECCA M. JONES, M.D.

INTRODUCTION

As W. B. Bean wrote, "At the frayed end of . . . [the human] spectrum is the fascinating derelict, human flotsam detached from its moorings, the peripatetic medical vagrant, the itinerant fabricator of nearly perfect facsimile of serious illness—the victim of Munchausen's Syndrome." According to the second edition of *Webster's International Dictionary* "factitious" means artificial, a sham; what is "made by art, in distinction from what is produced in nature." Factitious disorders, with the classically named Munchausen syndrome being the best studied, represent some of the most disturbing, bewildering, and frustrating presentations in psychiatric or medical practice. They also represent patients who are capable of arousing in many physicians a complex reaction of intense contempt, anger, and betrayal, as the doctor-patient relationship is turned on its head.

The disorders involve persons who intentionally cause themselves to be ill, sometimes desperately so, for the sole purpose of becoming a patient. Those persons feign or produce illness in such a manner that the charade is rigorously concealed, and in the process they mislead the treating physicians as to what interventions are needed. Not infrequently those patients place themselves in situations of great risk, with unnecessary, potentially dangerous procedures being performed. As part of the simulation, those patients often fabricate or greatly exaggerate a medical history or produce actual physical findings through self-infliction of various lesions or conditions. When the medically prescribed interventions inevitably do not work, or even do harm, or when the physician suspects and confronts the fabrications, the apparently desperate need for care turns to rage and withdrawal. The physician is often left feeling duped, helpless, and inadequate.

Examples of self-produced conditions include urinalyses contaminated with blood or feces, obtained through urethral self-laceration or a piece of the patient's own stool; acceptance of a radiographic contrast injection with a clear past history of an anaphylactic reaction; surreptitious self-administration of epinephrine resulting in headaches, tremor, tachycardia, and hypertension; surreptitious injection of insulin resulting in hypoglycemia; self-inoculation of bacteria resulting in fever; self-insertion of gas, needles, or metallic fragments in joint areas resulting in arthritic symptoms; and simulated symptoms of human immunodeficiency virus (HIV) infection, including self-description as HIV-positive, fever, diarrhea, and loss of weight. Numerous case reports in the literature describe such induced signs and symptoms and attest to the grimly determined and self-punishing creativity of many of the patients. All of those actions appear to be voluntary in that the person is fully aware of the deception and often goes to great lengths to protect it, yet there is a sense that the person is out of control in a compulsively self-destructive way. The actions, which can be extraordinarily bizarre, are deliberate, thought out, and intentional, yet appear to be beyond the patient's immediate power to control.

DEFINITION

The fourth edition of *Diagnostic and Statistical Manual of Mental Disorders* (DSM-IV) has made a number of changes from the revised third edition (DSM-III-R) in the classification and criteria for factitious disorders. DSM-III-R outlined separate criteria sets for factitious disorder with physical symptoms and factitious disorder with psychological symptoms, and required the use of the not otherwise specified category for persons who present with mixed pictures. DSM-IV has merged the disorders into a single criteria set, labeled factitious disorder, and has delineated three subtypes: factitious disorder with predominantly psychological signs and symptoms, factitious disorder with predominantly physical signs and symptoms, and factitious disorder with combined psychological and physical signs and symptoms when neither predominates. The diagnostic criteria for factitious disorder appears in Table 19-1. The factitious disorder not otherwise specified category includes disorders with factitious symptoms that do not meet the criteria for the other factitious disorders. The DSM-IV diagnostic criteria for factitious disorder not otherwise specified are outlined in Table 19-2.

An example of factitious disorder not otherwise specified is factitious disorder by proxy. It includes situations in which one person produces symptoms in another, typically a parent creating symptoms in a child, for the purpose of indirectly assuming the sick role (by proxy). The only current data on factitious disorder by proxy is empirical, involving approximately 68 case reports in the literature, but it is associated with substantial morbidity and mortality. The research criteria for factitious disorder by proxy are outlined in Table 19-3. The diagnosis is given to the person inducing the symptoms, not to the person in whom the symptoms are induced. If there is evidence that the person in whom the symptoms are induced has participated in the production of symptoms, than he or she is given the diagnosis of factitious disorder, and the person primarily responsible for the symptom induction is given the diagnosis of factitious disorder not otherwise specified or factitious disorder by proxy.

HISTORY

"Here is described a common syndrome which most doctors have seen, but about which little has been written. Like the famous Baron von Munchausen, the persons affected have always traveled widely; and their stories, like those attributed to him, are both dramatic and untruthful." Richard Asher coined the term "Munchausen syndrome" in 1951 to describe a special pattern of factitious disorder which was characterized by recalcitrant chronicity and the tendency of the patients to migrate from hospital to hospital, and from doctor to doctor, dramatically fabricating ("a matrix of fantasy and falsehood") different illnesses. Cases of self-induced or feigned illness have been described in the literature since the second century, when Galen wrote a treatise on the subject. In 1863, while studying "feigned and factitious diseases" in Great Britain, Gavin described an intriguing group of patients "who assume the semblance of disease from some inexplicable cause." Asher described a man who "is found to have attended, and deceived, an astounding number of other hospitals; and he nearly always discharges himself against advice, after quarreling violently with both

TABLE 19-1
Diagnostic Criteria for Factitious Disorder

A. Intentional production or feigning of physical or psychological signs or symptoms.
B. The motivation for the behavior is to assume the sick role.
C. External incentives for the behavior (such as economic gain, avoiding legal responsibility, or improving physical well-being, as in malingering) are absent.

Code based on type:
- **With predominantly psychological signs and symptoms:** if psychological signs and symptoms predominate in the clinical presentation
- **With predominantly physical signs and symptoms:** if physical signs and symptoms predominate in the clinical presentation
- **With combined psychological and physical signs and symptoms:** if both psychological and physical signs and symptoms are present but neither predominates in the clinical presentation

Table from DSM-IV, *Diagnostic and Statistical Manual of Mental Disorders,* ed 4. Copyright American Psychiatric Association, Washington, 1994. Used with permission.

TABLE 19-2
Diagnostic Criteria for Factitious Disorder Not Otherwise Specified

This category includes disorders with factitious symptoms that do not meet the criteria for factitious disorder. An example is factitious disorder by proxy: the intentional production or feigning of physical or psychological signs or symptoms in another person who is under the individual's care for the purpose of indirectly assuming the sick role.

Table from DSM-IV, *Diagnostic and Statistical Manual of Mental Disorders,* ed 4. Copyright American Psychiatric Association, Washington, 1994. Used with permission.

TABLE 19-3
Research Criteria for Factitious Disorder by Proxy

A. Intentional production or feigning of physical or psychological signs or symptoms in another person who is under the individual's care.
B. The motivation for the perpetrator's behavior is to assume the sick role by proxy.
C. External incentives for the behavior (such as economic gain) are absent.
D. The behavior is not better accounted for by another mental disorder.

Table from DSM-IV, *Diagnostic and Statistical Manual of Mental Disorders,* ed 4. Copyright American Psychiatric Association, Washington, 1994. Used with permission.

doctors and nurses.'' Asher observed three main subtypes of Munchausen syndrome: what he described as the most common acute abdominal type or ''laparotomophilia migrans,'' who presents with severe abdominal pain and evidence of multiple past surgical procedures; the hemorrhagic type, or ''haemorrhagica histrionica,'' who ''specializes in bleeding from the lungs or stomach . . . colloquially known as 'haemoptysis merchants' and 'haematemesis merchants'; ''and the neurological type, or ''neurologica diabolica,'' who presents with ''paroxysmal headache, loss of consciousness, and peculiar fits.'' Asher's diagnosis was made on the basis of what he termed ''useful pointers,'' including:

''1. A multiplicity of scars, usually abdominal.
2. A mixture of truculence and evasiveness in manner.
3. An immediate history which is always acute and harrowing, yet not entirely convincing—overwhelmingly severe abdominal pain of uncertain type, cataclysmal blood loss unsupported by corresponding pallor, dramatic loss of consciousness, and so forth.
4. A wallet or handbag stuffed with hospital attendance cards, insurance claim forms, and litigious correspondence.''

Asher stressed that despite the deceptive nature of those conditions, ''fragments of complete truth are surprisingly embedded.'' He emphasized that the patients are often quite ill psychologically, and even potentially medically, ''although their illness is shrouded by duplicity and deception,'' and concluded that research is needed to find an explanation which ''might lead to a cure of the psychological kink which produces the disease.'' In a 1968 article, H. R. Spiro chronicled the terminology used to describe factitious disorders since Asher's first description, concluding that it ''is better noted for its color than for its clarity,'' and that it was ''symptomatic of the mixture of bemusement, bewilderment, contempt, and anger that these patients arouse in their physicians.'' Spiro posed the question, ''In an era of modern psychiatry, how does a symptom complex earn an epithet like Munchausen's syndrome instead of a legitimate diagnosis?'' Examples given of such terms, other than Asher's original ones, included such language as J. S. Chapman's ''dermatitis autogenica'' and ''hyperpyrexia figmentatica,'' E. Clark and S. C. Melnick's ''hospital hoboes,'' and J. C. Barker's ''hospital addiction.'' Spiro suggested that those terms are ''misnomers,'' inducing most physicians to ''regard these people simply as tricksters, liars, and swindlers,'' and that a more ''impersonal nomenclature'' should be adopted. Spiro proposed that those patients should receive a primary psychiatric diagnosis, be it, in his words, neurotic, psychotic, or characterologic; the qualifying phrase ''with chronic factitious symptomatology'' would then be added as a ''more descriptive, nonepithetical appellation.'' Many articles and letters to the editor followed both Asher's and Spiro's papers, with most containing case reports of the most severe form of the disorder (the classic Munchausen syndrome) in which there is a dramatic picture of factitious physical symptoms and a history of multiple hospitalizations. For nearly four decades those reports greatly influenced the classification and thinking about factitious disorders among physicians and in the official nomenclature, with the term ''Munchausen syndrome'' being used incorrectly to designate all cases of factitious disorders. The designation clouded the real distinctions existing among patients and tended negatively to affect the attitudes of hospital staff toward all patients with factitious disorders.

COMPARATIVE NOSOLOGY

As new data emerged, thinking about factitious disorders began gradually to change, although the third edition of DSM (DSM-III) still placed great emphasis on chronic factitious disorder with physical symptoms as the major prototype for all factitious disorders. DSM-III-R advanced the conceptualization of factitious disorders, with the new nomenclature reflecting the emerging evidence that factitious disorders have varying degrees of chronicity and function, that episodic disorders do occur, as do both exclusively psychiatric presentations and mixed ones. DSM-IV carries the newly realized conceptualization even further with the designation of an overall category of factitious disorder, subdivided as appropriate with one of three equally presented subtypes: with predominantly physical symptoms, with predominantly psychological symptoms, and with combined psychological and physical symptoms when neither predominates. The inclusion in DSM-IV of research criteria for factitious disorder by proxy, first described by R. Meadow in 1977, gives increased status to an important variation of the classically described factitious disorders.

EPIDEMIOLOGY

It is apparent that factitious disorders encompass a wide variety of patients, varying in their presentation and induction of symptoms, as well as in the chronicity of their course and their associated psychopathology. As a result of the difficulty in diagnosing the disorder, as well as in obtaining reliable historical or psychological information in diagnosed patients, systematic epidemiological data has been hard to obtain. The frequency of identifying factitious disorders in the medical setting is dependent on a number of factors, including the diagnostic criteria applied, the threshold of suspicion, the particular setting studied, and the nature of the patient population. It is well known that factitious disorders are found in greater numbers by those researchers who specifically look for them among selected patients.

For instance, one study investigating the frequency of the

factitious disorder diagnosis among 343 patients referred to the National Institute for Allergy and Infectious Disease because of fever of undetermined origin, diagnosed 32 cases of factitious disorder, or 9.3 percent of the cases. On the other hand, a recent literature review of factitious disorder with psychological symptoms reported only a 0.5 percent admission rate to psychiatric hospitals, and a 1990 study of 1,288 patients consecutively referred to the psychiatric consultation-liaison service of a tertiary-care general hospital, reported the diagnosis of factitious disorder being made in 10, or 0.8 percent, of the patients. The 1990 study concluded that the percentage reported most likely represented only a small proportion of all factitious disorders in that setting, due to the fact that ''medical practitioners often do not detect psychiatric illness in patients with physical symptoms,'' and thus do not think to refer them to psychiatry.

The age range of patients diagnosed with factitious disorder has been reported to be approximately the same in various studies, ranging in one study between 19 and 64 (median age 26), and in another between 16 and 57 (median age 33). The median age of onset of factitious disorder is generally reported to be in early adulthood, usually the early 20s.

Although traditionally factitious disorders have been thought to be most common among men (probably secondary to the emphasis on the classic description of the middle-aged man suffering from Munchausen syndrome), a number of both older and more recent reviews have indicated a preponderance of female patients. In one 10-year retrospective study of hospitalized patients, 39 of 41 patients diagnosed with factitious disorder were women, and in the study of 1,288 patients referred to a consultation-liaison service, 7 of the 10 cases diagnosed with factitious disorder were women.

No genetic familial pattern has been established, although it has been reported that factitious disorders may run in families, and a large number of persons diagnosed with factitious disorders may have other underlying psychiatric diagnoses which have been established as being in part genetically influenced (for example, mood disorders, personality disorders, substance-related disorders, and others). It has been suggested that children who develop induced factitious symptoms as the result of factitious disorder by proxy in a parent, may themselves develop factitious disorder later in life.

Most studies of factitious disorder report that the diagnosis is closely associated with persons employed in or intimately familiar with medically related occupations, including nurses, medical technicians, medical secretaries, hospital volunteers, and physicians. Typical of those reports is the study describing 41 diagnosed cases of factitious disorder over a 10-year period in one hospital. Of those 41 cases, 28 worked in medically related jobs, 15 as nurses.

ETIOLOGY

Asher wrote, ''The most remarkable feature of the syndrome is the apparent senselessness of it. Unlike the malingerer, who may gain a definite end, these patients often seem to gain nothing except the discomfiture of unnecessary investigations and operations.'' Many investigators have attempted to make sense out of the ''apparent senselessness'' of factitious disorders, and all have concluded that complex forces are at work to produce the bizarre presentation of a simulated patient compulsively deceiving hospital staffs and self-inflicting harm. One of the particularly fascinating aspects of the disorders is that, in Spiro's conceptualization, the patients know when they are ''acting,'' but even with that knowledge cannot stop, and thus ''seemingly willful acts are determined by unconscious factors and environmental cues to produce a psychiatric illness of profound dimensions.'' Asher postulated that perhaps ''a desire to be the center of interest and attention'' was the motivating factor, with the persons ''suffering in fact from the Walter Mitty syndrome, but instead of playing the dramatic part of the surgeon, they submit to the equally dramatic role of the patient.'' Asher also hypothesized ''a grudge against doctors and hospitals, which is satisfied by frustrating or deceiving them'' as a possible determinant.

More sophisticated recent analyses of the psychodynamics of factitious disorders have focused on the choice of the medical world as the stage upon which to enact dramatic scenes, the unattached and nonintimate nature of relationships among the patients, and the aggressively masochistic, self-punishing style of their interactions with others. Many patients have a history of major organic illness or have experienced major illness among significant people. For some, the earlier experience of being a patient may have been the only source of nurturance they received in their lives, and they are compelled to repeat the experience as the only way to feel valued. Many patients report having had an intimate relationship with a physician, either as a child with a parent, or as a lover in a relationship, which is perceived as having been ultimately rejecting or otherwise unsatisfying. It has been suggested that those patients need to reenact, and thus hopefully to master, previous experiences where medical personnel or hospitals played a traumatic role in personality development. In many cases, the relationship with the physician is a reenactment of the perceived relationships with the parents. The aggressive acting out of the patient role allows the individual both to seek love and approval from an idealized rescuer and to wreak revenge on a devalued tormenter through deception and hostility. Often the person resorts to the simulated patient role by a frustrating triggering event in daily life that revives feelings of inadequacy, rejection, or helplessness. By acting out the role of patient, the person can feel symbolically in control of a situation which either currently or once felt out of control: in Spiro's words, ''he creates the illness and thus he can terminate it.'' Where once the feelings were those of helplessness and fear, the feelings now are those of superiority, power, and contempt.

The hostility of patients with factitious disorder can be unmistakable; beneath the ostensible helplessness, bitterness and resentment toward physicians may be palpable. It is probably in part that hostility which induces physicians unconsciously to respond aggressively to those patients with painful, dangerous, and unnecessary procedures. In the process, all of the patient's conflicts are acted out at once: he or she is cared for and nurtured by the physician, controls and unmasks the physician, and is inevitably rejected and punished by the physician. When the patient begins to feel out of control in the hospital, as when the staff begins to suspect that something is not right or when dangerous procedures are recommended which the patient does not want, the patient reasserts control by angrily walking out of the hospital against medical advice, usually accusing the physicians of incompetence and malpractice. Some have explained the choice of medically related careers by many of those patients as a mixture of identification with the aggressor, as merger with an ego-ideal, and as a need to acquiesce and cater to an ambivalently viewed authority. Others have understood those patients to be attempting psychologically to use the hospital, with, in Spiro's words, its ''mixture of care and pain, of attention and fear, of dependency and rejection'' as a more effective substitute for a confusing parental figure. Still others have emphasized the self-infliction of pain as a masochistic attempt to diminish unconscious guilt, deriving from intense reactions to intolerable childhood experiences.

DIAGNOSIS AND CLINICAL FEATURES

FACTITIOUS DISORDER WITH PREDOMINANTLY PSYCHOLOGICAL SIGNS AND SYMPTOMS The essential feature is intentional production or feigning of psychological symptoms, motivated solely by a psychological need to assume the sick role. Individuals may claim to be severely depressed and suicidal, often as the result of unverifiable tragic events (for example, the death of a spouse); psychotic symptoms, such as hallucinations or delusions; cognitive deficits, such as memory loss; dissociative symptoms, such as amnesia; and conversion symptoms, such as pseudoblindness or pseudoparalysis. Persons may adopt symptoms exhibited by other patients on a ward and may ultimately receive large doses of psychoactive medication or even electroconvulsive therapy (ECT), which invariably do not work. Whichever symptoms are described, they tend to be worse when the patient is aware of being observed, and they rarely conform to any established diagnostic categories.

Histories given are often dramatic, graphic, and self-aggrandizing. Associated features include the phenomenon of *vorbeireden,* in which the patient gives approximate answers or talks past the point, including answers which are near misses of the actual answer (''6 times 5'' becomes ''31''). *Vorbeireden* is not specific to factitious disorder and may be seen in persons with schizophrenia and those without mental illness who are tired or stressed. Patients may ingest such substances as stimulants, opioids, hallucinogens, and hypnotics, to induce simulated psychiatric symptoms.

The disorder is concomitant with a severe personality disorder in the vast majority of persons. The Minnesota Multiphasic Personality Inventory (MMPI) may help to confirm a diagnosis of factitious disorder with predominantly psychological signs and symptoms. An invalid test profile and elevations of all clinical scales indicate an attempt to appear more disturbed than is the case (''fake bad''). Patients with factitious illness in general (with either psychological or physical presentations) most often demonstrate a normal or above-average intelligent quotient (I.Q.); an absence of a formal thought disorder; a poor sense of identity; poor sexual adjustment; poor frustration tolerance; strong dependency needs, and narcissism. Diagnoses based on personality tests have most commonly been of borderline personality disorder, histrionic personality disorder, and depressive disorders.

J.P. was a muscular, 24-year-old man who presented himself to the admitting office of a state hospital. He told the admitting physician that he had taken 30 200-mg tablets of chlorpromazine (Thorazine) in the bus on the way over to the hospital. After receiving medical treatment for the ''suicide attempt,'' he was transferred to the inpatient ward.

On mental status examination, the patient told a fantastic story about his father's being a famous surgeon who had a patient die in surgery. The patient's husband then killed J.P.'s father. J.P. stalked his father's murderer several thousand miles across the United States and, when he found him, was prevented from killing him, at the last moment, by the timely arrival of his 94-year-old grandmother. He also related several other intriguing stories involving his $64,000 sports car, which had a 12-cylinder diesel engine, and about his children, two sets of identical triplets. All those stories had a grandiose tinge, and none of them could be confirmed. The patient claimed that he was hearing voices, as on the TV or in a dream. He answered affirmatively to questions about thought control, thought broadcasting, and other unusual psychotic symptoms; he also claimed depression. He was oriented and alert and had a good range of information except that he kept insisting that it was the Iranians (not the Iraquis) who had invaded Kuwait (referring to the Gulf War that took place in 1992–1993). There was no evidence of any associated features of mania or depression, and the patient did not seem either elated, depressed, or irritable when he related those stories.

It was observed on the ward that J.P. bullied the other patients and took food and cigarettes from them. He was very reluctant to be discharged, and whenever the subject of his discharge was brought up, he renewed his complaints about ''suicidal thoughts'' and ''hearing voices.'' It was the opinion of the ward staff that the patient was not truly psychotic but merely feigned his symptoms whenever the subject of further disposition of his case came up. They thought that he wanted to remain in the hospital primarily so that he could bully the other patients and be a ''big man'' on the ward.

Discussion Although the patient would have doctors believe that he was psychotic, his story, almost from the start, seemed to conform to no recognizable psychotic syndrome. That his symptoms are not genuine was confirmed by the observation of the ward staff that he seemed to feign them whenever the subject of discharge was brought up.

Why did this fellow try so hard to act crazy? His motivation was not to achieve some external incentive, such as, for example, avoiding the draft, as would be the case in malingering; his goal of remaining a patient was understandable only with knowledge of his individual psychology (the suggestion that he was motivated to assume the sick role because he derived satisfaction from being the ''big man'' on the ward). The diagnosis was, therefore, factitious disorder with predominantly psychological signs and symptoms. (From *DSM-IV Casebook.* Used with permission).

FACTITIOUS DISORDER WITH PREDOMINANTLY PHYSICAL SIGNS AND SYMPTOMS The essential feature is the intentional production or feigning of physical signs and symptoms, motivated solely by a psychological need to assume the sick role. The presentation of symptoms runs a spectrum from total fabrication, as in assertions that one is HIV-positive; to self-infliction, as in the surreptitious self-administration of epinephrine or insulin; to an exaggeration or exacerbation of a preexisting physical condition, such as acceptance of a treatment to which one has a known allergy. Evidence of earlier medical procedures, such as laparotomy scars, venous cutdown scars, cranial burr holes, or signs of recent cardioversion, testify to an extensive history of past hospitalizations.

Common clinical presentations include generalized rashes, abscesses, fevers of undetermined origin, bleeding secondary to ingestion of anticoagulants, and severe right lower quadrant pain. The ''gridiron'' abdomen resulting from multiple surgical procedures is a classic example of the most severe form of the disorder formerly known as Munchausen syndrome. The symptoms presented are shaped by the patient's level of medical knowledge and familiarity with medical language (which may be substantial), as well as by previous experiences with medical care.

There is invariably a lack of overt anxiety when confronted with the prospect of painful or life-threatening procedures. Many patients demand specific treatments, and complaints of severe pain are common. Medical and personal histories are often delivered in a dramatic manner, filled with flamboyant, grandiose, and outrageously untrue details, a phenomenon known as pseudologia fantastica. Hospitalized patients rarely have visitors of any kind, and totally resist any attempts to confirm details of their stories. When confronted with evidence or suspicions of deception, patients often indignantly deny the allegations and leave the hospital immediately. Those with histories of multiple hospitalizations often travel to new cities, states, and countries in an attempt to find hospitals where they will not be recognized. Associated features include psychoactive substance abuse, especially of prescribed analgesics and sedatives.

An orthopedic surgeon in Seattle requested a psychiatric consultation on Peggy S., a 28-year-old, single, graduate student who was recovering from a recent spinal fusion, because he thought she was not complying with physical therapy.

The psychiatrist noted that Ms. S. was an attractive young woman with a below-the-knee amputation of her left leg. She was oddly ingratiating and cheerful, and she didn't seem to be appropriately troubled by her deteriorating medical condition. She reported that five years previously she had been thrown to the ground by a boyfriend, injuring her back. Over the next two years she had multiple surgical procedures on her back. Finally, a fusion left her pain free until six months ago, when she was diagnosed with spinal degenerative changes and was referred for physical therapy.

Amazed that she didn't volunteer any information about her amputation, the psychiatrist asked how it happened and learned that shortly after the original surgery to her back, she had been in a motorcycle accident, sustaining burns to her left ankle. That became a chronic injury and ultimately led to amputation of her leg a year and a half ago. She reported that calmly and denied any distress over the disfigurement or disability. She also calmly reported that fluctuating swelling of her stump and recurrent ulcers had interfered with her being successfully fitted with a prosthesis. Thus, she had remained in a wheelchair. She had also been hospitalized several times many years earlier for colitis and kidney stones.

The psychiatrist called the surgeon who had performed her amputation. He reported that the original burn had quickly progressed to a chronic injury, with chronic pain and swelling of the left leg. When the leg proved unresponsive to medical management, the patient received a series of skin grafts, all of which failed because of infection and edema. She was instructed to keep her leg elevated but did not comply, and her leg continued to deteriorate. She saw many doctors and was followed in a pain clinic, but she continued to experience pain, massive edema, and recurrent infections. Ms. S. repeatedly urged her surgeon to amputate her leg, claiming that it was painful and of no use to her. Ultimately he complied.

The surgeon who performed the amputation also reported that Ms. S. had recently had several admissions for left-sided weakness and numbness. Physical findings were inconsistent, the workup was negative, and she was discharged with a diagnosis of conversion disorder. It was shortly thereafter that her back pain recurred. The surgeon also commented that various physicians involved in the management of her leg injury had raised the possibility that her symptoms might be self-induced.

Ms. S. was an only child, born to a middle-class family. By her own account, after graduating from college, she moved from job to job for a number of years, generally leaving because of medical problems and repeated hospitalizations. At the time of admission, she was a part-time graduate student, being supported by social security. No one had accompanied her to the hospital, and she had no visitors during her hospitalization. She asked that her doctors not contact her family.

Ms. S. was transferred to an inpatient rehabilitation unit, where she quickly developed a string of largely unexplained medical problems, including a urinary tract infection, gastroenteritis with diarrhea and fever, painful swelling of the right hand and wrist, a rash on her back and torso, and atypical mental status changes, including difficulty doing rudimentary calculations and inconsistent memory deficits. Meanwhile, she repeatedly refused to comply with safety procedures on the unit, leaving her wheelchair unlocked and her bed rail down, despite constant reminders by the staff. Over time she generated a good deal of anger and frustration among most staff members, although a few found her a particularly sad and pathetic case.

After her previous surgeon had been contacted, the staff became suspicious about the role that she might be playing in the development of her symptoms. Ms. S's room was searched, and furosemide (a diuretic), cathartics, and an exercise band that could serve as a tourniquet were found. Those were believed possibly to explain many of her symptoms as well as the unexplained metabolic abnormalities that had been noted in her chart. Careful review of her chart revealed that her urinary tract infection had been diagnosed on the basis of positive cultures in the absence of cells in the urine, most consistent with a fecal contaminant. It remained unclear if or how she might have factitiously elevated her temperature, even while observed, or how she might have induced the bitelike lesions on her back and torso.

Discussion When a clinician attempts to obtain a history from a patient, there is a basic assumption that the patient is doing the best that he or she can do to provide accurate information. In this case, the referral was triggered by noncompliance with the surgeon's therapeutic recommendation. The first suggestion that things might not be as they appeared was the patient's striking nonchalance about her disability (the leg amputation)—referred to as *la belle indifférence*. Suspicions were further raised when additional history became available from her previous surgeon. Finally, compelling evidence was obtained that indicated that she had deliberately produced many of her puzzling physical symptoms and metabolic abnormalities, suggesting a diagnosis of either factitious disorder or malingering.

The distinction between these two conditions depends on the underlying motivation. In malingering, there are clear external incentives—for example, the man who, in order to avoid military service, puts sugar in his urine to simulate diabetes. In contrast, in factitious disorder the motivation is presumed to be a psychological need to assume the sick role. In this case there did not appear to be any clear external incentives, and one can only presume that, for unknown reasons, Ms. S. had a pathological need to perpetuate being a medical patient. Because her symptoms are primarily physical, the Axis I diagnosis would be factitious disorder with predominantly physical signs and symptoms, a disorder that was first called Munchausen syndrome, after an 18-century baron who wrote many fantastic tales.

People with factitious disorder are also assumed to have severe personality disturbance. However, in the absence of any specific information about this patient's long-term personality functioning, diagnosis deferred on Axis II would be noted. On Axis III the left leg amputation and recent spinal fusion would be listed. Undoubtedly, Ms. S. had multiple psychosocial problems, but because of lack of any specific information, deferred would be noted on Axis IV. Her Axis V GAF rating of 33 reflected her major impairment in her thinking and judgment.

Multiaxial evaluation

Axis I Factitious disorder with predominantly physical signs and symptoms
Axis II Diagnosis deferred
Axis III Left leg amputation, recent spinal fusion
Axis IV Deferred
Axis V GAF = 33 (current)

Follow-up A team meeting was convened, and Ms. S. was told that it was suspected that she had factitious symptoms, implying that she was actively involved in inducing at least some of her symptoms. She was informed that it is a serious and potentially life-threatening mental illness, and that inpatient psychiatric hospitalization was recommended for further evaluation and management. She did not comment on the diagnosis, appeared unconcerned, and agreed to transfer to a psychiatric ward.

Ms. S. was in an acute psychiatric unit for four months. During that time she developed no new medical problems and made no complaints of pain or physical discomfort. Instead, she developed a series of psychiatric symptoms. She initially presented with rapid alternations of mood, appearing first hypomanic, racing around the unit in her wheelchair and claiming to be up all night, then depressed, curling up on her bed with the lights out, refusing to eat or interact with others. Her presentation was thought by some staff members to result from factitious bipolar disorder, whereas others attributed her symptoms to genuine affective instability or true dissociative phenomena.

Ms. S.'s behavior on the unit was provocative and impulsive. She was labile and suspicious. She split staff, threw tantrums, said she was suicidal, and barricaded herself in her room. She improved on an anticonvulsive medication and an antipsychotic, but nevertheless spent the second half of her hospitalization refusing to participate in activities and with restricted privileges because of her threats of self-destructive behavior if she was allowed to leave the unit.

In psychotherapy, she gradually revealed a history of daily physical abuse at the hands of her parents throughout childhood and early adolescence. Her therapist believed that the history was genuine and diagnosed a dissociative disorder on the basis of the symptoms she described. Other staff members remained unconvinced of the veracity of her story of childhood abuse, but were impressed with the array of features characteristic of borderline personality disorder.

Ms. S. agreed to a voluntary transfer to long-term hospitalization. One day before the planned transfer, she changed her mind, saying she wanted to "get on with my life," and submitted a sign-out letter. She went to court, where she was granted discharge by the judge. She signed out against medical advice, and was lost to follow-up. (From *DSM-IV Casebook*. Used with permission.)

FACTITIOUS DISORDER WITH COMBINED PSYCHOLOGICAL AND PHYSICAL SIGNS AND SYMPTOMS

In combined forms of factitious disorder, both psychological and physical signs and symptoms are present. If neither type predominates in the clinical presentation, a diagnosis of factitious disorder with combined psychological and physical signs and symptoms should be made (Table 19-1).

FACTITIOUS DISORDER NOT OTHERWISE SPECIFIED

Some patients with factitious signs and symptoms do not meet the DSM-IV criteria for a specific factitious disorder and should be classified as having factitious disorder not otherwise specified (Table 19-2). The most notable example of the diagnosis is factitious disorder by proxy, which is also included in a DSM-IV appendix (Table 19-3).

The essential feature of factitious disorder by proxy is the production or feigning of physical signs or symptoms in another person who is under the person's care, motivated solely by the psychological need to indirectly assume the sick role. The person who presents with physical signs or symptoms induced by a caregiver with the diagnosis of factitious disorder by proxy is considered to be suffering from a form of induced factitious symptoms. Factitious disorder by proxy is considered to be a form of child abuse, which unsuspecting care providers exacerbate when they perform potentially dangerous and unnecessary tests in an attempt to discover a diagnosis. A 9 percent mortality rate has been reported. The key to the diagnosis is the disappearance of symptoms whenever the child is removed from the parent's proximity.

It has been reported that the mother is the perpetrator of symptom induction in over 95 percent of the cases, with the father being most often described as passive and uninvolved, and the relationship between the mother and father being characterized as typically emotionally distant. Sometimes the father may be the perpetrator, either alone or in collaboration with the mother, or the perpetrator may be another caregiver, such as a babysitter. Profiles of the typical parent involved in factitious disorder by proxy include descriptions of the person as intelligent and articulate, with a medical sophistication and level of knowledge often based on professional experience in the health or child care fields. The hospital staff involved in the care of the child often initially describe the parent as unusually devoted to the child, and understanding about the need for diagnostic procedures, a view that gradually begins to shift to the feeling that the parent is excessively involved and inappropriately demanding about the need for particular treatments. Personality disorders, depression, and factitious disorder itself have been reported among the perpetrating parents, but no specific pattern of psychopathology has been described. A common presentation is a mother who refuses ever to leave her child alone with caregivers, who insists on always speaking for the child, who refuses to allow anyone other than herself to administer medications or procedures, and who insists on using medications or other supplies from her own sources rather than from the hospital source. When confronted with the consequences of what they are doing, the perpetrators may become suicidal and depressed, or they may become angry and insist on taking the child out of the hospital against medical advice. Perpetrators may face criminal charges, which can range from abuse to murder. Those parental features are often associated in the child with a puzzling, recurrent, "one of a kind" that which has not responded to conventional therapy. The presentation is also typically associated with a lack of documentation of prior diagnoses, despite detailed verbal histories, usually reported to be the result of inadvertently lost medical records. Usually only one child at a time is involved, although siblings and other persons may have already been abused or will be abused. Table 19-4 summarizes the most common presentations of factitious disorder by proxy as reported by D. A. Rosenberg. It has been postulated that the etiology of factitious disorder by proxy is psychodynamically very similar to the etiology of factitious disorder in general, with several additional ideas specific to this diagnosis. For instance, it has been suggested that certain basic needs of the mother are potentially met, including the esteem in which she is held by the hospital staff, the authority and involvement of the physician in her life, an attempt to save a failing marriage or shift attention away from a bad relationship, and the projection of the mother's own factitious disorder onto her child. Victimized children are at increased risk for developing factitious disorder themselves as they mature.

Paula P. brought her 9-year-old daughter, Cynthia, to the emergency room three times in three weeks. Cynthia had a fever and rash that were not responding to treatment for viral and bacterial illnesses. By the third visit, Cynthia was irritable and lethargic, and was admitted to the hospital for evaluation of her unusual syndrome. Soon after admission she was found to be in renal failure and was transferred to a large hospital center for dialysis. Ms. P. suggested that Cynthia might have mercury poisoning because her maternal grandmother had once had mercury poisoning. An extensive laboratory search was undertaken to explain Cynthia's renal failure, and several consultations were obtained to diagnose and manage Cynthia's illness and its complications. A diagnosis of acute interstitial nephritis secondary to mercury toxicity was eventually made, based on drastically elevated mercury levels.

When questioned, Ms. P. explained that she felt Cynthia's school had a vendetta against her family, beginning with her own mother who had been poisoned by the same teacher there. In fact, she wouldn't let Cynthia have friends over to visit because she was afraid they might be part of the evil conspiracy and would try to poison the food with mercury. Cynthia also believed she had been poisoned with mercury by her teacher. Ms. P. believed that other students had also been poisoned. The school, the Department of Social Service for Children, the police, and the district attorney were contacted, but Ms. P.'s claims could not be substantiated.

In further discussion, Ms. P. alleged other incidents that she felt were related to the vendetta. Cynthia had reportedly been sexually abused in the past at two different day-care centers, and Ms. P. had herself been sexually abused as a child in one of those same centers. In one instance involving her daughter, Ms. P. reported the allegation, but no basis for it was found. In the other instance, she did not report it, thinking she would not be believed.

Cynthia had developed normally, had briefly had some behavioral problems in school, but was in a gifted class before her illness. Cynthia's father was in prison intermittently and rarely saw his child. Ms. P.'s sister had been hospitalized in a state hospital and was treated with antipsychotics. She was said to be mentally retarded, violent, and self-mutilating. Ms. P. had been healthy, completed a general equivalency diploma, and had trained as a nurse's aide. She had no psychiatric history, did not feel depressed, denied hallucinations, and did not use alcohol or drugs.

During Cynthia's hospitalization, Ms. P. remained attentive and devoted, and the staff found her very personable. However, she became agitated about the plan to treat her daughter with prednisone (Deltasone), which she believed was evil and had made her mother ill in the past. Because the staff had by now become convinced that Ms. P. had somehow been poisoning her daughter, she was restricted to supervised visits only and was not permitted to bring her daughter any food. After two months, Cynthia became well enough to leave the hospital and was placed in foster care. Her mother was mandated by the court to enter psychiatric treatment. In treatment she continued to insist that various evil people were responsible for her daughter's illness.

Discussion For many years doctors have recognized that there are rare cases in which a person will intentionally produce or feign symptoms of a physical or mental illness when there is no apparent external incentive. That has been called Munchausen syndrome. More recently, an even rarer syndrome, called Munchausen by proxy, has been described, in which a person, almost always a mother, produces symptoms in her child, as apparently happened in this case. There have also been reports of cases in which a caretaker produced symptoms in a dependent elderly person.

In DSM-IV, factitious disorder by proxy is classified as factitious disorder not otherwise specified, a diagnosis given to the mother. (The child had no psychiatric diagnosis, but was identified with the V code, physical abuse of child.)

This case was typical in that usually the conclusion that the mother actually produced the symptoms was based on circumstantial evidence, the mother almost never acknowledging what she has done. Cynthia's mother was not typical in that her poisoning of her daughter was apparently a symptom of a delusional disorder, paranoid type, whereas most people with factitious disorder by proxy are not psychotic and seem to be motivated by the desire either to experience the sick role indirectly through their child or to be part of the system that takes care of their child. Factitious disorder by proxy, like factitious disorder itself, occurs more frequently in people who have had some long-term connection with the health-care system, either as providers or as patients. In this case, Ms. P. was trained as a nurse's aide.

Clinicians should be alert to the possibility of this condition when there is a discrepancy between the mother's complaint and the appearance of the child, when the child has been taken to see many different doctors, and when the child inexplicably gets better after being separated from the mother. Unfortunately, those mothers rarely accept treatment themselves, and the management therefore almost always requires separating the child from the mother. (From *DSM-IV Casebook.* Used with permission.)

TABLE 19-4
Presenting Complaint in Cases of Munchausen Syndrome by Proxy (in percent)

Bleeding	44
Seizures	42
Central nervous system depression	19
Apnea	15
Diarrhea	11
Vomiting	10
Fever	10
Rash	9

Table from D A Rosenberg: Web of deceit: A literature review of Munchausen syndrome by proxy Child Abuse Negl 11: 547, 1987. Used with permission.

DIFFERENTIAL DIAGNOSIS

FACTITIOUS DISORDER WITH PREDOMINANTLY PHYSICAL SIGNS AND SYMPTOMS

True physical illness Psychiatrists are often asked to confirm a diagnosis of factitious disorder with predominantly physical signs and symptoms. The first step must involve as much as possible ruling out any true physical disorder. Patients diagnosed with factitious disorders often also suffer from associated true medical complications. A patient who presents with septicemia secondary to self-injection of saliva, for example, still must be treated for sepsis. Multiple hospitalizations frequently lead to iatrogenically induced physical problems. Examples include abdominal adhesions from repeated surgeries and allergic reactions to drugs and contrast material. Many patients have histories of significant childhood illness or disability, for which they may have had extensive treatment. Residual sequelae or complications from earlier illness experiences may be present, and in fact may serve as the focal point for feigned symptoms. Once true physical conditions have been ruled out or treated, the psychiatrist must attempt to verify all the facts presented by the patient concerning prior hospitalization and medical care. Although often tedious and time-consuming, that process is essential, because interviews with reliable outside sources often reveal the false nature of the patient's illness.

Somatoform disorders A number of investigators have suggested that a useful way to think about the differential diagnosis of factitious disorder with predominately physical signs and symptoms is to consider the diagnosis along a spectrum, ranging between somatoform disorders at one end and malingering at the other.

In somatoform disorders, such as somatization disorder, conversion disorder, hypochondriasis, and pain disorder, the patient complains of physical symptoms which are excessive or for which there is no demonstrable organic basis, and there is a tendency to experience emotional distress physically. Unlike factitious disorder, the production of symptoms in somatoform disorders is unconscious and unintentional; the person is not simulating or feigning illness, but believes fully that the illness is real.

In malingering, symptoms are fabricated to achieve an overt and tangible goal, such as to seek compensation, obtain shelter, avoid work, or evade the police. Symptom production is fully conscious and intentional with obvious secondary gain, and symptoms disappear when they are no longer practically useful. Factitious disorders fall in the middle of the spectrum, with symptoms being intentionally but compulsively feigned, for largely unconscious motivations. In clinical practice, it is not always easy to distinguish definitively among those three conditions, and in fact many patients may show overlapping presentations suggesting that the disorders should not be thought of as mutually exclusive. Whether the association reflects a true continuum of illness behavior or a blurring of distinctions between conscious and unconscious behavior leading to unreliable diagnoses, is unclear.

Antisocial personality disorder Antisocial personality disorder may be incorrectly but commonly diagnosed, based on the clinical presentation of dramatic lying (pseudologia fantastica), lack of intimate relationships, hostile and provocative manner, and commonly associated substance-abuse histories.

Factitious disorder tends to have a later age of onset than antisocial personality disorder and a very different classic pattern of multiple hospitalizations and willingness to undergo the patient role as a way of life. If, however, the patient fits the criteria for both antisocial personality disorder and factitious disorder, both the Axis II and Axis I diagnoses may be made.

Borderline personality disorder Borderline personality disorder is often correctly diagnosed as an underlying Axis II condition existing concomitantly with factitious disorder. The diagnosis of borderline personality disorder may be made on the basis of the person's chaotic life-style, substance abuse, volatile interpersonal relationships, unstable sense of self, self-mutilating practices, and self-destructive manipulations.

Schizophrenia Schizophrenia may be incorrectly diagnosed based on the patient's life-style and behavior, which can appear to be nearly psychotic in its bizarreness. The patient's apparently unshakable conviction of illness can at times be mistaken for delusional thinking. However, few patients with factitious disorder show evidence of true delusions, hallucinations, or severe thought disorder.

FACTITIOUS DISORDER WITH PREDOMINANTLY PSYCHOLOGICAL SIGNS AND SYMPTOMS Differentiating the diagnosis of factitious disorder with predominantly psychological signs and symptoms, from true psychiatric disorder is extremely difficult and is only done often after prolonged investigation or observation. Even then, those involved with the care of the patient may never feel completely secure in their assessment of the situation. Complicating the picture is the assumption that virtually all patients with this type of factitious disorder have at least an underlying personality disorder (usually borderline, histrionic, or antisocial personality disorder), which means that feigned psychiatric illness coexists with severe, true psychiatric illness. Other psychiatric conditions which have been reported as being associated with factitious disorders include depressive disorders, substance-related disorders, somatization disorders, and dissociative disorders, including dissociative identity disorder. The clinician's level of suspicion that a factitious disorder is present must be raised by a number of factors, for instance, if the total clinical picture does not correspond to any recognized psychiatric disorder, but rather to the patient's perception of psychiatric disorder; if the patient's symptoms are only present or are worsened under the impression of being observed; if new symptoms continually arise that are incongruous with the already diagnosed condition; if new symptoms are produced that are similar to symptoms evidenced by other patients on the ward; if there is consistently and historically no response to standard treatment; if the presentation of the psychiatric history includes graphic, dramatic, flamboyant, or bizarre details that cannot be verified; if the psychiatric history is overly vague and inconsistent. Psychological testing (for example, projective tests, Bender Gestalt Test) may be helpful in distinguishing between factitious and true disorder.

COURSE AND PROGNOSIS

Factitious illness typically begins in early adulthood, although it has been reported during childhood and adolescence, and may be initially insidious in onset. The actual onset of episodes may follow a real illness, loss, or abandonment. As the disorder progresses, the patient becomes increasingly medically knowledgeable and sophisticated. Reviews of the literature indicate a shift from the older conceptualization of factitious disorders as invariably chronic and intractable to a newer vision of those disorders as having a range of outcomes in terms of chronicity and overall prognosis. Outcomes vary from lifelong, multiple hospitalizations with severe incapacitation to the resolution of the behavior after one or two brief episodes. Other possible outcomes include the development of new factitious symptomatology after the apparent resolution of previously described symptoms, psychotic decompensation, and suicide. Patients who wander from hospital to hospital, and thus are less compliant with treatment, appear to have a worse prognosis than other patients, as do patients who feign psychotic symptoms rather than other psychiatric presentations. The current state of understanding concerning the differential prognoses is limited. More systematic studies are needed.

TREATMENT

Wide-ranging and at times conflicting assumptions about the etiology of factitious disorders have led to a number of proposed treatment interventions, although there has been no systematic study of general efficacy or outcome. The treatment tends to be very difficult, with full resolution of symptoms rare. A number of case reports indicate that once a diagnosis is established, some factitious disorders may respond favorably to a combined medical and psychotherapeutic approach. Most investigators believe that early psychiatric consultation is helpful, particularly in preventing unneeded medical procedures. However, there is disagreement both about what psychotherapeutic intervention is most effective, and about whether and how the patient should be informed of the provisional diagnosis.

Most investigators recommend some form of confrontation of the patient (that is, in a supportive, nonaccusatory manner, coupled with assurances that care and treatment will continue, letting the patient know that the caregiving team believes the disorder to result from factors other than primarily medical ones). When undertaken in a nurturing, emphatic way, that method of confrontation ideally does not force the patient to ''lose face,'' and there is less likelihood of undesirable consequences, such as psychotic decompensation, rageful flight, or even suicide. Once the patient has been informed of the diagnosis, most researchers recommend psychiatric hospitalization. Treatment recommendations most often include psychodynamic, insight-oriented approaches in combination with behavioral techniques, with an emphasis on the concomitant treatment of any other, associated psychiatric disorder (for example, depressive disorders, borderline personality disorder, substance-related disorder).

A somewhat different technique is not to inform the patient of the team's suspicions, but rather to take the patient's symptoms seriously and at face value, and to give them a logical-scientific explanation. As part of the technique, some form of mildly aversive treatment is provided on a daily basis, with a single attending physician following the patient. Intrinsic to the approach, and applicable to others, is the belief that making the patient admit that there is no true physical disorder only serves to solidify the need to appear sick.

As with any complex disorder, the more chronic and deeply ingrained the pattern of behavior, and the more profound the psychological need to assume the sick role, the less likely the syndrome is to be modified by any intervention. An essential aspect of any treatment, regardless of chronicity, is the recognition that patients are driven by unconsciously compulsive, self-destructive impulses. The hostile and contemptuous responses patients provoke in their caregivers reflect how difficult it is to remember that they are often desperately disturbed persons willing to go to extraordinary extremes to maintain the illusion of being ill. For many of them, being a patient is the only remotely stable and gratifying identity they know.

FACTITIOUS DISORDER BY PROXY Factitious disorder by proxy presents additional challenges in treatment. The disorder is considered a form of child abuse and must be managed as such. R. M. Kravitz and R. W. Wilmott have suggested that treatment consist of three parts: (1) preventing the continued abuse of the child; (2) care of the affected child; and (3) counseling of the perpetrator. Prevention can only occur once the diagnosis is recognized, and that recognition is often delayed due in large part to the difficulty the medical team has in believing that an apparently caring parent could subject a healthy child to such potentially harmful interventions. Health care providers need to be fully informed about the nature of the disorder and the profile of the perpetrators so that they will be more readily and quickly able to identify those at high risk for that behavior. Once the diagnosis of factitious disorder by proxy is strongly suggested, the parents must be informed. Meadow recommends nonthreatening, direct confrontation, with involvement of all appropriate caregivers, including a support team of psychiatrists and child protection workers. Most studies indicate that getting the mother to admit her involvement is difficult, if not impossible. The need for denial and concealment is intense. Involving the mother with a psychiatrist both before and after confrontation is crucial in providing support. A high percentage of mothers have been reported to become acutely depressed or suicidal following confrontation.

Care of the child depends on the age and type of abuse. Some older children actually come to believe that they have the illnesses their mothers attribute to them. Children with induced factitious symptoms may go on to develop actual factitious disorders later in life if they are not properly treated. A number of investigators recommend removal of the child from the family, at least temporarily, while an intensive inpatient psychiatric evaluation is performed to determine the feasibility of eventually returning the child to the family. Long-term outcome studies of the illness indicate a generally poor prognosis due to the severity of the mother's psychopathology, and many children suffer repeated unnecessary hospitalizations and treatments.

SUGGESTED CROSS-REFERENCES

Chapter 20 is devoted to dissociative disorders. Chapter 18 discusses somatoform disorders. Section 28.2 treats malingering. Personality disorders are the subject of Chapter 25. Information on behavioral therapy is set forth in Section 31.2, and on insight-oriented psychotherapy in Section 31.1. Psychological testing is discussed in Sections 9.5 and 9.6.

REFERENCES

Amos R S, Bax D E, Bourne J T, Winfield J, Sheehan N J: Arthritis artefacta: Factitious disease in rheumatology. Br J Rheumatol *30:* 455, 1991.

*Asher R: Munchausen's syndrome. Lancet *1:* 339, 1951.

Banerjee A: Factitious disorders presenting as acute emergencies. Postgrad Med J *70:* 68, 1994.

Barker J C: The syndrome of hospital addiction (Munchausen syndrome). A report on the investigation of seven cases. J Ment Sci *108:* 167, 1962.

Bean W B: Munchausen's syndrome. Perspect Biol Med 2: 347, 1959.

Chapman, J S: Peregrinating problem patients—Munchausen's syndrome. JAMA *165:* 927, 1957.

Clark E, Melnick S C: The Munchausen syndrome or the problem of hospital hoboes. Am J Med *25:* 6, 1958.

Coons P M: Use of the MMPI to distinguish genuine from factitious multiple personality disorder. Psychol Rep *73:* 401, 1993.

Dalby J T: Detecting faking in the pre-trial psychological assessment. Am J of Forensic Psychol *6:* 49, 1988.

Dooley D P, Hodges S D, Kelly J W: Factitious infections in orthopedic patients. Orthopedics *16:* 816, 1993.

Evans G A, Gill M J: Factitious AIDS. N Engl J Med *319:* 1605, 1988.
Fonseca E, Rubio G: Factitious systemic lupus erythematosus. Lupus 2: 195, 1993.
Ford C V, Hollender M H: Lies and liars: Psychiatric aspects of prevarication. Am J Psychiatry *145:* 554, 1988.
Gavin H: *Feigned and Factitious Diseases, Chiefly of Soldiers and Seamen.* J & A Churchill, London, 1863.
Goldberg D P, Bridges K: Somatic presentations of psychiatric illness in primary care setting. J Psychosom Res *32:* 137, 1988.
Grinker R Jr: Imposture as a form of mastery. Arch Gen Psychiatry *5:* 449, 1961.
Humphries S R: Munchausen syndrome: Motives and the relation to deliberate self-harm. Br J Psychiatry *152:* 416, 1988.
Kaufman K L, Coury D, Pickrel E: Munchausen syndrome by proxy: A survey of professional's knowledge. Child Abuse Negl *13:* 141, 1989.
Keiser H R: Surreptitious self-administration of epinephrine resulting in pheochromocytoma. JAMA *266:* 1553, 1991.
Kravitz R M, Wilmott R W: Munchausen syndrome by proxy presenting as factitious apnea. Clin Pediatrics *85:* 22, 1990.
Makar A F, Squier P J: Munchausen syndrome by proxy. Father as perpetrator. Pediatr *85:* 370, 1990.
McGuire T L, Feldman K W: Psychologic morbidity of children subjected to Munchausen syndrome by proxy. Pediatrics *83:* 289, 1989.
Meadow R: Management of Munchausen syndrome by proxy. Arch Dis Child *60:* 385, 1985.
*Meadow R: Munchausen syndrome by proxy: The hinterland of child abuse. Lancet 2: 343, 1977.
Miller M, Cabeza-Stradi S: Addiction to surgery: A nursing dilemma. Crit Care Nurse *14:* 44, 1994.
Neighbour R, Middleton J, d'Ardenne P: Feigned infertility. Practitioner *237:* 727, 1993.
Prescott M V: Hospital hoppers—jumping to conclusion? Arch Emerg Med *10:* 362, 1993.
Reich P, Gottfried L A: Factitious disorders in a teaching hospital. Ann Intern Med *99:* 240, 1983.
*Rosenberg D A: Web of deceit: A literature review of Munchausen syndrome by proxy. Child Abuse Negl *11:* 547, 1987.
Schoen M: Resistance to health: When the mind interferes with the desire to become well. Am J Clin Hypn *36:* 47, 1993.
Sno H N, Storosum J G, Wortel C H: Psychogenic "HIV infection." Int J Psychiatry Med *21:* 93, 1991.
Solyom C, Solyom L: A treatment program for functional paraplegia/Munchausen syndrome. J Behav Ther Exp Psychiatry *21:* 225, 1990.
*Spiro H R: Chronic factitious illness: Munchausen's syndrome. Arch Gen Psychiatry *18:* 569, 1968.
Spivak H, Rodin G, Sutherland A: The psychology of factitious disorders. A reconsideration. Psychosomatics *35:* 25, 1994.
Stern T A: Munchausen's syndrome revisited. Psychosomatics *21:* 329, 1980.
Sullivan C A, Francis G L, Bain M W, Hartz J: Munchausen syndrome by proxy: 1990. A portent for problems? Clin Pediatr *30:* 112, 1991.
*Sutherland A J, Rodin G M: Factitious disorders in a general hospital setting: Clinical features and a review of the literature. Psychosomatics *31:* 532, 1990.
Toth E L, Baggaley A: Coexistence of Munchausen's syndrome and multiple personality disorder: Detailed report of a case and theoretical discussion. Psychiatry *54:* 1110, 1991.
Weston W A, Dalby T: A case of pseudologia fantastica with antisocial personality disorder. Can J Psychiatry *36:* 637, 1991.

CHAPTER 20 DISSOCIATIVE DISORDERS

JOHN C. NEMIAH, M.D.

INTRODUCTION

Modern interest in the dissociative disorders has been sparked in recent years by a renewed preoccupation with patients suffering from multiple personality disorders, and modern clinicians are now engaged in a voyage of rediscovery of what a century ago were well-charted waters.

HISTORY

MORTON PRINCE The publication in 1906 of Morton Prince's book *The Dissociation of a Personality* marked the apogee of early investigations of dissociative phenomena. The saga of Sally Beauchamp—"The Saint, the Devil, the Woman," as Prince ambivalently called the patient he examined in almost infinite detail—is among the most renowned of multiple personalities. In the book devoted to her biography, Prince summarized the essence of her clinical problem in a brief paragraph that delineates the characteristics of the disorder as it is known today.

"In addition," he wrote, "to the real, original or normal self, the self that was born and which she was originally intended to be, she may be any one of three different persons. I say three different because although making use of the same body, each, nevertheless, has a distinctly different character, a difference manifested by different trains of thought, by different views, beliefs, ideals, and temperament, and by different acquisitions, tastes, habits, experiences, and memories. Each varies in these respects from the other two, and from the original Miss Beauchamp. Two of these personalities have no knowledge of each other or of the third, excepting such information as may be obtained by inference or second hand, so that in the memory of these two there were blanks which correspond to the times when the others are in the flesh. Of a sudden one or the other wakes up to find herself, she knows not where, and ignorant of what she has said or done a moment before. Only one has knowledge of the lives of the others, and this one presents such a bizarre character, so far removed from the others in individuality, that the transformation from one of the other personalities to herself is one of the most striking and dramatic features of the case. The personalities come and go in kaleidoscopic succession, many changes often being made in the course of twenty-four hours. And so it happens that Miss Beauchamp, if I may use the name to designate several distinct people, at one moment says and does and plans and arranges something to which a short time before she most strongly objected, indulges in tastes which a moment before would have been abhorrent to her ideals, and undoes what she had just laboriously planned and arranged."

EUGÈNE AZAM Although perhaps the most dramatic member of the family of multiple personality disorders, Miss Beauchamp was only one of a number of patients with a variety of strange disruptions of memory and striking changes in personality whose histories were recounted throughout the Victorian and Edwardian eras. The account of Félida X. by Eugène Azam holds a place of particular historical importance. Suffering from the classical symptoms of multiple personality disorder, Félida consulted Azam in the 1850s. Although a surgeon by profession, Azam was fascinated by what he termed her "doubling of personality" and undertook an extensive course of treatment, which he subsequently described in the first French publications about the disorder. As a part of his therapeutic program, Azam applied the hypnotic techniques developed by James Braid a decade or two earlier in England. Azam's introduction of Braid's concepts and procedures into France met with a cool reception from his colleagues at a time when hypnotism and mesmerism were considered mere charlatinism. Not until 30 years later did Azam receive due appreciation, when Jean-Martin Charcot, whose investigations of hysteria rehabilitated hypnotic phenomena, recognized him publicly as a pioneer in the field.

PIERRE JANET Charcot's work had widespread ramifications, but perhaps its most important influence was on an obscure young professor of philosophy at the Lyceum in Le Havre during the 1880s. Working toward his *doctorat en philosophie,* Pierre Janet chose to focus his attention on pathological psychology. Through the kindness of two local physicians, Dr. Gibert and Dr. Powilewicz, he was able to study a series of hysterical patients, using the hypnotic techniques that Charcot had established as tools of observation and experimentation. In that setting and subsequently at the Salpêtrière in Charcot's clinic, Janet developed the concept of mental dissociation, a term that not only lends its name to the current nosological category of dissociative disorders but remains the bedrock of modern understanding of their clinical manifestations. Janet's observations and theoretical formulations are set forth in the first two of the many volumes he wrote during his lifetime, *L'automatisme psychologique* and *The Mental State of Hystericals.*

Intellectual background Despite his rustication in the provinces, Janet was not working in an intellectual vacuum. His uncle, Paul Janet, was a distinguished philosopher; he had for models contemporary savants like Hippolyte Taine and Théodule Ribot, whose writings were establishing the basis of pathological psychology; and he was significantly influenced by the investigations of Frederic W. H. Myers and Edmund Gurney, who were engaged in studies of hypnosis and automatic writing under the auspices of the Society for Psychical Research in England. Janet's own clinical investigations, however, carried from the start the stamp of his unique creative imagination that later made him preeminent in the field.

Hypnosis Following Charcot's lead, Janet used hypnosis as a primary investigative technique in his study of well over 100 patients during his sojourn at Le Havre and later in Paris. In his hands hypnosis became a sophisticated procedure that enabled him to uncover complex mental elements ordinarily unavailable to his patients' conscious awareness. In particular, it allowed him to restore to consciousness long-forgotten, buried memories of traumatic events that were significantly related to his patients' clinical symptoms.

Marie In the numerous detailed case histories that fill the pages of his early writings, Janet demonstrated the role of memories in the psychogenesis and the treatment of hysterical disorders. Marie, for example, a young woman of 19, had suffered from numbness of the left side of her face and blindness in her left eye for as long as she could remember. Although Marie maintained that the symptoms had existed from the time of her birth, it was, as Janet reported, "easy to demonstrate in hypnotic somnabulism that she was mistaken. If one changed her into a small child of five by the usual procedure [that is, hypnotic age-regression], she recovered the sensation that she had had at that age, and one could observe that she saw very well with both eyes. It was when she was six that the blindness had begun. What were the circumstances? Marie persisted in stating, when she was awake, that she had absolutely no idea. During hypnotic trance, however, in which I caused her to relive the significant events of her life at that period, I determined that the blindness had begun at a specific moment in connection with a trifling incident. She had been forced, despite her screams of protest, to sleep with a child of her own age *the left side of whose face was covered with impetiginous scabs* [italics in the original]. Some time afterward Marie herself developed similar scabs in the same location. These occurred annually at the same time of year for several years and then disappeared completely. No one, however, noticed that from that point on *the left side of her face was anesthetic and she was blind in her left eye* [italics in the original]. She has always since retained this anesthesia."

Janet then proceeded to describe his treatment. "I brought her back [in hypnosis] to the time of the episode with the child of whom she had such horror. I caused her to believe that the child was very attractive and had no impetiginous lesions, but she was only half convinced.

After two repetitions of the scene I was successful, and she fearlessly caressed the imaginary child. The sensation in the left side of her face reappeared without difficulty, and when I woke her up, Marie saw clearly with her left eye.'' By changing the cognitive content of the patient's memories, a maneuver similar to the guiding principle of modern cognitive therapy, Janet succeeded in removing symptoms that had been continuously present for more than a decade—a therapeutic result that persisted, as Janet commented in a follow-up note, for at least five months.

Marie's history shows the basic clinical observations that underlay Janet's conceptualization of dissociation, a mental process central to the psychological understanding of hysterical symptoms that is as vital and valid today as it was when Janet described it 100 years ago. First and foremost is the fact that memories of an early traumatic event are unavailable to Marie's voluntary recall; as a result, the memories are excluded from her conscious awareness and are totally separated (''dissociated'' in Janet's terminology) from Marie's personal consciousness of herself as an individual human being possessing a life history and a personality of her own. At the same time, despite the dissociation of Marie's mental organization, the interrelated mental events divorced from and unavailable to her personal consciousness are not obliterated. On the contrary, they remain intact and persist indefinitely in an unconscious state with a life and a consciousness of their own. As Janet's friend and colleague Alfred Binet phrased it, they constituted a ''secondary consciousness'' beneath the surface.

Although Marie had no access to that unconscious complex of interrelated mental events, the memories could be uncovered and exposed to observation by hypnosis, to which patients with dissociative disorders are particularly responsive. Hypnotic procedures enable the hypnotist to produce artificial dissociative states in which it is possible to raise into consciousness dissociated elements ordinarily unavailable to the person's consciousness. During hypnotic trance Marie could recall early traumatic memories of which she usually had no knowledge and that disappeared again, beyond her conscious voluntary control, when she awoke from the induced trance state.

Ordinarily excluded from her conscious awareness, Marie's traumatic memories significantly affected her everyday functioning by inducing symptoms that represented and reproduced the form and content of the memories. Marie had no awareness of the connection, but, once the dissociated memories were recovered under hypnosis, it was self-evident that the frightening image of her friend's impetiginous lesions was literally and graphically reflected in the site and the distribution of her conversion symptoms.

Early influence of Janet's ideas Although Janet never became the center of a school or a movement, his writings and ideas influenced many clinicians in France, England, and the United States, who pursued clinical experiments with hypnosis and added clinical data that substantiated and extended Janet's concept of dissociation. As the focal psychopathological process at work in hysterical patients, dissociation provided a simple and useful explanation for the variety of clinical forms that hysteria manifested. The disappearance of dissociated memories from conscious awareness and voluntary recall produced clinical amnesia, whereas the dissociative disappearance of sensations and patterns of movements led to sensorimotor conversion symptoms, such as anesthesias and paralyses. Such negative symptoms resulting from the loss of functions were matched by positive symptoms when the underlying dissociated contents exerted a direct effect on surface functioning; thus, the partial return of dissociated sensations or ideas of motor movements produced hallucinations or abnormal movements and muscular spasms that were ego-alien if the personal consciousness remained intact. By contrast, if the returning dissociated mental elements overwhelmed and replaced the personal consciousness, abnormal trance states resulted, and the patient appeared to relive and to reenact the intruding, often traumatic memories. In its ultimate form the intruding mental elements led to the total replacement of the ordinary personal consciousness by an emerging alternative personality, resulting in the characteristic clinical manifestations of multiple personality disorder (now called dissociative identity disorder).

The complexity of the hysterical symptoms and the usefulness of the concept of dissociation for understanding their genesis and variety were fully recognized by early investigators. Morton Prince, for example, commented some 70 years ago in his major work, *The Unconscious*: ''As a result of dissociation, systems of thoughts, ideas, memories, emotions, and dispositions previously habitual in the individual may cease to take part in the affected person's mental processes. Examination of recorded cases shows that besides mental memories, physiological functions may be involved in dissociation. Thus, there may be a loss of sensation in its various forms, and of the special senses, or of the power of movement (paralyses), or of visceral functions (gastric, sexual, etc.). Dissociation may, then, involve quite large parts of the personality, including very precise and definite physiological and psychological functions.''

ETIOLOGY

DISSOCIATION, HYPNOSIS, AND THE UNCONSCIOUS

The dissociative process is central to the genesis of the disorders that bear its name. Of equal importance for the understanding of symptom formation is the existence of the related underlying unconscious mental elements that help determine the form and the nature of the surface clinical syndromes. Furthermore, any consideration of dissociation would be incomplete without the recognition of its essential relation to hypnosis. In Janet's hands hypnosis became a vital experimental tool for exploring dissociative phenomena. Not only could hypnosis raise into consciousness those mental elements rendered unconscious by the dissociative process, but it could also produce many of the phenomena that occurred clinically as dissociative symptoms. Amnesias, trance states, and a variety of localized paralyses, anesthesias, paresthesias, and hallucinations induced by hypnotic suggestion were indistinguishable from those occurring symptomatically in hysterical patients. Dissociation and hypnosis, in other words, are but two sides of the same coin, a fact further attested to by the high degree of hypnotizability of persons with dissociative disorders.

JANET AND *LA MISÈRE PSYCHOLOGIQUE* If, as Janet commented, dissociation and unconscious mental elements are empirically demonstrated facts, it remains to be explained how and why dissociative processes occur in the first place. Janet postulated that dissociation results from what he termed *la misère psychologique*—that is, a pathological, presumably genetic poverty or deficiency of the basic mental energy that enables healthy persons to combine the various mental functions (sensations, memories, volitions) into a stable, unified psychological structure under the conscious domination and control of the personal self or ego. If, either spontaneously or as the result of the emotional expenditure of mental energy in the face of psychological trauma, the quantum of energy is lowered below a critical point, the binding power of the personal self is seriously impaired, and the various psychological functions escape from its control (that is, they are dissociated, with all the potential pathological consequences that have been described).

FREUD AND PSYCHOLOGICAL CONFLICT Sigmund Freud, like Janet, based his initial psychological explanation of the psychogenesis of hysteria (particularly in its manifestations as conversion symptoms) on the occurrence of a dissociative disappearance from consciousness of mental contents that, although now unconscious, can influence the form and the distribution of hysterical symptoms. ''Hysterics,'' as Freud wrote, ''suffer mainly from reminiscences.'' When, however, he came to explain the origin of the basic phenomenon of dissociation, Freud parted company with Janet. Unlike Janet, who tended to shy away from the emotional aspects of the human psyche, Freud from the earliest days of his psychological investigations viewed them as a central factor in mental disorders. Impressed by the painful quality of traumatic memories, he postulated that the traumatized person actively dissociated or, in his terminology, ''repressed'' the painful memories from conscious awareness and, by a continuation of that repression, maintained them over time in an unconscious state to prevent the conscious experiencing of the painful emotions associated with them. In other words, whereas Janet adhered to a deficit model of psychic functioning in which the ego is too weak to retain control of the psychic elements, Freud proposed a conflict model in which a strong ego vigorously protects itself from psychological pain through the operation of the defensive mechanism of repression—a process manifested phenomenologically as dissociation.

PSYCHOLOGICAL TRAUMA Regardless of the differences in their theoretical models of psychological functioning, both Freud and Janet initially emphasized the importance of traumatic events and their painful memory traces as a central factor in the formation of symptoms. Freud later shifted his attention from painful memories of actual traumatic events to the existence of painful, developmentally derived inner sexual and hostile drives and fantasies as the source of psychological conflict—a change in view that ultimately overshadowed Janet's observations and formulations as psychoanalytic theory became a dominant force in the development of 20th-century psychiatry.

Freud's and Janet's concern with psychological trauma is mirrored in the modern recognition of the importance of traumatic events in the genesis of dissociative disorders. That recognition derives in part from the study of posttraumatic stress disorder in Vietnam War veterans and in the victims of civilian disasters and in part (and perhaps most significantly) from the frequent reports of childhood physical and sexual abuse in patients with dissociative identity disorder.

MODERN VIEWS Despite the early recognition of the central role of dissociation in the panoply of hysterical symptoms, its importance has often been lost sight of by later generations of psychiatrists, who have tended to emphasize the distinction between the physical and the mental manifestations of hysterical illness. A significant impetus toward that separation came from Sigmund Freud, whose initial psychoanalytic studies of hysteria were focused on its somatic symptoms, the formation of which, he proposed, resulted from the specific psychological mechanism of conversion. Subsequent nosological classifications of the neuroses, although generally retaining the overall category of hysteria, divided it into conversion hysteria and dissociative hysteria. With the publication of the first edition of the American Psychiatric Association's *Diagnostic and Statistical Manual of Mental Disorders* (DSM-I) in 1952, the two were separated into the seemingly unrelated categories of conversion reaction and dissociative reaction. Although the breach was temporarily healed with the publication of the second edition of DSM (DSM-II) in 1968, which referred to hysterical neurosis, conversion type, and hysterical neurosis, dissociative type, the two categories were drastically torn apart in the radical revision of psychiatric nosology set forth in the third edition (DSM-III) in 1980 and its subsequent revision in 1985 (DSM-III-R). In the last two editions, conversion disorder is listed as a type of somatoform disorders, a major nosological category totally distinct from the equally major category of dissociative disorders, a distinction that is retained in the fourth edition (DSM-IV).

The motivation behind the current classification is understandable and is based in part on a valid concern. Over the centuries hysteria has been wanton in the partners it has taken into its bed, and the term eventually had so many referents that it verged on the useless as a diagnotic category. A mélange of somatic symptoms, a variety of alterations of consciousness, a diversity of character traits, a specific psychodynamic mechanism (conversion), phobic behavior (anxiety hysteria)—all huddled promiscuously under the covers and were commonly referred to, singly or collectively, as hysteria.

The current classificatory scheme attempts to bring order out of chaos by separating the protean symptoms labeled hysterical into what seem to be naturally related clusters or syndromes. In so doing, it appropriately draws attention to the predisposition in many patients to somatization, a process that has been inadequately studied and remains poorly understood. In its zeal for empiricism, however, DSM-IV and its immediate predecessors have perhaps overshot the mark in separating conversion disorder from the dissociative disorders and in overlooking the psychogenetic role of dissociation common to them all. Although there are clearly phenomenological grounds for making the diagnostic distinction (which, in conformity with the classificatory scheme of DSM-IV, is followed in the description of the dissociative disorders that follows), one does well to keep firmly in mind the clinical and historical origins of the term "dissociation," which designates a process underlying the genesis of both the somatic and the mental symptoms of the disorder traditionally referred to as hysteria.

CLINICAL SYNDROMES

Following the nosological scheme established by DSM-III, DSM-IV applies the term *"dissociative disorders"* to symptomatic disturbances of memory, consciousness, and personal identity. Sharing the underlying process of dissociation, the disorders are distinguished nosologically by phenomenological variations that are determined by the range of the patient's state of awareness and the extent and the nature of the intrusion of the dissociated mental elements into consciousness.

DISSOCIATIVE AMNESIA The central feature of dissociative amnesia, as the term implies, is a loss of memory, frequently sudden in onset, of personal experiences and events that are often physically and emotionally traumatic.

Epidemiology The prevalence, the incidence, and the sexual distribution of dissociative amnesia have not been adequately determined. In general clinical practice it is perhaps most commonly seen in general hospital emergency departments, where patients suffering from the disorder are taken by the police after being found wandering confusedly in the street. Recent studies of populations subjected to obviously traumatic situations (combat, civilian disasters, and mass abductions, for example) indicate that dissociative amnesia is a common short-term reaction to such stress in both men and women.

Etiology Emotional trauma is a frequent causative factor in the production of amnesia, perhaps potentiated by a person's predisposition to dissociation. The amnesia is the manifest result of the dissociative process as it acts to exclude mental contents from conscious awareness. Although the amnesia is the predominant symptom of the disorder, careful examination often reveals secondary clinical phenomena, such as conversion symptoms, that represent the return to consciousness of isolated, ego-alien fragments of dissociated mental contents, such as the hallucinatory visions observed in the case of Barbara M., described below.

Diagnosis and clinical features In its most common form the amnesia is localized; patients are unable to recall any of the events that have occurred during a specific period of time extending over a few hours to days. The traumatic event is the focal point of the amnesia, but the events leading up to that central point and after it are often forgotten as well. Far less frequently, the amnesia extends over the events of the person's entire life (generalized amnesia). Occasionally, the amnesia is restricted to selected memories, involving, for example, only those related to a specific person (selective or systematic amnesia); even more rarely, patients manifest a *continuous amnesia,* which causes them to forget ongoing, successive events as they occur from moment to moment. The DSM-IV diagnostic criteria for dissociative amnesia are given in Table 20-1.

In the earliest phase of an amnestic episode, a patient may forget aspects of identity, such as name and address, but that phenomenon is transitory, and personal identity characteristically remains unaltered and uncompromised throughout the duration of the amnesia. Despite the seriousness and the extent of the memory loss, patients generally appear remarkably unconcerned about the deficit. The memory loss is explicit or episodic (that is, it affects the recall only of discrete autobiographical events and experiences; the implicit or semantic memory of language, of learned skills, of general factual information, and of customary patterns of social behavior remains entirely intact). The case of Barbara M. illustrates many of those clinical features.

Barbara M. was a young unmarried mother of a 3-year-old son. Early one evening the police took her to the emergency ward of a large general hospital. Although aware of her identity, she could remember nothing of the events of the preceding eight hours. Pressed to recollect them, she was aware only of a vivid, hallucinatory vision of a parking lot full of cars and "someone running to someone for help," a scene to which she could attach no meaning or relation with herself.

Admitted to the psychiatric unit, she continued to be amnestic, despite all the therapeutic attempts to revive her hidden memories. She could, however, recount in detail the events of a short but troubled life. Some years earlier, her parents had separated because of her mother's flagrant promiscuity. The patient initially lived with her mother; she was witness to her mother's many affairs and was on occasion sexually approached by her mother's male visitors. At 17 she gave birth to a boy after being jilted by the infant's father. After a painful rift with her mother, the patient went to live with her father, but the change brought her little peace or security, and her life was punctuated by bitter arguments with both her father and her brother. The two weeks before the onset of her amnesia had been particularly quarrelsome, and the patient found herself growing increasingly disturbed. Her only source of comfort was a new boyfriend, Frank, to whom she had become deeply attached. Despite seeing him daily, she experienced mounting anxiety, headaches, fatigue, insomnia, depression, and despair. On the day her amnesia began, she had been on her way to her doctor because of her increasingly distressing symptoms. Her last memory was of boarding a bus to reach his office.

When her amnesia had not lifted by the end of a week in the hospital, it was decided to use hypnosis to retrieve her lost memories. The patient responded readily to trance induction, and, when questioned about the events covered by the amnestic interval, she was able to recount the details with a considerable show of emotion. At her doctor's office she found to her dismay that he was unavailable. Wondering what to do, she suddenly thought of Frank and impulsively decided to visit him at his place of work. As she approached the parking lot of the factory where he was employed, she saw his car in the distance and Frank himself walking toward it to go home. She ran to catch him but in vain. He did not see her and drove off, leaving her behind in despair. Suddenly, she felt dizzy, frightened, disappointed, angry, abandoned, and confused, and, as she said, "I just gave up." Not knowing where to turn, she wandered in a daze along the street, where the police found her and took her to the hospital.

When the patient was wakened from hypnosis, she retained all the painful memories that she had recovered in the trance state, with no subsequent recurrence of the amnesia. From that point on she had no further dissociative symptoms, and she was able to confront her emotional difficulties directly in outpatient psychotherapy.

TABLE 20-1
Diagnostic Criteria for Dissociative Amnesia

A. The predominant disturbance is one or more episodes of inability to recall important personal information, usually of a traumatic or stressful nature, that is too extensive to be explained by ordinary forgetfulness.
B. The disturbance does not occur exclusively as a symptom of dissociative identity disorder, dissociative fugue, posttraumatic stress disorder, acute stress disorder, or somatization disorder and is not due to the direct physiological effects of a substance (e.g., a drug of abuse, a medication) or a neurological or other general medical condition (e.g., amnestic disorder due to head trauma).
C. The symptoms cause clinically significant distress or impairment in social, occupational, or other important areas of functioning.

Table from DSM-IV, *Diagnostic and Statistical Manual of Mental Disorders,* ed 4. Copyright American Psychiatric Association, Washington, 1994. Used with permission.

Differential diagnosis When one is confronted with a patient with amnesia, the basic task in the differential diagnosis is to determine whether the absence of memories is the result of dissociative mechanisms or of gross physiological disturbances in brain function secondary either to external factors, such as trauma to the head, or to an internal pathological state, such as epileptic foci or vascular disease. Head trauma may occur at any age and is usually readily ascertained by the history and the physical evidence of injury, by a period of unconsciousness after the trauma, and by a persisting retrograde amnesia. The diagnosis of epilepsy may be established by a history of repeated epileptic seizures, supported by the evidence of characteristic electroencephalographic tracings. Transient global amnesia is found mainly in elderly patients with vascular disease, which leads to transient ischemic episodes affecting the limbic midline brain structures that produce both anterograde amnesia and retrograde amnesia.

In amnesia due to gross disturbances in cerebral function, the amnesia is permanent, and no memories can be retrieved by the usual techniques, hypnotic and otherwise, used to raise dissociated memories into consciousness. Dissociative amnesia appears to result from a dysfunction in the process of memory recall, whereas the amnesia due to brain disease involves a disturbance in the neurophysiological processes underlying the registration of memory traces. A patient observed by Romolo Righetti in a study of amnesia undertaken early in the 20th century accentuates that distinction.

"On the morning of the second of December, 1912," Righetti reported "Joseph P., an unmarried travelling salesman of about 23 years of age, for personal reasons, fired a pistol shot at his sister-in-law, causing a slight wound in her lumbar region; then suddenly turning the revolver on himself, he fired several shots point blank in the direction of his right auditory canal. As X-rays later confirmed, one bullet penetrated the cranial cavity through the petrous bone, injuring the brain substance of the right temporal pole and the contiguous portion of the frontal lobe of the same side. As an immediate consequence of the wound, the patient fell face down on the ground with a serious hemorrhage from his right auditory meatus and lost complete consciousness for a period of about an hour. Taken to the hospital, the injured man during the initial phase of the treatment deliriously uttered a few words ("that whore"), alluding to the lady at whom he had shot."

For three days thereafter the patient remained in shock and was semistuporous, after which he began to recover rapidly. His mental functioning was tested from that time on at regular intervals and consistently showed a marked, although circumscribed, loss of memory that was completely blank for a period that extended back to a month before his homocidal-suicidal act and forward in time to 40 days after the event.

Two years and three months after the injury, "on the night of the 13th of March, 1915," Righetti reported, "the patient had a dream in which he found himself in an insane asylum, without being able to discover the reason for his being there. All of a sudden there reappeared in his mind (in the dream) the episode of the 2nd of December with all of its particulars. He awoke with a start, the dream image remained in his consciousness, and from that moment on the patient retained a clear memory of the passionate scene that had transpired between himself and his sister-in-law up until the instant he had lost consciousness as a result of the revolver shot aimed at himself." Thereafter he recovered all his lost memories of events before and after the injury, except that, as the clinical account concluded, "There persisted a short gap in memory corresponding to the period of post-traumatic confusion."

Joseph P. had two kinds of amnesia. In one, the memories that were absent pertained to the short period immediately after the injury when the patient was semistuporous. Memory for that brief period appeared to be irrevocable. In the other, the absent memories were of events that extended over many weeks before and after the injury; during that time the patient was mentally alert and responded normally to his environment. Memories of that period, although unavailable for two years and three months after the shooting, were not permanently lost but returned at the end of that time with every detail intact. Furthermore, they returned suddenly and dramatically, irrupting into the patient's conscious awareness in the form of a vivid dream.

Similarly, the term *''unconscious''* is used in connection with the two sets of phenomena, again in two senses. In the first sense, the patient is unconscious, with the implication that the functioning of the brain is so grossly impaired that the patient is totally unaware of external stimuli and unable to respond to them. As a result of the disturbance in brain function, permanent memory traces of environmental events cannot be recorded; on regaining consciousness, the patient has a lasting amnesia for the period of impaired brain function. In that context, the words ''unconscious'' and ''amnesia'' are used to refer to events and processes that have a physiological frame of reference.

In the second sense, the memories are unconscious, with the implication that, although unavailable to consciousness by voluntary recall, they do not lack an underlying neural registration but are potentially accessible to conscious awareness, given the proper circumstances. Here, ''amnesia'' and ''unconscious'' refer to events and processes in a psychological frame of reference.

Course and prognosis Episodes of dissociative amnesia are generally short and self-limited, and the outlook for the recovery of the lost memories is good, particularly if appropriate therapeutic measures are applied. However, the tendency of patients with such a disorder to resort to dissociative mechanisms when they are under environmental or instinctual pressure remains a continuing liability.

Treatment The clinician must restore the lost memories to consciousness as soon as possible. In some cases one can get at the dissociated mental contents in one or two interviews by allowing patients to free-associate or by encouraging them to give their associations to a specific fragment of the dissociated material that has returned to consciousness in the form of a waking mental image, dream, or hallucination. At other times active measures, such as hypnosis and intravenous thiopental (Pentothal), may be required to mobilize the underlying memories. Once the memories are obtained, the clinician should suggest that the memories will be retained in consciousness after the patient has returned to normal consciousness. After that initial therapeutic intervention, extensive psychotherapy is often indicated to help the patient deal with the psychological conflicts that precipitated the amnestic episode.

DISSOCIATIVE FUGUE

Dissociative fugue is characterized by a sudden loss of personal identity and of the memory of one's entire past life, by the assumption of a new identity, and by a tendency to wander far from home to take up a new residence, occupation, and life.

Epidemiology Although its incidence and prevalence are unknown, dissociative fugue appears to be a rare disorder and to occur mainly in men. The dramatic features of the disorder compel widespread human interest, and accounts of persons found suffering from it are frequently published in the lay press.

Etiology The disorder usually occurs in the context of heightened emotional tension arising from conflicts in one's personal or professional life. It may also begin after stressful exposure to civilian catastrophes or military combat. As in the other dissociative disorders, the process of dissociation is the central causative factor in symptom formation. It results in the exclusion from consciousness of the patient's personal identity and memories of the past.

Diagnosis and clinical features Despite the magnitude and the extent of their dissociated memories and the loss of their customary personal identity, patients are unaware of the dramatic changes that have taken place (Table 20-2). After establishing a new residence, occupation, and identity, they not only have no recollection of their past but have no awareness that their memories of it are missing. They generally lead quiet, prosaic, somewhat seclusive lives, work at simple occupations, live modestly, and do nothing to draw to themselves the attention or the suspicions of their neighbors and acquaintances. Except for the distressed relatives of the missing person, no one, including the patient, is aware that anything is amiss. Only when, sometimes after many weeks, such patients suddenly revert to being their former selves do they become aware, often with great emotional distress, of an amnestic gap in their memories for the periods occupied by the fugue state. The amnesia may often be reversed by hypnotic procedures.

Perhaps the most renowned victim of dissociative fugue is the Reverend Mr. Ansel Bourne, who derives his fame from the fact that William James recorded his history in *The Principles of Psychology*.

> ''On January 17, 1887,'' recounted James, ''he drew 551 dollars from a bank in Providence with which to pay for a certain lot of land in Greene, paid certain bills, and got into a Pawtucket horsecar. This is the last incident which he remembers. He did not return home that day, and nothing was heard of him for two months. On the morning of March 14th, however, at Norristown, Pennsylvania, a man calling himself A. J. Brown, who had rented a small shop six weeks previously, stocked it with stationery, confectionery, fruit and small articles, and carried on his quiet trade without seeming to any one unnatural or eccentric, woke up in a fright and called the people of the house to tell him where he was. He said that his name was Ansel Bourne, that he was entirely ignorant of Norristown, that he knew nothing of shopkeeping, and that the last thing he remembered—it seemed only yesterday—was drawing the money from the bank, etc., in Providence. He would not believe that two months had elapsed.''
>
> After his return to Providence, Bourne was completely amnesic for the two months of his absence. No information was available about the two weeks in which he had traveled from his home to Norristown, but his neighbors there described him (as James reports it) ''as taciturn, orderly in his habits, and in no way queer. He went to Philadelphia several times; replenished his stock; cooked for himself in the back shop, where he slept; went regularly to church; and once at a prayer meeting made what was considered by the hearers a good address, in the course of which he related an incident which he had witnessed in his natural state of Bourne.''

TABLE 20-2
Diagnostic Criteria for Dissociative Fugue

A. The predominant disturbance is sudden, unexpected travel away from home or one's customary place of work, with inability to recall one's past.
B. Confusion about personal identity or assumption of a new identity (partial or complete).
C. The disturbance does not occur exclusively during the course of dissociative identity disorder and is not due to the direct physiological effects of a substance (e.g., a drug of abuse, a medication) or a general medical condition (e.g., temporal lobe epilepsy).
D. The symptoms cause clinically significant distress or impairment in social, occupational, or other important areas of functioning.

Table from DSM-IV, *Diagnostic and Statistical Manual of Mental Disorders,* ed 4. Copyright American Psychiatric Association, Washington, 1994. Used with permission.

Not until 1890 did James have the opportunity to examine the patient. Under hypnosis it was possible to revive the lost memories, which were readily recovered in the trance state—"so much so indeed," commented James, "that it proved quite impossible to make him whilst in the hypnosis remember any of the facts of his normal life. He had heard of Ansel Bourne but 'didn't know as he had ever met the man.' When confronted with Mrs. Bourne, he said that he had 'never seen the woman before.' On the other hand he told of his peregrinations during the lost fortnight, and gave all sorts of details about the Norristown episode. The whole thing was prosaic enough, and the Brown personality seems to be nothing but a rather shrunken, dejected, and amnesic extract of Bourne himself. I had hoped by suggestions to run the two personalities into one, and make the memories continuous, but no artifice would avail to accomplish this, and Mr. Bourne's skull to-day still covers two distinct personal selves."

Differential diagnosis Patients with dissociative amnesia have no lasting loss of personal identity or tendency to wander; the amnestic gap covers a restricted set of memories and a limited period of time; and the patients are aware of the hiatus in their memories. Patients with dissociative identity disorder usually have several distinct personalities, which are different from one another and which alternate in dominating consciousness with considerable frequency and fluidity. The primary personality is aware of an amnestic gap for the period when an alternate personality is in the ascendancy, and often one secondary personality is aware not only of itself but also of the existence and the mental contents of the primary and other personalities. Unlike patients in a fugue state, patients with dissociative trance disorder manifest an alteration in their behavior and state of consciousness that is readily detectable by observers and that distinguishes them from patients with fugue and other forms of dissociative disorders.

Course and prognosis Whether the fugue state is of short or long duration, it tends to remit spontaneously and rarely recurs.

Treatment The memories of events occurring during the period of the fugue may be recalled under hypnosis, although, as the case of Ansel Bourne suggests, the patient may have difficulty in retaining those memories when the hypnotic procedure is terminated. If the patient is seen during the fugue state itself, hypnosis may be helpful in restoring the personal identity and the memories of the past associated with the patient's customary self. For patients whose disorder has arisen in the setting of conflicts over their personal lives and relationships, prolonged psychotherapy after the termination of the fugue state may be helpful in resolving the precipitating conflicts.

DISSOCIATIVE IDENTITY DISORDER (MULTIPLE PERSONALITY DISORDER) After a century of existence, multiple personality disorder has succumbed to its own disease and emerges in DSM-IV as its alter, dissociative identity disorder. Like Proteus of the ancient seas, patients with dissociative identity disorder elusively assume many forms as clinicians try to grasp the essence of their origins. Such patients characteristically manifest two or more distinct, complexly woven personalities, each often designated by an identifying name. The personalities alternate kaleidoscopically with one another in dominating and controlling consciousness, and they exhibit varying degrees of amnesia for the existence and the mental contents of the other personalities.

Epidemiology Of all the dissociative disorders, dissociative identity disorder holds center stage in modern clinical interest—a rise to stardom that has occurred only during the past decade. As noted earlier, Victorian and Edwardian clinicians were well aware of the condition, but it was deemed rare and achieved notoriety mainly through a handful of lengthy, detailed, and dramatically written clinical biographies. During most of the 20th century it remained retiringly in the wings. In the 1970s an increasing number of reports began to appear in the literature, and the disorder became the focus of attention of a growing group of clinicians who collected extensive data on its prevalence and psychopathological features. More than 1,000 new cases have now been documented. The syndrome is found predominantly in women, and, in several series of patients examined with structured diagnostic interviews, it constitutes 3 to 5 percent of several different populations of patients with a variety of mental disorders.

The reasons for the surge in the prevalence of a disorder previously considered rare are not clear. Perhaps the basic underlying factors are the revival of interest in recent years in the psychological trauma associated with military combat and civilian disasters and with child abuse and the recognition that dissociative mechanisms play a vital part in coping with such traumas. Since both dissociative mechanisms and a history of child abuse are prominent features of dissociative identity disorder, clinicians have been sensitized to the existence of the syndrome and may include it more actively than in the past in their diagnostic considerations. Thus alerted, they now search for the existence of dissociative phenomena, about which patients are often secretive unless encouraged to reveal them by a sympathetic examiner. As a result, the diagnosis is less frequently overlooked than it once was. Whatever the reasons for its occurrence, the revived interest in dissociative identity disorder has brought about a renewal of psychiatric attention to the psychological dimensions of mental illness.

Etiology The fundamental mechanism leading to the genesis of dissociative identity disorder is (as with the other dissociative disorders) the process of psychological dissociation. It differs from the other dissociative syndromes in the fact that the dissociated unconscious mental elements in patients with dissociative identity disorder achieve a structure, complexity, and organization that constitute an autonomously functioning personality with distinctive characteristics and a separate personal identity of its own. In contrast, in the other dissociative disorders (save for dissociative fugue) the dissociated mental elements are only fragments of an otherwise intact, single, unitary personality.

As in all the dissociative disorders, the mechanism of dissociation serves a psychological defensive function by protecting the patient from the painful conscious awareness of emotionally disturbing mental contents, which may be either memories of traumatic events or the experiencing of the fantasies, emotions, and impulses associated with sexual and aggressive drives that the patient finds personally undesirable and unacceptable. Modern clinical investigators generally emphasize the causative role of traumatic memories; a history of childhood physical and sexual abuse in patients with dissociative identity disorder occurs in 90 percent of patients in some clinical series.

Some investigators have cautioned against a too ready acceptance of reports of child abuse, since the reports generally derive from the recollections of adult patients of long-past periods of early life. Although a history of abuse has not infrequently been independently verified, such verification is often lacking. In at least one study an extensive independent investigation of several reports of abuse in satanic cults could find no evidence of the occurrence of the reported events. The question is further confounded by the often marked propensity of patients with strong dissociative tendencies to have a firm conviction of the reality of ideas suggested to them by others. In the light of those uncertainties, the final determination of the role of child abuse in the genesis of dissociative identity disorder must await further scientific examination. At the same time, from a pragmatic clinical point of view, recollections of abuse, whether fact or fantasy or a mixture of both, are deeply troubling, profoundly anxiety-provoking, and terrifying to the patients who hold them. Therapists must explore the recollections with respectful acceptance, compassionate concern, and understanding sensitivity.

Clinical features Although patients with dissociative identity disorder may not appear to be abnormal when they are seen in passing during the presence of any one of their personality states, prolonged contact with them soon discloses the alternation of personalities that characterizes the syndrome. The shift from one personality (or *alter* as the individual personalities are now commonly called) is often sudden, and the shift dramatically changes the patient's entire demeanor. Such a change may frequently be observed during a clinical interview when the interviewer asks to talk to a specific alter. A depressed, retiring, somber, moralistic woman with multiple somatic complaints may in the twinkling of an eye (often marked by a momentary mental absence) become gay, effervescent, outgoing, and fun-loving, entirely free of somatic complaints, and caustically disparaging of the sick person she had been a moment before. When the clinician attempts to recall dissociated anxiety-provoking memories, the patient may abruptly switch to any of a variety of alters that represent an identification with one or another of the actors in the original traumatic episode. One alter, for example, may be hostile and threateningly aggressive in imitation of the perpetrator of a traumatic assault, or it may be a kindly helper in identification with a protecting older figure during the period of the early traumatic events. In some alternate states patients assume the role of the victim, with a marked propensity for self-harm and self-mutilation, such as cutting or burning themselves.

The alters are to a varying degree separated by an amnestic barrier. Personality A, for example, has no memory of the events that occurred while personality B was in the ascendancy; A, in other words, exhibits a dissociative amnesia for B, which A experiences as a perplexing discontinuity of consciousness—often referred to as "losing time." B, when dominating consciousness, is not only aware of its own identity but is fully cognizant of A's thoughts, feelings, memories, and existence. Usually, one alter has full knowledge of all the others, although the recognition is not reciprocated.

In some instances the alter endowed with the widest range of memories, although not at the moment dominating conscious awareness and behavior, is simultaneously fully aware of its own train of thought and of the thoughts and actions of the alter in the ascendancy—a phenomenon termed *"co-consciousness."* In an autobiographical account published by Morton Prince, his patient B.C.A. described such a double state of consciousness as follows:

> When I am not here as an alternating personality, my thoughts still continue during the lives of A. and C., although they are not aware of them. That is to say, my mental life continues independently of theirs. I think my own thoughts, which are different from theirs, and at the same time I know their thoughts and what they do. . . . My train of thought may be, and usually is, quite different from C.'s. When C. is ill, for instance, she is thinking about her headache, and how hard life seems and how glad she will be when it is over, and I am thinking how tiresome it is to lie in bed when I am just aching to go for a long tramp or do something gay. We rarely have the same opinion about any book we are reading, though we may both like it. C., however, enjoys some writers whom I find very tiresome, Maeterlinck, for example. She considers him very inspiring and uplifting, and I think he writes a lot of nonsense and is extremely depressing.

Certain alters may manifest classical conversion symptoms and other forms of somatization that disappear when they switch to another personality. That phenomenon and many other clinical features of dissociative identity disorder are clearly evident in the case of Martha B.

> Martha B., a 35-year-old married woman, was admitted to a hospital because she had been unable to walk for the past six months. Three years previously she had joined an evangelical religious sect and had given up "partying and dancing" because "the Lord didn't like those things." Six months before admission she had suffered a minor injury to her back in a car accident and had thereafter been confined to her bed—unable to walk and generally feeling chronically tired, sick, cold, and achy. A physical examination revealed no abnormalities whatsoever, save for a loss of all sensation in both legs from her hips down. As she commented: "My legs—there's no legs there. I don't know whether I have legs. I have to keep looking to see that they're there. There's no feeling, you know." Although she could stand with support, she could not take any steps. Otherwise, all her motor functions were intact. A diagnosis of conversion disorder was made.
>
> In addition to her physical symptoms, the patient complained of "hearing a terrible voice" that urged her constantly to "say and do mean things." During an interview shortly after her initial evaluation, the patient complained that the voice was particularly troublesome and threatened "to take me over completely." When the interviewer asked, "Why don't you let it take over?" the patient's response was immediate and dramatic. She closed her eyes, threw back her head, clenched her fists, and rocked back and forth, appearing to be momentarily out of contact with her environment. Suddenly, she opened her eyes, looked around with a smile, and, with a brightness and alertness in her manner and tone of voice that had previously been absent, she exclaimed, "We've got rid of that other one who stays sick all the time!" Her name, she said, was Harriet, and she proceeded to heap scorn on Martha for her chronic physical complaints and for her righteous, pious life. "We like different things," Harriet said bitterly. "I like to go out partying and dancing, and she likes to go to church, and I don't!" When asked if she could dance, she replied, "Sure, I can dance!" and (to the surprise of the observers) stood up and walked back and forth in the office without difficulty.
>
> Shortly thereafter, the interviewer suggested that it was time for Martha to return. After a mild protest, Harriet assented, and once again the patient appeared to lose contact with her environment as she rocked to and fro, clenched her fists, and muttered "No! No!" as if undergoing an internal struggle. On regaining consciousness, the patient remarked, "Oh, I've been asleep on you." It was evident that she had complete amnesia for the period in which Harriet had been in the ascendancy and that she had no awareness of the secondary personality she harbored inside. Furthermore, she once again had all her sensorimotor symptoms and complained in a plaintive, suffering voice, "I'm tired and cold, and my back's aching." Sick Martha had returned.

Diagnosis Since patients with dissociative identity disorder are either unaware of the dissociative fragmentation of their personality structures or tend to hide it, the diagnosis may not be evident in an initial interview unless an alter suddenly makes a spontaneous appearance in the course of the examination (Table 20-3). Clinicians must, therefore, not only be aware of the relative frequency with which the disorder occurs in modern

TABLE 20-3
Diagnostic Criteria for Dissociative Identity Disorder

A. The presence of two or more distinct identities or personality states (each with its own relatively enduring pattern of perceiving, relating to, and thinking about the environment and self).
B. At least two of these identities or personality states recurrently take control of the person's behavior.
C. Inability to recall important personal information that is too extensive to be explained by ordinary forgetfulness.
D. The disturbance is not due to the direct physiological effects of a substance (e.g., blackouts or chaotic behavior during alcohol intoxication) or a general medical condition (e.g., complex partial seizures). **Note:** In children, the symptoms are not attributable to imaginary playmates or other fantasy play.

Table from DSM-IV, *Diagnostic and Statistical Manual of Mental Disorders,* ed 4. Copyright American Psychiatric Association, Washington, 1994. Used with permission.

patients but also actively search for the subtle indications of dissociative disturbances of consciousness.

The clinician should ask patients about the existence of amnestic gaps in their memories, such as the subjective experience of losing time, and about other indications that an alternate personality has at some point dominated their consciousness. Have they suddenly found themselves in a strange place without knowing how they got there? Have they been recognized by people who are strangers to them? Have they found personal possessions missing or mysteriously altered? The presence of conversion symptoms and other forms of somatization may be clues that unconscious personalities are indirectly invading conscious awareness. If the clinician suspects that the presenting symptoms are the result of dissociated personalities, the patient's responsiveness to hypnosis should be determined; patients with dissociative identity disorder achieve extremely high scores on standard scales of hypnotizability, and hypnotic procedures usually disclose the presence of underlying alters.

Differential diagnosis Although dissociative amnesia, dissociative fugue, and dissociative identity disorder share the basic mechanism of dissociation, they may be distinguished from one another by the characteristic differences in their clinical manifestations.

Patients with dissociative amnesia have no significant disturbance in their personal identity, and their dissociated mental elements are not organized into separate, distinct personalities.

The alteration of personal identity that is a central feature of patients with dissociative fugue states generally occurs as an isolated episode, and such patients lack the multiplicity of personalities and the fluidity of change that characterize those with dissociative identity disorder.

The irruption of visual and auditory hallucinations in the course of dissociative identity disorder may lead the unwary clinician to conclude that the patient is suffering from schizophrenia. Careful observation, however, reveals the presence of dissociative mechanisms and the high degree of hypnotizability in patients with dissociative identity disorder that are absent in those with schizophrenia and the absence in the former of the thought disorder and disturbances in affect that are cardinal features of patients with schizophrenia.

The behavior and the patterns of relationships of patients with dissociative identity disorder often have a marked similarity to what is observed in persons with borderline personality disorder, but the latter lack the telltale presence of distinct, alternating personalities separated by an amnestic barrier that is the hallmark of the former. Electroencephalographic evidence of a temporal lobe dysrhythmia in some patients with the symptoms of dissociative identity disorder suggests the presence of temporal lobe epilepsy as a contributing factor.

Course and prognosis The symptoms of dissociative identity disorder often begin in adolescence and run a long, fluctuating course. Some personalities adapt better than others to their social environment, but the frequency and the unpredictability of the changes in identity make life a perplexing, hazardous affair for patients, their families, and their friends.

Treatment Extended psychotherapy is the principal approach to treatment. The goal is to achieve a merging of the alters into a stable, unified personality. In current practice, therapists attempt to unify the personality by exploring all the alters, often under hypnosis, to uncover traumatic memories and induce a cathartic expression of the emotions associated with them. At the same time, they try to facilitate communication among all the personalities by removing the amnestic barriers between them; the aim is to bring their various compartmentalized mental contents together under the domination of a single, persisting self that can deal with external and internal conflicts without the need for defensive dissociation and fragmentation.

Throughout the long therapeutic journey, patients require the continuous support of a steady therapeutic relationship, hospitalization during periods of disruptive behavior and exacerbation of symptoms, and often the shelter of such facilities as halfway houses. Within such structured management, patients may ultimately achieve a degree of stability that enables them to undertake steady employment and to lead a relatively effective and comfortable existence.

DEPERSONALIZATION DISORDER As defined in modern clinical terminology, the word "*depersonalization*" refers to the experience of feeling detached from one's mental processes or body, as if one were an external observer of those phenomena. Frequently found as a symptom in a variety of other disorders, depersonalization is viewed as being a specific disorder in its own right when it is the sole or predominant disturbance in function.

Epidemiology As an occasional isolated experience, depersonalization is a common phenomenon and, as such, is not considered pathological. Studies of its occurrence in normal college students indicate that transient depersonalization may be found in as many as 50 percent of a given population, without a significant difference in frequency in men and women. It is a frequent phenomenon in children as they develop the capacity for self-awareness, and adults may experience a temporary sense of unreality when they travel to new and strange places. As George Eliot wrote in *Silas Marner:*

> Even people whose lives have been made various by learning, sometimes find it hard to keep a fast hold on their habitual views of life or their faith in the invisible—nay, on the sense that their past joys and sorrows are a real experience, when they are suddenly transported to a new land, where the beings around them know nothing of their history, and share none of their ideas—where their mother earth shows another lap, and human life has other forms than those on which their souls have been nourished. Minds that have been unhinged from their old faith and love have perhaps sought this Lethean influence of exile, in which the past becomes dreamy because its symbols have all vanished, and the present too is dreamy because it is linked to no memories.

Information about the epidemiology of depersonalization as a pathological disorder is scanty. It is apparently rare as a pure syndrome but is frequently found as a symptom in association with anxiety and depressive disorders and with schizophrenia. As a distinct syndrome, it occurs at least twice as often in women as in men and is a disorder of young people, rarely being observed in those over 40 years of age.

Etiology Even though a number of clinical investigators have focused their attention on depersonalization, its cause remains obscure. Many physiological, psychodynamic, and ego psychological theories have been proposed, but their proponents agree on little about the mechanisms involved.

The experience of depersonalization may be associated with a variety of factors affecting the function of the brain, such as epilepsy and other diseases of the central nervous system and the ingestion of psychotomimetic drugs like mescaline and lysergic acid diethylamide (LSD). L. Dugas and F. Moutier, for example, cited a patient with an ultimately fatal brain tumor whose initial symptoms were attacks of altered perception in which, as the patient complained, "I am completely impersonal. . . . I see the world as if it were a photograph. . . . I feel myself outside of life."

In other cases the causative factors are clearly psychological, especially when depersonalization occurs in the face of traumatic events. David Spiegel described how in a prison riot "one hostage was kicked in the head, back, ribs, and testicles. Eventually he 'saw' all these things happening to him, but he did not feel anything. Another hostage said, 'I could see my body moving so I knew that I had been kicked, but I didn't feel anything.' "

Diagnosis and clinical features In what is still probably the most penetrating clinical treatise on the disorder, although it was written nearly a century ago, Dugas and Moutier summarized the salient clinical features of depersonalization as follows:

> Consider a person in the ordinary circumstances of life. He receives the sensory impressions of objects, marshals his memories, recalls images, forms and combines ideas, judges, reasons, carries out actions, is affected by pleasure and pain: he is aware of all of these and of their connections with himself. Suppose that the same person experiences identical states, but ceases to have an awareness of them as being his own; he will witness "his life as a performance presented by another" [Fromentin]; he will continue to perceive sensations, colors and forms, touches, smells, etc., but it will seem to him that these sensory impressions do not affect him any more. He will continue to have memories, but it will appear to him that the past they recall escapes him and is no longer his own. He will still think, reason, act, even be moved by feelings, but it will seem to him that it is not he who thinks, reasons, acts, or feels pleasure or pain. Although nothing in his life will be different, yet everything about it will appear changed. He will no longer know himself, will be amazed that he is still alive, and will be outside of his experiences.

As that passage suggests, the central characteristic of depersonalization is the quality of unreality and estrangement that colors conscious experience. Inner mental processes and external events go on exactly as before, yet everything is different and seems no longer to have any relation or meaning to the person who is aware of them. In describing those phenomena, some clinicians make a distinction between depersonalization and derealization. They apply the term *"depersonalization"* to the feeling that one's body or one's personal self is strange and unreal; they use the term *"derealization"* to denote the experience of perceiving objects in the external world as having the same quality of unreality and estrangement. Strictly speaking, that distinction provides a more accurate description of the phenomena than does lumping them together under the category of depersonalization alone. If a single term is to be used, "derealization" is the more inclusive and appropriate one, since it refers to a characteristic change in the perception of objects that is common to them all—to self, body, or objects in the external environment—whereas "depersonalization," being restricted to the perception of the one's personal self and body alone, has a limited scope. In the clinical descriptions that follow, however, the variegated individual symptoms are presented as the manifestations of depersonalization disorder in order to conform to the accepted modern terminology.

BODILY PERCEPTIONS Individual parts of one's body or one's entire physical being may appear foreign. One of Dugas's and Moutier's patients who experienced an attack of depersonalization while riding one night in a train exclaimed:

> I look at my hands, which are writing this; how odd it is! Are they really concerned with what they are doing? I look at my reflection in the window, and find myself to be strange, novel. For a moment I was almost afraid of the image the window pane returned to me—of this phantom of myself.

MENTAL AND BEHAVIORAL PERCEPTIONS All one's personal mental operations and behavior may feel alien. Said another of Dugas's and Moutier's correspondents:

> Is this really I who am at this moment receiving visitors in my drawing-room, speaking commonplace words, asking people about their health, laughing with them, while my real self follows another train of thought and is entirely under the sway of a tremendous change that has taken over my life? Yes, without doubt, I see myself, hear myself, and yet I witness what I am doing as if it involves someone else. I have the impression of strangeness and of the unknown in the face of actual reality.

EMOTIONAL PERCEPTIONS A common and particularly troublesome manifestation is a loss of the capacity to experience emotions, even though the patient appears to express them. Dugas and Moutier cited the plight of a woman who, separated from her family by hospitalization, vociferously complained of her inability to feel any emotion:

> "I wish," she said, "that I had some feeling of sorrow for my husband and son." At this point she cried and continued, "You see, sir, that I am crying, but it does not touch me. I feel nothing." Her husband came to visit her in the hospital. She was told to kiss him and did so. "That, sir, affects me as much as if I were to kiss this table."

PERCEPTIONS OF OTHERS Similar feelings of unreality and strangeness may invade patients' perceptions of the objects and the people in the world around them. One of Janet's patients complained:

> Things don't look the way they used to. Everything I see, even the decorations on the wall of my room, seem strange to me. It's as if I were seeing everything for the first time. Everything appears unreal to me. When I go out, it seems to me that the street is not the same. It's like a city I haven't seen for a long time. Suddenly everything around me gives me the effect of having become odd. It's as though reality were deformed.

ANXIETY Depersonalization is often accompanied by considerable anxiety, and patients are frequently afraid that the symptom is a sign that they are going insane. Even though they complain of being emotionally dead, patients frequently become greatly upset by the sense of that deadness. Indeed, all the manifestations of depersonalization are often highly unpleasant; they not only motivate patients to seek medical help but drive them to vigorous activity or to intense self-stimulation to break through the prison walls of their unreality. A patient described by M. Krishaber reported:

> I seemed to be dreaming and no longer the same person. The sensation of being in a dream was the most painful part for me. I would touch things around me hundreds of times, or would speak in a very loud voice in order to restore the reality of the external world and my own identity, but then my illusions became even more marked. The sound of my voice was absolutely insupportable, and touching things did nothing to restore my impressions to normal.

INSIGHT No matter how widespread and intense the sense of unreality, reality testing itself is unimpaired, and patients retain a keen self-awareness of their incapacitation. A chronic sufferer from the disorder, the Swiss diarist Henri-Frédéric Amiel, wrote in his *Journal Intime:*

> I find myself regarding existence as though from beyond the tomb, from another world; all is strange to me; I am, as it were, outside my own body and individuality; I am *depersonalized,* detached, cut adrift.—Is this madness? No. Madness means the impossibility of recovering one's normal balance after the mind has thus played truant among alien forms of being, and followed Dante to invisible worlds. Madness means incapacity for self-judgment and self-control.

Amiel's perceptive introspection revealed to him a clinical truth about depersonalization that remains a central element of the modern concept of the disorder: the patient's insight remains intact.

CLASSIFICATION The fact that depersonalization may occur during a traumatic experience suggests that dissociative processes are an important factor in its production and has led to the inclusion of depersonalization disorder in the general category of dissociative disorders in modern nosology. However, a careful and perceptive reading of the accounts that patients provide of their experiences of depersonalization indicates certain differences from the common phenomena of the other dissociative disorders. In the other disorders, sensations, memories, and a sense of identity are divorced from conscious awareness, with all that that entails in the way of symptoms. In depersonalization those mental functions remain intact, and what is lost to consciousness is the subtle function of the sense of reality and meaning. It is not, in other words, a loss of basic mental contents but a change in the quality of the patient's perception of those contents.

The fact that depersonalization, like other dissociative phenomena, is often a response to psychological trauma is perhaps sufficient reason on clinical grounds for including it among the dissociative disorders, but that commonality should not cause clinicians to lose sight of the special characteristics of depersonalization, which need far more careful consideration and investigation than they have yet received.

The DSM-IV diagnostic criteria for depersonalization disorder are given in Table 20-4.

Course and prognosis In the majority of patients, the symptoms begin abruptly. The disorder usually starts between the ages of 15 and 30, but it has been seen in children as young as 10; it begins infrequently after age 30 and almost never in the late decades of life. A few follow-up studies indicate that, in more than half the cases, depersonalization tends to be a long-lasting, chronic condition. In many patients the symptoms run a steady, unremitting course without significant fluctuations in intensity, but in some the symptoms occur in repeated attacks interspersed with symptom-free intervals.

Differential diagnosis Depersonalization may occur as a symptom in numerous other psychiatric disorders. Its common occurrence in patients with depression and schizophrenia should alert the clinician to the possibility that the patient who initially complains of feelings of unreality and estrangement may actually be suffering from those common disorders. A history and a mental status examination should in most cases disclose the characteristic features of those two illnesses.

Because of the frequency with which psychotomimetic drugs induce often long-standing changes in the sense of the reality of oneself and one's environment, the clinician should inquire about the use of such substances.

The nature of other clinical phenomena in patients complaining of unreality establishes the diagnosis of the primary disorder, of which depersonalization is a secondary symptom. The label "depersonalization disorder" should be reserved for those conditions in which depersonalization constitutes the predominant difficulty. The fact that depersonalization phenomena may result from a disease of the brain underscores the necessity for careful neurological evaluation, especially when the depersonalization is not accompanied by other more common and more obvious psychiatric symptoms.

Treatment Patients with depersonalization disorder have long been known to be notoriously refractory to treatment. When depersonalization is a symptom secondary to another psychiatric illness, the effective treatment of the primary disorder often eliminates the complaint of a disturbance in the sense of reality. A variety of medications have been used to treat the disorder itself, but controlled and uncontrolled trials provide little evidence of their effectiveness. Similarly, psychotherapeutic measures have generally proved to have little or no effect on the course or the severity of the symptoms.

In patients in whom depersonalization is clearly related to psychological trauma, the recovery of unconscious traumatic memories and the cathartic discharge of the emotions connected with them may prove therapeutic. Some patients obtain a degree of relief from the anxiety associated with the feeling of depersonalization by talking to a therapist about their symptoms and by discovering that they are not alone in their suffering or in danger of going insane. A supportive therapeutic relationship may moderate their distress, but specific recommendations for the management of the disorder must await more extensive clinical investigation.

TABLE 20-4
Diagnostic Criteria for Depersonalization Disorder

A. Persistent or recurrent experiences of feeling detached from, and as if one is an outside observer of, one's mental processes or body (e.g., feeling like one is in a dream).
B. During the depersonalization experience, reality testing remains intact.
C. The depersonalization causes clinically significant distress or impairment in social, occupational, or other important areas of functioning.
D. The depersonalization experience does not occur exclusively during the course of another mental disorder, such as schizophrenia, panic disorder, acute stress disorder, or another dissociative disorder, and is not due to the direct physiological effects of a substance (e.g., a drug of abuse, a medication) or a general medical condition (e.g., temporal lobe epilepsy).

Table from DSM-IV, *Diagnostic and Statistical Manual of Mental Disorders,* ed 4. Copyright American Psychiatric Association, Washington, 1994. Used with permission.

DISSOCIATIVE TRANCE DISORDER In dissociative trance disorder the affected persons exhibit an altered state of conscious awareness of their surroundings, during which they may have vivid hallucinatory recollections of an emotionally traumatic event or feel themselves taken over or possessed by an alien spirit who controls their minds and bodies. They generally retain no memories of the experiences during the ordinary waking state. In DSM-IV the disorder is included in Appendix B, "Criteria Sets and Axes Provided for Further Study."

Epidemiology The clinical study of dissociative trance disorder is limited and provides insufficient data from which to draw conclusions about its incidence, prevalence, or relative occurrence in men and women. Anthropological investigations offer a wealth of observations indicating the widespread existence of dissociative trance disorder phenomena throughout the world, especially in less developed cultures. And historical research reveals the recurrent waves, often in epidemic form, of similar phenomena throughout the history of Western civilization, beginning with the oracular sibyls in the mists of classical antiquity and encompassing the witch crazes of the 16th and 17th centuries, the spiritualist movement of the second half of the 19th century, and the modern preoccupation with diabolic cults and the phenomena of reported abductions by aliens from other worlds.

Although many of the persons who have undergone such dissociative trance experiences cannot necessarily be deemed clinically disordered, they frequently appear to have been markedly disposed to psychological dissociation. Some have certainly found their lives seriously compromised by the intrusiveness of the invading spirits that have possessed them.

Etiology In the handful of clinical cases reported by psychiatric clinicians, dissociative mechanisms are central causative factors in the production of the disorder. Although the form and the content of the surface manifestations, especially when they occur in epidemic proportions, may be strongly influenced by the specific characteristics of the surrounding cultural and social milieu, their origin in individual patients is generally found in unconscious memories and psychological conflicts that have been excluded from consciousness by dissociation.

Diagnosis and clinical features

TRANCE The central feature of dissociative trance disorder is an alteration in the patient's state of consciousness that may be easy to detect but is hard to describe (Table 20-5). In the abnormal state, patients are out of contact with their environment; appear to be preoccupied with a private, inner world; and are uncommunicative with those around them. They often appear emotionally distressed, speak excitedly in words or sentences that are hard to understand, and exhibit repetitious, complex patterns of behavior that derive from a hallucinatory reexperiencing of emotionally traumatic events. The episodes occur in discrete attacks and alternate with periods of normal consciousness and behavior in which the patient is amnesic for the trance state itself and the events associated with it.

Janet recorded his observations of a number of patients with this form of dissociative disorder. In *The Major Symptoms of Hysteria,* for example, he described the clinical condition of a young woman, Gib:

TABLE 20-5
Research Criteria for Dissociative Trance Disorder

A. Either (1) or (2):
  (1) trance, i.e., temporary marked alteration in the state of consciousness or loss of customary sense of personal identity without replacement by an alternate identity, associated with at least one of the following:
    (a) narrowing of awareness of immediate surroundings, or unusually narrow and selective focusing on environmental stimuli
    (b) stereotyped behaviors or movements that are experienced as being beyond one's control
  (2) possession trance, a single or episodic alteration in the state of consciousness characterized by the replacement of customary sense of personal identity by a new identity. This is attributed to the influence of a spirit, power, deity, or other person, as evidenced by one (or more) of the following:
    (a) stereotyped and culturally determined behaviors or movements that are experienced as being controlled by the possessing agent
    (b) full or partial amnesia for the event
B. The trance or possession trance state is not accepted as a normal part of a collective cultural or religious practice.
C. The trance or possession trance state causes clinically significant distress or impairment in social, occupational, or other important areas of functioning.
D. The trance or possession trance state does not occur exclusively during the course of a psychotic disorder (including mood disorder with psychotic features and brief psychotic disorder) or dissociative identity disorder and is not due to the direct physiological effects of a substance or a general medical condition.

Table from DSM-IV, *Diagnostic and Statistical Manual of Mental Disorders,* ed 4. Copyright American Psychiatric Association, Washington, 1994. Used with permission.

> [She] abruptly hears one day some disastrous news. Her niece, who lives next door, has just died in dreadful circumstances. She rushes out and comes unhappily in time to see the body of the young girl lying in the street. She had thrown herself out of the window in a fit of delirium. Gib., although very much moved, remains to all appearance calm, helping to make everything ready for the funeral. She goes to the funeral in a very natural way. But from that time on she grows more and more gloomy, her health fails, and we may notice the beginning of the following singular symptoms. Nearly every day, at night and during the day, she enters into a strange state; she looks as if she were in a dream, she speaks softly with an absent person she calls Pauline (the name of her lately deceased niece), and tells her that she admires her fate and her courage and that her death has been a beautiful one. She rises, goes to the windows and opens them, then shuts them up again, tries them one after the other, climbs on the window sill, and if her friends did not stop her, she would without doubt throw herself out of the window. She must be stopped, looked after incessantly, until she shakes herself, rubs her eyes and resumes ordinary business as if nothing had happened.

POSSESSION In other patients the internal trance imagery, rather than being a reproduction of traumatic memories, represents the experience of being possessed by vividly hallucinated figures who are either kindly, guiding mentors or terrifying diabolical beings. Benign possessions were commonly witnessed in 19th-century spirit mediums, whose guides or controls were often famous historical figures or imaginary powerful, exalted personages who introduced the entranced person to awesome, exhiliratingly beautiful new worlds and at times dictated lengthy, usually tedious philosophical or religious tracts. A striking example of that kind of possession is that of Mlle. Hélène Smith, whose exploration of life on the planet Mars under the guidance of her control Leopold was extensively studied and reported by the famous Swiss psychologist Théodore Flournoy at the turn of the century. The cameras of modern space exploration have exposed the errors of Mlle. Smith's romantic productions, but they remain an enigma to the explorer of the inner world.

The experience of being possessed by evil spirits occurs in patients with guilt-laden conflicts over personal transgressions that set in motion pathogenic dissociative processes. Janet described such a disorder in his lengthy clinical report of Achille.

> A happily married, cheerful businessman, Achille was entirely well until, at the age of 33, his wife noted a striking change in his personality after he returned home from a lengthy business trip. In contrast to his previous demeanor, he was depressed, withdrawn, and uncommunicative. He became increasingly agitated, began to worry that he had a variety of serious bodily illnesses, and finally took to his bed, where he lapsed into a state of apparent unconsciousness so extreme that his family thought he was dying. Suddenly, however, he awoke from that state to exhibit a new pattern of behavior. He was alert and in contact with his surroundings but insisted that he was possessed by the Devil, who caused him to utter terrible blasphemies.
>
> From that point on Achille alternated between two states of consciousness. In one he entered a trancelike phase in which he appeared to hallucinate and, with great terror, cried out that he was surrounded by the Devil and a host of leering demons, who threatened him with horrible tortures and forced him to curse God and the saints. In the other state he was subdued and in contact with his family but remained convinced that he was possessed by the Devil, who impelled him from within to utter sacrilegious blasphemies. In that state Achille had no recollection of the events that had occurred during his business trip or of the early stages of his illness. Janet gave a graphic description of Achille's behavior in one of the second states: "This poor man, small in stature, with haggard eyes and pitiful appearance murmured blasphemies in a muffled, sober voice. 'Cursed be God,' he would say. 'Damn the Trinity and damn the Virgin.' Then in a shriller voice, with tears in his eyes: 'It's not my fault if my voice utters these horrors. It's not me! It's not me! I tighten my lips so that the words won't escape them and be spoken aloud, but it does no good. The Devil speaks these words inside of me. I can clearly hear him speak them and make my tongue move despite me.' "
>
> Undaunted by the power of his diabolical adversary, Janet induced in Achille a hypnotic trance, during which he recovered the memories of the business trip and its immediate sequelae, for which Achille was

amnestic. In a brief moment of indiscretion during that trip, Achille had been unfaithful to his wife, a lapse for which, as Janet commented, "he was cruelly punished." On his return home Achille was suddenly overcome with remorse for his infidelity and was seized by a fear that, if he talked, he would reveal his peccadillo to his wife—hence his withdrawal into uncommunicative isolation. His guilt became worse with the passing days; he became convinced that he had a number of serious illnesses, and he began to have vivid dreams that he had died and was surrounded by a host of demons in hell. Those were initially nightmares but then merged into daytime dissociative trance states in which he vividly hallucinated hellfire and a satanic crew of tormentors. The episodes, as noted earlier, developed into a pattern of alternation with more normal states of consciousness, in which he was in contact with his surroundings but was amnesic for the precipitating events and was convinced that he was possessed by the Devil.

Armed with those new facts, Janet was able by hypnotic suggestion to allay the patient's anxious guilt with the subsequent relief of all his symptoms—a successful therapeutic result that, as Janet reported eight years later, had been fully maintained.

Differential diagnosis The central feature of an altered state of consciousness that characterizes an episode of trance distinguishes it from the other dissociative disorders. Although the sudden alteration of personality that occurs in an episode of possession is similar to the equally dramatic change of alters in patients with dissociative identity disorder, in possession the manifestation of the new personality is accompanied by the characteristic trancelike alteration of consciousness; patients with dissociative identity disorder are fully alert during their secondary states. The altered consciousness of a trance state differs from the unconsciousness that follows a head injury or an epileptic seizure; in the latter the obtunding of consciousness is severe, the recovery of consciousness is gradual, and, after returning to normal consciousness, patients manifest a permanent loss of memories that cannot be recovered by hypnosis or other measures capable of raising dissociated mental events into conscious awareness.

Treatment Few reports deal specifically with the treatment of patients with dissociative trance disorder. The basic therapeutic approach is similar to that for the other dissociative disorders. The therapist should attempt to explore the dissociated mental contents with hypnotic and other techniques designed to raise into consciousness the underlying traumatic memories and psychological conflicts and to achieve a therapeutic catharsis of the painful emotions associated with them. Therapy must proceed slowly and cautiously in the context of a supportive therapeutic relationship to keep patients from being overwhelmed by the often disruptive anxiety aroused by the emergence of the unconscious mental elements into conscious awareness. Gradually, over a series of treatment sessions, patients are able to work through their conflicts and to achieve a permanent conscious synthesis of the previously dissociated pathogenic elements. Once that has been accomplished, they are able to deal with their formerly intolerable memories, fantasies, and emotions.

DISSOCIATIVE DISORDERS NOT OTHERWISE SPECIFIED This category of dissociative disorders is designed to marshal those clinical stragglers with dissociative symptoms that do not fulfill the designated criteria for the specific syndromes listed above (Table 20-6). It includes patients with conditions resembling dissociative identity disorder in which the alter is not sharply defined, patients with derealization unaccompanied by depersonalization, patients with dissociativelike symptoms after prolonged torture or brainwashing, and patients with trancelike alterations of consciousness, such as koro and amok, that are indigenous to specific cultures or peoples.

Ganser's syndrome may be present in association with a variety of dissociative symptoms. Found mainly in men, especially those imprisoned in penal institutions, the syndrome is characterized by a quality of pseudostupidity in the person's speech and behavior; for example, although alert and oriented, the person gives inappropriate and even ridiculous answers to simple questions—replying "Five," for instance, when asked, "How much is two and two?"

The clinician who is alert to the existence of dissociative mechanisms occasionally recognizes their presence in patients whose confusing clinical presentations may not conform to the diagnostic criteria of the usual dissociative syndromes.

TABLE 20-6
Diagnostic Criteria for Dissociative Disorder Not Otherwise Specified

This category is included for disorders in which the predominant feature is a dissociative symptom (i.e., a disruption in the usually integrated functions of consciousness, memory, identity, or perception of the environment) that does not meet the criteria for any specific dissociative disorder. Examples include

1. Clinical presentations similar to dissociative identity disorder that fail to meet full criteria for this disorder. Examples include presentations in which (a) there are not two or more distinct personality states, or (b) amnesia for important personal information does not occur.
2. Derealization unaccompanied by depersonalization in adults.
3. States of dissociation that occur in individuals who have been subjected to periods of prolonged and intense coercive persuasion (e.g., brainwashing, thought reform, or indoctrination while captive).
4. Dissociative trance disorder: single or episodic disturbances in the state of consciousness, identity, or memory that are indigenous to particular locations and cultures. Dissociative trance involves narrowing of awareness of immediate surroundings or stereotyped behaviors or movements that are experienced as being beyond one's control. Possession trance involves replacement of the customary sense of personal identity by a new identity, attributed to the influence of a spirit, power, deity, or other person, and associated with stereotyped "involuntary" movements or amnesia. Examples include *amok* (Indonesia), *bebainan* (Indonesia), *latab* (Malaysia), *pibloktoq* (Arctic), *ataque de nervios* (Latin America), and possession (India). The dissociative or trance disorder is not a normal part of a broadly accepted collective cultural or religious practice.
5. Loss of consciousness, stupor, or coma not attributable to a general medical condition.
6. Ganser syndrome: the giving of approximate answers to questions (e.g., "2 plus 2 equals 5") when not associated with dissociative amnesia or dissociative fugue.

Table from DSM-IV, *Diagnostic and Statistical Manual of Mental Disorders,* ed 4.

Alice W., a young woman of 17, entered a general hospital psychiatric unit after a year of multiple admissions to another institution for intractable symptoms of rapid mood swings, outbursts of agitation and assaultive behavior, suicidal preoccupations with at least one serious suicidal attempt, and recurrent hallucinations of shadowy figures who urged her to kill herself. Classified as having bipolar mood disorder, rapid-cycling type, she had been unsuccessfully treated with at least six different medications over a 12-month period.

During her evaluation at the new hospital, the examining physician was struck by the patient's composure in the diagnostic interview, the warmth with which she related, and the articulateness with which she described her symptoms and previous clinical course. Her symptoms, she revealed, had started after her father had been hospitalized for severe depression two years earlier, an event that troubled her deeply. Although increasingly preoccupied with her father's illness, she managed to continue with her studies and other activities and, indeed, was elected president of her high school class during the academic year. Gradually, however, she found it harder and harder to pay attention to her class work, she became increasingly forgetful, and she noted that she would often come to with no memory of what had occurred for the previous hour or two. Struck by that fact and by the discrepancy between the disorganized, psychotic character of her affective symptoms and hallucinations on the one hand and, on the other hand, by her relatively successful functioning at school and her warm, composed, rational behavior in the interview, the evaluating psychiatrist suspected that dissociative mechanisms were playing a role in the production of her symptoms and referred her for a diagnostic hypnotic trance induction.

The patient proved to be highly hypnotizable and in the first trance state spontaneously reproduced her hallucinatory visions, which, it turned out on further questioning, had been central to her repeated episodes of disturbed mood and behavior during the previous year. Of particular importance was the fact that in subsequent hypnotic sessions the patient learned by self-hypnosis to induce and dispel the troublesome visions herself, thereby bringing them under her voluntary control. That was the key to a therapeutic program that allowed her to avoid further spontaneous dissociative episodes and hospitalizations as she pursued a course of outpatient psychotherapy.

Although her clinical disorder was hard to classify in a neat phenomenological pigeonhole, the recognition of the role of dissociation in her symptoms was central to understanding and treating her illness.

SUGGESTED CROSS-REFERENCES

Further descriptions of the nature and the function of dissociative mechanisms are found in Chapters 6, 7, and 8, dealing with the theories of personality and psychopathology, and in Chapter 11, dealing with the classification of mental disorders. The diagnostic distinction between dissociative disorders and other mental disorders is clarified in Chapter 14 on schizophrenia and in Section 17.4 on posttraumatic stress disorder. Chapter 18, on the somatoform disorders, provides a detailed description of the somatic symptoms that in this chapter are viewed as manifestations of dissociation. Expanded descriptions of the various psychotherapeutic approaches appear in Chapter 31, which is devoted to psychotherapies.

REFERENCES

Amiel H-F: *The Journal Intime of Henri-Frédéric Amiel.* Macmillan, London, 1893.

Azam E: *Hypnotisme et double conscience.* Alcan, Paris, 1893.

"B": An introspective analysis of co-conscious life, by a personality (B) claiming to be co-conscious. J Abnorm Psychol *3:* 311, 1908–1909.

Binet A: *Alterations of Personality.* Appleton, New York, 1896.

Braun B, editor: *Treatment of Multiple Personality Disorder.* American Psychiatric Press, Washington, 1986.

*Breuer J, Freud S: Studies on hysteria. In *Standard Edition of the Complete Psychological Works of Sigmund Freud,* vol 2, p 3. Hogarth Press, London, 1955.

Carlson E, Putnam F: An update on the dissociative experiences scale. Dissociation *6:* 16, 1993.

Coons P: Dissociative disorder not otherwise specified: A clinical investigation of 50 cases with suggestions for typology and treatment. Dissociation *5:* 187, 1992.

Dugas L, Moutier F: *La dépersonnalisation.* Alcan, Paris, 1911.

Ellenberger H: *The Discovery of the Unconscious.* Basic Books, New York, 1970.

Flournoy T: *From India to the Planet Mars.* Harper, New York, 1900.

Frankel F: Adult reconstruction of childhood events in the multiple personality literature. Am J Psychiatry *150:* 954, 1993.

Frankel F: *Trance as a Coping Mechanism.* Plenum, New York, 1976.

Ganaway G: Historical truth versus narrative truth: Clarifying the role of exogenous trauma in the etiology of multiple personality disorder and its variants. Dissociation *2:* 205, 1989.

James W: *The Principles of Psychology.* Holt, New York, 1890.

Janet P: *L'automatisme psychologique.* Alcan, Paris, 1889.

*Janet P: *The Major Symptoms of Hysteria.* Macmillan, New York, 1907.

Janet P: *The Mental State of Hystericals.* Putnam's, New York, 1901.

Janet P: *Névroses et idées fixes,* ed 2. Alcan, Paris, 1904.

*Kluft R, editor: *Childhood Antecedents of Multiple Personality.* American Psychiatric Press, Washington, 1985.

Kluft R: Multiple personality disorder. In *Review of Psychiatry,* A Tasman, editor, vol 10, p 161. American Psychiatric Press, Washington, 1991.

Kluft R: The treatment of dissociative disorder patients: An overview of discoveries, successes, and failures. Dissociation *6:* 87, 1993.

Krishaber M: *De la névropathic cérébro-cardiaque.* Masson, Paris, 1873.

Loewenstein R: Psychogenic amnesia and psychogenic fugue: A comprehensive review. In *Review of Psychiatry,* A Tasman, editor, vol 10, p 189. American Psychiatric Press, Washington, 1991.

Nemiah J: Dissociation, conversion, and somatization. In *Review of Psychiatry,* A Tasman, editor, vol 10, p 248. American Psychiatric Press, Washington, 1991.

Nemiah J: Dissociative amnesia: A clinical and theoretical reconsideration. In *Functional Disorders of Memory,* J Kihlstrom, editor, p 303. Erlbaum, Hillsdale, NJ, 1979.

*Prince M: *The Dissociation of a Personality.* Longmans, Green, New York, 1906.

Prince M: *The Unconscious,* ed 2. Macmillan, New York. 1924.

Putnam F: Diagnosis and clinical phenomenology of multiple personality disorder: A North American perspective. Dissociation *6:* 80, 1993.

*Putnam F: *Diagnosis and Treatment of Multiple Personality Disorder.* Guilford, New York, 1989.

Putnam F: Dissociative phenomena. In *Review of Psychiatry,* A Tasman, editor, vol 10, p 145. American Psychiatric Press, Washington, 1991.

Righetti R: Contributo allo studio delle amnesie lacunari. RW Patol Nerv Ment *25:* 261, 1920.

Spiegel D: *Dissociation: Culture, Mind, and Body.* American Psychiatric Press, Washington, 1994.

Spiegel D: Dissociation and trauma. In *Review of Psychiatry,* A Tasman, editor, vol 10, p 261. American Psychiatric Press, Washington, 1991.

Steinberg M: The spectrum of depersonalization: Assessment and treatment. In *Review of Psychiatry,* A Tasman, editor, vol 10, p 223. American Psychiatric Press, Washington, 1991.

Steinberg M: *Structured Clinical Interview for DSM-IV Dissociative Disorders (Scid-D),* American Psychiatric Press, Washington, 1993.

Steinberg M, Cicchetti D: Clinical assessment of dissociative symptoms and disorders: The Structured Clinical Interview for DSM-IV Dissociative Disorders (SCID-D). Dissociation *6:* 3, 1993.

Steingard S, Frankel F: Dissociation and psychotic symptoms. Am J Psychiatry *142:* 953, 1985.

Wilbur C, Kluft R: Multiple personality disorder. In *Treatments of Psychiatric Disorders,* p 2197. American Psychiatric Association, Washington, 1989.

Yates A: False and mistaken allegations of sexual abuse. In *Review of Psychiatry,* A Tasman, editor, vol 10, p 320. American Psychiatric Press, Washington, 1991.

CHAPTER 21 NORMAL HUMAN SEXUALITY AND SEXUAL AND GENDER IDENTITY DISORDERS

21.1 NORMAL HUMAN SEXUALITY

21.1a NORMAL HUMAN SEXUALITY AND SEXUAL DYSFUNCTIONS

VIRGINIA A. SADOCK, M.D.

INTRODUCTION

The study of human sexuality deals with everything that relates to or is affected by sex; the organs of sex and their functions; the sex impulses, instincts, and drives; and all those thoughts, feelings, and behaviors connected with sexual gratification and reproduction, including the attraction of one person to another.

Sexual behavior is diverse and determined by a complex interaction of factors. It is affected by one's relationships with others, by life circumstances, and by the culture in which one lives. A person's sexuality is enmeshed with other personality factors, with his or her biological makeup, and with a general sense of self. It includes the perception of being male or female, and it reflects developmental experiences with sex throughout the life cycle. A rigid definition of normal sexuality is difficult to draw and is clinically impractical. It is easier to define abnormal sexuality—that is, sexual behavior that is destructive to oneself or others, that cannot be directed toward a partner, that excludes stimulation of the primary sex organs, and that is inappropriately associated with guilt and anxiety.

HISTORY

Cultural mores regarding sexual behavior have varied throughout the history of Western civilization. Attitudes have oscillated between the liberal and the puritanical, between the acceptance and the repression of human sexuality. During the past several decades, the prevalent attitudes toward sex in the United States have been markedly liberal. However, recent studies indicate a trend toward accepting more conservative values. That shift is attributed largely to the fear of acquired immune deficiency syndrome (AIDS). A recent poll reported that 40 percent of Americans are concerned that they will contract AIDS and are altering their sexual behavior because of that fear. The greatest concern was expressed by young adults who are now more likely to use condoms as a precaution and to choose their sexual partners with greater care. Conservative segments of society emphasize abstinence before marriage as the answer to the fear of AIDS. The recurrence of conservative attitudes in response to the threat of illness has parallels in history. The sexual liberality of the Renaissance ended when syphilis swept the European continent and became a major argument for chastity among proponents of the Reformation. Other factors that predispose to more restrictive mores are periods of economic recession that tend to bring people to more puritanical positions and limited gratification when sexual freedom is used as a substitute for intimate relationships. Few of these issues have been resolved definitively in the form of new social mores, however, and the legacies of the sexual revolution of the 1960s and 1970s exert a strong effect on current sexual behavior.

That particular sexual revolution derived from social and scientific sources. The Kinsey reports of 1948 and 1953 made public the degree, type, and frequency of sexual activity occurring in the United States, bringing sexual practices from the realm of inference and secrecy into accepted, if still private, reality. In the early 1970s, the Presidential Commission on Pornography advised against sexual repression, encouraging the candid discussion of sexuality in society, and the acceptance of frank and sexually stimulating material. The recommendations of the report, however, were disregarded by that presidential administration. The advent of effective birth control methods and legalized abortion clearly differentiated the pleasure of sexual activity from its procreative function. The feminist movement attacked the double standard in what was considered acceptable sexual behavior for men and women, encouraged women to accept sexual responsibility for the gratification of their needs, and challenged society to reevaluate stereotyped male and female roles. The women's movement also focused attention on rape and incest. Gerontologists and elderly people alike have drawn attention to the sexual needs of the aged. Middle-class adolescents became sexually active and gay rights groups urged acceptance of their sexual orientations, and, in 1973, succeeded in having homosexuality dropped as a diagnostic category in the third edition of the American Psychiatric Association's *Diagnostic and Statistical Manual of Mental Disorders* (DSM-III).

Concurrent with the cultural changes of the sexual revolution there was growth in scientific research into sexual physiology and sexual dysfunctions. William Masters and Virginia Johnson published their pioneering work on the physiology of sexual response in 1966 and reported on their program for treating sexual complaints in 1970. Most medical centers now have programs specifically geared to the treatment of sexual dysfunctions.

Historically, problems of sexual conflict and sexual dysfunction have always been the province of psychiatry. Such pioneers as Havelock Ellis (Figure 21.1a-1), Richard Krafft-Ebing (Figure 21.1a-2), and Sigmund Freud focused broadly on human sexuality. More recent workers have focused more intensively on sexual physiology and dysfunctions. Problems of dysfunction are particularly distressing to patients and have often been resistant to treatment. The current approach to sexual dysfunctions reflects the cultural and scientific developments of recent years, the development of specific techniques for the treatment of these problems, the historical interest of psychiatry in this area, and the recognition of its importance in psychiatric practice.

SEX IN AMERICA A 1994 study conducted by the University of Chicago is the latest sex survey and the most authoritative. Based on a representative United States population between the ages of 18 and 59, it found the following:

1. Eighty-five percent of married women and 75 percent of married men are faithful to their spouses.
2. Forty-one percent of married couples have sex twice a week or more compared with 23 percent of single persons.

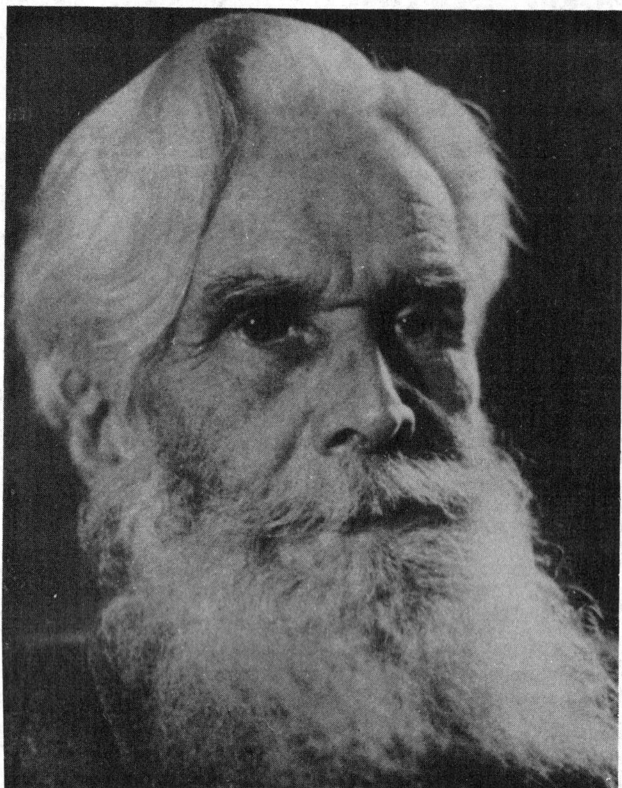

FIGURE 21.1a-1 *Havelock Ellis, 1859-1939. In his book* Studies in the Psychology of Sex *(1896), Ellis recorded examples of normal and abnormal sexuality. It remains a classic in the field of sexology. (Figure courtesy of New York Academy of Medicine.)*

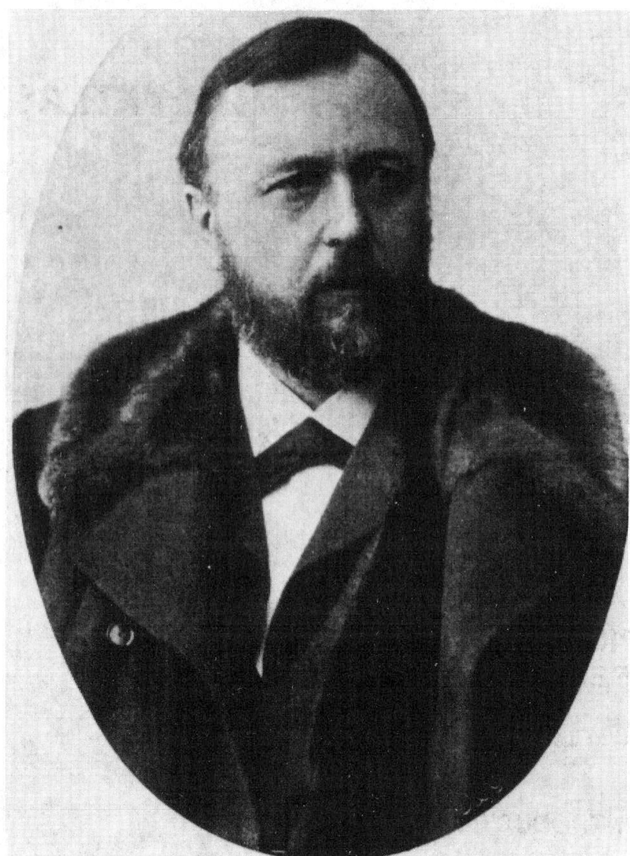

FIGURE 21.1a-2 *Richard von Krafft-Ebing (1840-1903) was a psychiatrist who published a classic text called* Psychopathia Sexualis *(1898) in which he documented every variation in sexuality, including zoophilia, necrophilia, urolagnia, and lust murder, among others. Case reports were so lurid and detailed that early editions were published in Latin. (Figure courtesy of New York Academy of Medicine.)*

3. Cohabiting single persons have the most sex of all, twice a week or more.
4. The median number of sexual partners over a lifetime for men is six; for women it is two.
5. A homosexual orientation was reported by 2.8 percent of men and 1.4 percent of women, with 9 percent of men and 5 percent of women reporting that they had at least one homosexual experience after puberty.
6. Vaginal intercourse was preferred by 83 percent of men and 78 percent of women as the most appealing type of sexual experience.
7. Among marriage partners, 93 percent are of the same race, 82 percent are of similar educational level, 78 percent are within five years of each other's age, and 72 percent are of the same religion.
8. Both men and women who, as children, had been sexually abused by an adult were more likely, as adults, to have had more than 10 sex partners, to engage in group sex, to report a homosexual or bisexual identification, and to be unhappy.
9. Less than 8 percent of the participants reported having sex more than four times a week. About two thirds said they had sex a few times a month or less, and about three in 10 have sex a few times a year or less.
10. About one man in 4 and one woman in 10 masturbates at least once a week, and masturbation is less common among those 18 to 24 years of age than among those who are 24 to 34 years old.
11. Three quarters of the married women said they usually or always had an orgasm during sexual intercourse, compared with 62 percent of the single women. Among men, 95 percent said they usually or always had an orgasm, married or single.
12. More than half of the men said they thought about sex every day, or several times a day, as compared with only 19 percent of the women.
13. More than four in five Americans had only one sexual partner, or no partner, in the past year. Generally, African Americans reported the most sexual partners and Asian Americans the fewest.

NORMAL SEXUALITY

ANATOMICAL AND PHYSIOLOGICAL BASES A discussion of the organs of sexuality and the normal physiological sequence of male and female response is necessary for an informed understanding of the sexual dysfunctions. In fact, the trend over the past decade has been to place greater emphasis on the genetic, neuroanatomical, and neurochemical model of human sexuality than on psychological and social factors.

Anatomy of the male The external genitalia of the normal adult male include the penis, scrotum, testes, epididymus, and parts of the vas deferens. Internal components include the vas deferens, seminal vesicles, ejaculatory ducts, and prostate gland.

Freud referred to the penis as the executive organ of sexuality. Since antiquity, culture after culture has represented the penis in a variety of art forms. In ancient Greece, the cults of Dionysus, Priapus, and the satyrs used the phallus as a recurrent symbol of fertility and rejuvenation. The word "penis" has been traced from the Latin, meaning variously "tail" or "to hang," and refers to the pendant position of the organ in its resting or flaccid state. The size of the penis varies within a fairly constant range, but sex researchers over the years have disagreed on the dimensions of the range. All agree, however, that concern over the size of the penis is practically universal among men. Masters and Johnson report a range of 7 to 11 cm in the flaccid state and 14 to 18 cm in the erect state. Of particular interest was their observation that the flaccid dimension bears little relation to the erect dimension: the smaller penis erects to a proportionally greater size than does the larger penis.

Circumcision, in which the prepuce is surgically removed, has been practiced for centuries as a religious rite by Jews and Moslems and is a common medical procedure in the United States today. It was once believed that the circumcised penis, with its exposed glans, was less sensitive due to cornification of the epithelium. In laboratory studies, however, researchers have found no difference in tactile threshold between the circumcised penis and the uncircumcised penis. Intravaginally, they have found, the prepuce of the uncircumcised penis remains retracted behind the glans during penile thrusting, dispelling the myth that premature ejaculation may be more common in uncircumcised men because of increased stimulation caused by preputial movements.

Ejaculation is the forceful propulsion of semen and of seminal fluid from the epididymis, vas deferens, seminal vesicles, and prostate into the urethra. The dilation of the prostatic urethra and the passage of fluid into the penile urethra provide the man with a sensation of impending climax. That is the emission phase of the ejaculatory process. Indeed, once the prostate contracts, ejaculation is inevitable. The ejaculate is also propelled through the penile urethra by contractions of the striated pelvic and perineal muscles. That phase of ejaculation is essentially under somatic efferent control. The ejaculate consists of about 1 teaspoon (2.5 mL) of fluid and contains about 120 million sperm cells. It is believed that the larger the bolus of ejaculate, the more pleasurable is the orgasm—but that belief is highly subjective.

Anatomy of the female The external genitalia of the normal female are also called the vulva and include the mons pubis, major and minor lips, clitoris, glans, vestibule of the vagina, and vaginal orifice. The internal system includes the ovaries, fallopian tubes, uterus, and vagina.

The word "vagina" comes from the Latin word meaning "sheath." The vagina is usually in a collapsed state, a potential rather than an actual space. About 8 cm long, the vagina extends from the cervix of the uterus above to the vestibule of the vagina or the vaginal opening below. In most virgins a membranous fold, the hymen, separates the vestibule and opening from the rest of the vaginal canal. The mucous membrane lining the vaginal walls rests in numerous transverse folds. To accommodate the penis during sexual intercourse, the vagina expands in both length and width. After menopause, due to decreased circulating estrogen levels, the vagina loses much of its elasticity.

Hippocrates first described the clitoris in the medical literature, referring to it as the site of sexual excitation. Masters and Johnson described the clitoris as the primary female sexual organ, because orgasm depends physiologically on adequate clitoral stimulation. Anatomically, the clitoris has a nerve net that is proportionally three times as large as that of the penis.

Kinsey found that, when women masturbate, most prefer clitoral stimulation to any other. That finding was refined further by Masters and Johnson, who reported that women prefer the shaft of the clitoris to the glans, because the glans is hypersensitive if stimulated excessively.

An important anatomical finding is that the clitoral prepuce is contiguous with the labia minora and that during coitus the penis does not stimulate the clitoris directly. Rather, penile thrusting exerts traction on the minor lips, which in turn stimulates the clitoris sufficiently for orgasm to occur. During heightened excitement, just before orgasm, the clitoris retracts under the clitoral hood as a result of the contraction of the ischiocavernosi muscles. Retracting thus, the clitoris moves away from the vaginal barrel, which makes clitoral-penile contact impossible. The size of the clitoris varies considerably and is unrelated to the degree of sexual responsiveness of a particular female.

G SPOT In 1950 Ernst Graefenberg described an area surrounding the female urethra in the anterior wall of the vagina that has come to be called the G spot. It is about 0.5 to 1 cm in size and becomes engorged during sexual stimulation. Many women report that stimulation of the area is highly pleasurable and can induce orgasm. Grafenburg believed that the tissue here was analogous to the prostate and may account for the spurt of fluid during orgasm reported by some women, similar to male ejaculation.

Innervation of the sex organs Innervation of the organs of sexuality is mediated primarily through the autonomic nervous system (ANS). It is generally assumed that the parasympathetic (cholinergic) system activates the process of erection via impulses that pass through the pelvic splanchnic nerves (S_2, S_3, and S_4), which cause the smooth muscles of the penile arteries to dilate. Blood flows into the sinuses of the corpora cavernosa and blood outflow from the penis is inhibited and erection results. Clitoral engorgements also occur as a result of parasympathetic stimulation that increases blood flow to clitoral tissue.

Adrian Zorgniotti has compared the erection phenomenon that results from increased penile blood inflow and decreased blood outflow to the functioning of an automobile tire because it requires an inflow of air and an intact casing to achieve inflation.

Recent evidence implicates the sympathetic (adrenergic) system as being responsible for ejaculation. Through its hypogastric plexus the adrenergic impulses innervate the urethral crest, the muscles of the epididymis, and the muscles of the vas deferens, seminal vesicles, and prostate. Stimulation of the plexus causes emission. In women the sympathetic system facilitates smooth muscle contraction of the vagina, urethra, and uterus that occurs during orgasm.

The ANS functions outside of voluntary control and is influenced by external events (for example, stress, drugs) and internal events (hypothalamic, limbic, and cortical stimuli). It is not surprising, therefore, that erection and orgasm are so vulnerable to dysfunction.

Recent studies on the role of nitric oxide, which has a relaxant effect on peripheral vascular smooth muscle, revealed that the tissue of the corpus cavernosum is very sensitive to that substance and relaxes under its influence. It is released in response to acetylcholine.

Endocrinology From the time of conception, hormones play a major role in human sexual development (Figure 21.1a-3). Unlike the fetal gonads, which are under chromosomal influence, the fetal external genitalia are very susceptible to hor-

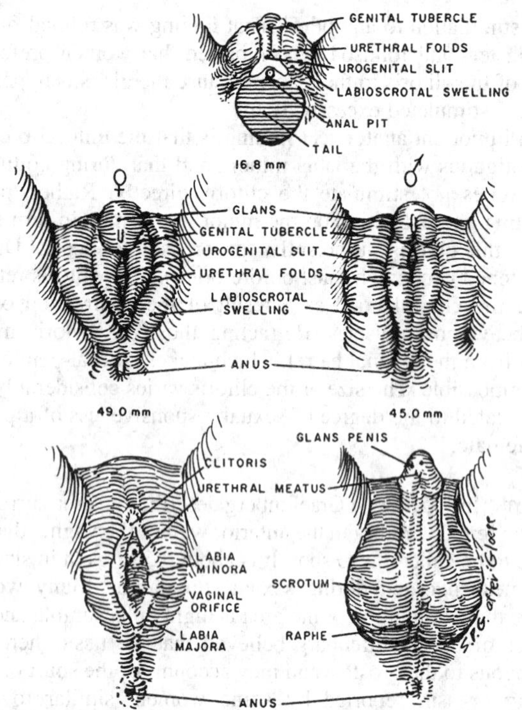

FIGURE 21.1a-3 *Differentiation of male and female external genitalia from indifferent primordia. Male differentiation occurs only in the presence of androgenic stimulation during the first 12 weeks of fetal life. (Figure from Van Wyk and Grumbach, 1968. From J R Brobeck, editor:* Best & Taylor's Physiological Basis of Medical Practice, *ed 9. Williams & Wilkins, Baltimore, 1973. Used with permission.)*

mones. Recently, however, a gene was found on the X chromosome that is believed capable of disrupting the normal development of male genitals. The finding requires replication.

Exogenous hormonal administration can cause external genital development inconsistent with the fetal sex gland development. For instance, if the pregnant mother receives sufficient exogenous androgen, a female fetus possessing an ovary can develop external genitalia resembling those of a male. Fetal, maternal, or exogenous hormones administered to a pregnant woman may all affect the development of external genitalia of the fetus. Deprived of male and female gonads and the respective hormones testosterone and estrogen, the human adult does not develop normal secondary sexual characteristics, is incapable of reproduction, and, in the case of the female does not develop a menstrual cycle.

Testosterone is the hormone believed to be connected with libido in both men and women. In men there is an inverse correlation between stress and the testosterone blood level. Other factors, such as sleep, mood, and life-style, influence circulating levels of the hormone. The administration of androgens to patients complaining of sexual dysfunction is usually futile if normal hormonal function is present. Androgen administered to men complaining of loss of potency and loss of libido has usually been unsuccessful unless testosterone levels are below normal, and administration to women results in disturbing virilizing side effects. Many clinicians correct the hormone deficiency of the postmenopausal period with estrogen replacement therapy. Testosterone has been used in combination with estrogens in women who do not respond to estrogen alone. The combination is especially useful in treating headache, depression, and reduced libido when present. Oxytocin, secreted by the hypothalamus, stimulates lactation and uterine contractions. It may play a role as an enhancer of sexual activity. Before ejaculation oxytocin blood levels rise in men.

Diethylstilbestrol Diethylstilbestrol (DES) is an androgenic steroid that was prescribed in the 1950s and 1960s for pregnant women with threatened abortion. However, the drug had untoward effects on the children (especially female children) born to mothers so treated. Reports of cervical and uterine abnormalities were reported in women and reproductive tract disorders in men. The children (called DES daughters and sons) organized a National DES Education Program sponsored by the National Cancer Institute to provide information on the potential medical problems confronting those born to DES mothers.

THE BRAIN AND SEXUAL BEHAVIOR Experimentation with animals has demonstrated that the limbic system is directly involved with elements of sexual functioning. In all mammals the limbic system is involved in behavior required for self-preservation and the preservation of the species.

Chemical or electrical stimulation of various sites of the limbic system—the lower part of the septum and the contiguous medial preoptic area, the fimbria of the hippocampus, the mammillary bodies, and the anterior thalamic nuclei—have all elicited penile erection. The hippocampus is believed to influence genital tumescence and affect the regulation of the release of gonadotropins.

The stimulation of the amygdala in primates initiates first oral (chewing, lip smacking) and then genital (penile erection) behavior. Researchers have stated that the closeness of those functions may derive from the evolutionary fact that the olfactory sense was strongly involved in both feeding and mating. They speculate that the evolution of the third subdivision of the limbic system may reflect a shift in importance from olfactory contact to visual communication in sociosexual behavior.

Brain neurotransmitters A vast array of neurotransmitters are produced by the brain. They include dopamine, epinephrine, norepinephrine, and serotonin. All have effects on sexual function. For example, an increase in dopamine is presumed to increase libido. Serotonin produced in the upper pons and midbrain is presumed to have an inhibitory effect on sexual function. Basic science and clinical research on brain neurotransmitters and their effects on behavior (including sex) is one of the most rapidly expanding fields. Some of those findings are summarized in Table 21.1a-1.

SEXUAL LEARNING AND MASTURBATION Sexual learning begins in childhood. In a broad sense, that learning occurs through parent-child interaction, including the meeting of the infant's physical needs, cuddling, the reinforcement or discouragement of gender-associated activities, and the establishment by the age of 2 of gender identity. The elaboration of gender roles continues throughout one's lifetime.

Genital self-stimulation is a normal activity of babies. It is particularly pronounced between the ages of 15 and 19 months and is part of the general interest of the child in his or her body. The activity is reinforced by the pleasurable sensations it produces. As the child grows older, that exploration and stimulation are extended to other children in "doctor" games. The child is socialized not to masturbate in public, but unless he or she is unduly shamed, self-stimulation usually continues as a pleasurable, private experience.

With the hormonal acceleration of puberty and the physiological changes of adolescence, masturbation serves additional

TABLE 21.1a-1
Responses of Sex Organs to Autonomic Nerve Impulses

	Adrenergic impulses		Cholinergic impulses
Effector organs	Receptor Type[2]	Responses	Responses
Urinary Bladder			
Detrusor	β_2	Relaxation (usually) +	Contraction +++
Trigone and sphincter	α_1	Contraction ++	Relaxation ++
Ureter			
Motility and tone	α_1	Increase	Increase (?)
Uterus	α_1; β_2	Pregnant: contraction (α_1); relaxation (β_2). Nonpregnant: relaxation (β_2)	Variable[10]
Sex Organs, Male	α_1	Ejaculation +++	Erection +++
Skin			
Pilomotor muscles	α_1	Contraction ++	—
Sweat glands	α_1	Localized secretion[11] +	Generalized secretion +++

Table from *Goodman and Gilman's The Pharmacological Basis of Therapeutics,* ed 8, A Goodman Gilman, T W Rall, A S Nies, P Taylor, editors, p 89. Pergamon, New York, 1990. Used with permission.

functions. At that time it is frequently accompanied by coital fantasies and acts as preparation for adult interaction with a partner. Also, it provides an acceptable release for the adolescent who must establish his or her sexual identity, but who frequently has no outlet for his or her heightened sexual impulses.

Masturbation usually continues to some degree through the life cycle. Even after a permanent sexual relationship has been established, masturbation remains a healthy sexual activity during the illness or absence of a partner. Only when it is a compulsive activity or when it is preferred to partner interaction should it be considered maladaptive. Even the punitive and inhibitory myths that surround masturbation—that it causes blindness, impotence, illness, or sterility—have not prevented it from being a nearly universal practice. Kinsey reported that nearly all men and three fourths of women masturbate sometime during their lives. In the study conducted by the University of Chicago, men were found to masturbate more than women, masturbation was not positively correlated with a lack of partnered sex, persons who masturbated frequently were most likely to usually or always experience an orgasm with that act, and approximately 50 percent of men and women who masturbated felt guilty after doing so.

Physiological responses Normal men and women experience a sequence of physiological responses to sexual stimulation. In the first detailed description of these responses, Masters and Johnson observed that the physiological process involves increasing levels of vasocongestion and myotonia (*tumescence*) and the subsequent release of the vascular activity and muscle tone as a result of orgasm (*detumescence*). Table 21.1a-2 and Table 21.1a-3 describe the male and female sexual response cycles respectively. The fourth edition of DSM (DSM-IV) defines a four-phase response cycle: Phase I—Desire; Phase II—Excitement; Phase III—Orgasm; Phase IV—Resolution.

PHASE I: DESIRE The phase is distinct from any identified solely through physiology and reflects the psychiatrist's fundamental concern with motivations, drives, and personality. It is characterized by sexual fantasies and the desire to have sexual activity.

PHASE II: EXCITEMENT The phase is brought on by psychological stimulation (fantasy or the presence of a love object), physiological stimulation (stroking or kissing), or a combination of the two. It consists of a subjective sense of pleasure. The excitement phase is characterized by penile tumescence leading to erection in the man and vaginal lubrication in the woman. The nipples of both sexes become erect, although nipple erection is more common in women than in men. The woman's clitoris becomes hard and turgid, and her labia minora become thicker as a result of venous engorgment. Initial excitement may last several minutes to several hours. With continued stimulation, the man's testes increase in size 50 percent and elevate. The woman's vaginal barrel shows a characteristic constriction along the outer third known as the orgasmic platform. The clitoris elevates and retracts behind the symphysis pubis. As a result the clitoris is not easily accessible. As the area is stimulated, however, traction on the labia minora and the prepuce occurs, and there is intrapreputial movement of the clitoral shaft. Breast size in the woman increases 25 percent. Continued engorgement of the penis and vagina produces specific color changes, particularly in the labia minora, which become bright or deep red. Voluntary contractions of large muscle groups occur, rate of heartbeat and respiration increases, and blood pressure rises. Heightened excitement lasts 30 seconds to several minutes.

PHASE III: ORGASM The phase consists of a peaking of sexual pleasure, with release of sexual tension and rhythmic contraction of the perineal muscles and pelvic reproductive organs. A subjective sense of ejaculatory inevitability triggers the man's orgasm. The forceful emission of semen follows. The male orgasm is also associated with four to five rhythmic spasms of the prostate, seminal vesicles, vas, and urethra. In the woman orgasm is characterized by 3 to 15 involuntary contractions of the lower third of the vagina and by strong sustained contractions of the uterus, flowing from the fundus downward to the cervix. Both men and women have involuntary contractions of the internal and external sphincter. Those and the other contractions during orgasm occur at intervals of 0.8 second. Other manifestations include voluntary and involuntary movements of the large muscle groups, including facial grimacing and carpopedal spasm. Blood pressure rises 20 to 40 mm (both systolic and diastolic), and the heart rate increases up to 160 beats a minute. Orgasm lasts from 3 to 25 seconds and is associated with a slight clouding of consciousness.

PHASE IV: RESOLUTION Resolution consists of the disgorgement of blood from the genitalia (detumescence), and that detumescence brings the body back to its resting state. If orgasm occurs, resolution is rapid; if it does not occur, resolution may take two to six hours and be associated with irritability and discomfort. Resolution through orgasm is characterized by a

TABLE 21.1a-2
Female Sexual Response Cycle*

Organ	Excitement Phase	Orgasmic Phase	Resolution Phase
	Lasts several minutes to several hours; heightened excitement before orgasm, 30 seconds to 3 minutes	3 to 15 seconds	10 to 15 minutes; if no orgasm, ½ to 1 day
Skin	Just before orgasm: sexual flush inconsistently appears; maculopapular rash originates on abdomen and spreads to anterior chest wall, face, and neck; can include shoulders and forearms	Well-developed flush	Flush disappears in reverse order of appearance; inconsistently appearing film of perspiration on soles of feet and palms of hands
Breasts	Nipple erection in two thirds of women, venous congestion and areolar enlargement; size increases to one fourth over normal	Breasts may become tremulous	Return to normal in about ½ hour
Clitoris	Enlargement in diameter of glans and shaft; just before orgasm, shaft retracts into pupuce	No change	Shaft returns to normal position in 5 to 10 seconds; detumescence in 5 to 30 minutes; if no orgasm, detumescence takes several hours
Labia majora	Nullipara: elevate and flatten against perineum Multipara: congestion and edema	No change	Nullipara: increase to normal size in 1 to 2 minutes Multipara: decrease to normal size in 10 to 15 minutes
Labia minora	Size increase two to three times over normal; change to pink, red, deep red before orgasm	Contractions of proximal labia minora	Return to normal within 5 minutes
Vagina	Color change to dark purple; vaginal transudate appears 10 to 30 seconds after arousal; elongation and ballooning of vagina; lower third of vagina constricts before orgasm	3 to 15 contractions of lower third of vagina at intervals of 0.8 second	Ejaculate forms seminal pool in upper two thirds of vagina; congestion disappears in seconds or, if no orgasm, in 20 to 30 minutes
Uterus	Ascends into false pelvis; laborlike contractions begin in heightened excitement just before orgasm	Contractions throughout orgasm	Contractions cease, and uterus descends to normal position
Other	Myotonia A few drops of mucoid secretion from Bartholin's glands during heightened excitement Cervix swells slightly and is passively elevated with uterus	Loss of voluntary muscular control Rectum: rhythmical contractions of sphincter Hyperventilation and tachycardia	Return to baseline status in seconds to minutes Cervix color and size return to normal, and cervix descends into seminal pool

*A desire phase consisting of sex fantasies and desire to have sex precedes excitement phase.

subjective sense of well-being, general relaxation, and muscular relaxation.

After orgasm men have a refractory period that may last from several minutes to many hours; in that period they cannot be stimulated to further orgasm. The refractory period does not exist in women who are capable of multiple and successive orgasms.

Sexual response is a true psychophysiological experience. Arousal is triggered by both psychological and physical stimuli, levels of tension are experienced both physiologically and emotionally, and, with orgasm, there is normally a subjective perception of a peak of physical reaction and release. Psychosexual development, psychological attitude toward sexuality, and attitudes toward one's sexual partner are directly involved with and affect the physiology of human sexual response.

ABNORMAL SEXUALITY AND SEXUAL DYSFUNCTIONS

INTRODUCTION Seven major categories of sexual dysfunction are listed in DSM-IV: (1) sexual desire disorders, (2) sexual arousal disorders, (3) orgasm disorders, (4) sexual pain disorders, (5) sexual dysfunction due to a general medical condition, (6) substance-induced sexual dysfunction, and (7) sexual dysfunction not otherwise specified.

DEFINITION In DSM-IV sexual dysfunctions are categorized as Axis I disorders. The syndromes listed are correlated with the sexual physiological response. The sexual response cycle is divided into four phases: desire (called appetitive in the revised third edition of DSM [DSM-III-R]), excitement, orgasm, and resolution. The essential feature of the sexual dysfunctions is inhibition in one or more of the phases, including disturbance in the subjective sense of pleasure or desire or disturbance in the objective performance (Table 21.1a-4 and Table 21.1a-5). Either type of disturbance can occur alone or in combination. Sexual dysfunctions are so diagnosed only when such disturbances are a major part of the clinical picture. They can be lifelong or acquired, generalized or situational, and due to psychological factors or due to combined factors. If they are attributable entirely to a general medical condition, substance use, or adverse effects of medication, then sexual dysfunction due to a general medical condition or substance-induced sexual dysfunction is diagnosed.

With the possible exception of premature ejaculation, sexual dysfunctions rarely are found separate from other psychiatric syndromes. Sexual disorders may lead to or result from rela-

TABLE 21.1a-3
Male Sexual Response Cycle*

Organ	Excitement Phase	Orgasmic Phase	Resolution Phase
	Lasts several minutes to several hours; heightened excitement before orgasm, 30 seconds to 3 minutes	3 to 15 seconds	10 to 15 minutes; if no orgasm, ½ to 1 day
Skin	Just before orgasm: sexual flush inconsistently appears; maculopapular rash originates on abdomen and spreads to anterior chest wall, face, and neck and can include shoulders and forearms	Well-developed flush	Flush disappears in reverse order of appearance; inconsistently appearing film of perspiration on soles of feet and palms of hands
Penis	Erection in 10 to 30 seconds caused by vasocongestion of erectile bodies of corpus cavernosa of shaft; loss of erection may occur with introduction of asexual stimulus, loud noise; with heightened excitement, size of glans and diameter of penile shaft increase further	Ejaculation; emission phase marked by three to four contractions of 0.8 second of vas, seminal vesicles, prostate; ejaculation proper marked by contractions of 0.8 second of urethra and ejaculatory spurt of 12 to 20 inches at age 18, decreasing with age to seepage at 70	Erection: partial involution in 5 to 10 seconds with variable refractory period; full detumescence in 5 to 30 minutes
Scrotum and testes	Tightening and lifting of scrotal sac and elevation of testes; with heightened excitement, 50% increase in size of testes over unstimulated state and flattening against perineum, signaling impending ejaculation	No change	Decrease to baseline size because of loss of vasocongestion; testicular and scrotal descent within 5 to 30 minutes after orgasm; involution may take several hours if no orgasmic release takes place
Cowper's glands	2 to 3 drops of mucoid fluid that contain viable sperm are secreted during heightened excitement	No change	No change
Other	Breasts: inconsistent nipple erection with heightened excitement before orgasm Myotonia: semispastic contractions of facial, abdominal, and intercostal muscles Tachycardia: up to 175 a minute Blood pressure: rise in systolic 20 to 80 mm; in diastolic 10 to 40 mm Respiration: increased	Loss of voluntary muscular control Rectum: rhythmical contractions of sphincter Heart rate: up to 180 beats a minute Blood pressure: up to 40 to 100 mm systolic; 20 to 50 mm diastolic Respiration: up to 40 respirations a minute	Return to baseline state in 5 to 10 minutes

*A desire phase consisting of sex fantasies and desire to have sex precedes excitement phase.

TABLE 21.1a-4
DSM-IV Phases of the Sexual Response Cycle and Associated Sexual Dysfunctions*

Phases	Characteristics	Dysfunction
1. Desire	This phase is distinct from any identified solely through physiology and reflects the patient's motivations, drives, and personality. The phase is characterized by sexual fantasies and the desire to have sex.	Hypoactive sexual desire disorder; sexual aversion disorder; hypoactive sexual desire disorder due to a general medical condition (male or female); substance-induced sexual dysfunction with impaired desire
2. Excitement	This phase consists of a subjective sense of sexual pleasure and accompanying physiological changes. All the physiological responses noted in Masters and Johnson's excitement and plateau phases are combined and occur in this phase.	Female sexual arousal disorder; male erectile disorder (may also occur in stage 3 and in stage 4); male erectile disorder due to a general medical condition; dyspareunia due to a general medical condition (male or female); substance-induced sexual dysfunction with impaired arousal
3. Orgasm	This phase consists of a peaking of sexual pleasure, with release of sexual tension and rhythmic contraction of the perineal muscles and pelvic reproductive organs.	Female orgasmic disorder; male orgasmic disorder; premature ejaculation; other sexual dysfunction due to a general medical condition (male or female); substance-induced sexual dysfunction with impaired orgasm
4. Resolution	This phase entails a sense of general relaxation, well-being, and muscle relaxation. During this phase men are refractory to orgasm for a period of time that increases with age, whereas women are capable of having multiple orgasms without a refractory period.	Postcoital dysphoria; postcoital headache

*DSM-IV consolidates the Masters and Johnson excitement and plateau phases into a single excitement phase, which is preceded by the desire (appetitive) phase. The orgasm and resolution phases remain the same as originally described by Masters and Johnson.

TABLE 21.1a-5
Sexual Dysfunction Not Correlated with Phases of the Sexual Response Cycle

Category	Dysfunctions
Sexual pain disorders	Vaginismus (female) Dyspareunia (female and male)
Other	Sexual dysfunctions not otherwise specified. Examples: 1. No erotic sensation despite normal physiological response to sexual stimulation (e.g., orgasmic anhedonia) 2. Female analogue of premature ejaculation 3. Genital pain occurring during masturbation

tional problems, and patients invariably develop an increasing fear of failure and self-consciousness about their sexual performance. Sexual dysfunctions are frequently associated with other mental disorders, such as depressive disorders, anxiety disorders, personality disorders, and schizophrenia. In many instances, sexual dysfunctions may be diagnosed in conjunction with the other psychiatric disorders. In some cases, however, it is but one of many signs or symptoms of the psychiatric disorder.

A sexual disorder can be symptomatic of biological problems, intrapsychic conflicts, interpersonal difficulties, or a combination of these factors. The sexual function can be affected by stress of any kind, by emotional disorders, and by a lack of sexual knowledge.

TAKING A SEXUAL HISTORY As with all psychiatric interviews, the sexual history taking not only is an information-gathering time but permits the development of a positive doctor-patient relationship. Essential to the development of confidence and rapport is an accepting atmosphere and a nonjudgmental attitude on the part of the therapist toward the patients' sexual values, ideas, and practices.

The taking of the sexual history is more structured than the rest of the psychiatric interview, although patients are encouraged to take their own lead in areas having great personal significance. In general, the therapist structures the interview so that both recent and early sexual histories are covered. The therapist must ascertain the specific current sexual complaint, the person's sexual practices and pattern of interaction with partners, the person's sexual goal and fantasies, the masturbatory history, the presence or extent of extramarital relationships, and the degree of commitment to the marriage and the partner. Patients describe their view of the problem and when it began. The courtship, honeymoon, and reproductive history are examined in detail. Premarital expectations, mutual physical attraction, periods of separation, the type of contraception used, and the effect of children on the couple's sexual life are covered. The satisfying aspects of the marriage must also be discussed. The patient is particularly asked to evaluate the partner's contribution to the present distress.

Early sexual development and education are also thoroughly discussed. The interviewer asks for the patient's view of the parents' marriage as seen in retrospect and as perceived in childhood. Relationships to peers, siblings, and important familial figures other than parents are also explored. Particular attention is paid to ways in which affection was expressed in the family and the degree of physical contact between family members. The sexual climate in which the patient grew up is seen through reported parental attitudes, memories of sexual games played as a child, the way in which the patient learned sexual facts, the specifics of religious training, reactions to masturbation and nocturnal emissions or the menarche, dating patterns, an adolescent rebellious phase, and any significant premarital involvements. Ethnic background and the socioeconomic level of the patient's primary family are also taken into account. As the interview progresses, the patient's self-image emerges. The interviewer must be sensitive to any event that was exceptional in the patient's sexual life in either a destructive or a highly pleasant manner and should take particular note of those people who contributed to the patient's sexual education, identity, and mores.

The interviewer must also ask specific questions to elicit information that may be outside the patient's view of the socially acceptable, such as premarital and extramarital affairs, group sex, homosexual involvements, and abortions.

The sexual orientation of the person being interviewed should be ascertained and questions related to same-sex interactions explored. In all interviews high-risk sexual behavior should be reviewed, regardless of sexual orientation since transmission of the human immunodeficiency virus (HIV) is increasing rapidly among all groups.

It should be kept in mind that similar disorders exist among both homosexual and heterosexual partners, with variations imposed by anatomical differences. For example, although penile-vaginal dysfunction cannot be described among homosexuals, penile-anal dysfunction may occur. In spite of sexual orientation each phase of the sex cycle applies equally to same-sex and heterosexual partners and the methods and principles for treatment are essentially similar.

SEXUAL DESIRE DISORDERS In DSM-IV sexual desire disorders are divided into two classes: hypoactive sexual desire disorder, characterized by a deficiency or the absence of sexual fantasies and desire for sexual activity (Table 21.1a-6), and sexual aversion disorder, characterized by an aversion to and avoidance of genital sexual contact with a sexual partner (Table 21.1a-7). The former condition is more common than the latter.

Hypoactive sexual desire disorder Hypoactive sexual desire disorder is experienced by both men and women; however, they may not be hampered by any dysfunction once they are involved in the sex act. Conversely, hypoactive desire may be used to mask another sexual dysfunction. Lack of desire may

TABLE 21.1a-6
Diagnostic Criteria for Hypoactive Sexual Desire Disorder

A. Persistently or recurrently deficient (or absent) sexual fantasies and desire for sexual activity. The judgment of deficiency or absence is made by the clinician, taking into account factors that affect sexual functioning, such as age and the context of the person's life.
B. The disturbance causes marked distress or interpersonal difficulty.
C. The sexual dysfunction is not better accounted for by another Axis I disorder (except another sexual dysfunction) and is not due exclusively to the direct physiological effects of a substance (e.g., a drug of abuse, a medication) or a general medical condition.

Specify type:
Lifelong type
Acquired type
Specify type:
Generalized type
Situational type
Specify:
Due to psychological factors
Due to combined factors

Table from DSM-IV, *Diagnostic and Statistical Manual of Mental Disorders,* ed 4. Copyright American Psychiatric Association, Washington, 1994. Used with permission.

TABLE 21.1a-7
Diagnostic Criteria for Sexual Aversion Disorder

A. Persistent or recurrent extreme aversion to, and avoidance of, all (or almost all) genital sexual contact with a sexual partner.
B. The disturbance causes marked distress or interpersonal difficulty.
C. The sexual dysfunction is not better accounted for by another Axis I disorder (except another sexual dysfunction).

Specify type:
Lifelong type
Acquired type
Specify type:
Generalized type
Situational type
Specify:
Due to psychological factors
Due to combined factors

Table from DSM-IV, *Diagnostic and Statistical Manual of Mental Disorders,* ed 4. Copyright American Psychiatric Association, Washington, 1994. Used with permission.

be expressed by decreased frequency of coitus, perception of the partner as unattractive, or overt complaints of lack of desire. In some cases there are biochemical correlates associated with hypoactive desire. A recent study found markedly decreased levels of serum testosterone in men complaining of this dysfunction when they were compared with normal controls in a sleep-laboratory situation. Also, a central dopamine blockage is known to decrease desire (Table 21.1a-6).

The need for sexual contact and satisfaction varies among different persons, as well as in the same person over time. In a group of 100 couples with stable marriages, 8 percent reported having intercourse less than once a month. In another group of couples, one third reported lack of sexual relations for periods averaging eight weeks. In a survey of a general medical practice in England, 25 percent of that sample reported no sexual activity the majority of the time. It has been estimated that 20 percent of the total population have hypoactive sexual desire disorder. The complaint is more common among women.

Patients with desire problems often have good ego strengths and use inhibition of desire in a defensive way to protect against unconscious fears about sex. Lack of desire can also be the result of chronic stress, anxiety, or depression. Abstinence from sex for a prolonged period sometimes results in suppression of the sexual impulse. It may also be an expression of hostility or the sign of a deteriorating relationship.

The presence of desire depends on several factors: biological drive, adequate self-esteem, previous good experiences with sex, the availability of an appropriate partner, and a good relationship in nonsexual areas with one's partner. Damage to any of those factors may result in diminished desire.

Hypoactive sexual desire disorders often become manifest during puberty and may remain a lifelong condition. A general medical workup is always indicated to rule out a medical cause, which would be diagnosed as male or female sexual desire disorder due to a general medical condition according to DSM-IV. Table 21.1a-6 presents the DSM-IV diagnostic criteria for hypoactive sexual desire disorder.

Mr. and Ms. B. have been married for 14 years and have three children, ages 8 through 12. They are both bright and well educated. Both are from Scotland, from which they moved 10 years ago because of Mr. B.'s work as an industrial consultant. They present with the complaint that Ms. B. has been able to participate passively in sex as a duty, but has never enjoyed it since they have been married.

Before their marriage, although they had intercourse only twice, Ms. B. had been highly aroused by kissing and petting and felt she used her attractiveness to seduce her husband into marriage. She did, however, feel intense guilt about their two episodes of premarital intercourse; during their honeymoon, she began to think of sex as a chore that could not be pleasing. Although she periodically passively complied with intercourse, she had almost no spontaneous desire for sex. She never masturbated, had never reached orgasm; thought of all variations, such as oral sex, as completely repulsive; and was preoccupied with a fantasy of how disapproving her family would be if she ever engaged in any of those activities.

Ms. B. is almost totally certain that no woman she respects in any older generation has enjoyed sex, and that despite the "new vogue" of sexuality, only sleazy, crude women let themselves act like animals. Those beliefs have led to a pattern of regular, but infrequent, sex that at best is accommodating and gives little or no pleasure to her or her husband. Whenever Ms. B. comes close to having a feeling of sexual arousal, numerous negative thoughts come into her mind, such as "What am I, a tramp?" "If I like this, he'll just want it more often." or "How could I look myself in the mirror after something like this?" Those thoughts almost inevitably are accompanied by a cold feeling and an insensitivity to sensual pleasure. As a result, sex is invariably an unhappy experience. Almost any excuse, such as fatigue or being busy, is sufficient for her to rationalize avoiding intercourse.

Yet, intellectually Ms. B. wonders, "Is something wrong with me?" She is seeking help to find out whether or not she is normal. Her husband, although extraordinarily tolerant of the situation, is very unhappy about their sex life and is very hopeful that help may be forthcoming.

Discussion This couple seeks help for the wife's long-standing sexual problem. Clearly this woman's sexual difficulties stem from her many negative attitudes toward sexuality, and cannot be accounted for by a nonsexual Axis I disorder, such as major depressive disorder. The diagnosis of sexual aversion disorder needs to be considered. Although she certainly has a persistent extreme aversion to genital sexual contact and might like to avoid sexual activity, she does, in fact, have regular although infrequent intercourse. The persistent absence of sexual fantasies and desire for sexual activity justify the diagnosis of hypoactive sexual desire disorder, due to psychological factors, lifelong, generalized type. When she does have sexual intercourse, she probably does not become sexually excited, so the additional diagnosis of female sexual arousal disorder should be considered. The diagnosis of inhibited female orgasm would be added only if there were many occasions when during sexual activity she failed to have an orgasm, but had no disturbance in sexual excitement—extremely unlikely in this case.

The absence of any significant complaint on the part of the husband is reflected in the notation "no diagnosis or condition on Axis I" for him. (From *DSM-IV Casebook.* Used with permission.)

Sexual aversion disorder That category of sexual disorder is defined in DSM-IV as a "persistent or recurrent and extreme aversion to, and avoidance of, all or almost all, genital sexual contact with a sexual partner." Some researchers consider the line between hypoactive desire disorder and sexual aversion disorder blurred, and in some cases both diagnoses are appropriate. Low frequency of sexual interaction is a symptom common to both disorders. From a clinician's perspective, it is helpful to think of the words "repugnance" and "phobia" in relation to the patient with sexual aversion disorder.

Sigmund Freud conceptualized sexual aversion as the result of inhibition during the phallic psychosexual phase and unresolved oedipal conflicts. Some men, fixated at the phallic stage of development, are fearful of the vagina, believing that they will be castrated if they approach it, a concept Freud called *vagina dentata,* because they believe unconsciously that the vagina has teeth. Hence they avoid contact with the female genitalia entirely.

The disorder may result from a traumatic sexual assault, such as rape or childhood abuse, from repeated painful experiences with coitus, and from early developmental conflicts that have left the patient with unconscious connections between the sexual impulse and overwhelming feelings of shame and guilt. The disorder may also be a reaction to a perceived psychological assault by the person's partner and to relationship difficulties.

The DSM-IV criteria for several aversion disorder appear in Table 21.1a-7.

A 33-year-old stockbroker sought treatment because of "impotence." Five months previously, a close male friend had died of a coronary occlusion, and within the following week the patient developed anxiety about his own cardiac status. Whenever his heart beat fast because of exertion, he became anxious that he was about to have a heart attack. He had disturbing dreams from which he would awaken anxious and unable to get back to sleep. He stopped playing tennis and running.

The patient began to avoid sexual intercourse, presumably because of his anxiety about physical exertion. That caused difficulties with his wife, who felt that he was deliberately depriving her of sexual outlets and was also preventing her from becoming pregnant, which she very much desired. In the past month, although no longer worried about his heart, the patient had avoided sexual intercourse entirely. He claimed to still have some desire for sex, but when the situation arose, he could not bring himself to do it. He became so upset about his sexual difficulties that he began to have trouble concentrating at work. He felt himself to be a failure, both as a husband and as a man.

Before his marriage the patient had had no sexual experience, and had masturbated by rubbing his penis against the beddings, without ever manually touching it. Four years previously, at 29 and after three years of marriage, he had presented himself for treatment with the complaint that he had never attempted to have sexual intercourse with his wife. Sexual activity consisted of his obtaining an erection without either his wife or himself touching his penis, and ejaculation occurred by rubbing his penis on his wife's abdomen. He was unable to touch his wife's genitalia with his hands or allow his penis to be placed anywhere near his wife's genitalia.

Treatment had consisted of two weeks of intensive couples therapy, using the techniques developed by Masters and Johnson, with dramatic success. Sexual activity became frequent, with vaginal penetration and ejaculation. The husband began to display flirtatious sexuality toward other females, which led to some embarrassing social situations, but not to promiscuity. His wife's anxiety about her own sexuality and the adoption of a more passive role led her to seek treatment in her own right. After one year of psychotherapy, her anxieties were allayed; sexual intercourse and interpersonal relationships between the patient and his wife had been at a satisfactory level until the present problem arose.

Discussion The man's reaction to the death of his friend five months previously involved severe anxiety and restriction in his physical activities because of fear that he might have a heart attack; had he been evaluated at that time, an appropriate diagnosis would have been adjustment disorder with anxious mood. What then happened was that his anxiety affected his sexual functioning, and it is the sexual difficulties that have persisted and occasioned this evaluation.

His current sexual problem is a recurrence of the problem that caused him to seek sex therapy four years earlier: avoidance of sexual intercourse because of the anxiety associated with it. Although he refers to his problem as "impotence," the diagnosis of male erectile disorder presumes that there is sexual activity during which a man fails to attain or maintain an erection until completion of the sexual activity. However, what this man demonstrates is avoidance of sexual intercourse. Persistent or recurrent extreme aversion to, and avoidance of, all or almost all genital sexual contact with a partner is diagnosed as sexual aversion disorder, due to psychological factors, acquired. (From *DSM-IV Casebook*. Used with permission).

SEXUAL AROUSAL DISORDERS The sexual arousal disorders are divided by DSM-IV into (1) female sexual arousal disorder, characterized by the persistent or recurrent partial or complete failure to attain or maintain the lubrication-swelling response of sexual excitement until the completion of the sexual act, and (2) male erectile disorder, characterized by the recurrent and persistent partial or complete failure to attain or maintain an erection until the completion of the sex act. The diagnosis takes into account the focus, the intensity, and the duration of the sexual activity in which the patient engages (Tables 21.1a-8 and 21.1a-9). If sexual stimulation is inadequate in focus, intensity, or duration, the diagnosis should not be made.

Female sexual arousal disorder Women who have excitement-phase dysfunction often have orgastic problems as well. In one series of relatively happily married couples, 33 percent of the women described difficulty in maintaining sexual excitement.

Numerous psychological factors are associated with female sexual inhibition. Those conflicts may be expressed through inhibition of excitement or orgasm and are discussed under orgasmic phase dysfunctions. In some women arousal disorders are associated with dyspareunia or with lack of desire.

TABLE 21.1a-8
Diagnostic Criteria for Female Sexual Arousal Disorder

A. Persistent or recurrent inability to attain, or to maintain until completion of the sexual activity, an adequate lubrication-swelling response of sexual excitement.
B. The disturbance causes marked distress or interpersonal difficulty.
C. The sexual dysfunction is not better accounted for by another Axis I disorder (except another sexual dysfunction) and is not due exclusively to the direct physiological effects of a substance (e.g., a drug of abuse, a medication) or a general medical condition.

Specify type:
Lifelong type
Acquired type
Specify type:
Generalized type
Situational type
Specify:
Due to psychological factors
Due to combined factors

TABLE 21.1a-9
Diagnostic Criteria for Male Erectile Disorder

A. Persistent or recurrent inability to attain, or to maintain until completion of the sexual activity, an adequate erection.
B. The disturbance causes marked distress or interpersonal difficulty.
C. The erectile dysfunction is not better accounted for by another Axis I disorder (other than a sexual dysfunction) and is not due exclusively to the direct physiological effects of a substance (e.g., a drug of abuse, a medication) or a general medical condition.

Specify type:
Lifelong type
Acquired type
Specify type:
Generalized type
Situational type
Specify:
Due to psychological factors
Due to combined factors

Less research has been done on physiological components of dysfunction in women than in men, and there have been conflicting results. Masters and Johnson found normally responsive women to be particularly desirous of sex premenstrually. In a recent study dysfunctional women tended to be more responsive immediately following their periods. A third group of dysfunctional women felt the greatest sexual excitement at the time of ovulation. There is some evidence that dysfunctional women are less aware of the physiological responses of their bodies such as vasocongestion, during arousal.

There are some organic etiologies for female sexual arousal disorder. Alterations in testosterone, estrogen, prolactin, and thyroxin levels have been implicated. Medications with antihistaminic or anticholinergic properties cause lessened vaginal lubrication and interfere with arousal. Also, postmenopausal women require a longer period of stimulation for lubrication to occur, and there is generally less vaginal transudate after menopause. An artificial lubricant is frequently useful in that situation.

Table 21.1a-8 presents the diagnostic criteria for female sexual arousal disorder.

Male erectile disorder Male erectile disorder is also called erectile dysfunction and impotence. A man with lifelong male erectile disorder has never been able to obtain an erection sufficient for vaginal insertion. In acquired male erectile disorder the man has successfully achieved vaginal penetration at some time in his sexual life but is later unable to do so. In situational male erectile disorder the man is able to have coitus in certain circumstances but not in others; for example, a man may function effectively with a prostitute but be impotent with his wife.

It was estimated by Kinsey that a few men (2 to 4 percent) are impotent at age 35, but 77 percent are impotent at age 80. Ten percent of the men in the University of Chicago study reported an experience with impotence in the past year, and between 15 and 20 percent experienced anxiety about performing. More recently it was estimated that the incidence of impotence in young men is about 8 percent. However, that sexual dysfunction may first appear later in life. Masters and Johnson reported a fear of impotence in all men over 40, which the researchers believed reflects the masculine fear of loss of virility with advancing age. (As it happens, however, impotence is not a regularly occurring phenomenon in the aged; having good health and an available sexual partner are more closely related to continuing potency in the aging man than is age per se.) The percentage of all men treated for sexual disorders who have impotence as the chief complaint ranges from 35 to 50 percent.

The incidence of psychological as opposed to organic impotence has been the focus of many recent studies. Physiologically, impotence may be due to a variety of medical causes (Table 21.1a-10). In the United States it is estimated that two million men are impotent because they suffer from diabetes mellitus; an additional 300,000 are impotent because of other endocrine diseases; 1.5 million are impotent as a result of vascular disease; 180,000 because of multiple sclerosis; 400,000 because of traumas and fractures leading to pelvic fractures or spinal cord injuries; and another 650,000 as a result of radical surgery, including prostatectomies, colostomies, and cystectomies. In addition, the clinician should be aware of the possible pharmacological effects of medication on sexual functioning. The increased incidence of organic etiologies for this dysfunction in the past 15 years may, in part, reflect the increased use of psychotropic and antihypertensive medications. Statistics indicate that 20 to 50 percent of men with erectile dysfunction have a medical basis for their problem.

Paul and Petula Petersen have been living together for the past six months and are contemplating marriage. Petula describes the problem that has brought them to the sex therapy clinic.

"For the last two months he hasn't been able to keep his erection after he enters me."

The psychiatrist turns to Paul and asks him how he sees the problem. Paul, embarrassed, agrees with Petula and adds, "I just don't know why."

The psychiatrist learns that Paul, age 26, is a recently graduated lawyer, and that Petula, age 24, is a successful buyer for a large department store. They both grew up in educated, middle-class, suburban families. They met through mutual friends, and started to have sexual intercourse a few months after they met and had no problems at that time.

Two months later Paul moved from his family home into Petula's apartment. It was her idea, and Paul was unsure that he was ready for such an important step. Within a few weeks Paul noticed that although he continued to be sexually aroused and wanted intercourse, as soon as he entered his partner, he would begin to lose his erection and could not stay inside. They would try again, but by then his desire had waned, and he was unable to achieve another erection.

After the first few times this happened, Petula became so angry that she began punching him in the chest and screaming at him. Paul, who weighs 200 pounds, would simply walk away from his 98-pound lover, which would infuriate her even more.

The psychiatrist learned that sex was not the only area of contention in the relationship. Petula complained that Paul did not spend enough

TABLE 21.1a-10
Diseases and Other Medical Conditions Implicated in Male Erectile Disorder

Infectious and parasitic diseases
- Elephantiasis
- Mumps

Cardiovascular disease*
- Atherosclerotic disease
- Aortic aneurysm
- Leriche's syndrome
- Cardiac failure

Renal and urological disorders
- Peyronie's disease
- Chronic renal failure
- Hydrocele and varicocele

Hepatic disorders
- Cirrhosis (usually associated with alcohol dependence)

Pulmonary disorders
- Respiratory failure

Genetics
- Klinefelter's syndrome
- Congenital penile vascular and structural abnormalities

Nutritional disorders
- Malnutrition
- Vitamin deficiencies

Endocrine disorders*
- Diabetes mellitus
- Dysfunction of the pituitary-adrenal-testis axis
- Acromegaly
- Addison's disease
- Chromophobe adenoma
- Adrenal neoplasia
- Myxedema
- Hyperthyroidism

Neurological disorders
- Multiple sclerosis
- Transverse myelitis
- Parkinson's disease
- Temporal lobe epilepsy
- Traumatic and neoplastic spinal cord diseases*
- Central nervous system tumor
- Amyotrophic lateral sclerosis
- Peripheral neuropathy
- General paresis
- Tabes dorsalis

Pharmacological contributants
- Alcohol and other dependence-inducing substances (heroin, methadone, morphine, cocaine, amphetamines, and barbiturates)
- Prescribed drugs (psychotropic drugs, antihypertensive drugs, estrogens, and antiandrogens)

Poisoning
- Lead (plumbism)
- Herbicides

Surgical procedures*
- Perineal prostatectomy
- Abdominal-perineal colon resection
- Sympathectomy (frequently interferes with ejaculation)
- Aortoiliac surgery
- Radical cystectomy
- Retroperitoneal lymphadenectomy

Miscellaneous
- Radiation therapy
- Pelvic fracture
- Any severe systemic disease or debilitating condition

*In the United States an estimated two million men are impotent because they suffer from diabetes mellitus; an additional 300,000 are impotent because of other endocrine diseases; 1.5 million are impotent as a result of vascular disease; 180,000 because of multiple sclerosis; 400,000 because of traumas and fractures leading to pelvic fractures or spinal cord injuries; and another 650,000 are impotent as a result of radical surgery, including prostatectomies, colostomies, and cystectomies.

time with her and preferred to go to baseball games with his male friends. Even when he was home, he would watch all the sports events that were available on TV, and was not interested in going to foreign movies, museums, or the theater with her. Despite those differences, Petula was eager to marry Paul and was pressuring him to set a date.

Physical examination of the couple revealed no abnormalities, and there was no evidence that either partner was persistently depressed.

Discussion Paul and Petula have many problems that a family-oriented clinician would want to focus on, such as Paul's ambivalence about committing himself to a relationship with Petula and her frantic efforts to obtain that commitment. The effect of these problems on Paul's sexual functioning is clear: he is unable to maintain his erection until the completion of sexual activity.

When there is no evidence that the disturbance is caused exclusively by a general medical condition (such as by diabetic neuropathy or certain medications), the diagnosis of male erectile disorder, due to psychological factors, is made. We note that the disorder is acquired (recent onset), not lifelong. (*Note:* When an erectile dysfunction is caused by a general medical condition, the medical condition would be coded as a physical disorder on Axis III.)

Follow-up Neither partner was willing to discuss nonsexual problems. They were treated with Masters and Johnson's sensate focus exercises over the next several months. In these exercises, the couple explored nongenital ways of giving physical pleasure to each other without the psychological demands of demonstrating sexual competence. Petula continually pressured Paul to translate the therapy into action. She saw herself as a therapist and teacher, and Paul as patient and pupil. Paul passively avoided doing the exercises on many occasions; but over a period of eight months, Paul's problem with maintaining an erection was gradually resolved. They were married within three months after treatment ended.

The Petersens sought treatment twice more over the next 8 years. On both occasions the underlying issue was again Paul's ambivalence about further committing himself to the relationship (buying a house, having children). Paul had a recurrence of erectile problems and, in addition, a complaint of premature ejaculation on the rare occasions when he could maintain an erection intravaginally. During the treatment, greater attention was given to their relationship rather than simply focusing on the sexual problem. At last report they had two children, had bought a house in the suburbs, and the sexual problem had again been resolved. (From *DSM-IV Casebook.* Used with permission.)

SEXUAL DYSFUNCTION DUE TO A GENERAL MEDICAL CONDITION The category covers sexual dysfunction that results in marked distress and interpersonal difficulty when there is evidence from the history, the physical examination, or the laboratory findings of a general medical condition judged to be causally related to the sexual dysfunction (Table 21.1a-11).

Male erectile disorder due to a general medical condition

The incidence of psychological as opposed to organic male erectile disorder has been the focus of many studies. Statistics indicate that 20 to 50 percent of men with erectile disorder have an organic basis for the disorder. The medical causes of male erectile disorder are listed in Table 21.1a-10. Side effects of medication may impair male sexual functioning in a variety of ways. Castration (removal of the testes) does not always lead to sexual dysfunction, depending on the person. Erection may still occur after castration. A reflex arc, fired when the inner thigh is stimulated, passes through the sacral cord erectile center to account for the phenomenon.

PHYSIOLOGICAL TEST A number of procedures, benign and invasive, are used to help differentiate medically caused impotence from psychogenic impotence. The procedures include monitoring nocturnal penile tumescence (erections that occur during sleep), normally associated with rapid eye movement; monitoring tumescence with a strain gauge; measuring blood pressure in the penis with a penile plethysmograph or an ultrasound (Doppler) flow meter, both of which assess blood flow in the internal pudendal artery; and measuring pudendal nerve latency time. Neurological impairment of penile function may be indicated if vibratory perception is decreased in the penis. Other diagnostic tests that delineate organic bases for impotence include glucose tolerance tests, plasma hormone assays, liver and thyroid function tests, prolactin and follicle-stimulating hormone (FSH) determinations, and cystometric examinations. Invasive diagnostic studies include penile arteriography, infusion cavernosography, and radioactive xenon penography. Invasive procedures require expert interpretation and are used only for patients who are candidates for vascular reconstructive procedures.

TABLE 21.1a-11
Diagnostic Criteria for Sexual Dysfunction Due to a General Medical Condition

A. Clinically significant sexual dysfunction that results in marked distress or interpersonal difficulty predominates in the clinical picture.
B. There is evidence from the history, physical examination, or laboratory findings that the sexual dysfunction is fully explained by the direct physiological effects of a general medical condition.
C. The disturbance is not better accounted for by another mental disorder (e.g., major depressive disorder).

Select code and term based on the predominant sexual dysfunction:

Female hypoactive sexual desire disorder due to a general medical condition: if deficient or absent sexual desire is the predominant feature.
Male hypoactive sexual desire disorder due to a general medical condition: if deficient or absent sexual desire is the predominant feature.
Male erectile disorder due to a general medical condition: if male erectile dysfunction is the predominant feature.
Female dyspareunia due to a general medical condition: if pain associated with intercourse is the predominant feature.
Male dyspareunia due to a general medical condition: if pain associated with intercourse is the predominant feature.
Other female sexual dysfunction due to a general medical condition: if some other feature is predominant (e.g., orgasmic disorder) or no feature predominates.
Other male sexual dysfunction due to a general medical condition: if some other feature is predominant (e.g., orgasmic disorder) or no feature predominates.

Coding note: Include the name of the general medical condition on Axis I, e.g., male erectile disorder due to diabetes mellitus; also code the general medical condition on Axis III.

Table from DSM-IV, *Diagnostic and Statistical Manual of Mental Disorders,* ed 4. Copyright American Psychiatric Association, Washington, 1994. Used with permission.

MEDICAL VERSUS PSYCHOGENIC CAUSES A good history is crucial in determining the etiology of the male erectile disorder. If a man reports having spontaneous erections at times when he does not plan to have intercourse, having morning erections or only sporadic erectile dysfunction, or having good erections with masturbation or with partners other than his usual one, then organic causes for his impotence can be considered negligible, and costly diagnostic procedures can be avoided. In those cases in which a medical basis for impotence is found, psychological factors often contribute to the dysfunction, and psychiatric treatment may be helpful. In some diabetics, for instance, erectile dysfunction may be psychogenic.

In general, the psychological conflicts that cause impotence are related to an inability to express the sexual impulse because of fear, anxiety, anger, or moral prohibition. Lifelong impotence is a more serious, but less common, condition than acquired impotence, and the former is less amenable to treatment.

Many developmental factors have been cited as contributing to erectile disorder. Any experience that hinders the ability to be intimate, that leads to a feeling of inadequacy or distrust, or that develops a sense of being unloving or unlovable may result in impotence. In an ongoing relationship erectile dysfunction may reflect difficulties between the partners, particularly if the person cannot communicate his or her needs or angry feelings in a direct and constructive way. Successive episodes of impotence are reinforcing, with the man becoming increasingly anxious about his next sexual encounter. Regardless of the original etiology of the dysfunction, his anticipatory anxiety about achieving and maintaining an erection interferes with his pleasure in sexual contact and with his ability to respond to stimulation, thus perpetuating the problem.

Dyspareunia due to a general medical condition An estimated 30 percent of all surgical procedures on the female genital area result in temporary dyspareunia. In addition, of women with the complaint who are seen in sex therapy clinics, 30 to 40 percent have pelvic pathology.

Organic abnormalities leading to dyspareunia and vaginismus include irritated or infected hymenal remnants, episiotomy scars, Bartholin's gland infection, various forms of vaginitis and cervicitis, and endometriosis. Postcoital pain has been reported by women with myomata and endometriosis and is attributed to the uterine contractions during orgasm. Postmenopausal women may have dyspareunia resulting from thinning of the vaginal mucosa and reduced lubrication.

Dyspareunia can also occur in men, but it is uncommon and is usually associated with an organic condition, such as Peyronie's disease, which consists of sclerotic plaques on the penis that cause penile curvature.

Hypoactive sexual desire disorder due to a general medical condition Desire commonly decreases after major illness or surgery, particularly when the body image is affected after such procedures as mastectomy, ileostomy, hysterectomy, and prostatectomy. Illnesses that deplete a person's energy, chronic conditions that require physical and psychological adaptation, and serious illnesses that may cause the person to become depressed can all result in a marked lessening of sexual desire in both men and women.

In some cases, biochemical correlates are associated with hypoactive sexual desire disorder (Table 21.1a-12). A recent study found markedly decreased levels of serum testosterone in men complaining of low desire when they were compared with normal controls in a sleep-laboratory situation. Drugs that depress the central nervous system (CNS) or decrease testosterone production can decrease desire.

Other male sexual dysfunction due to a general medical condition The category is used when some other dysfunctional feature is predominant (for example, orgasmic disorder) or no feature predominates.

Male orgasmic disorder may have physiological causes and can occur after surgery on the genitourinary tract, such as prostatectomy. It may also be associated with Parkinson's disease and other neurological disorders involving the lumbar or sacral sections of the spinal cord. The antihypertensive drug guanethidine monosulfate (Ismelin), methyldopa (Aldomet), the phenothiazines, the tricyclic drugs, and fluoxetine (Prozac), among others, have been implicated in retarded ejaculation. Male orgasmic disorder must also be differentiated from retrograde ejaculation, in which ejaculation occurs but the seminal fluid passes backward into the bladder. Retrograde ejaculation always has an organic cause. It can develop after genitourinary surgery and is also associated with medications that have anticholinergic side effects, such as the phenothiazines.

Other female sexual dysfunction due to a general medical condition The category is used when some other feature (for example, orgasmic disorder) is predominant or when no feature predominates.

Some medical conditions—specifically, such endocrine diseases as hypothyroidism, diabetes mellitus, and primary hyperprolactinemia—can affect a woman's ability to have orgasms. Also, a number of drugs affect some women's capacity to have orgasms. Antihypertensive medications, CNS stimulants, tricyclic drugs, fluoxetine, and, frequently, monoamine oxidase (MAO) inhibitors have interfered with female orgasmic capacity (Table 21.1a-13). However, one study of women taking MAO inhibitors found that, after 16 to 18 weeks of pharmacotherapy, that side effect of the medication disappeared, and the women were able to reexperience orgasms, although they continued taking an undiminished dosage of the drug.

ORGASMIC DISORDERS Female orgasmic disorder (also known as inhibited female orgasm [*anorgasmia*]) is defined as the recurrent and persistent inhibition of the female orgasm, as becomes manifest by the absence or delay of orgasm after a normal sexual excitement phase that the clinician judges to be adequate in focus, intensity, and duration. Women who can achieve orgasm with noncoital clitoral stimulation but are unable to experience it during coitus in the absence of manual clitoral stimulation are not necessarily categorized as anorgasmic.

Physiological research regarding the female sexual response has demonstrated that orgasms caused by clitoral stimulation and those caused by vaginal stimulation are physiologically identical. Freud's theory that women must give up clitoral sensitivity for vaginal sensitivity in order to achieve sexual maturity is now considered misleading, although some women say that they gain a special sense of satisfaction from an orgasm precipitated by coitus. Some workers attribute that to the psychological feeling of closeness engendered by the act of coitus,

TABLE 21.1a-12
Neurotransmitter Effects on Sex Function

	Dopamine	Serotonin	Adrenergic	Cholinergic	Clinical Correlation
Erection	++	+/−	α, β − +	+/−	Antipsychotics (dopamine receptor antagonists) may lead to erectile dysfunction: dopaminergic drug agonists may lead to enhanced erection and libido; priapism with trazodone (α_1 block); β-blockers may lead to impotence.
Ejaculation and orgasm	+/−	+	+ α_1	+/−	α_1-Blockers (tricyclic drugs, MAOIs, thioridazine) may lead to impaired ejaculation; serotonergic agents may inhibit orgasm.

Table adapted from R Segraves: Psychiatric Times, 1990. Used with permission.
+/− minimal or no effect
\+ facilitates effect
− inhibiting effect

but others maintain that the coital orgasm is a physiologically different experience. Many women achieve orgasm during coitus by a combination of manual clitoral stimulation and penile vaginal stimulation.

Lifelong female orgasmic disorder exists when the woman has never experienced orgasm by any kind of stimulation. Acquired orgasmic dysfunction exists if the woman has previously experienced at least one orgasm regardless of the circumstances or means of stimulation, whether by masturbation or during sleep while dreaming. Kinsey found that the proportion of married women over 35 years of age who had never achieved orgasm by any means was only 5 percent. The incidence of orgasm increases with age. According to Kinsey, the first orgasm occurs in late adolescence in about 50 percent of women. The rest usually experience orgasm by some means as they get older. Lifelong female orgasmic disorder is more common among unmarried women than among married women; 39 percent of the unmarried women over age 35 in Kinsey's study had never experienced orgasm. Increased orgasmic potential in women over 35 has been explained on the basis of less psychological inhibition, greater sexual experience, or both. Also, orgasmic consistency has been correlated with marital happiness, although cause and effect have not been determined. In the University of Chicago study, three quarters of the married female respondents usually or always experienced orgasm during sex compared with two thirds of the single women. One woman out of 10 complained of difficulty in achieving orgasm.

Lola, a 25-year-old laboratory technician, has been married to a 32-year-old cab driver for five years. The couple has a 2-year-old son, and the marriage appears harmonious.

The presenting complaint is Lola's lifelong inability to experience orgasm. She has never achieved orgasm, although during sexual activity she has received what should have been sufficient stimulation. She has tried to masturbate, and on many occasions her husband has manually stimulated her patiently for lengthy periods of time. Although she does not reach climax, she is strongly attached to her husband, feels erotic pleasure during lovemaking, and lubricates copiously. According to both of them, the husband has no sexual difficulty.

Exploration of her thoughts as she nears orgasm reveals a vague sense of dread of some undefined disaster. More generally, she is anxious about losing control over her emotions, which she normally keeps closely in check. She is particularly uncomfortable about expressing any anger or hostility.

Physical examination reveals no abnormality.

Discussion Lola's sexual difficulties are limited to the orgasm phase of the sexual response cycle (she has no difficulty in desiring sex or in becoming excited). During lovemaking there is what would ordinarily be an adequate amount of stimulation. The report of a "vague sense of dread of some undefined disaster" as she approaches orgasm is evidence that her inability to have orgasms represents a pathological inhibition. There is no suggestion of any other Axis I disorder or any physical disorder that could account for the disturbance. Thus, the diagnosis is of a sexual dysfunction orgasm disorder, female orgasmic disorder (inhibited female orgasm), due to psychological factors, lifelong, generalized.

If with treatment it became apparent that the fear of loss of control was a symptom of a personality disorder, such as obsessive-compulsive personality disorder, the diagnosis of a sexual dysfunction would still be made. However, if the sexual dysfunction occurred exclusively during the course of another Axis I disorder, such as major depressive disorder, then the sexual disturbance would be assumed to be a symptom of the Axis I disorder, and the diagnosis of a sexual dysfunction would not be made. (From *DSM-IV Casebook*. Used with permission.)

Acquired female orgasmic disorder is a common complaint in clinical populations. One clinical treatment facility described nonorgasmic women as about four times more common in its practice than patients with all other sexual disorders. In another study 46 percent of the women complained of difficulty in reaching orgasm, and 15 percent described an inability to have orgasm. The overall prevalence of inhibited orgasm in women is estimated at 30 percent.

Numerous psychological factors are associated with female sexual inhibition. They include fears of impregnation, rejection by the sexual partner, or damage to the vagina; hostility toward men; and feelings of guilt regarding sexual impulses. For some women orgasm is equated with loss of control or with aggressive, destructive, or violent behavior. Fear of those impulses may be expressed through inhibition of excitement or orgasm. The expression of orgasmic inhibition varies. Some women feel unentitled to gratify themselves and are unable to masturbate to climax. Others enjoy self-stimulation but are unable to reach orgasm with a partner present. Cultural expectations and societal restrictions on women are also relevant. Nonorgastic women may be otherwise symptom-free or may experience frustration in a variety of ways, including such pelvic complaints as lower abdominal pain, itching, and vaginal discharge, as well as increased tension, irritability, and fatigue. The diagnostic criteria for female orgasmic disorder are presented in Table 21.1a-14.

Male orgasmic disorder In male orgasmic disorder (previously inhibited male orgasm and called *retarded ejaculation*) the man achieves climax during coitus with great difficulty, if at all. A man suffers from lifelong orgasmic disorder if he has never been able to ejaculate during coitus. The disorder is diagnosed as acquired if it develops after previous normal functioning.

Some workers suggest that a differentiation should be made between orgasm and ejaculation. Certainly, inhibited orgasm must be differentiated from retrograde ejaculation, in which ejaculation occurs but the seminal fluid passes backward into the bladder. The latter condition always has an organic cause. Retrograde ejaculation can develop after genitourinary surgery and is also associated with medications that have anticholiner-

TABLE 21.1a-13
Some Psychiatric Drugs Implemented in Inhibited Female Orgasm*

Tricyclic antidepressants
Imipramine (Tofranil)
Clomipramine (Anafranil)
Nortriptyline (Aventyl)
Monoamine oxidase inhibitors
Tranylcypromine (Parnate)
Phenelzine (Nardil)
Isocarboxazid (Marplan)
Dopamine receptor antagonists
Thioridazine (Mellaril)
Trifluoperazine (Stelazine)
Selective serotonergic receptor inhibitors
Fluoxetine (Prozac)
Paroxetine (Paxil)
Sertraline (Zoloft)

*The interrelationship between female sexual dysfunction and pharmacological agents has been less extensively evaluated than have male reactions. Oral contraceptives are reported to decrease libido in some women, and some drugs with anticholinergic side effects may impair arousal as well as orgasm. Benzodiazepines have been reported to decrease libido, but in some patients the diminution of anxiety caused by those drugs enhances sexual function.

Both increase and decrease in libido have been reported with psychoactive agents. It is difficult to separate those effects from the underlying condition or from improvement of the condition. Sexual dysfunction associated with the use of a drug disappears when the drug is discontinued.

TABLE 21.1a-14
Diagnostic Criteria for Female Orgasmic Disorder

A. Persistent or recurrent delay in, or absence of, orgasm following a normal sexual excitement phase. Women exhibit wide variability in the type or intensity of stimulation that triggers orgasm. The diagnosis of female orgasmic disorder should be based on the clinician's judgment that the woman's orgasmic capacity is less than would be reasonable for her age, sexual experience, and the adequacy of sexual stimulation she receives.
B. The disturbance causes marked distress or interpersonal difficulty.
C. The orgasmic dysfunction is not better accounted for by another Axis I disorder (except another sexual dysfunction) and is not due exclusively to the direct physiological effects of a substance (e.g., a drug of abuse, a medication) or a general medical condition.

Specify type:
Lifelong type
Acquired type
Specify type:
Generalized type
Situational type
Specify:
Due to psychological factors
Due to combined factors

Table from DSM-IV, *Diagnostic and Statistical Manual of Mental Disorders,* ed 4. Copyright American Psychiatric Association, Washington, 1994. Used with permission.

gic side effects, such as the phenothiazines, particularly thioridazine (Mellaril).

The incidence of male orgasmic disorder is much lower than that of premature ejaculation and impotence. Masters and Johnson reported only 3.8 percent in one group of 447 sex-dysfunction cases. This problem is more common among men with obsessive-compulsive disorders than among others. Inhibited male orgasm may have physiological causes and can occur after surgery of the genitourinary tract, such as prostatectomy. It may also be associated with Parkinson's disease and other neurological disorders involving the lumbar or sacral sections of the spinal cord. The antihypertensive drugs guanethidine monosulfate (Esimil) and methyldopa (Aldomet) have been implicated in retarded ejaculation. Phenothiazines have also been associated with the disorder. Transient retarded ejaculation may occur with excessive alcohol intake or with hyperglycemia, whether caused by drugs or by a pituitary adenoma. Strictly organic cases and problems that are symptomatic of other Axis I psychiatric syndromes are not to be included in the diagnosis.

Primary inhibited male orgasm is indicative of more severe psychopathology. The man often comes from a rigid, puritanical background: he perceives sex as sinful and the genitals as dirty, and he may have conscious or unconscious incest wishes and guilt. There are usually difficulties with closeness that extend beyond the area of sexual relations.

In an ongoing relationship, secondary ejaculatory inhibition frequently reflects interpersonal difficulties. The disorder may be the man's way of coping with real or fantasized changes in the relationship. Those changes may include plans for a pregnancy about which the man is ambivalent, the loss of sexual attraction to the partner, or demands by the partner for greater commitment as expressed by sexual performance. In some men the inability to ejaculate reflects unexpressed hostility toward women.

In a version of the dysfunction, some men experience partial inhibition of ejaculation. Those men experience a slow dribbling of ejaculate (not related to age) rather than an ejaculatory spurt. They usually do not experience the pleasurable sensations of orgasm.

The DSM-IV diagnostic criteria for male orgasmic disorder are listed in Table 21.1a-15.

A 33-year-old college professor presented with the complaint that he had never been able to ejaculate while making love. He had no trouble in attaining and maintaining an erection and no difficulties in stimulating his partner to her orgasm, but he could never be stimulated himself to ejaculation and would finally give up in boredom. He has always been able to reach ejaculation by masturbation, which he does about twice a week, but he has never been willing to allow a partner to masturbate him to orgasm. Previously he resisted all of his girlfriend's attempts to persuade him to seek medical or psychological help, as he felt that intravaginal ejaculation was unimportant unless one wanted children.

The patient's current relationship is in jeopardy because his girlfriend is eager to marry and have children. He has never wanted to have children and is reluctant to become a father, but the pressures from his girlfriend have forced him to seek therapy. Throughout the interview his attitude toward the problem is one of distance and disdain. He describes the problem as though he were a neutral observer, with little apparent feeling.

Discussion The professor has an unusual sexual problem. He is able to have an erection without any difficulty, has no problem in sustaining the erection during intercourse (as would be the case in male erectile disorder), but is unable to have an orgasm during intercourse. Significantly, he has no trouble having an orgasm when he masturbates, which excludes the possibility that a general medical condition accounts for the problem. Persistent inhibition of the male orgasm phase not caused exclusively by an general medical condition or medication (such as a side effect of certain antidepressants) is called male orgasmic disorder (inhibited male orgasm). It is noted that the condition is due to psychological factors, lifelong (not acquired after a period of normal functioning) and generalized (not limited to a specific situation).

There is a suggestion of coldness and hyperintellectualization, traits often present in men with the disorder. Perhaps on the basis of more information, a diagnosis of obsessive-compulsive personality disorder might also be warranted. (From *DSM Casebook.* Used with permission.)

Premature ejaculation In *premature ejaculation* the man recurrently achieves orgasm and ejaculation before he wishes to do so. There is no definite time frame within which to define the dysfunction. The diagnosis is made when the man regularly ejaculates before or immediately after entering the vagina or following minimal sexual stimulation. The clinician should consider factors that affect duration of the excitement phase, such as age, novelty of the sexual partner, and the frequency and duration of coitus. Masters and Johnson conceptualized the dis-

TABLE 21.1a-15
Diagnostic Criteria for Male Orgasmic Disorder

A. Persistent or recurrent delay in, or absence of, orgasm following a normal sexual excitement phase during sexual activity that the clinician, taking into account the person's age, judges to be adequate in focus, intensity, and duration.
B. The disturbance causes marked distress or interpersonal difficulty.
C. The orgasmic dysfunction is not better accounted for by another Axis I disorder (except another sexual dysfunction) and is not due exclusively to the direct physiological effects of a substance (e.g., a drug of abuse, a medication) or a general medical condition.

Specify type:
Lifelong type
Acquired type
Specify type:
Generalized type
Situational type
Specify:
Due to psychological factors
Due to combined factors

Table from DSM-IV, *Diagnostic and Statistical Manual of Mental Disorders,* ed 4. Copyright American Psychiatric Association, Washington, 1994. Used with permission.

order in terms of the couple and consider a man a premature ejaculator if he cannot control ejaculation for a sufficient length of time during intravaginal containment to satisfy his partner in at least one half of their episodes of coitus. That definition assumes that the female partner is capable of an orgasmic response. As with the other dysfunctions, the disturbance is diagnosed only if it is not caused exclusively by medical factors or is not symptomatic of any other Axis I syndrome.

Premature ejaculation is more common today among college-educated men than among men with less education and is thought to be related to their concern for partner satisfaction. It is estimated that 30 percent of the male population have the dysfunction, and about 40 percent of men treated for sexual disorders have premature ejaculation as the chief complaint.

Difficulty in ejaculatory control may be associated with anxiety regarding the sex act or with unconscious fears about the vagina. It may also result from negative cultural conditioning. The man who has most of his early sexual contacts with prostitutes who demand that the sex act proceed quickly or in situations in which discovery would be embarrassing, such as in an apartment shared with roommates or in the parental home, may become conditioned to achieving orgasm rapidly. In ongoing relationships the partner has been found to have great influence on the premature ejaculator. A stressful marriage exacerbates the disorder. The developmental background and dynamics found in the disorder and in impotence are similar.

Table 21.1a-16 gives the diagnostic criteria for premature ejaculation.

Other orgasmic disorders Data on female premature orgasm are lacking; no separate category of premature orgasm for women is included in DSM-IV. However, in the University of Chicago study 10 percent of women felt they reached orgasm too quickly.

SEXUAL PAIN DISORDERS

Dyspareunia *Dyspareunia* refers to recurrent and persistent pain during intercourse in either the man or the woman. In women the dysfunction is related to and often coincides with vaginismus. Repeated episodes of vaginismus may lead to dyspareunia and vice versa, but in either case somatic causes must be ruled out. Dyspareunia should not be diagnosed as such when a medical basis for the pain is found, or when, in a woman, it is associated with vaginismus or with lack of lubrication.

TABLE 21.1a-16
Diagnostic Criteria for Premature Ejaculation

A. Persistent or recurrent ejaculation with minimal sexual stimulation before, on, or shortly after penetration and before the person wishes it. The clinician must take into account factors that affect duration of the excitement phase, such as age, novelty of the sexual partner or situation, and recent frequency of sexual activity.
B. The disturbance causes marked distress or interpersonal difficulty.
C. The premature ejaculation is not due exclusively to the direct effects of a substance (e.g., withdrawal from opioids).

Specify type:
Lifelong type
Acquired type
Specify type:
Generalized type
Situational type
Specify:
Due to psychological factors
Due to combined factors

Table from DSM-IV, *Diagnostic and Statistical Manual of Mental Disorders,* ed 4. Copyright American Psychiatric Association, Washington, 1994. Used with permission.

The true incidence of dyspareunia is unknown, but it has been estimated that 30 percent of surgical procedures on the female genital area result in temporary dyspareunia. Additionally, of women with the complaint who are seen in sex therapy clinics, 30 to 40 percent have pelvic pathology. Chronic pelvic pain is a more common complaint in women with a history of rape or childhood sexual abuse.

Structural or medical conditions leading to dyspareunia and vaginismus include irritated or infected hymenal remnants, episiotomy scars, Bartholin's gland infection, various forms of vaginitis and cervicitis, endometriosis, and other pelvic disorders. Dyspareunia prior to coitus may occur as a concomitant of sexual excitement when the woman has an irritation of her external genitalia. The vasocongestion that is intrinsic to the excitement phase may result in increased sensitivity and discomfort in the affected area. Postcoital pain sometimes has been attributed to intense uterine contractions during orgasm in women with myomata or endometriosis. The postmenopausal woman may develop dyspareunia resulting from thinning of the vaginal mucosa and lessened lubrication in most cases of dyspareunia. Dynamic factors are usually considered causative although situational factors probably account more for secondary dysfunctions. Painful coitus may result from tension and anxiety about the sex act that cause the woman to involuntarily tense her vaginal muscles. The pain is real and makes intercourse unbearable or unpleasant. The anticipation of further pain may cause the woman to avoid coitus altogether. If the partner proceeds with intercourse regardless of the woman's state of readiness, the condition is aggravated. Dyspareunia can also occur in men, but it is uncommon and is usually associated with a medical condition, such as Peyronie's disease, prostatitis, or gonorrheal or herpetic infections. Vasocongestion during sexual activity without orgasmic release also may lead to discomfort. Rarely, some men experience pain upon ejaculation (postejaculatory pain disorder). That pain results from an involuntary spasm of the perineal muscles that may be due to psychological conflicts about the sex act or that occurs as a side effect of some antidepressant medications. Table 21.1a-17 lists the diagnostic criteria for dyspareunia. In DSM-IV dyspareunia due to a general medical condition is a diagnostic category used when the medical condition is the sole or major etiological factor.

Vaginismus *Vaginismus* is an involuntary and persistent constriction of the outer one third of the vagina that prevents

TABLE 21.1a-17
Diagnostic Criteria for Dyspareunia

A. Recurrent or persistent genital pain associated with sexual intercourse in either a male or a female.
B. The disturbance causes marked distress or interpersonal difficulty.
C. The disturbance is not caused exclusively by vaginismus or lack of lubrication, is not better accounted for by another Axis I disorder (except another sexual dysfunction), and is not due exclusively to the direct physiological effects of a substance (e.g., a drug of abuse, a medication) or a general medical condition.

Specify type:
Lifelong type
Acquired type
Specify type:
Generalized type
Situational type
Specify:
Due to psychological factors
Due to combined factors

Table from DSM-IV, *Diagnostic and Statistical Manual of Mental Disorders,* ed 4. Copyright American Psychiatric Association, Washington, 1994. Used with permission.

penile insertion and intercourse. The response may be demonstrated during a gynecological examination when involuntary vaginal constriction prevents introduction of the speculum into the vagina, although some women only have vaginismus during coitus. The diagnosis is not made if the dysfunction is caused exclusively by medical or surgical factors or if it is symptomatic of another Axis I psychiatric syndrome (Table 21.1a-18). Vaginismus is less prevalent than anorgasmia. It most often afflicts highly educated women and those in the higher socioeconomic groups. A milder form of the dysfunction, where there is some degree of vaginal tightness that makes penile entry difficult, is experienced by a greater number of women on an intermittent or chronic basis.

The woman suffering from vaginismus may consciously wish to have coitus, but she unconsciously prevents penile entrance into her body. A sexual trauma, such as rape, may result in vaginismus. Women who have experienced pain with nonsexual bodily traumas, through accidents or because of illness or surgery, may become sensitized to the idea of penetration. Women with psychosexual conflicts may perceive the penis as a dangerous weapon. In some women pain or the anticipation of pain at the first coital experience causes vaginismus. A strict religious upbringing that associates sex with sin is frequently noted in such cases. For others there are problems in the dyadic relationship: If the woman feels emotionally abused by her partner, she may protest in that nonverbal fashion.

SEXUAL DYSFUNCTION AND SEXUAL DISORDER NOT OTHERWISE SPECIFIED DSM-IV uses two categories—sexual dysfunction not otherwise specified (NOS) and sexual disorder NOS. The diagnostic criteria are listed in Table 21.1a-19 and Table 21.1a-20. The distinction between the two categories is unclear, however, and there is overlap between them.

TABLE 21.1a-18
Diagnostic Criteria for Vaginismus

A. Recurrent or persistent involuntary spasm of the musculature of the outer third of the vagina that interferes with sexual intercourse.
B. The disturbance causes marked distress or interpersonal difficulty.
C. The disturbance is not better accounted for by another Axis I disorder (e.g., somatization disorder) and is not due exclusively to the direct physiological effects of a general medical condition.

Specify type:
Lifelong type
Acquired type

Specify type:
Generalized type
Situational type

Specify:
Due to psychological factors
Due to combined factors

Table from DSM-IV, *Diagnostic and Statistical Manual of Mental Disorders,* ed 4. Copyright American Psychiatric Association, Washington, 1994. Used with permission.

TABLE 21.1a-19
Diagnostic Criteria for Sexual Dysfunction Not Otherwise Specified

This category includes sexual dysfunctions that do not meet criteria for any specific sexual dysfunction: Examples include.
1. No (or substantially diminished) subjective erotic feelings despite otherwise normal arousal and orgasm
2. Situations in which the clinician has concluded that a sexual dysfunction is present but is unable to determine whether it is primary, due to a general medical condition, or substance induced

Table from DSM-IV, *Diagnostic and Statistical Manual of Mental Disorders,* ed 4. Copyright American Psychiatric Association, Washington, 1994. Used with permission.

TABLE 21.1a-20
Diagnostic Criteria for Sexual Disorder Not Otherwise Specified

This category is included for coding a sexual disturbance that does not meet the criteria for any specific sexual disorder and is neither a sexual dysfunction nor a paraphilia. Examples include
1. Marked feelings of inadequacy concerning sexual performance or other traits related to self-imposed standards of masculinity or femininity
2. Distress about a pattern of repeated sexual relationships involving a succession of lovers who are experienced by the individual only as things to be used
3. Persistent and marked distress about sexual orientation

Table from DSM-IV, *Diagnostic and Statistical Manual of Mental Disorders,* ed 4. Copyright American Psychiatric Association, Washington, 1994. Used with permission.

Examples include persons who experience the physiological components of sexual excitement and orgasm but report no erotic sensation or even anesthesia, and the male experience of orgasm with a flaccid penis. The orgasmic female who desires but has not experienced multiple orgasms can be classified under that heading as well. Also, disorders of excessive rather than inhibited function, such as compulsive masturbation, might be diagnosed under atypical dysfunctions. There are other sexual practices that are not listed in DSM-IV but exist nonetheless. An example would be behaviors that attempt to enhance sexual arousal by oxygen deprivation (hypoxyphilia) or by other deviant methods.

Atypical dysfunctions also might be used to cover complaints engendered by couple, rather than individual, dysfunction. An example is a couple of whom one partner prefers morning sex and one functions more readily at night; another example is a couple with unequal frequencies of desire.

Sex addiction The concept of sex addiction developed over the past two decades to refer to persons who compulsively seek out sexual experiences and whose behavior becomes impaired if they are unable to gratify their sexual impulses. The concept of sex addiction derived from the model of addiction to such drugs as heroin, or addiction to behavioral patterns, such as gambling. Addiction implies psychological dependence, physical dependence, and the presence of a withdrawal syndrome if the substance (for example, the drug) is unavailable or the behavior (for example, gambling) is frustrated.

In DSM-IV the term "sex addiction" is not used, nor is it a disorder that is universally recognized or accepted. Nevertheless, the phenomenon of a person whose entire life revolves around sex-seeking behavior and activities, who spends an excessive amount of time in such behavior, and who often tries to stop such behavior but is unable to do so is well known to clinicians. Such persons show repeated and increasingly frequent attempts to have a sexual experience, of which deprivation gives rise to symptoms of distress. In the author's view sex addiction is a useful concept heuristically in that it can alert the clinician to seek an underlying cause for the manifest behavior.

DIAGNOSIS Sex addicts are unable to control their sexual impulses, which can involve the entire spectrum of sexual fantasy or behavior. Eventually, the need for sexual activity increases and the person's behavior is motivated solely by the persistent desire to experience the sex act. The history usually reveals a long-standing pattern of such behavior, which the person repeatedly has tried to stop, but without success. Although there may be feelings of guilt and remorse after the act, they are not sufficient to prevent its recurrence. The patient may report that the need to act out is most severe during stressful periods or when angry, depressed, anxious, or otherwise dysphoric. Most acts culminate in a sexual orgasm, although a sense of excitement (a high) usually accompanies the sex-seeking behavior even in the absence of orgasm. Eventually, the sexual activity interferes with the person's social, vocational, or marital life, which begins to deteriorate.

The signs of sexual addiction are listed in Table 21.1a-21.

TYPES OF BEHAVIORAL PATTERNS The paraphilias constitute the behavioral patterns most often found in the sex addict. As defined in DSM-IV, the essential features of a paraphilia are recurrent intense sexual urges or behaviors, including exhibitionism, fetishism, frotteurism, sadomasochism, cross-dressing, voyeurism, and pedophilia. Paraphilias are associated with clinically significant distress and almost invariably interfere with interpersonal relationships, and they often lead to legal complications. In addition to the paraphilias, however, sex addiction can also include behavior that is considered normal, such as coitus and masturbation, except that it is promiscuous and uncontrolled.

In the 19th century the psychiatrist Richard von Krafft-Ebing reported on several cases of abnormally increased sexual desire. One was that of a 36-year-old married teacher, the father of seven children, who masturbated repeatedly while sitting at his desk in front of his pupils, after which he was "penitent and filled with shame." He indulged in coitus three or four times a day in addition to his repeated masturbatory acts. In another case a young woman masturbated almost incessantly and was unable to control her impulses. She had frequent coitus with many men, but neither coitus nor masturbation was sufficient, and she eventually was placed in an institution. Krafft-Ebing referred to the condition as sexual hyperaesthesia, which he believed could occur in otherwise normal persons.

In many cases sex addiction is the final common pathway of a variety of other disorders. In addition to the paraphilias that are almost always present, there may be an associated major mental disorder, such as anxiety disorder, depressive disorder, bipolar disorder, or schizophrenia. Antisocial personality disorder and borderline personality disorder are common.

COMORBIDITY Comorbidity (dual diagnosis) refers to the presence of an addiction that coexists with another psychiatric disorder. For example, about 50 percent of patients with substance-use disorder also have an additional psychiatric disorder. Similarly, many sex addicts have an associated psychiatric disorder. Dual diagnosis implies that the psychiatric illness and the addiction are separate disorders; one does not cause the other. The diagnosis of comorbidity is often difficult to make because addictive behavior (of all types) can produce extreme anxiety and severe disturbances in mood and affect, especially while the addictive behavior is treated. If, after a period of abstinence, symptoms of a psychiatric disorder remain, the comorbid condition is more easily recognized and diagnosed than during the addictive period. Finally, there is a high correlation between sex addiction and substance-use disorders (up to 80 percent in some studies), which not only complicates the task of diagnosis, but also complicates treatment.

TABLE 21.1a-21
Signs of Sexual Addiction

1. Out-of-control behavior
2. Severe adverse consequences (medical, legal, interpersonal) due to sexual behavior
3. Persistent pursuit of self-destructive or high-risk sexual behavior
4. Repeated attempts to limit or stop sexual behavior
5. Sexual obsession and fantasy as a primary coping mechanism
6. The need for increasing amounts of sexual activity
7. Severe mood changes related to sexual activity (for example, depression, euphoria)
8. Inordinate amount of time spent in obtaining sex, being sexual, or recovering from sexual experience
9. Interference of sexual behavior in social, occupational, or recreational activities

Data from P Carnes: *Don't Call It Love*. Bantam Books, New York, 1991.

MANAGEMENT Self-help groups based on the 12-step concept used in Alcoholics Anonymous (AA) have been employed successfully with many sex addicts. They include such groups as Sexaholics Anonymous (SA), Sex and Love Addicts Anonymous (SLAA), and Sex Addicts Anonymous (SAA). The groups differ in that some are for men or women or for married persons or couples. All advocate some degree of abstinence from either the addictive behavior or sex in general. Should a substance-use disorder also be present, the patient often requires referral to AA or Narcotics Anonymous (NA) as well. The patient may enter an inpatient treatment unit, when he or she lacks sufficient motivation to control his or her behavior on an outpatient basis or may be a danger to self or others. Additionally, there may be severe medical or psychiatric symptoms that require careful supervision and treatment that are best carried out in a hospital.

A 42-year-old married businessman with two children was considered to be a model of virtue in his community. He was active in his church and on the boards of several charitable organizations. He was living a secret life, however, in that he would visit a local video store where he would watch pornographic videotapes while masturbating. In addition, he would lie to his wife, telling her that he was at a board meeting when he was actually visiting massage parlors for paid sex. He eventually was engaging in the behavior four or five times a day, and although he tried to quit many times, he was unable to do so. He knew that he was harming himself by putting his reputation and marriage at risk.

The patient presented himself to the psychiatric emergency room, stating that he would prefer to be dead rather than continue the behavior described. He was admitted with a diagnosis of major depressive disorder and started on a daily dose of 20 mg of fluoxetine. In addition, he received 100 mg of medroxyprogesterone acetate (Provera) intramuscularly once a day. He experienced a marked diminution in his need to masturbate, which ceased entirely on the third hospital day, as did his mental preoccupation with sex. The medroxyprogesterone was discontinued on the sixth day, when he was discharged. He was continued on fluoxetine, enrolled in a local SA group, and entered individual and couples psychotherapy. His addictive behavior eventually stopped, he was having satisfactory sexual relations with his wife, and he was no longer suicidal or depressed.

PSYCHOTHERAPY Insight-oriented psychotherapy may help patients understand the dynamics of their behavioral patterns. Supportive psychotherapy can help repair the interpersonal, social, or occupational damage that occurs. Cognitive behavioral therapy helps the patient to recognize dysphoric states that precipitate sexual acting out. Marital therapy or couples therapy can aid the patient in regaining self-esteem, which is severely impaired by the time a treatment program is begun. Finally, psychotherapy may be of help in the treatment of any associated psychiatric disorder.

PHARMACOTHERAPY Most specialists in general addiction avoid the use of pharmacological agents, especially in the early stages of treatment. Substance-dependent persons have a tendency to abuse those agents, especially agents with a high abuse potential, such as the benzodiazepines. Pharmacotherapy is of use in the treatment of associated psychiatric disorders, such as major depressive disorder and schizophrenia.

Certain medications may be of use to the sex addict, however, because of their specific effects on reducing the sex drive. Fluoxetine and other serotonin-specific reuptake inhibitors

(SSRIs) reduce libido in some persons, a side effect that is used therapeutically. Compulsive masturbation is an example of a behavioral pattern that may benefit from such medication. Medroxyprogesterone acetate diminishes libido in men and thus enables the person better to control sexually addictive behavior.

The use of antiandrogens in women to control hypersexuality has not been sufficiently tested, but since androgenic compounds contribute to the sex drive in women, antiandrogens could be of benefit. Antiandrogen agents (cyproterone acetate) are not available in the United States but are used in Europe with varying success.

Postcoital dysphoria Postcoital dysphoria is not listed in DSM-IV. It occurs during the resolution phase of sexual activity, when the person normally experiences a sense of general well-being and muscular and psychological relaxation. Some persons, however, experience postcoital dysphoria. After an otherwise satisfactory sexual experience, they become depressed, tense, anxious, and irritable and show psychomotor agitation. They often want to get away from the partner and may become verbally or even physically abusive. The incidence of the disorder is unknown, but it is more common in men than in women. The causes are several and relate to the attitude of the person toward sex in general and toward the partner in particular. It may occur in adulterous sex and with prostitutes. The fear of acquired immune deficiency syndrome (AIDS) causes some persons to experience postcoital dysphoria. Treatment requires insight-oriented psychotherapy to help patients understand the unconscious antecedents to their behavior and attitudes.

Couple problems At times, a complaint must be viewed in terms of the spousal unit or the couple, rather than as an individual dysfunction. An example is a couple in which one prefers morning sex while the other functions more readily at night; another example is a couple with unequal frequencies of desire.

Unconsummated marriage A couple involved in an unconsummated marriage have never had coitus and are typically uninformed and inhibited about sexuality. Their feelings of guilt, shame, or inadequacy are increased by their problem, and they experience conflict between their need to seek help and their need to conceal their difficulty. Couples present with the problem after having been married several months or several years. William Masters and Virginia Johnson reported an unconsummated marriage of 17 years' duration.

Frequently, the couple does not seek help directly, but the woman may reveal the problem to her gynecologist on a visit ostensibly concerned with vague vaginal or other somatic complaints. On examining her, the gynecologist may find an intact hymen. In some cases though, the wife may have undergone a hymenectomy to resolve the problem. That surgical procedure is another stress and often increases the feelings of inadequacy in the couple. The wife may feel put on, abused, or mutilated, and the husband's concern about his manliness may increase. The hymenectomy usually aggravates the situation without solving the basic problem. The inquiry of a physician who is comfortable in dealing with sexual problems may be the first opening to a frank discussion of the couple's distress. Often, the pretext of the medical visit is a discussion of contraceptive methods or—even more ironically—a request for an infertility workup. Once presented, the complaint can often be successfully treated. The duration of the problem does not significantly affect the prognosis or the outcome of the case.

The causes of unconsummated marriage are varied: lack of sex education, sexual prohibitions overly stressed by parents or society, problems of an oedipal nature, immaturity in both partners, overdependence on primary families, and problems in sexual identification. Religious orthodoxy, with severe control of sexual and social development or the equation of sexuality with sin or uncleanliness, has also been cited as a dominant cause. Many women involved in an unconsummated marriage have distorted concepts about their vaginas. They may fear that the vagina is too small or too soft, or they may confuse the vagina with the rectum, leading to feelings of being unclean. The man may share in those distortions about the vagina and, in addition, perceive it as dangerous to himself. Similarly, both partners may have distortions about the man's penis, perceiving it as a weapon, as too large, or as too small. Many patients can be helped by simple education about genital anatomy and physiology, by suggestions for self-exploration, and by correct information from a physician. The problem of the unconsummated marriage is best treated by seeing both members of the couple. Dual-sex therapy involving a male-female cotherapist team has been markedly effective. However, other forms of conjoint therapy, marital counseling, traditional psychotherapy on a one-to-one basis, and counseling from a sensitive family physician, gynecologist, or urologist are all helpful.

Body image problems Some persons are ashamed of their bodies and experience feelings of inadequacy related to self-imposed standards of masculinity or femininity. They may insist on sex only during total darkness, not allow certain body parts to be seen or touched, or seek unnecessary operative procedures to deal with their imagined inadequacies. Body dysmorphic disorder should be ruled out.

Don Juanism Some men who appear to be hypersexual, as shown by their need to have many sexual encounters or conquests, use their sexual activities to mask deep feelings of inferiority. Some have unconscious homosexual impulses, which they deny by compulsive sexual contacts with women. After having sex, most Don Juans are no longer interested in the woman. The condition is also referred to as satyriasis or a form of sex addiction.

Nymphomania Nymphomania signifies excessive or pathological desire for coitus in a woman. There have been few scientific studies of the condition. Those patients who have been studied usually have had one or more sexual disorders, usually including female orgasmic disorder. The woman often has an intense fear of her loss of love. The woman attempts to satisfy her dependence needs, rather than to gratify her sexual impulses through her actions. It is sometimes classified as a form of sex addiction.

Fantasies Other atypical disorders are found in persons who have one or more sexual fantasies about which they obsess, feel guilty, or are otherwise dysphoric. As indicated in Table 21.1a-22, however, the range of common sexual fantasies is broad.

Persistent and marked distress about sexual orientation Distress about sexual orientation is characterized by a dissatisfaction with homosexual arousal patterns, a desire to increase heterosexual arousal, and strong negative feelings about being homosexual. Occasional statements to the effect that life would be easier if the person were not homosexual do not constitute persistent and marked distress about sexual orientation.

Treatment of sexual orientation distress is controversial. One study reported that, with a minimum of 350 hours of psycho-

TABLE 21.1a-22
Common Sexual Fantasies*

Men	Women
Heterosexual	
Replacement of established partner	Replacement of established partner
Forced sexual encounters with woman	Forced sexual encounters with man
Observing sexual activity	Observing sexual activity
Sexual encounters with man	Idyllic encounters with unknown man
Group sex	Sexual encounters with woman
Homosexual	
Images of male anatomy	Forced sexual encounters with women
Forced sexual encounters with men	Idyllic encounters with established partner
Sexual encounters with women	Sexual encounters with man
Idyllic encounters with unknown men	Memories of past sexual experiences
Group sex	Sadistic imagery

*Most frequent listed in order of occurrence. A 1994 study found that one in five persons experienced a same-sex sexual fantasy at some time in their lives.

Table adapted from W Masters, M Schwartz: The Masters and Johnson treatment program for dissatisfied homosexual men. Am J Psychiatry *141:* 173, 1984. Used with permission. (Courtesy of *The New York Times.*)

analytic therapy, about a third of about 100 bisexual and homosexual men achieved a heterosexual reorientation at a five-year follow-up, but that study has been challenged and was never replicated. Behavior therapy and avoidance conditioning techniques have also been used, but a basic problem with behavioral techniques is that the behavior may be changed in the laboratory setting but not outside the laboratory. Prognostic factors weighing in favor of heterosexual reorientation for men include being under 35 years of age, having some experience of heterosexual arousal, and having a high motivation for reorientation.

Another style of intervention is directed at enabling the person with persistent and marked distress about sexual orientation to live comfortably as a homosexual without shame, guilt, anxiety, or depression. Gay counseling centers are engaged with patients in such treatment programs. At present, outcome studies of such centers have not been reported in detail.

As for the treatment of women with persistent and marked distress about sexual orientation, few data are available, and those are primarily single-case studies with variable outcomes.

Postcoital headache Postcoital headache is characterized by headache immediately after coitus that may last for several hours. It is usually described as throbbing, and it is localized in the occipital or frontal area. The cause is unknown. There may be vascular, muscle contraction (tension), or psychogenic causes. Coitus may precipitate migraine or cluster headaches in predisposed persons.

Orgasmic anhedonia Orgasmic anhedonia is a condition in which the person has no physical sensation of orgasm, even though the physiological component (for example, ejaculation) remains intact. Medical causes, such as sacral and cephalic lesions that interfere with afferent pathways from the genitalia to the cortex, must be ruled out. Psychic causes usually relate to extreme guilt about experiencing sexual pleasure. Those feelings produce a type of dissociative response that isolates the affective component of the orgasmic experience from consciousness.

Masturbatory pain In some cases persons may experience pain during masturbation. Organic causes should always be ruled out. A small vaginal tear or early Peyronie's disease may produce a painful sensation. The condition should be differentiated from compulsive masturbation. People may masturbate to the extent that they do physical damage to their genitals and eventually experience pain during subsequent masturbatory acts. Such cases constitute a separate sexual disorder and should be so classified.

Certain masturbatory practices have resulted in what has been called autoerotic asphyxiation. The practices may involve masturbating while hanging by the neck to heighten erotic sensations and the intensity of the orgasm through the mechanism of mild hypoxia. Although they intend to release themselves from the noose after orgasm, an estimated 500 to 1,000 persons a year accidentally kill themselves by hanging. Most who indulge in the practice are men; transvestism is often associated with the habit, and the majority of deaths occurs among adolescents. Such masochistic practices are usually associated with severe mental disorders, such as schizophrenia and major mood disorders.

PHARMACOLOGICAL AGENTS IMPLICATED IN SEX DYSFUNCTION Almost every pharmacological agent, particularly those used in psychiatry, has been associated with an effect on sexuality. In men those effects include decreased sex drive, erectile failure (impotence), decreased volume of ejaculate, and delayed or retrograde ejaculation. In women decreased sex drive, decreased vaginal lubrication, inhibited or delayed orgasm, and decreased or absent vaginal contractions may occur. Drugs may also enhance the sexual response and increase the sex drive, but that effect is less common than are adverse effects.

Psychotherapeutic drugs

ANTIPSYCHOTIC DRUGS Most of those drugs are dopamine receptor antagonists and also block adrenergic and cholinergic receptors, thus accounting for adverse sex effects. Chlorpromazine (Thorazine), thioridazine (Mellaril), and trifluoperazine (Stelazine) are potent anticholinergics and impair erection and ejaculation in men and inhibit vaginal lubrication and orgasm in women. Thioridazine has a particular side effect of causing retrograde ejaculation in which the seminal fluid backs up into the bladder rather than being propelled through the penile urethra. Patients still have a pleasurable sensation of orgasm, but it is dry. When urinating after orgasm, the urine may be milky white since it contains the ejaculate. The condition is startling but harmless, and may occur in up to 50 percent of patients taking the drug. Paradoxically, some rare cases of priapism have been reported with antipsychotics.

Antidepressant drugs The drugs may be subdivided into heterocyclic antidepressants, such as imipramine (Tofranil); the SSRIs, such as fluoxetine; and the MAO inhibitors, such as phenelzine (Nardil).

The cyclic antidepressants have anticholinergic effects that interfere with erection and delay ejaculation. Since the anticholinergic effects vary among the cyclic antidepressants, those with the least effects (for example, desipramine [Norpramin]) produce the least sexual side effects. The effects in women of the heterocyclics have not been documented sufficiently; however, few women seem to complain of any effects. Deprenyl (Segiline) is a selective MAO_B inhibitor reported to increase sex drive, possibly by dopaminergic activity and increased production of norepinephrine.

Some men report an increased sensitivity of the glans that is pleasurable and that does not interfere with erection, although it delays ejaculation. In some cases, however, the tricyclic causes a painful ejaculation, perhaps as the result of interference with seminal propulsion caused by, in turn, interference with urethral, prostatic, vas, and epididymal smooth muscle contractions. Clomipramine (Anafranil) has been reported as increasing sex drive in some persons.

The SSRIs most often have adverse effects because of the rise in serotonin levels. A lowering of the sex drive and a difficulty in reaching orgasm occur in both sexes. Reversal of those negative effects has been achieved with cyproheptadine (Periactin), an antihistamine with antiserotonergic effects, and with methylphenidate (Ritalin), which has adrenergic effects.

The MAO inhibitors affect biogenic amines broadly. Accordingly, they produce impaired erection, delayed or retrograde ejaculation, vaginal dryness, and inhibited orgasm. Tranylcypromine (Parnate) has a paradoxical sexually stimulating effect in some persons, possibly as a result of its amphetaminelike properties.

GENERAL EFFECTS Since depression is associated with a decreased libido, varying levels of sexual dysfunction and anhedonia are part of the disease process. Some patients report improved sexual functioning as their depression improves as a result of antidepressant medication. That phenomenon makes the evaluation of sexual side effects in patients taking the drugs difficult. Finally, many of the sexual side effects disappear with time, perhaps as a result of a biogenic amine homeostatic mechanism's coming into play.

Lithium Lithium regulates mood and in the manic state may reduce hypersexuality, possibly by a dopamine antagonist activity. In other cases, impaired erection has been reported.

Psychostimulants Such drugs are sometimes used in the treatment of depression and include amphetamine, methylphenidate, and pemoline (Cylert), which raise the plasma levels of norepinephrine and dopamine. Libido is increased; however, with prolonged use, men may experience a loss of desire and erections.

α-Adrenergic and β-adrenergic receptor antagonists Such drugs are used in the treatment of hypertension, angina, and certain cardiac arrhythmias. They diminish tonic sympathetic nerve outflow from vasomotor centers in the brain. As a result, they can cause impotence, decrease the volume of ejaculate, and produce retrograde ejaculation. Changes in libido have been reported in both sexes.

Suggestions have been made to use the side effects of drugs therapeutically. Thus a drug that delays or interferes with ejaculation (such as fluoxetine) might be used to treat premature ejaculation.

Anticholinergics These drugs block cholinergic receptors and include such drugs as amantadine (Symmetrel) and benztropine (Cogentin). They produce dryness of the mucous membranes (including that of the vagina) and impotence.

Antihistamines Drugs such as diphenhydramine (Benadryl) have anticholinergic activity and are mildly hypnotic. They may inhibit sexual function as a result. Cyproheptadine, although an antihistamine, also has potent activity as a serotonin antagonist. It is used to block the serotonergic sexual side effects produced by SSRIs, such as delayed orgasm and impotence.

Antianxiety agents The major class of drugs in the antianxiety category is the benzodiazepines (for example, diazepam [Valium]). They act on the γ-aminobutyric acid (GABA) receptors, which are believed to be involved in cognition, memory, and motor control. Because they decrease plasma epinephrine concentrations, they diminish anxiety, and as a result they improve sexual function in those persons inhibited by anxiety.

Alcohol Alcohol suppresses CNS activity generally and can produce erectile disorders in men as a result. Alcohol has a direct gonadal effect that decreases testosterone levels in men; paradoxically, it can produce a slight rise in testosterone levels in women. The latter finding may account for women reporting increased libido after drinking small amounts of alcohol. The long-term use of alcohol reduces the ability of the liver to metabolize estrogenic compounds. In men that produces signs of feminization (for example, gynecomastia as a result of testicular atrophy).

Opioids Opioids, such as heroin, have adverse sexual effects, such as erectile failure and decreased libido. The alteration of consciousness may enhance the sexual experience in occasional users.

Hallucinogens The hallucinogens include lysergic acid diethylamide (LSD), phencyclidine (PCP), psilocybin (from some mushrooms), and mescaline (from peyote cactus). In addition to inducing hallucinations, the drugs cause loss of contact with reality and an expanding and heightening of consciousness. Some users report that the sexual experience is similarly enhanced, but others experience anxiety, delirium, or psychosis, which clearly interferes with sex function.

Cannabis The altered state of consciousness produced by cannabis may enhance sexual pleasure for some persons. Its prolonged use depresses testosterone levels.

Barbiturates and similarly acting drugs The drugs are sedative-hypnotics and may enhance sexual responsiveness in persons who are sexually unresponsive as a result of anxiety. They have no direct effect on the sex organs; however, they do produce an alteration in consciousness that some persons find pleasurable. They are subject to abuse and may be fatal when combined with alcohol or other CNS depressants.

Methaqualone (Quaalude) acquired a reputation as a sexual enhancer, which had no biological basis in fact. It is no longer marketed in the United States.

SUBSTANCE-INDUCED SEXUAL DYSFUNCTION The diagnosis is used when there is evidence from the history, the physical examination, or the laboratory findings of substance intoxication or withdrawal. Distressing sexual dysfunction occurs within a month of significant substance intoxication or withdrawal (Table 21.1a-23). Specified substances include alcohol; amphetamines or related substances; cocaine; opioids; sedatives, hypnotics, or anxiolytics; and other or unknown substances.

Abused recreational substances affect sexual function in various ways. In small doses many of the substances enhance sexual performance by decreasing inhibition or anxiety or by causing a temporary elation of mood. However, with continued use, erectile, orgasmic, and ejaculatory capacities become impaired. The abuse of sedatives, anxiolytics, hypnotics, and particularly opiates and opioids nearly always depresses desire. Alcohol may foster the initiation of sexual activity by removing inhi-

TABLE 21.1a-23
Diagnostic Criteria for Substance-Induced Sexual Dysfunction

A. Clinically significant sexual dysfunction that results in marked distress or interpersonal difficulty predominates in the clinical picture.
B. There is evidence from the history, physical examination, or laboratory findings that the sexual dysfunction is fully explained by substance use as manifested by either (1) or (2):
   (1) the symptoms in criterion A developed during, or within a month of, substance intoxication
   (2) medication use is etiologically related to the disturbance
C. The disturbance is not better accounted for by a sexual dysfunction that is not substance induced. Evidence that the symptoms are better accounted for by a sexual dysfunction that is not substance induced might include the following: the symptoms precede the onset of the substance use or dependence (or medication use); the symptoms persist for a substantial period of time (e.g., about a month) after the cessation of intoxication, or are substantially in excess of what would be expected given the type or amount of the substance used or the duration of use; or there is other evidence that suggests the existence of an independent non-substance-induced sexual dysfunction (e.g., a history of recurrent non-substance-related episodes).

Note: This diagnosis should be made instead of a diagnosis of substance intoxication only when the sexual dysfunction is in excess of that usually associated with the intoxication syndrome and when the dysfunction is sufficiently severe to warrant independent clinical attention.

Code: [Specific substance]-induced sexual dysfunction:
(alcohol, amphetamine [or amphetaminelike substance]; cocaine; opioid; sedative, hypnotic, or anxiolytic; other [or unknown] substance)

Specify if:
With impaired desire
With impaired arousal
With impaired orgasm
With sexual pain

Specify if:
With onset during intoxication: if the criteria are met for intoxication with the substance and the symptoms develop during the intoxication syndrome

Table from DSM-IV, *Diagnostic and Statistical Manual of Mental Disorders,* ed 4. Copyright American Psychiatric Association, Washington, 1994. Used with permission.

bition, but it impairs performance. Cocaine and amphetamines produce similar effects. Although no direct evidence indicates that sexual drive is enhanced, the user initially has a feeling of increased energy and may become sexually active. Ultimately, dysfunction occurs. Men usually go through two stages: prolonged erection without ejaculation, and then a gradual loss of erectile capacity.

Recovering substance-dependent patients may need therapy to regain sexual function. In part, that is one piece of psychological readjustment to a nondependent state. Many substance abusers have always had difficulty with intimate interactions. Others have missed the experiences that would have enabled them to learn social and sexual skills because they spent their crucial developmental years under the influence of some substance.

TREATMENT OF SEXUAL DYSFUNCTION

Various corrective therapies are now used to treat sexual dysfunctions. Psychiatrists are eminently well qualified to incorporate the techniques of sex therapy into their treatments. That practice simply follows the general history of psychiatry, which has modified and absorbed any number of specialized techniques into its treatment repertoire. Where the dysfunction occurs alone, an unmodified sex-therapy approach seems to be the treatment of choice. For patients with accompanying personality disorders or medical conditions, it is but one of many techniques to be considered.

In addition to making the determination of which type of therapy to use, the clinician must evaluate whether or not the disorder has a physiological cause. It is assumed that prior to entering psychotherapy, the patient will have had a thorough medical evaluation, including a medical history, physical examination, and appropriate laboratory studies when necessary. If a medical cause for the disorder is found, treatment should be directed toward ameliorating the cause of the dysfunction.

Prior to 1970 the most common treatment of sexual dysfunction was individual psychotherapy. Classic psychodynamic theory considers sexual inadequacy to have its roots in early developmental conflicts, and the sexual disorder is treated as part of a more pervasive emotional disturbance. Treatment focuses on the exploration of unconscious conflicts, motivation, fantasy, and various interpersonal difficulties. One of the assumptions of therapy is that the removal of the conflicts will allow the sexual impulse to become structurally acceptable to the patient's ego and thereby find appropriate means of satisfaction in the environment. Unfortunately, the symptom of sexual dysfunction frequently becomes secondarily autonomous and continues to persist when other problems evolving from the patient's pathology have been resolved. The addition of behavioral techniques is often necessary to cure the sexual problem.

Four treatment modalities that emphasize behavioral approaches—dual-sex therapy, hypnotherapy, behavior therapy, and group therapy—will be discussed, as well as analytically oriented sex therapy, which integrates the tenets of psychoanalysis with behavioral techniques. Biological therapies will also be reviewed.

DUAL-SEX THERAPY The theoretical basis of the dual-sex therapy approach is the concept of the marital unit or dyad as the object of therapy. The method of dual-sex therapy was originated and developed by Masters and Johnson. In dual-sex therapy there is no acceptance of the idea of a sick half of a patient couple. Both are involved in a relationship in which there is sexual distress, and both, therefore, must participate in the therapy program.

The sexual problem often reflects other areas of disharmony or misunderstanding in the marriage. The marital relationship as a whole is treated, with emphasis on sexual functioning as a part of that relationship. Improved communication in sexual and nonsexual areas is a specific goal of treatment. Psychological and physiological aspects of sexual functioning are discussed, and an educative attitude is used. Suggestions are made for specific sexual activity, and those suggestions are followed in the privacy of the couple's home.

Initial histories are taken to determine suitability for that type of treatment. When there is evidence of major underlying psychopathology, further psychiatric evaluation is suggested, and participation in the program may be deferred until the patient seems better able to benefit from it. Concurrent psychotherapy with a psychiatrist while participating in dual-sex therapy is sometimes recommended.

Each patient is interviewed individually early in the course of treatment. A complete sexual history is obtained, and that history is later reflected back to the couple, with the aim of helping them understand their present problem. The individual sessions also enable the therapist to understand the patients' life-style and to make suggestions that fit into that life-style.

Behavioral exercises Treatment is short term and is behaviorally oriented. Specific exercises are prescribed for the couple to help them with their particular problem. Sexual dysfunction often involves a fear of inadequate performance. The couples are, therefore, specifically prohibited from any sexual play other than that prescribed by the therapist. Initially, intercourse is interdicted, and couples learn to give and receive bodily pleasure without the pressure of performance. Beginning exercises usually focus on heightening sensory awareness to touch, sight, sound, and smell.

During those exercises, which are called *sensate focus exercises,* the couple is given much reinforcement to lessen anxiety. The patients are urged to use fantasies to distract them from obsessive concerns about performance, which is termed spectatoring. The needs of both the dysfunctional partner and the nondysfunctional partner are considered. If either partner becomes sexually excited by the exercises, the other is encouraged to bring him or her to orgasm by manual or oral means. That procedure is important to keep the nondysfunctional partner from sabotaging the treatment. Open communication between the partners is urged, and the expression of mutual needs is encouraged. Resistances, such as claims of fatigue or not enough time to complete the exercises, are common and must be dealt with by the therapist. Genital stimulation is eventually added to general body stimulation. The couple is instructed sequentially to try various positions for intercourse, without necessarily completing the act, and to use varieties of stimulating techniques before they are instructed to proceed with intercourse.

The specific exercises vary with differing presenting complaints, and special techniques are used to treat the various dysfunctions. In cases of vaginismus, for instance, the woman is advised to dilate her vaginal opening with her fingers or with size-graduated vaginal dilators as part of the therapy.

In cases of premature ejaculation an exercise known as the *squeeze technique* is used to raise the threshold of penile excitability. In that exercise the man or the woman stimulates the erect penis until the earliest sensations of impending orgasm and ejaculation are felt. Penile stimulation is then stopped abruptly, and the coronal ridge of the penis is forcibly squeezed for several seconds. The technique is repeated several times. A variation is the *stop-start technique* in which stimulation is interrupted for several seconds but no squeeze is applied. Masturbation to the point of imminent orgasm raises the threshold of excitability to a more tolerant stimulation level. Communication between the partners is improved, because the man must let his partner know the degree of his sexual excitement so that she can squeeze the penis before the ejaculatory process has started. Sex therapy has been most successful in the treatment of premature ejaculation.

A man with a sexual desire disorder or erectile disorder is sometimes told to masturbate to demonstrate that full erection and ejaculation are possible. In cases of lifelong female orgasmic disorder the woman is directed to masturbate, sometimes using a vibrator. Kegel's exercises to strengthen the pubococcygeal muscles may be introduced; that is, the woman is instructed to contract her vagina voluntarily. The woman is also encouraged to contract her abdominal and perineal muscles during masturbation and coitus. When a man is impotent, the woman may be instructed to stimulate or tease his penis. The same technique is used with men who suffer from retarded ejaculation, and, in that case, stimulation sometimes involves a vibrator. Retarded ejaculation is managed by extravaginal ejaculation initially and gradual vaginal entry after stimulation to the point of near ejaculation.

Treatment goals The overall goal of treatment always is to initiate an educational process, to diminish the fears of performance felt by both sexes, and to facilitate communication within the marital unit in sexual and nonsexual areas. Therapy sessions follow each new exercise period, and problems and satisfactions, both sexual and in other areas of the couple's lives, are discussed. Specific instructions and the introduction of new exercises geared to the individual couple's progress are reviewed in each session. Gradually, the couple gains confidence and learns or relearns to communicate verbally and sexually. Dual-sex therapy is most effective when the sexual dysfunction exists apart from other psychopathology.

HYPNOTHERAPY Hypnotherapists focus specifically on the anxiety-producing symptom—that is, the particular sexual dysfunction. The successful use of hypnosis enables the patient to gain control over the symptom that has been lowering self-esteem and disrupting psychological homeostasis. The cooperation of the patient is first obtained and encouraged during a series of nonhypnotic sessions with the therapist. The discussions permit the development of a secure doctor-patient relationship, a sense of physical and psychological comfort on the part of the patient, and the establishment of mutually desired treatment goals. During that time, the therapist assesses the patient's capacity for the trance experience. The nonhypnotic sessions also permit the clinician to take a careful psychiatric history and do a mental status examination before beginning hypnotherapy. The focus of treatment is on symptom removal and attitude alteration. In a trance state, the patient is able to entertain ideas incongruent with his or her usual (nonhypnotized) perceptions of reality. The patient is instructed in developing alternative means of dealing with the anxiety-provoking situation, which is the sexual encounter.

For example, a woman suffering from vaginismus is given the posthypnotic suggestion that she will not feel pain during intercourse and that she will be able to relax the muscles surrounding her vagina. If compliance with the suggestion is successful, the patient is able to deal with the anxiety produced by the sex act. She is also taught new attitudes, such as being entitled to sexual pleasure. Under hypnosis her fear or anger at sexual contact can be examined, and she learns how her emotions are expressed by involuntary spasms of her vagina.

Some patients respond particularly well to the use of self-hypnosis and to indirect suggestion. Those techniques allow them to retain a greater sense of control over their situation. Typically, patients are instructed to conjure up images and develop ideas that are antithetical to their dysfunctional responses. For example, a woman with an arousal disorder may first agree to concentrate on imagery that causes her to salivate. Then she is told that just as she has made her mouth water by focusing on stimulating images, she can affect the lubricating response of her vagina by focusing on images she finds erotic or romantic. At the same time, the therapist helps her deal with her anxieties about a positive sexual response. Patients are also taught relaxing techniques to use on themselves before sexual relations. With those methods to alleviate anxiety, the physiological responses to sexual stimulation can more readily result in pleasurable excitation and discharge. Hypnosis may be added to a basic individual psychotherapy program to accelerate the impact of psychotherapeutic intervention.

BEHAVIOR THERAPY Behavior therapists assume that sexual dysfunction is learned maladaptive behavior. Behavioral approaches were initially designed for the treatment of phobias. In cases of sexual dysfunction the therapist sees the patient as phobic of sexual interaction. Using traditional techniques, the therapist sets up a hierarchy of anxiety-provoking situations for the patient, ranging from the least threatening to the most threatening situation. Mild anxiety may be experienced at the thought of kissing, and massive anxiety may be felt when imagining penile penetration. The behavior therapist enables the patient to master the anxiety through a standard program of systematic desensitization. The program is designed to inhibit the learned anxious response by encouraging behaviors antithetical to anxiety. The patient first deals with the least anxiety-producing situation in fantasy and progresses by steps to the greatest anxiety-producing situation. Medication, hypnosis, or special training in deep-muscle relaxation is sometimes used to help with the initial mastery of anxiety.

Assertiveness training is also used and is helpful in teaching the patient to express his or her sexual needs openly and without fear. Exercises in assertiveness are given in conjunction with sex therapy, and the patient is encouraged both to make sexual requests and to refuse to comply with requests perceived as unreasonable. Sexual exercises may be prescribed for the patient to perform at home, and a hierarchy may be established, starting with those activities that have proved most pleasurable and successful in the past.

One treatment variation involves the participation of the patient's sexual partner in the desensitization program. The partner, rather than the therapist, presents the hierarchical items to the patient. In such situations a cooperative partner is necessary to help the patient carry gains made during treatment sessions to sexual activity at home.

Behavior therapy techniques have been found to be particularly effective in the treatment of women with severe inhibition of excitement and orgasm when such feelings were accompanied by strong feelings of anxiety, anger, or disgust.

GROUP THERAPY Methods of group therapy have been used to examine both intrapsychic and interpersonal problems in patients with sexual disorders. The therapy group provides a strong support system for a patient who feels ashamed, anxious, or guilty about a particular sexual problem. It is a useful forum in which to counteract sexual myths, correct misconceptions, and provide accurate information regarding sexual anatomy, physiology, and varieties of behavior.

Groups for the treatment of sexual disorders can be organized in several ways. Members may all share the same problem, such as premature ejaculation; members may all be of the same sex with different sexual problems; or groups may be composed of both men and women who are experiencing different sexual problems. Group therapy may be an adjunct to other forms of therapy or the prime mode of treatment. Groups organized to cure a particular dysfunction are usually behavioral in approach. For example, patients suffering from anorgasmia may participate with others suffering from the same problem in a short-term, intensive group experience. Sexual histories, feelings of inadequacy, and concerns about body image are shared. Specific physiological information, sometimes with the aid of audiovisual materials, is presented to the group members. Members are given homework assignments. For instance, they may be instructed to masturbate. A combination of group support and group pressure helps some of the participants complete assignments they might otherwise want to avoid. As the short-term group process nears termination, members are encouraged to talk about their experiences with their partners.

Groups have also been effective when composed of sexually dysfunctional married couples. The group provides the opportunity to gather accurate information, provides consensual validation of individual preferences, and enhances self-esteem and self-acceptance. Such techniques as role playing and psychodrama may be used in treatment. Such groups are not indicated for couples when one partner is uncooperative, when a patient is suffering from a severe depression or psychosis, when there is a strong repugnance for explicit sexual audiovisual material, or when there is a strong fear of groups.

INTEGRATED SEX THERAPY One of the most effective treatment modalities is the use of sex therapy integrated with supportive, psychodynamic, or insight-oriented psychotherapy. The addition of psychodynamic conceptualizations to the behavioral techniques used to treat sexual dysfunctions allows for the treatment of patients with sex disorders associated with other psychopathology. Also, the therapy is appropriate for patients suffering from hypoactive desire disorders. Insight-oriented therapy helps them deal with problems in their interpersonal relationships or with conflicts on an intrapsychic level that frequently are at the root of the problem.

The themes and dynamics that emerge in patients in analytically oriented sex therapy are the same as those seen in psychoanalytic therapy, such as relevant dreams, fear of punishment, aggressive feelings, difficulty with trusting the partner, fear of intimacy, oedipal feelings, and fear of genital mutilation.

A 34-year-old widow presented for therapy with a chief complaint of vaginismus. Her marriage of three years, which had been unconsummated, ended when her husband was killed in a car accident. Approximately one year after she lost her husband, the patient became involved with a married man. She was very attracted to him and became highly aroused during their sexual encounters. Although she could reach orgasm through manual or oral stimulation, she could not tolerate penetration. She was motivated to seek help for her problem—although she never considered therapy when she was married, in spite of her husband's requests to do so—because she felt sure her lover would leave his wife for her if they could have a more complete sexual experience together.

The patient's vaginismus was partly the result of unresolved developmental conflicts. Her parents had been loving but rigid people who came from different socioeconomic backgrounds. Their values often conflicted and they frequently fought over their daughter as she entered adolescence: the mother insisted that she take an academic course in high school to prepare for college, whereas the father pushed a more practical business program. The patient sided with her mother and felt that her father, whom she had always perceived as cold, became more distant than before. Some of her difficulties were due to unresolved oedipal problems: Both her husband and her lover were more than 20 years older than she was, and her lover, reflecting her parental situation, was married to a woman who was more successful than he was. In addition, she had identified with some of her mother's negative feelings about men. The mother had once expressed to the patient the hope that she would be spared marriage. Her vaginismus protected the patient from the closeness with men that she consciously wanted but that she unconsciously perceived as hurtful and dangerous.

Another patient, a 56-year-old man, came for treatment because of an erectile disorder. In general, he was better able to function in extramarital affairs than in his marriage. Although he loved his wife and felt that she was an attractive woman, he believed that she was not interested in sex. He was rarely able to achieve an erection with her and he gradually stopped approaching her sexually. His wife felt deprived by their lack of sexual relations and indulged in frequent masturbation.

The patient had been a sickly child, with a mother he described as devoted but smothering. He remembered her cuddling him in bed until he was 8 years old, and he felt that she was inappropriately affectionate in general; "she embarrassed me." At the same time, he remembered his father as an earthy man and had a childhood recollection of hearing his mother ask the father, "How could you, how could you?" The patient believed that it had been his mother's response to a sexual overture or act. In part, his disorder derived from his unconscious oedipal associations to his wife, which made her taboo for him as a sex partner. The women to whom he responded had to be blatantly sexual and signal their acceptance of him before he would risk an advance. Therapy involved both individual sessions with the patient and joint sessions with him and his wife. Communication, which had been strained partly because of the sexual distance between them, was encouraged, and a behavioral approach was used to reestablish some physical interaction. Individual work focused on his deeper psychological problems.

The dynamics and the emotional difficulties evident in the

vignettes are those seen every day by the psychiatrist. Psychiatrists are readily able to absorb the techniques of sex therapy into their treatment armamentarium, just as they have modified and absorbed any number of specialized techniques, from classic analytic dynamic formulations to the use of pharmacotherapy, group therapy techniques, and behavioral and other directive modalities.

The combined approach of individual and sex therapy is used by the general psychiatrist, who carefully judges the optimal timing of sex therapy and the ability of patients to tolerate the directive approach that focuses on their sexual difficulties.

BIOLOGICAL TREATMENT METHODS Biological forms of treatment, including pharmacotherapy and surgical treatment, may have some application in specific cases of sexual disorder. Coexisting physical and psychiatric problems should receive appropriate treatment as necessary.

Pharmacotherapy A variety of drugs have been explored in the treatment of sexual dysfunction. Intravenous methohexital sodium (Brevital) has been used in desensitization therapy. Antianxiety agents may have some application in tense patients, although those drugs can also interfere with the sexual response. Sometimes the side effects of such drugs as thioridazine (Mellaril), haloperidol (Haldol), lorazepam (Ativan), the MAO inhibitors, and the tricyclic antidepressants are used to prolong the sexual response in various conditions, such as premature ejaculation. The use of tricyclics has also been advocated in the treatment of patients who are phobic of sex and in patients with a posttraumatic stress disorder following rape. The risks of taking such medications must be carefully weighed against the possible benefits they provide, particularly when the sexual problems may respond to nonpharmacological means.

A number of substances have popular standing as aphrodisiacs. Examples of those are ginseng root and yohimbine (Yocon). However, studies have not confirmed that they have any aphrodisiac properties. Yohimbine is an α-adrenergic blocking agent and may cause dilation of the penile artery by that mechanism. Also, many recreational drugs, including cocaine, amphetamines, alcohol, and cannabis, are considered enhancers of sexual performance. Although they may provide the user with an initial benefit because of their tranquilizing, disinhibiting, or mood-elevating effects, consistent or prolonged use of any of those substances impairs sexual functioning.

Ginseng has been reported to have androgenic effects. One report described the case of a mother who ingested large amounts of ginseng during her pregnancy, resulting in androgenization of the neonate, who was born with pubic hair and enlarged testes.

Dopaminergic agents have been reported to increase libido and improve sex function. Those drugs include L-dopa, a dopamine precursor, and bromocriptine, a dopamine agonist. The antidepressant bupropion (Wellbutrin) has dopaminergic effects and has increased sex drive in some patients. Selegiline (Eldepryl, Deprenyl) is an MAO inhibitor, which is selective for MAO_B and is dopaminergic. It improves sexual functioning in older persons.

Penile injections A variety of injectable vasoactive substances have been studied for use in cases of erectile dysfunction. They produce a transient increase in penile blood flow, which allows the patient to become tumescent or gain an erection. The physician usually administers a test dose of the drug, and if the patient responds favorably, he is then taught to inject himself. The drugs are injected into the cavernosa of the penis. The substance most frequently used in this country is a mixture of papaverine HCL (Cerespan) and phentolamine mesylate (Regitine). Sometimes prostaglandin E is added to the mixture. Usually a urologist teaches the patient to inject himself in a series of training sessions. Erections occur immediately and last for hours. However, there are possible hazardous sequelae, including priapism and sclerosis of the small veins of the penis. Another substance being tried is vasoactive intestinal polypeptide (VIP). Intracavernous injection of VIP causes erection and has a parasympathomimetic effect. Some researchers speculate that the substance, which has been found in the hypothalamus and the female genital organs, is an essential factor in male and female arousal. In Europe phenoxybenzamine (Dibenzyline) is used to produce erections by injection into the penis. Serious side effects include priapism and pain accompanying the injection, and the drug is not allowed as a therapy in the United States.

Hormone therapy Androgens increase the sex drive in women and in men with low testosterone levels. Women may experience virilizing effects, some of which are irreversible (for example, deepening of the voice). In men the prolonged use of androgens produces hypertension and prostatic enlargement. Testosterone is most effective when given parenterally; however, effective oral and transdermal preparations are available.

Gonadotrophic releasing hormone (GnRH), also known as luteinizing hormone-releasing hormone (LHRH), stimulates the release of luteinizing hormone (LH), which increases testosterone secretion in both sexes. GnRH is used as an inhalant in Europe. It stimulates desire and increased potency. Since GnRH is released normally in a pulsatile fashion, portable infusion pumps have been developed that simulate pulsatile delivery. An excess of GnRH suppresses estrogen and testosterone; the therapeutic use of GnRH is limited by a narrow therapeutic window.

Women who use estrogens for replacement therapy or for contraception may report decreased libido; in such cases a combined preparation of estrogen and testosterone has been used effectively.

Pheromones are sexual scents that are found in animals and may be present in humans. They produce dramatic sex-seeking behavioral patterns in animals (for example, male deer following female deer in estrus and mounting behavior in primates). Human pheromones are believed to be short-acting fatty acids present in vaginal secretions and male sweat. In one study women were consistently attracted to items impregnated with a chemical derived from male sweat (α-androstenol) as compared with control items.

Antiandrogens and antiestrogens Estrogen and progesterone are antiandrogens and have been used to treat compulsive sexual behavior in men. Clomiphene (Clomid) and tamoxifen (Nolvadex) are both antiestrogenic and both stimulate GnRH (LHRH) secretion and increase testosterone, thereby increasing libido. Women being treated for breast cancer with tamoxifen report an increased libido.

Cyprosterone acetate is a strong antiandrogen used in male sex offenders. At doses of 100 to 200 mg a day, the sex drive disappears within two weeks. It is available in Europe but is in the investigational stage in the United States.

STEAL SYNDROME In male patients with arteriosclerosis (especially of the distal aorta, known as Leriche's syndrome) the loss of erection may occur during active pelvic thrusting. The need for increased blood in the gluteal muscles and others served by the ilial or hypogastric arteries takes blood away (steals) from the pudendal artery, thus interfering with penile blood flow. Relief may be obtained by decreasing pelvic thrusting, which is also aided by the woman's superior coital position.

SURGICAL TREATMENT

Male prosthesis Surgical treatment is rarely advocated, but improved penile prosthetic devices are available for men with inadequate erectile response who are resistant to other treatment methods or who have medically caused deficiencies. There are two main types of prostheses: a semirigid rod prosthesis that produces a permanent erection that can be positioned close to the body for concealment, and an inflatable type that is implanted together with its own reservoir and pump for inflation and deflation. The latter type is designed to mimic normal physiological functioning. Placement of a penile prosthesis in a man who has lost the ability to ejaculate or to have an orgasm as a result of medical causes will not enable him to recover those functions. Men with prosthetic devices have generally reported satisfaction with their subsequent sexual functioning. Their wives, however, report much less satisfaction than do the men. Presurgical counseling is strongly recommended so that the couple has a realistic expectation of what the prosthesis can do for their sex lives. Postsurgical counseling may also be necessary to help the couple adapt to their rediscovered ability to have intercourse. They may experience a high level of anxiety if their sex life had been inactive for a prolonged period before surgery. Prosthetic devices have been associated with severe side effects in some cases, including perforation, infection, urinary retention, and persistent pain.

Some surgeons are attempting revascularization of the penis as a direct approach to treating erectile dysfunction resulting from vascular disorders. In patients with corporal shunts that allow normally entrapped blood to leak from the corporal spaces, leading to inadequate erections (steal phenomenon), such surgical procedures are indicated. There are limited reports of prolonged success with the technique. Endarterectomy can be of benefit if aortoiliac occlusive disease is responsible for erectile dysfunction.

Another medical treatment that is being studied is electrostimulation to the base of the penis. The technique is being tested as a treatment for erectile disorders. Initial reports indicate minimal physical discomfort on the part of patients subjected to the therapy. However, response to treatment is inconsistent, and a problem exists in terms of maintaining erections. At the present time, the treatment seems to have no benefits.

Finally, vacuum pumps can also be used by patients without vascular disease to obtain erections but they are not very satisfactory.

Female procedures Surgical approaches to female dysfunctions include hymenectomy in the case of dyspareunia in an unconsummated marriage, vaginoplasty in multiparous women complaining of lessened vaginal sensations, or freeing of clitoral adhesions in women with inhibited excitement. Such surgical treatments have not been carefully studied and should be considered with great caution.

RESULTS OF TREATMENT The reported effectiveness of various treatment methods for problems of sexual dysfunction varies from study to study. Demonstrating the effectiveness of traditional outpatient psychotherapy is just as difficult when therapy is oriented to sexual problems as it is in general. In some cases the patient improves in all areas except the sexual area. The more severe the psychopathology associated with a problem of long duration, the more adverse the outcome is likely to be.

The more difficult treatment cases involve couples with severe marital discord. Cases involving problems of fear of intimacy, excessive dependency, or excessive hostility are also complex. Other challenges are posed by patients with lack of desire, impulse disorders, unresolved homosexual conflicts, or fetishistic defenses. Patients phobic of sex also present treatment difficulties.

When behavioral approaches are used, empirical criteria that are supposed to predict outcome are more easily isolated. Using those criteria, for instance, it appears that couples who regularly practice assigned exercises have a much greater likelihood of successful outcome than do more resistant couples or couples whose interaction involves sadomasochistic or depressive features or mechanisms of blame and projection. Flexibility of attitude is also a positive prognostic factor. Overall, younger couples tend to complete sex therapy more often than do older couples. Those couples whose interactional difficulties center on their sex problems, such as inhibition, frustration, or fear of performance failure, are also likely to respond well to therapy.

In general, methods that have proved effective singly or in combination include training in behavioral-sexual skills, systematic desensitization, directive marital counseling, traditional psychodynamic approaches, and group therapy. Although treating a couple for sexual dysfunctions is the mode preferred by most workers, treatment of individual persons has also been successful.

Masters and Johnson have reported positive results for their dual-sex therapy approach. They studied the failure rates of their patients (failure is defined as the failure to initiate reversal of the basic symptom of the presenting dysfunction). They compared initial failure rates with five-year follow-up findings for the same couples. Although some have criticized their definition of the percentage of presumed successes, other studies have confirmed the effectiveness of their approach. The use of one therapist, however, seems to be nearly as effective as the male-female therapy team that Masters and Johnson use.

SUGGESTED CROSS-REFERENCES

Homosexuality is discussed in Section 21.1b, paraphilias in Section 21.2, and gender identity disorders in Section 21.3. The neuropsychological and neuropsychiatric aspects of HIV infection are covered in Section 29.2a. Couples therapy is discussed in Section 31.7 and yohimbine and other pharmacological therapies are discussed in Section 32.27. The physical and sexual abuse of children, including incest, is the subject of Section 47.3.

REFERENCES

Araoz D L: Uses of hypnosis in the treatment of psychogenic sexual dysfunctions. Psychiatr Ann *16:* 2, 102, 1986.
Brady J P: Behavior therapy and sex therapy. Am J Psychiatry *133:* 896, 1976.
Chessick R D: Thirty unresolved psychodynamic questions pertaining to feminine psychology. Am J Psychother *42:* 86, 1988.
Diego B L, Magni G: Sexual side effects of anti-depressants. Psychosomatics *24:* 12, 1983.
Ellis A: *Studies in the Psychology of Sex,* 2 vols. Preston House, New York, 1936.
Furlow W L: Prevalence of impotence in the United States. Med Aspects Human Sex: 1985.
Herman J, LoPiccolo J: Clinical outcome of sex therapy. Arch Gen Psychiatry *40:* 443, 1983.

Koren G: Maternal ginseng use associated with neonatal androgenization. JAMA *264:* 2866, 1990.
Kegeles S M, Adler N E, Irwin C E: Sexually active adolescents and condoms: Changes over one year in knowledge, attitudes and use. Am J Publ Health *78:* 460, 1988.
Koppelman M, Parry B L, Hamilton J A, Alogna S W, Loreaux P L: Effect of bromocriptine on affect and libido in hyperprolactinemia. Am J Psychiatry *144:* 1037, 1987.
Krafft-Ebing R: *Psychopathia Sexual* ed. 12, Berlin 1906.
*Laughman E, Gagnon J, Michael R, Michaels S: Sex in America, University of Chicago Press, Chicago, 1994.
Leitenberg H, Detzer M, Srebnik D: Gender differences in masturbation and the relation of masturbation experience in preadolescence and/or early adolescence to sexual behavior and sexual adjustment in young adulthood. Arch Sex Behav 22(2): 87, 1993.
Loosen P T, Purdon S E, Pavlou S N: Effects on behavior of modulation of gonadal function in men with gonadotropin-releasing hormone antagonists. Am J Psychiatry *151:* 271, 1994.
LoPiccolo J, Lobitz W: The role of masturbation in the treatment of sexual dysfunction. Arch Sex Behav *2:* 163, 1972.
*Masters W H, Johnson V E: *Human Sexual Response*. Little, Brown, Boston, 1970.
*Masters W H, Johnson V E: *Human Sexual Inadequacy*. Little, Brown, Boston, 1970.
*Masters W H, Johnson V E, Kolodny R C: *Heterosexuality*. Harper Collins, New York, 1994.
Nunberg G H, Levine P E: Spontaneous remission of MAOI-induced anorgasmia. Am J Psychiatry *144:* 805, 1987.
Offit A K: *The Sexual Self*. Lippincott, Philadelphia, 1977.
Ottesen B: Vasoactive intestinal polypeptide as a neurotransmitter in the female genital tract. Am J Obstet Gynecol *147:* 208, 1983.
*Purnine D M, Carey M P, Jorgensen R S: *Gender differences regarding preferences for specific heterosexual practices*. J Sex Marital Ther *20:* 271, 1994.
Sadock V A: The treatment of psychosexual dysfunctions: An overview. In *Psychiatry 1982. The American Psychiatric Association Annual Review,* L Grinspoon, editor, American Psychiatric Press, Washington, 1982.
Sadock V A: Group psychotherapy of psychosexual dysfunctions. In *Comprehensive Group Psychotherapy*. H I Kaplan, B J Sadock, editors, Williams & Wilkins, Baltimore, 1983.
Segraves R T: Female orgasm and psychiatric drugs. J Sex Educ Ther *11:* 69, 1985.
Semans J H: Premature ejaculation: A new approach. South Med J *49:* 353, 1956.
Shrainer-Engel P, Schiavi R: Lifetime psychopathology in individuals with low sexual desire. J Nerv Ment Dis *174:* 646, 1986.
Small J G, Small I F: Psychosexual dysfunctions. In *Comprehensive Textbook of Psychiatry*. H I Kaplan, A M Freedman, B J Sadock, editors, ed 3, p 1783. Williams & Wilkins, Baltimore, 1980.
Stein D J, Hollander E, Anthony D T, Schneier F R: Serotonergic medications for sexual obsessions, sexual addictions, and paraphilias. J Clin Psychiatry *53:* 267, 1992.
Thase M, Reynolds C, Glanz L, Jennings J R, Sewitz D E, Kupper D J, Frank E: Nocturnal penile tumescence in depressed men. Am J Psychiatry *144:* 89, 1987.
Wise N T: Sexual dysfunctions in the medically ill. Psychosomatics *24:* 9, 1982.
Zorgniotto A W, Lefleur R S: Autoinjection of corpus cavernosium with vasoactive drug combination for vasculogenic impotence. J Urol *133:* 39, 1985.

21.1b HOMOSEXUALITY AND HOMOSEXUAL ACTIVITY

WARREN J. GADPAILLE, M.D.

INTRODUCTION

It is currently politically incorrect to look for or even to imply a cause for homosexuality. The position of gay activist groups and of many psychiatrists is that, if one is homosexual, that is just the way one is; one was simply born that way, and it should occasion no more curiosity or concern than the color of one's hair. However, even the issue of being born that way can lead to politically treacherous areas; for example, adult preferential or obligatory homosexuality is a minority orientation. Could that mean that the atypical genetic components or the fetal biological milieu is somehow disordered, so that the biological explanations still do not escape the possibility of pathology? Even the format of this section in the fifth edition of this textbook—using such headings as epidemiology, etiology, differential diagnosis, and so on—has drawn criticism from both gay and straight colleagues because of its implication of illness.

Political correctness is no more defensible when applied to scientific inquiry and the study of sexual orientation than it was during the generations of its misuse in Soviet psychiatry to subordinate the scientific pursuit of knowledge to political ideology. What is equally indefensible, however, is any effort to pervert an understanding of the cause or causes of homosexuality into a justification for stigmatization, persecution, or discrimination.

All human behavior has causes and reasons, whether the behavior is arbitrarily regarded as normal or abnormal. Homosexuality is best conceptualized as a final common pathway—sexual activity that represents many different sources, some conflict-based, some not conflict-based, and many about which only speculation is yet possible. This section makes no attempt at political correctness; it cannot avoid controversial areas, points of view, or data, and it does not resolve emotionally held conflicting opinions.

DEFINITIONS

The prefix ''homo'' comes from the Greek word for ''same,'' and ''homosexuality'' generically refers to any sexual activity between persons of the same sex. ''Lesbianism'' is frequently used to designate female homosexuality. The words ''gay'' and ''straight'' are the most commonly used terms to mean homosexual and heterosexual, respectively. ''Gay'' can be used for both sexes, but it is most frequently used for male homosexuals. ''Gay'' has also come to imply a particular group of homosexuals—those who are openly and proudly homosexual—and the life-style available to those who ignore and defy stigmatization. The terms ''nongay homosexual'' and ''ego-dystonic homosexual'' are sometimes used for those in conflict or still in the closet and specifically for those who recognize the conflictual basis of their orientation and are not proud of it.

''Homosexuality,'' when used correctly or incorrectly as a diagnostic term, is misleading; it implies a unity of meaning or of sexual activities that is not valid. Homosexual activity occurs in a broad variety of emotional and life circumstances that make the activity conceptually and qualitatively distinct, even though the anatomical and genital behaviors may be identical. Homosexuality and heterosexuality are not always lifelong, mutually exclusive orientations; a large proportion of people have had some of both kinds of experiences at some times in their lives.

The word ''homosexuality'' is used here for the sexual pattern of preferential or exclusive erotic attraction or sexual activity between persons of the same sex, regardless of the availability of willing heterosexual partners. ''Preferential'' is not to be misunderstood as implying a conscious choice between equally psychologically available and sexually arousing options. The preference is consciously known, but the direction of sexual orientation, whether heterosexual or homosexual, is something one simply discovers in oneself; one had no original choice in one's erotic orientation. Terms like ''homosexual activity'' and ''homosexual behavior'' are used for the many other forms of homosexual interaction, which involve a large number of people. "Homosexuality" as defined here commands the greatest social and sometimes clinical interest and is the principal focus of this section. But many of the other forms can also have clinical relevance and are discussed when appropriate.

HOMOSEXUALITY AS A DIAGNOSTIC CATEGORY

The official status of homosexuality as a diagnosis of mental disorder has changed markedly since the 1960s. In the first edition of *Diagnostic and Statistical Manual of Mental Disorders* (DSM-I), published in 1952 by the American Psychiatric Association, homosexuality was listed under the sociopathic personality disturbances as a sexual deviation involving pathological behavior. In the second edition (DSM-II), published in 1968, the category of sociopathic personality disturbances no longer appeared, but homosexuality remained under sexual deviations, and those with the deviations were described as unable to substitute normal sexual behavior for their deviant practices.

In 1973, after a great deal of gay activist agitation and protest and the support of many psychiatrists, the American Psychiatric Association Board of Trustees decided to remove homosexuality as a diagnosis of mental illness. That decision aroused considerable controversy, and the issue was submitted to a vote by the membership, which decided by a 58 percent majority (slightly more than 10,000 voting) to uphold the decision of the board. The issue was not settled for many psychiatrists, however, as shown by a poll conducted by the journal *Medical Aspects of Human Sexuality* in 1977; of the first 2,500 out of 10,000 polled psychiatrists who responded, 69 percent regarded homosexuality as a pathological adaptation, as opposed to a normal variation. The official action remained, however, and in the third edition (DSM-III), published in 1980, homosexuality as a diagnosis no longer appeared. The term "ego-dystonic homosexuality" appeared in the general category of psychosexual disorders. The reasoning was that only in those troubled by their homosexuality did it constitute a psychological disorder. The diagnostic criteria essentially required that the homosexual orientation be a persistent inner concern of the patient; mild dissatisfaction and conflict solely between one's homosexuality and society do not qualify for the diagnosis.

The tenth revision of the World Health Organization's *International Classification of Diseases and Related Health Problems* (ICD-10) lists a category of ego-dystonic sexual orientation under the heading of psychological and behavioral disorders associated with sexual development and orientation. That heading is followed by a note that sexual orientation alone is not to be regarded as a disorder. The ego-dystonic category is defined: The gender identity or sexual preference is not in doubt, but the person wishes it were different because of associated psychological or behavioral disorders, and may seek treatment to change it. However, in the revised third edition and the fourth edition of DSM (DSM-III-R and DSM-IV, respectively), ego-dystonic homosexuality is no longer a diagnostic term. Under sexual disorders not otherwise specified, one of three categories is persistent and marked distress about sexual orientation. No further comments or diagnostic criteria appear, and presumably the condition could include heterosexuals who are distressed with their heterosexuality and persistently wish to be homosexual.

Although the social and humanitarian thrust of the changes is clear, whether the changes reflect an advance in medical-psychiatric science is less clear. Categorizing homosexuality as a unitary sexual state of being is no longer scientifically tenable. The relevance of mental disorders in homosexual interactions is controversial and at least demands major reconceptualization. However, the implication that ego-syntonicity necessarily rules out psychopathology is patently invalid. Delusions and hallucinations are often ego-syntonic, and an entire category of mental disorders, character pathology, is defined in part by the characteristic of ego-syntonicity. Truth cannot be determined by vote, even by supposed authorities. The history of scientific issues that become highly charged emotionally is not distinguished by clear thought and the rational weighing of data.

CROSS-CULTURAL PREVALENCE OF HOMOSEXUALITY AND HOMOSEXUAL ACTIVITY

Homosexual activity of some form occurs in most if not all human cultures. One study of 76 non-Western cultures for which relevant data regarding men were available found that homosexual behavior was disapproved but not necessarily absent in only 36 percent; 64 percent of the cultures regarded homosexual activity as normal and socially acceptable for some members of society. Other studies of other cultures have generally supported that prevalence data, but they question the complete absence of homosexual activity in those cultures that deny its existence. The first study found only 17 non-Western cultures for which data on female homosexual activity existed; although their data are not quantified, the report describes both approving and disapproving cultures.

The most common homosexual interaction cross-culturally is anal intercourse. Homosexual activity ranges from experimental acts between children and adolescents, to enforced periods of homosexual relations for adolescent boys with married men, to a frequent form in which a man adopts the dress and the role of a woman and may marry a heterosexually active man who may have a female wife. Adult preferential or exclusive homosexuality is not the rule in any society for which adequate data are available.

One must be cautious about equating cultural acceptance of certain forms or periods of homosexual behavior with cultural approval of adult homosexuality. Even in ancient Greece and Rome, where nonexclusive homosexual activity in both sexes was widespread and generally tolerated and where homosexuality was extrolled in philosophical writings as the highest form of love, adult preferential homosexuality was also derided and caricatured in literary and historical commentaries. Most cultures have been and are more accepting of all forms of homosexual behavior than is Western culture. But an extensive historical and cross-cultural review indicates that adult homosexuality has universally been regarded as deviant, even in cultures in which accepted institutionalized roles exist for homosexuals.

Judeo-Christian culture was not originally fiercely antihomosexual. Adultery is the only sexual act forbidden by the Ten Commandments. In later pre-Christian times, Jews increasingly condemned homosexuality, both because of its association with pagan worship and because it was believed to be against God's law for a man to expend semen nonprocreatively. Leviticus 20:13 states, "If a man also lie with mankind, as he lieth with a woman, both of them have committed an abomination: they shall surely be put to death; their blood shall be upon them." Emerging Christian doctrine continued the Hebrew trend of increasing hostility toward homosexuality and shaped both secular law and the personal values of most people in Western culture. Homosexuality became a capital offense in some areas. Although legal sanctions against homosexual acts of all kinds have moderated greatly or disappeared throughout Western culture, social attitudes most often remain mildly to intensely negative.

In that social climate, preferential homosexuality exists as a minority but widespread orientation. The first major study of its incidence, by Alfred C. Kinsey in 1948, suggested that 10 percent of men were homosexual; for women, the figure was 5 percent. Kinsey also found that 37 percent of people reported a homosexual experience at some time in their lives, which included adolescent sexual experiences. Since then, numerous surveys have revised these figures significantly downward. A 1988 survey by the United States Census Bureau (sample 50,000 men) concluded that the male prevalence rate for homosexuality was 2 to 3 percent. A 1989 University of Chicago study (sample 1,537 sexually active adults over 18) found less than 1 percent of both sexes were exclusively homosexual; lifetime homosexual experiences for both sexes since age 18 was 4.9 to 5.6 percent. Most recently (1993) the Alan Guttmacher Institute (sample 3,321 men, age 20 to 39) found that 1 percent of men were exclusively homosexual in the previous year, and 2 percent reported any lifetime homosexual experience.

Since sex surveys are considered unreliable generally, there are no accurate data available, but Kinsey's figures are no longer used for national projections of homosexual behavior by government agencies like the Center for Disease Control. Table 21.1b-1 presents the worldwide estimates of homosexual behavior.

POSSIBLE BASES OF HOMOSEXUALITY

BIOLOGICAL FACTORS The following discussion is a simplified but generally valid summary of the sex-specific differentiation of the central nervous system (CNS). Most of the experimental data derive from rodents and, to a smaller extent, from primates.

The evidence indicates that various aspects of sociosexual behavior and possibly of sexual object choice are determined or influenced by the presence or the absence of fetal gonadal androgenic substances during the species-specific critical period for the differentiation of the brain for male or female characteristics. The presence of adequate fetal androgens organizes the CNS, principally portions of the hypothalamus and related structures for, among other things, the mediation of sexual and social behaviors typical of the species males, including sexual object choice and male copulatory behavior. The absence of androgenization results in the organization of somewhat different areas of the same CNS structures to mediate the complementary female behaviors, including the preference for male sex partners and female copulatory behaviors. In experimental deandrogenization of male fetuses and androgenization of female fetuses during their critical periods, cross-sex organization of the CNS occurs. The androgenized genetic females display male sexual and social behaviors and prefer female sexual partners; the deandrogenized males show comparable female patterns. One possible environmental cause of inadequate androgenization of male fetuses is that severe stress to the pregnant female may impair or delay the production of fetal gonadal androgens.

In nonhuman primates, portions of the anterior hypothalamus have been implicated in the generation of male-typical sexual behavior. Microscopic study of the human hypothalamus demonstrated that two specific groups of neurons were significantly larger in men than in women, suggesting that the neurons may be involved in the differentiation between male-typical sexual behavior and female-typical sexual behavior. In a postmortem study of the hypothalamic nuclei in women, men presumed to be heterosexual, and homosexual men, one of the nuclei was found to be more than twice as large in heterosexual men than it was in women and in homosexual men. Since that nucleus is dimorphic for sexual orientation, at least in men, it suggests a biological component in human sexual orientation.

TABLE 21.1b-1
Estimates of Homosexual Behavior (Worldwide)

Country	Sample	Findings
Canada	5,514 first-year college students under age 25.	98.0% heterosexual 1.0% bisexual 1.0% homosexual
Norway	6,155 adults age 18–60	3.5% of men and 3.0% of women reported any lifetime homosexual experience.
France	20,055 adults	Exclusive homosexuality 0.7% men 0.6% women Lifetime homosexual experience 4.1% males 2.6% females
Denmark	3,178 adults age 18–59	Less than 1% exclusive male homosexuality 2.7% lifetime homosexual intercourse
Britain	18,876 adults age 16–59	6.1% of men report any lifetime homosexual experience

Data from *Wall Street Journal* (March 31, 1993) and *New York Times* (April 15, 1993) from research studies on homosexual behavior.

Hormonal studies The extrapolation of the animal data noted above to humans is speculative at best. The evidence for comparable fetal hormonal influences on sex-dimorphic CNS organization rests principally on the occurrence of pathological conditions that to some extent parallel the animal experiments.

Sexual dimorphism in childhood play is remarkably parallel with that in rhesus monkeys. In that species, males and androgenized females threaten more, attempt mounting more often, engage in rough-and-tumble play more often, initiate play more, and withdraw less from threat than do females and deandrogenized males. The naturally occurring difference is best explained by the status of prenatal androgenization because, between 6 months and 3 years of age, no circulating androgens can be detected in rhesus males. The comparable dimorphic patterns of interests and attitudes in human childhood and adulthood are also mediated by the presence or the absence of prenatal androgens. The masculine traits are statistically high in studies of females with hyperadrenocorticism and with progestin-induced hermaphroditism; both conditions are produced by pathological androgenization in fetal development. Women with hyperadrenocorticism become bisexual or homosexual in greater proportions than do the general population. In the androgen-insensitivity syndrome, in which the tissues (including the CNS) of a genetic male are unresponsive to androgens, gender identity and psychosexual development, if not iatrogenically disrupted, are unequivocally female.

The gap between such observations and postulating a hormonal cause for homosexuality is too great to be bridged by current knowledge. Hyperadrenocorticism is a lifelong condition even when treated from birth, and influences other than fetal androgenization cannot be ruled out as playing a role in the high level of lesbianism in women with the condition. Studies that have reported differences in adult sex hormone levels between homosexuals and heterosexuals have not stood the test of replication by different researchers. The one type of experiment that was thought to reflect a difference in fetal CNS organization, a delayed surge of luteinizing hormone after estrogen injection in homosexual men (typical and more pronounced in heterosexual women, absent in heterosexual men) has also not held up uniformly in all studies. In addition, recent research has cast substantial doubt on the premise that the regulation of gonadotropin secretion in primates is in all manifestations determined by prenatal hormonal sex differentiation.

The maternal stress hypothesis is an intriguing one for the neurohormonal causation theory of homosexuality. Little evidence exists regarding what may trigger an atypical fetal hormone status. The studies of possible genetic differences are not conclusive. And differences in severe maternal stress during pregnancy could be one possible explanation for homosexual and heterosexual persons in the same sibship. But there, too, the findings are not uniform across studies; they vary from a highly significant correlation between male homosexuality and serious maternal stress to no correlation at all in differently designed studies.

On the basis of research data, some writers have proposed an essentially biological cause of homosexuality. But if the sole cause of homosexuality were a spontaneously occurring abnormality of critical-period CNS organization, one would expect that similar atypical or pathological hormonal conditions would occur in other mammalian species, resulting in some percentage of naturally occurring adult preferential homosexuality in other species. That is never the case. However, the evidence is cumulatively compelling that the early hormonal milieu probably plays some role, perhaps a variable one, in the development of human heterosexual or homosexual orientation, at least in some persons.

Genetic factors Franz Kallmann's original study of male monozygotic twin pairs (presumably reared together), one of whom was homosexual, found an astounding 100 percent concordance for homosexuality in the other twin. Methodological problems, stated bias, and puzzling familial data (for example, none of the fathers was homosexual) limit the usefulness of those findings. Recent and more carefully designed studies of homosexuality in male twin pairs reared together do not find full concordance but do find higher concordance in monozygotic twins than in dizygotic twins. In the largest study to date (115 male twin pairs and 46 males with adoptive brothers), 52 percent of the monozygotic cotwins, 22 percent of the dizygotic cotwins, and 11 percent of the adoptive brothers were concordant for homosexuality. The same investigators have presented preliminary data for female homosexuality that reveal a similar differential concordance for lesbianism in monozygotic and dizygotic cotwins and in adoptive sisters. Those findings clearly suggest a genetic component in at least some instances of homosexuality and just as clearly indicate that genetic factors do not act alone. Studies of homosexuality in monozygotic twins reared apart from birth, which would carry more weight than studies of monozygotic twins reared together, are few and report on only one or a few pairs. The studies find concordance in some twins and discordance in others; discordance was found in all four reported pairs of monozygotic female twins reared apart. Concordance in even one monozygotic twin pair reared apart, however, is suggestive of some genetic influence. In monozygotic twins reared together the intense and unique bond characteristic of such children could conduce toward homosexual feelings.

A number of recent studies have found a statistically higher prevalence of homosexuality in the brothers of homosexual males and in the sisters of homosexual females than in the general population. One study found that 33 of 40 pairs of homosexual brothers shared a genetic marker on the bottom half of the X chromosome. However, that study requires replication. Familiality of a trait can be related to genetic factors, but it is also amenable to prenatal hormone, biochemical, or rearing influences. The maternal stress hypothesis should result in similar concordance rates in both monozygotic and dizygotic twins. No definitive studies have been conducted yet, but the evidence indicates the likelihood of some genetic factor in the origin of homosexuality in at least some persons.

Evolutionary studies A few authorities have questioned the relevance of mammalian and primate sexual data for the understanding of human sexuality, but that position is difficult to support. It is reasonable to assume that analogous biological conditions and species behaviors are continuous, rather than discontinuous, in evolutionally related species unless proved otherwise. Therefore, evidence of such continuity is relevant to the biological underpinnings of human heterosexual and homosexual behavior, although the mechanisms responsible are not understood. As previously stated, homosexual behavior has been observed in every mammalian species for which it has been studied. As in humans, it is always more common in juveniles than in adults, and in most species it is more common in males than in females. In some primate species, however, homosexual interaction in which sexual arousal appears to be an important component may be more frequent in females than in males. Among adult males, homosexual activity occurs most often among those who are peripheral or subordinate to the group.

Despite the probable ubiquity of some homosexual behavior in other mammalian species, no evidence exists that homosexual interactions among adults in the wild is primarily motivated by or accompanied by sexual arousal, although it may be a secondary factor in bonding. In laboratory populations, anal intromission and ejaculation have been reported for only two species of primates and only when deprived of female partners; no such behavior continues once the males return to a mixed group. Evidence of female orgasm has been reported in only one species of macaque. There are no similar reports regarding any species in natural environments. Adult homosexual behavior is often stimulated in the immediate context of heterosexual excitement among others, but its most frequent context is that of dominance-submission interactions. In both sexes the dominant animal usually assumes the male mounting position. Those interactions help regulate the social hierarchy and the various behaviors and intragroup distinctions inherent in the hierarchy. Evidence of sexual motivation or pleasure is absent.

Various experiments with deprivation rearing of primates (usually rearing in isolation or same-sex rearing) have produced homosexual behavior that appears to have a sexual-arousal component in the partners while they remain isolated. The same-sex pairing does not remain a preference once opposite-sex partners are available, although the capacity for and the incidence of normal heterosexual copulation may remain impaired. Only one instance has been reported of a male pair whose unique same-sex rearing produced a preference for sexual interaction with each other, even in the presence of a female. Even in that pair, there was no evidence of sexual release between the partners, and each could copulate normally with females. No instances of adult preferential or obligatory homosexuality in any social context have been reported for any nonhuman mammalian species in the wild. Adult homosexuality as defined in this section is an exclusively human phenomenon.

FAMILIAL AND SOCIAL FACTORS Until recently, most theories of the causes of homosexuality have focused on a pathogenic family environment. In the best known theory, based on studies of male homosexual psychoanalytic patients, the predominant family pattern is that of a close-binding, seductive mother who devalues and dominates a passive, distant, sometimes hostile father. That constellation encourages defensive identification with the mother and undermines both the father's availability as an acceptable object for identification and the boy's masculinity for fear of losing the mother's love. Although that was the prevalent pattern in the study, the background of some of the patients showed other deleterious patterns. Other researchers have found a comparable pattern in the families of most lesbian patients.

Many studies and replicative attempts have focused on the early family milieus of homosexual persons and have explored the backgrounds of nonpatient samples. In virtually every study the common denominator of an overinvolved mother and a distant or hostile father prevailed in the families of most American homosexual men. The one well-known study from the Kinsey Institute that purported to disprove the existence of a pathogenic family constellation actually demonstrates the classic pattern at statistically significant levels when the published raw data are studied. The researchers apparently based their negative conclusions on statistical manipulations that attempted to turn their retrospective study into one that mimics a prospective study.

Recent advances in behavioral and sexual research have taken a biopsychosocial point of view and have focused broadly on all three kinds of influences—biological, psychological, and social—that are operative at various biologically timed critical or optimal periods that unfold throughout development from fetal life on. That approach looks at interacting influences, rather than unitary causes, although specific causes can and do exist. Throughout gender differentiation and psychosexual development, both continuing and varying influences from all three spheres influence one's ultimate sexual identity and orientation. Prospective and retrospective studies find that gender-disordered children, most of whom become homosexual, come from disturbed families, and the psychodynamics of their sexual conflicts and behaviors can often be clearly correlated with pathogenic parental influences. But even that research cannot address the possible influence of some biologically predisposed effeminate or nonmasculine behavior in some boys, for example, on the responses of the family toward them.

Social learning theories have also been proposed to explain homosexuality. Most of those theories are simplistic and generally discount biological species norms and deny the importance of early childhood experiences and unconscious psychodynamics in the shaping of adult sexuality. The majority of the theories postulate that sexual orientation is learned primarily postpubertally as one experiences the attitudes and mores of one's social milieu; the most important sexually functioning people at that stage of development are more likely to be friends than parents.

The biopsychosocial model also assumes the importance of social influences throughout development. For some homosexual males, the prepubertal years of trying and failing to fit with, to be like, and to be accepted by typical boys and men may play an important part in the psychodynamic genesis of their orientation. But for most homosexual adolescents, their peer social milieu is solidly and even pugnaciously heterosexual, and that milieu rarely helps them learn to be internally heterosexual. The simplistic position of most social learning theories regarding nature versus nurture is not scientifically tenable.

One special case of family and social trauma can apparently act as a determinant to bring about homosexuality, along with much nonsexual pathology: sexual abuse. Although severe abuse is usually a form of family pathology, it can occur outside the family; what the child learns in either social interaction can have the same consequences. Studies of male and female victims of sexual abuse that also inquire into sexual orientation are essentially uniform in finding a higher prevalence of homosexuality in those victims than in the general population.

The general consensus in the voluminous research into family pathogenesis supports the validity of the findings. However, important caveats are as relevant as are the positive correlations. One caveat is that most of the studies are retrospective, and correlations are not necessarily causations.

A second caveat is that a very small percentage of homosexual adults have been studied in the uncovering detail of psychoanalysis, where one can become confident of whatever pathogenic experiences emerge. Even though the studies of nonpatient populations have revealed a consistent pattern of dysfunctional families, the question of whether such parental patterns had the same influence on the vast majority of nonpatient homosexuals remains unanswered.

A third caveat is that many groups of homosexual persons have shared characteristics that vary from group to group, so one cannot expect any one type of influence to have the same power or necessarily even to be a factor in their sexual orientation.

A fourth caveat is that the same parental pathology does not always result in homosexuality. Siblings are not uniformly homosexual, and the same family patterns can be found in the backgrounds of some heterosexual persons with no homosexual siblings. In such families the same pathogenic patterns can and do take their toll in other ways. Of course, some children are treated by their parents differently from their siblings. Research makes it likely that family patterns sometimes strongly influence the sexual orientation of the children, but those forces probably do not act in all cases of homosexuality or do not act alone in most cases where they do exert an influence.

PSYCHODYNAMIC FACTORS Every developmental line follows an innate timetable. The unfolding sequence of developmental stages and the readiness for successive maturational levels is biologically determined and innate to each species. The developmental imperatives exist independently of the child's familial and cultural environment. The infant and child bring that developing intrapsychic self to parent-child interactions; by means of that self, the child responds to, interprets, and integrates experiences. Neither the sequence nor the nature of the developmental potentials is environmentally dependent, but the accomplishment of those potentials is environmentally dependent within the constraints of biological predisposition.

In the gradual organization of sexual identity, of which sexual orientation is but one component, developmental stages contribute different elements to the eventual outcome. In the intimate body contact, nurturing, and caretaking in infancy, infants are programmed to develop the most basic attitudes toward their own and others' bodies. Appropriate parenting of a biologically normal infant results in the firm sense that one's own body is good and pleasureful and that physical closeness to others can be trusted to be good and is worth seeking.

Toddlers become cognitively able to appreciate the difference between the sexes at about the same time they are working to accomplish a sense of separateness and individuality. Part of being separate is being the sex one is. Intrapsychically, the child must integrate the experience of its own particular self and body within its unique parental environment. Optimally, the child comes to feel safe to be separate and good to be the sex and only the sex that it is, with all the implicit but yet unconceptualized qualities and potentials of that specific sex. Out of that, one's core gender identity—the unshakable sense of being male or female—is consolidated by the age of 2 to 2½ years.

In the oedipal period the child forms a sexually tinged attachment to the parent of the opposite sex and develops rivalry with and fear of the same-sex parent. The child's intrapsychic self, regardless of what the parents are like, conjures up fantasies of replacing and destroying the rival and elaborates awesome fears of retaliation—castrative and, therefore, more intense for boys than for girls. Reality—the reality of the parents' qualities and personalities and the child's growing capacity for reality testing—largely determines the resolution of the dilemma. The situation that permits the fullest ultimate achievement of developmental potential is one in which the child identifies with the same-sex parent and relinquishes the wish for sexual possession of the other parent. At the same time, whatever fearful and aggressive fantasies may exist are not so overwhelming that the child cannot in the future desire partners of the opposite sex and be willing to compete with same-sex rivals for them.

One investigator posits that sexual imagery, the basis of future erotic arousal and attachment, differentiates as heterosexual, bisexual, or homosexual during the years between the oedipal period and adolescence and that it is a phase-specific process. For boys, the imagery differentiation occurs in the context of social interactions with male peers and significant men, including the father. Boys who share the same interests, attitudes, and activities of the heterosexual male world around them develop heterosexual erotic imagery. In boys who perceive themselves as unmasculine for any reason, their failure to fit in with and to be accepted by that world influences their erotic imagery to develop in a homosexual or bisexual direction. After puberty that same-sex imagery fuses with the lustful drive and becomes resistant to change.

Such dynamics are related to those involved in what researchers have called *pseudohomosexuality*. It has been described chiefly in men, but the complementary dynamics may exist in women. The conflicts center on power and dependence, associated respectively with masculinity and femininity. Adolescent and adult men who perceive themselves as weak, submissive, or inadequate compared with other men may unconsciously make the equation "I am nonmasculine=I am feminine=I am homosexual." Those men tend to conceptualize themselves as homosexual in a pejorative sense, rather than to feel strong erotic attraction to other men. That self-perception is most often associated with fear and self-loathing and can escalate into homosexual panic with violence or suicidality. Others, however, act out a passive homosexual role, and their homosexuality may develop an erotic component.

In each of the developmental phases, there is the potential for innumerable resolutions and outcomes, from the most optimal to the most crippling. They all play a role in the ultimate sexual identity, and all exert some degree of influence on sexual orientation.

AN INTEGRATION The attempt to understand the roots of sexual orientation is all-encompassing; it does not focus on homosexuality while assuming that heterosexuality needs no explanation. Biology, family-cultural environment, and intrapsychic psychodynamics are together and variably determinant of all aspects of life, not only of sexual orientation. With respect to homosexuality, no one influence acts necessarily or usually alone or in an invariable way. Biological predisposition may help determine a person's vulnerability or resistance to parental influences. It may play a role in the relative potency of intrapsychic conflict versus environmental reality. The power of parental influences may override predisposition to either heterosexuality or homosexuality. The positive or negative qualities in a preadolescent boy's same-sex peer and adult relationships may overcome an unmasculine self-concept or be a further influence toward a homosexual orientation. It is incontrovertible among mammalian species that species-typical biology and rearing conditions result in adult preferential heterosexuality. With that perspective, adult preferential homosexuality represents an adaptation—often unchallengeably successful—to differentiation and developmental conditions of any nature that render species-typical heterosexuality unavailable or unacceptable.

THE QUESTION OF PSYCHOPATHOLOGY

This issue is controversial and emotionally charged, but the forms that the controversies take often miss the point and create confusion. The questions usually focus on whether homosexuality is by definition psychopathological and whether homosexuality is, therefore, sick and heterosexuality is healthy. It should be obvious that heterosexuality conveys no special protection against psychopathology.

At any point along any developmental line, biological, interpersonal, or intrapsychic conditions may impair progress toward or achievement of phase-specific developmental potential. Symptoms and character pathology represent the defensive and adaptive or maladaptive compromises that the developing person had to make under those circumstances. That principle holds for all people. Sexual identity is one group of the many developmental lines.

All families and all environments are fallible and distortive to some degree. The fact that the families of most homosexual persons have a common dysfunctional pattern does not indicate that such families are any more or less pathogenic than are the families of most heterosexuals. Heterosexual persons are as likely as homosexual persons to have encountered impediments to optimal development in various areas and to have made symptomatic compromises. The only difference by definition between homosexual and heterosexual persons is that the species norm of adult preference for opposite-sex erotic partners is not one of the potentials impaired by compromise formation in heterosexuals, whereas it is in homosexuals.

A proportion of children may be biologically so strongly predisposed toward homosexuality that no postnatal influences are necessary for the development of that orientation, nor could they modify that developmental direction. In such instances homosexuality and the achievement of psychological health in a generally hostile social milieu represent adaptive triumphs. Whether those species-atypical biological determinants reflect pathology in any or all instances remains unknown because, even if a biologically determined subgroup exists, investigators have no knowledge yet about the mechanisms of the biological influences.

An overall assessment of psychological health and maturity considers total function. Although homosexuality can be a symptom of pathogenic influences or conflicts, it is not per se indicative of psychiatric illness. Studies using psychological testing of nonpatient homosexual and heterosexual samples are consistent in finding no differences in psychiatric health or illness between the two groups.

The relative degree of psychopathology in homosexuals and heterosexuals was a major focus in one study. The investigators found that male homosexuals were less well-adjusted intrapsychically, interpersonally, and socially along a number of dimensions than were the heterosexual controls. Lesbians were closer than the men in psychological adjustment measures to heterosexuals but were still less well-adjusted than heterosexual women along some of the same dimensions.

The researchers were clearly cognizant, however, of the nonhomogeneity of their homosexual sample. They devised a typology into which about 70 percent of the homosexual sample could be subdivided: The "coupled" lived in quasi marriage with one partner. Of their total sample of 686 men, the "close-coupled" (9.8 percent) desired monogamy and closeness. The "open-coupled" (17.5 percent) regarded a regular partner important for sex and affection but agreed to outside sexual encounters, despite considerable jealousy. The "functionals" (14.9 percent) had a high level of sexual activity, with more partners than the other groups; had little regret about their homosexuality; and had few sexual problems. The "dysfunctionals" (12.5 percent) had more sexual problems and more regret about their homosexuality than did the other groups. The "asexuals" (16 percent) had many sexual problems, little sexual interest or activity, and few partners. A similar percentage of the lesbians studied were also classifiable, but, compared with the men, the lesbians had about three times as many close-coupled and far fewer functionals, dysfunctionals, and asexuals.

Rating the categories separately, the investigators found pathology in the male homosexuals to be most concentrated in the dysfunctionals and asexuals; the remaining three groups were closer in psychological variables to the controls; in all groups, however, a greater degree of pathology was reported by the homosexuals than by heterosexuals. Among the lesbians the pathology was concentrated in the open-coupled, dysfunctionals, and asexuals; the pathology in the remaining two groups was roughly the same as in the heterosexual women.

The problems with the study are serious enough to negate the usefulness of any of the findings. There is obvious merit in recognizing the crucial differences between different psychologically functioning types of homosexuals. However, the researchers did not divide the heterosexual sample into comparable groups; each homosexual group was compared with the total heterosexual sample. Had parallel groups been compared, the differences might have been more comparable in each group. The results would certainly have been different and would have better contributed to the understanding of similarities and differences.

A more profound failing was that no data were provided for the 30 percent of the homosexual sample who did not fit into the typology. In all comparisons, 70 percent of one sample were compared with 100 percent of the other sample. That renders any statistical findings meaningless; one has no idea of the psychological and psychopathological variables in the missing 30 percent or what effects they had on any valid homosexual-heterosexual comparisons.

If it is reasonable not to anticipate significant, consistently greater psychopathology in homosexuals than in heterosexuals, the data require explanation. Perhaps the differences are secondary to social disapproval and stigmatization. Homosexuals typically learn a pathogenic self-concept in this culture. Those who believe that homosexuality is biologically innate postulate that the familial interactions are reversed: the child's built-in atypicality produces parental discord and rejection, rather than being caused by it. However, the one study that compared homosexual men in discriminatory and nondiscriminatory societies found more psychological problems in homosexuals than in heterosexuals in both milieus and failed to find that nondiscrimination made a significant difference.

In contrast with psychological test data, anamnestic studies are relatively consistent in finding a greater prevalence of psychopathology in preferential homosexual persons compared with heterosexual persons, the discrepancy being greater for males than for females. Whether the differences are inherent in homosexuality or secondary to familial-social pressures is an issue for which definitive data do not yet exist.

HOMOSEXUALITY AS A SYMPTOM OF PATHOGENESIS

Pathogenesis is relevant to homosexuality as an orientation in one specific, limited way: what influences kept species-typical heterosexuality from developing, and what influences helped determine the homosexual compromise? In whatever proportion biological predisposition plays the determining role, little or no conflict basis may be found. In other instances, nonbiological influences can be found in persons who allow themselves to be studied in depth.

With reference to patients in psychoanalysis, the range of pathology in the developmental line of sexual orientation is broad and can vary from minor to severe. The earlier the pathogenesis, the more primitive are the defenses and compromises, and the more global are the consequences. The compromises show up in many other aspects of a person's overall psychiatric status and may or may not be relevant to the homosexuality. Indeed, a strongly homosexually predisposed child could be born into a severely pathogenic family environment, and its homosexuality might exist independently of massive conflict-based or deficit-based psychopathology.

Patients who fail to establish basic bodily trust are crippled in their capacity for intimacy with anyone, man or woman, whether they are heterosexual or homosexual. Closeness engenders fear of annihilation, and sexuality, if the person is active at all, is often chaotic because orientation and even core gender identity are not firmly fixed.

Deficits at the level of separation-individuation leave men unconsciously terrified of engulfment by women; they are revolted by the prospect of a female sex partner. Internalized part objects remain unfused, and relationships with other men are primitive and infantile, often focusing on only a body part, the genitals or the anus, never the whole person. Women are not as avoidant of symbiosis with a mother figure because that symbiosis does not threaten their gender identity, but the fantasies and the needs acted out in the relationship are equally primitive.

Oedipal pathogenesis can leave much or most of ego development less compromised and the constrictions far less crippling than early pathogenesis. Sexual object choice is determined by castration anxiety in boys, who relinquish sexual relations with women to the fathers (heterosexual, dangerous men), although they can retain nonerotic closeness with women, and they eroticize their interactions with men. In oedipally damaged women, the conviction of genital inferiority fuels the sexual avoidance of men and the erotized turn toward women (the mother) with the fantasy of eventual genital restoration. Nonsexual relations with men can often be untroubled.

If an important origin of homosexuality occurs as a result of the differentiation of same-sex erotic imagery in feminine or nonmasculine boys during latency and prepuberty, there may be little developmental compromise other than in sexual orientation. The nonmasculinity itself may reflect a biological bent or may be conflict-based or deficit-based in a pathogenic family.

Heterosexual persons can and do suffer impaired development at all levels, and the impairments can and do lead to symptomatic compromises in areas of sexuality other than orientation, to say nothing of other nonsexual areas of psychological function. The various forms of sexual pathology are by no means preferable simply because the object choice remains heterosexual. Sexual pathology includes all forms of heterosexual paraphilia; heterosexual rape; and all the less dramatic, neurotically and characterologically guilt-ridden, unfulfilling, and destructive interactions between heterosexual partners.

In homosexual persons in analysis, the psychodynamic pathology can become apparent whether or not the sexual orientation is initially regarded as ego-dystonic.

A 25-year-old professional woman entered therapy because of increasing personality disorganization and deteriorating function in most areas of life. She spent much time withdrawn into solitary camping trips, sleeping in her car, and sitting in trees. Psychological testing indicated schizophrenia, but in retrospect she was functioning at a primitive level of borderline personality organization. She was technically bisexual, married to a man who had erectile dysfunction and little sexual interest and with whom coitus occurred rarely. However, she had a history of preferring homosexual play since early childhood. When therapy began, she had had an intense sexual and emotional involvement for more than a year with a woman about 20 years her senior, with whom she felt fully sexually fulfilled. Her lesbianism was not seen as a problem; rather, it was fully ego-syntonic and was her main source of joy and self-affirmation.

The patient was obese and sloppily butch. Her behavior during the early periods of therapy was often infantile to the extent of curling up or sitting on the floor and communicating only through drawings. She was the only child of an emotionally unavailable father and a controlling, intrusive mother with whom she recalled an eroticized relationship. She had a large, mostly female, overclose extended family.

Partly because she did not question her homosexuality and partly because of her overriding disintegration, therapy did not focus on her sexuality until she had begun to mobilize her considerable but unavailable ego strength and was able to withstand psychoanalysis. She began to discover that she had chosen a lover with a character pathology markedly similar to that of her mother and that her relationship with her lover was a fantasied reliving of a masochistic symbiosis with her mother. She hoped to gain her mother's love by giving her sexual pleasure; her own pleasure was intense but motivationally secondary to her infantile needs.

Through a turbulent, complex, and lengthy analysis, she resolved her infantile dependence and was able to progress to and resolve the oedipal issues. She divorced her husband, made her delayed adolescent sexual explorations, and entered into a loving, stable, and heterosexually fulfilling marriage, meanwhile functioning as a successful professional woman. Follow-up after more than 20 years found the marriage and all areas of function stable and rewarding.

It may never be possible to determine to everyone's satisfaction whether the various kinds of pathology evident in adequately studied patients can be extrapolated to that vast majority of homosexual people who never become patients. No one is immune to the causal influences that are part of the human condition and that determine health or illness and more or less achievement of potential. Developmental influences, good and bad, leave their fingerprints on people's lives as signs that can often be seen by any observer. But similar causes for similar signs can generally be only inferred; medicine has a long history of inferring the wrong causal relationships on seemingly logical bases.

One generalization that helps define virtually all preferential homosexuals is that they did not identify with the sexual orientation of their same-sex parent. Except in possible instances of biological predisposition, that pattern reflects conflict with and hostility toward that parent, which tends to extend to others of the same sex. Studies of nonpatient homosexual men find that hostility toward other men is characteristic. If such built-in hostility contaminates male-male relationships, it could help explain the great difficulty homosexual men have in forging long-term, committed, monogamous relationships. That hypothesis, however, leaves unexplained the fact that lesbians are much more successful than are male homosexuals in forming relationships, despite the same failure in identification. Perhaps one explanation is that lesbians are able to retain their early, deep, pregenital identifications with their mothers; little boys do not usually have that kind of identification with their fathers to retain.

CASUAL MULTIPARTNER SEX Casual sex with a multitude of strangers is considered symptomatic of pathology, as much in heterosexuals as in homosexuals, at least in this culture. To what extent that is a culture-bound definition of pathology is not clear. In some cultures, sexual partners are normally expected to be unlimited for the unmarried. Those cultures known to the author involve small population groups in which no partners are or remain strangers in the sense used here. In this culture, such casual sexual encounters with strangers is an expression of narcissistic, impersonal, often compulsively driven genital-oriented sex, rather than person-oriented sex, and of impaired capacity for intimacy and commitment.

Available studies find that pattern more typical of homosexuals, especially men, than of heterosexuals, although it is by no means limited to them. The biological constraints of pregnancy, the social constraints of marriage and children, and the lack of social support for open homosexuality and homosexual pairing may explain the lower incidence of that pattern of promiscuity in heterosexual persons. The pattern and the psychopathology are not unusual among straights who make a life-style of going to singles bars. In a study of the ultimate anonymity of public rest room sex, where the partner is not even seen, 38 percent of the recipients (not the providers) of sexual release, usually fellatio, were heterosexual men. At present, the data are insufficient to explain the greater incidence of pathological promiscuity among homosexuals or to support or refute the sociological hypotheses for it.

ATTITUDE OF THE UNITED STATES MILITARY SERVICES The current Pentagon policy toward homosexual persons in the military continues to regard homosexual acts as crimes of sufficient magnitude to warrant separation of the offender from service. While the wording of the policy does not refer to psychopathology or mental illness, the implication is clear that homosexuality is grossly deviant from the norm, and its overt expression is damaging to military effectiveness and to the well-being of heterosexual members of the services. The full text of the recent policy appears in Table 21.1b-2.

VARIETIES OF HOMOSEXUALITY

ADULT PREFERENTIAL HOMOSEXUALITY Homosexual persons express the same variety of erotic and sensual behaviors as do heterosexual persons—kissing, caressing, mutual masturbation, mouth-genital stimulation, and anal intercourse. Only the lack of complementary genitalia limits their activities; anal intercourse is much more common among male homosexuals than among heterosexual couples, and some uncommon homosexual practices, such as inserting one's fist in the partner's anus, are essentially absent in heterosexuals. The imitation of heterosexual intercourse by lesbians through the use of dildos is rare in this culture. Anal intercourse is imitative of coitus, but it may be enforced by anatomical limitations as often as it is expressive of male-female roles and of dominance-submission interactions. Homosexual persons, like heterosexual persons, have individual preferences for some practices over others, and some prefer or limit themselves to the active or the passive, the inserter or the insertee role. Most switch roles at least part of the time, and many express little preference.

Homosexual persons have no characteristic self-presentation. Probably no more than 20 percent are markedly or exaggeratedly effeminate among the men or hypermasculine and butch among the women. Both men and women are found in every professional and occupational field, even those most sterotypically heterosexual (for example, professional athletes, truck drivers, nurses, and models).

Relationship patterns are as varied among homosexuals as among heterosexuals. Homosexual relationships are not impoverished in their quality of interaction. William Masters and Virginia Johnson studied committed and functional homosexual and heterosexual couples and found that the homosexual couples were more egalitarian, communicated more freely about their sexual feelings and sensations, spent more time in total body sensuality and foreplay, and were more sensitive to the partners' needs and responses than were the heterosexual couples.

Even among those who are preferentially or exclusively homosexual at any given time, experience with heterosexual intercourse at some time in life is the rule, rather than the exception. Studies of homosexuals have found that from 33 to more than 65 percent of the men and 60 to 85 percent of the women experienced coitus, and a significant minority continued to have some degree of heterosexual activity. Many had been married, and 50 to 75 percent of those had children.

Homosexuals, in this culture at least, differ most from heterosexuals and male and female homosexuals differ most from each other in the number and the nature of their sexual partnerships. One study found that 72 percent of the male homosexuals reported more than 100 sexual partners, 41 percent reported more than 500 partners, and 27 percent reported more than 1,000 partners; 74 percent stated that more than half their partners were strangers, and 65 percent had sex only once with more than half of their partners. In contrast, only 8 percent of lesbians reported 50 or more partners, and only 6 percent stated that more than half of their partners were strangers. Comparative partnership data for their heterosexual controls were not provided. Another study compared homosexuals with heterosexuals in the number of partners, finding that homosexuals of both sexes change partners more frequently than do heterosexuals and that the difference is greatest between homosexual and heterosexual men. Parallel with that degree of activity, about 66 percent of the men but less than 1 percent of the women had had venereal disease at least once. Recent concern about acquired immune deficiency syndrome (AIDS) is reported to have cut down the number of indiscriminate liaisons, but no research data have yet shown that reduction.

OTHER VARIETIES OF HOMOSEXUAL BEHAVIOR Although adult preferential or exclusive homosexuality is the chief focus of both lay and scientific interest, it is not the only variety with potential clinical relevance, nor does it account for the majority of people involved in homosexual behavior. Along with pseudohomosexuality, the following types may require clinical recognition and attention.

Developmental behavior Homoerotic activity can occur in both boys and girls at any immature stage of development. It is usually part of normal development and is not prognostic of adult homosexuality. Alfred Kinsey found that it was more common than heteroerotic play in girls up to age 13 and in boys up to age 15 and that 33 percent of women and 50 percent of men reported such play by age 15. It is rarely a problem for the youngsters involved unless it is made so by their parents or other adults, who are usually deeply concerned that it may indi-

TABLE 21.1b-2
Text of Pentagon's New Policy Guidelines on Homosexuals in the Military*

Accession Policy
Applicants for military service will no longer be asked or required to reveal if they are homosexual or bisexual, but applicants will be informed of the conduct that is prescribed for members of the armed forces, including homosexual conduct.

Discharge Policy
Sexual orientation will not be a bar to service unless manifested by homosexual conduct. The military will discharge members who engage in homosexual conduct, which is defined as a homosexual act, a statement that the member is homosexual or bisexual, or a marriage or attempted marriage to someone of the same gender.

Investigations Policy
No investigations or inquiries will be conducted solely to determine a service member's sexual orientation. Commanders will initiate inquiries or investigations when there is credible information that a basis for discharge or disciplinary action exists. Sexual orientation, absent credible information that a crime has been committed, will not be the subject of a criminal investigation. An allegation or statement by another that a service member is a homosexual, alone, is not grounds for either a criminal investigation or a commander's inquiry.

Activities
Bodily contact between service members of the same sex that a reasonable person would understand to demonstrate a propensity or intent to engage in homosexual acts (e.g., handholding or kissing in most circumstances) will be sufficient to initiate separation.

Activities such as association with known homosexuals, presence at a gay bar, possessing or reading homosexual publications or marching in a gay rights rally in civilian clothes will not, in and of themselves, constitute credible information that would provide a basis for initiating an investigation or serve as the basis for an administrative-discharge under this policy. The listing by a service member of someone of the same gender as the person to be contacted in case of an emergency, as an insurance beneficiary, or in a similar context, does not provide a basis for separation or further investigations.

Speech within the context of priest-penitent, husband-wife or attorney-client communications remains privileged.

Off-Base Conduct
No distinction will be made between off-base and on-base conduct.

From the time a member joins the service until discharge, the service member's duty and commitment to the unit is a 24-hour-a-day, seven-day-a-week obligation. Military members are required to comply with both the Uniform Code of Military Justice, which is Federal law, and military regulations at all times and in all places. Unacceptable conduct, homosexual or heterosexual, is not excused because the service member is not "at work."

Investigations and Inquiries
Neither investigations nor inquiries will be conducted solely to determine an individual's sexual orientation.

Commanders can initiate investigations into alleged homosexual conduct when there is credible information of homosexual acts, prohibited statements, or homosexual marriage.

Commanders will exercise sound discretion regarding when credible information exists, and will evaluate the information's source and all attendant circumstances to assess whether the information supports a reasonable belief that a service member has engaged in proscribed homosexual conduct. Commanders, not investigators, determine when sufficient credible information exists to justify a detail of investigative resources to look into allegations.

Credible Information
Credible information of homosexual conduct exists when the information, considered in light of its source and all attendant circumstances, supports a reasonable belief that a service member has engaged in such conduct. It requires a determination based on articulable facts, not just a belief or suspicion.

Security Clearances
Questions pertaining to an individual's sexual orientation are not asked on personnel security questionnaires. An individual's sexual conduct, whether homosexual or heterosexual, is a legitimate security concern only if it could make an individual susceptible to exploitation or coercion, or indicate a lack of trustworthiness, reliability, or good judgment that is required of anyone with access to classified information.

The Threat of Extortion
As long as service members continue to be separated from military service for engaging in homosexual conduct, credible information of such behavior can be a basis for extortion. Although the military cannot eliminate the potential for the victimization of homosexuals through blackmail, the policy reduces the risk to homosexuals by making certain categories of information largely immaterial to the military's initiation of investigations.

Only credible information that a service member engaged in homosexual conduct will form the basis for initiating an inquiry or investigation of a service member; suspicion of an individual's sexual orientation is not a basis, by itself, for official inquiry or action.

Extortion is a criminal offense, under both the O.C.M.S. and United States Code, and offenders will be prosecuted. A service member convicted of extortion risks dishonorable discharge and up to three years confinement. Civilians found guilty of blackmail under the U.S. Code may be subject to a $2,000 fine and one year imprisonment. The risk of blackmail will be addressed by educating all service members on the policy and by emphasizing the significant criminal sanctions facing convicted extortionists.

Outing
A mere allegation or statement by another that a service member is a homosexual is not grounds for official action. Commanders will not take official action against members based on rumor, suspicion or capricious allegations.

However, if a third party provides credible information that a member has committed a crime or act that warrants discharge, e.g., engages in homosexual conduct, the commander may, based on the totality of the circumstances, conduct an investigation or inquiry, and take non-judicial or administrative action or recommend judicial action, as appropriate.

Commanders are responsible for initiating an investigation when credible information exists that a crime or basis for discharge has been committed. The commander examines the information and decides whether an investigation by the service investigative agency or a commander inquiry is warranted, or if no action should be taken.

Harassment
Commanders are responsible for maintaining good order and discipline.

All service members will be treated with dignity and respect. Hostile treatment or violence against a service member based on a perception of his or her sexual orientation will not be tolerated.

*While a Federal appeals court in November, 1993 would not consider the constitutionality of the policy, the court did say that the equal protection guarantee of the Fifth Amendment did not permit members of the military to be removed merely because they said they were homosexual. Table from the U S Department of Defense.

cate future homosexuality. In most instances a knowledgeable clinician can reassure both the adults and the children, but a minority of the children do progress to homosexuality.

Situational homosexual activity The absence of opposite-sex partners in some environments—such as unisex boarding schools, prisons, and some armed services stations— induces some preferential heterosexuals to turn to same-sex partners until they return to normal environments. Some have regarded it as a healthy adaptation; for mutually consenting persons it is usually not harmful. However, for people who are unaware of deep insecurities about their sexual identities or who possess powerful moral taboos, tremendous turmoil and emotional conflict may ensue.

Exploitative and enforced homosexual behavior As in heterosexual rape, the penis can be used as a weapon and as an assertion of dominance and power against other men. Homosexual rape is frequent in prison populations but is not limited to places where violence is endemic; those with the power to intimidate often coerce the weak and fearful into being recipient sexual partners, usually in anal intercourse and sometimes in fellatio. Sexual release is not the main emotional goal. Sexual exploitation is also common in women's prisons. The exploit-ers, particularly the men, do not consider themselves homosexual. As in some cultures and subcultural groups where there is a sharp dichotomy between inserter (male) and insertee (female) roles, the inserter does not lose status and is not regarded as homosexual within the group. The clinical import of the behavior bears almost exclusively on the exploited, although none question the severe character pathology of the exploiter. The trauma to an exploited partner's sexual and social self-concept can be shattering. Coerced homosexual compliance causes a true psychiatric emergency, often in settings where it cannot be properly addressed. Such experiences usually do not result in subsequent homosexuality, but in some cases the victims became homosexual, even though they had no prior awareness of homosexual feelings.

Bisexuality and ambisexuality Homosexuals usually also have heterosexual experiences. Those who have some degree of ongoing coital experience are often regarded as bisexual, but close attention to their erotic fantasies and differential arousal responses generally reveals that their erotic preference is homosexual. True *ambisexuality*—equal arousal and pleasure with partners of either sex—has been described, but it is apparently rare. Its clinical significance is rarely psychiatric; rather, it is medical for the men in terms of exposure to conditions that are common in homosexual populations. For example, venereal disease and hepatic carcinoma caused by hepatitis B are more common in homosexual men then in heterosexual men; pharyngeal and rectal syphilitic chancres may be unrecognized or not checked for during examinations of heterosexually functioning men whose bisexuality is not known; and anal receptive intercourse greatly heightens the risk of AIDS virus transmission to either sex. As long as AIDS is more common in homosexual men then in heterosexual men, both male and female partners of bisexual men are at high risk.

Ideological homosexuality Occurring principally among militant feminists, ideological homosexuality constitutes an angry repudiation of any need for men; it is, at times, an effort to deny innate masculine-feminine differences or complementarity. Sexual conflicts may masquerade as ideology; however, by definition, psychopathology is denied by those persons. Nonetheless, reports are appearing in the literature of such women seeking psychotherapy as they discover that conscious efforts to manipulate their sexual orientation do not solve their sexual relationship problems and may do violence to their basic sexual identities. It is a form of pseudohomosexuality in women.

DIFFERENTIATION FOR PURPOSES OF CLINICAL RELEVANCE

Adult preferential or obligatory homosexuals are distinguished simply by the conscious awareness of greater or exclusive sexual arousal by persons of the same sex. They need not be sexually active; persons of either homosexual or heterosexual orientation may be sexually inactive yet be clearly aware of their arousal patterns. In preferential or obligatory homosexuality, the sexual motivation is primarily erotic, genital, and affectional; regardless of its causes, the homosexual arousal is not secondary to some other motivation, and it is not sexual behavior used transparently in the service of some nonsexual goal.

Homosexuality may occur in the context of or even secondary to a major psychiatric illness, such as schizophrenia or bipolar disorder, in which the primary condition takes precedence and the sexual activity may never emerge as a treatment issue. Homosexuals who cross-dress must be differentiated from fetishistic *transvestites* (typically heterosexual men who are sexually aroused by donning female clothing) and *transsexuals* (persons who believe that they are members of the opposite sex who are trapped in the wrong bodies).

The primacy of homoerotic arousal allows its differentiation from other expressions of homosexual behavior with the possible exception of ambisexuality. In *pseudohomosexuality* the primary conflicts concern power and dependence. Although the patient may have homosexual dreams or fantasies, they typically involve not positively perceived erotic excitement and eagerness but, rather, issues of dominance and submission. The same is true if homosexual behavior occurs. In *situational homosexuality,* orgasmic pleasure and sexual release occur, but the participants are in no doubt about the substitutive nature of the same-sex activity. The motives of power, domination, and humiliation are primary in *exploitative homosexual activity;* motivationally, sexual release is secondary. Powerful, vicious, and violent homosexuals can (for example, in a prison setting) also use their sexuality for the same nonsexual purposes. For that small minority, positive erotic drive is also subordinate, as in heterosexual rape, although the sexual release achieved may be pleasureful if the partner happens to be of the preferred sex. In *ideological homosexuality* the choice of partner is reactive, rationalized, consciously defensive, and defiant. Except in those who have not yet recognized or accepted their lesbianism, the motivation is not primarily and spontaneously erotic, although, after the fact, the erotic superiority is often strongly proclaimed.

CHILDHOOD PREHOMOSEXUALITY Special problems are present in the differentiation of childhood prehomosexuality from developmental homosexual activity. In the case of highly effeminate boys (characterized by occasional to frequent cross-dressing; persistent preferences for girls' toys and activities, girl playmates, and the company of female adults; fear of physical injury and the avoidance of body-contact sports and other rough play with boys; feminine identification in family role play; and expressed cross-gender wishes), follow-up studies in the aggregate show that the majority, but not 100 percent, become homosexual, bisexual, or transsexual. Inquiries into the families of the boys reveal a pattern of pathogenic influences on sexual identity development. Not as much is known about equally masculine girls. Their pattern seems to be a mirror image of the effeminate boys, and they are more likely than feminine-identified girls to become lesbian or transsexual. However, tomboyism per se is not as prognostic of lesbianism as effeminacy in boys is of male homosexuality.

Most often, the youthful behavior that a physician is asked to evaluate is not so blatant as that just described. Most often, the parents are concerned, although the youngsters may become concerned, too. Often, the youngster is not clearly conscious of a preference for the pleasure derived from sex play with same-sex or opposite-sex partners, although that situation changes in early adolescence. The expression of a strong erotic homosexual preference by an adolescent is usually predictive of adult homosexuality. The homoerotic behaviors can be identical, whether prehomosexual or not. Mutual masturbation is the most common activity for both sexes, although fellatio, cunnilingus, and anal intercourse may occur in purely developmental play. Preoccupation with one of the less common behaviors may be prehomosexual, but it is not a reliable criterion. An older youngster who is involved in homosexual activity and who has a history of persistent cross-gender behavior in early childhood is likely to be prehomosexual. Purely developmental activity typically occurs between age peers; the child who is willingly erotically involved with a same-sex adult and the child who is erotically in love with someone of the same sex is possibly prehomosexual. Predominantly homosexual masturbatory fantasies are strongly predictive of homosexual development.

INTERNAL DISTRESS In patients who present with dysphoria over their homosexuality, the source of that distress must be explored. Often, the distress is external; a court, a spouse, parents, or others may be pressuring the patient. Such pressure may be strong enough to cause deep conflict and make the patient question or regret the homosexual orientation. Unless the dysphoria is truly internal, however, wishes or therapy for shifting orientation are likely to be neither effective nor appropriate. But such patients may need therapy, for example, to deal with the pressure or to learn how to curb illegal or criminal behavior, as in homosexual pedophilia.

Internal distress cannot be taken at face value. Growing up in a homosexually negative family or social milieu can produce guilt and self-derogation in someone who otherwise would not be motivated to change. The distinction between a genuine wish to be heterosexual and a reactive shame over homosexuality can be difficult to make. Contrary to the position of many gay activist spokesmen, some homosexuals of both sexes genuinely wish to be heterosexual and can accomplish the shift. The realities of life in a heterosexual world and the facts of relinquished reproductive and procreative potential are not always false pressures toward heterosexuality. The inner conviction of having experienced distorting developmental influences and of the constrictions of consequent compromise formations are valid awarenesses in those who have them. Whether to try to form a working alliance to accept homosexuality or to shift to heterosexuality depends on the evaluation of the nature and the sources of the ego-dystonicity. Because the distinctions may be unclear, the direction of therapy may, in fact, depend on the prognosis for or against change.

ISSUES OF THERAPY

The majority of homosexuals who deserve the attention of psychiatrists do not come into treatment because of a wish or a need to change their sexual orientation. Either their psychopathology is not dynamically related to their orientation, or it is due to the familial and social conflicts engendered by their homosexuality in a society that devalues and persecutes them. In the former case, therapy is essentially whatever is indicated for any patient with a similar pathology. In the latter case the goals involve undoing the self-devaluation and its effects on the patients' function and achieving an acceptance of and pleasure in their homosexuality.

Some homosexual psychiatrists and other mental health professionals are so militant against any implication of illness in homosexuality that they refuse to honor homosexuals' requests for therapy aiming at change and refuse to refer homosexuals to anyone who would undertake such a therapeutic effort. Their position is that no gay person would wish to change, were society not so repressive and punitive. They even place possibly prehomosexual children and adolescents in groups aimed at making homosexual development easier and more acceptable for the youngsters, with no effort to differentiate those for whom their orientation is conflict-based or deficit-based.

The author believes that such a stance is unethical—indeed, a form of malpractice—and equivalent to trying to force a change of orientation on those who do not wish it. Some gay patients yearn to be straight and may be able to make the change; their wishes must be respected. Furthermore, prehomosexual indicators may show up in childhood, when therapy may be genuinely preventive. Enlightened people know that homosexuality is neither bad nor evil, but they also know that it confers few benefits and many disadvantages in this culture. A majority of adult homosexuals, when polled on this issue, stated that they would prefer any children of their own not be homosexual, because of the problems encountered.

CHILDHOOD PREHOMOSEXUALITY Although it is unwise to try to convince adults to enter therapy, it is appropriate to urge therapy for prehomosexual children. Children cannot cognitively appreciate the future consequences of sexual orientation and cannot give, in effect, informed consent to a developmental direction that could eventuate in homosexuality. Ideally, therapy should involve the family, as well as the child, to try to modify the influences that may be impairing heterosexual development. Special attention should be given to nonmasculine boys, even when their overt function may not be seriously disturbed, on the principle of preventing unnecessary social disadvantages for several reasons. One reason is that many perfectly functional heterosexual males do not fit a simplistic masculine stereotype. Such boys may be helped to accept themselves as equally valid males without having to assume that homosexual orientation must necessarily accompany those differences. Therapy may accomplish that end, even in some boys with a small degree of biological predisposition. Another reason to give special attention to nonmasculine boys is that their nonmasculine personalities may be conflict-based symptomatic compromises caused by pathogenic parental influences; their capacity to fit in with typical boys and men may be therapeutically fostered.

Rationally, one may wish to apply the same principles to adolescents as to children, although sexual orientation as an intrapsychic state is more firmly fixed by adolescence than in childhood. Theoretically, the younger a person is, the more amenable to modification are his or her patterns. In reality, the dynamics of normal adolescence include a strong need to distance oneself from adults and to overcome dependence on adult parental figures. Forming a therapeutic alliance with an adolescent that is strong enough to withstand the emotional intensity of transference issues and long-term depth therapy is usually too difficult.

OUTSIDE PRESSURES Adults who present themselves for therapy because of outside pressure are poor prospects for change. Even when they have some ambivalence about their own homosexuality, their resentment of the pressure becomes a resistance that cannot usually be overcome. Sometimes, their sexual behavior is driven to the point that the compulsiveness is ego-dystonic, even though the orientation is not; the behavior may be criminal, as in homosexual pedophilia. Psychotherapy or medication, such as with medroxyprogesterone acetate (Provera) or cyproterone acetate (compounds with antiandrogen properties), can be helpful in reducing the intensity of the sexual drive in men to manageable levels, so that they can make full use of psychotherapy, in some cases to the degree that medication can be discontinued. Fluoxetine (Prozac) has also been effective in controlling compulsive paraphilic behavior.

SPECIAL PROBLEMS Homosexuals who come into therapy for emotional difficulties other than their homosexuality present a special problem. They may have conflicts in interpersonal relations with their lovers or with others, they may have neurotic or characterological pathology, or they may have sexual dysfunctions within their homosexual liaisons. Like anyone with such problems, many can benefit from psychotherapy that never focuses on their sexual orientation. But unless the therapy is specifically problem-oriented or behavior-oriented, material pertaining to sexual orientation will emerge if the patient remains long enough in any exploratory therapy. The emergence can be threatening and may cause termination. The author has found it helpful to discuss that eventuality in advance, when the goals and the treatment procedures are being decided on; that approach can sometimes help prevent termination so premature that even the nonorientation conflicts remain less well-resolved than would be possible.

A 36-year-old successful clergyman who was exclusively homosexual presented with sexual dysfunction within his monogamous relationship and with guilt-producing but highly exciting sadomasochistic (master-slave) masturbatory fantasies. He had been fetishistic for Western leatherware since early childhood. He was anorgasmic in his sexual relationship, although he had occasional retarded ejaculation, but was easily orgasmic with the masturbatory fantasies. The fantasies could allow him to be orgasmic during anal intercourse or fellatio, but they caused too much guilt for him to use them. He wanted therapy only to improve his homosexual relationship.

He was the only son of a sexually prohibitive mother (who died when he was 12 years old) and a father with whom he had a warm, seductive, and consciously erotic, though not actively incestuous, relationship. His father had remarried during the patient's teens, and his stepmother had originally been very nice to him but then suddenly became totally rejecting in his early 20s for reasons be claimed never to understand. He had never acknowledged his homosexuality to his father.

Therapy used a combination of behavior modification and uncovering techniques. Through behavior therapy he was able to use his fantasies to achieve successful physical closeness with his partner and then to replace the fantasy imagery with that of his lover. At the same time, he was discovering his negative oedipal attraction to his father—the father always wore Western clothing and boots—and eventually he came to recognize his father as the master in his fantasies. He also recognized his fear of women and of their anger and his conviction that women would always be right and he always wrong and guilty. His goal of orgasmic response with his partner was achieved at about the time he began to have dreams of heterosexual arousal to women. He was consciously threatened by the implications of that material and terminated therapy—fortunately, after the successful accomplishment of his original goal.

SHIFT TO HETEROSEXUALITY For those who wish to work toward heterosexuality and whose orientation is conflict-based or deficit-based, therapy can be effective to a greater degree than is often realized. About one third in most published surveys achieve a true shift to heterosexuality, and another third become heterosexually arousable and functional without losing their homosexual responsivity. One large center has reported a 79 percent reorientation rate by using intense behavior modification techniques, but, to this author's knowledge, that work has neither been reported in therapeutic detail nor replicated.

Some authors have questioned or qualified the change rates. Some simply deny the validity or the honesty of the published studies and claim that any effort to shift orientation damages the patient. This author knows from professional experience that that need not be true, although therapeutic efforts at change can be harmful when they are misapplied. Others have suggested that only those homosexuals who have always had some capacity for heterosexual arousal, however little or unacknowledged, are capable of becoming heterosexual. That may be true, but it is difficult to prove because it could be inferred ex post facto after successful therapy for conflict-based or deficit-based homosexuality. The author has one case of a man who had no awareness of heterosexual interest throughout years of active homosexuality until he fell in love with a woman.

Most therapeutic modalities—including psychoanalysis and psychoanalytically oriented psychotherapy, analytic group therapy, and behavior modification techniques involving conditioning, desensitizing, reconditioning, and aversive techniques—report roughly comparable results. Whether the outcomes are truly comparable in terms of the involvement of the whole person in coming to grips with the complexities of sexual intimacy and commitment is not clear. Nonanalytic techniques focus on increasing arousal and response to heterosexual stimuli and fantasies while decreasing homosexual arousal. The author has seen frequent resistance to and rejection of such therapy in otherwise well-motivated patients when the unconscious motivation compelling homoerotic responses has not yet been resolved. Data on the ability to carry those changes into real life and on the permanency of the shift to heterosexuality are inconclusive. Some follow-up studies of psychoanalytically treated patients show changes in all facets of heterosexual involvement that hold up well over time. In addition, some deep and well-defended conflicts cannot be uncovered and resolved by any less arduous approach.

Prognosis for change For those who genuinely wish to change, the prognosis is difficult to ascertain, and the indicators are not always either clear or clearly known. Strong motivation to change is most important, but it is insufficient in itself. Ego strength is of major prognostic import. Primitive levels of ego development, as in psychotic and borderline patients, make such major changes as sexual orientation unlikely. Patients with severe character pathology are less likely to reach their major therapeutic goals than are patients with essentially normal neurotic levels of ego development. Ego development can be assessed with psychological tests, especially the projective tests, and some sense of strength can be determined by assessing function in other appropriate areas of life, such as school performance, occupational function, interpersonal relations, and level of involvement in sports, hobbies, and cultural interests. Ego development affects not only the prognosis for various treatment goals but also the choice of treatment modality. Low levels of ego development argue against the rigors of psychoanalysis and for less threatening and more supportive or more mechanical therapies.

Relative youth argues for a good prognosis, but one cannot assume that the young have good ego flexibility and that the mature do not. Some history of heterosexual arousal and experience and the relative recency of beginning homosexual activity improve the prognosis, as does sex-appropriate role behavior. Marked effeminacy in a man and hypermasculine behavior in a woman—especially if continuous from chronic cross-gender behavior in childhood—are poor prognostic signs for change. The better the relationship, past or present, with an emotionally healthy same-sex parent and the more qualities that parent had that deserve respect, even if the patient was never able to acknowledge them, the greater is the potential of weathering the negative transference and achieving same-sex identification.

Therapy that aims at modifying the object of erotic arousal or the conditions for erotic arousal involves an added built-in difficulty. Even when homosexuality is strongly ego-dystonic, it is associated with intense physical pleasure. Sexual excitement and orgasm are powerful reinforcers of the behaviors that produce them. Although some homosexuals can achieve the shift to heterosexuality if they are so motivated, even more cannot or stop short of that goal, even when they personally chose it. A psychiatrist who works with ego-dystonic homosexuals should be prepared to help them be realistic about their goals when it appears that a shift is unlikely. The focus should appropriately change to accepting themselves and their homosexuality without shame and self-hatred, withstanding the social opprobrium, and functioning with the productivity and the maturity of which they are capable.

OTHER CONSIDERATIONS All the scientific questions about sexual orientation await definitive answers. Only because heterosexuality is the species norm, as in all mammalian species, do some persons seem to think that being straight requires no explanation, whereas being gay or any other deviation from heterosexuality does require an explanation. But one cannot validly try to understand one orientation without inevitably having to try to understand all. There are reasons why the norm exists, just as there are reasons for deviations. But that understanding is in its scientific infancy.

Some things are known. It is know that rearing pressures can help shape psychosexual development and sexual identity, including orientation; it is not known how broadly applicable is the knowledge derived from patients. It is known that biological factors play some role in the development of sexual identity; it is not known to what extent or in what ways those factors operate, how variably influential they are, and what determines that variability. It is known that most homosexuals who want or need psychiatric help have no interest in shifting orientation; the conditions for which they need therapy can be as successfully addressed in them as in heterosexual patients without concomitant efforts to shift homosexuals toward heterosexuality; they deserve that therapy, along with therapeutic respect for their homosexuality, although it is not known in how many the conflictual issues underlying their orientation may arise spontaneously. It is known that, since postnatal interpersonal influences can affect sexual orientation, interpersonal therapeutic influences can help bring about a shift in orientation in a significant proportion of those who want it and who are willing and able to withstand the emotional rigors of the effort.

Most notably, perhaps, it is known that homosexuality, whatever brings it about, is not a sign of degeneracy or evil or inferiority. It appears to be human to recoil unthinkingly from those who are different. That response has no place among thinking people—most particularly, not among psychiatrists.

SUGGESTED CROSS-REFERENCES

Normal human sexuality and sexual disorders are discussed in Section 21.1a, and gender identity disorders are discussed in Section 21.3. Normal child and adolescent development is discussed in Sections 33.2 and 33.3, and the sexual abuse of children is discussed in Section 47.3. Psychoneuroendocrinology is discussed in Section 1.11. Theories of personality and psychopathology are discussed in Chapters 6, 7, and 8. Psychotherapies are discussed in Chapter 31.

REFERENCES

Bailey J M, Pillard R C: A genetic study of male sexual orientation. Arch Gen Psychiatry *48:* 1089, 1991.

Bailey J M, Pillard R C, Neale M, Agyein Y: Heritable factors influencing sexual orientation in women. Arch Gen Psychiatry *50:* 217, 1993.

Bell A P, Weinberg M S: *Homosexualities.* Simon & Schuster, New York, 1978.

Bell A P, Weinberg M S, Hammersmith S K: *Sexual Preference.* Indiana University Press, Bloomington, 1981.

*Bieber I, Dain H J, Dince P R, Drellich M G, Grand H G, Grundlach R H, Kremer M W, Rifkin A H, Wilbur C B, Bieber T B: *Homosexuality.* Basic Books, New York, 1962.

Buhrich N J, Baily J M, Martin N G: Sexual orientation, sexual identity, and sex-dimorphic behaviors in male twins. Behav Genet *21:* 75, 1991.

Byne W: The scientific evidence challenged. Sci Am *270:* 50, 1994.

Byne W, Parsons B: Human sexual orientation: the biologic theories reappraised. Arch Gen Psychiatry *50:* 228, 1993.

Eckert E D, Bouchard T J, Bohlen J, Heston L L: Homosexuality in monozygotic twins reared apart. Br J Psychiatry *148:* 421, 1986.

Ehrhardt A A, Meyer-Bahlberg H F L: Effects of prenatal sex hormones on gender-related behavior. Science *211:* 1312, 1981.

Endelman R: New light on deviance and psychopathology?: The case of *Homosexualities* and *Sexual Preference.* J Psychoanal Anthropol *7:* 75, 1984.

Ford C S, Beach F A: *Patterns of Sexual Behavior.* Harper & Row, New York, 1951.

*Friedman R C: *Male Homosexuality: A Contemporary Psychoanalytic Perspective.* Yale University Press, New Haven, CT, 1988.

Friedman R C, Downey J: Neurobiology and sexual orientation: Current relationships. J Neuropsychiatr Clin Neurosci *5:* 131, 1993.

Friedman R C, Downey J: Psychoanalysis, psychobiology, and homosexuality. JAMA *41:* 1159, 1993.

*Gadpaille W J: Biological factors in the development of human sexual identity. Psychiatr Clin North Am *3:* 3, 1980.

*Gadpaille W J: Cross-species and cross-cultural contributions to understanding homosexual activity. Arch Gen Psychiatry *37:* 349, 1980.

Gadpaille W J: Research into the physiology of maleness and femaleness. Arch Gen Psychiatry *26:* 193, 1972.

Gooren I: Biomedical theories of sexual orientation: A critical examination. In *Homosexuality/Heterosexuality: Concepts of Sexual Orientation,* D P McWhirter, S A Sanders, J M Reinisch, editors, p 71. Oxford University Press, New York, 1990.

Green R: *The "Sissy Boy Syndrome" and the Development of Homosexuality.* Yale University Press, New Haven, 1987.

Hamer D H, Hu S, Magnuson V L, Hu N, Pattatucci A M L: A linkage between DNA markers on the X chromosome and male sexual orientation. Science *261:* 321, 1993.

Hooker E: Reflections of a 40-year exploration: A scientific view on homosexuality. Am Psychol *48:* 450, 1993.

Isay R A: *Being Homosexual: Gay Men and Their Development.* Farrar, Straus, Giroux, New York, 1989.

Kallman F J: Comparative twin study on the genetic aspects of male homosexuality. J Nerv Ment Dis *115:* 283, 1952.

*Karlen A: *Sexuality and Homosexuality.* Norton, New York, 1971.

Kinsey A C, Pomeroy W B, Martin C E: *Sexual Behavior in the Human Male.* Saunders, Philadelphia, 1948.

Kinsey A C, Pomeroy W B, Martin C E, Gebhard P H: *Sexual Behavior in the Human Female.* Saunders, Philadelphia, 1953.

LeVay S: A difference in hypothalamic structure between heterosexual and homosexual men. Science *253:* 1034, 1991.

LeVay S, Hamer D H: Evidence for a biological influence in male homosexuality. Sci Am *270:* 44, 1994.

Masters W H, Johnson V E: *Homosexuality in Perspective.* Little, Brown, Boston, 1979.

Nadler R D: Homosexual behavior in nonhuman primates. In *Homosexuality/Heterosexuality: Concepts of Sexual Orientation,* D P McWhirter, S A Sanders, J M Reinisch, editors, p 138. Oxford University Press, New York, 1990.

Nicolosi J: *Reparative Therapy of Male Homosexuality.* Aronson, Northvale, N J, 1991.

Ovesey L: *Homosexuality and Pseudohomosexuality.* Science House, New York, 1969.

Pillard R C: The Kinsey scale: Is it familial? In *Homosexuality/Heterosexuality: Concepts of Sexual Orientation,* D P McWhirter, S A Sanders, J M Reinisch, editors, p 88. Oxford University Press, New York, 1990.

Saghir M T, Robins E: *Male and Female Homosexuality.* Williams & Wilkins, Baltimore, 1973.

Schafer S: Sociosexual behavior in male and female homosexuals: A study of sex differences. Arch Sex Behav *6:* 355, 1977.

Stoller R J, Herdt G H: Theories of origins of male homosexuality: A cross-cultural look. Arch Gen Psychiatry *42:* 399, 1985.

Whitam F L, Diamond M, Martin J: Homosexual orientation in twins: A report on 61 pairs and three triplet sets. Arch Sex Behav *22:* 187, 1993.

Zucker K J, Green R, Garofano C, Bradley S J, Williams K, Rebach H M, Sullivan C B: Prenatal gender preference of mothers of feminine and masculine boys: Relation to sibling sex composition and birth order. J Abnorm Child Psychol *22:* 1, 1994.

21.2 PARAPHILIAS

JON K. MEYER, M.D.

INTRODUCTION

Paraphilias are characterized by specialized sexual fantasies, masturbatory practices, sexual props, and requirements of the sexual partner. The core fantasy, with its unconscious and conscious components, is the pathognomonic element. Arousal and orgasm are dependent to some degree on the playing out of that fantasy mentally and behaviorally. While the fantasy and its behavioral elaborations have a primary effect on eroticism, they also pervade the person's life far beyond the sexual sphere.

Paraphilias occupy an important position on the continuum between health and illness. In pure form, they are clinically distinct and unique. Some persons are so completely integrated with their paraphilia that it is a major component of their identity and way of life. They cannot imagine themselves without it. Paraphilias may merge with other conditions. At one end of the spectrum, paraphilias shade into the psychoses and gender identity disorders, and at the other, they gradually become repressed in the neuroses. Overall, paraphilias share much common ground with borderline character disorders.

Early in the 20th century, the discovery of childhood sexual fantasies, elucidation of their development, and the investigation of their contributions to both normal and deviant adult sexuality prepared the way for a better understanding of paraphilia. From a developmental point of view, paraphilias are created from common elements of experience and adaptation. Stated another way, a perversion is a recognizable human product of an individual developmental pathway. The titillation of perverse fantasies and practices, so intriguing in daydreams, in pornography, and in foreplay, testifies to the ubiquitous interest in paraphiliac sexuality. Under the cloak of secrecy and disguise, even everyday erotic fantasies manipulate dramatic elements of mystery, romance, and tragedy. Those processes, common to everyone, are simply recognizable in bold relief in the perversions. Paraphilias may therefore be approached with understanding and empathy.

DEFINITION

The fourth edition of *Diagnostic and Statistical Manual of Mental Disorders* (DSM-IV) specifies that paraphilias are characterized by intense sexual urges and sexual fantasies that involve nonhuman subjects, children, or nonconsenting persons, or the actual suffering or humiliation of oneself or a partner. In the nomenclature, diagnosis is critically dependent upon the duration of those fantasies, urges, or behaviors, which must be present for at least six months, and on the level of distress or impairment of function they cause. In general terms, the severity of a condition is usually dependent on the degree of enactment and level of distress: in a mild condition, the individual may be distressed by the imagery but have never acted on it; in a moderate condition, imagery may have occasionally been transformed into action, and social or occupational functioning may be impaired; and in a severe condition, the urges may have repeatedly been acted on, and other functioning may be preempted by the presentation with the perversion. Other clinical considerations include the degree to which perverse imagery is necessary for arousal, the harmfulness of the enactments, and associated psychological or social impairments.

HISTORY

Nonnormative sexual interests and practices have been known since antiquity. Not until the 19th and 20th centuries, however, have there been efforts to categorize and explicate them. Three well-known works published at about the same time began that process: Richard Krafft-Ebing's *Psychopathia Sexualis* in 1886, Havelock Ellis's *Studies in the Psychology of Sex* in 1904, and Sigmund Freud's *Three Essays on the Theory of Sexuality* in 1905. Each contributed a different perspective which is still reflected in current work. The cataloguing and descriptive efforts of Krafft-Ebing are mirrored in current descriptive efforts, including DSM. The anthropological and biological speculations of Ellis are reflected in modern sociological and cultural theories. Freud's developmental and dynamic approach is reflected in current work on genesis and treatment. All three authors confronted the Victorian era with an aspect of sexuality denied by the mores of the time. Freud's ideas and observations, however, were particularly scandalous to *fin-de-siècle* society since he suggested that there were sexual impulses in children, that childhood sexuality was characterized by "perverse" elements, and that those elements did not just go away but, consciously or unconsciously, were part of the adult repertoire.

COMPARATIVE NOSOLOGY

Paraphilias have also been referred to as sexual deviations and perversions, the three terms representing different points of view. The term "paraphilia" emphasizes the unusual quality or nature of the sexual object (for example, a child, an animal, or a shoe). "Sexual deviation" refers to nonnormative sexual activity in a statistical or cultural sense (for example, men dressing in women's clothes in order to achieve orgasm). "Perversion" refers to a developmental shift in eroticism, so that what is ordinarily a minor theme becomes a major theme (for example, the childhood fantasy that the anus functions as a genital organ may be elaborated into adult coprolagnia).

In the American nomenclature there has been an evolution in the classification of paraphilias with changing official and cultural perspectives. In 1952, the first edition of DSM (DSM-I) placed sexual deviations under "Sociopathic Personality Disturbance": illness primarily in terms of lack of conformity with society and prevailing cultural milieu, not just in terms of personal relationships and discomfort. While sociopathic reactions were generally considered symptomatic of underlying personality disorder, neurosis, or psychosis, the "Sexual Deviation" diagnosis—which included "homosexuality"—was reserved for unusual sexuality that was "not symptomatic of more extensive syndromes such as schizophrenia and obsessional reactions."

In 1968, the second edition of DSM (DSM-II) classified sexual deviations as part of "Personality Disorders." Deviations were defined in terms of erotic interests that preempted normal sexual activity and were directed toward objects other than people of the opposite sex, toward sexual acts not usually associated with coitus, and toward coitus performed under bizarre circumstances. As might be expected from that definition, homosexuality was included as a sexual deviation. The nomenclature was subsequently amended, however, removing homosexuality from the paraphilias and placing it in a separate category as "Sexual Orientation Disturbance," a diagnosis used only when the individual was disturbed by his or her homophiliac orientation.

In the third edition of DSM (DSM-III), published in 1980, paraphilia was placed in a new and major classification, "Psychosexual Disorders,'' which also included gender identity disorders, psychosexual dysfunctions, and ego-dystonic homosexuality. The subcategories of paraphilias included fetishism, transvestism, zoophilia, pedophilia, exhibitionism, voyeurism, sexual masochism, sexual sadism, and a residual category for other disorders. DSM-III, which focused on descriptive rather than dynamic or psychogenetic factors, considered the essential features to be involuntarily repetitive, unusual, or bizarre imagery or acts related to sexual excitement. To be considered paraphiliac, the sexual activity had to be characterized by preference for the use of nonhuman objects in achieving sexual arousal, by imposed sexual humiliation or suffering, or by sexual involvement with nonconsenting partners. The ninth edition of the *International Classification of Diseases and Related Health Problems* (ICD-9-CM), which is of the same vintage as the DSM-III, is roughly comparable to the latter, although it displaces fetishism, voyeurism, and sexual sadism and masochism into a less important category of ''Other Specified Psychosexual Disorders.''

In the revised DSM-III (DSM-III-R), the major aspects of the paraphilia category were retained while the declassification of homosexuality was completed and it disappeared from the nomenclature. In the paraphilia category per se, zoophilia was removed to the category ''not otherwise specified'' while frotteurism was reclassified as a major diagnostic entity. In 1994, DSM-IV retained the basic classification of the DSM-III-R with only minor changes in some specific categories.

Under the best of circumstances nosologies are arbitrary, because the clinical situation has more shades of gray than black and white dichotomies. For example, self-report and phallometric data suggest that exhibitionism, voyeurism, obscene phone calls, and frotteurism are closely related courtship disorders involving the pretactile or early tactile phases of sexual object approach. Recent psychometric studies have complemented clinical impressions by demonstrating that along major personality dimensions paraphilias are more similar to one another than to other sexual dysfunctions or to normal sexuality. Even though individual paraphilias are phenomenologically distinguishable, paraphilias as a group are clinically related by common dynamic and developmental roots. Descriptive nomenclatures, such as the DSM and ICD, emphasize the differences between patients in order to categorize them. By contrast, dynamic viewpoints emphasize the similarities among patients to provide the best possible clinical guide.

An example of classification conflicting with clinical observation was a suggestion that paraphilias, homosexuality, and gender identity disorders could be distinguished on the grounds that admixed perversions are routinely found in paraphilias but not in gender identity disorders and homosexuality. Clinical experience reveals, however, that both chronic and intercurrent paraphiliac practices may also exist in transsexualism and homosexuality. Homosexual sadomasochism and pedophilia and transsexual fetishism are particularly well recognized.

EPIDEMIOLOGY

Epidemiological information on perversions is notoriously poor despite the fact that perversions are, in principle, operationally defined and observable. In general, cases are noted only if treatment is sought or if there are legal entanglements. Even when treatment is sought, however, an adequate treatment register is not likely, because paraphilias are rarely diagnosed even though they may be relatively common. There are several reasons for that fact: (1) the diagnosis is often missed; (2) the condition may be ego-syntonic so that the patient reports no distress; and (3) the paraphiliac may conceal his or her practices.

While paraphilias are practiced by a small percentage of the population, the insistent, repetitive nature of the disorders may result in a high frequency of paraphiliac acts, so that a larger proportion of the population than one might suspect may have been affected by persons with paraphilias. More than 50 percent of paraphilias have their onset before age 18 and, over a lifetime, persons may manifest three to five paraphilias, either concurrently or at different times. The occurrence of paraphiliac behavior seems to peak between ages 15 and 25 and then gradually to decline, so that in men of 50, public paraphiliac acts are rare even when they continue in isolation or with a cooperative partner. There may be significant outbursts of paraphiliac activity at certain points in older life, especially during psychosocial developmental crises (Table 21.2-1).

Since most statistics come from the legal system, samples are biased toward impulsive persons and public nuisance or dangerous paraphilias. Among legal cases, pedophilia is common, because a child is involved and the act is taken more seriously. A greater effort is spent tracking down the offender. As many as 10 to 20 percent of children may have been molested by age 18. Child pornography—''kiddie porn''—has been one of the fastest growing areas of pornographic commerce despite the tightening of federal statutes and better enforcement. Exhibitionists are also commonly apprehended since they may expose themselves to young girls. Voyeurs may be apprehended, but their risk is not great. As many as 20 percent of women may have been the targets of exhibitionism and voyeurism. Sexual masochism and sadism are underrepresented because the former receives attention only when the degree of tolerable suffering is miscalculated with tragic results, and the latter in sensational cases of rape, brutality, or lust murder. As recent sensational cases have shown, necrophilia may also be associated with lust murder. Transvestites may be arrested occasionally on disturbing-the-peace misdemeanors if they are obviously men dressed in women's clothes, but that behavior is more common among the gender identity disorders. Frotteurs are seldom apprehended because the touch may be so slight or so fleeting that, while the victim may be aware of something unwelcome, the event is not of sufficient duration or definition to allow a response. The victim may also be embarrassed to raise a commotion in a public place. Fetishists ordinarily do not attract legal attention.

The excretory perversions are scarcely reported since the activity usually takes place between consenting adults or between prostitute and client. Zoophilia as a true paraphilia is

TABLE 21.2-1
Frequency of Paraphiliac Acts Committed by Paraphiliac Patients Seeking Outpatient Treatment

Diagnostic Category	Paraphiliac Patients Seeking Outpatient Treatment (%)	Paraphiliac Acts per Paraphiliac Patient (*)
Pedophilia	45	5
Exhibitionism	25	50
Voyeurism	12	17
Frotteurism	6	30
Sexual masochism	3	36
Transvestic fetishism	3	25
Sexual sadism	3	3
Fetishism	2	3
Zoophilia	1	2

*Median number.
Table by Gene G. Abel, M.D. Used with permission.

probably quite rare, accounting for its de-emphasis between DSM-III and the DSM-III-R. (One case was identified only because the young female zoophile was frightened that fellating her pet dog had given rise to herpetic oral lesions.) Individuals in equilibrium with their paraphilias are underrepresented in all samples.

ETIOLOGY

Three major factors influence personality development: biology, environment, and the mind's synthetic-integrative functions. Since the formation of psychopathology is a subset of personality development, those three factors are also central in the formation of paraphilia. Biology refers to constitutional and acquired physically based cognitive and emotional properties. Environment refers to the physical and psychological medium which nurtures the developing human. The synthetic-integrative function refers to the mental faculty that takes biological and environmental constraints and potentials and melds the parts into a coherent personality. A synthetic-integrative function implies that work is done to make something out of available capacities and impacting events. While the effects of biology, environment, and integrative processes may be separately emphasized, the influence of all three is required to produce the perverse personality.

In the expression of something so fundamental as sexuality, it seems likely that constitutionally determined biological factors would play a role. There is evidence that gender identity and sexual object preference may have constitutional components, but no specific factor has been identified for paraphilias although an association between poorly controlled, aggressive paraphilias and elevated plasma testosterone levels has been suggested. Reduction of testosterone levels by medroxyprogesterone has been associated with improved behaviors. While the neuron is affected by the endocrine system, the neuron also affects the endocrine system. Whether elevated testosterone is the cause of paraphilia or a consequence of driven mental imagery remains to be clarified. There is little to suggest that acquired biological conditions are significant contributors to paraphilias.

On the experiential side, there is a greater primate need for environmental priming than for most animals, and in all the primates inadequate mothering and peer contact seem causally related to aberrant sexuality. On the clinical side, histories characteristically reveal disordered nuclear families. In general, the more gross and disorganized the family milieu, the more gross and disorganized the paraphilia. Yet while few would doubt that the environment has profound effects on the genesis of paraphilia, it remains uncertain whether an abnormal environment is sufficient to cause a deviation without the personal interpretation of those experiences.

Presumably, few would doubt that mental factors contribute to idiosyncratic arousal stimuli. Something mental must account for the erotic quality of ropes, leather, rubber, shoes, animals, corpses, or children. The mental factors appear to be generated as specific, personal responses to the universal conflicts of separation-individuation and the dyadic and triadic relationships of power and sex found in the family.

BIOLOGICAL FACTORS

Constitution As long as it has been known that the organogenesis of the reproductive tract follows a bisexual pattern, there has been the tantalizing possibility that biological factors play a fundamental role in sexual aberrations. The possibility of biological factors in paraphilias was further strengthened by the discovery of the pivotal role of androgen in mammalian sexual organ differentiation. In addition, hormones and behavior-mediating brain sites were linked by evidence that sexual behavior in rodents may be profoundly influenced by small, accurately timed fetal or neonatal androgen or estrogen doses. Much thought and effort have been devoted to investigating possible biological roots of gender identity modifications (transsexualism) and sexual identity modifications (homosexuality). Less effort has been devoted to the modifications of eroticism (the paraphilias).

Observations and follow-up on intersex children, accidental and iatrogenic manipulations of fetal hormones, investigations of brain-hormone feedback loops, a review of brain lateralization findings, and extrapolations from human and infrahuman mammalian research have produced suggestive evidence but as yet no definitive links between biology and paraphiliac eroticism. The efficacy of antiandrogen medication in the control of driven or violent sexual behaviors suggests that the behavior is centrally mediated and androgen sensitive. However, the fact that many patients electively stopped their medication and returned to their previous deviations suggests that the behavior was also motivated by nonandrogen-sensitive areas of the brain. In at least one study, the antiandrogen cyproterone acetate was found to have more effect on rapid eye movement (REM)-related nocturnal penile tumescence (NPT) than on awake, motivated erections.

One reason for the linking of androgen with paraphilias is the apparently striking sex ratio in those disorders. The sexual perversions seem largely to be male conditions. It has been suggested that because the human fetus is basically female, making a male means jury-rigging the system so that modified sexual identity and eroticism emerge. Although much has been made of the innate femaleness of the fetus, a review of fetal development suggests that the viewpoint is a teleological misinterpretation of an efficient decision tree, in which there is one automatic pattern (female) and one hormone-mediated pattern (male). Furthermore, there are important questions about male preponderance in the paraphilias: Is it possible that the different incidence between males and females is more apparent than real? Are men simply more obvious about paraphiliac behavior? Might perversity among women be expressed in different forms? Since feminine integration ordinarily lends itself to complemental receptivity, are women more quietly perverse? Might consensual female partners in perverse activity, for example, be preferentially perverse in a truly feminine way? Is it conceivable that prostitution is the quintessential female perversion?

It is probable that constitutional factors are involved in sexual behavior but most likely as multiple feedback loops acting in concert from different loci. The capacity to form a sexual identity and some masculine or feminine predisposition are likely to be the legacy of fetal life; what is done with that legacy appears to be determined during postnatal development.

Organic findings There are some data—including from twin studies—suggesting temporal lobe abnormalities in persons who have committed sadistic rape, and those who practice transvestism, fetishism, pedophilia, and other perversions. A number of investigations of paraphiliac patients referred to large medical centers have identified abnormal organic findings. Of those patients with positive organic findings, 74 percent had abnormal hormone levels, 27 percent had hard or soft neurological signs, 24 percent had chromosomal abnormalities, 9 percent had seizures, 4 percent had abnormal electroencephalograms (EEGs) without seizures, 4 percent had major mental disorders, and 4 percent were mentally retarded. Of course, the question is whether those abnormalities were merely incidental or causally related to paraphilic interests.

ENVIRONMENT While a diagnosable paraphilia often has its onset before age 18, softer and subtler signs and symptoms of the perversion are common in childhood. As for so many psychiatric conditions, the crucial milieu for the development of the perversions is the family. At a more superficial level, familial factors contribute to the form and substance of paraphilia. It is not rare to see cases of father-son pursuit of identical or closely related perversions.

As a blatant example, it is estimated that from one third to one half of child molesters were themselves abused as children. More subtly, in transvestic households the parents usually have an uneasy adaptation to the paraphilia. The father's feminine wardrobe, wigs, and pornography are hidden, and cross-dressing is limited to when the children are in school or kept behind locked doors, but despite these precautions, the mother's or sister's missing garments may be discovered under a son's mattress. Reactions to the discovery may include parental guilt, depression, threats of separation or divorce, and, occasionally, the pursuit of sex reassignment by the father.

While it is possible to hide paraphiliac practices and paraphernalia, it is not possible to mask perverse preoccupations, emotional investments, and affective changes. More specifically, libidinal and aggressive undercurrents communicated in handling, feeding, clothing, and training children; uneasiness in both intimacy and separation; magical investment in talisman objects; tacit interdictions and seductions; and mythology about the differences between the sexes, procreation, and birth are emotionally alive in the paraphiliac household and cannot be kept from the children. Sons and daughters form emotional resonances to their family's unspoken wishes and unconscious needs.

The creation of a paraphilia occurs in the early developmental phases of self and identity formation and the conflicts around the family triangle. The following summarizes a complex developmental sequence.

In the first few months of life, the substrate for psychological development is an empathic and stable relationship between mother and child. A mother-infant relationship of that quality serves as the feeling basis for the growth of comfortable and trusting intimacy. Stemming from that relationship is the sense that needs and tensions are acceptable and will call forth an intuitively sensitive response. In perverse individuals that basic sense is often impaired, with the result that all intimacy suffers, and sexuality is marred by an insatiable emptiness and perpetual efforts to extract sustenance from others. The hopeless inadequacy of any response to those attempts leads to efforts to exact revenge. Emptiness, envy, and rage become the vehicles of sexual expression.

The specific sexual cast to the paraphilia often seems related to conflicts surrounding the dyadic and triadic sexualized relationships of the oedipal phase, as influenced by earlier flaws in separation-individuation. As development proceeds, the child normally independently moves away from and dependently returns to mother, establishing against her grid the capacity to relate as a separate and individual person. When that developmental task is poorly handled, separation comes to be experienced as abandonment and closeness as engulfment. Father, as a familiar and caring person outside of mother's immediate orbit, is important in fostering separateness from mother. When father is absent, uncaring, effeminate, devalued, or dominated by mother, disidentification from mother and establishment of appropriate object choices are impaired. Paraphiliac patients often have separation problems and histories of disparaged fathers.

Typically, families of paraphiliac persons have been blind to the increasingly desperate turmoil inside the child and have been unable to respond effectively. In one case the child left disturbed underwear in his mother's bureau as clear evidence of his fetishistic interests, but nothing was ever said.

SYNTHESIS AND INTEGRATION While family dynamics may be necessary to cause a perversion, they are not sufficient because of the crucial nature of intrapsychic factors. For example, in the same household one child may become perverse while another is unscathed (or has a different psychopathology) because of different integrations of family dynamics. The synthesized and integrated unique personality is more than the sum of biology and experience. The complexity of the neocortex in humans insures that 100 billion neurons will find a personal way to organize constitution and experience into an erotic substrate. In fact, what is incredible is not that there is such diversity in human sexual expression, but that it is all so similar. The similarity is undoubtedly related to common developmental processes and milestones.

DEVELOPMENTAL THEORIES

Early formulations At the time Freud began his work, the paraphilias were widely regarded as products of degeneracy. Freud, however, recognized the precursors of such conditions in the fantasies and preoccupations of children. He also discovered that perverse wishes and fantasies were unconscious in neurotic persons, whose symptoms were, in part, reactions to them. In 1905 Freud hypothesized that perversion was produced by the direct extension of childish libidinal currents into adult life, the infantile sexuality having failed to succumb to repressive forces that would convert it into neurotic symptoms. Subsequently, it became obvious that perversions were themselves defensive formations. Repression might be partially successful against especially strong components of childhood sexuality at the price of sanctioning some lesser part. The sanctioned aspect of infantile sexuality was suitable because it was unchallenged by parental representations in the superego. In that way, family dynamics were expressed in the perversion.

In addition to the role of perversion as a symptomatic compromise between drive and conscience, Freud noted that perversion had an important ego-sustaining function, patching over flaws in the sense of reality. Later observations reemphasized the complexity of the perverse formations in terms of the conscious and unconscious components, the role of guilt and conscience, the contributions of both aggression and libidinal interests, the symbolic representation of developmental missteps, and the adaptive functions.

Later formulations More recently, ego psychology, developmental observations, and object relations theory have suggested other important factors. For example, a phase of body-genital schematization was noted at 18 months of age around the onset of the rapprochement crisis of separation-individuation. It is characterized by heightened sexual and aggressive drives as manifested in object-directed masturbation and aggression. A time of incomplete discrimination between self and others, that phase is concurrent with gender identity formation, and related period-specific problems have been implicated in the etiology of paraphilia. During that phase, recognition of anatomical sexual distinctions has an important emotional impact. An impaired mother-child relationship leaves the child vulnerable to anxiety about sexual differences, body image, aggression, separation, and gender.

A poorly defined and unstable body image is a frequently noted feature of perversion. In addition to its localization and orientation functions, body image has emotional components consisting of the positive or negative investments in the body and its parts. In the proto-perverse situation, aggression is heightened and poorly differentiated, with the result that body appendages are more invested with aggression than usual. If an emotionally solid, stable body image is not established in childhood, body parts are ambivalently invested and feel in constant danger of coming apart. For example, the stress-related compulsive masturbation associated with perversion serves not only to discharge anxiety through orgasm, but also to alleviate aggression and combat feelings of bodily dissolution.

In disturbed children, the maturing sexual drives are distorted in the interest of bolstering body image, lending libidinal relationships more narcissistic than object-related value. Castration anxiety starts earlier and has a different quality from the normal, being much more involved with compensatory body narcissism. If the early relationship with mother lacks uncomplicated empathy and affection, a wish develops to compel through force what is not given through love. In that way, aggressive drives are further exaggerated in the service of narcissistic needs. Envy, spite, possessiveness, and derogation of one or both parents play a larger part in the precursors of paraphilias than in the healthier jealousies of other children. Given the instability of body image, the anxious body narcissism, and the exaggeration of aggressive drives, it is easy to imagine the severity of the oedipal crisis in the perversion-vulnerable child. Under such circumstances, infantile sexuality may feel like a safe haven from oedipal dangers.

Sexuality arrested at that level is characterized by perverse trends infiltrated with sadomasochism. Coincidentally, there is exquisite sensitivity to engulfment or abandonment with an uneasy oscillation in the degree of intimate contact permitted. In an effort to cope, devices such as fetishes, which are simultaneously bridging and distancing part objects, may be incorporated into sexuality. In certain respects a fetish may be viewed as a perversion of the normal transitional object.

Unconscious components of fantasy life contribute to the perverse outcome. At the heart of the perverse fantasy, anatomical differences between the sexes are recognized but their significance is denied—they are neither the cause nor the condition of sexual desire. A corollary to that negation is denial of the sexual relationship between the parents, of the complementarity of parental genitalia, and of mutual parental desire. A further, subsidiary denial is the wish not to grasp the reality of how babies are made and where they come from. A common clinical observation is that the pressure to have a child or the birth of a baby unbalances a compensated perversion, leading to serious acting out or depression.

While the above factors contribute to the difficulties which may be solved in a perverse way, the presence of such features is not necessarily specific. Similar guilt, anxiety, and aggression color the psychology and relationships of borderline individuals, so that the frequent overlapping of borderline and paraphiliac conditions is not surprising. The major difference is that in perversion those features are more clearly sexualized.

PARENTAL IDENTIFICATIONS Perverse fantasies are predicated upon and maintained by a sexualized but infantile attachment to mother. In fantasy, the relationship between the boy and his mother is a closed circuit from which father is excluded. The boy nourishes a fantasy that, with his infantile sexual capacities and yearnings, he is the perfect partner for his mother and has nothing to envy in his father. In some instances, the fantasy may be encouraged and stimulated by the child's mother. That creates a double problem since it facilitates the boy's feminine identification and precludes his masculine identification (which is ordinarily stimulated by his mother's attachment to her husband). Idealization and envy of father are vital constituents of masculine identification, and their lack arrests the development of the young man. While contact with the father may not be totally lost in the paraphilias, his representation may be elaborated in unusual ways. For example, the fantasized presence of an anonymous spectator may represent the father. In the transference, the anonymous spectator is often the psychiatrist. Other patients have represented the father in fantasized relationships with important personages or deified figures.

In paraphilias, female genitalia are frightening because of strong maternal identification and the boy's conscious or unconscious desire to sacrifice his penis to be like her. That identification and the associated wishes further threaten the child's brittle male identification and narcissistic investment in his phallus. The child destined to become perverse is caught in a developmental trap. The extraordinary incorporation of mother and identification with her which are adopted to meet separation crises undermine the adequate resolution of castration crises. He cannot win. Never having had a sufficiently conflict-free relationship with her, he cannot give up the identification, which, essential to his shaky psychological integrity, constantly undermines his masculinity.

Those identifications and fantasy constructs are virtually identical in the paraphilias and the gender identity disorders. The difference depends upon the degree to which the fantasy can be symbolized and the degree to which it must be made concrete. To the degree the child can symbolically deny the distinctions between the sexes and cope with castration anxiety, the more likely he is to be perverse; to the degree his symbolic capacities fail, or castration seems inescapable, the more likely he is to have a gender identity disorder. Perversion expresses the fantasy by symbolism and ritual; in transsexualism, the fantasy is often converted into reality.

Castration As the organ around which so much fantasy is spun, the importance of the phallus and potential threats to it can scarcely be overestimated. In fact, the dramatized denial of castration is common to all perversion, usually through denial of female genitalia and the fantasy of a female phallus. One important function of the fetish, for example, is as a magical phallus. In that role the fetish serves as a hedge against castration anxiety by reassuring the patient that women have not been genitally injured, that castration does not happen, and that he too is safe.

In the perverse ritual both male and female participants usually set out to prove the existence of the female phallus.

Female perversion Daughters as well as sons are born to parents and into households that promote perversion. Clinical experience also indicates that perversionlike developments occur in girls as well as boys. Boys at risk are in constant peril from impulses to yield up their penises in identification with mother. Vulnerable girls snub female genitalia as inadequate, intensify demands on mother for restitution, develop a complementary sense of hostile indebtedness to her, exclude father from the dyadic maternal preoccupation, and only superficially shift their love object to males. Their genitals become the focus of all their ambivalence and anxiety. Girls at risk have wishes to incorporate a penis or to develop an illusory one, not just for its own sake but to make themselves worthwhile in their own and their mother's eyes, erasing the stigma that prevents a more satisfactory union. To the extent that the girl can create or incorporate a symbolic penis she will be perverse; to the extent that she must confirm the fantasy in action, she will be transsexual.

Throughout the realm of sexual dysfunction (except for problems of childbirth), men's sexual problems are more concrete and external, whereas female sexuality is more inwardly oriented and visceral. Intrusiveness and receptivity, respectively, connote the differences in orientation. Male perversions are often flamboyant structures with concrete props that tell the story of triumph over castration threats. Female perversions are more unobtrusive, being revealed by a particular willingness to accommodate to the perversion of their partners. Fueled by castration resentment, female paraphilias represent a clandestine insurgence against a sense of genital inferiority. Hidden in male paraphiliac imagery and practice (including dominance and sadism) are extreme castration anxiety and feminine identification. Perverse women recognize those vulnerabilities and put them to use. There is a complementarity to the perverse man, in which he is repeatedly humiliated by virtue of his helpless dependence on the perversion, in general, and the role of his partner, in particular. His shakiness repeatedly demonstrates the loose attachment of his genital, bolsters the paraphiliac's denial of sexual distinctions, and gratifies her fantasies of phallic interchangeability and incorporability. Female perversity is satisfied by an illusory penis, which may be represented by rituals or props or, more commonly, by the incorporation of the phallus of a man whose enormous castration anxiety lends the act particular satisfaction.

DIAGNOSIS AND CLINICAL FEATURES

Clinical features are divisible into those common to the whole class of disorders and those specific to a given subclass. A common feature is the dependence of arousal and orgasm upon fantasies which attenuate the linkages among human contact, sexual expression, and genital congress. Subclasses of paraphilias are characterized by the particular nature of the fantasy and by specialized behaviors—for example, cross-dressing with arousal in transvestic fetishism, erotization of pain in sadomasochism, and sepulchral dramas in necrophilia. Although not all of a paraphiliac's sexual activity may be modified, typically perverse sexuality is exciting while normal sexuality is pedestrian.

Both clinical features and treatability are substantially influenced by ego strength, one hallmark of which is psychological flexibility. Relative flexibility is associated with health, some inflexibility with neurosis, rigidity with borderline characters, and brittleness with psychosis. Paraphiliac persons often show a borderline rigidity. At the far end of the ego-strength spectrum, where the patient constantly battles with psychosis, perverse practices polymorphously blend and merge. With a modicum of ego strength, a more stable perversion may be created, which then further stabilizes and fixes character. In that situation, there may be complete dependency on the perversion for arousal, orgasm, and protection from psychic fragmentation. Still greater ego capacities generally decrease the servitude to the perversion, and, at yet higher levels of ego strength, perverse elements are largely unconscious in neurosis.

Paraphilias may also be viewed in terms of the quality of object relations. It has been suggested that perverse imagery and arousal requirements are sufficiently atypical or bizarre to preclude consensual relationships, an assertion that has been overly generalized. It is true only for the more seriously disturbed paraphiliacs, who have no choice but totally to dehumanize any partner. For those less disturbed and capable of object attachments, stable relationships may develop. Durable transvestic, sadomasochistic, scopophiliac, scatological, and fetishistic marriages are well known. Nevertheless, various paraphilias do show a tendency to arrange themselves along an object-relations gradient. In fetishism, sadism, masochism, and transvestism, there is the potential for maintaining contact with adult objects. Contact of a sort is maintained in pedophilia, but with immature objects. In frotteurism, the object is usually an adult, but there is no relationship except with the part object (for example, buttocks or flanks). With exhibitionism and voyeurism, the contact is strained and largely autistic. In urolagnia and coprophilia, there may be involvement with a partner, but it is likely that the more meaningful contact is with the excremental part object. In perverse rape, the partner is important only in that she is humiliated, degraded, and brutalized. In zoophilia and necrophilia, the object is even further degraded and dehumanized.

Table 21.2-2 outlines the dynamic features of paraphilias.

FETISHISM Table 21.2-3 outlines the DSM-IV diagnostic criteria for fetishism. In fetishism, sexual activity may be directed toward the fetish itself, such as masturbation with or into a shoe, or the fetish may be incorporated into sexual congress. For example, it may be necessary that the woman wear high-heeled shoes, rubber garments, a belt, and so on. In one survey, 58 percent of fetishist persons used clothing articles, 23 percent rubber, 15 percent footwear, and 10 percent leather. Clearly, there was overlap, with some persons using more than one type of article. In the same survey, similarly overlapping behaviors toward the fetish included wearing it (44 percent), stealing it (38 percent), adorning someone else with it (23 percent), gazing at it (12 percent), placing it in the rectum (13 percent), hoarding it (12 percent), fondling it (8 percent), and sucking it (4 percent).

While fetishistic elements are common in the arousal phase of normal sexual activity, in the paraphilias the focus throughout the sexual response cycle is on relatively indestructible,

TABLE 21.2-2
Dynamic Features in Paraphilias

Essential Features	Important Features
(1) The nuclear perversion grows out of a blurring of sexual and generational differences and a poor infant-mother demarcation, particularly in the realm of the genitalia.	(1) There are persistent, repetitive, or intrusive sexual fantasies of an unusual nature.
(2) There is impairment in gender and reality sense.	(2) The fantasies are for the most part ego-syntonic although they are recognized as unusual.
(3) The paraphilia serves to cover flaws in the sense of bodily integrity and in the sense of reality.	(3) Sexual arousal and orgasm are often completely dependent upon those fantasies.
(4) The paraphilia protects against both castration and separation anxieties.	(4) The perverse fantasy is a powerful organizing motif in the patient's life.
(5) The paraphilia provides an outlet for aggressive as well as sexual drives.	(5) There is general psychopathology often characteristic of the spectrum of borderline disorders.
(6) The perverse fantasy and behavior are symptomatic compromise formations growing out of developmental conflict and distress.	

TABLE 21.2-3
Diagnostic Criteria for Fetishism

A. Over a period of at least six months, recurrent, intense sexually arousing fantasies, sexual urges, or behaviors involving the use of nonliving objects (e.g., female undergarments).
B. The fantasies, sexual urges, or behaviors cause clinically significant distress or impairment in social, occupational, or other important areas of functioning.
C. The fetish objects are not limited to articles of female clothing used in cross-dressing (as in transvestic fetishism) or devices designed for the purpose of tactile genital stimulation (e.g., a vibrator).

TABLE 21.2-4
Diagnostic Criteria for Transvestic Fetishism

A. Over a period of at least six months, in a heterosexual male, recurrent, intense sexually arousing fantasies, sexual urges, or behaviors involving cross-dressing.
B. The fantasies, sexual urges, or behaviors cause clinically significant distress or impairment in social, occupational, or other important areas of functioning.

Specify if:
With gender dysphoria: if the person has persistent discomfort with gender role or identity

inanimate objects associated with the human body. The fetish is unconsciously linked with important people of childhood and has qualities associated with those loved, needed, and traumatizing persons. Because of those associations and other meanings and functions, the fetish tends to remain constant over time. It serves as a magical (hence, ''fetish'') bridge to relatedness, as a binder of aggression, and as a representation of the female phallus. In some views, fetishization is considered to represent a more general process of ''dehumanization,'' in which the fetish stands for the human, *pars pro toto,* rather than solely for the maternal phallus. The fetish also compensates for the gap in reality sense left by disavowal of the sexual distinctions.

TRANSVESTIC FETISHISM The diagnostic criteria for transvestic fetishism are outlined in Table 21.2-4. The condition is marked by fantasized or actual dressing in female clothes for purposes of arousal and orgasm. As the name suggests, transvestism is fetishistic cross-dressing and dynamically a subcategory of fetishism. Usually more than one article of clothing and, not infrequently, an entire wardrobe, is involved. When cross-dressed the person's appearance of femininity may be quite striking, although not usually to the degree found in transsexualism. When not dressed in women's clothes, transvestic men may be hypermasculine in appearance and occupation. Cross-dressing exists on a gradient from solitary, depressed, guilt-ridden rituals to ego-syntonic, sociable membership in a transvestic subculture. Anxiety may be experienced about the acceptability of cross-dressing, but is seldom associated with cross-dressing per se unless it is failing as a defense.

Cross-dressing has been reported to begin in boys before their first birthday, when it reflects an extraordinary degree of identification with the mother. The cross-dressing in early childhood may consist of tottering around in mother's high-heeled shoes, wearing a towel to simulate a dress, wearing mother's wig, and using makeup and jewelry as a preferential pattern of behavior. (Cross-dressing, in the sense of refusal to wear dresses and girl's clothes, is also observed in girls but seems to start later.) The few long-term follow-ups suggest that some of those boys do become transvestic fetishists, although others become homosexual, transsexual, asexual, and heterosexual. Outcomes among girls are not as clear, but have included homosexuality, heterosexuality, and transsexualism. Children with early cross-dressing, however, are more likely to become homosexual rather than transvestic. A recognizably transvestic syndrome, with excitement and arousal initiated and sustained by feminine clothes, usually develops in latency. Reports from self-designated transvestites suggest that from 50 to 75 percent had cross-dressed by age 10.

Transvestic practices begin with attempts to control threatened ego and body dissolution through primitive (that is, childlike) magical acts and fantasies. Given enough ego strength, that desperate child's alchemy is refined into the highly condensed, elaborate, and finely tuned fantasy and behavior of the adult transvestite. Dynamically, cross-dressing serves two functions, expressing both feminine identification and triumph over it. The first serves to relieve separation anxiety by symbolic merger with mother. The desire for merger and identification, however, intensifies castration anxiety. Sexualization of castration anxiety and erection (proof of the continued presence of the penis) mark the battle against feminine identification. Temporary victory comes with orgasm.

The women of a transvestite's fantasies are often imagined to have control over him through a variety of stratagems and, therefore, may compel his feminization. Nevertheless, the patient secretly knows that the efforts toward subjugation, control, and feminization are, in fact, the most potent part of eroticism and bring him the most powerful erection and orgasm. At the moment of apparent subjugation—with his almost total feminization—the transvestite converts defeat into triumph through orgasm. Men are most often excluded from the transvestite's fantasy world, and any erotic fantasy into which they are insinuated is quickly aborted. In the psychotherapeutic transference, the male psychiatrist may be dealt with as an anonymous spectator or otherwise disavowed. Although the sex of the psychiatrist ordinarily does not make much difference, it may matter in transvestism. While it is difficult for the male psychiatrist to achieve access to fantasies, it may be impossible for a female psychiatrist to work with the eroticized defenses of subjugation and feminization by women.

Occasionally a transvestic man recollects having been punitively cross-dressed by a female relative, giving rise at that moment to the perversion. There is no doubt boys are punished in that way, just as there is no doubt children are seduced. However, since the fantasy of being forced by women to cross-dress is an important compromise formation in the transvestic person's eroticism, there is the distinct possibility that the ''recollection'' is a screen memory.

As transvestic persons age, relief of separation anxiety sometimes predominates over sexual arousal as the motivation for cross-dressing. There is a subgroup of transvestic men for whom the polarization between merger and masculine individuation is most acute. Under pressure of the losses and debility of aging, vulnerability to separation and abandonment becomes insurmountable, and masculinity is sacrificed to total feminine identification. Those cases begin to look more like gender identity disorders, and affected persons may gravitate toward sex reassignment surgery.

SEXUAL SADISM AND SEXUAL MASOCHISM The diagnostic criteria for sexual masochism are outlined in Table 21.2-5. The criteria for sexual sadism are outlined in Table 21.2-6.

It is notable that both conditions involve intense fantasies,

TABLE 21.2-5
Diagnostic Criteria for Sexual Masochism

A. Over a period of at least six months, recurrent, intense sexually arousing fantasies, sexual urges, or behaviors involving the act (real, not simulated) of being humiliated, beaten, bound, or otherwise made to suffer.
B. The fantasies, sexual urges, or behaviors cause clinically significant distress or impairment in social, occupational, or other important areas of functioning.

TABLE 21.2-6
Diagnostic Criteria for Sexual Sadism

A. Over a period of at least six months, recurrent, intense sexually arousing fantasies, sexual urges, or behaviors involving acts (real, not simulated) in which the psychological or physical suffering (including humiliation) of the victim is sexually exciting to the person.
B. The fantasies, sexual urges, or behaviors cause clinically significant distress or impairment in social, occupational, or other important areas of functioning.

urges, or behaviors of inflicting pain and humiliation. The only difference is the object of the torment, oneself in the case of the masochist versus the partner in the case of the sadist. A common clinical observation is that the subject-object distinction breaks down. Furthermore, aggression and hatred in sadistic or masochistic form are common to all perversions. Put another way, although officially considered separate diagnoses, sadism and masochism represent two polar but related aspects of the personality. For that reason, the two conditions are considered here under the same heading and are frequently referred to generically as sadomasochism. The power of sadomasochistic fantasies derives from poorly compensated fears of injury and reactive narcissistic rage. Triumph over fear of injury (equivalent to fear of feminine identification and castration) and expression of narcissistic rage (equivalent to reassertion of bodily integrity) provide the motivation for constant reenactment of actuations of power and dominance.

In sexual masochism, excitement is linked with the *passive* experience of physical or emotional subjugation, humiliation, discomfort, danger, abuse, or torture (any of which may be simulated or real). Sexual sadism is the reciprocal, excitement being linked to the *active* infliction, in fantasy or reality, of danger, humiliation, subjugation, abuse, or torture. (Some consider necrophilia the most extreme form of sexual sadism, since the power to resist is nullified and the subjugation of the sexual object is complete.) A useful definition is that sadomasochism consists of repeated fantasies and behaviors characterized by a wish to control (or be controlled) by domination, denigration, or pain in order to achieve sexual arousal and release.

Although relatively pure sadistic or masochistic persons exist, the most common finding is that the active or passive perversion is preferential but not exclusive. Sadists also indulge in masochistic fantasies or practices, and the subjugated, compliant masochist is often quite able to take the opposite role with arousal and pleasure. Neither condition is exclusive to men or women, although masochistic practices are more common among women and sadistic among men.

A stable, married couple illustrate a number of features of sadomasochism. His sexual arousal was dependent on inflicting pain in various ways but preferably by pulling out her hair. Hair pulling had gone to the point that wigs, heavy eyebrow pencil, and general cosmesis were required. The patient showed a tolerance to his ritual like that of an addict to his drug. Habituation of arousal resulted in more elaborate hair-pulling rituals, sadistic preoccupation, and more extreme acts, so that murder in the pursuit of an erection and orgasm became a possibility. Although the female partner participated willingly and was erotically responsive, after sex she was contemptuous of her husband. The male partner, sadistic and dominant during foreplay, was humble and submissive postcoitally. Although there was a risk that *she* would be killed during foreplay, *he* had asked her to kill him after intercourse. It was frightening to her that she could entertain sadistically enjoyable visions of doing just that. His hospitalization was required to interrupt the cycle. It is also worth noting that he suffered from ejaculatory incompetence, which could only be relieved through the perversion. Although it has not received much attention, there is often a connection between ejaculatory incompetence and sadism.

In another case, a 25-year-old female graduate student asked for a consultation because of depression and marital discord. The patient had been married for five years, during which time both she and her husband were in school. For the past three years, her academic performance had been consistently better than his, and she attributed their frequent, intense arguments to that. She noted that she experienced a feeling of sexual excitement when her husband screamed at her or hit her in a rage. Sometimes she would taunt him until he had sexual intercourse with her in a brutal fashion, as if she were being raped. She experienced the brutality and sense of being punished as sexually exciting.

One year before the consultation, the patient had found herself often ending arguments by storming out of the house. On one such occasion she went to a "singles' bar," picked up a man, and got him to slap her as part of their sexual activity. She found the "punishment" sexually exciting and subsequently fantasized about being beaten during masturbation to orgasm. The patient then discovered that she enjoyed receiving physical punishment at the hands of strange men more than any other type of sexual stimulus. In a setting in which she could be whipped or beaten, all aspects of sexual activity, including the quality of orgasms, were far in excess of anything she had previously experienced.

That sexual preference was not the reason for the consultation, however. She complained that she could not live without her husband, yet could not live with him. She had suicidal fantasies stemming from the fear that he would leave her.

She recognized that her sexual behavior was dangerous to herself and felt mildly ashamed of it. She was unaware of any possible reasons for its emergence and was not sure she wished treatment for it, because it gave her so much pleasure.

Discussion Fantasies of being humiliated, beaten, bound, or otherwise made to suffer may increase sexual excitement for some people whose sexual life is in all other respects unremarkable. However, when sexually arousing fantasies of that kind are acted out (as in this case) or are markedly distressing, the diagnosis of sexual masochism is made.

With the limited information available, it is not possible to determine if the patient's marital problem was primarily (1) a symptom of the sexual masochism (for example, did she provoke arguments in order to be sexually aroused?); (2) a symptom of a personality disorder; or (3) a problem unrelated to a mental disorder for which the V code partner relational problem would be appropriate. (From *DSM-IV Casebook.* Used with permission.)

EXHIBITIONISM AND VOYEURISM Exhibitionism is defined in DSM-IV according to the criteria represented in Table 21.2-7. Voyeurism is defined as in Table 21.2-8.

Although to comply with the nomenclature, exhibitionism

TABLE 21.2-7
Diagnostic Criteria for Exhibitionism

A. Over a period of at least six months, recurrent, intense sexually arousing fantasies, sexual urges, or behaviors involving the exposure of one's genitals to an unsuspecting stranger.
B. The fantasies, sexual urges, or behaviors cause clinically significant distress or impairment in social, occupational, or other important areas of functioning.

TABLE 21.2-8
Diagnostic Criteria for Voyeurism

A. Over a period of at least six months, recurrent, intense sexually arousing fantasies, sexual urges, or behaviors involving the act of observing an unsuspecting person who is naked, in the process of disrobing, or engaging in sexual activity.
B. The fantasies, sexual urges, or behaviors cause clinically significant distress or impairment in social, occupational, or other important areas of functioning.

Table from DSM-IV, *Diagnostic and Statistical Manual of Mental Disorders,* ed 4. Copyright American Psychiatric Association, Washington, 1994. Used with permission.

and voyeurism must be diagnosed independently; like sadism and masochism they are in many respects paired opposites. Exhibitionism involves acts of exposing the genitals to a stranger or unsuspecting person. Voyeurism, conversely, involves repetitively seeking out situations in which unsuspecting women may be observed while disrobing, grooming, or copulating. In both situations, sexual excitement occurs in anticipation of the exposure or observation, and orgasm is brought about by masturbation during or after the event.

Exhibitionism and voyeurism, showing and looking, define opposite positions along the scopophiliac axis and have related dynamics. The preferential object—young girls, women with large breasts, brunettes, and so on—is selected because of attributes which facilitate her substitution for mother in reenacting the struggle over separation and castration. In exhibitionism the presence and power of the phallus is reasserted by watching the confronted woman's reaction (fright, surprise, awe, or disgust). The exhibitionist both identifies with his victim and feels contemptuously superior to her. The voyeur watches a woman to note the true nature of her genitals and identifies with her. However, he reassures himself through masturbation that his penis is intact and that he is superior.

Although exhibitionists and voyeurs may marry, the importance of the relationship often lies in the wife's maternal qualities. Sexual performance is usually lackadaisical—a frequent wives' complaint—because real excitement is limited to showing or looking.

A 27-year-old engineer requested consultation because of irresistible urges to exhibit his penis to female strangers.

The patient, an only child, had been reared in an orthodox Jewish environment. Sexuality was strongly condemned by both parents as being "dirty." His father, a schoolteacher, was authoritarian and punitive, but relatively uninvolved in the home. His mother, a housewife, was domineering, controlling, and intrusive. She was preoccupied with cleanliness and bathed the patient until he was 10. The patient remembers that he feared he might have an erection in his mother's presence during one of his baths; however, that did not occur. His mother was opposed to his meeting and dating girls during his adolescence. He was not allowed to bring girls home; according to his mother, the proper time to bring a woman home was when she was "his wife, and not before." Despite his mother's antisexual values, she frequently walked about the house partially disrobed in his presence. To his shame, he found himself sexually aroused by that stimulation, which occurred frequently throughout his development.

As an adolescent the patient was quiet, withdrawn, and studious; teachers described him as a "model child." He was friendly, but not intimate, with a few male classmates. Puberty occurred at age 13, and his first ejaculation occurred at that age during sleep. Because of feelings of guilt, he resisted the temptation to masturbate, and between the ages of 13 and 18 orgasms occurred only with nocturnal emissions.

He did not begin to date women until he moved out of his parents' home, at the age of 25. During the next two years he dated from time to time, but was too inhibited to initiate sexual activity.

At age 18, for reasons unknown to himself, during the week before final exams, he first experienced an overwhelming desire to engage in exhibitionism, for which he now sought consultation. He sought situations in which he was alone with a woman he did not know. As he would approach her, he became sexually excited. He would then walk up to her and display his erect penis. He found that her shock and fear further stimulated him, and usually he would then ejaculate. At other times he fantasized past encounters while masturbating.

He felt guilty and ashamed after exhibiting himself and vowed never to repeat it. Nevertheless, the desire often overwhelmed him, and the behavior recurred frequently, usually at periods of tension. He felt desperate, but was too ashamed to seek professional help. Once, when he was 24, he had almost been apprehended by a policeman, but managed to run away.

For the previous three years, the patient had managed to resist his exhibitionistic urges. Then he met a woman, who fell in love with him and was willing to have intercourse with him. Never having had intercourse before, he felt panic lest he fail in the attempt. He liked and respected his potential sex partner, but also condemned her for being willing to engage in premarital relations. He once again started to exhibit himself and feared that, unless he stopped he would eventually be arrested.

Discussion One could discuss at great length the childhood experiences that may have contributed to the development of this disorder in this patient. Regarding the diagnosis, however, there can be little speculation. Recurrent intense sexual urges and sexually arousing fantasies involving the exposure of one's genitals to a stranger, acted upon or causing marked distress, establish the diagnosis of exhibitionism.

Many clinicians would assume that there was also a coexisting personality disorder, but without more information about the patient's personality functioning, such a diagnosis cannot be made. (From *DSM-IV Casebook.* Used with permission.)

PEDOPHILIA The diagnostic criteria for pedophilia are outlined in Table 21.2-9.

Pedophilia involves preferential sexual activity with children, either in fantasy or actuality. Adult sexual activities or fantasies involving prepubertal children, the essential behavior in pedophilia, may be exclusively homosexual or heterosexual, or a mixture of both, and may occur within the family, among acquaintance groups, or between strangers. Incestuous pedophilia is a problematic concept in that incest almost always begins in childhood but is often carried well past puberty into adolescence. In incest, the issue may not be so much a preference for children as an enactment of the sexual and aggressive tensions within the family. Incest victims tend to be somewhat older than victims of pedophilia, and incest offenders do not tend to show pedophiliac inclinations otherwise, although there are exceptions. One stereotype that needs to be dismantled in either type of child molestation is that of the seductive child who "invited" the sexual advance of the adult. Most data indi-

TABLE 21.2-9
Diagnostic Criteria for Pedophilia

A. Over a period of at least six months, recurrent, intense sexually arousing fantasies, sexual urges, or behaviors involving sexual activity with a prepubescent child or children (generally age 13 years or younger).
B. The fantasies, sexual urges, or behaviors cause clinically significant distress or impairment in social, occupational, or other important areas of functioning.
C. The person is at least age 16 years and at least 5 years older than the child or children in Criterion A.
Note: Do not include an individual in late adolescence involved in an ongoing sexual relationship with a 12- or 13-year-old.

Specify if:
Sexually attracted to males
Sexually attracted to females
Sexually attracted to both

Specify if:
Limited to incest

Specify type:
Exclusive type (attracted only to children)
Nonexclusive type

Table from DSM-IV, *Diagnostic and Statistical Manual of Mental Disorders,* ed 4. Copyright American Psychiatric Association, Washington, 1994. Used with permission.

cate that the so-called seductiveness is in the eye of the beholder and serves mainly as a convenient rationalization.

Pedophiliac perversions vary in their most conspicuous elements. In some, seduction predominates: the pedophiliac person plays games with the child, slowly steering the game's contingencies into sexual areas. Not uncommonly, the child is involved in a version of strip poker, leading to genital exposure. The pedophiliac person ordinarily feels excited and triumphant at that accomplishment and masturbates surreptitiously while the child is present or openly once the child has gone. In that form, the game, the stratagems to overcome the child's hesitations, and the looking are the exciting elements. In other variations, the child is induced to allow manipulation of his or her genitals or to manipulate the adult's. In all instances, the pedophile luxuriates in prepubescent or pubescent sexuality.

Although it is commonly stated that only a small percentage of pedophiliac encounters results in injury or death, aggression and sadism are inherent in the paraphilia. Pedophilia not only involves narcissistic identification with the child but also domination over the child. Children serve as an alternative to frightening adult partners, presenting the opportunity to terrify rather than be terrified. The pedophiliac person's physical superiority fosters the erotically tinged aggression so important in arousal. The aggression may be under control or may be out of awareness, but it is never far away. Where the sexual partner is a child and comparatively helpless, injury may be inflicted in passion, in panic, or in cold blood.

A cold, isolated, paranoid professional man described himself as a ''chicken hawk,'' a slang term for homophiliac pedophiles. (Young boys are the ''chickens.'') An unmarried man, he had befriended a divorced woman and her two sons, feigning interest in her in order to be near them. He found contact with them—holding them on his lap, reading bedtime stories, and so forth—highly arousing. The arousal, however, was associated with an increasing rage. The aggressive affect troubled him because earlier in his life, he had ''raped'' and killed animals and was afraid of losing control. Another patient, brought for consultation by his parents, acknowledged an interest in boys but steadfastly maintained that his predilections were under control. He was subsequently charged with the kidnapping, sexual abuse, and murder of boys in several states. He was tried, convicted of first-degree murder, and executed.

FROTTEURISM The diagnostic criteria for frotteurism are outlined in Table 21.2-10. Frotteurism is a sexual preference that involves a fantasy or activity of fondling or rubbing against an unfamiliar woman in public places. The fondling or rubbing may be so fleeting as to be virtually subliminal or may be so blatant as to be almost assaultive. Usually, the frotteur flees as soon as he is discovered, and the sexual act is completed by surreptitious masturbation. Sometimes, however, the excitement may lead to instant ejaculation.

Dynamically, contact and fondling often represent eroticized maternal contact which elicits both merger and castration fears. For that reason the contact is brief and orgasm necessary to reassert bodily integrity.

TABLE 21.2-10
Diagnostic Criteria for Frotteurism

A. Over a period of at least six months, recurrent, intense sexually arousing fantasies, sexual urges, or behaviors involving touching and rubbing against a nonconsenting person.
B. The fantasies, sexual urges, or behaviors cause clinically significant distress or impairment in social, occupational, or other important areas of functioning.

Table from DSM-IV, *Diagnostic and Statistical Manual of Mental Disorders,* ed 4. Copyright American Psychiatric Association, Washington, 1994. Used with permission.

Charles was 45 when he was referred for psychiatric consultation by his parole officer following his second arrest for rubbing up against a woman in the subway. According to Charles, he had a ''good'' sexual relationship with his wife of 15 years when he began, 10 years ago, to touch women in the subway. A typical episode would begin with his decision to go into the subway to rub against a woman, usually in her 20s. He would select the woman as he walked into the subway station, move in behind her, and wait for the train to arrive at the station. He would be wearing plastic wrap around his penis so as not to stain his pants after ejaculating while rubbing up against his victim. As riders moved on to the train, he would follow the woman he had selected. When the doors closed, he would begin to push his penis up against her buttocks, fantasizing that they were having intercourse in a normal, noncoercive manner. In about half of the episodes, he would ejaculate and then go on to work. If he failed to ejaculate, he would either give up for that day, or change trains and select another victim. According to Charles, he felt guilty immediately after each episode, but would soon find himself ruminating about and anticipating the next encounter. He estimated that he had done this about twice a week for the last 10 years, and thus had probably rubbed up against approximately a thousand women.

During the interview, Charles expressed extreme guilt about his behavior and often cried when talking about fears that his wife or employer would find out about his second arrest. However, he had apparently never thought about how his victims felt about what he did to them.

His personal history did not indicate any obvious mental problems other than being rather inept and unassertive socially, especially with women.

Discussion The recurrent touching and rubbing up against a nonconsenting person for the purpose of sexual arousal and gratification is called frotteurism and is classified as one of the paraphilias. In some classic textbooks frotteurism (rubbing) is distinguished from toucherism (fondling), but both are included in the DSM-IV category of frotteurism. No cases of the disorder have ever been reported in females.

Charles's behavior is typical of that seen in the disorder. A crowded place where there is a wide selection of victims is selected (for example, subway, sports event, mall). In such a setting the initial rubbing of the woman may not be immediately noticed; the victim usually does not protest because she is not absolutely sure what has happened. That probably explains why Charles was arrested only twice.

What is not known is the kind of sexual fantasies that Charles had for years before he actually engaged in the acts of frotteurism. However, as is common in the disorder, while he engaged in the act he fantasized about a loving sexual relationship with the victim. (From *DSM-IV Casebook.* Used with permission.)

PARAPHILIA NOT OTHERWISE SPECIFIED The classification of paraphilia not otherwise specified (NOS) includes varied paraphilias that do not meet the criteria for any of the aforementioned categories (Table 21.2-11).

Coprophilia, klismaphilia, and urophilia Coprophilia refers to erotic excitement related to defecating and feces, klismaphilia to enemas, and urophilia to urine. Together they constitute an important group of excretory perversions. Although analization is characteristic of all perversions, intrinsic to this closely allied group are fascination with dirtiness and soiling and eroticized overinvestment in excretory processes. The unifying feature is the incorporation of excretory functions, excreta, or their close substitutes into sexual activity (including derivative practices such as lewdness or obscenity during intercourse).

TABLE 21.2-11
Diagnostic Criteria for Paraphilia Not Otherwise Specified

This category is included for coding paraphilias that do not meet the criteria for any of the specific categories. Examples include, but are not limited to, telephone scatologia (obscene phone calls), necrophilia (corpses), partialism (exclusive focus on part of body), zoophilia (animals), coprophilia (feces), klismaphilia (enemas), and urophilia (urine).

Table from DSM-IV, *Diagnostic and Statistical Manual of Mental Disorders,* ed 4. Copyright American Psychiatric Association, Washington, 1994. Used with permission.

As a general perverse phenomenon, anality reflects developmental dilemmas and serves important functions. As noted previously, antecedents of perversion occur during separation-individuation concurrently with toilet training and the anal phase. A peculiar child-mother relationship which contributes to poor integration of body image also exaggerates a developmental focus on bodily part objects, such as the fecal mass. To a vulnerable child, separation from his or her stool during defecation may be frightening (reflected in the way some children fight against being placed on the toilet). In some children, such anxiety leads to unusual aggressive investment in elimination manifested either as retention with constipation or expulsion with encopresis. Later, if oedipal strivings and castration anxiety are dealt with regressively, the fecal bolus may become invested with qualities and anxieties more appropriate to the phallus. Under those circumstances the special characteristic of the stool, that it is eliminated but will reform, allows the reenactment of loss and reunion, castration and regeneration.

Telephone scatologia Obscene phone calls are in some ways related to exhibitionism and voyeurism with their central themes of looking or showing. For example, in obscene phone calling tension and arousal begin in anticipation of phoning, an unsuspecting partner is involved, the recipient listens while the caller verbally "exposes" his preoccupations or aurally "observes" her sexual activity, and the conversation is accompanied by masturbation (which is often completed after the contact is interrupted).

Telephone scatologia is also related to the excretory perversions through the lewdness and "dirty talk."

Zoophilia In zoophilia, animals are preferentially incorporated in arousal fantasies or sexual activity. The animal may also be trained to participate. Zoophilia as an organized perversion is rare, while sensual relations with animals are common. For a number of people, animals provide a major source of relatedness, so it is not surprising that some are used sensually or sexually.

Sexual relations with animals may occasionally be an outgrowth of availability or convenience, especially in parts of the world where rigid conventions preclude premarital sexuality or in situations of enforced isolation. Masturbation, however, is available in such situations, so one may suspect some predisposition for animal contact even in "opportunistic" zoophilia.

Hypoxyphilia Another important paraphilia is hypoxyphilia whether accomplished through hanging, use of a plastic bag, or a partner who manipulates gradients of suffocation or strangulation. Fatalities may be deliberate but are often the result of erotic efforts going beyond the narrow envelope of safety. The paraphilia takes an unfortunate toll of solitary adolescents who, given time to develop, might evolve toward partnered, consensual bondage.

A woman heard a man shouting for help and went to his apartment door. Calling through the door, she asked the man inside if he needed help.

"Yes," he said. "Break the door down."

"Is this a joke?"

"No."

The woman returned with her two sons, who broke into the apartment. They found the man lying on the floor, his hands tied behind him, his legs bent back, and his ankles secured to his hands. A mop handle had been placed behind his knees. He was visibly distraught, sweating, and short of breath, and his hands were turning blue. He had defecated and urinated in his trousers. In his kitchen the woman found a knife and freed him.

When police officers arrived and questioned the man, he stated that he had returned home that afternoon, fallen asleep on his couch, and awakened an hour later only to find himself hopelessly bound. The officers noted that the apartment door had been locked when the neighbors broke in. The man continued his story. As far as he knew, he had no enemies, and certainly no friends capable of that kind of practical joke. The officers questioned him about the rope. The man explained that, because he had considered moving in the near future, he kept a bag of rope in his bedroom. Near the couch lay a torn bag, numerous short lengths of thin rope, and a steak knife.

When the officers filed their report, they noted that "this could possibly be a sexual deviation act." Interviewed the next day, the man confessed to binding himself in the position in which he was found.

A month later, the police were called back to the same man's apartment. A building manager had discovered him face down on the floor in his apartment. A paper bag covered his head like a hood. When the police arrived, the man was breathing rapidly with a satin cloth stuffed in his mouth. Rope was stretched around his head and mouth and wrapped his chest and waist. Several lengths ran from his back to his crotch, and ropes at his ankles had left deep marks. A broom handle locked his elbows behind his back. Once freed, the man explained, "While doing isometric exercises, I got tangled up in the rope."

Police interviewed the man's employer, and the employer subsequently advised him to seek counseling. When the man agreed to follow through on a referral to a private psychiatrist, his boss supported his assertion that the incident, although unfortunate, had been unique and would not recur.

Two years passed and the man moved on to another job. He failed to appear for work one Monday morning. A fellow employee found him dead in his apartment.

During their investigation, police were able to reconstruct the man's final minutes. On the preceding Friday, he had bound himself in the following manner: sitting on his bed and crossing his ankles, left over right, he had bound them together with twine. Fastening a tie around his neck, he then secured the tie to an 86-inch pole behind his back. Aligning the pole with his left side, the upper end crossing the front of his left shoulder, he placed his hands behind his bent legs and there, leaving his wrists 4 inches apart, secured them with a length of rope. He then tied the rope that secured his wrists to the pole and to an electric cord girdling his waist. Thus bound, he lay on his bed on his back and stretched his legs. By thus applying pressure to the pole, still secured to the tie around his neck, he strangled himself. In order to save himself, he might have rolled over onto his side and drawn up his legs; but the upper end of the pole pressed against the wall. He was locked into place.

Discussion This man aroused himself sexually by depriving himself of oxygen while masturbating, thereby risking death. Such bizarre sexual behavior has to be regarded as a paraphilia, a sexual disorder in which the person is aroused by stimuli that are not part of normative arousal-activity patterns and that in varying degrees may interfere with the capacity for reciprocal, affectionate sexual activity.

This particular paraphilia, hypoxyphilia (hypoxy = lack of oxygen), is not common enough to be included as a specific paraphilia in DSM-IV and therefore is coded as a paraphilia not otherwise specified. The case was one of the few that has come to psychiatric attention before the death of the patient. When people with the disorder seek treatment, it is usually for depression, and they are unlikely to reveal their sexual practices unless a therapist takes a very careful sexual history. The most commonly associated paraphilias are sexual masochism and transvestic fetishism.

An estimated 500–1,000 people die annually in the United States from autoerotic asphyxiation; almost all (96 percent) are male. Deaths occur among persons from adolescence through the 70s, the greatest frequency being in the 20s. A complication of hypoxyphilia, other than death, is anoxic brain damage. (From P E Dietz, A W Burgess, R R Hazelwood: Autoerotic asphyxia, the paraphilias, and mental disorder. In *Autoerotic Fatalities,* R R Hazelwood, P E Dietz, A W Burgess, editors, p 83. Lexington Books, Lexington, MA, 1983.)

Necrophilia Necrophilia is erotic interest in the dead or near-dead and may involve sexual intercourse or masturbation in or around corpses or the dying. It is not clear how many murders associated with rape are committed in order to provide a sexual object that is either dead or dying, but some are perpetrated for precisely that reason.

Partialism Partialism devotes exclusive focus on a part of the body, such as a foot, rather than the whole person, as a source of sexual excitement and release. Part object substitution for human intimacy is characteristic of paraphilia.

DIFFERENTIAL DIAGNOSIS

Descriptive diagnosis is based on the presence of signs and symptoms meeting the DSM-IV criteria. In brief, criteria include the presence of the pathognomonic fantasy and its behavioral elaboration, providing that they have been present for at least six months and have been disturbing. The fantasy includes unusual sexual material, which is relatively fixed but may show occasional variations. The achievement of arousal and orgasm is dependent on mental elaboration or behavioral playing out of the fantasy. Sexual activity is ritualized or stereotyped and makes use of degraded, reduced, or dehumanized objects. Paraphiliacs regularly show earmarks of borderline personality disorder (for example, affect intolerance, rigidity in relationships, preambivalent orientation, inability to grieve, and use of primitive defenses, such as splitting, projection, and denial). They have symptoms that appear dynamically rooted in separation-individuation and phallic-narcissistic difficulties, such as dyadic object relations, body image instability, aggressivization of body parts and functions, and separation and castration anxieties.

The paraphilias must be differentiated from gender identity disorders, anxiety disorders, personality disorders, schizophrenia and other psychotic disorders, and normal experimentation. The gender identity disorders are characterized by a conscious sense of inappropriateness in the anatomically congruent sex role, a feeling that improvement would occur with role reversal, homoerotic interest, and heterosexual inhibition, and a desire for surgical intervention. Castration wishes growing out of feminine identification are handled concretely, such that bodily integrity is not protected through symbolization. In paraphilias the cross-sexual identification and the wish for role reversal are largely unconscious and, unless defenses fail, do not emerge with much power. In fact, paraphiliac fantasies and rituals help to maintain repression and symbolization so that physical integrity is preserved.

Paraphilias share many psychogenetic, characterological, and defensive features with borderline character disorder, and, reciprocally, borderline characters regularly show perverse trends. If those trends organize as the central defensive structure, the diagnosis shifts from borderline personality disorder to paraphilia. Deviant sexual currents are also found in schizophrenia, but are poorly organized, rapidly shifting attempts at discharge. Paraphilias may decay into psychosis, but in the majority of such cases soft signs of schizophrenia were already present. Perverse fantasies are universal in the anxiety disorders, but are unconscious and seldom acted upon. Furthermore, such fantasies in a neurotic person do not carry the same prognosis as an active perversion in a person with borderline personality disorder.

In the sexual dysfunctions, occasional perversity may be present without being obligatory or persistent. On the other hand, sexual dysfunction (for example, ejaculatory incompetence) may complicate a paraphilia. Since "paraphiliac" fantasies are common in foreplay, there may be occasional behaviors reflecting those fantasies in normal sexual activity. The fantasies and activities, however, are experimental rather than compulsive, preemptory, and obligatory.

PSYCHIATRIC EXAMINATION The findings on psychiatric examination reflect the descriptive, developmental, and dynamic features described in the preceding sections and tables. To obtain necessary diagnostic material, however, may be difficult. The task is to encourage the patient to share enough for a genuine clinical evaluation, since the perversion may be largely ego-syntonic but protected from inquiry by guilt, shame, or fear of humiliation. Experienced clinicians agree that a vital history requires an unhurried pace, careful attention to the sequencing and direction of the patient's associations, the use of questions that broaden the field of inquiry rather than foreclosing it, and curiosity about realms of human experience conspicuously omitted from associations.

Despite the concerns mentioned above, most patients are interested in telling their stories and will do so unless impediments are put in their way. One impediment is the one-hour (or even briefer) evaluation. One hour is seldom enough to get over the anxiety and reserve the patient justifiably feels at discussing his or her life. Three hours set aside for evaluation (assuming the situation is not complicated by the strictures of managed care), the hours separated by several days or a week, allow some familiarity and comfort to develop and give recall a chance to work. Since issues of separation and loss are important in the perversions, a facet of the extended evaluation is that it allows the patient to see that separation is compensated for by reappearance at the agreed-on time and place. The disappearance of extreme symptomatology—suicidal impulses, panic, and driven masturbation—during an evaluation is not unusual and is a good prognostic sign.

Another impediment to the psychiatric evaluation is the structured history, an often abused device. The place for a structured interview is in the psychiatrist's head, where it may serve as an internal, logical outline against which the patient's version of his or her history may be quietly and unobtrusively checked. Patients do not organize their histories in an obviously logical way (although they often follow internal logic) and they should not be straitjacketed. What is important is the way in which the patient tells the story: his or her sequencing, connections, emphasis, omissions, and so forth.

In extended evaluations, unstructured by the psychiatrist but structured by the patient, fantasies and behaviors emerge in the context of historical events, defensive maneuvers, superego constraints, and ego operations, which make the history come alive in a way essential for treatment selection.

In the first evaluation interview, a young man reported compulsive masturbation and frequent and risky obscene telephoning following a loss. He also recalled that his father died when he was eight years old. In the second interview, he remembered a period of driven masturbation after his father's death, associated in time with arguments with his mother. In the third interview, he recalled being taken to see a child psychiatrist to whom he confided a fear for his mother's safety. He had a vague memory that he had some rituals designed to protect her from harm. As an adolescent and adult, the patient was solicitous of his mother and had never dated. His only eroticism was occasional masturbation and rare obscene phone-calling. While it is impossible to make a definitive formulation, the nature and sequence of the material would allow the following hypothesis (among others). The death of the patient's father heightened fears about rivalry and competitive impulses. Related castration anxieties were partially dealt with by compulsive masturbation. By itself, that method was insufficient to handle his anger, guilt, and fear so that the patient became regressively identified with and attached to his mother. That attachment, however, increased his erotic interest, his castration anxiety, and fear for his masculinity. The "victory" in possessing mother solely for himself was undercut by fear, hostility, and guilt leading to preoccupation with her death. With the heightened drive tensions of adolescence, the correspondingly increased anxiety required the safeguard of sexual asceticism (albeit with the occasional breakthrough of paraphiliac sexuality). When he experienced another significant loss, childhood and adolescent anxieties were revivified, and he regressed to infantile conflicts, heightened drive tensions, and perverse attempts at stabilization. Over time, of course, that formulation would be subjected to the clinical test and modified as necessary.

One almost universal factor in evaluation is the patient's insistence that the perversion itself is not troublesome and is no cause for concern. The perversion is often depicted not as the culprit but as the one positive joy in life, any symptoms or inhibitions being viewed as unrelated. In fact, if totally honest, the paraphiliac person might add that his or her erotic preferences were superior to the humdrum sexuality of others. Only in intensive psychotherapy or psychoanalysis might it be recognized that the magical grandeur of the perversion was purchased at the price of maturation in the currency of sadness, isolation, and frustration.

PSYCHOLOGICAL TESTING For some patients psychological testing is useful. It is often useful to have an assessment of intelligence and general psychopathology in the evaluation of paraphilias. The Minnesota Multiphasic Personality Inventory (MMPI), the NEO-Personality Inventory, and the Brief Symptom Inventory are general tests that have frequently been used in clinical studies of paraphilias and therefore offer a broad base for interpretation. Another frequently employed but specialized test is the Derogatis Sexual Function Inventory (DSFI), an omnibus instrument with several scales that are valuable in assessing paraphilia, including experience (varieties of behavior), androgyny (masculine and feminine identifications), and fantasy (including paraphiliac fantasies). Although not often mentioned in more recent research studies, the utility of projective testing should not be overlooked.

UNSETTLED ISSUES There are a variety of unsettled issues. One is symptom choice, that is, the selection of a given perverse theme from among all the possibilities. Since the central constructs appear to be shared, what factors differentiate a transvestite from a zoophile? The best answer is that symptom choice appears determined by the dynamically important subsidiary goals: for example, transvestism may serve those whose maternal identification is strongest and are most vulnerable to separation anxiety, while zoophilia may be elaborated when the greatest need is to express hostile degradation of threatening human objects.

Another matter is the apparent specificity of the perversions as virtually a male domain. In fact, however, female sadists, masochists, exhibitionists, fetishists, and pedophiles do exist so that the exclusivity is more apparent than real. Men have a need to erect conspicuous clinical edifices to deny the possibility of castration. Perversion in females is expressed in a more subtle form in which the essential ingredient often being the manipulation and use of a vulnerable man. The old saw that if a man stops by a window to watch a woman undress, he is arrested for peeping and that if a woman stops by a window to watch a man undress, he is arrested for exposure reflects both the subtlety of and the cultural tolerance for what in some women is the female equivalent of paraphiliac activities.

Another controversial issue is the degree of psychopathology. The paraphilias are often considered wholly pathological because they are "inherently disadvantageous." Some authors have questioned that assumption, and have argued that the reasons for declassifying homosexuality apply in large measure to the paraphilias. For others, however, the arguments turn on the capacity for affectionate relationships: affectionate and loving relations are considered possible in homosexuality or heterosexuality but not in the paraphilias. Nonetheless, affection and love may develop in paraphilias as in homosexuality or heterosexuality. Conversely, in heterosexuality, homosexuality, and paraphilia there may be total absence of affectionate attachment. For some homosexual men the entire criterion of a satisfactory liaison is the availability and size of a partner's penis, and for some heterosexual men the size of a partner's breasts may be critical, relationships as fundamentally dehumanized as the relationship of a fetishist to his partner's feet. The capacity for affectionate attachment is not dependent upon the specific sexual preference but upon the degree of ego strengths.

The paraphilias are a composite product of psychological development that has suffered serious interference. There may be the capacity for affectionate ties or the object relations may be of the most degraded or tenuous sort. Psychopathology may run from the near-psychotic to the near-neurotic. The person may feel quite well, be enthusiastic about his or her practices, and be unable to imagine himself or herself as different even though sexuality and often generativity have been wrenched out of place. Certainly, treatment cannot prevail without the patient's sincerest efforts.

COURSE AND PROGNOSIS

While prognosis in the treatment of paraphilia is generally guarded, pessimism is not always justified. Prognosis varies according to ego strengths, the quality of object relationships, the rigidity and nature of defensive operations, the tolerance for anxiety and other affects, and the age of the patient. In some persons, many of those factors are positive.

The treatment of impulsive and driven paraphilias is somewhat more hopeful than formerly because of the use of antiandrogens. Enthusiasm for the treatment must be tempered, however, by the fact that a majority of treatment completers relapse during follow-up.

While no good data are available, the degree of compulsion in the paraphilias appears to decrease as the patient ages, along with a general decline in sexual preoccupations. In a number of paraphilias, the natural course of the condition is characterized by intermittent manifestations, so that for long periods deviant behavior may be absent. Spontaneous recovery, however, is unlikely.

TREATMENT

Treatment of paraphilias is subject to the same conditions and constraints as other areas of psychiatry or medicine. The fundamental task is to select the technique that will maximize the patient's chances for recovery and optimal health, respecting both the inroads of the disease and latent strengths.

Treatment selection depends on an assessment of tolerance for regression, synthetic and sublimatory capacities, and motivation. When those factors are sufficient, there is the opportunity to examine and unseat the illness through psychoanalysis. Psychoanalysis is effective through the transferential resurrection of the passions and relationships condensed in the perversion and their reexamination through the eyes of an adult ego. Such elemental forces are not to be reawakened without due concern for the patient's ability to withstand them, but with sufficient strengths the freeing up of stymied potentials leads to personal renovation. When fewer ego strengths are available, dynamic psychotherapy is likely to be beneficial in reducing and stabilizing pressures from the perversion and in freeing other aspects of life from its interference.

Cognitive and behavioral approaches, singly or in combination, have also been useful in modifying thought patterns and behaviors in a number of paraphilias. Sex therapy techniques are basically cognitive or behavioral methods and are included within this category. Suggested techniques have included covert sensitization, imaginal desensitization, thought stopping, masturbatory reconditioning, and aversive conditioning. In some instances, phallometric assessment has provided an important independent measure of change. In general terms, those approaches are designed to decrease paraphiliac interest and behavior, increase nondeviant behavior, and manage untoward consequences of paraphiliac thoughts and actions. Behavior modification techniques also have their place in detoxifying severe, compulsive, and driven perversions. The addictlike development of tolerance to ritual has been emphasized by so-called sexual addiction programs. Those methods, based on ones developed by Alcoholics Anonymous, may help stabilize driven or compulsive paraphilias, although their narrow focus often leads to correspondingly limited results.

Psychotropic agents, including major tranquilizers, may also be used in those perversions that are acutely or dangerously compulsive. Recently, there have been case reports of the use of lithium carbonate (Eskalith), imipramine (Tofranil), and especially fluoxetine (Prozac) in the treatment of a wide variety of paraphilias. The reports have been generally positive in terms of relief of paraphiliac compulsivity and improvement in the broader symptom picture. Antiandrogens, such as medroxyprogesterone acetate (Provera), have been used in treating perversions with good results in carefully selected cases. Medroxyprogesterone appears to be particularly beneficial for those patients whose driven hypersexuality (for example, constant masturbation, frantic sexual contact, or assaultive sexuality) is out of control. The possible adverse effects of long-term use, (for example, hypertension, diabetes, and gallbladder dysfunction) must be monitored.

Although far from unique to the treatment of paraphilias, special problems are posed in contemporary treatment by the managed care climate. While it may present ethical dilemmas for the psychiatrist, it is tragic for the patient with a complex perversion—threatening marriage, family, livelihood, and freedom—to be referred for diagnosis and treatment within a few sessions. No treatment modality—pharmacological, behavioral, dynamic, or otherwise—is likely to be effective in paraphilias without extended treatment contact.

SUGGESTED CROSS-REFERENCES

Topics relevant to the paraphilias include gender identity disorders (Section 21.3), personality disorders (Chapter 25), and sexual dysfunctions (Section 21.1a). Also germane are the discussions of pervasive developmental disorders (Chapter 37) and separation anxiety disorder in children (Section 43.1).

REFERENCES

Arndt W Jr: *Gender Disorders and the Paraphilias.* International Universities Press, Madison, CT, 1991.
Bak R C: The phallic woman: The ubiquitous fantasy in perversion. Psychoanal Study Child *23:* 15, 1968.
Blanchard R, Collins P I: Men with sexual interest in transvestites, transsexuals, and she-males. J Nerv Ment Dis *181:* 570, 1993.
Bradford J M, Pawlak A: Double-blind placebo crossover study of cyproterone acetate in the treatment of the paraphilias. Arch Sex Behav *22:* 383, 1993.
Bradford J M, Pawlak A: Effects of cyproterone acetate on sexual arousal patterns of pedophiles. Arch Sex Behav *22:* 629, 1993.
Chalkley A, Powell E: The clinical description of forty-eight cases of sexual fetishism. Br J Psychiatry *142:* 292, 1983.
Coates S, Friedman R C, Wolfe S: The etiology of boyhood gender identity disorders: A model for integrating temperament, development, and psychodynamics. Psychoanal Dial *1:* 481, 1991.
Cooper A: Progestogens in the treatment of male sex offenders: A review. Can J Psychiatry *31:* 73, 1986.
Cooper A, Cernovovsky Z: The effects of cyproterone acetate on sleeping and waking penile erections in pedophiles: Possible implications for treatment. Can J Psychiatry *37:* 33, 1992.
Ellis H: *Studies of the Psychology of Sex. Analysis of the Sexual Impulse; Love and Pain; The Sexual Impulse in Women.* Davis, Philadelphia, 1904.
Fagan P, Wise T, Schmidt C Jr, Ponticas Y, Marshall R, Costa P: A comparison of five-factor personality dimensions in males with sexual dysfunction and males with paraphilia. J Pers Assess *57:* 434, 1991.
*Freud S: Three essays on the theory of sexuality. In *Standard Edition of the Complete Psychological Works of Sigmund Freud,* J Strachey, editor, Vol 7, p 135. Hogarth, London, 1953.
Freund K, Blanchard R: The concept of courtship disorder. J Sex Marital Ther *12:* 79, 1986.
Freund K, Kuban M: Deficient erotic gender differentiations in pedophilia: A follow-up. Arch Sex Behav *22:* 619, 1993.
Grossman L: The perverse attitude toward reality. Psychoanal Q *62:* 422, 1993.
Hawton K: Behavioural approaches to the management of sexual deviations. Br J Psychiatry *143:* 248, 1983.
Kafka M: Successful treatment of paraphilic coercive disorder (a rapist) with fluoxetine hydrochloride. Br J Psychiatry *158:* 844, 1991.
Kaplan, L: *Female Perversions: The Temptations of Madame Bovary.* Doubleday, New York, 1991.
Kaul, A: Sex offenders—cure or management? Med Sci Law *33:* 207, 1993.
Krafft-Ebing R von: *Psychopathia Sexualis.* Stein and Day, New York, 1978.
Langevin R, Day D, Handy L, Russon A: Are incestuous fathers pedophilic, aggressive, and alcoholic? In *Erotic Preference, Gender Identity and Aggression in Men,* R Langevin, editor, p 137. Erlbaum, Hillsdale, NJ, 1985.
Laws D, Marshall W: Masturbatory reconditioning with sexual deviates: An evaluative review. Adv Behav Res Ther *13:* 13, 1991.
Lebegue B: Paraphilias in U.S. pornography titles: "Pornography made me do it" (Ted Bundy). Bull Am Acad Psychiatry Law *19:* 43, 1991.
Levine S B: Gender-disturbed males. J Sex Marital Ther *19:* 131, 1993.
Mancia M: The absent father: His role in the sexual deviations and in transference. Int J Psychoanal *74:* 941, 1993.
McDougall J: Primal scene and sexual perversion. Int J Psychoanal *53:* 371, 1972.
McDougall J: The anonymous spectator: A clinical study of sexual perversion. Contemp Psychoanal *10:* 289, 1974.
*Meyer J: The theory of gender identity disorders. J Am Psychoanal Assoc *30:* 381, 1982.
Meyer W 3d, Walker P, Emory L, Smith E: Physical, metabolic, and hormonal effects on men of long-term therapy with medroxyprogesterone acetate. Fertil Steril *43:* 102, 1985.
Meyer-Bahlburg H: Psychoendocrine research on sexual orientation. Current status and future options. Prog Brain Res *61:* 375, 1984.
Nabokov V: *The Annotated Lolita.* McGraw-Hill, New York, 1970.
Perilstein R, Lipper S, Friedman L: Three cases of paraphilia responsive to fluoxetine treatment. J Clin Psychiatry *52:* 169, 1991.
*Sachs H (1923): On the genesis of perversion. Psychoanal Q *55:* 477, 1986.
Simon W: Deviance as history: The future of perversion. Arch Sex Behav *23:* 1, 1994.
Socarides C W: *The Preoedipal Origin and Psychoanalytic Therapy of Sexual Perversions.* International Universities Press, Madison, CT, 1988.
*Stoller R J: *Pain and Passion.* Plenum, New York, 1991.
*Stoller R J: *Perversion: The Erotic Form of Hatred.* Pantheon, New York, 1975.
Waites E: Fixing women: Devaluation, idealization, and the female fetish. J Am Psychoanal Assoc *30:* 435, 1982.
Wise T, Fagan P, Schmidt C Jr, Ponticas Y, Costa P: Personality and sexual functioning of transvestic fetishists and other paraphilics. J Nerv Ment Dis *179:* 694, 1991.
Young G R, Wagner E E: Behavioral specificity in the Rorschach human movement response: A comparison of strippers and models. J Clin Psychol *49:* 407, 1993.
Zubenko G, George A, Soloff P, Schulz P: Sexual practices among patients with borderline personality disorder. Am J Psychiatry *144:* 748, 1987.

21.3 GENDER IDENTITY DISORDERS

RICHARD GREEN, M.D., J.D.,
RAY BLANCHARD, Ph.D.

INTRODUCTION

The differentiation of transvestism (called transvestic fetishism in the fourth edition of *Diagnostic and Statistical Manual of*

Mental Disorders [DSM-IV]) from homosexuality, and the differentiation of gender identity disorders from both of these are relatively recent advances in psychiatry. The phenomenological similarities and differences of these entities are still being investigated. For practical, clinical purposes, however, the distinctions are clear-cut. Unlike transvestism or homosexuality, gender identity disorders virtually always involve distress to the person, and that characteristic places them squarely within the purview of psychiatry.

DEFINITIONS

DSM-IV defines gender identity disorders as a heterogeneous group of disorders whose common feature is a strong and persistent preference for the status and role of the opposite sex. Those disorders may be manifested verbally, in assertions that one properly belongs to the opposite sex, or nonverbally, in cross-sex behavior. The affective component of gender identity disorders is commonly referred to as *gender dysphoria,* which may be defined as discontent with one's biological sex, the desire to possess the body of the opposite sex, and the wish to be regarded as a member of the opposite sex. The extreme forms of gender identity disorders, collectively referred to as *transsexualism* in the third edition of DSM (DSM-III) and revised third edition of DSM (DSM-III-R), commonly involve attempts to pass as a member of the opposite sex in society and to obtain hormonal and surgical treatment to simulate the phenotype of the opposite biological sex.

HISTORY

In 1960 the first author cowrote a paper describing behaviors in children that were consistent with the later described gender identity disorder of childhood, and in 1974 he published a text describing several dozen boys with sexual identity conflict. Drawing on this and related work, the psychosexual disorders advisory committee for the *Diagnostic and Statistical Manual of Mental Disorders* that was to become DSM-III, on which the first author served, introduced the diagnostic entity gender identity disorder of childhood in 1980.

Interest in the disorder grew from several sources. The range of behaviors that distinguish children of the two sexes has been a focus of developmental psychologists studying normal patterns of psychosexual differentiation. Work with sexually atypical adults, including transsexuals and homosexuals, who recalled extensive cross-gender behavior in childhood, brought clinical interest to the area. Work by medical psychologists with anatomically intersexed (for example, pseudohermaphroditic) children also documented the significance of gender identity as it emerged in early childhood.

Transsexualism became popularly known with the sex change of George Jorgensen into Christine Jorgensen in 1952. The 1966 professional book by Harry Benjamin, the pioneer who evaluated or treated hundreds of patients, and the introduction of sex-reassignment surgery at the Johns Hopkins Hospital in 1966 legitimized its treatment.

COMPARATIVE NOSOLOGY

DSM CLASSIFICATION SCHEMES Gender identity disorders first entered the American Psychiatric Association's official nomenclature in DSM-III, reflecting the growth of that area of human sexuality in psychiatry since DSM-II.

Nosological position of gender identity disorders In DSM-III, gender identity disorders were included in the category of psychosexual disorders along with the paraphilias and sexual dysfunctions. In DSM-III-R, the gender identity disorders were placed in the section on disorders usually first evident in infancy, childhood, or adolescence.

The location of gender identity disorders in DSM-III-R may have resulted in more notice of those conditions by child psychiatrists. However, its juxtaposition to attention-deficit disorders, conduct disorder, eating disorders, mental retardation, language problems, tics, and so on, was not entirely coherent. Furthermore, although adult transsexuals, whose cross-gender identification often begins in childhood, were placed in that category, persons with various other disorders, which might also extend from childhood behaviors, were not. A final problem with that nosological placement is that some adult men who meet the diagnostic criteria for gender identity disorder in adulthood may not have satisfied the diagnostic criteria for gender identity disorder during childhood.

The solution for DSM-IV was to place gender identity disorders in a separate section called sexual and gender identity disorders. The heading has the same status as mood disorders, anxiety disorders, and other major classifications.

Number of major categories In DSM-III two specific categories of gender identity disorders were coded, each with its own diagnostic criteria: transsexualism and gender identity disorder of childhood. DSM-III-R added a third category, gender identity disorder of adolescence or adulthood, nontranssexual type (GIDAANT), which appears to apply to persons with mild or fluctuating gender dysphoria.

DSM-IV reversed the trend toward greater differentiation by reducing the number of major diagnostic categories to just one, gender identity disorders. The main objective of the change was to unify the diagnostic criteria for children, adolescents, and adults. Inspection of the DSM-IV diagnostic criteria (Table 21.3-1) shows, however, that that goal was only partially realized. The diagnostic criteria for children do not fully parallel those for adults.

Subtypes DSM-III and DSM-III-R, following a long tradition of classifying cross-gender syndromes according to the patient's sexual orientation, listed three subtypes of gender identity disorder: The heterosexual subtype is attracted to members of the opposite genetic sex, the homosexual subtype to members of their own genetic sex, and the asexual subtype to neither. DSM-IV continues the tradition while avoiding the customary labels for those orientations. It also added a fourth subtype, bisexual, based on evidence that among gender dysphoric men the bisexual subtype is at least as common as the heterosexual or asexual subtypes. DSM-IV subtypes are (1) sexually attracted to males, (2) sexually attracted to females, (3) sexually attracted to both, and (4) sexually attracted to neither.

DSM-IV diagnostic criteria The current diagnostic criteria for both children and adults (Table 21.3-1) are organized under two main headings, cross-gender identification and discomfort with the assigned sex. A potential problem is that the arrangement promotes a questionable distinction between the two categories of symptoms. Criterion A for children, for example, includes the intense desire to participate in the games and pastimes of the other sex, while criterion B includes rejection of sex-conventional toys.

For all ages the presence of a nonpsychiatric medical condition, such as hermaphroditism, precludes the diagnosis. DSM-IV requires diagnosis of gender identity disorder not to be concurrent with a physical intersex condition (for example, hermaphroditism). That criterion assumes, not always correctly, that when the symptoms of gender identity disorder are manifested by a child with some intersex status, the behaviors are due to that status. It also assumes that children without obvious intersex status have no physiological basis for their disorder, which also may ultimately be proved false.

ICD CLASSIFICATION SCHEMES In the ninth revision of the *International Classification of Diseases and Related Health*

TABLE 21.3-1
Diagnostic Criteria for Gender Identity Disorder

A. A strong and persistent cross-gender identification (not merely a desire for any perceived cultural advantages of being the other sex).
   In children, the disturbance is manifested by four (or more) of the following:
   (1) repeatedly stated desire to be, or insistence that he or she is, the other sex
   (2) in boys, preference for cross-dressing or simulating female attire; in girls, insistence on wearing only stereotypical masculine clothing
   (3) strong and persistent preferences for cross-sex roles in make-believe play or persistent fantasies of being the other sex
   (4) intense desire to participate in the stereotypical games and pastimes of the other sex
   (5) strong preference for playmates of the other sex
   In adolescents and adults, the disturbance is manifested by symptoms such as a stated desire to be the other sex, frequent passing as the other sex, desire to live or be treated as the other sex, or the conviction that he or she has the typical feelings and reactions of the other sex.
B. Persistent discomfort with his or her sex or sense of inappropriateness in the gender role of that sex.
   In children, the disturbance is manifested by any of the following: in boys, assertion that his penis or testes are disgusting or will disappear or assertion that it would be better not to have a penis, or aversion toward rough-and-tumble play and rejection of male stereotypical toys, games, and activities; in girls, rejection of urinating in a sitting position, assertion that she has or will grow a penis, or assertion that she does not want to grow breasts or menstruate, or marked aversion toward normative feminine clothing.
   In adolescents and adults, the disturbance is manifested by symptoms such as preoccupation with getting rid of primary and secondary sex characteristics (e.g., request for hormones, surgery, or other procedures to physically alter sexual characteristics to simulate the other sex) or belief that he or she was born the wrong sex.
C. The disturbance is not concurrent with a physical intersex condition.
D. The disturbance causes clinically significant distress or impairment in social, occupational, or other important areas of functioning.

Code based on current age:
Gender identity disorder in children
Gender identity disorder in adolescents or adults
Specify if (for sexually mature individuals):
Sexually attracted to males
Sexually attracted to females
Sexually attracted to both
Sexually attracted to neither

Problems (ICD-9), gender identity disorders, without diagnostic criteria, were placed in the section on sexual deviations and disorders. As in DSM-III, ICD-9 had two major categories of gender identity disorders: transsexualism, and disorders of psychosexual identity. The latter corresponded to DSM-III's gender identity disorder of childhood.

In the 10th revision of ICD (ICD-10), gender identity disorders are placed in the section on disorders of adult personality and behavior. Three main categories are included: transsexualism, dual role transvestism, and—strangely, given the section heading—gender identity disorder of childhood. The description associated with dual role transvestism appears to be appropriate for transvestites whose erectile response to cross-dressing has declined.

EPIDEMIOLOGY

PREVALENCE IN CHILDREN The prevalence of the gender identity disorder of childhood can only be estimated because no epidemiological studies have been published. A rough estimate can be obtained from two items on Thomas Achenbach's Child Behavior Checklist that are consistent with components of the diagnosis: behaves like opposite sex and wishes to be of opposite sex. Among a sample of 4- to 5-year-old boys referred for a range of clinical problems, the reported desire to be of the opposite sex was 15 percent. Among 4- to 5-year-old boys not referred for behavioral problems, it was only 1 percent. For ages 6 to 7, the rates were 2.7 and 0 percent; for ages 8 to 9, 5.1 and 0 percent; and for ages 10 to 11, 1.1 and 2.3 percent. For clinically referred girls, there was more uniformity across the ages, with the highest being 8 percent at age 9, and the low 4 percent. For nonreferred girls, the highest rate was 5 percent at ages 4 to 5, and then less than 3 percent for other ages.

Parents reported cross-gender behavior for 16 percent of the clinically referred boys at ages 4 to 5, and for about 10 percent with the other age groups. Among the nonreferred boys the rates were about 5 percent. With clinically referred girls, nearly 19 percent reportedly showed cross-gender behaviors at ages 4 to 5, as did between 9 and 14 percent of girls in the other age groups. With the nonreferred girls the rate was about 11 percent for all ages.

Those data offer only an approximation for gender identity disorder in children because they do not assess the longitudinal persistence of the reported behavior and do not elucidate what constitutes "behaves like opposite sex."

Another way to estimate the prevalence of gender identity disorders in children is to use the percentage of adults with a predominant or exclusive homosexual orientation. The adult rates can then be compared with the percentage of homosexual men and women in various studies who report childhood cross-gender behavior. Predominant or exclusive homosexuality is estimated at 4 percent for men and 1½ to 2 percent for women. Estimates for homosexual men recalling childhood cross-gender behavior are between 50 and 65 percent and for homosexual women perhaps 50 percent. A methodological problem is that the behaviors in those retrospective reports are contaminated by time and different from study to study. Further, they rarely address the key item of wanting to be the opposite sex as a young child. Based on those imprecise assumptions, an estimate is reached of about 3 percent for boys and less than 1 percent for girls.

SEX RATIO IN CHILDREN As many as five boys are referred for each girl referred. Several explanations are possible. First, there is greater parental concern with sissiness than with tomboyism, and greater peer group stigma attaches to substantial cross-gender behavior in boys. Thus, there may be an equal prevalence of gender identity disorder in boys and girls but a differential referral rate. Another possibility is that a genuine disparity results from the male's more perilous developmental course. The fundamental mammalian state is female. No sex hormones are required for prenatal female anatomical development (XO children with gonadal dysgenesis [Turner's syndrome] appear female at birth). Sex hormones are required at critical developmental times for male anatomical differentiation. If the mechanisms of behavioral development track anatomical development, then the masculine behavioral system requires adequate levels of hormone at the appropriate time for normative expression. Finally, the psychodynamic developmental model explaining the disparate referral rates sees both boys and girls initially identifying with the female parent, with only boys needing to make the developmental shift for later normative identification.

AGE OF ONSET IN CHILDREN Most children with a gender identity disorder are referred for clinical evaluation in early grade school. Parents typically report that cross-gender behaviors were apparent before age 3.

PREVALENCE IN ADULTS There is no basis for estimating the proportion of adults who would qualify for a DSM-IV diagnosis of gender identity disorder. The only relevant data are for transsexuals, who comprise only a subgroup of gender dysphoric adults, and even those figures may be underestimates. The available data (from the United Kingdom, Sweden, and Australia) place the prevalence rate of transsexualism at about 1 case per 50,000 adults.

SEX RATIO IN ADULTS Recent data suggest that the sex ratio of adults with sufficient gender dysphoria to present at a gender identity center is about two males for each female. Many factors undoubtedly influence sex ratios at inception of treatment, including the greater publicity given to male-to-female transsexuals and the greater cosmetic and functional success of vaginoplasty compared with phalloplasty. Another factor is that gender dysphoric females nearly all belong to the homosexual subtype, whereas gender dysphoric males include an equal number of homosexuals and a large contingent, which has no comparable counterpart among the females of nonhomosexual (heterosexual, bisexual, and asexual) individuals.

AGE OF ONSET IN ADULTS Most gender dysphoric adults of the homosexual subtype would have qualified for a DSM-IV diagnosis of gender identity disorder in childhood, with their adult behavior simply being a continuation of their childhood disorder. Both males and females of that subtype tend first to present for clinical attention in their mid-20s.

Nonhomosexual gender dysphoric adults (virtually all of whom are males) typically seek help for their disorder in their mid-30s—a striking difference from the homosexual subtype. If the age of onset is considered to be the point at which those first qualify for a DSM-IV diagnosis of gender identity disorder, then they generally have an adolescent or adult onset. However, in most cases prodromes of the disorder were present before puberty.

ETIOLOGY

The etiology of gender identity disorder can be approached from two perspectives. The first applies only to the homosexual subtype of gender identity disorder. It assumes a developmental continuity with homosexuality and is based on theories of same-sex erotic attraction. The other perspective is based on the typical processes of psychosexual development.

BIOLOGICAL THEORIES Theories of homosexual development, notably in males, have taken on an increasingly biological basis, as opposed to an experiential one.

Genetic Theories The Franz Kallmann twin study of the 1950s found a 100 percent concordance for homosexuality between presumably monozygotic male twins. Further research identified discordant pairs, and methodological critiques of the Kallmann study resulted in a general decline of interest in the genetic basis. However, in recent years, twin studies and other family studies of sexual orientation have promoted new interest.

A 1991 study of 50 male monozygotic 56 pairs of twins raised together found a 52 percent concordance for homosexuality compared with 22 percent for 54 dizygotic pairs. A 1992 study found that, with 71 female monozygotic twin pairs, 48 percent were concordant for homosexuality or bisexuality compared with 16 percent for 37 dyzgotic pairs.

Monozygotic twins separated at birth, although rare, provide a better model for testing the relative influences of environment and genetics than do twins reared together, where the two factors are confounded. A report of two pairs of males separated at birth argues for an inherited influence on homosexual orientation. In one pair, both men were homosexually oriented. In the second pair, one twin was homosexual, and the other, while heterosexually married, had had a three-year homosexual relationship in adolescence. By contrast, in four pairs of separated female-female twins, where one twin in each pair was lesbian, none of the co-twins was lesbian.

Family studies of nontwin siblings of homosexual men and women also lend support to a genetic basis, although the confound of a similar environment is considerable. Two studies found higher rates of homosexuality in brothers than is expected in the general male population. No corresponding increase in the number of lesbian siblings was reported.

Hormonal influences Evidence for a hormonal influence on gender identity disorder derives from several research sources. One possible source is congenital virilizing adrenal hyperplasia. Girls with congenital virilizing adrenal hyperplasia overproduce adrenal androgen from before birth. They are more rough-and-tumble, less interested in doll play, and more likely to be considered tomboys than girls without the condition. Conversely, there is limited evidence that prenatal exposure of males to estrogenic or progestational agents may reduce the expression of conventional boy-type behaviors.

Atypical levels of sex-typed hormones before birth, and the attendant effects on specific sex-typed behaviors, can modify substantially the child's early social experiences. Boys who are disinclined to rough-and-tumble play or who play with dolls have different father-son and mother-son relationships and a different peer group experience from more conventionally masculine boys. Similarly, girls who prefer rough-and-tumble activity and sports to doll play have a different early socialization experience with parents and peers from girls who are conventionally feminine.

Reported neuroendocrine and neuroanatomical differences also suggest an inborn contribution to sexual orientation, particularly in men.

One phenomenon tested is the feedback response on luteinizing hormone (LH) after an intravenous pulse of estradiol. In women there is a marked rebound after an initial drop (the hormonal basis of ovulation). The original research found an attenuated femalelike response in homosexual men, which theoretically reflected a deficiency in prenatal androgenization of the central nervous system. In another study using the same methodology, more than half of a sample of homosexual men showed a response more like that of the heterosexual women than of the heterosexual men in the study. However, a subsequent study, which used a different approach to elicit the LH feedback phenomenon, found no significant group difference, and another study with a methodology similar to that used in the original research also failed to confirm a difference.

A related phenomenon that suggests that a deficiency in male hormone in utero leads to a homosexual orientation in men derives from the prenatal stress theory.

Stressing pregnant rodents results in feminized behavior in male offspring, owing either to the competition between adrenal stress steroids and testicular androgens or to the mistiming in testicular androgen secretion as a result of stress. In one study, a higher than average rate of homosexuality was found in men who were born in Germany between 1941 and 1946, the stressful years of World War II. However, an environmental explanation is also possible, because fathers were more likely to be away from their sons during the war. A second study, based on retrospective reports by homosexual, bisexual, and heterosexual men describing stress in their mothers, found more stress during the pregnancies of the homosexual men's mothers.

Other research has been less supportive of an association between stress and homosexuality. Some research found no connection. One American study found a marginally significant relationship, based on the reports of mothers of college students. Another found a low correlation between reported pregnancy stress and lesbianism, but not with male homosexuality. No prospective studies are available.

Although medical histories given by parents of children with gender identity disorder do not provide a basis for grossly abnormal hormone levels before birth, a neuroendocrine base may still be posited at a more subtle level. If the range of prenatal androgen levels is as wide as that in adult life, the fetus may also be exposed to a wide range of androgen. Another factor is the androgen surge that occurs in boys between about three weeks and three months of age.

Brain and central nervous system involvement A difference in a nucleus of the anterior hypothalamus may represent a central nervous system difference related to sexual orientation. The area known as interstitial nucleus of the anterior hypothalamus-3 (INAH-3) was compared, in autopsy, between homosexual men, heterosexual men, and heterosexual women. Although there was some overlap between the size of the nucleus between the groups, it was smaller on average in the homosexual men and women compared with the heterosexual men. All the homosexual men and some of the heterosexual men and women had died of acquired immune deficiency virus (AIDS), but death from AIDS was not a factor. No homosexual women were studied to determine whether the size of their nucleus was similar to that of the heterosexual men. INAH-3 is embedded in the hypothalamic area that appears to be related to some aspects of sexual behavior in male nonhuman primates. Another finding, of a larger suprachiasmatic nucleus in a sample of homosexual men, may be less relevant, because that area is not known to be associated with sexual behavior. It may, however, be related to endocrine function.

PSYCHOSOCIAL THEORIES Psychodynamic and behaviorial influences may lead to extensive cross-gender identification. Boys with an excessive mother-son symbiosis in the early years, replete with extensive mother-son skin-to-skin contact, appear later to manifest significant feminine behavior. That is attributed to the inability to differentiate psychologically from the mother. Male-identified females have been reported to have mothers who were removed in affect from their children, frequently by depression, and fathers who did not support their daughters' femininity. The girl becomes a substitute husband to treat the mother. Other reports describe traumatic psychological losses to boys and girls in the earliest years that appear related to the onset of cross-gender behavior.

Research by the first author with a sample of 66 boys with gender identity disorder found a positive correlation between the extent to which parents supported cross-gender behaviors in their sons and the extent of that cross-gender behavior. In most of the families, at least initially, there was no discouragement of cross-gender behaviors. In more limited work with girls with gender identity disorder, initial parental reactions were similar.

Social learning theories Social learning theories typically focus on the differential reinforcement by parents of sex-typed behaviors, starting shortly after birth. That reinforcement shapes conduct into conventional masculinity or femininity. Cause and effect are hard to distinguish here. On the one hand, sex differences are reported early in life, probably before any major differential impact of parental reinforcement. On the other hand, mothers and fathers apparently treat male and female newborns differently.

In Baby X experiments, adults are told, sometimes incorrectly, the sex of a clothed child and asked to describe the child's attributes or to provide it with toys. Perceived boys are encouraged more to physical action and are given more whole-body stimulation than perceived girls. Perceived girls are initially offered a doll; perceived boys are offered a hammer. When 6-month-old children were similarly clothed, toy choice by adults was related to perceived gender of the child. Boys were presented with footballs, girls with dolls. Strong bald babies were seen as male, soft fragile ones as female.

At 1 year, boys may be more exploratory and active and toy preferences may differ. Girls were found to prefer soft toys and dolls, whereas boys preferred transportation toys and robots. A preference for same-sex playmates emerges early. When 3½- to 4½-year-olds were shown photographs of boys and girls and asked to select those with whom they would like to play, boys preferred boys and girls preferred girls. By age 2 to 3 years, boys appear to be more aggressive toward peers and to show more rough-and-tumble play. Fathers are equally likely to give a 1-year-old daughter a truck as a doll but more likely to give the son a truck. However, when children are given dolls, boys play with them less than girls. Fathers more than mothers give negative responses to boys playing with dolls. Boys receive more positive responses for playing with blocks, and girls receive more positive responses for playing with dolls.

Imitative and vicarious learning pervade general theories of social learning of sex typing. In imitative learning, behaviors are adopted that stimulate those of a significant other person, the model. In vicarious learning, if something happens to a model the viewer's behavior is modified to resemble the model because the child perceives the model as possessing desirable attributes or obtaining desirable goals. The cognitive developmental theory, by contrast, sees the child first labeling itself as male or female and then finding the behaviors associated with that label rewarding.

Nature versus nurture The classic research on intersexed, or hermaphroditic, children points to the early life emergence of gender identity as being influenced primarily by environment and irreversible. In the studies by John Money, Joan Hampson, and John Hampson, a range of anatomical features discordant with the gender of rearing were found to be less relevant to the adoption of a male or female gender identity than the gender of rearing.

Studies of matched pairs, for example, demonstrate that with the syndrome of congenital virilizing adrenal hyperplasia (CAH), the newborn female, if considered to be male and designated male, matures with a male identity in spite of having the XX female chromosomal pattern, ovaries, and a uterus. However, questions have been raised about the generalizability of those findings to nonintersexed children because of the atypical prenatal endocrine environment and other atypical genetic influences of intersexed children.

Studies of children born with normal sex characteristics who undergo gender reassignment early in life may be a more relevant test of nature versus nurture. The tragedy of penile amputation, usually through negligent circumcision, has provided such a model. In one celebrated case, a reassigned male monozygotic twin who was apparently being raised successfully as a girl, has failed to incorporate a female identity. No other long-term follow-up reports have been published.

PSYCHOANALYTIC THEORIES As in other areas of psychopathology, psychoanalytic theories about gender identity disorders constitute a tradition distinct from biological and other nonbiological approaches.

One influential theory is that of Ethel Person and Lionel Ovesey, who advanced the hypothesis that transsexualism in males originates from unresolved separation anxiety during the separation-individuation phase of infantile development. To cope with this anxiety, the child resorts to a reparative fantasy of symbiotic fusion with his mother. Adult transsexualism may be understood as an attempt to master that anxiety through sex reassignment surgery, through which the transsexual acts out his unconscious fantasy and symbolically becomes his mother.

According to that hypothesis, male transsexuals vary in the directness with which they proceed to the transsexual resolution. Some individuals never develop any other psychosexual phenomena as defenses against separation anxiety, and they proceed to the transsexual outcome in a straightforward manner. Others develop transvestism or effeminate homosexuality as initial defenses. When those defenses fail in the face of various stressors, the individual regresses to the primitive fantasy of symbiotic fusion with his mother and begins to experience transsexual impulses.

The other major psychoanalytic theory was developed by Robert Stoller to explain the etiology of transsexualism in a specific group of biological males, who would fall within the DSM-IV category of gender identity disorder, sexually attracted to males. Stoller called those males true transsexuals.

The theory begins with the grandmother of the future transsexual, who treats her daughter coldly and neither encourages nor models femininity for her. The grandfather has a closer relationship with the daughter, but he encourages masculinity in her. In consequence the mother of the future transsexual develops a mild gender identity disorder of her own. In adolescence, however, she abandons her conscious transsexual wishes of someday being male and adopts a heterosexual facade. At the unconscious level she nevertheless retains a strong penis envy.

The transsexual's mother eventually enters an empty marriage with a passive and withdrawn husband, who is psychologically if not physically absent from the household. The final pathogenic process becomes operative when the mother gives birth to an infant son whom she perceives as particularly beautiful and graceful. The boy, who represents her feminized phallus, fulfills her lifelong wish for a penis. The mother-son interaction, described by Stoller as a blissful symbiosis, includes excessively close and prolonged body contact, sometimes with the infant's nude body cradled against the mother's nude body. The mother's behavior expresses her need to treat her son as an extension of her own body.

The transsexual's early experiences, especially the continuous skin-to-skin contact, produce an overidentification with his mother, a blurring of ego boundaries, and eventually a feminine gender identity. The transsexual boy never develops a heterosexual relationship with his mother and therefore never develops an oedipal conflict. His femininity is produced nonconflictually and remains a nonconflictual, autonomous form of behavior.

DIAGNOSIS AND CLINICAL FEATURES

CHILDREN The first author's longitudinal study of 66 boys provides a picture of gender identity disorders in children. The age range at the initial evaluation was 4 to 12 years. One third of the boys frequently stated their wish to be girls and three fifths did so occasionally. Three quarters cross-dressed frequently. The age of onset of cross-dressing was before the fifth birthday with 90 percent. A female-type doll, such as Barbie, was the favorite toy for one fifth of the boys and a frequently played with toy for another two fifths. Three fifths of the boys took a female role when playing house. Over four fifths had a primarily female peer group. Three fifths of the boys were rejected by other children or were voluntary loners.

The full prepubertal age range for evaluating gender identity disorders in children yields a variety of presenting behaviors. Younger children, 3 to 5, may believe that they are of the other sex or that they can easily become the other sex. At older ages, 6 to 9, the children's gestures and mannerisms may be cross-sex stereotypes. Older children have often been subjected to increased peer teasing and so may have gone underground with their cross-gender behaviors, particularly cross-dressing.

A 7-year-old boy was brought for evaluation by his mother because he had been saying intermittently since age 4 that he wanted to be a girl. He was demonstrating a range of girl-type play interests and behaviors and had an extensive interest in dress-up dolls like Barbie since age 2½. The mother had wanted a girl during her second pregnancy but claimed that she quickly became reconciled shortly after his birth to having another son.

When the boy was old enough to draw pictures, they were of princesses with large, flowing gowns. Characters imitated from the media were heroines. When playing mother-father games, he would be the mother. Recently, he had begun to display feminine gestures, particularly with his hands and wrists, and when he spoke he emphasized certain words in a manner that the mother described as effeminate. Although he had no girls' clothing, he would improvise long, flowing gowns, and at nursery school he preferred girls' and women's dress-up costumes. At a subsequent interview, the father acknowledged some of those cross-gender behaviors but felt that they were of little consequence. He reported that he did not spend nearly as much time with that boy as he did with the boy's older brother. The older brother and father had been closer since birth and were involved together in athletic activities.

At initial evaluation the boy confirmed that he wished that he had been born a girl and acknowledged that "I am a boy but playing with dolls makes me happy." He also expressed the fantasy that he had been a girl before he was born. Toy preferences were decidedly cross-gendered: "It hits me to be a girl every time I go to the toy store." He imagined that he was a girl: "Sometimes I talk to myself and say that I'm a girl."

A 5-year old boy was brought by both parents for the initial evaluation. From age 2½ he had preferentially role-played as females, starting with Dorothy in "The Wizard of Oz." He had an intense interest in Barbie doll play and would say, "I love the smell of them, I like their hair, I like to dress them, I like the way they talk." When asked by his parents what makes him happiest, he said, "When I'm a girl and when I wear dresses and heels." The parents had initially considered these behaviors to be a normal passing phase when he was between 2½ and 4, but now that the behaviors had not subsided, they expressed concern.

A 9-year-old girl's extensive cross-gender identification was described from age 4, when she would go into the boys' bathroom and void into the urinal. After age 5 she refused to wear dresses. She would tell people that she was a boy and told her parents, "I'm going to be a boy; I'll have an operation when I'm older." The parental attitude at the onset of these behaviors was that it was "a normal thing." Other children began to tease her a lot, but she said, "I don't care. I want to be a boy, and that's it." When asked why she wanted to be a boy, she said, "Because boys get to love girls." She would draw pictures of people with penises. She said, "I want to be like a boy. I want to have what they have. I want to do what they do."

A 6-year-old girl said since she was two that she did not want to be a girl. At 18 months she told her mother to go to the store and buy her a penis. She thought she may have been a boy in her mother's belly but that her penis had fallen off. She showed no interest in Barbie doll play, hated to wear girl's clothes, and imitated only male characters from television and books. Most of her friends were boys. At age 4 she said, "I am a boy," but when she knew that she was not a boy she still wanted "to be a boy." She thought that boys were "better, have more fun, and get to do better things." Most pictures she drew were of males. She refused to stand in the girls' line at school and told strangers that she was a boy.

Associated features Boys with gender identity disorder have been shown in some reports to evidence greater general psychopathology than nonclinical control boys. Using the Child Behavioral Checklist, a study at the second author's institution found that boys with gender identity disorder had indices of psychopathology similar to a clinic-referred group used in the instrument's standardization. However, another report by the same investigator did not find more behavioral problems on the checklist than among concurrently assessed, demographically comparable clinical controls.

The first author's clinical experience argues that much of the behavioral problem seen in gender-atypical boys is secondary to discomfort over gender and the consequent social ostracism and teasing. That social ostracism is the basis of psychopathology in cross-gendered boys is supported by the finding that checklist symptom scores increase with the age of the child (when stigma increases).

Some clinicians have found separation anxiety disorder in boys with gender identity disorder. They claim that separation anxiety disorder precedes feminine behavior, with cross-gender behavior emerging to restore the emotional tie with a mother who is perceived as unavailable. A recent study using liberal criteria for diagnosing separation anxiety disorder found a correlation between that disorder and gender identity disorder. In the absence of convincing data demonstrating that separation anxiety disorder precedes gender identity disorder and because most children with separation anxiety disorder do not have a gender identity problem, the connection is still problematic.

Psychological tests No psychological test is diagnostic of the gender identity disorder in children. However, the first author has demonstrated that two tests, the It-Scale for Children and the Draw-A-Person test, discriminate boys with gender identity disorder from gender-typical boys.

The It-Scale presents a child with a neuter stick figure (It). "It" then selects from a series of cards depicting gender-typed accessories and activities. Cross-gendered boys more often select feminine or girl-type cards. The Draw-A-Person test in its basic format requires a child to draw a person. Most gender-typical children draw a person of their sex. By contrast, the majority of cross-gendered boys drew a female first. Conversely, with a sample of nonclinical tomboys, the majority drew a male first, in contrast to a matched sample of nontomboys. Those tests can be used as ancillary evaluation procedures. The Draw-A-Person, in particular, is a good technique for making a child comfortable during the initial interview.

ADULTS Virtually all adults who present complaining of gender dysphoria are self-referred. In most cases, the relevant diagnostic question is not whether the patient is gender dysphoric but how severe the condition is.

Central features of gender identity disorders in adults are the persistent sense that one was born into the wrong sex, the belief that one would have been happier as the opposite sex, and the conviction that one has the typical feelings and reactions of the opposite sex. The discontent extends to the social, interpersonal, and somatic realms of the person's existence, although the relative emphases differ from case to case.

Social realm At the social level, there is a consistent indifference to, or distaste for, roles and activities traditionally associated with the original sex, together with recurrent desires to live in society as a part-time or full-time member of the opposite sex. In response to these longings, the gender dysphoric person begins cross-dressing in the company of friends or attempting to pass as a member of the opposite sex in public. Those behaviors may stabilize as intermittent activities or expand to permanent adoption of the cross-gender role, depending in part on the intensity of the gender dysphoria and the person's success in simulating the appearance and manner of the opposite sex.

Interpersonal factors The enjoyment of relationships—especially romantic ones—is significantly diminished by the conflict between the person's subjective feelings of masculinity or femininity and the discrepant perceptions of others. A female-to-male transsexual, for example, may reject an otherwise acceptable female partner if that partner clearly regarded the transsexual as essentially female and the relationship as a lesbian one. Efforts to find sexual or romantic partners who perceive the gender dysphoric person as a member of the opposite sex may lead the person into dangerous circumstances. For example, adolescent gender dysphoric women sometimes pass themselves off as men when first dating or courting potential girlfriends. Male-to-female transsexuals sometimes complete entire sexual encounters with unsuspecting men, discouraging interest in coitus with the excuse of menstruation and offering fellatio instead.

Somatic factors The gender dysphoric person often fails to value the primary and secondary sexual characteristics of his or her body, in many cases developing a positive aversion to those characteristics. A male-to-female transsexual, for example, may describe his penis as an ugly growth and avoid touching it as much as possible. Somatic dysphoria is usually accompanied by the desire for some or all of the physical characteristics of the opposite sex. Gender dysphoric persons use various means to simulate the desired phenotype. Women, for example, commonly flatten their breasts with elastic binding to produce a masculine chest contour. Eventually, transsexuals of both sexes seek hormonal and surgical treatment to complete the transformation.

A 37-year-old man presented with a request for sex reassignment surgery. He was dressed as a man, and he was masculine in his physical appearance and mannerisms.

The patient had not been observably effeminate in boyhood. He had, however, been attracted to and fascinated by feminine activities from an early age. He particularly recalled having liked to watch women apply makeup. He began cross-dressing around puberty. During adolescence he sometimes stole women's underwear from clotheslines. At that stage he preferred women's clothes that had been worn because he felt that they were somehow infused with femininity. Cross-dressing was sexually arousing from puberty until his early 30s, when sexual excitement yielded to feelings of comfort and naturalness.

The patient married at age 25. He initially hoped that marriage would cure his cross-dressing, but that hope soon proved false. The couple's sex life was poor, and the marriage dissolved after eight years. The patient began another heterosexual relationship a few years after his divorce, but that relationship also failed in the face of his growing gender dysphoria.

Following his clinical assessment, the patient began making systematic plans to move into the female role, and he commenced living and going to work as a woman full-time at age 39. The attempt to live as a woman proved successful, and the patient underwent surgical sex reassignment at age 41.

After moving into the female role, the patient (at that point, she) went on a few dates with men but found that she could not really develop an interest in them. After surgery she began moving in lesbian social circles and having sexual relationships with women. She was content with her life in general and had no regrets about her decision to undergo sex reassignment.

A 21-year-old woman complained that she felt uncomfortable with her body, that she should have been a male, and that she wanted to be a male. She presented in the female role, but all of her clothes (jeans, shoes, shirt, vest) were men's style. Her mannerisms and her voice were convincingly masculine.

The patient recounted a childhood history typical of gender identity disorder in girls. Her dissatisfaction with her sex intensified at puberty. She hated her menses and her developing breasts, which she began hiding with jackets, sweatshirts, and so on. The last time she wore a dress was at her eighth grade graduation.

The patient had no sexual experience with men. Her first homosexual relationship occurred in high school and lasted about two years. Her second was with her current partner, a divorcee 10 years older than she. She was currently cohabiting with her partner and her two young children. Their sexual relationship was reported by both partners to be satisfactory although it was one-sided; the patient brought her partner to orgasm but would not allow her own breasts or vulva to be touched because it reminded her of her anatomical sex.

The patient regarded herself as gay in high school but eventually came to realize that she was transsexual. Her goal at clinical presentation was to undergo sex reassignment, to marry her partner, and to be a father to her partner's children.

Associated features Gender identity disorders are not always associated with character pathology. Clinical authors sometimes assert that gender identity disorder patients tend to have narcissistic or borderline personality disorders, perhaps because a significant minority of patients impress as self-absorbed, demanding, unempathic, selfish, inconsiderate, or interpersonally shallow. It is likely that only a fraction of these, however, would meet DSM-IV criteria for a formal diagnosis of narcissistic personality disorder or borderline personality disorder. It is possible that, in some cases, the labels "narcissistic" and "borderline" are simply used as the closest available description for personality patterns that, in fact, may be specifically associated with gender identity disorders.

Associated features vary markedly for different subtypes. Gender dysphoric women exhibit the least associated psychopathology, and what they do exhibit appears to fall into no particular category. The sexually attracted to male subtype of males includes a notable proportion of persons with histories of drug abuse, property offenses, and prostitution. Prostitution is usually carried out in the female role, or, more precisely, in women's attire; the customers are frequently men specifically seeking transsexual prostitutes in preference to biological female prostitutes. There are no data to suggest how many of these cases would warrant a formal diagnosis of antisocial personality disorder.

The majority of men with nonhomosexual subtypes of gender identity disorder report past histories of erotic arousal in association with cross-dressing, and some qualify for a concurrent diagnosis of transvestic fetishism. Careful questioning usually reveals that they are more aroused by the thought or image of themselves as women (autogynephilia) than by items of clothing per se. Therefore, the label "fetishism," applied to their sexual behavior, may be somewhat misleading.

DIFFERENTIAL DIAGNOSIS

CHILDREN Gender atypical children without a gender identity disorder must be distinguished from those with a diagnosable disorder. Tomboys without gender identity disorder prefer functional and casual clothing or gender-neutral clothing. By contrast, gender identity disorder girls refuse to wear girl's clothes and usually reject gender-neutral clothes. Many girls prefer shirts and pants to dresses, enjoy rough-and-tumble play or sports, and show little interest in doll play. They may say it is better to be a boy because of perceived social advantages. Those girls do not necessarily have a gender identity disorder. What distinguishes girls who do is their repeated statements of being or wanting to be a boy and wanting to grow up to be a man, along with repeated cross-sex fantasy play and a marked aversion to traditional feminine dress and activities.

With boys the differential diagnosis must distinguish those who do not conform to traditional masculine sex-typed expectations but who do not show extensive cross-gender identification and who are not discontent with their anatomical sex. It is not uncommon for boys to reject rough-and-tumble play or sports, to prefer sedentary or aesthetic activities, or occasionally to role-play as a girl, to play with a doll, or to dress up in a girl's or woman's costume. Such boys do not necessarily have a gender identity disorder. That fact must be stressed to parents, especially to fathers who may have vigorous athletic expectations for their sons. What distinguishes those boys who do have a gender identity disorder is the stated preference for being a girl and for growing up to become a woman, along with repeated cross-sex fantasy play, a strong preference for traditionally female-type activities, including cross-dressing, and a female peer group.

The clinician may sometimes see boys with repetitive cross-dressing but no other observable evidence of cross-gender identification. Those boys are often brought by parents when they discover their son cross-dressed, usually in his mother's underclothes. Such children would not satisfy the diagnostic criteria for gender identity disorder in children, although it is possible or even likely that some of them will warrant a diagnosis of gender identity disorder by the time they are grown. Monosymptomatic cross-dressing of this nature is sometimes recalled by adults with transvestic fetishism, but no studies are available predicting the sexual outcome of early isolated cross-dressing.

Because the diagnosis of gender identity disorder excludes children with anatomical intersex, a careful family medical history needs to be taken, with a focus on any suggestion of hermaphroditism in the child, such as an unusual appearance of the genitalia. When there is doubt, referral to a pediatric endocrinologist is indicated for appropriate hormonal and cytological examinations.

ADULTS Psychotic persons rarely develop the delusion that their sex is changing. A male patient, for example, may claim that he can feel his breasts growing or his penis shrinking. Such beliefs are never expressed by adult patients with gender identity disorder, who understand that sex reversal does not occur spontaneously. In any event there are other signs (for example, hallucinations, ideas of reference) to aid in the differential diagnosis.

A more difficult diagnostic problem is posed by some late-adolescent patients who report that they were extreme sissies (or tomboys) as children, that they have always felt like members of the opposite sex, that they are uncomfortable with their bodies, and so on, but who go on to say that they feel guilty about their attraction to members of their own sex, that they believe that homosexuality is worse than transsexualism, and that they want sex reassignment so that they can lead normal heterosexual lives. It can be difficult, at initial assessment, to determine how much of the patient's behavior is driven by true gender dysphoria and how much by internalized homophobia. Fortunately, the diagnosis becomes clearer when such patients are followed into young adulthood.

COURSE AND PROGNOSIS IN CHILDREN

In the first author's 15-year prospective study, 44 of 66 cross-gendered boys, most of whom would be diagnosed today with gender identity disorder, were followed to adolescence or young adulthood. Sexual orientation was determined by interviews tapping erotic fantasies and erotic behaviors. Fantasies were determined from questioning about masturbation content, erotic nocturnal dreams, and experiences of arousal when seeing pornography or attractive persons. Behaviors were assessed by reports of interpersonal genital sexuality.

On the dimension of erotic fantasy, 33 of 44 (75 percent) previously gender-atypical boys were bisexual to homosexual (rated 2 to 6 on the Kinsey 7-point scale of sexual orientation, where 0 is exclusive heterosexuality and 6 is exclusive homosexuality). With behavior, 24 of 30 (80 percent) were bisexual to homosexual. One boy at 18 years was transsexual. None of the boys were sexually aroused by cross-dressing.

Behavioral changes were evident in the boys during the years prior to the determination of sexual orientation. There was a general lessening of specific cross-gender behaviors and a denial by all but one of the continued desire to be female.

There are several possible reasons for the considerable behavioral change from the time of initial evaluation to adolescence, with or without formal treatment. When deciding to seek professional counsel, parents have usually concluded, or may conclude after consultation, that their child's extensive cross-gender behaviors should be limited or eliminated. The child is also receiving negative reactions from age-mates for obviously cross-gendered activities. The developmental course of activity preferences in typical children also dictates change. Because even typical girls play less with dress-up dolls as they get older, cross-gendered boys can also be expected to show less interest.

There have been no large studies of atypical females evolving into adolescence. A community-based sample of 50 tomboys was generated by the first author, in which the girls shared some (but not all) features with girls with gender identity disorder. Because federal research funding was not forthcoming, no follow-up data are available for this unique sample.

COURSE AND PROGNOSIS IN ADULTS

BIOLOGICAL MALES SEXUALLY ATTRACTED TO MALES AND BIOLOGICAL FEMALES SEXUALLY ATTRACTED TO FEMALES Biological males sexually attracted to males and biological females sexually attracted to females are similar in course and prognosis. In many regards, the characteristics of the one group are mirror images of the characteristics of the other.

Course Adult homosexual gender dysphoric persons primarily represent that fraction of gender identity disorder children who did not normalize in gender identity by the end of adolescence. The course of the disorder is continuous, although certain manifestations of it may be driven underground in late childhood or early teens. A feminine boy, for example, may cross-dress frequently in connection with fantasy play; cease cross-dressing entirely from junior high school to early adulthood, as he attempts to fit into society or at least to minimize conflicts with family and peers; and then resume cross-dressing in his 20s with the intention of pursuing sex reassignment surgery.

Homoerotic feelings begin in puberty. Some adolescents label themselves initially as homosexual and seek companionship in a gay crowd. They find they do not really fit in there either, although some adolescent male transsexuals continue to socialize in the homosexual drag circuit simply because it offers the only available supportive environment. Eventually, homosexual gender dysphoric persons of both sexes begin to label their erotic attractions in terms of their subjective gender identity. Thus, for example, a female-to-male transsexual will assert that her romantic interest in another woman is heterosexual not lesbian, because inside she is really a man.

In young adulthood, there is often an increase in cross-dressing and in attempts to pass as the opposite sex. Quite often, patients have already moved into the cross-gender role full-time by the time they present for clinical attention. Those developments reflect freedom from parental controls and increased opportunities for self-expression more than intensification of the gender dysphoria. The homosexual type (biological male sexually attracted to males and biological female sexually attracted to females) of gender identity disorder does not have the character of a progressive disorder. In young males, adoption of the female role is sometimes accompanied by withdrawal from society at large into a subculture consisting mostly of other male-to-female transsexuals.

At initial presentation, female patients more often than males are involved in love relationships with same-sex partners. The female partner typically concurs with the patient's self-evaluation that she is really a man and reports that she perceives her lover as a man without a penis. Such partners are often anxious to be part of the transsexual's evaluation.

Prognosis Young adults who are still living in the original gender role when they first present sometimes relinquish the desire for sex reassignment and make a satisfactory adjustment to a homosexual lifestyle. In most cases, however, the disorder is chronic.

Impairment and complications Peer ostracism often makes school attendance so difficult for biological males with gender identity disorder, sexually attracted to males, that they drop out of high school without graduating. Lack of education and job skills contribute to chronic unemployment and further marginalization of the individual in society. Societal rejection and its sequelae may lead to prostitution or to drug and alcohol abuse. Gender identity disorder has fewer such consequences for women, possibly because of society's greater tolerance of cross-gender behavior in girls and women.

BIOLOGICAL MALES SEXUALLY ATTRACTED TO FEMALES, BOTH SEXES, OR NEITHER SEX There are marked and probably qualitative differences between the type of gender identity disorder that may occur in homosexual males and females (biological males sexually attracted to males and biological females sexually attracted to females) and the types that occur in nonhomosexual males (biological males sexually attracted to females, sexually attracted to both, and sexually attracted to neither). The differences in their natural histories suggest that homosexual and nonhomosexual gender identity disorders are etiologically different conditions.

Course In terms of observable symptoms, nonhomosexual gender identity disorders may be characterized as progressive disorders with an insidious onset. The course is fairly continuous in some cases; in others, the intensity of symptoms fluctuates to the point that the course might be called episodic. The subjective experience is of a lifelong struggle with feminine longings that change their focus from time to time and may temporarily recede in the face of conflicting desires, but which have always been present in one form or another from early consciousness.

In most cases, the first outward manifestation of the disorder is surreptitious cross-dressing in childhood (for example, in mother's or sister's clothing). Many men also report that they first began wishing they were female during that period. The boyhood behavior does not, however, exhibit the pervasive pattern of effeminacy required for a childhood diagnosis of gender identity disorder. At puberty, cross-dressing begins to elicit penile erection, and for the next few years or decades, the individual may qualify for a diagnosis of transvestic fetishism. In his 20s or 30s, the person's penile response to cross-dressing begins to wane, while at the same time his desire to have a woman's body grows stronger and more insistent. In general, the cross-gender wishes attain the highest intensity by the mid-30s and remain about the same thereafter. It must be stressed, however, that the course is highly variable.

Most men with gender identity disorder, sexually attracted to females, sexually attracted to both, or sexually attracted to neither establish relationships with women at some point in their lives, and many marry and father children. Those who fall in love with a woman often report that, during the early days of the romance, they lose their interest in cross-dressing or surgical sex reassignment. When the relationship becomes routine and the initial excitement subsides, however, their desire to dress or live as women reasserts itself.

The course of nonhomosexual gender identity disorders may also be punctuated by periods of increased symptomatology.

Men of that type occasionally present during an episode of intensified gender dysphoria, with anguished longings to be female accompanied by frustration and despair at their male state.

Prognosis The disorder tends to be chronic. Its tendency towards cyclical variation in many cases may mislead the patient (or his therapist) into thinking that the patient has been cured when he would be better regarded as in remission. As a group, nonhomosexual gender dysphoric patients are less likely than homosexual gender dysphoric patients to pursue surgical sex reassignment to completion. Many simply learn to live with their feelings. Acute episodes of intensified gender dysphoria usually resolve to the preepisode level after a few months, and patients should be discouraged from taking steps toward establishing themselves as females during such periods.

Impairment and complications Nonhomosexual gender identity disorders tend to interfere with heterosexual relationships. Feelings of sexual interest aroused by the sight of a beautiful woman may turn, in the next instant, into feelings of envy. Heterosexual intercourse may require the person to fantasize that he is the woman and his partner is the man, or that he and his partner are two women having lesbian relations; even with the help of such autogynephilic fantasies, erectile problems are common.

Gender identity disorders commonly result in marital breakdown, either because the husband wishes to be free to pursue sex reassignment, or because the wife can no longer tolerate her husband's cross-dressing or other cross-gender behaviors. Men contemplating or undergoing divorce often feel considerable guilt about the effect of their behavior on their children and anxiety about their prospects for continued access to them. Those concerns are often part of the clinical picture in patients of the nonhomosexual type first presenting for assessment.

TREATMENT

CHILDREN Evaluating the effects of intervention is difficult. Whereas short-term behavioral changes toward more conventional gender-typed activities are described, few data are available about adult sexuality. In the first author's prospective study, a subsample of boys with gender identity disorder were treated by a variety of approaches from several therapists, including psychoanalysis, family therapy, individual psychotherapy, and behavior modification. With each intervention, the boys showed lessening of cross-gender behaviors. At follow-up none expressed the desire to be female. However, the rates of homosexual or bisexual orientation did not differ from those boys who had no formal treatment, who also showed a lessening of cross-gender behaviors.

At present there is no convincing evidence from any controlled research that psychiatric or psychological intervention with children with gender identity disorder affects the direction of subsequent sexual orientation. Transsexualism, however, may be affected. Transsexuals are unable to cope socially as persons of their anatomical sex. The treatment of gender identity disorder in children is directly largely at developing social skills and comfort in the sex role dictated at birth. To the extent that treatment is successful, transsexual development is interrupted. The low prevalence of transsexualism in the general population, however, even in the special population of cross-gendered children, thwarts the testing of this assumption.

The most systematic attack on specific cross-gender behaviors is the behaviorist approach. Specific cross-gender behaviors in boys have been substantially reduced by the use of a token economy or differential social reinforcement. To the extent that such changes reduce stigma and enhance the boy's self-image, the results can be considered positive. However, one goal of George Rekers, the principal proponent of that type of intervention, appears not to be realized. Rekers wished to prevent the boy from yielding to "homosexual temptation" with homosexuality having "been sold to the unwary public as a right between consenting adults." At least two graduates of that program are bisexual. Systematic follow-up of adult sexual orientation on the others in that series has not been reported, although it is about two decades since many were treated.

The first author's current treatment approach is eclectic. It addresses the child's interaction with each parent, the child's social environment out of the home, the child's perception of sex roles, and the child's relations with peers.

For a period of a year or more, parents have observed behaviors in their child that constitute gender identity disorder. During that time, one parent may have taken a firmer stand against some of the behaviors, but for the most part the children have not been interrupted in these activities. Parents have typically been uncertain or ambivalent about its meaning, and until recently, if at all, the child has not been aware that his or her parents object to the atypical behavior. A child may interpret a parent's neutral stance to atypical behaviors as positive. Some parents may have begun to be concerned, but they have been advised by preschool teachers that the behaviors are normal and should not be discouraged. A parent who is concerned about the excessive nature of the child's cross-gender behaviors may have difficulty convincing the school of that child's special needs, notwithstanding any ideal of androgyny. A grandparent or housekeeper may be supportive of the child's cross-gender activities, or at least not discourage them, again undermining a concerted effort at behavioral change at least toward gender-neutral activities. Initial limit-setting by parents usually meets with considerable resistance and testing by the child. It may result in behaviors continuing in secret. Some children will relabel the cross-gender behaviors as gender-appropriate. For example, a long, flowing robe that was previously a princess gown is now a Superman cape.

One strategy of therapy looks to the child's level of cognitive development. Young children paint the world in black and white. In the area of gender, there are no grays. A child who does not like the activities he or she associates exclusively with that child's sex concludes that being of the other sex is the only solution. A girl will say that only boys play sports, or a boy will say boys play too rough. Grays must be introduced. Boys need to know that they can participate in sedentary play with other children, both boys and girls. Girls needs to know that girls play sports and can be as good as or better than many boys. Parents should find children who demonstrate those behaviors to play with their own.

Goals with parents should be set early. Many parents are motivated to the initial evaluation by fears that their children will become transsexual or homosexual. Parents should be redirected from hypothetical concerns of decades ahead to the immediacy of the child's life. At present, the child is unhappy being a boy or a girl, and the focus should be on making the child content with who he or she is. In the immediate term, the child is experiencing social stigma. The child should be integrated more effectively into the peer group.

The first author has demonstrated that by ages 4 to 5 boys and girls differ in their manners of walking, running, throwing a ball, and narrating a story. Cross-gender gestures and mannerisms should be pointed out to the child. The reason given to the child and parents for intervention is that otherwise the child will be teased. Children are often unaware of cross-gender mannerisms, but consistent alerting will help bring them into consciousness and under control.

A boy with gender identity disorder typically has a strained relationship with his father. The first author's study of cross-gendered boys found the extent of father-son involvement in the early years to be related to later sexual orientation. The association emerged not only between the two groups of boys studied (gender identity disorder and control) but within the subgroup of boys with gender identity disorder. Thus, for the clinically referred boys, the less time the father and son shared in the preschool years, the higher the later Kinsey score for homosexuality.

Identifying cause and effect in the distant father-son relationship is difficult. Some fathers were not available to their sons in the earliest years, and the boy gravitated toward his mother's activities. Then the father found that the boy did not respond to his belated attempts to engage him in sports or other activities. Alternatively, a father may have been available from the outset, but the child was temperamentally attuned to his mother's activities. The father became discouraged and his attention focused elsewhere, perhaps to another sibling with whom he shared interests. The need for a positive father-son experience must be emphasized to fathers. Nonathletic activities can be mutually enjoyable. Taking the son to work provides a better image of who father is. Board games, video games, and a shared father-son activity, such as Indian Guides, a program that emphasizes crafts and camping, can be helpful. Father's busy work schedule must be compromised lest the best years of their relationship be sacrificed, irrespective of any influence on any later sexual orientation. Whatever the outcome of the boy's sexuality, a more positive father-son relationship is to be sought; it is good for father and son.

The child may believe that the parents wanted a child of the other sex. Sometimes parents did and conveyed the wish to the child. Parents and therapists must convey the message to the child that this is not so (if it ever was) and that they are happy having a child of that sex.

Children should know that sex is irreversible. Not yet having achieved gender constancy at ages 4 to 6, they may think that by cross-dressing or changing hair length they change their sex. They should know the anatomical differences between the sexes and that superficial change will not achieve their goal. Older children, aware of genital differences, and cognitively more advanced, may also be sophisticated about sex-change surgery. The parade of transsexuals on television has educated children, so that the clinician's statement of irreversibility of sex can be challenged. One 10-year-old girl in treatment by the first author began to abandon hopes for surgery to male status only when she was convinced that the cosmetic and functional results of phalloplasty are poor.

The same treatment strategies used for boys with gender identity disorder are applicable to girls. Parental responses that have been supportive of behaviors causing the girl to be stigmatized should be interrupted. Same-sex peer group experiences are to be encouraged. Where a swagger has evolved, and teasing results, it should be modified as are the extensive feminine mannerisms in a boy.

No hormonal or psychopharmacological treatments for gender identity disorders in childhood have been identified.

ADOLESCENTS Young persons whose previous gender identity disorder has normalized (with or without treatment) by the end of puberty may experience new conflicts when homosexual feelings emerge in adolescence. Although homosexuality is not a psychiatric disorder, it may be a source of anxiety to the adolescent and cause intrafamily conflict. Teenagers should be reassured about the prevalence and the nonpathological aspects of a same-sex partner preference. Those who are bisexual may be reassured about the fluidity of sexual orientation in adolescence. Parents must also be informed of the nonpathological nature of a same-sex orientation. They must be dissuaded from obsessing over (or even asking) the question, "Where did I go wrong?" The goal of family intervention is to keep the family stable and to provide a supportive environment for the adolescent.

Adolescents whose gender identity disorders have persisted beyond puberty present quite different treatment problems. One problem in treating adolescent transsexuals is how to manage the rapid emergence of unwanted secondary sex characteristics. Legal issues may confront the clinician who would prescribe contrasex hormones or hormone-inhibiting substances to thwart that development, even with parental approval. Social cross-gender living is a possible alternative. Some schools have permitted teenagers to enroll as opposite-sex students.

ADULTS Adult patients with gender identity disorders present with various agendas. Some are seeking help in suppressing their cross-gender feelings, some are gathering information about gender identity disorders and treatment options, and still others come with straightforward requests for surgical sex reassignment. For all of the patients seeking a cure or information, and many of those seeking surgery, the first consideration should be to help the patient reconcile to the original gender role or at least learn to function reasonably well in it.

Psychotherapy At present, only psychological therapies are available to help patients accept their biological sex. No drug treatment has been shown to be effective in reducing cross-gender desires per se.

There are no general guidelines for individual psychotherapy with gender dysphoric patients. Some authorities recommend that, when treating patients with unrealistic hopes of sex reassignment surgery, it is best not to confront the patient on that point directly. Patients may be more open to critical examination of their goals and alternatives if they perceive the therapist as open-minded about the surgical option. There are exceptions: Some patients are relieved to be told frankly by an experienced professional that they are not suitable—or ready—for sex reassignment surgery, and they drop the idea without quarrel.

Gender identity disorder patients are often amenable to group therapy, especially if the group is homogeneous. Mixing patients who are attempting to become reconciled to their original gender roles with patients who are pursuing sex reassignment may make it more difficult to promote group cohesion.

Medical treatment When the patient's gender dysphoria is severe and intractable, sex reassignment may be the best solution. The first medical intervention in this process is hormone therapy, which should be supervised by an endocrinologist. Biological males are usually treated with daily doses of oral estrogens. That produces breast enlargement, which continues for about two years at any given dose. The final amount of gynecomastia varies greatly among patients. The other major effects of estrogen treatment are testicular atrophy, decreased libido, and diminished erectile capacity. There may be a slight decrease in the growth of facial and body hair together with arrest of male-pattern baldness.

Biological females are treated with biweekly or monthly intramuscular injections of testosterone enanthate or testosterone cypionate. Because the effects of (exogenous) testosterone are more profound than those of estrogen clinicians should be more conservative about commencing females on hormone treatment. The pitch of the voice drops permanently into the male range as the vocal cords thicken. The clitoris enlarges to about three times its pretreatment length, with a growth plateau of one year; that is often accompanied by increased libido. Hair growth changes to the male pattern, and a full, thick beard often develops. Male-pattern baldness may also develop. Ovarian function is suppressed, with the menses ceasing within four months of the start of treatment.

The second major stage in the medical treatment of transsexualism is sex reassignment surgery. All major gender identity clinics in North America and Western Europe require their patients to live full-time in the cross-gender role for some time—usually one to two years—prior to surgery. Most gender identity clinics further require that patients either work or attend school in the cross-gender role during the probationary period. The latter requirement is intended to demonstrate that the patient is capable of interacting successfully with members of the general public in the cross-gender role.

Sex reassignment surgery for biological males consists principally of vaginoplasty. Operative techniques vary, mainly in the method of obtaining material to line the neovagina. One technique uses a section of the rectosigmoid colon. The standard methods involve lining the neovagina with penile skin flaps, scrotal skin flaps, and free grafts from the thigh, in various combinations. Occasional postoperative complications include urethral strictures, caused by retraction of the urethra, and rectovaginal fistulas. Vaginal stenosis sometimes occurs; this is usually caused by inadequate postoperative care of the neovagina by the patient. Inadequate vaginal width or depth may make penile penetration difficult or impossible.

Surgical reassignment procedures for females are more variable. Construction of a male chest contour is virtually always performed. Panhysterectomy and bilateral salpingo-oophorectomy are usually carried out, although some patients, satisfied with the menstrual suppression produced by testosterone therapy, do not request those procedures. Phalloplasty is the least commonly performed, partly because it is relatively expensive, and partly because it is not as successful, cosmetically or functionally, as vaginoplasty. Surgical techniques for phalloplasty have recently improved, however, so that picture may be changing.

The best technique for constructing a male chest contour varies according to the size of the patient's breasts. For small-breasted females, the surgeon may perform a subcutaneous mastectomy through a keyhole incision without disturbing the nipple-areola complex. Large-breasted patients require breast amputation and replacement of the nipple as a free graft. Postoperative complications of the latter procedure include obvious chest scars and widening of the nipple-areola grafts.

Additional plastic surgeries are commonly sought by biological males, rarely or never by biological females. Male patients most often undergo thyroid cartilage shave (Adam's apple reduction), rhinoplasty (to create a more feminine nose), and breast implants.

Treatment outcome Numerous studies have investigated the postoperative adjustment of reassigned transsexuals, primarily among patients assessed and approved for surgery by established gender identity clinics. The findings are generalizable only to properly screened patients. The most reliable conclusion is that the overwhelming majority of postoperative transsexuals are contented with their decision to undergo sex reassignment.

Outcome studies as a whole suggest that surgical sex reassignment produces additional improvements in psychosocial adjustment. The main areas of benefit are interpersonal relationships and psychological symptomatology, especially morale and mood. It should be noted that only one outcome study has included random assignment to surgically treated and (waiting-list) control groups. Its findings bolster the conclusion that postoperative improvements in social integration, sexual adjustment, and psychological symptomatology can be attributed to the surgical intervention.

The available evidence for socioeconomic improvement is weaker perhaps because most studies fail to look at outcome variables for males and females separately. Studies that have examined socioeconomic change separately for male and female transsexuals have found that the socioeconomic status of biological females improves when they move into the male role, whereas the socioeconomic status of males worsens when they adopt the female role.

It has been shown that in male-to-female transsexuals the cosmetic and functional adequacy of surgical interventions affects the self-image of transsexuals and the degree to which they and their partners are reminded of the sex-reassigned status. Thus, the better the surgical result—other things being equal—the better the postoperative adjustment.

It should be noted, finally, that sex reassignment surgery has little or no effect on major mental illness or serious character pathology. Patients with preoperative histories of psychiatric hospitalization for depression or multiple suicide attempts are liable to be at risk for further episodes after surgery.

INTERSEX DISORDERS

Patients who present with uncertainty or confusion about their correct gender or discontent with the gender in which they have been living may have an intersexed physiological status. Differences between gender identity patients with and without physical intersexuality suggest distinct etiologies of gender identity complaints in the two groups. There are, on the other hand, occasional patients (for example, adult men with Klinefelter's syndrome) who appear similar in their clinical presentations to otherwise comparable men with normal karyotypes. For this reason, there is continuing discussion among specialists about whether the presence of intersexuality should preclude the diagnosis of gender identity disorder. For research purposes, intersexed patients should be excluded from gender-dysphoric samples. According to DSM-IV, intersex conditions are an example of a gender identity disorder not otherwise specified (Table 21.3-2). The most common intersex conditions will be described briefly.

TABLE 21.3-2
Diagnostic Criteria for Gender Identity Disorder not Otherwise Specified

This category is included for coding disorders in gender identity that are not classifiable as a specific gender identity disorder. Examples include

1. Intersex conditions (e.g., androgen insensitivity syndrome or congenital adrenal hyperplasia) and accompanying gender dysphoria.
2. Transient, stress-related cross-dressing behavior.
3. Persistent preoccupation with castration or penectomy without a desire to acquire the sex characteristics of the other sex.

CONGENITAL VIRILIZING ADRENAL HYPERPLASIA Formerly called adrenogenital syndrome, the disorder is characterized by an enzymatic defect in the production of cortisol by the adrenal gland. As a result, excessive androgenic adrenal hormone production begins prenatally. At birth, affected females show varying degrees of genital virilization. After birth, excessive androgen production can be controlled by cortisone.

With diagnosis of congenital virilizing adrenal hyperplasia neonatally, male or female children appear to develop a gender identity consistent with their chromosomal and gonadal sex and sex of rearing. Girls may show more than typical boy-type play behaviors. In earlier cases before the diagnosis was made neonatally and when the diagnosis for a woman was not made in childhood and socialization was as a man, a male identity typically evolved. There may be higher rates of homosexual behavior in affected women, whether or not treated with cortisone in childhood.

TURNER'S SYNDROME One sex chromosome is missing in Turner's syndrome, so that the sexual karyotype is simply X (designated XO). Affected children have poorly developed ovaries and possibly other anomalies, including an unusual appearance of the chest and neck. Their genitalia are female at birth. They develop into short women who require replacement estrogen for female secondary sex characteristics. Identity is usually female and gender identity conflict is rare, but they may experience psychosexual conflict over infertility.

KLINEFELTER'S SYNDROME An additional X chromosome is present here along with the typical XY male pattern. At birth affected infants appear to be normal males. There may be excessive gynecomastia in adolescence, and the testes are small, usually without spermatogenesis. Testosterone levels are low and the body habitus is eunichoid. A higher rate of gender identity disorder has been suggested in affected persons, but unrepresentative sampling clouds the issue.

5-α-REDUCTASE DEFICIENCY An enzymatic defect here prevents the conversion of testosterone to dihydrotestosterone, which is required for prenatal virilization of the genitalia. Thus, the XY-affected individual is born with female-appearing genitalia, although there is some evidence of abnormality. At puberty extensive virilization occurs from testosterone and some dihydrotestosterone; there is phallic growth and a male chest pattern.

Gender identity development is the subject of controversy. Many of the earliest described cases were raised as girls who with virilization during adolescence evolved a male identity. They were later heterosexually active as men. That transition was variously interpreted from neuroendocrine and social learning perspectives. It was posited that testosterone organized the prenatal central nervous system to mediate a later male identity, although that hormone was inadequate to virilize the genitalia in utero. Alternatively, it was posited that social pressures on these male-appearing adolescents to act like men and avoid the stigma of homosexuality forced them into their masculine heterosexual status. Subsequent generations born with the disorder are recognized as those who will virilize at puberty and so are raised with that hermaphroditic identity. When raised as men, perhaps with androgen supplementation, they function as relatively normal men, although their phallus is not entirely normal. When castrated in infancy and raised as girls, they may be markedly tomboyish in childhood. Insufficient numbers of cases are available for predicting their adult psychosexual status, but some appear to be feminine heterosexual women.

ANDROGEN INSENSITIVITY SYNDROME Formerly called testicular feminization, androgen insensitivity syndrome is a disorder of metabolism in the XY individual where tissue cells are unable to use testosterone or other androgens. Consequently, the person appears to be a normal female at birth. Testes are undescended, and no internal female reproductive structures are present. Puberty brings female-type breast development (from the conversion of testosterone to estradiol). A vagina needs to be constructed.

Gender identity usually evolves as female, with a sexual interest in males. There may be psychosexual conflict over the absence of menses and infertility.

SUGGESTED CROSS-REFERENCES

Related discussions include Section 21.1a on normal human sexuality and sexual dysfunctions, Section 21.1b on homosexuality, Section 33.2 on normal child development, and Section 33.3 on normal adolescent development. Transvestic fetishism is discussed in Section 21.2 on paraphilias. Intersex disorders are discussed in Section 26.6 on endocrine and metabolic disorders.

REFERENCES

Bailey R, Pillard R: A genetic study of male sexual orientation. Arch Gen Psychiatry *48:* 1089, 1991.

Benjamin H: *The Transsexual Phenomenon.* Julian Press, New York, 1966.

Blanchard R: Partial versus complete autogynephilia and gender dysphoria. J Sex Marital Ther *19:* 301, 1993.

Blanchard R: The she-male phenomenon and the concept of partial autogynephilia. J Sex Marital Ther *19:* 69, 1993.

Blanchard R: Varieties of autogynephilia and their relationship to gender dysphoria. Arch Sex Behav *22:* 241, 1993.

Blanchard R, Clemmensen L H, Steiner B W: Heterosexual and homosexual gender dysphoria. Arch Sex Behav *16:* 139, 1987.

Blanchard R, Collins P I: Men with sexual interest in transvestites, transsexuals, and she-males. J Nerv Ment Dis *181:* 570, 1993.

*Blanchard R, Steiner B W, editors: *Clinical Management of Gender Identity Disorders in Children and Adults.* American Psychiatric Press, Washington, 1990.

Coates S, Person E: Extreme boyhood femininity: Isolated behavior or pervasive disorder. J Am Acad Child Psychiatry *24:* 702, 1985.

Diamond M: Sexual identity, monozygotic twins reared in discordant sex roles and a BBC follow-up. Arch Sex Behav *11:* 181, 1982.

Dixen J M, Maddever H, Van Maasdam J, Edwards P W: Psychosocial characteristics of applicants evaluated for surgical gender reassignment. Arch Sex Behav *13:* 269, 1984.

Dörner G, Rohde W, Stahl F: A neuroendocrine predisposition for homosexuality in men. Arch Sex Behav *4:* 1, 1975.

Dörner G, Geiser T, Ahrens L: Prenatal stress and possible aetiogenic factor for homosexuals in human males. Endocrinologie *75:* 365, 1980.

Green R: Atypical psychosexual development. In *Child and Adolescent Psychiatry,* ed 3, M Rutter, L Hersov, E Taylor, editors. Blackwell Scientific, London, 1994.

*Green R: *Sexual Identity Conflict in Children and Adults.* Basic Books, New York, 1974.

*Green R: *The "Sissy Boy Syndrome" and the Development of Homosexuality.* Yale University Press, New Haven, 1987.

Green R, Fleming D T: Transsexual surgery follow-up: Status in the 1990s. Annu Rev Sex Research *1:* 63, 1990.

Green R, Money J: Incongruous gender role: Nongenital manifestation in prepubertal boys. J Nerv Ment Dis *131:* 160, 1960.

Green R, Money J, editors: *Transsexualism and Sex Reassignment.* Johns Hopkins Press, Baltimore, 1969.

LeVay S: A difference in hypothalamic structure between heterosexual and homosexual men. Science *253:* 1034, 1991.

Maccoby E, Jacklin C: *The Psychology of Sex Differences.* Stanford University Press, Stanford, CA, 1974.

*Mate-Kole C, Freschi M, Robin A: A controlled study of psychological and social change after surgical gender reassignment in selected male transsexuals. Br J Psychiatry *157:* 261, 1990.

Meyer-Bahlburg H F L: Intersexuality and the diagnosis of gender identity disorder. Arch Sex Behav *23:* 21, 1994.

Money J, Hampson J, Hampson J: An examination of some basic sexual concepts. Bull Johns Hopkins Hosp *97:* 301, 1955.

Person E, Ovesey L: The transsexual syndrome in males. I. Primary transsexualism. Am J Psychother *28:* 4, 1974.

Person E, Ovesey L: The transsexual syndrome in males. II. Secondary transsexualism. Am J Psychother *28:* 174, 1974.

Rekers G: *Shaping Your Child's Sexual Identity.* Baker Book House, Grand Rapids, MI, 1982.

Ross M W, Walinder J, Lundstrom B, Thuwe I: Cross-cultural approaches to transsexualism: A comparison between Sweden and Australia. Acta Psychiatr Scand *63:* 75, 1981.

Sidocowic L, Lunney G: Baby X revisited. Sex Roles *6:* 67, 1980.

Smith P, Connally K: Patterns of play and sexual interaction in preschool children. In *Ethological Studies of Child Behaviour,* N Jones, editor. Cambridge University Press, Cambridge, 1972.

Stoller R: *Sex and Gender,* Science House, New York, 1968.

Stoller R: *Sex and Gender. Vol* 2, *The Transsexual Experiment.* Aronson, New York, 1975.

Ward I: The prenatal stress syndrome. Psychoneuroendocrinology *9:* 3, 1984.

Williams K, Green R, Goodman M: Patterns of sexual identity development: A preliminary report on the "tomboy." In *Research in Community and Mental Health,* R Simmons, editor, p 321. JAI Press, Greenwich, CT, 1979

Zucker K J, Bradley S J, Lowry Sullivan C B, Kuksis M, Adams A, Mitchell J N: A gender identity interview for children. J Pers Assess *61:* 443, 1993.

*Zucker K, Green R: Gender identity disorders in children and adolescents. In *Child and Adolescent Psychiatry,* M Lewis, editor, p 604. Williams & Wilkins, Baltimore, 1991.

Zucker K J, Green R: Psychological and familial aspects of gender identity disorder. In *Child and Adolescent Psychiatric Clinics of North America. Sexual and Gender Identity Disorders,* A Yates, editor, p 513. Saunders, Philadelphia, 1993.

Zucker K, Green R, Garofano C, Bradley S, Williams K, Rebach M, Sullivan C: Prenatal gender preference of mothers of feminine and masculine boys: Relation to sibling sex compositions and birth order. J Abnorm Child Psychol *22:* 1, 1994.

INDEX

Page numbers in **boldface** type indicate major discussions; those followed by *t* or *f* indicate tables or figures, respectively.

C

E

H

I

M

O

Q

R

U

V

W

X

Y

Z